STROKE

STROKE

Pathophysiology, Diagnosis, and Management

5TH EDITION

J.P. Mohr, MD, MS
Daniel Sciarra Professor of Neurology
Department of Neurology
Columbia University
New York, New York

Philip A. Wolf, MD
Professor of Neurology, Medicine, and Public Health
Boston University School of Medicine
Principal Investigator
Framingham Heart Study
Boston, Massachusetts

James C. Grotta, MD
Professor of Neurology
Chairman
Department of Neurology
Director
Vascular Neurology Program
University of Texas Medical School at Houston
Houston, Texas

Michael A. Moskowitz, MD
Professor of Neurology
Harvard-MIT Division of Health Science and Technology
Boston, Massachusetts

Marc R. Mayberg, MD
Executive Director
Seattle Neuroscience Institute at Swedish Medical Center
Seattle, Washington

Rüdiger von Kummer, MD, FAHA
Professor of Diagnostic Radiology/Neuroradiology
Head
Department of Neuroradiology
Technische Universität Dresden
Director
Dresden University Stroke Centre
Dresden, Germany

ELSEVIER
SAUNDERS

1600 John F. Kennedy Blvd.
Ste 1800
Philadelphia, PA 19103-2899

STROKE: PATHOPHYSIOLOGY, DIAGNOSIS, AND MANAGEMENT   ISBN 978-1-4160-5478-8
Copyright © 2011, 2004, 1998, 1986 by Saunders, an imprint of Elsevier Inc.

Notice

Knowledge and best practice in this field are constantly changing. As new research and experience broaden our understanding, changes in research methods, professional practices, or medical treatment may become necessary.

Practitioners and researchers must always rely on their own experience and knowledge in evaluating and using any information, methods, compounds, or experiments described herein. In using such information or methods they should be mindful of their own safety and the safety of others, including parties for whom they have a professional responsibility.

With respect to any drug or pharmaceutical products identified, readers are advised to check the most current information provided (i) on procedures featured or (ii) by the manufacturer of each product to be administered, to verify the recommended dose or formula, the method and duration of administration, and contraindications. It is the responsibility of practitioners, relying on their own experience and knowledge of their patients, to make diagnoses, to determine dosages and the best treatment for each individual patient, and to take all appropriate safety precautions.

To the fullest extent of the law, neither the Publisher nor the authors, contributors, or editors, assume any liability for any injury and/or damage to persons or property as a matter of products liability, negligence or otherwise, or from any use or operation of any methods, products, instructions, or ideas contained in the material herein.

Library of Congress Cataloging-in-Publication Data

Stroke : pathophysiology, diagnosis, and management / [edited by] J.P. Mohr . . . [et al.]—5th ed.
  p. ; cm.
Includes bibliographical references and index.
ISBN 978-1-4160-5478-8 (hardcover : alk. paper) 1. Cerebrovascular disease. I. Mohr, J. P.
[DNLM: 1. Stroke. WL 355]
RC388.5.S8528 2011
616.8′1—dc22
                                                                    2011003851

Acquisitions Editor: Charlotta Kryhl
Developmental Editor: Joan Ryan
Publishing Services Manager: Patricia Tannian
Team Leader: Radhika Pallamparthy
Senior Project Manager: Linda Van Pelt
Project Manager: Anitha Sivaraj
Design Direction: Ellen Zanolle

Printed in the United States of America.

Last digit is the print number: 9 8 7 6 5 4 3 2 1

This book is dedicated to
Joan Mohr, Kathryn Dreyfus, Mary Lou Weir,
and Barbara Wolf, whose forbearance is herewith
acknowledged with gratitude, and to our stroke
patients and their families who consented to
participate in the clinical research protocols that
have provided us with so much of the information
that is contained in this book.

CONTRIBUTORS

Takato Abe, MD
Division of Neurobiology
Department of Neurology and Neuroscience
Weill Cornell Medical College
New York, New York
Cerebral Ischemia and Inflammation

Harold P. Adams, Jr., MD
Professor and Director
Division of Cerebrovascular Disorders
University of Iowa Stroke Center
Iowa City, Iowa
Antithrombotic Therapy for Treatment of
    Acute Ischemic Stroke
Clinical Scales to Assess Patients with Stroke

Opeolu Adeoye, MD
Assistant Professor of Emergency Medicine
    and Neurosurgery
Department of Emergency Medicine
University of Cincinnati
Cincinnati, Ohio
Prehospital and Emergency Department Care of the
    Patient with Acute Stroke

Sachin Agarwal, MD
Resident
Department of Neurology
Columbia University Medical Center
New York, New York
Collagen Vascular and Infectious Diseases

Maria I. Aguilar, MD
Assistant Professor
Division of Cerebrovascular Disease
Department of Neurology
Mayo Clinic Arizona
Phoenix, Arizona
Secondary Prevention of Cardioembolic Stroke

Lama Al-Khoury, MD
Department of Neurology
University of California, San Diego, School of Medicine
San Diego, California
Intravenous Thrombolysis

Adrià Arboix, MD, PhD
Associate Professor of Neurology
Cerebrovascular Division
Department of Neurology
Hospital Universitari del Sagrat Cor
University of Barcelona
Barcelona, Spain
Microangiopathies (Lacunes)

Roland N. Auer, MD, PhD
Department of Pathology and Laboratory Medicine
University of Calgary Health Science Center
Calgary, Alberta, Canada
Histopathology of Cerebral Ischemia

Issam A. Awad, MD, MSc, FACS, MA (hon)
Professor and Director
Neurovascular Surgery Program
Biological Sciences Division
University of Chicago
Chicago, Illinois
Cerebral Cavernous Malformations and Venous Anomalies:
    Diagnosis, Natural History, and Clinical Management
Dural Arteriovenous Malformations

Alison E. Baird, MD
Professor of Neurology, Physiology, and Pharmacology
Director
Division of Cerebrovascular Disease and Stroke
State University of New York Downstate Medical Center
Brooklyn, New York
Magnetic Resonance Imaging of Cerebrovascular Diseases

Selva Baltan, MD, PhD
Associate Professor of Neurology
Department of Neurology
University of Washington
Seattle, Washington
Molecular Pathophysiology of White Matter Anoxic-
    Ischemic Injury

Henry J.M. Barnett, MD, FRCPC, FACP
Scientific Director and Co-founder
The John P. Robarts Research Institute
London, Ontario, Canada
Spinal Cord Ischemia

H. Hunt Batjer, MD
Professor and Chair
Department of Neurological Surgery
Feinberg School of Medicine
Northwestern University
Chicago, Illinois
Cerebral Cavernous Malformations and Venous Anomalies:
    Diagnosis, Natural History, and Clinical Management

Oscar R. Benavente, MD, FRCPC
Professor and Research Director of Stroke
University of British Columbia
Vancouver, British Columbia, Canada
Antiplatelet Therapy for Secondary Prevention of Stroke
Secondary Prevention of Cardioembolic Stroke

Bernard R. Bendok, MD
Associate Professor of Neurological Surgery and Radiology
Northwestern University Feinberg School of Medicine
Northwestern Medical Faculty Foundation
Chicago, Illinois
Interventional Neuroradiologic Therapy of
    Atherosclerotic Disease and Vascular Malformations

Eric M. Bershad, MD
Vascular Neurology and Neurocritical Care
Baylor College of Medicine
Houston, Texas
Aneurysmal Subarachnoid Hemorrhage

Jeffrey R. Binder, MD
Professor of Neurology and Biophysics
Director
Stroke and Neurobehavior Programs
Department of Neurology
Medical College of Wisconsin
Milwaukee, Wisconsin
Posterior Cerebral Artery Disease

Alan S. Boulos, MD
Chairman
Division of Neurosurgery
Herman and Sunny Stall Chair of Endovascular
    Neurosurgery
Associate Professor of Surgery and Radiology
Albany Medical College and Hospital
Albany, New York
Interventional Neuroradiologic Therapy of
    Atherosclerotic Disease and Vascular Malformations

Marie-Germaine Bousser, MD
Service de Neurologie
Université Hôpital Lariboisière–Fernand Widal
Paris, France
CADASIL: Cerebral Autosomal Dominant Arteriopathy
    with Subcortical Infarcts and Leukoencephalopathy

Frank J. Bova, PhD
Department of Neurological Surgery
University of Florida
Gainesville, Florida
Radiosurgery for Arteriovenous Malformations

Michael Brainin, MD, PhD, FESO, FAHA
Professor of Neurology
Chairman and Director
Department of Clinical Neurosciences
Donau-Universität Krems
Head
Department of Neurology
Landesklinikum Donauregion
Tulln, Austria
Classification of Ischemic Stroke

Jonathan L. Brisman, MD
Neurological Surgery, PC
Long Island, New York
Indications for Carotid Endarterectomy in Patients with
    Symptomatic Stenosis

Wendy Brown, MD
Department of Neurology
University of California, San Diego, School of Medicine
San Diego, California
Intravenous Thrombolysis

John C.M. Brust, MD
Professor of Clinical Neurology
Columbia University College of Physicians and Surgeons
New York, New York
Anterior Cerebral Artery Disease
Stroke and Substance Abuse

Patrícia Canhão, MD, PhD
Department of Neurosciences
Hospital de Santa Maria
University of Lisbon
Lisbon, Portugal
Cerebral Venous Thrombosis

Louis R. Caplan, MD
Professor of Neurology
Harvard Medical School
Senior Member
Division of Cerebrovascular Disease
Beth Israel Deaconess Medical Center
Boston, Massachusetts
Intracerebral Hemorrhage
Vertebrobasilar Disease

Mar Castellanos, MD
Section of Neurology
Hospital Universitari Doctor Josep Trueta
Girona, Spain
Antiplatelet Therapy for Secondary Prevention of Stroke

Hugues Chabriat, MD, PhD
Service de Neurologie
Université Paris
Hôpital Lariboisière–Fernand Widal
Paris, France
CADASIL: Cerebral Autosomal Dominant Arteriopathy
    with Subcortical Infarcts and Leukoencephalopathy

Angel Chamorro, MD, PhD, FESO
Director
Comprehensive Stroke Center
Hospital Clinic of Barcelona
University of Barcelona and Institut d'Investigacions
  Biomediques August Pi i Sunyer (IDIBAPS)
Barcelona, Spain
Anterior Cerebral Artery Disease

Jae H. Choi, MD
Assistant Professor of Neurology
Columbia University Medical Center
New York, New York
Arteriovenous Malformations and Other Vascular
  Anomalies

Michael Chopp, PhD
Scientific Director
Neuroscience Research
Henry Ford Health System
Detroit, Michigan
Enhancing Brain Reorganization and Recovery
  of Function after Stroke

E. Sander Connolly, MD, FACS
Bennett M. Stein Professor of Neurological Surgery
Vice Chairman of Neurosurgery
Director
Cerebrovascular Research Laboratory
Surgical Director
Neuro-Intensive Care Unit
Department of Neurological Surgery
Columbia University Medical Center
New York, New York
Surgical Decision Making, Techniques, and Periprocedural
  Care of Cerebral Arteriovenous Malformations

Bruce M. Coull, MD
Professor of Neurology and Medicine
Associate Dean of Clinical Affairs, COM
Chief Medical Officer, UPH Plans
The University of Arizona
Tucson, Arizona
Coagulation Abnormalities in Stroke

Brett L. Cucchiara, MD
Assistant Professor
Department of Neurology
Hospital of the University of Pennsylvania
Philadelphia, Pennsylvania
Treatment of "Other" Stroke Etiologies

Turgay Dalkara, MD, PhD
Professor of Neurology
Department of Neurology
Faculty of Medicine
Director
Institute of Neurological Sciences and Psychiatry
Hacettepe University
Ankara, Turkey
Apoptosis and Related Mechanisms in Cerebral Ischemia

Krishna A. Dani, MRCP
Clinical Lecturer
Institute of Neuroscience and Psychology
University of Glasgow
Glasgow, Scotland
Magnetic Resonance Imaging of Cerebrovascular Diseases

Mark J. Dannenbaum, MD
Fellow
Cerebrovascular and Skull Base Surgery
Department of Neurosurgery
Brigham and Women's Hospital
Harvard Medical School
Boston, Massachusettts
Surgical Management of Posterior Circulation Aneurysms

Shervin R. Dashti, MD, PhD
Fellow, Cerebrovascular and Skull Base Surgery
Neurosurgical Institute of Kentucky
Norton Neuroscience Institute
Louisville, Kentucky
Spinal Arteriovenous Malformations

Patricia H. Davis, MD
Professor
University of Iowa Stroke Center
Iowa City, Iowa
Antithrombotic Therapy for Treatment of Acute Ischemic
  Stroke

Ted M. Dawson, MD, PhD
Leonard and Madlyn Abramson Professor in
  Neurodegenerative Diseases
Scientific Director
Institute for Cell Engineering
Professor
Departments of Neurology and Neuroscience
Johns Hopkins University School of Medicine
Baltimore, Maryland
Intracellular Signaling: Mediators and Protective
  Responses

Valina L. Dawson, PhD
Professor
Departments of Neurology, Neuroscience, and Physiology
Director
Neuroregeneration and Stem Cell Programs
Institute for Cell Engineering
Johns Hopkins University School of Medicine
Baltimore, Maryland
Intracellular Signaling: Mediators and Protective
  Responses

Arthur L. Day, MD
Director of Cerebrovascular Center
Brigham and Women's Hospital
Boston, Massachusetts
Surgical Management of Posterior Circulation Aneurysms

Michael J. De Leo III, MD
New England Center for Stroke Research
Department of Radiology
University of Massachusetts Medical School
Worcester, Massachusetts
Endovascular Treatment of Cerebral Aneurysms

Gregory J. del Zoppo, MD
Professor of Medicine (in Hematology)
Adjunct Professor of Neurology
University of Washington School of Medicine
Harborview Medical Center
Seattle, Washington
The Cerebral Microvasculature and Responses
    to Ischemia
Mechanisms of Thrombosis and Thrombolysis

Jennifer Diedler, MD
Department of Neurology
University of Heidelberg
Heidelberg, Germany
Critical Care of the Patient with Acute Stroke

Hans C. Diener, MD
Professor of Neurology and Chairman
Department of Neurology
University Duisburg-Essen
Essen, Germany
Migraine and Stroke

Marco R. Di Tullio, MD
Professor of Medicine
Division of Cardiology
Associate Director
Cardiovascular Ultrasound Laboratories
Columbia University Medical Center
New York, New York
Atherosclerotic Disease of the Proximal Aorta

Bruce H. Dobkin, MD, FRCP
Neurologic Rehabilitation and Research Director
University of California Los Angeles Stroke Center
Los Angeles, California
Rehabilitation and Recovery of the Patient with Stroke

Kendra Drake, MD
Department of Neurology
The University of Arizona
Tucson, Arizona
Coagulation Abnormalities in Stroke

Rose Du, MD, PhD
Assistant Professor of Surgery
Department of Neurosurgery
Harvard Medical School
Brigham and Women's Hospital
Boston, Massachusetts
Surgical Management of Posterior Circulation
    Aneurysms

Anne Ducros, MD, PhD
Emergency Headache Centre and Department of
    Neurology
University Hospital Lariboisière
Paris, France
Reversible Cerebral Vasoconstriction Syndromes

Imanuel Dzialowski, MD
Department of Neurology
Dresden University Stroke Centre
Technical University of Dresden
Dresden, Germany
Computed Tomography–Based Evaluation
    of Cerebrovascular Disease

Christopher S. Eddleman, MD, PhD
Department of Neurological Surgery
Feinberg School of Medicine
Northwestern University
Chicago, Illinois
Cerebral Cavernous Malformations and Venous Anomalies:
    Diagnosis, Natural History, and Clinical Management

Mohamed Samy Elhammady, MD
Department of Neurosurgery
University of Miami Miller School of Medicine
Lois Pope LIFE Center
Miami, Florida
Surgical Management of Asymptomatic Carotid Stenosis

Mitchell S.V. Elkind, MD, MS, FAAN
Associate Professor of Neurology and Epidemiology
Associate Chairman of Neurology for Clinical Research
    and Training
Departments of Neurology and Epidemiology
Columbia University Medical Center
New York, New York
Collagen Vascular and Infectious Diseases

J. Paul Elliott, MD
Neurosurgeon
Colorado Brain and Spine Institute, LLC, PC
Englewood, Colorado
Dural Arteriovenous Malformations

José M. Ferro, MD, PhD
Director and Full Professor
Department of Neurosciences
Hospital de Santa Maria
University of Lisbon
Lisbon, Portugal
Cerebral Venous Thrombosis

J. Max Findlay, MD, PhD, FRCSC
Division of Neurosurgery
University of Alberta
Edmonton, Alberta, Canada
Intraventricular Hemorrhage

William A. Friedman, MD
Chairman
Department of Neurosurgery
University of Florida
McKnight Brain Institute
Gainesville, Florida
Radiosurgery for Arteriovenous Malformations

Karen L. Furie, MD
Neurology Stroke Service
Massachusetts General Hospital
Boston, Massachusetts
Cardiac Diseases

Anthony J. Furlan, MD
Professor and Chairman of Neurology
Gilbert W. Humphrey Chair in Neurology
Case Western Reserve School of Medicine
University Hospitals–Case Medical Center
Cleveland, Ohio
Intraarterial Thrombolysis in Acute Ischemic Stroke

Sasikhan Geibprasert, MD
Department of Medical Imaging
The Hospital for Sick Children
Toronto, Ontario, Canada
Interventional Therapy of Brain and Spinal Arteriovenous
    Malformations

Y. Pierre Gobin, MD
Professor of Radiology in Neurology and Neurosurgery
Director
Interventional Neurology
Weill Cornell Medical Center
New York Presbyterian Hospital
New York, New York
Cerebral Angiography

Mark P. Goldberg, MD
Professor and Chair
Department of Neurology
University of Texas Southwestern Medical Center
Dallas, Texas
Molecular Pathophysiology of White Matter Anoxic-
    Ischemic Injury

Larry B. Goldstein, MD
Professor of Medicine
Division of Neurology
Department of Medicine
Director
Duke Stroke Center
Duke University
Durham, North Carolina
Primary Prevention of Stroke

Nicole R. Gonzales, MD
Assistant Professor of Neurology
Department of Neurology
University of Texas Medical School at Houston
Houston, Texas
Pharmacologic Modification of Acute Cerebral Ischemia

Matthew J. Gounis, PhD
Director
New England Center for Stroke Research
Assistant Professor
Department of Radiology
University of Massachusetts Medical School
Worcester, Massachusetts
Endovascular Treatment of Cerebral Aneurysms

Steven M. Greenberg, MD, PhD
Professor of Neurology
Harvard Medical School
Director
Hemorrhagic Stroke Research Program
Massachusetts General Hospital
Boston, Massachusetts
Intracerebral Hemorrhage

David M. Greer, MD, MA, FCCM
Dr. Harry M. Zimmerman and Dr. Nicholas and Viola
    Spinelli Associate Professor of Neurology
Vice Chairman
Department of Neurology
Yale School of Medicine
New Haven, Connecticut
Cardiac Diseases

Barbara A. Gregson, PhD
Principal Research Associate
Director of the Surgical Trial in Intracerebral
    Haemorrhage II (STICH II)
Newcastle University
Newcastle upon Tyne, United Kingdom
Surgery for Intracerebral Hemorrhage

James C. Grotta, MD
Professor of Neurology
Chairman
Department of Neurology
Director
Vascular Neurology Program
University of Texas Medical School at Houston
Houston, Texas
Pharmacologic Modification of Acute Cerebral Ischemia

Werner Hacke, MD, PhD
Professor and Chairman
Department of Neurology
University of Heidelberg
Heidelberg, Germany
Cerebral Infarction: Surgical Treatment
Critical Care of the Patient with Acute Stroke

John Hallenbeck, MD
Senior Investigator
Stroke Branch
National Institute of Neurological Disorders and Stroke
Bethesda, Maryland
Cerebral Ischemia and Inflammation

Gerhard F. Hamann, MD
Department of Neurology
Horst-Schmidt-Kliniken
Wiesbaden, Germany
The Cerebral Microvasculature and Responses to
    Ischemia

Andreas Hartmann, MD
Associate Professor of Neurology
Charité Berlin
Department of Neurology
Klinikum Frankfurt (Oder)
Oder, Germany
Arteriovenous Malformations and Other Vascular
    Anomalies

Michael Hennerici, MD, PhD
Professor of Neurology
Chairman
Department of Neurology
University of Heidelberg
Mannheim, Germany
Ultrasonography

Roberto C. Heros, MD
Department of Neurosurgery
University of Miami School of Medicine
Lois Pope LIFE Center
Miami, Florida
Surgical Treatment of Asymptomatic Carotid Stenosis

Randall Higashida, MD
Clinical Professor of Radiology, Neurological Surgery,
    Neurology, and Anesthesiology
Chief
Division of Neurointerventional Radiology
University of California, San Francisco, Medical Center
San Francisco, California
Intraarterial Thrombolysis in Acute Ischemic Stroke

Shunichi Homma, MD
Margaret Milliken Hatch Professor of Medicine
Associate Chief
Cardiology Division
Director
Noninvasive Cardiac Imaging
Columbia University Medical Center
New York, New York
Atherosclerotic Disease of the Proximal Aorta
Cardiac Diseases

Kazuhiro Hongo, MD
Department of Neurosurgery
Shinshu University School of Medicine
Matsumoto, Japan
Cerebellar Infarction and Hemorrhage

L. Nelson Hopkins, MD, FACS
Professor and Chairman of Neurosurgery
Professor of Radiology
University of Buffalo
Director
Toshiba Stroke Research Center State University
    of New York
Department of Neurosurgery
Millard Fillmore Gates Hospital
Kaleida Health
Buffalo, New York
Interventional Neuroradiologic Therapy of
    Atherosclerotic Disease and Vascular Malformations

Tetsuyoshi Horiuchi, MD
Department of Neurosurgery
Shinshu University School of Medicine
Matsumoto, Japan
Cerebellar Infarction and Hemorrhage

George Howard, DrPH
Department Chair
Biostatistics
School of Public Health
University of Alabama at Birmingham
Birmingham, Alabama
Distribution of Stroke: Heterogeneity by Age,
    Race, and Sex

Virginia J. Howard, PhD
Associate Professor of Epidemiology
School of Public Health
University of Alabama at Birmingham
Birmingham, Alabama
Distribution of Stroke: Heterogeneity by Age,
    Race, and Sex

Daniel Huddle, DO
Interventional Neuroradiologist
Colorado Brain and Spine Institute, LLC, PC
Englewood, Colorado
Dural Arteriovenous Malformations

Costantino Iadecola, MD
Cotzias Distinguished Professor of Neurology
    and Neuroscience
Chief
Division of Neurobiology
Weill Cornell Medical College
New York, New York
Cerebral Ischemia and Inflammation

Anne Joutel, MD
Laboratoire de Génétique
Université Hôpital Lariboisière–Fernand Widal
Paris, France
CADASIL: Cerebral Autosomal Dominant Arteriopathy
    with Subcortical Infarcts and Leukoencephalopathy

Eric Jüttler, MD, MSc
Junior Professor of Neurology
Center for Stroke Research Berlin
Charité—Universitätsmedizin Berlin
Berlin, Germany
Cerebral Infarction: Surgical Treatment

Udaya K. Kakarla, MD
Division of Neurological Surgery
Barrow Neurological Institute
St. Joseph's Hospital and Medical Center
Phoenix, Arizona
Spinal Arteriovenous Malformations

Mary A. Kalafut, MD
Co-Director
Vascular Laboratory
The Scripps Research Institute
La Jolla, California
Mechanisms of Thrombosis and Thrombolysis

William B. Kannel, MD, MPH
Senior Investigator
Framingham Heart Study
Professor Emeritus
Boston University School of Medicine
Framingham, Massachusetts
Epidemiology of Stroke

Carlos S. Kase, MD
Professor of Neurology
Boston University School of Medicine
Neurologist-in-Chief
Boston Medical Center
Boston, Massachusetts
Intracerebral Hemorrhage

Scott E. Kasner, MD, MSCE
Professor
Department of Neurology
University of Pennsylvania
Philadelphia, Pennsylvania
Treatment of "Other" Stroke Etiologies

Markku Kaste, MD, PhD, FAHA, FESO
Professor of Neurology Emeritus
Chair of Department of Neurology Emeritus
Head of Clinical Stroke Research
Department of Neurology
Helsinki University Central Hospital
University of Helsinki
Helsinki, Finland
General Stroke Management and Stroke Units

Alexander Khaw, MD
Director of Stroke Research and Neurovascular
    Laboratory
Department of Neurology
University of Greifswald
Greifswald, Germany
Arteriovenous Malformations and Other Vascular
    Anomalies

Chelsea S. Kidwell, MD
Professor of Neurology
Medical Director of Georgetown Stroke Center
Georgetown University Medical Center
Washington, D.C.
Magnetic Resonance Imaging of Cerebrovascular Diseases

Helen Kim, PhD
Assistant Professor
Departments of Anesthesia and Perioperative Care, and
    Epidemiology and Biostatistics
Center for Cerebrovascular Research
Institute for Human Genetics
University of California, San Francisco
San Francisco, California
Genetics and Vascular Biology of Brain Vascular
    Malformations

Louis J. Kim, MD
Assistant Professor of Neurological Surgery
University of Washington School of Medicine
Attending Neurosurgeon
Harborview Medical Center
Seattle, Washington
Spinal Arteriovenous Malformations

Stanley H. Kim, MD
Neurosurgeon
Neurosurgery, Endovascular, and Spine Center
Austin, Texas
Interventional Neuroradiologic Therapy of
    Atherosclerotic Disease and Vascular Malformations

Catharina J.M. Klijn, MD, PhD
Department of Neurology
Rudolf Magnus Institute of Neuroscience
University Medical Center Utrecht
Utrecht, The Netherlands
Genetics of Aneurysms and Arteriovenous Malformations

Shigeaki Kobayashi, MD
Department of Neurosurgery
Stroke and Brain Center
Aizawa Hospital
Matsumoto, Japan
Cerebellar Infarction and Hemorrhage

Ricardo J. Komotar, MD
Department of Neurological Surgery
Neurological Institute
Columbia University Medical Center
New York, New York
Surgical Decision Making, Techniques, and Periprocedural
    Care of Cerebral Arteriovenous Malformations

Timo Krings, MD, PhD, FRCP(C)
Professor of Radiology—Neuroradiology
Division of Neuroradiology
Joint Department of Medical Imaging
Toronto Western Hospital
University Health Network and Hospital for Sick Children
University of Toronto
Toronto, Ontario, Canada
Interventional Therapy of Brain and Spinal Arteriovenous
    Malformations

Alexander Kunz, MD
Division of Neurobiology
Department of Neurology and Neuroscience
Weill Cornell Medical College
New York, New York
Cerebral Ischemia and Inflammation

Tobias Kurth, MD, ScD
Director of Research
Inserm Unit 708—Neuroepidemiology
Paris, France
Migraine and Stroke

Catherine Lamy, MD
Department of Neurology
Hôpital Sainte-Anne
Paris Descartes University
Paris, France
Hypertensive Encephalopathy

Ronald M. Lazar, PhD, FAAN, FAHA
Professor of Clinical Neuropsychology in Neurology and
    Neurological Surgery
Director
Levine Cerebral Localization Laboratory
Neurological Institute
Columbia University
New York, New York
Middle Cerebral Artery Disease

Elad I. Levy, MD, FACS, FAHA
Director of Neuroendovascular Fellowship
Professor of Neurosurgery
Professor of Radiology
University of Buffalo Neurosurgery
Co-director
Toshiba Stroke Research Center
Department of Neurosurgery
Millard Fillmore Gates Hospital
Kaleida Health
Buffalo, New York
Interventional Neuroradiologic Therapy of
    Atherosclerotic Disease and Vascular Malformations

David S. Liebeskind, MD
Professor of Neurology
Director
Stroke Imaging
Director
Vascular Neurology Residency
Co-Director
Cerebral Blood Flow Laboratory
Associate Director
UCLA Stroke Center
David Geffen School of Medicine at UCLA
University of California, Los Angeles
Los Angeles, California
Cerebral Angiography

Patrick D. Lyden, MD, FAAN, FAHA
Chairman
Department of Neurology
Carmen and Louis Warschaw Chair in Neurology
Cedars-Sinai Medical Center
Los Angeles, California
Intravenous Thrombolysis

Joanne Markham, MS
Research Associate Professor of Radiology
Division of Radiological Sciences
Washington University Medical School
St. Louis, Missouri
Cerebral Blood Flow and Metabolism in Human
    Cerebrovascular Disease

Randolph S. Marshall, MD
John and Elizabeth Katte Harris Professor of Neurology
Division Head
Stroke and Cerebrovascular Division
Columbia University
New York, New York
Middle Cerebral Artery Disease

J.L. Marti-Vilalta, MD
Director
Cerebrovascular Unit
Department of Neurology
Hospital de la Santa Creu i Sant Pau
Barcelona, Spain
Microangiopathies (Lacunes)

Jean-Louis Mas, MD
Professor of Neurology
Department of Neurology
Hôpital Sainte-Anne
Paris Descartes University
Paris, France
Hypertensive Encephalopathy

Henning Mast, MD
Adjunct Associate Professor of Neurology
Stroke Unit, Neurological Institute
Columbia University
New York, New York
Arteriovenous Malformations and Other Vascular Anomalies
Carotid Artery Disease

Junichi Masuda, MD
Department of Laboratory Medicine
Shimane Medical University
Shimane, Japan
Moyamoya Disease

Colin Mathers, PhD
Coordinator
Mortality and Burden of Disease
Innovation, Information, Evidence and Research
    Cluster (IER)
World Health Organization
Geneva, Switzerland
The Global Burden of Stroke

Marc R. Mayberg, MD
Executive Director
Seattle Neuroscience Institute at Swedish Medical Center
Seattle, Washington
Indications for Carotid Endarterectomy in Patients with
    Symptomatic Stenosis

Stephen Meairs, MD
Professor of Neurology
Coordinator of European Stroke Network
University of Heidelberg
Mannheim, Germany
Ultrasonography

Alexander David Mendelow, MD, PhD
Department of Neurosurgery
Newcastle General Hospital
Newcastle upon Tyne, United Kingdom
Surgery for Intracerebral Hemorrhage

James F. Meschia, MD, FAAN
Professor of Neurology
Mayo Clinic
Jacksonville, Florida
Stroke Genetics

Alyson A. Miller, PhD
National Health and Research Council of Australia Career
    Development Award Fellow
Department of Pharmacology
Monash University
Clayton, Victoria, Australia
Vascular Biology and Atherosclerosis of Cerebral Arteries

Takahiro Miyawaki, MD
Department of Neuroscience
Albert Einstein College of Medicine
Bronx, New York
Molecular and Cellular Mechanisms of Ischemia-Induced
    Neuronal Death

J Mocco, MD, MS
Department of Neurosurgery
Toshiba Stroke Research Center
School of Medicine and Biomedical Sciences
State University of New York at Buffalo
Department of Neurosurgery
Millard Fillmore Gates Hospital
Kaleida Health
Buffalo, New York
Interventional Neuroradiologic Therapy of
    Atherosclerotic Disease and Vascular Malformations

J.P. Mohr, MD, MS
Daniel Sciarra Professor of Neurology
Department of Neurology
Columbia University
New York, New York
Arteriovenous Malformations and Other Vascular
    Anomalies
Carotid Artery Disease
Classification of Ischemic Stroke
Collagen Vascular and Infectious Diseases
Columbia University
Daniel Sciarra Professor of Neurology
Department of Neurology
Intracerebral Hemorrhage
Microangiopathies (Lacunes)
Middle Cerebral Artery Disease
New York, New York
Posterior Cerebral Artery Disease
Spinal Cord Ischemia
Ultrasonography
Vertebrobasilar Disease

Jacques J. Morcos, MD, FRCS(Eng), FRCS(Ed)
Professor
Departments of Neurosurgery and Otolaryngology
Co-Director
Microsurgery Training Center
University of Miami
Miller School of Medicine
Lois Pope LIFE Center
Miami, Florida
Surgical Treatment of Asymptomatic Carotid Stenosis

Lewis B. Morgenstern, MD
Professor
Neurology, Emergency Medicine, and Neurosurgery
Director
Stroke Program
University of Michigan School of Public Health
Ann Arbor, Michigan
Medical Therapy of Intracerebral and Intraventricular
    Hemorrhage

Michael A. Moskowitz, MD
Professor of Neurology
Harvard-MIT Division of Health Science and Technology
Boston, Massachusetts
Apoptosis and Related Mechanisms in Cerebral Ischemia

Brian V. Nahed, MD
Department of Neurosurgery
Massachusetts General Hospital
Boston, Massachusetts
Anterior Circulation Aneurysms

David W. Newell, MD
Executive Director
Swedish Neuroscience Institute
Seattle, Washington
Extracranial to Intracranial Bypass for Cerebral Ischemia

Dimitry Ofengeim, MD
Department of Neuroscience
Albert Einstein College of Medicine
Bronx, New York
Molecular and Cellular Mechanisms of Ischemia-Induced
    Neuronal Death

Jun Ogata, MD
Multiple Handicapped Children's Hospital
Hirakata Ryoikuen
Tsuda-higashi
Hirakata, Osaka, Japan
Moyamoya Disease

Christopher S. Ogilvy, MD
Robert G. and A. Jean Ojemann Professor of Surgery
    (Neurosurgery)
Director
Endovascular and Operative Neurovascular Surgery
Harvard Medical School
Attending Neurosurgeon
Massachusetts General Hospital
Boston, Massachusetts
Anterior Circulation Aneurysms

Yuko Y. Palesch, PhD
Professor
Department of Medicine
Division of Biostatistics and Epidemiology
Medical University of South Carolina
Charleston, South Carolina
Conduct of Stroke-Related Clinical Trials

Arthur Pancioli, MD
Robert C. Levy Professor and Chair
Department of Emergency Medicine
University of Cincinnati College of Medicine
Cincinnati, Ohio
Prehospital and Emergency Department Care of the
    Patient with Acute Stroke

Min S. Park, MD
Division of Neurological Surgery
Barrow Neurological Institute
St. Joseph's Hospital and Medical Center
Phoenix, Arizona
Spinal Arteriovenous Malformations

Ludmila Pawlikowska, PhD
Assistant Professor
Department of Anesthesia and Perioperative Care
Center for Cerebrovascular Research
University of California, San Francisco
San Francisco, California
Genetics and Vascular Biology of Brain Vascular
    Malformations

John Pile-Spellman, MD
Adjunct Professor of Radiology and Neurosurgery
Columbia University Medical Center
New York, New York
Arteriovenous Malformations and Other Vascular
    Anomalies

William J. Powers, MD
H. Houston Merritt Distinguished Professor and Chairman
Department of Neurology
University of North Carolina, Chapel Hill
Chapel Hill, North Carolina
Cerebral Blood Flow and Metabolism in Human
    Cerebrovascular Disease

Volker Puetz, MD
Department of Neurology
Dresden University Stroke Centre
Technical University of Dresden
Dresden, Germany
Computed Tomography–Based Evaluation
    of Cerebrovascular Disease

Bruce R. Ransom, MD, PhD
Warren and Jermaine Magnuson Professor and Chair of
    Neurology
Adjunct Professor of Physiology and Biophysics
University of Washington School of Medicine
Seattle, Washington
Molecular Pathophysiology of White Matter
    Anoxic-Ischemic Injury

Risto O. Roine, MD, PhD
Associate Professor
Department of Neurology
Helsinki University Central Hospital
University of Helsinki
Helsinki, Finland
General Stroke Management and Stroke Units

Ynte M. Ruigrok, MD, PhD
Department of Neurology
Rudolf Magnus Institute of Neuroscience
University Medical Center Utrecht
Utrecht, The Netherlands
Genetics of Aneurysms and Arteriovenous Malformations

Tatjana Rundek, MD, PhD
Associate Professor of Neurology
Department of Neurology
Miller School of Medicine
University of Miami
Miami, Florida
Prognosis after Stroke

Ralph L. Sacco, MS, MD, FAAN, FAHA
Adjunct Professor
Department of Neurology
Columbia University
New York, New York
Professor and Chairman
Department of Neurology
Miller School of Medicine
University of Miami
Miami, Florida
Prognosis after Stroke
Primary Prevention of Stroke
Classification of Ischemic Stroke

Ronald J. Sattenberg, MD
Assistant Professor of Radiology
Department of Radiology
University of Louisville Hospital
Louisville, Kentucky
Cerebral Angiography

Jeffrey L. Saver, MD, FAHA, FAAN
Professor of Neurology
David Geffen School of Medicine at UCLA
Director, UCLA Stroke Center
University of California, Los Angeles
Los Angeles, California
Cerebral Angiography

Sean I. Savitz, MD
Associate Professor of Neurology
University of Texas Medical School at Houston
Houston, Texas
Enhancing Stroke Recovery with Cellular Therapies

Sudha Seshadri, MD
Associate Professor
Department of Neurology
Boston University School of Medicine
Investigator, The Framingham Heart Study
Boston, Massachusetts
Vascular Dementia and Vascular Cognitive Decline

Jitendra Sharma, MD
Fellow
Interventional Neurology
Case Western Reserve School of Medicine
Cleveland, Ohio
Intraarterial Thrombolysis in Acute Ischemic Stroke

Gerald Silverboard, MD
Atlanta Family Neurology
Atlanta, Georgia
Arterial Dissections and Fibromuscular Dysplasia

Aneesh B. Singhal, MD
Neurology Stroke Service
Massachusetts General Hospital
Boston, Massachusetts
Reversible Cerebral Vasoconstriction Syndromes

Christopher G. Sobey, PhD
National Health and Medical Research Council of Australia
    Senior Research Fellow
Department of Pharmacology
Monash University
Clayton, Victoria, Australia
Vascular Biology and Atherosclerosis of Cerebral Arteries

Robert F. Spetzler, MD
Director
J. N. Harber Chair of Neurological Surgery
Barrow Neurological Institute
Phoenix
Professor
Department of Surgery
Section of Neurosurgery
University of Arizona College of Medicine
Tuscon, Arizona
Spinal Arteriovenous Malformations

Christian Stapf, MD
Adjunct Assistant Professor of Neurology
Division of Stroke
Department of Neurology
Columbia University Medical Center
New York, New York
Arteriovenous Malformations and Other Vascular
    Anomalies

Robert M. Starke, BS
Department of Neurological Surgery
Neurological Institute
Columbia University Medical Center
New York, New York
Surgical Decision Making, Techniques, and Periprocedural
    Care of Cerebral Arteriovenous Malformations

Michael F. Stiefel, MD
Division of Neurological Surgery
Barrow Neurological Institute
St. Joseph's Hospital and Medical Center
Phoenix, Arizona
Spinal Arteriovenous Malformations

Kathleen Strong, MD
Monitoring and Evaluation
UNITAID
Geneva, Switzerland
The Global Burden of Stroke

José I. Suarez, MD
Head
Vascular Neurology and Neurocritical Care
Professor
Neurology and Neurosurgery
Baylor College of Medicine
Houston, Texas
Aneurysmal Subarachnoid Hemorrhage

Marek Sykora, MD
Department of Neurology
University of Heidelberg
Heidelberg, Germany
Department of Neurology
Comenius University Bratislava
Bratislava, Slovakia
Critical Care of the Patient with Acute Stroke

Gilda Tafreshi, MD
Department of Neurology
Scripps Mercy Medical Center
San Diego, California
Intravenous Thrombolysis

Karel ter Brugge, MD, FRCP
Professor of Radiology and Surgery
The David Braley and Nancy Gordon Chair in
     Interventional Neuroradiology
University of Toronto
Head of Neuroradiology
University Health Network and the Mount Sinai and
     Women's College Hospitals
Toronto Western Hospital
Toronto, Ontario, Canada
Interventional Therapy of Brain and Spinal Arteriovenous
     Malformations

Barbara C. Tilley, MD, PhD
Lorne C. Bain Distinguished Professor and Director
Division of Biostatistics
The University of Texas Health Science Center at Houston
School of Public Health
Houston, Texas
Conduct of Stroke-Related Clinical Trials

Danilo Toni, MD, PhD
Professor of Neurology
Director of Emergency Department Stroke Unit
Department of Neurology and Psychiatry
Sapienza University of Rome
Rome, Italy
Classification of Ischemic Stroke

Elisabeth Tournier-Lasserve, MD
Laboratoire de Génétique
Université Hôpital Lariboisière–Fernand Widal
Paris, France
CADASIL: Cerebral Autosomal Dominant Arteriopathy
     with Subcortical Infarcts and Leukoencephalopathy

Marcelo D. Vilela, MD
Chief of Neurosurgery
Mater Dei Hospital
Belo Horizonte
Minas Gerais, Brazil
Affiliated Assistant Professor
Department of Neurological Surgery
University of Washington
Seattle, Washington
Extracranial to Intracranial Bypass for Cerebral Ischemia

Rüdiger von Kummer, MD, FAHA
Professor of Diagnostic Radiology/Neuroradiology
Head
Department of Neuroradiology
Technische Universität Dresden
Director
Dresden University Stroke Centre
Dresden, Germany
Computed Tomography–Based Evaluation of
     Cerebrovascular Disease

Ajay K. Wakhloo, MD, PhD
Professor of Radiology, Neurology, and Surgery
Director
Neuroimaging and Intervention
Director
Clinical Research
New England Center for Stroke Research
University of Massachusetts Medical School
Worcester, Massachusetts
Endovascular Treatment of Cerebral Aneurysms

Steven Warach, MD, PhD
Senior Investigator
Stroke Diagnostics and Therapeutic Section
National Institute of Neurological Disorders and Stroke
National Institutes of Health
Bethesda, Maryland
Magnetic Resonance Imaging of Cerebrovascular Diseases

Babette B. Weksler, MD, MS
Professor of Medicine
Weill Cornell Medical College
Weill Cornell Cancer Care and Blood Disorders
New York, New York
Antiplatelet Therapy for Secondary Prevention of Stroke

Joshua Z. Willey, MD, MS
Assistant Professor of Neurology
Division of Stroke
Columbia University Medical Center
New York, New York
Spinal Cord Ischemia

Max Wintermark, MD, MAS
Associate Professor of Radiology, Neurology, Neurological
     Surgery, and Biomedical Engineering
Chief of Neuroradiology
Department of Radiology
University of Virginia
Charlottesville, Virginia
Magnetic Resonance Imaging of Cerebrovascular Diseases

Philip A. Wolf, MD
Professor of Neurology, Medicine, and Public Health
Boston University School of Medicine
Principal Investigator
Framingham Heart Study
Boston, Massachusetts
Epidemiology of Stroke

Daniel Woo, MD, MS
Professor
Department of Neurology
University of Cincinnati College of Medicine
Cincinnati, Ohio
Stroke Genetics

Takenori Yamaguchi, MD, PhD
Professor Emeritus
National Cerebral and Cardiovascular Center
Osaka, Japan
Moyamoya Disease

Masahiro Yasaka, MD
Director
Department of Cerebrovascular Disease
National Hospital Organization
Kyusyu Medical Center
Kyushu, Japan
Moyamoya Disease

William L. Young, MD
James P. Livingston Professor and Vice Chair
Department of Anesthesia and Perioperative Care
Professor of Neurological Surgery and Neurology
Director
Center for Cerebrovascular Research
University of California, San Francisco
San Francisco, California
Genetics and Vascular Biology of Brain Vascular
    Malformations

Darin B. Zahuranec, MD
Assistant Professor of Neurology
University of Michigan Medical School
Ann Arbor, Michigan
Medical Therapy of Intracerebral and Intraventricular
    Hemorrhage

Allyson R. Zazulia, MD
Associate Professor
Department of Neurology
Section of Cerebrovascular Disease
Washington University School of Medicine
St. Louis, Missouri
Cerebral Blood Flow and Metabolism in Human
    Cerebrovascular Disease

Zheng Gang Zhang, MD, PhD
Department of Neurology
Henry Ford Health System
Detroit, Michigan
Enhancing Brain Reorganization and Recovery
    of Function after Stroke

R. Suzanne Zukin, PhD
F.M. Kirby Professor of Neural Repair and Protection
Dominick P. Pupura Department of Neuroscience
Director
Neuropsychopharmacology Center
Albert Einstein College of Medicine
New York, New York
Molecular and Cellular Mechanisms of Ischemia-Induced
    Neuronal Death

Richard M. Zweifler, MD
Chief of Neurology
Sentara Healthcare
Professor of Neurology and Eastern Virginia Medical
    School
Norfolk, Virginia
Arterial Dissections and Fibromuscular Dysplasia

PREFACE

The editors and the many contributors are grateful that their efforts have justified this, the fifth edition of this book, the first edition dating back 25 years. Further changes in the field of stroke are continuing to improve the knowledge of risk factors (modifiable or not); diagnosis, based not only on the clinical syndrome but also on greatly improved imaging; treatment to prevent the basic underlying disease and to stabilize and even to reverse the effects of acute stroke; and improvements in functional rehabilitation to improve the outcome.

Michael Moskowitz now edits the expanded section on pathophysiology. Philip A. Wolf continues as editor for the section on epidemiology and stroke prevention. J.P. Mohr continues as editor for clinical manifestations and specific medical diseases and stroke. Advances in the field have radically altered the number and length of the sections. A new editor, Rüdiger von Kummer, has taken charge of the section on diagnostic studies. The ever-enlarging subject of therapy has prompted further modifications of the book's structure. James C. Grotta continues as section editor for medical therapy. Reflecting the growing field of intravascular therapy and its multispecialty nature, Rüdiger von Kummer overlaps as section editor for interventional neuroradiology, and another new editor, Marc Mayberg, edits the section on neurosurgery.

We hope readers will be attracted to the important changes in scope of the subjects covered, with the inclusion of many new ones unknown or barely in existence when the original edition was brought forth. We continue the hope that the information contained in this edition makes for its rapid obsolescence, so great are our aspirations for continued rapid developments in our field.

J.P. MOHR, MD, MS

JAMES C. GROTTA, MD

MARC R. MAYBERG, MD

MICHAEL MOSKOWITZ, MD, PhD

RÜDIGER VON KUMMER, MD, FAHA

PHILIP A. WOLF, MD

CONTENTS

section four
Specific Medical Diseases and Stroke
J.P. MOHR

section five
Diagnostic Studies
RÜDIGER VON KUMMER

section six
Therapy
Part A: Medical Therapy
JAMES C. GROTTA

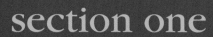

Pathophysiology

MICHAEL A. MOSKOWITZ

The science of stroke has progressed rapidly. Neurogenesis, angiogenesis, brain plasticity, and new stem cell technologies have emerged to turn the field toward longer term strategies for stroke recovery. This section focuses on many of these advances and summarizes key principles that affect the translational aspects of stroke science.

The basic science section focuses on vascular biology and atherosclerosis; the molecules and mechanisms that modulate vascular reactivity, vessel caliber, and ultimately blood flow; blood flow regulation, oxygen delivery and consumption, and hemodynamic and metabolic components that characterize brain before and after stroke; and pathologic conditions that modulate these mechanisms. Discussions of matrix molecules and responses of small blood vessels to stroke injury, as well as the biology of thrombus formation and clot lysis, are included.

Classic histopathology of stroke follows, including the underlying dynamics of cell death inferred from pathologic descriptions, the cell and tissue mechanisms contributing to ischemic injury and cell death, and the complexity of tissue response to injury and entryways into the cell death process. Reviewed is the comprehensive literature about ion channels, glutamate receptors, hydrogen ions, oxygen radicals, and ways in which molecular and cellular pathways can be harnessed during the preconditioning process to reduce injury in the vulnerable brain.

Vascular Biology and Atherosclerosis of Cerebral Arteries

ALYSON A. MILLER, CHRISTOPHER G. SOBEY

Cerebral perfusion is compromised by several pathophysiologic conditions that not only affect cerebrovascular reactivity and thrombosis but also are associated with an increased risk of stroke. Disease states may produce cerebrovascular abnormalities by a variety of mechanisms, including endothelial dysfunction, impaired relaxation of vascular muscle, and augmented vasoconstriction. Significant progress has been made in the understanding of mechanisms that normally regulate cerebral blood flow and abnormalities of cerebrovascular function in pathophysiologic states.

This chapter summarizes the current understanding of some important mechanisms of cerebrovascular function and dysfunction. We do not, however, address other aspects of vascular biology, including vascular proliferation, remodeling, and formation of collateral vessels.

Physiologic Regulation of Cerebrovascular Tone

Nitric Oxide and Cyclic Guanosine Monophosphate–Mediated Mechanisms

Endothelium modulates vascular tone by producing and releasing potent vasoactive substances.[1-3] One of these important substances is endothelium-derived nitric oxide (NO), which diffuses to vascular muscle and produces relaxation through activation of the soluble form of guanylyl cyclase, resulting in an increased intracellular concentration of cyclic guanosine monophosphate (cGMP) and relaxation. The NO–guanylyl cyclase mechanism represents a major mechanism of cerebral vasodilatation.

NO is a potent dilator of cerebral vessels and may be produced by one of three isoforms of NO synthase (NOS) (neuronal/type 1 or nNOS, immunologic/type 2 or iNOS, and endothelial/type 3 or eNOS), each of which uses L-arginine as a substrate.[1,2] In blood vessels, NO is generated under basal conditions in the endothelium by eNOS. Soluble guanylyl cyclase, which is cytosolic, can also be activated by pharmacologic agents, including nitroglycerin and sodium nitroprusside.[2,4] The activity of NOS can be further stimulated by increases in intracellular calcium levels that occur in response to many receptor-mediated agonists, such as acetylcholine, or in response to rises in shear stress that are associated with increases in the velocity of blood flow.[1]

Under normal conditions, NO is released both intraluminally and abluminally by endothelium. Endothelial release of both NO and prostacyclin, a product of arachidonic acid metabolism, into the vascular lumen contributes to the antithrombogenic properties of endothelium because both of these substances inhibit aggregation of platelets and adherence of leukocytes to endothelium.

Particulate guanylyl cyclase, the second form of guanylyl cyclase in vascular muscle, can be activated by members of the natriuretic peptide family: atrial natriuretic peptide, brain natriuretic peptide, and C-type natriuretic peptide.[5] Administration of exogenous atrial and brain natriuretic peptides produces relaxation of cerebral blood vessels, but it is not clear whether endogenously produced natriuretic peptides contribute to regulation of cerebrovascular tone.

Although the endothelial and neuronal isoforms of NOS are constitutively expressed in blood vessels, the inducible or "immunologic" isoform is probably not expressed under normal conditions; however, its expression may be induced in endothelium, vascular muscle, and other cell types in brain.[1] This inducible isoform of NOS can produce large amounts of NO in pathophysiologic conditions, such as ischemia–reperfusion, subarachnoid hemorrhage (SAH), and meningitis.

Cyclic Adenosine Monophosphate–Mediated Mechanisms

Activation of adenylate cyclase and production of cyclic adenosine monophosphate (cAMP) in vascular muscle mediate relaxation of blood vessels in response to a variety of endogenous substances, and this mediation represents a second major mechanism of vasodilatation in cerebral vessels. Stimuli that activate adenylate cyclase include prostanoids (prostacyclin and prostaglandin E_2), adenosine, calcitonin gene-related peptide (CGRP), vasoactive intestinal peptide, β-adrenergic agonists, pituitary adenylate cyclase activating peptide (PACAP), and adrenomedullin. A newer concept is that increases in intracellular cAMP in vascular muscle produce vasodilatation only in part by a direct effect and, in part, by activation of potassium ion (K^+) channels (see later).

K+ Channels and Endothelium-Derived Hyperpolarizing Factor (EDHF)

Vasodilator mechanisms also present in cerebral vessels involve activation of K+ channels and, apparently to a much lesser extent than in systemic vessels, the release of an EDHF. Increases in the activity of K+ channels ultimately result in membrane hyperpolarization of vascular muscle cells.[1,6,7] At least seven families of K+ channels are present in cerebral blood vessels: adenosine triphosphate (ATP)–sensitive K+ (K_{ATP}) channels; large-(BK_{Ca}), intermediate-(IK_{Ca}), and small-conductance (SK_{Ca}) calcium-activated K+ channels; voltage-dependent K+ (K_V) channels, inwardly rectifying K+ (K_{IR}) channels, and two-pore domain K+ (K_{2P}) channels.

K_{ATP} Channels

The activity of K_{ATP} channels is inhibited by intracellular ATP or an increased ratio of ATP to adenosine diphosphate (ADP). The intracellular concentration of ATP is normally sufficient to prevent opening of K_{ATP} channels, and in cerebrovascular muscle, these channels appear to be closed under normal conditions.[8] Because intracellular ATP levels are tightly regulated, it is likely that K_{ATP} channels are only rarely activated by reductions in ATP. Reductions in levels of intracellular pO_2 and pH also open these channels and produce vasorelaxation. Thus, the activity of K_{ATP} channels appears to reflect, at least in part, the metabolic state of cells.[6]

Several endogenous substances produce hyperpolarization and relaxation of cerebrovascular muscle that is mediated, either fully or partly, by activation of K_{ATP} channels. These substances include CGRP, norepinephrine, and increased intracellular concentration of cAMP.[7] The concept that K_{ATP} channels may be activated by higher concentrations of cAMP is supported by evidence that dilatation of the basilar artery in response to forskolin, a direct activator of adenylate cyclase, can be attenuated with glibenclamide, a selective inhibitor of K_{ATP} channels.[9,10] In contrast, vasodilators that increase cGMP in cerebral vessels are usually not inhibited by glibenclamide in most studies.[11,12]

Systemic hypoxia is a potent cerebral dilator, and relaxation of cerebral vessels during hypoxia appears to involve activation of K+ channels.[7,13] Relaxation during hypoxia of both large cerebral arteries in vitro and cerebral arterioles in vivo is inhibited by glibenclamide, suggesting that the response to hypoxia is mediated by activation of K_{ATP} channels.[8]

BK_{Ca} Channels

The activity of BK_{Ca} channels increases in response to elevations in intracellular calcium. In particular, this is now understood to be mediated by calcium sparks, which are transient local calcium-signaling events that deliver high (μM) local calcium levels from the opening of ryanodine-sensitive calcium release channels located in the sarcoplasmic reticulum to BK_{Ca} channels on the plasma membrane.[14] BK_{Ca} channels in blood vessels appear to act as a negative feedback mechanism during increases in intracellular concentrations of calcium; thus these channels open more frequently during increases in blood pressure and with membrane depolarization. The tone of cerebral vessels, particularly during elevations of arterial pressure, may potentially be influenced by the activity of BK_{Ca} channels (see later discussion of hypertension).[13] In contrast to K_{ATP} channels, BK_{Ca} channels may be active in large cerebral arteries under basal conditions, and selective inhibition of this channel (e.g., with tetraethylammonium [TEA] or iberiotoxin) leads to constriction of cerebral arteries.[15,16]

BK_{Ca} channels are responsive to other stimuli in addition to the intracellular concentration of calcium. Activation of BK_{Ca} channels appears to contribute to relaxation of cerebral arterioles in response to activation of adenylate cyclase and accumulation of cAMP.[17] Because a variety of endogenous vasoactive stimuli raise the concentration of cAMP in vascular muscle, activation of BK_{Ca} channels by cAMP may play a major role in regulation of cerebrovascular tone. There is similar evidence that increases in cGMP, or of NO independent of cGMP, can increase the activity of BK_{Ca} channels in cerebral vessels.[15,17]

IK_{Ca} and SK_{Ca} Channels and EDHF

Recent studies have established that both IK_{Ca} and SK_{Ca} channels are expressed in cerebral arteries.[18] Both of these channels are well known to be expressed in endothelial cells of systemic arteries, where they mediate K+ efflux and hyperpolarization, resulting in EDHF-mediated vasodilatation. However, studies to clarify the functional roles of IK_{Ca} and SK_{Ca} channels and, indeed, the existence and nature of EDHF-mediated responses have been much fewer in cerebral arteries. There is evidence that just as in systemic arteries, the functional importance of EDHF in endothelium-dependent relaxation becomes more prominent (with the role of endothelium-derived NO diminishing) in smaller arteries.[19] Although further study is clearly required in cerebral arteries, it appears that IK_{Ca} channel activation can fully mediate EDHF-dependent dilatation of the middle cerebral artery when NO is absent,[18,20,21] whereas SK_{Ca} channels can also contribute to endothelium-dependent hyperpolarization of this vessel only when NO synthesis is present.[18,21]

K_V Channels

Voltage-dependent K+ (K_V) channels are activated in response to membrane depolarization, but this process occurs independently of the intracellular calcium concentration. These K+ channels are also activated by elevations in arterial blood pressure and may thus modulate pressure-induced increases in cerebral artery tone.[22] Activation of K_V channels may also contribute directly to mechanisms that produce cerebral vasorelaxation in response to NO and EDHF.[23-25]

K_{IR} Channels

The name *inwardly rectifying K+ channels* is based on the channels' properties that enable conduction of K+ current into cells much more readily than K+ current out of cells.[6,26,27] At physiologic membrane potential, however, a small rise above the normal extracellular K+ (≈3 mM in cerebrospinal fluid) leads to an increase in the resting outward K+ current through K_{IR} channels. Hence, a modest increase in extracellular K+ (e.g., by <10 mmol/L), as may occur during neuronal or muscle activation,[28,29] can paradoxically lead to substantial vascular hyperpolarization and vasorelaxation because of K^+ efflux through K_{IR} channels.[26]

K_{2P} Channels

Very recently, two-pore domain K^+ (K_{2P}) channels were found to be present in cerebral arteries.[30,31] These channels can be activated by unmetabolized arachidonic acid (i.e., their activation by arachidonic acid is not sensitive to inhibitors of enzymes such as cylooxygenases, lipoxygenases, and cytochrome P450)[30] or by polyunsaturated fatty acids, such as α-linoleic acid and docosahexanoic acid,[31] which leads to cerebral vasodilation. In mice, basilar but not carotid arteries express TREK-1, one of several forms of K_{2P} channels. Interestingly, α-linoleic acid and docosahexanoic acid dilate the mouse basilar, but not the carotid, artery; this vasodilator response is absent in mice deficient in TREK-1.[31]

Transient Receptor Potential Channels

The transient receptor potential (TRP) superfamily of cation channels is grouped into three major subfamilies: TRPV (vanilloid), TRPC (canonical), and TRPM (melastatin).[32,33] It has been proposed that some of these channels play a role in dilator and constrictor responses in the cerebral circulation.[34] For example, epoxyeicosatrienoic acids (EETs), compounds that are produced by the endothelium and have been proposed to be an EDHF, have been reported to activate TRPV4 channels in cerebrovascular smooth muscle cells.[35] Activation of these receptors leads to increased Ca^{2+} influx, Ca^{2+} sparks, and BK_{Ca} channel activity, thereby hyperpolarizing and relaxing the smooth muscle.[35] Recent evidence also suggests a role for TRP channels in receptor-mediated contraction of cerebral arteries. Uridine triphosphate (UTP) depolarizes and contracts cerebral vessels.[36] Downregulation of TRCP3 expression with the use of antisense oligonucleotides has been reported to reduce UTP-induced depolarization and vasoconstriction of cerebrovascular smooth muscle (VSM) cells.[37]

Reactive Oxygen Species

The parent reactive oxygen species (ROS) molecule superoxide (O_2^-) is generated by oxidases and other sources via the univalent reduction of molecular oxygen and is rapidly dismutated either spontaneously or catalyzed by endogenous O_2^- dismutases (SOD) to form hydrogen peroxide (H_2O_2). In contrast to noncerebral arteries, O_2^- has been reported to elicit both relaxation[38-41] and contraction[38,42] of cerebral arteries. At present it is unclear why O_2^- has variable effects on cerebrovascular tone; however, one possible explanation is that its effect is concentration dependent, in that relaxation occurs at low concentrations[38,39] and contraction occurs at higher concentrations.[38] TEA attenuates cerebral relaxation to O_2^-, which suggests that BK_{Ca} channels are involved in mediating the dilator effects of O_2^-.[38,40] O_2^- reacts with NO in a reaction that is so rapid that it is near diffusion-limited. Indeed,

the reaction of O_2^- with NO (6.7×10^9 mol/L^{-1} s^{-1}) is three times faster than the dismutation of O_2^- by SOD (2×10^9 mol/L^{-1} s^{-1}).[43] Because NO plays a pivotal role in regulating cerebrovascular tone under basal conditions,[1] a loss of NO bioavailability could cause constriction of cerebral vessels. O_2^- has also been reported to constrict endothelium-denuded canine basilar arteries,[44] which implies that O_2^- can directly constrict cerebral arteries independent of its effect on endothelial NO bioavailability.

It has been demonstrated extensively that H_2O_2 elicits cerebral vasodilatation in vitro and in vivo in a number of different species.[40,45-52] Opening of K^+ channels is thought to be a major mechanism by which H_2O_2 elicits cerebral vasodilatation. For example, dilatation of rat cerebral arterioles to exogenous H_2O_2 is mediated by activation of BK_{Ca} channels.[49] Similarly, direct electrophysiologic recordings have shown that ROS can increase the activity of BK_{Ca} channels in cerebral arteries via Ca^{2+} sparks.[53-55] Some recent work suggests that eNOS produces O_2^- under normal physiologic conditions and that the subsequent generation of H_2O_2 mediates endothelium-dependent vasodilatation.[56] However, many other studies suggest that endothelium-dependent responses in cerebral vessels in numerous species are mediated by NO[1] and not ROS.

The levels of O_2^- and H_2O_2 within vascular cells and thus their effect on vascular tone depend not only on their rate of production but also on their rate of metabolism by antioxidant enzymes. Inhibition of CuSOD with the use of the copper chelator diethyldithiocarbamate (DETCA) elicits a large increase in levels of cerebrovascular O_2^-.[46,47,57] In addition, genetic deletion of SOD1 augments O_2^- levels and impairs NO-mediated dilatation in the cerebral circulation.[58] Taken together, these findings suggest that CuZn-containing SODs play a pivotal role in regulating levels of O_2^- and H_2O_2 in the cerebral circulation.

Sources of vascular ROS include the mitochondrial electron transport chain, the arachidonic acid metabolizing enzymes (cyclooxygenase [COX] and lipoxygenase), the cytochrome P450s, xanthine oxidase, NADPH (reduced form of nicotinamide adenine dinucleotide phosphate) oxidases, and NOS under special circumstances. Compelling evidence suggests that NADPH oxidase–derived ROS are functionally important in the regulation of cerebrovascular function in both physiology and pathophysiology.[59] (See later discussion of pathophysiologic alterations.) These enzymes are similar but not identical in structure to the phagocytic NADPH oxidases and comprise membrane (Nox and p22phox) and cytosolic subunits (p47phox, p67phox, and Rac). The catalytic domain resides in the Nox subunit, of which four isoforms appear to be important for vascular ROS production: Nox1, Nox2, Nox4, and Nox5.[59] Interestingly, the activity of NADPH oxidase is profoundly higher in cerebral versus systemic arteries.[46] Activation of NADPH oxidase using its substrate, NADPH, elicits profound cerebral vasodilatation in several animal species.[38,39,46,47,60] The identity of the NADPH oxidase–derived ROS molecule responsible for mediating cerebral vasodilatation is not well-defined and appears to be species dependent. For example, NADPH-induced vasodilatation of rat basilar arteries in vivo is inhibited by catalase (H_2O_2 scavenger) and DETCA.[47] In contrast, O_2^-, and not H_2O_2, is partially responsible for the increase in cerebral blood flow to NADPH in mice.[39] Neither ROS scavengers,[48,49] NADPH oxidase inhibitors,[38,39,47] or gene knockdown approaches[39] alter the resting tone of cerebral arteries or cerebral blood flow in rat, mouse, and rabbit models, which suggests that at least in these animals, the output of ROS by NADPH oxidase is not sufficient to modulate basal cerebral artery tone. Nevertheless, recent evidence suggests that NADPH oxidase–derived ROS serve as important physiologic molecules in cerebral endothelial and smooth muscle cells for increasing cerebral blood flow in response to humoral[46] and physical stimuli.[61]

Arachidonic acid elicits dilatation of cerebral arterioles that can be completely inhibited by indomethacin or scavengers of ROS, which suggests a key role for COX-derived ROS in mediating vasodilator responses to arachidonic acid.[48,49,62-64] Furthermore, catalase abolishes the dilator effects of bradykinin on cerebral arterioles,[49] which suggests that ROS may play a role in endothelium-dependent vasodilator responses to bradykinin in the cerebral circulation.

Regulation of Myogenic Tone: TRP Channels and RhoA/Rho Kinase

Myogenic tone, an inherent property of smooth muscle, is prominent in cerebral arteries and arterioles and plays an important role in the development of basal vascular tone and blood flow autoregulation. A number of studies suggest that TRP channels are important mediators of the myogenic vasoconstrictor response to increases in intravascular pressure. For example, downregulation of the TRPC6 channel with the use of antisense oligonucleotides decreases cerebral VSM depolarization and vasoconstriction induced by elevated intraluminal pressure.[65] These results suggest that membrane stretching activates a TRPC6-dependent depolarizing cation current that contributes to constriction of cerebral arteries.[34] A role for TRPM4 channels in the myogenic contractile response of cerebral arteries has also been reported. In vivo administration of TRPM4 antisense oligonucleotides to mice significantly reduced pressure-induced depolarization of isolated cerebral arteries and compromised autoregulatory function in vivo.[66]

Inhibition of myosin light chain phosphate (MLCPh) enhances the sensitivity of the VSM contractile apparatus to intracellular Ca^{2+}, a process known as Ca^{2+} sensitization. Activation of the RhoA/Rho-kinase (ROK) pathway results in phosphorylation of MLCPh, which renders it inactive and leads to increased vascular contractility.[67] The ROK pathway appears to play an important role in regulating smooth muscle contractility and hence may contribute to the myogenic response.[68] Consistent with this, RhoA can be activated by stretching,[69] and studies have found that the Rho-kinase inhibitor Y-27632 inhibits pressure-induced constriction of isolated cerebral arteries.[70,71] Moreover, administration of Y-27632 in vivo has been reported to cause dilatation of cerebral arteries[72,73] and arterioles.[74]

Pathophysiologic Alterations in Cerebral Vessel Function

Platelets and Leukocytes

Activated platelets release potent vasoactive substances, including ADP (an endothelium-dependent vasodilator), serotonin (either a vasoconstrictor or an endothelium-dependent vasodilator, depending on the vascular bed and vessel size) and thromboxane A_2 (a vasoconstrictor). In normal vessels, the vasomotor response to platelet products therefore may potentially be dilatation, constriction, or little net effect, depending on the relative influence of individual mediators. Under pathophysiologic conditions in which endothelial function is impaired, release of NO in response to ADP is reduced, and a greater portion of the net vasomotor response to platelet products is shifted to vasoconstrictor influences.

Polymorphonuclear leukocytes and monocytes also produce a variety of vasoactive agents, but the identity and conditions for release of many of these mediators are still poorly understood. In general, it is uncertain whether vasoconstrictor or vasodilator responses prevail in response to leukocytes.[75] Endothelium appears to either mediate dilator responses or attenuate constrictor responses to leukocytes (as well as platelets) in some vascular preparations. In contrast to platelets, however, leukocytes produce endothelium-dependent constriction of normal arteries.[75,76] The mechanism of this latter effect appears to be through inactivation or inhibition of NO that is released under basal conditions. The effect of endothelial dysfunction on vascular responses to leukocytes is therefore difficult to predict; evaluation of vasoactive influences of leukocytes on cerebral vessels under specific pathophysiologic conditions is an important issue.

Atherosclerosis

Endothelium-Dependent Relaxation in Atherosclerosis

Basal- and agonist-induced release or activity of NO is impaired in extracranial blood vessels by atherosclerosis.[77-79] SOD improves endothelium-dependent relaxation in atherosclerotic arteries,[78] which suggests that the mechanism of impairment involves excess generation of O_2^- and inactivation of NO. In advanced atherosclerotic lesions, however, impairment of relaxation may also be related to reduced production of NO.

The effect of atherosclerosis on endothelium-dependent relaxation of cerebral vessels is less clear. Atherosclerosis seems to develop in intracranial vessels much more slowly than in extracranial vessels.[80] Relaxation of cerebral vessels in response to endothelium-dependent stimuli can be normal in the same atherosclerotic animals that exhibit marked impairment of endothelium-dependent relaxation in the aorta.[80,81] In contrast, some studies suggest that atherosclerosis or hypercholesterolemia produces cerebral endothelial dysfunction. For example, hypercholesterolemia is associated with impaired endothelium-dependent relaxation of the rabbit basilar artery.[82] In a genetic model of hypercholesterolemia and atherosclerosis (apolipoprotein E–deficient mice; $ApoE^{-/-}$), endothelium-dependent relaxation of common carotid arteries[83] and cerebral arterioles[84] is impaired. In cerebral arteries from atherosclerotic monkeys, exogenous dilator responses to NO were found to be intact, whereas the basal activity of soluble guanylyl cyclase appeared to be diminished.[85] The mechanisms underlying cerebral vasomotor dysfunction are not completely understood. Administration of L-arginine, the substrate for NO synthesis, restores dilator responses of the rabbit basilar artery to acetylcholine to normal, which suggests that L-arginine deficiency may contribute to the dysfunction.[82] Alternatively, there is evidence that increased levels of asymmetrical dimethylarginine, which competes with L-arginine for binding to NOS, may also contribute to this phenomenon.[86] Finally, increased generation of cerebrovascular O_2^- may contribute to decreased NO bioavailability. Indeed, in ApoE$^{-/-}$ mice, dilator responses of cerebral arterioles to acetylcholine are enhanced by either the SOD mimetic tempol or the NADPH oxidase inhibitor apocynin,[84] which suggests that increased NADPH oxidase activity may contribute to endothelial dysfunction during hypercholesterolemia and atherosclerosis.

Some studies now indicate that endothelial dysfunction is predictive of cardiovascular events.[87,88] It will be of great interest to determine whether endothelial dysfunction is predictive of stroke.

Cerebrovascular Responses to Platelet and Leukocyte Products in Atherosclerosis

In the carotid and other large arteries supplying the brain, constrictor responses to serotonin and thromboxane A_2 are enhanced in the presence of atherosclerosis.[77,89-92] Collagen, which activates platelets, increases carotid blood flow normally but produces reductions in blood flow in the presence of atherosclerosis.[77] The normal increase in carotid blood flow produced by collagen is probably due largely to endothelium-dependent vasodilatation mediated by release of NO from small cerebral arteries in response to ADP,[93,94] a major product of platelet activation. Because NO normally inhibits constrictor responses of large cerebral arteries to serotonin, impairment of release or activity of NO may contribute to augmented vasoconstrictor responses during atherosclerosis.[95,96] Endothelial dysfunction alone, however, does not appear to be sufficient to account for all of the increases in constrictor responsiveness of large cerebral arteries to serotonin.[89,90]

Analogous results have been obtained concerning effects of leukocytes on cerebral arteries during atherosclerosis.[75] Leukocytes in vitro induce greater contraction of atherosclerotic arteries than of normal vessels.[75] Intravascular activation of leukocytes leads to prolonged contraction of cerebral arteries of the atherosclerotic monkey, whereas in normal animals, the constrictor effects of activated leukocytes are trivial.[92] Leukocytes from hypercholesterolemic rabbits release greater amounts of at least one unidentified contracting factor that inhibits NO-dependent vascular relaxation.[97]

Most transient ischemic attacks (TIAs) are thought to be produced by platelet adhesion, aggregation, and embolization from plaques in large extracranial arteries.[98] Release of serotonin during aggregation of platelets, coupled with augmented constrictor responses to serotonin

in atherosclerotic arteries, may produce pronounced vasoconstriction and perhaps contribute to cerebral ischemia.[89]

Importantly, vasoactive effects of platelets and leukocytes are likely to be closely interdependent. When leukocytes and platelets are activated together, there appears to be enhanced release of vasoactive products, and activation of leukocytes inhibits vasodilatation in response to platelets.[99] Furthermore, there is synergism in the action of platelet- and leukocyte-derived vasoconstrictors on vascular tone.[75] Abnormal cerebrovascular responses to activated platelets, and possibly leukocytes, may thus contribute to the pathophysiology of TIAs and cerebral ischemia in the presence of atherosclerosis.[90]

Effects of Therapy to Lower Plasma Cholesterol Levels

Hypercholesterolemia is a major risk factor for coronary vascular events, but plasma cholesterol has been thought to have only a small effect on susceptibility to cerebrovascular events. Reduction in dietary cholesterol levels produces regression of atherosclerosis and restores endothelium-dependent relaxation of extracranial arteries toward normal in experimental animals.[78,79] Susceptibility to vasoconstriction in response to activation of platelets and leukocytes is reduced or abolished by regression of atherosclerosis.[100]

Augmented constrictor responses of large cerebral arteries to serotonin are also restored largely to normal during regression of atherosclerosis.[77,90] Significant functional improvement appears to precede structural regression and occurs within only a few months of dietary treatment of hypercholesterolemia in cerebral and noncerebral arteries of atherosclerotic monkeys.[77,101] Thus, the benefits of cholesterol-lowering therapy may occur relatively rapidly. Hypercholesterolemia alters platelets as well as blood vessels, and part of the rapid improvement in vascular responses during treatment of hypercholesterolemia may be related to normalization of platelet function.[102]

Of considerable interest is the finding that in patients with coronary heart disease who received a cholesterol-lowering agent for approximately 5 years, reduction of cholesterol levels decreased cerebrovascular events by one third.[103] The finding has been confirmed in other large trials using HMG (3-hydroxy-3-methylglutaryl)–coenzyme A reductase inhibitors. Pharmacologic lowering of plasma cholesterol levels with the use of HMG–coenzyme A reductase inhibitors (i.e., statins) appears to provide additional benefits for vascular function, including increased expression of endothelial NOS and decreased activity of NADPH oxidase and Rho-kinase.[104-106] The response to statins is described as a "pleiotropic" effect; some effects also occur in normocholesterolemic animals and are not due to a reduction in plasma cholesterol levels (Fig. 1-1).[107] Upregulation of endothelial NOS by statins enhances cerebral blood flow and reduces stroke damage after cerebral ischemia.[104,105,107] Thus, statins not only reduce cerebrovascular events but also improve vascular function, by both cholesterol lowering with regression of atherosclerosis and a pleiotropic effect that is not related to reduction of the cholesterol level.

Chronic Hypertension

Chronic hypertension is a major risk factor for numerous cardiovascular disorders and, for reasons that are not clear, is even more strongly associated with stroke than with myocardial infarction.[108] Hypertension may have profound deleterious effects on cerebrovascular function, the underlying mechanisms of which are still not well understood.

Endothelial Function in Chronic Hypertension

Endothelium-dependent relaxation is impaired in the cerebral circulation during chronic hypertension (Fig. 1-2). Dilatation of cerebral arterioles and the basilar artery in response to endothelium-dependent agonists such as acetylcholine and ADP is impaired in the chronically hypertensive rat.[1] Cerebral vasodilatation in response to endothelium-independent agonists (which act directly on vascular muscle) such as NO, nitroglycerin, and adenosine is not impaired during chronic hypertension, which suggests that endothelial function is impaired but vascular muscle relaxation is preserved.[1] Thus, the cAMP and cGMP mechanisms appear to be relatively normal during chronic hypertension.

Altered responses of cerebral arterioles to endothelium-dependent agonists (acetylcholine and serotonin) in chronic hypertension may impair cerebral vasodilatation in response to vasoactive substances released by platelets. It is possible that when platelets aggregate at plaques in the carotid arteries and release serotonin, impairment of endothelium-dependent responses during chronic hypertension may predispose to cerebral ischemia and stroke. Evidence consistent with that possibility is that serotonin produces greater constriction of large cerebral arteries in spontaneously hypertensive stroke prone (SHRSP) rats than in Wistar Kyoto (WKY) rats.[109]

Mechanisms that account for impaired endothelium-dependent relaxation during chronic hypertension are not fully defined and appear to be different in cerebral arterioles than in the basilar artery. In cerebral arterioles, this impairment may be related to release of an endothelium-derived contracting factor (EDCF) that counteracts the normal dilator effects of NO (see Fig. 1-2).[110] This EDCF appears to be a prostanoid (and not, for example, endothelin) because indomethacin restores responses to endothelium-dependent agonists to or toward normal.[110] Impaired endothelium-dependent relaxation of the basilar artery, unlike that of the cerebral arterioles, does not appear to be due to production of an EDCF and is restored by L-arginine in SHRSP rats.[111,112]

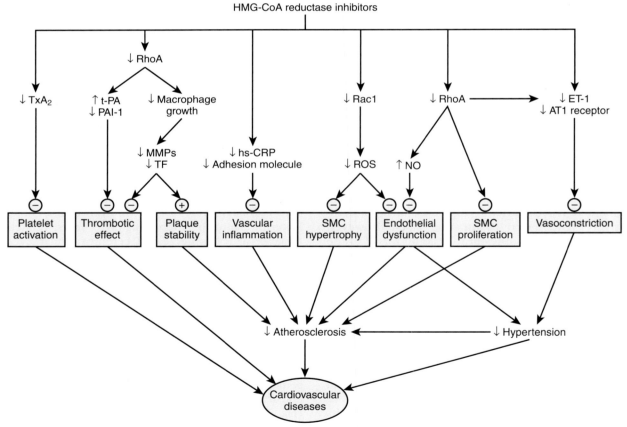

Figure 1-1 HMG–CoA reductase inhibitors (statins) have multiple effects on blood vessels. Many of the effects are not produced by reduction of plasma cholesterol. AT1 receptor, angiotensin type 1 receptor; ET-1, endothelin-1; hs-CRP, C-reactive protein; MMPs, matrix metalloproteinases; NO, nitric oxide; PAI-1, plasminogen activator inhibitor-1; ROS, reactive oxygen species; SMC, smooth muscle cell; TF, tissue factor; t-PA, tissue-type plasminogen activator; TxA_2, thromboxane A_2. (Adapted from Laufs U, Gertz K, Huang P, et al: Atorvastatin upregulates type III nitric oxide synthase in thrombocytes, decreases platelet activation, and protects from cerebral ischemia in normocholesterolemic mice. *Stroke* 31:2442-2449, 2000, with permission.)

Oxidative Stress and Endothelial Function

Since 2000, it has become apparent that levels of ROS in both systemic and cerebral arteries are increased during hypertension, which leads to a condition known as *oxidative stress*. In spontaneously hypertensive rats, relaxation of the carotid artery in response to acetylcholine is impaired and is associated with enhanced levels of O_2^-.[113] Moreover, treatment of rats with a recombinant adenovirus expressing SOD3 improves endothelial function and reduces levels of vascular O_2^-.[113] Similarly, polyethylene glycol SOD (PEG-SOD) treatment of the basilar artery in hypertensive transgenic mice overexpressing human renin and angiotensinogen reverses endothelial dysfunction.[114] Thus, increased inactivation of endothelium-derived NO by O_2^- appears to be an important underlying mechanism for cerebrovascular endothelial dysfunction in hypertension. Genetic eNOS deficiency and a subsequent loss of endothelium-derived NO lead to hypertrophy of cerebral vessels.[115] Thus, a loss of NO bioavailability during hypertension could have profound effects on the structure of cerebral arteries, in that thickening could ultimately impair maximal vasodilator capacity. In addition to impairing endothelial-dependent responses, other vasodilator mechanisms may be inhibited by O_2^-, including neurovascular coupling,[116] responses to glutamate,[117] hypercapnia,[118] and hypoxia.[119]

There are likely to be multiple vascular sources of O_2^- in hypertension. In noncerebral arteries, it has been suggested that decreased availability of eNOS substrate (L-arginine) or cofactor (tetrahydrobiopterin; BH$_4$) during hypertension leads to eNOS "uncoupling" and subsequent O_2^- generation.[120] It has been extensively demonstrated that the generation of O_2^- by vascular NADPH oxidases in systemic and cerebral vessels is enhanced in spontaneous (genetic) and pharmacologic or surgical models of hypertension.[59] Moreover, this is associated with an increase in expression of its catalytic subunits, Nox1, Nox2, and Nox4, as well as p22phox.[59] Furthermore, in experimental hypertension, mice genetically deficient in NADPH oxidase subunits have lower blood pressures and show

no evidence of impaired endothelial function.[59] Interestingly, recent studies have reported that interference with peroxisome proliferator-activated receptor-γ (PPARγ) signaling leads to increased O_2^- production, endothelial dysfunction, and vascular remodeling in the cerebral circulation.[121] Moreover, administration of PPARγ agonists (rosiglitazone and pioglitazone) to hypertensive mice and rats reduces O_2^- and improves endothelial function.[122,123]

Rho-Kinase Pathway

Dilator responses of the basilar artery to the Rho-kinase inhibitor Y-27632 in vivo are enhanced in experimental models of hypertension.[72,124,125] Similarly, Y-27632 inhibits the pressure-induced vasoconstriction of cerebral arteries to a greater extent in SHR than in WKY rats.[125] Taken together, these findings suggest that the activity of Rho-kinase in cerebral arteries may be increased during hypertension.

K+ Channels

Chronic hypertension has been the most extensively studied cardiovascular disease state in relation to changes to K$^+$ channel expression and function in cerebral arteries. There is evidence of abnormal function of several K$^+$ channel types in blood vessels during hypertension; this evidence has been reviewed.[1,7,126]

K$_{ATP}$ Channels

Dilator responses of cerebral arteries in chronically hypertensive rats are impaired with regard to activation of K$_{ATP}$ channels (see Fig. 1-2).[127] Because K$_{ATP}$ channels are important mediators of vasodilator responses to hypoxia and hypotension, one might speculate that cerebral dilator responses to hypoxia and hypotension are impaired in chronic hypertension.[8]

BK$_{Ca}$ Channels

Specific inhibitors of BK$_{Ca}$ channels produce greater contraction of cerebral vessels in hypertensive animals than in normotensive animals. Thus, basal activity of

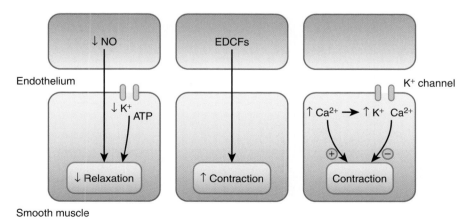

Figure 1-2 Some abnormalities in cerebral vessels during chronic hypertension. Decreased production or activity of nitric oxide (NO) may occur during chronic hypertension. Activity of ATP-sensitive potassium channels (K$_{ATP}$) may also be reduced during hypertension. Production of endothelium-derived contracting factors (EDCFs) may occur and counteract normal vasodilator mechanisms. Activity of large conductance calcium-activated K$^+$ channels appears to be increased during chronic hypertension, perhaps in response to increased levels of intracellular calcium.

BK_{Ca} channels appears to be increased in cerebral arteries during chronic hypertension.[16] Deficiency in expression of the BK_{Ca} channel may itself result in cerebral artery dysfunction and systemic hypertension. Targeted deletion of the β1 subunit of the BK_{Ca} channel, which renders the channel largely nonfunctional under physiologic conditions, produces hypertension (≈15 to 20 mm Hg higher than normal) in mice.[128,129] In addition, cerebral arteries constrict to a greater extent at a given pressure in BKβ1-deficient mice than in controls.[129] Thus, the normal function of BK_{Ca} channels appears to reduce cerebral artery tone as well as systemic blood pressure.

Consistent with such a function, studies in other experimental models of hypertension have also demonstrated that expression and activity of BK_{Ca} channels are increased in several vessels, including the carotid artery[130,131] and intracranial vessels.[16,132] Because of its role in limiting vasoconstriction, BK_{Ca} channel function may be increased in vascular muscle as a protective negative feedback mechanism against increases in blood pressure. Such a mechanism would act to limit pressure-induced vasoconstriction and preserve local blood flow. The potential clinical relevance of these findings may include the targeting of BK_{Ca} channels with therapeutic approaches to treat hypertension and also investigating whether mutations in genes encoding components of BK_{Ca} channels contribute to some types of human hypertension.

Subarachnoid Hemorrhage

Function of Endothelium and Soluble Guanylyl Cyclase

SAH produces several abnormalities of vascular function (Fig. 1-3). After SAH, cerebrovascular muscle is partially depolarized.[133] Depolarization of vascular muscle contributes to cerebral vasospasm, which often occurs after SAH.[134] Several mechanisms, including endothelial function, may contribute to vasospasm. Endothelium-dependent relaxation is impaired in large cerebral arteries in experimental models of SAH.[135] Similar impairment has been observed in the basilar artery from humans after SAH.[136]

Several mechanisms have been proposed to account for the impairment of endothelium-dependent relaxation after SAH.[134] Both the amount and activity of endothelial NOS protein are relatively unchanged in large cerebral arteries after SAH.[137,138] These findings are consistent with previous reports that release of NO is normal after SAH.[137,139,140]

Some findings suggest that impaired endothelium-dependent relaxation after SAH is due to reduction of protein levels, reduction of activity of soluble guanylyl cyclase, or both (see Fig. 1-3).[138,140,141] Increased phosphodiesterase activity and impaired K_V channel function in cerebral arteries after SAH could also contribute to this phenomenon.[142,143] In contrast, other studies report that vasorelaxation in response to nitrovasodilators is unaltered.[144,145]

The presence of hemoglobin in the cerebrospinal fluid may contribute to vasospasm after SAH by inactivation of NO. Hemoglobin avidly binds NO and thus may prevent diffusion of NO from endothelium to smooth muscle. In addition, hemoglobin may destroy NO through generation of O_2^-.[134] Spasm of large cerebral arteries after experimental SAH is attenuated by overexpression of SOD1 in mice[146] and by injection of adenovirus expressing human SOD3 into the cisterna magna of rabbits.[147] Furthermore, inhibitors of NADPH oxidase have been reported to attenuate cerebral vasospasm,[148,149] which suggests that NADPH oxidase–derived O_2^- may directly contribute to the pathogenesis of cerebral vasospasm after SAH. Thus, several mechanisms may contribute to impairment of endothelium-dependent relaxation of cerebral arteries after SAH.

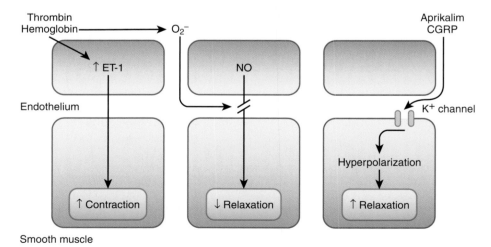

Figure 1-3 Some abnormalities in cerebral vessels after subarachnoid hemorrhage. Thrombin and hemoglobin cause increased gene expression for endothelin-1 (ET-1), a potent vasoconstrictor. Superoxide anion (O_2^-) may be formed from hemoglobin, inactivate nitric oxide (NO), and thus impair relaxation. Vasodilatation in response to activation of ATP-sensitive K^+ channels (K_{ATP}) appears to be augmented after subarachnoid hemorrhage. This latter mechanism, in contrast to the first two, has implications for treatment of vasospasm after subarachnoid hemorrhage. CGRP, calcitonin gene-related peptide.

Bilirubin Oxidized Products (BOXes)

It has recently been proposed that ROS generated in blood clots surrounding cerebral vessels may oxidize bilirubin, biliverdin, and possibly heme to produce BOXes.[150] BOXes constrict cerebral arteries in vivo and in vitro,[150] and there is a correlation between the clinical occurrence of vasospasm and the concentration of BOXes in cerebrospinal fluid of patients with SAH.[150]

Endothelin

Endothelin is a vasoconstrictor peptide that is produced by endothelial cells and is thus an EDCF. It is not clear whether endothelin plays a role in physiologic regulation of the cerebral circulation.[1] Because endothelin-mediated constriction is long-lasting, it seems unlikely that endothelin contributes to the fine, short-term regulation of cerebral blood flow. Topical application of endothelin receptor antagonists does not alter the diameter of cerebral vessels in vivo, which suggests that endothelin does not contribute to basal cerebrovascular tone.[151,152]

Several findings indicate that endothelin may contribute to cerebral vasospasm after SAH (see Fig. 1-3).[135] Hemoglobin and thrombin, which are present in cerebrospinal fluid after SAH, can enhance endothelin gene expression and endothelin release (see Fig. 1-3).[153,154] Concentrations of endothelin in the basilar artery and in cerebrospinal fluid are increased after SAH.[153-156] Intracisternal administration of endothelin-A (ET_A) receptor antagonists reduces vasospasm after SAH.[152,154,157-159] In contrast, other studies report no correlation between cerebrospinal fluid endothelin levels and cerebral vasospasm[160] and failure of ET_A receptor antagonists to reverse cerebral vasospasm.[161] However, most evidence is consistent with the concept that endothelin and activation of ET_A receptors contribute to the onset or maintenance of cerebral vasospasm after SAH.

Rho-Kinase Pathway

The activity and expression of Rho-kinase in cerebral arteries is enhanced after SAH.[162,163] Furthermore, experimental studies have found that inhibition of Rho-kinase with the use of Y-27632 prevents narrowing of the canine basilar artery after SAH.[164] Similarly, intravenous injection of another Rho-kinase inhibitor HA1077 (also known as fasudil) attenuates vasoconstriction of the canine basilar artery after SAH.[165] There is evidence that both hemoglobin and endothelin-1 may partially cause vasospasm by activating the Rho-kinase pathway.[68] Fasudil is used clinically in Japan for the treatment of vasospasm after SAH. Some clinical benefit has been found using fasudil; however, vasospasm development is not eliminated, which suggests that several major candidates play a role in mediating cerebral vasoconstriction after SAH.[68]

K+ Channel Function after Subarachnoid Hemorrhage

Another mechanism that may contribute to vasospasm after SAH may involve changes in the activity of K^+ channels in cerebral vessels. Partial depolarization of cerebrovascular muscle after SAH appears to be due to diminished membrane conductance of K^+.[133,143] Depolarization and vasospasm can be inhibited by nicorandil,[166] a vasodilator that activates both K^+ channels and soluble guanylyl cyclase.[133] These findings suggest that activators of K^+ channels in vascular muscle may have beneficial effects during vasospasm after SAH (see Fig. 1-3).

Consistent with these findings are reports that dilatation of the basilar artery in response to openers of K_{ATP} channels is enhanced after SAH (see Fig. 1-3).[167,168] Interestingly, K_{ATP} channel–mediated dilatation of large cerebral vessels may be especially enhanced after SAH during chronic hypertension.[168] Thus, augmented responses to activation of K^+ channels despite the presence of hypertension are unusual and potentially therapeutically useful.

Hyperhomocysteinemia

Moderate elevation of the plasma homocysteine level appears to be an independent risk factor for stroke and is associated with peripheral vascular disease and myocardial infarction.[169] Like hypercholesterolemia, hyperhomocysteinemia is caused by both genetic and dietary factors, and it may possibly contribute to vascular disease in a large number of patients.[170] Moderate elevations of the plasma homocysteine level can be decreased by dietary supplementation with folic acid, which is a finding that suggests that hyperhomocysteinemia may be a treatable risk factor for stroke and other vascular diseases.

Hyperhomocysteinemia produces vascular dysfunction, in both the carotid artery and the cerebral circulation. For example, acute elevation in homocysteine in the presence of copper (Cu^{2+}) inhibits NO-mediated cerebrovascular responses.[118] More modest but chronic hyperhomocysteinemia produces endothelial dysfunction.[171-175] Both plasma levels of homocysteine and the extent of endothelial dysfunction are strongly influenced by the content of folate in the diet.[174] It is not entirely clear, however, to what extent vascular dysfunction is due to elevated homocysteine levels, folate deficiency, or other mechanisms. Importantly, a 2001 study suggests that endothelial dysfunction occurs in mice deficient in cystathionine β-synthase even in the absence of folate deficiency and is associated with increased *S*-adenosylmethionine levels.[171] These results suggest that altered *S*-adenosylmethionine-dependent methylation may contribute to the vascular pathophysiology of hyperhomocysteinemia.[171] In addition, studies with pharmacologic scavengers and genetically altered mice suggest that vascular dysfunction during hyperhomocysteinemia is at least partly mediated by oxidative stress.[172,176]

Diabetes Mellitus

Endothelial dysfunction also occurs in cerebral vessels during diabetes mellitus.[177-180] Mechanisms that account for impairment in diabetes appear to be similar to those observed during chronic hypertension. Altered responses of cerebral arterioles to endothelium-dependent agonists are probably due to production of an EDCF that activates a prostaglandin H_2–thromboxane A_2 receptor[179] with activation of protein kinase C.[177] In the basilar artery, impaired responses to endothelium-dependent stimuli are not due to production of a cyclooxygenase-derived EDCF.[178]

There is some evidence that the expression and activity of the Rho-kinase pathway may be enhanced in cerebral arteries during diabetes. For example, in the basilar artery from streptozotocin-injected (i.e., type 1 diabetic) rats, levels of mRNA for RhoA are greater than in control rats.[181] Functionally, dilator responses of cerebral arterioles to Y-27632 appear to be enhanced in type 2 diabetic versus control mice.[74]

As in chronic hypertension, the activity of K_{ATP} channels in diabetes appears to be altered. Dilatation of the basilar artery in response to aprikalim, an activator of K_{ATP} channels, is reduced in diabetic rats, suggesting that function of K_{ATP} channels may be abnormal in diabetes mellitus.[182]

Other findings indicate that hyperglycemia per se may produce impairment of endothelium-dependent dilatation of cerebral arterioles. This impairment of endothelium-dependent vasodilatation during acute elevations of glucose appears to involve activation of protein kinase C.[183]

Summary

Abnormalities of cerebrovascular function occur in many disease states. Although the mechanisms are complex and multifactorial, a greater understanding of several mechanisms of cerebral vessel dysfunction is being achieved. Many abnormalities of vasomotor function compromise regulation of cerebral blood flow and thus increase the risk of stroke. Therapy for cerebrovascular dysfunction focuses primarily on treatment of risk factors and, in addition, may involve pharmacologic or dietary interventions.

Acknowledgments

The authors would like to acknowledge the contributions by authors of previous editions of this chapter: Dr Frank M. Faraci and Dr Donald D. Heistad.

REFERENCES

1. Faraci FM, Heistad DD: Regulation of the cerebral circulation: Role of endothelium and potassium channels, *Physiol Rev* 78:53-97, 1998.
2. Moncada S, Palmer RM, Higgs EA: Nitric oxide: Physiology, pathophysiology, and pharmacology, *Pharmacol Rev* 43:109-142, 1991.
3. Faraci FM, Brian JE Jr: Nitric oxide and the cerebral circulation, *Stroke* 25:692-703, 1994.
4. Schlossmann J, Feil R, Hofmann F: Signaling through NO and cGMP-dependent protein kinases, *Ann Med* 35:21-27, 2003.
5. Wong SK, Garbers DL: Receptor guanylyl cyclases, *J Clin Invest* 90:299-305, 1992.
6. Nelson MT, Quayle JM: Physiological roles and properties of potassium channels in arterial smooth muscle, *Am J Physiol* 268:C799-822, 1995.
7. Faraci FM, Sobey CG: Role of potassium channels in regulation of cerebral vascular tone, *J Cereb Blood Flow Metab* 18:1047-1063, 1998.
8. Kitazono T, Faraci FM, Taguchi H, Heistad DD: Role of potassium channels in cerebral blood vessels, *Stroke* 26:1713-1723, 1995.
9. Kitazono T, Faraci FM, Heistad DD: Effect of norepinephrine on rat basilar artery in vivo, *Am J Physiol* 264:H178-182, 1993.
10. Kitazono T, Heistad DD, Faraci FM: Role of ATP-sensitive K+ channels in CGRP-induced dilatation of basilar artery in vivo, *Am J Physiol* 265:H581-585, 1993.
11. Onoue H, Katusic ZS: Role of potassium channels in relaxations of canine middle cerebral arteries induced by nitric oxide donors, *Stroke* 28:1264-1270, 1997.
12. Faraci FM, Heistad DD: Role of ATP-sensitive potassium channels in the basilar artery, *Am J Physiol* 264:H8-13, 1993.
13. Nelson MT, Cheng H, Rubart M, et al: Relaxation of arterial smooth muscle by calcium sparks, *Science* 270:633-637, 1995.
14. Wellman GC, Nelson MT: Signaling between SR and plasmalemma in smooth muscle: Sparks and the activation of Ca^{2+}-sensitive ion channels, *Cell Calcium* 34:211-229, 2003.
15. Sobey CG, Faraci FM: Effect of nitric oxide and potassium channel agonists and inhibitors on basilar artery diameter, *Am J Physiol* 272:H256-262, 1997.
16. Paterno R, Heistad DD, Faraci FM: Functional activity of Ca^{2+}-dependent K+ channels is increased in basilar artery during chronic hypertension, *Am J Physiol* 272:H1287-1291, 1997.
17. Paterno R, Faraci FM, Heistad DD: Role of Ca^{2+}-dependent K+ channels in cerebral vasodilatation induced by increases in cyclic GMP and cyclic AMP in the rat, *Stroke* 27:1603-1607, 1996.
18. McNeish AJ, Sandow SL, Neylon CB, et al: Evidence for involvement of both IK$_{Ca}$ and SK$_{Ca}$ channels in hyperpolarizing responses of the rat middle cerebral artery, *Stroke* 37:1277-1282, 2006.
19. You J, Johnson TD, Marrelli SP, et al: Functional heterogeneity of endothelial P$_2$ purinoceptors in the cerebrovascular tree of the rat, *Am J Physiol* 277:H893-900, 1999.
20. Marrelli SP, Eckmann MS, Hunte MS: Role of endothelial intermediate conductance K$_{Ca}$ channels in cerebral EDHF-mediated dilations, *Am J Physiol Heart Circ Physiol* 285:H1590-1599, 2003.
21. McNeish AJ, Garland CJ: Thromboxane A$_2$ inhibition of SK$_{Ca}$ after NO synthase block in rat middle cerebral artery, *Br J Pharmacol* 151:441-449, 2007.
22. Knot HJ, Nelson MT: Regulation of arterial diameter and wall [Ca^{2+}] in cerebral arteries of rat by membrane potential and intravascular pressure, *J Physiol* 508(Pt 1):199-209, 1998.
23. Sobey CG, Faraci FM: Inhibitory effect of 4-aminopyridine on responses of the basilar artery to nitric oxide, *Br J Pharmacol* 126:1437-1443, 1999.
24. Petersson J, Zygmunt PM, Hogestatt ED: Characterization of the potassium channels involved in EDHF-mediated relaxation in cerebral arteries, *Br J Pharmacol* 120:1344-1350, 1997.
25. Dong H, Waldron GJ, Cole WC, et al: Roles of calcium-activated and voltage-gated delayed rectifier potassium channels in endothelium-dependent vasorelaxation of the rabbit middle cerebral artery, *Br J Pharmacol* 123:821-832, 1998.
26. Chrissobolis S, Sobey CG: Inwardly rectifying potassium channels in the regulation of vascular tone, *Curr Drug Targets* 4:281-289, 2003.
27. Quayle JM, Nelson MT, Standen NB: ATP-sensitive and inwardly rectifying potassium channels in smooth muscle, *Physiol Rev* 77:1165-1232, 1997.
28. Iadecola C: Regulation of the cerebral microcirculation during neural activity: Is nitric oxide the missing link? *Trends Neurosci* 16:206-214, 1993.
29. Caesar K, Akgoren N, Mathiesen C, et al: Modification of activity-dependent increases in cerebellar blood flow by extracellular potassium in anaesthetized rats, *J Physiol* Oct 1 (520 Pt 1):281-292, 2000.
30. Bryan RM Jr, You J, Phillips SC, et al: Evidence for two-pore domain potassium channels in rat cerebral arteries, *Am J Physiol Heart Circ Physiol* 291:H770-780, 2006.
31. Blondeau N, Petrault O, Manta S, et al: Polyunsaturated fatty acids are cerebral vasodilators via the TREK-1 potassium channel, *Circ Res* 101:176-184, 2007.
32. Clapham DE: TRP channels as cellular sensors, *Nature* 426:517-524, 2003.
33. Inoue R, Jensen IJ, Shi J, et al: Transient receptor potential channels in cardiovascular function and disease, *Circ Res* 99:119-131, 2006.
34. Brayden JE, Earley S, Nelson MT, et al: Transient receptor potential (TRP) channels, vascular tone and autoregulation of cerebral blood flow, *Clin Exp Pharmacol Physiol* 35:1116-1120, 2008.
35. Earley S, Heppner TJ, Nelson MT, et al: TRPV4 forms a novel Ca^{2+} signaling complex with ryanodine receptors and BK$_{Ca}$ channels, *Circ Res* 97:1270-1279, 2005.
36. Welsh DG, Brayden JE: Mechanisms of coronary artery depolarization by uridine triphosphate, *Am J Physiol Heart Circ Physiol* 280:H2545-2553, 2001.
37. Reading SA, Earley S, Waldron BJ, et al: TRPC3 mediates pyrimidine receptor-induced depolarization of cerebral arteries, *Am J Physiol Heart Circ Physiol* 288:H2055-2061, 2005.

38. Didion SP, Faraci FM: Effects of NADH and NADPH on superoxide levels and cerebral vascular tone, *Am J Physiol Heart Circ Physiol* 282:H688–695, 2002.

39. Park L, Anrather J, Zhou P, et al: Exogenous NADPH increases cerebral blood flow through NADPH oxidase-dependent and -independent mechanisms, *Arterioscler Thromb Vasc Biol* 24:1860–1865, 2004.

40. Wei EP, Kontos HA, Beckman JS: Mechanisms of cerebral vasodilation by superoxide, hydrogen peroxide, and peroxynitrite, *Am J Physiol* 271:H1262–1266, 1996.

41. Wei EP, Christman CW, Kontos HA, et al: Effects of oxygen radicals on cerebral arterioles, *Am J Physiol* 248:H157–162, 1985.

42. Cosentino F, Sill JC, Katusic ZS: Role of superoxide anions in the mediation of endothelium-dependent contractions, *Hypertension* 23:229–235, 1994.

43. Thomson L, Trujillo M, Telleri R, et al: Kinetics of cytochrome c^{2+} oxidation by peroxynitrite: Implications for superoxide measurements in nitric oxide-producing biological systems, *Arch Biochem Biophys* 319:491–497, 1995.

44. Tosaka M, Hashiba Y, Saito N, et al: Contractile responses to reactive oxygen species in the canine basilar artery in vitro: Selective inhibitory effect of MCI-186, a new hydroxyl radical scavenger, *Acta Neurochir (Wien)* 144:1305–1310, 2002.

45. Miller AA, Drummond GR, Mast AE, et al: Effect of gender on NADPH-oxidase activity, expression, and function in the cerebral circulation: Role of estrogen, *Stroke* 38:2142–2149, 2007.

46. Miller AA, Drummond GR, Schmidt HHHW, et al: NADPH oxidase activity and function are profoundly greater in cerebral versus systemic arteries, *Circ Res* 97:1055–1062, 2005.

47. Paravicini TM, Chrissobolis S, Drummond GR, et al: Increased NADPH-oxidase activity and Nox4 expression during chronic hypertension is associated with enhanced cerebral vasodilatation to NADPH in vivo, *Stroke* 35:584–589, 2004.

48. Sobey CG, Heistad DD, Faraci FM: Potassium channels mediate dilatation of cerebral arterioles in response to arachidonate, *Am J Physiol* 275:H1606–1612, 1998.

49. Sobey CG, Heistad DD, Faraci FM: Mechanisms of bradykinin-induced cerebral vasodilatation in rats. Evidence that reactive oxygen species activate K^+ channels, *Stroke* 28:2290–2295, 1997.

50. Leffler CW, Busija DW, Armstead WM, et al: H_2O_2 effects on cerebral prostanoids and pial arteriolar diameter in piglets, *Am J Physiol* 258:H1382–1387, 1990.

51. Iida Y, Katusic ZS: Mechanisms of cerebral arterial relaxations to hydrogen peroxide, *Stroke* 31:2224–2230, 2000.

52. You J, Golding EM, Bryan RM Jr: Arachidonic acid metabolites, hydrogen peroxide, and EDHF in cerebral arteries, *Am J Physiol Heart Circ Physiol* 289:H1077–1083, 2005.

53. Cheranov SY, Jaggar JH: Mitochondrial modulation of Ca^{2+} sparks and transient K_{Ca} currents in smooth muscle cells of rat cerebral arteries, *J Physiol* 556:755–771, 2004.

54. Cheranov SY, Jaggar JH: TNF-alpha dilates cerebral arteries via NAD(P)H oxidase-dependent Ca^{2+} spark activation, *Am J Physiol Cell Physiol* 290:C964–971, 2006.

55. Xi Q, Cheranov SY, Jaggar JH: Mitochondria-derived reactive oxygen species dilate cerebral arteries by activating Ca^{2+} sparks, *Circ Res* 97:354–362, 2005.

56. Drouin A, Thorin-Trescases N, Hamel E, et al: Endothelial nitric oxide synthase activation leads to dilatory H_2O_2 production in mouse cerebral arteries, *Cardiovasc Res* 73:73–81, 2007.

57. Didion SP, Hathaway CA, Faraci FM: Superoxide levels and function of cerebral blood vessels after inhibition of CuZn-SOD, *Am J Physiol Heart Circ Physiol* 281:H1697–1703, 2001.

58. Didion SP, Ryan MJ, Didion LA, et al: Increased superoxide and vascular dysfunction in CuZnSOD-deficient mice, *Circ Res* 91:938–944, 2002.

59. Miller AA, Drummond GR, Sobey CG: Novel isoforms of NADPH-oxidase in cerebral vascular control, *Pharmacol Ther* 111:928–948, 2006.

60. Miller AA, De Silva TM, Jackman KA, et al: Effect of gender and sex hormones on vascular oxidative stress, *Clin Exp Pharmacol Physiol* 34:1037–1043, 2007.

61. Paravicini TM, Miller AA, Drummond GR, et al: Flow-induced cerebral vasodilatation in vivo involves activation of phosphatidylinositol 3-kinase, NADPH-oxidase, and nitric oxide synthase, *J Cereb Blood Flow Metab* 26:836–845, 2006.

62. Kontos HA, Wei EP, Povlishock JT, et al: Oxygen radicals mediate the cerebral arteriolar dilation from arachidonate and bradykinin in cats, *Circ Res* 55:295–303, 1984.

63. Ellis EF, Police RJ, Yancey L, et al: Dilation of cerebral arterioles by cytochrome P-450 metabolites of arachidonic acid, *Am J Physiol* 259:H1171–1177, 1990.

64. Rosenblum WI: Hydroxyl radical mediates the endothelium-dependent relaxation produced by bradykinin in mouse cerebral arterioles, *Circ Res* 61:601–603, 1987.

65. Welsh DG, Nelson MT, Eckman DM, et al: Swelling-activated cation channels mediate depolarization of rat cerebrovascular smooth muscle by hyposmolarity and intravascular pressure, *J Physiol* Aug 15 (527 Pt 1):139–148, 2000.

66. Reading SA, Brayden JE: Central role of TRPM4 channels in cerebral blood flow regulation, *Stroke* 38:2322–2328, 2007.

67. Budzyn K, Marley PD, Sobey CG: Targeting rho and rho-kinase in the treatment of cardiovascular disease, *Trends Pharmacol Sci* 27:97–104, 2006.

68. Chrissobolis S, Sobey CG: Recent evidence for an involvement of rho-kinase in cerebral vascular disease, *Stroke* 37:2174–2180, 2006.

69. Numaguchi K, Eguchi S, Yamakawa T, et al: Mechanotransduction of rat aortic vascular smooth muscle cells requires rhoA and intact actin filaments, *Circ Res* 85:5–11, 1999.

70. Gokina NI, Park KM, McElroy-Yaggy K, et al: Effects of rho kinase inhibition on cerebral artery myogenic tone and reactivity, *J Appl Physiol* 98:1940–1948, 2005.

71. Lagaud G, Gaudreault N, Moore ED, et al: Pressure-dependent myogenic constriction of cerebral arteries occurs independently of voltage-dependent activation, *Am J Physiol Heart Circ Physiol* 283:H2187–2195, 2002.

72. Chrissobolis S, Sobey CG: Evidence that rho-kinase activity contributes to cerebral vascular tone in vivo and is enhanced during chronic hypertension: Comparison with protein kinase C. *Circ Res* 88:774–779, 2001.

73. Chrissobolis S, Budzyn K, Marley PD, et al: Evidence that estrogen suppresses rho-kinase function in the cerebral circulation in vivo, *Stroke* 35:2200–2205, 2004.

74. Didion SP, Lynch CM, Baumbach GL, et al: Impaired endothelium-dependent responses and enhanced influence of rho-kinase in cerebral arterioles in type II diabetes, *Stroke* 36:342–347, 2005.

75. Akopov S, Sercombe R, Seylaz J: Cerebrovascular reactivity: Role of endothelium/platelet/leukocyte interactions, *Cerebrovasc Brain Metab Rev* 8:11–94, 1996.

76. Sobey CG, Woodman OL: Myocardial ischaemia: What happens to the coronary arteries? *Trends Pharmacol Sci* 14:448–453, 1993.

77. Sobey CG, Faraci FM, Piegors DJ, et al: Effect of short-term regression of atherosclerosis on reactivity of carotid and retinal arteries, *Stroke* 27:927–933, 1996.

78. Mugge A, Elwell JH, Peterson TE, et al: Chronic treatment with polyethylene-glycolated superoxide dismutase partially restores endothelium-dependent vascular relaxations in cholesterol-fed rabbits, *Circ Res* 69:1293–1300, 1991.

79. Faraci FM, Orgren K, Heistad DD: Impaired relaxation of the carotid artery during activation of ATP-sensitive potassium channels in atherosclerotic monkeys, *Stroke* 25:178–182, 1994.

80. Kanamaru K, Waga S, Tochio H, et al: The effect of atherosclerosis on endothelium-dependent relaxation in the aorta and intracranial arteries of rabbits, *J Neurosurg* 70:793–798, 1989.

81. Kitagawa S, Yamaguchi Y, Sameshima E, et al: Differences in endothelium-dependent relaxation in various arteries from watanabe heritable hyperlipidaemic rabbits with increasing age, *Clin Exp Pharmacol Physiol* 21:963–970, 1994.

82. Rossitch E Jr, Alexander E 3rd, Black PM, et al: L-Arginine normalizes endothelial function in cerebral vessels from hypercholesterolemic rabbits, *J Clin Invest* 87:1295–1299, 1991.

83. d'Uscio LV, Smith LA, Katusic ZS: Hypercholesterolemia impairs endothelium-dependent relaxations in common carotid arteries of apolipoprotein E-deficient mice, *Stroke* 32:2658–2664, 2001.

84. Kitayama J, Faraci FM, Lentz SR, et al: Cerebral vascular dysfunction during hypercholesterolemia, *Stroke* 38:2136–2141, 2007.

85. Didion SP, Heistad DD, Faraci FM: Mechanisms that produce nitric oxide-mediated relaxation of cerebral arteries during atherosclerosis, *Stroke* 32:761–766, 2001.

86. Tsikas D, Boger RH, Sandmann J, et al: Endogenous nitric oxide synthase inhibitors are responsible for the L-arginine paradox, *FEBS Lett* 478:1-3, 2000.

87. Schachinger V, Britten MB, Zeiher AM: Prognostic impact of coronary vasodilator dysfunction on adverse long-term outcome of coronary heart disease, *Circulation* 101:1899-1906, 2000.

88. Suwaidi JA, Hamasaki S, Higano ST, et al: Long-term follow-up of patients with mild coronary artery disease and endothelial dysfunction, *Circulation* 101:948-954, 2000.

89. Tamaki K, Armstrong M, Heistad D: Effects of atherosclerosis on cerebral vessels: Hemodynamic and morphometric studies, *Stroke* 17:1209-1214, 1986.

90. Heistad DD, Breese K, Armstrong ML: Cerebral vasoconstrictor responses to serotonin after dietary treatment of atherosclerosis: Implications for transient ischemic attacks, *Stroke* 18:1068-1073, 1987.

91. Faraci FM, Williams JK, Breese KR, et al: Atherosclerosis potentiates constrictor responses of cerebral and ocular blood vessels to thromboxane in monkeys, *Stroke* 20:242-247, 1989.

92. Faraci FM, Lopez AG, Breese K, et al: Effect of atherosclerosis on cerebral vascular responses to activation of leukocytes and platelets in monkeys, *Stroke* 22:790-796, 1991.

93. Vanhoutte PM, Houston DS: Platelets, endothelium, and vasospasm, *Circulation* 72:728-734, 1985.

94. Hardebo JE, Kahrstrom J, Owman C: P1- and P2-purine receptors in brain circulation, *Eur J Pharmacol* 144:343-352, 1987.

95. Faraci FM, Heistad DD: Endothelium-derived relaxing factor inhibits constrictor responses of large cerebral arteries to serotonin, *J Cereb Blood Flow Metab* 12:500-506, 1992.

96. Brian JE Jr, Kennedy RH: Modulation of cerebral arterial tone by endothelium-derived relaxing factor, *Am J Physiol* 264:H1245-1250, 1993.

97. Hart JL, Sobey CG, Woodman OL: Cholesterol feeding enhances vasoconstrictor effects of products from rabbit polymorphonuclear leukocytes, *Am J Physiol* 269:H1-6, 1995.

98. Barnett HJ: Progress towards stroke prevention: Robert Wartenberg lecture, *Neurology* 30:1212-1225, 1980.

99. Kaul S, Waack BJ, Padgett RC, Brooks RM, Heistad DD: Interaction of human platelets and leukocytes in modulation of vascular tone, *Am J Physiol* 266:H1706-1714, 1994.

100. Padgett RC, Heistad DD, Mugge A, et al: Vascular responses to activated leukocytes after regression of atherosclerosis, *Circ Res* 70:423-429, 1992.

101. Benzuly KH, Padgett RC, Kaul S, et al: Functional improvement precedes structural regression of atherosclerosis, *Circulation* 89:1810-1818, 1994.

102. Kaul S, Waack BJ, Padgett RC, et al: Altered vascular responses to platelets from hypercholesterolemic humans, *Circ Res* 72:737-743, 1993.

103. Randomised trial of cholesterol lowering in 4444 patients with coronary heart disease: The Scandinavian Simvastatin Survival Study (4S), *Lancet* 344:1383-1389, 1994.

104. Laufs U, Endres M, Stagliano N, et al: Neuroprotection mediated by changes in the endothelial actin cytoskeleton, *J Clin Invest* 106:15-24, 2000.

105. Laufs U, Gertz K, Huang P, et al: Atorvastatin upregulates type III nitric oxide synthase in thrombocytes, decreases platelet activation, and protects from cerebral ischemia in normocholesterolemic mice, *Stroke* 31:2442-2449, 2000.

106. Erdos B, Snipes JA, Tulbert CD, et al: Rosuvastatin improves cerebrovascular function in Zucker obese rats by inhibiting NAD(P)-H oxidase-dependent superoxide production, *Am J Physiol Heart Circ Physiol* 290:H1264-1270, 2006.

107. Takemoto M, Liao JK: Pleiotropic effects of 3-hydroxy-3-methylglutaryl coenzyme A reductase inhibitors, *Arterioscler Thromb Vasc Biol* 21:1712-1719, 2001.

108. Warlow CP: Epidemiology of stroke, *Lancet* 352 (Suppl 3): SIII1-4, 1998.

109. Mayhan WG: Responses of the basilar artery to products released by platelets during chronic hypertension, *Brain Res* 545:97-102, 1998.

110. Mayhan WG: Role of prostaglandin H_2-thromboxane A_2 in responses of cerebral arterioles during chronic hypertension, *Am J Physiol* 262:H539-543, 1992.

111. Mayhan WG: Impairment of endothelium-dependent dilatation of basilar artery during chronic hypertension, *Am J Physiol* 259:H1455-1462, 1990.

112. Kitazono T, Faraci FM, Heistad DD: L-Arginine restores dilator responses of the basilar artery to acetylcholine during chronic hypertension, *Hypertension* 27:893-896, 1996.

113. Chu Y, Alwahdani A, Iida S, et al: Vascular effects of the human extracellular superoxide dismutase R213G variant, *Circulation* 112:1047-1053, 2005.

114. Faraci FM, Lamping KG, Modrick ML, et al: Cerebral vascular effects of angiotensin II: New insights from genetic models, *J Cereb Blood Flow Metab* 26:449-455, 2005.

115. Baumbach GL, Sigmund CD, Faraci FM: Structure of cerebral arterioles in mice deficient in expression of the gene for endothelial nitric oxide synthase, *Circ Res* 95:822-829, 2004.

116. Kazama K, Anrather J, Zhou P, et al: Angiotensin II impairs neurovascular coupling in neocortex through NADPH oxidase-derived radicals, *Circ Res* 95:1019-1026, 2004.

117. Arrick DM, Sharpe GM, Sun H, et al: nNOS-dependent reactivity of cerebral arterioles in type 1 diabetes, *Brain Res* 1184:365-371, 2007.

118. Zhang F, Slungaard A, Vercellotti GM, et al: Superoxide-dependent cerebrovascular effects of homocysteine, *Am J Physiol* 274: R1704-1711, 1998.

119. Phillips SA, Sylvester FA, Frisbee JC: Oxidant stress and constrictor reactivity impair cerebral artery dilation in obese Zucker rats, *Am J Physiol Regul Integr Comp Physiol* 288:R522-530, 2005.

120. Alp NJ, Channon KM: Regulation of endothelial nitric oxide synthase by tetrahydrobiopterin in vascular disease, *Arterioscler Thromb Vasc Biol* 24:413-420, 2004.

121. Beyer AM, Baumbach GL, Halabi CM, et al: Interference with PPARgamma signaling causes cerebral vascular dysfunction, hypertrophy, and remodeling, *Hypertension* 51:867-871, 2008.

122. Nakamura T, Yamamoto E, Kataoka K, et al: Pioglitazone exerts protective effects against stroke in stroke-prone spontaneously hypertensive rats, independently of blood pressure, *Stroke* 38:3016-3022, 2007.

123. Ryan MJ, Didion SP, Mathur S, et al: PPAR(gamma) agonist rosiglitazone improves vascular function and lowers blood pressure in hypertensive transgenic mice, *Hypertension* 43:661-666, 2004.

124. Kitazono T, Ago T, Kamouchi M, et al: Increased activity of calcium channels and rho-associated kinase in the basilar artery during chronic hypertension in vivo, *J Hypertens* 20:879-884, 2002.

125. Jarajapu YP, Knot HJ: Relative contribution of rho kinase and protein kinase C to myogenic tone in rat cerebral arteries in hypertension, *Am J Physiol Heart Circ Physiol* 289:H1917-1922, 2005.

126. Sobey CG: Potassium channel function in vascular disease, *Arterioscler Thromb Vasc Biol* 21:28-38, 2001.

127. Kitazono T, Heistad DD, Faraci FM: ATP-sensitive potassium channels in the basilar artery during chronic hypertension, *Hypertension* 22:677-681, 1993.

128. Pluger S, Faulhaber J, Furstenau M, et al: Mice with disrupted BK channel beta1 subunit gene feature abnormal Ca(2+) spark/stoc coupling and elevated blood pressure, *Circ Res* 87:E53-60, 2000.

129. Brenner R, Perez GJ, Bonev AD, et al: Vasoregulation by the beta1 subunit of the calcium-activated potassium channel, *Nature* 407:870-876, 2000.

130. Kolias TJ, Chai S, Webb RC: Potassium channel antagonists and vascular reactivity in stroke-prone spontaneously hypertensive rats, *Am J Hypertens* 6:528-533, 1993.

131. Asano M, Masuzawa-Ito K, Matsuda T, et al: Functional role of Ca(2+)-activated K^+ channels in resting state of carotid arteries from SHR, *Am J Physiol* 265:H843-851, 1993.

132. Liu Y, Hudetz AG, Knaus HG, et al: Increased expression of Ca^{2+}-sensitive K^+ channels in the cerebral microcirculation of genetically hypertensive rats: Evidence for their protection against cerebral vasospasm, *Circ Res* 82:729-737, 1998.

133. Harder DR, Dernbach P, Waters A: Possible cellular mechanism for cerebral vasospasm after experimental subarachnoid hemorrhage in the dog, *J Clin Invest* 80:875-880, 1987.

134. Cook DA: Mechanisms of cerebral vasospasm in subarachnoid haemorrhage, *Pharmacol Ther* 66:259-284, 1995.

135. Sobey CG, Faraci FM: Subarachnoid haemorrhage: What happens to the cerebral arteries? *Clin Exp Pharmacol Physiol* 25:867-876, 1998.

136. Hatake K, Wakabayashi I, Kakishita E, et al: Impairment of endothelium-dependent relaxation in human basilar artery after subarachnoid hemorrhage, *Stroke* 23:1111-1116, 1992.

137. Kim P, Lorenz RR, Sundt TM Jr, et al: Release of endothelium-derived relaxing factor after subarachnoid hemorrhage, *J Neurosurg* 70:108-114, 1989.

138. Kasuya H, Weir BK, Nakane M, et al: Nitric oxide synthase and guanylate cyclase levels in canine basilar artery after subarachnoid hemorrhage, *J Neurosurg* 82:250-255, 1995.

139. Kim P, Sundt TM Jr, Vanhoutte PM: Alterations of mechanical properties in canine basilar arteries after subarachnoid hemorrhage, *J Neurosurg* 71:430-436, 1989.

140. Kim P, Schini VB, Sundt TM Jr, Vanhoutte PM: Reduced production of cGMP underlies the loss of endothelium-dependent relaxations in the canine basilar artery after subarachnoid hemorrhage, *Circ Res* 70:248-256, 1992.

141. Chen AF, O'Brien T, Tsutsui M, et al: Expression and function of recombinant endothelial nitric oxide synthase gene in canine basilar artery, *Circ Res* 80:327-335, 1997.

142. Sobey CG, Quan L: Impaired cerebral vasodilator responses to NO and PDE V inhibition after subarachnoid hemorrhage, *Am J Physiol* 277:H1718-1724, 1999.

143. Quan Y, Sobey CG: Selective effects of subarachnoid hemorrhage on cerebral vascular responses to 4-aminopyridine in rats, *Stroke* 31:2460-2465, 2000.

144. Katusic ZS, Milde JH, Cosentino F, et al: Subarachnoid hemorrhage and endothelial L-arginine pathway in small brain stem arteries in dogs, *Stroke* 24:392-399, 1993.

145. Kanamaru K, Weir BK, Findlay JM, et al: Pharmacological studies on relaxation of spastic primate cerebral arteries in subarachnoid hemorrhage, *J Neurosurg* 71:909-915, 1989.

146. Kamii H, Kato I, Kinouchi H, et al: Amelioration of vasospasm after subarachnoid hemorrhage in transgenic mice overexpressing CuZn-superoxide dismutase, *Stroke* 30:867-871, 1999.

147. Watanabe Y, Chu Y, Andresen JJ, et al: Gene transfer of extracellular superoxide dismutase reduces cerebral vasospasm after subarachnoid hemorrhage, *Stroke* 34:434-440, 2003.

148. Kim DE, Suh YS, Lee MS, et al: Vascular NAD(P)H oxidase triggers delayed cerebral vasospasm after subarachnoid hemorrhage in rats, *Stroke* 33:2687-2691, 2002.

149. Zheng JS, Zhan RY, Zheng SS: Inhibition of NADPH oxidase attenuates vasospasm after experimental subarachnoid hemorrhage in rats, *Stroke* 36:1059-1064, 2005.

150. Clark JF, Sharp FR: Bilirubin oxidation products (BOXes) and their role in cerebral vasospasm after subarachnoid hemorrhage, *J Cereb Blood Flow Metab* 26:1223-1233, 2006.

151. Kitazono T, Heistad DD, Faraci FM: Enhanced responses of the basilar artery to activation of endothelin-b receptors in stroke-prone spontaneously hypertensive rats, *Hypertension* 25:490-494, 1995.

152. Foley PL, Caner HH, Kassell NF, et al: Reversal of subarachnoid hemorrhage-induced vasoconstriction with an endothelin receptor antagonist, *Neurosurgery* 34:108-112, 1994.

153. Kraus GE, Bucholz RD, Yoon KW, et al: Cerebrospinal fluid endothelin-1 and endothelin-3 levels in normal and neurosurgical patients: A clinical study and literature review, *Surg Neurol* 35:20-29, 1991.

154. Hirose H, Ide K, Sasaki T, et al: The role of endothelin and nitric oxide in modulation of normal and spastic cerebral vascular tone in the dog, *Eur J Pharmacol* 277:77-87, 1995.

155. Suzuki H, Sato S, Suzuki Y, et al: Increased endothelin concentration in CSF from patients with subarachnoid hemorrhage, *Acta Neurol Scand* 81:553-554, 1990.

156. Masaoka H, Suzuki R, Hirata Y, et al: Raised plasma endothelin in aneurysmal subarachnoid haemorrhage, *Lancet* 2:1402, 1989.

157. Zuccarello M, Lewis AI, Rapoport RM: Endothelin ETa and ETb receptors in subarachnoid hemorrhage-induced cerebral vasospasm, *Eur J Pharmacol* 259:R1-2, 1994.

158. Zuccarello M, Romano A, Passalacqua M, et al: Endothelin-1-induced endothelin-1 release causes cerebral vasospasm in-vivo, *J Pharm Pharmacol* 47:702, 1995.

159. Clozel M, Watanabe H: BQ-123, a peptidic endothelin ETa receptor antagonist, prevents the early cerebral vasospasm following subarachnoid hemorrhage after intracisternal but not intravenous injection, *Life Sci* 52:825-834, 1993.

160. Cosentino F, McMahon EG, Carter JS, et al: Effect of endothelinA-receptor antagonist BQ-123 and phosphoramidon on cerebral vasospasm, *J Cardiovasc Pharmacol* 22 (Suppl 8): S332-335, 1993.

161. Gaetani P, Rodriguez y Baena R, et al: Endothelin and aneurysmal subarachnoid haemorrhage: A study of subarachnoid cisternal cerebrospinal fluid, *J Neurol Neurosurg Psychiatry* 57:66-72, 1994.

162. Sato M, Tani E, Fujikawa H, et al: Involvement of rho-kinase-mediated phosphorylation of myosin light chain in enhancement of cerebral vasospasm, *Circ Res* 87:195-200, 2000.

163. Miyagi Y, Carpenter RC, Meguro T, et al: Upregulation of rho A and rho kinase messenger RNAs in the basilar artery of a rat model of subarachnoid hemorrhage, *J Neurosurg* 93:471-476, 2000.

164. Obara K, Nishizawa S, Koide M, et al: Interactive role of protein kinase C-delta with rho-kinase in the development of cerebral vasospasm in a canine two-hemorrhage model, *J Vasc Res* 42:67-76, 2005.

165. Kim I, Leinweber BD, Morgalla M, et al: Thin and thick filament regulation of contractility in experimental cerebral vasospasm, *Neurosurgery* 46:440-446, 2000.

166. Asano M, Masuzawa-Ito K, Matsuda T: Charybdotoxin-sensitive K^+ channels regulate the myogenic tone in the resting state of arteries from spontaneously hypertensive rats, *Br J Pharmacol* 108:214-222, 1993.

167. Sobey CG, Heistad DD, Faraci FM: Effect of subarachnoid hemorrhage on dilatation of rat basilar artery in vivo, *Am J Physiol* 271:H126-132, 1996.

168. Sobey CG, Heistad DD, Faraci FM: Effect of subarachnoid hemorrhage on cerebral vasodilatation in response to activation of ATP-sensitive K^+ channels in chronically hypertensive rats, *Stroke* 28:392-396, 1997.

169. Boushey CJ, Beresford SA, Omenn GS, et al: A quantitative assessment of plasma homocysteine as a risk factor for vascular disease. Probable benefits of increasing folic acid intakes, *JAMA* 274: 1049-1057, 1995.

170. Stampfer MJ, Malinow MR: Can lowering homocysteine levels reduce cardiovascular risk? *N Engl J Med* 332:328-329, 1995.

171. Dayal S, Bottiglieri T, Arning E, et al: Endothelial dysfunction and elevation of *S*-adenosylhomocysteine in cystathionine beta-synthase-deficient mice, *Circ Res* 88:1203-1209, 2001.

172. Eberhardt RT, Forgione MA, Cap A, et al: Endothelial dysfunction in a murine model of mild hyperhomocyst(e)inemia, *J Clin Invest* 106:483-491, 2000.

173. Symons JD, Mullick AE, Ensunsa JL, et al: Hyperhomocysteinemia evoked by folate depletion: Effects on coronary and carotid arterial function, *Arterioscler Thromb Vasc Biol* 22:772-780, 2002.

174. Lentz SR, Erger RA, Dayal S, et al: Folate dependence of hyperhomocysteinemia and vascular dysfunction in cystathionine beta-synthase-deficient mice, *Am J Physiol Heart Circ Physiol* 279:H970-975, 2000.

175. Lentz SR, Sobey CG, Piegors DJ, et al: Vascular dysfunction in monkeys with diet-induced hyperhomocyst(e)inemia, *J Clin Invest* 98:24-29, 1996.

176. Weiss N, Zhang YY, Heydrick S, et al: Overexpression of cellular glutathione peroxidase rescues homocyst(e)ine-induced endothelial dysfunction, *Proc Natl Acad Sci U S A* 98:12503-12508, 2001.

177. Pelligrino DA, Koenig HM, Wang Q, et al: Protein kinase C suppresses receptor-mediated pial arteriolar relaxation in the diabetic rat, *Neuroreport* 5:417-420, 1994.

178. Mayhan WG: Impairment of endothelium-dependent dilatation of cerebral arterioles during diabetes mellitus, *Am J Physiol* 256:H621-625, 1989.

179. Mayhan WG, Simmons LK, Sharpe GM: Mechanism of impaired responses of cerebral arterioles during diabetes mellitus, *Am J Physiol* 260:H319-326, 1991.

180. Mayhan WG: Impairment of endothelium-dependent dilatation of the basilar artery during diabetes mellitus, *Brain Res* 580:297-302, 1992.

181. Miao L, Calvert JW, Tang J, et al: Upregulation of small GTPase rhoA in the basilar artery from diabetic (mellitus) rats, *Life Sci* 71:1175-1185, 2002.

182. Mayhan WG: Effect of diabetes mellitus on response of the basilar artery to activation of ATP-sensitive potassium channels, *Brain Res* 636:35-39, 1994.

183. Mayhan WG, Patel KP: Acute effects of glucose on reactivity of cerebral microcirculation: Role of activation of protein kinase C, *Am J Physiol* 269:H1297-1302, 1995.

The Cerebral Microvasculature and Responses to Ischemia

GREGORY J. DEL ZOPPO, GERHARD F. HAMANN

Anatomy of the Cerebral Vasculature

Regulation of vascular tone and circulatory hemostasis are important components of cerebral vascular physiology that are disrupted by ischemia. The cerebral vasculature has unique features for protection of neuronal cells and preservation of their function through shifting of blood flow to regions of activation on demand and maintenance of an intravascular antithrombotic milieu.

The overall vascular strategy for protection of cortical and deep brain structures consists of the interconnection of territories of brain-supplying arteries via collateral anastomoses of the cerebral hemispheres and the circle of Willis. Pial and cortical penetrating arteries consist of (1) an endothelial cell layer, the basal lamina derived from the extracellular matrix (ECM), (2) layers of smooth muscle cells encased in ECM (myointima), and (3) an adventitia derived from the leptomeninges.[1] In the cortex, an extension of the subarachnoid space forms the Virchow-Robin space, which surrounds cortical penetrating arterioles until it "disappears" into the *glia limitans*. The abluminal boundary of the glia limitans is formed by the astrocyte end-feet. With further arborization of the microvasculature, the glia limitans at the capillary level fuses with the thin basal lamina. There is still discussion whether the glia limitans at the capillary level contains a virtual Virchow-Robin space and whether the basal lamina has a special organization. The ECM composition of the basal lamina suggests that these theories are likely. Cerebral capillaries are unique in that the endothelium and astrocyte end-feet are in close apposition, the adventitia being absent. Astrocytes serve both microvessels and neurons in this setting and may be considered the vascular portion of the neurovascular unit. The postcapillary venule network bears close ultrastructural resemblance to the capillaries, except for the presence of a limited myointimal layer. Another unique feature of the cerebral capillary is the permeability barrier, which prevents contact of the neuropil with the blood and its plasma constituents.

During normal blood flow not all capillaries are perfused.[2] Observations also suggest the presence of a cerebrovascular reserve that can be recruited on short notice but that does not involve neovascularization.[2,3] In contrast, direct measurements indicate that all capillaries of the pial and cortical circulation have plasma flow and that there is no capillary recruitment during forebrain ischemia.[4,5] Hence, the existence of a nascent microvascular bed that can be recruited in the early moments of focal ischemia remains uncertain.

The Neurovascular Unit

Control and modulation of regional and local blood flow under conditions of normoxia depend on neurovascular coupling.[6-8] The proximity of microvascular endothelial cells to the circumferential astrocyte end-feet of capillaries, which are separated from the endothelium only by the basal lamina matrix, and the support of neurons by astrocytes suggest that communication could also be directed from microvessels to the neurons they supply.[9,10] It has been hypothesized that neuron-microvascular interactions can be described by a "neurovascular unit," which consists of microvessels (endothelial cells, extracellular matrix, astrocyte end-feet, and pericytes), astrocytes, and neurons and their axons in addition to the supporting cells (e.g., microglia and oligodendroglia).[11] This unit construct provides a framework for considering the bidirectional actions of neurons and their supply microvessels via the intervening astrocytes. It also provides a structural framework for considering the elements of the unit in their responses to flow reduction or cessation. The resilience of the unit in the setting of focal ischemia is unknown, although the responses of the unit components to ischemia, hypoxia, inflammation, and other processes are described.

The Blood-Brain Barrier and Matrix Integrity

The permeability barrier characteristics of the cerebral microvasculature are represented by (1) interendothelial cell tight junctions (the blood-brain barrier) and (2) cell adhesion to the intact subtending basal lamina. Both the permeability barrier and the basal lamina derive from the concerted interaction of the endothelial cells and astrocytes.[12-15] Cerebral microvessel endothelial cells display regional functional specialization along the microvascular axis.[16-19] In vitro coculture studies suggest that this specialization depends on the interaction of its cellular components.[20,21] The proximity of the cellular components of intact cerebral capillaries implies ready communication between endothelial cells and astrocytes, and between astrocytes and neurons.[1,7] Flow alterations can be initiated by neuron stimulation or by metabolic demand during arousal.[1]

The blood-brain barrier, the primary permeability barrier, is formed by endothelial cell tight junctions and limited endothelial cell pinocytosis, and it relies on the interactions of endothelial cells and astrocytes, as demonstrated by elegant xenograft experiments.[22] The primary barrier may involve adhesion of endothelial cells and astrocytes to the intervening matrix (basal lamina).[23,24] Astrocytes promote many microvessel blood-brain barrier properties, including endothelial cell tight junctions, exclusion of Evans blue dye from the neuropil, and generation of the protein HT7-neurothelin.[25,26] It has been postulated that soluble factors generated by astrocytes maintain the endothelial characteristics of the blood-brain barrier, including the tight junctions, transendothelial resistance, and glucose–amino acid transport polarity.[22,27]

The secondary barrier involves both an intact basal lamina and receptor-associated cell adhesion to the matrix components. The intact barrier protects the brain parenchyma from hemorrhage.[23,28-32] The basal lamina separates the specialized endothelium from the astrocytes and from their connections to neurons. The cerebral vascular basal lamina contains laminins, type IV collagen, fibronectin, and other components, including heparan sulfate proteoglycans (HSPGs; e.g., perlecan), entactin, and nidogen. Developmental interrelationships between the endothelium and astrocytes highlight the close functional association of endothelial cells and astrocytes in cerebral capillaries.[33]

Adhesion of both endothelial cells and astrocytes to the subtending basal lamina requires the interaction of cellular integrin receptors to their matrix ligands.[28,29] Haring et al[29] described expression patterns of integrin subunits in normal central nervous system (CNS) microvessel subclasses. Integrin $\alpha_1\beta_1$ on endothelial cells appears on all cerebral microvessels, including cerebral capillaries.[29,31,34-37] Integrins $\alpha_3\beta_1$ and $\alpha_6\beta_1$ are also expressed by cerebral endothelial cells. Integrin $\alpha_6\beta_4$ is expressed on astrocyte end-feet around select microvessels, whereas integrin $\alpha_1\beta_1$ is found on their fibers.[30,31] $\alpha\beta$-Dystroglycan, the sole member of a separate family of matrix adhesion receptors, is expressed predominantly by astrocyte end-feet and is possibly the principal means of binding end-feet to the basal lamina.[38] Adhesion receptor–matrix relationships are perturbed during middle cerebral artery occlusion (MCAO), which coincides with the detachment of astrocyte end-feet from the basal lamina. Little is known, yet, about the signaling functions of the adhesion receptors expressed in cerebral microvessels.

Cerebral Microvessel Responses to Focal Ischemia

During focal cerebral ischemia, a series of metabolic and morphologic alterations occur in the ischemic microvasculature, in concert with responses of the glial and neuron components of the "unit."[39,40] Injury to neurons in the target area reflects both characteristics of the neurons ("selective vulnerability")[41-44] and the distance of neurons from their neighboring microvessels.[45]

At least five responses of microvessels can be seen after cerebral ischemia; they are (1) loss of the barrier to endothelial cell permeability with subsequent edema development, (2) loss of basal lamina and extracellular matrix, with subsequent hemorrhagic transformation, (3) alterations in microvessel cell–matrix adhesion, (4) loss of microvessel patency, and (5) generation of endothelial cell leukocyte adhesion receptors (Figs. 2-1 and 2-2). These events lead to the extravascular accumulation of fluid as edema, decreased basal lamina integrity, extravasation of blood elements as hemorrhage, and the activation of inflammatory responses.[9,46]

The capillary permeability barrier function is lost as early as 30 minutes after focal cerebral ischemia. This loss is associated with ultrastructural changes within the microvasculature, including swelling of the endothelium and of astrocytes, with their cytoplasmic reorganization.[47-49] Garcia et al[50] have also demonstrated that capillaries can expand and rupture. One consequence of the loss of endothelial barrier function is the accumulation of transudate (edema) in the extravascular intercellular space: albumin, immunoglobulins, and fibrinogen pass into these spaces in the neuropil.[51] In both clinical and experimental settings, edema within the region of injury follows leakage of the vascular permeability barrier shortly after the onset of focal ischemia.[24,52-55] Loss of selective K^+ channels is associated with the swelling of astrocyte end-feet.[51,52,56,57] Sulfonyl urea receptor-1 (SUR-1) channels, which facilitate water transit into the injured tissue, are expressed on astrocytes during focal ischemia.[58,59] Swelling of the cellular compartments contributes to the focal "no-reflow" phenomenon.[60] There is evidence that the loss of the blood-brain barrier and the microvascular ECM results from the actions of bradykinin,[61,62] vascular endothelial growth factor (VEGF),[63,64] thrombin,[53,62] active matrix metalloproteinases (MMPs),[65] cysteine proteases,[66] proteases released by activated leukocytes,[67-70] and other enzyme activities.[71] Blockade of bradykinin receptors has been associated with reduced injury and edema formation,[72] as has blockade of sulfonylurea receptor-1 channels.[58] Thrombin can increase edema formation through direct action on the cerebral microvascular endothelium.[62,73,74] VEGF disrupts the interendothelial cell tight junctions, which involve the gap junction complex containing connexin 43.[75]

The second functional microvascular barrier is the basal lamina, which prevents leakage of blood elements into the surrounding brain tissue. A gradual local decrease in the expression of the major vascular matrix components laminin-1 and laminin-5, collagen IV, and cellular fibronectin follows focal ischemia.[28,76] Hamann et al[76] found a significant association between regional loss of microvascular matrix and the extravascular accumulation of hemoglobin (hemorrhagic transformation) within the regions of ischemic injury. The loss of microvascular ECM is also associated with the loss of endothelial cell reactivity during focal ischemia. Endothelial cell P-selectin and E-selectin and expression of β_1 integrins within the ischemic territory occur only on those microvessels with an intact basal lamina.[77,78]

Separate studies suggest that β_1 integrins, through their participation in cell matrix adherence, may play a role in preventing transudation and edema formation, in conjunction with other contributors to the intact blood-brain

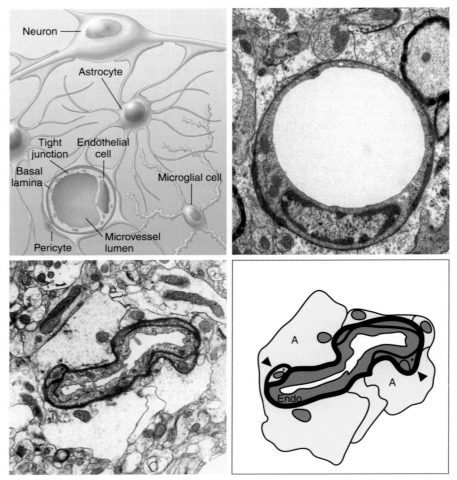

Figure 2-1 Characteristics of cerebral microvessels under normoxic conditions. *Upper left panel,* Depiction of neurovascular unit displaying relationships between neurons and their supply capillaries. (From del Zoppo GJ: Stroke and neurovascular protection. *N Engl J Med* 354:553-555, 2006.) *Upper right panel,* Capillary from rat inferior colliculus. Note endothelial cell, basal lamina matrix, and surrounding astrocyte end-foot. 4.5-5.0 μm diameter. (Courtesy of Dr. C. Willis.) *Lower left panel,* Post-capillary venule from rat cortex. ≈10 μm diameter. (Courtesy of J. H. Heo.) *Lower right panel,* Key to the *lower left* panel, indicating the endothelium (endo), basal lamina matrix *(arrowheads),* astrocyte and astrocyte end-feet (A), and pericytes (*).

barrier, and might be disturbed during ischemia by action of cytokines locally generated by microglia and astrocytes.[79-81] It has also been shown that αβ-dystroglycan is lost from astrocyte end-feet within the first 2 hours of focal ischemia.[38] This finding correlates with the detachment of the end-feet from their basal lamina following onset of ischemia.[50,82]

All of these events begin shortly after the onset of focal ischemia, indicating that microvessel functional integrity and ultrastructure can be rapidly affected. Studies of vascular integrin and dystroglycan expression responses indicate that certain responses fall within regions of microvessel activation bounded by regions of normal-appearing microvessels.[31]

Focal Cerebral Ischemia and Proteolysis of the Microvascular Matrix

Alterations in the immunoreactivity of the microvascular ECM can be explained by local proteolysis or conformational changes. Attention has focused on the expression and activity of MMPs and plasminogen activators (PAs) after experimental MCAO.[65,71,83-85] Loss of the basal lamina matrix in the primate ischemic striatum follows a rapid increase in the regional expression of pro-MMP-2, urokinase-type (u-PA), and plasminogen activator inhibitor-1 (PAI-1).[65,71,83,85] Note that endogenous tissue-type PA (t-PA) does not increase in the ischemic territory.[71] Pro-MMP-2 is rapidly generated by the microvasculature, and by nonvascular cells during ischemia.[65,71,86-89] In the primate, increased pro-MMP-9 expression within the ischemic tissue is associated with hemorrhagic transformation.[65] Rosenberg et al[89-91] have described a temporal correlation between pro-MMP-9 "activity" and edema formation in rat strains after MCAO. In contrast, in the nonhuman primate, early extravasation of plasma constituents coincides with expression of pro-MMP-2, u-PA, and PAI-1, but not pro-MMP-9, by the cerebral microvasculature in the ischemic core.[65,71] Although it has been hypothesized that members of the PA and MMP families contribute to matrix degradation, consistent proof of pro-MMP activation is not yet available, and the manner of

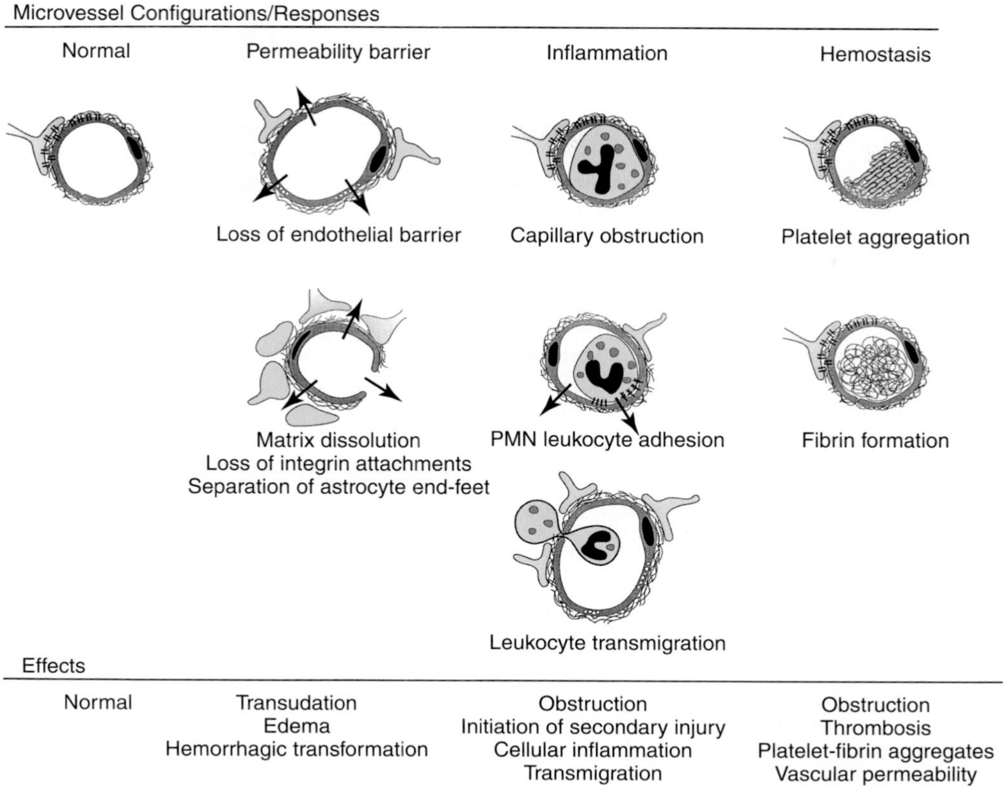

Microvessel Configurations/Responses

Figure 2-2 Early responses of cerebral microvessels in the target territory to focal ischemia. Not indicated are the appearance of activation antigens and the signal proteins and receptors associated with neogenesis (see text). PMN, polymorphonuclear leukocyte; *arrows*, leakage of plasma or blood.

protease compartmentalization has not yet been defined. Rosenberg et al[83,89] have shown that MMP-2 antigen rests in select astrocytes around microvessels in the ischemic rat brain.

Proteins known to participate in the activation pathways of pro-MMP-2, including MT1- and MT3-MMPs. appear simultaneously in the same regions of injury.[92] The expression of EMMPRIN, a transmembrane MMP inducer protein that affects the synthesis of several MMPs, was shown to increase following focal ischemia-reperfusion in a rodent model, in parallel with increases in MMP-2 and MMP-9 content and the number of EMMPRIN-immunoreactive microvessels.[93] The meaning of this association is not entirely clear, but points to a causal role of EMMPRIN in the activation and generation of MMPs following focal cerebral ischemia and reperfusion and also to relationships of MMP expression with other vascular elements.

Significant alterations in the plasminogen activator axis also occur after MCAO.[71] In rodent species, alterations in u-PA, PAI-1, and t-PA have been reported.[83,84] In the primate striatum, the very rapid increase in u-PA and PAI-1, and early regional increase in t-PA/PAI-1 complex (with transient decrease in free t-PA), are consistent with rapid changes in other gene products in the microvasculature.[63,71] Secretion of u-PA has been attributed to stimulated endothelial cells, astrocytes, neurons, and microglia in vivo or in vitro,[94-98] and PAI-1 can be generated by endothelial cells, astrocytes, and neurons.[94-97,99,100] The differential upregulation of u-PA/PAI-1 and t-PA in the ischemic parenchyma can be explained by stimulation by tumor necrosis factor-α (TNF-α), transforming growth factor-β (TGF-β), or interleukin-1β (IL-1β), none of which promotes endothelial cell t-PA synthesis or secretion.[95,97,101] The increase in u-PA and PAI-1 in both plasma and cerebral tissue after ischemia is consistent with an endothelial cell source.[71]

Together, these observations suggest that proteases that could contribute to vascular and parenchymal matrix degradation are generated shortly after MCAO in the striatum and that microvascular cells are a likely local source of pro-MMP-2, u-PA, PAI-1, cathepsin L, and heparinase. Because protease generation could contribute to loss of cerebral microvessel integrity, strategies designed to protect basal lamina structures may be of benefit. There is interest in the possibility that inhibitors of matrix-degrading Zn^{2+} metalloproteases might provide a reduction in consequences of ischemic injury to the microvascular cells, including total hemorrhage.[102-105] Unresolved issues include the combined effects of members of these several protease families, the relative specificities of protease family inhibitors, and the impact of active proteases on hemostasis and intravascular cell interactions.

An interesting parallel clinical situation to focal ischemia is provided by thrombotic occlusion of the sagittal or transverse cerebral sinuses. Local edema and hemorrhagic change can occur, which are compatible with the responses of cerebral tissues to focal ischemia. Vosko et al[106] characterized microvascular damage in a rodent model of cerebral venous thrombosis, including loss of laminin within the vascular basal lamina. Because hemorrhagic transformation is regularly seen in sinus venous thrombosis, the alterations in microvascular matrix integrity could be of relevance.

Focal Cerebral Ischemia and Microvessel Cell Adhesion

Cell adhesion receptors link the abluminal surfaces of the endothelium and astrocytes with the basal lamina. The immunoreactivity of endothelial cell β_1 integrins and of astrocyte $\alpha_6\beta_4$ and $\alpha\beta$-dystroglycan rapidly decreases after MCAO in the regions of neuron injury.[30,31,38] Within the ischemic core, microvessel-related β_1 integrin expression decreases to 20% of baseline, also implying continued endothelial cell synthesis of β_1 integrins.[31] The rapid fall and plateau of integrin expression could reflect injury to both endothelial cells and astrocytes initiated by ischemia, alterations of the matrix by processes involving microvessel endothelium or astrocytes with secondary changes in integrin expression, or both. Downregulation of β_1 integrin expression in microvessels is in part due to shutdown of its transcription.[31] In the ischemic core, these changes are reflected topographically as multiple subregions of increased microvessel-associated β_1 integrin messenger RNA (mRNA) surrounding islands devoid of vascular β_1 integrin messenger RNA.[31] The β_1 subunit transcripts appear prominently over noncapillary microvessels. Importantly, the dynamic nature of microvessel β_1 integrin responses confirms the reactivity of viable microvascular endothelial cells within the ischemic core.

Despite widespread loss of microvessel matrix adhesion receptor immunoreactivity, injury is not yet complete by 2 hours, in contrast to the commonly held view that permanent striatal injury after MCAO is rapid. Furthermore, the spatial distribution of altered microvessel adhesion receptor expression is not homogeneous.[30,31,63] Early changes in β_1 integrins and integrin $\alpha_6\beta_4$ expression are heterogeneously interspersed among microvessels displaying apparently normal expression of these integrins.[30,31] Furthermore, increased integrin $\alpha_v\beta_3$ expression by microvessels indicates that the early tissue injury within the ischemic core, where neuron injury is observed, is not homogeneous. Therefore, microvessels with apparently normal features may persist long after ischemia has been initiated, even in the most vulnerable territory, in contrast to evidence of neuron injury.

Pharmacologic Modulation of Microvascular Matrix-Adhesion Interactions

Growing experience in the experimental setting has focused on how agents employed in the clinic might affect microvessel matrix content, matrix protease generation, and injury during focal cerebral ischemia. Limited information indicates that pretreatment with a statin, a class of pleiotropic lipid-lowering agents that also decrease inflammation and alter membrane composition, can preserve microvessel basal lamina in the ischemic region.[107] Doxycycline, a tetracycline class antibiotic with multiple effects (e.g., anti-inflammatory and antileukocyte properties) also reduces the loss in basal ganglia constituents following focal ischemia.[108] This effect has been attributed

to reductions in MMP-2 and MMP-9 activity that can occur with doxycycline exposure.[108-110] Moderate hypothermia, with reduction in brain temperature to 32° to 34° C, produced a 50% reduction in microvessel basal lamina loss, decreasing hemorrhage and generation of MMPs.[111] Each strategy was associated with decreased injury development in focal ischemia rodent models. As here, experimental pretreatment strategies with statins and doxycycline are to be differentiated from those strategies that might reduce injury when applied early after stroke onset (e.g., plasminogen activators, hypothermia). The pretreatment approaches might be evaluated (as medical interventions) for use during procedures with associated stroke risk, including carotid artery surgery or coronary artery bypass graft placement.

The Focal No-Reflow Phenomenon and Secondary Injury

Transient occlusion of a brain-supplying artery significantly reduces the patency of the distal microvascular bed, causing the focal "no-reflow" phenomenon.[112-114] This finding accords with the demonstration by carbon tracer techniques of regions of territorial vascular compromise after transient MCAO.[112-115] Although attributed initially to extrinsic compression from edema, endothelial cell swelling, and endothelial microvillus formation,[116] intravascular obstruction also occurs with the local activation of platelets, leukocytes, and coagulation (fibrin).[112] A differential effect on flow or patency appears between cortical regions and the basal ganglia that are subject to ischemia.[117] Garcia et al[118] emphasized that swelling of astrocytes after ischemia may contribute to secondary neuronal death, although the time delays observed suggest that the relation must be complex.[118] Others have hypothesized that reactive astrocytes might contribute to impairment of microvessel perfusion in rodents, but technical issues needed to substantiate these claims have not been resolved.[119,120] It has been proposed that expansion of the regions of "no-reflow" by secondary injury recruits the peripheral zones into the ischemic core.[31]

Initiation of Cellular Inflammation

After ischemia, the microvasculature is a staging platform for secondary injury processes associated with cellular inflammation and thrombosis. The interface between the vascular wall and the plasma compartment is significantly and swiftly altered, promoting microvascular obstruction by leukocyte (and platelet) activation and adhesion. Endothelial cell leukocyte adhesion receptors respond to local ischemia in a rapid and orderly way. Transmigration of polymorphonuclear (PMN) leukocytes from microvessels in the ischemic core occurs as early as 1 hour after MCAO.[63,112] The appearance of P-selectin, intercellular adhesion molecule-1 (ICAM-1), and E-selectin on the microvessel endothelium, together with their counter-receptors (e.g., P-selectin ligand glycoprotein-1 [PSGL-1], the β_2 integrin CD18) on PMN leukocytes, accompanies the initial movement of inflammatory cells into the ischemic regions.[78,121,122] Observations in rodent models of focal cerebral ischemia have confirmed the appearance of leukocyte adhesion receptors on microvessels, but the details vary.[123,124]

The proinflammatory cytokines TNF-α and interleukin-1β are expressed in ischemic brain and influence the microvascular responses.[125-127] In anesthetized rodent models, evidence of interleukin-1β and TNF-α transcription is seen by 6 hours after MCAO.[127] The leukocyte adhesion receptors P-selectin, intercellular adhesion molecule-1, and E-selectin are stimulated by either TNF-α or interleukin-1β.[128,129] The actions of the cytokines can be pleiotropic, contributing to leukocyte adherence and transmigration, secondary injury, and protective processes.[125-127] For instance, although TNF-binding protein (TNF-bp) or neutralizing antibodies to TNF-α can reduce injury in rodent models of focal ischemia,[130,131] TNF-α has been shown to contribute to ischemic tolerance in similar rodent models.[132,133] Whether the microvascular responses to these cytokines contribute to both their beneficial and injurious properties in the CNS is unclear at this time.

PMN leukocyte adhesion requires the interaction of leukocyte β_2 integrin (CD18) with the endothelial cell receptor intercellular adhesion molecule in the CNS, as elsewhere.[121,122] Platelet-leukocyte interactions are mediated by platelet P-selectin–PMN leukocyte P-selectin ligand glycoprotein-1 binding, whereas platelet-fibrin binding requires the integrin $\alpha_{IIb}\beta_3$ on activated platelets.[134,135] The activation of PMN leukocytes may contribute to the focal "no-reflow" phenomenon.[112] Activated platelets begin to accumulate within the microvasculature of the ischemic territory within hours of MCAO.[121] Interference with either interaction by specific interventions against the β_2 integrin CD18 or integrin $\alpha_{IIb}\beta_3$ before reperfusion significantly increases residual microvessel patency (decreases focal "no-reflow").[122,136] Separate work with knockout preparations and specific inhibitors has demonstrated that inhibition of the platelet-fibrin interactions can reduce microvessel obstruction and decrease tissue injury.[137,138] Monocytoid cells and lymphocytes also adhere and transmigrate following PMN leukocytes,[139-141] processes that also require receptor activation. These interactions can contribute (1) to the loss of microvessel patency[112] and (2) to proteolysis of basal lamina matrix proteins.[116]

Fibrin Formation and Deposition

Activated platelets and fibrin(ogen) contribute to microvascular obstructions in both capillaries and postcapillary venules of the ischemic bed.[53,112,121,142] Fibrin is deposited in a growing proportion of microvessels with time after MCAO.[53,143] The accumulation of fibrin in the vascular lumen implies the intravascular generation of thrombin.[53] Tissue factor (TF), which is present preferentially in perivascular gray matter,[142] catalyzes fibrin formation when plasma fibrinogen is exposed to the TF that resides around noncapillary microvessels.[142,144,145] This process requires interaction of TF with circulating factor VII. Blockade of the TF–factor VIIa complex significantly reduces fibrin deposition within the microvessel lumen and modestly increases microvessel patency in ischemic regions.[53] Luminal fibrin implies locally increased permeability of the ischemic microvasculature.[53,146-148] Heparin

has also been shown to improve outcome after experimental stroke; the underlying mechanisms may vary and may include increased intravascular patency.[149,150]

Hemostasis and the Microvessel Wall

Cellular elements within the neurovascular unit modulate hemostasis in at least two general ways: (1) by expression of activators and inhibitors of thrombosis in the microvessel wall and (2) by cross-talk between the vascular cell components. As noted previously, TF, expressed by astrocytes around noncapillary microvessels, is the principal activator of coagulation in the CNS but is protected from the plasma column by the intact permeability barrier.[142,144,151] In addition, pericytes can express TF on their surfaces.[152] The expression of the principal endogenous inhibitor, tissue factor pathway inhibitor (TFPI), is lowest in the brain among all organs.[153] Craniocerebral injury decreases both circulating TF and TF pathway inhibitor levels.[154] There is little information about the interactions between TF and TF pathway inhibitor outside the circulation in the CNS.

Located in the perivascular space, protease nexin-1 (PN-1) presumably reduces exposure of the neuropil to low concentrations of thrombin, by direct interaction.[155-157] Thrombin, which is toxic to neurons, is generated when the permeability barrier is breached.

Angiogenesis

The formation of new microvessels from existing vessels (*angiogenesis*) is a hallmark tissue adaptation to injury[158-160] and involves some of the immediate microvessel responses already mentioned.[63,161] The general observation is that immediately after MCAO, the cerebral microvasculature expresses select receptors and their ligands known to promote angiogenesis in other biologic systems. Later, as after MCAO, the surviving microvasculature provides a scaffold for receptors and their ligands known to promote angiogenesis. New conduits are not formed immediately after MCAO,[4,5,162] but new capillaries begin to appear within the ischemic bed by 7 days after MCAO.[163,164]

It has been proposed that induction of angiogenesis following MCAO results from local hypoxia. Low tissue O_2 leads to inhibition of the degradation of hypoxia-inducible factor-1 (HIF-1). Hypoxia-inducible factor prolyl hydroxylase results in sustained expression, thereby stimulating expression of VEGF and integrin $\alpha_v\beta_3$.[165] VEGF is first synthesized by pericytes in response to hypobaric or normobaric hypoxia.[166] VEGF promotes microvessel proliferation, which requires the expression of the two endothelial cell receptors flt-1 (VEGFR-1) and flk/KDR (VEGFR-2).[167-170] Their interaction results in endothelial cell expression of integrin $\alpha_v\beta_3$. Integrin $\alpha_v\beta_3$ is necessary for angiogenesis, neovascularization in organ development, and tissue remodeling.[171,172] Endothelial cell migration and proliferation are stimulated by VEGF via VEGF receptor-1,[167] but only smooth muscle cells and pericytes migrate in response to VEGF.[173,174]

There is a robust literature on pericyte migration during angiogenesis. Destabilization of the microvessel with loss of basal lamina matrix at the leading edge in the early stages of angiogenesis is required for sprout formation.[175] However, if recovery is inhibited at the termination of angiogenesis by increased VEGF, then vascular regression can occur.

VEGF expression has been associated with increased microvascular permeability.[170,176,177] After MCAO, all of these elements are set in motion. In addition, focal cerebral ischemia stimulates the release of endothelial precursor cells (EPCs) into the circulation,[178-180] and the migration of neuroblasts from the subventricular zone.[181]

Activation of cerebral microvessel cells in precapillary arterioles occurs within 1 to 2 hours of MCAO within the ischemic territory of the primate striatum.[63] Okada et al[161] first demonstrated the differential upregulation of angiogenesis-related elements, including integrin $\alpha_v\beta_3$ but not integrin $\alpha_v\beta_5$, on microvessels within the ischemic territory immediately after MCAO. Integrin $\alpha_v\beta_3$ expression on cerebral microvessels is significantly and continuously associated with the intravascular deposition of fibrin.[161] Abumiya et al[63] demonstrated highly significant coexpression of VEGF, proliferating cell nuclear antigen (PCNA), and integrin $\alpha_v\beta_3$ in microvessels consistent with precapillary arterioles immediately after MCAO.[63] Other nonvascular sources of VEGF transcripts are leukocytes and microglia.[63] Kovacs et al[182] and Hayashi et al[183] described the appearance of VEGF on endothelial cells, neurons, and glial cells after MCAO in rodent models. It has also been demonstrated that VEGF can associate with neurons.[184] The coordination of VEGF expression and receptor binding among cellular elements of the neurovascular unit is not worked out.

In the boundary of the ischemic neocortex following MCAO in the rodent, hypoxia-induced VEGF expression precedes neovascularization.[185] VEGF expression has also been found to increase in both microvessels and neurons by 24 hours, most prominently in the peri-infarct regions. Under those conditions, VEGF receptor-1 (flt-1) increased in endothelial cells, neurons, and glial cells, and VEGF receptor-2 (flk/KDR) appeared in glial cells and endothelial cells.[186] Those findings indicate that the specific receptors for VEGF are expressed in concert with the ligand VEGF.

A similar relationship of microvessel VEGF and integrin α_v with hypoxia-inducible factor-1α transcription has also been noted (T. Abumiya and G. J. del Zoppo, unpublished observations, 1999).

Other receptors associated with vasculogenesis appear in response to focal ischemia. Both angiopoietin-1 and angiopoietin-2 appear in vascular endothelial cells in the ischemic territory with some delay after MCAO in the rodent.[187,188] Microvessels express both stroma-derived factor-1 (SDF-1) and angiopoietin-1 in response to ischemia.[181] Similarly, the tyrosine kinase receptors tyrosine kinase with immunoglobulin-like and epidermal growth factor–like domains–1 (tie-1) and tie-2 are expressed in the ischemic cortex, with tie-2 appearing on capillary-like structures in the outer cortical layers and tie-1 detected in layers II through IV.[189] Notably, under the conditions of focal cerebral ischemia, microvascular density can increase further in response to estradiol[190] and to diet-induced ketosis.[191,192]

One group of researchers has asserted that the neural adaptive response to injury (hypoxia) leads to induced physiologic angiogenesis associated with an increase in microvascular density.[193,194] Dysregulation of this response can lead to pathologic angiogenesis. Regulation of physiologic angiogenesis is central to cell-cell communication within the neurovascular unit. A central role for pericytes in the regulation of angiogenesis has been proposed. During the very early phases of angiogenesis, VEGF and VEGF receptor are expressed in pericytes within 24 to 45 hours of exposure to moderately low O_2.[195] Pericytes also express cell surface proteases and cytokines that activate the endothelium[196] and lead to pericyte migration from its capillary location.[175,194,197,198] Decreased pericyte-to–endothelial cell ratios are characteristic of angiogenic vessels, and these ratios return to normal at the maturation of angiogenesis. If pericyte coverage is disrupted at this latter stage, vascular integrity is reduced.[166] In physiologic angiogenesis, renewal of the hypoxic signal leads to vascular regression. This is supported by evidence that platelet-derived growth factor (PDGF) and VEGF can induce vascular instability and alter pericyte function.[199]

Proof of how the entire process proceeds and how it affects microvessel integrity, neovascularization, and outcome after focal cerebral ischemia is still lacking. Also, whether the observed alterations lead to functional microvessels and recovery, or are a function cul-de-sac, is still unclear.

Amyloid Deposition and Lipohyalinosis

Infiltration of cerebral microvessels can result from local insults, leading to impairment of their structural and functional integrity. Remodeling of vascular wall components may be a consequence.[200]

Amyloid precursor protein (APP) can accumulate within the cerebral vessel wall. APP messenger RNA has been detected in vascular endothelial cells, smooth muscle cells, and adventitial cells of cerebral vessels, and also in pericytes and perivascular cells.[201] Focal ischemia alters APP deposition in cerebral vessels. Cells that survive a focal ischemic insult or global cerebral hypoperfusion display an increased accumulation of APP.[202-204] The regional distribution of APP accumulation and its correlation with the reduction of cerebral blood flow reduction during cerebral ischemia have suggested the hypothesis that APP can contribute to selective neuronal vulnerability following ischemia.[205,206] APP has been shown to accumulate in the temporal neocortex, which is known to be sensitive to ischemia. However, APP also accumulates in the more resistant white matter tracts.[207,208] The age of rodents undergoing reversible focal cerebral ischemia influences the accumulation of APP, particularly by microglial cells. Accumulation of APP in astrocytes is greater in older rodents.[209] The vascular deposition of APP during ischemia is characterized by an increase in its Kunitz protease inhibitor-bearing isoform (KPI-APP) but a decrease in APP.[12,99] The shift between the different APP isoforms might explain neuron-degenerative processes resulting from cerebral ischemia.[210]

Work in transgenic models has demonstrated that mice overexpressing APP have profound impairment in the endothelium-dependent cerebrovascular responses. These changes can be reproduced by infusion of the APPβ-derived peptide Aβ 1-40, but not Aβ 1-42, in normal mice.[211] Therefore, the isoform Aβ 1-40 may contribute to functional impairment of cerebral vessels. Those animals overexpressing APP are also prone to development of severe ischemic lesions.[212] Reduced endothelium-dependent relaxation is thought to be an explanation for the greater susceptibility of this murine line to ischemia. Mice overexpressing APP are more likely to have spontaneous hemorrhagic stroke, mimicking the findings in human cerebral amyloid angiopathy.[213] Clinical risk factors for the development of hemorrhagic complications include advanced age, signs of severe microangiopathy (lacunar strokes, confluent white matter lesions), severe hypertension, diabetes mellitus, and vasculitides. Deposition of amyloid in the vessel wall (amyloid angiopathy) also leads to loss of vascular wall integrity, leakage, and, later, hemorrhagic changes.[214] The relative contributions of Aβ deposition to microvessel integrity could depend on β amyloid clearance.[215]

Lipohyalinosis or *fibrinoid microangiopathy* associated with hypertension has been classified into the following three states of severity: (1) sclerotic and hyalinotic thickening of the vessel wall, which primarily affects arterioles 100 to 200 μm in diameter, (2) disorganization of the vessel wall and disruption of the internal elastic lamina with occasional foam cell infiltration, and (3) fibrinoid degeneration of the vessel wall with thrombosis.[216] Most experimental models of focal cerebral ischemia do not mimic these age-dependent vascular disturbances, a lack that may also explain the relatively less frequent occurrence of large hemorrhages in small animal focal ischemia models than in humans. However, prolonged periods of ischemia or extended reperfusion can contribute to microvessel damage.

In neurologically normal individuals, increases in cerebral vessel wall thickness in comparison with luminal diameter have been observed with age.[217] An association of white matter microangiopathy with dilatative arteriopathies of the cerebral supply has been descrubed.[218] Also, Wardlaw et al[219] have described a general disorder of blood-brain barrier integrity within white matter microvessels in patients with microangiopathy. Gould et al[220] have suggested potential roles for basal lamina composition in white matter microangiopathy. Mutations within the *COL4a1* gene (encoding the procollagen type IVα1 protein) have been associated with retinal microvessel abnormalities, increased cerebral hemorrhagic risk, and lacunar infarction.[220]

Summary

Cerebral microvessels not only serve as conduits of blood but also respond dynamically to focal ischemia, initiating mechanisms important for cellular inflammation, secondary injury events, and potentially for vascular and tissue remodeling. The microvasculature is both a target and a platform for the interrelated processes of ischemia, thrombosis, and inflammation. All three processes stimulate protease secretion and activity. Consequences of their actions appear to be (1) loss of the primary blood-brain barrier, (2) alterations and degradation of the microvascular matrix (basal lamina), the second barrier, (3) microvascular hemorrhage, (4) edema formation, and (5) secondary alterations in the neuropil. Within select microvessels, immediately after thrombotic occlusion of the arterial supply, receptors important for the adhesion of endothelial cells and astrocyte end-feet to the basal lamina matrix are altered or lost, leukocyte adhesion receptors on endothelial cells of select vessels appear, leukocytes adhere and emigrate, and fibrin deposits and activated platelets accumulate. Activation of precapillary arterioles is accompanied by the expression of specific markers that presage angiogenesis. In the early moments after the onset of focal ischemia, these microvessel-dependent events occur together, distributed in a heterogeneous fashion adjacent to apparently normal microvessels throughout the ischemic region.

REFERENCES

1. Peters A, Palay SL, Webster HD: *The fine structure of the nervous system: neurons and their supporting cells*, ed 3, New York, 1991, Oxford University Press, pp 352-353.
2. Milner R, Campbell IL: The integrin family of cell adhesion molecules has multiple functions within the CNS, *J Neurosci Res* 69:286-291, 2002.
3. Weeks JB, Todd MM, Warner DS, et al: The influence of halothane, isoflurane, and pentobarbital on cerebral plasma volume in hypocapnic and normocapnic rats, *Anesthesiology* 73:461-466, 1990.
4. Pinard E, Engrand N, Seylaz J: Dynamic cerebral microcirculatory changes in transient forebrain ischemia in rats: Involvement of type I nitric oxide synthase, *J Cereb Blood Flow Metab* 20: 1648-1658, 2000.
5. Seylaz J, Charbonne R, Nari K, et al: Dynamic in vivo measurement of erythrocyte velocity and flow in capillaries and of microvessel diameter in the rat brain by confocal laser microscopy, *J Cereb Blood Flow Metab* 19:863-870, 1999.
6. Iadecola C: Neurovascular regulation in the normal brain and in Alzheimer's disease, *Nat Rev Neurosci* 5:347-360, 2004.
7. Zonta M, Angulo M, Gobbo S, et al: Neuron-to-astrocyte signaling is central to the dynamic control of brain microcirculation, *Nat Neurosci* 6:43-50, 2003.
8. Nedergaard M, Ransom BR, Goldman SA: New roles for astrocytes: Redefining the functional architecture of the brain, *Trends Neurosci* 26:523-530, 2003.
9. del Zoppo GJ, Mabuchi T: Cerebral microvessel responses to focal ischemia, *J Cereb Blood Flow Metab* 23:879-894, 2003.
10. del Zoppo GJ, Milner R: Integrin-matrix interactions in the cerebral microvasculature, *Arterioscler Thromb Vasc Biol* 26:1966-1975, 2006.
11. del Zoppo GJ: Stroke and neurovascular protection, *N Engl J Med* 354:553-555, 2006.
12. Janzer RC, Raff MC: Astrocytes induce blood-brain barrier properties in endothelial cells, *Nature* 325:253-257, 1987.
13. Nagano N, Aoyagi M, Hirakawa K: Extracellular matrix modulates the proliferation of rat astrocytes in serum-free culture, *Glia* 8:71-76, 1993.
14. Tagami M, Yamagata K, Fujino H, et al: Morphological differentiation of endothelial cells co-cultured with astrocytes on type-I or type-IV collagen, *Cell Tissue Res* 268:225-232, 1992.
15. Webersinke G, Bauer H, Amberger A, et al: Comparison of gene expression of extracellular matrix molecules in brain microvascular endothelial cells and astrocytes, *Biochem Biophys Res Commun* 189:877-884, 1992.
16. Spatz M, Bacic F, McCarron RM, et al: Human cerebromicrovascular endothelium: Studies in vitro, *J Cereb Blood Flow Metab* 9:S393, 1989.
17. Micic D, Swink M, Micic J, et al: The ischemic and postischemic effect on the uptake of neutral amino acids in isolated cerebral capillaries, *Experientia* 15:625-626, 1993.
18. McCarron RM, Merkel N, Bembry J, et al: Cerebrovascular endothelium in vitro: Studies related to blood-brain barrier function, *Proceedings of the XIth International Congress of Neuropathy* (Suppl 4):785-787, 1991:June.

19. Honkanen RA, McBath H, Kushmerick C, et al: Barbiturates inhibit hexose transport in cultured mammalian cells and human erythrocytes and interact directly with purified GLUT-1, *Biochemistry* 34:535-544, 1995.

20. Tran ND, Schreiber SS, Fisher M: Astrocyte regulation of endothelial tissue plasminogen activator in a blood-brain barrier model, *J Cereb Blood Flow Metab* 18:1316-1324, 1998.

21. Wang L, Tran ND, Kittaka M, et al: Thrombomodulin expression in bovine brain capillaries: Anticoagulant function of the blood-brain barrier, regional differences, and regulatory mechanisms, *Arterioscler Thromb Vasc Biol* 17:3139-3146, 1997.

22. Hurwitz AA, Berman JW, Rashbaum WK, et al: Human fetal astrocytes induce the expression of blood-brain barrier specific proteins by autologous endothelial cells, *Brain Res* 625:238-243, 1993.

23. Risau W, Wolburg H: Development of the blood-brain barrier, *Trends Neurosci* 13:174-178, 1990.

24. Risau W, Esser S, Engelhardt B: Differentiation of blood-brain barrier endothelial cells, *Pathol Biol* 46:171-175, 1998.

25. Schlosshauer B, Herzog KH: Neurothelin: An inducible cell surface glycoprotein of blood-brain barrier specific endothelial cells and distinct neurons, *J Cell Biol* 110:1261-1274, 1990.

26. Lobrinus JA, Juillerat-Jeanneret L, Darekar P, et al: Induction of the blood-brain barrier specific HT7 and neurothelin epitopes in endothelial cells of the chick chorioallantoic vessels by a soluble factor derived from astrocytes, *Brain Res Dev Brain Res* 70:207-211, 1992.

27. Estrada C, Bready JV, Berliner JA, et al: Astrocyte growth stimulation by a soluble factor produced by cerebral endothelial cells in vitro, *J Neuropathol Exp Neurol* 49:539-549, 1990.

28. Hamann GF, Okada Y, Fitridge R, et al: Microvascular basal lamina antigens disappear during cerebral ischemia and reperfusion, *Stroke* 26:2120-2126, 1995.

29. Haring H-P, Akamine P, Habermann R, et al: Distribution of integrin-like immunoreactivity on primate brain microvasculature, *J Neuropathol Exp Neurol* 55:236-245, 1996.

30. Wagner S, Tagaya M, Koziol JA, et al: Rapid disruption of an astrocyte interaction with the extracellular matrix mediated by integrin alpha 6 beta 4 during focal cerebral ischemia/reperfusion, *Stroke* 28:858-865, 1997.

31. Tagaya M, Haring H-P, Stuiver I, et al: Rapid loss of microvascular integrin expression during focal brain ischemia reflects neuron injury, *J Cereb Blood Flow Metab* 21:835-846, 2001.

32. Hamann GF, Liebetrau M, Martens H, et al: Microvascular basal lamina injury after experimental focal cerebral ischemia and reperfusion in the rat, *J Cereb Blood Flow Metab* 22:526-533, 2002.

33. Barone FC, Hillegass LM, Tzimas MN, et al: Time-related changes in myeloperoxidase activity and leukotriene by receptor binding reflect leukocyte influx in cerebral focal stroke, *Mol Chem Neuropathol* 24:13-30, 1995.

34. Kramer RH, Cheng Y-F, Clyman R: Human microvascular endothelial cells use beta$_1$ and beta$_3$ integrin receptor complexes to attach to laminin, *J Cell Biol* 111:1233-1243, 1990.

35. Paulus W, Baur I, Schuppan D, et al: Characterization of integrin receptors in normal and neoplastic human brain, *Am J Pathol* 143:154-163, 1993.

36. Gehlsen KR, Klier FG, Dickerson K, et al: Localization of the binding site for a cell adhesion receptor in laminin, *J Biol Chem* 264:19034-19038, 1989.

37. Korhonen M, Ylanne J, Laitinen L, et al: The alpha 1 and alpha 6 subunits of integrins are characteristically expressed in distinct segments of developing and adult human nephron, *J Cell Biol* 111:1245-1254, 1990.

38. Milner R, Hung S, Wang X, et al: The rapid decrease in astrocyte-associated dystroglycan expression by focal cerebral ischemia is protease-dependent, *J Cereb Blood Flow Metab* 28:812-823, 2008.

39. Dietrich WD: Neurobiology of stroke, *Int Rev Neurobiol* 42:55-101, 1998.

40. Dirnagl U, Iadecola C, Moskowitz MA: Pathobiology of ischaemic stroke: An integrated view, *Trends Neurosci* 22:391-397, 1999.

41. Francis A, Pulsinelli W: The response of GABAergic and cholinergic neurons to transient cerebral ischemia, *Brain Res* 243:271-278, 1982.

42. Gonzales C, Lin RCS, Chesselet MF: Relative sparing of GABAergic interneurons in the striatum of gerbils with ischemia-induced lesions, *Neurosci Lett* 135:53-58, 1992.

43. Nitsch C, Goping G, Klatzo I: Preservation of GABAergic perikarya and boutons after transient ischemia in the gerbil hippocampal CA1 field, *Brain Res* 495:243-252, 1989.

44. Nyberg P, Waller S: Age-dependent vulnerability of brain choline acetyltransferase activity to transient cerebral ischemia in rats, *Stroke* 20:495-500, 1989.

45. Mabuchi T, Lucero J, Feng A, et al: Focal cerebral ischemia preferentially affects neurons distant from their neighboring microvessels, *J Cereb Blood Flow Metab* 25:257-266, 2005.

46. del Zoppo GJ, Becker KJ, Hallenbeck JM: Inflammation after stroke: Is it harmful? *Arch Neurol* 58:669-672, 2001.

47. Naganuma Y: Changes of the cerebral microvascular structure and endothelium during the course of permanent ischemia, *Keio J Med* 39:26-31, 1990.

48. Dietrich WD, Busto R, Ginsberg MD: Cerebral endothelial microvilli: Formation following global forebrain ischemia, *J Neuropathol Exp Neurol* 43:72-83, 1984.

49. Okumura Y, Sakaki T, Hiramatsu K, et al: Microvascular changes associated with postischaemic hypoperfusion in rats, *Acta Neurochir (Wien)* 139:670-676, 1997.

50. Garcia JH, Lowry SL, Briggs L, et al: Brain capillaries expand and rupture in areas of ischemia and reperfusion. In Reivich M, Hurtig HI, editors: *Cerebrovascular diseases*, New York, 1983, Raven Press, pp 169-182.

51. Maxwell K, Berliner JA, Cancilla PA: Stimulation of glucose analogue uptake by cerebral microvessel endothelial cells by a product released by astrocytes, *J Neuropathol Exp Neurol* 48:69-80, 1989.

52. Chan PH, Chu L: Mechanisms underlying glutamate-induced swelling of astrocytes in primary culture, *Acta Neurochir Suppl* 51:7-10, 1990.

53. Okada Y, Copeland BR, Fitridge R, et al: Fibrin contributes to microvascular obstructions and parenchymal changes during early focal cerebral ischemia and reperfusion, *Stroke* 25:1847-1853, 1994.

54. Olesen S-P: Rapid increase in blood-brain barrier permeability during severe hypoxia and metabolic inhibition, *Brain Res* 368:24-29, 1986.

55. Gotoh O, Asano T, Koide T, et al: Ischemic brain edema following occlusion of the middle cerebral artery in the rat. I: The time courses of the brain water, sodium and potassium contents and blood-brain barrier permeability to ^{125}I-albumin, *Stroke* 16:101-109, 1985.

56. Petito CK, Babiak T: Early proliferative changes in astrocytes in postischemic noninfarcted rat brain, *Ann Neurol* 11:510-518, 1982.

57. Bender AS, Norenberg MD: Calcium dependence of hypoosmotically induced potassium release in cultured astrocytes, *J Neurosci* 14:4237-4243, 1994.

58. Simard JM, Chen M, Tarasov KV, et al: Newly expressed SUR1-regulated NC(Ca-ATP) channel mediates cerebral edema after ischemic stroke, *Nat Med* 12:433-440, 2006.

59. Simard M, Arcuino G, Takano T, et al: Signaling at the gliovascular interface, *J Neurosci* 23:9254-9262, 2003.

60. Ames A, Wright LW, Kowada M, et al: Cerebral ischemia. II: The no-reflow phenomenon, *Am J Pathol* 52:437-453, 1968.

61. Kamiya T, Katayama Y, Kashiwagi F, et al: The role of bradykinin in mediating ischemic brain edema in rats, *Stroke* 24:571-575, 1993.

62. Aschner JL, Lum H, Fletcher PW, et al: Bradykinin- and thrombin-induced increases in endothelial permeability occur independently of phospholipase C but require protein kinase C activation, *J Cell Physiol* 173:387-396, 1997.

63. Abumiya T, Lucero J, Heo JH, et al: Activated microvessels express vascular endothelial growth factor and integrin alpha(v) beta3 during focal cerebral ischemia, *J Cereb Blood Flow Metab* 19:1038-1050, 1999.

64. Zhang ZG, Zhang L, Jiang Q, et al: VEGF enhances angiogenesis and promotes blood-brain barrier leakage in the ischemic brain, *J Clin Invest* 106:829-838, 2000.

65. Heo JH, Lucero J, Abumiya T, et al: Matrix metalloproteinases increase very early during experimental focal cerebral ischemia, *J Cereb Blood Flow Metab* 19:624-633, 1999.

66. Fukuda S, Fini CA, Mabuchi T, et al: Focal cerebral ischemia induces active proteases that degrade microvascular matrix, *Stroke* 35:998-1004, 2004.

67. Garcia JH, Liu KF, Yoshida Y, et al: Influx of leukocytes and platelets in an evolving brain infarct (Wistar rat), *Am J Pathol* 144:188-199, 1994.

68. Armao D, Kornfeld M, Estrada EY, et al: Neutral proteases and disruption of the blood-brain barrier in rat, *Brain Res* 767:259-264, 1997.

69. Opdenakker G, Van den Steen PE, Dubois B, et al: Gelatinase B functions as regulator and effector in leukocyte biology, *J Leuk Biol* 69:851-859, 2001.

70. Hasty KA, Pourmotabbed TF, Goldberg GI, et al: Human neutrophil collagenase: A distinct gene product with homology to other matrix metalloproteinases, *J Biol Chem* 265:11421-11424, 1990.

71. Hosomi N, Lucero J, Heo JH, et al: Rapid differential endogenous plasminogen activator expression after acute middle cerebral artery occlusion, *Stroke* 32:1341-1348, 2001.

72. Relton JK, Beckey VE, Hanson WL, et al: CP-0597, a selective bradykinin B$_2$ receptor antagonist, inhibits brain injury in a rat model of reversible middle cerebral artery occlusion, *Stroke* 28:1430-1436, 1997.

73. Lee KR, Kawai N, Kim S, et al: Mechanisms of edema formation after intracerebral hemorrhage: Effects of thrombin on cerebral blood flow, blood-brain barrier permeability, and cell survival in a rat model, *J Neurosurg* 86:272-278, 1997.

74. Kubo Y, Suzuki M, Kudo A, et al: Thrombin inhibitor ameliorates secondary damage in rat brain injury: Suppression of inflammatory cells and vimentin-positive astrocytes, *J Neurotrauma* 2:163-172, 2000.

75. Suarez S, Ballmer-Hofer K: VEGF transiently disrupts gap junctional communication in endothelial cells, *J Cell Sci* 114:1229-1235, 2001.

76. Hamann GF, Okada Y, del Zoppo GJ: Hemorrhagic transformation and microvascular integrity during focal cerebral ischemia/reperfusion, *J Cereb Blood Flow Metab* 16:1373-1378, 1996.

77. Cowan DH, Haut JJ: Platelet function in acute leukemia, *J Lab Clin Med* 79:893-905, 1972.

78. Haring H-P, Berg EL, Tsurushita N, et al: E-selectin appears in non-ischemic tissue during experimental focal cerebral ischemia, *Stroke* 27:1386-1392, 1996.

79. Liu T, McDonnell PC, Young PR, et al: Interleukin-1beta mRNA expression in ischemic rat cortex, *Stroke* 24:1746-1751, 1993.

80. Buttini M, Appel K, Sauter A, et al: Expression of tumor necrosis factor alpha after focal cerebral ischaemia in the rat, *Neuroscience* 71:1-16, 1996.

81. Loddick SA, Rothwell NJ: Neuroprotective effects of human recombinant interleukin-1 receptor antagonist in focal cerebral ischaemia in the rat, *J Cereb Blood Flow Metab* 16:932-940, 1996.

82. Garcia JH, Cox JV, Hudgins WR: Ultrastructure of the microvasculature in experimental cerebral infarction, *Arch Neuropathol (Berlin)* 18:273-285, 1971.

83. Rosenberg GA, Navratil M, Barone F, et al: Proteolytic cascade enzymes increase in focal cerebral ischemia in rat, *J Cereb Blood Flow Metab* 16:360-366, 1996.

84. Ahn MY, Zhang ZG, Tsang W, et al: Endogenous plasminogen activator expression after embolic focal cerebral ischemia in mice, *Brain Res* 837:169-176, 1999.

85. Rosenberg GA: Matrix metalloproteinases in neuroinflammation, *Glia* 39:279-291, 2002.

86. Mackay AR, Corbitt RH, Hartzler JL, et al: Basement membrane type IV collagen degradation: Evidence for the involvement of a proteolytic cascade independent of metalloproteinases, *Cancer Res* 50:5997-6001, 1990.

87. Saksela O, Rifkin DB: Cell-associated plasminogen activation: regulation and physiological functions, *Annu Rev Cell Dev Biol* 4:93-126, 1988.

88. Vassalli JD, Sappino AP, Belin D: The plasminogen activator/plasmin system, *J Clin Invest* 88:1067-1072, 1991.

89. Rosenberg GA, Cunningham LA, Wallace J, et al: Immunohistochemistry of matrix metalloproteinases in reperfusion injury to rat brain: Activation of MMP-9 linked to stromelysin-1 and microglia in cell cultures, *Brain Res* 893:104-112, 2001.

90. Rosenberg GA, Dencoff JE, McGuire PG, et al: Injury-induced 92-kilodalton gelatinase and urokinase expression in rat brain, *Lab Invest* 71:417-422, 1994.

91. Rosenberg GA, Navratil M: Metalloproteinase inhibition blocks edema in intracerebral hemorrhage in the rat, *Neurology* 48:921-926, 1997.

92. Chang DI, Hosomi N, Lucero J, et al: Activation systems for matrix metalloproteinase-2 are upregulated immediately following experimental focal cerebral ischemia, *J Cereb Blood Flow Metab* 23:1408-1419, 2003.

93. Burggraf D, Martens HK, Wunderlich N, et al: Rt-PA causes a significant increase in endogenous u-PA during experimental focal cerebral ischemia, *Eur J Neurosci* 20:2903-2908, 2004.

94. Nakajima K, Tsuzaki N, Shimojo M, et al: Microglia isolated from rat brain secrete a urokinase-type plasminogen activator, *Brain Res* 577:285-292, 1992.

95. van Hinsbergh VW, van den Berg EA, Fiers W, et al: Tumor necrosis factor induces the production of urokinase-type plasminogen activator by human endothelial cells, *Blood* 75:1991-1998, 1990.

96. Masos T, Miskin R: Localization of urokinase-type plasminogen activator mRNA in the adult mouse brain, *Brain Res Mol Brain Res* 35:139-148, 1996.

97. Schleef RR, Bevilacqua MP, Sawdey M, et al: Cytokine activation of vascular endothelium: Effects on tissue-type plasminogen activator and type 1 plasminogen activator inhibitor, *J Biol Chem* 263:5797-5803, 1988.

98. Vivien D, Buisson A: Serine protease inhibitors: Novel therapeutic targets for stroke? *J Cereb Blood Flow Metab* 20:755-764, 2000.

99. Vincent VA, Lowik CW, Verheijen JH, et al: Role of astrocyte-derived tissue-type plasminogen activator in the regulation of endotoxin-stimulated nitric oxide production by microglial cells, *Glia* 22:130-137, 1998.

100. Levin EG, del Zoppo GJ: Localization of tissue plasminogen activator in the endothelium of a limited number of vessels, *Am J Pathol* 144:855-861, 1994.

101. Docagne F, Nicole O, Marti HH, et al: Transforming growth factor-beta$_1$ as a regulator of the serpins/t-PA axis in cerebral ischemia, *FASEB J* 13:1315-1324, 1999.

102. Rosenberg GA, Kornfeld M, Estrada E, et al: TIMP-2 reduces proteolytic opening of blood-brain barrier by type IV collagenase, *Brain Res* 576:203-207, 1992.

103. Abilleira S, Montaner J, Molina CA, et al: Matrix metalloproteinase-9 concentration after spontaneous intracerebral hemorrhage, *J Neurosurg* 99:65-70, 2003.

104. Montaner J, Alvarez-Sabin J, Molina CA, et al: Matrix metalloproteinase expression is related to hemorrhagic transformation after cardioembolic stroke, *Stroke* 32:2762-2667, 2001.

105. Montaner J, Molina CA, Monasterio J, et al: Matrix metalloproteinase-9 pretreatment level predicts intracranial hemorrhagic complications after thrombolysis in human stroke, *Circulation* 107:598-603, 2003.

106. Vosko MR, Rother J, Friedl B, et al: Microvascular damage following experimental sinus-vein thrombosis in rats, *Acta Neuropathol* 106:501-505, 2003.

107. Trinkl A, Vosko MR, Wunderlich N, et al: Pravastatin reduces microvascular basal lamina damage following focal cerebral ischemia and reperfusion, *Eur J Neurosci* 24:520-526, 2006.

108. Burggraf D, Trinkl A, Dichgans M, et al: Doxycycline inhibits MMPs via modulation of plasminogen activators in focal cerebral ischemia, *Neurobiol Dis* 25:506-513, 2007.

109. Jantzie LL, Cheung PY, Todd KG: Doxycycline reduces cleaved caspase-3 and microglial activation in an animal model of neonatal hypoxia-ischemia, *J Cereb Blood Flow Metab* 25:314-324, 2005.

110. del Zoppo GJ, Milner R, Mabuchi T, et al: Microglial activation and matrix protease generation during focal cerebral ischemia, *Stroke* 38:646-651, 2007.

111. Hamann GF, Burggraf D, Martens HK, et al: Mild to moderate hypothermia prevents microvascular basal lamina antigen loss in experimental focal cerebral ischemia, *Stroke* 35:764-769, 2004.

112. del Zoppo GJ, Schmid-Schönbein GW, Mori E, et al: Polymorphonuclear leukocytes occlude capillaries following middle cerebral artery occlusion and reperfusion in baboons, *Stroke* 22:1276-1284, 1991.

113. Little JR, Kerr FWL, Sundt TM Jr: Microcirculatory obstruction in focal cerebral ischemia: Relationship to neuronal alterations, *Mayo Clin Proc* 50:264-270, 1975.

114. Little JR, Kerr FWL, Sundt TMJ: Microcirculatory obstruction in focal cerebral ischemia: An electron microscopic investigation in monkeys, *Stroke* 7:25-30, 1976.

115. Sundt TM Jr, Grant WC, Garcia JH: Restoration of middle cerebral artery flow in experimental infarction, *J Neurosurg* 31:311-322, 1969.

116. del Zoppo GJ: Microvascular changes during cerebral ischaemia and reperfusion, *Cerebrovasc Brain Metab Rev* 6:47-96, 1994.

117. Wang CX, Todd KG, Yang Y, et al: Patency of cerebral microvessels after focal embolic stroke in the rat, *J Cereb Blood Flow Metab* 21:413-421, 2001.

118. Garcia JH, Liu KF, Yoshida Y, et al: Brain microvessels: Factors altering their patency after the occlusion of a middle cerebral artery (Wistar rat), *Am J Pathol* 145:728-740, 1994.

119. Zhang ZG, Bower L, Zhang RL, et al: Three-dimensional measurement of cerebral microvascular plasma perfusion, glial fibrillary acidic protein and microtubule associated protein-2 immunoreactivity after embolic stroke in rats: A double fluorescent labeled laser-scanning confocal microscopic study, *Brain Res* 844:55-66, 1999.

120. Zhang ZG, Davies K, Prostak J, et al: Quantitation of microvascular plasma perfusion and neuronal microtubule-associated protein in ischemic mouse brain by laser-scanning confocal microscopy, *J Cereb Blood Flow Metab* 19:68-78, 1999.

121. Okada Y, Copeland BR, Mori E, et al: P-selectin and intercellular adhesion molecule-1 expression after focal brain ischemia and reperfusion, *Stroke* 25:202-211, 1994.

122. Mori E, del Zoppo GJ, Chambers JD, et al: Inhibition of polymorphonuclear leukocyte adherence suppresses no-reflow after focal cerebral ischemia in baboons, *Stroke* 23:712-718, 1992.

123. Zhang RL, Chopp M, Li Y, et al: Anti-ICAM-1 antibody reduces ischemic cell damage after transient middle cerebral artery occlusion in the rat, *Neurology* 44:1747-1751, 1994.

124. Zhang R, Chopp M, Zhang Z, et al: The expression of P- and E-selectins in three models of middle cerebral artery occlusion, *Brain Res* 785:207-214, 1998.

125. Siren AL, Heldman E, Doron D, et al: Release of proinflammatory and prothrombotic mediators in the brain and peripheral circulation in spontaneously hypertensive and normotensive Wistar-Kyoto rats, *Stroke* 23:1643-1651, 1992.

126. Wang X, Barone FC, Aiyar NV, et al: Increased interleukin-1 receptor and receptor antagonist gene expression after focal stroke, *Stroke* 28:155-161, 1997.

127. Wang X, Yue T-L, Barone FC, et al: Concomitant cortical expression of TNF-α and IL-1β mRNA following transient focal ischemia, *Mol Chem Neuropathol* 23:103-114, 1994.

128. Wang X, Siren AL, Liu Y, et al: Upregulation of intercellular adhesion molecule 1 (ICAM-1) on brain microvascular endothelial cells in rat ischemic cortex, *Mol Brain Res* 26:61-68, 1994.

129. Wang X, Yue T-L, Barone FC, et al: Demonstration of increased endothelial-leukocyte adhesion molecule-1 mRNA expression in rat ischemic cortex, *Stroke* 26:1665-1669, 1995.

130. Dawson DA, Martin D, Hallenbeck JM: Inhibition of tumor necrosis factor-alpha reduces focal cerebral ischemic injury in the spontaneously hypertensive rat, *Neuroscience Lett* 218:41-44, 1996.

131. Nawashiro H, Martin D, Hallenbeck JM: Neuroprotective effects of TNF-binding protein in focal cerebral ischemia, *Brain Res* 778:265-271, 1997.

132. Nawashiro H, Tasaki K, Ruetzler CA, et al: TNF-alpha pretreatment induces protective effects against focal cerebral ischemia in mice, *J Cereb Blood Flow Metab* 17:483-490, 1997.

133. Tasaki K, Ruetzler C, Ohtsuki T, et al: Lipopolysaccharide pretreatment induces resistance against subsequent focal cerebral ischemic damage in spontaneously hypertensive rats, *Brain Res* 748:267-270, 1997.

134. Shattil SJ: Function and regulation of the beta 3 integrins in hemostasis and vascular biology, *Thromb Haemost* 74:149-155, 1995.

135. Shattil SJ: Signaling through platelet integrin alpha IIb beta 3: Inside-out, outside-in, and sideways, *Thromb Haemost* 82:318-325, 1999.

136. Abumiya T, Fitridge R, Mazur C, et al: Integrin alpha(IIb)beta(3) inhibitor preserves microvascular patency in experimental acute focal cerebral ischemia, *Stroke* 31:1402-1410, 2000.

137. Walder CE, Green SP, Darbonne WC, et al: Ischemic stroke injury is reduced in mice lacking a functional NADPH oxidase, *Stroke* 28:2252-2258, 1997.

138. Choudhri TF, Hoh BL, Zerwes HG, et al: Reduced microvascular thrombosis and improved outcome in acute murine stroke by inhibiting GP IIb/IIIa receptor-mediated platelet aggregation, *J Clin Invest* 102:1301-1310, 1998.

139. Becker K, Kindrick D, Relton J, et al: Antibody to the alpha4 integrin decreases infarct size in transient focal cerebral ischemia in rats, *Stroke* 32:206-211, 2001.

140. McCarron RM, Racke M, Spatz M, et al: Cerebral vascular endothelial cells are effective targets for in vitro lysis by encephalitogenic T lymphocytes, *J Immunol* 147:503-508, 1991.

141. de Jong AL, Green DM, Trial JA, et al: Focal effects of monoclonuclear leukocyte transendothelial migration: TNF-alpha production by migrating monocytes promotes subsequent migration of lymphocytes, *J Leukoc Biol* 60:129-136, 1996.

142. del Zoppo GJ, Yu J-Q, Copeland BR, et al: Tissue factor localization in non-human primate cerebral tissue, *Thromb Haemost* 68:642-647, 1992.

143. Thomas WS, Mori E, Copeland BR, et al: Tissue factor contributes to microvascular defects following cerebral ischemia, *Stroke* 24:847-853, 1993.

144. Mackman N, Morrissey JA, Fowler B, et al: Complete sequence of the human tissue factor gene, a highly regulated cellular receptor that initiates the coagulation protease cascade, *Biochemistry* 28:1755-1762, 1989.

145. Ruf W, Rehemtulla A, Morrissey JH, et al: Phospholipid independent and dependent interactions required for tissue factor receptor and cofactor function, *J Biol Chem* 266:2158-2166, 1990.

146. Mabuchi T, Kitagawa K, Ohtsuki T, et al: Contribution of microglia/macrophages to expansion of infarction and response of oligodendrocytes after focal cerebral ischemia in rats, *Stroke* 31:1735-1743, 2000.

147. Kitagawa K, Matsumoto M, Ohtsuki T, et al: The characteristics of blood-brain barrier in three different conditions—infarction, selective neuronal death and selective loss of presynaptic terminals—following cerebral ischemia, *Acta Neuropathol* 84:378-386, 1992.

148. Nordborg C, Sokrab TE, Johansson BB: The relationship between plasma protein extravasation and remote tissue changes after experimental brain infarction, *Acta Neuropathol* 82:118-126, 1991.

149. Li PA, He QP, Siddiqui MM, et al: Posttreatment with low molecular weight heparin reduces brain edema and infarct volume in rats subjected to thrombotic middle cerebral artery occlusion, *Brain Res* 801:220-223, 1998.

150. Quartermain D, Li Y, Jonas S: Enoxaparin, a low molecular weight heparin decreases infarct size and improves sensorimotor function in a rat model of focal cerebral ischemia, *Neurosci Lett* 288:155-158, 2000.

151. Eddleston M, de la Torre JC, Oldstone MB, et al: Astrocytes are the primary source of tissue factor in the murine central nervous system: A role for astrocytes in cerebral hemostasis, *J Clin Invest* 92:349-358, 1993.

152. Bouchard BA, Shatos MA, Tracy PB: Human brain pericytes differentially regulate expression of procoagulant enzyme complexes comprising the extrinsic pathway of blood coagulation, *Arterioscler Thromb Vasc Biol* 17:1-9, 1997.

153. Bajaj MS, Kuppuswamy MN, Manepalli AN, et al: Transcriptional expression of tissue factor pathway inhibitor, thrombomodulin and von Willebrand factor in normal human tissues, *Thromb Haemost* 82:1047-1052, 1999.

154. Tohgi H, Utsugisawa K, Yoshimura M, et al: Local variation in expression of pro- and antithrombotic factors in vascular endothelium of human autopsy brain, *Acta Neuropathol* 98:111-118, 1999.

155. Cunningham DD, Donovan FM: Regulation of neurons and astrocytes by thrombin and protease nexin-1: Relationship to brain injury, *Adv Exp Med Biol* 425:67-75, 1997.

156. Vaughan PJ, Cunningham DD: Regulation of protease nexin-1 synthesis and secretion in cultured brain cells by injury-related factors, *J Biol Chem* 268:3720-3727, 1993.

157. Vaughan PJ, Su J, Cotman CW, et al: Protease nexin-1, a potent thrombin inhibitor, is reduced around cerebral blood vessels in Alzheimer's disease, *Brain Res* 668:160-170, 1994.

158. Hynes RO: A reevaluation of integrins as regulators of angiogenesis, *Nat Med* 8:918-921, 2002.

159. Carmeliet P: Mechanisms of angiogenesis and arteriogenesis, *Nat Med* 6:389-395, 2000.

160. Dvorak HF, Brown LF, Detmar M, et al: Vascular permeability factor/vascular endothelial growth factor, microvascular hyperpermeability, and angiogenesis, *Am J Pathol* 146:1029-1039, 1995.

161. Okada Y, Copeland BR, Hamann GF, et al: Integrin alpha(v)beta3 is expressed in selected microvessels after focal cerebral ischemia, *Am J Pathol* 149:37–44, 1996.

162. Keyeux A, Ochrymowicz-Bemelmans D, Charlier AA: Induced response to hypercapnia in the two-compartment total cerebral blood volume: Influence on brain vascular reserve and flow efficiency, *J Cereb Blood Flow Metab* 15:1121–1131, 1995.

163. Tsutsumi K, Shibata S, Inoue M, et al: Experimental cerebral infarction in the dog. Ultrastructural study of microvessels in subacute cerebral infarction, *Neurol Med Chir (Tokyo)* 27:73–77, 1986.

164. Tsutsumi K: Experimental cerebral infarction in the dog. Scanning electron microscopy with vascular endocasts of the microvessels in the ischemic brain, *Neurol Med Chir (Tokyo)* 26:595–600, 1986.

165. Namiki A, Brogi E, Kearney M, et al: Hypoxia induces vascular endothelial growth factor in cultured human endothelial cells, *J Biol Chem* 270:31189–31195, 1995.

166. Dore-Duffy P, Balabanov R, Beaumont T, et al: Endothelial activation following prolonged hypobaric hypoxia, *Microvasc Res* 57:75–85, 1999.

167. Nicosia RF, Lin YJ, Hazelton D, et al: Endogenous regulation of angiogenesis in the rat aorta model: Role of vascular endothelial growth factor, *Am J Pathol* 151:1379–1386, 1997.

168. Straume O, Akslen LA: Expression of vascular endothelial growth factor, its receptors (FLT-1, KDR) and TSP-1 related to microvessel density and patient outcome in vertical growth phase melanomas, *Am J Pathol* 159:223–235, 2001.

169. Chan AS, Leung SY, Wong MP, et al: Expression of vascular endothelial growth factor and its receptors in the anaplastic progression of astrocytoma, oligodendroglioma, and ependymoma, *Am J Surg Pathol* 22:816–826, 1998.

170. Shibuya M: Differential roles of vascular endothelial growth factor receptor-1 and receptor-2 in angiogenesis, *J Biochem Mol Biol* 39:469–478, 2006.

171. Brooks PC, Montgomery AM, Rosenfeld M, et al: Integrin a_vb_3 antagonists promote tumor regression by promoting apoptosis of angiogenic blood vessels, *Cell* 79:1157–1164, 1994.

172. Varner JA, Brooks PC, Cheresh DA: The integrin a_vb_3: Angiogenesis and apoptosis, *Cell Adhes Commun* 3:367–374, 1995.

173. Wang Z, Castresana MR, Newman WH: Reactive oxygen and NF-kappaB in VEGF-induced migration of human vascular smooth muscle cells, *Biochem Biophys Res Commun* 285:669–674, 2001.

174. Grosskreutz CL, Anand-Apte B, Duplaa C, et al: Vascular endothelial growth factor-induced migration of vascular smooth muscle cells in vitro, *Microvasc Res* 58:128–136, 1999.

175. Nehls V, Denzer K, Drenckhahn D: Pericyte involvement in capillary sprouting during angiogenesis in situ, *Cell Tissue Res* 270:469–474, 1992.

176. Esser S, Wolburg K, Wolburg H, et al: Vascular endothelial growth factor induces endothelial fenestrations in vitro, *J Cell Biol* 140:947–959, 1998.

177. Al Ahmad A, Gassmann M: Ogunshola OO: Maintaining blood-brain barrier integrity: Pericytes perform better than astrocytes during prolonged oxygen deprivation, *J Cell Physiol* 218:612–622, 2009.

178. Yip HK, Chang LT, Chang WN, et al: Level and value of circulating endothelial progenitor cells in patients after acute ischemic stroke, *Stroke* 39:69–74, 2008.

179. Asahara T, Masuda H, Takahashi T, et al: Bone marrow origin of endothelial progenitor cells responsible for postnatal vasculogenesis in physiological and pathological neovascularization, *Circ Res* 85:221–228, 1999.

180. Taguchi A, Matsuyama T, Moriwaki H, et al: Circulating CD34-positive cells provide an index of cerebrovascular function, *Circulation* 109:2972–2975, 2004.

181. Ohab JJ, Fleming S, Blesch A, et al: A neurovascular niche for neurogenesis after stroke, *J Neurosci* 26:13007–13016, 2006.

182. Kovacs Z, Ikezaki K, Samoto K, et al: VEGF and flt: Expression time kinetics in rat brain infarct, *Stroke* 27:1865–1872, 1996.

183. Hayashi T, Abe K, Suzuki H, et al: Rapid induction of vascular endothelial growth factor gene expression after transient middle cerebral artery occlusion in rats, *Stroke* 28:2039–2044, 1997.

184. Stowe AM, Plautz EJ, Nguyen P, et al: Neuronal HIF-1 alpha protein and VEGFR-2 immunoreactivity in functionally related motor areas following a focal M1 infarct, *J Cereb Blood Flow Metab* 28:612–620, 2008.

185. Marti HJ, Bernaudin M, Bellail A, et al: Hypoxia-induced vascular endothelial growth factor expression precedes neovascularization after cerebral ischemia, *Am J Pathol* 156:965–976, 2000.

186. Lennmyr F, Ata KA, Funa K, et al: Expression of vascular endothelial growth factor (VEGF) and its receptors (Flt-1 and Flk-1) following permanent and transient occlusion of the middle cerebral artery in the rat, *J Neuropathol Exp Neurol* 57:874–882, 1998.

187. Beck H, Acker T, Wiessner C, et al: Expression of angiopoietin-1, angiopoietin-2, and tie receptors after middle cerebral artery occlusion in the rat, *Am J Pathol* 157:1473–1483, 2000.

188. Lin TN, Wang CK, Cheung WM, et al: Induction of angiopoietin and Tie receptor mRNA expression after cerebral ischemia-reperfusion, *J Cereb Blood Flow Metab* 20:387–395, 2000.

189. Lin TN, Nian GM, Chen SF, et al: Induction of Tie-1 and Tie-2 receptor protein expression after cerebral ischemia-reperfusion, *J Cereb Blood Flow Metab* 21:690–701, 2001.

190. Ardelt AA, Anjum N, Rajneesh KF, et al: Estradiol augments peri-infarct cerebral vascular density in experimental stroke, *Exp Neurol* 206:95–100, 2007.

191. Puchowicz MA, Zechel JL, Valerio J, et al: Neuroprotection in diet-induced ketotic rat brain after focal ischemia, *J Cereb Blood Flow Metab* 28:1907–1916, 2008.

192. Puchowicz MA, Xu K, Sun X, et al: Diet-induced ketosis increases capillary density without altered blood flow in rat brain, *Am J Physiol Endocrinol Metab* 292:E1607–E1615, 2007.

193. Xu K, LaManna JC: Chronic hypoxia and the cerebral circulation, *J Appl Physiol* 100:725–730, 2006.

194. Dore-Duffy P, LaManna JC: Physiologic angiodynamics in the brain, *Antioxid Redox Signal* 9:1363–1371, 2007.

195. Dore-Duffy P, Balabanov R, Beaumont T, et al: The CNS pericyte response to low oxygen: Early synthesis of cyclopentenone prostaglandins of the J-series, *Microvasc Res* 69:79–88, 2005.

196. Dore-Duffy P, Owen C, Balabanov R, et al: Pericyte migration from the vascular wall in response to traumatic brain injury, *Microvasc Res* 60:55–69, 2000.

197. Díaz-Flores L, Gutierrez R, Varela H: Angiogenesis: An update, *Histol Histopathol* 9:807–843, 1994.

198. Nehls V, Schuchardt E, Drenckhahn D: The effect of fibroblasts, vascular smooth muscle cells, and pericytes on sprout formation of endothelial cells in a fibrin gel angiogenesis system, *Microvasc Res* 48:349–363, 1994.

199. Greenberg JI, Shields DJ, Barillas SG, et al: A role for VEGF as a negative regulator of pericyte function and vessel maturation, *Nature* 456:809–813, 2008.

200. Gibbons GH, Dzau VJ: The emerging concept of vascular remodeling, *N Engl J Med* 330:1431–1438, 1994.

201. Natte R, de Boer WI, Maat-Schieman ML, et al: Amyloid beta precursor protein-mRNA is expressed throughout cerebral vessel walls, *Brain Res* 828:179–183, 1999.

202. Stephenson DT, Rash K, Clemens JA: Amyloid precursor protein accumulates in regions of neurodegeneration following focal cerebral ischemia in the rat, *Brain Res* 593:128–135, 1992.

203. Kalaria RN, Bhatti SU, Lust WD, et al: The amyloid precursor protein in ischemic brain injury and chronic hypoperfusion, *Ann N Y Acad Sci* 695:190–193, 1993.

204. Kalaria RN, Bhatti SU, Palatinsky EA, et al: Accumulation of the beta amyloid precursor protein at sites of ischemic injury in rat brain, *Neuroreport* 4:211–214, 1993.

205. Lin B, Schmidt-Kastner R, Busto R, et al: Progressive parenchymal deposition of beta-amyloid precursor protein in rat brain following global cerebral ischemia, *Acta Neuropathol (Berlin)* 97:359–368, 1999.

206. Shi J, Panickar KS, Yang SH, et al: Estrogen attenuates over-expression of beta-amyloid precursor protein messenger RNA in an animal model of focal ischemia, *Brain Res* 810:87–92, 1998.

207. Dietrich WD, Kraydieh S, Prado R, et al: White matter alterations following thromboembolic stroke: A beta-amyloid precursor protein immunoctyochemical study in rats, *Acta Neuropathol (Berlin)* 95:524–531, 1998.

208. Yam PS, Takasago T, Dewar D, et al: Amyloid precursor protein accumulates in white matter at the margin of a focal ischaemic lesion, *Brain Res* 760:150–157, 1997.

209. Popa-Wagner A, Schroder E, Schmoll H, et al: Upregulation of MAP1B and MAP2 in the rat brain after middle cerebral artery occlusion: Effect of age, *J Cereb Blood Flow Metab* 19:425–434, 1999.

210. Kim HS, Lee SH, Kim SS, et al: Post-ischemic changes in the expression of Alzheimer's APP isoforms in rat cerebral cortex, *Neuroreport* 16:533–537, 1998.

211. Niwa K, Carlson GA, Iadecola C: Exogenous A beta 1-40 reproduces cerebrovascular alterations resulting from amyloid precursor protein overexpression in mice, *J Cereb Blood Flow Metab* 20:1659–1668, 2000.

212. Zhang F, Eckman C, Younkin S, et al: Increased susceptibility to ischemic brain damage in transgenic mice overexpressing the amyloid precursor protein, *J Neurosci* 17:7655–7661, 1997.

213. Winkler DT, Bondolfi L, Herzig MC, et al: Spontaneous hemorrhagic stroke in a mouse model of cerebral amyloid angiopathy, *J Neurosci* 21:1619–1627, 2001.

214. Vinters HV, Wang ZZ, Secor DL: Brain parenchymal and microvascular amyloid in Alzheimer's disease, *Brain Pathol* 6:179–195, 1996.

215. Herzig MC, Van Nostrand WE, Jucker M: Mechanism of cerebral beta-amyloid angiopathy: Murine and cellular models, *Brain Pathol* 16:40–54, 2006.

216. Brun A, Fredriksson K, Gustafson L: Pure subcortical atherosclerotic encephalopathy (Binswanger disease): A clinicopathological study, *Cerebrovasc Dis* 2:87–92, 1992.

217. Uspenskaia O, Liebetrau M, Herms J, et al: Aging is associated with increased collagen type IV accumulation in the basal lamina of human cerebral microvessels, *BMC Neurosci* 5:37, 2004.

218. Pico F, Labreuche J, Seilhean D, et al: Association of small-vessel disease with dilatative arteriopathy of the brain: Neuropathologic evidence, *Stroke* 38:1197–1202, 2007.

219. Wardlaw JM, Farrall A, Armitage PA, et al: Changes in background blood-brain barrier integrity between lacunar and cortical ischemic stroke subtypes, *Stroke* 39:1327–1332, 2008.

220. Gould DB, Phalan FC, van Mil SE, et al: Role of COL4A1 in small-vessel disease and hemorrhagic stroke, *N Engl J Med* 354: 1489–1496, 2006.

3 Mechanisms of Thrombosis and Thrombolysis

GREGORY J. DEL ZOPPO, MARY A. KALAFUT

The processes of thrombosis—thrombus growth, dissolution, and migration—are inextricably connected. Thrombus formation involves activation of platelets, activation of the coagulation system, and the processes of fibrin dissolution. The central feature of each of these contributions is the generation of thrombin. Thrombin, in turn, generates the fibrin network from circulating fibrinogen. Excess vascular fibrin formation or excess fibrin degradation can contribute to thrombus growth or hemorrhage, respectively. Plasminogen activators have been exploited to dissolve significant (symptomatic) thrombi; however, all substances that promote plasmin formation retain the potential to increase the risk of hemorrhage.

The use of plasminogen activators (PAs), when applied in the acute setting, has been associated with detectable clinical improvement in selected patients with symptoms of focal cerebral ischemia.[1-9] Thrombolysis has thus attained a place in the acute treatment of ischemic stroke. Currently, recombinant tissue-type plasminogen activator (rt-PA) is licensed in the United States, Japan, Europe, and many other countries for the treatment of ischemic stroke within 3 hours of onset.[6] Both early studies and a later phase III prospective trial suggest that extension of the treatment window is possible with strict limitations on patient selection.[3-5,9]

The development of agents that promote fibrin degradation in the clinical setting stems from observations in the 19th century of the spontaneous liquefaction of clotted blood and the dissolution of fibrin thrombi.[10] A growing understanding of plasma proteolytic digestion of fibrin paralleled inquiry into the mechanisms of streptococcal fibrinolysis.[11,12] Streptokinase was first employed to dissolve closed-space (intrapleural) fibrin clots,[13] but purified preparations were required for lysis of intravascular thrombi.[14] The development of PAs for therapeutic lysis of vascular thrombi has progressed along with insights into the mechanisms of thrombus formation and degradation.

Thrombus Formation

The relative platelet-fibrin composition of a specific thrombus depends on the vascular bed, the local development of fibrin, platelet activation, and regional blood flow or shear stress.[15] Pharmacologic inhibition of the platelet activation and coagulation processes can also alter thrombus composition and volume. At arterial flow rates thrombi are predominantly platelet rich, whereas at lower shear rates characteristic of venous flow, activation of coagulation seems to predominate. It has been suggested that the efficacy of pharmacologic thrombus lysis depends on (1) the relative fibrin content and (2) the extent of fibrin cross-linking, which may reflect thrombus age, and thrombus remodeling. The latter may vary with location within a vascular bed (e.g., arterial, capillary, or venular).[16,17]

Thrombin (factor IIa) is the central player in clot formation (Fig. 3-1). Thrombin, a serine protease, cleaves fibrinogen to generate fibrin, which forms the scaffolding for the growing thrombus.[18] Inter–fibrin strand cross-linking requires active factor XIII, a transglutaminase bound to fibrinogen that is itself activated by thrombin. Factor XIIIa stabilizes the fibrin network (Fig. 3-2).[19-21] Thrombin-mediated fibrin polymerization leads to the generation of fibrin I and fibrin II monomers and to the release of fibrinopeptide A (FPA) and fibrinopeptide B (FPB).

Platelet activation is required for thrombus formation under arterial flow conditions and accompanies thrombin-mediated fibrin formation. Platelet membrane receptors and phospholipids form a workbench for the generation of thrombin through both the intrinsic and extrinsic coagulation pathways.[22] Platelets promote activation of the early stages of intrinsic coagulation by a process that involves the factor XI receptor and high-molecular-weight kininogen (HMWK) (see Fig. 3-1).[23] Also, factors V and VIII interact with specific platelet membrane phospholipids (receptors) to facilitate the activation of factor X to Xa (the "tenase complex") and the conversion of prothrombin to thrombin (the "prothrombinase complex") on the platelet surface.[24] Platelet-bound thrombin-modified factor V (factor Va) serves as a high-affinity platelet receptor for factor Xa.[25] These mechanisms accelerate the rate of thrombin generation, further catalyzing fibrin formation and the fibrin network.

This process also leads to the conversion of plasminogen to plasmin and to the activation of *endogenous* fibrinolysis. Thrombin provides one direct connection between thrombus formation and plasmin generation, through the localized release of tissue-type plasminogen activator (t-PA) and single-chain urokinase (scu-PA) from endothelial cells. Active thrombin has been shown in vitro and in vivo to markedly stimulate t-PA release from endothelial stores.[25-27] In one experiment, infusion of factor

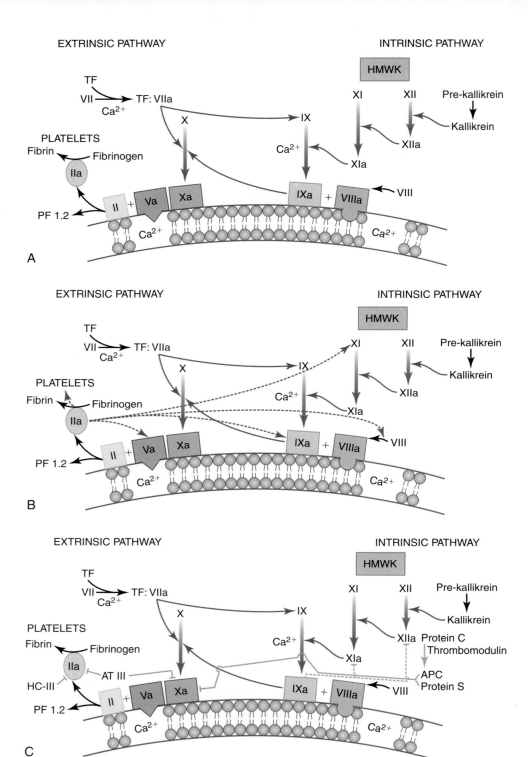

Figure 3-1 Intrinsic and extrinsic coagulation pathways (see text). Phospholipid-containing membranes (e.g., platelets) provide the scaffold for acceleration of coagulation pathway activation. Both intrinsic and extrinsic pathways lead to prothrombin (factor II) activation, with fibrin generation from circulating fibrinogen. The extrinsic pathway initiates coagulation through the interaction of factor VII with tissue factor (TF) in the vascular adventitia, in brain perivascular parenchyma, and on activated monocytes. The TF:VIIa complex catalyzes activation of factor X and acceleration of thrombin generation. The intrinsic system involves activation of components within the vascular lumen. Initiation of coagulation through this pathway involves pre-kallikrein, kallikrein, high-molecular-weight kininogen (HMWK), and factors XI and XII. A, Thrombin generation. The intrinsic system activates factor X through the "tenase" complex (factors VIIIa and IXa, and Ca^{2+} on phospholipid). Both intrinsic and extrinsic pathways activate prothrombin through the common "prothrombinase" complex (factors Xa and Va, and Ca^{2+}). The platelet surface has receptors for factors Va and VIIIa. Cleavage of prothrombin generates the prothrombin fragment 1.2 (PF 1.2) and thrombin (factor IIa). B, Thrombin has multiple stimulatory positive feedback effects. It catalyzes activation of factors XI and VIII as well as the activities of the tenase and prothrombinase complexes. Thrombin also stimulates activation of platelets and granule secretion via specific thrombin receptors on their surfaces. C, Coagulation activation is regulated by interleaving inhibitor pathways. The effects of factors Va, Xa, and VIIIa are modulated by the protein C pathway. Activated protein C (APC), generated by the action of the endothelial cell receptor thrombomodulin on protein C, along with its cofactor, protein S, inhibits the action of factor V. AT III, antithrombin-III; HC-III, heparin cofactor-III.

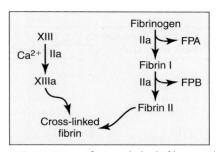

Figure 3-2 Generation of cross-linked fibrin. Fibrinogen is cleaved successively to form fibrin I and fibrin II by thrombin (factor IIa) with the release of fibrinopeptides A and B (FPA and FPB). Thrombin activates factor XIII to the active transglutaminase, which promotes cross-linking of fibrin and stabilization of the growing thrombus.

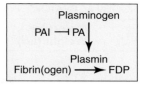

Figure 3-3 Plasminogen activation and fibrin(ogen)olysis. Degradation of fibrinogen and fibrin is catalyzed by plasmin. Plasminogen activators (PAs), including tissue-type PA (t-PA), urokinase-type PA (u-PA), and novel constructs, cleave plasminogen to the active plasmin. Characteristic products of fibrin and fibrinogen degradation (FDP) are generated (see text). PAI, plasminogen activator inhibitor.

Xa and phospholipid into nonhuman primates resulted in a pronounced increase in circulating t-PA activity, suggesting that significant vascular stores of this PA can be released by active components of coagulation.[28] Other vascular and cellular stimuli also augment PA release (see later), thereby pushing the hemostatic balance toward thrombolysis.

Development of arterial or venous thrombi requires abrogation of the constitutive antithrombotic characteristics of endothelial cells.[29] In addition to both the antithrombotic properties of the endothelial cell and the circulating anticoagulants and their cofactors (i.e., activated protein C, protein S), thrombus growth is limited by the *endogenous* thrombolytic system. Thrombus organization (or remodeling) results from the preferential conversion of plasminogen to plasmin on the thrombus surface. There, fibrin binds t-PA in proximity to its substrate (fibrin-bound) plasminogen, thereby accelerating local plasmin formation. In concert with local shear stress, these processes may also promote embolization into the downstream cerebral vasculature.[30] However, little is known about the endogenous generation and secretion of PAs within cerebral vessels.[31] *Exogenous* application of pharmacologic doses of PAs can accelerate conversion of thrombus-bound plasminogen to plasmin and thereby prevent thrombus formation and promote thrombus dissolution. This is discussed later.

Fibrinolysis

Plasmin formation is central to the lysis of vascular thrombi. The endogenous fibrinolytic system comprises plasminogen, scu-PA, urokinase (u-PA), and t-PA, and their inhibitors. Hence, plasmin degrades fibrin (and fibrinogen). Plasminogen, its activators, and their inhibitors contribute to the balance between vascular thrombosis and hemorrhage (Fig. 3-3; Tables 3-1 and 3-2).

Plasmin formation occurs (1) in the plasma, where it can cleave circulating fibrinogen and fibrin into soluble products,[17,32] and (2) on reactive surfaces (e.g., thrombi or cells). The fibrin network provides the scaffold for plasminogen activation, whereas various cells, including polymorphonuclear (PMN) leukocytes, platelets, and endothelial cells, express receptors for plasminogen to bind.[32] Specific cellular receptors concentrate

plasminogen and specific activators (e.g., urokinase-type plasminogen activator [u-PA]) on the cell surface, thereby enhancing local plasmin production. Similar receptors on tumor cells (e.g., the urokinase plasminogen activator receptor [u-PAR], which concentrates u-PA) also facilitate dissolution of basement membranes and matrix, promoting metastases. Both u-PA and the urokinase plasminogen activator receptor are expressed by microvessels and neurons in the ischemic bed.[33,34] Plasmin can also cleave various basal lamina and extracellular matrix (ECM) ligands (e.g., laminins, type IV collagen, perlecan) found in the basal lamina of microvessels of the central nervous system (CNS), and in other organs.[35-37]

Plasminogen

The naturally circulating PAs, single-chain t-PA and scu-PA (also known as pro-UK), catalyze plasmin formation.[38-42] Plasmin derives from the zymogen plasminogen, a glycosylated, single-chain, 92-kd serine protease.[43,44] Structurally, plasminogen contains five kringles and a protease domain, two of which (K1 and K5) mediate the binding of plasminogen to fibrin through characteristic lysine-binding sites (Fig. 3-4).[43,45,46] Glu-plasminogen has an NH_2-terminal glutamic acid, and lys-plasminogen, which lacks an 8-kd peptide, has an NH_2-terminal lysine. Plasmin cleavage of the NH_2-terminal fragment of glu-plasminogen generates lys-plasminogen.[47,48] Glu-plasminogen has a plasma clearance half-life ($t_{1/2}$) of about 2.2 days, whereas that of lys-plasminogen is 0.8 days.[14] Both t-PA and u-PA catalyze the conversion of glu-plasminogen to lys-plasmin through either of two intermediates, glu-plasmin or lys-plasminogen.[49] The lysine-binding sites of plasminogen mediate the binding of plasminogen to α_2-antiplasmin, thrombospondin, components of the vascular extracellular matrix, and histidine-rich glycoprotein (HRG).[44] α_2-Antiplasmin prevents binding of plasminogen to fibrin by this mechanism.[49] Partial degradation of the fibrin network enhances the binding of glu-plasminogen to fibrin, promoting further local fibrinolysis.

Plasminogen Activation

Plasminogen activation is tied to activation of the coagulation system and can involve secretion of physiologic PAs (extrinsic activation). It has been suggested that kallikrein, factor XIa, and factor XIIa, in the presence of

TABLE 3-1 PLASMINOGEN ACTIVATORS

Plasminogen Activators	Molecular Weight (kd)	Chains	Plasma Concentration (mg/dL)	Plasma Concentration Half-Life (t$_{1/2}$)	Substrates
Endogenous					
Plasminogen	92	2	20	2.2 days	(Fibrin)
Tissue-type PA (t-PA)	68 (59)	1→2	5×10^{-4}	5-8 min	Fibrin/plasminogen
Single-chain urokinase-type PA (scu-PA)	54 (46)	1→2	$2-20 \times 10^{-4}$	8 min	Fibrin/plasmin(ogen)
Urokinase-type PA (u-PA)	54 (46)	2	8×10^{-4}	9-12 min	Plasminogen
Exogenous					
Streptokinase	47	1	0	41 and 30 min	Plasminogen, fibrin(ogen)
Anisoylated plasminogen-streptokinase activator complex (APSAC)	131	Complex	0	70-90 min	Fibrin(ogen)
Staphylokinase	16.5		0		Plasminogen

TABLE 3-2 PLASMIN AND PLASMINOGEN ACTIVATOR INHIBITORS

Inhibitor	Molecular Weight (kd)	Chains	Plasma Concentration (mg/dL^{-1})	Plasma Concentration Half-Life (t$_{1/2}$)	Inhibitor Substrates
Plasmin inhibitors					
α_2-Antiplasmin	65	1	7	3.3 min	Plasmin
α_2-Macroglobulin	740	4	250		Plasmin (excess)
Plasminogen activator inhibitors (PAIs)					
PAI-1	48-52	1	5×10^{-2}	7 min	t-PA, u-PA
PAI-2	47, 70	1	$<5 \times 10^{-4}$	24 hr	t-PA, u-PA
PAI-3	50				u-PA, t-PA

t-PA, tissue-type plasminogen activator; u-PA, urokinase-type plasminogen activator.

HMWK, can directly activate plasminogen.[49,50] Several lines of evidence suggest that scu-PA activates plasminogen under physiologic conditions.[51-53] Tissue-type PA, which is secreted from the endothelium and other cellular sources, appears to be the primary PA in the vasculature.[14] Thrombin, generated by either intrinsic or extrinsic coagulation, stimulates secretion of t-PA from endothelial stores.[25,54,55]

Several serine proteases can convert plasminogen to plasmin by cleaving the arg[560]-val[561] bond.[43,56,57] Serine proteases have common structural features, including an NH$_2$-terminal "A" chain with substrate-binding affinity, a COOH-terminal "B" chain with the active site, and intrachain disulfide bridges. Plasminogen-cleaving serine proteases include the coagulation proteins factor IX, factor X, and prothrombin (factor II), protein C, chymotrypsin and trypsin, various leukocyte elastases, the plasminogen activators u-PA and t-PA, and plasmin itself.[43] Activation of plasminogen by t-PA is accelerated in a ternary complex with fibrin.[58,59] In the circulation, plasmin binds rapidly to the inhibitor α_2-antiplasmin and is thereby inactivated. Activation of thrombus-bound plasminogen also protects plasmin from the inhibitors α_2-antiplasmin and α_2-macroglobulin.[43] Here, the lysine-binding sites and the catalytic site of plasmin are occupied by fibrin, thereby blocking its interaction with α_2-antiplasmin.[43,59] Furthermore, fibrin and fibrin-bound plasminogen render t-PA relatively inaccessible to inhibition by other circulating plasma inhibitors.[60]

Thrombus Dissolution

Fibrinolysis occurs predominantly within the thrombus and at its surface but may be augmented by contributions from local blood flow.[61-64] During thrombus consolidation, plasminogen bound to fibrin and to platelets allows local release of plasmin.[65] In the *circulation*, plasmin cleaves the fibrinogen Aα chain appendage, generating fragment X (DED), Aα fragments, and Bβ 1-42. Further cleavage of fragment X leads to the generation of fragments DE, D, and E. By contrast, degradation of the fibrin network generates YY/DXD, YD/DY, and the unique DD/E (fragment X = DED and fragment Y = DE).[17,61,66] Cross-linkage of DD with fragment E is vulnerable to further cleavage, producing D-dimer fragments. The measurement of D-dimer levels has clinical utility, in that the absence of circulating D-dimer correlates with the absence of massive thrombosis.[67] Ordinarily, in the setting of focal cerebral ischemia, the thrombus load is small and the meaning of D-dimer elevations uncertain. The generation of the degradation products has the following two consequences: (1) Incorporation of some of these products into the forming thrombus destabilizes the fibrin network and (2) reduced circulating

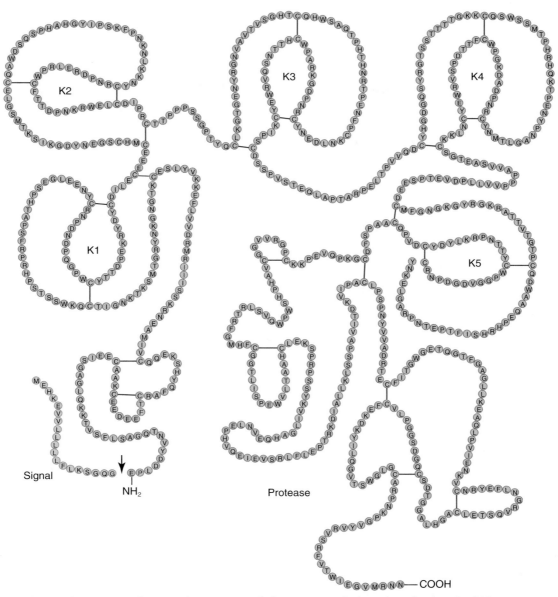

Figure 3-4 The secondary structure of plasminogen, which contains five kringles (Ks).

fibrinogen and the generation of breakdown products of fibrin(ogen) limit the protection from hemorrhage by hemostatic thrombi.

Plasminogen Activators

All fibrinolytic agents are obligate plasminogen activators (see Table 3-1). Tissue-type PA, scu-PA, and u-PA are *endogenous* plasminogen activators involved in physiologic fibrinolysis. Recombinant t-PA, scu-PA, and u-PA, as well as streptokinase (SK), acylated plasminogen streptokinase activator complex (APSAC), staphylokinase, PAs from *Desmodus* species, and other newer novel agents in clinical use (e.g., reteplase [r-PA] and tenecteplase [TNK-t-PA]), are termed *exogenous* plasminogen activators.[62-64] Tissue-type PA, scu-PA, and a number of novel agents have relative fibrin and thrombus specificity.[41,67]

Endogenous Plasminogen Activators

Tissue-Type Plasminogen Activator

Tissue-type PA is a 70-kd, single-chain glycosylated serine protease that has four distinct domains—a finger (F-) domain, an epidermal growth factor (EGF) domain (residues 50-87), two kringle regions (K1 and K2), and a serine protease domain (Fig. 3-5).[56,68,69] The COOH-terminal serine protease domain contains the active site for plasminogen cleavage, and the finger and K_2 domains are responsible for fibrin affinity.[41,69,70] The two kringle domains are homologous to the kringle regions of plasminogen.

The single-chain form is converted to the two-chain form by plasmin cleavage of the arg[275]-isoleu[276] bond. Both single-chain and two-chain species are enzymatically active and have relatively fibrin-selective

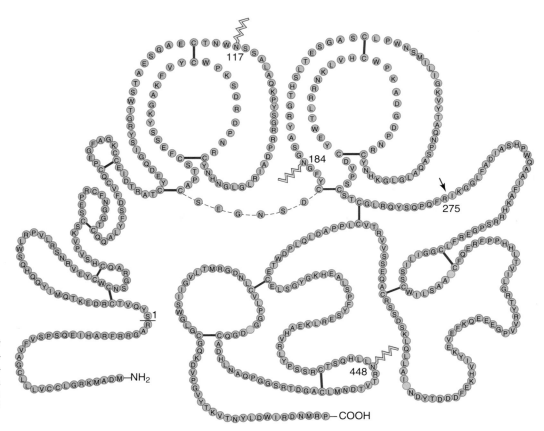

Figure 3-5 The secondary structure of tissue-type plasminogen activator (t-PA). Conversion of single-chain t-PA to two-chain t-PA by plasmin occurs at the arg[275]-isoleu[276] bond (arrow).

properties. Infusion studies in humans indicate that both single-chain t-PA and two-chain t-PA have circulating plasma $t_{1/2}$ values of 3 to 8 minutes,[41] although the biologic $t_{1/2}$ values are longer. Tissue-type PA is considered to be fibrin selective because of its favorable binding constant for fibrin-bound plasminogen and its activation of plasminogen in association with fibrin.[41,68] Significant inactivation of circulating factors V and VIII does not occur with infused rt-PA, and an anticoagulant state is generally not produced.[41] However, if sufficiently high dose rates are employed, clinically measurable fibrinogenolysis and plasminogen consumption can be produced.

Secretion of t-PA from cultured endothelial cells is stimulated by thrombin,[54,55,71] activated protein C (APC),[72] histamine,[54] phorbol myristate esterase, and other mediators.[73-77] Physical exercise and certain vasoactive substances produce measurable increases in circulating t-PA levels, and 1-deamino(8-D-arginine) vasopressin (DDAVP) may produce a threefold to fourfold increase in t-PA antigen levels within 60 minutes of parenteral infusion in some patients.[78-80] Both t-PA and u-PA have been reported to be secreted by endothelial cells, neurons, astrocytes, and microglia in vivo and in vitro.[31,81-88] The reasons for this broad cell expression are not known, however.

Urokinase-Type Plasminogen Activator

Single-chain urokinase-type PA is a 54-kd glycoprotein synthesized by endothelial and renal cells as well as by certain malignant cells (Fig. 3-6).[32] This single-chain proenzyme of u-PA is unusual in that it has fibrin-selective plasmin-generating activity[89,90] and has also been synthesized by recombinant techniques.[41,91]

The relationship of scu-PA to u-PA is complex: Cleavage or removal of lys[158] from scu-PA by plasmin produces 54-kd, two-chain u-PA. This PA consists of an A chain (157 residues) and a glycosylated B chain (253 residues), which are linked by the disulfide bridge between cys[148] and cys[279]. Further cleavages at lys[135] and arg[156] produce low-molecular-weight (31-kd) u-PA.[69] Both high- and low-molecular-weight species are enzymatically active.

The 54-kd urokinase (u-PA) activates plasminogen by first-order kinetics.[62,91] The two forms of u-PA exhibit measurable fibrinolytic and fibrinogenolytic activities in vitro and in vivo and have plasma $t_{1/2}$ values of 9 to 12 minutes.[92,93] When infused as an *exogenous* therapeutic agent, u-PA leads to plasminogen consumption and inactivation of factors II (prothrombin), V, and VIII. The latter changes constitute the systemic lytic state.

It has been postulated that t-PA is primarily involved in the maintenance of hemostasis through the dissolution of fibrin, whereas u-PA is involved in generating pericellular proteolytic activity by cells expressing the u-PA receptor, which are needed for degradation of the extracellular matrix for migration. The roles of these two PAs in CNS cell function are not yet fully understood.

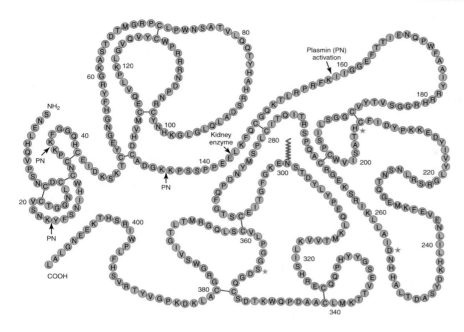

Figure 3-6 The secondary structure of single-chain urokinase-type plasminogen activator (scu-PA; 54 kd). Activation by plasmin (PN) takes place at the 158-159 bond (*arrow*). The *zigzag line* represents the glycosylation site.

Exogenous Plasminogen Activators

Streptokinase

Streptokinase is a 47-kd, single-chain polypeptide derived from group C β-hemolytic streptococci.[94] The active [SK-plasminogen] complex converts circulating plasminogen directly to plasmin and undergoes further activation to form SK-plasmin. The SK-plasminogen, SK-plasmin, and plasmin species circulate together.[95] The SK-plasmin complex (not bound by the inhibitor α₂-antiplasmin), and free circulating plasmin degrade both fibrinogen and fibrin and inactivate prothrombin, factor V, and factor VIII.[65] The kinetics of SK elimination are complex. Antistreptococcal antibodies formed from antecedent infections neutralize infused SK and arise maximally by 4 to 7 days after initiation of an SK infusion. Therefore, the doses of SK required to achieve steady-state plasminogen activation must be individualized. Plasminogen depletion through conversion to plasmin and by as yet poorly understood clearance mechanisms for the SK-plasminogen complex can lead to hypoplasminogenemia. Generation of plasmin is limited at both low and high SK infusion dose rates because of inadequate plasminogen conversion and depletion of plasminogen, respectively.

APSAC (e.g., anistreplase) is an artificial activator construct consisting of plasminogen and SK bound noncovalently. Fibrin selectivity relies on the fibrin-attachment properties of the plasminogen kringles.[41] The activity of APSAC depends on the deacylation rate of the acyl-plasminogen component. Hydrolytic activation of the acyl-protected active site of plasminogen allows plasmin formation by SK within the complex in the presence of fibrin. From those observations and on the basis of the terminal $t_{1/2}$ of SK and the $t_{1/2}$ for APSAC deacylation, APSAC has a longer circulation time than streptokinase.[96,97] However, despite these clinically favorable characteristics APSAC has not found a place in the treatment of vascular thrombosis.

Staphylokinase

Staphylokinase (STK) is a 16.5-kd polypeptide derived from certain strains of *Staphylococcus aureus*.[97-99] It combines stoichiometrically (1:1) with plasminogen to form an irreversible complex that activates free plasminogen. The binding of staphylokinase to plasmin has been worked out in detail.[97,99,100] Recombinant staphylokinase has been prepared from the known gene nucleotide sequence, has been tested in the setting of acute myocardial infarction, and has undergone preliminary testing in the setting of ischemic stroke.

Plasminogen Activators Derived from Desmodus rotundus

Recombinant PAs identical to those derived from the saliva of *Desmodus* species are fibrin dependent. The α form of *Desmodus* salivary PA (DSPA-α; desmoteplase) and vampire bat salivary plasminogen activator (bat-PA) are more fibrin-dependent than t-PA and may be superior to t-PA in terms of sustained recanalization without fibrinogenolysis.[101-105] The plasma $t_{1/2}$ of desmoteplase is significantly longer than that of rt-PA.[101] A program of studies of desmoteplase as acute treatment for ischemic stroke has so far failed to demonstrate improved outcomes in patients.[106,107] Significant issues in trial design are under discussion, and a phase III study is under way.

Novel Plasminogen Activators

Efforts to alter the stability and thrombus selectivity of endogenous PAs have led to a lengthening list of possible pharmacologic agents. Point and deletion mutations in t-PA and u-PA have provided molecules with unique specificities.[108,109] For instance, t-PA sequences lacking the K1 and K2 domains possess fibrin specificity, normal specific activity, but reduced inhibition by PA inhibitor-1 (PAI-1).[70] In theory, the increased fibrin selectivity might provide greater thrombolytic effect; however, in studies of the use of this agent in coronary artery thromboses, significant advantages were not evident.

For the clinical target of myocardial ischemia, several t-PA mutants with prolonged $t_{1/2}$ and delayed clearance have been devised that may have benefit when infused as a single bolus.[110-112] Reteplase, a nonglycosylated PA consisting of the K2 and protease domains of t-PA, has a 4.5- to 12.3-fold longer $t_{1/2}$ owing in part to lower affinity for the hepatic cell t-PA receptor.[112,113] It also possesses lower fibrin selectivity. Tenecteplase (TNK-t-PA) differs from t-PA at three mutation sites (T103N, N117Q, and KHRR[296-299]AAAA), thereby altering two glycosylation sites and increasing fibrin selectivity. The changes also result in decreased clearance and prolonged $t_{1/2}$.[114,115] Another t-PA mutant with greater $t_{1/2}$, lanoteplase (n-PA), derives from deletion of the fibronectin finger and epidermal growth factor domains and mutation of asn[117] to gln[117].[110,111] In addition to enhanced fibrin selectivity, TNK has relative resistance to inhibition by PAI-1.[116] A t-PA-like construct with moderate fibrin selectivity is monteplase (E6010).[117] This molecule differs from t-PA in the location and organization of disulfide bridges and the complexity of glycosylation. In contrast, the fibrin selectivity and specific activity of pamiteplase (YM866) are nearly identical to those of t-PA, but pamiteplase has a longer $t_{1/2}$.[118,119] These mutants have been developed for bolus infusion application in the setting of myocardial infarction (MI). Application of TNK to clinical ischemic stroke has been formally tested in a small trial[120] based on limited experimental studies; but clinical testing in ischemic stroke has been suspended as of this writing. What advantage delayed clearance or prolonged $t_{1/2}$ may have in acute application in ischemic stroke is yet to be demonstrated.[121] Dose-adjustment studies in patients with stroke have not been reported. One unproven concern with long $t_{1/2}$ molecules is that they may augment the intercerebral hemorrhage risk in the setting of ischemic stroke.

A similar situation obtains for other novel PA constructs. These have included single-site mutants and variants of rt-PA and recombinant scu-PA, t-PA/scu-PA and t-PA/u-PA chimerae, u-PA/antifibrin monoclonal antibodies, u-PA/antiplatelet monoclonal antibodies, bifunctional antibody conjugates, and scu-PA deletion mutants.[122-126]

Regulation of Endogenous Fibrinolysis

Endogenous fibrinolysis is modulated by several families of inhibitors of plasmin and of the PAs.

In the circulation, α_2-antiplasmin is the primary inhibitor of fibrinolysis, inhibiting plasmin directly. Excess plasmin is inactivated by α_2-macroglobulin. The potential risk of vascular thrombosis then depends on the balance between plasminogen activation and plasmin activity and their respective inhibitors in the circulation. Thrombospondin interferes with fibrin-associated plasminogen activation by t-PA.[127] Inhibitors of the contact activation system and complement (C1 inhibitor) have an indirect effect on fibrinolysis. Histidine-rich glycoprotein is a competitive inhibitor of plasminogen. Generally, though, these physiologic modulators of plasmin activity are overwhelmed by pharmacologic concentrations of PAs.

For streptokinase, APSAC, and staphylokinase, circulating neutralizing antibodies appear that directly inhibit their activation of plasminogen.

α_2-Antiplasmin and α_2-Macroglobulin

Circulating plasmin generated in the plasma during fibrinolysis is bound by α_2-antiplasmin. The two forms of α_2-antiplasmin are (1) the native form, which binds plasminogen, and (2) a second form that cannot bind plasminogen.[128] Ordinarily, α_2-antiplasmin is found in either plasminogen-bound or free circulating form.[129] Fibrin-bound plasmin is protected because of its interaction with fibrin and because α_2-antiplasmin is already occupied. Excess free plasmin is bound by α_2-macroglobulin. α_2-Macroglobulin is a relatively nonspecific inhibitor of fibrinolysis that inactivates plasmin, kallikrein, t-PA, and u-PA.[129]

Inhibitors of Plasminogen Activators and Fibrinolysis

PAIs also reduce the activities of t-PA, scu-PA, and u-PA by binding directly to their substrates (see Table 3-2).

PAI-1 specifically inhibits both plasma t-PA and u-PA. PAI-1 is derived from both endothelial cell and platelet sources.[130-132] Several lines of evidence indicate that the K2 domain of t-PA is responsible for the interaction between t-PA and PAI-1 and that this interaction is altered by the presence of fibrin.[133] PAI-1 is also an acute-phase reactant,[134] and deep venous thrombosis, septicemia, and type II diabetes mellitus, for instance, are associated with elevated plasma PAI-1 values.

PAI-2, which is found in a 70-kd form and a 47-kd low-molecular-weight form, has a lower inhibition constant (K_i) for u-PA and two-chain t-PA. PAI-2 is derived from placental tissue, granulocytes, monocytes/macrophages, and histiocytes.[135,136] This inhibitor probably plays little role in the physiologic antagonism of t-PA and is most important in the uteroplacental circulation.[137] The kinetics of PA inhibition by PAI-2 differs from those for PAI-1.

PAI-3 is a serine protease inhibitor of u-PA, t-PA, and activated protein C found in plasma and urine.[138,139]

Thrombin-activable fibrinolysis inhibitor (TAFI) is an endogenous inhibitor of glu-plasminogen and, therefore, fibrinolysis.[139] This inhibitor is a precursor of plasma carboxypeptidase B and, when activated by thrombin in the plasma, produces an antifibrinolytic effect.

Impact of Plasmin Generation on Microvascular Integrity

Plasminogen generation is confined to discrete regions of the CNS.[140] Early during focal ischemia, activators of plasminogen are expressed by microvessels and adjacent neurons (e.g., u-PA[34]); however, there is little evidence yet that plasmin activity *per se* is generated in the ischemic territory. The loss of basal lamina components and density is compatible with its action.[37,141] In addition, evidence of local plasminogen activation has been shown by in situ zymography.[142,143] Proteolytic fragments of matrix constituents (e.g., laminin) have been associated with enhanced excitotoxicity in the CNS in experimental settings[144] but have yet to be evaluated in postischemic states. A role for t-PA, even though it is not overtly upregulated in nonhuman primate ischemia,[34] has been implicated in neuron survival and injury.[145]

Consequences of Therapeutic Plasminogen Activation

Plasminogen activators given at pharmacologic doses significantly alter hemostasis. Urokinase-type PA, SK, and occasionally t-PA produce systemically detectable fibrinogen degradation, measured by a fall in fibrinogen concentration, and a reduction in circulating plasminogen and α_2-antiplasmin (through binding of the plasmin generated). Both u-PA and SK inactivate factors V and VIII, which contribute to the "systemic lytic state" or "anticoagulant state."[146] Fragments of fibrin(ogen) interfere with fibrin multimerization and contribute to thrombus destabilization, whereas the circulating fragments, hypofibrinogenemia, and factor depletion produce a transient anticoagulant state that limits thrombus formation and extension. The clinical consequences of u-PA or SK infusion include a progressive decrease or depletion of circulating plasminogen and fibrinogen, prolongation of the activated partial thromboplastin time due to significant fibrinogen reduction, and inactivation of factors V and VIII.

Platelet function can also be affected. Clinical studies of rt-PA have demonstrated prolongation of standardized template bleeding times.[147] In experimental systems, infusion of rt-PA produces greater hemorrhage.[148,149] Furthermore, t-PA is known to cause disaggregation of human platelets through selective proteolysis of intraplatelet fibrin, which is inhibitable by α_2-antiplasmin.[150] Lys-plasminogen and glu-plasminogen can potentiate the platelet disaggregatory effect of rt-PA.[151] It is likely that the risk of intracerebral hemorrhage that attends PA infusion involves disruption of sustained platelet aggregation and lysis of fibrin formed at the site of vascular injury.

Limitations on the Clinical Use of Fibrinolytic Agents

The clinical setting in which PAs are used is an important and relevant variable for both their efficacy and the reduction of hemorrhage risk. Intracerebral hemorrhage is a known risk of the clinical use of PAs. The use of fibrinolytic agents in pharmacologic doses in the acute setting of ischemic stroke must conform to the original report,[6] as confirmed subsequently.[152] An abbreviated summary of the strict contraindications to the use of fibrinolytic agents is as follows: (1) a history of previous intracranial hemorrhage, (2) septic embolism, (3) malignant hypertension or sustained diastolic or systolic blood pressure in excess of 180 mm Hg sysolic/110 mm Hg diastolic, (4) conditions consistent with ongoing parenchymal hemorrhage

(e.g., gastrointestinal source), (5) pregnancy or parturition, (6) a history of recent trauma or surgery, and (7) known acquired (e.g., from anticoagulant use) and inherited hemorrhagic diatheses. These contraindications currently apply to the use of rt-PA in selected patients with ischemic stroke less than 3 hours after symptom onset as well as other approved clinical indications for the use of rt-PA, u-PA, or SK.

Plasminogen Activators in Cerebral Tissue

Although current clinical interests focus on the use of PAs as therapeutic agents for vascular reperfusion, cerebral tissue also generates and uses PAs. PA activity has been associated with brain tissue development, vascular remodeling, cell migration, neuron viability, tumor development, and vascular invasion in the CNS. In normal cerebral tissue, t-PA antigen is associated with microvessels similar in size to those of the vasa vasorum of the aorta.[30] Expression of PA activity has been reported in nonischemic tissues of mice, spontaneously hypertensive and Wistar-Kyoto rats, and primates.[153,154] Tissue-type PA and u-PA are secreted by endothelial cells, neurons, astrocytes, and microglia in vivo or in vitro.[81-88] Urokinase-type PA messenger RNA is expressed in neurons and oligodendrocytes during process outgrowth in the rodent brain.[140] Although t-PA is expressed by neurons in many brain regions, extracellular proteolysis seems confined to specific, discrete brain regions. Studies suggesting that t-PA mediates hippocampal neurodegeneration during excitotoxicity or following focal cerebral ischemia[155] have opened a discussion about whether PAs play roles in cellular viability outside the fibrinolytic system.[155] Conflicting evidence of greater injury by t-PA in the hippocampus has been balanced against credible reports of no effect or of infarct volume reduction in rodent models of focal cerebral ischemia (see later).[155,156]

Plasminogen Activators in Experimental Cerebral Ischemia

A limited number of experimental studies have tested the ability of PAs to increase arterial recanalization. Improved clinical (behavioral and/or neurologic) outcomes have been reported in rodent models of focal cerebral ischemia treated with PAs (mostly rt-PA) very soon after thromboembolism.[157-160] Early infusion of rt-PA in a rabbit multiple-thromboembolism model demonstrated significant improvement in clinical outcome in comparison with untreated controls.[156] The use of rt-PA with putative inhibitors of polymorphonuclear leukocyte adhesion supports this notion, although differences among rt-PA cohorts were observed in various experimental sets.[160-162] In an rt-PA dose-rate study in a nonembolic nonhuman primate model of stroke, no significant difference in neurologic outcome (motor-weighted) from that in controls was observed.[163,164] However, another study demonstrated a significant reduction in infarction volume after reperfusion of the middle cerebral artery (MCA) territory in a single model.[165]

Focal cerebral ischemia rapidly increases the endogenous expression of u-PA and PAI-1 within striatal tissue of the primate.[34,166] Endogenous t-PA decreases transiently as it binds PAI-1 but otherwise does not change. Urokinase-type PA is an indirect activator of pro-matrix metalloproteinase-2, which is also generated early after middle cerebral artery occlusion.[33] The appearance of these proteases coincides with degradation of the extracellular matrix of the ischemic microvascular bed.[33,34,37,167,168] It has been postulated that loss of basal lamina integrity contributes to hemorrhagic transformation of the evolving infarction.[37,167] Whether exogenous PAs contribute to the loss in microvessel integrity is under study.

Plasminogen Activators and Recanalization in Ischemic Stroke

Experimental and clinical studies indicate that timely restoration of blood flow to the ischemic cerebral parenchyma is required for improved clinical outcome. The substrate and condition requirements of plasminogen activators have supported their potential use in cerebrovascular ischemia. Angiographic studies have provided valuable information about the anatomy of the vasculature, the magnitude of thrombus burden, and the success of recanalization with PAs.[3,169-173] Urokinase-type PA and rt-PA appear to contribute to arterial reperfusion, as anticipated from their known activities (Table 3-3).

The frequency of arterial recanalization appears to be greater when the PA is administered intraarterially than intravenously (see Table 3-3). That observation is consistent with the notion that enhanced efficacy may be due to the higher local concentration of the PA at the thrombus surface.

Only a handful of studies have prospectively compared recanalization rates in PA-treated patients with a control group.[4,169,174,175] In those studies, recanalization was significantly greater in patients receiving the PA for angiographically proven occlusion of the middle cerebral artery than in the control group. In a phase II study of recombinant scu-PA (pro-UK), the recanalization frequency was significantly improved by the co-administration of a heparin dose,[169] and was confirmed in a follow-on open phase III study.[174] Many, but not all, subjects in those studies in whom early recanalization was documented experienced clinical improvement. Lack of clinical improvement despite recanalization may be influenced by poor collateralization or increased time to reperfusion, although this issue is unproven.

Mechanical disruption with either catheter-type devices or ultrasonography has been employed to enhance recanalization in limited clinical series. High ultrasound frequencies have been shown to alter the properties of the fibrin network to increase transport of rt-PA into the structure,[176] thrombus penetration,[177] rt-PA binding to fibrin,[178] and flow through fibrin gel in in vitro systems.[176] Fibrin disaggregation can also occur.[179] It has been postulated that such high frequencies would also cause injury to the brain parenchyma and to the vessel wall structure.[180]

Plasminogen Activators and Cerebral Hemorrhage

Administration of PAs in the acute period can be complicated by the development of symptomatic parenchymal hemorrhage. A number of randomized studies have documented the greater risk of symptomatic hemorrhagic transformation associated with intravenous infusion of plasminogen activators.[6-8,181] Rates of

TABLE 3-3 PLASMINOGEN ACTIVATORS IN ACUTE ISCHEMIC STROKE: CAROTID TERRITORY

Study	Year	Agent	Patients (n)	Δ (T–0)* (hr)	Recanalization (%)	Total Hemorrhage (%)	Symptomatic Hemorrhage (%)
Intraarterial delivery							
del Zoppo et al[1]	1988	SK/u-PA	20	<24	90.0	20.0	0.0
Mori et al[2]	1988	u-PA	22	<7	45.5	18.2	9.1
Matsumoto et al[189]	1991	u-PA	39	<24	59.0	33.3	—
del Zoppo et al (PROACT)[169]	1997	scu-PA/h	26	<6	57.7	42.3	15.4
		C/h	14	<6	14.3	7.1	7.1
Gönner et al[190]	1998	u-PA	33	<6	58.0	21.2	6.1
Furlan et al (PROACT II)[174]	1999	scu-PA/h	121	<6	65.7	35.2	10.2
		—/h (IV)	59	<6	18.0	13.0	1.8
Intravenous delivery							
Yamaguchi[191]	1991	rt-PA	58	<6	43.1	20.7	—
del Zoppo et al[3]	1992	rt-PA	93 (104)†	<8	34.4	30.8	9.6
Mori et al[4]	1992	rt-PA	19	<6	47.4	52.6	—
		C	12		16.7	41.7	—
von Kummer and Hacke[192]	1992	rt-PA	32	<6	53.1	37.5	9.4
Yamaguchi et al[5]	1993	rt-PA	47 (51)	<6	21.3	47.1	7.8
		C	46 (47)		4.4	46.8	10.6

*Time from symptom onset to treatment.
†Intention-to-treat analysis.
C, control or placebo; h, heparin; IV, intravenous; rt-PA, recombinant tissue-type plasminogen activator; scu-PA, single-chain urokinase-type plasminogen activator; SK, streptokinase; u-PA, urokinase-type plasminogen activator.

symptomatic hemorrhage for hemispheric stroke in the cerebral artery territory range from 3.3% to 9.6% in this setting.[3,7,8,151,169,182] In addition, the development of symptomatic hemorrhage in rt-PA–treated patients contributed to mortality in properly controlled trials, including the National Institute of Neurological Disorders and Stroke (NINDS) study[6-8] and European-Australasian Acute Stroke Study III.[182] Overall, however, those well-designed trials showing benefit from the use of systemic parenteral rt-PA have demonstrated also risk factors for hemorrhage.

Clinical features that have been associated with higher risk of intracerebral hemorrhage include advancing age and signs of early infarction on initial cranial computed tomography. Early signs of infarction may reflect otherwise undetectable injury to the matrix of the microvascular bed.[6-8] Increased time to treatment, low body mass (higher relative rt-PA dose), diastolic hypertension, older age, early signs of ischemia, and the use of rt-PA are associated with the risk of intracerebral hemorrhage.[3,183-186] Additional insight has been obtained from clinical series employing magnetic resonance (MR) imaging techniques that can distinguish perfusion defects by perfusion-weighted imaging (PWI) and diffusion-weighted imaging (DWI).[107,187] From those recent studies subgroups of patients receiving rt-PA have been identified for whom the risk of hemorrhage is increased.[107] This is compatible with evidence that the depth and duration of focal ischemia is a contributor to the ultimate cerebral hemorrhage risk during exposure to plasminogen activators.[188]

Despite the higher risk of hemorrhage associated with rt-PA, a robust clinical benefit has been demonstrated with proper use of this agent.[6] However, both tissue injury and pharmacologic interventions can augment the risk of hemorrhage. The results of two randomized trials of intraarterial recombinant scu-PA are consistent with the effect of anticoagulation (heparin) to increase the risk of symptomatic cerebral hemorrhage.[169,174] Heparin dosage was lowered in the early stages of the phase II trial before a significant excess of symptomatic hemorrhages would have been observed.[169] A significant increase in recanalization rate also occurred in patients receiving the higher heparin dose. Nonetheless, there is no evidence that the increase in hemorrhage associated with the use of PAs was related to greater recanalization. Early infusion of a PA in selected patients is associated, however, with a decrease in hemorrhage risk.[3]

The experimental and clinical experience supports the view that careful intervention with PAs immediately after the onset of symptoms of focal ischemia can result in significant functional recovery, despite a possible increase in hemorrhagic transformation. This body of clinical evidence is consistent with the known pharmacologic properties of plasminogen activators.

REFERENCES

1. del Zoppo GJ, Ferbert A, Otis S, et al: Local intra-arterial fibrinolytic therapy in acute carotid territory stroke: A pilot study, *Stroke* 19:307-313, 1988.
2. Mori E, Tabuchi M, Yoshida T, et al: Intracarotid urokinase with thromboembolic occlusion of the middle cerebral artery, *Stroke* 19:802-812, 1988.
3. del Zoppo GJ, Poeck K, Pessin MS, et al: Recombinant tissue plasminogen activator in acute thrombotic and embolic stroke, *Ann Neurol* 32:78-86, 1992.
4. Mori E, Yoneda Y, Tabuchi M, et al: Intravenous recombinant tissue plasminogen activator in acute carotid artery territory stroke, *Neurology* 42:976-982, 1992.
5. Yamaguchi T, Hayakawa T, Kikuchi H: Intravenous tissue plasminogen activator ameliorates the outcome of hyperacute embolic stroke, *Cerebrovasc Dis* 3:269-272, 1993.
6. The NINDS and Stroke rt-PA Stroke Study Group: Tissue plasminogen activator for acute ischemic stroke, *N Engl J Med* 333:1581-1587, 1995.
7. Hacke W, Kaste M, Fieschi C, et al: Intravenous thrombolysis with recombinant tissue plasminogen activator for acute hemispheric stroke. The European Cooperative Acute Stroke Study (ECASS), *JAMA* 274:1017-1025, 1995.
8. Hacke W, Kaste M, Fieschi C, et al: Randomised double-blind placebo-controlled trial of thrombolytic therapy with intravenous alteplase in acute ischaemic stroke (ECASS II), *Lancet* 352:1245-1251, 1998.
9. Hacke W, Kaste M, Bluhmki E, et al: Thrombolysis with alteplase 3 to 4.5 hours after acute ischemic stroke, *N Engl J Med* 359:1317-1329, 2008.
10. Sherry S: The history and development of thrombolytic therapy. In Comerota AJ, editor: *Thrombolytic therapy for peripheral vascular disease*, Philadelphia, 1995, JB Lippincott, pp 67-86.
11. Christensen LR, MacLeod CM: A proteolytic enzyme of serum: Characterization, activation, and reaction with inhibitors, *J Gen Physiol* 28:559-583, 1945.
12. Kaplan MH: Nature and role of the lytic factor in hemolytic streptococcal fibrinolysis, *Proc Soc Exp Biol Med* 57:40-43, 1944.
13. Tillett WS, Sherry S: The effect in patients of streptococcal fibrinolysis (streptokinase) and streptococcal deoxyribonuclease on fibrinous, purulent and sanguineous pleural exudations, *J Clin Invest* 28:173-190, 1949.
14. Johnson AJ, Tillett WS: Lysis in rabbits of intravascular blood clots by the streptococcal fibrinolytic system (streptokinase), *J Exp Med* 95:449-464, 1952.
15. Masuda J, Yutani C, Ogata J, et al: Atheromatous embolism in the brain: A clinicopathologic analysis of 15 autopsy cases, *Neurology* 44:1231-1237, 1994.
16. Schwartz ML, Pizzo SV, Hill RL, et al: Human factor XIII from plasma and platelets. Molecular weight, subunit structures, proteolytic activation and cross-linking of fibrinogen and fibrin, *J Biol Chem* 248:1395-1407, 1973.
17. Gaffney PJ, Lane DA, Kakkar VV, et al: Characterization of a soluble D-dimer-E complex in cross-linked fibrin digests, *Thromb Res* 7:89-99, 1975.
18. Hermans J, McDonagh J: Fibrin: Structure and interactions, *Semin Thromb Hemost* 8:11-24, 1982.
19. Davie EW, Fujikawa K, Kisiel W: The coagulation cascade: Initiation, maintenance, and regulation, *Biochemistry* 30:10363-10370, 1991.
20. Nossel HL: Relative proteolysis of fibrin B-beta chain by thrombin and plasmin as a determinant of thrombosis, *Nature* 291:754-762, 1981.
21. Alkjaersig N, Fletcher AP: Catabolism and excretion of fibrinopeptide A, *Blood* 60:148-156, 1982.
22. Majerus PW, Miletich JP, Kane WP, et al: The formation of thrombin on the platelet surface. In Mann KG, Taylor FB, editors: *The regulation of coagulation*, New York, 1980, Elsevier/North Holland, pp 215.
23. Kaplan AP: Initiation of the intrinsic coagulation and fibrinolytic pathways of man: The role of surfaces, Hageman factor, prekallikrein, high molecular weight kininogen, and factor XI, *Prog Hemost Thromb* 4:127-175, 1978.
24. Nesheim ME, Hibbard LS, Tracy PB, et al: Participation of factor Va in prothrombinase. In Mann KG, Taylor FB, editors: *The regulation of coagulation*, New York, 1980, Elsevier/North Holland, pp 145-159.
25. Levin EG, Marzec U, Anderson J, et al: Thrombin stimulates tissue plasminogen activator release from cultured human endothelial cells, *J Clin Invest* 74:1988-1995, 1984.

26. van Hinsbergh VW: Regulation of the synthesis and secretion of plasminogen activators by endothelial cells, *Haemostasis* 18:307–327, 1988.

27. Liesi P, Kirkwood T, Vaheri A: Fibronectin is expressed by astrocytes cultured from embryonic and early postnatal rat brain, *Exp Cell Res* 163:175–185, 1986.

28. Giles AR, Nosheim ME, Herring SW, et al: The fibrinolytic potential of the normal primate following the generation of thrombin in vivo, *Thromb Haemost* 63:476–481, 1990.

29. Nawroth PP, Stern DM: Endothelial cells as active participants in procoagulant reactions. In Gimbrone MA, editor: *Vascular endothelium in hemostasis and thrombosis*, Edinburgh, 1986, Churchill Livingstone, pp 31–32.

30. Collen D, de Maeyer L: Molecular biology of human plasminogen. I: Physiocochemical properties and microheterogeneity, *Thromb Diath Haemorrh* 34:396–402, 1975.

31. Levin EG, del Zoppo GJ: Localization of tissue plasminogen activator in the endothelium of a limited number of vessels, *Am J Pathol* 144:855–861, 1994.

32. Plow EF, Felez J, Miles LA: Cellular regulation of fibrinolysis, *Thromb Haemost* 66:132–136, 1991.

33. Chang DI, Hosomi N, Lucero J, et al: Activation systems for matrix metalloproteinase-2 are upregulated immediately following experimental focal cerebral ischemia, *J Cereb Blood Flow Metab* 23:1408–1419, 2003.

34. Hosomi N, Lucero J, Heo JH, et al: Rapid differential endogenous plasminogen activator expression after acute middle cerebral artery occlusion, *Stroke* 32:1341–1348, 2001.

35. Whitelock JM, Murdoch AD, Iozzo RV, et al: The degradation of human endothelial cell-derived perlecan and release of bound basic fibroblast growth factor by stromelysin, collagenase, plasmin, and heparanases, *J Biol Chem* 271:10079–10086, 1996.

36. Lijnen HR: Plasmin and matrix metalloproteinases in vascular remodeling, *Thromb Haemost* 86:324–333, 2001.

37. Hamann GF, Okada Y, Fitridge R, et al: Microvascular basal lamina antigens disappear during cerebral ischemia and reperfusion, *Stroke* 26:2120–2126, 1995.

38. Bachmann F, Kruithof IE: Tissue plasminogen activator: Chemical and physiological aspects, *Semin Thromb Hemost* 10:6–17, 1984.

39. Aoki N, Harpel PC: Inhibitors of the fibrinolytic enzyme system, *Semin Thromb Hemost* 10:24–41, 1984.

40. Collen D, Lijnen HR: New approaches to thrombolytic therapy, *Arteriosclerosis* 4:579–585, 1984.

41. Verstraete M, Collen D: Thrombolytic therapy in the eighties, *Blood* 67:1529–1541, 1986.

42. Forsgren M, Raden B, Israelsson M, et al: Molecular cloning and characterization of a full-length cDNA clone for human plasminogen, *FEBS Lett* 213:254–260, 1987.

43. Bachmann F: Molecular aspects of plasminogen, plasminogen activators and plasmin. In Bloom AL, Forbes CD, Thomas DP, Tuddenham EGD, editors: *Haemostasis and thrombosis*, Edinburgh, 1994, Churchill Livingstone, pp 575–613.

44. Peterson LC, Serenson E: Effect of plasminogen and tissue-type plasminogen activator on fibrin gel structure, *Fibrinolysis* 5:51–59, 1990.

45. Tran-Thang C, Kruithof EK, Atkinson J, et al: High-affinity binding sites for human glu-plasminogen unveiled by limited plasmic degradation of human fibrin, *Eur J Biochem* 160:559–604, 1986.

46. Wallen P, Wiman B: Characterization of human plasminogen. II: Separation and partial characterization of different molecular forms of human plasminogen, *Biochim Biophys Acta* 257:122–134, 1973.

47. Holvoet P, Lijnen HR, Collen D: A monoclonal antibody specific for lys-plasminogen: Application to the study of the activation pathways of plasminogen *in vivo*, *J Biol Chem* 260:12106–12111, 1985.

48. The European Stroke Prevention Study (ESPS-2) Working Group: Secondary stroke prevention: Aspirin/dypyridamole combination is superior to either agent alone and to placebo, *Stroke* 27:195, 1996.

49. Miles LA, Greengard JS, Griffin JH: A comparison of the abilities of plasma kallikrein, beta-factor XIIa, factor XIa and urokinase to activate plasminogen, *Thromb Res* 29:407–417, 1983.

50. Kluft C, Dooijewaard G, Emeis JJ: Role of the contact system in fibrinolysis, *Semin Thromb Hemost* 13:50–68, 1987.

51. Wun TC, Ossowski L, Reich E: A proenzyme of human urokinase, *J Biol Chem* 257:7262–2768, 1982.

52. Wun TC, Schleuning E, Reich E: Isolation and characterization of urokinase from human plasma, *J Biol Chem* 257:3276–3287, 1982.

53. Ichinose A, Fujikawa K, Suyama T: The activation of pro-urokinase by plasma kallikrein and its inactivation by thrombin, *J Biol Chem* 261:3486–3489, 1986.

54. Hanss M, Collen D: Secretion of tissue-type plasminogen activator and plasminogen activator inhibitor by cultured human endothelial cells: Modulation by thrombin endotoxin and histamine, *J Lab Clin Med* 109:97–104, 1987.

55. Levin EG, Stern DM, Nawrath PP, et al: Specificity of the thrombin-induced release of tissue plasminogen activator from cultured human endothelial cells, *Thromb Haemost* 56:115–119, 1986.

56. Robbins KC, Summaria L, Hsieh B, et al: The peptide chains of human plasmin, *J Biochem* 242:2333–2342, 1967.

57. Robbins KC: The plasminogen-plasmin system. In Comerota AJ, editor: *Thrombolytic therapy for peripheral vascular disease*, Philadelphia, 1995, JB Lippincott, pp 41–65.

58. Wiman B, Lindahl T, Almqvist A: Evidence for a discrete binding protein of plasminogen activator in plasma, *Thromb Haemost* 59:392–395, 1988.

59. Collen D: On the regulation and control of fibrinolysis, *Thromb Haemost* 43:77–89, 1980.

60. Wun TC, Capuano A: Initiation and regulation of fibrinolysis in human plasma at the plasminogen activator level, *Blood* 69:1354–1362, 1987.

61. Bloom AL, Thomas DP: *Haemostasis and thrombosis*, Edinburgh, 1987, Churchill-Livingstone.

62. Kakkar VV, Scully MF: Thrombolytic therapy, *Br Med Bull* 34:191–199, 1978.

63. Sharma GVRK, Cella G, Parish AF, et al: Drug therapy: Thrombolytic therapy, *N Engl J Med* 306:1268–1276, 1982.

64. Verstraete M: Biochemical and clinical aspects of thrombolysis, *Semin Hematol* 15:35–54, 1978.

65. Castellino FJ: Biochemistry of human plasminogen, *Semin Thromb Hemost* 10:18–23, 1984.

66. Yasaka M, Yamaguchi T, Miyashita T, et al: Regression of intracardiac thrombus after embolic stroke, *Stroke* 21:1540–1544, 1990.

67. Bounameaux H, de Moerloose P, Perrier A, et al: Plasma measurement of D-dimer as diagnostic aid in suspected venous thromboembolism: An overview, *Thromb Haemost* 71:1–6, 1994.

68. Pennica D, Holmes WE, Kohr WJ, et al: Cloning and expression of human tissue-type plasminogen activator cDNA in E. coli, *Nature* 301:214–221, 1983.

69. Rijken DC: Structure/function relationships of t-PA. In Kluft C, editor: *Tissue type plasminogen activator (t-PA): physiological and clinical aspects*, Vol 1, Boca Raton, FL, 1988, CRC Press, pp 101–122.

70. Ehrlich HJ, Bang NW, Little SP, et al: Biological properties of a kringleless tissue plasminogen activator (t-PA) mutant, *Fibrinolysis* 1:75–81, 1987.

71. Gelehrter TD, Sznycer-Laszuk R: Thrombin induction of plasminogen activator-inhibitor in cultured human endothelial cells, *J Clin Invest* 77:165–169, 1986.

72. Sakata Y, Curriden S, Lawrence D, et al: Activated protein C stimulates the fibrinolytic activity of cultured endothelial cells and decreases antiactivator activity, *Proc Natl Acad Sci U S A* 82:1121–1125, 1985.

73. Moscatelli D: Urokinase-type and tissue-type plasminogen activators have different distributions in cultured bovine capillary endothelial cells, *J Cell Biochem* 30:19–29, 1986.

74. Bulens F, Nelles L, Van den Panhuyzen N, et al: Stimulation by retinoids of tissue-type plasminogen activator secretion in cultured human endothelial cells: Relations of structure to effect, *J Cardiovasc Pharmacol* 19:508–514, 1992.

75. Thompson EA, Nelles L, Collen D: Effect of retinoic acid on the synthesis of tissue-type plasminogen activator and plasminogen activator inhibitor-I in human endothelial cells, *Eur J Biochem* 201:627–632, 1991.

76. Saksela O, Moscatelli D, Rifkin DB: The opposing effects of basic fibroblast growth factor and transforming growth factor beta on the regulation of plasminogen activator activity in capillary endothelial cells, *J Cell Biol* 105:957–963, 1987.

77. Levin EG, Marotti KR, Santell L: Protein kinase C and the stimulation of tissue plasminogen activator release from human endothelial cells: Dependence on the elevation of messenger RNA, *J Biol Chem* 264:16030-16036, 1989.

78. Smith D, Gilbert M, Owen WG: Tissue plasminogen activator release *in vivo* in response to vasoactive agents, *Blood* 66:835-839, 1985.

79. Brommer EJP: Clinical relevance of t-PA levels of fibrinolytic assays. In Kluft C, editor: *Tissue-type plasminogen activator (t-PA): physiological and clinical aspects*, Part 2, Boca Raton, FL, 1988, CRC Press, pp 89.

80. Agnelli GE: *Thrombolysis yearbook 1995*, Amsterdam, 1995, Excerpta Medica.

81. Krystosek A, Seeds NW: Normal and malignant cells, including neurons, deposit plasminogen activator on growth substrata, *Exp Cell Res* 166:31-46, 1986.

82. Pittman RN: Release of plasminogen activator and a calcium-dependent metalloprotease from cultured sympathetic and sensory neurons, *Dev Biol* 110:91-101, 1985.

83. Vincent VA, Lowik CW, Verheijen JH, et al: Role of astrocyte-derived tissue-type plasminogen activator in the regulation of endotoxin-stimulated nitric oxide production by microglial cells, *Glia* 22:130-137, 1998.

84. Toshniwal PK, Firestone SL, Barlow GH, et al: Characterization of astrocyte plasminogen activator, *J Neurol Sci* 80:277-287, 1987.

85. Tsirka SE, Rogove AD, Bugge TH, et al: An extracellular proteolytic cascade promotes neuronal degeneration in the mouse hippocampus, *J Neurosci* 17:543-552, 1997.

86. Masos T, Miskin R: Localization of urokinase-type plasminogen activator mRNA in the adult mouse brain, *Brain Res Mol Brain Res* 35:139-148, 1996.

87. Tranque P, Naftolin F, Robbins R: Differential regulation of astrocyte plasminogen activators by insulin-like growth factor-I and epidermal growth factor, *Endocrinology* 134:2606-2613, 1994.

88. Nakajima K, Tsuzaki N, Shimojo M, et al: Microglia isolated from rat brain secrete a urokinase-type plasminogen activator, *Brain Res* 577:285-292, 1992.

89. Lijnen HR, Zamarron C, Blaber M, et al: Activation of plasminogen by pro-urokinase. I: Mechanism, *J Biol Chem* 261:1253-1258, 1986.

90. Petersen LC, Bjorn SE, Nordfang O: Effect of leukocyte proteinases on tissue factor pathway inhibitor, *Thromb Haemost* 67:537-541, 1992.

91. White FW, Barlow GH, Mozen MM: The isolation and characterization of plasminogen activators (urokinase) from human urine, *Biochemistry* 5:2160-2169, 1966.

92. Fletcher AP, Alkjaersig N, Sherry S, et al: The development of urokinase as a thrombolytic agent. Maintenance of a sustained thrombolytic state in man by its intravenous infusion, *J Lab Clin Med* 65:713-731, 1965.

93. Stump DC, Mann KH: Mechanisms of thrombus formation and lysis, *Ann Emerg Med* 17:1138-1147, 1988.

94. Davies MC, Englert ME, De Rezo EC: Interaction of streptokinase and human plasminogen observed in the ultracentrifuge under a variety of experimental conditions, *J Biol Chem* 239:2651-2656, 1964.

95. Reddy KN, Marcus B: Mechanisms of activation of human plasminogen by streptokinase, *J Biol Chem* 246:1683-1691, 1972.

96. Standing R, Fears R, Ferres H: The protective effect of acylation on the stability of APSAC (Eminase) in human plasma, *Fibrinolysis* 2:157, 1988.

97. Lijnen HR, de Cock F, Matsuo O, et al: Comparative fibrinolytic and fibrinogenolytic properties of staphylokinase and streptokinase in plasma of different species in vitro, *Fibrinolysis* 6:33-37, 1992.

98. Collen D: Staphylokinase: A potent, uniquely fibrin-selective thrombolytic agent, *Nat Med* 4:279-282, 1998.

99. Jespers L, Vanwetswinkel S, Lijnen HR, et al: Structural and functional basis of plasminogen activation by staphylokinase, *Thromb Haemost* 81:479-484, 1999.

100. Lijnen HR, Van Hoef B, Matsuo O, et al: On the molecular interactions between plasminogen-staphylokinase, α_2-antiplasmin and fibrin, *Biochim Biophys Acta* 1118:144-148, 1992.

101. Witt W, Maass B, Baldus B, et al: Coronary thrombosis with *Desmodus* salivary plasminogen activator in dogs: Fast and persistent recanalization by intravenous bolus administration, *Circulation* 90:421-426, 1994.

102. Hare TR, Gardell SJ: Vampire bat salivary plasminogen activator promotes robust lysis of plasma clots in a plasma milieu without causing fluid phase plasminogen activation, *Thromb Haemost* 68:165-169, 1992.

103. Bergum PW, Gardell SJ: Vampire bat salivary plasminogen activator exhibits a strict and fastidious requirement for polymeric fibrin as its cofactor, unlike human tissue-type plasminogen activator: A kinetic analysis, *J Biol Chem* 267:17726-17731, 1992.

104. Mellot MJ, Stabilito II, Holahan MA, et al: Vampire bat salivary plasminogen activator promotes rapid and sustained reperfusion without concomitant systemic plasminogen activation in a canine model of arterial thrombosis, *Arterioscler Thromb* 12:212-221, 1992.

105. Witt W, Baldus B, Bringmann P, et al: Thrombolytic properties of *Desmodus rotundus* (vampire bat) salivary plasminogen activator in experimental pulmonary embolism in rats, *Blood* 79:1213-1217, 1992.

106. Hacke W, Albers G, Al-Rawi Y, et al: The Desmoteplase in Acute Ischemic Stroke Trial (DIAS): A phase II MRI-based 9-hour window acute stroke thrombolysis trial with intravenous desmoteplase, *Stroke* 36:66-73, 2005.

107. Albers GW, Thijs VN, Wechsler L, et al: Magnetic resonance imaging profiles predict clinical response to early reperfusion: The Diffusion and Perfusion Imaging Evaluation For Understanding Stroke Evolution (DEFUSE) study, *Ann Neurol* 60:508-517, 2006.

108. Lijnen HR, Collen D: Development of new fibrinolytic agents. In Bloom AL, Forbes CD, Thomas DP, Tuddenham EGD, editors: *Haemostasis and thrombosis*, Edinburgh, 1994, Churchill-Livingstone, pp 625-637.

109. Van de Werf F: New thrombolytic strategies. *Aust N Z J Med* 23:763-765, 1993.

110. Smalling RW: Pharmacological and clinical impact of the unique molecular structure of a new plasminogen activator, *Eur Heart J* 18:F11-F16, 1997.

111. Benedict CR, Refino CJ, Keyt BA, et al: New variant of human tissue plasminogen activator (TPA) with enhanced efficacy and lower incidence of bleeding compared with recombinant human TPA, *Circulation* 92:3032-3040, 1995.

112. Kohnert U, Horsch B, Fischer S: A variant of tissue plasminogen activator (t-PA) comprised of the kringle 2 and the protease domain shows a significant difference in the in vitro rate of plasmin formation as compared to the recombinant human t-PA from transformed Chinese hamster ovary cells, *Fibrinolysis* 7:365-372, 1993.

113. Fischer S, Kohnert U: Major mechanistic differences explain the higher clot lysis potency of reteplase over alteplase: Lack of fibrin binding is an advantage for bolus application of fibrin-specific thrombolytics, *Fibrinolysis and Proteolysis* 11:129-135, 1997.

114. Refino CJ, Paoni NF, Keyt BA, et al: A variant of t-PA (T103N, KHRR 296-299 AAAA) that, by bolus, has increased potency and decreased systemic activation of plasminogen, *Thromb Haemost* 70:313-319, 1993.

115. Paoni NF, Keyt BA, Refino CJ, et al: A slow clearing, fibrin-specific, PAI-1 resistant variant of t-PA T103N, KHRR 296-299 AAAA, *Thromb Haemost* 70:307-312, 1993.

116. Keyt BA, Paoni NF, Refino CJ, et al: A faster-acting and more potent form of tissue plasminogen activator, *Proc Natl Acad Sci U S A* 91:3670-3674, 1994.

117. Kawai C, Suzuki S: Monteplase: Pharmacological and clinical experience. In *New therapeutic agents in thrombosis and thrombolysis*, New York, 2002, Marcel Dekker, Inc., pp 525-540.

118. Katoh M, Suzuki Y, Miyamoto I, et al: Biochemical and pharmacokinetic properties of YM866, a novel fibrinolytic agent, *Thromb Haemost* 65:1193, 1991.

119. Katoh M, Shimizu Y, Kawauchi Y, et al: Comparison of clearance rate of various tissue plasminogen activator (t-PA) analogues, *Thromb Haemost* 62:542, 1989.

120. Haley EC Jr, Lyden PD, Johnston KC, et al: A pilot dose-escalation safety study of tenecteplase in acute ischemic stroke, *Stroke* 36:607-612, 2005.

121. Modi NB, Eppler S, Breed J, et al: Pharmacokinetics of a slower clearing tissue plasminogen activator variant, TNK-tPA, in patients with acute myocardial infarction, *Thromb Haemost* 79:134-139, 1998.

122. Runge MS, Bode C, Matsueda GR, et al: Antibody-enhanced thrombolysis: Targeting of tissue plasminogen activator *in vivo*, *Proc Natl Acad Sci U S A* 84:7659-7662, 1987.

123. Kasper W, Erbel R, Meinertz T, et al: Intracoronary thrombolysis with an acylated streptokinase-plasminogen activator (BRL 26921) in patients with acute myocardial infarction, *J Am Coll Cardiol* 4:357-363, 1984.

124. Pierard L, Jacobs P, Gheysen D, et al: Mutant and chimeric recombinant plasminogen activators, *J Biol Chem* 262:11771-11778, 1987.

125. Bode C, Meinhardt G, Runge MS, et al: Platelet-targeted fibrinolysis enhances clot lysis and inhibits platelet aggregation, *Circulation* 84:805-813, 1991.

126. Jones RD, Donaldson IM, Parkin PJ: Impairment and recovery of ipsilateral sensory-motor function following unilateral cerebral infarction, *Brain* 112:113-132, 1989.

127. Bachmann F, et al: Fibrinolysis. In Verstraete M, Vermylen J, Lijnen HR, editors: *Thrombosis and haemostasis*, Leuven, 1987, ISTH/University of Leuven Press, pp 227-265.

128. Kluft C, Los N: Demonstration of two forms of α_2-antiplasmin in plasma by modified crossed immunoelectrophoresis, *Thromb Res* 21:65-71, 1981.

129. Philips M, Juul AG, Thorsen S: Human endothelial cells produce a plasminogen activator inhibitor and a tissue-type plasminogen activator-inhibitor complex, *Biochim Biophys Acta* 802:99-110, 1984.

130. Loskutoff DJ, van Mourik JA, Erickson LA, et al: Detection of an unusually stable fibrinolytic inhibitor produced by bovine endothelial cells, *Proc Natl Acad Sci U S A* 80:2956-2960, 1983.

131. Thorsen S, Philips M, Selmer J, et al: Kinetics of inhibition of tissue-type and urokinase-type plasminogen activator by plasminogen-activator inhibitor type 1 and type 2, *Eur J Biochem* 175:33-39, 1988.

132. Wilhelm OG, Jaskunas SR, Vlahos CJ, et al: Functional properties of the recombinant kringle-2 domain of tissue plasminogen activator produced in *Escherichia coli*, *J Biol Chem* 265:14606-14611, 1990.

133. Juhan-Vague I, Moerman B, de Cock F, et al: Plasma levels of a specific inhibitor of tissue-type plasminogen activator (and urokinase) in normal and pathological conditions, *Thromb Res* 33:523-530, 1984.

134. Schleuning WD, Medcalf RL, Hession C, et al: Plasminogen activator inhibitor 2: Regulation of gene transcription during phorbol ester-mediated differentiation of U-937 human histiocytic lymphoma cells, *Mol Cell Biol* 7:4564-4567, 1987.

135. Kruithof EK, Tran-Thang C, Gudinchet A, et al: Fibrinolysis in pregnancy: A study of plasminogen activator inhibitors, *Blood* 69:460-466, 1987.

136. Bonnar J, Daly L, Sheppard BL: Changes in the fibrinolytic system during pregnancy, *Semin Thromb Hemost* 16:221-229, 1990.

137. Stump DC, Thienpont M, Collen D: Purification and characterization of a novel inhibitor of urokinase from human urine: Quantitation and preliminary characterization in plasma, *J Biol Chem* 261:12759-12766, 1986.

138. Heeb MJ, Espana F, Geiger M, et al: Immunological identity of heparin-dependent plasma and urinary protein C inhibitor and plasminogen activator inhibitor-3, *J Biol Chem* 262:15813-15816, 1987.

139. Marder VJ, Sherry S: Thrombolytic therapy: Current status, *N Engl J Med* 318:1512-1520, 1988.

140. Sappino AP, Madani R, Huarte J, et al: Extracellular proteolysis in adult murine brain, *J Clin Invest* 92:679-685, 1993.

141. Heo JH, Han SW, Lee SK: Free radicals as triggers of brain edema formation after stroke, *Free Radic Biol Med* 39:51-70, 2005.

142. Pfefferkorn T, Staufer B, Liebetrau M, et al: Plasminogen activation in focal cerebral ischemia and reperfusion, *J Cereb Blood Flow Metab* 20:337-342, 2000.

143. Sironi L, Maria CA, Bellosta S, et al: Endogenous proteolytic activity in a rat model of spontaneous cerebral stroke, *Brain Res* 974:184-192, 2003.

144. Chen ZL, Yu H, Yu WM, et al: Proteolytic fragments of laminin promote excitotoxic neurodegeneration by up-regulation of the KA1 subunit of the kainate receptor, *J Cell Biol* 183:1299-1313, 2008.

145. Tsirka SE: Tissue plasminogen activator as a modulator of neuronal survival and function, *Biochem Soc Trans* 30:222-225, 2002.

146. Gimple LW, Gold HK, Leinbach RC, et al: Correlation between template bleeding times and spontaneous bleeding during treatment of acute myocardial infarction with recombinant tissue plasminogen activator, *Circulation* 80:581-588, 1989.

147. Agnelli G, Buchanan MR, Fernandez F, et al: A comparison of the thrombolytic and hemorrhagic effects of tissue-type plasminogen activator and streptokinase in rabbits, *Circulation* 72:178-182, 1985.

148. Marder VJ, Shortell CK, Fitzpatrick PG, et al: An animal model of fibrinolytic bleeding based on the rebleed phenomenon: Application to a study of vulnerability of hemostatic plugs of different age, *Thromb Res* 67:31-40, 1992.

149. Loscalzo J, Vaughan DB: Tissue plasminogen activator promotes platelet disaggregation in plasma, *J Clin Invest* 79:1749-1755, 1987.

150. Chen LY, Muhta JL: Lys- and glu-plasminogen potentiate the inhibitory effect of recombinant tissue plasminogen activator on human platelet aggregation, *Thromb Res* 74:555-563, 1994.

151. Albers GW, Bates VE, Clark WM, et al: Intravenous tissue-type plasminogen activator for treatment of acute stroke: The Standard Treatment with Alteplase to Reverse Stroke (STARS) study, *JAMA* 283:1145-1150, 2000.

152. Danglet G, Vinson D, Chapeville F: Qualitative and quantitative distribution of plasminogen activators in organs from healthy adult mice, *FEBS Lett* 194:96-100, 1986.

153. Matsuo O, Okada K, Fukao H, et al: Cerebral plasminogen activator activity in spontaneously hypertensive stroke-prone rats, *Stroke* 23:995-999, 1992.

154. Dent MA, Sumi Y, Morris RJ, et al: Urokinase-type plasminogen activator expression by neurons and oligodendrocytes during process outgrowth in developing rat brain, *Eur J Neurosci* 5:633-647, 1993.

155. del Zoppo GJ: t-PA: A neuron buster, too? [editorial], *Nat Med* 4:148-150, 1998.

156. Zivin JA, Fisher M, DeGirolami U, et al: Tissue plasminogen activator reduced neurological damage after cerebral embolism, *Science* 230:1289-1292, 1985.

157. Overgaard K, Sereghy T, Boysen G, et al: Reduction of infarct volume and mortality by thrombolysis in a rat embolic stroke model, *Stroke* 23:1167-1174, 1992.

158. Hamann GF, del Zoppo GJ: Leukocyte involvement in vasomotor reactivity of the cerebral vasculature, *Stroke* 25:2117-2119, 1994.

159. Byrne JG, Smith WJ, Murphy MP, et al: Complete prevention of myocardial stunning, contracture, total low reflow and edema after heart transplantation by blocking neutrophil adhesion molecules during reperfusion, *J Thorac Cardiovasc Surg* 104:1589-1596, 1992.

160. Bowes MP, Rothlein R, Fagan SC, et al: Monoclonal antibodies preventing leukocyte activation reduce experimental neurologic injury and enhance efficacy of thrombolytic therapy, *Neurology* 45:815-819, 1995.

161. Husain S, Gurewich V, Lipinski B: Purification and partial characterization of a single-chain high-molecular-weight form of urokinase from human urine, *Arch Biochem Biophys* 220:31, 1983.

162. Kunkel EJ, Jung U, Bullard DC, et al: Absence of trauma-induced leukocyte rolling in mice deficient in both P-selectin and intercellular adhesion molecule 1, *J Exp Med* 183:57-65, 1996.

163. Spetzler RF, Selman WR, Weinstein P, et al: Chronic reversible cerebral ischemia: Evaluation of a new baboon model, *J Neurosurg* 7:257-261, 1980.

164. del Zoppo GJ, Copeland BR, Anderchek K, et al: Hemorrhagic transformation following tissue plasminogen activator in experimental cerebral infarction, *Stroke* 21:596-601, 1990.

165. Young AR, Touzani O, Derlon J-M, et al: Early reperfusion in the anesthetized baboon reduces brain damage following middle cerebral artery occlusion: A quantitative analysis of infarction volume, *Stroke* 28:632-637, 1997.

166. Heo JH, Lucero J, Abumiya T, et al: Matrix metalloproteinases increase very early during experimental focal cerebral ischemia, *J Cereb Blood Flow Metab* 19:624-633, 1999.

167. Hamann GF, Okada Y, del Zoppo GJ: Hemorrhagic transformation and microvascular integrity during focal cerebral ischemia/reperfusion, *J Cereb Blood Flow Metab* 16:1373-1378, 1996.

168. Fukuda S, Fini CA, Mabuchi T, et al: Focal cerebral ischemia induces active proteases that degrade microvascular matrix, *Stroke* 35:998-1004, 2004.

169. del Zoppo GJ, Higashida RT, Furlan AJ, et al: PROACT: a phase II randomized trial of recombinant pro-urokinase by direct arterial delivery in acute middle cerebral artery stroke. PROACT Investigators. Prolyse in Acute Cerebral Thromboembolism, *Stroke* 29:4–11, 1998.

170. Fieschi C, Argentino C, Lenzi GL, et al: Clinical and instrumental evaluation of patients with ischemic stroke within the first six hours, *J Neurol Sci* 91:311–321, 1989.

171. Solis OJ, Roberson GR, Taveras JM, et al: Cerebral angiography in acute cerebral infarction, *Revist Interam Radiol* 2:19–25, 1977.

172. Fieschi C, Bozzao L: Transient embolic occlusion of the middle cerebral and internal carotid arteries in cerebral apoplexy, *J Neurol Neurosurg Psychiatry* 32:236–240, 1969.

173. Irino T, Taneda M, Minami T: Angiographic manifestations in post-recanalized cerebral infarction, *Neurology* 27:471–475, 1977.

174. Furlan AJ, Higashida R, Wechsler L, et al: Intra-arterial prourokinase for acute ischemic stroke. The PROACT II Study: A randomized controlled trial, *JAMA* 282:2003–2011, 1999.

175. Yamaguchi T: Intravenous tissue plasminogen activator in acute thromboembolic stroke: A placebo-controlled, double-blind trial. In del Zoppo GJ, Mori E, Hacke W, editors: *Thrombolytic therapy in acute ischemic stroke II*, Heidelberg, 1993, Springer-Verlag, pp 59–65.

176. Siddiqi F, Blinc A, Braaten J, et al: Ultrasound increases flow through fibrin gels, *Thromb Haemost* 73:495–498, 1995.

177. Francis CW, Blinc A, Lee S, et al: Ultrasound accelerates transport of recombinant tissue plasminogen activator into clots, *Ultrasound Med Biol* 21:419–424, 1995.

178. Siddiqi F, Odrljin TM, Fay PJ, et al: Binding of tissue-plasminogen activator to fibrin: Effect of ultrasound, *Blood* 91:2019–2025, 1998.

179. Braaten JV, Goss RA, Francis CW: Ultrasound reversibly disaggregates fibrin fibers, *Thromb Haemost* 78:1063–1068, 1997.

180. Daffertshofer M, Hennerici M: Ultrasound in the treatment of ischaemic stroke, *Lancet Neurol* 2:283–290, 2003.

181. Clark WM, Wissman S, Albers GW, et al: Recombinant tissue-type plasminogen activator (Alteplase) for ischemic stroke 3 to 5 hours after symptom onset. The ATLANTIS Study: A randomized controlled trial. Alteplase Thrombolysis for Acute Noninterventional Therapy in Ischemic Stroke, *JAMA* 282:2019–2026, 1999.

182. Hacke W, Kaste M, Bluhmki E, et al: Thrombolysis with alteplase 3 to 4.5 hours after acute ischemic stroke, *N Engl J Med* 359:1317–1329, 2008.

183. The NINDS t-PA Stroke Study Group: Intracerebral hemorrhage after intravenous t-PA therapy for ischemic stroke, *Stroke* 28:2109–2118, 1997.

184. Larrue V, von Kummer RR, Muller A, et al: Risk factors for severe hemorrhagic transformation in ischemic stroke patients treated with recombinant tissue plasminogen activator: A secondary analysis of the European-Australasian Acute Stroke Study (ECASS II), *Stroke* 32:438–441, 2001.

185. Cocho D, Borrell M, Marti-Fabregas J, et al: Pretreatment hemostatic markers of symptomatic intracerebral hemorrhage in patients treated with tissue plasminogen activator, *Stroke* 37:996–999, 2006.

186. Larrue V, von Kummer R, del Zoppo GJ, et al: Hemorrhagic transformation in acute ischemic stroke: Potential contributing factors in the European Cooperative Acute Stroke Study, *Stroke* 28:957–960, 1997.

187. Singer OC, Humpich MC, Fiehler J, et al: Risk for symptomatic intracerebral hemorrhage after thrombolysis assessed by diffusion-weighted magnetic resonance imaging, *Ann Neurol* 63:52–60, 2008.

188. Ueda T, Hatakeyama T, Kumon Y, et al: Evaluation of risk of hemorrhagic transformation in local intra-arterial thrombolysis in acute ischemic stroke by initial SPECT, *Stroke* 25:298–303, 1994.

189. Matsumoto K, Satoh K: Topical intraarterial urokinase infusion for acute stroke. In Hacke W, del Zoppo GJ, Hirschberg M, editors: *Thrombolytic therapy in acute ischemic stroke*, Heidelberg, 1991, Springer-Verlag, pp 207–212.

190. Gönner F, Remonda L, Mattle H, et al: Local intra-arterial thrombolysis in acute ischemic stroke, *Stroke* 29:1894–1900, 1998.

191. Yamaguchi T: Intravenous rt-PA in acute embolic stroke. In Hacke W, del Zoppo GJ, Hirschberg M, editors: *Thrombolytic therapy in acute ischemic stroke*, Heidelberg, 1991, Springer-Verlag, pp 168–174.

192. von Kummer R, Hacke W: Safety and efficacy of intravenous tissue plasminogen activator and heparin in acute middle cerebral artery, *Stroke* 23:646–652, 1992.

4

Cerebral Blood Flow and Metabolism in Human Cerebrovascular Disease

ALLYSON R. ZAZULIA, JOANNE MARKHAM, WILLIAM J. POWERS

Methods of Measurement
Cerebral Blood Flow

Cerebral blood flow (CBF) is measured as volume of blood delivered to a defined mass of tissue per unit time, usually mL $\cdot$ 100 g^{-1} $\cdot$ min^{-1}. Quantitative CBF measurement methods employ indicators in the blood as tracers for flow to the brain. These indicators may be externally administered compounds that can be detected by imaging devices or, with some magnetic resonance or near infrared methods, an endogenous substance such as water or oxyhemoglobin. These tracer methods require a mathematical model that relates the measurement of the tracer to CBF. Although a growing number of mathematical techniques are used to measure CBF, most are based on one of three fundamental tracer kinetic principles: the Fick principle, the central volume principle, or the compartmental principle.

The Fick principle states that the change in the quantity of substance in an organ, $q(t)$, is equal to the arterial flow, F, times the arterial concentration, $C_A(t)$, minus the venous flow times the venous concentration, $C_V(t)$.[1,2] Since arterial flow equals venous flow, it follows:

$$\frac{dq(t)}{dt} = F\,[C_A(t) - C_V(t)] \qquad (1)$$

$q(T)$, the total amount of tracer taken up by the brain at time T, can be obtained by integration of equation 1. When $q(0) = 0$,

$$F = \frac{q(T)}{\displaystyle\int_0^T (C_A(t) - C_V(t))\, dt} \qquad (2)$$

With this equation, three quantities must be known to compute flow: $q(T)$, $C_A(t)$, and $C_V(t)$. The Fick principle was the basis for the first technique used to measure quantitative CBF in human subjects developed by Kety and Schmidt.[1] The Kety-Schmidt technique uses an inert inhaled gas (originally nitrous oxide in low concentration) as the tracer. Arterial and jugular venous concentrations are measured directly during the period of inhalation to determine the integral of the arterial-venous difference. Because Kety and Schmidt could not directly measure $q(T)$ in the living human brain, they used a clever alternative approach to determine its value. First they determined the value for the ratio of brain-to-blood nitrous oxide concentrations at equilibrium (the partition coefficient) in vitro. Then they multiplied the partition coefficient by the equilibrium blood concentration to determine $q(T)$ per unit brain volume.

The original Kety-Schmidt method permits only whole brain measurements in mL $\cdot$ 100 g^{-1} $\cdot$ min^{-1}. Different adaptations of the Fick principle can be used to derive regional CBF measurements. Microsphere methods use tracers that are physically or metabolically trapped in the tissue, so that $C_V(t)$ is 0. The arterial concentration integral is measured directly. Regional tracer quantity $q(T)$ is measured directly by organ dissection[3] or by external radiation detection systems like single-photon emission computed tomography (SPECT).[4]

Autoradiographic techniques employ radioactive inert tracers that freely diffuse out of the blood into the brain.[5] Assuming instantaneous equilibration of the tracer in venous space with tissue tracer, the venous concentration can be expressed in terms of the tissue concentration, $C_T(t)$, or amount, $q(t)$, by the following equation:

$$C_V(t) = C_T(t)/\lambda = q(t)/(V_T\lambda) \qquad (3)$$

where λ is the partition coefficient and V_T is the tissue volume. As with the microsphere method, the arterial time-radioactivity curve is measured directly, and the regional tracer quantity is measured by organ dissection or by an external radiation detection system like positron emission tomography (PET) or SPECT.

The central volume principle is based on the concept of transit time. If a bolus of a tracer is introduced into arterial blood flowing through tissue, the tracer particles will flow through and then out the venous drainage on the other side.[6] Because not all particles will take the same path, they will take different times to transit the tissue. The mean transit time, $\bar{t}$, for the tracer particles is determined by the volume in which the tracer is distributed, V_d, and the flow through the tissue, F, as follows:

$$\bar{t} = \frac{V_d}{F} \qquad (4)$$

The mean transit time can be determined by measuring the total amount of tracer injected, q_o, and the residue amount that remains in the tissue as a function of time, $q(t)$:

$$\bar{t} = \frac{\int_0^\infty q(t)dt}{q_0} \tag{5}$$

With radioactive tracers, the residue function in the brain can be measured with external radiation detection devices. The integral of the residue function over time is equal to the numerator in equation 5. If the volume of the tracer injection is small enough and the injection is fast enough, all the tracer going to the tissue region under study will be measured by the external detector during the initial portion of the residue curve before any exits. Thus, the initial height of the residue curve will be equal to q_o. External radiation detection devices do not measure all of the radioactivity emitted within the tissue; some is absorbed by the tissue and some exits the brain at angles not covered by the detector crystals. Thus, although the efficiency of detection, ε, varies for different volumes of tissue depending on the location of the volume of tissue under study relative to the detector, it is the same for any given volume of tissue as long as its spatial relationship to the external detector does not change. Thus, both the initial height and the remainder of the residue curve will be measured at the same efficiency, $\bar{t}$, so they can be measured accurately. This is the strategy used for measuring CBF by intracarotid bolus injection of freely diffusible tracers such as radioactive xenon.[7] In this case,

$$\bar{t} = \frac{\varepsilon \int_o^\infty q(t)dt}{\varepsilon q_O} = \frac{\text{Area}}{\text{Height}} = \frac{V_d}{\text{CBF}} \tag{6}$$

The area and initial height of the residue curve are determined experimentally. If the volume of distribution of the tracer in the brain is known from previous in vitro experiments, CBF can be determined. The central volume principle is valid for both diffusible and nondiffusible (intravascular) tracers. For intravascular tracers, V_d is the intravascular space or cerebral blood volume (CBV). Thus, the mean vascular transit time, $\bar{t}_v$, is described by the following equation:

$$\bar{t}_v = \frac{\text{CBV}}{\text{CBF}} \tag{7}$$

Calculation of the mean transit time from the following equation:

$$\bar{t} = \frac{\text{Area}}{\text{Height}} \tag{8}$$

is practical only for very limited conditions. Estimation of *Height* requires that all tracer be present in the region of interest at one time, and *Area* must be calculated over a relatively long time, a difficult requirement because of recirculation. Various techniques have been proposed for correcting the residue curve for the effects of recirculation, but none has been successful for all situations.[8]

The central volume principle is also valid for nonbolus dispersed intravenous injection. However, in this latter case, q_o cannot be measured from the initial height of the residue curve because not all the tracer is within the field of view of the detector at once. Determining the total quantity of tracer delivered to the tissue region under these circumstances is difficult and limits the use of the central volume principle. The mean transit time cannot be determined from residue curves alone without accurate measurement of q_o, so methods for deriving $\bar{t}_v$ solely on the basis of the residue curve of the intravenous injection do not yield accurate values.

It is important not to confuse residue detection with outflow detection in indicator dilution methods. The indicator dilution method is based on the measurement of the concentration of tracer in the venous outflow over time.[9] Equations for computation of mean transit time from outflow and from residue curves differ. Unfortunately, residue data are sometimes used in place of venous outflow data in these calculations. This substitution can lead to erroneous calculation of $\bar{t}$, CBV, and CBF.[10,11]

It is also important not to confuse the transit time with measures of the circulation time, such as the time from injection to peak tracer concentration. The transit time describes the time it takes for a substance to move through a defined volume of tissue. The time-to-peak (TTP) is a measure of how long after injection it takes the tracer to reach the defined volume of tissue.

Methods based on *compartmental models* differ from those based on the Fick and central volume principles because the former make certain assumptions about the behavior of the tracer in the tissue. Compartmental models consist of a finite number of homogeneous, well-mixed pools or compartments that interact by the exchange of material.[7,12] A fundamental assumption of compartmental models of tracer kinetics is that the concentration of the tracer is instantaneously the same everywhere once it is introduced into the compartment. The quantity of tracer at time t after introduction, $q(t)$, depends on the initial amount of tracer, q_o, the volume of distribution of the tracer within the compartment, V_d, and the flow, F, through the compartment, as follows:

$$q(t) = q_o \exp(-\kappa t) \tag{9}$$

where $\kappa = F/V_d$. One-compartment models are reasonable approximations of the behavior of freely diffusible tracers in the brain and thus can be used for calculations of CBF from a residue curve if V_d is known.[7] The behavior of intravascular tracers in the brain does not conform to compartmental principles. Thus, compartmental models cannot be used to derive CBF or CBV from intravascular agents.[10]

Doppler devices measure the velocity of red blood cells moving toward the device. The relationship of Doppler velocity to CBF can be given as follows:

$$\text{CBF} = \frac{\cos\theta \, V_m \, A}{M} \tag{10}$$

where θ is the angle between the Doppler device and the vessel, V_m is the mean velocity throughout the cardiac cycle of all red blood cells at a point in the vessel with cross-sectional area A, and M is the mass of brain perfused by the vessel. The angle θ is difficult to measure accurately. A is also difficult to measure accurately and varies as vessels dilate and constrict under the influence of changes in perfusion pressure and other stimuli. M may change as collateral channels develop. All of these factors mean that the measurement of red blood cell velocity with Doppler ultrasonography in a single artery is only indirectly related to CBF.[13] However, with careful technique, it is possible to determine the total volume of flow through both internal carotid arteries and both vertebral arteries and, thus, measure the total brain blood flow in mL $\cdot$ min^{-1}.[14]

Cerebral Metabolism

The Fick principle can be used together with measurements of CBF to calculate substrate metabolism, as follows:

$$CMR = CBF(C_A - C_V) \qquad (11)$$

where *CMR* (cerebral metabolic rate) is the steady-state rate of substrate utilization by the brain, *CBF* is the rate of cerebral blood flow in volume of blood per unit time, and $C_A - C_V$ is the steady-state difference in concentration of the substance in arterial and cerebral venous blood. Because the Kety-Schmidt CBF technique requires measurement of arterial and jugular venous tracer concentrations to determine CBF, it is straightforward to measure substrate concentrations and determine CMR as well. Regional CBF techniques can also be combined with arterial-jugular venous difference measurements to try to measure regional metabolism, but these are subject to error because the arterial-jugular venous differences may not be the same everywhere in the brain under pathologic conditions.[15]

The primary technique for measuring regional metabolism is PET. PET employs radiotracers and complicated mathematical models to measure both the cerebral metabolic rate of oxygen (CMRO$_2$) and the cerebral metabolic rate of glucose (CMRglc).[16,17] Quantitative magnetic resonance methods for measuring CMRO$_2$ are under development.[18-21]

Energy Metabolism and Normal Cerebral Hemodynamics

The metabolic requirements of brain cells are substantial, accounting for about 20% of the total body basal oxygen consumption. Energy in the brain is used for maintenance of membrane potentials, ionic transport, maintenance of cell structure, biosynthesis and transport of neurotransmitters, and biosynthesis and transport of cellular elements. The brain performs work at the expense of adenosine triphosphate (ATP) energy, which it obtains by degrading exogenous compounds with a high-energy content (primarily glucose) to simpler compounds with less energy content (CO$_2$ and H$_2$O). Because storage of substrates for energy metabolism in the brain is minimal, the brain is highly dependent on a continuous supply of oxygen and glucose from the blood for its functional and

structural integrity; it is exquisitely sensitive to even brief disturbances in this supply. Thus in cardiac arrest, for example, complete interruption of the cerebral circulation results in loss of consciousness within 10 seconds.[22]

Normal Values of CBF and CMR

On the basis of the Kety-Schmidt technique, healthy young adults have an average whole brain CBF of approximately 46 mL $\cdot$ 100 g^{-1} $\cdot$ min^{-1}, CMRO$_2$ of 3.0 mL $\cdot$ 100 g^{-1} $\cdot$ min^{-1} (134 µmol $\cdot$ 100 g^{-1} $\cdot$ min^{-1}), and CMRglc of 25 µmol $\cdot$ 100 g^{-1} $\cdot$ min^{-1}.[23-26] The CMRO$_2$/CMRglc molar ratio is 5.4, rather than 6.0 as expected for complete oxidation, because of the production of a small amount of lactate by glycolysis.[23,25,27] CBF in gray matter (80 mL $\cdot$ 100 g^{-1} $\cdot$ min^{-1}) is approximately four times higher than in white matter (20 mL $\cdot$ 100 g^{-1} $\cdot$ min^{-1}).[28]

In newborn infants, mean global CBF is low, ranging from 6 to 35 mL $\cdot$ 100 g^{-1} $\cdot$ min^{-1}.[29-34] In preterm infants with subsequently normal development at 6 months of age, CBF may be less than 10 mL $\cdot$ 100 g^{-1} $\cdot$ min^{-1}.[35] Global CMRO$_2$ in the normal newborn is also very low, with the majority of values less than 1.3 mL $\cdot$ 100 g^{-1} $\cdot$ min^{-1}.[29,36] This finding indicates that energy requirements in fetal and newborn brain are minimal or can be met by nonoxidative metabolism. Mean CMRglc in the newborn has been reported to be 4 to 19 µmol $\cdot$ 100 g^{-1} $\cdot$ min^{-1}.[37-39]

Beyond the neonatal period, global CBF, CMRO$_2$, and CMRglc progressively increase, reaching a maximum at age 3-10 years.[33,40-45] There is some disagreement about the magnitude of the peaks, with reports of CBF ranging from 60 to 140 mL $\cdot$ 100 g^{-1} $\cdot$ min^{-1}, CMRO$_2$ ranging from 4.3 to 6.2 mL $\cdot$ 100 g^{-1} $\cdot$ min^{-1}, and CMRglc ranging from 49 to 65 µmol $\cdot$ 100 g^{-1} $\cdot$ min^{-1}. By late adolescence, cerebral flow and oxygen and glucose metabolism decrease to adult levels.[33,41,42,45] Many studies report that CBF declines further from the third decade onward, albeit much more slowly than the decrease in adolescence.[15,46-48] The change in metabolic rate for oxygen and glucose with age is less clear, with several studies showing a decrease[46,47,49-51] and others showing no change.[52-54] Studies that have corrected for brain atrophy show lesser or no changes in CBF, CMRO$_2$, and CMRglc with increasing age.[50,55-57] Our own data corrected for brain atrophy from 23 normal subjects, aged 23 to 71 years, shows no significant change in CBF or CMRO$_2$, but a decline in CMRglc.

Control of Cerebral Blood Flow

Cerebral perfusion pressure (CPP) is equal to the difference between the arterial pressure driving blood into the brain and the venous backpressure. Venous backpressure is negligible unless there is elevated intracranial pressure (ICP) or obstruction of venous outflow. Thus, under most circumstances CPP is equal to the mean arterial pressure (MAP). CBF is regulated by CPP and the cerebrovascular resistance (CVR) as follows:

$$CBF = \frac{CPP}{CVR} \qquad (12)$$

Under conditions of constant CPP, any local or regional changes in CBF must occur as a result of changes in CVR.

CVR is determined by blood viscosity, vessel length, and vessel radius. The cerebrovascular bed is not a static system. Rather, resistance vessels (primarily arterioles) dilate and constrict in response to a variety of stimuli.

Response of Cerebral Blood Flow and Metabolism to Changes in Metabolic Demand

Under normal resting physiologic conditions, regional blood flow is closely matched to the resting metabolic rate of the tissue.[58-60] Thus, the fraction of available oxygen that is extracted by the brain (oxygen extraction fraction [OEF]) and glucose (glucose extraction fraction [GEF]) is uniform. Approximately one third of the oxygen and one tenth of the glucose delivered to the brain by the blood are metabolized.[58,59,61-63] When there is a primary reduction in the metabolic rate of the brain (e.g., by hypothermia or barbiturates), there is a secondary decline in CBF to a comparable degree with little or no change in OEF or GEF.[64-66]

During functional activation of brain, both regional CBF and CMRglc increase in the area of increased neuronal activity.[67] It was long assumed that similar increases in regional $CMRO_2$ would accompany the CBF increases. However, PET studies revealed that in humans, large, stimulus-induced increases in CBF and CMRglc (30% and 50%, respectively) were accompanied by only small increases in $CMRO_2$ (5%).[68,69] Subsequent experiments have produced substantial controversy and disagreement in this rapidly moving field. At this time, the original observation that CBF and CMRglc both increase more than $CMRO_2$ under conditions of physiologic brain activation remains sound, although many details of the underlying cellular mechanisms need to be worked out.

Response of Cerebral Blood Flow to Changes in Arterial Partial Pressure of CO_2

The sensitivity of the cerebral circulation to changes in arterial partial pressure of CO_2 has been well established. This relationship, in which a decrease in arterial P_{CO_2} to approximately 25 mm Hg via hyperventilation leads to a decrease in CBF of 30% to 35% and an increase in arterial P_{CO_2} to more than 50 mm Hg via CO_2 inhalation leads to an increase in CBF of about 75%, was initially described by Kety and Schmidt[70,71] and has been confirmed repeatedly.[72-74] The mechanism for the change in CBF is a change in CVR produced by vasodilation with increased P_{CO_2} and vasoconstriction with decreased P_{CO_2}.[71] When the perturbation in arterial P_{CO_2} is maintained for a prolonged time, CBF gradually returns toward normal values.[74] With passive hyperventilation, CBF decreases but there is no reduction in $CMRO_2$ or high-energy phosphate levels[75,76] despite the appearance of disturbances in consciousness[70]; however, with active hyperventilation, a slight increase in $CMRO_2$ has been reported.[70,71]

Response of Cerebral Blood Flow to Changes in Arterial Partial Pressure of Oxygen, Oxygen Content, Hemoglobin, and Blood Viscosity

The effect of P_{O_2} on the cerebral circulation has been investigated primarily through reductions in the inspired concentration of oxygen. In both humans and experimental animals, CBF does not increase until arterial P_{O_2} is reduced below about 30 to 50 mm Hg,[77,78] indicating that variations in P_{O_2} are unlikely to constitute an important mechanism for regulating CBF at physiologic levels of P_{O_2}. The arterial oxygen content, Ca_{O_2}, depends on the concentration of hemoglobin in the blood and the degree to which it is saturated with oxygen. Because of the sigmoid shape of the oxygen dissociation curve, a significant reduction in hemoglobin saturation and hence in Ca_{O_2} does not occur until arterial P_{O_2} falls to about 50 to 60 mm Hg.[77,79] The similarity between this number and the threshold for hypoxia-induced reduction in CBF suggests that it is primarily Ca_{O_2} and not P_{O_2} that determines CBF. Reductions in Ca_{O_2} due to hypoxemia or anemia cause vasodilation and compensatory increases in CBF.[23,71,77,80] Likewise, the increase in Ca_{O_2} with polycythemia is associated with a decrease in CBF.[81] In neither of these cases does cerebral metabolism change.[77,81] With long-term changes in Ca_{O_2}, there is a significant reciprocal inverse relationship between Ca_{O_2} and CBF throughout the range of oxygen content levels.[80] Short-term changes in Ca_{O_2} due to reduction in hemoglobin or P_{O_2} produce less of an increase in CBF than do long-term changes.[82,83] Thus, increases in CBF brought about by hemodilution, if they are simply reciprocal responses to changes in arterial oxygen content, have no effect on cerebral oxygen delivery.

Hematocrit is an important determinant of viscosity, and thus, viscosity often varies with Ca_{O_2}. Although an inverse relationship between viscosity and CBF has also been reported,[80,84] it is unlikely that viscosity is an independent determinant of CBF under most circumstances. In anemic, paraproteinemic subjects in whom reduced Ca_{O_2} is dissociated from changes in viscosity, there is no correlation between viscosity and CBF, but there is a highly significant inverse relationship between Ca_{O_2} and CBF.[85] In hematologically normal subjects, reduction of viscosity by plasma exchange without a concomitant change in hemoglobin concentration or Ca_{O_2} does not increase CBF.[86] Finally, reducing Ca_{O_2} via carbon monoxide inhalation without changing arterial P_{O_2} or viscosity has been shown to increase CBF.[87] On the basis of experimental data, viscosity may have a more prominent effect on cerebral perfusion in the presence of preexisting vasodilation. In rats with increased CBF due to hemodilution, hypercapnia, and hypoxia, doubling of the plasma viscosity reduced CBF by as much as half.[88,89] Similarly, in a middle cerebral artery (MCA) occlusion model in rats, CBF was lower in ischemic animals with decreased Ca_{O_2} and higher in ischemic animals who had decreased viscosity due to hemodilution but no change in Ca_{O_2}.[90] From these findings, it can be concluded that increases in blood viscosity induce compensatory vasodilation to maintain cerebral oxygen delivery. This compensatory mechanism may be exhausted when preexisting vasodilation impairs the ability of vessels to dilate further.[89]

Response of Cerebral Blood Flow to Changes in Blood Glucose Concentration

In contrast to the relationship of CBF to oxygen supply and demand, the balance between glucose supply and demand has little effect on CBF. In insulin clamp or bolus/infusion experiments, decreasing blood glucose concentration to 2.3 to 3 mmol/L in normal subjects has generally been reported to cause no change in CBF.[91-94] In a later study with greater measurement precision, a slight decrease in CBF, of 6% to 8%, has been reported at a blood glucose concentration of 3.0 mmol/L.[95] More severe reductions in blood glucose, down to 1.1 to 2.2 mmol/L, produced a modest but significant increase in CBF.[96-100] This increase likely does not represent a compensatory mechanism to maintain glucose delivery to the brain. A blood glucose level of 2 mmol/L is well below the level at which brain dysfunction and counterregulatory hormone response occur.[92] Furthermore, increases in CBF do not increase blood:brain glucose transport.[101,102] Because vascular responses to other stimuli are preserved, this increase in CBF is not simply due to a general loss of vascular tone.[103,104]

Response of Cerebral Blood Flow to Changes in Cerebral Perfusion Pressure

Changes in CPP over a wide range from 70 to 150 mm Hg have little effect on CBF. Known as autoregulation, this compensatory mechanism is mediated by changes in CVR. When CPP decreases, vasodilation of the small arteries or arterioles reduces CVR. When CPP increases, vasoconstriction of the small arteries or arterioles increases CVR.[105,106] This mechanism is effective at maintaining CBF in normal human subjects until MAP falls below the lower autoregulatory limit.[107,108] Chronic hypertension shifts both the lower and upper limits of autoregulation to higher levels. In subjects with chronic hypertension, the lower autoregulatory limit is 100 to 120 mm Hg MAP.[107,109] This limit is variably and unpredictably affected by long-term antihypertensive drug treatment. Thus, acute reductions in MAP or CPP that would be safe in normotensive subjects may precipitate cerebral ischemia in patients with chronic hypertension. Within the limits of autoregulation, a 10% decrease in MAP produces only a slight (2% to 7%) decrease in regional CBF.[110,111] Reductions of CPP below the autoregulatory limit produce a much steeper fall in CBF.

These observations of the effect of changes in CPP on CBF were made by changing MAP or ICP over minutes, then measuring CBF at the new stable pressure. These responses have been termed "static cerebral autoregulation" to differentiate them from measurements of CBF velocity with Doppler ultrasonography in response to more rapid and less marked fluctuations in MAP or ICP, termed "dynamic cerebral autoregulation."[112] The physiologic relation between static autoregulation and dynamic autoregulation is not clear. Abnormalities of dynamic cerebral autoregulation may be associated with normal or abnormal static autoregulation.[113,114]

As CPP falls below the autoregulatory limit and the maximal vasodilatory capacity of the cerebral circulation has been exceeded, CBF begins to decline and a progressive increase in the amount of oxygen extracted from the blood by the brain maintains oxygen metabolism.[115,116] Under normal circumstances, only 30% to 40% of oxygen delivered to the brain is used for energy production. With reductions in CBF, the extraction may increase by a factor

of 2 or even more.[115] When this mechanism becomes maximal and the increased OEF is no longer adequate to supply the energy needs of the brain, further reductions in CPP disrupt normal cellular metabolism and produce clinical evidence of brain dysfunction (see later).

When the cerebral blood vessels are already dilated in response to some other stimulus, they are less responsive to further vasodilation induced by reduced CPP. Therefore, the autoregulatory response is attenuated or lost in the setting of preexisting hypercapnia, anemia, or hypoxemia.[117,118]

Although reductions in CPP produce visible dilation of pial vessels, data regarding the response of CBV to reduced CPP are conflicting (Fig. 4-1).[105,119-121] CBV is composed of arterial, capillary, and venous segments. Veins account for some 80% to 85% of CBV, arteries for 10% to 15%, and capillaries for less than 5%.[122,123] Of these, arteries are the most responsive to autoregulatory changes in CPP. Veins respond less, and capillaries even less.[124,125] With experimental reductions in CPP, it is often possible to measure an increase in CBV that is presumed to be due to autoregulatory vasodilation.[126-128] However, this increase in CBV to reduced CPP is not always evident,[116,129] and a decrease in CBV in response to severe reductions in CPP has even been observed.[130] Failure to demonstrate increased CBV in the setting of reduced CPP has been ascribed to various possible mechanisms in various situations, including differential vasodilatory capacity of different vascular beds, passive collapse of vessels due to low intraluminal pressures, small vessel vasospasm, and resetting of vascular tone in

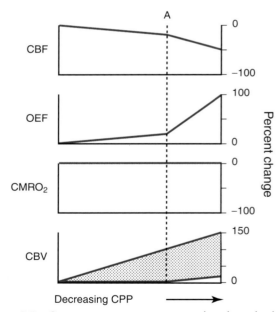

Figure 4-1 Compensatory responses to reduced cerebral perfusion pressure (CPP). As CPP falls, cerebral blood flow (CBF) is initially maintained (with only slight reduction) by arteriolar dilation. When vasodilatory capacity has been exceeded, cerebral autoregulation fails and CBF begins to decrease rapidly (A). A progressive increase in oxygen extraction fraction (OEF) preserves cerebral oxygen metabolism (CMRO$_2$). The response of cerebral blood volume (CBV) to reduced CPP is variable, ranging from a steady rise (of as much as 150%) to only a modest increase beginning at the point of autoregulatory failure.

response to a compensatory downregulation of $CMRO_2$.[131] The CBF/CBV ratio (or its reciprocal, the mean vascular transit time [MVTT]) has been proposed to be a more sensitive indicator of reduced CPP than CBV alone.[116,132] Although it may be more sensitive, this ratio is not reliable because it may decrease in low-flow conditions with normal perfusion pressure, such as hypocapnia.[133,134]

Hemodynamic Effects of Arterial Occlusive Disease
Hemodynamic Effect of Arterial Stenosis

Stenosis of the carotid artery produces no hemodynamic effect until a critical reduction of 60% to 70% in vessel lumen occurs. Even with this or greater degrees of stenosis, distal perfusion pressure is variable and may even remain normal with stenosis exceeding 90%.[135] The reason is that the hemodynamic effect of carotid artery stenosis depends not only on the degree of stenosis but also on the adequacy of the collateral circulation. The importance of collateral circulation pathways in the prediction of ischemic events among patients with carotid occlusive disease is debated. The patency of primary collateral pathways (anterior and posterior communicating and ophthalmic arteries) has been shown to be associated with a lower incidence of ipsilateral stroke,[136,137] and the presence of leptomeningeal collaterals with a higher incidence of ipsilateral stroke,[138] in some studies. However, the pattern of arteriographic collateral circulation to the MCA distal to an occluded carotid artery does not consistently differentiate those patients with poor cerebral hemodynamics[129,137,139,140] or predict stroke recurrence.[129,139] Vascular imaging techniques such as angiography and Doppler ultrasonography can identify the presence of these collateral vessels, but not necessarily the adequacy of the blood supply they provide.[139]

Determination of the hemodynamic effects of arterial stenosis or occlusion on the downstream perfusion pressure is of potential value in determining prognosis and in choosing or monitoring therapy for patients with cerebrovascular disease. Measurement of CBF alone is inadequate for this purpose. First, normal CBF may be found when perfusion pressure is reduced but flow is maintained by autoregulatory vasodilation of distal resistance vessels. Second, CBF may be low when perfusion pressure is normal, such as when the metabolic demands of the tissue are reduced, as in the destruction of normal afferent or efferent fibers by a remote lesion (see "Remote Metabolic Effects of Ischemia"). Current methods for assessment of local cerebral hemodynamics depend on the compensatory responses observed during global reductions in CPP due to systemic hypotension and increased ICP, as described previously. Similar responses are assumed to occur with local reductions in CPP due to focal arterial stenosis.

Methods to Measure the Hemodynamic Effects of Large Artery Occlusive Disease

Three strategies are commonly used clinically to determine hemodynamic status. The first relies on measurement of CBF at baseline and after application of a vasodilatory stimulus, such as CO_2 inhalation, breath holding, acetazolamide administration, or physiologic activity (e.g., hand movement). Impairment of the normal increase in CBF or Doppler blood flow velocity in response to vasodilatory stimuli is assumed to reflect existing autoregulatory vasodilation due to reduced CPP. Responses to vasodilatory stimuli have been categorized into the following three grades of hemodynamic impairment: (1) reduced augmentation (relative to contralateral hemisphere or normal controls), (2) absence of augmentation (same value as baseline), and (3) paradoxical reduction in regional blood flow compared with baseline measurement. This last category, also known as the "steal" phenomenon, can be identified only with quantitative CBF techniques.[141]

The second strategy entails the quantitative measurement of regional CBV either alone or in combination with measurement of CBF at rest to detect the presence of autoregulatory vasodilation. Increases in CBV or the CBV/CBF ratio relative to the range observed in normal control subjects is assumed to indicate hemodynamic compromise, but the sensitivity and specificity of these measurements in detecting reduced CPP are unknown.

The third strategy involves direct measurement of regional OEF as an indicator of local autoregulatory failure and currently is possible only with PET. MRI measurements using pulse sequences sensitive to deoxyhemoglobin, which is increased in regions with increased oxygen extraction, are being developed to provide similar information.[142,143]

Three-Stage Classification System of Cerebral Hemodynamics

On the basis of the known physiologic responses of CBF, CBV, and OEF to reductions in global CPP, a three-stage sequential classification system for local long-term hemodynamic status using noninvasive measurements has been proposed (Fig. 4-1).[144] Stage 0 consists of normal CPP with closely matched flow and metabolism such that OEF is normal. CBV and mean vascular transit time are not elevated, and the CBF response to vasodilatory stimuli is normal. Stage I, hemodynamic compromise, is manifested by autoregulatory vasodilation of arterioles to maintain a constant CBF. Consequently, CBV and the mean vascular transit time are increased, and the CBF response to vasodilatory stimuli is decreased, but OEF remains normal. In Stage II, hemodynamic failure, autoregulatory capacity is exceeded, and there is increased OEF because CBF has declined with respect to $CMRO_2$. $CMRO_2$ is preserved at a level that reflects the underlying energy demands of the tissue but may be lower than normal owing to the effects of previous neuronal loss.[145] Baron et al[146,147] have termed this stage "misery perfusion" (Fig. 4-2).

Although the three-stage classification scheme is conceptually useful, it is too simplistic. First, as discussed previously, increases in CBV and mean vascular transit time are not reliable indices of reduced CPP. Second, CBF responses to different vasodilatory agents may be impaired or normal in the same patient.[148-150] A normal vasodilatory response may occur in the setting of increased CBV.[151,152] Finally, according to the three-stage system, all patients with increased OEF should have increased CBV and poor

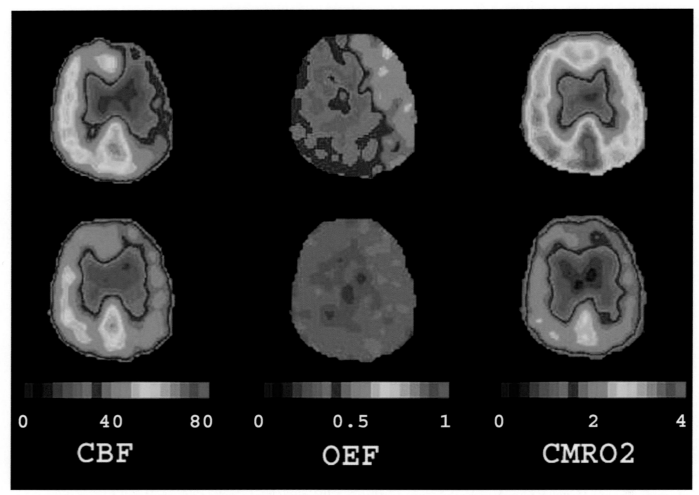

Figure 4-2 Normalization of oxygen extraction fraction (OEF) after extracranial-intracranial (EC-IC) bypass surgery in a 69-year-old man with symptomatic occlusion of the right carotid artery. The baseline positron emission tomographic images *(top row)* demonstrate reduced cerebral blood flow (CBF) and increased OEF in the right hemisphere. A second study performed 35 days after EC-IC bypass shows that ipsilateral CBF has improved and OEF has normalized *(bottom row)*. In all images, the right side of the brain is on the reader's right.

response to vasoactive stimuli; however, this increase in CBV is not always evident.[131]

Correlation of Cerebral Hemodynamics with Stroke Risk

Several studies have evaluated the prognostic value of measurements of cerebral hemodynamics on stroke risk in symptomatic carotid occlusion or MCA stenosis/occlusion. Data on vasomotor reactivity to acetazolamide or hypercapnia (stage I hemodynamic compromise) in predicting subsequent stroke have been inconsistent.[138,153-159] Because CBF responses may be different to different vasodilatory agents within the same patient (see earlier), this inconsistency is understandable. Evidence that hemodynamic impairment by one method of assessment predicts subsequent stroke risk does not prove the predictive value of a similar method. Different techniques rely on different physiologic mechanisms from which the presence of reduced perfusion pressure is inferred. For example, in a well-conducted prospective study, Ogasawara et al[157,158] showed that quantitative measurement of the ipsilateral CBF response to

acetazolamide with xenon-133 was significantly associated with the subsequent risk of stroke, whereas the use of the change in hemisphere asymmetry index was not.

In contrast, two independent studies have demonstrated that stage II hemodynamic failure, defined as increased OEF, is a powerful independent predictor of subsequent ipsilateral ischemic stroke.[129,160,161] When data were controlled for other factors, patients with symptomatic carotid artery occlusion with increased OEF were found to have a risk of ipsilateral ischemic stroke seven times greater than those with normal OEF.[129]

Acute Ischemic Stroke
Evolution of Infarction

The evolution of changes in flow and metabolism after acute ischemic stroke has been established through the study of patients at different time points after symptom onset and from experimental studies of cerebral arterial occlusion in large mammals.

The data from large mammals show an initial reduction in CBF that is most severe in the central perfusion

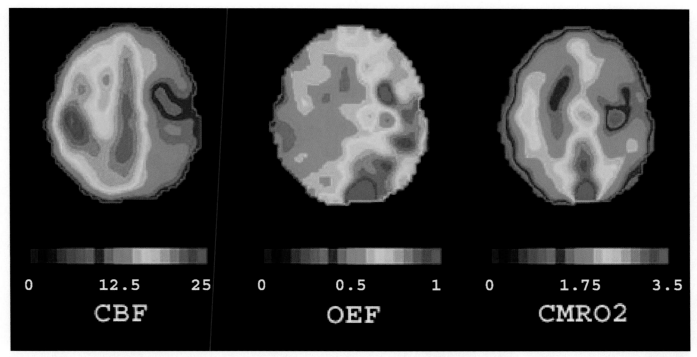

Figure 4-3 Positron emission tomography study in a 54-year-old woman in whom left hemiparesis due to vasospasm developed 9 days after subarachnoid hemorrhage. Right hemispheric cerebral blood flow (CBF) and oxygen metabolism ($CMRO_2$) are reduced, and oxygen extraction fraction (OEF) is increased, indicative of ischemia. In all images, the right side of the brain is on the reader's right.

territory of the artery and becomes increasingly less so in more peripheral areas, where collateral circulation from other arteries provides additional flow.[162] Accompanying this initial prominent reduction in CBF within 1 hour after occlusion, there is an increase in OEF. $CMRO_2$ is reduced somewhat initially but falls further over the subsequent 2 to 3 hours. CBF remains relatively stable, falling only slightly.[163-167] Reflecting the stably reduced CBF and further declining $CMRO_2$, the initially markedly increased OEF progressively decreases. By 24 hours, CBF in the center of the MCA territory reaches its nadir at less than 20% of baseline values, and $CMRO_2$ reaches 25% of baseline values. Also at this point, increased OEF is seen to develop outside the area of primary perfusion disturbance, in the tissue adjacent to the infarct core.[167] The volume of severely hypometabolic tissue remains stable between 1 and 7 hours after occlusion but increases by 24 hours and increases even further an average of 17 days after occlusion.[168] The fate of high-OEF regions in the core and surrounding regions is variable; some portions may go on to infarct and other portions may survive.[163]

Human data obtained at 2 to 24 hours after ictus show an area of reduced CBF, reduced $CMRO_2$, and high OEF (Figs. 4-3 and 4-4).[169,170] Over the subsequent days, CBF usually increases. Spontaneous reperfusion occurs in about three quarters of patients. It may take place within a few hours of infarction[171] but peaks at day 14.[172] This rise in CBF occurs without a concomitant rise in $CMRO_2$; rather, $CMRO_2$ generally falls further. Consequently, a decrease in regional OEF below normal values mirrors the rise in CBF. This state, termed "luxury perfusion,"[173] indicates that the normal coupling of CBF to oxygen metabolism in the resting brain is deranged. Luxury perfusion

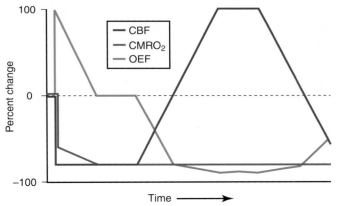

Figure 4-4 Pathophysiologic changes in cerebral infarction. At the onset of ischemia, the initial drop in regional cerebral blood flow (CBF; *purple line*) is mirrored by a rise in regional oxygen extraction fraction (OEF; *green line*). Because the increase in OEF is no longer able to maintain the energy needs of the brain, regional cerebral oxygen metabolism ($CMRO_2$; *red line*) falls to the level of oxygen delivery. With time, $CMRO_2$ falls further even though there is no further decrease in CBF, resulting in a decrease in OEF. Reperfusion via recanalization of the occluded artery or recruitment of collateral pathways results in an increase in CBF ("luxury perfusion") and a concomitant fall in OEF below baseline with no change in $CMRO_2$. With evolution to the stage of chronic infarction, CBF progressively declines, and OEF increases but often remains below baseline values.

may be absolute (Fig. 4-5A), with CBF values greater than normal. Alternatively, luxury perfusion may be relative (Fig. 4-5B), with low or normal CBF that is still in excess of that required to produce a normal OEF for the reduced $CMRO_2$.[174] Luxury perfusion is evident by 48 hours in one

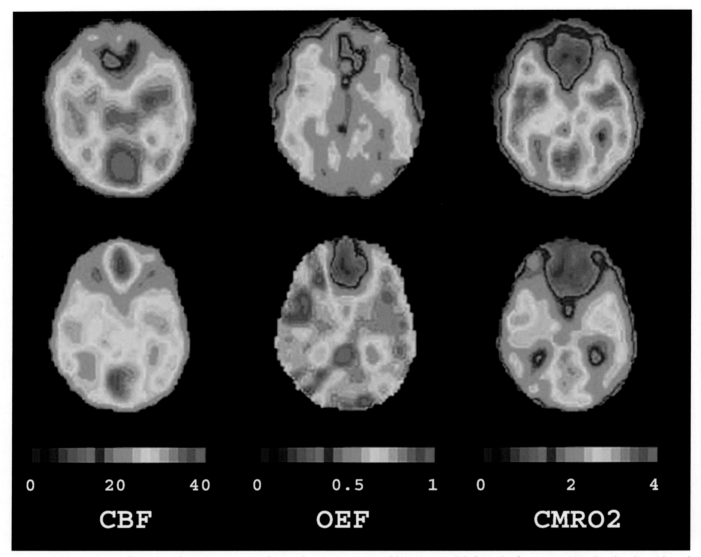

0   20   40   0   0.5   1   0   2   4

CBF   OEF   CMRO2

Figure 4-5   Sequential positron emission tomographic studies in a 22-year-old woman with bifrontal infarcts associated with subarachnoid hemorrhage–induced vasospasm demonstrating luxury perfusion. The first study, performed on day 6 after hemorrhage, reveals *relative* luxury perfusion (*top row*); cerebral blood flow (CBF) is reduced but is still in excess of oxygen requirements ($CMRO_2$), such that oxygen extraction fraction (OEF) is reduced. The second study, performed on day 20, shows increased CBF with reduced $CMRO_2$ and OEF, consistent with *absolute* luxury perfusion (*bottom row*).

third of patients[175,176] and peaks at 1 to 2 weeks, paralleling the time course of spontaneous reperfusion.[174] Following this subacute period, CBF progressively declines and OEF normalizes such that the chronic stable infarct demonstrates flow and metabolism values that are close to zero with OEF at or below baseline values (Fig. 4-6).[177] In the rim of tissue surrounding the infarct core, areas demonstrating reduced CBF and increased OEF with variable $CMRO_2$ can often be identified within hours after ictus and may persist for up to 16 hours. As with the animal data, the fate of high-OEF regions in the core and surrounding regions is variable; some go on to infarct and some do not.[178,179]

Determining the relationship between the metabolism of oxygen and glucose in acute ischemic stroke has been difficult because fluorine-18 fluorodeoxyglucose (^{18}FDG), the PET tracer used for this purpose, can produce artifactually high values for CMRglc under ischemic conditions.[180,181] Studies with ^{18}FDG have shown evidence for dissociation of oxidative and glucose metabolism,[59,63,170,175] with better preservation of CMRglc such that the $CMRO_2$/CMRglc ratio is one third that for normal brain.[63] This finding of relatively increased glycolysis in the presence of adequate oxygen delivery has been attributed to glycolytic activity in neutrophils and macrophages.[63] An alternative explanation for the increased glucose consumption is spreading depression,[182] which is a reversible, slow (≈ 3 mm/min) wave of depolarization accompanied by a marked change in interstitial ion concentrations that occurs spontaneously during ischemia in association with the sustained increase of extracellular potassium and glutamate.[183] The frequency and severity of this excitation-induced spreading depression correlate with the ultimate extent of structural injury in experimental models.[184]

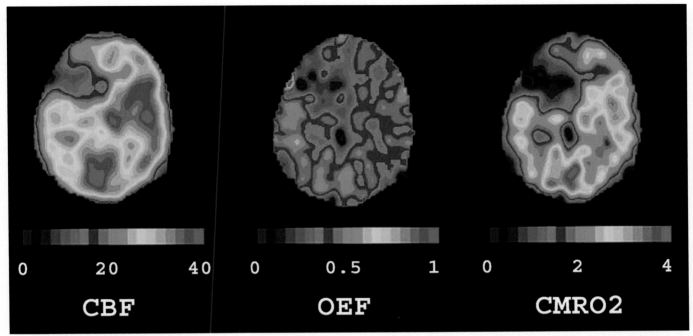

Figure 4-6 Positron emission tomographic study 5 months after left frontal infarct. Regional cerebral blood flow (CBF) and cerebral oxygen metabolism (CMRO$_2$) are severely reduced, and oxygen extraction fraction (OEF) is below normal. In all images, the left side of the brain is on the reader's left.

Autoregulation and Vasoreactivity

During the acute period following ischemic stroke, cerebrovascular control may be deranged. The normal CO$_2$ vasodilatory response may disappear, and autoregulation can be impaired. Abnormalities of CO$_2$ response and autoregulation may occur together or may be dissociated, and focal or global. Abnormalities of autoregulation occur in patients with and without persistent vessel occlusion. When autoregulation is impaired, changes in MAP within the normal autoregulatory range change CBF; induced arterial hypertension increases CBF, and blood pressure reduction decreases CBF.[185-187] Impaired autoregulation following ischemic stroke is not consistently found; it is most commonly described with increases in blood pressure.[185-187] There are several reports of preserved autoregulation when blood pressure is reduced in the first few days after ischemic stroke.[188-191]

Other abnormalities, such as intracerebral steal (decreased CBF in ischemic areas produced by vasodilation elsewhere), inverse steal (increased CBF in ischemic areas due to vasoconstriction elsewhere), and false autoregulation (decreased CBF in ischemic areas produced by increased CPP) also occur. These abnormalities in cerebrovascular control may persist for several weeks and even longer.[192,193]

Flow-Metabolism Thresholds of Tissue Function and Viability

When CBF rapidly declines below the level at which an increase in OEF can sustain normal metabolism, a series of functional and biochemical changes occur in response. The first is a progressive reduction in protein synthesis

that occurs when CBF falls below 50%. CMRglc increases at CBF values of 20 to 30 mL $\cdot$ 100 g^{-1} $\cdot$ min^{-1} and then declines as CBF falls below 20 mL $\cdot$ 100 g^{-1} $\cdot$ min^{-1}. At CBF of 15 to 20 mL $\cdot$ 100 g^{-1} $\cdot$ min^{-1}, normal cellular function and homeostasis is disrupted. Neuronal electrical activity is at first impaired and then abolished. Neurologic deficits appear. High-energy phosphate levels decline, pH drops, and lactate levels rise. With further declines in CBF below 10 mL $\cdot$ 100 g^{-1} $\cdot$ min^{-1}, potassium floods out of the cell into the extracellular space. If removal of arterial obstruction and reestablishment of blood flow occurs quickly enough, these changes are reversible. If CBF remains below 20 to 25 mL $\cdot$ 100 g^{-1} $\cdot$ min^{-1}, the cells may go on to die. The ability of brain cells to tolerate CBF below 20 to 25 mL $\cdot$ 100 g^{-1} $\cdot$ min^{-1} depends on both the magnitude and the duration of the CBF reduction. A CBF of 5 to 10 mL $\cdot$ 100 g^{-1} $\cdot$ min^{-1} may be tolerated for a period of less than 1 hour, whereas a CBF of 10 to 15 mL $\cdot$ 100 g^{-1} $\cdot$ min^{-1}may not produce cell death for 2 to 3 hours. The rapidity with which cell death occurs depends not only on the magnitude and duration of the CBF reduction but also on individual properties of the neurons. Some neurons may tolerate the same reduction in CBF for a period of time that is lethal to other cells. White matter is more tolerant than gray matter.[194-200] In a baboon model of transient MCA occlusion, evidence of reversibility manifested as immediate improvement in hemiparesis was observed in 14 of 14 subjects with occlusion less than 1 hour, 8 of 11 with occlusion lasting 2 to 4 hours, 1 of 3 with occlusion lasting 8 hours, and 1 of 6 with occlusion lasting 16 to 24 hours.[199,201-203]

Thus, in the early hours after cerebral arterial occlusion, the area of the brain with reduced blood flow consists of a mixture of cells that are already irreversibly damaged and destined for death along with some that exhibit abnormal biochemical changes and will go on to die later but may recover if the biochemical processes leading to cell death are interrupted by pharmacologic treatment or reestablishment of CBF. Irreversibly damaged cells are more common in the central areas with the greatest reduction of blood flow. whereas potentially salvageable cells are more common in the periphery, but there will be variation owing to the degree of heterogeneity of the individual cellular responses. A neuroimaging method to identify those patients with preventable infarction (i.e., with vulnerable brain cells that are still alive but whose natural history is to go on to die) would be a great advantage in first testing the efficacy of acute stroke interventions and then applying the interventions to the general population. To do so requires three neuroimaging signals that spatially match the three pathophysiologic tissue types in the brain with acute cerebral ischemia—already dead or irreversibly damaged (signal A), preventable infarction (signal B), and not at risk (signal C).[204] Defining cells that are already dead or irreversibly damaged involves determination of thresholds for CBF and/ or $CMRO_2$ below which spontaneous tissue survivability does not occur. Measurements of CBF alone perform poorly because of the importance of both magnitude and duration in determining cell death, the variable response of different cells, and the occurrence of high CBF in dead tissue (luxury perfusion; see earlier).[62,179,205] Thresholds for cell death based on early measurement of $CMRO_2$ have been shown to be more reliable. $CMRO_2$ thresholds for infarction have been reported from 0.87 to 1.7 mL • 100 g^{-1} • min^{-1}.[62,169,206,207] The values at the lower end of the ranges were derived from single-voxel measurements of both gray and white matter, whereas those at the higher end were determined from larger regions primarily in gray matter. All such attempts to determine thresholds suffer from a variety of technical problems, including small numbers of subjects, poor spatial resolution, lack of co-registration with CT, and poor counting statistics.

Identification of areas of preventable infarction by measurements of CBF and metabolism is much more difficult. Areas of preventable infarction have two simple characteristics—the cells in them will die if untreated and will live if treated. To demonstrate preventable infarction, therefore, requires an effective treatment. The biochemical and pathophysiologic (and, therefore, neuroimaging) characteristics that define preventable infarction may be different, depending on the treatment. For example, the cells that can be salvaged by a neuroprotective strategy that interferes with a specific biochemical pathway in the absence of reperfusion may be different from the cells salvaged by reperfusion.[204] Because tissue regions demonstrating increased OEF represent areas with reduced blood supply relative to oxygen demand but still with metabolically active cells, OEF has received much attention as the factor capable of predicting tissue viability, but it has been shown to be a poor predictor of tissue outcome.[163,179,205,208] The combination of $CMRO_2$ greater than 40% of normal and CBF less than 60% of normal has been shown to accurately identify areas of the brain that will go on to infarct if untreated and will live if treated, the treatment in these

studies being successful reperfusion.[62,163,168,205,207,209,210] These data represent a mix from humans and nonhuman primates with minimal human reperfusion data. Further human reperfusion studies are needed to demonstrate reliability of these criteria for identifying preventable infarction in clinically heterogeneous patient populations.

Thresholds for Ischemia in the Newborn Brain

Although it is generally accepted that the newborn brain is more resistant to ischemic injury than the adult brain, there have been no direct measurements of the tolerance of the newborn human brain to reductions in either blood flow or substrate supply. CBF as low as 5 mL • 100 g^{-1} • min^{-1} has been observed in newborns having normal neurodevelopmental outcome[35,211] and electroencephalographic (EEG) activity.[32] Most measurements of $CMRO_2$ in such newborns are below 1.3 mL • 100 g^{-1} • min^{-1}, which is indicative of infarction in adults with ischemic stroke, and virtual absence of $CMRO_2$ has been observed in newborns without evidence of parenchymal brain injury.[29,36]

Remote Metabolic Effects of Ischemia
Physiologic Basis

A common finding in many metabolic studies of stroke is the presence of areas of reduced blood flow and metabolism in structurally normal tissue distant from the site of infarction. Remote hypometabolism has been demonstrated for both oxygen consumption[174,212-214] and glucose utilization.[215,216] Metabolic values at these distant sites always remain greater than those within the ischemic core,[215] and flow is reduced to a slightly greater degree than metabolism, resulting in a slight increase in OEF.[217] Distinguished from "misery perfusion," this situation has been interpreted to represent primary metabolic depression with secondary reduction in perfusion.

The remote hypometabolism is typically ascribed to a decrease in neuronal activity caused by interruption of afferent or efferent fiber pathways by the ischemic lesion, a phenomenon often termed diaschisis.[212] This term is not strictly accurate, though, because *diaschisis* refers to an acute and reversible functional depression at sites distant from but connected with the site of injury,[218] whereas the remote effects of ischemia are often stable for months[213,219] and may be permanent. Transsynaptic neuronal degeneration has been proposed as an alternate explanation for the remote hypometabolism,[214] and the proposal is supported by the fact that contralateral $CMRO_2$ often declines between acute-period and chronic-period measurements,[220] but it is unlikely to account for all cases because hypometabolism can be seen within hours of stroke.[221] In all probability, demonstrations of remote hypometabolism encompass a variety of reversible and irreversible processes.

Contralateral Cerebellar Hypometabolism

The best-described remote metabolic effect of ischemia is contralateral cerebellar hypometabolism ("crossed cerebellar diaschisis"), which occurs in about 50% of patients with hemispheric lesions (Fig. 4-7).[214,221] Several

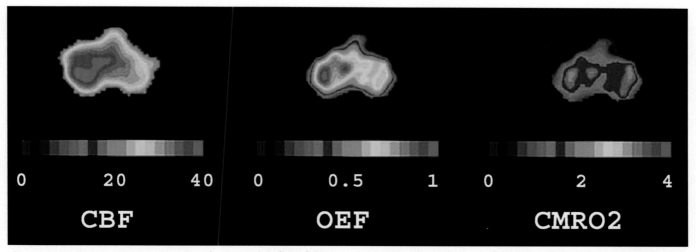

Figure 4-7   Positron emission tomography 5 months after left frontal infarct. Slices through the posterior fossa demonstrate crossed cerebellar hypometabolism with secondary hypoperfusion. In all images, the right side of the brain is on the reader's right.

factors have been reported to influence its occurrence, though data are not consistent among the studies. Such hypometabolism may be more profound with deep MCA infarcts,[214] infarcts involving the frontal[213] or parietal lobes,[174] and those encompassing more than one lobe.[214,216,222] Although Lenzi et al[174] found that "crossed cerebellar diaschisis was not evident in cases in which the dimensions of the infarct were small," Martin and Raichle[213] reported no relationship with infarct size. Cerebellar hypometabolism has been shown to correlate with the presence of,[177] but likely not the severity of,[213] hemiparesis. It also occurs in some patients having no motor deficit.[214,216] Although contralateral cerebellar $CMRO_2$ metabolism and CMRglc metabolism are reduced to the same degree acutely,[59] reduction of CMRglc is greater than that of $CMRO_2$ in chronic stroke (4 to 46 months), indicating an uncoupling of oxygen consumption and glucose utilization.[223]

Contralateral Cerebral Hypometabolism

Reduction in blood flow and metabolism in the hemisphere contralateral to cerebral infarction has also been described for both the homologous cortical area and the whole hemisphere.[174,224,225] Wise et al[226] found that although patients with recent infarction had lower contralateral $CMRO_2$ than normal control subjects, this difference vanished when the comparison group consisted of subjects with extracranial cerebrovascular disease but without previous cerebral infarction. Nonhuman primate models of cerebral ischemia have not revealed evidence for contralateral hemispheric hypometabolism either acutely[166] or at delayed measurement (>2 weeks).[208]

Ipsilateral Cerebral Hypometabolism

Ipsilateral cerebral hypometabolism has been observed in the cortex overlying subcortical stroke and in the basal ganglia, thalamus, and distant sites in the cortex after cortical stroke,[215,224,227,228] likely occurring in a delayed fashion (beyond 18 hours after clinical onset).[229] Because of the dense thalamocortical projections and interconnections between the thalamus and the brainstem, basal ganglia, and cerebellum, it is not surprising that this "intrahemispheric remote hypometabolism" is most frequently described with thalamic lesions.[215,230,231]

Clinical Relevance

The clinical correlate of these remote changes is unclear. Single case reports have suggested an association with focal neurologic deficits, including ataxia,[232,233] aphasia,[234,235] neglect,[236] and hemianopia,[224] but larger series of infarcts at various locations have revealed no such relationships.[214,237] In one study, stepwise regression analysis revealed that language performance depended mainly on parietotemporal metabolism irrespective of infarct location.[238] Impaired consciousness after stroke has been attributed to remote hypometabolism,[174,239] as has disordered higher cortical function.[240] Inconsistency of results may be at least partially explained by a failure to account for such confounding factors as patient age and lesion size and to match control subjects for cerebrovascular risk factors in some of the studies.

Similarly, the relation between remote metabolic effects seen acutely after stroke and eventual clinical outcome is uncertain. In one study, widespread metabolic disruption was a poor indicator of neurologic outcome (disability at 2 weeks to 3 months) regardless of CT findings.[240] In another, metabolism in structurally normal ipsilateral mesial-prefrontal tissue at 5 to 18 hours after MCA stroke was predictive of neurologic status at 3 weeks.[229] Furthermore, glucose metabolism in the left hemisphere 2 to 3 weeks after left MCA stroke predicted both short-term (4 months) and long-term (2 year) recovery from aphasia.[241,242] On the other hand, contralateral hemispheric or cerebellar $CMRO_2$ measured within 30 hours of MCA stroke did not correlate with either acute-stage neurologic deficit or recovery at 15 to 60 days.[220,221]

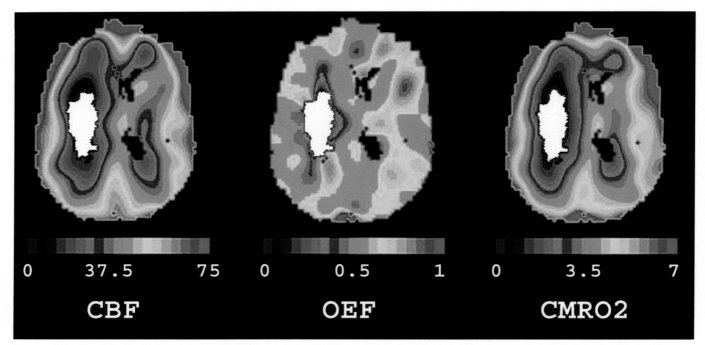

Figure 4-8 Partial volume-corrected positron emission tomographic images of a 44-year-old hypertensive man with a left putaminal hemorrhage studied 21 hours after onset. Periclot blood flow (CBF), cerebral oxygen metabolism (CMRO$_2$), and oxygen extraction fraction (OEF) are all reduced in comparison with the contralateral hemisphere, suggestive of primary metabolic depression. In all images, the left side of the brain is on the reader's left, and the hemorrhage is depicted in *white*.

Intracerebral Hemorrhage
Cerebral Blood Flow and Metabolism

Investigations of CBF and metabolic rate in intracerebral hemorrhage (ICH) have been less extensive than those in ischemic stroke. These have focused on the zone of tissue immediately surrounding the clot. Reduced CBF, determined by autoradiography or SPECT, has been demonstrated in this area in experimental models of ICH[243,244] and in patients with ICH,[245] but not always.[246,247] This reduction in CBF is often attributed to cerebral ischemia due to mechanical compression of the microvasculature surrounding the clot.[243,248] As in ischemic stroke, PET and SPECT studies of ICH suffer from the effect of partial volume averaging, which may cause regions of normal flow to appear reduced, depending on image resolution and the proximity to nonperfused tissue.[249,250] Unlike in ischemic stroke, a validated method exists permitting the correction for partial volume effects in ICH.[251] When this method is used, a zone of hypoperfusion is still evident surrounding acute ICH.[251,252] To determine whether this reduction in periclot flow indicates ischemia, evidence for increased OEF in perihematomal tissue has been sought. In 19 patients studied 5 to 22 hours after symptom onset, Zazulia et al[252] found that periclot CMRO$_2$ was reduced to a greater degree than CBF, resulting in decreased OEF rather than the increased OEF that occurs in ischemia. This pattern was suggestive of a primary metabolic depression, consistent with a subsequent report of perihematomal mitochondrial dysfunction (Fig. 4-8).[253] MRI studies performed within 6 hours of onset also have shown no evidence of very early perihematomal ischemia.[254] These regions of low

CBF adjacent to the hematoma disappear within the first week.[247,255]

Bilateral hemispheric blood flow reduction has been reported in subacute hypertensive hemorrhage accompanied by bihemispheric increase in OEF in patients with very large clots (> 40 mL), but not in those with smaller clots.[256] The increased hemispheric OEF in ICH may reflect the effects of chronic hypertension rather than increased ICP or other effects of the hematoma.[257]

Transient focal increases in glucose metabolism in the perihematomal region that occur 2 to 4 days after ICH have been described in 6 of 13 patients studied in the first week following ICH. The increases were resolving or had returned to baseline on repeat scans at 5 to 8 days (Fig. 4-9).[258] These focal increases are strikingly similar to the foci of hyperglycolysis observed following traumatic brain injury.[259,260] Their pathophysiologic basis and clinical import remain to be determined. Remote depression of CMRglc in morphologically intact brain structures in ICH has been compared to that in ischemic stroke. Remote hypometabolism has been found to depend on size and location, but not the underlying type of lesion.[261,262] When the patients studied within 3 weeks of ICH were compared with those studied more than 3 weeks after ICH, CMRglc in remote regions was found to have increased significantly with time.[262]

Autoregulation

Studies of CBF autoregulation in patients with recent ICH demonstrate that regional autoregulation and global autoregulation are preserved after acute ICH down to a lower

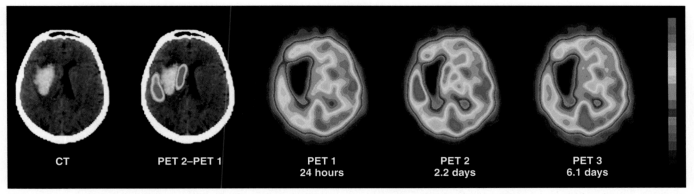

Figure 4-9 Co-registered CT and ^{18}F-fluorordeoxyglucose (FDG) positron emission tomography (PET) images normalized to mean activity in PET 1 from a 77-year-old woman with left putaminal hemorrhage studied 24 hours, 2.2 days, and 6.1 days after onset. PET 2–PET 1 represents the subtraction image of these two PET studies superimposed on the CT and demonstrates the region of increased glucose metabolism. The color scale is relative, with *blue* representing the lowest values and *red* the highest.

MAP limit, which averages 110 mm Hg or about 80% of the admission MAP but shows substantial individual variation. Reductions of MAP in excess of 20% or to less than 84 mm Hg may reduce CBF.[263] Calcium channel blockers and β-blockers have an equivalent minimal effect on CBF within the autoregulatory range of MAP; ganglionic blockers may have a more profound effect on CBF. None of the studies reporting these findings provided data on ICP and, with the exception of one in which hematoma size was not specified, all were carried out in patients with small to moderate hematomas. If ICP is elevated because of a large hematoma or hydrocephalus, then CPP will be below MAP and the level of MAP at which the lower limit of autoregulation occurs may be shifted to a higher value.

Arteriovenous Malformations

Cerebral arteriovenous malformations (AVMs) are high-flow vascular structures lacking capillaries between arteries and veins and, as such, may induce marked hemodynamic disturbances in the surrounding tissue. Many,[195,264-266] but not all,[267] physiologic studies have demonstrated regions of decreased blood flow in the tissue adjacent to the AVM or even far removed in the ipsilateral or contralateral hemisphere. It has been postulated that decreased perfusion around the AVM may be responsible for ischemic symptoms through an intracerebral "steal" syndrome, in which blood flow is disproportionately shunted through the low-resistance AVM and away from other areas of the brain. This concept is controversial, because there is no uniform clinical definition of *steal*. Stable, nonprogressive focal neurologic deficits or seizures are sometimes included along with transient or progressive deficits. Furthermore, there is no clear relationship between regional CBF patterns and symptoms.[268] Data linking the resolution of so-called steal-induced neurologic deficits after AVM obliteration with posttreatment resolution of hypoperfusion and return of normal vasoreactivity are rare.[269] Support for the "steal" hypothesis has been provided by PET studies, which show increases in OEF and CBV consistent with compensatory responses to reduced CPP in the perilesional area in comparison with remote ipsilateral and contralateral brain. The increases

in OEF in the perilesional region were more common in patients with high-flow AVMs, large AVMs, and progressive neurologic deficits.[270]

Similarly, it has been postulated that the occasionally encountered posttreatment complications of edema and hemorrhage are due to a sudden redistribution of previously shunted blood after AVM removal. This redistribution, termed *normal perfusion pressure breakthrough*,[271] assumes that (1) perfusion pressure is reduced below the lower limit of autoregulation by arterial hypotension and venous hypertension in neighboring vascular territories, (2) blood vessels in these territories are maximally dilated such that any decrease in perfusion pressure results in ischemia, (3) chronic hypoperfusion results in vasomotor paralysis and impaired autoregulatory capacity, and (4) reversal of arterial hypotension after treatment is not matched by a corresponding increase in CVR, leading to hyperemia and sometimes swelling and hemorrhage.[272-275] However, data counter to this theory have emerged, with several studies suggesting that autoregulation is intact in tissue adjacent to the AVM both before and after surgery[276,277] and that AVM removal may be associated with a decrease in regional CBF.[268] In addition, because feeding artery pressures are below the standard lower limit of autoregulation in the majority of patients with AVMs,[269] it would be expected that normalization of these pressures after AVM obliteration would result in a large number of "breakthrough" complications. Such complications are uncommon, however.[278-280] Finally, although there are some reports of impaired vascular reserve in tissue adjacent to and distant from the AVM,[281,282] others indicate that regional vasoreactivity may be preserved.[265,269] In fact, patients who experience hyperemic complications have been shown to exhibit *enhanced* vasoreactivity to acetazolamide.[265,280,282] Discrepant results may be partially explained by differing proportions of patients with prior AVM-associated hemorrhage, prior radiosurgery, and seizures, each of which may be associated with altered perfusion and impaired vasoreactivity.[282-285] The preceding facts notwithstanding, severely reduced regional perfusion and exhausted vasodilatory reserve occur in at least some patients with AVM,[269,281] but it is not clear that the abnormal hemodynamic pattern is reversed after AVM obliteration.[282]

Aneurysmal Subarachnoid Hemorrhage
Cerebral Blood Flow and Metabolism

Interpreting the alterations in CBF and metabolism that follow aneurysmal subarachnoid hemorrhage (SAH) is difficult because of the many different factors that can interact to produce the changes. Chief among these factors is the occurrence of large artery vasospasm. In contrast to acute ischemic stroke, in which the large artery flow reduction is caused by a single, sudden, well-timed event, large artery vasospasm occurs gradually over a period of days in different vessels at different times to variable degrees and resolves in the same gradual heterogeneous manner. Thus, at any given time the effect on CBF, CBV, $CMRO_2$, and OEF can be different in any given vascular territory and can correspond to any of the three stages in Figure 4-1 if the resultant reduction in CPP is not severe enough to produce infarction or to any of the time points in Figure 4-4 if CPP was severe enough at some previous time to produce infarction. Additional complicating factors that can affect cerebral hemodynamics and metabolism in this setting include medications, hydrocephalus, anemia, intracerebral hemorrhage, and injury due to brain retraction. Correlating CBF and $CMRO_2$ measurements at early times with subsequent clinical outcome or the development of tissue infarction is especially problematic because the severity of large vessel spasm can worsen, the duration can be protracted, and any of the other complicating factors may confound the association.

Several studies of patients performed within the first few days after aneurysm rupture have investigated the effects of SAH before vasospasm occurs. In one series of patients studied 1 to 4 days after aneurysmal SAH who had not undergone surgery and who did not have evidence of vasospasm, hydrocephalus, or ICH, there was a significant reduction in global $CMRO_2$ and CBF with normal OEF that did not correlate to the use of sedative drugs.[286] This finding was interpreted by the researchers as indicating that the initial aneurysm rupture produced a primary reduction in metabolism at this stage and the reduction in CBF occurred secondary to reduced metabolic demands. Another case series of 7 unsedated patients studied within the first 48 hours showed nonsignificant trends for a reduction in CBF and $CMRO_2$ and an increase in OEF. The investigators in this study did not posit a causal relationship.[287]

Vasospasm, defined as segmental or diffuse narrowing of the large arteries at the base of the brain, can be detected angiographically in up to 70% of patients beginning 4 to 12 days after aneurysm rupture.[288-290] This time course of angiographic vasospasm is paralleled by a progressive fall in CBF over the first 2 weeks and abnormally low CBF for at least 3 weeks after SAH.[291] Reduced CBF correlates well with angiographic vessel diameter in SAH when the blood flow study and angiogram are performed serially, preferably within 1 hour of each other.[292-296] However, in the case of focal angiographic vasospasm, the CBF reduction is often global rather than restricted to the distribution of the involved artery. Although this observation has been used to argue against vasospasm as the actual cause of the reduction in flow, these global changes may be due to the initial effects of the hemorrhage or other confounding factors noted previously.[295]

The degree of CBF reduction correlates well in general with the clinical severity of neurologic deficits after SAH, although there is a wide range of flows within each grade.[297-301] Patients with more severe neurologic deficits (Hunt and Hess grade III or IV) have a more marked reduction in regional CBF than patients with a more favorable clinical grade (Hunt and Hess I or II). Using regional CBF less than 20% of mean CBF as an indication of ischemia, Ishii[297] found foci of ischemia in 39% of measurements in patients with clinical grade I or II, 64% in those with clinical grade III, and 95% in those with clinical grade IV. Another study found that presence of ischemic foci is also correlated with outcome, being seen in only one quarter of the study patients who ultimately recovered but in two thirds of patients who died.[302] Yet another study showed a poor correlation between low CBF levels and the presence of hypodense lesions on CT or the occurrence of new focal deficit in patients evaluated from 1 to 13 days after aneurysm rupture. This finding likely represents the effects of infarcts with high flow due to luxury perfusion.[303]

There is a correlation between regional CBF and outcome. In two previously described studies, patients having a mean CBF of 41 to 42 mL $\bullet$100 g^{-1} $\bullet$ min^{-1} experienced an excellent outcome, and those with a mean CBF of 25 to 33 mL $\bullet$100 g^{-1} $\bullet$ min^{-1} suffered a poor outcome.[297,302]

Depression of CBF and $CMRO_2$ has been reported by several investigators, with OEF variably described as normal or elevated.[294,301,304-308] Reduced metabolism with normal OEF has been interpreted as evidence for nonischemic primary metabolic depression, with vasospasm as a secondary response to reduced metabolic demand. However, because OEF returns to normal within several hours or at most a few days after cerebral infarction, the findings of normal OEF with reduced CBF and $CMRO_2$ cannot be used to discard ischemic infarction as a cause of reduced metabolism (see preceding discussion and Fig. 4-4). Consistent with subacute cerebral infarction in which OEF had returned to normal, some investigators who have demonstrated reduced CBF and $CMRO_2$ with no change in OEF report subsequent cerebral infarction or moderate to severe disability in the majority of the patients.[301,306] To investigate whether large artery vasospasm causes ischemia without the confounding effects of subacute infarction, Carpenter et al[286] studied a group of patients with vasospasm who did not experience subsequent infarction. CBF was decreased, $CMRO_2$ was normal, and OEF was increased, consistent with ischemia.[286] Another study found that with resolution of vasospasm, CBF increases.[307]

Studies of CBV in patients with SAH likewise have yielded conflicting results. Grubb et al[294] reported a statistically significant increase in CBV in patients with angiographic vasospasm and Hunt and Hess clinical grade III or IV in comparison with normal volunteers. OEF values were not reported, but examination of the CBF and $CMRO_2$ data indicates that OEF was probably not higher in the patients with vasospasm than in those without it. In a PET study of SAH, Hino et al[306] reported a significant increase in CBV in regions of symptomatic angiographic vasospasm. They did not, however, observe an elevation in regional OEF. In another PET study, regional CBF was lower than normal in regions with and without vasospasm in patients with SAH as well as in patients with ipsilateral carotid occlusion.[309] Regional OEF was higher both during vasospasm and distal to carotid occlusion than in SAH without vasospasm or in normal volunteers. Regional CBV was lower than normal in regions with and without spasm, whereas it was increased ipsilateral to carotid occlusion. These findings of reduced parenchymal CBV during vasospasm under similar conditions of tissue ischemia that produce increased CBV in patients with carotid occlusion were interpreted as evidence that parenchymal vessels distal to arteries with angiographic spasm after SAH do not demonstrate normal autoregulatory vasodilation. The reason for the discrepancies among these studies in the measurement of CBV during vasospasm is not clear but it may reflect the variability of CBV changes during reduced CPP noted earlier.[131]

Surgical retraction of brain tissue may have profound effects on cerebral metabolism. A small PET study before and after right frontotemporal craniotomies for clipping of ruptured anterior circulation aneurysms showed a 45% reduction in regional $CMRO_2$ and a 32% reduction in regional OEF without significant change in CBF in the region of retraction, but no change in the other hemisphere.[310] These changes indicate a primary reduction in metabolism and uncoupling of flow and metabolism (luxury perfusion). They are not suggestive of vasospasm, which produces diffuse changes respecting large vascular territories; these changes were focal in the area of retractor blade placement. Other studies have shown a reduction in CBF in the area of retraction.[311,312] In one of these, xenon 133 (^{133}Xe) SPECT CBF measurements were made in patients with frontal lesions including infarction an average of 82 days after surgery.[311] In two other studies, CBF was measured with technetium Tc 99m (^{99m}Tc) hexamethylpropyleneamine oxime (HMPAO).[312,313] Because ^{99m}Tc HMPAO requires intact metabolism for radiotracer uptake, this technique may produce artifactually low CBF when metabolism is reduced.[314]

Autoregulation

In the absence of ICH, hydrocephalus, infarction, and vasospasm, static cerebral autoregulation of CBF in response to changes in CPP is probably preserved after SAH.[297,298,315,316] Static autoregulation is defective in the majority of patients with angiographic vasospasm of large arteries following aneurysmal SAH in response to both decreases[297,298,315,317] and increases[318,319] in systemic arterial pressure. Static autoregulation is impaired even in those patients with slight vasospasm (25% to 50% reduction of arterial caliber).[315] Studies of dynamic autoregulation of CBF velocity have described abnormalities in the early period after SAH prior to vasospasm.[316,320]

Transcranial Doppler Measurement of Cerebral Blood Flow Velocity

Transcranial Doppler (TCD) ultrasonography shows that flow velocity in the MCA progressively increases after SAH from normal values of 30 to 80 cm/sec,[321] peaking at 7 to 10 days and normalizing over the following 2 weeks.[322]

In patients with lateralized aneurysms, the increase is higher on the side of the ruptured aneurysm.[323] Velocities in excess of 200 cm/sec are assumed to indicate a reduction in angiographic caliber of more than 50%.[322] Correlation between TCD ultrasonography–detected flow velocity (TCD velocity) and angiographic vessel caliber is good when the velocity is either low (< 120 cm/sec) or very high (≥ 200 cm/sec), but intermediate velocities, which are seen in over half of the patients, do not reliably predict degree of angiographic vasospasm.[324] Measurement of flow velocity in the anterior and posterior cerebral arteries is limited because these vessels have less favorable angles of insonation and a greater degree of collateral flow than the MCA. Additionally, the sensitivity of TCD ultrasonography for detecting vasospasm in the anterior cerebral artery is poor because of the possibility of increased flow across the anterior communicating artery.[322]

Using TCD velocity to diagnose and monitor large artery vasospasm presumes that any changes in velocity are due to changes in cross-sectional area of the artery. This assumption is invalid if there are changes in the volume of flow through the artery. Factors that may affect the volume of flow through the artery and confound the interpretation of TCD velocity include reduced CBF due to downstream tissue infarction, changes in collateral circulation, and hemodilution.[325] In addition, with severe vasospasm, volume flow may be reduced, resulting in a decrease in velocity with further reduction in vessel diameter.[326] As a consequence of these factors, there is a poor correlation between TCD velocity and CBF.[303,327-329] These confounding factors are a particular problem when TCD velocity is used to monitor treatment of vasospasm; increased velocities may be due to either worsening spasm or successful improvement in volume flow.[330]

Conclusions

Measurements of CBF and CMR in ischemia and infarction have provided valuable insight into the pathophysiology of cerebrovascular disease. Much has been learned about the compensatory responses of the brain to reductions in perfusion pressure and in the evolution of changes in blood flow and metabolism that occur when these mechanisms fail. Knowledge of these changes can help guide therapy when multiple factors such as ischemia, hypoxemia, hypocarbia, and hypotension may affect cerebral blood flow. An understanding of the hemodynamic effects of arterial stenosis or occlusion on the downstream perfusion pressure has been instrumental in the design of new trials for treatment.[331] In acute ischemic stroke, measurements of CBF and metabolism have been used to define the "ischemic penumbra" and to predict both tissue and clinical outcomes, although the clinical utility of these markers of ischemia in distinguishing viable from irreversibly damaged tissue in the acute period still requires further study.

Blood flow and metabolic studies in ICH have documented the integrity of autoregulation and suggested that hematomas exert a primary depression of metabolism rather than inducing ischemia in the surrounding tissue. This finding has important implications for future consideration of therapeutic interventions in this disease. Studies in SAH have differentiated the primary effects of the hemorrhage on cerebral hemodynamics and metabolism from those of vasospasm and surgical retraction. In addition, vasospasm-induced ischemia has been demonstrated to be reversible.

In summary, defining the pathophysiologic changes in CBF and metabolism in human cerebrovascular disease has provided and will continue to provide the basic foundation for development and testing of new treatment strategies.

Acknowledgments

This work was supported by USPHS grants NS42167, NS35966, NS044885 and the H. Houston Merritt Professorship of Neurology at the University of North Carolina at Chapel Hill.

REFERENCES

1. Kety SS, Schmidt CF: The determination of cerebral blood flow in man by the use of nitrous oxide in low concentrations, *J Clin Invest* 143:53-66, 1945.
2. Kety SS, Schmidt CF: The nitrous oxide method for the quantitative determination of cerebral blood flow in man: theory, procedure, and normal values, *J Clin Invest* 27:476-483, 1948.
3. Marcus ML, Heistad DD, Ehrhardt JC, et al: Total and regional cerebral blood flow measurement with 7-10-, 15-, 25-, and 50-mum microspheres, *J Appl Physiol* 40:501-507, 1976.
4. Kuhl DE, Barrio JR, Huang SC, et al: Quantifying local cerebral blood flow by N-isopropyl-p- [123I]iodoamphetamine (IMP) tomography, *J Nucl Med* 23:196-203, 1982.
5. Kety SS: Blood-tissue exchange methods: theory of blood-tissue exchange and its application to measurement of blood flow. In Bruner HD, editor: *Methods in medical research*, Chicago, 1960, The Year Book Medical, pp 223-236.
6. Zierler KL: Equations for measuring blood flow by external monitoring of radioisotopes, *Circ Res* 16:309-321, 1965.
7. Hoedt-Rasmussen K, Sveinsdottir E, Lassen NA: Regional cerebral blood flow in man determined by intra-arterial injection of radioactive inert gas, *Circ Res* 18:237-247, 1966.
8. Larson KB, Snyder DL: Measurement of relative blood flow, transit-time distributions and transport-model parameters by residue detection when radiotracer recirculates, *J Theor Biol* 37:503-529, 1972.
9. Zierler KL: Theoretical basis of indicator-dilution methods for measuring flow and volume, *Circ Res* 10:393-407, 1962.
10. Axel L: Cerebral blood flow determination by rapid-sequence computed tomography: theoretical analysis, *Radiology* 137:679-686, 1980.
11. Weisskoff RM, Chesler D, Boxerman JL, et al: Pitfalls in MR measurement of tissue blood flow with intravascular tracers: which mean transit time? *Magn Reson Med* 29:553-558, 1993.
12. Larson KB, Markham J, Raichle ME: Tracer-kinetic models for measuring cerebral blood flow using externally detected radiotracers, *J Cereb Blood Flow Metab* 7:443-463, 1987.
13. Powers WJ: Hemodynamics and metabolism in ischemic cerebrovascular disease, *Neurol Clin* 10:31-48, 1992.
14. Scheel P, Ruge C, Schoning M: Flow velocity and flow volume measurements in the extracranial carotid and vertebral arteries in healthy adults: reference data and the effects of age, *Ultrasound Med Biol* 26:1261-1266, 2000.
15. Kety SS: Human cerebral blood flow and oxygen consumption as related to aging, *J Chron Dis* 3:478-486, 1956.
16. Baron JC, Frackowiak RS, Herholz K, et al: Use of PET methods for measurement of cerebral energy metabolism and hemodynamics in cerebrovascular disease, *J Cereb Blood Flow Metab* 9:723-742, 1989.
17. Powers WJ, Raichle ME: Positron emission tomography and its application to the study of cerebrovascular disease in man, *Stroke* 16:361-376, 1985.
18. Lu H, van Zijl PC: Experimental measurement of extravascular parenchymal BOLD effects and tissue oxygen extraction fractions using multi-echo VASO fMRI at 1.5 and 3.0 T, *Magn Reson Med* 53:808-816, 2005.
19. Lee JM, Vo KD, An H, et al: Magnetic resonance cerebral metabolic rate of oxygen utilization in hyperacute stroke patients, *Ann Neurol* 53:227-232, 2003.
20. Zhu XH, Zhang Y, Zhang N, et al: Noninvasive and three-dimensional imaging of CMRO(2) in rats at 9.4 T: reproducibility test and normothermia/hypothermia comparison study, *J Cereb Blood Flow Metab* 27:1225-1234, 2007.
21. Lin AL, Fox PT, Yang Y, et al: Evaluation of MRI models in the measurement of CMRO(2) and its relationship with CBF, *Magn Reson Med* 60:380-389, 2008.
22. Rossen R, Kabat H, Anderson JP: Acute arrest of cerebral circulation in man, *Arch Neurol Psychiatry* 50:510-528, 1943.
23. Cohen PJ, Alexander SC, Smith TC, et al: Effects of hypoxia and normocarbia on cerebral blood flow and metabolism in conscious man, *J Appl Physiol* 23:183-189, 1967.
24. Madsen PL, Holm S, Herning M, et al: Average blood flow and oxygen uptake in the human brain during resting wakefulness: a critical appraisal of the Kety-Schmidt technique, *J Cereb Blood Flow Metab* 13:646-655, 1993.
25. Gottstein U, Bernsmeier A, Sedlmeyer I: Der kohlenhydratstoffwechsel des menschlichen gehirns, *Klin Wochenschr* 41:943-948, 1963.
26. Scheinberg P, Stead EA: The cerebral blood flow in male subjects as measured by the nitrous oxide technique: normal values for blood flow, oxygen utilization, glucose utilization and peripheral resistance, with observations on the effect of tilting and anxiety, *J Clin Invest* 28:1163-1171, 1949.
27. Glenn TC, Kelly DF, Boscardin WJ, et al: Energy dysfunction as a predictor of outcome after moderate or severe head injury: indices of oxygen, glucose, and lactate metabolism, *J Cereb Blood Flow Metab* 23:1239-1250, 2003.
28. McHenry LC Jr, Merory J, Bass E, et al: Xenon-133 inhalation method for regional cerebral blood flow measurements: normal values and test-retest results, *Stroke* 9:396-399, 1978.
29. Altman DI, Perlman JM, Volpe JJ, et al: Cerebral oxygen metabolism in newborns, *Pediatrics* 92:99-104, 1993.
30. Meek JH, Tyszczuk L, Elwell CE, et al: Cerebral blood flow increases over the first three days of life in extremely preterm neonates, *Arch Dis Child Fetal Neonatal Ed* 78:F33-F37, 1998.
31. Pellicer A, Valverde E, Gaya F, et al: Postnatal adaptation of brain circulation in preterm infants, *Pediatr Neurol* 24:103-109, 2001.
32. Greisen G, Pryds O, Low CBF: Discontinuous EEG activity, and periventricular brain injury in ill, preterm neonates, *Brain Dev* 11:164-168, 1989.
33. Wintermark M, Lepori D, Cotting J, et al: Brain perfusion in children: Evolution with age assessed by quantitative perfusion computed tomography, *Pediatrics* 113:1642-1652, 2004.
34. Miranda MJ, Olofsson K, Sidaros K: Noninvasive measurements of regional cerebral perfusion in preterm and term neonates by magnetic resonance arterial spin labeling, *Pediatr Res* 60:359-363, 2006.
35. Altman DI, Powers WJ, Perlman JM, et al: Cerebral blood flow requirement for brain viability in newborn infants is lower than in adults, *Ann Neurol* 24:218-226, 1988.
36. Elwell CE, Henty JR, Leung TS, et al: Measurement of CMRO(2) in neonates undergoing intensive care using near infrared spectroscopy, *Adv Exp Med Biol* 566:263-268, 2005.
37. Powers WJ, Rosenbaum JL, Dence CS, et al: Cerebral glucose transport and metabolism in preterm human infants, *J Cereb Blood Flow Metab* 18:632-638, 1998.
38. Kinnala A, Suhonen-Polvi H, Aarimaa T, et al: Cerebral metabolic rate for glucose during the first six months of life: an FDG positron emission tomography study, *Arch Dis Child Fetal Neonatal Ed* 74:F153-F157, 1996.
39. Suhonen-Polvi H, Ruotsalainen U, Kinnala A, et al: FDG-PET in early infancy: simplified quantification methods to measure cerebral glucose utilization, *J Nucl Med* 36:1249-1254, 1995.
40. Kennedy C, Sokoloff L: An adaptation of the nitrous oxide method to the study of the cerebral circulation in children: normal values for cerebral blood flow and cerebral metabolic rate in childhood, *J Clin Invest* 36:1130-1137, 1957.

41. Chiron C, Raynaud C, Maziere B, et al: Changes in regional cerebral blood flow during brain maturation in children and adolescents, *J Nucl Med* 33:696-703, 1992.

42. Ogawa A, Nakamura K, Sugita Y, et al: Regional cerebral blood flow in children: normal values and regional distribution of cerebral blood flow in childhood, *J Cereb Blood Flow Metab* 5(Suppl 1): S97-S98, 1985.

43. Ogawa A, Sakurai Y, Kayama T, et al: Regional cerebral blood flow with age: changes in rCBF in childhood, *Neurol Res* 11:173-176, 1989.

44. Chugani HT, Phelps ME: Maturational changes in cerebral function in infants determined by [18]FDG positron emission tomography, *Science* 231:840-843, 1986.

45. Chugani HT, Phelps ME, Mazziotta JC: Positron emission tomography study of human brain functional development, *Ann Neurol* 22:487-497, 1987.

46. Leenders KL, Perani D, Lammertsma AA, et al: Cerebral blood flow, blood volume and oxygen utilization. Normal values and effect of age, *Brain* 113:27-47, 1990.

47. Pantano P, Baron JC, Lebrun-Grandie P, et al: Regional cerebral blood flow and oxygen consumption in human aging, *Stroke* 15:635-641, 1984.

48. Dastur DK: Cerebral blood flow and metabolism in normal human aging, pathological aging, and senile dementia, *J Cereb Blood Flow Metab* 5:1-9, 1985.

49. Kuhl DE, Metter EJ, Riege WH, et al: The effect of normal aging on patterns of local cerebral glucose utilization, *Ann Neurol* 15(Suppl):S133-S137, 1984.

50. Marchal G, Rioux P, Petit-Taboue MC, et al: Regional cerebral oxygen consumption, blood flow, and blood volume in healthy human aging, *Arch Neurol* 49:1013-1020, 1992.

51. Yamaguchi T, Kanno I, Uemura K, et al: Reduction in regional cerebral metabolic rate of oxygen during human aging, *Stroke* 17:1220-1228, 1986.

52. de Leon MJ, George AE, Ferris SH, et al: Positron emission tomography and computed tomography assessments of the aging human brain, *J Comput Assist Tomogr* 8:88-94, 1984.

53. Duara R, Margolin RA, Robertson-Tchabo EA, et al: Cerebral glucose utilization, as measured with positron emission tomography in 21 resting healthy men between the ages of 21 and 83 years, *Brain* 106:761-775, 1983.

54. Duara R, Grady C, Haxby J, et al: Human brain glucose utilization and cognitive function in relation to age, *Ann Neurol* 16:703-713, 1984.

55. Yoshii F, Barker WW, Chang JY, et al: Sensitivity of cerebral glucose metabolism to age, gender, brain volume, brain atrophy, and cerebrovascular risk factors, *J Cereb Blood Flow Metab* 8:654-661, 1988.

56. Meltzer CC, Cantwell MN, Greer PJ, et al: Does cerebral blood flow decline in healthy aging? A PET study with partial-volume correction, *J Nucl Med* 41:1842-1848, 2000.

57. Ibanez V, Pietrini P, Furey ML, et al: Resting state brain glucose metabolism is not reduced in normotensive healthy men during aging, after correction for brain atrophy, *Brain Res Bull* 63:147-154, 2004.

58. Lebrun-Grandie P, Baron JC, Soussaline F, et al: Coupling between regional blood flow and oxygen utilization in the normal human brain: A study with positron tomography and oxygen 15, *Arch Neurol* 40:230-236, 1983.

59. Baron JC, Rougemont D, Soussaline F, et al: Local interrelationships of cerebral oxygen consumption and glucose utilization in normal subjects and in ischemic stroke patients: a positron tomography study, *J Cereb Blood Flow Metab* 4:140-149, 1984.

60. Sette G, Baron JC, Mazoyer B, et al: Local brain haemodynamics and oxygen metabolism in cerebrovascular disease. Positron emission tomography, *Brain* 112:931-951, 1989.

61. Frackowiak RS, Lenzi GL, Jones T, et al: Quantitative measurement of regional cerebral blood flow and oxygen metabolism in man using [15]O and positron emission tomography: theory, procedure, and normal values, *J Comput Assist Tomogr* 4:727-736, 1980.

62. Powers WJ, Grubb RL Jr, Darriet D, et al: Cerebral blood flow and cerebral metabolic rate of oxygen requirements for cerebral function and viability in humans, *J Cereb Blood Flow Metab* 5:600-608, 1985.

63. Wise RJ, Rhodes CG, Gibbs JM, et al: Disturbance of oxidative metabolism of glucose in recent human cerebral infarcts, *Ann Neurol* 14:627-637, 1983.

64. Astrup J, Sorensen PM, Sorensen HR: Oxygen and glucose consumption related to Na^+-K^+ transport in canine brain, *Stroke* 12:726-730, 1981.

65. Bering EA Jr, Taren JA, McMurrey JD, et al: Studies on hypothermia in monkeys. II: The effect of hypothermia on the general physiology and cerebral metabolism of monkeys in the hypothermic state, *Surg Gynecol Obstet* 102:134-138, 1956.

66. Nilsson L, Siesjo BK: The effect of phenobarbitone anaesthesia on blood flow and oxygen consumption in the rat brain, *Acta Anaesthesiol Scand Suppl* 57:18-24, 1975.

67. Sokoloff L: Relationships among local functional activity, energy metabolism, and blood flow in the central nervous system, *Fed Proc* 40:2311-2316, 1981.

68. Fox PT, Raichle ME: Focal physiological uncoupling of cerebral blood flow and oxidative metabolism during somatosensory stimulation in human subjects, *Proc Natl Acad Sci U S A* 83:1140-1144, 1986.

69. Fox PT, Raichle ME, Mintun MA, et al: Nonoxidative glucose consumption during focal physiologic neural activity, *Science* 241:462-464, 1988.

70. Kety SS, Schmidt CF: The effects of active and passive hyperventilation on cerebral blood flow, cerebral oxygen consumption, cardiac output, and blood pressure of normal young men, *J Clin Invest* 25:107-119, 1946.

71. Kety SS, Schmidt CF: The effects of altered arterial tensions of carbon dioxide and oxygen on cerebral blood flow and cerebral oxygen consumption of normal young men, *J Clin Invest* 27:484-492, 1948.

72. Wollman H, Smith TC, Stephen GW, et al: Effects of extremes of respiratory and metabolic alkalosis on cerebral blood flow in man, *J Appl Physiol* 24:60-65, 1968.

73. Fencl V, Vale JR, Broch JA: Respiration and cerebral blood flow in metabolic acidosis and alkalosis in humans, *J Appl Physiol* 27:67-76, 1969.

74. Raichle ME, Posner JB, Plum F: Cerebral blood flow during and after hyperventilation, *Arch Neurol* 23:394-403, 1970.

75. Alexander SC, Smith TC, Strobel G, et al: Cerebral carbohydrate metabolism of man during respiratory and metabolic alkalosis, *J Appl Physiol* 24:66-72, 1968.

76. van Rijen PC, Luyten PR, van der Sprenkel JW, et al: ^{1}H and ^{31}P NMR measurement of cerebral lactate, high-energy phosphate levels, and pH in humans during voluntary hyperventilation: associated EEG, capnographic, and Doppler findings, *Magn Reson Med* 10:182-193, 1989.

77. Shimojyo S, Scheinberg P, Kogure K, et al: The effects of graded hypoxia upon transient cerebral blood flow and oxygen consumption, *Neurology* 18:127-133, 1968.

78. Buck A, Schirlo C, Jasinsky V, et al: Changes of cerebral blood flow during short-term exposure to normobaric hypoxia, *J Cereb Blood Flow Metab* 18:906-910, 1998.

79. Lassen NA: Cerebral blood flow and oxygen consumption in man, *Physiol Rev* 39:183-238, 1959.

80. Brown MM, Wade JP, Marshall J: Fundamental importance of arterial oxygen content in the regulation of cerebral blood flow in man, *Brain* 108:81-93, 1985.

81. Lambertsen CJ, Kough RH, Cooper DY, et al: Oxygen toxicity: Effects in man of oxygen inhalation at 1 and 3.5 atmospheres upon blood gas transport, cerebral circulation and cerebral metabolism, *J Appl Physiol* 5:471-486, 1953.

82. Todd MM, Wu B, Maktabi M, et al: Cerebral blood flow and oxygen delivery during hypoxemia and hemodilution: role of arterial oxygen content, *Am J Physiol* 267:H2025-H2031, 1994.

83. Mintun MA, Lundstrom BN, Snyder AZ, et al: Blood flow and oxygen delivery to human brain during functional activity: theoretical modeling and experimental data, *Proc Natl Acad Sci U S A* 98:6859-6864, 2001.

84. Thomas DJ, Marshall J, Russell RW, et al: Effect of haematocrit on cerebral blood-flow in man, *Lancet* 2:941-943, 1977.

85. Brown MM, Marshall J: Regulation of cerebral blood flow in response to changes in blood viscosity, *Lancet* 1:604-609, 1985.

86. Brown MM, Marshall J: Effect of plasma exchange on blood viscosity and cerebral blood flow, *Br Med J (Clin Res Ed)* 284:1733-1736, 1982.

87. Paulson OB, Parving HH, Olesen J, et al: Influence of carbon monoxide and of hemodilution on cerebral blood flow and blood gases in man, *J Appl Physiol* 35:111-116, 1973.

88. Tomiyama Y, Brian JE Jr, Todd MM: Plasma viscosity and cerebral blood flow, *Am J Physiol Heart Circ Physiol* 279:H1949-H1954, 2000.

89. Rebel A, Lenz C, Krieter H, et al: Oxygen delivery at high blood viscosity and decreased arterial oxygen content to brains of conscious rats, *Am J Physiol Heart Circ Physiol* 280:H2591-H2597, 2001.

90. Cole DJ, Drummond JC, Patel PM, et al: Effects of viscosity and oxygen content on cerebral blood flow in ischemic and normal rat brain, *J Neurol Sci* 124:15-20, 1994.

91. Powers WJ, Boyle PJ, Hirsch IB, et al: Unaltered cerebral blood flow during hypoglycemic activation of the sympathochromaffin system in humans, *Am J Physiol* 265:R883-R887, 1993.

92. Boyle PJ, Nagy RJ, O'Connor AM, et al: Adaptation in brain glucose uptake following recurrent hypoglycemia, *Proc Natl Acad Sci U S A* 91:9352-9356, 1994.

93. Gottstein U, Held K: The effect of insulin on brain metabolism in metabolically healthy and diabetic patients, *Klin Wochenschr* 45:18-23, 1967.

94. Boyle PJ, Kempers SF, O'Connor AM, et al: Brain glucose uptake and unawareness of hypoglycemia in patients with insulin-dependent diabetes mellitus, *N Engl J Med* 333:1726-1731, 1995.

95. Teves D, Videen TO, Cryer PE, et al: Activation of human medial prefrontal cortex during autonomic responses to hypoglycemia, *Proc Natl Acad Sci U S A* 101:6217-6221, 2004.

96. Tallroth G, Ryding E, Agardh CD: Regional cerebral blood flow in normal man during insulin-induced hypoglycemia and in the recovery period following glucose infusion, *Metabolism* 41:717-721, 1992.

97. Tallroth G, Ryding E, Agardh CD: The influence of hypoglycaemia on regional cerebral blood flow and cerebral volume in type 1 (insulin-dependent) diabetes mellitus, *Diabetologia* 36:530-535, 1993.

98. Neil HA, Gale EA, Hamilton SJ, et al: Cerebral blood flow increases during insulin-induced hypoglycaemia in type 1 (insulin-dependent) diabetic patients and control subjects, *Diabetologia* 30:305-309, 1987.

99. Kerr D, Stanley JC, Barron M, et al: Symmetry of cerebral blood flow and cognitive responses to hypoglycaemia in humans, *Diabetologia* 36:73-78, 1993.

100. Eckert B, Ryding E, Agardh CD: Sustained elevation of cerebral blood flow after hypoglycaemia in normal man, *Diabetes Res Clin Pract* 40:91-100, 1998.

101. Chen JL, Wei L, Acuff V, et al: Slightly altered permeability-surface area products imply some cerebral capillary recruitment during hypercapnia, *Microvasc Res* 48:190-211, 1994.

102. Chen JL, Wei L, Bereczki D, et al: Nicotine raises the influx of permeable solutes across the rat blood-brain barrier with little or no capillary recruitment, *J Cereb Blood Flow Metab* 15:687-698, 1995.

103. Derrer SA, Sieber FE, Saudek CD, et al: Cerebrovascular and metabolic responses to hypoxia during hypoglycemia in dogs, *Am J Physiol* 258:H400-H407, 1990.

104. Sieber FE, Koehler RC, Derrer SA, et al: Hypoglycemia and cerebral autoregulation in anesthetized dogs, *Am J Physiol* 258:H1714-H1721, 1990.

105. MacKenzie ET, Farrar JK, Fitch W, et al: Effects of hemorrhagic hypotension on the cerebral circulation. I: Cerebral blood flow and pial arteriolar caliber, *Stroke* 10:711-718, 1979.

106. Symon L, Pasztor E, Dorsch NW, et al: Physiological responses of local areas of the cerebral circulation in experimental primates determined by the method of hydrogen clearance, *Stroke* 4:632-642, 1973.

107. Strandgaard S: Autoregulation of cerebral blood flow in hypertensive patients: The modifying influence of prolonged antihypertensive treatment on the tolerance to acute, drug-induced hypotension, *Circulation* 53:720-727, 1976.

108. Schmidt JF, Waldemar G, Vorstrup S, et al: Computerized analysis of cerebral blood flow autoregulation in humans: validation of a method for pharmacologic studies, *J Cardiovasc Pharmacol* 15:983-988, 1990.

109. Strandgaard S, Olesen J, Skinhoj E, et al: Autoregulation of brain circulation in severe arterial hypertension, *Br Med J* 1:507-510, 1973.

110. Dirnagl U, Pulsinelli W: Autoregulation of cerebral blood flow in experimental focal brain ischemia, *J Cereb Blood Flow Metab* 10:327-336, 1990.

111. Heistad DD, Kontos HE: Cerebral circulation. In Shepherd JT, Aboud FM, editors: *Handbook of physiology, Sect 2,* Vol 3, Bethesda, MD, 1983, American Physiological Society, Pt 1, pp 137-182.

112. van Beek AH, Claassen JA, Rikkert MG, et al: Cerebral autoregulation: an overview of current concepts and methodology with special focus on the elderly, *J Cereb Blood Flow Metab* 28:1071-1085, 2008.

113. Dawson SL, Panerai RB, Potter JF: Serial changes in static and dynamic cerebral autoregulation after acute ischaemic stroke, *Cerebrovasc Dis* 16:69-75, 2003.

114. Steiner LA, Coles JP, Johnston AJ, et al: Assessment of cerebrovascular autoregulation in head-injured patients: a validation study, *Stroke* 34:2404-2409, 2003.

115. Powers WJ: Cerebral hemodynamics in ischemic cerebrovascular disease, *Ann Neurol* 29:231-240, 1991.

116. Schumann P, Touzani O, Young AR, et al: Evaluation of the ratio of cerebral blood flow to cerebral blood volume as an index of local cerebral perfusion pressure, *Brain* 121:1369-1379, 1998.

117. Maruyama M, Shimoji K, Ichikawa T, et al: The effects of extreme hemodilutions on the autoregulation of cerebral blood flow, electroencephalogram and cerebral metabolic rate of oxygen in the dog, *Stroke* 16:675-679, 1985.

118. Haggendal E, Johansson B: Effect of arterial carbon dioxide tension and oxygen saturation on cerebral blood flow autoregulation in dogs, *Acta Physiol Scand* 66:27-53, 1965.

119. Fog M: Cerebral circulation: The reaction of pial arteries to a fall in blood pressure, *Arch Neurol Psychiatry* 37:351-364, 1937.

120. Wolfe HG, Forbes HS: The cerebral circulation V: Observations of the pial circulation during changes in intracranial pressure, *Arch Neurol Psychiatry* 20:1035-1047, 1928.

121. Kato Y, Mokry M, Pucher R, et al: Cerebrovascular response to changes of cerebral venous pressure and cerebrospinal fluid pressure, *Acta Neurochir (Wien)* 109:52-56, 1991.

122. Wiedeman MP: Dimensions of blood vessels from distributing artery to collecting vein, *Circ Res* 12:375-378, 1963.

123. Hilal SK: Cerebral hemodynamics assessed by angiography. In Newton TH, Potts DG, editors: *Radiology of the skull and brain: angiography,* vol 2, book 1, St. Louis, 1974, CV Mosby.

124. Auer LM, Ishiyama N, Pucher R: Cerebrovascular response to intracranial hypertension, *Acta Neurochir (Wien)* 84:124-128, 1987.

125. Kato Y, Auer LM: Cerebrovascular response to elevation of ventricular pressure, *Acta Neurochir (Wien)* 98:184-188, 1989.

126. Grubb RL Jr, Phelps ME, Raichle ME, et al: The effects of arterial blood pressure on the regional cerebral blood volume by X-ray fluorescence, *Stroke* 4:390-399, 1973.

127. Grubb RL Jr, Raichle ME, Phelps ME, et al: Effects of increased intracranial pressure on cerebral blood volume, blood flow, and oxygen utilization in monkeys, *J Neurosurg* 43:385-398, 1975.

128. Ferrari M, Wilson DA, Hanley DF, et al: Effects of graded hypotension on cerebral blood flow, blood volume, and mean transit time in dogs, *Am J Physiol* 262:H1908-H1914, 1992.

129. Grubb RL Jr, Derdeyn CP, Fritsch SM, et al: Importance of hemodynamic factors in the prognosis of symptomatic carotid occlusion, *JAMA* 280:1055-1060, 1998.

130. Zaharchuk G, Mandeville JB, Bogdanov AA Jr, et al: Cerebrovascular dynamics of autoregulation and hypoperfusion: An MRI study of CBF and changes in total and microvascular cerebral blood volume during hemorrhagic hypotension, *Stroke* 30:2197-2204, 1999.

131. Derdeyn CP, Videen TO, Yundt KD, et al: Variability of cerebral blood volume and oxygen extraction: stages of cerebral hemodynamic impairment revisited, *Brain* 125:595-607, 2002.

132. Gibbs JM, Wise RJ, Leenders KL, et al: Evaluation of cerebral perfusion reserve in patients with carotid-artery occlusion, *Lancet* 1:310-314, 1984.

133. Powers WJ: Is the ratio of cerebral blood volume to cerebral blood flow a reliable indicator of cerebral perfusion pressure? *J Cereb Blood Flow Metab* 13(Suppl 1):S325, 1993.

134. Grubb RL Jr, Raichle ME, Eichling JO, et al: The effects of changes in $PaCO_2$ on cerebral blood volume, blood flow, and vascular mean transit time, *Stroke* 5:630-639, 1974.

135. Sillesen H, Schroeder T, Steenberg HJ, et al: Doppler examination of the periorbital arteries adds valuable hemodynamic information in carotid artery disease, *Ultrasound Med Biol* 13:177-181, 1987.

136. Henderson RD, Eliasziw M, Fox AJ, et al: Angiographically defined collateral circulation and risk of stroke in patients with severe carotid artery stenosis. North American Symptomatic Carotid Endarterectomy Trial (NASCET) Group, *Stroke* 31:128-132, 2000.

137. Vernieri F, Pasqualetti P, Matteis M, et al: Effect of collateral blood flow and cerebral vasomotor reactivity on the outcome of carotid artery occlusion, *Stroke* 32:1552-1558, 2001.

138. Klijn CJ, Kappelle LJ, van Huffelen AC, et al: Recurrent ischemia in symptomatic carotid occlusion: prognostic value of hemodynamic factors, *Neurology* 55:1806-1812, 2000.

139. Derdeyn CP, Shaibani A, Moran CJ, et al: Lack of correlation between pattern of collateralization and misery perfusion in patients with carotid occlusion, *Stroke* 30:1025-1032, 1999.

140. Yamauchi H, Kudoh T, Sugimoto K, et al: Pattern of collaterals, type of infarcts, and haemodynamic impairment in carotid artery occlusion, *J Neurol Neurosurg Psychiatry* 75:1697-1701, 2004.

141. Lassen NA, Palvolgyi R: Cerebral steal during hypercapnia and the inverse reaction during hypocapnia observed with the ^{133}xenon technique in man, *Scand J Clin Lab Invest* 22(Suppl 102):13D, 1968.

142. Oja JM, Gillen JS, Kauppinen RA, et al: Determination of oxygen extraction ratios by magnetic resonance imaging, *J Cereb Blood Flow Metab* 19:1289-1295, 1999.

143. An H, Lin W, Celik A, et al: Quantitative measurements of cerebral metabolic rate of oxygen utilization using MRI: a volunteer study, *NMR Biomed* 14:441-447, 2001.

144. Powers WJ, Press GA, Grubb RL Jr, et al: The effect of hemodynamically significant carotid artery disease on the hemodynamic status of the cerebral circulation, *Ann Intern Med* 106:27-34, 1987.

145. Kuroda S, Shiga T, Ishikawa T, et al: Reduced blood flow and preserved vasoreactivity characterize oxygen hypometabolism due to incomplete infarction in occlusive carotid artery diseases, *J Nucl Med* 45:943-949, 2004.

146. Baron JC, Bousser MG, Comar D, Kellershohn C: Human hemispheric infarction studied by positron emission tomography and the ^{15}O continuous inhalation technique. In Caille JM, Salamon G, editors: *Computerized tomography*, New York, 1980, Springer-Verlag, pp 231-237.

147. Baron JC, Bousser MG, Rey A, et al: Reversal of focal "misery-perfusion syndrome" by extra-intracranial arterial bypass in hemodynamic cerebral ischemia: A case study with ^{15}O positron emission tomography, *Stroke* 12:454-459, 1981.

148. Kazumata K, Tanaka N, Ishikawa T, et al: Dissociation of vasoreactivity to acetazolamide and hypercapnia: Comparative study in patients with chronic occlusive major cerebral artery disease, *Stroke* 27:2052-2058, 1996.

149. Inao S, Tadokoro M, Nishino M, et al: Neural activation of the brain with hemodynamic insufficiency, *J Cereb Blood Flow Metab* 18:960-967, 1998.

150. Pindzola RR, Balzer JR, Nemoto EM, et al: Cerebrovascular reserve in patients with carotid occlusive disease assessed by stable xenon-enhanced CT cerebral blood flow and transcranial Doppler, *Stroke* 32:1811-1817, 2001.

151. Hirano T, Minematsu K, Hasegawa Y, et al: Acetazolamide reactivity on ^{123}I-IMP single photon emission computed tomography in patients with major cerebral artery occlusive disease: correlation with positron emission tomography parameters, *J Cereb Blood Flow Metab* 14:763-770, 1994.

152. Nariai T, Suzuki R, Hirakawa K, et al: Vascular reserve in chronic cerebral ischemia measured by the acetazolamide challenge test: comparison with positron emission tomography, *AJNR Am J Neuroradiol* 16:563-570, 1995.

153. Webster MW, Makaroun MS, Steed DL, et al: Compromised cerebral blood flow reactivity is a predictor of stroke in patients with symptomatic carotid artery occlusive disease, *J Vasc Surg* 21:338-344, 1995.

154. Yokota C, Hasegawa Y, Minematsu K, et al: Effect of acetazolamide reactivity on long-term outcome in patients with major cerebral artery occlusive diseases, *Stroke* 29:640-644, 1998.

155. Vernieri F, Pasqualetti P, Passarelli F, et al: Outcome of carotid artery occlusion is predicted by cerebrovascular reactivity, *Stroke* 30:593-598, 1999.

156. Yonas H, Smith HA, Durham SR, et al: Increased stroke risk predicted by compromised cerebral blood flow reactivity, *J Neurosurg* 79:483-489, 1993.

157. Ogasawara K, Ogawa A, Terasaki K, et al: Use of cerebrovascular reactivity in patients with symptomatic major cerebral artery occlusion to predict 5-year outcome: comparison of xenon-133 and iodine-123-IMP single-photon emission computed tomography, *J Cereb Blood Flow Metab* 22:1142-1148, 2002.

158. Ogasawara K, Ogawa A, Yoshimoto T: Cerebrovascular reactivity to acetazolamide and outcome in patients with symptomatic internal carotid or middle cerebral artery occlusion: a xenon-133 single-photon emission computed tomography study, *Stroke* 33:1857-1862, 2002.

159. Vernieri F, Pasqualetti P, Matteis M, et al: Effect of collateral blood flow and cerebral vasomotor reactivity on the outcome of carotid artery occlusion, *Stroke* 32:1552-1558, 2001.

160. Yamauchi H, Fukuyama H, Nagahama Y, et al: Evidence of misery perfusion and risk for recurrent stroke in major cerebral arterial occlusive diseases from PET, *J Neurol Neurosurg Psychiatry* 61:18-25, 1996.

161. Yamauchi H, Fukuyama H, Nagahama Y, et al: Significance of increased oxygen extraction fraction in five-year prognosis of major cerebral arterial occlusive diseases, *J Nucl Med* 40:1992-1998, 1999.

162. Symon L, Branston NM, Strong AJ: Autoregulation in acute focal ischemia: an experimental study, *Stroke* 7:547-554, 1976.

163. Giffard C, Young AR, Kerrouche N, et al: Outcome of acutely ischemic brain tissue in prolonged middle cerebral artery occlusion: a serial positron emission tomography investigation in the baboon, *J Cereb Blood Flow Metab* 24:495-508, 2004.

164. Kuge Y, Yokota C, Tagaya M, et al: Serial changes in cerebral blood flow and flow-metabolism uncoupling in primates with acute thromboembolic stroke, *J Cereb Blood Flow Metab* 21:202-210, 2001.

165. Sakoh M, Ostergaard L, Rohl L, et al: Relationship between residual cerebral blood flow and oxygen metabolism as predictive of ischemic tissue viability: sequential multitracer positron emission tomography scanning of middle cerebral artery occlusion during the critical first 6 hours after stroke in pigs, *J Neurosurg* 93:647-657, 2000.

166. Pappata S, Fiorelli M, Rommel T, et al: PET study of changes in local brain hemodynamics and oxygen metabolism after unilateral middle cerebral artery occlusion in baboons, *J Cereb Blood Flow Metab* 13:416-424, 1993.

167. Heiss WD, Graf R, Wienhard K, et al: Dynamic penumbra demonstrated by sequential multitracer PET after middle cerebral artery occlusion in cats, *J Cereb Blood Flow Metab* 14:892-902, 1994.

168. Touzani O, Young AR, Derlon JM, et al: Sequential studies of severely hypometabolic tissue volumes after permanent middle cerebral artery occlusion: A positron emission tomographic investigation in anesthetized baboons, *Stroke* 26:2112-2119, 1995.

169. Ackerman RH, Lev MH, Mackay BC, et al: PET studies in acute stroke: Findings and relevance to therapy, *J Cereb Blood Flow Metab* 9(Suppl 1):S359, 1989.

170. Heiss WD, Huber M, Fink GR, et al: Progressive derangement of periinfarct viable tissue in ischemic stroke, *J Cereb Blood Flow Metab* 12:193-203, 1992.

171. Molina CA, Montaner J, Abilleira S, et al: Timing of spontaneous recanalization and risk of hemorrhagic transformation in acute cardioembolic stroke, *Stroke* 32:1079-1084, 2001.

172. Jorgensen HS, Sperling B, Nakayama H, et al: Spontaneous reperfusion of cerebral infarcts in patients with acute stroke: Incidence, time course, and clinical outcome in the Copenhagen Stroke Study, *Arch Neurol* 51:865-873, 1994.

173. Lassen NA: The luxury-perfusion syndrome and its possible relation to acute metabolic acidosis localised within the brain, *Lancet* 2:1113-1115, 1966.

174. Lenzi GL, Frackowiak RS, Jones T: Cerebral oxygen metabolism and blood flow in human cerebral ischemic infarction, *J Cereb Blood Flow Metab* 2:321-335, 1982.

175. Hakim AM, Pokrupa RP, Villanueva J, et al: The effect of spontaneous reperfusion on metabolic function in early human cerebral infarcts, *Ann Neurol* 21:279-289, 1987.

176. Marchal G, Serrati C, Rioux P, et al: PET imaging of cerebral perfusion and oxygen consumption in acute ischaemic stroke: relation to outcome, *Lancet* 341:925-927, 1993.

177. Baron JC, Bousser MG, Comar D, et al: Noninvasive tomographic study of cerebral blood flow and oxygen metabolism in vivo: Potentials, limitations, and clinical applications in cerebral ischemic disorders, *Eur Neurol* 20:273-284, 1981.

178. Furlan M, Marchal G, Viader F, et al: Spontaneous neurological recovery after stroke and the fate of the ischemic penumbra, *Ann Neurol* 40:216-226, 1996.

179. Shimosegawa E, Hatazawa J, Ibaraki M, et al: Metabolic penumbra of acute brain infarction: a correlation with infarct growth, *Ann Neurol* 57:495-504, 2005.

180. Hawkins RA, Phelps ME, Huang SC, et al: Effect of ischemia on quantification of local cerebral glucose metabolic rate in man, *J Cereb Blood Flow Metab* 1:37-51, 1981.

181. Gjedde A, Wienhard K, Heiss WD, et al: Comparative regional analysis of 2-fluorodeoxyglucose and methylglucose uptake in brain of four stroke patients: With special reference to the regional estimation of the lumped constant, *J Cereb Blood Flow Metab* 5:163-178, 1985.

182. Nedergaard M: Spreading depression as a contributor to ischemic brain damage, *Adv Neurol* 71:75-83, 1996.

183. Nedergaard M, Astrup J: Infarct rim: effect of hyperglycemia on direct current potential and [14C]2-deoxyglucose phosphorylation, *J Cereb Blood Flow Metab* 6:607-615, 1986.

184. Hossmann KA: Viability thresholds and the penumbra of focal ischemia, *Ann Neurol* 36:557-565, 1994.

185. Paulson OB, Lassen NA, Skinhoj E: Regional cerebral blood flow in apoplexy without arterial occlusion, *Neurology* 20:125-138, 1970.

186. Paulson OB: Regional cerebral blood flow in apoplexy due to occlusion of the middle cerebral artery, *Neurology* 20:63-77, 1970.

187. Agnoli A, Fieschi C, Bozzao L, et al: Autoregulation of cerebral blood flow: Studies during drug-induced hypertension in normal subjects and in patients with cerebral vascular diseases, *Circulation* 38:800-812, 1968.

188. Nazir FS, Overell JR, Bolster A, et al: Effect of perindopril on cerebral and renal perfusion on normotensives in mild early ischaemic stroke: a randomized controlled trial, *Cerebrovasc Dis* 19:77-83, 2005.

189. Nazir FS, Overell JR, Bolster A, et al: The effect of losartan on global and focal cerebral perfusion and on renal function in hypertensives in mild early ischaemic stroke, *J Hypertens* 22:989-995, 2004.

190. Pozzilli C, Di PV, Pantano P, et al: Influence of nimodipine on cerebral blood flow in human cerebral ischaemia, *J Neurol* 236:199-202, 1989.

191. Powers WJ, Zazulia AR, Diringer MN, et al: Effect of blood pressure reduction on regional cerebral blood flow in acute ischemic stroke, *Stroke* 38:506, 2007.

192. Fieschi C, Lenzi GL: Cerebral blood flow and metabolism in stroke patients. In Russell RWR, editor: *Vascular disease of the central nervous system*, New York, 1983, Churchill Livingstone, pp 101-127.

193. Meyer JS, Shimazu K, Fukuuchi Y, et al: Impaired neurogenic cerebrovascular control and dysautoregulation after stroke, *Stroke* 4:169-186, 1973.

194. Heiss WD, Rosner G: Functional recovery of cortical neurons as related to degree and duration of ischemia, *Ann Neurol* 14:294-301, 1983.

195. Marks MP, O'Donahue J, Fabricant JI, et al: Cerebral blood flow evaluation of arteriovenous malformations with stable xenon CT, *Am J Neuroradiol* 9:1169-1175, 1988.

196. Hossmann KA: Pathophysiology and therapy of experimental stroke, *Cell Mol Neurobiol* 26:1057-1083, 2006.

197. Crockard HA, Gadian DG, Frackowiak RS, et al: Acute cerebral ischaemia: concurrent changes in cerebral blood flow, energy metabolites, pH, and lactate measured with hydrogen clearance and 31P and 1H nuclear magnetic resonance spectroscopy. II: Changes during ischaemia, *J Cereb Blood Flow Metab* 7:394-402, 1987.

198. Astrup J, Symon L, Branston NM, et al: Cortical evoked potential and extracellular K+ and H+ at critical levels of brain ischemia, *Stroke* 8:51-57, 1977.

199. Marcoux FW, Morawetz RB, Crowell RM, et al: Differential regional vulnerability in transient focal cerebral ischemia, *Stroke* 13:339-346, 1982.

200. Sundt TM Jr, Sharbrough FW, Piepgras DG, et al: Correlation of cerebral blood flow and electroencephalographic changes during carotid endarterectomy: with results of surgery and hemodynamics of cerebral ischemia, *Mayo Clin Proc* 56:533-543, 1981.

201. Jones TH, Morawetz RB, Crowell RM, et al: Thresholds of focal cerebral ischemia in awake monkeys, *J Neurosurg* 54:773-782, 1981.

202. Morawetz RB, Crowell RH, DeGirolami U, et al: Regional cerebral blood flow thresholds during cerebral ischemia, *Fed Proc* 38:2493-2494, 1979.

203. Crowell RM, Marcoux FW, DeGirolami U: Variability and reversibility of focal cerebral ischemia in unanesthetized monkeys, *Neurology* 31:1295-1302, 1981.

204. Powers WJ: Imaging preventable infarction in patients with acute ischemic stroke, *AJNR Am J Neuroradiol* 29:1823-1825, 2008.

205. Frykholm P, Andersson JL, Valtysson J, et al: A metabolic threshold of irreversible ischemia demonstrated by PET in a middle cerebral artery occlusion-reperfusion primate model, *Acta Neurol Scand* 102:18-26, 2000.

206. Baron JC, Rougemont D, Bousser MG, et al: Local CBF, oxygen extraction fraction (OEF), and $CMRO_2$: Prognostic value in recent supratentorial infarction in humans, *J Cereb Blood Flow Metab* 3(Suppl 1):S1-S2, 1983.

207. Marchal G, Benali K, Iglesias S, et al: Voxel-based mapping of irreversible ischaemic damage with PET in acute stroke, *Brain* 122:2387-2400, 1999.

208. Young AR, Sette G, Touzani O, et al: Relationships between high oxygen extraction fraction in the acute stage and final infarction in reversible middle cerebral artery occlusion: an investigation in anesthetized baboons with positron emission tomography, *J Cereb Blood Flow Metab* 16:1176-1188, 1996.

209. Marchal G, Beaudouin V, Rioux P, et al: Prolonged persistence of substantial volumes of potentially viable brain tissue after stroke: a correlative PET-CT study with voxel-based data analysis, *Stroke* 27:599-606, 1996.

210. Young AR, Sette G, Touzani O, et al: Relationships between high oxygen extraction fraction in the acute stage and final infarction in reversible middle cerebral artery occlusion: an investigation in anesthetized baboons with positron emission tomography, *J Cereb Blood Flow Metab* 16:1176-1188, 1996.

211. Rosenbaum JL, Almli CR, Yundt KD, et al: Higher neonatal cerebral blood flow correlates with worse childhood neurologic outcome, *Neurology* 49:1035-1041, 1997.

212. Baron JC, Bousser MG, Comar D, et al: 'Crossed cerebellar diaschisis' in human supratentorial brain infarction, *Trans Am Neurol Assoc* 105:459-461, 1980.

213. Martin WR, Raichle ME: Cerebellar blood flow and metabolism in cerebral hemisphere infarction, *Ann Neurol* 14:168-176, 1983.

214. Pantano P, Baron JC, Samson Y, et al: Crossed cerebellar diaschisis: Further studies, *Brain* 109:677-694, 1986.

215. Kuhl DE, Phelps ME, Kowell AP, et al: Effects of stroke on local cerebral metabolism and perfusion: mapping by emission computed tomography of 18FDG and 13NH3, *Ann Neurol* 8:47-60, 1980.

216. Kushner M, Alavi A, Reivich M, et al: Contralateral cerebellar hypometabolism following cerebral insult: a positron emission tomographic study, *Ann Neurol* 15:425-434, 1984.

217. Yamauchi H, Fukuyama H, Kimura J: Hemodynamic and metabolic changes in crossed cerebellar hypoperfusion, *Stroke* 23:855-860, 1992.

218. Von Monakow C: Diaschisis. In Pribram KA, editor: *Brain and behavior I: mood, states and mind*, Baltimore, 1969, Penguin Books, pp 27-36.

219. Lenzi GL, Frackowiak RS, Jones T, et al: CMRO2 and CBF by the oxygen-15 inhalation technique: Results in normal volunteers and cerebrovascular patients, *Eur Neurol* 20:285-290, 1981.

220. Iglesias S, Marchal G, Rioux P, et al: Do changes in oxygen metabolism in the unaffected cerebral hemisphere underlie early neurological recovery after stroke? A positron emission tomography study, *Stroke* 27:1192-1199, 1996.

221. Serrati C, Marchal G, Rioux P, et al: Contralateral cerebellar hypometabolism: a predictor for stroke outcome? *J Neurol Neurosurg Psychiatry* 57:174-179, 1994.

222. Kim SE, Choi CW, Yoon BW, et al: Crossed-cerebellar diaschisis in cerebral infarction: technetium-99m-HMPAO SPECT and MRI, *J Nucl Med* 38:14-19, 1997.

223. Yamauchi H, Fukuyama H, Nagahama Y, et al: Uncoupling of oxygen and glucose metabolism in persistent crossed cerebellar diaschisis, *Stroke* 30:1424-1428, 1999.

224. Celesia GG, Polcyn RE, Holden JE, et al: Determination of regional cerebral blood flow in patients with cerebral infarction: Use of fluoromethane labeled with fluorine 18 and positron emission tomography, *Arch Neurol* 41:262-267, 1984.

225. Dobkin JA, Levine RL, Lagreze HL, et al: Evidence for transhemispheric diaschisis in unilateral stroke, *Arch Neurol* 46:1333–1336, 1989.

226. Wise R, Gibbs J, Frackowiak R, et al: No evidence for transhemispheric diaschisis after human cerebral infarction, *Stroke* 17:853–861, 1986.

227. Baron JC, Lebrun-Grandie P, Collard P, et al: Noninvasive measurement of blood flow, oxygen consumption, and glucose utilization in the same brain regions in man by positron emission tomography: concise communication, *J Nucl Med* 23:391–399, 1982.

228. Heiss WD, Pawlik G, Wagner R, et al: Functional hypometabolism of noninfarcted brain regions in ischemic stroke, *J Cereb Blood Flow Metab* 3(Suppl 1):S582–S583, 1983.

229. Iglesias S, Marchal G, Viader F, et al: Delayed intrahemispheric remote hypometabolism: Correlations with early recovery after stroke, *Cerebrovasc Dis* 10:391–402, 2000.

230. Wise RJ, Bernardi S, Frackowiak RS, et al: Serial observations on the pathophysiology of acute stroke: The transition from ischaemia to infarction as reflected in regional oxygen extraction, *Brain* 106:197–222, 1983.

231. Szelies B, Herholz K, Pawlik G, et al: Widespread functional effects of discrete thalamic infarction, *Arch Neurol* 48:178–182, 1991.

232. Sakai F, Aoki S, Kan S, et al: Ataxic hemiparesis with reductions of ipsilateral cerebellar blood flow, *Stroke* 17:1016–1018, 1986.

233. Giroud M, Creisson E, Fayolle H, et al: Homolateral ataxia and crural paresis: a crossed cerebral-cerebellar diaschisis, *J Neurol Neurosurg Psychiatry* 57:221–222, 1994.

234. Metter EJ, Kempler D, Jackson C, et al: Cerebral glucose metabolism in Wernicke's, Broca's, and conduction aphasia, *Arch Neurol* 46:27–34, 1989.

235. Karbe H, Herholz K, Szelies B, et al: Regional metabolic correlates of Token test results in cortical and subcortical left hemispheric infarction, *Neurology* 39:1083–1088, 1989.

236. Perani D, Vallar G, Cappa S, et al: Aphasia and neglect after subcortical stroke: A clinical/cerebral perfusion correlation study, *Brain* 110:1211–1229, 1987.

237. Feeney DM, Baron JC: Diaschisis, *Stroke* 17:817–830, 1986.

238. Karbe H, Szelies B, Herholz K, et al: Impairment of language is related to left parieto-temporal glucose metabolism in aphasic stroke patients, *J Neurol* 237:19–23, 1990.

239. Pappata S, Mazoyer B, Tran DS, et al: Effects of capsular or thalamic stroke on metabolism in the cortex and cerebellum: a positron tomography study, *Stroke* 21:519–524, 1990.

240. Kushner M, Reivich M, Fieschi C, et al: Metabolic and clinical correlates of acute ischemic infarction, *Neurology* 37:1103–1110, 1987.

241. Heiss WD, Kessler J, Karbe H, et al: Cerebral glucose metabolism as a predictor of recovery from aphasia in ischemic stroke, *Arch Neurol* 50:958–964, 1993.

242. Karbe H, Kessler J, Herholz K, et al: Long-term prognosis of poststroke aphasia studied with positron emission tomography, *Arch Neurol* 52:186–190, 1995.

243. Mendelow AD, Bullock R, Teasdale GM, et al: Intracranial haemorrhage induced at arterial pressure in the rat. Part 2: Short term changes in local cerebral blood flow measured by autoradiography, *Neurol Res* 6:189–193, 1984.

244. Nath FP, Jenkins A, Mendelow AD, et al: Early hemodynamic changes in experimental intracerebral hemorrhage, *J Neurosurg* 65:697–703, 1986.

245. Sills C, Villar-Cordova C, Pasteur W, et al: Demonstration of hypoperfusion surrounding intracerebral hematoma in humans, *J Stroke Cerebrovasc Dis* 6:17–24, 1996.

246. Qureshi AI, Wilson DA, Hanley DF, et al: No evidence for an ischemic penumbra in massive experimental intracerebral hemorrhage, *Neurology* 52:266–272, 1999.

247. Mayer SA, Lignelli A, Fink ME, et al: Perilesional blood flow and edema formation in acute intracerebral hemorrhage: a SPECT study, *Stroke* 29:1791–1798, 1998.

248. Nath FP, Kelly PT, Jenkins A, et al: Effects of experimental intracerebral hemorrhage on blood flow, capillary permeability, and histochemistry, *J Neurosurg* 66:555–562, 1987.

249. Hoffman EJ, Huang SC, Phelps ME: Quantitation in positron emission computed tomography. 1: Effect of object size, *J Comput Assist Tomogr* 3:299–308, 1979.

250. Mazziotta JC, Phelps ME, Plummer D, et al: Quantitation in positron emission computed tomography. 5: Physical–anatomical effects, *J Comput Assist Tomogr* 5:734–743, 1981.

251. Videen TO, Dunford-Shore JE, Diringer MN, et al: Correction for partial volume effects in regional blood flow measurements adjacent to hematomas in humans with intracerebral hemorrhage: implementation and validation, *J Comput Assist Tomogr* 23:248–256, 1999.

252. Zazulia AR, Diringer MN, Videen TO, et al: Hypoperfusion without ischemia surrounding acute intracerebral hemorrhage, *J Cereb Blood Flow Metab* 21:804–810, 2001.

253. Kim-Han JS, Kopp SJ, Dugan LL, et al: Perihematomal mitochondrial dysfunction after intracerebral hemorrhage, *Stroke* 37:2457–2462, 2006.

254. Schellinger PD, Fiebach JB, Hoffmann K, et al: Stroke MRI in intracerebral hemorrhage: is there a perihemorrhagic penumbra? *Stroke* 34:1674–1679, 2003.

255. Pascual AM, Lopez-Mut JV, Benlloch V, et al: Perfusion-weighted magnetic resonance imaging in acute intracerebral hemorrhage at baseline and during the 1st and 2nd week: a longitudinal study, *Cerebrovasc Dis* 23:6–13, 2007.

256. Uemura K, Shishido F, Higano S, et al: Positron emission tomography in patients with a primary intracerebral hematoma, *Acta Radiol Suppl* 369:426–428, 1986.

257. Zazulia AR, Diringer MN, Videen TO, et al: Effects of acute ICH on hemispheric blood flow and metabolism, *Stroke* 32:338, 2001.

258. Zazulia AR, Videen TO, Diringer MN, et al: Focal cortical hyperglycolysis in acute intracerebral hemorrhage, *Neurology* 68:A357, 2007.

259. Bergsneider M, Hovda DA, Shalmon E, et al: Cerebral hyperglycolysis following severe traumatic brain injury in humans: a positron emission tomography study, *J Neurosurg* 86:241–251, 1997.

260. Hattori N, Huang SC, Wu HM, et al: Acute changes in regional cerebral (18)F-FDG kinetics in patients with traumatic brain injury, *J Nucl Med* 45:775–783, 2004.

261. Heiss WD, Beil C, Pawlik G, et al: Non-traumatic intracerebral hematoma versus ischemic stroke: regional pattern of glucose metabolism, *J Cereb Blood Flow Metab* 5(Suppl 1):S5–S6, 1985.

262. Dal-Bianco P: Positron emission tomography of 2(18F)-fluorodeoxyglucose in cerebral vascular disease: clinicometabolic correlations in patients with nontraumatic spontaneous intracerebral hematoma and ischemic infarction. In Meyer JS, Lechner H, Reivich M, et al: *Cerebral vascular disease 6: proceedings of the World Federation of Neurology 13th international Salzburg conference*, Amsterdam, 1987, Excerpta Medica, pp 257–262.

263. Powers WJ, Zazulia AR, Videen TO, et al: Autoregulation of cerebral blood flow surrounding acute intracerebral hemorrhage, *Neurology* 57:18–24, 2001.

264. Batjer HH, Devous MD Sr, Seibert GB, et al: Intracranial arteriovenous malformation: contralateral steal phenomena, *Neurol Med Chir (Tokyo)* 29:401–406, 1989.

265. Batjer HH, Devous MD Sr: The use of acetazolamide-enhanced regional cerebral blood flow measurement to predict risk to arteriovenous malformation patients, *Neurosurgery* 31:213–217, 1992.

266. Homan RW, Devous MD Sr, Stokely EM, et al: Quantification of intracerebral steal in patients with arteriovenous malformation, *Arch Neurol* 43:779–785, 1986.

267. Tyler JL, Leblanc R, Meyer E, et al: Hemodynamic and metabolic effects of cerebral arteriovenous malformations studied by positron emission tomography, *Stroke* 20:890–898, 1989.

268. Van Roost D, Schramm J, Solymosi L, et al: Presence and removal of arteriovenous malformation: Impact of regional cerebral blood flow, as assessed with xenon/CT, *Acta Neurol Scand Suppl* 166:136–138, 1996.

269. Hacein-Bey L, Nour R, Pile-Spellman J, et al: Adaptive changes of autoregulation in chronic cerebral hypotension with arteriovenous malformations: an acetazolamide-enhanced single-photon emission CT study, *Am J Neuroradiol* 16:1865–1874, 1995.

270. Iwama T, Hayashida K, Takahashi JC, et al: Cerebral hemodynamics and metabolism in patients with cerebral arteriovenous malformations: an evaluation using positron emission tomography scanning, *J Neurosurg* 97:1314–1321, 2002.

271. Spetzler RF, Wilson CB, Weinstein P, et al: Normal perfusion pressure breakthrough theory, *Clin Neurosurg* 25:651–672, 1978.

272. Nornes H, Grip A: Hemodynamic aspects of cerebral arteriovenous malformations, *J Neurosurg* 53:456-464, 1980.

273. Takeuchi S, Kikuchi H, Karasawa J, et al: Cerebral hemodynamics in arteriovenous malformations: evaluation by single-photon emission CT, *Am J Neuroradiol* 8:193-197, 1987.

274. Barnett GH, Little JR, Ebrahim ZY, et al: Cerebral circulation during arteriovenous malformation operation, *Neurosurgery* 20:836-842, 1987.

275. Spetzler RF, Martin NA, Carter LP, et al: Surgical management of large AVM's by staged embolization and operative excision, *J Neurosurg* 67:17-28, 1987.

276. Young WL, Pile-Spellman J, Prohovnik I, et al: Evidence for adaptive autoregulatory displacement in hypotensive cortical territories adjacent to arteriovenous malformations, Columbia University AVM Study Project. *Neurosurgery* 34:601-610, 1994.

277. Young WL, Kader A, Prohovnik I, et al: Pressure autoregulation is intact after arteriovenous malformation resection, *Neurosurgery* 32:491-496, 1993.

278. Morgan MK, Johnston IH, Hallinan JM, et al: Complications of surgery for arteriovenous malformations of the brain, *J Neurosurg* 78:176-182, 1993.

279. Heros RC, Korosue K, Diebold PM: Surgical excision of cerebral arteriovenous malformations: late results, *Neurosurgery* 26:570-577, 1990.

280. Young WL, Kader A, Ornstein E, et al: Cerebral hyperemia after arteriovenous malformation resection is related to "breakthrough" complications but not to feeding artery pressure, The Columbia University Arteriovenous Malformation Study Project. *Neurosurgery* 38:1085-1093, 1996.

281. Tarr RW, Johnson DW, Rutigliano M, et al: Use of acetazolamide-challenge xenon CT in the assessment of cerebral blood flow dynamics in patients with arteriovenous malformations, *Am J Neuroradiol* 11:441-448, 1990.

282. Van Roost D, Schramm J: What factors are related to impairment of cerebrovascular reserve before and after arteriovenous malformation resection? A cerebral blood flow study using xenon-enhanced computed tomography, *Neurosurgery* 48:709-716, 2001.

283. Diehl RR, Henkes H, Nahser HC, et al: Blood flow velocity and vasomotor reactivity in patients with arteriovenous malformations: A transcranial Doppler study, *Stroke* 25:1574-1580, 1994.

284. Hasegawa S, Hamada J, Morioka M, et al: Radiation-induced cerebrovasculopathy of the distal middle cerebral artery and distal posterior cerebral artery—case report, *Neurol Med Chir (Tokyo)* 40:220-223, 2000.

285. Katayama S, Momose T, Sano I, et al: Temporal lobe CO_2 vasoreactivity in patients with complex partial seizures, *Jpn J Psychiatry Neurol* 46:379-385, 1992.

286. Carpenter DA, Grubb RL Jr, Tempel LW, et al: Cerebral oxygen metabolism after aneurysmal subarachnoid hemorrhage, *J Cereb Blood Flow Metab* 11:837-844, 1991.

287. Frykholm P, Andersson JL, Langstrom B, et al: Haemodynamic and metabolic disturbances in the acute stage of subarachnoid haemorrhage demonstrated by PET, *Acta Neurol Scand* 109:25-32, 2004.

288. Kassell NF, Sasaki T, Colohan AR, et al: Cerebral vasospasm following aneurysmal subarachnoid hemorrhage, *Stroke* 16:562-572, 1985.

289. Heros RC, Zervas NT, Varsos V: Cerebral vasospasm after subarachnoid hemorrhage: an update, *Ann Neurol* 14:599-608, 1983.

290. Suarez JI, Tarr RW, Selman WR: Aneurysmal subarachnoid hemorrhage, *N Engl J Med* 354:387-396, 2006.

291. Meyer CH, Lowe D, Meyer M, et al: Progressive change in cerebral blood flow during the first three weeks after subarachnoid hemorrhage, *Neurosurgery* 12:58-76, 1983.

292. Naderi S, Ozguven MA, Bayhan H, et al: Evaluation of cerebral vasospasm in patients with subarachnoid hemorrhage using single photon emission computed tomography, *Neurosurg Rev* 17:261-265, 1994.

293. Ohkuma H, Manabe H, Tanaka M, et al: Impact of cerebral microcirculatory changes on cerebral blood flow during cerebral vasospasm after aneurysmal subarachnoid hemorrhage, *Stroke* 31:1621-1627, 2000.

294. Grubb RL Jr, Raichle ME, Eichling JO, et al: Effects of subarachnoid hemorrhage on cerebral blood volume, blood flow, and oxygen utilization in humans, *J Neurosurg* 46:446-453, 1977.

295. Jakobsen M, Overgaard J, Marcussen E, et al: Relation between angiographic cerebral vasospasm and regional CBF in patients with SAH, *Acta Neurol Scand* 82:109-115, 1990.

296. James IM: Changes in cerebral blood flow and in systemic arterial pressure following spontaneous subarachnoid haemorrhage, *Clin Sci* 35:11-22, 1968.

297. Ishii R: Regional cerebral blood flow in patients with ruptured intracranial aneurysms, *J Neurosurg* 50:587-594, 1979.

298. Heilbrun MP, Olesen J, Lassen NA: Regional cerebral blood flow studies in subarachnoid hemorrhage, *J Neurosurg* 37:36-44, 1972.

299. Gelmers HJ, Beks JW, Journee HL: Regional cerebral blood flow in patients with subarachnoid haemorrhage, *Acta Neurochir (Wien)* 47:245-251, 1979.

300. Rosenstein J, Wang AD, Symon L, et al: Relationship between hemispheric cerebral blood flow, central conduction time, and clinical grade in aneurysmal subarachnoid hemorrhage, *J Neurosurg* 62:25-30, 1985.

301. Voldby B, Enevoldsen EM, Jensen FT: Regional CBF, intraventricular pressure, and cerebral metabolism in patients with ruptured intracranial aneurysms, *J Neurosurg* 62:48-58, 1985.

302. Geraud G, Tremoulet M, Guell A, et al: The prognostic value of noninvasive CBF measurement in subarachnoid hemorrhage, *Stroke* 15:301-305, 1984.

303. Minhas PS, Menon DK, Smielewski P, et al: Positron emission tomographic cerebral perfusion disturbances and transcranial Doppler findings among patients with neurological deterioration after subarachnoid hemorrhage, *Neurosurgery* 52:1017-1022, 2003.

304. Jakobsen M, Enevoldsen E, Bjerre P: Cerebral blood flow and metabolism following subarachnoid haemorrhage: cerebral oxygen uptake and global blood flow during the acute period in patients with SAH, *Acta Neurol Scand* 82:174-182, 1990.

305. Hayashi T, Suzuki A, Hatazawa J, et al: Cerebral circulation and metabolism in the acute stage of subarachnoid hemorrhage, *J Neurosurg* 93:1014-1018, 2000.

306. Hino A, Mizukawa N, Tenjin H, et al: Postoperative hemodynamic and metabolic changes in patients with subarachnoid hemorrhage, *Stroke* 20:1504-1510, 1989.

307. Powers WJ, Grubb RL Jr, Baker RP, et al: Regional cerebral blood flow and metabolism in reversible ischemia due to vasospasm: Determination by positron emission tomography, *J Neurosurg* 62:539-546, 1985.

308. Kawamura S, Sayama I, Yasui N, et al: Sequential changes in cerebral blood flow and metabolism in patients with subarachnoid haemorrhage, *Acta Neurochir (Wien)* 114:12-15, 1992.

309. Yundt KD, Grubb RL Jr, Diringer MN, et al: Autoregulatory vasodilation of parenchymal vessels is impaired during cerebral vasospasm, *J Cereb Blood Flow Metab* 18:419-424, 1998.

310. Yundt KD, Grubb RL Jr, Diringer MN, et al: Cerebral hemodynamic and metabolic changes caused by brain retraction after aneurysmal subarachnoid hemorrhage, *Neurosurgery* 40:442-450, 1997.

311. Rousseaux M, Huglo D, Steinling M: Cerebral blood flow in frontal lesions of aneurysms of the anterior communicating artery, *Stroke* 25:135-140, 1994.

312. Tranquart F, Ades PE, Groussin P, et al: Postoperative assessment of cerebral blood flow in subarachnoid haemorrhage by means of 99mTc-HMPAO tomography, *Eur J Nucl Med* 20:53-58, 1993.

313. Rosen JM, Butala AV, Oropello JM, et al: Postoperative changes on brain SPECT imaging after aneurysmal subarachnoid hemorrhage: A potential pitfall in the evaluation of vasospasm, *Clin Nucl Med* 19:595-597, 1994.

314. Ahn CS, Tow DE, Yu CC, et al: Effect of metabolic alterations on the accumulation of technetium-99m-labeled d, l-HMPAO in slices of rat cerebral cortex, *J Cereb Blood Flow Metab* 14:324-331, 1994.

315. Voldby B, Enevoldsen EM, Jensen FT: Cerebrovascular reactivity in patients with ruptured intracranial aneurysms, *J Neurosurg* 62:59-67, 1985.

316. Cossu M, Gennaro S, Rossi A, et al: Autoregulation of cortical blood flow during surgery for ruptured intracranial aneurysms, *J Neurosurg Sci* 43:99-105, 1999.

317. Nornes H, Knutzen HB, Wikeby P: Cerebral arterial blood flow and aneurysm surgery. Part 2: Induced hypotension and autoregulatory capacity, *J Neurosurg* 47:819-827, 1977.

318. Darby JM, Yonas H, Marks EC, et al: Acute cerebral blood flow response to dopamine-induced hypertension after subarachnoid hemorrhage, *J Neurosurg* 80:857-864, 1994.

319. Touho H, Ueda H: Disturbance of autoregulation in patients with ruptured intracranial aneurysms: mechanism of cortical and motor dysfunction, *Surg Neurol* 42:57-64, 1994.

320. Schmieder K, Moller F, Engelhardt M, et al: Dynamic cerebral autoregulation in patients with ruptured and unruptured aneurysms after induction of general anesthesia, *Zentralbl Neurochir* 67:81-87, 2006.

321. Aaslid R, Markwalder TM, Nornes H: Noninvasive transcranial Doppler ultrasound recording of flow velocity in basal cerebral arteries, *J Neurosurg* 57:769-774, 1982.

322. Macdonald RL, Weir BK: Radiology. In Macdonald RL, Weir BK, editors: *Cerebral vasospasm*, San Diego, 2001, Academic Press, pp 176-220.

323. Hutchison K, Weir B: Transcranial Doppler studies in aneurysm patients, *Can J Neurol Sci* 16:411-416, 1989.

324. Vora YY, Suarez-Almazor M, Steinke DE, et al: Role of transcranial Doppler monitoring in the diagnosis of cerebral vasospasm after subarachnoid hemorrhage, *Neurosurgery* 44:1237-1247, 1999.

325. Brass LM, Pavlakis SG, DeVivo D, et al: Transcranial Doppler measurements of the middle cerebral artery: Effect of hematocrit, *Stroke* 19:1466-1469, 1988.

326. Newell DW, Winn HR: Transcranial Doppler in cerebral vasospasm, *Neurosurg Clin North Am* 1:319-328, 1990.

327. Romner B, Brandt L, Berntman L, et al: Simultaneous transcranial Doppler sonography and cerebral blood flow measurements of cerebrovascular CO_2-reactivity in patients with aneurysmal subarachnoid haemorrhage, *Br J Neurosurg* 5:31-37, 1991.

328. Mizuno M, Nakajima S, Sampei T, et al: Serial transcranial Doppler flow velocity and cerebral blood flow measurements for evaluation of cerebral vasospasm after subarachnoid hemorrhage, *Neurol Med Chir (Tokyo)* 34:164-171, 1994.

329. Clyde BL, Resnick DK, Yonas H, et al: The relationship of blood velocity as measured by transcranial Doppler ultrasonography to cerebral blood flow as determined by stable xenon computed tomographic studies after aneurysmal subarachnoid hemorrhage, *Neurosurgery* 38:896-904, 1996.

330. Manno EM, Gress DR, Schwamm LH, et al: Effects of induced hypertension on transcranial Doppler ultrasound velocities in patients after subarachnoid hemorrhage, *Stroke* 29:422-428, 1998.

331. Adams HP Jr, Powers WJ, Grubb RL Jr, et al: Preview of a new trial of extracranial-to-intracranial arterial anastomosis: the carotid occlusion surgery study, *Neurosurg Clin North Am* 12:613-624, 2001.

5

Histopathology of Cerebral Ischemia

ROLAND N. AUER

The Biological Levels of Organization and Stroke

Numerous clinical stroke trials have failed, possibly because single molecular mechanisms only were addressed, whereas cerebral ischemia comprises a disease of blood flow, with damage at the tissue level. Hence, a brief review of the biological levels of organization is germane to the histopathology of cerebral ischemia.

The biological levels of organization (Table 5-1) range from molecules, to subcellular organelles, cells, tissues, organs, and organisms, to the biosphere. Although organ dysfunction (brain dysfunction) and deficits at the organism level are what primarily concern us as end results, such disease inevitably comes about from events gone awry at lower levels of biological organization. Pathology addresses damage mainly at the cellular and tissue levels. Diffuse cellular or subcellular (synaptic or chemical) lesions usually lead to behavioral deficits. Because of the extreme inhomogeneity of the brain compared with other organs, focal lesions in the brain, even minor ones in some critical locations, can also lead to either behavioral or homeostatic brain dysfunction. The pathology of brain ischemia thus lies squarely between the molecular and the clinical levels.

I note here that not all events at lower biological levels give rise to effects at higher levels. Thus, not all molecular events cause cellular dysfunction, and not all cellular or tissue lesions cause dysfunction of the organism. Stated differently, chemical changes can be silent at the cell or tissue level, and cytologic or histologic lesions can go undetected in the whole organism.

In this regard, it is important to remember that brain ischemia is not primarily a molecular dysfunction of the brain but, like brain trauma, is initiated by physical factors; in this case it is cessation of blood flow. Molecular events are invariable and follow the profound alterations in blood flow and cerebral metabolism, but the primary, initiating pathophysiologic event is at the tissue (not cellular, molecular, or whole organism) level. However, after being initiated by cessation of a fluid tissue (blood) flowing through a more formed tissue (brain), numerous potentially damaging molecular cascades are immediately set in motion. Which of these molecular events filters through to higher levels of biological organization, to damage cells and tissues, is not always known. I focus in this chapter on events that occur at the cell and tissue

levels and that are known to cause irreparable brain damage, teasing out only a few molecular mechanisms for which there is good evidence in the pathogenesis of ischemic brain damage.

One distinction deserves emphasis at the beginning: Behavioral tests in animals and clinical neurologic examination (or neuropsychologic testing) in humans all test the synapses of the brain. Classic neuropathology, in contrast, examines mainly the cell bodies of the brain, that is, the neuronal parenchyma in aggregate. This conceptual distinction is important. For example, ischemic brain damage may kill a few neurons in some places in the brain without causing a clinical neurologic deficit. This does not imply that neuronal death is not something to be avoided. It is insignificant or inconsequential by virtue of its location, not by the nature of the process.

Death of cells and tissues in the brain is always a serious event. Because the exact clinical consequences depend on the extent and precise location of the lesion, matters of pure chance (e.g., which arterial ramification receives an embolus) determine final end results, adding an unpredictable, stochastic element to ischemic brain damage. Clinical effects of lesions of roughly equal size are highly dependent on the location within the brain. Thus, silent frontal lobe infarcts in humans[1] are not to be regarded as inconsequential because, had they occurred in slightly more posterior locations, merely by chance, they would have the potential to produce major and catastrophic clinical deficits. In this way, the highly inhomogeneous brain gives rise to considerable clinical variability in both the severity and the nature of the deficit for lesions of identical size.

One implication of the preceding discussion is that focusing on lesion size rather than direct clinical benefit requires fewer subjects to ascertain differences.[2] This issue underscores the value of the tissue burden of disease (e.g., infarct size measured pathologically or neuroradiologically). These considerations have implications for clinical trials.

Selective Neuronal Necrosis versus Infarction

This discussion focuses on two grades of ischemic brain lesions: selective neuronal necrosis and infarction. Both kill neurons, and the former does so exclusively. The

TABLE 5-1 BIOLOGICAL LEVELS OF ORGANIZATION AND STROKE

Level	Tools Used
Terrome	—
Biome	—
Ecosystem	—
Community	Clinical
Organism	Clinical
Organ System	—
Organ	Gross observation, imaging
Tissue	Histopathology, imaging
Cell	Histopathology
Organelle [synapse]	Histopathology, E.M. [& Clinical]
Supramolecular aggregate	—
Molecule	Drugs
Atom	—

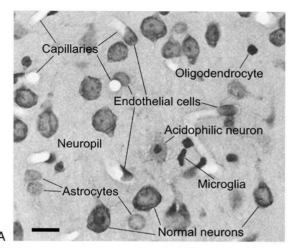

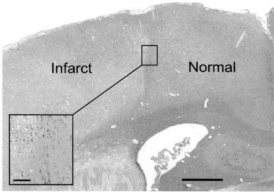

Figure 5-1 A, Normal central nervous system histologic appearance and a single necrotic (acidophilic) neuron, showing selective neuronal necrosis. This tissue lesion spares glia as well as neuropil. The square nucleus above the rod-shaped microglia is also probably a microglial cell, from its nuclear shape as well as its position between the vessel and the dead neuron, suggesting recent emigration from the vessel. Axons, dendrites, and glial processes constitute the unresolvable (on light microscopy), finely reticulated neuropil. Astrocytes show characteristically pale nuclei compared with oligodendroglia and microglia. Cortex, global ischemia, 1 week survival, rat. (Hematoxylin and eosin; bar = 20 μm.) B, One of the most remarkable features of infarction, rarely receiving emphasis, is its characteristically geographic, sharply demarcated border, seen here running vertically through the neocortex in the center of the picture. Early, patchy cysts are seen *(inset)* as infarcted tissue is resorbed. Although a few dark neurons *(inset, bottom)* are seen at the infarct rim, there is rapid transition to normal neuropil and normal neurons *(inset, right)*. Note that inflammation is not yet seen. Focal ischemia, 24 hours survival, rat. (Hematoxylin and eosin; bars = 2 mm and 400 μm *[inset]*.)

distinction rests on the physiologic severity of the lesion, in whatever brain location. Selective *neuronal necrosis* specifically denotes death of only neurons, sparing glia (Fig. 5-1A). *Infarction* refers to death of neurons *and* glia and is a much more serious tissue lesion (see Fig. 5-1B). The reason is that axonal sprouting, and any form of tissue regeneration, is precluded because all of the tissue dies. Infarction ultimately leaves a fluid-filled cyst, formed as a result of tissue breakdown and removal by macrophages. This cyst comes to contain only brain interstitial fluid, in direct exchange with cerebrospinal fluid (CSF).

It is important to remember that both grades of lesion severity can occur anywhere in the brain: in the brainstem, cerebellum, or forebrain. Selective neuronal necrosis and infarction denote a degree of brain damage, not a location in the brain.

Selective Vulnerability

The concept of two degrees of severity of damage (selective neuronal necrosis and infarction) must be clearly distinguished from the concept of selective vulnerability within the brain. The latter refers to the fact that the entire brain can be subjected to some primary insult, but only portions of the brain show damage. This is selective vulnerability and is the rule rather than the exception in neuropathology. It applies fully to brain damage in ischemia. Elucidation of the basis of selective vulnerability, when possible, gives valuable clues to the mechanism of tissue damage in ischemia. Likewise, elucidation of the mechanism of selective neuronal necrosis or infarction also yields information useful for understanding and ultimately preventing these two levels of tissue damage.

Selective Neuronal Necrosis

The concept of incomplete infarction has little support on close brain examination: it seems that either the entire local array of cells in the brain die en masse or only the neurons die, leaving the glia and neuropil intact. The neuropil is visible in histologic section as the finely reticulated or bubbly tissue that appears between cell bodies in central brain or spinal cord. Neuropil cannot be resolved at the light microscopic level. Electron microscopy,

however, reveals the neuropil to consist of axons, dendrites, and glial processes (Fig. 5-2).

Neuronal Acidophilia

At the cellular level, the pathology of cerebral ischemia has often focused on an ill-defined "ischemic cell change," which is, in essence, neuronal death. However, the hallmark of neuronal death at the light microscopic level is an increased affinity for acid dyes. The reason for this neuronal acidophilia (see Fig. 5-1A) is uncertain. Because

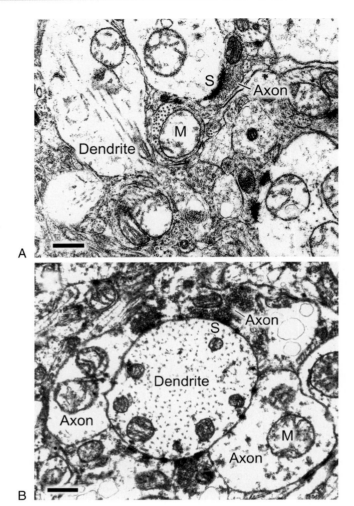

A

B

Figure 5-2 Contrasting features of excitotoxic and hypermetabolic pathology. A, Excitotoxicity shows dendritic swelling, sparing axons. Dendritic microtubules are hollow and serve to definitively identify the cell process around the central mitochondrion as a dendrite. (Hypoglycemia, hippocampus; bar = 1 μm.) (From Auer RN, Kalimo H, Olsson Y, Wieloch T: The dentate gyrus in hypoglycemia: Pathology implicating excitotoxin-mediated neuronal necrosis. *Acta Neuropathol [Berlin]* 67:279-288, 1985; © Springer-Verlag.) B, Hypermetabolism shows axonal swelling, sparing the central dendrite, which has axonal terminals surrounding it. Both the swollen axons and dendrites include swollen mitochondria (M). Synapses (S) are the darkest membranes in each picture because of embedded proteins in the membrane and can be seen to contain synaptic vesicles. (Epilepsy, substantia nigra, pars reticulata; bar = 1 μm.) (From Auer RN, Ingvar M, Nevander G, et al: Early axonal lesion and preserved microvasculature in epilepsy-induced hypermetabolic necrosis of the substantia nigra. *Acta Neuropathol [Berlin]* 71:207-215, 1985, © Springer-Verlag.)

hematoxylin and eosin stain is the stain routinely used in pathology, acidophilia is often commonly referred to as "eosinophilia." The reason nuclei are blue and cytoplasm is pink in conventionally stained sections is that hematoxylin is a base and eosin is an acid. Because each component of the acid–base pair stains its opposite element in the tissue (i.e., acids stain basic tissue components and bases stain acidic tissue components), death of neurons must be critically accompanied by some increase in

normal or altered chemically basic moieties of the molecular components of tissue. The nature of these basic tissue components that are revealed by acidic stains in neuronal death is uncertain but may involve binding of acid dyes to ε-amino groups of basic lysine residues in degenerating proteins.[3] Proteins constitute the bulk of stainable material in routine tissue sections and are, in fact, normally eosinophilic to some degree because of the basic amino acid groups (e.g., ε-amino of lysine, guanidino of arginine, and imidazole of histidine) in the residues of the polypeptide chain. This is the reason that neuropil and the cytoplasm of neuronal cell bodies between the RNA stain pink.

Alterations in protein are also suggested as the explanation for acidophilia because of the electron microscopic features of acidophilic neurons; mitochondrial flocculent densities (Fig. 5-3A) represent denatured protein.[4-6]

Conversely, nucleic acids stain blue because of their affinity for basic dyes, such as hematoxylin. The nucleic acid-containing parts of a cell—nucleoli, nucleus, and cytoplasmic Nissl substance (composed of RNA)—all stain blue because of the affinity of nucleic acids for basic dyes in routine staining. For these reasons, we see nuclei as blue and cytoplasm as pink in normal histopathologic sections. In ischemic neuronal death or, indeed, in any form of neuronal death, the acidophilia is not merely due to unmasking of basophilia by loss of nucleic acid staining.[3]

Neuronal acidophilia is not specific to neuronal death due to ischemia but merely indicates that the neuron has irreversibly succumbed from any cause. The etiology of cell death is clearly not revealed by the preceding description of acidophilic neurons, which have an identical acidophilic appearance whether cell death is caused by ischemia, hypoglycemia, epilepsy, or even neuronal infection by a virus. I thus decry the use of the term *ischemic cell change* for acidophilic neuronal death because this is simply the nonspecific appearance of an irreversibly damaged or dead neuron; the cell may not even have been exposed to ischemia.

Neurons Undergo a "Dendritic Death"

Electron microscopy gives some clue as to the nature of acidophilic neuronal death (see Fig. 5-2). Importantly, the neuropil surrounding neurons destined to die shows remarkably inhomogeneous damage to axons, dendrites, and glial processes. In the process of selective neuronal necrosis, dendrites swell selectively if attached to neurons destined to die, but intervening axons and glial processes are spared ultrastructurally (see Fig. 5-2A). This axon-sparing, dendritic lesion is the hallmark of the tissue action of endogenous excitatory amino acids or their chemical congeners. The selective dendritic swelling is due to the overwhelmingly dendritic location of excitatory amino acid receptors within the neuropil. Because excitatory amino acid receptors predominate on dendrites, ion and water fluxes are initiated there, and dendritic swelling results.

These axon-sparing, dendritic lesions are generally hard to find because an appropriate part of the neuropil surrounding the neurons must be examined (i.e., a part

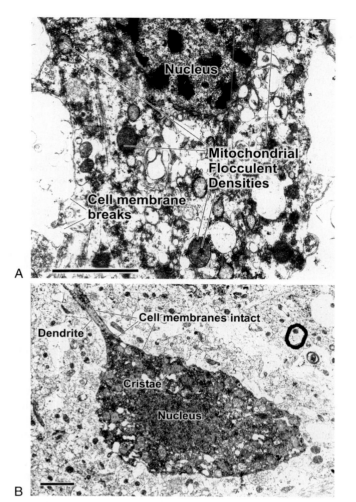

Figure 5-3 Contrasting features of necrotic and apoptotic morphology. A, Necrosis shows mitochondrial flocculent densities, representing denatured cytochrome proteins. The nucleus shows coarse, stippled chromatin. The cytoplasm shows few recognizable organelles, consisting mainly of amorphous debris and membranous whorls. (Bar = 5 μm.) B, Three weeks after a hypoglycemic injury. The neuron shown here, one of only two such neurons found in my entire experience, was located in the hippocampus. Mitochondrial cristae are still visible, and there is early blebbing of the cytoplasm, with intact membranes. The nucleus is homogeneous, as would be expected in apoptosis, and contrasts with necrosis. There is generalized condensation of both nucleus and cytoplasm that gives rise to increased electron density, a feature compatible with apoptosis. The rarity of this deserves emphasis. (Bar = 5 μm.) (From Auer RN, Kalimo H, Olsson Y, Siesjö B: The temporal evolution of hypoglycemic brain damage. II: Light- and electron-microscopic findings in the hippocampal gyrus and subiculum of the rat. *Acta Neuropathol [Berlin]* 67:25-36, 1985, © Springer-Verlag.)

of the neuropil containing dendrites that are activated by ischemia-released glutamate). Nevertheless, several independent laboratories have described axon-sparing dendritic lesions in ischemic neuronal death.[7,8] Although the excitatory amino acid released in ischemia is glutamate, identical dendritic swelling is seen in hypoglycemia,[9] in which aspartate[10] is released in greater quantities than glutamate. In epilepsy[11,12] and monosodium glutamate (MSG) neurotoxicity,[13] the neuropil has the same

appearance through a similar mechanism of excitatory compounds selectively binding to dendrites.

It seems that the stage of selective dendritic swelling and calcium entry is reversible[14] and may presage a more serious lesion: selective dendritic membrane breaks (see Figs. 5-2 and 5-4). This is evidenced by the entry of horseradish peroxidase (HRP) into the terminal dendrites in swollen ischemic neuronal cell processes.[15] HRP has a molecular weight of approximately 40,000 to 60,000 daltons, and its entry into neurons indicates holes of considerable size in the cell membrane. Neuronal death can thus be envisaged as a series of membrane breaches beginning in dendrites, with initial swelling developing into cell membrane breaks (see Figs. 5-3 and 5-4). Provided that these breaches are limited to the distal dendritic tree and are not large and confluent, the neuron can survive their presence.[15] However, extension of cell membrane breaks into large portions of the neuronal perikaryon constitutes a subcellular lesion that is clearly irreversible.

Concurrent with the appearance of large and confluent perikaryal membrane breaches is the appearance of mitochondrial flocculent densities (see Fig. 5-3A). These have been shown to represent trypsin-digestible proteins derived from the electron transport proteins of the mitochondrial matrix.[4-6] Mitochondrial flocculent densities and cell membrane breaks (in the neuronal perikaryon) constitute the electron microscopic counterpart of the acidophilic neuron seen at the light microscopic level.

Pannecrosis or Infarction

Although selective neuronal necrosis seems related to the selective neuronal actions of glutamate or its congeners, pannecrosis is a less discriminating cellular lesion that sweeps away neurons and glia alike. One can thus regard infarction, or pannecrosis, as a tissue-level lesion rather than a specific cellular lesion. The implication is that the cause of infarction is probably not related to the individually unique cytologic properties of the cells affected because they are affected so indiscriminately. This lack of discrimination contrasts sharply with selective neuronal necrosis, in which cellular properties of neurons are critical in determining neuronal death. Indeed, infarction must be considered a consequence of primary interruption of blood flow to a brain region below critical cerebral blood flow thresholds. If this interruption is permanent, tissue events simply resemble autolysis. Permanent focal ischemia can thus be conceptually termed *autolytic infarction*. The importance of restoring blood flow is obvious.

Hypermetabolism and Acidosis in Central Nervous System Tissue

There is, however, another mechanism for pannecrosis, or cerebral infarction. Massive productions of hydrogen ions have been shown experimentally to indiscriminately kill all cell types in central nervous system (CNS) tissue.[16] The fact that H+ ions, when injected into CNS tissue, can kill tissue components indiscriminately is only indirect evidence for acidosis-mediated tissue damage. However, there is more direct evidence from several

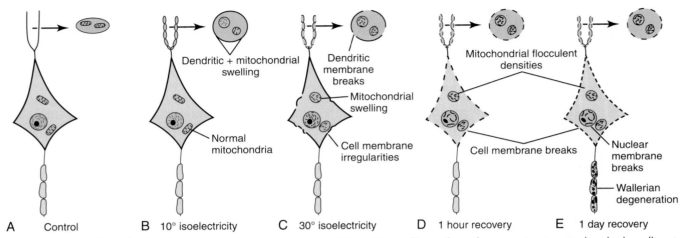

Figure 5-4 "Dendritic death" of neurons, beginning as segmental dendritic swelling only and progressing to mitochondrial swelling in the perikaryon. Cell membrane breaks begin in dendrites and, once they have spread to the perikaryon, signify irreversible cellular injury and death. Wallerian degeneration of the axon and karyorrhexis/cytolysis follow over days to weeks. (Adapted from Auer RN, Kalimo H, Olsson Y, Wieloch T: The dentate gyrus in hypoglycemia: Pathology implicating excitotoxin-mediated neuronal necrosis. *Acta Neuropathol [Berlin]* 67:279-288, 1985, © Springer-Verlag.)

CNS diseases that critical drops in pH cause pannecrosis. These diseases are Wernicke's encephalopathy,[17] necrosis of the substantia nigra, pars reticulata in epilepsy,[18,19] and ischemia itself,[20,21] in which the necrotizing effect of enhanced tissue acidosis is best revealed by expansion of infarction at high glucose levels, which promote acidosis.[22,23] It is important to note that focal acidosis in the brain can cause pannecrosis[17,18,24] even with adequate local blood flow.[19,25] As in selective neuronal necrosis, pannecrosis of identical appearance results from diverse initiating pathophysiologic states.

When experimental epilepsy is produced in rodents, high focal metabolic rates in the substantia nigra outstrip the capacity of the local blood supply to remove H+ ions from the tissue. A marked increase in tissue lactate ensues, with an accompanying drop in pH.[19,26] Pannecrosis occurs histologically, even though no hypoperfusion has taken place. The same process occurs in human encephalomyelopathies caused by mitochondrial abnormalities, in which acidotic brain infarcts occur in nonvascular distributions.[27,28]

In Wernicke's encephalopathy, there is a similar focal tissue acidosis due to thiamine deficiency.[17] The histologic appearance is noteworthy, consisting of selective necrosis of the neuropil, actually sparing cell bodies of all types. The sparing of neurons is especially remarkable. A similar histologic appearance is seen in Leigh's disease, another condition believed to be related to focal CNS acidosis.

In ischemia, pannecrosis has salient histologic features identical to those seen in other acidosis-related causes of CNS necrosis. Specifically, the neuropil can be selectively affected, which spares neurons at infarct borders. This may account for the very narrow rim of penumbra seen in many studies (see Fig. 5-1B).[29] The production of acid equivalents by the neuropil is due to the location of glycolytic metabolism in the neuropil as opposed to the neuronal cell bodies. This metabolic correlate of micronecrosis and pannecrosis in the neuropil derives from functional localization of glutamate-stimulated glycolysis[30,31]

predominantly to astrocytes and selective metabolism of lactate by neuronal processes in the neuropil.[32-34]

The finding that infarcts generally have a sharp, well-demarcated border, without always a rim of selective neuronal necrosis around an infarct (see Fig. 5-1B), implies that reduction of ischemic infarction may take place by shrinking of a relatively homogeneous area of tissue damage rather than through a decrease in grades of damage at the infarct border. This finding further supports the use of surrogate markers in clinical trials because infarcts can be sharply demarcated and their volumes determined neuroradiologically. In spite of graded reductions of cerebral blood flow as one progresses outward from the core of an infarct, the resulting pathology has an "all or none" feature, which suggests a threshold effect of pH. This pathology is consistent with acidosis below some critical threshold that gives rise to expanding pannecrosis at the sharp rim of CNS infarction in ischemia,[22,23,35] as it does in the other CNS diseases already reviewed.

Apoptosis in Ischemia

Since the description of apoptosis three decades ago,[36] an intense research effort has been made to demonstrate this phenomenon in adult nervous tissue subjected to ischemia. There are several reasons to believe that apoptosis is not a major occurrence in ischemia of the brain.

First, apoptosis is usually a counterforce to mitosis in biology. Thus, apoptosis balances mitosis in embryology, in tumors, and in normally proliferating epithelia of the body. Neurons lack mitosis, or a cell cycle. Indeed, it would be teleologically curious if apoptosis occurred in these important, postmitotic cells. Olfactory and dentate granule neurons of the hippocampus are salient exceptions.

Second, TUNEL labeling (terminal deoxyribonucleotidyl transferase [TDT]-mediated dUTP-digoxigenin nick end-labeling)[37] is often taken to support apoptosis, but results of TUNEL labeling are positive in not only

TABLE 5-2 CONSTRASTING FEATURES OF NECROSIS AND APOPTOSIS

Feature	Necrosis	Apoptosis
Acidophilia	Early	Late
Cell volume change	Swelling	Shrinkage
Cell membrane breaks	Early	Late
Mitochondrial flocculent densities	Early	Late
Inflammation	Prominent (depending on severity of tissue injury)	Absent

apoptosis but also necrosis and autolysis,[38,39] likely representing nonspecific DNA degradation.

Third, electron microscopic features of necrosis can be contrasted with those of apoptosis (Table 5-2) and are not seen in ischemia. Light microscopy is inadequate for resolving the features of the cell membrane and mitochondria. Thus, electron microscopy is required to determine the characteristic morphologic features of programmed cell death. Otherwise, karyorhectic and cytorhectic cell fragments may be mistaken for apoptotic bodies. In parts of the brain where there is a residuum of active neuronal regeneration, such as the dentate granule cell layer,[40] electron microscopic evidence of apoptotic neuronal death (in the dentate granule neurons of the hippocampus after adrenalectomy) has indeed been described.[41-43] Electron microscopic studies specifically looking for features of apoptosis in ischemia, under conditions theoretically favoring apoptosis, have not found them.[44-46]

Fourth, inflammation is absent in apoptosis yet forms a prominent component of ischemic histopathology. Attempts to dampen inflammation and ameliorate ischemic damage have generally met with positive results[47-51] but also some negative results.[52,53] Regardless of whether it plays a role in cell death, the vigorous inflammatory response of ischemia argues against apoptosis.

Fifth, apoptosis in ischemic stroke would require the simultaneous cell suicide of neurons and all types of glia, geographically demarcated across cell processes in the neuropil to form an infarct border. The signaling necessary to accomplish this geographic coordination of cell suicide seems far from clear. Furthermore, the sharp line of demarcation of infarcts across the neuropil (see Fig. 5-1*B*) would require apoptosis of processes of cells and is a feature also incompatible with apoptosis. A conceptual framework for apoptosis has been proposed.[54]

Epilogue

The histopathology of cerebral ischemia derives its importance from being the mediator of clinical neurologic deficits resulting from ischemia. Global ischemia clinically occurs in the setting of cardiac arrest and can be modeled by two-vessel occlusion,[55] four-vessel occlusion,[56] cardiac arrest, and aortic occlusion in animals. Focal cerebral ischemia is likewise easily modeled by either clip occlusion[57] or intraluminal occlusion models using an intraluminal suture[58] advanced into the middle cerebral artery

in experimental animals. This suture mimics thromboembolic stroke as opposed to cardiac arrest.

In both cardiac arrest encephalopathy and focal ischemic infarction, it is necrosis of cells and tissue that causes clinical neurologic deficits. In global cerebral ischemia, selective neuronal necrosis occurs in the selectively vulnerable CA1 pyramidal neurons of the hippocampus, the clinical counterpart of which is persistent amnesia after cardiac arrest.[59,60] Focal cerebral ischemia gives rise to a very rich spectrum of potential neurologic disabilities dependent on the location of the infarct in the telencephalon or brainstem–cerebellum. There is no precedent for acquired ischemic neurologic deficit without tissue necrosis of some kind. Thus, it is incumbent on the clinician treating stroke to understand the causes of selective neuronal necrosis and infarction when attempting to mitigate these two tissue lesions wherever they may occur in the brain.

REFERENCES

1. Norris JW, Zhu CZ: Silent stroke and carotid stenosis, *Stroke* 23:483–485, 1992.
2. de Courten-Myers GM, Kleinholz M, Wagner KR, Myers RE: Stroke assessment: Morphometric infarct size versus neurologic deficit, *J Neurosci Methods* 83:151–157, 1998.
3. Kiernan JA, Macpherson CM, Price A, Sun T: A histochemical examination of the staining of kainate-induced neuronal degeneration by anionic dyes, *Biotech Histochem* 73:244–254, 1998.
4. Trump BF, Goldblatt PJ, Stowell RE: Studies on necrosis of mouse liver in vitro: Ultrastructural alterations in the mitochondria of hepatic parenchymal cells, *Lab Invest* 14:343–371, 1965.
5. Trump BF, Strum JM, Bulger RE: Studies on the pathogenesis of ischaemic cell injury. I: Relation between ion and water shifts and cell ultrastructure in rat kidney slices during swelling at 0-4° C, *Virch Arch B Cell Pathol* 16:1–34, 1974.
6. Trump BF, McDowell EM, Arstila AU: Cellular reaction to injury. In Hill RB, LaVia MF, editors: *Principles of pathobiology*, ed 3, New York, 1980, Oxford University Press, pp 20–111.
7. Johansen FF, Jørgensen MB, von Lubitz DKJE, Diemer NH: Selective dendrite damage in hippocampal CA1 stratum radiatum with unchanged axon ultrastructure and glutamate uptake after transient cerebral ischemia in the rat, *Brain Res* 291:373–377, 1984.
8. Yamamoto K, Hayakawa T, Mogami H, et al: Ultrastructural investigation of the CA1 region of the hippocampus after transient cerebral ischemia in gerbils, *Acta Neuropathol* 80:487–492, 1990.
9. Auer RN, Kalimo H, Olsson Y, Wieloch T: The dentate gyrus in hypoglycemia: Pathology implicating excitotoxin-mediated neuronal necrosis, *Acta Neuropathol* 67:279–288, 1985.
10. Sandberg M, Butcher SP, Hagberg H: Extracellular overflow of neuroactive amino acids during severe insulin-induced hypoglycemia: In vivo dialysis of the rat hippocampus, *J Neurochem* 47:178–184, 1986.
11. Ingvar M, Morgan PF, Auer RN: The nature and timing of excitotoxic neuronal necrosis in the cerebral cortex, hippocampus and thalamus due to flurothyl-induced status epilepticus, *Acta Neuropathol* 75:362–369, 1988.
12. Griffiths T, Evans MC, Meldrum BS: Intracellular calcium accumulation in rat hippocampus during seizures induced by bicuculline or L-allylglycine, *Neuroscience* 10:385–395, 1983.
13. Olney JW, Sharpe LG, Feigin R: Glutamate-induced brain damage in infant primates, *J Neuropathol Exp Neurol* 31:464–488, 1972.
14. Griffiths T, Evans MC, Meldrum BS: Status epilepticus: The reversibility of calcium loading and acute neuronal pathological changes in the rat hippocampus, *Neuroscience* 12:557–567, 1984.
15. Diemer NH, von Lubitz DJKE: Cerebral ischaemia in the rat: Increased permeability of post-synaptic membranes to horseradish peroxidase in the early post-ischaemic period, *Neuropathol Appl Neurobiol* 9:403–414, 1983.
16. Kraig RP, Pulsinelli WA, Plum F: Carbonic acid buffer changes during complete brain ischemia, *Am J Physiol* 250:R348–R357, 1986.
17. Hakim AM: The induction and reversibility of cerebral acidosis in thiamine deficiency, *Ann Neurol* 16:673–679, 1984.

18. Ingvar M, Folbergrová J, Siesjö BK: Metabolic alterations underlying the development of hypermetabolic necrosis in the substantia nigra in status epilepticus, *J Cereb Blood Flow Metab* 7:103-108, 1987.

19. Ingvar M: Cerebral blood flow and metabolic rate during seizures, *Ann N Y Acad Sci* 462:194-206, 1986.

20. Hakim AM, Arrieta M: Cerebral acidosis in focal ischemia. I: A method for the simultaneous measurement of local cerebral pH with cerebral glucose utilization or cerebral blood flow in the rat, *J Cereb Blood Flow Metab* 6:667-675, 1986.

21. Hakim AM: Cerebral acidosis in focal ischemia. II: Nimodipine and verapamil normalize cerebral pH following middle cerebral artery occlusion in the rat, *J Cereb Blood Flow Metab* 6:676-683, 1986.

22. Nedergaard M: Transient focal ischemia in hyperglycemic rats is associated with increased cerebral infarction, *Brain Res* 408:79-85, 1987.

23. Nedergaard M, Diemer NH: Focal ischemia of the rat brain, with special reference to the influence of plasma glucose concentration, *Acta Neuropathol* 73:131-137, 1987.

24. Auer RN, Ingvar M, Nevander G, et al: Early axonal lesion and preserved microvasculature in epilepsy-induced hypermetabolic necrosis of the substantia nigra, *Acta Neuropathol* 71:207-215, 1986.

25. Hakim AM: Effect of thiamine deficiency and its reversal on cerebral blood flow in the rat: Observations on the phenomena of hyperperfusion, "no reflow," and delayed hypoperfusion, *J Cereb Blood Flow Metab* 6:79-85, 1986.

26. Folbergrová J, Ingvar M, Nevander G, Siesjö BK: Cerebral metabolic changes during and following flurothyl-induced seizures in ventilated rats, *J Neurochem* 44:1419-1426, 1985.

27. Kuriyama M, Umezaki H, Fukuda Y, et al: Mitochondrial encephalomyelopathy with lactate-pyruvate elevation and brain infarctions, *Neurology* 34:72-77, 1984.

28. Bogousslavsky J, Perentes E, Deruaz JP, Regli F: Mitochondrial myopathy and cardiomyopathy with neurodegenerative features and multiple brain infarcts, *J Neurol Sci* 55:351-357, 1982.

29. Nedergaard M, Gjedde A, Diemer NH: Focal ischemia of the rat brain: Autoradiographic determination of cerebral glucose utilization, glucose content, and blood flow, *J Cereb Blood Flow Metab* 6:414-424, 1986.

30. Pellerin L, Magistretti PJ: Glutamate uptake into astrocytes stimulates aerobic glycolysis: A mechanism coupling neuronal activity to glucose utilization, *Proc Natl Acad Sci U S A* 91:10625-10629, 1994.

31. Schurr A, Miller JJ, Payne RS, Rigor BM: An increase in lactate output by brain tissue serves to meet the energy needs of glutamate-activated neurons, *J Neurosci* 19:34-39, 1999.

32. Dringen R, Gebhardt R, Hamprecht B: Glycogen in astrocytes: Possible function as lactate supply for neighboring cells, *Brain Res* 623:208-214, 1993.

33. Sokoloff L, Takahashi S, Gotoh J, et al: Contribution of astroglia to functionally activated energy metabolism, *Dev Neurosci* 18:344-352, 1996.

34. Sokoloff L: Energetics of functional activation in neural tissues, *Neurochem Res* 24:321-329, 1999.

35. Anderson RE, Tan WK, Martin HS, Meyer FB: Effects of glucose and Pao$_2$ modulation on cortical intracellular acidosis, NADH redox state, and infarction in the ischemic penumbra, *Stroke* 30:160-170, 1999.

36. Kerr JFR: Shrinkage necrosis: A distinct mode of cellular death, *J Pathol* 105:13-20, 1971.

37. Charriaut-Marlangue C, Ben-Ari Y: A cautionary note on the use of the TUNEL stain to determine apoptosis, *Neuroreport* 7:61-64, 1995.

38. Grasl-Kraupp B, Ruttkay-Nedecky B, Koudelka H, et al: In situ detection of fragmented DNA (TUNEL assay) fails to discriminate among apoptosis, necrosis, and autolytic cell death: A cautionary note, *Hepatology* 21:1465-1468, 1995.

39. de Torres C, Munell F, Ferrer I, et al: Identification of necrotic cell death by the TUNEL assay in the hypoxic-ischemic neonatal rat brain, *Neurosci Lett* 230:1-4, 1997.

40. Palmer TD, Willhoite AR, Gage FH: Vascular niche for adult hippocampal neurogenesis, *J Comp Neurol* 425:479-494, 2000.

41. Sloviter RS, Valiquette G, Abrams GM, et al: Selective loss of hippocampal cells in the mature rat brain after adrenalectomy, *Science* 243:535-538, 1989.

42. Sloviter RS, Sollas AL, Dean E, Neubort S: Adrenalectomy-induced granule cell degeneration in the rat hippocampal dentate gyrus: Characterization of an in vivo model of controlled neuronal death, *J Comp Neurol* 330:324-336, 1993.

43. Sloviter RS, Dean E, Neubort S: Electron microscopic analysis of adrenalectomy-induced hippocampal granule cell degeneration in the rat: Apoptosis in the adult central nervous system, *J Comp Neurol* 330:337-351, 1993.

44. Deshpande J, Bergstedt K, Lindén T, et al: Ultrastructural changes in the hippocampal CA1 region following transient cerebral ischemia: Evidence against programmed cell death, *Exp Brain Res* 88:91-105, 1992.

45. Fukuda T, Wang H, Nakanishi H, et al: Novel non-apoptotic morphological changes in neurons of the mouse hippocampus following transient hypoxic-ischemia, *Neurosci Res* 33:49-55, 1999.

46. Colbourne F, Sutherland GR, Auer RN: Electron microscopic evidence against apoptosis as the mechanism of neuronal death in global ischemia, *J Neurosci* 19:4200-4210, 1999.

47. Bednar MM, Raymond S, McAuliffe T, et al: The role of neutrophils and platelets in a rabbit model of thromboembolic stroke, *Stroke* 22:44-50, 1991.

48. Bowes MP, Zivin JA, Rothlein R: Monoclonal antibody to the ICAM-1 adhesion site reduces neurological damage in a rabbit cerebral embolism stroke model, *Exp Neurol* 119:215-219, 1993.

49. Chen H, Chopp M, Bodzin G: Neutropenia reduces the volume of cerebral infarct after transient middle cerebral artery occlusion in the rat, *Neurosci Res Comm* 11:93-99, 1992.

50. Chopp M, Zhang RL, Chen H, et al: Postischemic administration of an anti-MAC-1 antibody reduces ischemic cell damage after transient middle cerebral artery occlusion in rats, *Stroke* 25:869-876, 1994.

51. Matsuo Y, Onodera H, Shiga Y, et al: Correlation between myeloperoxidase-quantified neutrophil accumulation and ischemic brain injury in the rat: Effects of neutrophil depletion, *Stroke* 25:1469-1475, 1994.

52. Schürer L, Grøgaard B, Gerdin B, et al: Leucocyte depletion does not affect post-ischaemic nerve cell damage in the rat, *Acta Neurochir (Wien)* 111:54-60, 1991.

53. Takeshima R, Kirsch JR, Koehler RC, et al: Monoclonal leukocyte antibody does not decrease the injury of transient focal cerebral ischemia in cats, *Stroke* 23:247-252, 1992.

54. Sloviter RS: Apoptosis: A guide for the perplexed, *Trends Pharmacol Sci* 23:19-24, 2002.

55. Smith M-L, Auer RN, Siesjö BK: The density and distribution of ischemic brain injury in the rat after 2-10 minutes of forebrain ischemia, *Acta Neuropathol* 64:319-332, 1984.

56. Pulsinelli WA, Brierley JB: A new model of bilateral hemispheric ischemia in the unanesthetized rat, *Stroke* 10:267-272, 1979.

57. Tamura A, Graham DI, McCulloch J, Teasdale GM: Focal cerebral ischemia in the rat. 1: Description of technique and early neuropathological consequences following middle cerebral artery occlusion, *J Cereb Blood Flow Metab* 1:53-60, 1981.

58. Longa EZ, Weinstein PR, Carlson S, Cummins R: Reversible middle cerebral artery occlusion without craniectomy in rats, *Stroke* 20:84-91, 1989.

59. Longstreth WT Jr, Inui TS, Cobb LA, Copass MK: Neurologic recovery after out-of-hospital cardiac arrest, *Ann Intern Med* 98:588-592, 1983.

60. Longstreth WT Jr, Inui TS: High blood glucose level on hospital admission and poor neurological recovery after cardiac arrest, *Ann Neurol* 15:59-63, 1984.

6 Molecular and Cellular Mechanisms of Ischemia-Induced Neuronal Death

DIMITRY OFENGEIM, TAKAHIRO MIYAWAKI, R. SUZANNE ZUKIN

Ischemia is the condition or state in which a tissue such as brain is subjected to hypoxia or low oxygen because of an obstruction of the arterial blood supply or inadequate blood flow. Brain ischemia can be broadly divided into two main classifications, global ischemia and focal ischemia. *Global ischemia* is the condition or state in which blood flow to the entire brain is transiently blocked, which results in delayed, selective neuronal death. *Focal ischemia* or cerebral infarction is the condition or state in which a specific area of brain tissue undergoes injury as a consequence of a temporary or permanent obstruction of local blood supply. Focal ischemia results in death of both neurons and nonneuronal cells in contiguous areas of brain, usually representing a single vascular territory. This chapter presents our current understanding of the molecular and cellular underpinnings of the neuronal death associated with brain ischemia.

Global Ischemia

Global or brain-wide ischemia arises most commonly in humans as a consequence of cardiac arrest, open-heart surgery, profuse bleeding, near-drowning, or carbon monoxide poisoning. Global ischemia associated with cardiac arrest affects 150,000 Americans each year and, in most cases, results in delayed onset of neurologic deficits (for review, see Liou et al,[1] Lo et al,[2] and Moskowitz et al[3]). The most common neurologic deficits are cognitive impairments, of which memory loss is most notable. Although all forebrain areas experience oxygen and glucose deprivation during the brief ischemic insult, only selected neuronal populations degenerate and die in humans and in animals subjected experimentally to global ischemia (for review, see Liou et al,[1] Lo et al,[2] and Moskowitz et al[3]). Pyramidal neurons in the hippocampal CA1 are particularly vulnerable. Other neurons that may be damaged are hilar neurons of the dentate gyrus; medium aspiny neurons of the striatum; pyramidal neurons in neocortical layers II, V, and VI; and Purkinje neurons of the cerebellum. The molecular mechanisms underlying the cell-specific pattern of global ischemia–induced neuronal death are not well understood.

Histologic evidence of degeneration, exhibiting characteristics of apoptosis and necrosis, is not observed until 2 to 3 days after ischemia in rats and 3 to 4 days in gerbils (for review, see Liou et al,[1] Lo et al,[2] Moskowitz et al,[3] and Schmidt-Kastner and Freund[4]). At 1 week after induction of transient global ischemia, virtually complete ablation of the CA1 pyramidal cell layer can be observed. During the ischemic episode, cells exhibit a transient early rise in intracellular Ca^{2+}, depolarize, and become inexcitable; ambient glutamate increases by approximately fourfold to approximately 2 μM. After reperfusion, cells appear morphologically normal, exhibit normal intracellular Ca^{2+}, and regain the ability to generate action potentials for 24 to 72 hours after the insult. Ultimately, there is a late increase in intracellular Ca^{2+} and Zn^{2+}, and death of CA1 pyramidal neurons ensues. Although the molecular mechanisms underlying ischemia-induced death are not yet completely understood, the substantial delay between insult and onset of death suggests that transcriptional changes play a critical role. Candidate transcription factors that are thought to direct programs of gene expression changes after global ischemia include the cyclic adenosine monophosphate (AMP) response element binding protein (CREB), nuclear factor-kappa B (NF-κB), the forkhead family of transcription factors, and repressor element 1 silencing transcription factor (REST), which is also known as neuron-specific silencing factor (NRSF) (see later).

Focal Ischemia

Focal or localized ischemia arises in humans most commonly as a result of stroke, cerebral hemorrhage, or traumatic brain injury (for review see Liou et al,[1] Lo et al,[2] and Moskowitz et al[3]). Most strokes are caused by clots that form at the site of occlusion in a cerebral artery or move there from the heart (classic stroke), whereas the remainder result from a weakened blood vessel in the brain that bursts and bleeds into the surrounding tissue (cerebral hemorrhage or traumatic brain injury). Stroke is the third leading cause of death in the United States and the primary cause of disabilities in adults. Of the approximately 600,000 new victims each year, nearly 30% die and 20%

to 30% become severely and permanently disabled. Others have paralysis; reduced coordination; abnormalities in motor strength, coordination, sensory function, and language abilities; and neurologic deficits including impaired cognition, visual disturbance, and loss of sensation. People older than age 65 experience almost three fourths of all strokes. The molecular and cellular mechanisms underlying cell death associated with a *brain attack* can be studied in animal models of focal ischemia (see later).

Tissues at risk of harm from occlusion of a cerebral artery are the *core* or center of the stroke, which contains cells that are highly dependent on the blocked artery and receive essentially no blood, and the *penumbra* or surrounding region, which contains cells that receive some blood from other arteries. Cells in the core die from several overwhelming causes and probably cannot be salvaged by any treatment short of immediate clot removal. Although the infarct starts in the core, at its maximum it encompasses both core and penumbra, generally by 6 to 24 hours after induction of permanent ischemia.[5] The duration of the ischemic episode determines the extent or grade of damage, assessed 1 to 2 days after reperfusion.[6] At 10 to 20 minutes after induction of focal ischemia, only a few scattered dead neurons are observed in the core. At 1 hour, infarct is observed in the core, and the infarct size is maximal. The mechanisms underlying death of cells in the core are complicated but most certainly include glutamate receptor–mediated necrotic cell death (see later). Brain edema (as studied by magnetic resonance imaging [MRI] and computed tomography) serves as one of the earliest markers for the ensuing pathophysiology and is a key determinant of whether a patient survives beyond the first few hours after a stroke.

Experimental Models of Global and Focal Ischemia

A number of experimental models are currently used to study brain ischemia. There are three main paradigms involving intact animals (in vivo ischemia): global ischemia, focal ischemia, and hypoxia/ischemia, a condition that shares properties with both focal and global ischemia. In vivo models of global ischemia enable neuronal death to mature in an intact animal in which neural circuitry is preserved. Therefore, these models have greater physiologic validity and clinical relevance to global ischemia associated with cardiac arrest in humans than do in vitro models. In vitro models involving primary cultures of neurons or organotypically cultured brain slices are particularly useful for knockdown or overexpression of genes of interest. In vitro models involving organotypically cultured brain slices are particularly useful in that they afford preservation of neural circuitry. Both in vivo and in vitro models are useful for examination of molecular and biophysical mechanisms of ischemia-induced neuronal death.

In Vivo Models

Global Ischemia

Global ischemic insults consist of brief but near-complete cessation of cerebral blood flow produced by permanent occlusion of the vertebral arteries and transient occlusion of the common carotid arteries (rats) or by transient occlusion of the common carotid arteries (gerbils and mice), followed by reperfusion.[7] The most commonly used models of global ischemia are (1) the four-vessel occlusion (4-VO) model in rats (Fig. 6-1A)[8,9]; (2) the two-vessel occlusion (2-VO, also known as temporary bilateral common carotid occlusion or BCCO) model in gerbils[10] or (less commonly) in mice[11,12]; and (3) two-vessel occlusion (2-VO) in combination with hypotension in rats[13]; for review, see Small and Buchan.[7] Global ischemia can also be induced in large mammals such as monkeys[14] or goats.[15] Global ischemic insults are typically short (on the order of 5 to 20 minutes). During the ischemic episode, blood flow to the entire brain is reduced (to <1%) essentially immediately and remains blocked until reperfusion. As a consequence, adenosine triphosphate (ATP) is depleted in cells throughout the brain but recovers to near-physiologic levels by the time of reperfusion (see later).

The 4-VO model in rats and the 2-VO model in gerbils differ from more severe models involving hypotension in that neuronal death is highly delayed and highly specific. Although all forebrain areas experience oxygen and glucose deprivation during a brief ischemic insult, neuronal death elicited by a brief episode (10 minutes for 4-VO in rats; 5 minutes for 2-VO in gerbils) is largely restricted to pyramidal neurons of the hippocampal CA1 and hilar neurons (for review, see Schmidt-Kastner and Freund[4]) (Fig. 6-1B). Inhibitory interneurons of the CA1 and most neurons in the nearby CA2 or transition zone, CA3, and dentate gyrus survive. With the exception of a few scattered hilar neurons and/or pyramidal neurons in the cortex, no other neurons exhibit cell death. Although these models afford virtual ablation of the hippocampal CA1 by 7 days, the onset of histologically detectable neuronal death is not manifested until more than 48 hours in rats[16] or more than 72 hours in gerbils.[10] Longer insults induce more widespread damage that includes medium aspiny striatal neurons; pyramidal neurons in neocortical layers II, V, and VI; and cerebellar Purkinje neurons.[10,16]

Advantages of the in vivo models of global ischemia are (1) the clinical relevance to global ischemia associated with cardiac arrest in humans; (2) the preservation of neural circuitry; (3) a substantial delay between insult and neuronal death, which enables detailed molecular studies; (4) specificity of cell death, which enables comparison of molecular changes in CA1 with those in CA3; (5) complete blockage of the cranium (rather than reduction by hypotension) rendering monitoring of blood flow unnecessary; and (6) no obvious behavioral manifestations exhibited by animals, and low mortality rate. The rare animals that exhibit obvious behavioral manifestations (e.g., abnormal vocalization when handled, generalized convulsions, loss of greater than 20% body weight by 3 to 7 days, and hypoactivity) are excluded from the study.

Four-vessel occlusion (4-VO) model in rats. Four-VO provides a well-established model of global ischemia in which neuronal death is largely restricted to pyramidal neurons of the hippocampal CA1 and does not manifest itself until 3 to 4 days after insult.[8,9] Age-matched male Sprague Dawley or Wistar rats weighing 100 to 125 grams are fasted overnight, and on the next day, they are anesthetized with halothane. The vertebral arteries are

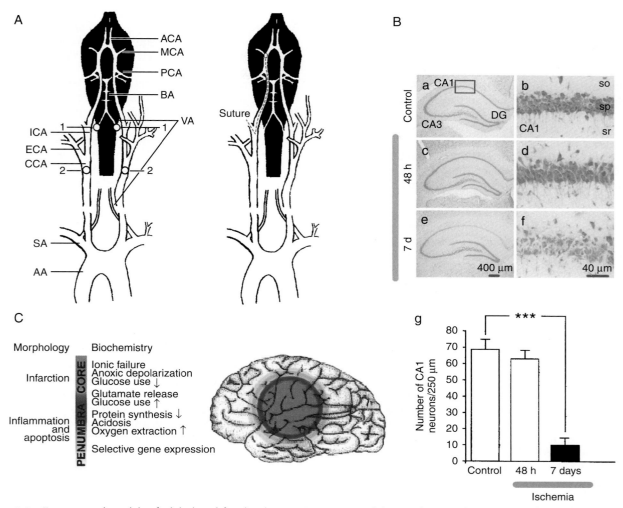

Figure 6-1 Experimental models of global and focal ischemia. A, Diagram of the cerebrovascular anatomy of the rat, illustrating the permanent electrocauterization of the vertebral arteries *(1)* and the position of the surgical clips in the common carotid arteries *(2)* in 4-VO model *(left)* and the intraluminal suture during occlusion in the temporary focal ischemia model *(right)*. AA, Arch of the aorta; ACA, anterior cerebral artery; BA, basilar artery; CCA, common carotid artery; ECA, external carotid artery; ICA, internal carotid artery; MCA, middle cerebral artery; PCA, posterior cerebral artery; SA, subclavian artery; VA, vertebral artery. B, Toluidine blue staining of coronal brain sections at the level of the dorsal hippocampus from control *(a, b)* and experimental male rats subjected to global ischemia at 48 hours *(c, d)* and 7 days *(e, f)* after ischemia. At 48 hours after global ischemia, there was no histologically detectable neuronal death in any hippocampal subfield. At 7 days after ischemia, the pyramidal cell layer of CA1 exhibited dramatic loss of neurons, whereas CA3 and dentate gyrus showed no damage. Scale bars: lower magnification, 400 μm; higher magnification, 40 μm. *(g)* Quantitation of cell counts from brain sections illustrated in *(a-f)*. For assessment of hippocampal injury, the number of surviving neurons per 250-μm length in the pyramidal cell layer of the medial CA1 were counted under a light microscope at 40× magnification in sections. Neuronal counts from a minimum of four microscopic sections per animal were analyzed; comparisons among group means were made using the Student *t*-test (***, $P < 0.001$). C, The core and penumbra of ischemia are induced by focal blockade of cerebral arteries. A brain region of low perfusion in which cells have lost their membrane potential terminally ("core") is surrounded by an area in which intermediate perfusion prevails ("penumbra") and cells depolarize intermittently ("peri-infarct depolarization"). Note that from the onset of the focal perfusion deficit, the core and penumbra are dynamic in space and time. Perfusion thresholds exist below which certain biochemical functions are impeded (color-coded scale). (A, Adapted from Longa EZ, Weinstein PR, Carlson S, et al: Reversible middle cerebral artery occlusion without craniectomy in rats. *Stroke* 20:84-91, 1989. B, Reprinted with permission from Calderone A, Jover T, Noh K-M, et al: Ischemic insults de-repress the gene silencer rest in neurons destined to die. *J Neurosci* 23:2112-2121, 2003. C, Reprinted with permission from Dirnagl U, Iadecola C, Moskowitz MA: Pathobiology of ischaemic stroke: an integrated view. *Trends Neurosci* 22:391-397, 1999.)

exposed by a small incision in the neck and subjected to permanent electrocauterization. The common carotid arteries are exposed and isolated with a 3-0 silk thread, and the wound is sutured. Twenty-four hours later, the wound is reopened and the common carotid arteries are subjected to temporary occlusion with surgical clasps (4 minutes for sublethal ischemia and 10 minutes for global

ischemia); anesthesia is discontinued. At the time of occlusion of the carotid arteries, blood flow is typically reduced to less than 3% of normal in the hippocampus, striatum, and neocortex.[9] The electroencephalogram (EEG) generally becomes flat, and spontaneous cortical activity is abolished within 1 minute.[9,17] For sham operation, animals are subjected to the same anesthesia and surgical exposure procedures, except that the carotid arteries are not occluded. Although anesthesia is typically administered until occlusion of the carotid arteries, it is not essential to the surgical procedure.

Two-vessel occlusion (2-VO) with hypotension in rats. An alternative model of global ischemia in rats involves ligation of the common carotid (but not vertebral) arteries, together with systemic hypotension (50 mm Hg).[13] Under these conditions, blood flow falls to 1% in the hippocampus, striatum, and neocortex, and the EEG becomes isoelectric within 15 to 25 seconds.[13] Animals are subjected to anesthesia for the entire duration of the ischemic episode. Models of global ischemia involving systemic hypoxia and/or hypotension are more severe than the 4-VO model. These models cause a more rapid onset of generalized neuronal death (pan-necrosis)—particularly in the cortex, striatum, and hippocampus—more severe behavioral manifestations, and considerable rates of mortality in animals.

Two-vessel occlusion (2-VO) in gerbils. The use of gerbils is advantageous in studies of global ischemia because gerbils lack the posterior communicating arteries (structures that in humans and rats is necessary to complete the circle of Willis and permit collateral blood flow). Thus, global ischemia can be induced in gerbils by the relatively simple 2-VO model. In gerbils, 2-VO (5 minutes) elicits highly selective, highly delayed neuronal death, and the pattern of cell specificity is virtually identical to that in rats; neuronal death is not manifested until after 72 hours.[10] Two-VO is the most frequently used model of global ischemia for testing neuroprotective agents. Within 20 seconds of 2-VO, blood flow falls to 1% in neocortex and to 4% in hippocampus; EEG failure occurs.[18] Anesthesia is not used during this type of ischemia.

Two-vessel occlusion (2-VO) in mice. Mice offer advantages in that some strains (C57/BL6 and related strains) exhibit global ischemia in response to the relatively simple 2-VO model and enable comparisons between animals with null mutations in a gene of interest and their wild-type littermates. However, strain differences in vulnerability to ischemic damage can complicate results.[19] In mice, 2-VO (20 minutes) elicits somewhat selective, delayed cell death. At 72 hours after ischemia, the majority of mice exhibit no detectable cell loss in the hippocampus; approximately 17% of mice exhibit minor cell loss, and approximately 17% exhibited moderate cell loss in the CA1.[12] At 7 days after ischemia, nearly all animals exhibited marked loss in the pyramidal cell layer of CA1. In the majority of animals, CA3 exhibited, at most, slight cell loss, and the dentate gyrus exhibited no cell loss at 7 days.

Focal Ischemia

Focal ischemia is the animal model that most nearly approximates stroke or cerebral infarction in humans.[20] Focal ischemia is produced experimentally by occlusion of the middle cerebral artery. Arterial occlusion can be permanent (arterial blockade maintained throughout the experiment) or temporary (occlusion for up to 3 hours, followed by reperfusion) and either proximal or distal (see later). These procedures induce a necrotic core of cells that are irreversibly damaged and a penumbra of cells that can be revived; lesions are of similar size and

time course of progression (Fig. 6-1C). Focal ischemia is typically performed in rodents such as rats or mice. For rats, a preferred strain is the spontaneously hypertensive rat, which exhibits reduced collateral circulation during the ischemic episode.

Proximal occlusion. In the case of proximal occlusion, the middle cerebral artery is subjected to occlusion (MCAO) close to its branching from the internal carotid, before the origin of the lenticulostriate arteries. Proximal MCAO is most commonly induced by ligation of the common carotid and external carotid arteries, followed by insertion of a suture into the internal carotid artery at the bifurcation of the common carotid and external carotid arteries. The suture is advanced intraluminally beyond the origin of the posterior communicating artery and past the origin of the MCAO.[21] After MCAO, blood flow is nonuniformly reduced throughout the affected region. The center of the stroke or core is defined as the region in which blood flow is reduced to less than 15% and encompasses the lateral portion of the caudate putamen and the parietal cortex. The penumbra, defined as the region in which blood flow is reduced to less than 40%, encompasses the remainder of the neocortex, the entorhinal cortex, and medial caudate-putamen.

Distal occlusion. In distal MCAO, blood flow to the basal ganglia is not interrupted; thus, damage is restricted to the neocortex. This type of occlusion can be induced surgically by means of a clip or by inducing thrombotic clots in combination with transient unilateral occlusion of the common carotid arteries.[22,23] The reduction of blood flow achieved in the core and penumbra is similar to that achieved in the proximal model.

Hypoxia/Ischemia

This ischemic model involves transient unilateral occlusion of the common carotid artery in combination with systemic hypoxia, such that oxygen flow to the brain is reduced to 3% in adults or to 8% in neonates.[24,25] After 15 to 30 minutes of hypoxia, delayed neuronal death occurs in the hippocampal CA1 and CA3, striatum, and layer V of the neocortex of adults. Young rats show delayed development of infarct, which can be induced by subjecting them to reduced oxygen (8% of normal) for 60 minutes.

In Vitro Models

Oxygen-glucose deprivation (OGD) of cell cultures or brain slices provides an in vitro model of global ischemia (for review, see Goldberg and Choi[26] and Martin et al[27]) (Fig. 6-2). In vitro models require longer periods of oxygen and glucose deprivation to induce cell death, and ATP levels do not fall as much as with in vivo models. The absence of blood vessels and blood flow simplifies interpretation of the results but renders the model less relevant than that of the intact animal. Advantages of the in vitro OGD model are (1) its amenability to more precise manipulations of the microenvironment, (2) amenability to patch-clamp recording and detailed electrophysiologic analyses, (3) prolonged survival of cultures, which permits molecular and genetic manipulations, (4) ease of antisense knockdown of a protein of interest by administration of antisense oligonucleotides and adaptability for

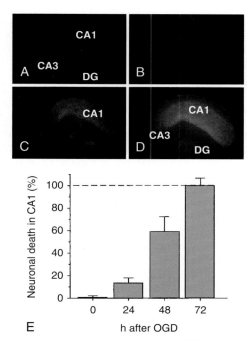

Figure 6-2 Oxygen-glucose deprivation (OGD), an in vitro model of global ischemia. Organotypically cultured hippocampal slices are maintained for 14 to 21 days in vitro and subjected to OGD by exposure to serum-free medium devoid of glucose and saturated with 95% N_2/5% CO_2 for 30 to 60 minutes. Slices are then transferred to oxygenated, serum-free medium containing glucose and propidium iodide. OGD (20- to 30-minute insult) elicits delayed, selective neuronal death, primarily of CA1 neurons, as occurs after transient global ischemia in the intact animal. Cell death is assessed by propidium iodide uptake due to breakdown of the integrity of the plasma membrane as cells enter the initial stages of cell death. A, A control slice shows no uptake of propidium iodide. B, C, D, Time course of neuronal death in the CA1 subfield at 24 hours (B), 48 hours (C), and 72 hours (D) after OGD. DG, dentate gyrus. E, Quantitation of data like those shown in B-D. (Adapted from Calderone A, Jover T, Noh K-M, et al: Ischemic insults de-repress the gene silencer rest in neurons destined to die. J Neurosci 23:2112-2121, 2003.)

optically monitoring changes in the same slice over days, and (5) internal control of a number of slices that can be obtained from the same animal.

OGD of Dissociated Neurons in Culture

In vitro OGD is performed in primary cultures of neurons/glia from the neocortex, hippocampus, cerebellum, and hypothalamus of embryonic or early postnatal rats or mice. Mixed neocortical cultures containing both neurons and glia are typically cultured from embryonic day 15 (E15) rats.[28] At 14 days in vitro (DIV), the culture medium is exchanged with deoxygenated, glucose-free salt solution so that OGD can be induced. Cultures are deprived of oxygen and glucose for 90 to 100 minutes and then transferred to oxygenated serum-free medium containing glucose and propidium iodide. Cell death is assayed at 24 and 48 hours.

OGD in Cultured Hippocampal Slices

Ischemic damage is also studied in organotypic hippocampal slice cultures from perinatal rats. Typically, hippocampal slices are obtained from rat pups (postnatal day 8 or P8) and maintained in vitro for 14 to 21 days.[28] Briefly, hippocampi are removed from rat brains, and transverse slices are cut with a tissue chopper in a sterile environment. Isolated slices are placed in ice-cold Hanks' balanced salt solution supplemented with glucose and amphotericin B (Fungizone) and then transferred to humidified semiporous membranes. Slices are maintained in culture medium at 37°C and 95% air/5% CO_2. At 14 to 21 DIV, hippocampal slices are subjected to OGD by exposure to serum-free medium devoid of glucose and saturated with 95% N_2/5% CO_2 for 30 to 60 minutes and transferred to oxygenated serum-free medium containing glucose and propidium iodide; cell death is assayed at 48 and 72 hours. A 30-minute insult elicits selective death of CA1 neurons by 48 hours (Fig. 6-2). Neuronal death is typically assessed by permeability to dyes such as trypan blue or propidium iodide.[29] In vitro ischemia impairs synaptic transmission, protein synthesis, ATP production, and neuron morphologic features.

Modalities of Ischemic Cell Death

Injurious stimuli such as ischemic insults activate multiple death cascades. There are three main classifications of mammalian cell death: apoptosis, necrosis, and autophagy, each of which exhibits a distinct histologic and biochemical signature (for review, see Kroemer et al[30]). *Apoptosis* is an evolutionarily conserved process of cell death by an internally programmed series of events mediated by a dedicated set of gene products (for review, see Kroemer et al,[30] Green,[31] Galluzzi et al,[32] and Wang and Youle[33]). *Necrosis* was traditionally thought to be a nonprogrammed, accidental form of cell death in response to overwhelming stress that is incompatible with cell survival (for review, see Kroemer et al[30] and Galluzi et al[34]). However, recent evidence indicates that necrosis can also be tightly regulated and that cells such as neurons can die by a form of necrosis, termed *necroptosis* or *programmed necrosis*.[35-37] Necroptosis is characterized by necrotic cell death morphology and activation of autophagy.[38-40] An additional modality of cell death is that of autophagy, an evolutionarily conserved catabolic process whereby cells generate energy and metabolites by digesting their own organelles and macromolecules via the lysosomal pathway.[30,41] *Autophagy* is a tightly regulated process that is essential to embryonic development, tissue homeostasis, and cell survival, helping to maintain a balance between the synthesis, degradation, and subsequent recycling of cellular products.[41] Autophagy is protective in that it allows an energy-deprived cell to survive during starvation by reallocating nutrients from unnecessary processes to more essential processes; however, it also functions in dying cells to mediate cell death.[39-41] Although recent evidence indicates that autophagy may be activated in postischemic hippocampal neurons,[42] a role for autophagy in ischemic injury is not well delineated.[3,30,41]

Necrosis

Necrotic cell death or *necrosis* is morphologically characterized by cell swelling (oncosis) that culminates in the rupture of the plasma membrane, swelling of mitochondria and other organelles, loss of integrity of the plasma membrane, and subsequent loss (disorganized dismantling) of intracellular contents (for review, see Kroemer et al[30]). The nucleus exhibits pyknosis and irregular clumping of the chromatin (peripheral chromatolysis), a pattern that contrasts sharply with the sparse, regularly shaped and uniformly distributed aggregates of chromatin observed in apoptosis.[34] Necrotic cell death can be further classified as edematous death, characterized by organelle swelling or edema and ischemic or homogenizing cell death.[43] In the *edematous state*, although the nucleus appears essentially normal, there is irregular clumping of chromatin. The endoplasmic reticulum, the Golgi apparatus, and polysomes are fragmented and accumulate around the nucleus. Microtubules and other filamentous structures are absent, and the cytoplasm is almost clear. The edematous condition is observed in the final stages of delayed death in gerbil and rat global ischemia.[43] By contrast, the *ischemic state* is characterized by pyknosis; the plasma and nuclear membranes become highly irregular and exhibit blebbing, and the cell assumes a triangular shape. Cells undergoing ischemic cell death are acidophilic. Many other morphologic characteristics of necrotic cell death have been described, but little is known about the molecular events responsible for these specific morphologies.

Molecular hallmarks of programmed necrosis or necroptosis include activation of death receptors and receptor-interacting protein 1 (RIP1) kinase.[30] Necroptosis is one of the events that can be induced by binding of members of the tumor necrosis factor (TNF) family of cytokines to their cognate cell surface death domain–containing receptors (members of the TNF superfamily of cytokine receptors), for example, TNFR1, CD95-Fas, and TNF-related apoptosis-inducing ligand (TRAIL) receptor (TRAIL-R; for review, see Park et al,[44] Haase et al,[45] and Vandenabeele et al[46]). Activation of the Toll-like receptors (TLR3 and 4) also elicits necrosis, particularly evident in the presence of caspase inhibitors.[30] On ligand activation, the death domain receptors and TLRs engage intracellular signaling cascades that activate the obligatory serine/threonine kinase known as RIP1.[46] Although the mechanisms by which RIP1 elicits necrosis are not well delineated, an important downstream effector of RIP1 is c-*jun* N-terminal protein kinase or JNK. Activated RIP3 can steer TNF-induced apoptosis toward necroptosis or even full-blown necrosis, in part through disruption of energy metabolism, generation of reactive oxygen species (ROS) and nitroxidative stress by nitric acid,[3,47] increases in intracellular Ca^{2+}, activation of Ca^{2+}-dependent, non-caspase proteases such as calpains and cathepsins, activation of cyclophilin D, opening of the mitochondrial membrane transition pore, and mitochondrial release of poly(adenosine diphosphate [ADP]-ribose)polymerase-1 (PARP-1).[34,48,49] In the final stage of necrotic cell death, swollen cells are internalized by a process known as macropinocytosis, in which only parts of the cell are taken up by phagocytes.[35] Necrosis is now thought to be the predominant form of neuronal death in models of focal ischemia and ischemic stroke in humans.[3] Genetic ablation of cyclophilin D, which abolishes necrotic cell death,[50-52] or pharmacologic inhibition of necrosis by necrostatin 1

(Nec-1), a small-molecule inhibitor of RIP1,[53] affords significant reduction of infarct volume and improves neurologic outcome in animal models of focal ischemia. These observations implicate RIP1 as a potential therapeutic target in ischemic stroke.

Apoptosis

Apoptosis is an evolutionarily conserved process by which cells die as a result of an internally programmed series of events mediated by a family of intracellular cysteine proteases called caspases (for review, see Galluzzi et al,[32] Wang and Youle,[33] and Youle and Strasser[54]). Apoptotic cell death is essential for the normal development and homeostasis of the nervous system and, when dysregulated, can result in cancer, autoimmunity, or neuronal death. After maturation of the central nervous system (CNS), programmed cell death by apoptosis or other mechanisms is markedly attenuated. Injurious stimuli such as focal and global ischemia reactivate apoptosis in mature neurons. Apoptosis is morphologically characterized by shrinkage and rounding up of the cell, chromatin condensation (pyknosis) and nuclear fragmentation (karyorrhexis) into uniformly distributed and regularly shaped structures, formation of "apoptotic bodies," which are membrane bound and composed of nuclear and cytoplasmic materials, fragmentation of the mitochondria, and bead formation along the dendrites and dynamic plasma membrane blebbing (zeiosis, the process by which apoptotic bodies are thought to be formed) with maintenance of integrity of the plasma membrane until the final stages of cell death, followed by complete engulfment of apoptotic cells and apoptotic bodies by resident phagocytes (for review, see Kroemer et al[30]). Whereas necrotic cells (which swell) are internalized by a macropinocytotic mechanism in that only parts of the cell are taken up by phagocytes, apoptotic cells (which shrink) are engulfed completely by phagocytes.[35] Molecular hallmarks of apoptosis include exposure of phosphatidylserine at the cell surface (thought to be the signal for engulfment), activation of death receptors such as CD95-Fas and TRAIL, mitochondrial release of cytochrome *c*, activation of the caspase death cascade, and DNA fragmentation into discrete 180- to 200-base pair fragments (necessary but not sufficient for apoptotic classification), although activation of death receptors and DNA fragmentation are also observed in cells undergoing necrosis (for review, see Kroemer et al[30] and Galluzzi et al[32]).

The Caspase Death Cascade

Caspases are a family of structurally related cysteine proteases that cleave target proteins just after an aspartate residue and are the executioners of apoptosis (for review, see Galluzzi et al,[32] Cheng et al,[55] Bao and Shi,[56] Li and Yuan,[57] Kurokawa and Kornbluth,[58] and Pop and Salvesen[59]). The human genome encodes 13 to 14 distinct caspases; of these, caspases 2, 3, 6, 7, 8, 9, and 10 predominantly function in cell death, whereas the others are involved in regulating immune responses.[59] Caspases are classified as "initiator caspases" (caspases 2, 8, 9, and 10), which integrate upstream apoptotic stimuli, and "effector caspases" (caspases 3, 6, and 7), which are activated by initiator caspases and cleave an array of diverse cellular targets. Caspases are synthesized as procaspases that have little biological activity and are activated either by direct proteolytic cleavage by the effector caspases or by recruitment to a molecular signaling complex (death-inducing signaling complex [DISC], apoptosome, PIDDosome; see later) that is thought to induce conformational changes required for activation by the initiator caspases. Because caspases are constitutively expressed as biologically inactive precursors or procaspases that are thought to cleave their own procaspases (autoactivation) as well as other procaspases, the caspase cascade has been described as "self-amplifying."

The caspase cascade can be activated by either of two main pathways: an extrinsic death receptor–dependent route or an intrinsic pathway involving mitochondria. In the extrinsic or death receptor–dependent pathway, apoptosis is initiated when injurious stimuli such as ischemia lead to activation of CD95-Fas, a member of the TNF receptor–nerve growth factor superfamily of death domain receptors that includes TNF receptor 1 (TNFR1), CD95-Fas, and TRAIL receptor (for review, see Park et al,[44] Haase et al,[45] and Vandenabeele et al[46]) (Fig. 6-3). Within seconds of activation, CD95-Fas (receptor for CD95-Fas ligand) forms a cytosolic DISC, also known as Complex II, composed of CD95-Fas and the adapter proteins TNF receptor-associated death domain (TRADD) and Fas-associated death domain (FADD), which act via their death domains to bind CD95-Fas and via their death effector domain to recruit procaspase 8 (Fig. 6-4).[44-46,56] DISC may also contain additional cofactors and regulatory proteins such as c-FLIP. DISC catalyzes the cleavage and inactivation of RIP1 and RIP3 and activation of procaspase 8 to generate the "instigator" caspase 8. The extrinsic pathway can connect to the intrinsic pathway when caspase 8 cleaves the Bcl-2 family protein Bid to generate truncated tBid, which translocates to the mitochondria, where it initiates permeabilization of the outer mitochondrial membrane and initiates the mitochondrial pathway of apoptosis. In addition, caspase 8 activates the effector caspases 3, 6, and 7, which promote proteolytic cleavage and destruction of an array of cellular targets, including DNases, paving the way for apoptotic cell death.[58-60] Under other conditions, RIP1 is recruited to a large prosurvival signaling complex called Complex I.[46] Complex I is a large molecular signaling platform comprising liganded TNFR1 and TRADD, which, in turn, recruits RIP1, inhibitor of apoptosis (cIAP1), cIAP2, and TNFR-associated factor (TRAF)2 and 5. Together the complex stabilizes cIAP1 and 2, which catalyze polyubiquitination of RIP1 at lysine 63, which in turn serves as a scaffold to recruit the inhibitor κB kinase (IKK) and activate the prosurvival NF-κB pathway. Under these circumstances, RIP1 is resistant to caspase-dependent cleavage, and formation of the DISC or Complex II is suppressed.

In the intrinsic or mitochondrial pathway, apoptosis is initiated when cell death stimuli activate prodeath Bcl-2 family proteins that in turn permeabilize the mitochondrial membrane, which leads to the release of mitochondrial proteins such as cytochrome c, Smac (second mitochondria-derived activator of caspases)/DIABLO (direct IAP-binding protein with low pI), and AIF (apoptosis-inducing factor) into the cytoplasm, an event that is blocked by anti-apoptotic Bcl-2 family members (for review, see Galluzzi et al,[32] Wang and Youle,[33] and Youle and Strasser[54]) (Fig. 6-5). Once in the cytoplasm, cytochrome c binds ATP to activate the apoptotic protease activating factor 1 (Apaf-1), which oligomerizes and recruits procaspase 9 to form the caspase-activating complex or "apoptosome" (Fig. 6-6).[57,58,60,61] Activated caspase 9, in turn, cleaves procaspase 3 to generate the active "effector" caspase 3. Caspase 3 promotes cell death by proteolytic cleavage of downstream target proteins such as poly(ADP-ribose) polymerase, nuclear lamins, DNA-dependent protein kinase, ICAD (the inhibitory subunit of the DNA ladder-inducing endonuclease CAD), and many others, endowing cells with the morphologic characteristic of apoptosis. DNA fragmentation and other events result in cellular disintegration, followed by engulfment of fragmented cells by surrounding cells.[32,33,54] Thus, the apoptosome enables cytochrome c to jump-start a caspase cascade of proteolysis independently of ligand-activated death receptors.

Alternative Pathways of Caspase Activation

An additional pathway critical to activation of the initiator caspases such as caspase 2 is that of DNA damage. DNA damage promotes p53-dependent transcriptional upregulation of p53-induced protein with a death domain (PIDD).[62] In response to injurious stimuli, PIDD forms the PIDDosome death complex, a large (molecular weight >670 kDa) macromolecular signaling platform that in response to DNA damage and stress recruits and activates procaspase 2 (Fig. 6-7).[63] The PIDDosome contains PIDD, the adapter protein RIP-associated Ich-1/Ced-3-homologue protein with a death domain (RAIDD) and procaspase 2. PIDD interacts via its death domain to bind RAIDD and acts via its caspase-recruitment domain (CARD) to recruit procaspase 2.[64] Although the details of caspase 2 activation are not well delineated, the PIDDosome is thought to promote autocleavage of procaspase 2 to generate caspase 2.[56] On activation, caspase 2 acts upstream of mitochondria to promote proteolytic cleavage of the BH3-only protein Bid, translocation of Bax to the mitochondria, opening of the mitochondrial permeability transition pore and release of cytochrome c.[56,62] It is the only caspase that when added to purified mitochondria can directly induce cytochrome c release. A 2008 article by Chan et al[65] demonstrates that brief global ischemia promotes expression of a short cleaved fragment of PIDD (PIDD-CC), formation of the PIDDosome, PIDD-dependent activation of procaspase 2, cleavage of Bid, and neuronal death in the hippocampal CA1. These findings implicate the PIDDosome in global ischemia-induced neuronal death.

Recent evidence indicates that PIDD can act as a molecular switch, controlling the balance between cell survival and death in response to DNA damage.[66,67] Depending on the cellular conditions, PIDD can form a distinct prosurvival complex by assembly with the death domain–containing kinase RIP1 and the sumoylated form of NF-κB essential modulator (NEMO).[66] This complex, which resides in the nucleus, phosphorylates the inhibitor of NF-κB, IκB, and releases it from NF-κB. On activation,

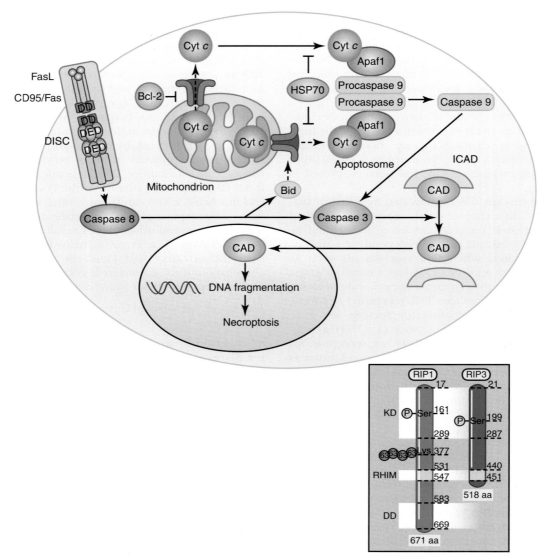

Figure 6-3 The extrinsic or death receptor pathway of caspase activation. In the extrinsic or death receptor–dependent pathway, apoptosis is triggered by stimulation of CD95-Fas, a member of the tumor necrosis factor (TNF) receptor–nerve growth factor superfamily of death domain receptors that includes TNF receptor 1 (TNFR1), CD95-Fas, and the TRAIL receptor. Within seconds of activation, CD95-Fas (receptor for CD95-Fas ligand) forms a cytosolic death-inducing signaling complex, DISC, which recruits procaspase 8. DISC activates procaspase 8 to generate the "instigator" caspase 8. The extrinsic pathway can connect to the intrinsic pathway when caspase 8 cleaves the Bcl-2 family protein Bid to generate truncated tBid, which translocates to the mitochondria, where it initiates permeabilization of the outer mitochondrial membrane and initiates the mitochondrial pathway of apoptosis. In addition, caspase 8 activates the effector caspases 3, 6, and 7, which promote proteolytic cleavage and destruction of an array of cellular targets, including DNases, paving the way for apoptotic cell death. *Arrows* indicate the activation of the targets, whereas *lines with blunt ends* indicate their inactivation. (Adapted from reference 46.)

NF-κB enters the nucleus, where it promotes transcription of mainly prosurvival genes. These findings, while greatly increasing our understanding of how PIDD controls cell survival, also raise important questions. What controls formation of the death signaling PIDDosome versus the prosurvival PIDDosome? It is known that PIDD undergoes proteolytic cleavage to a longer C-terminal cleavage product (PIDD-C), which favors formation of the prosurvival complex and a shorter cleavage product (PIDD-CC), which in turn favors formation of the death complex; the

cellular factors that shift the balance between the two are, however, as yet unclear. In addition to DNA damage, several studies implicate endoplasmic reticulum stress and the accumulation of misfolded proteins in activation of caspase 2.[68]

The Bcl-2 Family of Proteins

The Bcl-2 proteins are a family of structurally related proteins that serve as central regulators of intrinsic programmed cell death.[54,69-72] Bcl-2 family proteins are

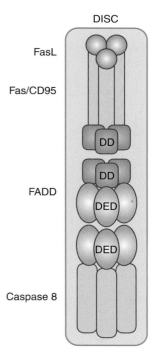

Figure 6-4 Structure of the death-inducing signaling complex (DISC). Adapter protein complexes, or apoptosomes, are responsible for the activation of initiator caspases. The activation of caspase 2 in mammalian cells is mediated by the DISC. DISC is assembled after binding of death ligand to its receptor and contains FADD and caspase 8 (or 10). (Adapted from Bao Q, Shi Y: Apoptosome: A platform for the activation of initiator caspases. *Cell Death Differ* 14:56-65, 2007.)

classified as either antiapoptotic or proapoptotic proteins. Antiapoptotic members (Bcl-x_L, Bcl-2, Bcl-w and Mcl-1) contain four Bcl-2 homology (BH1-4) domains. They localize to the cytosol and to the mitochondrial and endoplasmic reticulum membrane. Proapoptotic members are further classified as multidomain proteins that contain three BH domains: BH1-3 (Bak and Bax) and the "BH3-only" proteins (Bid, Bad, Bim, Puma, Noxa BIK, BMF, HKR/DP5) of unknown structure (except for Bid, which adopts the overall structure of the Bcl-2 family proteins).[54,69,70] Because they are thought to induce cell death by inhibiting the antiapoptotic family members, BH3-only proteins are divided into two groups: the "inactivators" or "indirect activators" (e.g., Bad, Noxa) and the "direct activators" (e.g., tBid and, possibly, also Bim and Puma), which bind transiently and activate the multidomain proteins Bax and Bak.[73] The balance between antiapoptotic and proapoptotic Bcl-2 family members has long been thought to determine the functional integrity of the mitochondrial outer membrane and commitment to cell death (see later).[33,54,72] When the abundance of Bax, Bim, Bad, and Bid exceeds that of antiapoptotic Bcl-2 family members, it promotes the release of cytochrome *c* and other apoptogenic factors from the mitochondria, which initiate apoptosis. More recent studies have focused on the affinities of the various BH3-only proteins for their respective antiapoptotic family members.[74,75] Cell death stimuli can shift this balance in favor of apoptosis by regulation of Bcl-2 protein abundance, post-translational modification, and activity.

Caspase activation by the intrinsic pathway is regulated by Bcl-2 proteins, a family of structurally related antiapoptotic and proapoptotic molecules.[54,69] A prevailing view is that under physiologic conditions, prosurvival Bcl-2 family members (Bcl-2, Bcl-x_L, Bcl-w and Mcl-1) bind and inhibit the proapoptotic direct-activator BH3-only proteins Bid and Bim and/or bind and inhibit the multidomain prodeath proteins Bax and Bak.[54,69] The association between the antiapoptotic proteins and the multidomain proapoptotic Bcl-2 proteins prevents the homooligomerization of Bax and Bak, which would otherwise permeabilize (form channels or pores in) the outer mitochondrial membrane. These pores are suggested by many (although universal agreement does not exist) to form the conduit through which cytochrome *c* passes when released into the cytoplasm. In addition, antiapoptotic Bcl-2 proteins such as Bcl-2 can directly bind the "effectors" Bax and Bak and inhibit channel/pore formation. In response to injurious stimuli, "inactivator" BH3-only proteins such as Bad bind and inhibit the antiapoptotic family members, liberating Bax and Bak and, possibly, "activator" BH3-only proteins Bid and Bim.[76] When unleashed, Bid and Bim trigger homooligomerization of Bak and Bax, which form channels in the outer mitochondrial membrane that permit the escape of apoptogenic proteins such as cytochrome *c*, Smac/DIABLO, and AIF.[54,69,70] On permeabilization of the outer mitochondrial membrane, caspase activation and apoptosis ensue, often within minutes.[72,77]

Recent studies challenge this canonical view of Bcl-2 proteins just described and reveal that in mature neurons, injurious stimuli such as ischemia promote proteolytic cleavage of the antiapoptotic protein Bcl-x_L to generate its proapoptotic counterpart, truncated Bcl-x_L or ΔN-Bcl-x_L.[76,78,79] Bcl-2 family proteins are substrates for caspases and other proteases, and cleavage generally results in the activation of their proapoptotic activities.[80-82] Application of the recombinant caspase cleavage fragment ΔN-Bcl-x_L activates Zn^{2+}-dependent, large conductance channels[76,78,79] that mimic the channel activity of mitochondria of postischemic neurons and promote release of cytochrome *c* in postischemic neurons.[76,83] Bcl-x_L not only influences neuronal survival but also modulates neuronal activity. Introduction of recombinant Bcl-x_L protein into the presynaptic terminal of the squid giant axon potentiates transmitter release and vesicle recycling after intense synaptic activity.[84,85] Expression of Bcl-x_L in hippocampal neurons increases the number and size of presynaptic vesicle clusters and miniature excitatory postsynaptic current (EPSC) amplitude and frequency.[86] Bcl-x_L is highly expressed in mature neurons after expression of many other Bcl-2 proteins such as Bax and Bcl-2 have declined.[87]

Until relatively recently, it was thought that permeabilization of the outer mitochondrial membrane and activation of the "effector" caspase, caspase 3, was a "point of no return" in the execution of apoptotic cell death of postischemic neurons and most other cell types.[77] Global ischemia promotes caspase 3 upregulation and activation within 1 to 2 hours after insult or 2 to 3 days before the onset of histologically detectable neuronal death.[88-90] The importance of early caspase 3 activation to global ischemia–induced neuronal death is underscored by the

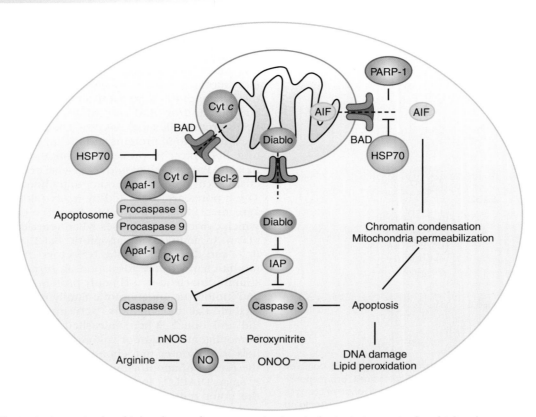

Figure 6-5 The intrinsic or mitochondrial pathway of caspase activation. In the intrinsic or mitochondrial pathway, apoptosis is initiated when injurious stimuli such as ischemia lead to activation of prodeath Bcl-2 family proteins that in turn permeabilize the mitochondrial membrane, leading to the release of mitochondrial proteins such as cytochrome *c*, second mitochondria-derived activator of caspases (Smac)/ direct IAP-binding protein with low pI (DIABLO), and apoptosis inducing factor (AIF) into the cytoplasm, an event that is blocked by antiapoptotic Bcl-2 family members. Once in the cytoplasm, cytochrome *c* binds ATP to activate the apoptotic protease activating factor 1 (Apaf-1), which oligomerizes and recruits procaspase 9 to form the caspase-activating complex or apoptosome. Activated caspase 9, in turn, cleaves procaspase 3 to generate active caspase 3. Caspase 3 promotes cell death by proteolytic cleavage of downstream target proteins such as poly (ADP-ribose) polymerase, nuclear lamins, DNA-dependent protein kinase, ICAD (the inhibitory subunit of the DNA ladder-inducing endonuclease CAD), and many others, endowing cells with the morphologic characteristic of apoptosis. Mitochondrial permeabilization and DNA fragmentation result in cell death, followed by engulfment by macrophages. Whereas cytochrome *c* activates Apaf-1, Smac/ DIABLO neutralizes the inhibitor of apoptosis proteins (IAPs). Heat shock protein 70 (Hsp70) inhibits apoptosis by preventing the release of cytochrome *c* and formation of the apoptosome and by inhibiting release of AIF. (Adapted from Zimmermann KC, Bonzon C, Green DR: The machinery of programmed cell death. *Pharmacol Ther* 92:57-70, 2001.)

finding that Z-DEVD-FMK, a selective caspase 3 inhibitor, is neuroprotective if administered at the time of ischemia but not at 24 hours or later.[89] Thus, the apoptotic machinery is engaged early in the postischemic period. However, it is now well established that neurons can survive cytochrome *c* release and caspase 3 activation.[90-92] These findings are consistent with the notion that caspase 3 activation is necessary but not sufficient to induce death of CA1 neurons. Moreover, a causal role for caspases or caspase substrates in global ischemia is challenged by the general consensus that adult neurons do not die by canonical apoptosis.[3,93]

Inhibitors of Apoptosis

Given that caspases are the key executioners of apoptotic cell death, there are surprisingly few direct inhibitors of caspases encoded by cells. The IAP proteins are a family of structurally related proteins that confer protection from death-inducing stimuli by inhibiting caspase activation; of these, only XIAP is a direct and potent inhibitor

of activated caspases.[94,95] IAP proteins, originally identified in the genome of baculoviruses based on their ability to suppress apoptosis in infected host cells, suppress apoptosis in mammalian cells by halting the caspase death cascade (for review, see Eckelman et al[94] and Gyrd-Hansen and Meier[95]). To date, eight human IAPs have been identified, including XIAP, c-IAP, c-IAP2, and survivin, which, unlike the other IAP family members, lack a C-terminal RING finger (E3 ubiquitin ligase) domain, and all exhibit antiapoptotic activity in cell culture. Perhaps the best-characterized IAP family member is the X-chromosome–linked IAP, XIAP. XIAP is a potent suppressor of apoptosis. XIAP binds caspase 3 and caspase 7 reversibly and with high affinity and suppresses caspase activity, at least in part by masking the caspase active site. The main functional unit in the IAPs is the BIR (or baculoviral IAP repeat) domain, which contains approximately 80 amino acids folded around a zinc atom. Most IAPs have multiple BIR domains, which mediate specialized functions such as direct binding to caspases. For example, BIR3 and

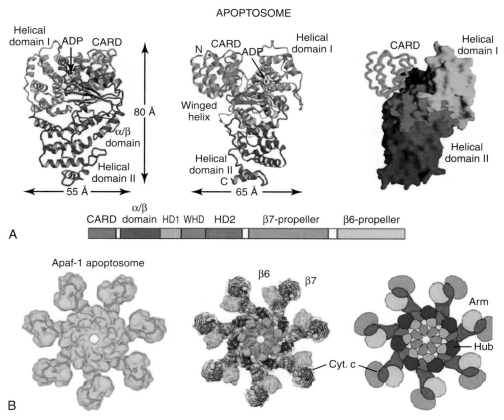

Figure 6-6 Structures of Apaf-1 and the apoptosome. A, Overall structure of the WD40-deleted Apaf-1. The *left* and *middle* panels display two perpendicular views of the ribbon diagram of the structure of Apaf-1 (residues 1591, bound to ADP). ADP binds to the hinge region between the α/β-fold and HD1 *(right arrow)* but is also coordinated by two critical residues from the WHD. The *right* panel shows the structure in surface representation except for the CARD domain. B, Domain organization in Apaf-1 apoptosome. *Left* panel shows a top view of the apoptosome. *Middle* panel shows the proposed domain organization in the apoptosome within semitransparent surfaces. *Right* panel shows a cartoon model of the apoptosome. Color-coding scheme for the panels is the same as in (A). In the presence of dATP or ATP, cytochrome *c* and Apaf-1 assemble into an approximately 1.4-MDa complex, termed the *apoptosome*. The apoptosome is composed of seven molecules of Apaf-1, which bind to cytochrome *c* in an ATP/dATP-dependent manner. Apaf-1 acts via its CARD domain to form a signaling platform known as the apoptosome. The apoptosome recruits and activates procaspase 9 to generate activated caspase 9. Thus, the apoptosome initiates apoptosis via the intrinsic mitochondrial pathway. (Reprinted with permission from Bao Q, Shi Y: Apoptosome: A platform for the activation of initiator caspases. *Cell Death Differ* 14:56-65, 2007.)

adjacent sequences in XIAP mediate inhibition of activated caspase 9, whereas the linker region between BIR1 and BIR2 selectively targets caspase 3.

Under physiologic conditions, IAPs are present in mammalian cells, where they act as buffers and/or dampeners that suppress spurious caspase activation. The actions of IAPs on neuronal survival are, however, not limited to caspase inhibition. Compelling data support additional roles for IAPs in protein degradation, cell-cycle regulation, and caspase-independent signaling cascades (for review, see Eckelman et al[94] and Gyrd-Hansen and Meier[95]). The presence of a zinc-binding motif or RING (E3 ubiquitin ligase) domain at the distal end of the carboxy-termini of a subset of IAPs confers protein degradation activity. These IAPs catalyze degradation of target proteins via ubiquitin-based proteasomal degradation. In this process, IAPs catalyze the sequential covalent addition of ubiquitin (a 76-amino-acid moiety) onto specific lysine residues within target proteins. The modified residues can form multimeric polyubiquitin chains, which tag the protein and mark it for destruction.

Injurious stimuli such as global ischemia elevate the expression of IAP proteins but at the same time promote the release of Smac/DIABLO from mitochondria, a factor that neutralizes the protective actions of IAPs and promotes neuronal apoptosis.[90] Smac/DIABLO is a mitochondrial protein that counteracts IAPs by promoting cIAP autoubiquitination and proteasomal degradation via the ubiquitin-based proteasomal pathway.[46] Whereas cytochrome *c* activates and assembles with Apaf-1 and procaspase 9 to form the apoptosome, Smac/DIABLO binds to IAP family members and neutralizes their antiapoptotic activity. Smac forms an elongated arch-shaped dimer, spanning over 130 Å in length; the N-terminus of Smac binds XIAP via its BIR2 and BIR3 domains.[94,95] Structural studies involving nuclear magnetic resonance and x-ray analyses reveal that the Smac N-terminal tripeptide (Ala-Val-Pro-Ile) recognizes a surface groove composed of highly conserved residues on the BIR3 domain.[94,95] The balance between the IAPs and Smac/DIABLO establishes a threshold for "lethal" caspase 3 activity. Only under conditions in which Smac/DIABLO is released from the

PIDDosome

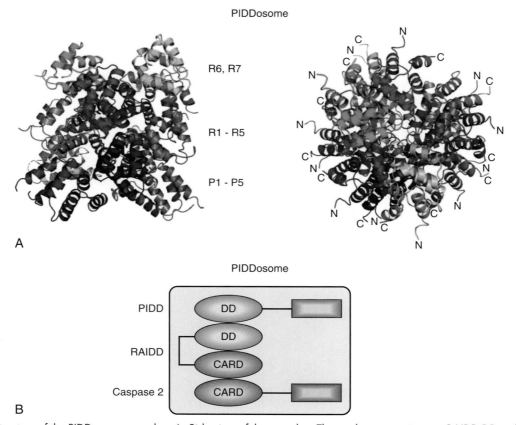

Figure 6-7 Structure of the PIDDosome complex. A, Side view of the complex. The top layer contains two RAIDD DD molecules (green and yellow). The middle layer contains five RAIDD DD molecules (red, purple, orange, magenta, and pink). The bottom layer contains five PIDD DD molecules (different shades of blue). B, Top view of the complex. (Reprinted with permission from Park HH, Logette E, Raunser S, et al: Death domain assembly mechanism revealed by crystal structure of the oligomeric PIDDosome core complex. *Cell* 128:533-546, 2007.)

mitochondria will activated caspase 3 be liberated from IAPs and be free to execute apoptotic cell death.

Caspase-Independent Programmed Cell Death

Classically, focal and global ischemia are thought to induce cell death by activation of caspases. However, an alternative pathway of cell death can occur in animal models of focal and global ischemia even in the presence of caspase inhibitors (for review see Kroemer and Martin,[62] Jaattela and Tschopp,[96] and Stefanis[97]). In this form of cell death, a rise in intracellular Ca^{2+} triggers permeabilization of the outer mitochondrial membrane and release of apoptogenic mitochondrial proteins. However, unlike the intrinsic pathway of caspase activation, which involves cytochrome *c* and formation of the apoptosome, the caspase-independent pathway of programmed cell death deploys the mitochondrial proteins AIF and endonuclease (Endo) G to induce neuronal death.[98,99] AIF is a mitochondrial protein essential to oxidative phosphorylation and the integrity of mitochondrial structure.[99] Endo G is a mitochondrial endonuclease that contains a nuclear localization sequence.[99] In response to injurious stimuli such as ischemia, AIF and Endo G are released from the mitochondria and translocate to the nucleus, where they promote DNA fragmentation and chromatin condensation.

A fundamental mechanism by which AIF is released from mitochondria to induce cell death is by overactivation of PARP-1.[100] PARP-1 is an abundant nuclear enzyme with approximately one molecule per 1000 DNA base pairs.[100-102] Under physiologic conditions, PARP-1 is involved in DNA surveillance, repair, and replication and gene transcription.[103] The obligatory trigger of PARP-1 activation is nicks and breaks in double-stranded DNA, which are recognized by PARP-1 via its DNA binding domain. PARP-1 catalyzes the conversion of β-nicotinamide adenine dinucleotide (NAD^+) into nicotinamide and poly(ADP-ribose). Once activated, PARP-1 transfers between 50 and 200 molecules of ADP-ribose to target proteins, which may activate or inhibit their function. Targets of PARP-1 include histones, DNA polymerases, topoisomerases I and II, and PARP-1 itself (for review, see Wang et al[102]). In the case of histones, poly-ADP-ribosylation promotes chromatin relaxation.

In response to death stimuli or stresses that are toxic to the genome, PARP-1 activity is markedly elevated. Overactivation of PARP-1 promotes excessive production of poly(ADP-ribose) and depletion of NAD^+, which together induce energy failure and signal the mitochondrial release of AIF (Fig. 6-8).[100-102] On release from the mitochondria, AIF is transformed into a powerful cytotoxin that rapidly translocates to the nucleus, where it promotes chromatin condensation and fragmentation. In addition, cytosolic AIF acts on the mitochondria to further compromise the

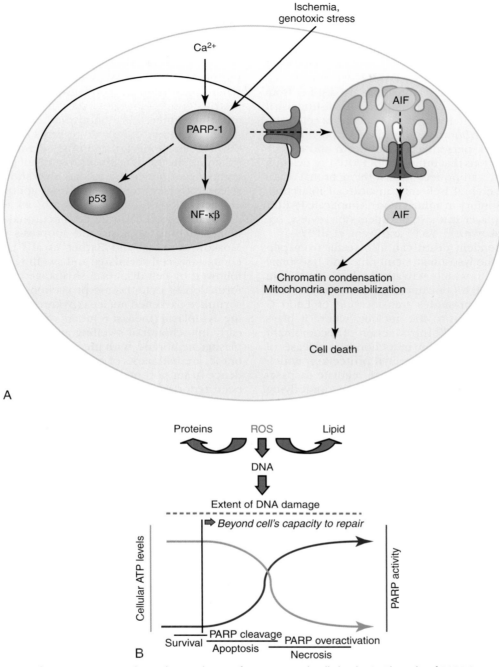

Figure 6-8 PARP-1 mediates a caspase-independent pathway of programmed cell death. A, The role of PARP-1 in apoptotic cell death. Insults to cells such as ischemia and stress can activate PARP-1, which promotes the release of AIF from the mitochondria. AIF can induce chromatin condensation and mitochondrial permeabilization independent of cytochrome *c*, thus triggering apoptotic cell death. PARP-1 can activate NF-κB, a transcription factor that has a crucial role in the regulation of genes involved in inflammatory responses. PARP-1 also transactivates p53, a transcription factor critical in the execution of apoptosis. On release from the mitochondria, AIF rapidly translocates to the nucleus, where it promotes chromatin condensation and fragmentation. In addition, cytosolic AIF promotes permeabilization of the mitochondria, releasing cytochrome *c* and other apoptogenic factors into the cytosol. ATP depletion inhibits caspase activation and shifts the balance of death cascades in favor of necrosis. B, A model of PARP-1 overactivation-mediated cytotoxicity. Reactive oxygen species (ROS) such as nitric oxide, O_2^-, or peroxynitrite are generated during inflammation or ischemia–reperfusion. ROS damages proteins, lipids, and DNA. DNA damage activates PARP-1, a DNA surveillance enzyme, which transforms NAD^+ into poly(ADP-ribose) and nicotinamide. Overactivation of PARP-1 promotes excessive production of poly(ADP-ribose) and depletion of NAD^+, which together induce energy failure and signal the mitochondrial release of AIF.

integrity of the outer mitochondrial membrane and initiate the release of cytochrome *c*, which activates caspase 3. PARP-1 is a critical downstream target of caspase 3. However, caspase activation is apparently not required for PARP-1–dependent cell death, because caspase inhibitors do not afford protection.[101] Moreover, PARP-1–dependent cell death exhibits morphologic features that are distinct from those of necrosis, apoptosis, and autophagy. To distinguish it from other forms of cell death, PARP-1–mediated cell death has been termed *parthanatos*, after the PAR polymer and Thanatos, the Greek personification of death and mortality.[102] The observations that inhibitors of PARP-1 or deletion of the *parp-1* gene can protect against the neuronal death associated with cerebral ischemia, myocardial infarction, and inflammatory injury in animal models implicate PARP-1 as an important player in these disorders (for review, see Chiarugi and Moskowitz,[100] Yu,[101] and Wang et al[102]).

Caspase-independent death can also result from permeabilization of the lysosomal membrane and lysosomal release of cathepsin, which activates Endo G.[104] OGD in primary cultures of hippocampal neurons, an in vitro model of ischemia, promotes translocation of Endo G from the mitochondrion to the nucleus, where it plays a role in neuronal death.[105] Introduction of recombinant Bcl-x$_L$ to neurons blocks the mitochondrial release of AIF and Endo G and affords neuronal protection, which suggests that Bcl-2 family members can regulate caspase-independent cell death. The mechanisms underlying caspase-independent cell death are as yet not well delineated, and recent studies bring into question its relation to ischemia-induced apoptotic cell death.

Autophagy

Macroautophagy is characterized by formation of vacuoles or autophagosomes, which sequester and engulf overly abundant, old, or damaged intracellular organelles and/or portions of the cytoplasm for bulk degradation by lysosomes.[39,40] The final stages of autophagy are marked by the fusion between autophagosomes and lysosomes to generate autolysosomes, in which the inner membrane of the autophagosome and its luminal contents are degraded by acidic lysosomal hydrolases. Autophagic cell death is morphologically characterized by the absence of chromatin condensation and by the presence of massive autophagic vacuoles or autophagosomes. Cells that die by autophagy have little or no association with phagocytes. Biochemically, autophagy is marked by the presence of Beclin-1 (also known as Atg6), a class III phosphoinositide 3-kinase and autophagy-related protein that initiates formation of vesicular structures such as autophagosomes, and by the redistribution of the ubiquitin-like protein LC3 (also known as Atg8) to autophagosomes and autolysosomes (for review, see Kroemer et al[30]).

Cell Death Pathways in Global and Focal Ischemia

Global ischemia induces neuronal death with hallmarks of both necrosis and apoptosis (for review, see Moskowitz et al[3] and Kroemer et al[30]). Ultrastructural studies of CA1 neurons undergoing delayed death in rat and gerbil models of global ischemia[106,107] and in humans who die as a consequence of cardiac arrest[108,109] exhibit many of the morphologic features of necrotic cell death (see later) and do not exhibit critical hallmarks of apoptosis, such as apoptotic bodies. Thus, apoptosis defined by stereotypic morphologic changes—especially evident in the nucleus, where the chromatin condenses to compact simple geometric figures—does not occur in global ischemia. These and other studies cast doubt whether global ischemia elicits any of the morphologic features of apoptosis. Strong evidence in support of apoptosis, defined as activation of specific cell-signaling events that result in cellular suicide, comes from molecular studies that show mitochondrial release of cytochrome *c* and other apoptogenic proteins and activation of the caspase death cascade (see later).

Focal ischemia also induces neuronal death with hallmarks of both necrosis and apoptosis (for review, see Moskowitz et al[3] and Barber et al[110]). Focal ischemia elicits early cell shrinkage and swelling of mitochondria, followed by cell dispersal, shrinkage of the nucleus, the formation of cytoplasmic projections, and, ultimately, a shrunken darkened nucleus (pyknosis) without surrounding cytoplasm (the last remnant of the dead neuron). The early mitochondrial swelling and loss of integrity of the plasma membrane, with preservation of the nuclear membrane, are hallmarks of necrotic cell death. Recently, evidence in support of apoptotic death in the penumbra has been reported, including DNA fragmentation, activation of death receptors, mitochondrial release of cytochrome *c*, and activation of the caspase death cascade (see later). Strong evidence in support of necrosis, defined as activation of specific signaling proteins, comes from genetic and pharmacologic studies that show a critical role for RIP1 and cyclophilin D and from biochemical studies that show disruption of energy metabolism, generation of ROS and nitroxidative stress by nitric acid, a rise in intracellular Ca^{2+}, activation of noncaspase proteases such as calpains and cathepsins, activation of cyclophilin D–dependent mitochondrial outer membrane permeabilization, and mitochondrial release of AIF (see previously).

Both focal and global ischemia trigger caspase activation in neurons destined to die. Global ischemia induces activation of death receptors such as CD95-Fas and TRAIL, effector caspases such as caspases 9 and 3, and DNA fragmentation factor, which promotes fragmentation of DNA.[89,90,111] Observations that global ischemia triggers early mitochondrial release of cytochrome *c*, activation of caspases 9 and 3, and relatively late activation of the death receptor CD95-Fas are consistent with the concept that caspases are activated in postischemic hippocampal neurons via the intrinsic or mitochondrial amplifying pathway. Focal ischemia promotes delayed neuronal death in the penumbra, with many of the features of apoptosis, including CD95-Fas receptor activation,[112] mitochondrial release of cytochrome *c*,[113] activation of caspase 3[114], and DNA fragmentation.[115-117]

Triggers of Ischemic Cell Death

Glutamate Excitotoxicity

Excitotoxicity refers to the form of cell death by which supraphysiologic levels of excitatory amino acids such as glutamate excessively activate excitatory amino acid receptors such as the N-methyl-D-aspartate (NMDA) receptor, leading to cytosolic Ca^{2+} overload and activation of lethal signaling pathways (for review, see Szydlowska and Tymianski[93]). Knowledge that glutamate is potentially toxic dates to observations by Lucas and Newhouse nearly a half century ago that glutamate administered to animals in vivo caused death of retinal neurons.[118] The concept of excitotoxic death was significantly advanced by Olney and Ho,[119] who used ultrastructural analysis to analyze the cytopathology of neurons exposed to glutamate. These studies revealed a characteristic pattern of glutamate-induced neuronal death in which postsynaptic structures such as dendrites and somata were destroyed, whereas axons, presynaptic terminals, and nonneuronal cells survived. Other excitatory amino acids and glutamate analogues induced neuronal death with a rank order of potency similar to that for their ability to elicit excitatory transmission. With the advent of selective excitatory amino acid receptor antagonists in the 1980s and their application to studies of glutamate actions, excitatory amino acids were accepted as the major excitatory transmitters of the CNS and, in high concentrations, as excitotoxins capable of excessive activation of excitatory amino acid receptors and excitotoxic cell death.

The concept that glutamate plays a critical role in the pathogenesis of global and focal ischemia originated with observations that raising extracellular magnesium levels markedly reduced the vulnerability of cultured hippocampal neurons to anoxia[120,121] and that glutamate antagonists reduced neuronal injury in in vitro and in vivo models of ischemia.[122,123] Over the past 15 to 20 years, mounting evidence has shown that glutamate antagonists afford neuroprotection in global and focal ischemia. It is now widely accepted that excitotoxicity plays a critical role in the neuronal death associated with ischemia and other neurologic disorders and diseases.

During the ischemic episode, anoxic depolarization activates voltage-sensitive Ca^{2+} channels, which trigger the massive release of synaptic glutamate (for review, see Szydlowska and Tymianski[93]). Synaptically released glutamate acts via the ionotropic glutamate receptors, N-methyl-D-aspartate receptors (NMDARs), α-amino-3-hydroxy-5-methyl-4-isoxazole-propionic acid receptors (AMPARs), and kainate receptors, to further depolarize the postsynaptic cell. In addition, NMDARs and GluR2-lacking AMPARs mediate a massive rise in cytosolic Ca^{2+} and depletion of Ca^{2+} from the extracellular space. Glutamate also activates metabotropic glutamate receptors (mGluRs), G-protein–coupled receptors that are enriched at excitatory synapses, where they act to regulate glutamatergic neurotransmission.[124-126] Group I mGluRs, mGluR1 and 5, engage the prosurvival ERK/MAPK and phosphatidylinositol 3-kinase (PI3K)/protein kinase B (Akt) signaling pathways. In addition, mGluR1/5 acts via phospholipase C and $Ins(1,4,5)P_3$ to trigger release of Ca^{2+} from intracellular stores. Depletion of Ca^{2+} from the endoplasmic reticulum triggers endoplasmic reticulum stress, which activates apoptosis. The massive rise in cytosolic Ca^{2+} causes cells to further depolarize and become inexcitable. Anoxic depolarization also drives the reverse operation of glutamate transporters in astrocytes, contributing to the rise in extracellular glutamate.[127]

Glutamate toxicity induces reverse operation of the Na^+/Ca^{2+} exchanger in neurons, exacerbating the buildup of intracellular Ca^{2+}.[128] During global ischemia, extracellular glutamate rises from approximately 0.6 μM to 1 to 2 μM.[129] During focal ischemia, glutamate rises to 16 to 30 μM in the core.[130,131] A major consequence of the rise in extracellular glutamate is activation of not only synaptic but also extrasynaptic ionotropic glutamate receptors (AMPARs, NMDAs, and kainate receptors), with consequent influx of toxic Ca^{2+} and shutoff of the CREB-initiated program of cell survival (see later).

NMDARs

For nearly two decades, intense interest focused on NMDARs as the candidate mediator of Ca^{2+} entry into neurons destined to die. NMDARs are glutamate-gated ion channels and play a pivotal role in the regulation of synaptic function in the brain (for review, see Carroll and Zukin,[132] Cull-Candy and Leszkiewicz,[133] Perez-Otono and Ehlers,[134] and Lau and Zukin[135]). NMDARs are heteromeric assemblies of NR1, NR2, and NR3 subunits that cotranslationally assemble in the endoplasmic reticulum to form functional channels with differing physiologic and pharmacologic properties. NMDAR-mediated Ca^{2+} influx is essential for synaptogenesis, experience-dependent synaptic remodeling, and long-lasting changes in synaptic efficacy such as long-term potentiation (LTP) and depression (LTD), cellular processes widely believed to underlie learning and memory.[136,137] Recent studies indicate that NMDARs not only serve as a trigger of synaptic plasticity but may also contribute to the expression of LTP and LTD.[135] NMDARs mediate the influx of toxic Ca^{2+} in a number of neurologic disorders, insults, and neurodegenerative diseases (for review, see Szydlowska and Tymianski[93] and Lau and Zukin[135]). Although it is well established that NMDARs are a critical player in focal ischemia–induced neuronal death, AMPARs appear to mediate the cell death associated with global ischemia. Although not completely understood, two factors are thought to reduce the contribution of NMDARs in postischemic neurons: (1) the rise in extracellular acidity, which inhibits NMDA functional activity, and (2) the rise in extracellular Zn^{2+}, which potentiates AMPAR currents and inhibits NMDAR currents.

Injurious stimuli such as hypoxia and focal ischemia cause overactivation of NMDARs, excessive Ca^{2+} influx, and excitotoxic cell death (see later). Targets of NMDAR-mediated Ca^{2+} influx include nNOS, JNK signaling, calpains and cathepsins, and Ca^{2+}-dependent transcription factors. NO is an important downstream mediator of NMDA-dependent neuronal signaling and synaptic plasticity and NMDA-induced excitotoxicity (see later).[93,135] NMDARs can also promote cell death in an nNOS-independent manner via activation of the JNK signaling pathway.[138] On activation, JNK phosphorylates and promotes mitochondrial translocation of Bim long (BimL), which promotes homooligomerization and formation of Bax channels that permeabilize the mitochondrial outer membrane.[139] JNK also phosphorylates and activates pyruvate dehydrogenase, which leads to ATP depletion.[140] In addition, JNK signaling contributes to neuronal death by promoting production of ROS.[141] A 2007 article[142] showed that calpain proteolytically cleaves the C-terminal domain of mGluR1 in an

NMDAR manner. Although truncated mGluR1 increases cytosolic Ca^{2+}, it cannot engage prosurvival PI3K/Akt signaling and thus promotes excitotoxicity. These findings suggest the existence of a positive feedback loop involving calpain and mGluR1 in excitotoxic cell death.

Findings by Hardingham et al reveal that the location of Ca^{2+} entry into cells critically influences the fate of neurons.[143,144] Whereas Ca^{2+} influx via synaptic NMDARs activates CREB, Ca^{2+} influx via extrasynaptic NMDARs elicits CREB shutoff (for review, see Szydlowska and Tymianski[93] and Lau and Zukin[135]). Synaptic NMDARs engage Ca^{2+}-calmodulin–dependent kinase IV (CaMKIV) and the Ca^{2+}-sensitive mitogen-activated protein kinase (MAPK) pathway, which in turn phosphorylate and activate CREB (see later). At extrasynaptic sites, Ca^{2+} influx via NMDARs activates the protein phosphatases phosphatase 1 (PP1) and PP2A, which dephosphorylate and inactivate CREB. Ca^{2+} influx via extrasynaptic NMDARs (and CREB shutoff) also causes breakdown of the mitochondrial membrane potential, ATP depletion, and necrotic cell death. Interestingly, contemporaneous activation of synaptic and extrasynaptic NMDARs by bath-applied NMDA also shuts off CREB, which suggests that extrasynaptic NMDARs act via a dominant, cell-death signal to override the CREB-promoting effects of synaptic NMDARs and/or L-type Ca^{2+} channels and protein kinase A (PKA).[143,144] Thus, the cellular penalty of excess Ca^{2+} entry through extrasynaptic NMDARs is impaired by not only CREB transcription but also neuronal death.

Two recent studies reveal important mechanisms that can enhance NMDA receptor activity and Ca^{2+} influx. Global ischemia induces the Cdk5-dependent phosphorylation of the NMDAR subunit at serine 1232; inhibition of endogenous Cdk5 affords protection against hippocampal injury, which suggests that an important role for this regulatory event is ischemia-induced neuronal death.[145] In addition, studies involving electrophysiology and two-photon laser scanning show that Ca^{2+} permeation through NMDARs is under the control of the cAMP/PKA signaling system.[146] Direct activation of PKA markedly enhances Ca^{2+} influx through NMDARs and NMDAR-mediated Ca^{2+} signaling in spines[146]; direct activation of γ-aminobutyric acid (GABA)$_B$ receptors, which negatively couple to cAMP/PKA signaling, strongly inhibits NMDAR-mediated Ca^{2+} signaling in spines in a PKA-dependent manner.[147] An important prediction of these findings is that extracellular signals that modulate cAMP or protein phosphatases at postsynaptic sites such as norepinephrine, dopamine, and GABA can bidirectionally regulate Ca^{2+} permeation through synaptic NMDARs and the induction of NMDAR-dependent LTP. Given the widespread distribution of NMDARs and PKA throughout the CNS, this represents a powerful mechanism for modulating Ca^{2+} signaling in neurons under physiologic and pathologic conditions.

An additional link between NMDARs and neuronal death is that of K^+ efflux. Mounting evidence indicates that K^+ efflux leads to reduced intracellular K^+ concentration, which is a possible trigger of apoptosis (for review, see Szydlowska and Tymianski[93]). NMDARs are an important route of K^+ efflux in cells undergoing apoptosis. Whereas NMDAR-mediated necrosis primarily involves influx of Na^+ and Ca^{2+}, NMDAR-mediated apoptosis primarily involves K^+ efflux. Under normal conditions, excessive activation of NMDARs in cultured cortical neurons triggers necrotic cell death, characterized by prominent acute swelling of cell bodies, little or no DNA laddering, and insensitivity to protein synthesis inhibitors. In contrast, under conditions of reduced extracellular Na^+ and Ca^{2+}, activation of NMDARs in the same cells induces apoptotic cell death, characterized by cell shrinkage, nuclear condensation, internucleosomal fragmentation, and sensitivity to protein synthesis inhibitors. The latter is particularly relevant in the face of low extracellular Na^+ and Ca^{2+}, as is observed after brain ischemia in vivo (for review, see Szydlowska and Tymianski[93]).

Functional NMDARs are expressed by not only neurons but also macroglia, astrocytes, and oligodendrocytes, glial cells that extend processes. Oligodendrocytes are essential to neuronal function and survival in that they produce myelin, which enwraps and insulates axons, thereby increasing conduction velocity.[148,149] In oligodendrocytes, NMDARs localize primarily to processes,[150] where they are activated in response to glutamate released from the nerve terminals of neighboring neurons under physiologic conditions and, under pathologic conditions, are overactivated in response to ischemia.[151] In oligodendrocytes, NMDARs localize to the cell processes that carry out myelination, which renders the processes more susceptible to excitotoxicity. Glial and neuronal NMDARs are permeable to Ca^{2+}, but they differ functionally and structurally: neuronal NMDARs are exquisitely sensitive to blockade by intracellular Mg^{2+}, but glial NMDARs are only weakly sensitive to Mg^{2+} blockade, presumably because of high expression of the NR3 subunit. In the cortex, astroglial NMDARs play a role in synaptic transmission under physiologic conditions. Activation of glial NMDARs in response to ischemia triggers Ca^{2+}-dependent damage of oligodendrocytes.[152] Ca^{2+} influx via glial NMDARs disrupts axoglial junctions and exposed juxtaparanodal K^+ channels, which results in impaired axonal conduction of neurons.[153] These findings suggest that analogous mechanisms of ischemic injury may be operative in gray and white matter. Oligodendrocyte injury and loss of myelination is a critical event in ischemia-induced neuronal death, and glial NMDARs represent an important new target for drug development in stroke.[148,149]

Ca^{2+}-Permeable AMPARs

AMPARs mediate fast synaptic transmission at excitatory synapses in the CNS. These receptors are tetrameric assemblies of subunits GluR1–4, which are encoded by separate genes, are differentially expressed throughout the CNS, and are crucial during neuronal development, synaptic plasticity, and structural remodeling (for review, see Liu and Zukin[154] and Isaac et al[155]). A critical feature of AMPARs lacking the GluR2 subunit is their permeability to Ca^{2+} and Zn^{2+}; presence of GluR2 in heteromeric AMPARs renders the channel impermeable to Ca^{2+} and Zn^{2+} and electrically linear.[154,155] The principal pyramidal neurons of the hippocampus abundantly express GluR2-containing Ca^{2+}-impermeable AMPARs. Because of the nature of these cells and their inability to handle high loads of Ca^{2+}, immediate loss of GluR2 would be expected to confer enhanced excitotoxicity of endogenous glutamate and vulnerability to neuronal insults.

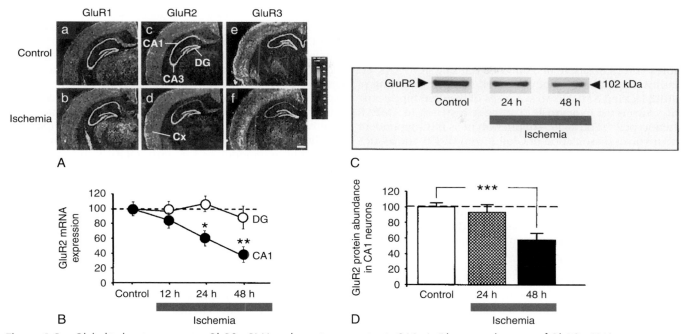

Figure 6-9 Global ischemia suppresses GluR2 mRNA and protein expression in CA1. A, Film autoradiograms of GluR2 mRNA expression, as detected by in situ hybridization, in the hippocampus of control and experimental rats at 12, 24, and 48 hours after global ischemia. B, Quantitative analysis of GluR2 mRNA expression in the pyramidal cell layer of the CA1 (• circles) and in the granule cell layer of the dentate gyrus (DG, ○ circles). Global ischemia induced a marked suppression of GluR2 mRNA expression specifically in the pyramidal neurons of the CA1 at 24 hours and was maximal at 48 hours. No changes were detected in the DG or CA3. Mean optical densities are reported after normalization to the corresponding control value for a given region as indicated in Methods. Statistical significance was assessed by ANOVA followed by Newman-Keuls test (*, $P < 0.05$; **, $P < 0.01$). C, Representative Western blots probed with a monoclonal antibody against a sequence within the N-terminal domain of the GluR2 subunit. D, Relative GluR2 subunit abundance (defined as the ratio of band densities of experimental versus control samples) for protein samples isolated from the CA1 of control and experimental rats at 24 and 48 hours after ischemia. GluR2 abundance was determined from band densities for GluR2 after normalization to the band densities for actin, which served as a loading control. Relative GluR2 subunit abundance was markedly decreased in CA1 at 48 hours. Bars are means ± SEMs. Statistical significance was assessed by means of the Student's unpaired t-test (***, $P < 0.001$). (A, Adapted from Pellegrini-Giampietro DE, Zukin RS, Bennett MV, et al: Switch in glutamate receptor subunit gene expression in CA1 subfield of hippocampus following global ischemia in rats. *Proc Natl Acad Sci U S A* 89:10499-10503, 1992. B, Reprinted with permission from Calderone A, Jover T, Noh K-M, et al: Ischemic insults de-repress the gene silencer rest in neurons destined to die. *J Neurosci* 23:2112-2121, 2003.)

Ca^{2+} permeable AMPARs play a critical role not only in synaptic plasticity but also in the excitotoxicity associated with a number of neurologic disorders and diseases (for review, see Liu and Zukin,[154] Sensi et al,[156] and Kwak and Weiss[157]). Under physiologic conditions, principal neurons of the hippocampus abundantly express GluR2-containing, Ca^{2+}-impermeable AMPARs (see earlier). Because these cells do not express high levels of Ca^{2+} binding proteins or fast local Ca^{2+} extrusion pumps, immediate loss of GluR2 would be expected to confer enhanced pathogenicity of endogenous glutamate and vulnerability to neuronal insults. Accordingly, ischemic insults trigger downregulation of GluR2 mRNA expression and protein abundance in selectively vulnerable CA1 neurons and induce a long-lasting switch in AMPAR phenotype from GluR2-containing to GluR2-lacking (Fig. 6-9).[158-165] By 24 hours after ischemia, AMPA EPSCs exhibit properties of Ca^{2+}/Zn^{2+}-permeable, GluR2-lacking AMPARs, including enhanced rectification of AMPA EPSCs, sensitivity to polyamines, and AMPAR-mediated Ca^{2+} influx.[162,164-166] In addition to their role in mediating Ca^{2+} entry, GluR2-lacking AMPARs are thought to mediate the late rise in toxic Zn^{2+}.[157]

It is now well established that Ca^{2+}-permeable, GluR2-lacking AMPARs are involved in the neuronal death associated with global ischemia (for review, see Liu and Zukin,[154] Sensi et al,[156] and Kwak and Weiss[157]). AMPAR antagonists, but not NMDAR antagonists, protect against global ischemia–induced cell death, even when administered hours after the ischemic insult[164,167] (but see also the study by Nurse and Corbett[168]). Immediate knockdown of GluR2 by antisense oligonucleotides, even in the absence of an ischemic insult, causes death of pyramidal neurons.[163] Overexpression of Ca^{2+}-permeable GluR2(Q) channels in vivo promotes ischemia-induced death of normally resistant CA3 pyramidal cells and dentate gyrus granule cells; overexpression of Ca^{2+}-impermeable GluR2(R) channels protects CA1 neurons against ischemic death.[165] The subunit-specific channel blockers N-naphthylspermine and philanthotoxin, which selectively inhibit GluR2-lacking AMPARs, afford neuroprotection in models of global ischemia.[164,169,170]

Recent studies document a role for the gene silencing transcription factor REST in the switch in AMPAR phenotype and highly selective neuronal death produced by global ischemia.[159] Ischemic insults trigger activation of the transcriptional repressor REST in selectively vulnerable CA1 neurons.[159] REST binds the GluR2 promoter and acts via epigenetic remodeling to suppress gene expression in neurons destined to die (see later). Emerging evidence indicates that not only GluR2 expression but also receptor trafficking and GluR2 RNA editing can be dysregulated in response to neuronal insults. For example, ischemia promotes internalization of GluR2-containing AMPARs via clathrin-dependent endocytosis and synaptic targeting of GluR2-lacking AMPARs to synapses of insulted hippocampal neurons via exocytosis, leading to a switch in AMPAR phenotype.[166] The switch in phenotype is PKC-dependent and involves dissociation of GluR2 from GRIP1 and association with PICK1. Global ischemia also inhibits activity of the RNA editing enzyme ADAR2 and disrupts Q/R editing of GluR2.[171] Direct delivery of ADAR2 or constitutively active CREB, which induces ADAR2 expression, restores Q/R editing and protects vulnerable neurons from cell death. Thus, reduced Q/R editing further contributes to neuronal vulnerability in brain ischemia.

Kainate Receptors

Kainate receptors are ionotropic glutamate receptors that mediate fast excitatory neurotransmission and are localized to the presynaptic and postsynaptic sides of excitatory synapses. Kainate receptors also localize to the presynaptic side of inhibitory synapses, where they are thought to modulate release of the inhibitory neurotransmitter GABA. A recent study implicates kainate receptors in global ischemia–induced neuronal death. The kainate-selective drug decahydroisoquinoline LY377770, a novel, soluble, and systemically active GluR5 antagonist, was found to afford protection of CA1 neurons against ischemia-induced death, even when administered after the ischemic event.[172] On activation, kainate receptors form a triheteromeric complex, GluR6-PSD-95-MLK3 in postischemic CA1, which engages and activates JNK signaling.[173,174] Because NMDAR antagonists have side effects including psychotomimetic effects, increased glucose utilization, and c-*fos* and hsp-70 expression[175] and produce morphologic changes in the rat cingulate cortex,[176] it has been suggested that non–NMDAR antagonists may represent neuroprotective agents that may be useful in the clinic.

Nonexcitotoxic Mechanisms

A role for NMDARs and AMPARs in the excitotoxicity associated with global ischemia is well established, but other channels are also implicated in ischemia-induced neuronal death. Two such channels are the transient receptor potential (TRP) channels and the acid sensing ion channels (ASIC).

TRP Channels

The TRP cation channel superfamily is a group of weakly voltage-sensitive, largely nonselective cation channels that sense and respond to changes in their local environments.[177,178] Structurally, TRP channels are typically homomeric or heteromeric tetramers composed of four subunits, each of which crosses the membrane six times. In the CNS, TRP channels participate in neurite outgrowth, maintain membrane excitability, integrate external signals, and regulate Ca^{2+}-sensitive intracellular signaling.[177,178] In mammals, there are more than 20 members of the TRP superfamily, many of which are

permeable to Ca^{2+}. The three major families of TRP genes are the canonical TRPC channels, the melastatin or long TRP (TRPM) channels, and vanilloid TRP (TRPV) V channels. Of these, TRPM2 and 7 are implicated in the cell death due to anoxia ROS and stroke (for review, see Aarts and Tymianski[179]).

TRPM7 channels are activated in response to a decrease in extracellular divalent cations, ROS, and extracellular activity, all of which occur in ischemia.[180] Recent studies indicate a role for TRPM7 in excitotoxicity and neuronal death in two models of ischemia. OGD, an in vitro model of ischemia, induces a decrease in extracellular Ca^{2+} concentration, which in turn activates a nonselective cation current with properties of the TRPM7 channel in cortical neurons.[180] The channel was identified as the TRPM7 based on its sensitivity to voltage-dependent blockade by Gd^{3+}, which blocks large, nonselective cationic channels, and by its potentiation by PIP_2 and ROS.[180] Pharmacologic blockers or small interfering RNA (siRNA) to TRPM7 suppressed the anoxia-induced current and afforded neuroprotection.[180] In addition to its role in anoxia-induced neuronal death, the TRPM7 channel plays a critical role in global ischemia–induced neuronal death.[181] Pharmacologic inhibition of TRP-mediated currents or suppression of TRPM expression affords protection from ischemia-induced cell death, in vivo.[181] Delivery of siRNA to TRPM7 directly into the hippocampus of living animals afforded protection against ischemia-induced neuronal death and synaptic and cognitive deficits.[181] TRP or TRP-like channels are activated by cellular stress and contribute to ischemia-induced membrane depolarization, intracellular Ca^{2+} accumulation, and cell swelling.[182] Based on these findings, the authors hypothesized that the neuroprotective effects of hypothermia might be mediated by closing of the temperature-sensitive TRPV3 and TRPV4 channels in response to lowering temperature.

Although TRPM2 and 7 are activated during the initial ischemic episode and promote ischemia-induced neuronal death, other members of the TRP family of cation channels have prosurvival actions. Two members of the TRP cation channel (TRPC) family, TRPC3 and 6, protect cerebellar granule neurons against serum deprivation–induced cell death in cultures and promote cerebellar granule neuron survival in rat brain.[183] Although pharmacologic blockade or siRNA to TRPC3 or TRPC6 suppressed a brain-derived neurotrophic factor (BDNF)–triggered rise in intracellular Ca^{2+}, CREB activation, and neuronal survival, overexpression of TRPC3 or 6 increased CREB-dependent gene transcription and prevented apoptosis in serum-deprived neurons.[183]

ASIC Channels

Another channel that contributes to the rise in Ca^{2+} associated with neuronal injury is the ASIC channel. ASICs are ligand-gated multimeric channels that belong to the epithelial sodium channel (DEG/ENaC) superfamily. They are Na^+-selective cation channels sensitive to amiloride, are expressed throughout the CNS, and can be activated by low pH, membrane stretching, lactate, arachidonic acid, and decreased extracellular Ca^{2+}.[184,185] In mammals there are four genes that encode six ASIC subunit proteins: ASIC1a, ASIC1b, ASIC2a, ASIC2b, ASIC3, and ASIC4.

The ASIC1a subunit is permeable to Ca^{2+}, a major excitotoxic ion, and contributes to acidosis-elicited neuronal injury.[186,187] ASICs are abundantly expressed in neurons throughout the brain including the cerebral cortex, cerebellum, hippocampus, amygdala, and olfactory bulb. Studies by Xiong et al point to a role for ASIC channels in ischemia-induced acidosis and neuronal death.[188] Acidosis occurring as a consequence of focal ischemia activates Ca^{2+}-permeable ASICs, which induce glutamate receptor independent, Ca^{2+}-dependent, neuronal injury.[188] Whereas cells lacking ASICs are resistant to acid injury, overexpression of the Ca^{2+}-permeable ASIC1a channel confers sensitivity to acidosis-induced cell death. Administration of ASIC1a blockers or knockout of the ASIC1a gene in living animals protects the brain from focal ischemia–induced brain injury and is more potent than glutamate antagonists.[188] Thus, acidosis injures the brain via membrane receptor–based mechanisms with resultant toxicity of $[Ca^{2+}]i$, which discloses new potential therapeutic targets for stroke. The ASIC1a subunit has two Ca^{2+}/calmodulin-dependent protein kinase II (CAMKII) phosphorylation sites.[189] Ischemia promotes association of CAMKII with ASIC1a, which in turn promotes phosphorylation of the ASIC1a subunit and enhanced ASIC1a-mediated currents. These effects require activation of NR2B-containing NMDARs.[189]

Calcium

Ca^{2+} is a neuronal signaling molecule that is critical to focal and global ischemia–induced neuronal death. During the ischemic episode, anoxic depolarization triggers the release of synaptic glutamate. Synaptically released glutamate acts via ionotropic and metabotropic receptors to induce a massive influx of Ca^{2+} from the extracellular space and mobilization of Ca^{2+} from intracellular stores. Depletion of Ca^{2+} from the endoplasmic reticulum initiates endoplasmic reticulum stress, which activates apoptosis (see earlier). Glutamate toxicity induces reverse operation of glutamate transporters in neurons and astrocytes,[127] exacerbating the buildup of glutamate in the extracellular space. In addition, glutamate induces reverse operation of the Na^+/Ca^{2+} exchanger, which exacerbates the buildup of cytosolic Ca^{2+} and elicits depletion of extracellular Ca^{2+} by more than 90%.[93] Ultimately, the massive rise in cytosolic Ca^{2+} causes cells to further depolarize and become inexcitable. After reperfusion, Ca^{2+} homeostasis is restored; cells appear morphologically normal, exhibit normal intracellular Ca^{2+}, and regain the ability to generate action potentials for 24 to 72 hours after the insult. Ultimately, ambient glutamate elicits a late rise in intracellular Ca^{2+} and Zn^{2+} (see later), and death of CA1 neurons ensues, exhibiting hallmarks of apoptosis and necrosis.

The massive rise in intracellular Ca^{2+} during the ischemic episode initiates a series of cytoplasmic and nuclear events that impairs cellular activity and damages tissue profoundly.[93] High cytosolic Ca^{2+} activates Ca^{2+}-dependent ATPase, which depletes the energy stores of the cell, and uncouples mitochondrial oxidative phosphorylation, causing immediate swelling of dendrites and cell bodies and subsequent cell death.[128] Additionally, the rise in intracellular Ca^{2+} activates phospholipases, endonucleases, and noncaspase proteases such as calpains and cathepsins, which destroy cytoskeletal proteins such as actin and spectrin and extracellular matrix proteins such as laminin, and Ca^{2+}-sensitive transcription factors.[190] Calpains are Ca^{2+}-dependent proteases with papain-like activity and are thought to be key players in the neurodegeneration associated with a number of neurologic disorders and diseases (for review, see Szydlowska and Tymianski[93]). Calpains and cathepsins also activate cyclophilin D–dependent mitochondrial outer membrane permeabilization and mitochondrial release of AIF (see earlier). In addition, high cytosolic Ca^{2+} induces excessive activation of nitric oxide synthase, which promotes generation of free radicals and oxidants. Other targets of calpains include the antiapoptotic Bcl-2 family member $Bcl-x_L$, which is cleaved to generate its proapoptotic counterpart $\Delta N-Bcl-x_L$[81] (see earlier), NMDARs and AMPARs, the Na^+/Ca^{2+} exchanger NCX, L-type Ca^{2+} channels, sarcoplasmic/endoplasmic reticulum Ca^{2+} ATPases, ryanodine receptors, and Ins $(1,4,5)P_3$, which regulates the release of Ca^{2+} from intracellular stores (for review, see Szydlowska and Tymianski[93]). Calpains can also cleave Ca^{2+}-dependent kinases and phosphatases associated with the NMDAR signaling complex such as Ca^{2+}/calmodulin-dependent protein kinase and the protein phosphatase calcineurin.

Neuronal homeostasis requires that the intracellular concentration of Ca^{2+} be maintained in the range of 50 to 300 nM (or approximately 4 times lower than that of extracellular Ca^{2+}). Aberrantly low cytosolic Ca^{2+} levels inactivate voltage-sensitive Ca^{2+} channels and induce apoptosis in otherwise healthy cells, but abnormally high Ca^{2+} levels promote neuronal death (the "calcium set-point hypothesis"). Whereas less severe insults elicit a more modest rise in intracellular Ca^{2+} levels and, like aberrantly low Ca^{2+} levels, trigger apoptosis, more severe insults elicit a more massive elevation in cytosolic Ca^{2+} levels, which inhibits apoptosis and shifts the balance to necroptosis or even full-blown necrosis.[34,37,49]

Zinc

The transition metal Zn^{2+}, like Ca^{2+}, is a neuronal signaling molecule and critical player in ischemic cell death (for review, see Sensi et al,[156] Kwak and Weiss,[157] and Frederickson et al[191]). In the brain, Zn^{2+} colocalizes with glutamate in presynaptic vesicles at a subset of excitatory synapses. In the hippocampus, Zn^{2+} is uniquely high in mossy fiber tracts, which project to the CA3 (Fig. 6-10). The zinc transporter 3 (ZnT-3) is localized to synaptic vesicle membranes within mossy fiber boutons and mediates loading of vesicular Zn^{2+}.[192] Zn^{2+} is coreleased with glutamate spontaneously and in an activity-dependent manner and achieves synaptic concentrations of 10 to 100 μM, but see Kay.[193] On release, synaptic Zn^{2+} modulates the activity of a number of postsynaptic receptors. Whereas Zn^{2+} inhibits NMDARs and $GABA_A$ receptors,[194-196] it potentiates AMPARs.[197,198] Zn^{2+} enters neurons via voltage-sensitive Ca^{2+} channels, NMDARs, GluR2-lacking AMPARs, and the Na^+/Zn^{2+} antiporter.[154,156,157] Of these, GluR2-lacking AMPARs exhibit highest permeability to Zn^{2+} but under

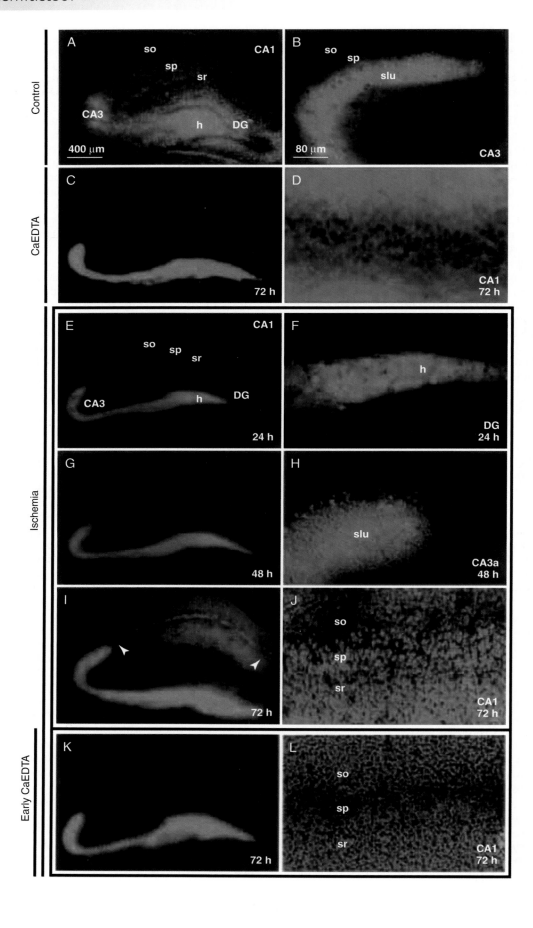

Figure 6-10 Global ischemia elicits a delayed rise in Zn^{2+} levels in selectively vulnerable CA1 neurons. Zn^{2+} fluorescence in TSQ–stained coronal brain sections from sham (A-D) and experimental animals subjected to global ischemia (E-L) or to CaEDTA, followed by global ischemia (K, L). CaEDTA injection at 30 minutes before surgery did not detectably alter the pattern of Zn^{2+} fluorescence in sham-operated control animals, assessed at 72 hours after surgery (C, D). In control hippocampus, TSQ labeling revealed intense fluorescence in the mossy fiber axon terminals of dentate granule neurons in the hilus and stratum lucidum of CA3 (B) and faint fluorescence in the stratum radiatum and stratum oriens of CA1 (A). Global ischemia induced a pronounced increase in Zn^{2+} fluorescence in the cell bodies of scattered hilar neurons, evident at 24 hours after insult (E, F). At 48 hours, Zn^{2+} fluorescence was visible in CA3a pyramidal neurons, extending into the CA1/CA3 transition zone but was not in CA1 (G, F, H). At 72 hours, Zn^{2+} fluorescence was pronounced in cell bodies of CA1 pyramidal neurons (I [*arrowheads*], J). Injection of CaEDTA 30 minutes before ischemia did not affect the increase in Zn^{2+} in the transition zone but attenuated the late rise in Zn^{2+} fluorescence in the CA1 (K, L). Scale bars: 400 μm in A, C, E, G, I, K; 80 μm in B, D, F, H, J, and L. slu, Stratum lucidum; so, stratum oriens; sp, stratum pyramidale; sr, stratum radiatum. (Reprinted with permission from Calderone A, Jover T, Mashiko T, et al: Calcium EDTA rescues hippocampal CA1 neurons from global ischemia-induced death. *J Neurosci* 24:9903–9913, 2004.)

physiologic conditions are expressed at low density on distal dendrites of hippocampal pyramidal neurons.[199-201] Within neurons, Zn^{2+} serves as a functionally important component of metalloenzymes and zinc finger-containing transcription factors. Synaptically released Zn^{2+} is thought to be essential for LTP induction at CA3 synapses,[202,203] but see Vogt et al.[204] Accordingly, Zn^{2+} deficiency causes cognitive impairment.[156]

The notion that Zn^{2+}, like glutamate, might be neurotoxic, emerged from findings that perforant path stimulation releases Zn^{2+} and that Zn^{2+} damages postsynaptic target hilar interneurons and CA3 pyramidal cells in vivo[205,206] and in vitro.[207] Exposure of cortical neurons in culture to 300 μM Zn^{2+} for 15 minutes or to 1 mM Zn^{2+} for 5 minutes kills virtually all neurons. Moreover, vulnerability to Zn^{2+} is substantially enhanced by concurrent membrane depolarization. Zn^{2+} at high concentrations is a critical mediator of the neuronal injury associated with global ischemia, seizures, traumatic brain injury, and other brain disorders.[154,156,157,208]

A striking feature of transient global or forebrain ischemia is an early rise in intracellular Ca^{2+} levels during the ischemic episode and a late rise in intracellular free Zn^{2+} in CA1 neurons at 24 to 48 hours after ischemia, just before onset of neuronal death (see Fig. 6-10).[164,209] Recent studies reveal a role for Zn^{2+} in the early postischemic period.[76,78,209] A hallmark event in the early postischemic period is permeabilization of the mitochondrial outer membrane, mitochondrial release of cytochrome *c*, and activation of the caspase death cascade in neurons destined to die. These studies demonstrate proteolytic cleavage of the antiapoptotic Bcl-2 family protein, Bcl-x_L, to generate its proapoptotic counterpart ΔN-Bcl-x_L and the formation of large, Zn^{2+}-dependent channels in the loss of mitochondrial functional integrity in postischemic neurons.[76,78] At late times (48 to 72 hours) after global ischemia, Zn^{2+} accumulates in degenerating hilar and selectively vulnerable CA1 neurons,[209,210] concurrent with p75[NTR] expression and DNA fragmentation.[209] Studies with Zn^{2+} indicator dyes show that intracellular Zn^{2+} levels may reach as high as 0.5 μM. Zn^{2+} enters postischemic neurons via GluR2-lacking AMPARs[164,209,211] and is released from intracellular stores.[212] The membrane-impermeant metal chelator CaEDTA, administered before ischemia, blocks the rise in Zn^{2+} and protects CA1 neurons. Ultimately, Zn^{2+} induces death of CA1 neurons, exhibiting the morphologic features of necrosis. Zn^{2+} may also play a role in the cell death associated with focal ischemia.

Zn^{2+} exerts its neurotoxic effects via several mechanisms, including potentiation of AMPAR-mediated currents,[197] generation of ROS,[213] and disruption of metabolic enzyme activity,[214] ultimately leading to apoptosis and/or necrosis.[156] In addition, Zn^{2+} impairs the ubiquitin-based proteasomal degradation pathway by promoting ubiquitination and inhibition of proteasomal enzyme activity.[215] The ability of Zn^{2+} to shift excitotoxic injury from NMDAR-mediated injury toward AMPAR-mediated injury is illustrated by preferential death of neurons with high NADPH diaphorase.[208] These neurons exhibit resistance to NMDA toxicity and high susceptibility to AMPA toxicity,[208] which is consistent with the presence of GluR2-lacking AMPARs.[154,157]

Mechanisms of Ischemic Cell Death

Metabolic Stress

A hallmark of cells undergoing ischemia is energy depletion and altered energy dynamics. Neurons and glia have relatively high consumption of oxygen and glucose and depend almost exclusively on oxidative phosphorylation for energy production. During the ischemic episode, obstruction of cerebral blood flow restricts the delivery of substrates, such as oxygen and glucose, and impairs the energetics required to maintain ionic gradients.[128] Anoxic depolarization triggers the release of synaptic glutamate, which acts via ionotropic and metabotropic receptors to induce a massive rise in cytosolic Ca^{2+} levels (see earlier) and a resultant loss of extracellular Ca^{2+} levels (for review, see Moskowitz et al[3] and Szydlowska and Tymianski[93]). Group I mGluRs activate phospholipase C and Ins(1,4,5)P_3, which promote release of Ca^{2+} from intracellular stores. Glutamate buildup in the cell drives the operation of glutamate transporters in neurons and astrocytes in reverse, exacerbating the buildup of glutamate in the extracellular space. In addition, glutamate drives reverse operation of the Na^+/Ca^{2+} exchanger, exacerbating the buildup of intracellular Ca^{2+}.[93] As a consequence, extracellular Ca^{2+} is depleted to less than 90% of its physiologic concentration. Moreover, Na^+ and Ca^{2+} influx drives a massive efflux of K^+, which flows out of neurons via NMDARs, leading to a rise in extracellular K^+ levels (see earlier). Ultimately, the massive rise in cytosolic Ca^{2+} levels causes cells to further depolarize and become inexcitable. After reperfusion, Ca^{2+} homeostasis is restored; cells appear morphologically normal, exhibit normal intracellular Ca^{2+}, and regain the ability to generate action potentials for 24 to 72 hours after the insult. Ultimately, ambient glutamate elicits a late rise in intracellular Ca^{2+} and Zn^{2+} levels (see earlier) and death of CA1 neurons ensues, exhibiting hallmarks of apoptosis and necrosis.

In global ischemia, high cytosolic Ca^{2+} during the ischemic event activates Ca^{2+}-ATPase, which depletes the energy stores of the cell, and uncouples mitochondrial oxidative phosphorylation, causing immediate swelling of dendrites and cell bodies and necrotic cell death (for review, see Galluzzi et al[32] and Nicotera et al[128]). ATP is depleted in cells throughout the brain but recovers to near physiologic levels by the time of reperfusion.[116,216] Low ATP levels encourage neurons to die by necrosis by inducing ion pump failure, depolarization, massive release of glutamate, reverse operation of glutamate transporters, swelling of cells (edema), and rupture of the plasma membrane.[128] Because ATP is required for formation of the apoptosome that activates the caspase death cascade, ATP depletion inhibits caspase activation and shifts the balance of death cascades in favor of necrosis.[128] Despite this, global ischemia activates caspase 3, which catalyzes cleavage and activation of downstream targets such as PARP-1. Excessive PARP-1 activation depletes the cell of NAD^+. NAD^+ depletion in mitochondria causes pronounced slowing of glycolysis, electron transport, and ATP formation, resulting in further energy failure and cellular demise (see earlier).[100-102,128]

Focal ischemia elicits different patterns of metabolic changes in the core and penumbra. Within 1 to 3 minutes, cells in the core exhibit a dramatic decline in ATP and anoxic depolarization, which triggers release of synaptic glutamate.[3,93] Na^+ enters neurons via NMDARs, AMPARs, and other channels permeable to monovalent ions. K^+ flows out of cells via NMDARs. Water follows passively, driven by the influx of Na^+ and Cl^-, which greatly exceeds the efflux of K^+. At the same time, as cells lose energy, energy-requiring pumps that normally force ions into and out of the cell in an attempt to maintain a concentration gradient fail or operate in reverse. These factors induce a rise in extracellular K^+ and a reduction in extracellular Ca^{2+}. By 2 hours of temporary focal ischemia, extracellular K^+ is restored to a physiologic concentration. The ensuing edema negatively affects perfusion of cells in the penumbra and affects more remote regions via long-range changes, including intracranial pressure, vascular compression, and herniation (for review, see Moskowitz et al[3] and Szydlowska and Tymianski[93]). In contrast, cells in the penumbra experience a decline in energy but do not exhibit anoxic depolarization or the rise in extracellular K^+.[128] Here, low ATP concentrations promote necrosis by inducing reverse operation or failure of ion pumps, swelling of cells, and rupture of the plasma membrane. At the same time, ATP depletion inhibits formation of the apoptosome and opposes caspase activation, yet apoptosis ensues in the penumbra. As in global ischemia, activated caspase 3 activates PARP-1, leading to NAD^+ depletion and further energy failure.

Mitochondrial Permeabilization

Mitochondria house not only proteins involved in oxidative phosphorylation but also proapoptotic proteins including cytochrome c. Under physiologic conditions, cytochrome c is localized to the outer compartment of the mitochondria, where it serves as an electron carrier and participates in oxidative phosphorylation. Apoptotic and necrotic stimuli converge on high cytosolic Ca^{2+}, which disrupts the integrity of the outer mitochondrial membrane, enabling the release of cytochrome c and other apoptogenic factors.[93] Once in the cytoplasm, cytochrome c binds dATP to form the apoptosome, a molecular signaling platform that recruits and transactivates procaspase 9 to generate activated caspase 9. The Bcl-2 proteins are a family of structurally related proteins that serve as central regulators of intrinsic programmed cell death.[54,69-72] For example, addition of proapoptotic Bcl-2 family members such as Bax to isolated mitochondria is sufficient to induce cytochrome c release, and addition of antiapoptotic Bcl-2 family members such as Bcl-x_L is sufficient to prevent it (see earlier).

Injurious stimuli such as ischemia trigger high intracellular Ca^{2+} levels, which promote activation of the serine-threonine phosphatase calcineurin.[32] Calcineurin dephosphorylates Bad, which translocates to the mitochondria, where it binds Bcl-2 and Bcl-xL and liberates Bak and Bax. On release, Bax and Bak homooligomerize and form channels in the mitochondrial membrane that promote permeabilization of the mitochondrial membrane and initiate apoptosis (see earlier). Growth factors such as BDNF and IGF and other prosurvival factors engage the PI3K/Akt signaling cascade and oppose the actions of prodeath stimuli.[217] Akt phosphorylates Bad, which promotes binding to 14-3-3, which, in turn, sequesters Bad in the cytosol, blocking its proapoptotic actions. A recent study showed that global ischemia in intact rats triggers expression and activation of the potent and selective endogenous inhibitor of Akt, carboxyl-terminal modulator protein (CTMP), in vulnerable hippocampal neurons and binds and extinguishes Akt activity.[218] Although ischemia induces a marked phosphorylation and nuclear translocation of Akt, phosphorylated Akt is not active in postischemic neurons, as assessed by kinase assays and phosphorylation of the downstream targets GSK-3β and FOXO-3A. RNA interference-mediated depletion of CTMP in a clinically relevant model of stroke restores Akt activity and rescues hippocampal neurons.[218] These findings indicate that CTMP is important in the neurodegeneration that is associated with stroke and identify CTMP as a therapeutic target for the amelioration of hippocampal injury and cognitive deficits. Dysregulation of Akt signaling is important in a broad range of diseases that includes cancer, diabetes, and heart disease. This study adds neurodegenerative disorders to the growing list of diseases involving aberrant Akt signaling.

Nitric Oxide

Nitric oxide (NO) is a small, diffusible signaling molecule. NO is an "aberrant transmitter" in that it is released by one cell and acts on another, although it is not released from vesicles and does not act via classic membrane receptors (for review, see Hara and Snyder[219] and Gadalla and Snyder[220]). NO is synthesized by the neuronal isoform of nitric oxide synthetase (nNOS), an enzyme that converts arginine to NO and citrulline. nNOS is expressed in neurons throughout the CNS, with particularly high density in the accessory olfactory bulb and cerebellar granule cells. At excitatory synapses, nNOS is physically anchored to NMDARs in the postsynaptic membrane via the scaffolding protein, postsynaptic density (PSD) protein-95 (PSD-95)/synapse-associated protein-90 (SAP-90). Activation of NMDARs triggers a rise in postsynaptic Ca^{2+} levels and activation of Ca^{2+}-dependent calmodulin, which rapidly activates nNOS and stimulates production of NO.[219,220]

NO is an important downstream mediator of NMDA-dependent neuronal signaling and synaptic plasticity and NMDA-induced excitotoxicity.[93,221] Injurious stimuli such as hypoxia and focal ischemia cause overactivation of NMDARs, excessive Ca^{2+} influx, and excitotoxic cell death. Overproduction of NO is a major mediator of excitotoxicity and focal ischemia–induced neuronal death. The free radical form of NO and the superoxide anion are implicated in the oxidative damage of cellular DNA, lipid peroxidation, and excitotoxic cell death (for review, see Liu et al[222]). NO diffuses from the mitochondria and cytoplasm to the nucleus, where it is cleaved to form hydroxyl radicals or singlet oxygen. NO reacts with the superoxide anion ($•O^{2-}$) to form peroxynitrite (ONOO−) (see later). In addition, NO interferes with superoxide dismutase, thereby reducing its antioxidant action, and complexes with nonheme iron within enzymes critical to DNA replication and mitochondrial energy production, thereby inhibiting their activity (see later). Recent evidence indicates that excessive Ca^{2+}-induced NO generation leads to the formation of S-nitrosylated dynamin-related protein 1, which causes abnormal mitochondrial fragmentation and impairs synaptic function.[221] Important evidence that NO is a critical mediator of neuronal death comes from studies that show that mice lacking nNOS or treated with the nNOS inhibitor 7-nitroindazole are protected against neuronal death in experimental models of stroke (for review, see Nakamura and Lipton[221] and Pacher et al[223]).

Free Radicals and Lipid Peroxidation

Neuronal insults and other types of environmental stress induce the formation of free radicals such as the superoxide anion, hydroxyl radical, singlet oxygen, and radical nitric oxide and oxidants such as peroxynitrite. Collectively, these agents (termed *reactive oxygen species* or ROS) are critical mediators of neuronal injury (for review, see Nakamura and Lipton,[221] Pacher et al,[223] and Niizuma et al[224]). Free radicals disrupt the membrane potential by inhibition of critical membrane proteins, initiate lipid peroxidation, damage DNA, and induce neuronal death with morphologic features of apoptosis and necrosis. NMDAR-mediated Ca^{2+} influx promotes free radical production by stimulation of NO, which reacts with superoxide free radical ($•O_2^-$) to form peroxynitrite. Peroxynitrite is a cytotoxic oxidant that induces DNA damage, thereby triggering apoptosis.[223,225] In addition to causing DNA damage, ROS such as peroxynitrite oxidize key mitochondrial enzymes such as mitochondrial cytochrome *c* oxidase, promote formation of the mitochondrial transition

pore and mitochondrial release of AIF, which activates PARP-1, and initiate lipid peroxidation by reaction with unsaturated fatty acids in membranes.[223,224] In addition, ROS activates Ca^{2+}-permeable TRPM7 channels.[179] Peroxynitrite also nitrosylates cysteine residues in target proteins such as NMDARs, thereby impairing synaptic transmission.

NMDAR-mediated Ca^{2+} influx promotes superoxide production, which is essential to normal functioning of the cell under physiologic conditions (for review, see Nakamura and Lipton,[221] Pacher et al,[223] and Niizuma et al[224]). Overactivation of NMDARs leads to excessive superoxide production and neuronal death. An important source of NMDA-induced superoxide production is the cytoplasmic enzyme NADPH oxidase. NMDAR-mediated Ca^{2+} influx also activates phospholipase A_2. Phospholipase A_2 liberates arachidonic acid, an unsaturated fatty acid, and promotes free radical production via activation of the lipoxygenase and cyclooxygenase pathways. Cyclooxygenase catalyzes the addition of two molecules of O_2 to arachidonic acid to produce prostaglandin G, which is rapidly peroxidized to prostaglandin H with concomitant release of $•O_2^-$. Metabolism of free arachidonic acid is thought to be a major source of $•O_2^-$. Zn^{2+} influx via GluR2-lacking AMPARs also promotes production of free radicals, such as mitochondrial superoxide, in injured neurons.[156,157]

In neurons, free radicals inactivate and damage critical membrane proteins such as Na^+ and Ca^{2+} pumps, creatine kinase, and mitochondrial dehydrogenases and promote oxidation of the Na^+–K^+–ATPase exchanger, rendering it susceptible to calpain-mediated proteolysis.[226] A fundamental mechanism by which free radicals damage proteins is by oxidation of side chains and disulfide bonds. Free radicals also damage DNA by causing single-and double-strand breaks, chemically modifying nucleic acid bases, breaking the glycosylic bond between ribose and individual bases, and cross-linking protein to DNA (for review, see Adibhatla and Hatcher[227]). If not repaired, oxidative damage impairs DNA elongation, replication, and gene transcription, which further contributes to cell death (for review, see Adibhatla and Hatcher[227]).

Free radicals also oxidize and damage unsaturated fatty acids. *Lipid peroxidation* is the oxidative deterioration of membrane unsaturated fatty acids and is caused by reaction of free radicals with unsaturated bonds in the side chains of polyunsaturated fatty acids.[227] These reactions spark a chain reaction leading to formation of peroxides, hydroperoxides, and aldehydes. Although $•O_2^-$ is not itself a potent oxidizer, it promotes oxidation of ferric ion and release of ferrous iron from ferritin.[228] In the presence of transition metals such as copper or ferrous iron, these chain reactions can expand geometrically. Ultrastructural studies reveal that excessive generation of oxygen radicals, followed by lipid peroxidation, accelerates the structural damage of neurons. Lipid peroxidation compromises the integrity of the neuronal plasma membrane by altering membrane permeability and fluidity and allowing ions such as Ca^{2+} to leak into the cell; disruption of the membrane compromises the function of receptors, channels, transporters, and ion exchangers, adding further to the demise of injured cells.[227]

Epigenetic Mechanisms and Transcriptional Regulation

Injurious stimuli such as ischemia trigger a number of transcriptional pathways. Candidate transcription factors that are thought to direct programs of gene expression changes after global ischemia include CREB and NF-κB, which direct prosurvival programs, and the forkhead family of transcription factors and REST/NRSF, which direct prodeath pathways in adult neurons.

The Transcription Activator CREB

CREB is a stimulus-induced transcription factor and activates transcription of prosurvival (and proadaptive) target genes in response to a wide array of external stimuli including NMDAR-mediated Ca^{2+} influx at synaptic sites (for review, see Lau and Zukin[135] and Hardingham[144]). Immediate-early genes, such as c-fos, Bcl-2, the IAPs, nNOS, and BDNF are important to neuronal survival and are gene targets of CREB (for review, see Lonze et al[229]). On activation, CREB plays an important role in promoting neuronal survival and adaptation in response to environmental cues. Consistent with this notion, targeted deletion of the genes encoding CREB and the cAMP-response modulatory protein (CREM) in neurons of the developing CNS elicits apoptosis. Postnatal ablation of CREB and CREM results in progressive neuronal degeneration in the adult brain (for review, see Mayr and Montminy[230] and Lonze and Ginty[231]).

CREB is a member of the leucine-zipper superfamily of transcription factors and is activated in response to external stimuli that activate intracellular signaling cascades, which culminate in phosphorylation of CREB. On phosphorylation, CREB forms a functionally active dimer that binds the cis-acting CRE element within the promoters of target genes (for review, see Mayr and Montminy[230] and Lonze and Ginty[231]). Findings by Hardingham et al[143,144] indicate that synaptic and extrasynaptic NMDARs signal through different intracellular signaling cascades (see earlier). Ca^{2+} influx via synaptic NMDARs promotes the activation of CaMKIV and ERK/MAPK (p42/44) signaling through which it sends a synapse to nuclear signal to phosphorylate and activate CREB.[135] On activation, MAPK phosphorylates and activates the pp90 ribosomal S6 kinases (Rsks), the "synapse to nuclear signal." Rsks translocate from the synapse to the nucleus, where they regulate gene expression by phosphorylation and activation of transcription factors such as CREB. Rsks act in a coordinated manner to promote robust, sustained phosphorylation of CREB at Ser133 and CREB activation. Whereas CaMKIV mediates the early phase of Ser133 phosphorylation, the ERK/MAPK pathway mediates late, prolonged phosphorylation of CREB (for review, see Mayr and Montminy[230] and Lonze and Ginty[231]). In addition, CaMKIV phosphorylates and activates the coadapter protein, CREB binding protein, at Ser301. On activation, CREB recruits phosphorylated CREB binding protein (CBP) to the promoters of CREB target genes, where it promotes epigenetic modifications and active gene transcription.[232]

Considerable evidence indicates that phosphorylation of Ser142 and Ser143 also contributes to CREB activation but inhibits the interaction of CREB with CBP.[230,231]

Nuclear Factor-κB: A Balance between Neuronal Survival and Death

NF-κB is expressed in nearly all mammalian cells. Under physiologic (resting) conditions, NF-κB exists as an inactive form composed of a dimeric form of the transcription factor and its binding partner, IκB, which maintains NF-κB in an inactive form (for review, see Mattson and Camandola[233]). NF-κB is activated in response to a diverse range of external stimuli including the cytokine TNF-α, neurotrophic factors such as nerve growth factor (NGF), neurotransmitters such as glutamate, cell adhesion molecules, and various types of stress. These stimuli activate NF-κB by inducing phosphorylation and proteasomal degradation of IκB, which releases active, dimeric NF-κB. On activation, NF-κB translocates to the nucleus, where it binds to upstream regulatory elements in κB-responsive genes. These include the Ca^{2+}-binding protein calbindin, cytokines such as TNF-α and interleukin 2κ manganese superoxide dismutase (MnSOD), the anti-apoptotic proteins Bcl-x_L and Bcl-2, the IAPs, and BDNF (for review, see Mattson and Camandola[233]). On activation, NF-κB plays an important role in regulating cell survival and synaptic plasticity in neurons. Focal ischemia activates NF-κB and relocalizes it to the nucleus of ischemic neurons, where it binds target genes.[234] Targeted deletion of NF-κB significantly reduces ischemic damage, which suggests a role for NF-κB in focal ischemia–induced neuronal death.[234]

The Pro-Death Transcription Activator FOXO

Forkhead1 (FOXO-3A or FKHRL-1) is a member of the forkhead family of transcription factors (FOXO-3A, FOXO-1, and AFX) and induces expression of proapoptotic target genes (for review, see Brunet et al,[235] van der Horst and Burgering,[236] Fukunaga and Shioda,[237] and Hannenhalli and Kaestner[238]). In mammals, there are four evolutionarily conserved members of the forkhead family of transcription (FOXO-1, FOXO-3, FOXO-4, and FOXO-6) that are negatively regulated by the PI3K/protein kinase B (Akt) signaling pathway. Forkhead transcription factors are central to cellular functions such as cell cycle arrest at the G1-S and G2-M checkpoints, detoxification of ROS, repair of damaged DNA, and apoptosis (for review, see Brunet et al,[235] van der Horst and Burgering,[236] Fukunaga and Shioda,[237] and Hannenhalli and Kaestner[238]). It is thought that these functions of the forkhead family of transcription factors could be related to their ability to promote longevity.

Under physiologic conditions, FOXO-3A resides in the cytosol away from target genes and is thus inactive (Fig. 6-11). The neurotrophins NGF and BDNF and other growth factors such as IGF-I act via the PI3K/protein kinase B (Akt) pathway to promote FOXO-3A phosphorylation (for review, see Brunet et al[235]). FOXO-3A is a critical target of Akt phosphorylation and inactivation. PI3K promotes neuronal survival by phosphorylation and activation of the serine-threonine kinase Akt. Akt promotes

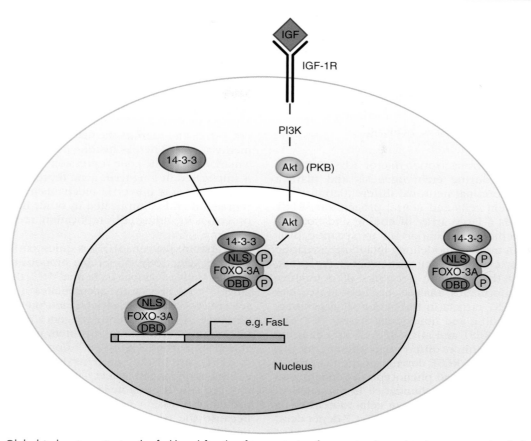

Figure 6-11   Global ischemia activates the forkhead family of transcription factors, implicated in longevity and cell death. Within the nucleus, FOXO-3A triggers apoptosis by transactivation of target genes such as Fas ligand (FasL) and TRAIL. FasL, in turn, activates the cell surface death receptor Fas, which initiates the caspase death cascade via the extrinsic pathway of apoptotic cell death. In the presence of survival factors, the serine/threonine kinase Akt phosphorylates FOXO-3A, leading to its association with 14-3-3 proteins and cytoplasmic retention and sequestration away from nuclear target genes. Ischemia promotes dephosphorylation (activation) of FOXO-3A in CA1, evident at 12 and 24 hours. Estrogen induces phosphorylation (inactivation) of FOXO-3A in control CA1 and attenuates ischemia-induced dephosphorylation of FOXO-3A. (Adapted from Burgering BM, Kops GJ: Cell cycle and death control: long live forkheads. *Trends Biochem Sci* 27:352-360, 2002.)

cell survival by phosphorylation and inactivation of target genes implicated in apoptotic cell death (for review, see Brunet et al[235]). FOXO-3A is a critical target of Akt phosphorylation and inactivation (for review, see Brunet et al,[235] van der Horst and Burgering,[236] Fukunaga and Shioda,[237] and Hannenhalli and Kaestner[238]). Phosphorylation of FOXO-3A promotes its binding to the retention factor 14-3-3, which retains FOXO-3A in the cytoplasm, away from target genes such as FasL. Injurious stimuli trigger FOXO-3A dephosphorylation and nuclear translocation. Putative targets of FOXO-3A are the cytokines TNF-α, CD95-Fas ligand, and TRAIL and their cognate death domain–containing TNF superfamily of receptors (for review, see Park et al[44] and Haase et al[45]). The death cytokines act via the extrinsic or death receptor–mediated pathway to initiate the caspase death cascade. Global ischemia triggers expression of CD95-Fas ligand, implicated in the extrinsic or death-receptor pathway of caspase activation.[44,45] CD95-Fas ligand triggers the activation of CD95-Fas, which rapidly recruits FADD and TRADD to form the DISC, which recruits and activates procaspase 8 to generate activated caspase 8 and initiate the caspase death cascade.

The Signal Transducer and Activator of Transcription 3 (STAT3)

Signal transducer and activator of transcription 3 (STAT3) is a transcription factor implicated in neuronal function and survival.[239-241] Cytokines, growth factors, and receptor and nonreceptor tyrosine kinases activate STAT signaling by phosphorylation of JAK2, a member of the Janus kinase (JAK) family of intracellular nonreceptor tyrosine kinases that transduce cytokine-mediated signals, at Tyr1138.[242,243] On activation, JAK2 promotes phosphorylation and activation of the transcription factor STAT3.[243] On activation, STAT3 dimerizes and translocates to the nucleus, where it acts by epigenetic remodeling to regulate transcription of target genes such as MnSOD, ERα, survivin, Bcl-2, and Bcl-x_L.[242] STAT3 can also be activated in a JAK-independent manner by receptor tyrosine kinases such as epidermal growth factor receptor and nonreceptor tyrosine kinases such as *src*. MnSOD is a mitochondrial antioxidant enzyme that scavenges free radicals. A 2009 article[241] shows that focal ischemia suppresses STAT3 expression and blocks recruitment of STAT3 to the MnSOD promoter and MnSOD transcription and that downregulation of MnSOD results in overproduction of superoxide anion ($\cdot O_2^-$). These findings suggest that STAT3 and its target MnSOD are critical to neuronal survival. In heart tissue, STAT3 promotes tissue survival in the face of myocardial infarction and is important in ischemic preconditioning.[244]

The Restrictive Element-1 Silencing Transcription Factor (REST)/Neuron Restrictive Silencing Factor (NRSF)

The gene silencing transcription factor REST/NRSF is widely expressed during embryogenesis and plays a strategic role in terminal neuronal differentiation.[245-247] In pluripotent stem cells and neural progenitors, REST actively represses a large array of coding and noncoding neuron-specific genes important to synaptic plasticity and structural remodeling including synaptic vesicle proteins, channels, neurotransmitter receptors, and microRNAs that regulate networks of nonneuronal genes. Bioinformatics analysis predicts more than 1000 putative REST targets in the mammalian genome, including both coding and noncoding genes.[248,249] The interplay between REST and microRNAs is an emerging topic. As neural progenitors differentiate and migrate out of the ventricular zone, REST downregulation is critical for acquisition of the neural phenotype. A fundamental mechanism by which REST abundance is regulated in the transition from pluripotent stem cells to neurons is via SCF (Skp1–Cul1–F-box protein)/β-TrCP-dependent, ubiquitin proteasomal degradation.[250,251] Perturbation of REST expression during embryogenesis causes cellular apoptosis, aberrant differentiation and patterning, and lethality.[245,246]

A fundamental mechanism by which REST silences target genes is that of epigenetic remodeling (for review, see Ballas and Mandel[245] and Ooi and Wood[246]). REST binds the RE1 element of target genes and recruits CoREST and mSin3A, corepressor platforms that, in turn, recruit histone deacetylases (HDACs)-1 and 2. HDACs deacetylate core histone proteins and effect dynamic and reversible gene silencing. REST mediates long-term gene silencing by association with the site-specific histone methyltransferase G9a, which promotes dimethylation of histone 3 at lysine 9 (H3K9me2) via CoREST-dependent and independent mechanisms, and with the site-specific histone demethylase LSD1, which removes methyl groups from H3 at K4 (H3K4). In addition, REST recruits methyl CpG binding protein 2 (MeCP2, a protein that reads epigenetic marks and recruits the machinery that mediates DNA methylation). Whereas histone deacetylation is primarily a mark of dynamic gene repression, cytosine methylation is implicated in long-term gene repression.[252] Chromatin remodeling is a universal mechanism of transcriptional repression and is implicated in other histone-modulated processes including DNA replication, recombination, and repair.

In mature neurons REST is quiescent but can be activated in selectively vulnerable hippocampal neurons by insults such as global ischemia[159,253] and epileptic seizures[254] and aberrantly accumulates in the nucleus of selectively vulnerable striatal neurons in Huntington's disease.[255] Global ischemia triggers a pronounced upregulation of REST mRNA and protein in selectively vulnerable CA1 neurons (Fig. 6-12).[159] Consistent with induction of REST, core histone proteins over the GluR2 promoter exhibit pronounced deacetylation, which is indicative of reduced GluR2 promoter activity, and GluR2 mRNA and protein expression are suppressed in CA1 neurons.[159] Because the GluR2 subunit governs AMPAR Ca^{2+} permeability and AMPARs are implicated in the excitotoxic death associated with global ischemia, these changes are expected to affect neuronal survival.[154,157] Consistent with this concept, immediate knockdown of the REST gene by antisense administration rescues neurons from ischemic death.[159] These findings suggest a causal relation between REST induction and neuronal death and implicate REST-dependent gene silencing and chromatin remodeling in transcriptional repression of GluR2 in insulted neurons. Dysregulation of REST and its target genes is also implicated in medulloblastomas, Down's

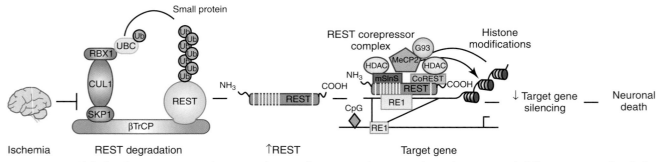

Figure 6-12 Global ischemia activates the gene silencing factor REST/NRSF, implicated in neuronal differentiation and cell death. The model shows the molecular mechanism by which transcriptional repression can play a role in cell death caused by ischemia. Global ischemia induces the neuronal repressor element-1 silencing transcription factor (REST), a member of the Gli-Krüppel family of zinc-finger transcriptional repressors containing nine noncanonical zinc finger motifs through which it binds the cis-acting RE-1 (neuronal repressor element) within the promoter region of target genes.[159] REST associates with the corepressors Sin3A and coREST, which in turn recruit histone deacetylases (HDAC) to the promoters of target genes, including the GluR2 gene subunit of the α-amino-3-hydroxy-5-methyl-4-isoxazole-propionic acid receptor (AMPAR).[159] Deacetylation of histone proteins and tightening of the core chromatin complex restrict access of the transcription machinery required for gene activation. Decreased expression of GluR2 protein increases the Ca^{2+} permeability of AMPA-type glutamate receptors, exacerbating excitotoxicity and increasing the severity of neuronal death (for review, see Liu and Zukin[154] and Kwak and Weiss.[157])

syndrome, Alzheimer's disease, and X-linked mental retardation (for review, see Ooi and Wood[246]).

Inflammation

Considerable evidence indicates that inflammation exacerbates ischemic injury (for review, see Moskowitz et al[3] and Kleinig and Vink[256]). Ischemia/hypoxia triggers activation of transcription factors such as NF-κB, hypoxia-inducible factor-1 (HIF-1), interferon regulatory factor-1, and STAT3. These, in turn, orchestrate expression of an array of proinflammatory target genes such as platelet-activating factor and the cytokines TNF-α and interleukin-1 beta (IL-1β) (for review, see Moskowitz et al,[3] Kleinig and Vink,[256] and Iadecola and Alexander[257]). Cytokines are critical mediators of inflammation and are expressed within the first 2 hours after ischemia. The first inflammatory response is the unleashing of resident immune cells such as microglia. Microglia become activated and exhibit characteristic ameboid morphologic features because of retraction of their processes by 24 hours.

Subsequently, invasion and infiltration of nonresident cells occurs. Ischemia/hypoxia triggers expression of adhesion molecules such as intercellular adhesion molecule-1 (ICAM-1), P-selectins, and E-selectins by endothelial cells on their luminal surface. The adhesion molecules interact with cognate receptors on neutrophils, guiding their migration across the vascular wall and inside the brain parenchyma to the site of injury. Neutrophils are present in high numbers in ischemic brain by 24 to 48 hours. Infiltration of lymphocytes, macrophages, and monocytes follows next. Lymphocytes release inflammatory cytokines such as TNF-α, which trigger production of chemokines such as interleukin-8 and monocyte chemoattractant protein-1, thereby initiating the inflammatory reaction (for review, see Moskowitz et al[3] and Kleinig and Vink[256]). Chemokines are a family of small, soluble adhesion molecules that rapidly recruit leukocytes (blood-borne inflammatory cells) from the circulation across the endothelial barrier to the site of injury by promoting their adhesion and chemotaxis. Macrophages appear in large quantity between 1 and 5 days after induction of focal ischemia by the MCAO model; by 5 to 7 days, they become the predominant cell type in the injured region, where they phagocytose dead cells. The triggering of inflammatory cascades and release of cytokines is thought to cause astrocyte death and exacerbate neuronal death (for review, see Moskowitz et al[3] and Kleinig and Vink[256]).

Critical evidence that inflammatory responses are involved in the pathogenesis of ischemia-induced neuronal death comes from studies that show that ischemic injury is attenuated by preischemic induction of systemic neutropenia, pharmacologic blockade of adhesion molecules or their receptors, deletion of the *Icam-1* gene, anti-inflammatory steroids, or antibody blockade of inflammatory mediators such as IL-1β or the transcription factor IFN regulatory factor-1 (for review, see Moskowitz et al[3] and Kleinig and Vink[256]). Mounting evidence indicates that, in addition to its role as perpetrator of neuronal death, NO is a catalyst for microglial activation (see earlier).

Acknowledgments

This work was supported by NIH grant NS 46742 (to R.S.Z.) and a generous grant from the F.M. Kirby Foundation. R. Suzanne Zukin is the F.M. Kirby Professor in Neural Repair and Protection.

REFERENCES

1. Liou AK, Clark RS, Henshall DC, et al: To die or not to die for neurons in ischemia, traumatic brain injury and epilepsy: a review on the stress-activated signaling pathways and apoptotic pathways, *Prog Neurobiol* 69:103–142, 2003.
2. Lo EH, Dalkara T, Moskowitz MA: Mechanisms, challenges and opportunities in stroke, *Nat Rev Neurosci* 4:399–415, 2003.
3. Moskowitz MA, Lo EH, Iadecola C: The Science of stroke: mechanisms in search of treatments, *Neuron* 67:181–198, 2010.
4. Schmidt-Kastner R, Freund TF: Selective vulnerability of the hippocampus in brain ischemia, *Neuroscience* 40:599–636, 1991.
5. Garcia JH, Yoshida Y, Chen H, et al: Progression from ischemic injury to infarct following middle cerebral artery occlusion in the rat, *Am J Pathol* 142:623–635, 1993.
6. Memezawa H, Smith ML, Siesjo BK: Penumbral tissues salvaged by reperfusion following middle cerebral artery occlusion in rats, *Stroke* 23:552–559, 1992.
7. Small DL, Buchan AM: Animal models, *Br Med Bull* 56:307–317, 2000.
8. Pulsinelli WA, Brierley JB: A new model of bilateral hemispheric ischemia in the unanesthetized rat, *Stroke* 10:267–272, 1979.
9. Pulsinelli WA, Buchan AM: The four-vessel occlusion rat model: method for complete occlusion of vertebral arteries and control of collateral circulation, *Stroke* 19:913–914, 1988.
10. Kirino T: Delayed neuronal death in the gerbil hippocampus following ischemia, *Brain Res* 239:57–69, 1982.
11. Kitagawa K, Matsumoto M, Yang G, et al: Cerebral ischemia after bilateral carotid artery occlusion and intraluminal suture occlusion in mice: evaluation of the patency of the posterior communicating artery, *J Cereb Blood Flow Metab* 18:570–579, 1998.
12. Oguro K, Jover T, Tanaka H, et al: Global ischemia-induced increases in the gap junctional proteins connexin 32 (Cx32) and Cx36 in hippocampus and enhanced vulnerability of Cx32 knockout mice, *J Neurosci* 21:7534–7542, 2001.
13. Dirnagl U, Thoren P, Villringer A, et al: Global forebrain ischaemia in the rat: controlled reduction of cerebral blood flow by hypobaric hypotension and two-vessel occlusion, *Neurol Res* 15:128–130, 1993.
14. Nemoto EM: Monkey model of complete global ischemia, *Stroke* 24:328–329, 1993.
15. Torregrosa G, Barbera MD, Centeno JM, et al: Characterization of the cortical laser-Doppler flow and hippocampal degenerative patterns after global cerebral ischaemia in the goat, *Pflugers Arch* 435:662–669, 1998.
16. Pulsinelli WA, Brierley JB, Plum F: Temporal profile of neuronal damage in a model of transient forebrain ischemia, *Ann Neurol* 11:491–498, 1982.
17. Raffin CN, Harrison M, Sick TJ, et al: EEG suppression and anoxic depolarization: influences on cerebral oxygenation during ischemia, *J Cereb Blood Flow Metab* 11:407–415, 1991.
18. Kirino T: Ischemic tolerance, *J Cereb Blood Flow Metab* 22:1283–1296, 2002.
19. Schauwecker PE, Steward O: Genetic determinants of susceptibility to excitotoxic cell death: implications for gene targeting approaches, *Proc Natl Acad Sci U S A* 94:4103–4108, 1997.
20. Braeuninger S, Kleinschnitz C: Rodent models of focal cerebral ischemia: procedural pitfalls and translational problems, *Exp Transl Stroke Med* 1:8, 2009.
21. Longa EZ, Weinstein PR, Carlson S, et al: Reversible middle cerebral artery occlusion without craniectomy in rats, *Stroke* 20:84–91, 1989.
22. Buchan AM, Xue D, Slivka A: A new model of temporary focal neocortical ischemia in the rat, *Stroke* 23:273–279, 1992.
23. Kilic E, Hermann DM, Hossmann KA: A reproducible model of thromboembolic stroke in mice, *Neuroreport* 9:2967–2970, 1998.

24. Taniguchi H, Andreasson K: The hypoxic-ischemic encephalopathy model of perinatal ischemia, *J Vis Exp* 21, 2008:(video article).

25. Ashwal S, Pearce WJ: Animal models of neonatal stroke, *Curr Opin Pediatr* 13:506-516, 2001.

26. Goldberg MP, Choi DW: Combined oxygen and glucose deprivation in cortical cell culture: calcium-dependent and calcium-independent mechanisms of neuronal injury, *J Neurosci* 13:3510-3524, 1993.

27. Martin RL, Lloyd HG, Cowan AI: The early events of oxygen and glucose deprivation: setting the scene for neuronal death? *Trends Neurosci* 17:251-257, 1994.

28. Pellegrini-Giampietro DE, Peruginelli F, Meli E, et al: Protection with metabotropic glutamate 1 receptor antagonists in models of ischemic neuronal death: time-course and mechanisms, *Neuropharmacology* 38:1607-1619, 1999.

29. Strasser U, Fischer G: Protection from neuronal damage induced by combined oxygen and glucose deprivation in organotypic hippocampal cultures by glutamate receptor antagonists, *Brain Res* 687:167-174, 1995.

30. Kroemer G, Galluzzi L, Vandenabeele P, et al: Classification of cell death: recommendations of the Nomenclature Committee on Cell Death 2009, *Cell Death Differ* 16:3-11, 2009.

31. Green DR: Apoptotic pathways: ten minutes to dead, *Cell* 121:671-674, 2005.

32. Galluzzi L, Blomgren K, Kroemer G: Mitochondrial membrane permeabilization in neuronal injury, *Nat Rev Neurosci* 10:481-494, 2009.

33. Wang C, Youle RJ: The role of mitochondria in apoptosis, *Annu Rev Genet* 43:95-118, 2009.

34. Galluzzi L, Aaronson SA, Abrams J, et al: Guidelines for the use and interpretation of assays for monitoring cell death in higher eukaryotes, *Cell Death Differ* 16:1093-1107, 2009.

35. Golstein P, Kroemer G: Cell death by necrosis: towards a molecular definition, *Trends Biochem Sci* 32:37-43, 2007.

36. Degterev A, Yuan J: Expansion and evolution of cell death programmes, *Nat Rev Mol Cell Biol* 9:378-390, 2008.

37. Christofferson DE, Yuan J: Necroptosis as an alternative form of programmed cell death, *Curr Opin Cell Biol* 22:263-268, 2010.

38. Degterev A, Huang Z, Boyce M, et al: Chemical inhibitor of nonapoptotic cell death with therapeutic potential for ischemic brain injury, *Nat Chem Biol* 1:112-119, 2005.

39. Baehrecke EH: Autophagy: dual roles in life and death? *Nat Rev Mol Cell Biol* 6:505-510, 2005.

40. Wong E, Cuervo AM: Autophagy gone awry in neurodegenerative diseases, *Nat Neurosci* 13:805-811, 2010.

41. Levine B, Kroemer G: Autophagy in aging, disease and death: the true identity of a cell death impostor, *Cell Death Differ* 16:1-2, 2009.

42. Adhami F, Liao G, Morozov YM, et al: Cerebral ischemia-hypoxia induces intravascular coagulation and autophagy, *Am J Pathol* 169:566-583, 2006.

43. Lipton P: Ischemic cell death in brain neurons, *Physiol Rev* 79:1431-1568, 1999.

44. Park SM, Schickel R, Peter ME: Nonapoptotic functions of FADD-binding death receptors and their signaling molecules, *Curr Opin Cell Biol* 17:610-616, 2005.

45. Haase G, Pettmann B, Raoul C, et al: Signaling by death receptors in the nervous system, *Curr Opin Neurobiol* 18:284-291, 2008.

46. Vandenabeele P, Declercq W, Van HF, et al: The role of the kinases RIP1 and RIP3 in TNF-induced necrosis, *Sci Signal* 3, 2010:re4.

47. Cho YS, Challa S, Moquin D, et al: Phosphorylation-driven assembly of the RIP1-RIP3 complex regulates programmed necrosis and virus-induced inflammation, *Cell* 137:1112-1123, 2009.

48. Schinzel AC, Takeuchi O, Huang Z, et al: Cyclophilin D is a component of mitochondrial permeability transition and mediates neuronal cell death after focal cerebral ischemia, *Proc Natl Acad Sci U S A* 102:12005-12010, 2005.

49. Hitomi J, Christofferson DE, Ng A, et al: Identification of a molecular signaling network that regulates a cellular necrotic cell death pathway, *Cell* 135:1311-1323, 2008.

50. Baines CP, Kaiser RA, Purcell NH, et al: Loss of cyclophilin D reveals a critical role for mitochondrial permeability transition in cell death, *Nature* 434:658-662, 2005.

51. Nakagawa T, Shimizu S, Watanabe T, et al: Cyclophilin D-dependent mitochondrial permeability transition regulates some necrotic but not apoptotic cell death, *Nature* 434:652-658, 2005.

52. Schneider MD: Cyclophilin D: knocking on death's door, *Sci STKE* 2005, 2005:e26.

53. Degterev A, Hitomi J, Germscheid M, et al: Identification of RIP1 kinase as a specific cellular target of necrostatins, *Nat Chem Biol* 4:313-321, 2008.

54. Youle RJ, Strasser A: The BCL-2 protein family: opposing activities that mediate cell death, *Nat Rev Mol Cell Biol* 9:47-59, 2008.

55. Cheng WC, Berman SB, Ivanovska I, et al: Mitochondrial factors with dual roles in death and survival, *Oncogene* 25:4697-4705, 2006.

56. Bao Q, Shi Y: Apoptosome: a platform for the activation of initiator caspases, *Cell Death Differ* 14:56-65, 2007.

57. Li J, Yuan J: Caspases in apoptosis and beyond, *Oncogene* 27:6194-6206, 2008.

58. Kurokawa M, Kornbluth S: Caspases and kinases in a death grip, *Cell* 138:838-854, 2009.

59. Pop C, Salvesen GS: Human caspases: activation, specificity, and regulation, *J Biol Chem* 284:21777-21781, 2009.

60. Riedl SJ, Salvesen GS: The apoptosome: signalling platform of cell death, *Nat Rev Mol Cell Biol* 8:405-413, 2007.

61. Qi S, Pang Y, Hu Q, et al: Crystal structure of the *Caenorhabditis elegans* apoptosome reveals an octameric assembly of CED-4, *Cell* 141:446-457, 2010.

62. Kroemer G, Martin SJ: Caspase-independent cell death, *Nat Med* 11:725-730, 2005.

63. Park HH, Logette E, Raunser S, et al: Death domain assembly mechanism revealed by crystal structure of the oligomeric PIDDosome core complex, *Cell* 128:533-546, 2007.

64. Tinel A, Tschopp J: The PIDDosome, a protein complex implicated in activation of caspase-2 in response to genotoxic stress, *Science* 304:843-846, 2004.

65. Niizuma K, Endo H, Nito C, et al: The PIDDosome mediates delayed death of hippocampal CA1 neurons after transient global cerebral ischemia in rats, *Proc Natl Acad Sci U S A* 105:16368-16373, 2008.

66. Janssens S, Tinel A, Lippens S, et al: PIDD mediates NF-kappaB activation in response to DNA damage, *Cell* 123:1079-1092, 2005.

67. Wu ZH, Mabb A, Miyamoto S: PIDD: a switch hitter, *Cell* 123:980-982, 2005.

68. Upton JP, Austgen K, Nishino M, et al: Caspase-2 cleavage of BID is a critical apoptotic signal downstream of endoplasmic reticulum stress, *Mol Cell Biol* 28:3943-3951, 2008.

69. Galonek HL, Hardwick JM: Upgrading the BCL-2 network, *Nat Cell Biol* 8:1317-1319, 2006.

70. Yip KW, Reed JC: Bcl-2 family proteins and cancer, *Oncogene* 27:6398-6406, 2008.

71. Hardwick JM, Youle RJ: SnapShot: BCL-2 proteins, *Cell* 138:404, 2009.

72. Chipuk JE, Moldoveanu T, Llambi F, et al: The BCL-2 family reunion, *Mol Cell* 37:299-310, 2010.

73. Cheng EH, Wei MC, Weiler S, et al: BCL-2, BCL-X(L) sequester BH3 domain-only molecules preventing BAX- and BAK-mediated mitochondrial apoptosis, *Mol Cell* 8:705-711, 2001.

74. Giam M, Huang DC, Bouillet P: BH3-only proteins and their roles in programmed cell death, *Oncogene* 27(Suppl 1):S128-S136, 2008.

75. Certo M, Del Gaizo Moore V, Nishino M, et al: Mitochondria primed by death signals determine cellular addiction to antiapoptotic BCL-2 family members, *Cancer Cell* 9:351-365, 2006.

76. Miyawaki T, Mashiko T, Ofengeim D, et al: Ischemic preconditioning blocks BAD translocation, Bcl-x_L cleavage, and large channel activity in mitochondria of postischemic hippocampal neurons, *Proc Natl Acad Sci USA* 105:4892-4897, 2008.

77. Albeck JG, Burke JM, Aldridge BB, et al: Quantitative analysis of pathways controlling extrinsic apoptosis in single cells, *Mol Cell* 30:11-25, 2008.

78. Bonanni L, Chachar M, Jover-Mengual T, et al: Zinc-dependent multi-conductance channel activity in mitochondria isolated from ischemic brain, *J Neurosci* 26:6851-6862, 2006.

79. Jonas EA, Hickman JA, Hardwick JM, et al: Exposure to hypoxia rapidly induces mitochondrial channel activity within a living synapse, *J Biol Chem* 280:4491-4497, 2005.

80. Cheng EH, Kirsch DG, Clem RJ, et al: Conversion of Bcl-2 to a Bax-like death effector by caspases, *Science* 278:1966-1968, 1997.

81. Clem RJ, Cheng EH, Karp CL, et al: Modulation of cell death by Bcl-XL through caspase interaction, *Proc Natl Acad Sci U S A* 95:554–559, 1998.
82. Li H, Zhu H, Xu CJ, et al: Cleavage of BID by caspase 8 mediates the mitochondrial damage in the Fas pathway of apoptosis, *Cell* 94:491–501, 1998.
83. Basanez G, Zhang J, Chau BN, et al: Pro-apoptotic cleavage products of Bcl-xL form cytochrome c-conducting pores in pure lipid membranes, *J Biol Chem* 276:31083–31091, 2001.
84. Jonas EA, Hoit D, Hickman JA, et al: Modulation of synaptic transmission by the BCL-2 family protein BCL-xL, *J Neurosci* 23:8423–8431, 2003.
85. Fannjiang Y, Kim CH, Huganir RL, et al: BAK alters neuronal excitability and can switch from anti- to pro-death function during postnatal development, *Dev Cell* 4:575–585, 2003.
86. Li H, Chen Y, Jones AF, et al: Bcl-xL induces Drp1-dependent synapse formation in cultured hippocampal neurons, *Proc Natl Acad Sci U S A* 105:2169–2174, 2008.
87. Krajewska M, Mai JK, Zapata JM, et al: Dynamics of expression of apoptosis-regulatory proteins Bid, Bcl-2, Bcl-X, Bax and Bak during development of murine nervous system, *Cell Death Differ* 9:145–157, 2002.
88. Sugawara T, Fujimura M, Morita-Fujimura Y, et al: Mitochondrial release of cytochrome c corresponds to the selective vulnerability of hippocampal CA1 neurons in rats after transient global cerebral ischemia, *J Neurosci* 19:RC39, 1999.
89. Chen J, Nagayama T, Jin K, et al: Induction of caspase-3-like protease may mediate delayed neuronal death in the hippocampus after transient cerebral ischemia, *J Neurosci* 18:4914–4928, 1998.
90. Tanaka H, Yokota H, Jover T, et al: Ischemic preconditioning: neuronal survival in the face of caspase-3 activation, *J Neurosci* 24:2750–2759, 2004.
91. McLaughlin B, Hartnett KA, Erhardt JA, et al: Caspase 3 activation is essential for neuroprotection in preconditioning, *Proc Natl Acad Sci U S A* 100:715–720, 2003.
92. Garnier P, Ying W, Swanson RA: Ischemic preconditioning by caspase cleavage of poly(ADP-ribose) polymerase-1, *J Neurosci* 23:7967–7973, 2003.
93. Szydlowska K, Tymianski M: Calcium, ischemia and excitotoxicity, *Cell Calcium* 47:122–129, 2010.
94. Eckelman BP, Salvesen GS, Scott FL: Human inhibitor of apoptosis proteins: why XIAP is the black sheep of the family, *EMBO Rep* 7:988–994, 2006.
95. Gyrd-Hansen M, Meier P: IAPs: from caspase inhibitors to modulators of NF-kappaB, inflammation and cancer, *Nat Rev Cancer* 10:561–574, 2010.
96. Jaattela M, Tschopp J: Caspase-independent cell death in T lymphocytes, *Nat Immunol* 4:416–423, 2003.
97. Stefanis L: Caspase-dependent and -independent neuronal death: two distinct pathways to neuronal injury, *Neuroscientist* 11:50–62, 2005.
98. Yu SW, Andrabi SA, Wang H, et al: Apoptosis-inducing factor mediates poly(ADP-ribose) (PAR) polymer-induced cell death, *Proc Natl Acad Sci U S A* 103:18314–18319, 2006.
99. Hangen E, Blomgren K, Benit P, et al: Life with or without AIF, *Trends Biochem Sci* 35:278–287, 2010.
100. Chiarugi A, Moskowitz MA: Cell biology. PARP-1—a perpetrator of apoptotic cell death? *Science* 297:200–201, 2002.
101. Yu S-W: Mediation of poly(ADP-ribose) polymerase-1-dependent cell death by apoptosis-inducing factor, *Science* 297:259–263, 2002.
102. Wang Y, Dawson VL, Dawson TM: Poly(ADP-ribose) signals to mitochondrial AIF: a key event in parthanatos, *Exp Neurol* 218:193–202, 2009.
103. D'Amours D, Desnoyers S, D'Silva I, et al: Poly(ADP-ribosyl)ation reactions in the regulation of nuclear functions, *Biochem J* 342(Pt 2):249–268, 1999.
104. Boya P, Kroemer G: Lysosomal membrane permeabilization in cell death, *Oncogene* 27:6434–6451, 2008.
105. Zhao ST, Chen M, Li SJ, et al: Mitochondrial BNIP3 upregulation precedes endonuclease G translocation in hippocampal neuronal death following oxygen-glucose deprivation, *BMC Neurosci* 10:113, 2009.
106. Colbourne F, Sutherland GR, Auer RN: Electron microscopic evidence against apoptosis as the mechanism of neuronal death in global ischemia, *J Neurosci* 19:4200–4210, 1999.
107. Pagnussat AS, Faccioni-Heuser MC, Netto CA, et al: An ultrastructural study of cell death in the CA1 pyramidal field of the hippocampus in rats submitted to transient global ischemia followed by reperfusion, *J Anat* 211:589–599, 2007.
108. Tsukada T, Watanabe M, Yamashima T: Implications of CAD and DNase II in ischemic neuronal necrosis specific for the primate hippocampus, *J Neurochem* 79:1196–1206, 2001.
109. Yamashima T: Implication of cysteine proteases calpain, cathepsin and caspase in ischemic neuronal death of primates, *Prog Neurobiol* 62:273–295, 2000.
110. Barber PA, Auer RN, Buchan AM, et al: Understanding and managing ischemic stroke, *Can J Physiol Pharmacol* 79:283–296, 2001.
111. Krajewski S, Krajewska M, Ellerby LM, et al: Release of caspase-9 from mitochondria during neuronal apoptosis and cerebral ischemia, *Proc Natl Acad Sci U S A* 96:5752–5757, 1999.
112. Martin-Villalba A: CD95 ligand (Fas-L/APO-1L) and tumor necrosis factor-related apoptosis-inducing ligand mediate ischemia-induced apoptosis in neurons, *J Neurosci* 19:3809–3817, 1999.
113. Fujimura M, Morita-Fujimura Y, Murakami K, et al: Cytosolic redistribution of cytochrome c after transient focal cerebral ischemia in rats, *J Cereb Blood Flow Metab* 18:1239–1247, 1998.
114. Namura S, Zhu J, Fink K, et al: Activation and cleavage of caspase-3 in apoptosis induced by experimental cerebral ischemia, *J Neurosci* 18:3659–3668, 1998.
115. Benveniste H, Drejer J, Schousboe A, et al: Elevation of the extracellular concentrations of glutamate and aspartate in rat hippocampus during transient cerebral ischemia monitored by intracerebral microdialysis, *J Neurochem* 43:1369–1374, 1984.
116. Cardell M, Koide T, Wieloch T: Pyruvate dehydrogenase activity in the rat cerebral cortex following cerebral ischemia, *J Cereb Blood Flow Metab* 9:350–357, 1989.
117. Tominaga T, Kure S, Narisawa K, et al: Endonuclease activation following focal ischemic injury in the rat brain, *Brain Res* 608:21–26, 1993.
118. Lucas DR, Newhouse JP: The toxic effect of sodium L-glutamate on the inner layers of the retina, *AMA Arch Ophthalmol* 58:193–201, 1957.
119. Olney JW, Ho OL: Brain damage in infant mice following oral intake of glutamate, aspartate or cysteine, *Nature* 227:609–611, 1970.
120. Kass IS, Lipton P: Mechanisms involved in irreversible anoxic damage to the in vitro rat hippocampal slice, *J Physiol* 332:459–472, 1982.
121. Rothman SM: Synaptic activity mediates death of hypoxic neurons, *Science* 220:536–537, 1983.
122. Rothman SM: The neurotoxicity of excitatory amino acids is produced by passive chloride influx, *J Neurosci* 5:1483–1489, 1985.
123. Simon RP, Swan JH, Griffiths T, et al: Blockade of N-methyl-D-aspartate receptors may protect against ischemic damage in the brain, *Science* 226:850–852, 1984.
124. Hermans E, Challiss RA: Structural, signalling and regulatory properties of the group I metabotropic glutamate receptors: prototypic family C G-protein-coupled receptors, *Biochem J* 359:465–484, 2001.
125. Ronesi JA, Huber KM: Metabotropic glutamate receptors and fragile X mental retardation protein: partners in translational regulation at the synapse, *Sci Signal* 1:e6, 2008.
126. Wang DO, Martin KC, Zukin RS: Spatially restricting gene expression by local translation at synapses, *Trends Neurosci* 33:173–182, 2010.
127. Swanson RA, Ying W, Kauppinen TM: Astrocyte influences on ischemic neuronal death, *Curr Mol Med* 4:193–205, 2004.
128. Nicotera P, Leist M, Fava E, et al: Energy requirement for caspase activation and neuronal cell death, *Brain Pathol* 10:276–282, 2000.
129. Meldrum B, Garthwaite J: Excitatory amino acid neurotoxicity and neurodegenerative disease, *Trends Pharmacol Sci* 11:379–387, 1990.
130. Baker AJ, Zornow MH, Scheller MS, et al: Changes in extracellular concentrations of glutamate, aspartate, glycine, dopamine, serotonin, and dopamine metabolites after transient global ischemia in the rabbit brain, *J Neurochem* 57:1370–1379, 1991.
131. Mitani A, Kataoka K: Critical levels of extracellular glutamate mediating gerbil hippocampal delayed neuronal death during hypothermia: brain microdialysis study, *Neuroscience* 42:661–670, 1991.

132. Carroll RC, Zukin RS: NMDA-receptor trafficking and targeting: implications for synaptic transmission and plasticity, *Trends Neurosci* 25:571-577, 2002.

133. Cull-Candy SG, Leszkiewicz DN: Role of distinct NMDA receptor subtypes at central synapses, *Sci STKE* 2004, 2004:re16.

134. Perez-Otano I, Ehlers MD: Homeostatic plasticity and NMDA receptor trafficking, *Trends Neurosci* 28:229-238, 2005.

135. Lau CG, Zukin RS: NMDA receptor trafficking in synaptic plasticity and neuropsychiatric disorders, *Nat Rev Neurosci* 8:413-426, 2007.

136. Collingridge GL, Isaac JT, Wang YT: Receptor trafficking and synaptic plasticity, *Nat Rev Neurosci* 5:952-962, 2004.

137. Malenka RC, Bear MF: LTP and LTD: an embarrassment of riches, *Neuron* 44:5-21, 2004.

138. Soriano FX, Martel MA, Papadia S, et al: Specific targeting of pro-death NMDA receptor signals with differing reliance on the NR2B PDZ ligand, *J Neurosci* 28:10696-10710, 2008.

139. Chen M, Xing D, Chen T, et al: BimL involvement in Bax activation during UV irradiation-induced apoptosis, *Biochem Biophys Res Commun* 358:559-565, 2007.

140. Zhou Q, Lam PY, Han D, et al: c-Jun N-terminal kinase regulates mitochondrial bioenergetics by modulating pyruvate dehydrogenase activity in primary cortical neurons, *J Neurochem* 104:325-335, 2008.

141. Ventura JJ, Cogswell P, Flavell RA, et al: JNK potentiates TNF-stimulated necrosis by increasing the production of cytotoxic reactive oxygen species, *Genes Dev* 18:2905-2915, 2004.

142. Xu W, Wong TP, Chery N, et al: Calpain-mediated mGluR1alpha truncation: a key step in excitotoxicity, *Neuron* 53:399-412, 2007.

143. Hardingham GE, Fukunaga Y, Bading H: Extrasynaptic NMDARs oppose synaptic NMDARs by triggering CREB shut-off and cell death pathways, *Nat Neurosci* 5:405-414, 2002.

144. Hardingham GE: Coupling of the NMDA receptor to neuroprotective and neurodestructive events, *Biochem Soc Trans* 37:1147-1160, 2009.

145. Wang J, Liu S, Fu Y, et al: Cdk5 activation induces hippocampal CA1 cell death by directly phosphorylating NMDA receptors, *Nat Neurosci* 6:1039-1047, 2003.

146. Skeberdis VA, Chevaleyre V, Lau CG, et al: Protein kinase A regulates calcium permeability of NMDA receptors, *Nat Neurosci* 9:501-510, 2006.

147. Chalifoux JR, Carter AG: GABA(B) receptors modulate NMDA receptor calcium signals in dendritic spines, *Neuron* 66:101-113, 2010.

148. Lipton SA: NMDA receptors, glial cells, and clinical medicine, *Neuron* 50:9-11, 2006.

149. Verkhratsky A, Kirchhoff F: NMDA receptors in glia, *Neuroscientist* 13:28-37, 2007.

150. Salter MG, Fern R: NMDA receptors are expressed in developing oligodendrocyte processes and mediate injury, *Nature* 438:1167-1171, 2005.

151. Karadottir R, Cavelier P, Bergersen LH, et al: NMDA receptors are expressed in oligodendrocytes and activated in ischaemia, *Nature* 438:1162-1166, 2005.

152. Micu I, Jiang Q, Coderre E, et al: NMDA receptors mediate calcium accumulation in myelin during chemical ischaemia, *Nature* 439:988-992, 2006.

153. Fu Y, Sun W, Shi Y, et al: Glutamate excitotoxicity inflicts paranodal myelin splitting and retraction, *PLoS One* 4:e6705, 2009.

154. Liu SJ, Zukin RS: Ca2+-permeable AMPA receptors in synaptic plasticity and neuronal death, *Trends Neurosci* 30:126-134, 2007.

155. Isaac JT, Ashby M, McBain CJ: The role of the GluR2 subunit in AMPA receptor function and synaptic plasticity, *Neuron* 54:859-871, 2007.

156. Sensi SL, Paoletti P, Bush AI, et al: Zinc in the physiology and pathology of the CNS, *Nat Rev Neurosci* 10:780-791, 2009.

157. Kwak S, Weiss JH: Calcium-permeable AMPA channels in neurodegenerative disease and ischemia, *Curr Opin Neurobiol* 16:281-287, 2006.

158. Pellegrini-Giampietro DE, Zukin RS, Bennett MV, et al: Switch in glutamate receptor subunit gene expression in CA1 subfield of hippocampus following global ischemia in rats, *Proc Natl Acad Sci U S A* 89:10499-10503, 1992.

159. Calderone A, Jover T, Noh K-M, et al: Ischemic insults de-repress the gene silencer rest in neurons destined to die, *J Neurosci* 23:2112-2121, 2003.

160. Opitz T, Grooms SY, Bennett MV, et al: Remodeling of alpha-amino-3-hydroxy-5-methyl-4-isoxazole-propionic acid receptor subunit composition in hippocampal neurons after global ischemia, *Proc Natl Acad Sci U S A* 97:13360-13365, 2000.

161. Weiss JH, Sensi SL: Ca2+-Zn2+ permeable AMPA or kainate receptors: possible key factors in selective neurodegeneration, *Trends Neurosci* 23:365-371, 2000.

162. Gorter JA, Petrozzino JJ, Aronica EM, et al: Global ischemia induces downregulation of Glur2 mRNA and increases AMPA receptor-mediated Ca2+ influx in hippocampal CA1 neurons of gerbil, *J Neurosci* 17:6179-6188, 1997.

163. Oguro K, Oguro N, Kojima T, et al: Knockdown of AMPA receptor GluR2 expression causes delayed neurodegeneration and increases damage by sublethal ischemia in hippocampal CA1 and CA3 neurons, *J Neurosci* 19:9218-9227, 1999.

164. Noh KM, Yokota H, Mashiko T, et al: Blockade of calcium-permeable AMPA receptors protects hippocampal neurons against global ischemia-induced death, *Proc Natl Acad Sci U S A* 102:12230-12235, 2005.

165. Liu S, Lau L, Wei J, et al: Expression of Ca(2+)-permeable AMPA receptor channels primes cell death in transient forebrain ischemia, *Neuron* 43:43-55, 2004.

166. Liu B, Liao M, Mielke JG, et al: Ischemic insults direct glutamate receptor subunit 2-lacking AMPA receptors to synaptic sites, *J Neurosci* 26:5309-5319, 2006.

167. Sheardown MJ: The pharmacology of AMPA receptors and their antagonists, *Stroke* 24:I146-I147, 1993.

168. Nurse S, Corbett D: Neuroprotection after several days of mild, drug-induced hypothermia, *J Cereb Blood Flow Metab* 16:474-480, 1996.

169. Ying HS, Weishaupt JH, Grabb M, et al: Sublethal oxygen-glucose deprivation alters hippocampal neuronal AMPA receptor expression and vulnerability to kainate-induced death, *J Neurosci* 17:9536-9544, 1997.

170. Carriedo SG, Yin HZ, Sensi SL, et al: Rapid Ca2+ entry through Ca2+-permeable AMPA/Kainate channels triggers marked intracellular Ca2+ rises and consequent oxygen radical production, *J Neurosci* 18:7727-7738, 1998.

171. Peng PL, Zhong X, Tu W, et al: ADAR2-dependent RNA editing of AMPA receptor subunit GluR2 determines vulnerability of neurons in forebrain ischemia, *Neuron* 49:719-733, 2006.

172. O'Neill MJ, Bogaert L, Hicks CA, et al: LY377770, a novel iGlu5 kainate receptor antagonist with neuroprotective effects in global and focal cerebral ischaemia, *Neuropharmacology* 39:1575-1588, 2000.

173. Pan J, Pei DS, Yin XH, et al: Involvement of oxidative stress in the rapid Akt1 regulating a JNK scaffold during ischemia in rat hippocampus, *Neurosci Lett* 392:47-51, 2006.

174. Zhang QG, Tian H, Li HC, et al: Antioxidant N-acetylcysteine inhibits the activation of JNK3 mediated by the GluR6-PSD95-MLK3 signaling module during cerebral ischemia in rat hippocampus, *Neurosci Lett* 408:159-164, 2006.

175. Hashimoto K, Tomitaka S, Bi Y, et al: Rolipram, a selective phosphodiesterase type-IV inhibitor, prevents induction of heat shock protein HSP-70 and hsp-70 mRNA in rat retrosplenial cortex by the NMDA receptor antagonist dizocilpine, *Eur J Neurosci* 9:1891-1901, 1997.

176. Ishimaru M, Fukamauchi F, Olney JW: Halothane prevents MK-801 neurotoxicity in the rat cingulate cortex, *Neurosci Lett* 193:1-4, 1995.

177. Moran MM, Xu H, Clapham DE: TRP ion channels in the nervous system, *Curr Opin Neurobiol* 14:362-369, 2004.

178. Kauer JA, Gibson HE: Hot flash: TRPV channels in the brain, *Trends Neurosci* 32:215-224, 2009.

179. Aarts MM, Tymianski M: TRPMs and neuronal cell death, *Pflugers Arch* 451:243-249, 2005.

180. Aarts M, Iihara K, Wei WL, et al: A key role for TRPM7 channels in anoxic neuronal death, *Cell* 115:863-877, 2003.

181. Sun HS, Jackson MF, Martin LJ, et al: Suppression of hippocampal TRPM7 protein prevents delayed neuronal death in brain ischemia, *Nat Neurosci* 12:1300-1307, 2009.

182. Lipski J, Park TI, Li D, et al: Involvement of TRP-like channels in the acute ischemic response of hippocampal CA1 neurons in brain slices, *Brain Res* 1077:187-199, 2006.

183. Jia Y, Zhou J, Tai Y, et al: TRPC channels promote cerebellar granule neuron survival, *Nat Neurosci* 10:559-567, 2007.

184. Immke DC, McCleskey EW: Lactate enhances the acid-sensing Na$^+$ channel on ischemia-sensing neurons, *Nat Neurosci* 4:869-870, 2001.

185. Immke DC, McCleskey EW: Protons open acid-sensing ion channels by catalyzing relief of Ca2$^+$ blockade, *Neuron* 37:75-84, 2003.

186. Yermolaieva O, Leonard AS, Schnizler MK, et al: Extracellular acidosis increases neuronal cell calcium by activating acid-sensing ion channel 1a, *Proc Natl Acad Sci U S A* 101:6752-6757, 2004.

187. Wang WZ, Chu XP, Li MH, et al: Modulation of acid-sensing ion channel currents, acid-induced increase of intracellular Ca2$^+$, and acidosis-mediated neuronal injury by intracellular pH, *J Biol Chem* 281:29369-29378, 2006.

188. Xiong ZG, Zhu XM, Chu XP, et al: Neuroprotection in ischemia: blocking calcium-permeable acid-sensing ion channels, *Cell* 118:687-698, 2004.

189. Gao J, Duan B, Wang DG, et al: Coupling between NMDA receptor and acid-sensing ion channel contributes to ischemic neuronal death, *Neuron* 48:635-646, 2005.

190. Higuchi M, Tomioka M, Takano J, et al: Distinct mechanistic roles of calpain and caspase activation in neurodegeneration as revealed in mice overexpressing their specific inhibitors, *J Biol Chem* 280:15229-15237, 2005.

191. Frederickson CJ, Koh JY, Bush AI: The neurobiology of zinc in health and disease, *Nat Rev Neurosci* 6:449-462, 2005.

192. Palmiter RD, Cole TB, Quaife CJ, et al: ZnT-3, a putative transporter of zinc into synaptic vesicles, *Proc Natl Acad Sci U S A* 93:14934-14939, 1996.

193. Kay AR: Evidence for chelatable zinc in the extracellular space of the hippocampus, but little evidence for synaptic release of Zn, *J Neurosci* 23:6847-6855, 2003.

194. Peters S, Koh J, Choi DW: Zinc selectively blocks the action of N-methyl-D-aspartate on cortical neurons, *Science* 236:589-593, 1987.

195. Westbrook GL, Mayer ML: Micromolar concentrations of Zn^{2+} antagonize NMDA and GABA responses of hippocampal neurons, *Nature* 328:640-643, 1987.

196. Christine CW, Choi DW: Effect of zinc on NMDA receptor-mediated channel currents in cortical neurons, *J Neurosci* 10:108-116, 1990.

197. Rassendren FA, Lory P, Pin JP, et al: Zinc has opposite effects on NMDA and non-NMDA receptors expressed in Xenopus oocytes, *Neuron* 4:733-740, 1990.

198. Bresink I, Ebert B, Parsons CG, et al: Zinc changes AMPA receptor properties: results of binding studies and patch clamp recordings, *Neuropharmacology* 35:503-509, 1996.

199. Lerma J, Morales M, Ibarz JM, et al: Rectification properties and Ca^{2+} permeability of glutamate receptor channels in hippocampal cells, *Eur J Neurosci* 6:1080-1088, 1994.

200. Toomim CS, Millington WR: Regional and laminar specificity of kainate-stimulated cobalt uptake in the rat hippocampal formation, *J Comp Neurol* 402:141-154, 1998.

201. Yin HZ, Sensi SL, Carriedo SG, et al: Dendritic localization of Ca(2+)-permeable AMPA/kainate channels in hippocampal pyramidal neurons, *J Comp Neurol* 409:250-260, 1999.

202. Lu YM, Taverna FA, Tu R, et al: Endogenous Zn(2+) is required for the induction of long-term potentiation at rat hippocampal mossy fiber-CA3 synapses, *Synapse* 38:187-197, 2000.

203. Li Y, Hough CJ, Frederickson CJ, et al: Induction of mossy fiber→Ca3 long-term potentiation requires translocation of synaptically released Zn^{2+}, *J Neurosci* 21:8015-8025, 2001.

204. Vogt K, Mellor J, Tong G, et al: The actions of synaptically released zinc at hippocampal mossy fiber synapses, *Neuron* 26:187-196, 2000.

205. Sloviter RS: A selective loss of hippocampal mossy fiber Timm stain accompanies granule cell seizure activity induced by perforant path stimulation, *Brain Res* 330:150-153, 1985.

206. Yanamoto H, Nagata I, Sakata M, et al: Infarct tolerance induced by intra-cerebral infusion of recombinant brain-derived neurotrophic factor, *Brain Res* 859:240-248, 2000.

207. Weiss JH, Hartley DM, Koh JY, et al: AMPA receptor activation potentiates zinc neurotoxicity, *Neuron* 10:43-49, 1993.

208. Koh JY: Zinc and disease of the brain, *Mol Neurobiol* 24:99-106, 2001.

209. Calderone A, Jover T, Mashiko T, et al: Late calcium EDTA rescues hippocampal CA1 neurons from global ischemia-induced death, *J Neurosci* 24:9903-9913, 2004.

210. Koh JY, Suh SW, Gwag BJ, et al: The role of zinc in selective neuronal death after transient global cerebral ischemia, *Science* 272:1013-1016, 1996.

211. Yin HZ, Sensi SL, Ogoshi F, et al: Blockade of Ca^{2+}-permeable AMPA/kainate channels decreases oxygen-glucose deprivation-induced Zn^{2+} accumulation and neuronal loss in hippocampal pyramidal neurons, *J Neurosci* 22:1273-1279, 2002.

212. Lee JY, Cole TB, Palmiter RD, et al: Accumulation of zinc in degenerating hippocampal neurons of ZnT3-null mice after seizures: evidence against synaptic vesicle origin, *J Neurosci* 20:RC79, 2000.

213. Sensi SL, Jeng JM: Rethinking the excitotoxic ionic milieu: the emerging role of Zn(2+) in ischemic neuronal injury, *Curr Mol Med* 4:87-111, 2004.

214. Dineley KE, Votyakova TV, Reynolds IJ: Zinc inhibition of cellular energy production: implications for mitochondria and neurodegeneration, *J Neurochem* 85:563-570, 2003.

215. Chen M, Chen Q, Cheng XW, et al: Zn^{2+} mediates ischemia-induced impairment of the ubiquitin-proteasome system in the rat hippocampus, *J Neurochem* 111:1094-1103, 2009.

216. Pulsinelli WA, Duffy TE: Regional energy balance in rat brain after transient forebrain ischemia, *J Neurochem* 40:1500-1503, 1983.

217. Datta SR, Brunet A, Greenberg ME: Cellular survival: a play in three Akts, *Genes Dev* 13:2905-2927, 1999.

218. Miyawaki T, Ofengeim D, Noh KM, et al: The endogenous inhibitor of Akt, CTMP, is critical to ischemia-induced neuronal death, *Nat Neurosci* 12:618-626, 2009.

219. Hara MR, Snyder SH: Cell signaling and neuronal death, *Annu Rev Pharmacol Toxicol* 47:117-141, 2007.

220. Gadalla MM, Snyder SH: Hydrogen sulfide as a gasotransmitter, *J Neurochem* 113:14-26, 2010.

221. Nakamura T, Lipton SA: Preventing Ca^{2+}-mediated nitrosative stress in neurodegenerative diseases: possible pharmacological strategies, *Cell Calcium* 47:190-197, 2010.

222. Liu PK, Grossman RG, Hsu CY, et al: Ischemic injury and faulty gene transcripts in the brain, *Trends Neurosci* 24:581-588, 2001.

223. Pacher P, Beckman JS, Liaudet L: Nitric oxide and peroxynitrite in health and disease, *Physiol Rev* 87:315-424, 2007.

224. Niizuma K, Endo H, Chan PH: Oxidative stress and mitochondrial dysfunction as determinants of ischemic neuronal death and survival, *J Neurochem* 109(Suppl 1):133-138, 2009.

225. Bolanos JP, Heales SJ, Land JM, et al: Effect of peroxynitrite on the mitochondrial respiratory chain: differential susceptibility of neurons and astrocytes in primary culture, *J Neurochem* 64:1965-1972, 1995.

226. Zolotarjova N, Ho C, Mellgren RL, et al: Different sensitivities of native and oxidized forms of Na$^+$/K(+)-ATPase to intracellular proteinases, *Biochim Biophys Acta* 1192:125-131, 1994.

227. Adibhatla RM, Hatcher JF: Phospholipase A(2), reactive oxygen species, and lipid peroxidation in CNS pathologies, *BMB Rep* 41:560-567, 2008.

228. Baimbridge KG, Celio MR, Rogers JH: Calcium-binding proteins in the nervous system, *Trends Neurosci* 15:303-308, 1992.

229. Lonze BE, Riccio A, Cohen S, et al: Apoptosis, axonal growth defects, and degeneration of peripheral neurons in mice lacking CREB, *Neuron* 34:371-385, 2002.

230. Mayr B, Montminy M: Transcriptional regulation by the phosphorylation-dependent factor CREB, *Nat Rev Mol Cell Biol* 2:599-609, 2001.

231. Lonze BE, Ginty DD: Function and regulation of CREB family transcription factors in the nervous system, *Neuron* 35:605-623, 2002.

232. Weeber EJ, Levenson JM, Sweatt JD: Molecular genetics of human cognition, *Mol Interv* 2:376-391, 2002:339.

233. Mattson MP, Camandola S: NF-kappaB in neuronal plasticity and neurodegenerative disorders, *J Clin Invest* 107:247-254, 2001.

234. Schneider A, Martin-Villalba A, Weih F, et al: NF-kappaB is activated and promotes cell death in focal cerebral ischemia, *Nat Med* 5:554-559, 1999.

235. Brunet A, Datta SR, Greenberg ME: Transcription-dependent and -independent control of neuronal survival by the PI3K-Akt signaling pathway, *Curr Opin Neurobiol* 11:297-305, 2001.

236. van der Horst A, Burgering BM: Stressing the role of FoxO proteins in lifespan and disease, *Nat Rev Mol Cell Biol* 8:440-450, 2007.

237. Fukunaga K, Shioda N: Pathophysiological relevance of forkhead transcription factors in brain ischemia, *Adv Exp Med Biol* 665:130-142, 2009.

238. Hannenhalli S, Kaestner KH: The evolution of Fox genes and their role in development and disease, *Nat Rev Genet* 10:233-240, 2009.

239. Dziennis S, Jia T, Ronnekleiv OK, et al: Role of signal transducer and activator of transcription-3 in estradiol-mediated neuroprotection, *J Neurosci* 27:7268-7274, 2007.

240. Guo Z, Jiang H, Xu X, et al: Leptin-mediated cell survival signaling in hippocampal neurons mediated by JAK STAT3 and mitochondrial stabilization, *J Biol Chem* 283:1754-1763, 2008.

241. Jung JE, Kim GS, Narasimhan P, et al: Regulation of Mn-superoxide dismutase activity and neuroprotection by STAT3 in mice after cerebral ischemia, *J Neurosci* 29:7003-7014, 2009.

242. Aaronson DS, Horvath CM: A road map for those who don't know JAK-STAT, *Science* 296:1653-1655, 2002.

243. Shuai K, Liu B: Regulation of JAK-STAT signalling in the immune system, *Nat Rev Immunol* 3:900-911, 2003.

244. Hattori R, Maulik N, Otani H, et al: Role of STAT3 in ischemic preconditioning, *J Mol Cell Cardiol* 33:1929-1936, 2001.

245. Ballas N, Mandel G: The many faces of REST oversee epigenetic programming of neuronal genes, *Curr Opin Neurobiol* 15:500-506, 2005.

246. Ooi L, Wood IC: Chromatin crosstalk in development and disease: lessons from REST, *Nat Rev Genet* 8:544-554, 2007.

247. Zukin RS: Eradicating the mediators of neuronal death with a fine-tooth comb, *Sci Signal* 3:e20, 2010.

248. Bruce AW: Genome-wide analysis of repressor element 1 silencing transcription factor/neuron-restrictive silencing factor (REST/NRSF) target genes, *Proc Natl Acad Sci U S A* 101:10458-10463, 2004.

249. Conaco C, Otto S, Han JJ, et al: Reciprocal actions of REST and a microRNA promote neuronal identity, *Proc Natl Acad Sci U S A* 103:2422-2427, 2006.

250. Westbrook TF, Hu G, Ang XL, et al: SCFbeta-TRCP controls oncogenic transformation and neural differentiation through REST degradation, *Nature* 452:370-374, 2008.

251. Guardavaccaro D, Frescas D, Dorrello NV, et al: Control of chromosome stability by the beta-TrCP-REST-Mad2 axis, *Nature* 452:365-369, 2008.

252. Borrelli E, Nestler EJ, Allis CD, et al: Decoding the epigenetic language of neuronal plasticity, *Neuron* 60:961-974, 2008.

253. Formisano L, Noh KM, Miyawaki T, et al: Ischemic insults promote epigenetic reprogramming of mu opioid receptor expression in hippocampal neurons, *Proc Natl Acad Sci U S A* 104:4170-4175, 2007.

254. Palm K, Belluardo N, Metsis M, et al: Neuronal expression of zinc finger transcription factor REST/NRSF/XBR gene, *J Neurosci* 18:1280-1296, 1998.

255. Zuccato C, Tartari M, Crotti A, et al: Huntington interacts with REST/NRSF to modulate the transcription of NRSE-controlled neuronal genes, *Nat Genet* 35:76-83, 2003.

256. Kleinig TJ, Vink R: Suppression of inflammation in ischemic and hemorrhagic stroke: therapeutic options, *Curr Opin Neurol* 22:294-301, 2009.

257. Iadecola C, Alexander M: Cerebral ischemia and inflammation, *Curr Opin Neurol* 14:89-94, 2001.

7

Apoptosis and Related Mechanisms in Cerebral Ischemia

TURGAY DALKARA, MICHAEL A. MOSKOWITZ

Pathways of Ischemic Cell Death

Research since 1970 has identified several mechanisms that can irreversibly damage brain tissue after ischemia, such as intracellular calcium overload, acidity, excitotoxicity, oxygen free radicals, excess nitric oxide (NO) and peroxynitrite formation, and protein aggregation.[1-3] It is now generally accepted that although some severely injured cells die exclusively by swelling and necrosis, other cells may activate apoptotic mechanisms and die through a combination of apoptosis and possibly regulated or secondary necrotic mechanisms.[4-8] The necrotic phenotype becomes more prevalent as the intensity and duration of ischemia increase (i.e., permanent focal ischemia and brief, transient focal ischemia form the two extremes of necrotic and apoptotic phenotypes, respectively). Recent studies also implicate autophagy as a cell death mechanism in ischemic neurons.[9,10] However, whether autophagy is an important cell death pathway in brain ischemia or simply a reaction to increased cellular catabolism is not well understood. Interestingly, autophagic activity may be cytoprotective in some disease models (e.g., polyglutamine expansions or in aging models), whereas in other disease states such as in neonatal hypoxic-ischemic models, autophagy reportedly promotes cell death.[11,12] Cell death phenotype is strongly age dependent; for instance, neonatal brain exhibits relatively more intense apoptotic activity as well as autophagy in hypoxic-ischemic models, and inhibition of apoptotic mechanisms or autophagy provides substantial neuroprotection.[13-15] Although several discrepancies remain to be resolved in cell death nomenclature, most agree that cell death pathways provide an important target for drug discovery in cerebral ischemia.[1]

Evidence now suggests, however, that apoptotic, autophagic, and necrotic cell death mechanisms are not entirely independent.[16-21] Early phases of cell death may involve common pathways; when energy levels are severely compromised, cells dying by apoptosis may divert to dying instead by necrosis. In fact, secondary necrosis is reportedly especially prevalent after transient focal ischemia.[4] Similarly, when cells dying by necrosis are incompletely treated, they may die by other cell death types including apoptosis. Substantial evidence indicates that programmed cell death (PCD) has more than one apoptotic phenotype as well as necrotic-like phenotypes, including the recently described necroptosis.[21,22] Both mitochondria and the death receptor have been implicated as major regulatory players in cell death cascades.[21-23] Mitochondria can trigger apoptotic and necrotic pathways, depending on the severity of insult.[24] After moderate but irreversible injury, mitochondria retain their membrane potential (at least partially) so they can continue synthesizing adenosine triphosphate (ATP), but they may release cytochrome c and other proapoptotic factors to initiate apoptosis. Severe injury leads to opening of the permeability transition pore, loss of mitochondrial membrane potential, and eventually swelling and rupture of the inner and outer mitochondrial membranes, collapse of oxidative phosphorylation, and, hence, necrosis. Opening of the mitochondrial permeability transition pore (MPT) triggers necrotic cell death through the loss of homeostasis and intramitochondrial milieu, whereas the role of MPT opening in inducing apoptosis by releasing mitochondrial macromolecules into cytoplasm is probably less important.[24-26] Activation of death receptors, on the other hand, can promote cell survival or induce apoptotic or necrotic cell death, depending on the coexisting signals.[27] For example, available levels of the Fas inhibitor protein FLIP in proximity to death receptors serve as a switch between cell proliferation and death.[28] Similarly, collapse of energy levels may divert the death receptor–mediated apoptosis to necroptosis.[21] Recently, receptor interacting protein 3 (RIP3), an energy metabolism regulator kinase, has been identified as being capable of switching the tumor necrosis factor (TNF)–induced cell death from apoptosis to necrosis.[29]

A considerable body of knowledge has now accumulated that establishes a role for oxidative/nitrative stress, calcium overload, NO and peroxynitrite, protein aggregation, cellular swelling, and inflammatory mediators in triggering apoptotic as well as necrotic pathways of cell death. In this chapter, we focus on the role of apoptosis and related mechanisms in ischemic cell demise within the brain. It should be noted that most of the literature reviewed in this chapter has focused on ischemic neuronal death. Nonneuronal brain cells may exhibit different combinations of cell death mechanisms after ischemia, and these pathways have not been as elaborately characterized in vivo as they have for neurons.[30]

Molecular Mechanisms of Apoptosis

Apoptosis, a form of PCD, is biochemically and morphologically distinct from necrotic cell death.[31-33] Apoptosis requires expression of a set of genes and proteins and is characterized by internucleosomal cleavage of DNA, margination and condensation of chromatin in the nucleus, shrinkage of cytoplasm, and preservation of membrane integrity and mitochondrial ultrastructure. Eventually, the cell disintegrates and forms apoptotic bodies, which are phagocytosed by neighboring cells, resident macrophages, and microglia without an overt inflammatory reaction. In contrast, necrotic cells die through swelling, rupture, loss of membrane integrity, leakage and active secretion of inflammatory molecules including cytokines to extracellular medium, and inflammation; DNA strands are randomly broken rather than precisely cleaved at internucleosomal linker points. The unregulated (accidental) form of *necrosis* (e.g., as seen after acute severe injury induced by heat, acidity, or crushing) is considered to be most probably a passive process, whereas necrotic death seen during physiologic or disease processes involves activation of constitutively expressed proteolytic enzymes such as calpains and cathepsins and a series of controlled events such as mitochondrial permeability transition, excessive generation of reactive oxygen species, ATP depletion, and early plasma and lysosomal membrane rupture, although damaged cells initially express some survival genes and proteins in an attempt to interrupt cell death.[20,22,34] Activation of lytic enzymes (e.g., cathepsins) disrupts plasmalemma integrity and promotes cell swelling and osmotic rupture. As already noted, necrotic mechanisms can be triggered by stimulation of specific membrane receptors (e.g., TNF-α) and downstream signal transduction cascades involving RIP1.[21] In addition to these primary necrotic events (also known as programmed necrosis or necroptosis), necrosis may follow apoptosis (secondary necrosis) on collapse of energy metabolism or when mechanisms for removal of apoptotic cell fragments become saturated.[8] ATP is required for apoptotic processes such as cell shrinkage, bleb formation, caspase activation, chromatin condensation, internucleosomal DNA fragmentation, nuclear fragmentation, exposure of engulfment signals, and apoptotic body formation. Cleavage of the Na^+Ca^{2+} exchanger, IP3 receptors, and the plasma membrane Ca^{2+} ATPases by caspase-3 may also aggravate cytoplasmic Ca^{2+} overload and lead to activation of calpains and lysosome rupture, all of which participate in plasma membrane damage and secondary necrosis.[8,35]

In addition to apoptotic (type I) and necrotic (type III) programmed cell death types as initially described based on morphology,[36] there is also an autophagic (type II) cell death characterized by a massive accumulation of two-membrane autophagic vacuoles in the cytoplasm and an increase in Beclin 1 together with associated changes in LC3-II. *Autophagy* is an energy-dependent process used by eukaryotes to degrade and recycle subcellular organelles; the process plays an important role in cellular catabolism but can also modify apoptotic and necrotic cell death pathways during cell stress.[11,21] The interaction is complex. For example, in some conditions such as metabolic stress, autophagy can postpone apoptotic cell death, whereas inactivation of autophagic survival mechanisms promotes necrotic cell death in vitro in cells with suppressed or defective apoptosis.[37] Nevertheless, two recent reports did find that genetic knockdown of *atg7*, a gene essential for induction of autophagy, or pharmacologic blockade with 3-methyl adenine, an autophagic inhibitor, decreases infarct size and the delayed neuronal appearance of autophagic and lysosomal activity markers (e.g., LC3II), particularly within the peri-infarct zone in neonatal models.[12,38]

Apoptosis is the main form of cell death during development.[31,39] A great number of cells are eliminated during fetal life in this way. Involution of tissues like the thymus and pineal gland in adults also occurs via apoptosis, as does the death of rapidly dividing cell populations such as intestinal villi.[26,40] For proliferative tissues to maintain a constant size, older cells die by apoptosis. Similarly, cells die by apoptosis during regression of hyperplastic tissues, such as after liver hyperplasia induced by various chemicals. There is substantial evidence to implicate apoptosis in neurodegenerative processes (e.g. Alzheimer's, Huntington's, and Parkinson's diseases; spinal muscular atrophy; amyotrophic lateral sclerosis),[41,42] although the extent of apoptosis in these pathologic processes is still a matter of considerable controversy. One factor contributing to the controversy is that apoptotic cell demise is difficult to detect in autopsy specimens because it possibly occurs rapidly over several hours. Given the longevity of neurons, cellular injury might build up over time to reach a threshold above which executioner programs are activated and promote the accelerated death of cells.[22]

Apoptosis may be triggered by developmental and environmental cues and is regulated by a complex balance between life- and death-promoting factors.[42] In the nematode *Caenorhabditis elegans*, the organism that has become a prototype for understanding apoptosis in mammalians and in which PCD has been extensively studied, apoptosis is regulated by a balance between the *ced-3* (cell *d*eath-3) and *ced-9* genes. The *ced-3* gene is indispensable for activating a cell death cascade, whereas the *ced-9* gene blocks PCD.[43,44] Another gene, *ced-4*, is also required for *ced-3* to execute cell death. *Caspases* are a family of Ced-3 homologues in mammalian cells that dismantle a group of proteins essential for cell survival.[45] The mammalian counterpart of the antiapoptotic *ced-9* gene is the *bcl-2* gene family, which has antiapoptotic as well as proapoptotic members.[46] In mammalian cells, each gene family is diversified, and several other pathways also trigger cell death. For example, death signals can be transduced from the extracellular medium into the cell via cell surface death receptors. Death-signaling cascades may also be initiated intracellularly from mitochondria, damaged DNA, or endoplasmic reticulum (ER). In mammalian cells, antiapoptotic Bcl-2 family members protect mitochondrial membrane integrity. In the presence of apoptotic signaling, sequestered apoptogenic proteins are released through membrane pores or breaches between the inner and outer mitochondrial membranes.[23]

Mitochondrial Pathway

The interactions between the proapoptotic and anti-apoptotic Bcl-2 family proteins on the outer mitochondrial membrane are believed to play an important role in making the life-or-death "decision."[24,26] Normally, anti-apoptotic members such as Bcl-2, Bcl-xL, Bcl-w, Mcl-1, and A1 are located on membranes of mitochondria, ER, and nucleus, and they protect mitochondria against several forms of injury, presumably by preventing release of apoptogenic mediators and, in some cases, opening of the permeability transition pore.[23,47] Members of the proapoptotic Bax group (Bax, Bak, and Bok) are structurally similar to Bcl-2 and contain 3 'BH' (Bcl-2 homology) domains, whereas the proapoptotic BH3-only proteins (Bim, Bad, Bid, Bik, Bmf, Puma, Noxa, and Hrk) have only the BH3 domain. The BH1, BH2, and BH3 domains form a hydrophobic cleft that serves as a heterodimerization interface for the BH3 domain of the other family members. The BH4 domain of antiapoptotic Bcl-2 family members inhibits apoptotic changes by interacting with a voltage-dependent anion channel on the mitochondrial membrane.[21,48] The BH3-only proteins can engage with antiapoptotic members by inserting the BH3 domain into the hydrophobic groove on their surface. This primes Bax and Bak oligomerization, which results in membrane permeabilization.[48] Bim, Puma, and tBid engage with all antiapoptotic Bcl-2 family members, whereas the remaining BH3-only proteins bind selectively only to subsets of the Bcl-2 family antiapoptotic proteins.

Proapoptotic Bcl-2 family members such as Bax, Bad, and Bid are normally situated in the cytoplasm and translocate to mitochondria on receiving death signals. Several mechanisms, such as dephosphorylation of Bad that is sequestered in the cytoplasm by the 14-3-3 protein and cleavage of Bid, may promote this translocation.[49,50] Activation of c-Jun N-terminal kinase (JNK) phosphorylates c-JUN, which in turn activates Bax via expression of DP5/Hrk, a Bcl-2 family protein.[42] p53 transcriptionally activates the proapoptotic Bcl-2 family members Puma and Noxa.[51] Caspases may also convert the antiapoptotic members to proapoptotic ones by cleaving their BH4 domain. The release of proapoptotic and antiapoptotic proteins from mitochondria is controlled by formation of pores on the outer mitochondrial membrane by homodimers and heterodimers of Bcl-2 family members. The released proteins include cytochrome c, apoptosis-inducing factor (AIF), endonuclease G (EndoG), and Smac/DIABLO.[23] Cytochrome c, deoxyadenosine triphosphate (dATP), and Apaf-1, the mammalian homologue of Ced-4, form the apoptosome complex and catalyze conversion of procaspase-9 to its active form (Fig. 7-1).[23,52] Activated caspase-9 in turn cleaves and activates procaspase-3. Neurons can survive release of cytochrome c if apoptosis inhibitor proteins (IAP, NAIP, XIAP, survivin),[53] which suppress the caspase system, are not inactivated by the mitochondrial protein Smac/DIABLO that is co-released with cytochrome.[23] AIF and EndoG translocate to the nucleus to degrade DNA.

How AIF initiates DNA fragmentation remains unclear, although recruited proteases and nucleases are speculated to cause the chromatin changes upon AIF–DNA binding.[23,54,55] AIF causes a lumpy and peripheral type of chromatin condensation and the formation of large DNA fragments that are independent of caspase activation; hence, AIF-induced PCD is called *caspase-independent apoptosis.* Strong chromatin compaction characteristic of caspase activity is not seen after AIF-induced apoptosis.[23,56] Deficiency of AIF has profound effects during animal development; in its absence, the apoptosis necessary for the cavitation of embryoid bodies, which is essential for mouse morphogenesis, does not occur.[57] Unlike caspase homologues, AIF homologues are found in all metazoan kingdoms (i.e., animal, plant, and fungi), which suggests that AIF could be one of the phylogenetically oldest death effectors known.[56] Yu and colleagues[57] reported that activation of the DNA repair enzyme poly(ADP-ribose) polymerase-1 (PARP-1) after damage to DNA triggers release of AIF and, hence, promotes PCD through a caspase-independent pathway (see also the study by Cipriani et al[58]).

Death Receptor–Mediated Pathway

Cell surface receptors mediate apoptosis in a diverse set of disease states ranging from autoimmunity and acquired immunodeficiency syndrome (AIDS) to cancer.[22,28,59] These receptors, which belong to the tumor necrosis factor receptor (TNFR) superfamily, include TNFR-1, Fas (CD95/Apo-1), and p75NTR. Death receptors share an evolutionarily conserved homologous amino acid sequence called the *death domain,* through which they bind to death domain–containing adapter molecules such as FADD (Fas-associated death domain protein) and TRADD (TNFR-associated death domain protein). Adapter proteins also contain another sequence called the *death-effector domain,* which binds to procaspase-8 by interacting with its death-effector domain.[60] On activation, Fas forms a death-inducing signaling complex (DISC) with FADD and procaspase-8 (see Fig. 7-1).[61,62] Binding of Fas ligand or TNF-α to their receptors leads to their oligomerization, which recruits and binds procaspase-8 and promotes its autoactivation. Active caspase-8 is released from the DISC and initiates downstream cleavage of caspase-3 by direct or mitochondrial-dependent mechanisms.[63] Bid, a cytosolic member of the Bcl-2 family of proapoptotic proteins, is cleaved by caspase-8 (see Fig. 7-1).[49,64] The truncated active form of Bid targets the outer mitochondrial membrane and induces release of cytochrome c by promoting pore formation via conformational changes in Bak and Bad within mitochondrial membranes.[65,66] In addition, activated caspase-3 may cleave procaspase-8, thereby amplifying the death process.[67]

Death receptors can also participate in necrosis.[21,22] That TNF-induced death can initiate either apoptosis or necrosis is well documented, and Fas receptor has also been shown to induce necrosis-like PCD.[22,68-70] As already noted, the Fas inhibitor protein FLIP serves as a switch between cell proliferation and death signaling: when FLIP levels are low, caspase-8 is recruited to the DISC on activation of Fas receptors.[28] In contrast, when FLIP levels are high, FLIP may outcompete procaspase-8 by preferentially binding to FADD and, hence, may divert signals toward cell proliferation via the ERK and nuclear factor (NF)-κB pathways. Activation of TNF-α in the presence of

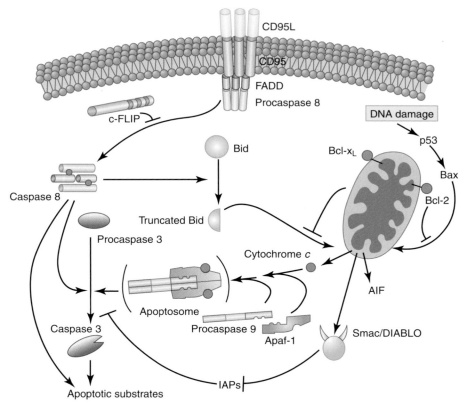

Figure 7-1 The mitochondrial pathway *(right)* is initiated through the activation of proapoptotic members of the Bcl-2 family, such as Bax, Bad, Bim, and Bid. On receiving proapoptotic signals, proapoptotic members translocate to the mitochondria from cytosol, where they interact with antiapoptotic members like Bcl-2 and Bcl-xL. This interaction leads to release of proteins such as cytochrome *c*, apoptosis-inhibiting factor (AIF), and Smac/DIABLO from the mitochondria. Cytochrome *c* associates with Apaf-1 and then procaspase 9 to form the apoptosome complex and activate caspase 9. Caspase 9, in turn, cleaves and activates procaspase 3. Caspase 3 activation and activity are antagonized by the inhibitors of apoptosis (IAPs), which themselves are inhibited by the Smac/DIABLO protein released from mitochondria. Active caspase-3 performs the ordered dismantling and removal of the cell.

The death receptor pathway is triggered by members of the death receptor superfamily, such as CD95/Fas. Binding of CD95/Fas ligand induces receptor clustering and formation of a death-inducing signaling complex (DISC). This complex recruits multiple procaspase 8 molecules via the adapter molecule FADD, resulting in caspase 8 activation. Caspase 8, in turn, cleaves and activates procaspase 3. Caspase 8 activation can be blocked by recruitment of the c-FLIP protein to the DISC.

Cross-talk between the death receptor and mitochondrial pathways is provided by Bid, a proapoptotic Bcl-2 family member. Caspase 8-mediated cleavage of Bid results in its translocation to mitochondria and release of cytochrome *c*. (Redrawn from Hengartner MO: The biochemistry of apoptosis. *Nature* 407:770-776, 2000.)

caspase inhibition (z-VAD-FMK) or low ATP levels causes a recently described form of α-necrotic PCD: necroptosis that utilizes the reciprocal kinase activity of the adapter molecules RIP1 and RIP3 to induce a regulated necrosis (Fig. 7-2).[21,27] RIP3 was recently proposed as an energy metabolism regulator capable of stimulating enzymes such as the glycogen degrading enzyme, glycogen phosphorylase, to steer TNF-induced apoptosis toward necrosis, in part through bursting energy metabolism and oxygen radical generation.[29]

Nuclear Pathway

DNA damage, if irreparable, may activate the apoptotic suicide program, especially in cells with high replicative capacity. Kinases such as ATM, DNA-PKcs, and ATR monitor and detect DNA damage.[71,72] On activation, ATM phosphorylates several cell cycle checkpoint proteins, including p53, to promote cell death.[73] In response to

DNA damage, p53 stops the cell cycle in dividing cells. If the DNA damage is irreparable, p53 triggers apoptosis in part by promoting Bax expression. The short half-life of p53 is prolonged upon ATM-induced phosphorylation. Phosphorylated p53 cannot bind to Mdm2, a major inhibitor of p53 that binds to it and targets it for ubiquitin-mediated degradation.[74] Stabilized p53 upregulates expression of several modulators of the cell cycle (e.g., p21, GADD45, 14-3-3 proteins) as well as proapoptotic proteins such as Bax, Puma, Noxa, Apaf-1, and death receptors; however, it represses expression of the *bcl-2* gene.[75]

DNA damage also leads to activation of the nuclear DNA repair enzyme PARP-1. PARP is a caspase substrate; however, studies on PARP knockout mice suggest that its cleavage is not essential for apoptosis.[76] Rapid activation of the enzyme in cells under stress depletes the cell of nicotinamide adenine dinucleotide (NAD) and ATP, which may result in cell death favoring a necrotic phenotype because of collapse of energy metabolism.[77]

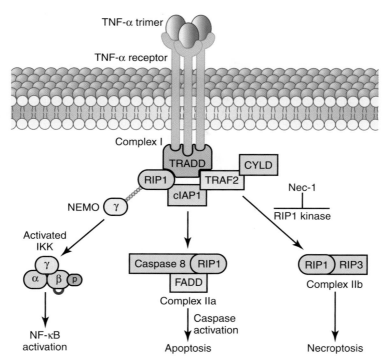

Figure 7-2 Stimulation of TNF-α may lead to NF-κB activation, apoptosis, or necroptosis. Stimulation of TNFR1 by TNF-α leads to the formation of an intracellular complex at the cytoplasmic membrane (complex I) that includes TRADD, TRAF2, RIP1, and cIAP1. Ubiquitination of RIP1 by cIAP1 leads to the recruitment of NEMO, a regulatory subunit of IKK complex that in turn activates NF-κB pathway. RIP1 is also involved in the formation of complex IIa including FADD and caspase 8 to activate a caspase cascade to mediate apoptosis. Under apoptosis-deficient conditions or when cells are infected by certain viruses, RIP1 interacts with RIP3 to form complex IIb, which is involved in mediating necroptosis. The formation of complex IIb requires the kinase activity of RIP1 that is inhibited by necrostatin-1 (Nec-1). (Redrawn from Christofferson DE, Yuan J: Necroptosis as an alternative form of programmed cell death. *Curr Opin Cell Biol* 22:263-268, 2010.)

Other evidence suggests, however, that PARP might also control the fate of cell death by regulating transcription factors such as NF-κB and p53 and by promoting release of mitochondrial AIF.[57,78,79] PARP signaling to mitochondria was reported to require RIP1, TNFR-associated factor 2 (TRAF2), and JNK1 pathway[80]; however, the relationship of these steps to necroptosis remains unclear.

Endoplasmic Reticulum Pathway

The ER is an essential organelle for protein synthesis and the site for calcium storage and release. Defective ER functioning—such as during cell stresses that include hypoxia-ischemia, disrupted calcium imbalance, and inhibition of protein glycosylation, among others—can cause the accumulation of unfolded or misfolded proteins within the ER lumen, which will initiate the unfolded protein response. This response includes both shutdown of translation at the initiation step of protein synthesis so that further accumulation of unfolded proteins is prevented and upregulation of genes required to restore normal ER functioning. Transient ischemia is a particularly effective stimulus for the ER stress response, and phosphorylation of eIF2 alpha, a key step at the initiation level, has been implicated in protein synthesis shutdown. One consequence of accumulated unfolded ER proteins is the formation of protein aggregates, which disrupts proteasomal function and, in turn, causes further ER stress. Cell death may result from the inability to restore protein synthesis, perhaps by activation of apoptotic pathways.[81]

A novel apoptotic pathway that is initiated within the ER was recently discovered.[82] Accumulation of misfolded proteins and altered calcium homeostasis in the ER leads to transcriptional upregulation of caspase-12, which is suggested to be the initiator caspase of this pathway.[82-84] Although this can activate downstream executioner caspases, the events that connect ER stress to caspase activation are not well known, and studies with caspase-12 knockout mice showed no noticeable developmental or behavioral defects, which indicates that this caspase is not essential for normal development or cell population homeostasis in the adult.[82] The role of the ER in calcium sequestration and as a source of released calcium suggests an important function for this organelle in cell death mechanisms that deserves additional investigation.

Cell Survival Pathways

Cell death and cell survival pathways converge and interact at several points. For example, overexpression of Bcl-2 not only inhibits apoptosis but also supports cell survival in response to a wide variety of insults as well as necrotic death.[85,86] Like all cells, neurons require trophic support for survival. Neuronal survival pathways are generally induced by the binding of neurotrophins (NTs) to tyrosine kinase receptors, which in turn activate phosphoinositide

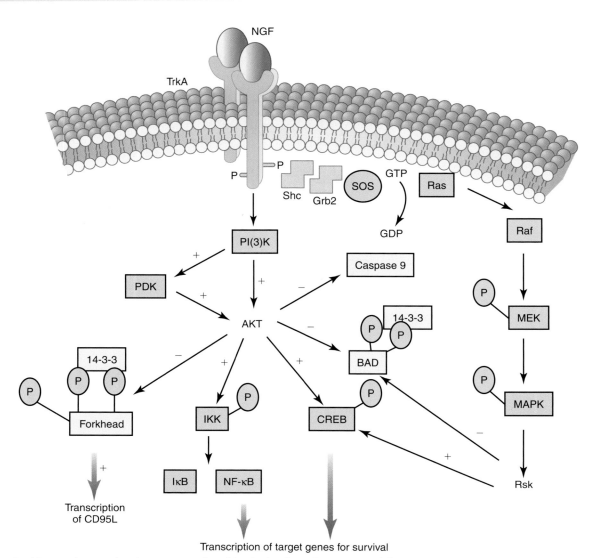

Figure 7-3 Neuronal survival pathways are induced by the binding of nerve growth factor (NGF) to its receptor TrkA (tyrosine kinase A). NGF induces the autophosphorylation of TrkA, which activates phosphoinositide 3-kinase [PI(3)K] and the adapter protein Shc. Activated PI(3)K phosphorylates Akt and phosphoinositide-dependent kinase (PDK), which in turn phosphorylates and activates Akt (protein kinase B). The phosphorylation of CREB and inhibitor of NF-κB kinase (IKK) stimulates the transcription of prosurvival factors, whereas the phosphorylation of Bad, forkhead transcription factor, and caspase 9 inhibits the proapoptotic pathway. The interaction of Shc-Grb2 and SOS activates the mitogen-activated protein kinase (MAPK) pathway, resulting in the activation of Rsk. Proteins Bad and CREB are also the targets of Rsk that might act synergistically with Akt. (Redrawn from Yuan J, Yankner B: Apoptosis in the nervous system. *Nature* 407:802-809, 2000.)

3-kinase (PI3K) and the mitogen-activated protein kinase (MAPK) pathway (Fig. 7-3).[42,87] Activated PI3K phosphorylates Akt (protein kinase B), which suppresses expression of proapoptotic genes such as Fas ligand by activating forkhead transcription factors. Akt phosphorylates and inactivates the proapoptotic factors Bad and procaspase 9.[88,89] Phosphorylation of transcription factor CREB and IκB kinase (IκB is the inhibitor of transcription factor NF-κB) stimulates the transcription of prosurvival factors such as Bcl-2. Triggering of the MAPK pathway by tyrosine kinase receptors leads to the activation of the pp90 ribosomal S6 kinase pathway (Rsk), which phosphorylates Bad and CREB and, hence, acts synergistically with Akt. For example, basic fibroblast growth factor (bFGF) hinders the release of the proapoptotic Bcl-2 family member Bad that is sequestered by cytoplasmic 14-3-3

protein.[89] In addition, bFGF prevents translocation of Bad to mitochondria via the neurotrophin receptor–PI3K–Akt pathway and the MAPK pathway. Basic FGF has also been shown to stimulate de novo synthesis of Bcl-xL through activation of MAPK by phosphorylation of CREB.[90,91]

The PI3K–Akt pathway can also promote cell survival by decreasing transcription of Fas receptor and activating the transcription factor.[87] On stimulation, NF-κB dissociates from IκB and translocates to the nucleus, where it activates antiapoptotic or proapoptotic genes, depending on the circumstances in which it is activated.[92] However, NTs may protect cells against death via more than a single mechanism. For instance, bFGF may decrease *N*-methyl-D-aspartate (NMDA) receptor–mediated influx and excitotoxicity of Ca^{2+} and may upregulate the expression of free radical scavenging enzymes.[93,94] The stimulus for necrosis is thus diminished, as is the development of apoptosis for those cells less severely affected.

Cell survival can also be affected by certain members of heat shock proteins (HSPs) by inhibiting cell death mechanisms at several critical steps. For example, HSP70 interacts with Apaf1 and may hinder apoptosome formation and subsequent caspase-9 activation.[95] HSP70 can antagonize AIF[96] and prevent Bax activation and AIF release. HSP70 has also been proposed to inhibit JNK activity and dephosphorylation.[34,97]

Apoptosis in Cerebral Ischemia

Linnik et al[98] provided early pharmacologic evidence for involvement of PCD in cerebral ischemia based on the ability of the protein synthesis inhibitor cycloheximide to reduce brain injury. Cellular features of apoptosis have been documented after focal and global ischemia, including cytoplasmic shrinkage, chromatin condensation, nuclear segmentation, and apoptotic bodies.[99-102] However, electron microscopic studies consistently indicate that ischemic neuronal death is characterized by a mixture of apoptotic and necrotic changes in ultrastructure.[103-106] Ischemic neuronal death has also been shown to exhibit combined biochemical and light microscopic features of apoptotic and necrotic pathways within the same cell and has been proposed to be mainly a necro-apoptotic form of cell death.[4] Recently, Degterev et al[5] emphasized that ischemic neuronal cell death displays characteristics of apoptotic, necrotic, and type II autophagic cell death and contains a substantial necrotic component involving activation of death receptors. Necroptosis is uniquely suppressed by necrostatin-1, a potent inhibitor of RIP1, identified by high throughput drug screening; it decreases ischemic cell injury in models of ischemia-reperfusion and improves neurologic outcomes (see Fig. 7-2).[21] Nevertheless, a substantial reduction in infarct volume after treatment by caspase inhibitors and in genetically engineered mice with caspase deletions indicates that the apoptotic cascade is significantly activated in injured surviving cells.[107,108] Recently, inhibition of the Apaf-1 signaling pathway, which transmits cell death signals after mitochondrial damage to effector caspases, has been shown to provide neuroprotection against neonatal hypoxic-ischemic brain injury.[14] Some biochemical markers conventionally thought to indicate necrosis (e.g., cathepsins and calpain) are also activated in ischemic cells, and inhibition of these enzymes confers resistance to ischemic injury, suggesting a complex interplay between apoptotic and necrotic death pathways in cerebral ischemia.[109,110,110a] Necrostatin-1 and the caspase inhibitor z-VAD-FMK synergistically reduce infarct size, which indicates that the simultaneous inhibition of several cell death pathways could provide optimal neuroprotection.[21,110a]

DNA laddering, a biochemical hallmark of apoptotic cell death, appears on gel electrophoresis of brain homogenate along with terminal deoxynucleotidyl transferase-mediated deoxyuridine triphosphate (dUTP)-biotin nick-end labeling (TUNEL) staining.[98,101,111-116] Several markers of DNA damage-induced apoptosis (i.e., upregulation of p53, growth arrest and DNA damage protein 45 [GADD45], and Mdm2) have also been detected in

ischemic brains.[117] PARP is activated, and NAD+ levels become depleted in ischemic brain within minutes of reperfusion after occlusion of the middle cerebral artery (MCA). Inhibition of PARP activation or disruption of the *parp* gene confers protection after brain ischemia.[118,119] Ischemic neurons attempt to reenter the cell cycle after the loss of control over mitotic machinery in these terminally differentiated cells.[120] Upregulation of Bax, downregulation of Bcl-2/Bcl-xL levels, and formation of Bax/Bcl-xL dimers have also been demonstrated in early hours of ischemia, which are findings that may account for the activation of the mitochondrial pathway.[99,121-123] Events that occur downstream of the formation of Bax/Bcl-xL dimers, such as release of cytochrome *c* from mitochondria and activation of caspase-9 and caspase-3, have also been detected.[124-127]

Caspase Activation during Focal and Global Ischemia

With few exceptions, apoptosis in mammalian cells depends on the activation of caspases.[22,26,42,128] As alluded to previously, activation of caspases can be mediated through several pathways encompassing death receptors, mitochondria, DNA, or ER. In all apoptotic pathways, a group of caspases called *executioner caspases* appear to dismantle several cellular structures by their proteolytic activity once they are activated. Most of the 14 caspases discovered are constitutively expressed as proenzymes (zymogens) in humans.[26,128] Caspases 1 through 3 and 7 through 9 have been detected in the brain. Caspase-1 (interleukin-converting enzyme [ICE]) family members—caspases 1, 4, and 5—are proinflammatory and proapoptotic. However, caspase-3 (CPP32) family members—caspases 2, 3, and 6 through 9—mediate apoptosis only. Caspases with death-effector domains (8 and 10) are activated after being recruited to death receptor complexes. Caspases with short prodomains (3, 6, and 7) are cleaved and activated by other caspases. The prodomains of activator and inflammatory caspases contain protein–protein interaction domains such as the caspase-recruitment domain (CARD; e.g., caspase-9) or the death-effector domain (DED; e.g., caspase-8) and are activated after binding to a molecular complex such as apoptosome or DISC.[21]

Caspase activity requires heterodimerization of the large and small cleavage products. Caspases have a catalytic site that contains a highly conserved amino acid sequence (QACXG) and cleave proteins at one or more sites but always after an aspartate residue.[128] They have a wide range of substrates, cleavage of which produces morphologic features characteristic of apoptosis. For example, caspase-mediated disintegration of the nuclear lamins may account for nuclear pyknosis and budding, whereas cleavage of cytoskeletal proteins like gelsolin, actin, and fodrin may cause cell shrinkage and cleavage of the kinase PAK2 may mediate blebbing.[26] Caspase-3 cleaves the inhibitory subunit of the caspase-activated DNase (CAD) by translocating to the nucleus from cytoplasm.[129] CAD cleaves DNA at internucleosomal linker points, yielding multiple integers of 180 base-pair fragments that form the DNA ladder seen on DNA gel electrophoresis.

A considerable body of evidence suggests that caspase-1 and caspase-3 are processed after focal cerebral ischemia.[108,130-132] Hara et al[130] found immunoreactive caspase-1 cleavage products (p20 and p10 bands) on Western blot analyses in a 2-hour reversible filament occlusion model of focal ischemic injury. They also reported that interleukin-1β (IL-1β) levels peaked in the brain 30 minutes to 1 hour after reperfusion and then decreased; this finding suggests that ICE (caspase-1) is transiently activated on reperfusion. In line with these findings, mutant mice that are deficient in *ice* gene expression or that express a dominant negative ICE mutation are more resistant to ischemia.[130,133] However, because IL-1β is proinflammatory, it was difficult to establish whether ICE inhibition of inflammation or apoptosis, or both, were protective in these experiments.

The role of caspase-3 has been more convincingly characterized in focal ischemic brain damage. Asahi et al[134] demonstrated upregulation of rat caspase-3 messenger RNA (mRNA) 1 hour after the induction of permanent ischemia. Namura et al[126] provided evidence for caspase-3 activation in the mouse brain subjected to 2-hour MCA occlusion. They detected caspase-3 and its cleavage products (p20) in ischemic brain tissue soon after reperfusion. Caspase-like enzyme activity was also elevated for the first 3 hours of reperfusion. Cleavage of gelsolin, a substrate of caspase-like proteases, was detected by 6 hours of reperfusion, along with DNA laddering and a positive response to TUNEL staining.[135] The p20 cleavage product (active caspase-3) was frequently visualized within TUNEL-positive cells, which is a finding that may account for CAD activation and DNA fragmentation. Cleavage of several other substrates of caspase activity (e.g., actin and PARP) has also been detected in brains after ischemia.[119,122,136] Hence, ischemia is accompanied by a time-dependent evolution of the mitochondrial apoptotic pathway, characterized by changes in Bcl-2 family proteins, cytochrome *c* release, caspase-like enzyme activation, and an associated increase in the cleaved active form (caspase-3 p20), which are followed several hours later by morphologic features of apoptosis and DNA fragmentation. The pace of caspase activation depends on the duration and severity of the insult. After brief periods of focal ischemia, caspase activation develops as late as 9 hours after reperfusion along with the appearance of the caspase-3–p20 immunoreactive cleavage product.[136]

Detection of the caspase-8 cleavage product in neurons suggests that death receptors are also activated on ischemic injury.[127,137] In line with these findings, inhibition of TNF and Fas directly blocks stroke-related damage in addition to reducing secondary inflammatory injury.[138] Mice expressing dysfunctional Fas (CD95) ligand and TNF knockout mice demonstrate smaller infarcts after MCA occlusion.[139,140] Strikingly, hybrid mice lacking both cytokines showed a 93% reduction in infarct volume. A similar protection was observed in wild-type mice treated with antibodies that neutralize Fas ligand and TNF.[138] These remarkable findings underscore the role of death receptors in ischemic cell death.[141]

Death receptors may be activated by cytokines released from granulocytes infiltrating the infarct or by microglia that are activated within the first hours of ischemia.[142]

The resistance of Bid knockout mice to ischemia suggests that there is cross-talk between the death receptor–induced and mitochondrial pathways during ischemic cell death.[143] Bid, after being cleaved by caspase-8, translocates to the outer mitochondrial membrane and induces conformational changes in Bak and Bax; by so doing, it initiates cytochrome *c* release and caspase-3–mediated apoptosis.[49,64,144] Caspase-11 is upregulated and cleaved 12 hours after permanent ischemia.[145] A murine caspase not found in humans, caspase-11, appears uniquely able to bind and cleave caspase-1 as well as caspase-3, hence promoting both cytokine maturation and apoptosis.[146] Studies using a positional scanning combinatorial library method found that the optimal cleavage site of caspase-11 is (Ile/Leu/Val/Pro)EHD, similar to that of upstream caspases such as caspase-8 and caspase-9.[146] Caspase-11 knockout mice showed reduced caspase-3 cleavage within the ischemic cortex.[146] Activation of caspase-12 secondary to ER stress and its colocalization with DNA fragmentation has also been demonstrated after transient MCA occlusion.[147] Contrary to activation of caspases 1, 3, 7, 8, and 9 with cerebral ischemia-reperfusion, caspase-2 protein levels remain unchanged after cerebral ischemia in the mouse. Also, mice deficient in caspase-2 are not protected from focal ischemic brain damage despite the finding that caspase-2 mRNA is upregulated after 8 hours of transient focal and transient global ischemia.[134,148,149] Most of the apoptotic changes described here have been observed in neurons but not in astrocytes in the adult brain, except an increased expression of caspase-12 in reactive astrocytes surrounding the ischemic area.[150] Although these observations led to the conclusion that astrocytes die by early swelling and necrosis even before neurons, recently it has convincingly been demonstrated that astrocytes are more resistant to ischemia than neurons and die by a delayed necrosis without activating apoptotic mechanisms.[30]

Similar changes have been reported in models of global ischemia. Caspase-3 is cleaved and activated, DNA laddering and a positive response to TUNEL staining appear, and cells are protected by caspase inhibition.[107,151,152] Bhat et al[153] found increases in caspase-1 mRNA and its corresponding protein within microglia of gerbil hippocampus several days after brief global ischemia. Other groups reported increased gene expression of caspases 2, 3, and 8 during the late stages of ischemia.[107,152,154-156] A change favoring Bax over Bcl-2 family proteins was convincingly documented in global ischemia.[99] Cytochrome *c* release was detected in hippocampal neurons after a global ischemic insult.[157-159] Caspase-9 activation and formation of apoptosome were also demonstrated.[125,160]

Apoptosis in Spinal Cord Ischemia

Cell death due to spinal cord ischemia is also mediated in part by apoptotic mechanisms. Matsushita et al[137] found that as early as 90 minutes after transient ischemia, activated caspase-8 (p18) appears within neurons in intermediate gray matter and in medial ventral horn. Cleaved caspase-8 appears before the activation of caspase-3, colocalized with Fas on motoneurons, possibly by formation of a DISC. The appearance of cytosolic cytochrome *c* and gelsolin cleavage along with numerous TUNEL-positive neurons containing cleaved forms of caspase-8 and caspase-3 was detected. These findings are consistent with the concept that transient spinal cord ischemia induces the formation of a DISC, which may participate in caspase-8 activation and sequential caspase-3 cleavage. DNA damage is significantly present from 1 to 6 hours after reperfusion in gray matter neurons of ischemic spinal cord. Caspase-3 is induced at 6 to 24 hours, and TUNEL reactivity peaked at 48 hours after reperfusion in spinal cord neurons.[161] Apoptosis signal-regulating kinase 1 (ASK1) and JNK pathways are activated in reperfused spinal cord and may play an important role in the apoptotic signaling mechanisms.[162]

Inhibition of Apoptotic Pathways Reduces Ischemic Damage

Overexpression of antiapoptotic proteins (e.g., Bcl-2) or knockout of genes that encode proapoptotic proteins (e.g., Bid, Bax, p53, caspase-3, and caspase-11) in transgenic animals confers resistance to ischemia,[85,146,163-165] which emphasizes the role of apoptotic mechanisms in ischemic cell death. Similarly, pharmacologic inhibition of caspase activity leads to a reduction in cell death in focal as well as global ischemia[107,108] and appears to be a promising therapeutic target. Loddick et al[132] and Hara et al[108] reported that z-VAD and z-DEVD, peptide inhibitors of caspases, protected brain tissue from ischemic injury and improved neurologic deficits in rats and mice. Peptide inhibitors given intraventricularly afforded protection against loss of cells in the CA1 subfield of the hippocampus during global ischemia, and treated animals displayed a better performance on memory tests.[107,166] Recently, it was demonstrated that z-DEVD could be effectively transported across the blood–brain barrier by nanospheres functionalized with antitransferrin antibody and that its systemic administration to mice afforded neuroprotection in a transient MCA model.[167,168]

Caspase inhibitors were effective if administered up to 1 hour after reperfusion following 2-hour MCA occlusion. After milder ischemia (30 minutes), z-DEVD-FMK protected the brain when injected up to 9 hours after restoration of blood flow.[136] The 9-hour treatment window corresponded to the onset of both DEVDase activation and caspase-3 cleavage, which suggests that activation of events downstream from caspase-3 may represent irreversible injury and that activation of execution caspases evolves slowly with delayed therapeutic opportunity in mild ischemia. In more severe ischemia (2 hours of occlusion), caspase inhibitors block cell death up to 2 hours after ischemia.[108,169] Although longer than for NMDA receptor antagonists, this time window is still shorter than desirable for clinical practice.

A synergy has been reported between an NMDA receptor antagonist and caspase inhibitors.[170] Not only did combination of subthreshold doses of the two agents protect against ischemia, but also the therapeutic window for caspase administration was extended. A similar synergy was also observed between a growth factor (bFGF) and caspase inhibitors.[171] The importance of interactions between survival factors and ischemic cell death is further exemplified by studies reporting that neurotrophin

4 (NT 4) and brain-derived neurotrophic factor (BDNF) exert a protective influence in cerebral ischemia because mice lacking one allele of BDNF or both alleles of NT 4 are more vulnerable to ischemic injury.[172] Exogenous administration of NT 4 or BDNF, both of which bind to the TrkB (tyrosine kinase B) receptor, is also found to be protective in models of cerebral ischemia.[173-176]

Apoptosis in Human Brain

Most apoptosis-related proteins are expressed in the normal human brain (Table 7-1), which suggests a potential role for these proteins in disease. It should be noted, however, that cell death phenotypes may significantly vary according to the species, age, cell type, triggering

TABLE 7-1 APOPTOSIS-RELATED PROTEINS DETECTED IN NORMAL HUMAN BRAIN

Protein	Study(ies) Reporting Detection
Bcl-2 family	
Bcl-2	Marshall et al (1997),[187] Su et al (1997),[188] Vyas et al (1997),[189] Yachnis et al (1997),[190] Desjardins and Ledoux, (1998),[191] Kitamura et al (1998),[192] Clark et al (1999),[193] Henshall et al (2000),[194] Jarskog and Gilmore (2000)[195]
Bcl-x	Yachnis et al (1997),[190] Kitamura et al (1998)[192]
Mcl-1	Desjardins and Ledoux (1998)[191]
Bax	Su et al (1997),[188] Desjardins and Ledoux (1998),[191] Kitamura et al (1998),[192] Tatton (2000),[196] Engidawork (2001),[197] Hartmann et al (2001)[198]
Bad	Kitamura et al (1998)[192]
Bak	Kitamura et al (1998)[192]
Bim	Engidawork et al (2001)[197]
Caspases	
Caspase 1	Clark et al (1999),[193] Henshall et al (2000),[194] Pompl et al (2003)[199]
Caspase 2	Pompl et al (2003)[199]
Caspase 3	Engidawork et al (2001),[200] Clark et al (1999),[193] Hartmann et al (2000),[201] Henshall et al (2000),[194] Pompl et al (2003),[199] Matsui et al (2006)[202]
Caspase 5	Pompl et al (2003)[199]
Caspase 6	Pompl et al (2003)[199]
Caspase 7	Pompl et al (2003),[199] Matsui et al (2006)[202]
Caspase 8	Rohn et al (2001),[203] Pompl et al (2003),[199] Matsui et al (2006)[202]
Caspase 9	Engidawork et al (2001),[200] Pompl et al (2003),[199] Matsui et al (2006)[202]
Others	
Apaf-1	Engidawork et al (2001)[200]
Fas	Nishimura et al (1995),[204] de la Monte et al (1997),[205] Ferrer et al (2001)[206]
FLIP	Engidawork et al (2001),[200] Gulesserian et al (2001)[207]
DR-3,4,5	Newman et al (2000),[208] Dorr et al (2002)[183]
p53	de la Monte et al (1997)[205]
DFF45	Engidawork et al (2001),[200] Gulesserian et al (2001)[207]

TABLE 7-2 APOPTOTIC BIOCHEMICAL ALTERATIONS DETECTED IN HUMAN BRAIN

Insultor Condition	Bcl-2 Family*	Caspase Activation†	DNA Fragmentation‡	Other§
Alzheimer's disease	O'Barr et al (1996)[209] Su et al (1997)[188]	Stadelmann et al (1999)[210] Rohn et al (2001)[203,213] Pompl et al (2003)[199] Matsui et al (2006)[202]	Su et al (1994)[211] Anderson et al (1996)[212] Su et al (1997)[188]	Anderson et al (1996)[212] **(c-Jun)** de la Monte et al (1997)[205] **(p53 & Fas)** Yang et al (1998)[214] **(cleaved actin)** Rohn et al (2001)[203,213] **(cleaved fodrin)** Newman et al (2000)[208] **(death receptor-3)**
Parkinson's disease	Marshall et al (1997)[187] Tatton (2000)[196] Hartmann et al (2001)[198]	Hartmann et al (2000)[201] Tatton (2000)[196] Hartmann et al (2001)[198]	Mochizuki et al (1996)[215] Tatton (2000)[196]	—
Huntington's disease	—	—	Dragunow et al (1995)[216] Portera-Cailliau et al (1995)[217] Butterworth et al (1998)[218]	—
Epilepsy	Henshall et al (2000)[194] Uysal et al (2003)[185] Yuzbasioglu et al (2009)[186]	Henshall et al (2000)[194] Uysal et al (2003)[185]	Henshall et al (2000)[194] Uysal et al (2003)[185]	
Acquired immunodeficiency syndrome	—	Garden et al (2002)[219]	Adle-Biassette et al (1995)[220] Shi et al (1996)[221]	—
Trauma (head injury)	Clark et al (1999)[193]	Clark et al (1999)[193] Williams et al (2001)[224]	Clark et al (1999)[193] Smith et al (2000)[223]	Qiu et al (2002)[222] **(Fas and DISC)**

*Alterations detected in various members of the Bcl-2 family.
†Cleaved active forms of one or more caspases detected.
‡Usually detected with TUNEL method.
§Several other biochemical markers of apoptosis detected; specified in parentheses.

factors, and coexisting conditions. Therefore, the biochemical characteristics of cell death in humans after ischemia, which may be different from that observed in experimental animals, need to be clarified. Love et al[177] examined the brains of 35 patients who died of focal ischemic stroke. The group detected an early increase in procaspase-3 immunoreactivity followed by appearance of TUNEL-positive neurons, especially at the edge of the infarcts. Despite findings suggesting PCD activation in brain infarcts, the morphologic changes they observed were not those of classic apoptosis. These researchers also showed that the TUNEL labeling they observed was probably mediated by the release of endogenous endonucleases during protease or microwave pretreatment of the damaged tissue. Another study has also reported colocalization of TNF-α with TUNEL staining in neurons from autopsy specimens collected from patients with stroke.[178] DNA fragmentation was also detected by in situ nick-end labeling in cerebellar granular cells after global ischemia in two autopsy cases.[179] Some of the biochemical steps of apoptosis may be activated in postmortem tissue, which suggests an important caveat in interpreting the aforementioned findings.[177] Cell death may also be triggered as a result of metabolic derangements during

the premortem period in vulnerable neurons.[180] Despite uncertainties in interpreting the data obtained from postmortem material, many studies performed on autopsy material have provided confirmation of findings, such as colocalization of apoptotic changes with specific disease in contrast to generalized nonspecific activation of cell death in diverse cellular groups (Table 7-2). Studies performed on brain biopsy specimens, which lack some of the problems encountered with postmortem tissue, have more convincingly demonstrated apoptotic cell death in human neurodegenerative diseases.[181-186] These and other studies indicate that human brain cells have the potential to die by apoptotic mechanisms.

REFERENCES

1. Dirnagl U, Iadecola C, Moskowitz MA: Pathobiology of ischaemic stroke: An integrated view, *Trends Neurosci* 22:391–397, 1999.
2. Lipton P: Ischemic cell death in brain neurons, *Physiol Rev* 79:1431–1568, 1999.
3. Lo EH, Dalkara T, Moskowitz MA: Mechanisms, challenges and opportunities in stroke, *Nat Rev Neurosci* 4:399–415, 2003.
4. Unal-Cevik I, Kilinc M, Can A, Gursoy-Ozdemir Y, Dalkara T: Apoptotic and necrotic death mechanisms are concomitantly activated in the same cell after cerebral ischemia, *Stroke* 35:2189–2194, 2004.

5. Degterev A, Huang Z, Boyce M, Li Y, Jagtap P, Mizushima N, Cuny GD, Mitchison TJ, Moskowitz MA, Yuan J: Chemical inhibitor of nonapoptotic cell death with therapeutic potential for ischemic brain injury, *Nat Chem Biol* 1:112-119, 2005.
6. Graham SH, Chen J: Programmed cell death in cerebral ischemia, *J Cereb Blood Flow Metab* 21:99-109, 2001.
7. Schulz JB, Weller M, Moskowitz MA: Caspases as treatment targets in stroke and neurodegenerative diseases, *Ann Neurol* 45:421-429, 1999.
8. Silva MT, do Vale A, dos Santos NM: Secondary necrosis in multicellular animals: An outcome of apoptosis with pathogenic implications, *Apoptosis* 13:463-482, 2008.
9. Rami A, Langhagen A, Steiger S: Focal cerebral ischemia induces upregulation of beclin 1 and autophagy-like cell death, *Neurobiol Dis* 29:132-141, 2008.
10. Adhami F, Schloemer A, Kuan CY: The roles of autophagy in cerebral ischemia, *Autophagy* 3:42-44, 2007.
11. Cuervo AM: Autophagy: In sickness and in health, *Trends Cell Biol* 14:70-77, 2004.
12. Puyal J, Vaslin A, Mottier V, Clarke PG: Postischemic treatment of neonatal cerebral ischemia should target autophagy, *Ann Neurol* 66:378-389, 2009.
13. Ginet V, Puyal J, Clarke PG, Truttmann AC: Enhancement of autophagic flux after neonatal cerebral hypoxia-ischemia and its region-specific relationship to apoptotic mechanisms, *Am J Pathol* 175:1962-1974, 2009.
14. Gao Y, Liang W, Hu X, Zhang W, Stetler RA, Vosler P, Cao G, Chen J: Neuroprotection against hypoxic-ischemic brain injury by inhibiting the apoptotic protease activating factor-1 pathway, *Stroke* 41:166-172, 2010.
15. Hu BR, Liu CL, Ouyang Y, Blomgren K, Siesjo BK: Involvement of caspase-3 in cell death after hypoxia-ischemia declines during brain maturation, *J Cereb Blood Flow Metab* 20:1294-1300, 2000.
16. Hirsch T, Marchetti P, Susin SA, Dallaporta B, Zamzami N, Marzo I, Geuskens M, Kroemer G: The apoptosis-necrosis paradox. Apoptogenic proteases activated after mitochondrial permeability transition determine the mode of cell death, *Oncogene* 15:1573-1581, 1997.
17. Martin LJ, Al-Abdulla NA, Brambrink AM, Kirsch JR, Sieber FE, Portera-Cailliau C: Neurodegeneration in excitotoxicity, global cerebral ischemia, and target deprivation: A perspective on the contributions of apoptosis and necrosis, *Brain Res Bull* 46:281-309, 1998.
18. Nicotera P, Leist M, Manzo L: Neuronal cell death: A demise with different shapes, *Trends Pharmacol Sci* 20:46-51, 1999.
19. MacManus JP, Buchan AM: Apoptosis after experimental stroke: Fact or fashion? *J Neurotrauma* 17:899-914, 2000.
20. Syntichaki P, Tavernarakis N: The biochemistry of neuronal necrosis: Rogue biology? *Nat Rev Neurosci* 4:672-684, 2003.
21. Degterev A, Yuan J: Expansion and evolution of cell death programmes, *Nat Rev Mol Cell Biol* 9:378-390, 2008.
22. Leist M, Jaattela M: Four deaths and a funeral: From caspases to alternative mechanisms, *Nat Rev Mol Cell Biol* 2:589-598, 2001.
23. Wang X: The expanding role of mitochondria in apoptosis, *Genes Dev* 15:2922-2933, 2001.
24. Kroemer G, Reed JC: Mitochondrial control of cell death, *Nat Med* 6:513-519, 2000.
25. Fiskum G: Mitochondrial participation in ischemic and traumatic neural cell death, *J Neurotrauma* 17:843-855, 2000.
26. Hengartner MO: The biochemistry of apoptosis, *Nature* 407:770-776, 2000.
27. Christofferson DE, Yuan J: Necroptosis as an alternative form of programmed cell death, *Curr Opin Cell Biol* 22:263-268, 2010.
28. Budd RC: Death receptors couple to both cell proliferation and apoptosis, *J Clin Invest* 109:437-441, 2002.
29. Zhang DW, Shao J, Lin J, Zhang N, Lu BJ, Lin SC, Dong MQ, Han J: RIP3, an energy metabolism regulator that switches TNF-induced cell death from apoptosis to necrosis, *Science* 325:332-336, 2009.
30. Gurer G, Gursoy-Ozdemir Y, Erdemli E, Can A, Dalkara T: Astrocytes are more resistant to focal cerebral ischemia than neurons and die by a delayed necrosis, *Brain Pathol* 19:630-641, 2009.
31. Kerr JF, Wyllie AH, Currie AR: Apoptosis: A basic biological phenomenon with wide-ranging implications in tissue kinetics, *Br J Cancer* 26:239-257, 1972.
32. Majno G, Joris I: Apoptosis, oncosis, and necrosis. An overview of cell death, *Am J Pathol* 146:3-15, 1995.
33. Wyllie AH, Kerr JF, Currie AR: Cell death: The significance of apoptosis, *Int Rev Cytol* 68:251-306, 1980.
34. Benn SC, Woolf CJ: Adult neuron survival strategies—slamming on the brakes, *Nat Rev Neurosci* 5:686-700, 2004.
35. Bano D, Young KW, Guerin CJ, Lefeuvre R, Rothwell NJ, Naldini L, Rizzuto R, Carafoli E, Nicotera P: Cleavage of the plasma membrane Na^+/Ca^{2+} exchanger in excitotoxicity, *Cell* 120:275-285, 2005.
36. Clarke PG: Developmental cell death: Morphological diversity and multiple mechanisms, *Anat Embryol (Berl)* 181:195-213, 1990.
37. White E: Autophagic cell death unraveled: Pharmacological inhibition of apoptosis and autophagy enables necrosis, *Autophagy* 4:399-401, 2008.
38. Koike M, Shibata M, Tadakoshi M, Gotoh K, Komatsu M, Waguri S, Kawahara N, Kuida K, Nagata S, Kominami E, Tanaka K, Uchiyama Y: Inhibition of autophagy prevents hippocampal pyramidal neuron death after hypoxic-ischemic injury, *Am J Pathol* 172:454-469, 2008.
39. Meier P, Finch A, Evan G: Apoptosis in development, *Nature* 407:796-801, 2000.
40. Renehan AG, Bach SP, Potten CS: The relevance of apoptosis for cellular homeostasis and tumorigenesis in the intestine, *Can J Gastroenterol* 15:166-176, 2001.
41. Mattson MP: Apoptosis in neurodegenerative disorders, *Nat Rev Mol Cell Biol* 1:120-129, 2000.
42. Yuan J, Yankner BA: Apoptosis in the nervous system, *Nature* 407:802-809, 2000.
43. Metzstein MM, Stanfield GM, Horvitz HR: Genetics of programmed cell death in *C. elegans*: Past, present and future, *Trends Genet* 14:410-416, 1998.
44. Yuan JY, Horvitz HR: The *Caenorhabditis elegans* genes ced-3 and ced-4 act cell autonomously to cause programmed cell death, *Dev Biol* 138:33-41, 1990.
45. Yuan J, Shaham S, Ledoux S, Ellis HM, Horvitz HR: The *C. elegans* cell death gene ced-3 encodes a protein similar to mammalian interleukin-1 beta-converting enzyme, *Cell* 75:641-652, 1993.
46. Joza N, Kroemer G, Penninger JM: Genetic analysis of the mammalian cell death machinery, *Trends Genet* 18:142-149, 2002.
47. Murphy AN, Fiskum G, Beal MF: Mitochondria in neurodegeneration: Bioenergetic function in cell life and death, *J Cereb Blood Flow Metab* 19:231-245, 1999.
48. Willis SN, Adams JM: Life in the balance: How BH3-only proteins induce apoptosis, *Curr Opin Cell Biol* 17:617-625, 2005.
49. Li H, Zhu H, Xu CJ, Yuan J: Cleavage of Bid by caspase 8 mediates the mitochondrial damage in the FAS pathway of apoptosis, *Cell* 94:491-501, 1998.
50. Wang HG, Pathan N, Ethell IM, Krajewski S, Yamaguchi Y, Shibasaki F, McKeon F, Bobo T, Franke TF, Reed JC: Ca^{2+}-induced apoptosis through calcineurin dephosphorylation of Bad, *Science* 284:339-343, 1999.
51. Puthalakath H, Strasser A: Keeping killers on a tight leash: Transcriptional and post-translational control of the pro-apoptotic activity of BH3-only proteins, *Cell Death Differ* 9:505-512, 2002.
52. Zou H, Henzel WJ, Liu X, Lutschg A, Wang X: Apaf-1, a human protein homologous to *C. elegans* ced-4, participates in cytochrome c-dependent activation of caspase-3, *Cell* 90:405-413, 1997.
53. Stennicke HR, Ryan CA, Salvesen GS: Reprieval from execution: The molecular basis of caspase inhibition, *Trends Biochem Sci* 27:94-101, 2002.
54. Susin SA, Lorenzo HK, Zamzami N, Marzo I, Snow BE, Brothers GM, Mangion J, Jacotot E, Costantini P, Loeffler M, Larochette N, Goodlett DR, Aebersold R, Siderovski DP, Penninger JM, Kroemer G: Molecular characterization of mitochondrial apoptosis-inducing factor, *Nature* 397:441-446, 1999.
55. Cande C, Cohen I, Daugas E, Ravagnan L, Larochette N, Zamzami N, Kroemer G: Apoptosis-inducing factor (AIF): A novel caspase-independent death effector released from mitochondria, *Biochimie* 84:215-222, 2002.
56. Lorenzo HK, Susin SA, Penninger J, Kroemer G: Apoptosis inducing factor (AIF): A phylogenetically old, caspase-independent effector of cell death, *Cell Death Differ* 6:516-524, 1999.
57. Yu SW, Wang H, Poitras MF, Coombs C, Bowers WJ, Federoff HJ, Poirier GG, Dawson TM, Dawson VL: Mediation of poly(ADP-ribose) polymerase-1-dependent cell death by apoptosis-inducing factor, *Science* 297:259-263, 2002.

58. Cipriani G, Rapizzi E, Vannacci A, Rizzuto R, Moroni F, Chiarugi A: Nuclear poly(ADP-ribose) polymerase-1 rapidly triggers mitochondrial dysfunction, *J Biol Chem* 280:17227-17234, 2005.

59. Eguchi K: Apoptosis in autoimmune diseases, *Intern Med* 40:275-284, 2001.

60. Itoh N, Nagata S: A novel protein domain required for apoptosis. Mutational analysis of human FAS antigen, *J Biol Chem* 268:10932-10937, 1993.

61. Kischkel FC, Hellbardt S, Behrmann I, Germer M, Pawlita M, Krammer PH, Peter ME: Cytotoxicity-dependent APO-1 (Fas/CD95)-associated proteins form a death-inducing signaling complex (DISC) with the receptor, *EMBO J* 14:5579-5588, 1995.

62. Medema JP, Scaffidi C, Kischkel FC, Shevchenko A, Mann M, Krammer PH, Peter ME: FLICE is activated by association with the CD95 death-inducing signaling complex (DISC), *EMBO J* 16:2794-2804, 1997.

63. Stennicke HR, Jurgensmeier JM, Shin H, Deveraux Q, Wolf BB, Yang X, Zhou Q, Ellerby HM, Ellerby LM, Bredesen D, Green DR, Reed JC, Froelich CJ, Salvesen GS: Pro-caspase-3 is a major physiologic target of caspase-8, *J Biol Chem* 273:27084-27090, 1998.

64. Luo X, Budihardjo I, Zou H, Slaughter C, Wang X: Bid, a Bcl2 interacting protein, mediates cytochrome c release from mitochondria in response to activation of cell surface death receptors, *Cell* 94:481-490, 1998.

65. Korsmeyer SJ, Wei MC, Saito M, Weiler S, Oh KJ, Schlesinger PH: Pro-apoptotic cascade activates BID, which oligomerizes BAK or BAX into pores that result in the release of cytochrome c, *Cell Death Differ* 7:1166-1173, 2000.

66. Wei MC, Zong WX, Cheng EH, Lindsten T, Panoutsakopoulou V, Ross AJ, Roth KA, MacGregor GR, Thompson CB, Korsmeyer SJ: Proapoptotic BAX and BAK: A requisite gateway to mitochondrial dysfunction and death, *Science* 292:727-730, 2001.

67. Slee EA, Harte MT, Kluck RM, Wolf BB, Casiano CA, Newmeyer DD, Wang HG, Reed JC, Nicholson DW, Alnemri ES, Green DR, Martin SJ: Ordering the cytochrome c-initiated caspase cascade: Hierarchical activation of caspases-2, -3, -6, -7, -8, and -10 in a caspase-9-dependent manner, *J Cell Biol* 144:281-292, 1999.

68. Vercammen D, Brouckaert G, Denecker G, Van de Craen M, Declercq W, Fiers W, Vandenabeele P: Dual signaling of the Fas receptor: Initiation of both apoptotic and necrotic cell death pathways, *J Exp Med* 188:919-930, 1998.

69. Holler N, Zaru R, Micheau O, Thome M, Attinger A, Valitutti S, Bodmer JL, Schneider P, Seed B, Tschopp J: Fas triggers an alternative, caspase-8-independent cell death pathway using the kinase RIP as effector molecule, *Nat Immunol* 1:489-495, 2000.

70. Khwaja A, Tatton L: Resistance to the cytotoxic effects of tumor necrosis factor alpha can be overcome by inhibition of a FADD/caspase-dependent signaling pathway, *J Biol Chem* 274:36817-36823, 1999.

71. Rich T, Allen RL, Wyllie AH: Defying death after DNA damage, *Nature* 407:777-783, 2000.

72. Zhou BB, Elledge SJ: The DNA damage response: Putting checkpoints in perspective, *Nature* 408:433-439, 2000.

73. Banin S, Moyal L, Shieh S, Taya Y, Anderson CW, Chessa L, Smorodinsky NI, Prives C, Reiss Y, Shiloh Y, Ziv Y: Enhanced phosphorylation of p53 by ATM in response to DNA damage, *Science* 281:1674-1677, 1998.

74. Maya R, Balass M, Kim ST, Shkedy D, Leal JF, Shifman O, Moas M, Buschmann T, Ronai Z, Shiloh Y, Kastan MB, Katzir E, Oren M: ATM-dependent phosphorylation of Mdm2 on serine 395: Role in p53 activation by DNA damage, *Genes Dev* 15:1067-1077, 2001.

75. Culmsee C, Mattson MP: p53 in neuronal apoptosis, *Biochem Biophys Res Commun* 331:761-777, 2005.

76. Leist M, Single B, Kunstle G, Volbracht C, Hentze H, Nicotera P: Apoptosis in the absence of poly-(ADP-ribose) polymerase, *Biochem Biophys Res Commun* 233:518-522, 1997.

77. Ha HC, Snyder SH: Poly(ADP-ribose) polymerase is a mediator of necrotic cell death by ATP depletion, *Proc Natl Acad Sci U S A* 96:13978-13982, 1999.

78. Chiarugi A: Poly(ADP-ribose) polymerase: Killer or conspirator? The 'suicide hypothesis' revisited, *Trends Pharmacol Sci* 23:122-129, 2002.

79. Chiarugi A, Moskowitz MA: Cell biology. PARP-1-a perpetrator of apoptotic cell death? *Science* 297:200-201, 2002.

80. Xu Y, Huang S, Liu ZG, Han J: Poly(ADP-ribose) polymerase-1 signaling to mitochondria in necrotic cell death requires RIP1/TRAF2-mediated JNK1 activation, *J Biol Chem* 281:8788-8795, 2006.

81. Paschen W: Shutdown of translation: Lethal or protective? Unfolded protein response versus apoptosis, *J Cereb Blood Flow Metab* 23:773-779, 2003.

82. Nakagawa T, Zhu H, Morishima N, Li E, Xu J, Yankner BA, Yuan J: Caspase-12 mediates endoplasmic-reticulum-specific apoptosis and cytotoxicity by amyloid-beta, *Nature* 403:98-103, 2000.

83. Morishima N, Nakanishi K, Takenouchi H, Shibata T, Yasuhiko Y: An endoplasmic reticulum stress-specific caspase cascade in apoptosis. Cytochrome c-independent activation of caspase-9 by caspase-12, *J Biol Chem* 277:34287-34294, 2002.

84. Rao RV, Castro-Obregon S, Frankowski H, Schuler M, Stoka V, del Rio G, Bredesen DE, Ellerby HM: Coupling endoplasmic reticulum stress to the cell death program. An Apaf-1-independent intrinsic pathway, *J Biol Chem* 277:21836-21842, 2002.

85. Li H, Yuan J: Deciphering the pathways of life and death, *Curr Opin Cell Biol* 11:261-266, 1999.

86. Tamatani M, Che YH, Matsuzaki H, Ogawa S, Okado H, Miyake S, Mizuno T, Tohyama M: Tumor necrosis factor induces Bcl-2 and Bcl-x expression through NFkappaB activation in primary hippocampal neurons, *J Biol Chem* 274:8531-8538, 1999.

87. Datta SR, Brunet A, Greenberg ME: Cellular survival: A play in three Akts, *Genes Dev* 13:2905-2927, 1999.

88. Cardone MH, Roy N, Stennicke HR, Salvesen GS, Franke TF, Stanbridge E, Frisch S, Reed JC: Regulation of cell death protease caspase-9 by phosphorylation, *Science* 282:1318-1321, 1998.

89. Datta SR, Dudek H, Tao X, Masters S, Fu H, Gotoh Y, Greenberg ME: Akt phosphorylation of Bad couples survival signals to the cell-intrinsic death machinery, *Cell* 91:231-241, 1997.

90. Bryckaert M, Guillonneau X, Hecquet C, Courtois Y, Mascarelli F: Both FGF1 and bcl-x synthesis are necessary for the reduction of apoptosis in retinal pigmented epithelial cells by FGF2: Role of the extracellular signal-regulated kinase 2, *Oncogene* 18:7584-7593, 1999.

91. Finkbeiner S: CREB couples neurotrophin signals to survival messages, *Neuron* 25:11-14, 2000.

92. Kaltschmidt B, Kaltschmidt C, Hofmann TG, Hehner SP, Droge W, Schmitz ML: The pro- or anti-apoptotic function of NF-kappaB is determined by the nature of the apoptotic stimulus, *Eur J Biochem* 267:3828-3835, 2000.

93. Mattson MP, Lovell MA, Furukawa K, Markesbery WR: Neurotrophic factors attenuate glutamate-induced accumulation of peroxides, elevation of intracellular Ca^{2+} concentration, and neurotoxicity and increase antioxidant enzyme activities in hippocampal neurons, *J Neurochem* 65:1740-1751, 1995.

94. Mattson MP, Scheff SW: Endogenous neuroprotection factors and traumatic brain injury: Mechanisms of action and implications for therapy, *J Neurotrauma* 11:3-33, 1994.

95. Saleh A, Srinivasula SM, Balkir L, Robbins PD, Alnemri ES: Negative regulation of the Apaf-1 apoptosome by Hsp70, *Nat Cell Biol* 2:476-483, 2000.

96. Ravagnan L, Gurbuxani S, Susin SA, Maisse C, Daugas E, Zamzami N, Mak T, Jaattela M, Penninger JM, Garrido C, Kroemer G: Heat-shock protein 70 antagonizes apoptosis-inducing factor, *Nat Cell Biol* 3:839-843, 2001.

97. Meriin AB, Yaglom JA, Gabai VL, Zon L, Ganiatsas S, Mosser DD, Sherman MY: Protein-damaging stresses activate c-Jun N-terminal kinase via inhibition of its dephosphorylation: A novel pathway controlled by HSP72, *Mol Cell Biol* 19:2547-2555, 1999.

98. Linnik MD, Zobrist RH, Hatfield MD: Evidence supporting a role for programmed cell death in focal cerebral ischemia in rats, *Stroke* 24:2002-2008, 1993:discussion 2008-2009.

99. Krajewski S, Mai JK, Krajewska M, Sikorska M, Mossakowski MJ, Reed JC: Upregulation of bax protein levels in neurons following cerebral ischemia, *J Neurosci* 15:6364-6376, 1995.

100. Li Y, Chopp M, Jiang N, Yao F, Zaloga C: Temporal profile of in situ DNA fragmentation after transient middle cerebral artery occlusion in the rat, *J Cereb Blood Flow Metab* 15:389-397, 1995.

101. Charriaut-Marlangue C, Margaill I, Represa A, Popovici T, Plotkine M, Ben-Ari Y: Apoptosis and necrosis after reversible focal ischemia: An in situ DNA fragmentation analysis, *J Cereb Blood Flow Metab* 16:186-194, 1996.

102. Chen J, Zhu RL, Nakayama M, Kawaguchi K, Jin K, Stetler RA, Simon RP, Graham SH: Expression of the apoptosis-effector gene, Bax, is up-regulated in vulnerable hippocampal CA1 neurons following global ischemia, *J Neurochem* 67:64-71, 1996.

103. Colbourne F, Sutherland GR, Auer RN: Electron microscopic evidence against apoptosis as the mechanism of neuronal death in global ischemia, *J Neurosci* 19:4200-4210, 1999.

104. Deshpande J, Bergstedt K, Linden T, Kalimo H, Wieloch T: Ultrastructural changes in the hippocampal CA1 region following transient cerebral ischemia: Evidence against programmed cell death, *Exp Brain Res* 88:91-105, 1992.

105. van Lookeren Campagne M, Gill R: Ultrastructural morphological changes are not characteristic of apoptotic cell death following focal cerebral ischaemia in the rat, *Neurosci Lett* 213:111-114, 1996.

106. Pagnussat AS, Faccioni-Heuser MC, Netto CA, Achaval M: An ultrastructural study of cell death in the CA1 pyramidal field of the hippocapmus in rats submitted to transient global ischemia followed by reperfusion, *J Anat* 211:589-599, 2007.

107. Chen J, Nagayama T, Jin K, Stetler RA, Zhu RL, Graham SH, Simon RP: Induction of caspase-3-like protease may mediate delayed neuronal death in the hippocampus after transient cerebral ischemia, *J Neurosci* 18:4914-4928, 1998.

108. Hara H, Friedlander RM, Gagliardini V, Ayata C, Fink K, Huang Z, Shimizu-Sasamata M, Yuan J, Moskowitz MA: Inhibition of interleukin 1beta converting enzyme family proteases reduces ischemic and excitotoxic neuronal damage, *Proc Natl Acad Sci U S A* 94:2007-2012, 1997.

109. Wang KK: Calpain and caspase: Can you tell the difference? *Trends Neurosci* 23:20-26, 2000.

110. Yamashima T: Implication of cysteine proteases calpain, cathepsin and caspase in ischemic neuronal death of primates, *Prog Neurobiol* 62:273-295, 2000.

110a. Kilinc M, Gürsoy-Özdemir Y, Gurer G, et al: Hysosomal rupture, necroapoptotic interactions and potential crosstalk between proteases in neurons shortly after focal ischemia. *Neurobiol Dis* 40:293-302, 2010.

111. Heron A, Pollard H, Dessi F, Moreau J, Lasbennes F, Ben-Ari Y, Charriaut-Marlangue C: Regional variability in DNA fragmentation after global ischemia evidenced by combined histological and gel electrophoresis observations in the rat brain, *J Neurochem* 61:1973-1976, 1993.

112. MacManus JP, Buchan AM, Hill IE, Rasquinha I, Preston E: Global ischemia can cause DNA fragmentation indicative of apoptosis in rat brain, *Neurosci Lett* 164:89-92, 1993.

113. Tominaga T, Kure S, Narisawa K, Yoshimoto T: Endonuclease activation following focal ischemic injury in the rat brain, *Brain Res* 608:21-26, 1993.

114. MacManus JP, Hill IE, Huang ZG, Rasquinha I, Xue D, Buchan AM: DNA damage consistent with apoptosis in transient focal ischaemic neocortex, *Neuroreport* 5:493-496, 1994.

115. Charriaut-Marlangue C, Margaill I, Plotkine M, Ben-Ari Y: Early endonuclease activation following reversible focal ischemia in the rat brain, *J Cereb Blood Flow Metab* 15:385-388, 1995.

116. Li Y, Chopp M, Jiang N, Zhang ZG, Zaloga C: Induction of DNA fragmentation after 10 to 120 minutes of focal cerebral ischemia in rats, *Stroke* 26:1252-1257, 1995:discussion 1257-1258.

117. Li Y, Chopp M, Powers C, Jiang N: Apoptosis and protein expression after focal cerebral ischemia in rat, *Brain Res* 765:301-312, 1997.

118. Eliasson MJ, Sampei K, Mandir AS, Hurn PD, Traystman RJ, Bao J, Pieper A, Wang ZQ, Dawson TM, Snyder SH, Dawson VL: Poly(ADP-ribose) polymerase gene disruption renders mice resistant to cerebral ischemia, *Nat Med* 3:1089-1095, 1997.

119. Endres M, Wang ZQ, Namura S, Waeber C, Moskowitz MA: Ischemic brain injury is mediated by the activation of poly(ADP-ribose)polymerase, *J Cereb Blood Flow Metab* 17:1143-1151, 1997.

120. Katchanov J, Harms C, Gertz K, Hauck L, Waeber C, Hirt L, Priller J, von Harsdorf R, Bruck W, Hortnagl H, Dirnagl U, Bhide PG, Endres M: Mild cerebral ischemia induces loss of cyclin-dependent kinase inhibitors and activation of cell cycle machinery before delayed neuronal cell death, *J Neurosci* 21:5045-5053, 2001.

121. Antonawich FJ, Krajewski S, Reed JC, Davis JN: Bcl-x(l) Bax interaction after transient global ischemia, *J Cereb Blood Flow Metab* 18:882-886, 1998.

122. Elibol B, Soylemezoglu F, Unal I, Fujii M, Hirt L, Huang PL, Moskowitz MA, Dalkara T: Nitric oxide is involved in ischemia-induced apoptosis in brain: A study in neuronal nitric oxide synthase null mice, *Neuroscience* 105:79-86, 2001.

123. Isenmann S, Stoll G, Schroeter M, Krajewski S, Reed JC, Bahr M: Differential regulation of Bax, Bcl-2, and Bcl-x proteins in focal cortical ischemia in the rat, *Brain Pathol* 8:49-62, 1998:discussion 62-43.

124. Fujimura M, Morita-Fujimura Y, Murakami K, Kawase M, Chan PH: Cytosolic redistribution of cytochrome c after transient focal cerebral ischemia in rats, *J Cereb Blood Flow Metab* 18:1239-1247, 1998.

125. Krajewski S, Krajewska M, Ellerby LM, Welsh K, Xie Z, Deveraux QL, Salvesen GS, Bredesen DE, Rosenthal RE, Fiskum G, Reed JC: Release of caspase-9 from mitochondria during neuronal apoptosis and cerebral ischemia, *Proc Natl Acad Sci U S A* 96:5752-5757, 1999.

126. Namura S, Zhu J, Fink K, Endres M, Srinivasan A, Tomaselli KJ, Yuan J, Moskowitz MA: Activation and cleavage of caspase-3 in apoptosis induced by experimental cerebral ischemia, *J Neurosci* 18:3659-3668, 1998.

127. Velier JJ, Ellison JA, Kikly KK, Spera PA, Barone FC, Feuerstein GZ: Caspase-8 and caspase-3 are expressed by different populations of cortical neurons undergoing delayed cell death after focal stroke in the rat, *J Neurosci* 19:5932-5941, 1999.

128. Thornberry NA, Lazebnik Y: Caspases: Enemies within, *Science* 281:1312-1316, 1998.

129. Zhang J, Xu M: Apoptotic DNA fragmentation and tissue homeostasis, *Trends Cell Biol* 12:84-89, 2002.

130. Hara H, Fink K, Endres M, Friedlander RM, Gagliardini V, Yuan J, Moskowitz MA: Attenuation of transient focal cerebral ischemic injury in transgenic mice expressing a mutant ICE inhibitory protein, *J Cereb Blood Flow Metab* 17:370-375, 1997.

131. Friedlander RM, Gagliardini V, Hara H, Fink KB, Li W, MacDonald G, Fishman MC, Greenberg AH, Moskowitz MA, Yuan J: Expression of a dominant negative mutant of interleukin-1 beta converting enzyme in transgenic mice prevents neuronal cell death induced by trophic factor withdrawal and ischemic brain injury, *J Exp Med* 185:933-940, 1997.

132. Loddick SA, MacKenzie A, Rothwell NJ: An ICE inhibitor, z-VAD-DCB attenuates ischaemic brain damage in the rat, *Neuroreport* 7:1465-1468, 1996.

133. Schielke GP, Yang GY, Shivers BD, Betz AL: Reduced ischemic brain injury in interleukin-1 beta converting enzyme-deficient mice, *J Cereb Blood Flow Metab* 18:180-185, 1998.

134. Asahi M, Hoshimaru M, Uemura Y, Tokime T, Kojima M, Ohtsuka T, Matsuura N, Aoki T, Shibahara K, Kikuchi H: Expression of interleukin-1 beta converting enzyme gene family and bcl-2 gene family in the rat brain following permanent occlusion of the middle cerebral artery, *J Cereb Blood Flow Metab* 17:11-18, 1997.

135. Endres M, Fink K, Zhu J, Stagliano NE, Bondada V, Geddes JW, Azuma T, Mattson MP, Kwiatkowski DJ, Moskowitz MA: Neuroprotective effects of gelsolin during murine stroke, *J Clin Invest* 103:347-354, 1999.

136. Fink K, Zhu J, Namura S, Shimizu-Sasamata M, Endres M, Ma J, Dalkara T, Yuan J, Moskowitz MA: Prolonged therapeutic window for ischemic brain damage caused by delayed caspase activation, *J Cereb Blood Flow Metab* 18:1071-1076, 1998.

137. Matsushita K, Wu Y, Qiu J, Lang-Lazdunski L, Hirt L, Waeber C, Hyman BT, Yuan J, Moskowitz MA: Fas receptor and neuronal cell death after spinal cord ischemia, *J Neurosci* 20:6879-6887, 2000.

138. Martin-Villalba A, Hahne M, Kleber S, Vogel J, Falk W, Schenkel J, Krammer PH: Therapeutic neutralization of CD95-ligand and TNF attenuates brain damage in stroke, *Cell Death Differ* 8:679-686, 2001.

139. Martin-Villalba A, Herr I, Jeremias I, Hahne M, Brandt R, Vogel J, Schenkel J, Herdegen T, Debatin KM: CD95 ligand (Fas-L/APO-1L) and tumor necrosis factor-related apoptosis-inducing ligand mediate ischemia-induced apoptosis in neurons, *J Neurosci* 19:3809-3817, 1999.

140. Rosenbaum DM, Gupta G, D'Amore J, Singh M, Weidenheim K, Zhang H, Kessler JA: Fas (CD95/APO-1) plays a role in the pathophysiology of focal cerebral ischemia, *J Neurosci Res* 61:686-692, 2000.

141. Mehmet H: Stroke treatment enters the Fas lane, *Cell Death Differ* 8:659-661, 2001.

142. Stoll G, Jander S, Schroeter M: Inflammation and glial responses in ischemic brain lesions, *Prog Neurobiol* 56:149-171, 1998.

143. Plesnila N, Zinkel S, Le DA, Amin-Hanjani S, Wu Y, Qiu J, Chiarugi A, Thomas SS, Kohane DS, Korsmeyer SJ, Moskowitz MA: Bid mediates neuronal cell death after oxygen/glucose deprivation and focal cerebral ischemia, *Proc Natl Acad Sci U S A* 98:15318-15323, 2001.

144. Wei MC, Lindsten T, Mootha VK, Weiler S, Gross A, Ashiya M, Thompson CB, Korsmeyer SJ: tBID, a membrane-targeted death ligand, oligomerizes BAK to release cytochrome c, *Genes Dev* 14:2060-2071, 2000.

145. Harrison DC, Davis RP, Bond BC, Campbell CA, James MF, Parsons AA, Philpott KL: Caspase mRNA expression in a rat model of focal cerebral ischemia, *Brain Res Mol Brain Res* 89:133-146, 2001.

146. Kang SJ, Wang S, Hara H, Peterson EP, Namura S, Amin-Hanjani S, Huang Z, Srinivasan A, Tomaselli KJ, Thornberry NA, Moskowitz MA, Yuan J: Dual role of caspase-11 in mediating activation of caspase-1 and caspase-3 under pathological conditions, *J Cell Biol* 149:613-622, 2000.

147. Shibata M, Hattori H, Sasaki T, Gotoh J, Hamada J, Fukuuchi Y: Activation of caspase-12 by endoplasmic reticulum stress induced by transient middle cerebral artery occlusion in mice, *Neuroscience* 118:491-499, 2003.

148. Bergeron L, Perez GI, Macdonald G, Shi L, Sun Y, Jurisicova A, Varmuza S, Latham KE, Flaws JA, Salter JC, Hara H, Moskowitz MA, Li E, Greenberg A, Tilly JL, Yuan J: Defects in regulation of apoptosis in caspase-2-deficient mice, *Genes Dev* 12:1304-1314, 1998.

149. Kinoshita M, Tomimoto H, Kinoshita A, Kumar S, Noda M: Upregulation of the Nedd2 gene encoding an ICE/Ced-3-like cysteine protease in the gerbil brain after transient global ischemia, *J Cereb Blood Flow Metab* 17:507-514, 1997.

150. Panickar KS, Norenberg MD: Astrocytes in cerebral ischemic injury: Morphological and general considerations, *Glia* 50:287-298, 2005.

151. Cheng Y, Deshmukh M, D'Costa A, Demaro JA, Gidday JM, Shah A, Sun Y, Jacquin MF, Johnson EM, Holtzman DM: Caspase inhibitor affords neuroprotection with delayed administration in a rat model of neonatal hypoxic-ischemic brain injury, *J Clin Invest* 101:1992-1999, 1998.

152. Gillardon F, Bottiger B, Schmitz B, Zimmermann M, Hossmann KA: Activation of CPP-32 protease in hippocampal neurons following ischemia and epilepsy, *Brain Res Mol Brain Res* 50:16-22, 1997.

153. Bhat RV, DiRocco R, Marcy VR, Flood DG, Zhu Y, Dobrzanski P, Siman R, Scott R, Contreras PC, Miller M: Increased expression of IL-1beta converting enzyme in hippocampus after ischemia: Selective localization in microglia, *J Neurosci* 16:4146-4154, 1996.

154. Gillardon F, Kiprianova I, Sandkuhler J, Hossmann KA, Spranger M: Inhibition of caspases prevents cell death of hippocampal CA1 neurons, but not impairment of hippocampal long-term potentiation following global ischemia, *Neuroscience* 93:1219-1222, 1999.

155. Ni B, Wu X, Su Y, Stephenson D, Smalstig EB, Clemens J, Paul SM: Transient global forebrain ischemia induces a prolonged expression of the caspase-3 mRNA in rat hippocampal CA1 pyramidal neurons, *J Cereb Blood Flow Metab* 18:248-256, 1998.

156. Ouyang YB, Tan Y, Comb M, Liu CL, Martone ME, Siesjo BK, Hu BR: Survival- and death-promoting events after transient cerebral ischemia: Phosphorylation of Akt, release of cytochrome c and activation of caspase-like proteases, *J Cereb Blood Flow Metab* 19:1126-1135, 1999.

157. Antonawich FJ, Federoff HJ, Davis JN: Bcl-2 transduction, using a herpes simplex virus amplicon, protects hippocampal neurons from transient global ischemia, *Exp Neurol* 156:130-137, 1999.

158. Nakatsuka H, Ohta S, Tanaka J, Toku K, Kumon Y, Maeda N, Sakanaka M, Sakaki S: Release of cytochrome c from mitochondria to cytosol in gerbil hippocampal CA1 neurons after transient forebrain ischemia, *Brain Res* 849:216-219, 1999.

159. Sugawara T, Fujimura M, Morita-Fujimura Y, Kawase M, Chan PH: Mitochondrial release of cytochrome c corresponds to the selective vulnerability of hippocampal CA1 neurons in rats after transient global cerebral ischemia, *J Neurosci* 19, 1999:RC39.

160. Perez-Pinzon MA, Xu GP, Born J, Lorenzo J, Busto R, Rosenthal M, Sick TJ: Cytochrome c is released from mitochondria into the cytosol after cerebral anoxia or ischemia, *J Cereb Blood Flow Metab* 19:39-43, 1999.

161. Lin R, Roseborough G, Dong Y, Williams GM, Wei C: DNA damage and repair system in spinal cord ischemia, *J Vasc Surg* 37:847-858, 2003.

162. Wang P, Cao X, Nagel DJ, Yin G: Activation of ASK1 during reperfusion of ischemic spinal cord, *Neurosci Lett* 415:248-252, 2007.

163. Chan PH: Reactive oxygen radicals in signaling and damage in the ischemic brain, *J Cereb Blood Flow Metab* 21:2-14, 2001.

164. Endres M, Hirt L, Moskowitz MA: Apoptosis and cerebral ischemia. In Rangnekar VM, editor: *Apoptosis: Role in disease, pathogenesis and prevention*, Amsterdam, 2001, Elsevier Science, pp 137-167.

165. Nakka VP, Gusain A, Mehta SL, Raghubir R: Molecular mechanisms of apoptosis in cerebral ischemia: Multiple neuroprotective opportunities, *Mol Neurobiol* 37:7-38, 2008.

166. Himi T, Ishizaki Y, Murota S: A caspase inhibitor blocks ischaemia-induced delayed neuronal death in the gerbil, *Eur J Neurosci* 10:777-781, 1998.

167. Aktas Y, Yemisci M, Andrieux K, Gursoy RN, Alonso MJ, Fernandez-Megia E, Novoa-Carballal R, Quinoa E, Riguera R, Sargon MF, Celik HH, Demir AS, Hincal AA, Dalkara T, Capan Y, Couvreur P: Development and brain delivery of chitosan-PEG nanoparticles functionalized with the monoclonal antibody OX26, *Bioconjug Chem* 16:1503-1511, 2005.

168. Karatas H, Aktas Y, Gursoy-Ozdemir Y, Bodur E, Yemisci M, Caban S, Vural A, Pinarbasli O, Capan Y, Fernandez-Megia E, Novoa-Carballal R, Riguera R, Andrieux K, Couvreur P, Dalkara T: A nanomedicine transports a peptide caspase-3 inhibitor across the blood-brain barrier and provides neuroprotection, *J Neurosci* 29:13761-13769, 2009.

169. Rothwell NJ, Loddick SA, Stroemer P: Interleukins and cerebral ischaemia, *Int Rev Neurobiol* 40:281-298, 1997.

170. Ma J, Endres M, Moskowitz MA: Synergistic effects of caspase inhibitors and MK-801 in brain injury after transient focal cerebral ischaemia in mice, *Br J Pharmacol* 124:756-762, 1998.

171. Ma J, Qiu J, Hirt L, Dalkara T, Moskowitz MA: Synergistic protective effect of caspase inhibitors and bFGF against brain injury induced by transient focal ischaemia, *Br J Pharmacol* 133:345-350, 2001.

172. Endres M, Fan G, Hirt L, Fujii M, Matsushita K, Liu X, Jaenisch R, Moskowitz MA: Ischemic brain damage in mice after selectively modifying BDNF or NT4 gene expression, *J Cereb Blood Flow Metab* 20:139-144, 2000.

173. Beck T, Lindholm D, Castren E, Wree A: Brain-derived neurotrophic factor protects against ischemic cell damage in rat hippocampus, *J Cereb Blood Flow Metab* 14:689-692, 1994.

174. Chan KM, Lam DT, Pong K, Widmer HR, Hefti F: Neurotrophin-4/5 treatment reduces infarct size in rats with middle cerebral artery occlusion, *Neurochem Res* 21:763-767, 1996.

175. Schabitz WR, Schwab S, Spranger M, Hacke W: Intraventricular brain-derived neurotrophic factor reduces infarct size after focal cerebral ischemia in rats, *J Cereb Blood Flow Metab* 17:500-506, 1997.

176. Tsukahara T, Yonekawa Y, Tanaka K, Ohara O, Wantanabe S, Kimura T, Nishijima T, Taniguchi T: The role of brain-derived neurotrophic factor in transient forebrain ischemia in the rat brain, *Neurosurgery* 34:323-331, 1994:discussion 331.

177. Love S, Barber R, Wilcock GK: Neuronal death in brain infarcts in man, *Neuropathol Appl Neurobiol* 26:55-66, 2000.

178. Sairanen T, Carpen O, Karjalainen-Lindsberg ML, Paetau A, Turpeinen U, Kaste M, Lindsberg PJ: Evolution of cerebral tumor necrosis factor-alpha production during human ischemic stroke, *Stroke* 32:1750-1758, 2001.

179. Hara A, Yoshimi N, Hirose Y, Ino N, Tanaka T, Mori H: DNA fragmentation in granular cells of human cerebellum following global ischemia, *Brain Res* 697:247-250, 1995.

180. Kingsbury AE, Mardsen CD, Foster OJ: DNA fragmentation in human substantia nigra: Apoptosis or perimortem effect? *Mov Disord* 13:877-884, 1998.

181. Anlar B, Soylemezoglu F, Elibol B, Dalkara T, Aysun S, Kose G, Belen D, Yalaz K: Apoptosis in brain biopsies of subacute sclerosing panencephalitis patients, *Neuropediatrics* 30:239-242, 1999.

182. Benjelloun N, Menard A, Charriaut-Marlangue C, Mokhtari K, Perron H, Hauw JJ, Rieger F: Case report: DNA fragmentation in glial cells in a cerebral biopsy from a multiple sclerosis patient, *Cell Mol Biol (Noisy-le-grand)* 44:579-583, 1998.

183. Dorr J, Bechmann I, Waiczies S, Aktas O, Walczak H, Krammer PH, Nitsch R, Zipp F: Lack of tumor necrosis factor-related apoptosis-inducing ligand but presence of its receptors in the human brain, *J Neurosci* 22:RC209, 2002.

184. Ferrer I: Nuclear DNA fragmentation in Creutzfeldt-Jakob disease: Does a mere positive in situ nuclear end-labeling indicate apoptosis? *Acta Neuropathol* 97:5–12, 1999.

185. Uysal H, Cevik IU, Soylemezoglu F, Elibol B, Ozdemir YG, Evrenkaya T, Saygi S, Dalkara T: Is the cell death in mesial temporal sclerosis apoptotic? *Epilepsia* 44:778–784, 2003.

186. Yuzbasioglu A, Karatas H, Gursoy-Ozdemir Y, Saygi S, Akalan N, Soylemezoglu F, Dalkara T, Kocaefe YC, Ozguc M: Changes in the expression of selenoproteins in mesial temporal lobe epilepsy patients, *Cell Mol Neurobiol* 29:1223–1231, 2009.

187. Marshall KA, Daniel SE, Cairns N, Jenner P, Halliwell B: Upregulation of the anti-apoptotic protein Bcl-2 may be an early event in neurodegeneration: Studies on Parkinson's and incidental Lewy body disease, *Biochem Biophys Res Commun* 240:84–87, 1997.

188. Su JH, Deng G, Cotman CW: Bax protein expression is increased in Alzheimer's brain: Correlations with DNA damage, Bcl-2 expression, and brain pathology, *J Neuropathol Exp Neurol* 56:86–93, 1997.

189. Vyas S, Javoy-Agid F, Herrero MT, Strada O, Boissiere F, Hibner U, Agid Y: Expression of Bcl-2 in adult human brain regions with special reference to neurodegenerative disorders, *J Neurochem* 69:223–231, 1997.

190. Yachnis AT, Powell SZ, Olmsted JJ, Eskin TA: Distinct neurodevelopmental patterns of bcl-2 and bcl-x expression are altered in glioneuronal hamartias of the human temporal lobe, *J Neuropathol Exp Neurol* 56:186–198, 1997.

191. Desjardins P, Ledoux S: Expression of ced-3 and ced-9 homologs in Alzheimer's disease cerebral cortex, *Neurosci Lett* 244:69–72, 1998.

192. Kitamura Y, Shimohama S, Kamoshima W, Ota T, Matsuoka Y, Nomura Y, Smith MA, Perry G, Whitehouse PJ, Taniguchi T: Alteration of proteins regulating apoptosis, Bcl-2, Bcl-x, Bax, Bak, Bad, ICH-1 and CPP32, in Alzheimer's disease, *Brain Res* 780:260–269, 1998.

193. Clark RS, Kochanek PM, Chen M, Watkins SC, Marion DW, Chen J, Hamilton RL, Loeffert JE, Graham SH: Increases in Bcl-2 and cleavage of caspase-1 and caspase-3 in human brain after head injury, *FASEB J* 13:813–821, 1999.

194. Henshall DC, Clark RS, Adelson PD, Chen M, Watkins SC, Simon RP: Alterations in bcl-2 and caspase gene family protein expression in human temporal lobe epilepsy, *Neurology* 55:250–257, 2000.

195. Jarskog LF, Gilmore JH: Developmental expression of Bcl-2 protein in human cortex, *Brain Res Dev Brain Res* 119:225–230, 2000.

196. Tatton NA: Increased caspase 3 and Bax immunoreactivity accompany nuclear GAPDH translocation and neuronal apoptosis in Parkinson's disease, *Exp Neurol* 166:29–43, 2000.

197. Engidawork E, Gulesserian T, Seidl R, Cairns N, Lubec G: Expression of apoptosis related proteins: RAIDD, ZIP kinase, Bim/BOD, p21, Bax, Bcl-2 and NF-kappaB in brains of patients with Down syndrome, *J Neural Transm Suppl* 61:181–192, 2001.

198. Hartmann A, Michel PP, Troadec JD, Mouatt-Prigent A, Faucheux BA, Ruberg M, Agid Y, Hirsch EC: Is Bax a mitochondrial mediator in apoptotic death of dopaminergic neurons in Parkinson's disease? *J Neurochem* 76:1785–1793, 2001.

199. Pompl PN, Yemul S, Xiang Z, Ho L, Haroutunian V, Purohit D, Mohs R, Pasinetti GM: Caspase gene expression in the brain as a function of the clinical progression of Alzheimer disease, *Arch Neurol* 60:369–376, 2003.

200. Engidawork E, Gulesserian T, Yoo BC, Cairns N, Lubec G: Alteration of caspases and apoptosis-related proteins in brains of patients with Alzheimer's disease, *Biochem Biophys Res Commun* 281:84–93, 2001.

201. Hartmann A, Hunot S, Michel PP, Muriel MP, Vyas S, Faucheux BA, Mouatt-Prigent A, Turmel H, Srinivasan A, Ruberg M, Evan GI, Agid Y, Hirsch EC: Caspase-3: A vulnerability factor and final effector in apoptotic death of dopaminergic neurons in Parkinson's disease, *Proc Natl Acad Sci U S A* 97:2875–2880, 2000.

202. Matsui T, Ramasamy K, Ingelsson M, Fukumoto H, Conrad C, Frosch MP, Irizarry MC, Yuan J, Hyman BT: Coordinated expression of caspase 8, 3 and 7 mRNA in temporal cortex of Alzheimer disease: Relationship to formic acid extractable abeta42 levels, *J Neuropathol Exp Neurol* 65:508–515, 2006.

203. Rohn TT, Head E, Nesse WH, Cotman CW, Cribbs DH: Activation of caspase-8 in the Alzheimer's disease brain, *Neurobiol Dis* 8:1006–1016, 2001.

204. Nishimura T, Akiyama H, Yonehara S, Kondo H, Ikeda K, Kato M, Iseki E, Kosaka K: Fas antigen expression in brains of patients with Alzheimer-type dementia, *Brain Res* 695:137–145, 1995.

205. de la Monte SM, Sohn YK, Wands JR: Correlates of p53- and Fas (CD95)-mediated apoptosis in Alzheimer's disease, *J Neurol Sci* 152:73–83, 1997.

206. Ferrer I, Puig B, Krupinsk J, Carmona M, Blanco R: Fas and Fas ligand expression in Alzheimer's disease, *Acta Neuropathol* 102:121–131, 2001.

207. Gulesserian T, Engidawork E, Yoo BC, Cairns N, Lubec G: Alteration of caspases and other apoptosis regulatory proteins in Down syndrome, *J Neural Transm Suppl* 61:1163–179, 2001.

208. Newman SJ, Bond B, Crook B, Darker J, Edge C, Maycox PR: Neuron-specific localisation of the TR3 death receptor in Alzheimer's disease, *Brain Res* 857:131–140, 2000.

209. O'Barr S, Schultz J, Rogers J: Expression of the protooncogene bcl-2 in Alzheimer's disease brain, *Neurobiol Aging* 17:131–136, 1996.

210. Stadelmann C, Deckwerth TL, Srinivasan A, Bancher C, Bruck W, Jellinger K, Lassmann H: Activation of caspase-3 in single neurons and autophagic granules of granulovacuolar degeneration in Alzheimer's disease. Evidence for apoptotic cell death, *Am J Pathol* 155:1459–1466, 1999.

211. Su JH, Anderson AJ, Cummings BJ, Cotman CW: Immunohistochemical evidence for apoptosis in Alzheimer's disease, *Neuroreport* 5:2529–2533, 1994.

212. Anderson AJ, Su JH, Cotman CW: DNA damage and apoptosis in Alzheimer's disease: Colocalization with c-Jun immunoreactivity, relationship to brain area, and effect of postmortem delay, *J Neurosci* 16:1710–1719, 1996.

213. Rohn TT, Head E, Su JH, Anderson AJ, Bahr BA, Cotman CW, Cribbs DH: Correlation between caspase activation and neurofibrillary tangle formation in Alzheimer's disease, *Am J Pathol* 158:189–198, 2001.

214. Yang F, Sun X, Beech W, Teter B, Wu S, Sigel J, Vinters HV, Frautschy SA, Cole GM: Antibody to caspase-cleaved actin detects apoptosis in differentiated neuroblastoma and plaque-associated neurons and microglia in Alzheimer's disease, *Am J Pathol* 152:379–389, 1998.

215. Mochizuki H, Goto K, Mori H, Mizuno Y: Histochemical detection of apoptosis in Parkinson's disease, *J Neurol Sci* 137:120–123, 1996.

216. Dragunow M, Faull RL, Lawlor P, Beilharz EJ, Singleton K, Walker EB, Mee E: In situ evidence for DNA fragmentation in Huntington's disease striatum and Alzheimer's disease temporal lobes, *Neuroreport* 6:1053–1057, 1995.

217. Portera-Cailliau C, Hedreen JC, Price DL, Koliatsos VE: Evidence for apoptotic cell death in Huntington disease and excitotoxic animal models, *J Neurosci* 15:3775–3787, 1995.

218. Butterworth NJ, Williams L, Bullock JY, Love DR, Faull RL, Dragunow M: Trinucleotide (CAG) repeat length is positively correlated with the degree of DNA fragmentation in Huntington's disease striatum, *Neuroscience* 87:49–53, 1998.

219. Garden GA, Budd SL, Tsai E, Hanson L, Kaul M, D'Emilia DM, Friedlander RM, Yuan J, Masliah E, Lipton SA: Caspase cascades in human immunodeficiency virus-associated neurodegeneration, *J Neurosci* 22:4015–4024, 2002.

220. Adle-Biassette H, Levy Y, Colombel M, Poron F, Natchev S, Keohane C, Gray F: Neuronal apoptosis in HIV infection in adults, *Neuropathol Appl Neurobiol* 21:218–227, 1995.

221. Shi B, De Girolami U, He J, Wang S, Lorenzo A, Busciglio J, Gabuzda D: Apoptosis induced by HIV-1 infection of the central nervous system, *J Clin Invest* 98:1979–1990, 1996.

222. Qiu J, Whalen MJ, Lowenstein P, Fiskum G, Fahy B, Darwish R, Aarabi B, Yuan J, Moskowitz MA: Upregulation of the Fas receptor death-inducing signaling complex after traumatic brain injury in mice and humans, *J Neurosci* 22:3504–3511, 2002.

223. Smith FM, Raghupathi R, MacKinnon MA, McIntosh TK, Saatman KE, Meaney DF, Graham DI: TUNEL-positive staining of surface contusions after fatal head injury in man, *Acta Neuropathol* 100:537–545, 2000.

224. Williams S, Raghupathi R, MacKinnon MA, McIntosh TK, Saatman KE, Graham DI: In situ DNA fragmentation occurs in white matter up to 12 months after head injury in man, *Acta Neuropathol* 102:581–590, 2001.

8

Molecular Pathophysiology of White Matter Anoxic-Ischemic Injury

BRUCE R. RANSOM, MARK P. GOLDBERG, SELVA BALTAN

Anoxia or ischemia of the mammalian central nervous system (CNS), including the secondary vascular embarrassment that frequently accompanies traumatic brain and spinal cord insults,[1,2] damages both gray and white matter (Fig. 8-1). In fact, about 20% of ischemic strokes involve predominantly white matter, as a result of occlusion of small penetrating arteries that supply the deep areas of the cerebral hemispheres (see Chapter 27).[3] Clinically, damage to white matter can result in serious disability, as seen in stroke, spinal cord and traumatic brain injury, some forms of vascular dementia, and hypoglycemia.[2,4,5] In spite of these facts, how white matter is injured by ischemia has received far less attention than is the case for gray matter. Two reasons are foremost in explanation of this neglect: first, the brain of rodents, which is most often used to study stroke, has far less white matter than the human brain, and second, there is a tendency to think that protection of neuron cell bodies alone is sufficient to rescue stroke-imperiled brain tissue.

Great progress has been made in understanding the pathophysiology of anoxic-ischemic white matter injury in the past decade, and the pace of this work is increasing. Models have been developed that allow white matter to be studied independently of gray matter. Basic knowledge about the ionic and molecular events initiated by ischemia in white matter is spawning testable hypotheses for protecting this unique part of the brain during stroke. Most significant, there is a growing awareness about the importance of this topic in achieving the goal of effective, early treatment of ischemic stroke. In this chapter, we review what is currently known about the cellular and molecular events triggered by anoxia or ischemia in white matter and how these events lead to loss of function and irreversible injury.

White Matter Anatomy and Physiology

White matter of the mammalian CNS consists of the afferent and efferent axonal tracts that interconnect cortical and neuronal cell body–containing nuclear areas of the brain and spinal cord. White matter contains no neuronal cell bodies or synapses. It consists of tightly packed glial cells and myelinated and unmyelinated axons; the presence of myelin lends a white appearance to this tissue. White matter regions vary widely with regard to the ratio of myelinated to unmyelinated axons; for example, all the axons of the optic nerve are myelinated, but only about 30% of those in the corpus callosum are myelinated.[6,7] The anatomy and physiology of myelinated axons are highly specialized and unique compared with those of unmyelinated axons.[8] It is not surprising, therefore, that regional differences have been noted in the pathophysiology of white matter injury.[9-11]

Most axons in cerebral white matter provide connections within cortical regions. These connections include short fiber bundles between adjacent cortical regions (U fibers) and longer axons projecting between contralateral hemispheres (callosal fibers) or distinct brain areas (association fibers). Output or input projections to basal ganglia, brainstem, or spinal cord are only a small proportion of total CNS axons. Because most white matter axons connect cortical regions, the massive growth in cortical area from small lissencephalic animals to animals with larger, gyrencephalic brains is associated with a great and disproportionate expansion in white matter volume (Fig. 8-2). White matter constitutes only a small fraction of forebrain volume in rodents (for mice, approximately 10% white matter; total forebrain volume 125 mm^3) but occupies a large proportion of the human brain (approximately 50%; total volume 1,000,000 mm^3) (see Fig. 8-2).[12] This massive, greater than fourfold expansion in the percent volume of brain occupied by white matter means that the human brain has far more white matter at risk during ischemia. It may also help explain why successful therapies in animal models of stroke have not proved successful in humans.[13]

Although the roles of glial cells in CNS functions continue to evolve,[14,15] it is clear that astrocytes are crucial for ionic homeostasis of brain extracellular space (ECS), glutamate uptake,[16] and synaptogenesis.[14] Astrocytes have a complicated but central role in supporting antioxidant synthesis in the brain.[17] Only astrocytes contain glycogen, and they can provide neurons and axons (and possibly oligodendrocytes) with usable energy substrate in the form of lactate when glucose is restricted.[18] Because

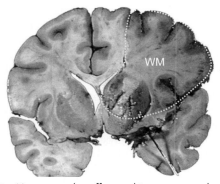

Figure 8-1 Human stroke affects white matter and gray matter. Subacute infarct in vascular distribution of the middle cerebral artery demonstrates damage of a large volume of white matter (WM), including subcortical white matter, centrum semiovale, and internal capsule, as well as gray matter structures such as neocortex and basal ganglia. (Image provided by Dr. Kevin A. Roth.)

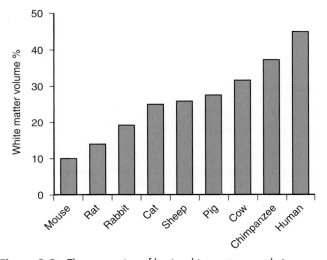

Figure 8-2 The proportion of brain white matter greatly increases as brain size enlarges. *Bars* show the percentage of cerebral hemisphere volume composed of white matter in several mammals, ranging from mouse to human. (Data calculated from Zhang K, Sejnowski TJ: A universal scaling law between gray matter and white matter of cerebral cortex. *Proc Natl Sci U S A* 97:5621–5626, 2000.)

It is essential to understand that an axon's energy metabolism is independent from that of its cell body of origin. Axons extend for great distances from their cell bodies and depend on local production of ATP to maintain ion gradients and sustain energy-consuming functions. This metabolic isolation also means that axons suffer energy deprivation in a manner that is independent of neuron cell bodies. The metabolic rate of white matter is about half that of gray matter on the basis of oxygen consumption.[21] Axons more than glial cells are calculated to contribute to this high metabolic rate.[22] The adult mammalian CNS is generally presumed to fail rapidly in the absence of oxygen. There are little actual data on this question because making an animal anoxic without compromising blood supply is challenging; Tekkök et al,[23] however, have shown that a high percentage of myelinated axons in young adult rodent optic nerve can function anaerobically. This finding implies that some axons in white matter could tolerate prolonged periods of pure anoxia without permanent injury.

Because white matter is less metabolically active than gray matter, it has a lower blood flow per volume of tissue. The blood flow in cerebral white matter averages 30 mL/100 mg per minute compared with 50 mL/100 mg per minute in gray matter. White matter has a much less dense capillary network than gray matter. Much of the cerebral white matter is perfused by penetrating arterioles that originate from larger pial vessels. Deeper regions of the subcortical white matter are supplied by the striate arteries that arise from the circle of Willis. The most important of these are the medial striate arteries, which arise directly from the internal carotid artery and supply much of the internal capsule as it courses through the basal ganglia. As white matter tracts descend through the brainstem, they are perfused by penetrating arteries from the vertebral and basilar arteries or their circumferential branches.

Different regions of white matter have distinct patterns of vascular supply (Fig. 8-3).[24] For example, in the centrum semiovale, the blood supply consists of long arterioles, which are characteristically terminal vessels with few anastomoses; occlusion of one of these vessels results in an area of ischemia that cannot be rescued by blood flow redistribution because there are no anastomotic connections with neighboring vessels. In contrast, the immediately subcortical association bundles (U fibers), corpus callosum, external capsule-claustrum, and extreme capsule are supplied by interdigitating arterioles derived from two or more pial vessels. Dual vascular supply may account for the relative resistance of these white matter areas to damage after anoxia or hypoperfusion.

Model Systems for Studying White Matter Ischemia

Research in white matter anoxia or ischemia requires experimental systems that appropriately model the cell biology and physiology of myelinated axons and glia. Improved understanding of the pathways leading to white matter injury can lead to therapeutic approaches that can be tested in progressively more complex in vitro and in vivo systems and, ultimately, in clinical trials. However,

astrocytes are natural anaerobes and contain glycogen, they are the only cells in the brain that are able to maintain enough adenosine triphosphate (ATP) to function, at least temporarily, during ischemia.[19,20] Oligodendrocytes provide myelin for CNS axons; conduction fails in myelinated axons with injury to oligodendrocytes or their myelin. Ischemia will, of course, eventually affect all the elements in white matter, leading to axon–glial interactions that are important for understanding how injury occurs. These complex cellular interactions during ischemia have just begun to be explored in white matter. For example, microglial cells are thought to produce damaging free radical species during ischemia, and astrocytes are the key cell type capable of defending against free radical–mediated injury.[16] Little is known, however, about these topics as they pertain to anoxic-ischemic injury in white matter.

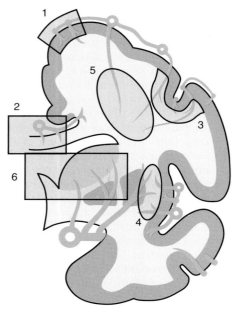

Figure 8-3 Distinct patterns of vascular supply to the supratentorial brain. Regions: *1*, cortex; *2*, corpus callosum; *3*, subcortical U fibers; *4*, external capsule/claustrum/extreme capsule; *5*, centrum semiovale; *6*, basal ganglia and thalamus. Microradiography studies demonstrate much denser capillary beds in gray matter than in white matter structures. The regions of highest vulnerability to anoxic or hypoperfusion damage (cortex, centrum semiovale, basal ganglia, thalamus) are supplied by isolated penetrating arterioles with minimal overlap, whereas more resistant areas (U fibers, external capsule) have interdigitating vessels from two or more arterial supplies. (Redrawn from Moody DM, Bell MA, Challa VR: Features of the cerebral vascular pattern that predict vulnerability to perfusion or oxygenation deficiency: An anatomic study. *AJNR Am J Neuroradiol* 11:431-439, 1990.)

it is important to understand the potential strengths and limitations of each model system and ensure that experiments appropriately examine specific facets of injury and recovery.

Cell Culture

Cell culture models provide the opportunity to examine individual cellular elements of white matter in isolation, separate from the effects of perfusion and vascular supply. Experiments in primary cultures allow assessment of enriched populations of brain cells to effects of energy deprivation, which is typically produced by transient removal of oxygen and glucose. Under these conditions, the relative vulnerabilities of cells, from greatest to least, are approximately as follows: neurons > oligodendrocytes = microglia > endothelial cells > astrocytes.[25-28] Within the oligodendrocyte lineage, immature oligodendrocytes are more vulnerable than slightly more mature cells to energy deprivation.[29] Reasons proposed for the high vulnerability of oligodendrocytes to ischemic damage include their high metabolic demands, poor resistance to oxidative stress, and vulnerability to extracellular glutamate.[30,31]

Cell culture models provide excellent systems for studying the molecular biology, pharmacology, and neurochemistry of ischemic injury, but important limitations must be considered. Most cultured cells are derived from brains of perinatal animals and so may reflect immature phenotypes not found in the adult brain. Relatively few studies of cultured central axons physically isolated from their neuronal cell bodies, as occurs in vivo, have been performed. More important, culture models generally exclude the important cell–cell interactions that characterize intact white matter. It is possible to address some of these concerns because systems for isolating axons are well described[32] and oligodendrocytes selectively myelinate axons in coculture.[33] With the use of such a compartmented chamber system, for example, it was possible to determine that ischemic injury to isolated axons (cell bodies in another compartment) is mediated primarily by influx of Ca^{2+} and Na^+ but is independent of glutamate receptor activation.[34]

In Vitro Tissue Models

Many of the limitations of cell cultures are avoided in models that use immediately isolated, perfused preparations of intact white matter. Considerable progress in understanding white matter injury comes from studies of the isolated rodent optic nerve,[35-40] a CNS white matter tract consisting solely of myelinated axons. Similarly, later studies have examined preparations of other CNS white matter regions, such as isolated spinal cord dorsal column[41] and brain slices, including corpus callosum.[9] These white matter tracts offer several advantages for studying the mechanisms of white matter injury, including the capacity to quantitatively assess axon function with the use of electrophysiology and perform confocal imaging of cellular components.[38,40] Most important, each white matter tract offers intact, three-dimensional interactions between glial cells and axons. The use of different white matter tracts facilitates detection of region-specific differences in the mechanisms of white matter injury.[9,40] Although these preparations are not suitable for studies of long-term outcomes after hypoxic or ischemic injury, the axons remain electrically functional for at least several hours in vitro, which allows assessment of short-term recovery. It is important to emphasize the importance of studying white matter injury at normal body temperature. Brain slices are commonly studied at several degrees below body temperature because they survive better at these cooler temperatures. Anoxic-ischemic injury of white matter, however, is very sensitive to temperature[42]; the degree of injury decreases markedly with cooling. The real pitfall is that lower temperatures alter injury mechanisms, which can lead to false conclusions.[43]

In Vivo Models

Hundreds of studies of focal ischemia in rodent models have been conducted, but the extent of white matter injury has been examined in only a handful (see Pantoni et al[44] and Dietrich et al[45-48]). This situation is, in part, due to the very small proportion of cerebral white matter in mice and rats (see Fig. 8-2); the most common outcome measure—infarct volume—is not significantly altered in such models regardless of whether white matter is injured.

Moreover, middle cerebral artery occlusion (MCAO), the most used model of focal ischemia, consistently spares the corpus callosum, one of the largest white matter tracts in rodents (reviewed by Ginsberg and Busto[49]). Furthermore, a frequently used method of infarct volume assessment in rodent models involves staining with a vital dye, triphenyltetrazolium chloride, which provides little labeling of intact white matter.[50] Careful examination of white matter injury requires special histologic techniques to identify injury of axons, myelin, and glial cells.

Current efforts to injure corpus callosum involve local injections of glutamate analogues,[26,51] demyelinating substances,[52] or vasoconstrictive agents.[53] These models do not mimic ischemia well and can cause confounding tissue injury due to trauma. Primate brain contains about 35% white matter volume and has an MCA perfusion territory closer to that of human brain. For these reasons, model systems of white matter injury based on the primate are attractive for further development.[54,55]

Effects of Ischemia on White Matter

One can monitor white matter function by electrically evoking a compound action potential (CAP) from constituent axons (Fig. 8-4A). Function (i.e., excitability) of CNS white matter fails rapidly during ischemia at 37° C.[9,38–40,56,57] In a completely myelinated white matter tract, the mouse optic nerve, the CAP begins to decline within 5 to 10 minutes of onset of ischemia and virtually disappears after 15 to 20 minutes (see Fig. 8-4B).[38,40] During reoxygenation after ischemia or anoxia, the CAP partially returns to a new stable level within 1 hour. The speed and magnitude of white matter recovery decrease as the duration of ischemia or anoxia increases. Even after 60 minutes of ischemia, however, the mean recovery of function is about 25%.[39,40] This result is interpreted to mean that about 75% of the axons in the tract have been irreversibly injured. Indeed, electron microscopic analysis shows that a majority of axons subjected to 60 minutes of ischemia or anoxia* have severe structural changes.[9,58,59] Large axons are more severely affected than small ones. In vitro experiments indicate that white matter recovers better from a given period of insult than gray matter.[57,60] The implication is that the therapeutic window for rescuing white matter from an ischemic insult is longer than that for gray matter. There are regional differences in the pattern of white matter dysfunction due to ischemia.[60] Ischemia causes a monophasic loss of function in both the optic nerve and the corpus callosum, but the pattern of CAP recovery is more complex in the corpus callosum (Fig. 8-5).[9] In the optic nerve, recovery of excitability is monophasic and stable after 30 to 60 minutes of restored glucose and oxygen.[38,40] The corpus callosum, however, recovers excitability in a multiphasic fashion and shows a late progressive decline (see Fig. 8-5C).[9] This difference provides evidence of differential susceptibility of white matter tracts to injury and suggests the possibility

that different pathologic mechanisms might operate in different regions.

Derangement of Transmembrane Ion Gradients

Rapid changes in brain extracellular ion concentrations occur with deprivation of oxygen, glucose, or both.[61] These changes reflect the metabolic state of local brain tissue[62] and can have direct effects on neural behavior. Elevated extracellular potassium concentration ($[K^+]_o$) depolarizes neuronal membranes, reducing and then blocking action potentials, causes uncontrolled transmitter release,[63] induces cell swelling,[64] and may affect cerebral blood flow.[65] Elevated $[K^+]_o$ does not, in and of itself, reduce electrogenic glial uptake of the excitotoxin glutamate,[66] as was anticipated.[67] Extracellular acidosis can have direct toxic effects on both neuronal and glial membranes,[68,69] alters ion channel function,[70] and blocks currents generated by activation of N-methyl-D-aspartate (NMDA) receptors.[71] In the case of white matter, the extracellular ionic changes produced by anoxia predispose to other ionic events that are critical for injury (see later).

In white matter, anoxia or ischemia causes rapid changes in the extracellular concentrations of K^+ and H^+ that are qualitatively similar to those seen in gray matter but smaller.[61,72,73] Within 3 or 4 minutes of the onset of anoxia, $[K^+]_o$ in the optic nerve begins to increase, reaching a final concentration of about 15 mM from a baseline of 3 mM. No spreading depression-like event occurs in white matter during anoxia, in contrast to most gray matter areas,[61,74] which partially explains why $[K^+]_o$ increases less in white matter than in gray matter.[73,75]

An acid shift in extracellular pH (pH_o) develops during anoxia and has a maximum value of about 0.3 pH units in standard physiologic solution.[73] After anoxia, pH_o returns slowly to its baseline level and exhibits a secondary acidification phase of unknown significance. The acid shifts in pH_o seen in white matter and gray matter during anoxia are probably the consequence of increased anaerobic metabolism leading to accumulation of extracellular lactic acid.[72,73,76] Lactic acid can exit cells by diffusion, in its undissociated form, or by a direct transport mechanism.[77] In vitro studies suggest that during anoxia, glial cells and neurons contain equivalent amounts of intracellular lactate but that glial cells transport more lactic acid to the ECS.[77] Astrocytes, but not neurons, contain glycogen,[18] which is broken down and anaerobically metabolized to lactate during ischemia. Astrocytes may therefore have an important role in producing the acid shift in pH_o seen with anoxia or ischemia.[73] Ischemia causes brain ATP to rapidly decline.[62,78] What is not well publicized is that the ATP decline appears to be significantly slower in white matter than in gray matter.[79] The simple hypothesis for the slower loss of white matter ATP during ischemia is the lower metabolic rate of this tissue compared with gray matter. The implication is that white matter may retain sufficient ATP to prolong the time it can endure ischemia without sustaining irreversible injury. Reduction of ATP causes energy-dependent ion pumps to fail, including the Na^+–K^+ and Ca^{2+}–ATPases, and this failure would affect both axons and

---

*For technical reasons, anoxia is essentially equivalent to ischemia in experiments on the rat optic nerve.[23] In this chapter, therefore, findings from anoxia experiments on rat optic nerve are considered relevant for ischemia.

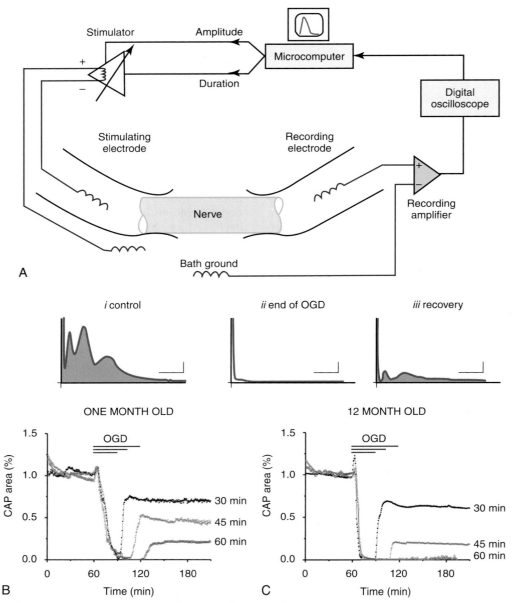

Figure 8-4 Quantifying mouse optic nerve (MON) function before and after ischemia. A, Diagram of recording arrangement. The MON is stimulated with a supramaximal voltage pulse via one suction electrode. The compound action potential (CAP) is recorded from the other end of the nerve with a second suction electrode; signals are amplified, digitized, and transferred to a microcomputer for processing and storage. B, Effects of ischemia on white matter function. The function of the MON was monitored as the area under the CAP (shaded areas). Examples are shown of the CAP before, during, and 60 minutes after ischemia (recovery). Changes in CAP area are shown graphically as percentage of the control CAP integral for young and very mature mice (1 and 12 months old, respectively). Ischemia lasting between 30 and 60 minutes was begun at 60 minutes on the time scale. CAP area rapidly declined, becoming virtually zero after 15 to 20 minutes of ischemia. After oxygen and glucose were reintroduced, CAP area gradually recovered to a mean of about 25% of control for the 60-minute insult and to a greater extent for shorter periods of ischemia. The extent of final injury was significantly worse in very mature, compared to young, animals for insults lasting 45 or 60 minutes. Calibration marks are 1 ms and 1 mV. (Modified from Stys PK, et al: Role of extracellular calcium in anoxic injury of mammalian central white matter. *Proc Natl Acad Sci U S A* 87:4212-4218, 1990; Baltan S, Besancon EF, Mbow B, et al: White matter vulnerability to ischemic injury increases with age because of enhanced excitotoxicity. *J Neurosci* 28:1479-1489, 2008.)

glial cells (see later). As a consequence, ions redistribute down their concentration gradients, which leads to membrane depolarization that activates voltage-gated ion channels. Other K^+ channels may be activated and contribute to the increase in $[K^+]_o$, including Ca^{2+}-dependent K^+ channels, ATP-dependent K^+ channels, and Na^+-dependent K^+ channels.[61,80] Anoxia or ischemia causes the volume of the

ECS of the rat optic nerve to decrease by as much as 20%,[81] probably because of glial swelling triggered by increases in $[K^+]_o$.[64] In animal experiments, gray matter appears to suffer more damage when ischemia occurs in the presence of higher-than-usual glucose concentrations.[82,83] It is not known whether this observation is also true for white matter. During anoxia, however, white matter is

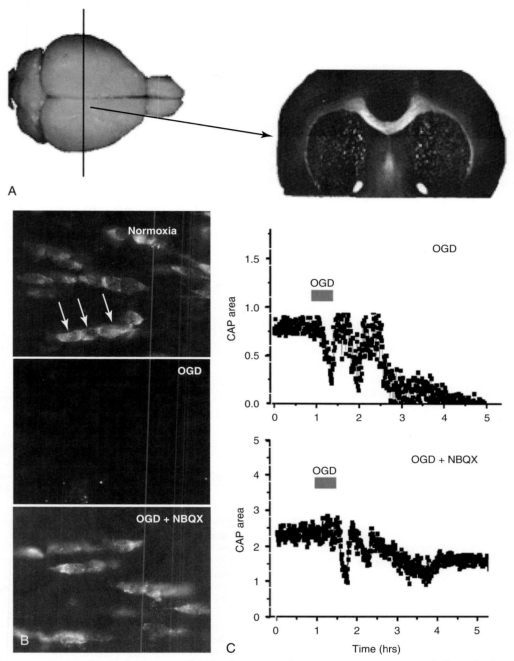

Figure 8-5 Glutamate receptor blockade protects oligodendrocytes and axons in an in vitro model of cerebral white matter injury. A, Acute coronal brain slices, 400 μM in thickness, are derived from adult mice. The slice includes subcortical white matter and intact corpus callosum. B, Immunofluorescence microscopy identifies oligodendrocyte cell bodies in the corpus callosum. Under normoxic perfusion conditions *(top panel)*, oligodendrocytes remain intact *(arrows)* for several hours. Oligodendrocytes die within 2 hours after exposure to oxygen and glucose deprivation (OGD) for 30 minutes *(middle panel)* but are preserved in OGD performed with the addition of a glutamate antagonist, NBQX *(bottom panel)*, which selectively inhibits the α-amino-3-hydroxy-5-methyl-4-isoxazole-propionic acid (AMPA) and kainate subtypes of glutamate receptors. C, Transient OGD disrupts axonal conduction in white matter, as demonstrated by loss of the stimulus-evoked compound action potential (CAP) recorded across the corpus callosum *(top)*. Addition of NBQX preserves the CAP *(bottom)* and prevents disruption of axonal morphology (not shown). These results suggest that glutamate receptor-mediated glial injury may contribute to axon damage under hypoxic-ischemic conditions. (Modified from Tekkök SB, Goldberg MP: AMPA/kainate receptor activation mediates hypoxic oligodendrocyte death and axonal injury in cerebral white matter. *J Neurosci* 21:4237-4248, 2001.)

functionally protected by elevated bath glucose,[73] even though it causes a greater extracellular acid shift, which is believed to worsen stroke outcomes.[84] Curiously, in vitro studies, in contrast to in vivo studies, indicate that gray matter and white matter are both protected from anoxic injury by elevated glucose concentrations.[73,85]

The Ca^{2+} Hypothesis and Anoxic-Ischemic White Matter Injury

The calcium hypothesis holds that unregulated increases in intracellular calcium concentration ($[Ca^{2+}]_i$) represent a "final common pathway" for cellular damage.[62,86] This hypothesis appears to be true in the case of white matter ischemic or anoxic injury, but not all the details are yet understood. In general, ischemia causes $[Ca^{2+}]_i$ to increase in axons within minutes of insult onset (see Nikolaeva et al[87]). Intracellular Ca^{2+} accumulation is the result of Ca^{2+} influx from the ECS and from Ca^{2+} release from intracellular stores. The relative importance of these two mechanisms appears to vary depending on animal age and possibly also on white matter region. The calcium hypothesis probably also applies to white matter glial cells, especially astrocytes and oligodendrocytes, but little is known about this.

Representative data indicating that extracellular Ca^{2+} is necessary for white matter injury in young adult animals are shown in Figure 8-6A.[38] White matter is severely injured by 60 minutes of ischemia (i.e., zero glucose and zero oxygen); about 80% of the axons are irreversibly damaged. In contrast, CAP area recovers to 100% of control after 60 minutes of ischemia when the insult is delivered during perfusion with zero $[Ca^{2+}]$ solution (see Fig. 8-6A). This recovery is stable for several hours, which indicates that the tissue is completely protected from an hour of total ischemia in the absence of extracellular Ca^{2+}. In young adult mice this effect is graded, and even modest reductions in $[Ca^{2+}]_o$ (i.e., 2 mM to 0.5 mM) during anoxia provide some benefit.[35] Anoxic-ischemic injury in other white matter preparations, specifically corpus callosum and spinal cord dorsal column, has similar dependencies on extracellular Ca^{2+}.[9,88] These findings indicate that in young adult animals the presence of extracellular Ca^{2+} is critical for the development of irreversible ischemic injury in white matter and suggest that the severity of injury is related to the transmembrane Ca^{2+} gradient. Extracellular Ca^{2+}, therefore, probably acts as a source for inward flux of Ca^{2+} into a cytoplasmic compartment. This is supported by the observation that $[Ca^{2+}]_o$ falls during anoxia and has a time course that fits well with the development of irreversible injury.[89]

Because white matter axons become dysfunctional during ischemia, on the basis of the loss of the CAP, a damaging increase in intraaxonal $[Ca^{2+}]$ seems likely. Indeed, 60 minutes of anoxia causes striking pathologic alterations within rat optic nerve axons.[58] Large vacuolar spaces appear between axons and their myelin sheaths, axoplasmic mitochondria are swollen and disrupted, and neurofilaments and microtubules disappear from the axoplasm (Fig. 8-7). Strengthening the argument that such changes are due to toxic increases in $[Ca^{2+}]_i$ is the observation that peripheral axons show similar ultrastructural abnormalities after a drug-induced increase in $[Ca^{2+}]_i$.[90] These changes are most prominent in large axons. Paranodal

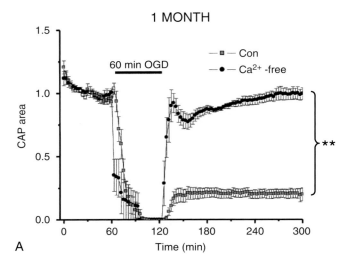

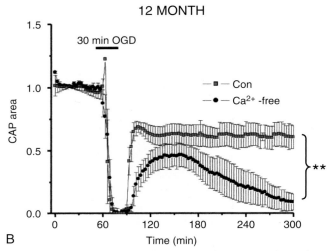

Figure 8-6 Ischemia-induced injury in white matter depends on the presence of extracellular Ca^{2+} in young adult animals but the situation is more complicated in older animals. Mouse optic nerves (MONs) were exposed to oxygen and glucose deprivation (OGD) in normal artificial cerebrospinal fluid (ACSF) (containing 2 mM Ca^{2+}) or in ACSF with no Ca^{2+} (plus 200 μM EGTA). Superfusion conditions were maintained starting 30 minutes before, during, and 30 minutes after OGD. A, Pretreatment with Ca^{2+}-free ACSF offered nearly complete recovery from 60 minutes OGD injury in 1-month-old MONs (95.6 ± 4.3%; n = 6). B, The compound action potential (CAP) area recovery in 12-month-old MONs failed to show improvement over control recovery when OGD was applied in the absence of Ca^{2+}. (From Tekkök S, Ye Z, Ransom BR: Excitotoxic mechanisms of ischemic injury in myelinated white matter. *J Cereb Blood Flow Metab* 27:1540-1552, 2007; and from Baltan S, Besancon EF, Mbow B, et al: White matter vulnerability to ischemic injury increases with age because of enhanced excitotoxicity. *J Neurosci* 28:1479-1489, 2008.)

myelin retracts from the node in some fibers, which is a change that may adversely affect saltatory conduction (see Fig. 8-7B, *arrow*). Although some of the ultrastructural changes seen after 60 minutes of anoxia can partially recover after 60 minutes of reoxygenation, neurofilament and microtubule damage persists. There is a partial restitution in many fibers of the normal relation between axon membrane and paranodal myelin, which might represent the ultrastructural substrate for some of the postanoxic

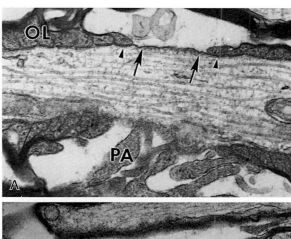

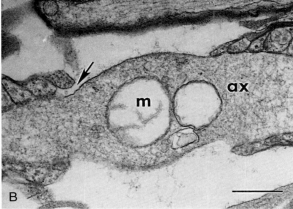

Figure 8-7 Electron micrographs showing ultrastructural changes at nodes of Ranvier in the anoxic optic nerve. A, In the control optic nerve, note the close opposition of terminating oligodendroglial loops *(OL)* to the axon in the paranode *(arrowheads)* and the dense undercoating of the normal axon membrane *(arrows)*. Perinodal astrocyte processes *(PA)* approach the node. The axoplasm contains a dense network of microtubules. B, In the anoxic optic nerve, there is occasional detachment of terminal myelin loops from the axon *(arrow)*. Mitochondria are swollen with distorted cristae *(m)*. There is destruction of microtubules within the axoplasm *(ax)*. A and B, ×40,000; *bar,* 0.5 microns. (Modified from Waxman SG, Black JA, Stys PK, et al: Ultrastructural concomitants of anoxic injury and early post-anoxic recovery in rat optic nerve. *Brain Res* 574:105-119, 1992.)

recovery that is measured as a partial return of the CAP (see Fig. 8-4B). We must emphasize, however, that the return of the CAP to a new steady level after anoxia is likely to be a multifactorial process and certainly involves the reestablishment of critical transmembrane ion gradients that are the basis of axonal excitability.[91]

If the nerve is exposed to anoxia in the absence of bath Ca^{2+}, the ultrastructural abnormalities previously described are not seen.[92] The correlation, therefore, between changes in axonal structure and changes in axonal function (i.e., CAP area) is excellent in young animals; in the presence of normal extracellular Ca^{2+}, anoxia disrupts both axonal structure and function, whereas in the absence of extracellular Ca^{2+}, anoxia does not produce long-term disruption of either. These ultrastructural observations were made on young adult optic nerves that suffered anoxia, not ischemia. While these observations are undoubtedly relevant to the pathophysiology of true ischemia, further ultrastructural studies are needed to verify this.

In young adult animals, the available evidence points to the conclusion that during anoxia, and probably ischemia as well, Ca^{2+} rushes into axonal cytoplasm—probably at the nodes of Ranvier, where the axon membrane is most exposed—leading to the loss of normal architecture and excitability.

In older adult animals, ischemia is more damaging, and the role of $[Ca^{2+}]_o$ in mediating injury is less certain (see Figs. 8-4B and 8-6B).[38] For a given period of ischemia, the extent of irreversible ischemic injury can be 50% greater in 12-month-old compared with 1-month-old animals.[38] In other words, white matter in older animals is intrinsically more susceptible to ischemic injury, completely independent of vascular factors such as vessel patency. In addition, the mechanisms of injury differ between young and old animals (see further on). These facts make two emphatic points: (1) animal age is a crucial variable in preclinical studies of stroke pathophysiology, and (2) it is likely that studies on older animals are most relevant in attempting to understand the cellular mechanisms of human ischemic stroke, a disease whose incidence increases greatly with age.

In 12-month-old mice, removal of extracellular Ca^{2+} during ischemia does not protect white matter from irreversible loss of function (see Fig. 8-6B).[38] After the insult in Ca^{2+}-free solution, the CAP makes a partial recovery and then deteriorates slowly over the next 2 hours. In spinal cord dorsal column, Ca^{2+}-free solution also fails to protect against ischemic injury.[93] A number of studies have directly measured axonal $[Ca^{2+}]_i$ and found it to increase with ischemia, even in Ca^{2+}-free extracellular solution.[87,93,94] As suggested by this finding, ischemia also causes intracellular Ca^{2+} release (see further on).

Ischemia also affects glial cells and myelin in white matter in a manner that can be Ca^{2+}-dependent.[9,88] In corpus callosum and dorsal column, oligodendrocytes and myelin are severely damaged according to histopathologic studies.[9,88] In general, the level of astrocyte injury seems relatively minor for the durations of ischemia that have been evaluated. This finding probably reflects the ability of astrocytes to anaerobically manufacture ATP from their glycogen stores for tens of minutes during ischemia.[18,19]

Mechanisms of White Matter Injury

Ca^{2+} Entry and Intracellular Ca^{2+} Release in Axons during Ischemia

The importance of Ca^{2+} influx in mediating anoxic-ischemic damage in neuron cell bodies[95] and axons[89] is well established, but in the case of white matter, Ca^{2+} influx appears to be a predominant mechanism only in younger animals.[38] As will become clear, however, it is difficult to judge the relative importance of a specific pathologic mechanism when it operates in parallel with other pathologic processes. In gray matter, where synapses abound, the predominant mechanism for Ca^{2+} entry into neurons is through NMDA-type glutamate receptors. White matter has no conventional synapses and appears to be resistant to prolonged application of high concentrations of glutamate[38,96] (but see Li et al[97]), which would quickly kill neuron cell bodies. However, the story of how white matter is disabled by ischemia has turned out to be more complicated and interesting than anticipated. Some early presumptions about white matter injury, most prominently that glutamate is not involved, have proved incorrect. There are still many unanswered questions about how white matter is injured, and the current model of ischemia-induced white matter injury will undoubtedly require major modifications. At present, there is good evidence that ischemia injures both axons and glial cells in white matter and does so by very different mechanisms. With this in mind, we discuss axon and glial injuries separately. The ionic mechanisms that mediate pathologic increases of $[Ca^{2+}]_i$ in axons during ischemia or anoxia are (1) reverse operation of the Na^+-Ca^{2+} exchanger, a ubiquitous (with the exception of red blood cells) membrane protein that normally operates to extrude cytoplasmic Ca^{2+} in exchange for Na^+ influx, (2) voltage-gated Ca^{2+} channels, and (3) Ca^{2+} release from intracellular stores.

Reversal of Na+–Ca2+ Exchange

The Na^+-Ca^{2+} exchanger does not consume ATP and is driven primarily by the transmembrane Na^+ gradient. The exchanger can function equally well in forward and reverse directions and is a high-capacity, relatively low-affinity transporter of Ca^{2+}.[98] The typical stoichiometry of this process is that three Na^+ ions exchange for each Ca^{2+} ion; this exchange ratio causes the process to be electrogenic, and in fact, membrane current is generated by its operation.[99] For this reason, the exchanger is also influenced by membrane potential[100]; membrane depolarization favors reverse exchange (i.e., Na^+ efflux and Ca^{2+} influx). The manner in which $[Ca^{2+}]_i$ can be modulated by changes in the transmembrane Na^+ gradient, membrane potential, or both can be calculated.[10] It is important to note that relatively small changes in $[Na^+]_i$ (intracellular $[Na^+]$) or membrane potential can markedly alter $[Ca^{2+}]_i$. Specifically, increases in $[Na^+]_i$ and membrane depolarization lead to large increases in $[Ca^{2+}]_i$.

The hypothesized sequence of events leading to ischemic injury of white matter axons is as follows. Ischemia causes a rapid drop in ATP with an increase in $[K^+]_o$ (see earlier), resulting in axonal depolarization. Na^+ influx through voltage-dependent Na^+ channels would lead to an increase in $[Na^+]_i$ because the Na^+ pump function would be impaired.[101,102] Both membrane depolarization and the increase in $[Na^+]_i$ favor reverse operation of the Na^+-Ca^{2+} exchanger, which would continue until a higher, steady-state $[Ca^{2+}]_i$ is reached. If reversal of Na^+-Ca^{2+} exchange mediates Ca^{2+} loading during ischemia in white matter, blocking the exchanger during ischemia should improve the outcome—and it does in young adult animals.[10,38] Inhibitors of this transporter (e.g., bepridil or KB-R 7943) markedly improve postischemic recovery. Additional proof that reverse operation of the Na^+-Ca^{2+} exchanger causes damaging Ca^{2+} influx into axons, at least during anoxia, is that the extent of $[Ca^{2+}]_o$ drop seen during anoxia is diminished by exchange inhibitors.[89] It follows from the preceding sequence that increases in $[Na^+]_i$ strongly propel reverse Na^+-Ca^{2+} exchange. Axons accumulate net amounts of Na^+ during disruption of energy metabolism as a result of activation of voltage dependent Na^+ channels (myelinated axons possess extremely high densities [$>10^3$/ mm^2] of nodal Na^+ channels).[8] Blocking Na^+ channels with tetrodotoxin (TTX) or removing Na^+ during the insult

significantly improves CAP recovery after anoxia.[103] In the optic nerve, entry of Na^+ during anoxia continues throughout the entire period of exposure.[10] Conventional Na^+ channels quickly inactivate with depolarization and would not be available to mediate persistent Na^+ influx. Some Na^+ channels, however, inactivate slowly or not at all.[104] Noninactivating Na^+ channels are present in optic nerve axons[103] and contribute to the pathologic Na^+ influx that leads to axonal dysfunction in white matter. Curiously, TTX fails to block CAP recovery after ischemia in mouse corpus callosum,[9] perhaps because of differences in the types of Na^+ channels expressed in these two white matter tracts.

Activation of Voltage-Gated Ca2+ Channels

Voltage-gated Ca^{2+} channels are known to participate in some models of energy-disruption injury.[105] Calcium channel blockers reduce the extent of this injury, presumably by preventing damaging influx of Ca^{2+} into neurons that are depolarized because of anoxia or ischemia.[105,106] Studies have clearly established that L-type Ca^{2+} channels are present on CNS myelinated axons[89] and mediate toxic Ca^{2+} influx during anoxia in CNS white matter.[89,107] Blockers of L-type Ca^{2+} channels applied during anoxia or ischemia improve functional recovery. L-type Ca^{2+} channels are also present on white matter astrocytes.[89] Astrocytes, however, continue to produce ATP during brief periods of anoxia or ischemia (see earlier discussion) and would not depolarize to the extent necessary to activate high threshold Ca^{2+} channels.

Reverse operation of the Na^+-Ca^{2+} exchanger and activation of Ca^{2+} channels may act in parallel to allow entry of Ca^{2+} into axons during anoxia or ischemia. Alternatively, Ca^{2+} influx may be initiated through Ca^{2+} channels, which leads to an increase in $[Ca^{2+}]_i$ that subsequently triggers reverse Na^+-Ca^{2+} exchange. For unclear reasons, higher-than-normal $[Ca^{2+}]_i$ is a necessary precondition for reversal of Na^+-Ca^{2+} exchange.[108] Axonal Ca^{2+} channels, therefore, might act to "kick-start" the phase of Ca^{2+} accumulation mediated by the Na^+-Ca^{2+} exchanger.

A summary diagram of how ischemia leads to Ca^{2+} accumulation in white matter axons is shown in Figure 8-8. In the presence of oxygen and glucose, sufficient ATP is generated to operate the Na^+ pump. The Na^+ pump maintains a low $[Na^+]_i$ and prevents large increases in $[Na^+]_i$ with nerve action potentials.[102] It is also responsible for the axon's high negative resting membrane potential. These two conditions—normal transmembrane Na^+ gradient and negative membrane potential—dictate that the Na^+-Ca^{2+} exchanger operates in the "forward" mode, extruding Ca^{2+} (see Fig. 8-8A). In the absence of oxygen and glucose, ATP drops sharply in 2 to 3 minutes. The Na^+ pump, which consumes about half of all the energy used in neurons,[101] is no longer able to maintain transmembrane gradients of K^+ and Na^+. Increases in $[Na^+]_i$ secondary to influx through Na^+ channels can no longer be corrected.[102] Myelinated axons may be especially susceptible to this cascade of events because their very high densities of Na^+ channels at nodes of Ranvier would predispose to large focal increases in $[Na^+]_i$. Increases in $[K^+]_o$ cause membrane depolarization and opening of noninactivating, voltage-dependent Na^+ channels[35] that elevate $[Na^+]_i$. Ca^{2+} channels would be open persistently under these conditions, and the resulting

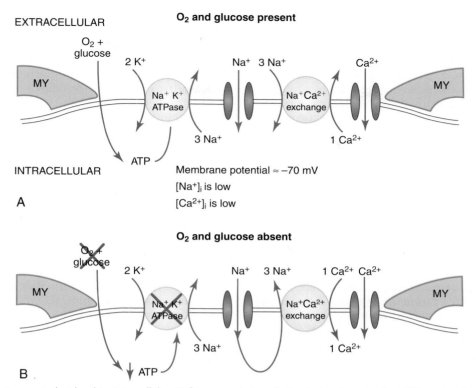

Figure 8-8 Key ionic events that lead to intracellular Ca^{2+} accumulation during ischemia at nodes of Ranvier of central nervous system axons. A, Under normal conditions, sufficient oxygen and glucose are present to generate enough adenosine triphosphate (ATP) to operate the necessary ion pumps for maintaining excitability. If $[Na^+]_i$ increases because of action potentials, this increase is easily compensated by enhanced Na^+ pump activity. The steep Na^+ gradient produced by the Na^+ pump in conjunction with high negative membrane potential drives the high-capacity Na^+–Ca^{2+} exchanger in the forward direction, helping to maintain low $[Ca^{2+}]_i$. There is reason to believe that both the Na^+ pump and the Na^+–Ca^{2+} exchanger might be preferentially located at the nodes because that is where activity-dependent ion fluxes occur in myelinated axons. Voltage-gated Ca^{2+} channels are also present but are not necessary for generation of action potentials. B, In the absence of oxygen and glucose, the generation of ATP is seriously reduced because it is now coming exclusively from glycolysis. The shortfall of ATP causes ion gradients to deteriorate, and the speed of deterioration is augmented by voltage-gated Na^+ channels, some of which are noninactivating, increasing the workload on the Na^+ pump. As the transmembrane Na^+ gradient falls and the membrane depolarizes, the Na^+–Ca^{2+} exchanger is driven to work in reverse and begins loading the axon with Ca^{2+}. Ca^{2+} also enters the axon by way of voltage-gated Ca^{2+} channels. The ultimate destruction of cellular integrity is probably mediated by Ca^{2+}-activated destructive enzymes, such as proteases and lipases, and the generation of free radicals. (Modified from Ransom BR, Stys PK, Waxman SG: Anoxic injury of central myelinated axons: Ionic mechanisms and pharmacology. In Waxman SG, editor: *Molecular and cellular approaches to the treatment of brain disease*, New York, 1993, Raven Press, pp 121-151.)

Ca^{2+} influx would lead to elevation of $[Ca^{2+}]_i$. The progressive deterioration of membrane potential and transmembrane Na^+ gradient, along with an increase in $[Ca^{2+}]_i$, causes reverse operation of the Na^+–Ca^{2+} exchanger, leading to a rapid rise in $[Ca^{2+}]_i$.[98] (see Fig. 8-8). This summary highlights the ionic disruptions that lead to increased $[Ca^{2+}]_i$ and ultimately to irreversible damage.[86] The downstream events promoted by increased $[Ca^{2+}]_i$ that are the ultimate cause of cell death[62,109,110] have yet to be defined in white matter. They are likely to include a set of biochemical reactions mediated by enzymes such as proteases and lipases, as well as the generation of free radicals.[111]

Activation of Intracellular Ca^{2+} Release

Axons exposed to ischemia show rapid increases in $[Ca^{2+}]_i$.[87,93] A significant portion of this increase occurs in the absence of extracellular Ca^{2+} and has been linked to Ca^{2+} release from intracellular stores, specifically from axonal endoplasmic reticulum (ER) and possibly also mitochondria.[93,94] The mechanisms of intracellular Ca^{2+} release during ischemia have proved complex. Axon depolarization can lead to activation of L-type Ca^{2+} channels[89] coupled to ryanodine receptors, leading to Ca^{2+} release from axonal ER.[93] Other pathways may also operate, including Ca^{2+} activation of second messenger cascades leading to nitric oxide formation and release of Ca^{2+} from mitochondria.[94] Pharmacologic blockade of these several pathways during ischemia improves functional outcome. Given the powerful effect that age has on ischemic injury mechanisms and outcomes in the rodent optic nerve,[38] it will be important to explore intracellular Ca^{2+} release mechanisms in older animals.

Excitotoxic Pathways Injure Glia in White Matter

Release of endogenous glutamate and activation of neuronal glutamate receptors (*excitotoxicity*) is a major pathway leading to gray matter injury in ischemic stroke.

Excitotoxicity was not expected to contribute to white matter injury because white matter lacks synapses and is devoid of the usual excitotoxic targets, neuronal cell bodies, and dendrites; however, this logic proved wrong.[13] During ischemia, glutamate is released in abundance from white matter[40] and mediates irreversible white matter injury, probably by activation of glutamate receptors on oligodendrocytes and their compacted membrane extensions, myelin.

Like neurons, astrocytes and oligodendrocytes express functionally active α-amino-3-hydroxy-5-methyl-4-isoxazole-propionic acid (AMPA) and kainate (KA) glutamate receptor subunits.[112-114] More recently, NMDA-type glutamate receptors were found on white matter oligodendrocytes during development[115-117] and in more mature animals.[38] The physiologic significance of these different glutamate receptors remains to be established. In culture, oligodendrocyte lineage cells are highly vulnerable to glutamate excitotoxicity, and they can be rescued from hypoxic injury by glutamate receptor blockade.[26,29,114,118]

These in vitro studies raised the hypothesis that activation of AMPA/KA receptors contributes to hypoxic-ischemic death of oligodendrocytes in vivo and, in so doing, is a crucial step in white matter injury. However, cultured oligodendrocytes differ from their in vivo counterparts in several important respects, including maturational state, receptor expression, and axonal–glial cellular interactions. Subsequent studies have confirmed a role for glutamate-mediated injury to oligodendrocytes in intact tissue preparations from mature white matter, including corpus callosum slices (see Fig. 8-5),[9] spinal cord white matter,[41] and mouse optic nerve.[38,40] In fact, the more severe ischemic injury seen in older animals is attributable to more intense excitotoxicity, related in part to earlier and more robust glutamate release.[38] Potential nonsynaptic sources for toxic glutamate release within ischemic white matter are axons,[41] astrocytes,[119,120] and oligodendrocytes.[29] While this question remains open, it is our opinion that astrocytes are the more probable source of glutamate. The release is mediated by reverse Na$^+$-dependent glutamate transport, and astrocytes are the cells with the highest density of these transporters.[38,40]

AMPA/KA-type glutamate receptors predominately mediate white matter excitotoxicity, but there is some variability in the subtype that is most important in different white matter regions.[38,121-124] Although NMDA receptors exist on oligodendrocytes, these receptors do not appear to participate in white matter injury in adult animals (e.g., see Baltan et al[38]), whereas they may do so during development.[116] In several experimental situations, AMPA/KA receptor blockade has been shown to protect axons as well as glial cells (e.g., see Tekkök and Goldberg[9]). Axons were not suspected of expressing functional glutamate receptors until recently[94] (see also Brand-Schieber and Werner[125]); still it seems likely that axonal protection associated with glutamate receptor blockade is mediated indirectly, through actions on associated glia.[9] These results support the hypothesis that glial cell injury mediated by glutamate and axon injury mediated by ion channels, ion exchangers, and intracellular Ca^{2+} release are parallel pathways that interact, in currently unknown ways, to enhance white matter

vulnerability to energy failure (Fig. 8-9). It is too early to conclude that this scheme applies to white matter everywhere in the brain. In fact, we predict that this will not be the case. It is logical to think that myelinated fibers would be more susceptible than unmyelinated fibers to failure and, perhaps, injury after oligodendrocyte and myelin damage, but this theory has not been critically tested. In addition, what about the comparative time courses of these parallel pathways? In other words, does one proceed more quickly than the other? Answers to these questions will be important in the development of therapeutic interventions.

Autoprotection in White Matter

Nerve fiber tracts in the CNS do not contain synapses, but they do contain neurotransmitters and their cognate receptors. In addition to glutamate and glutamate receptors (see earlier discussion), white matter contains the neurotransmitters γ-aminobutyric acid (GABA)[126] and adenosine[79] and their receptors.[127] Although the normal physiologic functions of GABA or adenosine in white matter are not known, both substances appear in extracellular fluid during ischemia.[126,128] Both GABA and adenosine, at very low concentrations, attenuate the severity of anoxia-induced white matter injury and therefore constitute a unique autoprotective system for this tissue.[129,130]

The effect of GABA on the extent of CAP recovery from a standard 60-minute period of anoxia is shown in Figure 8-10.[130] Application of GABA (1 mM) to the optic nerve during anoxia significantly enhances improvement. The beneficial effect of GABA was mediated by GABA-B-type receptors; thus, GABA-induced protection was duplicated by the selective GABA-B agonist baclofen and blocked by the GABA-B antagonist phaclofen. High concentrations of GABA or baclofen did not afford protection, probably because of receptor desensitization.[129] The GABA-B receptor blocker phaclofen significantly worsened outcomes from anoxia. This implied that GABA was being released from endogenous stores and was providing a protective action in the absence of bath application.[129] GABA-B receptors are known to act through G-proteins, and G-protein antagonists blocked the protective effect of GABA against anoxic injury.[129] The second messenger sequence of GABA's action was followed one step further and found to involve protein kinase C (PKC). Direct activation of PKC, in the absence of added GABA, mimicked the action of GABA, which is to say it was significantly protective.[129] Blockade of PKC prevented expression of GABA's protective action.

These findings suggest the following scheme. During ischemia-anoxia in white matter, GABA is released into the ECS, presumably from endogenous stores. The cellular origin of GABA under these conditions has not been determined, but glial cells contain GABA and have the capacity to release it if the ionic gradients that sustain uptake are degraded, as they would be during ischemia.[129] Once released, GABA acts at GABA-B receptors and through a G-protein/PKC pathway to partially protect the optic nerve from ischemia-induced injury. The protection is believed to be a result of the phosphorylation by

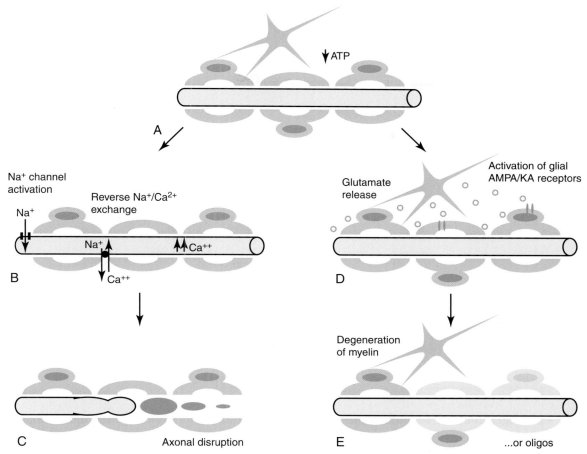

Figure 8-9 Proposed axon and glial injury pathways in hypoxic-ischemic white matter injury. Schematic shows myelinated axon, oligodendrocytes (attached to myelin), and astrocytes *(star-shaped)*. A, Hypoxia, ischemia, or glucose deprivation results in energy depletion and loss of adenosine triphosphate (ATP). B, Failure of Na/K-ATPase and depolarization leads to opening of noninactivating axon voltage-gated Na^+ channels. Ca^{2+} enters axons by reversal of Na–Ca exchange and activation of voltage-gated Ca^{2+} channels. Action potentials are halted reversibly by loss of ionic gradients. C, Excessive axoplasmic Ca^{2+} levels trigger destructive pathways, leading to degradation of axonal cytoskeleton and organelles, focal axonal swelling, and eventual interruption of axonal integrity. D, Another effect of energy deprivation is release of glutamate into the extracellular space from axons, astrocytes, and/or oligodendrocytes. Glutamate activates ionotropic AMPA/KA (α-amino-3-hydroxy-5-methyl-4-isoxazole-propionic acid/kainate) receptors on glial cells. E, Sustained glutamate receptor activation triggers excitotoxic damage of oligodendrocyte processes (myelin) and death of oligodendrocytes. Myelin damage might result in conduction delay or block. (From Tekkök SB, Goldberg MP: AMPA/kainate receptor activation mediates hypoxic oligodendrocyte death and axonal injury in cerebral white matter. *J Neurosci* 21:4237-4248, 2001.)

PKC of a critical protein within axons, but currently this target is not known. Phosphorylation and downregulation of the Na^+–Ca^{2+} exchanger would be one possibility. Curtailing the conductance of noninactivating Na^+ channels or voltage-gated Ca^{2+} channels are other possibilities that could serve to lessen the impact of a period of ischemia or anoxia.

Adenosine acts at specific receptors within white matter to reduce the extent of CAP loss associated with anoxic exposure and, in this way, closely mimics the behavior of GABA previously described.[129] In fact, GABA and adenosine act synergistically to protect white matter via the same G-protein/PKC pathway. Both are believed to be released at nanomolar concentrations during anoxia to recruit the "autoprotection" mechanism.[129] The extent to which this novel aspect of the pathophysiology of white matter damage can be pharmacologically manipulated remains to be investigated.

Strategies for Protecting White Matter from Anoxic-Ischemic Injury Are Diverse

The clinical importance and the pathophysiologic uniqueness of white matter ischemic injury have never seemed more obvious. The complexity of the injury process in white matter presents many potential strategies for therapeutic intervention. These injury cascades have not been completely explored, especially in older animals, but experiments with isolated white matter have shown that inhibitors of voltage-gated Na^+ channels, voltage-gated Ca^{2+} channels, the Na^+–Ca^{2+} exchanger, intracellular Ca^{2+} release, and AMPA/KA receptors are all protective against anoxic-ischemic injury.[9,38,89,93,103,131] Potentiation of the GABA–adenosine autoprotective system is also protective in isolated white matter.[129,130] These pharmacologic manipulations act to block events that occur relatively early in the injury cascade. For example,

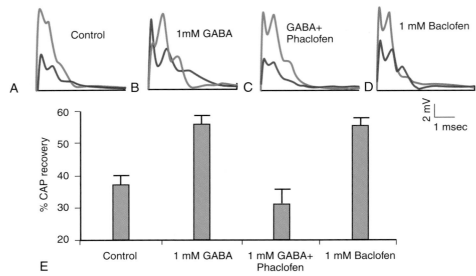

Figure 8-10 The inhibitory neurotransmitter γ-aminobutyric acid (GABA) acts at low concentrations to protect rat optic nerve axons from anoxia-induced damage. Superimposed preanoxic (green) and postanoxic (red) compound action potentials (CAPs) measured under control conditions and in the presence of various agents are shown along with a graphic summary of these results. A, Under control conditions, the mean postanoxic CAP recovery is 36.5 ± 2.9%. B, GABA at 1 mM significantly increased recovery to a mean of 55.7 ± 2.5%. C, The selective GABA-B antagonist phaclofen (500mM) blocked GABA's protective effect against anoxic injury. D, The selective GABA-B agonist baclofen (1 mM) protected against anoxic injury. E, Summarized results from numerous experiments like those shown in A through D. (Modified from Fern R, Waxman SG, Ransom BR: Endogenous GABA attenuates CNS white matter dysfunction after anoxia. *J Neurosci* 15:699-708, 1995.)

the Na⁺–Ca²⁺ exchanger inhibitor bepridil is protective because it prevents Ca^{2+} influx during anoxia, eliminating the downstream events that follow from high intracellular Ca^{2+}, such as the activation of destructive enzymes. In one sense this is advantageous because interrupting the chain of events during the early stages represents the best opportunity for complete arrest of the injury process. The disadvantage of these drugs is that they must be present either before or immediately after the onset of an anoxic-ischemic event if they are to have a significantly protective effect. Therefore, identification of high-risk patients for long-term treatment with prophylactic concentrations of drugs may represent the most effective way of reducing white matter ischemic injuries such as lacunar infarcts. To be justified for use in this preemptive way, such drugs would have to be very well tolerated and have few side effects.

The utility of a therapeutic strategy will therefore be governed by both its efficacy and the extent to which it is tolerated by patients. Within these constraints, two types of intervention seem most promising. A number of drugs currently in clinical use for other conditions have been shown to protect white matter from anoxic-ischemic injury as a result of blocking Na⁺ channels. They include antiarrhythmic drugs such as prajmaline and mexiletine[132,133] and the antiepileptic drugs phenytoin and carbamazepine.[134] Some of these drugs have been shown to protect isolated white matter from injury at concentrations below those in current clinical use. For example, phenytoin improves recovery from a 60-minute period of anoxia by about 80% at 1 μM, a concentration below that found in the cerebrospinal fluid of patients taking phenytoin to treat epilepsy.[134]

Drugs that interfere with GABA uptake and degradation represent a second way of interrupting the injury cascade with minimal side effects. These drugs, which include vigabatrin and gabapentin, have been developed to treat epilepsy and act by increasing the extracellular concentration of GABA.[135] Raising extracellular GABA levels is protective against anoxic injury in white matter,[129,130] which suggests a secondary use for these drugs in white matter ischemia. The relatively benign side effects of drugs such as gabapentin suggest that long-term treatment in patients at high risk of white matter injury may be possible.

Acknowledgments

Work in the authors' laboratories has been supported in part by grants from the National Institutes of Health (BRR, SB, MPG), Eastern Paralyzed Veterans Association (BRR), American Heart Association (MPG, SB), and the Juvenile Diabetes Research Foundation (MPG). Selva Baltan has published previously as Selva Tekkok.

REFERENCES

1. Young W: Blood flow, metabolic and neurophysiological mechanisms in spinal cord injury. In Becker D, Povlishock JT, editors: *Central nervous system trauma status report*, Bethesda, Md, 1985, NIH, NINCDS, p 463.
2. Loizou LA, Kendall BE, Marshall J: Subcortical arteriosclerotic encephalopathy: A clinical and radiological investigation, *J Neurol Neurosurg Psychiatry* 44(4):294–304, 1981.
3. Fisher CM: Capsular infarcts: the underlying vascular lesions, *Arch Neurol* 36(2):65–73, 1979.
4. McQuinn BA, O'Leary DH: White matter lucencies on computed tomography, subacute arteriosclerotic encephalopathy (Binswanger's disease), and blood pressure, *Stroke* 18(5): 900–905, 1987.

5. Ma JH, Kim YJ, Yoo WJ, et al: MR imaging of hypoglycemic encephalopathy: Lesion distribution and prognosis prediction by diffusion-weighted imaging, *Neuroradiology* 51(10):641-649, 2009.

6. Foster RE, Connors BW, Waxman SG: Rat optic nerve: Electrophysiological, pharmacological and anatomical studies during development, *Brain Res* 255(3):371-386, 1982.

7. Sturrock RR: Myelination of the mouse corpus callosum, *Neuropathol Appl Neurobiol* 6(6):415-420, 1980.

8. Waxman SG, Ritchie JM: Organization of ion channels in the myelinated nerve fiber, *Science* 228(4707):1502-1507, 1985.

9. Tekkök SB, Goldberg MP: AMPA/Kainate receptor activation mediates hypoxic oligodendrocyte death and axonal injury in cerebral white matter, *J Neurosci* 21(12):4237-4248, 2001.

10. Stys PK, Waxman SG, Ransom BR: Ionic mechanisms of anoxic injury in mammalian CNS white matter: Role of Na$^+$ channels and Na(+)-Ca^{2+} exchanger, *J Neurosci* 12(2):430-439, 1992.

11. Baltan S: Surviving anoxia: A tale of two white matter tracts, *Crit Rev Neurobiol* 18(1-2):95-103, 2006.

12. Zhang K, Sejnowski TJ: A universal scaling law between gray matter and white matter of cerebral cortex, *Proc Natl Acad Sci U S A* 97(10):5621-5626, 2000.

13. Ransom BR, Baltan SB: Axons get excited to death, *Ann Neurol* 65(2):120-121, 2009.

14. Barres BA: The mystery and magic of glia: A perspective on their roles in health and disease, *Neuron* 60(3):430-440, 2008.

15. Ransom B, Behar T, Nedergaard M: New roles for astrocytes (stars at last), *Trends Neurosci* 26(10):520-522, 2003.

16. Chen Y, Swanson RA: Astrocytes and brain injury, *J Cereb Blood Flow Metab* 23(2):137-149, 2003.

17. Swanson RA, Ying W, Kauppinen TM: Astrocyte influences on ischemic neuronal death, *Curr Mol Med* 4(2):193-205, 2004.

18. Wender R, Brown AM, Fern R, et al: Astrocytic glycogen influences axon function and survival during glucose deprivation in central white matter, *J Neurosci* 20(18):6804-6810, 2000.

19. Rose CR, Waxman SG, Ransom BR: Effects of glucose deprivation, chemical hypoxia, and simulated ischemia on Na$^+$ homeostasis in rat spinal cord astrocytes, *J Neurosci* 18(10):3554-3562, 1998.

20. Ransom BR, Fern R: Anoxic-ischemic glial cell injury: Mechanisms and consequences. In Haddad G, Lister G, editors: *Tissue oxygen deprivation*, New York, 1996, Marcel Dekker, Inc, pp 617-652.

21. Nishizaki T, Yamauchi R, Tanimoto M, Okada Y: Effects of temperature on the oxygen consumption in thin slices from different brain regions, *Neurosci Lett* 86:301-305, 1988.

22. Attwell D, Laughlin SB: An energy budget for signaling in the grey matter of the brain, *J Cereb Blood Flow Metab* 21(10):1133-1145, 2001.

23. Tekkök SB, Brown AM, Ransom BR: Axon function persists during anoxia in mammalian white matter, *J Cereb Blood Flow Metab* 23(11):1340-1347, 2003.

24. Moody DM, Bell MA, Challa VR: Features of the cerebral vascular pattern that predict vulnerability to perfusion or oxygenation deficiency: An anatomic study, *AJNR Am J Neuroradiol* 11(3):431-439, 1990.

25. Lyons SA, Kettenmann H: Oligodendrocytes and microglia are selectively vulnerable to combined hypoxia and hypoglycemia injury in vitro, *J Cereb Blood Flow Metab* 18(5):521-530, 1998.

26. McDonald JW, Althomsons SP, Hyrc KL, Choi DW, Goldberg MP: Oligodendrocytes from forebrain are highly vulnerable to AMPA/kainate receptor-mediated excitotoxicity, *Nat Med* 4(3):291-297, 1998.

27. Goldberg MP, Choi DW: Combined oxygen and glucose deprivation in cortical cell culture: Calcium-dependent and calcium-independent mechanisms of neuronal injury, *J Neurosci* 13(8):3510-3524, 1993.

28. Xu J, He L, Ahmed SH, et al: Oxygen-glucose deprivation induces inducible nitric oxide synthase and nitrotyrosine expression in cerebral endothelial cells, *Stroke* 31(7):1744-1751, 2000.

29. Fern R, Moller T: Rapid ischemic cell death in immature oligodendrocytes: A fatal glutamate release feedback loop, *J Neurosci* 20(1):34-42, 2000.

30. Oka A, Belliveau MJ, Rosenberg PA, Volpe JJ: Vulnerability of oligodendroglia to glutamate: Pharmacology, mechanisms, and prevention, *J Neurosci* 13(4):1441-1453, 1993.

31. Dewar D, Underhill SM, Goldberg MP: Oligodendrocytes and ischemic brain injury, *J Cereb Blood Flow Metab* 23(3):263-274, 2003.

32. Campenot RB: Local control of neurite development by nerve growth factor, *Proc Natl Acad Sci U S A* 74(10):4516-4519, 1977.

33. Lubetzki C, Demerens C, Anglade P, et al: Even in culture, oligodendrocytes myelinate solely axons, *Proc Natl Acad Sci U S A* 90(14):6820-6824, 1993.

34. Underhill SM, Goldberg MP: Hypoxic injury of isolated axons is independent of ionotropic glutamate receptors, *Neurobiol Dis* 25:284-290, 2007.

35. Stys PK, Ransom BR, Waxman SG, Davis PK: Role of extracellular calcium in anoxic injury of mammalian central white matter, *Proc Natl Acad Sci U S A* 87(11):4212-4216, 1990.

36. Ransom BR, Waxman SG, Stys PK: Anoxic injury of central myelinated axons: Ionic mechanisms and pharmacology, *Res Publ Assoc Res Nerv Ment Dis* 71:121-151, 1993.

37. Stys PK: Anoxic and ischemic injury of myelinated axons in CNS white matter: From mechanistic concepts to therapeutics, *J Cereb Blood Flow Metab* 18(1):2-25, 1998.

38. Baltan S, Besancon EF, Mbow B, et al: White matter vulnerability to ischemic injury increases with age because of enhanced excitotoxicity, *J Neurosci* 28:1479-1489, 2008.

39. Baltan S, Inman DM, Danilov CA, et al: Metabolic vulnerability disposes retinal ganglion cell axons to dysfunction in a model of glaucomatous degeneration, *J Neurosci* 30(16):5644-5652, 2010.

40. Tekkök SB, Ye Z, Ransom BR: Excitotoxic mechanisms of ischemic injury in myelinated white matter, *J Cereb Blood Flow Metab* 27(9):1540-1552, 2007.

41. Li S, Mealing GA, Morley P, Stys PK: Novel injury mechanism in anoxia and trauma of spinal cord white matter: Glutamate release via reverse Na(+)-dependent glutamate transport, *J Neurosci* 19(14):RC16, 1999.

42. Stys PK, Waxman SG, Ransom BR: Effects of temperature on evoked electrical activity and anoxic injury in CNS white matter, *J Cereb Blood Flow Metab* 12(6):977-986, 1992.

43. Li S, Jiang Q, Stys PK: Important role of reverse Na(+)-Ca(2+) exchange in spinal cord white matter injury at physiological temperature, *J Neurophysiol* 84(2):1116-1119, 2000.

44. Pantoni L, Garcia JH, Gutierrez JA: Cerebral white matter is highly vulnerable to ischemia, *Stroke* 27(9):1641-1646, 1996: discussion 1647.

45. Dietrich WD, Kraydieh S, Prado R, Stagliano NE: White matter alterations following thromboembolic stroke: A beta-amyloid precursor protein immunocytochemical study in rats, *Acta Neuropathol (Berl)* 95(5):524-531, 1998.

46. Schabitz WR, Li F, Fisher M: The N-methyl-D-aspartate antagonist CNS 1102 protects cerebral gray and white matter from ischemic injury following temporary focal ischemia in rats, *Stroke* 31(7):1709-1714, 2000.

47. Yam PS, Dunn LT, Graham DI, et al: NMDA receptor blockade fails to alter axonal injury in focal cerebral ischemia, *J Cereb Blood Flow Metab* 20(5):772-779, 2000.

48. Imai H, Masayasu H, Dewar D, et al: Ebselen protects both gray and white matter in a rodent model of focal cerebral ischemia, *Stroke* 32(9):2149-2154, 2001.

49. Ginsberg MD, Busto R: Rodent models of cerebral ischemia, *Stroke* 20(12):1627-1642, 1989.

50. Goldlust EJ, Paczynski RP, He YY, et al: Automated measurement of infarct size with scanned images of triphenyltetrazolium chloride-stained rat brains, *Stroke* 27:1657-1662, 1996.

51. Leroux P, Hennebert O, Legros H, et al: Role of tissue-plasminogen activator (t-PA) in a mouse model of neonatal white matter lesions: Interaction with plasmin inhibitors and anti-inflammatory drugs, *Neuroscience* 146(2):670-678, 2007.

52. Gadea A, Schinelli S, Gallo V: Endothelin-1 regulates astrocyte proliferation and reactive gliosis via a JNK/c-Jun signaling pathway, *J Neurosci* 28(10):2394-2408, 2008.

53. Sozmen EG, Kolekar A, Havton LA, Carmichael ST: A white matter stroke model in the mouse: Axonal damage, progenitor responses and MRI correlates, *J Neurosci Methods* 180(2):261-272, 2009.

54. Frykholm P, Andersson JL, Valtysson J, et al: A metabolic threshold of irreversible ischemia demonstrated by PET in a middle cerebral artery occlusion-reperfusion primate model, *Acta Neurol Scand* 102(1):18-26, 2000.

55. Enblad P, Frykholm P, Valtysson J, et al: Middle cerebral artery occlusion and reperfusion in primates monitored by microdialysis and sequential positron emission tomography, *Stroke* 32(7): 1574-1580, 2001.

56. Stys PK, Ransom BR, Waxman SG: Compound action potential of nerve recorded by suction electrode: A theoretical and experimental analysis, *Brain Res* 546(1):18-32, 1991.

57. Fern R, Davis P, Waxman SG, Ransom BR: Axon conduction and survival in CNS white matter during energy deprivation: A developmental study, *J Neurophysiol* 79(1):95-105, 1998.

58. Waxman SG, Black JA, Stys PK, Ransom BR: Ultrastructural concomitants of anoxic injury and early post-anoxic recovery in rat optic nerve, *Brain Res* 574(1-2):105-119, 1992.

59. Tekkok SB, Brown AM, Westenbroek R, et al: Transfer of glycogen-derived lactate from astrocytes to axons via specific monocarboxylate transporters supports mouse optic nerve activity, *J Neurosci Res* 81(5):644-652, 2005.

60. Tekkok SB, Ransom BR: Anoxia effects on CNS function and survival: regional differences, *Neurochem Res* 29(11):2163-2169, 2004.

61. Hansen AJ: Effect of anoxia on ion distribution in the brain, *Physiol Rev* 65(1):101-148, 1985.

62. Siesjo BK: Cell damage in the brain: a speculative synthesis, *J Cereb Blood Flow Metab* 1(2):155-185, 1981.

63. Benveniste H, Drejer J, Schousboe A, et al: Elevation of the extracellular concentrations of glutamate and aspartate in rat hippocampus during transient cerebral ischemia monitored by intracerebral microdialysis, *J Neurochem* 43(5):1369-1374, 1984.

64. Kimelberg HK, Ransom BR: Physiological and pathological aspects of astrocytic swelling. In Federoff S, Vernadakis A, editors: *Astrocytes*, Orlando, 1986, Academic Press, pp 129-166.

65. Paulson OB, Newman EA: Does the release of potassium from astrocyte endfeet regulate cerebral blood flow? *Science* 237(4817):896-898, 1987.

66. Longuemare MC, Rose CR, Farrell K, et al: K(+)-induced reversal of astrocyte glutamate uptake is limited by compensatory changes in intracellular Na(+), *Neuroscience* 93(1):285-292, 1999.

67. Schwartz EA, Tachibana M: Electrophysiology of glutamate and sodium co-transport in a glial cell of the salamander retina, *J Physiol (Lond)* 426:43-80, 1990.

68. Goldman SA, Pulsinelli WA, Clarke WY, et al: The effects of extracellular acidosis on neurons and glia in vitro, *J Cereb Blood Flow Metab* 9(4):471-477, 1989.

69. Kraig RP, Petito CK, Plum F, et al: Hydrogen ions kill brain at concentrations reached in ischemia, *J Cereb Blood Flow Metab* 7(4):379-386, 1987.

70. Tombaugh GC, Somjen GG: pH modulation of voltage-gated ion channels. In Kaila K, Ransom BR, editors: *pH and brain function*, New York, 1998, Wiley-Liss, pp 395-416.

71. Traynelis SF: pH modulation of ligand-gated ion channels. In Kaila K, Ransom BR, editors: *pH and brain function*, New York, 1998, Wiley-Liss, pp 417-446.

72. Kraig RP, Pulsinelli WA, Plum F: Hydrogen ion buffering during complete brain ischemia, *Brain Res* 342(2):281-290, 1985.

73. Ransom BR, Walz W, Davis PK, Carlini WG: Anoxia-induced changes in extracellular K(+) and pH in mammalian central white matter, *J Cereb Blood Flow Metab* 12(4):593-602, 1992.

74. Somjen GG, Aitken PG, Balestrino M, et al: Spreading depression-like depolarization and selective vulnerability of neurons. A brief review, *Stroke* 21(Suppl 11):III179-183, 1990.

75. Kraig RP, Nicholson C: Extracellular ionic variations during spreading depression, *Neuroscience* 3(11):1045-1059, 1978.

76. Kraig RP, Ferreira-Filho CR, Nicholson C: Alkaline and acid transients in cerebellar microenvironment, *J Neurophysiol* 49(3):831-850, 1983.

77. Walz W, Mukerji S: Lactate release from cultured astrocytes and neurons: a comparison, *Glia* 1(6):366-370, 1988.

78. Lowry OH, Passonneau JV, Hasselberger FH, et al: Effect of ischemia on known substrates and cofactors of the glycolytic pathway in brain, *J Biol Chem* 239:18-30, 1964.

79. Dohmen C, Kumura E, Rosner G, et al: Adenosine in relation to calcium homeostasis: comparison between gray and white matter ischemia, *J Cereb Blood Flow Metab* 21(5):503-510, 2001.

80. Haimann C, Bernheim L, Bertrand D, Bader CR: Potassium current activated by intracellular sodium in quail trigeminal ganglion neurons, *J Gen Physiol* 95(5):961-979, 1990.

81. Ransom BR, Yamate CL, Connors BW: Activity-dependent shrinkage of extracellular space in rat optic nerve: A developmental study, *J Neurosci* 5(2):532-535, 1985.

82. Li PA, He QP, Csiszar K, et al: Does long-term glucose infusion reduce brain damage after transient cerebral ischemia? *Brain Res* 912(2):203-205, 2001.

83. Plum F: What causes infarction in ischemic brain?: The Robert Wartenberg Lecture, *Neurology* 33(2):222-233, 1983.

84. Siesjo BK, Katsura KI, Kristian T, et al: Molecular mechanisms of acidosis-mediated damage, *Acta Neurochir Suppl (Wien)* 66: 8-14, 1996.

85. Schurr A, West CA, Reid KH, et al: Increased glucose improves recovery of neuronal function after cerebral hypoxia in vitro, *Brain Res* 421(1-2):135-139, 1987.

86. Schanne FA, Kane AB, Young EE, et al: Calcium dependence of toxic cell death: A final common pathway, *Science* 206(4419): 700-702, 1979.

87. Nikolaeva MA, Mukherjee B, Stys PK: Na+-dependent sources of intra-axonal Ca2+ release in rat optic nerve during in vitro chemical ischemia, *J Neurosci* 25:9960-9967, 2005.

88. Li S, Stys PK: Mechanisms of ionotropic glutamate receptor-mediated excitotoxicity in isolated spinal cord white matter, *J Neurosci* 20(3):1190-1198, 2000.

89. Brown AM, Westenbroek RE, Catterall WA, Ransom BR: Axonal L-type Ca2+ channels and anoxic injury in rat CNS white matter, *J Neurophysiol* 85(2):900-911, 2001.

90. Schlaepfer WW: Structural alterations of peripheral nerve induced by the calcium ionophore A23187, *Brain Res* 136(1):1-9, 1977.

91. Hodgkin AL: *The conduction of the nervous impulse*, London, 1964, Liverpool University Press.

92. Waxman SG, Black JA, Ransom BR, Stys PK: Protection of the axonal cytoskeleton in anoxic optic nerve by decreased extracellular calcium, *Brain Res* 614(1-2):137-145, 1993.

93. Ouardouz M, Nikolaeva MA, Coderre E, et al: Depolarization-induced Ca2+ release in ischemic spinal cord white matter involves L-type Ca2+ channel activation of ryanodine receptors, *Neuron* 40(1):53-63, 2003.

94. Ouardouz M, Coderre E, Basak A, et al: Glutamate receptors on myelinated spinal cord axons: I. GluR6 kainate receptors, *Ann Neurol* 65(2):151-159, 2009.

95. Choi DW: Calcium-mediated neurotoxicity: Relationship to specific channel types and role in ischemic damage, *Trends Neurosci* 11(10):465-469, 1988.

96. Ransom BR, Waxman SG, Davis PK: Anoxic injury of CNS white matter: Protective effect of ketamine, *Neurology* 40(9): 1399-1403, 1990.

97. Li PA, Shuaib A, Miyashita H, et al: Hyperglycemia enhances extracellular glutamate accumulation in rats subjected to forebrain ischemia, *Stroke* 31:183-192, 2000.

98. Blaustein MP: Calcium transport and buffering in neurons, *Trends Neurosci* 11(10):438-443, 1988.

99. Lagnado L, Cervetto L, McNaughton PA: Ion transport by the Na-Ca exchange in isolated rod outer segments, *Proc Natl Acad Sci U S A* 85(12):4548-4552, 1988.

100. Blaustein MP, Lederer WJ: Sodium/calcium exchange: Its physiological implications, *Physiol Rev* 79(3):763-854, 1999.

101. Ames AD, Li YY, Heher EC, Kimble CR: Energy metabolism of rabbit retina as related to function: High cost of Na+ transport, *J Neurosci* 12(3):840-853, 1992.

102. Rose CR, Ransom BR: Regulation of intracellular sodium in cultured rat hippocampal neurons, *J Physiol (Lond)* 499(Pt 3): 573-587, 1997.

103. Stys PK, Sontheimer H, Ransom BR, Waxman SG: Noninactivating, tetrodotoxin-sensitive Na+ conductance in rat optic nerve axons, *Proc Natl Acad Sci U S A* 90(15):6976-6980, 1993.

104. Taylor CP: Na+ currents that fail to inactivate, *Trends Neurosci* 16(11):455-460, 1993.

105. Lipton SA: Calcium channel antagonists in the prevention of neurotoxicity, *Adv Pharmacol* 22:271-297, 1991.

106. Weiss JH, Hartley DM, Koh J, Choi DW: The calcium channel blocker nifedipine attenuates slow excitatory amino acid neurotoxicity, *Science* 247(4949 Pt 1):1474-1477, 1990.

107. Fern R, Ransom BR, Waxman SG: Voltage-gated calcium channels in CNS white matter: role in anoxic injury, *J Neurophysiol* 74(1):369-377, 1995.

108. DiPolo R, Beauge L: Regulation of Na$^+$-Ca^{2+} exchange. An overview, *Ann N Y Acad Sci* 639:100–111, 1991.

109. Flamm ES, Demopoulos HB, Seligman ML, Poser RG, Ransohoff J: Free radicals in cerebral ischemia, *Stroke* 9(5):445–447, 1978.

110. Nicotera P, McConkey DJ, Dypbukt JM, et al: Ca2+-activated mechanisms in cell killing, *Drug Metab Rev* 20(2-4):193–201, 1989.

111. Garthwaite G, Goodwin DA, Neale S, et al: Soluble guanylyl cyclase activator YC-1 protects white matter axons from nitric oxide toxicity and metabolic stress, probably through Na(+) channel inhibition, *Mol Pharmacol* 61(1):97–104, 2002.

112. David JC, Yamada KA, Bagwe MR, Goldberg MP: AMPA receptor activation is rapidly toxic to cortical astrocytes when desensitization is blocked, *J Neurosci* 16(1):200–209, 1996.

113. Gallo V, Ghiani CA: Glutamate receptors in glia: new cells, new inputs and new functions, *Trends Pharmacol Sci* 21(7):252–258, 2000.

114. Matute C, Sanchez-Gomez MV, Martinez-Millan L, et al: Glutamate receptor-mediated toxicity in optic nerve oligodendrocytes, *Proc Natl Acad Sci U S A* 94:8830–8835, 1997.

115. Micu I, Jiang Q, Coderre E, et al: NMDA receptors mediate calcium accumulation in myelin during chemical ischaemia, *Nature* 439(7079):988–992, 2006.

116. Salter MG, Fern R: NMDA receptors are expressed in developing oligodendrocyte processes and mediate injury, *Nature* 438(7071):1167–1171, 2005.

117. Karadottir R, Cavelier P, Bergersen LH, Attwell D: NMDA receptors are expressed in oligodendrocytes and activated in ischaemia, *Nature* 438(7071):1162–1166, 2005.

118. Yoshioka A, Hardy M, Younkin DP, et al: Alpha-amino-3-hydroxy-5-methyl-4-isoxazolepropionate (AMPA) receptors mediate excitotoxicity in the oligodendroglial lineage, *J Neurochem* 64(6):2442–2448, 1995.

119. Anderson CM, Swanson RA: Astrocyte glutamate transport: Review of properties, regulation, and physiological functions. *Glia* 32(1):1–14, 2000.

120. Ye ZC, Wyeth MS, Baltan-Tekkok S, Ransom BR: Functional hemichannels in astrocytes: a novel mechanism of glutamate release, *J Neurosci* 23(9):3588–3596, 2003.

121. Wrathall JR, Choiniere D, Teng YD: Dose-dependent reduction of tissue loss and functional impairment after spinal cord trauma with the AMPA/kainate antagonist NBQX, *J Neurosci* 14(11 Pt 1): 6598–6607, 1994.

122. Kanellopoulos GK, Xu XM, Hsu CY, et al: White matter injury in spinal cord ischemia: protection by AMPA/kainate glutamate receptor antagonism, *Stroke* 31:1945–1952, 2000.

123. Follett PL, Rosenberg PA, Volpe JJ, et al: NBQX attenuates excitotoxic injury in developing white matter, *J Neurosci* 20(24): 9235–9241, 2000.

124. McCracken E, Fowler JH, Dewar D, et al: Grey matter and white matter ischemic damage is reduced by the competitive AMPA receptor antagonist, SPD 502, *J Cereb Blood Flow Metab* 22(9):1090–1097, 2002.

125. Brand-Schieber E, Werner P: AMPA/kainate receptors in mouse spinal cord cell-specific display of receptor subunits by oligodendrocytes and astrocytes and at the nodes of Ranvier, *Glia* 42(1):12–24, 2003.

126. Van der Heyden JA, de Kloet ER, Korf J, Versteeg DH: GABA content of discrete brain nuclei and spinal cord of the rat, *J Neurochem* 33(4):857–861, 1979.

127. Bowery NG, Hudson AL, Price GW: GABA(A) and GABA(B) receptor site distribution in the rat central nervous system, *Neuroscience* 20(2):365–383, 1987.

128. Shimada N, Graf R, Rosner G, Heiss WD: Ischemia-induced accumulation of extracellular amino acids in cerebral cortex, white matter, and cerebrospinal fluid, *J Neurochem* 60(1):66–71, 1993.

129. Fern R, Waxman SG, Ransom BR: Modulation of anoxic injury in CNS white matter by adenosine and interaction between adenosine and GABA, *J Neurophysiol* 72(6):2609–2616, 1994.

130. Fern R, Waxman SG, Ransom BR: Endogenous GABA attenuates CNS white matter dysfunction following anoxia, *J Neurosci* 15 (1 Pt 2):699–708, 1995.

131. Ransom BR, Philbin DM Jr: Anoxia-induced extracellular ionic changes in CNS white matter: The role of glial cells, *Can J Physiol Pharmacol* 70(Suppl):S181–189, 1992.

132. Stys PK: Protective effects of antiarrhythmic agents against anoxic injury in CNS white matter, *J Cereb Blood Flow Metab* 15(3):425–432, 1995.

133. Stys PK, Lesiuk H: Correlation between electrophysiological effects of mexiletine and ischemic protection in central nervous system white matter, *Neuroscience* 71(1):27–36, 1996.

134. Fern R, Ransom BR, Stys PK, Waxman SG: Pharmacological protection of CNS white matter during anoxia: Actions of phenytoin, carbamazepine and diazepam, *J Pharmacol Exp Ther* 266(3):1549–1555, 1993.

135. Sayin U, Timmerman W, Westerink BH: The significance of extracellular GABA in the substantia nigra of the rat during seizures and anticonvulsant treatments, *Brain Res* 669(1):67–72, 1995.

9

Cerebral Ischemia and Inflammation

COSTANTINO IADECOLA, TAKATO ABE, ALEXANDER KUNZ, JOHN HALLENBECK

Ischemic stroke triggers an inflammatory reaction in the affected area, which progresses for days to weeks after the onset of symptoms. There is evidence that selected aspects of such inflammatory processes contribute to the progression of ischemic brain injury, worsen the tissue damage, and exacerbate neurologic deficits. Therefore, interventions aimed at suppressing postischemic inflammation offer attractive therapeutic strategies for human stroke, with a potentially wide therapeutic window. On the other hand, inflammation can also have beneficial effects observed in the setting of ischemic tolerance and tissue repair (Fig. 9-1). A large body of work has addressed the inflammatory process in the postischemic brain.[1-5] In this chapter, we review the basic cellular and molecular features of postischemic inflammation, focusing on recent advances and insights on the potential mechanisms by which such inflammation influences stroke outcome. Furthermore, we examine the role of inflammatory mediators in the mechanisms of ischemic tolerance. Finally, we analyze the potential therapeutic implications of modulators of specific inflammatory targets from the perspective of near-future translational approaches.

Cerebral Ischemia, Cytokines, and Inflammation

Cerebral ischemia is associated with infiltration of inflammatory cells into ischemic territory (Fig. 9-2). Histopathologic studies, investigations using biochemical markers of leukocytes, and human studies using radioactive indium–labeled circulating leukocytes have demonstrated that early accumulation of blood-borne inflammatory cells in the ischemic brain persists for hours and even days after the initial insult.[5-8] The infiltration of hematogenous cells into the ischemic territory is the hallmark of the inflammatory reaction, which parallels activation of brain microglia and astrocytes (see Fig. 9-2).[4] Cytokines are important molecular signals in the inflammatory response to cerebral ischemia. In experimental models of stroke, ischemia induces expression of proinflammatory cytokines, such as tumor necrosis factor (TNF) and interleukin (IL)-6 and IL-1β, in the ischemic brain.[4] Increased production of cytokines has also been reported in patients with ischemic stroke.[7,9-11] Proinflammatory cytokines upregulate the expression of adhesion molecules such as intercellular adhesion molecule-1 (ICAM-1), selectins (especially E-selectin and P-selectin), and integrins on endothelial cells, leukocytes, and platelets.[4] Adhesion receptors mediate the interaction between endothelial cells and leukocytes that results in an initial "rolling" of leukocytes, which in turn leads to adhesion to the endothelium of venules, followed by leukocyte transmigration into the brain parenchyma.[7,12,13] Chemokines, the expression of which is upregulated in the ischemic territory, are believed to promote the infiltration of inflammatory cells toward the injured areas.[14]

Several lines of evidence suggest that postischemic inflammation has deleterious effects on the outcome of experimental cerebral ischemia (Tables 9-1 through 9-4). First, interventions aimed at reducing the number of circulating neutrophils ameliorate ischemic damage in most studies, as indicated by reduction in infarct volume and improvement in functional outcome (Table 9-1).[15-17] Second, antibodies blocking the action of adhesion molecules reduce the influx of neutrophils and lessen tissue damage (Table 9-2).[18-23] Third, genetically engineered mice lacking adhesion molecules, such as ICAM-1 and P-selectin, are less susceptible to ischemic damage (see Table 9-2).[24-26] Furthermore, compounds that block the interaction of E-selectin with Sleux—the counterpart adhesion molecule on leukocytes that binds to E-selectin—reduce ischemic brain damage.[21] Fourth, interventions that inactivate cytokines or block cytokine receptors lessen ischemic damage (Table 9-3).[27-34]

Mechanisms by Which Inflammation Contributes to Ischemic Brain Injury

The mechanisms by which postischemic inflammation contributes to cerebral ischemic damage are not well understood. Although infiltrating neutrophils and activated microglia may produce tissue damage by generating reactive oxygen species (ROS),[4] microvascular occlusion produced by intravascular neutrophils, lymphocytes, and platelets may also contribute by compromising microvascular flow.[1,3,13,35,36] However, a cause-and-effect relationship between the extent of neutrophil trafficking and the severity of ischemic damage has not been firmly established.[1,3] Although intravascular adhesion of neutrophils is a relatively early postischemic event, parenchymal accumulation is generally observed later, when most of the ischemic damage may have already occurred.[3] In addition, no consistent relationship has been found between the level of leukocyte infiltration and the extent of ischemic damage.[37] These observations raise questions about the role of neutrophils in the mechanisms of ischemic brain injury and suggest that our understanding of the mechanisms and pathophysiologic implications

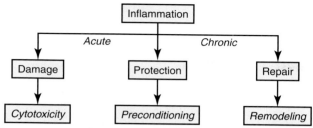

Figure 9-1 Beneficial and deleterious effects of inflammation. Inflammation leads to cytotoxicity in the acute setting but is also essential for brain protection in the setting of ischemic tolerance. Inflammation sets the stage for tissue repair and, as such, is beneficial during the recovery phase after stroke.

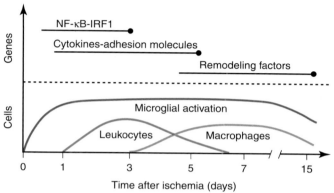

Figure 9-2 Temporal profile of the gene expression and associated cellular events that occur after focal cerebral ischemia in mice. Activation of inflammatory transcription factors leads to expression of cytokines and adhesion molecules. These molecular changes drive the trafficking of leukocytes (neutrophils and lymphocytes) and macrophages across the blood–brain barrier and into the brain. Microglia (i.e., resident brain macrophages) become activated and contribute to the inflammatory reaction. NF-κB, nuclear factor-kappa B; IRF-1, interferon regulatory factor-1. (Cell data modified from Schilling M, Besselmann M, Leonhard C, et al: Microglial activation precedes and predominates over macrophage infiltration in transient focal cerebral ischemia: a study in green fluorescent protein transgenic bone marrow chimeric mice. *Exp Neurol* 183:25-33, 2003.)

TABLE 9-1 EFFECTS OF LEUKOCYTE DEPLETION ON THE OUTCOME OF EXPERIMENTAL FOCAL CEREBRAL ISCHEMIA

Intervention	Outcome	Selected Chapter Reference
Mechlorethamine and vinblastine	Improved histologic or functional outcome in models of focal ischemia	15
Antineutrophilic antibodies	Reduction in infarct size or edema in a rat model of focal cerebral ischemia	16
Neutrophil inhibitory factor	Reduction in infarct size in rats with transient middle cerebral artery occlusion	17
Leukocyte depletion	No effect on brain injury	230

TABLE 9-2 ROLE OF ADHESION MOLECULES IN THE MECHANISMS OF EXPERIMENTAL FOCAL CEREBRAL ISCHEMIA

Intervention	Outcome	Selected Chapter Reference
Anti-ICAM-1 antibodies	Reduction in infarct size in rats with transient MCAO	18
ICAM-1-null mice	Reduction in infarct size in transient MCAO	26
Anti-CD18 monoclonal antibodies	Increased reflow in microvessels of different sizes in primates	19
Anti-CD11b monoclonal antibody	Reduction in infarct size in rats with transient MCAO	20
Mac-1 (CD11b/CD18)	Reduction in infarct size in rats with MCAO	25
CY-1503, analog of sialyl-Lewis (x)	Reduction in infarct size in rats with transient MCAO	21
Synthetic oligopeptide corresponding to the lectin domain of selectins	Reduction in infarct size in rats with MCAO	22
P-selectin-null mice	Reduction in infarct size with transient MCAO	24
Anti-P-selectin monoclonal antibody	Reduction in infarct size in rats with transient or permanent MCAO	23

Abbreviations: ICAM-1, intercellular adhesion molecule-1; Mac-1, macrophage-1 antigen complex; MCAO, middle cerebral artery occlusion.

of postischemic leukocyte trafficking is rather limited. There is also evidence that inhibition of adhesion molecules involved in lymphocyte trafficking, such as the very late activation antigen-4 (VLA-4) or the lymphocyte function antigen-1 (LIF-1), can reduce infarct volumes in preclinical stroke models.[38-41] These studies suggest that lymphocytes and monocytes, in addition to neutrophils, participate in postischemic brain inflammation.[42] However, the precise role that these cells have remains to be defined. While CD4+ and CD8+ T lymphocytes may contribute to focal ischemic injury,[36,43] regulatory T lymphocytes could have a protective effect by downregulating postischemic inflammation.[44,45]

New data have provided insight into additional mechanisms that may also play a role in the neurotoxicity of inflammation. In experimental models of stroke, TNF and IL-1β have been linked to the associated brain injury.[46-53] Intracerebral injection of TNF exacerbates ischemic injury, whereas anti-TNF monoclonal antibody or soluble TNF receptor (TNFR; TNF-binding protein) treatment reverses the effect.[54] Furthermore, the administration of IL-1 receptor antagonist (IL-1ra), a naturally occurring IL-1 inhibitor, or overexpression of IL-1ra in genetically engineered animals diminishes ischemic injury.[55-59] In addition, studies using IL-1 receptor I (IL-1RI) knockout mice

TABLE 9-3 EVIDENCE THAT CYTOKINES PLAY A ROLE IN THE MECHANISMS OF EXPERIMENTAL FOCAL CEREBRAL ISCHEMIA

Intervention	Outcome	Selected Chapter Reference(s)
TNF-α-soluble receptor type 1	Reduction in infarct size in rats and mice with permanent MCAO	27
Anti-TNF-α monoclonal antibody	Reduction in infarct size in rats and mice with MCAO	28, 54
IL-1β administration	Increase in infarct size in rats with transient MCAO	29
IL-1 receptor antagonist	Reduction in infarct size in rats with MCAO	30
IL-1 converting enzyme-null mice	Reduction in ICAM-positive vessels in mice with permanent MCAO	32
IL-6 administration	Reduction in infarct size in rats with permanent MCAO	31
Anti-IL-8 monoclonal antibody	Reduction in infarct size in rabbits with transient ischemia	33
Anti-CINC antibody	Reduction in infarct size in rats with transient MCAO	34
IL-IRI-null mice	Suppression of inflammation; reduced microglia activation; reduced IL-1, IL-6, ICAM-1, COX-2 expression	60

Abbreviations: CINC, cytokine-induced neutrophil chemoattractant; ICAM-1, intercellular adhesion molecule-1; IL, interleukin; MCAO, middle cerebral artery occlusion; TNF-α, tumor necrosis factor-α.

TABLE 9-4 iNOS AND COX-2 CONTRIBUTE TO CEREBRAL ISCHEMIC DAMAGE

Intervention	Outcome	Selected Chapter Reference(s)
iNOS inhibition/deletion		
Aminoguanidine, 1400W	Reduction in infarct size in rats with transient and permanent MCAO	81, 83
iNOS antisense	Reduction in infarct size in rats with transient MCAO	86
iNOS-null mice	Reduction in infarct size in permanent MCAO	85
COX-2 inhibition/deletion		
NS 398	Reduction in infarct size in rats and mice with permanent or transient MCAO	95, 99
SC236	Reduced behavioral deficits after spinal cord ischemia in rabbits	231
COX-2-null mice	Reduction in infarct size in permanent MCAO	100

Abbreviation: COX-2, cyclooxygenase-2; iNOS, inducible nitric oxide synthase; MCAO, middle cerebral artery occlusion.

suggest an involvement of this receptor in IL-1-mediated injury in brain trauma, possibly via microglia-macrophage activation as well as expression of cyclooxygenase-2 (COX-2), IL-1, and IL-6.[60] Interferon-γ (IFN-γ) produced after cerebral ischemia is also involved in tissue damage.[36,44] Consistent with a deleterious role of IFN-γ, mice lacking the interferon regulatory factor 1 (IRF1) are less susceptible to focal cerebral ischemia.[61] The mechanisms by which IFN-γ contribute to ischemic injury are multifactorial and include upregulation of adhesion molecules, prothrombotic effects, microglial activation, and formation of NADPH oxidase–derived ROS.[36,62]

There are instances in which cytokines ameliorate neuronal injury. For example, TNF can induce protection from subsequent ischemic injury (see section on ischemic preconditioning), and TNF receptor knockout mice have greater sensitivity to brain injury.[63,64] In the case of TNF preconditioning, TNF is presumed to act as a noxious stimulus that activates feedback control mechanisms and confers tolerance to subsequent ischemia by generating cell survival agonists and cell death inhibitors. The response of TNF receptor–deficient mice is more difficult to explain in light of the TNF inhibition studies just cited. One possible interpretation is that TNFRI/TNFRII-null

mice are exposed to long-term deprivation because of TNF homeostatic effects and may have developed compensatory mechanisms that render them different from wild-type mice that experience a sudden block of TNF activity. Such discrepancy may also be due to the specific TNF receptor involved in the process. For example, some studies indicate that different receptor subtypes (e.g., TNFRI and TNFRII) exert opposite roles in TNF-induced neuronal injury and survival.[65,66]

Another member of the TNF receptor superfamily, Fas, has been implicated in ischemic brain damage. Martin-Villalba et al[67] have reported that infarct volumes in both FasL (Fas ligand) and TNF knockout mice were 54% and 67% smaller, respectively, than those in controls. Hybrid mice lacking both cytokines showed a 93% reduction in infarct volume, and a combination of antibodies that neutralized FasL and TNF decreased infarct volume by 70%. Ligation of Fas by trimerized FasL leads to recruitment of adapter proteins that form the death-inducing signaling complex (DISC) and, eventually, apoptosis. TNFRI recruits the TNFR-associated death domain protein (TRADD), which can interact with both Fas-associated death domain protein (FADD) and TNFR-associated factor 2 (TRAF2) that can activate nuclear factor-κB (NF-κB). Accordingly, these receptors can activate both proinflammatory and apoptotic pathways, which is a feature that may account for the potency of their dual blockade in ischemia.

Recent work that has extended the compass of stroke-related inflammation beyond innate immune mechanisms to include adaptive immunity has been reviewed.[68] Disruption of the blood-brain barrier during acute stroke releases novel central nervous system (CNS) antigens that are normally sequestered in the brain and exposes them to the systemic immune system. Absent activation of the systemic immune system, autoimmune responses to these antigens do not seem to occur. However, cerebral ischemia induces a state of systemic immunodepression that predisposes to poststroke infections.[69,70] Stroke is frequently complicated by pulmonary or urinary tract infections; under these circumstances, T-effector lymphocytes can become primed to brain antigens and excite a CNS autoimmune response. Activated CD8+ T lymphocytes can secrete cytotoxic and proinflammatory cytokines and can also kill brain cells by direct lysis (e.g., perforin and granzyme) or by inducing apoptosis via the TNF family of receptors (e.g., Fas receptor and FasL).[62]

Nitric Oxide and Inducible Nitric Oxide Synthase

A growing body of evidence suggests that inducible nitric oxide synthase (iNOS) is a critical effector of the damage produced by postischemic inflammation.[71] Nitric oxide (NO), a free radical, acts as a signaling molecule in normal synaptic transmission as well as a neurotoxin in pathologic conditions.[72] The following three isoforms of NOS have been identified: neuronal (NOS1), inducible (iNOS, NOS2), and endothelial (NOS3) NOS. Both NOS1 and NOS3 are expressed constitutively, whereas NOS2 is induced in immune cells and neurons largely by stimuli such as lipopolysaccharide (LPS), cytokines, and pathogens. Sustained and robust production of NO by iNOS is thought to contribute to the cytotoxicity induced by inflammation.[71] The mechanisms by which NO and its derived chemical species exert their cytotoxic effects are diverse and include inhibition of adenosine triphosphate (ATP)–producing enzymes, DNA damage, and oxidative damage produced by peroxynitrite, a highly reactive chemical species formed by the reaction of NO with superoxide.[73,74]

The biosynthesis of NO is greatly enhanced in the setting of postischemic inflammation. After transient or permanent middle cerebral artery (MCA) occlusion in rodents, iNOS messenger RNA (mRNA) is upregulated, peaking at 12 to 48 hours after ischemia.[75-77] The increase in iNOS protein is associated with an increase in iNOS enzymatic activity[75,76] and NO production, as revealed by accumulation of NO-derived peroxynitrite.[78] Inducible NOS is strongly expressed in infiltrating neutrophils as well as cerebral blood vessels within the ischemic territory. Immunohistochemical localization of iNOS has also been documented after ischemic stroke in humans.[79] Immunoreactivity for nitrotyrosine, a marker of peroxynitrite, has also been observed in infiltrating neutrophils, suggesting that iNOS is catalytically active.[79] Furthermore, intrathecal levels of nitrate have been found to be elevated 3 months after a stroke, and the increase correlates with the infarct volume and the severity of the neurologic deficits.[80]

There is compelling evidence that iNOS is a critical component in ischemia-induced brain damage (Table 9-4). First, administration of the iNOS inhibitor aminoguanidine, starting 6 or 24 hours after MCA occlusion, attenuates postischemic iNOS activity and reduces the volume of the infarct by 30% to 40% (see Table 9-4).[76,81]

The reduction in histologic damage is associated with improvement in neurologic deficits and is not due to hemodynamic effects of aminoguanidine.[81,82] Second, delayed administration of 1400W, an iNOS inhibitor structurally unrelated to aminoguanidine, diminishes infarct volume in rats after MCA occlusion.[83] Third, iNOS-deficient mice have smaller infarcts after MCA occlusion and have better neurologic outcomes than wild-type controls. The effect is more pronounced in homozygous−/− than in heterozygous+/− null mice (see Table 9-4).[84] The reduction in injury volume is observed at 4 days but not at 1 day after ischemia, suggesting that iNOS plays a role in the later stages of the injury.[85] Fourth, administration of iNOS antisense downregulates iNOS expression and improves the outcome of cerebral ischemia in rats subjected to transient MCA occlusion.[86] In addition, suppression of iNOS expression has been implicated in the neuroprotection exerted by hypothermia, estrogen, and progesterone.[87-89] Collectively, these findings suggest that sustained NO production by iNOS is a critical factor in the delayed progression of ischemic damage and that the modulation of excessive NO production in a timely fashion may have a beneficial effect on the outcome of stroke.

Cyclooxygenase-2

COX-2 has also been implicated in the mechanisms of postischemic inflammation. Cyclooxygenase, an integral membrane glycoprotein, is the rate-limiting enzyme for the synthesis of prostaglandins and thromboxanes from arachidonic acid. Although COX-1, a constitutive isoform, is expressed in virtually all cell types and produces physiologic levels of prostanoids,[90,91] COX-2 is rapidly induced on activation by mitogens, inflammatory mediators, and hormones.[92,93] Several lines of evidence suggest that COX-2 participates in the progression of cerebral ischemic damage (see Table 9-4). First, COX-2 mRNA and protein expression are upregulated 12 to 24 hours after cerebral ischemia in rodents.[94,95-97] COX-2 expression in rodents is observed in neurons at the periphery of the infarct, in vascular cells, and in microglia.[94,95] COX-2 expression has also been demonstrated in the human brain after ischemic stroke.[96,98] As in rodents, COX-2 immunoreactivity in humans is observed in neurons at the border of ischemic territory as well as in neutrophils and vascular cells. In humans, as in rodents, the upregulation of COX-2 immunoreactivity is confined to the area of damage.[96] Administration of NS-398, a relatively selective COX-2 inhibitor, 6 hours after ischemia reduces the infarct volume by 20% to 30% in a model of focal ischemia in rats (see Table 9-4).[95,99] Moreover, mice with a targeted disruption of the COX-2 gene have been found to exhibit a significant reduction in the brain injury produced by occlusion of the MCA compared with wild-type littermates.[100] Interestingly, COX-2-null mice are also protected from the damage produced by direct microinjection of N-methyl-D-aspartate (NMDA) into the cerebral cortex. This observation indicates that COX-2 is also involved in the mechanisms of glutamate receptor–mediated brain damage, a process that occurs early in the ischemic cascade.[101,102]

The downstream mechanisms by which COX-2 exerts its deleterious effects on the ischemic brain have recently been investigated. The catalytic activity of COX-2 is associated with the production of the free radical superoxide and prostanoids.[103] Superoxide produced by COX-2 activity may react with NO to form the powerful oxidant peroxynitrite. Thus, increased COX-2 activity in inflammatory cells and neurons during acute and chronic inflammation could contribute to tissue damage through excessive generation of ROS and production of toxic prostanoids. However, data in mouse models of neurotoxicity and focal cerebral ischemia indicate that COX-2–derived ROS do not contribute to ischemic brain injury.[104,105] Rather, the evidence suggests that the deleterious effects of COX-2 in stroke are mediated by prostaglandin E_2 acting on its prostaglandin E_1 (EP1) receptor.[106,107] The mechanisms by which EP1 receptors contribute to neurotoxicity include enhancement of the Ca^{2+} dysregulation triggered by cerebral ischemia and suppression of the protective kinase Akt in the postischemic brain.[106,108]

Taken together, the evidence from studies of pharmacologic inhibition and genetic disruption of COX-2 suggests that this enzyme is involved in both the initiation and progression of ischemic injury and may be a valuable target in the treatment of human stroke. However, the results of several clinical trials have revealed an increased incidence of vascular complications in patients receiving long-term treatment with COX-2 inhibitors,[109] indicating that long-term COX-2 inhibition may not be safe in stroke patients. These complications have been attributed to the beneficial vascular effects of protective prostanoids, such as prostacyclin.[110] Therefore, targeting the downstream pathways that mediate COX-2–dependent neurotoxicity, such as the EP1 receptor, may be a more attractive strategy because the "beneficial" vascular effects of COX-2 reaction products (e.g., prostacyclin) would not be abrogated.

Danger Sensors: Scavenger Receptors and Toll-like Receptors

In a disorder such as stroke that results from multiple interacting mechanisms,[101,111-114] therapeutic targets that beneficially affect multiple mechanisms are arguably the most attractive. If the multifactorial progression of ischemic brain injury could be likened to a bad performance by a symphony orchestra, stopping the conductor should be far more effective than stopping the piccolo player. It is interesting in this regard to consider as possibly related to ischemic injury recently identified networks of ligands, receptors, transcription factors, and effector molecules that may function like "conductors" and orchestrate ongoing brain damage. Evolutionarily conserved pattern recognition receptors respond not only to pathogen-associated molecular patterns (PAMPs) but also to endogenous danger signals (termed either *alarmins* or *danger-associated molecular patterns* [DAMPs]) that can initiate responses to stresses such as ischemia.[115,116] Such receptor-mediated signaling may provide the first inkling to cells that they are in trouble. Examples of alarmins/DAMPs include cathelicidins,[117] high mobility group box protein 1 (HMGB1),[118] S100/calgranulins,[119] heparan sulfate, hyaluronic acid, cytochrome *c*, and advanced glycation end products (AGE).[120] Other endogenous ligands that may serve as stress signals are heat shock proteins

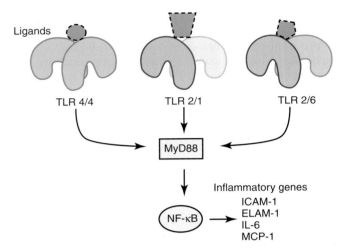

Figure 9-3 Toll-like receptors (TLR) are present as homodimers or heterodimers and, on ligand binding, lead to NF-κB activation through the adapter protein MyD88. NF-κB, Nuclear factor-kappa B; ICAM-1, intercellular adhesion molecule-1; ELAM-1, endothelial-leukocyte adhesion molecule-1; IL-6, interleukin-6; MCP-1, monocyte chemotactic protein-1. (Modified from *Stroke* 41:898-904, 2010.)

(HSPs), degraded extracellular matrix components, ROS, denatured proteins, and changes in lipid, carbohydrate, or protein moieties that are expressed on the outer cell membrane of stressed cells.[121] In addition, nucleic acids such as DNA and RNA and their metabolites (i.e., polynucleotides, oligonucleotides, nucleosides, free bases, and uric acid) that are normally sequestered can be released by injured cells and modify innate immune responses.[122]

Receptors for these stress molecules, which nucleate multiprotein signaling complexes, include toll-like receptor (TLR) and NACHT (domain present in neuronal apoptosis inhibitory protein)–leucine-rich repeat (NLR) receptor families on sentinel cells (macrophages, microglia, dendritic cells).[116,121] TLRs are key receptors of the innate immune system, comprising at least 12 families. On ligand binding, TLRs form homodimers (TLR4/4) or heterodimers (TLR2/6 or TLR2/1) (Fig. 9-3).[123] TLR2 forms functional heterodimers with TLR1 or TLR6[123,124] and recognizes a variety of PAMPs, including triacylated lipopeptides from bacteria, such as Pam3CSK4, peptidoglycan, diacylated lipopeptides such as Pam2CSK4, LPSs from gram-negative bacteria, fungal zymosan, and mycoplasma lipopeptides.[125] TLR4 predominantly recognizes LPS.[126] Activation of TLRs leads to NF-κB activation via the adapter protein MyD88 (see Fig. 9-3).[123] Recent expression studies have demonstrated that cerebral ischemia results in the upregulation of mRNA for TLR2, TLR4, and TLR9, and mice lacking TLR2 or TLR4 exhibit reduced infarct size after focal cerebral ischemic injury (Table 9-5).[127-132] The expression of IRF-1, iNOS, COX-2, and metalloproteinase-9 is reduced in TLR4-null mouse brains after MCA occlusion,[130] attesting to the key role of TLR4 in postischemic inflammation.

The receptor for advanced glycation end products (RAGE) and acute phase proteins of the pentraxin family (including C-reactive protein) can sense the presence of endogenous danger signals.[116,133] RAGE is a multiligand membrane receptor, and several of the established ligands

TABLE 9-5 ROLE OF SCAVENGER RECEPTORS AND TOLL-LIKE RECEPTORS IN THE MECHANISMS OF EXPERIMENTAL FOCAL CEREBRAL ISCHEMIA

Intervention	Outcome	Selected Chapter Reference
Scavenger receptors		
CD36-null mice	Reduction in infarct size in transient MCAO	149, 150, 232, 238
RAGE-null mice	Reduction in infarct size in permanent MCAO	138
TLRs		
TLR2-null mice	Reduction in infarct size in transient MCAO	127, 131, 238
TLR4-null mice	Reduction in infarct size in transient and permanent MCAO	127, 130

Abbreviations: MCAO, middle cerebral artery occlusion; RAGE, receptor for advanced glycation end products; TLR, toll-like receptor.

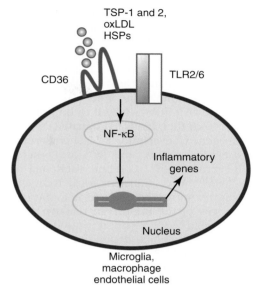

Figure 9-4 The scavenger receptor CD36 is present in microglia, macrophages, and endothelial cells. CD36 can signal independently or as part of a molecular cluster including TLR2/6, which is formed in response to a wide variety of ligands. On ligand binding, CD36 triggers inflammatory signaling through NF-κB activation. TSP-1 and -2, thrombospondin-1 and -2; oxLDL, oxidized low-density lipoprotein; HSPs, heat shock proteins; TLR, toll-like receptor; NF-κB, nuclear factor-kappa B.

may activate RAGE in cerebral ischemia. Administration of AGE, a RAGE ligand, increases ischemic injury in a rat model of focal cerebral ischemia.[134] Furthermore, HMGB1 is a well-known RAGE activator released from activated macrophages and neuronal and necrotic cells after cerebral ischemia.[135-137] A neutralizing anti-HMGB1 antibody and HMGB1 box A, an antagonist of HMGB1 at the receptor RAGE, ameliorates ischemic brain damage.[138] Consistent with a deleterious role of RAGE signaling, RAGE−/− mice have significantly smaller infarcts than controls (see Table 9-5).[138] Of note, TLR2 may also be needed for the inflammatory response triggered by necrotic cells.[139] However, it has not been established whether TLR2 plays a role in the effects of HMGB1.

Signal transduction from these receptors can lead to the formation of multiprotein complexes that nucleate on a scaffold protein, which characteristically has a region involved in ligand sensing, an oligomerization domain, and a domain involved in recruiting caspases.[140,141] The multiprotein complexes integrate cellular signals, promote activation of initiator caspases (caspase 2, 8, 9, or 10), and initiate signaling cascades that can lead to apoptosis and inflammation or cell survival. Examples of these multiprotein complexes are the apoptosome, the inflammasome, the DISC, and the PIDDosome.[142,143]

The class B scavenger receptor CD36 is a surface glycoprotein found in microglia, macrophages, microvascular endothelium, cardiac and skeletal muscle, adipocytes, and platelets.[144] CD36 recognizes a multitude of ligands, including oxidized low-density lipoprotein (LDL), long-chain fatty acids, thrombospondin-1, fibrillar-amyloid (Ab), and the membrane of cells undergoing apoptosis.[144-146] CD36 recognizes pathogen-associated molecular patterns and induces an inflammatory response through activation of NF-κB (Fig. 9-4).[147,148] Focal cerebral ischemia upregulates CD36 in the ischemic brain, and CD36-null mice have smaller infarcts and better neurologic outcomes after focal ischemia.[149] CD36 plays a key role

in focal cerebral ischemia because it is essential for postischemic NF-κB activation and for the full expression of the cellular and molecular signals driving postischemic inflammation.[150]

Three of the above complexes—inflammasome, DISC, and PIDDosome—as well as TLR, CD36, and RAGE[120,121,142] activate signal transduction pathways that induce nuclear translocation of a transcription factor, NF-κB, which serves as a critical nexus (a "conductor" perhaps) in the pathways regulating inflammation, cell death, and cell survival.

Transcription Factors Involved in Postischemic Inflammation

The molecular mechanisms that lead to activation of transcription of inflammatory genes in the postischemic brain are not fully understood. Gene expression is controlled by transcription factors, DNA-binding proteins that initiate mRNA transcription. Transcription factors that have been studied in the context of postischemic inflammation include NF-κB and IRF-1. NF-κB is a multifunctional switch that transactivates the expression of more than 150 target genes, of which some are potentially cytotoxic and others are potentially cytoprotective.[151,152] It functions in the negative feedback control of TNF cytotoxicity,[153,154] and it has been reported to be a key factor in the induction of tolerance to brain ischemia.[155,156] The activity of NF-κB proteins is regulated by hundreds of different stimuli in all cell types, and fine-tuning of NF-κB functional consequences involves posttranslational modification of the inhibitor of NF-κB (IκB) kinases (IKKs), the IκBs, or the NF-κB subunits themselves,[157] as well as various forms of epigenetic regulation.[158] Genes activated by NF-κB include those encoding for adhesion molecules, chemokines, iNOS, and COX-2.[154] In resting cells, two subunits of NF-κB, p65 and p50, are bound to the inhibitory factor IκB, and the complex is sequestered in the cytoplasm. Cell stimulation leads to degradation of IκB in the proteasome, unmasking a nuclear localization signaling sequence that allows NF-κB to be translocated to the nucleus. NF-κB then binds to cognate DNA sequences and activates gene transcription.[159] Ischemia-reperfusion, physical stress, cytokines, and ROS are potent stimuli for NF-κB activation.[154] Cerebral ischemia activates NF-κB.[150,154,160,161] After transient focal ischemia in the rat, greater immunoreactivity of p65 is found in neurons at the periphery of the infarct, in reactive glia, and in inflammatory cells.[162,163] NF-κB activation is observed 6 to 96 hours after ischemia, depending on experimental models and species.[162-164] Immunoreactivity for NF-κB is also observed in glial cells of human infarcts, particularly at the border of the zone between ischemic and nonischemic areas.[165]

Several studies have investigated the role of NF-κB in ischemic brain injury in vivo.[154] Thus, genetic deletion of the NF-κB subunit p50 reduces ischemic injury.[164,166] Similarly, expression of an NF-κB repressor[167] or deletion of the upstream kinase IKK[168] is neuroprotective. One study in which NF-κB was pharmacologically inhibited with diethyldithiocarbamate (DDTC) suggested a neuroprotective role of NF-κB.[169] However, this study has been questioned because of the lack of specificity of DDTC.[170,171] Currently, the weight of the evidence favors a deleterious role of NF-κB in acute focal ischemic injury. Although NF-κB and other inflammatory mediators may be protective in the setting of ischemic tolerance,[155,172,173] this is not surprising considering the well-established preconditioning effects of injurious stimuli.[174]

IRF-1 is a transcription factor that is thought to coordinate the expression of multiple inflammatory genes, including cytokines, adhesion molecules, iNOS, and COX-2.[175] Data now suggest that IRF-1 is also involved in the mechanisms of cerebral ischemia. In rodents, IRF-1 mRNA is upregulated after permanent MCA occlusion, reaching a peak 3 to 4 days after ischemia.[61,176] Cerebral ischemia increases IRF-1 binding activity, as demonstrated on gel-shift assays.[177] Furthermore, mice lacking IRF-1 have less brain damage and milder neurologic deficits after MCA occlusion.[61] The difference in infarct volume could not be attributed to differences in the reduction of cerebral blood flow produced by MCA occlusion.[61] These findings suggest that IRF-1-dependent gene expression plays a prominent role in the expression of ischemic brain injury. However, the cellular and molecular mechanisms responsible for the protection afforded by IRF-1 deletion remain to be defined.

CCAAT/enhancer binding protein β (C/EBPβ) is a leucine-zipper transcription factor that binds to CCAAT sequences in promoters of eukaryotic genes and regulates cell growth and differentiation.[178] C/EBPβ gene expression is significantly upregulated after MCA occlusion, and C/EBPβ-null mice have significantly smaller infarcts.[179] Also, in C/EBPβ-null mice brain after cerebral ischemia, numbers of ICAM-1 positive capillaries and infiltrated neutrophils and macrophages are reduced.[179] In addition, GeneChip analysis showed that the postischemic induction of many inflammatory and neuronal damage–inducing genes was less pronounced in the brains of C/EBPβ-null mice, suggesting a significant role for C/EBPβ in postischemic inflammation and brain damage.[179]

The peroxisome proliferator–activated receptors (PPARs) are the ligand-activated nuclear proteins, of which at least three subtypes exist (i.e., PPARα, PPARδ, and PPARγ).[180] PPARs regulate gene transcription by binding to conserved DNA sequences termed *peroxisome proliferator response elements* (PPREs) as heterodimers with the retinoic acid receptor (RXR).[181] Recent studies using animal stroke models suggest that PPARγ activation with thiazolidinediones (TZDs), which are potent PPARγ agonists,[182] is a potent therapeutic option for preventing inflammation and neuronal damage after stroke. TZDs, such as troglitazone, pioglitazone, or rosiglitazone, reduced infarct volume and resulted in a reduction of numbers of microglia/macrophages, myeloperoxidase (MPO) levels and activity, cytokine levels (TNF, IL-6, monocyte chemotactic protein-1 [MCP-1]), and decreased expression of COX-2, IL-1β, and iNOS mRNA or protein in the ischemic brain, which supported the link between anti-inflammatory effects of TZDs acting via PPARγ.[183-186] Treatment with the PPARγ antagonist T0070907 abrogates the protection.[187] Oral administration of the PPARα agonist fenofibrate reduced vascular cell adhesion molecule-1 (VCAM-1) and ICAM-1 expression and cortical infarction after transient MCA occlusion.[188] Furthermore, PPARα antagonist WY14643 decreased oxidative stress, iNOS, and ICAM-1 expression in a model of global ischemia.[189] These observations attest to a protective role of PPAR activation in ischemic injury. Given that PPARγ agonists are in clinical use for the treatment of type 2 diabetes, these agents could also have a therapeutic role in stroke. A recent meta-analysis indicated that the PPARγ agonist rosiglitazone increases the risk of ischemic myocardial events and cardiovascular deaths,[190] but the reliability of these findings has been questioned.[191] However, PPARγ agonists do cause fluid retention and increased incidence of heart failure,[191] which suggests that their potential use in stroke patients needs to be scrutinized further.

Inflammatory Mediators and Ischemic Preconditioning

As previously discussed, ischemic brain cells produce a large array of mediators that may participate in progression of ischemic brain injury. This is one factor that has complicated efforts to develop clinically effective therapies for stroke. Surprisingly, these inflammatory mediators, under certain conditions, can confer tolerance to cerebral ischemia. Study of the regulation of the endogenous neuroprotection associated with inflammatory mediators may enable investigators to guide the search for effective stroke therapy through the morass of interlaced injury mechanisms.

The earliest observations of tolerance were in the heart and involved preconditioning with brief sublethal ischemia. Preconditioning is the phenomenon whereby a stressful but sublethal stimulus sets in motion a cascade of molecular and biochemical events that renders cells, tissues, or the whole organism tolerant to a future more lethal stimulus. Myocardial ischemia preconditioning in animal models has been studied since the mid-1980s, and later clinical studies suggest that similar preconditioning may be operative in human coronary syndromes.[192-194] Murry et al[195] were the first to develop a preconditioning paradigm that reduced myocardial infarct size during a subsequent severe ischemia. Later, other groups attempted to replicate the preconditioned responses to ischemia observed in the myocardium in neurologic models. Kitagawa et al[196] showed that preconditioning with brief ischemia (2 minutes) protected against a later 5-minute episode of bilateral common carotid artery occlusion in gerbils that otherwise caused damage to pyramidal neurons in the CA1 region of the hippocampus, a region of brain selectively vulnerable to ischemia. Subsequently, many groups have demonstrated that diverse preconditioning strategies can induce tolerance to global or focal brain ischemia, and tolerance has been modeled in cell culture systems to facilitate the study of regulatory mechanisms. As with clinically relevant myocardial preconditioning, there is some clinical evidence for induction of neuroprotection after "preconditioning" that occurs from transient ischemic attacks.[197,198]

Proinflammatory cytokines IL-1 and TNF activate intracellular signaling pathways that mediate stress responses[199] and could, therefore, function in ligand-receptor interactions that induce the tolerant state. IL-1 has been observed to induce tolerance to global brain ischemia with protection of hippocampal CA1 neurons in the gerbil.[200] LPS is a potent stimulus for release of proinflammatory cytokines. Its administration in animal models has been reported to protect against ischemia in both the heart[201-203] and the brain.[204] NO, HSP70, and superoxide dismutase have been implicated in LPS-induced tolerance to brain ischemia.[205,206] A major cytokine elicited by LPS is TNF. Preconditioning with TNF has been reported to confer cytoprotection in an embryonic kidney cell line[207] and has also been reported to reduce injury in isolated perfused rat hearts subjected to ischemia[208] by increasing manganese superoxide dismutase. TNF preconditioning has also been shown to reduce infarct volumes in mice subjected to MCA occlusion[209] and to protect cultured neurons from severe hypoxic stress.[63] Downstream signaling in this pathway involves ceramide and the transcription factor NF-κB.[210] Such studies are moving toward points of intersection for multiple regulatory pathways and have the potential to identify molecular targets that can simultaneously affect multiple mechanisms of ischemic damage.

Important recent work has shown that tolerance to severe ischemia induced by preconditioning fundamentally involves reprogramming of the genetic response to injury.[211] During exposure to severe ischemia, both a high percentage of unique transcripts and widespread, gene-specific repression of gene expression have been found in brain samples that had been preconditioned by sublethal ischemia compared with samples from nonpreconditioned brains. Also, the profiles of gene expression during severe ischemia appear to differ depending on the nature of the preconditioning stimulus, as shown for ischemic preconditioning versus LPS preconditioning. These preconditioning-specific phenotypes appear to be adapted to counter the specific cytotoxicity mechanisms of the preconditioning stimulus. This suggests that multiple nonoverlapping pathways may subserve tolerance to brain ischemia.[211]

In addition, preconditioning protects cerebral blood vessels from the vasoparalysis induced by cerebral ischemia. Administration of LPS 24 hours before MCA occlusion reduced ischemic brain injury and prevented the dysfunction in cerebrovascular regulation induced by MCA occlusion, as demonstrated by normalization of the increase in cerebral blood flow produced by neural activity, hypercapnia, or the endothelium-dependent vasodilator acetylcholine.[173] These beneficial effects of LPS were not observed in mice lacking iNOS or the NOX2 subunit of the superoxide-producing enzyme NADPH oxidase.[173] LPS increased ROS and the peroxynitrite marker 3-nitrotyrosine in cerebral blood vessels of wild-type mice but not in NOX2 nulls, and the peroxynitrite decomposition catalyst 5,10,15, 20-tetrakis(4-sulfonatophenyl)porphyrinato iron (III) counteracted the beneficial effects of LPS, which suggests that the vasoprotective effects of LPS are mediated by peroxynitrite produced by the reaction of iNOS-derived NO with NOX2-derived superoxide.[173] As discussed by Kunz et al,[173] these findings are of interest because they indicate that peroxynitrite, in addition to its well-known deleterious vascular actions, can also protect cerebral blood vessels from the vascular dysregulation associated with cerebral ischemia.

From Bench to Bedside

As already discussed, data from animal stroke models provide a strong rationale for therapies directed at limiting the effects of certain components of inflammation in the postischemic period. Several clinical trials have used anti-inflammatory approaches to treat ischemic stroke, with mixed results (Table 9-6). A clinical trial using murine antibodies against ICAM-1 has failed to show a benefit in patients with ischemic stroke. This murine monoclonal antibody against ICAM-1 (enlimomab) was evaluated for clinical efficacy in a prospective, randomized, blinded, phase 3 trial in 625 patients presenting within 6 hours after onset of symptoms.[212] Treatment with anti–ICAM-1 antibodies was associated with a higher mortality rate and slightly larger infarct sizes.[213,214] Fever affected nearly twice as many patients treated with enlimomab as patients receiving placebo. The reasons for the failure of anti-ICAM antibodies to ameliorate ischemic stroke in humans are not entirely clear and have been the subject of extensive debates.[101,215] One likely possibility is that administration of heterologous antibodies leads to immunologic side effects, resulting in the worsening of tissue damage. This scenario is supported by the findings that enlimomab promotes activation of human neutrophils[214] and, in preclinical stroke models, was found to activate complement, induce anti-mouse antibodies, and enhance expression of the adhesion molecules P- and E-selectin as well as ICAM-1.[216,217] Furthermore, sensitization to enlimomab before induction of cerebral ischemia enhances infarct volume.[217] Therefore, future clinical studies

TABLE 9-6   SELECTED CLINICAL TRIALS OF ANTI-INFLAMMATORY TREATMENTS IN ISCHEMIC STROKE

Name of Trial	Phase	No. of Patients	Agent(s) Used	Time Window	Primary Endpoint	Effect	Reference
High-dose steroid treatment in cerebral infarction	2a	113	Dexamethasone	<48 h	Death at day 21, TSSS at days 2, 4, 6, 8, 10, 12, 21	No	233
EAST (Enlimomab Acute Stroke Trial)	3	625	Enlimomab (murine anti-ICAM-1 antibody)	<6 h	mRS at 90 days	No	213
HALT (Hu23F2G Phase 3 Stroke Trial)	3	400 (stopped)	LeukoArrest (Hu23F2G, humanized anti-Mac-1 antibody)	<12 h	—	No	234
ASTIN (Acute Stroke Therapy by Inhibition of Neutrophils)	3	966	rNIF (recombinant neutrophil inhibitory factor), UK-279, 276	<6 h	SSS at 90 days	No	220
Study of interleukin-1 receptor antagonist in acute stroke patients	2	34	IL-1ra (interleukin-1 receptor antagonist)	<6 h	Increase in NIHSS score >4 points within 72 h	Improved outcome	235
Minocycline treatment in acute stroke	2	152	Minocycline (inhibitor of microglial activation)	6-24 h	NIHSS at 90 days	Improved outcome	236
ONO-2506 in Acute Ischemic Stroke	2/3	757	Arundic acid (synonym: ONO-2506, MK0724; modulator of astrocytic activation)	<72 h	mRS at 90 days	N/A	Completed
RREACT (Rapid Response with an Astrocyte Modulator for the Treatment of Acute Cortical Stroke)	2	1320	Arundic acid (ONO-2506, MK0724; modulator of astrocytic activation)	<6 h	mRS at 90 days	N/A	Terminated
MINOS (Minocycline to Improve Neurologic Outcome Study)	2	60	Minocycline (inhibitor of microglial activation)	<6 h	Adverse events within 90 days	Safe and well tolerated alone or with rt-PA	239
APCAST (Activated Protein C in Acute Stroke Trial)	2	72	Activated protein C	<6 h	Adverse events (major ICH) at 36-48 h	N/A	Expected completion: Aug. 2011
Enoxaparin and/or Minocycline in Acute Stroke		64	Minocycline + Enoxaparin	<6 h	Indices of salvaged brain tissue	N/A	Expected completion: Sept. 2011

ICAM-1, intercellular adhesion molecule-1; ICH, intracranial hemorrhage; Mac-1, macrophage-1 antigen complex; mRS, modified Rankin Scale; N/A, not available; NIHSS, National Institutes of Health Stroke Scale; SSS, Scandinavian Stroke Scale; TSSS, Toronto Stroke Scoring system.

testing anti-inflammatory strategies based on heterologous proteins will have to take these factors into consideration to avoid deleterious immune-mediated side effects in patients with stroke.

The HALT stroke trial used humanized anti Mac-1 antibodies (Hu23F2G; LeukoArrest) in patients presenting within 12 hours after onset of symptoms. The trial was stopped after enrolling 400 patients because of lack of improvement of functional outcomes.[218] However, in preclinical studies, Hu23F2G was effective when administered 20 minutes after ischemia[219] and was not tested at the time window used in the clinical trial (12 hours after a stroke).[218] The ASTIN trial tested the recombinant neutrophil inhibitory factor (rNIF), a non-antibody small molecule, in acute stroke with a 6-hour time window. Patients presenting within 3 hours were also treated with tissue plasminogen activator (t-PA) or placebo. The trial was terminated prematurely after enrolling 966 patients because of lack of efficacy.[220] Notwithstanding the limitations of the ICAM-1 and rNIF trials, these clinical observations increase the possibility that modification of leukocyte trafficking by agents like enlimomab and NIF does not offer apparent benefit in human stroke. Therefore, therapeutic approaches based solely on prevention of leukocyte infiltration must be carefully reevaluated before further application in patients with stroke. In particular, clinical trials need to be based on rigorous preclinical studies designed to mimic as closely as possible the conditions of the trial (e.g., dosing, therapeutic window, sexually dimorphic effects, and effective brain concentrations). These efforts will be facilitated by new imaging approaches to monitor treatment effects by examination of the trafficking of inflammatory cells in the postischemic brain.[5] In contrast to these negative results, phase 2 trials with IL-1 receptor antagonists or with the broad-spectrum anti-inflammatory agent minocycline have reported improvement in functional outcomes (see Table 9-6). The outcomes of these trials suggest optimism in the quest for an effective treatment for stroke, but the findings need to be confirmed and expanded in larger double-blind trials.

Immunologic tolerance to antigens found in the brain or on luminal endothelium has found application in preclinical stroke models. Oral tolerance is a well-established model whereby immunologic tolerance is induced to a specific antigen through feeding of that antigen.[221] Orally administered antigen encounters the gut-associated lymphoid tissue (GALT), which forms a well-developed immune network. GALT has evolved to protect the host from ingested pathogens and, perhaps by necessity, has developed the inherent property of preventing the host from reacting to ingested proteins that are innocuous. The nature of the tolerance depends on the schedule and amount of antigen feeding. Clonal deletion of antigen-reactive T cells can occur after a single feeding of very high doses of antigen.[222] Active tolerance with production of regulatory T cells occurs after repetitive feedings of low doses of antigen.[223,224] On antigen restimulation, T cells made tolerant with a low-dose regimen secrete cytokines such as transforming growth factor β1 (TGF-β1) and IL-10, which suppress cell-mediated, or TH1, immune responses.[224] Although activation of these T cells is specific for the tolerance-causing antigen, the immunomodulatory cytokines secreted in response to activation have nonspecific effects. Thus, local immunosuppression occurs wherever the tolerance-causing antigen is present. This phenomenon, known as active cellular regulation or bystander suppression, leads to relatively organ-specific immunosuppression.[225] Other forms of mucosal tolerance have also been investigated, specifically the administration of antigen via the nasal or aerosol route. The nasal route appears equal in efficiency to, and in some instances even more effective than, the oral route in suppressing autoimmune diseases in animal models.[226] Controlling inflammation in the brain by inducing oral tolerance to the CNS antigen, myelin basic protein (MBP), has been reported to result in smaller infarcts after MCA occlusion in the rat.[227] Repetitive intranasal administration of E-selectin to induce mucosal tolerance in the spontaneously hypertensive, genetically stroke-prone rat with untreated hypertension has been observed to potently inhibit development of ischemic and hemorrhagic strokes.[228] Assessment of the clinical utility of these approaches requires further testing.

Another approach is to target the effector proteins that initiate the cellular changes and damage triggered by postischemic inflammation. Cytokines, their receptors, iNOS, and EP1 receptors would be suitable targets. An attractive feature of strategies based on iNOS or EP1 receptor inhibition is their extended therapeutic window ($\geq$6 hours). Considering that most patients with stroke reach medical attention more than 6 hours after onset of symptoms,[229] these agents could have an important therapeutic role. Furthermore, combination of thrombolysis with iNOS or EP1 receptor inhibition may enhance the benefits of early reperfusion and improve the overall outcome. EP1 receptor inhibition is particularly attractive because it may also attenuate glutamate-dependent brain damage, thereby counteracting pathogenic events that occur in both the early and late stages of cerebral ischemia. Other strategies, in addition to inhibition of synthesis of key mediators such as NO, prostaglandin E$_2$, and cytokine interaction with their receptors, also emerge. Interventions targeting more broadly inflammatory signaling might be an attractive opportunity. Such signaling elements may include the transcription factors IRF-1 and NF-κB and their activators, including TLRs and scavenger receptors. However, considering the double edged role of inflammation—destructive in the acute phase and beneficial in the repair phase—modulation of inflammatory signaling has to be carefully timed to the stage of evolution of the damage.

Conclusions

A growing body of evidence suggests that ischemia-induced inflammation might play an important role in various stages of cerebral ischemic injury. The use of anti-inflammatory strategies in ischemic stroke therapy is attractive because they have a wider therapeutic window than the now-predominant approaches based on reperfusion. Studies in animal stroke models indicate that interventions aimed at attenuating the infiltration of leukocytes may have a beneficial effect in ameliorating the progression of ischemic brain damage. However, clinical trials that utilize anti-leukocyte agents have failed to show benefits. Results of preclinical studies have recently revealed a previously unrecognized role for lymphocytes in ischemic brain injury. Therefore, modulation of the trafficking and/or function of specific lymphocyte subtypes might be a powerful new tool for influencing the outcome of ischemic brain injury. New strategies that create tolerance to selected brain antigens also offer the potential of considerable neuroprotection. However, additional translational studies are needed to develop strategies that would be suitable for application in stroke patients. Theoretically, given the multiplicity of the factors controlling postischemic inflammation, strategies targeted against upstream regulatory elements that control a wide array of inflammatory pathways, such as transcription factors or immunomodulatory cells, would be preferable to strategies targeting individual effectors of damage. However, because certain aspects of inflammation are needed for tissue repair, silencing specific effectors of damage at a certain time after the unfolding of the ischemic cascade should also be considered. A comprehensive therapeutic approach based on anti-inflammatory strategies will require a more complete understanding of the multifaceted effects of inflammation in the ischemic brain.

Acknowledgments

Supported by grants from the National Institutes of Health (NS34179 and NS35806). C.I. is the recipient of a Javits Award from the National Institute of Neurological Diseases and Stroke.

REFERENCES

1. Lipton P: Ischemic cell death in brain neurons, *Physiol Rev* 79:1431-1568, 1999.
2. Allan SM, Rothwell NJ: Cytokines and acute neurodegeneration, *Nat Rev Neurosci* 2:734-744, 2001.
3. Emerich DF, Dean RL 3rd, Bartus RT: The role of leukocytes following cerebral ischemia: Pathogenic variable or bystander reaction to emerging infarct? *Exp Neurol* 173:168-181, 2002.
4. Wang Q, Tang XN, Yenari MA: The inflammatory response in stroke, *J Neuroimmunol* 184:53-68, 2007.
5. Wunder A, Klohs J, Dirnagl U: Non-invasive visualization of CNS inflammation with nuclear and optical imaging, *Neuroscience* 158:1161-1173, 2009.
6. Barone FC, Feuerstein GZ: Inflammatory mediators and stroke: New opportunities for novel therapeutics, *J Cereb Blood Flow Metab* 19:819-834, 1999.
7. Frijns CJ, Kappelle LJ: Inflammatory cell adhesion molecules in ischemic cerebrovascular disease, *Stroke* 33:2115-2122, 2002.
8. Ogata J, Yamanishi H, Pantoni L: Chapter 5 neuropathology of ischemic brain injury, *Handb Clin Neurol* 92:93-116, 2008.
9. Kostulas N, Pelidou SH, Kivisakk P, Kostulas V, Link H: Increased IL-1beta, IL-8, and IL-17 mRNA expression in blood mononuclear cells observed in a prospective ischemic stroke study, *Stroke* 30:2174-2179, 1999.
10. Pelidou SH, Kostulas N, Matusevicius D, Kivisakk P, Kostulas V, Link H: High levels of IL-10 secreting cells are present in blood in cerebrovascular diseases, *Eur J Neurol* 6:437-442, 1999.
11. Suzuki S, Tanaka K, Suzuki N: Ambivalent aspects of interleukin-6 in cerebral ischemia: Inflammatory versus neurotrophic aspects, *J Cereb Blood Flow Metab* 29:464-479, 2009.
12. del Zoppo G, Ginis I, Hallenbeck JM, Iadecola C, Wang X, Feuerstein GZ: Inflammation and stroke: Putative role for cytokines, adhesion molecules and iNOS in brain response to ischemia, *Brain Pathol* 10:95-112, 2000.
13. Ritter LS, Orozco JA, Coull BM, McDonagh PF, Rosenblum WI: Leukocyte accumulation and hemodynamic changes in the cerebral microcirculation during early reperfusion after stroke, *Stroke* 31:1153-1161, 2000.
14. Peters EE, Feuerstein GZ: Chemokines and ischemic stroke. In Feuerstein GZ, editor: *Inflammation and stroke*, New York, 2001, Birkhauser, pp 155-162.
15. Heinel LA, Rubin S, Rosenwasser RH, Vasthare US, Tuma RF: Leukocyte involvement in cerebral infarct generation after ischemia and reperfusion, *Brain Res Bull* 34:137-141, 1994.
16. Matsuo Y, Onodera H, Shiga Y, Nakamura M, Ninomiya M, Kihara T, Kogure K: Correlation between myeloperoxidase-quantified neutrophil accumulation and ischemic brain injury in the rat, *Stroke* 25:1469-1475, 1994.
17. Jiang N, Moyle M, Soule HR, Rote WE, Chopp M: Neutrophil inhibitory factor is neuroprotective after focal ischemia in rats, *Ann Neurol* 38:935-942, 1995.
18. Zhang RL, Chopp M, Li Y, Zaloga C, Jiang N, Jones ML, Miyasaka M, Ward PA: Anti-ICAM-1 antibody reduces ischemic cell damage after transient middle cerebral artery occlusion in the rat, *Neurology* 44:1747-1751, 1994.
19. Mori E, del Zoppo GJ, Chambers JD, Copeland BR, Arfors KE: Inhibition of polymorphonuclear leukocyte adherence suppresses no-reflow after focal cerebral ischemia in baboons, *Stroke* 23:712-718, 1992.
20. Chen H, Chopp M, Zhang RL, Bodzin G, Chen Q, Rusche JR, Todd RF III: Anti-CD11b monoclonal antibody reduces ischemic cell damage after transient focal cerebral ischemia in rat, *Ann Neurol* 35:458-463, 1994.
21. Zhang RL, Chopp M, Zhang ZG, Phillips ML, Rosenbloom CL, Cruz R, Manning A: E-selectin in focal cerebral ischemia and reperfusion in the rat, *J Cereb Blood Flow Metab* 16:1126-1136, 1996.
22. Morikawa E, Zhang SM, Seko Y, Toyoda T, Kirino T: Treatment of focal cerebral ischemia with synthetic oligopeptide corresponding to lectin domain of selectin, *Stroke* 27:951-955, 1996.
23. Suzuki H, Hayashi T, Tojo SJ, Kitagawa H, Kimura K, Mizugaki M, Itoyama Y, Abe K: Anti-P-selectin antibody attenuates rat brain ischemic injury, *Neurosci Lett* 265:163-166, 1999.
24. Connolly ES Jr, Winfree CJ, Prestigiacomo CJ, Kim SC, Choudhri TF, Hoh BL, Naka Y, Solomon RA, Pinsky DJ: Exacerbation of cerebral injury in mice that express the P-selectin gene: Identification of P-selectin blockade as a new target for the treatment of stroke, *Circ Res* 81:304-310, 1997.
25. Soriano SG, Coxon A, Wang YF, Frosch MP, Lipton SA, Hickey PR, Mayadas TN: Mice deficient in Mac-1 (CD11b/CD18) are less susceptible to cerebral ischemia/reperfusion injury, *Stroke* 30:134-139, 1999.
26. Connolly ES Jr, Winfree CJ, Springer TA, Naka Y, Liao H, Yan SD, Stern DM, Solomon RA, Gutierrez-Ramos JC, Pinsky DJ: Cerebral protection in homozygous null ICAM-1 mice after middle cerebral artery occlusion. Role of neutrophil adhesion in the pathogenesis of stroke, *J Clin Invest* 97:209-216, 1996.
27. Dawson DA, Martin D, Hallenbeck JM: Inhibition of tumor necrosis factor-alpha reduces focal cerebral ischemic injury in the spontaneously hypertensive rat, *Neurosci Lett* 218:41-44, 1996.
28. Yang GY, Gong C, Qin Z, Ye W, Mao Y, Betz AL: Inhibition of TNFalpha attenuates infarct volume and ICAM-1 expression in ischemic mouse brain, *Neuroreport* 9:2131-2134, 1998.
29. Yamasaki Y, Matsuura N, Shozuhara H, Onodera H, Itoyama Y, Kogure K: Interleukin-1 as a pathogenetic mediator of ischemic brain damage in rats, *Stroke* 26:676-680, 1995.
30. Loddick SA, Rothwell NJ: Neuroprotective effects of human recombinant interleukin-1 receptor antagonist in focal cerebral ischemia in the rat, *J Cereb Blood Flow Metab* 16:932-940, 1996.
31. Loddick SA, Turnbull AV, Rothwell NJ: Cerebral interleukin-6 is neuroprotective during permanent focal cerebral ischemia in the rat, *J Cereb Blood Flow Metab* 18:176-179, 1998.
32. Yang GY, Schielke GP, Gong C, Mao Y, Ge HL, Liu XH, Betz AL: Expression of tumor necrosis factor-alpha and intercellular adhesion molecule-1 after focal cerebral ischemia in interleukin-1beta converting enzyme deficient mice, *J Cereb Blood Flow Metab* 19:1109-1117, 1999.
33. Matsumoto T, Ikeda K, Mukaida N, Harada A, Matsumoto Y, Yamashita J, Matsushima K: Prevention of cerebral edema and infarct in cerebral reperfusion injury by an antibody to interleukin-8, *Lab Invest* 77:119-125, 1997.
34. Yamasaki Y, Matsuo Y, Zagorski J, Matsuura N, Onodera H, Itoyama Y, Kogure K: New therapeutic possibility of blocking cytokine-induced neutrophil chemoattractant on transient ischemic brain damage in rats, *Brain Res* 759:103-111, 1997.
35. Del Zoppo GJ, Schmid-Schonbein GW, Mori E, Copeland BR, Chang CM: Polymorphonuclear leukocytes occlude capillaries following middle cerebral artery occlusion and reperfusion in baboons, *Stroke* 22:1276-1283, 1991.
36. Yilmaz G, Arumugam TV, Stokes KY, Granger DN: Role of T lymphocytes and interferon-gamma in ischemic stroke, *Circulation* 113:2105-2112, 2006.
37. Ahmed SH, He YY, Nassief A, Xu J, Xu XM, Hsu CY, Faraci FM: Effects of lipopolysaccharide priming on acute ischemic brain injury, *Stroke* 31:193-199, 2000.
38. Becker K, Kindrick D, Relton J, Harlan J, Winn R: Antibody to the alpha4 integrin decreases infarct size in transient focal cerebral ischemia in rats, *Stroke* 32:206-211, 2001.
39. Relton JK, Sloan KE, Frew EM, Whalley ET, Adams SP, Lobb RR: Inhibition of alpha4 integrin protects against transient focal cerebral ischemia in normotensive and hypertensive rats, *Stroke* 32:199-205, 2001.
40. Prestigiacomo CJ, Kim SC, Connolly ES Jr, Liao H, Yan SF, Pinsky DJ: CD18-mediated neutrophil recruitment contributes to the pathogenesis of reperfused but not nonreperfused stroke, *Stroke* 30:1110-1117, 1999.
41. Arumugam TV, Salter JW, Chidlow JH, Ballantyne CM, Kevil CG, Granger DN: Contributions of LFA-1 and Mac-1 to brain injury and microvascular dysfunction induced by transient middle cerebral artery occlusion, *Am J Physiol Heart Circ Physiol* 287:H2555-2560, 2004.

42. Campanella M, Sciorati C, Tarozzo G, Beltramo M: Flow cytometric analysis of inflammatory cells in ischemic rat brain, *Stroke* 33:586–592, 2002.

43. Hurn PD, Subramanian S, Parker SM, Afentoulis ME, Kaler LJ, Vandenbark AA, Offner H: T- and B-cell-deficient mice with experimental stroke have reduced lesion size and inflammation, *J Cereb Blood Flow Metab* 27:1798–1805, 2007.

44. Liesz A, Suri-Payer E, Veltkamp C, Doerr H, Sommer C, Rivest S, Giese T, Veltkamp R: Regulatory T cells are key cerebroprotective immunomodulators in acute experimental stroke, *Nat Med* 15:192–199, 2009.

45. Planas AM, Chamorro A: Regulatory T cells protect the brain after stroke, *Nat Med* 15:138–139, 2009.

46. Buttini M, Sauter A, Boddeke HW: Induction of interleukin-1 beta mRNA after focal cerebral ischaemia in the rat, *Brain Res Mol Brain Res* 23:126–134, 1994.

47. Liu T, McDonnell PC, Young PR, White RF, Siren AL, Hallenbeck JM, Barone FC, Feuerstein GZ: Interleukin-1 beta mRNA expression in ischemic rat cortex, *Stroke* 24:1746–1750, 1993.

48. Liu T, Clark RK, McDonnell PC, Young PR, White RF, Barone FC, Feuerstein GZ: Tumor necrosis factor-alpha expression in ischemic neurons, *Stroke* 25:1481–1488, 1994.

49. Wang X, Yue TL, Barone FC, White RF, Gagnon RC, Feuerstein GZ: Concomitant cortical expression of TNF-alpha and IL-1 beta mRNAs follows early response gene expression in transient focal ischemia, *Mol Chem Neuropathol* 23:103–114, 1994.

50. Minami M, Kuraishi Y, Yabuuchi K, Yamazaki A, Satoh M: Induction of interleukin-1 beta mRNA in rat brain after transient forebrain ischemia, *J Neurochem* 58:390–392, 1992.

51. Yabuuchi K, Minami M, Katsumata S, Yamazaki A, Satoh M: An in situ hybridization study on interleukin-1 beta mRNA induced by transient forebrain ischemia in the rat brain, *Brain Res Mol Brain Res* 26:135–142, 1994.

52. Saito K, Suyama K, Nishida K, Sei Y, Basile AS: Early increases in TNF-alpha, IL-6 and IL-1 beta levels following transient cerebral ischemia in gerbil brain, *Neurosci Lett* 206:149–152, 1996.

53. Uno H, Matsuyama T, Akita H, Nishimura H, Sugita M: Induction of tumor necrosis factor-alpha in the mouse hippocampus following transient forebrain ischemia, *J Cereb Blood Flow Metab* 17:491–499, 1997.

54. Barone FC, Arvin B, White RF, Miller A, Webb CL, Willette RN, Lysko PG, Feuerstein GZ: Tumor necrosis factor-alpha: A mediator of focal ischemic brain injury, *Stroke* 28:1233–1244, 1997.

55. Garcia JH, Liu KF, Relton JK: Interleukin-1 receptor antagonist decreases the number of necrotic neurons in rats with middle cerebral artery occlusion, *Am J Pathol* 147:1477–1486, 1995.

56. Relton JK, Rothwell NJ: Interleukin-1 receptor antagonist inhibits ischaemic and excitotoxic neuronal damage in the rat, *Brain Res Bull* 29:243–246, 1992.

57. Rothwell NJ, Relton JK: Involvement of interleukin-1 and lipocortin-1 in ischaemic brain damage, *Cerebrovasc Brain Metab Rev* 5:178–198, 1993.

58. Martin D, Chinookoswong N, Miller G: The interleukin-1 receptor antagonist (rhIL-1ra) protects against cerebral infarction in a rat model of hypoxia-ischemia, *Exp Neurol* 130:362–367, 1994.

59. Betz AL, Yang GY, Davidson BL: Attenuation of stroke size in rats using an adenoviral vector to induce overexpression of interleukin-1 receptor antagonist in brain, *J Cereb Blood Flow Metab* 15:547–551, 1995.

60. Basu A, Krady JK, O'Malley M, Styren SD, DeKosky ST, Levison SW: The type 1 interleukin-1 receptor is essential for the efficient activation of microglia and the induction of multiple proinflammatory mediators in response to brain injury, *J Neurosci* 22:6071–6082, 2002.

61. Iadecola C, Salkowski CA, Zhang F, Aber T, Nagayama M, Vogel SN, Ross ME: The transcription factor interferon regulatory factor 1 is expressed after cerebral ischemia and contributes to ischemic brain injury, *J Exp Med* 189:719–727, 1999.

62. Arumugam TV, Granger DN, Mattson MP: Stroke and T-cells, *Neuromolecular Med* 7:229–242, 2005.

63. Liu J, Ginis I, Spatz M, Hallenbeck JM: Hypoxic preconditioning protects cultured neurons against hypoxic stress via TNF-alpha and ceramide, *Am J Physiol Cell Physiol* 278:C144–153, 2000.

64. Bruce AJ, Boling W, Kindy MS, Peschon J, Kraemer PJ, Carpenter MK, Holtsberg FW, Mattson MP: Altered neuronal and microglial responses to excitotoxic and ischemic brain injury in mice lacking TNF receptors, *Nat Med* 2:788–794, 1996.

65. Yang L, Lindholm K, Konishi Y, Li R, Shen Y: Target depletion of distinct tumor necrosis factor receptor subtypes reveals hippocampal neuron death and survival through different signal transduction pathways, *J Neurosci* 22:3025–3032, 2002.

66. Fontaine V, Mohand-Said S, Hanoteau N, Fuchs C, Pfizenmaier K, Eisel U: Neurodegenerative and neuroprotective effects of tumor necrosis factor (TNF) in retinal ischemia: Opposite roles of TNF receptor 1 and TNF receptor 2, *J Neurosci* 22:RC216, 2002.

67. Martin-Villalba A, Hahne M, Kleber S, Vogel J, Falk W, Schenkel J, Krammer PH: Therapeutic neutralization of CD95-ligand and TNF attenuates brain damage in stroke, *Cell Death Differ* 8:679–686, 2001.

68. Becker KJ: Sensitization and tolerization to brain antigens in stroke, *Neuroscience* 158:1090–1097, 2009.

69. Prass K, Meisel C, Hoflich C, Braun J, Halle E, Wolf T, Ruscher K, Victorov IV, Priller J, Dirnagl U, Volk HD, Meisel A: Stroke-induced immunodeficiency promotes spontaneous bacterial infections and is mediated by sympathetic activation reversal by poststroke T helper cell type 1-like immunostimulation, *J Exp Med* 198:725–736, 2003.

70. Meisel C, Schwab JM, Prass K, Meisel A, Dirnagl U: Central nervous system injury-induced immune deficiency syndrome, *Nat Rev Neurosci* 6:775–786, 2005.

71. Murphy S, Gibson CL: Nitric oxide, ischaemia and brain inflammation, *Biochem Soc Trans* 35:1133–1137, 2007.

72. Garthwaite J: Concepts of neural nitric oxide-mediated transmission, *Eur J Neurosci* 27:2783–2802, 2008.

73. Beckman JS, Beckman TW, Chen J, Marshall PA, Freeman BA: Apparent hydroxyl radical production by peroxynitrite: Implications for endothelial injury from nitric oxide and superoxide, *Proc Natl Acad Sci U S A* 87:1620–1624, 1990.

74. Pacher P, Beckman JS, Liaudet L: Nitric oxide and peroxynitrite in health and disease, *Physiol Rev* 87:315–424, 2007.

75. Iadecola C, Zhang F, Xu X, Casey R, Ross ME: Inducible nitric oxide synthase gene expression in brain following cerebral ischemia, *J Cereb Blood Flow Metab* 15:378–384, 1995.

76. Iadecola C, Zhang F, Casey R, Clark HB, Ross ME: Inducible nitric oxide synthase gene expression in vascular cells after transient focal cerebral ischemia, *Stroke* 27:1373–1380, 1996.

77. Grandati M, Verrecchia C, Revaud ML, Allix M, Boulu RG, Plotkine M: Calcium-independent NO-synthase activity and nitrites/nitrates production in transient focal cerebral ischaemia in mice, *Br J Pharmacol* 122:625–630, 1997.

78. Hirabayashi H, Takizawa S, Fukuyama N, Nakazawa H, Shinohara Y: Nitrotyrosine generation via inducible nitric oxide synthase in vascular wall in focal ischemia-reperfusion, *Brain Res* 852:319–325, 2000.

79. Forster C, Clark HB, Ross ME, Iadecola C: Inducible nitric oxide synthase expression in human cerebral infarcts, *Acta Neuropathol* 97:215–220, 1999.

80. Tarkowski E, Ringqvist A, Rosengren L, Jensen C, Ekholm S, Wennmalm A: Intrathecal release of nitric oxide and its relation to final brain damage in patients with stroke, *Cerebrovasc Dis* 10:200–206, 2000.

81. Iadecola C, Zhang F, Xu X: Inhibition of inducible nitric oxide synthase ameliorates cerebral ischemic damage, *Am J Physiol* 268:R286–R292, 1995.

82. Nagayama M, Zhang F, Iadecola C: Delayed treatment with aminoguanidine decreases focal cerebral ischemic damage and enhances neurologic recovery in rats, *J Cereb Blood Flow Metab* 18:1107–1113, 1998.

83. Parmentier S, Bohme GA, Lerouet D, Damour D, Stutzmann JM, Margaill I, Plotkine M: Selective inhibition of inducible nitric oxide synthase prevents ischaemic brain injury, *Br J Pharmacol* 127:546–552, 1999.

84. Zhao X, Haensel C, Araki E, Ross ME, Iadecola C: Gene-dosing effect and persistence of reduction in ischemic brain injury in mice lacking inducible nitric oxide synthase, *Brain Res* 872:215–218, 2000.

85. Iadecola C, Zhang F, Casey R, Nagayama M, Ross ME: Delayed reduction in ischemic brain injury and neurological deficits in mice lacking the inducible nitric oxide synthase gene, *J Neurosci* 17:9157–9164, 1997.

86. Parmentier-Batteur S, Bohme GA, Lerouet D, Zhou-Ding L, Beray V, Margaill I, Plotkine M: Antisense oligodeoxynucleotide to inducible nitric oxide synthase protects against transient focal cerebral ischemia-induced brain injury, *J Cereb Blood Flow Metab* 21:15–21, 2001.

87. Han HS, Qiao Y, Karabiyikoglu M, Giffard RG, Yenari MA: Influence of mild hypothermia on inducible nitric oxide synthase expression and reactive nitrogen production in experimental stroke and inflammation, *J Neurosci* 22:3921–3928, 2002.

88. Coughlan T, Gibson C, Murphy S: Modulatory effects of progesterone on inducible nitric oxide synthase expression in vivo and in vitro, *J Neurochem* 93:932–942, 2005.

89. Park EM, Cho S, Frys KA, Glickstein SB, Zhou P, Anrather J, Ross ME, Iadecola C: Inducible nitric oxide synthase contributes to gender differences in ischemic brain injury, *J Cereb Blood Flow Metab* 26:392–401, 2006.

90. Vane JR, Bakhle YS, Botting RM: Cyclooxygenases 1 and 2, *Annu Rev Pharmacol Toxicol* 38:97–120, 1998.

91. Phillis JW, Horrocks LA, Farooqui AA: Cyclooxygenases, lipoxygenases, and epoxygenases in CNS: Their role and involvement in neurological disorders, *Brain Res Rev* 52:201–243, 2006.

92. Hurley SD, Olschowka JA, O'Banion MK: Cyclooxygenase inhibition as a strategy to ameliorate brain injury, *J Neurotrauma* 19:1–15, 2002.

93. Minghetti L: Role of COX-2 in inflammatory and degenerative brain diseases, *Subcell Biochem* 42:127–141, 2007.

94. Miettinen S, Fusco FR, Yrjanheikki J, Keinanen R, Hirvonen T, Roivainen R, Narhi M, Hokfelt T, Koistinaho J: Spreading depression and focal brain ischemia induce cyclooxygenase-2 in cortical neurons through *N*-methyl-D-aspartic acid-receptors and phospholipase A2, *Proc Natl Acad Sci U S A* 94:6500–6505, 1997.

95. Nogawa S, Zhang F, Ross ME, Iadecola C: Cyclo-oxygenase-2 gene expression in neurons contributes to ischemic brain damage, *J Neurosci* 17:2746–2755, 1997.

96. Iadecola C, Forster C, Nogawa S, Clark HB, Ross ME: Cyclooxygenase-2 immunoreactivity in the human brain following cerebral ischemia, *Acta Neuropathol* 98:9–14, 1999.

97. Nogawa S, Forster C, Zhang F, Nagayama M, Ross ME, Iadecola C: Interaction between inducible nitric oxide synthase and cyclooxygenase-2 after cerebral ischemia, *Proc Natl Acad Sci U S A* 95:10966–10971, 1998.

98. Sairanen T, Ristimaki A, Karjalainen-Lindsberg ML, Paetau A, Kaste M, Lindsberg PJ: Cyclooxygenase-2 is induced globally in infarcted human brain, *Ann Neurol* 43:738–747, 1998.

99. Nagayama M, Niwa K, Nagayama T, Ross ME, Iadecola C: The cyclooxygenase-2 inhibitor NS-398 ameliorates cerebral ischemic injury in wild-type mice but not in mice with deletion of the inducible nitric oxide synthase gene, *J Cereb Blood Flow Metab* 19:1213–1219, 1999.

100. Iadecola C, Niwa K, Nogawa S, Zhao X, Nagayama M, Araki E, Morham S, Ross ME: Reduced susceptibility to ischemic brain injury and NMDA-mediated neurotoxicity in cyclooxygenase-2 deficient mice, *Proc Natl Acad Sci U S A* 98:1294–1299, 2001.

101. Moskowitz MA, Lo EH, Iadecola C: The science of stroke: Mechanisms in search of treatments, *Neuron* 67:181–198, 2010.

102. Lo EH, Dalkara T, Moskowitz MA: Mechanisms, challenges and opportunities in stroke, *Nat Rev Neurosci* 4:399–415, 2003.

103. Candelario-Jalil E, Fiebich BL: Cyclooxygenase inhibition in ischemic brain injury, *Curr Pharm Des* 14:1401–1418, 2008.

104. Kunz A, Anrather J, Zhou P, Orio M, Iadecola C: Cyclooxygenase-2 does not contribute to postischemic production of reactive oxygen species, *J Cereb Blood Flow Metab* 27:545–551, 2007.

105. Manabe Y, Anrather J, Kawano T, Niwa K, Zhou P, Ross ME, Iadecola C: Prostanoids, not reactive oxygen species, mediate COX-2-dependent neurotoxicity, *Ann Neurol* 55:668–675, 2004.

106. Kawano T, Anrather J, Zhou P, Park L, Wang G, Frys KA, Kunz A, Cho S, Orio M, Iadecola C: Prostaglandin E(2) EP1 receptors: Downstream effectors of COX-2 neurotoxicity, *Nat Med* 12:225–229, 2006.

107. Ahmad AS, Saleem S, Ahmad M, Dore S: Prostaglandin EP1 receptor contributes to excitotoxicity and focal ischemic brain damage, *Toxicol Sci* 89:265–270, 2006.

108. Zhou P, Qian L, Chou T, Iadecola C: Neuroprotection by PGE2 receptor EP1 inhibition involves the PTEN/AKT pathway, *Neurobiol Dis* 29:543–551, 2008.

109. Iadecola C, Gorelick PB: The Janus face of cyclooxygenase-2 in ischemic stroke: Shifting toward downstream targets, *Stroke* 36:182–185, 2005.

110. McAdam BF, Catella-Lawson F, Mardini IA, Kapoor S, Lawson JA, FitzGerald GA: Systemic biosynthesis of prostacyclin by cyclooxygenase (COX)-2: The human pharmacology of a selective inhibitor of COX-2, *Proc Natl Acad Sci U S A* 96:272–277, 1999.

111. Hallenbeck JM, Frerichs KU: Secondary ischemic neuronal damage may involve multiple factors acting as an aggregate of minor causes. In Robertson JT, Nowak TS Jr, editors: *Frontiers in cerebrovascular disease: Mechanisms, diagnosis, and treatment*, Armonk, NY, 1998, Futura Publishing Company, Inc, pp 95–101.

112. Hallenbeck JM, Frerichs KU: Stroke therapy. It may be time for an integrated approach, *Arch Neurol* 50:768–770, 1993.

113. Iadecola C, Alexander M: Cerebral ischemia and inflammation, *Curr Opin Neurol* 14:89–94, 2001.

114. Lee YJ, Hallenbeck JM: Insights into cytoprotection from ground squirrel hibernation, a natural model of tolerance to profound brain oligaemia, *Biochem Soc Trans* 34:1295–1298, 2006.

115. Oppenheim JJ, Yang D: Alarmins: Chemotactic activators of immune responses, *Curr Opin Immunol* 17:359–365, 2005.

116. Zedler S, Faist E: The impact of endogenous triggers on trauma-associated inflammation, *Curr Opin Crit Care* 12:595–601, 2006.

117. Lehrer RI, Ganz T: Cathelicidins: A family of endogenous antimicrobial peptides, *Curr Opin Hematol* 9:18–22, 2002.

118. Kim JB, Sig Choi J, Yu YM, Nam K, Piao CS, Kim SW, Lee MH, Han PL, Park JS, Lee JK: HMGB1, a novel cytokine-like mediator linking acute neuronal death and delayed neuroinflammation in the postischemic brain, *J Neurosci* 26:6413–6421, 2006.

119. Foell D, Wittkowski H, Vogl T, Roth J: S100 proteins expressed in phagocytes: A novel group of damage-associated molecular pattern molecules, *J Leukoc Biol* 81:28–37, 2007.

120. Lin L: RAGE on the toll road? *Cell Mol Immunol* 3:351–358, 2006.

121. Akira S, Takeda K, Kaisho T: Toll-like receptors: Critical proteins linking innate and acquired immunity, *Nat Immunol* 2:675–680, 2001.

122. Ishii KJ, Akira S: Potential link between the immune system and metabolism of nucleic acids, *Curr Opin Immunol* 20:524–529, 2008.

123. Jin MS, Lee JO: Structures of the toll-like receptor family and its ligand complexes, *Immunity* 29:182–191, 2008.

124. Ozinsky A, Underhill DM, Fontenot JD, Hajjar AM, Smith KD, Wilson CB, Schroeder L, Aderem A: The repertoire for pattern recognition of pathogens by the innate immune system is defined by cooperation between toll-like receptors, *Proc Natl Acad Sci U S A* 97:13766–13771, 2000.

125. Horner AA, Redecke V, Raz E: Toll-like receptor ligands: Hygiene, atopy and therapeutic implications, *Curr Opin Allergy Clin Immunol* 4:555–561, 2004.

126. Arumugam TV, Okun E, Tang SC, Thundyil J, Taylor SM, Woodruff TM: Toll-like receptors in ischemia-reperfusion injury, *Shock* 32:4–16, 2009.

127. Tang SC, Arumugam TV, Xu X, Cheng A, Mughal MR, Jo DG, Lathia JD, Siler DA, Chigurupati S, Ouyang X, Magnus T, Camandola S, Mattson MP: Pivotal role for neuronal toll-like receptors in ischemic brain injury and functional deficits, *Proc Natl Acad Sci U S A* 104:13798–13803, 2007.

128. Ziegler G, Harhausen D, Schepers C, Hoffmann O, Rohr C, Prinz V, Konig J, Lehrach H, Nietfeld W, Trendelenburg G: TLR2 has a detrimental role in mouse transient focal cerebral ischemia, *Biochem Biophys Res Commun* 359:574–579, 2007.

129. Cao CX, Yang QW, Lv FL, Cui J, Fu HB, Wang JZ: Reduced cerebral ischemia-reperfusion injury in toll-like receptor 4 deficient mice, *Biochem Biophys Res Commun* 353:509–514, 2007.

130. Caso JR, Pradillo JM, Hurtado O, Lorenzo P, Moro MA, Lizasoain I: Toll-like receptor 4 is involved in brain damage and inflammation after experimental stroke, *Circulation* 115:1599–1608, 2007.

131. Lehnardt S, Lehmann S, Kaul D, Tschimmel K, Hoffmann O, Cho S, Krueger C, Nitsch R, Meisel A, Weber JR: Toll-like receptor 2 mediates CNS injury in focal cerebral ischemia, *J Neuroimmunol* 190:28–33, 2007.

132. Hua F, Ma J, Ha T, Xia Y, Kelley J, Williams DL, Kao RL, Browder IW, Schweitzer JB, Kalbfleisch JH, Li C: Activation of toll-like receptor 4 signaling contributes to hippocampal neuronal death following global cerebral ischemia/reperfusion, *J Neuroimmunol* 190:101–111, 2007.

133. Park IH, Yeon SI, Youn JH, Choi JE, Sasaki N, Choi IH, Shin JS: Expression of a novel secreted splice variant of the receptor for advanced glycation end products (RAGE) in human brain astrocytes and peripheral blood mononuclear cells, *Mol Immunol* 40:1203–1211, 2004.

134. Zimmerman GA, Meistrell M 3rd, Bloom O, Cockroft KM, Bianchi M, Risucci D, Broome J, Farmer P, Cerami A, Vlassara H, et al: Neurotoxicity of advanced glycation endproducts during focal stroke and neuroprotective effects of aminoguanidine, *Proc Natl Acad Sci U S A* 92:3744–3748, 1995.

135. Degryse B, Bonaldi T, Scaffidi P, Muller S, Resnati M, Sanvito F, Arrigoni G, Bianchi ME: The high mobility group (HMG) boxes of the nuclear protein HMG1 induce chemotaxis and cytoskeleton reorganization in rat smooth muscle cells, *J Cell Biol* 152:1197–1206, 2001.

136. Scaffidi P, Misteli T, Bianchi ME: Release of chromatin protein HMGB1 by necrotic cells triggers inflammation, *Nature* 418:191–195, 2002.

137. Qiu J, Nishimura M, Wang Y, Sims JR, Qiu S, Savitz SI, Salomone S, Moskowitz MA: Early release of HMGB-1 from neurons after the onset of brain ischemia, *J Cereb Blood Flow Metab* 28:927–938, 2008.

138. Muhammad S, Barakat W, Stoyanov S, Murikinati S, Yang H, Tracey KJ, Bendszus M, Rossetti G, Nawroth PP, Bierhaus A, Schwaninger M: The HMGB1 receptor RAGE mediates ischemic brain damage, *J Neurosci* 28:12023–12031, 2008.

139. Li M, Carpio DF, Zheng Y, Bruzzo P, Singh V, Ouaaz F, Medzhitov RM, Beg AA: An essential role of the NF-kappaB/toll-like receptor pathway in induction of inflammatory and tissue-repair gene expression by necrotic cells, *J Immunol* 166:7128–7135, 2001.

140. Martinon F, Tschopp J: Inflammatory caspases and inflammasomes: Master switches of inflammation, *Cell Death Differ* 14:10–22, 2007.

141. Tabuchi M, Inoue K, Usui-Kataoka H, Kobayashi K, Teramoto M, Takasugi K, Shikata K, Yamamura M, Ando K, Nishida K, Kasahara J, Kume N, Lopez LR, Mitsudo K, Nobuyoshi M, Yasuda T, Kita T, Makino H, Matsuura E: The association of C-reactive protein with an oxidative metabolite of LDL and its implication in atherosclerosis, *J Lipid Res* 48:768–781, 2007.

142. Lamkanfi M, Declercq W, Vanden Berghe T, Vandenabeele P: Caspases leave the beaten track: Caspase-mediated activation of NF-kappaB, *J Cell Biol* 173:165–171, 2006.

143. Wuerzberger-Davis SM, Nakamura Y, Seufzer BJ, Miyamoto S: NF-kappaB activation by combinations of NEMO SUMOylation and ATM activation stresses in the absence of DNA damage, *Oncogene* 26:641–651, 2007.

144. Silverstein RL, Febbraio M: CD36, a scavenger receptor involved in immunity, metabolism, angiogenesis, and behavior. *Sci Signal* 2:1–8, 2009.

145. Hirano K, Kuwasako T, Nakagawa-Toyama Y, Janabi M, Yamashita S, Matsuzawa Y: Pathophysiology of human genetic CD36 deficiency, *Trends Cardiovasc Med* 13:136–141, 2003.

146. Medeiros LA, Khan T, El Khoury JB, Pham CL, Hatters DM, Howlett GJ, Lopez R, O'Brien KD, Moore KJ: Fibrillar amyloid protein present in atheroma activates CD36 signal transduction, *J Biol Chem* 279:10643–10648, 2004.

147. Stuart LM, Deng J, Silver JM, Takahashi K, Tseng AA, Hennessy EJ, Ezekowitz RA, Moore KJ: Response to *Staphylococcus aureus* requires CD36-mediated phagocytosis triggered by the COOH-terminal cytoplasmic domain, *J Cell Biol* 170:477–485, 2005.

148. Triantafilou M, Gamper FG, Haston RM, Mouratis MA, Morath S, Hartung T, Triantafilou K: Membrane sorting of toll-like receptor (TLR)-2/6 and TLR2/1 heterodimers at the cell surface determines heterotypic associations with CD36 and intracellular targeting, *J Biol Chem* 281:31002–31011, 2006.

149. Cho S, Park EM, Febbraio M, Anrather J, Park L, Racchumi G, Silverstein RL, Iadecola C: The class B scavenger receptor CD36 mediates free radical production and tissue injury in cerebral ischemia, *J Neurosci* 25:2504–2512, 2005.

150. Kunz A, Abe T, Hochrainer K, Shimamura M, Anrather J, Racchumi G, Zhou P, Iadecola C: Nuclear factor-kappaB activation and postischemic inflammation are suppressed in CD36-null mice after middle cerebral artery occlusion, *J Neurosci* 28:1649–1658, 2008.

151. Ghosh S, Karin M: Missing pieces in the NF-kappaB puzzle, *Cell* 109 (Suppl):S81-96, 2002.

152. Pahl HL: Activators and target genes of Rel/NF-kappaB transcription factors, *Oncogene* 18:6853–6866, 1999.

153. Hallenbeck JM: The many faces of tumor necrosis factor in stroke, *Nat Med* 8:1363–1368, 2002.

154. Schwaninger M, Inta I, Herrmann O: NF-kappaB signalling in cerebral ischaemia, *Biochem Soc Trans* 34:1291–1294, 2006.

155. Blondeau N, Widmann C, Lazdunski M, Heurteaux C: Activation of the nuclear factor-kappaB is a key event in brain tolerance, *J Neurosci* 21:4668–4677, 2001.

156. Pradillo JM, Romera C, Hurtado O, Cardenas A, Moro MA, Leza JC, Davalos A, Castillo J, Lorenzo P, Lizasoain I: TNFR1 upregulation mediates tolerance after brain ischemic preconditioning, *J Cereb Blood Flow Metab* 25:193–203, 2005.

157. Perkins ND: Post-translational modifications regulating the activity and function of the nuclear factor kappa B pathway, *Oncogene* 25:6717–6730, 2006.

158. Vanden Berghe W, Ndlovu MN, Hoya-Arias R, Dijsselbloem N, Gerlo S, Haegeman G: Keeping up NF-kappaB appearances: Epigenetic control of immunity or inflammation-triggered epigenetics, *Biochem Pharmacol* 72:1114–1131, 2006.

159. Baeuerle PA, Baltimore D: NF-kappaB: Ten years after, *Cell* 87:13–20, 1996.

160. Salminen A, Liu PK, Hsu CY: Alteration of transcription factor binding activities in the ischemic rat brain, *Biochem Biophys Res Commun* 212:939–944, 1995.

161. Carroll JE, Hess DC, Howard EF, Hill WD: Is nuclear factor-kappaB a good treatment target in brain ischemia/reperfusion injury? *Neuroreport* 11:R1–4, 2000.

162. Gabriel C, Justicia C, Camins A, Planas AM: Activation of nuclear factor-kappaB in the rat brain after transient focal ischemia, *Brain Res Mol Brain Res* 65:61–69, 1999.

163. Stephenson D, Yin T, Smalstig EB, Hsu MA, Panetta J, Little S, Clemens J: Transcription factor nuclear factor-kappaB is activated in neurons after focal cerebral ischemia, *J Cereb Blood Flow Metab* 20:592–603, 2000.

164. Schneider A, Martin-Villalba A, Weih F, Vogel J, Wirth T, Schwaninger M: NF-kappaB is activated and promotes cell death in focal cerebral ischemia, *Nat Med* 5:554–559, 1999.

165. Terai K, Matsuo A, McGeer EG, McGeer PL: Enhancement of immunoreactivity for NF-kappaB in human cerebral infarctions, *Brain Res* 739:343–349, 1996.

166. Nurmi A, Lindsberg PJ, Koistinaho M, Zhang W, Juettler E, Karjalainen-Lindsberg ML, Weih F, Frank N, Schwaninger M, Koistinaho J: Nuclear factor-kappaB contributes to infarction after permanent focal ischemia, *Stroke* 35:987–991, 2004.

167. Xu L, Zhan Y, Wang Y, Feuerstein GZ, Wang X: Recombinant adenoviral expression of dominant negative IkappaBalpha protects brain from cerebral ischemic injury, *Biochem Biophys Res Commun* 299:14–17, 2002.

168. Herrmann O, Baumann B, de Lorenzi R, Muhammad S, Zhang W, Kleesiek J, Malfertheiner M, Kohrmann M, Potrovita I, Maegele I, Beyer C, Burke JR, Hasan MT, Bujard H, Wirth T, Pasparakis M, Schwaninger M: IKK mediates ischemia-induced neuronal death, *Nat Med* 11:1322–1329, 2005.

169. Hill WD, Hess DC, Carroll JE, Wakade CG, Howard EF, Chen Q, Cheng C, Martin-Studdard A, Waller JL, Beswick RA: The NF-kappaB inhibitor diethyldithiocarbamate (DDTC) increases brain cell death in a transient middle cerebral artery occlusion model of ischemia, *Brain Res Bull* 55:375–386, 2001.

170. Kim CH, Kim JH, Moon SJ, Hsu CY, Seo JT, Ahn YS: Biphasic effects of dithiocarbamates on the activity of nuclear factor-kappaB, *Eur J Pharmacol* 392:133–136, 2000.

171. Misra HP: Reaction of copper-zinc superoxide dismutase with diethyldithiocarbamate, *J Biol Chem* 254:11623–11628, 1979.

172. Ravati A, Ahlemeyer B, Becker A, Klumpp S, Krieglstein J: Preconditioning-induced neuroprotection is mediated by reactive oxygen species and activation of the transcription factor nuclear factor-kappaB, *J Neurochem* 78:909-919, 2001.

173. Kunz A, Park L, Abe T, Gallo EF, Anrather J, Zhou P, Iadecola C: Neurovascular protection by ischemic tolerance: Role of nitric oxide and reactive oxygen species, *J Neurosci* 27:7083-7093, 2007.

174. Gidday JM: Cerebral preconditioning and ischaemic tolerance, *Nat Rev Neurosci* 7:437-448, 2006.

175. Taniguchi T, Ogasawara K, Takaoka A, Tanaka N: IRF family of transcription factors as regulators of host defense, *Annu Rev Immunol* 19:623-655, 2001.

176. Paschen W, Gissel C, Althausen S, Doutheil J: Changes in interferon-regulatory factor-1 mRNA levels after transient ischemia in rat brain, *Neuroreport* 9:3147-3151, 1998.

177. Iadecola C, Alexander M, Nogawa S, Arachi E, Ross ME: Inflammation-related genes and ischemic brain injury. In Krieglstein J, Klumpp S, editors: *Pharmacology of cerebral ischemia 2000*, Stuttgart, 2000, Medpharm Scientific Publishers, pp 241-251.

178. Yi JH, Park SW, Kapadia R, Vemuganti R: Role of transcription factors in mediating post-ischemic cerebral inflammation and brain damage, *Neurochem Int* 50:1014-1027, 2007.

179. Kapadia R, Tureyen K, Bowen KK, Kalluri H, Johnson PF, Vemuganti R: Decreased brain damage and curtailed inflammation in transcription factor CCAAT/enhancer binding protein beta knockout mice following transient focal cerebral ischemia, *J Neurochem* 98:1718-1731, 2006.

180. Berger JP, Akiyama TE, Meinke PT: PPARs: Therapeutic targets for metabolic disease, *Trends Pharmacol Sci* 26:244-251, 2005.

181. Berger J, Moller DE: The mechanisms of action of PPARs, *Annu Rev Med* 53:409-435, 2002.

182. Lehmann JM, Moore LB, Smith-Oliver TA, Wilkison WO, Willson TM, Kliewer SA: An antidiabetic thiazolidinedione is a high affinity ligand for peroxisome proliferator-activated receptor gamma (PPAR gamma), *J Biol Chem* 270:12953-12956, 1995.

183. Sundararajan S, Gamboa JL, Victor NA, Wanderi EW, Lust WD, Landreth GE: Peroxisome proliferator-activated receptor-gamma ligands reduce inflammation and infarction size in transient focal ischemia, *Neuroscience* 130:685-696, 2005.

184. Luo Y, Yin W, Signore AP, Zhang F, Hong Z, Wang S, Graham SH, Chen J: Neuroprotection against focal ischemic brain injury by the peroxisome proliferator-activated receptor-gamma agonist rosiglitazone, *J Neurochem* 97:435-448, 2006.

185. Zhao Y, Patzer A, Gohlke P, Herdegen T, Culman J: The intracerebral application of the PPARgamma-ligand pioglitazone confers neuroprotection against focal ischaemia in the rat brain, *Eur J Neurosci* 22:278-282, 2005.

186. Chu K, Lee ST, Koo JS, Jung KH, Kim EH, Sinn DI, Kim JM, Ko SY, Kim SJ, Song EC, Kim KM, Roh JK: Peroxisome proliferator-activated receptor-gamma-agonist, rosiglitazone, promotes angiogenesis after focal cerebral ischemia, *Brain Res* 1093:208-218, 2006.

187. Victor NA, Wanderi EW, Gamboa J, Zhao X, Aronowski J, Deininger K, Lust WD, Landreth GE, Sundararajan S: Altered PPARgamma expression and activation after transient focal ischemia in rats, *Eur J Neurosci* 24:1653-1663, 2006.

188. Deplanque D, Gele P, Petrault O, Six I, Furman C, Bouly M, Nion S, Dupuis B, Leys D, Fruchart JC, Cecchelli R, Staels B, Duriez P, Bordet R: Peroxisome proliferator-activated receptor-alpha activation as a mechanism of preventive neuroprotection induced by chronic fenofibrate treatment, *J Neurosci* 23:6264-6271, 2003.

189. Collino M, Aragno M, Mastrocola R, Benetti E, Gallicchio M, Dianzani C, Danni O, Thiemermann C, Fantozzi R: Oxidative stress and inflammatory response evoked by transient cerebral ischemia/reperfusion: Effects of the PPAR-alpha agonist WY14643, *Free Radic Biol Med* 41:579-589, 2006.

190. Nissen SE, Wolski K: Effect of rosiglitazone on the risk of myocardial infarction and death from cardiovascular causes, *N Engl J Med* 356:2457-2471, 2007.

191. Zinn A, Felson S, Fisher E, Schwartzbard A: Reassessing the cardiovascular risks and benefits of thiazolidinediones, *Clin Cardiol* 31:397-403, 2008.

192. Bahr RD, Leino EV, Christenson RH: Prodromal unstable angina in acute myocardial infarction: Prognostic value of short- and long-term outcome and predictor of infarct size, *Am Heart J* 140:126-133, 2000.

193. Noda T, Minatoguchi S, Fujii K, Hori M, Ito T, Kanmatsuse K, Matsuzaki M, Miura T, Nonogi H, Tada M, Tanaka M, Fujiwara H: Evidence for the delayed effect in human ischemic preconditioning: Prospective multicenter study for preconditioning in acute myocardial infarction, *J Am Coll Cardiol* 34:1966-1974, 1999.

194. Ottani F, Galvani M, Ferrini D, Sorbello F, Limonetti P, Pantoli D, Rusticali F: Prodromal angina limits infarct size. A role for ischemic preconditioning, *Circulation* 91:291-297, 1995.

195. Murry CE, Jennings RB, Reimer KA: Preconditioning with ischemia: A delay of lethal cell injury in ischemic myocardium, *Circulation* 74:1124-1136, 1986.

196. Kitagawa K, Matsumoto M, Tagaya M, Hata R, Ueda H, Niinobe M, Handa N, Fukunaga R, Kimura K, Mikoshiba K, et al: "Ischemic tolerance" phenomenon found in the brain, *Brain Res* 528:21-24, 1990.

197. Weih M, Kallenberg K, Bergk A, Dirnagl U, Harms L, Wernecke KD, Einhaupl KM: Attenuated stroke severity after prodromal TIA: A role for ischemic tolerance in the brain? *Stroke* 30:1851-1854, 1999.

198. Moncayo J, de Freitas GR, Bogousslavsky J, Altieri M, van Melle G: Do transient ischemic attacks have a neuroprotective effect? *Neurology* 54:2089-2094, 2000.

199. Schobitz B, De Kloet ER, Holsboer F: Gene expression and function of interleukin 1, interleukin 6 and tumor necrosis factor in the brain, *Prog Neurobiol* 44:397-432, 1994.

200. Ohtsuki T, Ruetzler CA, Tasaki K, Hallenbeck JM: Interleukin-1 mediates induction of tolerance to global ischemia in gerbil hippocampal CA1 neurons, *J Cereb Blood Flow Metab* 16:1137-1142, 1996.

201. Song W, Furman BL, Parratt JR: Delayed protection against ischaemia-induced ventricular arrhythmias and infarct size limitation by the prior administration of *Escherichia coli* endotoxin, *Br J Pharmacol* 118:2157-2163, 1996.

202. Eising GP, Mao L, Schmid-Schonbein GW, Engler RL, Ross J: Effects of induced tolerance to bacterial lipopolysaccharide on myocardial infarct size in rats, *Cardiovasc Res* 31:73-81, 1996.

203. Rowland RT, Meng X, Cleveland JC Jr, Meldrum DR, Harken AH, Brown JM: LPS-induced delayed myocardial adaptation enhances acute preconditioning to optimize postischemic cardiac function, *Am J Physiol* 272:H2708-H2715, 1997.

204. Tasaki K, Ruetzler CA, Ohtsuki T, Martin D, Nawashiro H, Hallenbeck JM: Lipopolysaccharide pre-treatment induces resistance against subsequent focal cerebral ischemic damage in spontaneously hypertensive rats, *Brain Res* 748:267-270, 1997.

205. Puisieux F, Deplanque D, Pu Q, Souil E, Bastide M, Bordet R: Differential role of nitric oxide pathway and heat shock protein in preconditioning and lipopolysaccharide-induced brain ischemic tolerance, *Eur J Pharmacol* 389:71-78, 2000.

206. Bordet R, Deplanque D, Maboudou P, Puisieux F, Pu Q, Robin E, Martin A, Bastide M, Leys D, Lhermitte M, Dupuis B: Increase in endogenous brain superoxide dismutase as a potential mechanism of lipopolysaccharide-induced brain ischemic tolerance, *J Cereb Blood Flow Metab* 20:1190-1196, 2000.

207. Wong GH, Elwell JH, Oberley LW, Goeddel DV: Manganous superoxide dismutase is essential for cellular resistance to cytotoxicity of tumor necrosis factor, *Cell* 58:923-931, 1989.

208. Eddy LJ, Goeddel DV, Wong GH: Tumor necrosis factor-alpha pretreatment is protective in a rat model of myocardial ischemia-reperfusion injury, *Biochem Biophys Res Commun* 184:1056-1059, 1992.

209. Nawashiro H, Tasaki K, Ruetzler CA, Hallenbeck JM: TNF-alpha pretreatment induces protective effects against focal cerebral ischemia in mice, *J Cereb Blood Flow Metab* 17:483-490, 1997.

210. Ginis I, Jaiswal R, Klimanis D, Liu J, Greenspon J, Hallenbeck JM: TNF-alpha-induced tolerance to ischemic injury involves differential control of NF-kappaB transactivation: The role of NF-kappaB association with p300 adaptor, *J Cereb Blood Flow Metab* 22:142-152, 2002.

211. Stenzel-Poore MP, Stevens SL, King JS, Simon RP: Preconditioning reprograms the response to ischemic injury and primes the emergence of unique endogenous neuroprotective phenotypes: A speculative synthesis, *Stroke* 38:680-685, 2007.

212. Sherman DG, Investigators TEAST: The Enlimomab Acute Stroke Trial: Final results, *Neurology* 48:A270, 1997.

213. The Enlimomab Acute Stroke Trial Investigators: The Enlimomab Acute Stroke Trial: Final results, *Cerebrovasc Dis* 7(suppl 4):18, 1998.
214. Vuorte J, Lindsberg PJ, Kaste M, Meri S, Jansson SE, Rothlein R, Repo H: Anti-ICAM-1 monoclonal antibody R6.5 (enlimomab) promotes activation of neutrophils in whole blood, *J Immunol* 162:2353-2357, 1999.
215. Zhang RL, Zhang ZG, Chopp M: Thrombolysis with tissue plasminogen activator alters adhesion molecule expression in the ischemic rat brain, *Stroke* 30:624-629, 1999.
216. Zhang R, Powers C, Zhang Z, Chopp M: Infusion of intercellular adhesion molecule 1 antibody (18h) upregulates E- and P-selectin expression during focal embolic cerebral ischemia in rats [abstract], *Stroke* 29:282, 1998.
217. Furuya K, Takeda H, Azhar S, McCarron RM, Chen Y, Ruetzler CA, Wolcott KM, DeGraba TJ, Rothlein R, Hugli TE, del Zoppo GJ, Hallenbeck JM: Examination of several potential mechanisms for the negative outcome in a clinical stroke trial of enlimomab, a murine anti-human intercellular adhesion molecule-1 antibody: A bedside-to-bench study, *Stroke* 32:2665-2674, 2001.
218. Sughrue ME, Mehra A, Connolly ES Jr, D'Ambrosio AL: Anti-adhesion molecule strategies as potential neuroprotective agents in cerebral ischemia: A critical review of the literature, *Inflamm Res* 53:497-508, 2004.
219. Yenari MA, Kunis D, Sun GH, Onley D, Watson L, Turner S, Whitaker S, Steinberg GK: Hu23F2G, an antibody recognizing the leukocyte CD11/CD18 integrin, reduces injury in a rabbit model of transient focal cerebral ischemia, *Exp Neurol* 153:223-233, 1998.
220. Krams M, Lees KR, Hacke W, Grieve AP, Orgogozo JM, Ford GA: Acute stroke therapy by inhibition of neutrophils (ASTIN): An adaptive dose-response study of UK-279,276 in acute ischemic stroke, *Stroke* 34:2543-2548, 2003.
221. Weiner HL: Oral tolerance: Immune mechanisms and treatment of autoimmune diseases, *Immunol Today* 18:335-343, 1997.
222. Chen Y, Inobe J, Marks R, Gonnella P, Kuchroo VK, Weiner HL: Peripheral deletion of antigen-reactive T cells in oral tolerance, *Nature* 376:177-180, 1995.
223. Groux H, O'Garra A, Bigler M, Rouleau M, Antonenko S, de Vries JE, Roncarolo MG: A CD4+ T-cell subset inhibits antigen-specific T-cell responses and prevents colitis, *Nature* 389:737-742, 1997.
224. Chen Y, Kuchroo VK, Inobe J, Hafler DA, Weiner HL: Regulatory T cell clones induced by oral tolerance: Suppression of autoimmune encephalomyelitis, *Science* 265:1237-1240, 1994.
225. Faria AM, Weiner HL: Oral tolerance: Mechanisms and therapeutic applications, *Adv Immunol* 73:153-264, 1999.
226. Metzler B, Wraith DC: Mucosal tolerance in a murine model of experimental autoimmune encephalomyelitis, *Ann N Y Acad Sci* 778:228-242, 1996.
227. Becker KJ, McCarron RM, Ruetzler C, Laban O, Sternberg E, Flanders KC, Hallenbeck JM: Immunologic tolerance to myelin basic protein decreases stroke size after transient focal cerebral ischemia, *Proc Natl Acad Sci U S A* 94:10873-10878, 1997.
228. Takeda H, Spatz M, Ruetzler C, McCarron R, Becker K, Hallenbeck J: Induction of mucosal tolerance to E-selectin prevents ischemic and hemorrhagic stroke in spontaneously hypertensive, genetically stroke-prone rats, *Stroke* 33:2156-2163, 2002.
229. Alberts MJ, Bertels C, Dawson DV: An analysis of time of presentation after stroke, *JAMA* 263:65-68, 1990.
230. Hayward NJ, Elliott PJ, Sawyer SD, Bronson RT, Bartus RT: Lack of evidence for neutrophil participation during infarct formation following focal cerebral ischemia in the rat, *Exp Neurol* 139:188-202, 1996.
231. Lapchak PA, Araujo DM, Song D, Zivin JA: Neuroprotection by the selective cyclooxygenase-2 inhibitor SC-236 results in improvements in behavioral deficits induced by reversible spinal cord ischemia, *Stroke* 32:1220-1225, 2001.
232. Kim E, Tolhurst AT, Qin LY, Chen XY, Febbraio M, Cho S: CD36/ fatty acid translocase, an inflammatory mediator, is involved in hyperlipidemia-induced exacerbation of ischemic brain injury, *J Neurosci* 28:4661-4670, 2008.
233. Norris JW, Hachinski VC: High dose steroid treatment in cerebral infarction, *Br Med J (Clin Res Ed)* 292:21-23, 1986.
234. Becker KJ: Anti-leukocyte antibodies: LeukArrest (Hu23F2G) and enlimomab (R6.5) in acute stroke, *Curr Med Res Opin* 18 (suppl 2):s18-s22, 2002.
235. Emsley HC, Smith CJ, Georgiou RF, Vail A, Hopkins SJ, Rothwell NJ, Tyrrell PJ: A randomised phase II study of interleukin-1 receptor antagonist in acute stroke patients, *J Neurol Neurosurg Psychiatry* 76:1366-1372, 2005.
236. Lampl Y, Boaz M, Gilad R, Lorberboym M, Dabby R, Rapoport A, Anca-Hershkowitz M, Sadeh M: Minocycline treatment in acute stroke: An open-label, evaluator-blinded study, *Neurology* 69:1404-1410, 2007.
237. Schilling M, Besselmann M, Leonhard C, Mueller M, Ringelstein EB, Kiefer R: Microglial activation precedes and predominates over macrophage infiltration in transient focal cerebral ischemia: A study in green fluorescent protein transgenic bone marrow chimeric mice, *Exp Neurol* 183:25-33, 2003.
238. Abe T, Shimamura M, Jackman K, et al: Key role of CD36 in toll-like receptor 2 signaling in cerebral ischemia, *Stroke* 41:898-904, 2010.
239. Fagan SC, Waller JL, Nichols FT, et al: Minocycline to improve neurologic outcome in stroke (MINOS). A dose finding study, *Stroke* 41:2283, 2010.

10 Intracellular Signaling: Mediators and Protective Responses

VALINA L. DAWSON, TED M. DAWSON

The brain is arguably the most complex organ in the body. In the human brain there are billions of neurons that make trillions of connections necessary for daily normal brain function. Although the brain is only 2% of total body weight, it is the most metabolically active organ, consuming 25% of total body glucose and oxygen. This high level of energy metabolism generates oxidative stress in an organ with high levels of lipid and cells that are structurally elaborate with extensive processes. An expectation would be that the cells of the brain would be exquisitely sensitive to stress. However, neurons are terminally differentiated postmitotic cells with a limited capacity for replacement. Therefore, neurons have evolved powerful adaptive strategies to protect against the high level of oxidative stress produced during normal activity and possess a capacity for repair following injury. These neuroprotective and repair signaling pathways are largely not known but are an active area of scientific investigation. It is possible that the next generation of neuroprotective therapeutic targets will be derived from investigations into neuronal preconditioning.

Preconditioning

To uncover natural survival signaling pathways, the phenomenon of preconditioning is being investigated. Preconditioning of the brain and other organs is an adaptive response to a noxious but not lethal experience that activates an intracellular response rendering the tissue resistant to subsequent potentially lethal events.[1-3] There are two different temporal phases of preconditioning. One occurs immediately and is associated with posttranslational modifications of proteins. This *acute* preconditioning lasts for only a few hours at most (Fig. 10-1). The second phase of preconditioning is *delayed*. It requires new protein synthesis and the neuroprotection is sustained for several days. *Preconditioning* is a term applied to the noxious but not lethal event that activates the protective response. The state of enhanced resistance to subsequent lethal events is termed *tolerance*. The clinical utility of preconditioning, either acute or delayed, in the brain is not yet apparent. Retrospective studies in patients with a history of transient ischemic attack suggest that preconditioning and tolerance occur in human brain because these patients have a more favorable outcome with smaller infarct size, milder clinical impairment, and decreased morbidity following stroke.[4-9] Despite a more favorable outcome, patients who experience transient ischemic attack have a tenfold or higher increased risk of stroke[10,11] and these retrospective studies did not assess patients who did not survive their strokes. However, these data provide a provocative possibility that the human brain can be preconditioned and experience a state of tolerance. Thus understanding this process may provide new therapies targeted toward patients at risk for stroke.

Induction of Preconditioning

Preconditioning can be activated by nearly any stressful stimulus. In cell culture, preconditioning can be triggered by a wide variety of stimulations, including adenosine, norepinephrine, calcium, bradykinin, heat shock, mitochondrial uncouplers, chemical inhibition of oxidative phosphorylation, exposure to excitotoxins, cytokines, ceramide, nitric oxide (NO), potassium chloride, hypoxia, anoxia, and oxygen glucose deprivation. Several intracellular signaling pathways mediate preconditioning. The molecular events that mediate tolerance are an active area of investigation.

In vivo, preconditioning in the brain can also be experimentally induced by a variety of stimuli. Both global ischemia (occlusion of both common carotid arteries) and focal ischemia (occlusion of the middle cerebral artery) for short durations can activate tolerance within 24 hours. Placing animals in a chamber and exposing them to hypoxia for 1 to 6 hours induces tolerance to either transient or permanent focal ischemia 1 to 3 days following the hypoxic incident.[12,13] Small doses of lipopolysaccharide (LPS) injected into the peritoneal cavity are sufficient to induce tolerance within 2 to 3 days following injection that is sustained for approximately 7 days.[14-19] Inhibition of oxidative phosphorylation by the irreversible inhibitor of succinate dehydrogenase, 3-nitropropionic acid, activates preconditioning in gerbils and rats that develops over 1 to 4 days, providing protection against transient focal ischemia.[20-22] Exposure to cold or heat can trigger tolerance in experimental animals. Hypothermic (25° to 32° C)[23,24] or hyperthermic (42° to 43° C) temperatures[25,26] induce tolerance to focal ischemia 24 hours later. However, this preconditioning appears to have a shorter window of opportunity than other stressors, in which tolerance is sustained from 24 to 72 hours; temperature stress provides protection for between 18

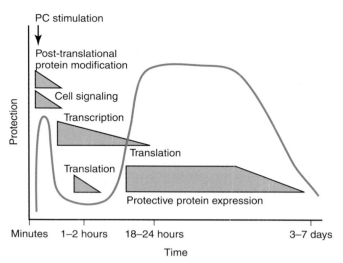

Figure 10-1 A preconditioning (PC) stimulation results in an acute transient period of neuroprotection lasting minutes to 1 to 2 hours and is due to posttranslational protein modifications. Subsequently, new gene transcription and protein translation occur, leading to the acquisition of neuroprotection that is stable for 24 to 48 hours and dissipates by 72 hours in most experimental models, although some models have described protection for up to 7 days.

and 24 hours but the protection resolves by 48 hours. Cortical spreading depression of slowly propagating waves of depolarization across the cortex can be triggered experimentally by the application of potassium chloride on the surface of the dura mater or the cortex. Cortical spreading depression induces a prolonged phase of ischemic tolerance that lasts 1 to 7 days,[27-29] providing protection against transient and permanent focal ischemia.

Surprisingly, inhalational anesthetics can chemically precondition the brain in experimental animal models. Isoflurane, sevoflurane, and halothane, when given to animals, provide protection against permanent or focal ischemia. In the case of isoflurane, the protective effects are immediate and last at least 24 hours, which suggest isoflurane can activate both acute and chronic preconditioning.[30] These observations introduce a significant factor in the exploration of preconditioning in animal models, because all experimental stroke studies are conducted with the subject under anesthesia.

Because preconditioning can be activated by a diverse set of stressors, the molecular mechanisms initiating and sustaining the protective response are active areas of investigation. It would be simple to understand if preconditioning altered cerebral blood flow in a positive manner. However, measurements of cerebral blood flow have shown that tolerance is not accompanied by an improvement of regional tissue perfusion during or after the ischemia that induces tolerance.[31,32] Thus, ischemic tolerance is likely a result of changes in the neurons, glia, and blood vessels of the brain at the cellular level in response to stress.

Cross-Tolerance

Numerous studies indicate that preconditioning can be activated by a wide range of insults, chemical, pharmacologic, or physical. Virtually any stimulus that can alter brain function appears to have the capacity to increase brain resistance to future injurious events. Furthermore, one stressor that activates preconditioning can induce tolerance toward a different injurious stressor, such as tolerance against ischemia being induced by lipopolysaccharide. This phenomenon is termed *cross-tolerance*. The degree of efficacy in cross-tolerance may be somewhat diminished in comparison with that of ischemic tolerance induced by ischemic preconditioning. Also the window for the development of tolerance may be altered. For example, in many models it takes between 2 and 3 days for maximal tolerance to be realized following injection of lipopolysaccharide rather than the 1 day needed for ischemic tolerance.[33]

Because tolerance is observed across organ systems and can be induced by a wide variety of stressors, it is logical but perhaps simplistic to presume that these stress signals would converge onto a final common pathway to promote cellular survival. Although very attractive, this hypothesis does not appear to be valid. A number of genetic analyses of tissue that have been exposed to different preconditioning stressors show that different gene sets are differentially expressed, depending on the nature of the preconditioning stimulus.[33,34] Studies of individual proteins and their involvement in preconditioning and tolerance support this observation as well.[3,33,35] Conceptually, potential mechanisms for improving cell maintenance through the stress response include both enhanced cellular defense functions and increased cellular surveillance. Evidence for both pathways exists. Preconditioning can arise both by posttranslational modification of proteins or by expression of new proteins. These newly expressed proteins and enhanced signaling cascades either can strengthen survival mechanisms or may inhibit cell death signaling. Activation of the cell stress response and synthesis of stress proteins will increase the capacity for general cell maintenance, allowing for proper cell function. The best-known stress response proteins are protein chaperones that unfold damaged or misfolded proteins to facilitate the disposal of these unneeded proteins by the cell. Whether these two strategies work in concert or independently is not yet known. It is curious, however, that in many experimental model systems, knockdown or knockout of a single preconditioning molecule is sufficient to block the development of preconditioning and the expression of a single molecule is often sufficient to provide protection. These observations would suggest some sort of a network response to provide protection, even if there is no final common pathway.

Cellular Defense

Reactive oxygen species (ROS): There is strong evidence that reactive oxygen species (ROS) are essential during the preconditioning response. Both in vitro and in vivo, nitric oxide generation following glutamate receptor stimulation activates preconditioning and tolerance[36,37] through the Ras, Raf, Mek, Erk signal cascade[37] to trigger gene transcription (Fig. 10-2). Superoxide anion production is also important because increasing levels of superoxide dismutase, the enzyme that degrades superoxide anion, is sufficient to block the development of tolerance in rats.[38] It is not surprising that ROS would be a strong

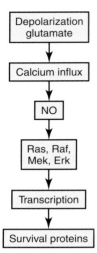

Figure 10-2 Neuronal depolarization leading to glutamate release and glutamate receptor stimulation activates production of nitric oxide (NO) and preconditioning and tolerance through the Ras, Raf, mitogen-activated protein kinase kinase (Mek), and extracellular signal-regulated kinase (Erk) signal cascade that triggers gene transcription and production of survival proteins.

inducer for preconditioning, considering the primary role ROS are considered to play in the pathogenesis of brain injury from ischemia. High levels of ROS are generated during both ischemia and reperfusion in all compartments of the brain, neurons, glia, and endothelial cells. Additionally, during reperfusion excessive NO generated during ischemia can be converted to peroxynitrite following the reaction with superoxide anion to generate highly toxic reactive nitrogen species. Thus one might expect that a component of the tolerance response would be the increased expression of antioxidant enzymes, including the superoxide dismutases, catalase, glutathione peroxidase, and thioredoxin. Both in vitro and in vivo, after ischemic preconditioning and some other stressors, significant induction of the superoxide dismutases (catalase, glutathione peroxidase, thioredoxin) has been observed. The development of tolerance has not been associated with the increased expression of these enzymes, indicating that increased antioxidant capacity can facilitate tolerance but is not essential for tolerance.

Neurotrophin support: Known survival-promoting molecules are often observed to be increased during the tolerance phase. Neurotrophins support survival and growth. Molecules that show increased expression include nerve growth factor,[39] brain-derived growth factor,[39,40] basic fibroblast growth factor,[41,42] insulin-like growth factor,[43] epidermal growth factor,[44,45] vascular endothelial growth factor,[12,46-49] and neuregulin.[50] Expression of these proteins provides protection against a variety of neurotoxic insults, and thus their increased expression following a preconditioning stimulation would reasonably provide resistance to subsequent injury. These growth factors are important in the maintenance and survival not only of neurons but also of glia and endothelial cells. Furthermore, these growth factors have been implicated in neurogenesis, vascular genesis, and remodeling events following ischemic injury and may play a similar role in the development of tolerance.

Survival kinases: Protein kinases phosphorylate proteins to activate signaling responses. The serine/threonine-specific protein kinase Akt (protein kinase B), when phosphorylated by phosphatidylinositol-3-kinase, is a key mediator of tolerance.[51] This protection appears to occur through Akt phosphorylation and activation of mixed-lineage kinase-3. However the role of Akt in tolerance as presented in the literature is unclear. In some model systems phospho-Akt is readily observed and mechanistic investigations can link it to neuronal survival.[52-54] In other studies investigators have not observed a role for Akt.[55,56] The discrepancy in these observations is likely due to differences in the experimental models used in these studies and reflects the diversity of tolerance pathways. Hypoxic preconditioning has been shown to involve phosphatidylinositol-3-kinase activation of Akt and subsequent phosphorylation of survivin to promote endothelial cell survival,[57] once again suggesting that an understanding of the role of Akt and its phosphorylation targets such as survivin may provide insight and therapeutic targets for protecting the brain from ischemic insult.

Erythropoietin: Erythropoietin (EPO) is an interesting molecule in the preconditioning and tolerance field (Fig. 10-3). EPO is a clinically approved glycoprotein hormone that is induced by ischemic preconditioning by activation of hypoxia-inducible factor-1α (HIF)-1α. Owing to the potential clinical utility of EPO, rapid progress has defined EPO signaling cascades, including the Janus kinase-2 pathway, the phosphoinositide-3 kinase,[58] Akt[59-61] pathway, and the extracellular signal-regulated kinase (ERK) and signal transducers and activators of transcription (STAT) pathways.[62] In part, the protective actions of EPO are thought to converge on the induction of Bcl-2 proteins to block cell death signaling. In experimental focal ischemia, EPO reduces infarct volume.[60] In a small phase I/II clinical stroke study, EPO was found to be safe, having penetrated into the brain and provided some improvement through reduced infarct size and better functional outcome.[63] These results are encouraging and suggest that EPO or EPO derivatives may be useful protective agents following stroke or as pretreatment agents for procedures that put the brain at risk.

Inhibition of cell death: Although death may be binary, pathways toward cell death are not. Many different forms of cell death are specialized by cell type and influenced by the local biochemical environment. In a heterogeneous structure such as the brain, which comprises many different types of cells, it is difficult to identify a single pathway of cell death. Neurons, glia, and endothelial cells are all susceptible to hypoxic-ischemic death but to different degrees, and the signaling events that result in cell demise vary with cell types. It is not uncommon to observe mixed forms of cell death in the brains of animals following experimental stroke. Of the different forms of cell death, the major forms in the brain described to date are extrinsic apoptosis, intrinsic apoptosis, necroptosis, paraptosis, parthanatos, unfolded-protein response (endoplasmic reticulum stress), and autophagy.[64]

Apoptosis has been widely studied and is defined as occurring through two primary signaling pathways, the extrinsic pathway, which originates through the

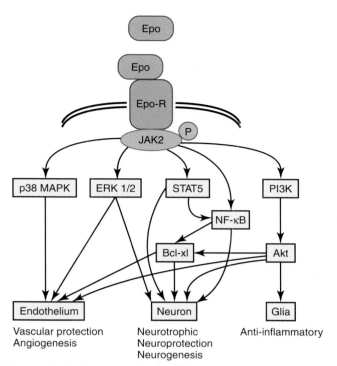

Figure 10-3 During conditions of low oxygen, the transcription factor hypoxia-inducible factor is stabilized, leading to the expression of erythropoietin (Epo), which binds to receptor (EpoR) on endothelial cells, neurons, and glia. Activation of the EpoR promotes phosphorylation of tyrosine kinase 2 (JAK2), triggering other signaling molecules including the mitogen-activated protein kinase p38 (p38 MAPK), extracellular signal-regulated kinase 1/2 (ERK1/2), signal transducer and activator of transcription 5 (STAT5), and phosphatidylinositol-3-kinase (PI3K). Additionally Akt and nuclear factor-κB (NF-κB) are activated. ERK1/2 is essential for Epo-mediated neuroprotection and angiogenesis. STAT5 may be involved in Epo-mediated NF-κB nuclear translocation but whether this involvement contributes to neuroprotection is not yet clear. Epo-mediated activation of PI3K/Akt phosphorylation is involved in prevention of inflammation, vascular protection, and angiogenesis. Through stimulating Bcl-xl, PI3K/Akt mediates Epo-dependent vascular protection and neuroprotection. The translocation of NF-κB to the nucleus triggers events leading to neurogenesis and neuroprotection.

activation of cell-surface death receptors resulting in the activation of caspase-8 or caspase-10, and the intrinsic pathway, which originates from mitochondrial release of cytochrome *c* and associated activation of caspase 9. A less well-characterized intrinsic pathway originating from the endoplasmic reticulum has also been found to result in the activation of caspase-9. Caspases are cysteine aspartyl–specific proteases that are the biochemical hallmark behind apoptosis. Through the action of these proteases, the cell is deconstructed and apoptotic bodies are formed.

Necroptosis is a form of cell death whereby features of both apoptosis and necrosis are observed. Paraptosis is a nonapoptotic form of cell death that is programmatic, because transcription and translation are required as are activation of extracellular signal-regulated kinase 2 and ASK-interacting protein-1. *Parthanatos* is cell death mediated by excess production of poly(ADP-ribose) (PAR) by PAR polymerase-1 (PARP-1). Parthanatos is

observed in many tissues throughout the body, including the brain, after hypoxic-ischemic insult. The generation of poly(ADP-ribose) leads to release of apoptosis-inducing factor (AIF) from the mitochondria that enters the nucleus, triggering chromosomal degradation, nuclear shrinkage, and cell death.

The *unfolded-protein response* is activated following cellular stress that leads to new protein expression to facilitate the efficiency of the endoplasmic reticulum and proper protein folding. This is a carefully choreographed response to prevent the accumulation of proteins in order to allow time for the elimination of unfolded proteins, and it reestablishes cellular homeostasis. However, if the stress cannot be resolved the system becomes overwhelmed and the cell dies. The exact mechanisms of cell death are not yet known but involve in part transcription factor regulation as well as activation of the caspase cascade. *Autophagy,* which is subdivided into macroautophagy, microautophagy, and chaperone-mediated autophagy, is a complementary pathway to the ubiquitin-proteasomal system to degrade proteins, protein aggregates, and organelles through the lysosome. It is generally thought that autophagy is a prosurvival response facilitating the clearance of damaged proteins and organelles, and data now show that interfering with autophagy results in neuronal demise while stimulating autophagy can improve survival.[65]

It is no surprise that induction of proteins that oppose these cell death signaling cascades would be part of the expression of tolerance. For the most part, the most-studied events are those involved in the apoptotic cascade, and most studies describe changes in protein expression, but the relative functional value of altered protein expression is not always apparent. In many cases it is likely that depressing cell death programs is part of a larger response that provides protection, survival, and restoration of function. For example, the tumor suppressor transcription factor protein, p53, which can mediate cell death, is suppressed in the tolerant brain.[66] Hippocampal cell cultures preconditioned with the K_{ATP} channel antagonist diazoxide express less p53 and are resistant to apoptosis.[67] Furthermore, overexpression of p53 exacerbates cell death. Taken together, these findings point to a role for p53 in regulating the degree of tolerance. Many investigators have explored the role of the Bcl family of proteins in preconditioning and tolerance because of their active role in promoting or preventing apoptosis.[68-76] Although there is some disparity in findings, most studies indicate that tolerance is associated with a persistent increase in the prosurvival Bcl-2 or Bcl-xl proteins. Less consistent are the observations of the prodeath Bax protein. Intriguingly there are reports that activation of caspase-3, an event most commonly associated with rapid and pronounced cell death, is important for the development of tolerance.[70,77] We do not yet know whether there is production of proteins that block the other forms of cell death that are observed in ischemic injury, such as blocking the ability of poly(ADP-ribose) to release apoptosis-inducing factor from the mitochondria. However, it is likely that the ability of preconditioning to reduce ischemic cell death probably involves networks of as yet unidentified proteins that have direct and unique cell survival functions. These novel proteins may not function entirely through existing proapoptotic or prodeath pathways.

Cellular Maintenance

Following a significant stressful event, cells respond by synthesizing a class of proteins called *stress proteins*. Increased expression of stress proteins can render cells resistant to subsequent potentially injurious stresses.[78] This stress response has been under investigation for several decades; the first studies analyzed the acquisition of tolerance to heat shock, from which these stress proteins were termed *heat shock proteins* (designated Hsps). Heat shock proteins can be divided into six subfamilies comprising many members[79-81] that facilitate the folding of newly synthesized polypeptides into functional proteins. Heat shock proteins also play an important role in maintaining properly folded protein folding as well as promoting protein-protein interactions and preventing protein aggregation. These actions are commonly referred to as *chaperone functions*. Through their interactions with cochaperones and client proteins, both constitutive and inducible Hsps regulate signal cascades.

Numerous reports on regulated expression of Hsp70 in response to preconditioning, tolerance, and cerebral ischemia have been published (Fig. 10-4).[82,83] A large body of published work describes a prominent role for Hsp70 in adaptive cytoprotection and tolerance and indicates that elevated expression of Hsp70 is neuroprotective. The roles that Hsp70 plays in the development and maintenance of tolerance are not entirely clear and are likely due to both the different stresses that trigger Hsp70 expression and the model systems studied. Hsp70 expression can be activated early and its increased expression sustained. In the early phase of expression it may facilitate preconditioning-induced activation of the transcription factor, nuclear factor-κB (NF-κB) that is well described as promoting preconditioning.[84] Hsp70 can also promote cell survival during the tolerance phase through maintenance of mitochondrial physiology. However, the direct actions of Hsp70 on the observed preservation of mitochondrial function are not yet understood. Hsp70 is a regulator of Bcl-2 expression in both normal and injured neurons.[85] Hsp70 can also bind to apoptosis protease–activating factor-1 (APAF-1), preventing the development of the apoptosome and subsequent caspase activation and cell death.[86] Importantly, Hsp70 both prevents mitochondrial release of apoptosis-inducing factor and sequesters apoptosis-inducing factor in the cytosol leading to degradation.[87,88] Because apoptosis-inducing factor is a primary mediator of ischemic injury, preventing its entry to the nucleus could have profound neuroprotective effects. Hsp70 and family members have been explored in brain ischemia, but the roles of the other Hsp family members in the development of preconditioning and tolerance or in response to ischemic injury are not well studied or developed yet. The strength of the data on Hsp70 as a neuroprotective molecule highlights the importance of understanding protein maintenance as a relevant therapeutic strategy.

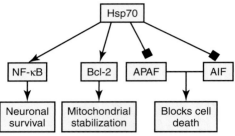

Figure 10-4 Heat shock proteins (Hsps) have been implicated in the development and maintenance of tolerance. Hsp70 expression can be activated early and may facilitate preconditioning-induced activation of the transcription factor and nuclear factor κB (NF-κB) as well as stabilizing mitochondrial function actions on Bcl-2. Hsp70 can block cell death signaling by binding to apoptosis protease–activating factor-1 (APAF-1), thereby preventing the development of the apoptosome, and by blocking mitochondrial release of apoptosis-inducing factor (AIF) and translocation to the nucleus.

Regeneration and Repair

For more than a century it was believed that the mature nervous system was the one organ system that lacked the capacity for renewal and repair. We have now come to appreciate that the brain has a limited capacity to replace and repair neural cells. This process of neurogenesis arises from progenitor or stem cells in specialized regions of the nervous system. The cells of the dentate gyrus and the subventricular zone have been the most intensively studied.[89,90] Ongoing studies are just defining the role these new cells play and how they integrate into the existing circuitry. From the limited literature currently available, it is reasonable to propose that the newly born cells are not just replacing old and damaged cells but may be important for the plasticity required to shape existing neural circuitry in response to experience in learning and memory, mood, and response to injury. Preconditioning produces enough stress to trigger plasticity and a neurogenesis response.[91-95] This neurogenesis corresponds with improved memory scores[94] and may be important in the development of tolerance[93]; the latter issue, however, is difficult to determine with currently available tools to block neurogenesis. Although a general focus of current research is to facilitate endogenous neurogenesis to replace cells lost to injury, it is also possible that these newly born cells may play an important role in remodeling the nervous system to resist further injury and loss of function. These possibilities await further scientific investigation.

Clinical Implications

With the failure of so many neuroprotective drug trials for the treatment of stroke,[96] investigators are looking for new approaches to development of effective therapies. Preconditioning and ischemic tolerance are particularly attractive phenomena because all compartments of the nervous system—neurons, glia, and endothelial cells—appear to be protected. The hope is that understanding the molecular events during preconditioning or those active during tolerance will provide a window through which we can discover new treatments. Functional and descriptive studies have facilitated the understanding of the initial cellular events that trigger gene transcription and lead to new protein translation resulting in the phenomena of preconditioning and tolerance. Genomic and proteomic experiments have generated large "laundry lists" of putative candidate proteins that may mediate the profound neuroprotection afforded by preconditioning. However, as our knowledge grows, it is becoming clear that these events set in motion a complicated network of signaling.

There are several challenges in harnessing preconditioning as a therapeutic tool. One is the observation that the most effective stressors in triggering preconditioning such as ischemia, glutamate, NO, and cytokines, also play important roles in acute stroke to promote ischemic tissue damage. For the development of new therapeutic strategies, it is important to separate the neuroprotective pathways from the neurotoxic pathways induced by these agents and to functionally identify the molecules that mediate neuroprotection. Another challenge is the possibility that combinatorial therapy is necessary to fully protect the nervous system from ischemic injury, because ischemic preconditioning is a complicated network of signaling events. It is possible that a chemical preconditioning drug could be found. The challenge is to identify a compound that will activate the stress response without itself being toxic as well as having a wide therapeutic window. The other challenge is to identify clinical populations that could measurably benefit from the treatment. Logically these might involve scenarios in which ischemic injury can occur, such as surgical settings. Coronary artery bypass surgery, although lifesaving, often has the adverse effects of neurologic damage and cognitive impairment from ischemic events. Preconditioning-directed therapies might be useful in this setting and other surgical settings. Depending on the treatment, there might also be a utility for treating the patient with an acute stroke during the period of maturation of the stroke. Our understanding of the plasticity of the nervous system is just emerging; harnessing the power of preconditioning and tolerance has promise as a new arena to develop novel therapies to protect the nervous system from ischemic injury.

REFERENCES

1. Dirnagl U, Meisel A: Endogenous neuroprotection: Mitochondria as gateways to cerebral preconditioning? *Neuropharmacology* 55:334–344, 2008.
2. Nandagopal K, Dawson TM, Dawson VL: Critical role for nitric oxide signaling in cardiac and neuronal ischemic preconditioning and tolerance, *J Pharmacol Exp Ther* 297:474–478, 2001.
3. Obrenovitch TP: Molecular physiology of preconditioning-induced brain tolerance to ischemia, *Physiol Rev* 88:211–247, 2008.
4. Arboix A, Cabeza N, Garcia-Eroles L, et al: Relevance of transient ischemic attack to early neurological recovery after nonlacunar ischemic stroke, *Cerebrovasc Dis* 18:304–311, 2004.
5. Fu Y, Sun JL, Ma JF, et al: The neuroprotection of prodromal transient ischaemic attack on cerebral infarction, *Eur J Neurol* 15:797–801, 2008.
6. Moncayo J, de Freitas GR, Bogousslavsky J, et al: Do transient ischemic attacks have a neuroprotective effect? *Neurology* 54:2089–2094, 2000.
7. Schaller B: Ischemic preconditioning as induction of ischemic tolerance after transient ischemic attacks in human brain: its clinical relevance, *Neurosci Lett* 377:206–211, 2005.
8. Wegener S, Gottschalk B, Jovanovic V, et al: Transient ischemic attacks before ischemic stroke: Preconditioning the human brain? A multicenter magnetic resonance imaging study, *Stroke* 35:616–621, 2004.
9. Weih M, Kallenberg K, Bergk A, et al: Attenuated stroke severity after prodromal TIA: A role for ischemic tolerance in the brain? *Stroke* 30:1851–1854, 1999.
10. Giles MF, Rothwell PM: Prediction and prevention of stroke after transient ischemic attack in the short and long term, *Expert Rev Neurother* 6:381–395, 2006.
11. Johnston SC, Gress DR, Browner WS, et al: Short-term prognosis after emergency department diagnosis of TIA, *JAMA* 284:2901–2906, 2000.
12. Bernaudin M, Nedelec AS, Divoux D, et al: Normobaric hypoxia induces tolerance to focal permanent cerebral ischemia in association with an increased expression of hypoxia-inducible factor-1 and its target genes, erythropoietin and VEGF, in the adult mouse brain, *J Cereb Blood Flow Metab* 22:393–403, 2002.
13. Miller BA, Perez RS, Shah AR, et al: Cerebral protection by hypoxic preconditioning in a murine model of focal ischemia-reperfusion, *Neuroreport* 12:1663–1669, 2001.
14. Ahmed SH, He YY, Nassief A, et al: Effects of lipopolysaccharide priming on acute ischemic brain injury, *Stroke* 31:193–199, 2000.
15. Dawson DA, Furuya K, Gotoh J, et al: Cerebrovascular hemodynamics and ischemic tolerance: Lipopolysaccharide-induced resistance to focal cerebral ischemia is not due to changes in severity of the initial ischemic insult, but is associated with preservation of microvascular perfusion, *J Cereb Blood Flow Metab* 19:616–623, 1999.
16. Furuya K, Zhu L, Kawahara N, et al: Differences in infarct evolution between lipopolysaccharide-induced tolerant and nontolerant conditions to focal cerebral ischemia, *J Neurosurg* 103:715–723, 2005.
17. Rosenzweig HL, Lessov NS, Henshall DC, et al: Endotoxin preconditioning prevents cellular inflammatory response during ischemic neuroprotection in mice, *Stroke* 35:2576–2581, 2004.
18. Tasaki K, Ruetzler CA, Ohtsuki T, et al: Lipopolysaccharide pretreatment induces resistance against subsequent focal cerebral ischemic damage in spontaneously hypertensive rats, *Brain Res* 748:267–270, 1997.
19. Zimmermann C, Ginis I, Furuya K, et al: Lipopolysaccharide-induced ischemic tolerance is associated with increased levels of ceramide in brain and in plasma, *Brain Res* 895:59–65, 2001.
20. Horiguchi T, Kis B, Rajapakse N, et al: Opening of mitochondrial ATP-sensitive potassium channels is a trigger of 3-nitropropionic acid-induced tolerance to transient focal cerebral ischemia in rats, *Stroke* 34:1015–1020, 2003.
21. Hoshi A, Nakahara T, Ogata M, et al: The critical threshold of 3-nitropropionic acid-induced ischemic tolerance in the rat, *Brain Res* 1050:33–39, 2005.
22. Wiegand F, Liao W, Busch C, et al: Respiratory chain inhibition induces tolerance to focal cerebral ischemia, *J Cereb Blood Flow Metab* 19:1229–1237, 1999.
23. Nishio S, Chen ZF, Yunoki M, et al: Hypothermia-induced ischemic tolerance, *Ann N Y Acad Sci* 890:26–41, 1999.
24. Urrea C, Danton GH, Bramlett HM, et al: The beneficial effect of mild hypothermia in a rat model of repeated thromboembolic insults, *Acta Neuropathol* 107:413–420, 2004.
25. Xu H, Aibiki M, Nagoya J: Neuroprotective effects of hyperthermic preconditioning on infarcted volume after middle cerebral artery occlusion in rats: Role of adenosine receptors, *Crit Care Med* 30:1126–1130, 2002.
26. Yang YL, Lin MT: Heat shock protein expression protects against cerebral ischemia and monoamine overload in rat heatstroke, *Am J Physiol* 276:H1961–H1967, 1999.
27. Chazot PL, Lawrence S, Thompson CL: Studies on the subtype selectivity of CP-101,606: Evidence for two classes of NR2B-selective NMDA receptor antagonists, *Neuropharmacology* 42:319–324, 2002.
28. Matsushima K, Hogan MJ, Hakim AM: Cortical spreading depression protects against subsequent focal cerebral ischemia in rats, *J Cereb Blood Flow Metab* 16:221–226, 1996.
29. Otori T, Greenberg JH, Welsh FA: Cortical spreading depression causes a long-lasting decrease in cerebral blood flow and induces tolerance to permanent focal ischemia in rat brain, *J Cereb Blood Flow Metab* 23:43–50, 2003.
30. Wang L, Traystman RJ, Murphy SJ: Inhalational anesthetics as preconditioning agents in ischemic brain, *Curr Opin Pharmacol* 8:104–110, 2008.

31. Barone FC, White RF, Spera PA, et al: Ischemic preconditioning and brain tolerance: Temporal histological and functional outcomes, protein synthesis requirement, and interleukin-1 receptor antagonist and early gene expression, *Stroke* 29:1937-1950, discussion, 1950-1931 1998.

32. Matsushima K, Hakim AM: Transient forebrain ischemia protects against subsequent focal cerebral ischemia without changing cerebral perfusion, *Stroke* 26:1047-1052, 1995.

33. Kirino T: Ischemic tolerance, *J Cereb Blood Flow Metab* 22:1283-1296, 2002.

34. Stenzel-Poore MP, Stevens SL, King JS, et al: Preconditioning reprograms the response to ischemic injury and primes the emergence of unique endogenous neuroprotective phenotypes: A speculative synthesis, *Stroke* 38(Suppl):680-685, 2007.

35. Shpargel KB, Jalabi W, Jin Y, et al: Preconditioning paradigms and pathways in the brain, *Cleve Clin J Med* 75(Suppl 2):S77-S82, 2008.

36. Gidday JM, Shah AR, Maceren RG, et al: Nitric oxide mediates cerebral ischemic tolerance in a neonatal rat model of hypoxic preconditioning, *J Cereb Blood Flow Metab* 19:331-340, 1999.

37. Gonzalez-Zulueta M, Feldman AB, Klesse LJ, et al: Requirement for nitric oxide activation of p21(ras)/extracellular regulated kinase in neuronal ischemic preconditioning, *Proc Natl Acad Sci U S A* 97:436-441, 2000.

38. Mori T, Muramatsu H, Matsui T, et al: Possible role of the superoxide anion in the development of neuronal tolerance following ischaemic preconditioning in rats, *Neuropathol Appl Neurobiol* 26:31-40, 2000.

39. Truettner J, Busto R, Zhao W, et al: Effect of ischemic preconditioning on the expression of putative neuroprotective genes in the rat brain, *Brain Res Mol Brain Res* 103:106-115, 2002.

40. Yanamoto H, Xue JH, Miyamoto S, et al: Spreading depression induces long-lasting brain protection against infarcted lesion development via BDNF gene-dependent mechanism, *Brain Res* 1019:178-188, 2004.

41. Matsushima K, Schmidt-Kastner R, Hogan MJ, et al: Cortical spreading depression activates trophic factor expression in neurons and astrocytes and protects against subsequent focal brain ischemia, *Brain Res* 807:47-60, 1998.

42. Sakaki T, Yamada K, Otsuki H, et al: Brief exposure to hypoxia induces bFGF mRNA and protein and protects rat cortical neurons from prolonged hypoxic stress, *Neurosci Res* 23:289-296, 1995.

43. Wang X, Deng J, Boyle DW, et al: Potential role of IGF-I in hypoxia tolerance using a rat hypoxic-ischemic model: Activation of hypoxia-inducible factor 1alpha, *Pediatr Res* 55:385-394, 2004.

44. Gustavsson M, Wilson MA, Mallard C, et al: Global gene expression in the developing rat brain after hypoxic preconditioning: Involvement of apoptotic mechanisms? *Pediatr Res* 61:444-450, 2007.

45. Mallard C, Hagberg H: Inflammation-induced preconditioning in the immature brain, *Semin Fetal Neonatal Med* 12:280-286, 2007.

46. Bernaudin M, Tang Y, Reilly M, et al: Brain genomic response following hypoxia and re-oxygenation in the neonatal rat. Identification of genes that might contribute to hypoxia-induced ischemic tolerance, *J Biol Chem* 277:39728-39738, 2002.

47. Ran R, Xu H, Lu A, et al: Hypoxia preconditioning in the brain, *Dev Neurosci* 27:87-92, 2005.

48. Ratan RR, Siddiq A, Aminova L, et al: Translation of ischemic preconditioning to the patient: Prolyl hydroxylase inhibition and hypoxia inducible factor-1 as novel targets for stroke therapy, *Stroke* 35(Suppl 1):2687-2689, 2004.

49. Wick A, Wick W, Waltenberger J, et al: Neuroprotection by hypoxic preconditioning requires sequential activation of vascular endothelial growth factor receptor and Akt, *J Neurosci* 22:6401-6407, 2002.

50. Xu Z, Ford GD, Croslan DR, et al: Neuroprotection by neuregulin-1 following focal stroke is associated with the attenuation of ischemia-induced pro-inflammatory and stress gene expression, *Neurobiol Dis* 19:461-470, 2005.

51. Miao B, Yin XH, Pei DS, et al: Neuroprotective effects of preconditioning ischemia on ischemic brain injury through down-regulating activation of JNK1/2 via *N*-methyl-D-aspartate receptor-mediated Akt1 activation, *J Biol Chem* 280:21693-21699, 2005.

52. Nakajima T, Iwabuchi S, Miyazaki H, et al: Preconditioning prevents ischemia-induced neuronal death through persistent Akt activation in the penumbra region of the rat brain, *J Vet Med Sci* 66:521-527, 2004.

53. Yano S, Morioka M, Fukunaga K, et al: Activation of Akt/protein kinase B contributes to induction of ischemic tolerance in the CA1 subfield of gerbil hippocampus, *J Cereb Blood Flow Metab* 21:351-360, 2001.

54. Gao X, Zhang H, Takahashi T, et al: The Akt signaling pathway contributes to postconditioning's protection against stroke, the protection is associated with the MAPK and PKC pathways, *J Neurochem* 105:943-955, 2008.

55. Namura S, Nagata I, Kikuchi H, et al: Serine-threonine protein kinase Akt does not mediate ischemic tolerance after global ischemia in the gerbil, *J Cereb Blood Flow Metab* 20:1301-1305, 2000.

56. Shibata M, Yamawaki T, Sasaki T, et al: Upregulation of Akt phosphorylation at the early stage of middle cerebral artery occlusion in mice, *Brain Res* 942:1-10, 2002.

57. Zhang Y, Park TS, Gidday JM: Hypoxic preconditioning protects human brain endothelium from ischemic apoptosis by Akt-dependent survivin activation, *Am J Physiol Heart Circ Physiol* 292:H2573-H2581, 2007.

58. Ruscher K, Freyer D, Karsch M, et al: Erythropoietin is a paracrine mediator of ischemic tolerance in the brain: Evidence from an in vitro model, *J Neurosci* 22:10291-10301, 2002.

59. Siren AL, Ehrenreich H: Erythropoietin—a novel concept for neuroprotection, *Eur Arch Psychiatry Clin Neurosci* 251:179-184, 2001.

60. Siren AL, Fratelli M, Brines M, et al: Erythropoietin prevents neuronal apoptosis after cerebral ischemia and metabolic stress, *Proc Natl Acad Sci U S A* 98:4044-4049, 2001.

61. Siren AL, Knerlich F, Poser W, et al: Erythropoietin and erythropoietin receptor in human ischemic/hypoxic brain, *Acta Neuropathol* 101:271-276, 2001.

62. Digicaylioglu M, Lipton SA: Erythropoietin-mediated neuroprotection involves cross-talk between Jak2 and NF-kappaB signalling cascades, *Nature* 412:641-647, 2001.

63. Ehrenreich H, Hasselblatt M, Dembowski C, et al: Erythropoietin therapy for acute stroke is both safe and beneficial, *Mol Med* 8:495-505, 2002.

64. Bredesen DE, Rao RV, Mehlen P: Cell death in the nervous system, *Nature* 443:796-802, 2006.

65. Levine B, Yuan J: Autophagy in cell death: An innocent convict? *J Clin Invest* 115(10):2679-2688, 2005.

66. Tomasevic G, Shamloo M, Israeli D, et al: Activation of p53 and its target genes p21(WAF1/Cip1) and PAG608/Wig-1 in ischemic preconditioning, *Brain Res Mol Brain Res* 70:304-313, 1999.

67. Huang L, Li W, Li B, et al: Activation of ATP-sensitive K channels protects hippocampal CA1 neurons from hypoxia by suppressing p53 expression, *Neurosci Lett* 398:34-38, 2006.

68. Brambrink AM, Schneider A, Noga H, et al: Tolerance-inducing dose of 3-nitropropionic acid modulates bcl-2 and bax balance in the rat brain: A potential mechanism of chemical preconditioning, *J Cereb Blood Flow Metab* 20:1425-1436, 2000.

69. Kato K, Shimazaki K, Kamiya T, et al: Differential effects of sublethal ischemia and chemical preconditioning with 3-nitropropionic acid on protein expression in gerbil hippocampus, *Life Sci* 77:2867-2878, 2005.

70. McLaughlin B, Hartnett KA, Erhardt JA, et al: Caspase 3 activation is essential for neuroprotection in preconditioning, *Proc Natl Acad Sci U S A* 21(100):715-720, 2003.

71. Meller R, Minami M, Cameron JA, et al: CREB-mediated Bcl-2 protein expression after ischemic preconditioning, *J Cereb Blood Flow Metab* 25:234-246, 2005.

72. Rybnikova E, Sitnik N, Gluschenko T, et al: The preconditioning modified neuronal expression of apoptosis-related proteins of Bcl-2 superfamily following severe hypobaric hypoxia in rats, *Brain Res* 1089:195-202, 2006.

73. Shimazaki K, Ishida A, Kawai N: Increase in bcl-2 oncoprotein and the tolerance to ischemia-induced neuronal death in the gerbil hippocampus, *Neurosci Res* 20:95-99, 1994.

74. Shimizu S, Nagayama T, Jin KL, et al: bcl-2 Antisense treatment prevents induction of tolerance to focal ischemia in the rat brain, *J Cereb Blood Flow Metab* 21:233-243, 2001.

75. Wu C, Fujihara H, Yao J, et al: Different expression patterns of Bcl-2, Bcl-xl, and Bax proteins after sublethal forebrain ischemia in C57Black/Crj6 mouse striatum, *Stroke* 34:1803-1808, 2003.

76. Wu LY, Ding AS, Zhao T, et al: Involvement of increased stability of mitochondrial membrane potential and overexpression of Bcl-2 in enhanced anoxic tolerance induced by hypoxic preconditioning in cultured hypothalamic neurons, *Brain Res* 999:149-154, 2004.

77. Miyawaki T, Mashiko T, Ofengeim D, et al: Ischemic precondition-ing blocks BAD translocation, Bcl-xL cleavage, and large channel activity in mitochondria of postischemic hippocampal neurons, *Proc Natl Acad Sci U S A* 105:4892-4897, 2008.

78. Daugaard M, Rohde M, Jaattela M: The heat shock protein 70 family: Highly homologous proteins with overlapping and distinct func-tions, *FEBS Lett* 581:3702-3710, 2007.

79. Jaattela M: Heat shock proteins as cellular lifeguards, *Ann Med* 31:261-271, 1999.

80. Balch WE, Morimoto RI, Dillin A, et al: Adapting proteostasis for disease intervention, *Science* 15:916-919, 2008.

81. Morimoto RI: Proteotoxic stress and inducible chaperone networks in neurodegenerative disease and aging, *Genes Dev* 22:1427-1438, 2008.

82. Giffard RG, Han RQ, Emery JF, et al: Regulation of apoptotic and inflammatory cell signaling in cerebral ischemia: The complex roles of heat shock protein 70, *Anesthesiology* 109:339-348, 2008.

83. Yenari MA, Liu J, Zheng Z, et al: Antiapoptotic and anti-inflamma-tory mechanisms of heat-shock protein protection, *Ann N Y Acad Sci* 1053:74-83, 2005.

84. Dirnagl U, Simon RP, Hallenbeck JM: Ischemic tolerance and endogenous neuroprotection, *Trends Neurosci* 26:248-254, 2003.

85. Kelly S, Zhang ZJ, Zhao H, et al: Gene transfer of HSP72 protects cornu ammonis 1 region of the hippocampus neurons from global ischemia: influence of Bcl-2, *Ann Neurol* 52:160-167, 2002.

86. Saleh A, Srinivasula SM, Balkir L, et al: Negative regulation of the Apaf-1 apoptosome by Hsp70, *Nat Cell Biol* 2:476-483, 2000.

87. Ravagnan L, Gurbuxani S, Susin SA, et al: Heat-shock protein 70 antag-onizes apoptosis-inducing factor, *Nat Cell Biol* 3:839-843, 2001.

88. Ruchalski K, Mao H, Li Z, et al: Distinct hsp70 domains mediate apoptosis-inducing factor release and nuclear accumulation, *J Biol Chem* 281:7873-7880, 2006.

89. Duan X, Kang E, Liu CY, et al: Development of neural stem cell in the adult brain, *Curr Opin Neurobiol* 18:108-115, 2008.

90. Ge S, Sailor KA, Ming GL, et al: Synaptic integration and plastic-ity of new neurons in the adult hippocampus, *J Physiol* 586: 3759-3765, 2008.

91. Lee SH, Kim YJ, Lee KM, et al: Ischemic preconditioning enhances neurogenesis in the subventricular zone, *Neuroscience* 146: 1020-1031, 2007.

92. Liu J, Solway K, Messing RO, et al: Increased neurogenesis in the dentate gyrus after transient global ischemia in gerbils, *J Neurosci* 18:7768-7778, 1998.

93. Maysami S, Lan JQ, Minami M, et al: Proliferating progenitor cells: A required cellular element for induction of ischemic tolerance in the brain, *J Cereb Blood Flow Metab* 28:1104-1113, 2008.

94. Naylor M, Bowen KK, Sailor KA, et al: Preconditioning-induced ischemic tolerance stimulates growth factor expression and neu-rogenesis in adult rat hippocampus, *Neurochem Int* 47:565-572, 2005.

95. Pourie G, Blaise S, Trabalon M, et al: Mild, non-lesioning tran-sient hypoxia in the newborn rat induces delayed brain neurogen-esis associated with improved memory scores, *Neuroscience* 140: 1369-1379, 2006.

96. Ford GA: Clinical pharmacological issues in the development of acute stroke therapies, *Br J Pharmacol* 153(Suppl 1):S112-S119, 2008.

11 Enhancing Brain Reorganization and Recovery of Function after Stroke

MICHAEL CHOPP, ZHENG GANG ZHANG

The ischemic brain has limited repair capacity that leads to some degree of functional recovery. The repair process is multifaceted and involves neurogenesis, angiogenesis, and axonal sprouting and synaptogenesis. Emerging preclinical data indicate that neurorestorative therapies facilitate and amplify these interwoven restorative events and thereby improve functional outcome after stroke. In this chapter, we first review stroke-induced neurogenesis, angiogenesis, and axonal remodeling as well as the coupling of these interacting remodeling events. We restrict discussion to neurogenesis in the subventricular zone (SVZ) of the lateral ventricle, because stroke primarily induces neuroblasts in the SVZ to migrate long distances to the ischemic boundary, where these cells likely contribute to the remodeling of cerebral tissue.[1-8] We then discuss the ways to amplify these events.

Neurogenesis in the Subventricular Zone

Neurogenesis in the adult mammalian brain has been investigated and well documented during the last 15 years, although neurogenesis was originally observed in the adult rat brain in the 1960s.[9] In the adult rodent brain, neurogenesis occurs in the SVZ of the lateral ventricle throughout the life of the animal.[1,2,10] Neural stem cells have capacity to undergo unlimited self-renewal and are multipotent, whereas neural progenitor cells exhibit limited self-renewal ability and generate differentiated cell types.[11,12] During developmental cortical neurogenesis in the rodent, neural stem cells reside in the ventricular zone (VZ) and generate cortical neurons.[13,14] The VZ is replaced by an ependymal layer while the SVZ shrinks and persists in the adult.[15] Radial glial cells located in the VZ and containing radial processes and astroglial properties are neural stem cells, and a subpopulation of radial glia transforms into SVZ astrocytes during early postnatal stage.[16-20] In adult SVZ, this astrocyte population forms neural stem cells (type B cells) that in turn produce neural progenitor cells that are transient amplifying cells (type C cells).[1,2,10,16,21] The neural progenitor cells differentiate into neuroblasts (type A cells) and oligodendrocytes.[1,2,10,21,22] More than 30,000 neuroblasts are generated daily in the adult rodent SVZ.[23,24] Neuroblasts generated in the SVZ travel through the rostral migratory stream (RMS) to the olfactory bulb, where they differentiate into granule and periglomerular neurons.[2,25] In the adult human brain, neural stem cells are present in a ribbon of SVZ astrocytes, and a rostral migratory stream is organized around a lateral ventricular extension to the olfactory bulb.[26-28]

During 2001 and 2002, using 5-bromo-2′-deoxyuridine (BrdU; labels new DNA in the S phase of the cell cycle) and antibodies against β-tubulin III (TuJ1, a marker of immature neurons) and doublecortin (DCX, a marker of neuroblasts), several groups demonstrated that experimental focal cerebral ischemia induces neurogenesis in the ipsilateral SVZ of the adult rodent.[4,29-31] Newly generated neuroblasts in the SVZ migrate to the ischemic boundary where they exhibit neuronal phenotypes.[4,29-31] Since then, many experimental studies have confirmed these findings.[32-36] Stroke-induced neurogenesis has also been demonstrated in the adult human SVZ and ischemic boundary, even in patients of advanced age.[37-39]

Proliferation of Neural Stem and Progenitor Cells after Stroke

In a rat model of focal cerebral ischemia, neural progenitor cell proliferation is increased starting 2 days after stroke. The proliferation reaches a maximum between 4 and 7 days after stroke and then decreases to levels observed 2 days after stroke.[40,41] These data indicate that proliferation of neural progenitor cells contributes to stroke-induced neurogenesis. Under physiologic conditions, proliferation of progenitor cells is tightly controlled by cell cycle kinetics.[42,43] The proportion of proliferating cells and the length of the cell cycle are two critical parameters of the cytokinetics for neocortical neurogenesis.[42-44] In the SVZ of the adult rat, approximately 15% to 21% of the neural progenitor cells are actively dividing with a cell cycle ranging from 18 to 21 hours.[40,45,46] Stroke transiently increases the percentage of dividing SVZ neural progenitor cells to 31%.[44] Analysis of cell cycle phases of actively proliferating SVZ neural progenitor cells reveals that the cell cycle length of these mitotic cells changes dynamically over a period of 2 to 14 days after stroke.[40,47] The cell cycle length reduces to 11 hours at 2 days after stroke, which is significantly shorter than the cell cycle length of 19 hours in nonischemic SVZ cells.[40,47] Reduction of the cell cycle induced by stroke likely results from a decrease of the G1 phase of the cell cycle because the G2, M, and S phases are unchanged. The length of the cell cycle returns to the nonstroke levels 14 days after stroke.[40,47] The reduction of the G1 phase is correlated with an increase in the dividing SVZ cell population, whereas an augmentation of the cell population that exits the cell cycle is associated with lengthening of the G1 phase.[40,47] The cells that exit the cell cycle differentiate into neuroblasts.[40,47] Thus, these data suggest that stroke triggers early expansion of the progenitor pool via shortening of the cell cycle length and a retention of daughter cells within the cell cycle, and the lengthening of G1 leads to exit of daughter cells from the cell cycle and their differentiation into neurons.

The stem cells in the SVZ of the adult rodent constitute approximately 2% of the total population of SVZ cells and are relatively quiescent with a cell cycle of approximately 15 days.[25,48] To allow investigation of the effect of stroke on neural stem cells, neural progenitor cells and neuroblasts in the SVZ are eliminated by infusion of an antimitotic agent (cytosine-β-D-arabiofuranoside [Ara-C]) for 7 days; this infusion does not ablate the relatively quiescent neural stem cells in the SVZ.[4,49,50] Seven days after termination of the Ara-C infusion, neural progenitor cells are entirely repopulated in the SVZ after stroke, whereas repopulation of neural progenitor cells in the SVZ takes 14 days in nonischemic SVZ.[4,49,50] These findings suggest that after stroke, neural stem cells accelerate the generation of neural progenitor cells, leading to augmentation of neurogenesis.

Gene profile analysis demonstrates that adult SVZ neural progenitor cells are actively proliferating.[51-56] The neural progenitor cells express many genes that are involved in the biologic processes of cell proliferation and cell cycle, which are not expressed by cells in the cerebral cortex, the hippocampus, and the olfactory bulb.[52] Among these genes are minichromosome maintenance (MCM) genes, cyclin-dependent kinases (CDKs), and CDK inhibitors.[52,53,57-60] MCM genes are essential for all dividing cells, and CDK and CDK inhibitors mediate the cell cycle during G1 phase.[52,53,57-61] Knockout of p21cip and p27kip genes results in increased proliferation of SVZ neural stem and progenitor cells, respectively.[61,62] Stroke substantially upregulates MCM2 expression and downregulates p27kip1 in neural progenitor cells.[40,61] These data provide clues for future analyses of the molecular mediators underlying stroke-induced neural progenitor cell proliferation.

Migration and Survival of Neuroblasts after Stroke

Neuroblasts generated in the ipsilateral SVZ migrate to the ischemic boundary.[3-7] Noninvasive MRI measurements show that intracisternally transplanted SVZ cells labeled by ferromagnetic particles selectively migrate into the ischemic boundary.[63] Among many molecules that regulate neuroblast migration, stroma-derived factor-1α (SDF-1α), a CXC chemokine, appears to play an important role

in mediating neuroblast migration to the ischemic boundary.[64] SDF-1α secreted by astrocytes and endothelial cells in the ischemic boundary attracts SVZ neuroblasts that express the SDF-1α receptor, CXCR4.[65,66] Blockage of either SDF-1α or CXCR4 suppresses neuroblast migration to the ischemic boundary.[65,67-69] In addition, vascular endothelial growth factor (VEGF), angiopoietin-1 (Ang1), and matrix metalloproteinases (MMPs) regulate neuroblast migration after stroke.[50,70-73] Thus, multiple factors in the ischemic brain may orchestrate neuroblast migration. Neuroblasts in the ischemic boundary exhibit phenotypes of mature neurons.[4,34] Studies using the patch-clamp technique show that the new neurons in the ischemic boundary have electrophysiologic characteristics of mature neurons, suggesting that neuroblasts mature into resident neurons and integrate into local neuronal circuitry.[74]

Angiogenesis

Vasculogenesis indicates that new vessels are formed by endothelial progenitor cells, whereas angiogenesis represents the sprouting of new capillaries from preexisting vessels.[75] Angiogenesis is a multistep process involving endothelial cell proliferation, migration, tube formation, branching, and anastomosis.[76,77] In the rodent, the cerebral vascular system develops primarily by angiogenesis.[75] The endothelial cells of cerebral capillaries differ functionally and morphologically from those of noncerebral capillaries.[75] The cerebral endothelial cells are linked by complex tight junctions that form the blood-brain barrier (BBB).[75,78] Under physiologic conditions, proliferation of the cerebral endothelial cells ceases and the turnover rate of endothelial cells is approximately 3 years in the adult rodent brain.[79,80] However, stroke induces angiogenesis in both adult human and rodent brains.[81,82] Angiogenesis is initiated at the border of the infarct areas, and sprouting capillaries develop into new vessels in the ischemic boundary during the first few weeks after the onset of stroke.[83,84] Analysis of gene expression reveals that stroke upregulates expression of VEGF, its receptor VEGFR2, Ang1 and Ang2 and their receptor, tyrosine kinase with immunoglobulin, and epidermal growth factor homology domains 2 (Tie2) in the ischemic boundary, suggesting that these genes are involved in development of angiogenesis in the ischemic brain.[81,84-86] Studies also indicate that angiogenesis in the ischemic boundary lasts for several months.[87,114] To examine whether newly formed cerebral vessels have function, temporal and spatial profiles of vascular permeability and cerebral blood flow (CBF) in the ischemic brain were analyzed by MRI indices.[88,89] Vascular permeability can be quantified and detected using T1 indices of brain-to-blood transfer constants of extrinsic contrast agents, such as gadolinium DTPA, as well as intrinsic magnetization contrast methods.[88,89] Cerebral blood flow can be measured by perfusion-weighted MRI. Analysis of these MRI indices reveals that the ischemic boundary exhibits the transient increase in vascular permeability 2 to 3 weeks after stroke, which leads to elevation of cerebral blood flow 6 weeks after stroke.[89] Areas with angiogenesis exhibit a remarkable correspondence of elevation of cerebral blood flow.[89] These data demonstrate that stroke induces functional new vessels in the ischemic brain.[89]

Coupling of Neurogenesis and Angiogenesis

Angiogenesis and neurogenesis are coupled.[90-96] Studies from Goldman's group[90,95] showed that migrating neuroblasts localize to angiogenic vessels within brain parenchyma. Palmer et al[91] demonstrated that new neurons are born in close proximity to blood vessels at angiogenic foci in the hippocampus. Shen et al[92] showed that endothelial cells release factors that stimulate the self renewal of both embryonic and adult neural stem cells. In vivo data from two 2008 studies show that under physiologic conditions, cerebral vasculature in the SVZ of adult mice secretes factors such as integrin $\alpha6\beta1$ that regulate neural stem and progenitor cell biologic function.[93,94] Coupling of angiogenesis and neurogenesis has also been observed in the adult human.[97] An MRI study showed that exercise specifically changes cerebral blood volume (CBV) in the adult human dentate gyrus, where exercise-induced neurogenesis has been demonstrated in the animal.[97] In the ischemic brain, neuroblasts are closely associated with cerebral vessels when neuroblasts migrate to the ischemic boundary.[34,72,87,98] Blockage of stroke-induced angiogenesis with systemic administration of endostatin substantially attenuates migration of neuroblasts newly born in the SVZ to the ischemic region.[33] Activated endothelial cells in the angiogenic areas secrete SDF-1α, MMPs, and Ang1 to attract neuroblasts.[70-73] Blockage of the SDF-1α/CXCR4, Ang1/Tie2, or MMP signaling suppresses neuroblast migration to the ischemic boundary.[65,68-73] To investigate the direct effect of endothelial cells on coupling with neural progenitor cells after stroke, coculture experiments were performed in which cerebral endothelial cells harvested from microvessels in the ischemic boundary were cultured with neural progenitor cells derived from the nonischemic SVZ. The endothelial cells activated by stroke increased neural progenitor cell proliferation by 38% and neuronal population by 44%,[98] suggesting that activated endothelial cells enhance neurogenesis. Symmetrically, neural progenitor cells isolated from ischemic SVZ promoted in vitro angiogenesis as measured by a capillary tube formation assay.[98,99] VEGF likely mediates this coupling because blockage of VEGFR2 with VEGFR2 antagonists suppresses coupling of angiogenesis with neurogenesis.[98] These in vitro data are further supported by in vivo gene profile analysis showing that ischemic neural progenitor cells isolated by laser capture microdissection in the SVZ express an array of angiogenic factors, including Ang2, VEGFR2, and fibroblast growth factor.[56] Collectively, these in vitro and in vivo findings indicate that induction of angiogenesis couples to and promotes neurogenesis and migration within the ischemic brain.

Angiogenesis, Neurogenesis, and Functional Recovery

Angiogenesis and neurogenesis are likely related to neurologic function. Experimental studies show that augmentation of angiogenesis enhances functional recovery and that blockage of angiogenesis exacerbates functional outcome.[33,81] Patients with stroke who have a higher cerebral blood vessel density appear to make better progress and survive longer than patients with a lower vascular density.[82,100,101] Reduction of neurogenesis after global ischemia results in impairment of functional recovery as measured by water-maze.[102] Patients with basal ganglia stroke have enhanced cognitive function 6 months after transplantation of neuronal cells.[103] However, there are currently no data to demonstrate the causality between angiogenesis and neurogenesis and functional recovery after stroke. Using tamoxifen-inducible Cre recombinase, one study has shown that conditional ablation of newborn neurons in the adult mouse results in olfactory bulb shrinkage and impairment of memory.[74] This transgenic mouse line may provide insight into the direct effect of neurogenesis on functional outcome during stroke recovery.

The Effect of Cell-Based and Pharmacologically Based Therapies on Angiogenesis and Neurogenesis

Angiogenesis and neurogenesis in response to stroke are limited during stroke recovery and many newborn neurons die,[4] which may contribute to incomplete functional recovery. Experimental studies show that cell-based and pharmacologic therapies targeting amplification of angiogenesis and neurogenesis substantially improve functional recovery after stroke.[104-110]

Among cell-based therapies, treatment of stroke with marrow stromal cells (MSCs) has been the most studied.[3,89,111-113] MSC therapy causes an improvement in neurologic function that lasts for at least 12 months when cells are administered days after stroke onset.[111,114-117] It is unlikely that the therapeutic benefits result from the replacement of cerebral tissue by administration of cells, because only a small fraction of MSCs in the host brain express parenchymal cell phenotypes.[111,114-117] We tested the hypothesis that MSCs induce changes within the parenchymal cells that lead to a remodeling of the intact noninfarcted brain, which thereby promotes functional improvement. Intravenous administration of MSCs increased angiogenesis and neurogenesis in the ischemic brain.[111,114-117] When they were administered to the ischemic rat, human MSCs induced a significant increase in rat VEGF levels in the ischemic brain, indicating that MSCs interact with parenchymal cells.[118] In addition to upregulation of VEGF in astrocytes and cerebral endothelial cells, MSCs induce astrocytes to secrete Ang1.[71] Thus, injected MSCs interact with cerebral parenchymal cells to produce VEGF, leading to angiogenesis, whereas Ang1 generated by MSC-stimulated astrocytes interacts with Tie2 receptor in the endothelial cells, promoting the maturation of newly formed vessels primarily in the ischemic boundary zone. This vascular niche not only enhances tissue perfusion but also attracts endogenous neuroblasts originating in the SVZ by the expression of chemotactic molecules such as VEGF, SDF-1α, and MMP9.[67,70-73,98,99] Furthermore, treatment of stroke with MSCs stimulates brain parenchymal cells to induce an array of neurotrophic factors, including basic fibroblast growth factor (bFGF) and brain-derived neurotrophic factor (BDNF), which promote neurogenesis and the survival of newly formed neurons.[119,120]

Pharmacologic therapies also foster endogenous angiogenesis and neurogenesis and improve functional outcome during stroke recovery. The pharmacologic agents are drugs that increase cyclic guanosine monophosphate (cGMP) (phosphodiesterase-5 inhibitors, such as sildenafil and tadalafil), statins, erythropoietin (EPO), granulocyte-colony stimulating factor (G-CSF), niacin extended-release tablets (Niaspan), and minocycline.[105,106,109,121-124] EPO interacts with its receptor, EPOR, to induce angiogenesis and neurogenesis.[125-127] Systemic administration of recombinant human EPO (rhEPO) augments angiogenesis and neurogenesis in the ischemic brain.[109,128,129] Cerebral endothelial cells activated by rhEPO secrete active forms of MMP2 and MMP9, which promote neuroblast migration.[72] Application of MMP inhibitors abolishes the endothelially enhanced neuroblast migration.[72] On the other hand, EPO elevates VEGF levels in neural progenitor cells, thereby augmenting in vitro angiogenesis.[72] Blockage of VEGFR2 with a VEGFR2 antagonist or small interfering RNA (siRNA) against VEGFR2 suppresses neural progenitor cell–increased angiogenesis.[72] These data indicate that MMPs and VEGF likely mediate coupling of EPO-enhanced angiogenesis and neurogenesis. Similar and complementary data demonstrating the coupling of neurogenesis and angiogenesis and functional recovery after stroke have been reported for statins, phosphodiesterase type 5 (PDE5) inhibitors, nitric oxide (NO) donors, granulocyte-colony stimulating factor, and agents that increase high-density lipoprotein.[105,106,109,121-124]

The Effect of Cell and Pharmacologically Based Therapies on Axonal Remodeling

In addition to angiogenesis and neurogenesis, cell-based and pharmacologically based therapies substantially remodel white matter in the ischemic brain.[130-133] Treatment of experimental stroke with MSCs, rhEPO, or sildenafil significantly increases axonal density encapsulating the ischemic lesion.[130-132] Dynamic changes of white matter structure along the ischemic boundary have been imaged in living animals by diffusion tensor imaging (DTI) and fractional anisotropy (FA) measurements.[132] Data from these MRI indices demonstrate that administration of rhEPO or sildenafil augments axonal remodeling and angiogenesis and that both of them are spatially and temporally correlated.[132,133] Nonmyelinating oligodendrocyte progenitor cells are present in the corpus callosum, the striatum, and the SVZ of the adult rodent brain.[22,134,135] These progenitor cells differentiate into mature oligodendrocytes to form myelin sheaths that encapsulate sprouting axons in the ischemic brain.[22,134,136] Administration of MSCs and rhEPO dramatically increased the number of oligodendrocyte progenitor cells in the corpus callosum, the striatum, and the SVZ of the ischemic hemisphere and mature oligodendrocytes in the ischemic boundary adjacent to myelinated axons.[130,136a] These findings suggest that cell-based and pharmacologically based therapies promote generation of oligodendrocyte progenitor cells

in the ischemic brain that migrate to target axons, where they extend their processes myelinating the axons.

Astrocytes constitute the largest population of cells in the central nervous system, constituting approximately 90% of human parenchymal cells.[137] Astrocytes are highly responsive to injury, undergoing rapid hyperplasia and hypertrophy.[138] Astrocytes act as physical and biochemical barriers to axonal regeneration by forming glial scars along ischemic lesions and producing axonal growth inhibitory proteglycans.[139] Administration of MSCs significantly attenuates the glial scar in the ischemic boundary and reduces expression of inhibitory proteins, such as Nogo.[131,140] Analysis of single-cell astrocytes isolated from the ischemic boundary by laser capture microdissection revealed that administration of MSCs dramatically downregulates neurocan, an axonal growth inhibitory proteoglycan.[140] Coculture of MSCs with astrocytes also substantially reduces neurocan expression in astrocytes activated by oxygen glucose deprivation.[140] These findings suggest that injected MSCs reduce physical and biochemical barriers of astrocytes, which also contribute to axonal and neurite outgrowth.

Conclusion

Brain undergoes dramatic remodeling in response to ischemic stroke. Induction of angiogenesis couples to and promotes neurogenesis. These interactive remodeling events create a microenvironment via the interaction with astrocytes and oligodendrocytes that foster axonal and neurite outgrowth and plasticity within the brain. These sets of interwoven restorative events can be amplified by the restorative cell and pharmacologic therapies that lead to improved functional outcome.

REFERENCES

1. Alvarez-Buylla A, Herrera DG, Wichterle H: The subventricular zone: Source of neuronal precursors for brain repair, *Prog Brain Res* 127:1-11, 2000.
2. Luskin MB, Zigova T, Soteres BJ, et al: Neuronal progenitor cells derived from the anterior subventricular zone of the neonatal rat forebrain continue to proliferate in vitro and express a neuronal phenotype, *Mol Cell Neurosci* 8:351-366, 1997.
3. Lindvall O, Kokaia Z, Martinez-Serrano A: Stem cell therapy for human neurodegenerative disorders—How to make it work, *Nat Med* 10(Suppl):S42-S50, 2004.
4. Arvidsson A, Collin T, Kirik D, et al: Neuronal replacement from endogenous precursors in the adult brain after stroke, *Nat Med* 8:963-970, 2002.
5. Zhang R, Zhang Z, Wang L, et al: Activated neural stem cells contribute to stroke-induced neurogenesis and neuroblast migration toward the infarct boundary in adult rats, *J Cereb Blood Flow Metab* 24:441-448, 2004.
6. Jin K, Sun Y, Xie L, et al: Directed migration of neuronal precursors into the ischemic cerebral cortex and striatum, *Mol Cell Neurosci* 24:171-189, 2003.
7. Jiang W, Gu W, Brannstrom T, et al: Cortical neurogenesis in adult rats after transient middle cerebral artery occlusion, *Stroke* 32:1201-1207, 2001.
8. Parent JM: Injury-induced neurogenesis in the adult mammalian brain, *Neuroscientist* 9:261-272, 2003.
9. Altman J: Autoradiographic and histological studies of postnatal neurogenesis. IV: Cell proliferation and migration in the anterior forebrain, with special reference to persisting neurogenesis in the olfactory bulb, *J Comp Neurol* 137:433-457, 1969.
10. Gage FH, Ray J, Fisher LJ: Isolation, characterization, and use of stem cells from the CNS, *Annu Rev Neurosci* 18:159-192, 1995.

11. Erlandsson A, Morshead CM: Exploiting the properties of adult stem cells for the treatment of disease, *Curr Opin Mol Ther* 8:331-337, 2006.

12. Morshead CM, van der Kooy D: Disguising adult neural stem cells, *Curr Opin Neurobiol* 14:125-131, 2004.

13. Hinds J, Ruffett T: Cell proliferation in the neural tube: An electron microscopic and Golgi analysis in the mouse cerebral vesicle, *Z Zellforsch Mikrosk Anat* 115:226-264, 1971.

14. Chenn A, McConnell SK: Cleavage orientation and the asymmetric inheritance of notch1 immunoreactivity in mammalian neurogenesis, *Cell* 82:631-641, 1995.

15. Morshead CM, Craig CG, van der Kooy D: In vivo clonal analyses reveal the properties of endogenous neural stem cell proliferation in the adult mammalian forebrain, *Development* 125:2251-2261, 1998.

16. Tramontin AD, Garcia-Verdugo JM, Lim DA, et al: Postnatal development of radial glia and the ventricular zone (VZ): A continuum of the neural stem cell compartment, *Cereb Cortex* 13:580-587, 2003.

17. Weissman T, Noctor SC, Clinton BK, et al: Neurogenic radial glial cells in reptile, rodent and human: From mitosis to migration, *Cereb Cortex* 13:550-559, 2003.

18. Miyata T, Kawaguchi A, Saito K, et al: Visualization of cell cycling by an improvement in slice culture methods, *J Neurosci Res* 69:861-868, 2002.

19. Noctor SC, Martinez-Cerdeno V, Ivic L, et al: Cortical neurons arise in symmetric and asymmetric division zones and migrate through specific phases, *Nat Neurosci* 7:136-144, 2004.

20. Anthony TE, Klein C, Fishell G, et al: Radial glia serve as neuronal progenitors in all regions of the central nervous system, *Neuron* 41:881-890, 2004.

21. Alvarez-Buylla A, Lim DA: For the long run: Maintaining germinal niches in the adult brain, *Neuron* 41:683-686, 2004.

22. Menn B, Garcia-Verdugo JM, Yaschine C, et al: Origin of oligodendrocytes in the subventricular zone of the adult brain, *J Neurosci* 26:7907-7918, 2006.

23. Alvarez-Buylla A, Garcia-Verdugo JM, Tramontin AD: A unified hypothesis on the lineage of neural stem cells, *Nat Rev Neurosci* 2:287-293, 2001.

24. Lledo PM, Alonso M, Grubb MS: Adult neurogenesis and functional plasticity in neuronal circuits, *Nat Rev Neurosci* 7:179-193, 2006.

25. Doetsch F, Garcia-Verdugo JM, Alvarez-Buylla A: Cellular composition and three-dimensional organization of the subventricular germinal zone in the adult mammalian brain, *J Neurosci* 17:5046-5061, 1997.

26. Curtis MA, Kam M, Nannmark U, et al: Human neuroblasts migrate to the olfactory bulb via a lateral ventricular extension, *Science* 315:1243-1249, 2007.

27. Quinones-Hinojosa A, Sanai N, Soriano-Navarro M, et al: Cellular composition and cytoarchitecture of the adult human subventricular zone: A niche of neural stem cells, *J Comp Neurol* 494:415-434, 2006.

28. Sanai N, Tramontin AD, Quinones-Hinojosa A, et al: Unique astrocyte ribbon in adult human brain contains neural stem cells but lacks chain migration, *Nature* 427:740-744, 2004.

29. Zhang RL, Zhang ZG, Zhang L, et al: Proliferation and differentiation of progenitor cells in the cortex and the subventricular zone in the adult rat after focal cerebral ischemia, *Neuroscience* 105:33-41, 2001.

30. Jin K, Minami M, Lan JQ, et al: Neurogenesis in dentate subgranular zone and rostral subventricular zone after focal cerebral ischemia in the rat, *Proc Natl Acad Sci U S A* 98:4710-4715, 2001.

31. Parent JM, Vexler ZS, Gong C, et al: Rat forebrain neurogenesis and striatal neuron replacement after focal stroke, *Ann Neurol* 52:802-813, 2002.

32. Iwai M, Sato K, Kamada H, et al: Temporal profile of stem cell division, migration, and differentiation from subventricular zone to olfactory bulb after transient forebrain ischemia in gerbils, *J Cereb Blood Flow Metab* 23:331-341, 2003.

33. Ohab JJ, Fleming S, Blesch A, et al: A neurovascular niche for neurogenesis after stroke, *J Neurosci* 26:13007-13016, 2006.

34. Yamashita T, Ninomiya M, Hernandez Acosta P, et al: Subventricular zone-derived neuroblasts migrate and differentiate into mature neurons in the post-stroke adult striatum, *J Neurosci* 26:6627-6636, 2006.

35. Kadam SD, Mulholland JD, McDonald JW, et al: Neurogenesis and neuronal commitment following ischemia in a new mouse model for neonatal stroke, *Brain Res* 1208:35-45, 2008.

36. Burns KA, Ayoub AE, Breunig JJ, et al: Nestin-Creer mice reveal DNA synthesis by nonapoptotic neurons following cerebral ischemia hypoxia, *Cereb Cortex* 17:2585-2592, 2007.

37. Jin K, Wang X, Xie L, et al: Evidence for stroke-induced neurogenesis in the human brain, *Proc Natl Acad Sci U S A* 103:13198-13202, 2006.

38. Macas J, Nern C, Plate KH, et al: Increased generation of neuronal progenitors after ischemic injury in the aged adult human forebrain, *J Neurosci* 26:13114-13119, 2006.

39. Minger SL, Ekonomou A, Carta EM, et al: Endogenous neurogenesis in the human brain following cerebral infarction, *Regen Med* 2:69-74, 2007.

40. Zhang RL, Zhang ZG, Lu M, et al: Reduction of the cell cycle length by decreasing G(1) phase and cell cycle reentry expand neuronal progenitor cells in the subventricular zone of adult rat after stroke, *J Cereb Blood Flow Metab* 26:857-863, 2006.

41. Zhang RL, Zhang ZG, Roberts C, et al: Lengthening the G(1) phase of neural progenitor cells is concurrent with an increase of symmetric neuron generating division after stroke, *J Cereb Blood Flow Metab* 28:602-611, 2008.

42. Caviness VS Jr, Goto T, Tarui T, et al: Cell output, cell cycle duration and neuronal specification: A model of integrated mechanisms of the neocortical proliferative process, *Cereb Cortex* 13:592-598, 2003.

43. Takahashi T, Nowakowski RS, Caviness VS Jr: Cell cycle parameters and patterns of nuclear movement in the neocortical proliferative zone of the fetal mouse, *J Neurosci* 13:820-833, 1993.

44. Nowakowski RS, Lewin SB, Miller MW: Bromodeoxyuridine immunohistochemical determination of the lengths of the cell cycle and the DNA-synthetic phase for an anatomically defined population, *J Neurocytol* 18:311-318, 1989.

45. Smith CM, Luskin MB: Cell cycle length of olfactory bulb neuronal progenitors in the rostral migratory stream, *Dev Dyn* 213:220-227, 1998.

46. Schultze B, Korr H: Cell kinetic studies of different cell types in the developing and adult brain of the rat and the mouse: A review, *Cell Tissue Kinet* 14:309-325, 1981.

47. Zhang RL, Zhang ZG, Roberts C, et al: Lengthening the G(1) phase of neural progenitor cells is concurrent with an increase of symmetric neuron generating division after stroke, *J Cereb Blood Flow Metab* 28:602-611, 2008.

48. Morshead CM, Reynolds BA, Craig CG, et al: Neural stem cells in the adult mammalian forebrain: A relatively quiescent subpopulation of subependymal cells, *Neuron* 13C 1994.

49. Doetsch F, Garcia-Verdugo JM, Alvarez-Buylla A: Regeneration of a germinal layer in the adult mammalian brain, *Proc Natl Acad Sci U S A* 96:11619-11624, 1999.

50. Chen J, Li Y, Zhang R, et al: Combination therapy of stroke in rats with a nitric oxide donor and human bone marrow stromal cells enhances angiogenesis and neurogenesis, *Brain Res* 1005:21-28, 2004.

51. Abramova N, Charniga C, Goderie SK, et al: Stage-specific changes in gene expression in acutely isolated mouse CNS progenitor cells, *Dev Biol* 283:269-281, 2005.

52. Lim DA, Suarez-Farinas M, Naef F, et al: In vivo transcriptional profile analysis reveals RNA splicing and chromatin remodeling as prominent processes for adult neurogenesis, *Mol Cell Neurosci* 31:131-148, 2006.

53. Gurok U, Steinhoff C, Lipkowitz B, et al: Gene expression changes in the course of neural progenitor cell differentiation, *J Neurosci* 24:5982-6002, 2004.

54. Bonnert TP, Bilsland JG, Guest PC, et al: Molecular characterization of adult mouse subventricular zone progenitor cells during the onset of differentiation, *Eur J Neurosci* 24:661-675, 2006.

55. Pennartz S, Belvindrah R, Tomiuk S, et al: Purification of neuronal precursors from the adult mouse brain: Comprehensive gene expression analysis provides new insights into the control of cell migration, differentiation, and homeostasis, *Mol Cell Neurosci* 25:692-706, 2004.

56. Liu XS, Zhang ZG, Zhang RL, et al: Stroke induces gene profile changes associated with neurogenesis and angiogenesis in adult subventricular zone progenitor cells, *J Cereb Blood Flow Metab* 27:564-574, 2007.

57. Maiorano D, Van Assendelft GB, Kearsey SE: Fission yeast cdc21, a member of the MCM protein family, is required for onset of s phase and is located in the nucleus throughout the cell cycle, *EMBO J* 15:861–872, 1996.

58. Maslov AY, Barone TA, Plunkett RJ, et al: Neural stem cell detection, characterization, and age-related changes in the subventricular zone of mice, *J Neurosci* 24:1726–1733, 2004.

59. Salim K, Guest PC, Skynner HA, et al: Identification of proteomic changes during differentiation of adult mouse subventricular zone progenitor cells, *Stem Cells Dev* 16:143–165, 2007.

60. Murray AW: Recycling the cell cycle: Cyclins revisited, *Cell* 116:221–234, 2004.

61. Doetsch F, Verdugo JM, Caille I, et al: Lack of the cell-cycle inhibitor p27kip1 results in selective increase of transit-amplifying cells for adult neurogenesis, *J Neurosci* 22:2255–2264, 2002.

62. Meletis K, Wirta V, Hede SM, et al: P53 suppresses the self-renewal of adult neural stem cells, *Development* 133:363–369, 2006.

63. Zhang Z, Jiang Q, Jiang F, et al: In vivo magnetic resonance imaging tracks adult neural progenitor cell targeting of brain tumor, *Neuroimage* 23:281–287, 2004.

64. Bajetto A, Bonavia R, Barbero S, et al: Chemokines and their receptors in the central nervous system, *Front Neuroendocrinol* 22:147–184, 2001.

65. Robin A, Zhang Z, Wang L, et al: Stromal-derived factor 1a mediates neural progenitor cell motility after focal cerebral ischemia, *Stroke* 35:272, 2004.

66. Tran PB, Ren D, Veldhouse TJ, et al: Chemokine receptors are expressed widely by embryonic and adult neural progenitor cells, *J Neurosci Res* 76:20–34, 2004.

67. Hill WD, Hess DC, Martin-Studdard A, et al: SDF-1 (CXCL12) is upregulated in the ischemic penumbra following stroke: Association with bone marrow cell homing to injury, *J Neuropathol Exp Neurol* 63:84–96, 2004.

68. Imitola J, Raddassi K, Park KI, et al: Directed migration of neural stem cells to sites of CNS injury by the stromal cell-derived factor 1alpha/CXC chemokine receptor 4 pathway, *Proc Natl Acad Sci U S A* 101:18117–18122, 2004.

69. Thored P, Arvidsson A, Cacci E, et al: Persistent production of neurons from adult brain stem cells during recovery after stroke, *Stem Cells* 24:739–747, 2006.

70. Chen J, Zhang ZG, Li Y, et al: Intravenous administration of human bone marrow stromal cells induces angiogenesis in the ischemic boundary zone after stroke in rats, *Circ Res* 92:692–699, 2003.

71. Zacharek A, Chen J, Cui X, et al: Angiopoietin1/Tie2 and VEGF/Flk1 induced by MSC treatment amplifies angiogenesis and vascular stabilization after stroke, *J Cereb Blood Flow Metab* 27:1684–1691, 2007.

72. Wang L, Zhang ZG, Zhang RL, et al: Matrix metalloproteinase 2 (MMP2) and MMP9 secreted by erythropoietin-activated endothelial cells promote neural progenitor cell migration, *J Neurosci* 26:5996–6003, 2006.

73. Lee SR, Kim HY, Rogowska J, et al: Involvement of matrix metalloproteinase in neuroblast cell migration from the subventricular zone after stroke, *J Neurosci* 26:3491–3495, 2006.

74. Hou SW, Wang YQ, Xu M, et al: Functional integration of newly generated neurons into striatum after cerebral ischemia in the adult rat brain, *Stroke* 39:2837–2844, 2008.

75. Risau W: Development and differentiation of endothelium, *Kidney Int Suppl* 67:S3–S6, 1998.

76. Risau W: Mechanisms of angiogenesis, *Nature* 386:671–674, 1997.

77. Carmeliet P: VEGF: gene therapy: Stimulating angiogenesis or angioma-genesis? *Nat Med* 6:1102–1103, 2000.

78. Rubin LL, Staddon JM: The cell biology of the blood-brain barrier, *Annu Rev Neurosci* 22:11–28, 1999.

79. Robertson PL, Du Bois M, Bowman PD, et al: Angiogenesis in developing rat brain: An in vivo and in vitro study, *Brain Res* 355:219–223, 1985.

80. Engerman RL, Pfaffenbach D, Davis MD: Cell turnover of capillaries, *Lab Invest* 17:738–743, 1967.

81. Zhang ZG, Zhang L, Jiang Q, et al: VEGF enhances angiogenesis and promotes blood-brain barrier leakage in the ischemic brain, *J Clin Invest* 106:829–838, 2000.

82. Krupinski J, Kaluza J, Kumar P, et al: Role of angiogenesis in patients with cerebral ischemic stroke, *Stroke* 25:1794–1798, 1994.

83. Garcia J, Cox J, Hudgins W: Ultrastructure of the microvasculature in experimental cerebral infarction, *Acta Neuropathol* 18:273–285, 1971.

84. Zhang ZG, Zhang L, Tsang W, et al: Correlation of VEGF and angiopoietin expression with disruption of blood-brain barrier and angiogenesis after focal cerebral ischemia, *J Cereb Blood Flow Metab* 22:379–392, 2002.

85. Beck H, Acker T, Wiessner C, et al: Expression of angiopoietin-1, angiopoietin-2, and tie receptors after middle cerebral artery occlusion in the rat, *Am J Pathol* 157:1473–1483, 2000.

86. Lin TN, Wang CK, Cheung WM, et al: Induction of angiopoietin and tie receptor mRNA expression after cerebral ischemia-reperfusion, *J Cereb Blood Flow Metab* 20:387–395, 2000.

87. Thored P, Wood J, Arvidsson A, et al: Long-term neuroblast migration along blood vessels in an area with transient angiogenesis and increased vascularization after stroke, *Stroke* 38:3032–3039, 2007.

88. Li L, Jiang Q, Zhang L, et al: Ischemic cerebral tissue response to subventricular zone cell transplantation measured by iterative self-organizing data analysis technique algorithm, *J Cereb Blood Flow Metab* 26:1366–1377, 2006.

89. Jiang Q, Zhang ZG, Ding GL, et al: Investigation of neural progenitor cell induced angiogenesis after embolic stroke in rat using MRI, *Neuroimage* 28:698–707, 2005.

90. Leventhal C, Rafii S, Rafii D, et al: Endothelial trophic support of neuronal production and recruitment from the adult mammalian subependyma, *Mol Cell Neurosci* 13:450–464, 1999.

91. Palmer TD, Willhoite AR, Gage FH: Vascular niche for adult hippocampal neurogenesis, *J Comp Neurol* 425:479–494, 2000.

92. Shen Q, Goderie SK, Jin L, et al: Endothelial cells stimulate self-renewal and expand neurogenesis of neural stem cells, *Science* 304:1338–1340, 2004.

93. Shen Q, Wang Y, Kokovay E, et al: Adult SVZ stem cells lie in a vascular niche: A quantitative analysis of niche cell-cell interactions, *Cell Stem Cell* 3:289–300, 2008.

94. Tavazoie M, Van der Veken L, Silva-Vargas V, et al: A specialized vascular niche for adult neural stem cells, *Cell Stem Cell* 3:279–288, 2008.

95. Louissaint A Jr, Rao S, Leventhal C, et al: Coordinated interaction of neurogenesis and angiogenesis in the adult songbird brain, *Neuron* 34:945–960, 2002.

96. Roitbak T, Li L, Cunningham LA, et al: Neural stem/progenitor cells promote endothelial cell morphogenesis and protect endothelial cells against ischemia via HIF-1alpha-regulated VEGF signaling, *J Cereb Blood Flow Metab* 28:1530–1542, 2008.

97. Pereira AC, Huddleston DE, Brickman AM, et al: An in vivo correlate of exercise-induced neurogenesis in the adult dentate gyrus, *Proc Natl Acad Sci U S A* 104:5638–5643, 2007.

98. Teng H, Zhang ZG, Wang L, et al: Coupling of angiogenesis and neurogenesis in cultured endothelial cells and neural progenitor cells after stroke, *J Cereb Blood Flow Metab* 28:764–771, 2008.

99. Wang L, Chopp M, Gregg SR, et al: Neural progenitor cells treated with EPO induce angiogenesis through the production of VEGF, *J Cereb Blood Flow Metab* 28:1361–1368, 2008.

100. Krupinski J, Kaluza J, Kumar P, et al: Prognostic value of blood vessel density in ischaemic stroke [letter; comment], *Lancet* 342:742, 1993.

101. Slevin M, Krupinski J, Slowik A, et al: Serial measurement of vascular endothelial growth factor and transforming growth factor-beta1 in serum of patients with acute ischemic stroke, *Stroke* 31:1863–1870, 2000.

102. Raber J, Fan Y, Matsumori Y, et al: Irradiation attenuates neurogenesis and exacerbates ischemia-induced deficits, *Ann Neurol* 55:381–389, 2004.

103. Stilley CS, Ryan CM, Kondziolka D, et al: Changes in cognitive function after neuronal cell transplantation for basal ganglia stroke, *Neurology* 63:1320–1322, 2004.

104. Zhang R, Wang L, Zhang L, et al: Nitric oxide enhances angiogenesis via the synthesis of vascular endothelial growth factor and CGMP after stroke in the rat, *Circ Res* 92:308–313, 2003.

105. Zhang R, Wang Y, Zhang L, et al: Sildenafil (Viagra) induces neurogenesis and promotes functional recovery after stroke in rats, *Stroke* 33:2675–2680, 2002.

106. Chen J, Zhang ZG, Li Y, et al: Statins induce angiogenesis, neurogenesis, and synaptogenesis after stroke, *Ann Neurol* 53:743-751, 2003.

107. Lu D, Goussev A, Chen J, et al: Atorvastatin reduces neurological deficit and increases synaptogenesis, angiogenesis, and neuronal survival in rats subjected to traumatic brain injury, *J Neurotrauma* 21:21-32, 2004.

108. Shyu WC, Lin SZ, Yang HI, et al: Functional recovery of stroke rats induced by granulocyte colony-stimulating factor-stimulated stem cells, *Circulation* 110:1847-1854, 2004.

109. Wang L, Zhang Z, Wang Y, et al: Treatment of stroke with erythropoietin enhances neurogenesis and angiogenesis and improves neurological function in rats, *Stroke* 35:1732-1737, 2004.

110. Jin K, Sun Y, Xie L, et al: Post-ischemic administration of heparin-binding epidermal growth factor-like growth factor (HB-EGF) reduces infarct size and modifies neurogenesis after focal cerebral ischemia in the rat, *J Cereb Blood Flow Metab* 24:399-408, 2004.

111. Chopp M, Li Y: Treatment of neural injury with marrow stromal cells, *Lancet Neurol* 1:92-100, 2002.

112. Chen J, Sanberg PR, Li Y, et al: Intravenous administration of human umbilical cord blood reduces behavioral deficits after stroke in rats, *Stroke* 32:2682-2688, 2001.

113. Zhang RL, Zhang ZG, Chopp M: Neurogenesis in the adult ischemic brain: Generation, migration, survival, and restorative therapy, *Neuroscientist* 11:408-416, 2005.

114. Chopp M, Li Y, Zhang J: Plasticity and remodeling of brain, *J Neurol Sci* 265:97-101, 2008.

115. Hess DC, Borlongan CV: Stem cells and neurological diseases, *Cell Prolif* 41(Supp 1):94-114, 2008.

116. Cramer SC, Riley JD: Neuroplasticity and brain repair after stroke, *Curr Opin Neurol* 21:76-82, 2008.

117. Parr AM, Tator CH, Keating A: Bone marrow-derived mesenchymal stromal cells for the repair of central nervous system injury, *Bone Marrow Transplant* 40:609-619, 2007.

118. Chen J, Li Y, Wang L, et al: Therapeutic benefit of intravenous administration of bone marrow stromal cells after cerebral ischemia in rats, *Stroke* 32:1005-1011, 2001.

119. Chaudhary LR, Hruska KA: The cell survival signal Akt is differentially activated by PDGF-BB, EGF, and FGF-2 in osteoblastic cells, *J Cell Biochem* 81:304-311, 2001.

120. Alessi DR, Andjelkovic M, Caudwell B, et al: Mechanism of activation of protein kinase B by insulin and IGF-1, *EMBO J* 15:6541-6551, 1996.

121. Zhang R, Zhang L, Zhang Z, et al: A nitric oxide donor induces neurogenesis and reduces functional deficits after stroke in rats, *Ann Neurol* 50:602-611, 2001.

122. Hossmann KA, Buschmann IR: Granulocyte-macrophage colony-stimulating factor as an arteriogenic factor in the treatment of ischemic stroke, *Expert Opin Biol Ther* 5:1547-1556, 2005.

123. Zhang L, Zhang Z, Zhang RL, et al: Tadalafil, a long-acting type 5 phosphodiesterase isoenzyme inhibitor, improves neurological functional recovery in a rat model of embolic stroke, *Brain Res* 1118:192-198, 2006.

124. Chen J, Cui X, Zacharek A, et al: Niaspan increases angiogenesis and improves functional recovery after stroke, *Ann Neurol* 62:49-58, 2007.

125. Nakano M, Satoh K, Fukumoto Y, et al: Important role of erythropoietin receptor to promote VEGF expression and angiogenesis in peripheral ischemia in mice, *Circ Res* 100:662-669, 2007.

126. Tsai PT, Ohab JJ, Kertesz N, et al: A critical role of erythropoietin receptor in neurogenesis and post-stroke recovery, *J Neurosci* 26:1269-1274, 2006.

127. Chen ZY, Asavaritikrai P, Prchal JT, et al: Endogenous erythropoietin signaling is required for normal neural progenitor cell proliferation, *J Biol Chem* 282:25875-25883, 2007.

128. Iwai M, Cao G, Yin W, et al: Erythropoietin promotes neuronal replacement through revascularization and neurogenesis after neonatal hypoxia/ischemia in rats, *Stroke* 38:2795-2803, 2007.

129. Li Y, Lu Z, Keogh CL, et al: Erythropoietin-induced neurovascular protection, angiogenesis, and cerebral blood flow restoration after focal ischemia in mice, *J Cereb Blood Flow Metab* 27:1043-1054, 2007.

130. Li Y, Chen J, Zhang CL, et al: Gliosis and brain remodeling after treatment of stroke in rats with marrow stromal cells, *Glia* 49:407-417, 2005.

131. Shen LH, Li Y, Chen J, et al: Intracarotid transplantation of bone marrow stromal cells increases axon-myelin remodeling after stroke, *Neuroscience* 137:393-399, 2006.

132. Jiang Q, Zhang ZG, Ding GL, et al: MRI detects white matter reorganization after neural progenitor cell treatment of stroke, *Neuroimage* 32:1080-1089, 2006.

133. Ding G, Jiang Q, Li L, et al: Magnetic resonance imaging investigation of axonal remodeling and angiogenesis after embolic stroke in sildenafil-treated rats, *J Cereb Blood Flow Metab* 28:1440-1448, 2008.

134. Gensert JM, Goldman JE: Endogenous progenitors remyelinate demyelinated axons in the adult CNS, *Neuron* 19:197-203, 1997.

135. Roy NS, Wang S, Harrison-Restelli C, et al: Identification, isolation, and promoter-defined separation of mitotic oligodendrocyte progenitor cells from the adult human subcortical white matter, *J Neurosci* 19:9986-9995, 1999.

136. Gregersen R, Christensen T, Lehrmann E, et al: Focal cerebral ischemia induces increased myelin basic protein and growth-associated protein-43 gene transcription in peri-infarct areas in the rat brain, *Exp Brain Res* 138:384-392, 2001.

136a. Zhang L, Chopp M, Zhang RL, et al: Erythropoietin amplifies stroke-induced oligodendrosis in the rat, *PLoS One* 5:e11016, 2010.

137. Bignami A: Glial cells in the central nervous system, *Discuss Neurosci* 8:1-45, 1991.

138. Pekny M, Nilsson M: Astrocyte activation and reactive gliosis, *Glia* 50:427-434, 2005.

139. Yiu G, He Z: Glial inhibition of CNS axon regeneration, *Nat Rev Neurosci* 7:617-627, 2006.

140. Shen LH, Li Y, Gao Q, et al: Down-regulation of neurocan expression in reactive astrocytes promotes axonal regeneration and facilitates the neurorestorative effects of bone marrow stromal cells in the ischemic rat brain, *Glia* 56:1747-1754, 2008.

Genetics and Vascular Biology of Brain Vascular Malformations

HELEN KIM, LUDMILA PAWLIKOWSKA, WILLIAM L. YOUNG

This chapter focuses on the vascular biology and genetics of two vascular malformations of the brain: arteriovenous (A-V) malformations and cavernous malformations. Other vascular malformations affecting the brain are also discussed more briefly. Despite their relative rarity, these malformations pose common challenges: they are resource-intensive to manage effectively, have a high probability of serious neurologic morbidity, and the biological mechanisms underlying them are poorly understood.

Each disease is characterized by the development of a distinct category of vascular malformations and a unique spectrum of clinical and phenotypic outcomes for which biological risk factors are either poorly understood or completely unknown. The identification of these risk factors would be of immediate significance for patient surveillance and for optimizing management. Further, there are no specific medical therapies for these diseases. Better understanding of the molecular etiology and pathophysiology holds promise for design of pharmacologic treatments. Most practically, appropriate treatment (efficacy) trials will require risk stratification for selection and surrogate outcomes for trial development. Therefore, better biomarkers are needed, especially for assessing the risk of spontaneous rupture.

Brain Arteriovenous Malformations

Brain arteriovenous malformations (AVMs) represent a relatively infrequent but important source of neurologic morbidity in relatively young adults.[1] Brain AVMs have a population prevalence of 10 to 18 per 100,000 adults[2,3] and a new detection rate of approximately 1.3 per 100,000 person-years.[4,5] The basic morphology is of a vascular mass, called the *nidus,* that directly shunts blood between the arterial and venous circulations without a true capillary bed. There is usually high flow through the feeding arteries, nidus, and draining veins. The nidus is a complex tangle of abnormal, dilated channels, not clearly artery or vein, with intervening gliosis.

Seizures, mass effect, and headache are causes of associated morbidity, but prevention of new or recurrent intracranial hemorrhage (ICH) is the primary rationale for treating AVMs, usually with some combination of surgical resection, embolization, and stereotactic radiotherapy. The risk of spontaneous ICH has been estimated in retrospective and prospective observational studies to range from approximately 2% to 4% per year.[6] Other than nonspecific control of symptoms (e.g., headache and seizures), primary medical therapy is lacking.

Etiology and Pathogenesis

The genesis of AVMs has been enigmatic. Unlike the association of antecedent head trauma or other injuries with the pathogenesis of dural arteriovenous fistulas (DAVFs), environmental risk factors for AVMs are unknown. In utero formation of AVMs does occur.[7] However, considering the high utilization of prenatal ultrasound, there is remarkably little evidence for the common belief that AVMs are congenital lesions arising during embryonic development (vein of Galen malformations are an interesting counterexample but probably represent a different disease process). In fact, the mean age at presentation (detection) is roughly 40 years of age, and the distribution is normal. Although it is possible that the lesions uniquely arise prenatally (and a small number do), it hardly seems to be an inference to the best explanation. There is indirect epidemiologic evidence that the hemorrhagic behavior of most AVMs undergoes some fundamental change during childhood. Examination of ICH rates from a large cohort of more than 1500 sporadic AVM cases suggests a biological change around 10 years of age influencing the ICH rate.[8]

Further, there have been multiple reports of AVMs that grow or regress and of local AVM regrowth after treatment.[9] AVMs have occasionally been shown to arise de novo after a normal angiogram and to regrow after resection, either de novo from a retained fragment[10-12] or from a lesion treated with radiotherapy.[12,13] Although such events are relatively rare in clinical practice (in the range of 1% to 5%; higher for radiotherapy), they support the hypothesis that active vascular changes are taking place in the lesion.[14] Perhaps these observations of regrowth or de novo appearance are extreme cases of a continuum of behaviors reflecting that AVMs are actively, albeit slowly, growing lesions. Consistent with this hypothesis, endothelial proliferation, estimated by Ki-67 immunohistochemical analysis, in surgically resected AVM tissue was sevenfold higher than in control tissue (structurally normal temporal lobe removed as part of epilepsy surgery).[14] The scarce clinical imaging data available on longitudinal assessment of AVM growth after detection suggests that approximately 50% of cases display interval growth.[14] The relationship of such growth with clinical risk profile (e.g., hemorrhagic risk) remains unknown. Because postnatal growth occurs, one plausible target for therapy might be to further slow lesion growth over time.

It remains obscure as to what initiates the AVM disease process. As will be developed further on, an underlying genetic predisposition may play a role, but some kind of inciting event or events appear necessary to complete the process.

Characterization of Lesional Tissue Removed at Surgery

Available evidence is more consistent with an active angiogenic and inflammatory lesion rather than with a static congenital anomaly. Several groups[15] have shown that a prominent feature of the AVM phenotype is relative overexpression of vascular endothelial growth factor (VEGF-A), at both the messenger RNA (mRNA) and protein level. VEGF may contribute to the hemorrhagic tendency of AVMs if one extrapolates from animal models.[16] Other upstream factors that may contribute to AVM formation include expression of homeobox (HOX) transcription factors, such as excess expression of proangiogenic HOXD3 or deficient expression of antiangiogenic HOXA5.[17,18] The vascular phenotype of AVM tissue may be explained, in part, by inadequate recruitment of periendothelial support structures, which is mediated by angiopoietins and TIE-2 signaling. For example, angiopoietin-2 (ANG-2), which allows loosening of cell-to-cell contacts, is overexpressed in the perivascular region in AVM vascular channels.[19]

A key downstream consequence of VEGF and ANG-2 signaling, contributing to the angiogenic phenotype, is matrix metalloproteinase (MMP) expression. MMP-9 expression, in particular, appears to be at least an order of magnitude higher in AVM than in control tissue,[20,21] and levels of naturally occurring MMP inhibitors, such as tissue inhibitor of metalloproteinases (TIMP)-1 and TIMP-3, are also increased but to a lesser degree. Additional inflammatory markers that are overexpressed include myeloperoxidase (MPO) and interleukin 6 (IL-6), both of which are highly correlated with MMP-9.[21,22] MMP-9 expression is correlated with the lipocalin–MMP-9 complex, which suggests neutrophils as a major source. In a subset of unruptured, nonembolized AVMs, neutrophils (MPO) and macrophages/microglia (CD68) were all prominent in the vascular wall and intervening stroma of AVM tissue, whereas T and B lymphocytes were present but rarely observed.[23] A recent report showed higher immunoglobulin levels in AVM tissue than in control brain.[24]

The extent to which progenitor cell populations influence AVM growth and development is an area in need of further exploration. For example, endothelial progenitor cells (EPCs) are present in the nidus of brain and spinal cord AVMs and may mediate pathologic vascular remodeling and impact the clinical course of AVMs. Hao et al demonstrated that both brain and spinal AVM tissues displayed more CD133, SDF-1, and CD68-positive signals than epilepsy and basilar artery control tissues. EPCs, identified as CD133 and KDR double stained–positive cells, were increased in the brain and spinal cord AVM nidus, mainly at the edge of the vessel wall. The expression of SDF-1 colocalized with CD31 and α-smooth muscle actin expression, predominantly found within the vessel wall.

More generally, based on several lines of evidence, circulating bone-marrow derived cells have a major role in both microcirculatory angiogenesis[25,26] and conductance vessel remodeling.[27,28] If AVM pathogenesis involves these two processes, it is reasonable to infer that bone-marrow derived cells may have an underappreciated role in lesion formation and growth.

Genetic Considerations Relevant to AVMs

The majority of brain AVMs are sporadic; however, some evidence supports a familial component to the AVM phenotype, and further evidence suggests that genetic variation is relevant to the disease course. Probably no more than 5% of AVMs occur in the context of rare inherited vascular disorders. Based on what is known from the mendelian forms of the disease, human tissue assays, and animal models (see next section), a simplified summary of potentially relevant pathways is shown in Fig. 12-1. The reader is referred to several more detailed reviews of the signaling pathways involved.[29-33]

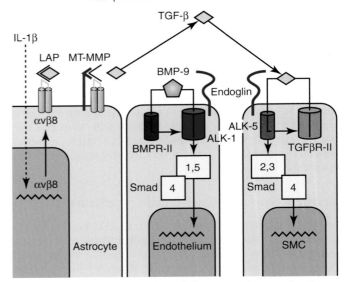

Figure 12-1 Transforming growth factor (TGF)-β superfamily signaling pathways relevant to arteriovenous malformation (AVM). Integrin αvβ8 is critical for liberation of TGF-β from latency-associated peptide (LAP); the β8-encoding gene, *ITGB8* has an interleukin (IL)-1β responsive element in its promoter in both humans and mice. TGF-β signaling involves both ALK-1 and ALK-5 receptors. ALK-5 receptors are expressed primarily on vascular smooth muscle cells, whereas ALK-1 is expressed in endothelial cells. BMP-9 may be an additional physiologic ligand for ALK-1 signaling. These signaling pathways have considerable cross-talk, the nature of which remains controversial. The ALK-1 signal is involved with endothelial cell migration and proliferation. Endoglin is an accessory receptor that can modulate both ALK-5 and ALK-1 signaling; ALK-1 and ALK-5 signal via distinct SMAD subtypes, all of which require the common co-SMAD, SMAD4, for translocation to the nucleus to effect downstream gene expression.

Mendelian Disease

Candidate genes and pathways for brain AVM pathogenesis have been suggested by mendelian disorders, which exhibit AVMs as part of their clinical phenotype. AVMs in various organs, including the brain, are highly prevalent in patients with hereditary hemorrhagic telangiectasia (HHT, OMIM#187300), an autosomal dominant disorder of mucocutaneous fragility. The two main subtypes of HHT (HHT1 and 2) are caused by loss-of-function mutations in two genes[34] originally implicated in transforming growth factor-beta (TGF-β) signaling pathways (see Fig. 12-1). The first is endoglin (ENG), which encodes an accessory protein of TGF-β receptor complexes. The second is activin-like kinase 1 (ALK-1, or ACVLR1), which codes for a transmembrane kinase also thought to participate in TGF-β signaling. There are hundreds of reported mutations in the ALK-1 and ENG genes[35]; the functional effect appears to be effective haploinsufficiency rather than a mutation-specific set of dysfunctions.

The exact signaling pathways for ALK-1 and endoglin are complex and interrelated, and the relative importance and cellular specificity are controversial.[30] Endoglin interacts with multiple TGF-β related signaling pathways and interacts with TGFBR-II (the type II TGF-β receptor) as well as with type I TGF-β receptors ALK-1 and ALK-5.[36] Endoglin can also bind ligands besides TGF-β, including activins and bone morphogenetic protein (BMP) family members.[37,38]

BMP-9 may represent a physiologically relevant *endothelial* signaling pathway for ALK-1; endoglin can potentiate the signal, which suggests a possible key interaction for HHT pathogenesis.[37,39] At the earliest stages of vascular development, mice lacking Alk-1 (Acvrl1) form systemic arteriovenous fistulas (AVFs) from fusion of major arteries and veins.[40] Endothelial cell (EC)–specific ablation of the murine Alk-1 gene causes vascular malformations to form during development, whereas mice harboring an EC-specific knockout of Alk-5 (the type I TGF-β receptor) or Tgfbr2 show neither vascular malformation nor any other perturbation in vascular morphogenesis.[41]

A third candidate gene for AVM pathogenesis is SMAD4, encoding a downstream participant in TGF-β and BMP signaling. SMAD4 is mutated in a combined syndrome of juvenile polyposis and HHT.[42] Two additional independent loci, termed HHT3 and HHT4, have been reported,[43,44] but the genes underlying these less common forms of HHT have yet to be identified.

In HHT, defects in either ENG or ALK-1 appear to affect a common set of signaling pathways. By inference, this common pathway may also contribute to sporadic brain AVM development. A potential *mechanism* for the role of this pathway in AVM pathogenesis would include the requirement of ALK-1 for normal EC maturation.[45,46] Disruption of this signaling pathway by mutation or as a downstream effect of physiologic perturbation would impair EC maturation, leading to inappropriate EC migration and proliferation. This is consistent with the view that aberrant EC migration and proliferation is an early stage in the development of an AVM. However, another view is that TGF-β/ALK-1 induces and TGF-β/ALK-5 inhibits cell migration and proliferation.[47] More work is needed with in vivo models to settle these apparent contradictions.

Levels of ENG and ALK-1 are reduced in ECs of HHT1 and HHT2 newborns. Both ALK-1 and ENG are expressed predominantly in ECs,[48,49,49a,49b] but ENG is also expressed in other cell types, notably in monocytes.[50] Monocytic ENG appears to be critical for vascular repair in other organs, for example, the heart.[51] ENG expression is grossly normal in both sporadic brain AVMs and those from HHT patients.[52] In one small series, ALK-1 expression was decreased in sporadic AVM.[53] The interaction or intersection of these pathways in postnatal brain needs more elucidation.[29,30,41,54,55]

Endoglin may contribute to disease formation via mechanisms other than the classical canonical TGF-β signaling pathway in endothelium or smooth muscle (or perhaps even in bone marrow–derived cells). Endoglin signaling may modulate endothelial nitric oxide synthase (eNOS) activation, thereby contributing to the local regulation of vascular tone and integrity.[56] Studies in $Eng^{+/-}$ mice suggest that impaired arterial myogenic responses and Eng-deficient ECs produce less nitric oxide (NO) and instead generate more eNOS-derived superoxide (O_2^-).[56a] Treatment with an O_2^- scavenger reversed the vasomotor abnormalities in $Eng^{+/-}$ arteries, which suggests that uncoupled eNOS activity and the resulting impaired myogenic response represent early events in HHT1 pathogenesis related to oxidative stress. A loss of local microvascular flow regulation may in and of itself lead to the development of arteriovenous shunts, as predicted by computational modeling studies.[57] There are conflicting data regarding the nature of the vasomotor response,[58] but this hemodynamic mechanism has been demonstrated in the pulmonary circulation[59]; detailed studies in the cerebrovascular setting have not been reported to date.

Recently, soluble ENG (sENG; cleaved extracellular domain of ENG) was shown to contribute to another vascular disease, preeclampsia.[60] That discovery led to the demonstration that sENG is elevated in human AVM lesional tissue; sENG overexpression, in the presence of VEGF overexpression, can induce vascular dysplasia in mice[61] (sENG is distinct from long [L] and short [S] form ENG, which have cytoplasmic tails of 47 and 14 amino acids, respectively.[62])

These sENG findings suggest the hypothesis that increased sENG might compete with membrane-bound ENG for ligand binding, thus decreasing downstream signaling. It is not clear how sENG is formed. The soluble form of a related type III TGF-β receptor, beta glycan, appears to be shed by a process mediated by MMP-1.[63] Expression of several different MMPs is increased in AVM nidal tissue.[21,22,64] Thus, an MMP-mediated proteolytic mechanism may contribute to the formation of sENG or sALK-1.[60] It is also possible that the soluble isoform could be formed via alternative splicing. AVMs seem to be characterized by a proinflammatory state.[21,22,65-67] Interestingly, TNF-α, implicated in AVM hemorrhage risk (discussed later), can induce release of sENG from normal placental villous explants.[68]

As a class, the inherited AVMs in HHT have distinguishing morphologic characteristics such as smaller size, higher incidence of single hole fistulas, and higher incidence of cortical location and lesion multiplicity. However, they are generally similar to the sporadic lesions and cannot be distinguished individually on the basis of their angioarchitecture.[69,70] There is a further distinction in that HHT brain AVMs are more frequently diagnosed before they have ruptured, but this probably reflects the more aggressive screening in HHT patients rather than an underlying biological difference. However, this remains to be tested.

Brain AVMs are approximately 10 times more common in patients with HHT1/*ENG* (≈20%) than in those with HHT2/*ALK-1* (≈2%).[71-73] Compared with the prevalence of sporadic lesions in the normal population, the presence of an *ENG* or *ALK-1* mutation results in approximately a 1000- and 100-fold increased risk, respectively, of developing a brain AVM. The greatly elevated risk of brain AVM development in the mendelian disorders raises the possibility that germline *sequence variants* of these and other genes in shared pathways may likewise pose a significant risk for *sporadic* brain AVM development.

Because the population prevalence of HHT is roughly 1/10,000, and approximately 10% of all HHT cases harbor brain AVMs,[71] an estimate of the population prevalence of HHT-related AVMs should be roughly 1/100,000. Given the total AVM population prevalence of 10 to 18 per 100,000 adults,[2,3] the fraction of HHT-AVMs in large referral series might be expected to be in the range of 5% to 10%. Interestingly, HHT accounts for less than 1% of the University of California–San Francisco (UCSF)[6] and Columbia[74] AVM databases (unpublished data). These epidemiologic inconsistencies need further clarification, and it may be the case that, for example, there is a systematic underestimation of undiagnosed HHT in the large AVM referral cohorts.

Familial Aggregation

Although rare, familial cases of AVM outside the context of HHT have been reported.[75,76] A recent review article examined all case reports and identified 53 patients without HHT in 25 families with AVMs, mostly of first-degree relationships (79%).[76] While no clear pattern of inheritance emerged from the pedigrees, the clinical characteristics in patients with familial AVM did not differ significantly from sporadic AVM, except for a younger age at diagnosis, which is consistent with a genetic influence. In addition, linkage and association analysis of six Japanese families, each with two affected relatives, was recently reported.[75] Linkage analysis revealed seven candidate regions, and the strongest signal was at chromosome 6q25 (LOD = 1.88; $P = 0.002$) under a dominant genetic model. However, the study was underpowered and did not reach genome-wide level of significance.

The lack of published population-based studies of AVM with family history information makes it difficult to assess familial aggregation. Evidence for a genetic component to AVMs can come from considering the excess risk of disease in relatives compared with that in the general population. A commonly used familial aggregation measure is the sibling recurrence risk ratio, lambda sibling ($\lambda_{sibling}$), defined as the risk of disease in siblings of an individual with disease ($K_{sibling}$), divided by the population prevalence of the disease (K).[77] A $\lambda_{sibling}$ value equal to 1.0 indicates no evidence for a genetic influence, whereas higher values suggest a greater genetic component to the pathogenesis of disease. For example, $\lambda_{sibling}$ values for complex diseases vary from 2.0 to 5.0 for ischemic stroke,[78] 58 for ankylosing spondylitis,[79] and 215 for autism.[80] Given the population prevalence of AVM of 0.018%, a sibling recurrence risk ($K_{sibling}$) even as low as 0.05% would yield a recurrence risk ratio to siblings compared with the general population ($\lambda_{sibling}$) of 2.78, which would support a genetic contribution to the disease.[81]

Taken together, there is modest evidence supporting familial aggregation for the AVM phenotype, although definitive proof is lacking. An increased relative risk to siblings would suggest a significant genetic influence, although this could also be the result of random chance, shared environmental factors, shared genetic factors, or any combination of these. The challenge is identifying enough non-HHT families with imaging-confirmed AVM cases and genetic data to perform classic familial aggregation and genetic studies.

Genetic Studies of Nonfamilial AVM

Candidate Gene Studies in AVM Patients

Regardless of whether true familial AVM cases exist, it is possible to perform candidate gene association studies to evaluate whether genetic variants in candidate genes are *associated* with disease or disease progression. An important consideration in any such discussion is care in the way one construes the nature of an "inherited disease."

The mechanism of AVM initiation is as yet unknown. However, even if it involves a structural aberration or mechanical insult—per se not a heritable trait—the subsequent growth and behavior of the lesion may still be influenced by genetic variation. For example, multiple genetic loci influence VEGF-induced angiogenesis.[82,83] Therefore, a pathogenesis that involves a response to injury at any level may be at least partially influenced by heritable aspects of such a response. Genetic influences on AVM pathobiology may then be evaluated in a case–control study design (comparing affected patients to normal control subjects) or in cohort designs (cross-sectional or longitudinal) so that genetic influences on the clinical course, such as propensity to rupture, can be investigated.

At least four general classes of candidates may be relevant to examine: (1) genes mutated in mendelian disorders affecting the cerebral circulation (e.g., *ALK1* and *ENG* in HHT); (2) genes in pathways known to be altered in AVM lesional tissue (e.g., inflammatory or angiogenic genes); (3) genes suggested by animal or in vitro models of relevant phenotypic variants; and (4) genes that may generally predispose to ICH, such as *APOE*. In all of these cases, common genetic polymorphisms may subtly alter protein function or expression, resulting in phenotypes relevant to the human disease.

For example, a common intronic variant of *ALK-1*, IVS3-35A>G, has been found to be associated with AVM.[84] This association was independently replicated by another group.[85,86] The functionality of this single nucleotide polymorphism (SNP) is unknown but it could affect mRNA splicing or represent a regulatory element. Thus, common variation in a gene that, when mutated, causes HHT may also contribute to the sporadic AVM phenotype.

One example of a candidate protein suggested by work in animal models is the astrocytic integrin αvβ8, an upstream regulator of TGF-β signaling. Integrin β8 abrogation in mice results in vascular instability leading to developmental ICH.[87] Preliminary data suggest that common genetic variants in *ITGB8* (encoding the integrin β8 subunit) are associated with AVM and with decreased αvβ8 expression in resected AVM tissue.[88] Polymorphisms in other candidate genes have also been associated with AVM susceptibility, including common promoter polymorphisms in IL-6 (*IL-6*-174 G>C)[89] among Hispanics and IL-1β (*IL-1β*-31 T>C and -511 C>T) among Caucasians.[67]

Genetic influences on the clinical course of AVM rupture resulting in ICH have been reported in three settings: presentation with ICH,[65,67] new ICH after diagnosis,[66,90] and ICH after treatment.[91]

The GG genotype of the IL-6 (*IL-6*-174G>C) promoter polymorphism was associated with clinical presentation of ICH.[65] The high-risk *IL-6*-174 GG genotype was also associated with the highest IL-6 mRNA and protein levels in AVM tissue.[22] Polymorphisms in the *EPHB4* gene, encoding a tyrosine kinase receptor involved in embryogenic arterial-venous determination, are also associated with increased risk of ICH presentation.[92]

The A allele of the *TNF-α*-238G>A promoter SNP was associated with new hemorrhages in the natural course of a sample of 280 AVM cases with a hazard ratio (HR) of 4.0 (95% confidence interval [CI], 1.3-12.3; P = 0.015), adjusted for initial ICH presentation, age, and race/ethnicity.[66] Apolipoprotein E (*APOE*) ε2 and ε4 alleles may predispose generally to ICH.[93,94] In AVM patients, the *APOE* ε2, but not *APOE* ε4, allele was associated with new hemorrhage after diagnosis (n = 284) in the natural course, with an adjusted HR of 5.1 (95% CI, 1.5-17.7; P = 0.01).[90] When examined together in a multivariate model, both the *APOE* ε2 and *TNF-α*-238 A alleles were independent predictors of ICH risk.[90] In addition to their association with spontaneous ICH in the natural, untreated course, both *APOE* ε2 and *TNF-α*-238 A alleles appear to confer greater risk for postradiosurgical and postsurgical hemorrhaging.[91] *IL-1β* polymorphism genotypes were also associated with increased risk of new ICH after diagnosis.[67]

The majority of these genetic association results await replication in independent AVM cohorts. Because AVMs are rare, this poses considerable challenges for accruing sufficiently large sample sizes so that this important goal may be accomplished; it will certainly require a level of international collaboration that has not yet been achieved. The large case series from referral centers that have examined phenotypic risk factors have generally not addressed genetic risk factors. However, there is indirect evidence of a genetic influence, in that race-ethnic background appears to influence the risk of spontaneous ICH during the natural history before treatment.[6] Further study is needed in this area as this association could also be explained by socioeconomic and environmental factors or a complex combination of these influences with genetics. It is interesting that no specific environmental factors have been identified in published case series, with the possible exception of essential hypertension.[95]

Beyond Candidate Gene Studies

A drawback of candidate gene studies is that although they are hypothesis driven, they represent, at best, an educated guess as to which genes are involved. An alternative is to conduct a genome-wide association (GWAS) study, which may be designed as a case-control or a cohort study, comparing cases and controls (disease susceptibility genes) or specific outcomes among cases (genetic modifiers of disease progression), respectively. This experimental approach relies on scanning all common variation in the human genome, utilizing microarrays that feature hundreds of thousands to millions of SNPs, which were selected based on the description of common human variation provided by the International HapMap project (www.hapmap.org).[96] GWAS can identify associated genes if the causative variants are common in the general population. An advantage of GWAS is that this approach can uncover completely novel biological mechanisms. A disadvantage is that given the very large number of variants tested, a large sample size (preferably in the 1000s) and replication in two or more independent cohorts is needed to determine and validate significant findings.[97] Furthermore, this approach addresses the "common disease–common variant" model and cannot uncover novel or rare SNPs associated with the disease. Nonetheless, the first such studies have been published in abstract form.[98]

What if the underlying genetic variants are not common but rare or unique to every affected individual, even if the same genes are affected in different AVM patients? To prove such a disease mechanism, it will be necessary to resequence the whole genome or select sets of candidate genes. Such whole-scale variation-discovery approaches will soon become feasible with the recent advent of massively high-throughput next-generation sequencing technology.

An Alternative Genetic Mechanism for Sporadic AVMs

An alternative hypothesis for sporadic AVM pathogenesis posits that the relevant genes and pathways are disrupted by *somatic* rather than *germline* mutations and thus are not inherited but arise de novo in development in a subset of the cells in each affected individual. This genetic mechanism would parallel that demonstrated recently for venous malformations, in which germline *TIE-2* mutations are found in autosomal dominant families with venous malformations[99,100] but somatic mutations are found in *tissue* isolated from sporadic venous malformations.[101,102] The same pattern has also been demonstrated in cerebral cavernous malformations (see CCM section further on).[103] The somatic mutation mechanism might also explain the rarity of families with AVMs outside the context of HHT. The occasional but rare familial occurrence of the usually sporadic AVM is similar to that found with other vascular traits such as Klippel-Trénaunay syndrome. This pattern has been termed *paradominant inheritance* and invokes a crucial role for both germline and somatic mutations for its underlying mechanism.[104,105] In the paradominant model, individuals heterozygous for a germline mutation are phenotypically normal, but germline homozygotes die during early embryogenesis. Thus the mutation rarely manifests as familial inheritance of a trait but instead is "silently" transmitted through many generations. However, the trait becomes manifest in an individual when a second, somatic mutation occurs in the same gene at a later stage of embryogenesis, giving rise to a mutant cell population either homozygous or hemizygous (if the somatic lesion is a deletion) for mutation in the gene. This clone of mutant cells has bypassed the developmental block, and these cells can now seed the development of the vascular anomaly. This intriguing hypothesis has yet to be explored for sporadic AVMs and will necessitate candidate gene (or in the future, whole genome) resequencing of DNA from AVM lesional tissue, preferably by isolating specific cell types that may have arisen from separate clonal populations in development.

Experimental AVM Models

Model systems for studying AVM are needed to test mechanistic hypotheses and develop novel therapies. Historically, "AVM" models have been largely based on extradural AVFs for the study of hemodynamic changes or for the development of platforms for technology.[106-124] These models have largely been developed by surgeons and endovascular therapists seeking to understand the pathophysiology of postoperative complications like "normal perfusion pressure breakthough"[125] or to develop embolic or radiotherapeutic methods.[126] With few exceptions,[123] the model lesions are extradural in nature. Such models are capable of inducing both hemodynamic[108] and histopathologic change.[124] However, they do not display the clinical syndrome of recurrent hemorrhage into the brain parenchyma or cerebrospinal fluid spaces. A *parenchymal* nidus is not formed, and nidus growth and hemorrhaging that mimic the human disease do not occur.

More recently, developmental biologists have taken an interest in the formation of vascular lesions in the brain that result in hemorrhages. Many different developmental gene defects result in antenatal or perinatal hemorrhages and, in some cases, display vascular structures reminiscent of the human disease. Some of the underlying proteins may be related to AVM biology. An example would be integrin $\alpha v \beta 8$, which is involved in modulating proteolytic cleavage of latency associated peptide (LAP) from the protein precursor of TGF-β, allowing liberation of the mature TGF-β molecule.[88]

The story becomes especially interesting when such models are focused on genes that are clearly related to the human disorder (e.g., the previously described genes that cause HHT). Both $Eng^{+/-}$[127] and $Alk-1^{+/-}$[128] adult mice develop vascular lesions in various organs, but spontaneous lesions in the brain, thus far, have only been observed with the use of scanning electron microscopy in $Eng^{+/-}$ mice.[129] Park et al[41,130] have developed several innovative inducible knockout systems using a novel endothelial Cre transgenic line. Alk-1-conditional deletion resulted in severe vascular malformations mimicking all pathologic features of HHT. Antenatal conditional deletion of Alk-1 causes severe cerebrovascular dysplasia and apparent fistula formation. Interestingly, conditional Alk-1 deletion in adult mice induced

AVFs and hemorrhage in the lung and gastrointestinal tract but not in skin or brain. Importantly, when the investigators induced skin wounding, Alk-1 deleted mice developed vascular dysplasia and direct A-V connections, suggesting an abnormal response to injury. These results suggest that physiologic or environmental factors in addition to the regional conditional genetic ablation are required for Alk-1-deficient vessels to develop vascular malformations in adult mice. Applying similar methods to the brain, Walker et al[131] described vascular dysplasia and apparent A-V shunting after focal VEGF stimulation in mice subjected to regional conditional Alk-1 deletion.

Milder forms of cerebrovascular dysplasia can be induced with the use of mice with heterozygous mutations in *Alk-1* or *Eng*.[132,133] These models use VEGF stimulation in an altered genetic background and result in enlarged, dysmorphic vascular structures at the capillary level, not the large vessels seen in the human disease. Even though the capillary level vascular dysplasia seen in these heterozygous murine models does not represent the intranidal vessels of the human disease, it is possible that it phenocopies the dysplastic capillaries that have been known for some time to inhabit the margins of the clinical lesions.[134-136]

Notch signaling appears important for the determination of arterial and venous fate, a process that seems to depend on local levels of VEGF.[137] Further, Notch appears to influence tip and stalk endothelial phenotypes during angiogenesis.[138] There is empirical evidence that proteins involved in Notch signaling, including the receptor, its ligands, and downstream signals, are expressed in excised surgical specimens.[139,140] Animal experiments support a potential link with the human disease. Using conditional endothelial expression, Murphy et al[141] used a tetracycline-responsive promoter to suppress overexpression during development and then, by withdrawal of doxycycline, caused overexpression of the intracellular signaling portion of Notch-4 (int3) in early postnatal mice. They observed a rapidly lethal phenotype, which mimicked aspects of human AVMs, including dysplastic posterior fossa vasculature with apparent A-V shunting. Upon retreatment with doxycycline, the lesions regressed,[141] although tetracyclines are well known to inhibit pathologic angiogenesis and vascular remodeling.[16,142,143] ZhuGe et al[139] described increased brain angiogenesis in adult rats treated with a Notch-1 activator and suggested that activation of Notch-1 in normal vasculature induces a proangiogenic state that may contribute to the development of vascular malformations.

Based on the aforementioned evidence, the Notch pathway merits further exploration.[144] Like other growth factors, Notch activation appears to be a fundamental part of the normal response to injury; in the brain this includes, for example, ischemia-induced neurogenesis.[145]

A caveat is worthy of mention here: many authors use the term *AVM* to describe their experimental models while referring to a wide range of morphologies and phenotypes, including various patterns of abnormal vessels, hemorrhagic lesions, and primitive fistulas between the developing great vessels in utero. We would prefer to reserve the name *arteriovenous malformation* for the human disease; models should bear the name of their specific morphologic features, such as *A-V fistula* or *vascular dysplasia.* To call such animal models *AVMs* confounds a rodent model phenotype and a human disease process. The human disease called *AVM* refers to a characteristic tangle of abnormal vessels that shunts blood and, although relatively stable, spontaneously ruptures at a generally predictable rate.

Several considerations can inform model development. Table 12-1 describes components of what would constitute an ideal AVM model, which would include anatomic, physiologic, biological, and clinical features resembling the human phenotype. It is reasonable to assume that

TABLE 12-1 PROPOSED COMPONENTS OF AN IDEAL EXPERIMENTAL AVM MODEL

Anatomic
Nidus of abnormal vessels of varying sizes
Both microcirculatory and macrocirculatory levels
Physiologic
A-V shunting
Hemodynamically significant (i.e., sufficient to decrease feeding artery or increase draining venous pressures)
Biological
Alterations in angiogenic and inflammatory protein expression
Involvement of or intersection with known genetic pathways
Clinical
Relative quiescence
Spontaneous hemorrhaging into the parenchyma or cerebrospinal fluid spaces

Abbreviations: AVM, Arteriovenous malformation; A-V, arteriovenous.

(1) polymorphic variation in *ALK1* or *ENG* or (2) more likely for sporadic AVMs, an upstream or downstream component of the pathway is involved in the human disease. This is speculative but rests on the unique nature of the human phenotype: there are no other inherited syndromes besides HHT with the peculiar vascular phenotype of a brain AVM, despite the existence of a number of other cerebrovascular malformations.

Further, an angiogenic phenotype seems likely. Clinically, environmental stimuli can result in an angiogenic response and fistula formation (i.e., trauma causing direct and indirect DAVFs).[146-148] Venous hypertension (VH) can induce DAVFs in rats,[112,115] and the fistulous material is angiogenic.[112] Resected human AVM specimens also induce angiogenesis in corneal transplant experiments. This response almost certainly involves VEGF, which is expressed in the human samples[149] and in the rodent brain VH models.[150,151]

High flow rates and VH are present in human AVM nidal vessels.[152] Such biophysical components of larger, more mature AVMs undoubtedly influence their biological behavior. Importantly, increased flow rates have been shown to interact with background genetic alterations: increased focal tissue perfusion (increased endothelial shear) and angiogenic factor VEGF stimulation had a synergistic effect on promoting capillary dysplasia in Alk-1 heterozygous mice.[133]

In the absence of an ideal animal model, model development might be reasonably focused on establishing an *intermediate or surrogate phenotype* that is relevant to the human disease and shares attributes of the human AVM lesional tissue (Fig. 12-2). Success in phenocopying

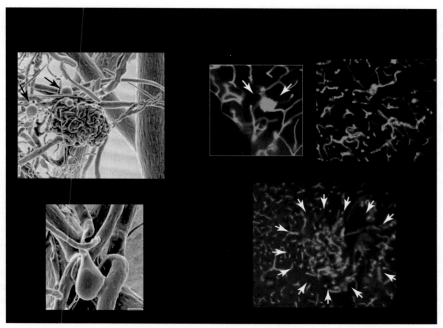

Figure 12-2 Vascular dysplasia in *Eng*[+/-] mice. Left panels are from unstimulated *Eng*[+/-] mouse brain (scanning electron microscopy); Right panels show green lectin-perfused vessels in vascular endothelial growth factor (VEGF)-stimulated *Eng*[+/-] mouse brain. Similar patterns are seen in both (small nidus or aneurysmal dilations), but VEGF stimulation increases the amount of dysplasia. (Left panel adapted from Satomi J, Mount RJ, Toporsian M, et al: Cerebral vascular abnormalities in a murine model of hereditary hemorrhagic telangiectasia. *Stroke* 34:783-789, 2003. Right panel adapted from Xu B, Wu YQ, Huey M, et al: Vascular endothelial growth factor induces abnormal microvasculature in the endoglin heterozygous mouse brain. *J Cereb Blood Flow Metab* 24:237-244, 2004.)

the clinical disorder will enable further work on novel therapeutic approaches of controlling pathologic angiogenesis and inflammation[16] to halt disease progression and decrease the risk of spontaneous hemorrhage.[153] An approach to model development is shown in Fig. 12-3.

Summary and Synthesis of Data Regarding Etiology and Pathogenesis of AVM

A prevailing hypothesis is that AVM pathophysiology is governed to a large extent by chronic hemodynamic derangements resulting from a congenital lesion. Based on the various lines of evidence just reviewed, an attractive alternative hypothesis to the notion of AVMs as a static congenital anomaly might be termed a *response-to-injury model of AVM pathogenesis*. Recent findings suggest that background genetic variation in angiogenic and inflammatory pathways may synergize with ongoing hemodynamic changes to influence this process.

Inciting event(s) that serve as copathogens might include the sequelae of even modest injury from an otherwise unremarkable episode of trauma, infection, inflammation, irradiation, or a mechanical stimulus such as compression. Perhaps these are superimposed on an

NORMAL GENETIC BACKGROUND

Quiescent — Stimulated (injury) *Normal angiogenic response* — Quiescent *Return to baseline*

A

ALTERED GENETIC BACKGROUND

Quiescent — Stimulated (injury) *Morphological dysplasia* — Disease progression *A-V shunting* — Disease progression *Rupture*

B

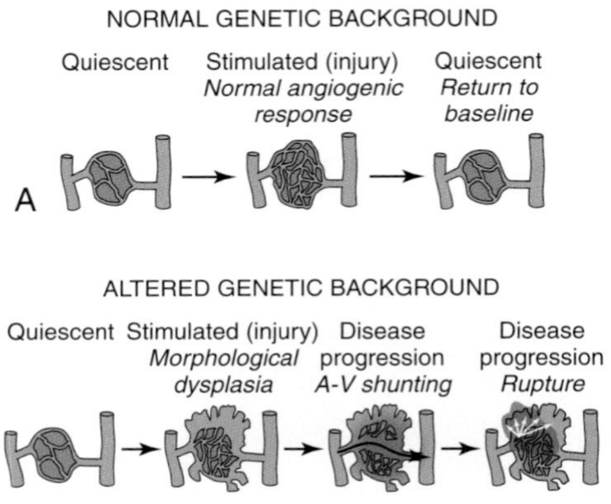

Figure 12-3 Arteriovenous malformation (AVM) model development. A, Against a normal genetic background, vascular endothelial growth factor (VEGF) stimulation increases capillary density, but the morphology is essentially normal and vascular density will regress to normal after stimulation ceases.[236] B, However, when VEGF-stimulation is performed against an altered genetic background, morphologic dysplasia results.[132] Altering hemodynamics further contributes to dysplasia.[133] Conditional knockout of relevant genes may play a key role in lesional development, especially arteriovenous (A-V) shunting.[41,130] Development of spontaneous hemorrhage, so that the human clinical course is mimicked, is a desirable component of phenocopying the human disease (see Table 12-1). (Data from Yang GY, Xu B, Hashimoto T, et al: Induction of focal angiogenesis through adenoviral vector mediated vascular endothelial cell growth factor gene transfer in the mature mouse brain. *Angiogenesis* 6:151-158, 2003; Xu B, Wu YQ, Huey M, et al: Vascular endothelial growth factor induces abnormal microvasculature in the endoglin heterozygous mouse brain. *J Cereb Blood Flow Metab* 24:237-244, 2004; Park SO, Lee YJ, Seki T, et al: ALK5- and TGFBR2-independent role of ALK-1 in the pathogenesis of hereditary hemorrhagic telangiectasia type 2 (HHT2). *Blood* 111:633-642, 2008; and Park SO, Wankhede M, Lee YJ, et al: Real-time imaging of de novo arteriovenous malformation in a mouse model of hereditary hemorrhagic telangiectasia. *J Clin Invest* 119:3487-3496, 2009.)

underlying structural defect, such as a microscopic developmental venous anomaly or some sort of venous outflow restriction in a microcirculatory bed. Two conceptual, speculative syntheses of available observations are shown in Fig. 12-4. We would suggest that a response-to-injury hypothesis is preferable to a two-hit hypothesis when describing this phenomenon because the latter is commonly used to identify a pure genetic mechanism, as has been demonstrated for cavernous malformations[103] and, furthermore, the disease mechanism might involve more than two factors.

One attractive line of inquiry would posit some degree of localized VH, which could result, for example, from microvascular thrombosis. A state of relative thrombophilia[154,154a] has been proposed as being operative in the pathophysiology of DAVF lesions. VH is a potentially angiogenic stimulus that can induce AVFs in model systems.[112,115] Interestingly, the proangiogenic effect appears to be mediated via hypoxia-inducible factor-1α (HIF-1α) and occurs even with modest, nonischemic levels of VH, which suggests some as yet unknown biomechanical signaling pathway.[150,151]

Elucidating these mechanisms offers promise for developing innovative treatments and better risk stratification for clinical management or clinical trial design. Further, study of brain AVMs may be a powerful platform from which to gain insights into general vascular biological mechanisms relevant to a wide variety of diseases affecting the vascular system.

Cerebral Cavernous Malformations

Overview

Cerebral cavernous malformations (CCMs) or cavernous angiomas (OMIM #116860) are rare vascular malformations that occur in the central nervous system, most often in the brain. In contrast to brain AVMs, CCMs are characterized as leaky, low-flow lesions that are angiographically occult. CCMs are clusters of enlarged capillary caverns lined with a single layer of endothelium without normal intervening brain parenchyma. Ultrastructural studies reveal abnormal or absent blood–brain barrier components, poorly formed tight junctions with gaps between ECs, lack of astrocytic foot processes, and few pericytes.[155]

The population prevalence of CCMs is estimated to be 0.1% to 0.5% based on MRI and autopsy studies[156,157] and represents 5% to 15% of all cerebral vascular malformations. CCMs can occur in a sporadic or a familial form; familial cases often present with multiple lesions that appear to grow in both number and size over time, which reflects the dynamic nature of these lesions.[158-162] The most common clinical sequelae include seizures (40% to 70%) and ICH (32% to 59%), resulting in acute or permanent focal neurologic deficits and even death.[160,163] Primary medical therapy is lacking for this disease.

CCM Genetics

Familial cases of CCM exhibit autosomal dominant inheritance with incomplete penetrance and account for approximately 10% to 50% of all cases. Disease-causing mutations

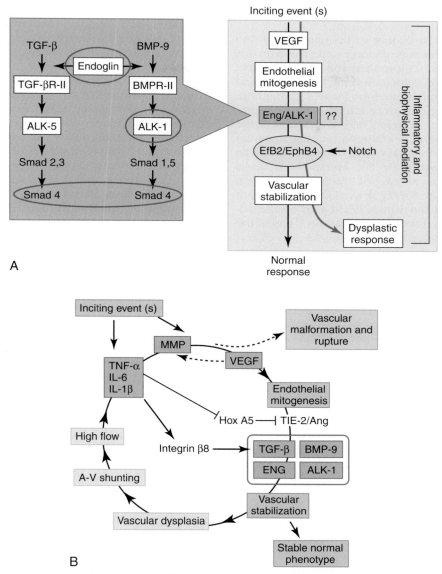

Figure 12-4   A, Speculative synthesis of pathways involved in arteriovenous malformation (AVM) pathogenesis. The blue shaded area is a simplified summary of presumed ALK-1 and ENG signaling via transforming growth factor (TGF)-β and BMP-9 in endothelial cells; the genes mutated in hereditary hemorrhagic telangiectasia (HHT) are circled. Main components of the scheme are (1) inciting event(s); (2) signaling aberration in ALK-1 and/or ENG, or in a closely related pathway (question marks); (3) ephrinB2 and EPHB4 imbalance, possibly through involvement of Notch signaling; and (4) modifier influences, potentially genetic and/or hemodynamic. Inflammation and involvement of circulating precursor cells may be relevant. **B,** Alternative depiction of speculative synthesis. This view suggests a circular or "reverberating" pathogenesis. After an inciting event, inflammatory or angiogenic activity (MMP, VEGF) initiates microvascular growth and remodeling, which are stabilized through interplay of pathways including TIE-2/ANG and TGF-β or BMP-9 signaling through the ALK-1/ENG pathway. Lack of integrin β8[88] and Hox A5,[18] an antiangiogenic transcription factor, may also play a role. Normal vessels stabilize, but an incipient AVM undergoes a dysplastic response. Arteriovenous (A-V) shunting and high flow rates synergize with the dysplastic response and with inflammatory signals, causing a vicious cycle in a localized area destined to become the nidus. Eventually, the human disease phenotype emerges. Genetic variation could influence any step of the cycle.

have been identified in *KRIT1* on 7q21-q22 (CCM1),[164-169] *MGC4067* on 7p13 (CCM2),[170-172] and *PDCD10* on 3q26-q27 (CCM3).[170-173] The majority of mutations identified in the three genes lead to loss of function of the gene product. Table 12-2 summarizes the known CCM genes, chromosome locations, and corresponding proteins. However, in 20-40% of individuals with familial CCM, mutations are not detected in any of the known CCM genes. A fourth CCM locus (CCM4) has been proposed on 3q26.3-q27.2, based on a large family showing linkage to CCM3 but with no mutations identified in PDCD10. The following paragraphs describe each of the known CCM genes in more detail, and Fig. 12-5[174] summarizes the signaling pathways involving the three known CCM proteins.

CCM1/KRIT1

The *KRIT1* gene has 16 coding exons encoding a 736 amino acid protein containing three ankyrin domains and one FERM domain.[175] More than 100 mutations have been identified in *KRIT1*, including microdeletions and nonsense and frameshift mutations located throughout the gene. Most of these mutations lead to premature protein termination, which suggests loss of function of the gene product. In addition, a common founder mutation has been identified in familial CCM1 Hispanic American cases of Mexican descent.[168,176,177] Mutational analysis originally identified this as a C-to-T transition in exon 6 at nucleotide 742 of the *KRIT1* gene (Q248X),[176] which was later assigned to exon 10 (Q455X) based on the discovery of four additional coding exons at the 5′ end of the gene.[175,178,179] The mutation substitutes a premature termination codon for glutamine. Virtually all cases of familial and sporadic CCM cases among Hispanic Americans are due to the inheritance of the same common founder mutation.[168,176]

KRIT1 was originally identified through a yeast two-hybrid screen as a novel binding partner of the Ras-family guanosine triphosphate (GTP)ase Rap1A[180,181] and has been shown to be a Rap1 binding protein regulating endothelial junction integrity by suppressing stress fibers and stabilizing cell–cell junctions.[182] Both Rap1 and KRIT1 act as inhibitors of canonical β-catenin signaling in multiple cell lineages, and loss of KRIT1 causes increased β-catenin signaling in mice.[183] Additionally, KRIT1 regulates integrin cytoplasmic domain-associated protein-1 (ICAP-1) alpha binding to integrin β1, which regulates cell adhesion and migration.[184,185] Both the integrin β1 cytoplasmic tail and KRIT1 N-terminus contain NPXY motifs that are critical for binding ICAP-1α.[184] Overexpression of KRIT1 diminishes the interaction between ICAP-1α and integrin β1.[185] Thus, impaired KRIT1 may interfere with integrin β1-dependent angiogenesis, which suggests that integrin signaling plays a role in CCM pathogenesis.

KRIT1 mRNA and protein have been detected in astrocytes, neurons, and epithelial cells in adults and in vascular ECs during early angiogenesis.[186-188] Mouse *Krit1−/−* knockouts die at mid-gestation because of abnormal vascular development associated with downregulation of arterial markers, such as *Efnb2*, *Dll4*, and *Notch4*.[189] In humans,

TABLE 12-2 CCM GENES, CHROMOSOMAL POSITION, AND CORRESPONDING PROTEIN NAME

Locus Name	Gene Symbol	Chromosomal Position	Protein Name
CCM1	*KRIT1*	7q21-q22	Krev interaction trapped 1
CCM2	*MGC4067*	7p13	Malcavernin
CCM3	*PDCD10*	3q26.1	Programmed cell death 10

CCM, Cerebral cavernous malformation.

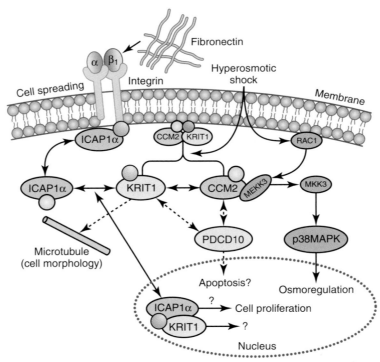

Figure 12-5 Schematic presentation of molecular pathways involving the cerebral cavernous malformation (CCM) proteins. ● NPxY motif; ○ phosphotyrosine binding (PTB) domain; dashed lines, hypothetical interactions. ICAP1α interacts with the β1 integrin cytoplasmic domain and controls cell spreading/cell proliferation on fibronectin. KRIT1 could modulate this pathway. KRIT1/CCM2/ICAP1α can form a ternary complex. ICAP1α and KRIT1 can go to the nucleus. It is not known if they go separately or together. A hyperosmotic environment stimulates in mammalian cells the Rac1–OSM(CCM2)–MEKK3–MKK3–p38MAPK pathway leading to osmoregulation. KRIT1/CCM2/MEKK3 form a ternary complex. (Reprinted with permission from Revencu N, Vikkula M: Cerebral cavernous malformation: New molecular and clinical insights. *J Med Genet* 43:716-721, 2006.)

NOTCH4 expression in arterioles associated with CCM is significantly reduced.[166,176] These results suggest that the basic defect in CCM1 involves abnormal arterial-venous specification, which, intriguingly, may also play a role in arteriovenous malformation pathogenesis as already discussed.[141]

CCM2/MGC4607

The *MGC4607* gene has 10 exons encoding the malcavernin protein, named for cavernous malformations, and mutations in this gene cause CCM2.[171,172] Mutations identified to date include nonsense, missense, frameshift, and splicing mutations, in addition to larger segmental deletions of the gene.

Ccm2 is expressed in the vasculature and is necessary for proper vacuolization leading to formation of endothelial tubes.[190,191] Kleaveland et al[192] studied the interaction of Ccm2 with heart of glass (HEG1) receptor in zebrafish and found preserved EC vacuolization and lumenization but defects in endothelial cell–cell association. In mice and zebrafish, *Ccm2$^{-/-}$* knockouts die early in embryonic development because of vascular defects.[193,194] Tissue-specific mutants show that selective deletion of *Ccm2* in the endothelium is sufficient to reproduce the vascular defects and timing of embryonic death seen in germline mutants, whereas mice lacking *Ccm2* in neural or smooth muscle cells develop normally.[190] Loss of Ccm2 results in activation of RHOA GTPase via loss of a CCM2-Smurf1 interaction, which localizes Smurf1 for RhoA degradation.[195] Treatment of *Ccm2$^{+/-}$* mice with simvastatin, a drug known to inhibit Rho GTPases, rescued the barrier function and cellular phenotype in vitro.[190] CCM2 also appears to mediate cell death signaling by tyrosine kinase (Trk) A receptor in neural cells (e.g., medulloblastoma or neuroblastoma).[196]

Malcavernin contains a phosphotyrosine binding domain (PTB), which interacts with KRIT1 to modulate the subcellular localization of KRIT1.[197] When overexpressed, malcavernin can sequester KRIT1 within the cytoplasm and form a molecular complex with MEKK3, a kinase involved in the activation of the p38 alpha pathway, and act as a scaffolding protein.[197] Mice deficient in Mekk3 or p38 Map kinase have significant defects in placental angiogenesis and blood vessel development, especially in the head region.[198,199] The only known in-frame deletion in the *CCM2* gene, which leads to deletion of 58 amino acids encoded by exon 2, was recently found to be critical for KRIT1 binding and for KRIT1-PDCD10 (CCM3) interaction.[200]

CCM3/PDCD10

PDCD10 has seven coding exons and three 5′ noncoding exons.[173] CCM3 mutations identified to date include nonsense and splice-site mutations, as well as larger macrodeletions including deletion of the entire gene in one case.[173] The protein PDCD10 (programmed cell death 10) has no known conserved functional domains or motifs. It was originally identified as a transcript showing increased expression in a myeloid cell line undergoing apoptosis[201] and, more recently, was shown to be both necessary and sufficient to induce apoptosis when overexpressed in cell culture.[202]

PDCD10 mRNA is highly expressed in arterial endothelium of neuronal cells during both embryonic and postnatal brain development.[203,204] Voss et al[205] demonstrated that PDCD10 coprecipitated and colocalized with CCM2. They hypothesized that PDCD10 is part of the CCM1–CCM2 protein complex through its interaction with CCM2 and therefore may participate in CCM1-dependent modulation of integrin β1 signaling.[205] An in-frame deletion in *CCM2* was found to inhibit formation of a CCM1–CCM2–CCM3 complex.[200]

CCM Pathogenesis

Several groups have hypothesized that the underlying pathogenesis of CCM might be due to somatic mutations in known CCM genes,[103,206,207] de novo germline mutations,[208] haploinsufficiency,[209,210] or paradominant inheritance as seen in other vascular malformations.[174] Because almost all mutations in CCM genes lead to loss of function, severe impairment of the respective protein is likely to underlie the pathogenesis of the disorder.

Evidence for Knudson's two-hit hypothesis has been demonstrated in both human CCM lesions[103,206,207] and murine models.[190,211] In the two-hit model, vascular cells with two mutations (either germline or somatic) would result in complete loss of functional protein; clonal expansion of the mutant cells would then seed formation of the CCM lesion. Both *Ccm1$^{+/-}$* and *Ccm2$^{+/-}$* heterozygous mice are viable and phenotypically normal.[193,211] However, in the background of homozygous knockout of the tumor suppressor gene *Trp53*, these transgenic mice (*Ccm1$^{+/-}$ Trp53$^{-/-}$* and *Ccm2$^{+/-}$ Trp53$^{-/-}$*) develop lesions resembling human CCM lesions.[211,212] *Trp53$^{-/-}$* mice are highly susceptible to spontaneous mutations, which suggests that a second genetic hit is involved in the pathogenesis of CCMs. In humans, both biallelic germline and somatic mutations have been identified in CCM lesions from all three forms of inherited CCMs,[103,206] with corresponding absence of CCM proteins in vascular EC lining the cavernous lesions.[213] The observation that de novo formation of lesions can occur after radiation therapy also lends indirect support to the two-hit hypothesis.[214-216] However, others have not observed somatic mutations or loss of heterozygosity in human CCM samples, which suggests that haploinsufficiency might be the underlying genetic mechanism for some cases.[209]

More recently, inflammatory or immune response has been hypothesized to play a role in the pathogenesis and progression of CCMs.[24,217] Microarray analysis of CCM lesions revealed upregulation of 10 immunoglobulin (Ig) genes compared with AVM tissue and normal superficial temporal arteries.[218] B cells were detected in CCM lesions, as was an oligoclonal pattern of IgG that was not observed in AVM or control brain specimens.[217] Maiuri et al[162] found that familial occurrence and more aggressive clinical behavior of cavernous angiomas were associated with higher expression of Ki-67, bcl-2, and TGF-β. The perilesional brain parenchyma showed significantly higher expression of TGF-β, platelet-derived growth factor, and tenascin, a glycoprotein of the extracellular matrix that is absent in the normal brain, in more aggressive cavernomas with larger size (>2 cm), mass effect, documented growth, or significant extralesional symptomatic hemorrhaging. Jung et al[219] found increased VEGF expression in a case of multiple cavernomas with a progressive course.

Genotype–Phenotype Correlation

With the identification of the specific genes and mutations underlying CCM1, CCM2, and CCM3, genotype–phenotype correlations between the three forms are beginning to emerge.[220] CCM1 mutation carriers appear to have a milder phenotype with regard to hemorrhage but may present with more seizures[221] and extraneurologic manifestations such as cutaneous vascular malformations.[222,223] In a consecutive series of 417 patients with familial CCM, 9% displayed the cutaneous vascular malformation phenotype, including hyperkeratotic cutaneous capillary–venous malformations (CCM1), capillary malformations (CCM1), and venous malformations (both CCM1 and CCM3).[222] CCM3 patients may have a more aggressive clinical course with an earlier age of onset of symptoms and greater risk of hemorrhagic events.[160] Retinal vascular malformations have been observed in all three familial forms with an estimated prevalence of 5%.[224] However, large prospective studies with better characterization of clinical symptoms are needed to firmly establish these phenotypic differences among different gene mutation carriers.

Summary of CCM Biology and Pathogenesis

There has been remarkable progress in elucidating the molecular genetics and biology of CCM pathogenesis over the past decade. Now that the genes and proteins have been identified, the specific mechanisms of how these proteins interact and function to cause CCM are under intense investigation. Better clinical characterization of CCM patients is needed to obtain more accurate estimates of genotype–phenotype correlations, clinical penetrance, frequency and severity of symptoms, progression, and response to treatments. Longitudinal studies are needed to determine the natural history and gain a better understanding of the progression of the disease in both sporadic and familial cases. Undoubtedly, additional modifier genes and other factors will emerge as important predictors of the variable expressivity of the disease and may shed light on the progression of related vascular malformations that operate via a common signaling pathway.

Other Vascular Malformations

Several other types of vascular malformations affecting blood and lymphatic vessels throughout the body exist; some but not all may also be found in the brain vasculature. For some of these rare anomalies, a genetic cause has been identified, and the resulting insight into their biological underpinnings can have relevance for studies of other vascular malformations, particularly where the genes affected participate in signaling via common pathways.

Patients with **capillary malformation–arteriovenous malformation (CM-AVM) syndrome,** an autosomal dominant disorder, have both cutaneous capillary malformations (also known as *port-wine stain*) and AVFs or AVMs that may affect other organs including the brain (e.g., intracranial AVMs and carotid AVFs). Linkage studies in families led to the identification of heterozygous inactivating mutations in *RASA1* (encoding p120-RasGTPase-activating protein, p120RasGAP).[225] Subsequent mutation screening showed that many of these mutations arise de novo.[226] p120RasGAP is a negative inhibitor of the Ras/MAPkinase signaling pathway in ECs, which mediates signaling from a wide range of growth factor receptors and affects several aspects of EC biology including cell motility and apoptosis. Mouse knockouts homozygous for *Rasa1* mutations die in embryo with defective angiogenesis and increased apoptosis, but heterozygotes are normal.[227] Phenotype variation and reduced penetrance of *RASA1* mutations in families suggest that a second hit, possibly a somatic mutation (see discussion of paradominant model in AVM and CCM sections) may be required.[226] Recently, both familial and de novo *RASA1* mutations have also been identified in CCM patients, who also have spinal AVMs or AVF lesions (conus or lumbosacral junction AVMs; cervical or cervicothoracic AVFs).[228]

Venous anomalies are slow-flow lesions further subclassified as **venous malformations (VMs),** including **cutaneomucosal VM (VMCM)** and **glomuvenous malformations (GVMs).** VMCMs show autosomal dominant inheritance and are caused by mutations in the gene encoding an EC-specific receptor tyrosine kinase, TIE2 (TEK).[99,100,229] The eight known mutations all appear to increase ligand-independent autophosphorylation of TIE2 to a variable level. TIE2 binds angiopoietins and signals via the PI3-kinase pathway and AKT to inhibit apoptosis and via the MAP-kinase pathways to mediate EC proliferation. As previously noted, somatic second-hit mutations have been identified in VMCM lesional tissue.[101,102]

Dural arteriovenous fistulas (DAVF) are neurovascular malformations comprising one or more arteriovenous shunts located in the dura mater.[230] They make up approximately one tenth of intracranial vascular malformations. DAVFs are similar to AVMs in that they involve active shunting of blood from the arterial to venous circulations, but one principal difference from AVMs is that DAVFs are typically supplied by extracranial arterial input. Several clinical characteristics of DAVFs are associated with a high risk of ICH, primarily related to a change in hemodynamics when venous drainage is shifted from extracranial to intracranial routes. VH is a hallmark of the disease process.[230]

Another difference from AVMs is that DAVFs are thought to be acquired lesions, resulting from some occurrence of, perhaps, unrecognized trauma. There is support for the view that the pathophysiology may involve venous thrombosis[146,231]; DAVFs can be induced in rodents by inducing VH.[111,112]

Given this hypothesis, genetic variation contributing to susceptibility to thrombosis has been evaluated for association with DAVFs.[232-235] In several small case series, thrombophilic mutations such as the factor V Leiden mutation (odds ratio [OR], 4.7; 95% CI, 1.24-17.69) and the prothrombin G20210A allele (OR, 10.9; 95% CI,

1.3-89.5) were associated with DAVF.[232] However, overall these mutations were only seen in a small minority of DAVF patients and require replication in larger cohorts. Finally, the same *ALK-1* (IVS3-35A>G) polymorphism found associated with brain AVMs[84] (see section on candidate gene studies) was also present at a higher frequency in DAVF cases compared with healthy control subjects.[85] Unlike for AVMs, this association has not yet been independently replicated for DAVFs but suggests possible commonalities in AVM and DAVF etiology, especially given the presence of A-V shunting in both types of malformation.

Acknowledgments

The authors gratefully acknowledge Douglas A. Marchuk, PhD, for his review of the chapter and helpful suggestions; the UCSF Brain AVM study project members (http://avm.ucsf.edu); the other Principal Investigators (Nancy Boudreau, Tomoki Hashimoto, Charles E. McCulloch, Stephen Nishimura, and Hua Su) of P01 NS044155 (Young), "Integrative Study of Brain Vascular Malformations"; and Voltaire Gungab for assistance in manuscript preparation. H.K. is supported in part by K23 NS058357.

REFERENCES

1. Arteriovenous Malformation Study Group: Arteriovenous malformations of the brain in adults, *N Engl J Med* 340:1812-1818, 1999.
2. Al-Shahi R, Fang JS, Lewis SC, et al: Prevalence of adults with brain arteriovenous malformations: A community based study in Scotland using capture-recapture analysis, *J Neurol Neurosurg Psychiatry* 73:547-551, 2002.
3. Berman MF, Sciacca RR, Pile-Spellman J, et al: The epidemiology of brain arteriovenous malformations, *Neurosurgery* 47:389-396, 2000.
4. Stapf C, Mast H, Sciacca RR, et al: The New York Islands AVM Study: Design, study progress, and initial results, *Stroke* 34:e29-e33, 2003.
5. Gabriel RA, Kim H, Sidney S, et al: Ten-year detection rate of brain arteriovenous malformations in a large, multiethnic, defined population, *Stroke* 41:21-26, 2010.
6. Kim H, Sidney S, McCulloch CE, et al: Racial/ethnic differences in longitudinal risk of intracranial hemorrhage in brain arteriovenous malformation patients, *Stroke* 38:2430-2437, 2007.
7. Potter CA, Armstrong-Wells J, Fullerton HJ, et al: Neonatal giant pial arteriovenous malformation: Genesis or rapid enlargement in the third trimester, *J Neurointervent Surg* 1:151-153, 2009.
8. Kim H, McCulloch CE, Johnston SC, et al: Comparison of two approaches for determining the natural history risk of brain arteriovenous malformation (BAVM) rupture, *Am J Epidemiol* 171:1317-1322, 2010.
9. Du R, Hashimoto T, Tihan T, et al: Growth and regression of an arteriovenous malformation in a patient with hereditary hemorrhagic telangiectasia: Case report, *J Neurosurg* 106:470-477, 2007.
10. Hino A, Fujimoto M, Iwamoto Y, et al: An adult case of recurrent arteriovenous malformation after "complete" surgical excision: A case report, *Surg Neurol* 52:156-158, 1999.
11. Kader A, Goodrich JT, Sonstein WJ, et al: Recurrent cerebral arteriovenous malformations after negative postoperative angiograms, *J Neurosurg* 85:14-18, 1996.
12. Klimo P Jr, Rao G, Brockmeyer D: Pediatric arteriovenous malformations: A 15-year experience with an emphasis on residual and recurrent lesions, *Childs Nerv Syst* 23:31-37, 2007.
13. Lindqvist M, Karlsson B, Guo WY, et al: Angiographic long-term follow-up data for arteriovenous malformations previously proven to be obliterated after gamma knife radiosurgery, *Neurosurgery* 46:803-808, 2000.
14. Hashimoto T, Mesa-Tejada R, Quick CM, et al: Evidence of increased endothelial cell turnover in brain arteriovenous malformations, *Neurosurgery* 49:124-131, 2001.
15. Hashimoto T, Lawton MT, Wen G, et al: Gene microarray analysis of human brain arteriovenous malformations, *Neurosurgery* 54:410-423, 2004.
16. Lee CZ, Xue Z, Zhu Y, et al: Matrix metalloproteinase-9 inhibition attenuates vascular endothelial growth factor-induced intracranial hemorrhage, *Stroke* 38:2563-2568, 2007.
17. Chen Y, Xu B, Arderiu G, et al: Retroviral delivery of homeobox d3 gene induces cerebral angiogenesis in mice, *J Cereb Blood Flow Metab* 24:1280-1287, 2004.
18. Zhu Y, Cuevas IC, Gabriel RA, et al: Restoring transcription factor HoxA5 expression inhibits the growth of experimental hemangiomas in the brain, *J Neuropathol Exp Neurol* 68:626-632, 2009.
19. Hashimoto T, Lam T, Boudreau NJ, et al: Abnormal balance in the angiopoietin-Tie2 system in human brain arteriovenous malformations, *Circ Res* 89:111-113, 2001.
20. Hashimoto T, Wen G, Lawton MT, et al: Abnormal expression of matrix metalloproteinases and tissue inhibitors of metalloproteinases in brain arteriovenous malformations, *Stroke* 34:925-931, 2003.
21. Chen Y, Fan Y, Poon KY, et al: MMP-9 expression is associated with leukocytic but not endothelial markers in brain arteriovenous malformations, *Front Biosci* 11:3121-3128, 2006.
22. Chen Y, Pawlikowska L, Yao JS, et al: Interleukin-6 involvement in brain arteriovenous malformations, *Ann Neurol* 59:72-80, 2006.
23. Chen Y, Zhu W, Bollen AW, et al: Evidence for inflammatory cell involvement in brain arteriovenous malformations, *Neurosurgery* 62:1340-1349, 2008.
24. Shenkar R, Shi C, Check IJ, et al: Concepts and hypotheses: Inflammatory hypothesis in the pathogenesis of cerebral cavernous malformations, *Neurosurgery* 61:693-702, 2007.
25. Hao Q, Liu J, Pappu R, et al: Contribution of bone marrow-derived cells associated with brain angiogenesis is primarily through leucocytes and macrophages, *Arterioscler Thromb Vasc Biol* 28:2151-2157, 2008.
26. Hao Q, Chen Y, Zhu Y, et al: Neutrophil depletion decreases VEGF-induced focal angiogenesis in the mature mouse brain, *J Cereb Blood Flow Metab* 27:1853-1860, 2007.
27. Ota R, Kurihara C, Tsou TL, et al: Roles of matrix metalloproteinases in flow-induced outward vascular remodeling, *J Cereb Blood Flow Metab* 29:1547-1558, 2009.
28. Nuki Y, Matsumoto MM, Tsang E, et al: Roles of macrophages in flow-induced outward vascular remodeling, *J Cereb Blood Flow Metab* 29:495-503, 2009.
29. ten Dijke P, Arthur HM: Extracellular control of TGFbeta signalling in vascular development and disease, *Nat Rev Mol Cell Biol* 8:857-869, 2007.
30. ten Dijke P, Goumans MJ, Pardali E: Endoglin in angiogenesis and vascular diseases, *Angiogenesis* 11:79-89, 2008.
31. Lebrin F, Mummery CL: Endoglin-mediated vascular remodeling: Mechanisms underlying hereditary hemorrhagic telangiectasia, *Trends Cardiovasc Med* 18:25-32, 2008.
32. Revencu N, Boon L, Vikkula M: Arteriovenous malformation in mice and men (Chapter 21). In Marmé D, Fusenig N, editors: *Tumor Angiogenesis, Part 2*, Berlin, 2008, Springer, pp 363-374.
33. Bernabeu C, Conley BA, Vary CP: Novel biochemical pathways of endoglin in vascular cell physiology, *J Cell Biochem* 102:1375-1388, 2007.
34. Marchuk DA, Srinivasan S, Squire TL, et al: Vascular morphogenesis: Tales of two syndromes, *Hum Mol Genet* 12:R97-R112, 2003.
35. Abdalla SA, Letarte M: Hereditary haemorrhagic telangiectasia: Current views on genetics and mechanisms of disease, *J Med Genet* 43:97-110, 2006.
36. Lux A, Attisano L, Marchuk DA: Assignment of transforming growth factor beta1 and beta3 and a third new ligand to the type I receptor ALK-1, *J Biol Chem* 274:9984-9992, 1999.
37. Scharpfenecker M, van Dinther M, Liu Z, et al: BMP-9 signals via ALK1 and inhibits bFGF-induced endothelial cell proliferation and VEGF-stimulated angiogenesis, *J Cell Sci* 120:964-972, 2007.
38. Barbara NP, Wrana JL, Letarte M: Endoglin is an accessory protein that interacts with the signaling receptor complex of multiple members of the transforming growth factor-beta superfamily, *J Biol Chem* 274:584-594, 1999.
39. David L, Mallet C, Mazerbourg S, et al: Identification of BMP9 and BMP10 as functional activators of the orphan activin receptor-like kinase 1 (ALK1) endothelial cells, *Blood* 109:1953-1961, 2007.

40. Urness LD, Sorensen LK, Li DY: Arteriovenous malformations in mice lacking activin receptor-like kinase-1, *Nat Genet* 26:328–331, 2000.

41. Park SO, Lee YJ, Seki T, et al: ALK5- and TGFBR2-independent role of ALK1 in the pathogenesis of hereditary hemorrhagic telangiectasia type 2 (HHT2), *Blood* 111:633–642, 2008.

42. Gallione CJ, Richards JA, Letteboer TG, et al: SMAD4 mutations found in unselected HHT patients, *J Med Genet* 43:793–797, 2006.

43. Bayrak-Toydemir P, McDonald J, Akarsu N, et al: A fourth locus for hereditary hemorrhagic telangiectasia maps to chromosome 7, *Am J Med Genet A* 140:2155–2162, 2006.

44. Cole SG, Begbie ME, Wallace GM, et al: A new locus for hereditary haemorrhagic telangiectasia (HHT3) maps to chromosome 5, *J Med Genet* 42:577–582, 2005.

45. Lamouille S, Mallet C, Feige JJ, et al: Activin receptor-like kinase 1 is implicated in the maturation phase of angiogenesis, *Blood* 100:4495–4501, 2002.

46. David L, Mallet C, Vailhe B, et al: Activin receptor-like kinase 1 inhibits human microvascular endothelial cell migration: Potential roles for JNK and ERK, *J Cell Physiol* 213:484–489, 2007.

47. Goumans MJ, Valdimarsdottir G, Itoh S, et al: Balancing the activation state of the endothelium via two distinct TGF-beta type I receptors, *EMBO J* 21:1743–1753, 2002.

48. Seki T, Yun J, Oh SP: Arterial endothelium-specific activin receptor-like kinase 1 expression suggests its role in arterialization and vascular remodeling, *Circ Res* 93:682–689, 2003.

49. Jonker L, Arthur HM: Endoglin expression in early development is associated with vasculogenesis and angiogenesis, *Mech Dev* 110:193–196, 2002.

49a. Abdalla SA, Pece-Barbara N, Vera S, et al: Analysis of ALK-1 and endoglin in newborns from families with hereditary hemorrhagic telangiectasia type 2, *Hum Mol Genet* 9(8):1227–1237, 2000.

49b. Cymerman U, Vera S, Pece-Barbara N, et al: Identification of hereditary hemorrhagic telangiectasia type 1 in newborns by protein expression and mutation analysis of endoglin, *Pediatr Res* 47:24–35, 2000.

50. Sanz-Rodriguez F, Fernandez LA, Zarrabeitia R, et al: Mutation analysis in Spanish patients with hereditary hemorrhagic telangiectasia: Deficient endoglin up-regulation in activated monocytes, *Clin Chem* 50:2003–2011, 2004.

51. van Laake LW, van den Driesche S, Post S, et al: Endoglin has a crucial role in blood cell-mediated vascular repair, *Circulation* 114:2288–2297, 2006.

52. Matsubara S, Bourdeau A, terBrugge KG, et al: Analysis of endoglin expression in normal brain tissue and in cerebral arteriovenous malformations, *Stroke* 31:2653–2660, 2000.

53. Chen GZ, Li TL, Quan W, et al: [Expression of TGFbeta1 and its type I receptors ALK1 and ALK5 mRNA in brain arteriovenous malformation], *Nan Fang Yi Ke Da Xue Xue Bao* 26:675–677, 2006.

54. Carvalho RL, Itoh F, Goumans MJ, et al: Compensatory signalling induced in the yolk sac vasculature by deletion of TGFbeta receptors in mice, *J Cell Sci* 120:4269–4277, 2007.

55. Yang LT, Li WY, Kaartinen V: Tissue-specific expression of Cre recombinase from the Tgfb3 locus, *Genesis* 46:112–118, 2008.

56. Toporsian M, Gros R, Kabir MG, et al: A role for endoglin in coupling eNOS activity and regulating vascular tone revealed in hereditary hemorrhagic telangiectasia, *Circ Res* 96:684–692, 2005.

56a. Toporsian M, Jerkic M, Zhou YQ, et al: Spontaneous adult-onset pulmonary arterial hypertension attributable to increased endothelial oxidative stress in a murine model of hereditary hemorrhagic telangiectasia, *Arterioscler Thromb Vasc Biol* 30:509–517, 2010.

57. Quick CM, Hashimoto T, Young WL: Lack of flow regulation may explain the development of arteriovenous malformations, *Neurol Res* 23:641–644, 2001.

58. Jerkic M, Rivas-Elena JV, Prieto M, et al: Endoglin regulates nitric oxide-dependent vasodilatation, *FASEB J* 18:609–611, 2004.

59. Belik J, Jerkic M, McIntyre BA, et al: Age-dependent endothelial nitric oxide synthase uncoupling in pulmonary arteries of endoglin heterozygous mice, *Am J Physiol Lung Cell Mol Physiol* 297:L1170–1178, 2009.

60. Venkatesha S, Toporsian M, Lam C, et al: Soluble endoglin contributes to the pathogenesis of preeclampsia, *Nat Med* 12:642–649, 2006.

61. Chen Y, Hao Q, Kim H, et al: Soluble endoglin modulates aberrant cerebral vascular remodeling, *Ann Neurol* 66:19–27, 2009.

62. Velasco S, Alvarez-Munoz P, Pericacho M, et al: L- and S-endoglin differentially modulate TGFbeta1 signaling mediated by ALK1 and ALK5 in L6E9 myoblasts, *J Cell Sci* 121:913–919, 2008.

63. Velasco-Loyden G, Arribas J, Lopez-Casillas F: The shedding of beta-glycan is regulated by pervanadate and mediated by membrane type matrix metalloprotease-1, *J Biol Chem* 279:7721–7733, 2004.

64. Hashimoto T, Matsumoto M, Li JF, et al: Suppression of MMP-9 by doxycycline in brain arteriovenous malformations, *BMC Neurol* 5:1, 2005.

65. Pawlikowska L, Tran MN, Achrol AS, et al: Polymorphisms in genes involved in inflammatory and angiogenic pathways and the risk of hemorrhagic presentation of brain arteriovenous malformations, *Stroke* 35:2294–2300, 2004.

66. Achrol AS, Pawlikowska L, McCulloch CE, et al: Tumor necrosis factor-alpha-238G>A promoter polymorphism is associated with increased risk of new hemorrhage in the natural course of patients with brain arteriovenous malformations, *Stroke* 37:231–234, 2006.

67. Kim H, Hysi PG, Pawlikowska L, et al: Common variants in interleukin-1-beta gene are associated with intracranial hemorrhage and susceptibility to brain arteriovenous malformation, *Cerebrovasc Dis* 27:176–182, 2009.

68. Cudmore M, Ahmad S, Al-Ani B, et al: Negative regulation of soluble Flt-1 and soluble endoglin release by heme oxygenase-1, *Circulation* 115:1789–1797, 2007.

69. Matsubara S, Mandzia JL, ter Brugge K, et al: Angiographic and clinical characteristics of patients with cerebral arteriovenous malformations associated with hereditary hemorrhagic telangiectasia, *AJNR Am J Neuroradiol* 21:1016–1020, 2000.

70. Maher CO, Piepgras DG, Brown RD Jr, et al: Cerebrovascular manifestations in 321 cases of hereditary hemorrhagic telangiectasia, *Stroke* 32:877–882, 2001.

71. Letteboer TG, Mager JJ, Snijder RJ, et al: Genotype-phenotype relationship in hereditary haemorrhagic telangiectasia, *J Med Genet* 43:371–377, 2006.

72. Bayrak-Toydemir P, McDonald J, Markewitz B, et al: Genotype-phenotype correlation in hereditary hemorrhagic telangiectasia: Mutations and manifestations, *Am J Med Genet A* 140:463–470, 2006.

73. Sabba C, Pasculli G, Lenato GM, et al: Hereditary hemorrhagic telangiectasia: Clinical features in ENG and ALK1 mutation carriers, *J Thromb Haemost* 5:1149–1157, 2007.

74. Mast H, Young WL, Koennecke HC, et al: Risk of spontaneous haemorrhage after diagnosis of cerebral arteriovenous malformation, *Lancet* 350:1065–1068, 1997.

75. Inoue S, Liu W, Inoue K, et al: Combination of linkage and association studies for brain arteriovenous malformation, *Stroke* 38:1368–1370, 2007.

76. van Beijnum J, van der Worp HB, Schippers HM, et al: Familial occurrence of brain arteriovenous malformations: A systematic review, *J Neurol Neurosurg Psychiatry* 78:1213–1217, 2007.

77. Risch N: Linkage strategies for genetically complex traits. I. Multilocus models, *Am J Hum Genet* 46:222–228, 1990.

78. Meschia JF, Brown RD Jr, Brott TG, et al: The Siblings With Ischemic Stroke Study (SWISS) protocol, *BMC Med Genet* 3:1, 2002.

79. Carter N, Williamson L, Kennedy LG, et al: Susceptibility to ankylosing spondylitis, *Rheumatology, (Oxford)*, 39:445, 2000.

80. Ritvo ER, Jorde LB, Mason-Brothers A, et al: The UCLA-University of Utah epidemiologic survey of autism: Recurrence risk estimates and genetic counseling, *Am J Psychiatry* 146:1032–1036, 1989.

81. Kim H, Marchuk DA, Pawlikowska L, et al: Genetic considerations relevant to intracranial hemorrhage and brain arteriovenous malformations, *Acta Neurochir* (Suppl) 105:199–206, 2008.

82. Rogers MS, D'Amato RJ: The effect of genetic diversity on angiogenesis, *Exp Cell Res* 312:561–574, 2006.

83. Shaked Y, Bertolini F, Man S, et al: Genetic heterogeneity of the vasculogenic phenotype parallels angiogenesis: Implications for cellular surrogate marker analysis of antiangiogenesis, *Cancer Cell* 7:101–111, 2005.

84. Pawlikowska L, Tran MN, Achrol AS, et al: Polymorphisms in transforming growth factor-β-related genes ALK1 and ENG are associated with sporadic brain arteriovenous malformations, *Stroke* 36:2278–2280, 2005.

85. Simon M, Franke D, Ludwig M, et al: Association of a polymorphism of the ACVRL1 gene with sporadic arteriovenous malformations of the central nervous system, *J Neurosurg* 104:945-949, 2006.

86. Simon M, Schramm J, Ludwig M, et al: Author reply to letter by Young WL, et al, "Arteriovenous malformation", *J Neurosurg* 106:732-733, 2007.

87. Cambier S, Gline S, Mu D, et al: Integrin alpha(v)beta8-mediated activation of transforming growth factor-beta by perivascular astrocytes: An angiogenic control switch, *Am J Pathol* 166:1883-1894, 2005.

88. Su H, Kim H, Pawlikowska L, et al: Reduced expression of integrin alphavbeta8 is associated with brain arteriovenous malformation pathogenesis, *Am J Pathol* 176:1018-1027, 2010.

89. Kim H, Hysi PG, Pawlikowska L, et al: Population stratification in a case-control study of brain arteriovenous malformation in Latinos, *Neuroepidemiology* 31:224-228, 2008.

90. Pawlikowska L, Poon KY, Achrol AS, et al: Apoliprotein E epsilon2 is associated with new hemorrhage risk in brain arteriovenous malformation, *Neurosurgery* 58:838-843, 2006.

91. Achrol AS, Kim H, Pawlikowska L, et al: Association of tumor necrosis factor-alpha-238G>A and apolipoprotein E2 polymorphisms with intracranial hemorrhage after brain arteriovenous malformation treatment, *Neurosurgery* 61:731-739, 2007.

92. Weinsheimer S, Kim H, Pawlikowska L, et al: EPHB4 gene polymorphisms and risk of intracranial hemorrhage in patients with brain arteriovenous malformations, *Circ Cardiovasc Genet* 2:476-482, 2009.

93. Woo D, Sauerbeck LR, Kissela BM, et al: Genetic and environmental risk factors for intracerebral hemorrhage: Preliminary results of a population-based study, *Stroke* 33:1190-1195, 2002.

94. O'Donnell HC, Rosand J, Knudsen KA, et al: Apolipoprotein E genotype and the risk of recurrent lobar intracerebral hemorrhage, *N Engl J Med* 342:240-245, 2000.

95. Langer DJ, Lasner TM, Hurst RW, et al: Hypertension, small size, and deep venous drainage are associated with risk of hemorrhagic presentation of cerebral arteriovenous malformations, *Neurosurgery* 42:481-486, 1998.

96. Frazer KA, Ballinger DG, Cox DR, et al: A second generation human haplotype map of over 3.1 million SNPs, *Nature* 449:851-861, 2007.

97. Schunkert H, Gotz A, Braund P, et al: Repeated replication and a prospective meta-analysis of the association between chromosome 9p21.3 and coronary artery disease, *Circulation* 117:1675-1684, 2008.

98. Kim H, Pawlikowska L, Weinsheimer S, et al: Genome-wide association study of intracranial hemorrhage in brain arteriovenous malformation (BAVM) patients [abstract], *Stroke* 41:e11, 2010:(P37).

99. Vikkula M, Boon LM, Carraway KL III, et al: Vascular dysmorphogenesis caused by an activating mutation in the receptor tyrosine kinase TIE2, *Cell* 87:1181-1190, 1996.

100. Calvert JT, Riney TJ, Kontos CD, et al: Allelic and locus heterogeneity in inherited venous malformations, *Hum Mol Genet* 8:1279-1289, 1999.

101. Brouillard P, Vikkula M: Genetic causes of vascular malformations, *Hum Mol Genet* 16(Spec No. 2):R140-R149, 2007.

102. Limaye N, Wouters V, Uebelhoer M, et al: Somatic mutations in angiopoietin receptor gene TEK cause solitary and multiple sporadic venous malformations, *Nat Genet* 41:118-124, 2009.

103. Akers AL, Johnson E, Steinberg GK, et al: Biallelic somatic and germline mutations in cerebral cavernous malformations (CCM): Evidence for a two-hit mechanism of CCM pathogenesis, *Hum Mol Genet* 18:919-930, 2009.

104. Happle R: Paradominant inheritance: A possible explanation for Becker's pigmented hairy nevus, *Eur J Dermatol* 2:39-40, 1992.

105. Happle R: Klippel-Trenaunay syndrome: Is it a paradominant trait? *Br J Dermatol* 128:465-466, 1993.

106. Spetzler RF, Wilson CB, Weinstein P, et al: Normal perfusion pressure breakthrough theory, *Clin Neurosurg* 25:651-672, 1978.

107. Scott BB, McGillicuddy JE, Seeger JF, et al: Vascular dynamics of an experimental cerebral arteriovenous shunt in the primate, *Surg Neurol* 10:34-38, 1978.

108. Bederson JB, Wiestler OD, Brustle O, et al: Intracranial venous hypertension and the effects of venous outflow obstruction in a rat model of arteriovenous fistula, *Neurosurgery* 29:341-350, 1991.

109. Chaloupka JC, Vinuela F, Robert J, et al: An in vivo arteriovenous malformation model in swine: Preliminary feasibility and natural history study, *AJNR Am J Neuroradiol* 15:945-950, 1994.

110. De Salles AAF, Solberg TD, Mischel P, et al: Arteriovenous malformation animal model for radiosurgery: The rete mirabile, *AJNR Am J Neuroradiol* 17:1451-1458, 1996.

111. Herman JM, Spetzler RF, Bederson JB, et al: Genesis of a dural arteriovenous malformation in a rat model, *J Neurosurg* 83:539-545, 1995.

112. Lawton MT, Jacobowitz R, Spetzler RF: Redefined role of angiogenesis in the pathogenesis of dural arteriovenous malformations, *J Neurosurg* 87:267-274, 1997.

113. Morgan MK, Anderson RE, Sundt TM Jr: A model of the pathophysiology of cerebral arteriovenous malformations by a carotid-jugular fistula in the rat, *Brain Res* 496:241-250, 1989.

114. Kutluk K, Schumacher M, Mironov A: The role of sinus thrombosis in occipital dural arteriovenous malformations—development and spontaneous closure, *Neurochirurgia (Stuttg)* 34:144-147, 1991.

115. Terada T, Higashida RT, Halbach VV, et al: Development of acquired arteriovenous fistulas in rats due to venous hypertension, *J Neurosurg* 80:884-889, 1994.

116. TerBrugge KG, Lasjaunias P, Hallacq P: Experimental models in interventional neuroradiology, *AJNR Am J Neuroradiol* 12:1029-1033, 1991.

117. Kailasnath P, Chaloupka JC: Mathematical modeling of AVM physiology using compartmental network analysis: Theoretical considerations and preliminary in vivo validation using a previously developed animal model, *Neurol Res* 18:361-366, 1996.

118. Massoud TF, Ji C, Vinuela F, et al: Laboratory simulations and training in endovascular embolotherapy with a swine arteriovenous malformation model, *AJNR Am J Neuroradiol* 17:271-279, 1996.

119. Massoud TF, Ji C, Vinuela F, et al: An experimental arteriovenous malformation model in swine: Anatomic basis and construction technique, *AJNR Am J Neuroradiol* 15:1537-1545, 1994.

120. Morgan MK, Anderson RE, Sundt TM Jr: The effects of hyperventilation on cerebral blood flow in the rat with an open and closed carotid-jugular fistula, *Neurosurgery* 25:606-611, 1989.

121. Murayama Y, Massoud TF, Vinuela F: Hemodynamic changes in arterial feeders and draining veins during embolotherapy of arteriovenous malformations: An experimental study in a swine model, *Neurosurgery* 43:96-104, 1998.

122. Nagasawa S, Kawanishi M, Kondoh S, et al: Hemodynamic simulation study of cerebral arteriovenous malformations. Part 2. Effects of impaired autoregulation and induced hypotension, *J Cereb Blood Flow Metab* 16:162-169, 1996.

123. Pietila TA, Zabramski JM, Thellier-Janko A, et al: Animal model for cerebral arteriovenous malformation, *Acta Neurochir (Wien)* 142:1231-1240, 2000.

124. Tu J, Karunanayaka A, Windsor A, et al: Comparison of an animal model of arteriovenous malformation with human arteriovenous malformation, *J Clin Neurosci* 17:96-102, 2010.

125. Young WL, Kader A, Ornstein E, et al: Cerebral hyperemia after arteriovenous malformation resection is related to "breakthrough" complications but not to feeding artery pressure. Columbia University AVM Study Project, *Neurosurgery* 38:1085-1093, 1996.

126. Massoud TF, Vinters HV, Chao KH, et al: Histopathologic characteristics of a chronic arteriovenous malformation in a swine model: preliminary study, *AJNR Am J Neuroradiol* 21:1268-1276, 2000.

127. Torsney E, Charlton R, Diamond AG, et al: Mouse model for hereditary hemorrhagic telangiectasia has a generalized vascular abnormality, *Circulation* 107:1653-1657, 2003.

128. Srinivasan S, Hanes MA, Dickens T, et al: A mouse model for hereditary hemorrhagic telangiectasia (HHT) type 2, *Hum Mol Genet* 12:473-482, 2003.

129. Satomi J, Mount RJ, Toporsian M, et al: Cerebral vascular abnormalities in a murine model of hereditary hemorrhagic telangiectasia, *Stroke* 34:783-789, 2003.

130. Park SO, Wankhede M, Lee YJ, et al: Real-time imaging of de novo arteriovenous malformation in a mouse model of hereditary hemorrhagic telangiectasia, *J Clin Invest* 119:3487-3496, 2009.

131. Walker E, Shen F, Halprin R, et al: Regional deletion of Smad4 plus VEGF stimulation leads to vascular dysplasia in the adult mouse brain [abstract], *Stroke* 41:e20, 2010:(#68).

132. Xu B, Wu YQ, Huey M, et al: Vascular endothelial growth factor induces abnormal microvasculature in the endoglin heterozygous mouse brain, *J Cereb Blood Flow Metab* 24:237-244, 2004.

133. Hao Q, Su H, Marchuk DA, et al: Increased tissue perfusion promotes capillary dysplasia in the ALK1-deficient mouse brain following VEGF stimulation, *Am J Physiol Heart Circ Physiol* 295:H2250-H2256, 2008.

134. McCormick WF: Pathology of vascular malformations of the brain. In Wilson CB, Stein BM, editors: *Intracranial Arteriovenous Malformations*, Baltimore, 1984, Williams & Wilkins, pp 44-63.

135. Attia W, Tada T, Hongo K, et al: Microvascular pathological features of immediate perinidal parenchyma in cerebral arteriovenous malformations: giant bed capillaries, *J Neurosurg* 98:823-827, 2003.

136. Sato S, Kodama N, Sasaki T, et al: Perinidal dilated capillary networks in cerebral arteriovenous malformations, *Neurosurgery* 54:163-168, 2004.

137. Zhang G, Zhou J, Fan Q, et al: Arterial-venous endothelial cell fate is related to vascular endothelial growth factor and Notch status during human bone mesenchymal stem cell differentiation, *FEBS Lett* 582:2957-2964, 2008.

138. Benedito R, Roca C, Sorensen I, et al: The notch ligands Dll4 and Jagged1 have opposing effects on angiogenesis, *Cell* 137:1124-1135, 2009.

139. ZhuGe Q, Zhong M, Zheng W, et al: Notch1 signaling is activated in brain arteriovenous malformation in humans, *Brain* 132:3231-3241, 2009.

140. Murphy PA, Lu G, Shiah S, et al: Endothelial Notch signaling is upregulated in human brain arteriovenous malformations and a mouse model of the disease, *Lab Invest* 89:971-982, 2009.

141. Murphy PA, Lam MT, Wu X, et al: Endothelial Notch4 signaling induces hallmarks of brain arteriovenous malformations in mice, *Proc Natl Acad Sci U S A* 105:10901-10906, 2008.

142. Lee CZ, Xu B, Hashimoto T, et al: Doxycycline suppresses cerebral matrix metalloproteinase-9 and angiogenesis induced by focal hyperstimulation of vascular endothelial growth factor in a mouse model, *Stroke* 35:1715-1719, 2004.

143. Lee CZ, Yao JS, Huang Y, et al: Dose-response effect of tetracyclines on cerebral matrix metalloproteinase-9 after vascular endothelial growth factor hyperstimulation, *J Cereb Blood Flow Metab* 26:1157-1164, 2006.

144. Niimi H, Pardali K, Vanlandewijck M, et al: Notch signaling is necessary for epithelial growth arrest by TGF-beta, *J Cell Biol* 176:695-707, 2007.

145. Wang X, Mao X, Xie L, et al: Involvement of Notch1 signaling in neurogenesis in the subventricular zone of normal and ischemic rat brain in vivo, *J Cereb Blood Flow Metab* 29:1644-1654, 2009.

146. Chaudhary MY, Sachdev VP, Cho SH, et al: Dural arteriovenous malformation of the major venous sinuses: An acquired lesion, *AJNR Am J Neuroradiol* 3:13-19, 1982.

147. Nabors MW, Azzam CJ, Albanna FJ, et al: Delayed postoperative dural arteriovenous malformations. Report of two cases, *J Neurosurg* 66:768-772, 1987.

148. Brown RD Jr, Flemming KD, Meyer FB, et al: Natural history, evaluation, and management of intracranial vascular malformations, *Mayo Clin Proc* 80:269-281, 2005.

149. Hashimoto T, Wu Y, Lawton MT, et al: Co-expression of angiogenic factors in brain arteriovenous malformations, *Neurosurgery* 56:1058-1065, 2005.

150. Zhu Y, Lawton MT, Du R, et al: Expression of hypoxia-inducible factor-1 and vascular endothelial growth factor in response to venous hypertension, *Neurosurgery* 59:687-696, 2006.

151. Gao P, Zhu Y, Ling F, et al: Nonischemic cerebral venous hypertension promotes a pro-angiogenic state through HIF-1 downstream genes and leukocyte-derived MMP-9, *J Cereb Blood Flow Metab* 29:1482-1490, 2009.

152. Young WL: Intracranial arteriovenous malformations: Pathophysiology and hemodynamics (Chapter 6). In Jafar JJ, Awad IA, Rosenwasser RH, editors: *Vascular Malformations of the Central Nervous System*, New York, 1999, Lippincott Williams & Wilkins, pp 95-126.

153. Frenzel T, Lee CZ, Kim H, et al: Feasibility of minocycline and doxycycline use as potential vasculostatic therapy for brain vascular malformations: Pilot study of adverse events and tolerance, *Cerebrovasc Dis* 25:157-161, 2008.

154. Singh V, Smith WS, Lawton MT, et al: Thrombophilic mutation as a new high-risk feature in DAVF patients [abstract], *Ann Neurol* 60:S30, 2006.

154a. Safavi-Abbasi S, Di Rocco F, Nakaji P, et al: Thrombophilia due to factor V and factor II mutations and formation of a dural arteriovenous fistula: Case report and review of a rare entity, *Skull Base* 18(2):135-143, 2008.

155. Clatterbuck RE, Eberhart CG, Crain BJ, et al: Ultrastructural and immunocytochemical evidence that an incompetent blood-brain barrier is related to the pathophysiology of cavernous malformations, *J Neurol Neurosurg Psychiatry* 71:188-192, 2001.

156. Otten P, Pizzolato GP, Rilliet B, et al: [131 cases of cavernous angioma (cavernomas) of the CNS, discovered by retrospective analysis of 24,535 autopsies], *Neurochirurgie* 35:82-83, 128-131, 1989.

157. Rigamonti D, Hadley MN, Drayer BP, et al: Cerebral cavernous malformations. Incidence and familial occurrence, *N Engl J Med* 319:343-347, 1988.

158. Labauge P, Laberge S, Brunereau L, et al: Hereditary cerebral cavernous angiomas: Clinical and genetic features in 57 French families. Societe Francaise de Neurochirurgie, *Lancet* 352:1892-1897, 1998.

159. Labauge P, Brunereau L, Laberge S, et al: Prospective follow-up of 33 asymptomatic patients with familial cerebral cavernous malformations, *Neurology* 57:1825-1828, 2001.

160. Denier C, Labauge P, Bergametti F, et al: Genotype-phenotype correlations in cerebral cavernous malformations patients, *Ann Neurol* 60:550-556, 2006.

161. Pozzati E, Acciarri N, Tognetti F, et al: Growth, subsequent bleeding, and de novo appearance of cerebral cavernous angiomas, *Neurosurgery* 38:662-669, 1996.

162. Maiuri F, Cappabianca P, Gangemi M, et al: Clinical progression and familial occurrence of cerebral cavernous angiomas: The role of angiogenic and growth factors, *Neurosurg Focus* 21:e3, 2006.

163. Denier C, Labauge P, Brunereau L, et al: Clinical features of cerebral cavernous malformations patients with KRIT1 mutations, *Ann Neurol* 55:213-220, 2004.

164. Dubovsky J, Zabramski JM, Kurth J, et al: A gene responsible for cavernous malformations of the brain maps to chromosome 7q, *Hum Mol Genet* 4:453-458, 1995.

165. Gunel M, Awad IA, Anson J, et al: Mapping a gene causing cerebral cavernous malformation to 7q11.2-q21, *Proc Natl Acad Sci U S A* 92:6620-6624, 1995.

166. Marchuk DA, Gallione CJ, Morrison LA, et al: A locus for cerebral cavernous malformations maps to chromosome 7q in two families, *Genomics* 28:311-314, 1995.

167. Johnson EW, Iyer LM, Rich SS, et al: Refined localization of the cerebral cavernous malformation gene (CCM1) to a 4-cM interval of chromosome 7q contained in a well-defined YAC contig, *Genome Res* 5:368-380, 1995.

168. Gunel M, Awad IA, Finberg K, et al: A founder mutation as a cause of cerebral cavernous malformation in Hispanic Americans, *N Engl J Med* 334:946-951, 1996.

169. Laberge S, Labauge P, Marechal E, et al: Genetic heterogeneity and absence of founder effect in a series of 36 French cerebral cavernous angiomas families, *Eur J Hum Genet* 7:499-504, 1999.

170. Craig HD, Gunel M, Cepeda O, et al: Multilocus linkage identifies two new loci for a mendelian form of stroke, cerebral cavernous malformation, at 7p15-13 and 3q25.2-27, *Hum Mol Genet* 7:1851-1858, 1998.

171. Liquori CL, Berg MJ, Siegel AM, et al: Mutations in a gene encoding a novel protein containing a phosphotyrosine-binding domain cause type 2 cerebral cavernous malformations, *Am J Hum Genet* 73:1459-1464, 2003.

172. Denier C, Goutagny S, Labauge P, et al: Mutations within the MGC4607 gene cause cerebral cavernous malformations, *Am J Hum Genet* 74:326-337, 2004.

173. Bergametti F, Denier C, Labauge P, et al: Mutations within the programmed cell death 10 gene cause cerebral cavernous malformations, *Am J Hum Genet* 76:42-51, 2005.

174. Revencu N, Vikkula M: Cerebral cavernous malformation: New molecular and clinical insights, *J Med Genet* 43:716-721, 2006.

175. Sahoo T, Goenaga-Diaz E, Serebriiskii IG, et al: Computational and experimental analyses reveal previously undetected coding exons of the KRIT1 (CCM1) gene, *Genomics* 71:123-126, 2001.

176. Sahoo T, Johnson EW, Thomas JW, et al: Mutations in the gene encoding KRIT1, a Krev-1/rap1a binding protein, cause cerebral cavernous malformations (CCM1), *Hum Mol Genet* 8:2325-2333, 1999.

177. Zhang J, Clatterbuck RE, Rigamonti D, et al: Mutations in KRIT1 in familial cerebral cavernous malformations, *Neurosurgery* 46:1272-1277, 2000.

178. Eerola I, McIntyre B, Vikkula M: Identification of eight novel 5'-exons in cerebral capillary malformation gene-1 (CCM1) encoding KRIT1, *Biochim Biophys Acta* 1517:464-467, 2001.

179. Zhang J, Clatterbuck RE, Rigamonti D, et al: Cloning of the murine Krit1 cDNA reveals novel mammalian 5' coding exons, *Genomics* 70:392-395, 2000.

180. Serebriiskii I, Estojak J, Sonoda G, et al: Association of Krev-1/rap1a with Krit1, a novel ankyrin repeat-containing protein encoded by a gene mapping to 7q21-22, *Oncogene* 15:1043-1049, 1997.

181. Kitayama H, Sugimoto Y, Matsuzaki T, et al: A ras-related gene with transformation suppressor activity, *Cell* 56:77-84, 1989.

182. Glading A, Han J, Stockton RA, et al: KRIT-1/CCM1 is a Rap1 effector that regulates endothelial cell cell junctions, *J Cell Biol* 179:247-254, 2007.

183. Glading AJ, Ginsberg MH: Rap1 and its effector KRIT1/CCM1 regulate beta-catenin signaling, *Dis Model Mech* 3:73-83, 2010.

184. Zhang J, Clatterbuck RE, Rigamonti D, et al: Interaction between krit1 and ICAP1alpha infers perturbation of integrin beta1-mediated angiogenesis in the pathogenesis of cerebral cavernous malformation, *Hum Mol Genet* 10:2953-2960, 2001.

185. Zawistowski JS, Serebriiskii IG, Lee MF, et al: KRIT1 association with the integrin-binding protein ICAP-1: A new direction in the elucidation of cerebral cavernous malformations (CCM1) pathogenesis, *Hum Mol Genet* 11:389-396, 2002.

186. Denier C, Gasc JM, Chapon F, et al: Krit1/cerebral cavernous malformation 1 mRNA is preferentially expressed in neurons and epithelial cells in embryo and adult, *Mech Dev* 117:363-367, 2002.

187. Guzeloglu-Kayisli O, Amankulor NM, Voorhees J, et al: KRIT1/cerebral cavernous malformation 1 protein localizes to vascular endothelium, astrocytes, and pyramidal cells of the adult human cerebral cortex, *Neurosurgery* 54:943-949, 2004:discussion 949.

188. Guzeloglu-Kayisli O, Kayisli UA, Amankulor NM, et al: Krev1 interaction trapped-1/cerebral cavernous malformation-1 protein expression during early angiogenesis, *J Neurosurg* 100:481-487, 2004.

189. Whitehead KJ, Plummer NW, Adams JA, et al: *Ccm1* is required for arterial morphogenesis: Implications for the etiology of human cavernous malformations, *Development* 131:1437-1448, 2004.

190. Whitehead KJ, Chan AC, Navankasattusas S, et al: The cerebral cavernous malformation signaling pathway promotes vascular integrity via Rho GTPases, *Nat Med* 15:177-184, 2009.

191. Boulday G, Blecon A, Petit N, et al: Tissue-specific conditional CCM2 knockout mice establish the essential role of endothelial CCM2 in angiogenesis: Implications for human cerebral cavernous malformations, *Dis Model Mech* 2:168-177, 2009.

192. Kleaveland B, Zheng X, Liu JJ, et al: Regulation of cardiovascular development and integrity by the heart of glass-cerebral cavernous malformation protein pathway, *Nat Med* 15:169-176, 2009.

193. Plummer NW, Squire TL, Srinivasan S, et al: Neuronal expression of the Ccm2 gene in a new mouse model of cerebral cavernous malformations, *Mamm Genome* 17:119-128, 2006.

194. Mably JD, Chuang LP, Serluca FC, et al: *santa* and *valentine* pattern concentric growth of cardiac myocardium in the zebrafish, *Development* 133:3139-3146, 2006.

195. Crose LE, Hilder TL, Sciaky N, et al: Cerebral cavernous malformation 2 protein promotes smad ubiquitin regulatory factor 1-mediated RhoA degradation in endothelial cells, *J Biol Chem* 284:13301-13305, 2009.

196. Harel L, Costa B, Tcherpakov M, et al: CCM2 mediates death signaling by the TrkA receptor tyrosine kinase, *Neuron* 63:585-591, 2009.

197. Zawistowski JS, Stalheim L, Uhlik MT, et al: CCM1 and CCM2 protein interactions in cell signaling: Implications for cerebral cavernous malformations pathogenesis, *Hum Mol Genet* 14:2521-2531, 2005.

198. Adams RH, Porras A, Alonso G, et al: Essential role of p38alpha MAP kinase in placental but not embryonic cardiovascular development, *Mol Cell* 6:109-116, 2000.

199. Yang J, Boerm M, McCarty M, et al: Mekk3 is essential for early embryonic cardiovascular development, *Nat Genet* 24:309-313, 2000.

200. Stahl S, Gaetzner S, Voss K, et al: Novel CCM1, CCM2, and CCM3 mutations in patients with cerebral cavernous malformations: Inframe deletion in CCM2 prevents formation of a CCM1/CCM2/CCM3 protein complex, *Hum Mutat* 29:709-717, 2008.

201. Wang H, Chen H, Xia N, et al: cDNA cloning and sequence analysis of hepatitis G virus genome isolated from a Chinese blood donor, *Chin Med J (Engl)* 112:747-749, 1999.

202. Chen L, Tanriover G, Yano H, et al: Apoptotic functions of PDCD10/CCM3, the gene mutated in cerebral cavernous malformation 3, *Stroke* 40:1474-1481, 2009.

203. Petit N, Blecon A, Denier C, et al: Patterns of expression of the three cerebral cavernous malformation (CCM) genes during embryonic and postnatal brain development, *Gene Expr Patterns* 6:495-503, 2006.

204. Tanriover G, Boylan AJ, Diluna ML, et al: PDCD10, the gene mutated in cerebral cavernous malformation 3, is expressed in the neurovascular unit, *Neurosurgery* 62:930-938, 2008:discussion 938.

205. Voss K, Stahl S, Schleider E, et al: CCM3 interacts with CCM2 indicating common pathogenesis for cerebral cavernous malformations, *Neurogenetics* 8:249-256, 2007.

206. Gault J, Shenkar R, Recksiek P, et al: Biallelic somatic and germ line CCM1 truncating mutations in a cerebral cavernous malformation lesion, *Stroke* 36:872-874, 2005.

207. Kehrer-Sawatzki H, Wilda M, Braun VM, et al: Mutation and expression analysis of the KRIT1 gene associated with cerebral cavernous malformations (CCM1), *Acta Neuropathol* 104:231-240, 2002.

208. Lucas M, Costa AF, Montori M, et al: Germline mutations in the CCM1 gene, encoding Krit1, cause cerebral cavernous malformations, *Ann Neurol* 49:529-532, 2001.

209. Marini V, Ferrera L, Pigatto F, et al: Search for loss of heterozygosity and mutation analysis of KRIT1 gene in CCM patients, *Am J Med Genet A* 130A:98-101, 2004.

210. Cave-Riant F, Denier C, Labauge P, et al: Spectrum and expression analysis of KRIT1 mutations in 121 consecutive and unrelated patients with cerebral cavernous malformations, *Eur J Hum Genet* 10:733-740, 2002.

211. Plummer NW, Gallione CJ, Srinivasan S, et al: Loss of p53 sensitizes mice with a mutation in Ccm1 (KRIT1) to development of cerebral vascular malformations, *Am J Pathol* 165:1509-1518, 2004.

212. Shenkar R, Venkatasubramanian PN, Wyrwicz AM, et al: Advanced magnetic resonance imaging of cerebral cavernous malformations: part II. Imaging of lesions in murine models, *Neurosurgery* 63:790-797, 2008:discussion 797-798.

213. Pagenstecher A, Stahl S, Sure U, et al: A two-hit mechanism causes cerebral cavernous malformations: Complete inactivation of CCM1, CCM2 or CCM3 in affected endothelial cells, *Hum Mol Genet* 18:911-918, 2009.

214. Detwiler PW, Porter RW, Zabramski JM, et al: Radiation-induced cavernous malformation, *J Neurosurg* 89:167-169, 1998.

215. Heckl S, Aschoff A, Kunze S: Radiation-induced cavernous hemangiomas of the brain: A late effect predominantly in children, *Cancer* 94:3285-3291, 2002.

216. Larson JJ, Ball WS, Bove KE, et al: Formation of intracerebral cavernous malformations after radiation treatment for central nervous system neoplasia in children, *J Neurosurg* 88:51-56, 1998.

217. Shi C, Shenkar R, Batjer HH, et al: Oligoclonal immune response in cerebral cavernous malformations. Laboratory investigation, *J Neurosurg* 107:1023-1026, 2007.

218. Shenkar R, Elliott JP, Diener K, et al: Differential gene expression in human cerebrovascular malformations, *Neurosurgery* 52:465-478, 2003.

219. Jung KH, Chu K, Jeong SW, et al: Cerebral cavernous malformations with dynamic and progressive course: Correlation study with vascular endothelial growth factor, *Arch Neurol* 60:1613-1618, 2003.

220. Labauge P, Denier C, Bergametti F, et al: Genetics of cavernous angiomas, *Lancet Neurol* 6:237-244, 2007.

221. Gault J, Sain S, Hu LJ, et al: Spectrum of genotype and clinical manifestations in cerebral cavernous malformations, *Neurosurgery* 59:1278-1284, 2006:discussion 1284-1285.

222. Sirvente J, Enjolras O, Wassef M, et al: Frequency and phenotypes of cutaneous vascular malformations in a consecutive series of 417 patients with familial cerebral cavernous malformations, *J Eur Acad Dermatol Venereol* 23:1066-1072, 2009.

223. Eerola I, Plate KH, Spiegel R, et al: KRIT1 is mutated in hyperkeratotic cutaneous capillary-venous malformation associated with cerebral capillary malformation, *Hum Mol Genet* 9:1351-1355, 2000.

224. Labauge P, Krivosic V, Denier C, et al: Frequency of retinal cavernomas in 60 patients with familial cerebral cavernomas: A clinical and genetic study, *Arch Ophthalmol* 124:885-886, 2006.

225. Eerola I, Boon LM, Mulliken JB, et al: Capillary malformation-arteriovenous malformation, a new clinical and genetic disorder caused by RASA1 mutations, *Am J Hum Genet* 73:1240-1249, 2003.

226. Revencu N, Boon LM, Mulliken JB, et al: Parkes Weber syndrome, vein of Galen aneurysmal malformation, and other fast-flow vascular anomalies are caused by RASA1 mutations, *Hum Mutat* 29:959-965, 2008.

227. Henkemeyer M, Rossi DJ, Holmyard DP, et al: Vascular system defects and neuronal apoptosis in mice lacking ras GTPase-activating protein, *Nature* 377:695-701, 1995.

228. Thiex R, Mulliken JB, Revencu N, et al: A novel association between RASA1 mutations and spinal arteriovenous anomalies, *AJNR Am J Neuroradiol* 31:775-779, 2010.

229. Wouters V, Limaye N, Uebelhoer M, et al: Hereditary cutaneomucosal venous malformations are caused by TIE2 mutations with widely variable hyper-phosphorylating effects, *Eur J Hum Genet* 18:414-420, 2010.

230. Singh V, Smith WS, Lawton MT, et al: Risk factors for hemorrhagic presentation in patients with dural arteriovenous fistulae, *Neurosurgery* 62:628-635, 2008:discussion 628-635.

231. Houser OW, Campbell JK, Campbell RJ, et al: Arteriovenous malformation affecting the transverse dural venous sinus—an acquired lesion, *Mayo Clin Proc* 54:651-661, 1979.

232. van Dijk JM, TerBrugge KG, Van der Meer FJ, et al: Thrombophilic factors and the formation of dural arteriovenous fistulas, *J Neurosurg* 107:56-59, 2007.

233. Gerlach R, Yahya H, Rohde S, et al: Increased incidence of thrombophilic abnormalities in patients with cranial dural arteriovenous fistulae, *Neurol Res* 25:745-748, 2003.

234. Kraus JA, Stuper BK, Muller J, et al: Molecular analysis of thrombophilic risk factors in patients with dural arteriovenous fistulas, *J Neurol* 249:680-682, 2002.

235. Singh V, Meyers PM, Halbach VH, et al: Dural arteriovenous fistula associated with prothrombin gene mutation, *J Neuroimaging* 11:319-321, 2001.

236. Yang GY, Xu B, Hashimoto T, et al: Induction of focal angiogenesis through adenoviral vector mediated vascular endothelial cell growth factor gene transfer in the mature mouse brain, *Angiogenesis* 6:151-158, 2003.

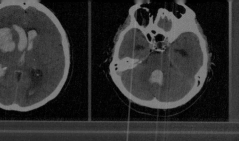

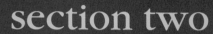

section two

Epidemiology and Prevention

PHILIP A. WOLF

In this edition, the epidemiology and prevention section has been expanded to provide comprehensive examination of stroke distribution according to age, race, and sex (Chapter 13); an overview of precursors and incidence of stroke (Chapter 14); outcomes following stroke (Chapter 15); current status of primary prevention of stroke (Chapter 16); the role of cerebrovascular disease and stroke in vascular dementia and vascular cognitive decline (Chapter 17); the current status of the role of genetics in stroke occurrence (Chapter 18); and a global perspective on the worldwide impact of stroke (Chapter 19). Expansion of the epidemiology and prevention section in this fifth edition reflects the increase in understanding and knowledge of the extent and distribution of stroke in populations as well as the factors predisposing to stroke occurrence and outcomes. Inclusion of a section on genetics recognizes the increasing appreciation of the role that genetic factors contribute to stroke, vascular dementia, and vascular cognitive decline. The increasing lifespan of much of the world's population will likely lead to increasing public health and financial burdens resulting from stroke and other consequences of cerebrovascular diseases, which will require strategies for prevention and management.

13

Distribution of Stroke: Heterogeneity by Age, Race, and Sex

VIRGINIA J. HOWARD, GEORGE HOWARD

Indices of Stroke Heterogeneity

Mortality, incidence, and *prevalence* are all indices that can be used to describe differences in the distribution or "risk" of stroke among selected populations. Each of these indices provides information that is of particular value to clinical or public health decision makers in addressing the burden of stroke. The use of an inappropriate index, however, can lead to inappropriate conclusions and decisions. There are also striking differences among these indices in the quantity and quality of the data available. For all of these reasons, the definitions and properties of these indices should be considered.

Stroke mortality reflects deaths from stroke. In the United States, the source of data underlying estimates of stroke mortality rates is the vital statistics system maintained by the National Center for Health Statistics.[1] The vital statistics system requires the reporting of all death events, with information on the "underlying" (primary) and "contributing" (secondary) causes as well as demographic descriptors such as age, sex, and ethnicity. The causes of death are locally coded, generally by nonphysicians, with the use of the codes in the World Health Organization's International Classification of Diseases (ICD).[2] The ICD codes have evolved over the years, and revision 10 is currently employed.

The *stroke mortality rate* is calculated by dividing the number of stroke deaths (with stroke coded as the underlying cause) occurring over a fixed time (normally a year) by the estimated population at risk. Intercensus estimates are obtained by adjustment of the census counts conducted each decade by regional reports of deaths and births (also part of the vital statistics reporting system). The major strength of stroke mortality rates as an index of the burden of stroke is the mandatory reporting of deaths. Because of this, estimates of stroke mortality rates can be made at the national level as well as for specific regions (e.g., county level) and for specific race or sex groups.

There are, however, shortcomings in the use of stroke mortality rates as an index of the burden of stroke. Among them is the inability to reliably report stroke death rates by stroke subtype, even at the level of distinguishing rates of death from infarction versus hemorrhage. The lack of detailed coding of causes of death requires estimates of the stroke mortality rates to be provided only for "all stroke." Specifically, Fig. 13-1*A* shows the distribution of

subtypes of 143,579 reported stroke deaths during 2005.[3] These data are striking in that 74,416 (52%) were reported "stroke, not specified as hemorrhage or infarction (ICD-10: I64)." In addition, deaths from "other cerebrovascular diseases (I67)" and "sequelae of cerebrovascular disease (I69)" likely include many stroke deaths, but these codes have been shown to not be as specific as other ICD codes.[4] The ICD system also provides for coding cause of death by detailed categories within the major stroke subtypes. On the surface, this coding potentially provides the possibility of distinguishing cerebral infarctions attributable to "thrombosis of cerebral arteries (I63.3)" from those attributable to "embolism of cerebral arteries (I63.4)." However, lack of coding detail also makes this distinction problematic, as within the 7563 deaths during 2005 from "cerebral infarction (I63)," Fig. 13-1*B* shows that 4564 (61%) of these deaths were reported only as "cerebral infarction, unspecified (I63.9)." For all of these reasons, the use of mortality rates generally must be limited to "all stroke" comparisons.

Decision makers must also be careful not to assume that differences among stroke mortality rates are attributable to differences in the number of stroke events, that is, incidence. Stroke mortality rates are a product of the stroke incidence and stroke case-fatality rates, and differences can be introduced from either of these sources. For example, many individuals considered the substantial 60% drop in stroke mortality occurring over the past decades to be largely attributable to a declining number of stroke events. Because recent reports suggest that a substantial component of the declining mortality rate is attributable to reductions in case-fatality rates rather than the number of incident events,[5-8] clinical and public health decisions made on this assumption may be ineffective. Hence, because the emphasis of decisions is frequently on reducing the number of stroke events in a population, the use of stroke mortality rates can potentially mislead decisions by providing an index that is a function of both the number of strokes occurring and the likelihood of dying of a stroke event.

The shortcomings of stroke mortality as an index of the distribution of disease are directly addressed by the use of the stroke incidence rate. The *stroke incidence rate* is defined as the number of new stroke events per population occurring over a fixed time (normally a year). Unfortunately, there are also

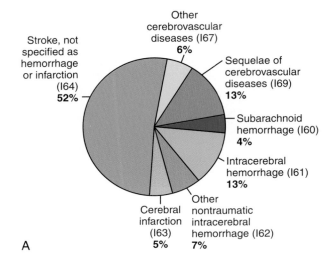

A

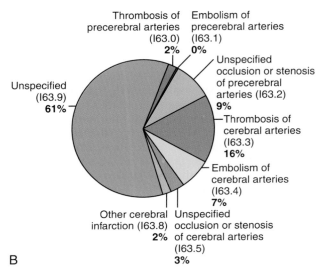

B

Figure 13-1 A, Stroke subtype by International Classification of Diseases-10 (ICD-10) code (in parentheses) for the 143,579 stroke deaths reported for 2005. B, Detailed stroke subtype by ICD-10 code (in parentheses) for the 7563 cerebral infarction deaths during 2005. (From the National Center for Health Statistics, Data Warehouse: Total deaths for each cause by 5-year age groups, United States, 2005: www.cdc.gov/nchs/datawh/statab/unpubd/mortabs/gmwki10.htm. Accessed February 28, 2009.)

shortcomings in the use of this index. Most important is that, unlike for cancer and selected sexually transmitted diseases, there is no required registry of stroke events. Without such a registry, no national data are available to describe the number of incident stroke events.[9] Current information on stroke incidence rates are based on (1) clinical reports in populations with tightly controlled referral patterns, most notably the Rochester Epidemiological Project (REP) in Olmsted County, Minnesota[10]; (2) funded stroke surveillance projects that capture admissions to medical facilities for a fixed geographic region, such as the Greater Cincinnati/Northern Kentucky stroke project (GCNKSS),[8] the Brain Attack Surveillance In Corpus Christi (BASIC) project,[11] the

Northern Manhattan Stroke Study (NOMASS),[12] and the Atherosclerosis Risk in Communities (ARIC) surveillance program[13]; or (3) large longitudinal epidemiologic cohort studies, such as the Framingham Study,[7] the Cardiovascular Health Study (CHS),[14] the ARIC cohort study,[15] the Strong Heart Study,[16] and the REasons for Geographic and Racial Differences in Stroke (REGARDS) study.[17] In general, both surveillance and cohort studies provide stroke incidence data for specific geographic regions, but many of the regions are in northern cities with predominantly white residents (e.g., Framingham, Massachusetts and Rochester, Minnesota). The first shortcoming of incidence data is in the assumptions required to generalize results from specific geographic and racial populations to provide either a national picture or a comparison of the disease burden between groups, such as between black people and white people. A second shortcoming is that the use of diagnostic technologies over time may differentially identify milder cases of stroke that previously would have been missed, raising the incidence rates (by adding to the numerator) while the case-fatality rate will be decreased because patients with mild strokes would tend to survive. A recent report from the GCNKSS, however, suggests that the advent of neuroimaging may actually exclude more suspected strokes rather than identify new mild strokes.[18] Regardless, changing technology is certainly a complicating factor in the interpretation of temporal changes in incidence. Although the potential effect of differential diagnostic evaluations will be most pronounced in examination of temporal patterns, one can also argue that populations with relatively lower average socioeconomic status, such as black people and persons in isolated or rural communities, may have been less likely to have had access to these newer technologies. Such a difference would introduce a bias toward reducing the magnitude of the differences in incidence and magnifying the differences in case-fatality rate in any contrast of black people versus white people or comparisons of residents from isolated or rural communities with residents from the rest of the nation.

Stroke is one of the leading causes of disability in the United States,[19] and survivors of stroke events carry this burden. The *prevalence of stroke* is defined as the proportion of the population that has survived a stroke. *Prevalence* is a proportion at a fixed point in time, which distinguishes it from incidence and mortality, which are rates (number of events per population per unit of time). Although the concept is initially counterintuitive, increases in stroke prevalence are not necessarily associated with poor health outcomes. Stroke prevalence can increase not only because of the "negative" effect of a rising stroke incidence but also because of the "positive" effect of a declining stroke case-fatality rate. Improvements in both emergency procedures and aggressive acute stroke management would be assumed to be associated with increasing stroke prevalence. Although changes in stroke prevalence are not necessarily an indication of desirable changes in the public health system, the understanding and prediction of stroke prevalence are critical to planning aspects of the health care delivery system, such as the number of nursing home beds, rehabilitation services, and efforts in secondary stroke prevention.

Distribution of Disease

Stroke Mortality

The Centers for Disease Control and Prevention (CDC) provides the most recent data (2005) for calculating age-specific stroke mortality rates for each of the major race/ethnic groups in the United States.[20] As shown in Fig. 13-2A, there is a striking rise in stroke mortality with increasing age in all race/ethnic groups.[20] However, at young ages, the stroke mortality rate for black people is substantially higher than the rates for other groups. For example, for the age group 35 to 44 years, the rate for black people is 12.5 (per 100,000) compared with 6.9 for American Indians, 4.6 for Hispanics, 3.9 for white people and 3.7 for Asian/Pacific Islanders. The mortality ratio for various ethnic groups compared with white people is shown in Fig. 13-2B. For the age group 35 to 44 years, the mortality ratio for black people is 3.2 (12.5/3.9). The highest mortality ratio is 3.6 (40.5/11.1) for the age group 45 to 54. Here, the mortality ratio for black people is strikingly different from those of other race/ethnic groups, for whom excess mortality rates are smaller. With increasing age, however, the race/ethnic disparity between black people and other groups tends to decrease so that by age 75, there are no substantial differences among race/ethnic groups in stroke mortality. This trend continues with age; among persons older than 85 years, white people carry the highest stroke mortality rate: 1171.8 per 100,000; the rates for other race/ethnic groups range from 574.9 per 100,000 for American Indians to 1122.3 per 100,000 for black people. [Of note, in 1996, a study by the Indian Health Service discovered that race had been misclassified for American Indians: 1.2% to 30.4% of American Indians who had died had been classified as another race.[21] Because this misreporting affects the numerator in the estimate of the deaths but not the denominator (the census estimates of the population size), previous stroke mortality statistics likely represent an underestimate of the burden of disease in this race/ethnic group.]

One natural focus of this pattern of excess rates is on the extraordinarily high stroke mortality rates for young black people. However, equal emphasis could be placed on the striking ethnic differences in the rate of increase in stroke mortality with increasing age. For example, between ages 35 to 44 and 45 to 54, black people had a larger increase in stroke mortality (from 12.5 to 40.5—a 3.2 times increase) than their white counterparts (from 3.9 to 11.1—a 2.8 times increase). However, between ages 45 to 54 and 55 to 64, this changed, and there was a slightly larger increase in stroke mortality for white people (11.1 to 26.9—a 2.4 times increase) than for black people (40.5 to 81.5—a 2.0 times increase). The increase in stroke mortality was substantially larger for white people than for black people when the rate of increase in stroke mortality was compared between all adjacent 10-year age strata above age 65. Specifically, between 55 to 64 and 65 to 74 there was a 3.9 times increase in white people and only a 2.3 times increase in black people; from 65 to 74 and 75 to 84 there

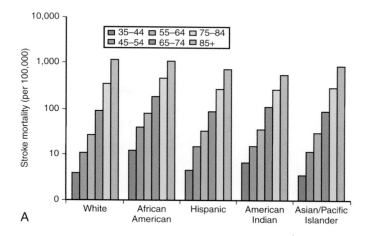

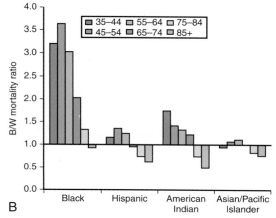

Figure 13-2 A, The U.S. stroke mortality for 2005 by age and ethnic group (on a log scale). B, The age-specific relative risk for each of the ethnic groups relative to that of white people. For example, the risk of stroke mortality is approximately three times greater for black people aged 35 to 44 years than for their white counterparts. (From National Center for Health Statistics, Data Warehouse: LCWK5 [Deaths, percent of total deaths, and death rates for the 15 leading causes of death in 10-year age groups, by Hispanic origin, race for non-Hispanic population and sex: United States, 1999-2005] for Hispanic, White and Black, and LCWK2 [Deaths, percent of total deaths, and death rates for the 15 leading causes of death in 10-year age groups, by race and sex: United States, 1999-2005] for American Indian and Asian/Pacific Islander: http://www.cdc.gov/nchs/nvss/mortality_tables.htm. Accessed February 28, 2009.)

was a 3.9 times increase in white people and a 2.6 times increase in black people; and between 75 to 84 and 85+ there was a 3.3 times increase in white people and a 2.4 times increase in black people. It is this more rapid increase in stroke mortality risk with increasing age that allows white people to "catch up and pass" black people in stroke death rates. The rate of increase in stroke risk with increasing age is intermediate between white people (generally the most rapidly increasing risk with age) and black people (generally the slowest increasing risk with age).

Fig. 13-3A shows the temporal pattern of age-adjusted (2000 standard) stroke mortality in the United States between 1979 and 2005 for white people and black people.[3] This figure shows both the remarkable success and the continuing failure of efforts to reduce the burden of

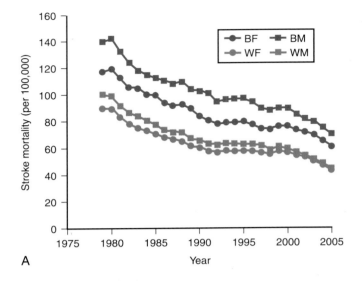

A

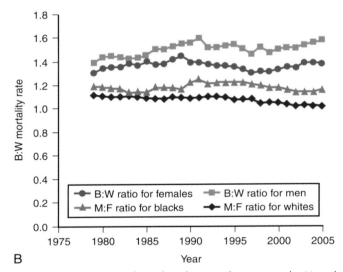

B

Figure 13-3 A, Age-adjusted stroke mortality rates in the United States, 1979 to 2005, by race and sex. B, Age-adjusted stroke mortality ratios in the United States, 1979 to 2005, by race and sex. Black-to-white ratios are shown in pink circles for women and in orange squares for men. Male-to-female ratios are shown in green triangles for black people and blue diamonds for white people.

stroke. The dramatic declines in stroke mortality that began as early as 1900[22] have continued. Fig. 13-3A shows stroke mortality declines from 1979 to 2005 as follows:

- From 100.4/100,000 to 44.7/100,000 for white men (−55%)
- From 89.9/100,000 to 44.0/100,000 for white women (−51%)
- From 139.6/100,000 to 70.5/100,000 for black men (−49%)
- From 117.5/100,000 to 60.7/100,000 for black women (−48%)

These dramatic declines are part of the reason that the CDC listed the declines in heart disease and stroke as one of the 10 great public health achievements of the twentieth century; it was the only accomplishment cited for which the disease was explicitly mentioned.[22]

The similarity of the percentage declines also reveals the continuing failure to reduce ethnic-racial and sex discrepancies in the burden of disease. The consistency of the burden is explicitly shown in Fig. 13-3B, in which the age-adjusted black-to-white stroke mortality ratio is shown for men and women, and the male-to-female stroke mortality ratio is shown for white people and black people.[3] For men, the age-adjusted black-to-white stroke mortality ratio was approximately 1.39 in 1979. This ratio rose in the 1980s and then showed a relative decline; however, the final level in 2005 was 1.58, representing a 48% increase in the magnitude of the relative racial disparity. Likewise, for women, the black-to-white stroke mortality ratio was approximately 1.31 in 1979 and increased to 1.45 in the late 1980s; by 2005, however, the ratio had returned to 1.38, still representing a 24% increase in the magnitude of the racial disparity. As can be seen in Fig. 13-3B, the male-to-female stroke mortality ratio has also proved to be relatively stable over this period for black people, in that black men have between a 13% to 25% excess risk compared with black women. This is in contrast to white people, in that men were at a 12% increased risk of death from stroke in 1979 but are now only at a 1% increased risk compared with women.

On the basis of preliminary mortality data for 2006 (the latest time period available at the time of this writing) in comparison to 2005 data, there was a 6.4% decline in overall age-adjusted stroke mortality (data not available by race/ethnic groups).[23]

Although mortality rates are low for the United States compared with many other countries, regional differences have long been recognized; in fact, the southeastern region of the country is called the *stroke belt*. This stroke belt, first identified in 1965 as a region of high stroke mortality,[24] is commonly defined as comprising eight southern states: North Carolina, South Carolina, Georgia, Tennessee, Mississippi, Alabama, Louisiana, and Arkansas. This region of excess stroke mortality has been shown to exist since at least 1940,[25] and despite relatively minor geographic shifts,[26] it still persists today according to the latest data available.[27,28] Furthermore, a "buckle" region along the coastal plains of North Carolina, South Carolina, and Georgia has been identified with stroke mortality even higher than that of the rest of the stroke belt.[29] The CDC's *Atlas of Stroke Mortality*, published in January 2003, presents a complete and extensive review of geographic variations in stroke mortality rates for 1991 to 1998 by race-ethnic group.[28] Fig. 13-4 is an update of these data to the most recent data available (2001-2004) and shows the excess mortality in the southeastern United States (with particularly high rates along the coastal plains of North Carolina, South Carolina, and Georgia) and the later-occurring high stroke mortality in the northwestern United States.[30] The atlas showing mortality (between 1991 and 1998) demonstrates a similar pattern of mortality for white people and black people (i.e., higher stroke mortality rates in the southeastern and northwestern United States). It also reveals substantial variations for Hispanics (with particularly high rates in west Texas and New Mexico), Asians (with particularly high rates in the Northwest, the Memphis area, and southern Nevada), and American Indians (with particularly high rates in the

STROKE DEATH RATES, 2000–2004
ADULTS AGES 35 YEARS AND OLDER BY COUNTY

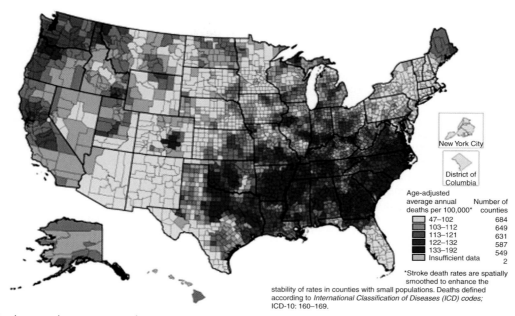

Age-adjusted average annual deaths per 100,000*	Number of counties
47–102	684
103–112	649
113–121	631
122–132	587
133–192	549
Insufficient data	2

*Stroke death rates are spatially smoothed to enhance the stability of rates in counties with small populations. Deaths defined according to *International Classification of Diseases (ICD) codes*; ICD-10: I60–I69.

Figure 13-4 Stroke mortality rates, United States, total population ages 35+ years, 2000 to 2004. Darkest colors represent areas with highest stroke mortality rates, and lightest colors represent areas with lowest rates. (From National Center for Health Statistics, Centers for Disease Control and Prevention. Division for Heart Disease and Stroke Prevention: *Stroke Fact Sheet*: www.cdc.gov/DHDSP/library/fs_stroke.htm. Accessed February 28, 2009.)

Carolinas, the Northwest, and the Northern Great Plains.) Comparisons of the total United States pattern of these racial-ethnic groups with white people and black people is difficult, however, because large areas of the United States lack sufficient representation of these race-ethnic groups for reliable estimates of stroke mortality.

Hence, ethnic differences in stroke mortality rates are dominated by the substantial excess risk for black people younger than 65 years. Although men are at higher risk of stroke death than women, the sex disparity is substantially less than the racial disparity observed between black people and white people. Although stroke mortality rates have shown remarkable declines over the past several decades, there has been virtually no progress in reducing the magnitude of the disparity in the risk of stroke death for black people.

Stroke Incidence

Information on the distribution of stroke as indexed by stroke incidence is available from the complementary approaches of cohort studies and community stroke surveillance studies. In cohort studies, incidence is estimated by the rate of new events in the cohort that is being prospectively followed. This approach has the strength of allowing the study of the role of risk factors that are measured before the stroke event. Because incident stroke is a relatively rare event in the general population, however, the use of a cohort design to describe incidence data has the notable shortcoming of relying on relatively few incident events. For example, the ARIC study followed up 15,792 individuals for an average of 7.2 years to obtain

267 incident stroke events.[15] Over the 51-year follow-up in the Framingham Study, 875 stroke events have occurred among the 4897 original cohort participants.[31] Although there are a larger number of strokes among more elderly cohorts, such as the CHS, whose participants were older than 65 years at baseline and where 5711 participants stroke-free at baseline were followed up for an average of 6.3 years to detect 399 stroke events,[14] much of the interest in the distribution of disease among racial groups is in younger age groups. The shortcoming of a relatively small number of events is overcome in community surveillance efforts that identify all stroke events in people who are then hospitalized in a geographically defined region. These approaches will have a substantially larger number of events (generally in the thousands), allowing much more precise description of racial/ethnic differences, temporal changes, and geographic differences than is possible from cohort studies (generally with a number of stroke events in the hundreds). However, because risk factors were not assessed before the stroke events, the surveillance approach is not optimal for evaluating the role of risk factors.

Several cohort studies have provided great insights into the racial and ethnic differences in the distribution of stroke as indexed by incidence rates. For example, the ARIC study showed a clear excess risk of incident ischemic stroke among black people: the black-to-white age-adjusted incidence rate ratio was 2.41 (95% confidence interval [CI], 1.85, 3.15) overall.[15] The study also revealed a greater relative risk for ischemic stroke for black people younger than 55 years (2.77) than for those older than 55 years (2.23), reflecting the larger racial disparities observed in mortality measures at younger ages. Racial differences in stroke were only partially mediated by adjustment for risk factors such as hypertension and diabetes and by further adjustment for education as a surrogate for socioeconomic status.[15] For all strokes combined (ischemic and hemorrhagic strokes), the age-adjusted black-to-white incidence rate ratio was 2.58 (95% CI, 2.02, 3.29).[15] The first National Health and Nutrition Examination Survey (NHANES I) Epidemiologic Follow-up Study (NHEFS) also used the cohort approach to document an age- and sex-adjusted relative risk of 2.3 for black people.[32] These observations of excess incidence among black people from cohort studies are supported by similar observations from several community surveillance studies. The most recent (2005) estimated stroke rates from the GCNKSS show a 1.74 black-to-white incidence ratio for ischemic stroke (280/100,000 versus 161/100,000), a 1.52 incidence ratio for subarachnoid hemorrhage (SAH) (47/100,000 versus 31/100,000), and 2.13 for SAH (17/100,000 versus 8/100,000).[33] The black excess risk for incident stroke is also supported by the surveillance data from the NOMASS: rates of 223 per 100,000 for black people and 93 for white people yielded an incidence rate ratio of 2.4.[12]

The NOMASS and the BASIC studies provide community surveillance data on stroke incidence rates for Hispanics and Mexican-Americans, the largest subgroup of Hispanics. For ischemic stroke, NOMASS data show that the annual age-adjusted incidence rate for Hispanics was 149/100,000 [95% CI, 132-165] compared with 88/100,000 [95% CI, 75-101] in white people, for a Hispanic-to-white incidence ratio of 1.69.[34] Likewise, the Corpus Christi stroke surveillance study (BASIC) showed an incidence rate of 168/100,000 in Mexican-Americans as compared with only 136/100,000 for white people, for a incidence ratio of 1.24 [95% CI, 1.12-1.37].[11] There are several potential explanations (each requiring further study) for the larger observed disparity for mortality than for incidence, specifically (1) perhaps the higher stroke incidence in Hispanics is offset by a lower case-fatality rate, resulting in a similar mortality rate, (2) perhaps the communities (northern Manhattan and Nueces County, Texas) are non-representative of white people or Hispanics nationally, or (3) perhaps the heterogeneity within the Hispanic ethnicity implies that the findings in Mexican-Americans in Nueces County and Puerto Rican populations in Northern Manhattan are not reflective of the larger Hispanic population.

Recent data from the Strong Heart Study, a population-based cohort study of cardiovascular disease in 13 American Indian tribes/communities throughout the United States, estimated the stroke incidence rate for the years 1989 to 2004 for American Indians to be 679/100,000.[16] This article notes that this incidence rate is higher than the reported rates for white people in Rochester (Minnesota) and black people in the Cincinnati region (data from the GCNKSS), which appears to be supported by a comparison of age-specific rates between American Indians and white people, but age-specific rates compared with black people appear largely equivalent. Specifically, at ages 45 to 54 incidence rates (per 100,000) were estimated to be 384 in American Indians compared with 63 in white people and 320 in black people; at ages 55 to 64

rates were 727, 273, and 637, respectively; and for ages 65 to 74 rates were 1002, 669, and 972, respectively. These comparisons should be interpreted with caution for at least two reasons: (1) the estimates of events in the American Indian population are from a cohort study, whereas the rates reported from both Rochester and Cincinnati are from surveillance studies, and differences in the detection rate for stroke events may differ in these approaches, and (2) the comparison groups differ not only by race but also by geographic location, which may also have a substantial impact on stroke incidence and/or mortality.

As observed in the previous section, there is a substantial difference in the magnitude of the racial disparity at younger compared with older ages, particularly for black people, who, at ages 35 to 64, have three to four times the risk of dying of stroke than do their white counterparts but have a similar risk by age 75 (see Fig. 13-2B). This interaction of age and stroke mortality naturally raises the question of whether a similar interaction exists between age and stroke incidence. The GCNKSS is uniquely positioned to provide insights into the black-to-white differences in the incidence of stroke across a broad age spectrum. The left panel of Fig.13-5A shows black and white incidence rates in 1993 to 1994 and higher stroke incidence rates for black people within each age strata[35]; however, the black-to-white incidence ratios for both 1993 to 1994 and 1999 are similar to that observed for mortality ratios (Fig. 13-5B).[8] Age-specific disparities in stroke mortality are not as large for Hispanics as for black people (see Fig. 13-2B); however, data from BASIC show that below age 65 Hispanics appear to have a greater risk of stroke incidence than their white counterparts but that little difference exists after age 75 (right panel of Fig. 13-5A).[11] There is also a declining magnitude of Hispanic-to-white disparity for incidence: Hispanics aged 45 to 59 are at nearly twice the risk of their white counterparts, which is approximately a 60% excess between ages 60 and 74, but have a similar risk after age 75 (right panel of Fig. 13-5B). Collectively, there is a similar pattern of excess stroke mortality and excess stroke incidence rates among black people, which suggests that racial difference in incidence (rather than case fatality) is the prime contributor to the disparities in stroke mortality in black people.

Unfortunately, there is no national reporting of stroke incidence rates to serve as the basis for a description of geographic variations in stroke incidence. Some geographic representation is provided by the studies already mentioned (Greater Cincinnati, ARIC). Using these studies as the basis of a description of geographic variations in stroke incidence is problematic because of (1) differences in study design and (2) the very focused geographic nature of these studies (e.g., using the ARIC study data from Forsyth County to describe stroke in North Carolina). As such, there is a substantial need for studies to provide nationally comparable, generalized data to describe the geographic variations in stroke incidence risk.

If one assumes that stroke case-fatality rates are similar across the nation, it is tempting (and perhaps reasonable) to use stroke mortality rates to provide a description of geographic variations in incidence. The compressed mortality files available from the CDC (through the CDC Wonder System) show that in 2005 there were 23,722

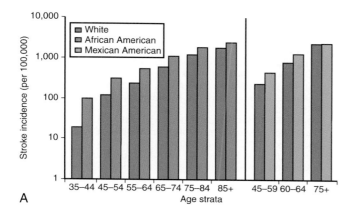

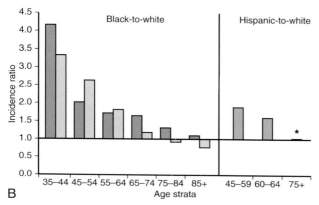

Figure 13-5 A, Left panel shows age-specific stroke incidence rates for 1993-1994 per 100,000 population from the Greater Cincinnati/Northern Kentucky Stroke Study (GCNKSS) by race and sex, and the right panel shows the stroke age-specific incidence rates for 2000-2002 per 100,000 population from the Brain Attack Surveillance in Corpus Christi (BASIC). (Data from Kissela B, Schneider A, Kleindorfer D, et al: Stroke in a biracial population: The excess burden of stroke among blacks. *Stroke* 35:426-431, 2004; and Morgenstern LB, Smith MA, Lisabeth LD, et al: Excess stroke in Mexican Americans compared with non-Hispanic whites: The Brain Attack Surveillance in Corpus Christi Project. *Am J Epidemiol* 160:376-383, 2004, respectively.) B, Left panel shows the age-specific black-to-white stroke incidence ratio for men and women for 1993-1994 (pink) and 1999 (yellow). Right panel shows the age-specific Mexican American to white incidence ratio for 2000-2002.

stroke deaths in the eight states frequently defined as the stroke belt (Alabama, Arkansas, Georgia, Louisiana, Mississippi, North Carolina, South Carolina, and Tennessee) that had an estimated population of 42,747,552, for a crude stroke mortality rate of 55.5/100,000.[20] In the same year there were 119,857 stroke deaths in the remaining 42 states and the District of Columbia that had a population of 253,759,509, for a crude stroke mortality rate of 47.2/100,000.[20] If the stroke mortality rate for the rest of the nation were applied to the population of the stroke belt states, there would be an expected 20,191 stroke events, which suggests that in 2005 the geographic disparity in stroke is responsible for approximately 3500 "extra" stroke deaths in the stroke belt. If one assumes the case-fatality rate for stroke to be 30%, these 3500 extra stroke deaths would be associated with 11,770

extra stroke events in the stroke belt during 2005 alone. In 1996, Taylor et al estimated that the lifetime cost of stroke was more than $90,000.[36] Between 1990 and 2009 the consumer price index has increased 1.62 times, and, although health care costs are increasing at a rate faster than the rest of the economy, this would suggest the lifetime cost of stroke is at least $157,000 ($90,000 × 1.62), and the cost of the disparity associated with the stroke belt is in excess of $1.8 billion.

Stroke Prevalence

Although one of the most quoted summary statistics is that stroke is one of the leading causes of disability among adults,[19] the focus of assessing the distribution of stroke seldom falls on the use of prevalence as an index. This is surprising because the burden of disability is borne by the survivors of stroke, which is directly indexed by measures of stroke prevalence. As important, substantial efforts in secondary stroke prevention have been or are being made through the performance of clinical trials.[37] These efforts are appropriate because the risk of subsequent stroke in patients who survive a stroke is perhaps as high as 10% per year[19]; however, any potential gain in reduction of stroke risk is available only to those with prevalent stroke.

The American Heart/Stroke Association estimates that there are 6,500,000 survivors of stroke alive today.[19] This estimate is based on cohort studies that reflect distinct ethnic and regional trends. For a description of differences across broad ages and by race and sex, it may be best to rely on national survey data, specifically the National Health Interview Survey.[38] The use of survey data has the strength of a substantial sample size; however, it has the weakness of dependence on self-reported conditions. With acknowledgment of this shortcoming, the prevalence rate of stroke is shown by sex and by age in Fig. 13-6A. The percent of the population with a history of stroke increases dramatically from 0.5% for those younger than age 45 to more than 11% for those 75 years or older. The higher stroke incidence rate in men likely underlies the higher prevalence of stroke in men also shown in Fig. 13-6A. However, because women have a greater life expectancy than men, the relationship between the percent of people with stroke and the absolute number of people with stroke is complex. Although the percent of individuals with stroke increases with age, Fig. 13-6B shows that the there are approximately 1.5 million individuals with stroke within the age strata 45 to 64, 65 to 74, and 75+. Because most individuals older than age 75 are women, there are also more women with a history of stroke than men (see Fig. 13-6B). While earlier publications from the CDC reported age–gender specific prevalence and percent with diseases, more recent publications report prevalence by age and gender separately.

Conclusions

The measures of stroke mortality, stroke incidence, and prevalence of stroke provide important insights into the description of the distribution of the disease. Each of these

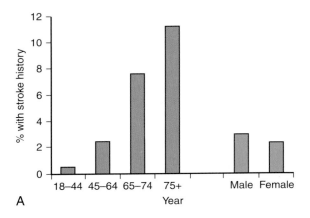

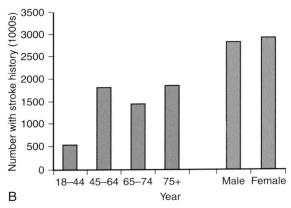

Figure 13-6 *A,* The 2006 stroke prevalence rate per 1000 population shown by age and by sex. *B,* Number of prevalent strokes (in 1000s) shown by age and by sex.

indices has important strengths and weaknesses, and the measures are of particular interest to specific users of the information. Overall, several recurring patterns are clear. Perhaps the most critical is the substantially higher risk of stroke (regardless of the index of measure) among black people, particularly young black people. Other important summary observations are the greater risk for men, again particularly for young men; however, the larger number of women in older age groups implies an absolutely larger number of women with stroke. In addition, at least by mortality measures, there is a substantial excess of stroke mortality among residents of the southeastern United States but few data to describe geographic variations in stroke incidence or prevalence.

REFERENCES

1. Technical Appendix from Vital Statistics of United States: 1995: Mortality, Hyattsville, Md, 1999, US Department of Health and Human Services, Public Health Service, Centers for Disease Control and Prevention, National Center for Health Statistics.
2. International Statistical Classification of Diseases and Related Health Problems, Geneva, Switzerland, 2007, World Health Organization, 10th revision.
3. National Center for Health Statistics. CDC Wonder. Available online at http://wonder.cdc.gov/ retrieved and compiled on March 1, 2009.
4. Iso H, Jacobs DR Jr, Goldman L: Accuracy of death certificate diagnosis of intracranial hemorrhage and nonhemorrhagic stroke: The Minnesota Heart Survey, *Am J Epidemiol* 132:993-998, 1990.
5. Shahar E, McGovern PG, Sprafka JM, et al: Improved survival of stroke patients during the 1980s. The Minnesota Stroke Survey, *Stroke* 26:1-6, 1995.
6. Howard G, Toole JF, Becker C, et al: Changes in survival following stroke in five North Carolina counties observed during two different periods, *Stroke* 20:345-350, 1989.
7. Wolf PA, D'Agostino RB, O'Neal MA, et al: Secular trends in stroke incidence and mortality. The Framingham Study, *Stroke* 23:1551-1555, 1992.
8. Kleindorfer D, Broderick J, Khoury J, et al: The unchanging incidence and case-fatality of stroke in the 1990s: A population-based study, *Stroke* 37:2473-2478, 2006.
9. Goff DC Jr, Brass L, Braun LT, et al: Essential features of a surveillance system to support the prevention and management of heart disease and stroke: a scientific statement from the AHA Councils on Epidemiology and Prevention, Stroke, and Cardiovascular Nursing and the Interdisciplinary Working Groups on Quality of Care and Outcomes Research and Atherosclerotic Peripheral Vascular Disease, *Circulation* 115:127-155, 2007.
10. Petty GW, Brown RD Jr, Whisnant JP, et al: Ischemic stroke subtypes: A population-based study of incidence and risk factors, *Stroke* 30:2513-2516, 1999.
11. Morgenstern LB, Smith MA, Lisabeth LD, et al: Excess stroke in Mexican Americans compared with non-Hispanic whites: The Brain Attack Surveillance in Corpus Christi Project, *Am J Epidemiol* 160:376-383, 2004.
12. Sacco RL, Boden-Albala B, Gan R, et al: Stroke incidence among white, black and Hispanic residents of an urban community: The Northern Manhattan Stroke Study, *Am J Epidemiol* 147:259-268, 1998.
13. White AD, Folsom AR, Chambless LE, et al: Community surveillance of coronary heart disease in the Atherosclerosis Risk in Communities (ARIC) Study: Methods and initial two years' experience, *J Clin Epidemiol* 49:223-233, 1996.
14. Lumley T, Kronmal RA, Cushman M, Manolio TA, Goldstein S: A stroke prediction score in the elderly: Validation and web-based application, *J Clin Epidemiol* 55:129-136, 2002.
15. Rosamond WD, Folsom AR, Chambless LE, et al: Stroke incidence and survival among middle-aged adults: 9-year follow-up of the Atherosclerosis Risk in Communities (ARIC) cohort, *Stroke* 30:736-743, 1999.
16. Zhang Y, Galloway JM, Welty TK, et al: Incidence and risk factors for stroke in American Indians: The Strong Heart Study, *Circulation* 118:1577-1584, 2008.
17. Howard VJ, Cushman M, Pulley L, et al: The REasons for Geographic And Racial Differences in Stroke (REGARDS) Study: Objectives and Design, *Neuroepidemiology* 25:135-143, 2005.
18. Kleindorfer D, Khoury J, Alwell K, et al: The impact of magnetic resonance imaging (MRI) on ischemic stroke detection and phenotyping: More strokes ruled out than ruled in [abstract], *Stroke* 40:38, 2009.
19. Lloyd-Jones D, Adams R, Carnethon M, et al: for the American Heart Association Statistics Committee and Stroke Statistics Subcommittee. Heart Disease and Stroke Statistics—2009 Update. A report from the American Heart Association Statistics Committee and Stroke Statistics Subcommittee, *Circulation* 119:e21-e181, 2009.
20. National Center for Health Statistics, Data Warehouse: LCWK5 (Deaths, percent of total deaths, and death rates for the 15 leading causes of death in 10-year age groups, by Hispanic origin, race for non-Hispanic population and sex: United States, 1999-2005) for Hispanic, White and Black, and LCWK2 (Deaths, percent of total deaths, and death rates for the 15 leading causes of death in 10-year age groups, by race and sex: United States, 1999-2005) for American Indian and Asian/Pacific Islander: http://www.cdc.gov/nchs/datawh/statab/unpubd/mortabs.htm. Accessed February 28, 2009.
21. Casper ML, Denny CH, Coolidge JN, et al: *Atlas of heart disease and stroke among American Indians and Alaska natives,* Atlanta, Ga, 2005, US Department of Health and Human Services, Centers for Disease Control and Prevention and Indian Health Services.
22. Centers for Disease Control and Prevention: Ten great public health achievements—United States, 1900-1999, *MMWR Morb Mortal Wkly Rep* 48:241-243, 1999.
23. Heron MP, Hoyert DL, Xu J, Scott C, Tejada-Vera B: Deaths: Preliminary data for 2006, *National vital statistics report,* vol 56, no 16. Hyattsville, Md, 2008, National Center for Health Statistics.

24. Borhani NO: Changes and geographic distribution of mortality from cerebrovascular disease, *Am J Public Health* 55:673–681, 1965.

25. Lanska DJ: Geographic distribution of stroke mortality in the United States: 1939-1941 to 1979-1981, *Neurology* 43:1839–1851, 1993.

26. Casper ML, Wing S, Anda RF, et al: The shifting stroke belt: Chances in the geographic pattern of stroke mortality in the United States, 1962 to 1988, *Stroke* 26:755–760, 1995.

27. Howard G, Howard VJ, Katholi C, et al: Decline in US stroke mortality: An analysis of temporal patterns by sex, race, and geographic region, *Stroke* 32:2213–2220, 2001.

28. Casper ML, Barnett E, Williams GI Jr, et al: *Atlas of stroke mortality: Racial, ethnic, and geographic disparities in the United States*, Atlanta, Ga, January 2003, US Department of Health and Human Services, Centers for Disease Control and Prevention.

29. Howard G, Anderson R, Johnson NJ, et al: Evaluation of social status as a contributing factor to the stroke belt of the United States, *Stroke* 28:936–940, 1997.

30. National Center for Health Statistics, Centers for Disease Control and Prevention. Division for Heart Disease and Stroke Prevention, *Stroke Fact Sheet*: www.cdc.gov/DHDSP/library/fs_stroke.htm. Accessed February 28, 2009.

31. Seshadri S, Beiser A, Kelly-Hayes M, et al: The lifetime risk of stroke: Estimates from the Framingham Study, *Stroke* 37:345–350, 2006.

32. Gillum RF: Coronary heart disease, stroke and hypertension in a U.S. national cohort: The NHANES I Epidemiologic Follow-up Study. National Health and Nutrition Examination Survey, *Ann Epidemiol* 6:259–262, 1996.

33. Kleindorfer D, Alwell K, Khoury J, et al: Stroke incidence is decreasing in whites, but stable in blacks: A preliminary population-based estimate of temporal trends in stroke incidence [abstract], *Stroke* 40:37, 2009.

34. White H, Boden-Albala B, Wang C, et al: Ischemic stroke subtype incidence among whites, blacks, and Hispanics: The Northern Manhattan Study, *Circulation* 111:1327–1331, 2005.

35. Kissela B, Schneider A, Kleindorfer D, et al: Stroke in a biracial population: The excess burden of stroke among blacks, *Stroke* 35:426–431, 2004.

36. Taylor TN, Davis PH, Torner JC, et al: Lifetime cost of stroke in the United States, *Stroke* 27:1459–1466, 1996.

37. Stroke Trials Registry (www.strokecenter.org/trials/) accessed April 4, 2009.

38. Pleis JR, Lethbridge-Cejku M: Summary health statistics for US adults: National Health Interview Survey, 2006. National Center for Health Statistics, *Vital Health Stat* 10(235), 2007.

14

Epidemiology of Stroke

PHILIP A. WOLF, WILLIAM B. KANNEL

Epidemiology is "the study of the distribution and determinants of disease frequency" in human populations.[1] Population research for stroke is concerned with learning in what particulars those who go on to have a stroke differ from those who stay free of the condition over long periods of follow-up. It is concerned with assessment of risk and seeking modifiable predisposing risk factors. Consideration of the distribution of stroke by geographic region, race-ethnicity, age, and gender has been dealt with comprehensively in Chapters 13 and 19. An exposition of outcomes after stroke, the other key determinant in stroke prevalence, morbidity, and mortality, is reviewed in detail in Chapter 15. This chapter will focus on the determinants of stroke: risk factors and predisposing conditions, including implications for stroke prevention. Although several medical and surgical therapies to reduce the damage from impending or recent-onset stroke have recently been shown to be effective in selected patients and deserve continued research and attention in practice, it seems likely that prevention will continue to be the most effective strategy for reducing the health and economic consequences of cerebrovascular disease in the general population. Prevention is facilitated by an understanding of predisposing host and environmental factors. The relative impact of each of these factors has become clearer, chiefly through prospective epidemiologic investigation. Controlled clinical trials have demonstrated the effectiveness of risk factor modification in stroke prevention. In this chapter, data obtained from a number of prospective observational studies of populations will be presented. In particular, assessment of risk factors measured systematically and prospectively in a variety of populations, before the appearance of disease, provides the least distorted picture of the influence of these host and environmental factors on stroke incidence.

Magnitude of the Problem

Stroke is the most common life-threatening neurologic disease and third leading cause of death in the United States, after heart disease and cancer. Among the elderly, the segment of the population in whom stroke occurs most frequently, it is a major cause of disability requiring long-term institutionalization.

Mortality

Stroke accounted for about one of every 18 deaths in the United States in 2006. About half of these deaths occurred out of hospital. Stroke ranks third among all causes of death, behind diseases of the heart and cancer (Centers for Disease Control and Prevention/National Center for Health Statistics). On average, someone dies of a stroke about every 4 minutes. The 2006 overall death rate per 100,000 for stroke was 43.6. Mortality rates per 100,000 were higher for black (67.1) than for white males (41.7); for white females it was 41.1, and for black females it was 57.0. Because women live longer than men, more women than men die of stroke each year. Women accounted for 60.6% of U.S. stroke deaths in 2006.[2]

Stroke case fatality rates are high: 8% to 12% of ischemic strokes and 37% to 38% of hemorrhagic strokes result in death within 30 days. From 1996 to 2006, the stroke death rate fell 33.5%; however, because of the aging population, the actual number of stroke deaths declined only 18.4%.[3]

Age-standardized mortality rates for SAH and IH as well as ischemic stroke are higher among black people than white people. Death rates from IH are also higher among Asian or Pacific Islanders than among white people. All minority populations have higher death rates from SAH than white people. Among adults, black people and American Indians or Alaska Natives have higher risk ratios than white people for all three stroke subtypes.[4]

Cost

The estimated direct and indirect cost of stroke for 2006 was $57.9 billion. In 2001, $3.7 billion ($6037 per discharge) was paid to Medicare beneficiaries discharged from short-stay hospitals for stroke. The mean lifetime cost of ischemic stroke in the United States is estimated at $140,048. This includes inpatient care, rehabilitation, and follow-up care necessary for lasting deficits. Inpatient hospital costs for an acute stroke account for 70% of first-year poststroke costs. Age, sex, and insurance status are unassociated with stroke cost. Severe strokes (National Institutes of Health Stroke Scale score, > 20) cost twice as much as mild strokes, despite similar diagnostic testing. Comorbidities such as ischemic heart disease and atrial fibrillation (AF) predict higher costs.[3]

Incidence of Stroke

The incidence of stroke should be ascertained by systematic evaluation of a population determined to be free of the disease at outset. Ideally, the population under study should be representative of a general population, although it is not possible to prospectively recruit and follow up a large number of individuals representative of

TABLE 14-1   ANNUAL INCIDENCE OF ATHEROTHROMBOTIC BRAIN INFARCTION (ABI) AND COMPLETED STROKES IN MEN AND WOMEN AGED 35 TO 94 YEARS

Age	*Men*		*Women*		*Men/Women Combined*	
	n	**Rate/1000**	**n**	**Rate/1000**	**n**	**Rate/1000**
ABI						
35-44	1	0.12	1	0.1	2	0.11
45-54	15	0.97	13	0.67	28	0.81
55-64	37	1.94	35	1.4	72	1.64
65-74	80	5.14	68	3	148	3.87
75-84	79	9.06	119	7.52	198	8.07
85-94	16	8.64	72	13.79	88	12.44
Total	228	*3.60	308	*2.90	536	3.21
Completed stroke						
35-44	3	0.37	3	0.3	6	0.33
45-54	25	1.61	20	1.04	45	1.29
55-64	60	3.15	60	2.41	120	2.73
65-74	127	8.16	115	5.08	242	6.33
75-84	126	14.45	203	12.83	329	13.41
85-94	30	16.21	121	23.18	151	21.35
Total	371	*5.89	522	*4.91	893	5.35

*Age-adjusted.
Data from the Framingham Heart Study: 55-year follow-up.

persons extant in the world, a nation, or even a smaller geographic locale such as a state or province. However, by accumulating data derived from a number of such general population samples a more complete picture of the incidence and distribution of a condition such as stroke may be ascertained.

The incidence of stroke was ascertained from prospective study over 55 years of follow-up of 5184 men and women, ages 30 to 62, who were free of stroke at entry to the Framingham Study in 1950. The population has been examined every 2 years, and follow-up has been satisfactory in that approximately 85% of subjects have participated in each examination. Study subjects suspected of having a stroke have been evaluated neurologically in the hospital at the time of the stroke since 1968, and the neurologic deficit was confirmed by the Framingham neurologist personally in more than half the cases. In the remainder, hospital records, including neurologists' evaluations, have usually provided confirmation. Since 1982, 91.5% have had at least one computed tomography (CT) or magnetic resonance imaging (MRI) scan of the brain and arteries; many have had more than one study. Other than confirmation or ruling out of a hemorrhage as the basis for the stroke, the stroke has been confirmed by CT/MRI study in 60.9% of cases. It has been possible, therefore, to clearly distinguish hemorrhage from infarction and to classify the ischemic stroke events into lacunar, large artery, and cardioembolic subtypes with a reasonable degree of assurance utilizing established criteria.[5] Over 40 years, since the study began, the neurologic deficit of the stroke was verified by a Framingham Study neurologist. Since 1981 when surveillance was intensified, the neurologic deficit was confirmed by a Framingham Study neurologist in 56.3% of cases. Follow-up of the population has been satisfactory; approximately 7% have been completely lost to follow-up because of death. After 55 years of follow-up

in the Framingham Study, there were 893 cases of initial completed strokes and 152 instances of isolated transient ischemic attacks (TIA). The average annual incidence of stroke events increased with age and approximately doubled in successive decades (Table 14-1). This was true for all cerebrovascular events combined, including isolated TIAs, atherothrombotic brain infarcts (ABI), and for *completed* strokes (ischemic strokes and hemorrhages combined) (see Table 14-1). Overall, the annual age-adjusted (ages 35 to 94 years) total initial completed stroke event rates were 5.89/1000 in men and 4.91/1000 in women; a 20% excess was seen in men (see Table 14-1). The annual age-adjusted (ages 35 to 94 years) incidence of isolated TIA also increased with age and was 1.207/1000 in men and 0.71/1000 in women. Perspective concerning incidence of symptomatic coronary heart disease (CHD) and stroke may be gained by a comparison of analogous manifestations, myocardial infarction (MI) (n = 1206), and ischemic stroke with no clear cardiac source for emboli, termed *ABI* (n = 536) (Fig. 14-1). When these two major manifestations of atherosclerotic disease are compared for men, the age-adjusted average annual incidence rate of MI was 4.1 times that of ABI; for women MI incidence was 1.6 times that of ABI. When incidence is compared with gender overall, MI developed 2.6 times more often in men than in women, whereas ABI was approximately 1.24 times more frequent in men. In both sexes, rates doubled with each advancing decade. The 20-year lag in incidence of MI in women was not seen for ABI, in that age-specific rates were similar for both men and women.

There is a curious inverse pattern of stroke incidence in relation to the occurrence of coronary disease in many populations. The "paradoxic" occurrence of high rates of stroke and low rates of CHD observed in Asian and other populations was investigated in the Hawaii Heart study with the use of accumulated clinical and autopsy

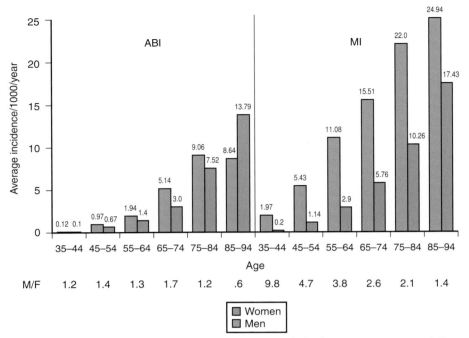

Figure 14-1 Incidence of atherothrombotic brain infarction (ABI) and myocardial infarction (MI); 50-year follow-up for the Framingham Heart Study. Data from the Framingham Heart Study.

data obtained during the long-term follow-up from 1965 to 1985 of cohorts of Japanese men living in Hawaii and Japan. The search for explanatory variables revealed three with the characteristic opposing patterns of associations with clinical stroke compared with CHD and of being more prevalent in Japan than in Hawaii. These variables were low serum cholesterol levels, high intake of alcohol, and some aspect of an Oriental diet characterized by low intake of fat and protein from animal sources. Analysis of associations of these variables with measures of atherosclerosis in coronary and cerebral arteries revealed no paradoxic differences, with the possible exception of some dietary variables. Associations with autopsy-measured myocardial infarctions, cerebral infarction, and hemorrhage, however, showed opposing patterns similar to those found for clinical disease. The investigators concluded that the main inference from this investigation is that the paradoxically high risk of stroke observed in populations with low risk of CHD is not due to atherosclerosis in the major cerebral arteries. Rather, it is more likely due to lesions in the small intracerebral arteries and appears to be related to low levels of serum cholesterol, high alcohol intake, and some aspect of a traditional Oriental diet.[6]

Frequency of Stroke by Type

The in-hospital assessment of stroke at Framingham by a study neurologist has helped document the stroke and determine stroke subtype as well as differentiate stroke from other neurologic diseases. Diagnosis of lacunar infarction was based on clinical and brain CT and MRI scan findings, whereas criteria for embolic infarction required a definite cardiac source for embolism. Distinction of cerebral infarction resulting from extracranial

versus intracranial arterial disease was made on clinical grounds relying on noninvasive carotid studies and magnetic resonance angiography. Contrast angiography was requested only infrequently by the study subjects' personal physicians, chiefly in cases of extracranial carotid stenosis before endarterectomy or with subarachnoid hemorrhage (SAH). The occurrence of TIA was obtained by systematic routine questioning on each biennial examination since 1971 and by scrutiny of physician records and hospital notes. This surveillance for TIA has been comprehensive, systematic, and extended over more than 25 years. In addition to the 15.1% of ABIs preceded by TIA, there were 148 persons whose initial cerebrovascular symptoms fulfilled criteria for TIA but who did not sustain a subsequent stroke. These isolated TIAs accounted for 14.8% of total cerebrovascular events in men and 12.7% of events in women.

The relative frequency of completed stroke by type was nearly identical in men and women (Table 14-2). ABI, which included infarction secondary to large vessel atherothrombosis, lacunar infarction, and infarct of undetermined cause, occurred most frequently: 61.5% in men and 60.0% in women. Intracranial hemorrhage accounted for 14.0% of completed strokes in men and 13.4% in women. Although a greater number of intracerebral hemorrhage (IH) and SAH occurred in women than in men, age-adjusted annual incidence rates of IH were higher in men than in women (0.52 versus 0.38 per 1000); rates of SAH were not appreciably different at 0.29 per 1000 in men and 0.28 in women. The relative frequency of IH and SAH varies according to the age of the population studied: SAH predominates below age 65 and is roughly equivalent at ages 65 to 74 years. At ages 75 to 84 years IH predominates: the incidence is 1.26 per 1000 annually compared with 0.29 per 1000 for SAH.

TABLE 14-2 FREQUENCY OF COMPLETED STROKE BY TYPE IN MEN AND WOMEN AGED 35 TO 94 YEARS

Completed Stroke	Men		Women		Total	
	n	%	n	%	n	%
Atherothrombotic brain infarction	228	61.5	308	59	536	60
Cerebral embolus	87	23.5	137	26.2	224	25.1
Subarachnoid hemorrhage	20	5.4	28	5.4	48	5.4
Intracerebral hemorrhage	32	8.6	42	8	74	8.3
Other	4	1.1	7	1.3	11	1.2
Total	371	100	522	100	893	100

Data from the Framingham Heart Study: 55-year follow-up.

Silent Stroke

It is now recognized that silent ischemic vascular insufficiency and infarction is a common occurrence in the peripheral and cerebral arterial vascular territories as well as in the heart. It is common to find CT scan evidence of a prior stroke without a history of such an event. In 1989, the Framingham Study reported the first population-based confirmation of the high prevalence (10% to 11%) of silent cerebral infarction that was later reported in the Stroke Data Bank investigation of hospitalized stroke patients from the National Institutes of Neurological and Communicative Disorders and Stroke.[7,8] MRI-defined infarcts were also similarly found to be associated with prevalent strokes in the population-based case-control Cardiovascular Health Study.[9] The likely reason for their being unrecognized is their small size and location in brain areas likely to evoke minimal symptoms. Their association with glucose intolerance, as has been established for silent MI, is noteworthy. Subcortical silent brain infarction has been found to be a risk for future clinically manifest strokes.[10] They have also been found in apparently healthy persons with hypertension and in patients with manifest atherosclerotic vascular disease.[11]

Recurrent Stroke

Recurrent stroke is common and likely to increase in frequency in the population as life expectancy increases and the stroke case fatality rates decline. The immediate period after a stroke is critical for recurrence. About one third of recurrent strokes within 2 years recorded by the Stroke Data Bank occurred within the first month.[12] The reported long-term cumulative recurrence rate for stroke was 14.1% in the Stroke Data Bank, which is close to the 25% recurrence rate over 5 years reported in the Northern Manhattan Stroke Study. Observed mortality from stroke recurrence exceeds that for an initial stroke.[13,14] Compared with data on risk factors for an initial stroke, information on risk factors for recurrent ischemic stroke is limited, and the reported rates of stroke recurrence vary because of methodologic differences in analysis or differences in age, gender, or coexistent morbidities among the cohorts studied. The Lehigh Valley Recurrent Stroke Study examined the frequency of a second stroke after an initial ischemic stroke in terms of five risk factors (i.e., hypertension, MI, cardiac arrhythmia, diabetes mellitus, and transient ischemic attacks).[15] Multivariable regression analysis was done with the use of the risk factor status at enrollment into the study and was adjusted for age and sex. Multiple risk factors were present in 57% of these patients: hypertension in 59%, cardiac arrhythmia in 47% (of which 16% had AF), diabetes mellitus in 30%, MI in 25%, and TIA in 18%. By the end of the 48-month study, 12% of the patients had a second stroke, 21% died, and 14% moved out of the study areas or refused further follow-up.

Of the selected risk factors tested individually for their influence on the likelihood of stroke recurrence, only history of hypertension and AF were associated with increased risk of second stroke independently and significantly ($P = 0.01$ and $P = 0.04$, respectively). However, when the treatment of diabetes mellitus was considered, diabetic patients treated with insulin had higher cumulative stroke recurrence rates than either diabetic patients not requiring insulin or nondiabetic patients. Ischemic stroke patients with a history of hypertension at initial stroke had a 1.9-fold (confidence interval [CI], 1.18–3.24) higher risk of subsequent stroke compared with those of the same age and sex without a history of hypertension. Patients with AF at baseline had 1.8-fold (CI, 1.04–3.06) higher risk compared with those without AF. Patients with both hypertension and AF at baseline had 3.5-fold higher risk of recurrent stroke compared with patients of the same age and gender without either of these risk factors. More studies of this type need to be undertaken to examine additional risk factors (e.g., lipid profile, obesity, insulin resistance, and smoking) for their effect on risk of stroke recurrence. The patient who is recovering from a mild stroke or who has had a recent TIA is at high risk of stroke recurrence, physical and intellectual disability, long-term institutionalization, and death. Furthermore, a patient with symptomatic cerebrovascular disease is likely to have other cardiovascular diseases or is more predisposed to them. Many of the same risk factors that predispose to initial strokes increase risk of recurrences. Known modifiable stroke risk factors include hypertension, smoking, obesity, heavy alcohol consumption, impaired glucose tolerance, and physical inactivity.

For example, hypertension and diabetes are significant factors associated with recurrent lacunar infarction in patients who have had a previous lacunar stroke. Multivariate analysis has shown that hypertension is a significant predictor of recurrence (odds ratio [OR], 2.01) as is diabetes (OR, 1.62). However, hyperlipidemia has been found to be associated with reduced risk (OR, 0.52).[16]

People who have just had their first ischemic stroke often have elevated inflammatory biomarkers in their blood that indicate an increased risk of dying or their likelihood of having another stroke.[17] These inflammatory markers are associated with long-term prognosis after a first stroke and may help guide clinical care for people who have had a first stroke. A Food and Drug Administration–approved biomarker called lipoprotein-associated phospholipase A2 (Lp-PLA2) predicts the risk of first stroke and was found to be a strong predictor of recurrent stroke risk. Elevated levels of high-sensitivity C-reactive protein (hs-CRP), a test commonly used to predict risk of heart disease, was also associated with more severe strokes and an increased risk of mortality.[17]

The occurrence of a stroke usually signifies diffuse vascular atherosclerosis. Atherothrombotic brain infarctions are associated with about a twofold excess risk of cardiac failure and coronary disease, presumably on the basis of diffuse atherosclerosis. Cardiac failure occurs in about 15% of stroke patients over a period of 10 years, at virtually identical rates in men and women (see Table 14-1). Coronary events can be expected in 44% of men and in 25% of women because of shared predisposing hypertension and diabetes. Various cardiac conditions increase the risk of developing a stroke.

Epidemiologic data indicate that development of a clinical atherosclerotic event in one arterial vascular territory is usually a hallmark of diffuse atherosclerosis and a heightened risk of clinical atherosclerotic events in other areas. The presence of cardiovascular risk factors common to all of the atherosclerotic cardiovascular disease outcomes suggests a universal pathogenesis promoting atherosclerosis in all vascular territories; however, some nontrivial differences exist. Although a better understanding of the reason for these differences is needed, it seems clear that measures taken against risk factors to prevent one atherosclerotic disease should carry a substantial bonus in also preventing atherosclerotic events in other vascular territories. Each of the standard risk factors has been shown to independently contribute to the occurrence of stroke and other atherosclerotic vascular disease, but the risk each imposes varies widely depending on the associated burden of other risk factors. This necessitates global risk evaluation with the use of multivariable risk formulations.

It is also important to recognize that the ultimate morbidity and mortality associated with a stroke is strongly affected by other cardiovascular events likely to make their appearance. For example, the risk of mortality is increased in persons with a stroke, but this mortality risk occurs not only from the stroke but also from cardiac failure and coronary disease. Not only do carotid bruits predict strokes, they also presage coronary disease, heart failure, and peripheral artery disease.

Vascular Bruits

Vascular bruits often signify the presence of diffuse as well as local vascular disease.[18,19] Because the femoral and carotid arteries are readily accessible for noninvasive assessment of the presence of obstructed blood flow, there is merit in detecting presymptomatic peripheral and cerebral arterial disease at a time when preventive measures can be effectively implemented to protect against occlusive clinical manifestations of atherogenesis in the brain. Although it is not surprising that femoral bruits are associated with a 20% to 30% prevalence of intermittent claudication, it is noteworthy that they are also associated with a significantly increased prevalence of atherothrombotic disease in other vascular territories.

Carotid bruits are indicators of vascular disease in the cerebral circulation and, as expected, are associated with a twofold to threefold increase in the risk of stroke. However, they are also associated with a twofold to threefold fold increase in the risk of developing peripheral artery disease (see Table 14-2). Detection of a carotid bruit is the most common finding leading to the diagnosis of asymptomatic carotid artery stenosis. A TIA is the most common expression of symptomatic carotid stenosis. Population-based data indicate that carotid bruits are present in 4% to 5% of persons older than 45 years and that its prevalence increases with age from 1% to 3% for those 45 to 54 years of age to 6% to 8% for persons older than 75 years.[19]

The Framingham Study population data indicate that it is associated with a stroke rate twice that expected for age and sex. However, more often than not, the brain infarction occurred in a vascular territory different from that of the carotid bruit, and lacunar infarction was the mechanism of stroke in nearly half the cases. Carotid bruit is clearly an indicator of increased risk of having a stroke but largely as a consequence of systemic vascular disease and not necessarily as a direct effect of the local stenosis.[19,20]

Race/Ethnicity

It has been established that death rates from stroke are at least twice as great in U.S. black people as in U.S. white people. Among persons ages 45 to 64 years, the stroke mortality rate for black people is 3 to 4 times higher than for white people, and there is a decreasing black-to-white mortality ratio with increasing age.[21] However, data on stroke rates in different race/ethnic groups are generally based on crude measures such as death certification. The limited population-based incidence data available confirm that stroke *incidence* rates in black people are more than double that of white people living in the same geographic region, such as northern Manhattan in New York City (Fig. 14-2) or Greater Cincinnati in Ohio/Northern Kentucky.[22,23]

There are more frequent subcortical infarctions and intracranial atherothromboses as the pathology for ischemic stroke in black patients versus extracranial atherothrombotic occlusion and cardiogenic embolism in white patients. Analysis of possible reasons for variation of stroke incidence in different ethnic or racial subgroups of the population requires taking into account place of birth, current geographic location, age, race/ethnicity, family history, personal habits such as cigarette smoking, physiologic characteristics, and disorders such as blood pressure, cardiac disease, diabetes, and many other risk factors. A possible explanation for the increased occurrence of lacunar and subcortical infarction in black people is the greater impact of hypertension, whereas cases of extracranial atherothrombosis and cardiogenic embolism in white people reflect more atherothrombotic disease. This would not explain the propensity for intracranial atherostenosis in blacks. It appears that influences associated with race/ethnicity above and beyond the current conventional risk factors for stroke are operating, and it is likely that these are mediated through genetic mechanisms.

Risk factors for increased stroke mortality in black people that have been explored are primarily a higher

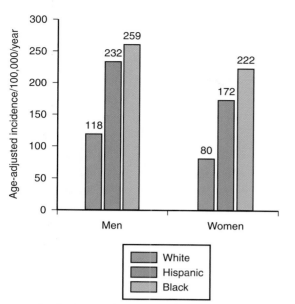

Figure 14-2 Stroke incidence according to race or ethnicity in the Northern Manhattan Stroke Study (NOMASS). (From Sacco RL, Boden-Albala B, Gan R, et al: Stroke incidence among whites, blacks and Hispanics from the same community of Northern Manhattan. *Am J Epidemiol* 147:260, 1998.)

prevalence of hypertension and diabetes and a lower socioeconomic status. They appear to explain only a fraction of this excess.[24] It is possible that elevated blood pressure and insulin resistance/diabetes affect black people more strongly, which suggests a genetic influence or susceptibility. It is also possible that black people do not comply with treatment of hypertension and diabetes as well as more affluent segments of society. A more complete understanding of the mechanisms underlying the race/ethnic differences in stroke subtype will likely depend on advances in genomics. These discoveries may point the way to more focused and, therefore, more effective treatment programs for persons with specific subtypes in specific race/ethnic groups.

Risk Factors for Stroke

It has been shown that risk factors differ between hemorrhagic and ischemic stroke and that the relative impact of risk factors operative in all ischemic stroke subtypes varies among its subtypes.[25] Identification of risk factors for stroke, awareness of the relative importance of each, and awareness of their interaction should facilitate stroke prevention. Because the pathogenetic process underlying the various stroke types differs, it is reasonable to expect that risk factors for infarction differ from risk factors for hemorrhage. Furthermore, precursors of intraparenchymatous bleeding are likely to differ from those for SAH. Risk factors for stroke from atherosclerosis of the carotid and vertebral arteries may well differ in their impact when compared with risk factors for stroke resulting from lacunar infarction. Precursors of embolic stroke are also likely to be different. Nevertheless, certain predisposing factors, particularly elevated blood pressure, are common to most stroke types.

Atherogenic Host Factors

The importance of the major atherogenic risk factors was assessed utilizing data from Framingham and other prospective epidemiologic studies. These risk factors include elevated blood pressure, blood lipid levels, diabetes, fibrinogen and other clotting factors, obesity, cardiac diseases (i.e., CHD, congestive heart failure [CHF], AF, left ventricular hypertrophy, and echocardiographic abnormalities), race, family history, and several recently recognized factors such as homocysteine levels and indices of inflammation.

Hypertension

Hypertension is the principal risk factor for ischemic stroke as well as for IH. Hypertension also predisposes to cardiac stroke precursors (notably MI and AF) that promote cerebral embolism. Elevated blood pressure also operates to increase the risk of SAH from aneurysm. Thus hypertension has the unique role of being a main risk factor for most types of stroke.

Hypertension and the risk of stroke. About 77% of people who have a first stroke, about 69% who have a first heart attack, and about 74% who have heart failure have blood pressures higher than 140/90 mm Hg (National Heart, Lung and Blood Institute unpublished estimates from Atherosclerosis Risk in Communities [ARIC], Cardiovascular Health Study, and Framingham Heart Study cohort and offspring studies). People with systolic blood pressures of 160 mm Hg or higher and/or diastolic blood pressures of 95 mm Hg or higher have a relative risk (RR) of stroke about 4 times greater than for those with normal blood pressures.[26] Hypertension is a powerful contributor to ABI in both sexes at all ages, including persons 75 to 84 years of age. It has been found to make a powerful and significant independent contribution to incidence of ABI even after age and other pertinent risk factors had been taken into account (Fig. 14-3).[27] There is little support for the widely held belief of a stronger relation of hypertension to hemorrhagic than ischemic stroke.

Although hypertension increases the incidence of stroke and ABI, the level of risk is clearly related to the *height* of the blood pressure throughout its range. When the Framingham cohort subjects are classified by the Joint National Committee VI systolic blood pressure categories, it is clear that the incidence of stroke increases with increasing blood pressure levels (see Fig. 14-3). However, more initial stroke events—hemorrhage as well as infarction—occurred in persons with mild hypertension (systolic blood pressure, 140 to 159 mm Hg) than in any other group (see Fig. 14-3). In fact, approximately half of the initial stroke events in Framingham occurred in subjects with pressures in the high normal (systolic pressure, 130 to 139 mm Hg) or in the mild hypertension categories (Fig. 14-4). On the basis of a combined analysis of nine major prospective (observational) studies of 420,000 individuals, a graded relationship between diastolic pressure and stroke and CHD incidence was apparent.[28]

Traditionally, greater importance has been ascribed to the diastolic than the systolic pressure level, and although most clinical trials of hypertension treatment have classified subjects by the diastolic level, evidence for the

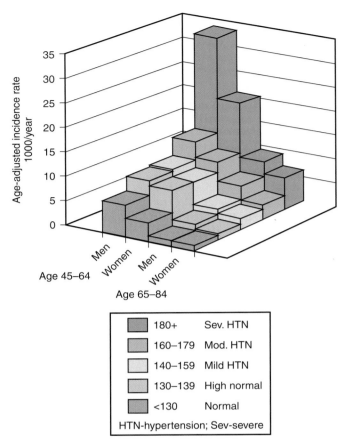

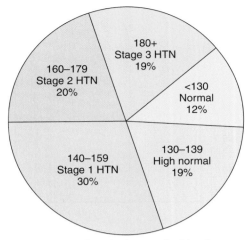

Figure 14-4 Percent of stroke by systolic blood pressure in subjects 45 to 64 years of age, the Framingham Study. (From Wolf PA: Cerebrovascular risk. In Izzo JL, Black HR, editors: *Hypertension primer, the essentials of high blood pressure*, ed 3, Philadelphia, 2003, Lippincott Williams & Wilkins, pp 239-242.)

Figure 14-3 Incidence of stroke and systolic blood pressure level according to Joint National Committee VI categories; 50-year follow-up for the Framingham Study. (From Wolf PA: Cerebrovascular risk. In Izzo JL, Black HR, editors: *Hypertension primer, the essentials of high blood pressure*, ed 3, Philadelphia, 2003, Lippincott Williams & Wilkins, pp 239-242.)

ascendancy of diastolic blood pressure over systolic is lacking. The opposite is probably true. With advancing age, systolic blood pressure continues to rise into the eighth decade, whereas diastolic pressures decline after reaching a plateau in the early 50s. Systolic blood pressure level is clearly directly related to risk of stroke, particularly after age 65 years.

Isolated systolic hypertension. In the elderly, isolated systolic hypertension (≥160/<90 mm Hg) becomes highly prevalent, affecting approximately 25% of persons older than 80 years. In Framingham, elderly subjects (65 to 84 years of age) with isolated systolic hypertension had a high risk of stroke; the risk was doubled for men and increased by 1.5-fold for women. Antihypertensive therapy in the very elderly (i.e., persons 80 years or older) was beneficial: a 30% reduction in fatal and nonfatal strokes was seen after 2 years. This was associated with a 21% reduction in the rate of death from any cause, a 23% reduction in the rate of death from cardiovascular causes, and a 64% reduction in the rate of heart failure. Further, significantly fewer serious adverse events were reported in the active treatment group.[29] This study of 3845 very elderly patients should finally and incontrovertibly dispel the long-held belief that reducing blood pressure,

particularly isolated systolic hypertension, in the elderly would precipitate stroke.

Long-term blood pressure and risk of stroke. Blood pressure stroke risk predictions are generally based on the measurement of current blood pressure. Clearly, the duration of the blood pressure elevation, as well as its height and other host factors, contributes to its cardiovascular risk. When 50 years of blood pressure data from the Framingham Study is used, it is evident that elevated midlife blood pressure during the prior 10 years increases the RR of stroke by 1.7-fold per standard deviation increment in women and by 1.9-fold per standard deviation increment in men at age 60 years.[30] Similar increases in RR by elevated antecedent pressures were also seen at age 70. These data confirm clinical experience as well as prior prospective epidemiologic data that, at any level of pressure, persons with evidence of prior elevated blood pressure such as left ventricular hypertrophy by electrocardiography or increased left ventricular mass (LVM) on echocardiography are at increased risk of stroke.

Blood Lipids

With increasing levels of total serum cholesterol, there is a steady increase in incidence of CHD in both sexes that declines with advancing age but persists after accounting for other risk factors. However, for stroke generally and for nonembolic ischemic stroke in particular, there is no clear or consistent relationship of their incidence to antecedent blood lipid levels. A recent report from the ARIC study found only weak and inconsistent associations between ischemic stroke and each of five lipid factors in the 305 subjects who had ischemic stroke after 10 years of prospective investigation.[31] The authors noted that the lack of relationship of these lipid factors to ischemic stroke is at odds with their well-known association with CHD.[31] These findings have been corroborated by analyses utilizing the Framingham Heart Study and Cardiovascular Health Study.[32] Furthermore, in a meta-analysis of 45 prospective epidemiologic studies comprising 450,000

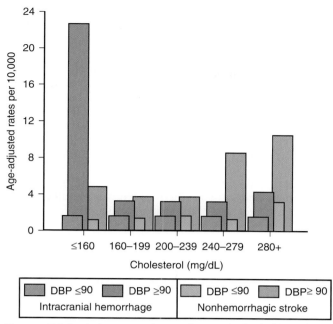

Figure 14-5 Ischemic stroke and intracerebral hemorrhage death rates in men with normal and elevated diastolic blood pressure (DBP) according to screening serum cholesterol level. (From Wolf PA, Cobb JL, D'Agostino RB: Epidemiology of stroke. In Barnett HJM, Mohr JP, Stein BM, Yatsu FM, editors: *Stroke: Pathophysiology, diagnosis, and management*, ed 2, New York, 1992, Churchill Livingstone, p 16.)

subjects among whom 13,000 strokes occurred, no significant association between total serum cholesterol level and total stroke incidence was seen.[33] Possible exceptions are the Honolulu Heart Study of Hawaiian men of Japanese ancestry and the Multiple Risk Factor Intervention Trial (MRFIT) screenees.[34] In Honolulu, the level of total cholesterol measured years before was directly related to the incidence of thromboembolism.[35] In MRFIT, the incidence of ischemic stroke, diagnosed on death certificates, was greater in those with the highest levels of serum total cholesterol obtained 6 years before (Fig. 14-5). A meta-analysis of the older cholesterol-lowering trials showed a definite benefit in reduction in MI but no significant impact on stroke occurrence.[36]

Although the impact of blood lipids on ischemic atherothrombotic stroke differs from their relationship to coronary artery atherosclerosis, serum total cholesterol and low-density lipoprotein (LDL) cholesterol levels have been directly related to the extent of extracranial carotid artery atherosclerosis; high-density lipoprotein (HDL) cholesterol levels exert a protective effect. These relationships also apply to extracranial carotid artery wall thickness.[37-39] Pravastatin was shown to reduce carotid artery plaque progression or promoted regression in an early study. This finding has also been corroborated for other statins.[40]

In view of the lack of association of blood lipid levels to incidence of ischemic stroke, the finding of a significant reduction in stroke incidence in a series of trials of statins in patients with clinical CHD was unexpected.[41-43] The 20% to 30% magnitude of the benefit was little different from the benefit for CHD endpoints.

All of these trials enrolled CHD patients, a small percentage of whom had sustained a cerebral infarct. More recently, in the Anglo-Scandinavian Cardiac Outcomes Trial—Lipid Lowering Arm (ASCOT-LLA),[44] 19,342 high-risk hypertensive patients without CHD were randomly assigned to 10 mg atorvastatin or placebo. After 3.3 years' mean follow-up, the trial was stopped; fatal and nonfatal stroke occurred in 89 atorvastatin assignees versus 121 placebo subjects (hazards ratio [HR], 0.73; $P = 0.024$).[44] This significant benefit for stroke prevention occurred in the absence of CHD in otherwise high-risk individuals and strongly suggests an indication for statins in the *primary prevention* of ischemic stroke. The lack of benefit observed in women in the trials may reflect the small number of women enrolled (18.8% of subjects) and the limited number of events among them. It has been speculated that the statin drugs alter the lipid composition of the plaque, reduce its tendency to rupture or fissure, reduce inflammation, and improve the hemorheologic environment. Pleotropic effects of statin therapy on platelet aggregation, endothelial function, and inflammation have also been postulated as operative.

Low total serum cholesterol levels have been found to be related to an increased incidence of IH.[45] This was first noted after World War II among rural Japanese who had very low serum cholesterol levels by Western standards (i.e., <160 mg/dL).[46] As nutrition improved, intake of animal fat increased, and sodium chloride intake fell, an increase in total serum cholesterol levels was seen in this population.[46] In both sexes aged 40 to 49, the total serum cholesterol levels rose from 155 mg/dL in 1963 to 1966, to 175 mg/dL in 1972 to 1975, and to 181 mg/dL in 1980 to 1983. Total serum protein levels and relative weight also rose significantly during these 20 years, whereas systolic and diastolic blood pressures declined. Accompanying these major changes in risk factor levels were similar substantial declines in the incidence of IH, which fell 65% in men ($P < 0.05$) and 94% in women ($P < 0.001$) between 1964–1968 and 1979–1983.[46] An etiologic link has been suggested by the recent confirmation of this relationship in other Asian populations, as well as in white men in the United States. In the 350,977 men aged 35 to 57 years who were screened for entry into the MRFIT, there were 83 deaths from IH and 55 deaths from SAH after 6 years of follow-up.[34] Compared with the lowest serum cholesterol category (<160 mg/dL), the risk factor–adjusted RR of intracranial hemorrhage at all higher levels of serum cholesterol was approximately 0.32. Death rates per 10,000 were 23.07 in the lowest serum cholesterol category (<160 mg/dL) and ranged from 3.09 to 4.83 in the four higher categories.[34] The mechanism by which a very low serum cholesterol level accompanied by elevated diastolic blood pressure promotes IH has been suggested to be an alteration in the cell membranes that weakens the endothelium of intracerebral arteries. However, despite early concerns, no significant increases in IH rates have been noted in the many trials using statins to reduce total and LDL cholesterol levels.

Diabetes

Diabetic patients are known to have an increased susceptibility to coronary, femoral, and cerebral artery atherosclerosis. Up to 80% of type 2 diabetic patients will have macrovascular disease or die of it. Hypertension is common in diabetic patients, affecting approximately 60%. Surveys of stroke patients and prospective investigations have confirmed the increased risk of stroke in diabetic patients. The Honolulu Heart Program found that increasing degrees of glucose intolerance conferred an increasing risk of thromboembolic stroke that was independent of other risk factors but found no relationship to hemorrhagic stroke (Fig. 14-6).[47] Evaluation of the impact of diabetes on stroke in a population-based cohort in Rancho Bernardo disclosed an RR of stroke that was 1.8 in men and 2.2 in women, even after adjustment for the effect of other pertinent risk factors.[48]

In the Framingham Study, peripheral artery disease with intermittent claudication occurs more than 4 times as often in diabetic patients; the coronary and cerebral arteries are also affected but to a lesser extent.[49] For ABI, the impact of indicators of diabetes (i.e., physician-diagnosed diabetes, glycosuria, or a blood sugar level more than 150 mg/100 mL) was significant as an independent contributor to incidence only in older women. However, later follow-up indicated that both men and women with glucose intolerance at all ages have approximately double the risk of ABI of those without diabetes.[50]

Because it has been shown that persons on their way to developing diabetes are at twofold increased risk compared with persons without diabetes, interest is now focusing on the prediabetic insulin resistant state. The Framingham Study found that the metabolic syndrome, an indicator of insulin resistance, carries a substantial risk of stroke.[50] Stroke risk was examined in men and women in relation to the metabolic syndrome alone, diabetes alone, and the presence of both. Over 14 years of follow-up, 75 men and 55 women had a first stroke; all but four events were ischemic. The RR of stroke in persons with both diabetes and metabolic syndrome (RR, 3.28; CI, 1.82-5.92) was higher than that for either condition alone (metabolic syndrome alone: RR, 2.10; CI, 1.37-3.22; diabetes alone: RR, 2.47; CI, 1.31-4.65). The population-attributable risk, because of its greater prevalence, was greater for metabolic syndrome alone than for diabetes alone (19% versus 7%), particularly in women (27% versus 5%). Thus, the metabolic syndrome is more prevalent than diabetes and a significant independent risk factor for stroke in people without diabetes. Prevention and control of the metabolic syndrome and its components, particularly the frequently associated hypertension, are likely to reduce stroke incidence (Fig. 14-7).

Obesity

Obese persons have higher levels of blood pressure, blood glucose, and atherogenic serum lipids; on that account alone, they would be expected to have an increased risk of stroke. Obesity (relative weight ≥30% above the median) was a significant independent contributor to ABI incidence in younger men and older women in the Framingham original cohort. However, in all age groups and in both sexes, obesity exerts an adverse influence on health status that is probably mediated through elevated blood pressure, impaired glucose tolerance, insulin resistance, and other mechanisms. However, in the Honolulu Heart Study, obesity was a risk factor for stroke that was independent of associated hypertension, glucose intolerance, and other covariates. In the Nurses Health Study, the incidence of stroke increased directly with body mass index

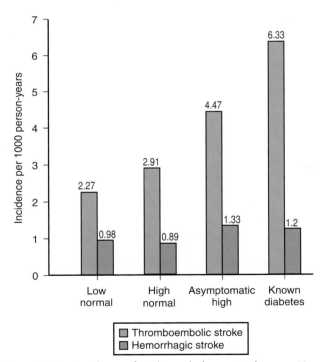

Figure 14-6 Incidence of stroke and glucose intolerance. Honolulu Heart Study; 22-year follow-up. (From Burchfiel CM, Curb JD, Rodriguez BL, et al: Glucose intolerance and 22-year stroke incidence. The Honolulu Heart Program. *Stroke* 25:951-957, 1994.)

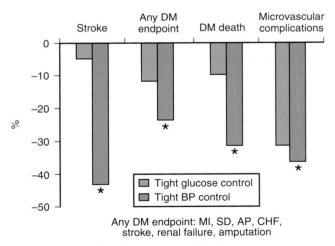

Figure 14-7 Effect of tight glucose control versus tight blood pressure control on cardiovascular disease outcomes in diabetic patients (United Kingdom Prospective Diabetes Study). (From United Kingdom Prospective Diabetes Study Group: Tight blood pressure control and risk of macrovascular and microvascular complication in type 2 diabetes: UKPDS 38. *BMJ* 317:703-713, 1998; and United Kingdom Prospective Diabetes Study Group: Efficacy of atenolol and captopril in reducing risk of macrovascular and microvascular complication in type 2 diabetes: UKPDS 39. *BMJ* 317:713-720, 1998.)

in women aged 30 to 55 years after adjustment for other risk factors, but no such relationship was seen in men aged 40 to 75 years, comprising the Health Professionals Follow-up Study. Abdominal or central obesity seems more closely related to adverse cardiovascular outcomes including stroke than overall elevated body mass index. In 28,643 male health professionals, the RR of stroke was significantly greater (RR, 2.33; 95% CI, 1.25–4.37) in those men with a waist to hip ratio in the uppermost quintile. Obesity as reflected in the body mass index was less strongly related than waist circumference was to stroke incidence, likely as a result of its closer relationship to insulin resistance.[51]

Family History of Stroke

Although family history of stroke is widely perceived to be an important marker of increased stroke risk, confirmation by epidemiologic study has, until recently, been lacking. Maternal history of death from stroke was significantly related to stroke incidence in a cohort of Swedish men born in 1913.[52] Maternal history of fatal stroke was independently related to stroke incidence in offspring, even after other significant risk factors such as hypertension, abdominal pattern of obesity, and fibrinogen level were taken into account.

In a study of familial predisposition to stroke in Framingham, there was no relationship between a *history* of stroke *death* in parents and documented stroke in subjects. However, definite nonfatal and fatal strokes in these cohort parents as determined by examination and systematic case review over decades were related to the observed *occurrence* of stroke in their children (members of the Framingham Offspring Study cohort). In these analyses, both maternal and paternal strokes by age 65 years were associated with approximately a 3.0-fold increased risk of stroke by age 65 years in their children, even after other risk factors were taken into account.[53]

These relationships were true for maternal and paternal strokes, total strokes, and ischemic stroke subtypes. This hereditability strongly suggests a genetic propensity to stroke in addition to or in combination with environmental factors (see Chapter 18; Stroke Genetics).

Fibrinogen, Clotting Factors, and Inflammation

An elevated fibrinogen level has been implicated in atherogenesis and in arterial thrombus formation. A number of epidemiologic studies have found a significant independent increase in cardiovascular disease incidence, including stroke, in relation to fibrinogen level. In a prospective study of 54-year-old Swedish men, fibrinogen level in combination with elevated systolic blood pressure was found to be a potent risk factor for stroke.[54] Level of fibrinogen, measured on the tenth biennial examination in Framingham, was also significantly related to incidence of cardiovascular disease, including stroke.[55]

However, fibrinogen is associated with many other risk factors for stroke including age, hypertension, hematocrit level, obesity, and diabetes.[56-58] Fibrinogen is also an acute-phase reactant to inflammation, so it seems likely that the atherogenic and procoagulant effects of inflammation reflected by elevated fibrinogen levels are responsible for its association with cardiovascular disease incidence, including stroke. In the Framingham original cohort, CRP level was found to be an independent risk marker for stroke and TIA incidence over 14 years of follow-up. For men, those with CRP levels in the upper quartile had double the risk of stroke and TIA of men in the bottom quartile; for women, risk in the CRP upper quintile was increased nearly threefold after other pertinent risk factors were taken into account.[59] CRP was also a potent independent risk marker for cardiovascular disease in the Women's Health Study and was said to be a stronger predictor than the LDL cholesterol level, making an independent contribution to cardiovascular disease risk prediction beyond that provided by the Framingham risk score.[60]

Blood Homocysteine Levels

In a number of cross-sectional studies and case-control studies and in a meta-analysis, elevated levels of plasma homocysteine (tHcy) were found to be associated with a higher incidence of CHD (OR, 1.6 per 5 µmol/L tHcy) and an increased incidence of stroke (OR, 1.5 per 5 µmol/L tHcy).[61] Level of tHcy is also directly related to many of the major components of the cardiovascular risk profile: male sex, increasing age, cigarette smoking, increased blood pressure, elevated blood cholesterol level, and lack of exercise.[62] However, even after adjustment for these factors, the risk of stroke was independently related to nonfasting tHcy level in the original Framingham cohort after 9.9 years of follow-up: the RR of 1.82 (CI, 1.14–2.91) was in quartile 4 compared with quartile 1, and a significant linear trend was seen across the quartiles (P < 0.001). A nested case-control study within the British Regional Heart Study cohort found a powerful and independent relationship between nonfasting tHcy level and stroke incidence. There was a graded increase in risk with increasing quartile levels of tHcy (Fig. 14-8) from an OR of 1.2 (<10.3 µmol/L) to 4.7 (≈15.4 µmol/L) in successive quartiles of tHcy (P = 0.03 for trend). Risk in the uppermost

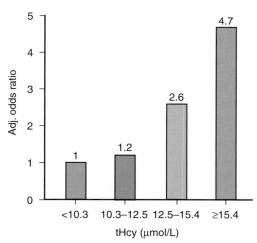

Figure 14-8 Homocysteine level and stroke risk in men; a case-control study. (From Wolf PA: Epidemiology and risk factor management. In Welch M, Caplan LR, Reis DJ, et al, editors: *Primer on cerebrovascular disease*, San Diego, 1997, Academic Press, pp 751-757.)

quartile was 4.7-fold greater than in the lowest quartile. This graded response with no threshold occurred after adjustment for serum creatinine level (associated with increased tHcy levels), age, social class, blood pressure, and other pertinent risk factors.[63]

However, in other large population studies (i.e., the ARIC study, Physicians Health Study, the Finnish Study, and MRFIT) no statistically significant relationship was found.[64,65] The ARIC study noted a strong independent relationship between fasting plasma tHcy concentrations and carotid artery intimal-medial wall thickening.[66] Increased levels of fasting plasma tHcy were also related to ultrasound-assessed extracranial common carotid artery stenosis of more than 25% in the Framingham cohort.[67] tHcy levels are inversely related to levels of dietary and plasma folic acid and vitamins B_{12} and B_6, which indicates a remedy for elevated tHcy levels.[67,68] The *fasting* tHcy level may miss persons with impaired tHcy metabolism because, in response to a methionine challenge, approximately 40% of persons with elevated tHcy levels, who are thought to be at increased cardiovascular risk, have normal fasting levels. Furthermore, tHcy level is like other physiologic measures such as blood pressure or serum cholesterol level in that it is a graded and continuous risk variable without clear threshold effect. Nevertheless, a number of large-scale clinical trials in stroke survivors have not demonstrated a beneficial effect of folate (with B_6 and B_{12}) supplementation on risk of stroke recurrence.[69] Supplementation did reduce the level of tHcy in the serum but did not result in lower rates of stroke or cardiovascular disease. The explanation for this puzzling finding includes current universal supplementation of grains and cereals with folate and a relationship to level of vitamin B_{12}, among others.[70]

Heart Disease and Impaired Cardiac Function

Cardiac diseases and impaired cardiac function predispose to stroke. Although hypertension is the preeminent risk factor for strokes of all types, at each blood pressure level, persons with impaired cardiac function have a significantly increased stroke risk.[71] The prevalence of these cardiac contributors to stroke increases with age (Fig. 14-9). After 36 years of follow-up, the prevalence of cardiovascular disease among stroke cases in the Framingham Study was found to be high: 80.8% had hypertension; 32.7% had prior CHD; 14.5% had prior heart failure; 14.5% had AF; and only 13.6% had none of these. Cardiac disease is an important precursor of stroke and is also dealt with in detail in several other chapters.

Coronary Heart Disease

In Framingham, CHD was ascertained prospectively on biennial examination as well as by monitoring of hospitalizations. It predisposes to stroke as a source for embolism from the heart; by virtue of shared risk factors; as an untoward effect of medical and surgical treatments for coronary atherosclerotic disease; and, less commonly, as a consequence of pump failure. In the 2-week period after an acute MI, stroke occurs at an estimated rate of 0.7% to 4.7%.[72] As expected, older age and ventricular dysfunction (decreased ejection fraction) after MI increases

stroke risk.[72] Treatment with aspirin and, particularly, with warfarin anticoagulation decreased the incidence of stroke in a large group of MI survivors, which is consistent with an embolic mechanism.[72,73] Stroke occurs most frequently after *anterior* wall MI (2% to 6% of cases). The mechanism is cerebral embolism principally from a left ventricular mural thrombus, which is demonstrable on echocardiographic studies in 40% of cases. Inferior wall MI is an infrequent basis for mural thrombus or stroke. Often, however, the mechanism of stroke in persons with CHD is less apparent. Persons with uncomplicated angina pectoris, non–Q wave infarction, and clinically silent MI also have an increased incidence of ischemic stroke. Recent data from Framingham suggest that silent or unrecognized MI survivors had a 10-year incidence of stroke of 17.8% in men and 17.3% in women, which is an incidence not that much less than the 19.5% in men and 29.3% in women seen after recognized MI.

Peripheral Artery Disease

The presence of peripheral artery disease often denotes widespread atherosclerotic vascular disease. In the Framingham study, 20% of persons 75 years or older had a low ankle brachial index denoting compromised peripheral arterial circulation. Among these, only 18% reported symptoms of intermittent claudication. In those with a low ankle brachial index, cardiovascular disease was present in 50%, among whom 15% had experienced a stroke.

During 4 years of follow-up, 13% of those with a low ankle brachial index had a stroke or TIA, which

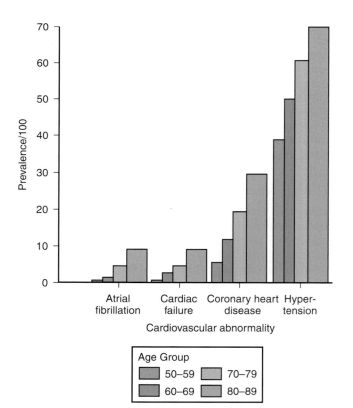

Figure 14-9 Prevalence of cardiovascular abnormality with increasing age, men and women combined; 34-year follow-up. Data from the Framingham Heart Study.

represented a twofold excess risk, and there was an increasing stroke hazard as the ankle brachial index decreased.[26]

As with peripheral arterial disease, persons with a low (<0.9) ankle brachial index have a high prevalence of associated cardiovascular disease, including stroke and CHD. The prevalence of these conditions increases inversely with the ankle brachial index (see Fig. 14-1). A low ankle brachial index was shown to be associated with a 2.2-fold increase in risk of a stroke, even after adjustment for associated cardiovascular risk factors.[74]

Atrial Fibrillation

It has long been acknowledged that AF in association with rheumatic heart disease and mitral stenosis predisposes to stroke. Chronic AF without valvular heart disease, which was previously considered to be innocuous, has since been shown to be associated with approximately a fivefold increase in stroke incidence. This is ominous because AF is also the most prevalent persistent cardiac arrhythmia in the elderly. In the Framingham Study, AF incidence has more than doubled in successive decades of follow-up. The incidence rises sharply with age from 0.2 per 1000 for ages 30 to 39 to 39.0 per 1000 for ages 80 to 89 years. AF is particularly important in the elderly because the proportion of total strokes associated with this arrhythmia increases steeply with age, reaching 36.2% for ages 80 to 89 years.[75] Although the prevalence of other cardiac contributors to stroke also increases with age, the increased incidence of stroke in persons with AF is more likely to be a consequence of the AF and not the associated CHD or CHF. This becomes apparent when age trends in AF risk of stroke are examined (Fig. 14-10).

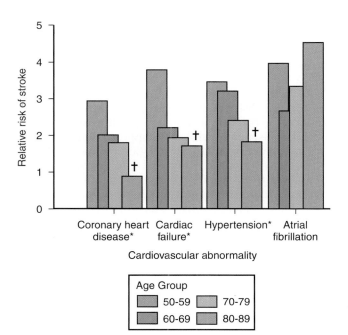

Figure 14-10 Estimated relative risk of stroke with advancing age according to the presence of coronary heart disease, cardiac failure, hypertension, and atrial fibrillation; 34-year follow-up. Data from the Framingham Heart Study. *Significant inverse trend for age (P < 0.05); †no significant excess of strokes.

Whereas risk of stroke attributable to AF increases with age, risk of stroke attributable to cardiac failure, CHD, and hypertension declines with age.[75] Notably, in the oldest age group, 80 to 89 years, the percent of stroke attributable to AF was 23.5%, which approaches that of hypertension (33.4%), a far more prevalent disorder. A dispute as to whether AF is an independent risk factor or merely a risk marker for other conditions predisposing to stroke raged for several years.[76,77] This issue has been settled by the remarkable concordance of a half dozen randomized clinical trials demonstrating a 68% stroke risk reduction after treatment with warfarin; treatment efficacy was more than 80%.[78,79]

A landmark study of untreated AF in 1983 by Sage et al provides insight on the gravity of the condition. AF is present in 24.6% of patients with ischemic stroke. These strokes with AF are more often in women, 80 years of age or older, and more often associated with coronary or peripheral artery disease. Recurrent strokes are frequent, occurring at a rate of 20% per year regardless of age, sex, previous MI, or whether the AF is chronic or intermittent. AF strokes are major strokes that have a high (32.5%) 30-day case fatality rate and a 1-year mortality rate of 49.5%. They are also associated with a higher stroke recurrence rate within the first year (6.6% versus 4.4%). They tend to be severe or moderately severe strokes.[80,81]

Much of the morbidity associated with AF is attributable to the fivefold increased risk of stroke that it imposes. However, the risk is variable, which has stimulated numerous investigations designed to define clinical criteria useful for classifying AF persons at high or low risk of stroke or excess mortality.[78,82-85] From a pooled analysis of five primary prevention trials, four risk factors were shown to increase AF stroke risk: increasing age, diabetes, hypertension, or a history of prior stroke or TIA.[78]

Such risk stratification is important for prognostication and the selection of candidates for anticoagulant therapy.[86] Most of the existing risk assessment tools for AF are derived from controlled trials containing more men than women and younger, healthier subjects than are encountered in the community. Management of AF needs to take into account the absolute risk of adverse outcomes because the therapy has potential hazards. The Framingham Study has provided a risk assessment profile that gives a more specific estimate of risk of stroke alone and stroke or death.[87]

Five-year risk of stroke or death varies over a wide range in relation to the cluster of accompanying independent risk factors identified in the Framingham cohort.[87] This suggests that risk assessment with the use of the risk factors specified could identify AF patients at low risk of stroke (e.g., 10% over 5 years) who may not achieve additional benefit from warfarin compared with aspirin and whose stroke risk may not exceed their risk of serious bleeding from warfarin therapy.[88] The Framingham Study has crafted a risk profile based on five independent predictors (i.e., age, sex, systolic blood pressure, diabetes status, and presence of prior stroke or TIA) (Table 14-3). Using this scoring scheme, one can estimate the 5-year conditional probability of a stroke in persons with AF.

Others have also identified risk factors for ischemic stroke and systemic embolism based on a collaborative analysis of five untreated control groups in primary prevention trials. Patients with AF in these trials had about a sixfold increased risk of thromboembolism compared with patients in sinus rhythm. Persons with a previous stroke or TIA had a 2.5-fold RR of stroke or systemic embolism, those with diabetes had a 1.7-fold risk, those with hypertension had a 1.6-fold risk, and those with heart failure had a 1.4-fold risk. Each decade increment of age was associated with a 1.4-fold risk.[78]

Cardiac Failure

AF and CHF frequently occur together, but there has been limited information regarding their temporal relations and the combined influence of these conditions on mortality. The Framingham Study investigators studied participants with new-onset AF or CHF using multivariable Cox proportional hazards models with time-dependent variables to evaluate whether mortality after AF or CHF was affected by the occurrence and timing of the other condition. HRs were adjusted for time period and cardiovascular risk factors. During the study period, 1470 participants developed AF, CHF, or both. Among 382 individuals with

both conditions, 38% had AF first, 41% had CHF first, and 21% had both diagnosed on the same day. The incidence of CHF among AF subjects was 33 per 1000 person-years, and the incidence of AF among CHF subjects was 54 per 1000 person-years. In AF subjects, the subsequent development of CHF was associated with increased mortality (men: HR, 2.7; 95% CI, 1.9–3.7; women: HR, 3.1; 95% CI, 2.2–4.2). Similarly, in CHF subjects, later development of AF was associated with increased mortality (men: HR, 1.6; 95% CI, 1.2–2.1; women: HR, 2.7; 95% CI, 2.0–3.6). Preexisting CHF adversely affected survival in individuals with AF, but preexisting AF was not associated with adverse chance of survival in those with CHF. Individuals with either AF or CHF who subsequently develop the other condition have a poor prognosis. Additional studies addressing the pathogenesis, prevention, and optimal management of the joint occurrence of AF and CHF appear warranted.[89]

Left Ventricular Hypertrophy

Left ventricular hypertrophy by electrocardiography increases in prevalence with age and blood pressure and the risk of ABI increases more than fourfold in men and sixfold in women with this electrocardiographic abnormality. The increased risk conferred persists even after the influence of age and other atherogenic precursors, including systolic blood pressure, are taken into account. The more sensitive and precise measure of cardiac hypertrophy, LVM, on echocardiography is also directly related to the incidence of stroke.[90] The estimated HR for stroke and TIA, when the uppermost quartile of LVM-to-height ratio is compared with the lowest, is 2.72 after adjustment for age, gender, and cardiovascular risk factors. There is a graded response with an HR of 1.45 for each quartile increment of LVM-to-height ratio. Clearly, echocardiography gives prognostic information beyond that provided by traditional risk factors.

Other Host Factors

Migraine

From clinical observations, case reports, and clinical series the notion evolved that migraine predisposes to stroke, particularly ischemic stroke. Complicated migraine with aura and migraine with neurologic concomitants seem to be the types most likely to be followed by stroke. Examples of the association between migraine and stroke occur in certain uncommon syndromes and instances. In cerebral autosomal dominant arteriopathy with subcortical infarcts and leukoencephalopathy, migraine headache is associated with white matter disease, dementia, and subcortical strokes.[91] Another migraine syndrome with increased stroke risk is said to occur in the antiphospholipid antibody syndrome.[91] Atypical migraine syndromes such as hemiplegic migraine are also associated with stroke but are quite rare.[92]

The relationship of stroke to the common migraine syndromes encompassing migraine with aura and migraine without aura has been investigated in two large case-control studies, the Italian National Research Council Study Group on Stroke in the Young and a substudy of the World Health Organization Collaborative Study of

TABLE 14-3 MULTIVARIABLE RISK ESTIMATION OF STROKE IN ATRIAL FIBRILLATION: FRAMINGHAM STUDY COHORTS—PREDICTED 5-YEAR RISK OF STROKE

	Points*	Total Points	5-Year Risk (%)
Age (years)		0–1	5
50-59	0	2-3	6
60-62	1	4	7
63-66	2	5	8
67-71	3	6–7	9
72-74	4	8	11
75-77	5	9	12
78-81	6	10	13
82-85	7	11	14
86-90	8	12	16
91-93	9	13	18
>93	10	14	19
Diabetes		15	21
No	0	16	24
Yes	5	17	26
Prior stroke or TIA		18	28
No	0	19	31
Yes	6	20	34
Systolic BP (mm Hg)		21	37
<120	0	22	41
120-139	1	23	44
140-159	2	24	48
160-179	3	25	51
>179	4	26	55
Sex		27	59
Male	0	28	63
Female	6	29	67
		30	71
		31	75

*Add points to determine the 5-year risk of stroke as indicated in the total point score.

Cardiovascular Disease and Steroid Hormone Contraception.[93] Migraine as a predisposing factor for stroke was also investigated in the Physicians Health Study. Migraine was associated with an increased risk of ischemic stroke in these aforementioned studies, and RRs or ORs ranged from 2.0 to 3.8.[92] The studies that distinguished between migraine with or without aura usually detected a higher risk for migraine with aura. The contribution of migraine to stroke risk decreases with increasing age.

Environmental Factors

Cigarette Smoking

Cigarette smoking, a powerful risk factor for MI and sudden death, has been clearly linked to brain infarction, as well as to IH and SAH.[94,95] A similar relationship between cigarette smoking and stroke has been seen in Hawaiian Japanese men after 10 years of follow-up in the Honolulu Heart Study, in which cigarette smoking made a significant independent contribution to cerebral infarction and intracranial hemorrhage risk.[96]

In the late 1970s, several studies of oral contraceptives (OCs) and stroke in young women identified cigarette smoking as an important risk factor. Surprisingly, the association between cigarette smoking, oral contraceptives, and stroke was primarily related to SAH. In the Royal College of General Practitioners Study of oral contraceptive use, the increased risk of SAH occurred principally in women older than 35 years, who were current or former OC users, and who smoked cigarettes.[97] In the Nurses' Health Study, a cohort of nearly 120,000 women were followed up prospectively for 8 years for the development of stroke. There was an increased risk of SAH as well as thrombotic stroke in cigarette smokers. The RR of SAH showed a dose–response relationship from fourfold in light smokers to 9.8-fold in smokers of 25 or more cigarettes daily.[97] Of note, in each smoking category the RR of SAH, regardless of whether other associated risk factors were taken into account, was twice as great as for thromboembolic stroke (Table 14-4).

The association between cigarette smoking and SAH from aneurysm was also found in men (as well as women) in Framingham[98] and in New Zealand[99] in case-control analyses. In a case-control study of 114 patients with SAH in a defined region in Finland, cigarette smoking was significantly more prevalent in case patients than in control subjects matched for age, sex, and domicile.[100] The RR of SAH in smokers, as compared with nonsmokers, was 2.7 in men and 3.0 in women. The authors suggested that smoking promoted a temporary increase in blood pressure, which, acting in concert with the "metastatic emphysema effect," was responsible for SAH from cerebral aneurysm. No more reasonable hypothesis has been promulgated to explain this powerful relationship.

The evidence that cigarette smoking increases the risk of thrombotic stroke and SAH is generally accepted, but the relationship of cigarette smoking to IH is less well-established. Data from the Honolulu Heart Program firmly links cigarette smoking in Hawaiian men of Japanese ancestry to stroke both "thromboembolic and hemorrhagic."[96] Risk of "hemorrhagic" stroke was significantly greater (RR, 2.5) in cigarette smokers than in nonsmokers,

and this excess risk persisted at an RR of 2.8, even after adjustment for the other associated risk factors of age, diastolic blood pressure, serum cholesterol level, alcohol consumption, hematocrit, and body mass index.

A meta-analysis of 32 separate studies, including those already cited, indicates that cigarette smoking *is* a significant independent contributor to stroke incidence in both sexes at all ages and is associated with about a 50% increased risk overall when compared with the risk seen for nonsmokers.[101] The risk of stroke generally and of ABI specifically rises as the number of cigarettes smoked per day increases, in both men and women.

Based on data from Framingham and the Nurses' Health Study it is clear that stroke risk in cigarette smokers is reduced by about 60% by stopping.[79,94] This reduction in risk occurs in a remarkably short time and is similar to the reduction in CHD risk, which decreases by approximately 50% within 1 year of smoking cessation and reaches the level of those who never smoked within 5 years. In men and women in the Framingham Study, risk of stroke in former cigarette smokers did not differ from that of persons who never smoked by the end of 5 years. There was no interaction with age, which suggests that cigarette smoking exerted a precipitating effect on stroke regardless of age or duration of smoking. Similar findings from the Nurses' Health Study show a sizable reduction of risk within 2 years (a reduction to an RR of 0.4) and the same risk as for women who never smoked (Fig. 14-11).[94] Because smoking confers an increase in stroke risk of 40% in men and 60% in women after all other pertinent risk factors have been taken into account, smoking cessation deserves a high priority as it may be expected to significantly reduce the risk of stroke.

Oral Contraceptives

In the 1970s, risk of stroke was found to be increased fivefold in women using OCs. This increased risk was most marked in women older than 35 years and was seen predominantly in those with other cardiovascular risk factors, particularly hypertension and cigarette smoking.[102] The RR of stroke was seen in OC users and former users, and the risk was concentrated in cigarette smokers older than 35 years. However, the mechanism of stroke in OC users is unclear. Their cerebral infarctions are more likely to be due to thrombotic disease than to atherosclerosis; it is known that clotting is enhanced by the OC-induced increased platelet aggregability and by its alteration of clotting factors to favor thrombogenesis. In young women with unexplained ischemic stroke, use of OCs is presumed to be the cause of the infarct; however, the stroke was attributed to OC use in no more than 10% of a series of carefully studied patients.[103]

There was no increase in stroke or other cardiovascular disease among former users of OCs in the Nurses' Health Study.[104] An international ischemic stroke and OC study assessed risk of stroke in women in Europe and in less developed countries.[105] Risk of stroke was increased for OC users (OR, 2.99; 95% CI, 1.65–5.40) and was lowest in younger nonsmokers without elevated blood pressure. Women with hypertension had an OR of 10.7 (95% CI, 2.04–56.6). In Europe, with current use of low-dose OCs (<50 μg estrogen), the OR was 1.53 (95% CI 0.71–3.31).[105]

TABLE 14-4 AGE-ADJUSTED RELATIVE RISKS OF STROKE (FATAL AND NONFATAL COMBINED), BY DAILY NUMBER OF CIGARETTES CONSUMED AMONG CURRENT SMOKERS

Event	Never Smoked	Former Smoker	Current Smoker	No. of Cigarettes Smoked per Day among Current Smokers			
				1–14	**15–24**	**25–34**	**35 or More**
Total stroke	1.00	1.35 (0.98–1.85)	2.73 (2.18–3.41)	2.02 (1.29–3.14)	3.34 (2.38–4.70)	3.08 (1.94–4.87)	4.48 (2.78–7.23)
Subarach-noid hem-orrhage	1.00	2.26 (1.16–4.42)	4.85 (2.90–8.11)	4.28 (1.88–9.77)	4.02 (1.90–8.54)	7.95 (3.50–18.07)	10.22 (4.03–25.94)
Ischemic stroke	1.00	1.27 (0.85–1.89)	2.53 (1.91–3.35)	1.83 (1.04–3.23)	3.57 (2.36–5.42)	2.73 (1.49–5.03)	3.97 (2.09–7.53)
Cerebral hemor-rhage	1.00	1.24 (0.64–2.42)	1.24 (0.64–2.42)	1.68 (0.34–5.28)	2.53 (0.71–6.05)	1.41 (0.39–5.05)	

Numbers in parentheses are 95% confidence intervals.
Relative risk: Adjusted for age in 5-year intervals, follow-up period (1976–1978, 1978–1980, 1980–1982, 1982–1984, 1984–1986, or 1986–1988), history of hypertension, diabetes, high cholesterol levels, body mass index, past use of oral contraceptives, postmenopausal estrogen therapy, and age at starting smoking.
Adapted with permission from Kawachi I, Colditz GA, Stampfer MJ: Smoking cessation and decreased risk of stroke in women. *JAMA* 269:233, 1993, Table 1.

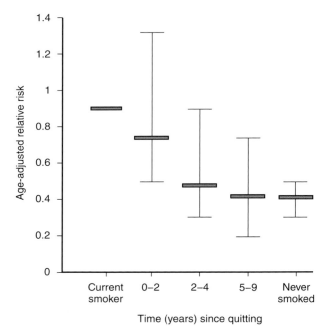

Figure 14-11 Smoking cessation and risk of stroke in women. (From Kawachi I, Colditz GA, Stampfer MJ, et al: Smoking cessation and decreased risk of stroke in women. *JAMA* 269:232-236, 1993.)

In the United States, a population-based case-control study from California Kaiser Permanente Medical Care Program was conducted of OC use in women with stroke in which the OC preparations contained the current low dose of estrogen.[106] Comparing current to former and never-users of OCs, the OR for ischemic stroke was 1.18 (95% CI, 0.54–2.59) after adjustment for other risk factors for stroke.[106] Thus, the risk of ischemic stroke is quite low in women of childbearing age and is definitely not increased in nonsmokers without hypertension.

A recent meta-analysis that included 16 studies published from 1960 to 1999 addressed the relationship of OC use with stroke. The overall RR of ischemic stroke across all preparations and study designs was 2.75 (95% CI, 2.24–3.38).[107] The RR in population-based studies of low-dose estrogen preparations in which adjustment was made for both smoking and hypertension was 1.93 (95% CI, 1.35–2.74). If these latter results are true, then low-dose oral contraceptive pills might lead to one stroke for every 24,000 women users, or 425 ischemic strokes in the United States each year. These results must be interpreted with caution because other studies did not find the same association between stroke and low-dose estradiol contraceptives.

With regard to SAH, of particular interest is the interaction between the older preparations of OCs (containing high doses of estrogens), cigarette smoking, and SAH. Prospective observation of more than 40,000 women, half of whom were taking OCs, showed an increased risk of fatal SAH (not cerebral infarction) in women taking OCs. The risk was increased fourfold in cigarette smokers older than 35 years, and most cases were confined to this group.[97]

The OR for hemorrhagic stroke in OC users in the California Kaiser Permanente Program study was not significantly increased.[106] There was a positive (nonsignificant) interaction for hemorrhage in current users who smoked (OR, 3.64; 95% CI, 0.95–13.87).[106] In the World Health Organization collaborative study, risk of hemorrhagic stroke was not increased in younger women and was only slightly increased in older women.[108] The bulk of these hemorrhages were subarachnoid (200 of 248 in Europe), and the risk was significantly increased in women older than 35 years. The OR for hemorrhage among current OC users older than 35 years who were current cigarette smokers was 3.91 (95% CI, 1.54–9.89).[108]

Hormone Replacement Therapy

Observational studies have either shown no influence of hormone replacement therapy (HRT) on stroke or a weak protective effect. The Women's Estrogen for Stroke Trial (WEST) of postmenopausal women randomly assigned to placebo or estradiol within 90 days of a TIA or non-disabling stroke found that after a mean 2.7-year follow-up there was no difference in the outcomes of nonfatal stroke or death.[109] This was consistent with previous findings of no protective impact of HRT on stroke incidence. However, the Women's Health Initiative randomized controlled trial, the largest trial to date that examined the issue of HRT and cardiovascular disease in 16,608 subjects randomly assigned to conjugated estrogens plus progesterone or placebo, was stopped after 5.2 years because of a global statistic that indicated that the risks of treatment exceeded the benefit. Women taking HRT had an increased risk of stroke with an RR of 1.41 (CI, 1.07–1.85).[110] Despite a large body of observational evidence supporting a preventive effect of HRT on CHD, women receiving treatment also had a significantly increased risk of CHD and stroke. Pending further evidence to the contrary, HRT increases stroke and other negative outcomes and cannot be recommended as a measure to prevent cardiovascular disease.

Alcohol Consumption

As in MI, the impact of alcohol consumption on stroke risk is related to the amount of alcohol consumed. Heavy alcohol use, either habitual daily heavy alcohol consumption or binge drinking, seems to be related to higher rates of cardiovascular disease. Light or moderate alcohol consumption, on the other hand, is inversely related to the incidence of CHD.[111] Light and moderate alcohol use tends to raise the HDL cholesterol level, whereas high levels of alcohol intake are linked to hypertension and hypertriglyceridemia and may, in this way, predispose to fatal and nonfatal CHD, which is a high risk condition for stroke.

The relationship of alcohol consumption to stroke occurrence per se is less clear.[112] Available evidence suggests that there is a U-shaped relationship between level of alcohol consumption and ischemic stroke risk. Minimal consumption or total abstinence and heavy alcohol consumption seem to increase ischemic stroke risk, whereas moderate alcohol use is associated with the lowest risk. Risk of stroke due to hemorrhage increases with the amount of alcohol consumed.[113]

In the Honolulu Heart Study of men of Japanese ancestry, there was a powerful dose–response relationship between alcohol consumption and incidence of IH and SAH. Increases in alcohol consumption were related to increasing levels of blood pressure, cigarette smoking, and to lower serum cholesterol levels, all of which are risk factors for IH. However, even after these factors were taken into account, alcohol consumption was independently related to the incidence of intracranial hemorrhage, both subarachnoid and intracerebral; no significant relationship was found between alcohol and thromboembolic stroke. The age-adjusted RR of IH for light drinkers (1 to 14 oz per month) as compared with nondrinkers was 2.1; for moderate drinkers (15 to 39 oz per month),

2.4; and for heavy drinkers (40+ oz per month), 4.0. After adjustment was made for the other associated risk factors, IH was 2.0, 2.0, and 2.4 times as frequent, respectively, in these alcohol consumption categories.[113] However, there was no significant relationship to thromboembolic stroke. Data from the Framingham Study also suggest an increased incidence of brain infarction and stroke with increased levels of alcohol use but only in men.[112] There are a number of mechanisms by which heavy alcohol consumption may predispose to stroke and moderate alcohol consumption may protect from stroke.[114] Cigarette smoking is more frequent in heavy drinkers and contributes to the hemoconcentration accompanying heavy alcohol consumption, which increases hematocrit and viscosity.[115] In addition, rebound thrombocytosis during abstinence has been observed. Cardiac rhythm disturbances, particularly AF, occur with alcohol intoxication, producing what has been termed *holiday heart*.[116] Acute alcohol intoxication has been invoked as a precipitating factor for thrombotic stroke and SAH in young people.[115,117] Others have found a relationship to acute intoxication; but a case-control study failed to find an effect that was independent of other risk factors, particularly cigarette smoking.[118]

Physical Activity

Vigorous exercise may exert a beneficial influence on risk factors for atherosclerotic disease by reducing elevated blood pressure, inducing weight loss, slowing the heart rate, raising HDL and lowering LDL cholesterol levels, improving glucose tolerance, and promoting a lifestyle conducive to favorably changing detrimental health habits such as cigarette smoking. However, only recently has physical activity been found to be associated with reduced stroke incidence.[119-124] In the Framingham Study, physical activity in subjects with a mean age of 65 years was associated with a reduced stroke incidence.[122] In men, the RR was 0.41 ($P = 0.0007$) after the effects of potential confounders were taken into account, including systolic blood pressure, serum cholesterol level, glucose intolerance, vital capacity, obesity, left ventricular hypertrophy on electrocardiogram, AF, valvular heart disease, CHF, CHD, and occupation. However, there was no evidence of a protective effect of physical activity on the risk of stroke in women. As in CHD, moderate physical activity conferred no less benefit than heavy activity levels. In a number of other population studies and in a series of case-control studies, low levels of physical activity were associated with increased incidence of stroke. Recently, a beneficial effect of exercise was found in women.[123]

A graded response to exercise was found in male British civil servants: the greatest benefit in reduced stroke incidence was derived from the most intense level of exercise, and an intermediate protective effect was derived from medium levels.[121] In the Honolulu Heart Study of Japanese men, higher levels of physical activity, after adjustment for other risk factors, was associated with lower rates of both ischemic and hemorrhagic stroke.[120] Recent data from the National Health and Nutrition Examination Survey 1 (NHANES 1) epidemiologic follow-up study disclosed a consistent association of low levels of physical activity and an increased risk of stroke in women as well as in men and in both black people and white people.[123]

Moderate levels of activity tended to provide an intermediate level of protection.[124]

Physical activity exerts a beneficial influence on standard risk factors for atherosclerotic disease by decreasing platelet aggregability, increasing insulin sensitivity, which improves glucose tolerance, and promoting a lifestyle conducive to changing diet and stopping cigarette smoking. Increased physical activity has now been convincingly associated with a reduced incidence of stroke. Moderate levels of recreational and nonrecreational physical activity provide substantial benefits and may be recommended as a sensible lifestyle modification for reduction of the risk of cardiovascular disease, including stroke.

Diet

Consumption of grains, fruits, vegetables, and fish has been associated with a reduced incidence of stroke in a number of studies. In the Nurses' Health Study of more than 75,000 women, the RR of ischemic stroke in the uppermost quintile of grain consumption was 0.69 relative to the lowest quintile, after adjustment for other stroke risk factors.[125] In an analysis combining the Nurses' Health Study and the Health Professionals Follow-up Study, fruit and vegetable consumption was also associated with a decreased risk of stroke (RR, 0.69; 95% CI, 0.52–0.92).[126]

Nurses in the Nurses' Health Study who consumed five or more servings of fish per week had an adjusted RR for stroke of 0.38 compared with women consuming less than 1 serving per month, which suggests a protective effect of omega-3 fatty acids.[127] Vitamins C or E levels have been related to stroke incidence, but the findings have been inconsistent. Based on 20 years of follow-up in the Shibata study, a prospective cohort of 880 men and 1241 women, the RR of stroke adjusted for all other risk factors was 0.71 in the subjects with the highest vitamin C levels relative to those with the lowest levels.[128] However, the Health Professionals Follow-up Study also examined this issue based on food frequency questionnaires administered to 43,738 men, aged 40 to 75 years. After 8 years of follow-up there were no significant relationships between consumption of vitamins C and E and the risk of stroke.[129] Consumption of fish, once a week or more frequently, was associated with an approximate 50% reduced stroke incidence in women and in black men. Stroke incidence was reduced by a nonstatistically significant 15% in white men who consumed fish compared with those who never ate fish.[130] (See Chapter 17.)

Identification of high-risk candidates for stroke prevention. (See Chapter 16, "Primary Prevention of Stroke.") Multivariable analysis, initially employed to gain insight into the underlying atherogenic process, also generated a set of independent risk factors useful for crafting multivariable risk equations to predict cardiovascular disease events. For use as a multivariable risk tool, it is compelled by the availability of reliable noninvasive tests for candidate risk factors, cost, and whether the risk factors used can be safely modified with expectation of benefit. This methodology implicitly recognizes that no known risk factor either inevitably leads to development of disease or confers immunity. The risk factors chosen for prediction depend on the purpose for assigning risk and the costs entailed. Framingham Study CHD multivariable

risk profiles have been tested in a variety of population samples and found to be reasonably accurate, except for those in areas where the cardiovascular disease rates are very low.[131-134]

However, even in these areas, high-risk persons can be distinguished from those at low risk, and if the intercept is adjusted, the true absolute risk can be estimated. The Framingham Study has crafted multivariable risk profiles for risk assessment of candidates for cardiovascular disease in general and stroke in particular.[135] These facilitate estimation of the conditional probability of these initial events with the use of ordinary office procedures. Epidemiologic investigation has long contended that atherosclerotic cardiovascular disease is of multifactorial etiology. Risk factors are related to cardiovascular disease occurrence in a continuous graded fashion, extending down into the perceived normal range, without indication of a critical value where normal leaves off. At any level of each risk factor, cardiovascular disease risk varies widely in accordance with the burden of accompanying risk factors. National guidelines are now linking treatment goals to global CHD risk. It has long been recognized that for any risk factor, predisposition to cardiovascular disease is markedly influenced by the associated burden of other risk factors. It is postulated that an insulin resistance syndrome is the metabolic basis for other atherogenic risk factors clustering with each of the major risk factors.

Cardiovascular disease risk factors seldom occur in isolation because they are metabolically linked, tending to cluster, the extent of which profoundly promotes components of the cluster of risk factors, characterized as the insulin-resistant metabolic influences on the cardiovascular disease hazard of any particular risk factor, such as weight gain leading to visceral adiposity syndrome The hazard of obesity varies widely depending on the burden of atherogenic risk factors that accompany it. When confronted with a patient with any particular cardiovascular disease risk factor, it is essential to test for the others that are likely to coexist with it. Such coexistence can be expected 80% of the time. Now that guidelines for dyslipidemia, hypertension, and diabetes recommend treating modest abnormality, candidates for treatment are best targeted by global risk assessment so that the number needed to treat to prevent one event is minimized.

To help identify persons at increased risk of stroke, the risk profile developed, utilizing 36 years of follow-up data from Framingham, allows physicians to determine a patient's conditional probability of having a stroke.[135] This can be done based only on information collected from a medical history and physical examination, plus an electrocardiogram. With the use of a risk factor scoring table that is sex-specific, the probability of a stroke occurring is determined by a point system, depending on the patient's age, systolic blood pressure, antihypertensive therapy use, and presence of diabetes, cigarette smoking, history of cardiovascular disease (CHD or CHF), and electrocardiographic abnormalities (left ventricular hypertrophy or AF). Stroke risk depending on the level of the aforementioned risk factors is distributed over a wide range and permits the physician to readily compare a particular patient's probability of stroke to that of an average person of the same age and sex.

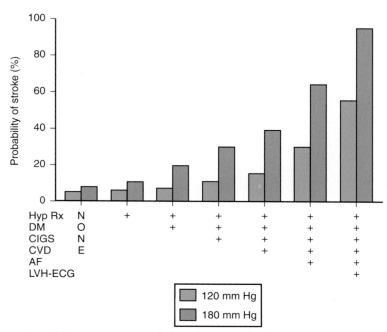

Figure 14-12 Probability of stroke in 10 years at two systolic blood pressure levels. Impact of other risk factors—70-year-old man. (From Wolf PA, D'Agostino RB, Belanger AJ, et al: Probability of stroke: A risk profile from the Framingham Study. *Stroke* 22:312-318, 1991.)

This assessment of global stroke risk will help the physician to identify which patients with borderline hypertension warrant pharmacologic treatment by virtue of an increased probability of stroke attributable to the presence of several other risk factor abnormalities that often accompany elevated blood pressure (Fig. 14-12). With the use of stroke risk profiles of a man age 70 years with either a systolic blood pressure level of 120 mm Hg or 180 mm Hg, it can be seen that the probability of a stroke in 10 years ranges from less than half the average level to nearly 100% depending on the associated risk factor burden. In the presence of multiple risk factor abnormalities, the probability of a stroke may actually be higher in the presence of a normal systolic blood pressure of 120 mm Hg than in a man with a pressure of 180 mm Hg who is free of diabetes and cardiovascular disease and who is a nonsmoker. The use of this risk profile provides a quantitative assessment of the level of risk and is particularly helpful in the presence of multiple borderline risk factor abnormalities. The graphic and percentage display provides the patient and his physician with a concrete estimate that the probability of stroke is below, at, or several-fold above average. It also can provide an illustration for patients of how treating certain of their risk factors that have been demonstrated to reduce stroke risk may be expected to result in a quantified decrease in stroke probability. Patients can be shown that reduction of their systolic blood pressure from 180 mm Hg to below 140 mm Hg by treatment, along with cessation of cigarette smoking and taking of warfarin anticoagulation if they have AF, may reduce their substantially elevated risk to nearly normal.[135]

The stroke profile may be used to select borderline hypertensive persons at high probability of stroke who warrant antihypertensive drug treatment. For example, by restricting drug treatment to persons with a borderline systolic blood pressure level who have two or more other risk factor abnormalities (not including age and male sex), it is possible to identify a group consisting of 22% of the men and 14% of women at high risk. In this group, approximately 40% of strokes will occur within the subsequent 10 years.[135]

Clearly, there are other settings not considered here when a patient can be identified to be at substantially increased risk of stroke: recent TIA, particularly in the presence of internal carotid artery stenosis greater than 70%; recent-onset AF; recent MI; during and immediately after cardiac surgery and cerebral angiography; and other situations dealt with elsewhere in this volume.

Acknowledgments

Supported in part by grants 2R01 NS17950 (National Institute of Neurological Disorders and Stroke, National Heart, Lung, and Blood Institute) and Contract N01-HC-25195 (National Heart, Lung, and Blood Institute).

REFERENCES

1. MacMahon B: *Epidemiologic methods*, ed 1, Boston, 1960, Little.
2. Lloyd-Jones D, Adams RJ, Brown TM, et al: Heart disease and stroke statistics—2010 update: A report from the American Heart Association, *Circulation* 121(7):e46–e215, 2010.
3. Rosamond WD, Folsom AR, Chambless LE, et al: Stroke incidence and survival among middle-aged adults: 9-year follow-up of the Atherosclerosis Risk in Communities (ARIC) cohort, *Stroke* 30(4): 736–743, 1999.
4. Ayala C, Greenlund KJ, Croft JB, et al: Racial/ethnic disparities in mortality by stroke subtype in the United States, 1995-1998, *Am J Epidemiol* 154(11):1057–1063, 2001.
5. Sacco RL, Ellenberg JH, Mohr JP, et al: Infarcts of undetermined cause: The NINCDS Stroke Data Bank, *Ann Neurol* 25(4):382–390, 1989.
6. Reed DM: The paradox of high risk of stroke in populations with low risk of coronary heart disease, *Am J Epidemiol* 131(4): 579–588, 1990.

7. Kase CS, Wolf PA, Chodosh EH, et al: Prevalence of silent stroke in patients presenting with initial stroke: The Framingham Study, *Stroke* 20(7):850-852, 1989.

8. Chodosh EH, Foulkes MA, Kase CS, et al: Silent stroke in the NINCDS Stroke Data Bank, *Neurology* 38(11):1674-1679, 1988.

9. Manolio TA, Kronmal RA, Burke GL, et al: Magnetic resonance abnormalities and cardiovascular disease in older adults. The Cardiovascular Health Study, *Stroke* 25(2):318-327, 1994.

10. Vermeer SE, Prins ND, den Heijer T, et al: Silent brain infarcts and the risk of dementia and cognitive decline, *N Engl J Med* 348(13):1215-1222, 2003.

11. Giele JL, Witkamp TD, Mali WP, et al: Silent brain infarcts in patients with manifest vascular disease, *Stroke* 35(3):742-746, 2004.

12. Sacco RL, Foulkes MA, Mohr JP, et al: Determinants of early recurrence of cerebral infarction. The Stroke Data Bank, *Stroke* 20(8):983-989, 1989.

13. Sacco RL, Wolf PA, Kannel WB, et al: Survival and recurrence following stroke. The Framingham Study, *Stroke* 13(3):290-295, 1982.

14. Sacco RL, Shi T, Zamanillo MC, et al: Predictors of mortality and recurrence after hospitalized cerebral infarction in an urban community: The Northern Manhattan Stroke Study, *Neurology* 44(4):626-634, 1994.

15. Brott T, Marks MP, Patel SC, et al: Acute Ischemic Stroke: New Concepts of Care 1998-1999: www.strokecenter.org.

16. Arboix A, Font A, Garro C, et al: Recurrent lacunar infarction following a previous lacunar stroke: A clinical study of 122 patients, *J Neurol Neurosurg Psychiatry* 78(12):1392-1394, 2007.

17. Elkind MS, Tai W, Coates K, et al: High-sensitivity C-reactive protein, lipoprotein-associated phospholipase A2, and outcome after ischemic stroke, *Arch Intern Med* 23;166(19):2073-2080, 2006.

18. Fuster V, Topol EJ, Nabel EG: *Atherothrombosis and coronary artery disease*, ed 2, Philadelphia, 2005, Lippincott Williams & Wilkins.

19. Wolf PA, Kannel WB, Sorlie P, et al: Asymptomatic carotid bruit and risk of stroke. The Framingham study, *JAMA* 245(14):1442-1445, 1981.

20. Sacco RL, Benjamin EJ, Broderick JP, et al: American Heart Association Prevention Conference. IV. Prevention and Rehabilitation of Stroke. Risk factors, *Stroke* 28(7):1507-1517, 1997.

21. Howard G, Labarthe DR, Hu J, et al: Regional differences in African Americans' high risk for stroke: The remarkable burden of stroke for Southern African Americans, *Ann Epidemiol* 17(9):689-696, 2007.

22. Sacco RL, Boden-Albala B, Gan R, et al: Stroke incidence among white, black, and Hispanic residents of an urban community: The Northern Manhattan Stroke Study, *Am J Epidemiol* 147(3):259-268, 1998.

23. Kissela B, Schneider A, Kleindorfer D, et al: Stroke in a biracial population: The excess burden of stroke among blacks, *Stroke* 35(2):426-431, 2004.

24. Bravata DM, Wells CK, Gulanski B, et al: Racial disparities in stroke risk factors: The impact of socioeconomic status, *Stroke* 36(7):1507-1511, 2005.

25. Petty GW, Brown RD Jr, Whisnant JP, et al: Ischemic stroke subtypes: A population-based study of incidence and risk factors, *Stroke* 30(12):2513-2516, 1999.

26. MacMahon S, Rodgers A: The epidemiological association between blood pressure and stroke: Implications for primary and secondary prevention, *Hypertens Res* 17(suppl 1):S23-S32, 1994.

27. The Sixth Report of the Joint National Committee on Prevention: Detection, evaluation, and treatment of high blood pressure, *Arch Intern Med* 157(21):2413-2446, 1997.

28. Collins R, Peto R, MacMahon S, et al: Blood pressure, stroke, and coronary heart disease. Part 2, Short-term reductions in blood pressure: Overview of randomised drug trials in their epidemiological context, *Lancet* 335(8693):827-838, 1990.

29. Beckett NS, Peters R, Fletcher AE, et al: Treatment of hypertension in patients 80 years of age or older, *N Engl J Med* 358(18):1887-1898, 2008.

30. Seshadri S, Wolf PA, Beiser A, et al: Elevated midlife blood pressure increases stroke risk in elderly persons: The Framingham Study, *Arch Intern Med* 161(19):2343-2350, 2001.

31. Shahar E, Chambless LE, Rosamond WD, et al: Plasma lipid profile and incident ischemic stroke: The Atherosclerosis Risk in Communities (ARIC) study, *Stroke* 34(3):623-631, 2003.

32. Wolf PA, D'Agostino RB, Belanger AJ, et al: Are blood lipids risk factors for stroke? *Stroke* 22(1):26, 1991.

33. Cholesterol, diastolic blood pressure, and stroke: 13,000 strokes in 450,000 people in 45 prospective cohorts. Prospective studies collaboration, *Lancet* 346:1647-1653, 1995.

34. Iso H, Jacobs DR Jr, Wentworth D, et al: Serum cholesterol levels and six-year mortality from stroke in 350,977 men screened for the multiple risk factor intervention trial, *N Engl J Med* 320(14): 904-910, 1989.

35. Benfante R, Yano K, Hwang LJ, et al: Elevated serum cholesterol is a risk factor for both coronary heart disease and thromboembolic stroke in Hawaiian Japanese men. Implications of shared risk, *Stroke* 25(4):814-820, 1994.

36. Atkins D, Psaty BM, Koepsell TD, et al: Cholesterol reduction and the risk for stroke in men. A meta-analysis of randomized, controlled trials, *Ann Intern Med* 119(2):136-145, 1993.

37. Fine-Edelstein JS, Wolf PA, O'Leary DH, et al: Precursors of extracranial carotid atherosclerosis in the Framingham Study, *Neurology* 44(6):1046-1050, 1994.

38. Wilson PWF, Hoeg JM, Belanger AJ, et al: Cholesterol-years, blood pressure-years, pack-years and carotid stenosis, *Circulation* 92(8):1-519, 1995.

39. O'Leary DH, Polak JF, Kronmal RA, et al: Thickening of the carotid wall. A marker for atherosclerosis in the elderly? Cardiovascular Health Study Collaborative Research Group, *Stroke* 27(2):224-231, 1996.

40. Furberg CD, Adams HP Jr, Applegate WB, et al: Effect of lovastatin on early carotid atherosclerosis and cardiovascular events. Asymptomatic Carotid Artery Progression Study (ACAPS) Research Group, *Circulation* 90(4):1679-1687, 1994.

41. Randomised trial of cholesterol lowering in 4444 patients with coronary heart disease: The Scandinavian Simvastatin Survival Study (4S), *Lancet* 344(8934):1383-1389, 1994.

42. Sacks FM, Pfeffer MA, Moye LA, et al: The effect of pravastatin on coronary events after myocardial infarction in patients with average cholesterol levels. Cholesterol and Recurrent Events Trial investigators, *N Engl J Med* 335(14):1001-1009, 1996.

43. Prevention of cardiovascular events and death with pravastatin in patients with coronary heart disease and a broad range of initial cholesterol levels. The Long-Term Intervention with Pravastatin in Ischaemic Disease (LIPID) Study Group, *N Engl J Med* 339(19):1349-1357, 1998.

44. Sever PS, Dahlof B, Poulter NR, et al: Prevention of coronary and stroke events with atorvastatin in hypertensive patients who have average or lower-than-average cholesterol concentrations, in the Anglo-Scandinavian Cardiac Outcomes Trial—Lipid Lowering Arm (ASCOT-LLA): A multicentre randomised controlled trial, *Lancet* 361(9364):1149-1158, 2003.

45. Yano K, Reed DM, MacLean CJ: Serum cholesterol and hemorrhagic stroke in the Honolulu Heart Program, *Stroke* 20(11):1460-1465, 1989.

46. Shimamoto T, Komachi Y, Inada H, et al: Trends for coronary heart disease and stroke and their risk factors in Japan, *Circulation* 79(3):503-515, 1989.

47. Burchfiel CM, Curb JD, Rodriguez BL, et al: Glucose intolerance and 22-year stroke incidence. The Honolulu Heart Program, *Stroke* 25(5):951-957, 1994.

48. Barrett-Connor E, Khaw KT: Diabetes mellitus: An independent risk factor for stroke? *Am J Epidemiol* 128(1):116-123, 1988.

49. Kannel WB, McGee DL: Diabetes and cardiovascular disease. The Framingham study, *JAMA* 241(19):2035-2038, 1979.

50. Najarian RM, Sullivan LM, Kannel WB, et al: Metabolic syndrome compared with type 2 diabetes mellitus as a risk factor for stroke: the Framingham Offspring Study, *Arch Intern Med* 166(1):106-111, 2006.

51. Walker SP, Rimm EB, Ascherio A, et al: Body size and fat distribution as predictors of stroke among US men, *Am J Epidemiol* 144(12):1143-1150, 1996.

52. Welin L, Svardsudd K, Wilhelmsen L, et al: Analysis of risk factors for stroke in a cohort of men born in 1913, *N Engl J Med* 317(9):521-526, 1987.

53. Seshadri S, Beiser A, Pikula A, et al: Parental occurrence of stroke and risk of stroke in their children: The Framingham Study, *Circulation* 121(11):1304-1312, 2010.

54. Wilhelmsen L, Svardsudd K, Korsan-Bengtsen K, et al: Fibrinogen as a risk factor for stroke and myocardial infarction, *N Engl J Med* 311(8):501-505, 1984.

55. Kannel WB, Wolf PA, Castelli WP, et al: Fibrinogen and risk of cardiovascular disease. The Framingham Study, *JAMA* 258(9):1183-1186, 1987.

56. Kannel WB, D'Agostino RB, Belanger AJ: Fibrinogen, cigarette smoking, and risk of cardiovascular disease: insights from the Framingham Study, *Am Heart J* 113(4):1006-1010, 1987.

57. Folsom AR, Qamhieh HT, Flack JM, et al: Plasma fibrinogen: Levels and correlates in young adults. The Coronary Artery Risk Development in Young Adults (CARDIA) Study, *Am J Epidemiol* 138(12):1023-1036, 1993.

58. Lee AJ, Lowe GD, Woodward M, et al: Fibrinogen in relation to personal history of prevalent hypertension, diabetes, stroke, intermittent claudication, coronary heart disease, and family history: The Scottish Heart Health Study, *Br Heart J* 69(4):338-342, 1993.

59. Rost NS, Wolf PA, Kase CS, et al: Plasma concentration of C-reactive protein and risk of ischemic stroke and transient ischemic attack: The Framingham Study, *Stroke* 32(11):2575-2579, 2001.

60. Ridker PM, Rifai N, Rose L, et al: Comparison of C-reactive protein and low-density lipoprotein cholesterol levels in the prediction of first cardiovascular events, *N Engl J Med* 347(20):1557-1565, 2002.

61. Boushey CJ, Beresford SA, Omenn GS, et al: A quantitative assessment of plasma homocysteine as a risk factor for vascular disease. Probable benefits of increasing folic acid intakes, *JAMA* 274(13):1049-1057, 1995.

62. Nygard O, Vollset SE, Refsum H, et al: Total plasma homocysteine and cardiovascular risk profile. The Hordaland Homocysteine Study, *JAMA* 274(19):1526-1533, 1995.

63. Perry IJ, Refsum H, Morris RW, et al: Prospective study of serum total homocysteine concentration and risk of stroke in middle-aged British men, *Lancet* 346(8987):1395-1398, 1995.

64. Stampfer MJ, Malinow MR, Willett WC, et al: A prospective study of plasma homocyst(e)ine and risk of myocardial infarction in US physicians, *JAMA* 268(7):877-881, 1992.

65. Verhoef P, Hennekens CH, Malinow MR, et al: A prospective study of plasma homocyst(e)ine and risk of ischemic stroke, *Stroke* 25(10):1924-1930, 1994.

66. Malinow MR, Nieto FJ, Szklo M, et al: Carotid artery intimal-medial wall thickening and plasma homocyst(e)ine in asymptomatic adults. The Atherosclerosis Risk in Communities Study, *Circulation* 87(4):1107-1113, 1993.

67. Selhub J, Jacques PF, Bostom AG, et al: Association between plasma homocysteine concentrations and extracranial carotid-artery stenosis, *N Engl J Med* 332(5):286-291, 1995.

68. Selhub J, Jacques PF, Wilson PW, et al: Vitamin status and intake as primary determinants of homocysteinemia in an elderly population, *JAMA* 270(22):2693-2698, 1993.

69. Toole JF, Malinow MR, Chambless LE, et al: Lowering homocysteine in patients with ischemic stroke to prevent recurrent stroke, myocardial infarction, and death: The Vitamin Intervention for Stroke Prevention (VISP) randomized controlled trial, *JAMA* 291(5):565-575, 2004.

70. Armitage JM, Bowman L, Clarke RJ, et al: Effects of homocysteine-lowering with folic acid plus vitamin B_{12} vs placebo on mortality and major morbidity in myocardial infarction survivors: a randomized trial, *JAMA* 303(24):2486-2494, 2010.

71. Wolf PA, Kannel WB, McNamara PM, et al: The role of impaired cardiac function in atherothrombotic brain infarction: The Framingham Study, *Am J Public Health* 63(1):52-58, 1973.

72. Loh E, Sutton MS, Wun CC, et al: Ventricular dysfunction and the risk of stroke after myocardial infarction, *N Engl J Med* 336(4):251-257, 1997.

73. Smith P, Arnesen H, Holme I: The effect of warfarin on mortality and reinfarction after myocardial infarction, *N Engl J Med* 323(3):147-152, 1990.

74. Murabito JM, Evans JC, Larson MG, et al: The ankle-brachial index in the elderly and risk of stroke, coronary disease, and death: The Framingham Study, *Arch Intern Med* 163(16):1939-1942, 2003.

75. Wolf PA, Abbott RD, Kannel WB: Atrial fibrillation: A major contributor to stroke in the elderly. The Framingham Study, *Arch Intern Med* 147(9):1561-1564, 1987.

76. Chesebro JH, Fuster V, Halperin JL: Atrial fibrillation—risk marker for stroke, *N Engl J Med* 323(22):1556-1558, 1990.

77. Wolf PA, Abbott RD, Kannel WB: Atrial fibrillation as an independent risk factor for stroke: The Framingham Study, *Stroke* 22(8):983-988, 1991.

78. Risk factors for stroke and efficacy of antithrombotic therapy in atrial fibrillation: Analysis of pooled data from five randomized controlled trials, *Arch Intern Med* 154:1449-1457, 1994.

79. Laupacis A, Albers G, Dalen J, et al: Antithrombotic therapy in atrial fibrillation, *Chest* 114(Suppl 5):579S-589S, 1998.

80. Sage JI, Van Uitert RL: Risk of recurrent stroke in patients with atrial fibrillation and non-valvular heart disease, *Stroke* 14(4):537-540, 1983.

81. Marini C, De Santis F, Sacco S, et al: Contribution of atrial fibrillation to incidence and outcome of ischemic stroke: Results from a population-based study, *Stroke* 36(6):1115-1119, 2005.

82. Patients with nonvalvular atrial fibrillation at low risk of stroke during treatment with aspirin: Stroke Prevention in Atrial Fibrillation III Study. The SPAF III Writing Committee for the Stroke Prevention in Atrial Fibrillation Investigators, *JAMA* 279(16):1273-1277, 1998.

83. Predictors of thromboembolism in atrial fibrillation: I. Clinical features of patients at risk. The Stroke Prevention in Atrial Fibrillation Investigators, *Ann Intern Med* 116(1):1-5, 1992.

84. Gage BF, Waterman AD, Shannon W, et al: Validation of clinical classification schemes for predicting stroke: Results from the National Registry of Atrial Fibrillation, *JAMA* 285(22):2864-2870, 2001.

85. van Walraven C, Hart RG, Wells GA, et al: A clinical prediction rule to identify patients with atrial fibrillation and a low risk for stroke while taking aspirin, *Arch Intern Med* 163(8):936-943, 2003.

86. Hart RG, Halperin JL: Atrial fibrillation and thromboembolism: A decade of progress in stroke prevention, *Ann Intern Med* 131(9):688-695, 1999.

87. Wang TJ, Massaro JM, Levy D, et al: A risk score for predicting stroke or death in individuals with new-onset atrial fibrillation in the community: The Framingham Heart Study, *JAMA* 290(8):1049-1056, 2003.

88. Fihn SD, Callahan CM, Martin DC, et al: The risk for and severity of bleeding complications in elderly patients treated with warfarin. The National Consortium of Anticoagulation Clinics, *Ann Intern Med* 124(11):970-979, 1996.

89. Wang TJ, Larson MG, Levy D, et al: Temporal relations of atrial fibrillation and congestive heart failure and their joint influence on mortality: The Framingham Heart Study, *Circulation* 107(23):2920-2925, 2003.

90. Bikkina M, Levy D, Evans JC, et al: Left ventricular mass and risk of stroke in an elderly cohort. The Framingham Heart Study, *JAMA* 272(1):33-36, 1994.

91. Chabriat H, Vahedi K, Iba-Zizen MT, et al: Clinical spectrum of CADASIL: A study of 7 families. Cerebral autosomal dominant arteriopathy with subcortical infarcts and leukoencephalopathy, *Lancet* 346:934-939, 1995.

92. Buring JE, Hebert P, Romero J, et al: Migraine and subsequent risk of stroke in the Physicians' Health Study, *Arch Neurol* 52(2):129-134, 1995.

93. Carolei A, Marini C, De Matteis G: History of migraine and risk of cerebral ischaemia in young adults. The Italian National Research Council Study Group on Stroke in the Young, *Lancet* 347:1503-1506, 1996.

94. Wolf PA, D'Agostino RB, Kannel WB, et al: Cigarette smoking as a risk factor for stroke. The Framingham Study, *JAMA* 259(7):1025-1029, 1988.

95. Colditz GA, Bonita R, Stampfer MJ, et al: Cigarette smoking and risk of stroke in middle-aged women, *N Engl J Med* 318(15):937-941, 1988.

96. Abbott RD, Yin Y, Reed DM, et al: Risk of stroke in male cigarette smokers, *N Engl J Med* 315(12):717-720, 1986.

97. Further analyses of mortality in oral contraceptive users: Royal College of General Practitioners' Oral Contraception Study, *Lancet* 317:541-546, 1981.

98. Sacco RL, Wolf PA, Bharucha NE, et al: Subarachnoid and intracerebral hemorrhage: natural history, prognosis, and precursive factors in the Framingham Study, *Neurology* 34(7):847-854, 1984.

99. Bonita R: Cigarette smoking, hypertension and the risk of subarachnoid hemorrhage: A population-based case-control study, *Stroke* 17(5):831–835, 1986.

100. Fogelholm R, Murros K: Cigarette smoking and subarachnoid haemorrhage: A population-based case-control study, *J Neurol Neurosurg Psychiatry* 50(1):78–80, 1987.

101. Shinton R, Beevers G: Meta-analysis of relation between cigarette smoking and stroke, *BMJ* 298(6676):789–794, 1989.

102. Stadel BV: Oral contraceptives and cardiovascular disease (second of two parts), *N Engl J Med* 305(12):672–677, 1981.

103. Adams HP Jr, Butler MJ, Biller J, et al: Nonhemorrhagic cerebral infarction in young adults, *Arch Neurol* 43(8):793–796, 1986.

104. Stampfer MJ, Willett WC, Colditz GA, et al: A prospective study of past use of oral contraceptive agents and risk of cardiovascular diseases, *N Engl J Med* 319:1313–1317, 1988.

105. Ischaemic stroke and combined oral contraceptives: results of an international, multicentre, case-control study. WHO Collaborative Study of Cardiovascular Disease and Steroid Hormone Contraception, *Lancet* 348:498–505, 1996.

106. Petitti DB, Sidney S, Bernstein A, et al: Stroke in users of low-dose oral contraceptives, *N Engl J Med* 335(1):8–15, 1996.

107. Gillum LA, Mamidipudi SK, Johnston SC: Ischemic stroke risk with oral contraceptives: A meta-analysis, *JAMA* 284(1):72–78, 2000.

108. Haemorrhagic stroke, overall stroke risk, and combined oral contraceptives: results of an international, multicentre, case-control study. WHO Collaborative Study of Cardiovascular Disease and Steroid Hormone Contraception, *Lancet* 348:505–510, 1996.

109. Viscoli CM, Brass LM, Kernan WN, et al: A clinical trial of estrogen-replacement therapy after ischemic stroke, *N Engl J Med* 345(17):1243–1249, 2001.

110. Rossouw JE, Anderson GL, Prentice RL, et al: Risks and benefits of estrogen plus progestin in healthy postmenopausal women: Principal results from the Women's Health Initiative randomized controlled trial, *JAMA* 288(3):321–333, 2002.

111. Stampfer MJ, Colditz GA, Willett WC, et al: A prospective study of moderate alcohol consumption and the risk of coronary disease and stroke in women, *N Engl J Med* 319(5):267–273, 1988.

112. Djousse L, Ellison RC, Beiser A, et al: Alcohol consumption and risk of ischemic stroke: The Framingham Study, *Stroke* 33(4):907–912, 2002.

113. Donahue RP, Abbott RD, Reed DM, et al: Alcohol and hemorrhagic stroke. The Honolulu Heart Program, *JAMA* 255(17):2311–2314, 1986.

114. Camargo CA Jr: Moderate alcohol consumption and stroke. The epidemiologic evidence, *Stroke* 20:1611–1626, 1989.

115. Hillbom M, Kaste M, Rasi V: Can ethanol intoxication affect hemocoagulation to increase the risk of brain infarction in young adults? *Neurology* 33(3):381–384, 1983.

116. Ettinger PO, Wu CF, De La Cruz C Jr, et al: Arrhythmias and the "Holiday Heart": alcohol-associated cardiac rhythm disorders, *Am Heart J* 95(5):555–562, 1978.

117. Taylor JR, Combs-Orme T: Alcohol and strokes in young adults, *Am J Psychiatry* 142(1):116–118, 1985.

118. Gorelick PB: The status of alcohol as a risk factor for stroke, *Stroke* 20(12):1607–1610, 1989.

119. Manson JE, Stampfer MJ, Willett WC, et al: Physical activity and incidence of coronary heart disease and stroke in women [abstract], *Circulation* 91:927, 1995.

120. Abbott RD, Rodriguez BL, Burchfiel CM, et al: Physical activity in older middle-aged men and reduced risk of stroke: The Honolulu Heart Program, *Am J Epidemiol* 139(9):881–893, 1994.

121. Wannamethee G, Shaper AG: Physical activity and stroke in British middle aged men, *BMJ* 304:597–601, 1992.

122. Kiely DK, Wolf PA, Cupples LA, et al: Physical activity and stroke risk: The Framingham Study, *Am J Epidemiol* 140(7):608–620, 1994.

123. Gillum RF, Mussolino ME, Ingram DD: Physical activity and stroke incidence in women and men. The NHANES I Epidemiologic Follow-up Study, *Am J Epidemiol* 143(9):860–869, 1996.

124. Lee IM, Hennekens CH, Berger K, et al: Exercise and risk of stroke in male physicians, *Stroke* 30(1):1–6, 1999.

125. Liu S, Manson JE, Stampfer MJ, et al: Whole grain consumption and risk of ischemic stroke in women: A prospective study, *JAMA* 284(12):1534–1540, 2000.

126. Joshipura KJ, Ascherio A, Manson JE, et al: Fruit and vegetable intake in relation to risk of ischemic stroke, *JAMA* 282:1233–1239, 1999.

127. Iso H, Rexrode KM, Stampfer MJ, et al: Intake of fish and omega-3 fatty acids and risk of stroke in women, *JAMA* 285(3):304–312, 2001.

128. Yokoyama T, Date C, Kokubo Y, et al: Serum vitamin C concentration was inversely associated with subsequent 20-year incidence of stroke in a Japanese rural community: the Shibata Study, *Stroke* 31:2287–2294, 2000.

129. Ascherio A, Rimm EB, Hernan MA, et al: Relation of consumption of vitamin E, vitamin C, and carotenoids to risk for stroke among men in the United States, *Ann Intern Med* 130(12):963–970, 1999 Jun 15.

130. Gillum RF, Mussolino ME, Madans JH: The relationship between fish consumption and stroke incidence. The NHANES I Epidemiologic Follow-up Study (National Health and Nutrition Examination Survey), *Arch Intern Med* 156(5):537–542, 1996.

131. Wilson PW, D'Agostino RB, Levy D, et al: Prediction of coronary heart disease using risk factor categories, *Circulation* 97(18):1837–1847, 1998.

132. Leaverton PE, Sorlie PD, Kleinman JC, et al: Representativeness of the Framingham risk model for coronary heart disease mortality: A comparison with a national cohort study, *J Chronic Dis* 40(8):775–784, 1987.

133. Brand RJ, Rosenman RH, Sholtz RI, et al: Multivariate prediction of coronary heart disease in the Western Collaborative Group Study compared to the findings of the Framingham study, *Circulation* 53(2):348–355, 1976.

134. Kannel WB, Gordon T: National Heart Institute (U.S.). *The Framingham Study; an epidemiological investigation of cardiovascular disease*, Bethesda, Md, 1968, U.S. Dept. of Health, Education, and Welfare, National Institutes of Health; US Government Printing Office, Washington, DC.

135. Wolf PA, D'Agostino RB, Belanger AJ, et al: Probability of stroke: A risk profile from the Framingham Study, *Stroke* 22(3):312–318, 1991.

15 Prognosis after Stroke

TATJANA RUNDEK, RALPH L. SACCO

Stroke is a common and debilitating disease that continues to have a great impact on the public health as the second most common cause of death in the world[1,2] and as a major cause of long-term disability.[2-4] In the United States each year, about 780,000 people experience new or recurrent strokes.[5] About 600,000 of these are first strokes and 180,000 are recurrent strokes. Preliminary data from 2005 indicate that stroke accounted for about one of every 17 deaths in the United States. On average, every 40 seconds someone in the United States has a stroke.

Stroke accounts for the greatest number of hospitalizations for neurologic disease.[3] The estimated direct and indirect cost of stroke in the Unites States for 2008 is $65.5 billion.[5] The mean lifetime cost of ischemic stroke in the United States is estimated at $140,048. This includes inpatient care, rehabilitation, and follow-up care necessary for lasting deficits. It is projected that the total cost of stroke from 2005 to 2050 will be more than $2 trillion, and loss of earnings is expected to be the highest cost contributor. Despite the expanding knowledge about novel strategies of stroke prevention, including the results from recent randomized clinical trials of antiplatelets and blood pressure- and lipid-lowering drugs for the risk reduction of initial and recurrent stroke,[4,6-12] the real challenge still remains: to successfully implement evidence-based practices in stroke prevention programs worldwide.

Much is known about the prevalence, incidence, and risk factors for stroke, but less is known about the outcomes after stroke, although these are often devastating for stroke survivors, their families, and society. The importance of recurrent stroke, functional disability, quality of life (QOL), depression, and dementia after stroke will increase as more patients experience and survive a first stroke. The recent trends have showed a decline in stroke mortality. The actual number of stroke deaths declined about 7% from 1994 to 2004.[5] Success of the secondary stroke prevention programs relies on understanding the outcomes after stroke, factors associated with increased risks for these outcomes, implementation of evidence-based preventive interventions and strategies, and a comprehensive public health approach.

The majority of strokes are cerebral infarcts. This chapter focuses on the prognosis after ischemic stroke. The prognosis after subarachnoid and intracerebral hemorrhages is addressed in separate chapters. In this chapter, the most recent epidemiologic evidence on ischemic stroke mortality, recurrence, functional disability, QOL, and depression after stroke is discussed. Cognitive decline and dementia after stroke are discussed in Chapter 17.

Mortality after Ischemic Stroke

Stroke is the third leading cause of death, behind heart disease and cancer. Stroke is estimated to be responsible for 9.5% of all deaths and 5.1 million of the 16.7 million cardiovascular disease deaths worldwide. About two thirds or more of stroke deaths occur in the developing world. Stroke accounts for approximately 1 of every 17 deaths in the United States.[5] On average, every 3 to 4 minutes, someone dies of a stroke. Approximately 54% of stroke deaths in 2004 occurred out of the hospital.[13] Death rates from stroke, however, have been declining.[14] From 1994 to 2004, the stroke death rate fell 24%, and the actual number of stroke deaths declined 6.8%.[5] Some of the improvement in stroke mortality may be the result of improved acute stroke care, but most is thought to be the result of improved detection and treatment of hypertension.[15] However, public awareness of risk factors and major stroke warning signs has not improved, despite numerous national stroke public awareness campaigns; prevention of first and recurrent strokes is still inadequate.[16-18]

Early Mortality after Ischemic Stroke

The greatest risk of mortality for patients with cerebral infarction occurs in the first 30 days, and case-fatality rates range from 8% to 20%.[19-21] In the Framingham Study the 30-day case-fatality rate for patients with atherothrombotic infarction was 15%. It was similar in men and women and increased directly with age.[22] During this early period, death was more likely caused by the stroke itself or cardiopulmonary complications.[23] In the Atherosclerosis Risk in Communities (ARIC) study, 8% to 12% of ischemic strokes resulted in death within 30 days among persons 45 to 64 years of age.[24] In a study of persons older than 65 years recruited from a random sample of Health Care Financing Administration Medicare Part B eligibility lists in four U.S. communities, the 1-month ischemic stroke case-fatality rate was 8.1%.[25] In Rochester, Minnesota, the risk of death after first cerebral infarction was 7% at 7 days and 14% at 30 days.[26] In the Northern Manhattan Stroke Study (NOMASS), the 30-day mortality decreased from 7.7% in the 1980s (1983 to 1988) to 5.0% in the 1990s (1990 to 1997).[27] The 30-day cumulative mortality risk of 5% in the northern Manhattan cohort was lower than reported in the other cohorts, possibly because of inclusion of younger patients, exclusion of prior strokes, a higher proportion of lacunar infarcts, and less severe strokes at onset (Table 15-1).

TABLE 15-1 STROKE MORTALITY AND RECURRENCE RATES (PERCENT)

	Stroke Mortality	Stroke Mortality in NOMASS	Stroke Recurrence	Stroke Recurrence in NOMASS
30-day	3-20	5	1-6	2
1-year	20-35	16	5-25	8
5-year	38-75	41	15-40	16

Abbreviation: NOMASS, Northern Manhattan Stroke Study.

In the United States, stroke hospitalization rates increased 18.6% between 1988 and 1997, and the increase was largely in elderly patients 65 years or older.[28] A decline, however, in the in-hospital case-fatality rate from stroke during the same time period was observed. The decline in the case-fatality rate suggested that there have been general improvements in the management of patients with acute stroke, decreases in the severity of strokes, or detection of milder cases of stroke secondary to greater use of neuroimaging technology. A decline in case-fatality rates was also observed in other countries.[29-31] "Jubilation" over the decline in stroke case-fatality rates should be tempered by the recognition that part of the decline may have been due to the shorter lengths of stay resulting in more out-of-hospital deaths.[30] In addition, new disparities in stroke mortality rates have emerged. Higher rates of in-hospital mortality were described for patients with acute strokes who arrived on weekends compared with regular workdays. In the Get With The Guidelines (GWTG) stroke program, which included data from 187,669 acute ischemic stroke admissions from 857 hospitals, the in-hospital case fatality rate was 6% for off-hour presentation compared with 5% for on-hour presentation.[32] Although this absolute effect was small, it was significantly associated with an increased risk of dying in-hospital, and it represents a potential target for quality improvement efforts.

However, questions still remain as to how much of the improved survival rates after ischemic stroke are due to (1) improved acute management and therefore a decrease in the 30-day case-fatality rate, (2) the decreasing proportion of severe strokes, or (3) a reduction in mortality rates among 30-day survivors.

Causes of Early Death after Ischemic Stroke

The immediate cause of death in more than 60% of stroke cases was related to the stroke itself.[14,33,34] Death within 30 days after a first stroke due to incident stroke was found in 91% of patients in the Oxfordshire Community Stroke Project and in 85% of patients in the Perth Community Stroke Study.[35,36] After 1 month cardiovascular pathology, stroke, and diseases resulting from stroke were the causes of death in up to 80% of the patients, which is substantially greater than in the age- and gender-matched general population.[34] In the German Stroke Registry of 13,440 ischemic stroke patients from 104 academic centers, in-hospital mortality was 5%, and increased intracranial pressure had the highest attributable risk, accounting for 94% of deaths among patients with that condition.[37] In the entire stroke population, pneumonia had the highest attributable risk of death, accounting for about a third of all deaths. More than half of all in-hospital deaths were attributable to either serious medical or neurologic complications. Impaired consciousness on admission, posterior circulation infarcts, and transtentorial herniation are the most important neurologic causes of death during the first week after stroke onset.[38] Thereafter, cardiac causes, pneumonia, pulmonary embolism, sepsis, and other medical complications account for the majority of deaths within the first month after stroke onset. Excess mortality related to cardiovascular disease has also been described among young adults. Among the 30-day survivors from the Helsinki Young Stroke Registry of 711 patients, the cause of death was stroke in 21%, cardioaortic and other vascular causes in 36%, malignancies in 12%, and infections in 9%.[39] In NOMASS, the proportion of 30-day deaths after a first ischemic stroke was 75%.[33] Incident (53%) or recurrent (4%) stroke caused early deaths in 57% of patients. It has been reported that cardiac causes of early death were higher among black people than among other race-ethnicities.[40,41] Of the 292 black and 801 white patients in the Trial of ORG 10172 in Acute Stroke Therapy (TOAST), there was a trend toward a higher rate of unfavorable outcomes in black people at 7 days.[42] Excess mortality related to cardiovascular disease has been described among young black people and Caribbean-Hispanics.[21,33]

Late Mortality after Ischemic Stroke

Longitudinal studies among patients with ischemic stroke have demonstrated that the risk of death at 5 years ranged from 40% to 60%, including early fatalities.[35,43] The average annual mortality rate in 30-day stroke survivors ranges from 8% to 9%, and the risk of death is two to three times higher than that of the age- and sex-matched general population.[35,43] In the National Survey of Stroke, only 53% of stroke patients who survived the initial 6 months lived for 5 years.[44] The 5-year survival rate was 75% in those younger than 65 and fell to 23% in those 85 or older. In the Oxfordshire Community Stroke Project, the stroke mortality rate was 10% at 30 days, 23% at 1 year, and 51% at 5 years.[35] In Rochester, Minnesota, the risk of death after first cerebral infarction was 27% at 1 year and 53% at 5 years.[26] In the Monitoring Trends and Determinants in Cardiovascular Disease (MONICA) Project, the estimated cumulative risks of death were 41% at 1 year after stroke and 60% at 5 years.[45] In NOMASS the lifetable cumulative risk of ischemic stroke mortality was 5% at 30 days, 16% at 1 year, and 41% at 5 years after stroke (see Table 15-1).[33] In the Framingham Study, 5-year mortality rates after atherothrombotic brain infarction were 44% for men and 36% for women and were similar to the standard population.[22] In the same cohort, however, stroke survivors for 20 years or more had a greater mortality rate than age- and sex-matched control subjects.[46] It is still not clear how much the long-term survival after ischemic stroke is influenced by the initial or recurrent stroke or by other associated comorbidities. Among young adults, the overall cumulative mortality risks are low (i.e., 1% to 4.0% at 1 month, 3% to 6% at 1 year, and 10% to 12% at 5 years). However, those older than 45 years of age have lower probabilities of survival.[39]

Stroke mortality has been declining, especially since the 1970s. Although the observed reduction in stroke mortality has been attributed to declining stroke incidence, new evidence is showing a secular trend in declining stroke severity.[26,35,47] Stroke with severe neurologic deficits decreased in later decades, and a decrease was seen in rates of severe stroke cases in which patients were unconscious on admission to the hospital.[47] Despite the encouraging decline in stroke incidence, there is evidence of a recent increase in mean blood pressure in young people in the United States and United Kingdom, prompting concern that favorable trends in stroke risk may not be maintained.[48] Recent data from the Framingham Study suggest that the lifetime risk of stroke is very high.[49] The same has been observed in other western countries; therefore monitoring cardiovascular risk factors in communities is of utmost importance for public health.

Predictors of Death after Ischemic Stroke

For early and late mortality, predictors of death after ischemic stroke may differ (Table 15-2). Most of them, however, affect both early and late mortality, and a clear distinction cannot be made. Early recognition of predictors of death after stroke onset is of special importance when relevant clinical variables are accounted for within

TABLE 15-2 DEFINITE AND POTENTIAL PREDICTORS OF DEATH AFTER ISCHEMIC STROKE

	Definite Predictors	Potential Predictors
Demographics	Age	Gender Race-ethnicity
Clinical parameters	Initial severity of stroke (NIHSS)	Other cardiac disease
	Decreased consciousness	Previous stroke
	Infarct size	
	Large hemispheric or basilar syndrome	Prestroke disability
	Ischemic stroke subtype	
	Fever	
	Hypertension	
	Atrial fibrillation	
	Congestive heart failure	
Biochemical parameters	Hyperglycemia	Type 2 diabetes
	C-reactive protein	Erythrocyte sedimentation rate
		Fibrinogen
		White blood cell count
		Uric acid/creatinine
		Microalbuminuria
		LpPLA2

Abbreviation: LpPLA2, Lipoprotein-associated phospholipase A2.

the first 72 hours after a stroke. Although the prediction of stroke outcome could probably be improved by including variables that are assessed later, the practical value would be limited, as the prediction cannot be given as early. In addition, a development of early prediction models taking into account only variables that are evaluated within the first 6 hours after onset would be interesting for designing acute stroke interventional clinical trials. Among 30-day survivors of ischemic stroke, determinants of death are less understood. Stroke-related deaths continue to be a problem during the years after an ischemic stroke, especially in patients who are functionally dependent at 6 months after onset.[50] Stroke risk factors, which are less important during the early period, may have a greater impact on long-term outcome. Therefore, better short-term treatments to reduce dependency and adequate secondary prevention remain high priorities.

Age, Gender, and Race-Ethnicity

Nonmodifiable factors such as age, gender, and race-ethnicity have been identified as potential determinants of stroke outcome.[45,51-54]

Age is an independent prognostic factor of both early and late stroke mortality.[51,54-59] Elderly patients have a higher risk of subsequent complications and therefore lower chances of recovery from stroke.

It has frequently been found that the age-standardized case-fatality rates are greater for women than for men.[51] These reports do not offer any explanation for the gender difference in case-fatality. In the Danish MONICA study, women had a higher risk of death than men for up to 1 year after the stroke, even after adjustment was made for age.[45] In contrast, in the Framingham Study, women had a better survival rate than men after stroke.[46] Many studies have reported poorer stroke outcomes in women and suggest that women are less likely to receive thrombolytic therapy and lipid testing and more likely to have urinary tract infections.[60] Further studies are needed to explore gender differences in stroke mortality.

Differences in mortality rates between various race-ethnic groups were observed in several cohorts.[33,61] In the Cardiovascular Health Study (CHS) cohort of patients 65 years of age or older, black people had a greater risk of death than other groups after ischemic stroke.[61] In a cohort of veterans with stroke living in the southeastern United States, non-Hispanic black people had significantly higher mortality rates than did non-Hispanic white people in 38 months of follow-up.[62] In NOMASS, 5-year cumulative lifetable mortality estimates after stroke differed only slightly among the three race-ethnic groups.[33] Disparities in the incidence of stroke risk factors (e.g., atrial fibrillation [AF], diabetes mellitus, and hypertension) and socioeconomic status between black, Hispanic, and white patients may, in part, explain the disproportionate mortality rates among Hispanic, black, and white patients after stroke.[63] However, the majority of the excess burden of stroke mortality is borne by relatively young black people and by black people living in the southeastern United States.[64] While overall stroke mortality rates have been rapidly declining for both black people and white people, the magnitude of the relative increased risk of dying from a stroke among black people, as compared with white people, has remained largely unchanged. As such, efforts to reduce ethnic disparities in stroke mortality have been unsuccessful. Further studies will determine how much of the possible differences in outcome by race-ethnic disparities may be explained by differences in stroke risk factors and subtype.

Initial Stroke Severity

The initial severity of a stroke, often measured by the National Institutes of Health Stroke Scale (NIHSS),[52,65] remains one of the major predictors of poor outcome, including mortality, after stroke.[46,51,54-67] In the TOAST trial, the baseline NIHSS score strongly predicted mortality and functional outcome, and one additional point on the NIHSS decreased the likelihood of survival and excellent outcomes at 7 days by 24% and at 3 months by 17%.[53] An NIHSS score of 16 or greater predicted a high probability of death or severe disability, whereas a score of 6 or less predicted a good recovery. Among patients with infarcts in the carotid artery territory arriving at the hospital within 6 hours, the severity of the neurologic deficit was the strongest indicator of both the 30-day and the 6-month prognosis.[65,68-71]

Markers of initial stroke severity such as depressed consciousness, infarct size, the severity of the neurologic deficit, and the type of admitting syndrome have been reported as clinical predictors of early outcome.[72-76] In the NOMASS cohort, patients in a coma had the worst prognosis and a greater likelihood of herniation from the mass effect or cerebral edema associated with the size of the infarct. Of the 1754 prospectively collected records of patients with acute ischemic stroke in the German Stroke Database, orientation, limb paresis, trunk ataxia, and dysphagia were independent predictors of early death after stroke.[55]

The type of initial stroke syndrome has been found to be another important clinical determinant of mortality. In NOMASS, patients seen with a major hemispheric or basilar syndrome had the worst early mortality rates, patients with minor hemispheric syndromes had an associated intermediate survival rate, and those with a lacunar syndrome had the best prognosis. In the Oxfordshire cohort, patients with total anterior cerebral infarcts had the worst survival rate.[77]

Fever

Pyrexia after stroke onset is associated with a marked increase in morbidity and mortality. Admission body temperature is considered to be a major determinant of short-term as well as long-term mortality after stroke.[78-80] During the first days after acute stroke, a fever or subfebrile temperature elevation develops in one fifth to almost one half of patients.[81-84] Subfebrile temperatures (37.5°C to 39°C) and fever (>39°C) after a stroke are associated with relatively large infarct volumes, high case-fatality rates, and poor functional outcomes, even after adjustment for initial stroke severity.[82-86] Hyperthermia within the first 12 or 24 hours after stroke onset may be more predictive of outcome than delayed fever.[86] The significant stroke prognostic influence of initial body temperature was confirmed by a metaanalysis of nine studies with 3790 patients.[87] A fever of more than 38°C within 3 days

after stroke was among the most important predictors of mortality or functional dependence after stroke.[55,78,83,88] In the recent pooled analyses covering 14,431 patients with stroke and other brain injuries, fever was consistently associated with worse outcomes across multiple outcome measures.[89]

In the Copenhagen Stroke Study, the mortality rate at 60 months after stroke was greater for patients with hyperthermia on admission (73% versus 59%).[80] A 1°C increase of admission body temperature independently predicted a 30% relative increase (95% confidence interval [CI], 4%-57%) in long-term mortality risk. An association between admission body temperature and stroke mortality was noted independent of stroke severity. The relative risk for 1-year mortality of hyperthermic versus normothermic patients was 3.4 (95% CI, 1.6-7.3).[78]

In patients with acute ischemic stroke, a pharmacologic reduction of body temperature or body cooling procedures may improve functional outcome.[90-92]

Ischemic Stroke Subtypes and Stroke Mortality

Ischemic stroke subtype is an important determinant of mortality in many prospective community stroke studies and clinical trials, including cohorts from Rochester, Minnesota; the NINDS Stroke Data Bank; Perth, Australia; Erlangen Stroke Project, Germany; NOMASS, Oxfordshire Community Stroke Project; TOAST; and CHS. The chance of survival was significantly better for patients with lacunar infarcts compared with nonlacunar infarcts.[26,53,61,77,93-96]

In the northern Manhattan cohort (Fig. 15-1), presentation with a lacunar syndrome was associated with a significantly better 5-year survival rate. Recent data on long-term outcomes in patients with lacunar stroke have shown that, for the first few years after lacunar infarct, the risk of death was similar to that of the general population.[97] However, a clear excess of death was observed later, indicating that the long-term prognosis in lacunar infarction appears less favorable than previously reported.[97,98]

Ischemic stroke subtype according to the TOAST criteria[99] was a significant predictor of stroke survival after adjustment for age and sex.[95] The highest mortality rate was reported for cardioembolic and large atherothrombotic strokes, and the lowest was for lacunar strokes. In the Rochester Epidemiology Project,[96] the case-fatality rates

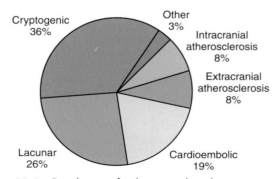

Figure 15-1 Distribution of ischemic stroke subtypes among 992 stroke patients in the Northern Manhattan Stroke Study.

for cardioembolic stroke at 1 month (30.3%), 1 year (53%), and 2 years (61.4%) were higher than reported in other cohorts, which was most likely due to the older patients in the cohort (mean age for cardioembolic stroke, 80 years).[18] In CHS, the most lethal ischemic stroke subtype was also cardioembolic.[61] Patients with cardioembolic stroke were nearly four times more likely to be dead 30 days after the stroke than patients with stroke due to large-vessel atherosclerosis with stenosis and 2.5 times more likely to be dead 5 years later. In the New England Medical Center Posterior Circulation Registry, a low mortality rate at 30 days after stroke onset (3.6%) was observed among patients with vertebrobasilar occlusive strokes.[100] A poor outcome was associated with basilar artery involvement, embolic stroke mechanism, and multiple posterior circulation intracranial territory involvement.

Blood Pressure, Atrial Fibrillation, and Heart Failure

Elevated blood pressure in stroke survivors increases the risk of death.[101,102] Blood pressure reduction after stroke recovery with the use of diuretics and/or angiotensin-converting enzyme inhibitors reduces stroke mortality and recurrence.[7,103,104]

Three quarters of patients with acute ischemic stroke have elevated blood pressure at presentation.[105] Blood pressure declines spontaneously over the first week after stroke onset and returns to prestroke levels in two thirds of patients. Most studies have found that high blood pressure, whether measured as casual or 24-hour ambulatory readings, in the acute phase of stroke is associated with a poor outcome.[101,106] Although the theory is not proven, high blood pressure in acute stroke might promote early recurrence, hemorrhagic transformation, or cerebral edema.[107]

In the International Stroke Trial of 17,398 stroke patients, both high and low blood pressure were independent prognostic factors for 6-month poor outcome after stroke.[101] Early death increased by 3.8% for every 10 mm Hg above 150 mm Hg and by 17.9% for every 10 mm Hg below 150 mm Hg. In the Multicenter rt-PA Stroke Survey of 1205 patients treated in routine clinical practice with intravenous rt-PA within 3 hours of stroke symptom onset, elevated pretreatment mean blood pressure was a main attribute associated with increased case-fatality and intracranial hemorrhage rates.[108]

Cardiac disease was a prominent predictor of survival in multiple studies. Cardiac failure is the most robust predictor of death within 1 to 5 years after stroke, secondary only to increasing age.[109] In Rochester, Minnesota, independent risk factors for death after first cerebral infarction were congestive heart failure, persistent AF, and ischemic heart disease.[26] In the Perth Community Stroke Study, predictors of death within 1 year included cardiac failure and AF.[36] In a 14-year follow-up study from Sweden, heart failure and history of diabetes were predictors of long-term mortality.[110] Stroke survivors with cardiac disease had a poorer 1-year survival rate in the Community Hospital-based Stroke Programs and a decreased 10-year survival in Framingham.[111]

AF is the most prevalent chronic cardiac arrhythmia in the elderly and has a well-documented impact on the prognosis of first-ever stroke.[34,112-115] In the Framingham cohort, 30-day mortality and stroke severity in the AF subjects was 25% versus 14% in non-AF subjects.[114] The other studies reported 30-day mortality of 23% to 35% in AF subjects versus 7% to 14% in non-AF subjects.[34,112,113,115] In a Swedish Stroke Registry of 105,074 patients, of whom 30% had documented AF, the age- and sex-adjusted relative risk of death was 46% greater for AF versus non-AF patients.[116] The difference in mortality between AF and non-AF subjects was more evident in the extreme elderly. Half of the strokes in AF subjects 75 years of age or older were either severe or fatal because of the contribution of AF to death.

Congestive heart failure is also a significant predictor of stroke severity and case-fatality rates.[27,34,112] Patients with dilated cardiomyopathy have a high incidence of left ventricular thrombus formation and are at increased risk of embolic complications.[117] In the Framingham Study, heart failure was ranked second in cardiogenic stroke risk, with a twofold to threefold relative risk.[118,119] Congestive heart failure is associated with high rates of mortality: a 15-year mortality rate is estimated at 39% for women and 72% for men.[120] In the Finland study, the presence of congestive heart failure doubled the age- and sex-adjusted risk of death from all causes, and quadrupled the risk of death from stroke and cardiovascular diseases during 4-year follow-up.[121] In the northern Manhattan cohort, congestive heart failure was an independent predictor of 5-year death among 30-day survivors.

Hyperglycemia and Diabetes

Abnormalities on admitting blood tests have also been evaluated as clinical predictors of early mortality. The most frequently studied abnormality has been hyperglycemia, which has been associated with an increased mortality rate after stroke, in both patients with and without diabetes.[122-127] Hyperglycemia during acute ischemic stroke may augment brain injury, predispose to intracerebral hemorrhage, or both.[128] Alternatively, the effect of hyperglycemia may be confounded by the acute stress reaction secondary to an infarct.[123-125] In the NINDS rt-PA Stroke Trial, higher admission glucose levels were associated with significantly lower odds for desirable clinical outcomes regardless of rt-PA treatment.[128] In northern Manhattan, hyperglycemia was associated with a poor prognosis after stroke, independent of the size or severity of the ischemic stroke.

Diabetes mellitus was found to be a prognostic variable for death in several studies.[55,57,59] This could be due to greater preexisting comorbidity of diabetic patients as well as to greater neuronal damage of ischemic tissue in hyperglycemia. In the prospective observational study of 4585 patients with type 2 diabetes in England, Scotland, and Northern Ireland, each 1% reduction in the mean HbA1c level was associated with reductions in risk of 21% for deaths related to diabetes, 14% for myocardial infarction (MI), and 37% for microvascular complications including stroke.[129] Early mortality after stroke in patients with type 2 diabetes was 28%. Recently, in a European Union Concerted Action involving seven countries and 4537 patients hospitalized for a first-time stroke (21% with diabetes), the case-fatality rates were not higher in the diabetic group in comparison with the nondiabetic group at 3 months after stroke onset.[130] The functional outcome including handicap and disability, however, was significantly worse in stroke patients with diabetes.

Inflammatory Markers and Other Biochemical Blood Parameters

Inflammatory biomarkers, such as C-reactive protein (CRP) and lipoprotein-associated phospholipase A2 (Lp-PLA2), predict not only development of atherothrombotic events but also long-term mortality after acute ischemic stroke.[17,131-135] Elevated admission CRP levels within 12 to 72 hours of stroke were associated with an increased risk of death.[135-139] Individuals with increased CRP levels may have a twofold increased risk of death compared with those with low CRP levels after stroke.[140] The relationship between CRP and poststroke mortality may in part reflect inflammation-induced endothelial cell dysfunction and platelet activation. Also, levels of CRP increase with stroke severity and may be associated with mortality to a greater degree than recurrence, whereas Lp-PLA2 may be a stronger predictor of recurrent stroke risk.[141] Lp-PLA2 is a leukocyte-derived enzyme involved in the metabolism of low-density lipoprotein cholesterol to proinflammatory mediators and was shown to predict incident stroke[142] and recurrent stroke.[143]

Several studies have shown that fibrinogen, erythrocyte sedimentation rate, and leukocyte count are increased after ischemic stroke and are independently associated with the risk of stroke mortality and recurrence.[135,139,144-147] In NOMASS, elevated leukocyte count at the time of ischemic stroke was a significant independent predictor of short-term (30-day) as well as long-term (5-year) combined vascular outcomes after stroke.[148] Further clarification of these biochemical parameters in the prediction of stroke risk is needed.

Uric acid and other parameters of chronic kidney disease have been associated with poor long-term survival rates after stroke. There is a well-recognized link between serum urate levels and increased cardiovascular risk. The serum urate level was associated with a threefold increase in relative risk of cardiac death within 5 years after stroke.[149] Serum urate measured within the first 24 hours after hospital admission for acute stroke was an independent marker of poor outcome in a large study from Scotland.[150] Although the role of urate in stroke pathophysiology remains uncertain, intervention to lower urate levels may be worth considering.[151] Other measures of renal dysfunction, even to a subtle degree, have also been noted to be a prognostic indicator of overall mortality rates in many patient groups.[152-154] In a Scottish, 7-year follow-up study of 2042 stroke patients, reduced admission creatinine clearance, raised serum creatinine and urea concentrations, and raised ratios of urea to creatinine were significant predictors of increased mortality.[115,152]

Soluble biomarkers may have a potential role in risk stratification, but their clinical utility and the clinical relevance of reducing their levels in reducing the risk of stroke outcomes need to be studied further.

Recurrence after Ischemic Stroke

Recurrent stroke is a major cause of morbidity and mortality among stroke survivors. With improved survival rates after first ischemic stroke, stroke recurrence may account for a greater share of the future annual cost of stroke-related health care.[5] Despite advances in stroke prevention strategies and treatments, stroke recurrence is still the major threat to any stroke survivor.

Large prospective, community-based studies indicate that the risk of recurrence after stroke varies from 1% to 4% in the first 30 days, 6% to 13% in the first year, and 5% to 8% per year for the next 2 to 5 years, which culminates in a cumulative risk of recurrence within 5 years of 19% to 42%.[26,57,155-158] Lower recurrent stroke rates have been observed among selected groups of patients in large clinical trials such as TOAST, International Stroke Trial (IST), WARSS, and PRoFESS[11,99,101,159] and also in some prospective community studies.[20,27,77,96] The reasons for the differences in recurrence rates between various studies may reflect the study design (hospital-based versus community), sociodemographics of the study population, definitions of recurrent stroke, and the use of preventive medications such as antiplatelets. Several studies reported recurrent stroke rates for individual subtypes of ischemic stroke.[96,160-163] Higher early recurrence rates for ischemic stroke due to large-vessel atherosclerosis have been consistently reported.[96,161,162,164]

In Rochester, Minnesota, the risk of recurrent stroke after first cerebral infarction was 2% at 7 days, 4% at 30 days, 12% at 1 year, and 29% at 5 years.[26,160] In the Stroke Data Bank, 3.3% of the hospitalized cohort had a stroke recurrence within 30 days, and this accounted for 30% of the recurrent strokes in 2 years of follow-up.[163] In Framingham, cumulative recurrence rates at 5 years after an infarction were 42% for men and 24% for women. Rates were lower in Rochester, Minnesota: 19.3% at 5 years and 28.8% at 10 years.[160] In the Perth Community Stroke Study of 343 patients with first-ever stroke, approximately one in six survivors (15%) of a first-ever stroke experienced a recurrent stroke over 5 years, of which 25% were fatal within 28 days.[157] The cumulative risks of first recurrent stroke were 23% at 5 years and 43% at 10 years.[165] In the northern Manhattan cohort of 992 patients with first-ever ischemic stroke, the cumulative lifetable estimated risks of recurrent stroke were 2.0% at 30 days, 8% at 1 year, and 16% at 5 years (Fig. 15-2).[162] At 30 days, the risk of recurrent stroke was approximately 2.5 times the risk of MI or fatal cardiac events, although this ratio fell to about twice the risk of MI or fatal cardiac event by 5 years.[54] Thus, risk of recurrent stroke predominated even at 5 years among stroke survivors. Other population-based epidemiologic studies have also found that early mortality after stroke is usually related to stroke or recurrent stroke, but that mortality at later time points is more often related to cardiovascular causes.[166,167] The occurrence of nonfatal strokes, although they do not result in death, leads to mounting disability as deficits from repeated strokes accumulate over time.

Predictors of Recurrence after Ischemic Stroke

Prognostic factors for recurrent stroke are clinically important because they help to identify high-risk patients and provide insights into ways to modify outcomes. Factors

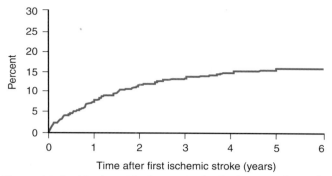

Figure 15-2 Northern Manhattan Stroke Study. Overall cumulative risk of recurrent stroke.

TABLE 15-3 RECURRENCE RISK BY ISCHEMIC STROKE SUBTYPE IN THE NORTHERN MANHATTAN STROKE STUDY

Stroke Subtype	30-Day	1-Year	5-Year
All stroke	2%	8%	16%
Extracranial atherosclerotic	9%	11%	23%
Intracranial atherosclerotic	8%	12%	16%
Cardioembolic	4%	7%	21%
Lacunar	1.4%	10%	14%
Cryptogenic	0.4%	6%	15%

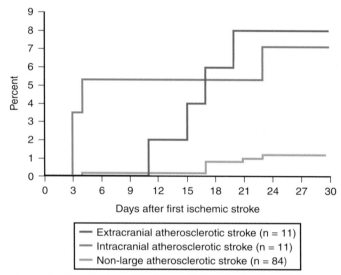

— Extracranial atherosclerotic stroke (n = 11)
— Intracranial atherosclerotic stroke (n = 11)
— Non-large atherosclerotic stroke (n = 84)

Figure 15-3 Northern Manhattan Stroke Study. Thirty-day cumulative risk of recurrence.

that have been associated with an increased risk of recurrent stroke in community-based and hospital-based series include increasing age[26,162,168-170]; male sex[171,172]; female sex[173]; clinical stroke syndrome[174]; history of transient cerebral ischemic attack[68,175]; hypertension[65,68,113,171,175-177]; initial elevated blood pressure[101,176,178,179]; low blood pressure[101,180]; cigarette smoking[174]; alcohol abuse and diabetes mellitus[26,176]; elevated blood glucose levels[173]; history of coronary heart disease[169,174]; AF[115,162,172,181] and other cardiac diseases such as valvular heart disease, congestive heart failure, patent foramen ovale (PFO), and aortic arch atheroma[173,182-188]; abnormal initial brain CT[57,176]; and dementia after stroke.[161]

Predictors of Early Stroke Recurrence

Predictors of recurrent stroke may be time specific and therefore may differ between early and late recurrence. Early after stroke, recurrent stroke tends to predominate, whereas at later points cardiac events begin to increase in relative importance and are the major cause of mortality.[189]

Ischemic stroke subtype was shown to be a predictor of early stroke recurrence. In the Rochester Epidemiology Project, ischemic stroke due to large-vessel atherosclerosis with stenosis had an elevated risk of early recurrence.[96] More than 18% of patients with this subtype had a recurrent stroke within 30 days of the first stroke, which was greater than the range of 8% to 14% reported in previous population- and hospital-based studies.[161,162,190] The variations in recurrence rates may be due to demographic and clinical characteristics of the study subjects and the methodologic differences between the studies. In NOMASS, a high 30-day recurrence risk for stroke due to large artery atherosclerotic disease was also found (Table 15-3 and Fig. 15-3). Estimated rates of recurrent stroke were greater for extracranial atherosclerotic infarcts (9%) and intracranial atherosclerotic infarcts (8%) than for cardioembolic (4%), lacunar (1.4%), and cryptogenic infarcts (0.4%). Patients with large atherosclerotic infarcts were seven times more likely to have recurrence 30 days after the index stroke than those with other ischemic stroke subtypes. Clinical trials have also provided indirect evidence that rates of recurrent stroke are higher among patients with carotid or intracranial atherosclerosis as a

cause of the stroke, as compared with other mechanisms of stroke, although treatment effects are likely to change these rates.[191]

Early stroke recurrence in cardioembolic stroke was reported to be low in several studies.[162,192] The frequent use of anticoagulants may prevent early cardioembolic events and therefore reduce the risk of early recurrence. Stroke due to large-artery stenotic disease is particularly prone to procedure-related cerebral ischemia, which may partly account for the higher risk of early recurrent stroke in this stroke subtype.[193]

Infarct subtype is usually not yet determined on admission; rather it depends on the diagnostic in-patient evaluation. In formulating predictors of early recurrence the best method would be to rely on factors that can be classified readily on first encounter with the patient through the clinical history, examination, and initial neuroimaging and laboratory testing.

In NOMASS besides ischemic stroke subtype, the most significant predictors associated with early stroke recurrence were AF (relative risk [RR], 4.0; 95%CI, 1.1-14.6), alcohol consumption (2-4 drinks per day versus none; RR, 6.8; 95%CI, 1.2-39.9), and hypercholesterolemia (RR, 0.15; 95%CI, 0.1-0.7).[162] Other studies have also identified AF and the presence of a potential cardioembolic source as predictors of early recurrent stroke.[194-196] In the IST, data from 17,398 patients with acute stroke and high or low systolic blood pressure were associated with increased stroke recurrence within 14 days after stroke onset.[101] The rate of recurrent ischemic stroke within 14 days increased by 4.2% for every 10-mm Hg increase in systolic blood pressure, and this association was present in both fatal and nonfatal recurrence. Also, relatively low blood pressure (systolic blood pressure, <120 mm Hg), although an uncommon clinical finding (5% of patients) was also associated with poor outcome. Both relationships appeared to be independent of age, stroke severity, level of consciousness, and AF. This may provide an explanation for a worsening of outcome after the use of calcium channel blockers in some of the acute ischemic stroke studies, most likely because of a reduction of cerebral perfusion.[197,198]

Predictors of Late Stroke Recurrence

Some nonmodifiable and modifiable predictors of late recurrence after ischemic stroke have been identified. Among nonmodifiable predictors, age was the most important predictor of survival after stroke but has not consistently been found to be a determinant of recurrence.

The lack of a significant association between age and stroke recurrence has been observed in several studies.[26,164,168,170] Most studies have found similar stroke recurrence rates for men and women. Fewer studies have evaluated stroke recurrence in different race-ethnic groups. Stroke recurrence was slightly more frequent among black people and Hispanics in northern Manhattan, but these differences failed to reach statistical significance.

In the Rochester study, ischemic stroke due to atherosclerosis with stenosis was associated with fewer recurrent strokes than cardioembolic stroke,[96] whereas in NOMASS the late recurrence risk did not significantly differ between the large atherosclerotic and non-large atherosclerotic stroke subtype (see Table 15-3 and Fig. 15-4).[162,177]

Modifiable predictors of late recurrence after ischemic stroke have not been uniformly established. Even the effect of hypertension has been debated. Some have found no effect of hypertension, while others have suggested that hypertension increased recurrence after stroke.[3,6,175,179,199] This failure to identify hypertension as a predictor of recurrence may reflect the phenomenon that the high risk among patients who already have the disease overwhelms any effect of a specific risk factor. Alternatively, it could serve as an indication that the thresholds for defining these risk factors dichotomously need to be adjusted for the population of patients who have already experienced stroke. In a sense, for a patient who has had a stroke, even a "normal" blood pressure may be too high.[200] Also, as hypertension is very prevalent among stroke patients, the degree of blood pressure control may be more important. High baseline, maximum, mean level, and variability of systolic blood pressure profiles were each inversely associated with favorable outcome in the European Cooperative Acute Stroke Study (ECASS-II) trial.[201] The recommended optimal level of

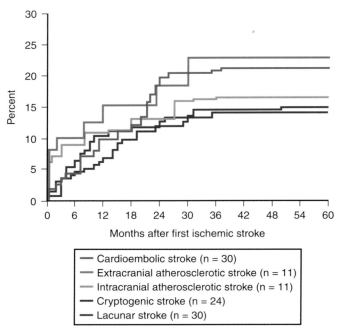

Figure 15-4 Northern Manhattan Stroke Study. Cumulative risk of recurrence by ischemic stroke subtype.

blood pressure reduction to achieve good control has been lowered to <120/80 mm Hg.[202] A J-shaped relation between blood pressure and stroke in treated hypertensive patients has been suggested.[203,204] In the Lehigh Valley Stroke Study, the risk of recurrent stroke was reduced when diastolic blood pressure was below 80 mm Hg.[205] This is consistent with a metaanalysis of antihypertensive medication intervention trials in which blood pressure-lowering drug interventions reduced the risk of stroke recurrence.[206] In PROGRESS, a randomized controlled trial among individuals with previous stroke or transient ischemic attack (TIA), a blood pressure-lowering regimen with perindopril and indapamide reduced the risk of recurrent stroke by more than a quarter.[7] Over 4 years, annual stroke recurrence was reduced from 3.8% to 2.7%. Importantly, stroke risk was also reduced among those patients classified as nonhypertensive (with a mean blood pressure at entry of 136/79 mm Hg). Therefore in all stroke patients, blood pressure may need to be treated more aggressively so that targets are lower. Clinical trials, such as the Secondary Prevention of Small Subcortical Strokes (or SPS3) trial, which randomly assigns patients with lacunar stroke to usual versus aggressive blood pressure targets, are addressing this question.[207]

Cardiac disease has also been found to be a determinant of recurrence after ischemic stroke. In Rochester, cardiac valvular disease and congestive heart failure were independent predictors of recurrent stroke. In the Lehigh Valley, the odds ratio associated with stroke recurrence was approximately 8.0 for either MI or other coronary disease.[208] In the Oxfordshire Community Stroke Project, AF was not associated with a recurrent stroke within the first 30 days and there was only a mild increase in the average annual risk of recurrent stroke from 8.2% with normal sinus rhythm to 11% with AF.[115] AF markedly curtails life expectancy after a stroke, but an independent effect on late recurrence needs further investigation.

Diabetes has been found to be a determinant of stroke recurrence. The data supporting diabetes as a risk factor for recurrent stroke, however, are sparse. In the Rochester study, age and diabetes mellitus were the only significant independent predictors of recurrent stroke.[26] In the Oxfordshire Stroke Project, diabetes was one of two factors independently associated with stroke recurrence, and it was estimated that 9% of the recurrent strokes were attributable to diabetes.[209] In the Stroke Data Bank for 2-year stroke recurrence, patients at the lowest risk had no history of diabetes. Because hyperglycemia at stroke onset is more common among diabetic patients and has been found to predict stroke recurrence, some of the effect of hyperglycemia may be dependent on the presence of diagnosed or undiagnosed diabetes. Further clarification is needed to determine how much control of diabetes after stroke is associated with a reduction in stroke recurrence.

There is a paucity of data on the effect of smoking and alcohol on stroke recurrence, particularly because these risk factors were not well established during the design of earlier stroke epidemiologic studies. Whether smoking is a risk factor for recurrent stroke is still contradictory.[210] Cohort studies have suggested that cessation of smoking after MI is associated with a significant decrease in mortality.[211] Knowledge regarding modification of smoking habits after stroke is nevertheless scant.[212] Whether cessation of smoking after stroke reduces the risk of new, major vascular events is still unknown. Despite current lack of proof, advice on cessation of smoking is included in the strategy for secondary prevention in patients with stroke.[213] Stroke recurrence was significantly increased among those with prior heavy alcohol use in the northern Manhattan cohort. Nearly half of those with a history of heavy alcohol use had a recurrent stroke within 5 years compared with 22% with no history of heavy alcohol use. The effect of alcohol was observed in smokers, nonsmokers, black people, and Hispanics but not among white people. Ethanol could theoretically increase recurrent stroke risk through numerous mechanisms that include hypertension, hypercoagulable states, cardiac arrhythmias, and cerebral blood flow reduction.[214] Ethanol consumption rarely has been identified as a predictor of outcome after stroke except for aneurysmal subarachnoid hemorrhage.[215-218] Because both alcohol and cigarette smoking are modifiable behaviors, it is important to determine their impact on stroke recurrence. In urban populations these behaviors may be more prevalent and may demand greater attention in stroke recurrence prevention programs.

Some new predictors of recurrent stroke have been suggested, including rheumatic mitral valve disease,[186] aortic atheromas,[182,188] and PFO,[183-185,187,219] but require further research.[220] Recurrent embolism occurs in 30% to 65% of patients with rheumatic mitral valve disease who have a history of a previous embolic event.[220] Between 60% and 65% of these recurrences develop within the first year, and most develop within 6 months. Mitral valvuloplasty does not seem to eliminate this risk; therefore these patients require long-term anticoagulation. In the French Study of Aortic Plaques in Stroke, atherosclerotic plaques of 4 mm thick or more in the aortic arch were significant predictors of recurrent brain infarction and other vascular events.[221] In a large cohort of 360 stroke patients enrolled in the PFO in Cryptogenic Stroke Study (PICSS)[219] with a prevalence of PFO of 33.8%, there was no significant difference in the rate of recurrent stroke or death over 2 years between those with PFO (14.8%) of any size and those without PFO (15.4%). In a 4-year follow-up study of 267 cryptogenic stroke patients younger than 55 years with PFO, a 4.5% recurrent stroke rate was reported.[219] Also in PICSS, aortic arch plaques thickness and morphology were associated with a significant increased risk of recurrent stroke and death, despite treatment with warfarin or aspirin.[222] This risk was exceptionally high in patients with cryptogenic stroke.

The evidence for the relationship between stroke recurrence and inflammatory and hemostatic markers has been accumulating.[223-225] Possible biochemical and clinical predictors of recurrent stroke include levels of CRP, Lp-PLA2, cholesterol, fibrinogen, hematocrit, protein C, lupus anticoagulant, anticardiolipin antibodies, and homocysteine and white blood cell count, the albumin–globulin ratio, free protein S deficiency, and obesity.[226-232] Although some markers had some predictive ability, none of the studies was able to demonstrate that the biomarker added predictive power to a validated clinical model. The clinical usefulness of blood biomarkers for predicting prognosis in the setting of ischemic stroke has yet to be established.

Worsening after Ischemic Stroke

The term *worsening after ischemic stroke* encompasses a broad range of causes with a variable starting period of onset, durations, and course.[233,234] Ideally, physicians should attempt to alter a declining course of illness that begins at the time of symptom onset. Worsening during the first few hours often has quite different explanations than worsening during hours 12 to 48. Unfortunately, it is often difficult to quantify deficits present before the patient is seen by medical personnel with the use of only the accounts of the patient and observers. There are three main categories of worsening: (1) neurologic deterioration—gradual or stepwise progression of neurologic focal deficits while the patient usually remains alert and free of medical complications, (2) brain edema—a complication of mostly large strokes, especially hemorrhages that are accompanied by headaches and decreased alertness, and (3) medical complications—especially febrile illnesses, which affect the patient systemically and may also lead to increased brain ischemia. Other medical complications include deep vein thrombosis and pulmonary embolism, and the risk ranges from less than 1% to 30% depending on stroke severity and the degree of immobility of the patient during the subacute phase of recovery.[235,236]

Neurologic deterioration is reported to occur in 20% to 58% of patients with acute stroke regardless of modern supportive care.[233,237,238] The frequency of clinical worsening after hospitalization varies depending on the mix of stroke patients and their time delay between symptom onset and entry into the hospital. In the Harvard Stroke

Registry, 20% of stroke patients progressed after stroke onset.[239] Progression was most common in patients with lacunar infarcts (37%) and large-artery occlusive disease (33%) and least frequent in patients with embolism (7%). In the Barcelona Stroke Registry, among more than 3500 patients, 37% worsened after onset.[240] In the Lausanne Stroke Registry, among more than 3000 patients, worsening after admission occurred in 29% of all stroke patients and in 34% of patients with noncardioembolic ischemic strokes.[241] Among the noncardioembolic stroke patients who worsened, 58% progressed during the first 24 hours. In a Japanese study, among 350 stroke patients, 25% progressed after admission and 26% had lacunar stroke.[242] When worsening occurred after acute ischemic stroke, the majority of the time it was due to stroke evolution. In the NINDS Stroke Data Bank, among 1271 ischemic stroke patients, 72% of those who worsened during their hospitalization did so because of stroke evolution.

The causes of neurologic deterioration have not been clearly identified, although several variables were associated with deterioration. Progression of thrombosis or recurrent embolism has attracted some attention. Variables reported as predictive of neurologic deterioration include high systolic blood pressure, hyperglycemia on admission, and carotid territory involvement.[243,244] Deterioration within 4 days after stroke onset mainly occurred in cases in which arterial occlusion led to large infarctions and secondary edema was found on brain CT studies.[238] Studies using magnetic resonance technology show that patients whose perfusion-weighted images (PWI) show a larger area of involvement than the diffusion-weighted images (DWI) and who have persistent occlusive lesions on magnetic resonance angiography develop larger infarcts and more severe clinical deficits than those patients with open arteries and no PWI–DWI mismatching.[245,246] In the cases of stenosis or occlusion of large arteries or penetrating artery disease, severe flow reduction to ischemic brain areas may occur. Hypoperfusion and distal embolization are likely the most important mechanisms that lead to progressive infarction.

Severe stroke has been shown to be an important predictor of clinical worsening.[174] In the Copenhagen Study, patients with neurologic deterioration had more severe strokes than patients without deterioration.[247] In ECASS, coronary heart disease, diabetes, and early signs of infarction on CT scans were predictive of deterioration within 24 hours, whereas age, severe stroke, and brain swelling were predictive of deterioration from 24 hours to 7 days.[243] Worsening after stroke is most often related to the stroke subtype. Although hemodynamic infarction from large artery occlusion or stenosis carries a great risk of worsening, small vessel lacunar infarcts may also be associated with a risk of worsening. A number of studies focused on progression and worsening in series of patients with lacunar strokes.[248-250] In the Neurological Institute's subpopulation of the Stroke Data Bank, a pure motor syndrome had a better outcome in terms of improvement of motor deficits than did the other lacunar syndromes.[251] In a German study, 24% of patients had a worsening of motor deficits after hospitalization, predominantly those with lacunar strokes.[250] Progression

of deficits in patients with lacunar strokes, even evolving within days after onset, has been noted many times in the past. Mohr, in a 1982 review of lacunar infarcts, commented that "a surprisingly leisurely mode of onset characterizes many lacunar strokes."[248]

The causes of clinical worsening are diverse and commonly include brain edema, seizures, collateral failure, reocclusion, and systemic medical complications. Because most causes of worsening can be treated effectively, the deteriorating stroke patient merits a swift and incisive diagnostic and therapeutic response.

Cardiac Events after Stroke

After a stroke, the risk of MI is increased by a factor of 2 to 3 compared with the stroke-free population.[252] MI is the most frequent cause of death in stroke survivors. In an older unselected series of 843 cases of cerebral thrombosis followed for 9 to 19 years, 41% of the initial survivors died of recurrent strokes and 30% died of heart disease.[106] In Rochester, stroke survivors died of heart disease twice as often as they died of recurrent stroke.[158] The annual risk of vascular death after a minor or a major stroke was estimated from various clinical trials to be 3.2% to 3.5%.[19,253] Forty percent of patients with a history of ischemic stroke or TIA have concomitant coronary artery disease.[254]

Overall, the risk of MI itself after stroke is probably relatively low in the short term, that is, up to 2 years. MI occurred in 2.5% of patients enrolled in the Second European Stroke Prevention Study (ESPS-2) during 2 years of follow-up.[255] MI occurred as the first event during almost 2 years of follow-up in only 1.5% of patients with stroke enrolled in another secondary prevention trial.[256] Data from administrative databases similarly suggest a risk of MI of about 2% to 3% during the first 2 years after ischemic stroke of noncardioembolic origin.[257]

The risk of MI over the long term after stroke, however, is significant and may increase in a nonlinear fashion. For example, in a retrospective study of 1044 patients with cerebral infarction, the 10-year risk of MI or sudden death was increased compared with the age-matched population at 5 years, but a divergence in risk curves was noted after 6 months.[258] The probability of MI or sudden death was only 0.8% at 6 months, but it was already 10.6% at 5 years, which was twice the expected rate. In NOMASS, the 5-year risk of MI or vascular death was 17%.[54] In Rochester, Minnesota, from 1960 to 1979,[258] the cumulative incidence of MI or "sudden unexpected death" after first stroke was 1.4% at 1 year, 11% at 5 years, and 17% at 10 years.

The cardiovascular risk in some patient populations with stroke may be lower than in others. Patients with lacunar strokes had a lower risk of subsequent MI and vascular death in northern Manhattan and other populations. In a group of patients with incident lacunar strokes in Portugal, for example, only 3% had MI after a median follow-up of 39 months.[259] In a large, randomized, secondary prevention trial in black people, in which two thirds of patients enrolled had lacunar strokes at baseline, the risk of MI and fatal vascular events was low (approximately 3% over 2 years).[51,260] Even if the vascular risk after a stroke is considered to be "low," all of these data provide evidence that the cardiovascular risk in stroke survivors is about 2% per year, which would place stroke in "coronary risk equivalents."[261]

Other abnormalities such as depolarization and ischemic-like electrocardiographic (ECG) changes observed during the acute phase of stroke are quite common. Ischemic-like ECG changes and/or QT prolongation were present in more than 90% of unselected patients with ischemic stroke and intracerebral hemorrhages and most often represent preexisting coronary artery disease.

Stroke Outcome Prediction Models

The discrepancies in identifying predictors of stroke outcome including mortality and recurrence have been observed across studies. They may result from the age and stroke subtype composition of the cohorts, the definition of the predictors used in the study, the duration of follow-up, the timing of the outcome of interest, and the relative contribution of other predictors.

The great variability of outcome seen in stroke patients has led to an interest in identifying predictors of outcome with the use of prediction models. The combination of clinical and imaging variables as predictors of stroke outcome in a multivariable risk adjustment model may be more powerful than either alone. Age and the severity of the presenting clinical deficit are consistently found to be predictive of outcome.[56,57,66,96] Many other predictors have been reported to have a univariable relationship with outcome, but their multivariable relationship to outcome is less clear.[57]

Several stroke mortality prediction models have been reported. In a model of 1-year survival after ischemic stroke from the Perth Community Stroke Study, coma, urinary incontinence, cardiac failure, severe paresis, and AF were the most important predictors.[36] The sensitivity, specificity, and negative predictive value for predicting death were 90%, 83%, and 95%, respectively. In the northern Manhattan cohort, independent determinants of 5-year mortality among 30-day survivors were age, major hemispheric or basilar syndrome, congestive heart failure, and admission glucose level. In the Helsinki Young Stroke Registry of young adult patients (ages 15 to 49 years), increasing age, malignancy, heart failure, heavy drinking, infection, type 1 diabetes, and large artery atherosclerosis independently predicted 5-year mortality.[39]

In the Randomized Trial of Tirilazad Mesylate in Acute Stroke (RANTTAS),[262] the baseline NIHSS score, small-vessel infarct, history of previous stroke, history of diabetes, history of prestroke disability, and infarct volume at 7 to 10 days were significant predictors of survival and excellent outcome as determined by the NIHSS score of 1 at 3 months.[57] For very poor outcomes, including death, only infarct volume was a significant predictor of an NIHSS score of 20 or death at 3 months. Other studies have also combined clinical and imaging variables for predicting stroke outcomes.[176,180,263] They suggested that because the final size of an infarct cannot be detected on CT for several days after the event, the infarct volume does not improve the predictive ability of such models. MR imaging techniques, such as diffusion-weighted MRI (DWI), that identify lesion volume in the acute setting may improve our ability to quickly predict stroke outcomes.[264-267] Recently, interest has focused on combining clinical and neuroimaging data to develop multivariable risk adjustment models of stroke outcome. Such models may provide greater discriminatory power to predict clinical outcomes than clinical or neuroimaging information alone. DWI is able to demonstrate areas of cerebral infarction within hours of symptom onset, and several studies of early DWI have found a strong association with outcome[268,269]; however, others have not supported a strong relation.[270-272] In the hours to days after a stroke, DWI lesions are dynamic, and early changes in DWI infarct volume after a stroke are an important predictor of outcome. Some have shown that growth in DWI lesion volume greater than 10 cm^3 in the first 5 days after a stroke of mild to moderate severity was significantly associated with a poor outcome,[273] but these data await further validation. If these results are replicated in larger trials, the incorporation of measures of change in early DWI lesion volume may improve the prognostic accuracy of stroke predictive models.

Stroke Prognostic Risk Scores

Risk stratification as a tool to determine optimal secondary prevention after a stroke requires consideration of levels of overall absolute vascular risk in patients with stroke rather than the risk of recurrent stroke alone. Those who experience a first ischemic stroke have a high relative risk as well as an absolute risk of a subsequent cardiovascular event. The subsequent event is more likely to be a stroke than an MI, but other manifestations of vascular disease, including MI and vascular death, are common potential outcomes. The risk of cardiovascular outcomes after TIA, even in the first 90 days, is as high as 25% and is not limited to stroke.[274] Predictive scores are important tools for stratifying patients based on the risk of future vascular events and for selecting potential prevention therapy. Several scores have been suggested for risk stratification in secondary stroke prevention including *Stroke Prognostic Instrument II*,[275] and *Essen Stroke Risk Score* (ESRS), derived from cerebrovascular patients in the Clopidogrel versus Aspirin in Patients at Risk of Ischemic Events (CAPRIE) trial.[276] ESRS was recently validated with the use of the data set of the ESPS-2[277] and in a large cohort of 15,605 outpatients with previous TIA or stroke from the REduction of Atherothrombosis for Continued Health (REACH) Registry.[278] In the ESRS, one point was given to each of the eight predictors including age, hypertension, diabetes, smoking, history of previous MI, other cardiac events excluding AF, peripheral artery disease, and TIA or stroke. In NOMASS, a weighted scoring system was developed using seven significant predictors of 5-year recurrent stroke (i.e., age, NIHSS, AF, peripheral artery disease, heavy alcohol use, physical inactivity, and high-density lipoprotein cholesterol level <40).

These scores include readily available patient demographic and clinical data and are therefore easy to calculate, may be applicable to a broad population of stroke patients, and can aid in prediction of recurrent stroke and other vascular outcomes for direction of treatment strategies.

Functional Disability and Handicap after Stroke

Functional disability, the lack of ability to perform an activity or task in the range considered normal for an individual, is an important outcome after a nonfatal stroke. Reliable and valid scales have been developed to determine activities of daily living and other indices for measuring functional dependence. Two of the most used are the Barthel Activities of Daily Living (ADL)[279,280] and the modified Rankin Scale.[281] These instruments are simple, reliable, and reasonably sensitive for assessing disability. The approximate proportion of stroke survivors who are independent at 6 months ranges from 40% to 65%, depending on the characteristics of the study population. A high ADL score at hospital discharge is a good predictor of a favorable functional prognosis.[282] Functional activity measured by ADL score has been often used as a primary outcome in randomized acute stroke clinical trials. In the GAIN (Glycine Antagonist in Neuroprotection) Americas trial, 38% of patients were functionally independent with the use of the ADL score (ADL of 95 to 100) and 27% were functionally independent with the use of the Rankin score (0 or 1) at 3 months after an acute onset of ischemic stroke.[283]

Once the patient has survived the immediate stroke, the potential for recovery and the likelihood of long-term survival free of dependence on others are the concerns for stroke patients, their families, and health care professionals. This information should be based on predictive models derived from data sets that include complete follow-up of cases of first-ever stroke from large, community-based cohorts with the standard diagnostic criteria and clinical assessments of disease severity, comorbidities, and sociodemographic factors and standardized measures of functional outcome. There are several studies of long-term functional outcome after stroke, but only a few reliable estimates of the long-term functional outcome after first-ever ischemic stroke are available.[280,284-300] The largest studies are summarized in Table 15-4. In a recent systematic review of the literature and despite the lack of uniformity of long-term outcome results among studies, the overall evidence supporting the use of the Barthel Index and modified Rankin Scale as prognostic tools is quite strong.[301]

One of the largest functional outcome studies was the Auckland Stroke Study, in which information on disability and health-related QOL (HRQOL) was available on nearly all of the 639 six-year survivors (36%) of the

TABLE 15-4 STUDIES OF DISABILITY OR HANDICAP AT LEAST 3 MONTHS AFTER STROKE

Study	Strokes, N	Mean Age or Range, yr	Follow-up Time	Outcomes Measured	Outcome Independence/ Survival, %
Community based					
Auckland, New Zealand	1761	71	6 yr	Disability (ADL)/SF-36	39
	680	70	6 mo	Disability (Katz Scale)	76
Rochester, Minnesota	292	72	5 yr	Disability (ADL)/SF-36	39
				Disability (Katz Scale)	76
Perth, Western Australia	492	73	5 yr	Disability (Barthel Index)	38
				Survival	59
Newcastle, UK	229	82	3 yr	Disability (Barthel Index)	45
Oxfordshire, UK	675	72	1 yr	Handicap (Rankin)	71
				Survival	49
Melbourne, Australia	264	72	1 yr	Handicap (Rankin)	65
				Survival	77
South England, UK	456	65	1 yr	Disability (Barthel Index)	71
L'Aquila, Italy	819	75	1 yr	Disability (Barthel Index)	76
				Survival	64
Bristol, UK	976	75	6 mo	Disability (Barthel Index)	64
				Survival	63
Tartu, Estonia	519	70	6 mo	Disability (undefined)	24
				Survival	63
NOMASS	395	69	6 mo	Disability (ADL)	33
				Survival	59
Hospital based					
Iowa Young Adults	296	15-45	16 yr	Disability (Barthel Index)	49
				Survival	79
Southeast London, UK	291	71	5 yr	Disability (Barthel Index)	34
				Handicap (Rankin)	36
				Survival	42
Hong Kong, China	303	70	20 mo	Disability (Barthel Index)	57
				Survival	58
GAIN Americas	1367	70	3 mo	Disability (Barthel Index)	38
				Handicap (Rankin)	27
				Survival	80

Abbreviations: ADL, Activities of daily living; NOMASS, Northern Manhattan Stroke Study; GAIN, Glycine Antagonist in Neuroprotection.

original cohort of 1761 patients registered in 1991 to 1992.[286] In this study, 42% of patients were dependent in at least one aspect of ADLs 6 years after stroke. In the Perth Community Stroke Study among 30-day survivors of initial stroke, one third remained disabled, and one in seven were in permanent institutional care.[287] The major predictors of poor long-term outcome were a low level of activity before the stroke, subsequent recurrent stroke, older age, baseline disability defined by the Barthel Index score, and severe stroke at onset. In NOMASS, functional outcome was assessed by ADLs at two time points: at 7 to 10 days and 6 months after stroke onset.[302] Among 359 stroke survivors, 35% were independent, 37% were moderately dependent, and 28% were dependent 7 to 10 days after first ischemic stroke (Fig.15-5). Six months later, 55% of patients were independent on the ADL scale. In the multivariate model, only ADLs assessed at 7 to 10 days were predictive of 6-month functional independence, which indicates that long-term functional independence was strongly influenced by early functional recovery after stroke.

Handicap is the disadvantage for an individual resulting from an impairment or disability that limits or prevents the fulfillment of a role (depending on age, sex, and social and cultural factors) that is normal for that individual.[303] Although poststroke disability has been the subject of much discussion in the literature, handicap has received little attention. Handicap is an important target of rehabilitation. Some domains of handicap are potentially modifiable, but knowledge of which aspects of handicap are most affected in stroke survivors is limited.[304] In the Melbourne Stroke Study, stroke survivors were found to be handicapped over a wide range of domains.[295] The most disadvantages occurred in the domains of physical independence and occupation. Handicap increased with the severity of disability. Patients with total anterior circulation infarcts were the most disabled and handicapped 3 and 12 months after stroke.[305] Using the modified Rankin Scale, the Oxfordshire Community Stroke Project and the Perth Community Stroke Study found that patients with total anterior circulatory infarcts had a low likelihood of living independently 12 months after stroke.[77,306] Patients with lacunar infarcts were least disabled. Similarly, in the Rochester Epidemiology Project, patients with lacunar infarcts had the best functional outcomes: more than 80% had minimal or no functional impairment 1 year after stroke. Patients with cardioembolic stroke had poorer

prestroke functional status, more severe neurologic deficits at the time of stroke, and poorer functional outcomes compared with patients with other subtypes.[96]

Some limitations of the ADL and Rankin scales need to be noted. One of them is the "ceiling effect" of the ADL scales. Patients who are functionally independent on the ADL scales (with the highest score) may continue to improve after stroke, and this improvement cannot be detected with the current ADL scales. The modified Rankin Scale, although easy to use and widely adopted as a measure of handicap in stroke clinical trials, is a fairly nonspecific instrument that measures a mix of impairment, disability, and handicap when natural history data and the effects of interventions on outcomes are assessed.[307] Furthermore, summary scores based on aggregated data may hide wide intraindividual variations. Some patients make a rapid, early recovery; others have a more prolonged recovery. Continuing improvement may also be minimized by the effects of aging and the development of other disabilities that may or may not be stroke related. Several new approaches to analysis of stroke outcome scales have recently been adopted, including the global statistic, responder analysis, and shift analysis.[308] Each of these approaches offers distinctive benefits and drawbacks. The choice of primary endpoint and analytical technique should be tailored to the study population, expected treatment response, and study purpose. Shift analysis, also known as analysis of distributions or rank analysis, generally provides the most comprehensive index of a treatment's clinical impact and has been a preferable choice of stroke outcome analysis in recent clinical trials.[309]

Stroke disability outcome scales rate patients across multiple ranks; for example, the modified Rankin Scale divides global disability into seven strata, and the Barthel Index rates functional ADLs among 20 levels; stroke-related QOL scales have, however, finer gradations that substantially reduce ceiling and floor effects.

Quality of Life after Stroke

QOL is another important outcome after stroke. Recreational and social activities are reduced for most stroke survivors after they return home, regardless of whether they have made a complete functional recovery.[310-312] There is no single accepted definition of HRQOL. It is assumed to be a broad, multidimensional construct that assesses some measurement of physical status, mental and psychological status, social activity status, and functional status.[313] A substantial proportion of stroke survivors have very poor HRQOL. In the community-based North East Melbourne Stroke Incidence Study (NEMESIS), 8% of patients had HRQOL assessed as equivalent to or worse than death and almost 25% had an overall poor outcome 2 years after stroke.[314]

Numerous instruments have been developed and applied to the evaluation of prognosis after stroke including the Stroke Impact Scale (SIS), Sickness Impact Profile, the Social Functioning subscale of the Short Form-36 (SF-36), the Nottingham Profile, Euroqual, and the Quality of Well Being (QWB).[315-322] All scales provide multidimensional assessment but vary in the number and combination

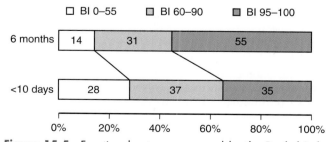

Figure 15-5 Functional outcome assessed by the Barthel Index (BI) at 6 months and less than 10 days after the onset of a first ischemic stroke among 359 stroke survivors in the Northern Manhattan Stroke Study.

of dimensions. All include assessment of physical functioning and most incorporate concepts, such as psychological well-being, social well-being, and role activities. The assessment of outcomes including QOL in individuals after stroke is important for both clinical practice and research, yet there is no consensus on the best measures of stroke outcome in either clinical practice or research. Existing measures have not been sensitive to change in patients with mild strokes.[320] There are very few studies that have quantitated the impact of stroke on QOL. However, no stroke-specific outcome measure has been developed that assesses other dimensions of HRQOL (e.g., emotion, communication, memory and thinking, and social role function).

The SIS has been developed as a stroke-specific outcome measure, especially for mild to moderate strokes.[323] The measure was developed from the perspective and input of both the patient and caregiver, and it incorporates contemporary standards of instrument development. This new, stroke-specific outcome measure seems to be comprehensive, reliable, valid, and sensitive to change. However, more studies are required to evaluate the SIS in larger and more heterogeneous populations and to evaluate the feasibility and validity of proxy responses for the most severely impaired patients.

In the northern Manhattan population-based case-control study of 207 patients older than 39 years with first cerebral infarction, the QWB scale was used to assess QOL after stroke. In the comparison with the prestroke QWB score, the 6-month QWB score decreased by 27%.[324] Even among those patients who were functionally independent at 6 months (Barthel ADL ≥ 70), there was still a 12% decrease in QWB.

The SF-36 is the most widely used generic instrument for measuring QOL, although it is not specific to stroke patients.[325] The instrument is translated into numerous languages, and the validity of the eight subscales is confirmed in general populations and in a wide variety of patient groups in more than 2000 articles. In view of the current evidence that the subscales of the SF-36 are psychometrically sound for measuring QOL in a range of patient populations, the SF-36 may be a useful measure of QOL in stroke.[325,326]

Stroke-specific QOL scores and patient impairments predict patient-reported overall HRQOL after stroke.[326] Disease-specific HRQOL measures are more sensitive to meaningful changes in poststroke HRQOL and may thus aid in identifying specific aspects of poststroke function that clinicians and "stroke trialists" can target to improve patients' HRQOL after stroke. In a recent review of the HRQOL scales, one generic (Sickness Impact Profile) and two stroke-specific scales (SIS and Stroke-Specific Quality of Life Scale) seemed most comprehensive.[327] Whether any of these assessments are sufficient to describe HRQOL after stroke in its entirety is unclear.

Several limitations of the QOL scales need to be emphasized. Most existing stroke QOL outcome measures suffer from floor and/or ceiling effects, and the summary scores may inadequately reflect the patient's physical and mental health.[328-330] When traditional multi-item instruments such as the SF-36 are used, summated scores are dependent on the number of various items included in the different instruments; therefore, it is impossible to compare scores obtained on different instruments. Furthermore, the clinical interpretation of summated scores is not straightforward. For example, the clinical meaning of a mean score of 47.6 on SF-36 in a stroke patient would be unclear for most neurologists. This problem is amplified by the ordinal nature of summated scores; that is, a given difference in scores at one point on the scale does not necessarily represent the same amount of functional change at another point on the scale. Following growing dissatisfaction with the classic scales, the alternative Item Response Theory (IRT) method has been introduced.[331] This statistical paradigm uses a logistic regression analysis to model the responses of the patients to the individual items. Therefore, the items can be placed on the same hierarchical continuous scale, which helps assessment and interpretation of the scales. Despite recent interest in IRT in clinical outcome measurement, these methods need to be developed in stroke research as a useful supplement to the traditional QOL approach.[332]

No single outcome measure can describe or predict all dimensions of recovery and disability after stroke, and each scale has a potential role in patient care and outcome research. Composite measures may be useful in determining the multiple dimensions of outcomes after stroke, and ongoing attempts are being made to incorporate patients' perspectives, as these ultimately are critical measures of either a high QOL or failure.

Depression after Stroke

Major depression is a common occurrence after stroke.[333-335] Pooled estimates from a recent metaanalysis suggest an incidence of poststroke depression of 33%.[336] This rate is relatively constant across the short and long term after stroke. The incidence, however, appears to vary widely across individual studies, ranging from 6% to 63%. The studies that have compared the poststroke incidence of depression with appropriately matched community control subjects have found that the risk of depression is at least doubled after stroke compared with what would be expected in the general population.[334] In addition to the emotional well-being of the stroke survivor, the recognition and treatment of depression is important because depression is associated with disability,[337] cognitive impairment,[338,339] suicide, and mortality.[340] Depression has been associated with excess stroke disability,[333,341-347] poor rehabilitation outcomes[348,349] morbidity and mortality,[350,351] and suicidal thoughts and plans.[344] In the vast majority of patients the detection of depression during standard stroke care is still overlooked by treating physicians.[352]

If standard diagnostic criteria (either the *Diagnostic and Statistical Manual of Mental Disorders* [DSM] or Research Diagnostic Criteria) is used to establish the presence of a major depressive episode, depression occurs, at least temporarily, in up to 30% to 40% of stroke survivors.[335] Although, the term *poststroke depression* has already been established in the literature, standardized criteria for this diagnosis do not exist. In most cases the DSM-IV or International Classification of Diseases system is applied. Other investigators used various psychiatric rating scales. In addition to diagnosis based on psychiatric interview and the DSM criteria, a variety of self-rating mood scales (e.g., Beck Depression Inventory [BDI])[353] and interviewer-administered scales (e.g., Hamilton Rating Scale for Depression [HRSD][354] are used. These measures are not specifically designed for patients with stroke, who typically have a variety of physical and cognitive impairments that may introduce difficulties in the use of these instruments. The BDI and the HRSD in patients with stroke have been acceptable screening instruments in the assessment of poststroke depression, but their specificity seems to be too low to provide a basis for diagnosis of depression.[355]

It is generally acknowledged that there is a high prevalence of depression after stroke. The occurrence of depression after stroke is, however, underdiagnosed and often left untreated. In addition, little is known about the course of major depression after a stroke. Prevalence clearly varies over time; depression has an apparent peak 3 to 6 months after a stroke and a subsequent decline in prevalence at 1 year to about 50% of initial rates.[356]

Treatment or prevention of depression after stroke is greatly dependent on understanding the pathophysiologic mechanism linking stroke and depression. Even though the DSM-IV classification implies that strokes "cause" depression through a direct biological mechanism, the nature of the mechanism linking stroke and depression remains debated in the literature.[335] Some propose a primary biological mechanism according to which ischemic insults directly affect neural circuits involved in mood regulation, while others propose a psychosocial mechanism according to which the social and psychological stressors associated with a stroke are considered the primary cause of depression.[357-359]

Stroke survivors in active rehabilitation programs have been shown to have lower rates of depression.[360] It has also been reported that depressed stroke survivors with cognitive impairment had greater chronicity of depression than depressed stroke survivors without significant cognitive impairment.[361] Furthermore, left anterior ischemic lesions were associated with cognitive impairment in stroke survivors with major depression. This finding indicates that ischemic lesions in the area of the striato-frontal circuit identified on brain imaging are associated with increased cognitive impairment and chronicity of depression.[362]

Depression after stroke is a common occurrence associated with excess disability, cognitive impairment, and mortality. Poststroke depression does not appear to be the result of "pure" biological versus psychological causes; instead it seems to be multifactorial in origin and consistent with the biopsychosocial model of mental illness. The relative effects of disability and reduced neurotransmitter system activity on poststroke depression remain uncertain. Similarly, the role of antidepressants has been demonstrated[363] but has not yet consistently been confirmed. A metaanalysis reported significant effect of antidepressants across 10 studies with a duration of treatment ranging from 4 to 52 weeks.[364] Some studies, however, were designed for prophylaxis, whereas other studies were short-term treatment studies. A better understanding of pathomechanism, incidence, prevalence, and factors associated with depression after stroke is needed.

REFERENCES

1. Murray CJL, Lopez AD: Mortality by cause for 8 regions of the world: Global burden of disease study, *Lancet* 349:1269-1276, 1997.
2. Murray CJL, Lopez AD: Global mortality, disability and the contribution of risk factors: Global burden of disease study, *Lancet* 349:1436-1442, 1997.
3. Wolf AP, Clagett P, Easton JD, et al: Preventing ischemic stroke in patients with prior stroke and TIA. A statement for healthcare professionals from the Stroke Council of the American Heart Association, *Stroke* 30:1991-1994, 1999.
4. Collins R, MacMahon S: Blood pressure, antihypertensive drug treatment and risk of stroke and coronary heart disease, *Br Med Bull* 50:272-298, 1994.
5. Rosamond W, Flegal K, Furie K, et al: Heart disease and stroke statistics—2008 update: A report from the American Heart Association Statistics Committee and Stroke Statistics Subcommittee, *Circulation* 117:e25-146, 2008.
6. Blood Pressure Lowering Treatment Trialists' Collaboration: Effects of ACE inhibitors, calcium antagonists and other blood pressure lowering drugs: Results of the prospective designed overviews of randomised trials, *Lancet* 356:1955-1964, 2000.
7. PROGRESS Collaborative Group: Randomized trial of perindopril-based blood-pressure-lowering regimen among 6105 individuals with previous stroke or transient ischemic attack, *Lancet* 358:1033-1041, 2001.
8. Heart Outcomes Prevention Evaluation (HOPE) Study Investigators: Effects of an angiotensin-converting-enzyme inhibitor, ramapril, on cardiovascular events in high-risk patients, *N Engl J Med* 342:145-153, 2000.
9. Amarenco P, Bogousslavsky J, Callahan A III, et al: Stroke Prevention by Aggressive Reduction in Cholesterol Levels (SPARCL) Investigators. High-dose atorvastatin after stroke or transient ischemic attack, *N Engl J Med* 355(6):549-559, 2006.
10. Diener HC, Bogousslavsky J, Brass LM, et al: On behalf of the MATCH investigators. Aspirin and clopidogrel compared with clopidogrel alone after recent ischaemic stroke or transient ischaemic attack in high-risk patients (MATCH): Randomized, double-blind, placebo-controlled trial, *Lancet* 364:331-337, 2004.
11. Sacco RL, Diener HC, Yusuf S, et al: PRoFESS Study Group. Aspirin and extended-release dipyridamole versus clopidogrel for recurrent stroke, *N Engl J Med* 359(12):1238-1251, 2008.
12. Romano JG, Sacco RL: Progress in secondary stroke prevention, *Ann Neurol* 63(4):418-427, 2008.
13. National Center for Health Statistics. *Vital Statistics of the United States, Data Warehouse.* Available at: http://www.cdc.gov/nchs/data/dvs/MortFinal2003_WorkTable307.pdf. Accessed October 29, 2006.
14. US Department of Health and Human Services: *Healthy People 2010: Understanding and improving health*, ed 2, Washington DC, November 2000, US Government Printing Office.
15. Luepker RV, Arnett DK, Jacobs DR Jr, et al: Trends in blood pressure, hypertension control, and stroke mortality: The Minnesota Heart Survey, *Am J Med* 119:42-49, 2006.
16. Kleindorfer D, Khoury J, Broderick JP, et al: Temporal trends in public awareness of stroke: Warning signs, risk factors, and treatment, *Stroke* 40(7):2502-2506, 2009.
17. Gorelick PB: Stroke prevention therapy beyond antithrombotics: Unifying mechanisms in ischemic stroke pathogenesis and implications for therapy, An invited review, *Stroke* 33:862-875, 2002.
18. Sacco RL, Wolf PA, Gorelick PB: Risk factors and their management for stroke prevention: Outlook for 1999 and beyond, *Neurology* 53(Suppl 4):S15-S24, 1999.
19. Wilterdink JL, Easton JD: Vascular event rates in patients with atherosclerotic cerebrovascular disease, *Arch Neurol* 49:857-863, 1992.
20. Sacco RL: Current Epidemiology of Stroke. In Fisher M, Bogousslavsky J, editors: *Current review of cerebrovascular disease*, Philadelphia, 1993, Current Medicine.
21. Sacco RL: Prognosis of Stroke. In Bogousslavsky J, Ginsberg MD, editors: *Cerebrovascular disease—Pathophysiology, diagnosis and management.* Malden, Mass, 1998, Blackwell Science, pp 879-891.

22. Sacco RL, Wolf PA, Kannel WB, McNamara PM: Survival and recurrence—The Framingham Study, *Stroke* 13:290-295, 1982.

23. Howard G, Evans GW, Murros KE, et al: Cause specific mortality following cerebral infarction, *J Clin Epidemiol* 42:45-51, 1989.

24. Rosamond WD, Folsom AR, Chambless LE, et al: Stroke incidence and survival among middle-aged adults: 9-year follow-up of the Atherosclerotic Risk in Communities (ARIC) cohort, *Stroke* 30:736-774, 1999.

25. El-Saed A, Kuller LH, Newman AB, et al: Geographic variations in stroke incidence and mortality among older populations in four US communities, *Stroke* 37:1975-1979, 2006.

26. Petty GW, Brown RD Jr, Whisnant JP, et al: Survival and recurrence after first cerebral infarction: A population-based study in Rochester, Minnesota, 1975 through 1989, *Neurology* 50(1):208-216, 1998.

27. Sacco RL, Shi T, Zamanillo MC, Kargman D: Predictors of mortality and recurrence after hospitalized cerebral infarction in an urban community: The Northern Manhattan Stroke Study, *Neurology* 44:626-634, 1994.

28. Fang J, Alderman MH: Trend of stroke hospitalization, United States, 1988-1997, *Stroke* 32(10):2221-2226, 2001.

29. D'Alessandro G, Bottacchi E, Di Giovanni M, et al: Temporal trends of stroke in Valle d'Aosta, Italy: incidence and 30-day fatality rates, *Neurol Sci* 21:13-18, 2000.

30. Mayo NE, Neville D, Kirkland S, et al: Hospitalization and case-fatality rates for stroke in Canada from 1982 through 1991: The Canadian Collaborative Study Group of Stroke Hospitalizations, *Stroke* 27:1215-1220, 1996.

31. Truelsen T, Gronbaek M, Schnohr P, Boysen G: Stroke case fatality in Denmark from 1977-1992: The Copenhagen City Heart Study, *Neuroepidemiology* 21(1):22-27, 2002.

32. Reeves MJ, Smith E, Fonarow G, et al: GWTG-Stroke Steering Committee & Investigators. Off-hour admission and in-hospital stroke case fatality in the Get With The Guidelines stroke program, *Stroke* 40(2):569-576, 2009.

33. Hartmann A, Rundek T, Mast H, Paik MC, Boden-Albala B, Mohr JP, Sacco RL: Mortality and causes of death after first-ischemic stroke: The Northern Manhattan Stroke Study, *Neurology* 57:2000-2005, 2001.

34. Loor HI, Groenier KH, Limburg M, et al: Risks and causes of death in a community-based stroke population: 1 month and 3 years after stroke, *Neuroepidemiology* 18:75-84, 1999.

35. Dennis MS, Burn JPS, Sandercock PAG, et al: Long-term survival after first-ever stroke: The Oxfordshire Community Stroke Project, *Stroke* 24:796-800, 1993.

36. Ward G, Jamrozik K, Stewart-Wynne E: Incidence and outcome of cerebrovascular disease in Perth, Western Australia, *Stroke* 19:1501-1506, 1988.

37. Heuschmann PU, Kolominsky-Rabas PL, Misselwitz B, et al: German Stroke Registers Study Group. Predictors of in-hospital mortality and attributable risks of death after ischemic stroke: the German Stroke Registers Study Group, *Arch Intern Med* 164(16):1761-1768, 2004.

38. van der Worp HB, Kappelle LJ: Complications of acute ischemic stroke, *Cerebrovasc Dis* 8:124-132, 1998.

39. Putaala J, Curtze S, Hiltunen S, et al: Causes of death and predictors of 5-year mortality in young adults after first-ever ischemic stroke. The Helsinki Young Stroke Registry, *Stroke* 40:2698-2703, 2009.

40. Karter AJ, Gazzaniga JM, Cohen RD, et al: Ischemic heart disease and stroke mortality in African-American, Hispanic, and non-Hispanic white men and women, 1985 to 1991, *West J Med* 169:139-145, 1998.

41. Sung JF, Harris-Hooker SA, Schmid G, et al: Racial differences in mortality from cardiovascular disease in Atlanta, 1979-1985, *J Natl Med Assoc* 84:259-263, 1992.

42. Hassaballa H, Gorelick PB, West CP, et al: Ischemic stroke outcome: racial differences in the trial of danaparoid in acute stroke (TOAST), *Neurology* 57:691-697, 2001.

43. Lai SM, Alter M, Friday G, Sobel E: Prognosis for survival after an initial stroke, *Stroke* 26:2011-2015, 1995.

44. Baum HM, Robins M: National Survey of Stroke: Survival and prevalence, *Stroke* 12(2 Pt 2 Suppl):159-168, 1981.

45. Bronnum-Hansen H, Davidsen M, Thorvaldsen P: Danish MONICA Study Group. Long-term survival and causes of death after stroke, *Stroke* 32:2131-2136, 2001.

46. Gresham GE, Kelly-Hayes M, Wolf PA, et al: Survival and functional status 20 or more years after first stroke. The Framingham Study, *Stroke* 29:793-797, 1998.

47. Wolf PA, D'Agostino RB, O'Neal MA, et al: Secular trends in stroke incidence and mortality. The Framingham Study, *Stroke* 23(11):1551-1555, 1992.

48. McCarron MO, Davey Smith G, McCarron P: Secular stroke trends: early life factors and future prospects, *QJM* 99(2):117-122, 2006.

49. Seshadri S, Beiser A, Kelly-Hayes M, et al: The lifetime risk of stroke: estimates from the Framingham Study, *Stroke* 37:345-350, 2006.

50. Slot KB, Berge E, Sandercock P, et al: Oxfordshire Community Stroke Project; Lothian Stroke Register; International Stroke Trial (UK). Causes of death by level of dependency at 6 months after ischemic stroke in 3 large cohorts, *Stroke* 40(5):1585-1589, 2009.

51. WHO MONICA Project (prepared by Thorvaldsen P, Asplund K, Kuulasmaa K, Rajakangas AM, Schroll M). Stroke incidence, case fatality, and mortality in the WHO MONICA Project: World Health Organization monitoring trends and determinants in cardiovascular disease, *Stroke* 26: 361-367, 1995.

52. Lyden P, Brott T, Tilley B, et al: for the NINDS TPA Stroke Study Group: Improved reliability of the NIH stroke scale using video training, *Stroke* 25:2220-2226, 1994.

53. Adams HP Jr, Davis PH, Leira EC, et al: Baseline NIH Stroke Scale score strongly predicts outcome after stroke: A report of the Trial of Org 10172 in Acute Stroke Treatment (TOAST), *Neurology* 53(1):126-131, 1999.

54. Dhamoon MS, Tai W, Boden-Albala B, et al: Risk of myocardial infarction or vascular death after first ischemic stroke: the Northern Manhattan Study, *Stroke* 38(6):1752-1758, 2007.

55. Weimar C, Ziegler A, König IR, Diener H-C: on behalf of the German Stroke Study Collaborators: Predicting functional outcome and survival after acute ischemic stroke, *J Neurol* 249:888-895, 2002.

56. Henon H, Godefry O, Leys D, et al: Early predictors of death after acute cerebral ischemic event, *Stroke* 26(3):392-398, 1995.

57. Johnston KC, Connors AF, Wagner DP, et al: A predictive risk model for outcomes of ischemic stroke, *Stroke* 31(2):448-455, 2000.

58. Macciocchi SN, Diamond PT, Alves WM, Mertz T: Ischemic stroke: Relation of age, lesion location, and initial neurologic deficit to functional outcome, *Arch Phys Med Rehabil* 79(10):1255-1257, 1998.

59. Sankai T, Iso H, Imano H, et al: Survival and disability in stroke by stroke subtype based on computed tomographic findings in three rural Japanese communities, *Nippon Koshu Eisei Zasshi* 45(6):552-563, 1998.

60. Gargano JW, Wehner S, Reeves M: Sex differences in acute stroke care in a statewide stroke registry, *Stroke* 39(1):24-29, 2008.

61. Longstreth WT Jr, Bernick C, Fitzpatrick A, et al: Frequency and predictors of stroke death in 5,888 participants in the Cardiovascular Health Study, *Neurology* 56(3):368-375, 2001.

62. Ellis C, Zhao Y, Egede LE: Racial/ethnic differences in stroke mortality in veterans, *Ethn Dis* 19(2):161-165, 2009.

63. Gentile NT, Seftchick MW: Poor outcomes in Hispanic and African American patients after acute ischemic stroke: Influence of diabetes and hyperglycemia, *Ethn Dis* 18(3):330-335, 2008.

64. Howard G, Howard VJ: REasons for Geographic And Racial Differences in Stroke (REGARDS) Investigators. Ethnic disparities in stroke: the scope of the problem, *Ethn Dis* 11(4):761-768, 2001.

65. The National Institute of Neurological Disorders and Stroke rt-PA Stroke Study Group: Tissue plasminogen activator for acute ischemic stroke, *N Engl J Med* 333:1581-1587, 1995.

66. Moroney JT, Bagiella E, Paik MC, et al: Risk factors for early recurrence after ischemic stroke: The role of stroke syndrome and subtype, *Stroke* 29(10):2118-2124, 1998.

67. Weimar C, König IR, Kraywinkel K, et al: German Stroke Study Collaboration: Age and National Institutes of Health Stroke Scale Score within 6 hours after onset are accurate predictors of outcome after cerebral ischemia: development and external validation of prognostic models, *Stroke* 35(1):158–162, 2004.

68. Censori B, Camerlingo M, Casto L, et al: Prognostic factors in first-ever stroke in the carotid artery territory seen within 6 hours after onset, *Stroke* 24:532–535, 1993.

69. Albers GW, Bates V, Clark WM, et al: Intravenous tissue-type plasminogen activator for treatment of acute stroke: the Standard Treatment with Alteplase to Reverse Stroke (STARS) study, *JAMA* 283:1145–1150, 2000.

70. Jansen O, Schellinger P, Fiebach J, et al: Early recanalisation in acute ischaemic stroke saves tissue at risk defined by MRI, *Lancet* 353:2036–2037, 1999.

71. Adams HP Jr, Bendixen BH, Leira E, et al: Antithrombotic treatment of ischemic stroke among patients with occlusion or severe stenosis of the internal carotid artery: A report of the Trial of Org 10172 in Acute Stroke Treatment (TOAST), *Neurology* 53(1):122–125, 1999.

72. Rasmussen D, Kohler O, Worm-Petersen S, et al: Computed tomography in prognostic stroke evaluation, *Stroke* 23:506–510, 1992.

73. Scmidt EV, Smirnov VE, Ryabova VS: Results of the seven-year prospective study of stroke patients, *Stroke* 19:942–949, 1988.

74. Bonita R, Ford MA, Stewart AW: Predicting survival after stroke: a three-year follow-up, *Stroke* 19:669–673, 1988.

75. Howard G, Walker MD, Becker C, et al: Community hospital-based stroke programs: North Carolina, Oregon, and New York. III. Factors influencing survival after stroke: proportional hazards analysis of 4219 patients, *Stroke* 17:294–299, 1986.

76. Smithard DG, O'Neill PA, Parks C, Morris J: Complications and outcome after acute stroke: Does dysphagia matter? *Stroke* 27(7):1200–1204, 1996.

77. Bamford J, Sandercock P, Dennis M, et al: Classification and natural history of clinically identifiable subtypes of cerebral infarction, *Lancet* 337:1521–1526, 1991.

78. Wang Y, Lim LL, Levi C, et al: Influence of admission body temperature on stroke mortality, *Stroke* 31(2):404–409, 2000.

79. Maher J, Hachinski V: Hypothermia as a potential treatment for cerebral ischemia, *Cerebrovasc Brain Metab Rev* 5:277–300, 1993.

80. Kammersgaard LP, Jorgensen HS, Rungby JA, et al: Admission body temperature predicts long-term mortality after acute stroke: The Copenhagen Stroke Study, *Stroke* 33(7):1759–1762, 2002.

81. Przelomski MM, Roth RM, Gleckman RA, Marcus EM: Fever in the wake of a stroke, *Neurology* 36:427–429, 1986.

82. Castillo J, Martinez F, Leira R, et al: Mortality and morbidity of acute cerebral infarction related to temperature and basal analytic parameters, *Cerebrovasc Dis* 4:66–71, 1994.

83. Azzimondi G, Bassein L, Nonino F, et al: Fever in acute stroke worsens prognosis: A prospective study, *Stroke* 26:2040–2043, 1995.

84. Hindfelt B: The prognostic significance of subfebrility and fever in ischaemic cerebral infarction, *Acta Neurol Scand* 53:72–79, 1976.

85. Castillo J, Davalos A, Marrugat J, Noya M: Timing for fever-related brain damage in acute ischemic stroke, *Stroke* 29:2455–2460, 1998.

86. Reith J, Jorgensen HS, Pedersen PM, et al: Body temperature in acute stroke: Relation to stroke severity, infarct size, mortality, and outcome, *Lancet* 347:422–425, 1996.

87. Hajat C, Hajat S, Sharma P: Effects of poststroke pyrexia on stroke outcome: A meta-analysis of studies in patients, *Stroke* 31:410–414, 2000.

88. Schwab S, Georgiadis D, Berrouschpt J, et al: Feasibility and safety of moderate hypothermia after massive hemispheric infarction, *Stroke* 32(9):2033–2035, 2001.

89. Greer DM, Funk SE, Reaven NL, et al: Impact of fever on outcome in patients with stroke and neurologic injury: A comprehensive meta-analysis, *Stroke* 39(11):3029–3035, 2008.

90. Dippel DW, van Breda EJ, van Gemert HM, et al: Effect of paracetamol (acetaminophen) on body temperature in acute ischemic stroke: a double-blind, randomized phase II clinical trial, *Stroke* 32(7):1607–1612, 2001.

91. Georgiadis D, Schwarz S, Aschoff A, Schwab S: Hemicraniectomy and moderate hypothermia in patients with severe ischemic stroke, *Stroke* 33(6):1584–1588, 2002.

92. Georgiadis D, Schwarz S, Kollmar R, Schwab S: Endovascular cooling for moderate hypothermia in patients with acute stroke: First results of a novel approach, *Stroke* 32(11):2550–2553, 2001.

93. Sacco SE, Whisnant JP, Broderick JP, et al: Epidemiological characteristics of lacunar infarcts in a population, *Stroke* 22:1236–1241, 1991.

94. Ward G, Jamrozik K, Stewart-Wynne E: Incidence and outcome of cerebrovascular disease in Perth, Western Australia, *Stroke* 19:1501–1506, 1988.

95. Kolominsky-Rabas PL, Weber M, Gefeller O, et al: Epidemiology of ischemic stroke subtypes according to TOAST criteria, Incidence, recurrence, and long-term survival in ischemic stroke subtypes: a population-based study, *Stroke* 32:2735–2740, 2001.

96. Petty GW, Brown RD Jr, Whisnant JP, et al: Ischemic stroke subtypes: a population-based study of functional outcome, survival, and recurrence, *Stroke* 31:1062–1068, 2000.

97. Staaf G, Lindgren A, Norrving B: Pure motor stroke from presumed lacunar infarct: Long-term prognosis for survival and risk of recurrent stroke, *Stroke* 32(11):2592–2596, 2001.

98. de Jong G, van Raak L, Kessels F, Lodder J: Stroke subtype and mortality. a follow-up study in 998 patients with a first cerebral infarct, *J Clin Epidemiol* 56(3):262–268, 2003.

99. Adams HP Jr, Bendixen BH, Kappelle LJ, et al: Classification of subtype of acute ischemic stroke. Definitions for use in a multicenter clinical trial. TOAST. Trial of Org 10172 in Acute Stroke Treatment, *Stroke* 24(1):35–41, 1993.

100. Glass TA, Hennessey PM, Pazdera L, et al: Outcome at 30 days in the New England Medical Center Posterior Circulation Registry, *Arch Neurol* 59(3):369–376, 2002.

101. Leonardi-Bee J, Bath PM, Phillips SJ, Sandercock PA: Blood pressure and clinical outcomes in the International Stroke Trial, *Stroke* 33(5):1315–1320, 2002.

102. Rodgers A, MacMahon S, Gamble G, et al: Blood pressure and risk of stroke in patients with cerebrovascular disease. The United Kingdom Transient Ischaemic Attack Collaborative Group, *BMJ* 313(7050):147, 1996.

103. PATS Collaborating Group: Post-stroke antihypertensive treatment study. A preliminary result, *Chin Med J (Engl)* 108(9):710–717, 1995.

104. Yusuf S, Sleight P, Pogue J, et al: Effects of an angiotensin-converting-enzyme inhibitor, ramipril, on cardiovascular events in high-risk patients. The Heart Outcomes Prevention Evaluation Study Investigators, *N Engl J Med* 342(3):145–153, 2000.

105. Britton M, Carlsson A, de Faire U: Blood pressure course in patients with acute stroke and matched controls, *Stroke* 17(5):861–864, 1986.

106. Robinson T, Waddinton A, Ward-Close S, et al: The predictive role of 24-hour compared to casual blood pressure levels on outcome following acute stroke, *Cerebrovasc Dis* 7:264–272, 1997.

107. Bath FJ, Bath PMW: What is the correct management of blood pressure in acute stroke? The Blood Pressure in Acute Stroke Collaboration, *Cerebrovasc Dis* 7:205–213, 1997.

108. Tanne D, Kasner SE, Demchuk AM, et al: Markers of increased risk of intracerebral hemorrhage after intravenous recombinant tissue plasminogen activator therapy for acute ischemic stroke in clinical practice: The Multicenter rt-PA Stroke Survey, *Circulation* 105(14):1679–1685, 2002.

109. Hankey GJ: Long-term outcome after ischaemic stroke/transient ischaemic attack, *Cerebrovasc Dis* 16(Suppl 1):14–19, 2003.

110. Eriksson SE, Olsson JE: Survival and recurrent strokes in patients with different subtypes of stroke: A fourteen-year follow-up study, *Cerebrovasc Dis* 12(3):171–180, 2001.

111. Howard G, Anderson R, Johnson NJ, et al: Evaluation of social status as a contributing factor to the stroke belt region of the United States, *Stroke* 28(5):936–940, 1997.

112. Appelros P, Nydevik I, Seiger A, Terent A: Predictors of severe stroke: Influence of preexisting dementia and cardiac disorders, *Stroke* 33(10):2357-2362, 2002.

113. Jorgensen HS, Nakayama H, Reith J, et al: Acute stroke with atrial fibrillation. The Copenhagen Stroke Study, *Stroke* 27(10):1765-1769, 1996.

114. Lin HJ, Wolf PA, Kelly-Hayes M, et al: Stroke severity in atrial fibrillation. The Framingham Study, *Stroke* 27(10):1760-1764, 1996.

115. Sandercock P, Bamford J, Dennis M, et al: Atrial fibrillation and stroke: Prevalence in different types of stroke and influence on early and long term prognosis (Oxfordshire Community Stroke Project), *BMJ* 305(6867):1460-1465, 1992.

116. Henriksson KM, Farahmand B, Johansson S, et al: Survival after stroke—The impact of CHADS(2) score and atrial fibrillation, *Int J Cardiol* 141:18-23, 2010.

117. Gottdiener JS, Gay JA, VanVoorhees L, et al: Frequency and embolic potential of left ventricular thrombus in dilated cardiomyopathy: Assessment by 2-dimensional echocardiography, *Am J Cardiol* 52(10):1281-1285, 1983.

118. Al-Khadra AS, Salem DN, Rand WM, et al: Warfarin anticoagulation and survival: A cohort analysis from the Studies of Left Ventricular Dysfunction, *J Am Coll Cardiol* 31(4):749-753, 1998.

119. Kannel WB, Wolf PA, Verter J: Manifestations of coronary disease predisposing to stroke. The Framingham Study, *JAMA* 250(21):2942-2946, 1983.

120. Pullicino PM, Halperin JL, Thompson JL: Stroke in patients with heart failure and reduced left ventricular ejection fraction, *Neurology* 54(2):288-294, 2000.

121. Kupari M, Lindroos M, Iivanainen AM, et al: Congestive heart failure in old age: Prevalence, mechanisms and 4-year prognosis in the Helsinki Ageing Study, *J Intern Med* 241(5):387-394, 1997.

122. Candelise L, Landi G, Orazio EN, Boccardi E: Prognostic significance of hyperglycemia in acute stroke, *Arch Neurol* 42(7):661-663, 1985.

123. Kiers L, Davis SM, Larkins R, et al: Stroke topography and outcome in relation to hyperglycaemia and diabetes, *J Neurol Neurosurg Psychiatry* 55(4):263-270, 1992.

124. Melamed E: Reactive hyperglycaemia in patients with acute stroke, *J Neurol Sci* 29(2-4):267-275, 1976.

125. Oppenheimer SM, Hoffbrand BI, Oswald GA, Yudkin JS: Diabetes mellitus and early mortality from stroke, *Br Med J (Clin Res Ed)* 291(6501):1014-1015, 1985.

126. Pulsinelli WA, Levy DE, Sigsbee B, et al: Increased damage after ischemic stroke in patients with hyperglycemia with or without established diabetes mellitus, *Am J Med* 74(4):540-544, 1983.

127. Williams LS, Rotich J, Qi R, et al: Effects of admission hyperglycemia on mortality and costs in acute ischemic stroke, *Neurology* 59(1):67-71, 2002.

128. Bruno A, Levine SR, Frankel MR, et al: Admission glucose level and clinical outcomes in the NINDS rt-PA Stroke Trial, *Neurology* 59(5):669-674, 2002.

129. Stratton IM, Adler AI, Neil HA, et al: Association of glycaemia with macrovascular and microvascular complications of type 2 diabetes (UKPDS 35): prospective observational study, *BMJ* 321(7258):405-412, 2000.

130. Megherbi SE, Milan C, Minier D, et al: Association between diabetes and stroke subtype on survival and functional outcome 3 months after stroke: data from the European BIOMED Stroke Project, *Stroke* 34(3):688-694, 2003.

131. Chamorro A, Vila N, Ascaso C, et al: Early prediction of stroke severity. Role of the erythrocyte sedimentation rate, *Stroke* 26(4):573-576, 1995.

132. Di Napoli M, Papa F, Bocola V: C-reactive protein in ischemic stroke: An independent prognostic factor, *Stroke* 32(4):917-924, 2001.

133. Pearson TA, Mensah GA, Alexander RW, et al: Markers of inflammation and cardiovascular disease: application to clinical and public health practice: A statement for healthcare professionals from the Centers for Disease Control and Prevention and the American Heart Association, *Circulation* 107(3):499-511, 2003.

134. Rost NS, Wolf PA, Kase CS, et al: Plasma concentration of C-reactive protein and risk of ischemic stroke and transient ischemic attack: the Framingham Study, *Stroke* 32(11):2575-2579, 2001.

135. Winbeck K, Poppert H, Etgen T, et al: Prognostic relevance of early serial C-reactive protein measurements after first ischemic stroke, *Stroke* 33(10):2459-2464, 2002.

136. Beamer NB, Coull BM, Clark WM, et al: Persistent inflammatory response in stroke survivors, *Neurology* 50(6):1722-1728, 1998.

137. Di Tullio MR, Sacco RL, Homma S: Atherosclerotic disease of the aortic arch as a risk factor for recurrent ischemic stroke, *N Engl J Med* 335(19):1464-1465, 1996.

138. Lagrand WK, Visser CA, Hermens WT, et al: C-reactive protein as a cardiovascular risk factor: More than an epiphenomenon? *Circulation* 100(1):96-102, 1999.

139. Ridker PM, Cushman M, Stampfer MJ, et al: Inflammation, aspirin, and the risk of cardiovascular disease in apparently healthy men, *N Engl J Med* 336(14):973-979, 1997.

140. Shantikumar S, Grant PJ, Catto AJ, et al: Elevated C-reactive protein and long-term mortality after ischaemic stroke: Relationship with markers of endothelial cell and platelet activation, *Stroke* 40(3):977-979, 2009.

141. Elkind MS, Tai W, Coates K, et al: High-sensitivity C-reactive protein, lipoprotein-associated phospholipase A2, and outcome after ischemic stroke, *Arch Intern Med* 166(19):2073-2080, 2006.

142. Packard CJ, O'Reilly DS, Caslake MJ, et al: Lipoprotein-associated phospholipase A2 as an independent predictor of coronary heart disease. West of Scotland Coronary Prevention Study Group, *N Engl J Med* 343(16):1148-1155, 2000.

143. Elkind MS, Tai W, Coates K, et al: Lipoprotein-associated phospholipase A2 activity and risk of recurrent stroke, *Cerebrovasc Dis* 27(1):42-50, 2009.

144. Gussekloo J, Schaap MC, Frolich M, et al: C-reactive protein is a strong but nonspecific risk factor of fatal stroke in elderly persons, *Arterioscler Thromb Vasc Biol* 20(4):1047-1051, 2000.

145. Kannel WB, Anderson K, Wilson PW: White blood cell count and cardiovascular disease. Insights from the Framingham Study, *JAMA* 267(9):1253-1256, 1992.

146. Qizilbash N: Fibrinogen and cerebrovascular disease, *Eur Heart J* 16(Suppl A):42-45, 1995.

147. Tuttolomondo A, Pedone C, Pinto A, et al: Predictors of outcome in acute ischemic cerebrovascular syndromes: The GIFA study, *Int J Cardiol* 125(3):391-396, 2008.

148. Elkind MS, Cheng J, Rundek T, et al: Leukocyte count predicts outcome after ischemic stroke: The Northern Manhattan Stroke Study, *J Stroke Cerebrovasc Dis* 13(5):220-227, 2004.

149. Wong KY, MacWalter RS, Fraser HW, et al: Urate predicts subsequent cardiac death in stroke survivors, *Eur Heart J* 23(10):788-793, 2002.

150. Weir CJ, Muir SW, Walters MR, Lees KR: Serum urate as an independent predictor of poor outcome and future vascular events after acute stroke, *Stroke* 34(8):1951-1956, 2003.

151. Daskalopoulou SS, Athyros VG, Elisaf M, Mikhailidis D: The impact of serum uric acid on cardiovascular outcomes in the LIFE study, *Kidney Int* 66(4):1714-1715, 2004.

152. MacWalter RS, Wong SY, Wong KY, et al: Does renal dysfunction predict mortality after acute stroke? A 7-year follow-up study, *Stroke* 33(6):1630-1635, 2002.

153. Wannamethee SG, Shaper AG, Perry IJ: Serum creatinine concentration and risk of cardiovascular disease: A possible marker for increased risk of stroke, *Stroke* 28(3):557-563, 1997.

154. Yahalom G, Schwartz R, Schwammenthal Y, et al: Chronic kidney disease and clinical outcome in patients with acute stroke, *Stroke* 40(4):1296-1303, 2009.

155. Nadeau SE, Jordan JE, Mishra SK, Haerer AF: Stroke rates in patients with lacunar and large vessel cerebral infarctions, *J Neurol Sci* 114(2):128-137, 1993.

156. Burn J, Dennis M, Bamford J, et al: Long-term risk of recurrent stroke after a first-ever stroke. The Oxfordshire Community Stroke Project, *Stroke* 25(2):333-337, 1994.

157. Hankey GJ, Jamrozik K, Broadhurst RJ, et al: Long-term risk of first recurrent stroke in the Perth Community Stroke Study, *Stroke* 29(12):2491-2500, 1998.

158. Matsumoto N, Whisnant JP, Kurland LT, Okazaki H: Natural history of stroke in Rochester, Minnesota, 1955 through 1969: An extension of a previous study, 1945 through 1954, *Stroke* 4(1):20-29, 1973.

159. Mohr JP, Thompson JL, Lazar RM, et al: A comparison of warfarin and aspirin for the prevention of recurrent ischemic stroke, *N Engl J Med* 345(20):1444-1451, 2001.

160. Meissner I, Whisnant JP, Garraway WM: Hypertension management and stroke recurrence in a community (Rochester, Minnesota, 1950-1979), *Stroke* 19(4):459-463, 1988.

161. Moroney JT, Bagiella E, Paik MC, et al: Risk factors for early recurrence after ischemic stroke: The role of stroke syndrome and subtype, *Stroke* 29(10):2118-2124, 1998.

162. Rundek T, Elkind MS, Chen X, et al: Increased early stroke recurrence among patients with extracranial and intracranial atherosclerosis: The Northern Manhattan Stroke Study, *Neurology* (Suppl 4):A75, 1998:S09.001.

163. Sacco RL, Foulkes MA, Mohr JP, et al: Determinants of early recurrence of cerebral infarction. The Stroke Data Bank, *Stroke* 20(8):983-989, 1989.

164. Hier DB, Foulkes MA, Swiontoniowski M, et al: Stroke recurrence within 2 years after ischemic infarction, *Stroke* 22(2):155-161, 1991.

165. Hardie K, Hankey GJ, Jamrozik K, et al: Ten-year risk of first recurrent stroke and disability after first-ever stroke in the Perth Community Stroke Study, *Stroke* 35(3):731-735, 2004.

166. Peltonen M, Stegmayr B, Asplund K: Time trends in long-term survival after stroke: the Northern Sweden Multinational Monitoring of Trends and Determinants in Cardiovascular Disease (MONICA) study, 1985-1994, *Stroke* 29(7):1358-1365, 1998.

167. Hankey GJ, Jamrozik K, Broadhurst RJ, et al: Five-year survival after first-ever stroke and related prognostic factors in the Perth Community Stroke Study, *Stroke* 31(9):2080-2086, 2000.

168. Broderick J, Brott T, Kothari R, et al: The Greater Cincinnati/Northern Kentucky Stroke Study: Preliminary first-ever and total incidence rates of stroke among blacks, *Stroke* 29(2):415-421, 1998.

169. Lefkovits J, Davis SM, Rossiter SC, et al: Acute stroke outcome: Effects of stroke type and risk factors, *Aust N Z J Med* 22(1):30-35, 1992.

170. Wade DT, Wood VA, Hewer RL: Recovery after stroke—the first 3 months, *J Neurol Neurosurg Psychiatry* 48(1):7-13, 1985.

171. Jongbloed L: Prediction of function after stroke: a critical review, *Stroke* 17(4):765-776, 1986.

172. Jorgensen HS, Nakayama H, Reith J, et al: Stroke recurrence: predictors, severity, and prognosis. The Copenhagen Stroke Study, *Neurology* 48(4):891-895, 1997.

173. Saver JL, Johnston KC, Homer D, et al: Infarct volume as a surrogate or auxiliary outcome measure in ischemic stroke clinical trials. The RANTTAS Investigators, *Stroke* 30(2):293-298, 1999.

174. DeGraba TJ, Hallenbeck JM, Pettigrew KD, et al: Progression in acute stroke: Value of the initial NIH stroke scale score on patient stratification in future trials, *Stroke* 30(6):1208-1212, 1999.

175. Hornig CR, Lammers C, Buttner T, et al: Long-term prognosis of infratentorial transient ischemic attacks and minor strokes, *Stroke* 23(2):199-204, 1992.

176. Henon H, Godefroy O, Leys D, et al: Early predictors of death and disability after acute cerebral ischemic event, *Stroke* 26(3):392-398, 1995.

177. Rundek T, Chen X, Steiner MM, et al: Predictors of 1-year stroke recurrence: The Northern Manhattan Stroke Study, *Cerebrovasc Dis* (Suppl 7):1-88, 1997.

178. Fiorelli M, Alperovitch A, Argentino C, et al: Prediction of long-term outcome in the early hours following acute ischemic stroke. Italian Acute Stroke Study Group, *Arch Neurol* 52(3):250-255, 1995.

179. Alter M, Sobel E, McCoy RL, et al: Stroke in the Lehigh Valley: Risk factors for recurrent stroke, *Neurology* 37(3):503-507, 1987.

180. Toni D, Fiorelli M, Bastianello S, et al: Acute ischemic strokes improving during the first 48 hours of onset: predictability, outcome, and possible mechanisms. A comparison with early deteriorating strokes, *Stroke* 28(1):10-14, 1997.

181. Secondary prevention in non-rheumatic atrial fibrillation after transient ischaemic attack or minor stroke: EAFT (European Atrial Fibrillation Trial) Study Group, *Lancet* 342(8882):1255-1262, 1993.

182. Amarenco P, Cohen A, Tzourio C, et al: Atherosclerotic disease of the aortic arch and the risk of ischemic stroke, *N Engl J Med* 331(22):1474-1479, 1994.

183. Comess KA, DeRook FA, Beach KW, et al: Transesophageal echocardiography and carotid ultrasound in patients with cerebral ischemia: Prevalence of findings and recurrent stroke risk, *J Am Coll Cardiol* 23(7):1598-1603, 1994.

184. Di Tullio M, Sacco RL, Gopal A, et al: Patent foramen ovale as a risk factor for cryptogenic stroke, *Ann Intern Med* 117(6):461-465, 1992.

185. Lechat P, Mas JL, Lascault G, et al: Prevalence of patent foramen ovale in patients with stroke, *N Engl J Med* 318(18):1148-1152, 1988.

186. Orencia AJ, Petty GW, Khandheria BK, et al: Mitral valve prolapse and the risk of stroke after initial cerebral ischemia, *Neurology* 45(6):1083-1086, 1995.

187. Webster MW, Chancellor AM, Smith HJ, et al: Patent foramen ovale in young stroke patients, *Lancet* 2(8601):11-12, 1988.

188. Di Tullio MR, Sacco RL, Gersony D, et al: Aortic atheromas and acute ischemic stroke: A transesophageal echocardiographic study in an ethnically mixed population, *Neurology* 46(6):1560-1566, 1996.

189. Dhamoon MS, Sciacca RR, Rundek T, et al: Recurrent stroke and cardiac risks after first ischemic stroke: The Northern Manhattan Study, *Neurology* 66(5):641-646, 2006.

190. Beneficial effect of carotid endarterectomy in symptomatic patients with high-grade carotid stenosis: North American Symptomatic Carotid Endarterectomy Trial Collaborators, *N Engl J Med* 325(7):445-453, 1991.

191. Chimowitz MI, Lynn MJ, Howlett-Smith H, et al: Comparison of warfarin and aspirin for symptomatic intracranial arterial stenosis, *N Engl J Med* 352(13):1305-1316, 2005.

192. Grau AJ, Weimar C, Buggle F, et al: Risk factors, outcome, and treatment in subtypes of ischemic stroke: the German stroke data bank, *Stroke* 32(11):2559-2566, 2001.

193. Petty GW, Brown RD Jr, Whisnant JP, et al: Ischemic stroke subtypes: a population-based study of incidence and risk factors, *Stroke* 30(12):2513-2516, 1999.

194. Hart RG, Coull BM, Hart D: Early recurrent embolism associated with nonvalvular atrial fibrillation: A retrospective study, *Stroke* 14(5):688-693, 1983.

195. Sage JI, Van Uitert RL: Risk of recurrent stroke in patients with atrial fibrillation and non-valvular heart disease, *Stroke* 14(4):537-540, 1983.

196. Sherman DG, Hart RG, Easton JD: The secondary prevention of stroke in patients with atrial fibrillation, *Arch Neurol* 43(1):68-70, 1986.

197. Ahmed N, Nasman P, Wahlgren NG: Effect of intravenous nimodipine on blood pressure and outcome after acute stroke, *Stroke* 31(6):1250-1255, 2000.

198. Squire IB, Lees KR, Pryse-Phillips W, et al: The effects of lifarizine in acute cerebral infarction: A pilot study, *Cerebrovasc Dis* 6:156-160, 1996.

199. Hypertension-Stroke Cooperative Study Group: Effect of antihypertensive treatment on stroke recurrence, *JAMA* 229(4):409-418, 1974.

200. Elkind MS: Outcomes after stroke: risk of recurrent ischemic stroke and other events, *Am J Med* 122(4 Suppl 2):S7-S13, 2009.

201. Yong M, Kaste M: Association of characteristics of blood pressure profiles and stroke outcomes in the ECASS-II trial, *Stroke* 39(2):366-372, 2008.

202. The sixth report of the Joint National Committee on Prevention: Detection, Evaluation, and Treatment of High Blood Pressure, *Arch Intern Med* 157(21):2413-2446, 1997.

203. Irie K, Yamaguchi T, Minematsu K, Omae T: The J-curve phenomenon in stroke recurrence, *Stroke* 24(12):1844-1849, 1993.

204. Voko Z, Bots ML, Hofman A, et al: J-shaped relation between blood pressure and stroke in treated hypertensives, *Hypertension* 34(6):1181-1185, 1999.

205. Friday G, Alter M, Lai SM: Control of hypertension and risk of stroke recurrence, *Stroke* 33(11):2652-2657, 2002.

206. Gueyffier F, Boissel JP, Boutitie F, et al: Effect of antihypertensive treatment in patients having already suffered from stroke. Gathering the evidence. The INDANA (INdividual Data ANalysis of Antihypertensive intervention trials) Project Collaborators, *Stroke* 28(12):2557-2562, 1997.

207. Pergola PE, White CL, Graves JW, et al: Reliability and validity of blood pressure measurement in the Secondary Prevention of Small Subcortical Strokes study, *Blood Press Monit* 12(1):1-8, 2007.

208. Sobel E, Alter M, Davanipour Z, et al: Stroke in the Lehigh Valley: Combined risk factors for recurrent ischemic stroke, *Neurology* 39(5):669-672, 1989.

209. Hillen T, Coshall C, Tilling K, et al: Cause of stroke recurrence is multifactorial: patterns, risk factors, and outcomes of stroke recurrence in the South London Stroke Register, *Stroke* 34(6):1457-1463, 2003.

210. Bak S, Sindrup SH, Alslev T, et al: Cessation of smoking after first-ever stroke: A follow-up study, *Stroke* 33(9):2263-2269, 2002.

211. Wilson K, Gibson N, Willan A, Cook D: Effect of smoking cessation on mortality after myocardial infarction: Meta-analysis of cohort studies, *Arch Intern Med* 160(7):939-944, 2000.

212. Redfern J, McKevitt C, Dundas R, et al: Behavioral risk factor prevalence and lifestyle change after stroke: A prospective study, *Stroke* 31(8):1877-1881, 2000.

213. Boysen G, Truelsen T: Prevention of recurrent stroke, *Neurol Sci* 21(2):67-72, 2000.

214. Gorelick PB: Alcohol and stroke, *Stroke* 18(1):268-271, 1987.

215. Camargo CA Jr: Moderate alcohol consumption and stroke. The epidemiologic evidence, *Stroke* 20(12):1611-1626, 1989.

216. Gill JS, Zezulka AV, Shipley MJ, et al: Stroke and alcohol consumption, *N Engl J Med* 315(17):1041-1046, 1986.

217. Gorelick PB, Rodin MB, Langenberg P, et al: Weekly alcohol consumption, cigarette smoking, and the risk of ischemic stroke: Results of a case-control study at three urban medical centers in Chicago, Illinois, *Neurology* 39(3):339-343, 1989.

218. Klatsky AL, Armstrong MA, Friedman GD: Alcohol use and subsequent cerebrovascular disease hospitalizations, *Stroke* 20(6):741-746, 1989.

219. Homma S, Sacco RL, Di Tullio MR, et al: Effect of medical treatment in stroke patients with patent foramen ovale: Patent foramen ovale in Cryptogenic Stroke Study, *Circulation* 105(22):2625-2631, 2002.

220. Sacco RL, Adams R, Albers G, et al: Guidelines for prevention of stroke in patients with ischemic stroke or transient ischemic attack: a statement for healthcare professionals from the American Heart Association/American Stroke Association Council on Stroke: co-sponsored by the Council on Cardiovascular Radiology and Intervention: The American Academy of Neurology affirms the value of this guideline, *Stroke* 37(2):577-617, 2006.

221. The French Study of Aortic Plaques in Stroke Group: Atherosclerotic disease of the aortic arch as a risk factor for recurrent ischemic stroke, *N Engl J Med* 334(19):1216-1221, 1996.

222. Di Tullio MR, Russo C, Jin Z, et al: Aortic arch plaques and risk of recurrent stroke and death, *Circulation* 119(17):2376-2382, 2009.

223. Di Napoli M, Papa F: Inflammation, hemostatic markers, and antithrombotic agents in relation to long-term risk of new cardiovascular events in first-ever ischemic stroke patients, *Stroke* 33(7):1763-1771, 2002.

224. Feinberg WM, Erickson LP, Bruck D, Kittelson J: Hemostatic markers in acute ischemic stroke. Association with stroke type, severity, and outcome, *Stroke* 27(8):1296-1300, 1996.

225. Tohgi H, Konno S, Takahashi S, et al: Activated coagulation/fibrinolysis system and platelet function in acute thrombotic stroke patients with increased C-reactive protein levels, *Thromb Res* 100(5):373-379, 2000.

226. Beamer N, Coull BM, Sexton G, et al: Fibrinogen and the albumin-globulin ratio in recurrent stroke, *Stroke* 24(8):1133-1139, 1993.

227. Hankey GJ, Eikelboom JW: Homocysteine levels in patients with stroke: clinical relevance and therapeutic implications, *CNS Drugs* 15(6):437-443, 2001.

228. Kittner SJ, Gorelick B: Antiphospholipid antibodies and stroke: an epidemiological perspective, *Stroke* 23(Suppl 2):I19-I22, 1992.

229. Mayer SA, Sacco RL, Hurlet-Jensen A, et al: Free protein S deficiency in acute ischemic stroke. A case-control study, *Stroke* 24(2):224-227, 1993.

230. Sacco RL, Owen J, Mohr JP, et al: Free protein S deficiency: A possible association with cerebrovascular occlusion, *Stroke* 20(12):1657-1661, 1989.

231. Anticardiolipin antibodies are an independent risk factor for first ischemic stroke: The Antiphospholipid Antibodies in Stroke Study (APASS) Group, *Neurology* 43(10):2069-2073, 1993.

232. Whiteley W, Chong WL, Sengupta A, Sandercock P: Blood markers for the prognosis of ischemic stroke: A systematic review, *Stroke* 40(5):E380-E389, 2009.

233. Caplan LR: Worsening in ischemic stroke patients: Is it time for a new strategy? *Stroke* 33(6):1443-1445, 2002.

234. Ali LK, Saver JL: The ischemic stroke patient who worsens: New assessment and management approaches, *Rev Neurol Dis* 4(2):85-91, 2007.

235. Bromfield EB, Reding MJ: Relative risk of deep venous thrombosis or pulmonary embolism post-stroke based on ambulatory status, *Neurorehabil Neural Repair* 2:51-57, 1988.

236. Sherman DG, Albers GW, Bladin C, et al: The efficacy and safety of enoxaparin versus unfractionated heparin for the prevention of venous thromboembolism after acute ischaemic stroke (PREVAIL Study): an open-label randomised comparison, *Lancet* 369(9570):1347-1355, 2007.

237. Fisher CM: The use of anticoagulants in cerebral thrombosis, *Neurology* 8(5):311-332, 1958.

238. Toni D, Fiorelli M, Gentile M, et al: Progressing neurological deficit secondary to acute ischemic stroke. A study on predictability, pathogenesis, and prognosis, *Arch Neurol* 52(7):670-675, 1995.

239. Mohr JP, Caplan LR, Melski JW, et al: The Harvard Cooperative Stroke Registry: a prospective registry, *Neurology* 28(8):754-762, 1978.

240. Marti-Vilalta JL, Arboix A: The Barcelona Stroke Registry, *Eur Neurol* 41(3):135-142, 1999.

241. Yamamoto H, Bogousslavsky J, van Melle G: Different predictors of neurological worsening in different causes of stroke, *Arch Neurol* 55(4):481-486, 1998.

242. Tei H, Uchiyama S, Ohara K, et al: Deteriorating ischemic stroke in 4 clinical categories classified by the Oxfordshire Community Stroke Project, *Stroke* 31(9):2049-2054, 2000.

243. Davalos A, Cendra E, Teruel J, et al: Deteriorating ischemic stroke: risk factors and prognosis, *Neurology* 40(12):1865-1869, 1990.

244. Jorgensen HS, Nakayama H, Raaschou HO, Olsen TS: Effect of blood pressure and diabetes on stroke in progression, *Lancet* 344(8916):156-159, 1994.

245. Parsons MW, Barber PA, Chalk J, et al: Diffusion- and perfusion-weighted MRI response to thrombolysis in stroke, *Ann Neurol* 51(1):28-37, 2002.

246. Thijs VN, Adami A, Neumann-Haefelin T, et al: Clinical and radiological correlates of reduced cerebral blood flow measured using magnetic resonance imaging, *Arch Neurol* 59(2):233-238, 2002.

247. Christensen H, Boysen G, Johannesen HH, et al: Deteriorating ischaemic stroke: Cytokines, soluble cytokine receptors, ferritin, systemic blood pressure, body temperature, blood glucose, diabetes, stroke severity, and CT infarction-volume as predictors of deteriorating ischaemic stroke, *J Neurol Sci* 201(1-2):1-7, 2002.

248. Mohr JP: Lacunes, *Stroke* 13:3-11, 1982.

249. Norrving B, Cronqvist S: Clinical and radiologic features of lacunar versus nonlacunar minor stroke, *Stroke* 20(1):59-64, 1989.

250. Steinke W, Ley SC: Lacunar stroke is the major cause of progressive motor deficits, *Stroke* 33(6):1510-1516, 2002.

251. Libman RB, Sacco RL, Shi T, Mohr JP: Spontaneous improvement in pure motor stroke: implications for clinical trials, *Neurology* 42:1713-1716, 1992.

252. Alberts MJ: Secondary prevention of stroke and the expanding role of the neurologist, *Cerebrovasc Dis* 1(Suppl 13):12-16, 2002.

253. MRC/BHF Heart Protection Study of cholesterol lowering with simvastatin in 20,536 high-risk individuals: A randomised placebo-controlled trial, *Lancet* 360(9326):7-22, 2002.

254. McDermott MM, Lefevre F, Arron M, et al: ST segment depression detected by continuous electrocardiography in patients with acute ischemic stroke or transient ischemic attack, *Stroke* 25(9):1820-1824, 1994.

255. Diener HC, Cunha L, Forbes C, et al: European Stroke Prevention Study. 2. Dipyridamole and acetylsalicylic acid in the secondary prevention of stroke, *J Neurol Sci* 143(1-2):1-13, 1996.

256. A randomised, blinded, trial of clopidogrel versus aspirin in patients at risk of ischaemic events (CAPRIE): CAPRIE Steering Committee, *Lancet* 348(9038):1329-1339, 1996.

257. Vickrey BG, Rector TS, Wickstrom SL, et al: Occurrence of secondary ischemic events among persons with atherosclerotic vascular disease, *Stroke* 33(4):901-906, 2002.

258. Dexter DD Jr, Whisnant JP, Connolly DC, O'Fallon WM: The association of stroke and coronary heart disease: A population study, *Mayo Clin Proc* 62(12):1077–1083, 1987.

259. Salgado AV, Ferro JM, Gouveia-Oliveira A: Long-term prognosis of first-ever lacunar strokes. A hospital-based study, *Stroke* 27(4):661–666, 1996.

260. Gorelick PB, Richardson D, Kelly M, et al: Aspirin and ticlopidine for prevention of recurrent stroke in black patients: A randomized trial, *JAMA* 289(22):2947–2957, 2003.

261. Executive summary of The Third Report of The National Cholesterol Education Program (NCEP) Expert Panel on Detection, Evaluation, And Treatment of High Blood Cholesterol in Adults (Adult Treatment Panel III), *JAMA* 285(19):2486–2497, 2001.

262. The RANTTAS Investigators: A randomized trial of tirilazad mesylate in patients with acute stroke (RANTTAS), *Stroke* 27(9):1453–1458, 1996.

263. Harrell FE Jr, Lee KL, Mark DB: Multivariable prognostic models: issues in developing models, evaluating assumptions and adequacy, and measuring and reducing errors, *Stat Med* 15(4):361–387, 1996.

264. Baird AE, Benfield A, Schlaug G, et al: Enlargement of human cerebral ischemic lesion volumes measured by diffusion-weighted magnetic resonance imaging, *Ann Neurol* 41(5):581–589, 1997.

265. Fisher M, Albers GW: Applications of diffusion-perfusion magnetic resonance imaging in acute ischemic stroke, *Neurology* 52(9):1750–1756, 1999.

266. Singer MB, Chong J, Lu D, et al: Diffusion-weighted MRI in acute subcortical infarction, *Stroke* 29(1):133–136, 1998.

267. Warach S, Gaa J, Siewert B, et al: Acute human stroke studied by whole brain echo planar diffusion-weighted magnetic resonance imaging, *Ann Neurol* 37(2):231–241, 1995.

268. Baird AE, Dambrosia J, Janket S, et al: A three-item scale for the early prediction of stroke recovery, *Lancet* 357(9274):2095–2099, 2001.

269. Thijs VN, Lansberg MG, Beaulieu C, et al: Is early ischemic lesion volume on diffusion-weighted imaging an independent predictor of stroke outcome? A multivariable analysis, *Stroke* 31(11):2597–2602, 2000.

270. Hand PJ, Wardlaw JM, Rivers CS, et al: MR diffusion-weighted imaging and outcome prediction after ischemic stroke, *Neurology* 66(8):1159–1163, 2006.

271. Wardlaw JM, Keir SL, Bastin ME, et al: Is diffusion imaging appearance an independent predictor of outcome after ischemic stroke? *Neurology* 59(9):1381–1387, 2002.

272. Johnston KC, Wagner DP, Wang XQ, et al: Validation of an acute ischemic stroke model: does diffusion-weighted imaging lesion volume offer a clinically significant improvement in prediction of outcome? *Stroke* 38(6):1820–1825, 2007.

273. Barrett KM, Ding YH, Wagner DP, et al: Change in diffusion-weighted imaging infarct volume predicts neurologic outcome at 90 days: Results of the Acute Stroke Accurate Prediction (ASAP) trial serial imaging substudy, *Stroke* 40(7):2422–2427, 2009.

274. Johnston SC, Gress DR, Browner WS, Sidney S: Short-term prognosis after emergency department diagnosis of TIA, *JAMA* 284(22):2901–2906, 2000.

275. Kernan WN, Viscoli CM, Brass LM, et al: The stroke prognosis instrument II (SPI-II): A clinical prediction instrument for patients with transient ischemia and nondisabling ischemic stroke, *Stroke* 31(2):456–462, 2000.

276. Diener HC, Ringleb PA, Savi P: Clopidogrel for the secondary prevention of stroke, *Expert Opin Pharmacother* 6(5):755–764, 2005.

277. Diener HC: Modified-release dipyridamole combined with aspirin for secondary stroke prevention, *Aging Health* 1:19–26, 2005.

278. Weimar C, Diener HC, Alberts MJ, et al: The Essen stroke risk score predicts recurrent cardiovascular events: a validation within the REduction of Atherothrombosis for Continued Health (REACH) registry, *Stroke* 40(2):350–354, 2009.

279. Wade DT, Collin C: The Barthel ADL Index: a standard measure of physical disability? *Int Disabil Stud* 10(2):6467, 1988.

280. Wade DT, Hewer RL: Functional abilities after stroke: Measurement, natural history and prognosis, *J Neurol Neurosurg Psychiatry* 50(2):177–182, 1987.

281. Rankin J: Cerebral vascular accidents in patients over the age of 60. II. Prognosis, *Scott Med J* 2(5):200–215, 1957.

282. Granger CV, Hamilton BB, Gresham GE, Kramer AA: The stroke rehabilitation outcome study: Part II. Relative merits of the total Barthel index score and a four-item subscore in predicting patient outcomes, *Arch Phys Med Rehabil* 70(2):100–103, 1989.

283. Sacco RL, DeRosa JT, Haley EC Jr, et al: Glycine antagonist in neuroprotection for patients with acute stroke: GAIN Americas: A randomized controlled trial, *JAMA* 285(13):1719–1728, 2001.

284. Dennis MS, Burn JP, Sandercock PA, et al: Long-term survival after first-ever stroke: the Oxfordshire Community Stroke Project, *Stroke* 24(6):796–800, 1993.

285. Dombovy ML, Basford JR, Whisnant JP, Bergstralh EJ: Disability and use of rehabilitation services following stroke in Rochester, Minnesota, 1975-1979, *Stroke* 18(5):830–836, 1987.

286. Hackett ML, Duncan JR, Anderson CS, et al: Health-related quality of life among long-term survivors of stroke: Results from the Auckland Stroke Study, 1991-1992, *Stroke* 31(2):440–447, 2000.

287. Hankey GJ, Jamrozik K, Broadhurst RJ, et al: Long-term disability after first-ever stroke and related prognostic factors in the Perth Community Stroke Study, 1989-1990, *Stroke* 33(4):1034–1040, 2002.

288. Kojima S, Omura T, Wakamatsu W, et al: Prognosis and disability of stroke patients after 5 years in Akita, Japan, *Stroke* 21(1):72–77, 1990.

289. Bamford J, Sandercock P, Dennis M, et al: A prospective study of acute cerebrovascular disease in the community: The Oxfordshire Community Stroke Project—1981-86. 2. Incidence, case fatality rates and overall outcome at one year of cerebral infarction, primary intracerebral and subarachnoid haemorrhage, *J Neurol Neurosurg Psychiatry* 53(1):16–22, 1990.

290. Bonita R, Beaglehole R: Recovery of motor function after stroke, *Stroke* 19(12):1497–1500, 1988.

291. Carolei A, Marini C, Di Napoli M, et al: High stroke incidence in the prospective community-based L'Aquila registry (1994-1998). First year's results, *Stroke* 28(12):2500–2506, 1997.

292. Greveson GC, Gray CS, French JM, James OF: Long-term outcome for patients and carers following hospital admission for stroke, *Age Ageing* 20(5):337–344, 1991.

293. Kappelle LJ, Adams HP Jr, Heffner ML, et al: Prognosis of young adults with ischemic stroke. A long-term follow-up study assessing recurrent vascular events and functional outcome in the Iowa Registry of Stroke in Young Adults, *Stroke* 25(7):1360–1365, 1994.

294. Korv J, Roose M, Haldre S, Kaasik AE: Registry of first-ever stroke in Tartu, Estonia, 1991 through 1993: Outcome of stroke, *Acta Neurol Scand* 99(3):175–181, 1999.

295. Sturm JW, Dewey HM, Donnan GA, et al: Handicap after stroke: How does it relate to disability, perception of recovery, and stroke subtype? The North East Melbourne Stroke Incidence Study (NEMESIS), *Stroke* 33(3):762–768, 2002.

296. Taub NA, Wolfe CD, Richardson E, Burney PG: Predicting the disability of first-time stroke sufferers at 1 year. 12-month follow-up of a population-based cohort in southeast England, *Stroke* 25(2):352–357, 1994.

297. Wilkinson PR, Wolfe CD, Warburton FG, et al: A long-term follow-up of stroke patients, *Stroke* 28(3):507–512, 1997.

298. Wolfe CD, Taub NA, Bryan S, et al: Variations in the incidence, management and outcome of stroke in residents under the age of 75 in two health districts of southern England, *J Public Health Med* 17(4):411–418, 1995.

299. Woo J, Yuen YK, Kay R, Nicholls MG: Survival, disability, and residence 20 months after acute stroke in a Chinese population: Implications for community care, *Disabil Rehabil* 14(1):36–40, 1992.

300. Lo RS, Cheng JO, Wong EM, et al: Handicap and its determinants of change in stroke survivors: One-year follow-up study, *Stroke* 39(1):148–153, 2008.

301. Huybrechts KF, Caro JJ: The Barthel Index and modified Rankin Scale as prognostic tools for long-term outcomes after stroke: A qualitative review of the literature, *Curr Med Res Opin* 23(7):1627–1636, 2007.

302. Rundek T, Boden-Alabalam B, DeRosam J, et al: Functional outcome 6 months after ischemic stroke: The influence of discharge destination after acute care hospitalization, 123rd Annual Meeting of the American Neurological Association, Montreal, Canada T205:79–80, 1998.

303. World Health Organization International classification of impairments, disabilities and handicaps, Geneva, Switzerland, 1980, WHO.

304. Walker MF, Gladman JR, Lincoln NB, et al: Occupational therapy for stroke patients not admitted to hospital: A randomised controlled trial, *Lancet* 354(9175):278-280, 1999.

305. Jenkinson C, Mant J, Carter J, et al: The London handicap scale: A re-evaluation of its validity using standard scoring and simple summation, *J Neurol Neurosurg Psychiatry* 68(3):365-367, 2000.

306. Anderson CS, Taylor BV, Hankey GJ, et al: Validation of a clinical classification for subtypes of acute cerebral infarction, *J Neurol Neurosurg Psychiatry* 57(10):1173-1179, 1994.

307. Wolfe CD, Taub NA, Woodrow EJ, Burney PG: Assessment of scales of disability and handicap for stroke patients, *Stroke* 22(10):1242-1244, 1991.

308. Saver JL: Novel end point analytic techniques and interpreting shifts across the entire range of outcome scales in acute stroke trials, *Stroke* 38(11):3055-3062, 2007.

309. Bath PM, Gray LJ, Collier T, et al: Can we improve the statistical analysis of stroke trials? Statistical reanalysis of functional outcomes in stroke trials, *Stroke* 38(6):1911-1915, 2007.

310. Angeleri F, Angeleri VA, Foschi N, et al: The influence of depression, social activity, and family stress on functional outcome after stroke, *Stroke* 24(10):1478-1483, 1993.

311. Labi ML, Phillips TF, Greshman GE: Psychosocial disability in physically restored long-term stroke survivors, *Arch Phys Med Rehabil* 61(12):561-565, 1980.

312. Lawrence L, Christie D: Quality of life after stroke: A three-year follow-up, *Age Ageing* 8(3):167-172, 1979.

313. Guyatt GH, Feeny DH, Patrick DL: Measuring health-related quality of life, *Ann Intern Med* 118(8):622-629, 1993.

314. Sturm JW, Donnan GA, Dewey HM, et al: Quality of life after stroke: the North East Melbourne Stroke Incidence Study (NEMESIS), *Stroke* 35(10):2340-2345, 2004.

315. The EuroQOl Group: EuroQOl—a new facility for the measurement of health-related quality of life, *Health Policy* 16(3):199-208, 1990.

316. Bergner M, Bobbitt RA, Kressel S, et al: The sickness impact profile: conceptual formulation and methodology for the development of a health status measure, *Int J Health Serv* 6(3):393-415, 1976.

317. Duncan PW, Lai SM, Tyler D, et al: Evaluation of proxy responses to the Stroke Impact Scale, *Stroke* 33(11):2593-2599, 2002.

318. Kaplan RM, Bush JW: Health-related quality of life measurement for evaluation research and policy analysis, *Health Psychol* 1: 61-67, 1982.

319. McEwen MJ: The Nottingham Health Profile. In Walker SR, Rosser RM, editors: *Quality of Life: Assessment and application.* Lancaster, England, 1988, MTp Press.

320. Roberts L, Counsell C: Assessment of clinical outcomes in acute stroke trials, *Stroke* 29(5):986-991, 1998.

321. Ware JE Jr, Sherbourne CD: The MOS 36-item short-form health survey (SF-36). I. Conceptual framework and item selection, *Med Care* 30(6):473-483, 1992.

322. Kasner SE: Clinical interpretation and use of stroke scales, *Lancet Neurol* 5(7):603-612, 2006.

323. Duncan PW, Wallace D, Lai SM, et al: The stroke impact scale version 2.0. Evaluation of reliability, validity, and sensitivity to change, *Stroke* 30(10):2131-2140, 1999.

324. Sacco RL, Boden-Albala B, Kargman DE, Gu Q: Quality of life after ischemic stroke: The Northern Manhattan Stroke Study, *Ann Neurol* 38:322, 1995.

325. de Haan RJ: Measuring quality of life after stroke using the SF-36, *Stroke* 33(5):1176-1177, 2002.

326. Williams LS, Weinberger M, Harris LE, Biller J: Measuring quality of life in a way that is meaningful to stroke patients, *Neurology* 53(8):1839-1843, 1999.

327. Salter KL, Moses MB, Foley NC, Teasell RW: Health-related quality of life after stroke: What are we measuring? *Int J Rehabil Res* 31(2):111-117, 2008.

328. Simon GE, Revicki DA, Grothaus L, Vonkorff M: SF-36 summary scores: are physical and mental health truly distinct? *Med Care* 36(4):567-572, 1998.

329. Taft C, Karlsson J, Sullivan M: Do SF-36 summary component scores accurately summarize subscale scores? *Qual Life Res* 10(5):395-404, 2001.

330. Wilson D, Parsons J, Tucker G: The SF-36 summary scales: problems and solutions, *Soz Praventivmed* 45(6):239-246, 2000.

331. Van der Linden WJ, Hambleton RK: *Handbook of modern item response theory,* New York, 1997, Springer.

332. Fayers PM, Machin D: *Quality of life: Assessment, analysis and interpretation,* London, England, 2000, John Wiley & Sons, pp 85-87.

333. Burvill PW, Johnson GA, Jamrozik KD, et al: Prevalence of depression after stroke: The Perth Community Stroke Study, *Br J Psychiatry* 166(3):320-327, 1995.

334. House A, Dennis M, Mogridge L, et al: Mood disorders in the year after first stroke, *Br J Psychiatry* 158:83-92, 1991.

335. Whyte EM, Mulsant BH: Post stroke depression: epidemiology, pathophysiology, and biological treatment, *Biol Psychiatry* 52(3):253-264, 2002.

336. Hackett ML, Yapa C, Parag V, Anderson CS: Frequency of depression after stroke: A systematic review of observational studies, *Stroke* 36(6):1330-1340, 2005.

337. Lenze EJ, Rogers JC, Martire LM, et al: The association of late-life depression and anxiety with physical disability: A review of the literature and prospectus for future research, *Am J Geriatr Psychiatry* 9(2):113-135, 2001.

338. Austin MP, Mitchell P, Goodwin GM: Cognitive deficits in depression: possible implications for functional neuropathology, *Br J Psychiatry* 178:200-206, 2001.

339. Butters MA, Becker JT, Nebes RD, et al: Changes in cognitive functioning following treatment of late-life depression, *Am J Psychiatry* 157(12):1949-1954, 2000.

340. Schulz R, Beach SR, Ives DG, et al: Association between depression and mortality in older adults: The Cardiovascular Health Study, *Arch Intern Med* 160(12):1761-1768, 2000.

341. Astrom M, Adolfsson R, Asplund K: Major depression in stroke patients. A 3-year longitudinal study, *Stroke* 24(7):976-982, 1993.

342. Herrmann N, Black SE, Lawrence J, et al: The Sunnybrook Stroke Study: A prospective study of depressive symptoms and functional outcome, *Stroke* 29(3):618-624, 1998.

343. Kauhanen M, Korpelainen JT, Hiltunen P, et al: Poststroke depression correlates with cognitive impairment and neurological deficits, *Stroke* 30(9):1875-1880, 1999.

344. Pohjasvaara T, Leppavuori A, Siira I, et al: Frequency and clinical determinants of poststroke depression, *Stroke* 29(11):2311-2317, 1998.

345. Singh A, Black SE, Herrmann N, et al: Functional and neuroanatomic correlations in poststroke depression: The Sunnybrook Stroke Study, *Stroke* 31(3):637-644, 2000.

346. Vataja R, Pohjasvaara T, Leppavuori A, et al: Magnetic resonance imaging correlates of depression after ischemic stroke, *Arch Gen Psychiatry* 58(10):925-931, 2001.

347. Hackett ML, Anderson CS: Predictors of depression after stroke: A systematic review of observational studies, *Stroke* 36(10): 2296-2301, 2005.

348. Gillen R, Tennen H, McKee TE, et al: Depressive symptoms and history of depression predict rehabilitation efficiency in stroke patients, *Arch Phys Med Rehabil* 82(12):1645-1649, 2001.

349. Paolucci S, Antonucci G, Grasso MG, et al: Post-stroke depression, antidepressant treatment and rehabilitation results. A case-control study, *Cerebrovasc Dis* 12(3):264-271, 2001.

350. House A, Knapp P, Bamford J, Vail A: Mortality at 12 and 24 months after stroke may be associated with depressive symptoms at 1 month, *Stroke* 32(3):696-701, 2001.

351. Parikh RM, Robinson RG, Lipsey JR, et al: The impact of poststroke depression on recovery in activities of daily living over a 2-year follow-up, *Arch Neurol* 47(7):785-789, 1990.

352. Schubert DS, Taylor C, Lee S, et al: Detection of depression in the stroke patient, *Psychosomatics* 33(3):290-294, 1992.

353. Beck AT, Ward CH, Mendelson M, et al: An inventory for measuring depression, *Arch Gen Psychiatry* 4:561-571, 1961.

354. Hamilton M: A rating scale for depression, *J Neurol Neurosurg Psychiatry* 23:56-62, 1960.

355. Salter K, Bhogal SK, Foley N, et al: The assessment of poststroke depression, *Top Stroke Rehabil* 14(3):1-24, 2007.

356. Robinson RG, Bolduc PL, Price TR: Two-year longitudinal study of poststroke mood disorders: Diagnosis and outcome at one and two years, *Stroke* 18(5):837-843, 1987.

357. Beblo T, Wallesch CW, Herrmann M: The crucial role of frontostri-atal circuits for depressive disorders in the postacute stage after stroke, *Neuropsychiatry Neuropsychol Behav Neurol* 12(4): 236–246, 1999.

358. Gainotti G, Azzoni A, Marra C: Frequency, phenomenology and anatomical-clinical correlates of major post-stroke depression, *Br J Psychiatry* 175:163–167, 1999.

359. Katz I: Presidential address: On the inseparability of mental and physical health in aged persons: Lessons from depression and medical comorbidity, *Am J Geriatr Psychiatry* 4(1):1–16, 1996.

360. Kotila M, Numminen H, Waltimo O, Kaste M: Depression after stroke: Results of the FINNSTROKE Study, *Stroke* 29(2):368–372, 1998.

361. Downhill JE Jr, Robinson RG: Longitudinal assessment of depres-sion and cognitive impairment following stroke, *J Nerv Ment Dis* 182(8):425–431, 1994.

362. Alexopoulos GS, Meyers BS, Young RC, et al: Clinically defined vascular depression, *Am J Psychiatry* 154(4):562–565, 1997.

363. Robinson RG, Jorge RE, Moser DJ, et al: Escitalopram and prob-lem-solving therapy for prevention of poststroke depression: A randomized controlled trial, *JAMA* 299(20):2391–2400, 2008.

364. Chen Y, Patel NC, Guo JJ, Zhan S: Antidepressant prophylaxis for poststroke depression: A meta-analysis, *Int Clin Psychopharma-col* 22(3):159–166, 2007.

Primary Prevention of Stroke

LARRY B. GOLDSTEIN, RALPH L. SACCO

Although there have been substantial improvements in the treatment of patients with acute ischemic stroke, primary prevention remains the most effective means for reducing its public health burden. Advances in the identification of the high-risk or stroke-prone individual help select persons for risk factor modification interventions. Many strategies are available to manage a number of risk factors that increase the risk of a first stroke. Numerous randomized clinical trials have been conducted, allowing for the development of comprehensive, evidence-based guidelines for the management of risk factors to prevent first stroke.[1] Successful implementation of these recommendations remains a great challenge worldwide.

This chapter provides an overview of primary prevention of stroke. Approaches to improve the identification of the stroke-prone individual are reviewed, including the use of stroke prediction models. The major focus is given to discussion of the management of modifiable stroke risk factors, including lifestyle behaviors such as smoking, alcohol use, physical inactivity, and obesity and the management of hypertension, diabetes, dyslipidemia, atrial fibrillation (AF), and the use of platelet antiaggregants in primary stroke prevention. Carotid artery stenosis is addressed in Chapter 75. The discussion of less well-documented risk factors such as inflammation, infection, and hypercoagulable disorders is beyond the scope of this chapter.

Assessing the Risk for a First Stroke

Approaches to predict an individual's stroke risk can aid health care professionals in identifying the stroke-prone individual. Many different independent risk factors can contribute to stroke risk, and most individuals have more than one risk factor. Several stroke risk assessment tools are available for use in primary stroke prevention screening programs.[2] These risk estimation tools are generally focused on combining several major vascular risk factors to compute a predicted probability of stroke risk. Currently, the Framingham-based models are the most widely studied tools for predicting the risk of developing coronary heart disease,[3] stroke,[4,5] and cardiovascular disease.[6] The Framingham Stroke Profile (FSP) is among the most widely utilized and includes the following variables: age, systolic blood pressure, hypertension, diabetes mellitus, current smoking, established cardiovascular disease (any one of myocardial infarction [MI], angina or coronary insufficiency, congestive heart failure, or intermittent claudication), AF, and left ventricular hypertrophy

on electrocardiogram. The FSP provides gender-specific 1-, 5-, or 10-year cumulative stroke risks and has been updated to include the use of antihypertensive therapy and the risk of stroke or death among individuals with AF (Table 16-1).[7] Despite the assessment tool's widespread use, the validity of the FSP among individuals of different age ranges and race-ethnic groups has not been fully studied. Although alternative risk prediction models have been developed in other cohorts, their validity has not been well tested.[8-10]

In the American Stroke Association guidelines for the prevention of stroke, the use of risk assessment tools is recommended to help identify individuals who could benefit from therapeutic interventions and who may not be treated on the basis of any one risk factor.[1] Despite the existence of various risk tools, none have been accepted or widely used in clinical settings. Validation of stroke risk assessment tools is needed in different age, gender, and race-ethnic groups. Emerging risk factors also may need to be considered in newer stroke risk assessment tools. There is a need for simple risk scores that can be easily integrated in primary care settings to help health care providers predict risk and monitor the effects of changing risk behaviors. The ultimate public health benefit, however, will depend on not only identification of stroke risk but also assessment and reduction of global vascular risk.[9]

Lifestyle Modification

Modification of a variety of lifestyle factors can lower the risk of stroke (Table 16-2).

Cigarette Smoking

Cigarette smoking is a well-recognized, modifiable risk factor for ischemic and hemorrhagic stroke.[11-14] The risk of ischemic stroke has been estimated to be twofold higher for smokers versus nonsmokers and threefold higher for subarachnoid hemorrhage.[15] The risk of stroke is reduced among those who quit.[12] Smoking cessation is associated with a reduction in the risk of stroke within 2 to 5 years to a level that approaches the risk of those who never smoked.[16,17] Sustained smoking cessation, however, is often difficult to achieve.

Effective smoking cessation programs often require a combination of social support, behavioral treatments such as hypnosis, and pharmacotherapies including nicotine replacement (see Table 16-2).[18] Three major

TABLE 16-1 MODIFIED FRAMINGHAM STROKE RISK PROFILE

Risk Factor Points	0	1	2	3	4	5	6	7	8	9	10
Age (years)	54-56	57-59	60-62	63-65	66-68	69-71	72-74	75-77	78-80	81-83	84-86
SBP (mm Hg)	95-105	106-116	117-126	127-137	138-148	149-159	160-170	171-181	182-191	192-202	203-213
SBP Rx	No		Yes								
DM	No		Yes								
CS	No			Yes							
CHD	No			Yes							
AF	No				Yes						
LVH	No						Yes				

AF, Atrial fibrillation; CHD, coronary heart disease; CS, cigarette smoking; DM, diabetes mellitus; LVH, left ventricular hypertrophy on electrocardio-gram; SBP, systolic blood pressure; SBP Rx, treated systolic blood pressure.
Modified from Wang TJ, Massaro JM, Levy D, et al: A risk score for predicting stroke or death in individuals with new-onset atrial fibrillation in the community: The Framingham Heart Study. *JAMA* 290:1049-1056, 2003.

TABLE 16-2 AMERICAN HEART ASSOCIATION MANAGEMENT RECOMMENDATIONS FOR LIFESTYLE RISK FACTORS

Factor	Goal	Recommendation
Cigarette smoking	Cessation	Abstention from cigarette smoking and (for current smokers) smoking cessation are recommended (Class I, Level of Evidence B). The use of counseling, nicotine replacement, and oral smoking-cessation medications has been found to be effective for smokers and should be considered (Class IIa, Level of Evidence B).
Physical activity	≥30 minutes of moderate activity/day	Increased physical activity is recommended because it is associated with a reduction in the risk of stroke (Class I, Level of Evidence B). Exercise guidelines of regular exercise as part of a healthy lifestyle as recommended by the Centers for Disease Control and Prevention and the National Institutes of Health (≥30 minutes of moderate-intensity activity daily) are reasonable (Class IIa, Level of Evidence B).
Obesity	Body mass index <25 kg/m²	Weight reduction is recommended because it lowers blood pressure (Class I, Level of Evidence A) and may thereby reduce the risk of stroke.
Diet/nutrition	Well-balanced diet	A reduced intake of sodium and increased intake of potassium are recommended to lower blood pressure (Class I, Level of Evidence A), which may thereby reduce the risk of stroke. The recommended sodium intake is ≤2.3 g/d (100 mmol/d), and the recommended potassium intake is ≥4.7 g/d (120 mmol/d). The DASH diet, which emphasizes fruit, vegetables, and low-fat dairy products, is reduced in saturated and total fat and also lowers blood pressure, is recommended (Class I, Level of Evidence A). A diet that is rich in fruits and vegetables may lower the risk of stroke and may be considered (Class IIb, Level of Evidence C).
Alcohol	Moderation	For those who consume alcohol, a recommendation of ≤2 drinks per day for men and ≤1 drink per day for nonpregnant women best reflects the state of the science for alcohol and stroke risk (Class IIb, Level of Evidence B).
Drug abuse	Cessation	Successful identification and management of drug abuse can be challenging. When a patient is identified as having a drug addiction problem, referral for appropriate counseling may be considered (Class IIb, Level of Evidence C).

Modified from Goldstein LB, Adams R, Alberts MJ, et al: Primary prevention of ischemic stroke: A guideline from the American Heart Association/American Stroke Association Stroke Council. *Stroke* 37:1583-1633, 2006.

pharmacotherapies that have demonstrated efficacy, especially when combined with behavioral support, are nicotine replacement therapy (NRT), bupropion, and varenicline.[19] Multiple commercially available forms of NRT (e.g., gum, transdermal patch, nasal spray, inhaler, and sublingual tablets/lozenges) are helpful in smoking cessation, increasing quitting rates by 50% to 70%.[20] Bupropion improves smoking cessation rates relative to placebo for both confirmed 7-day point-prevalence abstinence and self-reported prolonged abstinence.[21] Varenicline is a novel smoking-cessation agent that acts as a partial nicotinic receptor agonist and is superior to the current standard patch in achieving abstinence and in reducing withdrawal phenomena such as urges to smoke and withdrawal symptoms.[22,23] Further studies of varenicline are needed to evaluate the long-term efficacy of smoking cessation. The most effective preventive measure is to never smoke, as well as to minimize exposure to environmental tobacco smoke.

Physical Activity

Physical inactivity is a well-established and modifiable risk factor for stroke.[24-26] The protective effects of physical activity are present across different age groups, for men and women, and among different race-ethnic groups.[27,28] In the Northern Manhattan Stroke Study, a protective effect was noted with a dose-response relationship showing that more intense physical activity had additional benefits compared with light to moderate physical activity. The protective effect is likely partially mediated through the control of other vascular risk factors including blood pressure, body weight, lipid levels, and diabetes.[29]

Although no clinical trials have specifically addressed the effects of physical activity for stroke prevention, the evidence from epidemiologic studies and from a few clinical trials in other chronic diseases is very supportive of a beneficial effect. Clinical trials show that exercise reduced not only the risk of falls resulting in injury among the elderly but also systolic blood pressure and diastolic blood pressure and had beneficial effects on blood lipid levels without any reported harm.[30] The benefits of physical activity have been highlighted in the Centers for Disease Control and Prevention (CDC), the National Institutes of Health, and the American Heart Association guidelines that recommend moderate exercise for at least 30 minutes per day (see Table 16-2).[31-33] Despite these recommendations, most communities still have prevalence rates as great as 60% for adults not meeting the minimum physical activity recommendations.[34] Increasing physical activity could yield major public health gains in the prevention of cardiovascular disease and stroke.

Weight Management and Diet

Obesity is a risk factor for both stroke and cardiovascular disease and is associated with multiple other stroke risk factors including hypertension, dyslipidemia, hyperinsulinemia, and glucose intolerance. Greater weight during young adulthood and weight gain thereafter is associated with an increased stroke risk.[35] Measures of abdominal obesity, such as waist-to-hip ratio or waist circumference, are also stroke risk factors.[36] An increased waist circumference is a component of the metabolic syndrome, which is also a risk factor for stroke.[37] Drugs that reduce insulin resistance are being evaluated in primary and secondary stroke prevention.[38]

What makes obesity of even greater public health concern is its alarming increase in prevalence. Approximately one in three adults in the United States are obese, and nearly two thirds of US adults are classified as either overweight or obese.[39] Moreover, the prevalence of obesity has been steadily increasing among all US population groups, but especially among children and women.[40,41] It is projected that if these trends continue, by 2030, 86.3% of adults will be overweight or obese and 51.1% will be obese.[42]

Losing weight is associated with a reduction of other risk factors, possibly leading to a reduction in stroke risk. Although specific clinical trials evaluating the effects of weight reduction on stroke risk are lacking, the beneficial effects of weight reduction on blood pressure is well documented. In a meta-analysis of 25 clinical trials, blood pressure was reduced by 3.6 to 4.4 mm Hg with an average weight loss of 5.1 kg.[43] Weight reduction is a key component of the lifestyle measures recommended by the Seventh Report of the Joint National Committee on Prevention, Detection, Evaluation, and Treatment of High Blood Pressure (JNC 7) and Adult Treatment Panel III (ATP III) guidelines for control of high blood pressure and dyslipidemia, respectively.[44,45]

Multiple dietary components are associated with the risk of stroke. Diets with increased fruit and vegetable content are associated with a dose-related reduction in the risk of stroke.[46] The risk of stroke was reduced by 6% in the Nurses' Health Study and the Health Professionals' Follow-Up Study for each 1-serving/day increment in fruit and vegetable intake.[47] Diets with greater sodium and lower potassium content are also associated with an increased risk of stroke, possibly because they are mediated through blood pressure dependent mechanisms.[48]

Randomized trials have assessed the effects of diets rich in fruits and vegetables on lowering blood pressure but have not had sufficient follow-up to evaluate clinical events. The Dietary Approaches to Stop Hypertension (DASH) diet, which includes high consumption of fruits, vegetables, and low-fat dairy products and a reduced intake of total and saturated fat, reduces blood pressure.[49,50] A Mediterranean dietary pattern, which incorporates the consumption of fruits and vegetables, whole grains, folate, and fatty fish, as well as legumes and olive oil, may also prevent stroke.[51,52] Dietary trials specifically focused on reducing the risk of stroke are needed.

Alcohol and Drug Abuse

Epidemiologic evidence associating alcohol consumption and stroke risk has suggested a J-shaped relationship.[53,54] For ischemic stroke, as compared with nondrinkers, moderate drinkers (one to two drinks a day) have between a 0.3 and 0.5 stroke risk, whereas persons consuming three or more drinks per day have a greater stroke risk.[55] In a meta-analysis of 35 observational studies, consumption of less than one drink per day (one drink is defined as 12 g of alcohol), but not abstention, was associated with a 20% reduced risk of stroke. Consumption of one to two drinks per day was associated with a 28% risk reduction.[56] As compared with nondrinkers, those who drank more than five drinks per day had a 69% increased stroke risk. No protective relationship has been found for hemorrhagic stroke, and the relative increased risk varies from 2 to 4.[57] Light-to-moderate alcohol consumption (for women ≤1 drink/day and for men ≤2 drinks/day) can increase high-density lipoprotein (HDL) cholesterol, reduce platelet aggregation, and lower plasma fibrinogen concentration.[58] The deleterious consequences of heavy alcohol consumption include hypertension, hypercoagulability, reduced cerebral blood flow, and a greater likelihood of AF and other arrythmias.[59]

Despite the potential benefit of moderate alcohol consumption, there are other adverse health consequences related to excess alcohol use. Alcoholism remains a major public health problem in the United States. More than 10 million adults have alcoholism and alcohol-related diseases such as hypertension and cirrhosis.[60] Given the health risks associated with excessive alcohol use, it is not prudent to encourage alcohol consumption for stroke prevention. Reduction of alcohol consumption in heavy drinkers is recommended.[61] For those who drink alcohol, suggested consumption is ≤2 drinks per day for men and ≤1 drink per day for nonpregnant women (see Table 16-2).

Drug abuse including heroin, cocaine, and amphetamines is associated with an increased risk of ischemic and hemorrhagic strokes.[62-64] These drugs can cause hematologic and metabolic derangements, including increased platelet aggregation, fluctuations in blood pressure, and vasculopathy, and cerebral embolization from secondary cardiac conditions or endocarditis.[65] Identification and management of drug abuse can be very challenging. When a patient is identified as having a drug addiction problem, referral for appropriate counseling is recommended.[66] Various strategies are needed and often require a long-term commitment, medication, and psychological counseling. Community outreach programs are needed to prevent drug abuse and to reduce the prevalence of drug dependency.

Management of Well-Documented Modifiable Risk Factors for Preventing a First Stroke

Evidence-based guidelines are available for the management of several modifiable risk factors for a first stroke. Selected, well-documented, modifiable risk factors are discussed below.

Hypertension

Hypertension is one of the most important modifiable risk factors for prevention of a first stroke.[67] The most comprehensive review of evidence-based treatment of hypertension is provided in JNC 7.[45] The classification and treatment scheme for elevated blood pressure is outlined in Table 16-3.

JNC 7 guidelines recommend lowering blood pressure to less than 140/90 mm Hg (or <130/80 mm Hg in individuals with diabetes). Optimal blood pressure target levels for the most effective prevention of primary and recurrent stroke are part of the specific aims of ongoing randomized trials. Meta-analyses of numerous

randomized clinical trials show 35% to 44% reductions in the incidence of stroke across various antihypertensive regimens.[68] There are several classes of antihypertensive medications that have been evaluated for reducing stroke including thiazide diuretics, angiotensin-converting enzyme inhibitors (ACEIs), angiotensin receptor blockers (ARBs), β-adrenergic receptor blockers, and calcium channel blockers. In JNC-7 thiazide-type diuretics are often recommended as the preferred initial drugs for treatment of hypertension in most patients.[45] Differential efficacy of some of these classes of antihypertensive agents has been suggested by individual trials, as well as meta-analyses.[69] A meta-analysis of 18 long-term randomized trials found that both diuretics (hazard ratio [HR], 0.49; 95% confidence interval [CI], 0.39 to 0.62) and β-blockers (HR, 0.71; 95% CI, 0.59 to 0.86) are effective in preventing stroke.[70] Several other classes of blood pressure–lowering agents such as ACEIs and ARBs are recommended next.

Some individual trials provide evidence of the efficacy of antihypertensives for stroke prevention in specific patient subgroups. For patients older than 60 years with isolated systolic hypertension, the Systolic Hypertension in the Elderly Program (SHEP) found a 36% reduction in the incidence of stroke after treatment with a thiazide diuretic with or without a β-blocker.[71] The Antihypertensive and Lipid-Lowering Treatment to Prevent Heart Attack Trial (ALLHAT) demonstrated the superiority of diuretic-based over α-blocker-based antihypertensive treatment for the prevention of stroke and cardiovascular events in a randomized, double-blind, active, controlled clinical trial including 24,355 participants.[72]

There is conflicting evidence regarding the efficacy of calcium channel blockers for stroke prevention. In the Systolic Hypertension in Europe (Syst-Eur) Trial, a 42% stroke risk reduction was found among patients with isolated systolic hypertension treated with a calcium channel blocker (nitrendipine) compared with placebo.[73] Data from the Controlled ONset Verapamil INvestigation of Cardiovascular Endpoints (CONVINCE) trial, however, did not find benefit for cardiovascular risk reduction for another calcium channel blocker (verapamil) compared

TABLE 16-3 CLASSIFICATION AND TREATMENT OF BLOOD PRESSURE

Classification	Blood Pressure (mm Hg)	No Convincing Antihypertensive Indication*	With Convincing Antihypertensive Indication*
Normal	<120/80	No drug	No drug
Prehypertension	121/81 to <140/90	No drug	Drugs for the compelling indication
Stage 1 hypertension	141/91 to <159/99	Thiazide-type diuretics; may consider ACEIs, ARBs, β-blockers, calcium channel blockers, or combination	Drugs for the compelling indication; other drugs (diuretics, ACEIs, ARBs, β-blockers, calcium channel blockers) as needed
Stage 2 hypertension	≥160/100	Two-drug combination for most (usually thiazide-type diuretic and ACEI or ARB or β-blocker or calcium channel blocker)	Drugs for the compelling indication and other drugs as needed

*Lifestyle modifications are encouraged for all and include (1) weight reduction if overweight, (2) limitation of ethyl alcohol intake, (3) increased aerobic physical activity (30–45 minutes daily), (4) reduction of sodium intake (<2.34 g), (5) maintenance of adequate dietary potassium (>120 mmol/d), (6) smoking cessation, and (7) DASH diet (rich in fruit, vegetables, and low-fat dairy products and reduced in saturated and total fat). Compelling indications include (1) congestive heart failure, (2) myocardial infarction, (3) diabetes, (4) chronic renal failure, and (5) prior stroke.
Initial combined therapy should be used cautiously in those at risk of orthostatic hypotension.
Abbreviations: ACEI, Angiotensin-converting enzyme inhibitor; ARB, angiotensin receptor blocker.
Modified from Chobanian AV, Bakris GL, Black HR, et al: The seventh report of the Joint National Committee on Prevention, Detection, Evaluation, and Treatment of High Blood Pressure: The JNC 7 Report. *JAMA* 289:2560-2571, 2003.

with a diuretic or β-blocker treatment.[74] In the Anglo-Scandinavian Cardiac Outcomes Trial—Blood Pressure Lowering Arm (ASCOT-BPLA) trial, a combination of atenolol (β-blocker) with a thiazide prevented more major cardiovascular events and was associated with less diabetes than amlodipine (a calcium channel blocker) with perindopril (an ACEI).[75]

Some of the most convincing evidence regarding the benefits of ACEIs comes from the Heart Outcomes Prevention Evaluation (HOPE) study that demonstrated that ramipril (an ACEI) reduced the risk of cardiovascular events by approximately 20% compared with placebo in patients at risk of cardiovascular events without heart failure.[76] A substudy, the Study to Evaluate Carotid Ultrasound Changes in Patients Treated with Ramipril and Vitamin E (SECURE), also found that ramipril reduced carotid atherosclerosis.[77] Other ACEIs have not fared as well. Among 10,985 patients in the Captopril Prevention Project (CAPPP), no difference in efficacy was found between an ACE inhibitor–based therapeutic regimen (captopril) compared with conventional antihypertensive therapy (i.e., diuretics, β-blockers) in preventing cardiovascular morbidity and mortality.[78]

Angiotensin II type 1 receptor antagonists (ARBs) have been proposed as being better tolerated than ACEIs. The Losartan Intervention for Endpoint Reduction in Hypertension (LIFE) study found a substantial reduction in stroke risk among 9193 participants aged 55 to 80 years with essential hypertension and left ventricular hypertrophy by electrocardiogram treated with an ARB compared with conventional therapy with atenolol (β-blocker) for a similar reduction in blood pressure.[79]

The hypothesis that combined treatment with both an ACEI and ARB may be beneficial was assessed in the Ongoing Telmisartan Alone and in Combination with Ramipril Global Endpoint Trial (ONTARGET).[80] This large trial compared the benefits of ACEI treatment, ARB treatment, and treatment with an ACEI and ARB together. In the parallel study, Telmisartan Randomized Assessment Study in ACEI Intolerant Patients with Cardiovascular Disease (TRANSEND), patients unable to tolerate an ACEI were randomly assigned to receive an ARB (telmisartan) or placebo. The results of these landmark trials show that telmisartan, a second-generation ARB, was as effective as the current standard, ramipril (ACEI), in reducing the risk of stroke, MI, cardiovascular death, and hospitalization for congestive heart failure in a broad spectrum of high-risk cardiovascular patients. The combination of an ACEI (ramipril) and an ARB (telmisartan), however, did not show any advantages compared with single blockade.

Combinations of an ACEI and calcium channel blocker have also been assessed. In the Avoiding Cardiovascular events through Combination therapy in Patients Living with Systolic Hypertension (ACCOMPLISH) trial, the effects of two forms of antihypertensive combination therapy (benazepril plus hydrochlorothiazide and amlodipine plus benazepril) were compared for the reduction of major fatal and nonfatal cardiovascular events in 11,454 hypertensive patients at high cardiovascular risk.[81] The study was terminated early because combination ACEI plus the calcium channel blocker was more effective than combination treatment with ACEI plus the diuretic.

Treatment of hypertension is beneficial for older patients as well as younger patients. In the Hypertension in the Very Elderly Trial (HYVET), among 3845 individuals 80 years of age or older with a sustained systolic blood pressure of 160 mm Hg or more, a 30% reduction in the rate of fatal or nonfatal stroke and a 39% reduction in the rate of death from stroke was achieved with active treatment (the diuretic indapamide with addition of the ACEI perindopril, if needed, to achieve the target blood pressure of 150/80 mm Hg) in comparison with placebo.[82] In another meta-analysis of 31 trials, among 190,606 participants, the benefits of blood pressure reduction were found in adults, both younger (<65 years) and older (≥65 years), with no strong evidence that protection against stroke and other vascular events varies substantially with age.[83]

For secondary stroke prevention, the Perindopril Protection Against Recurrent Stroke Study (PROGRESS) trial confirmed that treatment with perindopril (an ACEI) in combination with a diuretic reduced the risk of recurrent stroke.[84] Combination therapy produced greater blood pressure reductions and led to larger stroke reductions than monotherapy with perindopril alone. Effects were observed among those with or without a previous history of hypertension.

It is well established that blood pressure lowering is effective for the primary prevention of stroke and other cardiovascular disorders. Although pharmacotherapies have helped achieve blood pressure control in most patients, the majority require combination therapy, often with more than two antihypertensive medications.[85] Despite the evidence from clinical trials, blood pressure levels are adequately controlled in less than 25% of the hypertensive population worldwide.[86] Many more strokes could be prevented with more effective treatment of hypertension. Lack of diagnosis and inadequate treatment are of particular importance among minority populations and in the elderly.[45,87]

Current American Heart Association (AHA) guidelines for primary stroke prevention call for regular screening for hypertension (at least every 2 years in most adults and more frequently in minority populations and the elderly) and appropriate management (Class I, Level of Evidence A), including dietary changes, lifestyle modification, and pharmacologic therapy.[1] The choice of a specific regimen must be individualized, but reduction in blood pressure is probably more important than the specific agent used to achieve this goal. Specific classes of antihypertensive drugs may offer special protection against stroke in addition to their blood pressure–lowering effects.

Diabetes

Diabetes increases the risk of stroke nearly threefold and disproportionately affects the elderly and minority populations.[88] Although generally considered a disease having pathophysiologic effects related to impaired blood glucose control, there remains no evidence that tight control of blood glucose levels reduces the risk of stroke or cardiovascular events in diabetic patients. The hypothesis was directly tested in several clinical trials.

The Action to Control Cardiovascular Risk in Type 2 Diabetes (ACCORD) study randomly assigned 10,251 patients with a median glycated hemoglobin level of 8.1% to intensive blood glucose control (target glycated hemoglobin, <6%) or standard control (glycated hemoglobin, 7.0 to 7.9%).[89] The study was stopped early because of higher mortality rates in the intensive control group (HR, 1.22; 95% CI, 1.01 to 1.46; P = 0.04). There was no difference in the risk of nonfatal stroke (HR, 1.06; 95% CI, 0.75 to 1.50; P = 0.74). The Action in Diabetes and Vascular Disease: Preterax and Diamicron Modified Release Controlled Evaluation (ADVANCE) trial randomly assigned 11,140 patients with diabetes to intensive blood glucose control (target glycated hemoglobin, <6.5%) or standard therapy.[90] Although there was a treatment-related reduction in nephropathy, there was no reduction in macrovascular events (HR, 0.94; 95% CI, 0.84 to 1.06; P = 0.32) including no reduction in nonfatal stroke (relative risk reduction, −2%; 95% CI, −24% to 15%). The United Kingdom Prospective Diabetes Study (UKPDS) had also found that newly diagnosed patients with type 2 diabetes had a lower risk of microvascular complications with intensive therapy.[91] Post-trial 10-year follow-up found that although the initial difference in glycated hemoglobin was not evident after the first year, reduction in microvascular complications persisted, and reductions in the rate of MI and death emerged over time.[92] There was, however, not a significant reduction in stroke (risk ratio, 0.80; 95% CI, 0.50 to 1.27; P = 0.35). The Veterans Affairs Diabetes Trial (VADT) randomly assigned 1791 veterans who had diabetes for a mean of 11.5 years but who had a suboptimal response to treatment (40% had a cardiovascular event) to intensive blood glucose control or standard therapy.[93] There was no effect of intensive control (mean glycated hemoglobin, 6.9% versus 8.4%) on the occurrence of major cardiovascular events (HR, 0.88; 95% CI, 0.74 to 1.05; P = 0.14), again including no impact on stroke (HR, 0.78; 95% CI, 0.48 to 1.28; P = 0.32). Therefore, evidence that intensive blood glucose control decreases the risk of stroke or other cardiovascular events in persons with diabetes is lacking.

Despite these disappointing results, treatments other than intensive blood glucose control have been associated with reductions in the risk of stroke in patients with diabetes. The UKPDS compared the effects of tight blood pressure control (target, <150/85 mm Hg; mean achieved, 144/82 mm Hg) with less tight control (mean, 154/87 mm Hg) in 1148 hypertensive patients with type 2 diabetes and found that tight control led to a 44% reduction (relative risk, 0.56; 95% CI, 0.35 to 0.89; P = 0.01) in the risk of stroke over a median of 8.4 years.[94] The between-group difference in blood pressures became insignificant after the trial was completed, and benefits decreased over time; by 10 years the reduction in stroke was reduced by half and was no longer significant (relative risk, 23%; P = 0.12), which suggests that tight blood pressure control needs to be sustained.[95] SHEP found that antihypertensive treatment of elderly diabetic patients led to a 34% (relative risk, 0.66; 95% CI, 0.46 to 0.94) reduction in major cardiovascular events that included a 22% (relative risk, 0.78; 95% CI, 0.45 to 1.034) reduction in stroke.[96] A substudy of 3577 diabetic patients with a previous cardiovascular event or an additional cardiovascular risk factor enrolled in the HOPE trial (of a total population of 9541

participants in the HOPE study) found that the addition of an ACEI to other antihypertensive drugs reduced a combined outcome of MI, stroke, and cardiovascular death by 25% (95% CI, 12 to 36; P = 0.0004) and stroke by 33% (95% CI, 10 to 50; P = 0.0074).[76] A prespecified subanalysis of the LIFE study compared the effects of an angiotensin II type-1 receptor blocker with a β-adrenergic receptor blocker in diabetic patients with essential hypertension (160-200/95-115 mm Hg) and electrocardiographically determined left ventricular hypertrophy.[97] There was a 24% (relative risk, 0.76; 95% CI, 0.58 to 0.98) reduction in major vascular events and a nonsignificant 21% (relative risk, 0.79; 95% CI, 0.55 to 1.14) reduction in stroke among those treated with the ARB. The available data suggest that patients with diabetes benefit from careful treatment of hypertension, which may also include a reduction in the risk of a first stroke.

Persons with diabetes may also benefit from treatment with an HMG-CoA reductase inhibitor (statin). The MRC/BHF Heart Protection Study (HPS) found that the addition of a statin to existing treatments resulted in a 22% (95% CI, 13% to 30%) reduction in major vascular events (regardless of cholesterol levels) and a 24% (95% CI, 6% to 39%; P = 0.01) reduction in strokes among 5963 patients with diabetes.[98] Consistent with these results, the Collaborative Atorvastatin Diabetes Study (CARDS) found that treatment with a statin in subjects with type 2 diabetes, a low-density lipoprotein-cholesterol (LDL-C) level less than 160 mg/dL, and at least one additional risk factor (i.e., retinopathy, albuminuria, current smoking, or hypertension) led to a 48% (95% CI, 11% to 69%) reduction in the risk of a first stroke.[99]

Lipid-Lowering Therapy

Unlike coronary heart disease, there is only a weak relationship between lipid levels and stroke risk. Meta-analyses found no significant reduction in stroke risk with a variety of lipid-lowering therapies including diet (10 trials; risk ratio [RR], 0.99; 95% CI, 0.85 to 1.15), fibrates (11 trials; RR, 1.04; 95% CI, 0.92 to 1.19), resins (4 trials; RR, 1.03; 95% CI, 0.54 to 2.00), or omega-3 fatty acids (8 trials; RR, 0.91; 95% CI, 0.56 to 1.48).[100] In contrast, several meta-analyses found that treatment of patients with a history of coronary heart disease or other high risk conditions with statins reduces the risk of a first stroke.[100-106] The most recent of these meta-analyses included 121,285 subjects enrolled in 42 trials and found that statin therapy resulted in a 16% (relative risk, 0.84; 95% CI, 0.79 to 0.91) reduction in stroke risk as well as a 12% (relative risk, 0.88; 95% CI, 0.83 to 0.93) reduction in all-cause mortality.[106] There was no effect of statin treatment on the risk of hemorrhagic stroke (11 trials; n = 54,334; relative risk, 0.94; 95% CI, 0.68 to 1.30).

These trials focused on statin treatment in patients with coronary heart disease and other high-risk conditions. The Justification for the Use of Statins in Primary Prevention: an Interventional Trial Evaluating Rosuvastatin (JUPITER) trial randomly assigned 17,802 cardiovascular disease-free men older than age 55 and women older than age 65 with an LDL-C level less than 130 mg/dL but evidence of systemic inflammation based on an elevated high-sensitivity C-reactive protein level of more than 2 mg/L to statin therapy or placebo.[107] Treatment resulted in a 44% (HR, 0.56; 95% CI, 0.46 to 0.69; $P < 0.00001$) reduction in the time to a combined cardiovascular endpoint that included a 48% (HR, 0.52; 95% CI, 0.34 to 0.79; $P = 0.002$) reduction in the risk of stroke. Further work will need to be done to determine the usefulness of wide-scale population screening for identifying patients who might benefit from treatment.[108]

Atrial Fibrillation

Nonvalvular AF is an important, treatable risk factor for stroke. Depending on patient age, the population-attributable risk varies from 1.5% to 23.5% with relative risks from approximately 2.5 to 4.5.[1] A systematic literature review identified 29 randomized trials that included more than 28,000 subjects and evaluated the impact of antithrombotic therapy in patients with AF.[109] Treatment with antiplatelet drugs reduced the risk of stroke by 22% (95% CI, 6% to 35%), whereas dose-adjusted warfarin reduced the risk by 64% (95% CI, 49% to 74%); warfarin was more efficacious than antiplatelet therapy (relative risk reduction, 39%; 95% CI, 22% to 52%). These reductions included the risk of antithrombotic-related intracranial hemorrhage.

The risk of stroke and therefore the benefits versus risks of antithrombotic therapy are not uniform for all patients with nonvalvular AF. As already noted, the population-attributable and relative risks of AF-related stroke increase with advancing age. A systematic review assessed the impact of a series of potential factors on the risk of stroke in patients with AF based on studies using multivariable regression analyses.[110] Increasing age (relative risk, 1.5 per decade; 95% CI, 1.3 to 1.7; absolute rate, 1.5% to 3% per year for age older than 75), a history of hypertension (relative risk, 2.0; 95% CI, 1.6 to 2.5; absolute rate, 1.5% to 3% per year), and diabetes mellitus (relative risk, 1.7; 95% CI, 1.4 to 2.0; absolute rate, 2.0 to 3.5% per year) were the strongest, most consistent independent risk factors.

There have been more than 12 schemes developed and published that stratify the stroke risk of patients with AF.[10] The rates of stroke predicted by these schemes vary widely. A systematic review found that observed rates for those categorized as low risk ranged from 0% to 2.3% per year, and rates for those categorized as being at high risk ranged from 2.5% to 7.9% annually.[10] When these schemes were applied to the same cohorts, the proportions of patients categorized as low risk varied from 9% to 49%, and those categorized as high-risk varied from 11% to 77%.[10] Although the CHADS2 score (congestive heart failure, hypertension, age older than 75 years, and diabetes equal 1 point each; stroke or TIA equals 2 points) is commonly used and predicts stroke risk (score: 0-1, low risk, stroke rate, ≈1% per year; score: 2, moderate risk, 2.5% per year; score: ≥3, high risk, >5% per year), it includes a history of prior stroke or transient ischemic attack.[111] In the absence of specific contraindications, the benefits of warfarin generally outweigh the risks when the predicted annual stroke rate is more than 4%.[1] The systematic review, however, concluded that, "additional

research to identify an optimum scheme for primary prevention"[10] was necessary.

There is a common concern among physicians about the risk of warfarin in the elderly. Advancing age, however, is associated with increasing risk of AF-related stroke. A small, open-label, safety study in patients with AF age 80 to 89 years found dose-adjusted warfarin was better tolerated than 300 mg of aspirin daily.[112] The Birmingham Atrial Fibrillation Treatment of the Aged (BAFTA) study was an open-label, randomized comparison of dose-adjusted warfarin versus 75 mg of aspirin daily in patients with AF older than 75 years.[113] Based on a treatment-masked assessment of outcomes, the risk of stroke was reduced by nearly half with warfarin (annual risk, 1.8% vs. 3.8%; relative risk, 0.48; 95% CI, 0.28 to 0.80; $P = 0.003$). The annual risks of extracranial hemorrhage were 1.4% for warfarin compared with 1.6% for aspirin. These results suggest that concern about the risk of warfarin-associated hemorrhage in the elderly may be overestimated and that the benefits outweigh the risks in the absence of specific contraindications.

Aspirin

There is no evidence that platelet antiaggregants reduce the risk of stroke in persons at low risk.[114-116] Because the risk of coronary heart disease generally outweighs the risk of stroke, coronary heart risk generally drives recommendations for the use of aspirin. The U.S. Preventive Services Task Force recommends 75 mg of aspirin per day for cardiac prophylaxis for persons whose 5-year coronary heart disease risk is 3% or greater.[114] AHA guidelines for the primary prevention of cardiovascular disease and stroke recommend aspirin if the patient has 10% or more risk per 10 years rather than more than 3% risk over 5 years.[117] AHA Primary Stroke Prevention Guidelines suggest that aspirin be considered for cardiovascular prophylaxis in patients with a 10-year risk of cardiovascular disease of 6% to 10%.[1] This excludes patients with AF (already discussed) and patients who have had a carotid endarterectomy.[118]

The majority of patients included in the studies on which these recommendations were based were men. The Women's Health Study (WHS) randomly assigned 39,876 initially asymptomatic women 45 years of age or older to receive 100 mg of aspirin on alternate days or placebo (combined primary endpoint was nonfatal MI, nonfatal stroke, or cardiovascular death).[119] There was a nonsignificant reduction in the primary endpoint with aspirin (relative risk, 0.91; 95% CI, 0.80 to 1.03; $P = 0.13$) but a significant reduction in the risk of stroke (relative risk, 0.83; 95% CI, 0.69 to 0.99; $P = 0.04$; 0.11% per year in aspirin-treated patients and 0.13% per year in placebo-treated patients; absolute risk reduction, 0.02% per year; number needed to treat, 5000). Gastrointestinal hemorrhaging requiring transfusion was more frequent in the aspirin group (relative risk, 1.40; 95% CI, 1.07 to 1.83; $P = 0.02$). Subgroup analyses showed the most consistent benefit with treatment was in women having a 10-year cardiovascular risk of 10% or greater (relative risk, 0.54; 95% CI, 0.30 to 0.98; $P = 0.04$). Similar to the previous recommendations, the 2007 Update of the AHA Evidence-Based Guidelines for Cardiovascular Disease Prevention in Women recommended that women be considered for aspirin therapy for primary stroke prevention depending on the balance of risks and benefits.[120]

REFERENCES

1. Goldstein LB, Adams R, Alberts MJ, et al: Primary prevention of ischemic stroke: A guideline from the American Heart Association/American Stroke Association Stroke Council, *Stroke* 37:1583-1633, 2006.
2. Grundy SM, Pasternak R, Greenland P, et al: Assessment of cardiovascular risk by use of multiple-risk-factor assessment equations: A statement for healthcare professionals from the American Heart Association and the American College of Cardiology, *J Am Coll Cardiol* 34:1348-1359, 1999.
3. Wilson PWF, D'Agostino RB, Levy D, et al: Prediction of coronary heart disease using risk factor categories, *Circulation* 97:1837-1847, 1998.
4. Wolf PA, D'Agostino RB, Belanger AJ, Kannel WB: Probability of stroke: A risk profile from the Framingham Study, *Stroke* 22:312-318, 1991.
5. D'Agostino RB, Wolf PA, Belanger AJ, Kannel WB: Stroke risk profile: adjustment for antihypertensive medication. The Framingham Study, *Stroke* 25:40-43, 1994.
6. D'Agostino RB, Vasan RS, Pencina MJ, et al: General cardiovascular risk profile for use in primary care: The Framingham Heart Study, *Circulation* 117:743-753, 2008.
7. Wang TJ, Massaro JM, Levy D, et al: A risk score for predicting stroke or death in individuals with new-onset atrial fibrillation in the community: The Framingham Heart Study, *JAMA* 290:1049-1056, 2003.
8. Lumley T, Kronmal RA, Cushman M, et al: A stroke prediction score in the elderly: Validation and web-based application, *J Clin Epidemiol* 55:129-136, 2002.
9. Sacco RL: The 2006 William Feinberg Lecture: Shifting the paradigm from stroke to global vascular risk estimation, *Stroke* 38:1980-1987, 2007.
10. Hart RG, Pearce LA, Halperin JL, et al: Comparison of 12 risk stratification schemes to predict stroke in patients with nonvalvular atrial fibrillation, *Stroke* 39:1901-1910, 2008.
11. Wolf PA, D'Agostino RB, Kannel WB, et al: Cigarette smoking as a risk factor for stroke. The Framingham Study, *JAMA* 259:1025-1029, 1988.
12. Manolio TA, Kronmal RA, Burke GL, et al: Short-term predictors of incident stroke in older adults: The Cardiovascular Health Study, *Stroke* 27:1479-1486, 1996.
13. Broderick JP, Viscoli CM, Brott T, et al: Major risk factors for aneurysmal subarachnoid hemorrhage in the young are modifiable, *Stroke* 34:1375-1381, 2003.
14. Surgeon General of the United States: The Centers for Disease Control, *The Surgeon General's 1989 Report on Reducing the Health Consequences of Smoking: 25 Years of Progress, MMWR Morb Mortal Wkly Rep*, 38(Suppl 2):1-32, 1989.
15. Shinton R, Beevers G: Meta-analysis of relation between cigarette smoking and stroke, *BMJ* 298:789-794, 1989.
16. Fagerstrom K: The epidemiology of smoking: health consequences and benefits of cessation, *Drugs* 62(Suppl 2):1-9, 2002.
17. Kawachi I, Colditz GA, Stampfer MJ, et al: Smoking cessation and decreased risk of stroke in women, *JAMA* 269:232-236, 1993.
18. Fiore MC: U.S. Public Health Service Clinical Practice Guideline: treating tobacco use and dependence, *Respir Care* 45:1200-1262, 2000.
19. Galanti LM: Tobacco smoking cessation management: Integrating varenicline in current practice, *Vasc Health Risk Manag* 4:837-845, 2008.
20. Stead LF, Perera R, Bullen C, et al: Nicotine replacement therapy for smoking cessation, *Cochrane Database Syst Rev* 23, 2008:CD000146.
21. McCarthy DE, Piasecki TM, Lawrence DL, et al: A randomized controlled clinical trial of bupropion SR and individual smoking cessation counseling, *Nicotine Tob Res* 10:717-729, 2008.
22. Aubin H-J, Bobak A, Britton JR, et al: Varenicline versus transdermal nicotine patch for smoking cessation: Results from a randomised open-label trial, *Thorax* 63:717-724, 2008.
23. Cahill K, Stead LF, Lancaster T: Nicotine receptor partial agonists for smoking cessation, *Cochrane Database Syst Rev* 16, 2008:CD006103.
24. Fletcher GF: Exercise in the prevention of stroke, *Health Rep* 6:106-110, 1994.
25. Wendel-Vos GCW, Schuit AJ, Feskens EJM, et al: Physical activity and stroke. A meta-analysis of observational data, *Int J Epidemiol* 33:787-798, 2004.
26. Lee CD, Folsom AR, Blair SN: Physical activity and stroke risk: A meta-analysis, *Stroke* 34:2475-2481, 2003.
27. Gillum RF, Mussolino ME, Ingram DD: Physical activity and stroke incidence in women and men: The NHANES I Epidemiologic Follow-up Study, *Am J Epidemiol* 143:860-869, 1996.
28. Sacco RL, Gan R, Boden-Albala B, et al: Leisure-time physical activity and ischemic stroke risk: The Northern Manhattan Stroke Study, *Stroke* 29:380-387, 1998.
29. Shinton R, Sagar G: Lifelong exercise and stroke, *BMJ* 307:231-234, 1993.
30. Karmisholt K, Gyntelberg F, Gøtzche PC: Physical activity for primary prevention of disease. Systematic reviews of randomised clinical trials, *Dan Med Bull* 52:86-89, 2005.
31. NIH develops consensus statement on the role of physical activity for cardiovascular health, *Am Fam Physician* 54:763-767, 1996.
32. Pate RR, Pratt M, Blair SN, et al: Physical activity and public health: A recommendation from the Centers for Disease Control and Prevention and the American College of Sports Medicine, *JAMA* 273:402-407, 1995.
33. Eyre H, Kahn R, Robertson RM, et al: Preventing cancer, cardiovascular disease, and diabetes: A common agenda for the American Cancer Society, the American Diabetes Association, and the American Heart Association, *Circulation* 109:3244-3255, 2004.
34. Ramsey F, Ussery-Hall A, Garcia D, et al: Prevalence of selected risk behaviors and chronic diseases. Behavioral Risk Factor Surveillance System (BRFSS), 39 steps communities, United States, 2005, *Morb Mortal Wkly Rep Surveill Summ* 57:1-20, 2008.
35. Heyden S, Hames CG, Bartel A, et al: Weight and weight history in relation to cerebrovascular and ischemic heart disease, *Arch Intern Med* 128:956-960, 1971.
36. Suk S-H, Sacco RL, Boden-Albala B, et al: Abdominal obesity and risk of ischemic stroke: The Northern Manhattan Stroke Study, *Stroke* 34:1586-1592, 2003.
37. Boden-Albala B, Sacco RL, Lee H-S, et al: Metabolic syndrome and ischemic stroke risk: Northern Manhattan Study, *Stroke* 39:30-35, 2008.
38. Kernan WN, Inzucchi SE, Viscoli CM, et al: Insulin resistance and risk for stroke, *Neurology* 59:809-815, 2002.
39. Hedley AA, Ogden CL, Johnson CL, et al: Prevalence of overweight and obesity among US children, adolescents, and adults, 1999-2002, *JAMA* 291:2847-2850, 2004.
40. Flegal KM, Carroll MD, Ogden CL, Johnson CL: Prevalence and trends in obesity among US adults, 1999-2000, *JAMA* 288:1723-1727, 2002.
41. Ford ES, Zhao G, Li C, et al: Trends in obesity and abdominal obesity among hypertensive and nonhypertensive adults in the United States, *Am J Hypertens* 21:1124-1128, 2008.
42. Wang Y, Beydoun MA, Liang L, et al: Will all Americans become overweight or obese? Estimating the progression and cost of the US obesity epidemic, *Obesity* 16:2323-2330, 2008.
43. Neter JE, Stam BE, Kok FJ, et al: Influence of weight reduction on blood pressure: A meta-analysis of randomized controlled trials, *Hypertension* 42:878-884, 2003.
44. Chobanian AV, Bakris GL, Black HR, et al: The Seventh Report of the Joint National Committee on Prevention, Detection, Evaluation, and Treatment of High Blood Pressure: The JNC 7 Report, *JAMA* 289:2560-2571, 2003.
45. Expert Panel on Detection, Evaluation, and Treatment of High Blood Cholesterol in Adults. Executive Summary of the Third Report of the National Cholesterol Education Program (NCEP) Expert Panel on Detection, Evaluation, and Treatment of High Blood Cholesterol in Adults (Adult Treatment Panel III), *JAMA* 285:2486-2497, 2001.

46. Steffen LM, Jacobs DR, Stevens J, et al: Associations of whole-grain, refined-grain, and fruit and vegetable consumption with risks of all-cause mortality and incident coronary artery disease and ischemic stroke: The Atherosclerosis Risk in Communities (ARIC) Study, *Am J Clin Nutr* 78:383-390, 2003.

47. Joshipura KJ, Ascherio A, Manson JE, et al: Fruit and vegetable intake in relation to risk of ischemic stroke, *JAMA* 282:1233-1239, 1999.

48. Khaw KT, Barrett-Connor E: Dietary potassium and stroke-associated mortality. A 12-year prospective population study, *N Engl J Med* 316:235-240, 1987.

49. Appel LJ, Moore TJ, Obarzanek E, et al: A clinical trial of the effects of dietary patterns on blood pressure, *N Engl J Med* 336:1117-1124, 1997.

50. John JH, Ziebland S, Yudkin P, et al: Effects of fruit and vegetable consumption on plasma antioxidant concentrations and blood pressure: A randomised controlled trial, *Lancet* 359:1969-1974, 2002.

51. Ding EL, Mozaffarian D: Optimal dietary habits for the prevention of stroke, *Semin Neurol* 26:11-23, 2006.

52. Serra-Majem L, Roman B, Estruch R: Scientific evidence of interventions using the Mediterranean Diet: A systematic review, *Nutr Rev* 64:S27-S47, 2006.

53. Sacco RL, Elkind MS, Boden-Albala B, et al: The protective effect of moderate alcohol consumption on ischemic stroke, *JAMA* 281:53-60, 1999.

54. Elkind MS, Sciacca R, Boden-Albala B, et al: Moderate alcohol consumption reduces risk of ischemic stroke: The Northern Manhattan Study, *Stroke* 37:13-19, 2006.

55. Bazzano LA, Gu D, Reynolds K, et al: Alcohol consumption and risk for stroke among Chinese men, *Ann Neurol* 62:569-578, 2007.

56. Reynolds K, Lewis LB, Nolen JDL, et al: Alcohol consumption and risk of stroke: A meta-analysis, *JAMA* 289:579-588, 2003.

57. Berger K, Ajani UA, Kase CS, et al: Light-to-moderate alcohol consumption and the risk of stroke among U.S. male physicians, *N Engl J Med* 341:1557-1564, 1999.

58. US Department of Health and Human Services, US Department of Agriculture. *Dietary Guidelines for Americans-2005.* Available at: http://www.healthierus.gov/dietaryguidelines/. Accessed Feb. 8, 2009.

59. Djoussé L, Levy D, Benjamin EJ, et al: Long-term alcohol consumption and the risk of atrial fibrillation in the Framingham Study, *Am J Cardiol* 93:710-713, 2004.

60. National Institute on Alcohol Abuse and Alcoholism: *Sixth Special Report to the US Congress on Alcohol and Health from the Secretary of Health and Human Services*, Washington, D.C., 1987, Government Printing Office (DHHS publication no. (ADM) 87-1519).

61. U.S. Preventive Services Task Force. Screening and Behavioral Counseling Interventions in Primary Care to Reduce Alcohol Misuse: Recommendation Statement. Agency for Healthcare Research and Quality. Available at: http://www.preventiveservices.ahrq.gov. Accessed Feb. 8, 2009.

62. Brust JCM: *Neurological Aspects of Substance Abuse*, Philadelphia, 2004, Butterworth-Heinemann.

63. Levine SR, Brust JC, Futrell N, et al: Cerebrovascular complications of the use of the "crack" form of alkaloidal cocaine, *N Engl J Med* 323:699-704, 1990.

64. Sloan MA, Marc F: *Illicit Drug Use/Abuse and Stroke. Handbook of Clinical Neurology*, Philadelphia, 2008, Elsevier, pp 823-840.

65. Neiman J, Haapaniemi HM, Hillbom M: Neurological complications of drug abuse: Pathophysiological mechanisms, *Eur J Neurol* 7:595-606, 2000.

66. Cami J, Farre M: Drug addiction, *N Engl J Med* 349:975-986, 2003.

67. Vasan RS, Beiser A, Seshadri S, et al: Residual lifetime risk for developing hypertension in middle-aged women and men: The Framingham Heart Study, *JAMA* 287:1003-1010, 2002.

68. Neal B, MacMahon S, Chapman N: Blood Pressure Lowering Treatment Trialists' Collaboration. Effects of ACE inhibitors, calcium antagonists, and other blood-pressure-lowering drugs: Results of prospectively designed overviews of randomised trials. Blood Pressure Lowering Treatment Trialists' Collaboration, *Lancet* 356:1955-1964, 2000.

69. Turnbull F: Effects of different blood-pressure-lowering regimens on major cardiovascular events: Results of prospectively-designed overviews of randomised trials, *Lancet* 362:1527-1535, 2003.

70. Psaty BM, Smith NL, Siscovick DS, et al: Health outcomes associated with antihypertensive therapies used as first-line agents. A systematic review and meta-analysis, *JAMA* 277:739-745, 1997.

71. SHEP Cooperative Research Group: Prevention of stroke by antihypertensive drug treatment in older persons with isolated systolic hypertension. Final results of the Systolic Hypertension in the Elderly Program (SHEP), *JAMA* 265:3255-3264, 1991.

72. ALLHAT Collaborative Research Group: Major outcomes in high-risk hypertensive patients randomized to angiotensin-converting enzyme inhibitor or calcium channel blocker vs diuretic: The Antihypertensive and Lipid-Lowering Treatment to Prevent Heart Attack Trial (ALLHAT), *JAMA* 288:2981-2997, 2002.

73. Staessen JA, Fagard R, Thijs L, et al: Randomised double-blind comparison of placebo and active treatment for older patients with isolated systolic hypertension, *Lancet* 350:757-764, 1997.

74. Black HR, Elliott WJ, Grandits G, et al: Principal results of the Controlled Onset Verapamil Investigation of Cardiovascular End Points (CONVINCE) Trial, *JAMA* 289:2073-2082, 2003.

75. Dahlöf B, Sever PS, Poulter NR, et al: Prevention of cardiovascular events with an antihypertensive regimen of amlodipine adding perindopril as required versus atenolol adding bendroflumethiazide as required, in the Anglo-Scandinavian Cardiac Outcomes Trial-Blood Pressure Lowering Arm (ASCOT-BPLA): a multicentre randomised controlled trial, *Lancet* 366:895-906, 2005.

76. Heart Outcomes Prevention Evaluation Study Investigators: Effects of ramipril on cardiovascular and microvascular outcomes in people with diabetes mellitus: Results of the HOPE study and MICRO-HOPE substudy, *Lancet* 355:253-259, 2000.

77. Lonn EM, Yusuf S, Dzavik V, et al: Effects of ramipril and vitamin E on atherosclerosis: The Study to Evaluate Carotid Ultrasound Changes in Patients Treated With Ramipril and Vitamin E (SECURE), *Circulation* 103:919-925, 2001.

78. Hansson L, Lindholm LH, Niskanen L, et al: Effect of angiotensin-converting-enzyme inhibition compared with conventional therapy on cardiovascular morbidity and mortality in hypertension: The Captopril Prevention Project (CAPPP) randomised trial, *Lancet* 353:611-616, 1999.

79. Dahlöf B, Devereux RB, Kjeldsen SE, et al: Cardiovascular morbidity and mortality in the Losartan Intervention For Endpoint reduction in hypertension study (LIFE): A randomised trial against atenolol, *Lancet* 359:995-1003, 2002.

80. The ONTARGET Investigators: Telmisartan, ramipril, or both in patients at high risk for vascular events, *N Engl J Med* 358:1547-1559, 2008.

81. Weber MA, Bakris GL, Dahlöf B, et al: Baseline characteristics in the Avoiding Cardiovascular events through Combination therapy in Patients Living with Systolic Hypertension (ACCOMPLISH) trial: A hypertensive population at high cardiovascular risk, *Blood Press* 16:13-19, 2007.

82. Beckett NS, Peters R, Fletcher AE, et al: Treatment of hypertension in patients 80 years of age or older, *N Engl J Med* 358:1887-1898, 2008.

83. Turnbull F, Neal B, Ninomiya T, et al: Effects of different regimens to lower blood pressure on major cardiovascular events in older and younger adults: meta-analysis of randomised trials, *BMJ* 336:1121-1123, 2008.

84. PROGRESS Collaborative Group: Randomised trial of a perindopril-based blood-pressure-lowering regimen among 6105 individuals with previous stroke or transient ischaemic attack, *Lancet* 358:1033-1041, 2001.

85. Cushman WC, Ford CE, Cutler JA, et al: Success and predictors of blood pressure control in diverse North American settings: The antihypertensive and lipid-lowering treatment to prevent heart attack trial (ALLHAT), *J Clin Hypertens* 4:393-404, 2002.

86. Cutler DM, Long G, Berndt ER, et al: The value of antihypertensive drugs: A perspective on medical innovation, *Health Aff* 26:97-110, 2007.

87. Douglas JG, Bakris GL, Epstein M, et al: Management of high blood pressure in African Americans: Consensus statement of the Hypertension in African Americans Working Group of the International Society on Hypertension in Blacks, *Arch Intern Med* 163:525-541, 2003.

88. Air EL, Kissela BM: Diabetes, the metabolic syndrome, and ischemic stroke: Epidemiology and possible mechanisms, *Diabetes Care* 30:3131-3140, 2007.

89. Action to Control Cardiovascular Risk in Diabetes Study Group: Effects of intensive glucose lowering in type 2 diabetes, *N Engl J Med* 358:2545-2559, 2008.

90. Advance Collaborative Group: Intensive blood glucose control and vascular outcomes in patients with type 2 diabetes, *N Engl J Med* 358:2560-2572, 2008.

91. UK Prospective Diabetes Study Group: Intensive blood-glucose control with sulphonylureas or insulin compared with conventional treatment and risk of complications in patients with type 2 diabetes (UKPDS 33), *Lancet* 352:837-853, 1998.

92. Holman RR, Paul SK, Bethel MA, et al: 10-year follow-up of intensive glucose control in type 2 diabetes, *N Engl J Med* 359:1577-1589, 2008.

93. Duckworth W, Abraira C, Moritz T, et al: Glucose control and vascular complications in veterans with type 2 diabetes, *N Engl J Med* 360:129-139, 2009.

94. UK Prospective Diabetes Study Group: Tight blood pressure control and risk of macrovascular and microvascular complications in type 2 diabetes: UKPDS 38, *BMJ* 317:703-713, 1998.

95. Holman RR, Paul SK, Bethel MA, et al: Long-term follow-up after tight control of blood pressure in type 2 diabetes, *N Engl J Med* 359:1565-1576, 2008.

96. Curb JD, Pressel SL, Cutler JA, et al: Effect of diuretic-based antihypertensive treatment on cardiovascular disease risk in older diabetic patients with isolated systolic hypertension. Systolic Hypertension in the Elderly Program Cooperative Research Group, *JAMA* 276:1886-1892, 1996.

97. Lindholm LH, Ibsen H, Dahlof B, et al: Cardiovascular morbidity and mortality in patients with diabetes in the Losartan Intervention For Endpoint reduction in hypertension study (LIFE): A randomised trial against atenolol, *Lancet* 359:1004-1010, 2002.

98. Heart Protection Study Collaborative Group: MRC/BHF Heart Protection Study of cholesterol-lowering with simvastatin in 5963 people with diabetes: A randomized placebo-controlled trial, *Lancet* 361:2005-2016, 2003.

99. Colhoun HM, Betteridge DJ, Durrington PN, et al: Primary prevention of cardiovascular disease with atorvastatin in type 2 diabetes in the Collaborative Atorvastatin Diabetes Study (CARDS): Multicentre randomised placebo-controlled trial, *Lancet* 364:685-696, 2004.

100. Briel M, Studer M, Glass TR, Bucher HC: Effects of statins on stroke prevention in patients with and without coronary heart disease: A meta-analysis of randomized controlled trials, *Am J Med* 117:596-606, 2004.

101. Blauw GJ, Lagaay AM, Smelt AH, Westendorp RG: Stroke, statins, and cholesterol. A meta-analysis of randomized, placebo-controlled, double-blind trials with HMG-Co-A reductase inhibitors, *Stroke* 28:946-950, 1997.

102. Corvol JC, Bouzamondo A, Sirol M, et al: Differential effects of lipid-lowering therapies on stroke prevention: A meta-analysis of randomized trials, *Arch Intern Med* 163:669-676, 2003.

103. Amarenco P, Labreuche J, Lavallee P, Touboul PJ: Statins in stroke prevention and carotid atherosclerosis. Systematic review and up-to-date meta-analysis, *Stroke* 35:2902-2909, 2004.

104. Cholesterol Treatment Trialists' (CTT) Collaborators: Efficacy and safety of cholesterol-lowering treatment: prospective meta-analysis of data from 90,056 participants in 14 randomised trials of statins, *Lancet* 366:1267-1278, 2005.

105. Thavendiranathan P, Bagai A, Brookhart MA, Choudhry NK: Primary prevention of cardiovascular diseases with statin therapy: A meta-analysis of randomized controlled trials, *Arch Intern Med* 166:2307-2313, 2006.

106. O'Regan C, Wu P, Arora P, et al: Statin therapy in stroke prevention: A meta-analysis involving 121,000 patients, *Am J Med* 121:24-33, 2008.

107. Ridker PM, Danielson E, Fonseca FAH, et al: Rosuvastatin to prevent vascular events in men and women with elevated C-reactive protein, *N Engl J Med* 359:2195-2207, 2008.

108. Goldstein LB: JUPITER and the world of stroke medicine, *Lancet Neurol* 8:130-131, 2009.

109. Hart RG, Pearce LA, Aguilar MI: Meta-analysis: Antithrombotic therapy to prevent stroke in patients who have nonvalvular atrial fibrillation, *Ann Intern Med* 146:857-867, 2007.

110. Hart RG, Pearce LA, Albers GW, et al: Independent predictors of stroke in patients with atrial fibrillation: A systematic review, *Neurology* 69:546-554, 2007.

111. Gage BF, Waterman AD, Shannon W, et al: Validation of clinical classification schemes for predicting stroke: Results from the National Registry of Atrial Fibrillation, *JAMA* 285:2864-2870, 2001.

112. Rash A, Downes T, Portner R, et al: A randomised controlled trial of warfarin versus aspirin for stroke prevention in octogenarians with atrial fibrillation (WASPO), *Age Ageing* 36:151-156, 2007.

113. Mant J, Hobbs FD, Fletcher K, et al: Warfarin versus aspirin for stroke prevention in an elderly community population with atrial fibrillation (the Birmingham Atrial Fibrillation Treatment of the Aged Study, BAFTA): A randomised controlled trial, *Lancet* 370:493-503, 2007.

114. Hayden M, Pigone M, Phillips C, Mulrow C: Aspirin for the primary prevention of cardiovascular events: A summary of the evidence for the US Preventive Services Task Force, *Ann Intern Med* 136:161-172, 2002.

115. Antiplatelet Trialists' Collaboration: Collaborative overview of randomised trials of antiplatelet therapy-I: Prevention of death, myocardial infarction, and stroke by prolonged antiplatelet therapy in various categories of patients, *BMJ* 308:81-106, 1994.

116. Hart RG, Halperin JL, McBride R, et al: Aspirin for the primary prevention of stroke and other major vascular events: Meta-analysis and hypotheses, *Arch Neurol* 57:326-332, 2000.

117. Pearson TA, Blair SN, Daniels SR, et al: AHA guidelines for primary prevention of cardiovascular disease and stroke: 2002 update, *Circulation* 106:388-391, 2002.

118. Taylor DW, Barnett HJM, Haynes RB, et al: Low-dose and high-dose acetylsalicylic acid for patients undergoing carotid endarterectomy: A randomised controlled trial, *Lancet* 353:2179-2184, 1999.

119. Ridker PM, Cook NR, Lee I-M, et al: A randomized trial of low-dose aspirin in the primary prevention of cardiovascular disease in women, *N Engl J Med* 352:1293-1304, 2005.

120. Mosca L, Banka CL, Benjamin EJ, et al: Evidence-based guidelines for cardiovascular disease prevention in women: 2007 update, *Circulation* 115:1481-1501, 2007.

17 Vascular Dementia and Vascular Cognitive Decline

SUDHA SESHADRI

Current projections suggest that the United States will have 80 million people older than 65 years of age by 2030, a greater than 10-fold increase in a century. In this older population, having one or more vascular risk factors is the norm rather than the exception. Thus, in the community-based Framingham Heart Study (FHS) sample, the lifetime risk for development of hypertension is more than 90%.[1] Not surprisingly, the burden of age-related neurologic illness has increased in parallel with lengthening life expectancy. A 2006 analysis of data from the FHS sample predicted that 1 in 3 people currently aged 65 and free of stroke and dementia would experience one or both of these conditions during their lifetimes.[2] It is generally acknowledged that exposure to vascular risk factors adversely affects cognitive function, although there is uncertainty about the extent and the mechanisms. However, the concept of what constitutes "vascular dementia" remains an evolving one.[3] There has been growing emphasis on identifying persons with early cognitive impairment due to vascular pathology, because these individuals are at maximal risk for development of vascular dementia (VD) and might benefit the most from preventive measures.

Historical Evolution of the Concept of Vascular Dementia

The evolution of the concept of vascular dementia has been elegantly summarized by Roman.[4] At the start of the 7th century, Saint Isadore, the Archbishop of Seville, used the term dementia (from the Latin root "demens," meaning out of one's mind) to describe a slowly progressive dullness or dotage. In 1672, Willis described the fairly sudden development of "dullness of mind and forgetfulness" accompanying a "half palsie" (hemiplegia) in his book *De Anima Brutorum*. Alzheimer's disease (AD) was described in 1904 but was considered a rare presenile form of dementia. In his 1910 *Lehrbuch der Psychiatrie*, Kraeplin, who has been called the Linnaeus of psychiatry, separated a presenile form of dementia from senile dementias and concluded that most senile dementia was arteriosclerotic insanity, which later became attributed to "progressive hardening of the arteries leading to slow ischemic neuronal loss." This remained a widely accepted viewpoint until 1970, when Tomlinson et al[5] established through careful autopsy studies that the pathology underlying most cases of dementia was, in fact, the plaques and

tangles associated with Alzheimer's disease. The definition of vascular dementia became restricted to "multi-infarct" dementia; it was argued that vascular pathology resulted in dementia largely through the occurrence of multiple small or large cerebral infarcts.[6] In the next 20 years careful clinical studies did establish that single infarcts could result in dementia if they were strategically located, and CT scans showed that among persons with a similar number and location of strokes, concomitant cortical atrophy increased the risk of symptomatic dementia.[7] With the emergence of brain MRI, covert brain infarcts (CBIs) and white matter hyperintensities (WMHs) were found to be widespread and to be associated with an increased risk of cognitive impairment.[8,9] In the past decade the concept of "mild cognitive impairment (MCI)" as a prodromal stage of Alzheimer's disease emerged, and, in parallel, a broader concept of vascular cognitive impairment (VCI) was solidified that included both dementia and mild cognitive impairment secondary to vascular pathology (VMCI).[3,10]

Diagnostic Criteria for Vascular Dementia

Since the 1970s, several sets of diagnostic criteria have been formulated in attempts to standardize the definition of VD. Such criteria are essential for use as diagnostic tools in clinical practice, to compare prevalence and incidence in different population samples, to uncover risk factors, and to recruit homogeneous cohorts for drug trials. These criteria range from the entirely clinical Hachinski Ischemic Score (HIS) to the strict National Institute for Neurological Diseases and Stroke–Association Internationale pour la Recherche et l'Enseignement en Neurosciences (NINDS-AIREN) criteria,[11] formulated largely for use in research settings, to the more clinical and epidemiologically applicable *Diagnostic and Statistical Manual* (DSM-III, IIIR, IV) criteria, the International Classification of Disease 10th revision (ICD-10) criteria, and the California Alzheimer's Disease Diagnostic and Treatment Centers (ADDTC) criteria.[12-14] The Hachinski Ischemic Score does not classify dementia but seeks to predict the dominant underlying pathology. It is based entirely on the history of vascular risk factors and on the clinical signs; in an abbreviated version, a score of 7 or more out of a possible 12 points is considered diagnostic of VD, whereas a score less than 4 is thought to exclude VD. The NINDS-AIREN and ADDTC criteria additionally consider CT or MRI data. Each broadly requires clinical and/or imaging documentation of strokes or vascular brain injury (such as extensive WMH), a temporal profile linking the vascular damage and the dementia (for example, abrupt onset or onset within 3 months after stroke, a stuttering or stepwise progression) and focal neurologic signs (for example, homonymous hemianopia, facial weakness, dysarthria, emotional lability [pseudobulbar affect], weakness of an extremity, exaggerated deep tendon reflexes, extensor plantar responses, gait abnormalities, and sensory deficit) if thought to be of vascular etiology and assigns a degree of certainty to the diagnosis, "probable" or "possible." When each of the different criteria is applied to a single sample, a varying, only partially overlapping set of subjects are categorized as having vascular dementia.[15] When pathology is used as a "gold standard," the sensitivity and specificity of the different clinical criteria have been noted to vary from 0.2 to 0.7 (possible VD as defined by the ADDTC being the most sensitive criterion) and from 0.78 to 0.93 (probably VD by the NINDS-AIREN criteria being the most specific), respectively. Thus, most of these criteria emphasize specificity over sensitivity; less than 50% of all persons with moderately severe vascular pathology at autopsy are diagnosed during life as having VD.[16] The various criteria have been summarized and compared in prior publications.[17] There is as yet no consensus on the best set of criteria to describe vascular dementia, and none of the criteria categorize cognitive impairment not amounting to dementia (CIND), which may occur in the presence of vascular risk factors.

Dementia following Stroke

The risk of new-onset dementia in patients who have had stroke is approximately twice the risk in age- and sex-matched controls and averages about 10% after the first stroke,[18,19] depending on the location, volume of damaged brain tissue, clinical severity, and presence of early poststroke complications (seizure, delirium, hypoxia, hypotension) as well as on prestroke cognitive status and concomitant imaging abnormalities such as CBI, WMH, and medial temporal lobe atrophy.[7,20-23] A 2009 review identified older age, less education, prestroke cognitive impairment, diabetes, and atrial fibrillation as factors that increased the risk, but the single strongest predictor of cognitive decline after an initial stroke was the occurrence of a second stroke.[22] In persons with recurrent stroke, the risk of dementia rose to approximately 30%, regardless of the number and severity of vascular risk factors they had been exposed to prior to the stroke.

The newly described concept of *vascular cognitive impairment*, outlined by the NINDS in collaboration with the Canadian Stroke Network (CSN), in a statement advising harmonization standards for data collection, is broad.[24] It includes but is not restricted to dementia following stroke. The term "vascular cognitive impairment" may be used to describe any syndrome of cognitive and behavioral impairment that is thought to be due to vascular factors affecting the brain. Thus, it could range from the subtle cognitive deficits seen in persons with diabetes when compared with their nondiabetic peers, through

the multifocal cognitive deficits that may accompany the presence of multiple brain infarcts or hemorrhages to clinical VD. The last requires the presence of cognitive or behavioral problems severe enough to affect social or occupational functioning (i.e., amounting to "dementia"), the documentation of disease affecting the blood vessels or blood flow to part or all of the brain, and clinical or radiologic evidence of structural damage to the brain due to these vascular factors.[3] There have also been efforts to define diagnostic clinical criteria for subcortical VD syndromes, conditions that have been described as Binswanger's syndrome: extensive WMHs and cognitive slowing in the absence of clinical strokes or CT/MRI infarcts and hemorrhages.[25,26] The criteria proposed in the fifth edition of the *Diagnostic and Statistical Manual* (DSM5; www.dsm5.org) replace the potentially stigmatizing term "dementia" with "major neurocognitive disorder," and the prodromal stage of MCI or VMCI is called "minor neurocognitive disorder."

Overlap of Vascular and Neurodegenerative Pathologies

The various criteria for VD and AD define "probable AD" and "probable VD" but do not address the large number of persons with mixed AD and VD.[27-29] The current consensus among clinicians and epidemiologists is to independently decide on the presence or absence of clinically probable AD and VD without requiring the presence of one condition to exclude the other diagnosis.

Epidemiology

When a similar set of criteria are used, the age-adjusted prevalence of VCI may be lower in developing countries that are still in the process of demographic transition.[30] However, it is these countries that may see the fastest increase in the prevalence of VCI. The incidence of vascular dementia in the U.S. among persons older than 65 years has been estimated at 14.6 per 1000 person-years.[31] The proportion of all cases of dementia that is vascular appears to vary by age, ethnicity (VD may be more common in Asians), geography, and definition used.[32] Mixed AD and VD may be the most common explanation for cognitive impairment in the elderly.[33] The ideal way to define the complete spectrum of cerebrovascular disease appears to be to prospectively follow epidemiologic cohorts exposed to vascular risk factors to define the full range of structural and cognitive changes associated with these vascular risk factors and also to determine which of these intermediate phenotypes results in clinical disease (Fig. 17-1). This approach is feasible because a number of studies of cardiovascular disease have incorporated brain imaging and cognitive testing in the past two decades,[34-39] and a few have additionally initiated brain banks to permit clinical imaging–pathologic correlations.[40]

Clinical Diagnosis

The VCI syndrome is best diagnosed and characterized by identifying the presence and quantifying the extent of (1) the cognitive deficits (and presence or absence of VD and

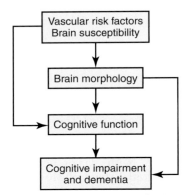

Figure 17-1 How to develop diagnostic and prognostic criteria and define the complete clinical spectrum.

VMCI) by clinical and formal neuropsychological testing *and* (2) the vascular brain injury through neuroimaging supplemented by cerebral and systemic vascular imaging as indicated. The term "VCI" can be used for cognitive disorders associated with varying forms of vascular brain injury: atherothrombotic, cardioembolic, hemorrhagic, and rare genetic vascular disorders.

The clinical neurologic profile of VD can be extremely varied depending on the underlying pathology, patient age and education, and presence or absence of concomitant AD pathology. However, patients with VD are typically younger and more likely to be male. Some clinical symptoms and signs that are more frequently seen in persons with VD than in persons with typical AD are a pattern of multifocal rather than global deficits, presence of focal neurologic signs (including gait abnormalities) as described previously, an early and disproportionately severe involvement of executive dysfunction (unlike the early verbal memory loss in AD), and relatively preserved recognition (improved performance when categorical or phonemic clues are offered) in comparison with spontaneous recall.[41,42] Depression and emotional lability are also more frequently seen. The frequently considered differential diagnoses for VD include AD, frontotemporal dementia, normal-pressure hydrocephalus, dementia with Lewy bodies, and dementia associated with cerebral infections such as HIV. The finding of cerebral vascular brain injury on CT or MRI can help establish a clinical diagnosis of VD.

Vascular Mild Cognitive Impairment

Community-based data have shown that even before the occurrence of an initial stroke, persons who subsequently experience a stroke do worse on global tests of cognition such as the mini–mental state examination (MMSE) than do age- and sex-matched controls.[43] This feature may represent a subtle effect of cumulated exposure to vascular risk factors over the preceding years;

indeed, a pattern of VCI can be defined that is associated with covert or subclinical brain injury and that doubles the risk of subsequent stroke.[44,45] Conversely, in a community-based series of subjects with MCI, a significant proportion have relative preservation of memory function and disproportionate involvement of attention, processing speed, and executive function domains. They are more likely to have vascular risk factors, imaging evidence of covert vascular brain injury, and a higher risk for subsequent stroke than persons with the predominantly amnestic MCI that seems to precede clinical AD; hence, these subjects may be considered to have VMCI. Therefore, the current nomenclature for MCI is much broader and may be categorized along multiple axes as single or multiple domain, predominantly amnestic or nonamnestic, and pathologically as likely vascular or neurodegenerative.[46-49] On follow-up, any sample of persons with VMCI includes persons who revert to normal (either they recover from the effects of a vascular insult such as a stroke or their clinical picture was due to a reversible cause such as depression), others who go on to demonstrate VD, and yet others who have typical AD. The MCI and subtype definitions are applied in research studies and also provide a useful interim category for classifying patients in clinical practice.

Neuropsychological Assessments of Vascular Cognitive Impairment

The neuropsychological assessment of patients with suspected VCI requires a comprehensive cognitive battery, which should include tests sensitive to executive function abnormalities, a salient feature of the condition.[50] Thus, the Montreal Cognitive Assessment (MOCA) has been recommended in place of the MMSE, also called the Folstein test,[51] because the former is more sensitive for the detection of executive function abnormalities. The 2006 NINDS-CSN VCI harmonization guidelines described several neuropsychological test protocols of varying length (30 minutes and 60 minutes), each of which covers the domains of frontal executive function (animal naming and phonemic fluency, digit-symbol substitution +/− trail-making test), visual perception and organization (a figure-copying task such as using the Rey-Osterreith figure), a verbal learning and memory task (such as the Hopkins verbal learning test), a lexical retrieval task (such as the Boston naming test), and a questionnaire-based screen for neuropsychiatric and depressive symptoms (using the neuropsychiatric inventory [NPI] and the Center for Epidemiological Studies–Depression [CES-D] Scale). They also suggest the MOCA as a 5-minute battery for use in patients with suspected VCI.[24] Detailed discussion of these protocols is beyond the scope of this chapter, but the tests listed have been well standardized and are referenced in the NINDS-CSN guidelines. Other batteries that cover these domains have been used in existing epidemiologic studies and in clinics.[34,38] The MOCA and trail-making test are also part of a cognitive test panel recommended by a National Human Genetics Research Institute (NHGRI) panel convened to suggest tests for use by phenotypic nonexperts conducting genome-wide association studies (www.phenxtoolkit.org).

Pathophysiology of Vascular Cognitive Impairment

Changes in the Neurovascular Unit

Neurons, glial cells, vascular smooth muscle, and adventitial and endothelial cells collectively form a *neurovascular unit* that maintains the cerebral microenvironment, which in turn is critical to optimal functioning of the brain.[52,53] The neurovascular unit regulates blood flow, constitutes the blood-brain barrier, and secretes neurotrophic and immunomodulatory factors. Neural activity induces an increase in cerebral blood flow (CBF), also termed functional hyperemia, that is detected by fluorodeoxyglucose positron emission tomography (PET) scans. This neurovascular unit is disrupted in VCI and AD, both of which are associated with structural changes that are visible on pathologic examination.[53,54] The detectable pathologies are microvascular changes (lipohyalinosis, amyloid angiopathy) and changes in the neuropil (reactive gliosis, demyelination, microinfarcts, and neuronal loss). The microvascular changes in turn blunt cerebral autoregulation and functional hyperemia, leading to more changes.

Cerebral Amyloid Angiopathy

Cerebral amyloid angiopathy (CAA)[55-58] is characterized by deposition of an amyloid (here, β-amyloid) in the walls of the arterioles and capillaries within the leptomeninges and in the penetrating vessels of the cerebral and cerebellar cortex. It is detected in more than 80% of all persons with clinical AD and in approximately 10% to 30% of any unselected brain autopsy series from older persons. Extensive amyloid deposition is accompanied by fibrinoid necrosis of the vessel wall, perivascular leakage, loss of smooth muscle, and the development of microaneurysms, all of which explain the high risk of cerebral microhemorrhages and macrohemorrhages associated with pathologic CAA. MRI shows microhemorrhages, microinfarcts, and WMHs, and a diagnosis of "probable CAA" can be made on the basis of imaging findings of multiple cortical hemorrhages and microhemorrhages in the absence of other causes, such as head trauma, tumor, and anticoagulant use. T2*-weighted gradient-echo MRI sequences performed on a 1.5 T or 3 T machine and three-dimensional (3D) sequences increase the sensitivity for detection of cerebral microbleeds. The clinical picture can be varied and may range from a subtle impairment of cognitive function involving multiple domains to clinical VD (typically associated with concomitant AD pathology but not necessarily so). It can include multiple discrete hemorrhagic and ischemic strokes of varying severity or a progressive accrual of neurologic deficits as seen in primary cerebral vasculitides. Management comprises controlling concomitant risk factors such as hypertension and avoiding antiplatelet and especially anticoagulant medication if possible; if anticoagulant therapy is to be used, tight regulation to avoid supratherapeutic International Normalized Ratios (INRs) is crucial.

Other Genetic Small Vessel Syndromes

The most commonly encountered hereditary cause of VCI is CADASIL (cerebral autosomal dominant arteriopathy with subcortical infarcts and leukoencephalopathy).[59]

These and other genetic vasculitides that can manifest as VCI, including familial CAA due to mutations in the β-amyloid precursor protein (*APP*) gene,[60,61] and CARASIL (cerebral autosomal recessive arteriopathy with subcortical infarcts and leukoencephalopathy), are discussed in the section on genetics.

Imaging Correlates of Vascular Cognitive Impairment

VCI may also be defined as a constellation of cognitive and functional impairments associated with the structural cerebrovascular brain injury (CVBI) noted on imaging (in vivo) or at autopsy. CVBI on imaging includes clinically symptomatic *large and small artery infarcts and hemorrhages*. However, clinically asymptomatic (covert) brain infarction is even more common, and the full spectrum of CVBI also includes *WMHs and total and regional brain atrophy*.[36,62-64] The relationship between CVBI on brain imaging and cognitive impairment is not simple or linear and remains inadequately understood. Partly, the prevalence and extent of CVBI detected vary with the imaging protocol used. Furthermore, many changes that could be attributed to ischemia (such as generalized and lobar atrophy, hippocampal sclerosis, and, to a lesser extent, WMHs) have also been associated with AD and other neurodegenerative pathologies. Finally, in most elderly persons both vascular and nonvascular pathologies coexist, making it difficult to attribute the cognitive impairment or dementia detected to a specific etiology. Quantifying the extent of AD pathology through in vivo imaging also remains difficult, although newer amyloid imaging techniques such as PET using Pittsburgh compound B (PiB) and 18F-FDNNP (2-(1-(6-[(2-[^{18}F]fluoroethyl)(methyl)amino]-2-naphthyl)ethylidene)malono nitrile) are steps in that direction. Studies combining these modalities (volumetric MRI and amyloid PET) are under way in clinical and epidemiologic settings.[65]

Because of these caveats, neuroimaging is currently used to describe the vasculature and CVBI rather than to diagnose VCI or VD. The NINDS-CSC VCI harmonization guidelines suggest that in a research setting, a minimal imaging dataset should include an MRI (≥1 T) with 3D T1-weighted, T2-weighted, fluid-attenuated inversion recovery (FLAIR), and gradient echo (GRE) sequences. Diffusion-weighted images (for acute stroke), diffusion tensor imaging (DTI) for assessing the state of the white matter tracts (abnormal DTI [lower fractional anisotropy] in normal-appearing white matter was associated with poorer executive function),[66] PET for β-amyloid, and noninvasive assessment of the cerebral vasculature (carotid ultrasound and/or MR angiogram) are encouraged. The minimum set of measurements recommended are: number, size and location of infarcts and hemorrhages, extent on a quantitative or validated semiqualitative scale of WMH volume,[35,67,68] and measures of total brain (or ventricular) and hippocampal volumes.

Prevalence of Cerebrovascular Brain Injury

Covert or incidentally detected infarcts (CBIs) are five times as common as symptomatic infarcts. Estimates of the prevalence of MRI brain infarction (CBI) in community-based samples have varied between 5.8% and 17.7%, depending on age, ethnicity, presence of comorbidities, and imaging techniques.[69] On average, CBI is present in approximately 11% of individuals in middle or late life. Most have a single lesion, and the infarcts are most often located in the basal ganglia (52%), followed in frequency by other subcortical (35%) and cortical areas (11%).[69] Risk factors for CBI are generally the same as those for clinical stroke.[69,70] WMHs are present to some degree in most individuals older than 30 years[7] and increase in volume with increasing age and with exposure to vascular risk factors.[35,67,68,71] Age-specific definitions of extensive WMHs can be created and can be useful for defining persons at higher than average risk of VCI.[72] Cerebral microbleeds are also common with increasing age, and their prevalence rises with greater sensitivity of the imaging technique used.[73-76]

Association of Cerebrovascular Brain Injury with Cognitive Changes

The presence of CBI at baseline more than doubled the risk of dementia (and tripled the risk of stroke) at about 4 years of follow-up of Rotterdam study participants, even after adjustment of data for extent of WMHs and degree of atrophy.[8] Similar results were noted on follow-up of the younger FHS Offspring Study sample.[77] There is convincing data from population-based samples that a higher WMH volume is associated with poorer cognitive function in cross-sectional studies, and an enlargement of WMH on serial MRI is an even better predictor of cognitive decline than a single estimate of WMH.[72,78-80] The location of the WMH may also be important, with periventricular, but not subcortical, WMH associated with an increased risk of dementia.[81] In addition to CBI and WMH, measures of cerebral gray matter and hippocampal volume have both been associated with decline in memory even among individuals clinically diagnosed with probable VD according to NINDS-AIREN criteria.[242]

Summary

The clinical presentation and course of CVBI are highly variable, with the classic phenotype of stepwise decline seen in association with stroke being a relatively uncommon presentation for VCI. Structural MRI provides a fairly sensitive and specific marker for CVBI, but the relationship between CVBI and cognitive impairment is confounded by the frequent presence of AD changes of the brain. It is recommended that a careful record of the following aspects be made at baseline and at each follow-up imaging assessment: (1) description of the severity and type of extracranial and intracranial vessel disease; (2) definition of the volume and location of infarcts or hemorrhages (total volumes >100 mL, bilateral lesions, and lesions involving the thalamus, caudate, and basal forebrain being considered more likely to explain VCI and VD), (3) the volume and location of white matter disease, and (4) the volume of total supratentorial brain parenchyma and of hippocampal lobes. In clinical situations, the same measures should be recorded qualitatively at baseline imaging, but the indications for follow-up imaging are unclear; such imaging might be indicated if sudden deterioration raises the possibility of an acute infarct or hemorrhage. How to integrate CVBI on brain MRI with PET measures of blood flow and amyloid burden remains under study.[24]

Neuropathologic Aspects

Defining the range and severity of pathologies underlying VCI has remained difficult. Infarcts and hemorrhages, the most obvious signs of vascular brain injury, can vary in size, location, and number (the number of infarcts, especially small infarcts, detected can vary depending on how carefully the brain is examined) and are prevalent among cognitively normal, community-dwelling persons. Such lesions may or may not have been accompanied by clinical symptoms or signs of a stroke, although covert and overt lesions may be equally significant in causing VCI. Further, there is associated AD pathology in a significant percentage of brains examined.[54,82-87]

Conceptually, it is generally acknowledged that the pathologic substrate of VCI and VD likely includes focal infarction in key areas (both cortical and deep nuclear areas critical to aspects of cognition, and disrupting key association pathways in the white matter), high total volume of tissue damaged (again typically thought to be larger than 100 mL), and extent of demyelination and gliosis. However, defining a typical pattern of lesions or pathologic criteria for VD that include a minimum amount of damage necessary for the diagnosis and/or a maximum amount sufficient to cause VCI has proved difficult because the pathologic substrate of VCI is highly heterogeneous.[24,88,89]

The most important cerebrovascular pathology that contributes to cognitive impairment is cerebral infarcts.[90] Cerebral infarcts are discrete regions of tissue loss observed by the naked eye (macroscopic) or under the microscope (microscopic). Perimortem infarcts are of uncertain clinical significance, but chronic macroscopic infarcts occur in about one third to one half of older persons. Including other measures of vascular brain pathology, such as microscopic infarcts, small vessel disease, and white matter changes, increases the frequency of cerebrovascular disease in older persons to more than 75%.[33,86]

In clinical-pathologic studies, larger volumes[34,43] and higher numbers of macroscopic infarcts[10,11,34,47,48] are associated with an increased likelihood of dementia. However, determining a volume or number of CBIs *necessary* for a clinical diagnosis of VCI or dementia has proved difficult; and unlike for AD and other neurodegenerative diseases, there are no currently accepted neuropathologic criteria to confirm a clinical diagnosis of VCI. Indeed, although Tomlinson et al[5] described 100 mL of tissue loss as sufficient to cause VD, persons with much lower volumes of infarcted tissue can have VD.[5] Infarcts, even small and single lesions, in certain locations, such as the thalamus, angular gyrus, and basal ganglia, are more likely to result in cognitive impairment. However, not all infarcts in these regions cause dementia, and small infarcts in other cortical and subcortical regions have also been associated with clinical dementia. Finally, multiple *microscopic* infarcts have been associated with an increased risk of dementia, even after the volume of macroscopic infarcts is accounted for.[83] This could be secondary to a cumulative large volume of tissue (neuronal and axonal pathway) damage from microscopic infarcts. However, it could just be a marker of other forms of vascular brain injury such as diffuse hypoxia or disruption in the blood brain-barrier. Other factors governing whether infarcts are related to impairment may include variation in cognitive reserve[56] and coexisting pathologies (see later).

Infarcts frequently coexist with AD pathology in the brains of older persons, and vascular disease may increase the risk of clinical dementia in two ways: (1) through an additive or synergistic effect of two pathologies on the clinical picture and (2) through a potentiation of the AD pathologic process. Snowdon et al[91] showed that after adjustment of data for age and extent of AD pathology, persons with subcortical infarcts and, to a lesser extent, persons with large cortical infarcts were several-fold more likely to have clinical symptoms and signs of dementia than persons without concomitant vascular pathology. Further, in mouse models of AD, concomitant ischemia induced presenilin 1 (*ps1*) gene expression and levels of amyloid precursor protein.[92]

Other Vascular Pathologies

Other vascular pathologies commonly seen in the elderly include white matter degeneration, cerebral microbleeds, lipohyalinosis, atherosclerosis, and CAA, but there is little data on how to incorporate these additional pathologies into pathologic diagnostic criteria for VCI and VD. Pathologic assessment in persons with suspected VCI/VD is most useful in detecting and quantifying microscopic infarcts and in characterizing the extent and severity of neurodegenerative pathologies (AD and Lewy-body pathology, traumatic encephalopathy, argyrophilic grain disease, hippocampal sclerosis) that may be contributing to the cognitive status that was observed antemortem. These microinfarcts and neurodegenerative changes are not easy to detect antemortem. Prospective quantitative clinical-pathologic-neuroimaging studies are ongoing that should help clarify the complex interactions between vascular and AD pathologies in the evolution of VCI, VD, and clinical AD.

Prevention of Vascular Cognitive Impairment

Association of Vascular Risk Factors with Vascular Cognitive Impairment and Vascular Dementia

Vascular risk factors and biomarkers that increase the risk of stroke would also be expected to increase the risk of VCI and VD.[93] There are, however, several difficulties with interpreting data relating vascular risk factors with the risk of VCI and VD. Cross-sectional studies cannot determine whether the observed association preceded or followed the onset of cognitive decline. Further, epidemiologic studies cannot prove causality.

Genetic factors: The apolipoprotein E ε4 (APOE-ε4) allele has been associated with an increased risk of all-cause dementia and VD in some but not all studies. There are several other candidate genes, such as *MTHFR* and *VLDLR*, but to date no whole genome–wide association studies have been published for the specific phenotype of VD. Specific genes have been identified through genome-wide association studies as being related to the risk of overt and covert brain infarcts, but the role of these genes in determining the risk of VCI and VD has not yet been studied.[94-96]

Lifestyle factors: The following lifestyle factors affect the risk of VCI and VD:

Lower **education** has been associated with an increased risk for VD. However, cognitive test performance is generally better in persons with greater education. Also poor educational status may reflect lower socioeconomic status that is also associated with a less healthy lifestyle.

Several **dietary** factors have been associated with a lower risk of dementia in general, although few studies have specifically addressed the risk of VD. These studies are difficult to perform because diet assessments are subject to recall bias and because dietary patterns rather than intake of individual items may be important.

Antioxidants (including vitamins E, C, and beta carotene, fruits, and vegetables) have been associated with a lower risk of cognitive impairment in some studies, but an interventional study showed no benefit.[97-99]

Intake of **n-3 polyunsaturated fatty acids (PUFAs)** found in fish oils and weekly intake of **fish** have been associated with better cognitive function and a lower risk of cognitive decline and dementia in most but not all studies.[100,101] This is also true of circulating and red blood cell membrane levels of PUFAs.[102,103] PUFAs may be beneficial through their antioxidant and anti-inflammatory properties, but their levels as components of membrane phospholipids could also directly impact neuronal function. Unfortunately, early randomized trials of fish oil did not show a benefit; larger trials are ongoing.[104]

Vitamin D deficiency is an emerging factor in increasing the risk of cardiovascular disease and stroke. Several studies have described an association of lower circulating vitamin D levels with poorer cognitive function, but there have been no randomized trials assessing the effect of vitamin D supplementation on cognitive decline.[105-107]

Homocysteine elevation is a risk factor for vascular damage.[108] Cross-sectional and longitudinal studies consistently show that rising levels of plasma total homocysteine (tHcy) are associated with poorer performance in global as well as multiple cognitive domains.[109-115] Elevated plasma tHcy values have also been associated with MRI evidence of CVBI and smaller brain volumes, suggesting that some of this cognitive decline is mediated through vascular pathways.[116-118] Folic acid and vitamins B$_{12}$ and B$_6$ are key components of the pathways leading to the production and metabolism of homocysteine. Results of clinical trials on the impact of vitamin B supplementation on the risk of cognitive decline have been largely disappointing; a large meta-analysis of data from all these trials is ongoing.

Physical activity may be beneficial in preventing strokes and maintaining cognitive function. Long-term regular physical activity has been consistently associated with higher levels of cognitive function and a lower risk of VCI and VD.[119-122] There is little data on the type and frequency of physical activity required, although the American Heart Association recommends 30 minutes of moderate-intensity exercise at least three or four times a week. These benefits might accrue through improvements in vascular risk factor profiles (improved blood pressure [BP], weight, and insulin sensitivity), decreased inflammation, and increased levels of neurotrophic factors such as brain-derived neurotrophic factor (BDNF).[123,124] Several clinical trials of exercise intervention on cognitive function (as a primary or secondary outcome) are ongoing (http://www.clinicaltrials.gov).[124-126]

Although heavy drinking has been associated with smaller brain volumes and an increased risk of cognitive decline, moderate **alcohol intake** might be beneficial, perhaps because of an effect of resveratrol.[127-130] A few studies, however, did find that even moderate alcohol intake was associated with smaller brain volumes,[131] suggesting that the association needs to be explored in further detail; there may be subgroups (either genetic or based on gender or patterns of alcohol use) that are likely to benefit from mild to moderate alcohol intake, whereas others might be at risk of cognitive decline in relation to the same exposures.

Obesity, particularly midlife obesity, has been associated with an increased risk of dementia and separately with an increased risk of stroke.[132-135] Hence it is likely to also be associated with an increased risk of VCI. The association is stronger for central obesity (as assessed by the waist circumference, waist-to-hip ratio, or sagittal abdominal diameter) than for overall body mass index.[136] In the Framingham Offspring Study, waist-to-hip ratio was inversely associated with cognitive function as measured 12 years later; a synergistic interaction with hypertension was noted.[137] Abdominal CT scans showed an association of visceral but not subcutaneous fat with total brain volume assessed on MRI.[138] In the Health, Aging and Body Composition study, CT measures of total body fat were associated with global cognitive decline.[139] These associations persisted after adjustment of data for concomitant levels of BP but could be mediated by inflammation, insulin resistance, or lower physical activity or through the action of adipokines such as leptin and adiponectin.[140]

Smoking increases the risk of stroke[93] and atrial fibrillation, accelerates systemic atherosclerosis, and increases systemic inflammation and hence would be expected to raise the risk of VCI. However, nicotine is an agonist at acetylcholine receptors in the hippocampus and hence could also be expected to improve cognition. Although initial case-control studies suggested a possible beneficial effect of smoking on the risk of dementia, this suggestion was likely a bias related to survival.[141] Several prospective studies have shown a higher risk for cognitive decline and VD in smokers than in nonsmokers.[142-144]

Blood pressure: High BP, especially levels of systolic, mean, or pulse pressure, has long been recognized as a major modifier of stroke risk.[93] Midlife hypertension ranks as an important modifiable risk factor for late-life cognitive decline and VD, an association that seems fairly consistent in a majority of observational studies, including cohort studies with follow-up spanning several decades.[145-151] Results of studies on BP measured in late life in relation to dementia are less consistent, most studies finding no association with hypertension or even a higher risk associated with lower systolic BPs.[152-154] This may be due to a parallel decrease in weight and BP in the decade preceding the onset of dementia and the impact of coexisting morbidities such as stroke and cardiovascular disease.

Of the **observational studies** on antihypertensive drugs and the risk of dementia, several longitudinal studies have assessed the impact of antihypertensive drug use on the risk of dementia and observed some benefit.[155] A longer duration of treatment and lower age at onset of treatment were associated with a stronger protective effect. Most studies suggest that it is the BP lowering rather than a particular class of drugs that is helpful. However, two population-based observational studies suggested that diuretics were more helpful than other antihypertensive drugs.[156,157] In a U.S. Veterans Affairs database study, men taking angiotensin receptor blockers (ARBs) were found to have a lower risk of dementia than those treated with lisinopril, an angiotensin-converting enzyme (ACE) inhibitor, and with other cardiovascular drugs.[158] These findings could represent bias by indication.

To date, five large randomized **clinical trials** of antihypertensive medication have also assessed cognitive function; of these, only one suggested a benefit of treatment. However, these studies, large as they were, remained insufficiently powered to assess the risk of dementia, because the differences in BP between the treatment and placebo arms were small and the studies were discontinued for ethical reasons once the treatment was shown to reduce the risk of stroke or other cardiovascular events. The "negative" studies include (1) the Systolic Hypertension in the Elderly Program (SHEP), which compared treatment with a diuretic and/or β-blocker to treatment with placebo[159,160]; (2) the Study on Cognition and Prognosis in the Elderly (SCOPE), which compared a combination of an angiotensin receptor blocker and a diuretic with usual treatment[161]; (3) the Perindopril Protection Against Recurrent Stroke Study (PROGRESS) trial, wherein patients with a prior stroke or transient ischemic attack (TIA) were randomly assigned to receive either an ACE inhibitor with a diuretic or a placebo (there was a benefit for the combined endpoint of stroke and dementia)[162]; and (4) the Hypertension in the Very Elderly–Cognitive Assessment (HYVET-COG) study, in which hypertensive persons older than 80 years were treated with slow-release indapamide and either perindopril or placebo.[163] The only study that did suggest a benefit of BP lowering on dementia risk was the Systolic Hypertension in Europe (Syst-Eur) trial comparing nitrendipine treatment with placebo.[164] There is incontrovertible evidence that lowering BP prevents stroke and that initial and subsequent strokes increase the risk of vascular dementia, whereas there is no compelling evidence that lowering BP increases the risk of dementia; hence antihypertensive treatment does appear to be indicated in persons with cognitive impairment if financial and logistic considerations permit its safe administration.

Hyperglycemia, insulin resistance, metabolic syndrome, and diabetes: Insulin resistance and hyperglycemia can lead to vascular and neuronal damage by promoting atherosclerosis and stroke, by directly promoting AD pathology, oxidative stress, and inflammation, and through other mechanisms. It may also, through an additive or synergistic effect with AD-related cognitive decline or through an ascertainment bias consequent to more frequent medical care, lead to earlier diagnosis. Diabetes itself and its component states of chronic hyperglycemia, insulin resistance, hyperinsulinemia, and the metabolic syndrome have each been associated with poorer cognitive function,[36,165-169] with cognitive decline in a pattern consistent with VCI,[165,170-173] as well as with VD in numerous studies.[174-180] This effect is accentuated by increased systemic inflammation. Patients with a longer duration of diabetes were at highest risk of cognitive decline.

Careful control of hyperglycemia might reduce vascular damage but has not been shown to reduce the risk of stroke, cognitive decline, or VCI or VD. Moreover there is a suggestion that repeated episodes of hypoglycemia may also cause persistent cognitive impairment, hence the need for caution when attempting aggressive glycemic control.[181] The results of the ongoing Action To Control Cardiovascular Risk in Diabetes–Memory in Diabetes (ACCORD-MIND) trial should help clarify whether improved diabetic control has a beneficial effect on cognitive function.[182] In the Action in Diabetes and Vascular Disease: Preterax and Diamicron Modified Release Controlled Evaluation (ADVANCE) trial, cognitive function status did not alter the benefit of controlling hypertension in reducing stroke and mortality risk.[183] Overall, the most beneficial intervention to reduce the risk of initial or continuing cognitive decline in persons with type 2 diabetes mellitus may remain the effective control of concomitant vascular risk factors such as hypertension, hypercholesterolemia, and smoking.

Lipids: In several large cohort studies and in the Kaiser Permanente database, midlife measures of total cholesterol predicted later cognitive impairment.[146,184-186] However, late-life or lifetime cumulated measures of serum cholesterol have not been consistently associated with an increased risk of clinical dementia in older cohorts.[187]

Treatment with *statins* has been associated with a lower risk of stroke and, in observational studies, with a lower risk of VCI and of dementia including VD.[188,189] The Pravastatin in Older Persons at risk for cardiovascular disease (PROSPER) trial found no difference in cognitive decline between the placebo and treatment arms.[190]

Inflammation and markers of endothelial function: Inflammation is a key process linking several cardiovascular risk factors to vascular and neuronal damage. It has been associated with an increased risk of stroke, smaller brain volumes, and an increased risk of dementia.[191,192] Plasma levels and peripheral blood monocyte production of inflammatory proteins, especially interleukin-6 (IL-6), α_1-antichymotrypsin, and C-reactive protein (CRP), were found to be increased prior to the onset of VD in several studies,[193] and in the Conselice Study of Brain Aging, the combination of high CRP and high IL-6 was associated with a nearly three-fold increase in the risk of VD.[194-203] Plasma levels of asymmetric dimethyl arginine (ADMA),

a modulator of endothelial function, have been associated with CBI on MRI and an increased risk of stroke and VCI.[204]

Association of Vascular Disease Severity Measures with Vascular Cognitive Impairment

A number of imaging markers indicating the severity of systemic or cerebral *atherosclerosis* (such as coronary calcium, tonometric measures of aortic wall stiffness, carotid stenosis), of systemic *arteriosclerosis* (such as carotid intima-medial thickness [IMT]), and of cumulated exposure to higher BP or other vascular risk factors (such as echocardiographic left ventricular mass) have been associated with poorer cognitive function and a higher risk of VCI and VD.

The relationship between carotid IMT and cognitive function has been analyzed cross-sectionally and longitudinally in a few studies.[205-208] Overall a significant inverse relationship was observed in each of these studies between carotid IMT and cognitive function—the greater the wall thickness, the poorer the cognitive performance. This relationship was significant after data were controlled for age, education, and, in some studies, concomitant levels of cardiovascular risk factors. It is not clear whether this association is mediated by a parallel impact of vascular risk factors on both the carotid wall and on the brain or it is a direct result of changes in the cerebral circulation secondary to changes in the carotid artery.

Aortic stiffness is best assessed by measuring the carotid-femoral pulse wave velocity (CFPWV) and more crudely by assessing pulse pressure (systolic BP − diastolic BP) or mean arterial pressure. An inverse association between CFPWV and cognitive function has been reported both cross-sectionally (for example, in the Maine-Syracuse study)[209] and longitudinally[210,211] and persists after adjustment of data for age and BP.[209,212] CFPWV has also been associated with WMH volume.[213] Echocardiographic left ventricular mass, remodeling, and hypertrophy have been associated with a higher frequency and severity of subclinical brain injury and poorer cognition as well as an increased risk of dementia.[214,215]

Retinal vessels, assessed at funduscopy or by scanning laser flowmetry, reflect cerebral arterioles, and narrowing of these vessels has been associated with increased arterial stiffness, cerebral small vessel disease, stroke, and poorer cognitive function.[154-156]

Association of Common Clinical Disease States with Vascular Cognitive Impairment

Coronary artery disease: In the Cardiovascular Health Study (CHS)[216] and the Age, Gene/Environment Susceptibility Reykjavik Study,[217] CT coronary artery calcium (CAC), a measure of coronary atherosclerosis severity, was associated with a higher risk of cognitive impairment. There was a simultaneous increased risk of WMHs and CBIs in persons with higher CAC scores, and after adjustment of data for these lesions, cerebral microbleeds and brain volumes attenuated the observed association between CAC and cognition, implicating various vascular mechanisms. Coronary artery disease has also been identified as an independent risk factor for vascular dementia.[218] Coronary artery bypass grafting (CABG) has been associated with poorer initial cognitive function and identified as a marker of late-life dementia risk. However, at 1-, 3-, and 6-year follow-up, the cognitive decline in these patients was no different from that observed in controls with an equivalent burden of CAD who opted for medical treatment or for percutaneous intervention.[219-221]

Chronic kidney disease (CKD): Severe chronic renal insufficiency has been associated with metabolic (uremic) and hypertensive encephalopathy, accelerated atherosclerosis, hyperhomocysteinemia, and an increased risk of stroke.[222] Data from the Heart Estrogen/Progestin Replacement Study (HERS), the Health Aging and Body Composition (Health ABC) Study, the Third National Health and Nutrition Examination Survey (NHANES III), the Reasons for Geographic and Racial Differences in Stroke (REGARDS) study, and the Maine-Syracuse study suggest that among all persons with severe and moderate CKD (estimated glomerular filtration rate [eGFR] less than 30 and less than 60 mL/min/1.73m², respectively) there is a graded continuous increase in the prevalence of cognitive impairment affecting the cognitive domains of attention and learning, memory, orientation, and visuospatial organization.[223-227] Recent results from the Northern Manhattan Stroke (NOMAS) study extended this observation to persons with mild renal dysfunction (eGFR higher than 60 but lower than 90 mL/min/1.73m²) using a global measure of cognition, the Telephone Interview for Cognitive Status (TICS-m).[228] The role of CKD in modifying the risk for clinical dementia is less certain; in the CHS, moderate CKD was related to risk of incident vascular dementia but not to the risk of incident AD.[229]

Atrial fibrillation: Atrial fibrillation, if not treated with adequate anticoagulation, is a strong risk factor for stroke.[93] In several large community-based samples and in a large prospectively studied registry of all persons undergoing cardiac catheterization within a geographic area, atrial fibrillation was found to be an independent risk factor for poorer cognitive performance and risk of vascular dementia,[230-233] even after adjustment of data for associated cardiovascular risk factors and for interim clinical stroke. The mechanism may be through the independent association of atrial fibrillation with subclinical vascular brain injury (WMH and CBI) or hippocampal atrophy.[234,235] However, a few studies did not observe an association of atrial fibrillation with dementia.[236,237] Some of these differences could be related to age (effect being less consistent in older persons), sex (stronger effects were observed in men), and the prevalence and effectiveness of anticoagulation therapy.

Peripheral arterial disease: In the Honolulu–Asia Aging Study (HAAS) and the CHS, a low ankle-brachial index, a measure of peripheral arterial disease, was associated with an increased risk of vascular dementia.[238,239]

Heart failure and cardiac output: In case series, persons with clinical heart failure show deficits in attention and executive function and this appears to be an independent correlate of the severity of functional disability in these patients.[240-242] In persons with bradycardia, pacing has been shown to improve cognition in parallel with the observed improvement in cardiac output. In the Framingham Offspring Study it was shown that subclinical variation

in cardiac output, insufficient to cause clinical heart failure, is also associated with a lower MRI brain volume (but not with lower cognitive function). It is possible that this finding represents an early change and that on follow-up, subjects with a lower cardiac output will be at greater risk for clinical dementia, but this issue remains uncertain.

Depression: Depression has been associated with an increased risk of incident stroke and dementia, even after accounting for concomitant levels of vascular risk factors.[243-246] In addition, depression can impact cognitive performance. The effects may be mediated by poor effort, by residual effects of vascular risk factors, by lifestyle changes associated with depression such as decreased social networking and physical and cognitive activity, by changes in levels of neurotrophic factors, or through other mechanisms.

Thrombosis and antiplatelets: Fibrinogen and D-dimer levels have been associated with an increased risk of stroke and VD. Aspirin reduces stroke risk, and some observational studies have suggested an additional beneficial effect of a daily aspirin on cognition. In the Aspirin or Asymptomatic Atherosclerosis (AAA) trial, 3350 participants aged 50 to 75 years were randomly assigned to receive 100 mg of enteric-coated aspirin or placebo; over a 5-year follow-up, no difference in cognitive abilities was noted between the aspirin and the placebo arms.[247] In the Prevention Regimen for Effectively Avoiding Second Strokes (PRoFESS) trial, more than 20,000 patients with ischemic stroke were randomly assigned in a two-by-two factorial design to receive either 25 mg aspirin and 200 mg extended-release dipyridamole twice a day or 75 mg clopidogrel once a day, and either 80 mg telmisartan or placebo once per day, to assess effectiveness in preventing a second stroke. Cognitive decline was assessed as a secondary endpoint. After a median follow-up of 2.4 years, no difference was observed between the two antiplatelet regimens as to change in MMSE scores.[248]

Treatment of Persons with Clinical Vascular Dementia

Management of vascular risks and symptomatic pharmacotherapy targeting VD has been the primary approach to treat patients with VD.[249] Standardized screening and monitoring to document baseline status, disease trajectory, and treatment response are essential. This should be supplemented with a detailed medical history and assessment of social and daily functioning, and as appropriate with additional blood tests and vascular and brain imaging. Also, factors that exacerbate clinical disease manifestations (e.g., sleep disorders, pain, stress) should be addressed. Cognitive and behavioral interventions for the patient, social support, respite care, and caregiver support are as important for VD as they are for AD, because these measures are critical to ensure optimal quality of life for patients and caregivers.

Control of Vascular Risk Factors

Currently, in the absence of definitive data or guidelines, clinicians should ideally use screening tools to detect cognitive impairment in persons with higher levels of vascular risk factors and in those who have had one or more strokes. The vascular risks should be treated according to nationally accepted guidelines for prevention of stroke and cardiac events.[250] In individual patients, distinguishing the relative contributions of vascular and AD pathology to the observed cognitive deficits is difficult. It is advisable to accurately assess and record baseline cognitive function across multiple domains, detect and address all vascular risk factors, and monitor rate of decline, again in a global as well as domain-specific manner. Prevention of additional strokes is the most effective intervention to reduce risk and rate of cognitive decline.

Pharmacologic Treatment of Cognitive Impairment

There is pathologic and clinical evidence of cholinergic compromise in VCI as there is in AD, and double-blind, placebo-controlled, randomized clinical trials have tested the efficacy of cholinesterase inhibitors in improving cognitive, global, and daily functioning in patients with VD, including the subgroup with VCI due to CADASIL.[251,252] Overall, the studies showed some benefit, particularly in tests of executive function, but a later meta-analysis concluded that the results were insufficient to recommend the routine use of these drugs in VCI.[253] VD has not been approved by the U.S. Food and Drug Administration (FDA) as an indication for the use of these drugs. The presence of concomitant VD need not, however, exclude a patient with AD from receiving a trial of these medications, unless there is a cardiac contraindication to their use, such as bradycardia or hypotension.

Similarly studies of memantine, an *N*-methyl-D-aspartate (NMDA) antagonist, showed minimal cognitive improvement in a few domains insufficient to effect any functional benefit. Trials of other putative disease-modifying agents, such as gingko, piracetam, and huperzine A, have shown no benefit. Symptomatic treatment of apathy with selective serotonergic agents is based on anecdotal reports but has not been validated by clinical trials. Assessment and management of behavioral problems in patients are similar to those described for patients with AD.[252]

Summary

Vascular risk factors contribute to the cognitive impairment and dementia that are common among older adults. A broad concept of VCI is currently used to describe the whole range of cognitive impairment that may be associated with various forms of CVBI, ranging from clinical VD to mild cognitive difficulties that are evident only on cognitive testing, to VMCI. Determining the contribution of vascular disease to an observed syndrome of cognitive impairment or dementia can be difficult and is greatly facilitated by sensitive neuroimaging studies such as MRI, which can show WMH and CBI. The neuropathology of cognitive impairment in later life is often a mixture of AD and vascular pathology, which may overlap and synergize to heighten risk of cognitive impairment (Fig. 17-2). Risk markers for VCI are largely the same as traditional risk

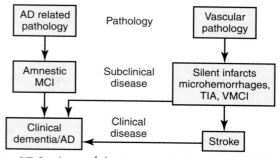

Figure 17-2 Axes of brain aging interact. AD, Alzheimer's disease; MCI, mild cognitive impairment; TIA, transient ischemic attack; VMCI, mild cognitive impairment secondary to vascular pathology.

factors for stroke. These risks may include but are not limited to atrial fibrillation, hypertension, and diabetes. Currently, no specific treatments for VCI have been approved by the FDA. Neurobehavioral and psychiatric symptoms that may be common are treated by the usual drugs and supportive strategies. Finally, standard stroke preventive measures are recommended for most patients with VCI. There is a need for further prospective studies integrating genetic, risk factor, quantitative clinical, and neuroimaging and pathologic data to improve our understanding of the clinical syndromes of VCI and VD.

REFERENCES

1. Vasan RS, Beiser A, Seshadri S, et al: Residual lifetime risk for developing hypertension in middle-aged women and men: The Framingham Heart Study, *JAMA* 287:1003–1010, 2002.
2. Seshadri S, Beiser A, Kelly-Hayes M, et al: The lifetime risk of stroke: Estimates from the Framingham Study, *Stroke* 37:345–350, 2006.
3. Hachinski V, Iadecola C, Petersen RC, et al: National Institute of Neurological Disorders and Stroke-Canadian Stroke Network vascular cognitive impairment harmonization standards, *Stroke* 37:2220–2241, 2006.
4. Roman G: Vascular dementia: A historical background, *Int Psychogeriatr* 15(Suppl 1):11–13, 2003.
5. Tomlinson BE, Blessed G, Roth M: Observations on the brains of demented old people, *J Neurol Sci* 11:205–242, 1970.
6. Hachinski VC, Lassen NA, Marshall J: Multi-infarct dementia. A cause of mental deterioration in the elderly, *Lancet* 2(7874):207–210, 1974.
7. Tatemichi TK, Foulkes MA, Mohr JP, et al: Dementia in stroke survivors in the Stroke Data Bank cohort. Prevalence, incidence, risk factors, and computed tomographic findings, *Stroke* 21:858–866, 1990.
8. Vermeer SE, Prins ND, den Heijer T, Hofman A, Koudstaal PJ, Breteler MM: Silent brain infarcts and the risk of dementia and cognitive decline, *N Engl J Med* 348:1215–1222, 2003.
9. Debette S, Beiser A, Decarli C, et al: Association of MRI markers of vascular brain injury with incident stroke, mild cognitive impairment, dementia, and mortality: The Framingham Offspring Study, *Stroke* 41:600–606, 2010.
10. Petersen RC, Smith GE, Waring SC, Ivnik RJ, Tangalos EG, Kokmen E: Mild cognitive impairment: Clinical characterization and outcome, *Arch Neurol* 56:303–308, 1999.
11. Roman GC, Tatemichi TK, Erkinjuntti T, et al: Vascular dementia: diagnostic criteria for research studies. Report of the NINDS-AIREN International Workshop, *Neurology* 43:250–260, 1993.
12. Chui HC, Victoroff JI, Margolin D, et al: Criteria for the diagnosis of ischemic vascular dementia proposed by the State of California Alzheimer's Disease Diagnostic and Treatment Centers, *Neurology* 42:473–480, 1992.
13. Wetterling T, Kanitz RD, Borgis KJ: The ICD-10 criteria for vascular dementia, *Dementia* 5:185–188, 1994.

14. American Psychiatric Association: *Diagnostic and statistical manual of mental disorders (DSM-IV)*, Washington, DC, 1994, American Psychiatric Association.

15. Pohjasvaara T, Mantyla R, Ylikoski R, et al: Comparison of different clinical criteria (DSM-III, ADDTC, ICD-10, NINDS-AIREN, DSM-IV) for the diagnosis of vascular dementia. National Institute of Neurological Disorders and Stroke-Association Internationale pour la Recherche et l'Enseignement en Neurosciences, *Stroke* 31:2952-2957, 2000.

16. Gold G, Bouras C, Canuto A, et al: Clinicopathological validation study of four sets of clinical criteria for vascular dementia, *Am J Psychiatry* 159:82-87, 2002.

17. Erkinjuntti T: Vascular dementia: Challenge of clinical diagnosis, *Int Psychogeriatr* 9(Suppl 1):51-58, 1997.

18. Ivan CS, Seshadri S, Beiser A, et al: Dementia after stroke: The Framingham Study, *Stroke* 35:1264-1268, 2004.

19. Kokmen E, Whisnant JP, O'Fallon WM, et al: Dementia after ischemic stroke: A population-based study in Rochester, Minnesota (1960-1984), *Neurology* 46:154-159, 1996.

20. Henon H, Pasquier F, Durieu I, et al: Medial temporal lobe atrophy in stroke patients: Relation to pre-existing dementia, *J Neurol Neurosurg Psychiatry* 65:641-647, 1998.

21. Henon H, Durieu I, Guerouaou D, et al: Poststroke dementia: Incidence and relationship to prestroke cognitive decline, *Neurology* 57:1216-1222, 2001.

22. Pendlebury ST, Rothwell PM: Prevalence, incidence, and factors associated with pre-stroke and post-stroke dementia: A systematic review and meta-analysis, *Lancet Neurol* 8:1006-1018, 2009.

23. Tatemichi TK, Desmond DW, Mayeux R, et al: Dementia after stroke: Baseline frequency, risks, and clinical features in a hospitalized cohort, *Neurology* 42:1185-1193, 1992.

24. Hachinski V, Iadecola C, Petersen RC, et al: National Institute of Neurological Disorders and Stroke-Canadian Stroke Network vascular cognitive impairment harmonization standards, *Stroke* 37:2220-2241, 2006.

25. Roman GC: Senile dementia of the Binswanger type. A vascular form of dementia in the elderly, *JAMA* 258:1782-1788, 1987.

26. Mathers SE, Chambers BR, Merory JR, Alexander I: Subcortical arteriosclerotic encephalopathy: Binswanger's disease, *Clin Exp Neurol* 23:67-70, 1987.

27. Chui HC, Victoroff JI, Margolin D, et al: Criteria for the diagnosis of ischemic vascular dementia proposed by the State of California Alzheimer's Disease Diagnostic and Treatment Centers, *Neurology* 42:473-480, 1992.

28. McKhann G, Drachman D, Folstein M, et al: Clinical diagnosis of Alzheimer's disease: report of the NINCDS-ADRDA Work Group under the auspices of Department of Health and Human Services Task Force on Alzheimer's Disease, *Neurology* 34:939-944, 1984.

29. Roman GC, Tatemichi TK, Erkinjuntti T, et al: Vascular dementia: diagnostic criteria for research studies. Report of the NINDS-AIREN International Workshop, *Neurology* 43:250-260, 1993.

30. Kalaria RN, Maestre GE, Arizaga R, et al: Alzheimer's disease and vascular dementia in developing countries: Prevalence, management, and risk factors, *Lancet Neurol* 7:812-826, 2008.

31. Fitzpatrick AL, Kuller LH, Ives DG, et al: Incidence and prevalence of dementia in the Cardiovascular Health Study, *J Am Geriatr Soc* 52:195-204, 2004.

32. Petrovich H, White LR, Ross GW, et al: Accuracy of clinical criteria for AD in the Honolulu-Asia Aging Study, a population-based study, *Neurology* 57:226-234, 2001.

33. Schneider JA, Aggarwal NT, Barnes L, Boyle P, Bennett DA: The neuropathology of older persons with and without dementia from community versus clinic cohorts, *J Alzheimers Dis* 18:691-701, 2009.

34. Au R, Seshadri S, Wolf PA, et al: New norms for a new generation: cognitive performance in the Framingham Offspring cohort, *Exp Aging Res* 30:333-358, 2004.

35. Decarli C, Massaro J, Harvey D, et al: Measures of brain morphology and infarction in the Framingham Heart Study: Establishing what is normal, *Neurobiol Aging* 2:491-510, 2005.

36. Seshadri S, Wolf PA, Beiser A, et al: Stroke risk profile, brain volume, and cognitive function: The Framingham Offspring Study, *Neurology* 63:1591-1599, 2004.

37. Price TR, Manolio TA, Kronmal RA, et al: Silent brain infarction on magnetic resonance imaging and neurological abnormalities in community-dwelling older adults. The Cardiovascular Health Study. CHS Collaborative Research Group, *Stroke* 28:1158-1164, 1997.

38. Harris TB, Launer LJ, Eiriksdottir G, et al: Age, Gene/Environment Susceptibility-Reykjavik Study: Multidisciplinary applied phenomics, *Am J Epidemiol* 165:1076-1087, 2007.

39. Hofman A, Breteler MM, van Duijn CM, et al: The Rotterdam Study: Objectives and design update, *Eur J Epidemiol* 22:819-829, 2007.

40. White L, Petrovitch H, Hardman J, et al: Cerebrovascular pathology and dementia in autopsied Honolulu-Asia Aging Study participants, *Ann N Y Acad Sci* 977:9-23, 2002.

41. Graham NL, Emery T, Hodges JR: Distinctive cognitive profiles in Alzheimer's disease and subcortical vascular dementia, *J Neurol Neurosurg Psychiatry* 75:61-71, 2004.

42. Lopez OL, Kuller LH, Becker JT, et al: Classification of vascular dementia in the Cardiovascular Health Study Cognition Study, *Neurology* 64:1539-1547, 2005.

43. Kase CS, Wolf PA, Kelly-Hayes M, et al: Intellectual decline after stroke: The Framingham Study, *Stroke* 29:805-812, 1998.

44. Decarli C: Mild cognitive impairment: prevalence, prognosis, aetiology, and treatment, *Lancet Neurol* 2:15-21, 2003.

45. Frisoni GB, Galluzzi S, Bresciani L, et al: Mild cognitive impairment with subcortical vascular features: Clinical characteristics and outcome, *J Neurol* 249:1423-1432, 2002.

46. Petersen RC, Smith GE, Waring SC, et al: Mild cognitive impairment: Clinical characterization and outcome, *Arch Neurol* 56:303-308, 1999.

47. Petersen RC, Stevens JC, Ganguli M, et al: Practice parameter: early detection of dementia: Mild cognitive impairment (an evidence-based review). Report of the Quality Standards Subcommittee of the American Academy of Neurology, *Neurology* 56:1133-1142, 2001.

48. Winblad B, Palmer K, Kivipelto M, et al: Mild cognitive impairment—beyond controversies, towards a consensus: Report of the International Working Group on Mild Cognitive Impairment, *J Intern Med* 256:240-246, 2004.

49. Petersen RC, Doody R, Kurz A, et al: Current concepts in mild cognitive impairment, *Arch Neurol* 58:1985-1992, 2001.

50. O'Brien JT, Erkinjuntti T, Reisberg B, et al: Vascular cognitive impairment, *Lancet Neurol* 2:89-98, 2003.

51. Folstein MF, Folstein SE, McHugh PR: "Mini-mental state." A practical method for grading the cognitive state of patients for the clinician, *J Psychiatr Res* 12:189-198, 1975.

52. Iadecola C: Cerebrovascular effects of amyloid-beta peptides: Mechanisms and implications for Alzheimer's dementia, *Cell Mol Neurobiol* 23:681-689, 2003.

53. Iadecola C, Goldman SS, Harder DR, et al: Recommendations of the National Heart, Lung, and Blood Institute working group on cerebrovascular biology and disease, *Stroke* 37:1578-1581, 2006.

54. Kalaria RN, Kenny RA, Ballard CG, et al: Towards defining the neuropathological substrates of vascular dementia, *J Neurol Sci* 226:75-80, 2004.

55. Vonsattel JP, Myers RH, Hedley-Whyte ET, et al: Cerebral amyloid angiopathy without and with cerebral hemorrhages: A comparative histological study, *Ann Neurol* 30:637-649, 1991.

56. Greenberg SM: Cerebral amyloid angiopathy: Prospects for clinical diagnosis and treatment, *Neurology* 51:690-694, 1998.

57. Johnson KA, Gregas M, Becker JA, et al: Imaging of amyloid burden and distribution in cerebral amyloid angiopathy, *Ann Neurol* 62:229-234, 2007.

58. Smith EE, Greenberg SM: Clinical diagnosis of cerebral amyloid angiopathy: Validation of the Boston criteria, *Curr Atheroscler Rep* 5:260-266, 2003.

59. Chabriat H, Joutel A, Dichgans M, et al: CADASIL, *Lancet Neurol* 8:643-653, 2009.

60. Grabowski TJ, Cho HS, Vonsattel JP, et al: Novel amyloid precursor protein mutation in an Iowa family with dementia and severe cerebral amyloid angiopathy, *Ann Neurol* 49:697-705, 2001.

61. Van Broeckhoven BC, Haan J, Bakker E, et al: Amyloid beta protein precursor gene and hereditary cerebral hemorrhage with amyloidosis (Dutch), *Science* 248:1120-1122, 1990.

62. Jeerakathil T, Wolf PA, Beiser A, et al: Stroke risk profile predicts white matter hyperintensity volume: The Framingham Study, *Stroke* 35:1857-1861, 2004.

63. Seshadri S: Methodology for measuring cerebrovascular disease burden, *Int Rev Psychiatry* 18:409–422, 2006.

64. Massaro JM, D'Agostino RB Sr, Sullivan LM, et al: Managing and analysing data from a large-scale study on Framingham Offspring relating brain structure to cognitive function, *Stat Med* 23:351–367, 2004.

65. Weiner MW, Aisen PS, Jack CR Jr, et al: The Alzheimer's disease neuroimaging initiative: Progress report and future plans, *Alzheimers Dement* 6:202–211, 2010.

66. Vernooij MW, Ikram MA, Vrooman HA, et al: White matter microstructural integrity and cognitive function in a general elderly population, *Arch Gen Psychiatry* 66:545–553, 2009.

67. Manolio TA, Kronmal RA, Burke GL, et al: Magnetic resonance abnormalities and cardiovascular disease in older adults. The Cardiovascular Health Study, *Stroke* 25:318–327, 1994.

68. Scheltens P, Erkinjunti T, Leys D, et al: White matter changes on CT and MRI: an overview of visual rating scales. European Task Force on Age-Related White Matter Changes, *Eur Neurol* 39:80–89, 1998.

69. Das RR, Seshadri S, Beiser AS, et al: Prevalence and correlates of silent cerebral infarcts in the Framingham Offspring study, *Stroke* 39:2929–2935, 2008.

70. Vermeer SE, den Heijer T, Koudstaal PJ, et al: Incidence and risk factors of silent brain infarcts in the population-based Rotterdam Scan Study, *Stroke* 34:392–396, 2003.

71. Bryan RN, Cai J, Burke G, et al: Prevalence and anatomic characteristics of infarct-like lesions on MR images of middle-aged adults: The Atherosclerosis Risk in Communities study, *AJNR Am J Neuroradiol* 20:1273–1280, 1999.

72. Au R, Massaro JM, Wolf PA, et al: Association of white matter hyperintensity volume with decreased cognitive functioning: The Framingham Heart Study, *Arch Neurol* 63:246–250, 2006.

73. Greenberg SM, Vernooij MW, Cordonnier C, et al: Cerebral microbleeds: A guide to detection and interpretation, *Lancet Neurol* 8:165–174, 2009.

74. Jeerakathil T, Wolf PA, Beiser A, et al: Cerebral microbleeds: Prevalence and associations with cardiovascular risk factors in the Framingham Study, *Stroke* 35:1831–1835, 2004.

75. Sveinbjornsdottir S, Sigurdsson S, Aspelund T, et al: Cerebral microbleeds in the population based AGES-Reykjavik study: Prevalence and location, *J Neurol Neurosurg Psychiatry* 79:1002–1006, 2008.

76. Vernooij MW, Van der Lugt A, Ikram MA, et al: Prevalence and risk factors of cerebral microbleeds: The Rotterdam Scan Study, *Neurology* 70:1208–1214, 2008.

77. Debette S, Beiser A, Decarli C, et al: Association of MRI markers of vascular brain injury with incident stroke, mild cognitive impairment, dementia, and mortality. The Framingham Offspring Study, *Stroke* 41:600–606, 2010.

78. Jokinen H, Kalska H, Ylikoski R, et al: MRI-defined subcortical ischemic vascular disease: Baseline clinical and neuropsychological findings. The LADIS Study, *Cerebrovasc Dis* 27:336–344, 2009.

79. Mosley TH Jr, Knopman DS, Catellier DJ, et al: Cerebral MRI findings and cognitive functioning: The Atherosclerosis Risk in Communities study, *Neurology* 64:2056–2062, 2005.

80. Prins ND, van Dijk EJ, den Heijer T, et al: Cerebral small-vessel disease and decline in information processing speed, executive function and memory, *Brain* 128:2034–2041, 2005.

81. Prins ND, van Dijk EJ, den Heijer T, et al: Cerebral white matter lesions and the risk of dementia, *Arch Neurol* 61:1531–1534, 2004.

82. Esiri MM, Wilcock GK, Morris JH: Neuropathological assessment of the lesions of significance in vascular dementia, *J Neurol Neurosurg Psychiatry* 63:749–753, 1997.

83. Esiri MM: Which vascular lesions are of importance in vascular dementia? *Ann N Y Acad Sci* 903:239–243, 2000.

84. Jellinger KA: Morphologic diagnosis of vascular dementia—a critical update, *J Neurol Sci* 270:1–12, 2008.

85. Savva GM, Wharton SB, Ince PG, et al: Age, neuropathology, and dementia, *N Engl J Med* 360:2302–2309, 2009.

86. Schneider JA, Arvanitakis Z, Bang W, Bennett DA: Mixed brain pathologies account for most dementia cases in community-dwelling older persons, *Neurology* 69:2197–2204, 2007.

87. Schneider JA, Aggarwal NT, Barnes L, et al: The neuropathology of older persons with and without dementia from community versus clinic cohorts, *J Alzheimers Dis* 18:691–701, 2009.

88. Jellinger KA: Morphologic diagnosis of "vascular dementia"—a critical update, *J Neurol Sci* 270:1–12, 2008.

89. Jagust WJ, Zheng L, Harvey DJ, et al: Neuropathological basis of magnetic resonance images in aging and dementia, *Ann Neurol* 63:72–80, 2008.

90. Schneider JA, Wilson RS, Cochran EJ, et al: Relation of cerebral infarctions to dementia and cognitive function in older persons, *Neurology* 60:1082–1088, 2003.

91. Snowdon DA, Greiner LH, Mortimer JA, et al: Brain infarction and the clinical expression of Alzheimer disease. The Nun Study, *JAMA* 277:813–817, 1997.

92. Sadowski M, Pankiewicz J, Scholtzova H, et al: Links between the pathology of Alzheimer's disease and vascular dementia, *Neurochem Res* 29:1257–1266, 2004.

93. Wolf PA, D'Agostino RB, Belanger AJ, Kannel WB: Probability of stroke: A risk profile from the Framingham Study, *Stroke* 22:312–318, 1991.

94. Debette S, Bis JC, Fornage M, et al: Genome-wide association studies of MRI-defined brain infarcts: Meta-analysis from the CHARGE Consortium, *Stroke* 41:210–217, 2010.

95. Ikram MA, Seshadri S, Bis JC, et al: Genomewide association studies of stroke, *N Engl J Med* 360:1718–1728, 2009.

96. Karvanen J, Silander K, Kee F, et al: The impact of newly identified loci on coronary heart disease, stroke and total mortality in the MORGAM prospective cohorts, *Genet Epidemiol* 33:237–246, 2009.

97. Morris MC, Evans DA, Tangney CC, et al: Associations of vegetable and fruit consumption with age-related cognitive change, *Neurology* 67:1370–1376, 2006.

98. Kang JH, Ascherio A, Grodstein F: Fruit and vegetable consumption and cognitive decline in aging women, *Ann Neurol* 57:713–720, 2005.

99. MRC/BHF Heart Protection Study of antioxidant vitamin supplementation in 20,536 high-risk individuals: A randomised placebo-controlled trial, *Lancet* 360(9326):23–33, 2002.

100. van de Rest O, Spiro A III, Krall-Kaye E, et al: Intakes of (n-3) fatty acids and fatty fish are not associated with cognitive performance and 6-year cognitive change in men participating in the Veterans Affairs Normative Aging Study, *J Nutr* 139:2329–2336, 2009.

101. van Gelder BM, Tijhuis M, Kalmijn S, Kromhout D: Fish consumption, n-3 fatty acids, and subsequent 5-y cognitive decline in elderly men: the Zutphen Elderly Study, *Am J Clin Nutr* 85:1142–1147, 2007.

102. Heude B, Ducimetiere P, Berr C: Cognitive decline and fatty acid composition of erythrocyte membranes—The EVA Study, *Am J Clin Nutr* 77:803–808, 2003.

103. Schaefer EJ, Bongard V, Beiser AS, et al: Plasma phosphatidylcholine docosahexaenoic acid content and risk of dementia and Alzheimer disease: The Framingham Heart Study, *Arch Neurol* 63:1545–1550, 2006.

104. van de Rest O, Geleijnse JM, Kok FJ, et al: Effect of fish oil on cognitive performance in older subjects: A randomized, controlled trial, *Neurology* 71:430–438, 2008.

105. Llewellyn DJ, Langa KM, Lang IA: Serum 25-hydroxyvitamin D concentration and cognitive impairment, *J Geriatr Psychiatry Neurol* 22:188–195, 2009.

106. Buell JS, Scott TM, Dawson-Hughes B, et al: Vitamin D is associated with cognitive function in elders receiving home health services, *J Gerontol A Biol Sci Med Sci* 64:888–895, 2009.

107. Annweiler C, Schott AM, Allali G, et al: Association of vitamin D deficiency with cognitive impairment in older women: Cross-sectional study, *Neurology* 74:27–32, 2010.

108. Seshadri S: Elevated plasma homocysteine levels: risk factor or risk marker for the development of dementia and Alzheimer's disease? *J Alzheimers Dis* 9:393–398, 2006.

109. Wright CB, Lee HS, Paik MC, et al: Total homocysteine and cognition in a tri-ethnic cohort: The Northern Manhattan Study, *Neurology* 63:254–260, 2004.

110. Miller JW, Green R, Ramos MI, et al: Homocysteine and cognitive function in the Sacramento Area Latino Study on Aging, *Am J Clin Nutr* 78:441–447, 2003.

111. Elias MF, Sullivan LM, D'Agostino RB, et al: Homocysteine and cognitive performance in the Framingham offspring study: Age is important, *Am J Epidemiol* 162:644–653, 2005.

112. Prins ND, den Heijer T, Hofman A, et al: Homocysteine and cognitive function in the elderly—The Rotterdam Scan Study, *Neurology* 59:1375–1380, 2002.

113. Morris MS, Jacques PF, Rosenberg IH, Selhub J: Hyperhomocysteinemia associated with poor recall in the third National Health and Nutrition Examination Survey, *Am J Clin Nutr* 73:927-933, 2001.

114. Schafer JH, Glass TA, Bolla KI, et al: Homocysteine and cognitive function in a population-based study of older adults, *J Am Geriatr Soc* 53:381-388, 2005.

115. Seshadri S, Beiser A, Selhub J, et al: Plasma homocysteine as a risk factor for dementia and Alzheimer's disease, *N Engl J Med* 346:476-483, 2002.

116. Den Heijer T, Vermeer SE, Clarke R, et al: Homocysteine and brain atrophy on MRI of non-demented elderly, *Brain* 126:170-175, 2003.

117. Seshadri S, Wolf PA, Beiser AS, et al: Association of plasma total homocysteine levels with subclinical brain injury: Cerebral volumes, white matter hyperintensity, and silent brain infarcts at volumetric magnetic resonance imaging in the Framingham Offspring Study, *Arch Neurol* 65:642-649, 2008.

118. Vermeer SE, van Dijk EJ, Koudstaal PJ, et al: Homocysteine, silent brain infarcts, and white matter lesions: The Rotterdam Scan Study, *Ann Neurol* 51:285-289, 2002.

119. Larson EB, Wang L, Bowen JD, et al: Exercise is associated with reduced risk for incident dementia among persons 65 years of age and older, *Ann Intern Med* 144:73-81, 2006.

120. Scarmeas N, Luchsinger JA, Schupf N, et al: Physical activity, diet, and risk of Alzheimer disease, *JAMA* 302:627-637, 2009.

121. Verghese J, Cuiling W, Katz MJ, et al: Leisure activities and risk of vascular cognitive impairment in older adults, *J Geriatr Psychiatry Neurol* 22:110-118, 2009.

122. Verghese J, Lipton RB, Katz MJ, et al: Leisure activities and the risk of dementia in the elderly, *N Engl J Med* 348:2508-2516, 2003.

123. Vaynman S, Gomez-Pinilla F: Revenge of the "sit": how lifestyle impacts neuronal and cognitive health through molecular systems that interface energy metabolism with neuronal plasticity, *J Neurosci Res* 84:699-715, 2006.

124. Aarsland D, Sardahaee FS, Anderssen S, Ballard C: Is physical activity a potential preventive factor for vascular dementia? A systematic review, *Aging Ment Health* 14:386-395, 2010.

125. Etgen T, Sander D, Huntgeburth U, et al: Physical activity and incident cognitive impairment in elderly persons: The INVADE study, *Arch Intern Med* 170:186-193, 2010.

126. Liu-Ambrose T, Eng JJ, Boyd LA, et al: Promotion of the mind through exercise (PROMoTE): A proof-of-concept randomized controlled trial of aerobic exercise training in older adults with vascular cognitive impairment, *BMC Neurol* 10:14, 2010.

127. Raval AP, Dave KR, Perez-Pinzon MA: Resveratrol mimics ischemic preconditioning in the brain, *J Cereb Blood Flow Metab* 26:1141-1147, 2006.

128. Ganguli M, Vander BJ, Saxton JA, et al: Alcohol consumption and cognitive function in late life: A longitudinal community study, *Neurology* 65:1210-1217, 2005.

129. Elias PK, Elias MF, D'Agostino RB, et al: Alcohol consumption and cognitive performance in the Framingham Heart Study, *Am J Epidemiol* 150:580-589, 1999.

130. Stott DJ, Falconer A, Kerr GD, et al: Does low to moderate alcohol intake protect against cognitive decline in older people? *J Am Geriatr Soc* 56:2217-2224, 2008.

131. Paul CA, Au R, Fredman L, et al: Association of alcohol consumption with brain volume in the Framingham study, *Arch Neurol* 65:1363-1367, 2008.

132. Gustafson D, Rothenberg E, Blennow K, et al: An 18-year follow-up of overweight and risk of Alzheimer disease, *Arch Intern Med* 163:1524-1528, 2003.

133. Gustafson DR, Backman K, Waern M, et al: Adiposity indicators and dementia over 32 years in Sweden, *Neurology* 73:1559-1566, 2009.

134. Kivipelto M, Ngandu T, Fratiglioni L, et al: Obesity and vascular risk factors at midlife and the risk of dementia and Alzheimer disease, *Arch Neurol* 62:1556-1560, 2005.

135. Whitmer RA, Gunderson EP, Quesenberry CP Jr, et al: Body mass index in midlife and risk of Alzheimer disease and vascular dementia, *Curr Alzheimer Res* 4:103-109, 2007.

136. Whitmer RA, Gustafson DR, Barrett-Connor E, et al: Central obesity and increased risk of dementia more than three decades later, *Neurology* 71:1057-1064, 2008.

137. Wolf PA, Beiser A, Elias MF, et al: Relation of obesity to cognitive function: Importance of central obesity and synergistic influence of concomitant hypertension. The Framingham Heart Study, *Curr Alzheimer Res* 4:111-116, 2007.

138. Debette S, Beiser A, Hoffmann U, et al: Visceral fat is associated with lower brain volume in healthy middle-aged adults, *Ann Neurol* 68:136-144, 2010.

139. Kanaya AM, Lindquist K, Harris TB, et al: Total and regional adiposity and cognitive change in older adults: The Health, Aging and Body Composition (ABC) study, *Arch Neurol* 66:329-335, 2009.

140. Lieb W, Beiser AS, Vasan RS, et al: Association of plasma leptin levels with incident Alzheimer disease and MRI measures of brain aging, *JAMA* 302:2565-2572, 2009.

141. Fratiglioni L, Wang HX: Smoking and Parkinson's and Alzheimer's disease: Review of the epidemiological studies, *Behav Brain Res* 113:117-120, 2000.

142. Peters R, Poulter R, Warner J, et al: Smoking, dementia and cognitive decline in the elderly, a systematic review, *BMC Geriatr* 8:36, 2008.

143. Ott A, Slooter AJ, Hofman A, et al: Smoking and risk of dementia and Alzheimer's disease in a population-based cohort study: The Rotterdam Study, *Lancet* 351(9119):1840-1843, 1998.

144. Ott A, Andersen K, Dewey ME, et al: Effect of smoking on global cognitive function in nondemented elderly, *Neurology* 62:920-924, 2004.

145. Elias MF, Wolf PA, D'Agostino RB, et al: Untreated blood pressure level is inversely related to cognitive functioning: The Framingham Study, *Am J Epidemiol* 138:353-364, 1993.

146. Kivipelto M, Helkala EL, Hanninen T, et al: Midlife vascular risk factors and late-life mild cognitive impairment: A population-based study, *Neurology* 56:1683-1689, 2001.

147. Launer LJ, Masaki K, Petrovitch H, et al: The association between midlife blood pressure levels and late-life cognitive function. The Honolulu-Asia Aging Study, *JAMA* 274:1846-1851, 1995.

148. Petrovitch H, White LR, Izmirilian G, et al: Midlife blood pressure and neuritic plaques, neurofibrillary tangles, and brain weight at death: The HAAS. Honolulu-Asia Aging Study, *Neurobiol Aging* 2:57-62, 2000.

149. Ruitenberg A, Skoog I, Ott A, et al: Blood pressure and risk of dementia: results from the Rotterdam study and the Gothenburg H-70 Study, *Dement Geriatr Cogn Disord* 12:33-39, 2001.

150. Swan GE, Decarli C, Miller BL, et al: Association of midlife blood pressure to late-life cognitive decline and brain morphology, *Neurology* 51:986-993, 1998.

151. Launer LJ, Hughes T, Yu B, et al: Lowering midlife levels of systolic blood pressure as a public health strategy to reduce late-life dementia: Perspective from the Honolulu Heart Program/Honolulu Asia Aging Study, *Hypertension* 55:1352-1359, 2010.

152. Skoog I, Lernfelt B, Landahl S, et al: 15-year longitudinal study of blood pressure and dementia, *Lancet* 347(9009):1141-1145, 1996.

153. Qiu C, Winblad B, Fratiglioni L: Low diastolic pressure and risk of dementia in very old people: A longitudinal study, *Dement Geriatr Cogn Disord* 28:213-219, 2009.

154. Nilsson SE, Read S, Berg S, et al: Low systolic blood pressure is associated with impaired cognitive function in the oldest old: Longitudinal observations in a population-based sample 80 years and older, *Aging Clin Exp Res* 19:41-47, 2007.

155. in't Veld BA, Ruitenberg A, Hofman A, et al: Antihypertensive drugs and incidence of dementia: The Rotterdam Study, *Neurobiol Aging* 22:407-412, 2001.

156. Guo Z, Fratiglioni L, Zhu L, et al: Occurrence and progression of dementia in a community population aged 75 years and older: Relationship of antihypertensive medication use, *Arch Neurol* 56:991-996, 1999.

157. Khachaturian AS, Zandi PP, Lyketsos CG, et al: Antihypertensive medication use and incident Alzheimer disease: The Cache County Study, *Arch Neurol* 63:686-692, 2006.

158. Li NC, Lee A, Whitmer RA, et al: Use of angiotensin receptor blockers and risk of dementia in a predominantly male population: Prospective cohort analysis, *BMJ* 340:5465, 2010.

159. Di Bari BM, Pahor M, Franse LV, et al: Dementia and disability outcomes in large hypertension trials: Lessons learned from the Systolic Hypertension in the Elderly Program (SHEP) trial, *Am J Epidemiol* 153:72-78, 2001.

160. Prevention of stroke by antihypertensive drug treatment in older persons with isolated systolic hypertension: Final results of the Systolic Hypertension in the Elderly Program (SHEP). SHEP Cooperative Research Group, *JAMA* 265:3255–3264, 1991.

161. Lithell H, Hansson L, Skoog I, et al: The Study on Cognition and Prognosis in the Elderly (SCOPE): principal results of a randomized double-blind intervention trial, *J Hypertens* 21:875–886, 2003.

162. Tzourio C, Anderson C: Blood pressure reduction and risk of dementia in patients with stroke: rationale of the dementia assessment in PROGRESS (Perindopril Protection Against Recurrent Stroke Study). PROGRESS Management Committee, *J Hypertens Suppl* 18:S21–S24, 2000.

163. Peters R, Beckett N, Forette F, et al: Incident dementia and blood pressure lowering in the Hypertension in the Very Elderly Trial Cognitive Function Assessment (HYVET-COG): A double-blind, placebo controlled trial, *Lancet Neurol* 7:683–689, 2008.

164. Forette F, Seux ML, Staessen JA, et al: Prevention of dementia in randomised double-blind placebo-controlled Systolic Hypertension in Europe (Syst-Eur) trial, *Lancet* 352(9137):1347–1351, 1998.

165. Fontbonne A, Berr C, Ducimetiere P, Alperovitch A: Changes in cognitive abilities over a 4-year period are unfavorably affected in elderly diabetic subjects: Results of the Epidemiology of Vascular Aging Study, *Diabetes Care* 24:366–370, 2001.

166. Knopman D, Boland LL, Mosley T, et al: Cardiovascular risk factors and cognitive decline in middle-aged adults, *Neurology* 56:42–48, 2001.

167. Verhaegen P, Borchelt M, Smith J: Relation between cardiovascular and metabolic disease and cognition in very old age: Cross-sectional and longitudinal findings from the Berlin Aging Study, *Health Psychol* 22(6):559–569, 2003.

168. Wu JH, Haan MN, Liang J, et al: Impact of diabetes on cognitive function among older Latinos: A population-based cohort study, *J Clin Epidemiol* 56:686–693, 2003.

169. Xiong GL, Plassman BL, Helms MJ, Steffens DC: Vascular risk factors and cognitive decline among elderly male twins, *Neurology* 67:1586–1591, 2006.

170. Elias PK, Elias MF, D'Agostino RB, et al: NIDDM and blood pressure as risk factors for poor cognitive performance. The Framingham Study, *Diabetes Care* 20:1388–1395, 1997.

171. Kanaya AM, Barrett-Connor E, Gildengorin G, Yaffe K: Change in cognitive function by glucose tolerance status in older adults: A 4-year prospective study of the Rancho Bernardo study cohort, *Arch Intern Med* 164:1327–1333, 2004.

172. Knopman DS, Mosley TH, Catellier DJ, Coker LH: Fourteen-year longitudinal study of vascular risk factors, APOE genotype, and cognition: the ARIC MRI Study, *Alzheimers Dement* 5:207–214, 2009.

173. Arvanitakis Z, Wilson RS, Bennett DA: Diabetes mellitus, dementia, and cognitive function in older persons, *J Nutr Health Aging* 10:287–291, 2006.

174. Hebert R, Lindsay J, Verreault R, et al: Vascular dementia: Incidence and risk factors in the Canadian study of health and aging, *Stroke* 31:1487–1493, 2000.

175. Ott A, Stolk RP, Hofman A, et al: Association of diabetes mellitus and dementia: The Rotterdam Study, *Diabetologia* 39:1392–1397, 1996.

176. Cukierman T, Gerstein HC, Williamson JD: Cognitive decline and dementia in diabetes—systematic overview of prospective observational studies, *Diabetologia* 48:2460–2469, 2005.

177. Arvanitakis Z, Schneider JA, Wilson RS, et al: Diabetes is related to cerebral infarction but not to AD pathology in older persons, *Neurology* 67:1960–1965, 2006.

178. Hassing LB, Johansson B, Nilsson SE, et al: Diabetes mellitus is a risk factor for vascular dementia, but not for Alzheimer's disease: A population-based study of the oldest old, *Int Psychogeriatr* 14:239–248, 2002.

179. MacKnight C, Rockwood K, Awalt E, McDowell I: Diabetes mellitus and the risk of dementia, Alzheimer's disease and vascular cognitive impairment in the Canadian Study of Health and Aging, *Dement Geriatr Cogn Disord* 14:77–83, 2002.

180. Luchsinger JA, Tang MX, Stern Y, et al: Diabetes mellitus and risk of Alzheimer's disease and dementia with stroke in a multiethnic cohort, *Am J Epidemiol* 154:635–641, 2001.

181. Whitmer RA, Karter AJ, Yaffe K, et al: Hypoglycemic episodes and risk of dementia in older patients with type 2 diabetes mellitus, *JAMA* 301:1565–1572, 2009.

182. Cukierman-Yaffe T, Gerstein HC, Williamson JD, et al: Relationship between baseline glycemic control and cognitive function in individuals with type 2 diabetes and other cardiovascular risk factors: The Action to Control Cardiovascular Risk in Diabetes-Memory in Diabetes (ACCORD-MIND) trial, *Diabetes Care* 32(2):221–226, 2009.

183. de Galan BE, Zoungas S, Chalmers J, et al: Cognitive function and risks of cardiovascular disease and hypoglycaemia in patients with type 2 diabetes: The Action in Diabetes and Vascular Disease: Preterax and Diamicron Modified Release Controlled Evaluation (ADVANCE) trial, *Diabetologia* 52:2328–2336, 2009.

184. Solomon A, Kivipelto M, Wolozin B, et al: Midlife serum cholesterol and increased risk of Alzheimer's and vascular dementia three decades later, *Dement Geriatr Cogn Disord* 28:75–80, 2009.

185. Elias PK, Elias MF, D'Agostino RB, et al: Serum cholesterol and cognitive performance in the Framingham Heart Study, *Psychosom Med* 67:24–30, 2005.

186. Trkanjec Z, Bene R, Martinic-Popovic I, et al: Serum HDL, LDL and total cholesterol in patients with late-life onset of Alzheimer's disease versus vascular dementia, *Acta Clin Croat* 48:259–263, 2009.

187. Tan ZS, Seshadri S, Beiser A, et al: Plasma total cholesterol level as a risk factor for Alzheimer disease: The Framingham Study, *Arch Intern Med* 163:1053–1057, 2003.

188. Jick H, Zornberg GL, Jick SS, et al: Statins and the risk of dementia, *Lancet* 356(9242):1627–1631, 2000.

189. Wolozin B, Kellman W, Ruosseau P, et al: Decreased prevalence of Alzheimer disease associated with 3-hydroxy-3-methyglutaryl coenzyme A reductase inhibitors, *Arch Neurol* 57:1439–1443, 2000.

190. Trompet S, van VP, de Craen AJ, et al: Pravastatin and cognitive function in the elderly. Results of the PROSPER study, *J Neurol* 257:85–90, 2010.

191. Jefferson AL, Massaro JM, Wolf PA, et al: Inflammatory biomarkers are associated with total brain volume: The Framingham Heart Study, *Neurology* 68:1032–1038, 2007.

192. Tan ZS, Beiser AS, Vasan RS, et al: Inflammatory markers and the risk of Alzheimer disease: The Framingham Study, *Neurology* 68:1902–1908, 2007.

193. Tan ZS, Seshadri S: Inflammation in the Alzheimer's disease cascade: culprit or innocent bystander? *Alzheimers Res Ther* 2:6, 2010.

194. Roberts RO, Geda YE, Knopman DS, et al: Association of C-reactive protein with mild cognitive impairment, *Alzheimers Dement* 5:398–405, 2009.

195. Sundelof J, Kilander L, Helmersson J, et al: Systemic inflammation and the risk of Alzheimer's disease and dementia: A prospective population-based study, *J Alzheimers Dis* 18:79–87, 2009.

196. Laurin D, David CJ, Masaki KH, et al: Midlife C-reactive protein and risk of cognitive decline: A 31-year follow-up, *Neurobiol Aging* 30:1724–1727, 2009.

197. Haan MN, Aiello AE, West NA, Jagust WJ: C-reactive protein and rate of dementia in carriers and non carriers of Apolipoprotein APOE4 genotype, *Neurobiol Aging* 29:1774–1782, 2008.

198. Ravaglia G, Forti P, Maioli F, et al: Blood inflammatory markers and risk of dementia: The Conselice Study of Brain Aging, *Neurobiol Aging* 28:1810–1820, 2007.

199. Weuve J, Ridker PM, Cook NR, et al: High-sensitivity C-reactive protein and cognitive function in older women, *Epidemiology* 17:183–189, 2006.

200. van Dijk EJ, Prins ND, Vermeer SE, et al: C-reactive protein and cerebral small-vessel disease: The Rotterdam Scan Study, *Circulation* 112:900–905, 2005.

201. Kuo HK, Yen CJ, Chang CH, et al: Relation of C-reactive protein to stroke, cognitive disorders, and depression in the general population: Systematic review and meta-analysis, *Lancet Neurol* 4:371–380, 2005.

202. Dik MG, Jonker C, Hack CE, et al: Serum inflammatory proteins and cognitive decline in older persons, *Neurology* 64:1371–1377, 2005.

203. Bruunsgaard H, Andersen-Ranberg K, Jeune B, et al: A high plasma concentration of TNF-alpha is associated with dementia in centenarians, *J Gerontol A Biol Sci Med Sci* 54:M357-M364, 1999.

204. Pikula A, Boger RH, Beiser AS, et al: Association of plasma ADMA levels with MRI markers of vascular brain injury: Framingham Offspring Study, *Stroke* 40:2959-2964, 2009.

205. Wendell CR, Zonderman AB, Metter EJ, et al: Carotid intimal medial thickness predicts cognitive decline among adults without clinical vascular disease, *Stroke* 40:3180-3185, 2009.

206. Komulainen P, Kivipelto M, Lakka TA, et al: Carotid intima-media thickness and cognitive function in elderly women: A population-based study, *Neuroepidemiology* 28:207-213, 2007.

207. Mathiesen EB, Waterloo K, Joakimsen O, et al: Reduced neuropsychological test performance in asymptomatic carotid stenosis: The Tromsø Study, *Neurology* 62:695-701, 2004.

208. Romero JR, Beiser A, Seshadri S, et al: Carotid artery atherosclerosis, MRI indices of brain ischemia, aging, and cognitive impairment: the Framingham study, *Stroke* 40:1590-1596, 2009.

209. Elias MF, Robbins MA, Budge MM, et al: Arterial pulse wave velocity and cognition with advancing age, *Hypertension* 53:668-673, 2009.

210. Scuteri A, Tesauro M, Appolloni S, et al: Arterial stiffness as an independent predictor of longitudinal changes in cognitive function in the older individual, *J Hypertens* 25:1035-1040, 2007.

211. Waldstein SR, Rice SC, Thayer JF, et al: Pulse pressure and pulse wave velocity are related to cognitive decline in the Baltimore Longitudinal Study of Aging, *Hypertension* 51:99-104, 2008.

212. Scuteri A, Brancati AM, Gianni W, et al: Arterial stiffness is an independent risk factor for cognitive impairment in the elderly: A pilot study, *J Hypertens* 23:1211-1216, 2005.

213. Henskens LH, Kroon AA, van Oostenbrugge RJ, et al: Increased aortic pulse wave velocity is associated with silent cerebral small-vessel disease in hypertensive patients, *Hypertension* 52:1120-1126, 2008.

214. Elias MF, Sullivan LM, Elias PK, et al: Left ventricular mass, blood pressure, and lowered cognitive performance in the Framingham Offspring, *Hypertension* 49:439-445, 2007.

215. Scuteri A, Coluccia R, Castello L, et al: Left ventricular mass increase is associated with cognitive decline and dementia in the elderly independently of blood pressure, *Eur Heart J* 30:1525-1529, 2009.

216. Rosano C, Naydeck B, Kuller LH, et al: Coronary artery calcium: associations with brain magnetic resonance imaging abnormalities and cognitive status, *J Am Geriatr Soc* 53:609-615, 2005.

217. Vidal JS, Sigurdsson S, Jonsdottir MK, et al: Coronary artery calcium, brain function and structure. The AGES-Reykjavik Study. *Stroke* 41:891-897, 2010.

218. Kuller LH, Lopez OL, Jagust WJ, et al: Determinants of vascular dementia in the Cardiovascular Health Cognition Study, *Neurology* 64:1548-1552, 2005.

219. McKhann GM, Grega MA, Borowicz LM Jr, et al: Is there cognitive decline 1 year after CABG? Comparison with surgical and nonsurgical controls, *Neurology* 65:991-999, 2005.

220. Selnes OA, Grega MA, Bailey MM, et al: Cognition 6 years after surgical or medical therapy for coronary artery disease, *Ann Neurol* 63:581-590, 2008.

221. Rosengart TK, Sweet JJ, Finnin E, et al: Stable cognition after coronary artery bypass grafting: comparisons with percutaneous intervention and normal controls, *Ann Thorac Surg* 82:597-607, 2006.

222. Brouns R, De Deyn PP: Neurological complications in renal failure: A review, *Clin Neurol Neurosurg* 107:1-16, 2004.

223. Kurella M, Chertow GM, Fried LF, et al: Chronic kidney disease and cognitive impairment in the elderly: The Health, Aging, and Body Composition Study, *J Am Soc Nephrol* 16:2127-2133, 2005.

224. Kurella M, Yaffe K, Shlipak MG, et al: Chronic kidney disease and cognitive impairment in menopausal women, *Am J Kidney Dis* 45:66-76, 2005.

225. Kurella TM, Wadley V, Yaffe K, et al: Kidney function and cognitive impairment in US adults: the Reasons for Geographic and Racial Differences in Stroke (REGARDS) Study, *Am J Kidney Dis* 5:227-234, 2008.

226. Elias MF, Elias PK, Seliger SL, et al: Chronic kidney disease, creatinine and cognitive functioning, *Nephrol Dial Transplant* 24:2446-2452, 2009.

227. Hailpern SM, Melamed ML, Cohen HW, Hostetter TH: Moderate chronic kidney disease and cognitive function in adults 20 to 59 years of age: Third National Health and Nutrition Examination Survey (NHANES III), *J Am Soc Nephrol* 18:2205-2213, 2007.

228. Khatri M, Nickolas T, Moon YP, et al: CKD associates with cognitive decline, *J Am Soc Nephrol* 20:2427-2432, 2009.

229. Seliger SL, Siscovick DS, Stehman-Breen CO, et al: Moderate renal impairment and risk of dementia among older adults: The Cardiovascular Health Cognition Study, *J Am Soc Nephrol* 15:1904-1911, 2004.

230. Bunch TJ, Weiss JP, Crandall BG, et al: Atrial fibrillation is independently associated with senile, vascular, and Alzheimer's dementia, *Heart Rhythm* 7:433-437, 2009.

231. Elias MF, Sullivan LM, Elias PK, et al: Atrial fibrillation is associated with lower cognitive performance in the Framingham offspring men, *J Stroke Cerebrovasc Dis* 15:214-222, 2006.

232. Kilander L, Andren B, Nyman H, et al: Atrial fibrillation is an independent determinant of low cognitive function: A cross-sectional study in elderly men, *Stroke* 29:1816-1820, 1998.

233. Ott A, Breteler MM, de Bruyne MC, et al: Atrial fibrillation and dementia in a population-based study. The Rotterdam Study, *Stroke* 28:316-321, 1997.

234. Das RR, Seshadri S, Beiser AS, et al: Prevalence and correlates of silent cerebral infarcts in the Framingham Offspring Study, *Stroke* 39:2929-2935, 2008.

235. Knecht S, Oelschlager C, Duning T, et al: Atrial fibrillation in stroke-free patients is associated with memory impairment and hippocampal atrophy, *Eur Heart J* 29:2125-2132, 2008.

236. Mead GE, Keir S: Association between cognitive impairment and atrial fibrillation: A systematic review, *J Stroke Cerebrovasc Dis* 10:35-43, 2001.

237. Miyasaka Y, Barnes ME, Petersen RC, et al: Risk of dementia in stroke-free patients diagnosed with atrial fibrillation: Data from a community-based cohort, *Eur Heart J* 28:1962-1967, 2007.

238. Laurin D, Masaki KH, White LR, Launer IJ: Ankle-to-brachial index and dementia: The Honolulu-Asia Aging Study, *Circulation* 116:2269-2274, 2007.

239. Newman AB, Fitzpatrick AL, Lopez O, et al: Dementia and Alzheimer's disease incidence in relationship to cardiovascular disease in the Cardiovascular Health Study cohort, *J Am Geriatr Soc* 53:1101-1107, 2005.

240. Hoth KF, Poppas A, Moser DJ, et al: Cardiac dysfunction and cognition in older adults with heart failure, *Cogn Behav Neurol* 21:65-72, 2008.

241. Jefferson AL, Poppas A, Paul RH, Cohen RA: Systemic hypoperfusion is associated with executive dysfunction in geriatric cardiac patients, *Neurobiol Aging* 28:477-483, 2007.

242. Temple RO, Putzke JD, Boll TJ: Neuropsychological performance as a function of cardiac status among heart transplant candidates: A replication, *Percept Mot Skills* 91:821-825, 2000.

243. Brommelhoff JA, Gatz M, Johansson B, et al: Depression as a risk factor or prodromal feature for dementia? Findings in a population-based sample of Swedish twins, *Psychol Aging* 24:373-384, 2009.

244. Camus V, Kraehenbuhl H, Preisig M, et al: Geriatric depression and vascular diseases: what are the links? *J Affect Disord* 81:1-16, 2004.

245. Castilla-Puentes RC, Habeych ME: Subtypes of depression among patients with Alzheimer's disease and other dementias, *Alzheimers Dement* 6:63-69, 2010.

246. Saczynski JS, Beiser A, Seshadri S, et al: Depressive symptoms and risk of dementia: the Framingham Heart Study, *Neurology* 75:35-41, 2010.

247. Price JF, Stewart MC, Deary IJ, et al: Low dose aspirin and cognitive function in middle aged to elderly adults: randomised controlled trial, *BMJ* 337:a1198, 2008.

248. Diener HC, Sacco RL, Yusuf S, et al: Effects of aspirin plus extended-release dipyridamole versus clopidogrel and telmisartan on disability and cognitive function after recurrent stroke in patients with ischaemic stroke in the Prevention Regimen for Effectively Avoiding Second Strokes (PRoFESS) trial: a double-blind, active and placebo-controlled study, *Lancet Neurol* 7:875-884, 2008.

249. Baskys A, Hou AC: Vascular dementia: pharmacological treatment approaches and perspectives, *Clin Interv Aging* 2:327-335, 2007.

250. Nyenhuis DL, Gorelick PB: Diagnosis and management of vascular cognitive impairment, *Curr Atheroscler Rep* 9:326–332, 2007.

251. Dichgans M, Markus HS, Salloway S, et al: Donepezil in patients with subcortical vascular cognitive impairment: a randomised double-blind trial in CADASIL, *Lancet Neurol* 7:310–318, 2008.

252. Burns A, O'Brien J, Auriacombe S, et al: Clinical practice with anti-dementia drugs: a consensus statement from British Association for Psychopharmacology, *J Psychopharmacol* 20:732–755, 2006.

253. Kavirajan H, Schneider LS: Efficacy and adverse effects of cholinesterase inhibitors and memantine in vascular dementia: a meta-analysis of randomised controlled trials, *Lancet Neurol* 6:782–792, 2007.

18 | Stroke Genetics

JAMES F. MESCHIA, DANIEL WOO

The basic terms and concepts of modern genetic epidemiology, reviewed in this introductory section, provide a framework for the chapter. Arguably, one of the most important accomplishments of the late 20th century was completion of the Human Genome Project. With the identification of millions of genetic variations comes the possibility of identifying genetic risk associations for numerous complex traits. This event has served as a catalyst for the field of genetics, which had previously struggled with complex but common traits such as atherosclerosis, diabetes, myocardial infarction, and stroke.

A simple trait refers to a disease (or phenotype) that has a classic mendelian (i.e., autosomal recessive, autosomal dominant, X-linked recessive, or X-linked dominant) or mitochondrial pattern of inheritance. Typically, a mutation in a single gene is both necessary and sufficient for a mendelian disorder to occur. Examples of simple traits are Huntington disease, myotonic dystrophy, and sickle cell disease. A complex trait, however, refers to a disease (or phenotype) that does not follow a simple pattern of inheritance and is the result of multiple factors, including genes. Stroke, cancer, and many other common diseases are highly complex, with multiple interacting genes and environmental risk factors. Other features of complex traits include genetic heterogeneity in which different genes lead to the same disease in different populations and phenotypic variation in which the same disease gene causes different phenotypes in different members of the family. It is this complexity that has made identification of risk genes difficult for these common diseases.

The central dogma of genetics is that DNA is transcribed into RNA, which is then translated into proteins. The genome refers to all the genetic information of an organism that is stored in DNA. Analogously, the transcriptome refers to all the messenger RNA that is transcribed from DNA, and the proteome refers to all the expressed proteins. Autosomes (non–sex chromosomes) are ordered by size, and chromosome 1 is the largest.

At any given location (or locus) in the genome, a genotype may refer to the sequences on the paternal and maternal chromosomes. A polymorphism indicates a genetic variation, and the different variations are called alleles. Numerous types of polymorphisms occur, including single base pair changes called single nucleotide polymorphisms (or SNPs) as well as insertions, deletions, or translocations of a single base pair or sections of DNA. Other types of polymorphisms include variable numbers of tandem repeats (VNTRs), which refer to consecutive repeats of the same nucleotide sequence. Examples of VNTR polymorphisms

are trinucleotide repeats such as those seen in Huntington disease. These are also called *microsatellites*. Although most microsatellites are nonpathogenic, they occur frequently and have multiple alleles. Thus, microsatellites are useful both for forensic identification of individuals and as markers for linkage analysis.

Copy number variations refer to sections of DNA that are copied onto the same section for variable numbers of times. A classic example in neurology occurs at the peripheral myelin protein 22 (*PMP22*) gene, in which the loss of one copy of the gene leads to hereditary neuropathy with liability to pressure palsies; the presence of an extra copy of the gene causes Charcot-Marie-Tooth disease. There may not be an actual variation in the sequence of the gene, but more or less than the usual number of that particular gene or gene segment is present. Several hundred thousand copy number variations have been identified in the genome, although their use as markers for disease has not yet been established.

Two classic methods of identifying risk genes are association studies and linkage studies. Association refers to a polymorphism and a particular phenotype occurring together more often than expected by chance alone. Association is not synonymous with causation, however, and may be related to chance, confounding, or linkage, with a causal variant. The major advantages of association studies are the ability to identify risks of small effect, the ease of collecting cases relative to collecting families, and the ease of genotyping methods.

The other major method for identifying risk genes is through linkage analysis (Fig. 18-1). Mendel's law of independent assortment states that the inheritance pattern of one trait is independent of the inheritance of another. This is true for traits that are on different chromosomes or appreciably separated in physical space on the same chromosome. However, loci that are physically close to one another on the same chromosome will not segregate independently and will instead be inherited together more often than expected by chance.

Evidence for Heritability for Stroke and Its Subtypes

Many lines of evidence support a familial component to stroke risk. A meta-analysis of 53 independent studies found that monozygotic twins were 65% more likely to be concordant for stroke (i.e., both twins having stroke) than dizygotic twins.[1] However, the confidence intervals were broad, and twin studies often failed to differentiate

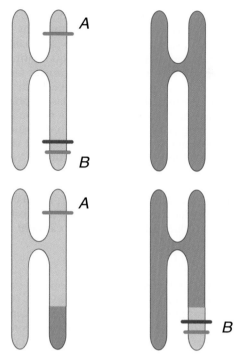

Figure 18-1 Parental chromosomes are shown above, and chromosomes after recombination are shown below. The assumption in this figure is that a stroke mutation occurs on the purple band, but it has not yet been identified. The locations of markers A and B are known. Because B is so much closer to the disease-causing locus than A, it will be inherited along with the trait of stroke more often than A will. Only a recombination event between B and the stroke mutation will lead to the marker not being linked with stroke. A classic example of linkage of traits is hemophilia and color blindness. Neither trait causes the other to occur, but they occur in the same individual more often than expected by chance because the genes responsible for each trait are physically adjacent to one another on the same chromosome. Using this basic phenomenon, one can examine a series of markers across the genome. Even if the marker itself does not lead to disease, if it is close enough to the actual disease-causing gene, it will be inherited more often than expected by chance alone.

ischemic from hemorrhagic stroke. Case–control studies showed that a positive family history of stroke increased the risk of stroke by 76%. One limitation of case–control studies is that case patients with severe strokes may not have survived to be included in the study (survivor bias). Furthermore, case patients might have had recall bias in which experiencing a stroke might trigger memories about family members who had a similar affliction (information bias). Finally, there may have been a tendency not to publish negative results (publication bias). Cohort studies have the advantage of not having the same risk of survivor bias or information bias as case–control studies. It is thus reassuring that cohort studies show that family history of stroke increases the risk of stroke by 30% (95% confidence interval, 20% to 50%).

Probands have a nearly linear increased risk of having a sibling history of stroke with age of the proband at the time of stroke from 55 to 80 years.[2] However, family history of stroke seems to be a greater risk factor for stroke in individuals younger than 70 years compared with older individuals.[1] An overview of 18 family history

TABLE 18-1 PHYSICAL EXAMINATION FINDINGS THAT ARE CLUES TO INHERITED DISORDERS ASSOCIATED WITH CEREBROVASCULAR DISEASES

System	Disease	Findings
Ophthalmologic findings	MELAS	Bilateral cataracts
	Fabry disease	Whorl-like corneal dystrophy
	CCM	Retinal vascular malformations
	Homocystinuria	Ectopia lentis, glaucoma
	Moyamoya disease	Morning glory optic disc
Dermatologic	Fabry disease	Angiokeratoma
Otologic	MELAS	Progressive bilateral sensorineural hearing loss

Abbreviations: CCM, Cerebral cavernous malformation; MELAS, mitochondrial encephalopathy, lactic acidosis, and stroke-like episodes.

studies found that women are more likely than men to have a parental history of stroke.[3] The difference may be explained by the excess maternal history of stroke in women. A positive maternal history of stroke increases the risk of stroke in women by nearly 50% relative to a positive paternal history of stroke. Whether these observations are attributable to genetic, epigenetic, or nongenetic factors is uncertain.

Inherited risk may differ depending on the type of ischemic stroke a patient sustains. A review of two population-based studies from Oxfordshire and three hospital-based studies found that family history of stroke was least frequent in patients with cardioembolic stroke compared with patients with large- or small-vessel stroke or stroke of unknown etiology.[4] Heritability seemed comparable among noncardioembolic etiologies of ischemic stroke. Notably, however, comparable rates of family history of conditions like large-vessel stroke and small-vessel stroke give insight into the magnitude of the heritable component to stroke risk, but these rates do not address whether genetic factors for the various types of ischemic stroke might differ qualitatively; that is, different genetic variants might predispose to different types of ischemic stroke.

Disorders Associated with Ischemic or Hemorrhagic Stroke

Several disorders have cerebrovascular disease as a prominent feature. Stroke is common and typically not associated with an obvious genetic disorder. This, combined with the fact that genetic disorders are so diverse, makes the task of precise diagnosis seem daunting. Targeted gene testing should be done after considering the constellation of physical findings (Table 18-1) and considering patterns of inheritance consistent with a detailed family history (Table 18-2).

Fabry Disease

Fabry disease, also known as angiokeratoma corporis diffusum, is an X-linked recessive disorder caused by reduced activity of the enzyme α-galactosidase. This

TABLE 18-2 PATTERNS OF INHERITANCE FOR DISEASES OR CONDITIONS ASSOCIATED WITH CEREBROVASCULAR DISEASES

Patterns of Inheritance	Disease/Condition
Autosomal dominant	CADASIL
	Cerebral cavernous malformations
	CCM1
	CCM2
	CCM3
	Cerebral amyloid angiopathy
	HCHWA-Dutch type
	HCHWA-Icelandic type
	FAP
	Polycystic kidney disease
	ADPKD 1
	ADPKD 2
Autosomal recessive	Sickle cell disease
	CARASIL
	Homocystinuria
X-linked recessive	Fabry disease
Mitochondrial	MELAS

Abbreviations: ADPKD, Autosomal dominant polycystic kidney disease; CADASIL, cerebral autosomal dominant arteriopathy with subcortical infarcts and leukoencephalopathy; CARASIL, cerebral autosomal recessive arteriopathy with subcortical infarcts and leukoencephalopathy; CCM, cerebral cavernous malformation; FAP, familial amyloid polyneuropathy; HCHWA, hereditary cerebral hemorrhage with amyloidosis; MELAS, mitochondrial encephalopathy, lactic acidosis, and stroke-like episodes.

enzyme is essential to the biodegradation of lipids, and its decreased activity leads to accumulation of lipids in lysosomes in endothelial and vascular smooth muscle cells, where cellular damage may lead to stroke.

Early in life, patients with Fabry disease may present with burning pain or acroparesthesia due to small-fiber sensory neuropathy, corneal clouding (cornea verticillata), or angiokeratomas. Because peripheral neuropathy typically involves only small fibers, it may be missed on routine electromyography. Later in life, the major sequelae of Fabry disease are symptoms of stroke, heart disease, and kidney disease from blood vessel ectasia. Grewal[5] reported a stroke prevalence of 24% in patients with cerebrovascular complications, and six of eight patients had strokes occur before 40 years of age.

Although Fabry disease has traditionally been classified as an X-linked recessive disorder in which males showed complete penetrance and women were carriers, the epidemiology of the disease may be more complex than originally thought. A recent study among 721 German adults aged 18 to 55 years with cryptogenic stroke found that 4.9% of male patients and, surprisingly, 2.4% of female patients had a biologically significant mutation of the α-galactosidase (*GLA*) gene.[6] Among the male patients with stroke, 38.1% demonstrated the typical dolichoectatic vertebrobasilar vessels. Fewer than half the patients studied showed angiokeratomas, acroparesthesia, or cornea verticillata, which suggests wide phenotypic variation. In a study of 103 young patients with cryptogenic stroke in a Belgian population, only three patients had low α-galactosidase activity, and none was found to have a mutation of the α-galactosidase gene.[7]

Diagnosis of Fabry disease can be made by different methods but is done most commonly by measurement of α-galactosidase activity. In some patients, the α-galactosidase level may be normal, and abnormally low activity of the enzyme is the key diagnostic factor. Two recombinant enzyme preparations have been approved for treatment of Fabry disease: agalsidase alpha or beta. Moore et al[8] demonstrated restoration of regional cerebral blood flow among patients treated with enzyme replacement, and subsequent studies demonstrated reversal of elevated cerebral blood flow velocities. In 2007, a randomized, double-blind, placebo-controlled trial demonstrated that intravenous infusion of agalsidase delayed the time to first clinical event (hazard ratio, 0.47; $P = 0.06$).[9] Some studies suggest that the development of antibodies to the treatment may reduce the efficacy of treatment.[10]

CADASIL

Cerebral autosomal dominant arteriopathy with subcortical infarcts and leukoencephalopathy (CADASIL) is caused by mutations of the *NOTCH3* receptor gene on chromosome 19 and is on the same locus as familial hemiplegic migraine. *NOTCH3* expression occurs almost exclusively in smooth muscle cells, and mutations of the receptor lead to accumulation of the protein. Pathologically, granular osmiophilic material accumulates in the smooth muscle of vessels, which leads to smooth muscle degeneration and, ultimately, subcortical leukoencephalopathy. Magnetic resonance imaging (MRI), positron emission tomography, and transcranial Doppler (TCD) studies have demonstrated reduced cerebral blood flow in the white matter.[11-14]

The mean age of onset of symptoms is in the later part of the fourth decade, although the condition may be detectable by MRI years earlier.[15] More than 85% of patients have migraine headaches, and transient ischemic attacks (TIAs) and mood disorders are also common at presentation. Classic lacunar stroke syndromes may occur in two thirds of patients. A patient with progressive leukoencephalopathy, particularly a young patient without hypertension or other reason for leukoencephalopathy, should prompt a search for CADASIL. In patients with CADASIL, brain MRI scans show T2-weighted hyperintensities occurring symmetrically in the white matter and deep gray nuclei. Small lacunar lesions immediately subcortical in the anterior temporal lobes have been reported to be 100% specific and 59% sensitive for CADASIL.[16]

Genetic testing is available but may require extensive sequencing of the large *NOTCH3* gene, which contains 33 exons. Identification of granular osmiophilic material in vascular tissue from biopsy specimens from skin, muscle, or peripheral nerves in the appropriate clinical setting of premature white matter ischemic strokes, dementia, and migraine may be sufficient to make the diagnosis.

No specific treatment is considered standard in patients with CADASIL, although some studies suggest that treatment with acetazolamide may improve cerebral hemodynamics.[11] An 18-week randomized, double-blind, placebo-controlled trial of donepezil at a daily dose of 10 mg was performed in the hope of enhancing cognition.[17] A total of 168 patients, mean age of 54.8 years, were enrolled. There was no significant improvement in the primary outcome, performance on the Vascular-Alzheimer's Disease Assessment Scale cognitive subscale (V-ADAS-cog). However, significant improvements were noted in Trail-Making Tests, parts A and B, and on the Executive Interview 25 (EXIT25).

CARASIL

Cerebral autosomal recessive arteriopathy with subcortical infarcts and leukoencephalopathy (CARASIL) is a distinct clinical entity that appears to predominantly affect individuals of Japanese ancestry, although a Chinese pedigree has been reported.[18] The condition is also known as Maeda syndrome. Subcortical encephalopathy leads to psychomotor deterioration when patients are in their 20s and 30s. Migraine is not a feature. Distinctive extracerebral manifestations of the disease that often predate the neurologic presentation include alopecia, herniation of vertebral disks, and spondylosis deformans. T2-weighted MRI shows extensive areas of hyperintensity in the hemispheric white matter and less dramatic changes in the thalami and pons.[19] The white matter changes occur without significant hypertension. Pathologically, there is severe widespread loss of arterial medial smooth muscle cells. Sclerotic changes are infrequent compared with CADASIL.[20] Also, unlike CADASIL, abnormal vessels are not periodic acid-Schiff stain–positive.[19]

Homocystinuria

The most common inherited form of elevated homocystine is attributable to cystathionine β-synthase deficiency and is referred to as homocystinuria. It should be noted that several conditions may lead to elevated homocystine levels. The trait is inherited in an autosomal recessive pattern; thus, both parents are typically asymptomatic carriers. It was first described in 1962 when elevated homocystine levels were identified in the serum and urine of mentally retarded patients; the enzymatic defect was reported several years later.[21-23]

Patients with homocystinuria are typically divided between those who respond to vitamin B_6 (pyridoxine) supplementation and those who do not. In 1985, Mudd et al[24] reported on 629 patients with homocystinuria; by the age of 10 years, 55% of vitamin B_6–responsive patients and 82% of vitamin B_6–unresponsive patients had dislocated lenses. Along with Marfan syndrome, syphilis, and trauma, homocystinuria is one of the major diagnostic considerations in a patient with dislocation of the lens of the eye.[24] Also similar to patients with Marfan disease, those with homocystinuria may develop skeletal abnormalities such as long limbs, tall height, pectus excavatum (caved chest) or pectus carinatum (pigeon chest), and arachnodactyly.

Classically, homocystinuria patients have the dermatologic features of thin blonde hair, a malar flush, and livedo reticularis. Without treatment, mental retardation may occur in two thirds of patients.[24] Elevated homocystine levels are associated with both thrombotic and embolic strokes, which occur by the age of 15 years in 12% of vitamin B_6–responsive patients and in 27% of vitamin B_6–unresponsive patients.[24] Stroke occurs in more than 60% of patients with homocystinuria by the age of 40 years.[24]

As already mentioned, diagnosis is typically made by identification of elevated levels of homocystine, and routine testing at birth can identify patients at an early age. Restriction of methionine and supplementation of vitamin B_6 are recommended as treatment.

MELAS

The syndrome of mitochondrial encephalopathy, lactic acidosis, and stroke-like episodes (MELAS) is caused by mutations in mitochondrial DNA. As with other mitochondrial disorders, it is inherited in a maternal pattern. Clinical criteria for making the diagnosis include stroke before the age of 40 years, encephalopathy characterized by seizures or dementia, and blood lactic acidosis or ragged red fibers on skeletal muscle pathologic examination.[25] Brain MRI typically shows lesions involving the occipital lobes. The lesions often do not respect the boundaries of named vascular territories. MELAS mutations cause impairment in the respiratory chain enzymes, particularly complex I. Eighty percent of cases are caused by a substitution mutation (A3243G) in the gene encoding for transfer RNA (tRNA)$^{Leu(UUR)}$. Other substitution mutations and deletions have also been described.[26,27]

There is no proven treatment for MELAS. However, seizures, which can be a manifestation of the condition, should not be treated with valproic acid because this agent has caused a paradoxic reaction in some patients.[28]

Sickle Cell Anemia

Sickle cell anemia is vital to recognize because it is a condition affecting the young for which there is overwhelming evidence of efficacious therapy. It is an autosomal recessive disorder, whereby valine is substituted for glutamic acid at position 6 of the β-polypeptide chain of hemoglobin.

The mutation causes polymerization or aggregation of abnormal hemoglobin within red blood cells, inducing the sickling change in the shape of the red cells. Patients typically have compensated hemolytic anemia, mild jaundice, and vaso-occlusive crises that cause excruciating pain in the back, chest, and extremities. Stroke is also a major complication of sickle cell disease.

The condition is most prevalent among patients of African origin. In untreated populations, sickle cell disease is seen with stroke, typically in elementary school–aged patients. In the Cooperative Study of Sickle Cell Disease (CSSCD), a multicenter cohort study of approximately 4000 patients followed up from the late 1970s to the late 1980s, the first incidence peak for stroke was between the ages of 2 and 5 years.[29] The cumulative risks of the first stroke were 11% by the age of 20 years and 24% by the age of 45 years. The proportion of ischemic stroke compared with hemorrhagic stroke varies according to patient age at presentation. In patients younger than 20 years, most strokes are ischemic; after the age of 20 years, most strokes are hemorrhagic.

Moyamoya syndrome is associated with sickle cell disease and is a risk factor for stroke. Accordingly, vasculopathy causing proximal intracranial arterial stenosis shows elevated velocities on TCD. The CSSCD identified dactylitis, severe anemia, and leukocytosis in very young children as risk factors for adverse outcomes, including death, stroke, and pain crises. However, these risk factors, when tested in a more current series of newborns and young children in the Dallas Newborn Cohort (DNC), were found to have poor clinical utility.[30] All children in the DNC received prophylactic penicillin, which may account for the different findings. Stroke remained the most frequent adverse event documented in both the DNC and the CSSCD. Neither cohort reflects the recent impact imparted by TCD screening on natural history.

The Stroke Prevention in Sickle Cell Disease trial, known as the STOP trial, definitively established that transfusion therapy dramatically reduces the risk of recurrent stroke in high-risk patients, where "high risk" was defined predominately by values on TCD studies.[31] In STOP, approximately 2000 children between the ages of 2 and 6 years old underwent TCD screening to detect blood flow velocities consistent with intracranial stenosis. Approximately 9% of those screened had time-averaged mean blood flow velocities in excess of 200 cm/s in either the middle cerebral artery or the internal carotid artery on either the right or the left side. Patients were randomly assigned either to episodic blood transfusion in accordance with the standard of care or to long-term transfusion therapy, intended to reduce hemoglobin S levels to a target of less than 30% of total hemoglobin. The aggressive transfusion protocol was clearly more efficacious, and, in fact, the study was stopped early as a result.

In the follow-up study known as STOP2, patients whose TCD blood flow velocities normalized after a 30-month transfusion program had a high rate of stroke and reversion to abnormal velocities with discontinuation of transfusion. Long-term aggressive transfusion therapy is not easily tolerated. Children must receive transfusions approximately once monthly to achieve the target hemoglobin S level consistent with the STOP study (<30% of total hemoglobin). Long-term transfusion therapy puts patients at risk of iron overload. Because of the complexities of transfusion therapy, patients typically are monitored by a pediatric neurologist and a pediatric hematologist with experience in treating patients with sickle cell disease. The efficacy of long-term transfusion therapy for preventing recurrent stroke has been less well studied. However, in defense of transfusion therapy as a means of secondary prevention, the STOP trial showed that transfusion therapy lowered the risk of new silent infarction or stroke in the 37% of patients who had clinically silent cerebral infarctions on baseline brain MRI.[32]

Other therapies beyond transfusion therapy have been tested with variable success. Myeloablative stem cell transplantation is an appealing alternative therapy.[33] In a series of 87 patients treated with allogeneic hematopoietic stem cell transplant, no individual who had successful engraftment developed stroke or silent ischemic lesions. Of further encouragement, arterial velocities were significantly reduced 1 year after transplantation. It should be noted, however, that patients who undergo such transplants are at risk of seizures and posterior reversible leukoencephalopathy as adverse effects of cyclosporine and corticosteroid therapy, and female children are at risk of ovarian failure.

Hydroxyurea has also been tested. Long-term observational follow-up in the multicenter study of hydroxyuria in sickle cell anemia showed that the risk of stroke was not substantially altered by treatment of hydroxyuria in adults with sickle cell anemia.[34] In contrast, hydroxyuria has been shown to reduce TCD velocities in children with sickle cell anemia.[35]

Fibromuscular Dysplasia

Fibromuscular dysplasia (FMD) is usually regarded as a sporadic condition that often remains subclinical. Cerebral angiography often shows the so-called stack-of-coins or string-of-beads appearance. Nevertheless, this nonatherosclerotic noninflammatory condition can lead to carotid dissection and stroke along with renovascular hypertension. Segregation analysis of pedigrees with renovascular FMD using echotracking of the carotid arteries found evidence supporting autosomal inheritance.[36] High-resolution echotracking can detect supernumerary interfaces, referred to as the triple signal pattern.[37] In one pediatric stroke series, FMD was associated with 7% of stroke cases. FMD may be a risk factor for both carotid dissection and its recurrence.[38] Stenting can be performed with minimal risk, but the long-term benefits of such a procedure remain to be established.[39]

FMD is also part of Grange syndrome. In the originally described pedigree with Grange syndrome, patients had stenosis or occlusion of renal, abdominal, and cerebral arteries, congenital cardiac defects, brachydactyly (particularly of the second and fifth digits), syndactyly, bone fragility, and learning disabilities.[40]

Collagen Type IV Alpha 1 Mutations

An autosomal dominant stroke syndrome causing small-vessel disease and cerebral hemorrhaging is caused by mutations in the collagen type IV alpha 1 (COL4A1) gene.[41] In addition to the stroke syndrome, mutations are associated with infantile spasms and porencephaly. Ophthalmoscopy may reveal tortuosity of retinal vessels. As in patients with CADASIL, brain MRI findings include leukoaraiosis, microbleeding on gradient imaging, and lacunes. Dilated perivascular spaces can also be prominent in COL4A1 disorders. Recurrent intracranial hemorrhages have been observed.[42] Early diagnosis is clinically advantageous because patients can be advised to avoid behaviors that would put them at risk of hemorrhaging. Putative risk factors include parturition, sports-related head trauma, and anticoagulation therapy.

Hypercoagulable Disorders

Because ischemic stroke is believed to be predominantly the result of thrombotic occlusion, it is not surprising that inherited thrombophilias have been studied in relation to stroke. Well-recognized thrombophilias include deficiency of protein C, deficiency of protein S, deficiency of antithrombin III, the factor V Leiden point mutation, and the prothrombin G20210A point mutation. Primary protein C, protein S, and antithrombin III deficiencies are challenging to diagnose in patients immediately after stroke. Acute measurements can be misleading. Warfarin and vitamin K deficiency lower protein C and protein S blood levels. Heparin lowers antithrombin III levels. Levels that are found to be low initially in the early poststroke period should be verified as persistently low more than 1 month after the stroke and in the absence of an active infection. Primary protein C, protein S, and antithrombin III deficiencies are uncommon and have only a tenuous association with adult ischemic stroke. Factor V Leiden (the most common cause of activated protein C deficiency) and prothrombin G20210A, determined by gene tests, can be measured with equal validity in the acute or chronic phases of stroke. A meta-analysis of candidate gene association studies shows that these genes likely impart a modest increased risk of ischemic stroke.[43] All of these thrombophilic states have been shown to have unequivocal association with venous thrombosis.

No clear guidelines describe the most appropriate time to perform these tests when a patient with stroke is evaluated. It is likely that the tests are overused. The tests have the highest yields in cases of pediatric stroke and cerebral venous thrombosis.[44]

Moyamoya Disease

Moyamoya disease, also known as spontaneous occlusion of the circle of Willis, is characterized by stenosis or occlusion of the temporal portions in the internal carotid artery bilaterally in the presence of an abnormal vascular network near the arterial occlusion. The disease has its highest prevalence in Japan. An epidemiologic study of moyamoya disease, based on *International Classification of Diseases, Ninth Revision* codes from Washington State and California, showed an overall incidence of 0.086 per 100,000 individuals.[45] Although this incidence was lower than the 0.35 per 100,000 rate found in the National Japanese Survey,[46] the incidence of moyamoya disease was comparable in Asian Americans in California and native Japanese. Racial-ethnic predilection of at least five chromosomal regions has been linked to moyamoya disease in Japanese populations.[47] These regions are 3p24.2-p26, 6q25, 8q23, 12p12, and 17q25. The genes that underlie these familial predilections remain to be defined.

Moyamoya disease is diagnosed on the basis of conventional angiographic findings. Other radiologic studies are helpful in delineating the extent of neovascularization and pathophysiologic disturbances in blood flow. High-field imaging such as 3.0-T time-of-flight magnetic resonance angiography (MRA) appears more sensitive in the detection of moyamoya vessels than 1.5-T imaging.[48] Steno-occlusive arteries show proliferation of smooth muscle cells and permanently tortuous, often-duplicated internal elastic lamina.[49]

MRI techniques can detect asymptomatic microbleeding in more than 40% of individuals with moyamoya disease.[50] Surgical pathology specimens of microbleeding indicate a correspondence to arteries and some arterioles with disrupted internal elastic lamina surrounding a small hemorrhage.[51] Computed tomographic angiography (CTA) can reveal a false "spot sign" in patients with moyamoya disease.[52]

A prospective study of 50 consecutive patients with moyamoya disease found that multiple instances of microbleeding detected on 3-T MRI scans successfully predicted the likelihood of subsequent intracranial hemorrhaging.[53] Surgical management consists of two different approaches: direct revascularization and indirect revascularization. Direct techniques include superficial temporal artery–to–middle cerebral artery bypass. Indirect techniques include pial synangiosis. Pial synangiosis generally carries a favorable prognosis in patients with recurrent stroke or in pediatric patients with TIA.[54]

No randomized clinical trial to study surgical intervention has yet been completed. However, the protocol for a Japanese multicenter, prospective, randomized clinical trial of extracranial-to-intracranial bypass to treat adult patients with moyamoya disease with several episodes of intracranial bleeding has been published.[55]

In addition to moyamoya disease, there is moyamoya syndrome, which occurs secondary to a systemic condition. Although the list of rare conditions associated with moyamoya vascular abnormalities is quite long, the most common include neurofibromatosis, tuberous sclerosis, and sickle cell anemia. In addition to these single-gene disorders, children with exposure to external-beam radiotherapy reportedly are at risk of developing moyamoya syndrome.[56]

The presence of moyamoya syndrome roughly doubles the risk of cerebrovascular events in patients with sickle cell disease.[57] Consensus does not exist regarding the screening of first-degree relatives of patients with moyamoya disease. A small study in Japan argued in favor of MRA screening of asymptomatic relatives of patients with moyamoya disease.[58] A multicenter Japanese study has shown that asymptomatic moyamoya disease is not benign; the study showed the annual risk for stroke was 3.2%.[59]

Asymptomatic patients may be seen with so-called morning glory disc anomaly, which is characterized by spoke-like vessels radiating outward from the edge of an anomalous optic disc. Typically, morning glory disc is seen unilaterally and is twice as common in females as it is in males. It has been argued that MRA or CTA should be performed in any patient, typically a child between the ages of 2 and 12 years, to detect vascular or structural brain abnormalities, including moyamoya disease.[60]

Mendelian CAAs

Cerebral amyloid angiopathy (CAA) is the chief manifestation of some rare single-gene disorders. Hereditary cerebral hemorrhaging with amyloidosis of the Dutch type (HCHWA-D) is an autosomal dominant condition caused by a point mutation in the amyloid precursor protein *(APP)* gene. A glutamine is substituted for glutamic acid at position 22 of *APP,* which is the result of a point mutation at base position number 693. Mutations within the coding region of the *APP* gene cause intracerebral hemorrhaging, whereas mutations in the noncoding region of the *APP* gene cause Alzheimer's disease (AD). About two thirds of HCHWA-D patients are seen with intracerebral hemorrhaging, and the remainder are seen with vascular dementia.

A mutation substituting glutamine for leucine at position 68 (C68Q) in the cystatin C (*CST3*) gene causes hereditary cerebral hemorrhaging with amyloidosis of the Icelandic type (HCHWA-I).[61] This amino acid substitution destabilizes α-helical structures, exposing tryptophan residue to a more polar environment. This mutant protein with a more open structure is more amyloidogenic, that is, more prone to form insoluble β-pleated sheets.[62] About 17% of patients in Iceland who have stroke before the age of 35 years have stroke due to HCHWA-I.[63] Most HCHWA-I patients experience their first stroke before the age of 30 years and die before the age of 50 years.

Mutations in the transthyretin (*TTR*) gene usually manifest as small fiber sensory and autonomic familial polyneuropathy. In rare instances, point mutations can result in cerebral hemorrhaging. A mutation of Phe64Ser causes oculoleptomeningeal amyloidosis and cerebral hemorrhaging.[64,65] Mutation Val30Met has caused intracerebral hemorrhaging in one autopsy-confirmed case.[66] Gly53glu caused recurrent subarachnoid hemorrhaging in siblings of one family.[67]

Mendelian Cerebral Cavernous Malformation Syndromes

Cerebral cavernous malformations (CCMs) can be sporadic or dominantly inherited. They have a prevalence of 0.1% to 0.5% in the general population. These lesions are often detected incidentally on MRI studies. They can act as an ictal focus or a nidus for cerebral hemorrhaging. Three familial CCM syndromes have been defined molecularly.

CCM1 is caused by various mutations in the *KRIT1* gene, which encodes for the Krev interaction trapped 1 protein. *KRIT1* mutations include frame shift, nonsense, missense, and splice-junction mutations. Frame shifts account for half the observed mutations. *KRIT1* is thought to be a tumor suppressor gene. The *KRIT1* mutations have high rates of incomplete clinical and radiographic penetrance. In a study of 33 *KRIT1* mutation carriers from several families, 57.6% had no symptoms.[68] Of symptom-free carriers, 82.3% had CCM lesions detected on MRI.

CCM2 is caused by mutations in the *CCM2* gene, which encodes for malcavernin, a phosphotyrosine binding protein. There is an intriguing potential pathophysiologic link between CCM1 and CCM2. Malcavernin binds to 2 NPXY motifs in the KRIT1 protein. NPXY stands for an amino acid motif of asparagine, proline, an undetermined/variable amino acid, and tyrosine.

CCM3 is caused by mutations in the programmed cell death 10 (*PDCD10*) gene.[69] A case of CCM3 with cerebral and multiple spinal cavernous malformations has been described.[70]

Autosomal Dominant Polycystic Kidney Disease

Neurologists need to be familiar with autosomal dominant polycystic kidney disease (ADPKD) because patients with ADPKD are at substantially increased risk of intracranial aneurysms relative to the general population. The prevalence of intracranial aneurysms in patients with ADPKD is 4% to 12% compared with about 1% in the general population. Furthermore, segregation analysis suggests that ADPKD is a risk factor for subarachnoid hemorrhaging due to ruptured aneurysm.[71] A consensus does not exist on the optimal imaging protocol for aneurysm screening. A study of Japanese patients with ADPKD found that serial MRA studies detected new intracranial aneurysms in 2 of 15 patients over the course of 18 to 72 months of follow-up.[72]

Hereditary Hemorrhagic Telangiectasia

Epistaxis, telangiectasia, and a positive family history are the clinical triad characterizing hereditary hemorrhagic telangiectasia (HHT), also known as Osler-Weber-Rendu syndrome. HHT is inherited as an autosomal dominant condition. HHT causes vascular malformations involving the lung, liver, brain, and gastrointestinal tract. Two types of HHT have been defined molecularly. HHT1 is caused by mutations in the endoglin (*ENG*) gene. HHT2 is caused by mutations in the activin A receptor type II–like 1 (*ACVRL1*) gene. Endoglin and ACVRL1 are cell surface receptors involved in the transforming growth factor-β pathway. Both types of HHT appear to be the result of haploinsufficiency. Mutations in the genes lead to a reduction in the number of wild-type receptors on vascular endothelial cells.

Interestingly, although HHT causes vascular malformations, ischemic cerebrovascular disease is more common than hemorrhaging in this population. In a series of more than 300 patients, just over 2% were seen with intracranial hemorrhages.[73] In contrast, nearly 30% had experienced either cerebral infarction or TIA. Acute ischemic cerebrovascular disease in this setting is often attributed to paradoxic embolism of thrombi or septic emboli by way of syndromic pulmonary arteriovenous malformations. Patients with infarction or TIA should be screened for pulmonary arteriovenous malformations, and if detected, these lesions should be considered as possible targets for ablation.

HERNS

Patients with HERNS, the syndrome of hereditary endotheliopathy, retinopathy, nephropathy, and stroke, are usually seen with visual impairment and renal dysfunction.[74] Findings on ophthalmologic examination include macular edema with capillary dropout and perifoveal microangiopathic telangectasias. Urinalysis may detect hematuria and proteinuria. Neurologically, patients can experience migraine headaches, strokes, and psychiatric symptoms. Contrast-enhancing subcortical lesions can be seen on brain imaging studies.

Genome-wide Association Studies

Genome-wide association studies (GWASs) use markers along the entire genome to identify risk genes and are known as hypothesis-free approaches. Single base pair changes or SNPs make up about 90% of all human genetic variation and occur frequently throughout the genome (1 in every 200 to 300 bases).[75] SNPs in physical proximity on the same chromosome are more likely to be inherited together than SNPs that are farther apart. Linkage disequilibrium is a measure of this nonrandom correlation between markers. Thus, if a disease-predisposing polymorphism is close to a SNP used as a marker, then the marker is associated with the disease proportional to the degree of linkage disequilibrium between them. With current technology, more than 90% of the genome among white people and black people is within a reasonable degree of linkage disequilibrium to available markers on standard genotyping sets.

GWASs aim to identify regions of interest throughout the genome that may harbor disease-predisposing polymorphisms, by comparing genotypes of case patients and control subjects at specific marker SNPs distributed across the genome. GWASs are based on two assumptions: (1) a patient with disease will carry a disease-predisposing polymorphism more commonly than will a control individual; and (2) specific alleles at nearby marker SNPs, inherited in conjunction with this disease-predisposing polymorphism, will also be more common in case patients than in control subjects. GWASs provide greater power to detect small-to-moderate disease-risk alleles than linkage study designs.

Several GWASs of ischemic stroke have identified isolated associations with ischemic stroke, including those at chromosome 12p13.[76] A review of eight stroke GWASs in 2010 noted that no single locus has been identified in two GWASs at a genome-wide significance level.[77] Larger studies and meta-analyses are ongoing, with the hope of developing new treatments and identifying novel risk factors that may increase the understanding of the biology of stroke.

Apolipoprotein E and Intracerebral Hemorrhage

Although once considered to be a rare cause of lobar hemorrhaging, CAA is now recognized as an important if not a predominant cause of lobar hemorrhaging in the elderly.[78-80] Its principal pathologic feature is the deposition of amyloid protein in the media and adventitia of leptomeningeal arteries, arterioles, capillaries, and, less often, veins.[78-82] CAA occurs in 50% to 79% of patients with AD.[83,84] A number of studies have associated apolipoprotein (Apo)E2, ApoE4, or both with CAA or lobar intracerebral hemorrhaging. McCarron and Nicoll[85] reported that the risk of ApoE2 with CAA occurred among subjects with and without AD, while the association of ApoE4 with CAA correlated with concomitant AD. This finding suggested that ApoE2 is a specific risk factor for CAA-related hemorrhaging, while ApoE4 is related to CAA in general.

When APP is cleaved by α-secretase, a transmembrane portion of the protein is left, ranging in length from 37 to 42 amino acids. Researchers have found that the β-amyloid 42 level is significantly elevated in AD patients and their first-degree relatives.[86] McCarron et al[87] reported that patients with CAA-related hemorrhaging were more reactive to β-amyloid 42. Rosand et al[88] reported an association of ApoE2 among 41 patients with warfarin-related intracerebral hemorrhaging compared with 66 control subjects in which 7 of 11 subjects had

pathologic evidence of CAA. In animal models, knock-in mice with human ApoE4 developed amyloid plaques as well as CAA, whereas ApoE3 knock-in mice resulted in almost no CAA or parenchymal plaques.[89]

Initial reports suggested that as many as 60% of lobar hemorrhage cases may have evidence of petechial hemorrhaging on gradient-echo MRI.[90] In addition, the technique detects new hemorrhages in 47% of cases of probable CAA.[91] Roob et al[92] reported that evidence of previous petechial hemorrhaging could be found in 6.4% of otherwise healthy elderly individuals and may therefore be a means of detecting early disease. In a study of 1062 persons from Rotterdam, the overall prevalence of microbleeding ranged from 17.8% among those aged 60 to 69 years to 38.3% for those older than 80 years, and ApoE4 carriers had more strictly lobar microbleeding than noncarriers.[93]

Despite the numerous reports of association, however, changes in management based on the results of genetic testing are not currently recommended, although some studies suggest that an increased risk of intracerebral hemorrhaging with anticoagulant treatment may occur, which may lead to eventual changes in management.[88]

Genetic Risk Factors for Common Ischemic Stroke

Clinical testing is available for gene variants associated recently with ischemic stroke. One example is a SNP-based test for variants on chromosome 4q25 that were first identified as associated with atrial fibrillation.[94] This locus was subsequently associated with ischemic stroke and most strongly associated with cardioembolic stroke. It has been postulated that identifying risk variants in individuals with ischemic stroke and sinus rhythm might justify long-term cardiac monitoring in an attempt to identify intermittent atrial fibrillation.[95]

Clinical testing is also available for gene variants on a locus on chromosome 9p21.3 that were first robustly associated with myocardial infarction. A meta-analysis involving 4645 patients with myocardial infarction or coronary artery disease showed that the risk allele (the C allele) of the lead SNP, rs1333049, increased the odds ratio per copy of the risk allele by 1.29.[96] Association of the chromosome 9p21.3 locus with ischemic stroke was demonstrated.[97] Studies are under way to determine whether the association of this locus with stroke is specific for large-vessel atherosclerotic stroke.

Genetics for Optimizing Drug Therapy

Genetic testing is likely to play a larger role in optimizing the care of patients at risk of stroke. Warfarin anticoagulation therapy is a highly effective means of preventing ischemic stroke in patients with atrial fibrillation. Genetic variants in the vitamin K epoxide reductase complex subunit 1 (*VKORC1*) and cytochrome P450, family 2, subfamily C, polypeptide 9 (*CYP2C9*) genes have been associated with the wide interindividual variability associated with warfarin dosing. Genomic studies predict that other genetic variants are unlikely to contribute in a major way to warfarin variability.[98] The finding that only two genes explain most of the variability of warfarin dosing should simplify converting knowledge of pharmacogenetics for warfarin into practical clinical tools. Small randomized trials show that multivariate gene-based warfarin dosing appears feasible and safe.[99,100] Larger studies are required to determine whether genetically refined dosing regimens translate into improved patient outcomes.[101]

Statins are effective for reducing risk of first-time and recurrent stroke. One potentially serious adverse effect is myopathy. Recently, a SNP in the *SLCO1B1* gene, rs4363657, has been associated with statin-induced myopathy.[102] The odds ratio for myopathy was 4.5 for each copy of the C allele. This allele is present in 15% of the population. Testing for this SNP could lead to avoidance of the complication of myopathy.

REFERENCES

1. Flossmann E, Schulz UG, Rothwell PM: Systematic review of methods and results of studies of the genetic epidemiology of ischemic stroke, *Stroke* 35:212-227, 2004.
2. Meschia JF, Atkinson EJ, O'Brien PC, et al: Familial clustering of stroke according to proband age at onset of presenting ischemic stroke, *Stroke* 34:e89-91, 2003.
3. Touze E, Rothwell PM: Sex differences in heritability of ischemic stroke: A systematic review and meta-analysis, *Stroke* 39:16-23, 2008.
4. Schulz UG, Flossmann E, Rothwell PM: Heritability of ischemic stroke in relation to age, vascular risk factors, and subtypes of incident stroke in population-based studies, *Stroke* 35:819-824, 2004.
5. Grewal RP: Stroke in Fabry's disease, *J Neurol* 241:153-156, 1994.
6. Rolfs A, Bottcher T, Zschiesche M, et al: Prevalence of Fabry disease in patients with cryptogenic stroke: A prospective study, *Lancet* 366:1794-1796, 2005.
7. Brouns R, Sheorajpanday R, Braxel E, et al: Middelheim Fabry Study (MiFaS): A retrospective Belgian study on the prevalence of Fabry disease in young patients with cryptogenic stroke, *Clin Neurol Neurosurg* 109:479-484, 2007.
8. Moore DF, Altarescu G, Herscovitch P, et al: Enzyme replacement reverses abnormal cerebrovascular responses in Fabry disease, *BMC Neurol* 2:4, 2002.
9. Banikazemi M, Bultas J, Waldek S, et al: Agalsidase-beta therapy for advanced Fabry disease: A randomized trial, *Ann Intern Med* 146:77-86, 2007.
10. Linthorst GE, Hollak CE, Donker-Koopman WE, et al: Enzyme therapy for Fabry disease: Neutralizing antibodies toward agalsidase alpha and beta, *Kidney Int* 66:1589-1595, 2004.
11. Chabriat H, Pappata S, Ostergaard L, et al: Cerebral hemodynamics in CADASIL before and after acetazolamide challenge assessed with MRI bolus tracking, *Stroke* 31:1904-1912, 2000.
12. Tuominen S, Miao Q, Kurki T, et al: Positron emission tomography examination of cerebral blood flow and glucose metabolism in young CADASIL patients, *Stroke* 35:1063-1067, 2004.
13. van den Boom R, Lesnik Oberstein SA, Ferrari MD, et al: Cerebral autosomal dominant arteriopathy with subcortical infarcts and leukoencephalopathy: MR imaging findings at different ages: 3rd-6th decades, *Radiology* 229:683-690, 2003.
14. Liebetrau M, Herzog J, Kloss CU, et al: Prolonged cerebral transit time in CADASIL: A transcranial ultrasound study, *Stroke* 33:509-512, 2002.
15. Dichgans M, Mayer M, Uttner I, et al: The phenotypic spectrum of CADASIL: Clinical findings in 102 cases, *Ann Neurol* 44:731-739, 1998.
16. van Den Boom R, Lesnik Oberstein SA, van Duinen SG, et al: Subcortical lacunar lesions: An MR imaging finding in patients with cerebral autosomal dominant arteriopathy with subcortical infarcts and leukoencephalopathy, *Radiology* 224:791-796, 2002.
17. Dichgans M, Markus HS, Salloway S, et al: Donepezil in patients with subcortical vascular cognitive impairment: A randomised double-blind trial in CADASIL, *Lancet Neurol* 7:310-318, 2008.
18. Zheng DM, Xu FF, Gao Y, et al: A Chinese pedigree of cerebral autosomal recessive arteriopathy with subcortical infarcts and leukoencephalopathy (CARASIL): clinical and radiological features, *J Clin Neurosci* 16:847-849, 2009.
19. Yanagawa S, Ito N, Arima K, et al: Cerebral autosomal recessive arteriopathy with subcortical infarcts and leukoencephalopathy, *Neurology* 58:817-820, 2002.
20. Oide T, Nakayama H, Yanagawa S, et al: Extensive loss of arterial medial smooth muscle cells and mural extracellular matrix in cerebral autosomal recessive arteriopathy with subcortical infarcts and leukoencephalopathy (CARASIL), *Neuropathology* 28:132-142, 2008.
21. Carson NA, Neill DW: Metabolic abnormalities detected in a survey of mentally backward individuals in Northern Ireland, *Arch Dis Child* 37:505-513, 1962.
22. Gerritsen T, Vaughn JG, Waisman HA: The identification of homocystine in the urine, *Biochem Biophys Res Commun* 9:493-496, 1962.
23. Mudd SH, Finkelstein JD, Irreverre F, et al: Homocystinuria: An enzymatic defect, *Science* 143:1443-1445, 1964.
24. Mudd SH, Skovby F, Levy HL, et al: The natural history of homocystinuria due to cystathionine beta-synthase deficiency, *Am J Hum Genet* 37:1-31, 1985.
25. Hirano M, Pavlakis SG: Mitochondrial myopathy, encephalopathy, lactic acidosis, and strokelike episodes (MELAS): Current concepts, *J Child Neurol* 9:4-13, 1994.
26. Ciafaloni E, Ricci E, Shanske S, et al: MELAS: Clinical features, biochemistry, and molecular genetics, *Ann Neurol* 31:391-398, 1992.
27. Goto Y, Nonaka I, Horai S: A new mtDNA mutation associated with mitochondrial myopathy, encephalopathy, lactic acidosis and stroke-like episodes (MELAS), *Biochim Biophys Acta* 1097:238-240, 1991.
28. Lam CW, Lau CH, Williams JC, et al: Mitochondrial myopathy, encephalopathy, lactic acidosis and stroke-like episodes (MELAS) triggered by valproate therapy, *Eur J Pediatr* 156:562-564, 1997.
29. Ohene-Frempong K, Weiner SJ, Sleeper LA, et al: Cerebrovascular accidents in sickle cell disease: Rates and risk factors, *Blood* 91:288-294, 1998.
30. Quinn CT, Lee NJ, Shull EP, et al: Prediction of adverse outcomes in children with sickle cell anemia: A study of the Dallas Newborn Cohort, *Blood* 111:544-548, 2008.
31. Adams RJ, McKie VC, Hsu L, et al: Prevention of a first stroke by transfusions in children with sickle cell anemia and abnormal results on transcranial Doppler ultrasonography, *N Engl J Med* 339:5-11, 1998.
32. Pegelow CH, Wang W, Granger S, et al: Silent infarcts in children with sickle cell anemia and abnormal cerebral artery velocity, *Arch Neurol* 58:2017-2021, 2001.
33. Bernaudin F, Socie G, Kuentz M, et al: Long-term results of related myeloablative stem-cell transplantation to cure sickle cell disease, *Blood* 110:2749-2756, 2007.
34. Steinberg MH, Barton F, Castro O, et al: Effect of hydroxyurea on mortality and morbidity in adult sickle cell anemia: Risks and benefits up to 9 years of treatment, *JAMA* 289:1645-1651, 2003.
35. Zimmerman SA, Schultz WH, Burgett S, et al: Hydroxyurea therapy lowers transcranial Doppler flow velocities in children with sickle cell anemia, *Blood* 110:1043-1047, 2007.
36. Perdu J, Boutouyrie P, Bourgain C, et al: Inheritance of arterial lesions in renal fibromuscular dysplasia, *J Hum Hypertens* 21:393-400, 2007.
37. Boutouyrie P, Gimenez-Roqueplo AP, Fine E, et al: Evidence for carotid and radial artery wall subclinical lesions in renal fibromuscular dysplasia, *J Hypertens* 21:2287-2295, 2003.
38. de Bray JM, Marc G, Pautot V, et al: Fibromuscular dysplasia may herald symptomatic recurrence of cervical artery dissection, *Cerebrovasc Dis* 23:448-452, 2007.
39. Assadian A, Senekowitsch C, Assadian O, et al: Combined open and endovascular stent grafting of internal carotid artery fibromuscular dysplasia: Long term results, *Eur J Vasc Endovasc Surg* 29:345-349, 2005.
40. Grange DK, Balfour IC, Chen SC, et al: Familial syndrome of progressive arterial occlusive disease consistent with fibromuscular dysplasia, hypertension, congenital cardiac defects, bone fragility, brachysyndactyly, and learning disabilities, *Am J Med Genet* 75:469-480, 1998.

41. Gould DB, Phalan FC, van Mil SE, et al: Role of *COL4A1* in small-vessel disease and hemorrhagic stroke, *N Engl J Med* 354: 1489-1496, 2006.

42. Vahedi K, Kubis N, Boukobza M, et al: *COL4A1* mutation in a patient with sporadic, recurrent intracerebral hemorrhage, *Stroke* 38:1461-1464, 2007.

43. Casas JP, Hingorani AD, Bautista LE, et al: Meta-analysis of genetic studies in ischemic stroke: Thirty-two genes involving approximately 18,000 cases and 58,000 controls, *Arch Neurol* 61: 1652-1661, 2004.

44. Rahemtullah A, Van Cott EM: Hypercoagulation testing in ischemic stroke, *Arch Pathol Lab Med* 131:890-901, 2007.

45. Uchino K, Johnston SC, Becker KJ, et al: Moyamoya disease in Washington State and California, *Neurology* 65:956-958, 2005.

46. Fukui M: Current state of study on moyamoya disease in Japan, *Surg Neurol* 47:138-143, 1997.

47. Meschia JF, Ross OA: Heterogeneity of moyamoya disease: After a decade of linkage, is there new hope for a gene? *Neurology* 70:2353-2354, 2008.

48. Fushimi Y, Miki Y, Kikuta K, et al: Comparison of 3.0- and 1.5-T three-dimensional time-of-flight MR angiography in moyamoya disease: preliminary experience, *Radiology* 239:232-237, 2006.

49. Fukui M, Kono S, Sueishi K, et al: Moyamoya disease, *Neuropathology* 20(Suppl):S61-64, 2000.

50. Fukui M: Research Committee on Spontaneous Occlusion of the Circle of Willis (Moyamoya Disease) of the Ministry of Health and Welfare, Japan: Guidelines for the diagnosis and treatment of spontaneous occlusion of the circle of Willis ('moyamoya' disease), *Clin Neurol Neurosurg* 99(Suppl 2):S238-240, 1997.

51. Kikuta K, Takagi Y, Nozaki K, et al: Histological analysis of microbleed after surgical resection in a patient with moyamoya disease, *Neurol Med Chir (Tokyo)* 47:564-567, 2007.

52. Gazzola S, Aviv RI, Gladstone DJ, et al: Vascular and nonvascular mimics of the CT angiography "spot sign" in patients with secondary intracerebral hemorrhage, *Stroke* 39:1177-1183, 2008.

53. Kikuta K, Takagi Y, Nozaki K, et al: The presence of multiple microbleeds as a predictor of subsequent cerebral hemorrhage in patients with moyamoya disease, *Neurosurgery* 62:104-111, 2008.

54. Scott RM, Smith JL, Robertson RL, et al: Long-term outcome in children with moyamoya syndrome after cranial revascularization by pial synangiosis, *J Neurosurg* 100:142-149, 2004.

55. Miyamoto S: Study design for a prospective randomized trial of extracranial-intracranial bypass surgery for adults with moyamoya disease and hemorrhagic onset: the Japan Adult Moyamoya Trial Group, *Neurol Med Chir (Tokyo)* 44:218-219, 2004.

56. Ullrich NJ, Robertson R, Kinnamon DD, et al: Moyamoya following cranial irradiation for primary brain tumors in children, *Neurology* 68:932-938, 2007.

57. Dobson SR, Holden KR, Nietert PJ, et al: Moyamoya syndrome in childhood sickle cell disease: A predictive factor for recurrent cerebrovascular events, *Blood* 99:3144-3150, 2002.

58. Houkin K, Tanaka N, Takahashi A, et al: Familial occurrence of moyamoya disease: Magnetic resonance angiography as a screening test for high-risk subjects, *Childs Nerv Syst* 10:421-425, 1994.

59. Kramer J, Abraham J, Teven CM, et al: Role of antiplatelets in carotid artery stenting, *Stroke* 38:14, 2007.

60. Lenhart PD, Lambert SR, Newman NJ, et al: Intracranial vascular anomalies in patients with morning glory disk anomaly, *Am J Ophthalmol* 142:644-650, 2006.

61. Revesz T, Holton JL, Lashley T, et al: Sporadic and familial cerebral amyloid angiopathies, *Brain Pathol* 12:343-357, 2002.

62. Calero M, Pawlik M, Soto C, et al: Distinct properties of wild-type and the amyloidogenic human cystatin C variant of hereditary cerebral hemorrhage with amyloidosis, Icelandic type, *J Neurochem* 77:628-637, 2001.

63. Olafsson I, Grubb A: Hereditary cystatin C amyloid angiopathy, *Amyloid* 7:70-79, 2000.

64. Uemichi T, Uitti RJ, Koeppen AH, et al: Oculoleptomeningeal amyloidosis associated with a new transthyretin variant Ser64, *Arch Neurol* 56:1152-1155, 1999.

65. Uitti RJ, Donat JR, Rozdilsky B, et al: Familial oculoleptomeningeal amyloidosis: Report of a new family with unusual features, *Arch Neurol* 45:1118-1122, 1988.

66. Sakashita N, Ando Y, Jinnouchi K, et al: Familial amyloidotic polyneuropathy (ATTR Val30Met) with widespread cerebral amyloid angiopathy and lethal cerebral hemorrhage, *Pathol Int* 51:476-480, 2001.

67. Ellie E, Camou F, Vital A, et al: Recurrent subarachnoid hemorrhage associated with a new transthyretin variant (Gly53Glu), *Neurology* 57:135-137, 2001.

68. Battistini S, Rocchi R, Cerase A, et al: Clinical, magnetic resonance imaging, and genetic study of 5 Italian families with cerebral cavernous malformation, *Arch Neurol* 64:843-848, 2007.

69. Guclu B, Ozturk AK, Pricola KL, et al: Mutations in apoptosis-related gene, *PDCD10*, cause cerebral cavernous malformation 3, *Neurosurgery* 57:1008-1013, 2005.

70. Lee ST, Choi KW, Yeo HT, et al: Identification of an Arg35X mutation in the *PDCD10* gene in a patient with cerebral and multiple spinal cavernous malformations, *J Neurol Sci* 267:177-181, 2008.

71. Belz MM, Hughes RL, Kaehny WD, et al: Familial clustering of ruptured intracranial aneurysms in autosomal dominant polycystic kidney disease, *Am J Kidney Dis* 38:770-776, 2001.

72. Nakajima F, Shibahara N, Arai M, et al: Intracranial aneurysms and autosomal dominant polycystic kidney disease: Followup study by magnetic resonance angiography, *J Urol* 164:311-313, 2000.

73. Maher CO, Piepgras DG, Brown RD Jr, et al: Cerebrovascular manifestations in 321 cases of hereditary hemorrhagic telangiectasia, *Stroke* 32:877-882, 2001.

74. Jen J, Cohen AH, Yue Q, et al: Hereditary endotheliopathy with retinopathy, nephropathy, and stroke (HERNS), *Neurology* 49:1322-1330, 1997.

75. Weiner AA, Zemnick C, Ganda K: Comparison of anxiety response levels in patients who are HIV-positive and patients who are not, *J Mass Dent Soc* 51:12-16, 2002.

76. Ikram MA, Seshadri S, Bis JC, et al: Genomewide association studies of stroke, *N Engl J Med* 360:1718-1728, 2009.

77. Lanktree MB, Dichgans M, Hegele RA: Advances in genomic analysis of stroke: What have we learned and where are we headed? *Stroke* 41:825-832, 2010.

78. Okazaki H, Whisnant JP: Clinical pathology of hypertensive intracerebral hemorrhage. In Mizukami M, Kogure K, Kanaya H, Yamori Y, editors: *Hypertensive intracerebral hemorrhage*, New York, 1983, Raven Press, pp 177-180.

79. Vinters HV: Cerebral amyloid angiopathy: A critical review, *Stroke* 18:311-324, 1987.

80. Vonsattel JP, Myers RH, Hedley-Whyte ET, et al: Cerebral amyloid angiopathy without and with cerebral hemorrhages: A comparative histological study, *Ann Neurol* 30:637-649, 1991.

81. Mandybur TI, Bates SR: Fatal massive intracerebral hemorrhage complicating cerebral amyloid angiopathy, *Arch Neurol* 35:246-248, 1978.

82. Maruyama K, Ikeda S, Ishihara T, et al: Immunohistochemical characterization of cerebrovascular amyloid in 46 autopsied cases using antibodies to beta protein and cystatin C, *Stroke* 21:397-403, 1990.

83. Glenner GG, Henry JH, Fujihara S: Congophilic angiopathy in the pathogenesis of Alzheimer's degeneration, *Ann Pathol* 1:120-129, 1981.

84. Olichney JM, Hansen LA, Galasko D, et al: The apolipoprotein E epsilon 4 allele is associated with increased neuritic plaques and cerebral amyloid angiopathy in Alzheimer's disease and Lewy body variant, *Neurology* 47:190-196, 1996.

85. McCarron MO, Nicoll JA: High frequency of apolipoprotein E epsilon 2 allele is specific for patients with cerebral amyloid angiopathy-related haemorrhage, *Neurosci Lett* 247:45-48, 1998.

86. Jensen M, Schroder J, Blomberg M, et al: Cerebrospinal fluid A beta42 is increased early in sporadic Alzheimer's disease and declines with disease progression, *Ann Neurol* 45:504-511, 1999.

87. McCarron MO, Nicoll JA, Stewart J, et al: Amyloid beta-protein length and cerebral amyloid angiopathy-related haemorrhage, *Neuroreport* 11:937-940, 2000.

88. Rosand J, Hylek EM, O'Donnell HC, et al: Warfarin-associated hemorrhage and cerebral amyloid angiopathy: A genetic and pathologic study, *Neurology* 55:947-951, 2000.

89. Fryer JD, Simmons K, Parsadanian M, et al: Human apolipoprotein E4 alters the amyloid-beta 40:42 ratio and promotes the formation of cerebral amyloid angiopathy in an amyloid precursor protein transgenic model, *J Neurosci* 25:2803-2810, 2005.

90. Greenberg SM, Finklestein SP, Schaefer PW: Petechial hemorrhages accompanying lobar hemorrhage: Detection by gradient-echo MRI, *Neurology* 46:1751-1754, 1996.

91. Greenberg SM, O'Donnell HC, Schaefer PW, et al: MRI detection of new hemorrhages: Potential marker of progression in cerebral amyloid angiopathy, *Neurology* 53:1135-1138, 1999.

92. Roob G, Schmidt R, Kapeller P, et al: MRI evidence of past cerebral microbleeds in a healthy elderly population, *Neurology* 52:991-994, 1999.

93. Vernooij MW, van der Lugt A, Ikram MA, et al: Prevalence and risk factors of cerebral microbleeds: The Rotterdam Scan Study, *Neurology* 70:1208-1214, 2008.

94. Gudbjartsson DF, Arnar DO, Helgadottir A, et al: Variants conferring risk of atrial fibrillation on chromosome 4q25, *Nature* 448:353-357, 2007.

95. Meschia JF: Decoding cryptogenic cardioembolism, *Ann Neurol* 64:364-366, 2008.

96. Schunkert H, Gotz A, Braund P, et al: Repeated replication and a prospective meta-analysis of the association between chromosome 9p21.3 and coronary artery disease, *Circulation* 117:1675-1684, 2008.

97. Matarin M, Brown WM, Singleton A, et al: Whole genome analyses suggest ischemic stroke and heart disease share an association with polymorphisms on chromosome 9p21, *Stroke* 39:1586-1589, 2008.

98. Cooper GM, Johnson JA, Langaee TY, et al: A genome-wide scan for common genetic variants with a large influence on warfarin maintenance dose, *Blood* 112:1022-1027, 2008.

99. Hillman MA, Wilke RA, Yale SH, et al: A prospective, randomized pilot trial of model-based warfarin dose initiation using CYP2C9 genotype and clinical data, *Clin Med Res* 3:137-145, 2005.

100. Anderson JL, Horne BD, Stevens SM, et al: Randomized trial of genotype-guided versus standard warfarin dosing in patients initiating oral anticoagulation, *Circulation* 116:2563-2570, 2007.

101. Lesko LJ: Personalized medicine: Elusive dream or imminent reality? *Clin Pharmacol Ther* 81:807-816, 2007.

102. Link E, Parish S, Armitage J, et al: *SLCO1B1* variants and statin-induced myopathy: A genomewide study, *N Engl J Med* 359:789-799, 2008.

19 | The Global Burden of Stroke

KATHLEEN STRONG, COLIN MATHERS

The 1990 Global Burden of Disease (GBD) study provided the first global estimates for the burden of 135 diseases. Cerebrovascular diseases ranked as the second leading cause of death globally after ischemic heart disease.[1] During the past two decades the coverage of death registration data has improved and has provided additional sources of information on causes of death. In addition, an increasing number of population studies on stroke epidemiology have been completed. We have used this increased availability to provide a more recent update on the global burden of stroke.

The World Health Organization (WHO) estimated that there were 9 million first-ever strokes worldwide in 2004; cerebrovascular disease accounted for 5.7 million deaths for this time period.[2] Given that there were 58 million total deaths in 2004, stroke accounted for nearly 10% of all deaths globally. Heart disease and stroke were the two leading causes of mortality in adults aged 15 years or older and the third and fourth leading causes of disease burden (as measured in disability-adjusted life years, DALYs) after human immunodeficiency virus/acquired immunodeficiency syndrome (HIV/AIDS) and unipolar depressive disorders.[2] Among adults aged 45 to 69 years, heart disease and stroke were the leading causes of DALYs lost and deaths globally. More than 85% of strokes were estimated to occur in low- and middle-income countries.

The burden of chronic, noncommunicable diseases, including stroke, has remained stable at about 85% of the total disease burden in high-income countries over the past 10 years. However, demographic and epidemiologic shifts have resulted in stroke becoming a major health problem in low- and middle-income countries. This increase can be attributed to population ageing and changes in the distribution of known, modifiable risk factors of cardiovascular diseases. These modifiable risk factors and the ways in which they contribute to premature deaths are known and well-documented. They include tobacco use, poor diet leading to overweight/obesity, raised blood pressure, increased cholesterol levels, and physical inactivity.[3]

Cerebrovascular diseases can be prevented by addressing known, modifiable risks. Public health initiatives that focus on these risks provide concrete actions to reduce the burden of stroke within a population. The GBD study has provided comprehensive and comparable estimates of incidence, mortality, and loss of health due to stroke at global, regional, and country levels, as well as estimates of the proportion of stroke burden attributable to known risk factors. These data are necessary for policy makers to define specific actions. This chapter gives an overview of the GBD studies, of the data and methods used in them, and of the most recent analyses of the global burden of stroke.

The Global Burden of Disease Studies

Governments and international agencies are faced with setting priorities for health research, investment in health systems, and health interventions in the contexts of increasing health care costs and increasing availability of effective interventions. Burden of disease studies aim to provide a framework and decision-making process to help governments and international agencies prioritize their actions and effectively use their resources to improve population health. Key inputs to decision making are detailed and comprehensive assessments of the causes of loss of health in populations. The optimal measure incorporates both causes of death and the main causes of nonfatal illnesses and their long-term sequelae. Broad evaluation of the effectiveness of health systems and major health programs and policies also requires assessments of the causes of loss of health that are comparable not only across populations but also over time.

The World Bank's 1993 World Development Report on *Investing in Health*[4] recommended cost-effective intervention packages for countries at different levels of development. Underpinning these analyses was the first GBD study, which generated a comprehensive and consistent set of estimates of mortality and morbidity by age, sex, and region of the world and introduced a new metric—the DALY. The DALY brings together and quantifies the burden of disease from premature mortality and the nonfatal consequences of more than 100 diseases and injuries.[5]

In recent years, WHO has undertaken a progressive reassessment of the GBD for the years 2000 to 2004, with consecutive revisions and updates published annually in WHO *World Health Reports* and in two recent books.[2,6] These updates have drawn on a wider range of data sources so that internally consistent estimates of incidence, severity, duration, and mortality could be developed for more than 130 major causes for 14 subregions of the world. The methods used in the WHO updates build on those used in the original GBD study and make use of substantial improvements in data availability and some new methods for dealing with incomplete and biased data.[7]

The DALY extends the concept of potential years of life lost owing to premature death to include equivalent years of "healthy" life lost by virtue of being in states of poor health or disability.[5] One DALY can be thought of as one lost year of "healthy" life, and the burden of disease can be thought of as a measurement of the gap between current health status and an ideal situation where everyone lives into old age, free of disease and disability.

DALYs for a disease or injury cause are calculated as the sum of the years of life lost (YLL) owing to premature mortality in the population and the years of life lost owing to disability (YLD) for incident cases of the disease or injury. YLL are calculated from the number of deaths at each age multiplied by a global standard life expectancy of the age at which death occurs.[8] YLD for a particular cause in a particular time period are estimated as follows: YLD = number of incident cases in that period × average duration of the disease × weight factor. The weight factor reflects the severity of the disease on a scale from 0 (perfect health) to 1 (death) and is discussed in more detail later on.

In the standard DALYs published by WHO, calculations of YLD used an additional 3% time discounting and nonuniform age weights that give less weight to years lived at young and older ages.[9] When discounting and age weights are used, a death in infancy corresponds to 33 DALYs, and deaths at ages 5 to 20 years correspond to about 36 DALYs.

Methods for Assessing Cause-Specific Mortality in the GBD

Lifetables specifying mortality rates by age and sex for 192 WHO member states were developed for 2004 from available death registration data (111 member states), sample registration systems (India, China), and data on child and adult mortality from censuses and surveys such as the Demographic and Health Surveys and UNICEF's Multiple Indicator Cluster Surveys (MICS). For countries without useable death registration data, estimated levels of child and adult mortality were input to a modified logit lifetable model to estimate the full lifetable for 2004.[10] For 55 countries, 42 of them in sub-Saharan Africa, no information was available on levels of adult mortality. Based on the predicted level of child mortality in 2004, the most likely corresponding level of adult mortality was selected, based on regression models of child versus adult mortality as observed in a set of almost 2000 lifetables judged to be of good quality. HIV and war deaths were separately estimated country-by-country.

Death registration data containing useable information on cause of death distributions were available for 111 countries, the majority of which were in the high-income group, Latin America and the Caribbean, Europe, and Central Asia. Deaths coded to International Classification of Diseases (ICD) codes for "symptoms, signs, and ill-defined conditions," as well as certain ill-defined codes within the cancer, cardiovascular disease, and injury chapters of ICD were redistributed across defined causes.[7] The percentage of deaths coded to these ill-defined causes varied from 4% in New Zealand to more than 30% in Sri Lanka and Thailand.[11]

For estimation of deaths by cause for populations without useable death registration data, improved models were developed for estimating broad cause-of-death patterns.[12] Regional patterns for detailed cause distributions within the broad cause groups were based on available death registration data within each region. For the 2004 estimates, the regional patterns were updated for African countries with a greater range of information on cause-of-death distributions in Africa than previously.[2]

Population-based epidemiologic studies, disease registers, and notification systems (in excess of 2700 datasets) also contributed to the estimation of mortality due to 21 specific causes of death, including HIV/AIDS, malaria, tuberculosis, childhood diseases preventable by immunization, schistosomiasis, trypanosomiasis, Chagas disease, cancers, drug dependence, war, and natural disasters. Almost one third of these datasets related to sub-Saharan Africa.

For China and India, causes of mortality were based on existing mortality registration systems, namely, the Disease Surveillance Points system (DSP) and the Vital Registration System of the Ministry of Health in China and the Medical Certificate of Cause of Death (MCCD) for urban India and the Annual Survey of Causes of Death (SCD) for rural areas of India.[2]

In terms of actual deaths recorded by registration systems, data are provided to WHO annually for about 18.6 million deaths, representing one third of all deaths estimated to occur in the world. If the sample registration systems in India and China are sufficiently representative to provide information on their whole populations, then information on mortality is available for around 72% of the world's population.[11]

GBD Estimates of Stroke Mortality at Global, Regional, and Country Level

Ischemic heart disease and cerebrovascular disease (stroke) were the leading causes of death in both middle- and high-income countries in 2004 and among the top five causes for low-income countries (Table 19-1). These two causes were together responsible for 22% of all deaths worldwide. Of the 5.7 million stroke deaths, 87% were in low- and middle-income countries (Fig. 19-1). The percentage of deaths from stroke coming from low- and middle-income countries rose to 94% for stroke deaths of persons younger than 70 years. In contrast, high-income countries contribute only 13% (all ages) and 6% (younger than 70 years) of deaths from stroke.

Figure 19-2 shows estimated regional stroke death rates for men and women aged 30 to 69 years in 2004. Stroke death rates for men and women younger than 70 years are generally similar in most regions but show a fivefold variation across regions, from around 50 per 100,000 in high-income countries to more than 200 per 100,000 in the low- and middle-income countries of Europe. This finding is further illustrated in Figure 19-3, which shows age-standardized stroke death rates among people aged 30 to 69 years for nine selected countries for which recent death registration data are available. Age-standardized death rates are highest in the Russian Federation and higher in most of the other low- and middle-income countries than in Canada or the United Kingdom. In terms of premature deaths and YLL, stroke is a greater problem in low- and middle-income countries than in high-income countries.

TABLE 19-1   TEN LEADING CAUSES OF DEATH: LOW, MIDDLE, AND HIGH INCOME COUNTRIES, 2004*

	Disease or injury	Deaths (Millions)	% Total Deaths		Disease or injury	Deaths (Millions)	% Total Deaths
World				**Low income countries**			
1	Ischemic heart disease	7.2	12.2	1	Lower respiratory infections	2.9	11.0
2	Cerebrovascular disease	5.7	9.7	2	Ischemic heart disease	2.5	9.4
3	Lower respiratory infections	4.1	7.0	3	Diarrheal diseases	1.8	6.8
4	COPD	3.0	5.1	4	HIV/AIDS	1.5	5.7
5	Diarrheal diseases	2.1	3.6	5	Cerebrovascular disease	1.5	5.6
6	HIV/AIDS	2.0	3.5	6	Malaria	1.0	3.7
7	Tuberculosis	1.5	2.5	7	COPD	0.9	3.6
8	Trachea, bronchus, lung cancers	1.3	2.3	8	Tuberculosis	0.9	3.5
9	Road traffic accidents	1.3	2.2	9	Neonatal infections[†]	0.9	3.4
10	Prematurity and low birth weight	1.2	2.0	10	Prematurity and low birth weight	0.8	3.2
Middle income countries				**High income countries**			
1	Cerebrovascular disease	3.5	14.2	1	Ischemic heart disease	1.3	16.3
2	Ischemic heart disease	3.4	13.9	2	Cerebrovascular disease	0.8	9.3
3	COPD	1.8	7.4	3	Trachea, bronchus, lung cancers	0.5	5.9
4	Lower respiratory infections	0.9	3.8	4	Lower respiratory infections	0.3	3.8
5	Trachea, bronchus, lung cancers	0.7	2.9	5	COPD	0.3	3.5
6	Road traffic accidents	0.7	2.8	6	Alzheimer and other dementias	0.3	3.4
7	Hypertensive heart disease	0.6	2.5	7	Colon and rectal cancers	0.3	3.3
8	Stomach cancer	0.5	2.2	8	Diabetes mellitus	0.2	2.8
9	Tuberculosis	0.5	2.2	9	Breast cancer	0.2	2.0
10	Diabetes mellitus	0.5	2.1	10	Stomach cancer	0.1	1.8

*Countries grouped by gross national income per capita: low income ($825 or less), high income ($10,066 or more). Note that these high-income groups differ slightly from those used in the Disease Control Priorities Project.
†This category also includes other noninfectious causes arising in the perinatal period, responsible for about 20% of deaths shown in this category.
COPD, Chronic obstructive pulmonary disease.
From the World Health Organization: *The global burden of disease: 2004 update,* Geneva, 2008, World Health Organization.

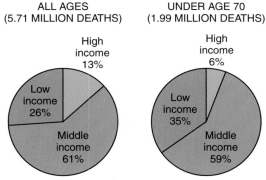

ALL AGES
(5.71 MILLION DEATHS)

UNDER AGE 70
(1.99 MILLION DEATHS)

Figure 19-1   Distribution of stroke deaths by World Bank income group for all ages and for people younger than 70 years, 2004. (World Health Organization: Global burden of disease estimates: http://www.who.int/evidence/bod. Accessed November 28, 2008.)

Age-adjusted mortality rates for cerebrovascular disease in persons aged 30 to 69 years ranged tenfold between countries, from around 25 per 100,000 in Canada and Switzerland to around 250 per 100,000 in Russia and Kyrgyzstan (Fig. 19-4). The highest premature death rates for

stroke are found in eastern Europe, northern Asia, central Africa, and the South Pacific, whereas the lowest rates are found in western Europe and North America. The high rates in eastern Europe reflect the substantial increases in adult male mortality and disability in the 1990s, leading to the highest male–female differential in disease burden in the world. A significant factor in this trend is thought to be increasing alcohol abuse, particularly among males, which has led to high rates of accidents, violence, and cardiovascular disease.[13,14] From 1991 to 1994, the risk of premature adult (15 to 59 years) death increased by 50% for Russian males. It improved somewhat between 1994 and 1998 but has increased significantly again in recent years.

Global Stroke Epidemiology: Data and Methods

The original GBD study based its estimates of incidence and hence the YLD component of the DALY on a back-estimation of incidence from its regional mortality estimates, using estimates of case fatality rates for high-income regions and simple assumptions that case fatality rates were up to 30% higher in developing regions. Since the GBD 1990 was completed, more stroke studies have become available, and the GBD 2000–2002 study developed a model for stroke based on available population data on case fatalities within 28 days for incident cases of first-ever stroke and on long-term survival in patients surviving this initial period, in whom the risk of mortality is highest.[15]

A consistent relationship between incidence, prevalence, and mortality was established with the use of data from the United States, and the resulting age- and sex-specific 28-day and survivor case fatality rates were used as the basis for subregional case fatality rates after adjustment for the observed relationship between gross national income per capita and the overall 28-day case

fatality rate in published studies from various countries. Estimated regional case fatality rates ranged from 14% and 16% for North American men and women to 40% and 42% for African men and women (Table 19-2). Consistent epidemiologic models for each subregion were then estimated with the use of these case fatality rates and observed mortality, after adjustment to account for the fact that the true excess risk of mortality in survivors is not fully reflected in deaths recorded as resulting from stroke in vital statistics.

For the GBD 2004, estimated prevalence rates for stroke survivors from this model were compared with results from available population studies. GBD estimates for stroke survivor prevalence rates were generally around 10% to 30% higher than prevalence rates reported in available studies from developing countries, but most of the studies dated from the 1980s or 1990s and may not

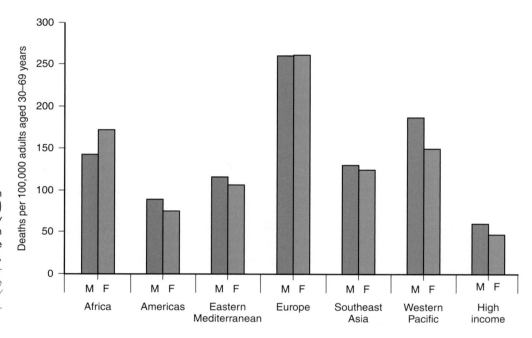

Figure 19-2 Estimated death rates from stroke (per 100,000) for ages 30 to 69 years, by World Health Organization region and sex; high income countries grouped separately, 2004. (World Health Organization: Global burden of disease estimates: *http://www.who.int/evidence/bod*. Accessed November 28, 2008.)

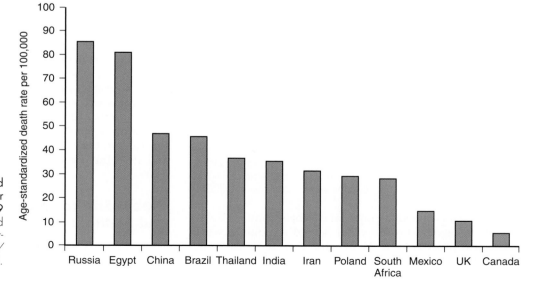

Figure 19-3 Age-standardized death rates from stroke (per 100,000) for ages 30 to 69 years, by country, 2004. (World Health Organization: Global burden of disease estimates: *http://www.who.int/evidence/bod*. Accessed November 28, 2008.)

have fully identified survivors of mild strokes without noticeable neurologic problems.

Two recent national burden of disease studies have made estimates of the prevalence of stroke survivors for Australia in 2003, a developed country population,[16] and for Thailand in 2004, a developing country population.[17] The Australian stroke estimates were based on detailed analysis of linked databases for Western Australia to identify incidence of first-ever stroke and mortality for cases. Provisional Thai stroke prevalence estimates were based on data from the Third National Health Examination Survey 2004.[18] Data from these studies were used to recalibrate the long-term case fatality rates for first-ever stroke survivors across all regions for the GBD 2004 estimates, resulting in a reduction in the estimated prevalence of stroke survivors from 50 million to 30 million and a 30% reduction in YLD for cerebrovascular disease compared with results published earlier for 2002.

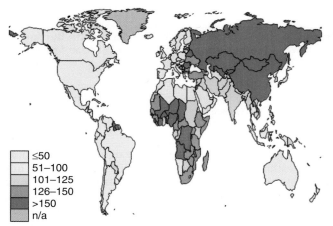

Figure 19-4 Age-standardized death rates from stroke (per 100,000) for ages 30 to 69 years, by country, 2004. (World Health Organization: Global burden of disease estimates: *http://www.who. int/evidence/bod.* Accessed November 28, 2008.) **Note:** Age-standardized using the WHO World Standard Population. (Ahmad O, Boschi-Pinto C, Lopez AD, et al: *Age standardization of rates: A new WHO standard.* GPE Discussion Paper No. 31, Geneva, 2001, World Health Organization.)

Legend:
≤50
51–100
101–125
126–150
>150
n/a

The GBD study estimated total incidence of first-ever stroke and prevalence of stroke survivors, regardless of whether disability was present (see Table 19-2). Although incidence, YLD, and DALYs were not calculated for stroke subtypes, a breakdown of DALYs by subtype was required for the risk factor analysis because the association of risks such as high blood pressure with stroke differ by type. In white populations approximately 80% of all strokes are ischemic, 10% to 15% are intracerebral hemorrhage, 5% are subarachnoid hemorrhage, and the rest are due to other causes.[19] Lawes et al[20] reviewed available studies as described elsewhere and estimated the proportion of ischemic and hemorrhagic strokes for the GBD subregions (see Table 19-2).

Because stroke patients with hemorrhagic stroke have higher short-term case fatality than patients with ischemic stroke events, the 28-day case fatality will be higher in populations with higher proportions of hemorrhagic strokes. In the present analyses this is reflected in the higher 28-day case fatality rates in other regions than the EME (see Table 19-2). Of the 5.7 million stroke deaths in 2004, an estimated 56% were due to ischemic stroke.

Assessing Disability Due to Stroke

The original GBD study brought to the attention of health policy makers the previously largely ignored burden of nonfatal illnesses, particularly mental disorders. It did this through the inclusion of "equivalent years of healthy life lost" or YLD, through living with states of less than full health after the incidence of disease or injury. Some national studies have considered the health states of stroke survivors in more detail. Table 19-3 outlines the health states considered in the Australian Burden of Disease study.[21]

The average loss of health for the health states of stroke survivors is estimated with the use of "health state preferences," commonly referred in the GBD literature as disability weights. The health state weights formalize and quantify social preferences for different states of health, thus allowing time (years of healthy life) to be used as the common currency for combining nonfatal health states and years of life lost owing to mortality. DALYs can thus

TABLE 19-2 ESTIMATED STROKE INCIDENCE, PREVALENCE (MILLIONS), 28-DAY CASE FATALITY RATE (%), AND TOTAL DEATHS BY STROKE SUBTYPE, BY WORLD HEALTH ORGANIZATION REGION, 2004

	World	Africa	The Americas	Eastern Mediterranean	Europe	Southeast Asia	Western Pacific
Incidence of first-ever stroke (millions)	9.0	0.7	0.9	0.4	2.0	1.8	3.3
Ischemic stroke	7.8	0.6	0.8	0.4	1.8	1.5	2.7
Hemorrhagic and other	1.3	0.1	0.1	0.1	0.2	0.2	0.6
28-Day case fatality rate (%)	31	40	24	32	28	34	32
Prevalence of stroke survivors (millions)	30.7	1.6	4.8	1.1	9.6	4.5	9.1
Total stroke deaths (millions)							
Ischemic stroke	3.21	0.24	0.29	0.15	0.91	0.60	1.02
Hemorrhagic and other	2.50	0.19	0.17	0.11	0.45	0.47	1.11

From World Health Organization, unpublished data.

TABLE 19-3 STROKE OUTCOMES IN THE AUSTRALIAN BURDEN OF DISEASE STUDY

Sequela/Stage/Severity Level	Health State Description
First-ever stroke—acute event	Acute stroke event and period immediately after. Severe pain, unable to self-care or carry out usual activities, severe mobility limitations. Likely cognitive and motor deficits. The average duration of this period for those who die within 28 days is around 6 days. Model this health state with duration of 6 days for all first strokes.
First-ever stroke with full recovery	After 1 year, no impairments or limitations in activities. The model assumes approximately 50% of long-term stroke survivors have full recovery.
First-ever stroke with long-term disability—mild	Permanent impairments and disability after 1 year. Motor impairment resulting in some problems with usual activities. Some pain and discomfort. Some depression or anxiety. No problems in self-care or cognition.
First-ever stroke with long-term disability—moderate	Permanent impairments and disability after 1 year. Cognitive or cognitive plus motor impairment resulting in some problems with mobility, usual activities. Some pain and discomfort, some depression or anxiety, and some problems in self-care.
First-ever stroke with long-term disability—severe	Severe permanent impairments and disability after 1 year. Severe cognitive problems, unable to perform usual activities or self-care. Severe pain or discomfort. Some problems in mobility and some depression or anxiety.

TABLE 19-4 DISABILITY WEIGHTS FOR CEREBROVASCULAR DISEASE

Stage/Sequela	Global Burden of Disease Study, 1990	Netherlands Study	Australian Burden of Disease Study
First-ever stroke with full recovery	0	0	0
First-ever stroke with long-term disability	0.224 (treated) 0.262 (untreated)	0.360 (mild) 0.630 (moderate) 0.920 (severe)	0.36 (younger ages) −0.58 (older ages)

also be thought of as a particular form of the more general concept of quality-adjusted life years (QALYs), widely used in economic evaluations for health interventions.

Health economists have developed a number of choice-based methods to measure preferences for health states, although there is considerable heterogeneity in the conceptualization of what the preferences relate to, ranging from health, through quality of life and well-being, to utility.[22] The original GBD study used two forms of the person trade-off method, and asked participants in weighting exercises to make a composite judgment about the severity distribution of the condition and the preference for time spent in each severity level.[8] This was largely necessitated by the lack of population information on the severity distribution of most conditions at the global and regional levels. The participants were not representative of general populations but were, for the most part, public health professionals involved either in a WHO meeting with representation from all regions or in training workshops held in several different regions.

A Dutch disability weight study attempted to address this problem by defining the distribution of health states associated with each sequela using the EuroQol health profile to describe the health states.[23] Using similar methodology to the original GBD study with three panels of public health physicians and one lay panel, this study concluded that it makes little difference whether the valuation panels are composed of medical experts or lay people, as long as accurate functional health state profiles are provided.

Different disability weights for cerebrovascular disease have been used in different studies (Table 19-4). The lack of

disability data from the vast majority of the world's regions made estimation of regional disability rates divided into level of severity impossible for the GBD study. It should be noted that the vast literature on impairment, disability, and handicap indicates the problems of developing a simple, easy, reliable, and valid measure of the outcome of a disease like stroke, which can have a wide spectrum of residual disability not covered in a simple measure of dependence on another person for daily activities. Different disability rating scales are likely to provide different estimates,[24] and scales that may provide an appropriate estimate of disability in one population may be inadequate in others.[25] The approach used in this study is a simplified method, but until more data and knowledge become available on how to assign disability for the world's regions, the WHO updates of the GBD have continued to use the same strategy as in the GBD 1990 study.

As used in the DALY, the term *disability* is essentially a synonym for health states of less than full health. The DALY is actually attempting to quantify loss of health, and the disability weights should thus reflect social preferences for health states, not broader valuations of "quality of life," "well-being," or "utility." Thus disability weights should reflect judgments about the "healthfulness" of defined states, not any judgments of quality of life or the worth of persons. A high disability weight for a health state then implies that people place a high social value on preventing such health states or on provision of treatment interventions that replace them by states closer to full health.

The original GBD study grouped disability weights into seven classes ranging from 0 to 0.02 for class I to 0.7

TABLE 19-5   ESTIMATED PREVALENCE OF MODERATE AND SEVERE DISABILITY (MILLIONS) FOR LEADING DISABLING CONDITIONS BY AGE, FOR HIGH-INCOME AND LOW- AND MIDDLE-INCOME COUNTRIES, 2004

	Disabling Condition†	High-Income Countries*		Low- and Middle-Income Countries		World
		0-59 years	60 years or older	0-59 years	60 years or older	All ages
11	Ischemic heart disease	1.0	2.2	8.1	11.9	23.2
16	Alzheimer and other dementias	0.4	6.2	1.3	7.0	14.9
18	Cerebrovascular disease	1.4	2.2	4.0	4.9	12.6

*High-income countries are those with 2004 gross national income per capita of $10,066 or more, as estimated by the World Bank.
†Global Burden of Disease disability classes III and above.
From *http://www.who1.net.*

to 1.0 for class VII and estimated the distribution across these seven classes of disability severity for each case and sequela. The GBD 2004 update used these estimates of disability weight distributions to estimate the prevalence of moderate and severe disability due to stroke (Table 19-5). An estimated 12 million people were moderately or severely disabled in 2004 owing to stroke, and 70% of these were in low- and middle-income countries; close to half in these countries were younger than 60 years.

The Global Burden of Stroke in 2004

The two leading causes of death globally—ischemic heart disease and cerebrovascular disease—remain among the top six causes of burden of disease (Table 19-6), but when measured by DALYs, nonfatal conditions such as depression are also among the leading causes of burden of disease. Stroke is the third leading cause of burden of disease in high-income countries and in middle-income countries. In low-income countries, it is pushed from the top 10 causes by HIV, tuberculosis, malaria, and a number of other infectious diseases. The DALY gives more weight to deaths at younger ages, thus giving somewhat less emphasis to stroke than mortality league tables.

Among the population aged 60 years or older, stroke accounted for 13% of the GBD in the population in 2004 and 38% of the burden due to cardiovascular diseases in the same age group. The total years of healthy life lost due to stroke, as measured by DALYs, are greater in those aged 0 to 59 years than for ages 60 to 69 years and ages beyond 70 years, although the DALY rate increases with age. In terms of numbers, two thirds of the burden of stroke occurs in people younger than 70 years.

Assessing the Contribution of Stroke Risk Factors

The major methodologic advance between the 2004 GBD update and the original GBD study was quantifying the contribution of risk factors to disease burden. Although the 1990 study estimated the attributable mortality and burden for 10 risk factors, there were serious concerns about the comparability of the estimates from the past to the present. For the WHO revisions to the GBD study, a new framework for risk factor quantification was defined: it calculated attributable fractions of disease due to a risk

TABLE 19-6   TEN LEADING CAUSES OF BURDEN OF DISEASE (DALYS), ALL AGES, 2004

	Disease or Injury	DALYs (millions)	Percent of Total DALYs
1	Lower respiratory infections	94.5	6.2
2	Diarrheal diseases	72.8	4.8
3	Unipolar depressive disorders	65.5	4.3
4	Ischemic heart disease	62.6	4.1
5	HIV/AIDS	58.5	3.8
6	Cerebrovascular disease	46.6	3.1
7	Prematurity and low birth weight	44.3	2.9
8	Birth asphyxia and birth trauma	41.7	2.7
9	Road traffic accidents	41.2	2.7
10	Neonatal infections and other*	40.4	2.7

*This category also includes other noninfectious causes arising in the perinatal period apart from prematurity, low birth weight, birth trauma, and asphyxia. These noninfectious causes are responsible for about 20% of DALYs shown in this category.
DALYs, Disability-adjusted life years.

factor based on a comparison of disease burden expected under the current estimated distribution of exposure with that expected if a counterfactual distribution of exposure had applied; it also took into account excess risk across the entire range of exposure for continuous exposures such as cholesterol level, blood pressure, and body mass index.[26] The counterfactual distribution was defined for each risk factor as the theoretically achievable population distribution of exposure that would lead to the lowest minimum levels of disease burden. The case of tobacco use is particularly clear because the theoretical minimum distribution would be 100% of the population being lifelong nonsmokers. For body mass index, it would be a population distribution of body mass index normally distributed with a mean and a standard deviation of 21 and 1 kg/m^2, respectively.[27]

Recently, WHO has updated estimates of stroke deaths and DALYs attributable to eight major cardiovascular risk factors.[3] WHO estimated that eight risk factors—alcohol use, tobacco use, high blood pressure, high body mass

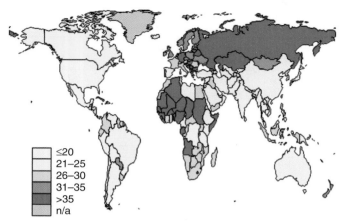

Figure 19-5 Age-standardized prevalence of high systolic blood pressure (>140 mm Hg), persons aged 30 years or older, 2004. (Strong KL, WHO Global Infobase Team: *The SuRF Report. Surveillance of chronic disease risk factors: Country level data and comparable estimates.* Geneva, 2005, World Health Organization.)

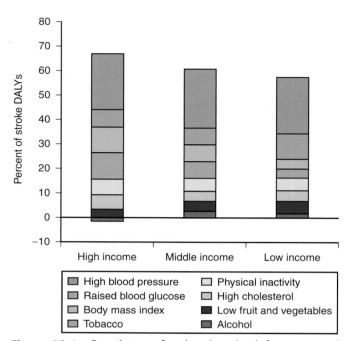

Figure 19-6 Contribution of eight selected risk factors to total stroke burden, by country income group, 2004. (World Health Organization: *Global health risks.* Geneva, 2009, WHO.)

index, high cholesterol level, high blood glucose level, low fruit and vegetable intake, and physical inactivity—accounted for 60% of loss of healthy life years (DALYs) from stroke and 55% of stroke deaths in 2004. The same risk factors together account for more than three quarters of deaths from ischemic and hypertensive heart disease.

Raised systolic blood pressure is by far the most important of these risks for stroke, causing an estimated 51% of stroke deaths. Figure 19-5 shows the age-standardized prevalence of systolic blood pressure greater than 140 mm Hg for WHO member states in 2004.

Data for the distributions of systolic blood pressure, serum cholesterol level, and body mass index were derived from the WHO Global Infobase.[28] Data sources and estimation methods for the other risk factors are described in the WHO report.[3]

Figure 19-6 shows the contributions of the eight risks to stroke burden measured in DALYs in high-, middle-, and low-income countries in 2004. The stroke DALYs attributable to individual risk factors are higher than shown in this figure, in which the contributions of individual risk factors have been scaled to sum to the estimated joint effects of all eight risk factors. The proportion of stroke deaths attributable to these eight risk factors ranges from 57% in low-income countries to 65% in high-income countries, in part because of the higher proportion of stroke deaths due to ischemic stroke in the high-income countries.

Projections of Stroke Mortality and Burden from 2004 to 2030

It is of interest to attempt to quantify how the future of global health might appear if there were to be no major changes to current disease control efforts and in the absence of major research breakthroughs that might lead to new, affordable, and implementable disease control technologies. WHO has prepared updated mortality projections from 2003 to 2030 using methods similar to those applied in the original GBD study. A set of relatively simple models were used to project future health trends for baseline, optimistic, and pessimistic scenarios, largely

on the basis of projections of economic and social development and with the use of historically observed relationships of these with cause-specific mortality rates.[29] The data inputs for the projection models take into account a greater number of countries reporting death registration data to WHO, especially low- and middle-income countries, as well as updated projections for HIV/AIDS and the tobacco-related epidemic.

For the projections reported here, historical death registration data for 107 countries between 1950 and 2002 were used to model the relationship between death rates for all major causes (excluding HIV/AIDS) and the following variables: average income per capita; the average number of years of schooling in adults; and time, a proxy measure for the impact of technological change on health status. Death rates were then projected with the use of World Bank estimates of income per capita and WHO projections of average years of schooling and smoking intensity.[29]

The mortality projections were also used as the basis for projections of the GBD from 2004 to the year 2030. For cerebrovascular disease projections, incidence rates were assumed to decline at half the rates projected for mortality.[29] In other words, projected trends in stroke mortality were assumed to be equally due to changes in incidence rates (reflecting changes in risk factor exposures and prevention activities) and changes in case fatality rates (reflecting improving treatment effectiveness).

As discussed earlier, there were an estimated 9 million first-ever strokes and 5.7 million stroke deaths in 2005. In the absence of additional population-wide interventions, these numbers are projected to rise to 10.5 million first-ever strokes and 6.6 million deaths in 2015, and to 13.2 million first-ever strokes and 8.2 million deaths by 2030. The projected stroke deaths and age-specific death rates for 2010, 2020, and 2030 under the baseline scenario are shown in

TABLE 19-7   PROJECTED DEATHS AND DALYS FOR STROKE: NUMBERS AND RATES BY AGE FOR 2010, 2020, AND 2030 UNDER THE BASELINE SCENARIO

	Number (millions)			Rate per 100,000		
	2010	**2020**	**2030**	**2010**	**2020**	**2030**
Deaths						
0-59	0.9	0.9	0.9	0.1	0.1	0.1
60-69	1.1	1.3	1.4	2.7	2.4	2.2
70+	4.2	4.8	5.9	12.2	11.4	10.6
All ages	6.1	7.0	8.2	0.90	0.93	1.0
DALYs						
0-59	20.7	20.8	20.5	0.3	0.3	0.3
60-69	11.3	13.6	15.1	28.3	25.4	22.9
70+	16.0	17.8	22.5	46.2	42.2	40.5
All ages	48.0	52.1	58.2	7.0	6.9	7.1

DALYs, Disability-adjusted life years.

Table 19-7. Although the age-specific death rates are projected to decline slightly between 2004 and 2030, population ageing worldwide will result in an overall increase in rates of death from stroke for all ages combined from 6.1 per 100,000 in 2004 to 8.2 per 100,000 in 2030. The projected increase in the total number of stroke deaths for the three World Bank groupings is shown in Figure 19-7. Stroke mortality is projected to increase faster in middle- and low-income countries than in high-income countries.

Projected age-specific DALY rates for 2030 are declining overall but are higher for all ages combined, reflecting global population ageing. The prevalence of stroke survivors, regardless of whether they are disabled as a result of the stroke, was estimated at 31 million globally in 2004 and is projected to rise to 36 million in 2030.

Discussion and Conclusions

Since the publication of the initial results of the first GBD study in 1993, there has been extensive interest by policy makers with national and international mandates for health development, as well as public health practitioners and researchers, in applying the methods and findings. This suggests that there is a very keen latent demand for comprehensive global, regional, and national assessments of disease and injury burden, of the factors that are primarily responsible for loss of healthy life, and of the likely impact of health interventions on future health.

Stroke caused an estimated 5.7 million deaths in 2004, and 87% of these deaths were in low- and middle-income countries. Without intervention, the number of global deaths is projected to rise to 8.2 million in 2030. The experience of high-income countries indicates that sustained interventions can achieve substantial reductions in stroke mortality in low- and middle-income countries.

There remains substantial uncertainty about the comparative burden of diseases and injuries in many parts of the world. In particular, for regions with limited death registration data such as the Eastern Mediterranean region, sub-Saharan Africa, and parts of Asia and the Pacific, there is considerable uncertainty in estimates of deaths by cause. It has been estimated that the 95% uncertainty intervals for stroke mortality range from around ±12% in developed

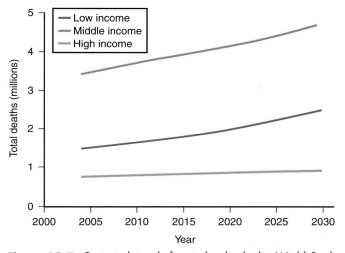

Figure 19-7   Projected trends for stroke deaths by World Bank income group, 2004–2030.

countries to ±18% in East Asia and the Pacific region, and ±30% in sub-Saharan Africa.[30] For some countries, only limited information on mortality is available from sources such as the Demographic and Health Surveys and from cause-specific mortality estimates for causes such as HIV/AIDS, malaria, tuberculosis, and vaccine-preventable diseases. The GBD approach included results for these regions, albeit with wider uncertainty ranges, based on the best possible assessment of the available evidence.[31]

The mortality and burden of disease projections are less firm than the base year assessments and provide "business-as-usual" projections under specified assumptions. Furthermore, the business-as-usual projections are driven, to a large extent, by World Bank projections of future growth in income per capita and do not specifically take account of trends in major stroke risk factors apart from tobacco smoking. The results depend strongly on the assumption that future mortality trends in poor countries will have the same relationship to economic and social development as has occurred in the higher income countries in the recent past. If this assumption is not correct, then the projections for low-income countries will be overoptimistic in the rate of decline of communicable diseases. The projections have also not taken explicit account of trends in major risk factors apart from tobacco smoking and, to a limited extent, overweight and obesity. If broad trends in risk factors are for worsening of risk exposures with development rather than the improvements observed in recent decades in many high-income countries, then, again, the projections for low- and middle-income countries presented here will be too optimistic.

The projections assumed equal contributions to the projected decline in mortality from improved incidence (primary prevention) and from prolonging lives after the acute event (secondary prevention resulting in improved case fatality). These assumptions were based on the findings from the WHO MONICA Project, which monitored the trends and determinants of stroke in 17 mostly European countries during the 1980s and 1990s.[32,33] Part of the explanation for the observed declines in case fatality could be a shift to stroke becoming more mild.[34] Despite the scientific progress made over the last few decades in imaging and other technologies, only the use of aspirin and management in stroke units is in widespread use.[35] Early aspirin treatment for ischemic stroke has been shown to reduce death or dependency by 12 per 1000 treated,[36] and coordinated care in stroke units has been shown to reduce death or dependency by 56 per 1000 receiving such treatment.[37] In low- and middle-income countries, where the bulk of strokes occur, health systems are already stretched and stroke units, with the gold standard of early management, may not be feasible. Aspirin, which is readily available, is not routinely administered in low- and middle-income countries.[38] To have any impact on stroke mortality, new technologies and new, immediate treatments will need to be widely diffused in low- and middle-income countries, where the majority of strokes occur. The major contribution to reduction in stroke deaths will therefore likely come from primary prevention. Greater efforts may need to be placed on integrated and comprehensive approaches within the context of improvements in the major risk factors common to stroke, heart disease, diabetes, and other chronic diseases.[39]

Primary and secondary prevention of stroke in the "western world" has reduced stroke mortality but has increased the number who require rehabilitation and admittance to long-term care facilities. If the prevalence and severity of disability among stroke survivors remains relatively constant over the next 10 to 20 years, then disability due to stroke and the demand for rehabilitation and long-term care will increase by around 24% between now and 2030, all of which have consequences for individuals, their families, and the societies in which they live.

Under the baseline projections, stroke death rates for the 60- to 69-year and 70- to 79-year age groups are projected to decline by an annual average of 3% and 2%, respectively, for high-income countries and by 2% and 1%, respectively, for low- and middle-income countries.

The experience of high-income countries clearly shows what can be achieved with sustained interventions. Stroke death rates for the 60- to 69-year age group in the 1990s declined by an annual average greater than 4% in a number of high-income countries including Australia, Germany, Israel, Italy, the Republic of Korea, and Spain. For the 70- to 79-year age group, average annual declines in stroke death rates exceeded 3% for a number of countries, including Austria, France, Germany, Israel, Italy, Portugal, the Republic of Korea, and Spain. Stroke death rates for persons aged 65 to 84 years in Australia have declined by 70% from 1970 to 2000, which represents an annual average decline of more than 4%.[40]

Estimates of the joint effects of the leading stroke risk factors (i.e., tobacco use, raised blood pressure, and poor diet) indicate that around 60% of stroke mortality in low- and middle-income countries, as well as high-income countries, is attributable to a relatively small number of modifiable risks, the most important of which is raised blood pressure.

Interventions to reduce the effects of the major risk factors on population-level disease burden and mortality have been shown to be effective in reducing risk of heart disease and stroke.[34,41] These include government actions to reduce tobacco use,[42,43] efforts to lower salt and saturated and trans fats[44,45] in both manufactured and home-cooked foods, and making fruit and vegetable intake[46] and physical activity[47] more attractive. These actions, although widely acknowledged in both medical journals and the popular press, are not widely used by national governments in all parts of the world, perhaps as a result of two common public health myths: that cardiovascular diseases, including stroke, are diseases of affluence and that stroke is a disease of people older than 70 years who will die soon anyway. Nothing could be farther from the truth. As we have demonstrated here, stroke is a leading cause of death and disability in low- and middle-income countries and in the global population younger than 70 years. This, in turn, has economic and social implications.

Acknowledgments

We wish to acknowledge the many WHO staff and external collaborators who have contributed to the GBD revisions for years 2000 and later, particularly Thomas Truelsen, Ruth Bonita, Steve Begg, and Steve Lim, who contributed to the analyses for stroke, and Gretchen Stevens, who carried out analyses of the burden of stroke attributable to risk factors. The authors alone are responsible for the views expressed in this publication, which do not necessarily reflect the decisions or the stated policy of WHO or of its member states.

REFERENCES

1. Murray CJL, Lopez AD: *The global burden of disease: 1*, Boston, 1996, Harvard School of Public Health.
2. World Health Organization: *The global burden of disease: 2004 update*, Geneva, 2008, World Health Organization.
3. World Health Organization: *Global health risks: mortality and burden of disease attributable to selected major risks*, Geneva, 2009, World Health Organization.
4. World Bank: *World development report 1993. Investing in health*, New York, 1993, Oxford University Press for the World Bank.
5. Murray CJL, Lopez AD: *The global burden of disease: a comprehensive assessment of mortality and disability from diseases, injuries and risk factors in 1990 and projected to 2020*, Cambridge, 1996, Harvard University Press.
6. Lopez AD, Mathers CD, Ezzati M, et al: *Global burden of disease and risk factors*, New York, 2006, Oxford University Press.

7. Mathers CD, Lopez AD, Murray CJL: The burden of disease and mortality by condition: Data, methods and results for 2001. In Lopez AD, Mathers CD, Ezzati M, Murray CJL, Jamison DT, editors: *Global burden of disease and risk factors*, New York, 2006, Oxford University Press, pp 45–240.

8. Murray CJL: Rethinking DALYs. In Murray CJL, Lopez AD, editors: *The global burden of disease*, Cambridge, 1996, Harvard School of Public Health on behalf of the World Health Organization and the World Bank, pp 1–98.

9. World Health Organization: *World health report 2004: Changing history*, Geneva, 2004, World Health Organization.

10. Murray CJL, Ferguson BD, Lopez AD, et al: Modified logit life table system: Principles, empirical validation and application, *Popul Stud* 57(2):1–18, 2003.

11. Mathers CD, Ma Fat D, Inoue M, et al: Counting the dead and what they died from: An assessment of the global status of cause of death data, *Bull World Health Organ* 83(March):171–177, 2005.

12. Salomon JA, Murray CJL: The epidemiologic transition revisited: Compositional models for causes of death by age and sex, *Popul Dev Rev* 28(2):205–228, 2002.

13. Shkolnikov V, McKee M, Leon D: Changes in life expectancy in Russia in the mid-1990s, *Lancet* 357:917–921, 2001.

14. McKee M, Shkolnikov V: Understanding the toll of premature death among men in eastern Europe, *BMJ* 323:1051–1055, 2001.

15. Truelsen T, Begg S, Mathers CD, Satoh T: *Global burden of cerebrovascular disease in the year 2000*, Geneva, 2002, World Health Organization. Available at. http://www.who.int/healthinfo/statistics/bod_cerebrovasculardiseasestroke.pdf. Accessed 8 June 2008. Global burden of disease 2000 working paper.

16. Begg S, Vos T, Barker B, et al: *The burden of disease and injury in Australia 2003*, Canberra, 2007, Australian Institute of Health and Welfare.

17. Lopez A, Phoolcharoen W, Vos T, et al: Burden of disease and cost-effectiveness of intervention options: Informing policy decisions and health system reform in Thailand. Wellcome Trust: NHMRC/Wellcome Trust International Collaborative Research Grant. Available at http://www.wellcome.ac.uk/doc_WTD003308.html. Accessed 29 Nov 2007. 2004.

18. Aekplakorn W, Abbott-Klafter J, Premgamone A, et al: Prevalence and management of diabetes and associated risk factors by regions of Thailand: Third National Health Examination Survey 2004, *Diabetes Care* 30(8):2007–2012, 2007.

19. Sudlow CLM, Warlow CP: Comparable studies of the incidence of stroke and its pathological types. Results from an international collaboration, *Stroke* 28:491–499, 1997.

20. Lawes CM, Vander Hoorn S, Law MR, et al: High blood pressure. In Ezzati M, Lopez A, Rodgers A, Murray CJL, editors: *Comparative quantification of health risks: Global and regional burden of disease attributable to selected major risk factors*, Geneva, 2004, World Health Organization, pp 281–390.

21. Mathers CD, Vos T, Stevenson C: *The burden of disease and injury in Australia*, Canberra, 1999, Australian Institute of Health and Welfare (AIHW).

22. Salomon JA, Murray CJL: A multi-method approach to estimating health state valuations, *Health Econ* 13(3):281–290, 2004.

23. Stouthard M, Essink-Bot M, Bonsel G, et al: *Disability weights for diseases in the Netherlands*, Rotterdam, 1997, Department of Public Health, Erasmus University.

24. Jette AM: How measurement techniques influence estimates of disability in older populations, *Soc Sci Med* 38(7):937–942, 1994.

25. Ali SM, Mulley GP: Is the Barthel scale appropriate in non-industrialized countries? A view of rural Pakistan, *Disabil Rehabil* 20:195–199, 1998.

26. Murray CJL, Lopez AD: On the comparable quantification of health risks: Lessons from the global burden of disease study, *Epidemiology* 10(5):594–605, 1999.

27. Ezzati M, Lopez AD, Rodgers A, Murray CJL: *Comparative quantification of health risks: Global and regional burden of disease attributable to selected major risk factors*, Geneva, 2004, World Health Organization.

28. Strong KL: *WHO Global Infobase Team: The SuRF Report. Surveillance of chronic disease risk factors: Country level data and comparable estimates*, Geneva, 2005, World Health Organization.

29. Mathers CD, Loncar D: Projections of global mortality and burden of disease from 2002 to 2030, *PLoS Med* 3(11):e442, 2006.

30. Mathers CD, Salomon JA, Ezzati M, et al: Sensitivity and uncertainty analyses for burden of disease and risk factor estimates. In Lopez AD, Mathers CD, Ezzati M, Murray CJL, Jamison DT, editors: *Global burden of disease and risk factors*, New York, 2006, Oxford University Press, pp 399–426.

31. Murray CJL, Mathers CD, Salomon JA: Towards evidence-based public health. In Murray CJL, Evans D, editors: *Health systems performance assessment: debates, methods and empiricism*, Geneva, 2003, World Health Organization, pp 715–726.

32. Asplund K: What MONICA told us about stroke, *Lancet Neurol* 4:64–68, 2005.

33. Truelsen T, Mahonen M, Tolonen H, et al: Trends in stroke and coronary heart disease in the WHO MONICA Project, *Stroke* 34:1346–1352, 2003.

34. Sarti C, Stegmayr B, Tolonen H, et al: Are changes in mortality from stroke caused by changes in stroke event rates or case fatality? Results from the WHO MONICA Project, *Stroke* 34:1833, 2003.

35. Whiteley W, Lindley R, Wardlaw J, Sandercock P: on behalf of the IST-3 Collaborative Group. Third International Stroke Trial, *Int J Stroke* 1:172–176, 2006.

36. Warlow C, Sudlow C, Dennis M, et al: Stroke, *Lancet* 362:2121–2122, 2003.

37. Chen ZM, Sandercock P, Pan HC, et al: Indications for early aspirin use in acute ischaemic stroke: A combined analysis of 40,000 randomised patients from the Chinese Acute Stroke Trial and the International Stroke Trial, *Stroke* 31:240–249, 2000.

38. Mendis S, Abegunde D, Usuf S, et al: WHO study on prevention of recurrences of myocardial infarction and stroke (WHO-PREMISE), *Bull World Health Organ* 83:820–829, 2005.

39. World Health Organization: *Preventing chronic diseases: A vital investment: WHO global report*, Geneva, 2005, World Health Organization.

40. Australian Institute of Health and Welfare: *Mortality over the twentieth century in Australia: Trends and patterns in major causes of death*, Canberra, 2006, Australian Institute of Health and Welfare (AIHW).

41. Murray CJL, Lauer J, Hutubessy R: Effectiveness and costs on interventions to lower systolic blood pressure and cholesterol: A global and regional analysis on reduction of cardiovascular disease risk, *Lancet* 361:717–725, 2003.

42. Sargent RP, Shepard RM, Glantz SA: Reduced incidence of admissions for myocardial infarction associated with public smoking ban: before and after study, *BMJ* 328:977–980, 2004.

43. Fichtenberg CM, Glantz SA: Association of the California tobacco control program with declines in cigarette consumption and mortality from heart disease, *N Engl J Med* 343(24):1772–1777, 2000.

44. Uusitalo U, Feskens EJM, Tuomilehto J, et al: Fall in total cholesterol concentration over five years in association with changes in fatty acid composition of cooking oil in Mauritius: cross sectional survey, *BMJ* 313:1044–1046, 1996.

45. Leth T, Jensen HG, Mikkelsen AE, Bysted A: The effects of regulation on *trans* fatty acid content in Danish food, *Atheroscler Suppl* 7:53–56, 2006.

46. Zatonski WA, McMichael AJ, Powles JW: Ecological study of reasons for sharp decline in mortality from ischaemic heart disease in Poland since 1991, *BMJ* 316(7137):1047–1051, 1998.

47. Dunn AL, Andersen RE, Jakicic JM: Lifestyle physical activity interventions. History, short-and long-term effects and recommendations, *Am J Prev Med* 15(4):398–412, 1998.

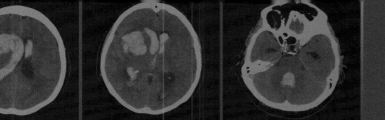

Clinical Manifestations

J. P. MOHR

This section continues the attempt to cover the
major syndromes of stroke, and, where possible,
to point to issues of pathophysiology that bear
on the diagnosis of stroke subtype, both
ischemic and hemorrhagic.

Evolving imaging information is offering
insight into functional reorganization following
acute stroke. The opportunities currently available for functional magnetic resonance imaging
in the hyperacute phase of stroke, even following transient ischemic attacks and in a setting of
impaired perfusion without obvious symptoms,
are clearly demonstrating the remarkable elasticity of brain function.

These advances have also prompted further
condensation of historical aspects of clinical
manifestations and diagnosis. Those seeking
more historical review than found in this edition
are encouraged to seek out copies of the earlier
editions.

Classification of Ischemic Stroke

DANILO TONI, RALPH L. SACCO, MICHAEL BRAININ, J.P. MOHR

Since 1990, advances in imaging technologies for the brain and blood vessels have improved the diagnostic accuracy of the classification of ischemic stroke. Infarct subtype used to be determined chiefly on clinical grounds; that is, there was heavy reliance on the clinical syndrome, neurologic findings, and coexisting risk factors. In the unfortunate patient who died, autopsy confirmation was often the basis of the classification. With the widespread application of computed tomography (CT), magnetic resonance imaging (MRI), duplex Doppler and transcranial Doppler (TCD) ultrasonography, single-photon emission computed tomography (SPECT), and other diagnostic studies, clinical impressions have been refined and supported by laboratory confirmation of the infarct subtype. Moreover, the evolution of acute stroke therapies aimed at saving brain tissue has provided the opportunity to differentiate stroke subtypes in the early hours after stroke onset, which is an important distinction because the treatment time window has been narrow.[1] The need for early differentiation of ischemic subtypes for specific therapies is exemplified by the demonstration of the delicate balance between striking improvement and the potentially disastrous hemorrhagic side effects with thrombolysis.[2-5] It has become important for the practicing physician to be able to exclude from therapy patients who have a high likelihood of spontaneous good functional recovery, such as those with some lacunar infarcts,[6-8] and to select appropriate thrombolytic approaches for patients with large artery thrombosis[9,10] and those with embolic occlusions of intracranial arteries.

Forms of Infarction: Bland and Hemorrhagic

When perfusion pressure falls to critical levels, ischemia develops, progressing to infarction if the effect persists long enough. Ischemic infarction is pathologically divided into bland infarction and hemorrhagic infarction. When the cause is thrombus, the usual occlusion persists, preventing reperfusion of the infarcted region and resulting in pale, anemic, or bland infarction.[11] In regions exposed to circulating blood, such as the edge of a bland infarct, widespread leukocyte infiltration occurs within days. For periods of up to several weeks, macrophages invade the infarct and are active for some months until all the products of infarction are carried off. Only scattered red cells are found.

Hemorrhagic infarction, in contrast to the bland form, occurs when varying amounts of red blood cells are found among the necrotic tissues.[12,13] In some cases, the concentration of red blood cells (RBCs) is enough to make a high-density appearance consistent with blood on CT or MRI, and at autopsy, the specimen shows hemorrhagic foci ranging from a few petechiae scattered through the infarct to a mass of confluent petechial foci having almost the appearance of frank hematoma. The timing of hemorrhagic infarction varies widely, from as early as a few hours to as late as 2 weeks or more after an arterial occlusion.

The explanation for hemorrhagic infarction has long been thought to result from reperfusion of the vascular bed of the infarct after relief of the occlusion, such as would occur after fragmentation and distal migration of an embolus[14] or after early reopening of a large vessel occlusion in the setting of an established large infarction.[15,16] Presumably, the renewed pressure of arterial blood into capillaries results in a diapedesis of RBCs through their hypoxic walls. The more intense the reperfusion and the more severely damaged the capillary walls, the more confluent the hemorrhagic infarction. Assuming that hemorrhagic infarction reflects restored lumen patency, it should be a consequence of spontaneous or thrombolytic recanalization of an embolic occlusion because the occlusion from thrombosis of an atherosclerotic stenosis would be more difficult to completely relieve. This hypothesis is supported by the greater frequency of hemorrhagic infarction found among cardioembolic infarcts.[12,17]

The simple explanation for hemorrhagic infarction previously given has been challenged by observations made by investigators using third-generation CT devices[18-20] and MRI.[21] These researchers have demonstrated that hemorrhagic infarction may frequently develop distal to the site of a persisting occlusion in the arterial bed exposed, at best, only to retrograde collaterals.[22,23] The severity of the hemorrhagic focus may differ from the more or less extended hematoma observed as a consequence of large artery recanalization. In these former cases, the occurrence of petechial, scattered hemorrhagic infarction may be related to surges in arterial blood pressure and the suddenness, severity, and size of the infarction.[12,19,23] It is presumed that edema initially surrounds the large infarct and compresses pial vessels. As edema subsides, retrograde reperfusion through pial collaterals ensues, leading to petechial hemorrhagic infarction.[18,19]

Problems in the Diagnosis of Infarction

Before modern neuroimaging was routinely available, many physicians persisted in believing that a definitive diagnosis as to stroke mechanism was merely a technical problem awaiting the proper laboratory procedures. In most circumstances the clinical features and CT or MRI findings suffice to differentiate acute intracerebral hemorrhage from infarction within the first hours after stroke onset. Clinical scores that have been developed to help differentiate infarct from hemorrhage rely on decreased consciousness, headache, and nausea and vomiting as predictors of hemorrhage.[24-28] The current utility of such scales would be to improve diagnoses in studies with no access to CT or to help with early mobilization of stroke teams who are alerted by emergency room personnel of a potential high-probability infarction case. Because small, deep, or lobar hematomas can manifest as circumscribed focal deficits and can easily lead those relying on the clinical syndrome alone to diagnose infarction mistakenly,[29] these scores can never be used to make a definitive diagnosis. The advent of CT and MRI has led to the correction of these potential misdiagnoses, resulting in a greater proportion of hemorrhages in stroke series[30] and elimination of the inadvertent use of anticoagulation in the case of a "masquerading" hemorrhage.[31] The prior concern regarding the limitations of acute MRI compared with CT in the diagnosis of intracerebral hemorrhage has also been eliminated with newer MRI protocols.[32]

The use of CT, MRI, noninvasive vascular imaging, and angiography has greatly improved our ability to diagnose ischemic stroke but has still left large issues unresolved. Ischemic strokes can now be classified into subtypes well enough to justify management decisions, but the classification is far from precise. Clinical grounds alone, with the use of age, risk factors, and so forth, have been the time-honored means of determining the subtype of infarction, such as separating embolism from thrombosis. However, it is often difficult to classify patients by different mechanism of cerebral infarction on clinical criteria alone. A thorough diagnostic evaluation is required because the presenting clinical syndromes are usually not distinctive enough to enable one to infer the cause. This is even more apparent in the acute setting, in which the common cognitive impairment, agitation, and poor cooperation of patients may hinder a thorough assessment of neurologic functions.

Even when strenuous efforts are made to establish the exact mechanism of infarction, the problem remains difficult. Duplex Doppler ultrasonography, MR angiography (MRA), and conventional angiography often fail to show either the expected arterial stenosis or occlusion; in addition, when a significant carotid stenosis is found, judging whether the clinical syndrome arose from an embolic or hemodynamic mechanism is often difficult.[33] The findings of brain imaging performed during the acute stage may suggest an occlusion of the middle cerebral artery (MCA), on the basis of the detection of a high-attenuation spot along the course of the artery, a finding in 30% to 50% of patients with angiographically proven arterial occlusion; such findings do not always settle the problem of the underlying mechanism. The identification of early signs of parenchymal damage and brain edema, proven to be useful as a prognostic index,[2,34-37] is not that helpful in the differentiation of ischemic pathogenetic mechanisms.

Few studies have collected detailed information on the clinical and radiologic characteristics of large

homogeneous subsets of patients with acute cerebral infarction. The Stroke Data Bank, created by the National Institute of Neurological Diseases and Stroke (NINDS), provided a large collection of prospectively collected information on patients with different subtypes of infarction.[38] A deliberate attempt was made to classify patients into distinct categories and to create new subsets on the basis of the presumed mechanism of infarction. This effort resulted in some changes in the large categories of stroke due to infarction. In particular, the atherothrombosis category was divided into two subgroups: large artery thrombosis with no evidence of embolic infarction and a form of artery-to-artery embolism arising from an atherosclerotic source. A separate category, infarct of undetermined cause, later characterized as "cryptogenic stroke,"[38a] was created to help ensure the homogeneity of the Stroke Data Bank diagnostic groups (Fig. 20-1).

Efforts to establish the diagnosis for the subtype of infarction proved remarkably difficult in a disappointingly high percentage of cases.[39] Despite efforts to arrive at the diagnosis with a CT scan or angiogram, it was apparent that the basis for the diagnosis in many of the cases was still a best clinical guess. When laboratory data were available, the results indicated that large artery atherosclerotic occlusive disease was a less common cause of stroke; that small vessel or lacunar and cardioembolic infarctions were relatively common; and that the cause of most cases of infarction could not be classified into these traditional diagnostic categories. The high frequency of surface infarcts in the setting of a normal or distal branch arterial occlusion led most investigators to regard these unexplained cerebral infarcts as examples of embolism with an undetected thrombotic source.[40] In the Stroke Data Bank, a separate diagnostic category was created for cases with unproven mechanisms of infarction: infarct of undetermined cause or cryptogenic infarction. Apart from a few common features, infarctions in this category are still poorly understood and have not yet been successfully characterized as a clinical group (Fig. 20-2).

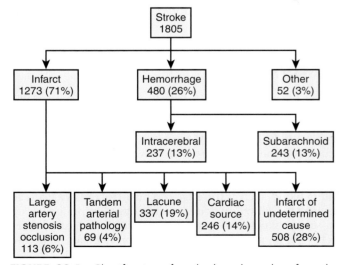

FIGURE 20-1 Classification of stroke based on data from the National Institute of Neurological Diseases and Stroke (NINDS) Stroke Data Bank (1983-1986).

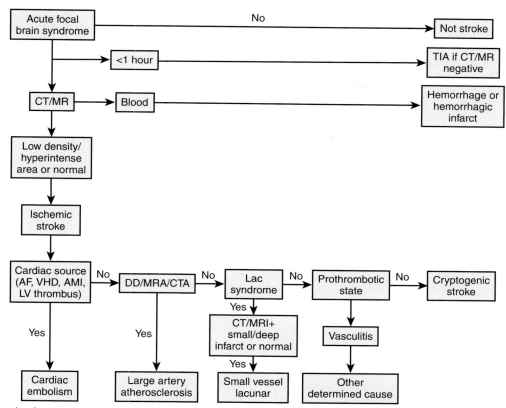

FIGURE 20-2 Stroke diagnostic algorithm. AF, Atrial fibrillation; AMI, acute myocardial infarction; DD, duplex and transcranial Doppler; lac syndrome, currently described classic lacunar syndromes, possibly including other syndromes from focal-deep infarction (e.g., cognitive changes from thalamic or caudate infarcts); LV, left ventricular; MRA, magnetic resonance angiography; TIA, transient ischemic attack; VHD, valvular heart disease.

Subtypes of Ischemic Stroke
Infarct with Large Artery Thrombosis

The classification of a stroke with an infarction due to large artery thrombosis was sometimes a diagnosis of exclusion in the days of less sophisticated laboratory investigations. Strokes were classified into one of three major diagnostic categories as follows: hemorrhage if the spinal fluid was bloody, embolism if atrial fibrillation or rheumatic heart disease was present, and thrombosis if none of the foregoing was present. Syndromes previously attributed to large artery atherosclerosis, when more closely evaluated with current technology, have been reclassified. The gradual decline in large artery thrombosis as a leading diagnosis has resulted from several factors. Among the most important are the more frequent use of duplex or TCD ultrasonography in the pursuit of stroke diagnosis; the recognition of several clinical subtypes of thrombosis, especially lacunes[6,41-43]; documentation proving that some ischemic strokes associated with large artery atherothrombosis are produced by artery-to-artery embolism (local embolism)[40,44-50]; and discontinuation of the casual classification of a stroke as atherothrombotic in favor of the additional category "undetermined."[39,51-54]

Many of the descriptions leading to the definition of this subtype stem from pathologic studies of the past.[55] Atherosclerotic lesions were found at bifurcations and curves of the larger vessels; the more proximal the location in the vascular tree, the more severe the atherosclerotic lesions.[56,57] Primary occlusion of the arteries distally located over the cerebral surface was less frequent.[58,59] Atherosclerotic plaque usually led to progressive stenosis, and the final large artery occlusion was due to thrombosis of the narrowed lumen. Intraplaque hemorrhaging sometimes led to accelerated occlusion,[60] although the frequency of this condition is more often a matter of speculation rather than confirmed in pathologic specimens.[61,62] The possibility of achieving an in vivo characterization of the carotid plaque with MRI has been suggested[63,64] but has still not entered into routine use.

Infarct Mechanism: Perfusion Failure

Stroke in the patient with atherothrombus was initially attributed to perfusion failure distal to the site of severe stenosis or occlusion of the major vessel.[59,65,66] In some instances, the major vessel occlusion was rather proximal in the arterial tree, and some degree of collateral flow was interposed between the occlusion and the cerebral territory at risk of infarction.[67] Some cases with interposed collateral were spared infarction of any kind, whereas in others the infarct was located mainly along the most distal brain regions originally supplied by the occluded vessel.[49,59,66,68-70] In the carotid territory, these regions were the suprasylvian frontal, central, and parietal portions of the hemisphere, and in the vertebrobasilar territory, they were the bilateral occipital poles. Internal borderzone regions have also been demonstrated in the white matter of the corona radiata supplied by both superficial MCA pial penetrators and lenticulostriate arteries.

The usually accepted mechanism of perfusion failure is more readily recognized in occlusive disease but becomes more difficult to define when, instead, the extracranial vessel is patent but highly stenotic. Some positron emission tomography–based studies have not found supportive evidence for selective hemodynamic impairment among patients with transient ischemic attacks (TIAs) and severe carotid stenosis.[33,71] The development of borderzone ischemia probably depends on multiple factors, not just on the severity of stenosis.[15,70,72]

Infarct Mechanism: Artery-to-Artery Embolism

In addition to vascular occlusion at the site of atherosclerosis, infarcts are produced by emboli arising from atheromatous lesions situated proximally to otherwise healthy branches located more distal in the arterial tree.[45] Embolic fragments may arise from extracranial arteries affected by stenosis or ulcer,[10,49,73-75] stenosis of any major cerebral artery stem,[47,76,77] or the basilar artery[78]; from the stump of the occluded internal carotid artery (ICA)[79]; and even from the intracranial tail of the anterograde thrombus atop an occluded carotid.[50,80] Nowadays embolism from a carotid source has become recognized as another, perhaps more common, cause of stroke in a setting of arterial stenosis and even occlusion.[40,44,46] In the Stroke Data Bank, this mechanism of infarction was labeled *tandem arterial pathology*. In later stroke series, borderzone infarcts appear to be less common than previously thought, which has led to the presumption that embolism was the actual mechanism even in the presence of ICA tight stenoses or occlusions. To add to the difficulty in distinguishing between these two mechanisms of infarction, cases of perfusion failure due to embolism have been demonstrated. Internal borderzone infarcts have been demonstrated after embolic occlusion of MCA pial branches.[81] This finding may be an example of an embolic stroke with a possible local hemodynamic effect as the final mechanism of the infarct.

Clinical Features

Focal cortical syndromes are usually found in patients with large artery thrombosis, but syndromes often attributed to lacunar disease, such as pure motor or sensorimotor stroke, can easily represent the first sign of impending flow failure.[35] Discriminating among infarct subtypes on clinical grounds alone is difficult. To determine some of these distinguishing clinical features in the Stroke Data Bank, investigators compared demographic, stroke risk, clinical, and radiologic features for 246 cardioembolic cerebral infarcts and 113 large vessel atherosclerotic cerebral infarcts.[82] The Stroke Data Bank definitions ensured more TIAs in atherosclerotic infarcts and more cardiac disease in cardioembolic infarcts, but the diagnosis was distinguished further. Cases with fractional arm weakness (shoulder different from the hand), hypertension, diabetes, and male gender occurred more frequently with atherosclerotic than with cardioembolic infarcts. Patients with atherosclerotic infarcts were more likely to have a fractional arm weakness, regardless of infarct size.

Distinguishing between the infarct mechanisms (hemodynamic versus embolism) in patients with large artery disease is quite difficult even for the most astute clinician. The sudden mode of onset may suggest, but does not confirm, a diagnosis of embolism.[83] Other clinical features may not enable such a distinction. Moreover, it is even more difficult to discriminate between emboli from a cardiac source and those from an arterial source. Comparisons in the NINDS Stroke Data Bank between the 246 patients with cardioembolic cerebral infarction and the 66 patients with arterial embolic cerebral infarction demonstrated some differences.[34] Even after the data were controlled for differences in the frequency of cardiac disease, TIAs, and carotid bruits, the probability of an artery-to-artery embolism was increased by the finding of a superficial infarct alone or by a higher hematocrit value. The probability of cardiac embolism was greater for patients who initially had decreased consciousness or for whom findings on first CT were abnormal. These findings suggested that these two embolic infarct subtypes differed as to the location and extent of the cortical infarction. Smaller and more distal infarction in an embolism from an arterial source compared with a cardiogenic embolism suggested a smaller embolic particle size. Clinical features observed at stroke onset can help distinguish cerebral infarction subtypes but are not reliable enough to lead to a definite determination of infarct subtype without confirmatory laboratory data.

Results of Diagnostic Tests

Brain Imaging

The only abnormalities on MRI or CT that are directly attributable to cerebral infarction from carotid artery thrombosis are those that can be interpreted to reflect the distal field effect along the borderzone between middle and anterior cerebral territories, especially on the middle cerebral side.[49,59,65,84] This topographic pattern involves the suprasylvian frontal and central regions, shading toward normal in the parietooccipital region, sparing the region of the sylvian fissure (operculum, insula) and the penetrating territories of the lenticulostriates. The centripetal spreading in more severe cases may involve so much of the hemisphere that a differentiation from embolism to the MCA stem is impossible.

CT and MRI are of help in supporting a diagnosis of embolism when (1) an infarct in the territories of large cerebral arteries or their branches is detected,[85] (2) a hyperdense spot along the course of the MCA is seen,[68] or (3) a scattered infarct pattern is seen on diffusion-weighted MRI.[86,87] However, none of the mentioned imaging techniques is of help in inferring embolism source from the neck. When occlusions involve the territories of the anterior, middle, or posterior cerebral artery or the basilar artery, brain imaging cannot distinguish between thrombosis and embolism if the scan or image shows low density only in the proximal fields of the arterial territory.

Vascular Imaging

In the clinical setting, for a diagnosis of large artery atherosclerotic occlusive disease, angiography, MRA, computed tomographic angiography (CTA), and Doppler ultrasonography remain the most important laboratory tests. On a conventional cerebral angiogram, the occlusion of the ICA at its origin or in the siphon has the appearance of a pencil point, blunt end, smooth end, or shoulder, and the intracranial portion of the internal carotid or major cerebral artery stems and branches are open.[88] Spiral occlusions of the extracranial portion of the internal carotid beyond 2 cm of its origin (a finding consistent with dissection)[89] help to indicate that the carotid lesion may be the source of the stroke but not by means of atherosclerosis. Because of the risks of cerebral angiography,[90-92] there has been increased reliance on duplex Doppler and TCD ultrasonography techniques to show no or highly resistant flow in the extracranial carotid with dampened pulsatility in the ipsilateral MCA.[91,93-98] MRA and CTA have became reliable diagnostic tools for the detection of extracranial and intracranial large artery stenosis,[99,100] which has led to less reliance on conventional angiography.[47]

No satisfactory criteria have yet been developed to certify that a stroke is caused by extracranial arterial disease through the mechanism of embolism. The mechanism is inferred when (1) the clinical syndrome suggests a cortical branch territory, (2) no obvious cardioembolic source is present and the extent of stenosis is less than 80% (which would not explain the stroke on the grounds of hemodynamic insufficiency), or (3) ulcerative plaque is imaged by noninvasive duplex Doppler ultrasonography, MRA, CTA, or cerebral angiogram.

On the other hand, angiographic evidence of intracranial occlusion above a carotid stenosis or ulcer is not proof of the source; however, when present, it serves to classify this type of stroke into the present category.[67] The frequency of occurrence of embolism of particles large enough to cause stroke and the variety or severity of carotid lesions giving rise to such embolization remain poorly understood. In a continuous series of patients who underwent angiography within the first 6 hours of stroke onset,[40] MCA stem or branch occlusion accounted for 60% of the cases.

Possible embolic sources included carotid plaque (19%), an occlusion of the ipsilateral ICA (14%), and a potential source of emboli both arterial and cardiac (27%). Conversely, 58% of patients with ICA occlusion had a tandem MCA occlusion. Despite a normal intracranial arterial tree, the remainder had a territorial infarct on CT, a finding that implied that an artery-to-artery embolism occurred with embolus fragmentation preceding angiography.

Intracranial atherosclerotic artery stem stenoses or occlusions may be due to arteriosclerotic thrombosis but are often difficult to distinguish from emboli of any extracerebral source.[101-103] If one or more appropriate TIAs occurred within the past 30 days, the diagnosis of thrombus may be correct, but the matter can be settled only if a widely patent lumen is subsequently found by serial TCD ultrasonography evaluations or a second angiogram.[104] The latter is diagnostic of embolism, whereas persistence of the occlusion leaves the mechanism unsettled.

Basilar occlusion on angiography is usually considered the mechanism for brainstem stroke even though, in many such cases, the clinical syndrome fits the criteria for lacune[78,105-107] because the territory of infarction, however small, is in the field of supply of a vessel thrombosed by the major basilar atheroma.[108] As for the carotid artery, the finding of stenosis of the basilar artery prevents a definite diagnosis regarding the mechanism of infarction because infarcts more distal in the vertebrobasilar territory might well be the result of distal embolization.[101,109] Atheromatous disease of the basilar artery often affects the vessel at sites where local branches directly supply brain tissue.[108,110] In the carotid artery, the atheroma involves the vessel proximal to the point where its branches supply the brain.[57] When the clinical syndrome of basilar stroke can be localized to the point of the stenosis, infarction may be caused by mural atheroma that only slightly stenoses the basilar artery but totally occludes a small penetrator departing from the basilar artery at that location. This point, established in a few instances by autopsy, can only be inferred in cases studied by angiography; CT scanning is usually not of technically high enough quality to detect the small brainstem infarcts. However, MRI has defined the lesion and permitted better delineation of such cases.

Blood flow techniques have also helped confirm the perfusion failure mechanism in patients with atherosclerotic stenosis or occlusive disease through SPECT,[111] xenon-enhanced CT,[112] regional cerebral blood flow measurements,[23] MRI,[113-115] and positron emission tomography.[33,116,117] The more widespread use of these techniques should allow for more accurate distinction between embolism and perfusion failure in the clinical setting.

Embolism Attributed to Cardiac Sources

Embolism from any source probably accounts for between 15% and 70% of all cases of ischemic stroke,[38,40,48,53,54,118] many of which occur from embolism into the territory of the MCA. Although the subject of embolism seems clear enough, in that a particle is swept through the blood stream until it jams in an artery too small to allow it to pass, the many complexities of the embolic process make it anything but easy to account for on a case-by-case basis.

The biggest clinical problem in arriving at a diagnosis of embolism is identifying the source. Embolism was diagnosed in earlier studies mainly when a cardiac source (atrial fibrillation with valvular disease) was obvious.[55] The results of later studies have shown that emboli, diagnosed angiographically from isolated branch occlusions, may occur despite all efforts to identify the source.[40,54,119,120] Given the many possibilities and given the traditional use of the term *embolism* to refer to a cardiac source,[121-124] the following discussion is limited to that subject.

Properties of Emboli

The instability of the embolic material is a point of prime importance in clinical and angiographic analysis of cases of embolism. Mural thrombi and platelet aggregates are the materials most commonly embolized to the brain. These materials are remarkably evanescent, as has been repeatedly inferred from findings on angiography. Embolic fragments are found in more than 75% of cases studied by angiography within 8 hours of the onset of the stroke,[40,125,126] whereas embolism is demonstrated in 40% of clinically identical cases in which angiography is delayed for up to 72 hours after the clinical onset of the stroke[127] and in only 15% of cases studied more than 72 hours after the onset. These decreasing proportions imply that embolic occlusions are liable to spontaneously recanalize in a sizable number of cases. Serial studies with TCD ultrasonography demonstrated a recanalization of MCA mainstem or branch occlusions in up to 52% of cases within the first 48 hours of stroke.[128-132] Second angiographic evaluations, performed in subsets of patients in whom arterial occlusion was demonstrated by an earlier angiogram, showed recanalization in 30% to 60% of cases.[40,104]

No reliable means have been developed thus far to identify which embolic occlusions will persist and which will disappear, although it is inferred that the more friable materials will disperse more rapidly. In one of the TCD ultrasonography studies mentioned, patients with an arterial source of emboli experienced recanalization of the vessel less commonly than those with a cardiac source, which suggests a different composition or size of emboli.[129] The size of the emboli is also probably responsible, at least in part, for the highest frequency of both spontaneous[129,130,132] and pharmacologic[9,133-135] recanalization in cases of distal MCA occlusion.

This evanescent quality of embolic material may explain the wide variation in the frequency with which embolism is diagnosed in retrospective or prospective studies of stroke. The size of the material embolized determines the site at which it initially comes to rest in the circulation but does not determine its final point of arrest. Embolic material stops where the lumen diameter is too small to permit it to pass. Bifurcations or foci of atheroma at curves in the artery are the two sites where emboli arrest. Fibrin–platelet complexes and those also laden with bacteria vary considerably in size; some are so huge that they have obstructed the stem of the MCA,[136] and others have been so small they have lodged asymptomatically in a sensitive region such as the rolandic branch of the MCA. Calcific plaques have only rarely been described as producing large embolic strokes[74,137]; more often, they seem to produce TIAs but not persisting cerebral deficits.[73] For noncompressible objects such as shotgun pellets, the site of embolus can easily be predicted from its size.[128] For the more common fibrin–platelet complexes, however, other factors are involved, especially the poorly understood compressibility of the mass and the time required to transit a certain point of narrowing in the arterial tree. The few cases that document the passage of fibrin–platelet emboli through the arterial tree[138] show considerable alteration in the length and width of the material at different points, which indicates that it possesses a remarkable elasticity and friability. What is sufficient lumen reduction to arrest the material may not be enough to keep it from changing shape or fragmenting within minutes to hours, leaving the site of the original embolic occlusion widely patent.

Embolic obstruction of an arterial lumen is most commonly cleared by recanalization with fibrinolysis. A column of blood develops between the embolus and the arterial wall, enlarges, and erodes the embolus until the lumen is finally cleared. The exact sequence of events is not fully understood in human material, but cases documented at different stages during the process make it clear that recanalization is accomplished within periods as short as hours to days.[134,138,139] The timetable for this process is also poorly understood. In some instances, the erosion takes enough time that noninvasive studies may document stenoses that create turbulences identical to those seen with atheroma. The angiographic appearance of the gradually eroding embolus is indistinguishable from that of atherostenosis. During this process, the lumen may appear stenotic.[140-142]

At the site of occlusion, opportunity exists for a thrombus to develop in anterograde fashion throughout the length of the vessel, but this event seems to occur only rarely. Lack of an anterograde thrombus implies either that an active flow is present proximal to the occlusion or that the occlusion was too short-lived to permit the development of the anterograde thrombus. At autopsy it is common to find the vessel distended by the embolus, yet the histologic appearance of the wall at that point usually shows no significant abnormalities. The frequent finding that the vessel wall itself is not significantly injured by the embolus argues against a role for endothelial injury, vasospasm, or necrotizing effects in the pathogenesis of the infarction from embolism.

Clinical Features

It was once taught that the sudden onset of a clinical deficit was typical of embolism and that a non-sudden onset would be more typical of thrombosis. Numerous case examples have now amply demonstrated that onset may be sudden in either condition. Non-sudden or fluctuating onset occurs in 5% to 6% of documented embolic strokes; the syndrome often requires about 36 hours to evolve.[59,143] A clinical diagnosis of multiple TIAs is often entertained. The reestablishment of flow, presumed further migration of embolic material, and subsequent repetition of these events are thought to be the mechanisms involved. Embolic material has even been documented to go to the same site on repeated occasions,[144] which is the opposite of traditional predictions.

In the past, many syndromes were considered almost specific for embolism. In each of these syndromes, it was assumed that the infarct was so focal and so far distal in the arterial tree that local atheroma was not a serious possibility. Hemianopia without hemiparesis or hemisensory disturbances, Wernicke's aphasia, ideomotor apraxia, and involvement of specific territories (e.g., the posterior division of the MCA, the anterior cerebral artery, the cerebellum, and multiple territories) were more commonly associated with the presence of a potential cardiac source of embolism in the Lausanne Stroke Registry.[17] CT and MRI have shown that any of these syndromes may arise from hematoma, and modern neurologists have become wary of administering anticoagulation therapy on the basis of clinical syndrome analysis alone.

One syndrome seems to have held its own as a sign of embolism, although it is met only rarely. A spectacular shrinking deficit can occur when the embolus is introduced into the ICA, causing a profound full hemispheral syndrome, after which it passes up the artery to its final resting place in, for example, the angular branch of the MCA, leaving only a mild aphasia after a few days or a week.[145] Especially characteristic of the MCA migratory embolism is the syndrome of fading hemiparesis with Wernicke's aphasia: the embolus lodges initially at the stem of the MCA, occluding the penetrating lenticulostriate branches long enough to produce scattered foci of infarction through the basal ganglia and internal capsule, of which the involvement of the latter produce the hemiparesis. Distal migration of the embolus then occurs, finally occluding the lower division of the MCA at the superior temporal plane and beyond. This infarct yields Wernicke's aphasia. Two separate foci of infarction occur, but they result from the same embolic event.

The cardiac history of the patient often provides important clues about a potential embolic source. In the Stroke Data Bank, besides a greater frequency of cardiac disease, patients with cardioembolic infarction were more often seen with reduced consciousness.[34,82] Cardioembolic infarcts were more likely to have nonfractional arm weakness, except for those with infarctions smaller than 20 mL, in which fractional weakness was more common. In a separate Stroke Data Bank analysis, a history of systemic embolism and an abrupt onset were historical features significantly associated with cardiac sources of embolism.[146] Clinical features observed at stroke onset help distinguish the cardioembolic group from other subtypes, but the diagnosis largely depends on confirmatory laboratory findings that suggest a definite cardiac source of embolism.[147]

Results of Diagnostic Tests

The role of CT and MRI in the diagnosis of embolism is limited. Only when the infarction is confined to the cerebral surface territory of a single branch can embolism be inferred from a scan or image. Infarcts involving branches of different divisions of major cerebral arteries strongly suggest that embolism explains at least some of the clinical strokes that have occurred. A diagnosis of embolism is suggested by a large zone of low density that encompasses what amounts to the entire territory of a major cerebral artery or its main divisions and is larger than one lobe. Embolism is also the leading diagnosis when hemorrhagic infarction is seen on brain imaging.[12,17] As already mentioned, this assumption is plausible in the presence of a more or less extended hematoma, but it may not be true for other cases displaying petechial, scattered high density along the margins or in the infarct zone.[18,19] In some 30% to 50% of cases, the CT scan (or MRI) may show the occlusion itself, as the presence of the hyperdense MCA sign. Finally, as mentioned previously, a scattered infarct pattern on diffusion-weighted MRI may suggest embolism from whatever source.[86,87,148]

Angiography was once considered sufficient to diagnose embolism from any source if the angiogram showed branch occlusion in the absence of other occlusive disease elsewhere.[104,149-151] This rule still holds for practical purposes, but isolated branch occlusions may occur in arteritis. Furthermore, growing evidence shows that intracranial atherosclerosis is common enough in some races, especially black people, that MCA stem occlusions may be atheromatous as well as embolic. Recanalizing embolus may mimic all the angiographic features of atherosclerosis.[140] Only when a second angiogram is performed within days of the angiogram demonstrating occlusion (and the initial occlusion is gone) can a diagnosis of embolism be made with confidence. Measures this extreme are impractical for the management of most patients.

In the presence of a cardiac source of embolism, the diagnosis is certain for all practical purposes. Establishing the cardiac source is not always a simple task. The most common sources of cardiac embolism are (1) valvular heart disease (e.g., mitral stenosis, mitral regurgitation, or rheumatic heart disease); (2) an intracardiac thrombus, particularly along the left ventricular wall (mural thrombus), after anterior myocardial infarction, or in the left atrial appendage in patients with atrial fibrillation; (3) ventricular or septal aneurysm; and (4) cardiomyopathies leading to stagnation of blood flow and a greater propensity for the formation of an intracardiac thrombus. A paradoxic embolus occurs when a thrombus crosses from the venous circulation to the left side of the heart, most often through a patent foramen ovale. Other possible causes of cardiac embolism are atrial myxoma, atrial septal aneurysm, spontaneous echo contrast, marantic endocarditis, and prolapse of the mitral valve. Finally, aortic arch plaques, particularly when they protrude and are complicated, have been identified as potentially active sources of emboli.[152-155]

The cardiac diagnostic evaluation starts with electrocardiography for identifying atrial fibrillation, acute myocardial infarction, or other arrhythmias. Holter monitoring for 24 hours is sometimes necessary to detect paroxysmal atrial fibrillation. Identification of the cardiac source depends most on transthoracic and transesophageal echocardiography, which has become more sensitive and has greatly improved the detection of sources of embolism. Bubble contrast is needed to diagnose a patent foramen ovale. Unfortunately, embolic material large enough to produce a focal stroke is so small that it may escape detection by echocardiography and all too often eludes all efforts at diagnosis. Future advances in cardiac imaging may help improve the sensitivity for detecting cardiac sources of embolism.

Lacunar Infarction

Cases of lacunar infarction represent a special group that warrants description because they often occur as a common set of clinical syndromes, angiographic findings are usually normal, and the zone of ischemia is confined to the territory of a single vessel, usually quite small. Lacunar infarctions are understood to reflect arterial disease of the vessels penetrating the brain to supply the capsule, basal ganglia, thalamus, and paramedian regions of the brainstem.[156] Only a handful have been studied by autopsy, and an even smaller number have been subjected to serial section.[157] The most common lesion is a tiny focus of microatheroma or lipohyalinosis stenosing one of the deep penetrating arteries. Less frequent causes are stenosis of the MCA stem[11,158] and microembolization to penetrant arterial territories.[159]

Histopathologic studies have rarely included patients with lacunar strokes because the in-hospital mortality of such patients is the lowest for all those with ischemic stroke. In one stroke registry, the in-hospital mortality for lacunar cases was only 2.9%.[160] A serial study of 100 autopsy cases with acute ischemic strokes has shown that hypoperfusion is an underestimated mechanism and was considered to be a definite cause of the infarct in five cases, whereas atheromatous causes were found in 10 cases. All infarcts were more than 10 mm in diameter, and no "classic" lacunes were seen as the corresponding infarcts, probably owing to the selection of cases reaching autopsy.[161] One single autopsied case study has shown a thrombus formation in the MCA as a convincing cause of striatocapsular infarction.[162]

Multiple infarcts in the centrum semiovale are rarely of lacunar origin, even if they do not exceed 1.5 cm in diameter. Mostly they represent consequences of hemodynamic failure and have been described to have a rosary-like appearance. For example, in an MRI study of 16 patients, centrum semiovale infarcts were thought to be caused by occluded or highly stenosed carotid vessels on the ipsilateral side.[163] One other pathologic study of centrum semiovale infarcts showed that in 10 of 12 consecutive cases, the underlying mechanism was thought to be either cardiogenic or due to large vessel disease.[164]

Because of the lack of autopsy data demonstrating lacunes, detailed MRI investigations have been undertaken. In one such study of nine patients with lacunar syndrome, the occluded perforator was visualized together with leaks of blood and fluid in the perivascular space.[165]

Investigators have used the term *lacunar hypothesis* to refer to the clinicopathophysiologic correlation of the condition. The hypothesis consists of two parts: (1) symptomatic lacunes are usually present with a small number of distinct lacunar syndromes and (2) lacunes are caused by a characteristic disease of the penetrating artery.[41] After satisfying both parts of the hypothesis, the stroke can be classified as a lacunar infarction. Lacunes were slow to gain clinical acceptance, but they are now considered to account for between 15% and 20% of all cases of stroke.[6,38,52,53,69,166]

Clinical Features

The diagnosis of lacunar strokes has long been based on clinical characteristics alone, a practice that has contributed little to their popularity among clinical researchers in the field. The term *lacunar syndrome* refers to the constellation of clinical features that may indicate, although not invariably, a lacune. The characteristic features of all these syndromes are their relative purity and their failure to involve higher cerebral functions such as language, praxis, behavior controlled by the nondominant hemisphere, memory, and vision.[167] The classic lacunar syndromes include pure motor, pure sensory, and sensorimotor syndromes; ataxic hemiparesis; clumsy hand dysarthria; and hemichorea/hemiballism. However, other combinations of findings may be attributed to small, deep infarcts due to a lacunar mechanism. Efforts to expand the diagnosis into new formulas that account for the presence of cognitive changes have shaken the earlier purity and confounded the appealing simplicity of the initial syndromes,[168] leading some to question the separate nosologic identity of lacunar infarcts.[169,170] Some skeptics have suggested the abolition of terms like *lacunar syndrome, lacune,* and *lacunar infarction* because of confusion. However, most of the investigations that have included analyses of clinical syndromes, results of diagnostic imaging, etiopathophysiologic correlations, and treatment implications justify the continued use of the term *lacune.*

The correspondence between lacunar syndrome and lacunar infarction depends on the timing of presentation and examination. The concordance is greatest among patients examined up to 96 hours after stroke onset[41,171] and is much less when patients are tested in the first few hours of stroke onset.[44,48,172-174]

There are clearly examples of thrombotic or embolic infarcts manifesting as pure motor hemiparesis or sensorimotor stroke, and, conversely, large lacunar infarcts in the caudate nucleus or thalamus that may initially manifest as impairment of higher cerebral functions. The latter syndromes are probably due to a reversible functional disconnection between the subcortical infarcted areas and their cortical projections.[175,176] In the acute setting, therefore, the reliance on clinical grounds alone for the identification of lacunar infarcts can be misleading for both prognostic estimates and therapeutic choices.[8]

Using data from the Northern Manhattan Stroke Study, Gan et al[177] were able to evaluate the value of lacunar syndromes in predicting radiologic lacunes as well as the value of clinicoradiologic lacunes in predicting lacunar infarction as a final stroke mechanism. Lacunar syndromes were found in 225 of 591 patients, and the proportions of lacunar infarction in black people and Hispanics were nearly twice that in white people. The positive predictive value for finding a small, deep infarct on brain imaging after a presenting lacunar syndrome was 87% and was best for pure sensory syndrome (100%) and ataxic hemiparesis (95%), intermediate for sensorimotor syndrome (87%), and least for pure motor hemiparesis (79%). Among the 195 patients who were seen with a lacunar syndrome and in whom radiologic evaluation confirmed a small deep infarct, 147 were classified with a final diagnosis of lacunar infarct mechanism (positive predictive value, 75%). Extracranial or intracranial atherosclerosis accounted for 16 cases (8%), cardioembolism for 10 (5%), cryptogenic causes for 19 (10%), and other causes for 3 (2%). These investigators concluded that lacunar syndromes, especially pure sensory syndrome and ataxic hemiparesis, were highly predictive of small deep infarcts; however, about one in four patients seen with lacunar syndromes that are confirmed radiologically may ultimately be proved to have a nonlacunar infarct mechanism. A complete diagnostic evaluation of large vessels and potential cardiogenic sources of embolism is warranted in these patients.

Results of Diagnostic Tests

CT scanning results are positive only for roughly half of cases of even the most common form of lacune: pure motor stroke.[6,42,178] Visualizing lacunes depends on their location, and MRI is clearly superior to CT in evaluating lesions, especially in the posterior fossa. Overall, MRI has improved the yield of finding a strategically placed, small deep infarct.[179] A complex diagnostic evaluation, including MRA and diffusion-weighted MRI, has been suggested to significantly improve the differential diagnosis among stroke subtypes when its findings are added to the Trial of Org 10172 in Acute Stroke Treatment (TOAST) or the Oxford Community Stroke Project (OCSP) clinical criteria of classification in patients seen within 24 hours of stroke onset. Particularly, the diagnosis of lacunar infarcts according to the TOAST criteria improved from 35% to 100% with addition of this evaluation, and that with the OCSP classification improved from 78% to 100%.[180]

In the Northern Manhattan Stroke Study, using either CT or MRI, Gan et al were able to radiologically detect small deep infarcts in appropriate locations in 84% of cases of lacunar syndromes.[177] The radiologic equivalent of a lacune was defined as a small deep lesion on brain imaging usually less than 1 cm in diameter with a density or signal consistent with an infarct located in the appropriate area of the brain to explain the syndrome or the absence of a responsible lesion despite a second evaluation. The latter definition is based on the fact that some lacunes are too small to be seen on CT or MRI despite a second scan.

Large deep infarcts, some of which have been called *super lacunes* or *giant lacunes,* may be seen on CT or MRI as a focal, deep site of infarction without involvement of the cerebral surface.[178] A problem arises in the interpretation of these deep lesions because an embolus may initially be arrested in the stem of the MCA, causing a large swath of infarction scattered through the lenticulostriate territories. When accompanied by a separate cerebral surface low-density area, such large deep infarcts are easily reclassified as examples of embolism, nonthrombotic infarction, or infarction of other cause. Therefore, most of these large, deep infarcts are really not lacunes.

In cases of pure motor hemiparesis, lacunes can be most commonly found in the internal capsule and corona radiata, but they have also been imaged in the basal ganglia, pons, and thalamus. Scan findings in the capsule, adjacent corona radiata, thalamus, or pons have been reported on occasion for the ataxic–hemiparesis, dysarthria–clumsy hand syndrome and hemiballism.[42,181] Pure sensory strokes have been reported from small thalamic infarcts, of which some were so small as to cause selective proprioceptive loss without pain or temperature deficits.[120] Reports of pure sensory stroke from low densities in the centrum semiovale are probably lacunar, although surface infarction has rarely been demonstrated.[182]

Because the vascular lesion lies in vessels some 200 to 400 μm in diameter, it is perhaps no surprise that conventional cerebral angiographic and MRA findings are normal. Incidental large vessel disease may be found in some series, but whether it is etiologically related to the site of infarction is often unclear.[42,173,174] An angiogram with normal findings could also be expected if microembolism was the cause of the deep infarction. Whether the outlook for stenosis of the MCA stem or the basilar artery differs if the syndrome is lacunar remains unsettled. Because some of the cases of pure motor stroke have been associated with MCA stenosis, the mere presence of such a syndrome has not been an indicator of the status of the major artery in question. TCD ultrasonography of the MCA stem or basilar artery has helped to establish the patency of these large vessels. MRA or CTA may be required to settle the matter in some cases, and it remains the preferred diagnostic technique when TCD ultrasonography is technically unsatisfactory and CT or MRI shows a large band of low density that spans several sections and whose abnormality is seen down to the base of the affected basal ganglia.[178] Such a large infarct is not easily accounted for by primary disease in the penetrating artery itself, which justifies angiography to seek stenosis of the MCA stem. The prognosis for later hemisphere symptoms in the patient with stem stenosis manifesting as a lacunar infarct is unknown.

Cryptogenic Infarction or Infarct of Undetermined Cause

Despite efforts to arrive at a diagnosis, the cause of the infarction may remain undetermined. A number of explanations can be offered. The first of the three major reasons for the failure is easily understood: no appropriate laboratory studies are performed. Advanced age, coexisting severe disease with a poor prognosis, and patient's or physician's unwillingness are only a few of the many reasons for deferring an evaluation. One reason no longer valid for this approach is that the mechanism of stroke has been diagnosed satisfactorily on clinical grounds alone. Among the syndromes attributed to ischemia, only the Wallenberg syndrome has yet to be reported from hematoma, and causes other than stroke have been so often reported with most of the classic focal brain syndromes that this point need not be labored.

A second common cause of failure to arrive at a diagnosis is improper timing of the appropriate laboratory studies. Angiography for embolism performed more than 48 hours after the ictus has a yield as low as 15% for evidence of the responsible occlusion.[125] Brain scans performed once only within a few hours of the onset of an ischemic stroke have a similarly low yield. Findings of brain scans performed no matter how often may remain negative in some cases of small lacunar infarction, if the lesion is below the limits of resolution of the scan technique.

As many as 40% of the cases of ischemic stroke of undetermined cause are in the third category, in which normal or ambiguous findings are reached despite appropriate laboratory studies performed at the appropriate time. This last group of cases poses special problems for research in stroke diagnosis. It would be comforting if most of these cases occurred in patients with the milder deficits, perhaps accounting for the normal laboratory findings by virtue of the relative insensitivity of such tests to smaller lesions. However, the scanty data on the subject indicate that this is not true; such cases are roughly as severe as ischemic strokes for which a cause is found.

In the Stroke Data Bank, a rigorous diagnostic scheme resulted in a high frequency of infarcts that were difficult to classify into the traditional subtypes. Despite considerable effort at evaluation, there remained a large proportion, fully 40% of patients, for whom the infarct mechanism escaped explanation and who were classified as having infarcts of undetermined cause.[38,39] Not all patients in the Stroke Data Bank underwent angiography, and when the procedure was performed, it was rarely in the first 48 to 72 hours after stroke. In other series in which patients underwent angiography within 6 hours of stroke onset,[40] the application of the same diagnostic scheme as that used in the Stroke Data Bank has led to a reduction in the number of cases labeled as strokes of undetermined cause to only 15%.

Clinical Features

Cases categorized as ischemic stroke of undetermined cause show no bruit or TIA ipsilateral to the hemisphere affected by stroke and have no obvious source of embolism; in short, the affected patients do not have the risk factors or prior history that help suggest a cardiac embolus or large artery thrombosis.[39,53] In the Stroke Data Bank, the mean age at stroke for patients with infarcts of undetermined cause studied by CT and angiography was 58 years.[39] Hemispheral syndromes predominated in 66%; basilar syndromes occurred in 15%. Very few patients had lacunar syndromes. Twenty-seven percent had worsening symptoms in the hospital, and 41% had a moderate to severe weakness score.

Results of Diagnostic Tests

Findings of CT or MRI performed within 7 days may be normal, may show an infarct limited to a surface branch territory, or may show a large zone of infarction affecting regions larger than that accounted for by a single penetrant arterial territory. In the Stroke Data Bank, among the cryptogenic infarcts fully evaluated, CT demonstrated clinically relevant infarcts in 57%; surface infarction was found in 40%.[39] Noninvasive vascular imaging failed to demonstrate an underlying large vessel occlusion or stenosis. No definite cardiac source of embolism was uncovered by echocardiography, electrocardiography, or Holter monitoring.

If angiography is performed, the findings may be normal or may show a distal branch occlusion or occlusion of a major cerebral artery stem or the top of the basilar artery. Because MCA stem or branch occlusions can have thrombotic or embolic causes, their demonstration does not settle the mechanism in all cases, particularly among black, Asian, and Hispanic patients, in whom intracranial atheroma has been more frequently detected.[166] In white patients, on the other hand, pathologic examination of MCA occlusion has rarely demonstrated an organized thrombus,[123,183] so the angiographic identification of an intracranial occlusion can usually be considered typical for embolism despite the absence of a source.[40] In the most extreme case, in which angiography is repeated and the original occlusion is no longer found, a definitive diagnosis of embolism can be made.

Potential Explanations for Cryptogenic Stroke

Some examples of the forms of stroke attributed to meningitis, migraine, lupus anticoagulant, arteritis, dissection, hypercoagulable states, and the like may be represented in the cryptogenic subgroup. Efforts should be made

in each case to establish the existence of these unusual causes, and all such instances should be identified and classified as cerebral infarction from *other determined cause*. Adding together all the estimated frequencies with which such unusual causes manifest without accompanying evidence of the underlying disease cannot remotely approach the high frequency of the cryptogenic subgroup of stroke documented in the Stroke Data Bank.

Emerging technologies have led to the suggestions that some of the cases of cryptogenic infarct may be explained by hematologic disorders causing hypercoagulable states from protein C, free protein S, lupus anticoagulant, or anticardiolipin antibody abnormalities and mutations of coagulation factors like factor II and factor V.[184-186]

Hyperhomocysteinemia, either acquired (environmental) or consequent to mutations of the *MTHFR* gene, has also received attention.[186-189] Other investigators have implicated paradoxic emboli through a patent foramen ovale[190-195] or emboli from the ascending tract of the aortic arch,[152,153] both of which have been better identified with the more widespread use of transesophageal echocardiography. The number of cases of cryptogenic infarction attributed to the lack of appropriate diagnostic examinations previously mentioned should diminish as newer and more sensitive diagnostic techniques are introduced.

One approach to dealing with this cohort of cases is their forced reclassification into the traditional categories of atherothrombosis, embolism, or lacune. The presentation of a hemispheral syndrome, a surface infarction shown by CT, and angiographic findings that either are normal or show a corresponding branch occlusion have long been considered suggestive of embolism. Nonthrombotic ischemia has been used to describe those cases with normal angiographic findings. Such findings could be inferred to represent emboli, even though no cardiac source for embolism is documented by clinical or laboratory criteria. There is ample evidence of many occult sources of emboli, the difficulty in proving their existence, and their role in the first or succeeding ischemic strokes. Reclassification of such cases (and others in which CT shows limited cerebral infarction) as embolism with unobvious source would add most of the patients with cryptogenic infarct to the embolism category, making embolism from all sources the largest subtype of stroke.[39,40] Alternatively, maintaining a separate category of cryptogenic strokes is useful for determining whether this group of cases differs in some way from those in which the mechanism of stroke is better defined and for encouraging the continued search for causes of brain infarction and precipitants of thromboembolism.

REFERENCES

1. Pulsinelli W: Pathophysiology of acute ischaemic stroke, *Lancet* 339:533–536, 1992.
2. Hacke W, Kaste M, Fieschi C, et al: Safety and efficacy of intravenous thrombolysis with a recombinant tissue plasminogen activator in the treatment of acute hemispheric stroke, *JAMA* 27:1017–1025, 1995.
3. The National Institute of Neurological Disorders and Stroke rt-PA Stroke Study Group: Tissue plasminogen activator for acute ischemic stroke, *N Engl J Med* 333:1581–1587, 1995.
4. Wardlaw JM, del Zoppo G, Yamaguchi T: Thrombolysis for acute ischaemic stroke, *Cochrane database syst rev* 2, 2000:CD000213.

5. Hacke W, Kaste M, Bluhmki E, et al: Alteplase compared with placebo within 3 to 4.5 hours for acute ischemic stroke, *N Engl J Med* 359:1317-1329, 2008.

6. Mohr JP: Lacunes. *Neurol Clin* 1:201-221, 1983.

7. Mohr JP: Lacunes. In Barnett HJM, Stein BH, Yatsu FM, editors: *Stroke: Pathophysiology, diagnosis and management*, New York, 1986, Churchill Livingstone, pp 475-496.

8. Toni D, Fiorelli M, De Michele M, et al: Clinical and prognostic correlates of stroke subtype misdiagnosis within 12 hours from onset, *Stroke* 26:1837-1840, 1995.

9. del Zoppo GJ, Poeck K, Pessin MS, et al: Recombinant tissue plasminogen activator in acute thrombotic and embolic stroke, *Ann Neurol* 32:78-86, 1992.

10. Von Kummer R, Forsting M, Sartor K, Hacke W: Intravenous recombinant tissue plasminogen activator in acute stroke. In Hacke W, del Zoppo GJ, Hirschberg M, editors: *Thrombolytic therapy in acute ischemic stroke*, Berlin, 1991, Springer-Verlag, pp 161-167.

11. Araki G: Small infarctions of the basal ganglia with special reference to transient ischemic attacks, *Nippon Ronen Igakkai Zasshi* 17(5):533-541, 1980.

12. Beghi E, Bogliun G, Cavaletti G, et al: Hemorrhagic infarction: Risk factors, clinical and tomographic features, and outcome: A case-control study, *Acta Neurol Scand* 80:226-231, 1989.

13. Gacs G, Fox AJ, Barnett HJM, Vinuela F: CT visualization of intracranial arterial thromboembolism, *Stroke* 14:756, 1983.

14. Fisher CM, Adams RD: Observations on brain embolism with special reference to the mechanism of hemorrhagic infarction, *J Neuropathol Exp Neurol* 10:92, 1951.

15. De Ley G, Weyne J, Demeester G, et al: Experimental thromboembolic stroke studied by positron emission tomography: Immediate versus delayed reperfusion by fibrinolysis, *J Cereb Blood Flow Metab* 8:539-545, 1988.

16. Sloan MA: Thrombolysis and stroke: Past and future, *Arch Neurol* 44:748-768, 1987.

17. Bogousslavsky J, Cachin C, Regli F, et al: Cardiac sources of embolism and cerebral infarction: Clinical consequences and vascular concomitants: The Lausanne Stroke Registry, *Neurology* 41:855-859, 1991.

18. Hornig CR, Dorndorf W, Agnoli AL: Hemorrhagic cerebral infarction—a prospective study, *Stroke* 17:179-185, 1986.

19. Toni D, Fiorelli M, Bastianello S, et al: Hemorrhagic transformation of brain infarct: Predictability in the first five hours from stroke onset and influence on clinical outcome, *Neurology* 46:341-345, 1996.

20. Paciaroni M, Agnelli G, Corea E, et al: Early hemorrhagic transformation of brain infarction: Rate, predictive factors, and influence on clinical outcome: results of a prospective multicenter study, *Stroke* 39:2249-2256, 2008.

21. Hornig CR, Bauer T, Simon C, et al: Hemorrhagic transformation in cardioembolic cerebral infarction, *Stroke* 24:465-468, 1993.

22. Mohr JP, Duterte DI, Oliveira VR, et al: Recanalization of acute middle cerebral artery occlusion, *Neurology* 38(Suppl):215, 1988.

23. Ogata J, Yutani C, Imakita M, et al: Hemorrhagic infarct of the brain without a reopening of the occluded arteries in cardioembolic stroke, *Stroke* 20:876-883, 1989.

24. Massaro AR, Sacco RL, Scaff M, Mohr JP: Clinical discriminators between acute brain hemorrhage and infarction—a practical score for early patient identification, *Arq Neuropsiquiatr* 60 (2-A):185-191, 2002.

25. Panzer RJ, Feibel JH, Barker WH, Griner PF: Predicting the likelihood of hemorrhage in patients with stroke, *Arch Intern Med* 145:1800-1803, 1985.

26. Sandercock PAG, Allen CMC, Corston RN, et al: Clinical diagnosis of intracranial haemorrhage using Guy's Hospital Score, *BMJ* 291:1675-1677, 1985.

27. Spitzer K, Thie A, Caplan LR, Kunze K: The MICRO-STROKE expert system for stroke type diagnosis, *Stroke* 20:1353-1356, 1989.

28. Von Arbin M, Britton M, de Faire U, et al: Accuracy of bedside diagnosis in stroke, *Stroke* 12:288-293, 1981.

29. Chen ZM, Sandercock P, Pan HC, et al: Indications for early aspirin use in acute ischemic stroke: A combined analysis of 40, 000 randomized patients from the Chinese Acute Stroke Trial and the International Stroke Trial. On behalf of the CAST and IST collaborative groups, *Stroke* 31:1240-1249, 2000.

30. Fieschi C, Carolei A, Fiorelli M, et al: Changing prognosis of primary intracerebral hemorrhage: Result of a clinical and computed tomographic study of 104 patients, *Stroke* 19:192-195, 1988.

31. Drurys I, Whisnant JP, Garraway WM: Primary intracerebral hemorrhage: Impact of CT on incidence, *Neurology* 34:653-657, 1984.

32. Chalela JA, Kidwell CS, Nentwich LM, et al: Magnetic resonance imaging and computed tomography in emergency assessment of patients with suspected acute stroke: A prospective comparison, *Lancet* 369(9558):293-298, 2007 Jan 27.

33. Powers WJ: Cerebral hemodynamics in ischemic cerebrovascular disease, *Ann Neurol* 29:231-240, 1991.

34. Timsit S, Sacco RL, Mohr JP, et al: Brain infarction severity differs according to cardiac or arterial embolic source: The NINDS Stroke Data Bank, *Neurology* 43:728-733, 1993.

35. Toni D, Fiorelli M, Gentile M, et al: Progressing neurological deficit secondary to acute ischemic stroke: Study on predictability, pathogenesis and prognosis, *Arch Neurol* 52:670-675, 1995.

36. von Kummer R, Meyding-Lamadi U, Forsting M, et al: Sensitivity and prognostic value of early CT in occlusion of the middle cerebral artery trunk, *AJNR Am J Neuroradiol* 15:9-15, 1994.

37. Pexman JH, Barber PA, Hill MD, et al: Use of the Alberta Stroke Program Early CT Score (ASPECTS) for assessing CT scans in patients with acute stroke, *AJNR Am J Neuroradiol* 22:1534-1542, 2001.

38. Foulkes MA, Wolf PA, Price TR, et al: The Stroke Data Bank: Design, methods, and baseline characteristics, *Stroke* 19:547-554, 1988.

38a. Mohr JP: Cryptogenic stroke [editorial], *N Engl J Med* 318:1197-1198, 1988.

39. Sacco RL, Ellenberg JA, Mohr JP, et al: Infarction of undetermined cause: The NINDS Stroke Data Bank, *Ann Neurol* 25:382-390, 1989.

40. Fieschi C, Argentino C, Lenzi GL, et al: Clinical and instrumental evaluation of patients with ischemic stroke within the first six hours, *J Neurol Sci* 91:311-321, 1989.

41. Bamford JM, Warlow CP: Evolution and testing of the lacunar hypothesis, *Stroke* 19:1074-1082, 1988.

42. Chamorro AM, Sacco RL, Mohr JP, et al: Lacunar infarction: Clinical-CT correlations in the Stroke Data Bank, *Stroke* 22:175-181, 1991.

43. Toni D, Del Duca R, Fiorelli M, et al: Pure motor hemiplegia and sensorimotor stroke: Accuracy of the very early clinical diagnosis of lacunar stroke, *Stroke* 25:92-96, 1994.

44. Edwards JH, Kricheff II, Riles T, Imparato A: Angiographically undetected ulceration of the carotid bifurcation as a cause of embolic stroke, *Radiology* 132:369, 1979.

45. Fisher CM, Karnes WE: Local embolism, *J Neuropathol Exp Neurol* 24:174, 1965.

46. Imparato AM, Riles TS, Gorstein F: The carotid bifurcation plaque: Pathologic findings associated with cerebral ischemia, *Stroke* 10:238, 1979.

47. Masuda J, Ogata J, Yutani C, et al: Artery to artery embolism from a thrombus formed in stenotic middle cerebral artery: Report of an autopsy case, *Stroke* 18:680-684, 1987.

48. Droste DW, Dittrich R, Kemeny V, et al: Prevalence and frequency of microembolic signals in 105 patients with extracranial carotid artery occlusive disease, *J Neurol Neurosurg Psychiatry* 67:525-528, 1999.

49. Tsiskaridze A, Devuyst G, de Freitas GR, et al: Stroke with internal carotid artery stenosis, *Arch Neurol* 58:605-609, 2001.

50. El-Mitwalli A, Saad M, Christou I, et al: Clinical and sonographic patterns of tandem internal carotid artery/middle cerebral artery occlusion in tissue plasminogen activator-treated patients, *Stroke* 33:99-102, 2002.

51. Bogousslavsky J, Van Melle G, Regli F: The Lausanne Stroke Registry: Analysis of 1000 consecutive patients with first stroke, *Stroke* 19:1083-1092, 1988.

52. Gross CR, Kase CS, Mohr JP, Cunningham SC: Stroke in south Alabama: Incidence and diagnostic features, *Stroke* 15:249, 1984.

53. Kunitz S, Gross CR, Heyman A, et al: The pilot stroke data bank: Definition, design, data, *Stroke* 15:740, 1984.

54. Mohr JP, Caplan LR, Melski JW, et al: The Harvard cooperative stroke registry: A prospective registry of cases hospitalized with stroke, *Neurology* 28:754, 1978.

55. Aring CD, Merritt HH: Differential diagnosis between cerebral hemorrhage and cerebral thrombosis, *Arch Intern Med* 56:435, 1935.

56. Fisher CM, Gore I, Okabe N, White PD: Atherosclerosis of the carotid and vertebral arteries: Extracranial and intracranial, *J Neuropathol Exp Neurol* 24:455, 1965.

57. Samuel KC: Atherosclerosis and occlusion of the internal carotid artery, *J Pathol Bacteriol* 71:391, 1956.

58. Fisher CM: Cerebral thromboangiitis obliterans, *Medicine (Baltimore)* 36:169, 1957.

59. Mohr JP: Neurologic complications of cardiac valvular disease and cardiac surgery. In Vinken PJ, Bruyn GW, editors: *Handbook of clinical neurology*, Vol. 34, Amsterdam, North Holland, 1979, pp 143.

60. Ogata J, Masuda J, Yutani C, Yamaguchi T: Rupture of atheromatous plaque as a cause of thrombotic occlusion of stenotic internal carotid artery, *Stroke* 21:1740-1745, 1990.

61. Lennihan L, Kupsky WJ, Mohr JP, et al: Lack of association between carotid plaque hematoma and ipsilateral cerebral symptoms, *Stroke* 18:879-881, 1987.

62. Ballotta E, Da Giau G, Renon L: Carotid plaque gross morphology and clinical presentation: A prospective study of 457 carotid artery specimens, *J Surg Res* 89:78-84, 2000.

63. Hatsukami TS, Ross R, Polissar NL, Yuan C: Visualization of fibrous cap thickness and rupture in human atherosclerotic carotid plaque in vivo with high-resolution magnetic resonance imaging, *Circulation* 102:959-964, 2000.

64. Yoshida K, Narumi O, Chin M, et al: Characterization of carotid atherosclerosis and detection of soft plaque with use of black-blood MR imaging, *AJNR Am J Neuroradiol* 29:868-874, 2008.

65. Bogousslavsky J, Regli F: Borderzone infarctions distal to internal carotid artery occlusion: Prognostic implications, *Ann Neurol* 20:346-350, 1986.

66. Hultquist GT: *Ueber Thrombose und Embolie der Arteria carotis und herbei vorkommende Gehirnveraenderungen: Eine pathologisch-anatomische Studie*, Stockholm, 1942, Gustav Fischer Verlag.

67. Pessin MS, Hinton RC, Davis KR, et al: Mechanisms of acute carotid stroke: A clinicoangiographic study, *Ann Neurol* 6:245, 1979.

68. Ring BA: Diagnosis of embolic occlusions of smaller branches of the intracerebral arteries, *Am J Roentgenol Radium Ther Nucl Med* 97:575, 1966.

69. Romanul FCA, Abramowicz A: Changes in brain and pial vessels in arterial borderzones, *Arch Neurol (Chic)* 11:40, 1964.

70. Torvick A: The pathogenesis of watershed infarcts in the brain, *Stroke* 15:221-223, 1984.

71. Carpenter DA, Grubb RL Jr, Powers WJ: Borderzone hemodynamics in cerebrovascular disease, *Neurology* 40:1587-1592, 1990.

72. Powers WJ, Tempel LW, Grubb RL Jr: Influence of cerebral hemodynamics on stroke risk: One year follow up of 30 medically treated patients, *Ann Neurol* 25:325-330, 1989.

73. Beal MF, Williams RS, Richardson EP, Fisher CM: Cholesterol embolism as a cause of transient ischemic attacks and cerebral infarction, *Neurology* 31:860, 1981.

74. David NJ, Gordon KK, Friedberg SJ, et al: Fatal atheromatous cerebral embolism associated with bright plaques in the retinal arterioles, *Neurology* 13:708, 1963.

75. Koennecke HC, Mast H, Trocio SS, et al: Frequency and determinants of microembolic signals on transcranial Doppler in unselected patients with acute carotid territory ischemia—A prospective study, *Cerebrovasc Dis* 8:107-112, 1998.

76. Adams HP, Gross CE: Embolism distal to stenosis of the middle cerebral artery, *Stroke* 12:228, 1981.

77. Segura T, Serena J, Castellanos M, et al: Embolism in acute middle cerebral artery stenosis, *Neurology* 56:497-501, 2001.

78. Castaigne P, Lhermitte F, Gautier J-C, et al: Arterial occlusions in the vertebro-basilar system: A study of forty-four patients with post-mortem data, *Brain* 96:133, 1973.

79. Barnett HJM, Peerless SJ, Kaufmann JCE: "Stump" of internal carotid artery—a source for further cerebral embolic ischemia, *Stroke* 9:448, 1978.

80. Russell RW: Atheromatous retinal embolism, *Lancet* 2:1354, 1963.

81. Angeloni U, Bozzao L, Fantozzi L, et al: Internal border zone infarction following acute middle cerebral artery occlusion, *Neurology* 40:1196-1198, 1990.

82. Timsit S, Sacco RL, Mohr JP, et al: Early clinical differentiation of atherosclerotic and cardioembolic infarction: Stroke Data Bank, *Stroke* 23:486-491, 1992.

83. Fieschi C, Sette G, Fiorelli M, et al: Clinical presentation and frequency of potential sources of embolism in acute ischemic stroke patients: The experience of the Rome Acute Stroke Registry, *Cerebrovasc Dis* 5:75-78, 1995.

84. Ringelstein EB, Zeumer H, Angelou D: The pathogenesis of strokes from internal carotid artery occlusion: Diagnostic and therapeutic implications, *Stroke* 14:867, 1983.

85. Ringelstein EB, Koschorke S, Holling A, et al: Computed tomographic patterns of proven embolic brain infarctions, *Ann Neurol* 26:759-765, 1989.

86. Ay H, Oliveira-Filho J, Buonanno FS, et al: Diffusion-weighted imaging identifies a subset of lacunar infarction associated with embolic source, *Stroke* 30:2644-2650, 1999.

87. Koennecke HC, Bernarding J, Braun J, et al: Scattered brain infarct pattern on diffusion-weighted magnetic resonance imaging in patients with acute ischemic stroke, *Cerebrovasc Dis* 11:157-163, 2001.

88. Pessin MS, Duncan GW, Davis KR, et al: Angiographic appearance of carotid occlusion in acute stroke, *Stroke* 11:485, 1980.

89. Quisling RG, Friedman WA, Rhoton AL: High cervical dissection: Spontaneous resolution, *AJNR Am J Neuroradiol* 1:463, 1980.

90. Dion JE, Gates PC, Fox AJ, et al: Clinical events following neuroangiography: A prospective study, *Stroke* 18:997-1004, 1987.

91. Hankey GJ, Warlow CP, Sellar RJ: Cerebral angiographic risk in mild cerebrovascular disease, *Stroke* 21:209-222, 1990.

92. Leow K, Murie JA: Cerebral angiography for cerebrovascular disease: The risks, *Br J Surg* 75:428-430, 1988.

93. Caplan LR, Brass LM, DeWitt LD, et al: Transcranial Doppler ultrasound: Present status, *Neurology* 40:696-700, 1990.

94. DeWitt LD, Wechsler LR: Transcranial Doppler, *Stroke* 19:915-921, 1988.

95. Grolimund P, Seiler RW, Aaslid R, et al: Evaluation of cerebrovascular disease by combined extracranial and transcranial Doppler sonography: Experience in 1,039 patients, *Stroke* 18:1018-1024, 1987.

96. Tatemichi TK, Chamorro A, Petty GW, et al: Hemodynamic role of ophthalmic artery collateral in internal carotid artery occlusion, *Neurology* 40:461-464, 1990.

97. Zanette EM, Fieschi C, Bozzao L, et al: Comparison of cerebral angiography and transcranial Doppler sonography in acute stroke, *Stroke* 20:899-903, 1989.

98. Zierler RE, Kohler TR, Strandness DE Jr: Duplex scanning of normal or minimally diseased carotid arteries: Correlation with arteriography and clinical outcome, *J Vasc Surg* 12:447-454, 1990.

99. Hirai T, Korogi Y, Ono K, et al: Prospective evaluation of suspected stenoocclusive disease of the intracranial artery: Combined MR angiography and CT angiography compared with digital subtraction angiography, *AJNR Am J Neuroradiol* 23:93-101, 2002.

100. Romero JM, Ackerman RH, Dault NA, Lev MH: Noninvasive evaluation of carotid artery stenosis: Indications, strategies, and accuracy, *Neuroimaging Clin N Am* 15:351-365, 2005.

101. Castaigne P, Lhermitte F, Gautier J-C: Role des lésions artérielles dans les accidents ischemiques cérébraux de l'athérosclerose, *Rev Neurol (Paris)* 113:1, 1965.

102. Castaigne P, Lhermitte F, Gautier J-C, et al: Internal carotid artery occlusion: A study of 61 instances in 50 patients with post-mortem data, *Brain* 93:231, 1970.

103. Torvik A, Jorgensen L: Thrombotic and embolic occlusions of the carotid arteries in an autopsy material. Part 2: Cerebral lesions and clinical course, *J Neurol Sci* 3:410, 1966.

104. Dalal PM, Shah PM, Aiyar RR: Arteriographic study of cerebral embolism, *Lancet* 2:358, 1965.

105. Caplan LR: Occlusion of the vertebral or basilar artery: Follow up analysis of some patients with benign outcome, *Stroke* 10:277, 1979.

106. Caplan LR: "Top of the basilar" syndrome, *Neurology* 30:72, 1980.

107. Castaigne P, Lhermitte F, Buge A, et al: Paramedian thalamic and midbrain infarcts: Clinical and neuropathological study, *Ann Neurol* 10:127, 1981.

108. Fisher CM: Bilateral occlusion of basilar artery branches, *J Neurol Neurosurg Psychiatry* 40:1182, 1977.

109. Voetsch B, DeWitt LD, Pessin MS, Caplan LR: Basilar artery occlusive disease in the New England Medical Center Posterior Circulation Registry, *Arch Neurol* 61:496-504, 2004.

110. Caplan LR: Intracranial branch atheromatous disease: A neglected, understudied, and underused concept, *Neurology* 39:1246-1250, 1989.

111. Heiss WD, Herholz K, Podreka I, et al: Comparison of ^{99m}Tc HMPAO SPECT with ^{18}F fluoromethane PET in cerebrovascular disease, *J Cereb Blood Flow Metab* 10:687-697, 1990.

112. Johnson DW, Stringer WA, Marks MP, et al: Stable xenon CT cerebral blood flow imaging: Rationale for and role in clinical decision making, *AJNR Am J Neuroradiol* 12:201-213, 1991.

113. Edelman RR, Mattle HP, Atkinson DJ, et al: Cerebral blood flow: Assessment with dynamic contrast enhanced T2*-weighted MR imaging at 1.5 T, *Radiology* 176:211-220, 1990.

114. Apruzzese A, Silvestrini M, Floris R, et al: Cerebral hemodynamics in asymptomatic patients with internal carotid artery occlusion: A dynamic susceptibility contrast MR and transcranial Doppler study, *AJNR Am J Neuroradiol* 22:1062-1067, 2001.

115. Nasel C, Azizi A, Wilfort A, et al: Measurement of time-to-peak parameter by use of a new standardization method in patients with stenotic or occlusive disease of the carotid artery, *AJNR Am J Neuroradiol* 22:1056-1061, 2001.

116. Baron JC, Frackowiak RS, Herholz K, et al: Use of PET methods for measurement of cerebral energy metabolism and hemodynamics in cerebrovascular disease, *J Cereb Blood Flow Metab* 9:723-742, 1989.

117. Sette G, Baron JC, Mazoyer B, et al: Local brain haemodynamics and oxygen metabolism in cerebrovascular disease: Positron emission tomography, *Brain* 112:931-951, 1989.

118. Kolominsky-Rabas PL, Weber M, Gefeller O, et al: Epidemiology of ischemic stroke subtypes according to TOAST criteria: Incidence, recurrence, and long-term survival in ischemic stroke subtypes: A population-based study, *Stroke* 32:2735-2740, 2001.

119. Caplan LR, Hier DB, D'Cruz I: Cerebral embolism in the Michael Reese Stroke Registry, *Stroke* 14:30, 1983.

120. Sacco RL, Bello JA, Traub RD, Brust JCM: Selective proprioceptive sensory loss from a thalamic lacunar stroke, *Stroke* 18:1160-1163, 1987.

121. Cardiogenic brain embolism: The second report of the Cerebral Embolism Task Force, *Arch Neurol* 46:727-743, 1989.

122. Hinton RC, Kistler JP, Fallon JT, et al: Influence of etiology of atrial fibrillation on incidence of systemic embolism, *Am J Cardiol* 40:509, 1977.

123. Lhermitte F, Gautier JC, Derouesne C, Guiraud B: Ischemic accidents in the middle cerebral artery territory (a study of the causes in 122 cases), *Arch Neurol* 19:248, 1968.

124. Santamaria J, Graus F, Rubio F, et al: Cerebral infarction of the basal ganglia due to embolism from the heart, *Stroke* 14:911, 1983.

125. Bozzao L, Fantozzi LM, Bastianello S, et al: Ischaemic supratentorial stroke: Angiographic findings in patients examined in the very early phase, *J Neurol* 236:340-342, 1989.

126. del Zoppo GJ, Higashida RT, Furlan AJ, et al: PROACT: A phase II randomized trial of recombinant pro-urokinase by direct arterial delivery in acute middle cerebral artery stroke, *Stroke* 29:4-11, 1998.

127. Fieschi C, Bozzao L: Transient embolic occlusion of the middle cerebral and internal carotid arteries in cerebral apoplexy, *J Neurol Neurosurg Psychiatry* 32:236-240, 1969.

128. Kase CS, White L, Vinson L, Eichelberger P: Shotgun pellet embolus to the middle cerebral artery, *Neurology* 31:458, 1981.

129. Zanette EM, Roberti C, Mancini G, et al: Spontaneous middle cerebral artery reperfusion in ischemic stroke: A follow-up study with transcranial Doppler, *Stroke* 26:430-433, 1995.

130. Toni D, Fiorelli M, Zanette EM, et al: Early spontaneous improvement and deterioration of ischemic stroke patients: A serial study with transcranial Doppler, *Stroke* 29:1144-1148, 1998.

131. Baracchini C, Manara R, Ermani M, Meneghetti G: The quest for early predictors of stroke evolution: Can TCD be a guiding light? *Stroke* 31:2942-2947, 2000.

132. Molina CA, Montaner J, Abilleira S, et al: Timing of spontaneous recanalization and risk of hemorrhagic transformation in acute cardioembolic stroke, *Stroke* 32:1079-1084, 2001.

133. Mori E, Yoneda Y, Tabuchi M, et al: Intravenous recombinant tissue plasminogen activator in acute carotid artery territory stroke, *Neurology* 42:976-982, 1992.

134. Ringelstein EB, Biniek R, Weiller C, et al: Type and extent of hemispheric brain infarctions and clinical outcome in early and delayed middle cerebral artery recanalization, *Neurology* 42:289-298, 1992.

135. Von Kummer R, Hacke W: Safety and efficacy of intravenous tissue plasminogen activator and heparin in acute middle cerebral artery stroke, *Stroke* 23:646-652, 1992.

136. Friedlich AL, Castleman B, Mohr JP: Case records of the Massachusetts General Hospital, *N Engl J Med* 278:1109, 1968.

137. Sacco RL, Owen J, Mohr JP, Tatemichi TK: Free protein S deficiency: A possible association with intracranial vascular occlusion, *Stroke* 20:1657-1661, 1989.

138. Liebeskind A, Chinichian A, Schechter MM: The moving embolus seen during serial cerebral angiography, *Stroke* 2:440, 1971.

139. Zatz LM, Iannone AM, Eckman PB, Hecker SP: Observations concerning intracerebral vascular occlusion, *Neurology* 15:390-401, 1965.

140. Irino T, Tandea M, Minami T: Angiographic manifestations in postrecanalized cerebral infarction, *Neurology* 27:471, 1977.

141. Little JR, Shawhan B, Weinstein M: Pseudo-tandem stenosis of the internal carotid artery, *Neurosurgery* 7:574, 1980.

142. Demchuk AM, Burgin WS, Christou I, et al: Thrombolysis in brain ischemia (TIBI) transcranial Doppler flow grades predict clinical severity, early recovery, and mortality in patients treated with intravenous tissue plasminogen activator, *Stroke* 32:89-93, 2001.

143. Fisher CM, Pearlman A: The non-sudden onset of cerebral embolism, *Neurology (Minneap)* 17:1025, 1967.

144. Whisnant JP: Multiple particles injected may all go to the same cerebral artery branch, *Stroke* 13:720, 1982.

145. Minematsu K, Yamaguchi T, Omae T: Spectacular shrinking deficit: Rapid recovery from a full hemispheral syndrome by migration of an embolus, *Neurology* 41(Suppl):329, 1991.

146. Kittner SJ, Sharkness CM, Price TR, et al: Infarcts with a cardiac source of embolism in the NINDS Stroke Data Bank: Historical features, *Neurology* 40:281-284, 1990.

147. Ramirez Lassepas M, Cipolle RJ, Bjok RJ, et al: Can embolic stroke be diagnosed on the basis of neurologic clinical criteria? *Arch Neurol* 44:87-89, 1987.

148. Wessels T, Röttger C, Jauss M, Kaps M, Traupe H, Stolz E: Identification of embolic stroke patterns by diffusion-weighted MRI in clinically defined lacunar stroke syndromes, *Stroke* 36:757-761, 2005.

149. Bladin PF: A radiologic and pathologic study of embolism of the internal carotid-middle cerebral arterial axis, *Radiology* 82:614, 1964.

150. Tomsick TA, Brott TC, Olinger CP, et al: Hyperdense middle cerebral artery: Incidence and quantitative significance, *Neuroradiology* 31:312-315, 1989.

151. David DO, Rumbaugh CL, Gilson JM: Angiographic diagnosis of small-vessel cerebral emboli, *Acta Radiol Diagn (Stockh)* 9:264, 1969.

152. Amarenco P, Duyckaerts C, Tzourio C, et al: The prevalence of ulcerated plaques in the aortic arch in patients with stroke, *N Engl J Med* 326:221-225, 1992.

153. Amarenco P, Cohen A, Tzourio C, et al: Atherosclerotic disease of the aortic arch and the risk of ischemic stroke, *N Engl J Med* 331:1474-1479, 1994.

154. The French Study of Aortic Plaques in Stroke Group: Atherosclerotic disease of the aortic arch as a risk factor for recurrent ischemic stroke, *N Engl J Med* 334:1216-1221, 1996.

155. Tenenbaum A, Fisman EZ, Schneiderman J, et al: Disrupted mobile aortic plaques are a major risk factor for systemic embolism in the elderly, *Cardiology* 89:246-251, 1998.

156. Fisher CM: Lacunes: Small deep cerebral infarcts, *Neurology (Minneap)* 15:774, 1965.

157. Tohgi H, Kawashima M, Tamura K, Suzuki H: Coagulation fibrinolysis abnormalities in acute and chronic phases of cerebral thrombosis and embolism, *Stroke* 21:1663-1667, 1990.

158. Hinton RC, Mohr JP, Ackerman RA, et al: Symptomatic middle cerebral artery stem stenosis, *Ann Neurol* 5:152, 1979.

159. Fisher CM: The arterial lesions underlying lacunes, *Acta Neuropathol* 12:1, 1969.

160. Moulin T, Tatu L, Vuillier F, et al: Role of a stroke data bank in evaluating cerebral infarction subtypes: Patterns and outcome of 1776 consecutive patients from the Besançon Stroke Registry, *Cerebrovasc Dis* 10:261-271, 2000.

161. MacKenzie JM: Are all cardioembolic strokes embolic? An autopsy study of 100 consecutive acute ischemic strokes, *Cerebrovasc Dis* 10:289-292, 2000.

162. Nishida N, Ogata J, Yutani C, et al: Cerebral artery thrombosis as a cause of striatocapsular infarction: A histopathological case study, *Cerebrovasc Dis* 10:151-154, 2000.

163. Krapf H, Widder B, Skalej M: Small rosarylike infarctions in the centrum semiovale suggest hemodynamic failure, *AJNR Am J Neuroradiol* 19:1479-1484, 1998.

164. Lammie GA, Wardlaw JM: Small centrum ovale infarcts: A pathological study, *Cerebrovasc Dis* 9:82-90, 1999.

165. Wardlaw JM, Dennis MS, Warlow CP, Sandercock PA: Imaging appearance of the symptomatic perforating artery in patients with lacunar infarction: Occlusion or other vascular pathology? *Ann Neurol* 50:208-215, 2001.

166. Sacco RL, Kargman DE, Gu Q, Zamanillo MC: Race-ethnicity and determinants of intracranial atherosclerotic cerebral infarction: The Northern Manhattan Stroke Study, *Stroke* 26:14-20, 1995.

167. Nelson RF, Pullicino P, Kendall BE, Marshall J: Computed tomography on patients presenting with lacunar syndromes, *Stroke* 11:256, 1980.

168. Fisher CM: Lacunar strokes and infarcts: A review, *Neurology* 32:871, 1982.

169. Landau WM: Clinical neuromythology VI. Au clair de lacune: Holy wholly, holey logic, *Neurology* 39:725-730, 1989.

170. Millikan C, Futrell N: The fallacy of the lacunar hypothesis, *Stroke* 21:1251-1257, 1990.

171. Bamford J, Sandercock P, Dennis M, et al: Classification and natural history of clinically identifiable subtypes of cerebral infarction, *Lancet* 337:1521-1526, 1991.

172. Chimowitz MI, Furlan AJ, Sila CA, et al: Etiology of motor or sensory stroke: A prospective study of the predictive value of clinical and radiological features, *Ann Neurol* 30:519-525, 1991.

173. Toni D: Hyperacute diagnosis of subcortical infarction. In Donnan G, Norrving B, Bamford J, Bogousslavsky J, editors: *Lacunar and other subcortical infarctions*, Oxford, UK, 2002, Oxford University Press.

174. Norrving B: No black holes in the brain are benign, *Pract Neurol* 8:222-228, 2008.

175. Perani D, Vallar G, Cappa S, et al: Aphasia and neglect after subcortical stroke: A clinical/cerebral perfusion study, *Brain* 110:1211-1229, 1987.

176. Takano T, Kimura K, Nakamura M, et al: Effect of small deep hemispheric infarction on the ipsilateral cortical blood flow in man, *Stroke* 16:64-69, 1985.

177. Gan R, Sacco RL, Kargman DE, et al: Testing the validity of the lacunar hypothesis: The Northern Manhattan Stroke Study experience, *Neurology* 48:1204-1211, 1997.

178. Rascol A, Clanet M, Manelfe C: Pure motor hemiplegia: CT study of 30 cases, *Stroke* 13:11, 1982.

179. Hommel M, Besson G, Le Bas JF, et al: Prospective study of lacunar infarction using magnetic resonance imaging, *Stroke* 21:546-554, 1990.

180. Lee LJ, Kidwell CS, Alger J, et al: Impact on stroke subtype diagnosis of early diffusion-weighted magnetic resonance imaging and magnetic resonance angiography, *Stroke* 31:1081-1089, 2000.

181. Sunohara N, Mukoyama M, Mano Y, Satoyoshi E: Action-induced rhythmic dystonia: An autopsy case, *Neurology (Cleveland)* 34:321, 1984.

182. Derouesne C, Mas JL, Bolgert AF, Castaigne P: Pure sensory stroke caused by a small cortical infarct in the middle cerebral artery territory, *Stroke* 15:660, 1984.

183. Jorgensen L, Torvik A: Ischaemic cerebrovascular diseases in an autopsy series. Part I: Prevalence, location and predisposing factors in verified thromboembolic occlusions, and their significance in the pathogenesis of cerebral infarction, *J Neurol Sci* 3:490-495, 1966.

184. Longstreth WT Jr, Rosendaal FR, Siscovick DS, et al: Risk of stroke in young women and two prothrombotic mutations: Factor V Leiden and prothrombin gene variant (G20210A), *Stroke* 29:577-580, 1998.

185. De Stefano V, Chiusolo P, Paciaroni K, et al: Prothrombin G20210A mutant genotype is a risk factor for cerebrovascular ischemic disease in young patients, *Blood* 91:3562-3565, 1998.

186. Dichgans M: Genetics of ischaemic stroke, *Lancet Neurol* 6:149-161, 2007.

187. Markus HS, Ali N, Swaminathan R, et al: A common polymorphism in the methylenetetrahydrofolate reductase gene, homocysteine and ischemic cerebrovascular disease, *Stroke* 28:1739-1743, 1997.

188. Arruda VR, von Zuben PM, Chiaparini LC, et al: The mutation Ala677Val in the methylene tetrahydrofolate reductase gene: A risk factor for arterial and venous thrombosis, *Thromb Haemost* 77:818-821, 1997.

189. Fletcher O, Kessling AM: MTHFR association with arteriosclerotic vascular disease? *Hum Genet* 103:11-21, 1998.

190. Di Tullio MR, Gopal AS, Sacco RL, et al: Prevalence of patent foramen ovale in older cryptogenic stroke patients assessed by contrast echocardiography, *J Am Soc Echocardiogr* 4:294, 1991.

191. Falk RH: PFO or UFO? The role of a patent foramen ovale in cryptogenic stroke [editorial], *Am Heart J* 121:1264-1266, 1991.

192. Lechat P, Mas JL, Lascault G, et al: Prevalence of patent foramen ovale in patients with stroke, *N Engl J Med* 318:1148-1152, 1988.

193. Homma S, Sacco RL: Patent foramen ovale and stroke, *Circulation* 112:1063-1072, 2005.

194. Di Tullio MR, Sacco RL, Sciacca RR, Jin Z, Homma S: Patent foramen ovale and the risk of ischemic stroke in a multiethnic population, *Stroke* 49:797-802, 2007.

195. Handke M, Harloff A, Olschewski M, Hetzel A, Geibel A: Patent foramen ovale and cryptogenic stroke in older patients, *N Engl J Med* 29:2262-2268, 2007.

21 Clinical Scales to Assess Patients with Stroke

HAROLD P. ADAMS, JR.

To expedite clinical research, management of patients, and communication among health care providers, several types of stroke scales have been developed. These scales are widely accepted and are now used extensively. As a result, it is important for physicians to have a working knowledge of the more commonly used stroke scales. However, physicians should be aware that the stroke scales cannot describe all the variations and nuances of the broad spectrum of the clinical features of stroke. All the stroke rating instruments involve some element of combining patients with different findings into groups. Thus, any stroke scale should be considered as an adjunct to a neurologic examination.

Some clinical rating instruments aid emergency care personnel and emergency physicians in their diagnosis of stroke (Table 21-1). Additional scales are used to differentiate hemorrhagic from ischemic stroke or to define the subtypes of ischemic stroke. Differentiation may be by vascular territory, size, and location of the brain injury or by the presumed etiology. Clinical scales are used to assess the types of neurologic impairments, which reflect the severity of brain injury and provide prognostic information. Other scales are used to assess patients' status after stroke including disability, handicap, global outcome, and quality of life. Many scales are complementary, and patients may be assessed at different points of their illness by the use of these rating instruments. For example, a patient may be first assessed by emergency medical services personnel using a scale such as the Cincinnati Prehospital Stroke Scale (CPHSS).[1] Then, physicians may evaluate the severity of the neurologic impairments through the use of the National Institutes of Health Stroke Scale (NIHSS).[2] These instruments also may be used to monitor for neurologic improvement or worsening during the immediate period after a stroke. Subsequently the patient's outcome may be rated by the score on the modified Rankin Scale (mRS) and the Barthel Index (BI).[3-5]

The most frequently used scales are those that rate impairments, disability, and global outcomes or handicap. Physicians, other health care providers, and the public have a reasonable understanding of the meanings of these terms, which are used in this chapter. However, the reader should be aware that the World Health Organization has developed terms (*body dimension, activities dimension,* and *participation dimension*) that generally correspond to the terms *impairment, disability,* and *handicap.* These terms likely will gain in popularity. This chapter will discuss some of the more commonly used stroke scales, but the reader should be aware that a large number of clinical rating instruments are available. In particular, rehabilitation specialists use a variety of instruments to measure responses to specific interventions.

Desired Qualities of Stroke Scales

Most currently used scales were originally developed to describe groups of subjects enrolled in clinical trials, but many instruments have been implemented in a broad variety of clinical settings. The results of a stroke scale should be clinically relevant and should be obvious to the variety of health care providers who will use the scale (face validity).[6-9] The aim of the scale should be clear. For a stroke scale to be useful it should be able to provide a numerical score or another categorization that is clinically relevant. The results should provide a clear impression of a patient's status. The derived information may affect decisions in diagnosis, treatment, or advice given to patients and their families.

The purpose of the scale and the proper time for its use should be obvious. For example, using an outcome scale such as the mRS at the time of admission for treatment of a stroke is not appropriate because this scale emphasizes functional outcomes that cannot be accurately assessed in the setting of an acute stroke. Many scales provide quantitative items that may be calculated with scores of individual items added to form a total score. In some scales that assess the severity of the neurologic illness, a higher score represents a more severe event, whereas in others, a higher score reflects a less severe brain illness. Unfortunately, direct translation of a score from one scale to another may be difficult. Thus, the clinician needs to understand the scoring system that is used for each individual rating instrument.

Scales should be evaluated in a manner that is similar to that used to validate a diagnostic test because, in fact, a stroke scale is an ancillary diagnostic test even if it is based on clinical findings.[10,11] The scale should be sensitive; it should be able to detect the findings that are of most interest. The scale should be specific; it should permit recognition and scoring of only those abnormalities that are important. As much as possible, the scale should not have high rates of false-positive or false-negative

TABLE 21-1 TYPES AND GOALS OF STROKE SCALES

Prehospital and emergency recognition of stroke
Differentiate hemorrhagic from ischemic stroke
Differentiate ischemic stroke syndrome
Differentiate etiology of ischemic stroke
Quantify severity of stroke and neurologic impairments
    Hemorrhagic stroke
    Ischemic stroke
Measure responses to specific rehabilitation therapies
Rate outcome after stroke
    Disability
    Handicap
Rate quality of life after stroke

results that would affect patient care. In summary, if possible, both the positive and negative predictive values of the scale should be determined with comparisons to a standard. These features are especially important for those clinical scales that are used to differentiate stroke from other acute neurologic illnesses, hemorrhagic from ischemic stroke, or the subtype of ischemic stroke. The standards to which these diagnoses are compared include subsequent clinical diagnoses, outcomes, and the results of diagnostic studies such as brain imaging. In summary, a scale must be accurate. Unfortunately, some scales, such as those differentiating hemorrhagic from ischemic stroke, have not met these criteria.

There is no single scale that provides information about the gamut of all the clinical aspects of stroke. In most circumstances, patients would be assessed by combinations of scales performed at different times. All the currently available stroke scales have individual strengths and weaknesses. For example, the widely used NIHSS has a bias toward higher scores being calculated when a stroke affects the left hemisphere.[12,13] Physicians and other health care providers need to know the idiosyncrasies and limitations of each scale.

A clinically useful scale should be easy to perform and germane to the clinical situation. In addition, scales that are used in an emergency situation should be able to be performed rapidly. Some of the rating instruments are based on the history obtained from the patient or observers, such as family members. The information may reflect performance, demographic findings (i.e., age), or the presence of risk factors for stroke. Other scales are based on the findings detected by a physical examination and place an emphasis on the findings from the neurologic assessment. Many scales, especially those used to rate the severity of neurologic impairments, include gradations in scoring; for example, some provide difference scores for the severity of motor signs or impairments in consciousness. The total score is important. For example, most health care providers have a mental image of a patient's illness if he or she has a Glasgow Coma Scale (GCS) score of less than 8.[14] In a similar way, the total score on the NIHSS provides important clinical information for physicians and staff in an emergency department. The total score provides information about prognosis, and it affects decisions about treatment. Some scores involve the addition of points to achieve a total score. In other instances, the score reflects subtraction from an initial baseline score; in such a case, a low score reflects a serious brain injury. Some scales use a numeric system of rating but are not based on adding scores from items contained in the scale. For example, the Hunt-Hess Scale for subarachnoid hemorrhage has five grades that are defined but do not include scoring of components to reach that grade.[15]

Some scales include weighting of different items. For example, in the Canadian Stroke (Neurological) Scale (CNS), the item scoring consciousness may be given more points than individual items rating language or arm motor function.[16,17] An even more elaborate rating system (the Japan Stroke Scale) was developed by Gotoh et al[18]; they selected 10 variables ranging from consciousness to pupillary abnormalities. The weighted factors ranged from consciousness (49.8%) to plantar reflex (2.2%) to sensory impairment (2.1%). Even though the Japan Stroke Scale has reasonable interrater and intrarater scores, the utility of this very complex approach that results in a wide range of scores has not been established. Regardless of the scale, the bottom line for its success is that the scale has credibility. Health care providers need to recognize the utility of the scale in their care of patients with stroke.

A few scales that have been used extensively for several years have considerable cachet. For example, the GCS, which was originally developed to define the severity of brain injury among patients with trauma, has become a worldwide standard for assessing a wide variety of critically ill patients with impairments of consciousness.[14]

A valid scale must have the attributes of a strong interrater agreement and intrarater reproducibility in scoring. These features are especially important for scales that describe subtypes of stroke or that measure the severity of neurologic impairments and outcomes. The goal is to achieve a score that is an accurate measure of the patient's neurologic status. A lack of agreement in diagnoses or assessments of the clinical findings presents a real problem for multicenter clinical trials. It also weakens the applicability of data obtained from these trials. For example, during the development of the Trial of Org 10172 in Acute Stroke Treatment (TOAST) classification, the researchers found that physicians often disagreed about the subtype of ischemic stroke even when presented with the same information.[19] Agreement was very high when a straightforward case was assessed but was disappointingly low for those cases with multiple possible explanations or for cases when some supporting data were limited. Thus, these researchers found that the kappa statistic (the degree of agreement above chance) was reasonably good for some subtypes of stroke but less acceptable for other cases. Measures to improve the agreement in these scales likely can be undertaken, but both researchers and clinicians in practice should recognize that no scale will probably ever achieve unanimity or perfection when a complex, multifactorial disease such as stroke is being considered.

To improve interrater agreement and reproducibility, developers of scales often use arbitrary rules to define the various grades of scored items. For scales that are based on historical information, specific questions to ask and specific answers to be sought are explained. For those scales that are primarily based on findings on the physical and neurologic examinations, the steps in performance of the examination and the methods to rate the findings are described. Some scales include scoring responses for contingencies such as an absent limb or severe comorbid disease. The scales that perform the best include detailed definitions for all the potential scores for items that are assessed. Still, even these definitions may not address the wide range of potential scenarios that can be found in a large group of patients with stroke. As an additional step to improve validity, researchers and other groups created programs to train clinicians on the use of these scales. The programs often are supplemented by a certification process that tests the clinician's ability to accurately use the rating instrument. Because the mRS and the NIHSS are the most widely used rating instruments in clinical trials, they have the most extensive educational and certification programs. The development of such programs has been a critical quality component of clinical trials in stroke.

Some multicenter clinical trials use the quality control measure of central adjudication or review of the results of diagnostic studies such as brain imaging. A similar strategy would be to improve the validity of clinical stroke trial measures, especially outcomes. The relevant data would be sent to an individual or panel that reviews the information collected from all subjects in a clinical trial. The group would improve consistency in the scoring of the scale. Although this measure may not be practical at the time of enrollment of a subject into a trial, subsequent review could be performed to reconfirm eligibility.

Emergency Medical Services Scales

Scales are available to help emergency medical services personnel in their assessment of patients with suspected stroke. Among the goals is the differentiation of stroke from other causes of acute neurologic impairment.

The GCS was developed to quantify the severity of neurologic impairments after craniocerebral trauma (Table 21-2).[14] Potential scores on the GCS range from 3 to 15 points and are based on the best verbal response, best motor response, and eye movement. For example, a patient with hemiparetic but volitional movement on the left and flexor posturing on the right would be rated as having 5 or 6 points for the motor item. In general, patients with scores less than 8 have a very serious brain injury and a poor prognosis. Although the GCS has not been tested for interrater agreement and intrarater reproducibility, it has strong predictive power. The GCS is used widely by emergency medical services personnel, physicians, and other health care providers. As the term *GCS* implies, the rating scale is most useful in assessment of patients with alterations in consciousness. Thus, its value will be greater among persons with hemorrhagic stroke than among those with cerebral infarctions.[20-24]

The World Federation of Neurological Surgeons (WFNS) Scale for measuring the severity of subarachnoid hemorrhage is based on the GCS.[25,26] The GCS is less helpful for evaluation of cases of suspected ischemic stroke because consciousness usually is not disturbed. Still, the best eye and verbal responses have been used to provide prognostic information among patients with ischemic stroke.[20]

TABLE 21-2 GLASGOW COMA SCALE

	Points
Best response—eye opening (range of scores 1-4 points)	
Eyes open spontaneously, not necessarily aware of environment	4
Eyes open to speech, not necessarily in response to command	3
Eyes open in response to painful stimuli	2
No eye opening in response to painful stimuli	1
Best response—motor (range of scores 1-6 points)	
Follows simple commands, may have paresis or hemiplegia	6
Responds to painful stimuli by attempting to remove source of pain	5
Withdraws to painful stimuli	4
Flexor (decorticate) posturing in response to painful stimuli	3
Extensor (decerebrate) posturing in response to painful stimuli	2
No motor response to painful stimuli	1
Best response—verbal (range of scores 1-5 points)	
Oriented to time, place, and person	5
Responds to conversation but is confused	4
Intelligible speech but no sustained sentences	
Incomprehensible sounds, moans, groans, but no words	2
No verbal response	1

Adapted from Jennett B, Teasdale G, Braakman R, et al: Prognosis of patients with severe head injury. *Neurosurgery* 4:283-289, 1979.

In addition, Tsao et al[27] found that the GCS score was a strong predictor of outcomes among patients with severe strokes in the posterior circulation. Overall, the GCS will continue to be an important component of assessment of patients in multiple patient care settings. The Japan Coma Scale also has been used to assess patients with impaired consciousness with a variety of acute neurologic illnesses; however, this scale is not widely used.[28]

Groups in Cincinnati, Los Angeles, and Miami independently developed scales that are used by paramedics and ambulance personnel to determine whether a patient has had a stroke.[29-32] A variation of the CPHSS called the FAST scale (Face, Arm, and Speech Test) was developed in the United Kingdom.[33] These rating instruments are used to collect information about patients with possible stroke that can be forwarded to a hospital emergency department. The Miami Emergency Neurologic Deficit (MEND) scale has two versions: one involves a brief examination performed on the scene, and the other involves a more extensive examination done while the patient is being transported to the hospital. The MEND does include information about severe headache or stiff neck that may point to an intracranial hemorrhage. These clinical rating instruments focus on a limited number of history and physical examination findings. For example, the MEND scale includes information that is directly related to possible exclusions for treatment with tissue plasminogen activator (t-PA), including the use of medications such as warfarin.[32] Screening for marked hyperglycemia or hypoglycemia is used to detect these abnormalities as the cause of the acute neurologic signs. The most commonly assessed features are language, facial weakness, and arm weakness (Tables 21-3 through 21-5). The assumption is that the finding of unilateral weakness points to a stroke. The scales may be performed rapidly and with a reasonable degree of accuracy. Kothari et al[31] compared the scores obtained by paramedics using the CPHSS with those obtained by physicians using the NIHSS. They found that an abnormality in any one of the three scale items was associated with 66% sensitivity and 87% specificity for identifying a stroke; the sensitivity was much higher for strokes in the anterior circulation than for strokes in the posterior circulation. The diagnoses of paramedics using the FAST scale were compared to the subsequent diagnoses of vascular neurologists.[34] Agreement was best for detection of arm weakness, but acceptable levels of concurrence were noted for facial weakness and speech disturbance. These scales have been validated by in-field tests, and educational programs are available to train emergency medical services personnel. The Los Angeles scale is being used by paramedics in that community to expedite enrollment of subjects into a clinical trial testing very early administration of magnesium in patients with stroke.[35] In addition, paramedics can also accurately and successfully assess a patient using the NIHSS while the patient is being transported to a hospital.[36]

A rating instrument that assists emergency medicine physicians in diagnosing stroke has also been developed (Recognition of Stroke in the Emergency Room [ROSIER] Scale).[24] The scale evaluates seven items with a total score ranging from −2 to +5 (Table 21-6). In general, a stroke is very unlikely if the total score is less than 0; scores of 4 or 5 are strongly correlated with the diagnosis of stroke. The aim is to differentiate stroke from other

TABLE 21-3 LOS ANGELES PREHOSPITAL STROKE SCALE

General screening	
Age >45 years	Yes ___, No ___, Unsure ___
No history of seizures	Yes ___, No ___, Unsure ___
Symptoms <24 hours	Yes ___, No ___, Unsure ___
Not in wheelchair/ bedridden	Yes ___, No ___, Unsure ___
Blood glucose >60 and <400	Yes ___, No ___, Unsure ___

Neurologic examination	
Facial smile	Normal ___, Right droop___ Left droop ___
Grip	Normal ___, Right weak ___, Right absent ___ Left weak ___, Left absent___
Arm strength	Normal ___, Right drift ___, Right falls ___ Left drift ___, Left falls ___
Has only unilateral weakness	Yes ___, No ___

Adapted from Kidwell CS, Starkman S, Eckstein M, et al: Identifying stroke in the field: Prospective validation of the Los Angeles Prehospital Stroke Screen (LAPSS). *Stroke* 31:71-76, 2000.

TABLE 21-4 CINCINNATI PREHOSPITAL SCALE

Facial weakness (patient is asked to smile or show teeth)
  Normal—both sides of face move equally
  Abnormal—one side of face does not move as well as other
Arm drift (patient extends both arms straight out for 10 seconds, eyes closed)
  Normal—both arms move the same or do not move at all
  Abnormal—one arm either does not move or drifts down compared with the other
Speech (patient is asked to repeat a sentence of at least seven words)
  Normal—says correct words without slurring
  Abnormal—slurs words, says wrong words, or does not speak

Adapted from Kothari RU, Pancioli A, Liu T, et al: Cincinnati Prehospital Stroke Scale: Reproducibility and validity. *Ann Emerg Med* 33:373-378, 1999.

TABLE 21-5 MIAMI EMERGENCY NEUROLOGIC DEFICIT (MEND) PREHOSPITAL CHECK LIST

Basic demographic information: Name, age, sex
Witness information (including contact telephone numbers)
Date and time of onset of stroke (last normal)
Exclusions for treatment with t-PA—head injury or seizure at onset, use of warfarin, past history of bleeding, brain hemorrhage
Examination

Blood pressure, heart rate and rhythm	Normal __, Abnormal __	
Mental status		
Level of consciousness	Normal __, Abnormal __	
Speech (slurred, wrong words)	Normal __, Abnormal __	
Questions (age, month)	Normal __, Abnormal __	
Commands (close, open eyes)	Normal __, Abnormal __	
Cranial nerves		
Facial droop (show teeth, smile)	Right __, Left __ Normal __, Abnormal __	
Visual fields (four quadrants)	Right __, Left __ Normal __, Abnormal __	
Horizontal gaze (side to side)	Right __, Left __ Normal __, Abnormal __	
Limbs		
Arm drift (hold out both arms)	Right __, Left __ Normal __, Abnormal __	
Leg drift (lift each leg)	Right __, Left __ Normal __, Abnormal __	
Sensory (touch or pinch)	Right __ Left __ Normal __, Abnormal __	
Coordination (finger to nose)	Right __, Left __	

Adapted from Gordon DL, Issenberg SB, Gordon MS, et al: Stroke training of prehospital providers: An example of simulation-enhanced blended learning and evaluation. *Med Teach* 27:114-121, 2005.

TABLE 21-6 RECOGNITION OF STROKE IN THE EMERGENCY ROOM (ROSIER) SCALE

Time of onset of symptoms	Date ___, Time ___
Time of examination	Date ___, Time ___
Glasgow Coma Scale score	
Eye movement ___, Motor response ___, Verbal response ___,	
Blood pressure ___, Blood glucose level ___,	
Correct glucose urgently if <3.5 mmol/L, then reassess	
Loss of consciousness/syncope	−1 Yes ___, 0 No ___
Presence of seizure activity	−1 Yes ___, 0 No ___
New onset (including awakening)	
Asymmetric facial weakness	+1 Yes ___, 0 No ___
Asymmetric arm weakness	+1 Yes ___, 0 No ___
Asymmetric leg weakness	+1 Yes ___, 0 No ___
Speech disturbance	+1 Yes ___, 0 No ___
Visual field defect	+1 Yes ___, 0 No ___

Adapted from Nor AM, Davis J, Sen B, et al: The Recognition of Stroke in the Emergency Room (ROSIER) scale: Development and validation of a stroke recognition instrument. *Lancet Neurol* 4:727-734, 2005.

mimics including seizures, syncope, or other acute neurologic illness. The ultimate goal is to facilitate selection of patients who may be treated with emergency interventions such as t-PA. The scale was tested in a prospective study and showed a sensitivity of 93% (95% confidence interval [CI], 89% to 97%), a specificity of 83% (95% CI, 77% to 89%), a positive predictive value of 90% (95% CI, 85% to 95%) and a negative predictive value of 88% (95% CI, 83% to 93%.) Singer et al[37] developed a simple system involving measurement of consciousness, gaze, and motor function. Each of the three items assessed is given a score from 0 (normal) to 2 (severe). The authors found that the scoring would predict proximal occlusion of the middle cerebral artery with reasonable accuracy. They proposed that the tool be used for triage of patients with suspected stroke.

Scales to Differentiate Hemorrhagic Stroke from Ischemic Stroke

Clinical rating instruments that could be used by emergency medical services and physicians to differentiate cases of hemorrhagic stroke from ischemic stroke have been constructed. The goal is to provide a diagnosis that would obviate the need for brain imaging before treatment. Such a scale would be most useful in initiation of therapies that might be associated with an increased risk of bleeding, for example, intravenous thrombolysis, and that would be contraindicated if the patient already had a hemorrhage. The current scales include historical information, blood pressure values, and findings on the neurologic examination.[38] Several groups tested these rating instruments and found that the scales have not reached adequate levels of either sensitivity or specificity for use in either clinical trials or patient care.[39-45] At present, these scales should not be used in lieu of modern brain imaging. Still, development of a clinical scale that could be used by emergency medical services personnel and physicians to differentiate hemorrhagic from ischemic stroke with a reasonable degree of accuracy would be very helpful.

Differentiation of Ischemic Stroke Syndromes

A patient's neurologic findings vary depending on the location and size of the ischemic lesion. Clinical manifestations are diverse and often idiosyncratic to individual patients. Each patient has his or her own clinical pattern of ischemic stroke. Still, there are general features that may be aggregated and correlated with specific patterns or stroke syndromes. These general features may be classified in groupings that could be useful in addressing questions about prognosis, etiology of stroke, acute treatment, and long-term management. For example, most isolated infarctions affecting the cerebral cortex are secondary to branch occlusions from embolism, either from the heart or from major intracranial or extracranial arteries. Patients with cortical infarctions generally have a good prognosis for survival from the acute stroke. Patients with small deep infarctions restricted to deep hemispheric strokes, such as the internal capsule or basal ganglia, usually have small artery disease and their acute prognosis for survival also is good. On the other hand, patients with major hemispheric infarctions with involvement of both deep and cortical structures usually have occlusions of major intracranial or extracranial arteries. These are the patients at greatest risk of malignant brain edema and death. The most widely used rating system, the Oxford Community Stroke Project (OCSP) Classification, categorizes ischemic stroke into four categories: (1) total anterior circulation infarction (TACI)—a large cerebral infarction, usually due to occlusion of a major intracranial artery, (2) partial anterior circulation infarction (PACI)—a smaller cerebral infarction primarily affecting the cortex, usually due to embolic occlusion of a pial/cortical branch artery, (3) lacunar infarction (LACI)—a small infarction involving structures deep in the cerebral hemisphere, usually due to occlusion of a small penetrating artery, and (4) posterior circulation infarction (POCI)—an infarction involving primarily the brainstem.[46] This scale is based on the patterns of neurologic impairments found on examination (Table 21-7). There is some uncertainty about some of the definitions for the categories included in the scale. For example, an isolated homonymous hemianopia, presumably secondary to occlusion of the posterior cerebral artery or calcarine artery, is categorized as a POCI lesion because the posterior cerebral artery is usually a branch of the basilar artery. It could also be considered a PACI because it is a restricted cortical infarction and patients with this infarction are more likely to behave similarly to patients with anterior circulation infarctions than those patients with brainstem strokes. Similarly, the definition of pure motor hemiparesis for the LACI category does not include dysarthria when many patients with these infarctions do have mild-to-moderate impairments in articulation. Although the OCSP classification was developed for differentiating patterns of infarction, Barber et al[47] also used the system to define patterns of clinical findings among patients with intracerebral hemorrhage.

Interrater agreement of the OCSP classification was tested by Lindley et al[48]; they found that agreement was moderate-to-good (kappa, 0.54; 95% CI, 0.39 to 0.68.) Another group found that agreement in the use of the

TABLE 21-7 OXFORD COMMUNITY STROKE PROJECT CLASSIFICATION OF ISCHEMIC STROKE SYNDROMES

Total anterior circulation (TACI) infarction
Presence of the following:
   Contralateral weakness of face, arm, and leg
   Contralateral homonymous hemianopia
   Behavioral or cognitive deficit (aphasia, neglect, etc.)

Partial anterior circulation (PACI) infarction
Presence of two of the following:
   Contralateral restricted weakness or sensory loss (face, arm, or leg)
   Contralateral homonymous hemianopia
   Behavioral or cognitive deficit (aphasia, neglect, etc.)

Lacunar (LACI) infarction
Presence of one of the following syndromes:
   Pure motor stroke
      Contralateral weakness of face, arm, and leg
      No other deficits
   Pure sensory stroke
      Contralateral sensory loss of face, arm, and leg
      No other deficits
   Ataxic hemiparesis
      Coexistent cerebellar and motor signs
      May have dysarthria
      No visual or cognitive deficits
   Sensorimotor stroke
      Contralateral sensory loss and motor signs of face, arm, and leg
      No visual or cognitive deficits

Posterior circulation (POCI) infarction
Presence of one or more of the following:
   Bilateral weakness or sensory loss
   Ipsilateral incoordination (cerebellar) not explained by weakness
   Diplopia with or without extraocular muscle palsy
   Crossed (ipsilateral face and contralateral body) weakness or sensory loss
   Isolated homonymous hemianopia

Adapted from Bamford J, Sandercock P, Dennis M, et al: Classification and natural history of clinically identifiable subtypes of cerebral infarction. *Lancet* 337:1521-1526, 1991.

OCSP classification between physicians and nurses was moderate (kappa, 0.31 to 0.45).[49] Because the classification seems straightforward, the relatively low agreement is somewhat surprising and disappointing. Pittock et al[50] found that the OCSP system identifies two major groups (TACI versus the other three categories) who behave differently. Patients with TACI have the poorest functional outcomes after stroke.[51,52] These results are not surprising given the extensive nature of the brain injury that occurs in this group of patients.

Wardlaw et al[53] compared the diagnoses obtained using the OCSP with the results of brain imaging. The classification predicted the site of stroke in 80 of 91 patients (88%, 95% CI, 77% to 92%). The OCSP classification was most successful for cases of large cortical infarctions and poorest for small subcortical infarctions. Using MRI as a control, a subsequent study found that the OCSP classification predicted the site of the lesion in approximately 75% of patients.[54] When early stroke diagnoses using the OCSP system were compared with subsequent brain imaging, Smith et al[55] found that the initial subtype diagnoses were accurate in 65% of cases. The sensitivity and specificity were highest for the POCI category (1.00 and 0.97, respectively) and lowest for the LACI category (0.33 and 0.88, respectively). On the other hand, early use of MRI and magnetic resonance angiography (MRA) may improve the diagnosis of subtype.[56] However, depending on the brain imaging to make the OCSP subtype diagnosis appears to defeat the original intent of the classification system, which was based on clinical findings alone. Based on findings of arterial imaging, Zhang et al[57] found that arterial narrowing of the extracranial internal carotid artery was correlated with the TACI category. On the other hand, the OCSP classification categories may not be associated with the site or presence of an intracranial arterial occlusion.[58,59]

Despite the apparent limitations of the OCSP classification, the rating instrument is used in clinical trials and in epidemiologic studies.[60-62] Overall, the OCSP system has advantages: it mimics the process that physicians use when assessing their patients, it is relatively simple, and it gives general information localizing the stroke. Its TACI category predicts poor outcomes. However, its utility in comparison with rating scales that directly quantify the severity of neurologic impairments is not obvious. In addition, the OCSP scale does not appear to predict the location of arterial pathology with sufficiently high frequency to be useful. It does not differentiate causes of stroke; for example, patients with PACI may have an embolus arising from either the heart or an extracranial artery; subsequent management of these underlying causes differs considerably. Overall, the role of the OCSP classification in general patient care seems to be limited.

Scales to Quantify the Severity of Hemorrhagic Stroke

The scales used to quantify the severity of primary intracerebral hemorrhage differ from the clinical scales that rate the severity of subarachnoid hemorrhage or ischemic stroke in that they include a limited amount of clinical information and are complemented by the results of brain imaging. Edwards et al[63] developed a scale that could be used to assess patients with either hemorrhagic or ischemic stroke. The scores of this scale, titled the Unified Neurological Stroke Scale, included assessments of consciousness; language; eye movements; face, arm, hand, leg, and foot power; and tone. The Intracerebral Hemorrhage (ICH) Scale score is based on the following variables: GCS score, age, infratentorial location of hemorrhage, volume of hemorrhage, and presence of intraventricular hemorrhage (Table 21-8).[64,65] The range of scores is 0 to 6. In one study, all patients with a score of 5 or greater died, and none of the patients with a score of 0 died. More recently, a variation of the instrument, called the ICH-GS, was used to predict outcomes in a large population of patients with primary intracerebral hemorrhage.[66] Modifying the scale to include an expanded range of points improved its ability to predict early mortality and functional outcomes. The severity of neurologic impairments after intracerebral hemorrhage has also been examined with the use of the CNS, Scandinavian Stroke Scale (SSS),

TABLE 21-8 INTRACEREBRAL HEMORRHAGE SCORE

Glasgow Coma Scale Score	
3-4	2 Points
5-12	1 Point
13-15	0 Point
Age	
80 Years or older	1 Point
Younger than 80	0 Point
Infratentorial location of hematoma	
Yes	1 Point
No	0 Point
Volume of hemorrhage	
30 cm^3 or greater	1 Point
Smaller than 30 cm^3	0 Point
Intraventricular hemorrhage	
Yes	1 Point
No	0 Point

Adapted from Hemphill JC, Bonovich DC, Besmertis L, et al: A simple, reliable grading scale for intracerebral hemorrhage. *Stroke* 32:891-897, 2001.

TABLE 21-9 HUNT-HESS CLASSIFICATION OF ANEURYSMAL SUBARACHNOID HEMORRHAGE

Grade	Description
1	Asymptomatic, mild headache, or possibly nuchal rigidity
2	Moderate-to-severe headache, nuchal rigidity, oculomotor nerve palsy but normal consciousness
3	Drowsy or confused, mild focal neurologic signs
4	Stupor, moderate-to-severe motor signs
5	Coma, moribund, and extensor posturing

Adapted from Hunt WE, Hess RM: Surgical risk as related to time of intervention in the repair of intracranial aneurysms. *J Neurosurg* 28:14-20, 1968.

TABLE 21-10 WORLD FEDERATION OF NEUROLOGICAL SURGEONS SUBARACHNOID HEMORRHAGE SCALE

Grade	Glasgow Coma Scale Score	Focal Signs
I	15	Absent
II	13-14	Absent
III	13-14	Present
IV	7-12	Present or absent
V	3-6	Present or absent

Adapted from Ogungbo B: The World Federation of Neurological Surgeons Scale for Subarachnoid Hemorrhage. *Surg Neurol* 25:236-238, 2003.

or the NIHSS.[47,67-70] These scales are being used to predict outcomes and to monitor for neurologic deterioration or improvement. Weimar et al[71] developed the Essen Intracerebral Hemorrhage Score based on the NIHSS. The scale includes scoring for patient age, the score on the level of consciousness item of the NIHSS, and an aggregate score based on ranges of total NIHSS scores. The authors found that this scale was useful in predicting outcomes. Still, experience with the NIHSS in assessing patients with hemorrhagic stroke is limited.

Scales to Quantify the Severity of Subarachnoid Hemorrhage

Two scales are commonly used to assess the severity of aneurysmal subarachnoid hemorrhage. A scale consisting of five grades ranging from minimally symptomatic to coma was developed by Hunt and Hess (Table 21-9).[15] The Hunt-Hess Scale is most useful in predicting outcomes among patients with severe neurologic impairments or coma.[72-74] The scale has not been tested for interrater agreement and intrarater reproducibility.

Because of perceived limitations of the Hunt-Hess Scale, the WFNS Scale was developed to rate the severity of subarachnoid hemorrhage. It is based on the scoring of the GCS (Table 21-10).[25,26,75] The scale has five grades that range from normal consciousness to major neurologic impairments and coma. It has strong and discriminatory prognostic value that appears to be superior to the Hunt-Hess Scale.[76-81] Although the WFNS Scale has not been tested widely for interrater agreement and reproducibility, it has largely replaced the Hunt-Hess Scale for evaluation of patients with aneurysmal subarachnoid hemorrhage in both clinical practice and clinical trials. Patients with poor grades (IV and V) have a high likelihood of unfavorable outcomes.[82] Rosen and Macdonald[83] proposed refining the WFNS Scale by the addition of clinical and imaging variables. However, these additions also increase the complexity of the scale. These modifications

have not been accepted by the community of physicians who treat subarachnoid hemorrhage.

Scales to Quantify the Severity of Ischemic Stroke

Several scales are available for assessing the severity of neurologic impairments among patients with acute ischemic stroke. In many ways, the scales are similar. All these scales are based on the findings detected on the neurologic examination. Most scales have gradations of scoring of these items to reflect the severity of the neurologic impairment. Some of these scales have not been widely used. Others have not been tested for validity, interrater reliability, and intrarater reproducibility.

The Mathew Scale includes most of the features of other ischemic stroke scales but also includes items such as scoring of muscle stretch reflexes that appears to provide limited prognostic information.[84] It also includes a global rating item that is not well-described and that is of limited usefulness in acute settings. The Mathew Scale generally functions similarly to other stroke scales.[85] However, it has not undergone the testing of other clinical rating instruments and is not widely used. The Orgogozo Scale includes an evaluation of consciousness, language, proximal and distal motor strength, and motor tone.[86] It does not test vision or articulation. The scoring of the Orgogozo Scale appears to correspond with the other acute stroke scales, but it has not undergone the testing of other rating instruments.[85] It is not widely used in either clinical trials or patient care situations. The Japanese Stroke Scale also has not been widely used.[18] The European Stroke Scale is a multiple-item clinical rating instrument that has been used to evaluate patients with stroke.[8] This scale includes an assessment of gait, which is a component of the neurologic examination that usually cannot be performed while an acutely ill patient with a recent stroke is being examined. This scale has not been widely used. The Orpington Prognostic Scale has been used to predict outcomes after rehabilitation; it has been used within 1 week of onset of stroke and was found to be equal to the NIHSS in predicting long-term outcomes.[87] The utility of the scale in the evaluation of patients with acute stroke, including those assessed in an emergency setting, has not been established.

The CNS has two variations that are scored depending on the patient's ability to comprehend commands.[16,17] The scale has been tested for validity, reliability, and reproducibility and has been used in several clinical trials.[9,17,88-90] The CNS includes assessments of consciousness, language, and motor function. It does not test vision, articulation, sensation, or right hemisphere cognitive impairments such as neglect (Table 21-11). The scores of the individual items are added; a high score generally predicts a favorable outcome. A total score of less than 6.5 points strongly predicts poor outcomes including mortality at 1 month and 1 year.[85,88,91] The CNS correlates well with other acute stroke scales, but it underestimates functional impairments in stroke survivors.[85] Conversion of the scores between the CNS and NIHSS is difficult, particularly among patients with severe stroke or aphasia.[92] Although it is not used as widely as the NIHSS or the SSS, the CNS remains a potentially useful clinical rating tool for both researchers and clinicians.

The SSS includes two different versions; an acute prognostic scale that has a range of 0 to 22 points and a convalescent scale that has a range of 0 to 48 points.[93,94] The two versions are used to examine patients at different points in the continuum of stroke. The components of the two versions differ; for example, the acute scale has an item that scores level of consciousness, whereas orientation and language are rated in the convalescent examination (Table 21-12). The validity and reliability of the SSS were tested by Barber et al.[95] They found strong agreement between face-to-face assessments and record reviews. The acute prognostic component of the SSS has been used in epidemiologic studies and clinical trials.[61,96-104] Christensen et al[105] reported that the SSS is useful in predicting outcomes among patients with mild ischemic stroke. A low score on the prognostic version of the SSS strongly predicts early neurologic worsening, poor outcomes, and a high mortality within 30 days of stroke.[101,106] The SSS score has been combined with other factors to predict mortality within 1 year among stroke survivors.[101] The scores on the SSS also correlate with the diagnosis of lacunar infarction.[100] In addition, the SSS has been used to describe neurologic findings in studies testing the utility of early brain imaging in the evaluation of patients with stroke.[107]

The convalescent SSS has not been tested extensively. The aphasia component of the SSS has been evaluated with mixed results. Davalos et al[106] found that the item

TABLE 21-11 CANADIAN NEUROLOGICAL (STROKE) SCALE

Level of consciousness	Alert	3	points
	Drowsy	1.5	points
Orientation	Oriented	1	point
	Disoriented, not applicable	0	point
Language	Normal	1	point
	Expressive deficit	0.5	point
	Receptive deficit	0	point
Motor function (scoring if normal comprehension)			
Face	No facial weakness	0.5	point
	Facial weakness is present	0	point
Proximal arm	No weakness	1.5	points
	Mild weakness	1	point
	Significant weakness	0.5	point
	Paralysis	0	point
Distal arm	No weakness	1.5	points
	Mild weakness	1	point
	Significant weakness	0.5	point
	Paralysis	0	point
Proximal leg	No weakness	1.5	points
	Mild weakness	1	point
	Significant weakness	0.5	point
	Paralysis	0	point
Distal leg	No weakness	1.5	points
	Mild weakness	1	point
	Significant weakness	0.5	point
	Paralysis	0	point
Motor function (scoring if impaired comprehension)			
Face	Symmetrical	0.5	point
	Asymmetrical	0	point
Arms	Equal	1.5	points
	Unequal	0	point
Legs	Equal	1.5	points
	Unequal	0	point

Adapted from Cote R, Hachinski VC, Shurvell BL, et al: The Canadian Neurological Scale: A preliminary study in acute stroke. *Stroke* 17:731-737, 1986.

had reasonable sensitivity and specificity. but they also noted that the positive predictive value was low. The latter finding was confirmed by Thommessen et al.[108] They reported that the aphasia score on the SSS results in a high rate of false-positive results and that this scoring could have an impact on epidemiologic studies in stroke.

The use of the SSS in clinical stroke trials is probably secondary to the use of the NIHSS in clinical trials for describing the severity of strokes among subjects in acute stroke treatment trials. SSS scores (low scores worse) can be compared with NIHSS scores (low scores better). Ali et al[109] found that the relationship between SSS and NIHSS scores is strong. They calculated an equation to convert the two scales: SSS = 50 − 2 times the NIHSS score. The acute prognostic component of the SSS will likely be used in future clinical trials.

The NIHSS was developed in the mid-1980s for the evaluation of neurologic impairments in patients being enrolled in pilot clinical trials testing therapies for treatment of acute ischemic stroke.[2] The scale was not originally designed to produce an aggregate score, but the initial

TABLE 21-12 SCANDINAVIAN STROKE SCALES

Item	Acute prognosis scale	Long-term convalescence scale
	Score (0-22 points)	Score (0-48 points)
CONSCIOUSNESS	Calculated	Not calculated
Fully conscious	6 points	
Somnolent, can awaken	4 points	
Reacts to verbal command	2 points	
ORIENTATION	Not calculated	Calculated
Correct for time, place, person		6 points
2 of the above correct		4 points
1 of the above correct		2 points
Completely disoriented		0 point
LANGUAGE	Not calculated	Calculated
No aphasia		10 points
Limited vocabulary		6 points
More than yes/no, no sentences		3 points
Only yes/no or less		0 point
EYE MOVEMENTS	Calculated	Not calculated
No gaze palsy	4 points	
Gaze palsy present	2 points	
Conjugate eye deviation	0 point	
AFFECTED ARM POWER	Calculated	Calculated
Raises arm, normal strength	6 points	6 points
Raises arm, reduced strength	5 points	5 points
Raises arm with elbow flexion	4 points	4 points
Can move, not against gravity	2 points	2 points
Paralysis	0 point	0 point
AFFECTED HAND POWER	Not calculated	Calculated
Normal hand strength		6 points
Reduced strength in full range		4 points
Some finger movement		2 points
Paralysis		0 point
AFFECTED LEG POWER	Calculated	Calculated
Raises leg, normal strength	6 points	6 points
Raises leg, reduced strength	5 points	5 points
Raises leg with knee flexion	4 points	4 points
Can move, not against gravity	2 points	2 points
Paralysis	0 point	0 point
FACIAL PALSY	Not calculated	Calculated
None or dubious		2 points
Facial palsy present		0 point
GAIT	Not calculated	Calculated
Walks 5 meters without aids		12 points
Walks with aids		9 points
Walks with person helping		6 points
Sits without support		3 points
Wheelchair or bedridden		0 point

Adapted from Scandinavian Stroke Study Group: Multicenter trial of hemodilution in ischemic stroke background and study protocol. *Stroke* 16:885-889, 1985.

testing found a strong correlation between the size of the ischemic lesion on CT and the total score.[110] Subsequently, it has become the most widely used rating instrument for assessing patients with ischemic stroke. It is the standard clinical assessment tool for rating the severity of stroke, monitoring for neurologic worsening or improvement, and forecasting outcomes after stroke. The NIHSS may be done within a few minutes, which is an advantage for a clinical assessment tool that is being used in an acute care situation.[2,36]

This scale includes 15 components that are scored independently.[2] Assessed items include consciousness, orientation, responses to commands, language, articulation, attention (neglect), visual fields, extraocular movements, facial strength, arm and leg strength, and coordination (Table 21-13). This scale includes items to test function of the right (nondominant) hemisphere and cerebellum. The NIHSS probably has been tested more extensively than any other stroke rating instrument. It has excellent inter-rater agreement and intrarater reproducibility, particularly if the users have been properly trained in the use of the scale.[111-114] The scale may also be used with high accuracy by nurses and other health care providers.[36] However, there is evidence that the NIHSS may not be reliable if raters have not been trained in its use.[115,116] A score may be calculated based on retrospective review of medical records; such retrospective review is not subject to bias, even when some elements of the examination may not be recorded.[117] This attribute is especially useful in epidemiologic studies. The scale has been adapted for use in evaluating Spanish-speaking patients and patients speaking other languages.[118-120] The scale is accompanied by detailed instructions on how to administer it and definitions about scoring each of the tested items. While the definitions of the items and potential scores are relatively straightforward, some of the rules of scoring are arbitrary. To improve compliance with administration of the NIHSS, instruction and certification programs have been developed.[121-123] However, the methods of certification of proficiency with the NIHSS may differ. On the basis of an analysis of one of the certification programs that included scoring by large numbers of physicians, Josephson et al[124] found that grading of the impairments and the total NIHSS scores were inconsistent. Bushnell et al[112] also reported that agreement in the scoring of the NIHSS is limited if not all the items are assessed. This scenario might happen in a community hospital, in which clinicians are not familiar with the scale.

Some items test impairments seen with left (dominant) hemisphere infarctions while others evaluate deficits seen with right (nondominant) hemisphere strokes.[13,125,126] The items of the NIHSS may function differently with strokes in the right hemisphere than with lesions of the left hemisphere.[127] In general, strokes in the left hemisphere are associated with higher scores than those vascular events affecting the right hemisphere.[12,13] The differences in scores between the right and left hemispheres affect prognosis and may influence decisions about acute management. Fink et al[128] reported that infarctions were larger among patients with infarctions of the right hemisphere than for patients with left hemisphere lesions that had comparable scores. Thus, there is a need to develop a

TABLE 21-13 NATIONAL INSTITUTES OF HEALTH STROKE SCALE

Level of consciousness	
Alert	0 point
Drowsy	1 point
Stupor	2 points
Coma	3 points
Orientation (responses to two questions)	
Knows age and current month	0 point
Answers one question correctly	1 point
Cannot answer either question correctly	2 points
Commands (responses to two commands)	
Follows two commands correctly	0 point
Follows one command	1 point
Cannot follow either command	2 points
Best gaze (movement of eyes to left and right)	
Normal full range of eye movements	0 point
Partial gaze paresis to one side	1 point
Forced gaze (deviation) to one side	2 points
Visual fields	
No visual loss	0 point
Partial homonymous hemianopia	1 point
Complete homonymous hemianopia	2 points
Bilateral visual loss	3 points
Facial motor function	
No facial weakness	0 point
Minor unilateral facial weakness	1 point
Partial unilateral facial weakness	2 points
Complete paralysis of one or both sides	3 points
Upper extremity motor function (arm extension)	
Right and left upper extremities scored independently (0-8 points)	
Normal movement	0 point
Drift of the arm	1 point

Some effort against gravity	2 points
No effort against gravity but moves limb	3 points
No movement of the arm	4 points
Lower extremity motor function (leg extension)	
Right and left lower extremities scored independently (0-8 points)	
Normal movement	0 point
Drift of the leg	1 point
Some effort against gravity	2 points
No effort against gravity but moves limb	3 points
No movement of the leg	4 points
Limb ataxia (cannot be tested in the presence of paresis)	
No limb ataxia	0 point
Ataxia present in one limb	1 point
Ataxia present in two limbs	2 points
Sensory function	
No sensory loss	0 point
Mild-to-moderate sensory loss	1 point
Severe-to-total sensory loss	2 points
Language	
Normal language	0 point
Mild-to-moderate aphasia	1 point
Severe aphasia	2 points
Mutism	3 points
Articulation	
Normal articulation	0 point
Mild-to-moderate dysarthria	1 point
Severe dysarthria	2 points
Extinction or inattention	
No neglect or extinction	0 point
Visual or sensory inattention or extinction	1 point
Profound visual and sensory inattention	2 points

Adapted from Brott T, Adams HP Jr, Olinger CP, et al: Measurements of acute cerebral infarction: A clinical examination scale. *Stroke* 20:864-870, 1989.

strategy to compensate for the differences in scoring the NIHSS for those patients with right (nondominant) hemisphere strokes and those with left (dominant) hemisphere events. Millis et al[127] proposed that individual targeted measures may be needed for strokes in either the right or left cerebral hemisphere. Although items to test for infarctions affecting the brainstem and cerebellum are included in the NIHSS (i.e., consciousness, dysarthria, facial weakness, extraocular movements, and ataxia), the scoring appears to be weighted toward infarctions of the hemisphere rather than toward strokes in the posterior circulation.[129]

Some items of the scale do not perform as well as others. For example, scoring of limb ataxia, articulation, or facial weakness may be difficult; interrater agreement may be poor.[111,114,126,130] Variations of the NIHSS that exclude some items have been proposed. In particular, consciousness, facial motor function, articulation, and limb ataxia were eliminated.[126,131] Elimination of these items would likely increase interrater agreement, but this modification has not been widely implemented. Elimination of items such as consciousness may also affect the prognostic features of the NIHSS.

The score on the baseline NIHSS evaluation is an important predictor of outcomes after ischemic stroke among a broad range of patients.[13,132-138] Both acute prognosis and long-term outcomes may be forecasted. In general, a patient with a baseline NIHSS score less than 5 has a high likelihood of a favorable outcome, whereas a score greater than 20 is often associated with a high probability of major disability or death. The NIHSS score may be a stronger predictor of outcomes among patients with subcortical hemispheric infarctions than among those with focal cortical lesions.[139] It is used in forecasting outcomes among patients with posterior circulation strokes.[140] The baseline NIHSS score is also associated with the size of the ischemic brain lesion.[110] Patients with multilobar cerebral infarctions generally have NIHSS scores greater than 15. Thus, the score may be used for forecasting the likelihood of major neurologic complications. For example, the risk of malignant brain edema and increased intracranial pressure is low among patients with a low NIHSS score.

An incongruity between a high NIHSS score that forecasts a multilobar infarction and brain imaging (CT or MRI) findings of a smaller ischemic lesion (clinical–imaging mismatch) may influence decisions about emergency treatment of patients with stroke.[141] The difference may predict those patients with a growth in the size of the infarction and neurologic worsening.[142] The utility of this relationship for selection of patients that need treatment with t-PA has not been established.[143] Choi et al[144] found that a mismatch between NIHSS score and CT findings is common but that this discrepancy did not predict responses to early administration of t-PA.

The baseline NIHSS score may also be used to predict responses to acute treatment, including thrombolytic therapy.[145,146] The baseline NIHSS score also forecasts the likelihood of symptomatic hemorrhagic transformation of the infarction and neurologic worsening after the use of interventions aimed at improving or restoring perfusion to the brain.[147-149]

Besides predicting mortality and the likelihood of a favorable outcome, changes in the NIHSS score may be used to assess responses to treatment, including a clinical response to recanalization after intraarterial or intravenous administration of thrombolytic agents.[150-153] Early improvement in the NIHSS score is associated with better outcomes. Conversely, deterioration in the score is associated with complications of the stroke or neurologic worsening, which is associated with poor outcomes. A change of 2 to 4 points on the NIHSS often is used as a sign of neurologic change.[154] One clinical trial used either a total deterioration of 4 points on the NIHSS or a decline of 1 point in the consciousness item as the clinical criteria for diagnosing symptomatic hemorrhagic transformation after reperfusion therapy.[155]

The NIHSS has also been used as a long-term outcome measure by clinical trials.[145] There are some limitations to this approach; as a rule, those patients who die are given the maximum score of 42 points, which may skew the results. In addition, patients generally have spontaneous improvement in their NIHSS score as they recover from their stroke, regardless of treatment. Still, there are advocates for the use of the NIHSS as an outcome measure. Bruno et al[150] believe that changes in NIHSS score would be an effective outcome measure because the changes are not completely linked to other outcome measures that often are analyzed with the use of a dichotomous or trichotomous methodology.

The NIHSS has been used in clinical trials testing numerous interventions for treatment of acute ischemic stroke.[145,148,155-164] Patient selection based on the baseline NIHSS score has been used to improve the efficiency of clinical trials.[165] Clinical trials often restrict enrollment of subjects with a low NIHSS score (generally <5 points) because of a generally favorable prognosis, and some have restricted enrollment of subjects with very high NIHSS score (usually >20 points) because of a poor prognosis and limited likelihood of success with treatment.[164,166-168] Unfortunately, this strategy has not been established as necessary, and it is possible that clinical trials are excluding subjects that might potentially respond to treatment. Another approach, which may be more statistically justifiable, uses the baseline NIHSS score as a stratification factor for enrollment in a clinical trial.[155,157,158,169-171] The baseline NIHSS may be used to forecast responses to treatment in clinical trials; the criterion for a successful response would be adjusted based on the baseline score.[172] A favorable outcome for a patient with a mild stroke (low NIHSS score) may be complete recovery, whereas a favorable response for a patient with a severe stroke (NIHSS score >15) may be avoidance of severe disability. Such an adjusted endpoint may allow therapeutic effects to be identified more easily.[156] Saver and Yafeh[173] used this strategy to reassess the results of the NINDS trials of thrombolysis and confirmed the utility of the medication in improving severity-adjusted outcome endpoints. The scale has also been used in epidemiologic studies.[174-176] The NIHSS is also described in the series of American guidelines for management of patients with acute ischemic stroke; in particular, it is used as a part of the initial assessment of patients who may be treated with thrombolytic therapy.[177-180]

Although the NIHSS does have limitations, it is a robust clinical rating instrument that assesses a broad range of neurologic deficits that occur in patients with stroke. This is an attribute for evaluating patients with a disease that has a diversity of clinical presentations. The scale is based solely on a neurologic examination that may, with training, be performed accurately and quickly by a broad spectrum of medical personnel. The rules for its use are straightforward, and educational programs to implement the use of the NIHSS are available. The validity of the scale is now established, and the NIHSS has become the standard way of assessing patients enrolled in clinical trials. It also is being used in community settings. Some modification of the NIHSS likely will occur in the future to address the previously noted weaknesses, but it will probably remain the usual way for clinicians and researchers to clinically rate the severity of ischemic stroke in acutely ill patients.

Because of the perceived limitations of the previously described scales for assessing the severity of stroke affecting the brainstem and cerebellum, the Israeli Vertebrobasilar Stroke Scale has been developed.[181] This scale has had limited testing, but it appears to correlate well with scores on the NIHSS and the mRS. Guidelines for the use of this scale and additional testing of the validity of this rating instrument are needed.

Systems to Differentiate the Cause of Ischemic Stroke

A variety of diseases affecting the blood vessels, the heart, and the coagulation system may produce ischemic stroke. Arterial diseases include large artery atherosclerosis, which affects the extracranial or intracranial vasculature, diseases of small penetrating arteries or arterioles, and nonatherosclerotic vasculopathies. Several diseases of the heart predispose to embolism or disorders of coagulation, including inherited or acquired hypercoagulable disorders, and may also lead to stroke. In some cases, no specific underlying cause for the stroke may be identified despite an extensive evaluation. The cause of the stroke does affect the short-term prognosis. The cause of the stroke also affects decisions about measures to prevent recurrent strokes. Thus, establishing the most likely cause of stroke is an important component of management.

The patient's history may influence the diagnosis of the subtype of ischemic stroke. For example, a history of a recent myocardial infarction or treatment for atrial fibrillation is supportive of a diagnosis of a cardioembolic cause of a stroke. A family or personal history of recurrent thromboembolic events, including venous thrombosis, may provide a clue that a hypercoagulable disorder is present. The presence of risk factors for atherosclerosis, including hypertension, diabetes mellitus, hyperlipidemia, and smoking, are also important in establishing an etiologic diagnosis. Unfortunately, clinical manifestations of ischemic stroke, including the pattern of neurologic impairments (OCSP scale) and the severity and types of neurologic deficits (NIHSS) often are not specific for a cause of stroke. For example, findings consistent with a branch cortical infarction (PACI) may occur with an embolic event of arterial or cardiac origin. On the other hand, the neurologic impairments with isolated deep hemisphere infarctions (lacunar strokes) often are relatively specific for the diagnosis of small vessel disease.

The location and size of the ischemic brain injury as detected by either CT or MRI may also provide clues about the likely cause. A small lesion deep in the hemisphere or brainstem suggests small vessel disease. A multilobar infarction portends an occlusion of a major artery, which is often affected by atherosclerosis. Multiple infarctions affecting different vascular territories usually point to cardioembolic events. Branch cortical infarctions restricted to the cerebral cortex are often associated with emboli that arise from the heart or proximal intracranial or extracranial arteries. In most cases, accurate diagnosis of the subtype of ischemic stroke also requires the performance of ancillary studies such as electrocardiography, cardiac imaging, vascular imaging, hematologic studies, coagulation tests, or assessment of metabolic risk factors or immunologic tests.

The investigators in the TOAST study developed a classification system to facilitate the diagnosis of subtypes of ischemic stroke.[182] The initial goal was to use this classification in clinical trials. Subsequently, the TOAST classification has been used extensively in epidemiologic and clinical studies in stroke performed around the world.[183-196] The scale has been used to help researchers examine special populations, such as young adults with stroke, study the impact of common risk factors on causes of stroke, evaluate genetic markers of stroke, validate brain imaging studies, and forecast long-term prognosis.[197-200] The results of the use of the TOAST classification affect decisions for future treatment. For example, Lovett et al[205] reported that the rate of early recurrent stroke was highest among patients with large artery atherosclerosis, and their findings suggested that this group of patients needed urgent carotid imaging and carotid endarterectomy. This scale has also been used in clinical trials testing interventions to treat acute ischemic stroke, and as such, it has been used almost as extensively as the NIHSS.[182]

The classification is based on the clinical findings, the results of brain imaging, and the results of ancillary diagnostic studies.[182] The diagnosis of subtype is categorized as probable or possible based on the strength of the supporting information, including the absence of alternative explanations (Table 21-14). The potential subtype categories are (1) large artery atherosclerosis, (2) cardiac embolism, (3) small artery occlusion, (4) other cause (most commonly nonatherosclerotic vasculopathy or a hypercoagulable disorder, or (5) stroke of undetermined cause. The latter category is used if the patient did not have ancillary diagnostic studies performed, if the

TABLE 21-14 TOAST/SSS-TOAST CLASSIFICATION

Large artery atherosclerosis
Clinical evidence of cerebral cortical or cerebellar infarction
Cerebral cortical, cerebellar, brainstem, subcortical infarction
  On CT or MRI, infarction is >1.5-2.0 cm in size
Stenosis or occlusion of major intracranial or extracranial artery
  Stenosis is >50%, occlusion of relevant artery
  Stenosis is ≤50% if ulceration or thrombus at site
No high-risk cardiac lesion found (for evident or probable diagnosis)

Small artery occlusion
Clinical evidence of one of the lacunar syndromes
Subcortical or brainstem infarction is <1.5-2.0 cm in size
No ipsilateral large artery atherosclerotic lesion found (for evident or probable diagnosis)
No high-risk cardiac lesion found (for evident or probable diagnosis)

Cardioembolism
Clinical evidence of cerebral cortical or cerebellar infarction
Cerebral cortical, cerebellar, brainstem, or cortical infarction
  On CT or MRI, infarction is >1.5-2.0 cm in size
Cardiac source for embolism found (high versus medium risk)
No ipsilateral large artery atherosclerotic lesion found (for evident or probable diagnosis)

Other demonstrated cause
Evaluation demonstrates another cause of stroke
  Presence of a specific disease in appropriate cerebral artery
  Presence of a specific hypercoagulable disorder
Other causes of stroke have been excluded

Undetermined cause (cryptogenic stroke)
Two or more causes identified, most likely not obvious
No abnormality found on evaluation
  Evidence of cryptogenic embolism
Evaluation incomplete

Adapted from Adams HP Jr, Bendixen BH, Kappelle LJ, et al: Classification of subtype of acute ischemic stroke. Definitions for use in a multicenter clinical trial. TOAST. Trial of Org 10172 in Acute Stroke Treatment. *Stroke* 24:35-41, 1993 and Ay H, Furie KL, Singhal A, et al: An evidence-based causative classification system for acute ischemic stroke. *Ann Neurol* 58:688-697, 2005.

evaluation did not demonstrate a likely explanation, or if the assessment found two or more potential causes that were equally as likely to have initiated the stroke. The diagnoses of subtype were influenced by the perceived risk of stroke from the underlying etiology. For example, atrial fibrillation complicating myocardial infarction was considered a "high-risk" cardiac source for embolism, whereas a patent foramen ovale was listed as a lower risk lesion. Some of the definitions are arbitrary; for example, the diagnosis of large artery atherosclerosis requires demonstration of an occlusion or stenosis in the relevant artery. Thus, fractured atherosclerotic plaque that does not cause narrowing greater than 50% would not be recognized as sufficient evidence for diagnosing large artery atherosclerosis as the cause of stroke. Because of the relatively rigid requirements for diagnosis with the use of the TOAST classification, especially for the diagnosis of stroke secondary to large artery atherosclerosis, the proportion of stroke of undetermined etiology in both epidemiologic studies and clinical trials has been relatively large.[194] The original definitions for the TOAST subtypes

TABLE 21-15 FUNCTIONAL INDEPENDENCE MEASURE

Category	Points
Personal care	
Total independence of all aspects of eating and drinking	4
Requires preparation of food or uses adaptive devices	3
Requires supervision or help while eating and drinking	2
Requires total assistance to eat or has enteral nutrition	1
Grooming	
Total independence—brushing teeth, washing face, grooming hair, shaving or applying make-up	4
Requires preparation, needs assistive devices, slow	3
Requires supervision or moderate assistance	2
Requires total assistance, cannot do alone	1
Bathing	
Total independence in bathing and drying body	4
Requires assistive devices, is slow, or unsafe	3
Requires supervision or moderate assistance	2
Requires total assistance, cannot do alone	1
Dressing upper body	
Total independence in dressing and undressing	4
Needs assistive devices or uses modified clothing	3
Requires supervision or moderate assistance	2
Requires total assistance, cannot do alone	1
Toileting	
Total independence in all aspects	4
Needs adaptive equipment or is slow	3
Requires supervision or moderate assistance	2
Requires total assistance, cannot do alone	1
Bladder control (urinary continence)	
Controls bladder, no incontinence	4
Requires catheter, bag, or medication, can use own	3
Requires supervision or moderate assistance	2
Requires total assistance, is incontinent despite devices	1
Bowel control (fecal continence)	
Controls bowels, no incontinence	4
Requires help including medications but no incontinence	3
Requires supervision or moderate assistance	2
Requires total assistance, is incontinent most days	1
Mobility (transfer to bed, chair, wheelchair)	
If walking, can sit down and rise without help, or if wheelchair can move to and from chair without help	4
Requires special assistance device to transfer	3
Requires supervision or moderate assistance	2
Requires total assistance	1
Mobility (transfer to toilet)	
If walking, can sit down and rise without help, or if wheelchair can move to and from toilet without help	4
Requires special assistance device or is unsafe	3

Category	Points
Requires supervision or moderate assistance	2
Requires total assistance	1
Mobility (transfer to shower or bath)	
If walking, can move into and out of bath/shower, or if wheelchair can approach and transfer safely	4
Requires special assistance devices or is unsafe	3
Requires supervision or moderate assistance	2
Requires total assistance	1
Locomotion	
Walks 50 meters without use of assistance devices	4
Walks 50 meters but needs devices or orthoses, or if wheelchair can maneuver at least 50 meters	3
Requires supervision or moderate assistance	2
Requires total assistance or cannot perform task	1
Stairs	
Goes up and down one flight of stairs without support	4
Goes up and down one flight of stairs with device	3
Requires supervision or moderate assistance	2
Requires total assistance or cannot go up or down stairs	1
Comprehension of language	
Comprehends spoken or written conversation	4
Has difficulty with spoken or written conversation	3
Does not follow conversation without cues or assistance	2
Does not follow spoken or written conversation	1
Expression of language	
Expresses complex ideas intelligibly and fluently	4
Expresses complex ideas with difficulty but may communicate basic wants and needs	3
Expresses thoughts in confused pattern or needs assistance	2
Does not express basic needs or wants	1
Social interactions	
Interacts appropriately with family members and others	4
Participates appropriately but in structured situations	3
Unpredictable or uncooperative behavior	2
Does not function in a family or group situation	1
Solving problems	
Is able to apply knowledge to initiate and complete task	4
Has difficulty in initiating task or correcting self	3
Needs help of another person to complete task	2
Is unable to solve problems	1
Memory	
Recognizes other people, remembers daily routines easily	4
Has memory difficulty but has self-initiated cues	3
Requires prompting from another person for memory	2
Does not recognize other people or remember routines	1

Adapted from Granger CV, Hamilton BB, Linacre JM, et al: Performance profiles of the Functional Independence Measure. *Am J Phys Med Rehabil* 72:84-89, 1993.

were determined before the widespread use of modern brain and vascular imaging. The results of transcranial Doppler ultrasonography, computed tomographic angiography, MRA, and modern MRI sequences may easily be incorporated in the TOAST classification. Using advances in the vascular and brain imaging that can be obtained early in hospitalization, Ay et al[206] were able to reduce the number of cases of stroke of undetermined etiology. In addition, there is some lumping of patients with stroke with undetermined etiology. This category includes those patients with an incomplete evaluation, those with negative findings on evaluation, and those with two or more likely causes of stroke. This latter group may need to be separated from the other two groups. This group of patients has demonstrated causes that need to be treated on a long-term basis. Decisions about management may be influenced by the causes that have been identified.

Recently, Ay et al[206,207] made adjustments in the TOAST classification in an attempt to improve the validity of the system by including a group called *evident,* which they titled SSS-TOAST. They also included the strength of current natural history data that shows the annual risk of stroke organized into higher and lower risk conditions. The revised classification also places aortic causes of embolism in the category of cardioembolism because the clinical findings overlap with those of emboli arising from the heart. The SSS-TOAST classification also includes cryptogenic embolism in the category of stroke of undetermined etiology. Still, the basic organization of the TOAST classification remains unchanged (Table 21-14).

The validity, interrater agreement, and intrarater reproducibility of TOAST classification has been tested extensively.[19,198,208,209] The levels of agreement and reproducibility are acceptable when rating physicians receive suitable training.[19] Goldstein et al[209] found that the TOAST classification could be applied with high reliability and reproducibility to the retrospective review of medical records. The SSS-TOAST version has also been tested for reliability and reproducibility; a kappa value for interrater agreement was 0.86, which is excellent.[207] Computerized algorithms have also been used.[207,209] In a paradigm that involved independent assessments by six physician reviewers, Meschia et al[198] found interrater agreements were highest for the subtypes of large artery atherosclerosis and cardioembolism. Fure et al[210] found that the TOAST classification was particularly helpful in differentiating stroke from small vessel disease from other causes when it was applied in an emergency situation; they found the sensitivity of the diagnosis to be 0.93 and the specificity to be 0.83. However, physicians continue to disagree about subtype diagnoses; these disagreements appear to reflect individual physician's sense of those findings that are the most important or reflect the physician's expertise. In particular, physicians seem reluctant to make the diagnosis of stroke of undetermined cause. Thus, physicians should be trained on how to use the TOAST classification with a reasonable degree of accuracy. In addition, clinical studies have used central adjudication of subtype diagnosis to increase the validity of the results.[148,157,198]

The TOAST classification is not easily used in the first hours after stroke when ancillary diagnostic studies may not be available. Thus, the initial subtype diagnosis often changes after the results of additional testing become available.[211] As a result, clinical trials testing interventions for stroke could not use the TOAST classification with sufficient accuracy to restrict enrollment to some specific subtypes. Some patients that truly would be eligible for treatment likely would be excluded. Conversely, other patients that would be ineligible would be enrolled. Fortunately, the advances in imaging of the brain and vasculature have eased some of these concerns. Wessels et al[203] found a strong relationship between stroke subtype and the pattern of imaging on diffusion-weighted imaging (DWI). They found that single corticosubcortical lesions and multiple bilateral lesions in the anterior and posterior circulations were strongly correlated with cardioembolic events. On the other hand, multiple unilateral lesions in the anterior circulation were correlated with large artery atherosclerosis. These associations, along with a test that would provide very early information about the location and extent of brain injury, would help the early diagnosis of subtype of ischemic stroke. If the MRI findings were combined with early MRA, the ability to establish an early subtype diagnosis may improve even more.[206,212] Lee et al[56] found that the combination of DWI and MRA improved the likelihood of agreement of TOAST subtype diagnoses considerably. Hence, the use of these emergency tests greatly strengthens the application of the TOAST and presumably the SSS-TOAST classification.

Han et al[213] recently developed a new classification system that they considered to be superior to the TOAST classification (Table 21-15). While the authors found the new method to be satisfactory, it has not been used outside the original institution. It is unclear whether this system will gain the widespread acceptance of the TOAST or SSS-TOAST classification. In addition, Hoffmann et al[214] concluded that the TOAST classification system included too much lumping of diagnoses into the system. In particular, they were concerned about the category of stroke of other demonstrated etiology that included a wide variety of disorders including prothrombotic disorders and nonatherosclerotic vasculopathy. They are correct in that those conditions are lumped together and the treatment of these disorders does differ. However, these conditions account for a small minority of patients in most clinical series, with the exception of studies that focus on the evaluation of children and young adults. Their expanded categorization would be as follows: (1) large vessel cerebrovascular disease (presumably atherosclerosis,) (2) small vessel cerebrovascular disease, (3) cardiogenic, (4) dissection, (5) hypercoagulable disorders, (6) migraine-induced, (7) cerebral venous thrombosis, (8) vasculitis, (9) other vasculopathy, (10) miscellaneous, and (11) unknown.[214] This classification includes cerebral venous thrombosis, which was not included in the TOAST classification. Besides having a different clinical profile than acute ischemic stroke and not being a specific cause of stroke, cerebral venous thrombosis is the result of several etiologies; it is not clear if strokes in patients with this diagnosis should be categorized by an alternative diagnosis such as a hypercoagulable disorder, which is the actual etiology of cerebral venous thrombosis. In addition, this classification also includes some lumping (e.g., both multisystem vasculitides and isolated central nervous system vasculitis are combined). The large number of categories will make determination of satisfactory interrater agreement difficult. This new rating system would need considerable testing to determine whether it is sufficiently useful for clinical research. This system likely is not superior to the TOAST or SSS-TOAST classification.

The TOAST classification has been criticized as not being useful, and suggestions have been made to discard it.[215] Still, critics have not proposed a viable alternative. The TOAST classification is already used widely and has gained international acceptance. The TOAST/SSS-TOAST classification has already passed the steps (i.e., reliability, reproducibility, validity, and accuracy) to ensure that it is a useful tool. Some of the recent modifications, which reflect the advances in diagnosis of patients with ischemic cerebrovascular disease, have strengthened the scale. Until another clinical rating instrument is developed that is superior to the TOAST/SSS-TOAST classification, it likely will continue to be used in a wide variety of stroke-related research projects.

The TOAST classification was developed to categorize subtypes of ischemic stroke in adults; its applicability to stroke in children is limited. As a result, Wraige et al[216] proposed modifications for a subtype classification system for the causes of stroke in children. These changes reflect the differences in diseases that lead to brain ischemia in children versus those found in adults. Atherosclerosis is not a common disease in children. The cardiac lesions that lead to embolism to the brain in children are at variance from those found in adults. Inherited or acquired disorders of coagulation or nonatherosclerotic vascular diseases constitute a relatively larger proportion of causes. The categories for the causes of pediatric ischemic stroke are as follows: (1) sickle cell disease, (2) cardioembolism, (3) moyamoya, (4) cervical arterial dissection, (5) stenoocclusive cerebral arteriopathy, (6) other determined cause, (7) multiple possible causes, and (8) undetermined cause. The utility of the pediatric subtype scale has not been extensively tested, but its components do reflect differences in causes of stroke found in children from those causes detected in adults.

Measures to Assess Responses to Rehabilitation Interventions

Rehabilitation specialists have developed several clinical instruments that are used to assess impairments and responses to individual rehabilitation interventions. Examples include the Modified Ashworth Scale for measuring spasticity, the Brunnstrom scale to assess upper extremity function, the ABILOCO questions to assess locomotion, the Dynamic Gait Index, the Wisconsin Gait Scale, and the Trunk Control Test.[217-226] Most nonrehabilitation physicians do not use these scales nor are they familiar with the nuances of these rating instruments. In-depth discussions of these rehabilitation rating scales are beyond the scope of this chapter.

Scales to Rate Outcomes (Disability) after Stroke

Disability after stroke may be assessed by a variety of rating tools. These scales may be used to monitor responses to rehabilitation and other interventions, to provide prognostic information, and to judge outcomes of immediate and subsequent treatment. Some outcome scales include assessments of the patient's ability to perform activities of daily living (ADLs). Some scales are based on historical information shared by the patient, family, or other observers. The scales usually include a series of relatively straightforward questions and may be performed through a telephone conversation. Patients' self reporting of perceived impairments appears to be valid.[227] Other scales require direct observation of the patient's performance; in some instances the scale assesses complex tasks or activities. Some scales emphasize physical independence and are weighted toward motor performance; others include observations about cognitive or other brain function. In general, the scales appear to have similar clinometric behavior.[228] The most commonly used scales are the BI, the Functional Independence Measure (FIM), Fugl-Myer Scale, the Katz index of ADL, the Frenchay Activities Index, and the Pulses Profile.[3,135,229-245] In addition, the Mini Mental State Examination (MMSE) is used to measure cognitive outcomes after stroke.[246-248]

The scores on the Fugl-Meyer assessment correlate with the score on the BI.[244] A validated, short form of the Fugl-Meyer scale is available.[249] Rabadi and Rabadi[250] found that the Fugl-Meyer assessment was sensitive to changes in motor function in patients having rehabilitation after stroke. The Frenchay Activities Index also has been used to assess outcomes among patients with a wide variety of neurologic diseases, including stroke.[246,251] These scales have not been used extensively in clinical trials in stroke or in general patient care.

The 17-item FIM scale tests motor and cognitive functions and has a range of scores of 1 to 4 points for each item (total 17 to 68 points) that may be calculated through retrospective review of medical records.[252-255] The results of the FIM have been correlated with quality-of-life outcomes and have been used to predict outcomes after stroke.[255-261] A FIM score less than 40 is generally associated with a low likelihood of independence after stroke. The FIM has been used to predict the length of stay for inpatient rehabilitation after stroke.[261] Sequential assessments of the FIM are used to monitor recovery during rehabilitation.[262,263] Stineman et al[259] found that the psychometric properties of the FIM compare favorably to most other clinical rating instruments. The FIM has demonstrated validity and reliability across a wide range of clinical settings, patients, and raters.[264-269]

A three-dimensional FIM tool including self-care, cognitive function, and toileting as the major grouping is useful for assessment of patients with stroke.[253,270] Mauthe et al[260] found that the items of bathing, bowel control, toileting, social interaction, dressing, and eating were the items that best predicted outcomes. Outcomes are most associated with cognitive, sphincter, ideomotor apraxia, and neglect items on the FIM. In addition, the scoring of the motor components of the FIM has been delineated from the total FIM.[271] Agreement and kappa values for scoring both the FIM and the BI are close.[272,273] Overall, the FIM and BI respond similarly.[271] The motor items from the FIM may be used to calculate the BI, but the FIM appears to have no advantage over the BI.[271,272] A derivative of the FIM, the FIM-Functional Assessment Measure, which has reasonable interrater agreement, has also been used to test patients with brain disease.[274] A pediatric version of the FIM called the WeeFIM shows good test–retest reliability. Individual items and subscale scores are also reliable for evaluating children with disabilities. The FIM is used in a wide spectrum of rehabilitation settings, but it has not been used in acute stroke trials.

The BI is used to evaluate disability and performance of ADLs in a variety of patients with a variety of acute and chronic diseases.[3,138,251] Presently, it is the most widely used clinical rating instrument to assess ADLs and stroke-related disability in clinical trials and epidemiologic studies on stroke.[6,135,145,148,171,230,232,275-281] Some trials have used the BI as a primary outcome measure.

Although it was used for assessment of American patients, the BI has been translated or adapted for use in other countries.[113,282-285] The patient or caregiver is asked a series of questions about 10 different components of ADLs (Table 21-16). Priority is given to mobility and continence.[286] The scores are rated as independent, partially independent, or dependent, and the definitions are straightforward. The BI is easy to administer, and scores are also easy to calculate; scores can range from 0 to 100. Generally a score of 60 or greater is associated with functional independence, although it is possible that a score of 100 may not be completely independent.[230,232,277,287] In general, higher scores are associated with shorter courses of acute care hospitalization and less need for intensive rehabilitation after stroke. The score on the BI also predicts long-term outcomes including mortality.

The minimally important difference in scores on the BI appears to be approximately 10 points.[249] In addition, dichotomous and trichotomous divisions of scoring, most commonly 0 to 55, 60 to 90, and 95 to 100, have been used to define poor, good, and excellent outcomes.[148,171] Song et al[288] recommended that mean values of the BI should be included along with the distribution of outcome scores so that they can be combined in meta-analyses. Another group suggested that the psychometric properties of the BI could be improved by focusing on the motor components of the scale.[289]

The BI does have some limitations. Because of its emphasis on motor recovery, patients with cognitive impairments, including aphasia or neglect, may have relatively high scores and still not be independent. It has ceiling and floor effects.[290-292] Because of the ceiling effect

and because important cognitive or behavioral impairments may be missed, the BI probably is not the best outcome measure to assess responses in clinical trials. It also has a floor effect, especially among seriously affected patients. Martinsson and Eksborg[293] recommended that additional measures of ADLs be added to further define outcomes. Still, the BI has excellent levels of agreement for the entire scale and for its constituents.[113] The BI has high interrater reliability, internal consistency, and validity.[277,294] Agreement with other measures of disability, including the mRS and FIM, is considerable.[286,295,296] A BI score of 95 generally correlates with an mRS score of 1, a BI score of 90 is comparable to an mRS of 2, and a BI score of 75 matches an mRS score of 3.[297] In addition, because of its simplicity and the utility of the scores on the BI, it is widely recognized by physicians treating patients with stroke. At present, the BI is the most important and commonly used measure to assess disability among patients enrolled in clinical trials testing therapies for acute stroke. A variation of the BI called the Extended BI has been developed to assess patients with recent stroke.[298]

Scales to Rate Outcomes (Global or Handicap) after Stroke

Several scales to measure global outcomes or handicap after stroke are available. These scales are relatively brief and include a few well-defined clinical grades. The most frequently used scales are the mRS and the Glasgow Outcome Scale (GOS).[4,299] They are efficient measures for assessing outcomes in large clinical trials after stroke and in epidemiologic studies.[85,281,300-302] These scales show a high degree of validity. The intrarater reproducibility is strong.[303] On the other hand, the definitions are somewhat arbitrary. Interrater agreement in differentiating adjacent scores, particularly among mildly affected patients, may be difficult.[304] The mRS has shown moderate interrater reliability that improves with structured interviews.[303] Training in the use of the scales also improves their reliability.[291] The fine distinctions in scoring may be taught to raters of varying backgrounds. Educational programs are available so that investigators may be certified in their proficiency in the use of the mRS.

The mRS is the most widely used global outcome scale in clinical trials for stroke.[155-158,305,306] The mRS is also associated with long-term outcome prediction after stroke.[295]

TABLE 21-16 BARTHEL INDEX

Component	Independent	Partially Independent	Dependent
Walking	15 points	5/10 points	0 points
Climbing stairs	10 points	5 points	0 points
Chair/bed transfers	15 points	5/10 points	0 points
Toilet transfers	10 points	5 points	0 points
Grooming	5 points	0 points	0 points
Dressing	10 points	5 points	0 points
Bathing	5 points	0 points	0 points
Eating	10 points	5 points	0 points
Bowel control	10 points	5 points	0 points
Bladder control	10 points	5 points	0 points

Adapted from Mahoney FI, Barthel DW: Functional evaluation: The Barthel Index. *Md State Med J* 14:61-65, 1965.

It was originally developed for a clinical trial in 1957.[4] It was modified to its current format by an expansion of the scale to six categories (Table 21-17).[5] The score of 0 may be difficult to achieve because a patient must have absolutely no symptoms related to stroke. This strict definition is problematic because a patient may have made an excellent recovery, but if minimal symptoms are present, a score of 1 must be rated. As a result, the score of 1 covers a broad spectrum of patients. Generally, clinical trials have used a dichotomous or trichotomous division of scores in that scores of 0-1 are considered very favorable, scores of 2-3 are favorable, and scores of 4-6 are rated as unfavorable. In some cases, a score of 2 would be considered a favorable response and 3 would be rated as an unfavorable outcome. Adams et al[172] recommended adjusting the definitions of favorable outcomes on the mRS by the baseline severity of neurologic impairments as rated by the NIHSS. In addition, Saver[307] advocated using a shift of the numbers of subjects in each of the groups on the mRS as a way to assess the success of treatment. This approach has been criticized.[308]

The construct validity of the mRS is demonstrated by its strong relationships with other indicators of severity of stroke including NIHSS scores and brain imaging.[303] The mRS should not be considered as being a pure handicap scale but as a global measure of health that has an emphasis on physical limitations.[85]

The GOS is a companion rating instrument to the GCS. It was used first to rate outcomes among patients with head injuries.[299,309] It contains five grades with some subdivision within the three highest grades (Table 21-18). Separating the scores of 2 (moderate disability) and 3 (severe disability) is difficult. Still, the GOS has very good interrater and intrarater agreement, reproducibility, and reliability. The validity of the GOS has been established in research in craniocerebral trauma. The GOS has also been used in clinical trials testing therapies for ischemic stroke and subarachnoid hemorrhage.[148,310-314] In general, the utility of the GOS seems to be best for subarachnoid hemorrhage because of the link of the GCS with the WFNS scale, which is used to assess the baseline severity of the vascular event. The spectrum of grades on the GOS may reflect serious diffuse or multifocal brain injury and includes the grade of a persistent vegetative state. This outcome is not especially common among survivors of ischemic stroke. In addition, the GOS does not differentiate between some of the more mildly affected patients.

Thus, the role of the GOS has declined in ischemic stroke trials as the mRS has become more widely used.

The global outcome measures involve some lumping of groups of patients with a wide spectrum of neurologic sequelae. As a result, some clinicians object to the use of the mRS or GOS because they cannot adequately define many subtle or diverse but important neurologic consequences of ischemic stroke. However, these scales are relatively simple to use, and their validity has been shown through their use in large clinical trials. Physicians dealing with patients with stroke are familiar with these instruments, and as a result, they are commonly used. Other outcome scales have been proposed, but these have not been used extensively.[310,315] Until better outcome scales to measure handicap or global functioning among stroke survivors are developed, these scales, particularly the mRS, will continue to be used in stroke trials.

Cramer et al[316] have proposed that new scales be developed that monitor responses to therapies aimed at promoting recovery after stroke. These scales are not yet available. Presumably, such scales would include measures of specific impairments, disability, and global outcomes.

Scales to Assess the Quality of Life after Stroke

There is considerable interest in the quality of life among survivors of stroke. Although the term *quality of life* is difficult to explain, most persons have their own definitions. McKevitt et al[317] concluded that the term *quality of life* might be translated as happiness and contentment. However, the term probably covers more than emotional responses and includes many other areas of functioning that interact. Stroke is a life-changing disease; most patients do not consider themselves as being better off after having had a stroke.[318] In addition, stroke affects interactions among family members and may affect the

TABLE 21-17 MODIFIED RANKIN SCALE

Findings	Score
No symptoms present at all	0
No disability despite some symptoms	1
Slight disability but does not require assistance	2
Moderate disability but can walk	3
Moderately severe disability	4
Severe disability, usually bedridden	5
Dead	0

Adapted from van Swieten JC, Koudstaal PJ, Visser MC, et al: Interobserver agreement for the assessment of handicap in stroke patients. *Stroke* 19:604-607, 1988.

TABLE 21-18 GLASGOW OUTCOME SCALE

	Grade
GOOD RECOVERY	5
(A) Full recovery without symptoms or signs	
(B) Capable of resuming normal activities but has minor complaints	
MODERATE DISABILITY	4
Independent but disabled	
(A) Signs present but can resume most former activities	
(B) Independent in activities of daily living but cannot resume previous activities	
SEVERE DISABILITY	3
Conscious but dependent	
(A) Partial independence in activities of daily living but cannot return to previous activities	
(B) Total or almost total dependency for activities of daily living	
VEGETATIVE STATE	2
DEATH	1

Adapted from Jennett B, Bond M: Assessment of outcome after severe brain damage. A practical scale. *Lancet* 305:480-484, 1975.

family's fiscal status.[319-323] Many stroke survivors report a lack of meaningful activity, severe depression, or a sense of their health being poor.[324] Thus, reductions in quality of life may be expected among stroke survivors of all age groups. The cause of stroke appears not to have a major impact, but the severity of the neurologic impairments is a major predictor of unsatisfactory responses.[323,325] Not surprisingly, those patients with severe impairments that require assistive devices and the help of family members or friends rate their quality of life as poor.[326] Quality of life measures also are lower among women than among men; these changes may reflect their older age and the higher rate of women living alone.[326] Other predictors of poor outcomes after stroke include overall functional status, residual upper extremity dysfunction, and educational level.[247] Because many of the long-term sequelae of stroke produce many of the problems seen with a chronic condition and because these outcomes affect not only the patient but also their family members and society at large, determination of the quality of an individual's life is important. After a severe stroke, many survivors need the assistance of family members or caregivers, and this also affects quality of life.[327-329] On the other hand, patients that had a minor ischemic stroke often rate their quality of life as relatively good.[330] Measures of quality of life should be able to detect reductions in changes in physical and psychological functioning.[328] Because each person has his or her own perception about the quality of life after stroke, ratings that evaluated outcomes in large populations may not be applicable to each individual.[331] In addition, quality-of-life scales have also been used to assess responses among family members of persons with stroke.[332]

Patel et al[258] looked at the quality of life, disability, and handicap of long-term stroke survivors. They found that patients had low perceptions of their physical health, although their mental health perception was considered satisfactory. They suggested that health-related quality of life (HRQL) measures be added to assessments of disability and handicap to have a broader assessment of outcomes after stroke. These measures have been developed to differentiate patients' health status from other aspects of their lives.[327,333] These rating instruments include components for assessing physical, social, psychological, and overall health as affected by the individual person's beliefs, perceptions, experiences, and expectations. Several scales are available for providing HRQL measurements among patients with stroke. This is a difficult task because there is probably no scale that is able to properly define all the components of quality of life. The scales are designed to cover symptoms, conditions, and social roles that are important for patients with stroke and that could be affected either positively or negatively by an intervention or the disease.[333] Scales that have these properties are designated as having good coverage. Still, these instruments need to be tested in the same vigorous manner as the acute stroke scales and other clinical tools.[85,300,334-336] Most of the currently available HRQL scales have not been evaluated extensively for sensitivity, specificity, reliability, reproducibility, or validity. Thus, this is an area that warrants considerable research.

Some stroke-specific HRQL scales have been created but are not fully validated. For example, Hamedani et al[337] evaluated patients surviving hemorrhagic stroke, using a specific 54-item quality-of-life instrument. They found reproducibility and validity and did not find ceiling effects that are found with some other outcome measures. This scale has not been tested by other researchers. Other scales also have had limited testing.[323,336,338-341]

Other stroke HRQL scales have been adapted from other instruments used to evaluate outcomes of patients with other chronic diseases.[334,336] These scales include the Nottingham Health Profile, the Medical Outcomes Short Form-36 (SF-36) or Short Form-12, and the Sickness Impact Profile (SIP).[102,242,247,315,342,343] The World Health Organization Quality of Life Measure also has been used.[284] Hacking et al[344] tested three generic HRQL status questionnaires among patients with stroke. They found that the results of the scales were not mutually interchangeable. They concluded that the SF-36 was the most appropriate for most patients with stroke (Table 21-19). Suenkeler et al[345] discovered that the levels assessed by global and domain-specific measures of the SF-36 continued to deteriorate during the first year after a stroke. On the other hand, others found that SF-36 had limited validity for assessing quality of life among survivors of stroke.[342] Thus, the utility of the SF-36 has not been established.

Hobart et al[342] also reported that five of the eight components of the SIP had limited validity in evaluating the quality of life among survivors of stroke. Conversely, another study found the SIP30 to have satisfactory performance for evaluation of physical and psychosocial dimensions.[346] In a similar way, the SIP30 was found to have internal consistent and convergent validity.[346] The SIP30 has been adapted to the Stroke-Adapted Sickness Impact Profiles (SA-SIP).[63] Among patients with mild stroke, the emotional well-being and activity participation components of the SA-SIP detected the most obvious quality-of-life problems.[347] The Stroke-Specific Quality of Life (SS-QOL) scale and the SIP30 have been translated into other languages and have been modified for other cultures.[346,348]

Williams et al[349,350] developed the SS-QOL. This scale is available in American and European versions.[256] This scale measures a wide range of sequelae from stroke including language and behavior impairments (Table 21-20).[348,350,351] It has been validated and is shown to have good associations with lower scores on the NIHSS, higher scores on the BI, and severity of depression.[341,349] The SS-QOL is a reliable instrument for measuring self-reported HRQL among persons with mild-to-moderate stroke.[341,348,352] The SS-QOL is becoming one of the more widely used tools for rating quality of life among persons who have had a stroke.

The EuroQOL scale is also widely used to assess quality of life issues in patients with a variety of medical diseases, including stroke.[353] The EuroQOL is being used by a large number of groups to test the cost-utility of health interventions in the United States.[318] For example, the EuroQOL scores are not affected by the duration from the onset of the illness.[354] The scale includes two components. Patients are asked about mobility, self-care, usual activities, pain or discomfort, or symptoms of anxiety or depression.

TABLE 21-19 SHORT FORM HEALTH SURVEY (SF-36)

Physical health
Physical functioning
   Limited doing vigorous activities
   Limited doing moderate activities
   Limited lifting or carrying groceries
   Limited climbing several flights of stairs
   Limited bending, kneeling, or stooping
   Limited walking more than one mile
   Limited walking one-half mile
   Limited walking 100 yards
   Limited bathing or dressing
Physical role
   Reduced amount of time spent at work
   Accomplished less than would like
   Limited in the kind of work
   Difficulty performing work
Pain
   Magnitude (severity) of pain
   Interference with work

General health
Overall general health
   Overall rating of general health
   I seem to get sick easier than others
   I am as healthy as anyone I know
   I expect my health to get worse
   My health is excellent

Mental health
Vitality
   Did you feel full of life?
   Did you have a lot of energy?
   Did you feel worn out?
   Did you feel tired?
Social functioning
   Extent of limitations
   Time of limitations
Emotional role
   Cut down time spent working
   Accomplished less than would like
   Did not work as carefully as usual
Overall mental health
   Have you been a nervous person?
   Have you felt down in the dumps?
   Have you felt calm and peaceful?
   Have you felt downhearted and low?
   Have you been a happy person?

Adapted from McHorey CA, Ware JE Jr., Lu LF, Sherbourne CD: The MOS 36-item short form health survey (SF-36) III. Tests of data quality, scaling assumptions, reliability across diverse groups. *Med Care* 32: 40-66, 1994.

TABLE 21-20 STROKE-SPECIFIC QUALITY OF LIFE SCALE

Tested Items	Number of Questions
Energy	4
Family role	8
Language	7
Mobility	12
Mood	8
Personality	4
Self-care	8
Social roles	7
Thinking	4
Upper extremity function	9
Vision	4
Work and productivity	3

Adapted from Williams LS, Weinberger M, Harris LE, et al: Measuring quality of life in a way that is meaningful to stroke patients. *Neurology* 53:1839-1843, 1999.

For each category, patients are given the option of three choices: no problem, moderate problem, severe problem. In addition, patients are asked to rate the state of their health on a range from 0 (worst) to 100 (best). The scale has been used to assess patients with stroke. Dorman et al[355,356] found that the EuroQOL had acceptable validity for measurement of HRQL among patients with stroke and that it functioned similarly to the SF-36. Because many patients with stroke may not be able to give the information directly, Dorman et al[357] looked at the utility of proxy assessments. Although the patients actually scored quality of life better than did the proxies, overall the tactic of using proxy ratings was considered acceptable. Because it contains a limited number of questions and because it can be performed by patients or proxies, the EuroQOL has become an increasingly used tool for assessment of HRQL among survivors of stroke.

The Stroke and Aphasia Quality of Life Scale-39 was developed to rate outcomes of stroke survivors with language impairments in physical, psychosocial, communication, and energy domains.[351,358] This scale needs additional testing, but it seems to have reasonable reliability and validity. The Katz Index has shown validity and a high level of interrater agreement.[359] The Stroke Impact Scale was developed to rate outcomes after stroke from the perspective of the patient, and it has been used in clinical trials.[135,360,361] The scale includes measures of ADLs. The scale appears to be valid and does differentiate stroke survivors, particularly through the use of the physical domain.[362] Lai et al[362] compared the SF-36 and the Stroke Impact Scale for detection of important outcomes after stroke and found the latter to be superior. The Health Utilities Index has also been used to evaluate quality of life after stroke.[363] This scale also appears to have validity and internal consistency.[364,365] British investigators have tried a very simple approach to asking patients about their quality of life by using two questions.[366] Patients are asked if they have fully recovered from the stroke and whether they have needed assistance from others in ADLs in the previous 2 weeks. This tactic has many potential advantages, and it appears to be valid; however, it has not gained much support from other investigators.

Depression has a major impact on outcomes after stroke; it affects both quality of life and the individual's handicaps.[227,247,283,367] Many of the quality of life scales have components dealing with poststroke depression. Diagnostic scales to assess for depression among persons with aphasia have been developed.[368] Any measure of quality of life after stroke needs sections that address the presence and severity of poststroke depression.

Despite the efforts to develop a quality-of-life measure that effectively rates outcomes among stroke survivors, problems persist. Critics have concluded that these scales do not provide data that are truly useful in conducting clinical trials testing therapies to treat acute stroke.[325,369] The selection of a HRQL scale should depend on the goal of the clinical trial and the specific intervention that is being tested.[365] Additional development of HRQL scales is needed to overcome some of the problems that have been identified.[370] Stroke researchers need valid scales that can reliably rate the HRQL outcomes among survivors of stroke. These scales need to be tested in the same way as other scales used to assess patients with stroke.

REFERENCES

1. Kothari R, Hall K, Brott T, Broderick J: Early stroke recognition: Developing an out-of-hospital NIH Stroke Scale, *Acad Emerg Med* 4:986–990, 1997.
2. Brott T, Adams HP Jr, Olinger CP, et al: Measurements of acute cerebral infarction: A clinical examination scale, *Stroke* 20:864–870, 1989.
3. Mahoney FI, Barthel DW: Functional evaluation: The Barthel Index, *Md State Med J* 14:61–65, 1965.
4. Rankin J: Cerebral vascular accidents in patients over the age of 60, *Scott Med J* 2:200–215, 1957.
5. van Swieten JC, Koudstaal PJ, Visser MC, Schouten HJA, van Gijn J: Interobserver agreement for the assessment of handicap in stroke patients, *Stroke* 19:604–607, 1988.
6. Lyden PD, Lau GT: A critical appraisal of stroke evaluation and rating scales, *Stroke* 22:1345–1352, 1991.
7. Boysen G: Stroke scores and scales, *Cerebravasc Dis* 2:239–247, 1992.
8. Hantson L, De Keyser J: Neurological scales in the assessment of cerebral infarction, *Cerebrovasc Dis* 4(Suppl 2):7–14, 1994.
9. D'Olhaberriague L: A reappraisal of reliability and validity studies in stroke, *Stroke* 27:2331–2336, 1996.
10. Feinstein AR, Josephy BR, Wells CK: Scientific and clinical problems in indexes of functional disability, *Ann Intern Med* 18:413–442, 1986.
11. Asplund K: Clinimetrics in stroke research, *Stroke* 18:528–530, 1987.
12. Woo D, Broderick J, Kothari R, et al, and the NINDS tPA Stroke Study Group: Does the National Institutes of Health Stroke Scale favor left hemisphere strokes, *Stroke* 30:2355–2359, 1999.
13. Lyden P, Claesson L, Havstad S, et al: Factor analysis of the National Institutes of Health Stroke Scale in patients with large strokes, *Arch Neurol* 61:1677–1680, 2004.
14. Jennett B, Teasdale G, Braakman R, et al: Prognosis of patients with severe head injury, *Neurosurgery* 4:283–289, 1979.
15. Hunt WE, Hess RM: Surgical risk as related to time of intervention in the repair of intracranial aneurysms, *J Neurosurg* 28:14–20, 1968.
16. Cote R, Hachinski VC, Shurvell BL, et al: The Canadian Neurological Scale: A preliminary study in acute stroke, *Stroke* 17:731–737, 1986.
17. Cote R, Battista RN, Wolfson SK, et al: The Canadian Neurological Scale: Validation and reliability assessment, *Neurology* 39:638, 1989.
18. Gotoh F, Terayama Y, Amano T: Development of a novel, weighted, quantifiable stroke scale, *Stroke* 32:1800–1807, 2001.
19. Gordon DL, Bendixen BH, Adams HP Jr, et al: Interphysician agreement in the diagnosis of subtypes of acute ischemic stroke: Implications for clinical trials. The TOAST Investigators, *Neurology* 43:1021–1027, 1993.
20. Weir CJ, Bradford AP, Lees KR: The prognostic value of the components of the Glasgow Coma Scale following acute stroke, *QJM* 96:67–74, 2003.
21. McNarry AF, Goldhill DR: Simple bedside assessment of level of consciousness: comparison of two simple assessment scales with the Glasgow Coma Scale, *Anaesthesia* 59:34–37, 2004.
22. Mayer SA, Brun N, Broderick J, et al: Safety and feasibility of recombinant factor VIIa for acute intracerebral hemorrhage, *Stroke* 36:74–79, 2005.
23. Mendelow AD, Gregson BA, Fernandes HM, Murray GD: Early surgery versus initial conservative treatment in patients with spontaneous supratentorial intracerebral haematomas in the International Surgical Trial In Intracerebral Haemorrhage (STICH): a randomised trial, *Lancet* 365:387–397, 2005.
24. Nor AM, Davis J, Sen B, et al: The Recognition of Stroke in the Emergency Room (ROSIER) Scale: Development and validation of a stroke recognition instrument, *Lancet Neurol* 4:727–734, 2005.
25. Oshiro EM, Walter KA, Piantadosi S, et al: A new subarachnoid hemorrhage grading system based on the Glasgow Coma Scale: A comparison with the Hunt and Hess and World Federation of Neurological Surgeons Scales in a clinical series, *Neurosurgery* 41:140–147, 1997.
26. Ogungbo B: The World Federation of Neurological Surgeons Scale for Subarachnoid Hemorrhage, *Surg Neurol* 25:236–238, 2003.
27. Tsao JW, Hemphill JC, Johnston SC, et al: Initial Glasgow Coma Scale score predicts outcome following thrombolysis for posterior circulation stroke, *Arch Neurol* 62:1126–1129, 2005.
28. Takagi K, Aoki M, Ishii T, et al: Japan Coma Scale as a grading scale of subarachnoid hemorrhage: A way to determine the scale, *No Shinkei Geka* 26:509–515, 1998.
29. Kidwell CS, Saver JL, Schubert GB, et al: Design and retrospective analysis of the Los Angeles Prehospital Stroke Screen (LAPSS), *Prehosp Emerg Care* 2:267–273, 1998.
30. Kidwell CS, Starkman S, Eckstein M, et al: Identifying stroke in the field. Prospective validation of the Los Angeles Prehospital Stroke Screen (LAPSS), *Stroke* 31:71–76, 2000.
31. Kothari RU, Pancioli A, Liu T, et al: Cincinnati Prehospital Stroke Scale: Reproducibility and validity, *Ann Emerg Med* 33:373–378, 1999.
32. Gordon DL, Issenberg SB, Gordon MS, et al: Stroke training of prehospital providers: An example of simulation-enhanced blended learning and evaluation, *Med Teach* 27:114–121, 2005.
33. Harbison J, Hossain O, Jenkinson D, et al: Diagnostic accuracy of stroke referrals from primary care, emergency room physicians, and ambulance staff using The Face Arm Speech Test, *Stroke* 34:71–76, 2003.
34. Nor AM, McAllister C, Louw SJ, et al: Agreement between ambulance paramedic- and physician-recorded neurological signs with Face Arm Speech Test (FAST) in acute stroke patients, *Stroke* 35:1355–1359, 2004.
35. Saver JL, Kidwell CS, Eckstein M, Starkman S: Prehospital neuroprotective therapy for acute stroke. Results of the field administration of stroke therapy-magnesium (FAST-MAG) pilot trial, *Stroke* 34:e106–e108, 2004.
36. Powers DW: Assessment of the stroke patient using the NIH stroke scale, *Emerg Med Serv* 30:52–56, 2001.
37. Singer OC, Dvorak F, du Mesnil de Rochemont R, et al: A simple 3-item stroke scale. Comparison with the National Institutes of Health Stroke Scale and prediction of middle cerebral artery occlusion, *Stroke* 36:773–776, 2005.
38. Sandercock PA, Allen CM, Corston RN, et al: Clinical diagnosis of intracranial haemorrhage using Guy's Hospital Score, *BMJ* 291:1675–1677, 1985.
39. Weir CJ, Murray GD, Adams FG, et al: Poor accuracy of stroke scoring systems for differential clinical diagnosis of intracranial haemorrhage and infarction, *Lancet* 344:999–1002, 1994.
40. Besson G, Robert C, Hommel M, Perret J: Is it clinically possible to distinguish nonhemorrhagic infarct from hemorrhagic stroke? *Stroke* 26:1205–1209, 1995.
41. Hui AC, Tang SK: Lack of clinical utility of the Siriraj Stroke Score, *Intern Med J* 32:311–314, 2002.
42. Badam P, Paik M, Solao V, Kalantri SP: Poor accuracy of the Siriraj and Guy's Hospital stroke scores in distinguishing haemorrhagic from ischaemic stroke in a rural, tertiary care hospital, *Armed Forces Med J India* 16:8–12, 2003.
43. Soman A, Joshi SR, Tarvade S, Jayaram S: Greek Stroke Score, Siriraj Score and Allen Score in clinical diagnosis of intracerebral hemorrhage and infarct: validation and comparison study, *Indian J Med Sci* 58:417–422, 2004.
44. Connor MD, Modi G, Warlow CP: Accuracy of the Siriraj and Guy's Hospital Stroke Scores in urban South Africans, *Stroke* 38:62–68, 2007.
45. Hawkins GC, Bonita R, Anderson NE: Inadequacy of clinical scoring systems to differentiate stroke subtypes in population-based studies, *Stroke* 26:1338–1342, 1995.
46. Bamford J, Sandercock P, Dennis M, et al: Classification and natural history of clinically identifiable subtypes of cerebral infarction, *Lancet* 337:1521–1526, 1991.
47. Barber M, Roditi G, Stott DJ, Langhorne P: Poor outcome in primary intracerebral haemorrhage: Results of a matched comparison, *Postgrad Med J* 80:89–92, 2004.
48. Lindley RI, Warlow CP, Wardlaw JM, et al: Interobserver reliability of a clinical classification of acute cerebral infarction, *Stroke* 24:1801–1804, 1993.

49. Dewey H, Macdonell R, Donnan G, et al: Inter-rater reliability of stroke sub-type classification by neurologists and nurses within a community-based stroke incidence study, *J Clin Neurosci* 8:14-17, 2001.

50. Pittock SJ, Meldrum D, Hardiman O, et al: The Oxfordshire Community Stroke Project classification: Correlation with imaging, associated complications, and prediction of outcome in acute ischemic stroke, *J Stroke Cerebrovasc Dis* 12:1-7, 2003.

51. Dewey HM, Sturm J, Donnan GA, et al: Incidence and outcome of subtypes of ischaemic stroke: Initial results from the North East Melbourne Stroke Incidence Study (NEMSIS), *Cerebrovasc Dis* 15:133-139, 2003.

52. Dennis MS, Burn JPS, Sandercock PAG, et al: Long-term survival after first-ever stroke: The Oxfordshire Community Stroke Project, *Stroke* 24:796-800, 1993.

53. Wardlaw JM, Dennis MS, Lindley RI, et al: The validity of a simple clinical classification of acute ischaemic stroke, *J Neurol* 243:274-279, 1996.

54. Mead GE, Lewis SC, Wardlaw JM, et al: How well does the Oxfordshire Community Stroke Project classification predict the site and size of the infarct on brain imaging? *J Neurol Neurosurg Psychiatry* 68:558-562, 2000.

55. Smith CJ, Emsley HCA, Libetta CM, et al: The Oxfordshire Community Stroke Project classification in the early hours of ischemic stroke and relation to infarct site and size on cranial computed tomography, *J Stroke Cerebrovasc Dis* 10:205-209, 2001.

56. Lee LJ, Kidwell CS, Alger J, et al: Impact on stroke subtype diagnosis of early diffusion-weighted magnetic resonance imaging and magnetic resonance angiography, *Stroke* 31:1081-1089, 2000.

57. Zhang H, Liu X, Zhang R, Yin Q, Zhu W: Arterial stenosis detected by digital subtraction angiography and its relationship with the Oxford Community Stroke Project classification, *J Int Med Res* 35:113-117, 2007.

58. Thomassen L, Waje-Andreassen U, Naess H, et al: Combined carotid and transcranial ultrasound findings compared with clinical classification and stroke severity in acute ischemic stroke, *Cerebravasc Dis* 21:86-90, 2006.

59. Li H, Wong KS, Kay R: Relationship between the Oxfordshire Community Stroke Project classification and vascular abnormalities in patients with predominantly intracranial atherosclerosis, *J Neurol Sci* 207:65-69, 2003.

60. Markus HS, Khan U, Birns J, et al: Differences in stroke subtypes between black and white patients with stroke: The South London Ethnicity and Stroke Study, *Stroke* 38:2157-2164, 2007.

61. Lyden P, Shuaib A, Ng K, et al: Clomethiazole Acute Stroke Study in Ischemic Stroke (CLASS-I): final results, *Stroke* 33:122-128, 2002.

62. Schulz UGR, Rothwell PM: Differences in vascular risk factors between etiological subtypes of ischemic stroke. Importance of population-based studies, *Stroke* 34:2050-2059, 2003.

63. Edwards DF, Chen Y-W, Diringer MN: Unified Neurological Stroke Scale is valid in ischemic and hemorrhagic stroke, *Stroke* 26:1852-1858, 1995.

64. Hemphill JC, Bonovich DC, Besmertis L, et al: The ICH Score: A simple, reliable grading scale for intracerebral hemorrhage, *Stroke* 32:891-897, 2001.

65. Hemphill JC III, Farrant M, Neill TA Jr.: Prospective validation of the ICH score for 12-month functional outcome, Neurology 73:1088-1094, 2009.

66. Ruiz-Sandoval JL, Chiquete E, Romero-Vargas S, et al: Grading scale for prediction of outcome in primary intracerebral hemorrhages, *Stroke* 38:1641-1644, 2007.

67. Leira R, Dávalos A, Silva Y, et al: Early neurologic deterioration in intracerebral hemorrhage: Predictors and associated factors, *Neurology* 63:461-467, 2004.

68. Castellanos M, Leira R, Tejada J, et al: Predictors of good outcome in medium to large spontaneous supratentorial intracerebral haemorrhages, *J Neurol Neurosurg Psychiatry* 76:691-695, 2005.

69. Cheung RTF, Zou L-Y: Use of the original, modified, or new intracerebral hemorrhage score to predict mortality and morbidity after intracerebral hemorrhage, *Stroke* 34:1717-1722, 2003.

70. Todd MM, Hindman BJ, Clarke WR, Torner JC, Hypothermia Intraoperative: for Aneurysm Surgery Trial (IHAST) Investigators: Mild intraoperative hypothermia during surgery for intracranial aneurysm, *N Engl J Med* 352:135-145, 2005.

71. Weimar C, Benemann J, Diener HC: Development and validation of the Essen Intracerebral Hemorrhage Score, *J Neurol Neurosurg Psychiatry* 77:601-605, 2006.

72. Cedzich C, Roth A: Neurological and psychosocial outcome after subarachnoid hemorrhage, and the Hunt and Hess scale as a predictor of clinical outcome, *Zentralbl Neurochir* 66:112-118, 2005.

73. Bonilha L, Marques EL, Carelli EF, et al: Risk factors and outcome in 100 patients with aneurysmal subarachnoid hemorrhage, *Arq Neuropsiquiatr* 59:676-680, 2001.

74. Soehle M, Chatfield DA, Czosnyka M, Kirkpatrick PJ: Predictive value of initial clinical status, intracranial pressure and transcranial Doppler pulsatility after subarachnoid haemorrhage, *Acta Neurochir (Wien)* 149:575-583, 2007.

75. Ogungbo B: Application of the World Federation of Neurological Surgeons Grading Scale for subarachnoid hemorrhage with GCS 13-14, *Br J Neurosurg* 16:312, 2002.

76. Katati MJ, Santiago-Ramajo S, Perez-Garcia M, et al: Description of quality of life and its predictors in patients with aneurysmal subarachnoid hemorrhage, *Cerebrovasc Dis* 24:66-73, 2007.

77. van Heuven AW, Dorhout Mees SM, Algra A, Rinkel GJE: Validation of a prognostic subarachnoid hemorrhage grading scale derived directly from the Glasgow Coma Scale, *Stroke* 39:1347-1348, 2008.

78. Sano K: Grading and timing of surgery for aneurysmal subarachnoid haemorrhage, *Neurol Res* 16:23-26, 1994.

79. Gnanalingham KK, Apostolopoulos V, Barazi S, O'Neill K: The impact of the International Subarachnoid Aneurysm Trial (ISAT) on the management of aneurysmal subarachnoid haemorrhage in a neurosurgical unit in the UK, *Clin Neurol Neurosurg* 108:117-123, 2006.

80. Chiang VL, Claus EB, Awad IA: Toward more rational prediction of outcome in patients with high-grade subarachnoid hemorrhage, *Neurosurgery* 46:28-35, 2000.

81. Cavanagh SJ, Gordon VL: Grading scales used in the management of aneurysmal subarachnoid hemorrhage: A critical view, *J Neurosci Nurs* 34:288-295, 2002.

82. Nieuwkamp DJ, De Gans K, Algra A, et al: Timing of aneurysm surgery in subarachnoid haemorrhage: An observational study in the Netherlands, *Acta Neurochir (Wien)* 147:815-821, 2005.

83. Rosen DS, Macdonald RL: Grading of subarachnoid hemorrhage: modification of the World Federation of Neurosurgical Societies scale on the basis of data for a large series of patients, *Neurosurgery* 54:566-575, 2004.

84. Mathew NT, Rivera VM, Meyer JS, et al: Double-blind evaluation of glycerol therapy in acute cerebral infarction, *Lancet* 2:1327-1329, 1972.

85. De Haan R, Horn J, Limburg M, et al: A comparison of five stroke scales with measures of disability, handicap, and quality of life, *Stroke* 24:1178-1181, 1993.

86. Orgogozo J-M: A unified form of neurological scoring of hemispheric stroke with motor impairment, *Stroke* 23:1678, 1992.

87. Wright CJ, Swinton LC, Green TL, Hill MD: Predicting final disposition after stroke using the Orpington Prognostic Score, *Can J Neurol Sci* 31:494-498, 2004.

88. Stavem K, Lossius M, Ronning OM: Reliability and validity of the Canadian Neurological Scale in retrospective assessment of initial stroke severity, *Cerebrovasc Dis* 16:286-291, 2003.

89. Goldstein LB, Chilukuri V: Retrospective assessment of initial stroke severity with the Canadian Neurological Scale, *Stroke* 28:1181-1184, 1997.

90. Hagen S, Bugge C, Alexander H: Psychometric properties of the SF-36 in the early post-stroke phase, *J Adv Nurs* 44:461-468, 2003.

91. Castillo J, Martinez F, Leira R, et al: Mortality and morbidity of acute cerebral infarction related to temperature and basal analytic parameters, *Cerebrovasc Dis* 4:66-71, 1994.

92. Muir KW, Weir CJ, Murray GD, et al: Comparison of neurological scales and scoring systems for acute stroke prognosis, *Stroke* 27:1817-1820, 1996.

93. Scandinavian Stroke Study Group: Multicenter trial of hemodilution in ischemic stroke background and study protocol, *Stroke* 16:885-889, 1985.

94. Lindenstrom E, Boysen G, Waage Christiansen L, et al: Reliability of Scandinavian Neurological Stroke Scale, *Cerebrovasc Dis* 1:103-107, 1991.

95. Barber M, Fail M, Shields M, et al: Validity and reliability of estimating the Scandinavian Stroke Scale Score from medical records, *Cerebrovasc Dis* 17:224-227, 2004.

96. Andersen MN, Andersen KK, Kammersgaard LP, Olsen TS: Sex differences in stroke survival: 10-year follow-up of the Copenhagen Stroke Study Cohort, *J Stroke Cerebrovasc Dis* 14:215-220, 2006.

97. Kammersgaard LP, Jorgensen HS, Reith J, et al: Early infection and prognosis after acute stroke: The Copenhagen Stroke Study, *J Stroke Cerebrovasc Dis* 10:217-221, 2001.

98. Wahlgren NG, Bornhov S, Sharma A, et al, for the CLASS study group: The Clomethiazole Acute Stroke Study (CLASS): Efficacy results in 545 patients classified as total anterior circulation syndrome (TACS), *Cerebrovasc Dis* 8:231-239, 1999.

99. Sprigg N, Gray LJ, Bath PMW, et al: Early recovery and functional outcome are related with causal stroke subtype: Data from the Tinzaparin in Acute Ischemic Stroke Trial, *J Stroke Cerebrovasc Dis* 16:180-184, 2007.

100. Sprigg N, Gray LJ, Bath PM, et al: Investigators Stroke: Severity, early recovery and outcome are each related with clinical classification of stroke: Data from the 'Tinzaparin in Acute Ischaemic Stroke Trial' (TAIST), *J Neurol Sci* 254:54-59, 2007.

101. Williams GR, Jiang JG: Development of an ischemic stroke survival score, *Stroke* 31:2414-2420, 2000.

102. Stavem K, Ronning OM: Quality of life 6 months after acute stroke: impact of initial treatment in a stroke unit and general medical wards, *Cerebrovasc Dis* 23:417-423, 2007.

103. Roden-Jullig A, Britton M: Effectiveness of heparin treatment for progressing ischaemic stroke: before and after study, *J Intern Med* 248:287-291, 2001.

104. Steiner T, Bluhmki E, Kaste M, et al: The ECASS 3-hour cohort, *Cerebrovasc Dis* 8:198-203, 1998.

105. Christensen H, Boysen G, Truelsen T: The Scandinavian Stroke Scale predicts outcome in patients with mild ischemic stroke, *Cerebrovasc Dis* 20:46-48, 2005.

106. Davalos A, Toni D, Iweins F, et al: Neurological deterioration in acute ischemic stroke: Potential predictors and associated factors in the European Cooperative Acute Stroke Study (ECASS), *Stroke* 30:2631-2636, 1999.

107. Rohl L, Geday J, Ostergaard L, et al: Correlation between diffusion- and perfusion-weighted MRI and neurological deficit measured by the Scandinavian Stroke Scale and Barthel Index in hyperacute subcortical stroke (< or = 6 hours), *Cerebravasc Dis* 12:203-213, 2001.

108. Thommessen B, Thoresen GE, Bautz-Holter E, Laake K: Validity of the aphasia item from the Scandinavian Stroke Scale, *Cerebrovasc Dis* 13:184-186, 2002.

109. Ali K, Cheek E, Sills S, et al: Development of a conversion factor to facilitate comparison of National Institute of Health Stroke Scale scores with Scandinavian Stroke Scale scores, *Cerebrovasc Dis* 24:509-515, 2007.

110. Brott T, Marler JR, Olinger CP, et al: Measurements of acute cerebral infarction: lesion size by computed tomography, *Stroke* 20:871-875, 1989.

111. Goldstein LB, Bertels C, Davis JN: Interrater reliability of the NIH stroke scale, *Arch Neurol* 46:660-662, 1989.

112. Bushnell CD, Johnston DCC, Goldstein LB: Retrospective assessment of initial stroke severity: comparison of the NIH Stroke Scale and the Canadian Neurological Scale, *Stroke* 32:656-660, 2001.

113. de Caneda MA, Fernandes JG, de Almeida AG, Mugnol FE: Reliability of neurological assessment scales in patients with stroke, *Arq Neuropsiquiatr* 64:690-697, 2006.

114. Goldstein L, Samsa G: Reliability of the National Institutes of Health Stroke Scale, *Stroke* 28:307, 1997.

115. Andre C: The NIH stroke scale is unreliable in untrained hands, *J Stroke Cerebrovasc Dis* 11:43-46, 2002.

116. Schmulling S, Grond M, Rudolf J, Kiencke P: Training as a prerequisite for reliable use of NIH Stroke Scale, *Stroke* 29:1258-1259, 1998.

117. Williams LS, Yilmaz EY, Lopez-Yunez AM: Retrospective assessment of initial stroke severity with the NIH Stroke Scale, *Stroke* 31:858-862, 2000.

118. Montaner J, Alvarez-Sabin J: NIH stroke scale and its adaptation to Spanish, *Neurologia* 21:192-202, 2007.

119. Dominguez RO: Adapted and validated Spanish version of National Institutes of Health Stroke Scale, *Rev Neurol* 43:191-192, 2006.

120. Dominguez R, Vila JF, Augustovski F, et al: Spanish cross-cultural adaptation and validation of the National Institutes of Health Stroke Scale, *Mayo Clin Proc* 81:476-480, 2006.

121. Albanese MA, Clarke WR, Adams HP Jr, Woolson RF: Ensuring reliability of outcome measures in multicenter clinical trials of treatments for acute ischemic stroke. The program developed for the Trial of Org 10172 in Acute Stroke Treatment (TOAST), *Stroke* 25:1746-1751, 1994.

122. Lyden P, Brott T, Tilley B, et al: Improved reliability of the NIH stroke scale using video training, *Stroke* 25:2220, 1994.

123. Lyden P, Raman R, Liu L, et al: NIHSS training and certification using a new digital video disk is reliable, *Stroke* 36:2446-2449, 2005.

124. Josephson SA, Hills NK, Johnston SC: NIH stroke scale reliability in ratings from a large sample of clinicians, *Cerebravasc Dis* 22:389-395, 2006.

125. Lyden P, Lu M, Jackson C, et al: Underlying structure of the National Institutes of Health Stroke Scale: results of factor analysis, *Stroke* 30:2347, 1999.

126. Lyden PD, Lu M, Levine S, et al: A modified National Institutes of Health Stroke Scale for use in stroke clinical trials. Preliminary reliability and validity, *Stroke* 32:1310-1317, 2001.

127. Millis SR, Straube D, Iramaneerat C, et al: Measurement properties of the National Institutes of Health Stroke Scale for people with right- and left-hemisphere lesions: further analysis of the Clomethiazole for Acute Stroke Study-Ischemic (Class-I) Trial, *Arch Phys Med Rehabil* 88:302-308, 2007.

128. Fink JN, Selim MH, Kumar S, et al: Is the association of National Institutes of Health Stroke Scale scores and acute magnetic resonance imaging stroke volume equal for patients with right- and left-hemisphere ischemic stroke? *Stroke* 33:954-958, 2002.

129. Linfante I, Llinas RH, Schlaug G, et al: Diffusion-weighted imaging and National Institutes of Health Stroke Scale in the acute phase of posterior-circulation stroke, *Arch Neurol* 58:621-628, 2001.

130. Dewey HM, Donnan GA, Freeman EJ, et al: Interrater reliability of the National Institutes of Health Stroke Scale: rating by neurologists and nurses in a community-based stroke incidence study, *Cerebrovasc Dis* 9:323-327, 1999.

131. Meyer BC, Hemmen TM, Jackson C, Lyden PD: Modified National Institutes of Health Stroke Scale for the use in stroke clinical trials, *Stroke* 33:1261-1266, 2002.

132. Adams HP Jr, Davis PH, Leira EC, et al: Baseline NIH Stroke Scale score strongly predicts outcome after stroke, *Neurology* 53:126-131, 1999.

133. Schlegel D, Kolb SJ, Luciano JM, et al: Utility of the NIH Stroke Scale as a predictor of hospital disposition, *Stroke* 34:134-137, 2003.

134. Schlegel DJ, Tanne D, Demchuk AM, et al: Prediction of hospital disposition after thrombolysis for acute ischemic stroke using the National Institutes of Health Stroke Scale, *Arch Neurol* 61:1061-1064, 2004.

135. Kasner SE: Clinical interpretation and use of stroke scales, *Lancet Neurol* 5:603-612, 2006.

136. Appelros P, Terént A: Characteristics of the National Institutes of Health Stroke Scale: Results from a population-based stroke cohort at baseline and after one year, *Cerebrovasc Dis* 17:21-27, 2004.

137. Odderson IR: The National Institutes of Health Stroke Scale and its importance in acute stroke management, *Phys Med Rehabil Clin N Am* 10:787-800, 1999.

138. Jeng JS, Huang SJ, Tang SC, Yip PK: Predictors of survival and functional outcome in acute stroke patients admitted to the stroke intensive care unit, *J Neurol Sci* 270:60-66, 2008.

139. Glymour MM, Berkman LF, Ertel KA, et al: Lesion characteristics, NIH Stroke Scale, and functional recovery after stroke, *Am J Phys Med Rehabil* 86:725-733, 2007.

140. Arnold M, Nedeltchev K, Schroth G, et al: Clinical and radiological predictors of recanalisation and outcome of 40 patients with acute basilar artery occlusion treated with intra-arterial thrombolysis, *J Neurol Neurosurg Psychiatry* 75:857-862, 2004.

141. Tei H, Uchiyama S, Usui T: Clinical-diffusion mismatch defined by NIHSS and ASPECTS in non-lacunar anterior circulation infarction, *J Neurol* 254:340-346, 2007.

142. Davalos A, Blanco M, Pedraza S, et al: The clinical-DWI mismatch. A new diagnostic approach to the brain tissue at risk of infarction, *Neurology* 62:2187-2192, 2004.

143. Messe SR, Kasner SE, Chalela JA, et al: CT-NIHSS mismatch does not correlate with MRI diffusion-perfusion mismatch, *Stroke* 38:2079-2084, 2007.

144. Choi JY, Pary JK, Alexandrov AV, et al: Does clinical-CT 'mismatch' predict early response to treatment with recombinant tissue plasminogen activator? *Cerebravasc Dis* 22:384-388, 2006.

145. The National Institute of Neurological Disorders and Stroke rt-PA Stroke Study Group: Tissue plasminogen activator for acute ischemic stroke, *N Engl J Med* 333:1581-1587, 1995.

146. The NINDS t-PA Stroke Study Group: Generalized efficacy of t-PA for acute stroke. Subgroup analysis of the NINDS t-PA Stroke Trial, *Stroke* 28:2119-2125, 1997.

147. The NINDS t-PA Stroke Study Group: Intracerebral hemorrhage after intravenous t-PA therapy for ischemic stroke, *Stroke* 28:2109-2118, 1997.

148. The Publications Committee for the Trial of ORG 10172 in Acute Stroke Treatment (TOAST) Investigators: Low molecular weight heparinoid, ORG 10172 (danaparoid), and outcome after acute ischemic stroke: A randomized controlled trial, *JAMA* 279:1265-1272, 1998.

149. Derex L, Hermier M, Adeleine P, et al: Clinical and imaging predictors of intracerebral haemorrhage in stroke patients treated with intravenous tissue plasminogen activator, *J Neurol Neurosurg Psychiatry* 76:70-75, 2005.

150. Bruno A, Saha C, Williams LS: Using change in the National Institutes of Health Stroke Scale to measure treatment effect in acute stroke trials, *Stroke* 37:920-921, 2006.

151. Wityk RJ, Pessin MS, Kaplan RF, Caplan LR: Serial assessment of acute stroke using the NIH Stroke Scale, *Stroke* 25:362-365, 1994.

152. Kasner SE, Chimowitz MI, Lynn MJ, et al: Predictors of ischemic stroke in the territory of a symptomatic intracranial arterial stenosis, *Circulation* 113:555-563, 2006.

153. Mikulik R, Ribo M, Hill MD, et al: Accuracy of serial National Institutes of Health Stroke Scale scores to identify artery status in acute ischemic stroke, *Circulation* 115:2660-2665, 2007.

154. Grotta JC, Welch KM, Fagan SC, et al: Clinical deterioration following improvement in the NINDS rt-PA Stroke Trial, *Stroke* 32:661-668, 2001.

155. Adams HPJ, Effron MB, Torner J, et al: Emergency administration of abciximab for treatment of patients with acute ischemic stroke: results of an international phase III trial: Abciximab in Emergency Treatment of Stroke Trial (AbESTT-II), *Stroke* 39:87-99, 2008.

156. Young FB, Lees KR, Weir CJ, et al: Improving trial power through use of prognosis-adjusted end points, *Stroke* 36:597-601, 2005.

157. Abciximab Emergent Stroke Treatment Trial (AbESTT) Investigators: Emergency administration of abciximab for treatment of patients with acute ischemic stroke. Results of a randomized phase 2 trial, *Stroke* 36:880-890, 2005.

158. The Abciximab in Ischemic Stroke Investigators: Abciximab in acute ischemic stroke: A randomized, double-blind, placebo-controlled, dose-escalation study, *Stroke* 31:601-609, 2000.

159. Lees KR, Zivin JA, Ashwood T, et al: NXY-059 for acute ischemic stroke, *N Engl J Med* 354:588-600, 2006.

160. Shuaib A, Lees KR, Lyden P, et al: NXY-059 for the treatment of acute ischemic stroke, *N Engl J Med* 357:562-571, 2007.

161. Ginsberg MD, Hill MD, Palesch YY, et al: The ALIAS Pilot Trial: A dose-escalation and safety study of albumin therapy for acute ischemic stroke—I: Physiological responses and safety results, *Stroke* 37:2100-2106, 2006.

162. Ginsberg MD, Palesch YY, Hill MD: The ALIAS (Albumin In Acute Stroke) phase III randomized multicentre clinical trial: design and progress report, *Biochem Soc Trans* 34:1323-1326, 2006.

163. Palesch YY, Hill MD, Ryckborst KJ, et al: The ALIAS Pilot Trial: A dose-escalation and safety study of albumin therapy for acute ischemic stroke. II: Neurologic outcome and efficacy analysis, *Stroke* 37:2107-2114, 2006.

164. Furlan AJ, Eyding D, Albers GW, et al: Dose Escalation of Desmoteplase for Acute Ischemic Stroke (DEDAS): Evidence of safety and efficacy 3 to 9 hours after stroke onset, *Stroke* 37:1227-1231, 2006.

165. Weimar C, Ho TW, Katsarava Z, et al: Improving patient selection for clinical acute stroke trials, *Cerebrovasc Dis* 21:386-392, 2006.

166. Palesch YY, Tilley BC, Sackett DL, et al: Applying a phase II futility study design to therapeutic stroke trials, *Stroke* 36:2410-2414, 2005.

167. Hill MD, Moy CS, Palesch YY, et al: The Albumin In Acute Stroke Trial (ALIAS); design and methodology, *Int J Stroke* 2:214-219, 2007.

168. The IMS Study Investigators: Combined intravenous and intra-arterial recanalization for acute ischemic stroke: The International Management of Stroke Study, *Stroke* 35:904-912, 2004.

169. DeGraba TJ, Hallenbeck JM, Pettigrew KD, et al: Progression in acute stroke: value of the initial NIH stroke scale score on patient stratification in future trials, *Stroke* 30:1208-1212, 1999.

170. Savitz SI, Lew R, Bluhmki E, et al: Shift analysis versus dichotomization of the Modified Rankin Scale outcome scores in the NINDS and ECASS-II trials, *Stroke* 38:3205-3212, 2007.

171. Sacco RL, DeRosa JT, Haley EC Jr, et al: Glycine antagonist in neuroprotection for patients with acute stroke: GAIN Americas: A randomized controlled trial, *JAMA* 285:1719-1728, 2001.

172. Adams HP Jr, Leclerc JR, Bluhmki E, et al: Measuring outcomes as a function of baseline severity of ischemic stroke, *Cerebrovasc Dis* 18:124-129, 2004.

173. Saver JL, Yafeh B: Confirmation of tPA treatment effect by baseline severity-adjusted end point reanalysis of the NINDS-tPA Stroke Trials, *Stroke* 38:414-416, 2007.

174. Meschia JF, Case LD, Worrall BB, et al: Family history of stroke and severity of neurologic deficit after stroke, *Neurology* 67:1396-1402, 2006.

175. Kimura K, Kazui S, Minematsu K, Yamaguchi T: Analysis of 16,922 patients with acute ischemic stroke and transient ischemic attack in Japan. A hospital-based prospective registration study, *Cerebrovasc Dis* 18:47-56, 2004.

176. Bokura H, Kobayashi S, Yamaguchi S, et al: Clinical characteristics and prognosis in stroke patients with diabetes mellitus: Retrospective evaluation using the Japanese Standard Stroke Registry database (JSSRS), *No To Shinkei* 58:135-139, 2006.

177. Adams HP Jr, Brott TG, Furlan AJ, et al: Guidelines for thrombolytic therapy for acute stroke: A supplement to the guidelines for the management of patients with acute ischemic stroke, *Stroke* 27:1711-1718, 1996.

178. Adams HP, Adams RJ, Brott T, et al: Guidelines for the early management of patients with ischemic stroke. A scientific statement from the stroke council of the American Stroke Association, *Stroke* 34:1056-1083, 2003.

179. Adams HP Jr, Adams R, del Zoppo G, Goldstein LB: Guidelines for the early management of patients with ischemic stroke. 2005 Guidelines update. A scientific statement from the Stroke Council of American Heart Association/American Stroke Association, *Stroke* 36:916-921, 2005.

180. Adams HP Jr, del Zoppo G, Alberts MJ, et al: Guidelines for the early management of adults with ischemic stroke: a guideline from the American Heart Association/American Stroke Association Stroke Council, Clinical Cardiology Council, Cardiovascular Radiology and Intervention Council, and the Atherosclerotic Peripheral Vascular Disease and Quality of Care Outcomes in Research Interdisciplinary Working Groups: The American Academy of Neurology affirms the value of this guideline as an educational tool for neurologists, *Stroke* 38:1655-1711, 2007.

181. Gur AY, Lampl Y, Gross B, et al: A new scale for assessing patients with vertebrobasilar stroke—the Israeli Vertebrobasilar Stroke Scale (IVBSS): Inter-rater reliability and concurrent validity, *Clin Neurol Neurosurg* 109:317-322, 2007.

182. Adams HP Jr, Bendixen BH, Kappelle LJ, et al: Classification of subtype of acute ischemic stroke. Definitions for use in a multicenter clinical trial. TOAST. Trial of Org 10172 in Acute Stroke Treatment, *Stroke* 24:35-41, 1993.

183. Pinto A, Tuttolomondo A, Di Raimondo D, et al: Cerebrovascular risk factors and clinical classification of strokes, *Semin Vasc Med* 4:287-303, 2004.

184. Pinto A, Tuttolomondo A, Di Raimondo D, et al: Risk factors profile and clinical outcome of ischemic stroke patients admitted in a Department of Internal Medicine and classified by TOAST classification, *Int Angiol* 25:261-267, 2006.

185. Nedeltchev K, der Maur TA, Georgiadis D, Arnold M: Ischaemic stroke in young adults: Predictors of outcome and recurrence, *J Neurol Neurosurg Psychiatry* 76:191-195, 2005.

186. Paradowski B, Maciejak A: TOAST classification of subtypes of ischaemic stroke: Diagnostic and therapeutic procedures in stroke, *Cerebravasc Dis* 20:319-324, 2005.

187. Ghandehari K, Izadi Z: The Khorasan Stroke Registry: Results of a five-year hospital-based study, *Cerebrovasc Dis* 23:132-139, 2007.

188. Ghandehari K, Moud ZI: Incidence and etiology of ischemic stroke in Persian young adults, *Acta Neurol Scand* 113:121-124, 2006.

189. Liu X, Xu G, Wu W, et al: Subtypes and one-year survival of first-ever stroke in Chinese patients: The Nanjing Stroke Registry, *Cerebrovasc Dis* 22:130-136, 2006.

190. Tuttolomondo A, Pinto A, Di Raimondo D, et al: Decreasing incidence of lacunar vs other types of cerebral infarction in a Japanese population, *Neurology* 68:311a-312a, 2007.

191. Alzamora MT, Sorribes M, Heras A, et al: Ischemic stroke incidence in Santa Coloma de Gramenet (ISISCOG), Spain. A community-based study, *BMC Neurol* 8:5, 2008.

192. Zhou H, Wang YJ, Wang SX, Zhao XQ: TOAST subtyping of acute ischemic stroke, *Zhonghua Nei Ke Za Zhi* 43:495-498, 2004.

193. Kolominsky-Rabas PL, Weber M, Gefeller O, et al: Epidemiology of ischemic stroke subtypes according to TOAST criteria: Incidence, recurrence, and long-term survival in ischemic stroke subtypes: A population-based study, *Stroke* 32:2735-2740, 2001.

194. Lee BI, Nam HS, Heo JH, et al: Team Yonsei Stroke Registry. Analysis of 1,000 patients with acute cerebral infarctions, *Cerebravasc Dis* 12:145-151, 2001.

195. Saposnik G, Gonzalez L, Lepidi S, et al: Southern Buenos Aires Stroke Project, *Acta Neurol Scand* 104:130-135, 2001.

196. Saposnik G, Caplan LR, Gonzalez LA, et al: Differences in stroke subtypes among natives and Caucasians in Boston and Buenos Aires, *Stroke* 31:2385-2389, 2000.

197. Telman G, Kouperberg E, Sprecher E, et al: Distribution of etiologies in patients above and below age 45 with first-ever ischemic stroke, *Acta Neurol Scand* 117:311-316, 2008.

198. Meschia JF, Barrett KM, Chukweudelunzu F, et al: Interobserver agreement in the TOAST classification of stroke based on retrospective medical record review, *J Stroke Cerebrovasc Dis* 15:266-272, 2006.

199. Hoffmann M: Stroke in the young: The multiethnic prospective Durban Stroke Data Bank results, *J Stroke Cerebrovasc Dis* 7:404-413, 1998.

200. Han SW, Nam HS, Kim SH, et al: Frequency and significance of cardiac sources of embolism in the TOAST classification, *Cerebravasc Dis* 24:463-468, 2007.

201. Ortiz G, Koch S, Romano JG, et al: Mechanisms of ischemic stroke in HIV-infected patients, *Neurology* 68:1257-1261, 2007.

202. Wiklund PG, Brown WM, Brott TG, et al: Lack of aggregation of ischemic stroke subtypes within affected sibling pairs, *Neurology* 68:427-431, 2007.

203. Wessels T, Wessels C, Ellsiepen A, et al: Contribution of diffusion-weighted imaging in determination of stroke etiology, *AJNR Am J Neuroradiol* 27:35-39, 2006.

204. Kristensen B, Malm J, Carlberg B, et al: Epidemiology and etiology of ischemic stroke in young adults aged 18 to 44 years in northern Sweden, *Stroke* 28:1702-1709, 1997.

205. Lovett JK, Coull AJ, Rothwell PM: Early risk of recurrence by subtype of ischemic stroke in population-based incidence studies, *Neurology* 62:569-573, 2004.

206. Ay H, Furie KL, Singhal A, et al: An evidence-based causative classification system for acute ischemic stroke, *Ann Neurol* 58:688-697, 2005.

207. Ay H, Benner T, Murat Arsava E, et al: A computerized algorithm for etiologic classification of ischemic stroke: The causative classification of stroke system, *Stroke* 38:2979-2984, 2007.

208. Zhou H, Wang YJ: The reliability of ischemic stroke subtype classification using the TOAST criteria, *Zhonghua Nei Ke Za Zhi* 44:825-827, 2005.

209. Goldstein LB, Jones MR, Matchar DB, et al: Improving the reliability of stroke subgroup classification using the Trial of ORG 10172 in Acute Stroke Treatment (TOAST) criteria, *Stroke* 32:1091-1098, 2001.

210. Fure B, Wyller TB, Thommessen B: TOAST criteria applied in acute ischemic stroke, *Acta Neurol Scand* 112:254-258, 2005.

211. Madden KP, Karanjia PN, Adams HP Jr, Clarke WR: Accuracy of initial stroke subtype diagnosis in the TOAST study. Trial of ORG 10172 in Acute Stroke Treatment, *Neurology* 45:1975-1979, 1995.

212. Rovira A, Grive E, Alvarez-Sabín J: Distribution territories and causative mechanisms of ischemic stroke, *Eur Radiol* 15:416-426, 2007.

213. Han SW, Kim SH, Lee JY, et al: A new subtype classification of ischemic stroke based on treatment and etiologic mechanism, *Eur Neurol* 57:96-102, 2007.

214. Hoffmann M, Chichkova R, Ziyad M, Malek A: Too much lumping in ischemic stroke—a new classification, *Med Sci Monit* 10:CR285-CR287, 2007.

215. Landau WM, Nassief A: Editorial comment—time to burn the TOAST, *Stroke* 36:902-904, 2005.

216. Wraige E, Pohl KRE, Ganesan V: A proposed classification for subtypes of arterial ischaemic stroke in children, *Dev Med Child Neurol* 47:252-256, 2005.

217. Yavuzer G, Selles R, Sezer N, et al: Mirror therapy improves hand function in subacute stroke: A randomized controlled trial, *Arch Phys Med Rehabil* 89:393-398, 2008.

218. Pizzi A, Carlucci G, Falsini C, et al: Gait in hemiplegia: Evaluation of clinical features with the Wisconsin Gait Scale, *J Rehabil Med* 39:170-174, 2007.

219. Caty GD, Arnould C, Stoquart GG, et al: ABILOCO: A Rasch-built 13-item questionnaire to assess locomotion ability in stroke patients, *Arch Phys Med Rehabil* 89:284-290, 2008.

220. Jonsdottir J, Cattaneo D: Reliability and validity of the dynamic gait index in persons with chronic stroke, *Arch Phys Med Rehabil* 88:1410-1415, 2007.

221. Verheyden G, Nieuwboer A, Van de Winckel A, De Weerdt W: Clinical tools to measure trunk performance after stroke: A systematic review of the literature, *Clin Rehabil* 21:387-394, 2007.

222. Shaughnessy M, Resnick BM, Macko RF: Reliability and validity testing of the short self-efficacy and outcome expectation for exercise scales in stroke survivors, *J Stroke Cerebrovasc Dis* 13:214-219, 2004.

223. Yabe I, Matsushima M, Soma H, et al: Usefulness of the Scale for Assessment and Rating of Ataxia (SARA), *J Neurol Sci* 266:164-166, 2008.

224. Blum L, Korner-Bitensky N: Usefulness of the Berg Balance Scale in stroke rehabilitation: A systematic review, *Phys Ther* 88:559-566, 2008.

225. Ng MF, Tong RK, Li LS: A pilot study of randomized clinical controlled trial of gait training in subacute stroke patients with partial body-weight support electromechanical gait trainer and functional electrical stimulation: six-month follow-up, *Stroke* 39:154-160, 2008.

226. Chou CY, Chien CW, Hsueh IP, et al: Developing a short form of the Berg Balance Scale for people with stroke, *Phys Ther* 86:195-204, 2006.

227. Wilz G: Predictors of subjective impairment after stroke: Influence of depression, gender and severity of stroke, *Brain Inj* 21:39-45, 2007.

228. Salter K, Jutai JW, Teasell R, et al: Issues for selection of outcome measures in stroke rehabilitation: ICF activity, *Disabil Rehabil* 27:315-340, 2005.

229. Katz S, Ford AB, Moskowitz RW, et al: The index of ADL: A standardized measure of biological and psychosocial function, *JAMA* 185:914, 1963.

230. Granger CV, Dewis LS, Peters NC, et al: Stroke rehabilitation: Analysis of repeated Barthel Index measures, *Arch Phys Med Rehabil* 60:14, 1979.

231. Granger CV, Hamilton BB, Linacre JM, et al: Performance profiles of the Functional Independence Measure, *Am J Phys Med Rehabil* 72:84-89, 1993.

232. Wade DT, Collin C: The Barthel ADL Index: A standard measure of physical disability? *Int Disabil Stud* 10:64, 1988.

233. Wade DT, Hewer RL: Functional abilities after stroke: Measurement, natural history and prognosis, *J Neurol Neurosurg Psychiatry* 50:177-182, 1987.

234. Granger CV, Hamilton BB, Gresham GE, Kramer AA: The stroke rehabilitation outcome study: Part II. Relative merits of the total Barthel Index score and a four-item subscore in predicting patient outcomes, *Arch Phys Med Rehabil* 70:100, 1989.

235. Gresham GE, Duncan PW, Stason WB, et al: *Post-Stroke Rehabilitation*, Rockville, MD, 1995, U.S. Department of Health and Human Services.

236. Sulter G, Steen C, De Keyser J: Use of the Barthel Index and Modified Rankin Scale in acute stroke trials, *Stroke* 30:1538-1541, 1999.

237. Appelros P, Viitanen M: What causes increased stroke mortality in patients with prestroke dementia? *Cerebravasc Dis* 19:323-327, 2005.

238. van Wijk I, Lindeman E, Kappelle LJ, et al: Functional status and use of healthcare facilities in long-term survivors of TIA or minor ischaemic stroke, *J Neurol Neurosurg Psychiatry* 77:1238-1243, 2006.

239. Ferrucci L, Bandinelli S, Guralnik JM, et al: Recovery of functional status after stroke. A postrehabilitation follow-up study, *Stroke* 24:200-205, 1993.

240. de Jong LD, Nieuwboer A, Aufdemkampe G: The hemiplegic arm: Interrater reliability and concurrent validity of passive range of motion measurements, *Disabil Rehabil* 29:1442-1448, 2007.

241. Duncan P, Richards L, Wallace D, et al: A randomized, controlled pilot study of a home-based exercise program for individuals with mild and moderate stroke, *Stroke* 29:2055-2060, 1998.

242. Duncan PW, Lai SM, Keighley J: Defining post-stroke recovery: Implications for design and interpretation of drug trials, *Neuropharmacology* 39:835-841, 2000.

243. Duncan PW, Bode RK, Min Lai S, Perera S, Glycine Antagonist in Neuroprotection Americans Investigators: Rasch analysis of a new stroke-specific outcome scale: the Stroke Impact Scale, *Arch Phys Med Rehabil* 84:950-963, 2003.

244. de Oliveira R, Cacho EW, Borges G: Post-stroke motor and functional evaluations: A clinical correlation using Fugl-Meyer assessment scale, Berg balance scale and Barthel Index, *Arq Neuropsiquiatr* 64:731-735, 2006.

245. Santos M, Zahner LH, McKiernan BJ, et al: Neuromuscular electrical stimulation improves severe hand dysfunction for individuals with chronic stroke: A pilot study, *J Neurol Phys Ther* 30:175-183, 2006.

246. Appelros P: Characteristics of the Frenchay Activities Index one year after a stroke: A population-based study, *Disabil Rehabil* 29:785-790, 2007.

247. Ones K, Yilmaz E, Cetinkaya B, Caglar N: Quality of life for patients poststroke and the factors affecting it, *J Stroke Cerebrovasc Dis* 14:261-266, 2005.

248. Grace J, Nadler JD, White DA, et al: Folstein vs Modified Mini-Mental State Examination in geriatric stroke. Stability, validity, and screening utility, *Arch Neurol* 52:477-484, 1995.

249. Hsieh YW, Hsueh IP, Chou YT, et al: Development and validation of a short form of the Fugl-Meyer Motor Scale in patients with stroke, *Stroke* 38:3052-3054, 2007.

250. Rabadi MH, Rabadi FM: Comparison of the Action Research Arm Test and the Fugl-Meyer Assessment as measures of upper-extremity motor weakness after stroke, *Arch Phys Med Rehabil* 87:962-966, 2006.

251. Nagayoshi M, Takahashi M, Saeki S, Hachisuka K: Disability and lifestyle of subacute myelo-optico-neuropathy and stroke patients and elderly persons living at home: A comparison of the Barthel Index Score and the Frenchay Activities Index Score, *J Univ Occup Environ Health* 29:407-415, 2007.

252. Gabbe BJ, Sutherland AM, Wolfe R, et al: Can the Modified Functional Independence measure be reliably obtained from the patient medical record by different raters? *J Trauma* 63:1374-1379, 2007.

253. Linacre JM, Heinemann AW, Wright BD, et al: The structure and stability of the Functional Independence Measure, *Arch Phys Med Rehabil* 75:127-132, 1994.

254. Keith RA, Granger CV, Hamilton BB, Sherwin FS: The Functional Independence Measure: A new tool for rehabilitation, *Adv Clin Rehabil* 1:6-18, 1987.

255. Ring H, Feder M, Schwartz J, Samuels G: Functional measures of first-stroke rehabilitation inpatients: Usefulness of the Functional Independence Measure total score with a clinical rationale, *Arch Phys Med Rehabil* 78:630-635, 1997.

256. Ewert T, Stucki G: Validity of the SS-QOL in Germany and in survivors of hemorrhagic or ischemic stroke, *Neurorehabil Neural Repair* 21:161-168, 2007.

257. Sonoda S, Saitoh E, Nagai S, et al: Stroke outcome prediction using reciprocal number of initial Activities of Daily Living status, *J Stroke Cerebrovasc Dis* 14:8-11, 2005.

258. Patel AB, Kostis JB, Wilson AC, et al: Long-term fatal outcomes in subjects with stroke or transient ischemic attack: Fourteen-year follow-up of the systolic hypertension in the elderly program, *Stroke* 39:1084-1089, 2008.

259. Stineman MG, Shea JA, Jette A, et al: The Functional Independence Measure: tests of scaling assumptions, structure, and reliability across 20 diverse impairment categories, *Arch Phys Med Rehabil* 77:1101-1108, 1996.

260. Mauthe RW, Haaf DC, Hayn P, Krall JM: Predicting discharge destination of stroke patients using a mathematical model based on six items from the functional independence measure, *Arch Phys Med Rehabil* 77:10-13, 1996.

261. Heinemann AW, Linacre JM, Wright BD, et al: Prediction of rehabilitation outcomes with disability measures, *Arch Phys Med Rehabil* 75:133-143, 1994.

262. Dombovy ML, Sandok BA, Basford JR: Rehabilitation for stroke: A review, *Stroke* 17:363-369, 1986.

263. Cook L, Smith DS, Truman G: Using functional independence measure profiles as an index of outcome in the rehabilitation of brain-injured patients, *Arch Phys Med Rehabil* 75:390-393, 1994.

264. Heinemann AW, Roth EJ, Cichowski K, Betts HB: Multivariate analysis of improvement and outcome following stroke rehabilitation, *Arch Neurol* 44:1167-1172, 1987.

265. Ottenbacher KJ, Mann WC, Granger CV, et al: Inter-rater agreement and stability of functional assessment in the community-based elderly, *Arch Phys Med Rehabil* 75:1297-1301, 1994.

266. Ottenbacher KJ, Hsu Y, Granger CV, Fiedler RC: The reliability of the functional independence measure: A quantitative review, *Arch Phys Med Rehabil* 77:1226-1232, 1996.

267. Kidd D, Stewart G, Baldry J, et al: The Functional Indepedence Measure: A comparative validity and reliability study, *Disabil Rehabil* 17:10-14, 1995.

268. Hamilton BB, Laughlin JA, Fiedler RC, Granger CV: Interrater reliability of the 7-level Functional Independence Measure (FIM), *Scand J Rehabil Med* 26:115-119, 1994.

269. Segal ME, Ditunno JF, Staas WE: Interinstitutional agreement of individual Functional Independence Measure (FIM) items measured at two sites on one sample of SCI patients, *Paraplegia* 31:622-631, 1993.

270. Cavanagh SJ, Hogan K, Gordon V, Fairfax J: Stroke-specific FIM models in an urban population, *J Neurosci Nurs* 32:17-21, 2000.

271. van der Putten JJ, Hobart JC, Freeman JA, Thompson AJ: Measuring change in disability after inpatient rehabilitation: Comparison of the responsiveness of the Barthel Index and the Functional Independence Measure, *J Neurol Neurosurg Psychiatry* 66:480-484, 1999.

272. Nyein K, McMichael L, Turner-Stokes L: Can a Barthel score be derived from FIM? *Clin Rehabil* 13:56-63, 1999.

273. Kidd D, Stout RW: The assessment of acute stroke in general medical wards, *Disabil Rehabil* 18:205-208, 1996.

274. McPherson KM, Pentland B, Cudmore SF, Prescott RJ: An interrater reliability study of the functional assessment measure (FIM+FAM), *Disabil Rehabil* 18:341-347, 1996.

275. Olsen TS: Arm and leg paresis as outcome predictors in stroke rehabilitation, *Stroke* 21:247-251, 1990.

276. Dods TA, Martin DP, Stolov WC, Deyo RA: A validation of the functional independence measurement and its performance among rehabilitation inpatients, *Arch Phys Med Rehabil* 74:531-536, 1993.

277. Hsueh IP, Lin JH, Jeng JS, Hsieh CL: Comparison of the psychometric characteristics of the functional independence measure, 5 item Barthel Index, and 10 item Barthel Index in patients with stroke, *J Neurol Neurosurg Psychiatry* 73:188-190, 2002.

278. The IMS II Trial Investigators: The Interventional Management of Stroke (IMS) II study, *Stroke* 38:2127-2135, 2007.

279. Vibo R, Kõrv J, Haldre S, Roose M: First-year results of the Third Stroke Registry in Tartu, Estonia, *Cerebrovasc Dis* 18:227-231, 2004.

280. Hennerici MG, Kay R, Bogousslavsky J, et al: ESTAT investigators: Intravenous ancrod for acute ischaemic stroke in the European stroke treatment with ancrod trial: a randomised controlled trial, *Lancet* 368:1871-1878, 2006.

281. Lampl Y, Boaz M, Gilad R, et al: Minocycline treatment in acute stroke: An open-label, evaluator-blinded study, *Neurology* 69:1404-1410, 2007.

282. Oveisgharan S, Shirani S, Ghorbani A, et al: Barthel Index in a middle-east country: translation, validity and reliability, *Cerebravasc Dis* 22:350-354, 2006.

283. Lo RSK, Cheng JOY, Wong EMC, et al: Handicap and its determinants of change in stroke survivors: One-year follow-up study, *Stroke* 39:148-153, 2008.

284. Kwok T, Lo RS, Wong E, et al: Quality of life of stroke survivors: A 1-year follow-up study, *Arch Phys Med Rehabil* 87:1177-1182, 2006.

285. Leung SO, Chan CC, Shah S: Development of a Chinese version of the Modified Barthel Index—validity and reliability, *Clin Rehabil* 21:912-922, 2007.

286. Gresham GE, Phillips TF, Labi MLC: ADL status in stroke: Relative merits of three standard indexes, *Arch Phys Med Rehab* 61:355, 1980.

287. Granger CV, Albrecht GL, Hamilton BB: Outcome of comprehensive medical rehabilitation: Measurement by pulses profile and the Barthel Index, *Arch Phys Med Rehabil* 60:145, 1979.

288. Song F, Jerosch-Herold C, Holland R, et al: Statistical methods for analysing Barthel scores in trials of poststroke interventions: a review and computer simulations, *Clin Rehabil* 20:347-356, 2006.

289. van Hartingsveld F, Lucas C, Kwakkel G, Lindeboom R: Improved interpretation of stroke trial results using empirical Barthel item weights, *Stroke* 37:162-166, 2006.

290. Tilley BC: Global statistical tests for comparing multiple outcomes in rheumatoid arthritis trials, *Arthritis Rheum* 42:1879-1888, 1999.

291. Broderick J, Lu M, Kothari R, et al: Finding the most powerful measures of the effectiveness of tissue plasminogen activator in the NINDS stroke trial, *Stroke* 31:2335-2341, 2000.

292. The Ancrod Stroke Study Investigators: Ancrod for the treatment of acute ischemic brain infarction, *Stroke* 25:1755-1759, 1994.

293. Martinsson L, Eksborg S: Activity index—a complementary ADL scale to the Barthel Index in the acute stage in patients with severe stroke, *Cerebrovasc Dis* 22:231-239, 2006.

294. Lyden P, Broderick J, Yamaguchi T, et al: *Reliability of the Barthel Index outcome measure selected for the NINDS t-PA stroke trial,* Tokyo, 1995, Springer-Verlag, 327.

295. Huybrechts KF, Caro JJ: The Barthel Index and modified Rankin Scale as prognostic tools for long-term outcomes after stroke: A qualitative review of the literature, *Curr Med Res Opin* 23:1627-1636, 2007.

296. Gosman H, Svensson E: Parallel reliability of the Functional Independence Measure and the Barthel ADL index, *Disabil Rehabil* 22:702-715, 2000.

297. Uyttenboogaart M, Stewart M, Vroomen PCAJ, et al: Optimizing cutoff scores for the Barthel Index and the Modified Rankin Scale for defining outcome in acute stroke trials, *Stroke* 36:1984-1987, 2005.

298. Jansa J, Pogacnik T, Gompertz P: An evaluation of the Extended Barthel Index with acute ischemic stroke patients, *Neurorehabil Neural Repair* 18:37-41, 2004.

299. Jennett B, Bond M: Assessment of outcome after severe brain damage. A practical scale, *Lancet* 305:480-484, 1975.

300. De Haan R, Aaronson N, Limburg M, et al: Measuring quality of life in stroke, *Stroke* 24:320, 1993.

301. Wong KS, Chen C, Ng PW, et al: Low-molecular-weight heparin compared with aspirin for the treatment of acute ischaemic stroke in Asian patients with large artery occlusive disease: a randomised study, *Lancet* 6:407-413, 2007.

302. Ogawa A, Mori E, Minematsu K, et al for The MELT Japan Study Group Randomized Trial of Intraarterial Infusion of Urokinase Within 6 Hours of Middle Cerebral Artery Stroke: The Middle Cerebral Artery Embolism Local Fibrinolytic Intervention Trial (MELT) Japan, *Stroke* 38:2633-2639, 2007.

303. Banks JL, Marotta CA: Outcomes validity and reliability of the Modified Rankin Scale: implications for stroke clinical trials: A literature review and synthesis, *Stroke* 38:1091-1096, 2007.

304. Shinar D, Gross CR, Mohr JP, et al: Interobserver variability in the assessment of neurologic history and examination in the stroke data bank, *Arch Neurol* 42:557, 1985.

305. Young FB, Lees KR, Weir CJ: for the Glycine Antagonist in Neuroprotection (GAIN) International Trial Steering Committee and Investigators: Strengthening acute stroke trials through optimal use of disability end points, *Stroke* 34:2676-2680, 2003.

306. Weir CJ, Kaste M, Lees KR: for the Glycine Antagonist in Neuroprotection (GAIN) International Steering Committee and Investigators: Targeting neuroprotection clinical trials to ischemic stroke patients with potential to benefit from therapy, *Stroke* 35:2111-2116, 2004.

307. Saver JL: Novel endpoint analytic techniques and interpreting shifts across the entire range of outcome scales in acute stroke trials, *Stroke* 38:3055-3062, 2007.

308. Koziol JA, Feng AC: On the analysis and interpretation of outcome measures in stroke clinical trials: Lessons From the SAINT I Study of NXY-059 for Acute Ischemic Stroke, *Stroke* 37:2644-2647, 2006.

309. Teasdale GM, Pettigrew LE, Wilson JT, et al: Analyzing outcome of treatment of severe head injury: A review and update on advancing the use of the Glasgow Outcome Scale, *J Neurotrauma* 15:587-597, 1998.

310. Wahlgren NG, Romi F, Wahlgren J: Glasgow outcome scale and global improvement scale were at least as sensitive as the Orgogozo, Mathew and Barthel scales in the Intravenous Nimodipine West Stroke Trial (INWEST), *Cerebrovasc Dis* 5:225, 1995.

311. Haley EC Jr, Kassell NF, Alves WM, and the participants: Phase II trial of tirilazad in aneurysmal subarachnoid hemorrhage: A report of the Cooperative Aneurysm Study, *J Neurosurg* 82:786, 1995.

312. Yamaguchi T, Sano K, Takakura K, et al: Ebselen in acute ischemic stroke: A placebo-controlled, double-blind clinical trial: Ebselen Study Group, *Stroke* 29:12-17, 1998.

313. Kassell NF, Torner JC, Haley EC Jr, et al: The International Cooperative Study on the Timing of Aneurysm Surgery. Part 1: Overall management results, *J Neurosurg* 73:18-36, 1990.

314. Vermuelen M, van Gijn J, Hijdra A: Causes of acute deterioration in patients with a ruptured intracranial aneurysm, *J Neurosurg* 60:935-939, 1984.

315. Essink-Bot M, Krabbe P, Bonsel B, Aaronson N: An empirical comparison of four generic health status measures. The Nottingham Health Profile, the Medical Outcomes Study 36-item Short-Form Health Survey, the COOP/WONCA charts, and the EuroQoL instrument, *Med Care* 35:522-537, 1997.

316. Cramer SC, Koroshetz WJ, Finklestein SP: The case for modality-specific outcome measures in clinical trials of stroke recovery-promoting agents, *Stroke* 38:1393-1395, 2007.

317. McKevitt C, Refern J, La-Placa V, Wolfe CD: Defining and using quality of life: A survey of health care professionals, *Clin Rehabil* 17:865-870, 2003.

318. Xie J, Wu EQ, Zheng ZJ, et al: Impact of stroke on health-related quality of life in the noninstitutionalized population in the United States, *Stroke* 37:2567-2572, 2006.

319. Lawrence L, Christie D: Quality of life after stroke: A three-year follow-up, *Age Ageing* 8:167-172, 1979.

320. Kappelle LJ, Adams HP Jr, Heffner ML, et al: Prognosis of young adults with ischemic stroke. A long-term follow-up study assessing recurrent vascular events and functional outcome in the Iowa Registry of Stroke in Young Adults, *Stroke* 25:1360-1365, 1994.

321. Duncan PW, Samsa GP, Weinberger M, et al: Health status of individuals with mild stroke, *Stroke* 28:740-745, 1997.

322. Parker CJ, Gladman JR, Drummond AE: The role of leisure in stroke rehabilitation, *Disabil Rehabil* 19:1-5, 1997.

323. Sturm JW, Donnan GA, Dewey HM, et al: Quality of life after stroke. The North East Melbourne Stroke Incidence Study (NEMESIS), *Stroke* 35:2340-2345, 2004.

324. Mayo NE, Wood-Dauphinee S, Cote R, Durcan J: Activity, participation, and quality of life 6 months post stroke, *Arch Phys Med Rehabil* 83:1035-1042, 2002.

325. Tengs TO, Luistro E: Health-related quality of life after stroke: A comprehensive review, *Stroke* 32:964-972, 2001.

326. Gosman-Hedstrom G, Claesson L, Blomstrand C: Consequences of severity at stroke onset for health-related quality of life (HRQL) and informal care: A 1-year follow-up in elderly stroke survivors, *Arch Gerontol Geriatr* 47:79-91, 2008.

327. Smout S, Koudstaal P, Ribbers GM, et al: Struck by stroke: a pilot study exploring quality of life and coping patterns in younger patients and spouses, *Int J Rehabil Res* 24:261-268, 2001.

328. Bluvol A, Ford-Gilboe M: Hope, health, work and quality of life in families of stroke survivors, *J Adv Nurs* 48:322-332, 2004.

329. Li TC, Lin CC, Amidon RL: Quality of life of primary caregivers of elderly with cerebrovascular disease or diabetes hospitalized for acute care: Assessment of well-being and functioning using the SF-36 health questionnaire, *Qual Life Res* 13:1081-1088, 2004.

330. van Wijk I, Gorter JW, Lindeman E, et al: Mental status and health-related quality of life in an elderly population 15 years after limited cerebral ischaemia, *J Neurol* 254:1018-1025, 2007.

331. McPherson K, Myers J, Taylor WJ, et al: Self-evaluation and societal evaluations of health state differ with disease severity in chronic and disabling conditions, *Med Care* 42:1143-1151, 2004.

332. Bethoux F, Calmels P, Gautheron V, Minaire P: Quality of life of the spouses of stroke patients: A preliminary study, *Int J Rehabil Res* 19:291-299, 1996.

333. Testa MA, Simonson DC: Assessment of quality-of-life outcomes, *N Engl J Med* 334:835-840, 1996.

334. de Haan RJ: Measuring quality of life after stroke using the SF-36, *Stroke* 33:1176-1177, 2002.

335. Buck D, Jacoby A, Massey A, Ford G: Evaluation of measures used to assess quality of life after stroke, *Stroke* 31:2000, 2004.

336. Buck D, Jacoby A, Massey A, et al: Development and validation of NEWSQOL((R)), the Newcastle Stroke-Specific Quality of Life Measure, *Cerebrovasc Dis* 17:143-152, 2004.

337. Hamedani AG, Wells CK, Brass LM, et al: A quality-of-life instrument for young hemorrhagic stroke patients, *Stroke* 32:687-695, 2001.

338. Sturm JW, Osborne R, Dewey H, et al: Brief comprehensive quality of life assessment after stroke: The assessment of quality of life instrument in the North East Melbourne Stroke Incident Study (NEMESIS), *Stroke* 33:2888-2894, 2002.

339. Doyle PJ, McNeil MR, Prieto L, et al: The Burden of Stroke Scale (BOSS) provides valid and reliable score estimates of functioning and well-being in stroke survivors with and without communication disorders, *J Clin Epidemiol* 57:997-1007, 2004.

340. Fernandez-Concepcion O, Roman PY, Alvarez-Gonzalez MA, et al: The development of a scale to evaluate the quality of life in stroke survivors, *Rev Neurol* 39:915-923, 2004.

341. Muus I, Williams LS, Ringsberg KC: Validation of the Stroke Specific Quality of Life Scale (SS-QOL): test of reliability and validity of the Danish version (SS-QOL-DK), *Clin Rehabil* 21:620-627, 2007.

342. Hobart JC, Williams LS, Moran K, Thompson AJ: Quality of life measurement after stroke: Uses and abuses of the SF-36, *Stroke* 33:1348-1356, 2002.

343. Bergner M, Bobbitt RA, Carter WB, Gilson BS: The Sickness Impact Profile: Development and final revision of a health status measure, *Med Care* 19:787-805, 1981.

344. Hacking HGA, Post MWM, Schepers VPM, et al: A comparison of 3 generic health status questionnaires among stroke patients, *J Stroke Cerebrovasc Dis* 15:235-240, 2006.

345. Suenkeler IH, Nowak M, Misselwitz B, et al: Timecourse of health-related quality of life as determined 3, 6 and 12 months after stroke: Relationship to neurological deficit, disability and depression, *J Neurol* 249:1160-1167, 2002.

346. Carod-Artal F, Gonzalez-Gutierrez JL, Egido-Herrero JA, Varela de Seijas E: The psychometric properties of the Spanish version of the stroke-adapted 30-item Sickness Impact Profile (SIP30-AI), *Rev Neurol* 45:647-654, 2007.

347. Edwards DF, Hahn M, Baum C, Dromerick AW: The impact of mild stroke on meaningful activity and life satisfaction, *J Stroke Cerebrovasc Dis* 14:151-157, 2006.

348. Muus I, Ringsberg KC: Stroke specific quality of life scale: Danish adaptation and a pilot study for testing psychometric properties, *Scand J Caring Sci* 19:140-147, 2005.

349. Williams LS, Weinberger M, Harris LE, Biller J: Measuring quality of life in a way that is meaningful to stroke patients, *Neurology* 53:1839-1843, 1999.

350. Williams LS, Weinberger M, Harris LE, et al: Development of a stroke-specific quality of life scale, *Stroke* 30:1362-1369, 1999.

351. Hilari K, Byng S: Measuring quality of life in people with aphasia: The Stroke Quality of Life Scale, *Int J Lang Commun Disord* 36:86-91, 2001.

352. Marco E, Duarte E, Santos JF, et al: Short Form 36 health questionnaire in hemiplegic patients 2 years after stroke, *Neurologia* 21:348-356, 2006.

353. Haacke C, Althaus A, Spottke A, et al: Long-term outcome after stroke: Evaluating health-related quality of life using utility measurements, *Stroke* 37:193-198, 2006.

354. Myers JA, McPherson KM, Taylor WJ, et al: Duration of condition is unrelated to health-state valuation on the EuroQol, *Clin Rehabil* 17:209-215, 2003.

355. Dorman PJ, Waddell F, Slattery J, et al: Is the EuroQol a valid measure of health-related quality of life after stroke? *Stroke* 28:1876-1882, 1997.

356. Dorman PJ, Dennis M, Sandercock P: How do scores on the Euro-Qol relate to scores on the SF-36 after stroke? *Stroke* 30:2146-2151, 1999.

357. Dorman PJ, Waddell F, Slattery J, et al: Are proxy assessments of health status after stroke with the EuroQol questionnaire feasible, accurate, and unbiased? *Stroke* 28:1883-1887, 1997.

358. Hilari K, Byng S, Lamping DL, Smith SC: Stroke and aphasia quality of life scale-39 (SAQOL-39). Evaluation of acceptability, reliability, and validity, *Stroke* 34:1944-1950, 2003.

359. Brorsson B, Asberg KH: Katz Index of Independence in ADL. Reliability and validity in short-term care, *Scand J Rehabil Med* 16:125-132, 1984.

360. Duncan PW, Lai SM, Tyler D, et al: Evaluation of proxy responses to the stroke impact scale, *Stroke* 33:2593-2599, 2002.

361. Duncan PW, Lai SM, Bode RK, et al: Stroke Impact Scale-16: A brief assessment of physical function, *Neurology* 60:291-296, 2003.

362. Lai SM, Perera S, Duncan PW, Bode R: Physical and social functioning after stroke: Comparison of the Stroke Impact Scale and Short Form-36, *Stroke* 34:488-493, 2003.

363. Feeny D, Furlong W, Boyle M, Torrance GW: Multi-attribute health status classification systems. Health utilities index, *Pharmacoeconomics* 7:490-502, 1995.

364. Grootendorst P, Feeny D, Furlong W: Health utilities index mark 3: Evidence of construct validity for stroke and arthritis in a population health survey, *Med Care* 38:290-299, 2000.

365. Pickard AS, Johnson JA, Feeny DH: Responsiveness of generic health-related quality of life measures in stroke, *Qual Life Res* 14:207-219, 2005.

366. Dorman P, Dennis M, Sandercock P: Are the modified "simple questions" a valid and reliable measure of health related quality of life after stroke? United Kingdom Collaborators in the International Stroke Trial, *J Neurol Neurosurg Psychiatry* 69:487-493, 2005.

367. Lo RS, Cheng JO, Wong EM, et al: Handicap and its determinants of change in stroke survivors: One-year follow-up study, *Stroke* 39:148-153, 2008.

368. Townend E, Brady M, McLaughlan K: A systematic evaluation of the adaptation of depression diagnostic methods for stroke survivors who have aphasia, *Stroke* 38:3076-3083, 2007.

369. Mathias SD, Bates MM, Pasta DJ, et al: Use of the Health Utilities Index with stroke patients and their caregivers, *Stroke* 28:1888-1894, 1997.

370. Golomb BA, Vickrey BG, Hays RD: A review of health-related quality-of-life measures in stroke, *Pharmacoeconomics* 19:155-185, 2001.

Carotid Artery Disease

J.P. MOHR, HENNING MAST

Atherosclerotic disease of the common, internal, and external carotid arteries is usually centered in the bifurcation area; that is, it mainly involves the distal common carotid artery (CCA) as well as the proximal internal carotid artery (ICA). As in proximal coronary and lower extremity arterial disease, cigarette smoking is also a major risk factor for carotid atherosclerosis.[1] The carotid has been the focus of neurologic attention for more than half a century after the link between stenosis, occlusion, and embolism from this source and brain infarction became clear. The site of (spontaneous or traumatic) dissecting or neoplastic lesions is usually more distal along the course of the ICA. The CCA and extracranial ICA can be examined clinically and by sonographic, conventional angiographic, computer tomographic (CT), and magnetic resonance imaging (MRI). Surgical as well as endovascular approaches to stenoses have a long-standing tradition. By comparison, the intracranial ICA lends itself poorly to clinical examination and intervention; ultrasonography, CT and MRI, and conventional angiography, however, allow for reliable imaging and guidance for endovascular treatment.

Carotid artery disease accounts for approximately 15% of all focal ischemic lesions. The clinical weight of carotid stroke, however, goes beyond this rather small proportion. With subsequent territorial infarction embolism, the most frequent mechanism of symptomatic carotid stroke, carries a worse prognosis regarding disability than lacunar infarction, including the risk of progressive stroke and secondary brain swelling. The clinical management of symptomatic carotid disease with recurrent transient ischemic attack (TIA) and early recurrence of stroke is among the most challenging in stroke treatment; patients with carotid disease—frequently smokers with complication-prone concomitant cardiac macroangiopathy—are often younger than the average stroke population. Furthermore, decisions on the indication and the timing of invasive measures (e.g., endarterectomy or stenting) pose additional challenges different from those for lacunar or cardioembolic infarction. Given the well-established, high early stroke recurrence rate, the issue of early intervention and the use of anticoagulation is still unsettled.

Carotid Anatomy and Lesion Development

The anatomy of the cerebral artery tree is presented in Fig. 22-1. The bifurcation, classically assumed to lie at the level of C3–4, is present in only 55% of cases; the locations of the remainder are scattered from as high as C2–3 to as low as C5–6. In 85% of cases the location of the bifurcations occurs at the same height.[2]

Atherosclerosis of the Extracranial Common Carotid Bifurcation and Internal Carotid

Lesion Location

As already stated, the bulk of carotid atheromatous disease affects the length of the common carotid. It is most intense at the bifurcation and into the first few centimeters of the internal carotid, after which it fades toward normal, leaving the bulk of the distal extracranial internal carotid unaffected.[3]

Lesion Asymmetry

Far from being a symmetrical disease, carotid atheroma has considerable asymmetry in lesion intensity. No suitable explanation has yet emerged. When asymmetry of atheroma severity is found, the atheroma is more common in the smaller carotid,[4] the one more angulated,[5] and the one in which flow separation is more easily demonstrated.[6-9] However, notable exceptions exist. An analysis of 5395 angiograms from the European Carotid Surgery Trial (ECST) found "large individual differences" in measurements, including differences in a variety of measurements between the two sides of more than or equal to 25% in fully 17% of cases; however, the analysis was unable to show a direct effect of any of these variables in atheroma development.[10]

Tempo of Development of Carotid Stenosis Bifurcation Lesions

Remarkably little has appeared in recent years on the tempo of lesion development, besides the initial reports when duplex Doppler technology first appeared. By digital subtraction methods,[11] conventional angiography[12] or noninvasive techniques, atheromatous stenoses may be seen to develop swiftly over months; however, it is usually a very slow process, stretching over years, and, in many cases, may even remain static despite being hemodynamically significant.[13] For those with more than or equal to 50% stenosis initially, little progression was found by duplex Doppler every 6 months for 2 years, except for patients with diabetes or those who continued to smoke. At most, the authors advised annual screening.[14] Current efforts to alter the tempo with the use of a statin have thus far been disappointing after short-term follow-up.[15]

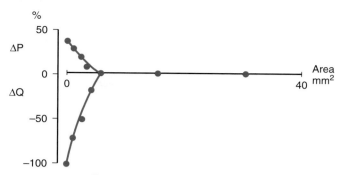

Figure 22-2 Effect of cross-sectional area on pressure and flow.

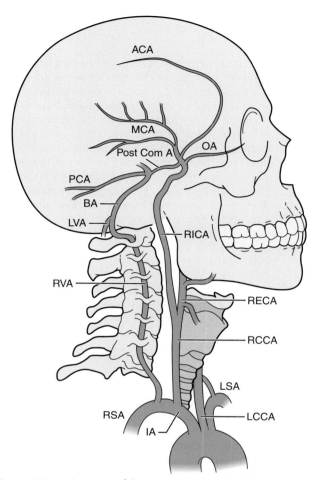

Figure 22-1 Anatomy of the extracranial cerebral-bound arteries and their main intracranial supplies, lateral view from the right. ACA, anterior cerebral artery; BA, basilar artery; IA, innominate artery; LCCA, left common carotid artery; LSA, left subclavian artery; LVA, left vertebral artery; MCA, middle cerebral artery; OA, ophthalmic artery; PCA, posterior cerebral artery; Post Com A, posterior communicating artery; RCCA, right common carotid artery; RECA; right external carotid artery; RICA, right internal carotid artery; RSA, right subclavian artery; RVA, right vertebral artery. The anterior choroidal artery is not depicted. (From Gautier JC, Mohr JP: Ischemic stroke. In Mohr JP, Gautier JC, editors: *Guide to clinical neurology*, New York, 1995, Churchill Livingstone, p 543.)

Hemodynamically Significant Extracranial Stenosis

Reduced cross-sectional area is the main factor in making a stenosis hemodynamically significant.[16-18] Hemodynamically important stenosis—one that limits flow intracranially—requires a cross-sectional area of 4 to 5 mm² along a length of 3 mm (Fig. 22-2); this area corresponds to less than 2 mm in the smallest two-dimensional profile seen on an angiogram[17] and occurs when 84% diameter stenosis and 96% area stenosis are achieved.[19] Ulceration is typically noncontributory and is strongly related to the degree of stenosis at the site of the ulcer. Other factors include the length of the stenosis,[16] blood flow velocity,[20] and blood viscosity.[21] No clear relationship has been found between the overall plaque volume and the degree of stenosis, which indicates a wide range of lengths and shapes for a stenosis that may be severe enough to be of hemodynamic importance.[22]

Angiography, once the gold standard for estimation of the severity of stenosis, has been superseded by modern duplex Doppler methods,[23] despite persisting impressions drawn from earlier clinical trials of endarterectomy based on angiographic assessment. Although largely outdated, several techniques previously used for estimates of stenosis created considerable controversy as to which measurement most accurately reflected stenosis. The North American Symptomatic Carotid Endarterectomy Trial (NASCET) formula [(1 − minimum residual lumen/normal distal cervical ICA diameter) × 100] differed somewhat from that of the Asymptomatic Carotid Atherosclerosis Study (ACAS). The controversy also illustrates the problems posed by the angiographic method, not to mention the difficulties of using a biplanar technique for a nonannular lesion. The method for selection of the sites in the vessel is shown in Fig. 22-3.[24] Interobserver agreement on measurements for digital subtraction angiograms and magnetic resonance angiograms have not been high. Practices also differ between continents: in the United States, a method of measuring the angiogram may yield a diagnosis of 60% stenosis, whereas the method used in Europe may produce a diagnosis of 75% stenosis from basically the same angiographic images.[25]

A long-standing controversy exists over whether stroke risk is tied mainly to the degree of stenosis, to ulcerations, or to both. The neuropathologic study of Fisher and Ojemann[26] challenged the embolic theory as the typical source of TIAs (see further on). The Consensus Conference for Carotid Plaque Morphology and Risk (Consensus sur la Morphologie et le Risque des Plaques Carotidiennes), held in December 1996 in Paris, determined that it is the *degree of stenosis* that is associated with stroke risk, not the ultrasonographic features of the plaque.[27] Undeterred, investigators continue their search for an embolic explanation for TIAs and stroke.

Plaque Rupture

Since the last edition of this book, advances in imaging technology,[28] including MRI, CT, and innovations in time-resolved laser-induced fluorescence spectroscopy,[29] have allowed documentation of the existence and rupture of carotid artery plaques. By MRI, wall shear stress is high at sites of ulceration, which suggests its role in prior plaque rupture.[30,31] The risk appears more related to plaque cap

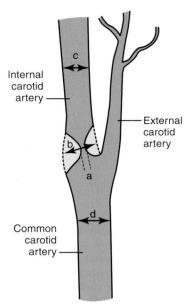

Figure 22-3 Position of measurements for stenosis. a, Site of maximum stenosis (regardless of whether in the carotid bulb); b, original internal carotid lumen; c, internal carotid distal to the stenosis; d, common carotid lumen. (From Young GR, Humphrey PR, Nixon TE, et al: Variability in measurement of extracranial internal carotid artery stenosis as displayed by both digital subtraction and magnetic resonance angiography: An assessment of three caliper techniques and visual impression of stenosis. *Stroke* 27:467, 1996, with permission.)

thickness[32] than to core composition.[33] On CT angiography, fissurization of carotid plaque caps is found more often in symptomatic patients.[34] MRI has also documented plaque wall hemorrhaging in 55% of patients with acute symptoms (50% with fibrous cap rupture) compared with 5% of asymptomatic patients (none showing rupture).[35] Readers remain frustrated by the terse descriptions of the cases, characterized in the acute symptom group only as "TIA or minor stroke," leaving unsettled the seriousness of the stroke event in those deemed to have had ruptured plaques. Individual case reports argue that an acute but minor syndrome may be associated with acute plaque rupture and prompt urgent endarterectomy.[36] However, the prevalence of unstable plaques compared with thrombotic or stable plaques may not be large. A large study (457 cases) of endarterectomy specimens found a distinct minority (16%) considered to be "vulnerable plaques" (i.e., thin cap fibroatheroma).[37] Some evidence argues that carotid plaques may stabilize and remodel over time after a stroke.[38] Prospective studies for stroke recurrence are underway.[39]

Initial enthusiasm decades ago for the concept that plaque rupture was caused by plaque hematoma faded when subsequent studies cast doubt not on its occurrence but on its importance.[40] Given the frustrating common failure to find a source of embolism in cases of cryptogenic stroke, hopes are raised once again that an innocent carotid lesion could be the cause. Nonetheless, the severity of stroke remains at issue and is surely a function of the size of the particle and density of organization being released into the distal circulation. Although these issues remain unsettled, discussion of them has been reopened by concerns for unstable plaque rupture (see later).

Carotid Disease Other than Atherosclerosis

Infection: Although atherosclerosis has been considered the basic disease process in the vast majority of cases, evidence is emerging that *Chlamydia pneumoniae* may have a role as a cause of relentlessly progressing arteriopathy that has the histologic appearance of atherosclerosis. Its presence in atheromatous arterial lesions is not in doubt and is related to a marker of inflammation. Real-time polymerase chain reaction assessment of bacterial loads in monocytes was found to correlate with carotid plaque disease and plaque rupture.[41] Progression of carotid artery disease tracked by Doppler has also been related to seropositivity,[42] but whether *C. pneumoniae* has a causative role in atheromatous-appearing lesions remains unsettled.[43,44] Treatment with antibiotics (Rifalazil) has been reported for peripheral vascular disease in *C. pneumoniae*–positive patients but has had disappointing results.[45]

Embolism: Prominent among the causes are embolism from cardiac or arterial sources and arterial dissection (see Chapter 20). A few additional causes are uncommon, some of which approach the status of medical curiosities.[46]

Fibromuscular dysplasia: Fibromuscular dysplasia is encountered in less than 0.6% of cases of ICA disease.[47] It may explain some kinks (see later) and is associated with separate intracranial aneurysm in almost 25% of cases of fibromuscular dysplasia (see later). Its clinical importance is unclear, but the disease has been the subject of publication often enough that it is discussed in a separate chapter (see Chapter 33).

Arterial kinks: Kinking of the ICA may achieve the same hemodynamic effects as atheromatous stenosis. It is an acquired condition and is not identical to coiling, which is believed to be congenital and of no clinical significance.[48,49] Kinking was thought to be caused by atherosclerosis or to occur as a complication of fibromuscular dysplasia, but recent studies argue that congenital dolichoectasia may play a larger role.[50] The stenotic effect of kinking can arise when positional head changes produce transient cerebral ischemia, a situation in which dramatic reductions in cerebral blood flow (CBF) have been documented, in some cases during intraoperative studies; as yet, the degree of stenosis observed angiographically has not proved to be an adequate basis for determining the need for corrective surgery without additional studies on the effect of head position change. Kinking caused by alteration in artery position appears to be a rare cause of TIAs. In one unusual example, Handa et al[51] described a patient who had undergone extracranial–intracranial bypass and then had experienced recurrent TIAs precipitated by yawning. The stretching and kinking of the donor artery by the mouth opening during the yawning was the alleged mechanism. A small randomized trial of medical versus surgical treatment found lower later stroke rates for those who had surgery.[52]

Primary tumors of the vascular structures: Primary tumors of vascular structures are uncommon, usually arising from mesoblastic and neural elements such as chemodectomas and paragangliomas.[53] Only 5% are bilateral.

Such masses grow slowly, manifesting as dysphagia and hoarseness, although dyspnea, Horner's syndrome, and facial pain may also occur.[54] The lesions produce metastases in only about 2% of cases. Local recurrence is uncommon and is usually delayed for many years.

Complications of head and neck cancer: Involvement of the extracranial carotid artery by direct extension of a local tumor is distinctly uncommon.[55] However, this complication occurs often enough in hospitals with a large oncology case load to warrant consideration here. Direct tumor invasion of the arterial wall from an extracranial site is well known,[56] but only rarely has involvement of parasellar tumors in the siphon been reported.[57] Surgical approaches to tumor resection that involve taking the carotid artery along with tumor are associated with stroke rates of up to 25%.[58,59] Interpositional grafting[60] is the usual approach, but saphenous vein grafting is preferred because of better patency than with the reversed graft.[61]

Radiation: The lesions from radiation to the head and neck, although typically delayed in onset, affect a longer segment of the artery than that affected by conventional atherosclerosis.[62] Radiation can induce or accelerate atherosclerosis, generally after an interval of several years,[56,63] and in some cases delays have been as long as 25 years.[64] Recurrence after stenting is higher in radiation-related stenoses.[65] Carotid rupture is a serious late complication of nasopharyngeal cancer and radiation treatment; management options are limited.[66]

Intracranial Internal Carotid Artery Disease

Despite painstaking anatomic–pathologic studies, there remains only limited agreement on the role of embolism alone, embolism in conjunction with existing stenosis, or atheromatous stenosis alone as the leading cause of disease. The intracranial ICA, especially the cavernous part, is the second site of predilection of atherosclerosis, but the extent and severity of the lesions are far behind those of the sinus. An undetermined number of atherosclerotic primary occlusive thromboses occur in the intracranial ICA.

There is no clear evidence to indicate that a siphon stenosis (tandem stenoses) increases the risk of occlusive thrombosis of a stenosis at the ICA origin or vice versa,[67-69] nor do tandem stenoses appear to raise the risk involved in carotid endarterectomy.[70]

Anterograde and retrograde secondary thromboses of the intracranial ICA are a subject for which only scanty literature exists. Pathologically well-studied instances of intracranial ICA thrombotic occlusion are rare, and the role of anterograde or retrograde extension of an associated thrombus is unclear.[67,71-73] Angiographic studies have shown a decline in the role of the siphon as time goes by.[74] Retrograde thrombi developing down to the ICA origin are probably not rare, and the angiographic appearance of the proximal end of carotid occlusion does not predict the age of the occlusion, at least within the first 6 days after stroke onset (Fig. 22-4).[75] Discontinuous occlusions (i.e., the presence of a patent segment of the ICA between the extracranial occluded ICA and the intracranial ICA) have been reported at autopsy, and it may be difficult or impossible to decide whether the distal plug is thrombotic or embolic, the lack of knowledge of which poses some difficulties for surgeons or interventionalists attempting removal of what is inferred to be an acute occlusion at the origin or the siphon of the ICA.[67,72,73,76]

Progressive occlusion of the siphon and distal intracranial ICA has been reported in a setting of essential thrombocythemia[77] and in mucormycosis, and investment by nasopalatine carcinoma (carcinoma of the fossa of Rosenmüller) and inflammatory pseudotumors[78] is also well-known.

Described in more detail in Chapter 44, transcranial Doppler technology has advanced enough to allow investigation of the orbit and siphon in many individuals, decreasing the former dependency on catheter angiography.[79] The calcium score correlates with atheromatous disease severity in the siphon.[80]

Pathophysiology of Carotid Artery Ischemia

The clinical syndromes that occur from disease involving the carotid artery itself result from two basic mechanisms: (1) arterial occlusion below the circle of Willis with inadequate compensatory collateral pathways available through the circle or retrograde over the convexity from adjacent cerebral arteries, or (2) perfusion failure due to inadequate collateral pathways distal to hemodynamically significant stenosis or occlusion (Fig. 22-5). Both mechanisms may even be operative in the same patient.[81,82] The first mechanism accounts for the larger or catastrophic carotid strokes, and the latter accounts for more limited clinical syndromes, of which some are mild enough that the demonstrated infarction and arterial occlusion confound the expectations of the clinicians.

Collateral Pathways

When the ICA is unable to supply its usual intracranial territory via its direct anterograde route, six major potential sources of collateral flow may develop, individually or in combination (Fig. 22-6).[83-85] Only in recent years, with the increased use of safely and readily repeatable studies of blood flow have the development and extent of such collateral pathways been found to mirror the severity of the carotid stenosis for which they are intended to compensate.[86]

Extracranial Pathways

Internal carotid–ophthalmic: The most readily recognized *extracranial* source is an anastomosis *via the external carotid artery (ECA) through the orbit*. Anterograde blood flow up the ECA via its facial branches to the orbit provides a ready link through the floor and roof of the orbit to the ophthalmic branch of the intracranial ICA. When blood flow is available in sufficient force, the direction of the ophthalmic artery flow can reverse, which provides a path to the siphon and thence, now anterograde, to the ipsilateral circle of Willis. These specific paths of anastomoses occur mainly between the maxillary branch of the ECA and the ophthalmic artery in the floor of the orbit. Smaller anastomoses occur over the roof of the orbit between the facial and frontal branches of the

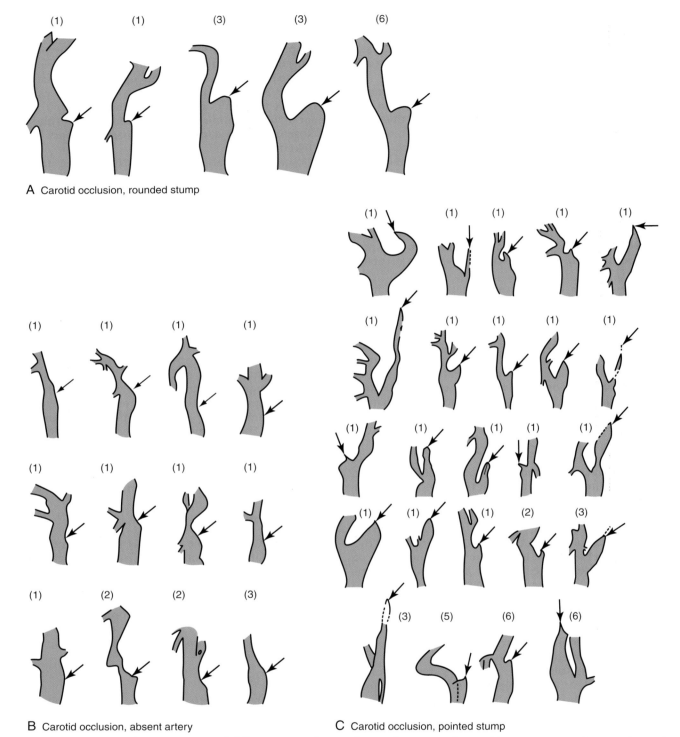

A Carotid occlusion, rounded stump

B Carotid occlusion, absent artery

C Carotid occlusion, pointed stump

Figure 22-4 Angiographic appearance of different types of internal carotid artery occlusion. Numbers in parentheses indicate days between stroke onset and angiography.

ECA and the supratrochlear and supraorbital branches of the ophthalmic artery. These latter paths were used for the classic "A, B, C" brow pulse test (CM Fisher), which determined the pulse direction at the edges of the orbit (angular brow, cheek): if compression of the facial artery branch along its periauricular course obliterated the pulse, then its source was extracranial, not, as normal, from intracranial flows directed by the ophthalmic artery. Collateral flow to the ophthalmic artery may come from meningeal branches of the ECA, not detectable by digital compression examination; rarely, the ophthalmic artery is not a branch of the ICA, instead receiving its entire flow from the meningeal artery, which is a linkage that offers little intracranial supply to the circle of Willis.

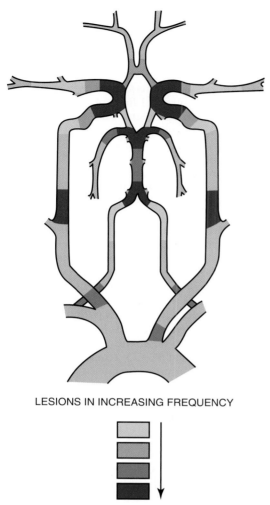

LESIONS IN INCREASING FREQUENCY

Figure 22-5 Distribution of lesions in the carotid territory.

Intracranial Pathways

The most important source of collateral circulation for a hemisphere comes from the *contralateral ICA via the circle of Willis*. In this case, blood flows anterograde up the opposite ICA and then across the circle of Willis via the anterior communicating artery, from which it has several potential paths to the affected hemisphere. The most useful is straight across the affected side of the circle directly into the middle cerebral artery (MCA). In addition, or, barring the patency of the path to the MCA, collateral flow may ascend along the cortical branches of the anterior cerebral artery (ACA), lacking direct supply from its own ICA, and then over the hemisphere and through borderzone links to the MCA, filling these MCA branches retrograde.

In like fashion the posterior cerebral artery (PCA), usually receiving its main flow from the basilar, may provide flow to the MCA via the posterior communicating artery or via anterograde flow in its cortical branches, linking to MCA branches through the borderzone anastomoses and retrograde through them into the MCA territory.

The circle of Willis, an arterial polygon, has many minor variations in its degree of completeness; in the most severe cases it has no links to the threatened ICA territory

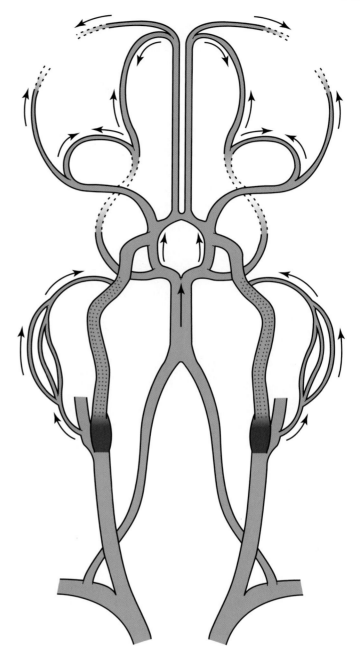

Figure 22-6 Sources of collateral flow for occlusion of the internal carotid territory (red, site of occlusion; stippled, distal flow failure) showing external carotid collateral to the ophthalmic (1) and intracranial collaterals via the basilar (2) through the posterior communicating arteries (3), the borderzone vessels linking the distal branches of the anterior-middle cerebral arteries (4) and posterior cerebral to anterior (5) and middle cerebral arteries (6). (From Gautier JC, Mohr JP: Ischemic stroke. In Mohr JP, Gautier JC, editors: *Guide to clinical neurology*, New York, 1995, Churchill Livingstone, p 543.)

via either the contralateral ACA or ipsilateral PCA. In such instances the territory of the affected ICA can be isolated; this is especially so if its ipsilateral ACA is not linked to the opposite side via the circle of Willis and its ipsilateral PCA is also supplied by the ICA (so-called fetal PCA, representing persistence of the early embryologic links

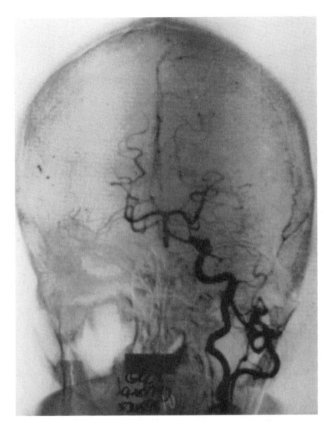

Figure 22-7 Example of a persistent trigeminal artery.

between these two vessels). In extreme cases, the ACA of the affected territory may have an azygous supply to both ACA territories, adding a portion of the fourth contralateral ACA territory to the areas at risk.

Rarely, the flow into the ICA territory from the basilar artery is by way of a persisting trigeminal artery, which usually reaches the ICA near the base of the skull (Fig. 22-7).

Borderzone collaterals: Flow retrograde from cerebral arteries *through the borderzones over the brain surface* may spare some or all of the cortical surface branches of the endangered arterial territories. In this setting, the anatomy of the circle of Willis plays a vital role: if the posterior communicating artery is too small to carry much collateral flow, then the distal ends of the cortical branches of the PCA may supply collateral flow to the ACA or MCA territories through the borderzone anastomoses over the hemisphere surface. If the stem of the ACA ipsilateral to the occluded ICA is likewise too small, the ACA may collateralize some or the entire middle cerebral surface branches through the borderzone. In such instances, the retrograde flow into the endangered territories ranges from full collateral flow all the way to the stem of the recipient vessel to little more than feeble flow into the distal cortical surface branches.

Other paths of collateral flow may develop under special circumstances, all of them so exceptional that they could not be counted on under normal conditions. Thus, cerebral surface vessels may anastomose with an extracranial arterial source through a craniotomy site (extracranial–intracranial [EC-IC] study), and extremely rare instances have been described in which the deep penetrating arteries (the lenticulostriates) have linked through the deep white matter to the cerebral convexity borderzones.

It has long been obvious that the mere angiographic demonstration of collateral flow bears little relationship to its physiologic effect. Using PET measurements (CBF, blood volume, and oxygen extraction fraction), Powers et al[87] found that neither the percent stenosis nor the residual lumen diameter of the extracranial ICA was a reliable predictor of the hemodynamic state of the cerebral circulation in patients. Hemodynamic insufficiency of the hemisphere correlated best with angiographic patterns of meningeal and ophthalmic arterial collateral paths. Similarly, transcranial Doppler (TCD) ultrasonography has shown that ophthalmic collateral flow is an insufficient source of supply to the brain and that its presence indicates that the more common sources of collateral flow are unavailable or incompetent. Prominent ophthalmic collateral flow is usually a poor prognostic sign, not a favorable one.[88,89] Nonetheless, we have a patient under observation since 1987 whose entire left hemisphere depends on transorbital collateral flow; the patient is clinically normal and shows normal 5% CO_2 reactivity.

Mechanisms of Ischemic Stroke

The problem in diagnosis and management of carotid artery disease lies mainly in (1) clarifying which one of these principles is at work in a given case, (2) identifying the source of an embolus, (3) determining the severity of the perfusion failure, and (4) predicting future events.

Most cases of carotid territory ischemia are broadly attributed to atherosclerosis, but a variety of mechanisms of infarction seem to be involved. For TIAs, these mechanisms could entail a temporary cessation of flow either in a distal branch artery from embolus or over the distal territories of the underperfused carotid artery during periods when systemic hypotension, bradyarrhythmia, or other causes of "low flow" exist. Examples are now well-described in instances of embolism clot extraction, where dramatic restoration of flow in a suitable timeframe has produced virtually complete restoration of function. With restoration of blood flow, the ischemic region of the brain quickly recovers, and the clinical deficits (TIA) vanish. For infarction, the processes would presumably be the same, but the effects of the occlusion would persist. That such events could occur with purely atheromatous stenosis leading to transient occlusions remains unproven but is the basis of much of the angioplasty and stenting literature.

Anterograde propagation of carotid thrombosis is the easiest of the effects of carotid artery occlusion to understand, although it is quite uncommon. Extension distally from the siphon to and beyond the circle of Willis involving the stems of the ACA and MCA usually creates devastating cerebral infarction (see later on).[82,90]

Embolism is a common cause of both TIA and stroke, whether into the carotid artery from a source proximal to the ICA (e.g., cardiac, aortic arch)[91-94] or from the carotid artery itself toward intracranial territories, arresting in

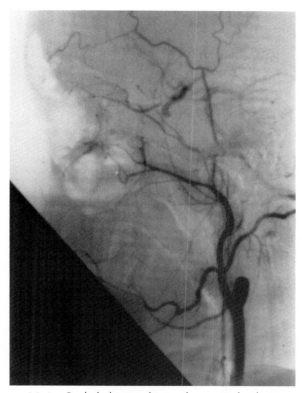

Figure 22-8 Occluded internal carotid artery with a large stump.

the siphon or the top of the intracranial carotid. The syndrome is typically acute and the deficit usually large[82]; the clinical features do not separate cardiogenic from local arterial sources of embolism.[95]

Although cardiogenic embolism into the carotid artery and its branches is well-established by pathologic studies, embolism *from* the carotid artery itself has long been assumed but has also been difficult to prove.[96] Examples of large particle embolism from the carotid appear to be rare; we have encountered a few in a setting of severe stenosis when the embolus appeared to have been too large to have passed through the stenosis from a cardiac cause. Early success with anticoagulant therapy supported the assumption that embolism was being prevented.[93,97,98] Proof of the embolic mechanism might be difficult to find because angiographic[99-103] and pathologic studies[91] have shown that cerebral emboli fragments may disappear promptly, leaving the affected vessel patent. Fisher[104] and, independently, Ross Russell[105] observed material passing through the retinal circulation during attacks of transient monocular blindness, documenting that migrating particles could be associated with transient symptoms but leaving unsettled whether the material seen was actually embolic in character or could be compared to the "cattle trucking" (i.e., spaces of clumped red cells alternating with spaces of plasma) seen in retinal vessels in a setting of hypotension associated with cardiac arrest. Evidence has also been presented for clinically asymptomatic cerebral embolization in patients suffering symptomatic transient monocular blindness.[106] Other case reports have been explained as embolism,[107,108] instances inferred to have passed up the

ophthalmic artery, having arisen from the patent "stump" proximal ICA (Fig. 22-8), which was a mechanism popular decades ago but set aside in recent years.[109] Embolism from cardiac or large artery sources has rarely been inferred to have reached the basilar from the carotid artery via a persistent trigeminal artery.[110]

Despite such claims, the findings of Fisher and Ojemann[26] in a study of 90 carotid endarterectomy specimens have challenged the embolic theory as the typical source of TIAs. They found that three clinical categories—hemispheric TIAs, transient monocular blindness, and asymptomatic, severe carotid obstruction producing near occlusion—led to hemodynamic insufficiency as the cause of the transient symptoms. Mural thrombus, present in many of the specimens, contributed to the overall obstructive process but had little independent serious consequences beyond this effect (Fig. 22-9).

Hopes for clear proof of a carotid origin for embolism are often confounded: Even the famous case of Chiari, dating from 1905,[111] the index case of inferred embolism from carotid ulcer (Fig. 22-10), involved a patient whose autopsy also showed a patent cardiac foramen ovale, which nowadays is regarded as equally or possibly more suspect as a source of stroke.

If one puts the issue of source aside, that of *particle size* is obviously of great importance. The size of embolic material sufficient to cause retinal ischemia (0 to 100 microns) may be too small to affect or block any but the tiny pial surface branches in the hemisphere and is unlikely to cause symptoms. Particle size remains an unsettled issue for carotid plaque cap rupture and ulceration. Small size may explain the usually asymptomatic state of cases in which cholesterol emboli are found in retinal vessels. However, once carotid territory embolism has occurred, no matter how small the particle size, no studies to date have avoided intervention to test recurrent embolism particle size, for fear subsequent emboli could be much larger, as indicated by a few discouraging cases.[90,103]

The possibility of a major stroke in a setting of presumably minor carotid artery disease is the dreaded complication that continues to dictate many management decisions. The mural hemorrhage thesis of Lusby et al[112] dating back several decades and recently resurrected by concepts of plaque rupture raised the worry that a small ulcer or modest atheroma may suffice to allow a subintimal dissection to develop. The inferred subintimal hemorrhage as the destabilizing cause received little support from observational studies or clinical trials in the years since its presentation.[26,40,113]

The embolic theory can account for different types of carotid territory TIAs on the basis of separate embolic material occluding different intracranial branches, and many TIAs may occur as a result of this short-lived embolic mechanism.[114] However, the clinical and angiographic details in many of these cases suggest that they are a variant type of TIA. Duration of the TIA deficit in embolic cases appears to be far longer (hours or more) than the usual brief period (minutes).[115] Later assessments of syndrome duration also support the notion that longer events relate to risk factors associated with embolism, in particular atrial fibrillation.[116]

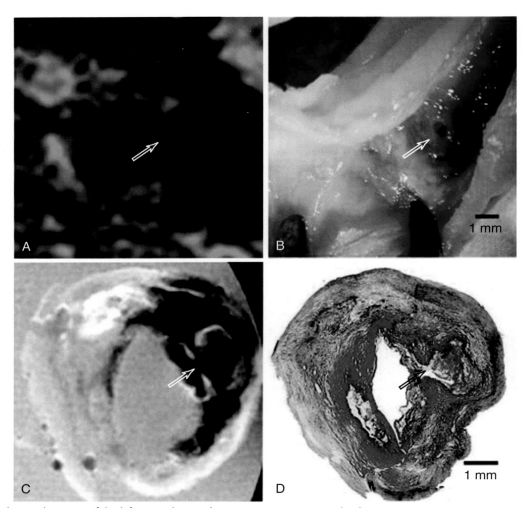

Figure 22-9 Plaque ulceration of the left internal carotid artery. A, In vivo T1-weighted MRI at 3T (repetition time, 1 RR of cardiac cycle; echo time, 10 ms; echo train, 9; 1 average and with heart rate of 50 bpm). B, Gross inspection of the carotid endarterectomy specimen. C, Ex vivo T1-weighted MRI at 11.7 T of the specimen. D, Trichrome-stained matched histology. *Arrows* in A through D indicate plaque ulceration and hemorrhage.

The classic *stereotypic TIAs* (see later on), in which attacks replicate themselves again and again, have proved difficult to document.[115] Their occurrence at any frequency is a major problem for the embolic theory, except for a single publication showing that artificial emboli injected into the carotid circulation in a dog model gathered in the same vessel.[117] In the published experience with aberrant embolization from polymeric silicone (Silastic) ball therapy used for arteriovenous malformations, several cases have been reported in which a similar syndrome occurred from embolism to a variety of different middle cerebral branches; the complaints included focal weakness of the arm[118] persisting for only a few minutes and transient dysesthesia of the contralateral hand, both of which are common symptoms of TIA. Such details are often lost on physicians from other specialties, as shown by studies indicating that many events that neurologists label as TIAs are not those of minor stroke and minor stroke is often included among the conditions labeled as TIAs by non-neurologists.[119]

Perfusion failure with distal insufficiency has long been recognized as a major mechanism that may account for cerebral ischemia. It explains the topography of cerebral infarcts, which in many cases of carotid occlusion closely mimics that found in obvious settings of hypotension such as cardiac arrest; in addition, the most reliable correlation with TIAs is severe stenosis. It implies decreased vascular perfusion in those areas of the brain parenchyma located at the greatest distance from the site of severe stenosis or occlusion.[120] In addition to impaired perfusion from low arterial pressure, stagnation thrombus has been observed in vessels at these distant sites,[121] and infarction follows. For the carotid system, if one assumes that collateral flow is available from the posterior cerebral for the lateral occipital and superior parietal areas, the regions at risk include the most distal segments of the cortical branches of the ACA and MCA, in particular the superior frontal and paracentral lobules.[122]

A lengthy list of publications documents the existence of infarction found along these regions in a setting of carotid occlusion or high-grade stenosis (Fig. 22-11).[123-131] In the 19th and early 20th centuries, common neuropathologic practice was to strip the pia-arachnoid off the brain, analogous to that for the kidney and liver, and for years

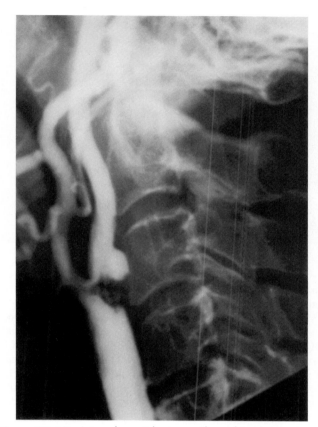

Figure 22-10 Internal carotid artery with combined stenosis and large ulceration.

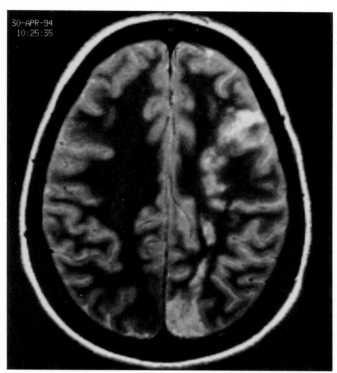

Figure 22-11 MRI scan of a distal-field (borderzone) infarction. (From Gautier JC, Mohr JP: Ischemic stroke. In Mohr JP, Gautier JC, editors: *Guide to clinical neurology*, New York, 1995, Churchill Livingstone, p 543.)

the role of vascular disease was unappreciated. The firm, pebbly, irregular surface of the naked brain earned names like *cirrhosis, granular atrophy,* and *cauliflower-like puckering* and was attributed to a number of processes, among them *infarct at a distance.* Such commentary is now the stuff of history, but interest in the mechanism of infarction became keen after Schneider's 1953 proposal of infarction by the process of distal insufficiency (so-called letzten Wiesen, or poorly supplied far fields—the metaphor being drawn from an agricultural irrigation system in which the pressure in the pump falls).[132] Despite the implied mechanism of transient hypotension, a high percentage of autopsy-documented cases with such infarct topography have been found to be associated with a thrombus or severe stenosis of the carotid artery.[26,107]

The advent of modern imaging studies, ranging from CT[127,131]—including xenon CT—to positron emission tomography (PET), has confirmed the correlation of a distal field topography with high-grade carotid stenosis or occlusion.[133-138] Lin et al[139] have not only teased from the case material a cohort of patients whose oxygen extraction fraction is increased, as shown by PET scanning, but also succeeded in correlating MRI and PET findings to assess CBF and have found a correlation with deep white matter infarct along the ventricular wall and low regional CBF as assessed by PET.[140] Known also as the "misery perfusion syndrome,"[141] this syndrome has been explained by reduced cerebral metabolism and has proved to be

surgically reversible from carotid stenosis and from intracranial angioplasty.[142]

Separate from PET studies, quantitative TCD ultrasonography has also been used to assess perfusion failure in carotid occlusive disease. Low reactivity of middle cerebral blood vessels in a setting of hypercapnia, a sign of fully dilated collateral vessels, has been documented by a number of groups to have a significant relationship ($P = 0.04$) to high-grade carotid stenosis.[143-145] The demonstration of such an extreme degree of sensitivity of cerebral flow to alterations in pCO_2 may help resurrect interest in notions of cerebral claudication,[146] which is a well-recognized clinical effect in the moyamoya disorder but is less well studied in carotid stenosis and occlusion.

Recently, CT perfusion techniques have even identified a "salvageable penumbra" capable of response to intraarterial thrombolytic therapy.[147]

The EC-IC bypass study met with disappointing results decades ago in part due to the inability to detect such perfusion failure by angiographic appearance alone. The concept has been revived in a clinical trial of those for whom oxygen extraction fraction as measured by PET detects such impaired metabolism and flow.[148] Many with carotid occlusion have ample replacement flow via the circle of Willis. Compared with the large numbers of cases deemed suitable for the original EC-IC study and based on the demonstration of carotid occlusion alone, special efforts have been needed to find those showing the required PET results.

There is also the possibility of *multimechanism infarction*. Modern imaging has allowed some assessment of the frequencies of embolism or signs of perfusion failure. A study of 102 consecutive cases with varying degrees of carotid stenosis found distal field lesions in approximately 50% of patients with high-grade carotid stenosis or occlusion and almost an equal number with "territorial infarctions" (i.e., inferred single-branch occlusions in those with occlusion). Of special interest was the observation that 77.8% of the cases with high-grade carotid stenosis had a perfusion-diffusion mismatch, that is, larger zones of impairment on perfusion-weighted MRI compared with the somewhat smaller lesions documented on diffusion-weighted MRI.[149]

Clinical Syndromes

The basic clinical features of extracranial carotid disease have been amply described for well over a century. The characteristic clinical syndrome of ICA occlusion has long been known to consist of "premonitory fleeting symptoms including paresthesias, paralysis, monocular blindness and aphasia," a description that preceded the concept later to be known as TIA.[150] It was the prospect of therapy that prompted so much interest in carotid disease. C.M. Fisher played a major role after World War II in the renewal of interest in the clinical importance of carotid disease first promulgated by Hvlquist, in a little noted work on the eve of World War II. In his early clinicopathologic studies, Fisher described the prodromal transient neurologic events frequently preceding stroke, discussed possible stroke mechanisms, and predicted the surgical treatment. Eastcott et al[151] were the first to reconstruct an extracranial ICA lesion successfully. Thus began the modern era in diagnosis and management of extracranial carotid artery disease.

Ischemic Stroke from Carotid Artery Disease
Ocular Infarction

Although both the eye and the brain are susceptible to ischemia from carotid disease, it is remarkable how infrequently the eye alone is the site of a permanent deficit. In textbook tables of frequencies, the eye and the brain are often listed as if they may show symptoms together, but simultaneous eye and brain infarction from hemodynamic carotid artery disease, known as the *opticocerebral syndrome* is distinctly rare: a mere 3 (0.5%) of 612 cases were found in one series of consecutive patients with carotid territory stroke.[152]

In natural history studies of transient monocular blindness (TMB, also known as amaurosis fugax—see later),[153] retinal infarction occurs in a small percentage of patients monitored over the long term. The presumed mechanism is embolic occlusion of either a retinal branch or the central retinal artery. Considerable controversy, however, has centered on the relationship between the embolic material and associated carotid artery disease as a potential source (see earlier discussion). *Cholesterol crystals* discovered in the retinal circulation are a known marker for systemic atherosclerosis, from the time of Hollenhorst's original 1961 report.[154] They are often noted incidentally

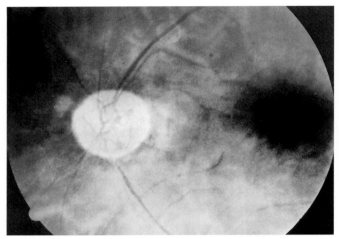

Figure 22-12 Attenuated retinal vessels.

on routine ophthalmologic examination in asymptomatic patients.[155,156]

The particulate matter explaining focal infarction has a wide range of causes. *Cholesterol emboli* may cause retinal branch occlusion,[105,157] but the embolic material is usually platelet debris. Pessin et al[158] found 42 instances of retinal cholesterol plaques, branch retinal artery occlusion, or central retinal artery occlusion in 39 patients; the incidence of carotid disease (56% to 60%) was not different for the groups with these separate types of retinal symptoms.

Central Retinal Artery Occlusion

Several large series of patients with central retinal artery occlusion who underwent cerebral angiography have documented ipsilateral carotid artery disease (i.e., ulcerative nonstenotic, stenotic without ulceration or irregularity, or occlusive) consistent with an embolic source in 50% to 70% of cases.[158-160] Carotid territory TIAs, including TMB, had occurred in many patients before central retinal artery occlusion. In all these instances, the particle size is small—on the order of 90 microns—and about the size of intracortical hemisphere microanastomoses.

Ischemic Optic Neuropathy

This disorder is widely acknowledged to be related to ischemia at the optic nerve head[161] and has a wide range of causes, including arteritis, carotid dissection, Takayasu's disease, carotid cavernous fistula, and many sources of embolism.[162] However, carotid stenosis is not high on the list, estimated to affect only 5% of patients in one of the early series[163] and 1.6% in a more recent one.[164]

The ocular abnormalities are (1) pupillary dilatation with poor light reaction, (2) neovascularization of the iris (rubeosis iridis), (3) elevated intraocular pressure with secondary glaucoma, and (4) proliferative retinopathy (Figs. 22-12 and 22-13) with microaneurysms, scattered flame-shaped hemorrhages, and prominent venous stasis.[163,165-168] Significant visual loss sometimes ending in blindness with optic atrophy makes this a serious condition. The presumed pathogenesis of reduced orbital blood flow has led some investigators to claim that the chronic changes of ocular ischemia may be reversible with EC-IC

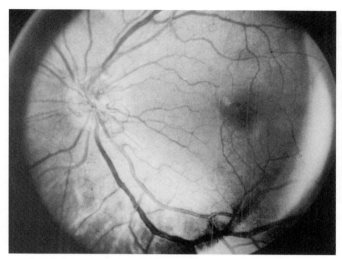

Figure 22-13 Neovascular proliferation affecting the disc.

arterial grafting,[168] coiling of a cavernous sinus fistula,[169] and even stellate ganglion block.[170]

Unusual Ocular Syndromes

A small series of cases have been described with symptoms and signs referable to the orbit in cases of carotid artery disease. For some, a variant of *migraine, Raeder's syndrome,* and the like have been described. Gelmers[171] described two cases with facial pain and ipsilateral oculosympathetic paresis, which he labeled the *pericarotid syndrome.* This researcher attributed the ocular disturbance to disease affecting the cervical portion of the ICA, as demonstrated angiographically.

The Anterior Choroidal Artery

The anterior choroidal artery (AChA) is a branch of the intracranial internal carotid, arising distal to the ophthalmic artery but below the circle of Willis. Its size compares with that of cerebral surface artery branches, but its location makes it an uncommon site of occlusion that causes stroke. A collateral path from the posterior choroidal system via the lateral geniculate body may explain clinical or imaging consequences from occlusion of the AChA near its origin. There is increasing awareness of the variety of syndromes from infarction in the AChA vascular territory, although for decades it was rarely considered among carotid artery syndromes. Accordingly, an anterior choroidal origin for stenoses or occlusion in the carotid siphon should be considered on the list that had been classically limited to the eye and the cerebral hemisphere.

Anatomic Aspects

In 1891, Kolisko[172] reported results of a pathologic series using injection techniques to determine the territory of the AChA, with clinical correlation; it was the first such description of a syndrome. He demonstrated that the AChA supplies the posterior two thirds of the posterior limb of the internal capsule, the retrolenticular fibers posterior to the internal capsule, the medial aspect of the pallidum, the uncus, the posterior portion of the optic tract, the tail of the caudate nucleus, the lateral choroid plexus, and

posterior and superficial areas of the thalamus. A decade later, Beevor[173] added the anterior portion of the cerebral peduncle, and in the 1930s Abbie[174] included a role in the supply of the lateral geniculate body. In the succeeding decades, similar findings from injection studies were made by Alexander[175] and Herman,[176] from microsurgical studies,[177] and from MRI and MR angiography.[178]

Autopsy Studies

Beginning with the article by Foix et al,[179] which some consider to be the first clinicoanatomic effort although earlier examples can be found,[180] such publications regularly showed a smaller territory on infarction. Irving S. Cooper[181] and, separately, Rand et al[182] undertook deliberate occlusion expecting to cause infarction of the peduncle of the midbrain with improvement in Parkinson symptoms but found only limited effects. From these observations came the common view that occlusion of this vessel would have few clinical effects. These findings might have been explained by retrograde collateral into the AChA from the posterior choroidal artery (PChA). Some reports argued otherwise.[183,184]

Imaging studies such as modern CT and MRI reawakened interest in the AChA. Helgason et al postulated a hemihypesthetic–ataxic syndrome,[185,186] drawing on the CT maps created by Damasio,[187] which prompted challenges from other authors. Based on these considerations, some reports argued such infarcts should be considered as the small, deep types labeled as *lacunes.*[188] Ambiguities in the location of the regions of supply prompted challenges from others concerned that infarcts long inferred to affect the lateral lenticulostriates—MCA origin—might be commingled with and considered due to occlusion of the AChA.[189] MRI of the infarct unambiguously, angiographically documented that AChA infarction affects the uncus, amygdaloid nucleus, genu and posterior limb of the internal capsule, globus pallidus, lateral geniculate body, and tail of the caudate nucleus.[190,191] Others consider that they have demonstrated the AChA as a cause of infarction affecting the posterior leg of the internal capsule and extending upward into the paraventricular corona.[192] The matter continues to attract interest and was discussed in detail as separate chapters in prior editions of this book.[193,194]

Causes

Mixed etiologies apply to the AChA, and the larger infarcts have a higher association with embolism.[195,196] That some of the larger ones are explained by occlusion along much of the AChA territory has been determined by unfortunate outcomes in a setting of glue embolism, where opportunities for retrograde collateral via the PChA are limited.[197] Autopsy documentation of AChA occlusion with involvement of the lateral geniculate has been rare. PChA disease with lateral geniculate infarction has also only been rarely diagnosed: one fully studied example by autopsy and serial section had embolism blocking the PCA at the origin of the choroidal artery branch.[198] In living patients, two examples showed angiographic stenosis of the PCA with MRI evidence of lateral geniculate infarction.[199,200] How embolism creates the large infarcts is unsettled.

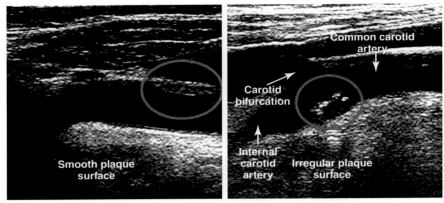

Figure 22-14 *Left panel,* Regular carotid plaque surface. *Right panel,* Irregular carotid plaque surface. (From Prabhakaran S, Rundek T, Ramas R, et al: Carotid plaque surface irregularity predicts ischemic stroke: The Northern Manhattan Stroke Study. *Stroke* 37:2696-2701, 2006, by permission.)

An AChA origin for small, deep arterial occlusion explained by microatheroma is increasingly being considered to be the explanation for the infarct affecting the deep basal ganglia and thalamus found by imaging. The neuropathologic basis for such a conclusion is slim, as is *distal field* infarction from intracranial ICA stenosis or occlusion. Nonetheless, the hemiparesis syndrome from AChA territory infarction can be among the most severe and persistent.

Clinical Syndromes

Considering the spectrum of sites affected by the AChA, it is perhaps no surprise that a wide range of syndromes have been attributed to occlusion along its course. These include pure motor stroke,[185] pure sensory stroke, sensorimotor stroke,[201] pseudobulbar state,[183] mutism,[202] possibly a form of neglect,[203] and remarkable visual field disturbances including homonymous hemianopia,[204] homonymous scotoma,[205] and quadrantic defects and sectoranopia.[198]

Cerebral Infarction

The number of instances of cerebral infarction in the territory of the ICA far exceeds the instances in which the mechanism of the stroke is determined.[55] Difficulties in determining whether the ICA is occluded, severely stenosed, slightly stenosed, ulcerated, or merely the conduit for the embolic material remain a major obstacle to progress in the analysis of cases of stroke in the carotid artery territory.

After a variable number of TIAs, the completed stroke that results from severe stenosis or occlusion of the ICA is explained by embolism, infarction from anterograde extension of carotid occlusion, embolization, or distal flow failure.[67,206] *Anterograde extension* is decidedly rare. Embolism is considered the most common mechanism and appears to account for virtually two thirds of strokes with ICA occlusion.[82] *Distal insufficiency* explains perhaps the other third. Simultaneous infarction of the eye and brain is rare.[207] The spectrum of clinical findings after carotid artery occlusion is wide, ranging from no symptoms to disastrous outcomes.[208]

Intracranial Internal Carotid Artery Embolism

Intracranial ICA embolism has also been commonly found in autopsy studies.[112,209-211] Embolism has also been the proposed mechanism in prior studies for some of the strokes that are delayed in onset after carotid artery occlusion.[3,67,109,212-214]

Embolism, regardless of whether its source is clarified, may be a common cause of stroke associated with carotid artery thrombosis. Pessin et al,[82] reporting fully 25 of the 64 cases evaluated angiographically, showed evidence of intracranial main stem or branch MCA occlusion, and another 17 had findings consistent with or suggestive of earlier embolization. The clinical picture in these 42 cases contrasted sharply with the 22 with no signs of embolism; less than half of the patients (17 of 42) had experienced prior TIAs, and 13 had strokes, which were moderately severe in 7 patients and mild in only 6. This difference in TIA frequency and stroke severity was the reverse of the pattern in the group whose symptoms were attributed to distal insufficiency. On clinical grounds of severity and topography of cerebral infarction, there appears to be no essential difference between the type and severity of the syndromes with carotid and cardiac sources.[82,127] In a recent report from the population-based Northern Manhattan Stroke Study, with a mean follow-up of 2.7 years for a stroke-free population of 1939 patients with carotid Doppler studies for whom plaque was visualized in 56% (irregular plaque in 5.5%), 69 had strokes during a 6-year follow-up. The unadjusted 5-year stroke rates were 1.3% for no plaque, 3.0% for regular plaque, and 8.5% for irregular plaque. In a multiple risk factor model, the odds ratio for plaque was 3.1 (95% confidence interval [CI], 1.1 to 8.5)[215] (Fig. 22-14). The clinical details of the stroke syndromes are discussed in the chapter on MCA disease (see Chapter 24).

Several sources of embolism can occur from the carotid, apart from cardiac, transcardiac (e.g., patent cardiac foramen ovale), or aortic arch sources (discussed in other chapters). *Anterograde propagation of the thrombosis intracranially* may result in a tail of thrombus that lies at the top of the ICA; the tail is then available to be swept distally via retrograde flow through the ophthalmic artery and into the middle and anterior cerebral arteries above.[105,216] Lethal hemispheric stroke has been encountered in one patient 3 days after angiographically documented occlusion of the ipsilateral cerebral ICA. The autopsy evidence was consistent with embolism from the distal intracranial tail of the propagated carotid thrombus. An infarct this large had not previously been reported.[216]

Embolization may also arise from the *stump of the ICA* that remains emanating from the bifurcation of the CCA after ICA occlusion; the Venturi effect of blood passing up the CCA to the ECA may sweep material from the stump distally to reach the intracranial arteries. First proposed by H.J.M. Barnett[197] and elaborated on with colleagues,[109] it appeared to be demonstrated in some dramatic case reports.[217,218] Stumpectomy and, more recently, isolation of the stump have been reported, but no clinical series has appeared.

Small-particle embolism appears by far to be the most common and is seen in those undergoing endovascular procedures[190]; most are asymptomatic for the patient.[195] Microembolism, that is, embolism inferred to be occurring in patients in whom high-intensity transient signals (HITS) are found at TCD ultrasonography and interpreted as evidence of platelet or plaque material but not regarded as harbingers or causes of stroke, was initially considered to be a potential cause of a dementia-like picture slowly emerging over time (see later).[219] However, the HITS relate more to degree of stenosis than they do to evidence of clinically important embolism.

Anterograde Extension of Thrombus

Pathologic studies of ICA thrombosis have documented anterograde extension of thrombus intracranially for varying distances; these are not so much a source of embolism as thrombotic occlusion of the circle of Willis. In a number of cases, extension occurred across the circle of Willis into the stems of the ACA and MCA, yielding devastating cerebral infarction.[6,67,123,124,212]

It is a source of the rare *telodiencephalic syndrome*,[220] featuring contralateral faciobrachial hemiplegia accompanied by homonymous hemianopia and aphasia (when the patient is able to be tested) and is associated with ipsilateral hemihypohidrosis and an ipsilateral Horner syndrome.[221] We consider it to be caused by an ischemic lesion of the crossed pathways descending from the cerebrum and the uncrossed hypothalamic–spinal sympathetic pathways.

Hemispheric Infarction with Distal Insufficiency

The clinical syndromes from cerebral infarction from this mechanism are characterized by a prominent visual field defect, aphasia or hemi-inattention features (from dominant or nondominant hemisphere involvement, respectively), and variable degrees of contralateral sensorimotor deficit. Based on now somewhat outmoded classic clinicopathologic correlations of the homunculus,[222] the latter should affect the proximal more than the distal segments of the upper limb, reflecting the location of the infarct along the upper portions of the frontal-parietal convexity.[120] Although the preceding constellation of symptoms is commonly found (bilaterally) in cases of cardiac arrest and hypotension with resulting bilateral distal field infarction, its unilateral occurrence from ICA atherothrombosis was not documented by CT scanning until the mid-1980s.[122]

Of diagnostic importance is that these syndromes are generally *less severe* than those attributed to embolism and feature a higher frequency of premonitory TIAs.[82] Although a possible explanation for recurrent stereotypic TIAs,[223] distal insufficiency has proved difficult to document as the source of cerebral infarction from ICA disease and depends on imaging evidence of either impaired perfusion or metabolism or both.

Numerous autopsy-documented studies have detailed findings and a relationship to the clinical picture in suprasylvian unilateral cerebral infarcts.[3,67,120,123,124,128,132,212] In many of the cases, the infarct developed in relation to carotid occlusion, under which circumstances the main bulk of the endangered territory lay between the ACA and MCA, causing softening in the upper frontal lobe.

The effects most commonly reported have been unilateral infarctions. Common symptoms are weakness, paralysis, dyspraxia, numbness and tingling, and stereo-dysnomia in one or more fingers or in the hand, wrist, or arm and leg. Grasp reflex has been observed. Transient impairment of ocular motility is often reported; in cases in which it is not reported, the meaning of the omission is unclear. Disturbances in higher cerebral function have included episodes of speechlessness and changes in personality,[121,124,220] as well as dysgraphia of both the paretic and dyspraxic types.[82,121,123-129,224]

A few well-known examples from the older literature indicate the long-standing recognition of the syndrome and remain landmarks of case descriptions. The patient reported by Elder in 1900 was a 69-year-old messenger who developed stepwise attacks of worsening right arm and leg paresis with slight dysarthria.[225] Sensation was said to be normal, and he had no hemianopia. His left eye was frequently painful. A right grasp was noted. The attacks progressed to hemiplegia, which spared his face. The patient's speech was intact, as were auditory comprehension and repetition. His writing was clumsy, large, and confined to his own name and a few letters; he found copying difficult. He named objects presented at sight easily. He was unable to read aloud and could manage only a few letters with frequent repetitions. At autopsy, white vessel and extensive infarction was observed extending from the upper frontal region to involve almost the entire lateral parietal and occipital regions. Spatz's famous case from 1935 occurred in a 43-year-old man whose problems began with attacks of headache and shimmering in the left eye.[129] He later experienced weakness in the right arm and disturbance of speech in which he often failed to find a word. A right homonymous hemianopia was observed. No tests of reading were reported. At autopsy, the suprasylvian territory of the left cerebral hemisphere from the frontal through posterior parietal regions was involved with "granular atrophy."

High-convexity infarction: The predominance of high-convexity infarction in carotid syndromes of distal insufficiency has yielded some distinctive syndromes (Fig. 22-15). Timsit et al[226] found examples of *fractional (different*

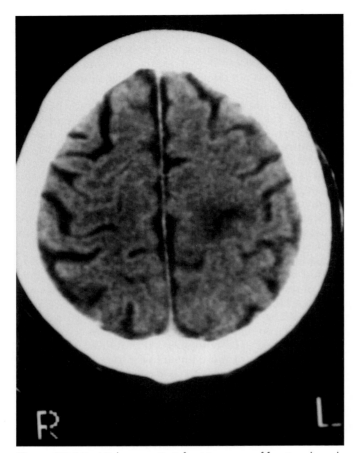

Figure 22-15 High-convexity infarct in a case of fractional weakness (see text).

degrees of) weakness in the shoulder versus the hand, which was thought to reflect the upper convexity infarction from distal insufficiency. Examples of embolism more often showed comparable degrees of weakness of the hand and shoulder, consistent with larger and lower convexity infarction. The probability of carotid artery disease rather than embolism was greater when fractional arm weakness (strength in the shoulder different from that in the hand) was present (odds ratio, 5.3; 95% CI, 3.1 to 9.0), which was a finding confirmed by the same group in another study.[227]

A preponderance of *leg weakness* has also been described in two separate reports.[210,228] The 19 patients described by Yanagihara et al[228] had episodic or progressive lower extremity weakness contralateral to severe extracranial ICA occlusive disease (16 patients) or carotid siphon stenosis (3 patients). Cerebral blood measurements, with the use of xenon-133 in some of the patients, corroborated reduced hemispheric flow on the appropriate side localized to the borderzone in the frontoparietal areas corresponding to motor function of the lower extremity.

Pure Dementia

Case reports continue to appear referring to dementia risk from arteriosclerosis in general[229] and, in a setting of stroke from occult repeated emboli,[230] showing high convexity, "distal field" infarction with high-grade carotid stenosis[231-233] or extracranial carotid disease and MRI evidence of brain infarction (this last from the Framingham Study).[234] Studies of mental function after carotid endarterectomy have used a battery of tests of memory and mental agility. Reports have appeared in which scores on tests conducted before and after successful endarterectomy indicate an initial improvement,[235] but thus far persistence of the improvement is open to question. Improvement has also been reported after EC-IC bypass,[235,236] as well as after stenting,[237] but some studies have not shown an improvement.[238] Data on the prevalence and course of dementia after surgery or endovascular procedures will be published from the Carotid Revascularization by Endarterectomy or Stent Trial (CREST).[238a]

Reversible Ischemic Neurologic Deficit

The usefulness of the older concept of reversible ischemic neurologic deficit has been questioned on the grounds that it has no prognostic value.[239,240] Arguments have now been put forward that a syndrome that clears slowly and requires more than 24 hours to do so is a sign of infarction, as has been corroborated many times by imaging.[95]

Some carotid-related strokes begin and progress in such a way that accumulation of neurologic deficit occurs over hours to a day or more, giving rise to the term *progressive stroke* or *evolving stroke*. The brain has clearly suffered infarction in this situation, but the patient may have only a submaximal neurologic deficit for the arterial territory affected. For example, if a patient has mild to moderate right arm and hand weakness but face, leg, speech, and visual field function are spared, the patient is considered to have a submaximal deficit for the territory involved, even though infarction may be present on a CT scan. The mechanism responsible for this deficit might recur, leading to further disability, unless treatment is offered. This approach, which stresses submaximal deficit rather than whether the brain has suffered infarction, allows for the opportunity of treatment (surgical or medical) in the hopes of preventing further disability.

Transient Ischemic Attacks

TIAs are defined as a focal, ischemic neurologic deficit of brief duration. For carotid territory TIAs in a setting of high-grade stenosis, their duration is typically 5 to 15 minutes.[241,242] Despite uncertainty regarding the origin of TIA as a syndrome of duration less than or equal to 24 hours, ample evidence supports TIA as a strong marker of stroke risk, mechanism, and source, namely—albeit not exclusively—embolism from the carotid arteries. For carotid stroke, the prognostic significance of TIA indicating stroke risk is clearly evident from the carotid surgery trials showing an almost tenfold higher risk of stroke in patients presenting with TIA and carotid stenosis as compared with cases with asymptomatic arterial narrowing. Further, recurrent TIAs with similar or identical clinical presentation clearly hint of an arterial obstruction, most frequently of the carotids. Most TIAs caused by carotid artery obstruction arise from embolism; however, hemodynamic failure presenting as brief spells of focal neurologic symptoms are well-known, and TIAs are not exclusively related to the carotid arteries. Cardiac embolism as well as lacunar syndromes may also present as abrupt-onset focal cerebral deficits lasting less than 24 hours. Last, but not least, other disease entities may present as brief spells of circumscribed cerebral dysfunction, the most frequent of which are migrainous aura and partial seizure.

How the notion of a 24-hour duration for TIAs became established has been difficult to determine. As best we can discover, far shorter durations were widely recognized during the years of the early Princeton Conferences.[243] The first citation suggesting such a long duration was that by Marshall,[244] whose review cited only a few instances of focal events lasting longer than a few minutes; nevertheless, he proposed 24 hours as a means to ensure not including in the definition cases in which the origin was not vascular. This expanded definition became widely accepted, based as it was on clinical criteria only in the days long before modern imaging.

When the subject has been studied through the use of actual case material, the 24-hour criterion has been recognized to be excessive.[115] The typical carotid territory TIAs are brief, typically lasting only some 7 to 10 minutes, as stated by patients in retrospective interviews. (TIAs are almost always assessed by interview, but in the attacks we have observed in patients, there is often a distortion of time in a patient's memory.) These brief spells have a higher correlation with angiographic evidence of tight carotid stenosis than do spells lasting an hour or longer. However, the prognosis for subsequent stroke appears to be the same regardless of whether the spell is brief or long.[239,245] More important, evidence has been demonstrated in the literature of brain infarction in patients whose syndromes last longer than an hour[246] with disturbed MR spectroscopy findings in the ipsilateral hemisphere.[247] Calls for a redefinition of TIA limited to an hour are thus not new.[248] An effort by a small consortium has attempted a reawakening of the definition of the TIA as lasting an hour or less, now cited as the "one-hour rule."[249]

The importance of carotid TIAs is highlighted when they are viewed from the perspective of carotid stroke. Patients who have a carotid stroke from extracranial carotid artery occlusion disease have a known prior TIA incidence of 50% to 75%.[115,250-252]

This situation contrasts sharply with the low incidence of TIAs (approximately 10%) associated with all types of stroke considered as a group and reinforces the strong relationship between these transient events and underlying atherothrombotic occlusive disease. The available data, both prospective and retrospective, indicate that TIAs may be impressive warnings of stroke in some patients, and their recognition provides the opportunity for therapeutic intervention.

Despite the large numbers of studies on TIAs, so many differences exist in definitions and methodology that all too many of the studies are disappointingly unhelpful. Few have focused on carotid territory TIAs alone, and even fewer have separated TMB from transient hemispheric attacks (THAs). Some studies emphasize incidence, and others describe prevalence. TIAs have been documented by various methods, including personal periodic examinations and searches of clinical records; questionnaires have also been used.[253-260]

The available data show a wide range in *prevalence and incidence.* The prevalence varies from 1.1 to 77 per 1000 persons, and the incidence rate varies from 2.2 to 8 per 1000 persons per year.[253,256,257] The stroke risk associated with TIAs is significant, although no well-designed, randomized controlled study has provided unequivocal information on the natural history of TIAs, nor is such a study likely to be done today. Past studies have assessed the stroke risk to be between 2% and 50%, which is a range so discrepant as to be useless in an individual case.[98,209,244,261-266] These studies suffer from several limitations, including ambiguity of TIA definition, lumping together of carotid and vertebral basilar TIAs, and, most important, no angiographic verification of underlying vascular disease. Despite the limitations of these early studies, the view emerged that a considerable stroke risk attends TIAs, namely, in the range of 35% over 5 years, or 5% to 6% a year.[256]

Many of the important questions relating TIAs to specific carotid lesion configurations, such as irregular plaques, ulcers, severe stenosis, and occlusion, remain unanswered, despite all the effort expended on the subject thus far.[267] At the least, the available evidence indicates that a serious stroke may follow a TIA in a discouraging number of patients; however, the factors contributing to the risks for individuals have remained elusive.

The argument of whether the outlook for TIA cases was too benign for endarterectomy to influence outcome favorably[13,268-270] has been settled by the dramatic results of the studies for symptomatic patients: both the NASCET and the European Cooperative Study showed a clear advantage of surgery over medical (aspirin) therapy (for further details, see Chapter 75 on endarterectomy). Neither trial tested surgery against anticoagulation, and the most striking of the positive findings were in those patients whose stenosis exceeded 70%. Over a period of 18 months in NASCET, of patients who were symptomatic with TIAs and who were found to have stenosis of 70% to 90%, 7% of the 300 who underwent surgery had a stroke or died, mostly in the perioperative period, whereas 24% of the 295 undergoing aspirin therapy had a stroke or died. This difference favoring surgery was highly significant ($P < 0.001$).[271] The risk of stroke was higher in patients with brain imaging showing "leukoaraiosis" than in those without such findings.[252] The outcomes and best management plans for those whose stenosis was in the 30% to 70% range were less striking: only modest or minimal benefits were seen with surgery.

Recent large cohort studies of management for TIA in a setting of intervention-eligible carotid stenosis support the long-standing bias toward intervention to avoid infarction.[272]

Differential Diagnosis of Transient Ischemic Attacks

Interobserver agreement on the diagnosis has remained a problem.[119,273] Many types of spells similar or even partly identical to TIAs have different pathogeneses and stroke prognoses.[223,273] The concept of TIA is based on an atherothrombotic mechanism, especially that of high-grade carotid stenosis, a preventable form of subsequent stroke, which makes the search for this cause well worth distinguishing TIAs from other types of spells.[243]

Seizures, migraine accompaniments, isolated vestibular syndromes, and transient memory disturbance are common conditions that may be confused with TIAs. Defying the definition of a focal encephalic deficit, rarely even episodes of syncope are falsely labeled "TIA." Even spells considered to meet the definition of TIAs may have an underlying vascular mechanism other than large artery atherothrombotic disease. TIAs may be related to small, penetrating arterial disease that causes lacunar infarction. They may occur as a flurry in the hours before stroke (so-called lacunar stutter or capsular warning syndrome) or as isolated events without stroke. The clinical features of lacunar TIAs may be indistinguishable from those of large artery TIAs, yet the diagnostic evaluation, treatment, and stroke risks are probably different. Also, rapidly fading cerebral embolism may give rise to a short-lived neurologic deficit consistent with the time criterion of TIA, but no atherothrombotic mechanism may exist. In one study,[115] such TIAs of a presumed embolic mechanism tended to be of longer duration, more than 1 hour, than TIAs from a carotid atheromatous cause.

All these variations should alert the clinician to the heterogeneous nature of TIAs. They are best viewed as symptoms, much like seizures and headaches, not as a homogeneous, pathogenic state. Further clarification of the underlying cerebrovascular mechanisms may lead to more rational therapy and more reliable prognostication.

Transient Ischemic Attacks with Intracranial Internal Carotid Artery Disease

TIAs can be expected to occur in atherosclerosis of the intracranial ICA, as in extracranial ICA disease. However, precise data are lacking. One reason is that most studies of TIAs have not isolated those specifically due to intracranial ICA lesions, and the few that did so have not dealt with symptoms, only with duration or prevalence. The common association is the occurrence of TIAs with lesions elsewhere, and the common occurrence of tandem lesions makes it difficult to sort out those TIAs that could specifically result from intracranial ICA disease.[68,69] Even though the ophthalmic artery arises from the intracranial ICA, amaurosis fugax (TMB) has been difficult to demonstrate in association with atherosclerosis in that portion of the vessel.[115,153,157,274-277] Very few specific cases have been recorded. Gerstenfeld[278] reported on a 30-year-old man who had many attacks of amaurosis fugax of the right eye. White streaks were seen in the retinal arterioles. Angiography disclosed an ICA occlusion above the level of the ophthalmic artery. In addition, the ophthalmic artery had an unusually early origin from the ICA because it arose from the infraclinoid part. It should be noted that a severe right frontal headache was mentioned, a very uncommon feature of amaurosis fugax, and in such a young patient, atherosclerosis would appear unlikely. Dyll et al[279] reported on a patient with four attacks of amaurosis fugax and roughening and narrowing of the uncoiled carotid siphon proximal to the origin of the ophthalmic artery. David[280] also described a case of amaurosis fugax with siphon lesions and a possible embolic mechanism.

Transient Monocular Blindness

TMB, also known as amaurosis fugax, has been recognized as an important manifestation of carotid artery disease since early reports.[281] TMB may be considered a brief monocular visual obscuration described by patients as a fog, blur, cloud, mist, and so forth. A shade or curtain effect occurs in only a minority of cases, approximately 15% to 20%, and is no more predictive of carotid artery disease than other variations of monocular visual loss.[223] The duration of visual impairment is brief, usually less than 15 minutes and rarely exceeding 30 minutes, and most patients are affected for only 1 to 5 minutes.[105,274,277,282,283]

Flashing lights, scintillations, colors, and fortification spectra rarely occur as TIA manifestations and usually signify a migrainous event.[283] However, the presence of visual phenomena during TMB in patients with greater than 75% stenosis has been recorded by Goodwin et al,[284] which makes differentiation from retinal migraine difficult on clinical grounds alone in some cases.

The number of TMB attacks that occur before a patient seeks medical attention varies greatly. Patients may experience a few or as many as 100 attacks of TMB over a span of several days to a year or more.[115] Vision is usually fully restored after an attack, although in long-term follow-up studies of affected patients,[153] a small number may sustain permanent visual loss from retinal infarction. TMB rarely occurs simultaneously with other neurologic deficits, and headache is not part of the disturbance. Hemisphere stroke is an infrequent sequel of TMB alone,[153,285,286] but careful studies of such cases occasionally reveal evidence of clinically unobvious cerebral embolism.[106] In most instances, clinically obvious stroke is preceded by one or more THAs. TMB tends to precede the first THA and can be documented with a careful history.

TMB poses endless diagnostic interpretation difficulties. The failure of the retinal arteries to show any abnormality during a period of TMB has been so often described that the normal appearance of the retinal arteries has been speculated to be a sign that the inferred embolic material or low-flow state applies to the choroidal circulation, which would not be visualized by the ophthalmoscope. However, experimental occlusion of the central retinal artery for up to 98 minutes was not revealed by ophthalmoscopic change, and no significant permanent neurologic damage was observed.[287] Occlusion for 105 minutes or longer, however, produced irreversible damage. Nonetheless, even then, no permanent injury was obvious in the retinal vascular bed. Only a transient leakage of fluorescein was observed 2.5 to 3 hours after the occlusion. These findings show that ophthalmoscopically normal vessels may be observed even in a setting of complete retinal artery occlusion.[276]

More than a century ago, Gowers[288] believed he had found intravascular material in his report on embolic material in the vessels supplying the eye. Cholesterol crystals, now known by his name (Hollenhorst plaques), were described by the Mayo Clinic ophthalmologist Hollenhorst.[154] He emphasized the association of the retinal material with systemic atherosclerosis and significant cardiovascular mortality, although he was uncertain about concomitant visual symptoms related to this particulate material.[154,289] He noted, however, that the embolic material in some cases was not necessarily associated with TMB. Reports prompted by the rare opportunity to observe a patient during an attack of TMB have described white or grayish material passing through the retinal circulation, presumably platelet complexes, perhaps mixed with fibrin.[104,105] This material is believed by many to be what is visualized by the ophthalmoscope in the rare instances of TMB studied during an attack.

Although he has been credited with the first description of such material observed during an attack, Fisher[104] was careful not to make too great a claim for how the material reached the vascular tree, and he left open the possibility that it may have been embolic or generated by local events such as sludging from inadequate perfusion. Gerstenfeld[278] found similar white bodies, but the disease in his reported cases was confined to the ICA above the origin of the ophthalmic artery. In other case reports, only pallor of the disc was found, even given a source for embolic material in the proximal ICA.[279] McBrien et al[290] succeeded in demonstrating a platelet origin for some of the embolic material seen in the retina of a 37-year-old man who had two episodes of blindness, of which the last left him with a permanent nasal field defect. Platelet material was found in a superior nasal branch (apparently serving a portion of the visual field that was clinically unaffected). In the rare instances of calcium emboli to the retinal artery, an opportunity was provided to document the visual loss associated with focal branch occlusions. Brockmeier et al[291] described four patients whose accompanying visual loss corresponded to the location of the retinal embolus. Transient visual loss of the type attributed to retinal branch occlusion with platelet aggregates was not encountered. These investigators suggested that the small size of the calcific emboli was sufficient to plug retinal arteries but insufficient to precipitate clinical symptoms in the cerebrum. However, Beal et al[92] documented several sites of cerebral infarction in a 69-year-old man who experienced numerous brief spells of numbness and weakness consistent with hemispheric TIAs, which indicates that some such particles can be large enough to precipitate symptoms. Cattle trucking, a sign described in agonal settings, has also been seen in the vessels during some attacks.[276]

A rare case of transient vertical monocular hemianopia has also been described: the attacks were attributed to an anomalous arteriolar pattern, in that both the superior and inferior nasal quadrants were supplied by the same arterial branch.[292] Microembolization to this common arteriolar trunk may have accounted for the six episodes of monocular vertical hemianopia occurring in a 3-day period in this case.

Winterkorn et al[293] described nine patients in whom TMB was associated with a variety of medical conditions unrelated to emboli or carotid hypoperfusion. This benign form was attributed to vasoconstriction of the retinal arterioles observed during funduscopic examination in several of their patients. The symptoms were responsive to calcium channel blockers. The clinical features show some variation from the TMB associated with carotid disease. Almost half of the patients in this report were older than 50 years and had had multiple attacks; some had had as

many as 40, often several a day over a brief period. Retro-orbital ache was noted in four of the nine patients. Several of the younger patients had a history of migraine or autoimmune conditions, but these features were not present in the older patients. In two older patients, temporal artery biopsy results were negative for temporal arteritis. This mechanism may partly explain the well-known clinical recognition of a benign form of TMB in younger patients.

Yet another variant of TMB has been reported by Furlan et al[294]; in five patients with high-grade ICA stenosis or occlusion, exposure to bright light (often sunlight) precipitated transient unilateral visual loss. All the patients also had typical, unprovoked TMB and reduced retinal artery pressure in the affected eye; three also had hemispheric TIAs. Hemodynamic insufficiency of the retinal circulation was the probable mechanism leading to reduced photochemical resynthesis of visual pigments by the retinal rods and cones. Donnan et al[295] recorded impairment of visual evoked responses in four patients with similar symptoms. Wiebers et al[296] extended these observations to include four patients with episodic bilateral visual blurring or dimming in response to bright light; all the patients had severe bilateral carotid occlusive disease. Apart from TMB, persisting visual deficit from ocular infarction may also occur (see later).

Compared with THA (see further on), TMB has a less malevolent prognosis for stroke; for the 198 cases of TMB in the nonsurgical treatment arm of the NASCET, the 3-year ipsilateral stroke rate was half that for the 417 medially treated cases of THA (adjusted hazard ratio, 0.53; 95% CI, 0.30 to 0.94).[297]

Transient Hemispheric Attacks

The symptoms reported for THAs have generally been weakness or numbness (or both) of part or all of the side of the body contralateral to the affected hemisphere, with the presence or absence of a speech disturbance, depending on whether the dominant hemisphere is affected.[97,150,197,244] An accurate history may be difficult to obtain because the episodes are brief and frightening to the patient, are not usually observed by another person, and may involve the right hemisphere, making the patient's report unreliable.

The most common constellation of symptoms involves motor and sensory dysfunction of the contralateral limbs, followed by pure motor dysfunction, pure sensory dysfunction, and lastly, isolated dysphasia.[115] The contralateral distal arm and hand are the body parts that most consistently suffer in the attack, and their symptoms may be the only manifestation. The deficit presumably reflects ischemia to a portion of the motor cortex in the distal field of the carotid circulation, by means of either embolism or perfusion failure.

Like occurrences of TMB, THAs are typically brief in duration (<15 minutes, with most lasting for 1 to 10 minutes). In one study, patients with THAs lasting for 1 hour or more tended to have wide open carotid arteries with evidence of intracranial branch occlusion, which suggests that the THAs reflected a short-lived cerebral embolus.[115] Patients may have one or many THAs before coming to medical attention; a few have 20 or more.[115] Most patients have

THAs over several weeks to a few months, but some may have a history spanning months to a year or, rarely, longer.

One distinctive if uncommon form of THA involves *limb shaking*.[150,299-305] Typically associated with severe carotid stenosis or occlusion, the attacks feature recurrent, involuntary, irregular, wavering movements of the contralateral arm or leg. The movements are described as shaking, trembling, twitching, flapping, or wavering. Limb shaking may be an initial form of THA, making distinction of THA from focal epilepsy an important differential point. In the limited number of patients reported to date, endarterectomy appears to be beneficial. The mechanism underlying the shaking TIAs is presumed to be hemodynamic insufficiency.

Nonsimultaneous Transient Monocular Blindness and Transient Hemispheric Attacks

Patients with carotid territory TIAs, depending on when they come to medical attention, may have had TMB, THA, or both types of TIA, although rarely simultaneously. There may be a stronger correlation with severe extracranial carotid artery disease in patients with a history of separate episodes of eye and hemispheric TIAs than in those with either type of spell alone.

Stroke Risk Associated with Transient Monocular Blindness and Transient Hemispheric Attacks

The NASCET provided important information on the stroke risk associated with the first clinically experienced (so-called first-ever) retinal versus hemispheric TIAs and high-grade (>70%) carotid stenosis.[306] Of the 129 medically treated patients, 59 had retinal TIAs, and 70 had hemispheric TIAs. Kaplan-Meier estimates of the risk of ipsilateral stroke at 2 years were 16.6% ± 5.6% for patients with retinal TIAs and 43.5% ± 6.7% for patients with hemisphere TIAs ($P = 0.002$). Patients with hemispheric TIAs were older and had a higher prevalence of most risk factors for stroke. In patients with TMB, the duration of delay before seeking medical treatment was longer. The researchers in this study speculated that TMB may reflect an earlier stage in the development of carotid atherosclerosis—a stage at which small thromboemboli may have a greater impact on sensitive retinal tissue but are of little consequence (because of size) to cortical tissue. An important feature not presented in this report that affects the conclusions is whether patients with TMB who had stroke had antecedent episodes of THAs.[307]

Angiographic Correlations with Transient Ischemic Attacks

A strong relationship exists between carotid territory TIAs (either TMB or THA) and extracranial carotid artery disease.[308-312] The correlation with severe stenosis is by no means a chance: it is prevalent in only 7% on autopsy in a population that is asymptomatic for carotid disease[6] and in less than 10% of patients with stroke due to another mechanism, such as hemorrhage.[238]

Apart from the degree of stenosis, no distinctive angiographic[313] or ultrasonographic[314] appearances have been found that separate symptomatic from asymptomatic patients who have the same severity of stenosis. Lesser degrees of stenosis do not have the same high correlation with TIA. However, misestimation of the stenosis is common when the imaging is based on conventional angiography. A severe stenosis found at surgery may be misread on an angiogram as a lesser degree of stenosis because of minor variations in lumen display or in the judgment of individuals (Fig. 22-16).[47,206] Oblique films of the carotid bifurcation, which should be obtained in addition to the standard anteroposterior and lateral views, disclose irregular or ulcerative lesions not appreciated on the standard views.

Transient Ischemic Attacks and Nonstenosing Carotid Lesions

Clinical impressions persist that any form of carotid atheromatous plaque can harbor thrombus and serve as a source of emboli causing TIAs, despite plaque's high correlation with severe stenosis. Early studies seemed to suggest that TIAs could be attributable to any degree of stenosis by means of microembolization.[113,114,309,312] Evidence in support of this view arose from individual case reports, to which whole series of cases were later added.[103,113,315-319] However, compared with stenosis and occlusion, ulcerations are not the common finding in patients with TIAs. With Doppler studies, it has been difficult—we would say thus far impossible—to predict the mechanism of stroke (perfusion failure or embolism) reliably from the ultrasonographic appearance of the plaque in cases of coexisting carotid stenosis.[316]

Despite the results of the NASCET and European Cooperative Study, debate continues on whether ulcers are important in stroke. Studies from individual centers continue to indicate that plaque morphology may have a predictive value in subsequent stroke risk.[320,321] It is sad to admit, however, that interrater reliability on the interpretation of carotid plaque morphology has not been high in any study,[322] which is an observation that may limit the value of single-center reports on correlations between plaque morphology and clinical events.

Ulcers are often found in surgical specimens.[315-317,323] The smaller ulcers are difficult to demonstrate angiographically, and considerable interobserver variation exists in the diagnosis of ulceration.[132] As many as 40% are missed on routine angiograms, and many ulcers are found at operation in "smooth, benign-appearing plaques...."[316] Ulceration may be an erroneous angiographic diagnosis for a lesion that is actually due to subintimal hemorrhage into a shallow plaque, which is a finding that may even resolve spontaneously.[324]

Fisher and Ojemann[26] studied pathologic carotid endarterectomy plaques and found no important clinical correlation with ulcerations or cul-de-sacs (defined as rounded pouches of diverticula protruding from the lumen into the plaque) in 90 patients who had hemispheric TIAs or TMB or who were asymptomatic, nor did they find correlations in a separate group of 51 patients with persistent neurologic deficit. Of 30 cases of ulceration and seven

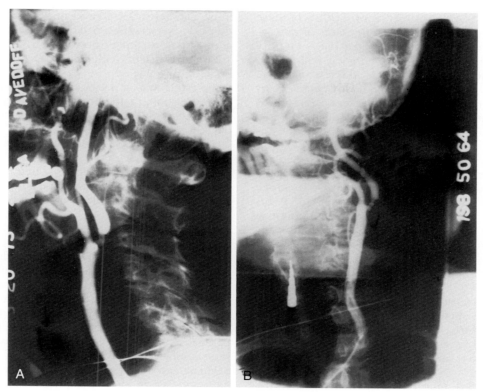

Figure 22-16 A and B, Two views of the same stenosis.

cul-de-sacs in the patients with TIAs, no definite examples of clinical embolic events had occurred. This point is underscored by the observation that nine ulcerations and five cul-de-sacs were found in 33 asymptomatic patients. Similarly, of 51 patients with persistent neurologic deficit signifying infarction, only 10 had ulcerations or cul-de-sacs, and six of these were associated with a severe stenosis (residual lumen < 1 mm). The remaining four patients, with widely patent lumens, had minor neurologic signs.

Opinions on the importance of ulceration per se have been changing over time.[325] The risk of TIA and stroke for complex, deep ulcers is still a subject of dispute, but the undeniable correlation with high-grade stenosis makes it difficult to perform a separate study of one of the two coexisting elements.

Asymptomatic Carotid Artery Disease

Asymptomatic Carotid Artery Occlusion

The documentation of carotid artery occlusion by a noninvasive study or angiography is fairly common, and the literature dates back several decades.[326] A series of studies attempted to use the case-control method to estimate stroke risk, the first and still the dominant of which was that conducted by Furlan and Whisnant,[327] in which the annual rate of 2% was derived from six cases among 138 that were evaluated angiographically and studied retrospectively. Similar event rates have been reported in other series from angiography.[81,328] The cohort studies reported by Sacquegna et al[329] consisted of a consecutive series of 100 patients with angiographically proven ICA occlusion,

68 of whom were monitored from 17 to 69 months; seven of the patients had new strokes, only three of which were in the territory of the occluded carotid artery, and four had TIAs during follow-up. The observed stroke rate was 4.7% at 1 year, 12.2% at 3 years, and 17.1% at 5 years.

Noninvasive Doppler ultrasonography provided the database for other studies. The early study by Bernstein and Norris[330] documented an annual stroke rate of 3.8%. Similar or higher rates have been published in other series, including the original EC-IC bypass study. In that study, 34 of 74 patients identified as having carotid artery occlusion were randomly assigned to undergo nonsurgical treatment and were followed up for a mean of 42 months. The annual stroke rate was 13% per patient-year; 50% of the survivors were symptom free or had minor disability.[331] More information on these outcomes is expected from publication of the CREST trial.[238a]

Asymptomatic Carotid Artery Stenosis

The risk of stroke in a setting of asymptomatic carotid artery stenosis, reported as case series in numerous publications,[13,268,332] was addressed in the largest study to date, the ACAS.[333] This trial randomly assigned all eligible patients with asymptomatic carotid stenosis consisting of 60% or greater lumen reduction to receive 325 mg of aspirin daily or to undergo carotid endarterectomy. All patients received appropriate counseling and treatment for risk factor reduction. The endpoints TIA and stroke in the distribution of the randomized arteries were used to assess the two treatments. Brott et al[334] reviewed 1132 patients in the ACAS and discovered 126 (15%) with what was characterized as silent infarct. For fully 72% of these patients, the infarcts were small, deep lesions often considered asymptomatic, but the remainder had convexity infarctions, of which some were as large as half a lobe. After a median follow-up of 2.7 years, the risk of ipsilateral stroke in the ACAS projected to occur over 5 years or of any perioperative stroke or death was 5.1% for surgically treated patients and 11.0% for medically treated patients. A low Mini-Mental State Examination score was correlated with a higher mortality rate.[335]

The favorable outcome for surgically treated patients was predicated on a remarkably low perioperative risk of stroke or death—2.3%. The 5-year reduction in stroke risk was different for men (67%) and women (17%); this difference was in part explained by a higher perioperative complication rate in women. The angiographically related stroke rate was 1.2% for the 414 patients who underwent arteriography before endarterectomy. Despite strong clinical opinions to the contrary, the severities of increasing stenosis (60% to 69%, 70% to 79%, and 80% to 99%) were not statistically related to reduction of the 5-year risk of the primary event. These data provide the first scientifically derived information on the stroke risk and benefits of carotid endarterectomy for asymptomatic carotid artery disease and are now the new benchmark for this condition.[333]

Since these studies appeared, additional evidence has accumulated indicating that the existence of intracranial perfusion impairment, as assessed by TCD ultrasonography—an evaluation not widely used in the ACAS—adds to the risk of TIA and stroke, when present. In a study of 114 patients with 80% to 99% stenosis of an extracranial ICA assessed by duplex Doppler ultrasonography, Hartmann et al[336] found that evidence of intracranial waveform blunting as assessed by TCD ultrasonography had a highly significant correlation with the symptomatic patients (odds ratio, 7.5; 95% CI, 3.1 to 18.1; $P < 0.001$). In a cohort of 153 patients studied by Blaser et al,[337] "exhausted" collateral vessels (i.e., blunted intracranial waveforms ipsilateral or bilateral atop ICA stenosis, inferred to be fully dilated because of not showing further dilation after CO_2 inhalation) were the principal independent risk factor for TIA and stroke.

Modern data on the advance in stenosis over time were summarized by the late D. Eugene Strandness, Jr.,[338] whose career spanned the development of Doppler ultrasonography. His advice was to recheck in 6-month intervals all patients with clinically asymptomatic stenosis of 50% to 79% but only annually for those with stenosis less than 50%. These observations are in general agreement with those of other large series.[339]

Asymptomatic Carotid Ulceration

The current literature shows considerable variation in the role of ulceration as a risk factor for stroke or for complications associated with interventions. Several recent reports found ulceration associated with no or low risk for endovascular or surgical carotid procedures.[340]

Ulceration was a risk factor but had wide confidence intervals (odds ratio, 2.08; 95% CI, 0.93 to 4.68) and a minor position among factors associated with unfavorable outcomes (stroke or death) in the report from a very large database (9308 procedures) from the New York Carotid Artery Surgery Study.[341] Other series found ulceration a risk for endarterectomy in a logistic regression analysis, sufficient to include it in a proposed risk scoring system.[342]

Investigations continue to accumulate on the imaging and ultrasonographic features of plaques; many show the more complex plaques to be associated with higher degrees of stenosis.[343]

Ulceration has been shown to increase Doppler evidence of turbulence.[344]

Poststenting assessment of ulceration has shown examples of healing.[345] Even an example of healing of an asymptomatic carotid ulcer has been reported.[346]

Asymptomatic Bruit

With widespread availability of Doppler studies, much of the earlier anxieties about whether bruits diagnose carotid stenosis, internal or external, or are augmentation flows in widely patent arteries have been replaced by results from readily-available duplex Doppler findings. A bruit in the neck is commonly encountered in routine clinical examination, found in as many as 4% to 5% of the population aged 45 to 80 years.[347,348] A local cervical bruit can be detected in approximately 70% to 89% of patients with an internal carotid stenosis of greater than or equal to 75% stenosis or less than or equal to 2 mm residual lumen.[349,350] The site of maximal intensity of the bruit usually corresponds to the carotid bifurcation area, in front of the upper portion of the thyroid cartilage. It can radiate into the ocular region, and its intensity usually decreases with the Valsalva maneuver. It was hoped that this simple test would differentiate the two sources, but it is disappointingly unreliable.[351] A bruit may also be absent in some patients whose stenosis has advanced to the point of distal flow impairment because of a slow-flow state through the stenotic artery.[350] Rarely, the bruit is due to a tight, diaphragm-like lesion not easily imaged by conventional angiography.[352]

Auscultation remains a useful tool: in a recent population-based study of a stroke-free cohort of 686 subjects with a mean age of 68.2 years, the prevalence of carotid stenosis greater than or equal to 60% detected by ultrasound was 2.2%; bruits had a prevalence of 4.1%. Bruit detection by auscultation had a sensitivity of 56%, a specificity of 98%, a positive predictive value of 25%, and a negative predictive value of 99%; the overall accuracy was 97.5%.[353]

Postendarterectomy Doppler Ultrasonography Findings

Despite the persisting hope that a successful endarterectomy has rid the patient of the risk of further disease at that site, recurrence is discouragingly frequent. The advice of the late D. Eugene Strandness was to undertake a study shortly after endarterectomy to confirm the success of the operation and provide a baseline.[338] This advice appears to apply even today, when the most recent report (CAVATAS) of carotid angioplasty, angioplasty and stenting, and surgical endarterectomy showed late (5-year cumulative) restenosis (≥70%) rates at 10.5% for endarterectomy and 30.7% for endovascular therapy; the rate was less for those whose angioplasty was associated with stent placement.[354] For those whose stenosis has reaccumulated, success rate for a second endarterectomy in experienced hands appears to approximate that for the first operation,[355,356] and similar results are seen for surgery or endovascular procedures.[357]

REFERENCES

1. Mast H, Thompson JLP, Hofmeister C, et al: Cigarette smoking as a determinant of high-grade carotid artery stenosis in Hispanic, black, and white patients with stroke or transient ischemic attack, *Stroke* 29:908-912, 1998.
2. Murie JA, Sheldon CD, Quin RO: Radiographic anatomy of the extracranial carotid artery, *J Cardiovasc Surg (Torino)* 26:143-146, 1985.
3. Fisher CM, Gore I, Okabe N, White PD: Atherosclerosis of the carotid and vertebral arteries—extracranial and intracranial, *J Neuropathol Exp Neurol* 24:455-476, 1965.
4. Caplan LR, Baker R: Extracranial occlusive vascular disease: Does size matter? *Stroke* 11:63, 1980.
5. Schneidau A, Harrison MJ, Hurst C: Predicting the normal dimensions of the internal carotid artery, *Eur J Vasc Surg* 2:273-274, 1988.
6. LoGerfo FW, Crawshaw HN, Nowak M, et al: Effect of flow split on separation and stagnation in a model vascular bifurcation, *Stroke* 12:660, 1981.
7. LoGerfo FW, Nowak MD, Quist WC, et al: Flow studies in a model of carotid bifurcation, *Arteriosclerosis* 1:235, 1981.
8. Wood CPL, Smith BR, McKinney CL, Toole JF: Non-invasive detection of boundary layer separation in the normal carotid artery bifurcation, *Stroke* 13:120, 1982.
9. Zarins CK, Giddens DP, Balasubramanian K, et al: Carotid plaques localized in regions of low flow velocity and shear stress, *Circulation* 64:44, 1981.
10. Schulz UG, Rothwell PM: Major variation in carotid bifurcation anatomy: A possible risk factor for plaque development? *Stroke* 32:2522-2529, 2001.
11. Schneidau A, Harrison MJ, Hurst C, et al: Arterial disease risk factors and angiographic evidence of atheroma of the carotid artery, *Stroke* 20:1466-1471, 1989.
12. Javid H, Ostermiller WE Jr, Hengesh JW, et al: Natural history of carotid bifurcation atheroma, *Surgery* 67:80, 1970.
13. Roederer GO, Langlois YE, Jager KA, et al: The natural history of carotid arterial disease in asymptomatic patients with cervical bruits, *Stroke* 15:605, 1984.
14. Jahromi AS, Clase CM, Maggisano R, et al: Progression of internal carotid artery stenosis in patients with peripheral arterial occlusive disease, *J Vasc Surg* 50:292-298, 2009.
15. Yamada K, Yoshimura S, Kawasaki M, et al: Effects of atorvastatin on carotid atherosclerotic plaques: A randomized trial for quantitative tissue characterization of carotid atherosclerotic plaques with integrated backscatter ultrasound, *Cerebrovasc Dis* 28:417-424, 2009.
16. Berguer R, Hwang NHC: Critical arterial stenosis: A theoretical and experimental solution, *Ann Surg* 180:39, 1974.
17. Brice JG, Dowsett DJ, Lowe RD: Haemodynamic effects of carotid artery stenosis, *Br Med J* 2:1363, 1964.
18. Shipley RE, Gregg DE: The effect of external constriction of a blood vessel on blood flow, *Am J Physiol* 141:389, 1944.
19. Archie JP, Feldtman RW: Critical stenosis of the internal carotid artery, *Surgery* 89:67, 1981.
20. Young DF, Cholvin NR, Kirkeeide RL, Roth AC: Hemodynamics of arterial stenoses at elevated flow rates, *Circ Res* 41:99, 1977.
21. Byar D, Fiddian RV, Quereau M, et al: The fallacy of applying the Poiseuille equation to segmental arterial stenosis, *Am Heart J* 70:216, 1965.
22. de Labriolle A, Mohty D, Pacouret G, et al: Comparison of degree of stenosis and plaque volume for the assessment of carotid atherosclerosis using 2-D ultrasound, *Ultrasound Med Biol* 35:1436-1442, 2009.
23. Kuntz KM, Skillman JJ, Whittemore AD, Kent KC: Carotid endarterectomy in asymptomatic patients—is contrast angiography necessary? A morbidity analysis, *J Vasc Surg* 22:706, 1995.
24. Gagne PJ, Matchett J, MacFarland D, et al: Can the NASCET technique for measuring carotid stenosis be reliably applied outside the trial? *J Vasc Surg* 24:449, 1996.
25. Bousser MG: Faut-il opérer les sténoses carotidiennes asymptomatiques? *Rev Neurol* 151:363, 1995.
26. Fisher CM, Ojemann RG: A clinico-pathologic study of carotid endarterectomy plaques, *Rev Neurol (Paris)* 142:573, 1986.
27. Mohr JP: *Plaques carotides: Diagnostic, evaluation, prognostic*, Paris, 1997, Sauramps, p 11.
28. Trivedi RA, Gillard JH, Kirkpatrick PJ: Modern methods for imaging carotid atheroma, *Br J Neurosurg* 22:350-359, 2008.
29. Marcu L, Jo JA, Fang Q, et al: Detection of rupture-prone atherosclerotic plaques by time-resolved laser-induced fluorescence spectroscopy, *Atherosclerosis* 204(1):156-164, 2009.
30. Tang D, Teng Z, Canton G, et al: Sites of rupture in human atherosclerotic carotid plaques are associated with high structural stresses: An in vivo MRI-based 3D fluid-structure interaction study, *Stroke* 40:3258-3263, 2009.
31. Li ZY, Taviani V, Gillard JH: The impact of wall shear stress and pressure drop on the stability of the atherosclerotic plaque, *Conf Proc IEEE Eng Med Biol Soc* 2008:1373-1376, 2008.
32. Redgrave JN, Gallagher P, Lovett JK, et al: Critical cap thickness and rupture in symptomatic carotid plaques: The Oxford Plaque Study, *Stroke* 39:1722-1729, 2008.
33. Gao H, Long Q: Effects of varied lipid core volume and fibrous cap thickness on stress distribution in carotid arterial plaques, *J Biomech* 41:3053-3059, 2008.
34. Saba L, Mallarini G: Fissured fibrous cap of vulnerable carotid plaques and symptomaticity: Are they correlated? Preliminary results by using multi-detector-row CT angiography, *Cerebrovasc Dis* 27:322-327, 2009.
35. Sadat U, Weerakkody RA, Bowden DJ, et al: Utility of high resolution MR imaging to assess carotid plaque morphology: A comparison of acute symptomatic, recently symptomatic and asymptomatic patients with carotid artery disease, *Atherosclerosis* 207:434-439, 2009.
36. Sallustio F, Di Legge S, Koch G, et al: Urgent carotid endarterectomy: the role of serial ultrasound studies in early detection of plaque rupture, *J Ultrasound Med* 28:239-243, 2009.
37. Mauriello A, Sangiorgi GM, Virmani R, et al: A pathobiologic link between risk factors profile and morphological markers of carotid instability, *Atherosclerosis* 208:572-580, 2010.
38. Peeters W, Hellings WE, de Kleijn DP, et al: Carotid atherosclerotic plaques stabilize after stroke: Insights into the natural process of atherosclerotic plaque stabilization, *Arterioscler Thromb Vasc Biol* 29:128-133, 2009.
39. Roquer J, Segura T, Serena J, et al: Endothelial dysfunction, vascular disease and stroke: The ARTICO study, *Cerebrovasc Dis* 27(Suppl 1):25-37, 2009.
40. Lennihan L, Kupsky WJ, Mohr JP, et al: Lack of association between carotid plaque hematoma and ipsilateral cerebral symptoms, *Stroke* 18:879, 1987.
41. Sessa R, Di Pietro M, Schiavoni G, et al: Measurement of *Chlamydia pneumoniae* bacterial load in peripheral blood mononuclear cells may be helpful to assess the state of chlamydial infection in patients with carotid atherosclerotic disease, *Atherosclerosis* 195:e224-e230, 2007.
42. Kim DK, Kim HJ, Han SH, et al: *Chlamydia pneumoniae* accompanied by inflammation is associated with the progression of atherosclerosis in CAPD patients: a prospective study for 3 years, *Nephrol Dial Transplant* 23:1011-1018, 2008.
43. Vikatmaa P, Lajunen T, Ikonen TS, et al: Chlamydial lipopolysaccharide (cLPS) is present in atherosclerotic and aneurysmal arterial wall—cLPS levels depend on disease manifestation, *Cardiovasc Pathol* 19:48-54, 2010.
44. Elkind MS, Luna JM, Moon YP, et al: High-sensitivity C-reactive protein predicts mortality but not stroke: The Northern Manhattan Study, *Neurology* 73:1300-1307, 2009.
45. Jaff MR, Dale RA, Creager MA, et al: Anti-chlamydial antibiotic therapy for symptom improvement in peripheral artery disease: Prospective evaluation of rifalazil effect on vascular symptoms of intermittent claudication and other endpoints in *Chlamydia pneumoniae* seropositive patients (PROVIDENCE-1), *Circulation* 119:452-458, 2009.
46. Fisher CM: Cerebral ischemia-less familiar types, *Clin Neurosurg* 18:267, 1971.

47. Croft RJ, Ellam LD, Harrison MJG: Accuracy of carotid angiography in the assessment of atheroma of the internal carotid artery, *Lancet* 315:997, 1980.

48. Cioffi FA, Meduri M, Tomasello F, et al: Kinking and coiling of the internal carotid artery, *J Neurosurg Sci* 19:15, 1975.

49. Correll JW, Quest DO, Carpenter DB: Nonatheromatous lesions of the extracranial cerebral arteries. In Smith RR, editor: *Stroke and the extracranial vessels*, Philadelphia, 1984, Lippincott-Raven, p 321.

50. Beigelman R, Izaguirre AM, Robles M, et al: Are kinking and coiling of carotid artery congenital or acquired? *Angiology* 61:107–112, 2010.

51. Handa J, Nakasu Y, Kidooka M: Transient cerebral ischemia evoked by yawning: An experience after superficial temporal artery–middle cerebral artery bypass operation, *Surg Neurol* 19:46, 1983.

52. Ballotta E, Thiene G, Baracchini C, et al: Surgical vs medical treatment for isolated internal carotid artery elongation with coiling or kinking in symptomatic patients: a prospective randomized clinical study, *J Vasc Surg* 42:838–846, 2005.

53. Merino MJ, Livolsi V: Malignant carotid body tumors, *Cancer* 47:1403, 1981.

54. Harrington HJ, Mayman CI: Carotid body tumor associated with partial Horner's syndrome and facial pain ("Raeder's syndrome"), *Arch Neurol* 40:564, 1983.

55. Grobe T: Diagnostik und Behandlungsmöglichkeiten extrakranieller Verschlussprozesse der Arteria carotis, *Fortschr Neurol Psychiatr* 49:335, 1981.

56. Huvos AG, Leaming RH, Moore OS: Clinicopathologic study of the resected carotid artery, *Am J Surg* 126:570, 1973.

57. Spallone A: Occlusion of the internal carotid artery by intracranial tumors, *Surg Neurol* 15:51, 1981.

58. Maves MD, Bruns MD, Keenan MJ: Carotid artery resection for head and neck cancer, *Ann Otol Rhinol Laryngol* 101:778, 1992.

59. Snyderman CH, D'Amico F: Outcome of carotid artery resection for neoplastic disease: A meta-analysis, *Am J Otolaryngol* 13:373, 1992.

60. Okamoto Y, Inugami A, Matsuzaki Z, et al: Carotid artery resection for head and neck cancer, *Surgery* 120:54, 1996.

61. Wright JG, Nicholson R, Schuller DE, Smead WL: Resection of the internal carotid artery and replacement with greater saphenous vein: A safe procedure for en bloc cancer resections with carotid involvement, *J Vasc Surg* 23:775, 1996.

62. Shichita T, Ogata T, Yasaka M, et al: Angiographic characteristics of radiation-induced carotid arterial stenosis, *Angiology* 60:276–282, 2009.

63. Piedbois P, Becquemin JP, Pierquin B, et al: Les sténoses artérielles après radiothérapie, *Bull Cancer Radiother* 77:3, 1990.

64. Levinson SA, Close MB, Ehrenfeld WK, et al: Carotid artery occlusive disease following external cervical irradiation, *Arch Surg* 107:395, 1973.

65. Shin SH, Stout CL, Richardson AI, et al: Carotid angioplasty and stenting in anatomically high-risk patients: Safe and durable except for radiation-induced stenosis, *J Vasc Surg* 50:762–767, 2009.

66. Luo CB, Teng MM, Chang FC, et al: Radiation carotid blowout syndrome in nasopharyngeal carcinoma: Angiographic features and endovascular management, *Otolaryngol Head Neck Surg* 138:86–91, 2008.

67. Castaigne P, Lhermitte F, Gautier JC, et al: Internal carotid artery occlusion: A study of 61 instances in 50 patients with post-mortem data, *Brain* 93:321, 1970.

68. Craig DR, Meguro K, Watridge C, et al: Intracranial internal carotid artery stenosis, *Stroke* 13:825, 1982.

69. Marzewski DJ, Furlan AJ, St. Louis P, et al: Intracranial internal carotid artery stenosis: Long term prognosis, *Stroke* 13:821, 1982.

70. Schuler JJ, Falnigan DP, Lim LT, et al: The effect of carotid siphon stenosis on stroke rate, death, and relief of symptoms following elective carotid endarterectomy, *Surgery* 92:1058, 1982.

71. Hutchinson EC, Yates PO: Caratico-vertebral stenosis, *Lancet* 269:2, 1957.

72. Torvik A, Jörgensen L: Ischemic cerebrovascular disease in an autopsy series. Part 1: Prevalence, location and predisposing factors in verified thrombo-embolic occlusion and their significance in the pathogenesis of cerebral infarction, *J Neurol Sci* 3:490, 1966.

73. Torvik A, Jörgensen L: Ischemic cerebrovascular disease in an autopsy series. Part 2: Prevalence, location, pathogenesis and clinical course of cerebral infarcts, *J Neurol Sci* 9:285, 1969.

74. Luessenhop AJ: Occlusive disease of carotid artery: Observations on the prognosis and surgical treatment, *J Neurosurg* 16:705, 1959.

75. Pessin MS, Duncan GW, Davis KR, et al: Angiographic appearance of carotid occlusion in acute stroke, *Stroke* 11:485, 1982.

76. Baud JM, De Bray JM, Delanoy P, et al: Reproductibilité ultrasonore dans la caractérisation des plaques carotidiennes, *J Echograph Med Ultrason* 17:377, 1996.

77. Mosso M, Georgiadis D, Baumgartner RW: Progressive occlusive disease of large cerebral arteries and ischemic events in a patient with essential thrombocythemia, *Neurol Res* 26:702–703, 2004.

78. Lu CH, Yang CY, Wang CP, et al: Imaging of nasopharyngeal inflammatory pseudotumours: Differential from nasopharyngeal carcinoma, *Br J Radiol* 83:8–16, 2010.

79. Alexandrov AV, Sloan MA, Wong LK, et al: American Society of Neuroimaging Practice Guidelines Committee. Practice standards for transcranial Doppler ultrasound: Part I—test performance, *J Neuroimaging* 17:11–18, 2007.

80. Taoka T, Iwasaki S, Nakagawa H, et al: Evaluation of arteriosclerotic changes in the intracranial carotid artery using the calcium score obtained on plain cranial computed tomography scan: Correlation with angiographic changes and clinical outcome, *J Comput Assist Tomogr* 30:624–628, 2006.

81. Bogousslavsky J, Regli F, Hungerbühler J-P, Chrzanowski R: Transient ischemic attacks and external carotid artery occlusion: A retrospective study of 23 patients with an occlusion of the internal carotid artery, *Stroke* 12:627, 1981.

82. Pessin MS, Hinton RC, Davis KR, et al: Mechanisms of acute carotid stroke, *Ann Neurol* 6:245, 1979.

83. Burnbaum MD, Selhorst JB, Harbison JW, Brush JJ: Amaurosis fugax from disease of the external carotid artery, *Arch Neurol* 34:532, 1977.

84. Krayenbühl H, Yasargil MG: *Die cerebrale Angiographie*, Stuttgart, 1965, George Thieme Verlag.

85. Van der Eecken HM: *Anastomoses between the leptomeningeal arteries of the brain*, Springfield, IL, 1959, Charles C Thomas.

86. Henderson RD, Eliasziw M, Fox AJ, et al: Angiographically defined collateral circulation and risk of stroke in patients with severe carotid artery stenosis: North American Symptomatic Carotid Endarterectomy Trial (NASCET) Group, *Stroke* 31:128–132, 2000.

87. Powers WJ, Press GA, Grubb RL, et al: The effect of hemodynamically significant carotid artery disease on the hemodynamic status of the cerebral circulation, *Ann Intern Med* 106:27, 1987.

88. Schneider PA, Rossman ME, Bernstein EF, et al: Noninvasive assessment of cerebral collateral blood supply through the ophthalmic artery, *Stroke* 22:31, 1991.

89. Tatemichi TK, Chamorro A, Petty GW, et al: Hemodynamic role of ophthalmic artery collateral in internal carotid artery occlusion, *Neurology* 40:461, 1990.

90. David NJ, Gordon KK, Friedberg SJ, et al: Fatal atheromatous cerebral embolism associated with bright plaques in the retinal arterioles, *Neurology* 13:708, 1963.

91. Adams RD, Fisher CM: Pathology of cerebral arterial occlusion. In Fields WS, editor: *Houston symposium on pathogenesis and treatment of cerebrovascular disease*, Springfield, IL, 1961, Charles C Thomas.

92. Beal MF, Williams RS, Richardson EP, Fisher CM: Cerebral embolism as a cause of transient ischemic attacks and cerebral infarction, *Neurology* 31:860, 1981.

93. Castaigne P, Lhermitte F, Gautier JC: Role des lésions artérielles dans les accidents ischémiques cérébraux de l'athérosclerose, *Rev Neurol (Paris)* 113:1, 1965.

94. Fisher CM: Clinical syndromes of cerebral thrombosis, hypertensive hemorrhage, and ruptured saccular aneurysm, *Clin Neurosurg* 22:117, 1975.

95. Waxman SG, Toole JF: Temporal profile resembling TIA in the setting of cerebral infarction, *Stroke* 14:433, 1983.

96. Gunning AJ, Pickering GW, Robb-Smith AHT, et al: Mural thrombosis of the internal carotid artery and subsequent embolism, *Q J Med* 33:155, 1964.

97. Millikan CH: The pathogenesis of transient focal cerebral ischemia, *Circulation* 32:438, 1965.

98. Olsson JE, Muller R, Berneli S: Long-term anticoagulant therapy for TIAs and minor strokes with minimum residuum, *Stroke* 7:444, 1976.

99. Delal PM, Shah PM, Aiyar RR: Arteriographic study of cerebral embolism, *Lancet* 286:358, 1965.

100. Liebeskind A, Chinichian A, Schechter MM: The moving embolus seen during serial cerebral angiography, *Stroke* 2:440, 1971.

101. Ring BA: Diagnosis of embolic occlusions of smaller branches of the intracerebral arteries, *Am J Roentgenol Radium Ther Nucl Med* 97:575, 1966.

102. Taveras JM, Wood EH: *Diagnostic neuroradiology*, ed 2, Vol 2, Sect 4: Vascular Diseases. Baltimore, Williams & Wilkins, 1976, p 850.

103. Zatz LM, Iannone AM, Eckman PB, Hecker SP: Observations concerning intracerebral vascular occlusion, *Neurology* 15:390, 1965.

104. Fisher CM: Observations of the fundus oculi in transient monocular blindness, *Neurology* 9:337, 1959.

105. Russell RW: Observations on the retinal blood vessels in monocular blindness, *Lancet* 278:1422, 1961.

106. Harrison MJG, Marshall J: Evidence of silent cerebral embolism in patients with amaurosis fugax, *J Neurol Neurosurg Psychiatry* 40:651, 1977.

107. Countee RW, Sapru HN, Vijayanathan T, Wu SZ: "Other syndromes" of the carotid bifurcation. In Smith RR, editor: *Stroke and the extracranial vessels*, Philadelphia, 1984, Lippincott-Raven, p 345.

108. Russell RW: Atheromatous retinal embolism, *Lancet* 282:1354, 1963.

109. Barnett HJM, Peerless SJ, Kaufmann JCE: The "stump" of internal carotid artery—a source for further cerebral embolic ischemia, *Stroke* 9:448, 1978.

110. Waller FT, Simons RL, Kerber C, et al: Trigeminal artery and micro-emboli to the brain stem: Report of two cases, *J Neurosurg* 46:104, 1977.

111. Chiari H: Ueber das Verhalten der Teilungswinkels der Carotid communis bei der Endarteritis chronica deformans, *Verh Dtsch Ges Pathol* 9:326, 1905.

112. Lusby RJ, Ferrell LD, Ehrenfeld WK, et al: Carotid plaque hemorrhage: Its role in production of cerebral ischemia, *Arch Surg* 117:1479, 1982.

113. Moore WS, Hall AD: Ulcerated atheroma of the carotid artery: A major cause of transient cerebral ischemia, *Am J Surg* 116:237, 1968.

114. Moore WS, Hall AD: Importance of emboli from carotid bifurcation in pathogenesis of cerebral ischemic attacks, *Arch Surg* 101:708, 1970.

115. Pessin MS, Duncan GW, Mohr JP, Poskanzer DC: Clinical and angiographic features of carotid transient ischemic attacks, *N Engl J Med* 296:358, 1977.

116. Mead GE, Lewis SC, Wardlaw JM, Dennis MS: Comparison of risk factors in patients with transient and prolonged eye and brain ischemic syndromes, *Stroke* 33:2383–2390, 2002.

117. Whisnant JP: Multiple particles injected may all go to the same cerebral artery branch, *Stroke* 13:720, 1982.

118. Wolpert SM, Stein BM: Catheter embolization of arteriovenous malformations as an aid to surgical excision, *Neuroradiology* 10:73, 1975.

119. Ferro JM, Falcao I, Rodrigues G, et al: Diagnosis of transient ischemic attack by a nonneurologist, *Stroke* 27:2225, 1996.

120. Mohr JP: Neurological complications of cardiac valvular disease and cardiac surgery including systemic hypotension. In Klawans HL, editor: *Neurological manifestations of systemic diseases (Handbook of clinical neurology, Vol 38)*, Amsterdam, 1979, North Holland Publishers, p 143.

121. Fisher CM: Cerebral thromboangiitis obliterans, *Medicine (Baltimore)* 36:169, 1957.

122. Bogousslavsky J, Regli F: Borderzone infarctions distal to internal carotid artery occlusion: Prognostic implications, *Ann Neurol* 20:346, 1986.

123. Fisher CM: Occlusion of the internal carotid artery, *AMA Arch Neurol Psychiatry* 69:346, 1951.

124. Fisher CM: Occlusion of the carotid arteries: Further experiences, *AMA Arch Neurol Psychiatry* 72:187, 1954.

125. Lindenberg R, Spatz F: Ueber die Thromboendarteritis obliterans der Hirngefässe, *Virchows Arch [A]* 305:531, 1940.

126. Pentschew A: Die granuläre Atrophie der Grosshirnrinde, *Arch Psychiatr Nervenkr* 101:80, 1934.

127. Ringelstein EB, Zeumer H, Angelou D: The pathogenesis of strokes from internal carotid artery occlusion, *Stroke* 14:867, 1983.

128. Romanul FCA, Abramowicz A: Changes in brain and pial vessels in arterial borderzones, *Arch Neurol (Chicago)* 11:40, 1964.

129. Spatz A: Uber die Beteiligung des Gehirns bei v. Winiwarter-Buergerische Krankheit, *Dtsch Z Nervenheilkd* 136:86, 1935.

130. Torvik A: The pathogenesis of watershed infarcts in the brain, *Stroke* 15:221, 1984.

131. Wodarz R, Ratzka M, Grosse D: Der Grenzzoneninfarkt als besondere Infarktkonstellation bei Karotisinsuffizienz, *Fortschr Geb Röntgenstr* 134:128, 1981.

132. Schneider M: Durchblutung und Sauerstoffversorgung des Gehirns, *Verh Dtsch Ges Kreislaufforsch* 19:3, 1953.

133. Carpenter DA, Grubb RL Jr, Powers WJ: Borderzone hemodynamics in cerebrovascular disease, *Neurology* 40:1587, 1990.

134. Leblanc R, Yamamoto YL, Tyler JL, et al: Borderzone ischemia, *Ann Neurol* 22:707, 1987.

135. Toyama H, Takeshita G, Takeuchi A, et al: SPECT measurement of cerebral hemodynamics in transient ischemic attack patients: Evaluation of pathogenesis and detection of misery perfusion, *Kaku Igaku* 26:1487, 1989.

136. Vorstrup S, Hemmingsen R, Henriksen L, et al: Regional cerebral blood flow in patients with transient ischemic attacks studied by xenon-133 inhalation and emission tomography, *Stroke* 14:903–910, 1983.

137. Raichle M, Discussion: In Reivich M, Hurtig H, editors: *Cerebrovascular disorders. XIIIth research (Princeton) conference*, Philadelphia, 1983, Lippincott-Raven.

138. Yamauchi H, Fukuyama H, Kimura J, et al: Hemodynamics in internal carotid artery occlusion examined by positron emission tomography, *Stroke* 21:1400, 1990.

139. Lin W, Celik A, Derdeyn C, et al: Quantitative measurements of cerebral blood flow in patients with unilateral carotid artery occlusion: A PET and MR study, *J Magn Reson Imaging* 14:659–667, 2001.

140. Derdeyn CP, Khosla A, Videen TO, et al: Severe hemodynamic impairment and border zone-region infarction: 1, *Radiology* 220:195–201, 2001.

141. Baron JC, Bousser MG, Rey A, et al: Reversal of focal "misery-perfusion syndrome" by extra-intracranial arterial bypass in hemodynamic cerebral ischemia, *Stroke* 12:454, 1981.

142. Derdeyn CP, Cross DT III, Moran CJ, Dacey RG Jr: Reversal of focal misery perfusion after intracranial angioplasty: Case report, *Neurosurgery* 48:436–439, 2001.

143. Marshall RS, Lazar RM, Young WL, et al: Clinical utility of quantitative cerebral blood flow measurements during internal carotid artery test occlusions, *Neurosurgery* 50:996–1004, 2002.

144. Levine RL, Dobkin JA, Rozental JM, et al: Blood flow reactivity to hypercapnia in strictly unilateral carotid disease: Preliminary results, *J Neurol Neurosurg Psychiatry* 54:204, 1991.

145. Markus H, Cullinane M: Severely impaired cerebrovascular reactivity predicts stroke and TIA risk in patients with carotid artery stenosis and occlusion, *Brain* 124:457–467, 2001.

146. Coakham HB, Duchen LW, Scaravilli F: Moyamoya disease: Clinical and pathological report of a case with associated myopathy, *J Neurol Neurosurg Psychiatry* 42:289, 1979.

147. Schaefer PW, Roccatagliata L, Ledezma C, et al: First-pass quantitative CT perfusion identifies thresholds for salvageable penumbra in acute stroke patients treated with intra-arterial therapy, *AJNR Am J Neuroradiol* 27:20–25, 2006.

148. Grubb RL Jr, Powers WJ, Derdeyn CP, et al: The Carotid Occlusion Surgery Study, *Neurosurg Focus* 14:e9, 2003.

149. Szabo K, Kern R, Gass A, et al: Acute stroke patterns in patients with internal carotid artery disease: A diffusion-weighted magnetic resonance imaging study, *Stroke* 32:1323–1329, 2001.

150. Fisher CM: Concerning recurrent transient cerebral ischemic attacks, *Can Med Assoc J* 86:1091, 1962.

151. Eastcott HG, Pickering GW, Rob CG: Reconstruction of internal carotid artery in a patient with intermittent attacks of hemiplegia, *Lancet* 264:994, 1954.

152. Bogousslavsky J, Regli F, Zografos L, Uske A: Optico-cerebral syndrome: Simultaneous hemodynamic infarction of optic nerve and brain, *Neurology* 37:263, 1987.

153. Marshall J, Meadows S: The natural history of amaurosis fugax, *Brain* 91:419, 1968.

154. Hollenhorst RW: Significance of bright plaques in the retinal arterioles, *JAMA* 178:23, 1961.

155. Bunt TJ: The clinical significance of the asymptomatic Hollenhorst plaque, *J Vasc Surg* 4:559, 1986.

156. Schwarcz TH, Eton D, Ellenby MI, et al: Hollenhorst plaques: Retinal manifestations and the role of carotid endarterectomy, *J Vasc Surg* 11:635, 1990.

157. Wilson LA, Warlow CP, Ross Russell RW: Cardiovascular disease in patients with retinal arterial occlusion, *Lancet* 313:292, 1979.

158. Pessin MS, Estol CJ, DeWitt LD, et al: Retinal emboli and carotid disease [abstract], *Neurology* 40(Suppl 1):249, 1990.

159. Douglas DJ, Schuler JJ, Buchbinder D, et al: The association of central retinal artery occlusion and extracranial carotid artery disease, *Ann Surg* 208:85, 1988.

160. Sheng FC, Quinones-Baldrich W, Machleder HI, et al: Relationship of extracranial carotid occlusive disease and central retinal artery occlusion, *Am J Surg* 152:175, 1986.

161. Hayreh SS: Acute ischemic disorders of the optic nerve: Pathogenesis, clinical manifestations and management, *Ophthalmol Clin North Am* 9:407–442, 1996.

162. Amick A, Caplan LR: Transient monocular visual loss, *Compr Ophthalmol Update* 8:91–98, 2007.

163. Kearns TP, Hollenhorst RW: Venous-stasis retinopathy of occlusive disease of the carotid artery, *Proc Staff Meet Mayo Clin* 38:304, 1963.

164. McCullough HK, Reinert CG, Hynan LS, et al: Ocular findings as predictors of carotid artery occlusive disease: Is carotid imaging justified? *J Vasc Surg* 40:279–286, 2004.

165. Magargal LE, Sanborn GE, Zimmerman A: Venous stasis retinopathy associated with embolic obstruction of the central retinal artery, *J Clin Neuroophthalmol* 2:113, 1982.

166. Fisher CM: Some neuro-opthalmological observations, *J Neurol Neurosurg Psychiatry* 30:383, 1967.

167. Hedges TR: Ophthalmoscopic findings in internal carotid artery occlusions, *Bull Johns Hopkins Hosp* 111:89, 1962.

168. Young LHY, Appen RE: Ischemic oculopathy: A manifestation of carotid artery disease, *Arch Neurol* 38:358, 1981.

169. Das S, Bendok BR, Novakovic RL, et al: Return of vision after transarterial coiling of a carotid cavernous sinus fistula: Case report, *Surg Neurol* 66:82–85, 2006.

170. Liu F, Xu G, Liu Z, et al: The effects of stellate ganglion block on visual evoked potential and blood flow of the ophthalmic and internal carotid arteries in patients with ischemic optic neuropathy, *Anesth Analg* 100:1193–1196, 2005.

171. Gelmers HJ: The pericarotid syndrome, *Acta Neurochir (Wien)* 57:37, 1981.

172. Kolisko A: *Ueber die Beziehung der Arteria choroidea anterior zum hinteren Schenkel der inneren Kapsel des Gehirns*, Wien, 1891, A. Hoelder.

173. Beevor CE: The cerebral artery supply, *Brain* 30:403–425, 1907.

174. Abbie AA: The blood supply of the lateral geniculate body, with a note of the morphology of the choroidal arteries, *J Anat* 67:491–527, 1933.

175. Alexander L: The vascular supply of the strio-pallidum, *Res Publ Assoc Res Nerv Ment Dis* 21:77–132, 1942.

176. Herman LH, Fernando OU, Gurdjian ES: The anterior choroidal artery: An anatomical study of its area of distribution, *Anat Rec* 154:95–102, 1966.

177. Rhoton AL Jr, Fujii K, Fradd B: Microsurgical anatomy of the anterior choroidal artery, *Surg Neurol* 12:171–187, 1979.

178. Wiesmann M, Yousry I, Seelos KC, Yousry TA: Identification and anatomic description of the anterior choroidal artery by use of 3D-TOF source and 3D-CISS MR imaging, *AJNR Am J Neuroradiol* 22(2):305–310, 2001.

179. Foix C, Chavany H, Hilleman P, et al: Obliteration de l'artere choroidienne anterieure: Ramollissement de son territoire cerebral: Hemiplegie, hemianesthesie, hemianopsie, *Bull Soc Opthalmol Fr* 27:221–223, 1925.

180. Poppi U: Sindrome talamo-capsulare per rammollimento nel territorio dell' arteria choroidea anteriore, *Riv Patol Nerv* 33:505–542, 1928.

181. Cooper IS: Surgical alleviation of parkinsonism: Effects of occlusion of the anterior choroidal artery, *J Am Geriatr Soc* 2:691–718, 1954.

182. Rand RW, Brown WJ, Stern WE: Surgical occlusion of anterior choroidal arteries in parkinsonism, *Neurology* 6:390–401, 1956.

183. Buge A, Escourolle R, Hauw J, et al: Syndrome pseudobulbaire aigu par infarctus bilateral limité du territoire des artères choroidiennes antérieures, *Rev Neurol (Paris)* 135:313–318, 1979.

184. Decroix JP, Graveleau PH, Masson M, Cambier J: Infarction in the territory of the anterior choroidal artery, *Brain* 109:1071–1085, 1986.

185. Helgason C, Capalan LR, Goodwin J, Hedges T III: Anterior choroidal artery-territory infarction, *Arch Neurol* 43:681–686, 1986.

186. Helgason C, Wilbur AC: Capsular hypesthetic ataxic hemiparesis, *Stroke* 21:24–33, 1990.

187. Damasio H: A computed tomographic guide to the identification of cerebral vascular territories, *Arch Neurol* 40:138–142, 1983.

188. Bruno A, Graff-Radford NR, Biller J, Adams HP: Anterior choroidal artery territory infarction: small vessel disease, *Stroke* 20:616–619, 1989.

189. Mohr JP, Steinke W, Timsit SG: The anterior choroidal artery does not supply the corona radiata and lateral ventricular wall, *Stroke* 22:1502–1507, 1991.

190. du Mesnil de Rochemont R, Schneider S, Yan B, et al: Diffusion-weighted MR imaging lesions after filter-protected stenting of high-grade symptomatic carotid artery stenoses, *AJNR Am J Neuroradiol* 27:1321–1325, 2006.

191. Ueda M, Morinaga K, Matsumoto Y, et al: [Infarction in the territory of the anterior choroidal artery due to embolic occlusion of the internal carotid artery—report of two cases], *No To Shinkei* 42:655–660, 1990.

192. Hupperts RMM, Lodder J, Heuts-van Raak EPM, Kessels F: Infarcts in the anterior choroidal artery territory. Anatomical distribution, clinical syndromes, presumed pathogenesis and early outcome, *Brain* 117:825–834, 1994.

193. Mohr JP, Timsit S, Yatsu FM: Choroidal artery disease. In Barnett HJM, Mohr JP, Stein BM, editors: *Stroke: Diagnosis, pathophysiology, and management*, ed 3, New York, 1998, Churchill Livingstone, pp 503–512.

194. Raymond MM, Hupperts RMM, Lodder J: The anterior choroidal artery. In Mohr JP, Choi DW, Grotta JC, Wier B, Wolf PA, editors: *Stroke: Diagnosis, pathophysiology, and management*, ed 4, New York, 2004, Churchill Livingstone, pp 193–206, pp 503–512.

195. Altaf N, Morgan PS, Moody A, et al: Brain white matter hyperintensities are associated with carotid intraplaque hemorrhage, *Radiology* 248:202–209, 2008.

196. Sterbini GL, Agatiello LM, Stocchi A, et al: CT of ischemic infarctions in the territory of the anterior choroidal artery: A review of 28 cases, *AJNR Am J Neuroradiol* 8:229–232, 1987.

197. Barnett HJ: Delayed cerebral ischemic episodes distal to occlusion of major cerebral arteries, *Neurology* 28:769–774, 1978.

198. Mohr JP, Sidman M, Stoddard LT, et al: Right hemianopia with memory and color deficits in circumscribed left posterior cerebral artery territory infarction, *Neurology* 21:1105–1113, 1971.

199. Wada K, Kimura K, Minematsu K, et al: Incongruous homonymous hemianopic scotoma, *J Neurol Sci* 163:179–182, 1999.

200. Shibata K, Nishimura Y, Kondo H, et al: Isolated homonymous hemianopsia due to lateral posterior choroidal artery region infarction: a case report, *Clin Neurol Neurosurg* 111:713–716, 2009.

201. Bogousslavsky J, Regli F, Delaloye B, et al: Hémiataxie et déficit sensitif ipsilateral. Infarctus du territoire de l'artère choroïdienne antérieure. Diaschisis cérébelleux croisé, *Rev Neurol* 142:671–676, 1986.

202. Helgason C, Wilbur A, Weiss A, et al: Acute pseudobulbar mutism due to discrete capsular infarction in the territory of the anterior choroidal artery, *Brain* 11:507–524, 1988.

203. Bogousslavsky J, Miklossy J, Regli F, et al: Subcortical neglect: Neuropsychological, SPECT and neuropathological correlations with anterior choroidal artery territory infarction, *Ann Neurol* 23:448–452, 1988.

204. Han SW, Sohn YH, Lee PH, et al: Pure homonymous hemianopia due to anterior choroidal artery territory infarction, *Eur Neurol* 43(1):35–38, 2000.

205. Nakae Y, Higashiyama Y, Kuroiwa Y: Case of brain infarction in the anterior choroidal territory with homonymous scotomas, *Brain Nerve* 61:979–982, 2009.

206. Chikos PM, Fisher LD, Hirsch JH, et al: Observer variability in evaluating extracranial carotid artery stenosis, *Stroke* 14:885, 1983.

207. Bogousslavsky J, Regli F: Cerebral infarction with transient signs (CITS): Do TIAs correspond to small deep infarcts in internal carotid artery occlusion? *Stroke* 15:536, 1984.

208. Macchi C, Molino LR, Miniati B, et al: Collateral circulation in internal carotid artery occlusion: A study by duplex scan and magnetic resonance angiography, *Minerva Cardioangiol* 50:695–700, 2002.

209. Frank G: Comparison of anticoagulation and surgical treatments of TIA: A review and consolidation of recent natural history and treatment studies, *Stroke* 2:369, 1971.

210. Chimowitz MI, Lafranchise EF, Furlan AJ, Awad IA: Ipsilateral leg weakness associated with carotid stenosis, *Stroke* 21:1362, 1990.

211. Karis R: Asymptomatic carotid artery disease [letter], *Stroke* 14:443, 1983.

212. Lhermitte F, Gautier JC, Derouesne C: Anatomie et physiopathologie des sténoses carotidiennes, *Rev Neurol (Paris)* 115:641, 1966.

213. Dandy WE: Results following ligation of the internal carotid artery, *Arch Surg* 45:521, 1942.

214. Fleming JFR, Petrie D: Traumatic thrombosis of the internal carotid artery with delayed hemiplegia, *Can J Surg* 11:166, 1968.

215. Prabhakaran S, Rundek T, Ramas R, et al: Carotid plaque surface irregularity predicts ischemic stroke: The Northern Manhattan Stroke Study, *Stroke* 37:2696–2701, 2006.

216. Finklestein S, Kleinman GM, Cuneo R, Baringer JR: Delayed stroke following carotid occlusion, *Neurology* 30:84, 1980.

217. Countee RW, Vijayanathan T: Intracranial embolization via external carotid artery: Report of a case with angiographic documentation, *Stroke* 11:465–468, 1980.

218. Watts C: External carotid artery embolus from the internal carotid artery "stump" during angiography. Case report, *Stroke* 13:515–517, 1982.

219. Russell D: Cerebral microemboli and cognitive impairment, *J Neurol Sci* 203-204(C):211–214, 2002.

220. Zülch KJ, Kleihues P: *Neuropathology of cerebral infarction: Thule international symposium*, Stockholm, 1957, Nordiska Bokhandlung Forlag, p 57.

221. Labar DR, Mohr JP, Nichols FT 3rd, et al: Unilateral hyperhidrosis after cerebral infarction, *Neurology* 38:1679–1682, 1988.

222. Mohr JP, Foulkes MA, Polis AB, et al: Infarct topography and hemiparesis profiles with cerebral convexity infarction: The Stroke Data Bank, *J Neurol Neurosurg Psychiatry* 56:344, 1993.

223. Duncan GW, Pessin MS, Mohr JP, Adams RD: Transient cerebral ischemic attacks, *Adv Intern Med* 21:1–20, 1976.

224. Liebers M: Alzheimerische Krankheit bei schwerer Gehirnarteriosklose, *Arch Psychiatr Nervenkr Z Gesamte Neurol Psychiatr* 124:639, 1932.

225. Elder W: The clinical varieties of visual aphasia (case 1), *Edinb Med J* 49:433, 1900.

226. Timsit SG, Sacco RL, Mohr JP, et al: Early clinical differentiation of atherosclerotic and cardioembolic infarction: The Stroke Data Bank (SDB). In: 1st European stroke conference, Duesseldorf, May 10-11, 1990.

227. Timsit S, Logak M, Manai R, Rancurel G: Evolving isolated hand palsy: A parietal lobe syndrome associated with carotid artery disease, *Brain* 120:2251–2257, 1997.

228. Yanagihara T, Sundt TM Jr, Piepgras DG: Weakness of the lower extremity in carotid occlusive disease, *Arch Neurol* 45:297, 1988.

229. van Oijen M, de Jong FJ, Witteman JC, et al: Atherosclerosis and risk for dementia, *Ann Neurol* 61:403–410, 2007.

230. Voshaar RC, Purandare N, Hardicre J, et al: Asymptomatic spontaneous cerebral emboli and cognitive decline in a cohort of older people: A prospective study, *Int J Geriatr Psychiatry* 22:794–800, 2007.

231. Rao R: The role of carotid stenosis in vascular cognitive impairment, *J Neurol Sci* 203-204(C):103–107, 2002.

232. Maeshima S, Terada T, Yoshida N, et al: Cerebral angioplasty in a patient with vascular dementia, *Arch Phys Med Rehabil* 78:666–669, 1997.

233. Hashiguchi S, Mine H, Ide M, Kawachi Y: Watershed infarction associated with dementia and cerebral atrophy, *Psychiatry Clin Neurosci* 54:163–168, 2000.

234. Romero JR, Beiser A, Seshadri S, et al: Carotid artery atherosclerosis, MRI indices of brain ischemia, aging, and cognitive impairment: The Framingham study, *Stroke* 40:1590–1596, 2009.

235. Jacobs LA, Ganji S, Shirley JG, et al: Cognitive improvement after extracranial reconstruction for the low flow-endangered brain, *Surgery* 93:683, 1983.

236. Tatemichi TK, Desmond DW, Prohovnik I, Eidelberg D: Dementia associated with bilateral carotid occlusions: Neuropsychological and haemodynamic course after extracranial to intracranial bypass surgery, *J Neurol Neurosurg Psychiatry* 58:633–636, 1995.

237. Sakoh M, Ueda T, Kumon Y, et al: [Bilateral carotid stenting for bilateral carotid artery stenosis improved vascular dementia], *No Shinkei Geka* 30:759–765, 2002.

238. Rabee HM, Saadani MK, Iqbal KM, Al Salman MM: Neurobehavioral effects of carotid endarterectomy, *Saudi Med J* 22:433–437, 2001.

238a. Brott TG, Hobson RWII, Howard G: Stenting versus endarterectomy for treatment of carotid artery stenosis. *N Engl J Med* 363:11–23, 2010.

239. Loeb C, Priano A, Albano C: Clinical features and long-term follow-up of patients with reversible ischemia attacks (RIA), *Acta Neurol Scand* 57:471, 1978.

240. Caplan LR: Are terms such as completed stroke or RIND of continued usefulness? *Stroke* 14:431, 1983.

241. Genton E, Barnett HJM, Fields WS, et al: Cerebral ischemia: The role of thrombosis and of antithrombotic therapy. Joint Committee for Stroke Resources, *Stroke* 8:147, 1977.

242. Heyman A, Leviton A, Nefzger D, et al: Transient focal cerebral ischemia: Epidemiological and clinical aspects, *Stroke* 5:277, 1974.

243. Fisher CM: Perspective: Transient ischemic attacks, *N Engl J Med* 347:1642–1644, 2002.

244. Marshall J: The natural history of transient ischemic cerebrovascular attacks, *Q J Med* 33:309, 1964.

245. Regli F: Die flüchtigen ischämischen zerebralen Attacken, *Dtsch Med Wochenschr* 96:526, 1971.

246. Kidwell CS, Alger JR, Di Salle F, et al: Diffusion MRI in patients with transient ischemic attacks, *Stroke* 30:1174–1180, 1999.

247. Bisschops RH, Kappelle LJ, Mali WP, van der Grond J: Hemodynamic and metabolic changes in transient ischemic attack patients: A magnetic resonance angiography and (1)H-magnetic resonance spectroscopy study performed within 3 days of onset of a transient ischemic attack, *Stroke* 33:110–115, 2002.

248. Mohr JP: Some clinical aspects of acute stroke: Excellence in Clinical Stroke Award Lecture, *Stroke* 28:1835–1839, 1997.

249. Albers GW, Caplan LR, Easton JD, et al: Transient ischemic attack—proposal for a new definition, *N Engl J Med* 347:1713–1716, 2002.

250. Mohr JP, Caplan LR, Melski JW, et al: The Harvard Cooperative Stroke Registry: A prospective registry, *Neurology* 28:754, 1978.

251. Russo LS: Carotid system transient ischemic attacks: Clinical, racial, and angiographic correlations, *Stroke* 12:470, 1981.

252. Streifler JY, Eliasziw M, Benavente OR, et al: Prognostic importance of leukoaraiosis in patients with symptomatic internal carotid artery stenosis, *Stroke* 33:1651–1655, 2002.

253. Boysen G, Jensen G, Schnor P: Frequency of focal cerebral transient ischemic attacks during a 12 month period, *Stroke* 10:533, 1979.

254. Karp HR, Heyman A, Heyden S, et al: Transient cerebral ischemia: Prevalence and prognosis in a biracial community, *JAMA* 225:125, 1973.

255. Ostfeld AM, Shekelle RB, Klawans HL: Transient ischemic attacks and risk of stroke in an elderly poor population, *Stroke* 4:980, 1973.

256. Whisnant JP, Matsumoto N, Elveback LR: The effect of anticoagulant therapy on the prognosis of patients with transient cerebral ischemic attacks in a community: Rochester, Minnesota, 1955 through 1969, *Mayo Clin Proc* 48:844, 1973.

257. Wilkinson WE, Heyman A, Burch JG, et al: Use of a self-administered questionnaire for detection of transient cerebral ischemic attacks: Survey of elderly persons living in retirement facilities, *Ann Neurol* 6:40, 1979.

258. Wolf PA, Dawber TR, Colton T, et al: Transient cerebral ischemic attacks and risk of stroke: The Framingham Study, *Cardiovasc Dis Epidemiol Newslett* 22:52, 1977.

259. Fratiglioni L, Arfaioli C, Nencini P, et al: Transient ischemic attacks in the community: Occurrence and clinical characteristics: A population survey in the area of Florence, Italy, *Neuroepidemiology* 8:87–96, 1989.

260. Dennis MS, Bamford JM, Sandercock PA, Warlow CP: Incidence of transient ischemic attacks in Oxfordshire, England, *Stroke* 20:333–339, 1989.

261. Baker RN, Ramseyer JG, Schwartz WS: Prognosis in patients with cerebral ischemic attacks, *Neurology* 18:1157, 1968.

262. Friedman GD, Wilson WS, Mosier JM, et al: Transient ischemic attacks in a community, *JAMA* 210:1428, 1969.

263. Link H, Lebram G, Johansson I, Radberg C: Prognosis in patients with infarction and TIA in carotid territory during and after anticoagulant therapy, *Stroke* 10:529, 1979.

264. Pearce JMS, Gubbay SS, Walton JN: Long-term anticoagulant therapy in transient cerebral ischemic attacks, *Lancet* 285:6, 1965.

265. Siekert RG, Whisnant JP, Millikan CH: Surgical and anticoagulant therapy of occlusive cerebrovascular disease, *Ann Intern Med* 58:637, 1963.

266. Ziegler DK, Hassanein RS: Prognosis in patients with transient ischemic attacks, *Stroke* 4:666, 1973.

267. Consensus sur la morphologie et la risque des plaques carotidiennes, *J Echograph Med Ultrason* 17:300, 1996.

268. Durward QJ, Ferguson GG, Barr HWK: The natural history of asymptomatic carotid bifurcation plaques, *Stroke* 13:459, 1982.

269. Kagan A, Popper J, Rhoads GG, et al: Epidemiologic studies on coronary artery disease and stroke in Japanese men living in Japan, Hawaii, and California: Prevalence of stroke. In Scheinberg P, editor: *Cerebrovascular diseases*, Philadelphia, 1976, Lippincott, p 267.

270. Shah AB, Coull BM, Howieson J, et al: Does natural history of transient ischemic attacks (TIAs) justify surgery [letter]? *Stroke* 14:828, 1983.

271. Haynes RB, Taylor DW, Sackett DL, et al: Prevention of functional impairment by endarterectomy for symptomatic high-grade carotid stenosis: North American Symptomatic Carotid Endarterectomy Trial Collaborators, *JAMA* 271:1256–1259, 1994.

272. Nano G, Dalainas I, Casana R, et al: Endovascular treatment of the carotid stump syndrome, *Cardiovasc Intervent Radiol* 29:140–142, 2006.

273. Koudstaal PJ, van Gijn J, Staal A, et al: Diagnosis of transient ischemic attacks: Improvement of interobserver agreement by a check-list in ordinary language, *Stroke* 17:723–728, 1986.

274. Adams HP Jr, Putnam SF, Corbett JJ, et al: Amaurosis fugax: The results of arteriography in 59 patients, *Stroke* 14:742, 1983.

275. DeBono DP, Warlow CP: Potential sources of emboli in patients with presumed transient cerebral or retinal ischemia, *Lancet* 317:343, 1981.

276. Gautier JC: Clinical presentation and differential diagnosis of amaurosis fugax. In Bernstein EF, editor: *Amaurosis fugax*, New York, 1990, Springer-Verlag.

277. Mungas JE, Baker WH: Amaurosis fugax, *Stroke* 8:232, 1977.

278. Gerstenfeld J: The fundus oculi in amaurosis fugax, *Am J Ophthalmol* 58:198, 1964.

279. Dyll LM, Margolis M, David NJ: Amaurosis fugax: Fundoscopic and photographic observations during an attack, *Neurology* 16:135, 1966.

280. David NJ: Amaurosis fugax and after. In Glaser JS, editor: *Neuroophthalmology*, St. Louis, 1979, CV Mosby.

281. Elschnig A: Ueber den Einfluss des Verschlusses der Arteria ophthalmica und der Carotis auf das Sehorgan, *Graefes Arch Clin Exp Ophthalmol* 39:151, 1893.

282. Fisher CM: Transient monocular blindness associated with hemiplegia, *AMA Arch Ophthalmol* 47:167, 1952.

283. Wagener HP: Amaurosis fugax: A specific type of transient loss of vision, *Ill Med J* January:21, 1957.

284. Goodwin JA, Gorelick PB, Helgason CM: Symptoms of amaurosis fugax in atherosclerotic carotid artery disease, *Neurology* 37:829, 1987.

285. Eisenberg RL, Mani RL: Clinical and arteriographic comparison of amaurosis fugax with hemispheric transient ischemic attacks, *Stroke* 9:254, 1978.

286. Hooshmand H, Vines FS, Lee HM, Grindal A: Amaurosis fugax: Diagnostic and therapeutic aspects, *Stroke* 5:643, 1974.

287. Hayreh SS, Weingeist TA: Experimental occlusion of the central artery of the retina. I: Ophthalmoscopic and fluorescein fundus angiographic studies, *Br J Ophthalmol* 64:896, 1980.

288. Gowers WR: On a case of simultaneous embolism of central retinal and middle cerebral arteries, *Lancet* 106:794, 1875.

289. Praffenbach DD, Hollenhorst RW: Morbidity and survivorship of patients with embolic cholesterol crystals in the ocular fundus, *Am J Ophthalmol* 75:66, 1973.

290. McBrien DJ, Bradley RD, Ashton N: The nature of retinal emboli in stenosis of the internal carotid artery, *Lancet* 281:697, 1963.

291. Brockmeier LB, Adolph RJ, Gustin BW, et al: Calcium emboli to the retinal artery in calcific aortic stenosis, *Am Heart J* 101:32, 1981.

292. Wolpow ER, Lupton RG: Transient vertical monocular hemianopsia with anomalous retinal artery branching, *Stroke* 12:691, 1981.

293. Winterkorn JMS, Kupersmith MJ, Wirtschafter JD, Forman S: Brief report: Treatment of vasospastic amaurosis fugax with calcium-channel blockers, *N Engl J Med* 329:396, 1993.

294. Furlan AJ, Whisnant JP, Kearns TP: Unilateral visual loss in bright light: An unusual symptom of carotid artery occlusive disease, *Arch Neurol* 36:675, 1979.

295. Donnan GA, Sharbrough FW, Whisnant JP: Carotid occlusive disease: Effect of bright light on visual evoked responses, *Arch Neurol* 39:687, 1982.

296. Wiebers DO, Swanson JW, Cascino TL, et al: Bilateral loss of vision in bright light, *Stroke* 20:554–558, 1989.

297. Benavente O, Eliasziw M, Streifler JY, et al: Prognosis after transient monocular blindness associated with carotid-artery stenosis, *N Engl J Med* 345:1084–1090, 2001.

298. Pessin MS, Duncan GW, Mohr JP, Poskanzer DC: Clinical and angiographic features of carotid transient ischemic attacks. *N Engl J Med* 296:358, 1977.

299. Baquis GD, Pessin MS, Scott RM: Limb shaking—a carotid TIA, *Stroke* 16:444, 1985.

300. Fisch BJ, Tatemichi TK, Prohovnik I, et al: Transient ischemic attacks resembling simple partial motor seizures [abstract], *Neurology* 38(Suppl):264, 1988.

301. Russell RW, Page NGR: Critical perfusion of brain and retina, *Brain* 106:419, 1983.

302. Tatemichi TK, Young WL, Prohovnik I, et al: Perfusion insufficiency in limb shaking transient ischemic attacks, *Stroke* 21:341, 1990.

303. Yanagihara T, Klass DW: Rhythmic involuntary movement as a manifestation of transient ischemic attacks, *Trans Am Neurol Assoc* 106:46, 1981.

304. Klempen NL, Janardhan V, Schwartz RB, Stieg PE: Shaking limb transient ischemic attacks: Unusual presentation of carotid artery occlusive disease: Report of two cases, *Neurosurgery* 51:483–487, 2002.

305. Radberg J, Sanner J, Bojo L, et al: [Limb-shaking—a rare manifestation of hemodynamic-related TIA], *Lakartidningen* 97:4313–4316, 2000.

306. Streifler JY, Eliasziw M, Fox AJ, et al: Angiographic detection of carotid plaque ulceration: Comparison with surgical observations in a multicenter study: North American Symptomatic Carotid Endarterectomy Trial, *Stroke* 25:1130, 1994.

307. Streifler JY, Eliasziw M, Bonavente OR, et al: The risk of stroke in patients with first-ever retinal vs. hemispheric transient ischemic attacks and high-grade carotid stenosis, *Arch Neurol* 52:246, 1995.

308. Eisenberg RL, Nemzek WR, Moore WS, Mani RL: Relationship of transient ischemic attacks and angiographically demonstrable lesions of carotid artery, *Stroke* 8:483, 1977.

309. Horenstein S, Hambrook G, Roat GW, et al: Arteriographic correlates of transient ischemic attacks, *Trans Am Neurol Assoc* 97:132, 1972.

310. Janeway R, Toole JF: Vascular anatomic status of patients with transient ischemic attacks, *Trans Am Neurol Assoc* 97:137, 1971.

311. Ramirez-Lassepas M, Sandok BA, Burton RC: Clinical indicators of extracranial carotid artery disease in patients with transient symptoms, *Stroke* 4:537, 1973.

312. Toole JF, Janeway R, Choi K, et al: Transient ischemic attacks due to atherosclerosis: A prospective study of 160 patients, *Arch Neurol* 32:5, 1975.

313. Rothwell PM, Salinas R, Ferrando LA, et al: Does the angiographic appearance of a carotid stenosis predict the risk of stroke independently of the degree of stenosis? *Clin Radiol* 50:830, 1955.

314. Hennerici M, Steinke W, Rautenberg W, Mohr JP: Symptomatic and asymptomatic high-grade carotid stenosis in Doppler color flow imaging, *Neurology* 42:131, 1992.

315. Blaisdell FW, Glickman M, Trunkey DD: Ulcerated atheroma of the carotid artery, *Arch Surg* 108:491, 1974.

316. Edwards JH, Kricheff II, Riles T, Imparato A: Angiographically undetected ulceration of the carotid bifurcation as a cause of embolic stroke, *Radiology* 132:369, 1979.

317. Kishore PRS, Chase NE, Kricheff II: Carotid stenosis and intracranial emboli, *Radiology* 100:351, 1971.

318. Meyer WW: Cholesterinkrystall emboli kleiner Organarterien und ihre Folgen, *Virchows Arch [A]* 314:616, 1947.

319. Wood EH, Correll JW: Atheromatous ulceration in major neck vessels as a cause of cerebral embolism, *Acta Radiol Diagn (Stockh)* 9:520, 1969.

320. Aburahma AF, Thiele SP, Wulu JT Jr: Prospective controlled study of the natural history of asymptomatic 60% to 69% carotid stenosis according to ultrasonic plaque morphology, *J Vasc Surg* 36:437–442, 2002.

321. Tegos TJ, Sohail M, Sabetai MM, et al: Echomorphologic and histopathologic characteristics of unstable carotid plaques, *AJNR Am J Neuroradiol* 21:1937–1944, 2000.

322. Hartmann A, Mohr JP, Thompson JL, et al: Interrater reliability of plaque morphology classification in patients with severe carotid artery stenosis, *Acta Neurol Scand* 99:61–64, 1999.

323. Imparato AM, Riles TS, Gorstein F: The carotid bifurcation plaque: Pathologic findings associated with cerebral ischemia, *Stroke* 10:238, 1979.

324. Kishore PRS, Dick AR: Spontaneous disappearance of carotid stenosis, *Radiology* 129:721, 1978.

325. Kroener JM, Dorn PL, Shoor PM, et al: Prognosis of asymptomatic ulcerating carotid lesions, *Arch Surg* 115:1387, 1980.

326. Dyken ML, Doepker JF, Kiovsky R, et al: Asymptomatic occlusion of an internal carotid artery in a hospital population: Determined by directional Doppler ophthalmosonometry, *Stroke* 5:714, 1974.

327. Furlan AJ, Whisnant JP: Long-term prognosis after carotid artery occlusion, *Neurology* 30:986, 1980.

328. Grillo P, Paterson RH: Occlusion of the carotid artery: Prognosis (natural history) and the possibilities of surgical revascularization, *Stroke* 6:17, 1975.

329. Sacquegna T, DeCarolis P, Pazzaglia P, et al: The clinical course and prognosis of carotid artery occlusion, *J Neurol Neurosurg Psychiatry* 45:1037, 1982.

330. Bernstein NM, Norris JW: Benign outcome of carotid occlusion, *Neurology* 39:6, 1989.

331. Wade JPH, Wong W, Barnett HJM, Vandervoort P: Bilateral occlusion of the internal carotid arteries: Presenting symptoms in 74 patients and a prospective study of 34 medically treated patients, *Brain* 110:667, 1987.

332. Hennerici M, Rautenberg W: Stroke risk from symptomless extracranial arterial disease, *Lancet* 320:1180, 1982.

333. Endarterectomy for asymptomatic carotid artery stenosis: Executive Committee for the Asymptomatic Carotid Atherosclerosis Study, *JAMA* 273:1421–1428, 1995.

334. Brott T, Tomsick T, Feinberg W, et al: Baseline silent cerebral infarction in the Asymptomatic Carotid Atherosclerosis Study, *Stroke* 25:1122, 1994.

335. Pettigrew LC, Thomas N, Howard VJ, et al: Low mini-mental status predicts mortality in asymptomatic carotid arterial stenosis: Asymptomatic Carotid Atherosclerosis Study investigators, *Neurology* 55:30–34, 2000.

336. Hartmann A, Mast H, Thompson JL, et al: Transcranial Doppler waveform blunting in severe extracranial carotid artery stenosis, *Cerebrovasc Dis* 10:33–38, 2000.

337. Blaser T, Hofmann K, Buerger T, et al: Risk of stroke, transient ischemic attack, and vessel occlusion before endarterectomy in patients with symptomatic severe carotid stenosis, *Stroke* 33:1057–1062, 2002.

338. Strandness DE Jr: Screening for carotid disease and surveillance for carotid restenosis, *Semin Vasc Surg* 14:200–205, 2001.

339. Lovelace TD, Moneta GL, Abou-Zamzam AM Jr, et al: Optimizing duplex follow-up in patients with an asymptomatic internal carotid artery stenosis of less than 60%, *J Vasc Surg* 33:56–61, 2001.

340. Sayeed S, Stanziale SF, Wholey MH, et al: Angiographic lesion characteristics can predict adverse outcomes after carotid artery stenting, *J Vasc Surg* 47:81–87, 2008.

341. Halm EA, Tuhrim S, Wang JJ, et al: Risk factors for perioperative death and stroke after carotid endarterectomy: Results of the New York Carotid Artery Surgery Study, *Stroke* 40:221–229, 2009.

342. Hofmann R, Niessner A, Kypta A, et al: Risk score for peri-interventional complications of carotid artery stenting, *Stroke* 37:2557–2561, 2006.

343. de Weert TT, Cretier S, Groen HC, et al: Atherosclerotic plaque surface morphology in the carotid bifurcation assessed with multidetector computed tomography angiography, *Stroke* 40:1334–1340, 2009.

344. Wong EY, Nikolov HN, Thorne ML, et al: Clinical Doppler ultrasound for the assessment of plaque ulceration in the stenosed carotid bifurcation by detection of distal turbulence intensity: a matched model study, *Eur Radiol* 19:2739–2749, 2009.

345. Kohyama S, Kazekawa K, Iko M, et al: Spontaneous improvement of persistent ulceration after carotid artery stenting, *AJNR Am J Neuroradiol* 27:151–156, 2006.

346. Qiao Y, Farber A, Semaan E, et al: Images in cardiovascular medicine. Healing of an asymptomatic carotid plaque ulceration, *Circulation* 118:e147–e148, 2008.

347. Heyman A, Wilkinson WE, Heyden S, et al: Risk of stroke in asymptomatic persons with cervical arterial bruits, *N Engl J Med* 302:838, 1980.

348. Wolf PA, Kannel WB, Sorlie P, McNamara P: Asymptomatic carotid bruit and the risk of stroke, *JAMA* 245:1442, 1981.

349. Gautier JC, Rosa A, L'hermitte F: Auscultation carotidienne: Correlations chez 200 patients avec 332 angiographies, *Rev Neurol (Paris)* 131:175, 1975.

350. Pessin MS, Panis W, Prager RJ, et al: Auscultation of cervical and ocular bruits in extracranial carotid occlusive disease: A clinical and angiographic study, *Stroke* 14:246, 1983.

351. Lees RS, Kistler JP: Carotid phonoangiography. In Bernstein E, editor: *Noninvasive diagnostic techniques in vascular disease*, St. Louis, 1978, CV Mosby, p 187.

352. Lipchik EO, DeWeese JA, Schenk EA, et al: Diaphragm-like obstructions of the human arterial tree, *Radiology* 113:43, 1974.

353. Ratchford EV, Jin Z, Di Tullio MR, et al: Carotid bruit for detection of hemodynamically significant carotid stenosis: The Northern Manhattan Study, *Neurol Res* 31:748–752, 2009.

354. Bonati LH, Ederle J, McCabe DJ, et al: on behalf of the CAVATAS Investigators: Long-term risk of carotid restenosis in patients randomly assigned to endovascular treatment or endarterectomy in the Carotid and Vertebral Artery Transluminal Angioplasty Study (CAVATAS): long-term follow-up of a randomised trial, *Lancet Neurol* 8:908–917, 2009.

355. Archie JP Jr: Reoperations for carotid artery stenosis: Role of primary and secondary reconstructions, *J Vasc Surg* 33:495–503, 2001.

356. O'Hara PJ, Hertzer NR, Karafa MT, et al: Reoperation for recurrent carotid stenosis: Early results and late outcome in 199 patients, *J Vasc Surg* 34:5–12, 2001.

357. Attigah N, Külkens S, Deyle C, et al: Redo surgery or carotid stenting for restenosis after carotid endarterectomy: Results of two different treatment strategies, *Ann Vasc Surg* 24:190–195, 2010.

23 Anterior Cerebral Artery Disease

JOHN C.M. BRUST, ANGEL CHAMORRO

Infarction in the territory of one or both anterior cerebral arteries (ACAs) can follow vasospasm after rupture of saccular aneurysms of the ACA or the anterior communicating artery (ACoA). When such cases are excluded, ACA infarcts represent 0.6% to 3% of acute ischemic strokes.[1-4] In most reports, ACA territory infarction is more often associated with internal carotid artery (ICA) atherosclerosis than with primary stenosis or thrombosis of the ACA itself.[5] In a series of 100 consecutive Korean patients with ACA infarction, however, 68 had local atherosclerosis of the vessel.[6] In another series of 27 patients, 17 (63%) had probable emboli from the ICA or the heart; other causes were isolated proximal ACA occlusion, paraneoplastic disseminated intravascular coagulation, ICA dissection with embolic occlusion of the opposite ACA, acute ethanol intoxication, and hypertensive occlusion of a small penetrating branch of the ACA. Six patients with no obvious cause were older than 50 years, five of whom had risk factors for atherosclerotic stroke.[1] In an autopsy series of 55 patients with ACA infarcts, 10 had probable cardiac emboli and only 5 had atherosclerosis primarily involving the ACA itself.[7] ACA territory infarction has resulted from vessel compression during transfalcial herniation.[8,9]

Dissecting aneurysms of the ACA affect either proximal or distal segments, produce both infarction and subarachnoid hemorrhage, and occur either spontaneously or after head trauma.[10-18] Case reports suggest embolic occlusion from small aneurysms of the distal ICA.[19]

A patient with transient ischemic attacks had fibromuscular dysplasia of both pericallosal arteries.[20] In another report, bilateral ACA infarction occurred in a patient with sickle cell trait during acute ethanol intoxication and withdrawal.[21] ACA infarction has also resulted from intracranial extension of Wegener's granulomatosis,[22] arteritis secondary to subarachnoid neurocysticercosis,[23,24] tuberculous meningitis,[24,25] and radiation vasculitis 19 years after cranial irradiation for acute lymphoblastic leukemia.[26] ACA territory infarction is also described in association with moyamoya disease,[27-29] migraine,[30] Takayasu disease,[31] and Susac's syndrome[32] and as a complication of intraarterial recombinant tissue plasminogen activator.[33]

Symptoms and signs, including weakness, sensory loss, and behavioral disturbance, vary widely among patients with ACA infarcts. To understand this variety, one must be familiar with the relevant anatomy.

Anatomy

The ACA can be divided into a proximal or A1 segment, from its origin as the medial component of the internal carotid bifurcation to its junction with the ACoA, and a distal or postcommunicating artery segment (Fig. 23-1).[34-36] The distal segment has been variably subdivided by different authorities[35,37-46]; for example, into an A2 segment beginning at the ACoA and passing in front of the lamina terminalis as far as the junction of the rostrum and genu of the corpus callosum, an A3 segment passing around the genu of the corpus callosum, an A4 segment from above the corpus callosum to just beyond the coronal suture, and an A5 segment extending to the artery's termination.[40] The A2 and A3 segments have together been referred to as the *ascending segment,* and the A4 and A5 segments have been referred to as the *horizontal segment.*[36]

The A1 segment passes over the optic chiasm (in 70% of cases) or optic nerve (30%), varying in length from 7.2 to 18 mm (average, 12.7 mm).[35] Its diameter ranges from 0.9 to 4.0 mm (average, 2.6 mm) and is greater than 1.5 mm in 90% of brains. In 74% of brains, both A1 segments are larger than the ACoA, the diameter of which ranges from 0.2 to 3.4 mm (average, 1.5 mm).[35]

The ACAs pass over the corpus callosum side by side in only a minority of cases, so the ACoA is most often directed obliquely or even anteroposteriorly; thus, it is often best seen with angiography on oblique projections.[35]

The recurrent artery of Heubner[47] arises either at the level of the ACoA or just proximal or distal to it; in different series, it was described as arising most often from the A1 segment,[48] from the A2 segment,[35] or at the level of the ACoA.[49-62] Usually the largest branch of the A1 or proximal A2 segment, Heubner's artery, doubles back on the ACA for a variable distance and then, either as a single trunk or with as many as 12 branches, penetrates the anterior perforated substance above the ICA bifurcation or lateral to it in the sylvian fissure; some branches enter the olfactory sulcus, the gyrus rectus, or more lateral inferior frontal areas.[35,53] Of obvious importance to the neurosurgeon[54-56] is the fact that Heubner's artery most consistently supplies the head of the caudate, the anterior inferior part of the internal capsule's anterior limb, the anterior globus pallidus, and parts of the uncinate fasciculus, olfactory regions, and anterior putamen and hypothalamus.[35,39,48,50,53,57-59]

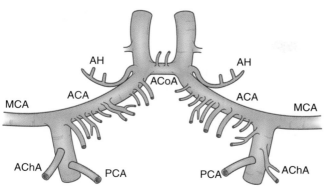

Figure 23-1 Diagram of the dorsal surface of the anterior circle of Willis, showing branches from the A1 segment of the anterior cerebral artery and from the anterior communicating artery. ACA, Anterior cerebral artery; AChA, anterior choroidal artery; ACoA, anterior communicating artery; AH, Heubner's artery; MCA, middle cerebral artery; PCA, posterior communicating artery. (From Dunker RO, Harris AB: Surgical anatomy of the proximal anterior cerebral artery. J Neurosurg 44:359, 1976.)

In addition to Heubner's artery, the A1 and A2 segments give off smaller basal perforating branches, up to 15 from each A1 segment[35,50] and up to 10 from each A2 segment.[35,36,54] One of these, called the short central artery, is considered more consistent than others, in some people supplying part of the caudate nucleus and anterior limb of the internal capsule.[61,62] Other proximal branches penetrate the anterior perforated substance and the optic tract and supply, variably, parolfactory structures, the medial anterior commissure, globus pallidus, caudate and putamen, and the anterior limb of the internal capsule; these vessels also commonly supply the genu and contiguous posterior limb of the internal capsule, part of the anterior nucleus of the thalamus, and most of the anterior hypothalamus.[50] More distal A1 penetrating branches are smaller and supply the optic nerve, chiasm, and tract[50,63]; gyrus rectus and inferior frontal lobe; anterior perforated substance; and suprachiasmatic area.[35] Additional supply to the anterior inferior striatum and anterior hypothalamus comes from A2 segment branches, which can arise either separately or from a larger common trunk (the pericallosal artery).[36] Similar penetrating branches from the ACoA, 13 or fewer in number,[50,64] supply the suprachiasmatic and parolfactory areas, dorsal optic chiasm, anterior perforated substance, inferior frontal lobe, septum pellucidum, columns of the fornix, corpus callosum, septal region, and anterior hypothalamus and cingulum.[34,35,63,64]

Vascular anastomoses are less functional in the diencephalon and basal ganglia than elsewhere in the cerebral hemispheres, and the territories supplied by these ACA penetrating end-zone arteries are no exception. Capillary anastomoses, which are difficult to demonstrate by standard perfusion techniques, exceed arterial anastomoses.[38,65-69]

The distal ACAs, deep in the interhemispheric fissure, are the only example of major cerebral arteries running side by side, although, as noted, one (usually the left) is often posterior to the other, and because of crossover of branches to the other hemisphere, occlusion of either artery can cause contralateral or bilateral infarction.[36]

Beyond the lamina terminalis, the main trunk of the ACA—the pericallosal artery—runs above the corpus callosum in the pericallosal cistern (or, less often, over the cingulate gyrus or in the cingulate sulcus[37]), passes around the splenium of the corpus callosum, and terminates in the choroid plexus of the third ventricle; its posterior extent depends on the anterior extent of the posterior cerebral artery (PCA).[36,70] Except most posteriorly, the pericallosal artery lies below the free edge of the falx cerebri and can therefore shift across the midline.

The pericallosal artery has been variably defined as beginning at the ACoA[46] or at the point where the ACA gives off the callosomarginal artery; however, the callosomarginal artery is absent in 18% to 60% of brains.[36,45] The callosomarginal artery has been defined as that branch of the ACA traveling in or near the cingulate sulcus and giving off at least two major cortical branches. It originates from just beyond the ACoA to the genu of the corpus callosum, most often from the A3 segment,[36] and can be of the same diameter, larger, or smaller than the pericallosal artery.[36] Any or all of the callosomarginal artery's usual branches can arise from the pericallosal artery[36]; these branches supply the inferior frontal lobe (including the gyrus rectus, the orbital part of the superior frontal gyrus, the medial part of the orbital gyri, and the olfactory bulb and tract), the medial surface of the hemisphere (including the cingulate gyrus, the superior frontal gyrus, the paracentral lobule, and the precuneus), and the superior 2 cm of the lateral convexity (including the superior frontal, precentral, central, and postcentral gyri), anastomosing there with branches of the middle cerebral artery (MCA).[37] (These border zones of shared arterial territory are of clinical importance: In a radionuclide study of 365 consecutive patients with stroke, infarction occurred in the "watershed" between the ACA and the MCA in 5% of patients compared with the MCA territory in 28% and the ACA territory in 1%.)[71-73] The band of lateral convexity supplied by the ACA is wider anteriorly than posteriorly and may extend into the middle frontal gyrus.

Although variable in number and in whether they arise directly from the pericallosal artery or from its callosomarginal branch, eight major cortical branches of the distal ACA can usually be defined.[36] The orbitofrontal artery arises from the A2 segment except, infrequently, when it shares a common trunk with the frontopolar artery or arises just proximal to the ACoA.[35] Running forward in the floor of the anterior fossa as far as the planum sphenoidale, the orbitofrontal artery supplies the gyrus rectus, olfactory bulb and tract, and orbital surface of the frontal lobe. The frontopolar artery arises from the A2 segment (or, uncommonly, from the callosomarginal artery), passes to the frontal pole along the medial hemispheric surface, and supplies parts of the medial and lateral surfaces of the frontal pole.

The anterior, middle, and posterior frontal arteries arise separately from the A2, A3, and A4 segments of the pericallosal artery or from the callosomarginal artery; infrequently they arise from a common stem.[36,45] They supply the anterior, middle, and posterior parts of the superior frontal gyrus and the cingulate gyrus. The paracentral artery, arising from A4 or the callosomarginal artery, supplies premotor, motor, and sensory areas of the paracentral lobule.

The superior parietal artery, arising anterior to the splenium of the corpus callosum from A4, A5, or the callosomarginal artery, passes through the marginal limb of the cingulate sulcus and supplies the superior part of the precuneus. The inferior parietal artery, subdivided by some authorities into the precuneal and parietooccipital arteries,[37,39] is the most commonly absent cortical branch of the ACA (36% of brains in one series[36]); it arises from the A5 segment (or rarely from the callosomarginal artery) just above the splenium of the corpus callosum and supplies the posterior inferior part of the precuneus and portions of the cuneus.

The rostrum, genu, body, and splenium of the corpus callosum are supplied by short callosal arteries, pericallosal artery branches that pass through the callosum to supply, additionally, the septum pellucidum, anterior pillars of the fornix, and anterior commissure.[36,37] Posteriorly, the pericallosal artery extends around the splenium of the corpus callosum (the posterior pericallosal artery) and then passes forward, ending on the inferior surface of the splenium or extending all the way to the foramen of Monro.[74]

Of obvious importance in interpreting symptoms and signs is the normal variability of the boundaries (or border zones) between the anterior, middle, and posterior cerebral arteries. Fig. 23-2, which is based on postmortem injection studies of 25 healthy brains, illustrates the range of cortical distribution of the ACA.[75] In those with the most extensive ACA distribution, the primary motor and sensory cortices were supplied by the ACA not only medially but also over the convexity as far as the inferior frontal sulcus. In those with the least extensive ACA distribution, the ACA supplied little or none of the primary motor cortex, even medially.

Anomalies and Species Differences

The anatomy of the anterior circle of Willis is so varied among otherwise healthy people that whether a variation should be called an anomaly is sometimes difficult to define. Especially common are hypoplastic A1 segments, from mildly narrow to nonfunctionally threadlike, with both distal ACAs filling from the larger A1 segment.[54,76-81] In one study, 7% of brains had a stringlike A1 segment, and 6% had a hypoplastic ACoA.[82] In another study, 22% of brains had A1 segment hypoplasia, which was severe in 8% of cases and was associated with additional anomalies of the ACA or the posterior cerebral, posterior communicating, or basilar arteries in 82%.[83] Such anomalies are associated with a greater frequency of saccular aneurysms, and ACA occlusion secondary to cardiac embolism is often accompanied by proximal hypoplasia of the contralateral ACA.[79,84-86]

A smaller ACA often occurs on the same side as a smaller ICA,[87] and a hypoplastic A1 segment tends to be associated with an ACoA of larger diameter than usual.[35,88] Small A1 segments are several times more common among patients with symptomatic cerebrovascular disease than in the general population.[59] Cerebral angiography in one young man with episodic vertigo, loss of consciousness, and left leg weakness showed absence of the ACAs; the MCAs and one intracavernous carotid artery provided collateral vessels to the patient's medial cerebral hemispheres.[89]

In 50 adult autopsy specimens, 60% had one ACoA, 30% two, and 10% three[35]; other investigators have also found doubling and tripling of this vessel, and some have found absence of the ACoA.[39,90,91] A1 segment duplication also occurs,[35] as well as a third or median ACA arising from the ACoA (arteria termatica), which is sometimes as large as the two other ACAs and may be the major supplier to the posterior medial hemispheres.[39,50,92]

The recurrent artery of Heubner rarely arises from the ICA at its bifurcation, from the MCA, from the ACoA, or from the orbitofrontal or frontopolar branches of the ACA.[35,93-95] Such anomalies increase the risk of infarction in the territory of the recurrent artery of Heubner during surgical treatment of aneurysms arising from the anterior circle of Willis.[96] Absence or doubling of Heubner's artery occurs.[53,97] Embryologically, this artery is a remnant of the primitive olfactory artery; thus a patient with a persistent primitive olfactory artery has no Heubner's artery.[98]

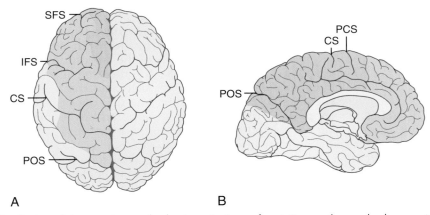

Figure 23-2 Cortical distribution of the anterior cerebral artery. A, Area of variation on the cerebral convexity. B, Area of variation on the cerebral medial surface. Combined pink and gray areas represent a composite of maximal extent. Gray areas represent a composite of minimal extent. CS, Central sulcus; IFS, inferior frontal sulcus; PCS, precentral sulcus; POS, parietooccipital sulcus; SFS, superior frontal sulcus. (From Van der Zwan A, Hillen B, Tulleken CAF, et al: Variability of the territories of the major cerebral arteries. *J Neurosurg* 77:927, 1992.)

Another well-recognized anomaly is a supernumerary vessel arising from the ICA at the level of the ophthalmic artery, coursing below the optic nerve, ascending in front of the optic chiasm, and terminating on the ipsilateral ACA near the ACoA. The A1 segment may be normal, hypoplastic, or absent[99-103]; in one instance both ACAs were absent.[104] Such an anomaly, which may be bilateral,[105] is commonly associated with ACA saccular aneurysm[100,102,104,106] and with other anomalies, such as duplication of the MCA,[107] median corpus callosum artery, distal moyamoya, aortic coarctation,[108] facial congenital defects, cerebral lipoma,[48] and absence of the ICA (in which the remaining carotid artery gives off a branch that passes beneath the optic nerve and divides into two ACAs while the other MCA arises from the PCA).[109] The anomalous vessel itself can cause visual symptoms from compression of the optic nerve or chiasm.[110]

The infraoptic ACA has been considered a remnant of the embryonic primitive maxillary artery, present in 3- to 4-mm embryos as an ICA branch and normally becoming a cavernous carotid branch, the inferior hypophyseal artery.[99,100,110-112] (The ACA normally arises from the primitive olfactory artery, eventually becoming the dominant vessel.)

Other anomalies, reported in an autopsied infant, include unilateral absence of the proximal MCA, ACA, and anterior choroidal artery, with much of the ipsilateral inferior frontal lobe supplied by branches from the opposite ACA, and secondary porencephaly of the orbital frontal lobe.[113] Autopsy of a neurologically healthy man showed a plexiform anterior communicating system connected to the left ICA by an anomalous vessel arising from the ICA near the ophthalmic artery, a single distal ACA, marked right A1 segment hypoplasia, and right plexiform vessels in the area of Heubner's artery, along with other anomalies of the posterior circulation.[114] Such anomalies, rare in combination, are not unusual individually. For example, in a series of 1250 consecutive autopsies, a plexiform anterior communicating system was found in 15% of subjects, hypoplastic ACAs were found in 4%, and fused distal ACAs were found in 4%; a plexiform Heubner artery was much less common.[114] An ophthalmic artery arising from the ACA has also been reported,[74,115-117] as has an accessory MCA arising from the A2 segment of the ACA.[118]

In a study of 381 brains, distal ACA anomalies were found in 25%.[37] Such anomalies include pericallosal artery triplication, absence of ACA pairing, branches from one ACA to the other hemisphere, and bihemispheric branches (Fig. 23-3).[36,39,76,90,92,119,120] Triplicate ACAs with a variably developed midline accessory artery arising from the ACoA and supplying little, much, or most of either or both hemispheres have been observed in up to 22% of autopsy specimens.[37,62,90,121-125] Also, a long callosal artery (medial artery of the corpus callosum, anterior MCA) can arise from the pericallosal artery and pass parallel to it, giving off callosal perforating branches.[36,37] At angiography these anomalies, like a hypoplastic A1 segment, produce apparent bilateral ACA filling after unilateral injection of a carotid artery.[38,44,126-128] Bihemispheric ACAs, with either ACA taking over the supply of part or all of the other hemisphere, have been reported in up to 64%

of brains.[36,38,125] (The highest value comes from a study in which any contralateral supply, however small, was included; brains in which most of both hemispheres are supplied by one of two ACAs are less common.[36])

In the fetus, there is gradual embryonic transition from one to two ACAs.[121,129] An unpaired or azygous ACA, arising through proximal union of the ACAs without an ACoA, occurs in 5% or less of adult brains.[37,90,91,121-124,130,131] Sometimes, the ACAs fuse for up to 3.9 cm, and an ACoA is absent.[89] Azygous ACAs are associated with a variety of other anomalies, including hydranencephaly, septum pellucidum defects, meningomyelocele, hydroencephalodysplasia, and vascular malformations,[132] and, like other ACA anomalies, with a higher frequency of saccular aneurysm.[133,134] In holoprosencephaly (fusion of the frontal neocortex and absence of the interhemispheric fissure), an azygous ACA courses just beneath the inner table of the skull.[108]

As noted, ACA anomalies are associated with an increased frequency of saccular aneurysms, especially at the ACoA, but also on distal or anomalous branches.[53,98,135-151] The embryonic prominence of the interhemispheric arterial plexus that develops into the ACoA is the most common site for the development of

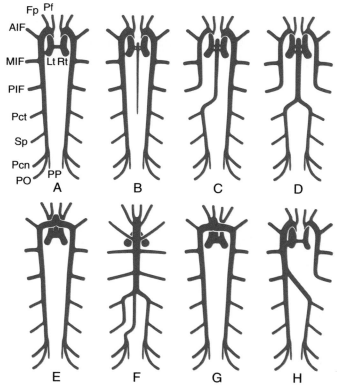

Figure 23-3 Variations in the distal anterior cerebral artery including patterns without (A) and with (B) a medial artery of the corpus callosum and variously developed accessory (C to E), unpaired (F), and bihemispheric lateral arteries (G and H). AIF, Anterior internal frontal; Fp, frontopolar; MIF, middle internal frontal; Pcn, precuneal; Pct, paracentral; Pf, prefrontal (orbitofrontal); PIF, posterior internal frontal; PO, parietooccipital; PP, posterior pericallosal; Sp, superior parietal. (From Baptista AG: Studies on the arteries of the brain. II: The anterior cerebral artery: Some anatomic features and their clinical implications. *Neurology* 13:825, 1963.)

intracranial aneurysms.[152] Of 206 patients with ACoA aneurysms in one study, 44 (21.4%) had ACA anomalies, especially a median artery of the corpus callosum and duplication of the ACoA.[140] Ruptured fusiform aneurysm of the A1 segment of the ACA has been reported.[153] Giant aneurysms have been found on azygous ACAs.[154,155] After subarachnoid hemorrhage, a congenitally narrow A1 segment may be mistaken for vasospasm. Furthermore, proximal ACA ligation in patients with surgically unclippable ACoA aneurysms is not a valid option if one A1 segment fills both distal ACAs or if, in the absence of cross-compression, the aneurysms fill well from either side.[77,156-159]

A common anomaly, ACA fenestration has no clinical significance except when it is mistaken for an aneurysm on angiography.[160] Vestibulocochlear symptoms developed in a 22-year-old patient with fenestration and ectasia of the left ACA and persistence of the right trigeminal artery.[161]

Species differences in the anatomy of the ACA (and other cerebral vessels) must be kept in mind when one is interpreting animal studies of cerebral ischemia and stroke. For example, birds, amphibians, and anteaters have paired arteries without an ACoA or other left-to-right anastomoses.[39] In most mammals, the two ACAs join to form a single pericallosal (azygous) artery, which may or may not bifurcate distally, and there is no ACoA.[39] In subhuman primates, several recurrent medial striate arteries (the equivalent of Heubner's artery in humans) supplying the anterior caudate, putamen, and globus pallidus have rich preparenchymal anastomoses with lateral lenticulostriate arteries from the MCA; the orbitofrontal artery, supplying most of the orbital surface of the frontal lobe, arises from the MCA and anastomoses with branches of the ACA, and extensive anastomoses exist between the ACA and the proximal MCA in the sylvian fissure.[58,162-165] In cats, the presence of an ACoA has been both claimed[166,167] and denied.[168] The feline ACA supplies the medial hemispheric cortex containing hind limb motor representation, but cerebral arterial occlusion tends to cause smaller and deeper infarcts than in higher primates.[169] In rats the rostral caudatoputamen is supplied by penetrating ACA branches and a vessel running alongside the lateral olfactory tract, and this area accounts for 25% of strokes in stroke-prone, spontaneously hypertensive rats.[170,171]

Symptoms and Signs

Weakness and Sensory Loss

ACA occlusion causes infarction of the paracentral lobule and, as a result, weakness and sensory loss in the contralateral leg (Fig. 23-4).[172-177] The deficit is usually greatest distally for the following two reasons: (1) the proximal leg is represented on the primary sensorimotor cortex either superiorly on the medial hemisphere or on the high convexity with, therefore, richer collateral vessels from the MCA and (2) proximal muscles have substantial representation in the ipsilateral hemisphere.[178] If infarction extends to the upper convexity, there may be proximal arm weakness or, as is usual with cortical lesions, clumsiness or slowness out of proportion to the actual loss of strength.

Paretic muscles are initially most often flaccid, becoming spastic over days or weeks; at the outset, tendon reflexes may be decreased, normal, or increased. (This common early dissociation between tone and tendon reflexes has been attributed to the loss of supraspinal influence on different kinds of muscle spindle afferents [e.g., phasic versus tonic].) Babinski's sign may be present.

The sensory modalities most often affected are discriminative (two-point discrimination, localization, stereognosis) and proprioceptive (position sense). Pain and temperature sensation and gross touch are usually only mildly decreased; the patient can tell sharp from dull, but the pinprick does not feel as sharp or as "normal" as on the unaffected side. Vibratory loss is variable. Depending on the posterior extent of the ACA and collaterals from the PCA, sensory loss may be mild or even absent in the presence of marked crural hemiparesis.[39] Sensation may be similarly spared when occlusion is not of the ACA or the pericallosal artery but of the paracentral branch.[39,179-182]

In the acute phase, the head and eyes may be deviated toward the side of the lesion.[39,183,184] Forced grasping and groping of the contralateral hand, regardless of whether it is weak, follows damage to the posterior superior frontal gyrus.[39,185-187] Such forced grasping has been considered "a type of limb-kinetic apraxia" and "only one aspect of a total change in behavior toward a compulsive exploration of the environment"[188]; foot grasping[189] can cause the lower limb to seem "glued to the floor"[188] on attempted walking. Patients with such findings also display sucking and biting,[188] "ansaugen" (a movement of the lips and tongue toward stimulation of the skin near the lower lip),[186] bradykinesia (or an "absence of movement intention"),[39,190,191] catalepsy,[192] and "tonic innervation" ("amorphous movements of a pseudospontaneous character")[39] on attempted voluntary action of the affected arm or leg.[189-191] During the first few days after ACA territory infarction, two patients displayed "hyperkinetic motor behaviors" (including head and eye movements, grimacing, chewing, rubbing body parts, rhythmically moving the fingers, and flexing and extending the thigh) on the nonparalyzed side.[193] It was suggested that such movements (which also occurred contralateral to hemiplegia after MCA territory infarction) signify "an active process induced by disinhibition in order to establish new compensatory pathways."

The "pusher syndrome," a disturbed control of upright body posture in which the patient suffers from a severe misperception of his body's orientation in the coronal plane, was described in a patient with a right ACA infarction, severe left hemiparesis, spatial neglect, visual and auditory extinction, and forced contraversive pushing away from the nonparalyzed side.[194,195]

Pronounced weakness of the arm and face in the presence of ACA occlusions has been attributed to involvement of Heubner's artery and its supply to the anterior limb and genu of the internal capsule (Fig. 23-5).[39] If the circle of Willis is complete, such proximal thrombosis must extend as far as the ACoA to produce complete hemiplegia, or the contralateral ACA takes over the supply of both medial hemispheres and weakness is limited to the face and arm. Paralysis of the right arm, paresis of the right face, and only slight weakness of the right

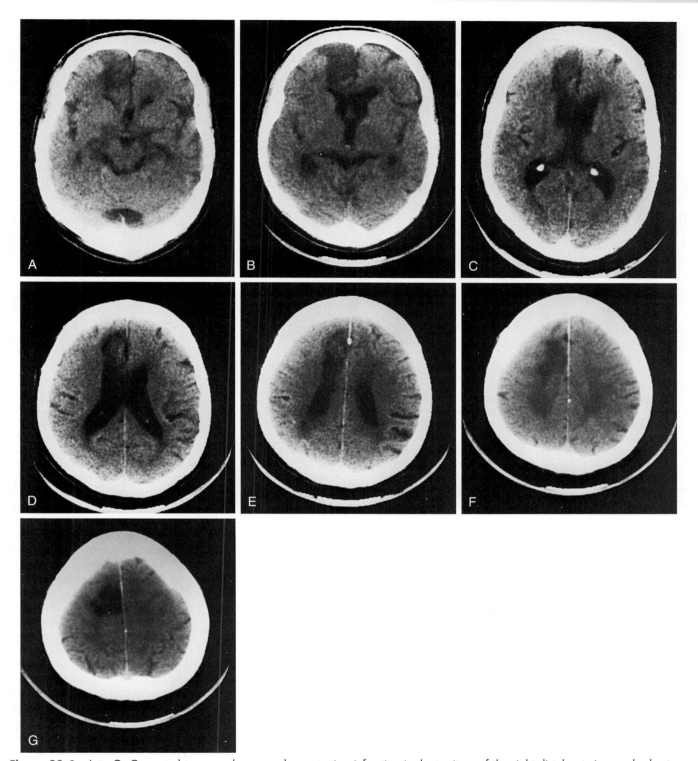

Figure 23-4   A to G, Computed tomography scans demonstrating infarction in the territory of the right distal anterior cerebral artery, including the orbitofrontal and medial and superior frontoparietal lobes. Diencephalic structures supplied by proximal anterior cerebral artery penetrating branches are not involved.

leg occurred in a man who at autopsy was found to have infarction of the left putamen, caudate, and anterior limb of the internal capsule, plus a "shrunken and occluded artery of Heubner."[39] (The leg weakness was attributed to additional softening in the territories of the ACA's middle and posterior internal frontal branches.)

Later anatomic studies have shown, however, that Heubner's artery supplies only the most anterior striatum and anterior limb of the internal capsule and is, therefore, probably uncommonly the responsible vessel when brachial or facial palsy accompanies ACA occlusion. The more likely possibility in such a situation is involvement

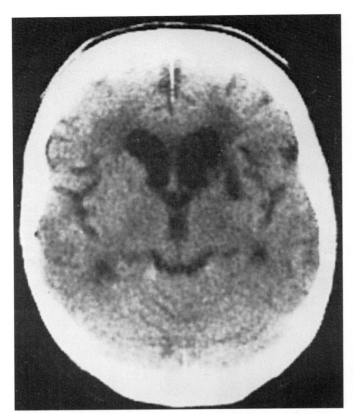

Figure 23-5 Computed tomography scan showing infarction in the territory of either the left artery of Heubner or another penetrating branch of the proximal anterior cerebral artery. Brain supplied by the distal anterior cerebral artery was radiographically normal, and at autopsy, infarction was found to be limited to the head of the caudate, the anterior part of the internal capsule's anterior limb, and the anterior putamen.

of penetrating branches arising from the most proximal ACA and the internal carotid bifurcation, which supply the genu and the anterior part of the internal capsule's posterior limb in addition to the hypothalamus and the rostral thalamus.[50] Moreover, caudate infarction can cause contralateral limb bradykinesia, clumsiness, and loss of associated movements mistakenly interpreted as weakness.[61] Dysarthria has followed unilateral infarction of either the left or right anterior limb of the internal capsule, and in one report, dysarthria occurred after infarction apparently confined to the caudate nucleus.[61] Five patients with unilateral capsular genu infarction had contralateral facial and lingual weakness with dysarthria, three had unilateral mastication-palatal-pharyngeal weakness, and one had unilateral vocal cord paresis; the only limb involvement was mild hand weakness in three patients.[196]

As previously noted, the ACA territory in some individuals encompasses a considerable portion of the upper cerebral convexity; in such a situation, infarction would include arm and hand representations on the primary motor (and sensory) cortex.[75,197] Conversely, in subjects with a smaller than usual ACA territory, leg weakness can be a consequence of MCA or PCA territory infarction. Of 63 patients in one series with acute stroke and "leg-predominant weakness," infarction occurred in 12 in the

ACA territory, in 9 in the MCA territory, in 2 in both territories (not "watershed"), in 18 in the internal capsule, in 10 in the brainstem, and in 2 in the thalamus.[198] Leg weakness was more lasting when infarction involved the motor cortex than when it involved the premotor cortex or supplementary area and spared the motor cortex.

Of 100 patients with "ataxic hemiparesis" after a first stroke, four had infarction of the contralateral ACA territory.[199] Pyramidal weakness was greatest in the leg, and ataxia of the cerebellar type was seen in the ipsilateral arm. Such ataxia has been attributed to involvement of frontopontocerebellar projections and also, on the basis of single-photon emission computed tomography (SPECT) studies, to transsynaptic dysfunction of the contralateral cerebellum (diaschisis).[200,201] A problem with the ataxic hemiparesis syndrome—regardless of the lesion's location—is that upper motor neuron lesions, as a rule, produce clumsiness out of proportion to weakness; determining whether the "ataxia" is qualitatively or quantitatively sufficient to label it "cerebellar" can be difficult.

The transient ischemic attack syndrome of limb shaking of the leg was described in a woman with an acute infarction on the right corpus callosum and cingulate gyrus secondary to focal stenosis of the right ACA. She had episodic shaking movements of the left leg 1 to 15 times per day, preceded by a brief sensation of weakness and elicited only when she arose from a sitting position.[202]

Infarction in the territories of both ACAs causes paraparesis, with or without sensory loss.[203] Paraparesis occurs most often as a consequence of bilateral ACA vasospasm after rupture of an ACA or ACoA aneurysm.[204,205] In thrombotic or embolic infarction, paraparesis is especially likely when there is a vascular anomaly, such as a hypoplastic A1 segment or an azygous distal ACA.[39,133,183,206-212] Particularly when symptoms are stutteringly progressive, spinal cord disease may be erroneously suspected.[36,37,213,214] Even if weakness is mild or absent, there may be severe gait disturbance, with inability to initiate the first step with either foot, to lift either foot off the ground, or to turn to either side ("slipping clutch syndrome").[215-217] Grasp reflexes of the feet (or hands) are not present in all affected patients, and although some can move their legs freely in the air (e.g., bicycling motions),[217] others cannot.[215] When severe, such medial prefrontal damage can produce a pronounced immobility of all four limbs, from bradykinesia to catatonic (perseverative) posturing with gegenhalten, sucking, and biting.[217] In one such report the patient had unexplained vertical gaze palsy (upward and downward), suggesting midbrain localization.[218]

The gait disability bears an obvious resemblance to that found with hydrocephalus and with the paraplegia in flexion of degenerative disease that mainly affects the frontal lobes[219]; in these conditions, the pathophysiology is not understood, and the possible roles of descending frontal and prefrontal fibers[220,221] or the globus pallidus[222] are uncertain. Pulsatile flow in the ACAs is decreased in infantile hydrocephalus,[223] and some researchers have suggested that secondary ACA ischemia may be the cause of lower extremity spasticity in hydrocephalic infants and may contribute to the gait disturbance seen in adult normal-pressure hydrocephalus.[224]

A man whose anomalous ACAs resulted in bilateral infarction restricted to the supplementary motor areas had what was considered gait apraxia; he had difficulty standing from a chair on command, rolling over in bed, starting or stopping walking, and maintaining stance. There were no elementary motor abnormalities, and the authors considered his disorder a "loss of monitoring of the automatic implementation of gait mechanisms."[225] Drop attacks and right-sided limb-shaking TIAs occurred in a man with left ICA stenosis and a left A1 segment of the ACA supplying both medial frontal lobes; symptoms resolved after endarterectomy.[226]

Callosal Disconnection Signs

In addition to either right or left leg weakness, ACA occlusion can cause left-sided apraxia, agraphia, and tactile anomia.[42,76,186,190,227-230] Early cases, however, are difficult to interpret.[231,232] For example, the patient reported by Liepmann and Maas[42] had right hemiplegia, including his arm, so it is uncertain whether the agraphia and apraxia were truly unilateral. The patient described by Goldstein[190] had left-sided weakness, greatest in the leg, with a pronounced left hand grasp reflex, which was itself another possible reason for left-sided motor difficulty.[217,233] Agraphia, apraxia, and tactile anomia have occurred, however, in otherwise normal left limbs of patients with ACA occlusion, right leg weakness, and normal right arms.[228,229,234,235]

After surgical occlusion of the left ACA, a patient described by Geschwind and Kaplan[231] had right hemiparesis that was worse in the leg, a marked grasp reflex in the right hand, and mild right proprioceptive loss. He also had left-handed agraphia, writing incorrectly and paragraphically both spontaneously and to dictation, and he could not perform written calculations with his left hand. He could not name objects, letters, or numbers placed in his left hand out of his sight, but he could identify them afterward with his left hand by pointing to them or demonstrating their use. Using either hand, he could not correctly select from a group of objects placed out of sight in the other hand. Finally, he had difficulty performing verbal commands with his left hand (e.g., draw a square, point to the examiner, show how to brush teeth). Despite the grasp reflex, his right hand could write normally, and his left hand could slavishly copy writing. Either hand could imitate the examiner's movements or manipulate objects. Following the lead of earlier investigators,[42] Geschwind and Kaplan[231] attributed their findings to anterior callosal destruction, with disconnection of the right hemisphere from the left or, more specifically, of the right sensorimotor cortex from the left language areas. (Earlier writers who claimed that callosal lesions could cause left astereognosis[190,236] were undoubtedly observing tactile anomia rather than true agnosia, although the ability of a patient to identify objects but not letters placed in the left hand is less easily explained.[237]) Preservation of the posterior corpus callosum was manifested by the ability of Geschwind and Kaplan's[231] patient to read words presented to either visual field. Retained ability to perform tasks requiring both hands, such as threading a needle, suggested that the two hemispheres could cooperate like two individuals on such visually guided activities.

A left-handed patient had a stroke with weakness of the right leg but not the right arm, plus loss of ability to write with the right but not the left hand; if he is presumed to have had right cerebral language dominance, callosal disconnection might explain the agraphic right hand.[238] Another patient, considered to have pure agraphia, may represent a similar example of ACA occlusion.[239]

Some patients with presumed ACA occlusion and anterior callosal damage have had difficulty not only in performing verbal commands with the left hand but also in imitating the examiner and using actual objects.[185,192,236,240] Inaccessibility of verbal information to the right sensorimotor cortex would not explain this type of apraxia. Some investigators have suggested that, in right-handed people, engrams for skilled movements (space–time or visuokinesthetic engrams)[241] reside in the left hemisphere and that callosal apraxia with impaired imitation and object use is the result of disconnection between these motor engrams and the right hemisphere.[241,242] In support of such a view is the observation, in a left-handed person, that dominance for language and dominance for skilled motor acts appeared to be in different hemispheres.[232] That some patients with ACA occlusion have impaired imitation and object use and some do not has been explained by the hypothesis that verbal motor programs may be transmitted to the right hemisphere across the genu of the corpus callosum, whereas visuokinesthetic engrams may be transmitted across the body.[241]

The alien hand syndrome consists of apparently purposeful movements of an upper extremity that a patient cannot control.[242-247] Different forms are described. A review of published cases concluded that damage to the medial prefrontal cortex of the dominant hemisphere and the anterior corpus callosum resulted in intermanual conflict and inability to perform bimanual tasks.[243] In another report, interfering movements of the alien hand were triggered by movements of the other hand and often had a mischievous quality. For example, a patient was about to hit a nail on a block with a hammer when his left hand pushed the block away, causing the hammer to miss the target. In that report patients with chronic symptoms had lesions of both the anterior corpus callosum and the contralateral medial frontal cortical and subcortical regions.[248] Patients express astonishment and frustration when conflict occurs, and they adopt avoidance behavior such as sitting on the alien hand. Involuntary masturbation by the alien hand has followed both unilateral and bilateral ACA territory infarction.[249,250]

The alien hand phenomenon is possibly related to other bizarre signs associated with callosal and/or medial frontal damage, including diagonistic apraxia (as one hand attempts to perform a voluntary action, the other performs the opposite; e.g., the patient puts on his glasses with his right hand, but his left hand then takes them off)[251] and utilization behavior (the patient cannot refrain from picking up and using an object, such as a toothbrush, placed in front of him).[252-254] A patient developed severe utilization behavior after bilateral infarcts that damaged both supplementary motor areas but spared the rest of the premotor cortices, the cingulate gyri, and the corpus callosum. The authors speculated that utilization behavior, reflecting disinhibition of responses to environmental stimuli, might be viewed as a bilateral alien hand syndrome.[255]

A woman with left ACA territory infarction had difficulty naming her left fingers and moving her named left fingers; she also had difficulty pointing to her own body parts with her left hand.[256] It was suggested that the patient's "body schema" was organized principally in her left cerebral hemisphere and was therefore, as a consequence of callosal infarction, disconnected from her right hemisphere.

Occlusion of an ACA that extends around the splenium of the corpus callosum can produce pure alexia in the left visual field or other visual anomic or agnostic problems.[36,241]

A problem in evaluating these patients is the extent to which they differ from those who have undergone surgical callosectomy. Left-sided apraxia to verbal commands occurs immediately after complete section of the corpus callosum and anterior commissure, usually with preserved ability to carry out the act in imitation of the examiner.[257,258] Right-sided movements, when governed by the right hemisphere (e.g., drawing an object seen only in the left visual field), are also impaired.[259] Such deficits tend to improve over days, however,[258] unless severe extracallosal brain damage is present.[257] A lasting deficit after callosal and commissural section is most likely to affect homolateral control of fingers (e.g., moving the left fingers to identify areas corresponding to regions stimulated on the right fingers or mimicking with the left hand postures shown pictorially to the right visual field). When left hemispheric damage occurs early in life, the minor hemisphere can comprehend spoken or written names of familiar objects[260-263] but, except in the setting of prolonged stimulus exposure[264] or in rare instances of unusual plasticity in speech organization,[265,266] usually cannot comprehend verbs or action nouns.[261,267,268] Such lack of comprehension accounts for the inability of a patient who has callosectomy to follow verbal commands with either hand when the information is given to the minor hemisphere. Recovery of all but the most distal and subtle apraxia when commands are given to the language hemisphere is explained by each hemisphere's control over homolateral as well as contralateral limbs.

A patient with anterior callosal hemorrhage and bilateral ACA vasospasm had alexia in the left hemifield, anomia for objects held in the left hand, and left-handed agraphia and apraxia (including imitation and object use).[269] She also had bilateral pseudoneglect: Visual or tactile line bisection produced left hemineglect with the right hand in the left hemispace and right hemineglect with the left hand in the right hemispace. A proposed explanation was disconnection of "the hemisphere important for directing attention–intention into the contralateral hemispace" from "the hemisphere important for controlling sensory motor processing of the limb."[269] By contrast, left hemispatial neglect "confined to right-hand and verbal responses" occurred in a patient with infarction of the posterior genu and whole trunk of the corpus callosum plus the left medial frontal and temporooccipital lobes.[270] These findings were consistent with the hypothesis that "the left hemisphere is only concerned with attending to the contralateral hemispace," whereas "the right hemisphere is specialized for attending to both sides of space." Also consistent with previous reports, hemineglect does not seem to occur with lesions restricted to the corpus callosum but requires additional destruction (e.g., medial frontal lobe) that blocks transmission through extracallosal commissures.[244,271]

In a right-handed patient who had undergone callosectomy but displayed unusually rich right hemispheric verbal comprehension, there was no left-sided apraxia to verbal information presented to the right hemisphere.[268] This finding argues against the notion that motor engrams reside solely in one hemisphere, language-dominant or not.[236,272-278] In other patients undergoing callosectomy, visual nonverbal stimulation has also produced normally coordinated contralateral motor acts.[278]

Consistent with the view that extracallosal damage is probably crucial to the appearance of anterior callosal disconnection syndrome after ACA occlusion is the finding that left tactile anomia, apraxia for verbal commands, and agraphia did not occur in two patients who underwent sectioning of the anterior commissure and only the anterior two thirds of the corpus callosum.[258] These patients, moreover, performed a variety of nonverbal cross-integration tasks, matching visual or tactile stimuli directed separately to each hemisphere.[279] Conversely, selective sectioning of the splenium, sparing the genu and body, does produce verbal deficits for left visual field and tactile stimuli[237,280] as well as for tactile-motor tasks requiring interhemispheric integration.[277,278] It appears that "the anterior commissure and the rostral callosum do not transfer either lateralized visual images that elicit motor activity or the specific motor program needed to carry out the appropriate movement."[278] An isolated 3-cm midcallosal section impairs interhemispheric transfer of tactile data but not of information obtained visually.[281] Section of the most posterior 1.5 cm of the callosum disrupts naming of visual stimuli in the left visual field,[280,282-284] and an additional 1.5-cm section further impairs sensorimotor integration and tactile naming.[278,285] What information is transferred across the rostral callosum (the part most often damaged after ACA occlusion) is unclear; it has been suggested that the anterior callosum transfers information after processing it into higher order abstraction.[278,286] Tomaiuolo et al[287] performed simple reaction times for interhemispheric transfer tasks in a patient with callosal lesions sparing the splenium and rostrum. They measured unimanual responses to simple lateralized visual displays presented tachistoscopically. The impaired responses, when compared with those of a patient with complete callosal section, led to the conclusion that "specific callosal channels mediate the basic visuomotor interhemispheric transfer times (ITTs), and these do not include the rostrum and/or the splenium of the corpus callosum." (After posterior callosal section, interhemispheric transfer of sensory information from the right hemisphere is lost, but transfer of semantic information is still possible; after complete section, neither sensory nor semantic information can be transferred.)[286]

Akinetic Mutism (Abulia)

Akinetic mutism is "a state of limited responsiveness to the environment in the absence of gross alteration of sensorimotor mechanisms operating at a more peripheral level."[288] Neither paralysis nor coma accounts for the symptoms. Patients may open their eyes and seem alert, and brief movement, speech, or even agitation may follow powerful stimuli; however, patients are otherwise "indifferent, detached, frozen, and apathetic."[288] The term *akinetic mutism* was used by Cairns et al[289] to describe such a state in association with a tumor of the third ventricle. Patients with such lesions often have ophthalmoparesis and fluctuating or continuous somnolence.[290,291]

Akinetic mutism also occurs with lesions of the anteromedial frontal lobes, including infarction.[286,292-297] Ophthalmoparesis (except for early gaze preference) is then not present, and the patient, whose open eyes may follow objects, is more obviously alert than the patient with mesencephalic or thalamic lesions; the patient may make brief, monosyllabic, but appropriate responses to questions. Striking dissociation occurs between spontaneous verbal communication, which is often totally absent, and solicited communication, which is often retained although restricted.[292] *Abulia* refers to a continuum of such abnormalities, from mild to severe, having in common decreased spontaneous movement and speech, latency in responding to verbal and other stimuli, and impersistence in responses and tasks.[108,296] Although verbal responses are "late, terse, incomplete, and emotionally flat," the patient who is sufficiently prodded sometimes reveals a cognitive capacity much more normal than expected.[61] When the patient is literally akinetic and mute, however, the condition must be differentiated from true stupor or coma, a locked-in state, extrapyramidal akinesia, catatonia, hysteria, and a persistent vegetative state. The two structures most often implicated in the production of abulia are the cingulate gyrus and the supplementary motor area (SMA).

Abulia has occurred after bilateral cingulate gyrus lesions. A woman had a sudden headache and then "lay staring at the ceiling, not asking for water or food, and never speaking spontaneously."[298] She was incontinent of urine, ate and drank when food or water was brought, comprehended spoken speech, answered questions monosyllabically, and did not display any emotional reaction. Right-sided hyperreflexia and bilateral Babinski's signs were present. At autopsy, embolic hemorrhagic infarction of the cingulate gyri bilaterally and of the corpus callosum was seen. A clinically and pathologically similar patient showed Babinski's signs but no hypertonus, and there were "no visible reactions to pain."[299] Inability to walk despite normal strength has been specifically mentioned in other reports.[300] In another report, however, unilateral cingulate infarction in two patients was followed by seizures in one and personality change in another, with no reduction in motor activity.[300] Akinetic mutism occurred in one patient with presumed unilateral cingulate (and pontine) damage, but autopsy findings were incomplete.[301] A patient with hemorrhage into the right medial frontal lobe had marked bradykinesia of the left limbs that improved when the limbs were placed in his right hemispace.[302] This disturbance was considered motor neglect ("a failure of the intentional systems that lead to preparation and activation of movement"), possibly secondary to SMA damage.[302] It is not unusual for patients with unilateral ACA territory infarction (or medial frontal lobe surgical ablation) to have

several days of abulia followed by return of verbal and ipsilateral motor responses, persistence of weakness in the contralateral leg, and a disinclination to move the contralateral arm. Motor neglect thus might be viewed as unilateral abulia.[39,189,303-306] Chamorro et al[177] demonstrated that motor neglect explains some of the apparent hemiparesis affecting the face, arm, and leg in infarction in the ACA territory, as revealed by computed tomography (CT) or magnetic resonance imaging (MRI) and, in one case, by autopsy correlation (Fig. 23-6). Before the report of these cases, the usual explanation for such face-arm-leg hemiparesis had been involvement of the primary motor cortex or the deeper pathways, neither of which was involved in this series of eight patients. Instead, defective supramotor planning, unilateral hypokinesia, and motor neglect were due to damage of medial premotor areas. Five of the patients had a total lack of voluntary movement in the contralateral limbs that prevented adequate testing of motor praxis and performance of bimanual tasks. Movement could not be elicited by the examiner despite strong verbal and gestural commands. Pain reaction was also defective or absent in the limbs contralateral to the lesion. Transcranial motor stimulation demonstrated absence of responses to cortical stimulation in the lower limbs of the affected side, interpreted as a sign of functional interruption of the corticospinal tract. In the upper limbs, the response to transcranial motor stimulation was normal; this finding indicated that the impaired voluntary function reflected impairment of circuits involved in motor planning or in the initiation of motor action.

With further improvement, signs can become increasingly subtle (e.g., difficulty with sequential movements involving different joints or coordinating the movements of both arms).[306,307] In one report there was inability to reproduce rhythms from memory,[308] and in another, in patients with bilateral SMA lesions, there was inability to perceive as separate two successive tactile stimuli applied to the body.[309] Observations such as these have led to the hypotheses that the SMA (and perhaps other premotor structures) is responsible for generating "sequences from memory that fit into a precise timing plan."[308]

Patients with abulia or motor neglect often display relative preservation of reflexic (externally stimulated) movements, in contrast to anticipated or willed movements. (A comparable dissociation is seen in parkinsonism.) Disinhibition of unanticipated complex motor movements as a result of SMA damage has been invoked to explain such phenomena as alien hand syndrome, diagonistic apraxia, and utilization behavior.[310]

A man with akinetic mutism after bilateral ACA territory infarction had bilateral independent periodic lateralized epileptiform discharges (BIPLEDs) frontally on electroencephalography (EEG).[311] A woman with akinetic mutism after bilateral infarcts that included the cingulate gyri and orbitofrontal structures had reduced striatal dopamine uptake that returned to normal as her symptoms resolved.[312] Anecdotal reports describe improvement in akinetic mutism from frontal lobe damage after treatment with levodopa.[313]

Cingulectomy in monkeys caused reduction of motor activity and "loss of social conscience"; the animals

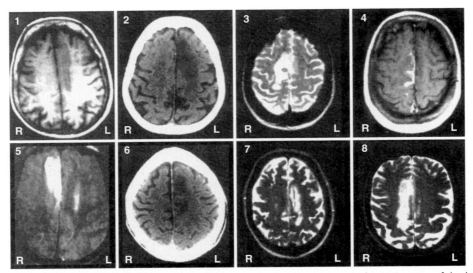

Figure 23-6 Representative axial magnetic resonance (MR) images and computed tomography (CT) scans of the brains of eight patients with anterior cerebral artery (ACA) infarctions. 1, T1-weighted axial MR image; 2, CT scan; 3, T2-weighted MR image; 4, T1-weighted MR image; 5, proton-density MR image; 6, CT scan; 7, T2-weighted MR image; 8, T2-weighted MR image. (From Chamorro A, Marshall RS, Valls-Sole J, et al: Motor behavior in stroke patients with isolated medial frontal ischemic infarction. *Stroke* 28:1755, 1997.)

treated their fellows as inanimate objects not to be feared.[165] Monkeys in which the medial temporal lobes were removed and with Klüver-Bucy syndrome (quietness, no fear, and increased curiosity with compulsive nosing and smelling of all objects) showed gradual clearing of symptoms, which returned after bilateral cingulectomy.[314] In cingulectomized cats, motor signs suggested catatonia.[314] The consequences of surgical cingulate ablation for psychiatric disturbance in humans are difficult to interpret because the amount of cingulate removed is usually small.[315]

The full syndrome of akinetic mutism or abulia has thus not been produced in animals by experimental cingulectomy or in humans by surgical cingulectomy, and even bilateral ACA ligation in humans has on occasion failed to cause the syndrome.[293] In an autopsy report of eight patients with akinetic mutism and bilateral cingulate destruction, no difference was seen in the clinical picture regardless of whether additional lesions existed in the medial orbital cortex or septal region.[300] Most reports, however, have emphasized additional lesions or diffuse compressive cerebral injury,[292,293] and electroencephalograms usually show bilateral cerebral slowing.[293] An angiographic study of patients with subarachnoid hemorrhage showed correlation of unilateral or bilateral ACA vasospasm with akinetic mutism, but it was unclear whether brain damage was limited to one hemisphere in the patients with unilateral vasospasm.[316]

Abulia has also followed unilateral or bilateral caudate infarction (most likely from occlusion of the recurrent artery of Heubner). In one series of unilateral caudate infarction in 17 patients, abulia was the most prominent feature in 10 patients (6 left, 4 right).[61] In four patients, CT showed the lesions to be restricted to the caudate; in others, the anterior limb of the internal capsule was involved. Three abulic patients had alternating restlessness and hyperactivity, and in four others, hyperactivity was present without abulia. In another report it was

proposed that abulia resulted from damage to the dorsolateral caudate (which connects to the dorsolateral frontal lobe) and disinhibition from damage to the ventromedial caudate (which connects to orbitofrontal areas).[317]

After surgical partial section of the anterior corpus callosum, acute akinetic mutism is often seen, but patients tend to recover over days.[318,319] Positron emission tomography studies in baboons have shown that the procedure causes transient depression of cortical metabolism in widespread areas of both frontal lobes (diaschisis).[320]

Language Disturbance

Unilateral ACA occlusion can produce language disturbance, but whether the disturbance is aphasic is uncertain.[321-323] Details are often lacking in case reports. In some patients, "reduction of spontaneous verbal expression"[303] or muteness, often in association with more global psychomotor bradykinesia,[303,324] seems to be a manifestation of abulia; in such patients, comprehension of spoken speech may be untestable.[325] Some investigators describe true impairment of speech comprehension,[326] word-finding difficulty, alexia,[42] and phonemic or verbal paraphasias on spontaneous speech, reading aloud, or writing.[326,327] Others, however, emphasize the absence of paraphasias[324,328,329] or consider the difficulty "partly defects of an aphasic order and partly those of a dysarthria."[39] A number of reports describe impairment of spontaneous speech with normal repetition and sometimes echolalia (transcortical aphasia),[325,328,330-333] and in one instance, echolalia and palilalia occurred without other evidence of aphasia.[183] A man with transcortical motor aphasia, although lacking echolalia and echopraxia, could not refrain from completing the sentences of others.[334] Some patients have had transcortical aphasia, with relative preservation of speech repetition and a strikingly greater impairment of list naming than of naming to confrontation,[328] or particularly impaired speech initiative, as in attempts to narrate stories or describe complex pictures.[334]

In one report, a patient with transcortical mixed aphasia had infarction of both the medial frontal and the medial parietal lobes, whereas two other patients with transcortical motor aphasia had infarction of only the medial frontal lobe.[333] After a large left ACA infarction, one patient had transcortical motor aphasia and mirror writing.[323] Another, who was right-handed, had left-handed mirror writing after infarction of the right medial frontal cortex sparing the corpus callosum, leading to the conjecture that the SMA is "responsible for nonmirror transformation of motor programs originating in the left hemisphere before execution by the primary motor area in the right hemisphere."[335] A woman with aphasia that included impairment of comprehension, repetition, reading, and writing had medial frontal infarction plus an old infarct over the rolandic convexity.[336]

In some patients, speech disturbance was transient, whereas paucity of other movements, including writing, persisted.[326] *Strategic infarct dementia* is a term also used to describe the paucity of speech and motor behavior, accompanied by long delays in response and poor scores on tests involving narrative and naming response. Deep infarcts in the anterior limb of the internal capsule or anterior thalamus are associated with this syndrome.[337,338]

Nearly all reports of severe language impairment after pathologically documented ACA occlusion have involved left-sided lesions[323] with one exception[339]: a right-handed woman with left hemiparesis, diffuse bradykinesia, speech limited to short replies to questions, and a tendency to echolalia; naming and comprehension of spoken or written language seemed impaired in this patient but were difficult to test. At autopsy, infarction was found in the territory of the right ACA, including the head of the caudate, the anterior limb of the internal capsule, the anterior putamen, the anterior cingulate and superior frontal gyri, and the entire SMA (Fig. 23-7). Several reports describe language disturbance after bilateral ACA occlusion,[325,340,341] including stuttering[342]; in one report with neither postmortem examination nor disclosure of the patient's handedness, the patient had occlusion of the right ACA.[303] Another report described two right-handed women with transient verbal output loss, normal writing and ability to comprehend spoken language, and infarction of the right anterior cingulate cortex. In these cases, impaired speech initiation was attributed to disruption of a signal transmission through the right anterior corpus callosum to the left language network.[343] A man with right SMA infarction had "aphemia": impaired articulation with normal repetition, auditory comprehension, reading, and writing. The author proposed that both SMAs participate in the initiation of articulatory movements, but only the left SMA affects linguistic aspects of speech.[344]

Most investigators, regardless of whether they consider these abnormalities to be truly aphasic, attribute them to damage to the SMA on the medial surface of the frontal lobe, anterior to the paracentral lobule, and between the cingulate and superior frontal gyri (i.e., the medial hemispheric part of Brodmann's area 6).[321,345-347] Of 10 right-handed patients with left ACA territory infarcts described

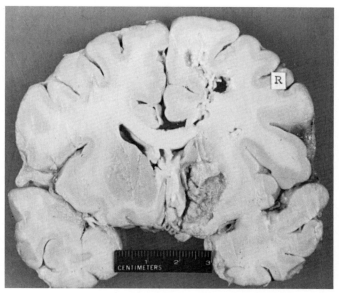

Figure 23-7 Autopsy specimen showing a coronal section of the anterior frontal and temporal lobes. There is infarction in the territories of both the proximal and distal portions of the right anterior cerebral artery. Affected areas include the caudate, putamen, internal capsule's anterior limb, cingulate gyrus, and supplementary motor area. (From Brust JCM, Plank C, Burke A, et al: Language disorder in a right-hander after occlusion of the right anterior cerebral artery. *Neurology* 32:492, 1982.)

in one report, four had transcortical motor aphasia, and in each, the SMA was involved. Three other patients with sparing of the SMA but involvement of the cingulate had only "alterations of verbal memory."[348] In monkeys, stimulation of this area causes arm and leg movements and head turning, and there seems to be rostral-caudal forelimb-hind limb somatotopy.[349-355] Unilateral ablation of the SMA in monkeys produces a deficit in tasks of bimanual coordination.[356] In humans, SMA stimulation induces bodily postures (e.g., turning of the head and eyes toward a contralaterally uplifted arm) or repetitive movements (e.g., stepping or hand-waving).[347] Such responses are often bilateral and can occur after ablation of area 4 (the primary motor cortex). SMA stimulation can also cause speech and movement arrest or vocalization.[357]

Although stimulation of the face region of area 4 causes vocalization of continuous vowel sounds,[357] SMA stimulation on either hemisphere[178] produces intermittently repeated words, syllables, or meaningless combinations of syllables (saccadic vocalization).[347] The repeated word might be a palilalia of what was being said at the onset of stimulation. Rhythmic mouth and jaw movements sometimes accompany the vocalization. Speech arrest, hesitation, or slowing also occurs, sometimes with mouth movements suggesting attempted speech or with arrest of other voluntary movement. Speech comprehension is usually preserved, but anomia and paraphasias have occurred.[178]

Such symptoms, with or without other motor, sensory, or autonomic phenomena, may be the manifestation of seizures caused by structural lesions affecting the SMA, especially meningiomas.[337,340,358-362] Although experimental stimulation of either the right or left SMA can cause speech arrest or repetition, seizures causing altered speech have only rarely occurred in right-handed persons with lesions of the right SMA.[363] Both stimulation and seizure phenomena raise the question of whether true aphasia is occurring and which brain structures are, in fact, responsible.

Destructive lesions, including infarction, are similarly problematic. Medial hemispheric structural lesions such as neoplasm, vascular malformation, subdural empyema, surgical ablation, and trauma not only can directly affect more regions than the SMA but also produce distant effects from edema or brain distortion. SMA excision for the treatment of epilepsy has led to language disturbance, but interpretation of such cases has varied. One group found that excision of the language hemisphere's SMA back to area 4 caused muteness, whereas excision of the language hemisphere's anterior SMA or the non-language hemisphere's entire SMA produced "no specific deficit."[364] Others found, after excision of either SMA, more lasting speech disturbances, although they seemed nonaphasic and secondary to bradykinesia.[365] Bilateral ideomotor apraxia without aphasia affected two patients with ACA infarction involving both the left SMA and the corpus callosum.[366]

The SMA receives afferents from the ipsilateral primary and secondary somatosensory cortex and has reciprocal connections to ipsilateral area 4, posterior parietal cortex, upper convexity premotor cortex (area 6), several thalamic nuclei, and, across the corpus callosum, the contralateral SMA and convexity area 6.[367-369] It has been suggested, therefore, that the SMA is "an area of sensory convergence."[349] Efferents project bilaterally to the cingulate gyrus and striatum[281,324,370,371]; ipsilaterally to the red nucleus, pontine nuclei, and dorsal column nuclei[349]; and contralaterally to area 4 and the midconvexity premotor region (area 8).[324] There are also SMA neurons that project to the spinal cord.[350,372,373] Regional cerebral blood flow (rCBF) increases in the SMA during automatic speech and during repetitive finger movement but not during isometric hand muscle contraction.[374-376] Cerebral blood flow also increases in the SMA during planning of sequential movements.[377-379] (By contrast, the cerebral blood flow of area 4 increases only during execution of such movements.[378]) In monkeys, medullary pyramidal section did not affect movements produced by SMA stimulation,[380] increased discharge of SMA neurons preceded stereotyped learned motor tasks of either the ipsilateral or contralateral extremities, and SMA neurons fired in response to sensory signals "only when the signal called for a motor response."[353] Neurons in the SMA are, however, less responsive to peripheral stimuli than those in area 4,[349,354] which suggest that part of the SMA's function may be "to 'gate' or suppress the afferent influences on area 4"[182] (perhaps accounting for the transient contralateral grasp reflex commonly seen after SMA ablation).[178,328,347,354,381] Such suppression would convert area 4's activity from a closed loop to an open loop mode,[354,382] consistent with the further notion that the SMA develops "a preparatory state" for impending movement[353,383] or that it elaborates "programs for motor subroutines necessary in skilled voluntary motion,"[384] including, with its "sequences of fast isolated muscular contraction," human speech.[378]

The often cited case described by Bonhoeffer[192] in 1914 may represent ACA occlusion causing language disturbance by a different mechanism. The patient experienced right hemiplegia, with the leg weaker than the arm, plus reduction of speech to one or two words, relatively preserved comprehension of spoken speech, alexia, agraphia, and apraxia (difficulty following commands, imitating, and handling objects) that was greater on the left than the right. Abnormalities at autopsy included infarction of the posterior left middle and superior frontal gyri, the anterior four fifths of the corpus callosum, the anterior limb of the left internal capsule, and a small part of the left posterior inferior parietal lobule. Bonhoeffer[192] (and Geschwind,[236] reviewing the case 50 years later) explained the left apraxia as that resulting from the callosal lesion and the aphasia from the combined callosal and capsular lesions, which in effect isolated Broca's area; the posterior parietal lesion probably contributed to the alexia, agraphia, and right apraxia. Neither writer discussed the possible contribution of SMA destruction to the language disturbance, which theoretically could have occurred without it.

Other Mental Abnormalities

Besides abulia, apraxia, and language impairment, patients with ACA occlusion can have a variety of other emotional or intellectual disturbances, usually attributed to involvement of structures supplied by branches of the proximal ACA (A1 segment or ACoA).[56,359,385] Anxiety, fear, insomnia, talkativeness, or agitation has occurred with or without weakness, bradykinesia, or grasp and suck reflexes.[39,183,300,359] A young woman, awakening from a coma after ACoA aneurysm rupture, had severe withdrawal with unprovoked agitation and screaming; autopsy demonstrated bilateral infarction of the orbital gyri, gyri recti, septal nuclei, cingulate gyri, hippocampal formations, and right amygdala.[386] Damage to hypothalamic or other limbic structures has also been considered responsible for these symptoms,[50] which, when they predominate, can suggest nonstructural neurotic or psychotic illness.[37] In any event, the notion that apathy and poor motivation predictably follow dorsolateral frontal lesions and that orbitofrontal damage causes disinhibited behavior appears to be an oversimplification.[203,387]

Confusion, disorientation, and memory loss, sometimes severe, also occur.[36,78,340,388-391] Retrograde and anterograde amnesia after ACoA aneurysm rupture may be subtle or severe,[392-395] with variable denial or confabulation.[188,396-398] In one report, a patient with bilateral infarction of both medial frontal lobes as well as the right inferior temporal lobe and pole had severely impaired recognition of previously presented words or pictures yet could spontaneously recall them.[399] In another report, five patients with lesions restricted to basal forebrain structures (sparing the hippocampus and temporal lobes) were able to recall particular stimuli (e.g., someone's name or face) but could not bring such differently learned components together as an integrated memory.[400] Structures that have been implicated in these amnestic syndromes include the hypothalamus, medial forebrain bundle, septum, nucleus of Meynert, nucleus accumbens, and fornix, with possible secondary dysfunction of medial temporal regions.[401-403] Bilateral infarction of the caudate nucleus and fornix resulted in impaired verbal working memory and "delayed recall."[404] Left caudate infarction in five patients resulted in impairment of both declarative memory and motor procedural memory.[405]

Functional neuroimaging studies implicate medial frontal structures in the ability of humans to attribute mental states to others ("mentalizing," "Theory of Mind").[406] Such a role was questioned in a study of a woman with bilateral ACA territory infarction who had impairments in planning and memory but who performed normally on Theory of Mind tasks.[407]

Of 251 patients examined 3 months after acute ischemic stroke, 66 had dementia. Infarction in the territory of the left ACA was more predictive of dementia than infarction in the MCA or PCA territory.[408]

Visuospatial disturbance with difficulty dressing, drawing, or copying or with left hemineglect has occurred after infarction of the caudate and anterior limb of the internal capsule. Primary dyscalculia was also reported after infarction in the territory of the left ACA.[409] Depression has been associated with left caudate lesions.[410]

Incontinence and Other Autonomic Changes

Urinary (and, less often, fecal) incontinence can occur with either unilateral or bilateral ACA occlusion.[37,39,59] Involvement of the paracentral lobule (presuming homuncular representation of motor and sensory components of micturition) has been offered as an explanation,[36,105] even though paracentral stimulation was found to produce only contralateral sensation without motor response in the penis.[411] Damage to the superior medial frontal lobe, especially the midportion of the superior frontal gyrus, the cingulate, and the white matter in between, is a more likely cause, because such damage (e.g., from frontal leukotomy) causes transient or permanent disturbance of urination and defecation, including urgency and incontinence.[219,412-414]

Cardiorespiratory alterations are common after stroke, regardless of whether limbic structures are specifically damaged.[415,416] Such changes seen after ACA occlusion are therefore open to interpretation, but it is not unreasonable to incriminate damage to the hypothalamus, cingulate gyrus, or other limbic areas. Fever not always related to infection, tachycardia, and unexpected death have followed cingulate infarction in humans.[299,300] Human and animal cingulate stimulation can produce altered respiration, bradycardia, temporary respiratory or cardiac arrest, hypertension or hypotension, pupillary dilatation, and piloerection.[299,417,418] Diabetes insipidus, perhaps from anterior hypothalamic infarction, has occurred after surgical occlusion of a proximal ACA for ACoA aneurysm.[39,56] Gastrointestinal bleeding after ACoA aneurysm rupture has also been blamed on hypothalamic damage.[419]

Miscellaneous Symptoms

Visual loss has followed compression of the optic nerve or chiasm by an ACA aneurysm or dolichoectasia.[420,421] Bitemporal hemianopia occurred from compression of the optic chiasm by an elongated right ACA.[422]

Inability to close the left eye on verbal command with otherwise preserved movement of left facial muscles followed right ACA territory infarction. The authors suspected an apraxia of eye closure from damage to the anterior corpus callosum.[423]

Generalized tonic-clonic seizures during menses arose from a region of the left frontal lobe supplied by an aberrant contralateral orbitofrontal artery. The authors speculated that increased progesterone levels during the luteal phase lowered blood pCO_2, leading to ischemia in the tenuously supplied region.[424]

Periventricular Leukomalacia of Infancy

Brains of infants dying within hours or months of birth may have necrotic foci along the lateral ventricles, considered by some investigators to be infarcts at border zones between the territories of the ACA, MCA, and PCA.[425] Others have stressed that the periventricular areas are more properly called end zones and are not in anastomotic areas but rather within a few millimeters of the ventricular wall "between the terminal distributions of ventriculopetal and ventriculofugal branches of small arteries that penetrate deeply into the brain,"[426] including those from the ACA passing through the cingulate gyrus.[427] Such lesions usually spare the cerebral cortex because the fetus has rich meningeal anastomoses between pial vessels and because the white matter in newborns has a relatively higher metabolic rate.[426] Hypotensive newborn dogs develop decreased white matter blood flow and lesions resembling those of periventricular leukomalacia.[428] Autopsy in infants with periventricular leukomalacia and no apparent perinatal asphyxia has shown poorly developed ventriculofugal branches.[427,429] Affected infants display lethargy, hypotonia, difficulty feeding, and seizures; survivors are usually mentally retarded, with spastic quadriparesis.

Because cerebral autoregulation is impaired in neonates with asphyxia, periventricular hemorrhage in the newborn may be the result of capillary dilatation and rupture in these same deep end zones.[425]

REFERENCES

1. Bogousslavsky J, Regli F: Anterior cerebral artery territory infarction in the Lausanne Stroke Registry: Clinical and etiological patterns, *Arch Neurol* 47:144, 1990.
2. Gacs G, Fox AJ, Barnett HJM, Vinuela F: Occurrence and mechanism of occlusion of the anterior cerebral artery, *Stroke* 14:952, 1983.
3. Kazui S, Sawada T, Kuriyama Y, et al: A clinical study of patients with cerebral infarction localized in the territory of anterior cerebral artery, *Jpn J Stroke* 9:317, 1987.
4. Hollander M, Bots ML, Del Sol AI, et al: Carotid plaques increase the risk of stroke and subtypes of cerebral infarction in asymptomatic elderly: The Rotterdam study, *Circulation* 105:2872, 2002.
5. Rodda RA: The arterial patterns associated with internal carotid disease and cerebral infarcts, *Stroke* 17:69, 1986.
6. Kang SY, Sim JS: Anterior cerebral artery infarction. Stroke mechanism and clinical-imaging study in 100 patients, *Neurology* 70:2386, 2008.
7. Castaigne P, Lhermitte F, Escourelle R, et al: Étude anatomo-pathologique de 74 infarcts de l'artère cérébrale antérieure (55 observations), *Rev Med Toulouse Suppl* 339, 1975.
8. Rothfus WE, Goldberg AL, Tabas JH, Deeb ZL: Callosomarginal infarction secondary to transfalcial herniation, *AJNR Am J Neuroradiol* 8:1073, 1987.

9. Sharma VK, Chan BPL: Involvement of the recurrent artery of Heubner with contralateral middle cerebral artery infarction, *J Neurol Neurosurg Psychiatry* 78:362, 2007.

10. Amagasa M, Sato S, Otabe K: Posttraumatic dissecting aneurysm of the anterior cerebral artery: Case report, *Neurosurgery* 23:221, 1988.

11. Araki T, Ouchi M, Ikeda Y: A case of anterior cerebral artery dissecting aneurysm, *No Shinkei Geka* 24:87, 1996.

12. Ishibashi A, Kubota Y, Yokokura Y, et al: Traumatic occlusion of the anterior cerebral artery—case report, *Neurol Med Chir (Tokyo)* 35:882, 1995.

13. Kidooka M, Okada T, Sonabe M, et al: Dissecting aneurysm of the anterior cerebral artery: Report of two cases, *Surg Neurol* 39:53, 1993.

14. Yano H, Sawada M, Shinoda J, Funakoshi T: Ruptured dissecting aneurysm of the peripheral anterior cerebral artery—case report, *Neurol Med Chir (Tokyo)* 35:450, 1995.

15. Wakabayashi Y, Nakano T, Isono M, et al: Dissecting aneurysm of the anterior cerebral artery requiring surgical treatment—case report 5, *Neurol Med Chir (Tokyo)* 40:624, 2000.

16. Ohkuma H, Suzuki S, Kikkawa T, et al: Neuroradiologic and clinical features of arterial dissection of the anterior cerebral artery, *AJNR Am J Neuroradiol* 24:691, 2003.

17. Kodera T, Hirose S, Takeuchi H, et al: Radiological findings for arterial dissection of the anterior cerebral artery, *J Clin Neurosci* 14:77, 2007.

18. Sakata N, Hamasaki M, Iwasaki H, et al: Dissecting aneurysms involving both anterior cerebral artery and aorta, *Pathol Int* 57:224, 2007.

19. Smrcka M, Ogilvy C, Koroshetz W: Small aneurysms as a cause of thromboembolic stroke, *Bratisl Lek Listy* 103:250, 2002.

20. Shimauchi M, Kaji Y, Goya T, Kinoshita K: A case report of fibromuscular dysplasia presenting symptoms like moyamoya disease: "String of beads" appearance of the pericallosal artery, *No Shinkei Geka* 17:981, 1989.

21. Swanson TH, Zinkel JL, Peterson PL: Bilateral anterior cerebral artery occlusion in an alcohol abuser with sickle cell trait, *Henry Ford Hosp Med J* 35:67, 1987.

22. Satoh J, Miyasaka N, Yamada T, et al: Extensive cerebral infarction due to involvement of both anterior cerebral arteries by Wegener's granulomatosis, *Ann Rheum Dis* 47:606, 1988.

23. Levy AS, Lillehei KO, Rubinstein D, Stears JC: Subarachnoid neurocysticercosis with occlusion of the major intracranial arteries: Case report, *Neurosurgery* 36:183, 1995.

24. Lee SI, Park JH, Kim JH, et al: Paradoxical progression of intracranial tuberculomas and anterior cerebral artery infarction, *Neurology* 71:68, 2008.

25. Kashiwagi S, Abiko S, Harada K, et al: [Ischemic cerebrovascular complication in tuberculous meningitis: A case of Fröhlich syndrome and hemiparesis], *No Shinkei Geka* 18:1141, 1990.

26. Foreman NK, Laitt RD, Chambers EJ, et al: Intracranial large vessel vasculopathy and anaplastic meningioma 19 years after cranial irradiation for acute lymphoblastic leukaemia, *Med Pediatr Oncol* 24:265, 1995.

27. Katayama W, Enomoto T, Yanaka K, Nose T: Moyamoya disease associated with persistent primitive hypoglossal artery: Report of a case, *Pediatr Neurosurg* 35:262, 2001.

28. Lim SM, Chae EJ, Kim MY, et al: Steal phenomenon through the anterior communicating artery in Moyamoya disease, *Eur Radiol* 17:61, 2007.

29. Lee JY, Kim KS, Song SK, et al: Atypical territorial infarction in moyamoya disease, *Neurology* 65:E28, 2005.

30. Frigerio R, Santoro P, Ferrarese C, et al: Migrainous cerebral infarction: Case reports, *Neurol Sci* 25(Suppl 3):S300, 2004.

31. Ha SW, Kim JS: Double infarcts in the anterior and posterior cerebral artery territories, *Eur Neurol* 54:120, 2005.

32. Lammouchi TM, Bouker SM, Grira MT, et al: Susac's syndrome, *Saudi Med J* 25:222, 2004.

33. King S, Khatri P, Carrozzella J, et al: Anterior cerebral artery emboli in combined intravenous and intra-arterial rtPA treatment of acute ischemic stroke in the IMS I and II trials, *AJNR Am J Neuroradiol* 28:1890, 2007.

34. Czochra M, Kozniewska H, Muszynski A, Trojanowski T: Surgical treatment of aneurysms of the anterior communicating artery using Yasargil's approach, *Neurol Neurochir Pol* 13:71, 1979.

35. Perlmutter D, Rhoton AL: Microsurgical anatomy of the anterior cerebral-anterior communicating-recurrent artery complex, *J Neurosurg* 45:259, 1976.

36. Perlmutter D, Rhoton AL: Microsurgical anatomy of the distal anterior cerebral artery, *J Neurosurg* 49:204, 1978.

37. Baptista AG: Studies on the arteries of the brain. II: The anterior cerebral artery: Some anatomic features and their clinical implications, *Neurology* 13:825, 1963.

38. Beevor CE: The cerebral arterial supply, *Brain* 30:403, 1907.

39. Critchley M: The anterior cerebral artery and its syndromes, *Brain* 53:120, 1930.

40. Fischer E: Die Lageabweichungen der vorderen Hirnarterie im Gefässbild, *Zentralbl Neurochir* 3:300, 1938.

41. Lazorthes G, Bastide G, Gomes FA: Les variations du trajet de la carotide interne d'après une étude artériographe, *Arch Anat Pathol* 9:129, 1961.

42. Liepmann H, Maas O: Fall von linksseitiger Agraphie und Apraxie bei rechtsseitiger Lähmung, *J Psychol Neurol* 10:214, 1907.

43. Marino R: The anterior cerebral artery. I: Anatomico-radiological study of its cortical territories, *Surg Neurol* 5:81, 1976.

44. Morris AA, Peck CM: Roentgenographic study of variation in normal anterior cerebral artery: One hundred cases studied in the lateral plane, *AJR Am J Roentgenol* 74:818, 1955.

45. Ring BA, Waddington MM: Roentgenographic anatomy of the pericallosal arteries, *AJR Am J Roentgenol* 104:109, 1968.

46. Snyckers FD, Drake CG: Aneurysms of the distal anterior cerebral artery: A report on 24 verified cases, *S Afr Med J* 47:1787, 1973.

47. Heubner O: Zur Topographie der Ernährungsgebiete der einzelnen Hirnarterien, *Zentralbl Med Wissenschaften* 10:817, 1872.

48. Ostrowski AZ, Webster JE, Gurdjian ES: The proximal anterior cerebral artery: An anatomic study, *Arch Neurol* 3:661, 1960.

49. Aydin IH, Onder A, Takei E, et al: Heubner's artery variations in anterior communicating artery aneurysms, *Acta Neurochir* 127:17, 1994.

50. Dunker RO, Harris AB: Surgical anatomy of the proximal anterior cerebral artery, *J Neurosurg* 44:359, 1976.

51. Gomes F, Dujouny M, Umansky F, et al: Microsurgical anatomy of the recurrent artery of Heubner, *J Neurosurg* 60:130, 1984.

52. Gorczyca W, Mohr G: Microvascular anatomy of Heubner's recurrent artery, *Neurol Res* 9:254, 1987.

53. Ahmed DS, Ahmed RH: The recurrent branch of the anterior cerebral artery, *Anat Rec* 157:699, 1967.

54. Falconer MA: The surgical treatment of bleeding intracranial aneurysms, *J Neurol Neurosurg Psychiatry* 14:153, 1951.

55. Gillingham FJ: The management of ruptured intracranial aneurysms, *Ann R Coll Surg Engl* 23:89, 1958.

56. Hegenholtz H, Morley TP: The results of proximal anterior cerebral artery occlusion for anterior communicating aneurysms, *J Neurosurg* 37:65, 1972.

57. Alexander MP, Freedman M: Amnesia after anterior communicating artery aneurysm rupture, *Neurology* 33(Suppl 2):104, 1983.

58. Gillilan LA: The arterial and venous blood supplies to the forebrain (including the internal capsule) of primates, *Neurology* 18:653, 1968.

59. Webster JE, Gurdjian ES, Lindner DW, Hardy WG: Proximal occlusion of the anterior cerebral artery, *Arch Neurol* 2:19, 1960.

60. Ghika JA, Bogousslavsky J, Regli F: Deep perforators from the carotid system: Template of the vascular territories, *Arch Neurol* 47:1097, 1990.

61. Caplan LR, Schmahmann JD, Kase CS, et al: Caudate infarcts, *Arch Neurol* 47:133, 1990.

62. Berman SA, Hayman LA, Hinck VC: Correlation of CT cerebral vascular territories with function. 1: Anterior cerebral artery, *AJR Am J Roentgenol* 135:253, 1980.

63. Dawson BH: The blood vessels of the human optic chiasma and their relation to those of the hypophysis and thalamus, *Brain* 81:207, 1958.

64. Crowell RM, Morawetz RB: The anterior communicating artery has significant branches, *Stroke* 8:272, 1977.

65. Abbie AA: The morphology of the forebrain arteries, with especial reference to the evolution of the basal ganglia, *J Anat* 68:433, 1934.

66. Alexander L: The vascular supply of the striopallidum, *Res Publ Assoc Res Nerv Ment Dis* 21:77, 1942.

67. Cobb S: The cerebral circulation. 13: The question of "end-arteries" of the brain and the mechanism of infarction, *Arch Neurol Psychiatry* 25:273, 1931.

68. Shellshear JC: The basal arteries of the forebrain and their functional significance, *J Anat* 55:27, 1920.

69. Van den Bergh R, Vander Eecken H: Anatomy and embryology of cerebral circulation, *Prog Brain Res* 30:1, 1968.

70. Zeal AA, Rhoton AL: Microsurgical anatomy of the posterior cerebral artery, *J Neurosurg* 48:534, 1978.

71. Booker J, Morris N, Huang C-Y: Cerebral radionuclide scintigraphy in the stroke syndrome, *Med J Aust* 1:625, 1978.

72. Waltz AG, Sundt TM: The microvascular and microcirculation of the cerebral cortex after arterial occlusion, *Brain* 90:681, 1967.

73. Watanabe O, Bremer AM, West CR: Experimental regional cerebral ischemia in the middle cerebral artery territory in primates. 1: Angioanatomy and description of an experimental model with selective embolization of the internal carotid artery bifurcation, *Stroke* 8:61, 1977.

74. Lasjaunias P, Vignaud J, Clay C: Radioanatomie de la vascularisation artérielle de l'orbite, à l'éxception du tronc de l'artère ophtalmique, *Ann Radiol* 18:181, 1975.

75. Van der Zwan A, Hillen B, Tulleken CAF, et al: Variability of the territories of the major cerebral arteries, *J Neurosurg* 77:927, 1992.

76. Alpers BJ, Berry RG, Paddison RM: Anatomical studies of the circle of Willis in normal brain, *Arch Neurol Psychiatry* 81:409, 1959.

77. Pool JL: Aneurysms of the anterior communicating artery: Bifrontal craniotomy and routine use of temporary clips, *J Neurosurg* 18:98, 1961.

78. Tindall GT: The treatment of anterior communicating aneurysms by proximal anterior cerebral artery ligation, *Clin Neurosurg* 21:134, 1974.

79. Wilson G, Riggs HE, Rupp C: The pathologic anatomy of ruptured cerebral aneurysms, *J Neurosurg* 11:128, 1954.

80. Uchino A, Nomiyama K, Takase Y, et al: Anterior cerebral artery variations detected by MR angiography, *Neuroradiology* 46:647, 2006.

81. Chuang Y-M, Liu C-Y, Pan P-J, et al: Anterior cerebral artery A1 segment hypoplasia may contribute to A1 hypoplasia syndrome, *Eur Neurol* 57:208, 2007.

82. Riggs HE, Rupp C: Variation in form of circle of Willis, *Arch Neurol* 8:8, 1963.

83. Marinkovic S, Kovacevic M, Milisavljevic M: Hypoplasia of the proximal segment of the anterior cerebral artery, *Anat Anz* 168:145, 1989.

84. Kirgis HD, Fisher WL, Llewellyn RC, Peebles EM: Aneurysms of the anterior communicating artery and gross anomalies of the circle of Willis, *J Neurosurg* 25:73, 1966.

85. Stebbens WE: Aneurysms and anatomic variation of cerebral arteries, *Arch Pathol* 75:45, 1963.

86. VanderArk GD, Kempe LC: Classification of anterior communicating aneurysms as a basis for surgical approach, *J Neurosurg* 32:300, 1970.

87. Lehrer HZ: Relative calibre of the cervical internal carotid artery: Normal variation with the circle of Willis, *Brain* 91:339, 1968.

88. Tindall GT, Kapp J, Odom GL, Robinson SC: A combined technique for treating certain aneurysms of the anterior communicating artery, *J Neurosurg* 33:41, 1970.

89. Kruyt RC: Aplasia of the anterior cerebral arteries: Angiographic study of a case, *Neurochirurgia* 14:172, 1971.

90. Windle BCA: On the arteries forming the circle of Willis, *J Anat Physiol* 22:289, 1888.

91. Kapoor K, Singh B, Dewan LI: Variations in the configuration of the circle of Willis, *Anat Sci Int* 83:96, 2008.

92. Blackburn IW: Anomalies of the encephalic arteries among the insane, *J Comp Neurol Psychol* 17:493, 1907.

93. Pearce JMS: Heubner's artery, *Eur Neurol* 54:112, 2005.

94. Loukas M, Louis RG, Childs RS: Anatomical examination of the recurrent artery of Heubner, *Clin Anat* 19:25, 2006.

95. Martinez F: Commentary: Anatomical examination of the recurrent artery of Heubner, *Clin Anat* 20:473, 2007.

96. Hashimoto Y, Tsushima S, Komeichi T, et al: Contralateral infarction in the territory of the recurrent artery of Heubner after anterior communicating artery aneurysm surgery, *No Shinkei Geka-Neurol Surg* 36:813, 2008.

97. Tao X, Yu XJ, Bhattori B, et al: Microsurgical anatomy of the anterior communicating artery complex in adult Chinese heads, *Surg Neurol* 65:155, 2006.

98. Tsuji T, Abe M, Tabuchi K: Aneurysm of a persistent primitive olfactory artery, *J Neurosurg* 83:138, 1995.

99. Brismar J, Ackerman R, Roberson G: Anomaly of anterior cerebral artery: A case report and embryologic considerations, *Acta Radiol Diagn (Stockh)* 18:154, 1977.

100. Isherwood I, Dutton J: Unusual anomaly of anterior cerebral artery, *Acta Radiol Diagn (Stockh)* 9:345, 1969.

101. Mercier P, Velvt S, Fournier D, et al: A rare embryologic variation: Carotid-anterior cerebral artery anastomosis or infraoptic course of the anterior cerebral artery, *Surg Radiol Anat* 11:73, 1989.

102. Nutic S, Dilence D: Carotid-anterior cerebral artery anastomosis: Case report, *J Neurosurg* 44:378, 1976.

103. Robinson LR: An unusual human anterior cerebral artery, *J Anat* 93:131, 1959.

104. Senter HJ, Miller DJ: Interoptic course of the anterior cerebral artery associated with anterior cerebral artery aneurysm: Case report, *J Neurosurg* 56:302, 1982.

105. Besson G, Leguyader J, Mimassi N, et al: Anomalie rare du polygone de Willis: Trajet sous-optique des deux artères cérébrales antérieures. Aneurysme associé de la bifurcation due tronc basilaire, *Neurochirurgie* 26:71, 1980.

106. Padget DH: The circle of Willis: Its embryology and anatomy. In Dandy WE, editor: *Intracranial arterial aneurysms*, Ithaca, NY, 1945, Comstock, p 67.

107. Milenkovic Z: Anastomosis between internal carotid artery and anterior cerebral artery with other anomalies of the circle of Willis in a fetal brain, *J Neurosurg* 55:701, 1981.

108. Lehmann G, Vincentelli F, Ebagosti A: Anomalies rares du polygone de Willis: Le trajet infraoptique des artères cérébrales antérieures, *Neurochirurgie* 26:243, 1980.

109. Turnbull I: Agenesis of the internal carotid artery, *Neurology* 12:588, 1962.

110. Bosma NJ: Infra-optic course of anterior cerebral artery and low bifurcation of internal carotid artery, *Acta Neurochir* 38:305, 1977.

111. Padget DH: The development of the cranial arteries in the human embryo, *Contrib Embryol* 32:205, 1948.

112. Peltier J, Fichten A, Havet E, et al: The infra-optic course of the anterior cerebral arteries: an anatomic case report, *Surg Radiol Anat* 29:389, 2007.

113. Stewart RM, Williams RS, Luhl P, Schoenen J: Ventral porencephaly: A cerebral defect associated with multiple congenital anomalies, *Acta Neuropathol* 42:231, 1978.

114. McCormick WF: A unique anomaly of the intracranial arteries of man, *Neurology* 10:77, 1969.

115. Hassler W, Zentner J, Voigt K: Abnormal origin of the ophthalmic artery from the anterior cerebral artery: Neuroradiological and intraoperative findings, *Neuroradiology* 31:85, 1989.

116. Islak C, Ogut G, Numan F, et al: Persistent nonmigrated ventral primitive ophthalmic artery, *J Neuroradiol* 21:46, 1994.

117. Maruyama N, Fukama A, Ihara I, et al: Unusual variant of the anterior cerebral artery, *Neurol Med Chir (Tokyo)* 45:246, 2005.

118. Tacconi L, Johnston FG, Symon L: Accessory middle cerebral artery: Case report, *J Neurosurg* 83:916, 1995.

119. Tubbs RS, Shoja MM, Shokouhi G, et al: Unusual origins of accessory pericallosal arteries in man: Case report, *Surg Radiol Anat* 29:313, 2007.

120. Kahilogullari G, Comert A, Arslan M, et al: Callosal branches of the anterior cerebral artery: An anatomical report, *Clin Anat* 21:383, 2008.

121. De Vriese B: Sur la signification morphologique des artères cérébrales, *Arch Biol* 21:357, 1904/05.

122. Fawcett E, Blachford JV: The circle of Willis: An examination of 700 specimens, *J Anat Physiol* 40:63a, 1905/06.

123. Kleiss E: Die verschiedenen Formen des circulus arteriosus cerebralis Willisi, *Anat Anz* 92:216, 1942.

124. Lazorthes G, Gaubert J, Poulhes J: La distribution centrale et corticale de l'artère cérébrale antérieure: Étude anatomique et incidences neuro-chirurgicales, *Neurochirurgie* 2:237, 1956.

125. Van der Eecken H: Discussion of "collateral circulation of the brain," *Neurology* 11:16, 1961.

126. Curry RW, Culbreth GC: The normal cerebral angiogram, *AJR Am J Roentgenol* 65:345, 1951.

127. Ruggiero G: Factors influencing the filling of the anterior cerebral artery in angiography, *Acta Radiol* 37:87, 1952.

128. Saita I, Shigeno T, Aritake K, et al: Vasospasm assessed by angiography and computerized tomography, *J Neurosurg* 51:466, 1979.

129. Lesem WW: The comparative anatomy of the anterior cerebral artery, *Postgrad Med* 20:445, 1905.

130. LeMay M, Gooding CA: The clinical significance of the azygous anterior cerebral artery (ACA), *AJR Am J Roentgenol* 98:602, 1966.

131. Szdzuy D, Lehmann R, Nickel B: Common trunk of the anterior cerebral arteries, *Neuroradiology* 4:51, 1972.

132. Niizuma H, Kwak R, Uchida K, Susuki J: Aneurysms of the azygous anterior cerebral artery, *Surg Neurol* 15:225, 1980.

133. Fujimoto K, Waga S, Kojima T, Shimosaka S: Aneurysm of distal anterior cerebral artery associated with azygous anterior cerebral artery, *Acta Neurochir* 59:79, 1981.

134. Katz RS, Horoupian DS, Zingesser L: Aneurysm of azygous anterior cerebral artery: A case report, *J Neurosurg* 48:804, 1978.

135. Friedlander RM, Oglivy CS: Aneurysmal subarachnoid hemorrhage in a patient with bilateral A1 fenestrations associated with an azygous anterior cerebral artery: Case report and literature review, *J Neurosurg* 84:681, 1996.

136. Hanakita J, Nagayasu S, Nishi S, Suzuki T: An aneurysm of the distal anterior cerebral artery with a remarkably anomalous configuration, *No Shinkei Geka* 16:781, 1988.

137. Klein SI, Gahbauer H, Goodrich I: Bilateral anomalous anterior cerebral artery and infraoptic aneurysm, *AJNR Am J Neuroradiol* 8:1142, 1987.

138. Mishima H, Kim YK, Shiomi K, et al: Ruptured anterior communicating artery aneurysm associated with inter-optic course of anterior cerebral artery: Report of a case and review of the literature, *No Shinkei Geka* 22:495, 1994.

139. Ogasawara H, Inagawa T, Yamamoto M, Kamiya K: Aneurysm in a fenestrated anterior cerebral artery—case report, *Neurol Med Chir* 28:575, 1988.

140. Ogawa A, Suzuki M, Sakurai Y, Yashimoto T: Vascular anomalies associated with aneurysms of the anterior communicating artery: Microsurgical observations, *J Neurosurg* 72:706, 1990.

141. Sakai K, Asari S, Fujisawa M, Katagi R: Ruptured aneurysm arising from the anomalous anterior cerebral artery—case report, *Neurol Med Chir (Tokyo)* 32:846, 1992.

142. Schick RM, Rumbaugh CL: Saccular aneurysm of the azygous anterior cerebral artery, *AJNR Am J Neuroradiol* 10(Suppl):S73, 1989.

143. Suzuki M, Onuma T, Sakurai Y, et al: Aneurysms arising from the proximal (A1) segment of the anterior cerebral artery: A study of 38 cases, *J Neurosurg* 76:55, 1992.

144. Tracy PT: Unusual intracarotid anastomosis associated with anterior communicating artery aneurysm: Case report, *J Neurosurg* 67:765, 1987.

145. Horie N, Tsutsumi K, Kaminogo M, et al: Agenesis of the internal carotid artery with transcavernous anastomosis presenting with an anterior communicating artery aneurysm—a case report and review of the literature, *Clin Neurol Neurosurg* 110:622, 2008.

146. Leyon JJ, Kaliaperumal C, Choudhari KA: Aneurysm at the fenestrated anterior cerebral artery: Surgical anatomy and management, *Clin Neurol Neurosurg* 110:511, 2008.

147. Kawashima M, Endo M, Kitahara T, et al: Unusual location of anterior communication artery aneurysm located on the planum sphenoidale due to long A1 segments, *Neurol Med Chir (Tokyo)* 48:254, 2008.

148. Bikmaz K, Erdem E, Kright A: Arteriovenous fistula originating from proximal part of the anterior cerebral artery, *Clin Neurol Neurosurg* 109:589, 2007.

149. Lehecka M, Lehto H, Niemela M, et al: Distal anterior cerebral artery aneurysms. Treatment and outcome analysis of 501 patients, *Neurosurgery* 62:590, 2008.

150. Morigaki R, Uno M, Matsubara S, et al: Choreoathetosis due to rupture of a distal accessory anterior cerebral artery aneurysm, *Cerebrovasc Dis* 25:285, 2008.

151. deOliveira JG, du Mesnil de Rochemont R, Beck J, et al: A rare anomaly of the anterior communicating artery complex hidden by a large broad-neck aneurysm and disclosed by three-dimensional rotational angiography, *Acta Neurochir* 150:279, 2008.

152. Truwit CL: Embryology of the cerebral vasculature, *Neuroimaging Clin North Am* 4:663, 1994.

153. Oba M, Suzuki M, Onuma T: Two cases of ruptured fusiform aneurysm of the proximal anterior cerebral artery (A1 segment), *No Shinkei Geka* 17:365, 1989.

154. Hashizume K, Nukui H, Horikoshi T, et al: Giant aneurysm of the azygous anterior cerebral artery associated with acute subdural hematoma: Case report, *Neurol Med Chir (Tokyo)* 32:693, 1992.

155. Shiokawa K, Tanikawa T, Satoh K, et al: Two cases of giant aneurysms arising from the distal segment of the anterior cerebral circulation, *No Shinkei Geka* 21:467, 1993.

156. Choudhury AR: Proximal occlusion of the dominant anterior cerebral artery for anterior communicating aneurysms, *J Neurosurg* 45:484, 1976.

157. Cuatico W: The phenomenon of ipsilateral innervation: One case report, *J Neurosurg Sci* 23:81, 1979.

158. Durity F, Logue V: The effect of proximal anterior cerebral occlusion on anterior communicating artery aneurysms: Postoperative radiological survey of 43 cases, *J Neurosurg* 35:16, 1971.

159. Nornes H, Wikeby P: Cerebral arterial blood flow and aneurysm surgery. 1: Local arterial flow dynamics, *J Neurosurg* 47:810, 1977.

160. Ito J, Washiyama K, Kim CH, Ibuchi Y: Fenestration of the anterior cerebral artery, *Neuroradiology* 21:277, 1981.

161. Tran-Dinh HD, Dorsch NW, Soo YS: Ectasia and fenestration of the anterior cerebral artery associated with persistent trigeminal artery: Case report, *Neurosurgery* 31:125, 1992.

162. Campbell JB, Forster FM: The anterior cerebral artery in the macaque monkey (*Macaca mulatta*), *J Nerv Ment Dis* 99:229, 1944.

163. Kaplan HA: Vascular supply of the base of the brain. In Fields WS, editor: *Pathogenesis and treatment of parkinsonism*, Springfield, IL, 1958, Charles C Thomas, p 138.

164. Molinari GF, Moseley JI, Laurent JP: Segmental middle cerebral artery occlusion in primates: An experimental method requiring minimal surgery and anesthesia, *Stroke* 5:334, 1974.

165. Ward AA: The anterior cingulate gyrus and personality, *Res Publ Assoc Nerv Ment Dis* 27:438, 1948.

166. Hayakawa T, Waltz AG: Immediate effects of cerebral ischemia: Evolution and resolution of neurological deficits after experimental occlusion of one middle cerebral artery in conscious cats, *Stroke* 6:321, 1975.

167. Hayakawa T, Waltz AG: On the importance of the anterior cerebral artery, *Stroke* 7:523, 1976.

168. Kamijyo Y, Garcia JH: Carotid arterial supply of the feline brain: Applications to the study of regional cerebral ischemia, *Stroke* 6:361, 1975.

169. Thompson FJ, Campbell ML: Arterial supply of the feline motor cortex, *Stroke* 12:233, 1981.

170. Rieke GK, Bowers DE, Penn P: Vascular supply pattern to rat caudatoputamen and globus pallidus: Scanning electron microscopic study of vascular endocasts of stroke-prone vessels, *Stroke* 12:840, 1981.

171. Yamori Y, Horie R, Akiguchi I, et al: Pathogenic mechanisms and prevention of stroke in stroke-prone spontaneously hypertensive rats, *Prog Brain Res* 47:219, 1977.

172. Brust JCM: Circulation of the brain. In Kandel ER, Schwartz JH, Jessel TM, editors: *Principles of neural science*, ed 4, New York, 2000, McGraw-Hill.

173. Brust JCM: Cerebral infarction. In Rowland LP, Pedley TA, editors: *Merritt's Neurology*, 12th ed, Philadelphia, 2009, Lippincott Williams & Wilkins.

174. Tichy F: The syndromes of the cerebral arteries, *Arch Pathol* 48:475, 1949.

175. Kumrai E, Bayulkem G, Evyapan D, et al: Spectrum of anterior cerebral artery territory infarction: Clinical and MRI findings, *Eur J Neurol* 9:615, 2002.

176. Maeder-Ingvar M, van Melle G, Bogousslavsky J: Pure monoparesis. A particular stroke subgroup? *Arch Neurol* 62:1221, 2005.

177. Chamorro A, Marshall RS, Valls-Sole J, et al: Motor behavior in stroke patients with isolated medial frontal ischemic infarction, *Stroke* 28:1755, 1997.

178. Penfield W, Jasper H: *Epilepsy and the functional anatomy of the human brain*, Boston, 1954, Little, Brown.

179. Long E: Contributions à l'étude des fonctions de la zone motrice du cerveau, *Rev Neurol* 15:1218, 1907.

180. Long E: Monoplegie crurale, par lésion du lobule paracentrale, *Nouv Icon Salpetr* 21:37, 1908.

181. Wilson G: Crural monoplegia, *Arch Neurol Psychiatry* 10:699, 1923.

182. Winkelman NW: Two brains showing the lesions producing cerebral monoplegia, *Arch Neurol Psychiatry* 12:241, 1924.

183. Baldy R: *Les syndromes de l'artère cérébrale antérieure*, Paris, 1927, Jouve.

184. Foix C, Hillemand P: Les syndromes de l'artère cérébrale antérieure, *Encephale* 20:209, 1925.

185. Lhermitte J, Schiff P, Curtois A: Le phénomène de la préhension forcée, expression d'un ramollissement complet de la première convolution frontale, *Rev Neurol* 15:1218, 1907.

186. Schuster P, Pinéas M: Weitere Beobachtungen über Zwangsgreifen u. Nachgreifen u. deren Beziehungen zu ahnlichen Bewegungsstörungen, *Dtsch Z Nervenheilkd* 91:16, 1926.

187. Seyffarth H, Denny-Brown D: The grasp reflex and the instinctive grasp reaction, *Brain* 71:9, 1948.

188. DeLuca J, Cicerone KD: Cognitive impairments following anterior communicating artery aneurysm, *J Clin Exp Neuropsychol* 11:47, 1989.

189. Landau WM, Clare MH: Pathophysiology of the tonic innervation phenomenon of the foot, *Arch Neurol* 15:252, 1966.

190. Goldstein K: Zur Lehre von der motorischen Apraxie, *J Psychol Neurol* 11(169):270, 1908.

191. Goldstein K: Der makroskopiesche Befund in meinem Fall v. Linksseiter motorischen Apraxie, *Zentralbl Neurol* 28:898, 1909.

192. Bonhoeffer K: Klischer u. anatomischer Befund zur Lehre von der Apraxie und der motorischen Sprachbahn, *Monatsschr Psychiatr Neurol* 35:113, 1914.

193. Ghika J, Bogousslavsky J, van Melle G, Regli F: Hyperkinetic motor behaviors contralateral to hemiplegia in acute stroke, *Eur Neurol* 35:27, 1995.

194. Karnath H-O: Pusher syndrome—a frequent but little-known disturbance of body orientation perception, *J Neurol* 254:415, 2007.

195. Karnath H-O, Suchan J, Johannsen L: Pusher syndrome after ACA territory infarction, *Eur J Neurol* 15:e84, 2008.

196. Bogousslavsky J, Regli F: Capsular genu syndrome, *Neurology* 40:1499, 1990.

197. Ugur HC, Kahilogullari G, Esmer AF, et al: A neurosurgical view of anatomical variations of the distal anterior cerebral artery: An anatomical study, *J Neurosurg* 104:278, 2006.

198. Schneider R, Gautier J-C: Leg weakness due to stroke: Site of lesions, weakness patterns and causes, *Brain* 117:347, 1994.

199. Moulin T, Bogousslavsky J, Chopard JL, et al: Vascular ataxic hemiparesis: A reevaluation, *J Neurol Neurosurg Psychiatry* 58:422, 1995.

200. Bogousslavsky J, Martin R, Moulin T: Homolateral ataxia and crural paresis: A syndrome of anterior cerebral artery territory infarction, *J Neurol Neurosurg Psychiatry* 55:1146, 1992.

201. Giroud M, Creisson E, Fayolle H, et al: Homolateral ataxia and crural paresis: A crossed cerebral-cerebellar diaschisis, *J Neurol Neurosurg Psychiatry* 57:221, 1994.

202. Han SW, Kim SH, Kim JK, et al: Hemodynamic changes in limb-shaking TIA associated with anterior cerebral artery stenosis, *Neurology* 63:1519, 2004.

203. Stuss DT, Benson DF: Neuropsychological studies of the frontal lobes, *Psychol Bull* 95:3, 1984.

204. Greene KA, Marciano FF, Dickman CA, et al: Anterior communicating artery aneurysm paraparesis syndrome: Clinical manifestations and pathologic correlates, *Neurology* 45:45, 1995.

205. Endo H, Shimizu H, Tominaga T: Paraparesis associated with ruptured anterior cerebral artery territory aneurysms, *Surg Neurol* 64:135, 2005.

206. Borggreve F, DeDeyn PP, Marien P, et al: Bilateral infarction in the anterior cerebral artery vascular territory due to an unusual anomaly of the circle of Willis, *Stroke* 25:1279, 1994.

207. Chimowitz MI, Lafranchise EF, Furlan AJ, Awad IA: Ipsilateral leg weakness with carotid stenosis, *Stroke* 9:1362, 1990.

208. Schuster P: Zwangsgreifen u. Nachgreifen, zweipost-hemisplegische Bewegungsstörungen, *Z Ges Neurol Psychiatr* 83:586, 1923.

209. Schuster P: Autoptische Befunde bei Zwangsgreifen u. Nachgreifen. *Z Ges Neurol Psychiatr* 108:751, 1927.

210. Yamaguchi K, Uchino A, Sawada A, et al: Bilateral anterior cerebral artery territory infarction associated with unilateral hypoplasia of the A1 segment: Report of two cases, *Radiat Med* 22:422, 2004.

211. Menezes BF, Cheserem B, Kandasamy J, et al: Acute bilateral anterior circulation stroke due to anomalous cerebral vasculature: A case report, *J Med Case Reports* 2:188, 2008.

212. Babu AN, Babu LA, Raden M, et al: Transient paraparesis due to right carotid stenosis with left anterior cerebral artery aplasia, *Neurology* 67:907, 2006.

213. Marie P, Foix C: Paraplégie en flexion d'origine cérébrale par nécrose sous épendymaire progressive, *Rev Neurol* 27:1, 1920.

214. Van Bogaert L, Ley R: Contribution à la connaissance de la paraplegie en flexion, type Babinski, d'origine cérébrale, *J Neurol Psychiatry* 26:547, 1926.

215. Meyer JS, Barron DW: Apraxia of gait: A clinicophysiological study, *Brain* 83:261, 1960.

216. Ueno E: Clinical and physiological study of apraxia of gait and frozen gait, *Rinsho Shinkeigaku* 29:275, 1989.

217. Denny-Brown D: The nature of apraxia, *J Nerv Ment Dis* 126:9, 1958.

218. Ferbert A, Thron A: Bilateral anterior cerebral artery territory infarction in the differential diagnosis of basilar artery occlusion, *J Neurol* 239:162, 1992.

219. Bradley WE, Timm GW, Scott FB: Innervation of the detrusor muscle and urethra, *Urol Clin North Am* 1:3, 1974.

220. Fisher CM: Hydrocephalus as a cause of disturbances of gait in the elderly, *Neurology* 32:1358, 1982.

221. Yakovlev PI: Paraplegias of hydrocephalics (clinical note and interpretation), *Am J Ment Defic* 51:561, 1947.

222. Yakovlev PI: Paraplegia in flexion of cerebral origin, *J Neuropathol Exp Neurol* 13:267, 1954.

223. Hill A, Volpe J: Decrease in pulsatile flow in the anterior cerebral arteries in infantile hydrocephalus, *Pediatrics* 69:4, 1982.

224. Mathew NT, Hartmann A, Meyer JS, et al: The importance of "CSF pressure-regulated cerebral blood flow dysregulation" in the pathogenesis of normal pressure hydrocephalus. In Lundberg N, Panton V, Brock M, editors: *Intracranial pressure, two: proceedings*, New York, 1975, Springer-Verlag, p 145.

225. Della S, Francescani A, Spinnler H: Gait apraxia after bilateral supplementary motor area lesion, *J Neurol Neurosurg Psychiatry* 72:77, 2002.

226. Gerstner E, Liberato B, Wright CB: Bi-hemispheric anterior cerebral artery with drop attacks and limb shaking TIAs, *Neurology* 65:174, 2005.

227. Levin HS, Goldstein FC, Ghostine SY, et al: Hemispheric disconnection syndrome persisting after anterior cerebral artery aneurysm rupture, *Neurosurgery* 21:831, 1987.

228. Maas O: Ein Fall von linksseitiger Apraxie und Agraphie, *Zentralbl Neurol* 26:789, 1907.

229. Van Vleuten CF: Linksseitige motorische Apraxie, *Z Psychiatr* 64:203, 1907.

230. Yamadori A, Osumi Y, Ikeda H, Kanazawa Y: Left unilateral agraphia and tactile anomia: Disturbances after occlusion of the anterior cerebral artery, *Arch Neurol* 37:88, 1980.

231. Geschwind N, Kaplan E: A human cerebral disconnection syndrome: A preliminary report, *Neurology* 12:675, 1962.

232. Hecaen H, Gimeno-Alava A: L'apraxie idéomotrice unilatérale gauche, *Rev Neurol* 102:648, 1960.

233. Bouman L, Grunbaum AA: Über motorische Momente der Agraphie, *Monatsschr Psychiatr Neurol* 77:223, 1930.

234. Geschwind N: The apraxias: Neural mechanisms of disorders of learned movement, *Am Sci* 63:188, 1975.

235. Schott B, Michel F, Michel D, Dumas R: Apraxie idéomotrice unilatérale gauche avec main gauche anomique: Syndrome de déconnection calleuse? *Rev Neurol* 120:359, 1969.

236. Geschwind N: Disconnection syndromes in animals and man, *Brain* 88:237, 1965.

237. Trescher JH, Ford FR: Colloid cyst of the third ventricle, *Arch Neurol Psychiatry* 37:959, 1937.

238. Nielsen JM: *Agnosia, apraxia, aphasia*, ed 2, New York, 1946, Hoeber.

239. Pitres A: Considerations sur l'agraphie, *Rev Med* 4:855, 1884.

240. Luria AR, Tsvetkova LS: Towards the mechanism of "dynamic aphasia, *Acta Neurol Belg* 67:1045, 1967.

241. Watson RT, Heilman KM: Callosal apraxia, *Brain* 106:391, 1983.

242. Goldberg G, Mayer NH, Toglia JU: Medial frontal cortex infarction and the alien hand sign, *Arch Neurol* 38:683, 1981.

243. Feinberg TE, Schindler RJ, Flanagan NG, Haber LD: Two alien hand syndromes, *Neurology* 42:19, 1992.

244. Gasquoine PG: Alien hand sign, *J Clin Exp Neuropsychol* 15:653, 1993.

245. Goldenberg G: Neglect in a patient with partial callosal disconnection, *Neuropsychologia* 24:397, 1986.

246. Trojano L, Crisci C, Lanzillo B, et al: How many alien hand syndromes? Follow-up of a case, *Neurology* 43:2710, 1993.

247. Della Sala S, Marchetti C, Spinnler H: Right-sided anarchic (alien) hand: A longitudinal study, *Neuropsychologia* 29:1113, 1991.

248. Brainin M, Seiser A, Matz K: The mirror world of motor inhibition: The alien hand syndrome in chronic stroke, *J Neurol Neurosurg Psychiatry* 79:246, 2008.

249. Hal BG, Odderson IR: Involuntary masturbation as a manifestation of stroke-related alien hand syndrome, *Am J Phys Med Rehabil* 79:4, 2000.

250. Bejot Y, Cailler M, Osseby G-V, et al: Involuntary masturbation after bilateral anterior cerebral artery infarction, *Clin Neurol Neurosurg* 110:190, 2008.

251. Tanaka Y, Iwasa H, Yoshida M: Diagonistic dyspraxia: Case report and movement-related potentials, *Neurology* 40:657, 1990.

252. Chan JL, Liu AB: Anatomical correlates of alien hand syndromes, *Neuropsychiatry Neuropsychol Behav Neurol* 12:149, 1999.

253. Fukui T, Hasegawa Y, Sugita K, Tsukagoshi H: Utilization behavior and concomitant motor neglect by bilateral frontal lobe damage, *Eur Neurol* 33:325, 1993.

254. Lhermitte F, Pillon B, Serdaru M: Human anatomy and the frontal lobes. Part I: Imitation and utilization behavior: A neuropsychological study of 75 patients, *Ann Neurol* 19:326, 1986.

255. Boccardi E, Della Salla S, Motto C, et al: Utilization behavior consequent to bilateral SMA softening, *Cortex* 38:289, 2002.

256. Nagumo T, Yamadori A: Callosal disconnection syndrome and knowledge of the body: A case of left hand isolation from the body schema with names, *J Neurol Neurosurg Psychiatry* 59:548, 1995.

257. Gazzaniga MS, Bogen JE, Sperry RW: Some functional effects of sectioning the cerebral commissures in man, *Proc Natl Acad Sci U S A* 48:1765, 1962.

258. Gazzaniga MS, Bogen JE, Sperry RW: Dyspraxia following division of the cerebral commissures, *Arch Neurol* 16:606, 1967.

259. Bogen JE, Gazzaniga MS: Cerebral commissurotomy in man: Minor hemisphere dominance for certain visuo-spatial functions, *J Neurosurg* 23:394, 1965.

260. Gazzaniga MS, Bogen JE, Sperry RW: Observations on visual perception after disconnection of the cerebral hemispheres in man, *Brain* 88:221, 1965.

261. Gazzaniga MS, Sperry RW: Language after section of the cerebral commissures, *Brain* 90:131, 1967.

262. Sperry RW, Gazzaniga MS: Language following surgical disconnection of the hemispheres. In Millikan CH, editor: *Brain mechanisms underlying speech and language*, New York, 1966, Grune & Stratton.

263. Sperry RW, Gazzaniga MS, Bogen JE: Interhemispheric relationships: The neocortical commissures: Syndromes of hemispheric disconnection. In Vinken PJ, Bruyn GW, editors: *Handbook of clinical neurology, vol 4, Disorders of speech, perception, and symbolic behaviour*, Amsterdam, 1969, Holland Publishing, pp 273-290.

264. Zaidel E: Unilateral auditory language comprehension on the Token test following cerebral commissurotomy and hemispherectomy, *Neuropsychologia* 15:1, 1977.

265. Gazzaniga MS, Volpe BT, Smylie CS, et al: Plasticity in speech organization following commissurotomy, *Brain* 102:805, 1979.

266. Sidtis JJ, Volpe BT, Wilson DH, et al: Variability in right hemisphere language function after callosal section: Evidence for a continuum of generative capacity, *J Neurosci* 1:323, 1981.

267. Gazzaniga MS, Hillyard SA: Language and speech capacity of the right hemisphere, *Neuropsychologia* 9:273, 1971.

268. Gazzaniga MS, LeDoux JE, Wilson DH: Language, praxis, and the right hemisphere: Clues to some mechanisms of consciousness, *Neurology* 27:1144, 1977.

269. Heilman KM, Bowers D, Watson RT: Pseudoneglect in a patient with partial callosal disconnection, *Brain* 107:519, 1984.

270. Kashiwagi A, Kashiwagi T, Nishikawa T, et al: Hemi-spatial neglect in a patient with callosal infarction, *Brain* 113:1005, 1990.

271. Sine RD, Soufi A, Shah M: Callosal syndrome: Implications for understanding the neuropsychology of stroke, *Arch Phys Med Rehabil* 65:606, 1984.

272. Heilman KM, Coyle JM, Gonyea EF, Geschwind N: Apraxia and agraphia in a left-hander, *Brain* 96:21, 1973.

273. Kimura D: Neuromotor mechanisms in the evolution of human communication. In Steklin HD, Raleigh MJ, editors: *Neurobiology of social communication in primates*, San Diego, Calif, 1979, Academic Press, p 197.

274. Kimura D, Archibald Y: Motor functions of the left hemisphere, *Brain* 97:337, 1974.

275. Kimura D, Archibald Y: Acquisition of a motor skill after left hemisphere damage, *Brain* 100:527, 1977.

276. Sabouraud O, Pecker J: Suspension de langage non-aphasique après intervention sur la region interhémisphérique, *Rev Otoneuroophthalmol* 1:42, 1960.

277. Volpe BT: Observation of motor control in patients with partial and complete callosal section: Implications for current theories of apraxia. In Reeves A, editor: *Epilepsy and the corpus callosum*, New York, 1983, Plenum Press.

278. Volpe BT, Sidtis JJ, Holzman JD, et al: Cortical mechanisms involved in praxis: Observations following partial and complete section of the corpus callosum in man, *Neurology* 32:645, 1982.

279. Gordon HW, Bogen JE, Sperry RW: Absence of disconnection syndrome in two patients with partial section of the neocommissures, *Brain* 94:327, 1971.

280. Maspes PE: Le syndrome expérimental chez l'homme de la section du splenium du corps calleux: Alexie visuelle pure hémianopique, *Rev Neurol* 80:100, 1948.

281. Jeeves MA, Simpson DA, Geffen G: Functional consequences of the transcallosal removal of intraventricular tumours, *J Neurol Neurosurg Psychiatry* 42:134, 1979.

282. Gazzaniga MS, Freedman H: Observations on visual processes after posterior callosal section, *Neurology* 23:1126, 1973.

283. Iwata M, Sugishita M, Toyokura Y, et al: Étude sur le syndrome de disconnection visuo-lingual après le transéction du splenium du corps calleux, *J Neurol Sci* 23:421, 1974.

284. Sugishita M, Iwata M, Toyokura Y, et al: Reading ideograms and phonograms in Japanese patients after partial commissurotomy, *Neuropsychologia* 16:417, 1978.

285. Damasio AR, Chui HC, Corbett J, Kassel N: Posterior callosal section in a non-epileptic patient, *J Neurol Neurosurg Psychiatry* 43:351, 1980.

286. Sidtis JJ, Volpe BT, Holtzman JD, et al: Cognitive interaction after staged callosal section: Evidence for transfer of semantic activation, *Science* 212:344, 1981.

287. Tomaiuolo F, Nocentini U, Grammaldo L, Caltagirone C: Interhemispheric transfer time in a patient with a partial lesion of the corpus callosum, *Neuroreport* 12:1469, 2001.

288. Segarra JM: Cerebral vascular disease and behavior. I: The syndrome of the mesencephalic artery (basilar artery bifurcation), *Arch Neurol* 22:408, 1970.

289. Cairns H, Oldfield RC, Pennybacker JB: Akinetic mutism with an epidermoid cyst of III ventricle, *Brain* 64:273, 1941.

290. Castaigne P, Buge A, Cambier J, et al: Démence thalamique d'origine vasculaire par ramollissement bilateral, limité au territoire du pedicule retromammilaire, *Rev Neurol* 114:89, 1966.

291. Lechi A, Marchi G: Nécrose méso-diencephalique au cours d'une méningo-encephalite subaiguë: Observation anatomoclinique, *Acta Neurol Belg* 67:475, 1967.

292. Buge A, Escourelle R, Rancurel G: "Mutisme akinétique" et ramollissement bilingulaire: Trois observations anatomoclinique, *Rev Neurol* 131:121, 1975.

293. Freeman FR: Akinetic mutism and bilateral anterior cerebral artery occlusion, *J Neurol Neurosurg Psychiatry* 34:693, 1971.

294. Gugliotta MA, Silvestri R, DeDomenico P, Galatioto S: Spontaneous bilateral anterior cerebral artery occlusion resulting in akinetic mutism: A case report, *Acta Neurol (Napoli)* 11:252, 1989.

295. Wolff V, Saint Maurice JP, Ducros A, et al: [Akinetic mutism and anterior bicerebral infarction due to abnormal distribution of the anterior cerebral artery], *Rev Neurol (Paris)* 158:377, 2002.

296. Fisher CM: Abulia minor versus agitated behavior, *Clin Neurosurg* 31:9, 1983.

297. Minager A, David NJ: Bilateral infarction in the territory of the anterior cerebral arteries, *Neurology* 52:886, 1999.

298. Nielsen JM, Jacobs LL: Bilateral lesions of the anterior cingulate gyri, *Bull Los Angeles Neurol Soc* 16:231, 1951.

299. Barris RW, Schuman HR: Bilateral anterior cingulate gyrus lesions. Syndrome of the anterior cingulate gyri, *Neurology* 3:44, 1953.

300. Amyes EW, Nielsen JM: Clinicopathologic study of vascular lesions of the anterior cingulate region, *Bull Los Angeles Neurol Soc* 20:112, 1955.

301. Skultety FM: Clinical and experimental aspects of akinetic mutism: Report of a case, *Arch Neurol* 19:1, 1968.

302. Meador KJ, Watson RT, Bowers D, Heilman KM: Hypometria with hemispatial and limb motor neglect, *Brain* 109:293, 1986.

303. Cambier J, Dehen H: Les syndromes de l'artère cérébrale antérieure, *Nouv Presse Med* 28:1137–1141, 1973.

304. Castaigne P, LaPlane D, Degos JD: Trois cas de negligence motrice par lesion frontal prerolandique, *Rev Neurol* 126:5, 1972.

305. Paillard J: À propos de la négligence motrice: Issues et perspectives, *Rev Neurol* 146:600, 1990.

306. Schell G, Hodge CJ, Cacayorin E: Transient neurological deficit after therapeutic embolization of the arteries supplying the medial wall of the hemisphere, including the supplementary motor area, *Neurosurgery* 18:353, 1986.

307. Dick JPR, Benecke R, Rothwell JC, et al: Simple and complex movements in a patient with infarction of the right supplementary area, *Mov Disord* 1:255, 1986.

308. Halsband U, Ito N, Tanji J, Freund H-J: The role of premotor cortex and the supplementary motor area in the temporal control of movement in man, *Brain* 116:243, 1993.

309. Lacruz F, Artieda J, Pastor MA, Obeso JA: The anatomical basis of somatesthetic temporal discrimination in humans, *J Neurol Neurosurg Psychiatry* 54:1077, 1991.

310. Paus T, Kalina M, Patockova L, et al: Medial vs lateral frontal lobe lesions and differential impairment of central-gaze fixation in man, *Brain* 114:2051, 1991.

311. Nicolai J, van Putten MJAM, Tavy DLJ: BIPLEDs in akinetic mutism caused by bilateral anterior cerebral artery infarction, *Clin Neurophysiol* 112:1726, 2001.

312. Yang C-P, Huang W-S, Shih HT, et al: Diminution of basal ganglia dopaminergic function may play an important role in the generation of akinetic mutism in a patient with anterior cerebral arterial infarct, *Clin Neurol Neurosurg* 109:602, 2007.

313. Combarros O, Infante J, Berciano J: Akinetic mutism from frontal lobe damage responding to levodopa, *J Neurol* 247:568, 2000.

314. Kennard M: The cingulate gyrus in relation to consciousness, *J Nerv Ment Dis* 121:34, 1955.

315. Whitty CWM, Duffield JE, Tow PM, Cairns H: Anterior cingulectomy in the treatment of mental disease, *Lancet* 1:475, 1952.

316. Fisher CM, Kistler JP, David JM: Relation of cerebral vasospasm to subarachnoid hemorrhage by computerized tomographic scanning, *Neurosurgery* 6:1, 1980.

317. Mendez MF, Adams NL, Lewandowski KS: Neurobehavioral changes associated with caudate lesions, *Neurology* 39:349, 1989.

318. Spencer SS: Corpus callosum section and other disconnection procedures for medically intractable epilepsy, *Epilepsia* 29(Suppl 2):S85, 1988.

319. Sussman NM, Gur RC, Gur RE, O'Connor MJ: Mutism as a consequence of callosectomy, *J Neurosurg* 59:514, 1983.

320. Yamaguchi T, Kunimoto M, Pappata S, et al: Effects of anterior corpus callosum section on cortical glucose utilization in baboons: A sequential positron emission tomography study, *Brain* 113:937, 1990.

321. Gelmers HJ: Non-paralytic motor disturbances and speech disorders: The role of the supplementary motor area, *J Neurol Neurosurg Psychiatry* 46:1052, 1983.

322. Jonas S: The supplementary motor region and speech emission, *J Commun Disord* 14:349, 1981.

323. Bogousslavsky J, Assal G, Regli F: Infarctus du territoire de l'artère cérébrale antérieure gauche. 2: Troubles du langage, *Rev Neurol* 143:121, 1987.

324. Damasio AR, Van Hoesen GW: Structure and function of the supplementary motor area, *Neurology* 30:359, 1980.

325. Kornyey E: Aphasie transcorticale et écholalie: Le problème de l'initiative de la parole, *Rev Neurol* 131:347, 1975.

326. Masdeu JC, Schoene WC, Funkenstein H: Aphasia following infarction of the left supplementary motor area: A clinical pathological study, *Neurology* 28:1220, 1978.

327. Van Stockert TR: Aphasia sine aphasia, *Brain Lang* 1:277, 1974.

328. Alexander MP, Schmitt MA: The aphasia syndrome of stroke in the left anterior cerebral artery territory, *Arch Neurol* 37:97, 1980.

329. Lhermitte J, Schiff P: Le phénomène de la préhension forcée, expression d'un ramollissement complet de la première circonvolution frontale, *Rev Neurol* 35:175, 1928.

330. Atkinson MS: Transcortical motor aphasia associated with left frontal lobe infarction, *Trans Am Neurol Assoc* 96:136, 1971.

331. Damasio AR, Kassel NF: Transcortical motor aphasia in relation to lesions of the supplementary motor area, *Neurology* 28:396, 1978.

332. Kertesz A, Lesk D, McCabe P: Isotope localization of infarcts in aphasia, *Arch Neurol* 34:590, 1977.

333. Ross ED: Left medial parietal lobe and receptive language functions: Mixed transcortical aphasia after left anterior cerebral artery infarction, *Neurology* 30:144, 1980.

334. Rubens AB: Aphasia with infarction in the territory of the anterior cerebral artery, *Cortex* 11:239, 1975.

335. Carrieri G: Sindrome da sofferenza dell'area supplementaria motoria sinistra nel corso di un meningioma parasaggitale, *Riv Patol Nerv Ment* 84:29, 1963.

336. Racy A, Jannotta FS, Lehner LH: Aphasia resulting from occlusion of the left anterior cerebral artery: Report of a case with an old infarct in the left rolandic region, *Arch Neurol* 36:221, 1979.

337. Tatemichi TK, Desmond DW, Prohovnik I: Strategic infarcts in vascular dementia: A clinical and brain imaging experience, *Arzneimittelforschung* 45:371, 1995.

338. Auchus AP, Chen CP, Sodagar SN, et al: Single stroke dementia: Insights from 12 cases in Singapore, *J Neurol Sci* 203-204:85–89, 2002.

339. Brust JCM, Plank C, Burke A, et al: Language disorder in a right-hander after occlusion of the right anterior cerebral artery, *Neurology* 32:492, 1982.

340. Hyland HH: Thrombosis of intracranial arteries: Report of three cases involving, respectively, the anterior cerebral, basilar and internal carotid arteries, *Arch Neurol Psychiatry* 30:342, 1933.

341. Masdeu JC: Language disturbance after mesial frontal infarction, *Neurology* 33 (Suppl 2):243, 1983.

342. Tsumoto T, Nishioka K, Nakakita K, et al: [Acquired stuttering associated with callosal infarction: A case report], *No Shinkei Geka* 27:79, 1999.

343. Chang CC, Lee YC, Lui CC, et al: Right anterior cingulate cortex infarction and transient speech aspontaneity, *Arch Neurol* 64:442, 2007.

344. Mandez MF: Aphemia-like syndrome from a right supplementary motor area lesion, *Clin Neurol Neurosurg* 106:337, 2004.

345. Iragui VJ: Ataxic hemiparesis associated with transcortical motor aphasia, *Eur Neurol* 30:162, 1990.

346. Penfield W, Welch K: The supplementary motor area in the cerebral cortex of man, *Trans Am Neurol Assoc* 74:179, 1949.

347. Penfield W, Welch K: The supplementary motor area of the cerebral cortex: A clinical and experimental study, *Arch Neurol Psychiatry* 66:289, 1951.

348. Bogousslavsky J, Regli F: Infarctus du territoire de l'artère cérébrale antérieure gauche. 1: Correlations clinico-tomodensitometriques, *Rev Neurol* 143:21, 1987.

349. Brinkman C, Porter R: Supplementary motor area in the monkey: Activity of neurons during performance of a learned motor task, *J Neurophysiol* 42:681, 1979.

350. Macpherson JM, Marangoz C, Miles TS, Wiesendanger M: Microstimulation of the supplementary motor area (SMA) in the awake monkey, *Exp Brain Res* 45:410, 1982.

351. Smith AM: The activity of supplementary motor area neurons during a maintained precision grip, *Brain Res* 172:315, 1979.

352. Tanji J, Kurata K: Neuronal activity in the cortical supplementary motor area related with distal and proximal forelimb movements, *Neurosci Lett* 12:201, 1979.

353. Tanji J, Kurata K: Comparison of movement-related activity in two cortical motor areas of primates, *J Neurophysiol* 48:633, 1982.

354. Wise SP, Tanji J: Supplementary and pre-central motor cortex: Contrast in responsiveness to peripheral input in the hindlimb area of the unanesthetized monkey, *J Comp Neurol* 195:433, 1981.

355. Woolsey CN, Settlage PH, Meyer DR, et al: Patterns of localization in precentral and "supplementary" motor areas, *Res Publ Assoc Res Nerv Ment Dis* 30:238, 1952.

356. Brinkman C: Lesions in supplementary motor area interfere with a monkey's performance of a bimanual coordination task, *Neurosci Lett* 27:267, 1981.

357. Penfield W, Rasmussen T: Vocalization and arrest of speech, *Arch Neurol Psychiatry* 61:21, 1949.

358. Arseni C, Botez MI: Speech disturbances caused by tumours of the supplementary motor area, *Acta Psychiatr Scand* 36:279, 1961.

359. Boudouresques J, Bonnal J: Les troubles psychiques des tumeurs frontales, *Rev Prat* 7:1375, 1957.

360. Castaigne P: Vocalisations itératives et crises palilaliques dans les lésions prérolandiques de la face interne du lobe frontal, *Neurologia* 9:39, 1964.

361. Guidetti B: Désordres de la parole associés à des lésions de la surface interhémisphérique frontale postérieure, *Rev Neurol* 97:121, 1957.

362. Talairach J, Bancaud J: The supplementary motor area in man, *Int J Neurol* 5:330, 1966.

363. Caplan LR, Zervas NT: Speech arrest in a dextral with a right mesial frontal astrocytoma, *Arch Neurol* 35:252, 1978.

364. Penfield W, Rasmussen T: *The cerebral cortex of man: a clinical study of localization of function,* New York, 1950, Macmillan.

365. Laplane D, Talairach J, Meininger J, et al: Clinical consequences of corticectomies involving the supplementary motor area in man, *J Neurol Sci* 34:301, 1977.

366. Watson RT, Fleet S, Gonzalez-Rothi L, Heilman KM: Apraxia and the supplementary motor area, *Arch Neurol* 43:787, 1986.

367. Jones EG, Coulter JD, Burton H, Porter R: Cells of origin and terminal distribution of corticostriatal fibers arising in the sensory-motor cortex of monkeys, *J Comp Neurol* 173:53, 1977.

368. Jones EG, Coulter JD, Hendry SHC: Intracortical connectivity of architectonic fields in the somatic sensory, motor, and parietal cortex of monkeys, *J Comp Neurol* 181:291, 1978.

369. Jones EG, Powell TPS: Connections of the somatic sensory cortex of the rhesus monkey. I: Ipsilateral cortical connections, *Brain* 92:477, 1969.

370. De Vito JL, Smith OA: Projections from the mesial frontal cortex (supplementary motor area) to the cerebral hemispheres and brain stem of the *Macaca mulatta, J Comp Neurol* 11:261, 1959.

371. Kunzle H: Bilateral projections from precentral motor cortex to the putamen and other parts of the basal ganglia: An autoradiographic study in *Macaca fascicularis, Brain Res* 88:195, 1975.

372. Biber MP, Kneisley LW, LaVail JH: Cortical neurons projecting to the cervical and lumbar enlargements of the spinal cord in young and adult rhesus monkeys, *Exp Neurol* 59:492, 1978.

373. Murray EA, Coulter JD: Organization of corticospinal neurons in the monkey, *J Comp Neurol* 195:339, 1981.

374. Ingvar DH, Schwartz MS: Blood flow patterns induced in the dominant hemisphere by speech and reading, *Brain* 97:273, 1974.

375. Larson B, Skinhoj E, Larsen NA: Variations in regional cortical blood flow in the right and left hemispheres during automatic speech, *Brain* 101:193, 1978.

376. Lassen NA, Roland PE, Larsen B, et al: Mapping of human cerebral functions: A study of the regional cerebral blood flow pattern during rest, its reproducibility and the activation seen during basic sensory and motor functions, *Acta Neurol Scand Suppl* 64:262, 1977.

377. Orgogozo JM, Larsen B: Activation of the supplementary motor area during voluntary movement in man suggests it works as a supramotor area, *Science* 206:847, 1979.

378. Roland PE, Larsen B, Lassen NA, Skinhoj E: Supplementary motor areas in organization of voluntary movements in man, *J Neurophysiol* 43:118, 1980.

379. Roland PE, Meyer E, Shibasaki T, et al: Regional cerebral blood flow changes in cortex and basal ganglia during voluntary movements in normal human volunteers, *J Neurophysiol* 48:467, 1982.

380. Woolsey CN: Cortical motor map of *Macaca mulatta* after chronic section of the medullary pyramid. In Zulch KJ, Creutzfeldt O, Galbraith GC, editors: *Cerebral localisation: an Otto Foerster Symposium,* Berlin, 1975, Springer-Verlag, p p 19.

381. Smith AM, Bourbonnais D, Blanchette G: Interaction between forced grasping and learned precision grip after ablation of the supplementary motor area, *Brain Res* 222:395, 1981.

382. Wiesendanger M, Ruegg DG, Lucier GE: Why transcortical reflexes? *Can J Neurol Sci* 2:295, 1975.

383. Tanji J, Taniguchi K, Saga T: Supplementary motor area: Neuronal responses to motor instructions, *J Neurophysiol* 43:60, 1980.

384. Roland PE, Skinhoj E, Lassen NA, Larsen B: Different cortical areas in man in organization of voluntary movements in extrapersonal space, *J Neurophysiol* 43:137, 1980.

385. Sengupta RP: Direct surgery of anterior communicating aneurysms and its effect on intellect and personality, *J Neurol Neurosurg Psychiatry* 38:406, 1975.

386. Faris AA: Limbic system infarction, *J Neuropathol Exp Neurol* 26:174, 1967.

387. Grafman J, Vance SC, Weingartner H, et al: The effects of lateralized frontal lesions on mood regulation, *Brain* 109:1127, 1986.

388. Davison C, Goodhart SP, Needles W: Cerebral localization in cerebrovascular disease, *Res Publ Assoc Res Nerv Ment Dis* 13:435, 1934.

389. Dimitri V, Victoria M: Sindrome de la arteria cerebral anterior, *Rev Neurol Buenos Aires* 1:81, 1936.

390. Larsson C, Forssell A, Ronnberg J, et al: Subarachnoid blood on CT and memory dysfunction in aneurysmal subarachnoid hemorrhage, *Acta Neurol Scand* 90:331, 1994.

391. Scott M: Ligation of an anterior cerebral artery for aneurysms of the anterior communicating artery complex, *J Neurosurg* 38:481, 1973.

392. Janowsky JS, Shimamura AP, Kritchevsky M, Squire LR: Cognitive impairment following frontal lobe damage and its relevance to human amnesia, *Behav Neurosci* 103:548, 1989.

393. Parkin AJ, Leng NRC, Stanhope N, Smith AP: Memory impairment following ruptured aneurysm of the anterior communicating artery, *Brain Cogn* 7:231, 1988.

394. Stuss DT, Alexander MP, Lieberman A, Levine H: An extraordinary form of confabulation, *Neurology* 28:1166, 1978.

395. Vilkki J: Amnestic syndromes after surgery of anterior communicating artery aneurysms, *Cortex* 21:431, 1985.

396. Talland GA, Sweet WH, Ballantine HT: Amnestic syndrome with anterior communicating artery aneurysm, *J Nerv Ment Dis* 145:179, 1967.

397. Volpe BT, Hirst W: Amnesia following rupture and repair of an anterior communicating artery aneurysm, *J Neurol Neurosurg Psychiatry* 46:704, 1983.

398. Youngjohn JR, Altman IM, Van Doren J: Amnesia following anterior communicating aneurysm surgery, *J Clin Exp Neuropsychol* 11:61, 1989.

399. Delbecq-Derouesné J, Beauvois MF, Shallice T: Preserved recall versus impaired recognition: A case study, *Brain* 113:1045, 1990.

400. Damasio AR, Graff-Radford NR, Eslinger PJ, et al: Amnesia following basal forebrain lesions, *Arch Neurol* 42:263, 1985.

401. Phillips S, Sangalang V, Sterns G: Basal forebrain infarction: A clinicopathologic correlation, *Arch Neurol* 44:1134, 1987.

402. Wolfe N, Linn R, Babikian VL, et al: Frontal system impairment following multiple lacunar infarcts, *Arch Neurol* 47:129, 1990.

403. Moudgil SS, Azzouz M, Al-Azzaz A, et al: Amnesia due to fornix infarction, *Stroke* 31:1418, 2000.

404. den Heijer T, Ruitenberg A, Bakker J, et al: Bilateral caudate nucleus infarction associated with variant in circle of Willis, *J Neurol Neurosurg Psychiatry* 78:1175, 2007.

405. Mizuta H, Motomura N: Mental dysfunction in caudate infarction caused by Heubner's recurring artery occlusion, *Brain Cogn* 61:133, 2006.

406. Frith V, Frith CD: Development and neurophysiology of mentalizing, *Philos Trans R Soc Lond B Biol Sci* 358:459, 2003.

407. Bird CM, Castelli F, Malik O, et al: The impact of extensive medial frontal lobe damage on "Theory of Mind" and cognition, *Brain* 127:914, 2004.

408. Tatemichi TK, Desmond DW, Patik M, et al: Clinical determinants of dementia related to stroke, *Ann Neurol* 33:568, 1993.

409. Lucchelli F, DeRenzi E: Primary dyscalculia after a medial frontal lesion of the left hemisphere, *J Neurol Neurosurg Psychiatry* 56:304, 1993.

410. Starkstein SE, Robinson RG, Berthier ML, et al: Differential mood changes following basal ganglia vs thalamic lesions, *Arch Neurol* 45:725, 1988.

411. Penfield W, Boldrey E: Somatic motor and sensory representation in cerebral cortex of man as studied by electrical stimulation, *Brain* 60:384, 1937.

412. Andrew J, Nathan PW: Lesions of the anterior frontal lobes and disturbances of micturition and defecation, *Brain* 87:233, 1964.

413. Andrew J, Nathan PW: The cerebral control of micturition, *Proc R Soc Med* 58:553, 1965.

414. Risso M, Poeck K, Creutzfeld O, Pilleri G: Katamnestische Untersuchungen nach frontaler Leukotomie. I: Klinische Beobachtungen. II. Anatomischklinische Korrelationen, *Bibl Psychiatr Neurol* 116:1, 1962.

415. Lloyd T Jr: Effect of stroke on lung function and the pulmonary circulation. In Price TR, Nelson E, editors: *Cerebrovascular diseases: proceedings of the Eleventh Research Conference*, Philadelphia, 1979, Lippincott-Raven, p 371.

416. Vincent GM: Cardiac electrophysiologic abnormalities in the stroke syndrome. In Price TR, Nelson E, editors: *Cerebrovascular diseases: proceedings of the Eleventh Research Conference*, Philadelphia, 1979, Lippincott-Raven, p 365.

417. Dunsmore RH, Lennox MA: Stimulation and strychninization of supracallosal anterior cingulate gyrus, *J Neurophysiol* 13:207, 1950.

418. Segundo JP, Naquet R, Buser P: Cortical stimulation in monkeys, *J Neurophysiol* 18:236, 1955.

419. Tanaka S, Mori T, Ohara H, et al: Gastrointestinal bleeding in cases of ruptured cerebral aneurysms, *Acta Neurochir* 48:223, 1979.

420. Craenen G, Brown SM, Freedman KA, et al: Rapid painless unilateral vision loss in a 37-year-old healthy woman, *Surv Ophthalmol* 49:343, 2004.

421. Rivet DJ, Dacey RG: Visual loss from a dolichoectatic anterior cerebral artery, *J Neurosurg* 102:576, 2005.

422. Chen CS, Gailloud P, Miller NR: Bitemporal hemianopia caused by an intracranial vascular loop, *Arch Ophthalmol* 126:274, 2008.

423. Korn T, Reith W, Becker G: Impaired volitional closure of the left eyelid after right anterior cerebral artery infarction. Apraxia due to hemispheric disconnection? *Arch Neurol* 61:273, 2004.

424. Maruyama N, Fukuma A, Ihara I, et al: Epilepsy and variation in the frontal lobe artery, *Epilepsy Res* 64:71, 2005.

425. Volpe JJ: Cerebral blood flow in the newborn infant: Relations to hypoxic-ischemic brain injury and periventricular hemorrhage, *J Pediatr* 94:170, 1979.

426. De Reuck J, Chatta AS, Richardson EP: Pathogenesis and evolution of periventricular leukomalacia in infancy, *Arch Neurol* 27:229, 1972.

427. Takashima S, Tanaka K: Development of cerebrovascular architecture and its relationship to periventricular leukomalacia, *Arch Neurol* 35:11, 1978.

428. Young RSK, Hernandez MJ, Yagel SK: Selective reduction of blood flow to white matter during hypotension in newborn dogs: A possible mechanism of periventricular leukomalacia, *Ann Neurol* 12:445, 1982.

429. Armstrong D, Norman MG: Periventricular leukomalacia in neonates: Complications and sequelae, *Arch Dis Child* 49:367, 1974.

24 Middle Cerebral Artery Disease

J.P. MOHR, RONALD M. LAZAR, RANDOLPH S. MARSHALL

The middle cerebral artery (MCA), the largest of the branches of the internal carotid, is also the most commonly affected artery in stroke syndromes.[1-6] The MCA supplies most of the convex surface of the brain, leaving to other cerebral arteries the frontal pole and its immediately adjacent lateral gyro, the extremes of the high parietal and very posterolateral aspects of the occipital gyri, and occipital pole. In the brain parenchyma its branches irrigate almost all of the basal ganglia and capsules (internal, external, and extreme capsule), claustrum, putamen, the upper parts of the globus pallidus, parts of the substantia innominata of Reichert, the posterior portion of the head and all of the body of the caudate nucleus, and all but the very lowest portions of the anterior and posterior limbs of the internal capsule. Supply to any portion of the thalamus has only rarely been demonstrated.[7]

The internal capsule, classically the MCA territory, has a complex arterial supply: Its anterior limb has some supply from a large branch of the anterior cerebral artery known as Heubner's artery, yet the MCA supplies the anterior limb in one third of cases; most of the posterior limb of the internal capsule and the corona radiata are fed by the deep, lenticulostriate branches of the MCA, whereas the lowest portion of the posterior limb, where it makes a transition to the peduncle of the midbrain, is supplied by the anterior choroidal artery, which usually arises from the internal carotid artery just proximal to the circle of Willis (see Chapter 22).[8]

Descriptive Terms

The anatomy of the MCA tree has been described by named branching and by the relationship between the vessel and the anatomic landmarks of the cerebral surface.

Names of Stem, Divisions, and Branches

The traditional terminology analogizes the vessel as a tree with a trunk and branches (Fig. 24-1), a clinically useful descriptive method that we employ throughout this chapter. The MCA regularly begins as a single trunk or stem. Its length varies from 18 to 26 mm. The diameter at its origin is roughly 3 mm, varying from 2.5 mm to 4.9 mm.[9,10] The stem gives rise to most of the lenticulostriate branches, so named because they penetrate the brain to supply the lentiform nucleus (putamen and pallidum), body of the caudate nucleus (together with the putamen known as the striatum), and the internal capsule.[9] (The claustrum and extreme capsule are supplied by vessels

from the surface, penetrating through the insula.)[11] The lenticulostriate arteries number from 5 to 17 branches, each of them end arteries and each supplying cones of varying size of adjacent tissue in their curvilinear (on coronal view) course to end in the corona radiata near the lateral ventricular wall. A few of the smaller lenticulostriate arteries may arise from the distal internal carotid artery, but the larger penetrating vessels do not.[10]

No clear correlations between the length of the MCA stem and the pattern or number of the lenticulostriate arteries has been shown, nor does the pattern on one side predict that on the other.[10] The lenticulostriate arteries arising more medially on the MCA stem are the smaller vessels (50 to 150 μm), whereas those arising more laterally are larger (some as large as 500 μm). Three patterns of origin of the lenticulostriate arteries from the MCA have been described.[10] In the most common variant (49%), one or more of the larger lenticulostriate branches arise just beyond the major bifurcation (in the territory of the upper division of the MCA—see further on). The next most common permutation (39%) features all the larger lenticulostriate arteries arising from the stem just proximal to its bifurcation. In the least commonly encountered pattern, some of the larger penetrators arise from the medial portion of the stem. These variations may explain differing patterns of infarction from occlusion of the MCA stem alone or its main divisions.

One important anatomic feature these arteries all share is the lack of anastomoses among themselves. There are almost no examples of actual branches of these small arteries nor anastomotic links to the cerebral surface vessels (see Chapter 5).

The cerebral surface, centrum semiovale, claustrum, extreme capsule, the hemispheral cortex, and white matter are supplied by those MCA branches that originate beyond (distal to) the lenticulostriate arteries. These cortical surface branches usually number 12 to 15. They arise from the MCA stem in a variety of patterns, and by far the most common (78%)[9] is two large branches (bifurcation pattern). Less often (12%) the 12 branches arise from three major trunks (trifurcation pattern). The least differentiated and least common (10% of cases) is the continuation of the stem with no major divisions, and each of the surface branches arises in turn from the common trunk until the primary vessel has given off 11 of the usual 12 branches, after which it terminates as the angular artery.[6]

In the bifurcation pattern the two main branches are referred to as the superior and inferior division, the superior division insula, frontal lobe, and rolandic regions and

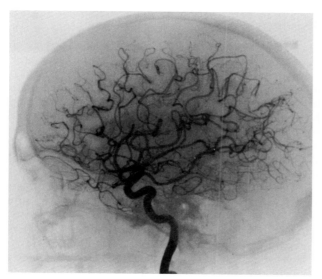

Figure 24-1   Lateral view of the middle cerebral artery anatomy.

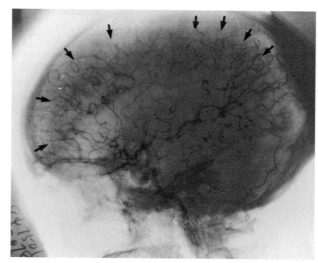

Figure 24-2   Anatomy of the borderzone anastomoses (individual anastomoses shown by *arrows*).

always contain the orbitofrontal and prefrontal branches. The inferior division reliably supplies the temporal polar, anterior temporal, and middle temporal branches. The distribution of the remaining branches in a given division varies. Although the central (rolandic) branch is almost always in the upper division, in a few cases it is included in the lower. Likewise, the posterior temporal branch is almost always in the lower division. The upper division is usually the source of the anterior parietal, posterior parietal, and angular branches, which arise in the middle of this fanlike array of vessels and have an almost equal chance of being in either division; the branches are orderly in their supply and do not appear to cross one another. No branch arising from the upper division irrigates brain regions that would be expected to be supplied from a branch of the lower division or vice versa

In the trifurcation pattern, the orbitofrontal, prefrontal, and precentral branches supplying the frontal lobe are regularly represented in the upper division. The middle division is made up of the central (rolandic), the anterior parietal, and the angular branches. Less often, the precentral branch is a member of this trunk on the frontal side, and in a few other instances, the temporooccipital and superior temporal branches are added on the inferior side. The inferior division regularly contains the temporal polar, anterior, and middle temporal branches, to which the posterior temporal and temporooccipital branches are less often added.

Other Anatomic Features

Regardless of the exact brain regions supplied by each branch, remarkable variations have been found in the exact position over gyri and sulci of individual branches within their section of the convexity. Variation in length is orderly: The smallest and the shortest branches supply the frontal lobe; the longest, the high parietal and lateral occipital.[12] Only 27% of the orbital frontal branches are as large as 1 mm in diameter.[9] The largest artery is usually the artery of the central (rolandic) sulcus. The more posterior regions of the brain are supplied by fewer arteries, which

are larger in diameter, give off fewer major branches, and have the longest course from the circle of Willis to their termination in a borderzone (Fig. 24-2). The temporooccipital artery is 1 mm in diameter in 90% of cases and more than 1.5 mm in up to 63% of cases. This large diameter and the ease with which it can be followed on the surface for long distances led surgeons to use this branch when the extracranial–intracranial anastomosis operation was in its heyday. The three vessels with the longest course on the cortical surface are the angular, posterior parietal, and temporooccipital arteries. Intraluminal diameters greater than 1 mm have been encountered in up to 86% of angular arteries, in 68% of temporooccipital arteries, and in 52% of posterior parietal arteries but in only 14% of central sulcus arteries.[13]

Arterial Segments in Relation to Anatomic Landmarks

Another method of classifying the branches of the MCA is based on the relationship of the artery with the major landmarks on the brain, especially the Sylvian fissure, the operculum, and the convex surface. This scheme, which has found its greatest use in angiographic descriptions of the MCA and its branches, divides the MCA into four major segments (Fig. 24-3).[9,14] The first sphenoidal segment, M1, occupies the space from the origin of the MCA to the limen insulae. The second segment, or M2, encompasses the branches of the upper and lower divisions that overlie the insula as it bends laterally. The lower division branches pass posterosuperiorly without supplying the insula and gain the convexity at the posterior end of the Sylvian fissure. The M3 segments are the continuation of these branches as they curve caudally along the undersurface of the operculum, most of which are upper division branches. The M4 segments describe those portions of the branches of the MCA over the convex surface of the brain.

The MCA branches that constitute the M3 or opercular segment follow the curve of the operculum back over the surface of the insula. Some of these branches

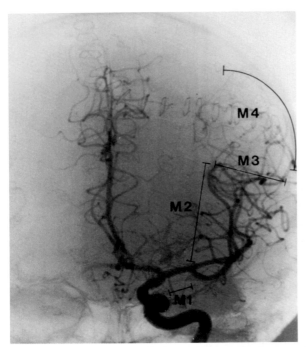

Figure 24-3 Classification of the middle cerebral artery by segments.

reverse course over as much as 180 degrees,[6] especially those ascending over the frontal and central operculum to gain access to the frontal half of the cerebral convexity. The branches passing over the parietal and temporal operculum make less striking reversals of direction, some turning only a few degrees before reaching the convex surface of the temporal and parietal regions. Finally, the M4 or cortical segments are those portions of the branches of the MCA after they emerge from the Sylvian fissure beyond the operculum and course along the sulci and gyri of the cerebral convexity. Considerable variation in their path is found from brain to brain. Upper division M4 branches typically follow a path mainly along the depths of a given sulcus, as do many of the lower division, but a few of them pass long distances over the surface of a gyrus, making them suitable for extracranial–intracranial bypass surgery recipients.

Anomalies

Anomalies of the MCA occur in no more than 3% of cases.[9,15,16] Some writers even dispute their occurrence.[10] *Duplication* of the MCA is more common, usually arising from the internal carotid artery and supplying the same regions that would otherwise have been supplied by the original MCA. An *accessory* MCA has also been described,[17] arising from the anterior cerebral artery, usually supplying frontal polar areas.

Borderzone Anastomoses

For each cerebral surface branch of the major cerebral arteries, the terminal twigs end in a narrow network of vessels that form the borderzone (see Chapter 22; Fig. 24-2) between the major arterial territories (see Chapter 22).[18-20]

Histology

The MCA contains the same intima, media, and adventitia as other arteries, but the relative thicknesses of these component parts differ from those in peripheral arteries of comparable size.[21] The differences begin even within the intracranial internal carotid artery, which changes the histologic character of the MCA in such a way that the two blend in a smooth continuum. Compared with extracranial vessels of similar size, the MCA has a narrower adventitia with little elastic tissue and few perivascular supporting structures; the media is also thinner, with some 20 circular muscle layers.[22,23] The internal elastic lamina is thicker[24] and finely fenestrated. The intima, although somewhat thin, seems essentially the same as that of comparably sized vessels elsewhere.[23] No evidence of vasa vasorum has been demonstrated to date.[23-25]

The thinner adventitia of intracranial vessels may be a sign of the lower exposure to stretching and trauma than is present in the extracranial arteries.[26] Elastic tissue is concentrated in the internal elastic lamina instead of being scattered through the vessel as in other arterial beds, perhaps making intracranial arteries more prone to dampen pulse waves.[24]

Pathology

Embolism

Embolism exceeds atheroma as the most common cause of disease of the major cerebral arteries beyond the circle of Willis, accounting for 15% to 30% of strokes,[27-29] most of which occur in the territory of the MCA.

Etiology

Occlusion by embolism has been appreciated since the time of Chiari.[30] These large ones have been traced to "paradoxical" embolus from a leg vein source,[31,32] atrial fibrillation,[33] mitral valve prolapse,[34,35] marantic embolus,[36,37] fragmented thrombus complexes from a nonobstructing internal carotid artery plaque,[38,39] shotgun pellet,[40] metal fragment from a penetrating neck wound,[41] traumatic dissection of the internal carotid artery,[42] internal carotid occlusion of various causes,[43] and automobile accident with angiographically normal ipsilateral internal carotid artery.[29,42] Recent striking images support aortic arch embolism, even in a setting of clinically important carotid stenosis.[44]

Embolism to the surface branches affecting one or more branches of the MCA may occur from almost any of these sources as well as others less well documented.[45,46] Sources include calcific material from the ipsilateral internal carotid (although the patient in Chiari's famous case also had a patent cardiac foramen ovale),[30] spontaneous dissection of the internal carotid artery from fibromuscular hyperplasia,[47] traumatic internal carotid dissection,[48] mucin and emulsified fat from breast metastasis,[49] endocarditis due to candida,[50] mitral valve prolapse,[34] cardiac myxoma,[51] marantic embolus,[36] arterial wall fragments after resuscitation,[52] giant fusiform MCA aneurysm,[53] internal carotid occlusion from various causes, and various types of transcardiac emboli via a patent cardiac foramen ovale.

Particle Size and Composition

A mere few millimeters in size is all that is needed for embolic material to arrest in the stem of the MCA. Rigid materials such as shotgun pellets[40] (first described by Leceve and Lhermitte in 1920 and later by computed tomographic [CT] imaging), catheter tips, and the like may be this large, as may some fresh or well-organized emboli, but occlusion of the length of the MCA stem from embolism is only infrequently demonstrated. The usual size is far smaller; some, less calcific plaques[54] are too small to block the stem[55] save for those calcific plaques arising from direct-puncture carotid arteriography and only rarely from carotid atheroma itself. Carotid plaque rupture as a cause of major middle cerebral stem occlusion has been difficult to demonstrate.[56,57] Rarely, large particle embolism may occur from fibrocartilaginous material.[58]

Most of the embolic material is a small fragment of a vessel or cardiac wall thrombus, alone or in bacterial endocarditis, mixed with bacteria.[4] Quite compressible,[59] such embolic fragments may alter their length and width as they pass through the arterial tree.

Distribution in the Middle Cerebral Artery Territory

Emboli follow preferential paths through the MCA system.[29,60] The lower division receives the larger share of the emboli. Occlusions also have different territorial effects in the two divisions. In the upper division, the serial arrangement of the major branches allows the entire division to be occluded by a large embolus blocking the first branch point. Small emboli often pass by the more anterior branches to lodge in those more posteriorly. The sharply angulated orbitofrontal branch is rarely occluded.[29,60-62] The lower division remains a single vessel as it passes over the insula until it reaches the superior temporal plane, where it gives off its three main branches within the space of 1 cm or less. As a result, even small particle embolization often results in the simultaneous occlusion of more than one or even all of the branches of the division.

Persistence of Material

Autopsies commonly show no occlusion, despite stem division or branch occlusion typical of embolism. Many emboli must be poorly organized, subject to spontaneous dissolution. For those vessels with persisting occlusion, the functional prognosis for the infarct is worse.[43,63-65] By imaging alone, such persistent occlusions may have all the features of in situ thrombi.[66] Transcranial Doppler ultrasonographic studies have shown recanalization in periods as short as minutes or indefinite persistence.[42]

Effects of Collateral Flow on Embolic Infarct Patterns

Unless adequate collateral flow is present, embolic occlusion of the MCA stem yields a gigantic infarct affecting both the superficial and deep territories of supply. When collateral flow is readily available, the territory distal to the occlusion may be remarkably spared.[67]

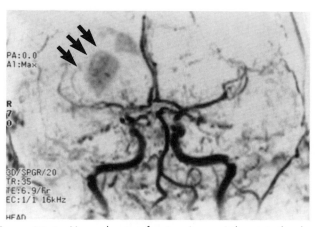

Figure 24-4 Hemorrhagic infarction *(arrows)* shown in the deep (lenticulostriate) territories of the middle cerebral artery on a coronal magnetic resonance image. (From Gautier JC, Mohr JP: Ischemic stroke. In Mohr JP, Gautier JC, editors: *Guide to clinical neurology,* New York, 1995, Churchill Livingstone, p 543.)

Clinical Syndromes of Embolism

A variety of temporal profiles occur in embolism to branches of the MCA (Fig. 24-4). In some instances, the deficits are only transient, even with angiographic evidence of persisting occlusion or brain image evidence of focal infarction that confounds traditional clinical definitions of transient ischemic attack (TIA), which raises the possibility that the nature of the material may play a role in the severity of the infarct.[68,69] In the days of polymeric silicone (Silastic) pellet therapy for arteriovenous malformations (AVMs), aberrant embolism was a well-recognized risk,[70] usually occurring near the end of the embolization procedure, when conditions initially favoring the entry of the pellets directly into the AVM vessels changed as the fistula became clogged with pellets.[70,71] In our personal series, one patient in whom two beads traveled into an angular branch of the MCA experienced 15 minutes of contralateral arm numbness—a complaint not entirely predicted by classic clinicopathologic correlation—and also showed immediate distal retrograde collateral flow; the pellet remained in place. Single beads occluded parietal branches of the MCA in two other patients and an ascending frontal branch in a third, none of whom experienced any deficits; in all patients, immediate collateral flow occurred retrograde into the embolized branch. We have found no other reported cases with clinical details.

Emboli initially occluding the MCA stem and then later migrating to the convexity branches may leave lesions in the deep and superficial territories as discontinuous multifocal infarction. The lack of collateral branches to the lenticulostriates makes these deep arterial territories especially vulnerable to infarction. The distally placed embolic fragment in a cortical branch is usually considerably smaller than the mass of which it was part that initially blocked the MCA stem; if ample collateral occurs retrograde through the borderzones linking to unaffected adjacent cerebral arteries, the infarct may be limited to a few centimeters distal to the site of occlusion. The initial

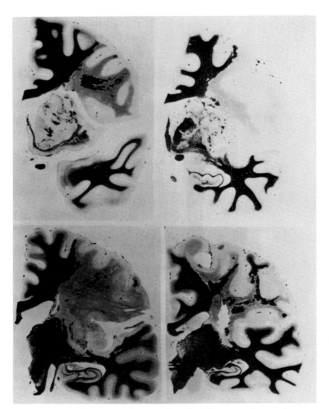

Figure 24-5 Deep and superficial infarction from the same embolic occlusion (myelin stain of celloidin section). (From Friedlich AL, Castleman B, Mohr JP: Case records of the Massachusetts General Hospital. *N Engl J Med* 278:1109, 1968.)

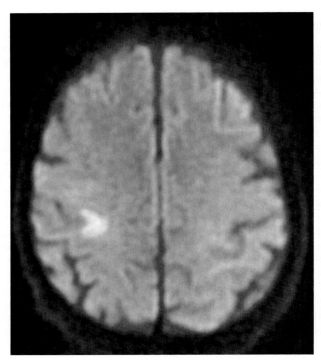

Figure 24-6 Brain imaging showing a high rolandic focal infarct in a patient with acute distal brachial plagia, normal after 1 month.

major hemispheral clinical syndrome may ameliorate to that of deep infarction affecting the penetrating vessels of the MCA stem. This clinical picture, dubbed *spectacular shrinking deficit,* described in earlier versions of this book and given the acronym SSS by Minematsu et al,[67] appears to be the consequence of thrombolysis or distal migration of both fragmentation and residual particles of an initial major occlusion. Also reported recently with MR imaging,[72] such cases often leave two separate foci of infarction, assumed to be from the same embolic event (Fig. 24-5).

Syndromes of nonsudden or fluctuating onset may also occur, reported in a small series in 5% to 6% of documented embolic strokes. In some instances the syndrome has required about 36 hours to evolve.[29,73] A clinical diagnosis of multiple TIAs is often entertained.

Thrombosis

Autopsy studies indicate that thrombotic occlusion accounts for only 2% of cases of ischemic events in the MCA territory.[29] Asymptomatic occlusion of the MCA stem is rare, regardless of the cause.[74,75]

Atherosclerosis

Primary arteriosclerotic occlusive thrombosis is an uncommon cause of symptomatic disease of the MCA,[29,76-79] even though this diagnosis is often made clinically. These findings lend support to the diagnosis of embolism for angiographically documented occlusions of the MCA and its branches unless shown to be otherwise at autopsy. Angiographically demonstrated MCA stenosis found above a normal internal carotid artery is also compatible with recanalizing embolism, preventing certain diagnosis unless follow-up studies are done seeking evidence of full recanalization.[65,80,81]

Although small, deep infarcts known as lacunes are usually explained by local microatheroma, some infarcts affecting the subinsula, external and extreme capsule, and upper corona radiata, which lie in the territory of several lateral lenticulostriates, create a curvilinear appearance on coronal imaging. They often spare the putamen, globus pallidus, capsule, and even the entry zone for the corona radiata (Fig. 24-6). Local atheromatous stenosis of the upper division is the usual cause but is not always easily demonstrated.[82]

Stenosis

Stenosis, familiar in the extracranial carotid artery, is uncommon anywhere in the MCA and, when found, is almost always in the stem (Fig. 24-7). The appearance is explained by incompletely developed atheroma, recent embolus undergoing recanalization, moyamoya disease, dissection, postradiation effects, metastatic tumors (including atrial myxoma), infection, and other causes. The clinical syndromes range from minor pure motor stroke,[83,84] minor focal hemispheral syndrome, and even TIA[75,80,83,85,86]; however, some have caused severe disability.[87,88]

Dissection

Autopsy diagnosis of MCA dissection has been rare. A wide variety of settings are recognized and include trauma,[89] strenuous physical exertion,[90] surgery,[91] fibromuscular

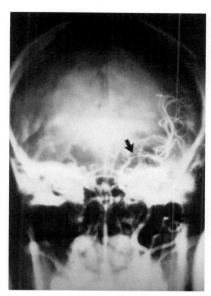

Figure 24-7 Angiogram showing middle cerebral artery stem stenosis *(arrow)*.

hyperplasia,[92] atherosclerosis,[84] mucoid degeneration of the media,[89] moyamoya disease,[93] split or frayed internal elastic lamina,[94] congenital defect of the media,[95] syphilis,[96] and even migraine.[97] The disorder has been most often reported in younger patients, of which many are children. The usual site is a short section of the stem, although adjacent branches may also be affected.[98] In some, symptoms have been delayed for minutes,[98] hours,[95] or up to 4 days.[99]

Other Diseases

The MCA, like other vessels, may fall victim to arteritis, fibromuscular hyperplasia, altered coagulation states, delayed effects of radiation, and other conditions. Reports in the literature remain too scant to enable determination of whether unique syndromes occur, and the reader is referred to the chapters in this book that deal with these topics individually.

Clinical Syndromes of Middle Cerebral Artery Territory Infarction

The textbook accounts, briefly reviewed here, assume total infarction in the territory at risk. Uncollateralized occlusion of the main trunk of the MCA causes softening of the basal ganglia and internal capsule within the substance of the hemisphere as well as a large portion of the cerebral surface and subcortical white matter.[4,100-103] The large infarct produces contralateral hemiplegia, deviation of the head and eyes toward the side of the infarct, hemianesthesia, and hemianopia. Foix and Levy[4] detailed the clinical elements almost a century ago. Major disturbances also occur in behavior: global aphasia occurs when the hemisphere dominant for speech and language is involved, whereas impaired awareness of the stroke is expected when the

nondominant hemisphere is affected. When the infarct is large, the hemianopia may be due to involvement of the visual radiations deep in the brain. More often, the hemianopia is part of a syndrome of hemineglect for the opposite side of the space and is accompanied by failure to turn toward the side of the hemiplegia in response to sounds from that side, which is a problem separate from the head and eye deviation toward the side of the infarct.

A variant of the syndrome of MCA stem occlusion, colorfully named *malignant infarction,*[104] applies mainly to those experiencing subsequent herniation. The time to severe decline is brief, between 2 and 5 days. Advances in treatment have allowed survival for some; however, most of the syndrome elements persist (Fig. 24-8).[105]

When the occlusion is restricted to the upper division, the sensorimotor syndrome mimics that from occlusion of the main trunk. Added to it is aphasia when the dominant hemisphere is involved or impaired awareness of the deficit when the other hemisphere is affected. However, the hemiparesis usually affects the face and arm more heavily than the leg, which is a picture opposite that in anterior cerebral artery disease. Because the occlusions usually affect the anterior branches of the upper division, the aphasia from dominant hemisphere infarction is usually of the motor (Broca's) type, whereas the disturbance in behavior from nondominant hemisphere infarction may be mild.

In the lower division syndromes, infarction typically spares the rolandic region, hemiparesis is mild or may not occur, head and eye deviations are rarely encountered, and even disorders of sensation are infrequent. When the infarct affects the dominant hemisphere, pure aphasia (Wernicke's type) is the rule, whereas in nondominant hemisphere infarction, the behavior disturbances may appear in relative isolation. Hemianopia may be a prominent sign.

When the involvement is limited to the territory of a small penetrating artery branch of the main stem, a small, deep infarct (lacune) occurs, affecting part or the entire internal capsule and producing a syndrome of pure hemiparesis unaccompanied by sensory, visual, language, or behavior disturbances.

Clinical Syndromes from Infarction of Either Hemisphere

Loss of Consciousness

Transient loss of consciousness is uncommon in all forms of ischemic stroke and is rare in MCA territory infarction. It occurs at onset in only 8.4% of carotid ischemic strokes[106] and in 5.7% of vertebrobasilar territory strokes. Delayed loss of consciousness is more common, often occurring 36 hours to 4 days after hemispheral infarcts ranging in size from the entire MCA territory to only the frontotemporal region.[107] The decline in consciousness is usually part of a larger clinical picture of impending cerebral herniation and seems not to be due to an injury to a specific brain region in the MCA territory controlling consciousness (see Fig. 24-8).

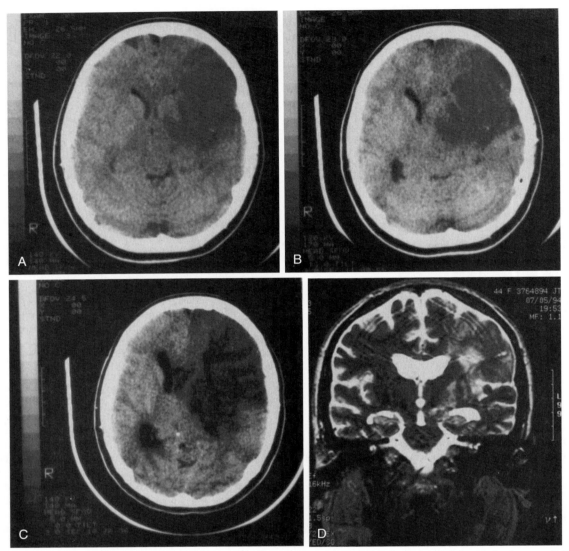

Figure 24-8 Four stages of midbrain compression. A, Viewed from an axial CT scan, the large middle cerebral artery (MCA) territory infarction has just begun to produce slight displacement a few hours after the acute stroke. B, By the second day, edema and "mass effect" have displaced the midbrain and thalamic structures slightly across the midline. C, By the fourth day, at the height of compression, the midline structures have been rotated and displaced considerably, during which time the patient appeared in a state of uncal herniation. D, A week later, a coronal T2-weighted MR image shows the midline structures back at their normal positions, and no lasting damage is evident from the displacement. (From Gautier JC, Mohr JP: Ischemic stroke. In Mohr JP, Gautier JC, editors: *Guide to clinical neurology,* New York, 1995, Churchill Livingstone, p 543.)

Hemiplegia and Hemiparesis

The terms *hemiplegia* and *hemiparesis* have been used rather loosely in many case reports, which makes a clear correlation between the severity of weakness and a given site of infarction difficult. In 150 years of reports, the number of cases that correlate the hemiparesis formula and imaging or autopsy findings remains disappointingly small, and some of them, despite an autopsy study, lack credibility.[108] Henschen's[109] massive review of the published autopsy literature on higher cerebral function before 1920 was typical of most writers: The occurrence of hemiparesis on a case-by-case basis was mentioned only in passing, and details of the syndrome were rarely given. This literature remains frustrating because of many surprising instances in which the motor deficit has shown considerable improvement. MCA stem occlusions affecting either side of the brain appear to produce the same basic motor deficit and can be described under the same heading. Such were the findings in the 488 cases of MCA territory infarction published in the pilot phase of the National Institute of Neurological and Communicative Disorders and Stroke (NINCDS) Stroke Data Bank project.[110] Eye deviation has been reported more often in right hemisphere infarcts.

Hemiplegia

The most reliable occurrence of hemiplegia follows *complete occlusion of the MCA at its stem* (Figs. 24-9 and 24-10). The typical picture consists of dense contralateral hemiplegia, hemianesthesia, homonymous hemianopia, and conjugate gaze deviation to the contralateral side.[4] The syndrome is more severe when the stem is affected.[4,75,111,112] Among the patients who die within days, contralateral hemiplegia is usually accompanied by hemianesthesia and hemianopia.[113]

The syndrome among survivors without hemicraniectomy seems similar.[81] While some have had only mild facial paresis,[114] distal functions of the limbs are much impaired, and hand and finger movements and the foot are often paralyzed. In some patients, movement of the shoulder and elbow may allow the arm to lift, and movement of the hip and knee may suffice for walking.

Hemiplegia from deep infarction alone features several different syndromes. Foix and Levy[4] described two types. In the first, massive hemiplegia occurred, and the appearance was the same as that observed when the infarct involved both the superficial and deep territories. Initial hemiplegia gave way to marked contracture. These investigators observed no instances of involuntary movements, choreoathetosis, parkinsonism, or disturbances in balance. The second type involved a more marked hemiplegia in the leg than in the arm, rendering the patient unable to walk. Contracture in this syndrome was more common in the leg and was often associated with a permanently flaccid hemiplegia. Later studies[115-117] and CT scans have reported a range of weakness, from profound hemiplegia to mild weakness, which underwent striking improvement despite persistence of the deep infarct.[118,119]

Hemiplegia from surface infarction is the third type. Infarction of the entire surface territory of the MCA produces a syndrome essentially identical to that found when the deep territory is also affected. A few instances of surface infarcts confined to the cortical surface of the insula and operculum have been described[120]; the syndrome involves hemiplegia with faciobrachial predominance that soon fades to a facial plegia with mild, predominantly distal paresis of the arm.

Individual branch occlusions seem only uncommonly to produce hemiplegia.[4] In most cases, either hemiparesis occurs or the syndrome of paralysis is incomplete and is confined to one or more body parts. The most reliable deficit is encountered among patients with occlusion of the ascending frontal branch.[50] Dramatic improvements within weeks are reported.[34] A large number of variables affect the outcome.[121] Efforts are under way to study a variety of treatment options, among them constraint therapy and transcranial magnetic stimulation[122] (see Chapter 56).

Syndromes of Partial Hemiparesis

The most commonly encountered pattern of hemiparesis seems to be one with equivalent weakness of the hand, shoulder, foot, and hip. This type occurred in 71.2% of the 488 unilateral hemisphere strokes studied during the pilot phase of the NINCDS Stroke Data Bank project.[110] A few other types of hemiparesis are also well known. Among them are the classic syndromes of distal predominance of the hemiparesis (often attributed to Broadbent,[123] although we have found no source among his writings), a faciobrachial paresis, and monoplegia. The main phase of the NINCDS Stroke Data Bank study provided data for 183 of 1276 patients with convexity infarction in the MCA territory and is still the largest cohort reported to date. Infarct size did not differ according to side, but the location of the main site of the infarct did. On the left side, the infarct was centered in the inferior parietal region,

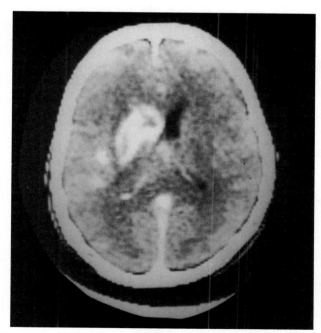

Figure 24-9 Large deep infarction of the middle cerebral artery lenticulostriate territories shown by CT scan.

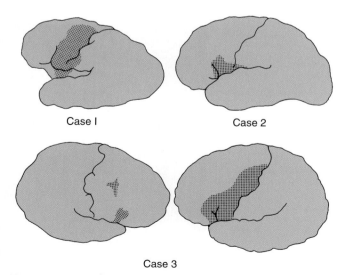

Case 1 Case 2

Case 3

Figure 24-10 Three examples of embolic infarction of Broca's area and surrounding cerebrum. (From Mohr JP: Broca's area and Broca's aphasia. In Whitaker H, editor: *Studies in neurolinguistics.* New York, 1976, Academic Press, p 201.)

but on the right, it was midfrontal. There was a good correlation between infarct size and level of weakness as estimated by overall motor function on one side, the arm, or the hand alone. There was poor correlation, however, for lesion location (lower third, middle third, or upper third on either side of the rolandic fissure) and any of the specific syndromes of focal weakness; no two cases shared the same lesion for the same syndrome, and several cases shared the same lesion with a different syndrome.

The findings indicated a difference in weakness syndromes between the two hemispheres and great individual variation of the acute syndrome caused by a given site of focal infarction along the rolandic convexity.[110]

When hemiparesis features *distal predominance,* it affects the lower face, fingers and forearm, and toes and lower leg, with relative sparing of the forehead, shoulder and upper arm, hip, and thigh, neck, and trunk. This lower facial and distal predominance of hemiparesis has been taken to represent the density of the homuncular representation over the hemispheral surface[124,125] but occurred in only 23.5% of the 488 patients with unilateral weakness affecting the cerebrum in the Stroke Data Bank.[110] In addition, it occurred with approximately the same frequency regardless of whether the infarct was confined to a single lobe or was as large as several lobes and whether the area involved was frontal, parietal, temporal, or opercular.

The syndrome of *faciobrachial paresis* also has a widely varying frequency.[75,120,125-127] Obvious weakness is present in the muscles of the jaw. Movements of the tongue and oropharynx show impairment of swallowing and occasionally impairment of vocalization. These lower face and oral pharyngeal disturbances may persist long after forehead movement has been restored. The initial appearance is sometimes similar to that of Bell's palsy, but the upper deviation of the eyes characteristic of peripheral facial palsy (Bell's phenomenon) is typically not present, even in the earliest stages. The involvement of the upper extremity is usually more obvious in the impaired movement of the fingers and hand.

Monoplegia

Although described in standard texts, detailed case reports are not easily found in the literature. von Monakow[128] made reference to the possibility of an isolated brachial plegia arising from a lesion confined to the middle of the second frontal gyrus, provided that the lesion is acute and does not extend too deeply into the white matter ("wenn sie akut einsetzt und nicht zu tief in das subcorticale Mark übergrieft"). Dejerine and Regnard[129] found a case with weakness limited to the muscles of the thenar, hypothenar, and interosseous muscles; they did not mention confirmation of the presumed vascular nature of the lesion. Garcin[130] described a monoparesis with weakness predominating in the flexor movements, mimicking median nerve palsy; the locus of the lesion was inferred in the absence of autopsy data. The only case of focal upper rolandic infarction with autopsy documentation (Fig. 24-11) of which we know was of an elderly woman, whose examination within hours of onset revealed normal power in the upper extremity, including the hands and fingers, sparing the limb entirely. The only clinical signs were slight right facial weakness with initial mutism. She was monitored for months, during which time the initial deficit improved, but no disturbance of limb power occurred at any time. Among recent publications was a well-documented example of "hand knob" infarction.[131] A recent example from our service was of a patient whose stroke began with complete plegia of the fingers and thumb; the patient was also incapable of dorsiflexion of the wrist. Within weeks all her testing results were normal.

Isolated brachial monoplegia has often been described as a clinical sign in carotid territory TIAs. It has also been encountered as a transient syndrome in aberrant emboli during pellet embolization in the treatment of AVMs, regardless of the MCA branch being embolized. These findings are of great interest but must be interpreted with caution because the setting (an angiogram

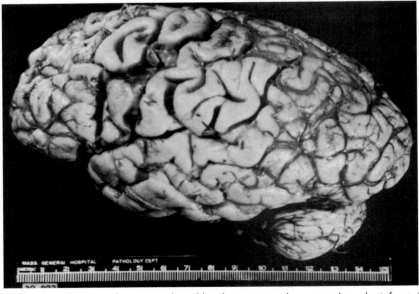

Figure 24-11   Small upper rolandic infarction. The pia-arachnoid has been stripped away to show the infarct. (Courtesy of J. M.C. Pearce.)

suite with the patient under a drape) does not lend itself to detailed evaluation of the leg and axial structures during the frantic period when the physicians are striving to reverse the acute deficit. Schneider and Gautier,[132] in an extensive review of 1575 patients with acute stroke and predominance of leg weakness, found that only 63 had predominance of leg weakness. Although 41 patients had hemispheric convexity lesions, the MCA territory was affected in only one. The NINCDS Pilot Stroke Data Bank project contained a mere 31 cases of monoplegia involving the arm among the 488 patients with cerebral stroke,[110] yet even this small number showed a significant correlation with infarct of a single lobe rather than multiple lobes ($P < 0.002$).

"Recovery" from Hemiparesis

The means by which improvement occurs in hemiparesis remains unclear but is persistently described as *recovery,* a term suggesting a restoration of the original function. Such may not be the case, but the term is too well embedded in usage for us to constantly point out the ambiguities and force readers to face alternative terms throughout this chapter.

"Recovery" after stroke-induced hemiparesis is the rule rather than the exception. Clinical and imaging factors have been put forward to predict who is likely to recover and to what extent. The degree and nature of recovery depends critically on the outcome measure chosen. Several commonly cited observational studies have demonstrated, for example, that the initial severity of hemiparesis and lesion volume are reasonably good at predicting scores on disability scales at 3 or 6 months.[133-137] Neurologic impairment can dissociate from disability assessments, however, allowing a patient to be deemed recovered by a disability score while still harboring a substantial, unaddressed neurologic deficit.[138] Because the approach of most stroke rehabilitation programs is to teach compensation for deficits, such as the nonparetic hand accomplishing a motor task, rather than to reverse the neurologic impairment, recovery may be reported after a course of rehabilitation; however, at the level of impairment, recovery may not have occurred. Other studies have used impairment of motor function as the primary outcome measure and have shown varying correlations with their independent variables.[139-141] Duncan et al[139] ran a widely cited study that serially evaluated the course of motor recovery among 104 hemiparetic stroke patients. Stratifying by severity of the motor impairment as measured by the standardized Fugl-Meyer (FM) stroke scale at day 1, the investigators followed the course of motor recovery at 5 days and at 1, 3, and 6 months. The investigators showed that the FM scores at day 1 accounted for only half of the variance in 6-month motor function ($r^2 = 0.53$, $P < 0.001$).[139]

Alternatively, if one defines recovery as the change in impairment score from the initial time point to 90 days later, prediction of recovery is more consistent. Newer evidence suggests that for patients who have mild-to-moderate deficits, there is a remarkably consistent course of recovery, and all patients achieve a specific proportion (approximately 70%) of the potential total remaining recovery.[142] For patients with severe deficits at onset,

prediction of recovery is much more difficult: some follow the same course of proportional recovery as their more mildly affected counterparts, but others show very little recovery. To distinguish those likely to recover from those who are not likely to recover, investigators recently showed that expression of a "recovery pattern" on functional magnetic resonance imaging (fMRI), obtained in the first few days after stroke, correlated well with the degree of subsequent recovery that then occurred.[143]

Functional imaging has also begun to reveal the dynamic process of brain reorganization after stroke. Neuronal activity in regions outside primary motor cortex after stroke-induced hemiparesis may appear both in the opposite hemisphere and in secondary motor areas in the ipsilesional hemisphere as early as 24 hours after stroke onset.[144,145] The appearance of this task-related activity suggests that alternative brain regions participate in the performance of motor function when a deficit is present, then revert to a more typical, contralateral pattern as recovery proceeds.[146-149] Physiologic measures of white matter tracts such as transcranial magnetic stimulation (TMS) also support the idea that a changing balance of cross-callosal inhibition between the two hemispheres plays a role in recovery. Loss of inhibition from the stroke hemisphere to the contralesional hemisphere may interfere with recovery of motor function through the increased inhibition back on the hemisphere with the stroke.[150] This competitive inhibition between hemispheres after stroke has led to the proposal of rehabilitation measures that restore physiologic balance between hemispheres through the use of TMS[151] and transcranial direct current stimulation (tDCS).[152]

Infarcts without Hemiparesis

Infarction confined to the lower division of the MCA is not expected to produce hemiparesis in any form because the site of the infarct lies so far posterior to the rolandic sulcus. This point also seems to apply to the postrolandic branches of the upper division. Occlusion of the ascending parietal branch is uncommonly reported, but the few cases documented have been remarkably free of focal motor deficit.[153] The pilot phase of the NINCDS Stroke Data Bank study[110] documented a handful of instances of hemiparesis after opercular infarction. Several notable cases exist with autopsy correlation in which weakness did not occur in either the face or the limbs at any time during an acute infarction affecting the inferior frontal region's anterior operculum.[154] Reports of infarction confined to the orbital frontal branch of the upper division are exceedingly rare. In one case,[13] a man's only motor deficit consisted of the grasp reflex and contralateral extensive planar response. The case was studied by angiography only. Rare reports of occlusion may be a result of the low frequency of embolism into this particular branch of the MCA.

Movement Disorders

Temporary or permanent movement disorders, including hemichorea, athetosis, and dystonia, are uncommon sequelae of MCA territory infarcts. Despite a large body of literature on the subject in children, few reports have appeared on adults.[155] Only one adult has been described with *chorea*.[156]

Dystonia has been the subject of the other reports. The one adult described in the series reported by Demierre and Rondot[118] was a 17-year-old with left hemiplegia that improved slightly within 4 weeks, by which time signs of dystonia had appeared. A large hypodensity affecting the putamen, anterior capsule, and caudate was seen on CT. Similar cases have been reported.[155]

Contraversive Eye and Head Deviation

Prevost[153] first described deviation of the head and eyes after a unilateral lesion in 1896. Ocular deviation is included as part of the National Institutes of Health Stroke Scale but is rarely cited with clinical correlation of the infarct focus.[157-160] It has long been held that deviation of the eyes represents disruption of the frontal eye fields in and around area 8 alpha, located in the premotor region of the superior frontal lobe,[157,158,161-163] but few examples exist.[164,165] In most cases, deviation of the head or eyes has been associated with large lesions more centrally located in the deeper MCA territory near the operculum or insula.

Types of Deviation

De Renzi et al[166] encountered three types of deviation in their 120 patients with ocular motility disorders. In the first group, the head and eyes were midline and moved spontaneously to either side in response to stimulus but were less complete to the side of the space served by the damaged hemisphere. In the second group, the head and eyes were found completely to one side with absence of spontaneous movements to the contralateral side and only fleeting voluntary deviation of the eyes into the side of the space served by the damaged hemisphere. In the most severely affected group, the head, eyes, or both were completely deviated away from the side of the space served by the damaged hemisphere and failed to turn in response to verbal or sensory stimuli; no spontaneous or voluntary movements were observed to the midline or beyond. Hemi-inattention or neglect of the contralateral side of the space usually accompanied cases with head and eye deviation.

Eye Deviation and Infarct Topography

Eye deviation is the expected finding after massive infarction of the entire MCA territory.[75] For upper division syndromes encountered in studies of Broca's aphasia, one of us (JPM) reported uncovering 10 autopsy cases from the Massachusetts General Hospital files[167]; all of the patients had experienced head and eye deviation to the site of the lesion that persisted for days and cleared within a week. Less frequent eye deviation has been found in opercular infarction. Ocular deviation with deep infarction has been reported in individual cases with autopsy correlation and has occurred from hemorrhage (thalamic, frontal, or frontotemporal location) and subdural hematoma.[117,160] From CT scan studies and in the NINCDS Stroke Data Bank study,[168] 86 cases (16%) of supratentorial-type conjugate ocular deviation occurred among the 531 cases of hemispheral stroke diagnosed according to clinical

or radiologic criteria. The occurrence of ocular deviation was significantly correlated with larger infarcts, but among the infarcts confined to single lobes, those involving the right side were more commonly associated with ocular deviation, which confirms the findings of De Renzi et al.[166] A frontal predominance over parietal infarcts was not found, and a parietal location was not the explanation for the effect of the right-sided stroke. The prevalence of frontal or parietal lobe location did not differ significantly in single-lobe infarcts. Ocular deviation occurred from infarction as low on the surface as the operculum.

Duration of the Deviation and Severity of Infarct

In the NINCDS Stroke Data Bank, gaze deviation of less than 5 days' duration did not correlate with lesion side, size, site, cause, or positive initial CT findings. However, the larger lesions predominated among the nine patients whose ocular deviation persisted beyond 20 days.

Some with infarction affecting the operculum and insula have shown what has been labeled *pseudoophthalmoplegia* for the first few days after the stroke.[120] Conjugate deviation of the head and eyes lasts for several days and then disappears. The lesion causing this condition is far away from area 8 alpha and is considered a reliable feature of infarcts of the insula and operculum.

Infarction with No Eye Movement Disturbances

De Renzi et al[166] reported one patient who was completely free of any gaze disturbance and who had a cortical–subcortical lesion (a frontal hematoma) on the left involving the areas of the rolandic fissure. The few cases with focal infarction confined to the superior frontal region, near area 8 alpha, have not confirmed the hypothesis that this region is vital for ocular motility.

Dizziness and Vertigo

Hemispheral infarcts have long been assumed to have a vertiginous component. A unique case reported by Brandt et al[169] provides a contrasting view. The patient had "well-demarcated infarction" in the right posterior insular region and had rotational vertigo, among other signs, for almost a week.

Sensory Disturbances

Although sensory disturbances have been assumed to be part of the hemispheral infarct syndrome, few details have been published concerning the syndrome elements, their lesion correlation, and duration. On the basis of the NINCDS Stroke Data Bank material, a disturbance in sensation carries an important indication of a large lesion when it accompanies hemiparesis; it is highly significant for infarcts greater than a single lobe in size ($P < 0.001$).[110]

Hemispherectomies and Sensory Disturbances

Late after surgery, a relative preservation of sensory function in the face seems common, whereas more blunted sensation to several modalities has been reported, occurring the more distally the test is performed in the arm.[114] Complete astereognosia is common. Vibration and position sense are heavily affected but not definite alteration of the body scheme. Recent reports focus on hemiplegia and hemianopia; mention of hemisensory changes is infrequent.[170] We await more detailed reports of the sensory disturbances in the massive "malignant" infarcts treated with hemicraniectomy.

Pure Sensory Deficits

Focal sensory deficits have been described in detail in only a handful of cases with autopsy correlation. One syndrome is a pseudoradicular pattern of sensory loss, with impairment of joint position sense, stereognosis, graphesthesia, and two-point discrimination.[127] The hand is the most severely affected, but two cases have been described with both hand and foot disturbances. Hemianesthesia has also been described in a few other cases.[4,13,171] These outlast the complaints of sensory impairment. In recent years few reports have appeared, but one of special interest documented contralateral loss of cold, cold pain, and pinprick perception; other sensory modalities were reported as normal.[172]

Hemisensory Deficits and Lesion Topography

Foix et al[173] are credited with demonstrating that an infarct affecting the anterior parietal region may produce a profound hemisensory loss (pseudothalamic syndrome) with little or no accompanying hemiparesis. Their patient had a large anterior parietal infarct that was so deep it created almost a cleft in the hemisphere to the ventricular wall. Only a few subsequent reports have appeared[171,174,175] and are in general agreement with the original publication.

Correlation of Sensory Disturbances with Motor Deficits

The few cases reported suggest that, for the same size lesion, the sensory disturbance may affect a far more circumscribed area of the face, limbs, or trunk than that affected by the accompanying motor disturbance.[176]

Visual Field Disturbances

There is little doubt that hemianopia to confrontation clinical testing accompanies the huge infarcts.[4] Before modern imaging provided ample contradictory evidence, hemianopia was often ascribed to involvement of the visual radiation, through a mechanism of edema, even though the MCA supplies only the upper half of the radiation.[177] For less global infarcts, hemianopia has been described with infarcts involving the frontal region, and some have been as low as the Sylvian fissure.[125] However, hemianopia has been absent in some instances of focal infarction, even when impaired opticokinetic nystagmus (OKN) was found.

It is difficult to sustain the notion that edema involving the radiations explains hemianopia when the infarct is far away from these structures. Instead of some reversible edema effect, it is likely that hemianopia as described is actually a disturbance in hemispatial response that is part

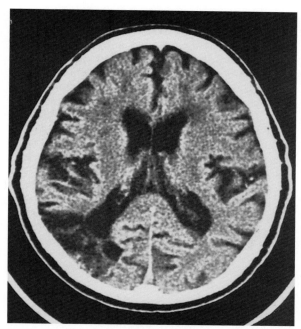

Figure 24-12 Axial CT scan showing a left parietal infarct in a patient with right inferior quadrantanopia.

of a hemineglect syndrome.[178] In such cases, other faulty responses to spatial stimuli are noted, such as the patient with a left hemispheral infarction turning toward the left in response to a voice from the right and a patient showing failure to blink in response to threat stimuli from the right.

Quadrantanopia

Parietal infarction deep enough to affect the fibers of the upper half of the visual radiation is presumably responsible for the infrequently described inferior quadrantanopia of MCA territory infarction (Fig. 24-12).[179] Case reports with lower quadrantanopia have eluded our search to date. The syndrome should indicate a deep cleft of infarction reaching the visual radiation, but it remains unsettled whether it may occur in a more superficial infarct.

Impairment of Opticokinetic Nystagmus

A test for OKN is assumed to detect disorders of the gaze mechanism mild enough that conjugate ocular gaze deviation is not present at rest. Considering the number of patients tested for OKN, it is remarkable that there is still considerable controversy over the usual locus of the lesion, the pathways injured, and even the nature of the disturbance. The early view was that OKN was a reflex activity of the cerebral cortex, that the slow component was initiated from the occipital region and the fast corrective phase from the frontal region, and that the OKN response was blunted by lesions at any point in the pathway.[180,181] However, the higher prevalence of abnormal OKN in parietal lesions has supported another view that the slow component from the occipital region passed directly to the brainstem through a pathway adjacent to the visual radiations organized in ipsilateral pathways.[182,183] Still another approach has argued that the pathway runs deep through the parietal region to the

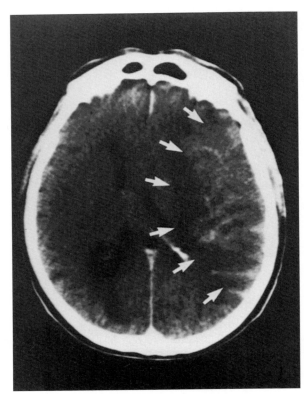

Figure 24-13 Coronal view of insular and upper opercular infarction from embolism to the upper division of the middle cerebral artery. (Myelin stain of celloidin section.)

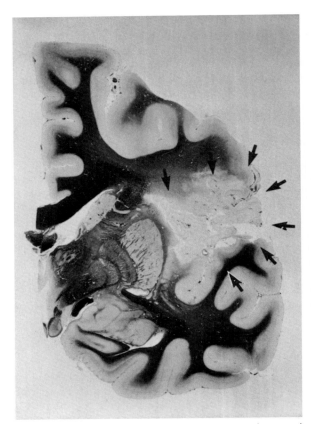

Figure 24-14 Non–contrast-enhanced CT scan showing hemorrhagic infarction of the entire middle cerebral artery territory *(arrows)*. Hemihyperhidrosis and distal arm edema were part of the clinical picture.

frontal lobe, crosses the posterior limb of the corpus callosum, and controls fast-phase components generated in the opposite frontal lobe.[180] Other arguments have been put forward for separate mechanisms controlling foveal and full-field pursuit.[184] These studies have shown the main disturbance to be in the slow component when targets were moved into the field of vision from the side of space served by the damaged hemisphere.

The actual documented sites vary considerably (and are not all in the parietal lobe) and demonstrate that clinically evident hemianopia need not occur. Impairment of OKN has been encountered in at least one patient with a small, high rolandic infarct whose visual fields were intact (see Fig. 24-11).[125] Baloh et al[184] also reported a patient with a large infarct apparently involving the posterior cerebral artery territory, accompanied by right hemianopia and alexia but no language disturbance.

Autonomic Disturbances

Excessive sweating contralateral to an MCA territory infarction is rarely encountered. Case reports show that patients have major syndromes of hemiparesis, hemisensory problems, hemianopia, and altered behavior states, indicating a large lesion affecting both the superficial and deep territories of the MCA (Fig. 24-13).[185] Sweating in these few cases affected the face, neck, axilla, and upper trunk contralateral to the infarct and faded to normal within days. Appenzeller[186] published an autopsy case for which the patient was described clinically as showing hyperhidrosis on the contralateral side of the body.

No further details were mentioned, not even the extent of the other clinical deficits. The published photographs show a site of small hemorrhagic infarction in the upper bank of the insula and adjacent orbital surface of the operculum. An MRI series describes hypertensive episodes in patients with infarcts restricted to the right insular cortex.[187] Contralateral rubbery edema of the affected hands and feet may also occur from large MCA territory infarction (Fig. 24-14). The syndrome usually becomes evident within a few hours and persists for up to 2 weeks. The exact anatomic correlates are unknown.

Syndromes Referable to Language-Dominant (Usually Left) Hemisphere Infarction

Aphasia

The cerebrum irrigated by the left MCA is of prime importance in language function. This function can be defined operationally for clinical purposes as a symbolic system in which the relations between meaningful elements (i.e., sounds, print, gestural signs) are purely arbitrary. Aphasia (or its more commonly less severe variant known as dysphasia) is thus regarded as a disorder caused by acquired brain injury that results in dysfunctional use of rule-governed, symbolic behavior.[188,189] The Sylvian fissure of the hemisphere dominant for speech and language is the region most likely to cause symptoms of dysphasia after a focal brain lesion. More than 95% of right-handed people and even most left-handed people have dominance for speech and language in the left hemisphere. Right hemisphere dominance for speech and language in a right-handed person is distinctly uncommon.

Many of the traditional clinicopathologic correlations of brain and language function have undergone revisions in the last few decades under the influence of modern imaging.[190,191] Among them has been that smaller focal brain lesions once thought to produce the major syndromes of aphasia are now known to cause less severe, minor, or even transient disturbances in production or comprehension of speech, sounds, and shapes. Much larger lesions are necessary to produce the lasting major disruptions in language function. Later work has also made it apparent that deeper structures, especially the thalamus, play vital roles in speech and language.[192] Nevertheless, there have been few additional gains over the past few years regarding the clinical characteristics of acute aphasia, and most new studies show that lesion location is still the main determinant of the language syndrome. The contributions of new work have centered on insights achieved with functional imaging during the course of stroke recovery, and the pharmacologic challenge has been targeted toward restitution of function.

Global or Total Aphasia

Few studies have indicated the different types of aphasia expected in a setting of acute stroke. In a survey of 850 patients, Brust et al[193] found that 177 (21%) had acute aphasia. Fifty-seven (32%) had "fluent" aphasia, and 120 (68%) had "nonfluent" (see later for definitions). Nonfluency was significantly correlated ($P < 0.01$) with a poor prognosis for mortality. Even highly significant mortality was found for patients with fluent and nonfluent aphasia who showed hemiparesis or a visual field disturbance. Similarly, Marquardson[194] reported 769 patients with acute stroke, 133 (33%) of whom showed aphasia in the acute state; hemiplegia was less likely to improve if accompanied by aphasia, and aphasia had a better outlook when unaccompanied by hemiplegia.

Clinical Features. Occlusion of the trunk of the MCA or its upper division produces a global disruption of language function. Its effect puts out of action virtually all the brain regions mainly responsible for language. The initial disturbance can be so profound that it goes by the term *total aphasia*. After the early period, clinicians and family sometimes observe some improvement in the patient's capacity to both understand context-related information (e.g., "Are you feeling better?") and participate in the give-and-take of simple communication. Within weeks or months, comprehension improves, especially for nongrammatical forms, and the patient shows more disturbances in speaking and writing than in listening and reading.[195] This emphasis on dysphasia more in speaking and writing is known as *Broca's aphasia* or *major motor aphasia*.

Lesion Size. With the advent of CT and MRI, a volumetric measure of the lesion became possible during life, permitting inquiry into the issues of not only the usual lesion size associated with the syndrome but also the minimal and maximal dimensions.[41,196] Naeser and Hayward,[197] relying on CT data, documented the lesion volume in two groups of patients: those identified as having *mixed aphasia*, a term that broadly encompasses the clinical picture of total aphasia, and those identified as having *global aphasia*, usually equated with total aphasia. The site of the lesion in seven cases of mixed aphasia reflected a large infarct affecting the Sylvian region and beyond, but in a few instances, Broca's or Wernicke's areas proper were not mapped in the scanned lesion. The lesion size in these cases was approximately 3.9 × 3.9 cm, and such a lesion was usually seen on five CT slices. The lesion volume in five cases of global aphasia was considerably larger, on the order of 5.8 × 5.8 cm. As with the mixed aphasia cases, the site of the minimal lesion lay in the Sylvian region, and the major contribution to the larger volume was its centrifugal spreading into the adjacent frontal, parietal, and temporal regions. An example of such a case is shown in Figure 24-15A. With time, such lesions may evolve, leaving a major syndrome associated with considerable postinfarction atrophy (Fig. 24-15B).

Advances in MRI, described in more detail elsewhere in this volume, have shown that "lesion" size is actually the total region of hemodynamically compromised tissue, encompassing areas of infarction and nearby ischemic zones still capable of recovery.[198,199] Asymmetries of Broca's area recording the left side have still not reliably been demonstrated.[200] Hillis et al have shown that aphasia severity correlates more strongly with the volume of abnormality on perfusion-weighted imaging (PWI), revealing both infarcted and ischemic regions, than does the volume of abnormality on diffusion-weighted imaging (DWI), which only shows the infarcted tissue.[201] This group also demonstrated that the volume of left-sided subcortical infarcts can underrepresent the extent of cortical hypoperfusion. Of 37 patients in one study with strictly left-sided subcortical strokes on DWI, 25 had aphasia with cortical hypoperfusion in the distal left MCA territory demonstrated on PWI. Six of these patients with cortical hypoperfusion and subcortical infarction then underwent treatment to restore blood flow, which resulted in at least partial cortical reperfusion after repeated PWI. Repeated language testing showed improvement in all of the subjects who had cortical reperfusion.[202]

Motor Aphasia

For more than 100 years, a syndrome has been recognized in which the ability to communicate by speaking or writing seems far more impaired than the comprehension of words heard or seen.[62] Although Boulliaud[203] deserves credit for popularizing the notion that a lesion of both frontal lobes disrupts the power of spoken speech, the surgeon Paul Broca, the friend of Boulliaud's son-in-law, has received most of the credit for the documentation that a left-sided Sylvian infarct more reliably causes the syndrome. Broca described two patients who appeared to have lost their memory of how to speak. Considerable controversy has persisted concerning whether this characterization is suitable for the findings and for the locus of the minimal lesion to precipitate the major syndrome and whether the effects are the same when the lesion is

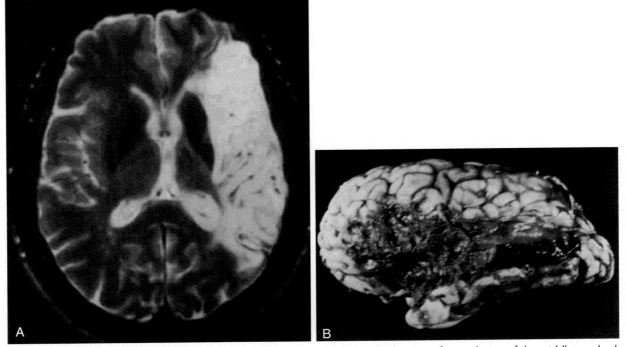

Figure 24-15 A, Complete infarction of the surface territory of the middle cerebral artery after occlusion of the middle cerebral artery. B, Appearance of another similar case at a later stage.

confined to the third frontal convolution, which Broca took to be the site causing the syndrome that bears his name. The actual lesion sizes were far larger, encompassing most of the Sylvian region and adjacent superior temporal lobe; lesions of this size nowadays would be expected to be associated with a syndrome of total aphasia (Fig. 25-16). Recent studies using MRI for Broca's two important cases confirm the large size of the lesions.[204] Efforts continue to explain the basis for the syndrome.[205]

Major motor aphasia. In its usual form, major motor aphasia appears to be an improvement of a syndrome of total aphasia and is a late sign in the course of the major Sylvian cerebral infarct. In such patients, there is a sharp contrast between the hesitant, agrammatical speech and the relatively better comprehension evident in conversational tests as long as the examiner keeps the sentences and questions simple.

In the initial period after the acute infarction, the speech and language disturbances are too severe to allow a distinction between speech and language production and comprehension.[125,127,167,206-208] With the passage of a few months and some improvements in testability, the syndrome of Broca's aphasia begins to appear.

Whether the motor aphasia that emerges is a disturbance confined to speaking and writing or contains a global disturbance in the brain's capacity to deal with grammatical functions has been argued for almost 150 years. Part of the argument stems from the terms used to substitute for Broca's aphasia: expressive dysphasia, efferent motor dysphasia,[209] motor dysphasia,[210] verbal dysphasia,[211] and, simply, nonfluency,[207] to name but a few. Despite the semantics, most investigators echo the impression of Liepmann[212] that symptoms of motor

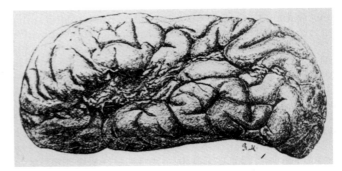

Figure 24-16 One of Broca's original cases.

aphasia predominate and the limited capacity for spoken expression conceals the deeper language disturbances that persist but are less obvious.

The *speech disturbance* is evident to a similar degree whether the utterances are produced in spontaneous conversation or during efforts to repeat aloud or read aloud; that is, they are obligatory. The spoken responses are hesitant, demonstrating impairment of skilled interaction (dyspraxia) between the settings of the oropharynx and the respiratory elements that permit smooth vocalization.[213] In the production of individual words, the transitions from sound to sound are accomplished only with difficulty,[209] which is especially obvious with polysyllabic words. The disturbance disrupts the usual clustering of words to form phrases, interfering with the normal melodic intonation that serves to indicate differences among exclamations, questions, and declarative statements. There is a high correlation between the degree of buccolingual dyspraxia and the extent of speech loss in patients with Broca's aphasia.[214]

Apart from these signs of *speech dyspraxia*, the structure of the spoken phrases may show a simplification of grammar, in that the language content consists largely of single words that function as predicative elements; this performance is formerly known as *telegraphic speech*, a term coined in the days when telegrams were an expensive form of communication charged by the word(s) sent. These grossly condensed utterances, lacking as they do normal sentence structure, have also been labeled *agrammatism*. In some cases, the utterances have been limited to a single word or phrase,[215] characterized as verbal stereotypes. The more limited the range of utterances, the more discouraging the prognosis for improvement.

Other disorders of language usage are part of the syndrome and seem independent of the difficulty in speaking aloud. They include difficulties responding to spoken or written material that features small grammatical words such as *the, are,* and *then* or involves spelling.[216] The poorest performance occurs when the meaning is highly dependent on grammatical features, especially when subject–object relations are based less on simple nouns (e.g., "John saw Jane") than on pronouns (e.g., "He saw it") or when the passive voice is used (e.g., "He was seen by her"). The disturbances observed extend beyond the acts of speaking or writing to comprehension of the material itself. Silent reading comprehension, which requires no overt vocalization, is usually only a little disturbed for single words that are pictureable nouns, but difficulties are encountered when the material to be read contains a particularly high density of such grammatical words. When it does, the comprehension may be strikingly abnormal. This condition has been termed *deep dyslexia* and has been described as a third form of dyslexia.[215] Similar disturbances can be documented in tests requiring the patient to point to visual displays containing single letters or grammatical words in response to hearing the names of the letters. Some have even shown faulty selection of a single letter among a visually presented display of letters when the test stimulus was a printed word whose pronounced sound (homophone) is identical to that of a given letter (i.e., "eye" to "I").[195] These examples are indicative of the global disturbances in language that occur and persist in patients with the major syndrome of Broca's aphasia.

The *clinicopathologic correlation* for the syndrome has evolved over the last century. Major motor or Broca's aphasia is not a syndrome expected from infarction restricted to Broca's area. It usually reflects a major infarction involving most of the territory of supply of the upper division of the left MCA, which was actually shown in Broca's original cases.[167] Accompanying disturbances in motor, sensory, and visual function usually makes the diagnosis easy. The usually large size of the Sylvian infarct sets the stage for contralateral hemiplegia.[217] At times, however, the main weight of the lesion may fall on the Sylvian region alone, which produces a surprisingly slight hemiparesis, considering the major effect on language function (Fig. 24-17).[218] In these cases, the hemiparesis may be limited to the face and hand. Ideomotor dyspraxia of the unaffected left upper extremity is the rule, as is bilateral buccofacial dyspraxia, which has been reported in 90% of patients.[214,219] Contralateral hemineglect to the right is the rule in the early stage.

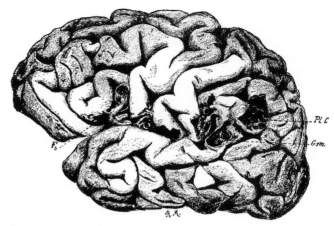

Figure 24-17 Lithograph of an example of infarction limited to the Sylvian lip. (From Moutier F: *L'aphasie de Broca.* Paris, 1908, Thèse Médicine.)

Autopsy documentation of the major syndrome of Broca's aphasia comes largely from the older literature[167]; living patients with the syndrome have been studied extensively by CT[220-222] and less frequently by MRI, given the extensive work already done earlier. The imaged lesions in patients with persistent Broca's aphasia were largely opercular and insular[223] and fronto-Sylvian, sparing the temporal lobe. The larger Sylvian lesions were associated with persistent nonfluency.[207] In cases with smaller lesions, destruction of the region taken to represent Broca's area was more often associated with transient deficits.

A few notable exceptions to the usual clinical picture accompanying Broca's aphasia may occur when the lesion is confined to the insula and adjacent operculum. Moutier's[224] patient Chissadon had a hemiplegia in the early period but in the chronic state had only the slightest motor deficit. A remarkably circumscribed infarct was found along the lip of the upper bank of the Sylvian fissure, which may have sufficed to interfere with language function and not with sensory motor function. A few cases of this type have been described with the use of Benson's term, the *Sylvian lip syndrome.*[215] One of Broca's patients was also described as having no detectable motor disturbance but was examined several years after the onset of his original deficit. The issue of the smallest lesion sufficient to produce the persisting syndrome of Broca's aphasia remains unresolved. To date, no known case of an infarct confined to Broca's area alone has produced lasting, severe Broca's aphasia,[225] save for the tersely described case cited by Van Gehuchten.[226]

The means by which clinical improvement occurs remains unclear. Like motor recovery, impairment reversal in aphasia appears to follow a proportional recovery pattern: nearly all patients achieve approximately 70% of their potential remaining recovery.[227] Work with metabolic imaging points to activation of tissue adjacent to the lesion site as instrumental in recovery, whereas activation in the opposite hemisphere, while supportive in the first few weeks,[228] is associated with a worse outcome when the activity is persistent (see further on).

Minor motor aphasia. Focal infarcts affecting the operculum produce a rather circumscribed syndrome lacking the full elements of Broca's aphasia.[125,167,196,225,229] In the acute stages, complete mutism with ideomotor and buccofacial dyspraxia is commonly encountered. Auditory and visual comprehension for language is virtually intact, and some patients are capable of writing properly with the unaffected left hand. Improvement from the initial mutism begins within hours or, at the least, days and, rarely, weeks later.[222,230] Any language deficit evident in speaking and writing is extremely transitory and often disappears before it can be tested in full detail. The accompanying bucco-linguo-facial and ideomotor limb dyspraxia likewise disappears quickly. The dyspraxia appears to contribute to most of the disturbances in speaking. The oral cavity positions closely approximate those desired to generate given sounds, but the slight inaccuracies strike the listener's ears as mispronunciations. Also, the dyspraxic disturbance in respiration interferes with the smooth flow of sounds and transition from syllable to syllable in running speech; this pattern has variously been called aphemia, oral–verbal apraxia, and apraxia of speech.[231] The disorder is not a result of weakness of the muscle serving articulation.

The initial mutism is usually accompanied by contralateral hemiparesis, but limitation of the weakness to the lower face and hand is not uncommon. Head and eye deviation have been documented but not often.[125] A few cases of Broca's infarction have manifested with no hint of motor paresis.[154,232] In those reports using the term *nonfluency*,[207] a similarly transient disturbance has been seen in the smaller lesions found on CT (Fig. 24-18).

The clinicopathologic correlation has shown few exceptions to the rule that Broca's area infarction does not precipitate either the acute or the chronic forms of Broca's aphasia, which is an observation made from the earliest days after Broca's original publication[233] and confirmed many times since.[167,222,234,235] The exceptions to this rule appear infrequent enough to warrant special comment. Van Gehuchten[226] described a 60-year-old man with sudden total loss of speech accompanied by paresis of the right upper limb and a small amount of facial involvement. The paresis diminished progressively, but the speech disturbance persisted unchanged until the man's death 1 year later. Van Gehuchten described the clinical picture as "pure motor aphasia with agraphia with no word blindness or deafness."[226] The patient was incapable of speaking. He uttered only a few sounds and sometimes a word or two. However, he could express himself adequately by gestures and writing some letters or ordinary words in response to dictation but was unable to write spontaneously or from dictation under more demanding circumstances. Autopsy revealed an infarct affecting the inferior half of the middle frontal gyrus from the top to the bottom of what was described as Broca's area. The accompanying photograph disclosed the infarct but did not indicate the involvement or sparing of the insula, nor whether the lesion extended deep into the brain.

Kleist[236] believed that the rare instances of a persistent and severe deficit associated with Broca's area infarction could be explained by an extension of the infarct

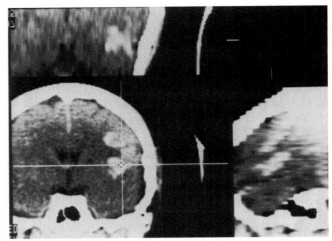

Figure 24-18 CT scan showing three views of an inferior frontal infarct, presenting as minor motor aphasia.

deep into the hemisphere, disrupting the white matter fibers that serve as projection and association pathways for Broca's area. Foix[237] made a similar inference earlier, referring to infarcts affecting the deeper branches of the MCA. Goldstein[210] also made similar suggestions but did not specify the vascular territory involved in these larger lesions.

Speech disturbances with lower rolandic infarction. Few cases of lower rolandic infarction have been reported since the days of Moutier,[224] whose studies suggested that infarcts in the region did not cause motor aphasia.[229,230] Levine and Sweet[238] cited a third case of rolandic infarction involving most of the precentral gyrus. The patient was only able to vocalize grunting or moaning sounds for the 10 days she was testable before her death. Autopsy disclosed a highly focal hemorrhage involving the midportion of the precentral gyrus that spared the frontal region in Broca's area.

The overlap of this syndrome with cases producing predominantly literal paraphasias has been noted by Luria[209] under the term *afferent motor aphasia*, attributed to faulty sensory feedback from a postrolandic lesion leading to inaccurate anatomic settings of the oropharynx, with resultant mispronunciations. Few instances have been reported to settle the inferred mechanism.

Speech disturbances from deep infarcts. Infarcts affecting the motor outflow of both sides have produced mutism as part of a syndrome of paralysis of both sides of the face, oropharynx, and tongue. However, a more interesting syndrome is that from a single deep infarct that has produced enough disturbance in speech and language to be described as an aphasic disorder. Bonhoeffer's[52] classic patient, unable to speak anything more than a few poorly formed vowels, had a large, deep infarct of the type described as a "giant lacune."[239] The giant lacune prevented innervation of the bulbar apparatus from ipsilateral pathways, and the anterior cerebral territory infarct cut off transcallosal projections. The basic pathophysiology is supported by a handful of other autopsy reports[236]; some have been from CT studies,[240,241] while others have shown impairment of frontal reactivity in studies of cerebral blood flow. Altogether the studies suggest that the disorder may be explained by damage to thalamofrontal pathways, and the diminished verbal behavior forms part of a syndrome of abulia.[242,243]

Sensory Aphasia

The syndrome known as Wernicke's aphasia is most commonly explained by occlusion of the lower division of the MCA and its branches, usually due to embolism. Because the lower division gives off its branches over an extremely short distance just at or distal to the posterior end of the Sylvian fissure, the occlusion at or near the point of take-off of these branches may give rise to several distinct variants in the size and topography of the infarction. There is a rough correlation between the extent of the language deficit and its intensity as a function of the lesion size, which is reflected in the text that follows.

Major sensory aphasia. An occlusion that blocks the trunk of the lower division or occludes all the branches, allowing no retrograde collateral flow from the posterior cerebral artery, causes a large infarct encompassing the whole posterior temporal, inferior parietal, and lateral temporooccipital regions (Fig. 24-19). Infarcts of such huge size generate a profound deficit in language function, classically known as Wernicke's aphasia but here described as major sensory aphasia.

In the early phase, in contrast to motor aphasia, patients with any degree of sensory aphasia show little or no disturbance in the ability to vocalize; they even make smooth transitions between syllables, assembling utterances in the form of phrases, and usually achieve intonations of utterances that sound like questions, replies, and declarative statements, regardless of the severity of the language disturbance reflected in the content of their speech.[206]

The extent of the language disturbance may often require prolonged conversation to document the full

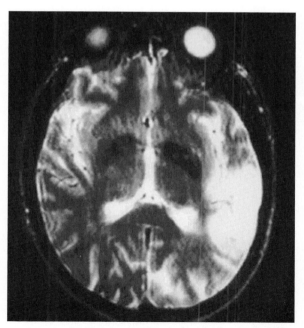

Figure 24-19 Large posterior hemispheral infarct with syndrome of major sensory (Wernicke's) aphasia.

range of errors. The casual or hurried examiner may find that the patient speaks easily, engages in simple conversational exchanges, and even appears to be making an effort at communication. Because the utterances often flow in a manner suggesting attempts at declarative statements, questions, or explanations and are accompanied by gestures of the face and limbs, the patient seems to be making efforts to communicate. At the extreme, the normal-appearing expressive tone during spontaneous discourse is such that if the patient were assumed to be speaking in an unfamiliar language, the listener might infer intact linguistic function. However, attempts to engage the patient in testing often fail to yield much evidence that the patient has understood the task and is attempting to respond. When the patient does not respond properly, the examiner is faced with the difficulty of deciding whether the fault lies in comprehension, in praxis, or in his/her own failure to make clear to the patient what is required.[244]

For the large infarcts, the disturbance in language content manifests as such gross disturbance in the *content* of spoken speech as to contain no understandable words, often occurring as isolated single or multiple syllables, a condition known as *jargon paraphasia*, commonly referred to by the laity by such terms as *word salad* or *gibberish*. The specific words expected to be uttered—the target words—are often distorted (but recognizable) in their phonetic structure (*literal paraphasia*) both in vowels and consonants or comprise other words in the same class (*verbal paraphasias*); in addition, these errors are occasionally accompanied by unwanted suffixes (e.g., "cold-ing"; less often prefixes) and are often also contaminated by the recurrence (*perseverations*) of previously uttered words or word fragments. The effects on language behavior are almost the reverse of those in the insular–opercular syndromes. The speech that is understandable is filled with small grammatical words but is missing the key words (the *predicative elements*) that contain the essence of the message (e.g., "I...you well"; the expected "know" is absent from the sentence).

Writing is usually disturbed in *content* but not in *form*, much like spoken speech. The cursive script is usually legible, but the language content reflected in the written letters and words has little communicative value. In some cases, writing and oral naming show striking differences in the severity of the language disorder, which some researchers have argued means that the two forms of expression are not under the same control.[245,246] The disturbance in *comprehension* of language for words heard or seen has long been assumed to be of the same type as that observed in spoken and written speech, claimed to be a sign of the essentially unitary nature of the disorder.[219] However, despite the assumption that the brain lesion on the superior temporal plane interferes with auditory comprehension, it has been difficult to demonstrate any such disturbance in phonemic processing.[230] Instead, the problem lies at the level of determining the linguistic significance of the adequately discriminated auditory stimuli.[247] It has likewise proved difficult to determine the extent to which disturbances in reading comprehension parallel those of auditory comprehension. A few patients with rather large lesions have shown a relative superiority in reading for comprehension compared with auditory comprehension.[245]

The phenomenology of major sensory aphasia has always been of interest to students of language abnormality, but the severe comprehension deficits during the acute syndrome usually preclude study[248] and often represent the insensitivity of the observer's methods.[249]

The *clinicopathologic correlation* in Wernicke's aphasia, as in Broca's aphasia, has been with a rather large lesion.[197,250] In our case material, some correlation seems to exist between lesion size and performance in special language studies comparing the spoken and written response to auditory and visual presentation of words, pictures, and sounds: patients with small lesions have been no better at oral response to words, sounds, or pictures of the same items (i.e., the disturbance was just as severe for words heard as words seen or for sounds heard as pictures seen). Other patients with smaller lesions have shown more limited disturbance in either auditory or visual comprehension but not both to the same degree.[245] Patients with protracted and exaggerated spontaneous speaking (logorrhea) have been those

with the larger infarcts; those with smaller infarcts rarely show this sign, which is a point that could be studied in more detail.

Exceptions exist: some patients with a large lesion across the lower division may not show a full clinical picture of Wernicke's aphasia at all. In some, the syndrome has been conduction aphasia (see further on).[251,252] In these cases, comprehension is so satisfactory that the main finding is difficulty in repeating aloud. A few cases have been reported in which either no detectable initial deficit in language occurred or the deficit was at most only slight and transient,[253-255] even though the patient had an infarct affecting the posterior superior temporal region that was large enough to have been expected to produce Wernicke's aphasia. One author (JPM) has had a similar case— that of an elderly right-handed woman whose cerebral embolism occurred while she was walking in her garden in the company of her internist son. She was immediately tested: she could read aloud and write correctly and could repeat and converse normally, but she experienced signs of a right hemianopia. Examination within days also failed to disclose language disturbance (Fig. 24-20). Cases of this sort serve to indicate the limitations of our present understanding of language organization in the brain.

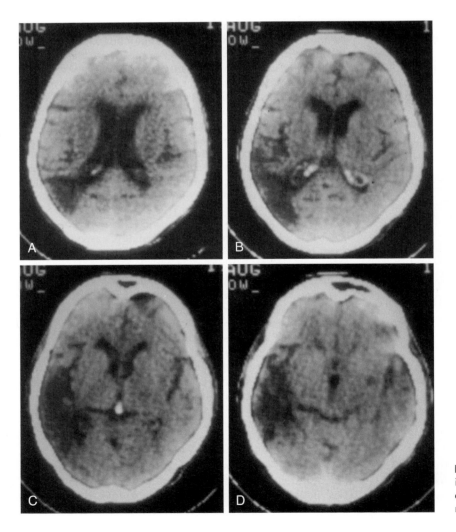

Figure 24-20 A to D, CT evidence of large infarct involving the lower division of the middle cerebral artery in a right-handed woman who had no aphasia.

Minor sensory aphasia and variants. Retrograde collateral flow established from the branches of the posterior cerebral artery may reduce the total infarct size; the ischemic zone may shrink in centripetal fashion toward the site of occlusion. How small a lesion is sufficient to precipitate the full syndrome of Wernicke's aphasia is still the subject of investigation.

An associated issue is the precise location and size of Wernicke's area.[256,257] Lesion mapping by CT or MRI has led to a Venn diagram of overlaps[258] but may be misleading because the site common to all cases is the posterior superior temporal plane, the usual site of the embolic vascular occlusion causing the syndrome. Cases of the fully developed, major Wernicke's aphasia with a lesion confined to the superior temporal plane appear to be remarkably rare.[109,209,223,237,259-261] Our personal literature search showed that only three superior temporal plane lesions have been found with Wernicke's aphasia among 89 published cases with autopsy correlation. Two of the cases are subject to criticisms that minimize their utility,[109] and the third is described too briefly to permit much analysis.[236] Henschen,[109] in a review of the literature up to the mid-1920s, concluded that a superior temporal plane lesion does not cause the full picture of Wernicke's aphasia (i.e., both "pure word deafness" and "alexia"). He based this opinion on a review of 35 patients with temporal lobe lesions, 20 of whom had "pure word deafness." In none was alexia present. Earlier, Bastian[262] had found alexia and sensory (Wernicke's) aphasia in only 5 of 16 cases of temporal lobe lesions, and in most, the lesion was large. Studies based on imaging have added no qualitatively new cases.[196,241]

There is no lack of superior temporal plane lesion cases, but there is a lack of such cases showing the full syndrome of Wernicke's aphasia. Many of the cases involving an infarct limited to less than the whole lower division territory appear to have been labeled conduction aphasia, pure word deafness, or alexia with agraphia.

Pure word deafness. More than 40 cases with CT or autopsy correlation are reported. According to the classic formulations, the only deficit should be auditory; spontaneous speech should be normal, as should reading comprehension and writing.[263] Eight well-known cases exist in which a unilateral lesion is confined to the superior temporal plane in the dominant hemisphere. In seven of these cases, paraphasic speaking was prominent, which is a clinical picture not permitted in the formulation of pure word deafness, which, by definition, should be free of a disturbance in speaking. In many cases, the elements of paraphasic speech cleared later.[264,265]

Many of the patients with bilateral lesions also experienced paraphasic speaking with poor comprehension during the early phase of the stroke.[251,266] In the famous case reported by Pick,[267] bilateral lesions, including a large left temporal plane lesion, rendered the patient paraphasic for 4 years.[251]

There is not even much current evidence that unilateral infarcts of the left temporal lobe create a state of impaired auditory discrimination.[206] Instead, small temporal lobe infarcts or parenchyma residue of an old slit hemorrhage (see Chapter 29) seem to create a transient form of Wernicke's aphasia, the major clinical feature of

which is a disturbance in auditory comprehension, such as in the aneurysm case we described earlier. The spontaneous speech contains many paraphasic errors, especially in the acute stages; the errors are frequent enough that the listener may make a preliminary diagnosis of Wernicke's aphasia. In addition, when taxed with reading aloud or comprehension tasks, patients with such lesions make enough errors that the notion of a pure disorder in auditory comprehension is not easily maintained.

Cortical deafness. At least one case report exists of an autopsied patient who was well studied clinically and was found to have deafness occasioned by an infarct confined to Heschl's transverse gyrus.[268] Bilateral infarcts affecting the temporal plane are a well-recognized cause of deafness, even though only a few reports have appeared.[269,270]

Alexia with agraphia. Alexia with agraphia as an isolated syndrome, absent any aphasic errors in speech or in auditory comprehension, is extremely rare. Henschen[109] found five "pure" cases among the more than 250 patients who had dyslexia and dysgraphia as part of larger clinical syndromes, noting that "almost all patients suffering alexia with agraphia have some degree of aphasia which ranges from a minimal degree of word-finding difficulty. The disturbance in reading comprehension and in the morphology and language content of writing far exceeds but does not occur in the absence of a disturbance in auditory comprehension or in spontaneous speech.[127,250,260,271,272,272a] Sidman et al[273,274] studied such a patient for many years; autopsy eventually showed a large lesion affecting much of the posterior left hemisphere (Fig. 24-21). His deficit began as sensory aphasia, affecting all forms of language and all conditions of testing. As time passed, the spoken response to auditory language stimuli improved, but the written response to any tests and the response to printed words remained impaired, which is a disturbance that could be classified grossly as dyslexia with dysgraphia.

The clinical problem is not whether dyslexia with dysgraphia exists but whether it is only a transient, acute disorder or one that occurs mainly as a long-term condition of an initially more severe Wernicke's aphasia. For

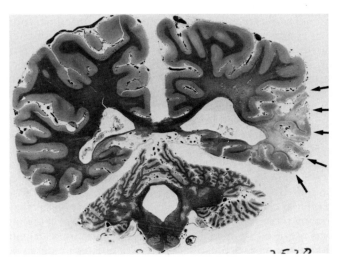

Figure 24-21 Coronal section from the posterior half of the brain in a patient with Wernicke's aphasia that evolved over years toward a syndrome of dyslexia with dysgraphia.

the syndrome to be dyslexia and dysgraphia, classic doctrine would require a circumscribed infarction beyond the superior temporal plane. Embolism is the only reliable source of such an infarct, apart from the focal form of vasculitis. In the unusual case in which the posterior cerebral artery takes its origin from the carotid artery, the main weight of the distal infarction could fall on the parietooccipital lobe, which happened in the case reported by Sidman et al,[274] but such an event would be most unusual. The available clinical data do not permit the determination of how quickly this syndrome can occur. The cases in the literature suggest that it is a late development from an earlier syndrome of more extensive deficits. The few cases of the syndrome from nonvascular causes do not have a bearing on this problem and are beyond the scope of this discussion.

Conduction Aphasia

Conduction aphasia occupies a special position in aphasiology, mainly because of its theoretical prediction rather than its isolated occurrence as a clinical entity. Wernicke,[275] who first defined the syndrome, offered the opinion that it represented the interruption of fiber pathways connecting the sensory language zone of the posterior half of the brain with the motor language zone in the frontal lobe. For Goldstein,[210] the disorder also represented disruption of a brain region located between the major sensory and motor centers, but for him the region mediated the interaction of both functions simultaneously. Neither theories account for the clinical features.[276] Modern efforts with tensor MR tractography have also not settled the issue,[277] and examples even exist with the syndrome and a left thalamic infarct by MRI.[278]

The term *conduction aphasia* has become accepted in clinical circles as applying to patients with poor repetition, mostly of phonemic errors (substitutions of one sound for the target sound), especially for unfamiliar material, and far better auditory and visual comprehension of language than that evident in their spontaneous spoken and written efforts. That spontaneous speech is often contaminated by paraphasic utterances is not emphasized. Although auditory and visual language comprehension is relatively preserved, neither function is normal at any stage of the disorder.[241] The ease with which disturbances in comprehension and the language content of speech are demonstrated has proved to be a major stumbling block to the satisfactory application of the label *conduction aphasia* when the physician encounters such a patient at the bedside. The disturbance in repeating aloud, on which great stress has been laid,[216,279] is not so useful a distinguishing point in the early stage of the syndrome because it also occurs in Wernicke's aphasia. In assessing the deficits in conversation, Burns and Canter[280] found a higher incidence of unwanted phonemes and intrusion of semantically related words among those patients classified as having Wernicke's aphasia than among those with conduction aphasia, but careful testing was required to make this distinction. Patients with conduction aphasia are also said to have a greater tendency to attempt self-correction than those with Wernicke's aphasia[260]; in our own experience, failure of self-correction efforts applies only to cases of Wernicke's aphasia with

the major syndrome. For ordinary clinical purposes, the distinction between the error patterns in speaking in the two types is not an easy one, except that semantic word substitutions are rare in conduction aphasia.[281,282] The syndrome, however named, often proves surprisingly evanescent when seen in an acute setting. More often, the initial syndrome is a Wernicke-type aphasia, evolving later into the picture of greater difficulty with pronunciation of words.[252]

Because the site of the infarct lies behind the rolandic region, there is usually no contralateral hemiparesis. Disturbances in eye movements and visual fields are also minor or not present. Bucco-linguo-facial dyspraxia is a common accompaniment, as is bimanual ideomotor dyspraxia. The dyspraxia of the latter state is different in the two limbs: the disorder in the limb served by the infarcted hemisphere takes the form of a de-afferentation[174] and that in the other limb conforms more to the picture expected in ideomotor dyspraxia.

The clinicopathologic correlation is also at odds with the theory. The classic hypothesis envisioned interruption of the arcuate fasciculus as the mechanism for the errors.[216,279] The interruption presumably prevents adequate control by the auditory system over the speech apparatus. Because this hypothesis hinges on a lesion interrupting the arcuate fasciculus, the findings expected on brain imaging or autopsy would be mainly subcortical. However, autopsy evidence in support of this hypothesis is surprisingly slight. The documented lesions have all been superficial infarcts whose penetration into the subcortical white matter has varied considerably.[215] In some instances, the infarction was completely superficial; in only a few has it been profound enough to produce a cleft deep enough to injure the arcuate fasciculus.[251] More than 20 cases with CT, MRI, or autopsy correlation are reported with this syndrome, and many show the lesion located in the same area usually attributed to Wernicke's aphasia. Naeser[223] found no difference in the lesion size per CT slice in cases with conduction or Wernicke's aphasia, but the mean percentage of left hemispheral tissue damage was larger in patients with Wernicke's aphasia than in those with conduction aphasia ($P < 0.01$). Electrical stimulation of the exposed brain has also shown disturbances in repeating aloud from surface stimulation of the superior temporal and supramarginal gyri.[283]

Another major hypothesis of the conduction aphasia theory considers the deficit to represent a disturbance in kinesthetic feedback. Luria[209] coined the term *afferent motor aphasia* to characterize this behavior. He assumed that the lesion lay in the Sylvian operculum posterior to the rolandic fissure, yielding a disturbance in pronunciation resulting from faulty anatomic oropharyngeal positionings. The words pronounced would contain sounds different from those intended. These errors, analogous to the typing errors of a novice typist, require considerable listener training for their detection, rather like the recognition of typing errors by those familiar with the typewriter keyboard. The novice listener may easily mistake them for language errors (paraphasias) and may assume that the speaker has a language disorder. Such an interpretation may be inaccurate, but it remains common medical practice to refer to errors of this type as "literal paraphasias."

This hypothesis assumes a surface lesion, such as would be expected from the embolic infarction that is almost invariably the responsible lesion. It matches with studies, which suggests that the major difficulty experienced by affected patients in repeating aloud can be considered to represent a disturbance in encoding accompanied by a disturbance in short-term memory.[284]

The question of whether the impairment in conduction aphasia represents mere phonologic mistargeting or is truly language based was raised for us again when we encountered a patient with dilated cardiomyopathy who experienced a syndrome of fluent conversational speech, normal auditory and reading comprehension, and repetition that was halting and effortful.[285] Nearly all of this patient's paraphasic errors—on naming, on repetition, on reading aloud, and on writing—were semantic substitutions. For example, "The quarterback threw the football down the field on Saturday" became "The quarterback through the baseball into the field." High-resolution MRI identified an infarct restricted to the posterior left insular cortex and intra-Sylvian parietal operculum (Fig. 24-22).

As a result of the more modern studies using brain imaging, it has been recognized for some time that the syndrome may occur from infarction in the lower division of the MCA, affecting the same territory producing Wernicke's aphasia.[236] We and others have considered the disturbance merely a mild form of sensory aphasia.[286]

"Transcortical" Aphasia

The observation of an aphasic syndrome with relatively intact ability to repeat dictated material aloud is attributed to Wernicke,[275,287] but Goldstein[210,288] has been recognized for his attempt to establish a separate entity characterized by an "isolation of the speech area." The traditional inference has been that the Sylvian region is preserved, as demonstrated by intact repetition skills, and that the responsible lesion for the aphasic disorder is elsewhere.

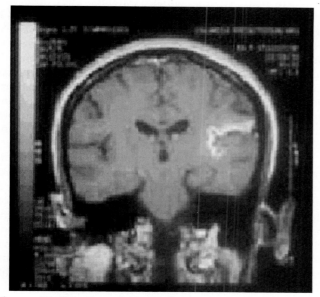

Figure 24-22 Coronal T1-weighted MR image with contrast enhancement showing a posterior insular cortex infarct in a patient with conduction aphasia featuring semantic errors.

The exact anatomic basis is less well-established than the term *transcortical* suggests, but three syndrome subsets have been described—motor, sensory, and mixed—corresponding to the major motor, major sensory, and global aphasias, respectively, except for the presence of otherwise preserved repetition.[289,290] Recent reports of such cases have shown some very large lesions.[291]

Transcortical motor aphasia (TCMA) resembles major motor aphasia (i.e., limited spontaneous speech and good comprehension) with relatively intact repetition,[276] although significant variations in the syndrome exist and have made it difficult to create any single underlying explanation. The language of some patients matches the classic behavioral description, but lesions have been found in the white matter anterolateral to the left frontal horn. They have been caused by infarction or hemorrhage in the upper division of the MCA. They demonstrate that the expected lesion location for TCMA produces varying degrees of impaired articulation, mild deficits in auditory comprehension, and stuttering. TCMA has also been described as a phase during the evolution of Broca's syndrome. It has also been observed that motor language syndromes with good repetition occur during the recovery process after infarction in the territory of the anterior cerebral artery, usually involving the supplementary motor area in the paramedian region of the frontal lobe.

Transcortical sensory aphasia (TCSA) resembles a major sensory syndrome consisting of fluent speech, impaired comprehension, alexia with agraphia, and paraphasic errors but relatively preserved repetition ability.[292] Patients often display compulsive repetition (echolalia), which suggests more linguistic competence than is actually the case. The responsible lesion is usually large, occurring in the territory of the posterior cerebral artery and involving the temporoparietooccipital junction[293]; occasionally an isolated thalamic infarct is present. The broad range of cognitive deficits often seen in conjunction with TCSA, including amnestic and attention disturbances,[294] has clouded its status as a separable aphasic disorder.

Mixed transcortical aphasia is the entity to which Goldstein[288] made reference in 1917 as "isolation of the speech." These patients have a global aphasia, except for retention of good repetition and virtually no other capacity for receptive or expressive propositional language. This is a very unusual syndrome. Only a small number of cases have been reported, mostly in patients with stroke, with the study of patients during the evolution of global aphasia or instances of recurrent stroke.[279] In the setting of acute stroke with no prior language disturbance, mixed transcortical aphasia has been said to occur from occlusion of the left internal carotid artery, resulting in simultaneous embolism in the anterior pial territory and perfusion failure in the terminal branches of the middle and posterior cerebral arteries.[295]

Functional Imaging in Aphasia

After infarction, regional changes in cerebral blood flow and metabolism can be identified by single-photon emission CT (SPECT), positron emission tomography (PET), or ultrafast MRI. Hypoperfusion and hypometabolism may extend into the peri-infarct area or may be seen at a site distant from the lesion itself.[296] With the ability to evaluate physiologic effects of structural lesions in regions adjacent to or remote from the territory of infarction has come a reexamination of some clinicopathologic correlations.

Patients with moderate to severe aphasia often show regions of hypometabolism encompassing large frontoparietal or temporoparietal areas, even in the presence of modest cortical or subcortical structural lesions.[248,289,297,298] Larger metabolic defects in the early phase of hemispheral stroke that extend beyond the borders of infarction[299,300] correlate with a worse initial clinical state and appear to predict poorer recovery from aphasia.[301,302] Reversal of cortical hypometabolism may correlate with clinical improvement when lesions are deep,[251,303] although in some cases of subcortical stroke, cortical hypometabolism may persist for at least 3 months despite good clinical recovery.[304]

A PET study by Metter et al[299] suggested that different aphasias may share common regions of hypometabolism regardless of lesion site. These researchers studied 44 aphasic patients with fluorodeoxyglucose (^{18}F) PET. Nineteen patients had "anomic," 10 had "Broca's," 8 had "conduction," 5 had "Wernicke's," 1 had "global," and 1 had "transcortical" aphasia. The researchers found that metabolic decreases were found in the left angular gyrus in 97% of patients, in the left supramarginal gyrus in 87%, and in the left posterior superior temporal gyrus in 85%. Taken all together, 100% of the patients had PET abnormalities in the left parietotemporal region. A greater degree of hypometabolism in the prefrontal region was the only imaging feature that distinguished patients with Broca's aphasia from those with Wernicke's aphasia. In functional imaging studies of normal control subjects performing language tasks, hyperperfusion or hypermetabolism has been demonstrated in certain brain regions. The superior temporal gyrus has been implicated both in the early acoustic processing of words and nonwords[305-307] and in the word-retrieval process required to generate verbs from noun stimuli.[308] The prefrontal region and supplementary motor area may also play a role in word selection and output.[307]

Functional imaging has also been used to explore the pathophysiology of atypical aphasias. Cappa et al[309] showed that, in two right-handed aphasic patients with right-sided lesions (periventricular corona radiata and lentiform nucleus), there was not only widespread hypometabolism in right cortical and subcortical structures but also decreased metabolism in the left frontal and parietal cortex, suggesting that the left hemisphere played a role in the aphasia even though the structural lesion was restricted to the right. Contralateral hemispheral contributions have also been evoked in cases of transcortical aphasias. When structural damage has unexpectedly included the left peri-Sylvian region, SPECT and ^{133}Xe regional cerebral blood flow studies have revealed extensive hypoperfusion throughout the left hemisphere but increased blood flow in the contralateral right temporal lobe.[289] Finally, in a patient with a conduction aphasia in which the paraphasic errors were nearly all semantic substitutions, MRI showed an infarct restricted to the posterior left insular cortex and intra-Sylvian parietal operculum, but SPECT revealed hypometabolism in the inferomedial and lateral left temporal lobe, suggesting a physiologic but nonischemic role for these regions in the syndrome.[310]

Important functional information can also be obtained by imaging aphasic patients while they are actively engaged in a language task. Such functional imaging studies have begun to elucidate the functional reorganization that is associated with recovery of stroke-induced deficits. Although some investigators have reported that contrahemispheral mirror locations correlate with the recovery process in mildly affected aphasic patients, others claim that peri-infarct and other ipsilateral regions are crucial for recovery and that activation in the contralateral hemisphere may correlate with persistence of aphasia.[311] Most of the evidence to date suggests that the right hemisphere contributes to recovery from aphasia, particularly in the early phase and that ultimate recovery depends on return of function in the left hemisphere.[228]

In a PET study of 12 aphasic patients with strokes in the left MCA territory, Heiss et al[312] observed unique activation during a word-repetition task 3 to 4 weeks after the patients had experienced stroke in the right supplementary motor area (SMA); this activation was not seen in 10 roughly age-matched control subjects. Then, in follow-up PET performed 18 months after the stroke, return of left superior temporal (Wernicke's area) activity was shown to be associated with good performance on an auditory comprehension task, which suggests that it was the return of left hemisphere function over time that was important in good recovery. Additional evidence that right hemisphere involvement in language was only the second-best mediator of recovery was demonstrated by the findings that (1) persistence of the right SMA activity was *inversely* correlated with performance on the language comprehension task and (2) persistence of right temporal activation was inversely correlated with recovery of left temporal activity. In a follow-up study, the same investigators performed PET imaging at 1 week and 8 weeks after cortical or subcortical stroke in 23 aphasic patients. They observed unique activation in the right inferior frontal region at 1 week. Good recovery of language correlated with activity in the left superior temporal region at 1 week, 8 weeks, or both and also with a disappearance of the right hemisphere activation. Patients with stroke whose original infarcts destroyed the left superior temporal region were not able to incorporate Wernicke's area back into a language network, and this was the reason, the investigators argued, that these patients had a worse prognosis for language recovery.[312]

Further evidence to support the functional significance of brain reorganization after stroke can be gained by performance of functional imaging before and after a specific rehabilitative intervention. Only a few studies of this type have been done to date. The right superior temporal gyrus and left precuneus were reported to be associated with improvements in language comprehension after brief, intense language therapy in a group of four patients with poststroke Wernicke's aphasia.[313] The study, however, did not contain a comparison group who did not receive the therapy. Ipsihemispheral translocation of language function has also been demonstrated in patients with AVMs in the posterior, dominant hemisphere,[314] but contralesional extension of function has been seen in right frontal AVM.[248] Whatever the mechanism, it seems clear that the brain is capable of reorganization. The pathophysiology of this process remains to be elucidated.

Epidemiology and Natural History of Aphasia

According to NINCDS, which is part of the National Institutes of Health, there are more than 1 million aphasia survivors in the United States.[315] Acquired disorders of language can arise from many causes, such as cerebrovascular disease, trauma, tumor, and most other causes of cerebral dysfunction,[314] but stroke represents by far the most frequent etiology of language-based disorders. Among those with acute stroke, 21% to 38% of patients are seen with aphasia,[316] and an ischemic event is the cause in about 80%.[317] As a group, 79% of patients with poststroke aphasia still have aphasic deficits at the end of 12 months; complete recovery is seen in 21% of patients compared with posttraumatic aphasias, in which about half of the patients achieve recovery. Engelter et al[318] showed that there is increasing risk of developing poststroke aphasia with advancing age. In their population-based study of first-ever stroke patients in Basel, Switzerland, the risk of aphasia increased by 1% to 7% per each year of age. Whereas every seventh patient younger than 65 years had aphasia, subjects older than 85 years were three times more likely to develop aphasia. Depression is common after stroke,[319] but studies have confirmed that 30% to 40% of patients with left hemisphere stroke and a nonfluent aphasia experienced profound depressive symptoms.[320]

Most patients who have had a stroke improve in function at least to some degree.[321] Although most improvement is detected within the first 3 months after a stroke,[322,323] longer term follow-up has shown that motor function improvement continues well beyond 6 months[324] and after 2 years for aphasia.[195] Pedersen et al[317] showed, however, that different initial syndromes appear to improve at different rates. In their series of 203 first-time stroke patients with aphasia, 32% had global aphasia and 25% had anomic aphasia. By the end of 1 year, however, nearly 40% of patients had anomic syndromes, and about one fourth had Wernicke's and Broca's aphasias, respectively. In general, older patients were likely to be seen with focal aphasias, whereas younger patients were more likely to be seen with global syndromes that evolved to more focal features.

Although long-term follow-up has shown considerable improvement—often described as recovery—after years,[195,325] the greatest degree of spontaneous improvement appears to occur within the first 3 months after a stroke.[326-329] Among the factors purported to determine language improvement after stroke, initial syndrome severity and lesion size have been reported to be important predictors.[330-334]

Many studies of the course of aphasia, however, did not collect baseline data until several days to weeks after admission, did not exclude patients with prior strokes, and reported data as mean values for patient groups based on initial aphasia diagnosis, which obscures potential variability across individual patients. The advantage of evaluating individual deficits rather than global characterizations (e.g., Wernicke's and Broca's aphasias) is that within each of these syndromes is a wide range of profiles and that disturbances can be highly idiosyncratic, especially when the lesions are smaller. Moreover, it has been shown in large studies of acute poststroke aphasia that only slightly more than half of patients have the classic syndromes that comprise aphasiology.[334]

We had the opportunity to follow the evolution of language in the Columbia Performance and Recovery in Stroke (PARIS) study, a prospective database of first-time stroke patients.[335] We chose comprehension, naming, and repetition because of their sensitivity to deficits that can arise from anterior or posterior lesions and because of their objectivity in measurement. The major aim of this study was to characterize the nature and extent of recovery of aphasic deficits from 24 to 72 hours after stroke onset through a 90-day follow-up. Twenty-two of 91 patients had language disorders. Initial syndrome scores were positively correlated with 90-days scores ($r = 0.60$) and negatively correlated with the change in score from baseline to follow-up ($r = -0.66$). Neither lesion size, age, nor education correlated with initial syndrome severity or with performance at 90 days. Level of education was not associated with the degree of recovery. A multiple regression model that combined lesion size, age and initial syndrome was significant ($P = 0.03$) but only explained 29% of the variance. Patients with severe deficits at baseline in individual language domains could improve close to normal, improve to a less severe deficit, or not improve at all. We concluded that there was significant variability in language improvement after first-time stroke, even in more severe, initial syndromes. Traditional predictors of poststroke language outcomes at the time of acute admission did not reliably predict function at 90 days. These data suggest that other factors have not yet been identified that account for functional stroke recovery.

Efficacy of Aphasia Therapy

It is widely agreed that in the clinical practice of speech-language pathology a comprehensive examination is appropriate.[329] Some of the commonly used aphasia batteries include the Boston Diagnostic Aphasia Examination[336] and the Western Aphasia Battery,[337] both of which assess functions such as spontaneous speech, comprehension, naming, reading, writing, and repetition. There are also more functionally based evaluation batteries, such as the Porch Index of Communicative Abilities[338] and the Communicative Abilities in Daily Living.[339]

An evaluation of aphasia therapy, however, depends on the choice of outcome measurements and the language assessment methodology. Two considerations include whether there should be a single outcome measure of global function (e.g., the Aphasia Severity Score of the Western Aphasia Battery) or a focus on particular outcome skills (e.g., Visual Confrontation Naming on the Boston Diagnostic Aphasia Examination). Outcomes can also be based on a group-design format or the use of single subjects as their own controls. Regardless of the analytic approach, the importance of treating aphasic patients is such that over the past 50 years, more than 600 articles have appeared in the literature examining treatment approaches.[340]

Among the first meta-analyses in the aphasia literature was Robey's inclusion of 21 studies that evaluated three classes of effect sizes: untreated aphasia recovery, treated aphasia recovery, and treated versus untreated recovery.[341] Excluding single-case studies and reports with incomplete information, he found that treatment in the early period yielded nearly twice the recovery of untreated individuals. Four years later, he added 34 additional studies to his database (N = 55) in which he analyzed four dimensions of treatment: amount of treatment, type of treatment, severity of aphasia, and type of aphasia.[327] To his inclusion criteria from 4 years earlier, he added quasiexperimental designs such as patients who were not randomly selected and studies in which there was no random treatment assignment. The main findings showed a positive outcome for (1) treated over untreated patients at all stages of recovery, with an average treatment effect size that was 1.83 times that for untreated patients in the early period, and (2) treatment longer than 2 hours per week inducing greater changes than treatment of shorter durations. The main conclusion was that intensive treatment over short periods of time provides better outcomes than less intensive regimens over a longer period of time.

In 2003, Bhogal et al evaluated the intensity of aphasia therapy in a meta-analytic evaluation of 10 studies from Medline.[342] They found that studies demonstrating a significant treatment effect provided 8.8 hours per week of therapy for 11.2 weeks. Studies failing to show a positive effect for aphasia treatment provided approximately 2 hours of therapy per week for 22.9 weeks. As Bethier has pointed out, however, these positive findings from the aphasia remediation literature are tempered when only randomized controlled trials (RCTs) are included. In a Cochrane review, Greener et al examined 60 RCTs in which only 12 satisfied selection criteria.[343] On the basis of the Cochrane analysis, it was concluded that "speech and language therapy for people with aphasia after a stroke has not been shown either to be clearly effective or clearly ineffective within an RCT. Decisions about management of patients must therefore be based on other forms of evidence."

It has been argued that many of the studies included in the analysis by Greener et al were not well-designed investigations and that, in recent years, there have been model-based interventions that have employed innovative methodologies using case-series approaches and multiple-baseline designs with subjects used as their own controls.[340,344] Using this kind of analysis for single-subject treatment effects, Moss and Nicholas[345] evaluated 23 studies that met criteria identifying subjects as those who received direct continuous therapy for spoken language deficits and whose changes in response to therapy were measurable. It was found that when subjects were grouped by years post onset, there was treatment by therapy and that there were no significant differences found over time. Thus treatment was capable of demonstrating benefit even years after stroke onset.

All of these language-based therapies, whether analyzed on an individual or group basis, occur in patients who have an admixture of factors that mediate the outcomes of intervention.[329] Factors such as nonlanguage cognitive status, affective status (e.g., depression), physical illness, concomitant medications, and support system have all been shown to affect long-term aphasia outcomes.

Innovative Aphasia Therapies

New therapies hold promise for increased benefits for patients with postinjury aphasia. Rather than being based on the traditional notion of compensating for deficits, more recent approaches have been based on principles of human learning and on theories of neural plasticity.

Based on the success of constraint-induced therapy for hemiparesis,[346] constraint-induced language therapy (CILT) involves the forced use of spoken communication with restraint of other modalities of communication, including gestures.[347,348] To determine whether there are corresponding neurophysiologic changes that would provide a mechanistic basis for improvement in behavioral function, Breier et al[348] showed that five patients who responded well to CILT exhibited a greater degree of late magnetoencephalographic (MEG) activation in posterior language areas of the left hemisphere and homotopic areas of the right hemisphere before therapy than those who did not respond well. Analogously, probes with TMS have also demonstrated functional reorganization after therapy.[349] Errorless learning procedures, derived from principles of operant conditioning, have also been studied.[350] Fillingham et al,[351] for example, showed that such techniques were as effective as more traditional, errorful approaches to enhance word-retrieval skills but that errorless procedures were greatly preferred by patients.

There are an increasing number of studies that suggest that intervention that combines behavioral techniques with a biological perturbation might improve overall outcomes, as was first demonstrated by Feeney et al studying the effects of amphetamines in an animal model of motor deficits.[352] Some efficacy in the administration of amphetamines combined with aphasia remediation to improve language outcomes has been shown.[353] TMS has also been paired with aphasia therapy to suppress the presumed inhibitory influence of activation in the right hemisphere. Naeser et al[354] found that picture naming was enhanced with stimulation over the right hemisphere, even 2 months later without intervening TMS or language therapy.

Another biological intervention involves the administration of pharmacologic agents. Early animal studies by Feeney et al,[352] for example, showed that administration of D-amphetamines given to rats 24 hours after surgical resection of the motor cortex produced acceleration of function. Later studies have shown these same facilitating effects in rats after experimenter-induced stroke.[355,356] After several pilot investigations in patients with poststroke weakness had positive results,[357,358] Walker-Batson et al[353] showed, in a double-blind, placebo-controlled study of 21 patients with aphasia, that dextroamphetamine produced greater improvement in language scores at 1 week, but the differences were not significant when corrected for multiple comparisons. Unfortunately, a recent review of 10 human poststroke studies involving 287 patients did not provide evidence that amphetamine treatment improved either neurologic function or activities of daily living.[359] Indeed, Gladstone et al showed in the largest double-blind study to date that amphetamines coupled with physical therapy given to patients in the early poststroke period provided no additional benefit in motor recovery compared with physiotherapy alone.[360] A concern regarding the use of amphetamines is that concomitant measurement of cardiovascular function during poststroke trials with amphetamines has demonstrated increases in both blood pressure and heart rate during treatment compared with placebo.[361,362] Perhaps such safety issues contribute to the lack of a sustainable amphetamine effect owing to the reluctance to increase the dose higher than the 10 mg used in human treatment protocols.

Others have sought to administer pharmacologic agents that target specific transmitter systems. There is some evidence that cholinergic mechanisms may also be important in stroke and that such agents may work both as a neuroprotectant and by independently promoting functional recovery.[363] While acetylcholine appears to induce plasticity as a facilitator of other mechanisms, such as N-methyl-D-aspartate receptor–dependent long-term potentiation, it has also been shown to be an independent initiator of plasticity in rats.[364] There are reports suggestive of the restorative effects of cholinergic therapy for the treatment of poststroke aphasia.[365-367] A recent small clinical trial of 26 patients compared aphasia recovery for those taking donepezil versus placebo. At the end of the 12-week treatment period, those taking active drug had greater language recovery, which, unfortunately, was not sustained 1 month after drug intervention had stopped.[368]

The administration of dopaminergic agents after stroke apparently has a role that combines controlling functions for both motor performance and cognition.[369] Studies in animals and humans report that the dopamine agonist bromocriptine has improved aphasia (left hemisphere function) and left hemineglect (right hemisphere function). With regard to restoration of language after stroke, bromocriptine has been most extensively studied for treatment of motor (nonfluent) aphasias. Positive results in poststroke patients in the initial study[370] were followed by negative findings in a second study,[101] although the patients in the latter study were described only as "brain-injured." Later work with a higher dose of bromocriptine in the first double-blind study involving patients whose strokes had occurred more than 1 year previously showed statistically significant improvement in verbal latency, repetition, reading comprehension, dictation, and free speech.[371,372] Bragoni et al[372] proposed that these findings result from dopamine's active role in neuronal projections from the midbrain to frontal brain regions, including SMAs and the cingulate gyrus.

We (RML, RSM) have sought to determine the importance of a transmitter system in stroke recovery through the demonstration that, once a function has significantly improved after infarction, former stroke or TIA deficits can be transiently reinduced with a targeted sedating agent. We administered the short-acting gamma-aminobutyric acid A (GABA_A) agonist midazolam to eight poststroke patients.[102] Those with left cerebral injury demonstrated

reemergence of aphasia, right-sided weakness, or both but never left-sided weakness or left hemineglect. Conversely, patients who had had a right cerebral stroke demonstrated left-sided weakness, hemineglect, or both but no aphasia or right-sided paresis. More recently, we were able to achieve greater specificity in the effects of GABA agonism on the restitution of poststroke dysfunction. In a series of seven recovered aphasic patients, we demonstrated in double-blinded fashion that midazolam reinduced former aphasia deficits, whereas the sedative scopolamine had no impact on language function in the same group of patients.[373] Moreover, neither midazolam nor scopolamine had any statistical effect on the language behavior of age-matched, healthy control subjects.

The data seem to suggest that remediation for aphasia is most effective when outcomes are specific and intervention is tailored to the nature of the deficits. Therapy appears most effective when initiated earlier rather than later, but there is evidence to indicate that therapy even years after stroke onset has benefit. Successful therapy seems to depend on many nonlanguage factors, such as cognitive function, emotional status, and medications. Advances in treatment will depend on combined biological and innovative behavioral techniques.

Apraxias

Apraxias are acquired disorders of execution. They represent an inability to perform a previously learned, skilled act that is unexplained by weakness, visual loss, incoordination, dementia, sensory loss, or aphasia. Liepmann[374,375] described apraxia as the "incapacity for purposive movement despite retained mobility." Apraxic patients are unable to perform skilled acts because they either have lost or cannot access the motor engrams (programs) that guide skilled acts. Because these deficits in skilled movement are rarely complete, the term *dyspraxia* is often used. Apraxic deficits may affect movements of the body, face, or limbs. Liepmann proposed that the left hemisphere possesses the motor engrams necessary for skilled movements, just as it possesses the linguistic engrams necessary for speech. A left hemisphere dominance for skilled motor activity has been proposed,[376] in part based on the overwhelming proportion of left hemisphere lesions in right-handed patients with motor apraxia,[377] and the absence of motor apraxia in those with right retrorolandic lesions.[378]

Ideomotor Apraxia

The most common type of motor apraxia, ideomotor apraxia, was speculated by Liepmann[374,375] to be a dissociation between the brain areas that contain the "ideas" for movements and the "motor" areas responsible for execution. The examiner tests for the disturbance by asking patients to show how they would salute, wave goodbye, hammer a nail, saw wood, and perform various other actions; only crude left-sided movement is observed in the most severe case. In milder cases, the actions are clumsy and lack precision. Performance may improve on imitation but typically is abnormal.[379] The best performance is elicited on actual use of the object.[219] Although aphasia commonly accompanies ideomotor apraxia, there is no close relationship between ideomotor apraxia and either the severity or the type of aphasia.[380-382] Heilman[383] suggested that the motor programs for skilled motor movements are stored in the left superior parietal lobe. Skilled motor activity would then depend on the transmission of these programs to the premotor area in the left frontal lobe. Ideomotor apraxia may then arise from either (1) direct destruction of motor programs in the left superior parietal lobe or (2) destruction of the pathways from the left superior parietal lobe to the premotor area of the left frontal lobe (i.e., disconnection).[384] Although ideomotor apraxia is more common with superficial than with deep lesions, large, deep lesions may produce ideomotor apraxia.[234] Ideomotor apraxia does not occur with smaller or deeper infarcts of the lacunar type. Little is known about the course of improvement, but it can be rapid in some cases.[219] Frontal lesions have a better prognosis than do posterior lesions.[380]

Ideational Apraxia

Ideational apraxia, a disorder of the sequencing and planning of complex motor acts,[385] bears an uncertain relation to ideomotor apraxia. The examiner can elicit it by asking the patient to demonstrate complex motor tasks, such as lighting a candle or mailing a letter. The literature is sparse in cases of stroke.[379] Sittig[386] believed that ideational apraxia is only a severe form of ideomotor apraxia, but others hold that they are distinct entities.[387,388] Ideational apraxia is generally observed after dominant hemisphere parietal lobe lesions. Associated findings may include a fluent aphasia (anomic, semantic, or Wernicke's), constructional apraxia, and elements of Gerstmann's syndrome. Dementia and confusion are noted in some cases. Bilateral parietal lesions are present in some cases,[378,389] but isolated right parietal lesions seem to produce ideational apraxia only in individuals with anomalous cerebral dominance.[390] Little is known about the improvement over time and whether there is "recovery" or simply a new strategy in responding.

Limb-Kinetic Apraxia

Limb-kinetic (also innervational or melokinetic) apraxia is manifested as a lack of rapidity, skill, and delicacy in the performance of learned motor movements.[377] Liepmann held that in limb-kinetic apraxia "the virtuosity which practice lends to movement is lost. Therefore the movements are...clumsy, without precision" (quoted by Kertesz[391]). The patient is clumsy in the execution of common motor acts, such as the manipulation of objects (e.g., eating utensils, combs, brushes, saws, hammers, and playing cards). Limb-kinetic apraxia is unilateral and affects the limb contralateral to the cerebral lesion. It may be difficult to distinguish between limb-kinetic apraxia and paresis in some cases. Commonly associated neurologic signs are ataxia, choreoathetosis, grasping, spasticity, weakness, and dystonic posturing. However, the clumsiness in using objects is out of proportion to these other deficits. The perseverative and conceptual disturbances that characterize ideational apraxia are not prominent. Patients with limb-kinetic apraxia respond poorly to commands or imitations. Performance may improve slightly with the use of the object, but patients often act as if they were somewhat unfamiliar with its use.

Limb-kinetic apraxia may occur after injury to either the right or left premotor cortex or subjacent white matter.[259] Slight weakness is usually present, which suggests that injury to the pyramidal pathways is an essential feature of limb-kinetic apraxia. However, injury limited solely to the pyramidal pathways does not produce limb-kinetic apraxia. Patients with pure motor hemiplegia due to lacunar infarction in the internal capsule do not manifest limb-kinetic apraxia. Thus, the elicitation of this sign is a useful indicator that the surface cortex or subjacent white matter has been injured. The diagnosis of limb-kinetic apraxia is rarely made, which reflects the doubts of some as to its validity as an apraxic entity discrete from either pyramidal weakness or ideomotor apraxia.

Callosal Apraxia

Callosal apraxia (sympathetic apraxia) represents a restricted form of ideomotor apraxia in which the apraxia is limited to the nondominant arm. Liepmann and Maas[286] first described a patient with right hemiplegia who was unable to perform skilled movements with his nonparetic left arm. Similar patients have been described.[392,393] Critical to the syndrome is disruption of the anterior portions of the corpus callosum. Infarction of the medial or anterior left frontal lobe with Broca's aphasia and right hemiplegia is often present, but these elements are not critical to the genesis of the apraxia.

The syndrome is unilateral and limited to the nondominant arm. The disturbance is similar to the bilateral apraxia that characterizes ideomotor apraxia: the movements are slow and lacking "lithness."[394] Two somewhat similar hypotheses have been offered to explain callosal apraxia; both cite a form of "disconnection": one from the dominant hemisphere's "speech area"[279,392] and the other[383] from the "motor engram centers" in the left hemisphere.

The lesion producing callosal apraxia is rare, given the low frequency of an isolated lesion of the corpus callosum. More commonly, the crossing callosal fibers are disrupted in the mesial left hemisphere by an infarction either in the left anterior cerebral artery territory or in the distribution of the anterior division of the left MCA. These anterior division left MCA territory infarctions are associated with right hemiplegia and Broca's aphasia. Injury to the corpus callosum rather than to the left supplementary motor cortex is critical to the syndrome.[395]

Oral-Bucco-Lingual Apraxia

Orofacial or oral-bucco-lingual apraxia is the inability to perform skilled movements with the oral and facial musculature on command.[217,385] Oral apraxia is unusual in cases of anomic or Wernicke's aphasia. Although oral apraxia is common in global aphasia, testing for oral apraxia may be difficult because of comprehension disturbances.[396]

Oral-bucco-lingual apraxia generally results from an inferior frontal lesion in the premotor cortex adjacent to the face area on the motor strip. Most lesions are cortical and superficial,[397] but some have been from large, deep lesions.[7]

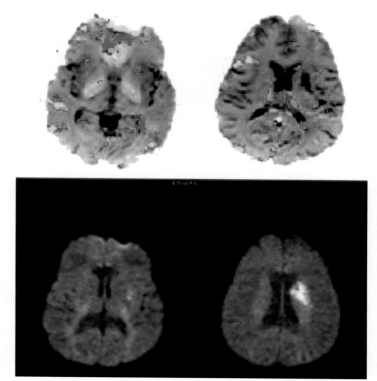

Figure 24-23 Aphasia recovery. Activation seen in the right frontal and temporal lobes in regions homologous to Broca's and Wernicke's areas. Infarct in left basal ganglia and periventricular white matter seen on diffusion-weighted MR image.

Syndromes of Infarction in the Hemisphere Nondominant for Speech and Language

A wide variety of behavioral abnormalities may follow stroke in the hemisphere nondominant for speech and language; this is the right hemisphere in most left-handed people. (For brevity of text, this hemisphere is referred to as the right in this chapter.)

The clinical syndromes observed are governed in general by several unifying observations. First, despite some rudimentary capacity to comprehend language, language plays no important role in the activities subserved by the right hemisphere. Second, the commitment of the cerebral cortex to a specific "higher cortical" function is less precise in the right hemisphere than in the left hemisphere. Although higher cortical functions in the left hemisphere appear to be governed by identifiable "centers" of function, higher cortical functions of the right hemisphere appear to be governed by far-flung "networks."

The right hemisphere is dominant for certain aspects of attention,[398] including directed attention, focused attention, and vigilance. This specialization for attention may be reflected in a variety of right hemisphere deficits, such as neglect, extinction, and impersistence. Many spatial and quasispatial operations are performed by the right hemisphere. This specialization for spatial operations may be reflected in such right hemisphere deficits as prosopagnosia,[399] topographic disorientation, constructional apraxia, and dressing apraxia. Confabulatory behaviors are more common after right than left hemisphere injury.[279] Both reduplicative paramnesia and anosognosia may be considered forms of confabulation that occur after right hemisphere stroke.

Patients lacking the syndromes from right hemispheral infarction fare better in rehabilitation than do patients with these deficits. Although some patients show a steady improvement (Fig. 24-23), others are left with persistent and disabling behavioral abnormalities, including constructional and dressing apraxias, left neglect, and motor impersistence. The size of the lesion, rather than its exact location, is a better predictor of behavioral deficits after right hemisphere damage (Fig. 24-24).

Neglect and Extinction

Extinction and neglect are two forms of impaired response to contralateral space, labeled *hemiinattention,* and may occur after right hemisphere stroke. Extinction implies that a "stimulus is not perceived only when a second stimulus is presented simultaneously—usually but not necessarily on the opposite side of the body."[400] Unilateral spatial neglect (USN) is a restricted syndrome in which patients fail to copy one side (usually the left) of a figure, fail to read one side of words or sentences, and bisect lines far to the right of center.

The term *neglect* indicates disturbances shown by patients in their responses to stimuli from the right side of space, including impairment of OKN, turning to the left in response to auditory stimuli from the right, and faulty performance in reading aloud or naming objects in the right side of space.[401,402]

It implies a more flagrant syndrome characterized by a failure of the patient to attend to new stimuli coming from one side (usually the left). Neglect is often trimodal (auditory, visual, and tactile). In left-sided

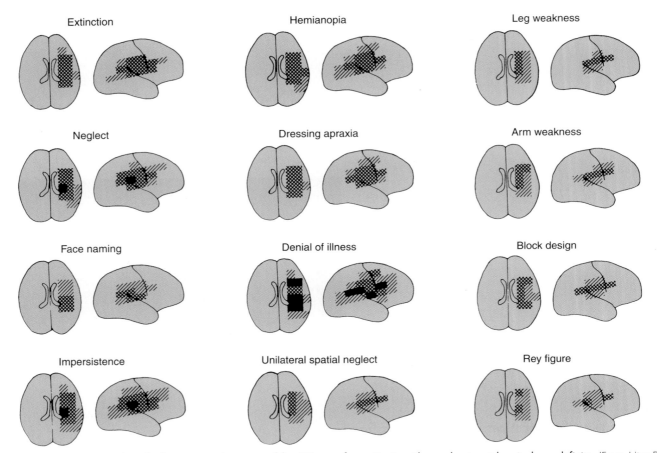

Figure 24-24 Topography of infarction as documented by CT scan for patients with nondominant hemisphere deficits. (From Hier DB, Mondlock J, Caplan LR: Behavioral abnormalities after right hemisphere stroke. *Neurology [NY]* 33:337, 1983.)

neglect, the patient may not explore the left side of space; the eyes and body may be turned tonically to the right.[182] Neglect is characterized by "a lack of responsivity to stimuli on one side of the body, in the absence of any sensory or motor deficit severe enough to account for the imperception,"[403] seen more often from right than left hemispheral lesions.[404-406] Marked neglect of the left side tends to occur in conjunction with other markers of severe right hemisphere damage, including anosognosia (i.e., implicit unawareness of illness and its clinical manifestations)[178] and motor impersistence. By contrast, USN may occur with smaller right hemisphere strokes, which usually have a good prognosis (Fig. 24-25). Failure to bisect a line using an optokinetic tape appears to be a common finding in posterior hemispheral lesions.[407,408]

Neglect has been traditionally attributed to injury in the vicinity of the right parietal lobe. However, neglect may follow injury to the right frontal lobe,[409] right cingulum,[410] right lenticular nucleus, or right thalamus.[407,411] Mesulam has postulated a "network" model to account for the lesions of a variety of cortical and subcortical structures that produce left neglect,[412] consisting of a reticular element (providing arousal and vigilance), a parietal element (providing sensory and spatial mapping), a frontal element (providing the motor programs for exploration), and a limbic element.

Neglect from Frontal Lesion

It has long been appreciated that a parietal lesion (from infarct or hemorrhage or even other causes) may be associated with an impaired response to stimuli from the opposite side of space, whether from a visual, auditory, or even somatosensory source.[413,414] These deficits are thought to reflect impaired input from sensory to motor regions. However, a similar disturbance occurs from frontal lesions as well,[409,415] whether cortical or subcortical.[416] Using positron emission transverse tomographic scanning, Deuel and Collins[417] found widespread metabolic suppression in the basal ganglia and thalamus after a unilateral frontal lesion, with little evidence of cortical hypometabolism beyond the immediate confines of the lesion. Their findings suggest that part of the syndrome might result from impaired activation of subcortical structures involved in planning motor movements. Corbetta et al, using fMRI showed that the spatial attention deficits in neglect (rightward bias and reorienting) after right frontal damage correlated with abnormal activation of structurally intact dorsal and ventral parietal regions that mediate related attentional operations in the normal brain.[418] An imbalance of parietal activity favoring the left hemisphere was associated with asymmetrical attention, and a recovery of this neglect phenomenon was associated with a restoration of the balance of activity between

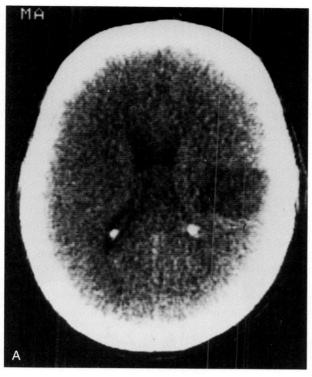

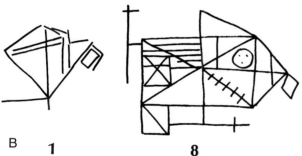

B **1**   **8**

Figure 24-25 A, CT scan of small right middle cerebral artery territory infarct. B, Drawings made by the patient with the infarct shown in A at 1 and 8 weeks after stroke.

the hemispheres. In the human, the signs of neglect from frontal lesions are remarkably transient, usually fading within a week in all patients except those with the largest infarcts.[419]

Motor Neglect

Motor neglect, said to be characterized by underutilization of one side without defects in strength reflex or sensibility, has been described by LaPlane and Degos.[420] Siekierka-Kleiser et al characterized it as an underutilization of the opposite side of the body.[421] This condition has a long history in clinical neurology. Under most circumstances of clinical examination, the patient with this syndrome appears to have a hemiparesis; with special efforts on examination, however, normal strength and dexterity can be demonstrated.

The usual features are (1) a lack of spontaneous placing reaction, such as failure to place the hand in the lap or on the arm of a chair when sitting, letting it instead drag down beside the body; (2) delayed or insufficient assumption of correct postures, resulting in heavy falls to the affected side with no attempts to minimize the effect of the fall by reaching out or correcting the balance; (3) impairment of automatic withdrawal reaction to pain; and (4) lack of excursions of the limb necessary to achieve a movement such as touching the nose; for example, the patient instead leans the head forward to compensate for failure to bring the finger far enough up. This disturbance may occur in the absence of a sensory disturbance or demonstrable hemiparesis. Hartmann[422] described an autopsy case with similar disturbances secondary to an infarct affecting the second frontal gyrus of the right frontal lobe. Animal studies in the monkey have demonstrated a similar transitory disturbance observed high over the prefrontal region after selective research.[423]

Neglect for Verbal Material

Leicester et al[424] described a form of visual neglect in which the occurrence and frequency of errors were determined by the verbal content of the test materials. When the patient was required to select from an array of choices displayed directly in front, errors were seen with those materials that the patient found the most difficult to name or write; in such instances, responses were made less frequently to choices on the right-hand side of the display. When the test materials were easily named, little or no evidence of neglect for the right side of space was noted. This form of neglect, which is commonly encountered in testing of patients with aphasia but not often reported as such, is not obligatory but is highly dependent on the verbal material in the test itself. It was explained neither by defective spatial responding nor by defective sensory function, and it occurred with left-sided but not right-sided lesions, which argues for an aphasic basis to the effect.

Anosognosia

This syndrome (i.e., unawareness of illness or its clinical manifestations) is more likely to be associated with severe as opposed to mild hemiparesis.[425-427] Anosognosia for either hemianopia or hemiparesis can be dissociated from elementary[103] neurologic deficits or neglect. Nonpersistence of the syndrome was evidenced in studies showing improvement toward normal within 22 weeks.[425,428] The lesion producing anosognosia is usually large (Fig. 24-26).[425] Involvement of the insula plays what could be an important role.[429] Although a hemispheral site is classic, a pontine infarct has reportedly caused such disturbance.[430]

Sensory loss, confusion, or dementia cannot adequately account for anosognosia. Gerstmann[431] has viewed anosognosia as a disorder of a hypothetical "body image." Although he believed that this body image is "mapped" into the left parietal lobe, input from the right parietal lobe is essential in updating the left parietal lobe as to the condition of the left side of the body. Injury to the right parietal lobe or to connecting pathways between the right and left parietal lobes could lead to anosognosia. It may be viewed as a variation of "neglect" or "inattention" in that the patient with anosognosia fails to "attend" to the hemiplegia.

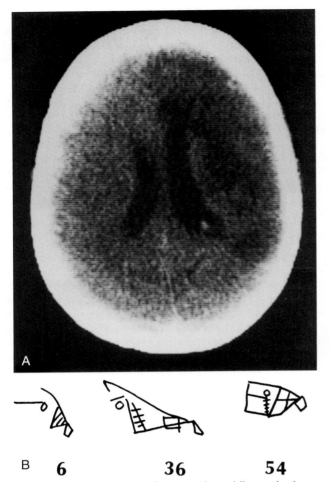

B   6   36   54

Figure 24-26 A, CT scan of large right middle cerebral artery territory infarct. B, Drawings done by the patient with the infarct shown in A at 6, 36, and 54 weeks after stroke.

Impersistence

In 1956, Fisher[432] introduced the term *impersistence* to characterize 10 patients with left hemiplegia who were unable to persist at a variety of willed acts, including eye closure, breath-holding, conjugate gaze deviation, tongue protrusion, and hand gripping. He noted that "mental impairment of some degree was always present" and that impersistence was "encountered almost exclusively in association with left hemiplegia." Many of the patients had accompanying left neglect, constructional apraxia, and anosognosia. Subsequent studies have found impersistence with both left and right hemispheral lesions individually.[428,433-436]

Impersistence has been correlated with the severity of the hemiparesis and with a poor prognosis for rehabilitation efforts, as well as with a variety of other deficits, including prosopagnosia, dressing apraxia, constructional apraxia, left neglect, and anosognosia.[425]

Dressing Apraxia

Brain[437] described "apraxia for dressing" in 1941. The syndrome appears with difficulty in the orientation of clothing during dressing.[438] There is a close association with constructional apraxia (see later).[439] In a setting of stroke, the syndrome occurs almost exclusively with lesions of the right hemisphere.

Loss of Topographic Memory and Disorientation for Place

This disorder is shown by an inability of patients to find their way in familiar surroundings, to recognize familiar surroundings, and to learn new routes in unfamiliar surroundings. Loss of topographic memory is somewhat different from disorientation to place, which refers to confusion about current location.[440,441] In milder cases, patients recognize surroundings as familiar; in more severe cases, even very familiar surroundings may seem strange. Loss of topographic memory is uncommon.[442] Although this is often considered a parietal lobe syndrome, right medial temporoparietal lesions may be the most common and may be in the territory of the posterior cerebral artery.[443] It can occur with unilateral stroke in either hemisphere.[444] The mechanism underlying loss of topographic memory is uncertain.[445,446]

Disorders of Spatial Localization

The right hemisphere plays a special role in the spatial localization of both visual and auditory stimuli. The most severe syndromes occur after posterior right hemisphere damage.[447,448] Short-term spatial memory (a skill analogous to the auditory short-term memory task of digit span) is a dominant function of the posterior right hemisphere.[447] Auditory localization of sounds in space also depends on an intact posterior right hemisphere.[103]

Confusion and Delirium

Acute confusion and delirium are states characterized by impaired orientation, diminished attention, and aberrant perception. Alertness is usually well-maintained, clarity and speed of thinking are diminished, and memories are poorly formed. Inattentiveness, poor concentration, and awareness of irrelevant stimuli are present. There is overlap between confusional and delirious states, and some investigators regard delirium as a subset of confusion. Delirium is characterized by disturbed perception with terrifying hallucinations, vivid dreams, fantasies, insomnia, and overactivity.

Acute confusional states have been reported after right MCA infarctions[449-451] and may be accompanied by retropulsion, unsteady gait, incontinence, difficulty in using common objects, and lack of concern for the illness. Mental agitation can evolve into a state of irritable sluggishness, inattention, and memory disorder. The disorder has been found in conjunction with parietal as well as temporal lesions.[410] Hallucinations, delusions, and agitation have also occurred.[400,452,453]

Caplan et al[454] found that posterior right temporal lesions were more likely to produce acute confusion than posterior right parietal lesions. The propensity of temporal lesions to produce confusional states may be explained by the proximity of these lesions to the underlying limbic system. Confusional states that follow brain infarction may result from one of two processes: disrupted modulation of affective responses in the limbic system or disruption of right hemisphere networks subserving attention.

Confabulation and Reduplicative Paramnesia

Confabulation, the unintentional production of inappropriate and fabricated information, is often associated with a failure to inhibit incorrect responses, poor error awareness, and poor self-correction abilities. Impaired memory, poor motivation, and anosognosia are often present. Although impairment of memory is often associated with confabulation, the two behaviors vary independently in severity.[455,456]

Reduplication is a special form of confabulation. It appears to reflect an attempt of brain-injured patients to fuse experiences from two disparate periods in their lives. In instances of reduplication for place, patients hold an inaccurate belief that two versions of a geographic location exist. Hospitalized patients may persist in believing that they are at home or at another hospital despite repeated attempts to orient them to current location.[457] Environmental reduplication occurs most commonly after right frontoparietal lobe injury. Reduplication of person (a false belief that two versions of an individual exist) may also occur after right hemisphere injury. Like reduplication of place, reduplication of person is a restricted form of confabulation.

Constructional Apraxia

In 1934, Kleist[236] defined constructional apraxia as "a disturbance which appears in formative activities (arranging, building, drawing) and in which a spatial part of the task is missed, although there is no apraxia of single movements." Clinically, the patients fail at tasks that require the manipulation of objects in space. A variety of tests have been utilized to identify constructional apraxia, including the copying of block designs, the copying of simple and complex figures, puzzle constructions, mental rotations, and three-dimensional model building. Constructional apraxia is synonymous with other terms, including apractognosia, constructional disability, and visual-spatial agnosia.

Constructional apraxia occurs after injury to either cerebral hemisphere.[458,459] Most lesions are parietal. The nature of constructional apraxia differs according to the hemisphere injured. Patients with left-sided lesions improve their drawings when aided by visual cues, whereas patients with right-sided lesions do not.[460] It is widely believed that the drawings of patients with left hemisphere damage are oversimplified and have reduced detail, whereas left unilateral neglect characterizes the drawings of patients with right hemisphere damage; however, Gainotti et al[461,462] were not able to distinguish right-sided from left-sided constructional apraxia. Lazar et al[463] reported the case of a 66-year-old woman with CT-verified infarction in the region of the right caudate nucleus and putamen who was tested with traditional clinical measures of perception, attention, and constructional apraxia, followed by the presentation of matching-to-sample procedures. The clinical measures first showed severe constructional apraxia

without hemineglect; the matching procedures then provided demonstrable evidence that she could not copy Greek letter forms that she could otherwise match with perfect accuracy, thereby eliminating perceptual dysfunction as a cause of her deficit.

Allesthesia

Allesthesia (also "allochiria") is the referral of a sensory stimulus (visual, tactile, or auditory) from one side of the body to the other.[17,414] Right hemisphere involvement with left-sided neglect is usually present. When the left side is touched, the sensation may be reported by the patient as occurring on the right side. Allesthesia may also occur in the setting of spinal cord injury or conversion hysteria.

Amusia

Amusia (loss of musical ability secondary to brain disease) has been an elusive deficit to study.[464-466] Brust[467] concluded that no simple relationship exists between the location of a lesion and the extent of musical disability. Case reports of expressive amusia after right hemisphere lesions are numerous. Affected patients are unable to sing or whistle, but their language function and melody recognition are preserved. Receptive amusia may also occur with right hemisphere lesions. Because of its complexity, the neural basis of music remains obscure. Amusia is an isolated phenomenon that may occur after right hemisphere lesions of varying location, size, and etiology. A remarkable case of a blind organist who had left hemispheral infarction with aphasia but without amusia (some of his poststroke compositions were published) suggests that a clear separation between the two entities is possible.[468]

Aprosody and Affective Agnosia

Monrad-Krohn[469] defined prosody as the musical quality of speech produced by "variations in pitch, rhythm, and stress of pronunciation." Buck and Duffy[470] reported that after right hemisphere damage, some patients are unable to intone affect into their speech; this deficit is known as aprosody. On the basis of their work and that of Heilman et al,[471] Ross and Mesulam[472] proposed that the right hemisphere was dominant for the modulation of affective language and that this modulation was organized in a fashion analogous to left hemisphere organization for propositional language. In a subsequent study, Ross[473] provided additional confirmatory evidence of the functional–anatomic organization of the affective components of language in the right hemisphere. By utilizing a combination of a bedside examination strategy analogous to a routine aphasia examination and CT mappings, he observed that the organization of affective language in the right hemisphere mirrored that of propositional language in the left hemisphere. The resulting disturbances of affective modulation were coined the aprosodias.

In analogy with the aphasias, Ross[473] proposed the existence of motor, sensory, global, conduction, and transcortical aprosodias. In motor aprosody, the patient is unable to utilize prosody to inject affect into speech, nor is the patient able to repeat the affect-laden prosody of others. However, the patient can comprehend the affect conveyed by the prosody of other speakers. The patient with sensory aprosody shows poor comprehension of affective prosody and cannot repeat affective prosody; however, the patient has normal spontaneous affective prosody in speech. Global aprosody is reflected in the drawing errors of apraxias. Hecaen and Albert[396] suggest that "constructional apraxia may result from a breakdown in different underlying neuropsychological mechanisms, depending on the hemisphere damaged."

Heilman and Van Den Abell,[474] noting that right temporoparietal lesions cause defects in the comprehension of affective speech, term this disorder *affective agnosia.* Tucker et al[475] observed that right temporoparietal lesions caused deficits both in affective comprehension and in evoking emotional intonation in a speech repetition task.

Treatment of Hemineglect

Proposed approaches to treat hemineglect have been available for more than 50 years, but positive results have been sparse with rare exceptions. For those whose neglect does not fade spontaneously, global inattention may impede necessary cooperation with treatment regimens. Most treatment trials have focused on altering the asymmetry of attention. One approach (called "top-down") uses external cues and guidance to engage the conscious and purposeful involvement of the patient. These treatments rely heavily on the participation of a therapist who provides continuous feedback, encouragement, and training. Cooperation and conscious effort on the part of the patient is required for success. Treatments that follow such an approach include visual scanning training,[418,476,477] sustained attention training,[478,479] and mental imagery training.[480] Alternatively, "bottom-up" approaches attempt to alter the attentional system by manipulating endogenous components of the neural axis, of which most is sensory input. This has been tried with prism glasses,[481] trunk rotation,[482,483] or by stimulation of the contralateral body with neck vibration,[484] limb movements,[485] or opticokinetic stimulation.[486,487] Combined top-down and bottom-up approaches include the moderately successful prism adaptation[488] method in which the patient wears prism glasses that shift the visual world further to the right (away from the neglected side). Training follows to move the attention leftward using a line bisection paradigm. Removal of the glasses may then produce a lasting shift of attention toward the neglected field.[489] A final approach has been to try to alter brain function directly, for example, with TMS to decrease overactive input from the contralateral parietal lobe.[490] Although this approach can result in an improved symmetry of attention at the time of the stimulus, the behavior reverts back to the hemiinattentive state once the stimulation stops.

REFERENCES

1. Abbie AA: The morphology of the forebrain arteries with especial reference to the evolution of the basal ganglia, *J Anat* 68:432, 1934.
2. Abbie AA: The vascular supply of the internal capsule, *Med J Aust*, 1934.
3. Beevor CE: On the distribution of the different arteries supplying the human brain, *Philos Trans R Soc Lond B Biol Sci* 200:1–55, 1909.
4. Foix C, Levy M: Les ramollissements sylviens, *Rev Neurol (Paris)* 11:51, 1927.
5. Shellshear JC: A contribution to our knowledge of the arterial supply of the cerebral cortex in man, *Brain* 50:236, 1927.
6. Lazorthes G, Gouaze A, Salomon G: *Vascularisation et circulation de l'encéphale,* Paris, 1976, Masson.
7. Mohr JP, Kase CS, Meckler RJ, Fisher CM: Sensorimotor stroke due to thalamocapsular ischemia, *Arch Neurol* 34:739, 1977.
8. Alexander L: The vascular supply of the striato-pallidum, *Res Publ Assoc Nerv Ment Dis* 21:77, 1941.
9. Gibo H, Carver CP, Rhoton AL, et al: Microsurgical anatomy of the middle cerebral artery, *J Neurosurg* 54:151, 1981.
10. Grand W: Microsurgical anatomy of the proximal middle cerebral artery and the internal carotid artery bifurcation, *Neurosurgery* 7:151, 1980.
11. Marinkovic R, Markovic L: The role of the middle cerebral artery in the vascularization of the claustrum, *Med Pregl* 43:361, 1990.
12. Amyes EW, Nielsen JM: Clinicopathologic study of vascular lesions of the anterior cingulate region, *Bull Los Angeles Neurol Soc* 20:112, 1955.
13. Waddington MM, Ring BA: Syndromes of occlusions of middle cerebral artery branches, *Brain* 91:685, 1968.
14. Fischer E: Die Lageabweichungen der vorden Hirnarterie im Gefaessbild, *Zentralbl Neurochir* 3:300, 1938.
15. Teal JS, Rumbaugh CL, Bergeron RT, et al: Anomalies of the middle cerebral artery: Accessory artery, duplication, and early bifurcation, *Am J Roentgenol Radium Ther Nucl Med* 118:567, 1973.
16. Umansky F, Dujovny M, Ausman JI, et al: Anomalies and variations of the middle cerebral artery: A microanatomical study, *Neurosurgery* 22:1023, 1988.
17. Jain KK: Some observations on the anatomy of the middle cerebral artery, *Can J Surg* 7:134, 1964.
18. Akelatis AJ: Symmetrical bilateral granular atrophy of the cerebral cortex of vascular origin: A clinico-pathologic study, *Am J Psychiatry* 99:447, 1942.
19. Brierley JB, Adams JH, Connor RCR, Triep CS: The effects of systemic hypotension upon the human brain, *Brain* 89:235, 1966.
20. Romanul FCA, Abramowicz A: Changes in brain and pial vessels in arterial borderzones, *Arch Neurol* 11:40, 1964.
21. Strong KC: A study of the structure of the media of the distributing arteries by the method of microdissection, *Anat Rec* 72:151, 1938.
22. Baker AB: Structure of the small cerebral arteries and their changes with age, *Am J Pathol* 13:453, 1937.
23. Stehbens WE: Focal intimal proliferation in the cerebral arteries, *Am J Pathol* 36:289, 1960.
24. Wolff HG: The cerebral blood vessels—anatomical principles, *Res Publ Assoc Res Nerv Ment Dis* 18:39, 1938.
25. Clower BR, Sullivan DM, Smith RR: Intracranial vessels lack vasa vasorum, *J Neurosurg* 61:44, 1984.
26. Maksimow AA, Bloom W: *A textbook of histology,* ed 4, Philadelphia, 1942, WB Saunders.
27. Gross CR, Kase CS, Mohr JP, et al: Stroke in south Alabama: Incidence and diagnostic features—a population based study, *Stroke* 15:249, 1984.
28. Kunitz S, Gross CR, Heyman A, et al: The pilot Stroke Data Bank: Definition, design, data, *Stroke* 15:740, 1984.
29. Lhermitte F, Gautier JC, Derouesne C: Nature of occlusions of the middle cerebral artery, *Neurology (Minneap)* 20:82, 1970.
30. Chiari H: Ueber das Verhalten des Teilungswinkels der Carotis communis bei der Endarteritis chronic deformans, *Verh Dtsch Ges Pathol* 9:326, 1905.
31. Friedlich AL, Castleman B, Mohr JP: Case records of the Massachusetts General Hospital, *N Engl J Med* 278:1109, 1968.
32. Gleysteen JJ, Silver D: Paradoxical arterial embolism: Collective review, *Am Surg* 36:47, 1970.
33. Fairfax AJ, Lambert CD, Leatham A: Systemic embolism in chronic sinoatrial disorder, *N Engl J Med* 275:190, 1976.
34. Barnett HJM, Jones MW, Boughner DR, Kostuk WJ: Cerebral ischemic events associated with prolapsing mitral valve, *Arch Neurol* 33:777, 1976.

35. Bluschke V, Hennerici M, Scharf RE, et al: Mitralklappenprolaps-Syndrom und Thrombozytenaktivität bei jungen Patienten mit zerebralen Ischämien, *Dtsch Med Wochenschr* 107:410, 1982.
36. Kooiker JC, MacLean JM, Sumi SM: Cerebral embolism, marantic endocarditis, and cancer, *Arch Neurol* 33:260, 1976.
37. Neufield HN, Cadman NL, Miller AW, Edwards JE: Embolism from marantic endocarditis as a manifestation of occult carcinoma, *Proc Staff Meet Mayo Clin* 35:292, 1960.
38. David NJ, Gordon KK, Friedberg SJ, et al: Fatal atheromatous cerebral embolism associated with bright plaques in the retinal arterioles, *Neurology* 13:708, 1963.
39. Wood EH, Correll JW: Atheromatous ulceration in major neck vessels as a cause of cerebral embolism, *Acta Radiol Diagn (Stockh)* 9:520, 1969.
40. Kase CS, White L, Vinson L, Eichelberger P: Shotgun pellet embolus to the middle cerebral artery, *Neurology* 31:458, 1981.
41. Kerbler S, Schober PH, Steiner H: Traumatische Embolisierung der Arteria cerebri media, *Z Kinderchir* 45:301, 1990.
42. Hollin SA, Silverstein A: Transient occlusion of the middle cerebral artery, *JAMA* 194:243, 1965.
43. Pessin MS, Duncan GW, Mohr JP, Poskanzer DC: Clinical and angiographic features of carotid transient ischemic attacks, *N Engl J Med* 296:358, 1977.
44. Moustafa RR, Izquierdo D, Weissberg PL, et al: Neurological picture. Identifying aortic plaque inflammation as a potential cause of stroke, *J Neurol Neurosurg Psychiatry* 79:236, 2008.
45. Caplan LR, Hier DB, D'Cruz I: Cerebral embolism in the Michael Reese Stroke Registry, *Stroke* 14:30, 1983.
46. Davis DO, Rumbaugh CL, Gilson JM: Angiographic diagnosis of small-vessel cerebral emboli, *Acta Radiol Diagn (Stockh)* 9:264, 1969.
47. Weiller C, Ringelstein EB, Reiche W, et al: The large striatocapsular infarct: A clinical and pathophysiological entity, *Arch Neurol* 47:1085, 1990.
48. Stringer WL, Kelly DL: Traumatic dissection of the extracranial internal carotid artery, *Neurosurgery* 6:123, 1980.
49. Deck JHN, Lee MA: Mucin embolism to cerebral arteritis: A fatal complication of carcinoma of the breast, *J Can Sci Neurol* 5:327, 1978.
50. Glew RH: Case records of the Massachusetts General Hospital, *N Engl J Med* 301:36, 1979.
51. Yufe R, Karpati G, Carpenter S: Cardiac myxoma: A diagnostic challenge for the neurologist, *Neurology* 26:1060, 1976.
52. Bonhoeffer K: Klinischer und anatomischer Befund zur Lehre von der Apraxie und der "motorische Sprachbahn," *Monatsschr Psychiatr Neurol* 35:113, 1914.
53. Cohen MM, Hemalatha CP, D'Addario RT, Goldman HW: Embolism from a fusiform middle cerebral artery aneurysm, *Stroke* 11:58, 1980.
54. Sylaja PN, Hill MD: Stroke due to calcific embolus following coronary angiography, *Neurology* 67:E16, 2006.
55. Steiner TJ, Rail DL, Rose FC: Cholesterol crystal embolization in rat brain: a model for atherosclerotic cerebral infarction, *Stroke* 11:184, 1980.
56. Edwards JH, Kricheff II, Riles T, Imparato A: Angiographically undetected ulceration of the carotid bifurcation as a cause of embolic stroke, *Radiology* 132:369, 1979.
57. Imparato AM, Riles TS, Gorstein F: The carotid bifurcation plaque: Pathologic findings associated with cerebral ischemia, *Stroke* 10:238, 1979.
58. Toro-Gonzalez G, Navarro-Roman L, Roman GC, et al: Acute ischemic stroke from fibrocartilaginous embolism to the middle cerebral artery, *Stroke* 24:738, 1993.
59. Liebeskind A, Chinichian A, Schechter MM: The moving embolus seen during serial cerebral angiography, *Stroke* 2:440, 1971.
60. Gacs G, Merei F, Bodosi M: Balloon catheter as a model of cerebral emboli in humans, *Stroke* 13:39, 1982.
61. Bladin PF: A radiologic and pathologic study of embolism of the internal carotid–middle cerebral arterial axis, *Radiology* 82:614, 1964.
62. Broca P: Remarques sur le siège de la faculté du langage articule, suivies d'une observation d'aphémie (perte de la parole), *Bull Soc Anat Paris* 6:330, 1861.
63. Zatz LM, Iannone AM, Eckman PB, Hecker SP: Observations concerning intracerebral vascular occlusion, *Neurology* 15:390, 1965.
64. Lhermitte F, Gautier JC, Derouesne C, Guiraud B: Ischemic accidents in the middle cerebral artery territory (a study of the causes in 122 cases), *Arch Neurol* 19:248, 1968.
65. Delal PM, Shah PM, Aiyar RR: Arteriographic study of cerebral embolism, *Lancet* 2:358, 1965.
66. Fisher CM, Gore I, Okabe N, White PD: Atherosclerosis of the carotid and vertebral arteries: Extracranial and intracranial, *J Neuropathol Exp Neurol* 24:455, 1965.
67. Minematsu K, Yamaguchi T, Omae T: "Spectacular shrinking deficit": Rapid recovery from a full hemispheral syndrome by migration of an embolus, *Neurology* 41(Suppl):329, 1991.
68. Donnan GA, Bladin PF, Berkovic SF, et al: The stroke syndrome of striatocapsular infarction, *Brain* 114:51, 1991.
69. Pessin MS, Hinton RC, Davis KR, et al: Mechanisms of acute carotid stroke, *Ann Neurol* 6:245, 1979.
70. Wolpert SM, Stein BM: Catheter embolization of intracranial arteriovenous malformations as an aid to surgical excision, *Neuroradiology* 10:73, 1975.
71. Kusske JA, Kelly WA: Embolization and reduction of the "steal" syndrome in cerebral AVMs, *J Neurosurg* 40:313, 1974.
72. Sakai T, Kuzuhara S: Diffusion-weighted magnetic resonance imagings at the acute stage in two patients with spectacular shrinking deficit due to cardioembolic stroke, *Rinsho Shinkeigaku* 46:122-127, 2006.
73. Fisher CM, Pearlman A: The non-sudden onset of cerebral embolism, *Neurology (Minneap)* 17:1025, 1967.
74. Fisher CM: Capsular infarcts, *Arch Neurol* 36:65, 1979.
75. Lascelles RG, Burrows EH: Occlusion of the middle cerebral artery, *Brain* 88:85, 1966.
76. Aring CD, Merritt HH: Differential diagnosis between cerebral hemorrhage and cerebral thrombosis, *Arch Intern Med* 56:435, 1935.
77. Fisher CM: Occlusion of the internal carotid artery, *AMA Arch Neurol Psychiatry* 69:346, 1951.
78. Blackwood W, Bratty P, Mair WGP: In Jakob H, editor: *Observations on occlusive vascular disease of the brain*, vol 3, Stuttgart, 1963, Thieme Verlag, p 146.
79. Fisher CM: Cerebral ischemia: less familiar types, *Clin Neurosurg* 18:267, 1971.
80. Hinton RC, Mohr JP, Ackerman RA, et al: Symptomatic middle cerebral artery stenosis, *Ann Neurol* 5:152, 1979.
81. Irino T, Tandea M, Minami T: Angiographic manifestations in postrecanalized cerebral infarction, *Neurology* 27:471, 1977.
82. Kumral E, Ozdemirkiran T, Alper Y: Strokes in the subinsular territory: clinical, topographical, and etiological patterns, *Neurology* 63:2429-2432, 2004.
83. Kawase T, Mizukami M, Tazawa T, Araki G: The significance of lenticulostriate arteries in transient ischemic attack: Neuroradiological and regional cerebral blood flow studies, *Brain Nerve* 31:1033, 1979.
84. Araki G: Small infarctions of the basal ganglia with special reference to transient ischemic attacks, *Recent Adv Gerontol* 469:161, 1978.
85. Feldmeyer JJ, Merendaz C, Regli F: Sténoses symptomatiques de l'artère cérébrale moyenne, *Rev Neurol (Paris)* 139:725, 1983.
86. Day AL: Anatomy of the extracranial vessels. In Smith RR, editor: *Stroke and the extracranial vessels*, New York, 1984, Raven Press, p 9.
87. Corston RN, Kendall BE, Marshall J: Prognosis in middle cerebral artery stenosis, *Stroke* 15:237, 1984.
88. Adams HP, Gross CE: Embolism distal to stenosis of the middle cerebral artery, *Stroke* 12:228, 1981.
89. Hyland HH: Thrombosis of intracranial arteries, *Arch Neurol Psychiatry* 30:342, 1933.
90. Wolman L: Cerebral dissecting aneurysms, *Brain* 82:276, 1959.
91. Bigelow NH: Intracranial dissecting aneurysms: An analysis of their significance, *Arch Pathol* 60:271, 1955.
92. Hirsch CS, Roessmann U: Arterial dysplasia with ruptured basilar artery aneurysm: Report of a case, *Hum Pathol* 6:749, 1975.
93. Yamashita M, Tanaka K, Matsuo T, et al: Cerebral dissecting aneurysms in patients with moyamoya disease, *J Neurosurg* 58:120, 1983.
94. Dratz HM, Woodhall B: Traumatic dissecting aneurysm of left internal carotid, anterior cerebral and middle cerebral arteries, *J Neuropathol Exp Neurol* 6:286, 1947.

95. Yonas H, Agamanolis D, Takaoka Y, et al: Dissecting intracranial aneurysms, *Surg Neurol* 8:407, 1977.

96. Turnbull HM: Alterations in arterial structures, and their relation to syphilis, *Q J Med* 8:201, 1915.

97. Sinclair W Jr: Dissecting aneurysm of the middle cerebral artery associated with migraine syndrome, *Am J Pathol* 29:1083, 1953.

98. Johnson AC, Graves VB, Pfaff JP Jr: Dissecting aneurysm of intracranial arteries, *Surg Neurol* 7:49, 1977.

99. Duman S, Stephans JW: Post-traumatic middle cerebral artery occlusion, *Neurology* 13:613, 1963.

100. Adams RD, Victor M: *Principles of neurology*, New York, 1984, McGraw-Hill.

101. Gupta SR, Mlcoch AG, Stolaro C, Montz T: Bromocriptine treatment of nonfluent aphasia, *Neurology* 45:2170, 1995.

102. Lazar RM, Fitzsimmons B-F, Marshall RS, et al: Midazolam challenge reinduces neurological deficits after transient ischemic attack, *Stroke* 34:794, 2003.

103. Bisiach E, Cornacchia L, Sterzi R, Vallar G: Disorder of perceived auditory lateralization after lesions of the hemisphere, *Brain* 107:37, 1984.

104. Hacke W, Schwab S, Horn M, et al: 'Malignant' middle cerebral artery territory infarction: Clinical course and prognostic signs, *Arch Neurol* 53:309, 1996.

105. Steiner T, Ringleb P, Hacke W: Treatment options for large hemispheric stroke, *Neurology* 57(Suppl 2):S61, 2001.

106. Bousser MG, Dubois B, Castaigne P: Pertes de connaissance brèves au cours des accidents ischemiques cérébraux, *Ann Med Interne (Paris)* 132:300, 1981.

107. Rengachary SS, Batnitzky S, Morantz RA, et al: Hemicraniectomy for acute mass of cerebral infarction, *Neurosurgery* 8:321, 1981.

108. Davison C, Goodhart SP, Needles W: Cerebral localization and cerebral vascular disease, *Arch Neurol Psychiatry* 30:749, 1933.

109. Henschen SE: *Klinische und Anatomische Beitrage zur Pathologie des Gehirns*, Stockholm, 1920, Nordiska.

110. Mohr JP, Foulkes MA, Polis AT, et al: Infarct topography and hemiparesis profiles with cerebral convexity infarction: The Stroke Data Bank, *J Neurol Neurosurg Psychiatry* 56:344, 1993.

111. Barat M, Constant P, Mazaux JM, et al: Corrélations anatomo-cliniques dans l'aphasie: Apport de la tomodensitometrie, *Rev Neurol (Paris)* 134:611, 1978.

112. Rondot P: Syndromes of central motor disorder. In Vinken PJ, Bruyn GW, editors: *Handbook of clinical neurology, vol 1: Disturbances of nervous function*, Amsterdam, 1969, North-Holland Publishing, p 169.

113. Gazengel JGL: *Etude de 276 emboles cérébrales d'origine cardiaque: Thèse Faculté de Médécine de Paris*, Paris, 1966, Editions AGEMP, p 123.

114. Obrador S: Nervous integration after hemispherectomy in man. In Schaltenbrand G, Woolsey CN, editors: *Cerebral localization and organization*, Madison, Wisc, 1964, University of Wisconsin Press, p 133.

115. Fisher CM, Curry HB: Pure motor hemiplegia of vascular origin, *Arch Neurol* 13:30, 1965.

116. Hanaway J, Torack R, Fletcher AP, Landau WM: Intracranial bleeding associated with urokinase therapy for acute ischemic hemispheral stroke, *Stroke* 7:143, 1976.

117. Healton EB, Navarro C, Bressman S, Brust JCM: Subcortical neglect, *Neurology (NY)* 32:776, 1982.

118. Demierre B, Rondot P: Dystonia caused by putamino-capsulo-caudate vascular lesions, *J Neurol Neurosurg Psychiatry* 46:404, 1983.

119. Santamaria J, Graus F, Rubio F, et al: Cerebral infarction of the basal ganglia due to embolism from the heart, *Stroke* 14:911, 1983.

120. Bruyn GW, Gathier JC: The operculum syndrome. In Vinken PJ, Bruyn GW, editors: *Handbook of clinical neurology, vol 2*, Amsterdam, 1976, North Holland Publishing, p 776.

121. Hinkle JL: Variables explaining functional recovery following motor stroke, *J Neurosci Nurs* 38:6–12, 2006.

122. Harvey RL, Winstein CJ: Everest Trial Group Design for the Everest Randomized Trial of Cortical Stimulation and Rehabilitation for Arm Function Following Stroke, *Neurorehabil Neural Repair* 23:32–44, 2009.

123. Broadbent WH: On the cerebral mechanism of speech and thought, *Trans R Med Chir Soc (Lond)* 55:145, 1872.

124. Phillips CG: Some thoughts on the organization of the motor cortex. In Eccles JC, editor: *The brain and conscious experience*, New York, 1966, Springer-Verlag.

125. Mohr JP: Rapid amelioration of motor aphasia, *Arch Neurol* 28:77, 1973.

126. Alajouanine T, Boudin G, Pertuiset B, Pepin B: Le syndrome operculaire unilatéral avec atteinte contralatérale du territoire des V, VII, IX, XI, XIIème nerfs craniens, *Rev Neurol (Paris)* 101:167, 1959.

127. Dejerine J: *Séméiologie des affections du système nerveux*, Paris, 1914, Masson.

128. von Monakow K: *Die Lokalisation im Grosshirn und der Abbau der Funktion durch Kortikale Herde*, Wiesbaden, 1914, JF Begman.

129. Dejerine J, Regnard M: Monoplegie brachiale gauche limitée aux muscles des eminences thenar, hypothenar et aux interosseux: Astereognosie, épilepsie jacksonienne, *Rev Neurol* 1:285, 1912.

130. Garcin R: Paralysie dissociée du median d'origine corticale (sur le caractère durement familial de certains accidents vasculaires cérébraux), *Médecine* 137, 1932.

131. Hall J, Flint AC: Neurological picture. Hand knob infarction, *J Neurol Neurosurg Psychiatry* 79:406, 2008.

132. Schneider R, Gautier JC: Leg weakness due to stroke: Site of lesions, weakness patterns and causes, *Brain* 117:347, 1994.

133. Saver JL, Johnston KC, Homer D, et al: Infarct volume as a surrogate or auxiliary outcome measure in ischemic stroke clinical trials, *Stroke* 30:293–298, 1999.

134. Johnston SC, Rothwell PM, Nguyen-Huynh MN, et al: Validation and refinement of scores to predict very early stroke risk after transient ischaemic attack, *Lancet* 369:283–292, 2007.

135. Finocchi C, Gandolfo C, Gasparetto B, et al: Value of early variables as predictors of short-term outcome in patients with acute focal cerebral ischemia, *Ital J Neurol Sci* 17:341–346, 1996.

136. Johnston KC, Barrett KM, Ding YH, et al: Clinical and imaging data at 5 days as a surrogate for 90-day outcome in ischemic stroke, *Stroke* 40:1332–1333, 2009.

137. Lyden PD, Lu M, Levine SR, et al: A modified National Institutes of Health Stroke Scale for use in stroke clinical trials: preliminary reliability and validity, *Stroke* 32:1310–1317, 2001.

138. Dhamoon M, Lazar R, Marshall R: Impairment versus activity limitation after incident ischemic stroke, *Int J Stroke* 5:132–133, 2010.

139. Duncan PW, Goldstein LB, Matchar D, et al: Measurement of motor recovery after stroke. Outcome assessment and sample size requirements, *Stroke* 23:1084–1089, 1992.

140. Schiemanck SK, Post MW, Kwakkel G, et al: Ischemic lesion volume correlates with long-term functional outcome and quality of life of middle cerebral artery stroke survivors, *Restor Neurol Neurosci* 23:257–263, 2005.

141. Crafton KR, Mark AN, Cramer SC: Improved understanding of cortical injury by incorporating measures of functional anatomy, *Brain* 126:1650–1659, 2003.

142. Prabhakaran S, Zarahn E, Riley C, et al: Inter-individual variability in the capacity for motor recovery after ischemic stroke, *Neurorehabil Neural Repair* 22:64–71, 2008.

143. Marshall RS, Zarahn E, Alon L, et al: Early imaging correlates of subsequent motor recovery after stroke, *Ann Neurol* 65:596–602, 2009.

144. Marshall RS, Perera GM, Lazar RM, et al: Evolution of cortical activation during recovery from corticospinal tract infarction, *Stroke* 31:656–661, 2000.

145. Dijkhuizen RM, Singhal AB, Mandeville JB, et al: Correlation between brain reorganization, ischemic damage, and neurologic status after transient focal cerebral ischemia in rats: A functional magnetic resonance imaging study, *J Neurosci* 23:510–517, 2003.

146. Ward NS, Brown MM, Thompson AJ, et al: Neural correlates of motor recovery after stroke: A longitudinal fMRI study, *Brain* 126:2476–2496, 2003.

147. Cao Y, D'Olhaberriague L, Vikingstad EM, et al: Pilot study of functional MRI to assess cerebral activation of motor function after poststroke hemiparesis, *Stroke* 29:112–122, 1998.

148. Feydy A, Carlier R, Roby-Brami A, et al: Longitudinal study of motor recovery after stroke: recruitment and focusing of brain activation, *Stroke* 33:1610–1617, 2002.

149. Calautti C, Leroy F, Guincestre JY, et al: Sequential activation brain mapping after subcortical stroke: Changes in hemispheric balance and recovery, *Neuroreport* 12:3883–3886, 2001.

150. Murase N, Duque J, Mazzocchio R, et al: Influence of interhemispheric interactions on motor function in chronic stroke, *Ann Neurol* 55:400–409, 2004.

151. Khedr EM, Ahmed MA, Fathy N, et al: Therapeutic trial of repetitive transcranial magnetic stimulation after acute ischemic stroke, *Neurology* 65:466–468, 2005.

152. Hummel F, Celnik P, Giraux P, et al: Effects of non-invasive cortical stimulation on skilled motor function in chronic stroke, *Brain* 128:490–499, 2005.

153. Prevost JL: *De la déviation conjuguée des yeux et de la rotation de la tête*, Paris, 1896, Thèse.

154. Bramwell B: A remarkable case of aphasia, *Brain* 21:343, 1898.

155. Grimes JD, Hassan MN, Quarrington AM, d'Alton J: Delayed-onset post hemiplegic dystonia: CT demonstration of basal ganglia pathology, *Neurology (NY)* 32:1033, 1982.

156. Austregesilo A, Borges-Forte A: Sur un cas de hemischorée avec lésion du noyau caude, *Rev Neurol (Paris)* 67:477, 1937.

157. Bizzi E: Discharge of frontal eye field neurons during saccadic and following eye movements in unanesthetized monkeys, *Exp Brain Res* 6:69, 1968.

158. Pederson RA, Troost BT: Abnormalities of gaze in cerebrovascular disease, *Stroke* 12:251, 1981.

159. Pierrot-Deseilligny C: Saccade and smooth-pursuit impairment after cerebral hemispheric lesions, *Eur Neurol* 34:121, 1994.

160. Tijssen CC: Contralateral conjugate eye deviation in acute supratentorial lesions, *Stroke* 25:1516, 1994.

161. Bizzi E: Discharge of frontal eye field neurons during eye movements in unanesthetized monkeys, *Science* 157:1588, 1967.

162. Daroff RB, Hoyt WF, et al: Supranuclear disorders of ocular control system in man: Clinical, anatomical and physiological correlates. In Bach-Y-Rita P, Collins CC, editors: *The control of eye movements*, New York, 1971, Academic Press, p 175.

163. Holmes G: The cerebral integration of the ocular movements, *BMJ* 2:108, 1938.

164. Bender MB: Brain control of conjugate horizontal and vertical eye movements: A survey of the structural and functional correlates, *Brain* 103:23, 1980.

165. Schiller PH, True SD, Conway JL: Effects of frontal eye field and superior colliculus ablations on eye movements, *Science* 206:590, 1979.

166. De Renzi E, Colombo A, Faglioni P, Gilbertoni N: Conjugate gaze paresis in stroke patients with unilateral damage, *Arch Neurol* 39:42, 1982.

167. Mohr JP: Broca's area and Broca's aphasia. In Whitaker H, editor: *Studies in neurolinguistics*, New York, 1976, Academic Press, p 201.

168. Mohr JP, Rubinstein LV, Kase CS, et al: Gaze palsy in hemispheral stroke: The NINCDS Stroke Data Bank. Presented at the Annual Meeting of the American Academy of Neurology, Boston, April 12, 1984.

169. Brandt T, Botzel K, Yousry T, et al: Rotational vertigo in embolic stroke of the vestibular and auditory cortices, *Neurology* 45:42, 1995.

170. Cukiert A, Cukiert CM, Argentoni M, et al: Outcome after hemispherectomy in hemiplegic adult patients with refractory epilepsy associated with early middle cerebral artery infarcts, *Epilepsia* 50:1381–1384, 2009.

171. Lhermitte F, Desi M, Signoret JL, Deloche G: Aphasie kinesthetique associée à un syndrome pseudothalamique, *Rev Neurol (Paris)* 136:675, 1980.

172. Birklein F, Rolke R, Müller-Forell W: Isolated insular infarction eliminates contralateral cold, cold pain, and pinprick perception, *Neurology* 65:1381, 2005.

173. Foix C, Chavany J-A, Levy M: Syndrome pseudo-thalamique d'origine pariétale: Lésion de l'artère du sillon interpariétal (Pa P1 P2 antérieurs, petit territoire insulo-capsulaire), *Rev Neurol (Paris)* 35:68, 1927.

174. Derouesne C, Mas JL, Bolgert AF, Castaigne P: Pure sensory stroke caused by a small cortical infarct in the middle cerebral artery territory, *Stroke* 15:660, 1984.

175. Paillard J, Michel F, Stelmach G: Localization without content: A tactile analogue of "blind sight," *Arch Neurol* 40:548, 1983.

176. Gacs G, Fox AJ, Barnett HJM, Vinuela F: CT visualization of intracranial arterial thromboembolism, *Stroke* 14:756, 1983.

177. Miller NR: *Walsh and Hoyt's clinical neuro-ophthalmology*, ed 4, Baltimore, 1983, Williams & Wilkins.

178. Weinstein EA, Kahn RL: The syndrome of anosognosia, *Arch Neurol Psychiatr* 64:772, 1950.

179. Bounds JV, Sandok BA, Barnhorst DA: Fatal cerebral embolism following aorto-coronary bypass graft surgery, *Stroke* 7:611, 1976.

180. Gay AJ, Newman NM, Keltner JL: *Eye movement disorders*, St. Louis, 1974, CV Mosby.

181. Smith JL: *Optokinetic nystagmus*, Springfield, Ill, 1963, Charles C Thomas.

182. Costa LD, Vaughan G Jr, Horwitz M, et al: Patterns of behavioral deficit associated with visual spatial neglect, *Cortex* 5:242, 1969.

183. Stenvers HW: Ueber die klinische Bedeutung des optischen Nystagmus für die zerebrale Diagnostik, *Schweiz Arch Neurol Psychiatr* 14:279, 1925.

184. Baloh RW, Yee RD, Honrubia V: Optokinetic nystagmus and parietal lobe lesions, *Ann Neurol* 7:269, 1980.

185. Labar DR, Mohr JP, Nichols FT, Tatemichi TK: Unilateral hyperhidrosis after cerebral infarction, *Neurology* 38:1679, 1988.

186. Appenzeller O: *The autonomic nervous system*, Amsterdam, 1970, North Holland Publishing.

187. Cereda C, Ghika J, Maeder P, Bogousslavsky J: Strokes restricted to the insular cortex 1, *Neurology* 59:2002, 1950.

188. Lazar RM, Marshall RS, Mohr JP: Aphasia and stroke. In Bogousslavsky J, Caplan L, editors: *Stroke syndromes*, New York, 1995, Cambridge University Press, p 118.

189. Weisenberg T, McBride K: *Aphasia: A clinical and psychological study*, New York, 1935, Hafner.

190. Brain WR: *Speech disorders*, London, 1962, Butterworths.

191. Brown JW: *Aphasia, apraxia, and agnosia*, Springfield, IL, 1972, Charles C Thomas.

192. Nadeau S, Crosson B: Subcortical aphasia, *Brain Lang* 58:355, 1997.

193. Brust JCM, Shafer SQ, Richter RW, Bruun B: Aphasia in acute stroke, *Stroke* 7:167, 1976.

194. Marquardson J: The natural history of acute cerebral vascular disease: A retrospective study of 769 patients, *Acta Neurol Scand Suppl* 38:45, 1969.

195. Mohr JP, Sidman M, Stoddard LT, et al: Evolution of the deficit in total aphasia, *Neurology* 23:1302, 1973.

196. Mazzocchi F, Vignolo LA: Localization of lesions in aphasia: Clinical-CT scan correlations in stroke patients, *Cortex* 15:627, 1979.

197. Naeser MA, Hayward RW: Lesion localization in aphasia with cranial computerized tomography and The Boston Diagnostic Aphasia Examination, *Neurology* 28:545, 1978.

198. Quast MJ, Huang NC, Hillman GR, Kent TA: The evolution of acute stroke recorded by multimodal magnetic resonance imaging, *Magn Reson Imaging* 11(4):465–471, 1993.

199. Schlaug G, Benfield A, Baird AE, et al: The ischemic penumbra: operationally defined by diffusion and perfusion MRI, *Neurology*. 53(7):1528–1537, 1999.

200. Keller SS, Crow T, Foundas A, et al: Broca's area: nomenclature, anatomy, typology and asymmetry, *Brain Lang* 109(1):29–48, 2009.

201. Hillis AE, Barker PB, Beauchamp NJ, et al: MR perfusion imaging reveals regions of hypoperfusion associated with aphasia and neglect, *Neurology* 55(6):782–788, 2000.

202. Lee A, Kannan V, Hillis AE: The contribution of neuroimaging to the study of language and aphasia, *Neuropsychol Rev* 16(4):171–183, 2006.

203. Boulliaud J: Recherches cliniques propres à demonstrer que la perte de la parole correspond à la lésion des lobules antérieurs du cerveau, et à confirmer l'opinion de M. Gall sur le siège de l'organe du langage articule, *Arch Gen Med* 8:25, 1825.

204. Dronkers NF, Plaisant O, Iba-Zizen MT, et al: Paul Broca's historic cases: high resolution MR imaging of the brains of Leborgne and Lelong, *Brain* 130(Pt 5):1432–1441, 2007.

205. Grodzinsky Y, Santi A: The battle for Broca's region, *Trends Cogn Sci* 12(12):474–480, 2008.

206. Albert ML, Goodglass H, Helm NA, et al: *Clinical aspects of dysphasia*, New York, 1981, Springer-Verlag.

207. Knopman DS, Selnes OA, Niccum N, et al: A longitudinal study of speech fluency in aphasia: CT correlates of recovery and persistent nonfluency, *Neurology (Cleve)* 33:1170, 1983.
208. Wernicke C: The symptom-complex of aphasia. In Church A, editor: *Modern clinical medical disease of the nervous system*, New York, 1908, Appleton.
209. Luria AR: *Higher cortical functions in man*, New York, 1966, Basic Books.
210. Goldstein K: *Language and language disturbances*, New York, 1948, Grune & Stratton.
211. Head H: *Aphasia and kindred disorders of speech*, London, 1926, Cambridge University Press.
212. Liepmann H: Diseases of the brain. In Barr CW, editor: *Curschmann's textbook of nervous diseases, vol 1*, Philadelphia, 1915, Blakiston, p 467.
213. Alajouanine T, Ombredane A, Durand M: *Le syndrome de désintégration phonétique dans l'aphasie*, Paris, 1939, Masson.
214. De Renzi E, Pieczuro A, Vignola L: Oral apraxia and aphasia, *Cortex* 2:50, 1966.
215. Benson DF: *Aphasia, alexia and agraphia*, New York, 1979, Churchill Livingstone.
216. Benson DF, Sheremata WA, Bouchard R, et al: Conduction aphasia, *Arch Neurol* 28:339, 1973.
217. Hughlings-Jackson J: On affections of speech from diseases of the brain, *Brain* 38:106, 1910.
218. Niessl von Mayendorf E: Ueber die sogenannter Brocasche Windung und ihre Angebliche Bedeutung für den motorischen Sprach, *Monatsschr Psychiatr Neurol* 61:129, 1926.
219. Goodglass H, Kaplan E: *The assessment of aphasia and related disorders*, Philadelphia, 1972, Lee & Febiger.
220. Barat M, Mazaux JM, Bioulac B, et al: Troubles de langage de type aphasique et lésions putamino-caudées, *Rev Neurol (Paris)* 137:343, 1981.
221. Kertesz A, Harlock W, Coates R: Computer tomographic localization, lesion size and prognosis in aphasia and nonverbal impairment, *Brain Lang* 8:34, 1979.
222. Mohr JP, Pessin MS, Finkelstein S, et al: Broca aphasia: Pathologic and clinical aspects, *Neurology* 28:311, 1978.
223. Naeser MA: CT scan lesion size and lesion locus in cortical and subcortical aphasias. In Kertesz A, editor: *Localization in neuropsychology*, New York, 1983, Academic Press, p 63.
224. Moutier F: *L'aphasie de Broca*, Paris, 1908, Thèse Médecine.
225. Levine DN, Sweet E: Localization in lesions in Broca's motor aphasia. In Kertesz A, editor: *Localization in neuropsychology*, New York, 1983, Academic Press, p 185.
226. Van Gehuchten P: *The scientific work of Arthur Van Gehuchten*, Louvain, 1974, Francqui Fondation, p 60.
227. Lazar RM, Minzer B, Antoniello D, et al: Improvement in aphasia scores after stroke is well predicted by initial severity, *Stroke* 41:1485–1488, 2010.
228. Saur D, Lange R, Baumgaertner A, et al: Dynamics of language reorganization after stroke, *Brain* 129:1371–1384, 2006.
229. LaCours AR, Lhermitte F: The "pure form" of the phonetic disintegration syndrome (pure anarthria): Anatomical-clinical report of a historical case, *Brain Lang* 3:88, 1976.
230. Tonkonogy J, Goodglass H: Language function, foot of the third frontal gyrus, and rolandic operculum, *Arch Neurol* 38:486, 1981.
231. Darley FL, Aaronson A, Brown J: *Motor speech disorders*, Philadelphia, 1975, WB Saunders.
232. Masdeu JC, O'Hara RJ: Motor aphasia unaccompanied by faciobrachial weakness, *Neurology (Cleve)* 33:519, 1983.
233. Chouppe: Ramollissement superficiel du cerveau intéressant surtout la troisième circonvolution frontale gauche, sans aphasie, *Bull Soc Anat Paris* 45:365, 1870.
234. Agostini E, Coletti A, Orlando G, Tredici G: Apraxia in deep cerebral lesions, *J Neurol Neurosurg Psychiatry* 46:804, 1983.
235. Levine DN, Mohr JP: Language after bilateral cerebral infarctions: Role of the minor hemisphere and speech, *Neurology* 29:927, 1979.
236. Kleist K: *Gehirnpathologie*, Barth, 1934, Leipzig.
237. Foix C, Aphasies: In Roger GH, Widal F, Teissier PJ, editors: *Nouveau traité de médecine, vol 18*, Paris, 1928, Masson, p 135.
238. Levine DN, Sweet E: The neuropathologic basis of Broca's aphasia and its implications for the cerebral control of speech. In Arbib M, Kaplan D, Marshall J, editors: *Neural models of language processes*, New York, 1982, Academic Press.
239. Rascol A, Clanet M, Manelfe C: Pure motor hemiplegia: CT study of 30 cases, *Stroke* 13:11, 1982.
240. Damasio AR, Damasio H, Rizzo M, et al: Aphasia with non-hemorrhagic lesions of the basal ganglia and the internal capsule, *Arch Neurol* 39:15, 1982.
241. Naeser MA, Alexander MP, Helm-Estabrooks N, et al: Aphasia with predominantly subcortical lesion sites, *Arch Neurol* 39:2, 1982.
242. Croisile B, Henry E, Trillet M, Aimard G: Loss of motivation for speaking with bilateral lacunes in the anterior limb of the internal capsule, *Clin Neurol Neurosurg* 91:325–327, 1989.
243. Laitinen LV: Loss of motivation for speaking with bilateral lacunes in the anterior limb of the internal capsule (letter), *Clin Neurol Neurosurg* 92:177–178, 1990.
244. Leicester J, Sidman M, Stoddard LT, Mohr JP: The nature of aphasic responses, *Neuropsychologia* 9:141, 1971.
245. Hier DB, Mohr JP: Incongruous oral and written naming: Evidence for a subdivision of the syndrome of Wernicke's aphasia, *Brain Lang* 4:115, 1977.
246. Mohr JP, Hier DB, Krishner HS: Modality bias in Wernicke's aphasia, *Neurology (NY)* 4:395, 1978.
247. Blumstein SE, Baker E, Goodglass H: Phonological factors in auditory comprehension in aphasia, *Neuropsychologia* 15:19, 1977.
248. Lazar RM, Marshall RS, Pile-Spellman J, et al: Interhemispheric transfer of language in patients with left frontal cerebral arteriovenous malformation, *Neuropsychologia* 38:1325, 2000.
249. Sidman M: *Tactics of scientific research*, New York, 1960, Basic Books.
250. Touche: Contribution a l'étude anatomo-clinique des aphasies, *Arch Gen Med* 6:326, 1901.
251. Damasio H, Damasio AR: Localization of lesions in conduction aphasia. In Kertesz A, editor: *Localization in neuropsychology*, New York, 1983, Academic Press, p 231.
252. Rothi LJ, McFarling D, Heilman KM: Conduction aphasia, syntactic alexia, and the anatomy of syntactic comprehension, *Arch Neurol* 39:272, 1982.
253. Boller F: Destruction of Wernicke's area without language disturbance: A fresh look at crossed aphasia, *Neuropsychologia* 11:243, 1973.
254. Kleist K: Gehirnpathologische und Lokalisatorische Ergebnisse über Hörstörungen: Gerauschtaubheiten und Amusie, *Monatsschr Psychiatr Neurol* 66:853, 1928.
255. Mazzuchi A, Marchini C, Budai R, et al: A case of receptive amusia with prominent timbre perception defect, *J Neurol Neurosurg Psychiatry* 445:644, 1982.
256. Bogen JE, Bogen GM: Wernicke's region—where is it?, *Ann N Y Acad Sci* 280:834, 1976.
257. Geschwind N: Problems in the anatomical understanding of the aphasias. In Benton AL, editor: *Contributions to clinical neuropsychology*, Chicago, 1969, Aldin.
258. Kertesz A: Localization of lesions in Wernicke's aphasia. In Kertesz A, editor: *Localization in neuropsychology*, New York, 1983, Academic Press, p 209.
259. Nielsen JM: *Agnosia, apraxia, aphasia*, New York, 1946, Hoeber.
260. Benson DF, Geschwind N: The aphasias and related disorders. In Baker AB, Baker LH, editors: *Clinical neurology, vol 1*, Hagerstown, Md, 1976, Harper & Row.
261. Kertesz A, Benson DF: Neologistic jargon: A clinical pathological study, *Cortex* 6:362, 1970.
262. Bastian HC: Some problems in connection with aphasia and other speech defects, *Lancet* 1:933, 1897.
263. Liepmann H, Storch E: Ein Fall Von Reiner Sprachtaubheit, *Psychiatr Abhandlung von Wernicke Hft 7/8*, 1898.
264. Schuster P, Taterka H: Beitrag zur Anatomie und Klinik der Reinen Wourttaubheit, *Z Neurol Psychiatr* 105:494, 1926.
265. Nielsen JM: The unsolved problems in aphasia, *Bull Los Angeles Neurol Soc* 162, 1939.
266. Coslett HB, Brashear HR, Heilman KM: Pure word deafness after bilateral primary auditory cortex infarcts, *Neurology (Cleve)* 34:347, 1984.
267. Pick A: *Studien uber Motorische Apraxie und ihre Mahestehende Erscheinungen*, Leipzig, 1905, Deuticke.
268. Leicester J: Central deafness and subcortical motor aphasia, *Brain Lang* 10:224, 1980.
269. Khurana RK, O'Donnell PP, Suter CM, Inayatullah M: Bilateral deafness of vascular origin, *Stroke* 12:521, 1981.

270. Leussink V, Andermann P, Reiners K, et al: Sudden deafness from stroke, *Neurology* 64:1817-1818, 2005.

272. Dejerine J: Des différentes variétés de cecite verbale, *Mem Soc Biol* 1:30, 1892.

272a. DeMassary J: L'alexie, *Encephale* 27:134, 1934.

273. Sidman M: The behavioral analysis of aphasia, *J Psychiatr Res* 8:413, 1971.

274. Sidman M, Stoddard LT, Mohr JP, Leicester J: Behavioral studies of aphasia: Methods of investigation and analysis, *Neuropsychologia* 9:119, 1971.

275. Wernicke C: Der Aphasische Symptomencomplex, Reprinted in *Gesammelte Aufsatze*, Breslau, Berlin, 1874, Fisher, 1893.

276. Levine DN, Calvanio R: Conduction aphasia. In Kirshner HS, Freemon FR, editors: *The neurology of aphasia*, 1982, Lisse, Swets & Zeitlinger, p 79.

277. Yamada K, Nagakane Y, Mizumo T, et al. MR tractography depicting damage to the arcuate fasciculus in a patient with conduction aphasia, *Neurology* 68:789, 2007 and Geldmacher DS, Quigg M, Elias WJ. MR tractography depicting damage to the arcuate fasciculus in a patient with conduction aphasia (letter), *Neurology* 69:321-322, 2007.

278. Weisman D, Hisama FM, Waxman SG, Blumenfeld H: Going deep to cut the link: cortical disconnection syndrome caused by a thalamic lesion, *Neurology* 60(11):1865-1866, 2003.

279. Geschwind N: Disconnection syndromes in animals and man, *Brain* 88:237, 1965.

280. Burns MS, Canter GJ: Phonemic behavior of aphasic patients with posterior cerebral languages, *Brain Lang* 4:492, 1977.

281. Ardila A, Rosselli M: Language deviations in aphasia: A frequency analysis, *Brain Lang* 44:165, 1993.

282. Stengel E: Lodge Patch IC: Central aphasia associated with parietal symptoms, *Brain* 78:401, 1955.

283. Quigg M, Geldmacher DS, Elias WJ: Conduction aphasia as a function of the dominant posterior perisylvian cortex. Report of two cases, *J Neurosurg* 104(5):845-848, 2006.

284. Shallice T, Warrington EK: The possible role of selective attention in acquired dyslexia, *Neuropsychologia* 15:31, 1977.

285. Marshall RS, Lazar RM, Mohr JP, et al: "Semantic" conduction aphasia from a posterior insular cortex infarction, *J Neuroimag* 6:189, 1996.

286. Liepmann H, Maas O: Fall von linksseitiger Agraphie und Apraxie bei rechtsseitiger Lähmung, *Z Psychol Neurol* 10:214, 1907.

287. Wernicke C: *Lehrbuch der Gehirnkrankheiten*, Kassel, 1881, Theodore Fischer.

288. Goldstein K: *Die Transkortikal Aphasien*, Jena, 1917, G Fischer.

289. Berthier ML, Starkstein SE, Leiguarda R, et al: Transcortical aphasia, *Brain* 114:1409, 1991.

290. Grossi D, Trohano L, Chiacchio L, et al: Mixed transcortical aphasia: Clinical features and neuroanatomical correlates: A possible role of the right hemisphere, *Eur Neurol* 31:204, 1991.

291. Warabi Y, Bandoh M, Kurisaki H, et al: Transcortical sensory aphasia due to extensive infarction of left cerebral hemisphere, *Rinsho Shinkeigaku* 46:317-321, 2006.

292. Alexander MP, Hiltbrunner B, Fischer RS: Distributed anatomy of transcortical sensory aphasia, *Arch Neurol* 46:885, 1989.

293. Kertesz A, Sheppard A, MacKenzie R: Localization in transcortical sensory aphasia, *Arch Neurol* 39:475, 1982.

294. Graff-Radford NR, Damasio AR: Disturbances of speech and language associated with thalamic dysfunction, *Semin Neurol* 4:162, 1984.

295. Bogousslavsky J, Regli F, Assal G: Acute transcortical mixed aphasia: A carotid occlusion syndrome with pial and watershed infarcts, *Brain* 111:631, 1988.

296. Rango R, Candelise L, Perani D, et al: Cortical pathophysiology and clinical neurologic abnormalities in acute cerebral ischemia, *Arch Neurol* 46:1318, 1989.

297. Karbe H, Szelies B, Herholz K, Heiss WD: Impairment of language is related to left parieto-temporal glucose metabolism in aphasic stroke patients, *J Neurol* 237:19, 1990.

298. Steckler T, Sahgal A: The role of serotonergic–cholinergic interactions in the mediation of cognitive behaviour, *Behav Brain Res* 67:165, 1995.

299. Metter EJ, Hanson WR, Hackson CA, et al: Temporoparietal cortex in aphasia: Evidence from positron emission tomography, *Arch Neurol* 47:1235, 1990.

300. Perani D, Vallar G, Cappa S, et al: Aphasia and neglect after subcortical stroke, *Brain* 110:1211, 1987.

301. Bushnell DL, Gupta S, Mlcoch AG, Barnes WE: Prediction of language and neurologic recovery after cerebral infarction with SPECT imaging using N-isopropyl-p-(I 123) iodoamphetamine, *Arch Neurol* 46:665, 1989.

302. Metter EJ, Kempler D, Jackson CA, et al: Are remote glucose metabolic effects clinically important? *J Cereb Blood Flow Metab* 7(Suppl 1):S196, 1987.

303. Vallar G, Perani D, Cappa SF, et al: Recovery from aphasia and neglect after subcortical stroke: Neuropsychological and cerebral perfusion study, *J Neurol Neurosurg Psychiatry* 51:1269, 1988.

304. Demeurisse G, Capon A, Verhas M, Attig E: Pathogenesis of aphasia in deep-seated lesions: Likely role of cortical diaschisis, *Eur Neurol* 30:67, 1990.

305. Binder JR, Rao SM, Hammeke TA, et al: Lateralized human brain language systems demonstrated by task subtraction functional magnetic resonance imaging, *Arch Neurol* 52:593, 1995.

306. McClelland JL, Rumelhart DE: An interactive activation model of context effects in letter perception. Part 1: An account of basic findings, *Psychol Rev* 88:375, 1981.

307. Petersen SE, Fox PT, Posner MI, et al: Positron emission tomographic studies of the cortical anatomy of single-word processing, *Nature* 331:585, 1988.

308. Wise R, Chollet F, Hadar U, et al: Distribution of cortical neural networks involved in word comprehension and word retrieval, *Brain* 114:1991, 1803.

309. Cappa SF, Perani D, Bressi S, et al: Crossed aphasia: A PET follow up study of two cases, *J Neurol Neurosurg Psychiatry* 56:665, 1993.

310. Marshall RS, Lazar RM, Binder JR, et al: Intrahemispheric localization of drawing dysfunction, *Neuropsychologia* 32:493, 1994.

311. Belin P, Van Eeckhout P, Zilbovicius M, et al: Recovery from nonfluent aphasia after melodic intonation therapy: A PET study, *Neurology* 47:1504, 1996.

312. Heiss WD, Kessler J, Thiel A, et al: Differential capacity of left and right hemispheric areas for compensation of poststroke aphasia, *Ann Neurol* 45:430, 1999.

313. Musso M, Weiller C, Kiebel S, et al: Training-induced brain plasticity in aphasia, *Brain* 122:1781, 1999.

314. Lazar RM, Marshall RS, Pile-Spellman J, et al: Anterior translocation of language in patients with left cerebral AVMs, *Neurology* 49:802, 1997.

315. NIDCDS: Aphasia. 2007. http://www.aphasia.org/.

316. Elman RJ, Olgar J, Elman SH: Aphasia: Awareness, advocacy, and activism, *Aphasiology* 14:455-459, 2000.

317. Pedersen PM, Vinter K, Olsen TS: Aphasia after stroke: type, severity and prognosis. The Copenhagen aphasia study, *Cerebrovasc Dis* 17(1):35-43, 2004.

318. Engelter ST, Gostynski M, Papa S, et al: Epidemiology of aphasia attributable to first ischemic stroke: Incidence, severity, fluency, etiology, and thrombolysis, *Stroke* 37(6):1379-1384, 2006.

319. Damush TM, Jia H, Ried LD, et al: Case-finding algorithm for poststroke depression in the Veterans Health Administration, *Int J Geriatr Psychiatry* 23:517-522, 2008.

320. Robinson RG, Bolduc PL, Price TR: Two-year longitudinal study of poststroke mood disorders: Diagnosis and outcome at one and two years, *Stroke* 18(5):837-843, 1987.

321. Gresham GE, Phillips TF, Wolf PA, et al: Epidemiologic profile of long-term stroke disability: The Framingham Study, *Arch Phys Med Rehabil* 60:487-491, 1979.

322. Kelly-Hayes M, Wolf PA, Kase C, et al: Time course of functional recovery after stroke, *J Neurol Rehabil* 3:65-70, 1989.

323. Skilbeck CE, Wade DT, Hewer RL, et al: Recovery after stroke, *J Neurol Neurosurg Psychiatry* 46(1):5-8, 1983.

324. Ferrucci L, Bandinelli S, Guralnik JM, et al: Recovery of functional status after stroke. A postrehabilitation follow-up study, *Stroke* 24:200-205, 1993.

325. Heiss WD, Thiel A, Kessler J, Herholz K: Disturbance and recovery of language function: correlates in PET activation studies, *Neuroimage* 20(Suppl 1):S42-49, 2003.

326. Demeurisse G, Demol O, Derouck M, et al: Quantitative study of the rate of recovery from aphasia due to ischemic stroke, *Stroke* 11(5):455-458, 1980.

327. Robey RR: A meta-analysis of clinical outcomes in the treatment of aphasia, *J Speech Lang Hear Res* 41(1):172-187, 1998.

328. Laska AC, Hellblom A, Murray V, et al: Aphasia in acute stroke and relation to outcome, *J Intern Med* 249(5):413-422, 2001.

329. Berthier ML: Poststroke aphasia: Epidemiology, pathophysiology and treatment, *Drugs Aging* 22(2):163-182, 2005.

330. Lendrem W, Lincoln NB: Spontaneous recovery of language in patients with aphasia between 4 and 34 weeks after stroke, *J Neurol Neurosurg Psychiatry* 48(8):743-748, 1985.

331. Mark VW, Thomas BE, Berndt RS: Factors associated with improvements in global aphasia, *Aphasiology* 6:121-134, 1992.

332. Kertesz A: What do we learn from recovery from aphasia? *Adv Neurol* 47:277-292, 1988.

333. Mohr JP, Lazar RM, Marshall RS, Hier DB: Middle cerebral artery disease. In Mohr JP, Choi DW, Grotta JC, Weir B, Wolf PA, editors: *Stroke: Pathophysiology, diagnosis, and management*, ed 4, Philadelphia, 2004, Churchill-Livingstone, pp 123-166.

334. Godefroy O, Dubois C, Debachy B, et al: Vascular aphasias: Main characteristics of patients hospitalized in acute stroke units, *Stroke* 33(3):702-705, 2002.

335. Lazar RM, Speizer AE, Festa JR, et al: Variability in language recovery after first-time stroke, *J Neurol Neurosurg Psychiatry* 79:530-534, 2008.

336. Goodglass H, Kaplan E: *Boston diagnostic aphasia examination*, Philadelphia, 1983, Lea & Febiger.

337. Kertesz A: *Western Aphasia Battery-Revised*, San Antonio, Tex, 2006, Harcourt Assessment.

338. Porch B: *The Porch Index of Communicative Abilities*, Palo Alto, Calif, 1982, Consulting Psychologists Press.

339. Holland A: *Communicative Abilities in Daily Living: A test for functional communication in aphasic adults*, Baltimore, 1980, University Park Press.

340. Beeson PM, Robey RR: Evaluating single-subject treatment research: lessons learned from the aphasia literature, *Neuropsychol Rev* 16(4):161-169, 2006.

341. Robey RR: The efficacy of treatment for aphasic persons: A meta-analysis, *Brain Lang* 47(4):582-608, 1994.

342. Bhogal SK, Teasell R, Speechley M: Intensity of aphasia therapy, impact on recovery, *Stroke* 34(4):987-993, 2003.

343. Greener J, Enderby P, Whurr R: Speech and language therapy for aphasia following stroke, *Cochrane Database Syst Rev* (2): CD000425, 2000.

344. Nickels L: Therapy for naming disorders: Revisiting, revising and reviewing, *Aphasiology* 16:935-975, 2002.

345. Moss A, Nicholas M: Language rehabilitation in chronic aphasia and time postonset: A review of single-subject data, *Stroke* 37:3043-3051, 2006.

346. Taub E: Harnessing brain plasticity through behavioral techniques to produce new treatments in neurorehabilitation, *Am Psychol* 59(8):692-704, 2004.

347. Meinzer M, Djundja D, Barthel G, et al: Long-term stability of improved language functions in chronic aphasia after constraint-induced aphasia therapy, *Stroke* 36(7):1462-1466, 2005.

348. Breier JI, Billingsley-Marshall R, Pataraia E, et al: Magnetoencephalographic studies of language reorganization after cerebral insult, *Arch Phys Med Rehabil* 87(12 Suppl 2):S77-83, 2006.

349. Devlin JT, Watkins KE: Stimulating language: insights from TMS, *Brain* 130(Pt 3):610-622, 2007.

350. Fillingham JK, Sage K, Ralph MA: Treatment of anomia using errorless versus errorful learning: are frontal executive skills and feedback important? *Int J Lang Commun Disord* 40(4):505-523, 2005.

351. Fillingham JK, Sage K, Lambon Ralph MA: The treatment of anomia using errorless learning, *Neuropsychol Rehabil* 16(2):129-154, 2006.

352. Feeney DM, Gonzalez A, Law WA: Amphetamine, haloperidol, and experience interact to affect rate of recovery after motor cortex injury, *Science* 217:855, 1982.

353. Walker-Batson D, Curtis S, Natarajan R, et al: A double-blind, placebo-controlled study of the use of amphetamine in the treatment of aphasia, *Stroke* 32(9):2093-2098, 2001.

354. Naeser MA, Martin PI, Nicholas M, et al: Improved picture naming in chronic aphasia after TMS to part of right Broca's area: An open-protocol study, *Brain Lang* 93(1):95-105, 2005.

355. Hurwitz BE, Dietrich WD, McCabe PM, et al: Amphetamine promotes recovery from sensory-motor integration deficit after thrombotic infarction of the primary somatosensory rat cortex, *Stroke* 22:648, 1991.

356. Stroemer RP, Kent TA, Hulsebosch CE: Enhanced neocortical neural sprouting, synaptogenesis, and behavioral recovery with D-amphetamine therapy after neocortical infarction in rats, *Stroke* 29:2381, 1998.

357. Crisostomo EA, Duncan PW, Propst M, et al: Evidence that amphetamine with physical therapy promotes recovery of motor function in stroke patients, *Ann Neurol* 23:94, 1988.

358. Grade C, Redford B, Chrostowski J, et al: Methylphenidate in early poststroke recovery: A double-blind, placebo-controlled study, *Arch Phys Med Rehabil* 79:1047, 1998.

359. Martinsson L, Hardemark H, Eksborg S: Amphetamines for improving recovery after stroke, *Cochrane Database Syst Rev* (1): CD002090, 2007.

360. Gladstone DJ, Danells CJ, Armesto A, et al: Physiotherapy coupled with dextroamphetamine for rehabilitation after hemiparetic stroke: A randomized, double-blind, placebo-controlled trial, *Stroke* 37(1):179-185, 2006.

361. Martinsson L, Wahlgren NG: Safety of dexamphetamine in acute ischemic stroke: A randomized, double-blind, controlled dose-escalation trial, *Stroke* 34(2):475-481, 2003.

362. Sprigg N, Willmot MR, Gray LJ, et al: Amphetamine increases blood pressure and heart rate but has no effect on motor recovery or cerebral haemodynamics in ischaemic stroke: A randomized controlled trial (ISRCTN 36285333), *J Hum Hypertens* 21(8):616-624, 2007.

363. Fisher M, Finklestein S: Pharmacological approaches to stroke recovery, *Cerebrovasc Dis* 9(Suppl 5):29-32, 1999.

364. Rasmussen D: The role of acetylcholine in cortical synaptic plasticity, *Behav Brain Res* 115:205-218, 2000.

365. Jacobs DH, Shuren J, Gold M, et al: Physostigmine pharmacotherapy for anomia, *Neurocase* 2:83-91, 1996.

366. Tanaka Y, Miyazaki M, Albert ML: Effects of increased cholinergic activity on naming in aphasia, *Lancet* 350:116-117, 1997.

367. Hughes JD, Jacobs DH, Heilman KM: Neuropharmacology and linguistic neuroplasticity, *Brain Lang* 71(1):96-101, 2000.

368. Berthier ML, Green C, Higueras C, et al: A randomized, placebo-controlled study of donepezil in poststroke aphasia, *Neurology* 67(9):1687-1689, 2006.

369. Cummings JL: Frontal-subcortical circuits and human behavior, *Arch Neurol* 50:873, 1993.

370. Albert ML, Bachman DL, Morgan A, et al: Pharmacotherapy for aphasia, *Neurology* 38:877, 1988.

371. Gold M, VanDam D, Silliman ER: An open-label trial of bromocriptine in nonfluent aphasia: A qualitative analysis of word storage and retrieval, *Brain Lang* 74:141, 2000.

372. Bragoni M, Altieri M, Dipiero V, et al: Bromocriptine and speech therapy in non-fluent chronic aphasia after stroke, *Neurol Sci* 21:19, 2000.

373. Lazar RM, Berman MB, Festa JR, et al: GABA-ergic but not anti-cholinergic agents re-induce former stroke deficits, *J Neurol Sci* 292:72-76, 2010.

374. Liepmann H: *Aufsätze aus den Apraxiegebeit*, Berlin, 1908, Karger.

375. Liepmann H: The syndrome of apraxia (motor asymboly) based on a case of unilateral apraxia. (Translated by Bohne WHO, Liepmann K, Rottenberg DA, from Monatsschr Psychiatr Neurol 8:15, 1900.) In Rottenberg DA, Hochberg FH, editors: *Neurological classics in modern translation*, New York, 1977, Hafner.

376. Kimura D, Archibald Y: Motor functions of the left hemisphere, *Brain* 97:337, 1974.

377. Heilbronner K: Die aphasischen, apraktischen und agnostischen Störungen. In Lewandowsky M, editor: *Handbuch der Neurologie, vol 1*, Berlin, 1910, Springer-Verlag, p 982.

378. Ajuriaguerra J, Hecaen H, Angelergues R: Les apraxies: Varietés cliniques et latéralisation lésionelle, *Rev Neurol (Paris)* 102:494, 1960.

379. Hecaen H, Gimeno A: L'apraxie idéomotrice unilatérale, *Rev Neurol* 102:648, 1960.

380. Basso A, Luzzatti C, Spinnler H: Is ideomotor apraxia the outcome of damage to well-defined regions of the left hemisphere? *J Neurol Neurosurg Psychiatry* 43:118, 1980.

381. Basso A, Capitani E, Luzzatti C, Spinnler H: Intelligence and left hemisphere disease: The role of aphasia, apraxia and size of lesion, *Brain* 104:721, 1981.

382. Lehmkuhl G, Poeck K, Willmes K: Ideomotor apraxia and aphasia: An examination of types and manifestations of apraxic symptoms, *Neuropsychologia* 21:199, 1983.

383. Heilman KM: Apraxia. In Heilman K, Valenstein E, editors: *Clinical neuropsychology*, New York, 1979, Oxford University Press.

384. Heilman KM, Rothi LJ, Valenstein E: Two forms of ideomotor apraxia, *Neurology (NY)* 32:342, 1982.

385. De Renzi E, Pieczuro A, Vignolo L: Ideational apraxia: A quantitative study, *Neuropsychologia* 6:41, 1968.

386. Sittig O: *Ueber Apraxie*, Berlin, 1931, Karger.

387. Arena R, Gainotti G: Constructional apraxia and visuo-perceptive disabilities in relation to laterality of cerebral lesions, *Cortex* 14:463, 1978.

388. Lehmkuhl G, Poeck K: A disturbance in the conceptual organization of actions in patients with ideational apraxia, *Cortex* 17:153, 1981.

389. De Renzi E, Lucchelli F: Ideational apraxia, *Brain* 198:1173, 1988.

390. Poeck P, Lehmkuhl G: Ideatory apraxia in a left-handed patient with right-sided brain lesion, *Cortex* 16:273, 1980.

391. Kertesz A: *Aphasia and associated disorders: taxonomy, localization and recovery*, New York, 1979, Grune & Stratton.

392. Geschwind N, Kaplan E: A human disconnection syndrome, *Neurology* 12:675, 1962.

393. Watson RT, Heilman KM: Callosal apraxia, *Brain* 106:391, 1983.

394. Verstichel P, Meyrignac C: Left unilateral melokinetic apraxia and left dynamic apraxia following partial callosal infarction, *Rev Neurol (Paris)* 156:274–277, 2000.

395. Graff-Radford NR, Welsh K, Godersky J: Callosal apraxia, *Neurology* 37:100, 1987.

396. Hecaen H, Albert ML: *Human Neuropsychology*, New York, 1978, John Wiley.

397. Whitty CWM, Newcombe F: Disabilities associated with lesions in the posterior parietal region of the non-dominant hemisphere, *Neuropsychologia* 3:175, 1965.

398. Mesulam M-M: Behavioral neuroanatomy. In Mesulam M-M, editor: *Principles of Behavioral and Cognitive Neurology*, Oxford, 2000, Oxford University Press, p 120.

399. Bodamer J: Die Prosop-Agnosie, *Arch Psychiatr Nervenkr* 179:6, 1947.

400. Mori E, Yamadori A: Acute confusional state and acute agitated delirium: Occurrence after infarction in the middle cerebral artery territory, *Arch Neurol* 4:1139, 1987.

401. Albert ML: A simple test for neglect, *Neurology* 23:658, 1973.

402. Bisiach E, Luzzatti C: Unilateral neglect of representational space, *Cortex* 14:129, 1978.

403. Schwartz AS, Marchok PL, Kreinick CJ, et al: The asymmetric lateralization of tactile extinction in patients with unilateral cerebral dysfunction, *Brain* 102:669, 1979.

404. Battersby WS, Bender MB, Pollack M: Unilateral spatial agnosia (inattention) in patients with cerebral lesions, *Brain* 79:68, 1956.

405. Schenkenberg T, Bradford DC, Ajax ET: Line bisection and unilateral visual neglect in patients with neurological impairment, *Neurology (NY)* 30:509, 1980.

406. Heilman KM, Valenstein E: Mechanisms underlying hemispatial neglect, *Ann Neurol* 5:166, 1979.

407. Binder JR, Marshall RS, Lazar RM, et al: Distinct syndromes of hemineglect, *Arch Neurol* 49:1187, 1992.

408. Rorden C, Fruhmann Berger M, Karnath HO: Disturbed line bisection is associated with posterior brain lesions, *Brain Res* 1080:17–25, 2006.

409. Damasio A, Damasio H, Chang Chi H: Neglect following damage to frontal lobe or basal ganglia, *Neuropsychologia* 18:123, 1980.

410. Mullally W, Huff K, Ronthal M, et al: Frequency of acute confusional states with lesions of the right hemisphere, *Ann Neurol* 12:113, 1982.

411. Heilman KM, Van Den Abell T: Right hemisphere dominance for attention: The mechanism underlying hemispheric asymmetries of inattention (neglect), *Neurology (NY)* 30:327, 1980.

412. Mesulam M-M: A cortical network for directed attention and unilateral neglect, *Ann Neurol* 10:309, 1981.

413. Birch HG, Belmont I, Karp E: Delayed information processing and extinction following cerebral damage, *Brain* 90:113, 1967.

414. Joanette Y, Brouchon M: Visual allesthesia in manual pointing: Some evidence for a sensorimotor cerebral organization, *Brain Cogn* 3:152, 1984.

415. Heilman K, Valenstein E: Frontal lobe neglect in man, *Neurology (Minneap)* 22:660, 1972.

416. Stein S, Volpe B: Classical "parietal" neglect syndrome after subcortical right frontal lobe infarction, *Neurology (Cleve)* 33:797, 1983.

417. Deuel RK, Collins RC: The functional anatomy of frontal lobe neglect in the monkey: Behavioral and quantitative 2-deoxyglucose studies, *Ann Neurol* 15:521, 1984.

418. Corbetta M, Kincade MJ, Lewis C, et al: Neural basis and recovery of spatial attention deficits in spatial neglect, *Nat Neurosci* 8:1603–1610, 2005.

419. Campbell DC, Oxbury JM: Recovery from unilateral visuo-spatial neglect, *Cortex* 12:303, 1976.

420. LaPlane D, Degos JD: Motor neglect, *J Neurol Neurosurg Psychiatry* 46:152, 1983.

421. Siekierka-Kleiser EM, Kleiser R, Wohlschläger AM, et al: Quantitative assessment of recovery from motor hemineglect in acute stroke patients, *Cerebrovasc Dis* 21:307–314, 2006.

422. Hartmann F: Beitrage zur Apraxielehre, *Monatsschr Psychiatr Neurol* 21:97, 1907.

423. Welch K, Stuteville P: Experimental production of unilateral neglect in monkeys, *Brain* 81:341, 1958.

424. Leicester J, Sidman M, Stoddard LT, Mohr JP: Some determinants of visual neglect, *J Neurol Neurosurg Psychiatry* 32:580, 1969.

425. Hier DB, Mondlock J, Caplan LR: Behavioral abnormalities after right hemisphere stroke, *Neurology (NY)* 33:337, 1983.

426. Willanger R, Danielsen VT, Ankerhus J: Denial and neglect of hemiparesis in right-sided apoplectic lesions, *Acta Neurol Scand* 64:310, 1981.

427. Willanger R, Danielsen UT, Ankerhus J: Visual neglect in right-sided apoplectic lesions, *Acta Neurol Scand* 64:327, 1981.

428. Hier DB, Mondlock J, Caplan LR: Recovery of behavioral abnormalities after right hemisphere stroke, *Neurology (NY)* 33:345, 1983.

429. Karnath HO, Baier B, Nägele T: Awareness of the functioning of one's own limbs mediated by the insular cortex? *J Neurosci* 25:7134–7138, 2005.

430. Assenova M, Benecib Z, Logak M: Anosognosia for hemiplegia with pontine infarction, *Rev Neurol (Paris)* 162:747–749, 2006.

431. Gerstmann J: Problem of imperception of disease and of impaired body territories with organic lesions, *Arch Neurol Psychiatry* 48:890, 1942.

432. Fisher CM: Left hemiplegia and motor impersistence, *J Nerv Ment Dis* 123:201, 1956.

433. Joynt RL, Benton AL, Fogel ML: Behavioral and pathological correlates of motor impersistence, *Neurology (NY)* 12:876, 1964.

434. Levin HS: Motor impersistence and proprioceptive feedback in patients with unilateral cerebral disease, *Neurology (NY)* 23:833, 1973.

435. Ben-Yishay Y, Diller L, Gerstman L, et al: The relationship between impersistence, intellectual function and outcome of rehabilitation in patients with left hemiplegia, *Neurology* 18:852, 1968.

436. Kertesz A, Nicholson I, Cancelliere A, Kassa K: Motor impersistence: A right-hemisphere syndrome, *Neurology* 35:662, 1985.

437. Brain WR: Visual disorientation with special reference to the lesions of the right hemisphere, *Brain* 64:244, 1941.

438. McFie J, Piercy MF, Zangwill OL: Visual spatial agnosia associated with lesions of the right cerebral hemisphere, *Brain* 73:167, 1950.

439. Roth M: Disorders of body image caused by lesions of the right parietal lobe, *Brain* 72:89, 1949.

440. Fisher CM: Topographic disorientation, *Arch Neurol* 19:33, 1982.

441. Critchley M: *The parietal lobes*, New York, 1953, Hafner.

442. Hecaen H, Angelergues R: Etude anatomoclinique de 280 lésions retrorolandiques unilatérales des hémisphères cérébraux, *Encephale* 6:533, 1961.

443. Landis T, Cummings JL, Benson DF, Palmer EP: Loss of topographic familiarity: An environmental agnosia, *Arch Neurol* 43:132, 1986.

444. Alsaadi T, Binder JR, Lazar RM: Pure topographic disorientation: A distinctive syndrome with varied localization, *Neurology* 54:1864, 2000.

445. Warrington EK, James M: An experimental investigation of facial recognition in patients with unilateral cerebral lesions, *Cortex* 3:317, 1967.

446. Ross ED: Sensory-specific and fractional disorders of recent memory in man: Isolated loss of visual recent memory, *Arch Neurol* 37:193, 1980.

447. De Renzi E, Faglioni P, Previdi P: Spatial memory and hemispheric locus of lesion, *Cortex* 13:424, 1977.

448. Meerwaldt JD, Van Harskamp F: Spatial orientation in right-hemisphere infarction, *J Neurol Neurosurg Psychiatry* 45:586, 1982.

449. Schmidley JW, Messing RO: Agitated confusional states: Patients with right hemisphere infarctions, *Stroke* 19:883, 1984.

450. Vighetto A, Aimard G, Confavreux C, et al: Une observation anatomo-clinique de fabulation (ou delire) topographique, *Cortex* 16:501, 1980.

451. Mesulam M-M, Waxman SG, Geschwind N, et al: Acute confusional states with right middle cerebral artery infarctions, *J Neurol Neurosurg Psychiatry* 39:84, 1976.

452. Levine DN, Finkelstein S: Delayed psychosis after right temporoparietal stroke or trauma: Relation to epilepsy, *Neurology (NY)* 32:267, 1982.

453. Dunne JW, Leedman PJ, Edis RH: Inobvious stroke: A cause of delirium and dementia, *Aust N Z J Med* 16:771, 1986.

454. Caplan LR, Kelly M, Kase CS, et al: Infarcts of the inferior division of the right middle cerebral artery: Mirror image of Wernicke's aphasia, *Neurology* 36:1015, 1986.

455. Benson DF, Gardner H, Meadows JC: Reduplicative amnesia, *Neurology* 26:147, 1976.

456. Mercer B, Wapner W, Gardner H, Benson DF: A study of confabulation, *Arch Neurol* 34:429, 1977.

457. Luria AR: *The working brain*, New York, 1976, Basic Books.

458. Piercy M, Hecaen H, de Ajuriaguerra J: Constructional apraxia associated with unilateral cerebral lesions: Left and right cases compared, *Brain* 83:225, 1960.

459. Arrigoni G, De Renzi E: Constructional apraxia and hemispheric locus of lesion, *Cortex* 1:170, 1964.

460. Warrington EK, James M, Kinsbourne M: Drawing disability in relation to laterality of cerebral lesion, *Brain* 89:53, 1966.

461. Gainotti G, Messerli G, Tissot R: Qualitative analysis of unilateral spatial neglect in relation to laterality of cerebral lesion, *J Neurol Neurosurg Psychiatry* 35:545, 1972.

462. Gainotti G, Tiacci C: The relationships between disorders of visual perception and unilateral spatial neglect, *Neuropsychologia* 9:451, 1971.

463. Lazar RM, Weiner M, Wald HS, Kula RW: Visuoconstructive deficit following infarction in the right basal ganglia: A case report and some experimental data, *Arch Clin Neuropsychol* 10:543, 1995.

464. Benton AL: The amusias. In Critchley M, Henson RA, editors: *Music and the brain*, London, 1977, Heinemann Medical.

465. Botez MI, Wertheim N: Expressive aphasia and amusia following right frontal lesion in a right-handed man, *Brain* 82:186, 1959.

466. Wertheim N: The amusias. In Vinken PJ, Bruyn GW, editors: *Handbook of clinical neurology, vol 4*, Amsterdam, 1969, North-Holland Publishing, p 195.

467. Brust JCM: Music and language, *Brain* 103:367, 1980.

468. Signoret JL, van Eeckhout P, Poncet M, Castaigne P: [Aphasia without amusia in a blind organist. Verbal alexia-agraphia without musical alexia-agraphia in braille], *Rev Neurol (Paris)* 143:172, 1987.

469. Monrad-Krohn GH: The prosodic quality of speech and its disorders, *Acta Psychiatr Neurol Scand* 22:255, 1947.

470. Buck R, Duffy RJ: Nonverbal communication of affect in brain-damaged patients, *Cortex* 16:331, 1980.

471. Heilman KM, Scholes R, Watson RT: Auditory affective agnosia: Disturbed comprehension of affective speech, *J Neurol Neurosurg Psychiatry* 38:69, 1975.

472. Ross ED, Mesulam M-M: Dominant language functions of the right hemisphere, *Arch Neurol* 36:144, 1979.

473. Ross ED: The aprosodias, *Arch Neurol* 38:561, 1981.

474. Heilman KM, Van Den Abell T: Right hemispheric dominance for mediating cerebral activation, *Neuropsychologia* 17:315, 1979.

475. Tucker DM, Watson RT, Heilman KM: Discrimination and evocation of affectively intoned speech in patients with right parietal disease, *Neurology (NY)* 27:947, 1977.

476. Antonucci G, Guariglia C, Judica A, et al: Effectiveness of neglect rehabilitation in a randomized group study, *J Clin Exp Neuropsychol* 17:383-389, 1995.

477. Fanthome Y, Lincoln NB, Drummond A, et al: The treatment of visual neglect using feedback of eye movements: A pilot study, *Disabil Rehabil* 17:413-417, 1995.

478. Robertson IH, Tegner R, Tham K, et al: Sustained attention training for unilateral neglect: theoretical and rehabilitation implications, *J Clin Exp Neuropsychol* 17:416-430, 1995.

479. Wilson FC, Manly T, Coyle D, et al: The effect of contralesional limb activation training and sustained attention training for self-care programmes in unilateral spatial neglect, *Restor Neurol Neurosci* 16:1-4, 2000.

480. Niemeier JP, Cifu DX, Kishore R: The lighthouse strategy: Improving the functional status of patients with unilateral neglect after stroke and brain injury using a visual imagery intervention, *Top Stroke Rehabil* 8:10-18, 2001.

481. Rossi PW, Kheyfets S, Reding MJ: Fresnel prisms improve visual perception in stroke patients with homonymous hemianopia or unilateral visual neglect, *Neurology* 40:1597-1599, 1990.

482. Wiart L, Come BS, Debelleix X, et al: Unilateral neglect syndrome rehabilitation by trunk rotation and scanning training, *Arch Phys Med Rehabil* 78:424-429, 1997.

483. Schindler I, Kerkhoff G: Head and trunk orientation modulate visual neglect, *Neuroreport* 8:2681-2685, 1997.

484. Johannsen L, Ackermann H, Karnath HO: Lasting amelioration of spatial neglect by treatment with neck muscle vibration even without concurrent training, *J Rehabil Med* 35:249-253, 2003.

485. Eskes GA, Butler B, McDonald A, et al: Limb activation effects in hemispatial neglect, *Arch Phys Med Rehabil* 84:323-328, 2003.

486. Kerkhoff G, Keller I, Ritter V, et al: Repetitive optokinetic stimulation induces lasting recovery from visual neglect, *Restor Neurol Neurosci* 24:357-369, 2006.

487. Pizzamiglio L, Fasotti L, Jehkonen M, et al: The use of optokinetic stimulation in rehabilitation of the hemineglect disorder, *Cortex* 40:441-450, 2004.

488. Pisella L, Rode G, Farne A, et al: Prism adaptation in the rehabilitation of patients with visuo-spatial cognitive disorders, *Curr Opin Neurol* 19:534-542, 2006.

489. Luaute J, Michel C, Rode G, et al: Functional anatomy of the therapeutic effects of prism adaptation on left neglect, *Neurology* 66:1859-1867, 2006.

490. Brighina F, Bisiach E, Oliveri M, et al: 1 Hz repetitive transcranial magnetic stimulation of the unaffected hemisphere ameliorates contralesional visuospatial neglect in humans, *Neurosci Lett* 336:131-133, 2003.

25 Posterior Cerebral Artery Disease

J.P. MOHR, JEFFREY R. BINDER

Anatomy

The posterior cerebral artery (PCA) usually arises from a terminal bifurcation of the basilar artery. Both posterior cerebral arteries arise from the basilar artery in 70% of cases. In the remainder, one or both maintain their embryologic "fetal" origin from the ipsilateral internal carotid artery by way of a large posterior communicating artery.

At its origin and along its initial course around the peduncle (Fig. 25-1), the PCA gives off small branches penetrating the midbrain and thalamus (so-called thalamoperforating arteries), which supply the midbrain en route to their supply for the thalamus. Distal to the peduncle, the artery gives rise to the medial and lateral posterior choroidal arteries. These vessels supply the posterior portion of the thalamus, a portion of the lateral geniculate body, and, finally, the choroid plexus. Distal to the peduncle, the PCA initially courses downward and backward in the ambient cistern immediately below the tentorium cerebelli, just above and slightly lateral to the superior cerebellar artery, then curves upward and medially in the quadrigeminal cistern. After crossing above the medial edge of the tentorium, the PCA reaches the medial surface of the occipital lobe near the anterosuperior border of the lingual gyrus just below the splenium of the corpus callosum. As it reaches the surface, it divides into two major divisions, one angling sharply forward, the other continuing posteriorly to become the calcarine artery.

The anterior division gives rise to the two inferior temporal arteries, the anterior and the posterior. These branches supply the ventral surface of the temporal and occipital lobes. They anastomose with the middle cerebral artery via a borderzone network that runs roughly along the margin of the hemisphere, where the ventral surfaces become convex. The sharp angulation of the anterior division from the PCA stem prevents most emboli from occluding it and its main branches.

The posterior division yields three major branches in sequence; the first bifurcation gives rise to the occipitotemporal artery and the calcarine artery, which then gives rise to the occipitoparietal artery. The calcarine artery supplies the calcarine cortex and medial surfaces of the occipital lobe as far distally as the occipital pole, anastomosing with terminal branches of the middle cerebral artery. The branches of the occipitoparietal artery supply the precuneus, and along a borderzone network, the terminal vessels anastomose with branches of the anterior cerebral artery. These branches are less acutely angulated from the PCA trunk than the anterior division and are more subject to embolic occlusion.

Brainstem and Thalamic Territory

The branches of the PCA that supply the midbrain and adjacent thalamus are considered to follow the general plan of the arteries of the brainstem.[1] They are divided into three major groups—paramedian penetrating, short circumferential, and long circumferential arteries.[2] The thalamoperforating arteries are the midbrain equivalent of the paramedian penetrating branches encountered lower in the brainstem and of the lenticulostriate arteries of the anterior circle of Willis. Measuring between 200 and 400 μm in diameter, the thalamoperforating arteries arise from the posterior communicating artery as well as from the proximal portions of the PCA. They are divided into three groups; the first two, the premammillary and the postmammillary, follow an upward curvilinear course into the anterior and ventromedial nuclei of the thalamus, and a third group, which pursues a horizontal course, supplies the cerebral peduncle.[3] In one variant, both left and right postmammillary thalamoperforating arteries arise mainly from a unilateral trunk branching from one of the proximal PCAs, referred to as the artery of Percheron.[4]

The arteries making up the midbrain-thalamic equivalent of the basilar artery's short circumferential group arise from the PCA as it winds around the stem. Measuring from 320 to 800 μm in diameter and numbering between eight and ten branches, these thalamogeniculate, posterior thalamic, and pulvinarian branches curve upward into the posterior portions of the thalamus, supplying the posterolateral nuclei and the pulvinar. One to three thalamogeniculate branches have been found in individual brains.[5]

The medial and lateral posterior choroidal arteries are the equivalent of the lower brainstem long circumferential group.[6] Both arise from the PCA in the circum-mesencephalic course. The posterolateral choroidal artery arises first. It follows the curve of the pulvinar, which it supplies only superficially, irrigates the posterior portion of the lateral geniculate body and a small portion of the medial temporal lobe, and then enters the choroidal fissure to supply the choroid plexus of the lateral ventricle.[7] In the terminal branches, the posterolateral choroidal artery anastomoses with the anterior choroidal artery (Fig. 25-2), and its collateral may suffice to irrigate the anterior choroidal artery's entire territory in the event of the latter's occlusion near its origin.

425

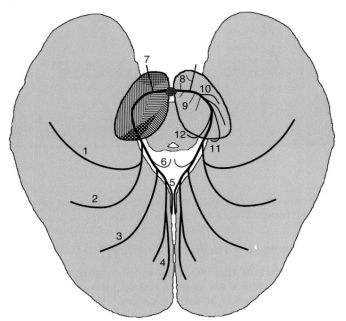

Figure 25-1 Schematic diagram of the posterior cerebral artery and its branches: 1, anterior inferior temporal artery; 2, posterior inferior temporal artery; 3, occipitotemporal artery; 4, calcarine arteries; 5, occipitoparietal artery; 6, splenial artery; 7, posterior communicating artery; 8, tuberothalamic arteries; 9, thalamoperforating arteries; 10, thalamogeniculate and posterior thalamic arteries; 11, posterolateral choroidal artery; 12, posteromedial choroidal artery. Arterial territories of the thalamus are indicated as follows: *horizontal hatching,* thalamoperforator territory; *vertical hatching,* thalamogeniculate territory; *cross-hatching,* tuberothalamic territory; *checkerboard pattern,* posterolateral choroidal territory; *diagonal hatching,* posteromedial choroidal territory.

The posteromedial choroidal artery arises a few millimeters behind the posterolateral choroidal artery, passing first over the medial and lateral geniculate bodies. This double-humped course gives the vessel the appearance of the number "3" on an angiogram.[3] Proximally, it supplies part of the upper midbrain and the peduncle. After entering the choroidal fissure, it supplies the choroid plexus of the third ventricle, the anterior aspect of the pulvinar, and the medial thalamus, this last supply accounting for some thalamic infarcts from occlusion of the proximal portion of the PCA. The terminal branches of the posteromedial choroidal artery supply the anterior nucleus of the thalamus. The last branch of the arteries supplying the deep territory is the posterior pericallosal or splenial artery.[3,7] Rarely, the thalamotuberal artery takes its origin from the middle cerebral artery instead of its more common origination from the posterior communicating artery.[8]

Cortical Territory

There remains considerable disagreement as to the names of the cortical branches (Fig. 25-3).[9] Specific names aside, three branches usually supply the entire ventral surface of the temporal and occipital lobes; a fourth, the calcarine region; and a fifth, more anterior regions of the medial occipital and parietal lobes (see Fig. 25-2).[10]

The anterior inferior temporal and the posterior inferior temporal arteries usually arise from a single trunk, separate from the occipitotemporal branch. Less often the three arise from a common trunk. The two anterior arteries supply the entire undersurface of the temporal lobe. The occipitotemporal branch separately supplies the undersurface of the occipital lobe, including the posterior portion of the fusiform and lingual gyri.

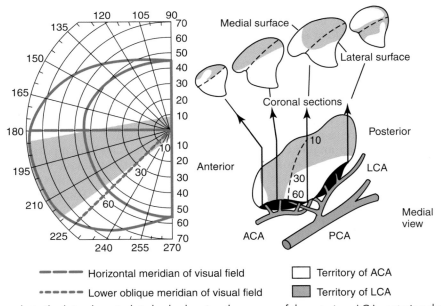

Figure 25-2 Arterial supply to the lateral geniculate body showing the course of the arteries. ACA, anterior choroidal artery; LCA, posterolateral choroidal artery. (From Frisen L, Holmegaard L, Rosencrantz M: Sectorial optic atrophy and homonymous horizontal sector anopia: A lateral choroidal artery syndrome? *J Neurol Neurosurg Psychiatry* 41:374, 1978.)

The calcarine artery may be single or double.[9] Its supply includes both banks of the calcarine cortex, inferiorly parts of the lingual gyrus, and superiorly the cuneus. Although the calcarine artery has been claimed to be the exclusive supply to the visual cortex in the calcarine fissure,[11] the striate area may at times be supplied in part by the occipitotemporal or occipitoparietal arteries.[12] The termination of the supply of the calcarine artery and its branches is far posterior along the occipital pole.[13] The supply commonly passes around the edge of the occipital pole and as far forward as 1 cm on the convex surface of the hemisphere, where anastomoses are formed with terminal branches of the middle cerebral artery. This arrangement means that almost the entire lateral surface of the brain is in the middle cerebral territory.

The final cortical surface branch, the occipitoparietal artery, typically courses up under the splenium of the corpus callosum, supplying the isthmus of the gyrus fornicati, splenium, and portions of the precuneus and cuneus.

Collateral Linkages

The PCA has abundant collateral connections with the middle and anterior cerebral arteries.[14] The collaterals occur in the borderzone, a narrow (usually 1-cm) strip separating two major arterial territories. Within this zone, anastomoses between end arteries occur freely in a variety of forms—end-to-end, side-to-side, and end-to-side. The actual size of the anastomosing vessels varies considerably, but most are on the order of 300 to 600 μm, only rarely as large as 1 mm. As a result, although a potential collateral vessel exists at any point along a borderzone, it is all but impossible to anticipate that a given terminal

branch will receive the immediate flow through the borderzone that it may need to prevent infarction when its territory is suddenly compromised.

The anastomoses with the anterior cerebral artery usually take place along a narrow borderzone of vessels on the surface of the precuneus between the transverse parietal sulcus and the parietooccipital fissure, extending from the isthmus of the gyrus fornicati inferiorly to the margin of the hemisphere superiorly. Three or four branches enter the borderzone.

With the middle cerebral artery, anastomoses occur from the orbital surface of the anterior tip of the temporal lobe inferolaterally along the inferolateral margin of the hemisphere as far back as the occipital pole.[15] Between five and eight such branches can be traced into the borderzones in most hemispheres.

Vascular Disease

Occlusion of the PCA or its branches is less common than that of the middle cerebral artery.[16] By autopsy reports, bilateral involvement has been reported in 16% to 25% of the cases.[17,18] Bilateral infarction of the entire deep and superficial territory of the PCA appears to be quite rare.[19] Infarction of individual branches, alone or in combination, is more common (Table 25-1), the calcarine artery leading the list.[18] Isolated occlusion of the anterior temporal artery is so rare that the range of clinical features is poorly known. Brain imaging by computed tomography (CT) and magnetic resonance imaging (MRI) has shown thalamic involvement in 19%[18,20] and 30% of cases, respectively.[17,18] Midbrain infarction is uncommon.[17,18]

Embolism

Embolism has long been considered to lead all other causes of PCA occlusion.[17-19] Its usual path is via the vertebral or basilar arteries, but some pass via the internal carotid artery. In their series of 44 autopsy studies,

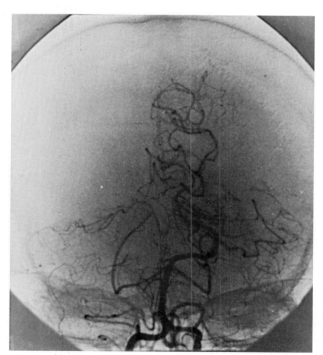

Figure 25-3 Anteroposterior view of the posterior cerebral artery territory showing the cerebral surface branches supplying the inferior surface branches, which in turn supply the inferior surface of the temporal lobe and the medial occipital region.

TABLE 25-1   REGIONAL DISTRIBUTION OF INFARCTS

Site(s)	Number
PCA	6
CA	7
PTA	7
ATA	1
POA	2
PTA + ATA	7
CA + POA	6
CA + PTA	10
CA + PTA + ATA	11
CA + PTA + POA	1
CA + PTA + POA + PPA	2

ATA, anterior temporal artery; CA, calcarine artery; PCA, posterior cerebral artery; POA, parieto-occipital artery; PPA, posterior pericallosal artery; PTA, posterior temporal artery.
Adapted from Kinkel WR, Newman RP, Jacobs L: Posterior cerebral artery branch occlusions: CT and anatomic considerations. In Berguer R, Bauer RB, editors: *Vertebrobasilar arterial occlusive disease: medical and surgical management.* Philadelphia, Lippincott-Raven, 1984, p 117.

Castaigne[16] attributed only one case of PCA occlusion to cardiac source embolism, whereas in 50% of the remaining cases, the source was plaques in the vertebral or basilar arteries. More recent series, based on imaging, attribute 25% to 40% of PCA occlusions to cardiogenic sources.[18,19] Because the PCA may be "fetal" from the carotid artery, examples exist with hemianopia as the initial presentation of carotid artery disease.[17,21] Bilateral PCA involvement is a common result of basilar embolism in which the particle(s) arrests at the top, occluding both PCA origins (Fig. 25-4).[22] Other common sites of arrest are the stem of the PCA where it winds around the brainstem, at the origin of the cortical surface branches, and along the course of the branches serving the occipital lobe. Embolic occlusions often produce incomplete infarction of the territory distal to the occluded site.[7,23-27] Complete infarction affecting the gray matter and subcortical white matter to the depths of the ventricular wall is rarely reported,[3] the lesions more typically being patchy.[26]

Thrombosis

Atheromatous thrombosis of the PCA accounts for only 5% to 15% of cases.[16-19] However, modern MRI is citing a higher percentage for thrombus than was common for autopsy series.[28] Atheroma usually affects the PCA along its course around the brainstem, at approximately the same sites where embolic materials stop (Fig. 25-5). It is uncommon more distally. Thrombus atop preexisting stenosis is rare.[16]

Occlusion from anterograde extension of thrombus from an occlusion of the upper basilar artery appears to account for half of the cases of bilateral PCA territory infarction.[29,30] The occipital lobes may suffer ischemia as a "distal field" effect from occlusion of the vertebral arteries bilaterally or the basilar artery itself.[31-34] No clinical features specifically distinguish thrombosis from embolic occlusion in the proximal PCA.

Few studies have been made of atherostenotic disease of the posterior cerebral stem.[35] The syndromes include diplopia, ipsilateral ptosis, and contralateral hemiataxia—the last syndrome reported as a mixture of Benedikt's syndrome with pupil-sparing oculomotor palsy, transient ischemic attacks (TIAs), and homonymous visual field defects. The TIAs were predominantly either visual disturbances in the contralateral half-field or sensory complaints in the form of paresthesias involving the arm and hand or, occasionally, the face and leg.

Other Causes of Infarction

Migraine, hypercoagulopathy, and brain herniation dominate this short list of other causes of PCA infarction. Many researchers accept the concept of vasospasm with infarction as a cause of ischemia,[18,19,36] but for some patients, the migraine is a secondary phenomenon.[37,38]

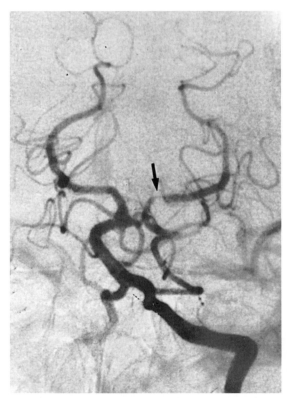

Figure 25-5 Anteroposterior view of a selective left vertebral angiogram with simultaneous compression of the left carotid artery. A high-grade stenosis *(arrow)* can be seen in the proximal left posterior cerebral artery just distal to its junction with the left posterior communicating artery. Compression of the left carotid artery eliminated the possibility of flow artifact created by nonpacified blood from the anterior circulation. (From Pessin MS, Kwan ES, DeWitt LD, et al: Posterior cerebral artery stenosis. *Ann Neurol* 21:85, 1987.)

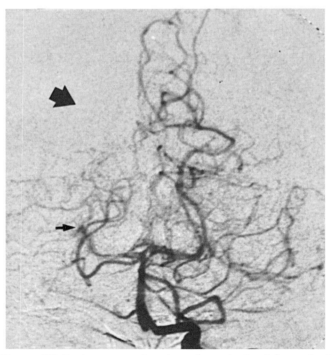

Figure 25-4 Anteroposterior view of a selective left vertebral angiogram. The ambient segment of the right posterior cerebral artery is occluded *(small arrow)*. There is no opacification of the terminal branches of this artery *(large arrow)*.

Hypercoagulopathic states may precipitate infarction in any vascular territory, that of the PCA included.[17-19] Transtentorial brain herniation is a well-recognized cause of PCA occlusion. The artery is usually compressed in its course around the midbrain between the herniated temporal lobe medially and the tentorium laterally.[39,40] Compression may also occur contralateral to the herniation because of lateral displacement of the brainstem against the contralateral tentorium.[41] Brucellosis has now been reported as a cause of PCA occlusion.[42]

Clinical Syndromes

Distal Basilar and Posterior Cerebral Artery Stem Occlusion

Occlusions affecting the top of the basilar artery are discussed in detail in Chapter 26. In this section, the discussion is confined to those syndromes in which the PCA is affected as part of the basilar occlusion.

In the autopsy series reported by Castaigne and associates,[29] four cases involved the red nucleus and the intralamellary, parafascicular, central, and median nuclei of the thalamus. Bilateral, symmetric infarcts in such cases may be due to distal basilar occlusion or to occlusion of an azygous thalamoperforating artery supply (artery of Percheron). Profound deficits occurred, particularly in bilateral cases, featuring obtundation, stupor or coma, disturbance in memory, hemiplegia, varying degrees of hemihypesthesia, and isolated instances of hemianopia or partial third nerve paresis. Other researchers have had similar experiences.[43,44] Occlusion of the PCA stem between the basilar artery and the junction with the posterior communicating artery is sufficient to precipitate a hemiparesis from peduncular infarct, ocular motility disorder from deeper infarction of the midbrain, and complex disturbances in

consciousness, memory, and even language for patients in whom infarcts penetrate deeper into medial thalamic structures. In some cases, hypersexuality and changes in appetite occur as well.

Unilateral occlusion of the PCA stem has also caused syndromes mimicking those from middle cerebral artery territory infarction (Fig. 25-6). Involvement of both the deep and superficial territories of the PCA (right side) has produced not only contralateral plegia, hemisensory syndrome, hemianopia, and behavioral effects but also Horner's syndrome and contralateral hyperhidrosis; these last two are explained by involvement of the thalamus and hypothalamus.[45] Four reports have described small case series with occlusion of the proximal PCA.[46,47]

Sensory Syndromes

Hypesthesia or anesthesia is explained by supply to the ventral tier nuclei of the thalamus in the territory of its penetrating branches.[43] Individual reports describing hypesthesia, and even "considerable anesthesia," include one from the pre-20th century literature with a large, autopsy-documented, dominant hemisphere occipital infarction but no lesions described in the thalamus (on gross inspection); the patient was described as complaining that "the whole right side of the body [felt] cold and heavy . . . the difference of sensation in the two sides being so marked he felt as if a plumb line down the middle of the head and trunk had divided him into two halves."[27]

The branches supplying the ventral tier nuclei of the thalamus come most regularly from the thalamogeniculate branch of the PCA and the posterolateral choroidal artery (Fig. 25-7), whose main target is the lateral geniculate nucleus. Frisen and coworkers[48] speculated that occlusion of the posterolateral choroidal artery could produce not only a somatosensory defect but also a hemianopia from involvement of the lateral geniculate body.

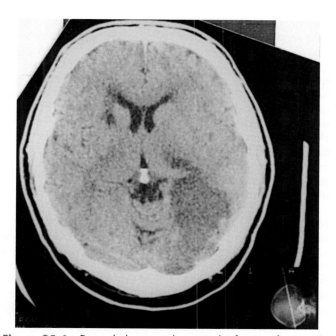

Figure 25-6 Deep thalamic and occipital infarction from occlusion of the posterior cerebral artery in a patient with severe sensory loss and dense hemianopia.

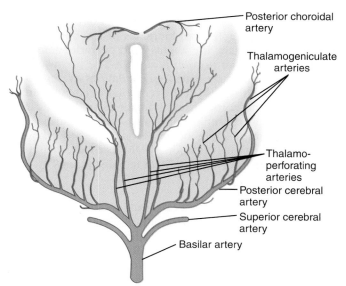

Figure 25-7 Thalamus with the usual arterial distribution. Note the multiple thalamogeniculate arteries.

A case studied by one of the authors (JPM) had hemianopia but no abnormality of sensation.[7]

The Déjerine-Roussy syndrome, dating from 1906, has been attributed to occlusion of the thalamogeniculate branch of the PCA.[49] The patients showed a syndrome of rapidly improving hemiparesis with choreic movements and ataxia, persisting hypesthesia, and initial and later-evolving severe paroxysmal pain in the hypesthetic side. The original pathologic and clinical correlations have been reconfirmed by others (see Chapter 27).[50-53]

Not usually classified among the sensory syndromes, dysgeusia has been related to unilateral ventroposterolateral and ventroposteromedial infarction in a series of cases.[54]

Motor Syndromes

Hemiparesis and even hemiplegia may also occur in the PCA syndrome,[46,47] attributed to involvement of the upper brainstem or ischemia on the edge of the internal capsule.[55] Hyperkinetic and dystonic syndromes involving limbs contralateral to the lesion, including "jerky dystonic unsteady hand" (three cases attributed to occlusion of the posterior choroidal arteries),[50] hemichorea-hemiballism,[49,56,57] "hyperkinesie volitionnelle,"[58] asterixis, and hemidystonia.[49,56,59] Delayed onset of contralateral limb and palatal myoclonus has been reported from unilateral thalamic infarction.[60] Links to specific thalamic nuclei have been described.[61]

Oculomotor and Pupillary Disturbances

Oculomotor and pupillary disturbances are described in more detail in the discussion of basilar artery occlusion (see Chapter 26). Unilateral mesencephalic infarction from PCA disease has been a documented cause.[62]

Visual Field Disturbances

The lower portions of the visual radiations lie in the territory of the PCA through their entire course. Much of the upper portion, running on the upper wall of the ventricle, receives some supply from branches of the middle cerebral artery, especially the angular and posterior temporal branches. The lower portion is all PCA. The pathway may suffer infarction at the lateral geniculate body, the radiations along their course in the temporal/occipital lobe, or at the calcarine cortex itself. Damage near the calcarine cortex may cause amblyopic disturbances featuring relative rather than absolute loss of vision. It has proved possible to track the visual radiation by MRI following infarction, showing changes in the external sagittal striatum.[63]

Bilateral Infarction

Complete Infarction. Bilateral blindness is an uncommon complication of cerebral arteriography, and in this setting it is fortunately rarely persistent, lasting hours to days, with recovery of vision usually all but complete.[64] This complication is usually ascribed to toxic effects of contrast agents, though embolism is also an occasional cause.

Complete destruction of both the visual cortices has only rarely been reported.[34,65-67] Brindley and Janota's[68] patient is still the best described. She remained blind, with no response to opticokinetic stimuli and no visual evoked potentials. Although unable to distinguish steady darkness from steady light, nor light moving in front of her, she consistently detected change by sudden darkening of a lighted room or sudden lighting of a darkened room. A similar patient, blind to clinical testing, had visual evoked potentials to pattern stimulation.[69] Goldenberg's patient,[66] shown by MRI to have all but complete bilateral destruction of the calcarine regions, denied blindness but was able to describe by recall the shapes of letters and colors typical of certain objects named by the examiners. This last case addresses the issue whether preservation of the primary visual cortex is necessary to generate conversationally tested recall of images.

The huge infarcts in such cases are often accompanied by severe amnestic states, amnestic aphasia, amnestic color dysnomia (failure to recall the name of the color typical for a given item, e.g., green for grass), topographic disorientation, and implicit unawareness of the extent of the deficit and perhaps even of its existence.[70] This last point suggests that the preservation or loss of awareness of the blindness is of little value in differentiating middle from posterior cerebral artery territory infarction.[22]

Incomplete Infarction. Incomplete bilateral infarction is better known and produces a remarkable variety of syndromes. Some cases have begun as complete blindness but improved somewhat within hours or days to less striking deficits.[32] During the time of complete blindness, patients commonly volunteer no complaints and are unaware of the deficit.[67] In some, detection of movement of objects in visual space was present and sufficient for localization, but there has been no discrimination of size or shape.[71]

In these cases superficial infarction may involve almost the whole of the calcarine cortex, but if it spares the occipital pole and the subcortical visual radiations, visual function for complex activities such as reading may be spared even if only a tiny portion of the central field remains.[33,34,65,72] Holmes[73] described a patient with a narrow wedge of preserved vision extending from the fixation point upward on either side of the vertical meridian, with its apex at the fixation point and its base at the periphery. Serial sections of the autopsy specimen from this patient showed total calcarine infarction except for a small region, nearly symmetric bilaterally, that extended along the inferior lip of the striate cortex from the anterior end to the pole. An upper homonymous paracentral quadrantanopic defect has been described by MRI to affect the lower calcarine area over the region considered the extrastriate area.[74]

Bilateral altitudinal hemianopia may result from incomplete bilateral occipital infarction, usually taking the form of inferior altitudinal anopia.[26,34,75,76] The number of reported cases remains small.[77] Autopsies have shown foci of infarction scattered through the calcarine cortex with varying subcortical involvement. In several reported cases the onset was preceded by hallucinations of lights, prismatic or geometric forms, and other phenomena suggestive of migrainous scintillations. After the hemianopias developed, associated visual disturbances included color dysnomias, difficulties with visual form discrimination, spatial disorientation, and disordered visual search behavior of the type encountered in Balint's syndrome. However, other patients have had little such disturbance.[26] In a personal case of one of the authors (JPM), a construction foreman was annoyed most by his inferior altitudinal hemianopia because it prevented his easy scanning of blueprints and caused difficulty in reaching for the floor-mounted gear shift in his pickup truck. He was implicitly unaware of his visual field disturbance. The visual field disturbances seemed more homogeneous than indicated by the discontinuous foci of infarction. The syndromes typically persist with little change.[68,70,78]

Unilateral Infarction

Isolated infarction of the visual radiation seems rare. In contrast to middle cerebral artery territory disease, infarctions of the PCA territory have often been reported in which the subcortical component was more evident than the infarction involving the cortical surface.[7,23,34] In most instances, the damage found subcortically affected the white matter of the lingual or fusiform gyrus, often sparing the visual radiations, which pass deeper and are adjacent to the ventricular wall. Infarcts in this deeper territory are rare unless they are the result of a complete infarction from the cortical surface to the ventricular wall forming a schizencephalic cleft.

Temporal crescent sparing has been described in a few instances of unilateral infarction with sparing of the anterior end of the calcarine cortex.[79,80] This pattern, which cannot be detected with standard automated perimetry, may nonetheless be of prognostic importance because of the usefulness of peripheral vision in daily activites.[80]

Macular sparing is frequently encountered in unilateral (and also in bilateral) infarction of the PCA territory. The most common explanation is that the collateral flow available from the middle cerebral artery territory spares the pole.[26,65,81] For macular vision to remain, the infarct must be superficial enough to spare the visual radiations; when they are involved, anatomic integrity of the occipital pole does not suffice to preserve central vision.[68] Infarcts limited to the middle fields of supply of the PCA involve the anterior portions of the calcarine cortex and lingual gyrus.[9,14] The most common finding in such instances is a homonymous hemianopia with macular sparing, the most consistent deficit involving visual field adjacent to the horizontal meridian.[9] Isolated macular hemianopia, the inverse of hemianopia with macular sparing, is less common and occurs when infarction is relatively confined to the occipital pole.[26,34,82]

Lateral Geniculate Infarction. The anterior choroidal artery supplies the anterior hilum and the anterior and lateral aspects of the nucleus. The lateral posterior choroidal artery supplies the remainder, including the crown. The two sources of supply do not anastomose before or in the nucleus and appear to be end arteries with no collaterals.

The visual field is represented in the following three parts in the nucleus: the anteromedial, which subserves inferior quadrant vision; the crown, serving macular vision; and the lateral, which serves upper quadrantic vision.

Autopsy-proven cases are rare (see Fig. 25-2).[7,48,83,84] The only pathologically documented infarcts produced a congruous, complete upper quadrantanopia involving the macula, with some involvement of the upper portion of the lower quadrant.[85] Brain imaging in living patients has shown inferred infarcts of the lateral geniculate to have clinically demonstrated wedge-shaped homonymous sectoranopia, congruent upper quadrantanopia, or a quadruple sectoranopia (one case).[86] Upper and lower homonymous sectoranopias have also been reported after ligation of the anterior choroidal artery but were documented only by CT.[87] A later case, also congruous, was documented by MRI.[88] An unusual bilateral infarct documented by MR imaging also showed homonymous hemianopias.[89]

Occlusion limited to the posterior choroidal artery yields a rather unusual syndrome: The artery supplies the lateral geniculate body, the fornix, the dorsomedial nucleus, and the posterior pulvinar. Infarction of these structures in one autopsied case studied by serial sections caused hemianopia, color dysnomia, and disturbance of memory.[6] A few patients with posterior choroidal artery occlusion imaged clinically had homonymous quadrantanopia or sectoranopia, with or without sensory disturbances, and a variety of behavioral disturbances, including memory disturbance and "transcortical aphasia."[86]

Hemiamblyopias

Hemiamblyopias represent disturbance of a subtype of visual function without complete loss of vision. Lesions in most of the cases involve extrastriate regions, most notably lingual and fusiform gyri, and spare the calcarine cortex. The disturbance may be a complete or relative loss of color perception, referred to as *dyschromatopsia* (see later), or a reduction in the perception of light or form. In mild cases, the visual field abnormality is detected only by testing with small targets. With more severe impairments, there may be no perception of stationary targets of any size, but awareness of moving stimuli may be preserved ("Riddoch phenomenon").[71,90] The pattern of loss of color perception with preserved motion perception is particularly well documented in patients with medial occipitotemporal lesions in the PCA territory.[91-93] One patient, with MRI-documented infarction of the right fusiform gyrus, was unable to discriminate colors, name objects, or discriminate grating orientations in the left upper quadrant but showed normal perception of coherently moving dots in the same location.[91] Such partial defects attest to the complexity of visual perception, which depends on parallel and largely independent processing pathways for color, motion, and form.[94]

Rare patients have had calcarine cortex lesions and what appeared to be typical dense, scotomatous field defects with no detection of moving stimuli, but they could localize in space stimuli they claimed not to see. The physiologic basis for this so-called blindsight phenomenon remains controversial,[95] with some researchers proposing a separate geniculocortical pathway that bypasses calcarine cortex and others favoring a mechanism based on small remnants of spared striate cortex.[96,97]

Clinical Course of Visual Field Abnormalities

Significant improvement is rare,[98,99] owing to the strictly unilateral representation of the primary visual pathway.[98] Those with infarcts with visual disturbance confined to the paracentral regions may show improvements during the first months after onset. Some improvement may occur for target detection, color discrimination, and form discrimination in the impaired field as well as shift of the scotoma border by a few degrees with daily computerized visual training,[98,100] in some but not all. The current authors have only one example of substantial improvement within months of onset for a focal partial anopia documented by formal visual fields shortly after onset and again after improvement. The MR image showed an infarct adjacent to the calcarine cortex, so the improvement could represent that theorized by Polyak[26] for the famous case involving the famous pathologist Tracy B. Mallory (see later).

The rare instances of lengthy clinical observation offer some insights into the visual system's pathophysiology.

The case of Tracy B. Mallory is the best known, as he was under observation for upwards of 30 years. He initially experienced a large visual field defect at an evening cocktail party after looking into the sunlight. It was said later to have "cleared up." As late as 1 year after its onset, he was examined by an ophthalmologist, who described a large hemianopic scotoma in the left upper fields "too far from the macula to cause him any disturbances in microscopic work." Twenty-four years later, this patient's formal visual fields were plotted on a tangent screen and showed a dense but highly circumscribed upper quadrantanopia confined to the macular region and extending some 20 degrees in the horizontal plane and 10 degrees in the vertical plane (Fig. 25-8). No comments were made on the disparity between the patient's comment that his vision had cleared up and the persisting visual field deficit.

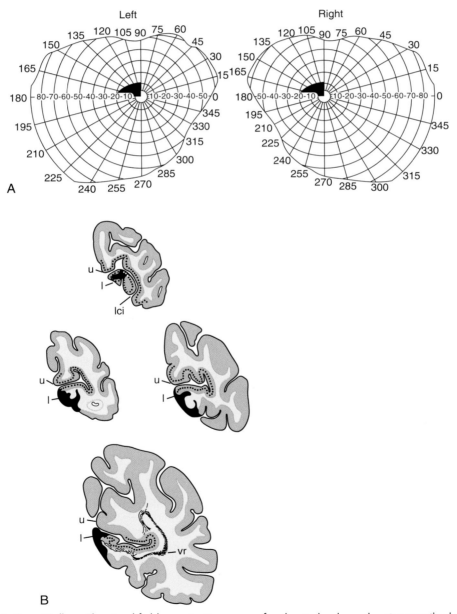

Figure 25-8 A and B, Case Mallory. The visual field examination years after the stroke showed a circumscribed upper quadrantanopia. (From Polyak SL: *The vertebrate visual system*, Chicago, 1957, University of Chicago.)

At autopsy years later, the only site of infarction affecting the calcarine cortex was a small wedge of the lower bank near the pole. However, a larger area of infarction had undermined much of the lingual gyrus and adjacent inferior bank of the calcarine cortex, within which the cellular elements were much reduced in number. The findings were interpreted by Polyak[26] as indicating that the surviving cells sufficed to permit the initial visual field defect to undergo functional resolution, a speculation that appears not to have been challenged.

Visual Agnosia

Extensive occipital infarction, bilateral or unilateral, is the usual cause of the rare disorder visual agnosia, which features an inability to "recognize" objects visually, usually tested by the patient's ability to name, describe uses for, or pantomime the use of visually presented objects. This syndrome differs from a more general aphasic disturbance in that with visual agnosias, the same objects that cannot be named from visual input are readily named after tactile presentation or after a verbal description of the object is provided. Visual agnosias may also be the residua of cardiac arrest or anoxia.

A great deal of effort has been expended in asserting[101,102] or denying[103-105] that such syndromes exist. Opponents of the notion argue that the deficits are a combination of a "primary" visual field defect, a secondary perceptual disorder, and some degree of dementia. Researchers in support of the notion admit that few cases have been fully described but that in those cases, the strict criteria have been met—intact primary visual function and no language disturbance. Two forms are said to exist: an apperceptive form, caused by "interference with the processing of primary visual sensory data,"[102] and an associative form, "caused by disorders affecting associative cortex where visual percepts are matched with previously processed sensory data for recognition."[102] Other, more detailed taxonomies based on modern studies of normal visual recognition have also been proposed.[106]

Closely related to the associative form of visual agnosia is a syndrome called *optic aphasia*,[107-109] in which patients are unable to name visually presented objects but otherwise show relatively intact knowledge by answering questions about the objects, categorizing them, or demonstrating their use through pantomime. The visual agnosia and optic aphasia syndromes have similar lesion localization and may simply represent ends of a continuum with varying deficit in knowledge retrieval.[110,111] The restriction of impairments to the visual modality has suggested to many investigators a functional disconnection between an intact visual perceptual system and an intact language system.[108,112,113] This formulation is supported by the frequent co-occurrence of associative visual agnosia with right homonymous hemianopia, which deprives the left hemisphere of direct visual input, and splenial damage, which interrupts the transfer of information from the intact right visual cortex to the left hemisphere. Patients typically have large infarcts affecting the left PCA territory.[107,108,111,112,114-118] Many patients with this profile have also had alexia (without writing impairment) and color dysnomia, both of which have also been attributed to visual-verbal disconnection.[119]

An unexplained but repeatedly observed feature of this syndrome is relatively preserved naming and "recognition" of actions in comparison with objects.[111,120-122] Objects whose use is demonstrated through action are also better named than those shown in stationary positions.[111,116,120]

Prosopagnosia

Prosopagnosia is a term used to describe the failure to "recognize" previously known faces at sight. Almost all cases of prosopagnosia have resulted from damage to ventral temporal or ventral temporo-occipital areas. Largely on the basis of cases of carbon monoxide poisoning, with bilateral lesions, prosopagnosia was long thought to require bilateral lesions,[123,124] as also reported from cases of infarction.[125] However, later case reports based on MRI indicate that unilateral right PCA territory infarct may suffice.[126,127] This intriguing syndrome may in some cases be but a component of "visual agnosia." Achromatopsia, dyslexia, and topographic disorientation are also often present,[108,123,128] and in a few instances, more striking disturbances of visual neglect or Balint's syndrome are found.

Functional imaging studies in healthy subjects implicate both posterior and anterior regions of the temporal lobe in face processing, particularly the right posterior fusiform gyrus, superior temporal sulcus, and temporal pole.[129-132] These results suggest a hierarchical face processing stream progressing posteriorly to anteriorly along much of the ventral temporal lobe, which may explain why prosopagnosia can occur from ventral temporal lobe lesions in a variety of locations.[133] When studied in detail, some patients with prosopagnosia show impairments in processing more general object features, such as curved surfaces and spatial configurations, that happen to be particularly important for discriminating faces.[134-136] When object agnosia is also present, the stimulus classes most affected are those with many perceptually similar members, such as cars, flowers, and buildings.[123,133,137] Some writers have argued that such deficient discrimination between similar members within a category, whether at a perceptual level or a semantic level, is the crucial deficit in prosopagnosia.[123,136]

Distortions of Visual Perception

Palinopsia

Palinopsia has been regarded as a bit of a curiosity and is not commonly a result of vascular disease.[138] It is often caused by metastatic lesions such as tumors, but some newer cases have been associated with use of the anticonvulsant drug topiramate.[139] When due to structural disease, the syndrome usually occurs in a patient who has an impaired visual field but is not entirely blind.[140] One autopsied patient with palinopsia had subcortical infarct undermining the right lingual and fusiform gyri that was several months old.[141] Another three patients, all studied by CT,[138] had infarct affecting the right side in two and the left in one, and all the infarcts were large. However, in two later cases, one with a small occipital arteriovenous malformation, another due to anteromedial periventricular occipital infarction, palinopsia occurred without visual field defects.[142]

Two clinical variants are described.[141] In one, there is a persistence of some or all of a visual image immediately after it has disappeared from the environment. In the other, the image reappears only some time later and persists for varying periods. This latter form is quite striking, because the time between the disappearance of the original stimulus and its reappearance may be hours or days, and the image may persist into the following day. A peculiar feature of the palinopic images is their tendency to be incorporated in the appropriate position into visual stimuli in the present environment, such as a cigar and beard appearing on the faces of all the people at a party. Frank hallucinations and illusions of visual movement are common accompaniments of both types.[143]

Micropsia

An unusual complaint, micropsia is a visual disorder in which objects appear smaller than expected. Yamada and associates[144] reported a 63-year-old man whose micropsia occurred suddenly and was associated with an acute amnestic state (as expected from large left PCA territory infarction), although his visual field disturbance was limited to a right upper quadrantanopia. CT and MRI showed an infarct in the left occipital lobe and hippocampus. All the clinical features improved within a month, save for the persistence of the quadrantanopia. Another patient with a migraine history was found at postmortem to have right inferolateral occipital infarction near the inferred borderzone shared by the middle and posterior cerebral arteries.[145] The syndrome started as left homonymous hemianopia with prominent prosopagnosia. As these complaints faded over a week's time, the patient noted that objects seemed somewhat shrunken and compressed in his left visual field, making the plotting of visual fields difficult and producing an awareness that pictures seemed asymmetric. He drew the left-hand side of a pattern larger than the right so it would look symmetric to him.

Metamorphopsia

In metamorphopsia, another unusual condition, objects and faces, and rarely other visual stimuli, appear distorted or differing in size. Difficulties exist in estimating size and shape but pictures of the same display can be selected correctly from among incorrect displays.[146] A patient reported in 2008 with unilateral infarction described the left-hand side of the faces of family members and people in the street as distorted ("They look like monsters"). Right temporooccipital infarction was found on MRI. The syndrome persisted for 3 years.[147]

Topographical Disorientation

Patients with topographical disorientation have a striking inability to find their way around (Fig. 25-9).[148] Infarction in the right hemisphere, left visual field defects, and, occasionally, a disorder in recognition of faces are among the usual accompanying signs. There are at least three distinct syndromes. In the first, patients have difficulty "recognizing" familiar environmental landmarks such as buildings and street corners.[149,150] This syndrome resembles and is often accompanied by prosopagnosia, and some investigators prefer the label *topographical agnosia* or *landmark agnosia*. In the second form of the syndrome, landmarks are "recognized" but do not evoke a sense of direction; the patient fails to utilize routes previously learned in going from one landmark to another.[151,152] Alternative terms for this type are *topographical amnesia, directional disorientation,* and *heading disorientation*.[148] In the third variant, the patient is able to "recognize" landmarks and follow familiar routes but is impaired in learning new routes.[153,154] The responsible lesions, though variable, often affect the right posterior medial temporal lobe or posterior cingulate gyrus.[149-151,155]

Disorders of Reading

Ischemic lesions in the territory of the PCA produce a variety of disorders labeled "alexia" or "dyslexia." Reading difficulty occurs to varying degrees in the majority of patients with dominant hemisphere PCA infarcts.[156] Writing and other language functions typically are completely or almost completely spared. Major infarction in the PCA territory of the hemisphere dominant for speech and language, usually the left, appears necessary to precipitate the striking disorder of global or absolute alexia.[112,119,156-161]

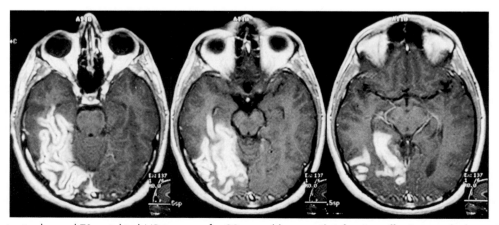

Figure 25-9 Contrast-enhanced T1-weighted MR images of a 32-year-old man with infarction affecting nearly the entire ventral occipito-temporal territory of the right posterior cerebral artery. The patient had mild topographical disorientation but no prosopagnosia.

Much of the literature dates back to Déjerine's[24] famous case. At autopsy, an old infarct was found to have damaged the inferior edge of the posterior portion of the corpus callosum as well as the cortex of the cuneus and adjacent calcarine region and completely penetrated the underlying white matter to the wall of the ventricle (Fig. 25-10). Although the patient in this case is commonly considered to have had hemianopia, the right visual field function was intact enough that Landolt's[162] original examination demonstrated only a hemiachromatopsia (see later discussion on color); the patient had full, albeit dim, vision in the right visual field to white targets. Déjerine proposed that the subcortical component of the infarct served to disrupt the projections to the angular gyrus (which he considered to be the site where the lexical information gained access to the language system) from both the ipsilateral calcarine cortex and the opposite side, this latter pathway via the corpus callosum. He made little mention of the callosal lesion, as did Vialet[161] in a thorough review of the case. In both instances, emphasis was placed on the deep periventricular lesion. Damasio and Damasio[157] resurrected these observations and drew attention to the likelihood that the inferior fibers of the forceps major, which cross in the inferior portion of the corpus callosum and terminate in the inferior visual association cortices, were the fibers of relevance for the conveyance of lexical information from the right to the left hemisphere.

The anatomic course of these fibers places them in the position to be caught in a deep infarct that penetrates to the wall of the ventricle. Like many others, our own case showed somewhat different infarcts (Fig. 25-11). Many other reports of severe alexia have also documented right hemianopia together with damage to the splenium or forceps major.[112,119,158,160,163] These studies suggest that the pathway from the right visual cortex to left language areas involved in reading is most vulnerable at the splenium and forceps major, before it fans out laterally over the top of the occipital horn to synapse in ventrolateral and anterior visual association areas.[156] This formulation is different from the more inferomedial location favored by several other writers.[157] An example of improved reading aloud despite large splenial and posterior cerebral infarction in a patient fluent in Arabic argues for some right hemispheric role in languages read from right to left.[164]

On the basis of these cases, an argument can be made that left visual association areas, particularly those lateral and anterior to the lingual gyrus, are critical components of the reading pathway and receive input from visual systems in both hemispheres. This interpretation is further supported by functional imaging studies in normal subjects demonstrating a "visual word-form" area in the left ventrolateral visual cortex (particularly fusiform gyrus), which responds more to letters, words, and word-like letter strings than to nonsense shapes.[165] Unlike the calcarine cortex and lingual gyrus, which are activated only by stimuli from the contralateral hemifield, this left hemisphere visual word-form area responds to graphemic stimuli presented to either hemifield, indicating that it receives transcallosal projections from the right visual cortex.[165]

Global Alexia

Global alexia is the most severe reading disorder syndrome. The patients can read no words aloud and are markedly inaccurate in naming aloud visually displayed single letters. When presented with lexical stimuli, a patient with global alexia may display no awareness that the responses are well off the mark. For example, Wyllie's[27] famous patient (Fig. 25-12) named the word "Dugald" as a series of single letters "k-a-n-i-o-i," similarly responded to the digit set "123456" as "i-r-e-i-u-e," and even named the mathematical symbols "+ − =" as "n-e-a." Such errors occur in this syndrome irrespective of whether the displays are typed, printed, or handwritten. Most patients cannot even read their own handwriting. They can, however, easily read aloud some words ordinarily presented in a distinctive form (e.g., the logo for well-known products like Coca-Cola, or the font used for certain newspaper names), as did Déjerine's patient for his favorite Paris newspaper, but the meaning of the words is derived from the shape of the logo, not from the meaning of the letters as a word. Despite this marked inability to name the letters, letters and digits are readily discriminated as separate from unfamiliar characters, such as lexical shapes from other languages. Evidence of familiarity with the shapes is seen as the patient readily and spontaneously re-orients letters presented in upside-down or rotated orientation. Musical notes and digits are

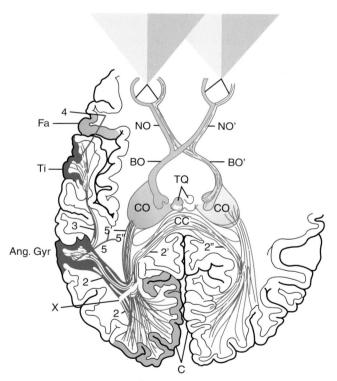

Figure 25-10 Diagram of the possible site (X) of interruption of the visual pathways linking the calcarine cortices (C) with the angular gyrus (Ang. Gyr). BO, left optic tract; BO′, right optic tract; CC, corpus callosum; CO, left lateral geniculate body; CO′, right lateral geniculate body; Fa, frontal operculum; NO, left optic nerve; NO′, right optic nerve; Ti, superior temporal gyrus. (Adapted from Déjerine J, Vialet N: Contribution à l'étude de la localisation anatomique de la cécité verbale pure. *C R Séances Soc Biol* 45:790, 1893.)

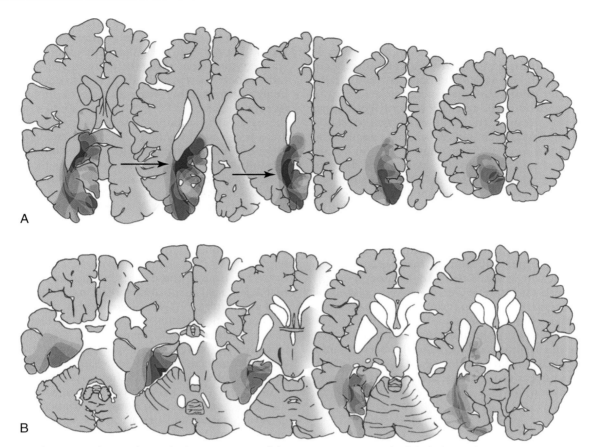

Figure 25-11 Lesion overlap analyses. A, Common areas of damage, in patients with global alexia, that were not damaged in normal readers with left posterior cerebral artery infarcts. B, Common areas of damage, in patients with verbal dyslexia (letter-by-letter reading), that were not damaged in normal readers with left posterior cerebral artery infarcts. *Arrows* denote sites of infarction.

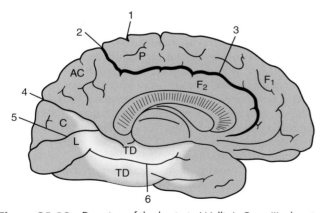

Figure 25-12 Drawing of the brain in Wyllie's Case III, showing the mesial left occipital infarction that produced global alexia. (From Wyllie J: *The disorders of speech,* Edinburgh, 1894, Oliver Boyd.)

classifiable separately from letters, but these items also fail to convey meaning. The first reported patient with global alexia was an accomplished musician who, in addition to losing the ability to name letters, lost the power to read musical scores after his stroke, although he retained the ability to play and sing from memory.[166] In some cases, the patient can name letters and digits when his or her hand is passively traced over the shapes (Willbrand's

sign), indicating that the problem is with the visual forms, not the forms per se. Writing, spelling aloud, and naming words heard in spelled form are usually spared.

This clinical picture is often accompanied by many other disorders indicative of a major left PCA territory infarction.[167] A dense right homonymous hemianopia is nearly always present. There may also be optic aphasia or visual agnosia, color dysnomia, amnestic aphasia, transcortical sensory aphasia, or memory disturbance.[112,119] In other patients, the deficits accompanying the alexia have been less spectacular.[157]

Verbal Dyslexia

Verbal dyslexia is a less severe impairment in which individual letter naming is preserved, but letters linked as words are not read aloud nor do they convey meaning. The patient can be taught to adopt a strategy of recognizing words by naming the letters one by one, and as (s)he spells them aloud, the letter strings heard prompt a spoken response (e.g., "c-a-t" "cat!"). This syndrome is the most common form of alexia without agraphia and has been by far the most studied, almost to the point of obscuring the existence of global alexia.[158] Many writers use *letter-by-letter reading* to denote the syndrome,[168,169] which has also been called *word-form dyslexia*[170] and *spelling dyslexia*.[156] Because the patient depends on sequential identification of letters, the time needed to read a word increases with word length.[168,170] The syndrome may initially manifest as global alexia, but within days to weeks after onset, the patient begins to read words by laboriously naming individual letters. Letter naming typically becomes fluent after weeks to months. We monitored five such patients and documented continued improvement in both reading accuracy and reading speed throughout the first year after stroke.[156] Some patients with verbal dyslexia have right upper quadrantanopia rather than a complete hemianopia.[156,157]

Dyslexia with No Visual Field Defect

Although it is exceedingly rare, the existence of dyslexia with no visual field defect challenges some theories of the lesions that explain dyslexia.[171] The first description of the syndrome was made without autopsy or imaging data and reported in France during late 1944; the patient, a 20-year-old woman, while walking in the street suddenly noticed she could not read the letters on a sign or the names of the subway stations.[11] Her alexia was described as complete for all varieties of reading tasks, including musical notes. The handful of autopsied or imaged cases of dyslexia have been due to tumors, arteriovenous malformations, hematomas, and the like, but rarely from infarction.[115,171,172] Most of the patients had relatively mild deficits, such as slowing or hesitation during reading, or transient dyslexia that rapidly cleared. The patients read very slowly and inaccurately and showed a marked drop in word recognition with increasing word length, suggesting a letter-by-letter reading strategy. Patients with severe deficits had large lesions of the left ventrolateral occipitotemporal cortex and lateral occipitotemporal convexity, the residue of lobar hemorrhages involving fusiform, inferior temporal, and lateral occipital gyri.[171,173] These regions are considered sites for interpretations of lexical displays; this function is separate from discrimination of visual displays mediated by the visual pathways and calcarine cortex.

Hemidyslexia

Wilbrand[174] described hemidyslexia as a macular hemianopic disturbance of reading (makulähemianopische Lesestörung). It is a frequent accompaniment of a homonymous hemianopia contralateral to infarction affecting the PCA territory of the hemisphere dominant for speech and language. In some instances, the hemianopia is limited to the right upper quadrant or the macular region, as demonstrated by Polyak's[26] patient Harry Kraft.

For most patients with such lesions, reading of connected text is more disturbed than reading of single words, owing to a disruption of the visuomotor coordination of saccadic eye movements during text reading.[175,176] Reading speed directly depends on the amount of spared macular vision in the right hemifield.[176,177] Reading of single words is often disturbed as well, manifested as both slowed recognition and misreading of the right-hand end of longer words. The time needed to read a word increases with word length, though not nearly as dramatically as in verbal dyslexia.[171] Errors occur whether the task is reading aloud or for comprehension and whether the words are printed or written, large or small, and isolated or embedded in text, as long as the words are lengthy (four letters or more). Errors occur less often when the right-hand end of the word is easily predicted by the left-hand end (e.g., "eight") and more often when the right-hand end has many possibilities not predicted by the left-hand end (e.g., "predator"). The term hemidyslexia is not quite accurate, because the errors do not begin at the midpoint of the stimulus but instead occur only at some point beyond the midline of the word.

Hemidyslexia affecting the left side of words occurs after sectioning of the corpus callosum.[178,179] The surgical section does no damage to the primary visual pathways but interrupts transmission of information from the right hemisphere to the left. Because the initial letters of a word fall within the left visual field during word fixation, they are transmitted first to the right hemisphere and are then misperceived because of the interhemispheric disconnection. Binder and coworkers[178] reported two patients with left hemidyslexia who also had macula-splitting right hemianopia. Both patients had left calcarine and splenial infarcts that occurred after treatment (embolization or resection) of left-sided retrosplenial arteriovenous malformations. Because visual input in these patients came only from the left visual field, the left-sided errors were taken as evidence that callosal transfer was weaker for letters presented farther to the left from the visual midline. This theory was confirmed by presentation of words in vertical orientation, which improved single-word reading accuracy from 55% to 93%. Left hemidyslexia has also been reported in association with Marchiafava-Bignami disease.[180]

Dyslexia for Numbers

Dyslexia for numbers, an isolated failure to read aloud numbers with preserved ability to read aloud letters and words, is distinctly rare. Passing anecdotal reference was made to "number alexia" (Zahlenalexie) in the 1930s *Bumpke-Förster Handbuch der Neurologie*. In later years, such a disturbance has been reported in a setting of initial aphasia and acalculia, the number alexia emerging as a late residue of the aphasia.[181] Where imaged, the infarcts have been large, involving the lateral parietal lobe,[182] in the middle cerebral artery, not PCA territory. The syndrome seems not to have a parallel to letter or word alexia.

Color Dysnomia and Dyschromatopsia

Some degree of faulty color discrimination may occur with dysfunction at any level along the visual pathway.[183,184] The lateral geniculate body is considered to play a role in color discrimination,[185] but deficits in color discrimination would be expected to occur only when the lesion is bilateral. However, when infarction is the cause of dyschromatopsia, it usually lies in the occipital lobe inferior to the calcarine cortex in the fusiform or lingual gyri, either with full-thickness infarction or with subcortical infarction that undermines the gyri. The lesion may be unilateral on either side[26,91,166,162,186,187] or bilateral.[25,92,93,183,186-190] In human functional imaging studies, the posterior fusiform gyrus responds more strongly to color stimuli than to luminance-matched grays,[188,191] suggesting that it may be the homologue of visual area V4 in the monkey, which is specialized for perception of color.[92,192]

Patients with bilateral color blindness from cerebral disease show impaired performance on tests of color discrimination (e.g., Ishihara color plates, Farnsworth-Munsell 100-hue test), although performance is usually far better than chance. Total absence of color perception (achromatopsia) appears to be rather rare.[193] Unilateral cases (hemidyschromatopsia) are best detected with color perimetry, because vision in the unimpaired hemifield is sufficient for normal performance on free-field tests such as the Ishihara plates. When the defect is quadrantic, the upper quadrants are affected, never the lower.[194] In typical cases, the colors in the affected field(s) are described as gray, pale, or washed out. At times, a given color is misnamed for another having a similar hue or brightness. This last finding is of little clinical value because it also occurs in patients whose color discrimination is intact (see later). Recall is normal for the color name characteristically associated with a given object (e.g., green with grass). Some improvement over time has been reported, even though an upper quadrantanopia might remain.[188,195] Prosopagnosia and topographical disorientation have been reported as associated findings in many patients with color blindness, particularly those with bilateral lesions.[25,92,93,183,186,189,194] Dyslexia often accompanies right hemidyschromatopsia. One among these cases[24,162,166] was explained by subsequent reviewers as a disconnection syndrome,[196] which would be expected to impair color naming but not color discrimination. Unfortunately, no details were provided about whether the color recognition impairment involved one or both fields or whether the patient was asked to name colors or simply discriminate between them.

Color and color-name disconnection describes a bidirectional impairment in relating a color to its name in the absence of deficits in color discrimination. The term color agnosia has also been used. The absence of deficits in color discrimination is revealed by normal performance on tests such as the Ishihara color plates. The bidirectional impairment in relating a color to its name is shown by errors in naming colors at sight and in matching color names heard or color names seen with color choices, and vice versa. Geschwind and Fusillo[119] applied *disconnection syndrome* to this type of case to stress the point that the lesion may have separated the adequately discriminated visual input in the right hemisphere from access to the language region of the left hemisphere. As a result, the patient presumably could not associate visual stimuli with their names, causing alexia (letters and words), defective naming of colors, and defective matching of color names to colors. In support of the disconnection notion, these researchers stressed that their patient "would answer at random" when shown an object and asked whether it was a certain color. This random quality of color naming has not been a feature in other reported patients with the disorder, however, even in some other patients with a bidirectional failure in relating colors to their names.

The infarct in the best-known case was in the distribution of the left PCA, destroying most of the gray matter and deep white matter of the medial occipital lobe, including the visual radiation, the inferior longitudinal fasciculus, and the crossing fibers through the splenium of the corpus callosum in the tapetum.[119] A subsequent case reported by Rubens and Benson[102] showed more circumscribed subcortical infarction underlying the left lingual gyrus. In another case used by these researchers in support of their thesis,[24,162,166] the patient appears to have had right hemidyschromatopsia; it is not clear from the details of the clinical case report that a disturbance as thoroughly documented as that by Geschwind and Fusillo[119] was present. Unfortunately, for most of the other reported patients whose deficits might represent bidirectional disconnection, precise documentation of a disconnection state was lacking.[189,197-201] In only a few was complete testing performed for color discrimination, impaired color naming, and impaired matching of colors with color names.[101,119,202] Clinically, these patients also showed a right homonymous hemianopia and dyslexia. The patient described by Zihl and von Cramon[203] exhibited intact color discrimination but impaired color naming restricted to the left visual field after splenial damage, consistent with a disconnection mechanism.

Color dysnomia is often considered synonymous with the bidirectional *color disconnection syndrome*. In the initial days after onset, a patient encountered by one of the authors (JPM) (Fig. 25-13) showed errors both in naming colors and in selecting the correct color from among an array of color choices when a color name was dictated aloud to him.[7] However, within several days, he became able to select a color from among several choices when its name was provided. He was easily able to recall the name of a color commonly associated with a given item and items commonly associated with a given color, yet he continued to have difficulties in naming a color shown to him. His naming errors were not random or of the confabulatory type. He often named a given color using the name of another color close to it on the spectrum of hue or brightness, such as green for blue, or yellow for orange. The errors were mild enough to be overlooked on casual testing and might have been attributed to dim light in less rigorous test settings. Casual explanations such as these probably account for the infrequency with which the dysnomia is reported in patients with an infarct in a similar locale. When sought in such cases, the deficit is often easily demonstrated. The infarct is often quite modest and may be confined to the subcortical structures of the lingual gyrus.

The syndrome of color dysnomia is also of interest because it may be present without dyslexia (i.e., with preserved reading). Although the two deficits frequently coexist, color dysnomia and alexia do not reflect a common mechanism; rather, they show that spatially proximate regions of the cerebrum serving different functions are susceptible to simultaneous involvement by the same lesion if it is large enough.[204]

Amnestic color dysnomia, a syndrome so rare that it is almost nonexistent, is a disturbance in the recall of the names of the colors that are characteristic of a given object (e.g., green for grass) and vice versa.[205] Tests of color discrimination and cross-matching of color with color names are said to be performed well.[206] No definite neuropathologic basis for this disorder has been established. We have seen three examples in a setting of lateral sinus thrombosis, all of which improved after the occlusion was recanalized and the occipital edema subsided.

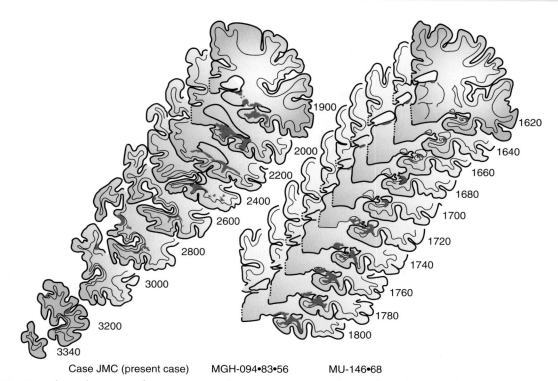

Case JMC (present case)   MGH•094•83•56   MU•146•68

Figure 25-13 Traced serial sections of a posterior cerebral artery territory infarct with involvement of the lateral geniculate body, hippocampus, and subcortical portions of the calcarine region. (From Mohr JP, Leicester J, Stoddard LT, Sidman M: Right hemianopia with memory and color deficits in circumscribed left posterior cerebral artery territory infarction. *Neurology* 21:1104, 1971.)

Other unusual disturbances in color naming or discrimination occur in cerebral disease.[207] However, none of them has as yet been related to a focal lesion. The delineation of most such disturbances requires the examiner to depend on the patient's subjective description of the altered appearance of color and of its relationship to the environment. The syndromes include illusory spread of color.

Aphasia

Aphasia and the Thalamus

Long ignored as a source of aphasia from focal infarction, the thalamus has been shown by electroencephalographic recordings to respond to syntactic and semantic elements in audiotorily presented language testing.[208,209] Rare cases exist in which an infarct in the pulvinar of the thalamus has produced an acute disturbance in semantic errors and word finding in a previously normal person.[210]

Transcortical Sensory Aphasia

That aphasia may occur with PCA territory lesions, including both cortical[167,211] and thalamic lesions,[212] is well documented. Transcortical sensory aphasia is an uncommon disturbance said to feature fluent speech, accurate repetition sometimes accompanied by echolalia, and impaired comprehension of both speech and text. Data on neuroanatomic correlation is somewhat lacking, and the term may not be as anatomically accurate as it is a reflection of former systems of classifying language disorders into cortical, subcortical, and transcortical forms.

There are several examples due to infarction in the middle cerebral artery territory or arterial borderzones.[213-215] Whether to place this syndrome among the consequences of PCA territory infarction is subject to argument, but it is discussed here because of the high frequency of accompanying hemianopia, visual object agnosia, and occipitotemporal low density seen on CT or MRI.[216,217]

The mechanism of these infarctions is unclear. Some could be the result of combined middle cerebral and posterior cerebral occlusion, or an internal carotid occlusion with distal field infarction affecting the parieto-occipital region in the unusual instances in which the PCA is a branch of the internal carotid artery. At least one patient had an arteriovenous malformation—a lesion suitable for such an unusual location, crossing as it does between two major arterial territories.[216]

Amnestic Aphasia

Amnestic (or anomic) aphasia is characterized by a failure to recall the names of people as well as many other individual nouns when the stimuli are presented in visual, tactile, or auditory form. The independence of the deficit from modality of sensory input distinguishes it from optic aphasia, in which anomia occurs only with visual presentation. Commonly, the expected response fails to occur, with the patient often falling silent or hesitating as if the name is about to be produced momentarily ("tip of the tongue" phenomenon). When the name fails to be given, it is rare for the patient to produce a neologism or other substitutive error. Instead, attributes of the item are described, indicating the patient's familiarity with the item in question. The failures in naming are often associated with circumlocutions, lame excuses for failure, and a general acceptance of the correct name when offered.[206] A category-specific form due to focal thalamic infarction has been described.[218]

Amnestic aphasia has been associated with lesions throughout the language-dominant hemisphere, but severe and isolated anomia has classically been considered a sign of deep temporal lobe[207] or lateral temporo-occipital damage.[219,220] The syndrome has been reported, often incidentally, in patients showing infarction limited to the territory of the dominant PCA.[27,112,167,189] Its features are different from phonemic and semantic errors mapped to lateral convexity cites.[221] Some writers have emphasized a correlation between the severity of anomia and the severity of dyslexia in patients with amnestic aphasia.[112,167] The exact pathologic correlation for naming deficits remains unclear, but one possibility is that amnestic aphasia appears when the temporal lobe component of the infarct extends sufficiently laterally (into fusiform and inferior temporal gyri) or deeply to involve lexical systems critical for name retrieval.

Memory Disorder Syndromes

PCA territory infarction may profoundly disrupt memory function[167,222,223] through damage to the hippocampus, the parahippocampus, or the efferents and afferents of these structures. As with surgical lesions of the medial temporal lobe, medial temporal infarcts produce impaired acquisition of new memories (anterograde amnesia), with relatively little effect on retrieval of memories encoded prior to onset of the lesion (retrograde amnesia). Amnestic disorders from occlusion of thalamoperforating arteries have also been reported, but in these cases, the possibility of simultaneous infarction of structures supplied by larger PCA branches is not easily ruled out.

On the basis of available literature, the occurrence of an amnestic state is no guide to whether the infarct is of thrombotic or embolic origin. Bilateral infarction has been the usual setting for severe memory disorders.[28,34,224-228] Both embolism and thrombus have been found to be responsible.[34] The occlusions have usually been found proximally in the PCA stem and precortical segment. The infarcts frequently spread along most of the undersurface of the cerebrum, involving the parahippocampus and lingual and fusiform gyri, some as far posteriorly as the cuneus[28]; others have been extensive enough to include the fornices and fimbria of the hippocampus.[227] The hippocampus is sometimes affected in amnestic cases, though PCA infarcts always involve other structures surrounding the hippocampus as well.

Bilateral infarcts with memory disturbance have been documented in a large literature. Much of it argues it is a necessary condition for amnesia to occur and to persist.[229] Numerous reports suggest that a bilateral disruption of the fornix though surgical section,[230-232] penetrating wounds,[233] or tumors[234] may achieve the same effect. In other similar cases, however, either no such deficits occurred[235,236] or memory impairments were transient.[237,238] The exact role of fornix damage in the occurrence and persistence of anterograde memory deficits has been difficult to determine because

instances of isolated bilateral fornix interruption are rare.[230,231,234-236,239-243]

Some cases of transient global amnesia (TGA) may represent bilateral medial temporal lobe ischemia. Single-photon emission CT (SPECT) scans performed during the amnestic ictus in TGA frequently show bitemporal hypoperfusion.[244] TGA is only rarely associated with embolism or thrombosis, however, and many cases with the association are probably caused by posterior circulation migraine[245] or venous congestion.[246]

Unilateral infarcts in the left PCA territory have also produced anterograde impairments of memory.[7,112,119,167,223,224,226,247,248] A patient described by one of the authors (JPM) showed a severe memory disorder from onset that persisted unchanged until his death on day 82.[7] On initial examination within 12 hours of onset, this patient also stated his name, failed to recall his exact age, and was unable to state his address or where he had been the evening of his stroke. He repeatedly asked many questions, such as "Where is my wife?" He accepted the examiner's answer but within seconds asked the question again. When his wife arrived hours after onset of the stroke and mentioned her brother by name, the patient asked, "Ed who?" He repeatedly attempted to learn the examiner's name, often wrote it on a note pad and, when the examiner reappeared, did not recall the name or consult the note pad. Weeks after discharge, when returning to the laboratory for reexamination, the patient regularly introduced himself to the staff whom he had met on every previous occasion and only rarely walked spontaneously in the correct direction toward the examining room. He showed a retrograde and anterograde amnesia for the events surrounding his admission, faulty retention of verbal material, impaired retention on a form discrimination test, and an amnestic dysnomia. Whether his deficit would have persisted over a longer period remains an open question. The pathologic findings indicated only unilateral infarction of the left hippocampus, with secondary degeneration of the left fornix and the precommissural bed nuclei of the septum (see Fig. 25-13).

Thalamic lesions have also been documented to produce anterograde amnestic syndromes, whether from Wernicke-Korsakoff syndrome,[249,250] trauma,[251] or infarction.[29,252,253] Lesions in the infarct cases have been unilateral but are usually bilateral and associated with a variety of etiologies.[254] They lie in the territory of the tuberothalamic or anterior paramedian perforators and involve anterior nuclei and the mamillothalamic tract.[255]

Klüver-Bucy Syndrome

Klüver-Bucy syndrome is described here because its cause is usually bilateral lesions in the territory of the PCAs. In the small number of reports of the syndrome, some not using this eponym,[256] the lesions have been very large, affecting most of the undersurface of the temporal lobes,[257-262] including the fusiform and lingual gyri, the parahippocampal gyri, and the hippocampal structures. Apart from video cases, few have been reported with lesion delineation in recent years.[262a] In addition to the fearless exploration of environment, the syndromes precipitated by these infarctions frequently include a prominent state of exaggerated motor activity; restlessness, agitation, delirium, crying out, and unwarranted excessive reaction to visual, auditory, or cutaneous stimuli may be the most striking features noted in the acute phase.[263] Within hours to days, these states usually subside.

REFERENCES

1. Lazorthes G, Salamon G: Étude anatomique et radio-anatomique de la vascularisation arterielle du thalamus, *Ann Radiol* 14:905, 1971.
2. Abbie AA: The blood supply of the visual pathways, *Med J Aust* 2:199, 1938.
3. Salamon G, Huang YP: *Radiologic anatomy of the brain*, Berlin, 1976, Springer-Verlag.
4. Percheron G: The anatomy of the arterial supply of the human thalamus and its use for the interpretation of the thalamic vascular pathology, *Z Neurol* 205:1–13, 1973.
5. Milisavljevic MM, Marinkovic SV, Gibo H, et al: The thalamogeniculate perforators of the posterior cerebral artery: The microsurgical anatomy, *Neurosurgery* 28:523, 1991.
6. Galloway JR, Greitz T: The medial and lateral choroidal arteries: An anatomic and roentgenographic study, *Acta Radiol (Stockh)* 53:353, 1960.
7. Mohr JP, Leicester J, Stoddard LT, et al: Right hemianopia with memory and color deficits in circumscribed left posterior cerebral artery territory infarction, *Neurology* 21:1104, 1971.
8. Ghika JA, Bogousslavsky J, Regli F: Deep perforators from the carotid system: Template of the vascular territories, *Arch Neurol* 47:1097, 1990.
9. Kaul SN, DuBoulay GH, Kendall BE, et al: Relationship between visual field defects and arterial occlusion in the posterior cerebral circulation, *J Neurol Neurosurg Psychiatry* 37:1033, 1974.
10. Margolis MT, Newton TH, Hoyt WF: Cortical branches of the posterior cerebral artery: Anatomic-radiologic correlation, *Neuroradiology* 2:127, 1971.
11. Peron N, Goutner V: Alexie pure sans hemianopsie, *Rev Neurol* 76:81, 1944.
12. Smith CG, Richardson WFG: The course and distribution of the arteries supplying the visual striate cortex, *Am J Ophthalmol* 61:1391, 1966.
13. Margolis MT, Smith CG, Richardson WF: The course and distribution of the arteries supplying the visual (striate) cortex, *Am J Ophthalmol* 61:1391, 1966.
14. Beevor CE: On the distribution of the different arteries supplying the human brain, *Philos Trans R Soc [Biol]* 200:1, 1909.
15. Shellshear JL: A contribution to our knowledge of the arterial supply of the cerebral cortex in man, *Brain* 50:236, 1927.
16. Castaigne P, Lhermitte F, Gautier JC, et al: Arterial occlusions in the vertebro-basilar system: A study of forty-four patients with post-mortem data, *Brain* 96:133, 1973.
17. Steinke W, Mangold J, Schwartz A, et al: Mechanisms of infarction in the superficial posterior cerebral artery territory, *J Neurol* 244:571, 1997.
18. Kinkel WR, Newman RP, Jacobs L: Posterior cerebral artery branch occlusions: CT and anatomic considerations. In Berguer R, Bauer RB, editors: *Vertebrobasilar arterial occlusive disease: medical and surgical management*, Philadelphia, 1984, Lippincott-Raven, p 117.
19. Pessin MS, Lathi ES, Cohen MB, et al: Clinical features and mechanism of occipital infarction, *Ann Neurol* 21:290, 1987.
20. Goto K, Takagawa K, Uemura K, et al: Posterior cerebral artery occlusion: Clinical computed tomographic and angiographic correlation, *Radiology* 132:357, 1979.
21. Pessin MS, Kwan ES, Scott RM, et al: Occipital infarction with hemianopia from carotid occlusive disease, *Stroke* 20:409, 1989.
22. Caplan LR: "Top of the basilar" syndrome, *Neurology* 30:72, 1980.
23. Benson DF, Segarra J, Albert ML: Visual agnosia-prosopagnosia, *Arch Neurol* 30:307, 1974.
24. Déjerine J: Contribution à l'étude anatomo-pathologique et clinique des différentes variétés de cécité verbale, *C R Séances Soc Biol* 44:61, 1892.
25. Lenz G: Zwei Sektionsfalle doppelseitigen zentraler Farbenhemianopsie, *Z Ges Neurol Psychiatr* 71:135, 1921.
26. Polyak SL: *The vertebrate visual system*, Chicago, 1957, University of Chicago Press.
27. Wyllie J: *The disorders of speech*, Edinburgh, 1894, Oliver, Boyd.
28. Lee E, Kang DW, Kwon SU, et al: Posterior cerebral artery infarction: Diffusion-weighted MRI analysis of 205 patients, *Cerebrovasc Dis* 28:298–305, 2009.
29. Castaigne P, Lhermitte F, Buge A, et al: Paramedian thalamic and midbrain infarcts: Clinical and neuropathological study, *Ann Neurol* 10:127, 1981.
30. Landis T, Regard M, Bliestle A, Kleihues P: Prosopagnosia and agnosia for noncanonical views: An autopsied case, *Brain* 111:1287, 1988.
31. Bohdiewicz P, Juni JE: Watershed ischemia demonstrated with acetazolamide enhanced Tc-99m HMPAO SPECT, *Clin Nucl Med* 19:452, 1994.
32. Melamed E, Abraham FA, Lavy S: Cortical blindness as a manifestation of basilar artery occlusion, *Eur Neurol* 11:22, 1974.
33. Riley HA, Yaskin JC, Riggs ME, et al: Bilateral blindness due to lesions in both occipital lobes, *N Y J Med* 43:1619, 1943.
34. Symonds C, Mackenzie I: Bilateral loss of vision from cerebral infarction, *Brain* 80:415, 1957.
35. Duncan GW, Weidling SM: Posterior cerebral artery stenosis with midbrain infarction, *Stroke* 26:900, 1995.
36. Fisher CM: The posterior cerebral artery syndrome, *Can J Neurol Sci* 13:232, 1986.
37. Lauritzen M: Pathophysiology of the migraine aura, *Brain* 117:199, 1994.
38. Olesen J, Friberg L, Olsen TS, et al: Ischaemia-induced (symptomatic) migraine attacks may be more frequent than migraine-induced ischaemic insults, *Brain* 116:187, 1993.
39. Meyer A: Herniation of the brain, *Arch Neurol Psychiatry* 4:387, 1920.
40. Ropper AH: Syndrome of transtentorial herniation: Is vertical displacement necessary? *J Neurol Neurosurg Psychiatry* 56:932, 1993.
41. Sato M, Tanaka S, Kohama A, Fujii C: Occipital lobe infarction caused by tentorial herniation, *Neurosurgery* 18:300, 1986.
42. Jochum P, Kliesch U, Both R, et al: Neurobrucellosis with thalamic infarction: A case report, *Neurol Sci* 29:481–483, 2008.
43. Sieben G, De Reuck J, Eecken HV: Thrombosis of the mesencephalic artery: A clinico-pathological study of two cases and its correlation with the arterial vascularization, *Acta Neurol Belg* 77:151, 1977.
44. Waterston JA, Stark RJ, Gilligan BS: Paramedian thalamic and midbrain infarction: The 'mesencephalothalamic syndrome'. *J Clin Exp Neurol* 24:45, 1987.
45. Bassetti C, Staikov IN: Hemiplegia vegetativa alterna (ipsilateral Horner's syndrome and contralateral hemihyperhidrosis) following proximal posterior cerebral artery occlusion, *Stroke* 26:702, 1995.
46. Hommel M, Besson G, Pollak P, et al: Hemiplegia in posterior cerebral artery occlusion, *Neurology* 40:1496, 1990.
47. Argentino C, De Michele M, Fiorelli M, et al: Posterior circulation infarcts simulating anterior circulation stroke: Perspective of the acute phase, *Stroke* 27:1306, 1996.
48. Frisen L, Holmegaard L, Rosencrantz M: Sectorial optic atrophy and homonymous horizontal sector anopia: A lateral choroidal artery syndrome? *J Neurol Neurosurg Psychiatry* 41:374, 1978.
49. Déjerine J, Roussy G: La syndrome thalamique, *Rev Neurol (Paris)* 14:521, 1906.
50. Ghika J, Bogousslavsky J, Henderson J, et al: The "jerky dystonic unsteady hand": A delayed motor syndrome in posterior thalamic infarctions, *J Neurol* 241:537, 1994.
51. Hayman LA, Berman SA, Hinck VC: Correlation of CT cerebral vascular territories with function. II: Posterior cerebral artery, *Am J Neuroradiol* 2:219, 1981.
52. Manfredi M, Curccu G: Thalamic pain revisited. In Loeb C, editor: *Studies in cerebrovascular-disease*, Milan, 1981, Masson Italia Editori, p 73.
53. Demasles S, Peyron R, Garcia Larrea L, et al: Central post-stroke pain, *Rev Neurol (Paris)* 164:825–831, 2008.
54. Fujikane M, Itoh M, Nakazawa M, et al: Cerebral infarction accompanied by dysgeusia—a clinical study on the gustatory pathway in the CNS, *Rinsho Shinkeigaku* 39:771–774, 1999.

55. Mohr JP, Case CS, Meckler RJ, et al: Sensorimotor stroke due to thalamocapsular ischemia, *Arch Neurol* 34:739, 1977.

56. Ghika-Schmid F, Ghika J, Regli F, et al: Hyperkinetic movement disorders during and after acute stroke: The Lausanne Stroke Registry, *J Neurol Sci* 146:109, 1997.

57. Lee MS, Marsden CD: Movement disorder following lesions of the thalamus or subthalamic region, *Mov Disord* 9:493, 1994.

58. Ferroir JP, Feve A, Khalil A, et al: Hyperkinesie volitionnelle et d'attitude d'un membre supérieur: Manifestation d'un accident ischemique dans le territoire de l'artère cérébrale postérieure, *Presse Med* 21:2104, 1992.

59. Gille M, Van den Bergh P, Ghariani S, et al: Delayed-onset hemidystonia and chorea following contralateral infarction of the posterolateral thalamus: A case report, *Acta Neurol Belg* 96:307, 1996.

60. Cerrato P, Grasso M, Azzaro C, et al: Palatal myoclonus in a patient with a lateral thalamic infarction, *Neurology* 64:924-925, 2005.

61. Lehéricy S, Grand S, Pollak P, et al: Clinical characteristics and topography of lesions in movement disorders due to thalamic lesions, *Neurology* 57:1055-1066, 2001.

62. Suzuki K, Odaka M, Tatsumoto M, et al: Case of unilateral thalamo-mesencephalic infarction with enlargement to bilateral vertical gaze palsy due to vertical one-and-a-half syndrome, *Brain Nerve* 60:92-96, 2008.

63. Kitajima M, Korogi Y, Takahashi M, et al: MR signal intensity of the optic radiation, *AJNR Am J Neuroradiol* 17:1379-1383, 1996.

64. Math RS, Singh S, Bahl V: An uncommon complication after a common procedure, *J Invasive Cardiol* 20:E301-E303, 2008.

65. Förster O: Ueber Rindenblindheit, *Graefes Arch Ophthalmol* 36:94, 1890.

66. Goldenberg G: Loss of visual imagery and loss of visual knowledge: A case study, *Neuropsychologia* 30:1081, 1992.

67. Spector RH, Glaser JS, David NJ, et al: Occipital lobe infarctions: Perimetry and computed tomography, *Neurology (NY)* 31:1198, 1981.

68. Brindley GS, Janota I: Observations on cortical blindness and on vascular lesions that cause loss of recent memory, *J Neurol Neurosurg Psychiatry* 38:459, 1975.

69. Celesia GG, Archer CR, Kuriowa Y: Visual function of the extrageniculo-calcarine system in man, *Arch Neurol* 37:704, 1980.

70. Bergman PS: Cerebral blindness, *Arch Psychiatry Neurol* 78:568, 1957.

71. Blythe IM, Kennard C, Ruddock KH: Residual vision in patients with retrogeniculate lesions of the visual pathways, *Brain* 110:887, 1987.

72. Meyer O: Ein- und doppleseitige homonyme Hemianopsia mit Orientirungsstörungen, *Monatsschr Psychiatr Neurol* 8:440, 1900.

73. Holmes G: *Selected papers of Sir Gordon Holmes*, London, 1956, Blackwell, p 195.

74. Lin SF, Kuo YT, Chang FL, et al: Homonymous central quadrantanopia caused by an extrastriate (v2/v3) infarction: A case report, *Kaohsiung J Med Sci* 24:430-435, 2008.

75. Heller-Bettinger I, Kepes JJ, Preskorn SH, et al: Bilateral altitudinal anopia caused by infarction of the calcarine cortex, *Neurology* 26:1176, 1976.

76. Newman RP, Kinkel WR, Jacobs L: Altitudinal hemianopia caused by occipital infarctions, *Arch Neurol* 41:413, 1984.

77. Papageorgiou E, Gatzioufas Z, Wilhelm H: Bilateral altitudinal visual field defects caused by occipital infarctions, *Klin Monatsbl Augenheilkd* 226:132-134, 2009.

78. Bogousslavsky J, Regli F, van Melle G: Unilateral occipital infarction: Evaluating the risks of developing bilateral loss of vision, *J Neurol Neurosurg Psychiatry* 46:78, 1983.

79. Benton S, Levy I, Swash M: Vision in the temporal crescent in occipital infarction, *Brain* 103:83, 1980.

80. Lepore FE: The preserved temporal crescent: The clinical implications of an "endangered" finding, *Neurology* 57:1918, 2001.

81. Holmes G, Lister WT: Disturbances of vision from cerebral lesions, with special reference to the cortical representation of the macula, *Brain* 39:34, 1916.

82. Isa K, Miyashita K, Yanagimoto S, et al: Homonymous defect of macular vision in ischemic stroke, *Eur Neurol* 46:126, 2001.

83. Luco C, Hoppe A, Schweitzer M, et al: Visual field defects in vascular lesions of the lateral geniculate body, *J Neurol Neurosurg Psychiatry* 55:12, 1992.

84. Miller NR: *Walsh and Hoyt's clinical neuro-ophthalmology*, vol 1, ed 4, Baltimore, 1982, Williams & Wilkins.

85. Mackenzie I, Meighan S, Pollock EN: On the projection of the retinal quadrants on the lateral geniculate bodies and the relationship of the quadrants to the optic radiations, *Trans Ophthalmol Soc U K* 53:142, 1933.

86. Neau J-P, Bogousslavsky J: The syndrome of posterior choroidal artery territory infarction, *Ann Neurol* 39:779, 1996.

87. Frisen L: Quadruple sector anopia and sectorial optic atrophy: A syndrome of the distal anterior choroidal artery, *J Neurol Neurosurg Psychiatry* 42:590, 1979.

88. Shibata K, Nishimura Y, Kondo H, et al: Isolated homonymous hemianopsia due to lateral posterior choroidal artery region infarction: A case report, *Clin Neurol Neurosurg* 111:713-716, 2009.

89. Mudumbai RC, Bhandari A: Bilateral isolated lateral geniculate body lesions in a patient with pancreatitis and microangiopathy, *J Neuroophthalmol* 27:169-175, 2007.

90. Riddoch G: Dissociation of visual perceptions due to occipital injuries, with especial reference to appreciation of movement, *Brain* 40:15, 1917.

91. Merigan W, Freeman A, Meyers SP: Parallel processing streams in human visual cortex, *Neuroreport* 8:3985, 1997.

92. Rizzo M, Nawrot M, Blake R, et al: A human visual disorder resembling area V4 dysfunction in the monkey, *Neurology* 42:1175, 1992.

93. Vaina L: Functional segregation of color and motion processing in the human visual cortex: Clinical evidence, *Cereb Cortex* 5:555, 1994.

94. Van Essen DC, Felleman DJ, DeYoe EA, et al: Modular and hierarchical organization of extrastriate visual cortex in the macaque monkey, *Cold Spring Harb Symp Quant Biol* 55:679, 1990.

95. Barton JJ, Sharpe JA: Smooth pursuit and saccades to moving targets in blind hemifields: A comparison of medial occipital, lateral occipital and optic radiation lesions, *Brain* 120:681-699, 1997.

96. Weiskrantz L: *Blindsight: a case study and implications*, Oxford, 1986, Clarendon.

97. Wessinger CM, Fendrich R, Gazzaniga MS: Islands of residual vision in hemianopic patients, *J Cogn Neurosci* 9:203, 1997.

98. Zihl J, von Cramon D: Visual field recovery from scotoma in patients with postgeniculate damage: A review of 55 cases, *Brain* 108:335, 1985.

99. Nelles G, Esser J, Eckstein A, et al: Compensatory visual field training for stroke patients with hemianopia after stroke, *Neurosci Lett* 306:189, 2001.

100. Kasten E, Wust S, Behrens-Baumann W, et al: Computer-based training for the treatment of partial blindness, *Nature Med* 4:1083, 1998.

101. Lissauer H: Ein fall von Seelenblindheit nebst einem Beitrage zur Theorie derselben, *Arch Psychiatr Nervenkr* 21:2, 1889.

102. Rubens AB, Benson DF: Associative visual agnosia, *Arch Neurol* 24:305, 1971.

103. Bay E: *Agnose und funktionswandel: eine hirnpathologische studie*, Berlin, 1950, Springer-Verlag.

104. Bender MB, Feldman M: The so-called visual agnosias, *Brain* 95:173, 1972.

105. Head H: Aphasia: An historical review, *Brain* 43:340, 1920.

106. Farah MJ: *Visual agnosia: disorders of object recognition and what they tell us about normal vision*, Cambridge, MA, 1990, MIT Press.

107. Freund CS: Ueber optische Aphasie und Seelenblindheit, *Archiv für Psychiatrie und Nervenkrankheiten* 20:276, 1889.

108. Lhermitte F, Beauvois MF: A visual speech disconnection syndrome: Report of a case with optic aphasia, agnosic alexia and colour agnosia, *Brain* 96:695, 1973.

109. Coslett HB, Saffran EM: Preserved object recognition and reading comprehension in optic aphasia, *Brain* 112:1091-1110, 1989.

110. De Renzi E, Saetti MC: Associative agnosia and optic aphasia: Qualitative or quantitative difference? *Cortex* 33:115, 1997.

111. Schnider A, Benson DF, Scharre DW: Visual agnosia and optic aphasia: Are they anatomically distinct? *Cortex* 30:445, 1994.

112. Michel F, Schott B, Boucher M, et al: Alexie sans agraphie chez un malade ayant un hémisphére gauche déafférenté, *Rev Neurol* 135:347, 1979.

113. Poeck K: Neuropsychological demonstration of splenial interhemispheric disconnection in a case of "optic anomia, *Neuropsychologia* 22:707, 1984.

114. Coslett HB, Saffran EM: Preserved object recognition and reading comprehension in optic aphasia, *Brain* 112:1091, 1989.

115. Carlesimo GA, Casadio P, Sabbadini M, et al: Associative visual agnosia resulting from a disconnection between intact visual memory and semantic systems, *Cortex* 34:563, 1998.

116. Greenblatt SH: Subangular alexia without agraphia or hemianopsia, *Brain Lang* 3:229, 1976.

117. Larrabee GJ, Levin HS, Huff FJ, et al: Visual agnosia contrasted with visual-verbal disconnection, *Neuropsychologia* 23:1, 1985.

118. Ohtake H, Fujii T, Yamadori A, et al: The influence of misnaming on object recognition: A case of multimodal agnosia, *Cortex* 37:175, 2001.

119. Geschwind N, Fusillo M: Color-naming defects in association with alexia, *Arch Neurol* 15:137, 1966

120. Ferreira CT, Guisiano B, Ceccaldi M, Poncet M: Optic aphasia: Evidence of the contribution of different neural systems to object and action naming, *Cortex* 33:499, 1997.

121. McCarthy R, Warrington EK: Visual associative agnosia: A clinico-anatomical study of a single case, *J Neurol Neurosurg Psychiatry* 49:1233, 1986.

122. Hillis AE, Caramazza A: Cognitive and neural mechanisms underlying visual and semantic processing: Implications from "optic aphasia," *J Cogn Neurosci* 7:457, 1995.

123. Damasio A, Damasio H, Van Hoesen GW: Prosopagnosia: Anatomic basis and behavioral mechanisms, *Neurology (NY)* 323:331, 1982.

124. Meadows JC: The anatomical basis of prosopagnosia, *J Neurol Neurosurg Psychiatry* 37:489, 1974.

125. Karnath HO, Rüter J, Mandler A, Himmelbach M: The anatomy of object recognition—visual form agnosia caused by medial occipitotemporal stroke, *J Neurosci* 29:5854–5862, 2009.

126. De Renzi E, Perani D, Carlesimo GA, et al: Prosopagnosia can be associated with damage confined to the right hemisphere: An MRI and PET study and a review of the literature, *Neuropsychologia* 32:893–902, 1994.

127. Steeves J, Dricot L, Goltz HC, et al: Abnormal face identity coding in the middle fusiform gyrus of two brain-damaged prosopagnosic patients, *Neuropsychologia* 47:2584–2592, 2009.

128. Michel F, Poncet M, Signoret JL: Les lésions responsables de la prosopagnosie: sont-elles toujours bilatérales? *Rev Neurol* 146:764, 1989.

129. Allison T, Puce A, Spencer DD, et al: Electrophysiological studies of human face perception. 1: Potentials generated in occipitotemporal cortex by face and non-face stimuli, *Cereb Cortex* 9:415, 1999.

130. Nakamura K, Kawashima R, Sato N, et al: Functional delineation of the human occipitotemporal areas related to face and scene processing, *Brain* 123:2000, 1903.

131. Leveroni C, Seidenberg M, Mayer AR, et al: Neural systems underlying the recognition of familiar and newly learned faces, *J Neurosci* 20:878, 2000.

132. Kanwisher N, McDermott J, Chun MM: The fusiform face area: A module in human extrastriate cortex specialized for face perception, *J Neurosci* 17:4302–4311, 1997.

133. Clark S, Lindemann A, Maeder P, et al: Face recognition and postero-inferior hemispheric lesions, *Neuropsychologia* 35:1555, 1997.

134. Laeng B, Caviness VS: Propagnosia as a deficit in encoding curved surface, *J Cogn Neurosci* 13:556, 2001.

135. Farah MJ, Wilson KD, Drain HM, et al: The inverted face inversion effect in prosopagnosia: Evidence for mandatory, face-specific perceptual mechanisms, *Vision Res* 35:2089, 1995.

136. Dixon MJ, Bub DN, Arguin M: Semantic and visual determinants of face recognition in a prosopagnosic patient, *J Cogn Neurosci* 10:362, 1998.

137. De Haan EHF, Young AW, Newcombe F: Covert and overt recognition in prosopagnosia, *Brain* 114:2575, 1991.

138. Michel EM, Troost BT: Palinopsia: Cerebral localization with computed tomography, *Neurology* 30:887, 1980.

139. Evans RW: Reversible palinopsia and the Alice in Wonderland syndrome associated with topiramate use in migraineurs, *Headache* 46:815–818, 2006.

140. Bender MB, Feldman M, Sobin AJ: Palinopsia, *Brain* 91:321, 1968.

141. Meadows JC, Munro SS: Palinopsia, *J Neurol Neurosurg Psychiatry* 40:5, 1977.

142. Ritsema ME, Murphy MA: Palinopsia from posterior visual pathway lesions without visual field defects, *J Neuroophthalmol* 27:115–117, 2007.

143. Critchley M: Types of visual perseveration: 'Palinopsia' and 'illusory visual spread,' *Brain* 74:267, 1951.

144. Yamada A, Miki H, Nishioka M: A case of posterior cerebral artery territory infarction with micropsia as the chief complaint, *Rinsho Shinkeigaku* 30:894, 1990.

145. Cohen L, Gray F, Meyrignac C, et al: Selective deficit of visual size perception: Two cases of hemimicropsia, *J Neurol Neurosurg Psychiatry* 57:73, 1994.

146. Nijboer TC, Ruis C, van der Worp HB, et al: The role of Funktionswandel in metamorphopsia, *J Neuropsychol* 2:287–300, 2008.

147. Kamikubo T, Abo M, Yatsuzuka H: Case of long-term metamorphopsia caused by multiple cerebral infarction, *Brain Nerve* 60:671–675, 2008.

148. Aguirre GK, D'Esposito M: Topographical disorientation: A synthesis and taxonomy, *Brain* 122:1613, 1999.

149. Cogan DG: Visuospatial dysgnosia, *Am J Ophthalmol* 88:361, 1979.

150. Takahashi N, Kawamura M: Pure topographical disorientation: The anatomical basis of landmark agnosia, *Cortex* 38:717, 2002.

151. Alsaadi T, Binder JR, Lazar RM, et al: Pure topographic disorientation: A distinctive syndrome with varied localization, *Neurology* 54:2000, 1864.

152. Luzzi S, Pucci E, Di Bella P, et al: Topographical disorientation consequent to amnesia of spatial location in a patient with right parahippocampal damage, *Cortex* 36:427, 2000.

153. Barrash J, Damasio H, Adolphs R, et al: The neuroanatomical correlates of route learning impairment, *Neuropsychologia* 38:820, 2000.

154. Epstein R, DeYoe EA, Press DZ, et al: Neuropsychological evidence for a topographical learning mechanism in parahippocampal cortex, *Cogn Neuropsychol* 18:481, 2001.

155. Habib M, Sirigu A: Pure topographical disorientation: A definition and anatomical basis, *Cortex* 23:73–85, 1987.

156. Binder JR, Mohr JP: The topography of transcallosal reading pathways: A case-control analysis, *Brain* 115:1807, 1992.

157. Damasio AR, Damasio H: The anatomic basis of pure alexia, *Neurology* 33:1573, 1983.

158. Dalmás JF, Dansilo S: Visuographemic alexia: A new form of a peripheral acquired dyslexia, *Brain Lang* 75:1, 2000.

159. Greenblatt SH: Alexia without agraphia or hemianopsia: Anatomical analysis of an autopsied case, *Brain* 96:307, 1973.

160. Foix C, Hillemand P: Role vraisemblable du splenium dans la pathogénie de l'alexie pure par lésion de la cérébrale postérieure, *Bull Mem Soc Med Hop Paris* 49:393, 1925.

161. Vialet N: *Les centres cérébraux de la vision et l'appareil nerveux visuel intra-cérébral*, Paris, 1893, Faculté de Medecine de Paris.

162. Landolt E: De la cécité verbale, *Neurol Cbl* 7:605, 1888.

163. Stommel EW, Friedman RJ, Reeves AG: Alexia without agraphia associated with spleniogeniculate infarction, *Neurology* 41:587, 1991.

164. el Alaoui-Faris M, Benbelaid F, Alaoui C, et al: Alexia without agraphia in the Arabic language: Neurolinguistic and MRI study, *Rev Neurol (Paris)* 150:771–775, 1994.

165. Cohen L, Lehéricy S, Chochon F, et al: Language-specific tuning of visual cortex? Functional properties of the visual word form area, *Brain* 125:1054, 2002.

166. Déjerine J, Vialet N: Contribution a l'étude de la localisation anatomique de la cécité verbale pure, *C R Séances Soc Biol* 45:790, 1893.

167. De Renzi E, Zambolin A, Crisi G: The pattern of neuropsychological impairment associated with left posterior cerebral infarcts, *Brain* 110:1099, 1987.

168. Patterson KE, Kay J: Letter-by-letter reading: Psychological descriptions of a neurological syndrome, *Q J Exp Psychol* 34A:411, 1982.

169. Shallice T, Saffran E: Lexical processing in the absence of explicit word identification: Evidence from a letter-by-letter reader, *Cogn Neuropsychol* 3:429, 1986.

170. Warrington EK, Shallice T: Word-form dyslexia, *Brain* 103:99, 1980.

171. Leff AP, Crewes H, Plant GT, et al: The functional anatomy of single-word reading in patients with hemianopic and pure alexia, *Brain* 124:510, 2001.

172. Vincent FM, Sadowsky CH, Saunders RL, et al: Alexia without agraphia, hemianopia, or color-naming defect: A disconnection syndrome, *Neurology* 27:689, 1977.

173. Henderson VW, Friedman RB, Teng EL, et al: Left hemisphere pathways in reading: Inferences from pure alexia without hemianopia, *Neurology* 35:962, 1985.

174. Wilbrand H: Ueber die makulär-hemianopische Lesestörung und die v Monakowsche Projektion der Makula auf die Sehspäre, *Klin Monatsbl Augenheilkd* 45:1, 1907.

175. Gassel MM, Williams D: Visual function in patients with homonymous hemianopia. Part II: Oculomotor mechanisms, *Brain* 86:1, 1963.

176. Zihl J: Eye movement patterns in hemianopic dyslexia, *Brain* 118:891, 1995.

177. McConkie G, Rayner K: Asymmetry of the perceptual span in reading, *Bull Psychonom Soc* 8:365, 1976.

178. Binder JR, Lazar RM, Tatemichi TK, et al: Left hemiparalexia, *Neurology* 42:562, 1992.

179. Levine DN, Calvanio R: Visual discrimination after lesion of the posterior corpus callosum, *Neurology* 30:21, 1980.

180. Berek K, Wagner M, Chemelli AP, et al: Hemispheric disconnection in Marchiafava-Bignami disease: Clinical, neuropsychological and MRI findings, *J Neurol Sci* 123:2–5, 1994.

181. Cipolotti L, Warrington EK, Butterworth B: Selective impairment in manipulating Arabic numerals, *Cortex* 31:73–86, 1995.

182. Marangolo P, Nasti M, Zorzi M: Selective impairment for reading numbers and number words: A single case study, *Europsychologia* 42:997–1006, 2004.

183. Green GJ, Lessell S: Acquired cerebral dyschromatopsia, *Arch Ophthalmol* 95:121, 1977.

184. Urechia CI, Cremene V, Popescu P: Hémianopsie avec chromoagnosie, *Rev Neurol (Paris)* 80:70, 1948.

185. LeGros Clark WE: The laminar pattern of the lateral geniculate nucleus considered in relation to color vision, *Doc Ophthalmol* 3:57, 1949.

186. Damasio A, Yamada T, Damasio H: Central achromatopsia: Behavioral and anatomic and physiologic aspects, *Neurology* 30:1064, 1980.

187. Ziehl-Lübeck: Ueber einem Fall von Alexia and Farbenhemiagnosie, *Verh Ges Dtsch Natur Aertze* 67:184, 1895.

188. Beauchamp MS, Haxby JV, Rosen AC, et al: A functional MRI case study of acquired cerebral dyschromatopsia, *Neuropsychologia* 38:1170, 2000.

189. Heidenhain A: Beitrag zur Kenntnis der Seelenblindheit, *Monatsschr Psychiatr Neurol* 66:61, 1927.

190. Pearlman AL, Birch J, Meadows JC: Cerebral color blindness: An acquired defect in hue discrimination, *Ann Neurol* 5:253, 1979.

191. Sakurai Y, Takeuchi S, Takada T, et al: Alexia caused by a fusiform or posterior inferior temporal lesion, *J Neurol Sci* 178:42, 2000.

192. Zeki S: A century of cerebral achromatopsia, *Brain* 113:1721, 1990.

193. Heywood CA, Wilson B, Cowey A: A case study of cortical colour "blindness" with relatively intact achromatic discrimination, *J Neurol Neurosurg Psychiatry* 50:22, 1987.

194. Meadows JC: Disturbed perception of colours associated with localized cerebral lesions, *Brain* 97:615, 1974.

195. Albert NL, Reches A, Silverberg R: Hemianopic colour blindness, *J Neurol Neurosurg Psychiatry* 38:546, 1975.

196. Geschwind N: Disconnection syndromes in animals and man, *Brain* 88:237, 1965.

197. Pötzl O: Ueber einige zentrale Probleme des Farbensehens, *Wien Klin Wochenschr* 61:706, 1949.

198. Schober H: Erworbene Farbenblindheit nach Schadeltrauma, *Graefes Arch Ophthalmol* 148:93, 1948.

199. Siemerling: Ein Fall sogenannter Seelenblindheit nebst anderweitigen cerebralen Symptomen, *Arch Psychiatr Nervenkr* 21:284, 1889.

200. Sittig O: Stoerungen in Verhalten gegenuber Farben bei Aphasischen, *Monatsschr Psychiatr Neurol* 49:63, 1921.

201. Stengel E: The syndrome of visual alexia without colour agnosia, *J Mental Sci* 94:46, 1948.

202. Lewandowsky M: Ueber Abspaltung des Farbensinnes, *Monatsschr Psychiatr Neurol* 23:488, 1908.

203. Zihl J, von Cramon D: Color anomia restricted to the left visual hemifield after splenial disconnection, *J Neurol Neurosurg Psychiatry* 43:719, 1980.

204. Pötzl O: Die zweite Gruppe der optischen Agnosien. In Aschaffenburg G, editor: *Handbuch der psychiatrie die aphasielehre i optische-agnostischen storungen*, Wien, 1928, Franz Deuticke, p 80.

205. Miceli G, Fouch E, Capasso R, et al: The dissociation of color from form and function knowledge, *Nat Neurosci* 4:662–667, 2001.

206. Goldstein K: *Language and language disturbances*, New York, 1948, Grune & Stratton.

207. Critchley M: Acquired disturbances of color perception of central origin, *Brain* 88:711, 1965.

208. Wahl M, Marzinzik F, Friederici AD, et al: The human thalamus processes syntactic and semantic language violations, *Neuron* 59:695–707, 2008.

209. Metz-Lutz MN, Namer IJ, Gounot D, et al: Language functional neuro-imaging changes following focal left thalamic infarction, *Neuroreport* 11:2907–2912, 2000.

210. Buckner CD, Moroney JT, Desmond DW, et al: Posterior thalamic infarction with cortical diaschisis as a basis for dementia, *Neurology* 48:3050 (Suppl 2), 1997.

211. Servan J, Verstichel P, Catala M, et al: Aphasia and infarction of the posterior cerebral artery territory, *J Neurol* 242:87, 1995.

212. McFarling D, Rothi W, Heilman KM: Transcortical aphasia from ischemic infarcts of the thalamus: A report of two cases, *J Neurol Neurosurg Psychiatry* 45:107, 1982.

213. Geschwind N, Quadfasel FA, Segarra JM: Isolation of the speech area, *Neuropsychologia* 6:327, 1968.

214. Heubner: Über Aphasie, cited in Goldstein K, editor: *Language and language disturbances.* New York, Grune & Stratton, 1948, p 303.

215. Otsuki M, Soma Y, Koyama A, et al: Transcortical sensory aphasia following left frontal infarction, *J Neurol* 245:69, 1998.

216. Kertesz A, Sheppard A, MacKenzie R: Localization in transcortical sensory aphasia, *Arch Neurol* 39:475, 1982.

217. Alexander MP, Hiltbrunner B, Fischer RS: Distributed anatomy of transcortical sensory aphasia, *Arch Neurol* 46:885, 1989.

218. Levin N, Ben-Hur T, Biran I, et al: Category specific dysnomia after thalamic infarction: A case-control study, *Neuropsychologia* 43:1385–1390, 2005.

219. Foundas A, Daniels SK, Vasterling JJ: Anomia: Case studies with lesion localisation, *Neurocase* 4:35, 1998.

220. Mills CK, McConnell JW: The naming centre, with the report of a case indicating its location in the temporal lobe, *J Nerv Ment Dis* 22:1, 1895.

221. Fridriksson J, Baker JM, Moser D: Cortical mapping of naming errors in aphasia, *Hum Brain Mapp* 30:2487–2498, 2009.

222. Nicolai A, Lazzarino LG: Acute confusional states secondary to infarctions in the territory of the posterior cerebral artery in elderly patients, *Ital J Neurol Sci* 15:91, 1994.

223. von Cramon DY, Hebel N, Schuri U: Verbal memory and learning in unilateral posterior cerebral infarction, *Brain* 111:1061, 1988.

224. Servan J, Verstichel P, Catala M, Rancurel G: Syndromes amnésiques et fabulations au cours d'infarctus du territoire de l'artère cérébrale postérieure, *Rev Neurol* 150:201, 1994.

225. Dide M: Botcazo: Amnesie continue, cécité verbale pure, perte du sens topographique, ramollissement double du lobe lingual, *Rev Neurol* 10:676, 1902.

226. Trillet M, Fischer C, Serclerat D, et al: Le syndrome amnésique des ischémies cérébrales postérieures, *Cortex* 16:421, 1980.

227. Victor M, Angevine JB, Mancall EL: Memory loss with lesions of the hippocampal formation, *Arch Neurol (Chicago)* 5:244, 1961.

228. Zola-Morgan S, Squire LR, Amaral DG: Human amnesia and the medial temporal region: Enduring memory impairment following a bilateral lesion limited to field CA1 of the hippocampus, *J Neurosci* 6:2950, 1986.

229. Milner B: Amnesia following operations on the temporal lobes. In Whitty CMW, Zangwill OL, editors: *Amnesia*, London, 1966, Butterworth, p 109.

230. Aggleton JP, McMackin D, Carpenter K, et al: Differential cognitive effects of colloid cysts in the third ventricle that spare or compromise the fornix, *Brain* 123:800, 2000.

231. Gaffan EA, Gaffan D, Hodges JR: Amnesia following damage to the left fornix and to other sites: A comparative study, *Brain* 114:1297, 1991.

232. Sweet WH, Talland GA, Ervin FR: Loss of recent memory following section of fornix, *Trans Am Neurol Assoc* 84:76, 1959.

233. D'Esposito M, Verfaellie M, Alexander MP, et al: Amnesia following traumatic bilateral fornix transection, *Neurology* 45:1546, 1995.

234. Heilman KN, Sypert GW: Korsakoff's syndrome resulting from bilateral fornix lesions, *Neurology* 27:490, 1997.

235. Akelaitis AJ: Study of language functions unilaterally following section of the corpus callosum, *J Neuropathol Exp Neurol* 2:226, 1943.

236. Woolsey RM, Nelson JS: Asymptomatic destruction of the fornix in man, *Arch Neurol* 32:566, 1975.

237. Milner B: Discussion of Sweet WH, Talland GA, Ervin FR (reference 305), *Trans Am Neurol Assoc* 84:78, 1959.

238. Zola-Morgan S, Squire LR, Amaral DG: Lesions of the hippocampal formation but not lesions of the fornix or mammillary nuclei produce long-lasting memory impairment in monkeys, *J Neurosci* 9:898, 1989.

239. Laplane D, Degos JD, Baulac M, et al: Bilateral infarction of the anterior cingulate gyri and of the fornices, *J Neurol Sci* 51:289, 1981.

240. Moudgil SS, Azzouz M, Abkulkader AA, et al: Amnesia due to fornix infarction, *Stroke* 31:1418, 2000.

241. Park SA, Hahn JH, Kim JI, et al: Memory deficits after bilateral anterior fornix infarction, *Neurology* 54:1379, 2000.

242. Gaffan D, Gaffan EA: Amnesia in man following transection of the fornix, *Brain* 114:2611, 1991.

243. Renou P, Ducreux D, Batouche F, et al: Pure and acute Korsakoff syndrome due to a bilateral anterior fornix infarction: A diffusion tensor tractography study, *Arch Neurol* 65:1252–1253, 2008.

244. Schmidtke K, Reinhardt M, Krause T: Cerebral perfusion during transient global amnesia: Findings with HMPAO SPECT, *J Nucl Med* 39:155, 1998.

245. Hodges JR, Warlow CP: The aetiology of transient global amnesia, *Brain* 113:639, 1990.

246. Akkawi NM, Agosti C, Anzola GP, et al: Transient global amnesia: A clinical and sonographic study, *Eur Neurol* 49:67–71, 2003.

247. Benson DF, Marsden CD, Meadows JC: The amnesic syndrome of posterior cerebral artery occlusion, *Acta Neurol Scand* 50:133, 1974.

248. Escourolle R, Gray F: Les accidents vasculaires du système limbique. In: *Proceedings of the VIIth International Congress of Neuropathology*, Amsterdam, 1975, Excerpta Medica, p 195.

249. Mair WGP, Warrington EK, Weiskrantz L: Memory disorder in Korsakoff's psychosis: A neuropathological and neuropsychological investigation of two cases, *Brain* 102:749, 1979.

250. Victor M, Adams RD, Collins GH: *The Wernicke-Korsakoff syndrome*, Philadelphia, 1971, FA Davis.

251. Squire LR, Amaral DG, Zola-Morgan S, et al: Description of brain injury in the amnesia patient N.A. based on magnetic resonance imaging, *Exp Neurol* 105:23, 1989.

252. Graff-Radford NR, Tranel D, Van Hoesen GW, et al: Diencephalic amnesia, *Brain* 113:1, 1990.

253. von Cramon DY, Hebel N, Schuri U: A contribution to the anatomical basis of thalamic amnesia, *Brain* 108:993, 1985.

254. Rahme R, Moussa R, Awada A, et al: Acute Korsakoff-like amnestic syndrome resulting from left thalamic infarction following a right hippocampal hemorrhage, *AJNR Am J Neuroradiol* 28:759–760, 2007.

255. Yoneoka Y, Takeda N, Inoue A, et al: Acute Korsakoff syndrome following mammillothalamic tract infarction, *AJNR Am J Neuroradiol* 25:964–968, 2004.

256. Suzuki T, Iwakuma A, Tanaka Y, et al: Changes in personality and emotion following bilateral infarction of the posterior cerebral arteries, *Jpn J Psychiatr Neurol* 46:897, 1992.

257. Horenstein S, Chamberlin W, Conomy J: Infarction of the fusiform and calcarine regions: Agitated delirium and hemianopia, *Trans Am Neurol Assoc* 92:85, 1967.

258. Medina JL, Chokroverty S, Rubino FA: Syndrome of agitated delirium and visual impairment: A manifestation of medial temporooccipital infarction, *J Neurol Neurosurg Psychiatry* 40:861, 1977

259. Conomy JP, Laureno R, Massarweh W: Transient behavioral syndrome associated with reversible vascular lesions of the fusiform-calcarine region in humans [Abstract], *Ann Neurol* 12:83, 1982.

260. Levine DN, Finklestein S: Delayed psychosis after right temporoparietal stroke or trauma: Relation to epilepsy, *Neurology* 32:267, 1982.

261. Lilly R, Cummings JL, Benson DF, et al: The human Klüver-Bucy syndrome, *Neurology (Cleve)* 33:1141, 1983.

262. Shraberg D, Weisberg L: The Klüver-Bucy syndrome in man, *J Nerv Ment Dis* 166:130, 1978.

262a. Chou CL, Yin YJ, Sheu YL, et al: Persistent Klüver-Bucy syndrome after bilateral temporal lobe infarction, *Acta Neurol Taiwan* 7:199–202, 2008.

263. Medina JL, Rubino FA, Ross E: Agitated delirium caused by infarctions of the hippocampal formation and fusiform and lingual gyri: A case report, *Neurology* 24:1181, 1974.

26 | Vertebrobasilar Disease

J.P. MOHR, LOUIS R. CAPLAN

Vascular disease of the vertebrobasilar system has a long history dating from the landmark descriptions by Henri Duret in 1873 and 1874.[1,2] Isolated cases of basilar artery (BA) occlusion, usually attributed to syphilitic endarteritis, had been described in the later 19th century.[3,4] Twentieth century studies by Marburg,[5] Pines and Gilinsky,[6] Stopford,[7,8] and Foix and colleagues[9-11] described basilar brainstem and branch occlusive syndromes, and diagnosable syndromes emerged in the 1930s[12] and 1940s[13] from clinical and autopsy correlations. By midcentury a role for extracranial occlusive disease became apreciated[14,15] and was soon confirmed by arteriography.[16] Transient clinical events associated with occlusive disease became recognized,[17-22] and the term *vertebrobasilar insufficiency* was born.[23] The literature in the last half century has reported efforts to prevent or reverse ischemic stroke.[24-55]

Anatomy

Embryology

For a period in the embryologic life of the fetus, the hindbrain structures receive much of their blood supply from the carotid circulation. This source and the linkage of embryologic elements give the vertebrobasilar system a high incidence of variations, anomalies, and persistent fetal vessels. The system forms a single larger trunk and from its tributaries and branches usually supplies the spinal cord below and the occipital lobes beyond the brainstem and cerebellum.

Vascular Anatomy

Vertebral Artery

The two vertebral arteries (VAs), which often differ considerably in size, can be thought of as constituting several segments (Fig. 26-1).[56-58] In the first segment, the artery courses directly cephalad from its origin as the first branch of the subclavian artery (SA), riding anterior to the transverse foramen until it enters the costotransverse foramen usually at C6 or C5. The second segment runs entirely within the transverse foramina from C5–6 to C2. The third segment emerges from the transverse foramen of C2 and has a complex course posteriorly and laterally toward the costotransverse foramen of the atlas. There it circles the posterior arch of C1 and passes between the atlas and occiput within the suboccipital triangle. During its course, the third segment of the VA is covered by muscles and nerves and is pressed against bone while

being covered by the atlantooccipital membrane. Its intracranial portion constitutes the fourth segment of the VA. It pierces the dura mater to enter the foramen magnum, where its adventitial and medial coats become less thick, and there is a gross reduction in elastic lamina.[59]

Intracranially, usually at the level of the pontomedullary junction, the two VAs merge to form the BA, but the exact site varies; the site is sometimes high enough on the brainstem for the VA to supply the middle and lower pons. The BA becomes somewhat smaller as it travels distally, frequently curving slightly away from the larger VA. It divides near the pontomesencephalic junction to form the two posterior cerebral arteries (PCAs).

Variations are relatively common. In approximately 8% of humans, the left VA originates directly from the aortic arch and not from the SA (in which case, the left VA would not fill from a left brachial injection). Rarely, the right VA arises as a separate branch from the innominate artery and not from the SA. The VAs are commonly asymmetrical (in 45% of people the left VA is larger, in 21% the right VA is larger, and in 24% the arteries are of equal size).

Cerebellar Arteries

It is the rostrally forward inclination of the brainstem that barely justifies the designation of posterior and anterior inferior cerebellar arteries. Less tradition-bound clinicians might well have referred to the *posterior inferior cerebellar artery* (PICA) as the posterior cerebellar artery and its rostral main branch the middle cerebellar artery, but the acronyms are well embedded in the literature.

PICA. The PICA, usually the largest branch of the VA, arises from its intradural segment approximately 1.5 cm from the origin of the BA. This site is an average of 8.6 mm above the foramen magnum, but extremes occur: it may originate from the VA as low as 24 mm below the foramen magnum.[11,60] The PICA arises extracranially and courses cephalad within the spinal canal.[61] Some examples are a branch of the ascending pharyngeal artery.[62]

Although a branch of the VA, the PICA may actually be its termination, in which case the VA segment distally is a hypoplastic link to the BA or even nonexistent. When the VA ends in the PICA, it is smaller than the contralateral VA.[63] The PICA has a medial branch, which also arises directly from the VA. Its lateral branch may be from the BA or, more commonly, from the anterior inferior cerebellar artery (AICA).[2]

One PICA is entirely lacking in 15% of individuals and is hypoplastic in 5%.[64] Other variations included posterior

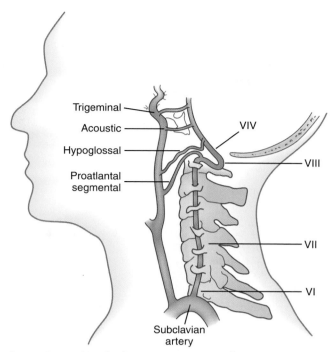

Figure 26-1 Vertebral artery segments and persisting primitive anastomotic connections within the carotid arterial tree (VI to VIV denote vertebral artery segments 1 to 4).

Labels on figure: Trigeminal, Acoustic, Hypoglossal, Proatlantal segmental, VIV, VIII, VII, VI, Subclavian artery

Superior Cerebellar Artery

The superior cerebellar artery (SCA) takes its origin from the rostral BA just before its bifurcation into the PCAs. When one or both PCAs are supplied mainly from the carotid system, the SCA may be misinterpreted as the PCA.

Each SCA has a short trunk that divides into two main branches, a medial (mSCA) branch and a lateral (lSCA) branch. These two branches sometimes arise separately from the BA. They follow the pontomesencephalic sulcus and pass around the superior cerebellar peduncle to ramify onto the rostral cerebellum (Fig. 26-3). The SCA courses along the anterosuperior margin of the cerebellum. The mSCA starts with a course parallel to that of the lSCA but turns medially to reach the lateral surface of the mesencephalon and the inferior colliculus; from there, the mSCA makes a rostral loop along the superior margin of the colliculus and then courses over the superior vermis (see Fig. 26-3). The SCA supplies the rostral half of the cerebellar hemispheres as well as the dentate nucleus.[72] Along the course of the SCA, branches supply the laterotegmental portion of the rostral pons (see Fig. 26-2).

Cerebellum and Its Arterial Supply

The cerebellum is supplied by the long, so-called basilar circumferential vessels (see Fig. 26-3).[11] The PICA course encircles the medulla and supplies the suboccipital surface in the caudal part of the cerebellum.

The PICA has a sinuous course with several loops (see Fig. 26-3). It travels dorsally, lateral to the medulla, below the roots of the ninth and tenth cranial nerves. From there, it courses inferiorly, makes the first (caudal) loop at a variable level, and goes up onto the posterior surface of the medulla in the sulcus, separating the medulla and the tonsil. At the top of the tonsil, the PICA makes a second (cranial) loop around the tonsil and then goes downward to the inferior part of the vermis. Sometimes the second loop occurs at the midpoint of the tonsil. Thus, the PICA has lateral medullary, dorsal medullary (ventral tonsillar), superior tonsillar, and dorsal tonsillar segments.

The PICA divides into two main branches, the medial (mPICA) and the lateral (lPICA).[73] The mPICA climbs along the inferior and dorsal surface of the vermis and the internal part of the hemispheres, making a third loop. The lPICA most often arises from the upper part of the dorsal medullary segment of the parent trunk, between the first and second loops, and then gives rise to several terminal branches to the caudal hemisphere.[74] Sometimes it arises from the first loop. The caudal loop is usually found at the level of the foramen magnum. It can be found below this level, but rami from the lPICA that supply the tonsil are always above the foramen magnum, except for instances of tonsillar herniation.[73] Rami from the cranial loop supply the choroid plexus of the fourth ventricle.

Two main areas of supply can be distinguished within the PICA territory.[75] The dorsomedial area is supplied by the mPICA, whose territory includes the dorsolateral portion of the medulla. The anterolateral area is supplied by the lPICA, which never supplies the medulla (see Fig. 26-2).

spinal arteries taking their origin from the PICA instead of the VA origin.[65]

The lateral medulla is rarely fed primarily from the PICA; in most cases, the major blood supply is from direct lateral medullary branches of the VA.[66-68] The only part of the medulla that the PICA constantly supplies is the dorsal tegmental area, and thus it supplies together with the posterior spinal arteries.[2,11,66] This region is supplied by rami from the medial PICA.[69]

PICA and AICA. The PICA and AICA are often reciprocally related in size; for example, a large PICA may supply most of the inferior surface of the cerebellum, and the AICA on the same side is quite small with little cerebellar supply. When the AICA on one side is large, the ipsilateral PICA is frequently small.

Anterior Inferior Cerebellar Artery

The AICA arises from the caudal third of the BA in 75% of people, sometimes from the middle third or, occasionally, from its inferior limit. Although not always easily demonstrated by noninvasive modern imaging, the AICA is absent in only 4% of individuals.[8,70] It can arise from the VA or the BA by a common trunk together with the PICA. Rarely, several small vessels arising directly from the BA or from the internal auditory artery replace the AICA. Because of its small size, the AICA supplies a small area of the anterior and medial cerebellum (i.e., the middle cerebellar peduncle and the flocculus).[70] Proximal branches of the AICA usually supply the lateral portion of the pons, including the facial, trigeminal, vestibular, and cochlear nuclei, the root of the seventh and eighth cranial nerves, and the spinothalamic tract (Fig. 26-2).[66,71]

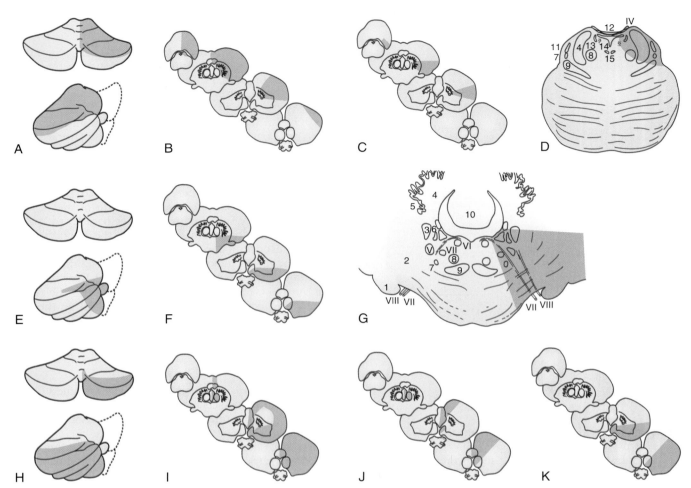

Figure 26-2 Anatomic drawings of the territory of cerebellar arteries and their branches at autopsy. A, Superior cerebellar artery (SCA) territory (superior, dorsal view; inferior, lateral view). B, SCA territory (sections from the rostral to the caudal cerebellum). C, Lateral SCA territory. D, Brainstem territory of SCA. E, Anterior inferior cerebellar artery (AICA) territory (dorsal and lateral views). F, AICA territory. G, Brainstem territory of AICA. H, Posterior inferior cerebellar artery territory (PICA) (dorsal and lateral views). I, PICA territory. J, Medial PICA territory. K, Lateral PICA territory. *1*, Flocculus; *2*, middle cerebellar peduncle; *3*, inferior cerebellar peduncle; *4*, superior cerebellar peduncle; *5*, dentate nucleus; *6*, vestibular nuclei; *7*, spinothalamic tract; *8*, central tegmental tract; *9*, medial lemniscus; *10*, nodulus; *11*, lateral lemniscus; *12*, decussation of trochlear nerve; *13*, mesencephalic trigeminal tract; *14*, locus ceruleus; *15*, medial longitudinal fasciculus. (Data from Amarenco P, Hauw J-J: Cerebellar infarction in the territory of the anterior and inferior cerebellar artery: A clinicopathological study of 20 cases. *Brain* 113:139, 1990; Amarenco P, Hauw J-J: Anatomie des artères cérébelleuses. *Rev Neurol* 145:267, 1989; and Amarenco P, Roullet E, Goujon C, et al: Infarction in the anterior rostral cerebellum (the territory of the lateral branch of the superior cerebellar artery). *Neurology* 41:253, 1991.)

The AICA winds around the lower pons and irrigates usually only the small ventral surface in the anteromedial part of the cerebellum.

The SCA supplies the tentorial surface (the rostral part of the cerebellum) after encircling the upper pons. When a large AICA is present on one side, the ipsilateral PICA is often hypoplastic, and the AICA territory encompasses the whole anterior inferior aspect of the cerebellum.

These three major arteries (the PICA, AICA, and SCA) and their branches are connected by numerous free anastomoses, which limit infarct size in patients who have cerebellar, vertebral, or basilar artery occlusions. Drawings of the territory of each cerebellar artery and their branches conform to the computed tomographic (CT) and magnetic resonance imaging (MRI) horizontal axial sections (Fig. 26-4).

Basilar Artery and Its Main Branches

The major branches of the BA are generally uniform; however, the most common variation is that the internal auditory artery, usually an AICA branch, may arise directly from the BA. The SCAs occasionally are duplicated or arise from the PCA. Even more uniform are the smaller penetrating branches of the vertebral and basilar arteries.[66,67,76-78]

The three groups of arterial penetrators (Fig. 26-5) are (1) median arteries, which usually take a slightly caudal course and then penetrate the brainstem and supply the paramedian basal and tegmental regions, (2) short lateral circumferential arteries, which give rise to branches that penetrate the brainstem and supply the intermediate tegmental and basal regions, and (3) long lateral circumferential arteries, which course around the brainstem and

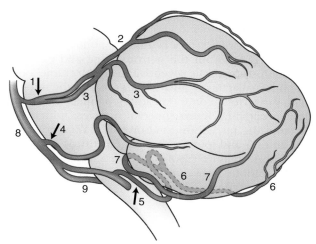

Figure 26-3 Lateral view of cerebellar arteries. *1,* Superior cerebellar artery (SCA); *2,* medial branch of the SCA; *3,* lateral branch of the SCA; *4,* anterior inferior cerebellar artery; *5,* posterior inferior cerebellar artery (PICA); *6,* medial branch of the PICA; *7,* lateral branch of the PICA; *8,* basilar artery; *9,* vertebral artery.

supply the lateral basal and tegmental regions.[57] There are also posterior branches, which arise from the long lateral circumferential cerebellar vessels (the SCA, PICA, and AICA), course in a horizontal and dorsoventral direction, and supply the lateral tegmentum (see Fig. 26-5). Penetrating vessels are usually less than 100 μm in diameter, and their size is roughly proportional to their length.[79]

The medial penetrating vessels arise from the anterior spinal, vertebral, and basilar arteries as well as from the AICA and PCA; lateral penetrators frequently enter the brainstem along the laterally emerging nerve roots and arise from the vertebral, PICA, AICA, basilar, SCA, and posterior choroidal arteries. The medial tegmental region has a prominent rich collateral supply, making it more resistant to ischemia than the base or lateral tegmentum.

The distal basilar segments are also the source of occasional variations. During early fetal life, the internal carotid artery (ICA) supplies the posterior hemispheres and brainstem via posterior communicating arteries. In one third of humans, this primitive vascular pattern persists, and the connecting segment from the BA to the PCA (variously called the basilar communicating artery or mesencephalic artery or P1 segment of the PCA) remains vestigial.[78-80] In these patients, the PCA may fill from carotid injection and not after VA opacification. In 2% of humans, this primitive circulatory pattern is bilateral; even more rarely, the BA may be hypoplastic in its distal segment and end in the SCAs.[80] Penetrating branches from the distal basilar communicating artery, SCA, and proximal PCA pass through the posterior perforating substance and supply the paramedian midbrain and diencephalon.

The paramedian mesencephalic arteries arise from the proximal portion of the basilar communicating artery to supply the cerebral peduncle and red nucleus.[6,7,11,73,81] The lateral midbrain is supplied by peduncular perforating branches arising from the proximal portion of the PCA and from its earliest main branches, the posterior choroidal arteries.[66,81] There are usually two separate paramedian

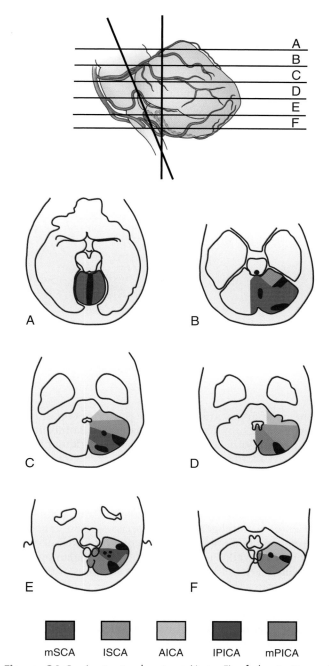

Figure 26-4 Anatomic drawings (A to F) of the territory of branches of the cerebellar arteries as they appear on computed tomography and magnetic resonance imaging. *AICA,* Anterior inferior cerebellar artery; *IPICA,* lateral branch of the posterior inferior cerebellar artery; *ISCA,* lateral branch of the SCA; *mPICA,* medial branch of the PICA; *mSCA,* medial branch of the superior cerebellar artery. (Data from Amarenco P, Kase CS, Rosengart A, et al: Very small [border zone] cerebellar infarcts: Distribution, mechanisms, causes and clinical features. *Brain* 116:161, 1993.)

thalamoperforating arteries[58,82-86]: (1) the polar artery (also called the tuberothalamic artery) and the preliminary pedicles[11,83,87] and (2) the thalamic–subthalamic arteries (also called the paramedian thalamic,[88] deep interpeduncular profunda,[83] and the thalamoperforating pedicle[11,87]).

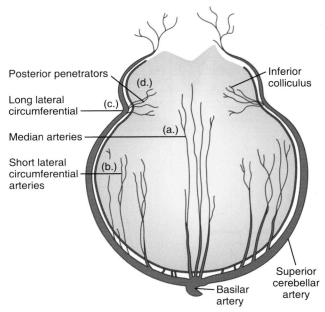

Figure 26-5 *Rostral pons with the usual arterial distribution. A, Median penetrating arteries. B, Short lateral circumferential arteries. C, Long lateral circumferential artery. D, Posterior penetrating arteries.*

The polar artery arises from the posterior communicating artery and supplies the anterolateral thalamus, including the mamillothalamic tract, the paraventricular region, and a part of the reticular nucleus.[83,89,90] Occasionally, the right and left thalamoperforating arteries arise from a common single trunk that originates from the P1 segment of the PCA on one side (Percheron's artery).[88]

The lateral portions of the thalamus are supplied by a series of thalamogeniculate arteries—often called the thalamogeniculate pedicle—and not a large vessel as was formerly believed (Fig. 26-6).[1,11,57,90] The thalamogeniculate pedicle arises from the ambient segment of the PCAs and penetrates the thalamus between the geniculate bodies.[91] These arteries supply the posterolateral and posteromedial ventral somatosensory nuclei, part of the ventralis lateralis, part of the centromedian nucleus, and the rostrolateral portion of the pulvinar.

The posterior choroidal arteries arise from the PCAs more laterally and supply portions of the medial nuclei, the habenular nucleus, and the rostromedial pulvinar.

Anastomotic Links

Occasionally, primitive connections from the ICA to the posterior circulation vessels persist into adult life.[12,57,58] The most common persisting channel is the trigeminal artery, which remains in 0.1% to 0.2% of adults.[92] The trigeminal artery arises from the ICA as it enters the cavernous sinus proximal to the carotid siphon, penetrates the sella turcica or the dura near the clivus, and joins the BA between the AICA and SCA branches. In such cases, the VAs and proximal BA are commonly small or hypoplastic.

Persistence of the hypoglossal artery is the next most common variant.[92-94] This vessel originates from the ICA in the neck, usually between C1 and C3, and courses posteriorly to enter the hypoglossal canal, from which it joins the BA.[94]

A persistent otic artery is a rarer anomaly; this vessel leaves the ICA within the petrous bone and enters the posterior fossa with the seventh and eighth cranial nerves at the internal acoustic meatus, later to join the mid-BA.

The rarest fetal communicating channels are the persistent proatlantal intersegmental arteries, which originate from the nuchal internal or external carotid artery at C2 and C3 and join the horizontal (third) segment of the VA suboccipitally.[95] Isolated reports have documented communications between the common or proximal ICA and the lower VAs.[96]

Pathology

Atherosclerosis

Atherosclerosis is by far the most common vascular condition responsible for posterior circulation ischemia. The histologic features do not differ qualitatively from atherosclerosis elsewhere.[97-103]

Ulceration in plaques is less common in the posterior circulation.[103,104] However, when it is present, the SA is the usual vessel, at the origin of the VA or in the most proximal portion of the VA in the neck.[103,105] The left and right VAs are approximately equally affected by atherosclerosis, but there is some indication that when the two vessels are unequal in diameter, the smaller vessel is more frequently occluded.[103,106]

As in the anterior circulation, thrombosis may occur in the absence of severe preexisting atherosclerosis of the vessel wall.[107] Plaque forms and may assume a ringlike extension from the SA to encircle the VA orifice.[108]

Although aortic arch ulcerated atherosclerotic plaques have been a source of posterior circulation ischemia,[109-111,111a] the most common site of atherosclerotic stenosis is at the origin of the VAs.[15,76,103,108-113] The intracranial VA after it pierces the dura is another site of occlusive disease.[76,108,112]

When thrombosis occurs within the extracranial vertebral artery (ECVA), the clot usually develops at a site of atherosclerotic stenosis and seldom forms a long anterograde or retrograde extension,[76,114] which differs from thrombus extension in the ICA. Extensive collateral channels in the VA system may explain the difference.[115] Thrombus formed within the intracranial VA (ICVA), however, frequently extends into the proximal BA.[76]

Within the BA, fatty sudanophilic plaques are more prevalent on the ventral surface and do not typically lead to napkin-ring or circumferential occlusive disease.[93] (Angioplasty and stenting may thus prove less likely to cause local mural atheromas to occlude basilar penetrating branches.) Stenosis or occlusion is common in the proximal 2 cm of the vessel.[34,76,100,116] Distal stenosis is more common in black people.[117]

At the distal end of the BA, the proximal PCAs are also sites of atherosclerotic lesions; however, such lesions are less common here than in the middle cerebral artery (MCA).[76,112] *Thrombi* within the BA also tend to have limited propagation,[87] frequently extending only to the orifice of the next long circumferential cerebellar artery (the AICA or SCA). *Embolic material* is most often found

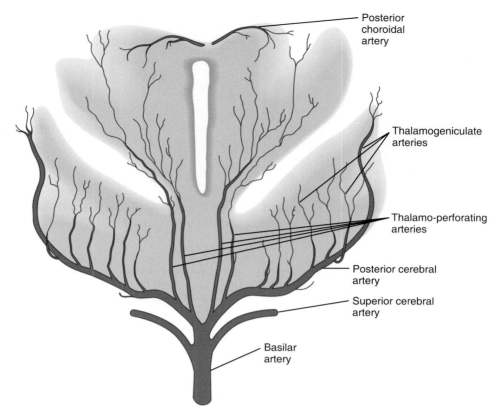

Posterior choroidal artery

Thalamogeniculate arteries

Thalamo-perforating arteries

Posterior cerebral artery

Superior cerebral artery

Basilar artery

Figure 26-6 Diagram of the thalamic arteries.

within the distal basilar tributaries, especially the PCA branches; less often, an embolus lodges in the more proximal vertebral or basilar arteries. This uncommon event is found more often at sites of luminal encroachment by preexisting atherosclerotic lesions.[13,53,76] Atherothrombosis in the aortic arch causing artery-to-artery embolism in the posterior circulation has probably been neglected until now because of the lack of clinical diagnostic tools.[118]

Autopsy and angiographic studies[16,119-121] have corroborated that the origins of the VA, the intradural VA,[122] the BA,[16] and the SA proximal to the VA origin are the most common sites of occlusive disease. The ECVA is affected less than half as much by atherosclerotic stenosis as the extracranial ICA.[103,104,108,112] Castaigne et al[76] reported that 60% of their patients with occlusions in the vertebrobasilar system had no serious occlusive disease within the anterior circulation. The frequency of atherosclerotic lesions in the subclavian and proximal VAs is different in men and women and in persons of different racial backgrounds.[117,123,124]

Atherosclerosis may also affect the branches of the vertebral and basilar arteries.[125] Because the origin of the AICA is situated in the basilar wall, AICA occlusions are atherothrombotic and in situ in most cases.[71,110,126] PICA occlusions, by contrast, are equally divided between in situ atherothrombosis and cardioembolism; SCA occlusions are most commonly cardioembolic.[110,127,128]

The smaller penetrating branches (approximately 0.5 mm in diameter) are vulnerable to occlusive disease. Fisher and Caplan[129] found four such small basilar branch occlusions in a serial section (Fig. 26-7). Two branches

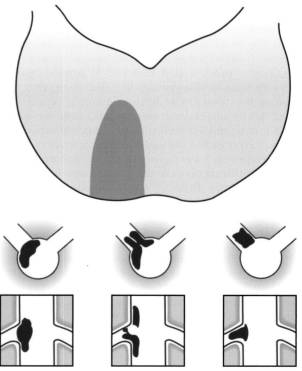

Figure 26-7 Diagrammatic representation of types of branch occlusion. *Left to right,* Luminal plaque blocking the orifice of a branch, junctional plaque spreading into a branch, and a clot in the proximal part of a branch.

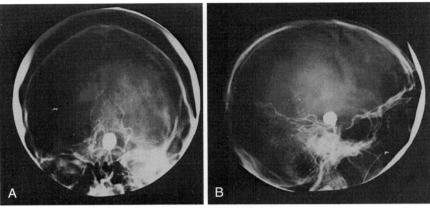

Figure 26-8 Basilar apex aneurysm. A, Anteroposterior view. B, Lateral view.

were blocked as they traversed the intramural portion of the parent BA; a foamy macrophage plaque caused blockage of the orifice of the branch in one. In the other two vessels, a junctional plaque extended from the parent BA into the proximal branch and occluded the branch lumen. Microatheromas as the cause of infarction in regions of the pons and diencephalon supplied by paramedian penetrating branches are found more often in patients with diabetes than in nondiabetic patients.[130] The morphology of the presumed branch disease in these patients has not been studied but could represent similar microatheromata.[125] Figure 26-7 depicts mechanisms of branch occlusion.

Lipohyalinosis

The pathology of smaller penetrating arteries (<200 μm) within the brainstem parenchyma is qualitatively quite different from atherosclerosis of larger vessels.[99,131-134] A distinctive process that Fisher[133,134] labeled *lipohyalinosis* can lead to disorganization and disruption of the lumen of the vessel. The hyaline material readily stains for fat, accumulates subintimally, and may weaken the wall, allowing aneurysmal dilations. Red blood cells may become extravasated through the disintegrating wall.

Lipohyalinosis leads to functional occlusion of the vessel by a subintimal process that obliterates the lumen and leads to ischemia distal to the lesion. Because the ischemic lesions are generally small and somewhat round, the term *lacune* (hole) has been applied. In addition, the same vascular process can lead to a break in the vessel wall and parenchymatous hemorrhage.[135] Most patients with lipohyalinosis and lacunar infarctions have or have had hypertension, although lipohyalinosis is not limited to patients with hypertension. The incidence of lipohyalinosis increases with the age of the patient but is not correlated with atheroma of larger vessels.

Aneurysms

Saccular Aneurysms

Saccular aneurysms are usually discovered during evaluation of subarachnoid hemorrhage (SAH). They account for only 3.6% (64 of 1769).[136] Their most common site in the

posterior circulation is the basilar apex (60%); less often, they are found in the vertebral–PICA junction (20%), the basilar–SCA junction (11%), and at the junction of the vertebral and basilar arteries (3%).[58,136,137]

Basilar apex aneurysms may grow quite large, some splaying the cerebral peduncle (Fig. 26-8)[138]; when these apex aneurysms leak, blood in the interpeduncular fossa may lead to spasm and infarction in the territory of vessels within the posterior perforated substance, which produces a complex clinical picture of rostral brainstem ischemia.

Despite their frequency, it is unusual for basilar apex aneurysms to manifest as isolated third nerve palsy, the classical sign of posterior communicating artery aneurysms.[139] In a case report of a large aneurysm at the junction of the BA and left PCA, paroxysmal hypertension occurred, closely simulating a pheochromocytoma[140]; blood pressure normalized after clipping of the aneurysm. Partially thrombosed giant basilar aneurysms are seen on CT scans as calcified, partially enhancing lesions, often near the cerebellopontine angle (Fig. 26-9).[141] However, MRI, magnetic resonance angiography (MRA), and CT angiography undoubtedly improve their detection.[142,143]

Ischemic stroke has been reported from blockage of the orifice of tributary vessels due to embolization from a clot within the aneurysm.[144]

Fusiform (Dolichoectatic) Aneurysms

Fusiform aneurysms often differ in embryology from saccular aneurysms. As suggested by their name, they are tortuous, elongated, ectatic variations of the normal arterial anatomy (see Fig. 26-9).[145] They are now increasingly identified by CT scanning or MRI and MRA, on which they appear as dilated enhancing channels crossing the cerebellopontine angle.

Symptoms occur either by compression and traction on posterior fossa structures[146,147] or by ischemia[148] from several mechanisms, including obstruction of blood flow related to atherosclerotic stenosis of the vertebrobasilar arteries, local embolism from in situ thrombus within the aneurysm, and compromise of the orifice of tributary vessels.[149-151] Occipital–nuchal headache is common. Cranial nerve compression and traction may result in neuropathies, usually affecting the seventh and eighth cranial

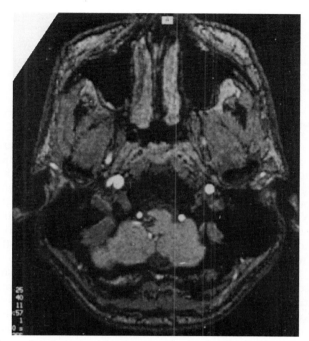

Figure 26-9 T1-weighted MR image showing a lateral medullary infarct sparing the cerebellum.

nerves; some manifest as hemifacial spasms, tinnitus, deafness, vertigo,[152-155] glossopharyngeal and trigeminal-like pain, hiccups, and even hypoglossal paralysis.[152] The larger BA aneurysms can even compress the basis pontis or cerebral peduncle (leading to spastic paraparesis[156]), may cause hydrocephalus,[151] or may manifest as cerebellopontine angle masses.[157,158] VA aneurysms have compressed the medulla[159] or upper brainstem.[151]

The pathogenesis of these aneurysms involves congenital, degenerative, and genetic influences, that is, underlying structural arterial defects, including connective tissue replacement and deficient elastin,[160] fibrous dysplasia and degeneration of internal elastic lamina,[161] and fibrous and collagen replacement of the media. In adults, atherosclerotic changes in the vessels may interact with congenital structural defects to result in fusiform aneurysm formation. A genetic deficiency in α-glucosidase was found in three adolescent brothers with fusiform basilar aneurysms, two of whom had ruptures of the aneurysms; the third had cerebellar infarction.[162] In some patients with structural defects, the arterial abnormalities are widespread, affecting other vessels.[153,163]

An association with aneurysms of the abdominal aorta occurs in up to 45% of patients with dolichoectatic basilar arteries.[164] One patient has been described as having a fusiform aneurysm in association with ulcerative colitis.[165]

Dolichoectatic VA and BA aneurysms are also readily visualized on MRI and MRA. The heterogeneity of echo densities and morphology of flow voids usually allow detection of a thrombus within the aneurysm. MRA accurately detects the vast majority of sizable saccular and fusiform aneurysms.[51,52,101] Angiography or metrizamide CT cisternography can confirm the diagnosis but is not usually needed if high-quality plain and contrast-enhanced CT or MRI has been performed with special attention to the posterior fossa or if MRA is available.[166] The pons appears to be the most common site,[167] and lacunar presentation predominates[168]; however, a wide range of syndromes can occur, including hydrocephalus, pseudotumor, cranial nerve dysfunction (all from compression), ischemic stroke, and even subarachnoid hemorrhage.[169]

Arterial Dissection

Dissection of the vertebral and basilar arteries has been increasingly recognized since the clinical and angiographic descriptions of ICA dissection.[170-176] The artery most commonly affected in the posterior circulation is the ECVA; dissection usually occurs well above the origin from the subclavian and below the intradural intracranial penetration of the vessel. The initial reports of ECVA dissection featured chiropractic or other neck manipulations, but some arise from minor trauma and even may be spontaneous.[177-183] Minor trauma causes of dissection include riding on a rollercoaster,[184] heavy coughing, falling on the back (not the neck) from a handstand, turning the head to back a car, and falling while waterskiing.

VA dissections have been associated with conditions such as Marfan's syndrome, Ehlers-Danlos syndrome, pseudoxanthoma elasticum, lentiginosis, systemic lupus erythematosus, fibromuscular dysplasia, congenital bicuspid aortic valves,[185-188] and arterial redundancy.[189,190] Simultaneous dissection of the carotid and vertebral arteries is a common angiographic finding, and simultaneous dissection of both cervical and renal arteries in a setting of fibromuscular dysplasia suggests an underlying morbid systemic process.[185]

Genetic factors may also predispose to dissection. Whereas the risk of recurrent dissection is 1% a year, it is as high as 50% in patients with a familial history of dissection.[191,192]

The most common symptom of VA dissection is pain in the head or neck. Usually, the pain is in the posterior neck with radiation to the occiput, sometimes to the shoulder.[176] Headache and neck pain may be the only complaints. Ischemic symptoms and signs may develop at the same time as the pain or after a delay of hours to a few days. The lateral medulla and cerebellum are the brainstem regions most susceptible to ischemia from ECVA dissection.[173-175] The clinical features usually correspond to a partial lateral medullary syndrome (see further on).

ICVA dissection is less common than ECVA dissection. Two major clinical presentations have been described: subarachnoid hemorrhage (SAH) and brainstem infarction.[193] Less commonly, the dissection may act as a mass lesion compressing posterior fossa structures.[193]

SAH as a complication of ICVA dissection reflects, in part, the differences in vessel morphology of intracranial and extracranial arteries. The intracranial arteries have thinner media and adventitial layers and only an internal elastic lamina; extracranial arteries have thicker media and adventitial layers and an external as well as an internal elastic lamina. If an intracranial dissection involves the media and spreads to the outer layers, rupture and SAH may occur. When the dissection occurs in the media and subintimal layers, obstruction to blood flow from a narrowing of the lumen or local embolism may lead to brainstem infarction. When SAH is present, its clinical effects are no different from SAH due to saccular aneurysm rupture.

Headache, often chronic, is common in all presentations of ICVA dissection. Acute headaches associated with prodromal leaks have also been suspected to be caused by dissection. As with SAH from saccular aneurysms, the outcome is poor. When brainstem infarction occurs, it is usually severe and is often fatal. Initially unilateral signs frequently become bilateral, and coma and quadriparesis ensue. Deficits limited to the lateral medulla, as in ECVA dissection, are unusual when the dissection involves the ICVA. Dissecting aneurysms of the ICVA may manifest as mass lesions without SAH or stroke. Headache, neck pain, and signs of progressive lower cranial nerve compression have been the hallmarks.[194-196]

Dissection of the BA and its major branches is very uncommon compared with VA dissection. Most dissections are described in isolated case reports and diagnosed at postmortem examination.[171,197-201] The most common clinical presentation is sudden coma with no history of preceding events. Major brainstem infarction correlates with the clinical findings. SAH as the initial presentation of basilar dissection has also been documented. Rare reports have described dissection beginning in the right ICVA and extending into the BA[140]; some of the cases have had remarkably mild initial syndromes.[197,198,200,202,203]

The principal features thought to distinguish carotid artery dissection from atherosclerotic occlusion are (1) local neck or jaw pain, (2) migrainous spells of scintillation, (3) relatively rapid onset with multiple spells (carotid allegro), and (4) Horner's syndrome.[171] Migraine has been found to be significantly associated with dissection.[204] Some investigators have proposed that migraine may predispose to dissection by producing edema of the media of vessels.[200,205]

VA dissections can be imaged at the C2 and C3 levels by means of high-quality color-flow ultrasonography.[206] MRA is also a useful screening test, but the sensitivity and specificity of this method is not yet as good for VA dissection as it is for carotid artery dissection.[207,208] Standard angiography combined with axial MR images of the arteries is still the best way to diagnose VA dissections.

Cervical Spondylosis

In 1960 Sheehan et al[209] popularized the idea that compression of the VA by osteophytes was a common cause of vertebrobasilar insufficiency. Spondylitic osteophytes project from the vertebral joints adjacent to the transverse foramina through which the VAs course. In cadavers, extreme neck turning can cut off VA flow, especially at C5 to C6.[210] Angiographic studies have shown stenosis to be common but occlusion rare at the point of maximal concavity. Clinical examples are decidedly uncommon.[211-213] In many cases, either the ECVA contralateral to the compressed VA is hypoplastic or previously occluded, or the ICVA ends in the PICA; thus, the compressed ECVA could be the major supply to the posterior circulation, even from an osteophyte.[211,213,214-217] Symptoms are often intermittent and may be precipitated by turning or rotation of

the neck during which the ECVA can become occluded; this is easily understood but rarely demonstrated.

Although spondylosis is common, it only rarely explains symptomatic vascular compression[76,103,108,112,218]; labyrinthine and other nonvascular mechanisms explain most cases.[219]

Neck Rotation or Trauma

In 1947, Pratt-Thomas and Berger[220] provided an account of two previously healthy individuals, a 32-year-old man and a 35-year-old woman, who became unconscious during chiropractic manipulation and died in less than 24 hours without regaining consciousness. Occlusion of the BA, left AICA, and right PICA with brainstem and bilateral cerebellar hemisphere softenings were found in one patient, and occlusion of the right vertebral and basilar arteries and left PICA were found in the other.

Since this original report, more than 50 additional patients have been described in whom posterior circulation stroke followed neck rotation or injury.[178,182,221-229] Most cases occur after chiropractic manipulation, but manipulation of the neck by a patient's wife,[178] neck turning while driving a car, wrestling,[226] and practicing archery and yoga[221] have also been implicated. Most of the patients have been young (average age, 37 years)[227] and have had no evidence of preexisting vascular disease.

The syndrome is typically unilateral, and ischemia is limited to the lateral medulla or pons and the ipsilateral cerebellum.[177,221,223-226] Pseudoaneurysm formation has been reported. Unilateral lesions occurring at the time of neck rotation often do not progress.[182] When initial findings indicate bilateral brainstem lesions, the course is often progressive. Symptoms appear at the time of neck rotation or injury in approximately one third of cases, symptoms develop minutes or days later in one third, and symptoms progress after the onset in one third.[227]

The third segment of the VA system is especially susceptible to injury during neck rotation, as it lies in relation to the atlas, axis, and atlantooccipital membrane. Injury to the intima activates clotting mechanisms and leads to the formation of thrombus in the VA, usually at the C2 to C1 region. Thrombus may propagate distally or may embolize to more rostral portions of the basilar arterial tree. Filling defects in the distal vascular bed are occasionally verified angiographically.[172,227] Perforation of the VA is rare.

Fibromuscular Dysplasia

Fibromuscular dysplasia (FMD) is characterized by hyperplasia of the intima and media of arteries, adventitial sclerosis, and breakdown of normal elastic tissue. Thickened septa and ridges protrude into the lumen. At postmortem examination, basilar occlusion with brainstem infarction has been documented; the BA has been severely ectatic and atherosclerotic with focal variations in wall thickness and aneurysm formation. Homonymous hemianopia has been reported with FMD of the PCA,[230,231] and cephalic FMD is strongly associated with an accompanying intracranial aneurysm.[199,230,232-235] Pseudoaneurysm formation is commonly described.[171]

Temporal Arteritis

Headache and visual loss, the most common clinical manifestations of temporal arteritis, are caused by giant cell granulomatous disease of the ophthalmic branches to the optic nerve and central retinal arteries and the superficial temporal and occipital branches of the external carotid artery (see Chapter 22). The most frequently described intracranial vessel disease in temporal arteritis is thrombus formation without local arteritis; it is probably due to embolization from extracranial arteritic occlusive disease.[236] Rarely, smaller intracranial vessels, including posterior circulation branches, may demonstrate granulomatous arteritis.[236] The related clinical findings are headache, cerebrospinal fluid pleocytosis, and multifocal cranial nerve and parenchymatous dysfunction, including some typically distinctive basilar branch syndromes such as one-and-a-half ocular palsies (see later)[237]; many such cases do not have clear histories of stroke.[236]

Other Diseases

Less common diseases affecting vascular structures of the posterior fossa are mentioned only briefly here because of their rarity and the lack of data on their special features within the posterior circulation.

Aspergillosis seems to have a special tropism for the posterior circulation vessels.[238] It involves the brain by infarction due to occlusion of distal branches in the cerebellum or occipital lobes. Infarctions are commonly small and hemorrhagic. Later, abscesses may develop at the borderzone of the infarcted area. Aspergillosis is usually a nosocomial fungal infection that disseminates via the blood route. Unlike cryptococcosis, another fungal infection, aspergillosis rarely occurs together with meningitis.[239] Mechanisms of arterial occlusion are (1) thromboangiitis with presence of aspergillosis in the arterial wall and in the thrombus and (2) embolic occlusion from an endocarditis due to *Aspergillus*.[238] Endocarditis is very difficult to diagnose, even with transesophageal echocardiography, but is found in as many as 50% of patients with aspergillosis at autopsy.[240]

The diagnosis of aspergillosis in the presence of brain infarctions is usually very difficult and is based on repeated serology, biopsy, and culture of an associated arthritis or spondylitis infection,[241] culture of a perfusion catheter, or presence of pneumonia due to *Aspergillus*, especially in severely ill patients in intensive care units, patients with chronic polyinfection, and drug users.[239,242]

Meningitis due to other fungal infections or tuberculosis commonly produces changes within vessels. Branches of the MCA and those traversing the interpeduncular fossa to penetrate the rostral brainstem are the most often affected. The exudate produces a reaction in the media of these vessels, usually referred to as Heubner's arteritis. Sudden stupor may be due to infarction of the brainstem, often with third cranial nerve palsies and bilateral pyramidal tract dysfunction. Headache, fever, cranial nerve palsies, and confusion dominate the clinical picture, and examination of the cerebrospinal fluid usually confirms the diagnosis.

Fibrous bands crossing the proximal VA before it enters the transverse foramina may constrict the vessel when the neck is turned.[217]

Sickle cell disease is associated with occlusion of small and larger vessels[243]; the larger vessels frequently show extensive intimal proliferation of fibrodysplasia, possibly related to abnormal flow mechanisms.[244] Stroke often occurs during a sickle cell crisis and is heralded by seizures. Few data are available concerning the findings related to posterior circulation occlusion in this group of patients; pseudobulbar signs are more common than bulbar paralysis.

Young women taking oral contraceptives may have occlusion of the ECVA, and for unclear reasons, BA occlusion occasionally occurs in the first two decades of life.

Syphilis can also produce an arteritis and can be associated with brainstem infarcts, usually in branch distribution.

Systemic lupus erythematosus and granulomatous angiitis affect cerebral blood vessels, but a strokelike picture is rarely found. CT or MRI shows very small infarcts often in borderzone areas of the cerebellum or occipital lobes.[245]

Rare causes of ischemic brainstem stroke have been related to homocystinuria, Marfan's syndrome, Ehlers-Danlos syndrome, pseudoxanthoma elasticum, polyarteritis nodosa, Kohlmeier-Degos disease, and Fabry's disease, but little is known of the incidence and site of involvement in the vertebrobasilar system in these diseases.

Takayasu's pulseless disease often involves the SA and VA orifices as well as the aorta.[246,247] Occasionally, the intracranial arteries also show intensive inflammation typical of Takayasu's arteritis.[248] Brainstem lesions are especially common in Behçet's syndrome.[249]

Behçet's disease was first described by a Turkish ophthalmologist; although rare, this disorder is more common in the Middle East and Mediterranean countries. Clinical findings include aphthous stomatitis and genital ulcers, uveitis, cells in the cerebrospinal fluid, and multifocal neurologic signs.[250,251] The neurologic symptoms often relate to the brainstem and can develop either quickly or gradually. CT usually shows a low-density abnormality, and T2-weighted MRI shows an area of hyperintense signal in the brainstem, cerebellum, or cerebral white matter that enhances acutely.[250] Mass effect may be seen. With time, enhancement is lost, and the patient stabilizes or improves. Angiography usually does not show arterial occlusions, but dural sinus occlusions are common. At necropsy, inflammatory lesions are seen with perivascular lymphocytic cuffing around capillaries and ventricles, especially in the brainstem.[250]

Neurofibromatosis has been rarely reported as a cause of basilar compression with stroke.[252]

Pathophysiology

Although posterior circulation ischemic stroke is expected to have a sudden onset, some few reports have considered its temporal course.[253,254] In major basilar occlusion, prior TIAs are common; fluctuations are common within the first week but unusual thereafter, and an alarming number show progressive deterioration, despite intense therapy. Postural changes may alter the course in

TABLE 26-1 PATHOPHYSIOLOGY OF TENUOUS EQUILIBRIUM AFTER OCCLUSION OF AN ARTERY

Factors Promoting Deficit	Factors Defending against Deficit
Blood flow to lesion diminished by stenosis of occlusion	Collateral circulation and autoregulation
Embolization from plaque or clot	Passing of emboli
Activation of clotting factors	Thrombolysis (?)

the early stages,[255,256] more so for vertebrobasilar than for carotid territory cases.[257]

Intraarterial Embolism

Although embolic occlusions are often considered unusual with vertebrobasilar infarction,[258] autopsy studies long ago showed them to be common,[76,259] especially at the top of the basilar, SCA, PICA, and distal VAs.[109,110,260] Initial syndromes are often severe.

The aortic arch leads the list of embolic sources, followed by the SA, VA origin, and distal VA[261,262]; ulcerated plaques are also a source.[105,262] Cardiac source emboli most often affect the cerebellar and occipital lobe territories.[110,128,263,264]

Worsening

Apart from an increase in the size of the territory subject to failing flow is the special problem of edema with cerebellar infarction. Although it is rare in SCA or AICA infarcts, where the territory at risk is not in a tight space, for PICA infarcts the pressure on the brainstem and ventricular pathways may prove fatal.[265] Amenable to surgical decompression, it is common for the initial syndrome to appear stable while brainstem compliance is steadily reduced until sudden failure triggers a near brain-death clinical syndrome with coma, fixed ocular position, apneustic breathing, and even fixed pupils. The peak period of risk is the first 3 days and is predicted by the size of the PICA infarct. As determined by imaging, total PICA infarction carries a high risk of fatal edema; infarcts limited to single branch are scarce.[266]

Lability of blood pressure and blood flow can result from lesions of the medulla and pons[267] and can be explained by involvement of the fastigial nucleus of the cerebellum[268] in altering cerebral blood flow. Stimulation of regions within the brainstem tegmentum can alter heart rate and rhythm.[267,269,270] Even unilateral lesions can be accompanied by tachycardia and lability of blood pressure.[271]

Clinical Findings in Patients with Vascular Lesions in Various Locations

Occlusion or Severe Stenosis of the Basilar Artery

Historical Aspects

Kubik and Adams,[13] in their landmark description of occlusion of the BA, summarized the findings: the onset is sudden and is not preceded by tangible causal factors.

The first symptom is usually a headache, dizziness, confusion, or coma. Difficulty in speaking and unilateral paresthesias occur in a large proportion of the cases. Common findings are pupillary abnormalities, disorders of ocular movement, facial palsy, hemiplegia, quadriplegia, or both, and bilateral extensor plantar reflexes. Cranial nerve palsies and contralateral hemiplegia may be combined. It is common for temporary improvement, lasting hours or days, to occur during the course of the illness. In the majority of cases, death takes place between 2 days and 5 weeks from onset. Rare cases have been reported in which the first symptom was deafness.[272] In the half century since, there has been little improvement in this description; instead, the main focus has been on determining what factors may mitigate the severe outcomes. Angiographically documented BA occlusion is associated with severe outcomes,[273] but some have escaped with only limited deficits,[21,97,274-277] which suggests that the angiographic findings are not fully predictive of the outcome.

Patterns of Infarction

One reason for the wide spectrum of syndrome severity from basilar occlusion is the spectrum of infarction. For some, the occlusion is quite limited and segmental, whereas in others, thrombosis can affect multiple segments or can even occlude the entire BA and extend into the VA and PCA.[76,278-280] Biemond[281] noted frequent tegmental sparing and sought to explain it by emphasizing that the tegmentum is supplied mainly by the SCA and its branches. The SCA is the most anatomically constant long circumferential branch vessel and often has a prominent anastomosis with the PCA. He followed small branches of the SCA and found that they formed a corona around the cranial part of the pontine tegmentum and anastomosed with the SCA branches of the other side. When a lateral branch of the SCA was injected, the tegmentum was stained bilaterally; when the BA was injected from the VA, the basis pontis was deeply stained but the tegmentum remained entirely clear. He also obtained little tegmental staining from injection of the AICA. Angiographic material in patients with BA occlusion reported by Caplan and Rosenbaum[282] also demonstrated retrograde filling of the PCA and SCA from carotid injection and the prominence of cerebellar artery anastomotic vessels that fill other lateral circumferential cerebellar artery branches. Tegmental involvement thus depends on the involvement of the distal BA and the adequacy of collateral vessels. Collateral circulation through the PICA is poor when the VA and BA are both obstructed. Archer and Horenstein[273] wondered whether hypertension, by reducing the number and adequacy of collateral vessels, might considerably affect prognosis.

Angiographic and MRI Diagnosis

MRI has been a great advance in mapping. Its demonstration of the tissue affected by various forms of BA and branch occlusion (Fig. 26-10) now allows better understanding of the effects of collateral flow and the range of different outcomes, as compared with studies initially limited to autopsy or angiography,[260] and helps explain why the lack of a uniform syndrome or outcome is applicable to all patients with BA occlusion.[283,284]

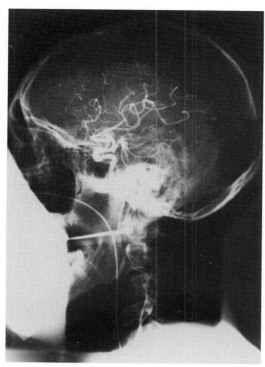

Figure 26-10 Carotid arteriogram demonstrating retrograde filling of the basilar artery and the posterior cerebral and superior cerebellar arteries. Note the midbasilar occlusion.

Clinical Tempo and Course

Information correlating the usual tempo of neurologic deficit acquisition with the location of vascular occlusion remains scanty.[13,279] Clinical studies often lack angiographic or pathologic confirmation,[22,253,254,274,285] as well as ample documentation of an unstable course characterized by progression or remission and relapses; most changes occur within the first 48 hours. Declining consciousness is an ominous sign. Sudden onset followed by stabilization and gradual onset with later progression are common patterns, and as many as 50% of patients may have some premonitory symptoms.[286] Vertigo and headache are especially common.

Clinical Syndromes of Basilar Occlusion

Coma

Unresponsiveness to external stimuli occurs in some patients with BA occlusion,[90] explained by bilateral damage to the medial pontine tegmentum. Those with unilateral tegmental damage usually remain alert or only "slightly obtunded." Lesions below the trigeminal nerve entry zone of the pons usually do not affect alertness in the experimental animal.[287]

Weakness

Occlusion begins with hemiplegia, and the other limbs are generally affected within 24 hours.[281] BA occlusion in which one side of the body is more affected than the other has been reported.[13] Crossed motor paralysis, ipsilateral

facial or conjugate gaze paralysis, and contralateral hemiparesis, tetraparesis, tetraplegia, and hemiparesis have also been seen in patients.[286]

Decerebrate Responses

Decerebrate responses are common in patients with extensive BA infarction; in some, the inferior extremity flexes as the arms extend, which is a response correlated with lesions at the level of the vestibular nuclei in the pontine tegmentum.[287] Some observers claim that the findings have the appearance of seizures in some patients, whereas in others, responses take the form of tonic-clonic movements, myoclonic jerks, or fasciculation, shivering, and generalized nonclonic shaking movements.[288]

Locked-in Syndrome

Kemper and Romanul[289] described a patient who, although paralyzed and speechless, could move his eyes horizontally and raise his eyebrows. Postmortem examination of this case showed extensive destruction of the pontine base and only slight encroachment on the ventral part of the pontine tegmentum unilaterally. These researchers sought to differentiate this paralytic state from akinetic mutism, a condition in which the patient could, under certain circumstances, speak and move. Plum and Posner[287] coined the term *locked-in syndrome* to describe a state in which severe paralysis prevents the usual means of gestural or vocal communication. In some patients with this condition, oral automatisms have been reported: chewing and sucking movements were reflex-induced by oral and perioral stimulation, indicating loss of voluntary control over bulbar masticatory function.[290] These patients have been likened to the character M. Noirtier de Villefort, in the Dumas novel *The Count of Monte Cristo*, who, while encased in armor, could not communicate except with his eyes.

The most common vascular lesion underlying the locked-in syndrome is BA occlusion with extensive destruction of the pontine base. Vertical eye movements are usually spared. Midbrain lesions may also produce a locked-in state.[291,292]

Ataxia

Ataxia is frequently hidden by weakness and has been difficult to analyze, although the location of necropsy findings would predict its presence. Nystagmus is common in patients with tegmental ischemia but may be overshadowed by nuclear, internuclear, or gaze paresis. Vertical nystagmus commonly accompanies internuclear ophthalmoplegia and pontine infarction. Dysarthria, dysphagia, and facile laughing and crying can be due to pseudobulbar paralysis and are present to some degree in most patients with moderate to severe limb paresis.

Palatal Myoclonus

Palatal myoclonus is a rhythmic involuntary jerking movement of the soft palate and pharyngopalatine arch, often involving the diaphragm and laryngeal muscles.[293]

It usually appears some time after the early brainstem process, which is most often an infarction. The locus and nature of the responsible vascular lesion have not been analyzed, but the parenchymatous lesion involves the dentate nucleus of the cerebellum, the red nucleus, the inferior olivary nucleus, or their connections (the Guillain-Mollaret triangle). The dentate nucleus and contralateral inferior olive are somatotopically related. Fibers from the dentate nuclei travel in the superior cerebellar peduncle and decussate in the midbrain to the region of the contralateral red nucleus, from which the central tegmental tract descends to the inferior olivary nucleus of the same side.[294] The pathologic lesion most often seen in patients with palatal myoclonus is hypertrophic degeneration of the inferior olive, often associated with a lesion of the ipsilateral central tegmental tract or the contralateral dentate nucleus. The olivary lesion consists of enlarged neurons, loss of the other neurons, and gliosis, usually with enlargement of the olive; these changes are thought to be transsynaptic and secondary to lesions of the neuronal system afferent to the inferior olivary nucleus.

The brachial movements may vary in rate (40 to 200 motions per min).[293] The patient may complain of an audible clicking noise due to movement of the eustachian tube, or the noise may be heard by the examiner applying a stethoscope to the lateral neck. The movements of the pharynx can be readily seen and are often accompanied by a fluttering of the diaphragm, which is usually obvious on chest fluoroscopy. Palatal myoclonus has surprisingly little effect on swallowing.

Neuroophthalmologic Observations

Ocular Bobbing

Fisher[295] introduced the term *ocular bobbing* to describe an unusual vertical movement of the eyes: "The eyeballs intermittently dip briskly downward through an arc of a few millimeters and then return to the primary position in a kind of bobbing action." He believed that this was a sign of "advanced pontine disease" and of little diagnostic importance because "the site of the disease process is usually obvious from the other ocular abnormalities" and clinical findings. His cases included two with pathologic documentation of BA occlusion and extensive infarction of the pontine base and tegmentum and one with a pontine hemorrhage. Nelson and Johnston[296] added four cases of bilateral ocular bobbing, of which all were in patients with pontine hemorrhage; one had a hemorrhage to the tegmentum and fourth ventricle.

The mechanism of ocular bobbing in pontine lesions[295,296] relates the bobbing to roving eye movements. In patients with coma due to bilateral supratentorial lesions, the eyes rove from side to side freely. In pontine lesions, horizontal gaze is lost but vertical gaze is preserved because the midbrain tegmentum is spared; therefore, the vertical vector of gaze is accentuated so that the eyes "bob" down. In addition, caloric irrigation increases the bobbing, acting as an afferent stimulus to gaze. Similarly, a unilateral bob (downward dip), when the affected eye is pointed toward the direction of paralytic lateral gaze, could evoke a downward movement. Some authors have disputed the basic findings, presenting

a case of "typical ocular bobbing" (referring to bilateral conjugate downward movements) from a large cerebellar hemorrhage with no extensive pontine lesion. The patient was in a deep coma and had distortion of the pons and a small unilateral Duret-type hemorrhage in the adjacent pontine tegmentum.[297] Other reports of ocular bobbing have been seen in cerebellar hemorrhage[298] and cerebellar infarction,[299] as well as in an unusual example[300] of a patient in a coma after cranial gunshot wounds. After removal of the necrotic temporal lobe, the patient initially had no spontaneous or reflex oculocephalic eye movements, but after the patient became alert, ocular bobbing appeared and was accentuated during voluntary eye movements, especially when he attempted fields of gaze with limitation of horizontal eye movements. The authors speculated that the vertical vectors could originate inferior to the lesion, for example, in the medulla or vestibular nuclei; they emphasized the possibility of recovery.

Skew Deviation

Skew deviation refers to an altered vertical position of the eyes, with one eye situated above the other and the vertical displacement remaining nearly constant in all planes of gaze. Skew is quite common in patients with brainstem infarction, especially those whose lesions are asymmetrical. When skew deviation is associated with a unilateral internuclear ophthalmoplegia, the elevated eye is usually ipsilateral to the lesion.[301] Asymmetrical lesions in the region of the vestibular nuclei, dorsolateral medulla, brachium pontis, cerebellum, and rostral midbrain may all produce skewing.

Internuclear Ophthalmoplegia

In the 1950s, Cogan et al[302-304] revised the nomenclature and described the usual findings in patients with internuclear ophthalmoplegia. Earlier investigators had originally designated two types of internuclear ophthalmoplegia: an anterior type, in which the medial rectus muscle is paralyzed for conjugate movements toward the side of the lesion but functions normally in convergence and the lateral rectus muscle operates normally on lateral gaze, and a posterior type, in which both internal recti function normally on convergence and lateral gaze movements but the extremus on the side of the lesion is paralyzed for voluntary conjugate movements even though it can function on labyrinthine stimulation.

Smith and Cogan,[304] stating that posterior internuclear ophthalmoplegia was merely a partial sixth cranial nerve palsy, proposed a new designation that is now in common usage. In their terminology, internuclear ophthalmoplegia always involves paralysis of the adducting eye; the posterior type designates cases in which the medial rectus works normally during convergence, and the anterior type consists of absence of medial rectus function in either convergence or conjugate lateral gaze. In either type, nystagmus of the abducting eye occurs, a phenomenon that had led other writers to designate internuclear ophthalmoplegia as *ataxic nystagmus,* a term still used in some regions.[305] Furthermore, analysis of 58 cases (29 unilateral and 29 bilateral) led Smith and Cogan[304] to assert that bilateral internuclear ophthalmoplegia was "invariably indicative of multiple sclerosis" and that unilateral internuclear ophthalmoplegia was most commonly vascular in etiology. A few authors have disputed these interpretations, documenting their findings from brainstem infarction.[306,307] Absence of associated convergence does not necessarily implicate the more rostral midbrain medial longitudinal fasciculus (MLF), as Cogan and associates[302,308] initially believed.

Although the eyes are generally conjugate at rest in patients with internuclear ophthalmoplegia, some patients have bilateral exotropia; this situation has been referred to as *wall-eyed bilateral internuclear ophthalmoplegia*.[309] Outward deviation of the eyes has been used as evidence of medial rectus nuclear involvement, and exotropia is to be anticipated with dysconjugate impairment of medial rectus function at any level, including the MLF.[302,307,308]

MRI studies of patients with internuclear ophthalmoplegia showed damage of the MLF and adjacent structures.[310]

Conjugate Horizontal Gaze Palsy

Fibers from the frontal eye fields affecting conjugate lateral gaze cross at or near the level of the abducens nucleus in the pons[284] and end in the reticular gray region in the neighborhood of the contralateral abducens nucleus.[311] This region is usually referred to as the *paramedian pontine reticular formation* (PPRF) or, by some, as the pontine lateral gaze center. Damage to the abducens nucleus can probably produce an ipsilateral gaze palsy for all lateral eye movements, voluntary and reflex (caloric or vestibuloocular).[312]

MRI shows that in patients with a unilateral abduction weakness (sixth cranial nerve palsy), the lesion invariably involves the intrapontine nerve fascicles and not the abducens nucleus.[98] Involvement of the PPRF leads to absence of voluntary lateral gaze to the side of the lesion with preservation of reflex movements.[312] The PPRF also mediates ipsilaterally directed saccades within the contralateral hemifield of movement. Bilateral lesions in the pontine tegmentum involving the abducens nucleus and PPRF produce paralysis of all horizontal eye movements, but the vertical gaze is spared because it is mediated at a more rostral level. MRI studies of patients with unilateral conjugate gaze palsy show lesions in the paramedian pons, including the abducens nucleus, the nucleus reticularis pontis oralis, and the lateral portion of the nucleus reticularis pontis caudalis. These latter two structures are identified in animals as being responsible for lateral gaze and contain burst neurons of the PPRF. Patients with bilateral horizontal gaze palsies usually have bilateral medial pontine lesions, but some have unilateral lesions that include the pontine tegmental raphe.[98] Patients with bilateral horizontal gaze palsies often also have slowness of vertical gaze saccades or limitation of upgaze. Horizontal gaze palsies are common in patients with BA occlusive disease.

One-and-a-Half Syndrome

Fisher[114] introduced the term *one-and-a-half syndrome* to refer to "a paralysis of eye movements in which one eye lies centrally and fails completely to move horizontally while the other eye lies in an abducted position and cannot be adducted past the midline." A unilateral pontine lesion involving the PPRF produces an ipsilateral conjugate gaze palsy and also affects the MLF on the same side, which leads to paralysis of adduction of the ipsilateral eye on conjugate gaze to the opposite side.[114,312] MRI has disclosed infarcts affecting the superior or inferior parts of the pons or widely scattered in the pons of patients with one-and-a-half syndrome.[313]

Ptosis

Common in patients with BA occlusion, ptosis is usually attributed to involvement of the descending sympathetic fibers in the lateral pontine tegmentum. However, even with severe bilateral ptosis, the pupils may not be miotic.[114] Pontine ptosis is often more severe than the ptosis that usually accompanies peripheral Horner's syndrome or Horner's syndrome found in patients with lateral medullary syndrome. Pontine ptosis is often modified by involvement of the seventh cranial nerve or a hemiparesis.[314] In patients with hemiparesis, whether brainstem or supratentorial, ptosis is often more severe on the hemiparetic side. A peripheral type of facial weakness diminishes the ptosis by paralyzing the orbicularis oculi muscle, widening the palpebral fissure. If BA occlusion produces infarction of a third nerve nucleus, complete bilateral ptosis is the rule.

Pontine Pupils

Pupillary disturbances from pontine infarction are frequently pinpoint,[114] but a reaction can be seen if a bright light and magnification are used.[287] When pontine and midbrain infarctions coexist, the pupils are often at midposition but poorly reactive. Lesions in the midbrain alone, with sparing of the pons, produce fixed, dilated pupils. Pupillary constriction is more severe with pontine infarction or hemorrhage than with peripheral Horner's syndrome, which may mean that parasympathetic irritation as well as a destructive sympathetic process explains the pinpoint pupils.

Nystagmus

Common in patients with basilar occlusion, vertical nystagmus is an important sign of pontine infarction. Rhythmic vertical nystagmus does not occur with higher brainstem lesions, although other disorders of vertical gaze are hallmarks of mesencephalic and diencephalic damage.[287]

Sensory Findings

Sensory findings are quite variable in BA occlusion, a fact that may be explained by the bias toward a medial location of infarction that allows the more laterally placed spinothalamic tracts to be spared. More rostrally, the main somatosensory lemnisci are supplied by lateral circumferential collaterals and are relatively spared.[286] Occasional patients with BA disease have bilateral, severe, unusual pain sensations in the face, said to be like the feeling of salt and pepper thrown on the face.[315] This symptom could be due to involvement of fibers crossing the midline from the trigeminal nuclei to join the medial border of the spinothalamic tracts. Alternatively, the symptoms could be explained by involvement of the nucleus raphe magnus in the periaqueductal gray matter. This nucleus has serotonergic projections to the spinal tracts of the fifth cranial nerve and their nuclei.

Abnormalities of Respiration

Abnormalities of respiration are also common, but their mechanism is difficult to determine because of the extensiveness of the infarction and the presence of general medical factors (e.g., aspiration, fever, and hypoventilation). Apneustic breathing with a hang-up of the inspiratory phase and grossly regular breathing (ataxic respirations) occasionally occur terminally in patients with BA occlusion and carry an ominous prognosis.[279,287,316,317]

Top of the Basilar Artery Occlusion

Occlusive lesions of the rostral tip of the BA lead to bilateral infarction of midbrain, thalamus, and occipital and medial temporal lobes. In this area, in addition to the major tributary branches of the basilar apex, the SCA, posterior communicating artery, and PCA, numerous smaller

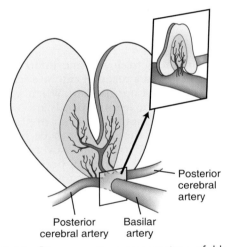

Posterior cerebral artery

Posterior cerebral artery   Basilar artery

Figure 26-11 Diagrammatic representations of blood supply from the distal basilar artery. Note the single midline vessel supplying the thalamus bilaterally. The area of infarction is the zone within the ellipse. *Inset,* Midbrain with shaded area of infarction.

perforating midbrain arteries and vessels course through the posterior perforating substance to feed the hypothalamus and paramedian diencephalic structures (Fig. 26-11). Atherosclerosis is generally most severe in the proximal BA; in the more cephalad portion, atherosclerotic stenosis is less common, and the vessel gradually tapers in size. Occlusions of the basilar apex are generally embolic,[110,215] but severe atherothrombosis is also reported.[318,319] Rostral basilar territory ischemia may also occur after posterior circulation angiography, and initial cortical blindness, agitated delirium, and an amnesic state are the cardinal features, usually with accompanying headache. The symptoms and signs reverse within 24 hours, leaving a permanent amnesia for the period of the angiography; the syndrome is attributed to contrast reaction.

Abnormalities of Alertness, Attention, and Behavior

The medial mesencephalon and diencephalon contain the most rostral portions of the reticular activating system. Infarcts in these regions frequently affect consciousness, sleep, and behavior[116,320,321] and have been attributed to occlusion of the perforating branches of the mesencephalic artery (the first portion of the PCA as it courses around the midbrain) (Fig. 26-12).[87]

Because the reticular gray matter is adjacent to the third cranial nerve nuclei and the vertical gaze regions near the posterior commissure, somnolence is invariably associated with pupillary abnormalities, third cranial nerve palsies, and defects of vertical gaze, although lateralized motor or sensory signs are often absent. A similar syndrome can occur after herniation, presumably as a result of extension pressure on these same vascular structures, caused by wedging of the mammillary bodies into the interpeduncular fossa, which is a situation that causes either median brainstem infarction[322] or Duret hemorrhages.[323]

Pupillary Abnormalities

When ischemia affects the medial midbrain tegmentum or medial diencephalon, pupillary reactivity is usually abnormal because the afferent limb of the pupillary

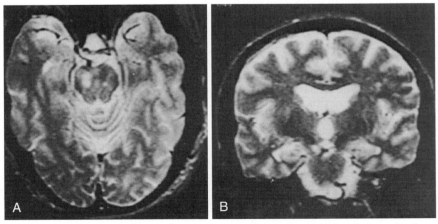

Figure 26-12 T2-weighted MR images of pontomesencephalic infarct. A, Axial plane. B, Coronal plane.

reflex arc is interrupted in its course from the optic tract of the Edinger-Westphal nucleus. Midbrain pupils are frequently eccentric (corectopia iridis) and may shift position severely.[324,325] If the lesion affects only the Edinger-Westphal nucleus, the pupils are generally fixed and dilated, but if rostral extension of the lesion occurs with resultant sympathetic paralysis, the deficit involves a midposition, fixed pupil. In some cases the pupil is oval, which is a phenomenon that is usually transient and most often found in patients with supratentorial vascular catastrophes that lead to tentorial herniation.[326] Occasionally a pupil becomes oval in a patient with midbrain infarction when a third cranial nerve paralysis is developing or recovering[326]; other pupillary sizes, shapes, or functions have also been reported.[319]

Oculomotor Dysfunction

Vertical gaze–vertical plane eye movements are voluntarily generated by bilaterally simultaneous activation of the frontal and parietal occipital conjugate gaze centers. Vertical gaze pathways then converge on the periaqueductal region beneath the collicular plate, near the interstitial nucleus of Cajal and the posterior commissure.[327-329] In this region in the monkey, there is a cluster of neurons important in vertical gaze; it is situated among fibers of the MLF and is generally referred to as the *rostral interstitial nucleus* of the MLF[330] or the *nucleus of the prerubral field.*[329]

Clinically, there is often a disparity between paralysis of voluntary vertical gaze and vertical eye movements reflex-induced by a vertical doll's-eyes maneuver, bilateral simultaneous caloric stimulation, or Bell's phenomenon, although the anatomic basis for the disparity is not clear. Most commonly, upgazes and downgazes are affected together. Debate still centers on the question of whether such dysfunctions occur only with bilateral lesions because unilateral stereotactic-placed lesions[331] or unilateral vascular[332] and metastatic[138] lesions have, on occasion, produced upward gaze paralysis. Selective paralysis of downward gaze is much rarer; when it occurs, the lesions usually border the red nucleus and lie more ventral and caudal, producing paralysis of upward gaze.[329,333,334] Some patients with unilateral lesions of the paramedian midbrain and caudal diencephalon have abnormal control of head and eye posture in the roll plane.[335] Some patients with mesodiencephalic infarcts have had vertical one-and-a-half syndrome.[336,337] Unilateral midbrain infarcts affecting the third nerve nucleus cause impaired upward gaze from the contralateral eye, explained by the crossing fibers controlling contralateral orbital elevation.[337a]

Abnormalities of Convergence

Ocular convergence is probably controlled in the medial midbrain tegmentum, although there is considerable debate as to whether a formal nuclear structure, such as the nucleus of Perlia, subserves this function. One or both eyes may rest in, and convergence vectors are frequently evident on attempted upward gaze. Rhythmic convergence nystagmus may be elicited if patients are told to follow a downgoing opticokinetic target with their eyes.

Convergence vectors may also modify lateral gaze. Voluntary lateral movements of the lateral rectus are balanced against convergence vectors, thus limiting abduction and giving the superficial appearance of a sixth cranial nerve palsy (pseudo-sixth nerve palsy).[259] Lid abnormalities are also a common sign of rostral brainstem disease. Unilateral infarction of a third cranial nerve nucleus can lead to complete bilateral ptosis.[314] Retraction of the upper lid, giving the eye a prominent stare (Collier's sign), is also common in tectal lesions.[338]

Hallucinations

Complaints of hallucination are also made by patients with rostral brainstem infarction, leading to application of the term *peduncular hallucinosis.*[339-341] The hallucinations occur at twilight or during the night, and all such patients also have sleep disorders (nocturnal insomnia or daytime hypersomnolence).[259] The hallucinations are usually vivid, are most commonly visual, and contain multiple colors, objects, and scenes. Blood and red hair, horses and green serpents against a red background, and brightly plumed parrots are examples. Occasionally, auditory or tactile hallucinations are associated. Similar hallucinations also accompany sleep deprivation or drug intoxication and may relate to dysfunction of the reticular activating system. Brainstem lesions have been large, making it difficult to relate the abnormality to any particular anatomic structure.[342]

Confabulations

Confabulations are often reported in patients with rostral brainstem infarcts.[343] They consist of descriptions of behavior or present whereabouts that are totally unrealistic and have many of the features described in the Wernicke-Korsakoff psychosis.

Hemiballism and Abnormal Movements

Long known clinically, involuntary movements occur from lesions affecting the subthalamic nucleus (corpus Luysii).[344,345] Attempts have been made[346] to differentiate *ballism*—that is, incessant, violent, limb-flinging proximal movements—from other types of adventitious movements such as chorea and clonic, athetoid, and myoclonic movements. Either type may be delayed in onset,[87] and both have a predilection for the face, arm, and thumb.

Basilar Branch and Lacunar Disease

A heterogeneous group of disorders, *basilar branch disease* involves all occlusive disease arising in small or larger branches of the basilar arteries. Convenient subdivisions, which are used in this discussion, are (1) intraparenchymatous occlusions resulting in lacunar infarctions due to hypertensive arteriolopathy, usually within the tiny penetrating parenchymatous vessels, (2) extraparenchymatous occlusion of small branches, such as median pontine or thalamogeniculate arteries, usually by miniature atherosclerotic plaques or junctional lesions involving the BA wall,[129,266] and (3) stenosis or occlusion of larger circumferential branches, such as the AICA and SCA (Fig. 26-13). The subject is discussed in more detail in Chapter 27.

Occlusion of Long Circumferential Branches of the Basilar Artery

The most common mechanism of occlusion of the circumferential (cerebellar) branches of the BA is embolism, atheroma, or thrombus in the parent BA that blocks the orifices of these branches. The nomenclature is a bit misleading, in that the three vessels are more easily described as superior, midline, and inferior, but because the brainstem and cerebellum lie in a forward angle, they have traditionally been broken into two groups, superior and inferior (anterior inferior and posterior inferior) (Figs. 26-14 and 26-15). Despite objections, it seems unlikely that any change will be achieved in this nomenclature. Because of the intimate association of the PICA with the lateral medullary syndrome and vertebral artery occlusion, the discussion that follows reviews cerebellar arterial occlusion in reverse order: superior, anterior inferior, and then posterior inferior.

Superior Cerebellar Artery Occlusions

SCA infarctions are among the most common of the cerebellar stroke syndromes.[127,128,263,347-349] SCA territory infarctions are characterized by the rarity of clinical involvement of the brainstem territory of the SCA and do not frequently manifest as the classic SCA syndrome.[127,128,264,349,350] They typically have partial

cerebellar involvement, a cardioembolic origin, and a relatively benign prognosis.[128,263,347,351-353] The SCA supplies the rostral surface of the cerebellum down to the great horizontal sulcus (see Fig. 26-3), including the lobulus centralis, culmen, clivus, folium, and tuber of the vermis; the anterior, simplex, and superior semilunar lobules of the cerebellar hemispheres; and, rarely, the upper part of the inferior semilunar lobules.[75] Hemispheric branches can be classified as *medial, intermediate* (both arising from mSCA), and *lateral* (arising from lSCA) groups (Fig. 26-16).[354]

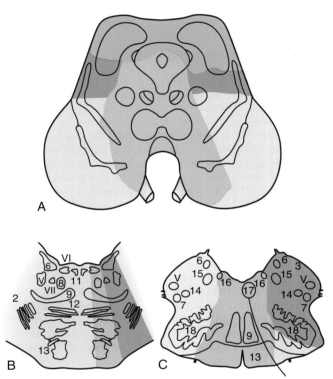

Figure 26-14 Drawing of the arterial territories in the (A) medulla, (B) pons, and (C) mesencephalon.

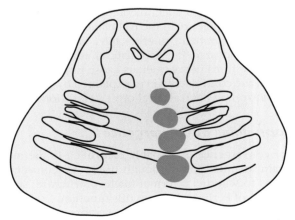

Figure 26-15 Infarcts en chapelet by Foix and Hillemand. (From Foix C, Hillemand P: Contribution à l'étude des ramollissements protubérantiels. *Rev Med* 43:287, 1926.)

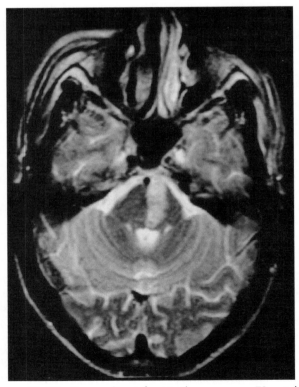

Figure 26-13 Paramedian infarct in the pons on a T2-weighted MR image. Note that the basilar artery is patent.

Causes

Arterial occlusions leading to strokes in the SCA distribution usually involve the distal tip of the BA, the ICVA, the ECVA at its origin, and, less frequently, the SCA itself.[110,127,263,349,350,353] However, in most patients with SCA strokes, no arterial occlusion is found. Presumably, the thromboembolus has moved on or has been lysed by the time of angiography or postmortem examination. Thus, the frequency of SCA occlusion is probably underestimated. Embolism is the leading cause.[9,127,128,263,349,351,353,355]

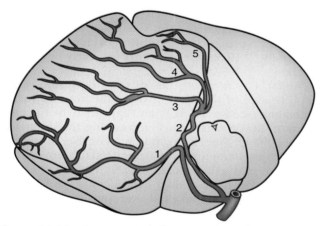

Figure 26-16 Superior cerebellar artery (SCA) branches (three-quarter view). The lateral branch of the SCA and medial branch of the SCA and its vermal branches, paravermal branches, and hemispheric branches.

Rare causes of SCA territory stroke in the young include SCA dissection and FMD,[356,357] migraine,[358,359] and transcardiac embolism from a patent foramen ovale during Valsalva's maneuver.[351]

A classic SCA territory infarction syndrome has been reported[355,360] since early in the 20th century, featuring ipsilateral limb ataxia, ipsilateral Horner's syndrome, contralateral loss of pain and temperature sensibility of the face, arm, leg, and trunk, and contralateral fourth nerve palsy.[127] A few have also had abnormal ipsilateral spontaneous involuntary movement.[127,350,361,362] Kase et al produced the landmark series.[349]

Partial territory SCA infarctions may be associated with rostral BA infarctions[127]; however, they more commonly involve the rostral cerebellum alone.[128,263,349,351,353] The brainstem territory of the SCA supplied by branches arising early from the parent trunk is usually unaffected in patients with partial territory SCA infarctions. Partial territory infarctions are the most common type of SCA infarction[128,263,347,349] and differ from full territory infarctions in that they have routinely benign outcomes.[128,349,351]

Six distinct clinical patterns exist (Table 26-2). The previously described classic SCA syndrome[361,363,364] is but rarely seen.[127,349,350] This syndrome develops with involvement of the brainstem territory of the SCA (see Fig. 26-2). Signs characteristic of the syndrome are ipsilateral limb dysmetria, ipsilateral Horner's syndrome, contralateral pain and temperature sensory loss, and contralateral fourth nerve palsy. Other signs less commonly reported are ipsilateral loss of emotional expression in the face,

TABLE 26-2 CEREBELLAR STROKE SYNDROMES

Location of Cerebellar Infarct	Associated Infarcts	Clinical Syndrome
Rostral (SCA)	Mesencephalon, subthalamic area, thalamus, occipitotemporal lobes	Rostral basilar artery syndrome or coma from onset ± tetraplegia
	Laterotegmental area of the upper pons	Dysmetria and Horner's syndrome (ipsilateral), temperature and pain sensory loss, and CN IV palsy (contralateral)
	—	Dysarthria, headache, dizziness, vomiting, ataxia, and delayed coma (pseudotumoral form)
Dorsomedial (mSCA)		Dysarthria
		Ataxia
Ventrolateral (lSCA)	—	Dysmetria, axial lateropulsion (ipsilateral) ataxia, and dysarthria
Medial (AICA)	Lateral area of the lower pons	CN V, VII, and VIII, Horner's syndrome, dysmetria (ipsilateral), temperature and pain sensory loss (contralateral)
	—	Pure vestibular syndrome
Caudal (PICA)	—	Vertigo, headache, vomiting, ataxia, and delayed coma (pseudotumoral form)
Dorsomedial (mPICA)	Dorsolateromedullary area	Wallenberg's syndrome
	—	Isolated vertigo or vertigo with dysmetria and axial lateropulsion (ipsilateral) and ataxia
Ventrolateral (lPICA)	—	Vertigo, ipsilateral limb dysmetria
Caudal and medial	Lateral area of the lower pons or lateromedullary area, or both	AICA syndrome ± delayed coma (pseudotumoral form)
Rostrocaudal	—	Vertigo, vomiting, headache, ataxia, dysarthria, and delayed coma (pseudotumoral form)
	Brainstem, thalamus, occipitotemporal lobes	Coma from onset ± tetraplegia

AICA, Anterior inferior cerebellar artery; CN, cranial nerve; lPICA, lateral branch of the PICA; lSCA, lateral branch of the SCA; mPICA, medial branch of the PICA; mSCA, medial branch of the SCA; PICA, posterior inferior cerebellar artery; SCA, superior cerebellar artery.

unilateral or bilateral hearing loss (possibly due to involvement of the lateral lemniscus), and sleep disorders (due to locus ceruleus damage).[364] Ipsilateral abnormal limb movements are more unusual.[350,360,365-367] Movement disorders occurring with classic SCA syndrome, described as choreiform[350] or athetotic,[360,365,367] consist of slow, undulatory movements[361,366] of large amplitude.[350,365,367] They appear with effort or emotion.[366] Movement disorders are presumed to arise from involvement of the dentate nucleus or damage to the superior cerebellar peduncle. A few weeks after ischemic injury, palatal myoclonus and contralateral hypertrophy of the inferior olivary nucleus may occur with dentate nucleus damage.[368] Palatal myoclonus is occasionally accompanied by synchronous myoclonic movements of the jaw, face,[368] tongue, and ipsilateral vocal cord, producing voice disorders.[367] Davison et al[360] described a patient with SCA infarction without palatal myoclonus who had myoclonus of the jaw and a coarse tremor of the hand.

The *rostral BA syndrome* is one of the most striking clinical presentations of SCA occlusion, occurring in about a quarter of the cases.[127] It features visual field defects, vomiting, dizziness, diplopia, paresthesia, clumsiness of limbs, weakness, and drowsiness. These signs and symptoms suggest occipitotemporal lobe damage. Some patients clearly have cortical blindness or hemianopia, memory loss or confusion, or paralysis of visual fixation (Balint's syndrome). Thalamomesencephalic involvement is manifest in other patients as multimodal sensory loss, contralateral Horner's syndrome, ipsilateral hemianopia, appendicular ataxia or pendular reflexes, behavioral changes, abulia, unilateral spatial neglect, memory loss, transcortical motor aphasia, and vertical gaze palsy. Subthalamic damage may produce hemiballism. Mesencephalic damage usually manifests as one of several syndromes: Benedikt's syndrome of third nerve palsy with contralateral limb movement disorders, Claude's syndrome with third nerve palsy and contralateral limb dysmetria, Weber's syndrome with contralateral limb weakness, or Parinaud's syndrome with vertical gaze paresis. Some individuals with mesencephalic damage have also had pseudo-sixth nerve palsy, tonic deviation of gaze, palpebral retraction, pupillary disturbances, drowsiness, hallucinosis, and confusion.[127,259,318] Additional signs are ipsilateral Horner's syndrome, limb dysmetria, hemiplegia, contralateral pain and temperature sensory loss, and internuclear ophthalmoplegia. Usually only two or three of these signs of rostral BA occlusion are present; in such circumstances, the SCA involvement is commonly difficult to recognize or is unexpectedly discovered on CT.[127,369]

A third syndrome features *coma from onset*, together with tetraplegia and oculomotor palsy. These clinical findings are included in the top-of-the-basilar syndrome (see earlier).[127]

SCA occlusion may be *clinically inapparent* if there is simultaneous embolic infarction in the distribution of the ICA with a resultant brachiofacial sensorimotor deficit and aphasia. This second infarction is identified in a small percentage of cases.[127]

Cerebellar and vestibular signs are the prominent presenting features in many clinical series.[128,264,347,349,351,353]

They are due to partial involvement of the SCA territory (see Fig. 26-4). Symptoms are headache, gait abnormalities, and, in about 35% of patients, dizziness and vomiting.[128,263,349,353] In a series of 30 patients with unilateral, isolated infarctions of the SCA territory as documented on CT,[273] patients most often were seen with appendicular ataxia (73%), gait ataxia (67%), nystagmus (50%), and brainstem signs (30%).[349] Nystagmus was horizontal and ipsilateral in 20% of patients, horizontal and contralateral in 3%, horizontal and bilateral in 20%, and vertical in 7%.[349] In an unselected CT series of 17 SCA infarctions, 15 patients had limb ataxia and 12 had truncal ataxia and dysarthria.[353] Dysarthria, one of the main symptoms of SCA infarction, seems to be the counterpart of the vertigo that typically develops with PICA infarctions.[351] Hemiparesis occurs in nearly one fourth of patients.[353]

The *lSCA syndrome*[351] arises from occlusion of the lateral branch of the SCA, involves the anterior rostral cerebellum (see Fig. 26-4),[351] and appears to be the most common of SCA infarctions, accounting for about half the cases.[128,370] The lSCA syndrome consists of dysmetria of the ipsilateral limbs, ipsilateral axial lateropulsion, dysarthria, and gait unsteadiness.[351] The findings can mimic the dysarthria–clumsy hand lacunar syndrome,[371] may manifest as isolated axial lateropulsion,[372] and may be associated with prominent dysmetria, nystagmus, or contrapulsion of saccades.[350,373] Occasionally, lSCA infarctions may manifest as transient symptoms (transient blurring of vision, unsteadiness of gait, and tinnitus lasting a few seconds) and no clinical neurologic signs.[72]

Clinical syndromes due to *dorsomedial infarction* of the rostral cerebellum in the territory of the mSCA have not been fully characterized, although some individual patients have been reported.[350,374,375] In large registries of cerebellar infarctions, mSCA infarcts represent 10% to 20% of all SCA infarctions,[127] but no specific clinical syndrome has been reported.[128,370] Among the individual patients who have been described, those in whom the most medial branches were involved have shown isolated unsteadiness of gait.[350] In those in whom the anterior cerebellar lobe (i.e., the lingula, central, culmen lobules of the vermis, and the anterior lobule of the hemisphere) was involved, some appendicular ataxia and spontaneous posturing of the neck, trunk, and limbs occurred.[375] With involvement of more lateral branches of the paravermal territory, isolated dysarthria was found.[374]

Prognosis

SCA territory infarctions can have a pseudotumoral presentation, a characteristic observed in 21% of autopsy cases.[127] However, the course and outcome of SCA infarctions are best evaluated in CT and MRI series of patients.[128,263,347,349,376] In the vast majority, the lesion is limited to the SCA territory with partial SCA involvement. Such patients have benign outcomes and are left minimally disabled or neurologically intact.[349] Only 7% of patients have a pseudotumoral pattern leading to coma and, occasionally, death.[349] This relatively benign course is seen with both lSCA and mSCA infarctions.

Anterior Inferior Cerebellar Artery Occlusions

Reported AICA infarctions were exceedingly rare[71] until the advent of MRI (see Fig. 26-4).[126] This type of pontocerebellar infarction differs strikingly from SCA and PICA infarctions in terms of brainstem signs associated with the clinical presentation.

The *cerebellar territory* of the AICA (see Fig. 26-2) varies as a function of its caliber (see the anatomy section earlier in the chapter). The artery nearly always supplies the flocculus, the only territory of the cerebellum usually vascularized solely by the AICA.[70] Although often ending in the flocculus,[70] it may follow the sulcus, separating the anterior lobule and the semilunar lobule, and give rise to terminal branches that supply the following neighboring lobules: anterior, simplex, superior semilunar, inferior semilunar, gracilis, and lobulus biventer.[70,377] The AICA can even replace the territory of a hypoplastic PICA, taking over the supply to most of the inferior surface of the cerebellum, including the anterolateral part of the tonsil but not the vermis. A balance in size exists between the AICA and PICA.[8,11,377-379] The terminal branches of the AICA anastomose with the ipsilateral SCA and the PICA at the borderzone areas of these arteries.

In its *pontine distribution*, the AICA (see Fig. 26-2)[66] always supplies the middle cerebellar peduncle, the lower third of the lateral pontine territory (in most cases), frequently its middle third, and, in a few individuals, the superior part of the lateral region of the medulla.

The paucity of autopsy reports[69,71] have been supplemented by CT and MRI.[126,380,381] These sources indicate most AICA infarcts involve a small territory restricted to the lateral region of the caudal pons and, in the cerebellum, to the middle cerebellar peduncle (100% of cases) and flocculus (69% of cases). Involvement of this region accounts for most of the clinical signs described for AICA occlusions.[71] Infarctions often also affect other cerebellar lobules (75% of cases) but usually remain limited in size.

Infarcts commonly involve a small part of the cerebellum comprising the central white matter, the flocculus, and a thin rim of cerebellar cortex located at the junction of the territories of the three major cerebellar arteries, as illustrated in Figure 26-3, but this involvement does not modify the clinical presentation. When the AICA is large (and the PICA is hypoplastic), the AICA territory encompasses the whole anterior inferior cerebellum. There is no significant clinical difference between the signs and symptoms initially observed after infarctions arising with relatively limited AICA involvement and those observed after infarctions arising in vascular systems in which both the AICA and the PICA come from a common trunk of the vertebral or basilar artery.[71]

In most AICA infarctions, the inferolateral pontine territory is involved, and the infarction sometimes extends up to the middle third of the lateral pons and down to the superior part of the lateral medulla. It involves neither the upper third of the lateral pons, which is supplied by the superior lateral pontine artery, a branch of the BA or a branch of the mSCA, nor the ventral aspect of the pons. AICA territory infarctions are associated with PICA and SCA infarcts in 35% of autopsy cases, and this association frequently occurs with ventromedian pontine infarction

and tonsillar herniation.[71] Other partial AICA infarctions involve at least the middle cerebellar peduncle, the core of the vessel's territory.

Cause

Atherosclerotic occlusion seems to be the most common mechanism,[71,110] but embolism has also been documented. Intracranial giant cell arteritis[382] and infarcts associated with migraine have also been reported.[358]

Clinical Aspects

Four distinct clinical pictures can be distinguished in patients with AICA occlusions (see Table 26-2).

The classic syndrome of the AICA, first described by Adams[383] in one patient, is the most common clinical picture described.[71] Symptoms are vertigo, vomiting, tinnitus, and dysarthria. Signs comprise ipsilateral facial palsy, hearing loss, trigeminal sensory loss, Horner's syndrome, appendicular dysmetria, and contralateral temperature and pain sensory loss over the limbs and trunk.[71,383] The AICA syndrome may also include ipsilateral conjugate lateral gaze palsy due to involvement of the flocculus rather than damage to the abducens nucleus, dysphagia due to extension of the infarction to the superior part of the lateral medulla, and ipsilateral limb weakness due to contralateral involvement of the corticospinal tract in the pons or mesencephalon.[71] Because some signs are crossed and some are similar to signs observed in Wallenberg's syndrome, an AICA occlusion is often misdiagnosed as lateral medullary infarction. However, signs unusual in Wallenberg's syndrome, such as severe facial palsy, deafness, tinnitus, and multimodal sensory impairment over the face, allow accurate clinicotopographic diagnosis.[71]

Coma with tetraplegia from onset occurred in 20% of cases of AICA that came to autopsy in one series.[71] It was due to massive ventromedial involvement of the basis pontis together with cerebellar infarction in the territory of all three cerebellar arteries.

Isolated vertigo, mimicking labyrinthitis, occurs in partial AICA territory infarcts[69,72,383,384] but is not often documented.[72,384-386] Oas and Baloh[387] reported on two patients with unilateral AICA territory infarcts in whom attacks of vertigo preceded the strokes by 12 months and 3 months, respectively. Each patient also had unilateral hearing loss. However, because of the extent of the territory usually supplied by the AICA, isolated vertigo as the sole clinical presentation is likely to be exceptional. AICA territory infarctions can also cause *isolated cerebellar signs*, as demonstrated in a clinical MRI report of an infarction in a child.[388]

Prognosis

Although most cases reported in the literature have been based on autopsies, clinical MRI reports that have been published depict patients with benign outcomes and minimal neurologic residua.[126,381,384] Descriptions of banal, isolated vertigo with a benign outcome suggest that partial AICA territory infarctions may be more frequent than has been recognized.[384,387] Alternatively, AICA occlusion may be a very rare cause of isolated vertigo,[384] and in some cases, AICA territory infarctions may herald massive BA thrombosis.[72,126]

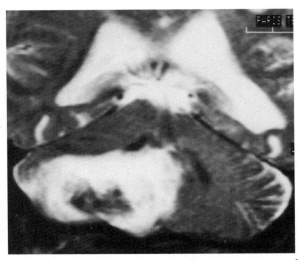

Figure 26-17 Posterior inferior cerebellar artery territory infarction on T2-weighted MR image.

Posterior Inferior Cerebellar Artery Infarctions

PICA infarcts arise from occlusion of the ICVA facing the PICA ostium or (directly) the main stem of the PICA; both sites have the same causes.[389]

Symptoms of *cerebellar infarction* are nonspecific, including vertigo, headache, vomiting, dysarthria, and gait unsteadiness. The major sign is gait and trunk ataxia, ipsilateral axial lateropulsion, or both, which usually prevent standing in an upright position. Usually patients able to walk or stand in tandem position are unlikely to have important cerebellar infarction.[390] Other signs are nystagmus, ipsilateral limb dysmetria, and dysarthria. Impairment of consciousness, ranging from drowsiness to deep coma, occurs in half the patients either at onset or later. More than half the patients have signs of *associated brainstem infarction* (facial palsy, trigeminal involvement, ocular motor abnormalities, motor weakness, and sensory loss) or occipitotemporal infarction (visual field defects, cortical blindness, memory loss).

The clinical presentation is similar to that of cerebellar hemorrhage, but unenhanced CT allows distinction between the two conditions.[298,391] MRI clearly delineates the increased signal on diffusion-weighted images, then on T2-weighted axial, coronal, and sagittal sections (Fig. 26-17).

The clinical *outcome* of cerebellar infarctions is usually benign and relatively good recovery is expected; however, large cerebellar infarctions can take a pseudotumoral form because of edema, cerebellar swelling, brainstem compression, obstruction of the fourth ventricle, and hydrocephalus (see later). In that case, life-saving surgery is needed if deterioration of consciousness appears.

PICA infarcts were formerly the most studied and were presumed to be the most common of all cerebellar infarctions. Most often the pseudotumoral form and the form associated with Wallenberg's syndrome have been emphasized. MRI has shown that tumoral forms of PICA infarcts are not common. Awareness of both presentations is very important because a patient with the pseudotumoral form may need life-saving surgical treatment and a patient with Wallenberg's syndrome may require gastrostomy. Other more common presentations have a benign course.

Clinicopathologic and clinicoradiologic series show that PICA infarcts are actually about as common as SCA infarcts.[128,263,347-349,389]

Historical Aspects

PICA infarcts were historically but partly erroneously associated closely with lateral medullary infarctions (i.e., Wallenberg's syndrome; see later). After the anatomic descriptions by Duret in 1873,[1] in which only the PICA was posited to supply the lateral region of the medulla, and Wallenberg's description[392,393] of a case of lateral medullary infarction due to PICA occlusion, every lateral medullary infarction was assumed to be due to a PICA occlusion,[394-399] even when no occlusion could be found.[395-397,399,400] In fact, necropsy showed that Wallenberg's original patient also had an ipsilateral ICVA occlusive lesion.

Subsequently, the lateral medullary syndrome was confused with the PICA syndrome. Further studies revealed that the lateral region of the medulla is supplied most often by three or four small branches arising from the distal ICVA between the PICA ostium and the origin of the BA and less commonly by small branches arising from the PICA.[67,111,401-403] PICA infarctions sparing the lateral medullary territory are the most common, and paradoxically, syndromes featuring occlusion of the PICA were not described until Duncan et al[404] emphasized the frequency of vertigo as the prominent presenting symptom. In summary, the PICA (1) sometimes participates in the supply of the lateral medullary area, usually together with branches from the VA but alone in 22% of individuals, and (2) usually participates in the supply of the dorsal medullary area together with the posterior spinal arteries.[405]

Topography of Infarction and Clinical Outcomes

The arterial occlusion primarily involves the intracranial portion of the VA facing the PICA ostium and the origin of the PICA. Embolism (arch ulceration included)[110] and atherosclerotic occlusion lead the list of causes[349,389]; other uncommon causes are VA dissection[128,349] and occlusion of the mPICA by tonsillar herniation due to raised posterior fossa pressure.[406]

Two different clinical situations occur, depending on whether the medulla is involved.[389] No lateral medullary infarction is seen without associated infarction in the dorsal medullary territory. PICA infarctions are much less frequently associated with other vertebrobasilar (pontine, mesencephalic, thalamic, or occipitotemporal) infarctions than AICA or SCA infarctions. The full PICA territory is rarely affected in isolation but is more routinely associated with SCA infarction, AICA infarction, or both (46%).[389] These combined infarctions are frequently edematous and produced brainstem compression.

Partial PICA territory infarctions were very common (46%) among the autopsy cases reported by Amarenco et al.[389] They usually involved the dorsomedial area of the

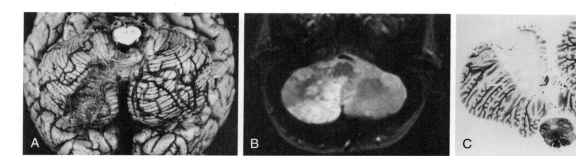

Figure 26-18 Infarctions in the territory of the medial branch of the posterior inferior cerebellar artery (A) at autopsy, (B) on a T2-weighted MR image, and (C) in a drawing.

caudal cerebellum—that is, the territory of the mPICA (32%)—and less frequently the lateral area, the territory of the lPICA (18%). Partial infarctions represented 75% of PICA infarctions in one clinical series[349] and two thirds in another series.[128] Such infarctions are never edematous. Thus, when restricted to branch PICA territory, they are often small and benign.[349] In the nine examples of brainstem compression reported among 36 PICA cases by Kase et al,[349] all had full PICA territory infarction. Seven of these patients had obstructive hydrocephalus, and four died from cerebellar swelling. No clinically significant differences exist between full PICA and mPICA territory lesions.[407]

Clinical Picture

PICA territory cerebellar infarcts are undoubtedly under-recognized and underdiagnosed.[408] Some estimates suggest that one fourth of elderly patients seen with severe vertigo and nystagmus may have PICA territory cerebellar infarcts.

The *dorsal lateral medullary syndrome*[67,69,392,393,409] occurred in 25% of one autopsy series[374] and in one third of a clinical series.[349] Because dorsal medullary infarctions are almost constantly associated with PICA infarctions and 13% of cases of lateral medullary infarctions occur together with dorsal medullary infarctions,[68] a PICA territory cerebellar infarction is estimated to exist in 13% of cases of lateromedullary infarction.[389] The Wallenberg syndrome accompanying the lateral medullary infarct can be complete or partial, with vertigo, nystagmus, loss of pain and temperature on the ipsilateral face, ninth and tenth cranial nerve palsies, ipsilateral Horner's syndrome, appendicular ataxia, and contralateral temperature and pain sensory loss.

Patients with *PICA territory infarctions sparing the medulla* usually are seen with vertigo, headache, gait ataxia, limb ataxia, and horizontal nystagmus.[349,410-413] Headache is cervical, occipital, or both, occasionally with periauricular or hemifacial–ocular radiation. Unilateral headaches are ipsilateral to the cerebellar infarction.[349] Nystagmus is the most common sign (75%) and is either horizontal (ipsilateral in 47% of patients, contralateral in 5%, bilateral in 11%) or vertical (11% of patients).[349] In addition to vertigo, one of the most striking findings in patients with PICA infarctions is ipsilateral axial lateropulsion, a phenomenon suggestive of a lateral displacement of the central representation of the center of gravity.[390] This sign is distinct from lateral deviation of the limbs

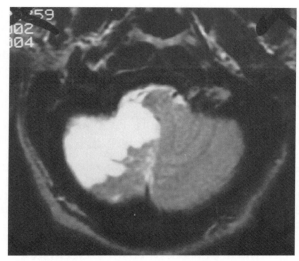

Figure 26-19 Infarction in the territory of the lateral branch of the PICA on T2-weighted MR image.

(i.e., past-pointing) and gait veering. A patient's attempts to stand or walk are usually associated with falling toward the side of the cerebellar infarction.[349]

The *isolated acute vertigo* form of PICA infarction, mimicking labyrinthitis, was first described clinicopathologically by Duncan et al.[404] The autopsy showed a recent medial and caudal cerebellar infarction with no other brain lesions. Additional cases have been reported,[385,414-416] some of which had dorsomedial infarction of the right caudal cerebellum in the territory of mPICA and normal brainstem (Fig. 26-18).[72,389] Normal caloric responses and direction-changing nystagmus on gaze to each side or after a patient changes head position or lies down are additional signs suggesting a pure vestibular syndrome explained by PICA territory infarction.[404,412] Vertigo occurs from involvement of the uvulonodular complex of the vermis, which is part of the vestibular portion of the cerebellum. Because the nodulus is supplied by the PICA and the flocculus by the AICA, these infarctions should not be labeled "flocculonodular."

Infarcts of the *lateral branch of the PICA* have been reported as chance autopsy findings[69,389] but are now known as a cause of isolated dysmetria ipsilateral to the infarct without dysarthria, nystagmus, or rotatory vertigo (Fig. 26-19).[72,417]

PICA territory infarctions associated with AICA or SCA infarctions are much more severe in clinical presentation than isolated PICA territory infarctions.[389] They often manifest a pseudotumoral pattern or with deep coma and tetraplegia.

Syndromes of the mPICA are now common MRI findings.[128,347,390,407,418] They appear on T2-weighted MRI axial sections as areas of increased signal in a triangular zone, dorsomedially directed with the dorsal base and the ventral point toward the fourth ventricle, consistent with the appearance on pathologic sections of the cerebellum at necropsy (see Fig. 26-18). Infarctions with occlusion of the medial branch may be clinically silent[389,407] or may manifest in one of three principal patterns[407]: (1) isolated vertigo, often misdiagnosed as labyrinthitis, (2) vertigo together with ipsilateral axial lateropulsion of the trunk and gaze[419] and dysmetria or unsteadiness, and (3) Wallenberg's syndrome in patients in whom the medulla is also involved. By contrast with PICA, only the mPICA gives rise to rami to the dorsolateral aspect of the medulla.

Prognosis

Clinical series have shown that PICA infarctions have a much more benign outcome than usually thought.[349] Kase et al[349] found signs of brainstem compression in one fourth of their 36 patients (all of whom had full PICA territory infarcts) and acute hydrocephalus in 7 patients; only 4 patients died from cerebellar swelling. Most full and partial PICA territory infarctions have a relatively benign course.[128,349,407]

Intracranial Vertebral Artery Occlusive Disease

Occlusive disease of the intracranial portion of the VA is much more serious than extracranial disease and is commonly associated with infarction of posterior circulation structures. When the occluded VA is responsible for supplying the major source of the blood flow (because the contralateral VA is tiny, previously occluded, severely narrowed, or ends in the PICA), the resulting syndrome is indistinguishable from that caused by occlusion of the BA. Fisher[420] used the term *basilarization* of the VA to describe the situation of dependence on one VA for maintenance of the posterior circulation. A clot formed within the distal VA may propagate into the proximal BA, again producing a syndrome indistinguishable from that seen with BA occlusion.

In the more common situation of bilaterally competent VAs, occlusion of a single VA may be asymptomatic or may be associated with one of the following clinical pictures: (1) lateral medullary infarction, (2) PICA infarction due to obstruction of the ostium of the PICA by an occlusive thrombus in the intracranial VA, (3) ischemia of the ipsilateral hemimedulla through obstruction of the ostia of the anterior spinal artery arising from the intracranial portion of the VA, (4) embolic occlusion in vessels of the distal basilar arterial tree, with the embolus originating from the VA clot, and (5) transient spells without infarction. Because these syndromes are common, quite distinct, and clinically important, they are considered separately in detail here.

Lateral Medullary Infarction

Anatomic Vascular Aspects

The issue of vascular supply from the vertebral or posterior inferior cerebellar artery in lateral medullary infarction has a long history dating from the Duret[1] report of 1873, supplemented by that of Dumenil[409] in 1875; in 1895, Wallenberg's report[392] emphasized the lateral medulla and focused on the PICA as the expected cause.[421] More than half a century later, Fisher et al[67] found sole involvement of the PICA in only two of their 17 cases of lateral medullary infarction, in 13 showing the vertebral artery occluded, and in one severely stenosed. They and, separately, Escourolle et al[111] demonstrated that not one (Foix's artery or the PICA, as stated by Wallenberg) but several small arteries from the VA usually supply the lateral medullary area. Foix et al probably described an infrequent arterial anomaly and Wallenberg probably described an unusual lateral medullary supply because the PICA participates in the supply of the lateral medulla in less than one third of cases. However, the mPICA always participates in the supply of the dorsal medulla along with branches from the posterior spinal arteries.[66] If indeed the intrinsic arterial distribution is usually fixed and divided into medial, lateral, and dorsal areas, the extrinsic arterial supply is extremely variable from one individual to the next.[11] Similar findings have subsequently been reported based on angiography,[422] noninvasive imaging including Doppler sonography,[423] and MRI.[424]

Infarct Topography

The infarct usually involves a wedge of the medulla extending from the lateral edge (see Fig. 26-9). It usually affects a portion of the olive ventrally and in some cases extends dorsally to involve the restiform body. Currier et al[425] divided the pattern of infarction into ventral, superficial, and dorsal lesions, indicating that the extent of infarction was quite variable. When the dorsal medulla is infarcted, the lesion is almost always accompanied by cerebellar infarction.[68] Because the lesion extends dorsally to the olive, the older terminology referred to the lesion as the "retro-olivary syndrome."[426] The zone of infarction usually extends 7 to 10 mm in a rostrocaudal dimension, occurring most commonly in the middle part of the olive but frequently extending into its upper or lower third[67]; some extend into the pontomedullary junction.[68] A similar distribution of infarcts has been documented by CT or MRI.[422-424,427]

Vascular Pathology

Vascular pathology also plays a role. Among the patients studied at necropsy by Fisher et al,[67] 14 were thought to have *atherostenotic thrombotic occlusions* and three were thought to have *embolic occlusions*. In the first reported case, described by Hallopeau, a patient studied at necropsy by Charcot was thought to have a distal VA embolus that arose from ulcerated atheromatous plaques in the aorta. Embolism also explained several famous earlier cases.[53,67,428] Foix et al[402] found in an autopsy case that the lateral medulla was supplied by a single lateral medullary artery that arose from the very proximal portion of the BA; they postulated that the syndrome was caused by occlusion of "the artery of the lateral sulcus of the medulla." This teaching persisted for decades, despite recent authors failing to find more than a handful of such examples in autopsy material.[69,111]

VA occlusion has been reported by a number of workers[389,429] and has been due to embolism[76,274,430] and VA stenosis; some patients showed basilar embolic occlusion inferred from a VA source.[65,431] One series had examples of extension of VA thrombus into the BA.[432] Figure 26-20 shows an example of VA intracranial occlusion with an embolus to the distal BA. In patients with distal BA territory infarction, scant data are available concerning the incidence of coincidentally discovered VA occlusion that might have provided an embolic source. Within the anterior circulation, occlusion of the ICA is commonly heralded by a distal embolus.

Symptoms

The symptoms of lateral medullary infarction are explained by the distinctive anatomy of the lesion (Fig. 26-21). The symptoms are described here in detail and specifically focus on those elements that separate the lateral medullary syndrome from other sites of occlusive vertebrobasilar disease.

Vertigo. The most common symptom is dizziness or vertigo, often accompanied by staggering and double vision. The syndrome may develop suddenly, but more commonly it progresses gradually over 24 to 48 hours. Fluctuations or stepwise deterioration frequently characterizes the first week after stroke onset but is less common thereafter and distinctly unusual after 2 weeks.

Facial pain. Facial pain is more diagnostic and is a cardinal feature of the syndrome, although it is also reported in other vertebrobasilar artery territory lesions.[315] The pain usually appears at onset and heralds other symptoms and signs.[425] Sharp, single stabs or jolts of pain are felt in the eye or face. Occasionally, these may occur in flurries. Sticking, burning, stinging, tingling, and numbness are other commonly used descriptive terms. The eye is the most commonly affected region, but the pain may be limited to the ear or isolated spots on the forehead or cheeks. Pain frequently affects the entire face, including the lips and inside the mouth, but is rarely if ever limited to the mandibular division of the trigeminal nerve.

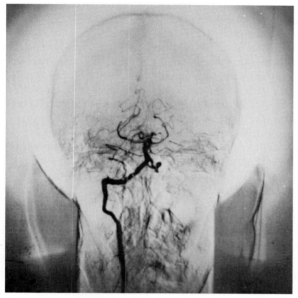

Figure 26-20 Vertebral angiogram showing right vertebral artery intracranial occlusion. The top of the basilar artery and posterior cerebral arteries are not opacified, probably because of embolus from the vertebral artery clot.

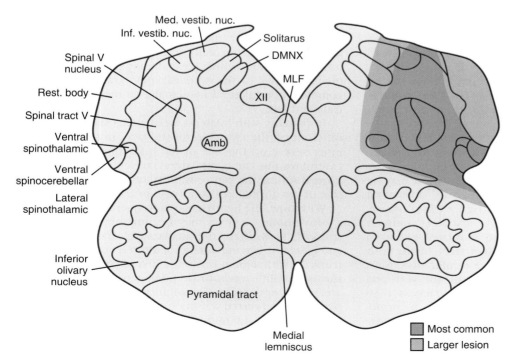

Figure 26-21 Lateral medullary infarction. The most common involvement and largest extent of the lesion are designated by the shaded areas, as described in the key. (Based on a figure in Currier R, Giles C, Dejong R: Some comments on Wallenberg's lateral medullary syndrome. *Neurology [NY]* 11:778, 1961.)

The coexistent contralateral hemianalgesia of the body is seldom mentioned but is usually evident to the patient only after pain or temperature testing. The striking contrast between the spontaneous sudden facial pain due to involvement, presumably, of the nucleus of the descending tract of the fifth cranial nerve and the lack of perception of the hemianalgesia related to ischemia of the spinothalamic tract may reflect that dysfunction of sensory neurons (either within the dorsal root ganglia or buried within the central nervous system, as in the nucleus of the tract of the fifth cranial nerve or in its main sensory nucleus) produces spontaneous pain, but lesions of white matter or nerves do not generally evoke pain as an early finding.[433]

Feelings of disequilibrium and ataxia. Vertigo or other feelings of disequilibrium described as feelings of swaying or falling, feeling seasick, or being off balance are nearly always present; less often, whirling or rotational turning is described. Alteration of vision, another common complaint, may even be described as diplopia (18 of 39 cases) or as the illusion that objects are oscillating or moving.[425] Occasionally, patients with lateral medullary infarction complain of tilting of the visual world; some have even described it as a sudden 90- to 180-degree inversion of the visual images, but the events are too brief for detailed description.[111]

Nausea and vomiting. Nausea and vomiting are also common[425,434] and are thought to be caused by vestibular dysfunction or involvement of the dorsal tegmentum—the *vomiting centers*[435]—in the floor of the fourth ventricle.[425]

Hiccups. Hiccups are common, usually developing some time after the onset. The lateral medullary infarct is typically complete and is usually not ventral or superficial.[425] No clear explanation exists.[425,436]

Dysphagia. Difficulty in swallowing is common (55 of the 74 total patients reported by Currier et al[425] and in other series[434]). Food or secretions may have unusually free influx into the air passages, which is a phenomenon unusual in patients with peripheral ninth and tenth cranial nerve involvement at the jugular foramen. Disturbances of the coordination of epiglottic closure and palatal and pharyngeal function may be more likely with a central lesion of the nucleus ambiguus. Food gets stuck in the piriform recess of the pharynx adjacent to the larynx; patients attempt to extricate the material by an unusual cough-like maneuver. This crowing-like cough is characteristic, and its presence in a patient with stroke is virtually diagnostic of lateral medullary infarction.

Hoarseness. Hoarseness is also common but may be absent in ventral or more superficial lesions.[437] Ipsilateral stuffy nose, altered taste, and dysarthria are less common.

Headache. Moderate or severe headache is common in lateral medullary infarction and is related either to involvement of the descending spinal tract of the fifth cranial nerve and its nucleus or to vascular distension produced by the occlusive process within the vertebral artery. This complaint was noticed as far back as 1836 in a report by Bright,[438] who called attention to posterior headache in vascular disease. He described a "gentleman past the meridian of life" who had apoplectic attacks and complained, "I feel completely knocked up and have much pain in the back of the head, like a rheumatic pain, generally at the same spot the right side of the back part of the head." Bright commented, "This pain would itself chiefly direct our suspicions to disease of the vertebral arteries."

Steady or, less commonly, pulsatile headaches are located most often in the occipital region and are unilateral in about half of cases.[420]

Signs

The signs accompanying lateral medullary infarction have been extensively reviewed.[425,434,436,437,439,440] This discussion is confined to a review of the seven main signs.

Diminished sensation in the ipsilateral face. Involvement of the descending tract of the fifth cranial nerve and its nucleus usually produces decreased pain and temperature sensation of the ipsilateral face. Almost invariably, the corneal reflex is lost or severely reduced. The forehead and rest of the ophthalmic division are more analgesic than the lower face. Pain and cold sensitivities are generally affected equally. At times, although single pinpricks feel less sharp and less discrete, there may be a dysesthetic quality, with spreading and persistence of the perceived stimulus. When the ipsilateral face is severely analgesic, the lower border does not usually conform to the limits of the peripheral mandibular division of the fifth cranial nerve but can be portrayed as a gentle curve sloping downward and medially from the tragus to the mandible, where the facial artery lies.[434] Touch may also be diminished in the analgesic face.[437] The sensory defect in the face usually clears more quickly than that on the contralateral body, although the loss of corneal reflex usually persists.[437]

Diminished pain and temperature sensation on the contralateral body. Ischemia of the lateral spinothalamic tract is responsible for diminished pain and temperature sensation on the side of the body contralateral to the infarct. The fibers within the spinothalamic tract are laminated, and the sacral fibers are most lateral and the arm is more medial. The arm and upper neck and trunk are spared in more superficial lesions. When the lesion extends far medially, it may even involve the quintothalamic fibers, which have already crossed to join the medial border of the spinothalamic tract, producing a complete contralateral hemianalgesia including the contralateral face.

In patients with bilateral facial analgesia, the pin feels different on the two sides of the face, in that the loss is more severe on the side of the infarction. Without very careful testing, the contralateral face could be assessed as normal unless the pin sensibility here is compared with that in the normal ipsilateral arm or trunk.

With time, the hemianalgesia frequently improves, and a pain–numbness level may become apparent over the trunk.[441] Less often, the analgesia clears both rostrally and caudally, leaving a band of altered sensibility on the trunk.[436] Although at onset the loss of pain and temperature sensibility tends to be homogeneous over affected areas, greater degrees of sensibility appear later; however, patches of perverted sensation remain. The analgesia usually extends to the midline at onset, but the paramedian region of the body often clears more in the front than in the back.[437]

At times, the loss of pain and temperature can be entirely crossed, occurring in the face, arm, trunk, and leg contralateral to the infarct. The lesions that cause this unilateral pattern of sensory loss are located more medially and involve the crossing fibers in the ventral trigeminal thalamic tract and the fibers in the crossed lateral spinothalamic tract. At times, the discomfort is severe and is comparable to thalamic pain, with which it probably shares a common mechanism. Rubbing of the involved part, the pressure of tight clothing, or excessive heat or cold may aggravate the discomfort. When pain makes a delayed appearance on the contralateral side of the body, the pain generally persists and is relatively resistant to pharmacologic treatments.[437]

Horner's syndrome. Sympathetic nervous system fibers course through the lateral reticular substance and are involved in most cases of lateral medullary infarction,[68] resulting in ipsilateral Horner's syndrome. Usually, the syndrome is incomplete; ptosis is the most common element and leads to drooping of the upper eyelid and some elevation of the lower lid, which narrows the palpebral fissure. Miosis is also very common, but the pupil usually retains its reactivity to light. Anhidrosis is the least common element of the Horner's syndrome in lateral medullary infarction.

Ataxia. Gait ataxia and limb ataxia are very important signs of lateral brainstem infarction and are due to ischemia of the restiform body or to associated infarction of the inferior cerebellum in the territory of the PICA. The gait ataxia seen in the lateral medullary syndrome is different from that seen with the vermal degeneration of alcoholism. Leaning, veering, falling, or toppling to the side when the patient is placed in an erect or sitting position is characteristic of medullary infarction and can be contrasted with the wide-based gait with truncal titubation seen in vermal lesions. The ipsilateral limbs are often called "weak" by the patient, and examination reveals striking rebound and finger-to-nose ataxia. The most sensitive test to elicit the cerebellar limb abnormality is to have the patient quickly lift or drop the arms and brake them suddenly; the affected limb overshoots.

When the cerebellum is infarcted, a posterior fossa pressure cone can develop and may lead to death unless medical or surgical decompression is instituted. The presence of cerebellar infarction thus alters the management and prognosis.

Nystagmus. The vestibular nuclei and their connections are affected in the lateral tegmentum and very frequently lead to nystagmus. The nystagmus is horizontal and frequently rotatory[67,425]; the quick component of the rotation usually moves the upper border of the iris toward the side of the lesion.[425] Vertical nystagmus is seldom if ever seen with ischemic lesions in the lateral medulla.[67] The eyes frequently drift away from the side of the lesion; small-amplitude, quick nystagmus is present on voluntary gaze to the contralateral side, and coarser, larger amplitude but slower nystagmus is present on ipsilateral gaze. In some cases, this pattern is reversed, with coarser horizontal nystagmus to the other side. The directional preponderance of nystagmus probably depends on the rostrocaudal location of the lesion.[442]

The nystagmus may even be torsional,[442] bearing away from the lesion side. Most often, lateral gaze is characterized by hypermetric saccades to the side of the lesion and hypometric saccades to the opposite side.[440] At times the eyes are forcibly deviated to the side of the lesion: so-called ocular lateropulsion.[443-445] Reflex and voluntary eye movements are full, but at rest the eyes may be deviated far to the side, closely mimicking conjugate eye deviation from a hemispheric lesion.[444]

Skewing and slight dysconjugacy (the abducting eye lagging on gaze to the ipsilateral side) may explain the patient's complaints of diplopia. Diplopia is relieved in some patients by tilting the head to the side of the lesion.[440,442,446-449]

Paralysis of the ipsilateral vocal cord and weakness of the ipsilateral palate. Involvement of the nucleus ambiguus is responsible for paralysis of the ipsilateral vocal cord and weakness of the ipsilateral palate. These signs are frequently absent in more superficial lesions that do not extend far medially. Unexplained tachycardia has accompanied lateral medullary infarction and could be due to involvement of vagal fibers arising from the dorsal motor nucleus of the vagus.

Slight weakness of the ipsilateral face. Although a common occurrence, a slight weakness of the ipsilateral face is difficult to explain because the lesion is below the facial nucleus. Dejerine and Roussy[450] commented on an aberrant corticobulbar tract that coursed dorsal to the other corticospinal and corticobulbar fibers and looped a bit caudally before traveling rostrally toward the facial nucleus. Kim et al[427] found a prominent contrast between rostral and caudal lateral medullary infarcts. In this series, patients with rostral lateral medullary infarcts invariably had dysphagia and hoarseness, and although vertigo and ataxia were common, nystagmus was not prominent. By contrast, patients with caudal lateral medullary infarcts had severe vertigo and gait ataxia but not dysphagia or hoarseness. Rostral medullary lesions tended to extend more deeply and involve the nucleus ambiguus, whereas caudal medullary lesions were more superficial.

Prognosis

Contralateral hemiparesis and Babinski's sign are not components of the lateral medullary syndrome; their presence indicates a wider zone of ischemia and, possibly, a more serious prognosis. In the patient with a pure lateral medullary syndrome, the prognosis is usually quite good.[451] However, death may ensue from cerebellar infarction with development of a *posterior fossa pressure cone,* as described earlier. Some patients with lateral medullary infarction do die unexpectedly without an obvious explanation, that is, either cerebellar infarct or a more extensive occlusion or ischemia.[67]

In 1991, Norrving and Cronqvist[422] reported a study of prognosis in 43 patients with lateral medullary infarcts whose data were collected as part of a population-based stroke registry in Lund, Sweden. During a 6-year period, 43 patients with lateral medullary infarcts were registered, representing 1.9% of all admissions for acute stroke during that period. Four patients died during the acute stroke, two from nocturnal apnea, one from an acute myocardial infarct, and one from myocardial infarction, pulmonary embolism, and aspiration pneumonia. Three other patients also had aspiration pneumonia. In two patients, new medullary infarcts occurred during the 2 weeks after the lateral medullary infarct; one was a medial medullary infarct that appeared during hypotension (the patient died 3 weeks later), and the other was an ipsilateral hemiparesis possibly from caudal spreading of the lateral medullary infarct. During follow-up, one patient with a VA occlusion experienced a medial medullary infarct, and one patient with severe bilateral VA occlusive disease with extension of thrombus into the BA had a fatal progressive brainstem infarct. Five patients, four of whom were known to have VA occlusions and one of whom had not been studied by angiography, had posterior circulation TIAs during follow-up. Two patients died of myocardial infarcts. The researchers concluded that prognosis depended heavily on the nature of the underlying vascular lesions and the coexistence of coronary artery disease.[422]

Bilateral lesions are the usual setting,[453,454] although rare instances of unilateral medullary infarcts have been reported. Levin and Margolis described a single patient with *failure of automatic respiration (Ondine's curse)*.[267,452]

Patients with lateral medullary infarcts may worsen because of *extension of ischemia*. One cause is distal embolization of thrombus from the VA to the top of the BA.[67] Embolization or thrombus extension occurs early in the course (<7 days) and is very rare after 2 weeks.

Transcranial MR images of the brainstem often define the location of lateral medullary infarcts; MRI is far superior to CT in sensitivity for detection of these lesions.[423,424,427,455]

Hemimedullary Infarction (Elements of Medial and Lateral Ischemia)

Although the lateral medulla and inferior cerebellum are the most common sites of infarction in patients with occlusion of a single intracranial VA, ischemia may extend more rostrally to affect the inferolateral pons.[67,456] Such extension involves the pyramidal tract; fifth, sixth, and seventh cranial nerves; and motor dysfunction of the fifth cranial nerve in the territory of the inferolateral pontine artery. This branch, usually from the AICA, may arise from the very proximal BA.[66,71] When infarction extends to the medial medulla as well as the lateral tegmentum,[67,68,456] it may cause the hemiparesis or Babinski's sign in the Babinski-Nageotte syndrome.[258,457,458] Paramedian arteries supplying the medial medullary territory arise from the anterior spinal arteries, which are branches of the V4 segments of the VAs.[66,68,458] Transient hemiparesis occurring in VA occlusion is presumably due to decreased flow in the medial medullary branches or to rostral brainstem ischemia.

The hemiparesis is usually contralateral to the infarct and on the same side as the body and limb pain and temperature loss. The anatomic basis for the hemiparesis is infarction of the medullary pyramid, a region supplied by the anterior spinal artery.[458,459] Occasionally, the hemiparesis is ipsilateral to the infarct, on the side of the cerebellar signs, and contralateral to pain loss,[460] but in at least one fatal case it was bilateral, with quadriplegia.

Medial Medullary Infarction

Each VA usually gives rise to one or several small paramedian anterior spinal branches, which join to form the anterior spinal artery. This disposition usually prevents spinal cord or medial medullary infarction in cases of unilateral VA occlusion.[66,68] Occasionally, however, unilateral occlusion of one anterior spinal branch can give rise to a paramedian medullary infarction involving the pyramid, medial lemniscus, and, at times, the hypoglossal nerve or nucleus.[68] Although the supply of anterior spinal branches is well-known and lesions are frequently postulated, documented occlusion of these vessels is extremely rare.[461-463]

Embolic occlusion of the anterior spinal artery territory may be more common than is currently recognized. MRI documentation of unilateral medial medullary infarction[464] and bilateral medial medullary infarcts[465,466] during life has been reported. Kase et al[467] described a 23-year-old woman with sudden-onset fibrocartilaginous disk embolization to the anterior spinal artery branches of the VAs, causing bilateral medial medullary and rostral spinal cord infarction. It is of interest that even though the most rostral level of infarction was below the pontomedullary junction, the patient had bilateral facial weakness, vertical nystagmus, and ocular bobbing in addition to a flaccid quadriplegia.

Flaccid or spastic quadriparesis and impaired control of respiration have been the most consistent clinical findings in patients with bilateral medial medullary infarcts.[465-471]

Transient Ischemic Attacks or No Deficit

As in the case of occlusive disease of other major vessels, some patients have an ICVA occlusion without permanent deficit. On some occasions, the occlusion may be totally silent or may produce only an occipital headache. The most common transient symptom is dizziness or vertigo (Fig. 26-22).

Extracranial Vertebral Artery Occlusive Disease

The ECVA is a common site of *atheromatous disease* and also exhibits an unusually high rate of congenital variability (i.e., asymmetry, small size, residual embryologic anastomosis, and termination in the PICA).[103,108,112,472]

Despite the high incidence of disease, serious brainstem or posterior circulation strokes have only rarely been caused by occlusive disease limited to an ECVA. During the 19th century, Alexander[473] treated epilepsy with apparent impunity by placing a ligature on the VA. Surgeons have ligated the VA as a treatment for subclavian steal, eliminating the siphonage through this vessel. Fisher[474] reported in detail five patients in whom bilateral occlusions of the proximal vertebral system could be demonstrated angiographically. All patients had transient ischemic episodes, but in only one was there a persisting

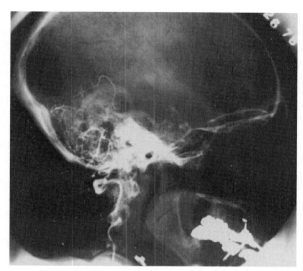

Figure 26-22 Vertebral angiogram. The vertebral artery does not fill past the posterior inferior cerebellar artery branch, and superior cerebellar artery branches fill from the posteroinferior cerebellar artery.

neurologic deficit; that patient also had an occlusion of the ICA at the siphon on the appropriate side to explain the findings.

Extensive collateral circulation may develop, especially if the VA occlusion occurs gradually. The occipital branch of the external carotid artery is a prominent source of collateral supply, often filling the deep muscular branches of the VA near the atlas.[428,474] The ascending cervical and transverse cervical branches of the thyrocervical trunk originating from the SA may also fill the VA in its midcervical course. Compensatory flow from the contralateral VA and retrograde flow down the BA from the carotid-posterior communicating system is also commonly visualized. The most common transient symptoms are dizziness, faintness, blurred vision, and imbalance. Fisher,[474] who was the unsigned author of the alliterative *New England Journal of Medicine* editorial "Subclavian Steal" (see further on), has argued that occlusion of the proximal VA, like subclavian steal, is usually a benign syndrome rarely accompanied by serious brainstem infarction.

Embolism has become increasingly recognized[105]; some instances arise from tight stenosis[76] but also from a previously occluded ECVA.[65,262,274,282,431,432]

Traumatic occlusions within the nuchal VA are clearly not as benign (see Chapter 33, Arterial Dissections).

There are still only a few systematic studies of the incidence of symptoms and signs and prognosis in untreated patients with occlusive disease of the proximal VAs. Headache and "cerebellovestibular" symptoms appear common,[475-477] and some have no neurovascular symptoms.[478]

Bilateral Vertebral Artery Occlusion

Occlusion of the *origins* of the VAs, even when bilateral, can be surprisingly well tolerated because of the potential plethora of available collateral vessels that may supply the more rostral cervical VAs and ICVAs. *Intracranial occlusion* of both VAs, by contrast, generally is poorly tolerated

by the patient and usually leads to severe cerebellar and brainstem infarction.[454,479] Few examples of bilateral ICVA occlusion have been reported in clinical detail. Roski et al[480] reviewed patients treated with occipital artery–PICA bypass, including six patients with bilateral ICVA occlusion. Three of these patients had only TIAs, one had a stroke, and two had both TIAs and strokes. Cerebellar, limb, and gait abnormalities were present in four patients, one had nystagmus, and one had normal neurologic findings. Bogousslavsky et al[481] monitored 10 patients with bilateral ICVA occlusions and reported a more benign prognosis. Four patients presented with TIAs only, four had nondevastating strokes, and only two had severe brainstem infarcts. During follow-up, no severe brainstem strokes occurred, and only one patient died of brainstem infarction.

In a clinicopathologic series of 64 patients with cerebellar infarction, five had bilateral ICVA occlusion.[71,127,389] Bilateral distal VA occlusion is usually considered rare; only one patient in a series of 115 consecutive patients with cerebellar infarction had this lesion.[128] The full neurologic deficit in this condition develops over a longer period than in BA occlusion, branch disease, lacunes, or embolic infarction. The principal pathogenesis of posterior circulation ischemia in this condition is inferred to represent chronically reduced vertebrobasilar perfusion.[482]

Several series have been published indicating improvement after bypass surgery.[480,483-485] The prognosis of bilateral ICVA occlusion is variable. Some patients, in whom adequate collateral circulation develops, survive without major subsequent infarction.[481] In others, ischemia progresses, and the prognosis is grave.

Subclavian-Innominate Artery Disease and Subclavian Steal

In a 1961 issue of the *New England Journal of Medicine*, Reivich et al[486] reported their observations of two patients with TIAs referable to the posterior circulation. Each patient had diminished pulse and blood pressure in the left arm. Attacks were precipitated by exercise in one patient and by change of head posture in the other. Angiography in each case revealed stenosis of the SA proximal to the origin of the left VA. In one patient, the left ICA was also occluded. Blood flowed from the normal right VA into the cranium and then down the left VA in a retrograde fashion and filled the distal left SA. These investigators then performed experiments in which they occluded the left SA of dogs and measured blood flow in the other great vessels. In this artificially induced situation, they documented a compensatory increase in flow through the right VA. In an editorial in the same issue (unsigned, as was the custom at the time), Fisher[487] coined the term *subclavian steal* to refer to the siphoning of blood away from its proper cranial destination toward the ischemic arm.

Within the next few years, angiography in similar groups of patients documented reversal of flow in the VA due to SA occlusive disease and showed that the phenomenon was not rare.[487-493] In the 50 years since the original report, a clearer definition of the clinical findings has been established and, with it, a lessening of the role of surgery. Patients with subsequently verified subclavian steal may be seen with one of several types of symptoms: (1) headache, (2) intermittent episodes of cerebral ischemia, or (3) claudication or pain in the ischemic arm. However, many are entirely asymptomatic from the subclavian lesion, as was the case in fully 74% of the 155 lesions evaluated by Hennerici et al.[494]

The usual slow development of the occlusion and the richness of collateral supply tend to make upper extremity ischemia a relatively minor problem unless the patient exercises the arm frequently, as has been the case in some noted golfers and baseball pitchers.[343,494-496]

Cerebral symptoms are common but usually transient, lasting seconds to minutes but often recurring over months or even years.[491,493] The source of the symptoms is difficult to discover.[486,491]

The most common cause of subclavian occlusive disease is atherosclerosis, although congenital lesions such as preductal coarctation of the aorta with patent ductus arteriosus,[274] atresia of the left SA,[497] and a pseudocoarctation of the aorta with kinked left SA[137] occasionally produce the syndrome. Sometimes, subclavian steal follows surgical manipulation of the SA, as in the Blalock-Taussig procedure for tetralogy of Fallot, in which the SA is anastomosed to the pulmonary artery. Traumatic injury, embolism, and arteritis (temporal arteritis and Takayasu's arteritis) may also cause subclavian steal. In the large series reported by North et al,[491] the left SA was affected alone in 33 cases, the right subclavian or innominate artery was affected in 13 cases, and 13 cases were bilateral.

The left SA is involved approximately three times more frequently than the right innominate or subclavian artery.[498] Stenosis or occlusion of the innominate artery is less common than SA disease.[499]

At one time innominate and SA occlusive disease was the province of angiography, but noninvasive testing now accurately documents it with a high degree of reliability.[42-44,46,48] Provocative tests such as decreasing peripheral resistance in the upper arm could cause temporary BA flow reversal, which can be insonated by TCD ultrasonography.[47,86]

Mobile Thrombus in the Aortic Arch

See Chapter 38 for a full discussion of this disorder.

Multiple Infarcts in the Posterior Circulation

BA occlusion often accompanies ICVA occlusion either on one or on both sides; PICA, AICA, SCA, or PCA occlusion is due to blockage of their origin by the occlusive thrombus in the parental artery or is due to artery-to-artery embolism. Patients with occlusion of the ICVAs and BA and patients with large emboli often have infarcts in multiple cerebellar artery territories. Penetrator branches at various levels (i.e., pontine, midbrain, or thalamosubthalamic level) may also be occluded. Massive multiple infarction may occur when there is no collateral anastomosis involving mainly the cerebellum, ventromedial

pons and midbrain, thalamus, and occipitotemporal lobes.[128,370,376,389] Embolism and thrombosis account for the middle + territory infarcts (i.e., proximal + middle, middle + distal, or proximal + middle + distal). Embolism is the predominant stroke mechanism for the proximal and distal territory cerebellar infarction (proximal + distal group). For this latter group, the infarcts are usually limited to the PICA and SCA cerebellum. The vascular lesion, when present, is usually on the side of the PICA territory infarct because the ECVA and ICVA supply only the ipsilateral PICA but can be the source of embolism to both SCA territories.

Unlike in the proximal + distal territory group, the most common cause for middle territory infarction is large artery intracranial occlusive disease. Embolism is a less common cause.

BA lesions are more often due to in situ occlusive disease of the BA itself or to propagation of thrombus from the ICVA. ICVA occlusive disease and BA occlusive disease often coexist.

Low-Flow States with Resultant Borderzone Ischemia in the Posterior Circulation

Occlusion of a blood vessel, whether due to in situ thrombosis or embolus, results in a region of infarction, usually within the center of distribution of that vessel. Collateral circulation is apt to supply the more peripheral zones and thus limit the centrifugal extent of the infarct. When, however, flow is diffusely diminished, for example, during shock due to blood loss or cardiogenic hypotension, the distribution of ischemia more often straddles the borderzone regions between major blood vessels.[500-505] Few examples of necropsy-confirmed posterior circulation borderzone infarction have been reported.[15,503] Reports of borderzone infarction in the posterior circulation mainly focused on borderzone ischemia in the cerebellum, and few reports concentrated on borderzone ischemia within the brainstem. Although claimed as a cause,[15,245,260,348,502] hypotension as the mechanism of borderzone ischemia in the cerebellum is probably uncommon, depending on underlying conditions with preexisting bilateral severe occlusive disease of VAs or occlusion of basilar arteries without refilling via the posterior communicating arteries because the P1 segments are hypoplastic; most cerebellar borderzone infarcts are due to cardiac or artery-to-artery embolism (Figs. 26-23 through 26-25).

Migraine

In 1961, Bickerstaff[506] reported a distinct symptom complex occurring in adolescent girls that consisted of repeated episodes of altered vision, vertigo, ataxia, dysarthria, and numbness and tingling of the limbs and sometimes face, followed by headache. The common family history of migraine and clearing of ischemic symptoms by the time the headache began stamped the disorder as migrainous for Bickerstaff, who called this disorder *basilar artery migraine*. Swanson and Vick[507] have corroborated the existence of this syndrome, noted its occasional onset in adult life, and described an occasional familial tendency.[508]

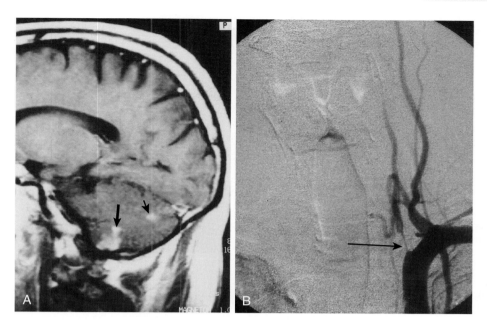

Figure 26-23 A and B, Cerebellar borderzone infarcts *(arrows)* and tight stenosis of the left vertebral artery. (The right vertebral artery was severely hypoplastic.)

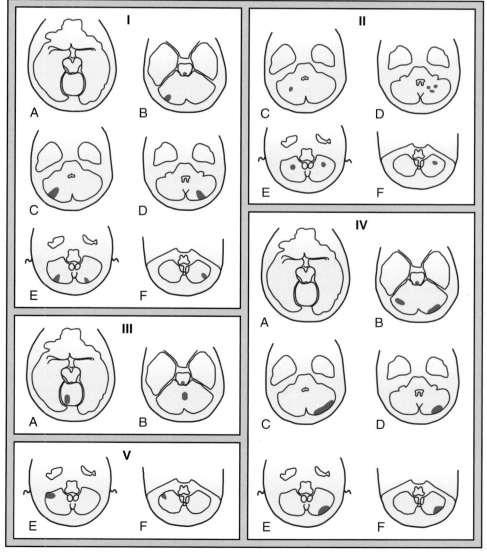

Figure 26-24 Pattern of distribution of cerebellar borderzone infarcts.

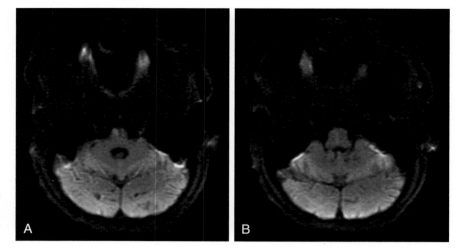

Figure 26-25 A 76-year-old man with brief episode of ataxia and arm weakness; syndrome resolved within days. Medullary pyramid DWI+.

The term *basilar artery migraine* is perhaps redundant because it has long been known, but not understood, that migraine tends to involve the BA and its branches. Visual scintillations are the most common accompaniments of migraine and are occipital (PCA) in origin. Examples of transient global amnesia are known in migraine, and the pathologic anatomy and physiology of memory suggest a dominant PCA localization.[509] Physiologic studies using xenon-133 have documented oligemia as an early finding or as occurring subsequent to focal hyperemia.[510,511] Blood flow changes are maximal in the occipitoparietal regions.[512] In addition, angiography performed during the prodromal phase of migraine has demonstrated filling of the PCA from carotid injection, suggesting low pressure in the basilar system. Any of these patients might fall within the usually accepted nosology of migraine.[509] Caplan[358] reviewed his experience with patients who had migraine (classic or common) and posterior circulation ischemic attacks and strokes and underwent angiography. Nine patients were presented. Men and women of widely varying ages were included. The clinical patterns involved just TIAs, single strokes, single stroke followed by attacks, and multiple strokes. In some patients, classic migraine developed only months or years later. CT and MRI confirmed infarctions in patients who had strokes with persistent neurologic deficits (seven of nine patients).[358] Angiography showed BA occlusions, severe diffuse narrowing of vertebrobasilar arteries (rather persistent in one patient), or normal posterior circulation vessels. The mechanism of infarction was not elucidated, but clearly, vasoconstriction, which was often protracted, and BA occlusion did occur. Caplan[358] posited that ischemia was due to protracted vasoconstriction or to vascular thrombosis precipitated by activation of platelet adhesion and agglutination and activation of the intrinsic and extrinsic coagulation pathways.

REFERENCES

1. Duret H: Recherches anatomiques sur la circulation de l'encéphale, *Arch Physiol Norm Pathol* 3:60, 1874.
2. Duret H: Sur la distribution des artères nourricières du bulbe rachidien, *Arch Physiol Norm Pathol* 2:97, 1873.
3. Hayem G: Sur la thrombose par artérite du tronc basilaire comme cause de mort rapide, *Arch Physiol Norm Pathol* 1:270, 1868.
4. Leyden E: Uber die Thrombose der basilar Arterie, *Z Klin Med* 5:165, 1882.
5. Marburg O: Uber die neuren Fortschritte in der topischen Diagnostic du Pons und Oblongata, *Dtsch Z Nervenheilkd* 41:41, 1911.
6. Pines L, Gilinsky E: Uber die Thrombose der Arteria basilaris und uber die Vascularization de Brucke, *Arch Psychiatr Nervenkr* 26:380, 1932.
7. Stopford J: The arteries of the pons and medulla oblongata. I, *J Anat Physiol* 50:131, 1915.
8. Stopford J: The arteries of the pons and medulla oblongata. II, *J Anat Physiol* 50:255, 1916.
9. Caplan LR: Charles Foix: The first modern stroke neurologist, *Stroke* 21:348, 1990.
10. Foix C, Hillemand P: Contribution à l'étude des ramollissements protubérantiels, *Rev Med* 43:287, 1926.
11. Foix C, Hillemand P: Les artères de l'axe encéphalique jusqu'au diencéphale inclusivement, *Rev Neurol* 32:705, 1925.
12. Lhermitte J, Trelles JO: L'artério-sclérose du tronc basilaire et ses conséquences anatomo-cliniques, *Jahrbücher Psychiatr Neurol* 51:91, 1934.
13. Kubik C, Adams R: Occlusion of the basilar artery: A clinical and pathologic study, *Brain* 69:73, 1946.
14. Fisher CM: Occlusion of the internal carotid artery, *Arch Neurol Psychiatry* 65:345, 1951.
15. Hutchinson E, Yates P: Carotico-vertebral stenosis, *Lancet* 269:2, 1957.
16. Meyer JS, Sheehan S, Bauer R: An arteriographic study of cerebrovascular disease in man: Stenosis and occlusion of the vertebral basilar arterial system, *Arch Neurol* 2:27, 1960.
17. Williams D: The syndromes of basilar insufficiency. In Garland H, editor: *Scientific aspects of neurology*, Baltimore, 1961, Williams & Wilkins, pp 202.
18. Williams D, Wilson T: The diagnosis of the major and minor syndromes of basilar insufficiency, *Brain* 85:741, 1962.
19. Denny-Brown D: Basilar artery syndromes, *Bull N Engl Med Cent* 15:53, 1953.
20. Fang H, Palmer J: Vascular phenomena involving brainstem structures, *Neurology (NY)* 6:402, 1956.
21. Millikan C, Siekert R: Studies in cerebrovascular disease: The syndrome of intermittent insufficiency of the basilar arterial system, *Proc Staff Meet Mayo Clin* 30:61, 1955.
22. Wolf J: *The classical brainstem syndromes*, Springfield, Ill, 1971, Charles C Thomas.
23. Denny-Brown D: Recurrent cerebrovascular episodes, *Arch Neurol* 2:194, 1960.
24. Millikan C, Siekert R, Shick R: Studies in cerebrovascular disease: The use of anticoagulant drugs in the treatment of insufficiency or thrombosis within the basilar arterial system, *Proc Staff Meet Mayo Clin* 30:116, 1955.
25. Millikan C, Siekert R, Whisnant J: Anticoagulant therapy in cerebrovascular disease: Current status, *JAMA* 166:587, 1958.
26. Browne T, Poskanzer D: Treatment of strokes, *N Engl J Med* 281:594, 1969.

27. Ausman JI, Diaz FG, Pearce JE, et al: Endarterectomy of the vertebral artery from C-2 to posterior inferior cerebellar artery intracranially, *Surg Neurol* 18:400, 1982.

28. Khodadad G, Singh R, Olinger C: Possible prevention of brainstem stroke by microvascular anastomosis in the vertebrobasilar system, *Stroke* 8:316, 1977.

29. Sundt T, Whisnant J, Piepgras D, et al: Intracranial bypass grafts for vertebral basilar ischemia, *Mayo Clin Proc* 53:12, 1978.

30. Imparato A, Riles T, Kim G: Cervical vertebral artery angioplasty for brainstem ischemia, *Surgery* 90:842, 1981.

31. McNamara J, Heyman A, Silver D, et al: The value of carotid endarterectomy in treating transient cerebral ischemia of the posterior circulation, *Neurology (NY)* 27:682, 1977.

32. Sundt T, Smith H, Campbell J, et al: Transluminal angioplasty for basilar artery stenosis, *Mayo Clin Proc* 55:673, 1980.

33. Hacke W, Zeumer H, Ferbert A, et al: Intra-arterial thrombolytic therapy improves outcome in patients with acute vertebrobasilar occlusive disease, *Stroke* 19:1216, 1988.

34. Pessin MS, del Zoppo GJ, Estol C: Thrombolytic agents in the treatment of stroke, *Clin Neuropharmacol* 13:271, 1990.

35. Zeumer H: Vascular recanalizing technique in interventional neuroradiology, *J Neurol* 231:287, 1985.

36. Zeumer H, Hacke W, Ringelstein EB: Local intraarterial thrombolysis in vertebrobasilar thromboembolic disease, *AJNR Am J Neuroradiol* 4:401, 1983.

37. Biller J, Yuh W, Mitchell GW: Early diagnosis of basilar artery occlusion using magnetic resonance imaging, *Stroke* 19:297, 1988.

38. Kistler JP, Buonnano FS, DeWitt LD, et al: Vertebral-basilar posterior cerebral territory stroke: Delineation by proton nuclear magnetic resonance imaging, *Stroke* 15:417, 1984.

39. Simmons Z, Biller J, Adams HP, et al: Cerebellar infarction: Comparison of computed tomography and magnetic resonance imaging, *Ann Neurol* 19:291, 1986.

40. Ackerstaff RG, Hoenefeld H, Slowikowski JM, et al: Ultrasonic duplex scanning in atherosclerotic disease of the innominate, subclavian and vertebral arteries: A comparative study with angiography, *Ultrasound Med Biol* 10:409, 1984.

41. Bluth EL, Merritt CR, Sullivan MA, et al: Usefulness of duplex ultrasound in evaluating vertebral arteries, *J Ultrasound Med* 8:229, 1989.

42. Ekestrom S, Eklund B, Liljequist L, et al: Noninvasive methods in the evaluation of obliterative disease of the subclavian or innominate artery, *Acta Med Scand* 206:467, 1979.

43. Hennerici M, Rautenberg W, Schwartz A: Transcranial Doppler ultrasound for the assessment of intracranial arterial flow velocity. II: Evaluation of intracranial arterial disease, *Surg Neurol* 27:523, 1987.

44. Liljequist L, Ekerstrom S, Nordhus O: Monitoring direction of vertebral artery blood flow by Doppler shift ultrasound in patients with suspected subclavian steal, *Acta Chir Scand* 147:421, 1981.

45. Touboul PJ, Bousser MG, Laplane D, et al: Duplex scanning of normal vertebral arteries, *Stroke* 17:97, 1986.

46. von Reutern GM, Budingen JH: *Ultraschalldiagnostik der Hirnversorgenden Arterien*, Stuttgart, 1989, Thieme.

47. Caplan LR, Brass LM, DeWitt LD, et al: Transcranial Doppler ultrasound: Present status, *Neurology (NY)* 40:696, 1990.

48. Hennerici M, Rautenberg W, Sitzer G, et al: Transcranial Doppler ultrasound for the assessment of intracranial arterial flow velocity. I: Examination of technique and normal values, *Surg Neurol* 27:439, 1987.

49. Tettenborn B, Estol C, DeWitt LD, et al: Accuracy of transcranial Doppler in the vertebrobasilar circulation, *J Neurol* 237:159, 1990.

50. Dumoulin CL, Hart HR: MR angiography, *Radiology* 161:717, 1986.

51. Edelman RR, Mattle HP, Atkinson DJ, et al: MR angiography, *AJR Am J Roentgenol* 154:937, 1990.

52. Zuccoli G, Guidetti D, Nicola F, et al: Carotid and vertebral artery dissection: Magnetic resonance findings in 15 cases, *Radiol Med* 104:466-471, 2002.

53. Caplan LR, Tettenborn B: *Embolism in the posterior circulation in vertebrobasilar disease*, St. Louis, 1991, Quality Medical Publishing, p 52.

54. Prognosis of patients with symptomatic vertebral or basilar artery stenosis: The Warfarin-Aspirin Symptomatic Intracranial Disease (WASID) Study Group, *Stroke* 29:1389, 1998.

55. Libman R, Benson R, Einberg K: Myasthenia mimicking vertebrobasilar stroke, *J Neurol* 249:1512, 2002.

56. Krayenbüll H, Yasargil M: Radiological anatomy and tomography of the cerebral arteries. In Vinken P, Bruyn G, editors: *Handbook of clinical neurology, vol. 2*, Amsterdam, 1972, North-Holland, pp 65.

57. Stephens R, Stilwell D: *Arteries and veins of the human brain*, Springfield, Ill, 1969, Charles C Thomas.

58. Takahashi S: *Atlas of vertebral angiography*, Baltimore, 1974, University Park Press.

59. Wilkinson I: The vertebral artery, *Arch Neurol* 27:392, 1972.

60. Lister J, Rhoton A, Matsushima T, et al: Microsurgical anatomy of the posterior inferior cerebellar artery, *Neurosurgery* 10:170, 1982.

61. Fankhauser H, Kamano S, Hanamura T, et al: Abnormal origin of the posterior inferior cerebellar artery, *J Neurosurg* 51:569, 1979.

62. Lasjaunias P, Guibert-Tranier F, Braun JP: The pharyngocerebellar artery or ascending pharyngeal artery origin of the posterior inferior cerebellar artery, *J Neuroradiol* 8:317, 1981.

63. Guillard A: Pathologie ischemique cérébrale et anomalie de terminaison intracrânienne de l'artère vertébrale, *Sem Hop Paris* 62:2755, 1986.

64. Margolis MT, Newton TH: The posterior inferior cerebellar artery. In Newton TH, Potts G, editors: *Radiology of the skull and brain: angiography*, vol 68, St. Louis, 1974, CV Mosby, pp 1710.

65. George B, Laurian C: Vertebro-basilar ischemia with thrombosis of the vertebral artery: Report of two cases with embolism, *J Neurol Neurosurg Psychiatry* 45:91, 1982.

66. Duvernoy HM: *Human brainstem vessels*, Heidelberg, 1978, Springer-Verlag.

67. Fisher CM, Karnes W, Kubik C: Lateral medullary infarction: The pattern of vascular occlusion, *J Neuropathol Exp Neurol* 20:323, 1961.

68. Hauw J-J, Der Agopian P, Trelles L, et al: Les infarctus bulbaires, *J Neurol Sci* 28:83, 1976.

69. Goodhart S, Davison C: Syndrome of the posterior inferior and anterior inferior cerebellar arteries and their branches, *Arch Neurol Psychiatry* 35:501, 1936.

70. Lazorthes G: *Vascularisation et Circulation Cérébrales*, Paris, 1961, Masson.

71. Amarenco P, Hauw J-J: Cerebellar infarction in the territory of the anterior and inferior cerebellar artery: A clinicopathological study of 20 cases, *Brain* 113:139, 1990.

72. Amarenco P, Hauw J-J, Caplan LR: Cerebellar infarctions. In Lechtenberg R, editor: *Handbook of cerebellar diseases*, New York, 1993, Marcel Dekker, pp 251.

73. Taveras JM, Wood EH: *Diagnostic neuroradiology, vol. II*, Baltimore, 1976, Williams & Wilkins, p 783.

74. Greitz T, Sjögren S: The posterior inferior cerebellar artery, *Acta Radiol* 1:284, 1963.

75. Amarenco P, Hauw J-J: Anatomie des artères cérébelleuses, *Rev Neurol* 145:267, 1989.

76. Castaigne P, Lhermitte F, Gautier J-C, et al: Arterial occlusions in the vertebral-basilar system, *Brain* 96:133, 1973.

77. Foix C, Hillemand P: Irrigation de la protubérance, *C R Soc Biol Paris* 42:35, 1925.

78. Gillian L: The correlation of the blood supply to the human brainstem with brainstem lesions, *J Neuropathol Exp Neurol* 23:78, 1964.

79. Gillian L: Anatomy and embryology of the arterial system of the brainstem and cerebellum. In Vinken P, Bruyn G, editors: *Handbook of clinical neurology*, vol 2, Amsterdam, 1972, North-Holland, pp 24.

80. Szdzuy D, Lehman R: Hypoplastic distal part of the basilar artery, *Neuroradiology* 4:118, 1972.

81. Hommel M, Besson G, Pollak P, et al: Hemiplegia in posterior cerebral artery occlusion, *Neurology (NY)* 40:1496, 1990.

82. Caplan LR: Vertebrobasilar system syndromes. In Vinken PJ, Bruyn GW, Klawans HL, editors: *Handbook of clinical neurology*, Amsterdam, 1988, North-Holland, pp 371.

83. Graff-Radford NR, Damasio H, Yamada T, et al: Non-haemorrhagic thalamic infarction, *Brain* 108:495, 1985.

84. Hopkins LN, Martin NA, Hadley MN, et al: Vertebrobasilar insufficiency. II: Microsurgical treatment of intracranial vertebrobasilar disease, *J Neurosurg* 66:662, 1987.

85. Percheron GMJ: *Etude anatomique du thalamus de l'homme adulte et de sa vascularisation artérielle*, Paris, 1966, Thesis.

86. von Cramm D, Hebel N, Schieri U: A contribution to the anatomical basis of thalamic amnesia, *Brain* 108:993, 1985.

87. Castaigne P, Lhermitte F, Buge A, et al: Paramedian thalamic and midbrain infarcts: clinical and neuropathological study, *Ann Neurol* 10:127, 1981.

88. Percheron G: Les artères du thalamus humain, *Rev Neurol (Paris)* 132:297, 1976.

89. Bogousslavsky J, Regli F, Assal G: The syndrome of unilateral tuberothalamic artery territory infarction, *Stroke* 17:434, 1986.

90. Chase T, Moretti L, Prensky A: Clinical and electro-encephalographic manifestations of vascular lesions of the pons, *Neurology (NY)* 18:357, 1968.

91. Caplan LR, DeWitt LD, Pessin MS, et al: Lateral thalamic infarcts, *Arch Neurol* 45:959, 1988.

92. Lie T: Congenital malformations of the carotid and vertebral arterial systems, including the persistent anastomoses. In Vinken P, Bruyn G, editors: *Handbook of clinical neurology,* vol 2, Amsterdam, 1972, North-Holland, pp 289.

93. Kingsley D, Radue E, DuBoulay E: Evaluation of computed tomography in vascular lesions of the vertebrobasilar territory, *J Neurol Neurosurg Psychiatry* 43:193, 1980.

94. Pinkerton J, Davidson K, Hibbard B: Primitive hypoglossal artery and carotid endarterectomy, *Stroke* 6:658, 1980.

95. Obayashi T, Furuse M: The proatlantal intersegmental artery, *Arch Neurol* 37:387, 1980.

96. Parkinson D, Reddy V, Ross R: Congenital anastomosis between the vertebral artery and internal carotid artery in the neck, *J Neurosurg* 51:697, 1979.

97. Asplund K, Wester P, Fodstad H, et al: Long time survival after vertebral/basilar occlusion, *Stroke* 11:304, 1980.

98. Bronstein AM, Morris J, DuBoulay G, et al: Abnormalities of horizontal gaze: Clinical, oculographic and magnetic resonance imaging findings. I: Abducens palsy, *J Neurol Neurosurg Psychiatry* 53:194, 1990.

99. Caplan LR: Lacunar infarction: A neglected concept, *Geriatrics* 3:71, 1976.

100. Cornhill J, Akins D, Hutson M, et al: Localization of atherosclerotic lesions in the human basilar artery, *Atherosclerosis* 35:77, 1980.

101. Echiverri HC, Rubino FA, Gupta SR, et al: Fusiform aneurysm of the vertebrobasilar arterial system, *Stroke* 20:1741, 1989.

102. Feigin I, Budzilovich G: The general pathology of cerebrovascular disease. In Vinken P, Bruyn G, editors: *Handbook of clinical neurology,* vol 2, Amsterdam, 1972, North-Holland, pp 128.

103. Schwartz C, Mitchell J: Atheroma of the carotid and vertebral arterial systems, *BMJ* 2:1057, 1961.

104. Fisher CM, Ojemann RG: A clinico-pathologic study of carotid endarterectomy plaques, *Rev Neurol (Paris)* 142:573, 1986.

105. Pelouze GA: Plaque ulcérée de l'ostium de l'artère vertébrale, *Rev Neurol* 145:478, 1989.

106. Caplan L, Baker R: Extracranial occlusive disease: Does size matter? *Stroke* 11:63, 1980.

107. Reznik M: Le ramollissement du tronc cérébral, *Acta Neurol Belg* 81:257, 1981.

108. Fisher C, Gore I, Okabe N, et al: Atherosclerosis of the carotid and vertebral arteries: Extracranial and intracranial, *J Neuropathol Exp Neurol* 24:455, 1965.

109. Amarenco P, Duyckarets C, Tzourio C, et al: The prevalence of ulcerated plaques in the aortic arch in patients with stroke, *N Engl J Med* 326:221, 1992.

110. Amarenco P, Hauw J-J, Gautier J-C: Arterial pathology in cerebellar infarction, *Stroke* 21:1299, 1990.

111. Escourolle R, Hauw J-J, Der Agopian P, et al: Les infarctus bulbaires, *J Neurol Sci* 28:103, 1976.

111a. DiTullio MR, Russo C, Jin Z, et al: Aortic arch plaques and risk of recurrent stroke and death, *Circulation* 119:2376–2382, 2009.

112. Moosy J: Morphology, sites and epidemiology of cerebral atherosclerosis, *Proc Assoc Res Nerv Ment Dis* 51:1, 1966.

113. Whisnant J, Martin M, Sayre G: Atherosclerotic stenosis of cervical arteries, *Arch Neurol* 5:429, 1961.

114. Fisher C: Some neuro-ophthalmological observations, *J Neurol Neurosurg Psychiatry* 30:383, 1967.

115. Fields WS: Collateral circulation in cerebrovascular disease. In Vinken P, Bruyn G, editors: *Handbook of clinical neurology,* vol 2, Amsterdam, 1972, North-Holland, pp 168.

116. Castaigne P, Buge A, Escourolle R, et al: Ramollissement pédonculaire médian, tégmentothalamique avec ophtalmoplégie et hypersomnie, *Rev Neurol* 106:357, 1962.

117. Caplan LR, Gorelick PB, Hier DB: Race, sex and occlusive cerebrovascular disease: A review, *Stroke* 17:648, 1986.

118. Tunick PA, Kronzon I: Protruding atherosclerotic plaque in the aortic arch of patients with systemic embolization: A new finding seen by transesophageal echocardiography, *Am Heart J* 120:658, 1990.

119. Bauer R, Sheehan S, Wechsler N, et al: Arteriographic study of sites, incidence and treatment of arteriosclerotic cerebrovascular lesions, *Neurology (NY)* 12:698, 1962.

120. Stein B, McCormick W, Rodriques J, et al: Incidence and significance of occlusive vascular disease of the extracranial arteries as documented by post-mortem angiography, *Trans Am Neurol Assoc* 86:60, 1961.

121. Ueda K, Toole J, McHenry L: Carotid and vertebrobasilar transient ischemia attacks: Clinical and angiographic correlation, *Neurology (NY)* 29:1094, 1979.

122. Thompson JR, Simmons C, Hasso A, et al: Occlusion of the intradural vertebrobasilar artery, *Neuroradiology* 14:219, 1978.

123. Feldmann E, Daneault N, Kwan E, et al: Chinese-white differences in the distribution of occlusive cerebrovascular disease, *Neurology (NY)* 40:1541, 1990.

124. Gorelick PB, Caplan LR, Hier DB, et al: Racial differences in the distribution of posterior circulation occlusive disease, *Stroke* 16:785, 1985.

125. Caplan LR: Intracranial branch atheromatous disease: A neglected, understudied and underused concept, *Neurology (NY)* 39:1246, 1989.

126. Amarenco P, Rosengart A, DeWitt LD, et al: Anterior inferior cerebellar artery territory infarcts: Mechanisms and clinical features, *Arch Neurol* 50:154, 1993.

127. Amarenco P, Hauw J-J: Cerebellar infarction in the territory of the superior cerebellar artery, *Neurology (NY)* 40:1383, 1990.

128. Amarenco P, Lévy C, Cohen A, et al: Causes and mechanisms of territorial and nonterritorial cerebellar infarcts in 115 consecutive cases, *Stroke* 25:105, 1994.

129. Fisher CM, Caplan L: Basilar artery branch occlusion: A cause of pontine infarction, *Neurology (NY)* 21:900, 1971.

130. Peress N, Kane WC, Aronson SM: Central nervous system findings in a tenth decade autopsy population, *Prog Brain Res* 40:473, 1973.

131. Fisher CM: Ataxic hemiparesis: A pathologic study, *Arch Neurol* 35:126, 1978.

132. Fisher CM: Cerebral ischemia: Less familiar types, *Clin Neurosurg* 18:267, 1971.

133. Fisher CM: The arterial lesions underlying lacunes, *Acta Neuropathol* 12:1, 1967.

134. Fisher CM: The vascular lesion in lacunae, *Trans Am Neurol Assoc* 90:243, 1965.

135. Fisher CM: Pathological observations in hypertensive cerebral hemorrhage, *J Neuropathol Exp Neurol* 30:536, 1971.

136. Bull J: Contribution of radiology to the study of intracranial aneurysms, *BMJ* 2:1701, 1962.

137. Lochaya S, Kaplan B, Shaffer AB: Pseudocoarctation of the aorta with bicuspid aortic valve and kinked left subclavian artery, a possible cause of subclavian steal, *Am Heart J* 73:369, 1967.

138. Auerbach S, De Piero T, Romanul F: Sylvian aqueduct syndrome caused by unilateral midbrain lesion, *Ann Neurol* 11:91, 1982.

139. Barnes KL, Ferrario CM: Role of the central nervous system in cardiovascular regulation. In Furlan A, editor: *The heart and stroke,* Heidelberg, 1987, Springer Verlag.

140. Emanuele M, Dorsch T, Scarff T, et al: BA aneurysm simulating pheochromocytoma, *Neurology (NY)* 31:1560, 1981.

141. Naheedy M, Tyler H, Wolf M, et al: Diagnosis of thrombotic giant basilar artery aneurysm on computed tomographic scan, *Arch Neurol* 39:64, 1982.

142. Aichner FT, Felber SR, Birhamer GG, Posch A: Magnetic resonance imaging and magnetic resonance angiography of vertebrobasilar dolichoectasia, *Cerebrovasc Dis* 3:280, 1993.

143. Schwartz A, Rautenberg W, Hennerici M: Dolichoectatic intracranial arteries: Review of selected aspects, *Cerebrovasc Dis* 3:273, 1993.
144. Barrows L, Kubik C, Richardson E: Aneurysms of the basilar and vertebral arteries: A clinicopathologic study, *Trans Am Neurol Assoc* 81:181, 1956.
145. Yu Y, Moseley I, Pullicino P, et al: The clinical pictures of ectasia of the intracerebral arteries, *J Neurol Neurosurg Psychiatry* 45:29, 1982.
146. Moseley I, Holland I: Ectasia of the basilar artery: The breadth of the clinical spectrum and the diagnostic value of computed tomography, *Neuroradiology* 18:83, 1979.
147. Pessin MS, Chimowitz MI, Levine SR, et al: Stroke in patients with fusiform vertebrobasilar aneurysms, *Neurology (NY)* 39:16, 1989.
148. Hirsh L, Gonzalez C: Fusiform basilar aneurysm simulating carotid transient ischemic attacks, *Stroke* 10:598, 1979.
149. DeBosscher J: Anévrysme de l'artère vertébrale gauche chez un homme 45 ans, *Acta Neurol Psychiatr Belg* 52:1, 1952.
150. Denny-Brown D, Foley J: The syndrome of basilar aneurysm, *Trans Am Neurol Assoc* 77:30, 1952.
151. Ekbom K, Grietz T, Kugelberg E: Hydrocephalus due to ectasia of the basilar artery, *J Neurol Sci* 8:465, 1969.
152. Kerber C, Margolis M, Newton T: Tortuous vertebrobasilar system: A cause of cranial nerve signs, *Neurocardiology* 4:74, 1972.
153. Nishizaki T, Tamikl N, Takeda N: Dolichoectatic basilar artery: A review of 23 cases, *Stroke* 17:1277, 1986.
154. Passerini A, Tagliabue G: Aneurysms of the vertebrobasilar system, *Radiol Clin Biol* 35:257, 1966.
155. Paulson G, Nashold B, Margolis G: Aneurysms of the vertebral artery, *Neurology (NY)* 9:590, 1959.
156. Milandre L, Bonnefoi B, Pestre P, et al: Dolichoectasies artérielles vertébrobasilaires: Complications et pronostique, *Rev Neurol (Paris)* 147:714, 1991.
157. Pollock M, Blennerhassett J, Clarke A: Giant cell arteritis and the subclavian steal syndrome, *Neurology* 23:653, 1973.
158. Rao K, Woodlief C: Stimulation of cerebellopontine tumor by tortuous vertebrobasilar artery, *AJR Am J Roentgenol* 132:602, 1979.
159. Maruyama K, Tanaka M, Ikeda S, et al: A case report of quadriparesis due to compression of the medulla oblongata by the elongated left vertebral artery, *Rinsho Shinkeigaku* 29:108, 1989.
160. Paulson G, Boesel C, Evans W: Fibromuscular dysplasia, *Arch Neurol* 35:287, 1978.
161. Hirsch CS, Roessmann U: Arterial dysplasia with ruptured basilar artery aneurysm: Report of a case, *Hum Pathol* 6:749, 1975.
162. Makos MM, McComb RD, Hart MN, et al: Alphaglucosidase deficiency and basilar artery aneurysm: Report of a sibship, *Ann Neurol* 22:629, 1987.
163. Little JR, St. Louis P, Weinstein M, et al: Giant fusiform aneurysm of the cerebral arteries, *Stroke* 12:183, 1981.
164. Gautier JC, Hauw JJ, Awada A, et al: Artères cérébrales dolichoectasiques: Association aux anévrysmes de l'aorte abdominales, *Rev Neurol (Paris)* 144:437, 1988.
165. Monge-Argiles J, et al: [Megadolicobasilar, ulcerative colitis and ischemic stroke], *Neurologia* 18:221, 2003.
166. del Zoppo GJ, Zeumer H, Harker LA: Thrombolytic therapy in stroke: Possibilities and hazards, *Stroke* 17:595, 1986.
167. Passero S, Filosomi G: Posterior circulation infarcts in patients with vertebrobasilar dolichoectasia, *Stroke* 29:653, 1998.
168. Ince B, et al: Dolichoectasia of the intracranial arteries in patients with first ischemic stroke: A population-based study, *Neurology* 50:1694, 1998.
169. de Oliveira R, Cardeal JO, Lima JG: [Basilar ectasia and stroke: Clinical aspects of 21 cases], *Arq Neuropsiquiatr* 55:558, 1997.
170. Alpert J, Gerson L, Hall R, et al: Reversible angiopathy, *Stroke* 13:100, 1982.
171. Fisher CM, Ojemann R, Roberson G: Spontaneous dissection of cervico-cerebral arteries, *J Can Sci Neurol* 5:9, 1978.
172. Caplan L, Young RR: EEG findings in certain lacunar stroke syndromes, *Neurology (NY)* 22:403, 1972.
173. Chiras J, Marciano S, Vega Molina J, et al: Spontaneous dissecting aneurysm of the extracranial vertebral artery (20 cases), *Neuroradiology* 27:327, 1985.
174. Mas JL, Bousser MG, Hasboun D, et al: Extracranial vertebral artery dissection: A review of 13 cases, *Stroke* 18:1037, 1987.
175. Mokri B, Houser OW, Sandok BA, Piepgras DG: Spontaneous dissections of the vertebral arteries, *Neurology* 38:880, 1988.
176. Silbert PL, Mokri B, Schievink W: Headache and neck pain in spontaneous internal carotid and vertebral artery dissections, *Neurology* 45:1517, 1995.
177. Easton JD, Sherman DG: Cervical manipulation and stroke, *Stroke* 8:594, 1977.
178. Ford F, Clark D: Thrombosis of the basilar artery with softenings in the cerebellum and brainstem due to manipulation of the neck, *Bull Johns Hopkins Hosp* 98:37, 1956.
179. Frumkin L, Baloh R: Wallenberg's syndrome following neck manipulation, *Neurology* 40:611, 1990.
180. Goldstein S: Dissecting hematoma of the cervical vertebral artery, *J Neurosurg* 56:451, 1982.
181. Houser OW, Baker H, Sandok B, et al: Cephalic arterial fibromuscular dysplasia, *Radiology* 101:605, 1971.
182. Kreuger B, Okazaki H: Vertebral-basilar distribution infarction following chiropractic cervical manipulation, *Mayo Clin Proc* 55:322, 1980.
183. Norris JW, Beletsky V, Nadareishvili ZG: Sudden neck movement and cervical artery dissection. The Canadian Stroke Consortium, *CMAJ* 163:38, 2000.
184. Biousse V, Chabriat H, Amarenco P, Bousser M-G: Roller-coaster-induced vertebral artery dissection, *Lancet* 346:767, 1995.
185. Amarenco P, Seux-Levieil M-L, Lévy C, et al: Carotid artery dissection with renal infarcts: Two cases, *Stroke* 25:2488, 1994.
186. Schievink WI, Michels VV, Mokri B, et al: A familial syndrome of arterial dissections with lentiginosis, *N Engl J Med* 332:576, 1995.
187. Schievink WI, Mokri B, Piepgras DG, Kuiper JD: Recurrent spontaneous arterial dissections: Risk in familial versus nonfamilial disease, *Stroke* 27:622, 1996.
188. Youl BD, Coutellier A, Dubois B, et al: Three cases of spontaneous extracranial vertebral artery dissection, *Stroke* 21:618, 1990.
189. Barbour PJ, Castaldo JE, Rae-Grant AD, et al: Internal carotid artery redundancy is significantly associated with dissection, *Stroke* 25:1201, 1994.
190. Ben Hamouda-M'Rad I, Biousse V, Bousser M-G, et al: Internal carotid artery redundancy is significantly associated with dissection, *Stroke* 26:1962, 1995.
191. Schievink WI, Mokri B: Familial aorto-cervicocephalic arterial dissections and congenitally bicuspid aortic valve, *Stroke* 26:1935, 1995.
192. Schievink WI, Mokri B, O'Fallon WM: Spontaneous recurrent cervical-artery dissection, *N Engl J Med* 330:393, 1994.
193. Caplan LR, Baquis G, Pessin MS, et al: Dissection of the intracranial vertebral artery, *Neurology (NY)* 38:868, 1988.
194. Alom J, Matias-Gurer J, Padeo L, et al: Spontaneous dissection of intracranial vertebral artery: Clinical recovery with conservative treatment, *J Neurol Neurosurg Psychiatry* 49:599, 1986.
195. Caplan L, Goodwin J: Hypertensive lateral tegmental brainstem hemorrhage, *Neurology (NY)* 32:252, 1982.
196. Deeb Z, Janetta P, Rosenbaum A, et al: Tortuous vertebrobasilar arteries causing cranial nerve syndromes: Screening by computed tomography, *J Comput Assist Tomogr* 3:774, 1965.
197. Alexander C, Burger P, Goree J: Dissecting aneurysms of the basilar artery, *Stroke* 10:294, 1979.
198. Escourolle R, Gautier J-C, Rosa A, et al: Anévrysme dissequant vertébrobasilaire, *Rev Neurol* 128:95, 1972.
199. Ringel S, Harrison S, Norenberg M, et al: Fibromuscular dysplasia: Multiple "spontaneous" dissecting aneurysms of the major cranial arteries, *Ann Neurol* 1:301, 1977.
200. Watson AJ: Dissecting aneurysm of arteries other than the aorta, *J Pathol Bacteriol* 72:439, 1956.
201. Lacour JC, et al: [Isolated dissection of the basilar artery], *Rev Neurol (Paris)* 156:654, 2000.
202. Endoh H, et al: [A case of vertebrobasilar dissection which was associated with progressing stroke and was successfully treated by intravascular surgery in the acute stage], *No Shinkei Geka* 26:1001, 1998.
203. Wolman L: Cerebral dissecting aneurysms, *Brain* 82:276, 1959.
204. D'Anglejan-Chatillon J, Ribeiro V, Mas J-L, et al: Migraine-risk factor for dissection of cervical arteries, *Headache* 29:560, 1989.

205. Yap C, Mayo C, Barron K: Ocular bobbing in palata: Myoclonus, *Arch Neurol* 18:304, 1968.
206. Touboul P-J, Mas J-L, Bousser M-G, Laplane D: Duplex scanning in extracranial vertebral artery dissection, *Stroke* 18:116, 1987.
207. Lévy C, Laissy J-P, Raveau V, et al: 3D-time-of-flight MR angiography and MR imaging versus angiography in carotid and vertebral artery dissections: A prospective study in 18 patients, *Radiology* 190:97, 1994.
208. Rother J, Schwartz A, Rautenberg W, Hennerici M: Magnetic resonance angiography of spontaneous vertebral artery dissection suspected on Doppler ultrasonography, *J Neurol (Germany)* 242:430, 1995.
209. Sheehan S, Bauer R, Meyer J: Vertebral artery compression in cervical spondylosis, *Neurology (NY)* 10:968, 1960.
210. Tatlow W, Bammer H: Syndrome of vertebral artery compression, *Neurology (NY)* 7:331, 1957.
211. Chin JH: Recurrent stroke caused by spondylitic compression of the vertebral artery, *Ann Neurol* 33:558, 1993.
212. Powers SR, Drislane TM, Nevins S: Intermittent vertebral artery compression: A new syndrome, *Surgery* 49:257, 1961.
213. Rosengart A, Hedges TR III, Teal PA, et al: Intermittent downbeat nystagmus due to vertebral artery compression, *Neurology* 43:216, 1993.
214. Dadsetan MR, Skeihut HEI: Rotational vertebrobasilar insufficiency secondary to vertebral artery occlusion from fibrous band of the longus colli muscle, *Neuroradiology* 32:514, 1990.
215. George B, Laurian C: Impairment of vertebral artery flow caused by extrinsic lesions, *Neurosurgery* 24:206, 1989.
216. Hardin CA, Poser CA: Rotational obstruction of the vertebral artery due to redundancy and extraluminal cervical fascial bands, *Ann Surg* 158:133, 1963.
217. Mapstone T, Spetzler R: Vertebrobasilar insufficiency secondary to vertebral artery occlusion from a fibrous band, *J Neurosurg* 56:581, 1982.
218. Radner S: Vertebral angiography by catheterization, *Acta Radiol [Suppl] (Stockh)* 87:1–133, 1951.
219. Fisher CM: Vertigo in cerebrovascular disease, *Arch Otolaryngol* 85:529, 1967.
220. Pratt-Thomas H, Berger K: Cerebellar and spinal injuries after chiropractic manipulation, *JAMA* 133:600, 1947.
221. Hanus S, Homer T, Harter D: Vertebral artery occlusion complicating yoga exercises, *Arch Neurol* 34:547, 1977.
222. Heros R: Cerebellar infarction resulting from traumatic occlusion of a vertebral artery, *J Neurosurg* 51:111, 1979.
223. Levy R, Dugan T, Bernat J, et al: Lateral medullary syndrome after neck injury, *Neurology (NY)* 30:788, 1980.
224. Mueller S, Sahs A: Brainstem dysfunction related to cervical manipulation, *Neurology (NY)* 26:547, 1976.
225. Robertson J: Neck manipulation as a cause of stroke, *Stroke* 12:1, 1981.
226. Rogers L, Sweeney P: Stroke: A neurological complication of wrestling, *Am J Sports Med* 7:352, 1979.
227. Sherman D, Hart R, Easton JD: Abrupt change in head position and cerebral infarction, *Stroke* 12:2, 1981.
228. Woolsey R, Chang H: Fatal basilar artery occlusion following cervical spine injury, *Paraplegia* 17:280, 1979.
229. Yates A, Guest D: Cerebral embolism due to an ununited fracture of the clavicle and subclavian thrombosis, *Lancet* 2:25, 1928.
230. Frens D, Petajan J, Anderson R, et al: Fibromuscular dysplasia of the posterior cerebral artery: Report of a case and review of the literature, *Stroke* 5:161, 1974.
231. Osborn A, Anderson R: Angiography spectrum of cervical and intracranial fibromuscular dysplasia, *Stroke* 8:617, 1977.
232. Corrin LS, Sandok BA, Houser W: Cerebral ischemic events in patients with carotid artery fibromuscular disease, *Arch Neurol* 38:616, 1981.
233. Handa J, Kamijo Y, Handa H: Intracranial aneurysms associated with fibromuscular hyperplasia of the renal and internal carotid arteries, *Br J Radiol* 43:483, 1970.
234. Mettinger K: Fibromuscular dysplasia and the brain. II: Current concepts of the disease, *Stroke* 13:53, 1982.
235. So EL, Toole JF, Dalal P, et al: Cephalic fibromuscular dysplasia in 32 patients: Clinical findings and radiologic features, *Arch Neurol* 38:619, 1981.
236. Goodwill J: Temporal arteritis. In Vinken P, Bruyn G, editors: *Handbook of clinical neurology,* vol 39, Amsterdam, 1980, North-Holland, pp 313.
237. Zamarbide ID, Maxit MJ: [Fisher's one and half syndrome with facial palsy as clinical presentation of giant cell temporal arteritis], *Medicina (B Aires)* 60:245, 2000.
238. Walsh TJ, Hier DB, Caplan LR: Aspergillosis of the central nervous system: Clinicopathological analysis of 17 patients, *Ann Neurol* 18:574, 1985.
239. Young RC, Bennett JE, Vogel CL, et al: Aspergillosis: The spectrum of the disease in 98 patients, *Medicine (Baltimore)* 49:147, 1970.
240. Walsh TJ, Hutchins GM, Bukley BH, Mendelsohn G: Fungal infections of the heart: Analysis of 51 autopsy cases, *Am J Cardiol* 45:357, 1980.
241. Tack KJ, Rhame FS, Brown B, Thompson RC: Aspergillus osteomyelitis: Report of four cases and review of the literature, *Am J Med* 83:295, 1982.
242. Caplan LR, Thomas C, Banks G: Central nervous system complications of addiction to T's and Blues, *Neurology* 32:623, 1982.
243. Wood D: Cerebrovascular complications of sickle cell anemia, *Stroke* 9:73, 1978.
244. Merkel K, Grinsberg P, Parker J, et al: Cerebrovascular disease in sickle cell anemia: A clinical, pathological, and radiological correlation, *Stroke* 9:45, 1978.
245. Amarenco P, Kase CS, Rosengart A, et al: Very small (border zone) cerebellar infarcts: Distribution, mechanisms, causes and clinical features, *Brain* 116:161, 1993.
246. Ishikawa K: Natural history and classification of occlusive thromboarteriopathy (Takayasu disease), *Circulation* 57:27, 1978.
247. Lupi-Herrera E, Sanchez-Torres G, Marcushamer J, et al: Takayasu's arteritis: Clinical study of 27 cases, *Am Heart J* 93:94, 1977.
248. Molnar P, Hegedus K: Direct involvement of intracerebral arteries in Takayasu's arteritis, *Acta Neuropathol (Berl)* 63:83, 1984.
249. McMenemy WH, Lawrence BJ: Encephalomyelopathy in Behçet's syndrome, *Lancet* 2:353, 1957.
250. Herskovitz S, Lipton RB, Lantos G: Neuro-Behçet's disease, *Neurology (NY)* 38:1714, 1988.
251. Seldarogiu P, Yazici H, Ozdemir C, et al: Neurologic involvement in Behçet's syndrome: A prospective study, *Arch Neurol* 46:265, 1989.
252. Piovesan EJ, et al: Neurofibromatosis, stroke and basilar impression: Case report, *Arq Neuropsiquiatr* 57:484, 1999.
253. Jones HE, Millikan C, Sandok B: Temporal profile (clinical course) of acute vertebrobasilar system cerebral infarction, *Stroke* 11:173, 1980.
254. Patrick B, Ramirez-Lassepas M, Snyder B: Temporal profile of vertebrobasilar territory infarction, *Stroke* 11:643, 1980.
255. Sundt TM, Piepgras D: Occipital to posterior inferior cerebellar artery bypass surgery, *J Neurosurg* 49:916, 1978.
256. Naritomi H, Sakai F, Meyer J: Pathogenesis of transient ischemic attacks within the vertebrobasilar arterial system, *Arch Neurol* 36:121, 1979.
257. Fisher CM: The "herald hemiparesis" of basilar artery occlusion, *Arch Neurol* 45:1301, 1988.
258. Babinski J, Nageotte J: Hémiasynergie, latéropulsion et myosis bulbaires avec hémianesthésie et croisées, *Rev Neurol* 10:358, 1902.
259. Caplan L: Top of the basilar syndrome: Selected clinical aspects, *Neurology (NY)* 30:72, 1980.
260. Amarenco P, Caplan LR: Vertebrobasilar occlusive disease: Review of selected aspects. 3: Mechanisms of cerebellar infarctions, *Cerebrovasc Dis* 3:66, 1993.
261. Caplan LR: Brain embolism, revisited, *Neurology* 43:1281, 1993.
262. Caplan LR, Amarenco P, Rosengart A, et al: Embolism from vertebral artery origin occlusive disease, *Neurology* 42:1505, 1992.
263. Chaves CJ, Caplan LR, Chung CS, et al: Cerebellar infarcts in the New England Medical Center Posterior Circulation Stroke Registry, *Neurology* 44:1385, 1994.
264. Chaves CJ, Pessin MS, Caplan LR, et al: Cerebellar hemorrhagic infarction, *Neurology* 46:346, 1996.
265. Lehrich J, Winkler G, Ojemann R: Cerebellar infarction with brainstem compression: Diagnosis and surgical treatment, *Arch Neurol* 22:490, 1970.

266. Fisher CM: Bilateral occlusion of basilar artery branches, *J Neurol Neurosurg Psychiatry* 40:1182, 1977.

267. Khurana R: Autonomic dysfunction in pontomedullary stroke, *Ann Neurol* 12:86, 1982.

268. Reis DJ, Iadecola C, Nakai M: Control of cerebral blood flow and metabolism by intrinsic neural systems in brain. In Plum P, Pulsinelli W, editors: *Cerebrovascular diseases: Proceedings of the Fourteenth (Princeton) Conference*, Philadelphia, 1985, Lippincott-Raven, p 1.

269. Barnes M, Hunt B, Williams I: The role of vertebral angiography in the investigation of third nerve palsy, *J Neurol Neurosurg Psychiatry* 44:1153, 1981.

270. Lindgren SO: Infarctions simulating brain tumors in the posterior fossa, *J Neurosurg* 13:575, 1956.

271. Bogousslavsky J, Khurana R, Deruaz JP, et al: Respiratory failure and unilateral caudal brainstem infarction, *Ann Neurol* 28:668, 1990.

272. Toyoda K, et al: Bilateral deafness as a prodromal symptom of basilar artery occlusion, *J Neurol Sci* 193:147, 2002.

273. Archer C, Horenstein S: Basilar artery occlusion: Clinical and radiological correlation, *Stroke* 8:383, 1977.

274. Caplan L: Occlusion of the vertebral or basilar artery, *Stroke* 10:277, 1979.

275. Fields W, Ratinov G, Weibel J, et al: Survival following basilar artery occlusion, *Arch Neurol* 15:463, 1966.

276. Moscow N, Newton T: Angiographic implications in diagnosis and prognosis of basilar artery occlusion, *AJR Am J Roentgenol* 119:597, 1973.

277. Pochaczevsky R, Uygur Z, Berman A: Basilar artery occlusion, *J Can Assoc Radiol* 22:261, 1971.

278. Labauge R, Pages M, Marty-Double C, et al: Occlusion du tronc basilaire, *Rev Neurol* 137:545, 1981.

279. Silverstein A: Acute infarctions of the brainstem in the distribution of the basilar artery, *Confin Neurol* 24:37, 1964.

280. Loeb C, Meyer JS: *Strokes Due to Vertebro-Basilar Disease*, Springfield, Ill, 1965, Charles C Thomas.

281. Biemond A: Thrombosis of the basilar artery and the vascularization of the brainstem, *Brain* 74:300, 1951.

282. Caplan LR, Rosenbaum A: Role of cerebral angiography in vertebrobasilar occlusive disease, *J Neurol Neurosurg Psychiatry* 38:601, 1975.

283. Pessin MS, Gorelick PB, Kwan ES, et al: Basilar artery stenosis: Middle and distal segments, *Neurology (NY)* 37:1742, 1987.

284. Ackerman E, Levinsohn M, Richards D, et al: Basilar artery occlusion in a 10-year-old boy, *Ann Neurol* 1:204, 1977.

285. Kase C, Maulsby G, De Juan C, et al: Hemichorea-hemiballism and lacunar infarction in the basal ganglia, *Neurology (NY)* 31:452, 1981.

286. Ferbert A, Bruckmann H, Drummen R: Clinical features of proven basilar artery occlusion, *Stroke* 21:1135, 1990.

287. Plum F, Posner J: *The diagnosis of stupor and coma*, ed 3, Philadelphia, 1980, FA Davis.

288. Saposnik G, Caplan LR: Convulsive-like movements in brainstem stroke, *Arch Neurol* 58:654, 2001.

289. Kemper T, Romanul F: State resembling akinetic mutism in basilar artery occlusion, *Neurology (NY)* 17:74, 1967.

290. Bauer G, Prugger M, Rumpl E: Stimulus evoked oral automatisms in the locked-in syndrome, *Arch Neurol* 39:435, 1982.

291. Karp J, Hurtig H: Locked-in state with bilateral midbrain infarcts, *Arch Neurol* 30:176, 1974.

292. Meienberg O, Mumenthaler M, Karbowski K: Quadriparesis and nuclear oculomotor palsy with total bilateral ptosis mimicking coma, *Arch Neurol* 36:708, 1979.

293. Tahmoush A, Brooks J, Keltner J: Palatal myoclonus associated with abnormal ocular and extremity movements, *Arch Neurol* 27:431, 1972.

294. Lapresle J: Ben Hamida M: The dentato-olivary pathway, *Arch Neurol* 22:135, 1970.

295. Fisher CM: Ocular bobbing, *Arch Neurol* 11:543, 1964.

296. Nelson J, Johnston C: Ocular bobbing, *Arch Neurol* 22:348, 1970.

297. Bosch E, Kennedy S, Aschenbrenner C: Ocular bobbing: The myth of its localizing value, *Neurology (NY)* 25:949, 1975.

298. Ott K, Kase C, Ojemann R, et al: Cerebellar hemorrhage: Diagnosis and treatment, *Arch Neurol* 31:160, 1974.

299. Susac J, Hoyt W, Daroff R, et al: Clinical spectrum of ocular bobbing, *J Neurol Neurosurg Psychiatry* 33:771, 1970.

300. Newman N, Gay A, Heilbrun M: Disconjugate ocular bobbing: Its relation to midbrain, pontine and medullary function in a surviving patient, *Neurology (NY)* 21:633, 1971.

301. Smith M, Launa J: Upward gaze paralysis following unilateral pretectal infarction, *Arch Neurol* 38:127, 1981.

302. Cogan D, Kubik C, Smith WL: Unilateral internuclear ophthalmoplegia, *Arch Ophthalmol* 44:783, 1950.

303. Cogan DG: Supranuclear connections of the ocular motor system. In *Neurology of the ocular muscles*, ed 2, Springfield, Ill, 1956, Charles C Thomas, p 84.

304. Smith JL, Cogan D: Internuclear ophthalmoplegia, *Arch Ophthalmol* 61:687, 1959.

305. Harris W: Ataxic nystagmus: A pathognomonic sign in disseminated sclerosis, *Br J Ophthalmol* 28:40, 1944.

306. Christoff N, Anderson P, Nathanson M, et al: Problems in anatomical analysis of lesions of the medial longitudinal fasciculus, *Arch Neurol* 2:293, 1960.

307. Gonyea E: Bilateral internuclear ophthalmoplegia: Association with occlusive cerebrovascular disease, *Arch Neurol* 31:168, 1974.

308. Cogan D: Internuclear ophthalmoplegia, typical and atypical, *Arch Ophthalmol* 84:583, 1970.

309. Daroff R, Hoyt W: Supranuclear disorders of ocular control systems in man. In Bach Y, Rita P, Collins C, editors: *The control of eye movements*, Orlando, Fla, 1977, Academic Press, pp 175.

310. Bronstein AM, Rudge P, Gresty MA, et al: Abnormalities of horizontal gaze: Clinical, oculographic and magnetic resonance imaging findings. II: Gaze palsy and internuclear ophthalmoplegia, *J Neurol Neurosurg Psychiatry* 53:200, 1990.

311. Crosby E, Yoss R, Henderson J: The mammalian midbrain and isthmus regions. II: The fiber connections. D: The pattern for eye movement in the frontal eye fields and the discharge of specific portions of this field to and through midbrain levels, *J Comp Neurol* 97:357, 1952.

312. Pierrot-Deseilligny C, Chain F, Serdaru M, et al: The one and a half syndrome, *Brain* 104:665, 1981.

313. de Seze J, Lucas C, Leclerc X, et al: One-and-a-half syndrome in pontine infarcts: MRI correlates, *Neuroradiology* 41:666, 1999.

314. Caplan L, Ptosis: *J Neurol Neurosurg Psychiatry* 37:1, 1974.

315. Caplan L, Gorelick P: 'Salt and pepper in the face' pain in acute brainstem ischemia, *Ann Neurol* 13:344, 1983.

316. Fisher CM: The neurological examination of the comatose patient, *Acta Neurol Scand* 45(Suppl 36):1, 1969.

317. Silverstein A: Pontine infarction. In Vinken P, Bruyn G, editors: *Handbook of clinical neurology,* vol 12, Amsterdam, 1972, North-Holland, p 13.

318. Mehler MF: The rostral basilar artery syndrome: Diagnosis, etiology, prognosis, *Neurology* 39:9, 1989.

319. Mehler MF: The neuro-ophthalmologic spectrum of the rostral basilar artery syndrome, *Arch Neurol* 45:966, 1988.

320. Facon E, Steriade M, Werthein N: Hypersomnie prolongée engendrée par des lésions bilatérales du système activateur médial: Le syndrome thrombotique de la bifurcation du tronc basilaire, *Rev Neurol* 98:117, 1958.

321. Segarra J: Cerebral vascular disease and behavior. I: The syndrome of the mesencephalic artery (basilar artery bifurcation), *Arch Neurol* 22:408, 1970.

322. Lindenberg R: Compression of brain arteries as a pathogenetic factor for tissue necrosis and their areas of predilection, *J Neuropathol Exp Neurol* 14:223, 1955.

323. Caplan L, Zervas N: Survival with permanent midbrain dysfunction after surgical treatment of traumatic sub-dural hematoma: The clinical picture of a Duret hemorrhage, *Ann Neurol* 1:587, 1977.

324. Selhorst J, Hoyt W, Feinsod M, et al: Midbrain corectopia, *Arch Neurol* 33:193, 1976.

325. Wilson SAK: Ectopia pupillae in certain mesencephalic lesions, *Brain* 29:524, 1906.

326. Fisher CM: Oval pupils, *Arch Neurol* 37:502, 1980.

327. Meissner I, Sapir S, Kokmen E, et al: The paramedian diencephalic syndrome: A dynamic phenomenon, *Stroke* 18:380, 1987.

328. Pedersen R, Troost BT: Abnormalities of gaze in cerebrovascular disease, *Stroke* 12:251, 1981.

329. Trojanowski J, Wray S: Vertical gaze ophthalmoplegia: Selective paralysis of downgaze, *Neurology (NY)* 30:605, 1980.

330. Buttner-Ennever J, Buttner U, Cohen B, et al: Vertical gaze paralysis and the rostral interstitial nucleus of the medial longitudinal fasciculus, *Brain* 105:125, 1982.

331. Nashold B, Seaber J: Defects of ocular mobility after stereotactic midbrain lesions in man, *Arch Ophthalmol* 88:245, 1972.

332. White DN, Ketelaars EJ, Cledgett PR: Non-invasive techniques for the recording of vertebral artery flow and their limitations, *Ultrasound Med Biol* 6:315, 1980.

333. Halmagyi G, Evans W, Hallinan J: Failure of downward gaze, *Arch Neurol* 35:22, 1978.

334. Jacobs L, Anderson P, Bender M: The lesion producing paralysis of downward but not upward gaze, *Arch Neurol* 28:319, 1973.

335. Halmagyi MB, Brandt T, Dieterich M, et al: Tonic contraversive ocular tilt reaction due to unilateral mesodiencephalic lesion, *Neurology (NY)* 40:1503, 1990.

336. Bogousslavsky J, Regli F: Upgaze palsy and monocular paresis of downgaze from ipsilateral thalamo-mesencephalic infarction: A vertical one-and-a-half syndrome, *J Neurol* 231:43, 1984.

337. Deleu D, Buisseret T, Ebinger G: Vertical one-and-a-half syndrome: Supranuclear downgaze paralysis with monocular elevation palsy, *Arch Neurol* 46:1361, 1989.

337a. Tatemichi T, Steinke W, Duncan C, et al: Paramedian thalamopeduncular infarction: Clinical syndromes and magnetic imaging, *Ann Neurol* 32:162, 1992.

338. Collier J: Nuclear ophthalmoplegia with especial reference to retraction of the lids and ptosis and to lesions of the posterior commissure, *Brain* 50:488, 1927.

339. Lhermitte J: Syndrome de la calotte du pédoncule cérébral: Les troubles psycho-sensoriels dans les lesions du mésocéphale, *Rev Neurol (Paris)* 38:1359, 1922.

340. Van Bogaert L: L'hallucinose pedonculaire, *Rev Neurol (Paris)* 43:608, 1927.

341. Van Bogaert L: Syndrome inferieure du noyau rouge, troubles psycho-sensoriels d'origine mésocéphalique, *Rev Neurol (Paris)* 40:416, 1924.

342. McKee AC, Levine DN, Kowall NW, et al: Peduncular hallucinosis associated with isolated infarction of the substantia nigra pars reticulata, *Ann Neurol* 27:500, 1990.

343. Strukel RJ, Garrick JG: Thoracic outlet compression in athletes: A report of four cases, *Am J Sports Med* 6:35, 1978.

344. Martin JP: Hemichorea resulting from a local lesion of the brain (the syndrome of the body of Luys), *Brain* 50:637, 1927.

345. Moersch F, Kernohan J: Hemiballismus, a clinicopathological study, *Arch Neurol Psychiatry* 41:365, 1939.

346. Whittier J: Ballism and the subthalamic nucleus, *Arch Neurol Psychiatry* 58:672, 1947.

347. Barth A, Bogousslavsky J, Regli F: The clinical and topographic spectrum of cerebellar infarcts: A clinical-magnetic resonance imaging correlation study, *Ann Neurol* 33:451, 1993.

348. Hinshaw D, Thompson J, Hasso A, et al: Infarction of the brainstem and cerebellum: A correlation of computed tomography and angiography, *Radiology* 137:105, 1980.

349. Kase CS, Norrving B, Levine SR, et al: Cerebellar infarction: Clinico-anatomic correlations, *Stroke* 24:76, 1993.

350. Kase CS, White JL, Joslyn N, et al: Cerebellar infarction in the superior cerebellar artery distribution, *Neurology (NY)* 35:705, 1985.

351. Amarenco P, Roullet E, Goujon C, et al: Infarction in the anterior rostral cerebellum (the territory of the lateral branch of the superior cerebellar artery), *Neurology* 41:253, 1991.

352. Macdonell RAL, Kalnins RM, Donnan GA: Cerebellar infarction: Natural history, prognosis, and pathology, *Stroke* 18:849, 1987.

353. Struck LK, Biller J, Bruno A, et al: Superior cerebellar artery territory infarction, *Cerebrovasc Dis* 1:71, 1991.

354. Lazorthes G, Gouazé A, Salamon G, et al: La vascularisation artérielle du cervelet. In Lazorthes G, Gouazé A, Salamon G, editors: *La vascularisation cérébrale*, Paris, 1978, Masson, pp 205–219.

355. Thompson GN: Cerebellar embolism, *Bull Los Angeles Neurol Soc* 9:140, 1944.

356. Kalyan-Raman UP, Kowalski RV, Lee RH, Fierer JA: Dissecting aneurysm of superior cerebellar artery, *Arch Neurol* 40:120, 1983.

357. Perez-Higueras A, Alvarez-Ruiz F, Martinez-Bermejo A, et al: Cerebellar infarction from fibromuscular dysplasia and dissecting aneurysm of the vertebral artery: Report of a child, *Stroke* 19:521, 1988.

358. Caplan LR: Migraine and vertebrobasilar ischemia, *Neurology (NY)* 41:55, 1991.

359. Titus F, Montalban J, Molins A, et al: Migraine-related stroke: Brain infarction in superior cerebellar artery territory demonstrated by nuclear magnetic resonance, *Acta Neurol Scand* 79:357, 1989.

360. Davison C, Goodhart S, Savitsky N: The syndrome of the superior cerebellar artery and its branches, *Arch Neurol Psychiatry* 33:1143, 1935.

361. Guillain G, Bertrand L, Péron N: Le syndrome de l'artère cérébelleuse supérieure, *Rev Neurol* 2:835, 1928.

362. Savoiardo M, Bracchi M, Passerini A, et al: The vascular territories in the cerebellum and brainstem: CT and MR study, *AJNR Am J Neuroradiol* 8:199, 1987.

363. Mills CK: Hemianesthesia to pain and temperature and loss of emotional expression on the right side with ataxia of the upper limb on the left, *J Nerv Ment Dis* 35:331, 1908.

364. Mills CK: Preliminary note on a new symptom complex due to lesion of the cerebellum and cerebello-rubro-thalamic system, the main symptoms being ataxia of the upper and lower extremities of one side, and the other side deafness, paralysis of emotional expression in the face, and loss of the senses of pain, heat, and cold over the entire half of the body, *J Nerv Ment Dis* 39:73, 1912.

365. Girard PF, Bonamour Garde E: Les syndromes de l'oblitération de l'artère cérébelleuse supérieure et du ramollissement global de la calotte protubérantielle dans son tiers supérieur: Participation du pathétique, *Rev Neurol (Paris)* 83:199, 1950.

366. Worster-Drought C, Allen I: Thrombosis of the superior cerebellar artery, *Lancet* 214:1137, 1929.

367. Cossa P, Richard S: Sur deux cas de syndrome de l'artère cérébelleuse supérieure (ou de ses branches), *Rev Neurol (Paris)* 92:633, 1955.

368. Freeman W, Jaffe D: Occlusion of the superior cerebellar artery, *Arch Neurol Psychiatry* 46:115, 1941.

369. Levine SR, Welch KMA: Superior cerebellar artery territory stroke [abstract], *Neurology* 38(Suppl 1):344, 1988.

370. Caplan LR, editor: *Posterior circulation disease*, Cambridge, UK, 1996, Blackwell Science.

371. Tougeron A, Samson Y, Schaison M, et al: Syndrome dysarthrie-main malhabile par infarctus cérébelleux, *Rev Neurol (Paris)* 144:596, 1988.

372. Bogousslavsky J, Régli F: Latéro-pulsion axiale isolée lors d'un infarctus cérébelleux flocculo-nodulaire, *Rev Neurol (Paris)* 140:140, 1984.

373. Ranalli PJ, Sharpe JA: Contrapulsion of saccades and ipsilateral ataxia: A unilateral disorder of the rostral cerebellum, *Ann Neurol* 20:311, 1986.

374. Amarenco P, Chevrie-Muller C, Roullet E, Bousser M-G: Paravermal infarct and isolated cerebellar dysarthria, *Ann Neurol* 30:211, 1991.

375. Ringer RA, Culberson JL: Extensor tone disinhibition from an infarction within the midline anterior cerebellar lobe, *J Neurol Neurosurg Psychiatry* 52:1597, 1989.

376. Tohgi H, Takahashi S, Chibra K, et al: Cerebellar infarction: Clinical and neuroimaging analysis in 293 patients, *Stroke* 24:1697, 1993.

377. Atkinson WJ: The anterior inferior cerebellar artery, *J Neurol Neurosurg Psychiatry* 12:137, 1949.

378. Takahashi S, Goto K, Fukasawa H, et al: Computed tomography of cerebral infarction along the distribution of the basal perforating arteries. II: Thalamic arterial group, *Radiology* 155:119, 1985.

379. Perneczky A, Perneczky G, Tschabitscher M, et al: The relationship between the caudolateral pontine syndrome and the anterior inferior cerebellar artery, *Acta Neurochir* 58:245, 1981.

380. Matsushita K, Naritomi H, Kazui S, et al: Infarction in the anterior inferior cerebellar artery territory: Magnetic resonance imaging and auditory brainstem responses, *Cerebrovasc Dis* 3:206, 1993.

381. Fisher CM: Lacunar infarct of the tegmentum of the lower lateral pons, *Arch Neurol* 46:566, 1989.

382. McLean CA, Gonzales MF, Dowling JP: Systemic giant cell arteritis and cerebellar infarction, *Stroke* 24:899, 1993.

383. Adams R: Occlusion of the anterior inferior cerebellar artery, *Arch Neurol Psychiatry* 49:765, 1983.

384. Amarenco P, Roullet E, Chemouilli P, Marteau R: Infarctus pontin inféro-latéral: Deux aspects cliniques, *Rev Neurol (Paris)* 146:433, 1990.

385. Rubenstein RL, Norman D, Schindler R, et al: Cerebellar infarction: A presentation of vertigo, *Laryngoscope* 90:505, 1980.

386. Amarenco P, Debroucker T, Cambier J: Dysarthrie et instabilité révélant d'un infarctus distal de l'artère cérébelleuse supérieure gauche, *Rev Neurol (Paris)* 144:459, 1988.

387. Oas JG, Baloh RW: Vertigo and the anterior inferior cerebellar artery syndrome, *Neurology* 42:2274, 1992.

388. Philips PC, Lorenstsen KJ, Shropshire LC, Ahn HS: Congenital odontoid aplasia and posterior circulation stroke in childhood, *Ann Neurol* 23:410, 1988.

389. Amarenco P, Hauw J-J, Henin D, et al: Les infarctus du territoire de l'artère cérébelleuse postéro-inférieure: Étude clinicopathologique de 28 cas, *Rev Neurol* 145:277, 1989.

390. Amarenco P: The spectrum of cerebellar infarctions, *Neurology* 41:973, 1991.

391. Heros R: Cerebellar hemorrhage and infarction, *Stroke* 13:106, 1982.

392. Wallenberg A: Acute bulbar affection, *Arch Psychiatr Nervenheilkd* 27:504, 1895.

393. Wallenberg A: Anatomischer Befund in einem als Acute Bulbäraffection (Embolie der art. cerebellar. post. inf. sinistr.?). Beschriebenem falle, *Arch Fr Psychiatr* 34:923, 1901.

394. Diggle FH, Stopford JSB: PICA and vertebral artery thrombosis, *Lancet* 225:1214, 1935.

395. Hall AJ, Eaves EC: Posterior inferior cerebellar thrombosis (autopsy), *Lancet* 224:975, 1934.

396. Hun H: Analgesia, thermic anesthesia, and ataxia, resulting from foci of softening in the medulla oblongata and cerebellum due to occlusion of the left PICA, *N Y Med J* 65:513, 1897.

397. Spiller WG: The symptom-complex of occlusion of PICA, *J Nerv Ment Dis* 35:365, 1908.

398. Thomas HM: Symptoms following the occlusion of the PICA, *J Nerv Ment Dis* 34:48, 1907.

399. Wilson G, Winkelman NW: Occlusion of the PICA, *J Nerv Ment Dis* 65:125, 1927.

400. Harris TH, Hauser A: Occlusion of the right posterior inferior cerebellar artery and right vertebral artery, *Arch Neurol Psychiatry* 26:396, 1931.

401. Breuer R, Marburg O: Zur Klinik und Pathologie der apoplektiformen Bulbärparalyse, *Arb Neurol Inst Wien Univ* 9:181, 1902.

402. Foix C, Hillemand P, Schalit I: Sur le syndrome latéral due bulbe et l'irrigation du bulbe supérieur: L'artère de la fossette latérale du bulbe, le syndrome de la cérébelleuse inférieure, territoire de ces artères, *Rev Neurol* 32:160, 1925.

403. Ramsbottom A, Stopford JSB: Occlusion of the PICA, *BMJ* 1:364, 1924.

404. Duncan G, Parker S, Fisher CM: Acute cerebellar infarction in the PICA territory, *Arch Neurol* 32:364, 1975.

405. Krayenbüll H, Yasargil MG: *Die vaskulären Erkrankungen im Gebiet der Arteria vertebralis und Arteria basilaris*, Stuttgart, 1957, George Thieme.

406. Amarenco P, Hauw J-J: Infarctus cérébelleux œdémateux: Etude clinico-pathologique de 16 cas, *Neurochirurgie* 36:234, 1990.

407. Anson JA, Spetzler RF: Endarterectomy of the intradural vertebral artery via the far lateral approach, *Neurosurgery* 33:804, 1993.

408. Norrving B, Magnusson M, Holtas S: Isolated acute vertigo in the elderly: Vestibular or vascular disease? *Acta Neurol Scand* 91:43, 1995.

409. Dumenil L: De la paralysie unilatérale du voile du palais d'origine centrale, *Arch Gen Med* 25:385, 1875.

410. Ho SU, Kim KS, Berenberg RA, Ho HT: Cerebellar infarction: A clinical and CT study, *Surg Neurol* 16:350, 1981.

411. Samson M, Milhout B, Onnient Y, et al: Les ramollissements cérébelleux: Données diagnostiques et pronostiques, *Sem Hop Paris* 62:2766, 1986.

412. Samson M, Milhout B, Thiebot J, et al: Forme bénigne des infarctus cérébelleux, *Rev Neurol* 137:373, 1981.

413. Tomaszek DE, Rosner MJ: Cerebellar infarction: Analysis of twenty-one cases, *Surg Neurol* 24:223, 1985.

414. Feely MP: Cerebellar infarction, *Neurosurgery* 4:7, 1979.

415. Guiang RL, Ellington OB: Acute pure vertiginous disequilibrium in cerebellar infarction, *Eur Neurol* 16:11, 1977.

416. Huang CY, Yu YL: Small cerebellar strokes may mimic labyrinthine lesions, *J Neurol Neurosurg Psychiatry* 48:263, 1985.

417. Barth A, Bogousslavsky J, Régli F: Infarcts in the territory of the lateral branch of the posterior inferior cerebellar artery, *J Neurol Neurosurg Psychiatry* 57:1073, 1994.

418. Amarenco P, Roullet E, Hommel M, et al: Infarction in the territory of the medial branch of the posterior inferior cerebellar artery, *J Neurol Neurosurg Psychiatry* 53:731, 1990.

419. Pierrot-Deseilligny C, Amarenco P, Roullet E, et al: Vermal infarct with pursuit eye movement disorders, *J Neurol Neurosurg Psychiatry* 53:519, 1990.

420. Fisher CM: Headache in cerebrovascular disease. In Vinken P, Bruyn G, editors: *Handbook of clinical neurology*, vol 5, Amsterdam, 1968, North-Holland, p 124.

421. Wilkins R, Brody I: Wallenberg's syndrome, *Arch Neurol* 22:379, 1970.

422. Norrving B, Cronqvist S: Lateral medullary infarction: Prognosis in an unselected series, *Neurology* 41:244, 1991.

423. Sacco RL, Freddo L, Bello JA, et al: Wallenberg's lateral medullary syndrome: Clinical-magnetic resonance imaging correlation, *Arch Neurol* 50:609, 1993.

424. Vuilleumier P, Bogousslavsky J, Regli F: Infarction of the lower brainstem: Clinical, aetiological and MR-topographical correlations, *Brain* 118:1013, 1995.

425. Currier R, Giles C, Dejong R: Some comments on Wallenberg's lateral medullary syndrome, *Neurology (NY)* 11:778, 1961.

426. Sheehan D, Smith G: A study of the anatomy of vertebral thrombosis, *Lancet* 2:614, 1937.

427. Kim JS, Lee JH, Suh DC, Lee MC: Spectrum of lateral medullary syndrome: Correlation between clinical findings and magnetic resonance imaging in 33 subjects, *Stroke* 25:1405, 1994.

428. Richter R: Collaterals between the external carotid artery and the vertebral artery in cases of thrombosis of the internal carotid artery, *Acta Radiol Diagn (Stockh)* 40:108, 1953.

429. McCusker E, Rudick R, Honch G, et al: Recovery from the locked-in syndrome, *Arch Neurol* 39:145, 1982.

430. Fisher CM, Karnes WE: Local embolism, *J Neuropathol Exp Neurol* 24:174, 1965.

431. Koroshetz WJ, Ropper AH: Artery-to-artery embolism causing stroke in the posterior circulation, *Neurology (NY)* 37:292, 1987.

432. Pessin MS, Daneault N, Kwan E, et al: Local embolism from vertebral artery occlusion, *Stroke* 19:112, 1988.

433. Fisher CM: Is pressure on nerves and roots a common cause of pain?, *Trans Am Neurol Assoc* 97:282, 1972.

434. Peterman A, Siekert R: The lateral medullary (Wallenberg) syndrome: Clinical features and prognosis, *Med Clin North Am* 44:887, 1960.

435. Borison H, Wang S: Physiology and pharmacology of vomiting, *Pharmacol Rev* 5:193, 1953.

436. Louis-Bar D: Sur le syndrome vasculaire de l'hémibulbe (Wallenberg), *Monatsschr Psychiatr Neurol* 112:53, 1946.

437. Soffin G, Feldman M, Bender M: Alterations of sensory levels in vascular lesions of lateral medulla, *Arch Neurol* 18:178, 1968.

438. Bright R: Cases illustrative of the effects produced when the arteries and brain are diseased, *Guys Hosp Rep* 1:9, 1836.

439. Merritt H, Finland M: Vascular lesions of the hindbrain (lateral medullary syndrome), *Brain* 53:290, 1930.

440. Estanol B, Lopez-Rios G: Neuro-otology of the lateral medullary infarct syndrome, *Arch Neurol* 39:176, 1982.

441. Matsumoto S, Okuda B, Imai T, et al: A sensory level on the trunk in lower lateral brainstem lesions, *Neurology (NY)* 38:1515, 1988.

442. Morrow MJ, Sharpe JA: Torsional nystagmus in the lateral medullary syndrome, *Ann Neurol* 24:390, 1988.

443. Bjewer K, Silkerskjold BP: Lateropulsion and imbalance in Wallenberg's syndrome, *Acta Neurol Scand* 44:91, 1968.

444. Kommerell G, Hoyt W: Lateropulsion of saccadic eye movements, *Arch Neurol* 28:313, 1973.

445. Meyer K, Baloh R, Krohel G, et al: Ocular lateropulsion: A sign of lateral medullary disease, *Arch Ophthalmol* 98:1614, 1980.

446. Keane JR: Ocular tilt reaction following lateral pontomedullary infarction, *Neurology* 42:259, 1992.

447. Brandt T, Dieterich M: Skew deviation with ocular torsion: A vestibular brainstem sign of topographic diagnostic value, *Ann Neurol* 33:528, 1993.

448. Dieterich M, Brandt T: Ocular torsion and tilt of subjective visual vertical are sensitive brainstem signs, *Ann Neurol* 33:292, 1993.

449. Dieterich M, Brandt T: Wallenberg's syndrome: Lateropulsion, cyclorotation, and subjective visual vertical in thirty-six patients, *Ann Neurol* 31:399, 1992.

450. Dejerine J, Roussy G: Le syndrome thalamique, *Rev Neurol* 14:521, 1906.

451. Currier R, Giles C, Westerberg M: The prognosis of some brain-stem vascular syndromes, *Neurology (NY)* 8:664, 1958.

452. Levin B, Margolis G: Acute failure of automatic respirations secondary to a unilateral brainstem infarct, *Ann Neurol* 1:583, 1977.

453. Devereaux M, Keane J, Davis R: Automatic respiratory failure associated with infarction of the medulla: Report of two cases with pathologic study of one, *Arch Neurol* 29:46, 1973.

454. Caplan L: Bilateral distal vertebral artery occlusion, *Neurology (NY)* 33:552, 1983.

455. Ross MA, Biller J, Adams HP, et al: Magnetic resonance imaging in Wallenberg's lateral medullary syndrome, *Stroke* 17:542, 1986.

456. Duffy P, Jacobs G: Clinical and pathologic findings in vertebral artery thrombosis, *Neurology (NY)* 8:862, 1958.

457. Babinski J, Nageotte J: Hémiasynergie, latéropulsion et myosis bulbaire, *Nouv Iconog Salpetriere* 15:492, 1902.

458. Marinesco G, Draganesco S: Hémisyndrome bulbaire relevant d'un ramollissement de l'étage moyen du bulbe, suite de thrombus de l'artère vertébrale droite, *Ann Med* 13:1, 1923.

459. Paulson GW, Yates AJ, Paltan-Ortiz JD: Does infarction of the medullary pyramid lead to spasticity?, *Arch Neurol* 43:93, 1986.

460. Dhamoon SK, Igbal J, Collins GH: Ipsilateral hemiplegia and the Wallenberg syndrome, *Arch Neurol* 41:179, 1984.

461. Ho K, Meyer K: The medial medullary syndrome, *Arch Neurol* 38:385, 1981.

462. Ropper A, Fisher CM, Kleinman G: Pyramidal infarction in the medulla: A cause of pure motor hemiplegia sparing the face, *Neurology (NY)* 29:91, 1979.

463. Kumral E, Afsar N, Kirbas D, et al: Spectrum of medial medullary infarction: Clinical and magnetic resonance imaging findings, *J Neurol* 249:85, 2002.

464. Sawada H, Seriu N, Udaka F, Kameyama M: Magnetic resonance imaging of medial medullary infarction, *Stroke* 21:963, 1990.

465. Kleineri G, Fazekas F, Kleinert R, et al: Bilateral medial medullary infarction: Magnetic resonance imaging and correlative histopathologic findings, *Eur Neurol* 33:74, 1993.

466. Toyoda K, Hasegawa Y, Yonehara T, et al: Bilateral medial medullary infarction with oculomotor disorders, *Stroke* 23:1657, 1992.

467. Kase C, Varakis J, Stafford J, et al: Medial medullary infarction from fibrocartilaginous embolism to the anterior spinal artery, *Stroke* 14:413, 1983.

468. Davison C: Syndrome of the anterior spinal artery of the medulla oblongata, *J Neuropathol Exp Neurol* 3:73, 1944.

469. Jagiella WM, Sung JH: Bilateral infarction of the medullary pyramids in humans, *Neurology* 39:21, 1989.

470. Milandre L, Habib M, Hassoun J, Khalil R: Bilateral infarction of the medullary pyramids, *Neurology* 40:556, 1990.

471. Mizutani T, Lewis R, Gonatas N: Medial medullary syndrome in a drug abuser, *Arch Neurol* 37:425, 1980.

472. Imparato A, Riles T, Kim G, et al: Vertebral artery reconstruction, *Stroke* 12:125, 1981.

473. Alexander A: The treatment of epilepsy by ligature of the vertebral arteries, *Brain* 5:170, 1882.

474. Fisher CM: Occlusion of the vertebral arteries, *Arch Neurol* 22:13, 1970.

475. Moufarrij NA, Little JR, Furlan AJ, et al: Basilar and distal vertebral artery stenosis: Long-term follow-up, *Stroke* 17:938, 1986.

476. Labauge R, Boukobza M, Pages M, et al: Occlusion de l'artère vertébrale, *Rev Neurol* 143:490, 1987.

477. Moufarrij NA, Little JR, Furlan AJ, et al: Vertebral artery stenosis: Long-term follow-up, *Stroke* 15:260, 1984.

478. Hennerici M, Aulich A, Sandmann W, et al: Incidence of asymptomatic extracranial arterial disease, *Stroke* 12:750, 1981.

479. Shin HK, Yoo KM, Chang HM, et al: Bilateral intracranial vertebral artery disease in the New England Medical Center, Posterior Circulation Registry, *Arch Neurol* 56:1353, 1999.

480. Roski R, Spetzler R, Hopkins L: Occipital artery to posterior inferior cerebellar artery bypass for vertebrobasilar ischemia, *Neurosurgery* 10:44, 1982.

481. Bogousslavsky J, Gates PC, Fox AJ, et al: Bilateral occlusion of vertebral artery, *Neurology (NY)* 36:1309, 1986.

482. Desmet Y, Brucher JM: L'infarctus bilatéral du territoire latéral du bulbe, *Acta Neurol Belg* 85:137, 1985.

483. Ausman J, Nicoloff D, Chou S: Posterior fossa revascularization anastomosis of vertebral artery to PICA with interposed radial artery graft, *Surg Neurol* 9:281, 1978.

484. Ausman J, Diaz F, de los Reyes RA, et al: Occipital artery to anterior inferior cerebellar artery anastomosis for vertebrobasilar junction stenosis, *Surg Neurol* 16:99, 1981.

485. Sundt T, Piepgras D, Houser O, et al: Interposition saphenous vein grafts for advanced occlusive disease and large aneurysms in the posterior circulation, *J Neurosurg* 56:205, 1982.

486. Reivich M, Holling E, Roberts B, et al: Reversal of blood flow through the vertebral artery and its effect on cerebral circulation, *N Engl J Med* 265:88, 1961.

487. Fisher CM: A new vascular syndrome: The subclavian steal [editorial], *N Engl J Med* 265:912, 1961.

488. Daves J, Treger A: Vertebral grand larceny, *Circulation* 29:911, 1964.

489. Fields WS, Lemak N: Joint study of extracranial arterial occlusion. VII: Subclavian steal, *JAMA* 222:1139, 1972.

490. Heyman A, Young W, Dillon M, et al: Cerebral ischemia caused by occlusive lesions of the subclavian or innominate arteries, *Arch Neurol* 10:581, 1964.

491. North R, Fields W, DeBakey M, et al: Brachial-basilar insufficiency syndrome, *Neurology (NY)* 12:810, 1962.

492. Patel A, Toole J: Subclavian steal syndrome: Reversal of cephalic blood flow, *Medicine (Baltimore)* 44:289, 1965.

493. Siekert R, Millikan C, Whisnant J: Reversal of blood flow in the vertebral arteries, *Ann Intern Med* 61:64, 1964.

494. Hennerici M, Klemm C, Rautenberg W: The subclavian steal phenomenon: A common vascular disorder with rare neurologic deficits, *Neurology (NY)* 38:669, 1988.

495. Fields WS: Neurovascular syndromes of the neck and shoulders, *Semin Neurol* 1:301, 1981.

496. Fields WS, Lemak NA, Ben-Menachem Y: Thoracic outlet syndrome: Review and reference to a stroke in a major league pitcher, *AJNR Am J Roentgenol* 7:73, 1986.

497. Gerber N: Congenital atresia of the subclavian artery producing subclavian steal syndrome, *Am J Dis Child* 113:709, 1967.

498. Berguer R, Higgins R, Nelson R: Non-invasive diagnosis of reversal of vertebral artery blood flow, *N Engl J Med* 302:1349, 1980.

499. Brewster DC, Moncure AC, Darling C, et al: Innominate artery lesions: Problems encountered and lessons learned, *J Vasc Surg* 2:99, 1985.

500. Zülch KJ: On circulatory disturbances in borderline zones of cerebral and spinal vessels. *Proceedings of the Second International Congress of Neurology*, London, 1955, Excerpta Medica.

501. Zülch KJ, Behrend R: The pathogenesis and topography of anoxia, hypoxia, and ischemia of the brain in man. In Meyer J, Gastaut H, editors: *Cerebral anoxia and the EEG*, Springfield, Ill, 1961, Charles C Thomas, p 144.

502. Romanul F: Examination of the brain and spinal cord. In Tedeschi CG, editor: *Neuropathology: methods and diagnosis*, Boston, Little, 1970, Brown, p p 131.

503. Romanul F, Abramowicz A: Changes in brain and pial vessels in arterial boundary zones, *Arch Neurol* 11:40, 1964.

504. Mohr JP: Neurological complications of cardiac valvular disease and cardiac surgery including systemic hypotension. In Vinken P, Bruyn G, editors: *Handbook of clinical neurology*, vol 38, Amsterdam, 1979, North-Holland, p 143.

505. Brierley JB: The neuropathology of brain hypoxia. In Critchley M, O'Leary J, Jennett B, editors: *Scientific foundations of neurology*, Philadelphia, 1972, FA Davis, p 243.

506. Bickerstaff E: Basilar artery migraine, *Lancet* 277:15, 1961.

507. Swanson J, Vick N: Basilar artery migraine, *Neurology (NY)* 28:782, 1978.

508. Caplan L: A tale of two brothers, *Headache* 17:49, 1977.

509. Caplan L, Chedru F, Lhermitte F, et al: Transient global amnesia and migraine, *Neurology (NY)* 31:1167, 1981.

510. Simard D: Cerebral vasomotor paralysis during migraine attack, *Arch Neurol* 29:207, 1973.

511. Skinhoj E: Hemodynamic studies within the brain during migraine, *Arch Neurol* 29:95, 1973.

512. Olesen J, Larsen B, Lauritzen M: Focal hyperemia followed by spreading oligemia and impaired activation of CBF in classic migraine, *Ann Neurol* 9:344, 1981.

27 Microangiopathies (Lacunes)

J.L. MARTÍ-VILALTA, ADRIÀ ARBOIX, J.P. MOHR

Microangiopathies or cerebral small vessel diseases are the cause of alterations in the microcirculation. Cerebral microcirculation, the small blood vessels, are formed by small terminal arteries (branches of large caliber arteries of the carotid and vertebrobasilar system), arterioles or capillaries, venules with their arteriovenous anastomoses (the structural unit in which metabolic changes between blood and tissues takes place), and terminal cerebral veins. The small blood vessels are found in the surface of the brain or in the inner or deep cerebral tissue. These are the small cortical arteries and arterioles and the penetrating arteries, including superficial or medullary and deep penetrating arteries. Deep penetrating arteries include lenticulostriate, thalamoperforating, and brainstem paramedian branches. Arteries of the microvasculature, especially penetrating arteries, are electively altered as a result of hypertension and sudden changes in cerebral perfusion because they are terminal branches without anastomoses. As a result, microatheromatosis, atherosclerosis, and lipohyalinosis occur, which give rise to arterial wall thickening with a decrease in the lumen, intimal fibrous proliferation, disruption (splitting) of the elastica interna, hyalinosis in the tunica media, and adventitial fibrosis (fibrosis and wall thinning).[1]

Brain areas mainly supplied by microcirculation are cortical and subcortical areas; distal zones of frontier territories; centrum semiovale; central and deep encephalic areas, such as the caudate nucleus, internal capsule, globus pallidus, putamen, and the middle line of the brainstem; and the cerebellum.

Small vessel diseases or microangiopathies can be of different types: degenerative, such as lipohyalinosis or atherosclerosis of lacunar infarcts; hereditary, such as cerebral autosomal dominant arteriopathy with subcortical infarcts and leukoencephalopathy (CADASIL); mitochondrial, such as mitochondrial encephalopathy, lactic acidosis, and stroke-like episodes (MELAS); due to deposition of substances in the vessel wall, such as amyloid in cerebral amyloidosis or ceramide in Fabry's disease; or due to a poorly defined cause or an immunologic, inflammatory, or toxemic cause, such as in Susac's syndrome, Eales disease, or pregnancy or postpartum vasculopathy.[2] Alterations of microcirculation may be also caused by pathologic modifications of the blood without lesions of the blood vessels. Polycythemia vera, hemoglobinopathies, or proteinopathies may increase blood viscosity, which produce an increase in blood flow resistance and aggregation of blood cell elements and give rise to cerebral ischemia. Rarely, small emboli can be the cause.

Of all small vessel diseases resulting from angiopathies that affect microcirculation, the most common clinical entity is lacunar infarct. White matter changes are common findings in patients with lacunes; the association of lacunar infarcts and white matter changes supports the concept of small vessel disease as the underlying mechanism of these two conditions. Cerebral microangiopathies account for an important part of ischemic and hemorrhagic cerebrovascular diseases, particularly ischemic events, and among them, cognitive decline or dementia. Between 20% and 30% of all strokes are due to cerebral microangiopathies.[3]

Historical Aspects

In 1838, Dechambre[4] used the term *lacune* for the first time with pathologic criteria. The entity was confused with other cavitary lesions in the brain such as état criblé (small bilateral, multiple lesions in the white matter described by Durand-Fardel[5] in 1842; Fig. 27-1), residual necrotic tissue of small infarcts or hemorrhages, enlarged perivascular spaces (Fig. 27-2), and porosis due to postmortem bacterial autolysis.

In 1901, Pierre Marie[6] used *lacune* as his descriptive term for 50 cases of capsular infarction and clearly established the concept and classification of different small cavities in the brain. Marie emphasized a capsular and lenticular location for the syndrome. Ferrand[7] claimed the next year that the same syndrome occurred whether the lesion was capsular or pontine in location.

During the first quarter of the 20th century, the German pathologists Cecil and Oscar Vogt[8] firmly established the ischemic etiology.

Lacunes began their modern comeback almost entirely through the efforts of C.M. Fisher. Fisher described pure motor hemiplegia,[9] pure sensory stroke,[10] homolateral ataxia and crural paresis (known mainly thereafter as ataxic hemiparesis),[11] dysarthria-clumsy hand syndrome,[12] sensorimotor stroke,[13] basilar branch syndromes,[14] and the vascular pathology underlying lacunes.[15] The position was so thoroughly developed that it triggered companion studies, of which many corroborated[13,16] and others enlarged on the clinical entities, vascular pathology, and clinicoradiologic correlations.[17-19] Other researchers attacked the basic principles[20-22]: some argued for other causes including embolism[23] and others recommended that the concepts be abandoned altogether.[24] However, the high frequency of publications worldwide[25] indicates that the subject has become

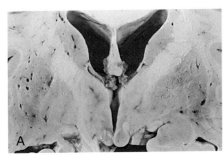
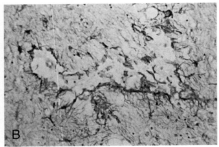

FIGURE 27-1   État criblé. A, Macroscopic coronal section. B, Microscopic pathologic specimen. (Glial fibrillary acidic protein [GFAP] stain.)

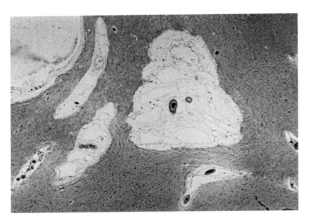

FIGURE 27-2   Multiple enlarged perivascular spaces in the putamen of a patient with marked small blood vessel disease. (Hematoxylin and eosin, ×40.) (From Garcia JH, Ho KL: Pathology of hypertensive arteriopathy. *Neurosurg Clin N Am* 3:487, 1992.)

firmly established among the syndromes of stroke. In some countries, notably China, the high frequency of deep infarcts has even been proposed to have a racial or ethnic basis.[26,27]

Numerous studies have claimed that the syndromes may have causes other than hypertensive arteriopathy.[11,28-31] Not long after the introduction of high-quality brain imaging, a wider range of locations of small, deep infarcts was found, together with an expansion of the syndromes associated with such lesions, now including the brainstem, parts of the thalamus, and other nuclei in the basal ganglia, corona radiata, centrum semiovale, and even some straddling of the thalamus and internal capsule; the concept was thus expanded to include syndromes overlapping with those caused by Binswanger's disease.[21,22,28,32,33] The earlier insistence on autopsy studies has largely been lost under the weight of publications based entirely on computed tomography (CT) or magnetic resonance imaging (MRI) findings. In recent years, it has been the exception, not the rule, to find a case report with autopsy correlation. Lamentably, *lacune* has passed into common use to refer to any small, deep lesion. Despite these shortcomings, *lacune* has become firmly established among the syndromes of stroke and is a useful term when it refers to a lacunar syndrome implying a variety of causes, topographies, and clinical features that need careful study by the clinician, not just a simple diagnosis at the bedside.

Definitions

As a term based on neuropathologic findings, *lacune* refers to a small, deep infarct attributable to a primary arterial disease that involves a penetrating branch of a large cerebral artery (Fig. 27-3). It should not be used to describe lesions of nonvascular origin, nor does it apply to deep infarction that is simply part of a larger stroke affecting the cerebral surface in continuity or separately, such as that which occurs in embolism affecting the middle cerebral artery. It is also inapplicable for describing deep infarction from disease involving the stems of the large cerebral arteries (such as the middle or anterior cerebral vessels) that affects the penetrating branches.

The low frequency of autopsy studies has forced modification of the definitions to include small, deep lesions found on brain imaging with CT or MRI. Numerous groups have attempted to define the term; most commonly, an attempt is made to distinguish among a small, deep infarct, the residue of a small hemorrhage, and dilated Virchow-Robin spaces; for those readers inclined to use numbers, these are types I, II, and III lacunes, respectively. In this chapter, we discuss first the autopsy-based material, then the studies based only on brain imaging, and finally the clinical studies.

Pathoanatomy

Table 27-1 summarizes the findings of pathologic series of lacunar infarcts.

Size

Most autopsy-documented lacunar infarcts are small, ranging from 0.2 to 15 mm^3 in size.[34] They vary according to the territory supplied by the occluded vessel feeding the infarct. In general, vessels are 100 to 400 μm[10] in size and serve territories varying from little more than a cylinder the size of the vessel itself to wedges as large as 15 mm on a side. Although the smallest infarcts are unresolved by CT scanners and occasionally even escape detection at autopsy,[18] the largest, the so-called super lacunes, are as large as 15 mm^3.[34] They are seen as obvious abnormalities at several levels on a CT scan. Thus, far fewer of these super lacunes have been examined at autopsy, and in some that were examined, no detailed search for the underlying vascular disorder was made. Embolism into the stem of the middle cerebral artery with occlusion of several of the lenticulostriate branches is a possible cause

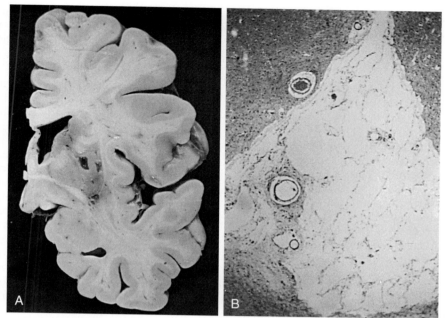

FIGURE 27-3 Lacunes in the basal ganglia. A, Macroscopic coronal section. B, Microscopic pathologic specimen. (Hematoxylin and eosin stain.)

TABLE 27-1 LACUNAR INFARCTS: PATHOLOGIC SERIES

Lacunar Series (Year)	Number of Cases	Number of Infarcts per Case	Topography	Risk Factors	Clinical Data	Causes of Death
Marie (1901)[6]	50	—	Lenticular nucleus	—	Pseudobulbar palsy; hemiparesis	—
Ferrand (1902)[7]	88	2.4	Lenticular nucleus	—	Pseudobulbar palsy	—
Hughes and Dodgson (1954)[343]	15	—	Lenticular nucleus (putamen/ caudate)	—	Pseudobulbar palsy	—
Fisher (1965)[28]	114	3	Putamen/pons/ thalamus	Hypertension (>90%)	Silent ischemic stroke	—
Fang (1972)[344]	51	—	Basal ganglia	—	—	—
De Reuck and van der Eecken (1976)[102]	75	4.4	Putamen/thalamus	—	—	—
Ishii et al (1986)[345]	30	12	Frontal white matter	Hypertension (86%)	Pseudobulbar palsy/ dementia	—
Mancardi et al (1988)[346]	51	2.02	Putamen/ thalamus/frontal white matter/ caudate	—	Pseudobulbar palsy	—
Tuszynski et al (1989)[88]	169	1.9	Basal ganglia/ internal capsule/ putamen/ thalamus	Hypertension (59%)	Pure motor hemiparesis (31%)	Ischemic heart disease/acute stroke
Dozono et al (1991)[347]	532	2.36	Frontal white matter/ putamen/pons	Hypertension (58%)	—	—
Arboix et al (1996)[348]	25	4.2	Putamen/pons/ frontal white matter	Hypertension (84%)	Silent ischemic stroke/pseudobulbar palsy/pure motor stroke	Respiratory events (pulmonary thromboembolism/lower respiratory tract infection)

of such infarcts, which do not deserve the name lacune except for their location in the depths of the brain.[35]

Location

Lacunes predominate in the basal ganglia, especially the putamen, the thalamus, and the white matter of the internal capsule and pons; they also occur occasionally in the white matter of the cerebral gyri. They are rare in the gray matter of the cerebral surface, as well as in the corpus callosum, visual radiations, centrum semiovale of the cerebral hemispheres, medulla, cerebellum, and spinal cord.[36] In general, the larger the series, the more widespread the lesions.[37] In the largest autopsy series reported thus far (169 found among 2859 patients), 81% of the lacunes seem to have been asymptomatic in life, which may indicate that many lacunes seen nowadays on brain imaging are of uncertain clinical significance.

Vascular Territories Involved

Most lacunes occur in the territories of the lenticulostriate branches of the anterior and middle cerebral arteries, the thalamoperforating branches of the posterior cerebral arteries, and the paramedian branches of the basilar artery. Their occurrence is rare in the territories of the cerebral surface branches.

The lenticulostriate vessels arise from the circle of Willis and the stems of the anterior and middle cerebral arteries to supply the putamen, globus pallidus, caudate nucleus, and internal capsule. They are composed of two main groups: those more medial, with diameters of 100 to 200 μm, and those more lateral, with diameters of 200 to 400 μm.[34] The thalamoperforating vessels arise from the posterior half of the circle of Willis and the stems of the posterior cerebral arteries to supply the midbrain and thalamus.[38] Their size varies from 100 to 400 μm. The paramedian branches of the basilar artery mainly supply the pons. Few branches have been measured, but sizes ranging from 40 to as large as 500 μm have been observed.[15,39] These arteries have in common both a tendency to arise directly from much larger arteries and an unbranching end-artery anatomy. The penetrators are all less than 500 μm in size and arise directly from the larger, 6- to 8-mm, internal carotid or basilar artery. Their small size and their points of origin rather proximal in the arterial network are thought to expose these vessels to forces that scarcely reach other arteries of similar size in the cerebral cortex.[40] These latter arteries are apparently protected by a gradual step-down in size from the 8-mm internal carotid, to the 3- to 4-mm middle cerebral, to the 1- to 2-mm surface branches, from which the intracortical vessels whose diameters are less than 500 μm arise. Perhaps this difference explains the low frequency of lacunes in the cerebral surface vessels.[41,42]

The lack of collateral circulation for the penetrators results in an infarct that spreads distally from the point of occlusion through the entire territory of the vessel affected. The exact volume of tissue supplied by each penetrating artery varies enormously.[15] Some arteries supply little more than a territory of the same diameter as the vessels,[34] whereas others arborize widely and leave an infarct shaped like a wedge or cone.[15] Most capsular

infarcts arise from arteries 200 to 400 μm in size and produce infarcts of about 2 to 3 mm[3]. These small infarcts are found regularly only on MRI with 1.5-Tesla strength, are commonly missed on CT scanning, and are easily overlooked at autopsy.[18]

The arterial occlusion usually occurs in the first half of the course of the penetrating vessel, which ensures that most such occlusions are quite small. These sites are not usually detected on angiography because the course of the individual vessels is difficult to plot, which makes it difficult to show that one is missing. However, in disease involving the stem of the cerebral artery from which the penetrator arises, or from one of the small number of large penetrators, a bigger infarction results. Occlusions at the ostium of a penetrator where it departs from the parent major cerebral artery may yield a swath of infarction some 15 mm large.[6] These so-called super lacunes[34] are large enough to produce a striking abnormality at several levels on the CT scan. In most instances, however, super lacunes result from occlusions of larger vessels and are not a sign of primary arteriopathy of the penetrating vessels.

Arteriopathies Underlying Lacunes

Microatheroma

Several distinct but related arteriopathies cause lacunes. Microatheroma is believed to be the most common mechanism of arterial stenosis underlying symptomatic lacunes (Fig. 27-4).[15,34,43] The artery is usually involved in the first half of its course. Microatheroma stenosing or occluding a penetrating artery was found in 6 of 11 capsular infarcts in the only published pathologic study on the cause of capsular infarcts,[34] and it was the cause of the only published case of a thalamic lacune.[10] The histologic characteristics of the microatheroma are identical to those affecting the larger arteries.

These tiny foci of atheromatous deposits are commonly encountered in chronic hypertension. In the usual nonhypertensive case, atheroma appears mostly in the extracranial internal carotid and basilar arteries but only rarely in the stems of the major cerebral arteries.[44,45] In hypertension, however, the lesions not only are more advanced for the patient's age but also are spread more distally in the arterial system, at times involving even some of the cerebral surface arteries. In patients with advanced hypertension, miniature foci of typical atherosclerotic plaques are found even in arteries as small as 100 to 400 μm in diameter, resulting in a stenosis or occlusion that sets the stage for a lacune. In a retrospective autopsy study of 70 brains with microscopic evidence of small vessel disease, the morphology of the vessel disease, the arteriolosclerosis, was similar in normotensive and hypertensive subjects. Lacunes were as prevalent in normotensive subjects (36%) as in hypertensive patients (40%), which suggests that the control of hypertension has modified the pathology of small vessel disease.[46]

Lipohyalinosis and Fibrinoid Necrosis

Other arterial disorders seem less common. Lipohyalinosis, formerly considered the most frequent cause of lacunes, affects penetrating arteries in a segmental fashion

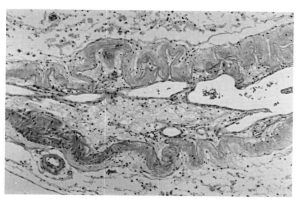

FIGURE 27-4 Intimal deposit of lipid-laden macrophages in a penetrating intracerebral artery that shows partial occlusion of the lumen. (Hematoxylin and eosin, ×100.) (Courtesy of J.H. Garcia, MD.)

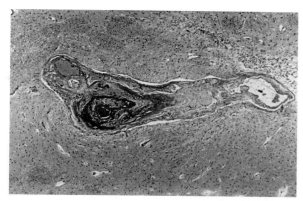

FIGURE 27-5 Terminal segment of a lenticulostriate artery showing marked mural changes (hyalinization and fibrinoid change) as well as occlusion of the lumen. (Hematoxylin and eosin, ×60.) (From Garcia JH, Ho KL: Pathology of hypertensive arteriopathy. *Neurosurg Clin N Am* 3:487, 1992.)

in chronic hypertension.[40] It was the cause attributed to 40 of 50 lacunes studied in serial section by Fisher[15] in four cases of stroke. It seems to occur most often in the smaller penetrating arteries, that is, in those less than 200 μm in diameter, and accounts for many of the smaller lacunes, especially those that are clinically asymptomatic. Lipohyalinosis has been thought to be an intermediate stage between the fibrinoid necrosis of severe hypertension and the microatheroma associated with more long-standing hypertension.[15,39,42]

Fibrinoid necrosis is a related condition found in arterioles and capillaries of the brain (Fig. 27-5), retina, and kidneys in a setting of extremely high blood pressure.[47] It appears histopathologically as a brightly eosinophilic, finely granular, or homogeneous deposit involving the connective tissue of blood vessels.[48] The mechanism is believed to involve disordered cerebrovascular autoregulation[49,50] and has a necrotizing consequence.[37] This thesis envisions that the thickened arterial walls are unable to constrict, which results in a resetting of cerebrovascular autoregulation at higher blood pressure levels. Continued high pressure produces increased capillary hydrostatic pressure and capillary damage. The overdistension[29,51] of these small arteries occurs in segmental fashion,[52] leading to vascular necrosis,[37,41,53] which allows red blood cells, plasma, and protein ultrafiltrates into the stretched segments of the wall.[52]

That other vessels are spared such injury is not easily explained. However, the arteriolar and capillary necrosis encountered in severe hypertension does not occur in renal arteries, which are protected from hypertension distal to an experimental arterial clamp or renal arterial stenosis. Larger vessels seem able to absorb enough in the subintima and in their thicker muscularis layer to resist such change, and the tiny cerebral cortical arteries of a size similar to the deep branches of the circle of Willis are protected by their more distal location.[29,37,42]

Fibrinoid necrosis shares some of the histochemical, electron microscopic,[29,54] and immunofluorescent[55] characteristics of lipohyalinosis,[56] another cause of lacunes. Both occur in the brain[15,34] in a setting of hypertension, and both occur in a segmental location along the course of the arteries.[15] The two conditions have also been labeled

hyalinosis, hyaline fatty change, hyaline arterionecrosis, angionecrosis, fibrinoid arteritis, plasmatic vascular destruction, atherosclerosis of small arteries, and segmental arterial disorganization. Although often considered identical,[15,34] segmental fibrinoid necrosis and lipohyalinosis differ histochemically in that fibrinoid necrosis is said to stain strongly for phosphotungstic acid hematoxylin, whereas lipohyalinosis does not.[47,52] In addition, lipohyalinosis is found most commonly in a setting of chronic, nonmalignant hypertension,[15,39] whereas fibrinoid necrosis is said to be found only with extreme blood pressure elevations[42,47] such as those that occur in hypertensive encephalopathy[42] and eclampsia.

Charcot-Bouchard Aneurysms

A long-standing, little noted controversy concerns whether lipohyalinosis or microatheroma is the precursor, is the result, or is even related to another commonly encountered arteriopathy in chronic hypertensive patients, Charcot-Bouchard aneurysms (Fig. 27-6).[15,31,57,58] The controversy also involves the following questions:

- Does the Charcot-Bouchard arteriopathy represent a true aneurysm formation, merely a dissection into the wall of a microatheroma, or twists, coils, and loops that are misdiagnosed as aneurysms?[59]
- Do both lipohyalinosis and Charcot-Bouchard aneurysms deserve consideration as pathologic processes separate from microatheroma of the penetrating arteries?
- Are these lesions simply variants along a spectrum of vascular effects of hypertension?

The available evidence suggests that lipohyalinosis is more significant than Charcot-Bouchard aneurysms in the development of lacunes.[15,58] No evidence has appeared to support an earlier suggestion that lipohyalinosis is the end stage of a preceding Charcot-Bouchard aneurysm.[31]

Other Causes

Microembolism has been inferred in a few serially sectioned lacunes shown to have normal arteries leading to the infarct.[34] Macroembolism is considered elsewhere, but

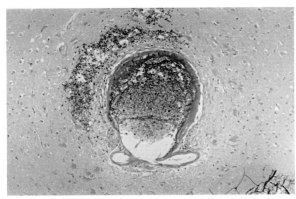

FIGURE 27-6 A saccular microaneurysm (Charcot-Bouchard aneurysm) with extravasated erythrocytes and reactive astrocytes. The longitudinally sectioned vessel is seen at the bottom. (Hematoxylin and eosin, ×33.) (From Garcia JH, Ho KL: Pathology of hypertensive arteriopathy. *Neurosurg Clin N Am* 3:487, 1992.)

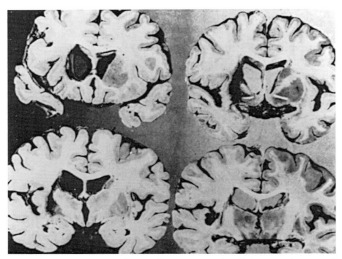

FIGURE 27-7 Large, deep infarct reported in the original series of pure motor stroke syndrome. (From Fisher CM, Curry HB: Pure motor hemiplegia of vascular origin. *Arch Neurol [Chic]* 13:30, 1965.)

one such case (case 10) is to be found among Fisher and Curry's[9] original descriptions of pure motor stroke (Fig. 27-7). Cholesterol emboli from atheromatous changes in the aortic arch have been shown occluding small arteries around multiple lacunar infarcts on pathologic examination.[60] Even polycythemia has been thought to be a cause of lacunes,[61] in that the small vessels may be obstructed by the sludged blood. Small, deep infarcts have been found in patients with antiphospholipid antibodies.[62] Dissection of a tiny artery may occur in the process leading to Charcot-Bouchard aneurysms.[63] Intracranial arterial dolichoectasia is considered to be an independent associated marker of small vessel disease such as lacunes.[64]

Attempts have been made[65] to relate severe extracranial carotid stenosis to deep infarcts on a hemodynamic basis when the lacunar infarct has been imaged on a brain scan. Although the mechanism has been presumed to be perfusion failure in the symptomatic deep territory,

the lack of autopsy data leaves unsettled the question of whether such infarction is from embolism from the carotid disease or is associated with severe stenosis of a penetrating artery.[66] Amyloid angiopathy related to aging can narrow the lumen of small arteries through deposition of amyloid in the adventitia and media and can produce small infarcts.[67] Varying forms of arteritis may also occur, especially that due to chronic meningitis (so-called Heubner's arteritis),[68,69] chronic neurosyphilis,[70,71] any severe granulomatous meningitis, and chronic fibrosing meningitis. Neurocysticercosis,[72] neuroborreliosis,[73] and acquired immunodeficiency syndrome (AIDS)[74] affecting small arteries can produce lacunar infarcts. Arteritides of unknown cause, such as polyarteritis nodosa and granulomatous angiitis, autoimmune disorders like lupus erythematosus,[75] and drug abuse, particularly of cocaine,[76] may produce small, deep infarcts. Lacunar strokes due to thrombotic microangiopathy, not vasculitis, in deep, small, or penetrating arteries is the main cause of early ischemia in patients with polyarteritis nodosa.[77]

Arteritis may have been a major cause of small, deep infarcts[78] when chronic neurosyphilis was in its heyday. However, two major works[69,79] on the subject contain no specific cases, even though the authors of one opined that "they undoubtedly occur."[69] This opinion was not shared by Pentschew,[71] who doubted whether "syphilitic endarteritis" was actually of syphilitic origin. In patients with first-ever stroke, chronic *Helicobacter pylori* infection detected by immunoglobulin (Ig) G antibodies was associated with a risk of small artery occlusion.[80] Pseudoxanthoma elasticum may also cause small deep infarcts.[81,82]

General Clinical Features

Lacunar infarctions share many risk factors, of which the most common are hypertension and diabetes mellitus. These two common accompaniments of lacunar disease have been present with comparable frequencies in those clinical series exceeding 100 patients collected over the last 20 years: 75% and 29%, respectively, of lacunar cases diagnosed in the Harvard Cooperative Stroke Registry;[33] 74% and 27%, respectively, of cases in the south Alabama population study[10]; and 72% and 28%, respectively, of the Barcelona series reported by Arboix et al,[82] in which only 26% of patients had cardiac disease. A high frequency of hypertension or left ventricular hypertrophy (93%) was found by Reimers et al,[83] whereas no clear correlation with blood pressure or hypertension was found in some of the smaller series.[84] In a prospective epidemiologic study of 3660 elderly people examined with cranial MRI, 23% had one or more lacunes; the lacunes were single in 66% of subjects and silent in 89%. Risk factors associated independently with lacunar infarcts were age, diastolic blood pressure, creatinine level, smoking, and carotid artery stenosis of more than 50%.[85] In other studies, the risk factors for silent lacunar infarcts were age, systolic blood pressure,[86] and plasma homocysteine level.[87]

The largest currently reported autopsy-based study was that of Tuszynski et al[88] (2859 patients), who found lacunar infarction in 169 patients (6%). Hypertension was present in 64%, diabetes in 34%, and smoking in 46% of patients, and there were no known risk factors for cerebrovascular disease in 18%. A correlation was found between high hematocrit value and hypertension in the patients with lacunar syndromes in a population-based study.[89] In the Barcelona Stroke Registry, 399 (11%) of the 3577 patients with acute stroke had a lacunar infarct.[90] In the Stroke Data Bank project of the National Institute of Neurological and Communicable Diseases and Stroke (NINCDS), 337 (27%) of the 1273 patients diagnosed as having infarction had typical lacunar syndromes. In this large cohort, no striking differences were found among the risk factors for each of the lacunar subtypes, but differences were found between lacunar syndrome stroke as a group and other types of infarcts.[91] Lacunar syndrome strokes shared risk factors with large vessel infarction, except for fewer transient ischemic attacks (TIAs) (13% versus 40%, respectively) and prior stroke (19% versus 39%). Compared with cardioembolism, lacunar syndrome strokes were more strongly associated with hypertension (75% for lacunar syndrome strokes versus 60% for cardioembolism) and diabetes (26% versus 17%) and less strongly associated with cardiac disease (24% versus 77%).[92] Lacunar syndrome strokes may be more common among black patients.[70] Diabetes and hyperlipidemia are associated independently with lacunes in patients with carotid artery stenosis.[93]

Atrial fibrillation, one of the hallmarks of embolism, has a low frequency of small, deep infarcts (5%),[94] similar to the frequency in the general population older than 60 years. In very elderly patients (older than 85 years), there is a high frequency of atrial fibrillation (28%) as a consequence of age.[95] In a series comparing patients with atrial fibrillation with control subjects, in which neither group was known to have symptomatic stroke, Kempster et al[96] found that all infarcts with atrial fibrillation were peripheral and consistent with embolism. In the control group, three asymptomatic infarcts were lacunes.

Prior TIAs are documented in approximately 20% of cases of lacunar infarcts, which is a frequency intermediate between embolism (5%) and large artery atherosclerosis (40%). No correlation has yet been documented among the type of lacune, severity of the clinical deficit, and occurrence of TIAs. Compared with TIAs in large vessel infarcts, TIAs in lacunar infarcts have a higher number of episodes, a longer duration of neurologic deficit in each TIA, and a shorter latency between the first and last TIA and the definitive infarction. Stepwise or stuttering onset is more common in lacunar infarcts with TIA than in those without. There is a positive correlation between the number of prior TIAs and the volume of the lacunar infarct.[97]

Compared with the sudden onset more typical of infarction in other territories, a leisurely mode of onset has occurred in many lacunar strokes, delayed over enough time that an opportunity often exists to determine the effects of intervention. In contrast to major atheromatous or embolic stroke, in which a gradual onset is encountered in less than 5% of cases, as many as 30% of lacunes develop over a period of up to 36 hours.[10,34,98,99] During this time, a mild weakness may evolve into total paralysis, usually by intensifying the initial deficit but occasionally by spreading into limbs not affected initially.[10] This smooth onset occurs with equal frequency in all types of lacunar syndromes. Sudden onset occurs in only 40% of cases.[99] The progression of initial motor deficit is associated with a poor functional outcome.[100] The rate of evolution of the stroke appears not to predict the severity of the eventual defect, but this matter has not yet received much detailed study. With respect to the circadian rhythm, the pattern of onset is uniform throughout the 24 hours.[101]

Lacunes typically manifest as the highly focal symptoms described later, but a few nonfocal symptoms have been reported in clinical series of patients with the typical motor or sensory syndromes. Lability of mood was once taken as a sign of multiple lacunes. This sign occurs in 26% of patients, with equal frequency regardless of whether single or multiple lacunes are visible on CT scanning.[102] It may simply be that multiple lacunes are present pathologically but are too small to be seen on the CT scan. To date, headaches (9% to 15%),[103,104] lightheadedness, hiccups, and asterixis do not occur in a predictable manner with a high frequency, nor has any symptom been correlated with the presence of a CT scan abnormality or with the size or location of the lacunes shown on the CT scan. In addition, none appears to predict the clinical outcome.

Clinical Syndromes

Lacunar State

For many years, lacunar state was what most clinicians understood was meant by the term *lacunes*. It was part of the original description by Marie.[6] His syndrome included a progressive decline in neurologic function punctuated by a few episodes of mild hemiparesis and followed by the appearance of dysarthria, imbalance, incontinence, pseudobulbar signs, and a short-step gait (marche à petits pas). Other clinical symptoms and neurologic signs are usually low mental speed, extrapyramidal symptoms (rigidity, hypokinesia), bilateral pyramidal signs (vivid reflex activity in the legs), positive masseter reflex, and dysphagia. Behavioral and psychiatric symptoms include depression, personality change, emotional lability, emotional bluntness, and mental slowness. This syndrome is also called *fronto-subcortical syndrome*.[105]

It was easy to envision that the small infarcts, widely scattered throughout the deep white matter, might accumulate gradually; each infarct is inconspicuous but the cumulative effect is devastating. Despite a few dissenting voices, matters have remained thus over the years.

Whether because of the effects of antihypertensive treatment or from some other undefined cause, the lacunar state is a rarity in modern times. One reason might be that the syndrome had been due to other causes. Fisher[63] pointed out that symptomatic occult hydrocephalus may have been the more common cause and that Marie's own published cases show such findings. He further noted that most lacunar infarcts are symptomatic and that the number of infarcts is small compared with the greatly deteriorated state of the patients. Earnest et al[106] and Koto et al[107] have observed a correlation between lacunar infarcts and hydrocephalus, suggesting that the infarcts may arise from the pressure on the white matter.

Pure Motor Stroke

Pure motor stroke is undoubtedly the most common of any lacunar form, accounting for between one half and two thirds of cases, depending on the series.[82,83,88,108] It was the first lacunar syndrome recognized clinically,[6,9] and its features have been the most thoroughly explored.

Clinicoanatomic Correlations

Pure motor stroke, also known as pure motor hemiparesis, has been reported from autopsied cases with focal infarction involving the corona radiata (Fig. 27-8),[102] internal capsule,[9,34] pons,[14] and medullary pyramid.[9,20,25] The most common correlations have been with capsular locations. Of the two ends of the capsule, the greater number of lacunes has been reported in the posterior limb (Fig. 27-9).

Posterior limb capsular lacunes usually involve the globus pallidus and posterior limb of the capsule,[109]

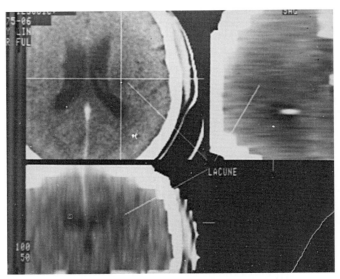

FIGURE 27-8   Lacune affecting the corona radiata.

which are supplied by the lenticulostriate branches of the middle cerebral artery. The vessels occluded vary in size from small, medially placed penetrators to the larger lateral lenticulostriate vessels. The infarcts range in location from the genu to the back of the posterior limb. It is in this group that most of the data referable to the classic views of a homunculus in the internal capsule are to be found. Lesions in this region, especially those affecting the corona radiata, have also produced the syndrome of ataxic hemiparesis.

Anterior limb capsular lacunes constitute a smaller number of cases and are smaller infarcts that may affect the caudate in addition to the anterior limb of the capsule.[18] Some of them are in the territory of supply of the anterior cerebral artery, including the largest of the penetrating vessels, the recurrent artery of Heubner. Syndromes of hemiparesis constitute only one of the many permutations of anterior capsular infarcts,[109,110] which also include ataxic hemiparesis[111] and some unusual speech and language disorders.[112,113]

Compared with the small number of cases with autopsy correlation, a steadily growing group of cases of pure motor stroke have been documented by CT scan alone. In the NINCDS Pilot Stroke Data Bank project, fully 45 of the 100 cases of lacunes were diagnosed with CT scans, most often as instances of pure motor stroke.[13] The pathology in such cases is rarely defined.

Other Causes of Pure Motor Syndromes

Nonlacunar pure motor syndromes have also been described, indicating that the clinical picture alone is not invariably due to deep infarction. Less than a year after Marie's description of lacunes, protests against his definitions were lodged. In an earlier thesis Abadie[114] contrasted the great frequency with which a capsular lesion was diagnosed clinically and the rarity with which such a lesion was found without other complaints accompanying the hemiparesis. His objection set the stage for many others down through the years.

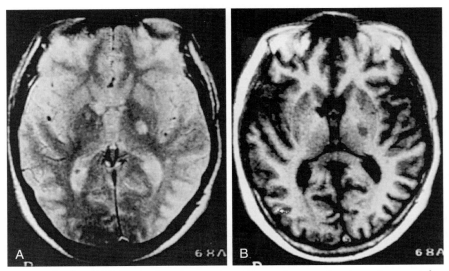

FIGURE 27-9   Axial (A) T2-weighted and (B) T1-weighted magnetic resonance images showing a lacunar infarct in the posterior limb of the internal capsule.

After Fisher and Curry's 1965 report[9] of pure motor stroke, several articles appeared, challenging the lacunar origin by detailing a similar syndrome due to a variety of other causes, including nocardial abscess of the motor cortex,[22] ischemia-edema after craniotomy for postoperative bleeding,[115] internal carotid artery occlusion in the neck,[116] and cerebral cortical surface infarction or ventromedial pontine infarction due to a propagating thrombosis of the basilar branch.[117] Lesions rostral to the capsule have been described in cases studied only by CT,[19] and the syndrome has also been encountered with both deep and superficial low-density lesions on CT that were inferred to be from infarction.[18] A few such cases have even been reported from hemorrhage.[109,118-122]

The clinical picture itself has also come under criticism. Richter et al[123] studied all cases of stroke that occurred in a single hospital and found that pure motor stroke occurred rarely, was not more prevalent among hypertensive patients, and did not usually have a good clinical outlook.

Even the most careful studies exploring the limits of the syndrome and its causes, however, have found a remarkably high percentage of cases with a clinical and radiologic picture conforming to the original syndrome described by Fisher and Curry[9]; Pullicino et al[18] studied 297 consecutive patients whose CT scans showed one or more foci of low density and found among them 42 single, small, deep lesions. Hypertension was more prevalent in this group than in the 122 patients with large lesions. Nine of the 42 (21%) with small lesions had a pure motor deficit, in contrast to only three of 122 (2%) with large lesions, a highly significant difference ($P < 0.0005$). Furthermore, in another 13 cases with isolated deep lesions, either the clinical deficit could not be related to the lesion or there was no clinical deficit at all, which is a point consistent with the observation that deep infarcts may spare the capsule.

Clinical Features

Pure motor stroke is most easily diagnosed when the stroke affects the face, arm, and leg equally on the same side, sparing sensation, vision, language, and behavior.[9] The complete syndrome, however, is somewhat uncommon. As a clinical rule, as long as the syndrome is purely motor, the diagnosis applies when the affected side involves one part more than the other. Some cases have been described in which the face is essentially spared; the best known is from pyramidal infarction.[124] In a series of 22 patients with a brachiofacial pure motor stroke, four had a cortical infarct in the superficial middle cerebral artery.[125] Pure motor monoparesis is almost never due to a lacunar infarct.[126] The term *pure motor stroke* was initially used to draw attention to the lack of expected accompanying sensory, visual, or behavior disturbances, especially considering the severity of the weakness. In this sense only is it "pure."

Pure motor stroke has been described in both capsular and pontine locations, producing a clinical picture essentially identical to that first suggested by Ferrand.[7] Some reports suggested that a case with capsular infarct might have an associated conjugate eye movement disturbance that would follow the hemispheral pattern (i.e., deviation of the eyes toward the side of the lesion) and that those involving the pons would have the opposite effect, the so-called wrong way eyes.[9,127] However, this finding occurs too infrequently to serve a useful function.[33]

Despite earlier opinions expressed by Ferrand[7] and by Foix and Levy,[128] it has become clear that pure motor stroke may be associated with considerable variations among the syndromes involving the face, arm, and leg. Fisher and Curry[9] found the arm severely affected in all 50 of their cases of pure motor stroke, but the lower the lesion occurred in the neuraxis, the less the face was involved.

When the lacune affects the internal capsule and corona radiata, the motor deficits encountered have shown considerable variety in both severity and form. Despite the many CT correlations with capsular lesions, only a handful of cases exists with a capsular infarct for which the syndrome was fully studied in life. Among this small group, there are remarkable variations. The most compact lesion with a hemiplegia was an autopsied case with an infarct confined to the third quarter of the posterior limb of the internal capsule.[129] This location corresponds to the approximate pathway of the motor fibers as inferred from whole brain anatomic dissections.[130] The clinical deficit had persisted for years, affecting the face, arm, and leg equally. In another autopsied case involving the same site in the posterior limb of the internal capsule, the deficit was less severe. Spastic hemiparesis developed over many hours and lasted for the remaining 9 months of the patient's life, paralyzing the tongue, palate, face, arm, and hand but only slightly affecting the leg.[47] In still another case, ischemia involving the posterior quarter of the internal capsule was associated with hemiparesis that only slightly affected the face.[33]

Most of the initial imaging studies were based on CT scans. Donnan et al[17] found hemiplegia involving the face, arm, and leg in equivalent fashion in all 36 patients with infarction involving the capsule, but 22 other patients in the same series had incomplete syndromes, the most common of which was paresis of the arm and leg that spared the face. The inferred lacune in these latter cases occurred more often in the fibers of the corona radiata or at the extreme ends of the capsule. One lacune with pure facial weakness was located at the genu, whereas another associated with pure leg weakness lay at the extreme posterior end of the capsule. Rascol et al[109] also found a spectrum of syndromes of hemiparesis that varied at one end from equal involvement of the face, arm, and leg to partial syndromes of faciobrachial weakness, and a few cases were purely crural[109]; similar incomplete formulas of hemiparesis occurred in the smaller capsulopallidal cases and also in the anterior capsulocaudate infarct cases. In both the NINCDS Pilot Stroke Data Bank project[108] and the population-based study of stroke conducted in southern Alabama,[131] lacunes located more posteriorly in the capsule produced a deficit greater in the leg than in the arm, but several varieties were encountered, including some in which the arm was worse than the leg. Lesions affecting the anterior limb and genu have also been a source of syndromes of partial hemiparesis, and a few cases have featured greater weakness of the face than of the leg.[17] In cases studied in the Stroke Data Bank, lesions seen in the corona radiata were associated with hemiparesis that took highly variable forms, whereas those located lower in the capsule produced a wide variety of syndromes (Fig. 27-10).[92] Taken together, the CT scan correlations with the syndromes of hemiparesis showed only slight support for the classic view of a homunculus in the internal capsule with the face, arm, and leg displayed in an anteroposterior distribution.

When these findings are taken together, it is no longer possible to infer the exact site and size of the lesion in the motor pathway using the clinical formulation based on the older dogma[132] that the motor fibers occupy a certain functionally reliable position in the posterior limb of the internal capsule. The case material only vaguely supports the traditional impression of a homunculus whose face is forward and whose leg is located posteriorly. These findings suggest that even more careful attention to the clinical details in future cases might permit a clearer understanding of the variability and reliability of the pathways that make up the capsule.[21,82,110,130] At the least, the findings thus far indicate that partial syndromes of hemiparesis

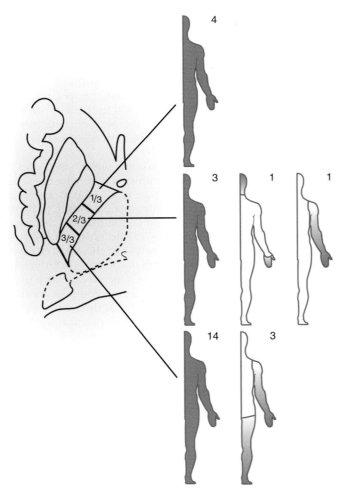

FIGURE 27-10 Hemiparesis formulas for capsular lesions of the anterior, middle, and posterior thirds of the posterior limb of the internal capsule. (From Chamorro AM, Saco RL, Mohr JP, et al: Lacunar infarction: Clinical–CT correlations in the Stroke Data Bank. *Stroke* 22:175, 1991.)

are common manifestations of lacunar infarction affecting the internal capsule and adjacent territory.

Associated Complaints

Although the main elements of the pure motor stroke syndromes are motor, other complaints are not rare, especially sensory disturbances, which occur initially in as many as 42% of cases.[17] These complaints usually are seen as numbness, heaviness, and loss of feeling. Only scant abnormalities are found on clinical examination. Given their vague character, they are all too easily brushed aside or ignored. However, complaints of undue coldness, at times confined to the distal arm, are less easily ignored, and, in a few cases personally observed by one of the authors, they have lasted for years.[33] The anatomic disorder of these complaints has not been resolved. These sensory complaints are thought to reflect slight involvement of the projections to the sensory cortex from occlusion of the larger lateral striate vessels, although few such cases have actually been documented by autopsy. When the perception threshold for temperature and thermal pain is measured, a significant thermal hypesthesia on the affected side is found. This semiologic finding has also been reported in pure motor and sensorimotor stroke.[133] No disturbance in visual field function has been described from such infarcts. Dysphasia, dyspraxia, and other disturbances of higher cerebral function have rarely been described.

Clinical Course

At clinical onset, the progression of the neurologic deficit is frequent, and lacunar stroke is the major cause of progressive motor dysfunction.[134] Improvement is seen in a high percentage of cases. It is usually more rapid and more complete than that after cerebral surface infarction with a similar initial motor deficit.[18] The syndromes of partial hemiparesis show the best prognosis, as do those with the smaller infarct size on CT scanning, but cases of complete plegia with virtually total recovery have been encountered. Rascol et al[109] found that all their patients regained the ability to walk. Fully 19 of the 30 patients experienced a favorable outcome, whereas another six were left with functional incapacity of the upper extremity. Thirty-five of the 42 patients documented in the pilot phase of the NINCDS Stroke Data Bank improved to a functionally useful level within a few months.[13] The improvement occurred regularly in the patients whose initial syndrome was incomplete. Unfortunately, of the seven patients initially paralyzed, only two experienced much improvement in the first few months, and both of them improved almost to normal. In five patients with pure motor hemiparesis, pontine (three) and capsular (two) functional MRI in the acute phase showed activation in the ipsilateral sensorimotor cortex and contralateral supplementary motor area and reduction in the contralateral sensorimotor cortex. After recovery, the activity normalized in the contralateral cortex.[135]

Pure Sensory Stroke

Pure sensory stroke is assumed to be due to infarction of the sensory pathway of the brainstem, thalamus, or thalamocortical projections. The thalamus is supplied by very small arteries susceptible to the effects of chronic hypertension.[38] Few autopsy-documented cases have been reported, and the syndrome was not noted in one large autopsy-based series.[88] In this small group, the most common location was the thalamus,[10,13,136] mostly in the ventral posterior tier nuclei, which is the main sensory relay nuclei to the cerebrum.[136] The only autopsied case with pure sensory stroke from a lesion outside the thalamus[137] consisted of a small hemorrhage that involved the corona radiata of the posterior limb of the internal capsule.

CT has been the basis of identification of the other sites associated with pure sensory stroke (Fig. 27-11). One case, inferred to be due to a lacune because of the small size of the lesion, affected the centrum semiovale, presumably with involvement of the thalamocortical

projection area.[138] Caution is necessary in this interpretation because lacunes in the centrum semiovale are distinctly uncommon in series based on autopsy data.[28,102] Involvement of subthalamic brainstem pathways has not yet been reported to be associated with pure sensory stroke. Pure sensory stroke due to a pontine tegmentum lesion can cause ipsilateral impairment of the smooth pursuit eye movements, which can be differentiated to thalamic topography.[139]

Observations of the arterial disease are confined to two cases. In one, a microatheroma was found narrowing the lumen of a small artery to the posterior thalamus,[15] which led to a lacunar infarct. The report did not mention whether the lacune was symptomatic. In the other case, a pure sensory syndrome was described clinically.[10] The 54-year-old patient was recovering from a right-sided pure motor hemiplegia when a feeling of pins and needles developed in the left lower lip, the left side of the mouth, and the fingers of the left hand; the sole of the left foot tingled and felt numb, dull, and swollen many hours later. No sensory deficit was evident on examination. Unpleasant paresthesias affected the left side of the face and the left foot. The CT scan findings were normal on the fourth day. At autopsy 6 months later, a lacune measuring 2 × 2 × 3.7 mm was found in the right ventral posterior nucleus, fed by four tiny arteries that arose from a single artery destroyed by lipohyalinosis.

The lacunes in both of the reported autopsied cases were quite small. If they are typical, it is easy to understand why many thalamic lacunes have thus far escaped detection by CT and require the higher grade image provided by MRI. Larger lesions may be seen with both techniques (Fig. 27-12). In a clinical series of 99 patients with pure sensory stroke that accounted for 17.4% of lacunar syndromes, a lacunar infarct on CT or MRI studies was observed in 84% of cases.[140]

Complete Hemisensory Syndromes

Typically, the disturbance in sensation extends over the entire side of the body, involving the face, proximal as well as distal limbs, and axial structures including the

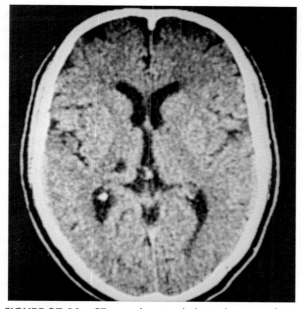

FIGURE 27-11 CT scan showing thalamic lacunar infarct.

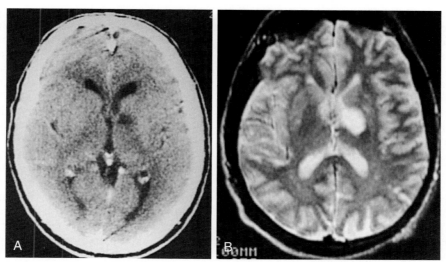

FIGURE 27-12 Anterior thalamic infarct seen on (A) CT scan and (B) MRI of the same patient.

scalp, neck, trunk, and genitalia right to the midline, even splitting the two sides of the nose, tongue, penis, and anus.[33,136] This remarkable midline split, especially when the trunk or abdomen is involved, may be unique to thalamic or thalamocortical pathway lesions. This type of hemisensory syndrome affected one patient with a thalamic infarction measuring $4 \times 4 \times 2$ mm.

In the earliest report of a patient with a complete hemisensory syndrome that was not attributed to a lacune, Wyllie[141] described the clinical picture as if a plumb had been dropped down the exact center of the patient's body so that exactly one half only was affected. In this case, the responsible thalamic infarct was not reported: Wyllie's main interest was the associated disturbances in higher cerebral function from the remainder of the large left posterior cerebral artery territory infarction. This complaint of total hemisensory loss has also been part of the syndrome in the small number of patients with the syndrome of sensorimotor stroke.

Incomplete Hemisensory Syndromes

Variants in the topography of pure sensory stroke have been reported that involve less than the entire side of the body. One patient, reported with autopsy correlation (case 9 in Fisher's original collection of pure sensory stroke[136]), suffered only TIAs affecting at one time the right fingers and at another time the right upper and lower lips, right side of the tongue, and the two medial toes of the right foot. At autopsy, a lacune 7 mm in diameter was found in the left ventral posterior nucleus. The complaints in other cases without autopsy documentation have involved the face, arm, and leg; head, cheek, lips, and hand; unilateral intraoral and perioral sites and fingers, the so-called cheiro-oral syndrome; face, fingers, and foot; shoulder tip and lower jaw; distal forearm alone; fingers alone; and leg alone.[36,136] How many permutations exist is a subject of some interest because establishing them might serve to determine the organization of a sensory homunculus in the ventral tier nuclei.

Lapresle and Haguenau[142] found partial sensory syndromes involving the face, the arms, the leg, the oral cavity, the peribuccal area and forearm, and the peribuccal area and radial edge of the forearm, of which all were from focal thalamic softening of lacunar size. As already mentioned, the patient in Fisher's case 9 suffered only TIAs affecting the right fingers at one time and the right upper and lower lips, the right side of the tongue, and the two medial toes of the right foot at another time.[10] A lacune 7 mm in diameter affecting the left ventral posterior nucleus was found at autopsy. In another autopsied case also previously described, a 54-year-old patient recovering from a right pure motor hemiplegia experienced a feeling of pins and needles in the left lower lip, the left side of the mouth, and the fingers of the left hand; the sole of the left foot tingled and felt numb, dull, and swollen many hours later. No sensory deficit was evident on examination. Unpleasant paresthesias affected the left side of the face and the left foot. CT scan results were normal on the fourth day. At autopsy 6 months later, a $2 \times 2 \times 3$-mm lacune was found in the right ventral posterior thalamus.[10] The complaints in other cases without autopsy documentation have involved the face, arm, and

leg; head, cheek, lips, and hand; face, fingers, and foot; shoulder tip and lower jaw; distal forearm alone; fingers alone; and leg alone. The full array of permutations has been subject to considerable study.[143] Incomplete hemisensory syndrome was present in 19 of 99 patients with pure sensory stroke (cheiro-oral in 12, cheiro-oral-pedal in six, and isolated oral in one).[140]

Electrophysiologic studies have found a well-organized topographic arrangement of the ventroposterolateral nucleus of the thalamus in animals, which has been confirmed in humans by single-unit studies of thalamic neurons. The location and size of the receptive field have been mapped, showing a high number of cells concentrated on perioral and digital sensation and only a few for the forearm and upper arm.[144] The organization of the cells is in the sagittal plane with cutaneous and deep stimuli aligned toward each other. The failure of the clinical syndromes from infarction to reflect this type of organization may be explained by the vascular anatomy. The small vessels, individually occluded, may cause an infarct that cuts across the functional anatomic fields of somatosensory projections, causing clusters of symptoms and signs from lesions that are at variance with the normal organization.

Nature of the Sensory Complaints

The patients complain of striking alterations in spontaneous sensations.[136,145] The parts feel stretched, hot, and sunburned, as if being stuck by pins, larger, smaller, or heavier. Contacts with the skin from eyeglasses, bedclothes, rings, watches, and sheets feel heavier on the affected side and may transiently aggravate the sensory disturbance. The stimulus seems to persist for a few seconds after its removal. In the patients with severe disturbances, the occurrence of a stimulus is better reported than its exact location. In a series of 21 cases, impairment of all sensory types (touch, pinprick, vibration, and position sense) was usually associated with large lacunes in the lateral thalamus; restricted sensory complaints suggest small lacunes at any level of the sensory pathway.[146]

The Dejerine-Roussy syndrome[147] is an uncommon accompaniment of lacunar infarction of the thalamus, although dysesthetic accompaniments are common in pure sensory stroke, as described previously. The full Dejerine-Roussy syndrome was originally described as the effect of occlusion of the thalamogeniculate branch of the posterior cerebral artery, with infarction of the ventral posterolateral and ventral posteromedial nuclei, largely sparing the remaining nuclei of the thalamus. Cases documented only by CT have shown a lesion small enough to qualify for a clinical diagnosis of lacunar infarction.[148] The initial deficit usually consists of hemiparesis and a hemisensory syndrome. The pain, which is an inconstant feature in cases with such infarcts, may begin at the onset of the syndrome or appear only later; delays of up to several months are common. The pains are intermittent or constant, appear spontaneously, or at other times are provoked by contact with the affected parts. They are usually accompanied by many other disturbances in sensation, including tingling, feelings of excessive weight, and feelings of cold, although a few cases exist in which the sensory function is normal on clinical testing. The special disturbance known as hyperpathia is particularly characteristic but not common: after a sensory stimulus, a disagreeable response occurs that is usually delayed in onset, may spread over a large area, persists after removal of the stimulus, and may even increase in intensity over several seconds. The syndrome may outlast other features of the original stroke syndrome and may even become permanent. Amitriptyline has been used with some success; treatment begins with doses of 10 mg at bedtime and increases to 25 mg after a week in most patients who tolerate the dry mouth; the doses can increase to even higher levels in some cases. A month or more may be required for benefit to appear in patients who show response to the therapy.

Associated Disturbances

Disturbances in motor function, language, and vision might be expected in a setting of thalamic infarction but have thus far been unreported, except for a single example of sensorimotor stroke due to a thalamic lacune (see later).[149] Given the anatomy of the thalamus and its widely varying projections to the cerebrum, such syndromes should be encountered but have thus far eluded the most careful diagnostic efforts of vascular neurologists.

Clinical Course

Improvement, often to normal within weeks, appears to be the rule.[143] The topography of the shrinking deficit may be rather unusual. Improvement in the trunk with persistence of deficit in the distal extremities, a pattern common in hemispheral disease, is only occasionally encountered. In one case, the deficit shrank to a vertical band from the axilla down the lateral trunk to the thigh,[98] which is a finding encountered by one of the authors (JPM) in several cases studied in southern Alabama.

Sensorimotor Stroke

Three autopsied cases of sensorimotor stroke have been reported to date,[13,119,141] but only one of which was published with "sensorimotor stroke" in the title.[13] Such cases, although rare, are important because they attest to the occurrence of a combined motor and sensory deficit from a small, deep infarct. Their vascular anatomy also helps clarify the vascular supply to the thalamus and adjacent internal capsule. The rarity of these cases should obviate any casual assumption that small, deep infarcts cause most cases of sensorimotor stroke.

The first case report that we found was published by Garcin and Lapresle[150] as part of a review of sensory disorders from thalamic infarction. The patient was a 65-year-old woman who suddenly developed left hemiparesis and a combination of hypesthesia and dysesthesia in the left peribuccal area and forearm. At autopsy, a small infarct was found straddling the intersection of the ventral posterior lateral and medial nucleus of the right thalamus. Involvement of the internal capsule was not mentioned.

The patient reported by Mohr et al[13] was a 61-year-old man. The sensory component preceded the motor component by several hours. The syndrome evolved smoothly and steadily over approximately a day and then stabilized for many days before beginning to improve. The sensory component involved the entire half of the body, including the neck, ear, and genitalia. The sensory and motor deficits each followed a temporal course and clinical profile typical of pure sensory stroke and pure motor stroke, respectively. Neither deficit faded completely with time, but both underwent considerable improvement. The hemihypalgesia shrank to a vertical band from the axilla down the lateral trunk to the thigh. At autopsy, a well-developed lacune 4 × 4 × 2 mm was found in the ventral lateral nucleus of the thalamus, and the adjacent internal capsule showed a slight pallor (Fig. 27-13). Efforts to track down the vascular supply to the infarct by means of serial sections were frustrated by the gross horizontal section made before embedding. The small artery found in the infarct was tracked downward toward its expected source from the posterior cerebral artery. Instead of gradually enlarging, however, the vessel gradually became smaller and vanished, leaving the investigators to infer that its origin was from above the infarct. Efforts to trace the artery upward also proved futile when the serial sections crossed the plane of the original gross section. Here the discontinuity was too great to permit matching of sections to map the course of the artery.

The third patient attracted more interest because of his action-induced rhythmic dystonia than because of the sensorimotor stroke.[151] The stroke occurred when the patient was 61 years old; he had had diabetes for 4 years. He fell suddenly, with left leg weakness. On examination, he was found to have a left hemiparesis "with loss of all sensory modalities." He improved within a week and was able to walk with support within a month. Involuntary movements began in the left leg by the fourth month. When examined by the investigators 4 years after the stroke, the

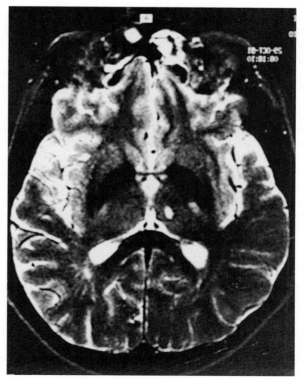

FIGURE 27-13   MRI showing a small thalamic lacune.

patient had slight lower facial weakness and slightly exaggerated left-sided reflexes but normal strength and sensation. Autopsy revealed an infarct 3 × 3 × 10 mm involving the ventral posterolateral nucleus of the right thalamus and adjacent internal capsule. No mention was made of the arterial anatomy of the lesion.

The neurovascular issues raised by the case are also of importance. Before such cases were documented, the vascular supply to the internal capsule was believed to be wholly separate from that to the thalamus. The lenticulostriate branches of the middle cerebral artery presumably supplied the capsule, and the thalamus was the artery presumed to receive its supply from the perforating branches of the posterior cerebral artery.[149] The extreme posterior nuclei of the thalamus received a few branches from the choroidal arteries.[38] However, three cases now exist showing that a single infarct may involve both the thalamus and the adjacent internal capsule. These cases suffice to overturn earlier claims and to reopen the issues of the boundary line between the middle and posterior cerebral artery territories.

At least 13 clinical examples of sensorimotor stroke have been documented by CT.[17,108,110,152] In these cases, the lesions were fairly large. Donnan et al[17] described one extending from the left putamen to the corona radiata, not obviously involving the thalamus. One of the authors (JPM) encountered two other examples in southern Alabama. The first case began as an incomplete pure motor stroke to which the hemisensory component was added within hours. This pattern was the reverse of the author's autopsy-documented case of sensorimotor stroke. In the series reported by Weisberg,[110] eight cases were described with "weakness and sensory disturbance and were found to have a hemiparesis and a decreased appreciation of pinprick, light-touch, vibration, and position sense involving the face, arm, and leg."[110] Large caudatoputaminal infarcts were seen on CT scans. It is presumed that these CT-documented cases affected the thalamocortical projections.

Sensorimotor stroke was caused by symptomatic intracranial small vessel disease in 69.5% of cases. However, other stroke subtypes were found in 30.5% of cases, a higher percentage than that observed in other lacunar syndromes. The striking similarity of risk factors and clinical features between sensorimotor stroke and other lacunar strokes and the important differences with non-lacunar sensorimotor stroke support the validity of the lacunar hypothesis.[153] However, apart from the cases reported by Groothius et al,[137] no autopsy-documented material has appeared to clarify the course followed by the thalamocortical fibers.

Ataxic Hemiparesis

The syndrome of ataxic hemiparesis has both cerebellar and pyramidal elements.[44] It was initially described as homolateral ataxia with crural paresis, which is its most familiar form.[11,154] The investigators of the original report speculated that the lesion might lie either in the anterior limb of the internal capsule or in the adjacent corona radiata. However, the first autopsied cases showed a pontine lesion of the small size typical of lacunar infarction.[44]

Since these early observations, numerous case reports have shown a low-density CT lesion lying in the corona radiata[155] or the posterior limb of the internal capsule, thalamus, lentiform nucleus, cerebellum, and frontal cortex.[44,99,102,110,156,157] These lesions have not been in the same site in each case and have been encountered as far forward as the head of the caudate and as far posterior as the posterior limb of the internal capsule.[102] Because the lesions in all these cases have been documented by CT scan alone, their exact correlation with the syndrome has been called into question by the disturbing case reported by Kistler et al.[158] The CT scan showed a corona radiata lesion; a nuclear MR scan revealed a recent pontine lesion that better explained the deficit. The pontine lesion was not seen on CT scanning because of the difficulty in averaging the bone densities adjacent to the brainstem. Because this effect prevents all but the largest pontine infarcts from being seen on CT scans, other cases may also have had a similar second lesion. In the series reported by Gorman et al,[159] 3% of patients with stroke fulfilled criteria for a diagnosis of ataxic hemiparesis. In another series, ataxic hemiparesis accounted for 4.1% of all lacunar infarcts, and the internal capsule was the most frequent lesional topography, followed by pons (13%) and corona radiata (9%).[160] In a series of 29 patients, diffusion-weighted MRI carried out within the first 4 days of stroke onset identified infarcts in 97% of patients; pontine lesions were the main topography followed by the internal capsule and corona radiata.[161]

Although the syndrome is best known to occur from infarction, it has also been reported from a tumor,[162] although not in as pure a form, or as intracerebral hemorrhage in the parasagittal part of the precentral area.[163]

The clinical features have been rather similar from case to case. The usual form manifests as a mild to moderate weakness of the leg, especially the ankle, with little or no weakness of the upper limb and face, accompanied by an ataxia of the arm and leg on the same side. In a few cases, a mild and transient hemisensory deficit may initially accompany the motor findings.[63,155] In one series of 100 patients with ataxic hemiparesis, sensory disturbances were frequently associated with the capsular location.[156] The syndrome commonly develops only gradually, requiring from hours to a day or more to reach its peak.[155] There are a few instances of a chronic state, but some degree of improvement within days or months is usual. In some cases, the syndrome changes: the hemiparesis clears but the ataxia remains.[155]

Efforts to separate a hemispheral location from a brainstem location have met with only limited success.[11,155] Patients with the former are said to have paresthesias when the lesion is in the thalamus, and those with the latter are said to have a slightly higher frequency of dysarthria and trigeminal weakness. In most instances, however, no distinctive features separate the cases of capsular or radiation origin from those involving the pons. The extent of weakness accompanying the ataxia is no guide to the location. In both the capsular and pontine cases, weakness may involve more structures than the leg, at times affecting the face and arm to almost the same extent. In all cases, the severity of ataxia is more striking than the weakness and exceeds that attributable to weakness alone.

Dysarthria-Clumsy Hand Syndrome

The dysarthria-clumsy hand syndrome has the advantage of emphasizing the distinctive elements of the stroke: In patients seen with the syndrome, the dysarthria and the ataxia of the upper limb appear to be the prominent components of the clinical deficit, but they do not occur in isolation. The syndrome usually also includes facial weakness, which at times may be profound; dysphagia; and some weakness of the hand and even of the leg. The reflexes on the affected side are usually exaggerated, and the plantar response is extensor. The clinical picture usually develops suddenly. The cases with autopsy correlation have shown no sensory deficit. In one case, the facial weakness was accompanied by impaired strength in opening the jaw.[164] In the case of pontine hemorrhage, several features differed from those reported with infarction: vomiting and lethargy occurred at onset; balance was impaired enough that the patient was unable to stand; and the facial weakness was mild. It was only after a week that the persisting deficit was reduced to dysarthria and a clumsy hand.

Some researchers have equated the dysarthria-clumsy hand syndrome with ataxic hemiparesis,[165] whereas Fisher,[63] the originator, has come to the view that it is a variant. The best-recognized association has been with lacunes of the anterior limb of the internal capsule.[28] Other sites have been reported less often: Spertell and Ransom[166] described a case with a low-density lesion near the genu, and two of Fisher's patients with anterior capsular infarcts had combinations of mild ataxia and dysarthria. In a few other cases, the lesion has been in the basis pontis or corona radiata.[167,168] The syndrome has also been reported from hemorrhage of the pons.[163] The outlook for functional recovery is good. Of 2500 acute stroke patients included in a hospital-based prospective stroke registry, 35 were identified as having dysarthria-clumsy hand syndrome, which accounted for 1.6% of all acute stroke, 1.9% of acute ischemic stroke, and 6.1% of lacunar syndromes.[168]

Atypical Lacunar Syndromes

In contrast to well-defined classic or typical lacunar syndromes, atypical lacunar syndromes (e.g., lateralized movement disorders; paucisymptomatic forms of a classic lacunar syndrome [e.g., pure dysarthria, isolated hemiataxia]; miscellaneous syndromes due to vertebrobasilar small infarcts or pure motor hemiparesis with transient subcortical aphasia) accounted for 6.8% of lacunar strokes in a clinical series.[169] In a comparative clinical study, risk factors and vascular concomitants were the same among classic lacunar syndromes and the miscellaneous group of lacunar strokes; thus this miscellaneous group of lacunar strokes may be included in lacunar strokes.[170]

Movement Disorders

Several types of movement disorders have been described with small, deep infarcts. Although the exact vascular occlusion has not been demonstrated in many of these cases, the small size of the infarct and its occurrence in territories fed by small penetrating arteries justify its possible inclusion among the lacunar syndromes. The disorder may appear as the only sign of the infarct or may develop later, after an initial syndrome, different in character, has resolved.

Hemichorea–Hemiballismus

Hemichorea–hemiballismus is the most commonly documented form of movement disorder, accounting for 68% in a series of 22 patients with movement disorders of vascular origin; lacunar infarcts are the most frequent cause.[171] The infarcts found in different parts of the striatum have been of lacunar size,[172,173] including those in the head of the caudate nucleus and adjacent corona radiata,[174] the subthalamic nucleus,[16,175] and the thalamus.[98,173,176] The onset is typically abrupt and is usually unaccompanied by other complaints. The chorea usually involves the forearm, hand, and fingers. In one case, it was accompanied by hemiparesis that faded within 3 months even though the chorea persisted unchanged.[174] In some cases, chorea has been delayed by some weeks or months after the initial occurrence of hemiparesis. One patient familiar to one of the authors (JPM), whose putaminal lesion was documented only by CT scan,[177] suffered choreic movements of the distal parts of the arm and leg that interfered with normal activity and prevented easy walking for more than 4 weeks. In this case the chorea improved, only to relapse a few weeks later. Rare ballistic movements were superimposed. The examination revealed normal strength, sensation, and reflexes.

Treatment with haloperidol is a common approach but has not been uniformly effective.[174] Doses as high as 5 mg three times daily have been required to suppress the chorea.[177]

Dystonia

Two types of dystonia have been described in cases of lacunes. Action-induced rhythmic dystonia has been documented by an autopsy study. In the case reported, the syndrome began as a sensorimotor stroke.[151] Both of the deficits improved within a month. By 3 months, the movement disorder began in the left leg, which had been the most severely affected part in the initial stroke. The disorder spread to involve the patient's entire left side. The fingers of the affected hand became flexed into the palm, leaving only the thumb free. When the patient was examined 4 years later, the hand was unchanged, but strength was otherwise normal. Voluntary movements of any parts of the body, including even eye closure, precipitated rhythmic dystonic extension and rotation of the left arm and leg (sparing the trunk) that subsided a few seconds after the voluntary movements ceased. Clonazepam and 5-hydroxytryptophan were successful in suppressing the involuntary movement disorder. At autopsy, an infarct 5 × 1 × 2 mm was found straddling the ventral posterolateral nucleus and the adjacent posterior limb of the internal capsule.

The other type is a focal dystonia. One patient has been described whose CT scan showed a low density in the right lenticular nucleus.[178] As with the cases of hemichorea and hemiballismus, the deficit appeared abruptly, unaccompanied by weakness or sensory disturbances.

Only the distal end of the upper extremity was affected. Although it was described as dystonic, the disorder featured changing postures: "The movements were slow and caused the patient's fingers to assume unusual positions. Activity exacerbated the movements...the left hand and forearm showed involuntary movements that produced an unusual posture, with hyperpronation and flexion at the wrist, extension of the fingers, and opposition of the thumb." Haloperidol, 1 mg three times daily, relieved much of the movement and posture disorder. Attempts to remove the medication more than 8 months later produced relapse, requiring reinstitution of therapy to suppress the disorder.

Pseudochoreoathetosis

The syndrome pseudochoreoathetosis, consisting of piano-playing movements of the fingers contralateral to the lesion and due to a loss of proprioception, has been described during the acute phase in three patients with lacunar thalamic infarcts.[179]

Asterixis and Tremor

The unilateral flapping tremor or asterixis affecting an upper extremity may be produced by a lacunar infarct in the basal ganglia, thalamus, internal capsule, or midbrain, although no cases with pathologic images have been published.[180,181] Unilateral tremor can appear several months after the initial lacunar infarction in the caudate nucleus or the thalamus.[182,183]

Speech and Language Disorders

Mutism, Aphonia, and Anarthria

Bilateral capsular lacunar infarctions have been a cause of mutism in the absence of any disturbance in language or praxis. One patient reported by Fisher,[34] in whom infarction was documented by microscopic vascular pathology, had no difficulty with speech after his first infarct but became mute with the second infarct, which involved the left internal capsule. The left capsular lacune was $4 \times 4 \times 5$ mm and lay at the genu. Marie[6] had earlier reported a case of unilateral stroke with "anarthria" and no aphasic symptoms, but the cause of the small, deep lesion was a putaminal hemorrhage.

In subsequent years, several such cases, in which the lesions were documented on brain imaging, have been reported. None of these patients with bilateral capsular infarcts have had aphasia apart from the disturbance in articulation. One of the author's (JPM) collection includes a case of an infarct affecting the posterior limb of the right internal capsule followed by an infarct affecting the left internal capsule at the genu.[108] This last infarct was so small that it was barely visible on the CT scan, yet it yielded virtual anarthria, severe dysphonia, and dysphagia but only a mild right arm weakness. Three others have been reported, each with bilateral capsular infarcts involving the genu or anterior limb of the capsule.[88,184,185]

Disorders of Language

Considerable doubt still remains as to whether aphasic disturbances per se occur from lacunes. At least one case indicates that they may.[63] In most instances, the cause is not the primary arteriopathy, but instead is embolism into the stem of the middle cerebral artery with involvement of many lenticulostriate vessels together. Fisher's patient is the only autopsy-verified patient to date reported with a language disorder from an infarct involving the territory of a lenticulostriate. The syndrome included a modified pure motor hemiparesis with "motor aphasia." It was attributed to a large infarct involving the genu and anterior limb of the internal capsule and adjacent white matter of the corona radiata. Speech initially was dysarthric, progressed later to mispronunciation of words and then to a state of utterance of single-syllable unintelligible sounds, and ended in mutism. Comprehension was reportedly intact. The accompanying weakness severely affected the right side of the face and moderately involved the right hand. This case is important not because of the large size of the infarct but because the underlying lesion was a thrombosis of a lenticulostriate artery.

One case diagnosed on CT scan only has also been associated with a small lesion.[186] It was but one among eight large, deep infarcts attributed to cardiac embolism; the patient was seen with an "expressive dysphasia." The disturbance was characterized by "nonfluent conversational speech, naming and reading difficulties, dysgraphia, and normal auditory comprehension." This case is of special interest, given the small size of the lesion demonstrated on the CT scan because a lacunar cause is in the differential diagnosis.

That unilateral, large, deep infarcts may disrupt language function to some extent has never been the subject of serious dispute (Fig. 27-14). Several well-known cases attest to the correlation. However, except for the case noted previously, in each case the infarct was quite large, of the super lacune category, well beyond the usual limits of the infarcts caused by primary disease of the penetrating arteries. Although it is described in more detail elsewhere in this volume, the subject is touched on here to settle the point of the larger size of the infarcts.

Two famous cases are on record with large infarctions documented by autopsy. Bonhoeffer's[187] classic case was associated with a large, deep lesion typical of the type I lacuna described by Rascol et al,[109] involving the caudate nucleus, internal capsule, and putamen as far laterally as the external capsule. The patient was unable to speak anything more than a few poorly formed vowels. The cause of the lesion was undetermined, but its large size suggested occlusion of the middle cerebral artery stem. An embolic mechanism was suggested by the second infarct, of fairly large size, affecting almost the entire anterior cerebral artery territory. Kleist[188] reported a case with an infarct of similar size and location (Bühlmeir case) featuring severe dysarthria, rare paraphasias, and only a slight disturbance in comprehension. No mention was made of the vascular pathology.

Thirteen other cases to date have been documented by CT scanning, all of which involved large, deep infarcts.[112,113,186] In the series reported by Naeser et al,[113] at least three patients had accompanying surface infarcts. That an accompanying surface infarct that is not obvious on CT scan might be the cause keeps the value of the reports based entirely on CT scans well below that of reports with autopsy documentation. These cases have

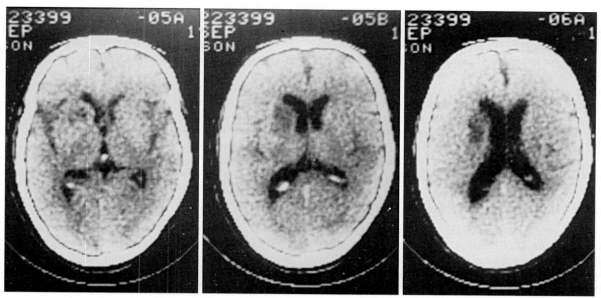

FIGURE 27-14 Large anterior capsular infarct with dysnomia.

been characterized by dysprosody, at times accompanied by dysarthria and a mixture of deficits in syntactic and semantic functions not typical of any of the classic syndromes of dysphasia.

Other Disorders of Higher Cerebral Function

A single instance of pure motor stroke with "confusion" has been reported, in which a 1.2-cm lacune affecting the anterior limb and the anterior portion of the posterior limb of the right internal capsule has been documented.[34] The behavior disorder was characterized as "acute onset of confusion and impairment of attention and memory." Later studies using brain imaging to document the lesion have found a few instances of deep infarction, usually affecting the genu or anterior limb of the internal capsule and causing a greatly reduced level of activity. In a study comparing 11 patients who had multiple lacunes with 11 control subjects, Wolfe et al[189] found that patients with lacunar infarcts showed neuropsychological signs of frontal system disturbance, although only 27% met clinical criteria for a diagnosis of dementia. The disturbances were described as "shifting mental set, response inhibition, and executive function," and the patients with these disturbances "were more often rated apathetic on a behavior-rating scale." Symptomatic supratentorial lacunar infarction, even single, can determine neuropsychological impairment, decreased performance for mental capacities, and, more often than in control subjects, emotional disturbances.[190] In a prospective series of 40 lacunar stroke patients studied within 1 month after stroke onset, 57% of them showed mild neuropsychological disturbances.[191] Some insight into the underlying mechanisms was provided in the study of one patient by Satomi et al,[192] who performed a single-photon emission computed tomogram (SPECT) study with ^{123}I iodoamphetamine; this study showed decreased vasoreactivity, predominantly to the frontal lobes. Tatemichi et al[193] studied a right-handed man whose infarct was limited to the genu of the capsule in the left hemisphere;

they suggested that the impaired SPECT reactivity could be from interruption of thalamofrontal projections passing below the genu, producing a syndrome of frontal lobe dysfunction without a direct lesion to the frontal lobe. This patient became the index case for a series subsequently reported with similar clinical features.

The literature continues to document disorders of language, memory, orientation, and activity after infarction of the paramedian thalamic nuclei. Except for two reports,[194,195] CT has been the basis for lesion localization. In many of these cases, including some of the autopsied material collected by Castaigne et al,[194] embolism to the top of the basilar artery or to the posterior cerebral artery stem or thrombosis of the basilar artery may have been the cause, rather than vascular disease of the lacunar type. Given the origin of these cases, CT might not reveal all the foci of infarction, which makes the correlation of clinical features with CT findings a bit unreliable.[23,196-198] In the few cases with autopsy documentation, the arterial disease has been rather unusual. Poirer et al,[195] for example, encountered a picture of thalamic dementia. Autopsy showed many small, deep infarcts of lacunar size. These researchers formed the impression that the lesion was an angiitis hitherto undefined. Among the cases documented only by CT, hypertension, a normal angiogram, several spells typical of TIAs before the final stroke, and then the emergence of a CT-positive low-density lesion have been documented in a few instances; this pattern seems consistent with the course expected of lacunar disease. The patient reported by Michel et al[23] is such an example, described as having a thalamic lacune. The initial deficit consisted of right hemiparesis with agitation, disorientation, and language disturbances. The language disorder was of the expressive type, with reduction in language, slowness in response, and some verbal paraphasias. Verbal memory was greatly disturbed and was the subject of a special investigation. The presence of the hemiparesis might mean that the scope of the lesion exceeded that seen on the CT scan, but this issue was not settled.

A single case of dysphasia with a small thalamic infarction documented by CT scan has been reported.[58] The infarct was large enough to include the ventral anterior and rostral ventral lateral nucleus, which might be too large for an infarct from primary disease of the thalamoperforating vessels. No cause of the infarct was found. In the other cases in the literature, the infarcts were bilateral or large enough to make it unlikely that they were due to primary arteriopathy of the penetrating vessels. These cases are detailed elsewhere in this book. The last word has not been written on the syndromes of deep infarction with disturbances in speech and language.

Infarcts in the Centrum Semiovale

The centrum ovale, or semiovale from Vieussens, is the region of cerebral hemispheres at the top of the brainstem. It includes the white matter with the projection and association fibers between the cortex and deep structures of the hemispheres, and its name is due to the oval appearance in horizontal sections of the brain. Perforating medullary arteries supply this region. These small arteries, without anastomosis, have their origin at the superficial or pial branches from the middle cerebral artery, until the lateral ventricle walls.

Infarcts due to small vessel disease can occur in the centrum semiovale, can be large or small, usually less than 1.5 cm in diameter, and with a round or ovoid shape. In a clinical study of 1800 consecutive admissions, 21 patients had an infarct in the centrum semiovale (1.2%); the majority of infarcts were small (<1.5 cm), and only 13% of patients were seen with large infarcts (>1.5 cm).[199] Arteriopathy of the medullary branches related to hypertension or diabetes is the main cause. Hypotension and embolic stroke involving the penetrating arteries or the parent vessel can also be the cause. Large vessel atherosclerosis with stenosis and distal perfusion failure is also possible.[200,201] Multiple infarcts in the centrum semiovale are rarely of lacunar origin, even if they do not exceed 1.5 cm in diameter; most are a consequence of hemodynamic failure and have a rosary-like appearance.[202]

In a pathologic series of 12 cases, of which six were symptomatic, there was evidence of small artery disease in all cases. Borderzone localization was seen in the centrum semiovale; the most commonly involved area was the zone between the middle and anterior cerebral artery territories.[203]

Small infarcts are either silent or not. Neurologic features are usually related to a lacunar, motor, or sensory syndrome. Because of the small size of the infarct and the amplitude of the connecting ascending or descending fibers at this region, the clinical picture, motor or sensory, can be frequently partial or nonsymmetrical in the two extremities.[204] CT or MRI studies can show the semioval infarct related to the clinical symptoms. The prognosis of the deficit in patients with infarct in the centrum ovale is usually good.

Microangiopathies in Vascular Dementia

Cerebrovascular diseases of different origins can be the cause of vascular cognitive impairment. This more wide and generic term allows the inclusion of different degrees of cognitive disturbances and causative vascular disorders and has replaced the term *multiinfarct dementia*.[205]

Cognitive impairment may be mild (i.e., mild cognitive impairment or cognitive impairment no dementia) or can affect daily living activities (i.e., vascular dementia). The vascular cause may coexist with degenerative alterations characteristics of Alzheimer's disease (i.e., mixed dementia).

Cognitive impairment of vascular etiology may be due to small vessel disease (microangiopathies) or large vessel disease, which is usually termed *poststroke dementia*. One third of patients with dementia show abnormalities of the cerebral vasculature in autopsy studies.[206]

Vascular Dementia

Impairment of cognitive function with interference of daily life activities secondary to cerebrovascular disease is vascular dementia. Vascular dementia includes the concepts of leukoaraiosis, subcortical dementia, multiinfarct dementia, and poststroke dementia. Vascular dementia due to alteration of the white matter may be of three types: atherosclerosis, amyloid angiopathy, and CADASIL.

Clinical recognition of vascular dementia requires the following data: medical history and a neurologic examination in which the presence of cognitive impairment, vascular risk factors, and possible cerebral abnormalities will be assessed; a neuropsychological study to confirm and quantify the degree of dementia; a neuroimaging study with MRI to assess the presence of vascular lesions; and etiologic, arterial, cardiac, or hematologic investigation of causes of the cerebrovascular disease.

Vascular dementia is the second cause of dementia.[207] Lacunar infarct is the most common stroke subtype that predisposes to vascular dementia.[208,209] In clinical studies, the proportion of vascular dementia caused by small vessel disease or subcortical vascular dementia ranges from 36% to 67%.[210] In three prospective studies, approximately 11% of patients with first-ever lacunes developed vascular dementia over the following 3 years, which translates into an annual incidence of about 3% to 5% per year.[211,212]

Cognitive impairment in patients with symptomatic lacunes is influenced by stroke recurrence, the presence of multiple infarcts (symptomatic or silent), and white matter abnormalities. The degree of preexisting white matter disease, infarct volume, and global and medial temporal lobe atrophy have been identified as some of the relevant neuroimaging determinants of poststroke dementia.[213]

In subcortical vascular dementia, the primary types of brain lesions are lacunar infarcts and ischemic white matter lesions; demyelination and loss of axons, a decreased number of oligodendrocytes, and reactive astrocytosis are seen. The primary lesion site is the subcortical region.[214,215] This type of vascular dementia includes the old entities *lacunar state* and *Binswanger's disease*. These are the two main pathophysiologic pathways involved in subcortical vascular dementia and often coexist in the same patient. In the first, occlusion of the arteriolar lumen due to atherosclerosis leads to the formation of lacunes, which results in a lacunar state (l'état lacunaire). In the second, critical stenosis and hypoperfusion of multiple medullary arterioles cause widespread incomplete infarction of deep white matter[216] with the clinical picture of Binswanger's disease.

Patients with subcortical vascular dementia often have a history of multiple vascular disorders, including hypertension, diabetes, and ischemic heart disease. The onset of dementia is insidious in more than half of the patients, and the course is usually continuous and slowly progressive but seldom stepwise.[217]

The typical cognitive syndrome in patients with subcortical vascular dementia is the *dysexecutive syndrome.* It includes slowed information processing, memory deficits, and behavioral and psychiatric symptoms,[218] as well as impairment in goal formulation, initiation, planning, organizing, executing, and abstracting.[219] The essential neuroimaging changes in subcortical vascular dementia include extensive ischemic white matter lesions and lacunar infarcts in the deep gray and white matter structures. These manifestations probably result from ischemic interruption of parallel circuits from the prefrontal cortex to the basal ganglia and the corresponding thalamocortical connections.[220]

Mild cognitive impairment of the vascular type was found in 22 of 40 consecutive patients with acute lacunar infarction. When voxel-based morphometry was used, both gray and white matter changes seemed to contribute to the cognitive impairment of such patients.[221] Furthermore, about 10% of patients with mild cognitive impairment related to cerebrovascular disease developed vascular dementia within 1 year.[222-225] However, some authors have reported a general functional improvement in 2.7% to 31.0% of these patients during the first year[222,223,226,227] or even the second year,[228] while others found a progressive decline of the cognitive impairment in general.[229,230]

Binswanger's Disease

In 1894, the Swiss physician Otto Ludwig Binswanger (1852-1929) described a form of vascular dementia with the name *encephalitis subcorticalis chronica progressiva,*[231] the disease that is currently known with his name. For the first time, a causal relationship between cerebrovascular disease and dementia was established. After stating the low frequency of presentation (eight cases over 11 years), Binswanger described salient clinical and pathologic features of the disease. Starting in the sixth decade of life, the clinical picture included progressive intellectual deterioration associated with focal neurologic signs, such as aphasia, hemiparesis, sensory loss on one side of the body, or hemianopsia. The disease had a fluctuating clinical course with periods of stabilization and worsening for about 10 years or more. Death of the patients was attributed to general causes, such as heart failure, infection, or an acute stroke episode.

Current criteria for the definition of Binswanger's disease include (1) dementia; (2) one of the following: (a) presence of a vascular risk factor or systemic vascular disease, such as cardiopathy, (b) evidence of cerebrovascular disease, or (c) evidence of subcortical cerebral dysfunction, such as parkinsonism; and (3) leukoaraiosis on the CT scan or multiple bilateral subcortical hyperintensity images greater than 2 × 2 mm on T2-weighted MRI scans.[232] The presence of severe dementia (Mini-Mental State Examination score, <10) or cortical lesions on CT or MRI scans invalidate the aforementioned criteria.

Arterial hypertension is a risk factor found in leukoaraiosis, lacunar infarcts, and Binswanger's disease. This association suggests that these entities form part of the same process: hypertensive microangiopathy. However, hypertension is not a uniform risk factor because it presents variations during the daytime and at night and may cause episodes of hypoperfusion, with alteration of the subcortical white matter substance. Ambulatory 24-hour blood pressure monitoring has shown more pronounced daytime blood pressure variations, although without statistical significance, in patients with Binswanger's than in patents with lacunar infarction. Changes in blood pressure are a risk factor for small vessel disease but not for the cognitive impairment of Binswanger's disease.[233]

Pathology. Binswanger described macroscopic findings in a single case. This was a patient with a history of syphilitic infection who, at the end of the fourth decade of life, presented a clinical picture of headaches, paresthesia in the right arm and leg, impairment of fine movements in the right hand, and speech disturbance with paraphasia, in association with calculation dysfunction, memory impairment, and intellectual deterioration. After a progressive clinical course with episodes of agitation and confusion, an infection was the cause of the patient's death. The necropsy study revealed alteration of the most posterior cerebral segments, with atrophy of the white matter mainly in the temporal and occipital lobes, dilatation of the ventricular system especially of the inferior horns, and minimal reduction of the frontal cortex volume. He did not mention the presence of cavitary lesions, focal abnormalities, or atherosclerotic changes in the basal arteries or vessels of small caliber. In this case, demential syndrome and an abnormality of the white matter substance were related for the first time. Binswanger later described two related clinical entities of acute onset, arteriosclerotic brain degeneration and dementia postapoplexiam, different from the initial report.

Alzheimer,[234] when analyzing mental abnormalities of cerebral atherosclerosis, that is, cognitive impairment of vascular origin, mentioned that two types may occur: those involving cerebral cortex by alteration of large arteries, and those involving the white matter by alteration of small arterial vessels. In Binswanger's disease, cerebral cortex is preserved, but there is reduction of the white matter volume and secondary degeneration foci in the internal capsule, lenticular nucleus, or thalamus. It was also stated that these abnormalities were due to severe atherosclerosis of arteries of the deep white matter cerebral hemispheres.

In an attempt to define pathologic criteria of Binswanger's disease, subsequent reports including the study of Bucholz[235] with five cases, Ladame[236] with one case, and Nissl[237] indicated that the disease was a severe form of cerebral atherosclerosis. Olszewski[238] added two new cases and proposed the term *subcortical arteriosclerotic encephalopathy* due to predominant involvement of the white matter and subcortical vessels. Biemond[239] suggested for the first time the possibility of making the diagnosis of the disease during life on the basis of clinical data only. De Reuk et al[240] described four new patients and concluded that lacunar infarcts in the thalamus and basal ganglia had an analogous substrate to abnormalities of periventricular white matter, which is the frontier area vascularized by penetrating arteries. Fisher[241] proposed lacunar infarcts as the morphologic basis of Binswanger's disease. Multiple lacunes and widespread white matter lesions are the main pathologic characteristic of Binswanger's disease.

Brain imaging. Brain CT scans show lacunar infarcts in the basal ganglia and a bilateral low attenuation area of the periventricular white matter substance in the centrum semiovale and corona radiata as characteristic findings. Same lesions in the form of more evident hyperintensities are observed on T2-weighted MRI scans.[242,243] Revesz et al[244] reported four cases with a clinical diagnosis of subcortical arteriosclerotic encephalopathy and a good correlation between the abnormal MRI signal and the pathologic changes. Microscopic signs of axonal and myelin loss with gliosis were found in the areas with signal abnormalities on MRI and were attributable to gliosis and an expanded extracellular space.

Binswanger's disease as an entity. In his era Binswanger contributed to the progression of our knowledge of vascular cerebral pathology and its relation to dementia; however, more than 100 years after his original description, it has not been ascertained whether there is a clinical, topographic, and, particularly, etiologic correlation with Binswanger's disease. We only know that Binswanger's disease is a clinical form of cerebral atherosclerosis with elective involvement of subcortical white matter penetrating arteries causing lacunar infarctions and leukoaraiosis in patients with hypertension; these patients have a progressive clinical course of subcortical dementia and pseudobulbar syndrome.[245]

In summary, Binswanger tried to establish a causal relationship between cerebrovascular disease and dementia. It is known that this disease is characterized by cognitive function impairment and cerebral vascular abnormality, probably causal, that is manifested on neuroimaging studies by alteration of the white matter in the form of leukoaraiosis and lacunar infarcts. Because of the lack of well-defined pathologic criteria and the unknown etiology of the disease, Binswanger's disease should be considered the starting point for a relationship, undoubtedly present, between dementia and cerebrovascular disease.

Strategic Infarcts

A strategic cerebral infarct presents with a series of clinical manifestations that are not specific to the necrosed cerebral tissue. The lesion of the strategic zone affects specific cortical functions. Clinical symptoms are due to a disruption of corticosubcortical circuits causing impairment of cortical functions. Strategic infarcts present a variety of clinical symptoms, one of which is dementia. The neuropsychological symptoms that lead to subcortical dementia

are mainly produced by a disruption of the deep cortical circuits, such as those in the thalamocortical path. Small-size infarcts localized in strategic areas may be caused by alterations of both large and small cerebral vessels.

Cognitive impairment and vascular dementia have been related, usually in single cases, to several topographic localizations of lacunar cerebral infarcts. The most specific locations include the angular gyrus, internal capsule, caudate nuclei, and thalamus.

Angular gyrus: Angular gyrus infarction produces aphasia with paraphasia, alexia, agraphia, and memory impairment, which may mimic Alzheimer's disease. Gerstmann syndrome with confusion of laterality of body, finger agnosia, agraphia, and acalculia may also be observed. Motor and sensory deficits may be absent.[246,247]

Internal capsule: Strategic small infarcts in the genu of the internal capsule can cause an acute confusional state, inattention, apathy, abulia, and memory loss; contralateral motor deficits can be absent or mild. After the acute phase, patients can show cognitive impairment with verbal memory loss, visuospatial memory defect, impairment of naming and verbal fluency with a dominant hemispheric lesion.[248]

Caudate nuclei: In the acute phase of infarctions in the caudate nuclei, anosognosia, auditory or visual hallucinations, and apraxia have been described.[249] Left more than right caudate infarcts can cause nonfluent aphasia, apraxia, and amnesia.[250]

Thalamus: The thalamus is related to several cortical functions through cortical connections (i.e., the thalamocortical network). The anterior and medial thalamus is related to the frontal cortex and is responsible for cognitive functions. Unilateral or bilateral thalamic infarctions can cause several changes in relation to frontal alterations such as memory or attention deficit, apathy, mood disorders, or dementia. Infarction in the thalamus has been associated, on the dominant side, with dysphasic symptoms and, on the nondominant side, with visuospatial and hemispatial neglect. In anterior nuclei lesions, impairment of memory may occur after the acute phase.[195,251]

Other possible topographies of the strategic infarcts are inferomesial temporal,[252] hippocampal, fornix, cingulate gyrus, basal forebrain, and globus pallidus.

Smaller infarcts in particular regions, for example, in the deep central gray matter, may have an important role in causing dementia.[253] Lacunar infarcts involving the thalamus, internal capsule, and basal ganglia are sometimes associated with widespread cognitive deficits, including confusion and memory impairment.[254] Infarcts involving the dorsomedial and anterior thalamus might also produce significant executive symptoms and important amnesia, which can persist in some cases.[255] Cognitive symptoms associated with strategic infarcts are often reversible by 12 months and therefore are not a common cause of persistent dementia.[256]

Laboratory Studies

Computed Tomography

Technical limitations of the most modern CT scanners prevent the resolution of most lacunes smaller than 2 mm in the internal capsule and almost all of those in the thalamus and brainstem[22,257] because of an obscuring artifact. For the lacunar syndromes documented in the NINCDS Stroke Data Bank, a lesion was found in 35% of cases on the first CT scan; most lesions were located in the posterior limb of the internal capsule and corona radiata.[92] Repeated CT scans increased the yield to 39%. Brainstem lesions were not often visualized. The mean infarct volume in this cohort was greater in pure motor and sensorimotor stroke syndromes than in ataxic hemiparesis, dysarthria-clumsy hand, and pure sensory stroke syndromes. In those patients with pure motor stroke and posterior capsule infarction, there was a correlation between lesion size and severity of hemiparesis, except for the small number of patients whose infarcts involved the lowest portion of the capsule, supplied by the anterior choroidal artery, where severe deficits occurred without regard for lesion size. Enhancement of small, deep infarcts on CT with intravenous contrast is seen in 13% to 40% of patients, mainly during the second and third weeks after onset.[257,258]

Magnetic Resonance Imaging

MRI has greatly changed the frequency with which small infarcts are demonstrated.[259] Although CT is still used, MRI has now surpassed it in sensitivity for detection of lacunes.[72,260] In their study of 227 patients with lacunar infarcts, Arboix et al[82] found that CT findings were positive in 100 patients (44%), whereas MRI findings were positive in 35 of 45 (78%). MRI was significantly better ($P < 0.001$) than CT for imaging lacunes, especially those located in either the pons ($P < 0.005$) or the internal capsule ($P < 0.001$). Motor stroke, pure or sensorimotor, has the highest positive rate on MRI, and pure sensory stroke has the lowest. This finding corresponds to the main volumes of the classic lacunar syndromes on MRI: sensorimotor, 1.7 mL; pure motor, 1.2 mL; ataxic hemiparesis, 0.6 mL; and pure sensory, 0.2 mL. Hommel et al[260] used MRI for 100 patients hospitalized with lacunar infarct syndrome and also found it more sensitive. MRI detected at least one lacune appropriate to the symptoms in 89 patients in whom 135 lacunes were found on imaging. MRI was more effective when it was performed a few days after the stroke.

The superiority of MRI over CT for detection of small lesions now seems generally accepted. Enhancement of small, deep infarcts on MRI with the use of an intravenous contrast agent (gadolinium) is seen in 67% of cases during the first week and in 100% by the second week; this finding is useful in differentiating the present lacune from old ones.[120,261] The hyperintense signals on T2-weighted images in MRI may be lacunar infarcts, état criblé (dilated perivascular spaces), wallerian degeneration, later stages of small hemorrhages, small artery ectasia, myelin loss, or other incidental white matter lesions, and they must be differentiated. In a pathologic study of small hyperintense foci in the basal ganglia on MRI, lesions with smooth margins and putaminal locations were mainly dilated perivascular spaces, whereas lesions with irregular margins and thalamic locations were mainly lacunes.[262] Echoplanar gradient-echo T2-weighted MRI is effective for the detection of small hypointense lesions due to lacunar hemorrhages; these lesions were found in 68% of patients with multiple lacunar infarcts.[263]

MRI may have a higher yield, as inferred from our experience, as well as the experience of Kistler et al.[158] To date, only a few lesions seen on MRI have been confirmed by autopsy. Autopsy correlations with CT findings indicate that CT overestimates lacunar size by as much as 100%.[17] The yield on scans performed within 2 days of the stroke is very low, but by 10 days, more than 50% of the lacunes that eventually show on CT can be detected.[17-19,108,110] The high yield in the study reported by Rascol et al[109] may have been an artifact of selection, but fully 29 of their 30 cases of hemiparesis were documented by CT. The population-based study conducted in southern Alabama noted that 13% of the strokes were due to lacunes; 40% of these were documented by fourth-generation CT.[131] Some of the lesions seen on MRI have been judged to be incidental.[264]

Microbleeds

Cerebral microbleeds are microangiopathies, defined as focal lesions visualized on MRI, especially in T2-weighted gradient-echo imaging, that are sequences highly sensitive for iron-containing compounds such as hemosiderin.[265] The lesions are seen as hypointense signal loss or dark imaging. The histopathologic analysis of microbleeds show perivascular hemosiderin deposits from red blood cells, leaked from small vessels, mainly angiopathic arterioles, and more frequently in amyloid angiopathy.[266,267] Other causes are possible and include head trauma, small cavernous hemangiomas, dense calcifications, or air bubbles after surgery. Numerous aspects of this new finding on imaging studies related to microcirculation are poorly studied. A prevalence of microbleeding between 20% and 70% in patients with symptomatic ischemic or hemorrhagic cerebrovascular disease, depending on sensitivity and MRI sequences used, has been reported.[268] Risk factors for microbleeding are poorly defined, although it is known that it is more frequent in older people and increases with age: 17.8% in subjects between 60 and 69 years of age and 39.3% in subjects older than 80 years. Microbleeding is more often found in patients with hypertension and other cardiovascular risk factors.[269] Lesions are distributed throughout the brain, corticosubcortical regions, basal ganglia, brainstem, and cerebellum. Microbleeding is a general marker of various types of cerebral microangiopathy; the types can be ischemic, as seen with lacunes or white matter damage, or hemorrghagic.[270] Cerebral white matter lesions are a predictor of microbleeding. An association between microbleeding located in the basal or infratentorial ganglia and the presence of lacunar infarcts and white matter abnormalities has been attributed to hypertension or atherosclerotic microangiopathy.[269] In addition, lobar microbleeding has been associated with lobar hemorrhages and cerebral amyloid angiopathy.[269] The current data do not support the general exclusion of patients from therapy based on the presence of cerebral microbleeding.[271]

Diffusion-Weighted Magnetic Resonance Imaging

Diffusion-weighted (DW) MRI is the most sensitive and specific imaging method for detection of acute subcortical ischemic lesions and can differentiate acute from nonacute lesions. Acute lacunar infarcts show a high value on DW MRI, appearing as a bright area of decreased apparent diffusion coefficient (ADC); a subacute lacunar infarct is seen as an area of decreased or normal ADC, and a chronic infarct is seen as with a normal or increased ADC.[272] In all or nearly all patients with clinical acute subcortical infarction, focal areas of high intensity appeared on DW MRI that correlated with all or part of the patients' clinical syndromes.[273,274]

DW MRI performed in 62 patients with well-defined lacunar syndrome during the first 3 days after onset showed the clinically relevant lesion in 68% of cases and additional simultaneous lesions in 16%. The diagnosis of lacunar syndrome can be expected to be inaccurate in one third of cases if it is based on clinical and CT findings.[275] In patients with lacunar syndrome, acute DW imaging can show a subcortical infarct as striatocapsular, and perfusion imaging can modify the final pathogenetic diagnosis, large artery or cardioembolism, based on simultaneous cortical infarcts.[276] These data confirm the need to investigate the etiology and possible embolic mechanism in every patient with a classic clinical picture of lacunar infarction.[277]

Magnetic Resonance Angiography

Magnetic resonance angiography (MRA) can detect intracranial large artery diseases, stenoses, or occlusions in 21% of patients meeting clinical and radiologic criteria for lacunar infarcts, but only in 10% is the artery disease related to the affected penetrating vessel.[278] In four of 11 patients with paramedian pontine infarction of lacunar type and a clinical lacunar syndrome in one study (10 with pure motor hemiparesis and one with ataxic hemiparesis), MRA disclosed a basilar artery stenosis.[279] Microvasculature of the brain as lenticulostriate arteries can be observed by 7.0-Tesla MRA.[280]

Angiography

Similar technical limitations apply to arteriography. Because the artery affected is usually in the range of 100 to 500 μm, conventional angiography does not often demonstrate abnormalities.[58] However, in the case of giant lacunes stenosis of the middle cerebral artery stem or, occasionally, one of the larger lateral lenticulostriate arteries may be documented.[109] In a series of young patients with lacunar infarcts (≤50 years old), conventional angiography was performed in 19 to search for unusual vascular disorders such as vasculitis and extracranial artery dissection; findings were normal in all cases.[66] Ipsilateral extracranial carotid stenosis has a low incidence in patients with lacunar infarcts (89%)[93] and an uncertain relationship.[281] Insufficient cases have been studied to determine how often angiography shows major extracranial or intracranial atheroma in classic lacunar syndromes (Fig. 27-15) and what prognostic interaction exists between such findings and the lacunar syndromes. Nowadays, angiography by MRA or CT can help in providing the true incidence of abnormalities in large extracranial or intracranial vessels in patients with lacunar stroke.

Transcranial Doppler Ultrasonography

In patients with lacunes, transcranial Doppler ultrasonography (TCD) can be used to determine whether the lacunar infarct is associated with stenosis of the middle cerebral artery or basilar artery. In these cases, if the origin of lenticulostriate or paramedian branches corresponds to the stenotic segment, the perfusion pressure could be reduced in the vessel's territories and a hemodynamic mechanism could be involved. One study has shown that the pulsatility indices measured by TCD can be elevated, reflecting increased vascular resistance.[282] In another study, the vascular resistance was higher in patients with silent lacunar infarcts.[283]

Echocardiography

Transesophageal echocardiography demonstrated atheromatous aortic plaques greater than 5 mm in 20% of patients with lacunar stroke and in 4% of control cases in one study.[284] In a prospective series, the main significant risk factor for recurrence was the cardioembolic source detected by transesophageal echocardiography.[285]

Neurophysiologic Studies

Electroencephalography

Their small size prevents most individual lacunes from disrupting enough of the general brain function to produce changes in the conventional electroencephalogram (EEG).[286] In the data from the NINCDS Pilot Stroke Data Bank, no significant EEG abnormalities were encountered, even in patients with positive CT findings.[108] EEG abnormalities were so uncommon in their 56 patients with lacunes that Falcone et al[287] considered a normal EEG a helpful sign suggesting a lacune. Quantitative analysis of

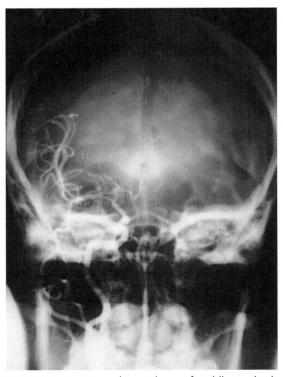

FIGURE 27-15 Angiographic evidence of middle cerebral artery stem stenosis in a patient with dysnomia. The CT scan of this patient is shown in Figure 27-14.

the different frequencies of the α- and μ-rhythms on the EEG has not been useful in the diagnosis and prognosis of lacunar infarcts.[108,286-288]

Evoked Cerebral Responses

A few studies of the somatosensory response have shown alterations in the waveform, suggesting a subclinical sensory impairment in clinically pure motor strokes. Efforts to find an abnormality in the sensory evoked potential were disappointing in a study by Mohr et al[124]; only patients with a large CT lesion and an accompanying motor deficit showed such abnormalities. Other even larger series have also failed to show the usefulness of evoked potentials, except in patients with the largest lesions and sensorimotor deficits.[289] As a test for brain image–negative lacunes, the evoked potential seems thus far to have little use.

Cerebral Blood Flow Measurement

The cerebral blood flow measured in the cortex of patients with lacunar infarcts after stroke is lower in those with multiple lacunes than in those with single lacunar infarcts. The changes induced in cerebral blood flow by intravenous injection of acetazolamide are also lower in multiple than in single lacunar infarctions. These data suggest that atherosclerosis is more advanced and widespread in patients with multiple lacunar infarctions.[290]

Genetic Study

It seems likely that the genetic component of stroke risk is modest and that many (probably hundreds) of genes are involved, each one contributing only a small increased risk. Much of the genetic risk of stroke seems likely to be mediated through already known risk factors, such as cholesterol and blood pressure levels.[291]

It is probable that the genetic background could be an important aspect of clinical or silent manifestations in patients with lacunar infarcts. The possible genetic predisposition to clinical symptoms in patients with lacunar infarctions has been studied.

The most common single gene disorder leading to ischemic stroke in CADASIL is the mutation in the notch 3 gene associated with arteriopathy that involves cerebral small vessels.[292]

The angiotensin-converting enzyme gene and the angiotensinogen gene were found to be associated with the presence of neurologic manifestations in lacunar infarctions.[293] Homozygosity for the G allele of the Glu-298Asp polymorphism in the endothelial constitutive nitric oxide synthetase gene is associated with brain infarction and, especially, with lacunar stroke.[294] The TPA-7351C/T polymorphism is an independent risk factor for lacunar stroke.[295] AGT gene M235T polymorphism may represent a risk factor for lacunar infarction.[296] An association between lacunar infarction and the genotype of the interleukin-6 polymorphism has been found. This association suggests a susceptibility of penetrating arteries to inflammatory damage mediated by interleukin-6.[297]

Patients with lacunar syndromes due to lacunar infarcts can have associated hyperintense signals on T2-weigthed images on MRI. In these cases, the angiotensin-converting enzyme insertion/deletion genotype is more frequent.[298]

Prognosis

In general, the patient with a lacunar infarction has a good early prognosis, which is a finding that Pierre Marie and Miller Fisher noted as one of the characteristics of lacunes. In comparison with other vascular processes (ischemic or hemorrhagic, hemispheric or in the brainstem), lacunes have the best early prognosis (not always, however, as good as we expect). The prognosis of lacunes is influenced by several factors. The presence of TIAs before the infarct indicates a poor prognosis, more recurrence, and coronary artery disease in the clinical evolution.[299] Generally, when the motor or sensory deficit is complete (affecting the face, arm, and leg), the prognosis is worse than with an incomplete deficit. The size of the lacunar infarction on CT or MRI is usually correlated with prognosis and is better for smaller lesions. Hyperglycemia, which is associated with a poor outcome in acute ischemic strokes because of large vessel atherothrombotic or cardioembolic disease, does not affect the prognosis in acute lacunar cerebral infarction.[300,301]

The prognosis in such vascular processes as lacunes implies four aspects: survival, recovery of deficits, general or neurologic complications in the acute phase, and recurrence. Survival is the rule during the acute phase. The possibility of death in this phase is related to other complications rather than the lacunar infarct itself. The risk of death after the acute phase is no different from that in the general population.[302,303]

Early neurologic deterioration in lacunar infarction, as well a poor outcome, has been associated with a high blood concentration of inflammatory markers such as interleukin-6, tumor necrosis factor-α, and intercellular adhesion molecule-1.[304] Recovery of deficits is generally good in the first few weeks after onset. Related functional outcomes of 94% of patients at 6 months[113] are independent.[305] Complications in the acute phase occur in 18% of patients, and urinary infections are the most common.[306] The prognosis for recurrence of stroke in lacunar infarcts at 1 year in hospital studies or community series is about 10%. The rate of recurrence in following years is similar[303,307]; the rate is 23.5%, however, with a follow-up of 10 years, as shown in one series of pure motor stroke from presumed lacunar infarction.[308]

Hypertension, diabetes mellitus, leukoaraiosis, and high hematocrit levels are the main risk factors associated with recurrence and multiple lacunar infarcts.[309,310] Recurrent strokes were more likely to be lacunar if the first event was lacunar.[311]

In patients with lacunar infarct, an angiographic study usually shows no occlusive lesion of the relevant artery or an occlusive lesion of the parent artery occluding the deep penetrating artery. Patients with an occlusive lesion of the parent artery have a recurrence rate similar to those with large artery disease.[312] Stroke recurrence is more frequent in patients with lacunar infarcts associated with ipsilateral large artery disease.[313]

Risk of Vascular Dementia

The incidence of vascular dementia has been related to the rate of stroke recurrence; demented patients had a significantly higher rate of stroke recurrence than patients who did not develop dementia. Vascular cognitive impairment is considered to increase the risk of death and institutionalization and progresses to dementia in approximately half of the cases.[222,314] In cognitive and functionally normal persons, the number of subcortical silent lacunes on MRI is the only significant predictor of poorer executive performance.[315] In these patients, cerebral white matter changes influence the executive function testing.[316] An autopsy study found that patients who had lacunes were more likely to be demented than those without infarcts, and fewer neuropathologic changes of Alzheimer disease were needed for clinical symptoms to be manifest.[208] In an autopsy series, gray matter lacunes (thalamic and basal ganglia) were related to ischemic vascular dementia more than white matter demyelination.[317] In patients with lacunar infarcts, ambulatory 24-hour blood pressure readings showed that nondipping status was one of the predictors of the development of dementia. High systolic blood pressure was a predictor for future vascular events.[318]

Progression of Asymptomatic Small Vessel Disease

Asymptomatic or silent lacunar infarcts are more frequent than symptomatic infarcts. Approximately 20% to 28% of the population aged 65 years or older has lacunes documented by MRI.[319] The presence of silent lacunar infarcts is a risk factor for both stroke recurrence and cognitive impairment. Patients with more than one silent lacunar infarct on CT have a worse prognosis for mortality, recurrent stroke, and functional outcome.[320]

Treatment

The use of thrombolytic therapy, intravenous thrombolysis with recombinant tissue plasminogen activator (rt-PA) within 3 hours of stroke onset, in patients in whom lacunar infarct is clinically suspected can be controversial, but the results of the NINDS study[100] as well as those of others,[321,322] in which three of every four patients with lacunar infarction had a favorable outcome, can support its indication.

The patient with a lacunar infarction may have had prior TIAs (20%) close to the infarct onset or a leisurely mode of onset (30%). In both cases anticoagulant therapy did not prove its efficacy. No specific treatment exists for the necrotic tissue of a small, deep infarct, but we can act on its causes and consequences. Atherosclerosis is the most important cause, usually affecting small vessels and less frequently affecting main intracranial or extracranial trunks; the current treatment is directed at correcting vascular risk factors such as hypertension, diabetes mellitus, and cigarette smoking. Specific drugs acting against platelet aggregation, such as aspirin, ticlopidine, and clopidogrel, can be used, but their efficacy has not been proven. Mohr et al[323] found that after the first-ever lacunar infarction, aspirin and warfarin do not show a difference in the prevention of recurrence during a 2-year period. Statins (3-hydroxy-3-methylglutaryl-coenzyme A reductase inhibitors) act to inhibit hydroxyl-methyl-glutaryl Co-A reductase, involved in the synthesis of a substrate for cholesterol and coenzyme Q10, and decrease

levels of cholesterol. There is biological evidence that statins have neuroprotective properties related to scavenged oxygen-derived free radicals.[324] Statins also have a beneficial effect on the vascular endothelium.[325] Statin treatment with atorvastatin, 80 mg daily, in patients with small vessel disease, reduces low-density lipoprotein cholesterol levels and is useful in prevention and treatment; it reduces the risk of a first clinical stroke and recurrence.[326]

Extracranial carotid stenosis must be regarded as asymptomatic, except in cases in which stenosis is the sole causative factor, which could produce lacunes hemodynamically or by embolism.

Hypertension must be treated similarly to other types of cerebral infarction, that is, not in the first days of the acute phase, when values are greater than 190 to 200 mm Hg systolic and 110 to 115 mm Hg diastolic. After the acute phase, hypertension must be accurately controlled.[66] The continuous control of blood pressure levels, during the day and night, can avoid the development of new silent lacunes.[327] Heart diseases (e.g., ischemia, atrial fibrillation, or valvulopathy) are regarded and treated as risk factors. Similarly, diabetes mellitus must be treated as a risk factor in all patients and occasionally is the cause of a lacune.

When an elevated hematocrit value (>45%) is the sole cause, phlebotomy may be indicated.[89] When arteritis is the cause of lacunes, as in chronic neurosyphilis, granulomatosis, cysticercosis, or tuberculosis, treatment with penicillin, steroids, praziquantel, or antituberculous drugs, respectively, is indicated. In relation to the symptoms of lacunar infarct, the treatment can be specific. In all patients with motor deficit, prevention of deep venous thrombosis with low-molecular-weight heparin (0.2 mL/day subcutaneously) is the rule. In a double-blind, crossover placebo study, the motor performance in patients with pure motor stroke was modulated by a single dose of fluoxetine, with hyperactivation in the primary motor cortex ipsilateral to the lesion as evaluated by functional MRI; this treatment enhanced motor performance.[328] Motor rehabilitation must be started as soon as possible. When hyperpathia is present in sensory stroke, amitriptyline, carbamazepine, gabapentin, or clonazepam has been used with an inconsistent response. Movement disorders such as hemichorea–hemiballismus or dystonia can be relieved with haloperidol, 1 to 5 mg three times a day,[29] but this treatment has not always been effective. Pallidotomy can be useful in reducing hemichorea.[329] When motor aphasia is present, speech therapy is started.

Although primary prevention of lacunes has not been investigated, the treatment of hypertension and other established risk factors, such as diabetes mellitus and cigarette smoking, is probably the best way to avoid lacunes in the symptomatic and asymptomatic forms.

Practical Approach

An acute or stuttering unilateral or focal deficit referable to the brain with motor, sensory, ataxic, or dysarthric deficits in the form of one of the five lacunar syndromes (pure motor, pure sensory, sensorimotor, ataxic hemiparesis, or dysarthria-clumsy hand) suggests the probability of a lacunar infarction. However, this diagnosis is only a possibility that must be confirmed. A patient with a motor deficit must be admitted to the hospital. All cases must be investigated with the aim of confirming the presumed diagnosis, establishing its cause, and starting the best treatment. The clinical picture can never be regarded as synonymous with a lacunar infarction.

The diagnosis of a lacunar syndrome has a 20% possibility of being explained by other processes, vascular or not. The clinical diagnosis of lacunar infarction has a sensitivity—that is, the proportion of patients with the same diagnosis at the initial examination and at the end of the study—between 81% and 95%. Specificity—or the proportion of patients with different final diagnoses who also had other initial diagnoses—is between 81% and 93%.[330-332]

The first step in the study of a patient is to confirm the lacunar infarction and differentiate it from other possible diagnoses. CT scanning excludes such other possibilities as intracerebral hemorrhage, tumor, metastasis, subdural hematoma, and abscess, with a positive rate in lacunes of between 15% and 58%,[333,334] but MRI is the best and most useful exploration, confirming lacunar infarction in 74% to 98% of cases.[335,336] MRI can also establish the topography (68%), diagnose silent infarcts (13%) in neurologically normal adults,[337] and differentiate a lacune from other small, deep hyperintensive signals.

Once the lacunar infarct is confirmed by MRI or is suspected because the clinical picture is appropriate and MRI findings are normal, the next step is the etiologic investigation. This is the most important work in the management of a patient with lacunar infarct, and hypertension can never be considered the sole cause of the infarct. Although carotid and other vascular lesions, cardioembolic disease, and hematologic alterations have a low etiologic incidence in patients with lacunar infarct, they must be investigated.[94,338-341] Etiologic study consists of looking for vascular risk factors (mainly hypertension and diabetes mellitus) and trying to find a vascular abnormality on TCD ultrasonography or MRA, a cardioembolic disease on EEG and echocardiography, and a hematologic process. Patients with lacunes have a risk of developing dementia in the next 4 years of 23%[342]; because of this it is important to perform a neuropsychological study as a reference point for the follow-up. Treatment of vascular risk factors, other possible causes, and the consequences of stroke is the next step.

Evidence shows that one in every five patients with ischemic stroke has a lacune; such evidence has good sensitivity and specificity in clinical diagnosis and good correlation with lacunar syndromes and with pathologic studies. Thus, small vessel disease producing lacunes is a well-established subtype of ischemic stroke; in one study at 28 medical centers, small vessel disease was the most common initial diagnosis (38%) in 479 patients with ischemic stroke.[332] In spite of this evidence, complete investigations must be performed in all patients seen with a lacunar syndrome due to this stroke subtype because the others have many problematic aspects in terms of etiology, pathology, topography, and treatment that deserve careful and exhaustive clinical study and research.[349]

REFERENCES

1. Moskalenko YE, editor: *Biophysical aspects of cerebral circulation*, Oxford, 1980, Pergamon Press.
2. Ringelstein EB, Nabavi DG: Cerebral small vessel diseases: Cerebral microangiopathies, *Curr Opin Neurol* 18:179-188, 2005.
3. Bamford J, Sandercock P, Jones L, et al: The natural history of lacunar infarction: The Oxfordshire community stroke project, *Stroke* 18:545-551, 1987.
4. Dechambre A: Mémoire sur la curabilité du ramollissement cérébral, *Gaz Med (Paris)* 6:305, 1838.
5. Durand-Fardel M: Mémoire sur une alteration particulière de la substance cérébrale, *Gaz Med (Paris)* 10:23, 1842.
6. Marie P: Des foyers lacunaire de désintegration et de différents autres états cavitaires du cerveau, *Rev Med* 21:281, 1901.
7. Ferrand J: *Essai sur l'hémiplegie des vieillards, les lacunes de désintegration cérébrale [thesis]*, Paris, 1902, Rousset.
8. Vogt C, Vogt O: Zur Lehre der Erkrankungen des striaren Systems, *J Psychol Neurol* 25:627, 1920.
9. Fisher CM, Curry HB: Pure motor hemiplegia of vascular origin, *Arch Neurol (Chic)* 13:30, 1965.
10. Fisher CM: Thalamic pure sensory stroke: A pathologic study, *Neurology* 28:1141, 1978.
11. Fisher CM, Cole M: Homolateral ataxia and crural paresis: A vascular syndrome, *J Neurol Neurosurg Psychiatry* 28:48, 1965.
12. Fisher CM: A lacunar stroke: The dysarthria-clumsy hand syndrome, *Neurology (Minneap)* 17:614, 1967.
13. Mohr JP, Kase CS, Meckler RJ, Fisher CM: Sensorimotor stroke, *Arch Neurol* 34:739, 1977.
14. Fisher CM, Caplan LR: Basilar artery branch occlusion: A cause of pontine infarction, *Neurology (Minneap)* 21:900, 1971.
15. Fisher CM: The arterial lesions underlying lacunes, *Acta Neuropathol* 12:1, 1969.
16. Melamed E, Korn Lubetzki I, Reches A, et al: Hemiballismus: Detection of focal hemorrhage in subthalamic nucleus by CT scan, *Ann Neurol* 4:582, 1978.
17. Donnan GA, Tress BM, Bladin PF: A prospective study of lacunar infarction using computerized tomography, *Neurology* 32:49, 1982.
18. Pullicino P, Nelson RF, Kendall BE, Marshall J: Small deep infarcts diagnosed on computed tomography, *Neurology* 30:1090, 1980.
19. Weisberg LA: Computed tomography and pure motor hemiparesis, *Neurology* 29:490, 1979.
20. Chokroverty S, Rubino FA, Haller C: Pure motor hemiplegia due to pyramidal infarction, *Arch Neurol* 2:647, 1975.
21. Rottenberg DA, Talman W, Chernik NL: Location of pyramidal tract questioned, *Neurology (Minneap)* 26:291, 1976.
22. Weintraub MI, Glaser GH: Nocardial brain abscess and pure motor hemiplegia, *N Y J Med* 70:2717, 1970.
23. Michel D, Laurent B, Foyatier N, et al: Infarctus thalamique paramedian gauche, *Rev Neurol (Paris)* 138:6, 1982.
24. Landau WM: Clinical neuromythology VI: Au clair de lacune: Holy, wholly, holey logic, *Neurology* 39:725, 1989.
25. Leestma JE, Noronha A: Pure motor hemiplegia, medullary pyramid lesion, and olivary hypertrophy, *Arch Neurol* 39:877, 1976.
26. Davis LE, Xie JG, Zou AH, et al: Deep cerebral infarcts in the People's Republic of China, *Stroke* 21:394, 1990.
27. Huang CY, Chan FL, Yu YL, et al: Cerebrovascular disease in Hong Kong Chinese, *Stroke* 21:230, 1990.
28. Fisher CM: Lacunes: Small deep cerebral infarcts, *Neurology (Minneap)* 15:774, 1965.
29. Goldblatt H: Studies on experimental hypertension. VII: The production of the malignant phase of hypertension, *J Exp Med* 67:809, 1938.
30. Nelson RF, Pullicino P, Kendall BE, Marshall J: Computed tomography on patients presenting with lacunar syndromes, *Stroke* 11:256, 1980.
31. Ross Russell RW: Observations on intracerebral aneurisms, *Brain* 86:425, 1963.
32. Loeb C: The lacunar syndromes, *Eur Neurol* 29:2, 1989.
33. Mohr JP, Caplan LR, Melski JW, et al: The Harvard Cooperative Stroke Registry, *Neurology* 28:754, 1978.
34. Fisher CM: Capsular infarcts, *Arch Neurol* 36:65, 1979.

35. Bokura H, Kobayashi S, Yamaguchi S: Distinguishing silent lacunar infarction from enlarged Virchow-Robin spaces: A magnetic resonance imaging and pathological study, *J Neurol* 245:116, 1998.

36. Combarros O, Polo JM, Pascual J, et al: Evidence of somatotopic organization of the sensory thalamus based on infarction in the nucleus ventralis posterior, *Stroke* 22:1445, 1991.

37. Byrom FB, Dodson LF: The causation of acute arterial necrosis in hypertensive disease, *J Pathol Bacteriol* 60:357, 1948.

38. Percheron SMJ: Les artères du thalamus humain, *Rev Neurol* 132:297, 1976.

39. Heptinstall RH: *Pathology of the kidney*, vol 1, 2nd ed. Boston, Little, Brown, 1974, pp 121.

40. Gautier JC: Cerebral ischemia in hypertension. In Ross Russell RW, editor: *Cerebral arterial disease*, London, 1978, Churchill Livingstone, pp 181.

41. Byrom FB: The pathogenesis of hypertensive encephalopathy and its relation to the malignant phase of hypertension, *Lancet* 2:201, 1954.

42. Chester EM, Agamanolis DP, Banker Q, Victor M: Hypertensive encephalopathy: A clinicopathologic study of 20 cases, *Neurology* 28:928, 1978.

43. Fisher CM: Bilateral occlusion of basilar artery branches, *J Neurol Neurosurg Psychiatry* 40:1182, 1977.

44. Fisher CM: Ataxic hemiparesis, *Arch Neurol* 35:126, 1978.

45. Fisher CM, Gore I, Okabe N, White PD: Atherosclerosis of the carotid and vertebral arteries: Extracranial and intracranial, *J Neuropathol Exp Neurol* 24:455, 1965.

46. Lammie GA, Brannan F, Slattery J, Warlow CH: Nonhypertensive cerebral small-vessel disease: An autopsy study, *Stroke* 28:2222, 1997.

47. Hanaway J, Young RR: Localization of the pyramidal tract in the internal capsule of man, *J Neurol Sci* 34:63, 1977.

48. Rosenberg EF: The brain in malignant hypertension: A clinico-pathological study, *Arch Intern Med* 65:545, 1940.

49. Ekstrom Jodal B, Haggendal E, Linder LE, et al: Cerebral blood flow autoregulation at high arterial pressures and different levels of carbon dioxide tension in dogs, *Eur Neurol* 6:6, 1972.

50. Skinhoj E, Strandgaard S: Pathogenesis of hypertensive encephalopathy, *Lancet* 1(7801):461, 1973.

51. Hill GS: Studies on the pathogenesis of hypertensive vascular disease: Effect of high pressure intraarterial injections in rats, *Circ Res* 27:657, 1970.

52. Giese J: The pathogenesis of hypertensive vascular disease, *Dan Med Bull* 14:259, 1967.

53. Byrom FB: *The hypertensive vascular crisis*, New York, 1969, Grune & Stratton.

54. Wiener J, Spiro D, Lattes RG: The cellular pathology of experimental hypertension. II: Arteriolar hyalinosis and fibrinoid change, *Am J Pathol* 47:457, 1965.

55. Paronetto F: Immunocytochemical observations on the vascular necrosis and renal glomerular lesions of malignant nephrosclerosis, *Am J Pathol* 46:901, 1965.

56. Feigin I, Prose P: Hypertensive fibrinoid arteritis of the brain and gross cerebral hemorrhage: A form of "hyalinosis," *Arch Neurol* 1:98, 1959.

57. Cole FM, Yates PO: Pseudo-aneurysms in relationship to massive cerebral haemorrhage, *J Neurol Neurosurg Psychiatry* 30:61, 1967.

58. Fisher CM: Cerebral ischemia: Less familiar types, *Clin Neurosurg* 18:267, 1971.

59. Challa VR, Moody DM, Bell MA: The Charcot-Bouchard aneurysm controversy: Impact of a new histologic technique, *J Neuropathol Exp Neurol* 51:264, 1992.

60. Laloux P, Broucher JM: Lacunar infarctions due to cholesterol emboli, *Stroke* 22:1440, 1991.

61. Pearce JMS, Chandrasekera CP, Ladusans EJ: Lacunar infarcts in polycythemia with raised packer cell volumes, *BMJ* 287:935, 1983.

62. Levine SR, Deegan MJ, Futrell N, et al: Cerebrovascular and neurologic disease associated with antiphospholipid antibodies: 48 cases, *Neurology* 40:1181, 1990.

63. Fisher CM: Lacunar strokes and infarcts: A review, *Neurology* 32:871, 1982.

64. Pico F, Labreuche J, Seilhean D, et al: Association of small-vessel disease with dilatative arteriopathy of the brain. Neuropathologic evidence, *Stroke* 38:1197–1202, 2007.

65. Waterston JA, Brown MM, Butler P, Swash M: Small deep cerebral infarcts associated with occlusive internal carotid artery disease: A hemodynamic phenomenon? *Arch Neurol* 47:953, 1990.

66. Luijckx GJ, Boiten J, Lodder J, et al: Cardiac and carotid embolism, and other rare definite disorders are unlikely causes of lacunar ischaemic stroke in young patients, *Cerebrovasc Dis* 6:28, 1996.

67. Loeb DJ, Biller J, Yuh WTC, et al: Leukoencephalopathy in cerebral amyloid angiopathy: MR imaging in four cases, *AJNR Am J Neuroradiol* 11:485, 1990.

68. Kribs M, Kleihues J: The recurrent artery of Heubner. In Zulch KJ, editor: *Cerebral Circulation and Stroke*, New York, 1971, Springer-Verlag, pp 40.

69. Merritt HH, Adams RD, Solomon HC: *Neurosyphilis*, New York, 1946, Oxford University Press.

70. Gorelick PB, Caplan LR: Racial differences in the distribution of anterior circulation occlusive disease, *Neurology* 34:54, 1984.

71. Pentschew A: Gibt es eine Endarteritis luica der kleinen Hirnrindengefässe (Nissl Alzheimer)? *Nervenartz* 8:393, 1935.

72. Barinagarrementeria F, Del Brutto OH: Lacunar syndrome due to neurocysticercosis, *Arch Neurol* 46:415, 1989.

73. Kohler J, Kern U, Kasper J, et al: Chronic central nervous system involvement in Lyme borreliosis, *Neurology* 38:863, 1988.

74. Park YD, Belman AL, Kim TS, et al: Stroke in pediatric acquired immunodeficiency syndrome, *Ann Neurol* 28:303, 1990.

75. Devinsky O, Petito CK, Alonso DR: Clinical and neuropathological findings in systemic lupus erythematosus: The role of vasculitis, heart emboli, and thrombotic thrombocytopenic purpura, *Ann Neurol* 23:380, 1988.

76. Fredericks RK, Leflowitz DS, Challa VR, et al: Cerebral vasculitis associated with cocaine abuse, *Stroke* 22:1437, 1991.

77. Reichart MD, Bogousslavsky J, Janzer RC: Early lacunar strokes complicating polyarteritis nodosa, *Neurology* 54:883, 2000.

78. Ho KL: Pure motor hemiplegia due to infarction of the cerebral peduncle, *Arch Neurol* 39:524, 1982.

79. Dattner B, Thomas EW, Wexler G: *The management of neurosyphilis*, New York, 1944, Grune & Stratton.

80. Heuschemann PU, Neureiter D, Gesslein M, et al: Association between infection with *Helicobacter pylori* and *Chlamydia pneumoniae* and risk of ischemic stroke subtypes: Results from a population-based case-control study, *Stroke* 32:2253, 2001.

81. Pavlovic AM, Zidverc-Trajkovic J, Milovic MM, et al: Cerebral small vessel disease and pseudoxanthoma elasticum: Three cases, *Can J Neurol Sci* 32:115–118, 2005.

82. Arboix A, Marti-Vilalta JL, Garcia JH: Clinical study of 227 patients with lacunar infarcts, *Stroke* 21:842, 1990.

83. Reimers J, de Wytt C, Seneviratne B: Lacunar infarction: A 12 month study, *Clin Exp Neurol* 24:28, 1987.

84. Lazzarino LG, Nicolai A, Poldelmengo P, et al: Risk factors in lacunar strokes: A retrospective study of 52 patients, *Acta Neurol (Napoli)* 11:265, 1989.

85. Longstreth WT, Bernick CH, Manolio TA, et al: Lacunar infarcts defined by magnetic resonance imaging of 3660 elderly people, *Arch Neurol* 55:1217, 1998.

86. Shintani S, Shiigai T, Arinami T: Silent lacunar infarction on magnetic resonance imaging (MRI): Risk factors, *J Neurol Sci* 160:82, 1998.

87. Toshifumi M, Arai H, Yuzuriha T, et al: Elevated plasma homocysteine levels and risk of silent brain infarction in elderly people, *Stroke* 32:1116, 2001.

88. Tuszynski MH, Petito CK, Levy DE: Risk factors and clinical manifestations of pathologically verified lacunar infarctions, *Stroke* 20:990, 1989.

89. LaRue L, Alter M, Lai SM, et al: Acute stroke, hematocrit, and blood pressure, *Stroke* 18:565, 1987.

90. Marti-Vilalta JL, Arboix A: The Barcelona Stroke Registry, *Eur Neurol* 41:135, 1999.

91. Mast H, Thompson JL, Lee SH, et al: Hypertension and diabetes mellitus as determinants of multiple lacunar infarcts, *Stroke* 26:30, 1995.

92. Chamorro AM, Sacco RL, Mohr JP, et al: Lacunar infarction: Clinical–computed tomographic correlations in the Stroke Data Bank, *Stroke* 22:175, 1991.

93. Inzitari D, Eliasziw M, Sharpe BL, et al: Risk factors and outcome of patients with carotid artery stenosis presenting with lacunar stroke, *Neurology* 54:660, 2000.

94. Arboix A, Marti-Vilalta JL: Presumed cardioembolic lacunar infarcts, *Stroke* 23:1992, 1841.

95. Arboix A, Garcia-Eroles L, Massons J, et al: Lacunar infarcts in patients aged 85 years and older, *Acta Neurol Scand* 101:25, 2000.

96. Kempster PA, Gerraty RP, Gates PC: Asymptomatic cerebral infarction in patients with chronic atrial fibrillation, *Stroke* 19:955, 1988.

97. Arboix A, Marti-Vilalta JL: Transient ischemic attacks in lacunar infarct, *Cerebrovasc Dis* 1:20, 1991.

98. Hyland HH, Forman DM: Prognosis in hemiballismus, *Neurology (Minneap)* 7:381, 1957.

99. Ichikawa K, Tsutsumishita A, Fujioka A: Capsular ataxic hemiparesis: A case report, *Arch Neurol* 39:585, 1982.

100. Nakamura K, Saku Y, Ibayashi S, Fujishima M: Progressive motor deficits in lacunar infarction, *Neurology* 52:29, 1999.

101. Arboix A, Marti-Vilalta JL: Acute stroke and circadian rhythm, *Stroke* 21:826, 1990.

102. De Reuck J, van der Eecken H: The topography of infarcts in the lacunar state. In Meyer JS, Lechner H, Reivich M, editors: *Cerebral Vascular Disease: 7th International Conference*, Salzburg. New York, 1976, Thieme Edition/Publishing Sciences Group, p 162.

103. Kumral E, Bogousslavsky J, Van Melle G, et al: Headache at stroke onset: The Lausanne Stroke Registry, *J Neurol Neurosurg Psychiatry* 58:490, 1995.

104. Vestergaard K, Andersen G, Nielsen MI, et al: Headache in stroke, *Stroke* 24:1621, 1993.

105. Wallin A, Sjögren M, Edman A, et al: Symptoms, vascular risk factors and blood-brain barrier function in relation to CT white matter changes in dementia, *Eur Neurol* 44:229–235, 2000.

106. Earnest MP, Fahn S, Karp JH, Rowland LP: Normal pressure hydrocephalus and hypertensive cerebrovascular disease, *Arch Neurol* 31:262, 1974.

107. Koto A, Rosenberg G, Zingesser LH, et al: Syndrome of normal pressure hydrocephalus: Possible relation to hypertensive and arteriosclerotic vasculopathy, *J Neurol Neurosurg Psychiatry* 40:73, 1977.

108. Mohr JP, Kase CS, Wolf PA, et al: Lacunes in the NINCDS Pilot Stroke Data Bank [abstract], *Ann Neurol* 12:84, 1982.

109. Rascol A, Clanet M, Manelfe C, et al: Pure motor hemiplegia: CT study of 30 cases, *Stroke* 13:11, 1982.

110. Weisberg LA: Lacunar infarcts, *Arch Neurol* 39:37, 1982.

111. Iragui VJ, McCutchen CB: Capsular ataxic hemiparesis, *Arch Neurol* 39:528, 1982.

112. Damasio AR, Damasio H, Rizzo M, et al: Aphasia with nonhemorrhagic lesions of the basal ganglia and internal capsule, *Arch Neurol* 39:15, 1982.

113. Naeser MA, Alexander MP, Helm Estabrooks N, et al: Aphasia with predominantly subcortical lesion sites, *Arch Neurol* 39:2, 1982.

114. Abadie JL: *Les localisations functionelles de la capsule interne* [thesis], Bordeaux, 1900.

115. Igapashi S, Mori K, Ishijima Y: Pure motor hemiplegia after recraniotomy for postoperative bleeding, *Arch Jpn Chir* 41:32, 1965.

116. Aleksie SN, George AE: Pure motor hemiplegia with occlusion of the extracranial carotid artery, *J Neurol Sci* 19:331, 1973.

117. Kaps M, Klostermann W, Wessel K, et al: Basilar branch diseases presenting with progressive pure motor stroke, *Acta Neurol Scand* 96:324, 1997.

118. Arboix A, García-Eroles L, Massons J, et al: Hemorrhagic lacunar stroke, *Cerebrovasc Dis* 10:229, 2000.

119. Misra UK, Kalita J: Putaminal haemorrhage leading to pure motor hemiplegia, *Acta Neurol Scand* 91:283, 1995.

120. Miyashita K, Naritomi H, Sawada T, et al: Identification of recent lacunar lesions in cases of multiple small infarctions by magnetic resonance imaging, *Stroke* 19:834, 1988.

121. Tapia JF, Kase CS, Sawyer RH, Mohr JP: Hypertensive putaminal hemorrhage presenting as pure motor hemiparesis, *Stroke* 14:505, 1983.

122. Arboix A, García-Eroles L, Massons J, et al: Haemorrhagic pure motor stroke, *Eur J Neurol* 14:219–223, 2007.

123. Richter RW, Brust JCM, Bruun B, Shafer SQ: Frequency and course of pure motor hemiparesis: A clinical study, *Stroke* 8:58, 1977.

124. Robinson RK, Richey ET, Kase CS, Mohr JP: Somatosensory evoked potentials in pure sensory stroke and allied conditions [abstract], *Neurology* 34:231, 1984.

125. Fraix V, Besson G, Hommel M, Perret J: Brachiofacial pure motor stroke, *Cerebrovasc Dis* 12:34, 2001.

126. Melo TP, Bogousslavsky J, Van Melle G, et al: Pure motor stroke: A reappraisal, *Neurology* 42:789, 1992.

127. Fisher CM: Some neuroophthalmologic observations, *J Neurol Neurosurg Psychiatry* 30:383, 1967.

128. Foix C, Levy M: Les ramollissements sylviens, *Rev Neurol* 11:1, 1927.

129. Englander RN, Netsky MG, Adelman LS: Location of human pyramidal tract in the internal capsule: Anatomic evidence, *Neurology* 25:823, 1975.

130. Ross ED: Localization of the pyramidal tract in the internal capsule by whole brain dissection, *Neurology* 30:59, 1980.

131. Gross CR, Kase CS, Mohr JP, Cunningham SC: Stroke in south Alabama: Incidence and diagnostic features, *Stroke* 15:249, 1984.

132. Dejerine J, Dejerine Klumpke H: *Anatomie des centres nerveux*, Vol 2, Paris, 1901, Rueff.

133. Samuelsson M, Samuelsson L, Lindell D: Sensory symptoms and signs and results of quantitative sensory thermal testing in patients with lacunar infarct syndromes, *Stroke* 25:2165, 1994.

134. Steinke W, Ley SC: Lacunar stroke is the major cause of progressive motor deficit, *Stroke* 33:1510–1516, 2002.

135. Lazar RM, Perera GM, Marshall RS, et al: The evolution of fMRI activation following pure motor stroke, *Neurology* 50:402, 1998.

136. Fisher CM: Pure sensory stroke involving face, arm and leg, *Neurology (Minneap)* 15:76, 1965.

137. Groothius DR, Duncan GW, Fisher CM: The human thalamocortical sensory path in the internal capsule: Evidence from a capsular hemorrhage causing a pure sensory stroke, *Ann Neurol* 2:328, 1977.

138. Rosenberg NL, Koller R: Computerized tomography and pure sensory stroke, *Neurology* 31:217, 1981.

139. Jokura K, Matsumoto S, Komiyama A, et al: Unilateral saccadic pursuit in patients with sensory stroke: Sign of pontine tegmentum lesion, *Stroke* 29:2377, 1998.

140. Arboix A, García C, Massons J, et al: Clinical study of 99 patients with pure sensory stroke, *J Neurol* 252:156–162, 2005.

141. Wyllie J: *The disorders of speech*, Edinburgh, 1894, Oliver & Boyd, pp 340.

142. Lapresle J, Haguenau S: Anatomico-clinical correlation in focal thalamic lesions, *Z Neurol* 205:29, 1973.

143. Fisher CM: Pure sensory stroke and allied conditions, *Stroke* 13:434, 1982.

144. Lenz FA, Dostrovsky JO, Tasker RR, et al: Single unit analysis of the human ventral thalamic nuclear group: Somatosensory responses, *J Neurophysiol* 59:299, 1988.

145. Mohr JP: Lacunes, *Neurol Clin* 1:201, 1983.

146. Kim JS: Pure sensory stroke: Clinical-radiological correlates of 21 cases, *Stroke* 23:983, 1992.

147. Dejerine J, Roussy G: La syndrome thalamique, *Rev Neurol (Paris)* 14:521, 1906.

148. Manfredi M, Cruccu G: Thalamic pain revisited. In Loeb C, ed: *Studies in cerebrovascular disease*, Milano, 1981, Masson Italiano, pp 73.

149. Plets C, De Reuck J, Vander Eecken H, et al: The vascularization of the human thalamus, *Acta Neurol Belg* 70:685, 1970.

150. Garcin R, Lapresle J: Syndrome sensitif de type thalamique et etopographie cheiro orale par lesion localisée du thalamus, *Rev Neurol* 90:124, 1954.

151. Sunohara N, Mukoyama M, Mano Y, Satoyoshi E: Action-induced rhythmic dystonia: An autopsy case, *Neurology (Cleve)* 34:321, 1984.

152. Gursahani RD, Khadilkar SV, Surya N, Singhal BS: Capsular involvement and sensorimotor stroke with posterior cerebral artery territory infarction, *J Assoc Physicians India* 38:939, 1990.

153. Arboix A, Oliveres M, García-Eroles L, et al: Risk factors and clinical features of sensorimotor stroke, *Cerebrovasc Dis* 16:448–451, 2003.

154. Perman GP, Racey A: Homolateral ataxic and crural paresis: Case report, *Neurology* 30:1013, 1980.

155. Huang CY, Lui FS: Ataxic hemiparesis: Localization and clinical features, *Stroke* 15:363, 1984.

156. Moulin T, Bogousslavsky J, Chopard JL, et al: Vascular ataxic hemiparesis: A re-evaluation, *J Neurol Neurosurg Psychiatry* 58:422, 1995.

157. Sage JI: Ataxic hemiparesis from lesions of the corona radiata, *Arch Neurol* 40:449, 1983.

158. Kistler JP, Buonanno FS, DeWitt LD, et al: Vertebral basilar posterior cerebral territory stroke delineation by proton nuclear magnetic resonance imaging, *Stroke* 15:417, 1984.

159. Gorman MJ, Dafer R, Levine SR: Ataxic hemiparesis: Critical appraisal of a lacunar syndrome, *Stroke* 29:2549, 1998.

160. Arboix A: Clinical study of 23 patients with ataxic hemiparesis, *Med Clin (Barc)* 122:342-344, 2004.

161. Hiraga A, Uzawa A, Kamitsukasa I: Diffusion weighted imaging in ataxic hemiparesis, *J Neurol Neurosurg Psychiatry* 78:1260-1262, 2007.

162. Bendheim PE, Berg BO: Ataxic hemiparesis from a midbrain mass, *Ann Neurol* 9:405, 1981.

163. Tjeerdsma HC, Rinkel GJE, van Gijn J: Ataxic hemiparesis from a primary intracerebral haematoma in the precentral area, *Cerebrovasc Dis* 6:45, 1996.

164. Sakai T, Murakami S, Ito K: Ataxic hemiparesis with trigeminal weakness, *Neurology* 31:635, 1981.

165. Tuhrim S, Yang WC, Rubinowitz H, Weinberger J: Primary pontine hemorrhage and the dysarthria-clumsy hand syndrome, *Neurology* 31:635, 1982.

166. Spertell RB, Ransom BR: Dysarthria-clumsy hand syndrome produced by capsular infarct, *Ann Neurol* 6:268, 1979.

167. Glass JD, Levey AI, Rothstein JD: The dysarthria-clumsy hand syndrome: A distinct clinical entity related to pontine infarction, *Ann Neurol* 27:487, 1990.

168. Arboix A, Bell Y, García-Eroles L, et al: Clinical study of 35 patients with dysarthria-clumsy hand syndrome, *J Neurol Neurosurg Psychiatry* 75:231-234, 2004.

169. Arboix A, López-Grau M, Casasnovas C, et al: Clinical study of 39 patients with atypical lacunar syndrome, *J Neurol Neurosurg Psychiatry* 77:381-384, 2006.

170. Besson G, Hommel M, Perret J: Risk factors for lacunar infarcts, *Cerebrovasc Dis* 10:387-390, 2000.

171. D'Olhaberriague L, Arboix A, Marti-Vilalta JL, et al: Movement disorders in ischemic stroke: Clinical study of 22 patients, *Eur J Neurol* 2:553, 1995.

172. Goldblatt D, Markesbery W, Reeves AG: Recurrent hemichorea following striatal lesions, *Arch Neurol* 31:51, 1974.

173. Martin JP: Hemichorea (hemiballismus) without lesions in the corpus Luysii, *Brain* 80:1, 1957.

174. Saris S: Chorea caused by caudate infarction, *Arch Neurol* 40:590, 1983.

175. Meyers R: Ballismus. In Vinken PJ, Bruyn GW, editors: *Handbook of clinical neurology*, vol 6, Amsterdam, 1968, North Holland, p 476.

176. Antin SP, Prockop LD, Cohen SM: Transient hemiballismus, *Neurology (Minneap)* 17:1068, 1967.

177. Kase CS, Maulsby GO, de Juan E, Mohr JP: Hemichorea hemiballism and lacunar infarction in the basal ganglia, *Neurology* 31:454, 1981.

178. Russo LS: Focal dystonia and lacunar infarction of the basal ganglia, *Neurology* 40:61, 1983.

179. Kim JW, Kim SH, Cha JK: Pseudochoreoathetosis in four patients with hypesthetic ataxic hemiparesis in a thalamic lesion, *J Neurol* 246:1075, 1999.

180. Massey EW, Goodman JC, Stewart C, et al: Unilateral asterixis: Motor integrative dysfunction in focal vascular disease, *Neurology* 29:1188, 1979.

181. Yagnik P, Dhopesh V: Unilateral asterixis, *Arch Neurol* 38:601, 1981.

182. Dethy S, Luxen A, Bidaut LM, et al: Hemibody tremor related to stroke, *Stroke* 24:2094, 1993.

183. Kim JS: Delayed onset hand tremor caused by cerebral infarction, *Stroke* 23:292, 1992.

184. Croisile B, Henry E, Trillet M, Aimard G: Loss of motivation for speaking with bilateral lacunes in the anterior limb of the internal capsule, *Clin Neurol Neurosurg* 91:325, 1989.

185. Laitinen LV: Loss of motivation for speaking with bilateral lacunes in the anterior limb of the internal capsule [letter], *Clin Neurol Neurosurg* 92:177, 1990.

186. Santamaria J, Graus F, Rubio F, et al: Cerebral infarction of the basal ganglia due to embolism from the heart, *Stroke* 14:911, 1983.

187. Bonhoeffer K: Klinischer und anatomischer Befund zur Lehre von der Apraxie und der "motorischen Sprachbahn." *Monatsschr Psychiatr Neurol* 35:113, 1914.

188. Kleist K: *Gehirnpathologie*, Leipzig, 1934, Barth, p 930.

189. Wolfe N, Linn R, Babikian VL, et al: Frontal systems impairment following multiple lacunar infarcts, *Arch Neurol* 47:129, 1990.

190. Van Zandvoort MJE, Kappelle LJ, Algra A, et al: Decreased capacity for mental effort after single supratentorial lacunar infarct may affect performance in everyday life, *J Neurol Neurosurg Psychiatry* 56:697, 1998.

191. Grau-Olivares M, Arboix A, Bartrés-Faz D, et al: Neuropsychological abnormalities associated with lacunar infarction, *J Neurol Sci* 257:160-165, 2007.

192. Satomi K, Terashima Y, Goto K, et al: Capsular pseudobulbar mutism in a patient of lacunar state, *Rinsho Shinkeigaku* 30:299, 1990.

193. Tatemichi TK, Desmond DW, Prohovnik I, et al: Confusion and memory loss from capsular genu infarction: A thalamocortical disconnection syndrome? *Neurology* 42:1966, 1992.

194. Castaigne P, Lhermitte F, Buge A, et al: Paramedian thalamic and midbrain infarcts: Clinical and neuropathologic study, *Ann Neurol* 10:127, 1981.

195. Poirer J, Barbizet J, Gaston A, Meyrignac C: Démence thalamique, *Rev Neurol (Paris)* 139:5, 1983.

196. Guberman A, Stuss D: The syndrome of bilateral paramedian thalamic infarction, *Neurology (Cleve)* 33:540, 1983.

197. Schott B, Maugiere F, Laurent B, et al: L'amnésie thalamique, *Rev Neurol (Paris)* 136:117, 1980.

198. Wallesch CW, Kornhuber HH, Kunz T, Brunner RJ: Neuropsychological deficits associated with small unilateral thalamic lesions, *Brain* 106:141, 1983.

199. Read SJ, Pettigrew L, Schimmel L, et al: White matter medullary infarcts: acute subcortical infarction in the centrum semiovale, *Cerebrovasc Dis* 8:289-295, 1998.

200. Boiten J, Rothwell PM, Slattery J, et al: Frequency and degree of carotid stenosis in small centrum ovale infarcts as compared to lacunar infarcts, *Cerebrovasc Dis* 7:138-143, 1997.

201. Leys D, Mounier-Vehier F, Rondepierre PH, et al: Small infarcts in the centrum ovale: Study of predisposing factors, *Cerebrovasc Dis* 4:83-87, 1994.

202. Krapf H, Widder B, Skalej M: Small rosarylike infarctions in the centrum semiovale suggest hemodynamic failure, *AJNR Am J Neuroradiol* 19:1479-1484, 1998.

203. Lammie GA, Wardlaw JM: Small centrum ovale infarcts. A pathological study, *Cerebrovasc Dis* 9:82-90, 1999.

204. Bogousslavsky J, Regli F: Centrum ovale infarcts: Subcortical infarction in the superficial territory of the middle cerebral artery, *Neurology* 42:1992-1998, 1992.

205. Hachinski V, Bowler J: Vascular dementia, *Neurology* 43:2159-2160, 1993.

206. Neuropathology Group: Medical Research Council cognitive function and aging study. Pathological correlates of late onset dementia in a multicentre, community-based population in England and Wales, *Lancet* 357:169-175, 2001.

207. Moorhouse P, Rockwood K: Vascular cognitive impairment: current concepts and clinical developments, *Lancet Neurol* 7:246-255, 2008.

208. Snowdon DA, Greiner LH, Mortimer JA: Brain infarction and the clinical expression of Alzheimer disease. The Nun Study, *JAMA* 277:813-817, 1997.

209. Tatemichi TK, Desmond D, Paik M, et al: Clinical determinants of dementia related to stroke, *Ann Neurol* 33:568-575, 1993.

210. Chui H: Dementia due to subcortical ischaemic vascular disease, *Clin Cornerstone* 3:40-51, 2001.

211. Miyao S, Takano A, Teramoto J, et al: Leukoaraiosis in relation to prognosis for patients with lacunar infarction, *Stroke* 23:1434-1438, 1992.

212. Tatemichi TK, Paik M, Bagiella E, et al: Risk of dementia after stroke in a hospitalized cohort: results of a longitudinal study, *Neurology* 44:1885-1891, 1994.

213. Pohjasvaara T, Mäntylä R, Ylikoski R, et al: How complex interactions of ischemic brain infarcts, white matter lesions and atrophy relate to poststroke dementia, *Arch Neurol* 57:1295-1300, 2000.

214. Wallin A, Blennow K, Gottfries CG: Subcortical symptoms predominate in vascular dementia, *Int J Geriatr Psychiatry* 6:137-146, 1991.

215. O'Brien JT, Erkinjuntti T, Reisberg B, et al: Vascular cognitive impairment, *Lancet Neurol* 2:89-98, 2003.

216. Englund E, Person B: Correlations between histopathologic white matter changes and proton MR relaxation times in dementia, *Alzheimer Dis Assoc Disord* 1:156-170, 1987.

217. Babikian V, Ropper AH: Binswanger's disease: A review, *Stroke* 18:2-12, 1987.

218. Erkinjuntti T: Vascular cognitive impairment and dementia. In Mohr JP, Choi DW, Grotta JC, Weir B, Wolf PhA, editors: *Stroke: Pathophysiology, diagnosis, and management*, Philadelphia, 2004, Churchill Livingstone, pp 648-660.

219. Cummings JL: Vascular subcortical dementias: Clinical aspects, *Dementia* 5:177-180, 1994.

220. Roman GC, Erkinjuntti T, Wallin A, et al: Subcortical ischaemic vascular dementia, *Lancet Neurol* 1:426-436, 2002.

221. Grau Olivares M, Bartrés-Faz D, Arboix A, et al: Mild cognitive impairment after lacunar infarction: Voxel-based morphometry and neuropsychological assessment, *Cerebrovasc Dis* 23:353-361, 2007.

222. Wentzel C, Rockwood K, MacKnight C, et al: Progression of the impairment in patients with vascular cognitive impairment without dementia, *Neurology* 57:714-716, 2001.

223. Tham W, Auchus AP, Thong M, et al: Progression of cognitive impairment after stroke: One year results from a longitudinal study of Singaporean stroke patients, *J Neurol Sci* 203-204:49-52, 2002.

224. Ingles JL, Wentzel C, Fisk JD, et al: Neuropsychological predictors of incident dementia in patients with vascular cognitive impairment without dementia, *Stroke* 33:1999-2002, 2002.

225. Ballard C, Rowan E, Stephens S, et al: Prospective follow-up study between 3 and 15 months after stroke, *Stroke* 34:2440-2445, 2003.

226. Kotila M, Waltimo O, Niemi ML, et al: The profile of recovery from stroke and factors influencing outcome, *Stroke* 15:1039-1044, 1984.

227. Patel M, Coshall C, Rudd AG, et al: Natural history of cognitive impairment after stroke and factors associated with its recovery, *Clin Rehabil* 17:158-166, 2003.

228. Rasquin SMC, Lodder J, Verhey FRJ, et al: Predictors of reversible mild cognitive impairment after stroke: A two-year follow-up study, *J Neurol Sci* 229-230:21-25, 2005.

229. Desmond DW, Moroney JT, Sano M: Incidence of dementia after ischemic stroke: Results of a longitudinal study, *Stroke* 33:2254-2260, 2002.

230. Sachdev PS, Brodaty H, Valenzuela MJ, et al: Progression of cognitive impairment in stroke patients, *Neurology* 63:1618-1623, 2004.

231. Binswanger OL: Die Abgrenzung der allgemeinen progressive paralyse, *Berl Klin Wochenschr* 31:1102-1105: 1137-1139, 1180-1186, 1894.

232. Bennet DA, Wilson RS, Gillen DW, et al: Clinical diagnosis of Binswanger's disease, *J Neurol Neurosurg Psychiatry* 53:961-965, 1990.

233. Martí-Fàbregas J, Valencia C, Lopez J, et al: Blood pressure variability in Binswanger's disease and isolated lacunar infarction, *Cerebrovasc Dis* 11:230-234, 2001.

234. Alzheimer A: Die seelenstörungen auf arteriosclerotischer grundlage, *Allgemeine Zeitschrift fur Psychiatrie* 59:695, 1902.

235. Bucholz: Ueber die Geistesstoerungen bei Arteriosklerose und ihre Beziehungen zu den psychischen Erkrankungen des Seniiums, *Arch Psychiatr Nervenkr* 39:499, 1905.

236. Ladame C: Encephalopathie sous-corticale chronique, *Encephale* 7:13, 1912.

237. Nissl: Zur Kasuistik der arteriosklerotischen Demenz (ein Fall von sogennanter "Encephalitis subcorticalis"), *Ges Neuro* 19:438, 1920.

238. Olszewski J: Subcortical arteriosclerotic encephalopathy: Review of the literature on the so-called Binswanger's disease and presentation of two cases, *World Neurol* 3:359, 1962.

239. Biemond A: On Binswanger's subcortical arteriosclerotic encephalopathy and the possibility of its clinical recognition, *Psychiatr Neurol Neurochir* 73:413-417, 1970.

240. De Reuck J, Crevits L, DeCoster W, et al: Pathogenesis of Binswanger's chronic progressive subcortical encephalopathy: A clinical and radiological investigation, *Neurology* 30:920-928, 1980.

241. Fisher C: Binswanger's encephalopathy: A review, *J Neurol* 236:65-79, 1989.

242. Lotz PR, Ballinger WE Jr, Quisling RG: Subcortical arteriosclerotic encephalopathy: CT spectrum and pathologic correlation, *AJR Am J Roentgenol* 147:1209-1214, 1986.

243. Mathers SE, Chambers BR, Meroy JR, et al: Subcortical arteriosclerotic encephalopathy: Binswanger's disease, *Clin Exp Neurol* 23:67-70, 1987.

244. Revesz T, Hawkins CP, du Boulay EP, et al: Pathological findings correlated with magnetic resonance imaging in subcortical arteriosclerotic encephalopathy (Binswanger disease), *J Neurol Neurosurg Psychiatry* 52:1337-1344, 1989.

245. Mast H, Mohr JP: Binswanger's disease and vascular dementia. In Mohr JP, Choi DW, Grotta JC, Weir B, Wolf PA, editors: *Stroke: Pathophysiology, Diagnosis and Management*, ed 4, Philadelphia, 2004, Churchill Livingstone, Chapter 31, pp 679-686.

246. Benson DF, Cummings JL, Tsai SY: Angular gyrus syndrome simulating Alzheimer's disease, *Arch Neurol* 39:616-620, 1982.

247. Cummings JL, Benson DF: *Dementia: A clinical approach*, Boston, 1992, Butterworth-Heinemann.

248. Tatemichi TK, Desmond DW, Prohovnik I: Strategic infarcts in vascular dementia. A clinical and brain imaging experience, *Drug Res* 45:371-385, 1995.

249. Mendez MF, Adams NL, Lewandowski KS: Neurobehavioral changes associated with caudate lesions, *Neurology* 39:349-354, 1989.

250. Kumral E, Evyapan D, Balkir K: Acute caudate vascular lesions, *Stroke* 30:100-108, 1999.

251. Tatemichi TK, Desmond DW, Mayeux R, et al: Dementia after stroke: Baseline frequency, risks, and clinical features in a hospitalized cohort, *Neurology* 42:1185-1193, 1992.

252. Ott B, Saver J: Unilateral amnesic stroke: Six new cases and a review of the literature, *Brain* 24:1033-1042, 1993.

253. Chui H: Neuropathology lesions in vascular dementia, *Alzheimer Dis Assoc Disord* 19:45-52, 2005.

254. Vermeer SE, Prins ND, den Heijer T, et al: Silent brain infarcts and the risk of dementia and cognitive decline, *N Engl J Med* 348:1215-1222, 2003.

255. Perren F, Clarke S, Bogousslavsky J: The syndrome of combined polar and paramedian thalamic infarction, *Arch Neurol* 62:1212-1216, 2005.

256. Madureira S, Guerreiro M, Ferro JM: A follow-up study of cognitive impairment due to inferior capsular genu infarction, *J Neurol* 246:764-769, 1999.

257. Pullicino P, Kendall BE: Contrast enhancement in ischaemic lesions. I: Relationship to prognosis, *Neuroradiology* 19:235, 1980.

258. Launay M, N'Diaye M, Bories J: X-ray computed tomography (CT) study of small, deep and recent infarcts (SDRIs) of the cerebral hemispheres in adults, *Neuroradiology* 27:494, 1985.

259. Arboix A, Marti-Vilalta JL, Pujol J, et al: Lacunar infarct and nuclear magnetic resonance: A review of sixty cases, *Eur Neurol* 30:47, 1990.

260. Hommel M, Besson G, Le Bas JF, et al: Prospective study of lacunar infarction using magnetic resonance imaging, *Stroke* 21:546, 1990.

261. Elster AD: MR contrast enhancement in brainstem and deep cerebral infarction, *AJNR Am J Neuroradiol* 12:1127, 1991.

262. Takao M, Koto A, Tanahashi N, et al: Pathologic findings of silent, small hyperintense foci in the basal ganglia and thalamus on MRI, *Neurology* 52:666, 1999.

263. Kinoshita T, Okudera T, Tamura H, et al: Assessment of lacunar hemorrhage associated with hypertensive stroke by echo-planar gradient-echo T2-weighted MRI, *Stroke* 31:1646, 2000.

264. Awad IA, Johnson PC, Spetzler RF, Hodak JA: Incidental subcortical lesions identified on magnetic resonance imaging in the elderly. II: Postmortem pathological correlates, *Stroke* 17:1090, 1986.

265. Offenbacher H, Fazekas F, Smith R, et al: MR of cerebral abnormalities concomitant with primary intracerebral hematomas, *AJNR Am J Neuroradiol* 17:573-578, 1996.

266. Fazekas F, Kleinert R, Roob G, et al: Histopathologic analysis of foci of signal loss on gradient-echo T2-weighted MR images in patients with spontaneous intracerebral hemorrhage: Evidence of microangiopathy-related microbleeds, *AJNR Am J Neuroradiol* 20:637–642, 1999.

267. Greenberg S, O'Donnell H, Schaefer P, et al: MRI detection of new hemorrhages: Potential marker of progression in cerebral amyloid angiopathy, *Neurology* 22:1135–1138, 1999.

268. Koennecke HC: Cerebral microbleeds on MRI: Prevalence, associations, and potential clinical implications, *Neurology* 66:165–171, 2006.

269. Vernooij MW, van der Lugt A, Ikram MA, et al: Prevalence and risk factors of cerebral microbleeds. The Rotterdam Scan Study, *Neurology* 70:1208–1214, 2008.

270. Roob G, Lechner A, Schmidt R, et al: Frequency and location of microbleeds in patients with primary intracerebral hemorrhage, *Stroke* 31:2665–2669, 2000.

271. Fiehler J: Cerebral microbleeds: Old leaks and new haemorrhages, *Int J Stroke* 1:122–130, 2006.

272. Noguchi K, Nagayoshi T, Watanabe N, et al: Diffusion-weighted echo-planar MRI of lacunar infarcts, *Neuroradiology* 40:448, 1998.

273. Schonewille WJ, Tuhrim S, Singer MB, et al: Diffusion-weighted MRI in acute lacunar syndromes: A clinical-radiological correlation study, *Stroke* 30:2066, 1999.

274. Singer MB, Chong J, Dongfeng L, et al: Diffusion-weighted MRI in acute subcortical infarction, *Stroke* 29:133, 1998.

275. Wessels T, Röttger C, Jauss M, et al: Identification of embolic stroke patterns by diffusion-weighted MRI in clinically defined lacunar stroke syndromes, *Stroke* 36:757–761, 2005.

276. Gerraty RP, Parsons MW, Barber A, et al: Examining the lacunar hypothesis with diffusion and perfusion magnetic resonance imaging, *Stroke* 33:2019–2024, 2002.

277. Ay H, Oliveira-Filho J, Buonanno FS, et al: Diffusion-weighted imaging identifies a subset of lacunar infarction associated with embolic stroke, *Stroke* 30:2644, 1999.

278. Sweeny R, Cheng EM, Kidwell CHS, et al: Incidence of intracranial large vessel disease in patients with radiologic lacunar stroke, *Neurology* 52(suppl 2):557, 1999.

279. Thompson DW, Cruz S, Eichholz KM: Magnetic resonance angiography in patients with paramedian pontine infarcts and a lacunar syndrome, *Neurology* 50:A-215, 1998.

280. Cho Z-H, Kang CK, Han J-Y, et al: Observation of the lenticulostriate arteries in the human brain in vivo using 7.0T MR angiography, *Stroke* 39:1604–1606, 2008.

281. Kapelle LJ, van Gijn J: Carotid angiography in patients with subcortical ischaemia. In Donnan GA, Norrving B, Bamford JM, Bogousslavsky J, editors: *Lacunar and other subcortical infarctions*, Oxford, 1995, Oxford University Press, p 80.

282. Kidwell CS, El-Saden S, Livshits Z, et al: Transcranial Doppler pulsatility indices as a measure of diffuse small-vessel disease, *J Neuroimag* 11:229, 2001.

283. Chamorro A, Saiz A, Vila N, et al: Contribution of arterial blood pressure to the clinical expression of lacunar infarction, *Stroke* 27:388, 1996.

284. Donnan GA, Kazui S, Levi CR, et al: Risk factors for lacunar stroke: A case-control transesophageal echocardiographic study, *Stroke* 31:284, 2000.

285. Kazui S, Levi CR, Jones EF, et al: Lacunar stroke: Transoesophageal echocardiographic factors influencing long-term prognosis, *Cerebrovasc Dis* 12:325, 2001.

286. Caplan LR, Young RR: EEG findings in certain lacunar stroke syndromes, *Neurology* 22:403, 1972.

287. Falcone N, Fensore C, Lanzetti A, et al: Clinical considerations and EEG-CT correlations in lacunar infarcts, *Rev Neurol* 56:396, 1986.

288. Kapelle LJ, van Huffelen AC: Electroencephalography in patients with small, deep infarcts. In Donnan GA, Norrving B, Bamford JM, Bogousslavsky J, editors: *Lacunar and other subcortical infarctions*, Oxford, 1995, Oxford University Press, p 87.

289. Labar DR, Petty GW, Emerson RG, Mohr JP, Pedley TA: Abnormal somatosensory evoked potentials in patients with motor deficits due to lacunar strokes, *Electroencephalogr Clin Neurophysiol* 67:74, 1987.

290. Mochizuki Y, Oishi M, Takasu T: Cerebral blood flow in single and multiple lacunar infarctions, *Stroke* 28:1458, 1997.

291. Matarin M, Brown WM, Scholtz S, et al: A genome-wide genotyping study in patients with ischaemic stroke: Initial analysis and data release, *Lancet Neurol* 6:414–420, 2007.

292. Joutel A, Corpechot C, Ducros A, et al: Notch 3 mutations in CADASIL, a hereditary adult-onset condition causing stroke and dementia, *Nature* 383:707–710, 1996.

293. Zhang J, Kohara K, Yamamoto Y, et al: Genetic predisposition to neurological symptoms in lacunar infarction, *Cerebrovasc Dis* 17:273–279, 2004.

294. Elbaz A, Poirier O, Moulin T, et al: Association between the Glu-298Asp polymorphism in the endothelial constitutive nitric oxide synthase gene and brain infarction. The GENIC investigators, *Stroke* 31:1634–1639, 2000.

295. Jannes J, Hamilton-Bruce MA, Pilotto L, et al: Tissue plasminogen activator -7351C/T enhancer polymorphism is a risk factor for lacunar stroke, *Stroke* 35:1090–1094, 2004.

296. Nakase T, Mizuno T, Harada S, et al: Angiotensinogen gene polymorphism as a risk factor for ischemic stroke, *J Clin Neurosci* 14:943–947, 2007.

297. Chamorro A, Revilla M, Obach V, et al: The -174G/C polymorphism of the interleukin 6 gene is a hallmark of lacunar stroke and not other ischemic stroke phenotypes, *Cerebrovasc Dis* 19:91–95, 2005.

298. Hassan A, Lansbury A, Catto AJ, et al: Angiotensin converting enzyme insertion/deletion genotype is associated with leuko-araiosis in lacunar syndromes, *J Neurol Neurosurg Psychiatry* 72:343–346, 2002.

299. Alpers BJ: *Clinical neurology*, Philadelphia, 1958, FA Davis.

300. Bruno A, Biller J, Adams HP Jr, et al: Acute blood glucose level and outcome from ischemic stroke, *Neurology* 52:280, 1999.

301. Chan RKT, Chong PN: Hyperglycemia is not associated with adverse outcome in patients with lacunar infarcts, *Neurology* 52(suppl 2):301, 1999.

302. Millikan C, Futrell N: The fallacy of the lacune hypothesis, *Stroke* 21:1251, 1990.

303. Sacco SE, Whisnant JP, Broderick J, et al: Epidemiological characteristics of lacunar infarcts in a population, *Stroke* 22:1236, 1991.

304. Castellanos M, Castillo J, García MM, et al: Inflammation-mediated damage in progressing lacunar infarctions. A potential therapeutic target, *Stroke* 33:982–987, 2002.

305. Boiten J: *Lacunar stroke: A prospective clinical and radiological study* [thesis], 1991, Maastricht.

306. Arboix A, Marti-Vilalta JL: Lacunar syndromes not due to lacunar infarcts, *Cerebrovasc Dis* 2:287, 1992.

307. Hier DB, Foulkes MA, Swiontoniowski M, et al: Stroke recurrence within 2 years after ischaemic infarction, *Stroke* 22:155, 1991.

308. Staaf G, Lindgren A, Norrving B: Pure motor stroke from presumed lacunar infarct: Long-term prognosis for survival and risk of recurrent stroke, *Stroke* 32:2592, 2001.

309. Arauz A, Murillo L, Cantú C, et al: Prospective study of single and multiple lacunar infarcts using magnetic resonance imaging. Risk factors, recurrence, and outcome in 175 consecutive cases, *Stroke* 34:2453–2458, 2003.

310. Arboix A, Font A, Garro C, et al: Recurrent lacunar infarction following a previous lacunar stroke: A clinical study of 122 patients, *J Neurol Neurosurg Psychiatry* 78:1392–1394, 2007.

311. Jackson C, Sudlow C: Comparing risks of death and recurrent vascular events between lacunar and non-lacunar infarction, *Brain* 128:2507–2517, 2005.

312. Bang OY, Joo SY, Lee PH, et al: The course of patients with lacunar infarcts and a parent arterial lesion. Similarities to large vs small artery disease, *Arch Neurol* 61:514–519, 2004.

313. Roquer J, Rodriguez A, Gomis M: Association of lacunar infarcts with small artery and large artery disease: A comparative study, *Acta Neurol Scand* 110:350–354, 2004.

314. Rockwood K, Wentzel C, Hachinski V, et al: Prevalence and outcomes of vascular cognitive impairment. Vascular Cognitive Impairment Investigators of the Canadian Study of Health and Aging, *Neurology* 54:447–451, 2000.

315. Carey CI, Kramer JH, Josephson SA, et al: Subcortical lacunes are associated with executive dysfunction in cognitive normal elderly, *Stroke* 39:397–402, 2008.

316. Wen HM, Mok VCT, Fan YH, et al: Effect of white matter changes on cognitive impairment in patients with lacunar infarcts, *Stroke* 35:1826–1830, 2004.

317. Gold G, Kövari E, Hermann FR, et al: Cognitive consequences of thalamic, basal ganglia, and deep white matter lacunes in brain aging and dementia, *Stroke* 36:1184-1188, 2005.

318. Yamamoto Y, Akiguchi I, Oiwa K, Hayashi M, Kasai T, Ozasa K: Twenty-four-hour blood pressure and MRI as predictive factors for different outcome in patients with lacunar infarct, *Stroke* 33:297-305, 2002.

319. Vermeer SE, Hollander M, van Dijk EJ, et al: Silent brain infarcts and white matter lesions increase stroke risk in the general population: The Rotterdam Scan Study, *Stroke* 34:1126-1129, 2003.

320. De Jong G, Kessels F, Lodder J: Two types of lacunar infarcts. Further arguments from a study on prognosis, *Stroke* 33:2072-2076, 2002.

321. Frey JL, Snider RM, Jahnke H, et al: rt-PA in lacunar infarction, *Neurology* 50:A-406, 1998.

322. Cocho D, Belvis R, Marti-Fàbregas J, et al: Does thrombolysis benefit patients with lacunar syndrome? *Eur Neurol* 55:70-73, 2006.

323. Mohr JP, Thompson JLP, Lazar RM, et al: A comparison of warfarin and aspirin for the prevention of recurrent ischemic stroke, *N Engl J Med* 345:1444, 2001.

324. DiNapoli P, Taccardi AA, Oliver M, et al: Statins and stroke: Evidence for cholesterol-independent effects, *Eur Heart J* 23:1908-1921, 2002.

325. Endres M, Laufs U: Effects of statins on endothelium and signaling mechanisms, *Stroke* 35(Suppl 1):2708-2711, 2004.

326. Amarenco P, Benavente O, Goldstein LB, et al: Atorvastatin is similarly effective in all ischemic stroke subtypes: Secondary analysis of the SPARCL trial, *Neurology* 70(Suppl 1):230, 2008.

327. Yamamoto Y, Akiguchi I, Oiwa K, et al: Adverse effect of night-time blood pressure on the outcome of lacunar infarct patients, *Stroke* 29:570, 1998.

328. Pariente J, Loubinoux I, Carel C, et al: Fluoxetine modulates motor performance and cerebral activation of patients recovering from stroke, *Ann Neurol* 50:718, 2001.

329. Hashimoto T, Morita H, Tada T, et al: Neuronal activity in the globus pallidus in chorea caused by striatal lacunar infarction, *Ann Neurol* 50:528, 2001.

330. Boiten J, Lodder J: Lacunar infarcts: Pathogenesis and validity of the clinical syndromes, *Stroke* 22:1374, 1991.

331. Gan R, Sacco RL, Kargman DE, et al: Testing the validity of the lacunar hypothesis: The Northern Manhattan Stroke Study experience, *Neurology* 48:1204, 1997.

332. Madden KP, Karanjia PN, Adams HP, et al: Accuracy of initial stroke subtype diagnosis in the TOAST study, *Neurology* 45:1975, 1995.

333. Rothrock JF, Lyden PD, Yee J, et al: "Crescendo" transient ischemic attacks: Clinical and angiographic correlations, *Neurology* 38:198, 1988.

334. Salgado ED, Weinstein M, Furlan AF, et al: Proton magnetic resonance imaging in ischaemic cerebrovascular disease, *Ann Neurol* 20:502, 1986.

335. Brown MM, Hesselink JR, Rothrock JF: MR and CT of lacunar infarcts, *AJNR Am J Neuroradiol* 9:477, 1988.

336. Rothrock JF, Lyden PD, Hesselink JR, et al: Brain magnetic resonance imaging in the evaluation of lacunar infarcts, *Stroke* 18:781, 1987.

337. Kobayashi S, Okada K, Yamashita K: Incidence of silent lacunar lesion in normal adults and its relation to cerebral blood flow and risk factors, *Stroke* 22:1379, 1991.

338. Horwitz DR, Tuhrim S, Weinberger JM: Mechanism in lacunar infarction, *Stroke* 23:325, 1992.

339. Kilpatrick TJ, Matkovic Z, Davis SM, et al: Hematologic abnormalities occur in both cortical and lacunar infarction, *Stroke* 24:1945, 1993.

340. Mast H, Thompson JL, Voller H, et al: Cardiac sources of embolism in patients with pial artery infarcts and lacunar lesions, *Stroke* 25:776, 1994.

341. Tegeler CH, Shi F, Morgan T: Carotid stenosis in lacunar stroke, *Stroke* 22:1124, 1991.

342. Loeb C, Gandolfo C, Croce R, et al: Dementia associated with lacunar infarction, *Stroke* 23:1225, 1992.

343. Hughes M, Dodgson MCH: Chronic cerebral hypertensive disease, *Lancet* 2:770, 1954.

344. Fang HCH: Lacunar infarction: Clinico-pathologic correlation study [abstract], *J Neuropathol Exp Neurol* 31:212, 1972.

345. Ishii N, Nishihara Y, Imamura T: Why do frontal lobe symptoms predominate in vascular dementia with lacunes? *Neurology* 36:340, 1986.

346. Mancardi GL, Romagnoli P, Tassinari T, et al: Lacunes and cribriform cavities of the brain: Correlations with pseudobulbar palsy and parkinsonism, *Eur Neurol* 28:11, 1988.

347. Dozono K, Ishii N, Nishihara Y, Horie A: An autopsy study of the incidence of lacunes in relation to age, hypertension, and arteriosclerosis, *Stroke* 22:993, 1991.

348. Arboix A, Ferrer I, Marti-Vilalta JL: Análisis clinico-anatomopatológico de 25 pacientes con infartos lacunares, *Rev Clin Esp* 196:370, 1996.

349. The National Institute of Neurological Disorders and Stroke: Rt-PA Stroke Study Group. Tissue plasminogen activator for acute ischemic stroke, *N Engl J Med* 333:1581, 1995.

28 | Cerebral Venous Thrombosis

JOSÉ M. FERRO, PATRÍCIA CANHÃO

Cerebral vein and dural sinus thrombosis (CVT) are less frequent than other types of strokes and have a quite different clinical presentation and involve different etiologic investigations. They rarely manifest as a stroke syndrome—that is, as the sudden onset of focal symptoms and signs in patients with classic vascular risk factors. The clinical features are rather diverse; hence CVTs are more challenging to diagnose than other types of stroke. Once considered a rare, often fatal disease related to the puerperium and to infections of the central nervous system (CNS), sinuses, and mastoid,[1] CVT is now recognized with increasing frequency. The clinical spectrum of CVT and associated conditions has widened considerably. The apparent rise in the frequency of CVT is related to increasing awareness of its diagnosis among neurologists and emergency physicians and to the use of magnetic resonance imaging (MRI) for the investigation of patients with headache, seizures, and unclear neurologic pictures. Because it can be the initial manifestation of or can complicate several systemic conditions, CVT is a disease of interest not only for neurologists but also for neurosurgeons; ear, nose, and throat (ENT) specialists; ophthalmologists; internists; rheumatologists; oncologists; hematologists; and obstetricians.

Epidemiology

No epidemiologic studies of CVT meet the current standards for a good-quality epidemiologic stroke study. Such a study would be difficult and expensive to perform because of the variable and often nonacute presentation of CVT. A large spectrum of neurologic complaints would need to be investigated by MRI to ascertain CVT cases ("hot" pursuit), and MRI reports, autopsy reports, and certificates of death would have to be reviewed ("cold" pursuit). The few epidemiologic studies available have methodologic limitations and probably underestimate the true incidence of CVT. They probably missed many of the mild, self-limited forms of CVT. A community study performed in England and Wales found an annual incidence of only 22 cases.[2] An autopsy study of 160 women who died during pregnancy found 10 cases (6%) of intracranial venous thrombosis.[3] In an autopsy study performed in the 1970s, the prevalence of CVT was 9%.[4] This high number could not be reproduced in a 2003 study,[5] which found a prevalence of only 1% in consecutive autopsies. Autopsy studies are biased because they reflect severe fatal cases of CVT, in particular those associated with intracranial infection, which are fortunately rare. In a nationwide hospital-based series in Portugal, including patients admitted to all neurology services in the country, 91 new cases of CVT were identified, corresponding to an incidence of 0.22/100,000/year.[6] In Hong Kong, the rate among admitted patients was 3.4/100,000/year.[7] In Isfahan, Iran, the annual frequency of CVT was 1.23/100,000/year.[8] A hospital discharge registry in the United States gave an incidence of CVT during pregnancy of 11.6 per 100,000 deliveries.[9] The incidence in the multicenter Canadian registry of CVT in infants and children younger than 18 years was 0.67/100,000.[10] In hospital-based series, CVT is more common in children than in adults. Among children, CVT is more common in neonates than in older children.[10] In adults, CVT affects patients who are younger than those with other types of strokes, and the incidence apparently decreases in older subjects. The median age in the International Study on Cerebral Vein and Dural Sinus Thrombosis (ISCVT) cohort was 37 years,[11] with only 8% of the patients older than 65. CVT is more common in females than in males (female-to-male ratio 2.9:1).[11]

A few studies addressed the chronobiology of CVT. In Portugal, CVTs were more frequent in autumn and winter, raising the hypothesis that upper respiratory infections are the trigger of CVT in prone individuals.[12] However, in Germany, CVTs were more frequent in winter and summer,[13] whereas in Iran the seasonal CVT rate was higher in autumn and lower in summer.[8]

Venous Anatomy

Blood of the brain is drained by the cerebral venous system, which consists of the cerebral veins and dural venous sinuses. Cerebral veins comprise the superficial venous system, deep venous system, and posterior fossa veins (Fig. 28-1). Superficial cerebral veins course over the surface of the brain, draining the major part of the cerebral cortex, with the exception of the inner face of temporal and occipital lobes, and a portion of the subjacent white matter. They are quite variable in number and location. They have no valves and are linked by several anastomoses, allowing the development of collateral circulation in the event of vein or sinus occlusion. Ascending superficial veins are named according to the area of cortex they drain. Anastomotic Trolard and Labbé's veins connect the sylvian or superficial middle cerebral veins with the superior sagittal sinus and the lateral sinus, respectively.

The deep venous system drains the inferior frontal lobe, most of the deep white matter of cerebral hemispheres, the corpus callosum, the basal ganglia, and the upper brainstem. It includes the internal cerebral and

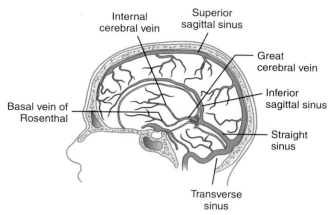

Figure 28-1 Sagittal view of the anatomy of superficial and deep cerebral veins and dural sinuses.

basal veins of Rosenthal that join to form the great cerebral vein of Galen, which drains into the straight sinus. Except for the anatomic variations of the basal veins, the deep venous system is relatively constant compared with the superficial cortical venous system. Posterior fossa veins are variable in their number and course. Three groups of veins may be recognized: superior veins draining into the great vein of Galen, anterior veins draining into the petrosal sinus, and posterior veins draining into the torcular Herophili or the straight or lateral sinuses.

Cerebral veins drain the blood into the dural sinuses, which are endothelium-lined channels without valves and enclosed in the leaves of the dura mater. There are two groups of dural sinuses, superior and inferior. The superior group, which collects the major part of blood of the brain and skull, comprises the superior and inferior sagittal sinus, and the straight, transverse, and sigmoid sinuses (see Fig. 28-1). Superficial veins drain into the superior sagittal and transverse sinuses, and the deep cerebral veins into the straight and transverse sinuses. The confluence of the sinuses (torcular Herophili) results from the junction of superior sagittal, straight, and transverse sinuses and is often asymmetrical. The inferior group drains the basal and medial parts of the undersurface of the brain, the orbits, and the sphenoparietal sinus and collects at the cavernous sinus. Cavernous sinuses connect with the lateral sinuses via superior and inferior petrosal sinuses and with the pterygoid plexus.

Most of the cerebral venous blood flows posteriorly, from the superior sagittal sinus or the straight sinus via the lateral sinuses into the internal jugular veins. A smaller proportion flows to the cavernous sinuses.

There are several anatomic variations of the dural sinuses. The most important are atresia of the anterior part of the superior sagittal sinus; duplication of the superior sagittal sinus, mainly in its posterior part; asymmetry of the transverse sinus with dominance of the right transverse sinus in the majority of cases; and aplasia or hypoplasia of the posteromedial segment of the left transverse sinus. The straight sinus may join the torcular, the right transverse sinus, the left transverse sinus, or all three. Owing to the variability of cerebral veins and anatomic variants of the dural sinus, the angiographic diagnosis

of vein or dural sinus thrombosis can occasionally be challenging.

Pathophysiology

Developments in imaging modalities, such as diffusion-weighted MRI (DWI) and perfusion-weighted MRI (PWI), have improved our knowledge of the pathophysiology of CVT and have established some differences between venous and arterial occlusion and infarction.[14-25] Nevertheless, results provided by these studies are still conflicting, and ultimately, the pathogenesis of parenchymal lesions due to venous occlusion remains insufficiently understood. There are few experiments in adequate animal models of CVT.[26] The variability of venous system anatomy makes the understanding of venous flow disturbances and mechanisms of lesion formation difficult.

At least two different mechanisms may contribute to the clinical features of CVT: the thrombosis of the cerebral veins or dural sinus, leading to cerebral lesions; and the occlusion of the dural sinus, resulting in disturbance of cerebrospinal fluid (CSF) absorption and increased intracranial pressure.

Venous or dural sinus occlusion may have different consequences in the brain: no detectable lesions, focal edema, or hemorrhage. Several mechanisms may be involved, namely vasogenic edema, cytotoxic edema, both vasogenic and cytotoxic edema, and hemorrhage. One of the first consequences of venous occlusion is the increase in venous pressure. At an early stage, the collateral pathways of venous drainage allow for significant compensation, and parenchymal lesions may not develop. Some animal experiments have shown that thrombosis of the cortical veins is required to induce brain lesions, but this may not be the case in human CVT. As venous and capillary pressure rise, dilatation of veins and capillaries occurs, followed by blood-brain barrier disruption with leakage of blood plasma into the interstitial space, resulting in vasogenic edema. This pattern is confirmed by diffusion-weighted MRI, which shows isointensity, hypointensity, or hyperintensity signal abnormality in the affected area without significantly lower apparent diffusion coefficient (ADC) values than in unaffected regions.[14,15,24] On perfusion-weighted MRI, relative cerebral blood volume (rCBV) and mean transit time (MTT) are increased in affected areas, with preserved relative cerebral blood flow (rCBF).[15,24] Experimental animal data suggest that vasogenic edema occurs earlier in venous stroke than in arterial stroke.[27] At this stage, if collateral pathways are efficacious or recanalization occurs, tissue perfusion may be possible, and swollen brain cells are potentially recoverable.[28] Further increase in intravenous pressure exacerbates cerebral edema and may lead to venous or capillary rupture, causing brain hemorrhage. In addition, elevation of intravenous pressure produces venous congestion, raises intravascular pressure, and lowers cerebral perfusion pressure. Cerebral blood flow may then fall below the penumbra or ischemic threshold, resulting in energetic failure, loss of the Na^+,K^+-ATPase pump activity, and intracellular entry of water, with consequent cytotoxic edema. MRI has confirmed a cytotoxic pattern of edema in patients with CVT, characterized by

TABLE 28-1 RISK FACTORS ASSOCIATED WITH CEREBRAL VENOUS THROMBOSIS

Prothrombotic condition
  Genetic
  Acquired (e.g., antiphospholipid syndrome)
Infection
  Central nervous system (e.g., abscess, empyema, meningitis)
  Ear, sinus, mouth, face and neck (e.g., otitis, mastoiditis, tonsillitis, stomatitis, sinusitis, skin)
  Systemic infectious disease (e.g., sepsis, endocarditis, tuberculosis, HIV)
Inflammatory disease
  Systemic lupus erythematosus
  Behçet's disease
  Sjögren's syndrome
  Wegener's granulomatosis
  Temporal arteritis
  Thromboangiitis obliterans
  Inflammatory bowel disease
  Sarcoidosis
Malignancy
  Central nervous system (meningioma, metastasis, glomus tumor, medulloblastoma)
  Solid tumor outside the central nervous system
  Hematologic (leukemias, lymphomas)
Hematologic condition
  Anemia
  Sickle cell disease or trait
  Iron deficiency
  Paroxysmal nocturnal hemoglobinuria
  Polycythemia (primary or secondary)
  Thrombocythemia (primary or secondary)
Pregnancy and puerperium
Other disorders
  Dehydration
  Nephrotic syndrome
  Congenital heart disease
  Diabetic ketoacidosis
  Thyroid disease (hyperthyroidism or hypothyroidism)
  Central nervous system disorder
    Dural fistula
    Arachnoid cyst
Other precipitants
  Head trauma
  Lumbar puncture, myelography, intrathecal steroids
  Neurosurgical procedures, irradiation
  Jugular catheter occlusion
  Drugs (oral contraceptives, hormone replacement therapy, androgens, medroxyprogesterone acetate, L-asparaginase, cyclosporine, tamoxifen, steroids, lithium, thalidomide, ecstasy, sildenafil)

TABLE 28-2 THROMBOPHILIA CONDITIONS ASSOCIATED WITH INCREASED RISK OF CEREBRAL VENOUS THROMBOSIS

Antiphospholipid antibody/anticardiolipin antibody (immunoglobulins G and M)
Protein S deficiency
Protein C deficiency
Antithrombin III deficiency
G20210A prothrombin gene mutation
Factor V Leiden mutation
Hyperhomocysteinemia (may or may not be caused by gene polymorphism TT homozygosity in methylene tetrahydrofolate reductase)
Homocystinuria
Increased coagulation factor VIII
Plasminogen deficiency

Besides parenchymal changes, dural sinus thrombosis may impair cerebrospinal fluid (CSF) circulation and cause intracranial hypertension. CSF absorption occurs mainly in the arachnoid villi and granulations (pacchionian bodies) contained in the superior sagittal sinus and other sinuses. Thrombosis of the sinuses leads to increased venous pressure, impaired CSF absorption, and, consequently, increased intracranial pressure. This process is more frequent with superior sagittal sinus occlusion, but it may also result from a rise in sinus pressure without thrombosis of the superior sagittal sinus, such as in lateral sinus or jugular vein thrombosis.

Etiology

A large number of conditions are known to cause or predispose to CVT (Table 28-1). At least one risk factor can be identified in more than 85% of patients with CVT, and multiple risk factors may be found in about half of patients.[11]

The more frequent risk factors are prothrombotic conditions (either genetic or acquired), oral contraceptive use, puerperium or pregnancy states, infection, and malignancy.[11] A patient's genetic background most likely determines the inherent individual risk. In the presence of some identified prothrombotic conditions, patients are at increased risk for development of CVT when exposed to CVT precipitants. Thrombophilic disorders are leading risk factors for CVT (Table 28-2). A prothrombotic condition was identified in 34% of the patients in the ISCVT cohort, being genetically determined in 22% of the patients.[11] The most frequent are G20210A prothrombin mutation (identified in 6% to 20% of patients with CVT),[31-34] factor V Leiden (10% to 24%),[32-38] and anticardiolipin/antiphospholipid antibodies (6% to 8%).[11,35] Less often, protein C, protein S, or antithrombin III deficiencies are identified (0 to 9%).[32-37] A systematic review confirmed the increased risk of CVT in patients with G20210A prothrombin mutation (odds ratio [OR, 9.27; 95% confidence interval [CI], 5.85-14.67), factor V Leiden (OR, 3.38; 95% CI, 2.27-5.05), and hyperhomocysteinemia (OR, 4.07; 95% CI, 2.54-6.52).[39] There are insufficient data to support the independent contribution of *MTHFR* (methylenetetrahydrofolate reductase) gene mutation as a risk factor for CVT.[40]

high signal intensity on DWI and low ADC values.[16,20,22,29] However, in comparison with arterial stroke, the lesions of venous stroke visible on DWI might be more capable of recovering.[22]

In summary, the pathogenesis of venous lesions is very different from that of arterial infarcts. Vasogenic edema predominates, and cytotoxic edema is far less common. After venous occlusion, large areas of the brain may be functionally and metabolically disturbed, but not irreversibly. Reversibility is very typical of venous lesions, reflected in both favorable clinical recovery and vanishing lesions on neuroimaging.[30]

The prevalence of selected thrombophilia disorders may be different in patients with CVT and in patients with lower extremity deep venous thrombosis (DVT). In the study carried out in the Mayo Clinic, the G20210A prothrombin mutation was more than twice as common in patients with CVT, whereas factor V Leiden and protein C deficiency were more common in patients with DVT.[41]

Infective causes of CVT have declined, being responsible for 6% to 12% in large series of adults with the disease.[1,11] In developing countries, systemic and nervous system infections may remain an important cause of CVT (18%).[42] Although uncommon, cavernous sinus thrombosis is caused predominantly by skin infections of the face.

Cancers account for 7.4% of all CVTs. Of these, 2.2% were associated with CNS malignancy, 3.2% with solid tumors outside the CNS, and 2.9% with hematologic disorders.[11] Sinus or venous thrombosis can result from local compression or invasion by the tumor, can be caused by a hypercoagulable state, or, less commonly, can be associated with local or systemic infections, can be therapy related, or can be paraneoplastic.[43] Many of the reported precipitants of CVT are systemic diseases or conditions known to predispose to venous thrombosis in other parts of the body, but others are peculiar to CVT. Among the latter are local causes such as brain tumors or arteriovenous malformations, major or minor head trauma,[44] spontaneous intracranial hypotension,[45] and some invasive procedures (e.g., neurosurgery, jugular catheterization, irradiation, and lumbar puncture with or without drug infusion) (see Table 28-1).

The risk of CVT varies throughout life. In the Canadian Pediatric Ischemic Stroke Study Group, a risk factor was identified in 98% of the children.[10] In neonates, acute systemic illness such as perinatal complications and dehydration were frequent, occurring in 84% of patients.[10] Head and neck disorders, mostly infections, and chronic systemic diseases (e.g., connective tissue diseases, hematologic disorders, and cancers) were common in older children. A prothrombotic state was found in 41% of the patients, most often in non-neonates.

The most common risk factor in young women is oral contraceptive use. Two case-control studies have shown an increased risk of sinus thrombosis in women who use oral contraceptives.[34,36] In their meta-analysis, Dentali and colleagues[39] pointed out that the risk of DVT in women taking oral contraceptives was almost six times higher than that of non-users of the agents (OR 5.59; 95% CI, 3.95-7.91).[39] The risk for women who use oral contraceptives and carry a prothrombotic defect is higher than that for women without such risk factors.[36] Another frequent setting related to CVT in women is pregnancy and the puerperium,[11,46,47] more common in less developed world regions with higher pregnancy rates.[48] CVT has also been diagnosed in association with the rare ovarian hyperstimulation syndrome resulting from in vitro fertilization protocol.[49]

In the ISCVT study, genetic or acquired thrombophilia, malignancies, and hematologic disorders such as polycythemia were the most common risk factors in elderly patients with CVT.[50] In 37% of elderly patients, no risk factors could be identified.

Despite extensive search, no underlying risk factor is found in almost 13% of adult patients with CVT. At times, the cause is revealed weeks or months after the acute phase. Therefore, in the case of CVT without known cause, it is recommended to monitor the patient and to continue searching for a cause (vasculitis, antiphospholipid syndrome, cancer).

Clinical Aspects

The clinical presentation of CVT is highly variable.[1] In more than half of patients the onset is subacute, with symptoms increasing in intensity and severity over several days. In a third of the patients the onset is acute, the full clinical picture being established within 24 hours, but onset is rarely apoplectic. A few cases have a protracted, chronic presentation. A patient with CVT manifesting as multiple transient ischemic attacks (TIAs) has also been reported.[51] Symptoms and signs of CVT can be grouped in three more frequent syndromes, as follows: (1) isolated intracranial hypertension syndrome, consisting of headache with or without vomiting, papilledema, and visual troubles,[52] (2) focal syndrome, including focal deficits, seizures, or both, and (3) encephalopathy, when bilateral or multifocal signs, delirium, or dysexecutive or consciousness disturbances occur.[1,6] Less frequent presentation syndromes include the cavernous sinus syndrome, consisting of orbital pain, oculomotor palsies, proptosis, and chemosis, and syndromes involving multiple palsies of the lower cranial nerves.

Clinical symptoms and signs depend on the following factors: (1) gender of the patient,[10,50] (2) age of the patient,[10,50] (3) interval from onset to presentation,[53,54] (4) presence of parenchymal lesions, and (5) site and number of occluded sinuses and veins. As in the general population, headaches are more frequent in women than in men with CVT. Symptoms of CVT differ in neonates and older children.[10] In neonates, presentation is often nonspecific, with seizures in more than half of the babies, respiratory distress syndrome or apnea, poor feeding, lethargy, and hypotonia or hypertonia.[55] Diffuse signs of brain damage, with coma and seizures, are also the main manifestations in younger children. Clinical manifestations in older children, such as headache with or without vomiting, papilledema, sixth nerve palsy, motor deficits, focal or generalized seizures, and disturbances of consciousness, are more similar to the adult presentation.[10,56-58] Elderly patients have a clinical picture distinct from that in younger adults: Decreased vigilance and mental symptoms are more common in the elderly, whereas headaches and isolated intracranial hypertension are less common.[50] The clinical picture also depends on the time elapsed from onset to presentation.[53] Patients with more severe clinical features, such as disturbance of consciousness or of mental status, seizures, or motor deficits, tend to present earlier.[54] Isolated intracranial hypertension and papilledema are more frequent in patients with a chronic presentation. As expected, if the admission neuroimaging shows either a hemorrhage or a venous infarct, the clinical picture is more severe. Coma and consciousness disturbances, paresis, aphasia, and seizures are more common in patients with such brain lesions than in subjects without them. Conversely, patients with brain lesions are less likely to present with isolated headache.

Up to 90% of patients with CVT complain of headache, which is the most frequent symptom of CVT and usually the initial one. In 9% of patients in the ISCVT, headache was the only symptom of CVT. As for other secondary headaches, headaches associated with CVT are more frequent in women and young patients. The localization of the headaches has no relationship with the localization of the occluded sinus or of the parenchymal lesions.[59,60] CVT-associated headaches are more severe and of more acute onset than other types of headaches requiring emergency care,[61] with the exception of subarachnoid hemorrhage. Headache is more frequently localized and continuous, with an acute-subacute onset of pain and moderate to severe intensity. The most frequent type of headache is the intracranial hypertension variety, a severe, generalized headache worsening with Valsalva's maneuvers and when the patient is lying down. Transient loss of vision can occur in association with spells of more intense headache. In CVT manifesting only as headache, the onset of the latter is usually progressive, and the pain is continuous. Headache is more often unilateral and ipsilateral to the occluded lateral sinus than it is diffuse.[62] A few cases of CVT manifesting only as sudden, explosive headache and neck stiffness,[63,64] mimicking subarachnoid hemorrhage, have been reported. In a minority of patients with headache and stiffness, the CSF is bloody, but in the majority, the headache meets the criteria of the thunderclap type.[65] Migraine with aura has also been reported.[66-68] Some of the conditions and precipitants associated with CVT also manifest as headache, thus increasing the challenge of the diagnosis of CVT complicating these conditions. This is the case for meningitis, meningiomas, dural arteriovenous fistulas, Behçet's disease, other vasculitides, and also low intracranial pressure. CVT must also be included as a possible cause of persisting headache after lumbar puncture.[69]

Some patients may complain of visual loss (13% of cases) or are found to have papilledema on funduscopy (28%), a finding more frequent in chronic cases.[53] Severe acute cases of CVT manifest as disturbances of consciousness, ranging from drowsiness to coma (14%), or mental troubles (22%), such as delirium, apathy, or dysexecutive syndrome. Unilateral or, less frequently, bilateral motor deficits, in the form of monoparesis or hemiparesis, are the most common focal deficits (37%). Aphasia can also occur (19%). Fluent aphasia is a manifestation of an occlusion of the left lateral sinus with a posterior temporal lobe lesion. Sensory deficits (5%) and visual field defects are less common. Seizures are more frequent in CVT than in other stroke types. They can be focal (20%) or generalized (30%) and may be complicated by status epilepticus, which can occur rarely from the onset. Seizures are more frequent in patients with brain lesions, motor or sensory deficits, and sagittal sinus and cortical vein thrombosis.[70,71]

The clinical presentation of CVT also varies according to the location of the occluded sinus or vein. In cavernous sinus thrombosis, which is rare and usually has an infectious cause, ocular signs dominate the clinical picture, consisting of headache, orbital pain, chemosis, proptosis, ptosis, diplopia, and oculomotor palsies. Isolated cortical vein thrombosis is probably underidentified, and its diagnosis is difficult to confirm. With use of traditional MRI sequences and MR angiography, the interobserver agreement for the diagnosis of cortical vein thrombosis is low.[72] The diagnostic accuracy is much improved by the use of T2 spin-echo (SE) sequences. Typically, cortical vein thrombosis produces motor or sensory deficits and seizures.[73-76] In occlusion of the sagittal sinus, motor deficits (46%) and focal (35%) and generalized (47%) seizures are frequent, but presentation as an isolated intracranial hypertension syndrome (17%) is infrequent. Bilateral motor deficits are not uncommon (7%). The opposite is found in patients with isolated thrombosis of the lateral sinus, who often at presentation have isolated intracranial hypertension (31% to 47%) but rarely have paresis (11% to 15%) or focal (9% to 12%) or generalized seizures (20% to 24%). Aphasia is frequent in left transverse sinus occlusion (40%). Multiple cranial nerve palsies (Collet-Sicard syndrome) are a rare manifestation of lateral sinus,[77] jugular, or posterior fossa vein thrombosis. A pulsating tinnitus may be the sole symptom of a jugular vein or lateral sinus thrombosis.[78,79] When the deep cerebral venous system is occluded, the clinical picture is often severe, with coma (67%), mental deficits (87%), and paresis (56%) that can be bilateral (11%).[80-82] In deep CVT, the severity of the clinical picture depends on the extent of the thrombosis in the deep veins and the territory of the involved vessels, the establishment of collaterals, and the duration of the occlusion. Limited thrombosis of the deep venous system can produce relatively mild symptoms without disturbances of consciousness.[83]

Diagnosis

The confirmation of the diagnosis of CVT depends on the demonstration of thrombi in the cerebral veins or sinuses by neuroimaging.

Computed Tomography

Computed tomography (CT) is usually the first investigation performed, particularly if patients are evaluated in an emergency setting. CT is useful to rule out other acute or subacute cerebral disorders that CVT may imitate, such as tumor, subdural hematoma, and abscess. CT is normal in up to 30% of cases of CVT, and most of the findings are nonspecific. CT signs are divided into direct and indirect. Direct signs of CVT, which can be found in about one third of cases, correspond to the visualization of thrombus itself (Fig. 28-2)[1,84]: the cord sign (thrombosed cortical or deep vein), the dense triangle sign (visualization of the clot inside the sinus), and the empty delta sign, visible after injection of a contrast agent as a contrast between the nonopacified thrombus inside the sinus and the collateral veins of the sinus wall. Indirect signs are more frequent and include intense contrast enhancement of falx and tentorium, dilated transcerebral veins, small ventricles, localized or diffuse white matter hypodensity without contrast enhancement, and

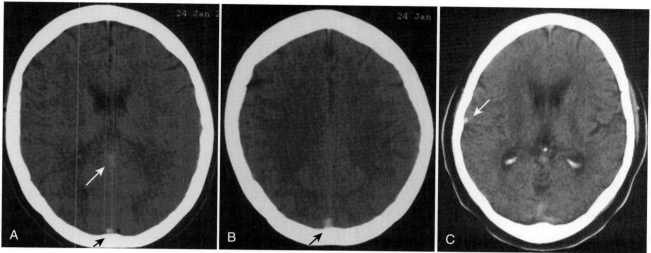

Figure 28-2 Unenhanced CT scans showing direct signs of cerebral thrombosis. A and B, The dense triangle sign—hyperdensities in the torcular Herophili (A, *black arrow*), the straight sinus (A, *white arrow*), and the superior sagittal sinus (B, *arrow*). C, The cord sign *(arrow).*

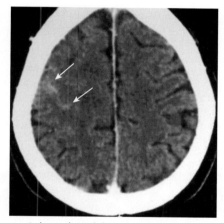

Figure 28-3 Subarachnoid hemorrhage as a manifestation of cerebral venous thrombosis *(arrows).*

hemorrhagic lesions. Parenchymal abnormalities may occur in 60% to 80% of cases, and some topographic lesions are suggestive of a specific sinus occlusion: bilateral parasagittal hemispheric lesions, temporooccipital lesions, and bilateral thalamic lesions, which are highly suspicious for thrombosis of the superior sagittal sinus, lateral sinus, and deep venous system, respectively. A small subdural hematoma or subarachnoid hemorrhage may rarely be demonstrated (Fig. 28-3).[63,64,85] In serial CT scans, new lesions may appear, and some may disappear ("vanishing infarcts").

CT Venography

Helical CT venography with bolus injection of contrast material provides excellent anatomic detail of venous circulation and can demonstrate filling defects in the dural sinus and cortical veins, sinus wall enhancement, and increased collateral venous drainage (Fig. 28-4).[86-89]

CT venography has several advantages over intraarterial angiography: it is less invasive and less expensive, and

the time to the initial diagnosis is shorter because it may be carried out immediately after brain CT. Visualization of the cavernous sinus, the inferior sagittal sinus, and the basal vein of Rosenthal with multiplanar reformatted images can be superior to that with conventional intraarterial angiography.[90] The following advantages of CT venography over MRI in visualization of CVT have been reported: rapid image acquisition, no contraindication to ferromagnetic devices, increased imaging resolution, and fewer equivocal imaging findings.[89] Furthermore, CT venography is more commonly able to image sinuses or cerebral veins with low flow than is MR venography.[87] Some limitations of CT venography are limited visualization of skull base structures in three-dimensional display, adverse reactions to iodinated contrast medium, and exposure to ionizing radiation, which may limit its use in pregnant women, children, and patients with renal failure.[89]

Magnetic Resonance Techniques

MRI combined with MR venography is currently the best method to confirm the diagnosis of CVT for the following reasons: It is noninvasive, allows the visualization of the thrombi and the occluded dural sinus or vein, and depicts parenchymal lesions (Figs. 28-5 and 28-6).[1,17,81,91,92] Even so, there are some limitations and diagnostic pitfalls with these techniques.[93,94] The primary finding of thrombosis is the absence of a flow void and the presence of altered signal intensity in the sinus. The combination of an abnormal signal in a sinus and a corresponding absence of flow on MR venography supports the diagnosis of CVT. Administration of contrast material and application of specific MR sequences and venographic techniques are often required for a confident diagnosis.

Magnetic Resonance Imaging

The signal intensity of the thrombus on T1- and T2-weighted MR images depends on the age of the thrombus: In the first 5 days, the signal is predominantly isointense on T1-weighted

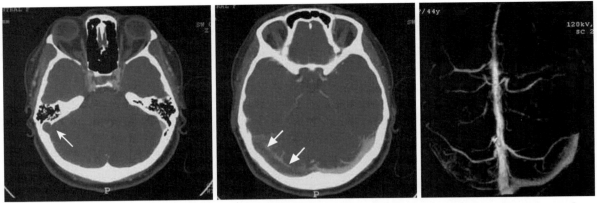

Figure 28-4 CT venograms in a patient with headache showing filling defects in the right lateral sinus *(arrows)*.

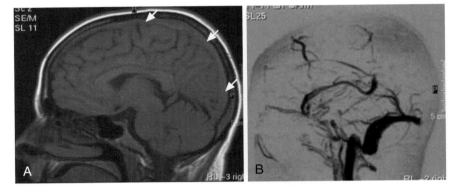

Figure 28-5 A, T1-weighted MR image discloses an isointense signal in the superior sagittal sinus *(arrows)*, corresponding to a thrombus. B, Magnetic resonance venogram showing the corresponding absence of flow.

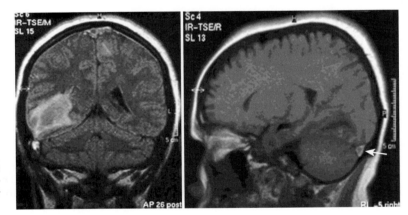

Figure 28-6 Lateral sinus thrombosis demonstrated as a hyperintense signal in T1- and T2-weighted FLAIR (fluid-attenuated inversion recovery) MR images. Concomitant hemorrhagic infarct can be seen *(arrow)*.

images and hypointense on T2-weighted images; after this time, the diagnosis becomes easier because of an increased signal on both T1- and T2-weighted images. After the first month, there is a variable pattern of signal, which may more frequently become isointense or hyperintense on T2-weighted images and hypointense or isointense on T1.[91,95,96] After gadolinium administration, marked contrast enhancement and flow voids may be observed within the thrombosed sinuses,[96,97] which could be related to organized thrombus with intrinsic vascularization, slow flow in dural and intrathrombus collateral channels, or recanalization. Echo-planar T2 susceptibility-weighted

imaging (T2*SW) sequences improve the diagnosis of CVT, enabling the identification of intraluminal thrombus as a hypointense area. T2*SW sequences are particularly useful in the acute stage of dural sinus thrombosis and in the diagnosis of isolated cortical venous thrombosis.[75,92,98,99] On diffusion-weighted MRI, hyperintense signals in veins or dural sinus can be observed.[17,21,100] Although the presence of such signals is a sign with low sensitivity for the acute detection of clot in CVT,[100] it may be predictive of a low rate of vessel recanalization.[100]

Besides the assessment of veins and sinuses, MRI is also useful in showing parenchymal lesions secondary to venous occlusion: brain swelling, focal or diffuse edema (which is demonstrated as a hypointense or isointense lesion on T1-weighted images and a hyperintense lesion on T2-weighted images), and hemorrhagic lesions, which appear as hyperintense lesions on both MRI sequences.

MR Venography

Several methods can assess venous or dural sinus flow: unenhanced two-dimensional time-of-flight (TOF) MR venography, three-dimensional TOF MR venography, and phase-contrast MR venography.[94] Contrast enhancement MR venography with elliptic centric ordering is a new method in which the paramagnetic effect of gadolinium is used to shorten T1 and provide positive intravascular contrast enhancement.[101] In comparison with TOF MR venography, this newer technique allows superior depiction of small vessels and dural sinuses.[94,101]

The most common method used is two-dimensional TOF MR venography, which typically demonstrates the absence of flow in the thrombosed vessel. Limitations of MR venography are diagnosis of cortical vein thrombosis, diagnosis of partial occlusion, and distinction between hypoplasia and thrombosis.

Intraarterial Angiography

At present, intraarterial angiography is rarely required for diagnosis. It may be performed mainly when the diagnosis of CVT is doubtful, namely, in the rare cases of isolated cortical vein thrombosis or when it is mandatory to exclude a dural arteriovenous fistula or distal aneurysm, such as in the presence of subarachnoid hemorrhage. Typical signs of CVT on angiography are partial or complete lack of filling of veins or sinuses, delayed emptying, dilated collaterals, and the sudden stopping of cortical veins surrounded by dilated and tortuous collateral "corkscrew veins" (Fig. 28-7). Anatomic variations may complicate the interpretation of angiography, such as hypoplasia of the anterior part of the superior sagittal sinus, duplication of the superior sagittal sinus, and hypoplasia or aplasia of the transverse sinuses.[1]

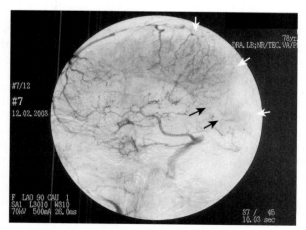

Figure 28-7 Intra-arterial angiogram showing typical signs of cerebral venous thrombosis: lack of filling of part of sagittal sinus (*white arrows*) and of the straight sinus (*black arrows*); nonfilling of the deep venous system; and dilated and tortuous collateral veins.

Interobserver Agreement on Neuroimaging Diagnosis of Cerebral Venous Thrombosis

The interobserver agreement on CVT diagnostic imaging is not perfect. The proportion of agreement is 62% for intraarterial angiography and 94% for MRI plus intraarterial angiography.[102] A study using MRI and MR venography suggested that the agreement between observers in the diagnosis of the location of CVT varies with the location of sinus or vein thrombosis. It is good or very good for most of the occluded sinus and veins, moderate to very good for the left lateral sinus and jugular vein, and poor to good for the cortical veins.[72]

Transcranial Doppler Ultrasonography

Transcranial Doppler ultrasonography[103,104] and transcranial power or color Doppler imaging, with or without the use of a contrast agent,[105-107] were reported as potential noninvasive techniques for the diagnosis or follow-up of CVT, but more studies are needed to determine the true clinical value of these methods.

D-Dimer Levels

In a 2009 systematic review, Haapaniemi and colleagues[108] examined published studies that had analyzed the value of measuring plasma levels of the fibrin degradation product D dimer in the diagnosis of patients with CVT.[109-113] Most such patients had increased D-dimer levels, but a few patients, mainly those presenting later after onset of symptoms or with isolated headache, exhibited normal D-dimer levels.[108,113] D-dimer levels had a significant positive correlation with the extent of CVT and a negative correlation with the duration of symptoms. The D-dimer assay demonstrated a high negative predictive value (95% to 100%) but a low sensitivity (83% to 95%). Although a normal D-dimer level makes CVT diagnosis unlikely, it cannot rule out the diagnosis, and, consequently, measurement of plasma D-dimer level is not a good screening test in patients with suspected CVT.

Prognosis

Traditionally, the prognosis of CVT was often considered to be ominous. Several prospective series,[114-119] and above all the large ISCVT cohort,[11] clarified the contemporary vital and functional prognosis of patients with acute CVT. The aggregate rate of death or dependency at the end of follow-up in these studies was 15%. In the ISCVT cohort, 79% of patients recovered completely. In a meta-analysis that also included retrospective studies, the overall rate of acute death was 5.6%, that of death at the end of follow-up was 9.4%, and that of complete recovery was 88%.[120] Predictors of poor long-term prognosis derived from the ISCVT cohort were CNS infection, malignancy, deep cerebral venous system thrombosis, hemorrhage on admission CT/MRI, Glasgow Coma Scale score on admission less than 9, mental status disorder, age older than 37 years, and male gender.[11] This predictive model was validated in two independent validation cohorts.[121]

Although in general, patients with CVT have a favorable prognosis, 4% die during the acute phase. Predictors of mortality at 30 days in the ISCVT cohort were depressed consciousness, mental status disorder, thrombosis of the deep cerebral venous system, right hemispheric hemorrhage, and posterior fossa lesions.[122] The main cause of death in acute CVT is transtentorial herniation secondary to a large hemorrhagic lesion.[122] Other causes of death are herniation due to multiple lesions or to diffuse brain edema, status epilepticus, medical complications, and pulmonary embolism.[123]

Among patients with CVT who have hemorrhagic lesions, 21% are dead or dependent at 6 months. Predictors of death or dependency in this subgroup of CVT patients are older age, male gender, thrombosis of the deep venous system or of the right lateral sinus, and motor deficit.[124] Prognosis is less favorable in patients at both extremes of age. One study found that the prognosis in adults older than 64 years is considerably worse than that in younger patients.[50] Only 47% of elderly patients made a complete recovery, whereas 27% died and 22% were dependent at the end of follow-up. In children, the death, dependency, and late complication rates are also higher than those in adults. The death rate ranges from 2% to 13%,[10,58,125,126] especially in neonates, whose mortality may be as high as 25%.[58] Only 22% of neonates survive free of any impairment.[55] Half of the deaths are a direct consequence of the venous thrombosis.[10] Sequelae of CVT include cognitive and motor impairments, seizures, and symptomatic persistent increased intracranial hypertension. Predictors of unfavorable outcome include coma, seizures, and venous infarcts,[10,58] whereas older age, anticoagulation, and transverse sinus involvement were predictors of good cognitive outcome, although the last item predicted isolated intracranial hypertension syndrome.[126]

Classically, the clinical course of CVT is unpredictable.[1] Clinical course after admission was prospectively investigated in the ISCVT cohort, with the following conclusions: About one fourth of the patients deteriorate in status after admission. Neurologic worsening may occur several days after admission and may consist of depressed consciousness, mental state disturbance, new seizures, worsening of a previous symptom or a new focal deficit, increase in headache severity, or visual loss. About one third of patients whose status deteriorates show new parenchymal lesions on "repeat" neuroimaging.[127] Patients with depressed consciousness on admission are more likely to deteriorate, and those with seizures at onset are more likely to have repeated seizures. Deterioration is less frequent but can occur in patients presenting with isolated headache or with isolated intracranial hypertension syndrome.

Patients who survive the acute phase of CVT are at risk for complications, especially further venous thrombotic events, seizures, and headaches. The underlying disease, in particular malignancies, may lead to death in the months or years following CVT. Headaches severe enough to require bed rest or hospital admission afflict 14% of patients with CVT.[11] MRI and MR venography are necessary to exclude recurrent CVT and other intracranial lesions and to document persistent cerebral venous occlusion, partial or complete sinus recanalization, or dural sinus stenosis.

Concerning new thrombotic events, recurrent CVT is rare and difficult to document. It is useful for the patient to undergo MRI/MR angiography 3 to 6 months after CVT to document the extent of recanalization. If new symptoms suggesting recurrence of CVT, such as new headaches or headaches increasing in severity, seizures, or a new focal sign, occur, MRI and MR venography should be performed and the images compared with original images. Other thrombotic events, specifically DVT of the limbs or pelvis and pulmonary embolism, occur in about 5% of patients. In the ISCVT cohort, 2.2% of patients had recurrent CVT and 4.3% had other thrombotic events. In the Mayo Clinic case series of 154 patients with CVT followed for a mean of 36 months, recurrent CVT occurred in 6.5%.[128] The rate of further venous thrombotic events is similar in children: In a European cohort of 396 children with CVT (median age 5.2 years) followed for a median of 36 months, recurrent venous thrombosis occurred in 22 (6%) children at a median of 6 months, including CVT in 13 children (3%).[125] There were no recurrences of CVT among children younger than 25 months. Absence of administration of anticoagulant therapy before relapse, persistent venous occlusion on "repeat" venous imaging, and heterozygosity for the prothrombin G20210A mutation[125] were independently associated with recurrent cerebral and systemic venous thrombosis in children.

Seizures may occur in up to 11% of the patients. Risk factors for these remote seizures are seizures during the acute phase, a hemorrhagic parenchymal lesion, and a motor deficit.[129]

Severe visual loss due to intracranial hypertension is very rare.[11,117,130] However, when evaluated by a neuroophthalmologist, a few CVT survivors may be found to have subnormal visual acuity or visual fields as well as esodeviation.[130]

In spite of the apparent generally good recovery, several studies pointed out that psychological and cognitive complaints are not uncommon among CVT survivors. About half of the survivors of CVT feel depressed or anxious[131] and demonstrate minor cognitive or language deficits,[132] which may preclude resumption of previous levels of professional activity.[133]

Pregnancy and puerperium are risk factors for CVT. For that reason, an important practical question is the outcome of future pregnancies in women who have had a CVT. Information to answer this question is available in six studies[11,47,115,117,134,135] involving a total of 855 women under observation, of whom 83 became pregnant after their CVTs, with a total number of 101 pregnancies. The large majority (88%) of the pregnancies ended in normal births, the remaining being prematurely terminated by voluntary or spontaneous abortion. The rate of spontaneous abortion was higher than expected. There were no instances of recurrent CVT and only two cases of DVT.

Recanalization of thrombosed cerebral vein and sinus occurs in 40% to 90% of patients after CVT, mostly within the first 4 months.[136] This process was confirmed by a systematic review that identified only five small studies evaluating recanalization after CVT. In the pooled population of these studies, recanalization rates at 3 months

(84%) and 1 year of follow-up (85%) were nearly identical. Recanalization is more common after thrombosis of the deep cerebral veins and of the cavernous sinuses, and less common in lateral sinus occlusion.[136]

Regarding the influence of recanalization on prognosis in adults, limited data suggest that recanalization of the occluded sinus is not related to outcome after CVT[137]; in children, however, nonrecanalization is associated with higher risk of recurrence.[125] The presence of hyperintensities in the veins or sinus on DWI sequences predicts a low chance of recanalization.[100]

Treatment

The treatment of CVT includes (1) antithrombotic treatment, (2) symptomatic treatment of intracranial hypertension, seizures, headache, and visual failure, and (3) etiologic treatment to manage the associated conditions and risk factors, which is beyond the scope of this chapter (Table 28-3). A guideline for the treatment of cerebral venous and sinus thrombosis was issued by the European Federation of Neurological Societies (EFNS) in 2006.[138]

The therapeutic priorities in the acute phase are to stabilize the hemodynamic and physiologic parameters, to prevent or reverse cerebral herniation, to stop seizures, and to treat infections or other associated condition needing urgent management.

Antithrombotic Treatment

The aims of antithrombotic treatment in CVT are (1) to recanalize the occluded sinus or vein, (2) to combat the propagation of the thrombus, namely to the bridging cerebral veins, thus preventing cerebral edema and infarct, (3) to prevent pulmonary embolism,[123] and (4) to treat the underlying prothrombotic state in order to prevent venous thrombosis in other parts of the body and the recurrence of CVT.

Two randomized controlled trials (RCTs) of anticoagulation in acute CVT have been performed in Europe.[139,140] Both have some methodologic problems, namely their modest sample size, selection, and measurement bias. The trial performed by Einhäupl and coworkers[140] in Berlin compared intravenous (IV) heparin with placebo. The trial was prematurely stopped because of excess deaths in the placebo arm. This trial showed a significantly better outcome for patients randomly assigned to the heparin arm. However, outcome was measured with a nonvalidated composite CVT severity scale. The Dutch trial, which compared subcutaneous (SC) nadroparin with placebo, excluded patients who would need lumbar punctures for the relief of intracranial pressure.[139] Despite randomization, the two arms were not balanced because there were more patients with isolated intracranial hypertension in the control group and more patients with infarcts in the nadroparin group. This trial showed a nonsignificant superiority of nadroparin over placebo. Two other trials were performed in India, but for these trials, outcome assessment was not blind, and the diagnosis of CVT was confirmed by CT alone.[141,142] One trial involved 57 patients and the other 40 patients. Results of

TABLE 28-3 TREATMENT OF CEREBRAL VENOUS THROMBOSIS (CVT): FUNDAMENTALS FOLLOWING EUROPEAN FEDERATION OF NEUROLOGICAL SOCIETIES GUIDELINES

Acute Phase
TREATMENT OF THE ETIOLOGY
Antithrombotic treatment
Subcutaneous low-molecular-weight heparin or intravenous heparin in therapeutic dosages
In experienced centers, if neurologic worsening occurs despite heparin and the best medical treatment and other causes of deterioration are excluded, local intravenous thrombolysis with/without mechanical thrombectomy is an option
Symptomatic treatment
Antiepileptics
In patients with acute seizures and supratentorial lesions
Consider as an option also for patients with either acute seizures or supratentorial lesions
Intracranial hypertension
Headache
Analgesics
Lumbar puncture, if there are no parenchymal lesions; perform before starting anticoagulation
Acetazolamide
Impairment of consciousness of herniation
Osmotic therapy
Sedation and hyperventilation
Hemicraniectomy
Threatened vision
Lumbar puncture, if there are no parenchymal lesions; perform before starting anticoagulation
Acetazolamide
Lumboperitoneal shunt
Optic nerve fenestration
Post–Acute Phase
TREATMENT OF THE ETIOLOGY
Antithrombotic treatment
Oral anticoagulants
For 3-6 months if CVT related to a transient risk factor
For 6-12 months if CVT idiopathic or related to "mild" hereditary thrombophilia
For life for recurrent CVT or "severe" hereditary thrombophilia
Symptomatic treatment
Antiepileptics
In patients with acute seizures or seizures in the post-acute phase and supratentorial lesions
Consider as an option also for patients without seizures but with either supratentorial lesions or motor deficits

both favored heparin: Maiti and Chakrabarti[141] reported fatality rates of 15% for heparin versus 40% for placebo; recovery in all heparin-treated patients contrasted with two deaths and one patient with residual hemiparesis in the control group of the trial conducted by Nagaraja and associates.[142] All four trials show an advantage of heparin over placebo. In addition, two cases of pulmonary embolism occurred in the placebo groups of the German and Dutch trials. The meta-analysis of the German and Dutch trials showed a relative risk of 0.46 (95% CI, 0.16–1.31) (60% relative risk reduction) of death or dependency after anticoagulant therapy in comparison with placebo.[143]

Regarding the safety of acute anticoagulant treatment, there is a theoretical concern because heparin might cause venous infarcts to become hemorrhagic or might increase bleeding in already existing hemorrhagic lesions. New or increased hemorrhage does indeed occur after heparin treatment for CVT, but the frequency is low. In case series, the risks of intracranial hemorrhage (<5%) and systemic hemorrhage (<2%) were also low, and such hemorrhages did not influence outcome.[144] Anticoagulants are also safe to use in patients with intracranial hemorrhages, either intracerebral or subarachnoid.[138] This finding is in accord with the fact that such intracranial hemorrhages are secondary to venous outflow blockage. Anticoagulant therapy is also safe in children.[145] Both the German and Dutch trials included patients with hemorrhagic infarcts on baseline scans, but there were no intracranial hemorrhagic complications and only one major extracranial bleed. These findings support the choice of full anticoagulation with intravenous heparin or subcutaneous high-dose low-molecular-weight heparin (LMWH) as the initial treatment for nearly all patients with acute or subacute sinus thrombosis. There is a large consensus on the use of heparin or LMWH in acute CVT. For instance, more than 80% of the patients in the ISCVT underwent anticoagulation.[146] The European Federation of Neurological Societies guidelines on the treatment of CVT recommended that patients with CVT but with no contraindications to anticoagulation should be treated either with APTT-adjusted IV heparin or with body weight–adjusted LMWH.[138]

Although antiplatelet drugs may be used as alternatives when anticoagulants are contraindicated, there is no evidence, even from uncontrolled series, regarding the efficacy and safety of antiplatelet agents in CVT.

Thrombolysis

The majority of patients with CVT experience a good outcome, but 4% die during the acute phase of CVT,[122] and the condition of some patients worsens despite anticoagulant therapy. Direct thrombolysis has been used as an alternative treatment in the latter case. Direct thrombolysis aims to dissolve the thrombus by delivering a thrombolytic substance (urokinase or recombinant tissue plasminogen activator [rt-PA]) within the occluded sinus (transverse, superior sagittal, or straight sinus) through an IV catheter. In some cases, mechanical endovascular disruption of the thrombus has also been used. Endovascular thrombolysis, when successful, can remove the thrombus from the major sinuses within hours. However, this procedure is complicated and expensive. The patient needs anesthesia and intensive care monitoring, and usually the catheter remains in the sinus for hours to days, with repeated applications of the thrombolytic agent and radiologic assessments.

Many case reports or case series describing the use of thrombolytics have been published, suggesting that these agents might be useful and safe, but no RCTs evaluating the efficacy and safety of systemic or local thrombolysis

in patients with CVT have yet been performed. In a systematic review of 169 patients treated with local thrombolysis, only 5% died during the acute phase of CVT, and 8% were dependent at discharge.[147] The results of this systematic review suggest a possible benefit of thrombolytics in cases of severe CVT, indicating that the agents may reduce the case fatality rate in critically ill patients. Intracranial hemorrhages were reported in 17% of cases but were associated with clinical deterioration in only 5%. Extracranial hemorrhages were reported in 19% of cases but were severe in only 2%. The case fatality was not higher in the 39 patients with CT/MRI evidence of hemorrhage (7%). Hemorrhagic complications were not significantly higher in patients with CT/MRI evidence of previous hemorrhage.

There is a potential publication bias in the literature for this issue, with possible underreporting of cases with poor outcome and complications. Treatment and evaluation were nonblinded, leading to bias in evaluating outcomes. In the ISCVT, 13 patients were treated with local thrombolysis. Five (38.5%) were dead or dependent 6 months after CVT. In a Dutch series of 20 patients treated with IV local thrombolysis, 12 recovered to independent living, and 6 died.[148] Local thrombolysis was not useful in patients with large infarcts and impending herniation. These results are worse than those in the previously published literature but may reflect the prevailing results in clinical practice. Currently, there is no evidence to support the routine use of thrombolysis. Endovascular thrombolysis may be performed in selected centers with expertise in interventional radiology as a therapeutic option in patients with a poor prognosis, such as those whose condition worsens despite best medical treatment and anticoagulation, provided that other causes of the worsening are excluded and treated. A randomized trial to compare endovascular treatment with heparin has been announced.

Prevention of Thrombotic Events after the Acute Phase

After the acute phase of CVT, recurrence of cerebral venous thrombosis can be detected in 2% to 7% of patients, and extracerebral venous thrombosis can occur in up to 5%. To prevent further thrombotic events, anticoagulation with warfarin is recommended. In the Rochester Mayo Clinic series, the likelihood of recurrent venous thrombosis was the same after CVT and lower extremity DVT. Recurrence of CVT was not influenced by warfarin therapy.[128] In children, nonadministration of anticoagulation predicts recurrent CVT or systemic venous thrombosis.[125] The optimal duration of anticoagulation is not known, because it was not addressed in RCTs. Anticoagulation is usually maintained for 3 to 12 months after acute CVT, aiming at an international normalized ratio (INR) of 2 to 3. The EFNS guidelines suggest that when CVT is related to a transient risk factor (e.g., pregnancy, infection), anticoagulants may be used for 3 months. In patients with idiopathic CVT or CVT associated with "mild" thrombophilia, the period of anticoagulation must be longer (6 to 12 months). In patients with "severe" thrombophilia (e.g., two or more prothrombotic abnormalities or antiphospholipid syndrome), anticoagulants should be given for life.

Symptomatic Treatment

Treatment of Intracranial Hypertension

In the acute phase, increased intracranial pressure (ICP) due to single or multiple large hemorrhagic lesions or infarcts or to massive brain edema may be fatal by causing transtentorial herniation. General recommendations to control acutely increased ICP include elevating the head of the bed, osmotic diuretics such as mannitol, intensive care unit admission with sedation, hyperventilation to a target $Paco_2$ of 30 to 35 mm Hg, and ICP monitoring.[138] Although corticosteroids may decrease vasogenic edema, they cannot be recommended routinely to decrease ICP. Steroid may even promote thrombosis. A case-control study failed to demonstrate any benefit of steroids even in patients with parenchymal lesions.[149] In patients with impending herniation due to unilateral hemispheric lesion, hemicraniectomy can be life-saving.[150,151] In patients with acute CVT who have severe headache with or without papilledema, intracranial hypertension can be reduced and symptoms relieved through a therapeutic lumbar puncture when not contraindicated by parenchymal lesions.

In patients with chronically increased intracranial pressure, treatment of intracranial hypertension is necessary to improve headache and prevent visual failure. A diagnostic/therapeutic lumbar puncture decreases the CSF pressure and offers headache relief. Although its efficacy is not proven, administration of a diuretic such as acetazolamide or furosemide is a therapeutic option. If severe headaches persist or if visual acuity is decreasing, repeated lumbar punctures, a lumboperitoneal shunt, stenting of a sinus stenosis,[152-154] or fenestration of the optic nerve sheath should be considered.[155,156]

Treatment and Prevention of Seizures

Acute seizures and supratentorial lesions are the risk factors for subsequent early seizures. Patients with both risk factors should be prescribed antiepileptic drugs. Prophylactic antiepileptics can also be considered in patients with one of the risk factors and should be avoided in patients with none of the risk factors.[70]

The long-term risk of remote seizures is approximately 11%.[11,71,129] The risk factors for remote seizures and post-CVT epilepsy are acute seizures, supratentorial hemorrhagic lesions, and motor deficits. Antiepileptics are recommended for patients with seizures in the acute phase of CVT and for those who experience a seizure after the acute phase. Antiepileptics can also be considered for patients without seizures but with either supratentorial hemorrhagic lesions or motor deficit. The optimal duration of antiepileptic treatment is unknown. General recommendations for the selection and withdrawal of antiepileptic drugs can be used as options. Valproate is preferred to phenytoin and carbamazepine because it causes less interference with oral anticoagulants and can be used intravenously. If valproate is not tolerated, a "new" antiepileptic (e.g., lamotrigine, topiramate, or levetiracetam) can be used. Patients with status epilepticus should be treated accordingly to guidelines for this epileptic condition.

Contraception and Future Pregnancies

Women of fertile age with past CVT should not become pregnant while taking an oral anticoagulant, because of its teratogenic effects. They should use contraceptive methods other than oral or parenteral contraceptives. Emergency contraception is also contraindicated.[157] Hormonal replacement therapy should also be stopped. CVT and pregnancy and puerperium-related CVT are not contraindications to future pregnancy. Although pregnancy and the puerperium are risk factors for CVT, the risk of complications during subsequent pregnancy among women who have a history of CVT is low.[11,47,115,134,135]

REFERENCES

1. Bousser MG, Russell RR: Cerebral venous thrombosis. In Warlow CP, Van Gijn J, editors: *Major problems in neurology*, vol 33. London, 1997, WB Saunders.
2. Kalbag RM, Woolf AL: *Cerebral venous thrombosis*, London, 1967, Oxford University Press.
3. Angelov A: Intracranial venous thrombosis in relation to pregnancy and delivery, *Pathol Res Pract* 185:843-847, 1989.
4. Towbin A: The syndrome of latent cerebral venous thrombosis: Its frequency and relation to age and congestive heart failure, *Stroke* 4:419-430, 1973.
5. Bienfait HP, van Duinen S, Tans JT: Latent cerebral venous and sinus thrombosis, *J Neurol* 250:436-439, 2003.
6. Ferro JM, Correia M, Pontes C, et al: for the Cerebral Venous Thrombosis Portuguese Collaboration Study Group (VENOPORT): Cerebral venous thrombosis in Portugal 1980-98, *Cerebrovasc Dis* 11:177-182, 2001.
7. Mak W, Mok KY, Tsoi TH, et al: Cerebral venous thrombosis in Hong Kong, *Cerebrovasc Dis* 11:282-283, 2001.
8. Janghorbani M, Zare M, Saadatnia M, et al: Cerebral vein and dural sinus thrombosis in adults in Isfahan, Iran: Frequency and seasonal variation, *Acta Neurol Scand* 117:117-121, 2008.
9. Lanska DJ, Kryscio RJ: Risk factors for peripartum and postpartum stroke and intracranial venous thrombosis, *Stroke* 31:1274-1282, 2000.
10. deVeber G, Andrew M, Adams C, et al: Canadian Pediatric Ischemic Stroke Study Group: Cerebral sinovenous thrombosis in children, *N Engl J Med* 345:417-423, 2001.
11. Ferro JM, Canhão P, Stam J, et al: ISCVT Investigators: Prognosis of cerebral vein and dural sinus thrombosis: Results of the International Study on Cerebral Vein and Dural Sinus Thrombosis (ISCVT), *Stroke* 35:664-670, 2004.
12. Ferro JM, Lopes GC, Rosas MJ, et al: VENOPORT Investigators: Chronobiology of cerebral vein and dural sinus thrombosis, *Cerebrovasc Dis* 14:265, 2002.
13. Stolz E, Klötzsch C, Rahimi A, et al: Seasonal variations in the incidence of cerebral venous thrombosis, *Cerebrovasc Dis* 16:455-456, 2003.
14. Corvol JC, Oppenheim C, Manai R, et al: Diffusion-weighted magnetic resonance imaging in a case of cerebral venous thrombosis, *Stroke* 29:2649-2652, 1998.
15. Keller E, Flacke S, Urbach H, et al: Diffusion- and perfusion-weighted magnetic resonance imaging in deep cerebral venous thrombosis, *Stroke* 30:1144-1146, 1999.
16. Manzione J, Newman GC, Shapiro A, et al: Diffusion- and perfusion-weighted MR imaging of dural sinus thrombosis, *AJNR Am J Neuroradiol* 21:68-73, 2000.
17. Chu K, Kang DW, Yoon BW, et al: Diffusion-weighted magnetic resonance in cerebral venous thrombosis, *Arch Neurol* 58:1569-1576, 2001.
18. Doege CA, Tavakolian R, Kerskens CM, et al: Perfusion and diffusion magnetic resonance imaging in human cerebral venous thrombosis, *J Neurol* 248:564-571, 2001.
19. Ducreux D, Oppenheim C, Vandamme X, et al: Diffusion-weighted imaging patterns of brain damage associated with cerebral venous thrombosis, *AJNR Am J Neuroradiol* 22:261-268, 2001.

20. Forbes KP, Pipe JG, Heiserman JE: Evidence for cytotoxic edema in the pathogenesis of cerebral venous infarction, *AJNR Am J Neuroradiol* 22:450–455, 2001.
21. Lövblad KO, Bassetti C, Schneider J, et al: Diffusion-weighted MR in cerebral venous thrombosis, *Cerebrovasc Dis* 11:169–176, 2001.
22. Peeters E, Stadnik T, Bissay F, et al: Diffusion-weighted MR imaging of an acute venous stroke, *AJNR Am J Neuroradiol* 22:1949–1952, 2001.
23. Yoshikawa T, Abe O, Tsuchiya K, et al: Diffusion-weighted magnetic resonance imaging of dural sinus thrombosis, *Neuroradiology* 44:481–488, 2002.
24. Makkat S, Stadnik T, Peeters E, et al: Pathogenesis of venous stroke: Evaluation with diffusion- and perfusion-weighted MRI, *J Stroke Cerebrovascular Dis* 12:132–136, 2003.
25. Mullins ME, Grant PE, Wang B, et al: Parenchymal abnormalities associated with cerebral venous sinus thrombosis: Assessment with diffusion-weighted MR imaging, *AJNR Am J Neuroradiol* 25:1666–1675, 2004.
26. Schaller B, Graf R: Cerebral venous infarction: The pathophysiological concept, *Cerebrovasc Dis* 18:179–188, 2004.
27. Gotoh M, Ohmoto T, Kuyama H: Experimental study of venous circulatory disturbance by dural sinus occlusion, *Acta Neurochir (Wien)* 124:120–126, 1993.
28. Frerichs KU, Deckert M, Kempski O, et al: Cerebral sinus and venous thrombosis in rats induces long-term deficits in brain function and morphology: Evidence for a cytotoxic genesis, *J Cereb Blood Flow Metab* 14:289–300, 1994.
29. Rother J, Waggie K, van Bruggen N, et al: Experimental cerebral venous thrombosis: Evaluation using magnetic resonance imaging, *J Cereb Blood Flow Metab* 16:1353–1361, 1996.
30. Röttger C, Trittmacher S, Gerriets T, et al: Reversible MR imaging abnormalities following cerebral venous thrombosis, *AJNR Am J Neuroradiol* 26:607–613, 2005.
31. Biousse V, Conard J, Brouzes C: Frequency of 20210 GA mutation in the 3'-untranslated region of the prothrombin gene in 35 cases of cerebral venous thrombosis, *Stroke* 29:1398–1400, 1998.
32. Reuner KH, Ruf A, Grau A, et al: Prothrombin gene G20210→A transition is a risk factor for cerebral venous thrombosis, *Stroke* 29:1765–1769, 1998.
33. Weih M, Vetter B, Castell S, et al: Hereditary thrombophilia in cerebral venous thrombosis, *Cerebrovasc Dis* 10:161–162, 2000.
34. Martinelli I, Sacchi E, Landi G, et al: High risk of cerebral-vein thrombosis in carriers of prothrombin-gene mutation and in users of oral contraceptives, *N Engl J Med* 338:1793–1797, 1998.
35. Deschiens MA, Conard J, Horellou MH, et al: Coagulation studies, factor V Leiden, and anticardiolipin antibodies in 40 cases of cerebral venous thrombosis, *Stroke* 27:1724–1730, 1996.
36. de Bruijn SF, Stam J, Koopman MM, et al: Case-control study of risk of cerebral sinus thrombosis in oral contraceptive users and in carriers of hereditary prothrombotic conditions, *BMJ* 316:589–592, 1998.
37. Ludemann P, Nabavi DG, Junker R, et al: Factor V Leiden mutation is a risk factor for cerebral venous thrombosis: A case-control study of 55 patients, *Stroke* 29:2507–2510, 1998.
38. Zuber M, Toulon P, Marnet L, et al: Factor V Leiden mutation in cerebral venous thrombosis, *Stroke* 27:1721–1723, 1996.
39. Dentali F, Crowther M, Ageno W: Thrombophilic abnormalities, oral contraceptives, and the risk of cerebral vein thrombosis: A meta-analysis, *Blood* 107:2766–2773, 2006.
40. Gouveia LO, Canhão P: Allele 677T MTHFR: Prothrombotic risk factor for cerebral venous thrombosis? A meta-analysis, *Cerebrovasc Dis* 25:152–153, 2008.
41. Wysokinska EM, Wysokinski WE, Brown RD, et al: Thrombophilia differences in cerebral venous sinus and lower extremity deep venous thrombosis, *Neurology* 70:627–633, 2008.
42. Khealani BA, Wasay M, Saadah M, et al: Cerebral venous thrombosis: A descriptive multicenter study of patients in Pakistan and Middle East, *Stroke* 39:2707–2711, 2008.
43. Grisold W, Oberndorfer S, Struhal W: Stroke and cancer: A review. *Acta Neurol Scand* 119:1–16, 2009.
44. Dalgiç A, Seçer M, Ergüngör F, et al: Dural sinus thrombosis following head injury: Report of two cases and review of the literature, *Turk Neurosurg* 18:70–77, 2008.
45. Savoiardo M, Armenise S, Spagnolo P, et al: Dural sinus thrombosis in spontaneous intracranial hypotension: Hypothesis on possible mechanisms, *J Neurol* 253:1197–1202, 2006.
46. Cantu C, Barinagarrementeria F: Cerebral venous thrombosis associated with pregnancy and puerperium; Review of 67 cases, *Stroke* 24:1880–1884, 1993.
47. Srinivasan K: Cerebral venous and arterial thrombosis in pregnancy and puerperium: A study of 135 patients, *Angiology* 34:731–746, 1983.
48. Canhão P, Bousser MG, Barinagarrementeria F, et al: ISCVT Collaborators: Predisposing conditions for cerebral vein thrombosis, *J Neurol* 249(Suppl 1):52, 2002.
49. Edris F, Kerner CM, Feyles V, et al: Successful management of an extensive intracranial sinus thrombosis in a patient undergoing IVF: Case report and review of the literature, *Fertil Steril* 88:705, e9-e14:2007.
50. Ferro JM, Canhão P, Bousser MG, et al: ISCVT Investigators: Cerebral vein and dural sinus thrombosis in elderly patients, *Stroke* 36:1927–1932, 2005.
51. Ferro JM, Falcão F, Melo TP, et al: Dural sinus thrombosis mimicking "capsular warning syndrome," *J Neurol* 247:802–803, 2000.
52. Biousse V, Ameri A, Bousser MG: Isolated intracranial hypertension as the only sign of cerebral venous thrombosis, *Neurology* 53:1537–1542, 1999.
53. Ferro JM, Lopes MG, Rosas MJ, et al: VENOPORT Investigators: Delay in hospital admission of patients with cerebral vein and dural sinus thrombosis, *Cerebrovasc Dis* 19:152–156, 2005.
54. Ferro JM, Canhão P, Bousser MG, et al: ISCVT Investigators: Delay in the diagnosis of cerebral vein and dural sinus thrombosis (CVT): Influence on outcome, *Cerebrovasc Dis* 25(Suppl 2):17, 2008.
55. Fitzgerald KC, Williams LS, Garg BP, et al: Cerebral sinovenous thrombosis in the neonate, *Arch Neurol* 63:405–409, 2006.
56. Lancon JA, Killough KR, Tibbs RE, et al: Spontaneous dural sinus thrombosis in children, *Pediatr Neurosurg* 30:23–29, 1999.
57. Heller C, Heinecke A, Junker R, et al: Childhood Stroke Study Group: Cerebral venous thrombosis in children: A multifactorial origin, *Circulation* 108:1362–1367, 2003.
58. Wasay M, Dai AI, Ansari M, et al: Cerebral venous sinus thrombosis in children: A multicenter cohort from the United States, *J Child Neurol* 23:26–31, 2008.
59. Ameri A, Bousser MG: Headache in cerebral venous thrombosis: A study of 110 cases, *Cephalalgia* 13(Suppl 13):110, 1993.
60. Lopes MG, Ferro J, Pontes C, et al: for the Venoport Investigators: Headache and cerebral venous thrombosis, *Cephalalgia* 20:292, 2000.
61. Iurlaro S, Ciccone E, Beghi A, et al: Headache in early diagnosis of cerebral venous thrombosis: Clinical experience in 59 patients, *Cerebrovasc Dis* 16(Suppl 4):109, 2003.
62. Cumurciuc R, Crassard I, Sarov M, et al: Headache as the only neurological sign of cerebral venous thrombosis: A series of 17 cases, *J Neurol Neurosurg Psychiatry* 76:1084–1097, 2005.
63. Sztajzel R, Coeytaux A, Dehdashti AR, et al: Subarachnoid hemorrhage: A rare presentation of cerebral venous thrombosis, *Headache* 41:889–892, 2001.
64. Oppenheim C, Domingo V, Gauvrit JY, et al: Subarachnoid hemorrhage as the initial presentation of dural sinus thrombosis, *Am J Neuroradiol* 26:614–617, 2005.
65. de Bruijn SF, Stam J, Kappelle LJ: Study Group CVST: Thunderclap headache as first symptom of cerebral venous sinus thrombosis, *Lancet* 348:1623–1625, 1996.
66. Newman DS, Levine SR, Curtis VL, et al: Migraine-like visual phenomena associated with cerebral venous thrombosis, *Headache* 29:82–85, 1989.
67. Martins IP, Sá J, Pereira RC, et al: Cerebral venous thrombosis may mimic migraine with aura, *Headache Q* 12:121–124, 2001.
68. Slooter A, Ramos L, Lapelle L: Migraine-like headache as the presenting symptom of cerebral venous sinus thrombosis, *J Neurol* 249:775–776, 2002.
69. Canhão P, Batista P, Falcão F: Lumbar puncture and dural sinus thrombosis: A causal or casual association? *Cerebrovasc Dis* 19:53–56, 2005.
70. Ferro JM, Canhão P, Bousser MG, et al: Investigators ISCVT: Early seizures in cerebral vein and dural sinus thrombosis: Risk factors and role of antiepileptics, *Stroke* 39:1152–1158, 2008.

71. Ferro JM, Correia M, Rosas MJ, et al: Cerebral Venous Thrombosis Portuguese Collaborative Study Group (VENOPORT): Seizures in cerebral vein and dural sinus thrombosis, *Cerebrovasc Dis* 15:78–83, 2003.

72. Ferro JM, Morgado C, Sousa R, et al: Interobserver agreement in the magnetic resonance location of cerebral vein and dural sinus thrombosis, *Eur J Neurol* 14:353–356, 2007.

73. Jacobs K, Moulin T, Bogousslavsky J, et al: The stroke syndrome of cortical vein thrombosis, *Neurology* 47:376–382, 1996.

74. Ahn TB, Roh JK: A case of cortical vein thrombosis with the cord sign, *Arch Neurol* 60:1314–1316, 2003.

75. Cakmak S, Hermier M, Montavon A, et al: T2*-weighted MRI in cortical venous thrombosis, *Neurology* 63:1698, 2004.

76. Duncan IC, Fourie PA: Imaging of cerebral isolated cortical vein thrombosis, *AJR Am J Roentgenol* 184:1317–1319, 2005.

77. Kuehnen J, Schwartz A, Neff W, et al: Cranial nerve syndrome in thrombosis of the transverse/sigmoid sinuses, *Brain* 121:381–388, 1998.

78. Utz N, Mull M, Kosinski C, et al: Pulsatile tinnitus of venous origin as a symptom of dural sinus thrombosis, *Cerebrovasc Dis* 7:150–153, 1997.

79. Waldvogel D, Mattle HP, Sturzenegger M, et al: Pulsatile tinnitus—a review of 84 patients, *J Neurol* 245:137–142, 1998.

80. Crawford SC, Digre KB, Palmer CA, et al: Thrombosis of the deep venous drainage of the brain in adults: Analysis of seven cases with review of the literature, *Arch Neurol* 52:1101–1108, 1995.

81. Lafitte F, Boukobza M, Guichard JP, et al: Deep cerebral venous thrombosis: Imaging in eight cases, *Neuroradiology* 41:410–418, 1999.

82. Lacour JC, Ducrocq X, Anxionnat R, et al: Les thromboses veineuses profondes de l'encéphale de l'adulte: aspects cliniques et approche diagnostique, *Rev Neurol (Paris)* 156:851–857, 2000.

83. Van den Bergh WM, van der Schaaf I, van Gijn J: The spectrum of presentations of venous infarction caused by deep cerebral vein thrombosis, *Neurology* 65:192–196, 2005.

84. Buonanno F, Moody DM, Ball MR, et al: Computed cranial tomographic findings in cerebral sino-venous occlusion, *J Comput Assist Tomogr* 2:281–290, 1978.

85. Chang R, Friedman DP: Isolated cortical venous thrombosis presenting as subarachnoid hemorrhage: A report of three cases, *AJNR Am J Neuroradiol* 25:1676–1679, 2004.

86. Casey SO, Alberico RA, Patel M, et al: Cerebral CT venography, *Radiology* 198:163–170, 1996.

87. Ozsvath RR, Casey SO, Lustrin ES, et al: Cerebral venography: Comparison of CT and MR projection venography, *AJNR Am J Neuroradiol* 169:1699–1707, 1997.

88. Majoie CB, van Straten M, Venema HW, et al: Multisection CT venography of dural sinuses and cerebral veins by using matched mask bone elimination, *AJNR Am J Neuroradiol* 25:787–791, 2004.

89. Rodallec MH, Krainik A, Feydy A, et al: Cerebral venous thrombosis and multidetector CT angiography: Tips and tricks, *Radio-Graphics* 26:S5–S18, 2006.

90. Wetzel SG, Kirsch E, Stock KW: Cerebral veins: Comparative study of CT venography with intra-arterial digital subtraction angiography, *Am J Neuroradiol* 20:249–255, 1999.

91. Dormont D, Anxionnat R, Evrard S, et al: MRI in cerebral venous thrombosis, *J Neuroradiol* 21:81–99, 1994.

92. Selim M, Fink J, Linfante I, et al: Diagnosis of cerebral venous thrombosis with echo-planar T2*-weighted magnetic resonance imaging, *Arch Neurol* 59:1021–1026, 2002.

93. Ayanzen RH, Bird CR, Keller PJ, et al: Cerebral MR venography: Normal anatomy and potential diagnostic pitfalls, *AJNR Am J Neuroradiol* 21:74–78, 2000.

94. Leach JL, Fortuna RB, Jones BV, et al: Imaging of cerebral venous thrombosis: Current techniques, spectrum of findings and diagnostic pitfalls, *RadioGraphics* 26(Suppl 1):S19–S43, 2006.

95. Isensee C, Reul J, Thron A: Magnetic resonance imaging of thrombosed dural sinuses, *Stroke* 25:29–34, 1994.

96. Leach JL, Wolujewics M, Strub WM: Partially recanalized chronic dural sinus thrombosis: Findings on MR imaging, time-of-flight MR venography, and contrast-enhancement venography, *AJNR Am J Neuroradiol* 28:782–789, 2007.

97. Dormont D, Sag K, Biondi A, et al: Gadolinium-enhancement MR of chronic dural sinus thrombosis, *AJNR Am J Neuroradiol* 16:1347–1352, 1995.

98. Fellner FA, Fellner C, Aichner FT, et al: Importance of T2*-weighted gradient-echo MRI for diagnosis of cortical vein thrombosis, *Eur J Neurol* 56:235–239, 2005.

99. Idbaih A, Boukobza M, Crassard I, et al: MRI of clot in cerebral venous thrombosis: High diagnostic value of susceptibility-weighted images, *Stroke* 37:991–995, 2006.

100. Favrole P, Guichard JP, Crassard I, et al: Diffusion-weighted imaging of intravascular clots in cerebral venous thrombosis, *Stroke* 35:99–103, 2004.

101. Farb RI, Scott JN, Willinsky RA, et al: Intracranial venous system: Gadolinium-enhanced three-dimensional MR venography with auto-triggered elliptic centric-ordered sequence—initial experience, *Radiology* 226:203–209, 2003.

102. de Bruijn SF, Majoie CB, Koster PA, et al: Interobserver agreement for MR-imaging and conventional angiography in the diagnosis of cerebral venous thrombosis. In de Bruijn SF, editor: *Cerebral venous sinus thrombosis: clinical and epidemiological studies*, Amsterdam, 1998, Thesis Publishers, pp 23–33.

103. Canhão P, Batista P, Ferro JM: Venous transcranial Doppler in acute dural sinus thrombosis, *J Neurol* 245:276–279, 1998.

104. Valdueza JM, Hoffmann O, Weih M, et al: Monitoring of venous hemodynamics in patients with cerebral venous thrombosis by transcranial Doppler ultrasound, *Arch Neurol* 56:229–234, 1999.

105. Becker G, Bogdahn U, Gehlberg C, et al: Transcranial color-coded real-time sonography of intracranial veins: Normal values of blood flow velocities and findings in superior sagittal sinus thrombosis, *J Neuroimaging* 5:87–94, 1995.

106. Ries S, Steinke W, Neff KW, et al: Echocontrast-enhanced transcranial color-coded sonography for the diagnosis of transverse sinus venous thrombosis, *Stroke* 28:696–700, 1997.

107. Stolz E, Kaps M, Dorndorf W: Assessment of intracranial venous hemodynamics in normal individuals and patients with cerebral venous thrombosis, *Stroke* 30:70–75, 1999.

108. Haapaniemi E, Tatlisumak T: Is D-dimer helpful in evaluating stroke patients? A systematic review, *Acta Neurol Scand* 119:141–150, 2009.

109. Tardy B, Tardy-Poncet B, Viallon A, et al: D-dimer levels in patients with suspected acute cerebral venous thrombosis, *Am J Med* 113:238–241, 2002.

110. Lalive PH, de Moerloose P, Lovblad K, et al: Is measurement of D-dimer useful in the diagnosis of cerebral venous thrombosis? *Neurology* 61:1057–1060, 2004.

111. Kosinski CM, Mull M, Schwarz M, et al: Do normal D-dimer levels reliably exclude cerebral sinus thrombosis? *Stroke* 35:2820–2825, 2004.

112. Cucchiara B, Messe S, Taylor R, et al: Utility of D-dimer in the diagnosis of cerebral venous sinus thrombosis, *J Thromb Haemost* 3:387–389, 2005.

113. Crassard I, Soria C, Tzourio C, et al: A negative D-dimer assay does not rule out cerebral venous thrombosis: A series of seventy-three patients, *Stroke* 36:1716–1719, 2005.

114. Rondepierre P, Hamon M, Leys D, et al: Thromboses veineuses cérébrales: étude de l'évolution, *Rev Neurol (Paris)* 151:100–104, 1995.

115. Preter M, Tzourio CH, Ameri A, et al: Long term prognosis in cerebral venous thrombosis: A follow-up of 77 patients, *Stroke* 27:243–246, 1996.

116. de Bruijn SF, de Haan RJ, Stam J: Cerebral Venous Sinus Thrombosis Study Group: Clinical features and prognostic factors of cerebral venous sinus thrombosis in a prospective series of 59 patients, *J Neurol Neurosurg Psychiatry* 70:105–108, 2001.

117. Ferro JM, Lopes MG, Rosas MJ, et al: Cerebral Venous Thrombosis Portuguese Collaborative Study Group (VENOPORT): Long-term prognosis of cerebral vein and dural sinus thrombosis: Results of the VENOPORT Study, *Cerebrovasc Dis* 13:272–278, 2002.

118. Breteau G, Mounier-Vehier F, Godefroy O, et al: Cerebral venous thrombosis: 3-year clinical outcome in 55 consecutive patients, *J Neurol* 250:29–35, 2003.

119. Cakmak S, Derex L, Berruyer M, et al: Cerebral venous thrombosis: Clinical outcome and systematic screening of prothrombotic factors, *Neurology* 60:1175–1178, 2003.

120. Dentali F, Gianni M, Crowther MA, et al: Natural history of cerebral vein thrombosis: A systematic review, *Blood* 108:1129–1134, 2006.

121. Ferro JM, Canhão P, Crassard I, et al: External validation of a prognostic model of cerebral vein and dural sinus thrombosis, *Cerebrovasc Dis* 19(Suppl 2):154, 2005.

122. Canhão P, Ferro JM, Lindgren AG, et al: ISCVT Investigators: Causes and predictors of death in cerebral venous thrombosis, *Stroke* 36:1720-1725, 2005.

123. Diaz JM, Schiffman JS, Urban ES, et al: Superior sagittal sinus thrombosis and pulmonary embolism: A syndrome rediscovered, *Acta Neurol Scand* 86:390-396, 1992.

124. Girot M, Ferro JM, Canhão P, et al: ISCVT Investigators: Predictors of outcome in patients with cerebral venous thrombosis and intracerebral hemorrhage, *Stroke* 38:337-342, 2007.

125. Kenet G, Kirkham F, Niederstadt T, et al: European Thromboses Study Group: Risk factors for recurrent venous thromboembolism in the European collaborative paediatric database on cerebral venous thrombosis: A multicentre cohort study, *Lancet Neurol* 6:595-603, 2007.

126. Sébire G, Tabarki B, Saunders DE, et al: Cerebral venous sinus thrombosis in children: Risk factors, presentation, diagnosis and outcome, *Brain* 128:477-489, 2005.

127. Crassard I, Canhão P, Ferro JM, et al: Neurological worsening in the acute phase of cerebral venous thrombosis in ISCVT (International Study on Cerebral Venous Thrombosis), *Cerebrovasc Dis* 16(Suppl 4):60, 2003.

128. Gosk-Bierska I, Wysokinski W, Brown RD Jr, et al: Cerebral venous sinus thrombosis: Incidence of venous thrombosis recurrence and survival, *Neurology* 67:814-819, 2006.

129. Ferro JM, Vasconcelos J, Canhão P, et al: Remote seizures in acute cerebral vein and dural sinus thrombosis (CVT): Incidence and associated conditions, *Cerebrovasc Dis* 23(Suppl 2):48, 2007.

130. Purvin VA, Trobe JD, Kosmorsky G: Neuro-ophthalmic features of cerebral venous obstruction, *Arch Neurol* 52:880-885, 1995.

131. Madureira S, Canhão P, Ferro JM: Cognitive and behavioural outcome of patients with cerebral venous thrombosis, *Cerebrovasc Dis* 11(Suppl 4):108, 2001.

132. Buccino G, Scoditti U, Patteri I, et al: Neurological and cognitive long-term outcome in patients with cerebral venous sinus thrombosis, *Acta Neurol Scand* 107:330-335, 2003.

133. de Bruijn SF, Budde M, Teunisse S, et al: Long-term outcome of cognition and functional health after cerebral venous sinus thrombosis, *Neurology* 54:1687-1689, 2000.

134. Lamy C, Hamon JB, Coste J, et al: Ischemic stroke in young women: Risk of recurrence during subsequent pregnancies. French Study Group on Stroke in Pregnancy, *Neurology* 55(269):274, 2000.

135. Mehraein S, Ortwein H, Busch M, et al: Risk of recurrence of cerebral venous and sinus thrombosis during subsequent pregnancy and puerperium, *J Neurol Neurosurg Psychiatry* 74:814-816, 2003.

136. Baumgartner RW, Studer A, Arnold M, et al: Recanalisation of cerebral venous thrombosis, *J Neurol Neurosurg Psychiatry* 74:459-461, 2003.

137. Strupp M, Covi M, Seelos K, et al: Cerebral venous thrombosis: Correlation between recanalization and clinical outcome—a long-term follow-up of 40 patients, *J Neurol* 249:1123-1124, 2002.

138. Einhäupl K, Bousser MG, de Bruijn SF, et al: EFNS guideline on the treatment of cerebral venous and sinus thrombosis, *Eur J Neurol* 13:553-559, 2006.

139. de Bruijn SF, Stam J, Study Group CVST: Randomized, placebo-controlled trial of anticoagulant treatment with low-molecular-weight heparin for cerebral sinus thrombosis, *Stroke* 30:484-488, 1999.

140. Einhäupl KM, Villringer A, Meister W, et al: Heparin treatment in sinus venous thrombosis, *Lancet* 338:597-600, 1991.

141. Maiti B, Chakrabarti I: Study on cerebral venous thrombosis with special reference to efficacy of heparin, *J Neurol Sci* 50:s147, 1997.

142. Nagaraja D, Rao B, Taly AB, et al: Randomized controlled trial of heparin in puerperal cerebral venous/sinus thrombosis, *Nimhans Journal* 13:111-115, 1995.

143. Stam J, de Bruijn SF, deVeber G: Anticoagulation for cerebral sinus thrombosis, *Cochrane Database Syst Rev* (4), 2002:CD002005.

144. Wingerchuk DM, Wijdicks EF, Fulgham JR: Cerebral venous thrombosis complicated by hemorrhagic infarction: Factors affecting the initiation and safety of anticoagulation, *Cerebrovasc Dis* 8:25-30, 1998.

145. deVeber G, Chan A, Monagle P, et al: Anticoagulation therapy in pediatric patients with sinovenous thrombosis: A cohort study, *Arch Neurol* 55:1533-1537, 1998.

146. Ferro JM, Bousser MG, Barinagarrementeria F, et al: and the ISCVT Collaborators: Variation in management of acute cerebral vein and dural sinus thrombosis, *Cerebrovasc Dis* 13(Suppl 3):60, 2002.

147. Canhão P, Falcão F, Ferro JM: Thrombolytics for cerebral sinus thrombosis: A systematic review, *Cerebrovasc Dis* 15:159-166, 2003.

148. Stam J, Majoie BLM, van Delden OM, et al: Endovascular thrombectomy and thrombolysis for severe cerebral sinus thrombosis: A prospective study, *Stroke* 39:1487-1490, 2008.

149. Canhão P, Cortesão A, Cabral M, et al: for the ISCVT Investigators: Are steroids useful to treat cerebral venous thrombosis? *Stroke* 39:105-110, 2008.

150. Keller E, Pangalu A, Fandino J, et al: Decompressive craniectomy in severe cerebral venous and dural sinus thrombosis, *Acta Neurochir* 94:177-183, 2005.

151. Armonda RA, Vo AH, Bell R, et al: Multimodal monitoring during emergency hemicraniectomy for vein of Labbé thrombosis, *Neurocrit Care* 4:241-244, 2006.

152. Higgins JN, Owler BK, Cousins C, et al: Venous sinus stenting for refractory benign intracranial hypertension, *Lancet* 359:228-230, 2002.

153. Owler BK, Parker G, Halmagyi GM, et al: Pseudotumor cerebri syndrome: Venous sinus obstruction and its treatment with stent placement, *J Neurosurg* 98:1045-1055, 2003.

154. Tsumoto T, Miyamoto T, Shimizu M, et al: Restenosis of the sigmoid sinus after stenting for treatment of intracranial venous hypertension: Case report, *Neuroradiology* 45:911-915, 2003.

155. Horton JC, Seiff SR, Pitts LH, et al: Decompression of the optic nerve sheath for vision-threatening papilledema caused by dural sinus occlusion, *Neurosurgery* 31:203-211, 1992.

156. Acheson JF: Optic nerve disorders: Role of canal and nerve sheath decompression surgery, *Eye* 18:1169-1174, 2004.

157. Horga A, Santamaria E, Quinlez A, et al: Cerebral venous thrombosis associated with repeated use of emergency contraception, *Eur J Neurol* 14:e5, 2007.

29 Intracerebral Hemorrhage

CARLOS S. KASE, STEVEN M. GREENBERG, J.P. MOHR, LOUIS R. CAPLAN

Intracerebral hemorrhage (ICH) occurs as a result of bleeding from an arterial source directly into the brain substance. Although its relative frequency in patients with stroke is subject to geographic and racial variations, values between 5% and 10% are most commonly quoted.[1-3] In a consecutive series of 938 patients with stroke entered into the National Institute of Neurological and Communicative Disorders and Stroke (NINCDS) Data Bank, primary ICH accounted for 10.7% of the cases.[4] Similar figures were obtained in population or community studies from Denmark (10.4%),[5] Holland (9%),[6] Oxfordshire, England (10%),[7] southern Alabama (8%),[8] and Italy (13.5%).[9] The incidence of ICH increases with advancing age,[3,10,11] which is a feature that applies to all types of stroke, both ischemic and hemorrhagic.

The incidence rates are relatively constant in predominantly white populations: rates range between 7 and 11 cases per 100,000 (Table 29-1).[10,12-15] The figures were higher in a U.S. population (southern Alabama) with a mixture of white and black people because the former had an incidence rate of 12 per 100,000; in black people, the rate was 32 per 100,000.[8] Similar comparisons between white and black people in Cincinnati, Ohio, yielded an overall age- and sex-adjusted incidence of ICH that was 1.4-fold higher in black people.[10] The difference in ICH incidence was even higher (2.3-fold) for black persons who were younger than 75 years. In addition, a Hispanic population in New Mexico had a high incidence of ICH (34.9/100,000), whereas non-Hispanic whites from the same population had an incidence rate (16.6/100,000) comparable to that of whites in other geographic locations.[16] Some series from Asian countries, such as that from Shibata, Japan,[17] report severalfold higher incidence rates of ICH (61/100,000).

Along with these differing incidence rates from various geographic locations, a general trend toward declining rates of ICH has been detected, starting in the 1960s with the initial observation in Göteborg, Sweden[18] and subsequently confirmed in the United States in a population from Rochester, Minnesota.[12,19] From analysis of data encompassing a 32-year period (1945 to 1976), Furlan et al[12] showed a significant decrease in incidence between the first and second parts of this period: 13.3 per 100,000 for 1945 to 1960 and 6.7 per 100,000 for 1961 to 1976. These figures correlated with a similar decline in the frequency and severity of hypertension in the population studied. A similarly declining trend in the incidence of ICH has been reported from Hisayama, Japan,[20] where it was also related to a decrease in the frequency of hypertension. However, recent figures from Gothenburg, Sweden, documented no changes in ICH incidence in men and women when comparing years 1987 to 1989, 1990 to 1994, and 1995 to 1999.

The role of hypertension as a leading risk factor is well-established, and its frequency has been estimated to be between 72%[2,12,21] and 81%.[2,12,21] The causative role of hypertension is supported by the high frequency of left ventricular hypertrophy in autopsy cases of ICH[22-24] and the significantly higher admission blood pressure readings in patients with ICH than in those with other forms of stroke.[25] The autopsy study by McCormick and Rosenfield[26] challenged the view that hypertension represents the main causative factor in ICH. Their series included a large number of cases of ICH due to blood dyscrasias, vascular malformations, and tumors, and hypertension was regarded as the sole basis for the bleeding in only 25% of the total. This difference from most reported series of ICH may reflect a referral pattern bias in this series as well as more stringent criteria for establishing a causal relationship between hypertension and ICH. However, clinical series have also questioned the validity of the concept of ICH as a condition most commonly related to hypertension. Brott et al[14] found a history of hypertension in only 45% of 154 patients, which is a figure that rose to only 56% when electrocardiographic or chest radiographic evidence of cardiomegaly was added to criteria for the diagnosis of hypertension. Similarly, Schütz et al[15] labeled only 59% of their cases of ICH as due to hypertension. Certain subgroups of hypertensive patients, however, appear to be at particularly high risk of ICH. They include subjects who are 55 years or younger, smokers, and those who have stopped taking their antihypertensive medications.[27] Finally, the beneficial effects of antihypertensive treatment with regard to risk of ICH have been documented in the Perindopril Protection Against Recurrent Stroke Study (PROGRESS) trial[28]: the combination of the angiotensin-converting enzyme inhibitor perindopril and the diuretic indapamide resulted in a 76% relative risk reduction of ICH in comparison with the placebo-treated group after 4 years of follow-up.

A number of other risk factors in addition to advancing age, hypertension, and race have been evaluated, including cigarette smoking, alcohol consumption, and serum cholesterol levels. Abbott et al[29] showed a higher risk of intracranial hemorrhage (both ICH and subarachnoid hemorrhage [SAH]) in cigarette-smoking Hawaiian men of Japanese ancestry. The risk of "hemorrhagic stroke" was 2.5 times higher in smokers, which was an effect

TABLE 29-1 INCIDENCE OF INTRACEREBRAL HEMORRHAGE IN STUDIES FROM VARIOUS GEOGRAPHIC LOCATIONS

Location	Chapter Reference	No. of Cases	Rate*
Rochester, Minnesota	13	81	7
Framingham, Massachusetts	3	58	10
Southern Alabama	8	13	12
Cincinnati, Ohio	14	154	11
Giessen, Germany	15	100	11
Shibata, Japan	17	97	61
L'Aquila, Italy	10	588	16
Bernalillo Co., New Mexico	16		
Non-Hispanic whites		47	17
Hispanics		39	35

*Per 100,000 population.

TABLE 29-2 ESTIMATED PREVALENCE OF CAA-RELATED ICH IN A CLINICAL SERIES OF ELDERLY PATIENTS

ICH Location (n = 355)	Percentage of Total*
Lobar	45.9 × 74%[†] = 34% of all primary ICHs in elderly due to CAA
Deep hemispheric	41.1
Brainstem	3.7
Cerebellum	8.5
Intraventricular	0.9

*Data from 355 consecutive patients age ≥55 presenting to Massachusetts General Hospital with spontaneous ICH.
[†]The estimated proportion of primary lobar ICH in the elderly caused by CAA, based on detection of advanced CAA in 29 of 39 consecutive pathology specimens of lobar ICH.
CAA, Cerebral amyloid angiopathy; ICH, intracerebral hemorrhage.

that was independent of other risk factors. However, the diagnosis of ICH was often made on clinical grounds, without verification by imaging or autopsy findings. In a study based on computed tomography (CT) diagnosis of ICH in Finland, Juvela et al[30] found that smoking was not an independent risk factor for ICH. However, recent data from the Physicians' Health Study and the Women's Health Study[31] documented a significant association[31] between cigarette smoking and both SAH and ICH risk in men and women.[31,32] After controlling for a number of vascular risk factors, investigators found that smoking 20 or more cigarettes per day was an independent risk factor for SAH (relative risk [RR], 3.22; 95% confidence interval [CI], 1.26–8.18) and ICH (RR, 2.06; 95% CI, 1.08–3.96) in a cohort of predominantly white male physicians.[32] Corresponding figures for women who smoked 15 or more cigarettes per day were RR of 4.02 (95% CI, 1.63–9.89) for SAH and 2.67 (95% CI, 1.04–6.90) for ICH in the Women's Health Study.[31]

The series reported by Donahue et al[33] and Juvela et al[30] also documented an increased risk of ICH in relation to alcohol ingestion, which was an effect that operated independently of other risk factors. Both studies showed a strong dose-response relationship between alcohol use and ICH. Juvela et al[30] documented a similar effect for alcohol ingestion within 24 hours and within 1 week before onset of ICH. Low serum cholesterol level, defined as serum cholesterol less than 160 mg/dL, has been shown to be associated with a higher risk of ICH in Japanese men[17] as well as in Hawaiian men of Japanese origin.[34] Other risk factors have been suggested in some studies. Cirrhosis was highly represented (15.5%) in the autopsy series of Boudouresques et al,[35] but its significance could not be assessed because comparison with a control autopsy series of the general population was not available. The occasional association of ICH with cirrhosis has been linked to thrombocytopenia and other abnormalities in coagulation.[36] The role of aspirin use in the risk of ICH is controversial. The Physicians' Health Study, which evaluated the effect of low-dose aspirin (325 mg every other day) in comparison with placebo in the primary prevention of coronary events,

documented a borderline-significant increase in the relative risk of hemorrhagic stroke (ICH and SAH) in the aspirin group.[37] Similarly, the Swedish Aspirin Low-Dose Trial (SALT), a secondary stroke prevention trial, documented a significantly higher frequency of hemorrhagic stroke in the group assigned to aspirin (75 mg/day) than in the group given placebo.[38] These data contrast with those from other secondary stroke prevention trials, in which various doses of aspirin did not lead to a higher risk of ICH.[39-44]

Cerebral amyloid angiopathy (CAA) is a diagnosis being recognized with increasing frequency. The difficulty of diagnosing CAA in living subjects makes precise figures on disease incidence or prevalence hard to ascertain. CAA *without* ICH is clearly a common phenomenon in the elderly brain. A review of published autopsy series suggests a prevalence for CAA of approximately 10% to 30% among unselected brains and 80% to 100% among brains with accompanying Alzheimer's disease (AD).[45] When these figures are compared with the annual rate for *all* types of ICH, approximately 0.1% among North American and European elderly,[12,15,16] it is clear that only a minority of pathologically advanced CAA results in hemorrhagic stroke.

Despite the low frequency of hemorrhage, those produced by CAA account for a substantial proportion of all spontaneous ICHs in elderly patients. Estimated rates of 11% to 15% emerged from autopsies of elderly patients with ICH (age ≥ 60 years) at the Japanese Yokufukai Geriatric Hospital between 1979 and 1990[46] and the Hawaiian Kuakini Hospital between 1965 and 1976.[47] Analysis of consecutively encountered clinical patients at the Massachusetts General Hospital (MGH) between 1994 and 2001 suggests an even greater proportion of hemorrhages, approximately 34%, attributable to CAA (Table 29-2). The apparently higher frequency of CAA in the MGH cohort might reflect either a lower incidence of hypertensive ICH in this Western population or secular improvements in blood pressure control as well as the methodologic differences between autopsy-based and clinic-based studies.

Examination of the clinical characteristics that predispose to CAA-related ICH (Table 29-3) suggests that its

TABLE 29-3 RISK FACTORS FOR CAA-RELATED ICH

Risk factors for CAA	Advanced age
	ApoE ε2 or ε4
	Alzheimer's disease
Risk factors for lobar ICH (not specifically linked to CAA)	Family history of ICH
	Frequent use of alcohol
	Previous ischemic stroke
	Low serum cholesterol

CAA, Cerebral amyloid angiopathy; ICH, intracerebral hemorrhage; ApoE, apolipoprotein E.

incidence is likely to rise with the aging of the population and is unlikely to be reduced through control of modifiable risk factors. *Advancing age* is the strongest clinical risk factor for CAA-related ICH, as predicted by the age dependence of the underlying disease.[45,48-50] There is no marked predilection for *gender* in either clinical (54% men, 46% women)[2] or pathologic (49% men, 51% women)[51] series.

Dementia has generally been considered a major risk factor for CAA-related ICH because of the close molecular relationship between CAA and AD. A pathologic study of 117 consecutive brains with AD demonstrated advanced CAA to be common; moderate to severe CAA was found in 25.6% of specimens and CAA-related hemorrhages were found in 5.1%.[52] Despite the frequent overlap of AD with CAA, approximately 60% to 80% of patients given diagnoses of CAA-related ICH do *not* show clinical symptoms of dementia before their initial hemorrhagic stroke.[51,53,54] It is thus unclear from a clinical standpoint whether the presence or absence of dementia is useful in making the diagnosis of CAA. The association of CAA and AD appears to be due in part to the shared genetic risk factor apolipoprotein E (ApoE) ε4, although there are substantial differences between the roles of ApoE in the two disorders.

Despite the clear importance of *hypertension* in promoting necrosis and rupture of the deep penetrating vessels,[55] there is little evidence for a similar role in CAA-related ICH. The estimated prevalence of hypertension in CAA is in the range of 32% (determined from pathologic cases[51]) to 49% (measured in clinical subjects[2]), which are figures not much greater than the expected rate of hypertension for the general elderly population. Hypertension is significantly less common in lobar ICH than in ICH of the deep hemispheres, cerebellum, or pons in most[15,54,56,57] though not all[27,58] studies of the elderly. Among other vascular factors, neither *diabetes mellitus* nor *coronary atherosclerosis* has demonstrated an elevated frequency in CAA.

Other clinical risk factors have been suggested for lobar ICH without specific evidence linking them to CAA. Midpoint analysis of the population-based Greater Cincinnati/Northern Kentucky study identified *family history of ICH*, *previous ischemic stroke*, and *frequent alcohol use* in addition to ApoE genotype as predictors of lobar ICH in a multivariable model.[59] *Low serum cholesterol* has been found to be associated with ICH in several other population-based studies.[60-62] The few studies that have analyzed ICH according to location or presumed etiology

have not indicated a specific relationship of cholesterol to CAA-related hemorrhages.[63]

CAA can also present clinically with nonhemorrhagic features. These include the following:

1. There is accumulating data to suggest that advanced CAA may sufficiently affect blood flow (possibly by the effects on vascular reactivity already described) to cause *ischemic brain injury* as well as ICH. Various types of ischemic lesions are reported in association with CAA, including punctate areas of gliosis in the cerebral cortex[64] and regions of myelin loss and focal gliosis in the white matter.[65] A histopathologic study of 73 postmortem brains found a correlation between white matter lesions and the proportion of amyloid-positive vessels but not with age or severity of Alzheimer pathology.[60] Similarly, magnetic resonance imaging (MRI) analysis of subjects with probable CAA demonstrated significantly greater volume of white matter T2-hyperintensity (median normalized volume, 19.8 cm^3) than similar-aged subjects with AD (11.1 cm^3) or mild cognitive impairment (10.0 cm^3).[61] Radiographic markers of white matter lesions in CAA appear to correlate with cognitive impairment,[62] which suggests that ischemic brain injury may be an important contributor to neurologic disability in these patients.

2. A subset of patients with CAA are seen with clinical and radiographic features related to *vascular inflammation*. Although some increase in inflammatory cells may be a common feature of advanced CAA,[53,66] a minority of patients demonstrate more robust reactions ranging from perivascular giant cells to frank vasculitis.[63,66,67] These patients are more likely to be seen with subacute cognitive decline or seizures than with symptomatic ICH. MRI often shows T2-hyperintensity that is asymmetrical, extends to subcortical white matter and the overlying cortex, and improves dramatically with courses of immunosuppressive agents such as high-dose corticosteroids or cyclophosphamide.[68] The clinical and radiographic response of many subjects to treatment suggests that CAA-related inflammation may be an important subtype to diagnose during life.

3. CAA can also manifest as *transient neurologic symptoms*,[69-71] another syndrome for which diagnosis during life is of particular practical importance. The neurologic symptoms can include focal weakness, numbness, paresthesias, or language abnormalities, often occurring in a recurrent and stereotyped pattern. Spells typically last for minutes and may spread smoothly from one contiguous body part to another during a single spell. Transient neurologic symptoms in CAA appear to be related to the hemorrhagic rather than the ischemic component of the disease because gradient-echo MRI commonly demonstrates otherwise asymptomatic hemorrhage in the cortical region corresponding to the spell.[69] Spells often cease with anticonvulsant treatment. The major practical issue is to differentiate these episodes by clinical or radiographic means from true transient ischemic attacks because administering anticoagulant agents in this setting may severely increase the risk of major ICH.

Genetics

The study of the genetics of cerebrovascular disease has focused mainly on ischemic stroke, but some researchers have also addressed ICH.[72] Alberts et al[73] addressed the issue of familial aggregation of cases of ICH. Their prospective study in North Carolina found that 10% of probands had a history of ICH. No significant clinical or demographic differences separated those with and without family history of ICH. Data reported by Woo et al[59] indicated that the presence of a first-degree relative is a risk for ICH of the lobar variety. These investigators also documented that the occurrence of lobar ICH is associated with the ε2 and ε4 alleles of the ApoE gene. These alleles, particularly ε4, have been identified as factors related to an increased risk of lobar ICH, presumably owing to the presence of CAA.[54] In addition, the presence of the ε4 allele was found to determine an earlier age of onset of ICH in its carriers compared with the age of presentation of CAA-related ICH in those without the allele.[54]

A potential association between a point mutation in codon 34 of exon 2 for factor XIII Val34Leu and ICH was suggested by Catto et al.[74] The suggested association was based on the known protective effect of this mutation for myocardial infarction (MI), as a result of its interfering with the formation of cross-linked fibrin. This last feature suggested the hypothesis that the mutation may result in an increased risk of ICH via the formation of weak fibrin structures. The study, which involved a large cohort of patients with stroke of both ischemic and hemorrhagic varieties, suggested that the mutation was significantly more common in subjects with ICH than in controls and in those with cerebral infarction.[74] However, a similar study from Korea did not show an association between factor XIII Val34Leu polymorphism and ICH.[75] These inconsistent observations may simply reflect the differences in the cohorts studied, and further data from other population samples will be required before a definitive statement can be made about the potential role of this mutation in the risk of ICH. Recently, a study in Chinese people of Han ancestry suggested an association between the 1425G/A single nucleotide polymorphism in the *PRKCH* gene in chromosome 14q22-q23 and increased incidence of ICH.[76]

Familial Cerebral Amyloid Angiopathy

Several familial forms of CAA have been identified in which a protein entirely unrelated to amyloid beta (Aβ) accumulates in vessels, assumes amyloid conformation,

and promotes vascular dysfunction. The clinical presentation of these familial CAAs differs from mutation to mutation, suggesting that each protein deposit provokes its own specific reaction. Substitution of glutamine for leucine at position 68 in the protease inhibitor cystatin C results in Icelandic CAA, which is characterized by very early deposition of a mutant protein fragment in vessel walls and symptomatic ICH by the third or fourth decade.[77] ICH is much less prominent in familial British dementia, a disorder caused by mutation in the *BRI* gene.[78] A single nucleotide substitution in the BRI stop codon causes cerebrovascular deposition of an abnormal carboxyl-terminus peptide fragment and a clinical syndrome of dementia and ataxia.[79] A third clinical presentation is associated with mutations in the transthyretin gene. When these mutations affect the central nervous system, they favor leptomeningeal and subependymal deposition, causing varying combinations of SAH, seizures, hydrocephalus, cognitive changes, ataxia, and hearing loss.[80]

The other major forms of familial CAA are caused by mutations or duplications of the *APP* gene. Interestingly, the APP mutations associated with CAA cluster within the Aβ-coding region of *APP* (Fig. 29-1) rather than flanking the Aβ-coding segment like the AD-associated mutations.[81] The Dutch-type hereditary CAA caused by substitution of glutamate to glutamine at Aβ position 22[82,83] manifests as recurrent lobar ICH in the fifth or sixth decade and progresses to an early mortality.[84] A similar clinical picture is produced by the Italian substitution of lysine at this position.[85,86] Dementia and AD-like neuritic pathology are more prominent features of duplication of the APP locus[87] and of two other CAA-associated APP mutations, the Flemish substitution of glycine at Aβ position 21[88] and the Iowa asparagine for aspartate substitution at residue 23.[89] Although differences have emerged among the various mutations in their effects on APP processing and Aβ bioactivity,[90,91] the precise mechanisms by which they predispose toward specific combinations of CAA and AD pathology remain unclear.

Sporadic Cerebral Amyloid Angiopathy

The genes associated with familial CAA do not appear to play major roles as risk factors for sporadic CAA. Among 55 patients with sporadic CAA-related ICH examined for the cystatin C Icelandic mutation,[92,93] only one positive finding has been reported. Similar searches for APP mutations at Aβ position 22 or 23 have yielded no instances in

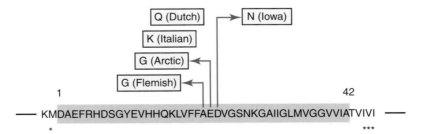

Figure 29-1 Mutations of the APP (β-amyloid precursor protein) gene associated with familial cerebral amyloid angiopathy (CAA). The boxed segment of APP contains the region representing Aβ42 as well as the amino acid substitutions at positions 21 to 23 associated with familial CAA (see text for references). Asterisks indicate the positions of some of the mutations linked with early-onset Alzheimer's disease.

111 reported patients with sporadic CAA.[89,92] ApoE has emerged as the strongest predictor of risk for sporadic CAA-related ICH. The ApoE ε2 and ε4 alleles appear to promote CAA-related ICH at two distinct steps in the disease's pathogenesis, as previously described.[94-96] Each of these alleles was overrepresented more than twofold among 182 reviewed pathologic cases of CAA-related ICH.[97] The general importance of ApoE to lobar ICH was further supported by the midpoint analysis of the Greater Cincinnati/Northern Kentucky cohort, in which the presence of ApoE ε2 or ε4 was associated with an adjusted odds ratio for lobar ICH of 2.3.[59] The ApoE alleles had an attributable risk for lobar ICH of 29% in this study, which is the largest proportion for any risk factor examined. ApoE ε2 and ε4 appear to associate with not only greater risk of ICH occurrence[94] but also a younger age at first hemorrhage[96] and a shorter time until ICH recurrence (see later).[98]

Pathologic Features and Pathogenesis

Spontaneous ICH occurs predominantly in the deep portions of the cerebral hemispheres. Its most common location is the putamen; this site accounts for 35% to 50% of the cases.[2,4,12,99-101] The second site of preference varies in different series; in most, it is the subcortical white matter,[2,12,23,100] and the frequency is 30%. The thalamus follows, with a uniform frequency of 10% to 15%.[2,4,12,100-104] Pontine hemorrhage accounts for 5% to 12% of cases of ICH.[2,4,12,100,102] The distribution figures in a series of 100 unselected cases of ICH are shown in Table 29-4.

The hemorrhages of putaminal, thalamic, and pontine location occur in the vascular distribution of small, perforating intracerebral arteries: the lenticulostriate, thalamoperforating, and basilar paramedian groups, respectively. Cerebellar hemorrhage occurs in the area of the dentate nucleus,[105,106] which is supplied by small branches of both the superior and the posterior–inferior cerebellar arteries.[105] Thus, most ICHs originate from the rupture of small, deep arteries[55] with diameters between 50 and 200 μm. The same arteries are recognized to be those occluded in cases of lacunar infarcts,[107] a form of stroke correlated primarily with chronic hypertension and diabetes.[108,109] Thus, it is apparent that these various groups of small arteries, located in well-defined anatomic areas, become the targets of chronic hypertension, and the result can be either occlusion or rupture, leading to lacunar infarcts or ICH, respectively.

Vascular Rupture

The actual mechanism of vascular rupture leading to ICH has been the subject of considerable interest, and several detailed pathologic studies[110-112] have addressed this point. Because hypertension is one of its main causative factors,[113] arterial changes associated with it have been commonly implicated in its pathogenesis. Since Charcot and Bouchard[114] described "miliary aneurysms" in brain specimens from patients with hypertensive ICH in 1868, these lesions have been the subject of extensive interest. Initially, they were thought to represent true dilatations of the arterial wall, and their preferential location deep in the hemispheres lent support to their pathogenic role. In the early twentieth century, however, with the use of a more precise histologic technique, Ellis[115] was able to show that miliary aneurysms represent "false aneurysms" and are actually made of blood collected outside the vessel wall, as "masses of blood" surrounded by either "remains of the vessel wall" or fibrin. His view of the pathogenesis of ICH implied a primary intimal lesion, with or without secondary involvement of the media and adventitia, and the former often led to passage of blood into the vessel wall and formation of a dissecting aneurysm. Either form of vascular abnormality (dissecting aneurysm or simple "weakening" of the vessel wall by extension of the primary intimal lesion into the media and adventitia) would then be responsible for rupture and hemorrhage.

Over the following years, miliary aneurysms in the brain of hypertensive patients were shown through the use of thick frozen sections[116] and x-ray imaging of brain specimens injected with radiopaque media.[117] Green[116] demonstrated three such lesions, two of which were associated with a fresh hemorrhage in the pons and frontal lobe. His view was that these lesions were mainly related to atherosclerosis and that they "may be responsible for some cases of cerebral hemorrhage." However, the definitive work that established the relationship between hypertension and miliary aneurysms was performed by Ross Russell,[117] who combined postmortem angiography with routine histologic study of brain specimens. He found miliary aneurysms in 15 of 16 brains of hypertensive patients and in 10 of 38 normotensive patients. The aneurysms were found mostly in the basal ganglia, internal capsule, and thalamus and less commonly in the centrum semiovale and cortical gray matter. Ross Russell[117] regarded these lesions as most likely acquired, strongly related to hypertension, and possibly causally related to ICH. He rejected the notion that aneurysms may be consequences rather than causes of ICH, as they were present in brains of hypertensive patients without ICH.

This study was followed by a series of observations reported by Cole and Yates[110,111,118] in a systematic analysis of 100 brains from hypertensive patients and an equal number of brains from normotensive persons. Miliary aneurysms were found in 46% of hypertensive brains but only in 7% of normotensive brains; furthermore, they occurred in 85% of the hypertensive patients with massive ICH and in all of those with small "slit" hemorrhages,

TABLE 29-4 DISTRIBUTION BY SITE OF 100 CASES OF ICH AT THE UNIVERSITY OF SOUTH ALABAMA MEDICAL CENTER

Type	No. of Cases
Putaminal	34
Lobar	24
Thalamic	20
Cerebellar	7
Pontine	6
Miscellaneous	
Caudate	5
Putaminothalamic	4

ICH, Intracerebral hemorrhage.

which suggested that small hemorrhages probably result from microaneurysmal "leaks."[110] These researchers did not, however, establish a relationship between microaneurysms and bleeding sites, thereby failing to prove that these leaks had a causal role in ICH.

In 1971, Fisher[55] reported the study of two brains containing three ICHs, one pontine and two putaminal, by serial sections of blocks of tissue containing the hemorrhage. In both putaminal hemorrhages, the primary arterial bleeding sites were identified along with multiple sites of secondary bleeding. The latter was thought to result from mechanical disruption and tearing of smaller vessels at the periphery of the enlarging hematoma. In the pontine ICH, only the secondary bleeding sites were recognized. No instances of microaneurysm formation were found in immediate relationship to the hematomas, whereas "lipohyalinosis" was a common abnormality of the walls of small arteries harboring the bleeding sites. Miliary aneurysms were identified in both hemorrhages, although not in relation to the bleeding points. Fisher[55] thought the aneurysms were unlikely to be sources of major hemorrhage and more probably the end result of old small sites of arterial rupture ("the end stage of a limited extravasation"). A year later, Fisher[119] reported a detail of the types of microaneurysms found in brains of hypertensive patients. He described "saccular," "lipohyalinotic," and "fusiform" varieties of microaneurysms and suggested that the lipohyalinotic form may be the process underlying ICH (as well as lacunar infarcts). He regarded the saccular and fusiform varieties as less likely to be important factors in the pathogenesis of ICH. On the basis of these two studies, Fisher[55,119] concluded that

hypertensive ICH most likely results from rupture of one or two lipohyalinotic arteries, followed by secondary arterial ruptures at the periphery of the enlarging hematoma in a cascade or avalanche fashion.

Active Bleeding

Early studies conducted before the wide availability of CT scanning suggested that the period of active bleeding in ICH is rather brief (<1 hour),[120] and the observation of clinical deterioration after admission was frequently attributed to the effects of brain edema,[2,120] although instances of continuous bleeding were occasionally reported.[121] A number of subsequent CT studies of the early phases of ICH have helped to clarify these concepts.

Broderick et al[122] evaluated eight patients with ICH by CT within 2.5 hours of onset and again several hours later (within 12 hours of onset in seven patients), documenting a substantial increase in hematoma size (mean percentage increase, 107%) (Fig. 29-2). This increase in the volume of the hemorrhage was accompanied by clinical deterioration in six of the eight patients, all of whom had a 40% increase in hematoma volume. In five patients, the clinical deterioration occurred with blood pressure measurements of 195 mm Hg or higher. These investigators suggested that a prolongation of active bleeding for several hours (up to 5 or 6 hours) after onset may not be uncommon as a mechanism of early clinical deterioration in ICH. Similarly, Fehr and Anderson[123] reviewed 56 cases of hypertensive ICH in the basal ganglia and thalamus and documented enlargement of the hematoma with CT in four (7%); in two of the four, the increase in hematoma

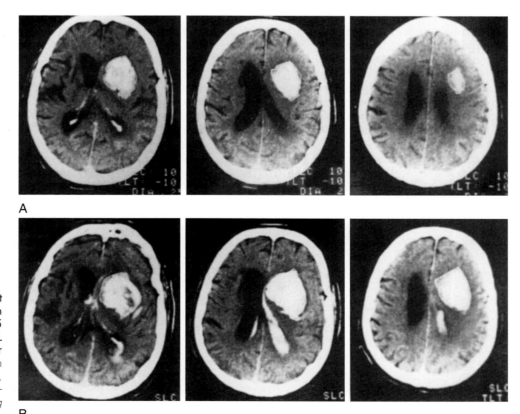

Figure 29-2 Enlargement of left putaminal hemorrhage (A) from 25 mL on CT scan performed 35 minutes after onset, to (B) 44 mL on scan obtained 70 minutes later (105 minutes after onset). (From Broderick JP, Brott TG, Tomsick T, et al: Ultra early evaluation of intracerebral hemorrhage. *J Neurosurg* 72:195, 1990.)

size was documented within 24 hours from onset, and in the other two, it was documented on days 5 and 6. Three of the patients had neurologic deterioration. In two who experienced deterioration within 24 hours, it occurred in the setting of poorly controlled hypertension, whereas the others had adequate blood pressure control. One of two patients with adequate blood pressure control was a chronic alcoholic, leading the investigators to suggest that alcoholism may be a risk factor for delayed progression of ICH.

Three subsequent studies further clarified the patterns of early enlargement of ICH. Fujii et al[124] studied 419 patients with ICH, in whom they performed the first CT within 24 hours of onset and the follow-up CT within 24 hours of admission, which showed hematoma enlargement in 60 patients (14.3%). Kazui et al[125] conducted sequential CT evaluations in 204 patients with acute ICH, documenting enlargement of at least 12.5 cm³, or by 40% of the original volume, in 20% of the cases. The highest frequency of detection of hematoma enlargement was seen in patients in whom the initial CT scan was performed within 3 hours of stroke onset (36%); the detection of enlargement declined progressively as the time from ICH onset to first CT increased, and there was no documentation of enlargement in those first scanned more than 24 hours after onset. These observations suggest that the period of hematoma enlargement can extend for a number of hours from onset as a result of active bleeding, which is a phenomenon that is frequently, but not always, associated with clinical deterioration. The study reported by Brott et al[126] involved 103 patients in whom first CT scans were obtained within 3 hours of ICH onset and follow-up CT scans were obtained 1 hour and 20 hours after the initial scans. ICH enlargement (>33% volume increase) was detected in 26% of patients at the 1-hour follow-up scan, and an additional 12% showed enlargement between the 1-hour and 20-hour CT scans. The change in hematoma volume was often associated with clinical deterioration, but there were exceptions. These researchers found no predictors of ICH enlargement, evaluating age, hemorrhage location, severity of initial clinical deficit, systolic and diastolic blood pressure at onset or history of hypertension, use of antiplatelet drugs, platelet counts, prothrombin time, and partial thromboplastin time.

Recent data suggest that the presence of small foci of contrast extravasation (the "spot sign"[127]) during CT angiography (CTA) in patients with acute ICH may predict subsequent hematoma enlargement.[127,128] The documentation of active bleeding by this technique (Fig. 29-3), especially when CTA is performed within the first few hours from symptom onset, has been correlated with a high frequency of hematoma enlargement (in up to 77% of patients with the spot sign) in comparison with patients without the sign (with only 4% showing hematoma expansion).[127] The following criteria for the definition of the spot sign have been outlined[129]: a spot-like or serpiginous focus of enhancement located within a parenchymal hematoma without connection to vessels outside the ICH, with a diameter greater than 1.5 mm, and with Hounsfield units (HU) at least double that of the background hematoma density. Further evidence for the

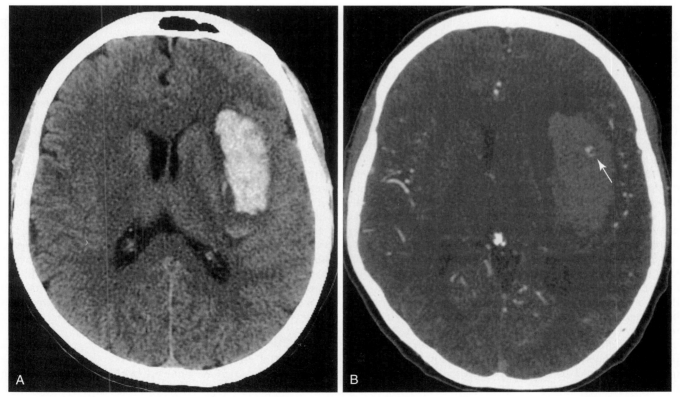

Figure 29-3 CT scan with right occipital hemorrhage (A), showing "spot sign" (B, *arrow*) on computerized tomographic angiogram (CTA), (B), corresponding to ongoing bleeding at that site.

value of the spot sign for predicting hematoma expansion includes its correlation with features such as number of spot signs (≥ 3), maximal diameter (≥ 5 mm), and maximal attenuation (HU ≥ 180), all of which were found to be independent predictors of hematoma expansion.[130]

Further studies are needed to identify potential risk factors of early ICH enlargement so that attempts can be made to prevent its associated neurologic morbidity and mortality. Such studies should be facilitated with the use of techniques of hematoma volume measurement that are easy to apply.[131-133] The "abc method"[132] uses the formula (a × b × c)/2, in which *a* is the largest diameter of the hematoma in the CT slice with the largest area of ICH; *b* is the largest diameter of the hemorrhage perpendicular to line *a*; and *c* is number of slices with hematoma times the slice thickness; this formula yields hematoma volume in cubic centimeters (Fig. 29-4). The use of these volumetric measurements of ICH should improve our understanding of the clinical consequences of early changes in hematoma size and their risk factors so that we may better define clinical and CT patterns of ICH evolution. The use of volumetric measurements of ICH in the early phase, along with techniques such as CTA documentation of ongoing bleeding, should serve as the background for new strategies of management of ICH and their eventual testing in randomized clinical trials; one such trial is the STOP-IT trial, which will evaluate hematoma growth in patients with ICH and a CTA-detected spot sign at baseline, with randomized treatment allocation to activated factor VII or placebo. It is expected that the study of patients with ICH at high risk of hematoma expansion will help identify treatments with potential for arresting this process.

Gross Pathologic Anatomy

The gross pathologic anatomy of ICH includes a number of features peculiar to the various locations of the hematomas.

Putaminal Hemorrhage

The common *putaminal* variety originates at the posterior angle of this nucleus and spreads in a concentric fashion but generally extends more in the anteroposterior than the transverse diameter.[102] The result is an ovoid mass of maximal anteroposterior diameter collected in the putamen and the structures located laterally to it, the external capsule and claustrum. The insular cortex is pushed laterally, whereas the internal capsule is either displaced medially or involved directly by the hematoma (Fig. 29-5). The origin of this form of ICH in the lateral-posterior aspect of the putamen is bleeding from a lateral branch of the striate arteries.[102] The lumens of these laterally placed middle cerebral artery perforating branches are between 200 and 400 μm wide at their entry to the brain,[117] and they supply the putamen, internal capsule, and head of the caudate nucleus. From its initial putaminal–claustral location, a sufficiently large hematoma may extend to other structures in the vicinities: medially into the internal capsule and lateral ventricle, superiorly into the corona radiata, and inferolaterally into the white matter of the temporal lobe (Fig. 29-6).

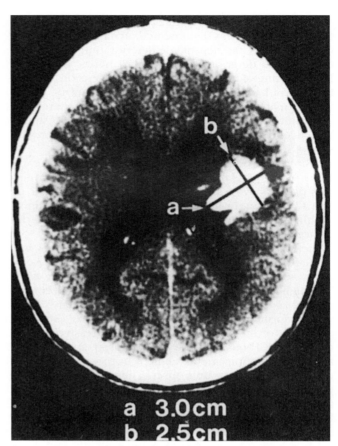

Figure 29-4 Method of calculating hematoma volume on CT, in which *a* is the largest diameter, *b* is the largest diameter perpendicular to *a*, and *c* is the number of slices with hematoma times the slice thickness. The formula [(a × b × c)/2] gives the hematoma volume in cubic centimeters. (From Broderick J, Brott TG, Duldner JE, et al: The ABCs of measuring of intracerebral hemorrhage volumes. *Stroke* 27:1304, 1996.)

These variations in the pattern of extension result in clinical variants of putaminal hemorrhage. The extension of the hemorrhage from its site of origin can follow several patterns, of which the most common is dissection along the course of adjacent white matter fibers. The common medial extension of the hematoma leads to communication with the lateral ventricle, through a process of slow leakage of blood rather than as direct communication between active bleeding site and ventricular system.[102] Direct communication of the hematoma with the ventricular system, at times with associated hydrocephalus, is more likely to result from bleeding at sites adjacent to the ventricular space, such as the thalamus[99] and the head of the caudate nucleus.[134] A putaminal hematoma that extends directly into the ventricle is usually large and thus is associated with high mortality.[135]

Caudate Hemorrhage

A variant of striatal hematomas is that occurring in the head of the *caudate* nucleus. Although the bleeding source is thought to be the same as in putaminal hemorrhage (the lateral group of striate arteries), this form of ICH is less common.[134] The recognized low frequency of

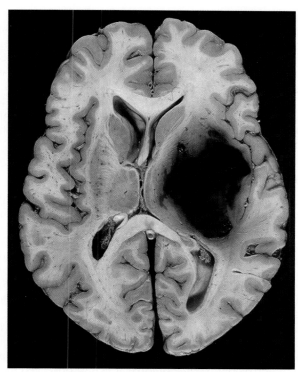

Figure 29-5 Passive right putaminal hemorrhage involving the posterior half of the putamen, globus pallidus, posterior limb of the internal capsule, and claustral area. Effacement of the ipsilateral lateral ventricle and midline shift are present.

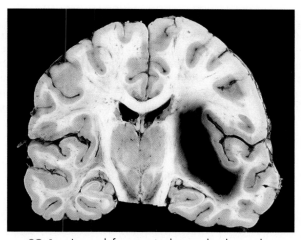

Figure 29-6 Large left putaminal–capsular hemorrhage, with tracking into the white matter of the temporal lobe.

this type of striatal hemorrhage in hypertensive patients leads the clinician to a search for a different underlying cause, such as an arteriovenous malformation (AVM) or aneurysm. This variation in the frequency of two types of striatal bleeding (putaminal and caudate) from the same arterial source is unexplained and may reflect a higher rate of arterial rupture at the more proximal segments of these arteries. This higher rate, in turn, may correlate with a higher frequency of "lipohyalinosis" or "microatheroma" at the more proximal segments of these vessels, as shown by Fisher[136] in serial studies of the underlying vascular

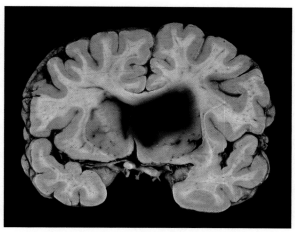

Figure 29-7 Hemorrhage originating from the head of the left caudate nucleus, with involvement of the anterior limb of the internal capsule and direct ventricular extension with formation of a ventricular cast.

lesions in cases of capsular infarcts. Fisher implied that the same basic vascular abnormality (lipohyalinosis or microatheroma) may be the basis for both lacunar infarcts and ICH in hypertensive patients.[102] The predominantly proximal location of these lesions could therefore explain the low frequency of caudate hemorrhage because it originates from the distal ends of these lateral striate branches. Caudate hemorrhage occurs most commonly in the head of this nucleus (Fig. 29-7), and ventricular entry is an early event; this component is sometimes many times larger than the parenchymal hematoma.[135] Involvement of the anterior limb of the internal capsule is the rule.

Thalamic Hemorrhage

Thalamic hemorrhages can involve most or the entire nucleus, and their extension is mostly in the transverse direction, into the third ventricle medially and the posterior limb of the internal capsule laterally (Fig. 29-8). Because the hemorrhage commonly extends transversely, it produces a pressure effect or extends directly inferiorly into the tectum and tegmentum of the midbrain. Moderate-sized and large thalamic hematomas often extend superiorly into the corona radiata and parietal white matter, following the orientation of their fibers.

Lobar (White Matter) Hematoma

White matter (*lobar*) hematomas collect along the fiber bundles of the cerebral lobes, most commonly at the parietal and occipital levels (Fig. 29-9).[100,137] Blood usually collects between the cortex and underlying white matter, separating them and often extending along the white matter pathways. These hematomas are close to the cortical surface, at a distance from the ventricular system and midline structures, and usually not in direct contact with deep hemispheric structures (e.g., internal capsule or basal ganglia).

Cerebellar Hemorrhage

Cerebellar hemorrhages usually occur on one hemisphere, originating in the area of the dentate nucleus (Fig. 29-10).[105,106] From here they extend into the hemispheric white matter as well as the cavity of the fourth ventricle. The adjacent brainstem (pontine tegmentum) is rarely involved directly by the hematoma but is often compressed by it, at times with resultant pontine necrosis. A variant of cerebellar hemorrhage, the midline hematoma originating from the cerebellar vermis is virtually always in direct communication with the fourth ventricle through its roof and frequently extends into the pontine tegmentum bilaterally. The bleeding artery in this variety usually corresponds to distal branches of the superior cerebellar artery. These two forms of cerebellar hemorrhage have distinct clinical and prognostic features.

Pontine Hemorrhage

In *pontine* hemorrhages, the bleeding sites correspond to small paramedian basilar perforating branches.[55] The result is a medially placed hematoma that extends symmetrically to involve the basis pontis bilaterally, with variable degrees of tegmental extension (Fig. 29-11). Tracking

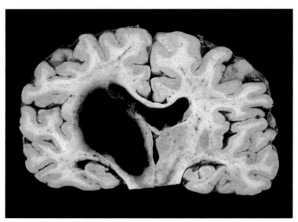

Figure 29-8 Right thalamic hemorrhage, involving most of this nucleus, with extension into the corona radiata as well as inferiorly into the subthalamic area, with compression of the dorsal midbrain.

of the hematoma into the middle cerebellar peduncle is rarely seen. A partial unilateral variety of pontine hematoma, predominantly tegmental in location, is recognized clinically and documented by CT scans.[138,139] These hypertensive hemorrhages result from rupture of distal tegmental segments of long circumferential branches of the basilar artery.[139] The hematomas usually communicate with the fourth ventricle, and they extend laterally and ventrally into the tegmentum and upper part of the basis pontis on one side.

Recurrence of Intracerebral Hemorrhage

The ICH of hypertensive patients is often a one-time event: in a group of 101 patients with ICH entered into the NINCDS Stroke Data Bank,[4] history of a prior hemorrhage was documented in only one instance. Long-term follow-up studies in patients with ICH have found a low frequency of recurrent bleeding,[140] which clearly differentiates ICH from aneurysms and AVMs, in which rebleeding is a prominent feature. In a study reported by Gonzalez-Duarte et al,[141] however, data showed ICH recurrence in approximately 6% of an unselected series of patients with ICH. Among hypertensive patients, the pattern of recurrence was that of repeated episodes of basal ganglionic ICH, whereas recurrence of lobar ICH was observed more often in nonhypertensive subjects, in whom the predominant putative mechanism of ICH was CAA. A similar rate of recurrence (5.4%) was documented by Bae et al[142] within a median interval of about 2 years from the first episode of ICH. The risk of ICH recurrence was significantly increased by poor hypertension control, which stresses the value of hypertension treatment in the prevention of ICH.

Occasionally, multiple simultaneous ICHs can occur.[143,144] In a series of 600 consecutive cases of ICH diagnosed by CT scan, Weisberg[144] found 12 patients (2%) with multiple hematomas. These double lesions were probably simultaneous (because of equal CT attenuation values) in 11 instances, and they occurred in the same

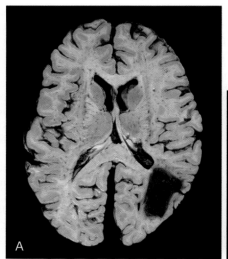
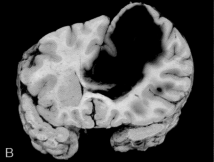
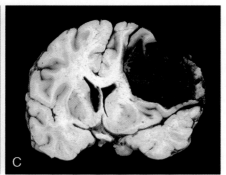

Figure 29-9 A, Right subcortical (white matter) occipital lobe hemorrhage, without extension into the ventricular system or midline shift. B, Large left frontal subcortical hemorrhage, with extension into the lateral ventricle and marked midline shift. C, Large left frontoparietal lobar hemorrhage, with cortical involvement and communication with the subarachnoid space; marked mass effect and midline shift.

intracranial compartment (supratentorial or infratentorial) in all patients but one, in whom thalamic and cerebellar hematomas coexisted. The incidence of hypertension was unusually low (2 of 12 patients) in this series, which suggests that cases of multiple spontaneous ICHs may frequently have other causative factors.

Cerebral Amyloid Angiopathy

Among the survivors of CAA-related ICH, the major neurologic risk is hemorrhage recurrence. A pooled analysis of patients monitored after lobar ICH reported a recurrence rate of 4.4% per year.[145] The value for cumulative ICH recurrence rate among the consecutive patients followed up at MGH was approximately 10% per year,[98] perhaps reflecting a higher prevalence of CAA among the patients with lobar ICH in this population. Recurrent hemorrhages, like the initial hemorrhages, are typically

lobar, although generally at a site distinct from that of the initial ICH (Fig. 29-12).

The strongest risk factors for CAA-related ICH recurrence are a history of previous recurrences, ApoE genotype, and number of hemorrhages (microbleeding plus macrobleeding) detected by gradient-echo MRI.[94,98] The prognosis for good functional outcome after a second CAA-related ICH appears to be relatively poor.[98] These observations highlight secondary hemorrhage prevention as an important treatment goal in CAA.

Histopathologic Studies

The studies on the histopathology of ICH have been mostly concerned with pathogenic issues. However, the main features of the microscopic anatomy of ICH and its changes with time are well-documented. The initial arterial rupture leads to local accumulation of blood, which in part destroys the parenchyma locally, displaces nervous structures in the vicinity, and dissects at some distance from the initial focus. The bleeding sites are at times difficult to locate, and serial sections are needed to show them.[55] The bleeding sites appear as round collections of platelets admixed with and surrounded by concentric lamellae of fibrin, so-called bleeding globes or fibrin globes.[55] These fibrin or bleeding globes at the primary and secondary sites are histologically identical, except that the fibrin globes are larger. The bulk of the hematoma is formed by a compact mass of red blood cells, and the bleeding sites are characteristically found at its periphery.

García et al[146] have described in detail the sequential histologic changes that take place in the hematoma. After hours or days, extracellular edema develops at the periphery of the hematoma, resulting in pallor and vacuolation of myelin sheaths. After 4 to 10 days, the red blood cells begin to lyse, eventually turning into an amorphous mass of methemoglobin. Cellular infiltration by polymorphonuclear leukocytes appears at the periphery of the hematoma as early as 2 days after onset, and the number of leukocytes peaks at 4 days.[147] This event is

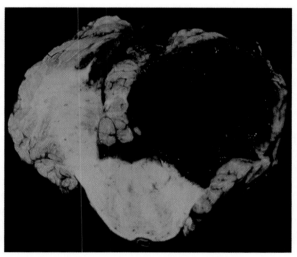

Figure 29-10 Left cerebellar hemorrhage with mass effect on the pontine tegmentum. (From Kase CS: Cerebellar hemorrhage. In Kase CS, Caplan LR, editors: *Intracerebral hemorrhage*, Boston, 1994, Butterworth-Heinemann, p 425.)

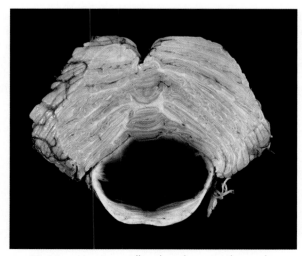

Figure 29-11 Massive midline basal pontine hemorrhage, with bilateral destruction of basis and tegmentum.

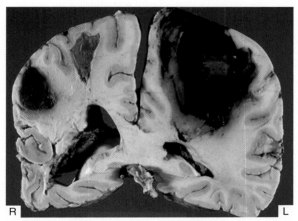

Figure 29-12 Multiple intracerebral hemorrhages of different ages in patient with autopsy-documented cerebral amyloid angiopathy: acute fatal left lobar, subacute right lateral parietal, and chronic (with ocher discoloration) right upper parietal locations.

followed by the arrival of microglial cells, which become foamy macrophages after the ingestion of cellular debris, including products of disintegration of myelin as well as blood-derived pigments, especially hemosiderin. The final stages of this process consist of the proliferation of astrocytes at the periphery of the hematoma, where these cells become enlarged and display prominent eosinophilic cytoplasm (gemistocytes), which at times contains hemosiderin granules. Once the late stage of hematoma reabsorption and repair has been reached, the astrocytes are replaced by abundant glial fibrils.

This histologic process is correlated with macroscopic changes in the hematoma, which initially becomes a soft, spongy mass of brick-red, altered blood (Fig. 29-13). After many months of slowly progressing phagocytosis, the residua of the hematoma is confined to a flat, collapsed cavity lined by reddish orange discoloration resulting from the accumulation of hemosiderin-laden macrophages (Fig. 29-14).[24]

Cerebral Amyloid Angiopathy

CAA appears on pathologic analysis as a variable combination of vascular amyloid deposition and vessel wall breakdown (Fig. 29-15). Affected vessels are the capillaries, arterioles, and small- and medium-sized arteries primarily of the cerebral cortex, overlying leptomeninges, and cerebellum; the white matter and deep gray structures are largely spared. The distribution of CAA is typically patchy and segmental, such that heavily involved vessel segments may alternate with essentially amyloid-free regions (see Fig. 29-15C).[67] In its mildest detectable form, congophilic material accumulates at the border of the vessel's media and adventitia (see Fig. 29-15A). Amyloid-lined vacuoles often seen at this stage[67] may represent former sites of vascular smooth muscle cells that have died in apparent response to the surrounding amyloid. In moderately severe segments of CAA, vascular amyloid extends throughout the media to replace essentially the entire smooth muscle cell layer (see Fig. 29-15B).

The most advanced extent of CAA is marked by not only severe amyloid deposition but also pathologic changes in the amyloid-laden vessel wall. These vasculopathic changes can include microaneurysms, concentric splitting of the vessel wall (see Fig. 29-15D), chronic perivascular or transmural inflammation, fibrinoid necrosis (see Fig. 29-15E), and even perivascular giant-cell reaction (Fig. 29-15F).[53,66-68] CAA-related vasculopathic changes are often associated with paravascular red cells or hemosiderin deposits, which suggests ongoing leakage of blood. It is this combination of extensive amyloid deposition and breakdown of the amyloid-laden vessel walls that appears to act as the substrate for symptomatic hemorrhagic strokes.[53,67,87,94]

The principal constituent of both vascular amyloid in CAA and plaque amyloid is the β-amyloid peptide (Aβ). The Aβ peptides are 39- to 43-amino acid proteolytic fragments of the 695- to 770-residue β-amyloid precursor protein (APP). The subset of Aβ peptides with carboxyl termini extending to position 42 or 43 (denoted Aβ42) appears to be an important trigger to amyloid aggregation in both vessels and plaques.[148] In support of Aβ42 deposition as an early step in initiation of CAA is the observation that mildly affected vessels can stain positive for Aβ42 but stain negative for the more common Aβ fragments terminating at position 39 or 40 (Aβ40).[149] It is Aβ40, however, that appears to be the predominant species in more heavily involved vessel segments.[150-152] Quantitative analysis of brains with mild and severe CAA suggests a progressive addition of Aβ40 to previously seeded vessel segments.[152] A variety of other proteins or protein fragments can also be detected as components of vascular amyloid, although the pathogenic role in the breakdown of the vessel wall is not known. These CAA-associated proteins include apoE, cystatin C, α-synuclein, heparan sulfate proteoglycan, amyloid P component, and several complement proteins.[153,154]

The relationship of the pathology of CAA and ApoE genotype provides an interesting insight into the importance of both Aβ deposition and vessel breakdown to the pathogenesis of CAA-related ICH. The ApoE ε2 and ε4 alleles, each a suggested risk factor for CAA-related ICH, appear to act at these two distinct stages of CAA to promote hemorrhage. ApoE ε4 associates in a dose-dependent manner with increased deposition of Aβ in vessels as it does in plaques[95]; ApoE ε2 appears instead to promote the CAA-related vasculopathic changes such as concentric vessel splitting and fibrinoid necrosis.[94,96] The mechanism for this unexpected effect of ApoE ε2 on vascular

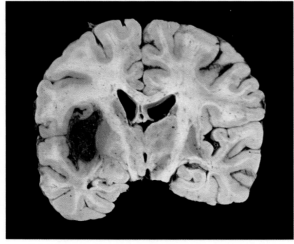

Figure 29-13 A 2-month-old right putaminal–insular hemorrhage, with partial cavitation, good demarcation from the adjacent parenchyma, and lack of signs of mass effect.

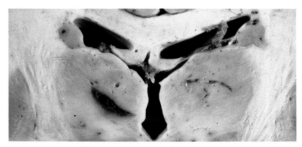

Figure 29-14 Old right thalamic hemorrhage reduced to a slit with hemosiderin-stained edges.

breakdown is unknown. The domain of the ApoE protein containing the ε2 determinant is present in both vessel and plaque amyloid deposits[154] but has not been linked to any specific pathogenic function.

One experimental approach to clarifying pathogenic mechanisms for CAA has been to study the effects of Aβ on vessel components in vitro. Aβ exerts toxic effects on a variety of vascular cells in culture, including cerebrovascular smooth muscle cells, endothelial cells, and pericytes.[90,155] Cell death is enhanced when the Aβ peptide used is either wild-type Aβ42 or mutant Aβ40 containing one of the amino acid substitutions associated with hereditary CAA,[85,91,156] which suggests that particular chemical properties of Aβ can specifically promote toxicity. Death of the cultured cerebrovascular smooth muscle cells appears to require a series of events on the cell surface, including assembly of Aβ into amyloid fibrils (Fig. 29-16) and accumulation of the secreted amino-terminal portion of APP.[157] Another in vitro property of Aβ is to stimulate tissue-type plasminogen activator (t-PA),[158] which raises the intriguing possibility that CAA might promote ICH through direct effects on the coagulation–thrombolysis cascade as well as on the integrity of the vessel wall.

The pathogenesis of CAA has also been studied in transgenic mouse models (Fig. 29-17). Substantial CAA develops at advanced ages in lines of mice expressing high levels of mutant APP.[159,160] Affected vessels in these animals can demonstrate several pathologic features reminiscent of human CAA, including disruption or loss of the vascular smooth muscle, microaneurysms, and perivascular cerebral hemorrhages.[159-161] Because the expression of human APP in these animals is virtually all neuronal, the occurrence of CAA demonstrates that Aβ produced by neurons is capable of reaching vascular sites of deposition, possibly via the interstitial fluid drainage pathway.[162] Once produced, Aβ may be cleared by proteolytic enzymes such as neprilysin[15,46] or insulin-degrading enzyme[47] or may exit the brain by receptor-mediated efflux across the blood–brain barrier.[48]

A further insight to come from these transgenic studies is the possibility that Aβ may have specific effects on vessel physiology. Investigations in mouse models of CAA using a variety of techniques to measure blood flow have indicated blunted vasodilatory response to pharmacologic or functional stimulation.[49-51] These hints of altered vascular physiology, raised as well by earlier studies of isolated vessel segments exposed to Aβ, have found important parallels

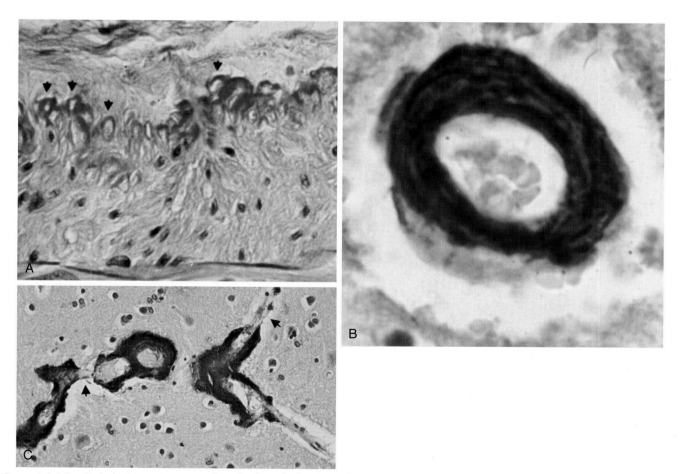

Figure 29-15   Pathologic appearances of cerebral amyloid angiopathy (CAA). A, Vessel in longitudinal section. In mild stages of disease, amyloid appears at the outer edge of the vessel media, creating vesicle-like structures *(arrows)* at sites believed to be previously occupied by smooth muscle cells. B, Further amyloid deposition replaces the media and all smooth muscle cells. C, Specimen taken from a brain with the Iowa APP mutation. Amyloid deposits can cause marked thickening of vessel wall segments that alternate with skipped areas of normal caliber *(arrows)*.

Continued

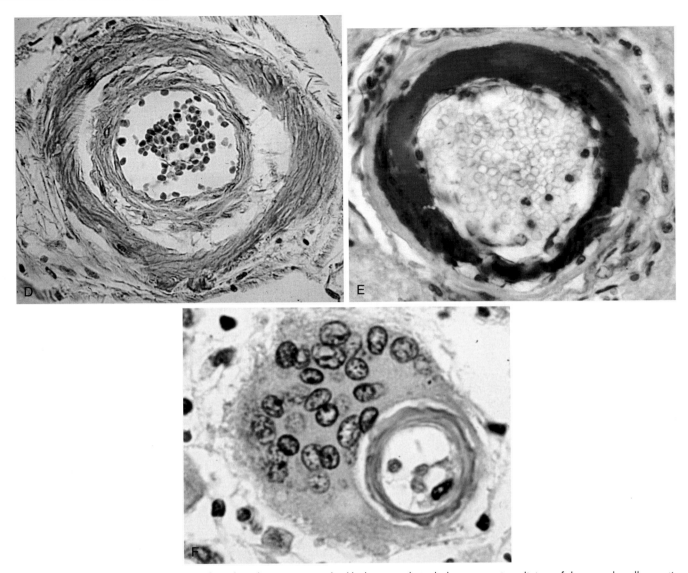

Figure 29-15, cont'd Further vasculopathic changes in amyloid-laden vessels include concentric splitting of the vessel wall, creating a vessel-in-vessel appearance (D) and fibrinoid necrosis (E), signifying entry of plasma components into the wall. F, Some instances of advanced CAA are accompanied by visible inflammatory changes such as perivascular giant cell reaction. (A, D, and F stained by Luxol fast blue–hematoxylin-eosin; B and C by anti-β-amyloid immunostain with hematoxylin counterstain; and E with phosphotungstic acid–hematoxylin.)

in studies of vascular reactivity to visual stimulation in humans with CAA.[52]

Nonhypertensive Causes of Intracerebral Hemorrhage

There are a number of instances in which ICH occurs in the absence of a history of long-standing hypertension. These mechanisms of ICH are (1) small vascular malformations, (2) sympathomimetic drugs, (3) brain tumors, (4) anticoagulants, (5) fibrinolytic agents, and (6) vasculitis. CAA, another mechanism of nonhypertensive ICH, is discussed in more detail in Chapter 34.

Small Vascular Malformations

Small vascular malformations, also referred to as angiomas, are commonly implicated in cases of ICH, especially lobar ICH.[163] Margolis et al[164] first called attention to these

lesions in 1951, when they reported four cases of fatal ICH in young patients, in whom pathologic examination disclosed small vascular malformations: one arteriovenous, two venous, and one probably cavernous. These researchers add two other cases in which malformations were incidentally found (not associated with ICH): a cavernous angioma and a telangiectasis. Margolis et al[164] stressed the need to consider such lesions in cases of nonhypertensive ICH, especially in the young.

Since that report, several researchers have shared this point of view.[165-167] Fisher[102] recorded 17 such lesions in his series of ICH and suggested that the hemorrhages they produce are less massive or slower to develop than most hypertensive ones.

Crawford and Russell[165,167] reported 21 examples of ICH due to small vascular malformations, 20 of which were arteriovenous and only 1 a cavernous angioma. The 20 arteriovenous lesions were located in the cerebral convexity

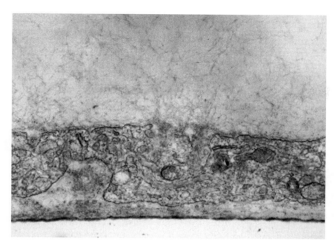

Figure 29-16 Deposition of β-amyloid (Aβ) on cerebrovascular smooth muscle cell. This transmission electron micrograph shows a cultured human cerebrovascular smooth muscle cell treated with Dutch-type mutant Aβ40 for 6 days. Under these conditions, Aβ assembles into amyloid fibrils on the cell surface (seen at top). (Courtesy of William E. Van Nostrand.)

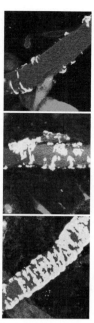

Figure 29-17 Cerebral amyloid angiopathy in a transgenic mouse. Mice transgenic for mutant β-amyloid (Aβ) precursor protein driven by the platelet-derived growth factor promoter demonstrate vessels with varying amounts of vascular Aβ deposition. Amyloid is visualized through topical application of thioflavine-S, and vessel lumens with intravenous Texas red-labeled dextran. In vivo imaging is performed by multiphoton fluorescent microscopy. (Courtesy of Bradley T. Hyman.)

(10 cases), deep portions of the hemispheres (four cases), and cerebellum (six cases). Because of their small size and the difficulties in diagnosing them in life, the term *cryptic* was proposed for these malformations. However, the term has become obsolete since the introduction of CT and especially MRI; the latter technique routinely demonstrates these small lesions, which were previously undetectable on cerebral angiography. Multiple series have now documented instances of ICH due to rupture of small vascular malformations that occur either sporadically[166,168-170] or on a familial basis.[171-175]

In the series of 18 cases reported by Becker et al,[168] the hemorrhages were predominantly lobar, reflecting the usually cortical location of the malformations. These investigators found a mean age at diagnosis of 23 years in their series and documented a female preponderance of 2.5:1, which was similar to the sex distribution of 42 cases previously reported in the literature.

Cavernous angiomas (Fig. 29-18) are thought to have a generally lower bleeding potential than the arteriovenous variety. However, they occasionally lead to progressive, subacute deficits that result from protracted bleeding or recurrent small hemorrhages, mimicking brainstem tumors[170] or even multiple sclerosis.[176] Natural history data suggest that bleeding from cavernous angiomas may be more common than previously recognized. Bleeding rates of 0.7%[177] and 1.1%[178] per year were recorded in two reports with follow-up periods of 2.2 years. In a third series, Kondziolka et al[179] found the bleeding risk on follow-up to differ according to the initial presentation. They documented bleeding rates of 0.6% per year for patients without a history of ICH and 4.5% per year for patients with prior ICH (Table 29-5).

The availability of MRI has greatly facilitated the diagnosis of cavernous angiomas (Fig. 29-19). They characteristically appear, on T2-weighted sequences, as irregular lesions with a central core of mixed (high and low) signal, surrounded by a halo of hypodensity corresponding

to hemosiderin deposits, which represent previous episodes of bleeding around the malformation.[180-182] Although these lesions generally occur in isolation and with a preference for the cortical and subcortical regions of the cerebral hemispheres and the pons,[180,183] occasional examples are multiple,[181] in which case a familial occurrence is likely.[184] The latter appears to be particularly common among individuals of Mexican-American descent,[184] in whom cavernous angiomas are inherited as an autosomal dominant pattern linked to a mutation that has been mapped to the short arm of chromosome 7.[185,186] Recent studies of subjects with cerebral cavernous malformations have identified mutations in one of three genes: *CCM1/KRIT1*, *CCM2/malcaverin*, or *CCM3/PDCD10*.[187] The authors have postulated a "two-hit" mechanism in the pathogenesis of cerebral cavernous malformations, in which the germline mutation requires a second, somatic mutation for the phenotype to be expressed. The somatic mutation has been identified in endothelial cells of the cavernous vessels,[187] which suggests that they are the primary substrate of disease expression.

On the basis of the preceding reports, it now seems well-established that small vascular malformations, both arteriovenous and cavernous, are likely to bleed and may be responsible for cases of nonhypertensive ICH. The frequency of this occurrence is difficult to establish, but one figure is available from the autopsy study by Russell,[167] who obtained 21 cases with vascular formations from a total of 461 cases of ICH, which yields a frequency of 4.5%.

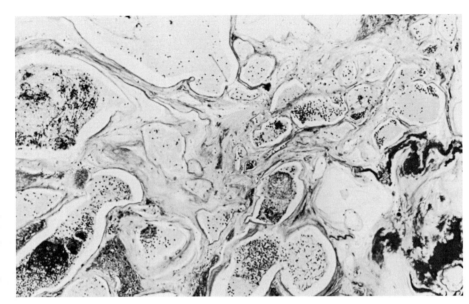

Figure 29-18 Incidentally found cavernous angioma in the subcortical white matter of the left frontal lobe, showing widely separated vascular channels with primitive walls and without intervening brain parenchyma. Areas of calcification are shown in the right lower corner. (Hematoxylin and eosin, ×48.)

TABLE 29-5 NATURAL HISTORY OF CAVERNOUS ANGIOMAS

Study	No. of Patients	Bleeding Rate per Year (%)
Robinson et al[177]	57	0.7
Zabramski et al[178]	31	1.1
Kondziolka et al[179]	122	2.63
Without prior intracerebral hemorrhage	61	0.6
With prior intracerebral hemorrhage	61	4.5

Sympathomimetic Drugs

ICH related to the use of *amphetamines* has been documented in several publications.[188-191] The preparation most commonly implicated has been intravenous methamphetamine,[188] but cases related to intranasal[190] or oral[189] use of this drug and amphetamine have also been reported. Another sympathomimetic drug, *pseudoephedrine*, has been associated with one reported instance of ICH.[191] In these cases, ICHs have developed usually within minutes (20 to 40) to a few hours (4 to 6) after the use of the drug; frequently, the ICH represents an established pattern of drug abuse for months beforehand, but at times it has followed a first-time use.[189] An association with transiently elevated blood pressure has been noticed in about 50% of cases, and most of the hematomas have been of lobar location.[190,191] Their pathogenesis has been related to either transient drug-induced elevation in blood pressure[189] or an arteritis-like vascular change histologically similar to periarteritis nodosa.[192] The latter is considered either a direct "toxic" effect of the drug on cerebral blood vessels or a hypersensitivity reaction to the drug or its vehicle.

The cerebral "arteritis" related to use of these drugs is characterized angiographically by beading (multiple areas of focal arterial stenosis or constriction) of medium-sized and large intracranial arteries,[190,191,193-195] which is an effect that has been shown to be reversible after use of steroids and discontinuation of drug abuse.[195] However,

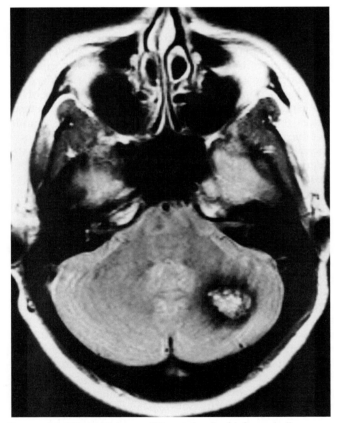

Figure 29-19 MR image (T2-weighted) of left cerebellar cavernous angioma, with mixed-signal central core and peripheral low-signal hemosiderin ring.

it is likely that these reversible vascular changes correspond not to a true vasculitis but rather to a nonspecific phenomenon of multifocal spasm related to the effects of the sympathomimetic drug on the vessel wall. In isolated instances, intravenous use of methamphetamine precipitated an ICH from a Sylvian-region AVM,[196] and oral use

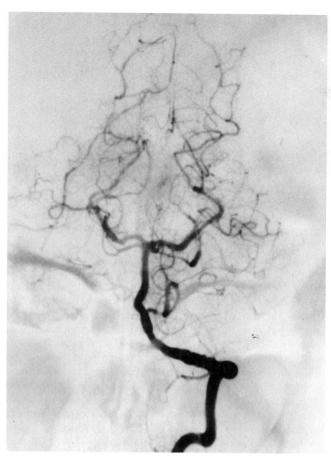

Figure 29-20   Multifocal areas of arterial constriction and dilatation ("beading") in the vertebrobasilar system after an episode of severe headache and transient hypertension (200/110 mm Hg), shortly after the ingestion of a phenylpropanolamine-containing nasal decongestant. (From Kase CS, Foster TE, Reed JE, et al: Intracerebral hemorrhage and phenylpropanolamine use. *Neurology* 37:399, 1987.)

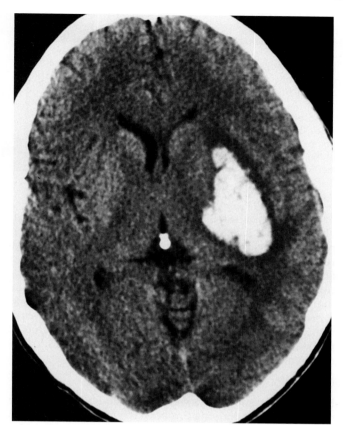

Figure 29-21   Left putaminal hemorrhage secondary to use of crack cocaine.

of dextroamphetamine was associated with SAH in the presence of a small middle cerebral artery aneurysm.[197] Most other reports of amphetamine-related ICH and SAH have not documented preexisting vascular malformations or mycotic aneurysms.

Other sympathomimetic agents have been related to episodes of ICH. *Phenylpropanolamine* (PPA) has been associated with instances of ICH and SAH. Most affected patients have been young (median age in the third decade), have been women more often than men, and generally have lacked other risk factors for ICH.[198] Results of a case-control study reported by Kernan et al[199] have suggested the potential association between PPA and ICH. These investigators found that women who used appetite suppressants containing PPA had a significantly higher risk of intracranial hemorrhage (odds ratio [OR], 16.58; 95% CI, 1.51–182.21; $P = 0.02$). The hemorrhages occur shortly after PPA ingestion (most between 1 and 8 hours).[198-204] The ICHs are most commonly of lobar location, and about two thirds of the patients that have undergone angiography have shown widespread beading of intracranial arteries (Fig. 29-20), without documentation

of other vascular lesions responsible for bleeding, such as AVM and aneurysm. Histologic examination of blood vessels from biopsy material has been nondiagnostic, except for one instance in which changes consistent with vasculitis were found.[205]

The pathogenesis of these PPA-related hemorrhages is obscure. Although rare patients have been previously hypertensive, transient hypertension was noted at presentation in about 50% of the reported cases.[198] This finding suggests that a possible mechanism of vascular rupture is drug-induced transient hypertension associated with multifocal arterial changes due to vasospasm or, less commonly, vasculitis. However, transient hypertension alone is an unlikely explanation for these hemorrhages because the hypertension has generally been modest, even in comparison with blood pressure rises documented under physiologic conditions.[206] These observations suggest that mechanisms other than transient hypertension must be present in order for intracranial hemorrhage to occur under these circumstances.

Cocaine is being increasingly reported as a cause of cerebral hemorrhage in young individuals, especially in its precipitate form, known as "crack." Instances of ICH and SAH have occurred within minutes to 1 hour from use of crack cocaine.[207] The ICHs are either lobar or deep ganglionic (Fig. 29-21); occasionally there are multiple hemorrhages in both locations.[208] The mechanism of these ICHs is unclear, although these lesions are, in many respects, similar to those related to the use

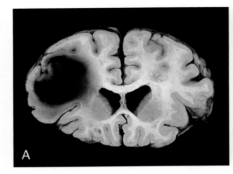
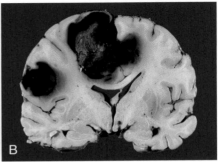

Figure 29-22 A, Large hemorrhage into a metastatic lesion (from bronchogenic carcinoma) in the right frontal subcortical white matter. A second, nonhemorrhagic metastasis is present in the white matter of the left frontal lobe. B, Hemorrhagic metastases from melanoma, with visible necrotic tumor at the center of the larger hemorrhage, extending into both medial parietal lobes.

of amphetamine or PPA; the angiographic beading that characterizes ICHs due to amphetamine or PPA use is relatively uncommon in cocaine-related ICHs, which, in turn, have shown a stronger association with AVMs or aneurysms as the bleeding mechanism.[207] This association suggests that the hypertensive response that commonly follows cocaine use may act in some instances as a precipitant of ICH in preexisting vascular malformations. In one case, ICH after cocaine use was related to pathologically documented vasculitis of a small intraparenchymal artery.[209]

Intracranial Tumors

Intracranial tumors are a well-recognized but uncommon cause of ICH. Underlying tumors have accounted for 1% to 2% of cases of ICH in autopsy series,[23] whereas rates of 6% to 10% have been found in clinical-radiologic series.[210,211] The great majority of the underlying neoplasms have been malignant, either primary or metastatic, but rarely, meningiomas[212] or oligodendrogliomas[210] have manifested as ICH. An example of a generally benign tumor with relatively high tendency to bleed is pituitary adenoma, which was associated with bleeding in 15% of the cases in one large series of brain tumors.[213] Among the primary malignant brain tumors causing ICH, glioblastoma multiforme predominates[210]; the metastatic tumors have been melanoma, choriocarcinoma, renal cell, and bronchogenic carcinoma.[211,214-217] The frequency of hemorrhagic metastases was estimated at 60% for germ cell tumors, 40% for melanoma, and 9% for bronchogenic carcinoma.[218]

The bleeding tendency in neoplasms is thought to be directly related to the richness of their vascular components and their pathologic, neoplastic character.[219] In the case of metastatic choriocarcinoma, these features are enhanced by the normal biological tendency of trophoblastic tissue to invade the walls of blood vessels.[215,220] The location of the hemorrhage relates to some extent to the type of neoplasm involved: Hemorrhages occurring in glioblastoma multiforme are frequently deep into the hemispheres, basal ganglia, or corpus callosum.[210] Hemorrhages due to metastatic tumors occur more often in the subcortical white matter (Fig. 29-22)[214] because metastatic nodules commonly deposit at the gray–white matter junction.

In approximately half of the reported instances of ICH within an intracerebral tumor, the hemorrhage was the first clinical manifestation of the neoplasm. The radiologic diagnosis by CT can be established easily in instances of multiple metastatic lesions,[214] but cases of ICH into a single tumor can be more difficult to diagnose. Such a diagnosis should be suspected with the finding of large areas of low-density edema surrounding the hematoma (Fig. 29-23) of an area of contrast enhancement at the periphery of the hematoma, frequently forming a ring pattern on initial presentation with ICH.[210,214] Because ring enhancement is not expected on presentation of spontaneous, hypertensive ICH,[220-223] its presence should strongly suggest the possibility of an underlying, previously asymptomatic primary or metastatic brain tumor. Other features suggesting ICH into a brain tumor are (1) finding of papilledema at presentation with acute ICH; (2) atypical location of the ICH, in areas such as the corpus callosum, which is rarely the site of "spontaneous" ICH and is commonly involved by malignant gliomas (Fig. 29-24); and (3) a ring-like high-density area corresponding to blood around a low-density center, resulting from bleeding by tumor vessels at the junction of tumor and adjacent brain parenchyma.[224] In addition, Iwama et al[225] have suggested that a low-density indentation of the periphery of an ICH on CT should raise the suspicion of an underlying tumor nodule. These clinical and radiologic features should prompt a search for a primary or metastatic brain tumor with MRI and cerebral angiography. If the results of these studies are inconclusive, biopsy of the hematoma cavity should be considered to establish the diagnosis of an underlying brain tumor because the therapeutic options and prognosis are radically different from those for spontaneous or hypertensive ICH.

Anticoagulant and Thrombolytic Therapy

Warfarin. Long-term oral anticoagulation with warfarin is often listed among the causes of ICH. In a consecutive series of 100 cases of ICH that Kase et al[226] observed over a 3-year period, warfarin anticoagulation was a factor in 9% of the cases. Boudouresques et al[35] reported that in their autopsy series of 500 cases of ICH, anticoagulation was implicated in 11%. After excluding cases due to trauma, ruptured aneurysm, or concomitant brain tumor, Rådberg et al[227] documented an anticoagulant-related mechanism in 14% of 200 consecutive patients with ICH. Furthermore, anticoagulation is second only to hypertension as a causative factor in series of cerebellar[228] and lobar[137] locations. The risk of ICH in patients undergoing long-term oral anticoagulation has been shown to be 8 to

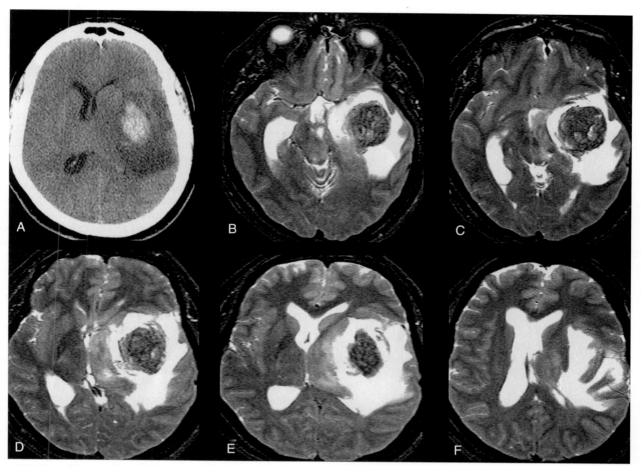

Figure 29-23   CT scan (A) and T2-weighted MR images (B to F) of acute hemorrhage into glioblastoma multiforme, showing the acute hematoma with marked edema extending well beyond the immediate vicinity of the acute hemorrhage.

11 times that in patients of similar age who are not receiving anticoagulants.[229-232]

The incidence of ICH in patients receiving warfarin after MI is approximately 1% per year.[230] A number of factors are known to contribute to a higher risk of ICH in these patients, including advanced age (>70 years),[233,234] hypertension,[226,232,233,235-237] and concomitant use of aspirin, which has been estimated to double the rate of ICH in comparison with individuals taking oral anticoagulants alone.[230,238]

Other features related to ICH in patients receiving anticoagulants are as follows:

Duration of Anticoagulation Therapy before Onset of ICH. In two series, most ICHs (70%,[226] 54%[227]) occurred during the first year after start of treatment. In another report, only one third of ICHs occurred after that period of time[229]; the other two thirds appeared between 2 and 18 years after the start of treatment.

Relationship between Intensity of Anticoagulant Effect and Risk of ICH. Excessive anticoagulant effect is now well-established as a powerful risk factor for ICH.[226,232-235,237,239] Hylek and Singer,[233] reporting data from an anticoagulant therapy unit, showed that the risk of ICH doubled with each 0.5-point increase in the prothrombin time ratio above the recommended limit of 2.0. Data from the Stroke Prevention in Reversible Ischemia

Trial,[240] a secondary stroke prevention trial in which patients with transient ischemic attack or minor ischemic stroke were randomly assigned to receive either aspirin (30 mg/day) or warfarin (to achieve an international normalized ratio [INR] of 3.0 to 4.5), add further evidence of the effect of excessive anticoagulation and frequency of ICH: the trial was stopped early, after the occurrence of 24 ICHs (14 fatal) in the warfarin group in comparison with only three ICHs (one fatal) in the aspirin group; there was a strong relationship between bleeding complications and rise in INR values.

Presence of Leukoaraiosis. Severe and confluent areas of leukoaraiosis were associated with a higher risk of ICH in warfarin-anticoagulated subjects in the Stroke Prevention in Reversible Ischemia Trial.[240] Similarly, data reported by Smith et al[237] documented CT-detected leukoaraiosis as an independent risk factor (OR, 12.9; 95% CI, 28–59.8) for ICH in subjects receiving anticoagulation therapy with warfarin after an episode of ischemic stroke.

Location of ICH. A high frequency of cerebellar location was found in some studies,[226,227,241] whereas others found no differences in location of ICH between patients who were and were not receiving anticoagulation therapy.[229,230,232]

Characteristics. Characteristics of these hemorrhages include a tendency to occur in the absence of signs of systemic bleeding, lack of relationship between the ICH and preceding cerebral infarction, frequent leisurely progression of the focal neurologic deficits (at times over periods as long as 48 to 72 hours), and high mortality (46% to 68%) related to hematoma size (the hematoma is generally larger than in hypertensive ICH).[227,229,230] In

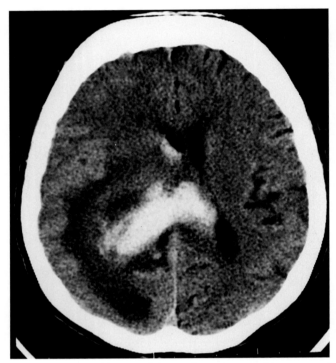

Figure 29-24   CT scan of hemorrhage into glioblastoma multiforme, with bleeding into the corpus callosum and adjacent thalamus and deep parietal lobe as well as extensive surrounding low-density edema.

addition, warfarin-related ICHs are associated with a high risk of hematoma expansion,[242] which in turn correlates with clinical deterioration (Fig. 29-25) and increased mortality. On CT scan, the hemorrhages often show blood-fluid levels, which result from "sedimentation" of red blood cells in a hematoma that does not clot because of the anticoagulation effect (Fig. 29-26).

The actual mechanism of ICH in patients undergoing anticoagulation is unknown, in part because of the lack of adequate pathologic studies with serial histologic sections aimed at identifying the type of bleeding vessel and the histopathologic abnormality at the bleeding site. Such studies should determine whether anticoagulant-related ICHs have different microscopic pathologic features from that of spontaneous ICH, in terms of the type of affected vessel as well as the eventual presence of local vascular disease (i.e., microaneurysm, fibrinoid necrosis, lipohyalinosis, or CAA) at the rupture site as a possible substrate for this complication of warfarin anticoagulation. Hart et al[230] have hypothesized that ICH in patients undergoing anticoagulation could result from enlargement of small, spontaneous hemorrhages that would otherwise occur without clinical consequence in individuals with normal coagulation function. The contributing role of local vascular disease, such as CAA, is favored by observation of a high frequency of this angiopathy in individuals with warfarin-related ICH. Rosand et al[243] documented CAA in brain tissue samples from 7 of 11 patients with warfarin-related ICH. In addition, these investigators found an overrepresentation of the ApoE ε2 allele, a marker of CAA, in patients with warfarin-related ICH in comparison with a control group.

Heparin. The occurrence of ICH during intravenous heparin anticoagulation represents a different situation because this complication generally occurs in the setting of preceding acute cerebral infarction (because ICH is

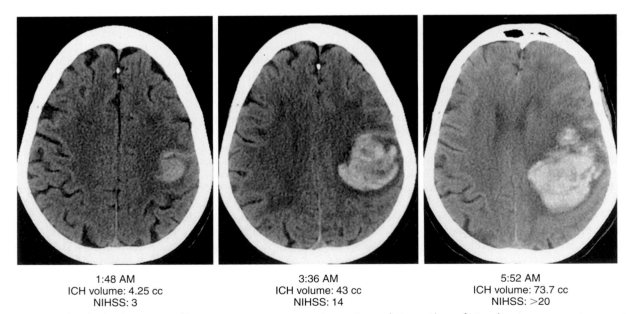

1:48 AM	3:36 AM	5:52 AM
ICH volume: 4.25 cc	ICH volume: 43 cc	ICH volume: 73.7 cc
NIHSS: 3	NIHSS: 14	NIHSS: >20

Figure 29-25   Gradual enlargement of hematoma in patient receiving anticoagulation with warfarin, showing progression over time of the volume of the hematoma and the corresponding neurologic deterioration, as measured by the National Institutes of Health Stroke Scale (NIHSS) score.

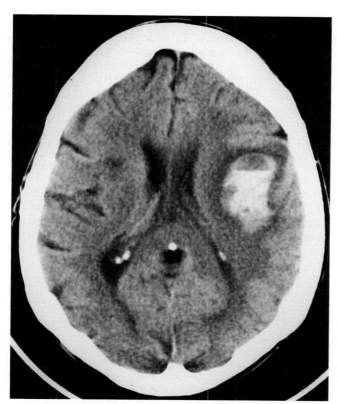

Figure 29-26 CT of acute intracerebral hemorrhage in left frontal white matter, with blood-fluid level.

extremely uncommon in patients receiving intravenous heparin for noncerebrovascular indications, such as deep vein thrombosis and MI[244,245]). Thus, a recent cerebral infarction with local ischemic blood vessels is a likely site for the occurrence of secondary ICH, especially in embolic infarcts, which tend to become hemorrhagic as part of their natural history.[246] ICH in this setting occurs within 24 to 48 hours of the start of heparin treatment,[247] and excessive prolongation of the activated partial thromboplastin time (aPTT) is common.[248,249] Other risk factors for ICH in the setting of intravenous heparin therapy for acute cerebral infarction are infarcts of large size and uncontrolled hypertension (blood pressure exceeding 180 mm Hg systolic/100 mm Hg diastolic).[250]

These findings have led to recommendations that the immediate use of intravenous heparin anticoagulation in acute nonseptic cerebral infarction be limited to those patients with subtotal infarcts in a given vascular territory but without uncontrolled hypertension (i.e., blood pressure <180/100 mm Hg) and that it be accompanied by close adherence to a prolongation of the aPTT value within the recommended therapeutic range (1.5 times the control value).[249] However, the immediate use of intravenous heparin after cerebral infarction has been questioned in view of the lack of data supporting the value of any parenteral antithrombotic agents in this setting.[251] Because intravenous heparin has not been properly tested in patients with acute ischemic stroke of nonlacunar type, a prospective, randomized clinical trial, the Rapid Anticoagulation Prevents Ischemic Damage (RAPID) trial,[252] was performed in Europe. The design involved the

comparison between aspirin and unfractionated heparin (administered within 12 hours of stroke symptom onset) given for 1 week, with regard to the primary endpoint of rate of favorable outcome, measured as a modified Rankin Scale (mRS) score of 2 or less at 90 days. Although the sample size for the study was 592 patients, the trial was stopped early because of low recruitment (only 67 patients had been recruited after 30 months from study onset). An analysis of the small sample of 67 patients showed no significant differences between the groups in terms of mRS, National Institutes of Health Stroke Scale (NIHSS) score < 1, mortality, ischemic stroke worsening, or stroke worsening related to hemorrhage, whereas a trend ($P = 0.09$) in favor of unfractionated heparin was detected for the secondary endpoint of ischemic stroke recurrence.[253] Based on these limited data, the authors planned to conduct a larger multicenter trial to test the hypothesis that early administration of unfractionated intravenous heparin may have a neuroprotective effect in patients with acute ischemic stroke.

Fibrinolytic agents. Fibrinolytic agents, especially t-PA, are used in the treatment of coronary, arterial, and venous thromboses in the limbs and pulmonary circulation. The ability of these agents to produce clot lysis and a relatively low level of systemic hypofibrinogenemia makes them ideal choices for the treatment of acute thrombosis. However, the major complication, although it is relatively infrequent, continues to be hemorrhage, in particular ICH. ICH has been reported in 0.4% to 1.3% of patients with acute MI treated with the single-chain t-PA alteplase.[254] The clinical and CT features of ICHs related to coronary thrombolysis with t-PA have been extensively reviewed.[255-259] The hemorrhages tend to occur early after start of t-PA treatment: In one study, 40% of the hemorrhages started during the infusion, and another 25% occurred within 24 hours of the start of treatment.[255] In 70% to 90% of cases, the hemorrhages are lobar. In about 30% of cases the hemorrhages are multiple[256]; the mortality for multiple hemorrhages is high (44% to 66%).[255-258]

The mechanism of bleeding in this setting is unknown. On several occasions, patients have had excessively prolonged aPTT values at the time of onset of intracranial hemorrhage, as a result of the use of intravenous heparin (aimed at preventing reocclusion of reperfused coronary arteries).[256-258] Other factors suggested as significant in raising the risk of ICH after the use of t-PA in acute MI are advanced age (>65 years), history of hypertension, and the use of aspirin before t-PA therapy[258]; in one study, however, none of these factors was found to be significantly different in patients with or without ICH.[257] A possible role for local cerebral vascular disease has been considered because examples of pretreatment head trauma[257] and concomitant CAA[259-261] have been documented in association with ICH after the use of t-PA. Other coagulation defects related to this treatment, such as hypofibrinogenemia and thrombocytopenia, have not been found to correlate with this complication.

In addition to their role in the treatment of acute MI, intravenous thrombolytic agents (t-PA) are the only approved therapy for patients with acute ischemic stroke. Initial pilot studies with the use of intraarterial agents, mainly urokinase and t-PA, yielded encouraging rates of reperfusion, on the order of 55% of patients treated, and hemorrhagic complications (i.e., hemorrhagic infarction and ICH) and neurologic deterioration occurred in about 11% of patients.[262] Attention has also been directed at the less invasive administration of intravenous t-PA and streptokinase. The initial experience with intravenous t-PA administered within 8 hours of stroke onset, reported by del Zoppo et al,[263] yielded angiographically documented rates of reperfusion at a disappointingly low level, in the range of 26% to 38%. Despite this low level of recanalization, hemorrhagic changes with neurologic deterioration occurred in 9% of patients. In addition, the study showed that the rate of hemorrhagic complications was significantly higher in patients to whom t-PA was administered more than 6 hours after stroke onset, in comparison with patients treated within 6 hours.[264]

Nonangiographic studies of intravenous t-PA in acute stroke, the European Cooperative Acute Stroke Study[265] and the National Institute of Neurological Diseases and Stroke (NINDS) rt-PA Stroke Study,[266] used entry windows (time after onset during which patients could be entered into the study) of 6 hours and 3 hours, respectively, and doses of alteplase of 1.1 mg/kg (to a maximum of 100 mg) and 0.9 mg/kg (to a maximum of 90 mg), respectively. Results of both studies were positive, especially those of the NINDS study, which showed an improved functional outcome at 3 months in the group treated with t-PA without a higher mortality due to hemorrhagic complications. Despite a tenfold increase in symptomatic ICH during the first 36 hours in patients treated with t-PA (6.4% versus 0.6% for the placebo group), a net benefit accrued for the t-PA–treated group as measured by three functional scales 3 months after treatment. The intracranial hemorrhages in the t-PA group occurred in both the lobar white matter and the deep gray nuclei (Fig. 29-27), and they carried a high mortality (45%).[267] The risk factors for intracranial hemorrhage after thrombolysis with intravenous t-PA within 3 hours of acute ischemic stroke onset include the severity of the neurologic deficit (as measured by the NIHSS score) and the presence of edema and mass effect in the baseline CT scan.[267] When intravenous t-PA was given between 3 and 6 hours from stroke onset, the size of the baseline infarct on diffusion-weighted MRI and evidence of early post–t-PA reperfusion were independent predictors of the risk of ICH.[268] Other potential factors associated with increased risk of postintravenous t-PA bleeding include hyperglycemia at baseline[269] and elevated serum levels of biomarkers indicative of vascular fragility or abnormal permeability of the blood–brain barrier such as matrix metalloproteinase-9,[270] cellular fibronectin,[271] endogenous activated protein C,[272] and markers of endogenous fibrinolysis.[273]

Three clinical trials of intravenous streptokinase in acute ischemic stroke have found an alarmingly high rate of ICH and mortality.[274-276] The use of 1.5 million IU of streptokinase within 4[274] or 6[275,276] hours from stroke onset resulted in rates of symptomatic ICH between 6%[275] and 21.2%,[274] with mortality rates of 19%[275] and 34%[276] at 10 days and 43.4%[274] at 90 days, resulting in the termination of the trials. It is possible that the higher rates of ICH after streptokinase therapy than after t-PA therapy in acute ischemic stroke may reflect a dose of streptokinase that is too high for this indication (as opposed to its safer profile in the treatment of patients with acute MI[277]). Additional possible reasons for such observations include a more pronounced and longer lasting systemic fibrinolytic effect with streptokinase than with t-PA.[278]

The use of intraarterial recombinant prourokinase (proUK) was tested in the PROlyse in Acute Cerebral Thromboembolism (PROACT) I[279] and II trials.[280] When given directly into a middle cerebral artery clot, proUK was associated with a recanalization rate of 66% (compared with 18% for the control group) in the PROACT II study.[280] This rate correlated with a significantly better functional outcome at 3 months for the treated group, without differences in mortality, even though the rate of symptomatic ICH was 10% in treated patients and only 2% in the control subjects. Virtually all proUK-related ICHs were massive (Fig. 29-28), and all occurred in the area of the qualifying acute infarct in the middle cerebral artery distribution.[281] Among a number of possible risk factors for post-proUK symptomatic ICH, only hyperglycemia at baseline was identified as being potentially associated with a higher risk.[281]

Anticoagulation and cerebral amyloid angiopathy. Iatrogenic ICH occurring during anticoagulation or thrombolysis is an especially important manifestation of CAA. Anticoagulation is hypothesized to promote ICH by allowing small leakages of blood to expand into large symptomatic hemorrhages and might thus be particularly risky in the setting of advanced CAA. This possibility is supported by demonstration of advanced CAA in individuals who have ICH after thrombolysis or during warfarin therapy. CAA may also have a role in ICH occurring with antiplatelet treatment, but the overall added risk conferred by antiplatelet agents in CAA appears to be relatively small.[59] These observations raise the important possibility that an individual's risk for CAA could ultimately be incorporated into the decision whether to treat with thrombolytic or anticoagulant therapy.

Vasculitis

The cerebral vasculitides generally result in arterial occlusion and cerebral infarction and are only rarely responsible for ICH. Most of these unusual examples of ICH secondary to cerebral arteritis have been secondary to *granulomatous angiitis of the nervous system* (GANS).[282] This primary cerebral vasculitis occurs in the absence of systemic involvement. Histologically, it is characterized by mononuclear inflammatory exudates with giant cells in the media and adventitia of small and medium-sized arteries and veins. This vascular inflammation is occasionally associated with the formation of microaneurysms. The cerebral disease evolves with chronic headache, progressive cognitive decline, seizures, and recurrent episodes of cerebral infarction.[283] Because of its primary cerebral location, systemic features such as malaise, fever, weight loss, arthralgias, myalgias, anemia, and elevated sedimentation rate are absent.[283,284] The diagnosis is favored by the finding of lymphocytic cerebrospinal fluid (CSF) pleocytosis with elevated protein levels, and angiography may show a beading pattern in multiple medium-sized and small intracranial arteries. The instances of ICH reported in patients with GANS have occurred in the setting of progressive

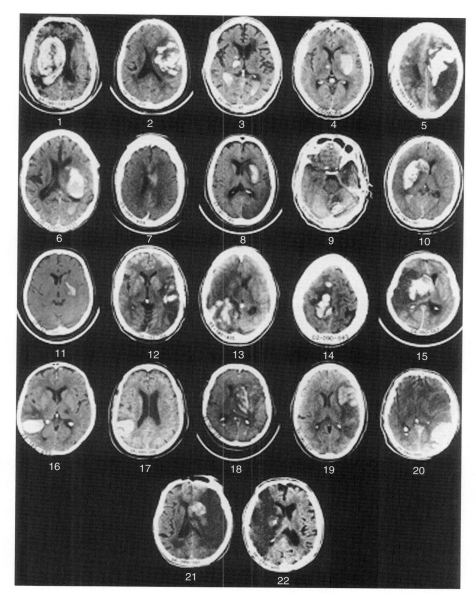

Figure 29-27 CT scans of hemorrhages from the National Institutes of Neurological Diseases and Stroke (NINDS) trial of tissue-type plasminogen activator (t-PA). Cases 1 through 20 are from the t-PA-treated group; cases 21 and 22 are from the control group. (From The NINDS t-PA Stroke Study Group: Intracerebral hemorrhage after intravenous t-PA therapy for ischemic stroke. *Stroke* 28:2109, 1997.)

encephalopathy or myelopathy,[285,286] although ICH has occasionally been the first manifestation of the condition.[287] The hemorrhages have been predominantly lobar in location, and in rare instances, histologic examination of cerebral vessels has shown the association of GANS with CAA,[288,289] which suggests that either vascular lesion could have been responsible for the episode of ICH.

Brain Imaging

The imaging aspects of ICH are discussed in Chapters 45, 46, and 47. This section only briefly highlights developments in this area.

The view that CT is superior to MRI for the diagnosis of acute ICH has been challenged by new observations. With the use of susceptibility-weighted (also known as gradient-echo) MRI sequences, Linfante et al[290] were able to document acute ICHs within periods as short as 30 minutes after symptom onset. Their observations, along with

those of others,[291,292] suggest that in the early phase of ICH, MRI protocols that include susceptibility-weighted sequences are as reliable as CT for diagnosis.

Microhemorrhages

An additional value of these MRI sequences is their ability to document areas of "microhemorrhage," detected as areas of low signal of up to 5 mm in diameter (Fig. 29-29), that correspond to deposits of hemosiderin as a sequelae from past episodes of minor bleeding.[293-295] The importance of these lesions stems from their potential role in instances of major hemorrhage in subjects receiving anticoagulants or after treatment with thrombolysis. The potential association between microhemorrhages and ICH after use of anticoagulants, thrombolytics, and antiplatelet agents is still controversial. Despite anecdotal reports of post-tPA ICH in sites of preexisting microhemorrhages,[296] prospective studies have failed to establish a

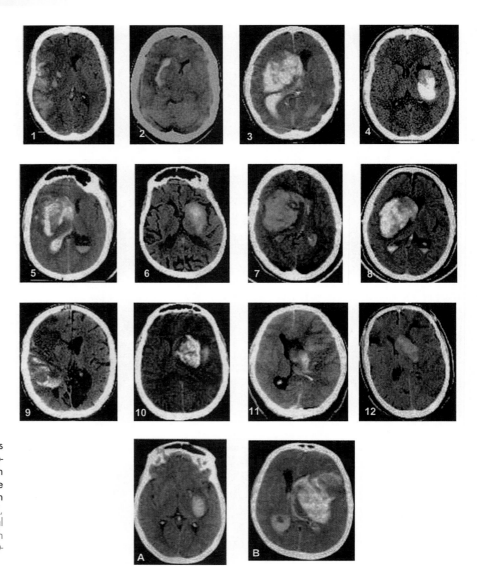

Figure 29-28 CT scans of hemorrhages from the PROlyse in Acute Cerebral Thromboembolism (PROACT) II trial. Cases 1 through 12 are from the recombinant pro-urokinase (r-proUK) group, and cases A and B are from the control group. (From Kase CS, Furlan AJ, Wechsler LR, et al: Symptomatic intracerebral hemorrhage after intra-arterial thrombolysis with prourokinase in acute ischemic stroke: The PROACT II trial. *Neurology 57*:1603, 2001.)

clear association because rates of post-tPA ICH have not differed in subjects with or without microhemorrhages in the baseline imaging studies.[297,298] Similar prospective studies are not currently available to assess the potential relationship between baseline frequency of microhemorrhages and risk of ICH in patients receiving oral anticoagulants. Although the known correlation between microhemorrhages, especially those located in cortical areas, and subsequently increased risk of spontaneous lobar ICH[299] raises a potential concern about the use of oral anticoagulants in patients with a heavy burden of cortical microhemorrhages, the currently available data suggest that a balance between this risk, on the one hand, and the expected benefits in the prevention of ischemic stroke, on the other, should drive this clinical decision in individual patients.[300] Finally, the data on antiplatelet agents (mainly aspirin) use derived from a population-based study in Rotterdam, The Netherlands, indicate that microhemorrhages may be more prevalent in subjects receiving aspirin than in those not receiving this agent,[301] but the relationship between this observation and the frequency of ICH has not been studied prospectively.

Data from a case-control study[302] suggest a relationship between aspirin treatment, microhemorrhages, and risk of ICH, but further prospectively collected data are required before these observations can be applied to clinical decisions in individual patients.

In addition, cerebral microhemorrhages may be markers of arteriopathies with potential for bleeding,[303] such as CAA.[304] Finally, their high prevalence in the aging population, estimated to be on the order of 16% for patients older than 75 years,[305] makes them a likely substrate for bleeding, either by reflecting the presence of CAA or by leading to major ICH in the setting of treatments that involve alterations of the coagulation system or platelet function.

General Clinical and Laboratory Features

The different forms of ICH share a number of clinical features that result from the progressive accumulation of a mass of blood in the parenchyma. These features include mode of onset as well as clinical manifestations reflecting increased intracranial pressure. ICH occurs

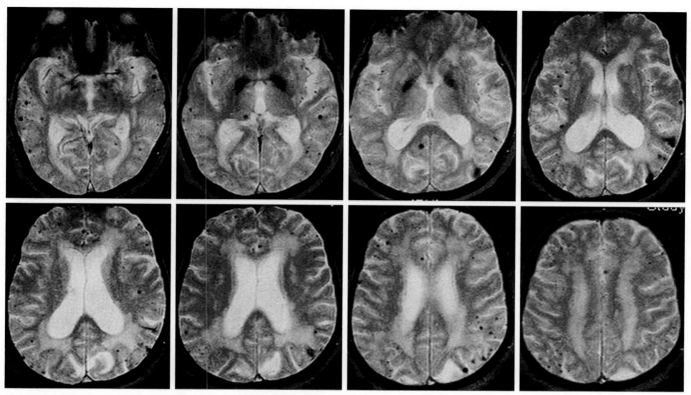

Figure 29-29   MRI, gradient-echo sequence, showing multiple microhemorrhages as small black round images corresponding to hemosiderin deposits. The microhemorrhages predominate in the cortical and subcortical areas in this patient with biopsy-documented cerebral amyloid angiopathy.

characteristically during activity,[55,106] and its onset during sleep is extremely rare.[306] It occurred in only one instance in the series reported by Fisher,[306] and in only 3% of ICH cases included in the NINDS Data Bank.[4] The type of onset, studied in 70 cases of ICH prospectively included in the Harvard Cooperative Stroke Registry, was found to be one of gradual and smooth progression in two thirds of the cases; the deficit was maximal at onset in the remainder.[2] No cases showed a regressive course in the early phase, which supports the clinical dictum that a definite improvement in the early hours of a stroke syndrome rules out ICH.[307] Along with a gradual onset over periods of 5 to 30 minutes, patients with ICH frequently show some decrease in alertness at the time of admission. The frequency and severity of this sign vary to some extent according to the location of the hemorrhage, but when all forms are considered, a decrease in alertness is present in at least 60% of cases[2,135]; in two thirds of them, the decrease is to a level of coma.[2,101] Coma has been correlated with ventricular extension of the hemorrhage,[101,293] large hematoma,[135] and poor vital prognosis.[101,135,308,309]

The clinical features of ICH associated with increased intracranial pressure are headache and vomiting. Although these features also vary widely in frequency with the location of hemorrhage, their overall diagnostic value at the onset of ICH is limited.[2] Of 54 patients alert enough to report the symptom, only 36% reported headache in the study by Mohr et al[2]; in Aring's[310] series, the frequency of headache was 23%. The reporting of vomiting at onset follows similar frequencies: 44%[2] and 22%[310] in two series.

These findings stress the important clinical point that absence of a headache or vomiting does not rule out ICH. On the other hand, when present, these signs suggest ICH (or SAH) as the most likely diagnosis because they are present in less than 10% of ischemic strokes.[2]

Seizures at the onset of ICH are uncommon. They have been reported at rates as low as 7%,[2] 11%,[12] and 14%[310] when all forms of ICH are considered together. In some groups, such as in patients with lobar hemorrhages, seizures have been reported with a frequency as high as 32%.[100]

In the general physical examination, a common abnormality is hypertension, found in as many as 91% of the cases in some series.[2] The high frequency of elevated blood pressure on admission in all forms of ICH correlates with other physical signs indicative of hypertension, such as left ventricular hypertrophy[311] and hypertensive retinopathy.[306] The examination of the ocular fundi in a case of suspected ICH serves the dual purpose of detecting signs of hypertensive retinopathy and allowing careful search for subhyaloid hemorrhages. The latter represent blood collections in the preretinal space, and their presence is virtually diagnostic of SAH[307] because they rarely occur in primary ICH.[137,228,307] Although an occasional case of massive primary ICH does show this sign,[312] its presence has a high correlation with ruptured aneurysm as the cause of the intracranial hemorrhage. The neurologic findings permit the differentiation of the different topographic varieties of ICH (see later).

Communication of the hematoma with the ventricular space accounts for the presence of bloody or xanthochromic

CSF in 70% to 90% of cases.[2,12,101,228,306,310,313] A somewhat lower frequency of bloody CSF (63%) has been reported in hematomas of lobar location,[137] probably reflecting the less frequent communication with the ventricular system[100] due to the subcortical location of the hematoma. The small percentages of cases with clear CSF in all series of ICH reflect hematomas of small size that do not reach the ventricular system even though located close to it. Furthermore, on account of the small size of such hematomas, the clinical presentation may not clearly indicate ICH; signs of increased intracranial pressure may be lacking in such cases, so differentiating them from ischemic strokes is difficult. It is in this particular group of strokes that CT scan has had its most dramatic impact.

In addition to simple inspection of the CSF for bloody or xanthochromic aspect, spectrophotometric CSF analysis can disclose blood products in virtually 100% of cases.[314] However, this technique is not routinely used because the two widely available anatomic means of diagnosis (CT and MRI) have made CSF examination unnecessary in establishing the presence of an ICH. Moreover, the uncommon but well-recognized precipitation of uncal or tonsillar herniation by lumbar puncture in supratentorial ICH[102,307,315] has contributed to the abandonment of this test for the diagnosis of ICH.

The use of angiography in the evaluation of cases of ICH has similarly declined since the introduction of CT and MRI. Angiography most commonly shows the nonspecific signs of mass effect at the site of the hematoma[316] and occasionally has detected extravasation of contrast medium.[317,318] The study by Mizukami et al[319] correlated the angiographic pattern of displacement of the lenticulostriate arteries with functional prognosis in putaminal hemorrhage. Because of the obvious advantages of CT and MRI in disclosing most of the anatomic features of ICH, angiography is now used only in selected instances. Its main role at present is in the evaluation of nonhypertensive forms of ICH, multiple ICHs, and ICHs located in atypical sites, to look for AVM, aneurysm, or tumor as the possible cause of the hemorrhage. Even this role for angiography is steadily diminishing with improvements in noninvasive brain imaging.

Supratentorial Intracerebral Hemorrhage

Most cases of ICH occur in the supratentorial compartment, usually involving the deep structures of the cerebral hemispheres, the basal ganglia, and the thalamus.[2,12,25,99-101] In addition, a substantial number of hemispheral ICHs occur in the subcortical white matter of the cerebral lobes, the so-called lobar hemorrhages.[100,137] These various forms of ICH have distinctive features in terms of clinical presentation, CT aspects, course, and therapy.

Putaminal Hemorrhage

The several clinical subtypes of putaminal hemorrhage, which is the most common form of ICH, are determined by the size and pattern of extension of the hematoma. Each of these variables in turn determines the prognosis. Overall, a mortality of 37% is expected,[135] which is a value

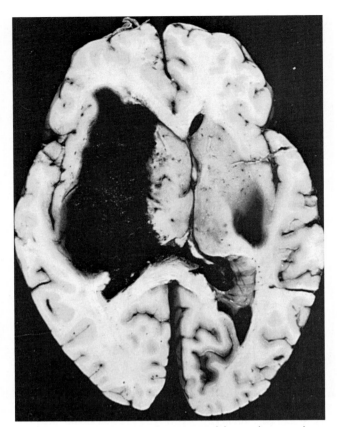

Figure 29-30 Massive right putaminal hemorrhage with ventricular extension. Incidental finding of a small hemorrhage on the posterior corner of the contralateral (left) putamen.

that is far lower than those quoted in the pre-CT literature,[320] which did not include the undiagnosed smaller cases.

The classic presentation of massive putaminal hemorrhage (Fig. 29-30) is with rapidly evolving unilateral weakness accompanied by sensory, visual, and behavioral abnormalities. Headache is common, as is vomiting, within a few hours of onset.[2] Although the onset is abrupt, there is often a gradual worsening of both the focal deficit and the level of consciousness in the following minutes or hours.[306,307] A "maximal from the onset" deficit is uncommon. Whether with sudden or gradual onset, medium-sized or large hematomas are invariably accompanied by a decreased level of alertness correlated with hematoma size. Once the syndrome is well developed, neurologic examination shows a dense flaccid hemiplegia with a hemisensory syndrome and homonymous hemianopia, with global aphasia if the hematoma is in the dominant hemisphere and hemi-inattention if it is in the nondominant hemisphere.[306,307] A horizontal gaze palsy, with the eyes conjugately deviated toward the side of the lesion, is usually found, which can be reversed momentarily by doll's head maneuver or ice-water caloric testing.[309] The pupillary size and reactivity are normal unless uncal herniation has occurred; if it has, signs of an ipsilateral third cranial nerve palsy are present.[306] These abnormalities in oculomotor function have a poor prognosis.[135] Total unilateral motor deficit, coma, and clinical progression after

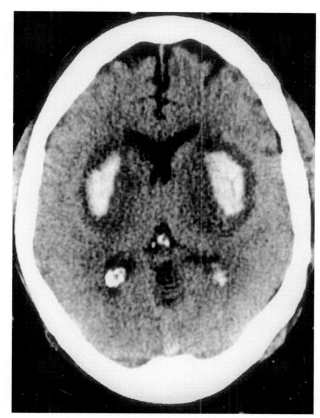

Figure 29-31   CT scan of bilateral, symmetric putaminal hemorrhages in a hypertensive subject. (From Silliman S, McGill J, Booth R: Simultaneous bilateral hypertensive putaminal hemorrhages. *J Stroke Cerebrovasc Dis* 12:44, 2003.)

admission all correlate with large hematoma size and poor functional and vital prognosis, as does ventricular extension of the hematoma by CT scan.[135]

The presence of two hypertensive putaminal hemorrhages, one recent and one old, has been described in pathologic material.[23,36,55,103] The occurrence of simultaneous fresh bilateral putaminal hemorrhages (Fig. 29-31), although occasionally reported,[321] is distinctly uncommon: it was observed in only 2 of 86 cases in Fisher's series[99] and in none of 42 hypertensive ICH cases from the series reported by McCormick and Schochet.[36] Multiple ICHs are rare unless due to bleeding diathesis associated with thrombocytopenia,[99,322] metastatic tumor,[214] or CAA.[323]

Syndromes Due to Small Hemorrhages

The availability of CT and MRI allows the diagnosis of a number of variations in the presentation of small putaminal ICHs, which in the pre-CT era would have been clinically diagnosed as small infarcts. They are as follows:

Pure motor stroke. Instances of pure motor stroke due to small putaminal–capsular hemorrhages have been rarely documented.[324,325] The clinical presentation in such cases has consisted of a mild and transient pure motor syndrome affecting the face and limbs, and the small hematomas originated from the posterior angle of the putamen, with impingement of the posterior limb of the internal capsule. At times, a small capsular hemorrhage

has manifested as pure motor stroke and dysarthria,[326] although the clinical syndrome has been more properly that of a "pure sensory-motor" stroke, related to a component of lateral thalamic compression accompanying the capsular lesion.

Pure sensory stroke. The syndrome of pure sensory stroke, related to thalamic lacunar infarction, has rarely been due to a small putaminal ICH. Three such cases were reported among a group of 152 patients with putaminal ICH.[327] All three patients had posteriorly located putaminal hemorrhages that were adjacent to the posterior limb of the internal capsule and the adjacent thalamus. The clinical syndrome was a contralateral hemisensory syndrome involving both superficial and deep sensory modalities, with more severe involvement of the leg than of the arm and face. The imaging studies demonstrated involvement of the dorsolateral thalamus or the ascending thalamocortical projections located in the posterior ("retrolenticular") portion of the posterior limb of the internal capsule.

Hemichorea–hemiballism. A unilateral dyskinetic syndrome, hemichorea–hemiballism is most commonly due to lacunar infarction in the basal ganglia, thalamus, or subthalamic nucleus but can rarely result from a small putaminal hemorrhage.[328,329] In both series reporting such cases, a right, laterally placed putaminal hemorrhage manifested as contralateral chorea and ballism in the absence of hemiparesis, hemisensory loss, gaze paresis, and hemineglect. The prognosis was excellent in both cases.

Clinical Syndromes in Relationship to the Location of Putaminal Hemorrhage

In a study of 100 patients with putaminal hemorrhage, Weisberg et al[330] established the following clinicoanatomic correlations:

1. *Medial hemorrhages* extended medially from the putamen and involved the genu and posterior limb of the internal capsule. This finding correlated with a contralateral hemisensory syndrome, but there were no abnormalities of ocular motility, visual fields, or level of consciousness. Affected patients generally had full clinical recovery.

2. *Lateral hemorrhages* originated from the lateral putamen and extended anteriorly along the external capsule. They produced a contralateral hemiplegia and sensory deficits. More than half the patients showed delayed neurologic deterioration, and persistent deficits were more common than full recovery.

3. *Putaminal hemorrhages with extension to the internal capsule and subcortical white matter* extended medially through the internal capsule and superiorly into the corona radiata, causing a more severe syndrome of hemiplegia and hemianesthesia, often but not always with homonymous hemianopia and conjugate ocular deviation. Most patients were left with persistent neurologic sequelae.

4. *Putaminal hemorrhages with subcortical and hemispheric extension* were large hematomas that extended into the white matter of adjacent cerebral lobes, causing mass effect on the lateral ventricle and frequently extending into the ventricular system. They

were clinically similar to those of the preceding group, except for having more prominent aphasia or parietal lobe findings and causing impaired consciousness. The mortality rate in this group was 16%, and the majority of the survivors had deficits that interfered with independent living.

5. *Putaminal-thalamic hematomas*, the largest group, extended from the putamen into the thalamus (through the internal capsule) and into the subcortical white matter. They all were accompanied by intraventricular hemorrhage. The clinical picture included impaired consciousness in all patients, frequently associated with hemiplegia, abnormalities of horizontal more than vertical gaze, and homonymous hemianopia. The mortality rate in this group was 79%.

These clinical–CT correlations allowed Weisberg et al[330] to characterize a number of clinically useful patterns as follows: (1) intraventricular hemorrhage was seen with large hematomas, and both features were associated with high mortality rates; (2) all patients had combined motor and sensory deficits; (3) the best functional outcome was seen in patients with medial or lateral putaminal hematomas that did not involve the internal capsule or the corona radiata; and (4) delayed neurologic deterioration occurred only in patients with hematomas that extended into the cerebral hemisphere or the thalamus.

Chung et al[326] analyzed the clinicoanatomic correlations in 192 patients with putaminal hemorrhage. They divided their cases into five anatomic types—middle, posteromedial, posterolateral, lateral, and massive—and related the outcomes to the presumed ruptured arterial branches leading to hematoma formation. The *middle* type (Fig. 29-32) was caused by rupture of medial lenticulostriate arteries, with bleeding into the medial putamen and globus pallidus; the result was a benign syndrome of mild contralateral hemiparesis and hemisensory loss, with a low frequency of impairment of consciousness and with transient conjugate ocular deviation toward the side of the hematoma. Intraventricular extension of the hemorrhage did not occur, and all patients survived. This group of lesions was equivalent to the medial putaminal hemorrhages described by Weisberg et al.[330]

The *posteromedial* type (Fig. 29-33) corresponded to small hematomas confined to the posterior limb of the internal capsule ("capsular" hemorrhages) and were associated with contralateral hemiparesis, hemisensory loss, and dysarthria. The small hematomas, which did not reach the ventricular system, were associated with excellent functional outcome and no mortality. The bleeding vessel in this type of hemorrhage is a branch of the anterior choroidal artery, which supplies a portion of the posterior limb of the internal capsule.[331]

The *posterolateral* type (Fig. 29-34) was a putaminocapsular hemorrhage caused by rupture of posterior branches of the lateral lenticulostriate arteries. These larger hematomas occasionally ruptured into the lateral ventricle and produced a more severe syndrome consisting of impaired consciousness, frequent conjugate ocular deviation toward the affected hemisphere, and constant and generally severe contralateral hemiparesis and hemisensory loss, along with aphasia or hemineglect, depending on hematoma location in the dominant or nondominant hemisphere, respectively.

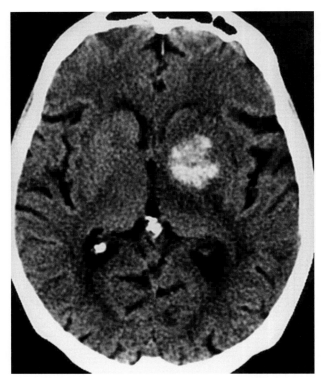

Figure 29-32 CT scan of the medial variety of striatocapsular (putaminal) hemorrhage with minimal mass effect on the frontal horn of the lateral ventricle. (From Chung C, Caplan LR, Yamamoto Y, et al: Striatocapsular haemorrhage. *Brain* 123:1850, 2000.)

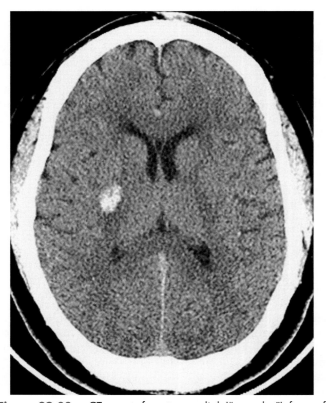

Figure 29-33 CT scan of posteromedial ("capsular") form of putaminal hemorrhage. This small hemorrhage is limited to the posterior limb of the internal capsule.

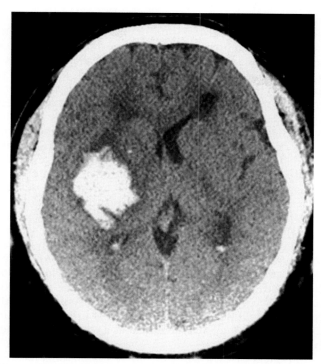

Figure 29-34 CT scan of posterolateral putaminal hemorrhage. Moderate-sized hematoma originating in the posterior putamen, with compression and medial displacement of the posterior limb of the internal capsule but without ventricular extension.

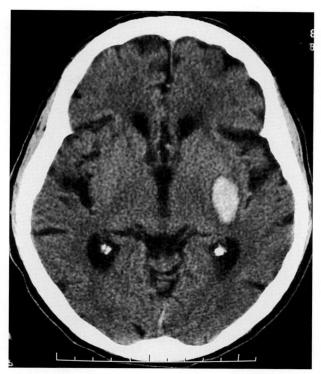

Figure 29-35 CT scan of lateral variety of putaminal hemorrhage. The small lens-shaped hematoma has collected between the insula and the posterior putamen without ventricular extension.

The *lateral* type of hematoma (Fig. 29-35) originated from rupture of the most lateral branches of the lenticulostriate arteries. It remained confined to an elliptical hematoma collected between the putamen and the insular cortex, producing contralateral hemiparesis, often without an associated hemisensory loss but frequently with either aphasia or hemineglect, depending on the side of the brain involved. The outcome was generally excellent, except in cases of large hematomas, which frequently ruptured into the ventricular system and often required surgical treatment, which in turn was generally associated with a good outcome. This lateral type of putaminal ICH in the dominant hemisphere is occasionally the cause of the syndrome of conduction aphasia.[332]

The *massive* type (Fig. 29-36) involved the entire striatocapsular area and probably resulted from rupture of the same branches (posteromedial branches of the lateral lenticulostriate arteries) that cause the posterolateral type of putaminal ICH. Affected patients had a depressed level of consciousness and hemiparesis, frequently associated with ipsilateral conjugate eye deviation, and often progressed to coma with brainstem involvement and death despite treatment with surgical drainage of the hematoma. This group corresponds to the "putaminal-thalamic" group described by Weisberg et al.[330]

In a separate study, Weisberg et al[333] analyzed 14 cases of massive putaminal–thalamic hemorrhage. All of their patients were young black people with hypertension who were seen with headache several hours before the onset of the focal deficit, and all became hemiplegic and comatose over periods of 4 to 12 hours. The hematomas were large, with marked mass effect and intraventricular extension.

All patients died within 72 hours of onset of symptoms despite treatment of hypertension and increased intracranial pressure.

Caudate Hemorrhage

Caudate hemorrhage represents approximately 5% to 7% of cases of ICH (see Table 29-4).[134] Most of the published series on caudate ICH have identified hypertension as the leading cause.[134,334,335] However, other causes not generally associated with deep spontaneous ICH are frequently identified, including cerebral aneurysms,[336] arteriovenous malformations,[168,337] and the basal vascular abnormalities associated with moyamoya disease.[334,338] The last mechanism is thought to lead to ICH through rupture of the anastomotic channels that develop in the area of the basal ganglia, including the head of the caudate, as a result of the progressive occlusion of trunks of the circle of Willis.[339]

The bleeding vessels correspond to deep penetrating branches of the anterior and middle cerebral arteries, which are vessels similar in diameter to those that supply the putamen and thalamus.[340] Because of its paraventricular location, the caudate also receives blood supply from ependymal arteries that flow outward from the ventricular surface into the parenchyma. These arteries originate beneath the ependymal surface as terminal branches of the anterior choroidal artery, posterior choroidal artery, and striatal rami of the middle cerebral artery.[341]

A number of reported cases of spontaneous hemorrhage in the caudate nucleus have delineated a relatively consistent clinical picture.[134,334-336,342,343] The onset has generally been abrupt, with headache and vomiting

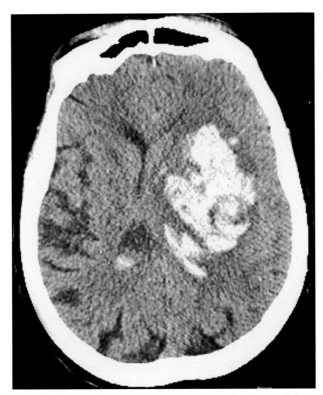

Figure 29-36   CT scan of massive type of putaminal hemorrhage, showing marked mass effect with midline shift and effacement of the lateral ventricle as well as intraventricular extension.

commonly followed by variably decreased level of consciousness, resembling the onset of SAH from aneurysmal rupture. Seizures at onset have been reported rarely[168] and were not encountered in the series of 12 patients reported by Stein et al.[134] Consistent physical findings have included neck stiffness and various types of behavioral abnormalities, of which the latter are most commonly abulia, impairment of memory (both short-term and long-term), and abnormalities of speech, especially verbal fluency.[134,334] These deficits are thought to occur as a result of interruption of cortical–subcortical tracts between the caudate nucleus and the frontal cortex.[334]

The neuropsychological abnormalities of caudate hemorrhage have been described in detail by Fuh and Wang[334] and by Kumral et al.[335] A common pattern is that of presentation with abulia, confusion, and disorientation at onset, followed by the development of a prominent amnestic syndrome, at times accompanied by language disturbances. The latter have most often included a nonfluent aphasia,[335] and occasional examples of transcortical motor aphasia have also been recorded.[331] Hematomas in the nondominant hemisphere generally do not produce unilateral disturbances of attention,[134,331] although one patient reported by Kumral et al[335] developed visuospatial neglect.

In approximately 50% of cases, the common clinical features are accompanied by others, which most often take the form of transient gaze paresis and contralateral hemiparesis and, rarely, features of an ipsilateral Horner's syndrome.[134] The abnormalities described in gaze

mechanisms have most often been horizontal gaze palsies with conjugate deviation or preference toward the side of the hemorrhage, with full correction by oculocephalic maneuvers. Less commonly, vertical gaze palsy has been described, either combined with a horizontal gaze palsy or, more commonly, as an isolated phenomenon. Occasionally, the motor deficit is accompanied by a transient hemisensory syndrome. In those cases in which hemiparesis is a feature, the weakness tends to be slight (never to the point of hemiplegia) and transient, resolving within days of the onset.[134,342] The generally small size and the localized character of caudate hemorrhage are the reasons why focal neurologic deficits such as transient hemiparesis are relatively uncommon (in 30% of the 23 cases studied by Chung et al[326]). The virtually consistent extension into the ventricular system accounts for the high frequency of headache and meningeal signs, which resemble those seen in SAH. Rare instances of bilateral caudate ICH[344] or hemorrhage associated with intraventricular extension with acute hydrocephalus[134] can have a more dramatic presentation, with coma and ophthalmoplegia; the latter is presumably due to oculomotor nuclei involvement as a result of aqueductal dilatation.[345]

In typical cases, a CT scan shows a hematoma located in the area of the head of the caudate nucleus (Fig. 29-37). Ventricular extension into the frontal horn of the ipsilateral ventricle is an invariable feature.[134] In approximately 75% of cases, mild to moderate hydrocephalus of the body and temporal horns of the lateral ventricles has been present.

Hemorrhages that are medium-sized or large are frequently accompanied by transient gaze palsies and hemiparesis, and those accompanied by an ipsilateral Horner's syndrome extend more inferiorly and laterally. Occasionally, the hematomas extend from the region of the head of the caudate nucleus into the anterior portions of the thalamus (Fig. 29-38). In those instances, the clinical syndrome has featured a prominent but transient short-term memory defect.[134] Before the introduction of CT, these cases of caudate ICH with consistent extension into the ventricular system may have been diagnosed as "subarachnoid hemorrhage with negative arteriography" or even as "primary intraventricular hemorrhage."[341] The latter is probably a rare condition,[25] in most instances reflecting a lack of documentation of the parenchymal or meningeal (in cases of ruptured aneurysm) site of origin of the hemorrhage rather than a hemorrhage truly confined to the ventricular space.

Caudate hemorrhage can be separated from putaminal and thalamic hemorrhage clinically and radiographically. Headache, nausea, vomiting, and stiff neck regularly accompany caudate hemorrhage[134] but are less common manifestations in putaminal hemorrhage.[135] Disorders of language are regular features of putaminal and thalamic hemorrhage in the dominant hemisphere,[104,135,346] whereas hemorrhages that remain confined to the caudate nucleus are only rarely associated with aphasia.[335] Furthermore, caudate hemorrhages in the nondominant hemisphere do not cause hemi-inattention and anosognosia, the behavioral abnormalities associated with thalamic[347-349] and putaminal[135] hemorrhages in that hemisphere.

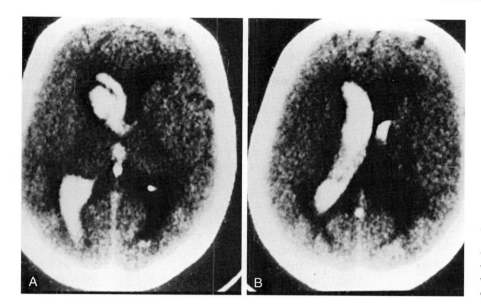

Figure 29-37 A, Hemorrhage originating in the head of the right caudate nucleus with extension into the anterior limb of the internal capsule and into the lateral ventricle and third ventricle. B, Extensive amount of intraventricular blood in the body of the lateral ventricles, primarily on the right side, associated with moderate hydrocephalus.

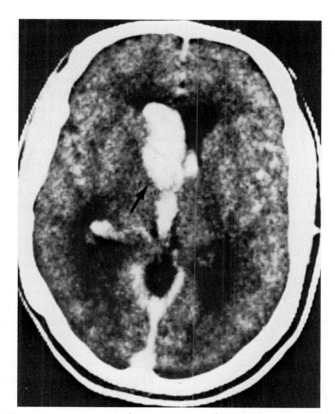

Figure 29-38 Hemorrhage originating from the head of the left caudate nucleus with extension into the anterior-dorsal aspect of the thalamus (arrow), lateral ventricle, and third ventricle.

Caudate hemorrhage must be distinguished from anterior communicating artery aneurysms that bleed into the brain parenchyma. In primary caudate hemorrhage, there is no accumulation of blood in the interhemispheric fissure, and most of the blood is located in the lateral ventricle adjacent to the involved caudate nucleus. In addition, extension of the hemorrhage into the basal frontal region, a feature invariably seen when hemorrhage into the

parenchyma results from ruptured anterior communicating aneurysm, is rarely present in caudate ICH.[134]

The outcome in caudate hemorrhage is usually benign, and most patients recover fully, without permanent neurologic deficits.[134] The accompanying hydrocephalus characteristically tends to disappear as the hemorrhage resolves, and ventriculoperitoneal shunting for persistent hydrocephalus is rarely required.[134] This generally benign outcome in caudate ICH occurs despite the virtually consistent ventricular extension of the hemorrhage.

Thalamic Hemorrhage

The thalamic form of ICH accounts for 10% to 15% of parenchymatous hemorrhages.[2,4,99-101,103,104] Its clinical and pathologic characteristics are well-recognized, and the spectrum of clinical variations reflects the size and pattern of extension of the hematoma. The mass originates in the thalamus and, if it enlarges, extends laterally (into the internal capsule), medially (into the third ventricle), inferiorly (into the subthalamus and dorsal midbrain), upward, and into the parietal white matter.[307,348,350]

The main cause of thalamic hemorrhage is hypertension, which accounts for 74% to 83% of cases.[350-352] Other reported mechanisms are the use of anticoagulant and thrombolytic agents,[353] use of cocaine,[350] rupture of posterior cerebral artery aneurysm,[354] and cavernous malformations.[355] The hemorrhages due to these mechanisms are not clinically different from those caused by hypertension, except for (1) the tendency toward recurrent bleeding in those due to cavernous angioma[355] and (2) the potential for multiple ICHs after use of cocaine[208] and after thrombolysis.[353]

The clinical picture has several distinctive features. They are listed in Table 29-6, which summarizes data from a total of 41 patients in two series.[104,356] A typical mode of presentation features a rapid onset of unilateral sensorimotor deficit, frequent occurrence of vomiting (about half the cases) but a low frequency of headache

TABLE 29-6 CLINICAL FEATURES OF THALAMIC HEMORRHAGE

	Walshe et al[104] (N = 18)	Barraquer-Bordas et al[356] (N = 23)
History		
Age (yr) (mean)	64	68
Headache	22%	30%
Vomiting	77%	48%
Physical findings		
Level of consciousness		
Alert	6%	21%
Drowsy	33%	40%
Stuporous	33%	18%
Comatose	28%	21%
Hemiplegia-hemiparesis	100%	100%
Hemisensory deficit	100%	100%
Homonymous hemianopia	—	18%
Aphasia	4/7*	4
Mutism	1	1
Anosognosia	2/3*	2
Upward gaze palsy	94%	35%
Horizontal ocular deviation		
Toward side of lesion	6	3
Opposite side of lesion	3	6
Pupillary abnormalities		
Miosis	100%	70%
Absence of light reflex	62%	13%
Mortality	50%	39%

*Number of patients with deficit/number of patients tested.

(less than one third of cases). In some, the onset was signaled by coma.[104] A slowly progressive initial course with headache preceding the focal deficits is distinctly uncommon,[307] and only 4 of 13 patients in the series reported by Walshe et al[104] experienced symptoms for 1 to 2 hours before hemiparesis occurred. In a few cases, unilateral sensory symptoms (numbness) precede the onset of hemiparesis and stupor.[104,357]

The physical findings include hemiparesis or hemiplegia in 95% of cases,[104,346,347,356] virtually all of which have an associated severe hemisensory syndrome (see Table 29-6). This syndrome usually appears as a decrease or loss of all sensory modalities over the contralateral limbs, face, and trunk.[352] The severity and distribution of the motor and sensory symptoms are similar to those of putaminal hemorrhage and therefore are not useful differentiating points. Homonymous hemianopia is an uncommon finding and tends to be transient,[102,306] probably reflecting the location of the lateral geniculate body below and lateral to the hematoma. This sign would be expected in large hemorrhages with extrathalamic extension, but these lesions also affect consciousness severely, generally precluding detection of the visual field defect.

The clinical presentation of thalamic hemorrhage has distinctive oculomotor findings. The most characteristic combination is one of upward gaze palsy with miotic, unreactive pupils[102,104,306,357] and elements of Parinaud's syndrome caused when the enlarging mass presses on the upper midbrain. The upward gaze palsy determines the ocular position at rest of conjugate downward deviation, sometimes associated with convergence, as if the eyes were peering at the tip of the nose.[102] In addition, nystagmus retractorius on attempted upward gaze and skew deviation are commonly present.[102,306] Other, less common oculomotor abnormalities reported in thalamic hemorrhage are downward gaze palsy[102,306]; anisocoria with ipsilateral miosis, sometimes associated with palpebral ptosis[306]; transient opsoclonus[358]; and ipsilateral[104,356] or contralateral[356,359] horizontal ocular deviation.

The classic combination of upward gaze palsy with miotic unreactive pupils has high diagnostic value, and it is due to compressive or destructive effects of the thalamic hematoma on the underlying midbrain tectum.[102,306,312,356] The precise anatomic structures involved in these oculomotor abnormalities have been delineated by experimental studies in monkeys[360,361] and a number of observations in humans.[362,363] The experimental observations of Pasik et al[361] established that involvement of the posterior commissure and the "nucleus interstitialis of the posterior commissure" were consistently associated with upward gaze palsy. Areas that were not essential for the development of the gaze palsy included the superior colliculi, the nucleus of Darkschewitsch and the interstitial nucleus of Cajal, and the medial thalamus. Christoff et al,[362,364] from their observations in human clinicopathologic material, concluded that most lesions producing upward gaze palsy required bilateral or midline involvement of the midbrain tectum, particularly when loss of pupillary light reflex was also present.[362] Denny-Brown and Fischer,[360] however, performed unilateral midbrain tegmental lesions in monkeys, which resulted in upward gaze palsy, skew deviation (with the ipsilateral eye in a higher position than the contralateral eye), and head tilt. In addition, after performing unilateral stereotactic lesions of the dorsolateral midbrain tegmentum in humans for the treatment of pain syndromes, Nashold and Seaber[363] recorded symmetrical upward gaze palsy in 13 of 16 subjects. In 10 subjects, downward gaze was also impaired but never without upward gaze palsy. Of their 16 patients, 15 had miotic nonreactive pupils, 11 had convergence paralysis, and 10 showed skew deviation; the ipsilateral eye was in a lower position in two thirds.

In summary, virtually all the oculomotor findings observed in thalamic hemorrhage have been described after unilateral tegmental midbrain lesions in humans. This fact supports the view that the oculomotor findings in this condition are due to compression or extension of the hemorrhage into the midbrain tegmentum. However, other observations suggest that CSF hypertension and hydrocephalus associated with the hemorrhage may play an additional role in the production of the oculomotor findings because ventricular shunting has been shown to reverse these manifestations.[357,365,366] In conclusion, a compressive effect on the tegmental–tectal portion of the midbrain, either directly from unilateral compression by the hematoma or indirectly through hydrocephalus, results in the classic oculomotor and pupillary abnormalities of thalamic hemorrhage.

Contralateral Conjugate Eye Deviation

Some patients with thalamic hemorrhage may show horizontal eye deviation, with or without the characteristic downward deviation at rest. This horizontal eye deviation is more commonly ipsilateral (toward the side of the lesion),[104] as is routinely observed in putaminal hemorrhage, but a contralateral conjugate deviation (toward the side of the hemiplegia) is occasionally observed.[104,356] This eye deviation occurs in the direction opposite that is expected in a supratentorial lesion and is thus labeled the "wrong-way eye deviation."[367] Although this peculiar sign has been recorded in instances of unilateral subarachnoid–Sylvian hemorrhage with frontal and insular extension[368] and in frontoparietal subcortical hematoma,[369] most reported cases have occurred in association with thalamic hemorrhage. The mechanism of the sign is obscure. Postdecussation involvement of horizontal oculomotor pathways by compression by the hematoma at the midbrain level has been suggested, and support exists from autopsy data.[369]

Aphasia in Dominant Hemisphere Thalamic Hemorrhage

Occasionally, left thalamic hemorrhages have been associated with a peculiar form of language disturbance.[104,306,356] The relatively low frequency reported for this disturbance is probably because its detection is restricted to cases of small dominant hemisphere hemorrhages, as large ones are likely to be accompanied by stupor or coma.[366] A detailed analysis of three cases by Mohr et al[346] stressed the main feature of this syndrome: fluctuating performance in language function from almost normal to a profusely paraphasic, fluent speech akin to a delirium. The almost "uncontrollable" character of the paraphasias, in conjunction with intact repetition, led these investigators to postulate the removal by the thalamic lesion of a controlling influence of that structure over the intact cerebral surface speech areas. Similar clinical observations were reported by Reynolds et al,[366] who commented on the frequency of aphasic abnormalities after left stereotactic thalamotomy and suggested that language disorders occurring after acute thalamic lesions may, to some extent, be mediated by disturbances in attention and recent memory.

A study by Alexander and LoVerme[370] involved nine cases of aphasia in left thalamic hematomas, in which the speech profile was a fluent, relatively well-articulated speech with poor naming, relatively good repetition, and prominent paraphasias. These researchers commented on the lack of distinctive features in aphasias from putaminal and thalamic hemorrhages. They also suggested a prominent role for memory and attention deficits in the production of the language disturbances.

Neglect in Thalamic Hemorrhage of the Nondominant Lobe

Syndromes of hemineglect are classically associated with lesions of the nondominant parietal lobe. Other areas, such as the frontal lobe, can rarely give rise to a similar set of symptoms.[371] Among ICHs, those in the putamen can be associated with this syndrome.[135] The occurrence of the syndrome in thalamic hemorrhage is rare. Reports by Walshe et al[104] and Barraquer-Bordas et al[356] each described two patients with anosognosia from right thalamic hemorrhages. Watson and Heilman[347] reported hemineglect in three patients with right thalamic hemorrhages. These patients exhibited prominent anosognosia and hemispatial agnosia, and two of them (cases 1 and 2) showed limb akinesia, manifested as lack of spontaneous movements of the left limbs despite only mild weakness. The patients in this study, particularly the two with limb akinesia, had relatively small thalamic hemorrhages that disrupted sensation only partially in case 1 and affected motor function partially, to a level of weakness only, in cases 1 and 2. In the third patient, a larger hemorrhage was associated with arm paralysis, marked leg weakness, absence of sensation, bilateral Babinski signs, and drowsiness, whereas patients 1 and 2 were alert and cooperative. These three cases illustrated a neglect syndrome similar to that observed in nondominant cortical surface disease, from documented medium-sized and small right thalamic hematomas.

Clinical Syndromes Related to the Topography of Thalamic Hemorrhage

Both Kumral et al[351] and Chung et al[350] delineated the clinical syndromes related to specific areas of involvement of the thalamus by hemorrhage. These two groups divided the thalamic hematomas into anterior, posteromedial, posterolateral, dorsal, and global, and related each location to the presumed arterial rupture within the thalamus.[350] The clinical features of hemorrhages in these various locations were as follows:

Anterior. Hematomas located in the most anterior portion of the thalamus, in the territory of the polar or tuberothalamic artery (Fig. 29-39), are often associated with ventricular extension and are clinically characterized by memory impairment and apathy, preservation of alertness, rare and transient sensory motor deficits, and absence of ophthalmologic findings.

Posteromedial. Posteromedial hemorrhages occur from rupture of thalamoperforating arteries. Hematomas are located in the medial aspect of the thalamus, with frequent rupture into the third ventricle and hydrocephalus, along with extension into the midbrain (Fig. 29-40). Small, localized hematomas result in memory disturbances and behavioral abnormalities, whereas larger lesions with downward extension into the midbrain are associated with early stupor or coma along with severe motor deficits and oculomotor disturbances.

Posterolateral. Posterolateral hemorrhages are due to rupture of thalamogeniculate arteries (Fig. 29-41). They are generally large and commonly extend into the internal capsule and ventricular space. Clinical features are severe sensory motor deficits as well as aphasia or hemineglect. Large hematomas also cause ipsilateral Horner's syndrome, a depressed level of consciousness, and ophthalmologic abnormalities.[351] Approximately one third of patients with posterolateral thalamic hemorrhage reported by Chung et al[350] showed delayed onset of a "thalamic pain syndrome." The aphasia of dominant

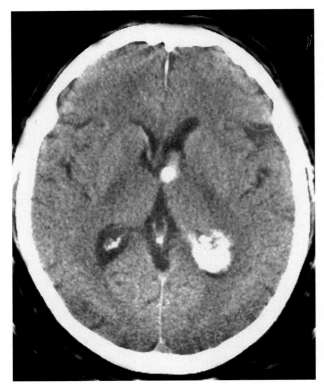

Figure 29-39   CT scan of anterior type of thalamic hemorrhage. Small hematoma confined to the most anterior aspect of the thalamus, with ventricular extension (blood in the atrium of the ipsilateral lateral ventricle).

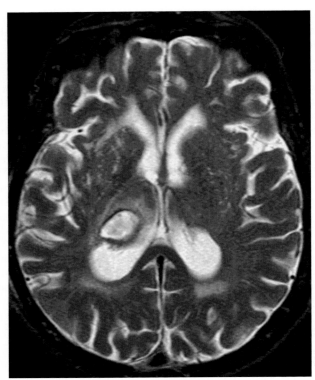

Figure 29-41   T2-weighted MR image of posterolateral form of thalamic hemorrhage, in which hematoma abuts the atrium of the lateral ventricle without ventricular extension.

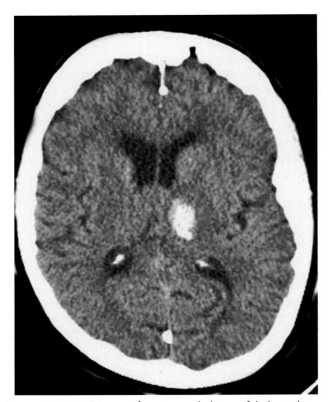

Figure 29-40   CT scan of posteromedial type of thalamic hemorrhage, with small hematoma along the medial aspect of the thalamus that does not extend into the third ventricle.

posterolateral thalamic hematomas has been most often described as "transcortical motor" type,[351,372] although in hematomas of the pulvinar nucleus, the aphasia can be so markedly paraphasic that it becomes jargon.[346] The syndromes of hemi-inattention in nondominant thalamic hemorrhage have included marked anosognosia,[372] in one instance with prominent associated mania,[373] and examples of motor neglect or "inertia" manifested as lack of use of limbs with normal strength.[374]

Dorsal. Rupture of branches of the posterior choroidal artery causes hematomas located high in the thalamus, with frequent extension into the parietal white matter and the ventricular space (Fig. 29-42). They are characterized clinically by mild and transient sensory motor deficits, generally without oculomotor disturbances, with rare confusion and memory abnormalities in hemorrhages located most posteriorly (in the area of the pulvinar nucleus).

Global. The global type corresponds to involvement of the whole thalamus by a large hematoma that commonly enters the ventricular system (with associated hydrocephalus) and extends into the suprathalamic hemispheric white matter (Fig. 29-43). The clinical features are stupor or coma, severe sensory motor deficits, and paralysis of upward more than downward gaze, skew deviation, and small and unreactive pupils.

Unusual Sensory Syndromes

Unusual sensory syndromes are infrequently encountered in thalamic hemorrhage. The best recognized is the *thalamic pain syndrome* described by Dejerine and

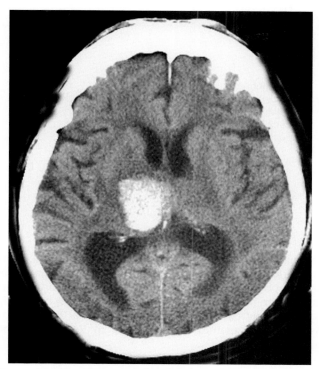

Figure 29-42 CT scan of dorsal thalamic hemorrhage, located in the medial portion of the upper thalamus, without ventricular extension.

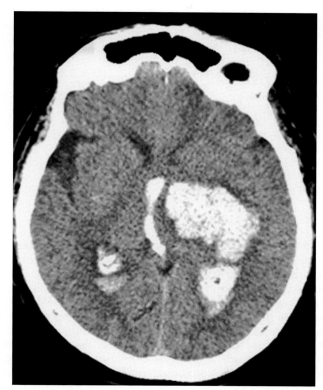

Figure 29-43 CT scan of large, global type of thalamic hemorrhage, with mass effect on the third ventricle and extension into the third and lateral ventricles.

Roussy,[375] which is usually regarded as a feature of thalamic infarction in the distribution of the perforating branches of the posterior cerebral artery.[376,377] The profoundly distressing dysesthesias and spontaneous pain characteristically arise days to weeks after onset. The occurrence of this syndrome after thalamic hemorrhage is variable: Alexander and LoVerme[370] commented on the presence of a central pain syndrome in six of their nine patients with thalamic hemorrhages; Chung et al[350] reported it in one third of their patients with the posterolateral form of thalamic hemorrhage. The relative rarity of this syndrome in the setting of hemorrhage has suggested that partial thalamic lesions of a precise lateral-posterior location are necessary to produce it.[377] This sensory syndrome is an uncommon feature of the usually more massive thalamic destruction due to hematoma.

A second unusual sensory syndrome is a form of *pure sensory stroke*, classically associated with small (lacunar) thalamic infarcts.[378] Small thalamic hemorrhages have occasionally presented as pure sensory stroke.[379-381] Thalamic hematomas of dorsal location have caused a pure hemisensory syndrome, with loss of sensation to pinprick predominating over that of vibration and joint position sense; motor strength was preserved, but coordination in the affected arm was abnormal with the eyes closed, reflecting the "sensory" rather than cerebellar character of the ataxia.[379] Paciaroni and Bogousslavsky[380] reported two patients with involvement of all sensory modalities affecting the face, arm, and leg contralaterally to a small hemorrhage in the center of the thalamus that involved all the ventral nuclei and the parvocellular and dorsocaudal nuclei but sparing the pulvinar. Shintani et al[381]

reported two patients with sensory loss in the arm and leg more than the face, with contralateral lesions in either the ventral-posterior-lateral (VPL) nucleus or the ventral-posterior-medial (VPM) nucleus; another patient with restricted "cheiro-oral" (affecting the hand and the corner of the mouth) dysesthesias with a "burning" quality in the absence of sensory loss to superficial or deep modalities had a small hematoma in the border between the VPL and VPM.

The syndrome of sensory ataxic hemiparesis has also been reported in the setting of small thalamic hemorrhages.[382] The clinical presentation differed from that of lacunar ataxic hemiparesis,[383] in that the ataxia of the patients with hemorrhages corresponded to proprioceptive sensory loss, as opposed to the cerebellar character of the ataxia in lacunar ataxic hemiparesis. The hematomas were small (mean volume, 7.2 mL), were located in the dorsolateral thalamus, and were associated with marked impairment of proprioception but preservation of superficial sensory modalities; the associated hemiparesis was transient and predominated in the leg.

The *CT aspects of thalamic hemorrhage* are shown in Table 29-7. Of interest are the high frequency of ventricular extension (reflecting the location of the hematoma adjacent to the third ventricle) and the resulting high rate (about 25%)[356] of hydrocephalus.

The *mortality rate* reported after thalamic hemorrhage has ranged from 25% to 52%,[350-352] and it is closely correlated to the volume of the hematoma, level of consciousness at presentation, and presence of intraventricular hemorrhage and hydrocephalus.[351,352,384]

TABLE 29-7 CT ASPECTS OF THALAMIC HEMORRHAGE

	Walshe et al[104]	Barraquer-Bordas et al[356]
	(N = 18)	(N = 23)
Side of hematoma Right/left	8/10	17/6
Size of hematoma		
<3.3 cm	11	—
>3.3 cm	7	—
Ventricular extension	66%	50%
Hydrocephalus	27%	21%

TABLE 29-8 LOCATION OF LOBAR ICH

Location	No.	
Frontal	4	
Parietal	3	
Temporoparietal	8	
Parietooccipital	2	18 (82%)
Parietotemporooccipital	1	
Parietofrontal	2	
Occipital	2	
Total	**22**	

ICH, Intracerebral hemorrhage.
From Kase CS, Williams JP, Wyatt DA, et al: Lobar intracerebral hematoma: Clinical and CT analysis of 22 cases. *Neurology* 32:1146, 1982.

When comparing patients with or without intraventricular hemorrhage who were otherwise comparable in regard to clinical features with prognostic significance, Steinke et al[352] found a significantly higher mortality rate for those with intraventricular extension. The finding suggests that this factor is an independent predictor of mortality. In addition, the different locations of hemorrhage within the thalamus have been associated with outcome: anterior and dorsal hematomas had a benign course, whereas posterolateral, posteromedial, and global hemorrhages were associated with higher mortality rates and higher levels of disability.[350] The functional motor outcome in survivors after thalamic hemorrhage is compromised by extension of the hematoma into the internal capsule, midbrain, or putamen. Cognitive impairment as a sequela correlates with initial disturbance of consciousness and ventricular extension of the hematoma.[384] Performance in activities of daily living is influenced by advanced age and hematoma size[384] as well as by the presence of unilateral spatial neglect, aphasia, and severity of paresis of the lower limb.[385]

White Matter (Lobar) Hemorrhage

The main clinical features of lobar hemorrhage were delineated in the last two decades,[57,100,137] and still there are no reliable criteria for a choice of therapy.[133,386]

Anatomy

Lobar hemorrhages occur in the subcortical white matter of the cerebral lobes, usually extending longitudinally in a plane parallel to the overlying cortex. As they become larger, their shape changes into the more common oval or round one. They occur in all cerebral lobes but have a predilection for the parietal, temporal, and occipital lobes (Table 29-8).[100,137] This predilection for the posterior half of the brain in lobar ICH is unexplained and is probably not a reflection of differences in relative lobe size because the ratio of 3:1 between parietotemporooccipital and frontal hematomas[100] is larger than the anatomic volumetric ratio between these two areas, which is 2:1 or 3:2. A possible explanation for this finding is the predilection of intracerebral microaneurysms for the parietooccipital area found by Cole and Yates.[118] These investigators found that the junction of cortical gray matter and white matter contained about 30% of the microaneurysms, and

the diagrams included in their article show a higher concentration of these lesions on the parietooccipital areas and proportionately smaller numbers of them in the frontal and temporal poles. Although the causal relationship between microaneurysms and ICH has not been established, these anatomic correlations in lobar ICH lend some support to it.

Etiology

The etiologic factors in lobar ICH may be somewhat different from those in other forms of ICH, particularly with regard to a less significant role of hypertension.[23,26,100,137,222] Ropper and Davis[137] reported chronic hypertension in only 31% of their cases of lobar ICH, and in the series reported by Kase et al,[100] only 50% of the patients had elevated blood pressure on admission; in half of this group high blood pressure had been documented before the hemorrhage. In Weisberg's[222] study, only 33% of the patients with lobar ICH had hypertension compared with 81% of the patients with deep (ganglionic–thalamic) ICHs. However, data reported by Broderick et al[58] suggest that hypertension contributes to lobar hemorrhage as much as it does to deep hemispheric, cerebellar, or pontine hemorrhages. These authors found hypertension to be the likely explanation of ICH in 67% of their patients with lobar ICHs and in 73% with deep hemispheric, 73% with cerebellar, and 78% with pontine hemorrhages. This predominance of the hypertensive mechanism in lobar ICH remained unchanged with advancing age, which argues against the notion that nonhypertensive mechanisms such as CAA may be the predominant cause of lobar ICH in elderly patients.

Etiologic factors other than hypertension that are relevant in lobar ICH include (1) AVMs, which occur at rates between 7% and 14%, (2) tumors, which occur in 7% to 9%, and (3) blood dyscrasias or anticoagulation, in 5% to 20% of the hemorrhages.[306] There is a large group of patients (22% in one series[100]) in whom the mechanism for ICH remains unknown. This fact raises the possibility that some etiologic factors may exist for white matter (lobar) ICH that are more common than in other forms of ICH. One such factor is CAA, which is being increasingly recognized as the substrate of recurrent, sometimes multiple ICHs in elderly nonhypertensive patients. In this CAA-related category of lobar hemorrhage, O'Donnell et al[98]

TABLE 29-9   COMPARISON OF CLINICAL FEATURES OF LOBAR ICH WITH ALL FORMS OF ICH

Feature	All Forms of ICH (%)*			Lobar ICH (%)*		
	HCSR[2]	Lausanne[388]	Kase et al[100]	Ropper and Davis[137]	Weisberg[387]	SDB[57]
Hypertension						
History	72		22	31	30	55
On admission	91	55†	66	46	56	?
Headache	33	40	61	46	72	60
Vomiting	51	?	33	61	32	29
Seizures	6	7	33	0	28	16
Coma	24	22	18	0.4	?	19

*Percentages rounded to the closest whole number (decimals from the original omitted).
†Not specified whether hypertension was diagnosed by history or at entry examination.
HCSR, Harvard Cooperative Stroke Registry; ICH, intracerebral hemorrhage; SDB, Stroke Data Bank; ?, information not provided.
From Kase CS: Lobar hemorrhage. In Kase CS, Caplan LR, editors: *Intracerebral hemorrhage.* Boston, 1994, Butterworth-Heinemann, p 363.

found that the presence of ε2 or ε4 alleles of the ApoE gene was associated with a high risk of recurrent ICH (28% at 2 years compared with 10% in patients with lobar ICH who did not have the ε2/ε4 alleles). An additional factor that is highly correlated with the risk of lobar ICH recurrence is the presence and number of microhemorrhages detected at the time of presentation with the initial lobar ICH.[299]

Clinical Features

The clinical manifestations of lobar ICH have been extensively analyzed, and a number of differences from other types of ICH have been noted.[57,100,137,387] The circumstances at onset are listed in Table 29-9, which compares series of lobar ICH with those including all forms of ICH.[2,57,100,137,387-389] The distinguishing features of lobar ICH are lower frequency of hypertension and coma on admission and higher frequency of headache and seizures. The higher frequency of headache at onset may reflect the larger number of patients with lobar ICH who are awake and can give a history. Ropper and Davis[137] described the headaches as located in and around the ipsilateral eye in occipital hematomas, around the ear in temporal hemorrhages, anteriorly in frontal hemorrhage, and anterior temporal (temple) in parietal lobe hematomas. The low incidence of coma on admission in lobar ICH is probably related to the peripheral location of the hematoma, at a distance from midline structures.[137]

Seizure as a common event at the onset of lobar ICH has been well-documented.[57,100,387,390-394] The mechanism of seizures in lobar hematomas may reflect the location of the hemorrhage in the gray matter–white matter interface, which creates a situation similar to the surgical isolation of cortex by subcortical injury that results in sustained paroxysmal activity from the isolated cortex.[395]

The neurologic deficits seen with lobar ICH depend on the location and size of the hematoma.[137] They include (1) sudden hemiparesis, worse in the arm, with retained ability to walk, in frontal hematoma, (2) combined sensory and motor deficits, the former predominating, and visual field defects in parietal hemorrhage, (3) fluent paraphasic speech with poor comprehension and relative sparing of repetition in left temporal lobe hematomas, and (4) homonymous hemianopia, occasionally accompanied by mild sensory changes (extinction to double simultaneous stimulation), in occipital lobe hemorrhages. In the group of 24 patients described by Kase et al,[100] hemiparesis and visual field defects were the most common abnormality, found in 60% and 30% of patients who were not comatose on admission, respectively. Those patients in whom the two signs coexisted had larger and more anteriorly placed hematomas, whereas those with hemianopia and no hemiparesis had posterior hemorrhages. From these data, the clinical presentation in a lobar parietooccipital hematoma emerges as sudden onset of headache, sometimes associated with vomiting, not uncommonly associated with seizure activity, with state of consciousness in the alert or obtunded level, associated with mild contralateral hemiparesis and visual field defect. Specific deficits in speech or spatial function are seen when the hematomas are of dominant frontotemporal or nondominant parietal location, respectively, mimicking the deficits seen with infarction.[396,397]

Cerebral Amyloid Angiopathy and Lobar Hemorrhage

The best recognized clinical manifestation of CAA is spontaneous ICH. The hemorrhages largely follow the distribution of the vascular amyloid, appearing with highest frequency in the corticosubcortical or lobar regions and less commonly in cerebellum, generally sparing the brainstem and deep hemispheric structures.[46,51] Lobar ICH in CAA is more likely to dissect into the subarachnoid space than into the lateral ventricles.[46,398,399] Despite extensive involvement of the leptomeningeal vessels, symptomatic subarachnoid hemorrhage due to CAA is rare.[398,400]

CAA-related lobar ICH presents much like other types of lobar ICH,[389] with early onset of neurologic symptoms and a variable combination of headache, seizures, and decreased consciousness according to hemorrhage size and location. Hemorrhagic lesions in CAA can also be small and clinically silent.[64] These small corticosubcortical "microbleeds" are well-visualized by gradient-echo or T2*-weighted MRI techniques, which enhance the signal dropout associated with deposited hemosiderin.[401] By detecting even old hemorrhagic lesions, gradient-echo MRI provides a clinical method for demonstrating an individual's lifetime history of hemorrhage and thus for identifying the pattern of multiple lobar lesions characteristic of CAA (Fig. 29-44). CAA-related microbleeds, like symptomatic "macrobleeds," occur typically in corticosubcortical locations[54] or at the superficial cortical surface.[55]

The Boston criteria for CAA codify the typical features of CAA-related ICH into the diagnostic categories "definite," "probable," and "possible" disease, as listed in Table 29-10.[54,402] Although diagnosis of definite CAA requires demonstration of advanced disease through postmortem examination, a clinical diagnosis of probable CAA can be reached during life through radiographic demonstration of at least two strictly lobar or corticosubcortical hemorrhagic lesions (either large symptomatic macrobleeds or smaller microbleeds) without other definite hemorrhagic process. In a small clinical-pathologic validation study, 13 of 13 subjects given a clinical diagnosis of probable CAA also had pathologic evidence of CAA,[402] which suggests that the criteria may be sufficiently specific to be useful in practice. In the same study, gradient-echo MRI detected the diagnostic pattern in 8 of 11 patients (73%) with pathologically documented CAA, providing an estimate for the sensitivity of the diagnosis. The Boston criteria propose a separate category of *probable CAA with supporting pathology* for patients with lobar ICH and an antemortem brain sample containing evidence of CAA (see Table 29-10). A validation study for this diagnosis suggested that CAA of at least moderate severity in a random tissue sample was a reasonably specific marker for severe CAA in the brain as a whole.[45]

For reasons that are poorly understood, CAA pathology[56,57] and CAA-related hemorrhagic lesions localize preferentially to posterior (parietooccipital or temporooccipital) cortical brain regions. In a study of 321 macrobleeds and microbleeds detected by gradient-echo MRI among 59 subjects with probable CAA, 26.5% of the lesions were in occipital cortex and 30.5% were in temporal cortex, which was significantly greater than the proportions (18.3% and 22.3%, respectively) predicted by the volumes of these cortical regions.[54] The posterior predilection of CAA has been further corroborated by the distribution of the amyloid-ligand Pittsburgh Compound B detected by positron emission tomographic imaging in subjects with probable CAA but without dementia.[27,58]

Prognosis for Lobar Hemorrhage

The prognosis in lobar hematomas is usually less grave than in other forms of ICH. The mortality rates reported have been between 11.5% and 29%,[100,137,222,403] all of which are lower than the rates for the other varieties of ICH. A low frequency (6%) has been reported in an autopsy series,[103] whereas in clinical series, the frequency

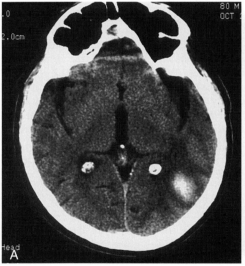 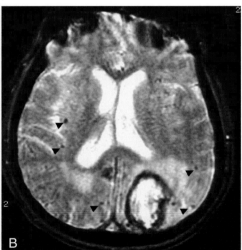

Figure 29-44 Recurrent intracerebral hemorrhage (ICH). A, The CT scan shows a left temporal ICH in an 80-year-old man with a history of previous cognitive decline. B, A gradient-echo MRI sequence obtained 2 years later demonstrates recurrent ICH in the left parietal lobe as well as multiple punctate hypointense lesions *(arrowheads)* consistent with chronic asymptomatic hemorrhages. The presence of two or more strictly lobar hemorrhagic lesions is consistent with a diagnosis of probable cerebral amyloid angiopathy (see Table 29-10).

TABLE 29-10 BOSTON CRITERIA FOR DIAGNOSIS OF CAA–RELATED ICH

Definite CAA	Full postmortem examination of brain shows lobar ICH, severe CAA (see ref 67), and no other diagnostic lesion
Probable CAA with supporting pathology	Clinical data and pathologic tissue (evacuated hematoma or cortical biopsy specimen) showing some lobar CAA in pathologic specimen, and no other diagnostic lesion
Probable CAA	Clinical data and MRI or CT demonstration of two or more hemorrhagic lesions restricted to lobar regions (cerebellar hemorrhage allowed), patient age ≥55yr, and no other cause of hemorrhage*
Possible CAA	Clinical data and MRI or CT demonstration of single lobar ICH, patient age ≥55yr, and no other cause of hemorrhage*

*Other causes of ICH defined as excessive anticoagulation (INR > 3.0), antecedent head trauma or ischemic stroke, CNS tumor, vascular malformation or vasculitis, blood dyscrasia or coagulopathy. INR > 3.0 or other nonspecific laboratory abnormalities permitted for diagnosis of *possible* CAA.
CAA, Cerebral amyloid angiopathy; CNS, central nervous system; CT, computed tomography; ICH, intracerebral hemorrhage; INR, international normalized ratio; MRI, magnetic resonance imaging.

is between 10% and 32%.[100,137,222] In addition, the functional outcome for survivors is generally better than in those with deep hemispheric ICHs; a good outcome was reported in 57% to 85% of patients.[403-405]

Computed Tomography Aspects

After the early phase of the ICH, lobar hematomas can adopt a number of residual patterns, as analyzed by Sung and Chu.[406] Frequently (27% of the time), the ICH leaves no CT-demonstrated residual, although a slit and a round cavity (34%) are the most common CT sequelae; rarely (3%), only calcification at the ICH site remains.

Ropper and Davis[137] provided two-dimensional measurements of 26 hematomas and commented on the tendency of these lesions to enlarge mostly in the transverse and anteroposterior planes of the CT section. In Weisberg's[222] series of 45 patients with lobar ICH, 10 were found to have intraventricular extension, a factor that did not affect the mortality rates in this group.

The CT features of the 22 cases reported by Kase et al[100] are shown in Table 29-11. The hematomas could be divided by volume into three main groups, which in turn correlated with the presence and severity of mass effect. Ventricular extension was a factor that correlated with location (proximity to ventricular system) rather than size of the hematoma. The outcome was in part a function of hematoma size; no patient with a hematoma larger than 60 mL survived, whereas all those with small hematomas (<20 mL) did. In the group with moderate-sized hematomas, 75% survived, and the functional level was, in general, poorer than in the group with small hematomas. These figures, in addition, give some indication of the possible role of surgical drainage as a therapeutic option in lobar ICH. Writers of some studies of lobar ICH have stated that surgery offers no advantage over medical therapy,[137,407] whereas results of the uncontrolled study reported by Kase et al[100] suggested a trend toward better outcome after surgery. Surgery as a possible option for lobar hematomas is further encouraged by the superficial location of the hemorrhage, which makes it more easily accessible.[408] This form of therapy is particularly indicated in patients with medium-sized or large hematomas who show signs of progressive neurologic deterioration after diagnosis.[25,100,409]

Flemming et al[410] have further analyzed the surgical management of lobar ICH. In a review of 61 patients, they found neurologic deterioration after admission in 16 patients (26%), and predictors of a deteriorating course were a decreased level of consciousness, ICH volume greater than 60 mL, and CT signs of mass effect. The main cause of neurologic decline was hematoma enlargement. These data further strengthen the view that early aggressive management, including hematoma evacuation, should be considered in patients with lobar ICH who meet the preceding criteria. In a subsequent analysis of Mayo Clinic data, Flemming et al[411] reported observations on 81 patients with lobar ICH. Volume larger than 40 mL on CT was associated with poor outcome; in patients with hemorrhage smaller than 40 mL, interval from symptom onset to hospital presentation of less than 17 hours and a Glasgow Coma Scale (GCS) score of 13 or less were predictive of a poor outcome. These data stress the importance of hematoma enlargement as a factor in the deterioration of patients who are seen early after onset of lobar ICH.

A more definitive assessment of the value of surgical drainage of lobar hematomas is likely to come from the results of the Surgical Trial in Intracerebral Haemorrhage (STICH). The initial STICH trial[412] compared surgical with nonsurgical treatment of patients with lobar or deep ICHs in a randomized multicenter international study and detected no differences among groups when the intervention occurred within 4 days from ICH symptom onset. In a prespecified subgroup analysis, a trend favorable to surgical treatment was observed for patients with lobar hemorrhages located at 1 cm or less from the cortical surface. Based on this observation, a second trial (STICH II) will include patients with lobar ICHs located within 1 cm from the cortical surface, without associated intraventricular hemorrhage (a factor that was highly correlated with poor prognosis in the initial STICH trial) and with hematoma volumes of 10 to 100 mL, who will be randomly assigned to hematoma evacuation within 48 hours from symptom onset versus nonsurgical treatment. This study will hopefully clarify the role of hematoma removal in this subgroup of patients with lobar hemorrhage.

Hemorrhage Affecting the Brainstem and Cerebellum

Cerebellar Hemorrhage

In a landmark article in 1959, Fisher et al[106] described the main clinical features of cerebellar hemorrhage. Especially important diagnostic features were the inability to walk, gaze palsy without hemiplegia, and the absence of unilateral limb paresis. These investigators found that surgical decompression could be lifesaving, occasionally even in patients in deep coma before surgery. More

TABLE 29-11 COMPUTED TOMOGRAPHY FEATURES AND OUTCOME OF LOBAR INTRACEREBRAL HEMATOMAS

Hematoma Size	No. of Cases	Midline Shift	Ventricular Extension	Outcome/Operated
Small (<20 mL)	5	1	0	5 improved/0
Moderate (20–40 mL)	7	6	1	6 improved/3 1 died/0
Massive (>40 mL)	10	10	7	4 improved/2 6 died/1
Total	22	17	8	

From Kase CS, Williams JP, Wyatt DA, et al: Lobar intracerebral hematomas: Clinical and CT analysis of 22 cases. *Neurology* 32:1146, 1982.

important, patients who had been treated surgically were often able to return to active lives without the overwhelming disability often retained by survivors of basal ganglionic hemorrhages. Although these diagnostic formulations were initially subject to dispute, CT scanning and MRI have made the detection of smaller cerebellar hematomas possible,[413,414] essentially confirming the initial observations of Fisher et al.[106]

Cerebellar hemorrhage appears at a rate variously quoted as between 5% and 15%.[99,105,415-418] The average rate is about 10%, which is also approximately the percentage of brain weight accounted for by the cerebellum. Although 10% is a relatively low frequency, the importance of establishing the diagnosis resides in the good prognosis after prompt surgical treatment.[99,228,419] Cerebellar hemorrhage usually occurs in one of the hemispheres, generally originating in the region of the dentate nucleus, from distal branches of the superior cerebellar artery[106] or occasionally the posterior-inferior cerebellar artery.[196] In the study by Fisher et al,[106] the left hemisphere was affected twice as often as the right. McKissock et al[420] also commented on a left hemisphere preponderance in cerebellar hemorrhage. Most other series do not report hemorrhage laterality.

The hematoma collects around the dentate and spreads into the hemispheral white matter, commonly extending into the cavity of the fourth ventricle as well (Fig. 29-45). The adjacent brainstem (pontine tegmentum) is rarely involved directly by the hematoma but is often compressed by it, which, at times, leads to pontine necrosis. The midline variant of cerebellar hemorrhage originates from the vermis and represents only about 5% of the cases.[106] It virtually always communicates directly with the fourth ventricle through its roof and frequently extends into the pontine tegmentum bilaterally (Fig. 29-46). The bleeding vessel in this variety corresponds to distal branches of the superior or the posterior-inferior cerebellar artery. These two forms of cerebellar hemorrhage have distinctive clinical and prognostic features.

Distribution of etiologic factors in cerebellar hemorrhage is similar to that in other forms of ICH, and hypertension is the leading cause.[106,228] AVMs are said to be common in the cerebellum[417,420]: they accounted for 5 of 15 cerebellar hematomas in the autopsy series reported by McCormick and Rosenfield[26]; in other series,[228] lower rates of AVMs (4%), similar to those for ICH at other sites, have been reported.[137] Anticoagulation is an important etiologic factor in cerebellar hemorrhage and was the second most common cause reported by Ott et al.[228] Among 24 ICHs in patients undergoing oral anticoagulation therapy,[226] nine occurred in the cerebellum. Three of these were of the less common vermian or midline variety. Fisher et al[106] commented on a relative female preponderance in their series (13:8); in other series, the female-to-male ratio was reported as 26:30,[420] 6:6,[105] 5:14,[421] and 17:17.[420]

Symptoms usually develop while the patient is active. Occasionally a single prodromal episode of dizziness or facial numbness may precede the hemorrhage. The most common symptom is *an inability to stand or walk*, which in many patients has been dramatic in onset. One man leaned against a fence while painting and could not right himself; another bumped downstairs on his bottom to call for help. Crawling or propelling oneself prone on the floor to get to the bathroom to vomit has been mentioned. Rare patients maintain their ability to walk a few steps, but scarcely any patient with a sizable hemorrhage (>2 cm) walks into the emergency room or physician's office.

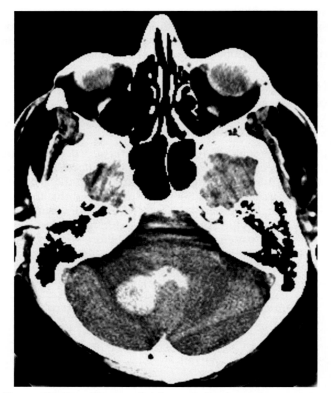

Figure 29-45 CT scan of right cerebellar hemorrhage originating in the area of the dentate nucleus, with extension into the adjacent fourth ventricle.

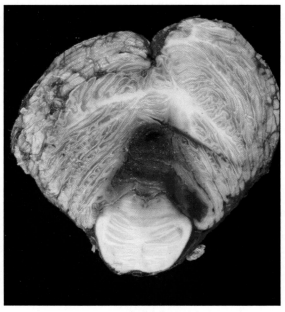

Figure 29-46 Vermian cerebellar hemorrhage with pressure on the pontine tegmentum.

Vomiting is also very common, being present in 42 of 44 patients,[228] 12 of 12 patients,[419] and 14 of 18 patients[106] in various series. Vomiting usually occurs soon after the onset in cerebellar and subarachnoid hemorrhage but often develops later, after other symptoms, in putaminal hemorrhage. *Dizziness* is also common, occurring in 24 of 44 patients,[228] 8 of 21 patients,[106] and 4 of 12 patients[419] in various series. More often the feeling is one of insecurity, a "drunken feeling," or wavering rather than true rotational vertigo.

Headache is also very common, occurring in 32 of 44 patients,[228] 10 of 21 patients,[106] and 12 of 12 patients[105] in various series. Most often the pain is occipital, but occasionally it can occur on the side of the head or frontally. At times the headache is abrupt and excruciating, closely mimicking SAH. In other patients the pain is located primarily in the neck or shoulder. Dysarthria, tinnitus, and hiccups occur but are less common. Loss of consciousness at onset is unusual,[228,422] and only one third of patients are obtunded by the time they reach the hospital.[228] Most patients show gradual worsening over 1 to 3 hours, as in other forms of ICH.[2]

The classic physical findings are a combination of a unilateral cerebellar deficit with variable signs of ipsilateral tegmental pontine involvement. These are detailed in Table 29-12, from an analysis of 38 noncomatose patients in the series reported by Ott et al.[228] Appendicular and gait ataxia occurred in 65% and 78%, respectively, of patients who were alert enough to cooperate for cerebellar function testing. Other patients lean to the side when placed upright. On the side of the hemorrhage, there usually is overshoot or inability to brake the limb quickly; this sign is more common than finger-to-nose or finger-to-object ataxia. Signs of involvement of the ipsilateral pontine tegmentum include peripheral facial palsy, ipsilateral horizontal gaze palsy, sixth cranial nerve palsy, depressed corneal reflex, and miosis. In some patients the hemorrhage presses laterally in the area of the cerebellopontine angle, producing peripheral facial palsy, deafness, and diminished corneal response.

From analysis of the relative frequency of signs in noncomatose patients reported by Ott et al,[228] a characteristic triad consisting of appendicular ataxia, ipsilateral gaze palsy, and peripheral facial palsy was suggested; at least two of the three signs were present in 73% of the patients tested for all three. Ocular skew deviation is also common.[415] Additional findings useful in differential diagnosis are hemiplegia and subhyaloid hemorrhages, both of which are uncommon enough in cerebellar hemorrhage that their presence essentially rules out the diagnosis.[228] The frequency of unilateral limb weakness in cerebellar hemorrhage has been a matter of controversy. In the study by Fisher et al,[106] hemiplegia was observed only in the setting of a prior stroke, and similar findings were recorded by Ott et al.[228] In two autopsy series, however, hemiplegia was reported in 50% and 20% of the cases,[417,419] and Richardson[418] noted contralateral hemiplegia in more than 50% of cases in his clinical series. Although in some instances reports of ipsilateral hemiplegia may have corresponded to decreased mobility of grossly ataxic limbs or decreased spontaneous movement, a contralateral hemiplegia cannot be explained on those bases, so one must assume involvement of the corticospinal tract in the ipsilateral basis pontis.

Other neurologic findings add little specific diagnostic data: the pupils are commonly small and reactive to light, dysarthria is present in two thirds of cases, and the respiratory rhythm is usually unaffected.[228] Unilateral involuntary eye closure has been occasionally observed,[367,423] the involved eye usually being contralateral to the hematoma. This sign has been interpreted as eye closure for avoidance of diplopia, but this interpretation is probably not always correct because the sign occurs in the absence of diplopia, in both infratentorial and supratentorial strokes.[367] Other less common oculomotor abnormalities, such as ocular bobbing, have occasionally been reported in cerebellar hemorrhage[228,424,425] but with a lower frequency than in pontine hemorrhage and infarction. Some patients have a head tilt. Neck stiffness and unwillingness to move the head or neck either actively or passively probably signify increased pressure in the posterior fossa.

Along with these focal neurologic manifestations, patients with cerebellar hemorrhage may be seen with variable levels of decreased alertness. Of the 56 cases reported by Ott et al,[228] 14 (25%) were alert, 22 (40%) were drowsy, 5 (9%) were stuporous, and 15 (26%) were comatose. That two thirds of the patients are responsive (alert or drowsy) on admission justifies the intensive efforts to diagnose this condition early because the surgical prognosis largely depends on the preoperative level of consciousness.

The clinical course in cerebellar hemorrhage is notoriously unpredictable: some patients who are alert or drowsy on admission can deteriorate suddenly to coma and death without warning,[106,228,426] whereas others with similar clinical status have an uneventful course with complete recovery of function. Of those patients who were not comatose on admission, only 20% had a smooth,

TABLE 29-12 NEUROLOGIC FINDINGS IN CEREBELLAR HEMORRHAGE FOR NONCOMATOSE PATIENTS

Neurologic Finding	No.	%
Appendicular ataxia	17/26	65
Truncal ataxia	11/17	65
Gait ataxia	11/14	78
Dysarthria	20/32	62
Gaze palsy	20/37	54
Cranial nerve findings		
Peripheral facial palsy	22/36	61
Nystagmus	18/35	51
Miosis	11/37	30
Decreased corneal reflex	10/33	30
Abducens palsy	10/36	28
Loss of gag reflex	6/30	20
Skew deviation	4/33	12
Trochlear palsy	0/36	—
Hemiparesis	4/35	11
Extensor plantar response	23/36	64
Respiratory irregularity	6/28	21
Nuchal rigidity	14/35	40
Subhyaloid hemorrhage	0/34	—

From Ott KH, Kase CS, Ojemann RJ, et al: Cerebellar hemorrhage: Diagnosis and treatment. *Arch Neurol* 31:160, 1974.

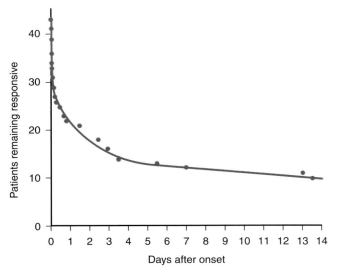

Figure 29-47 Coma in patients with cerebellar hemorrhage as a function of time after onset. (From Ott KH, Kase CS, Ojemann RG, et al: Cerebellar hemorrhage: Diagnosis and treatment. *Arch Neurol* 31:160, 1974.)

uneventful recovery in the series reported by Ott et al[228]; 80% deteriorated to coma, and in one fourth of them, this occurred within 3 hours of onset (Fig. 29-47). A similar frequency was observed in the study by Fisher et al,[106] in which only 2 of 18 patients had a benign course; the other 16 deteriorated to coma at variable intervals, mostly within a few hours after onset. Most patients deteriorate early in the course, but occasional patients have shown fatal decompensation at a later stage, even a month later, after being stable in the interim.[427]

Because prediction of the clinical course cannot be made on the basis of clinical variables on admission, Ott et al[228] recommended that surgical evacuation of the hematoma should be undertaken whenever the diagnosis is made within 48 hours of onset.[228] They justified the need for prompt diagnosis and emergency surgery by pointing to poor surgical outcome with worsening preoperative mental status: the surgical mortality was 17% for responsive and 75% for unresponsive patients.[228] These figures have proved generally accurate, despite occasional reports of good surgical results in comatose patients.[428]

The use of CT and MRI in cerebellar hemorrhage has permitted the recognition of many different aspects of these lesions, some of which are useful early predictors of clinical course.[413,414,429] Little et al[413] reported two groups of patients with cerebellar hemorrhage: one group had abrupt onset, a more severely depressed level of consciousness, and a tendency toward progressive deterioration, and the other had a more benign, stable course. The first group required surgical treatment, whereas the second group did well with a medical program. CT scans of the first group showed hematomas 3 cm or more in diameter, obstructive hydrocephalus, and ventricular extension of the hemorrhage; in the second group of patients, all of whom had hematomas less than 3 cm in diameter, the other two features were absent. These observations, along with those of others,[430] have identified a group of cerebellar hemorrhages with a benign course. It may be

possible to make accurate predictions from the combined analysis of clinical and CT data at the time of onset. Especially important is careful monitoring of the status of the patient. The development of obtundation and extensor plantar responses is ominous and is virtually always followed by a fatal outcome unless surgery is performed.

In an attempt to identify predictors of neurologic deterioration, St. Louis et al[426] analyzed a series of 72 patients with cerebellar hemorrhage. For the 33 patients (46%) with deterioration, independent predictors of such a course were a vermian location of the hemorrhage and hydrocephalus. On the basis of these data, St. Louis et al[426] suggested that patients with these features are likely to require neurosurgical treatment. The same group analyzed clinical factors predictive of poor outcome in a group of 94 patients. Poor outcome was predicted by admission systolic blood pressure higher than 200 mm Hg, hematoma diameter more than 3 cm, brainstem distortion, and acute hydrocephalus, and death was predicted by abnormal brainstem reflexes (corneal and oculocephalic), GCS score less than 8, acute hydrocephalus, and intraventricular hemorrhage.[431]

Kirollos et al[432] have made further refinements in the approach to the treatment of cerebellar hemorrhage. They evaluated 50 consecutive patients and used the level of mass effect in the fourth ventricle (graded as absent, compression, or complete obliteration), size of hematoma, GCS score, and hydrocephalus as the variables correlated with type of management and outcome. Their findings indicated that patients with an obliterated fourth ventricle, even if conscious on admission, had a high rate of subsequent neurologic deterioration (43%) and that surgical treatment with posterior fossa craniectomy for clot evacuation was recommended before these patients experienced neurologic deterioration. Of interest, 60% of subjects in whom hematoma diameter was more than 3 cm but who had only moderate compression or normal size of the fourth ventricle did not require surgery for clot evacuation.

The uncommon midline (vermian) cerebellar hematoma still represents a serious diagnostic challenge, and its outcome is generally poor. Its frequency in autopsy series has been 6% of all cerebellar hemorrhages.[105] Our experience has documented syndromes featuring relatively early onset of coma, ophthalmoplegia, and respiratory abnormalities, and the severity of bilateral limb weakness has been variable. Early extension of the vermian hematoma into the midline pontine tegmentum is probably responsible for the abrupt onset of coma and bilateral oculomotor signs (Fig. 29-48). This variant of cerebellar hematoma carries a poor prognosis, similar to that of primary pontine hemorrhage. At times, a relatively small hematoma in this location results in fatal brainstem compression.

Midbrain Hemorrhage

Spontaneous, nontraumatic mesencephalic hemorrhage is rare. In most instances the hemorrhage has dissected down from the thalamus or putamen, is part of a lesion originating in the cerebellum or pons, or arises from blood dyscrasias or AVMs.

Mesencephalic AVMs generally produce a stepwise progressive deterioration. Ataxia and ophthalmoplegia

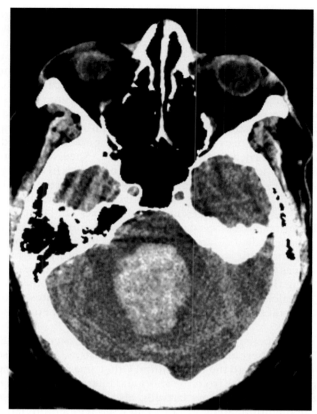

Figure 29-48   CT scan of large midline (vermian) cerebellar hemorrhage with extension into the fourth ventricle and compression of the tegmentum of the pons.

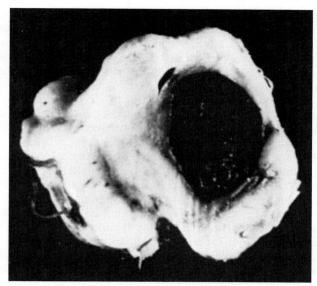

Figure 29-49   Midbrain hemorrhage in a patient with bleeding diathesis.

(especially third cranial nerve palsy and paralysis of upward gaze) are common. Aqueductal or third ventricular blockage or distension often leads to hydrocephalus. Bleeding diathesis can lead to isolated midbrain hemorrhage, as shown in Figure 29-49, a brain tissue specimen from an elderly woman with leukemia in whom a third cranial nerve palsy and contralateral intention tremor developed shortly before death. Hypertensive primary mesencephalic hemorrhage is very rare but does occur. One might predict that the hemorrhage would be in the tegmentum in the territory supplied by branches of the superior cerebellar arteries, as in the hypertensive patients reported by several groups.[433-435] The details of these cases follow.

Durward et al[434] described two patients with mesencephalic hematomas. Their first patient was a 71-year-old hypertensive man (blood pressure 230/130 mm Hg) who suddenly could not stand or open his eyes. Signs included bilateral third cranial nerve paralysis, bulbar weakness, and extensor plantar responses. CT scan revealed a 1-cm hematoma in the ventral tegmentum of the midbrain with rupture into the third ventricle. He experienced obstructive hydrocephalus, which was treated with a ventriculoperitoneal shunt, and survived with bilateral third cranial nerve palsies and poor balance with a tendency to fall backward. Arteriographic findings were normal. Although there was no pathologic confirmation, this case may represent a primary hypertensive mesencephalic tegmental hematoma. The second patient was a normotensive young

man who experienced Weber's syndrome (crossed third cranial nerve palsy and hemiparesis) after a week of prodromal headache. The CT scan showed a right midbrain hematoma. After further deterioration, the hematoma was surgically decompressed, and microscopic examination of the wall of the hematoma revealed an AVM. The patient survived but was grossly ataxic.

A 71-year-old patient reported by Morel-Maroger et al[435] had midbrain hemorrhage due to hypertension. After being treated for hypertension for 5 years, he suddenly lost consciousness and awakened confused and dizzy. He had a diffuse headache and vomited. Clinical findings included a right third cranial nerve palsy, left hemiparesis, and a cerebellar-type ataxia of the right limbs. Blood pressure was 290/110 mm Hg. CT scan documented a 12 × 16-mm hematoma in the right superior cerebellar peduncle. The patient recovered after antihypertensive therapy without surgical intervention.

Roig et al[433] described two patients with hypertensive mesencephalic hematomas detected on CT. One patient had an ipsilateral third cranial nerve paralysis with contralateral hemihypesthesia and limb ataxia. The hyperdense lesion was high in the right mesencephalic tegmentum near the midline, probably draining into the third ventricle. Vertebral angiographic findings were normal. A second patient had a right third cranial nerve palsy and left hemiparesis. The lesion was high in the right side of the midbrain. Both patients survived.

A 10-year-old boy reported by Humphreys[436] suddenly demonstrated right hemiparesis and confusion. Neuroophthalmologic findings were not given in detail. A CT scan showed a large hematoma in the basis pedunculi extending into the interpeduncular fossa. The lesion was drained surgically and was found to contain nuclear debris. The nature of the lesion is unknown, but it was likely a hemorrhage into an AVM or a benign tumor.

LaTorre et al[437] described a 38-year-old woman who, after complaining of headache and intermittent diplopia for 2 years, vomited and demonstrated bilateral sixth cranial nerve palsies and paralysis of upward gaze. CSF was found to contain blood, and ventriculography visualized a beaded aqueduct and hydrocephalus. Surgical exploration of the midbrain discovered an AVM of the quadrigeminal plate with a blood clot embedded in the aqueduct.

A single patient was reported by Scoville and Poppen.[438] The 44-year-old woman experienced an ataxic right hemiparesis in stepwise fashion over 1.5 years. Vomiting, bilateral third cranial nerve paralysis, stupor, and pinpoint pupils suddenly supervened. After a blood clot was drained from her left cerebral peduncle, the patient awakened. Normal blood pressure and coagulation values and the gradual onset favored an AVM in this patient.

A number of further observations have stressed the presentation of small midbrain hemorrhages with features of isolated forms of ophthalmoplegia.[439-441] These have included isolated fourth[439] and third[440,441] nerve palsies as well as various combinations of a dorsal midbrain syndrome.[442,443] Most of these cases were remarkable for the absence or paucity of signs of long-tract involvement, stressing the fact that small midbrain ICHs can present with isolated ophthalmoplegia.

Pontine Hemorrhage

The early clinicopathologic observations in pontine hemorrhage correspond to those made by Fang and Foley[444] and later by Dinsdale,[105] who reviewed the necropsies at Boston City Hospital and found 511 ICHs among 19,093 autopsies, of which 30 were pontine (6%). Two thirds of the patients in this autopsy series had been comatose when first seen, 13% vomited, and 78% were dead within 48 hours. One patient who survived for 23 days had a small hemorrhage in the right pontine tegmentum. All of the remainder had massive hemorrhages, usually in the midpons at the junction of the basis pontis and tegmentum that frequently spread rostrally into the midbrain; the hemorrhages almost never spread caudally to the medulla but frequently ruptured into the fourth ventricle.

In 1971 Fisher,[55] using serial sections from a patient with a massive fatal pontine hemorrhage, identified numerous small vessels with "fibrin globes," which he thought were related to the vascular rupture causing the hemorrhage. "From the gaping end of each of these torn vessels there protruded a large mass of platelets partially encircled by thin concentric layers of fibrin." He suggested that the primary hemorrhage led to pressure on surrounding vessels, which subsequently ruptured, causing a cascade or avalanche effect and producing gradual enlargement of the hematoma. Ross Russell[117] had demonstrated large asymptomatic fusiform enlargements on the penetrating vessels of the pons in patients with "atherosclerosis" and hypertensive vascular disease. Cole and Yates,[110] Rosenblum,[112] Fisher,[55] and Caplan[445] all explained bleeding in hypertensive patients as leakage from tiny penetrating vessels damaged by lipohyalinosis and containing small microaneurysms.

Kornyey[446] reported a patient whose pontine hemorrhage occurred during clinical observation; the slow march of signs was similar to the pattern of development seen in ganglionic and thalamic hemorrhages, providing support for Fisher's postulation of the slowly evolving avalanche. Kornyey's patient was a 39-year-old man referred for admission because of malignant hypertension. While his admission history was being taken, he complained of numb hands, weakness, and dizziness. His blood pressure was 245/170 mm Hg. He became restless and apprehensive and complained that he could not hear and had difficulty swallowing and breathing. A bilateral sixth cranial nerve palsy and dilated pupils developed, and his corneal reflexes disappeared. Speech became "bulbar," he was deaf, and he could not move his left leg. Within 15 minutes the patient was comatose; the pupils were small, and the eyes were converged. Bilateral bulbar palsy, stiff limbs with exaggerated reflexes, and extensor plantar responses were observed. Two hours after onset, the patient died. A large hemorrhage in the tegmentum of the pons, with some spreading into the right basis pontis, was found at necropsy.[446] In other patients observed during the onset of pontine hemorrhage, development of the deficit usually evolved gradually over minutes (1 to 30 minutes) and was not as instantaneous as aneurysmal SAH.

In the pons, the largest penetrating arteries enter medially, arise perpendicular to the basilar artery, and course from the base to the tegmentum. Other small penetrating arteries originate from the short and long circumferential vessels and enter more laterally, also coursing from base to tegmentum. Some arteries enter the tegmentum laterally and course horizontally across it.[139] Because vessels in all of these sites are potentially susceptible to hypertensive damage and lipohyalinosis, they could theoretically also be sites for pontine bleeding. Silverstein[447,448] reviewed the pathologic material from Philadelphia General Hospital and confirmed that these sites (Fig. 29-50) were the usual regions of pontine hemorrhage. Of 50 cases, 28 were massive central hemorrhages presumably arising from large paramedian penetrators; 11 were more lateralized, usually spreading from base to tegmentum; and 11 had a tegmental location, of which 4 remained unilateral and 7 involved the tegmentum bilaterally.

Not until the mid-1970s, when CT became available, was it possible to diagnose smaller nonfatal pontine hemorrhages accurately and to separate them positively from pontine infarction during life. MRI data, acquired through the use of gradient-echo sequences, indicate that pontine microhemorrhages tend to adopt a distribution similar to that of the large, symptomatic hemorrhages,[449] favoring the dorsal aspect of the basis pontis.

Large Paramedian Pontine Hemorrhage

Massive pontine hemorrhage results from rupture of parenchymal midpontine branches originating from the basilar artery. The bleeding vessel is thought to be a paramedian perforator in its distal portion,[105] causing initial hematoma formation at the junction of tegmentum and basis pontis,[105,448] from which the mass grows into its final round or oval shape and replaces most of both subdivisions of the pons (Fig. 29-51).The lesion usually begins in the middle of the pons and extends along the longitudinal axis of the brainstem into the lower midbrain. The hematoma may track into the middle cerebellar peduncles

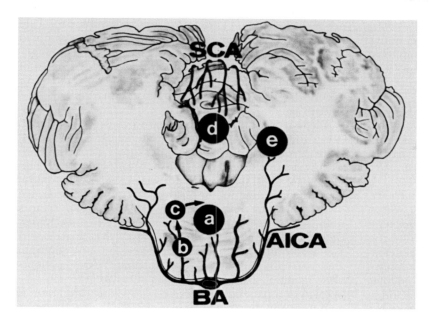

Figure 29-50 Schematic representation of common sites of hypertensive pontine and cerebellar hemorrhages: *a,* massive, paramedian pontine; *b,* basal pontine; *c,* lateral tegmental pontine; *d,* cerebellar vermian; *e,* cerebellar hemispheral. AICA, anterior–inferior cerebellar artery; BA, basilar artery; SCA, superior cerebellar artery.

but usually does not extend caudally beyond the ponto-medullary junction.[105] In the process of rapid hematoma expansion, destruction of tegmental and ventral pontine structures results, with the classic combination of signs caused by involvement of cranial nerve nuclei, long tracts, autonomic centers, and structures responsible for maintenance of consciousness. Large pontine hematomas also regularly rupture into the fourth ventricle.[105,447,448]

The classic form of pontine hemorrhage, bilateral and massive, is almost exclusively of hypertensive origin. Other etiologies, such as cryptic vascular malformation, account for 10% or less of the cases in most series.[105,448] Russell[167] regarded pontine hemorrhage as a form of ICH most likely to occur in patients with so-called malignant hypertension or hypertension associated with chronic nephropathy. Clinical presentation is characteristically one of rapid development of coma (80% of cases) without warning signs. Dana[450] recognized that some patients were conscious when first examined; in three different series, 4 of 19 patients (22%),[444] 10 of 30 patients (33.3%),[105] and 5 of 50 patients (10%)[447,448] were alert when initially seen. By 48 hours, approximately 80% were dead.[105,444] In some patients (30%), a complaint of severe occipital headache preceded by minutes the catastrophic onset of coma.[447,451] Vomiting was noted in 4 of 30 (13%)[105] and 4 of 19 (22%)[444] patients in two series, occasionally being a prominent early symptom.

The frequency of seizures at onset, estimated to be as high as 22%,[447] probably represents a combination of true convulsive phenomena in rare instances, along with episodes of spasmodic decerebrate posturing and even the sometimes violent shivering associated with autonomic dysfunction and rapidly evolving hyperthermia. Some patients are seen before the development of coma with focal pontine signs, such as facial or limb numbness, deafness, diplopia, bilateral leg weakness, or progressive hemiparesis. Physical examination often reveals an abnormal respiratory rhythm or apnea.[105,448,452] Steegmann[452] analyzed these respiratory abnormalities in detail and

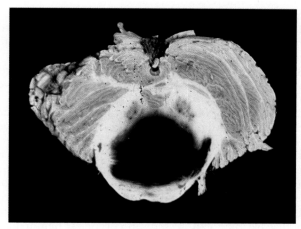

Figure 29-51 Massive pontine hemorrhage with dissection into brachium pontis and fourth ventricle.

reported a variety of abnormal respiratory patterns, including "inspiratory gasps of apneustic respiration," Cheyne-Stokes rhythm, slow and labored respirations, "gasping" respiration, and apnea. Two thirds of his 17 patients exhibited either apnea or severely abnormal patterns of hypoventilation. Hyperthermia frequently coexisted, with temperatures above 39°C in more than 80% of the patients,[451] in one fourth of whom it reached levels of 42°C to 43°C,[447] usually in the preterminal stages. Neurologic findings characteristically result from involvement of cranial nerve nuclei and long tracts; they include quadriplegia with decerebrate posturing, bilateral Babinski signs, absence of corneal reflexes, pinpoint miotic pupils, and various forms of ophthalmoplegia.[139,451,452]

The oculomotor findings include miotic pinpoint pupils, absence of horizontal eye movements, and ocular bobbing. *Miotic pinpoint pupils* are usually about 1 mm in diameter. They react to light if a strong light source is used, and a tiny constriction can be detected with a magnifying lens.[367,422] Pontine hemorrhage can be confused with opiate poisoning.[452] The pupillary abnormality probably results from bilateral interruption of descending sympathetic pupillodilator fibers.[367,422] Because pupillary dilatation preceded miosis in Kornyey's[446] patient, it is possible that early stimulation of these fibers could lead to transient pupillary dilatation.

Absence of horizontal eye movements, detected with reflex testing with the doll's head maneuver or ice-water caloric stimulation, reflects bilateral injury of the paramedian pontine reticular formation. This sign occurs in partial forms or variants such as the *one-and-a-half syndrome*,[367] also referred to as *paralytic pontine exotropia*,[453] which represents a combination of unilateral horizontal gaze palsy plus ipsilateral internuclear ophthalmoplegia, resulting in one immobile eye and abduction preserved only in the contralateral one. It is more commonly seen in the smaller unilateral lesions from infarcts,[367,453] partial hematomas,[138,454,455] AVMs,[453] or tumors,[453] which result in unilateral involvement of the paramedian pontine reticular formation and the dorsally located ipsilateral medial longitudinal fasciculus. In one of our patients with a hematoma limited to the basis pontis, there was no voluntary horizontal gaze, but reflex movements were preserved. This situation, which has been described by Halsey et al,[456] reflects damage to supranuclear fibers traveling with corticobulbar fibers in the pontine basis before they reach the tegmental paramedian pontine reticular formation.

Described by Fisher,[425] *ocular bobbing* denotes brisk movements of conjugate ocular depression, followed within seconds by a slower return to midposition. It occurs most commonly from a pontine lesion, either hemorrhage or infarction, although it has also been described in cerebellar hemorrhage.[228,425,457] Typically, it affects both eyes simultaneously and is accompanied by bilateral paralysis of horizontal gaze.[425] Atypical varieties include unilateral or markedly asymmetrical forms and those occurring when horizontal eye movements are still present.[425,457] The latter form is less strictly localizing to pontine disease, as it can be seen in cerebellar hemorrhage, SAH, and even coma of nonvascular mechanism.[425]

Weakness of pontine and bulbar musculature is invariable in the larger median hemorrhages but is difficult to assess because patients with bilateral tegmental damage are always comatose. Puffing of the cheeks with expiration, diminished eyelid tone, and pooling of secretions in the oropharynx are commonly observed. Deafness, dysarthria, dizziness, and facial numbness occasionally precede the development of coma. Facial weakness is often asymmetrical and may be associated with a crossed hemiplegia at the time the patient is first seen.[458]

Limb motor abnormalities are also always present in large tegmental–basal hemorrhages; usually it is quadriplegia with stiffness of all limbs. Hemiplegia was noted in four of 15 tegmental–basal hemorrhages by Goto et al[458] but was present in only three of 28 cases of bilateral hemorrhages reviewed by Silverstein.[447,448] The motor abnormality is usually bilateral with minor asymmetries. Asymmetries in decerebrate posturing, reflexes, or clonus are commonly detected. Tremor, shivering, restless limb movements, and dystonic postures have been common in our experience; patients may suddenly stiffen, giving the false impression of convulsive phenomena. Shivering

occurs as the patient's condition worsens and can indicate failing motor function. Decerebrate posturing was noted in 12 of 15 patients reported by Goto et al.[458] Surprisingly, only two of the 28 patients in Silverstein's[447,448] series of large bilateral pontine hematomas were reported to have decerebrate rigidity, but 13 had flaccid quadriplegia, and 10 had "generalized flaccidity."

Massive pontine hemorrhages are always fatal, although death does not come instantaneously. Steegmann[452] noted no deaths among 17 patients in less than 2 hours. Death usually occurs between 24 and 48 hours.[105,444,448,452] Survival for 2 to 10 days is not unusual and depends on the vigor of nursing and supportive care and the presence of complicating respiratory or urinary sepsis. Factors found to be early predictors of mortality include hyperthermia (temperature > 39°C), tachycardia (heart rate > 110 beats/min), CT evidence of extension into midbrain and thalamus, and acute hydrocephalus.[459] Some patients with medium-sized hemorrhages survive.[459,460] On rare occasions, a patient has survived the surgical removal of a pontine and fourth ventricular clot,[454,461] which usually has been due to bleeding from a pontine AVM. Because the development of such lesions is so rapid, it is unlikely that surgical treatment could be provided early enough in the larger hemorrhages to be helpful. No other medical or surgical therapy seems likely to help these grave lesions.

Unilateral Basal or Basotegmental Hemorrhages

Unilateral basal or basotegmental hemorrhages are less common than the large paramedian lesions already discussed. In his autopsy-based series, Silverstein[448] described 11 such lesions (22%); three were limited to the base, and eight were basotegmental. The larger lesions ruptured into the fourth ventricle. Reports based on CT scans have shown more restricted syndromes,[414,462] increasing the range of causes of a pure motor syndrome. Gobernado et al[463] described a hypertensive woman with the gradual development over 3 days of a pure motor hemiplegia affecting the right arm and leg, sparing the face. A CT scan defined a small hematoma limited to the base of the left pons. Another patient with a small hematoma confined to the right basis pontis had an "ataxic hemiparesis" of the left limbs.[464] Small unilateral hematomas limited to the base manifest as syndromes indistinguishable from lacunar infarction in the same region (Fig. 29-52). Tuhrim et al[465] reported a patient with dysarthria, limb ataxia, and extensor plantar response due to a small basal pontine hematoma; although they labeled this case dysarthria–clumsy hand syndrome, it more closely resembles ataxic hemiparesis.[109]

Bleeding originating from a pontine penetrating artery may start in the basis pontis but also frequently dissects dorsally into the tegmentum. When the lesion spreads to the tegmentum, an ipsilateral facial palsy and conjugate gaze or sixth cranial nerve palsy often accompanies the contralateral hemiplegia.[466] Larger unilateral lesions may rupture into the fourth ventricle after spreading within the tegmentum (Fig. 29-53). In Silverstein's series,[448] these larger unilateral basotegmental lesions usually lead to hemiplegia, coma, and death.

Lateral Tegmental Brainstem Hematomas

Lateral tegmental brainstem hematomas usually originate from vessels penetrating into the brainstem from long circumferential branches. They enter the tegmentum laterally and course medially. Small hematomas remain confined to the lateral tegmentum, and larger lesions spread across to the opposite side and can destroy the entire tegmentum. Neurologic examination reveals a predominantly unilateral tegmental lesion with variable degrees of basilar involvement.[138,139] Oculomotor abnormalities, especially the "one-and-a-half syndrome," horizontal gaze palsy, internuclear ophthalmoplegia, partial involvement of vertical eye movements, and ocular bobbing, have been described.[138,139,460,466-468] The tegmental location of the spinothalamic tract makes sensory symptoms common. Ataxia, either unilateral or bilateral, may also accompany the oculomotor signs.[138,139] Action tremor has developed as the transient hemiparesis improves; this observation can be possibly explained by involvement of the red nucleus or its connections.[139] Facial numbness, ipsilateral miosis, and hemiparesis have also been noted.[138,139] Two patients[138] developed Cheyne-Stokes respirations, one of the short-cycle type,[309,422] the other of the classic variety. Table 29-13 reviews some reported examples of tegmental pontine hematomas.[105,138,139,414,448,455,467]

We examined two patients with tegmental pontine hemorrhage, and Lawrence and Lightfoote[469] studied a patient with a pontine AVM; all three patients showed vertical pendular ocular oscillations with dizziness and vertical oscillopsia weeks after the hemorrhage. Delayed pain in the contralateral limbs, as in the thalamic pain syndrome, began during recovery from a unilateral tegmental hemorrhage in another patient. We have also observed "palatal myoclonus" as a sequela of lateral tegmental hematomas.

Medullary Hemorrhage

Hemorrhage into the medulla oblongata (Fig. 29-54) is even more rare than hemorrhage into the midbrain.

Arseni and Stanciu[470] described a 40-year-old woman with dizziness, vomiting, and headache with diplopia and right limb paresthesias. She suddenly became somnolent and ataxic, with a stiff neck, left hemiparesis, diminished pain and temperature sensation on the left side of the

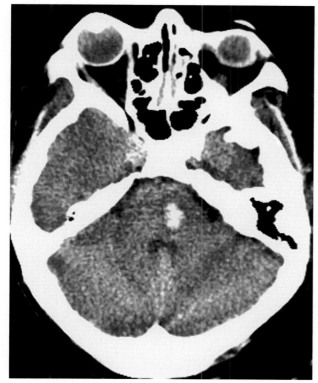

Figure 29-52 CT scan of a small left basal paramedian pontine hemorrhage.

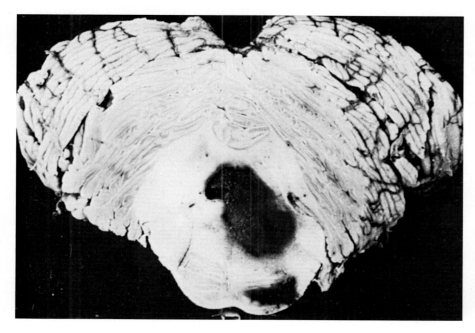

Figure 29-53 Unilateral basotegmental pontine hemorrhage with rupture into fourth ventricle.

TABLE 29-13 TEGMENTAL PONTINE HEMORRHAGES

Study	Extraocular Movements	Motor	Sensory	Other Cranial Nerves	Cerebellar
Computed tomography diagnosis					
Caplan and Goodwin[139]	No vertical, R gaze, R 6th, bilat. INO	L ↑ toe	L ↓ pin	R 7th, dysarthria, ptosis	Ataxia R > L
Caplan and Goodwin[139]	"1½," vertical nystagmus	L hemip, ↑↑ toes	L ↓ pin	R 7th, 8th, ptosis, dysarthria	Ataxia L > R
Müller et al[414]	R INO	L hemip, ↑↑ toes	L ↓ pin	R 5th, 7th	—
Kase et al[138]	"1½," No ↑ gaze	R hemip	R ↓ pin and joint position sense	Dysarthria, L 7th	Ataxia L
Kase et al[138]	L INO and 6th, R 4th, bobbing	R hemip	R ↓ pin	Dysphagia, L 7th	Ataxia R & L
Autopsy cases					
Caplan and Goodwin[139]	"1½," bobbing, OD ↓ & inward	L hemip, Babinski	L ↓ pin	Dysarthria	Ataxia R > L
Tyler and Johnson[467]	No horizontal or ↑ gaze, bobbing, skew	L hemip, ↑↑ toes	L ↓ pin	R 5th, 7th, dysarthria, dysphagia, ptosis	R tremor
Dinsdale[105]	R gaze palsy	L hemip	L ↓ pin	R 7th, 8th	—
Silverstein[448]	R gaze palsy	L hemip, ↑↑ toes	L ↓ pin	R 7th, ptosis, dysphagia	—
Pierrott-Deseilligny et al[455]	"1½"	L hemip, ↑↑ toes	L hemis	R 5th, 7th, 8th	Ataxia R arm

Hemip, hemiparesis; hemis, hemisensory syndrome; INO, internuclear ophthalmoplegia; OD, right eye; "1½," the "one-and-one-half" syndrome; R, right; L, left.

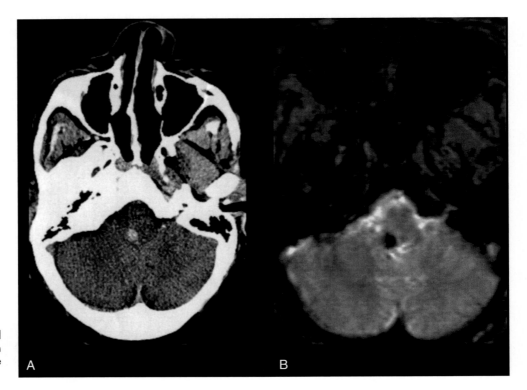

Figure 29-54 Right dorsolateral medullary hemorrhage on CT scan (A) and gradient-echo MR image (B).

face, left limb ataxia, nystagmus, dysphonia, and dysphagia. Surgical exploration found a hematoma on the floor of the fourth ventricle laterally. After drainage of the clot, the patient was said to do well.

Kempe[471] reported on a similar patient who had a lateral medullary hematoma. The 25-year-old woman noted diminished hearing on the left and then suddenly became ill with headache, vomiting, vertigo, and hiccups. She was ataxic and fell to the left. Findings included left nystagmus, diminished pain and temperature sensation on the left side of the face, and left facial weakness; the left ear was deaf and unreactive to caloric stimuli. Pneumoencephalography documented a defect in the rhomboid fossa of the fourth ventricle, which at surgical exploration was found to be a clot bulging through the floor of the fourth ventricle medial to the restiform body. Both this patient and the one described by Arseni and Stanciu[470] had findings similar to those in patients with lateral medullary infarcts, and each had a stepwise course. Arteriography was not performed, and CT and MRI were not available. We suspect that the underlying process in both patients was a cavernous angioma.

In another patient,[309] the explanation was an AVM. At age 37, the woman experienced weakness and decreased position sense in her left arm and leg. Right vocal cord and hypoglossal paralysis developed at age 60, and 2 years later, she became gradually and then abruptly worse and was hypertensive. Necropsy revealed a hemorrhage in the medial medullary tegmentum with spreading into the dorsal medulla and right lateral medulla.

Mastaglia et al[472] reported two cases of medullary hemorrhage with quite different clinical features. In one case, an 87-year-old hypertensive woman was found unconscious with a right gaze palsy, right facial weakness, and left hemiplegia. The hemorrhage was largest in the lateral pons and descended into the medullary pyramid. The cause seems to have been a pontine basal–tegmental hemorrhage with unusual caudal dissection, but its clinical picture did not differ from that already described in unilateral pontine hemorrhage. The other patient was hypertensive and had been undergoing anticoagulation with warfarin. She demonstrated an unusual clinical picture consisting of markedly decreased postural sensation and incoordination of her left arm and leg, diminished left arm reflexes, numbness over the right eye, and subjective numbness of the right limbs. Autopsy showed a hemorrhage into the rostral spinal cord with dissection into the left medullary pyramid. The most likely etiologic factor in this patient was anticoagulation, perhaps compounded by hypertension.

There is one well-documented case of medullary hemorrhage due to hypertension, but whether the hemorrhage arose in the medulla or arose in the caudal pontine tegmentum and dissected into the medulla is not certain.[430] The patient, a 56-year-old, previously hypertensive man, experienced difficulty swallowing, and examination found paralysis of the left side of the face, soft palate, vocal cord, and tongue. A left Horner's syndrome, deafness in the left ear, and paresthesias of the right limbs were also found. CT scan showed a left medullary tegmental hematoma, but the signs of deafness and facial palsy might indicate some pontine involvement.

Barinagarrementeria and Cantú[473] described four cases of their own and reviewed 12 others from the literature. The characteristic profile was one of sudden onset of headache, vertigo, dysphagia, dysphonia or dysarthria, and limb incoordination. Common findings on examination were palatal weakness (88%); nystagmus, cerebellar ataxia, or both (75%); limb weakness (68%); and hypoglossal nerve palsy (56%). Less common signs were facial palsy and Horner's syndrome. The mechanism of the medullary hemorrhage could be determined in only seven of the 16 patients, corresponding to ruptured vascular malformation (3), hypertension (3), and anticoagulation treatment (1). The mortality rate for the group was 19% (three of 16), and in most of the survivors, residual neurologic deficits were either mild (56%) or absent (19%).

Unusual presentations of medullary hemorrhage have included a patient with isolated hiccups from a small dorsal ICH,[474] and a second patient with dorsolateral hemorrhage into an area of infarction[475] who was seen initially with features of Wallenberg's syndrome.

REFERENCES

1. Kurtzke JF: *Epidemiology of cerebrovascular disease*, Berlin, 1969, Springer-Verlag.
2. Mohr JP, Caplan LR, Melski JW, et al: The Harvard Cooperative Stroke Registry: A prospective registry, *Neurology* 28:754, 1978.
3. Sacco RL, Wolf PA, Bharucha NE, et al: Subarachnoid and intracerebral hemorrhage: Natural history, prognosis, and precursive factors in the Framingham Study, *Neurology* 34:847, 1984.
4. Kunitz SC, Gross CR, Heyman A, et al: The Pilot Stroke Data Bank: Definition, design and data, *Stroke* 15:740, 1984.
5. Hansen BS, Marquardsen J: Incidence of stroke in Frederiksberg, Denmark, *Stroke* 8:663, 1977.
6. Herman B, Schulte BPM, Van Luijk JH, et al: Epidemiology of stroke in Tilburg, The Netherlands: The population-based stroke incidence register. 1: Introduction and preliminary results, *Stroke* 11:162, 1980.
7. Bamford J, Sandercock P, Dennis M, et al: A prospective study of acute cerebrovascular disease in the community: The Oxfordshire Community Stroke Project, 1981-86. 2: Incidence, case fatality rates and overall outcome at one year of cerebral infarction, primary intracerebral and subarachnoid haemorrhage, *J Neurol Neurosurg Psychiatry* 53:16, 1990.
8. Gross CR, Kase CS, Mohr JP, et al: Stroke in south Alabama: Incidence and diagnostic features—a population based study, *Stroke* 15:249, 1984.
9. Sacco S, Marini C, Toni D, et al: Incidence and 10-year survival of intracerebral hemaorrhage in a population-based registry, *Stroke* 40:394, 2009.
10. Broderick J, Brott T, Tomsick T, et al: The risk of subarachnoid and intracerebral hemorrhages in blacks as compared with whites, *N Engl J Med* 326:733, 1992.
11. Harmsen P, Wilhelmsen L, Jacobsson A: Stroke incidence and mortality rates 1987 to 2006 related to secular trends of cardiovascular risk factors in Gothenburg, Sweden, *Stroke* 40:2691, 2009.
12. Furlan AJ, Whisnant JP, Elveback LR: The decreasing incidence of primary intracerebral hemorrhage: A population study, *Ann Neurol* 5:367, 1979.
13. Drury I, Whisnant JP, Garraway WM: Primary intracerebral hemorrhage: Impact of CT on incidence, *Neurology* 34:653, 1984.
14. Brott T, Thalinger K, Hertzberg V: Hypertension as a risk factor for spontaneous intracerebral hemorrhage, *Stroke* 17:1078, 1986.
15. Schütz H, Bödeker R-H, Damian M, et al: Age-related spontaneous intracerebral hematoma in a German community, *Stroke* 21:1412, 1990.
16. Bruno A, Carter S, Qualls C, et al: Incidence of spontaneous intracerebral hemorrhage among Hispanics and non-Hispanic whites in New Mexico, *Neurology* 47:405, 1996.

17. Tanaka H, Ueda Y, Date C, et al: Incidence of stroke in Shibata, Japan, 1976-1978, *Stroke* 12:460, 1981.

18. Aurell M, Head B: Cerebral hemorrhage in a population after a decade of active anti-hypertensive treatment, *Acta Med Scand* 176:377, 1964.

19. Garraway WM, Whisnant JP, Drury I: The continuing decline in the incidence of stroke, *Mayo Clin Proc* 58:520, 1983.

20. Ueda K, Omae T, Hirota Y, et al: Decreasing trend in incidence and mortality from stroke in Hisayama residents, *Japan, Stroke* 12:154, 1981.

21. Qureshi AI, Suri MAK, Safdar K, et al: Intracerebral hemorrhage in blacks: Risk factors, subtypes, and outcomes, *Stroke* 28:961, 1997.

22. Brewer DB, Fawcett FJ, Horsfield GI: A necropsy series of non-traumatic cerebral haemorrhages and softenings, with particular reference to heart weight, *J Pathol Bacteriol* 96:311, 1968.

23. Mutlu N, Berry RG, Alpers BJ: Massive cerebral hemorrhage: Clinical and pathological correlations, *Arch Neurol* 8:74, 1963.

24. Stehbens WE: *Pathology of the Cerebral Blood Vessels,* St. Louis, 1972, CV Mosby.

25. Ojemann RG, Heros RC: Spontaneous brain hemorrhage, *Stroke* 14:468, 1983.

26. McCormick WF, Rosenfield DB: Massive brain hemorrhage: A review of 144 cases and an examination of their causes, *Stroke* 4:946, 1973.

27. Thrift AG, McNeil JJ, Forbes A, et al: Three important subgroups of hypertensive persons at greater risk of intracerebral hemorrhage, *Hypertension* 31:1223, 1998.

28. PROGRESS Collaboration Group: Randomised trial of a perindopril-based blood-pressure-lowering regimen among 6105 individuals with previous stroke or transient ischaemic attack, *Lancet* 358:1033, 2001.

29. Abbott RD, Yin Y, Reed DH, Yano K: Risk of stroke in male cigarette smokers, *N Engl J Med* 315:717, 1986.

30. Juvela S, Hillbom M, Palomaki H: Risk factors for spontaneous intracerebral hemorrhage, *Stroke* 26:1558, 1995.

31. Kurth T, Kase CS, Berger K, et al: Smoking and risk of hemorrhagic stroke in women, *Stroke* 34:2792, 2003.

32. Kurth T, Kase CS, Berger K, et al: Smoking and the risk of hemorrhagic stroke in men, *Stroke* 34:1151, 2003.

33. Donahue RP, Abbott RD, Reed DM, Yanko K: Alcohol and hemorrhagic stroke: The Honolulu Heart Program, *JAMA* 255:2311, 1986.

34. Ueshima H, Iida M, Shimamoto T, et al: Multivariate analysis of risk factors for stroke: Eight-year follow-up of farming villages in Akita, Japan, *Prev Med* 9:722, 1980.

35. Boudouresques G, Hauw JJ, Meininger V, et al: Étude neuropathologique des hémorragies intracraniennes de l'adulte, *Rev Neurol* 135:197, 1979.

36. McCormick WF, Schochet SS: *Atlas of cerebrovascular disease,* Philadelphia, 1976, WB Saunders, p 328.

37. Steering Committee of the Physicians' Health Study Research Group. Final report on the aspirin component of the ongoing Physicians' Health Study, *N Engl J Med* 321:129, 1989.

38. The SALT Collaborative Group. Swedish Aspirin Low-dose Trial (SALT) of 75 mg aspirin as secondary prophylaxis after cerebrovascular ischaemic events, *Lancet* 338:1345, 1991.

39. Bousser MG, Eschwege E, Haguenau M, et al: "AICLA" controlled trial of aspirin and dipyridamole in the secondary prevention of atherothrombotic cerebral ischemia, *Stroke* 14:5, 1983.

40. Canadian Cooperative Study Group: A randomized trial of aspirin and sulfinpyrazone in threatened stroke, *N Engl J Med* 299:53, 1978.

41. The American-Canadian Co-Operative Study Group: Persantine aspirin trial in cerebral ischemia. Part II: Endpoint results, *Stroke* 16:406, 1985.

42. The European Stroke Prevention Study (ESPS): Principal endpoints. The ESPS Group, *Lancet* 2:1351, 1987.

43. United Kingdom Transient Ischaemic Attack (UK-TIA) aspirin trial: Interim results. UK-TIA Study Group, *BMJ* 296:316, 1988.

44. Diener HC, Cunha L, Forbes C, et al: European Stroke Prevention Study. 2: Dipyridamole and acetylsalicylic acid in the secondary prevention of stroke, *J Neurol Sci* 143:1, 1996.

45. Greenberg SM, Vonsattel J-PG: Diagnosis of cerebral amyloid angiopathy: Sensitivity and specificity of cortical biopsy, *Stroke* 28:1418, 1997.

46. Itoh Y, Yamada M, Hayakawa M, et al: Cerebral amyloid angiopathy: A significant cause of cerebellar as well as lobar cerebral hemorrhage in the elderly, *J Neurol Sci* 116:135, 1993.

47. Lee SS, Stemmermann GN: Congophilic angiopathy and cerebral hemorrhage, *Arch Pathol Lab Med* 102:317, 1978.

48. Tomonaga M: Cerebral amyloid angiopathy in the elderly, *J Am Geriatr Soc* 29:151, 1981.

49. Vinters HV, Gilbert JJ: Cerebral amyloid angiopathy: Incidence and complications in the aging brain. II: The distribution of amyloid vascular changes, *Stroke* 14:924, 1983.

50. Masuda J, Tanaka K, Ueda K, et al: Autopsy study of incidence and distribution of cerebral amyloid angiopathy in Hisayama, Japan, *Stroke* 19:205, 1988.

51. Vinters HV: Cerebral amyloid angiopathy: A critical review, *Stroke* 18:311, 1987.

52. Ellis RJ, Olichney JM, Thal LJ, et al: Cerebral amyloid angiopathy in the brains of patients with Alzheimer's disease: The CERAD experience, Part XV, *Neurology* 46:1592, 1996.

53. Mandybur TI: Cerebral amyloid angiopathy: The vascular pathology and complications, *J Neuropathol Exp Neurol* 45:79, 1986.

54. Greenberg SM, Briggs ME, Hyman BT, et al: Apolipoprotein E ε4 is associated with the presence and earlier onset of hemorrhage in cerebral amyloid angiopathy, *Stroke* 27:1333, 1996.

55. Fisher CM: Pathological observations in hypertensive cerebral hemorrhage, *J Neuropathol Exp Neurol* 30:536, 1971.

56. Bahemuka M: Primary intracerebral hemorrhage and heart weight: A clinicopathologic case-control review of 218 patients, *Stroke* 18:531, 1987.

57. Massaro AR, Sacco RL, Mohr JP, et al: Clinical discriminators of lobar and deep hemorrhages: The Stroke Data Bank, *Neurology* 41:1881, 1991.

58. Broderick J, Brott T, Tomsick T, et al: Lobar hemorrhage in the elderly: The undiminishing importance of hypertension, *Stroke* 24:49, 1993.

59. Woo D, Sauerbeck LR, Kissela BM, et al: Genetic and environmental risk factors for intracerebral hemorrhage: Preliminary results of a population-based study, *Stroke* 33:1190, 2002.

60. Gatchev O, Rastam L, Lindberg G, et al: Subarachnoid hemorrhage, cerebral hemorrhage, and serum cholesterol concentration in men and women, *Ann Epidemiol* 3:403, 1993.

61. Lindenstrom E, Boysen G, Nyboe J: Influence of total cholesterol, high density lipoprotein cholesterol, and triglycerides on risk of cerebrovascular disease: The Copenhagen City Heart Study [see comments], *BMJ* 309:11, 1994:published erratum appears in BMJ 309:1619, 1994.

62. Iribarren C, Jacobs DR, Sadler M, et al: Low total serum cholesterol and intracerebral hemorrhagic stroke: Is the association confined to elderly men, *Stroke* 27:1996, 1993.

63. Segal AZ, Chiu RI, Eggleston-Sexton PM, et al: Low cholesterol as a risk factor for primary intracerebral hemorrhage: A case-control study, *Neuroepidemiology* 18:185, 1999.

64. Okazaki H, Reagan TJ, Campbell RJ: Clinicopathologic studies of primary cerebral amyloid angiopathy, *Mayo Clin Proc* 54:22, 1979.

65. Gray F, Dubas F, Roullet E, et al: Leukoencephalopathy in diffuse hemorrhagic cerebral amyloid angiopathy, *Ann Neurol* 18:54, 1985.

66. Yamada M, Itoh Y, Shintaku M, et al: Immune reactions associated with cerebral amyloid angiopathy, *Stroke* 27:1155, 1996.

67. Vonsattel JP, Myers RH, Hedley-Whyte ET, et al: Cerebral amyloid angiopathy without and with cerebral hemorrhages: A comparative histological study, *Ann Neurol* 30:637, 1991.

68. Vinters HV, Natte R, Maat-Schieman ML, et al: Secondary microvascular degeneration in amyloid angiopathy of patients with hereditary cerebral hemorrhage with amyloidosis, Dutch type (HCHWA-D), *Acta Neuropathol* 95:235, 1998.

69. Greenberg SM, Vonsattel JP, Stakes JW, et al: The clinical spectrum of cerebral amyloid angiopathy: Presentations without lobar hemorrhage, *Neurology* 43:2073, 1993.

70. Smith DB, Hitchcock M, Philpott PJ: Cerebral amyloid angiopathy presenting as transient ischemic attacks: Case report, *J Neurosurg* 63:963, 1985.

71. Yong WH, Robert ME, Secor DL, et al: Cerebral hemorrhage with biopsy-proved amyloid angiopathy, *Arch Neurol* 49:51, 1992.

72. Alberts MJ: Stroke genetics update, *Stroke* 34:342, 2003.

73. Alberts MJ, McCarron MO, Hoffman KL, et al: Familial clustering of intracerebral hemorrhage: A prospective study in North Carolina, *Neuroepidemiology* 21:18, 2002.

74. Catto AJ, Kohler HP, Bannan S, et al: Factor XIII Val 34 Leu: A novel association with primary intracerebral hemorrhage, *Stroke* 29:813, 1998.

75. Cho KH, Kim BC, Kim MK, et al: No association of factor XIII Val-34Leu polymorphism with primary intracerebral hemorrhage and healthy controls in Korean population, *J Korean Med Sci* 17:249, 2002.

76. Wu L, Shen Y, Liu X, et al: The 1425G/A SNP in *PRKCH* is associated with ischemic stroke and cerebral hemorrhage in a Chinese population, *Stroke* 40:2973, 2009.

77. Levy E, Lobez-Otin C, Ghiso J, et al: Stroke in Icelandic patients with hereditary amyloid angiopathy is related to a mutation in the cystatin C gene, an inhibitor of cysteine proteases, *J Exp Med* 169:1771, 1989.

78. Vidal R, Frangione B, Rostagno A, et al: A stop-codon mutation in the BRI gene associated with familial British dementia, *Nature* 399:776, 1999.

79. Mead S, James-Galton M, Revesz T, et al: Familial British dementia with amyloid angiopathy: Early clinical, neuropsychological and imaging findings, *Brain* 123:975, 2000.

80. Mascalchi M, Salvi F, Pirini MG, et al: Transthyretin amyloidosis and superficial siderosis of the CNS, *Neurology* 53:1498, 1999.

81. Selkoe DJ: The origins of Alzheimer disease: A is for amyloid, *JAMA* 283:1615, 2000.

82. Levy E, Carman MD, Fernandez Madrid IJ, et al: Mutation of the Alzheimer's disease amyloid gene in hereditary cerebral hemorrhage, Dutch type, *Science* 248:1124, 1990.

83. Van Broeckhoven C, Haan J, Bakker E, et al: Amyloid beta protein precursor gene and hereditary cerebral hemorrhage with amyloidosis (Dutch), *Science* 248:1120, 1990.

84. Bornebroek M, Westendorp RG, Haan J, et al: Mortality from hereditary cerebral haemorrhage with amyloidosis-Dutch type: The impact of sex, parental transmission and year of birth, *Brain* 120:2243, 1997.

85. Miravalle L, Tokuda T, Chiarle R, et al: Substitutions at codon 22 of Alzheimer's Abeta peptide induce diverse conformational changes and apoptotic effects in human cerebral endothelial cells, *J Biol Chem* 275:27110, 2000.

86. Tagliavini F, Rossi G, Padovani A, et al: A new βPP mutation related to hereditary cerebral haemorrhage, *Alzheimers Rep* 2:S28, 1999.

87. Natte R, Vinters HV, Maat-Schieman ML, et al: Microvasculopathy is associated with the number of cerebrovascular lesions in hereditary cerebral hemorrhage with amyloidosis, Dutch type, *Stroke* 29:1588, 1998.

88. Cras P, van Harskamp F, Hendriks L, et al: Presenile Alzheimer dementia characterized by amyloid angiopathy and large amyloid core type senile plaques in the APP 692Ala->Gly mutation, *Acta Neuropathol (Berl)* 96:253, 1998.

89. Grabowski TJ, Cho HS, Vonsattel JPG, et al: Novel amyloid precursor protein mutation in an Iowa family with dementia and severe cerebral amyloid angiopathy, *Ann Neurol* 49:697, 2001.

90. Wang Z, Natte R, Berliner JA, et al: Toxicity of Dutch (E22Q) and Flemish (A21G) mutant amyloid beta proteins to human cerebral microvessel and aortic smooth muscle cells, *Stroke* 31:534, 2000.

91. Van Nostrand WE, Melchor JP, Cho HS, et al: Pathogenic effects of D23N Iowa mutant amyloid beta-protein, *J Biol Chem* 276:32860, 2001.

92. Nagai A, Kobayashi S, Shimode K, et al: No mutations in cystatin C gene in cerebral amyloid angiopathy with cystatin C deposition, *Mol Chem Neuropathol* 33:63, 1998.

93. McCarron MO, Nicoll JA, Stewart J, et al: Absence of cystatin C mutation in sporadic cerebral amyloid angiopathy-related hemorrhage, *Neurology* 54:242, 2000.

94. McCarron MO, Nicoll JA, Stewart J, et al: The apolipoprotein E epsilon2 allele and the pathological features in cerebral amyloid angiopathy-related hemorrhage, *J Neuropathol Exp Neurol* 58:711, 1999.

95. Olichney JM, Hansen LA, Galasko D, et al: The apolipoprotein E epsilon 4 allele is associated with increased neuritic plaques and cerebral amyloid angiopathy in Alzheimer's disease and Lewy body variant, *Neurology* 47:190, 1996.

96. Greenberg SM, Vonsattel JP, Segal AZ, et al: Association of apolipoprotein E epsilon2 and vasculopathy in cerebral amyloid angiopathy, *Neurology* 50:961, 1998.

97. McCarron MO, Nicoll JAR: ApoE genotype in relation to sporadic and Alzheimer-related CAA. In Verbeek MM, de Waal MW, Vinters HV, editors: *Cerebral amyloid angiopathy in Alzheimer's disease and related disorders*, Dordrecht, 2000, Kluwer Academic Publishers, p 81.

98. O'Donnell HC, Rosand J, Knudsen KA, et al: Apolipoprotein E genotype and the risk of recurrent lobar intracerebral hemorrhage, *N Engl J Med* 342:240, 2000.

99. Fisher CM: The pathology and pathogenesis of intracerebral hemorrhage. In Fields WS, editor: *Pathogenesis and Treatment of Cerebrovascular Disease*, Springfield, IL, 1961, Charles C Thomas, p 295.

100. Kase CS, Williams JP, Wyatt DA, Mohr JP: Lobar intracerebral hematomas: Clinical and CT analysis of 22 cases, *Neurology* 32:1146, 1982.

101. Wiggins WS, Moody DM, Toole JF, et al: Clinical and computerized tomographic study of hypertensive intracerebral hemorrhage, *Arch Neurol* 35:832, 1978.

102. Fisher CM: The pathologic and clinical aspects of thalamic hemorrhage, *Trans Am Neurol Assoc* 84:56, 1959.

103. Freytag E: Fatal hypertensive intracerebral haematomas: A survey of the pathological anatomy of 393 cases, *J Neurol Neurosurg Psychiatry* 31:616, 1968.

104. Walshe TM, Davis KR, Fisher CM: Thalamic hemorrhage: A computed tomographic-clinical correlation, *Neurology* 27:217, 1977.

105. Dinsdale HB: Spontaneous hemorrhage in the posterior fossa: A study of primary cerebellar and pontine hemorrhage with observations on the pathogenesis, *Arch Neurol* 10:200, 1964.

106. Fisher CM, Picard EH, Polak A, et al: Acute hypertensive cerebellar hemorrhage: Diagnosis and surgical treatment, *J Nerv Ment Dis* 140:38, 1965.

107. Fisher CM: The arterial lesions underlying lacunes, *Acta Neuropathol* 12:1, 1969.

108. Fisher CM: Lacunes: Small, deep cerebral infarcts, *Neurology* 15:774, 1965.

109. Fisher CM: Cerebral ischemia: Less familiar types, *Clin Neurosurg* 18:267, 1971.

110. Cole FM, Yates PO: Intracranial microaneurysms and small cerebrovascular lesions, *Brain* 90:759, 1967.

111. Cole FM, Yates PO: Pseudo-aneurysms in relationship to massive cerebral hemorrhage, *J Neurol Neurosurg Psychiatry* 30:61, 1967.

112. Rosenblum WI: Miliary aneurysms and "fibrinoid" degeneration of cerebral blood vessels, *Hum Pathol* 8:133, 1977.

113. Cole FM, Yates PO: Comparative incidence of cerebrovascular lesions in normotensive and hypertensive patients, *Neurology* 18:255, 1968.

114. Charcot JM, Bouchard C: Nouvelles recherches sur la pathogénie de l'hémorragie cérébrale, *Arch Physiol Norm Pathol* 1:110, 1868.

115. Ellis AG: The pathogenesis of spontaneous cerebral hemorrhage, *Proc Pathol Soc* 12:197, 1909.

116. Green FHK: Miliary aneurysms in the brain, *J Pathol Bacteriol* 33:71, 1930.

117. Ross Russell RW: Observations on intracerebral aneurysms, *Brain* 86:425, 1963.

118. Cole FM, Yates PO: The occurrence and significance of intracerebral microaneurysms, *J Pathol Bacteriol* 93:393, 1967.

119. Fisher CM: Cerebral miliary aneurysms in hypertension, *Am J Pathol* 66:313, 1972.

120. Herbstein DJ, Schaumburg HH: Hypertensive intracerebral hematoma: An investigation of the initial hemorrhage and rebleeding using chromium Cr 51-labeled erythrocytes, *Arch Neurol* 30:412, 1974.

121. Kelley RE, Berger JR, Scheinberg P, Stokes N: Active bleeding in hypertensive intracerebral hemorrhage: Computed tomography, *Neurology* 32:852, 1982.

122. Broderick JP, Brott TG, Tomsick T, et al: Ultra-early evaluation of intracerebral hemorrhage, *J Neurosurg* 72:195, 1990.

123. Fehr MA, Anderson DC: Incidence of progression or rebleeding in hypertensive intracerebral hemorrhage, *J Stroke Cerebrovasc Dis* 1:111, 1991.

124. Fujii Y, Tanaka R, Takeuchi S, et al: Hematoma enlargement in spontaneous intracerebral hemorrhage, *J Neurosurg* 80:51, 1994.

125. Kazui S, Naritomi H, Yamamoto H, et al: Enlargement of spontaneous intracerebral hemorrhage: Incidence and time course, *Stroke* 27:1783, 1996.

126. Brott T, Broderick J, Kothari R, et al: Early hemorrhage growth in patients with intracerebral hemorrhage, *Stroke* 28:1, 1997.

127. Wada R, Aviv RI, Fox AJ, et al: CT angiography "spot sign" predicts hematoma expansion in acute intracerebral hemorrhage, *Stroke* 38:1257, 2007.

128. Goldstein JN, Fazen LE, Snider R, et al: Contrast extravasation on CT angiography predicts hematoma expansion in intracerebral hemorrhage, *Neurology* 68:889, 2007.

129. Thompson AL, Kosior JC, Gladstone DJ, et al: Defining the CT angiography 'spot sign' in primary intracereberal hemorrhage, *Can J Neurol Sci* 36:456, 2009.

130. Delgado Almandoz JE, Yoo AJ, Stone MJ, et al: Systematic characterization of the computed tomography angiography spot sign in primary intracerebral hemorrhage identifies patients at highest risk for hematoma expansion: the spot sign score, *Stroke* 40:2994, 2009.

131. Broderick J, Brott TG, Duldner JE, et al: Volume of intracerebral hemorrhage: A powerful and easy-to-use predictor of 30-day mortality, *Stroke* 24:987, 1993.

132. Kothari RU, Brott T, Broderick JP, et al: The ABCs of measuring intracerebral hemorrhage volumes, *Stroke* 27:1304, 1996.

133. Lisk DR, Pasteur W, Rhoades H, et al: Early presentation of hemispheric intracerebral hematoma: Prediction of outcome and guidelines for treatment allocation, *Neurology* 44:133, 1994.

134. Stein RW, Kase CS, Hier DB, et al: Caudate hemorrhage, *Neurology* 34:1549, 1984.

135. Hier DB, Davis KR, Richardson EP, Mohr JP: Hypertensive putaminal hemorrhage, *Ann Neurol* 1:152, 1977.

136. Fisher CM: Capsular infarcts, *Arch Neurol* 36:65, 1979.

137. Ropper AH, Davis KR: Lobar cerebral hemorrhages: Acute clinical syndromes in 26 cases, *Ann Neurol* 8:141, 1980.

138. Kase CS, Maulsby GO, Mohr JP: Partial pontine hematomas, *Neurology* 30:652, 1980.

139. Caplan LR, Goodwin JA: Lateral tegmental brainstem hemorrhages, *Neurology* 32:252, 1982.

140. Fieschi C, Carolei A, Fiorelli M, et al: Changing prognosis of primary intracerebral hemorrhage: Results of a clinical and computed tomographic follow-up study of 104 patients, *Stroke* 19:192, 1988.

141. González-Duarte A, Cantú C, Ruiz-Sandoval JL, et al: Recurrent primary cerebral hemorrhage: Frequency, mechanisms, and prognosis, *Stroke* 29:1998, 1802.

142. Bae H, Jeong D, Doh J, et al: Recurrence of bleeding in patients with hypertensive intracerebral hemorrhage, *Cerebrovasc Dis* 9:102, 1999.

143. Hickey WF, King RB, Wang A-M, et al: Multiple simultaneous intracerebral hematomas: Clinical, radiologic, and pathologic findings in two patients, *Arch Neurol* 40:519, 1983.

144. Weisberg L: Multiple spontaneous intracerebral hematomas: Clinical and computed tomographic correlations, *Neurology* 31:897, 1981.

145. Bailey RD, Hart RG, Benavente O, et al: Recurrent brain hemorrhage is more frequent than ischemic stroke after intracranial hemorrhage, *Neurology* 56:773, 2001.

146. García JH, Ho KL, Caccamo DV: Intracerebral hemorrhage: Pathology of selected topics. In Kase CS, Caplan LR, editors: *Intracerebral Hemorrhage*, Boston, 1994, Butterworth-Heinemann, p 45.

147. Jenkins A, Maxwell W, Graham D: Experimental intracerebral hematoma in the rat: Sequential light microscopic changes, *Neuropathol Appl Neurobiol* 15:477, 1989.

148. Jarrett JT, Berger EP, Lansbury PT: The carboxy terminus of the beta amyloid protein is critical for the seeding of amyloid formation: Implications for the pathogenesis of Alzheimer's disease, *Biochemistry* 32:4693, 1993.

149. Natte R, Yamaguchi H, Maat-Schieman ML, et al: Ultrastructural evidence of early non-fibrillar Abeta42 in the capillary basement membrane of patients with hereditary cerebral hemorrhage with amyloidosis, Dutch type, *Acta Neuropathol (Berl)* 98:577, 1999.

150. Castano EM, Prelli F, Soto C, et al: The length of amyloid-beta in hereditary cerebral hemorrhage with amyloidosis, Dutch type: Implications for the role of amyloid-beta 1-42 in Alzheimer's disease, *J Biol Chem* 271:32185, 1996.

151. Mann DM, Iwatsubo T, Ihara Y, et al: Predominant deposition of amyloid-beta 42(43) in plaques in cases of Alzheimer's disease and hereditary cerebral hemorrhage associated with mutations in the amyloid precursor protein gene, *Am J Pathol* 148:1257, 1996.

152. Alonzo NC, Hyman BT, Rebeck GW, et al: Progression of cerebral amyloid angiopathy: Accumulation of amyloid-β40 in already affected vessels, *J Neuropathol Exp Neurol* 57:353, 1998.

153. Vinters HV, Nishimura GS, Secor DL, et al: Immunoreactive A4 and gamma-trace peptide colocalization in amyloidotic arteriolar lesions in brains of patients with Alzheimer's disease, *Am J Pathol* 137:233, 1990.

154. Cho HS, Hyman BT, Greenberg SM, et al: Quantitation of apoE domains in Alzheimer disease brain suggests a role for apoE in Abeta aggregation, *J Neuropathol Exp Neurol* 60:342, 2001.

155. Eisenhauer PB, Johnson RJ, Wells JM, et al: Toxicity of various amyloid beta peptide species in cultured human blood-brain barrier endothelial cells: Increased toxicity of Dutch-type mutant, *J Neurosci Res* 60:804, 2000.

156. Melchor JP, McVoy L, Van Nostrand WE: Charge alterations of E22 enhance the pathogenic properties of the amyloid beta-protein, *J Neurochem* 74:2209, 2000.

157. Melchor JP, Van Nostrand WE: Fibrillar amyloid beta-protein mediates the pathologic accumulation of its secreted precursor in human cerebrovascular smooth muscle cells, *J Biol Chem* 275:9782, 2000.

158. Van Nostrand WE, Porter M: Plasmin cleavage of the amyloid beta-protein: Alteration of secondary structure and stimulation of tissue plasminogen activator activity, *Biochemistry* 38:11570, 1999.

159. Van Dorpe J, Smeijers L, Dewachter I, et al: Prominent cerebral amyloid angiopathy in transgenic mice overexpressing the London mutant of human APP in neurons, *Am J Pathol* 157:1283, 2000.

160. Christie R, Yamada M, Moskowitz M, et al: Structural and functional disruption of vascular smooth muscle cells in a transgenic mouse model of amyloid angiopathy, *Am J Pathol* 158:1065, 2001.

161. Winkler DT, Bondolfi L, Herzig MC, et al: Spontaneous hemorrhagic stroke in a mouse model of cerebral amyloid angiopathy, *J Neurosci* 21:1619, 2001.

162. Weller RO, Massey A, Newman TA, et al: Cerebral amyloid angiopathy: Amyloid beta accumulates in putative interstitial fluid drainage pathways in Alzheimer's disease, *Am J Pathol* 153:725, 1998.

163. Ruiz-Sandoval JL, Cantú C, Barinagarrementeria F: Intracerebral hemorrhage in young people: Analysis of risk factors, location, causes, and prognosis, *Stroke* 30:537, 1999.

164. Margolis G, Odom GL, Woodhall B, Bloor BM: The role of small angiomatous malformations in the production of intracerebral hematomas, *J Neurosurg* 8:564, 1951.

165. Crawford JV, Russell DS: Cryptic arteriovenous and venous hamartomas of the brain, *J Neurol Neurosurg Psychiatry* 19:1, 1956.

166. Krayenbühl H, Siebenmann R: Small vascular malformations as a cause of primary intracerebral hemorrhage, *J Neurosurg* 22:7, 1965.

167. Russell DS: The pathology of spontaneous intracranial haemorrhage, *Proc Soc Med* 47:689, 1954.

168. Becker DH, Townsend JJ, Kramer RA, et al: Occult cerebrovascular malformations: A series of 18 histologically verified cases with negative angiography, *Brain* 70:530, 1979.

169. Roberson GH, Kase CS, Wolpow ER: Telangiectases and cavernous angiomas of the brainstem: "Cryptic" vascular malformations, *Neuroradiology* 8:83, 1974.

170. Wakai S, Ueda Y, Inoh S, et al: Angiographically occult angiomas: A report of thirteen cases with analysis of the cases documented in the literature, *Neurosurgery* 17:549, 1985.

171. Bicknell JM, Carlow TJ, Kornfeld M, et al: Familial cavernous angiomas, *Arch Neurol* 35:746, 1978.

172. Clark JV: Familial occurrence of cavernous angiomata of the brain, *J Neurol Neurosurg Psychiatry* 33:871, 1970.

173. Kattapong VJ, Hart BL, Davis LE: Familial cerebral cavernous angiomas: Clinical and radiological studies, *Neurology* 45:492, 1995.

174. Labauge P, Brunereau L, Levy C, et al: The natural history of familial cerebral cavernomas: A retrospective MRI study of 40 patients, *Neuroradiology* 42:327, 2000.

175. Labauge P, Brunereau L, Laberge S, et al: Prospective follow-up of 33 asymptomatic patients with familial cerebral cavernous malformations, *Neurology* 57:1825, 2001.

176. Stahl SM, Johnson KP, Malamud N: The clinical and pathological spectrum of brainstem vascular malformations: Long-term course simulates multiple sclerosis, *Arch Neurol* 37:25, 1980.

177. Robinson JR, Awad IA, Little JR: Natural history of the cavernous angioma, *J Neurosurg* 75:709, 1991.

178. Zabramski JM, Wascher TM, Spetzler RF, et al: The natural history of familial cavernous malformations: Results of an ongoing study, *J Neurosurg* 80:422, 1994.

179. Kondziolka D, Lunsford LD, Kestle JR: The natural history of cerebral cavernous malformations, *J Neurosurg* 83:820, 1995.

180. Requena I, Arias M, Lopez-Ibor L, et al: Cavernomas of the central nervous system: Clinical and neuroimaging manifestations in 47 patients, *J Neurol Neurosurg Psychiatry* 54:590, 1991.

181. Rigamonti D, Drayer BP, Johnson PC, et al: The MRI appearance of cavernous malformations (angiomas), *J Neurosurg* 67:518, 1987.

182. Zimmerman RS, Spetzler RF, Lee KS, et al: Cavernous malformations of the brain stem, *J Neurosurg* 75:32, 1991.

183. Simard JM, Garcia-Bengochea F, Ballinger WE, et al: Cavernous angioma: A review of 126 collected and 12 new clinical cases, *Neurosurgery* 18:162, 1986.

184. Rigamonti D, Hadley MN, Drayer BP, et al: Cerebral cavernous malformations: Incidence and familial occurrence, *N Engl J Med* 319:343, 1988.

185. Gil-Nagel A, Dubovsky J, Wilcox KJ, et al: Familial cerebral cavernous angioma: A gene localized to a 15-cM interval on chromosome 7q, *Ann Neurol* 39:807, 1996.

186. Günel M, Awad IA, Finberg K, et al: A founder mutation as a cause of cerebral cavernous malformation in Hispanic Americans, *N Engl J Med* 334:946, 1996.

187. Akers AL, Johnson JE, Steinberg GK, et al: Biallelic somatic and germline mutations in cerebral cavernous malformations (CCMs): Evidence for a two-hit mechanism of CCM pathogenesis, *Hum Mol Genet* 18:919, 2009.

188. Delaney P, Estes M: Intracranial hemorrhage with amphetamine abuse, *Neurology* 30:1125, 1980.

189. D'Souza T, Shraberg D: Intracranial hemorrhage associated with amphetamine use (letter), *Neurology* 31:922, 1981.

190. Harrington H, Heller HA, Dawson D, et al: Intracerebral hemorrhage and oral amphetamine, *Arch Neurol* 40:503, 1983.

191. Loizou LA, Hamilton JG, Tsementzis SA: Intracranial hemorrhage in association with pseudoephedrine overdose, *J Neurol Neurosurg Psychiatry* 45:471, 1982.

192. Citron BP, Halpern M, McCarron M, et al: Necrotizing angiitis associated with drug abuse, *N Engl J Med* 283:1003, 1970.

193. Margolis MT, Newton TH: Methamphetamine ("speed") arteritis, *Neuroradiology* 2:179, 1971.

194. Rumbaugh CL, Bergeron RT, Fang HCH, et al: Cerebral angiographic changes in the drug abuse patient, *Radiology* 101:335, 1971.

195. Yu YJ, Cooper DR, Wellenstein DE, et al: Cerebral angiitis and intracerebral hemorrhage associated with methamphetamine abuse, *J Neurosurg* 58:109, 1983.

196. Lukes SA: Intracerebral hemorrhage from an arteriovenous malformation after amphetamine injection, *Arch Neurol* 40:60, 1983.

197. Matick H, Anderson D, Brumlik J: Cerebral vasculitis associated with oral amphetamine overdose, *Arch Neurol* 40:253, 1983.

198. Kase CS, Foster TE, Reed JE, et al: Intracerebral hemorrhage and phenylpropanolamine use, *Neurology* 37:399, 1987.

199. Kernan WN, Viscoli CM, Brass LM, et al: Phenylpropanolamine and the risk of hemorrhagic stroke, *N Engl J Med* 343:2000, 1826.

200. Barinagarrementeria F, Méndez A, Vega F: Hemorragia cerebral asociada al uso de fenilpropanolamina, *Neurología* 5:292, 1990.

201. Bernstein E, Diskant BM: Phenylpropanolamine: A potentially hazardous drug, *Ann Emerg Med* 11:311, 1982.

202. Fallis RJ, Fisher M: Cerebral vasculitis and hemorrhage associated with phenylpropanolamine, *Neurology* 35:405, 1985.

203. Kikta DG, Devereaux MX, Chandar K: Intracranial hemorrhages due to phenylpropanolamine, *Stroke* 16:510, 1985.

204. Stoessl AJ, Young GB, Feasby TE: Intracerebral haemorrhage and angiographic beading following ingestion of catecholaminergics, *Stroke* 16:734, 1985.

205. Glick R, Hoying J, Cerullo L, et al: Phenylpropanolamine: An over-the-counter drug causing central nervous system vasculitis and intracerebral hemorrhage, *Neurosurgery* 20:969, 1987.

206. MacDougall JD, Tuxen D, Sale DG, et al: Arterial blood pressure response to heavy exercise, *J Appl Physiol* 58:785, 1985.

207. Levine SR, Brust JCM, Futrell N, et al: Cerebrovascular complications of the use of the "crack" form of alkaloid cocaine, *N Engl J Med* 323:699, 1990.

208. Green RM, Kelly KM, Gabrielsen T, et al: Multiple intracranial hemorrhages after smoking "crack" cocaine, *Stroke* 21:957, 1990.

209. Tapia JF, Golden JA: Case records of the Massachusetts General Hospital (Case 27-1993), *N Engl J Med* 329:117, 1993.

210. Little JR, Dial B, Bellanger G, et al: Brain hemorrhage from intracranial tumor, *Stroke* 10:283, 1979.

211. Scott M: Spontaneous intracerebral hematoma caused by cerebral neoplasms: Report of eight verified cases, *J Neurosurg* 42:338, 1975.

212. Modesti LM, Binet EF, Collins GH: Meningiomas causing spontaneous intracranial hematomas, *J Neurosurg* 45:437, 1976.

213. Wakai S, Yamakawa K, Manaka S, et al: Spontaneous intracranial hemorrhage caused by brain tumors: Its incidence and clinical significance, *Neurosurgery* 10:437, 1982.

214. Gildersleve N, Koo AH, McDonald CJ: Metastatic tumor presenting as intracerebral hemorrhage, *Radiology* 124:109, 1977.

215. Gurwitt LJ, Long JM, Clark RE: Cerebral metastatic choriocarcinoma: A postpartum cause of "stroke," *Obstet Gynecol* 45:583, 1975.

216. Mandybur TI: Intracranial hemorrhage caused by metastatic tumors, *Neurology* 27:650, 1977.

217. Vaughan HG, Howard RG: Intracranial hemorrhage due to metastatic chorionepithelioma, *Neurology* 12:771, 1962.

218. Graus F, Rogers LR, Posner JB: Cerebrovascular complications in patients with cancer, *Medicine* 64:16, 1985.

219. Zülch KJ: Neuropathology of intracranial haemorrhage, *Prog Brain Res* 30:151, 1968.

220. Shuangshoti S, Panyathanya R, Wichienkur P: Intracranial metastases from unsuspected choriocarcinoma: Onset suggestive of cerebrovascular disease, *Neurology (NY)* 24:649, 1974.

221. Herold S, von Kumer R, Jaeger CH: Follow-up of spontaneous intracerebral haemorrhage by computed tomography, *J Neurol* 228:267, 1982.

222. Weisberg LA: Computerized tomography in intracranial hemorrhage, *Arch Neurol* 36:422, 1979.

223. Zimmerman RD, Leeds NE, Naidich TP: Ring blush associated with intracerebral hematoma, *Radiology* 122:707, 1977.

224. Kase CS: Intracerebral hemorrhage: Non-hypertensive causes, *Stroke* 17:590, 1986.

225. Iwama T, Ohkuma A, Miwa Y, et al: Brain tumors manifesting as intracranial hemorrhage, *Neurol Med Chir* 32:130, 1992.

226. Kase CS, Robinson RK, Stein RW, et al: Anticoagulant-related intracerebral hemorrhage, *Neurology* 35:943, 1985.

227. Rådberg JA, Olsson JE, Rådberg CT: Prognostic parameters in spontaneous intracranial hematomas with special reference to anticoagulant treatment, *Stroke* 22:571, 1991.

228. Ott KH, Kase CS, Ojemann RG, Mohr JP: Cerebellar hemorrhage: Diagnosis and treatment, *Arch Neurol* 31:160, 1974.

229. Franke CL, deJonge J, van Swieten JC, et al: Intracerebral hematomas during anticoagulant treatment, *Stroke* 21:726, 1990.

230. Hart RG, Boop BS, Anderson DC: Oral anticoagulants and intracranial hemorrhage, *Stroke* 26:1471, 1995.

231. Whisnant JP, Cartlidge NEF, Elveback LR: Carotid and vertebral-basilar transient ischemic attacks: Effect of anticoagulants, hypertension, and cardiac disorders on survival and stroke occurrence in a population study, *Ann Neurol* 3:107, 1978.

232. Wintzen AR, de Jonge H, Loeliger EA, Bots GTAM: The risk of intracerebral hemorrhage during oral anticoagulant treatment: A population study, *Ann Neurol* 16:553, 1984.

233. Hylek EM, Singer DE: Risk factors for intracranial hemorrhage in outpatients taking warfarin, *Ann Intern Med* 120:897, 1994.

234. Landefeld CS, Goldman L: Major bleeding in outpatients treated with warfarin: Incidence and prediction by factors known at the start of outpatient therapy, *Am J Med* 87:144, 1989.

235. Barron KD, Fergusson G: Intracranial hemorrhage as a complication of anticoagulant therapy, *Neurology* 9:447, 1959.

236. Dawson I, van Bockel JH, Ferrari MD, et al: Ischemic and hemorrhagic stroke in patients on oral anticoagulants after reconstruction for chronic lower limb ischemia, *Stroke* 24:1655, 1993.

237. Smith EE, Rosand J, Knudsen KA, et al: Leukoaraiosis is associated with warfarin-related hemorrhage following ischemic stroke, *Neurology* 59:193, 2002.

238. Hart RG, Pearce LA: In vivo antithrombotic effect of aspirin: Dose versus nongastrointestinal bleeding, *Stroke* 24:138, 1993.

239. Snyder M, Renaudin J: Intracranial hemorrhage associated with anticoagulation therapy, *Surg Neurol* 7:31, 1977.

240. The Stroke Prevention In Reversible Ischemia Trial (SPIRIT) Study Group: A randomized trial of anticoagulants versus aspirin after cerebral ischemia of presumed arterial origin, *Ann Neurol* 42:857, 1997.

241. Stroke Prevention in Atrial Fibrillation Investigators: Warfarin versus aspirin for prevention of thromboembolism in atrial fibrillation, *Lancet* 343:687, 1994.

242. Filibotte JJ, Hagan N, O'Donnell J, et al: Warfarin, hematoma expansion, and outcome of intracerebral hemorrhage, *Neurology* 63:1059, 2004.

243. Rosand J, Hylek EM, O'Donnell HC, et al: Warfarin-associated hemorrhage and cerebral amyloid angiopathy: A genetic and pathologic study, *Neurology* 55:947, 2000.

244. Drapkin A, Merskey C: Anticoagulant therapy after acute myocardial infarction: Relation of therapeutic benefit to patient's age, sex, and severity of infarction, *JAMA* 222:541, 1972.

245. Handley AJ, Emerson PA, Fleming PR: Heparin in the prevention of deep vein thrombosis after myocardial infarction, *BMJ* 2:436, 1972.

246. Fisher CM, Adams RD: Observations on brain embolism with special reference to the mechanism of hemorrhagic infarction, *J Neuropathol Exp Neurol* 10:92, 1951.

247. Camerlingo M, Casto L, Censori B, et al: Immediate anticoagulation with heparin for first-ever ischemic stroke in the carotid artery territories observed within 5 hours of onset, *Arch Neurol* 51:462, 1994.

248. Babikian VL, Kase CS, Pessin MS, et al: Intracerebral hemorrhage in stroke patients anticoagulated with heparin, *Stroke* 20:1500, 1989.

249. Chamorro A, Villa N, Saiz A, et al: Early anticoagulation after large cerebral embolic infarction: A safety study, *Neurology* 45:861, 1995.

250. Cerebral Embolism Study Group: Immediate anticoagulation of embolic stroke: Brain hemorrhage and management options, *Stroke* 15:779, 1984.

251. Adams HP: Emergent use of anticoagulation for treatment of patients with ischemic stroke, *Stroke* 33:856, 2002.

252. Chamorro A: Immediate anticoagulation in acute focal brain ischemia revisited: Gathering the evidence, *Stroke* 32:577, 2001.

253. Chamorro A, Busse O, Obach V, et al: The Rapid Anticoagulation Prevents Ischemic Damage study in acute stroke: Final results from the Writing Committee, *Cerebrovasc Dis* 19:402, 2005.

254. TIMI Study Group: Comparison of invasive and conservative strategies after treatment with intravenous tissue plasminogen activator in acute myocardial infarction: Results of the Thrombolysis in Myocardial Infarction (TIMI) phase II trial, *N Engl J Med* 320:618, 1989.

255. Gore JM, Sloan M, Price TR, et al: Intracerebral hemorrhage, cerebral infarction, and subdural hematoma after acute myocardial infarction and thrombolytic therapy in the Thrombolysis in Myocardial Infarction Study: Thrombolysis in myocardial infarction, phase II, pilot and clinical data, *Circulation* 83:448, 1991.

256. Kase CS, O'Neal AM, Fisher M, et al: Intracranial hemorrhage after use of tissue plasminogen activator for coronary thrombolysis, *Ann Intern Med* 112:17, 1990.

257. Kase CS, Pessin MS, Zivin JA, et al: Intracranial hemorrhage following coronary thrombolysis with tissue plasminogen activator, *Am J Med* 92:384, 1992.

258. O'Connor CM, Aldrich H, Massey EW, et al: Intracranial hemorrhage after thrombolytic therapy for acute myocardial infarction: Clinical characteristics and in-hospital outcome [abstract], *J Am Coll Cardiol* 15:213A, 1990.

259. Sloan MA, Price TR, Petito CK, et al: Clinical features and pathogenesis of intracerebral hemorrhage after rt-PA and heparin therapy for acute myocardial infarction: The Thrombolysis in Myocardial Infarction (TIMI) II pilot and randomized clinical trial combined experience, *Neurology* 45:649, 1995.

260. Pendlebury WW, Iole ED, Tracy RP, Dill BA: Intracerebral hemorrhage related to cerebral amyloid angiopathy and t-PA treatment, *Ann Neurol* 29:210, 1991.

261. Wijdicks EFM, Jack CR: Intracerebral hemorrhage after fibrinolytic therapy for acute myocardial infarction, *Stroke* 24:554, 1993.

262. Pessin MS, del Zoppo GJ, Estol CJ: Thrombolytic agents in the treatment of stroke, *Clin Neuropharmacol* 13:271, 1990.

263. del Zoppo GJ, Poeck K, Pessin MS, et al: Recombinant tissue plasminogen activator in acute thrombotic and embolic stroke, *Ann Neurol* 32:78, 1992.

264. Wolpert SM, Bruckmann H, Greenlee R, et al: Neuroradiologic evaluation of patients with acute stroke treated with recombinant tissue plasminogen activator: The rt-PA Acute Stroke Study Group, *AJNR Am J Neuroradiol* 14:3, 1993.

265. Hacke W, Kaste M, Fieschi C, et al: Intravenous thrombolysis with recombinant tissue plasminogen activator for acute hemispheric stroke: The European Cooperative Acute Stroke Study (ECASS), *JAMA* 274:1017, 1995.

266. The National Institute of Neurological Disorders and Stroke rt-PA Stroke Study Group: Tissue plasminogen activator for acute ischemic stroke, *N Engl J Med* 333:1581, 1995.

267. The NINDS t-PA Stroke Study Group: Intracerebral hemorrhage after intravenous t-PA therapy for ischemic stroke, *Stroke* 28:2109, 1997.

268. Lansberg MG, Thijs VN, Bammer R, et al: Risk factors of symptomatic hemorrhage after tPA therapy for acute stroke, *Stroke* 38:2275, 2007.

269. Bruno A, Levine SR, Frankel MR, et al: Admission glucose level and clinical outcomes in the NINDS rt-PA stroke trial, *Neurology* 59:669, 2002.

270. Montaner J, Molina CA, Monasterio J, et al: Matrix metalloproteinase-9 pretreatment level predicts intracranial hemorrhagic complications after thrombolysis in human stroke, *Circulation* 107:598, 2003.

271. Castellanos M, Leira R, Serena J, et al: Plasma cellular-fibronectin concentration predicts hemorrhagic transformation after thrombolytic therapy in acute ischemic stroke, *Stroke* 35:1671, 2004.

272. Mendioroz M, Fernández-Cadenas I, Alvarez-Sabín J, et al: Endogenous activated protein C predicts hemorrhagic transformation and mortality after tissue plasminogen activator treatment in stroke patients, *Cerebrovasc Dis* 28:143, 2009.

273. Ribo M, Montaner J, Molina CA, et al: Admission fibrinolytic profile is associated with symptomatic hemorrhagic transformation in stroke patients treated with tissue plasminogen activator, *Stroke* 35:2123, 2004.

274. Donnan GA, Davis SM, Chambers BR, et al: Trials of streptokinase in severe acute ischaemic stroke [letter], *Lancet* 345:578, 1995.

275. Multicentre Acute Stroke Trial-Italy (MAST-I) Group: Randomised controlled trial of streptokinase, aspirin, and combination of both in treatment of acute ischaemic stroke, *Lancet* 346:1509, 1995.

276. The Multicenter Acute Stroke Trial-Europe Study Group: Thrombolytic therapy with streptokinase in acute ischemic stroke, *N Engl J Med* 335:145, 1996.

277. GISSI-2: A factorial randomised trial of alteplase versus streptokinase and heparin versus no heparin among 12,490 patients with acute myocardial infarction. Gruppo Italiano per lo Studio della Sopravivenza nell' Infarto Miocardico, *Lancet* 336:65, 1990.

278. Clark WM, Lyden PD, Madden KP, et al: Thrombolytic therapy in ischemic stroke [letter], *N Engl J Med* 336:65, 1997.

279. Del Zoppo GJ, Higashida RT, Furlan AJ, et al: PROACT: A phase II randomized trial of recombinant pro-urokinase by direct arterial delivery in acute middle cerebral artery stroke, *Stroke* 29:4, 1998.

280. Furlan A, Higashida R, Wechsler L, et al: Intra-arterial prourokinase for acute ischemic stroke: The PROACT II Study: A randomized controlled trial, *JAMA* 282:1999, 2003.

281. Kase CS, Furlan AJ, Wechsler LR, et al: Symptomatic intracerebral hemorrhage after intra-arterial thrombolysis with prourokinase in acute ischemic stroke: The PROACT II trial, *Neurology* 57:1603, 2001.

282. Kolodny EH, Rebeiz JJ, Caviness VS, Richardson EP: Granulomatous angiitis of the central nervous system, *Arch Neurol* 19:510, 1968.

283. Moore PM, Cupps TR: Neurological complications of vasculitis, *Ann Neurol* 14:155, 1983.

284. Hankey GJ: Isolated angiitis/angiopathy of the central nervous system, *Cerebrovasc Dis* 1:2, 1991.

285. Clifford-Jones RE, Love S, Gurusinghe N: Granulomatous angiitis of the central nervous system: A case with recurrent intracerebral hemorrhage, *J Neurol Neurosurg Psychiatry* 48:1054, 1985.

286. De Reuck J, Crevits L, Sieben G, et al: Granulomatous angiitis of the nervous system: A clinicopathological study of one case, *J Neurol* 227:49, 1982.

287. Biller J, Loftus CM, Moore SA, et al: Isolated central nervous system angiitis first presenting as spontaneous intracranial hemorrhage, *Neurosurgery* 20:310, 1987.

288. Probst A, Ulrich J: Amyloid angiopathy combined with granulomatous angiitis of the central nervous system: Report on two patients, *Clin Neuropathol* 4:250, 1985.

289. Shintaku M, Osawa K, Toki J, et al: A case of granulomatous angiitis of the central nervous system associated with amyloid angiopathy, *Acta Neuropathol* 70:340, 1986.

290. Linfante I, Llinas RH, Caplan LR, et al: MRI features of intracerebral hemorrhage within two hours from symptom onset, *Stroke* 30:2263, 1999.

291. Schellinger PD, Jansen O, Fiebach JB, et al: A standardized MRI stroke protocol: Comparison with CT in hyperacute intracerebral hemorrhage, *Stroke* 30:765, 1999.

292. Patel MR, Edelman RR, Warach S: Detection of hyperacute primary intraparenchymal hemorrhage by magnetic resonance imaging, *Stroke* 27:2321, 1996.

293. Tanaka A, Ueno Y, Nakayama Y, et al: Small chronic hemorrhages and ischemic lesions in association with spontaneous intracerebral hematomas, *Stroke* 30:1637, 1999.

294. Roob G, Schmidt R, Kapeller P, et al: MRI evidence of past cerebral microbleeds in a healthy elderly population, *Neurology* 52:991, 1999.

295. Atlas SW, Thulborn KR: MR detection of hyperacute parenchymal hemorrhage of the brain, *Am J Neuroradiol* 19:1471, 1998.

296. Kidwell CS, Saver JL, Villablanca JP, et al: Magnetic resonance imaging detection of microbleeds before thrombolysis: An emerging application, *Stroke* 33:95, 2002.

297. Kakuda W, Thijs VN, Lansberg MG, et al: Clinical importance of microbleeds in patients receiving IV thrombolysis, *Neurology* 65:1175, 2005.

298. Derex L, Nighoghossuian N, Hermier M, et al: Thrombolysis for ischemic stroke in patients with old microbleeds on pretreatment MRI, *Cerebrovasc Dis* 17:238, 2004.

299. Greenberg SM, Eng JA, Ning MM, et al: Hemorrhage burden predicts recurrent intracerebral hemorrhage after lobar hemorrhage, *Stroke* 35:1415, 2004.

300. Koenneke H-C: Cerebral microbleeds on MRI: Prevalence, associations, and potential clinical implications, *Neurology* 66:165, 2006.

301. Vernooij MW, Haag MDM, van der Lugt A, et al: Use of antithrombotic drugs and the presence of cerebral microbleeds: The Rotterdam Scan Study, *Arch Neurol* 66:714, 2009.

302. Wong KS, Chan YL, Liu JY, et al: Asymptomatic microbleeds as risk factors for aspirin-associated intracerebral hemorrhages, *Neurology* 60:511, 2003.

303. Tsushima Y, Aoki J, Endo K: Brain microhemorrhages detected on T2-weighted gradient-echo MR images, *AJNR Am J Neuroradiol* 24:88, 2003.

304. Greenberg SM, Finklestein SP, Schaefer PW: Petechial hemorrhages accompanying lobar hemorrhage: Detection by gradient-echo MRI, *Neurology* 46:1751, 1996.

305. Jeerakathil TJ, Wolf PA, Beiser AB, et al: Gradient-echo cerebral microbleeds predict diminished cognitive function in a community-based sample: The Framingham Study [abstract], *Stroke* 33:345, 2002.

306. Fisher CM: Clinical syndromes in cerebral hemorrhage. In Fields WS, editor: *Pathogenesis and treatment of cerebrovascular disease*, Springfield, IL, 1961, Charles C Thomas, p 318.

307. Ojemann RG, Mohr JP: Hypertensive brain hemorrhage, *Clin Neurosurg* 23:220, 1976.

308. Portenoy RK, Lipton RB, Berger AR, et al: Intracerebral hemorrhage: A model for the prediction of outcome, *J Neurol Neurosurg Psychiatry* 50:976, 1987.

309. Tuhrim S, Dambrosia JM, Price TR, et al: Prediction of intracerebral hemorrhage survival, *Ann Neurol* 24:258, 1988.

310. Aring CD: Differential diagnosis of cerebrovascular stroke, *Arch Intern Med* 113:195, 1964.

311. Abu-Zeid HAH, Choi NW, Maini KK, et al: Relative role of factors associated with cerebral infarction and cerebral hemorrhage, *Stroke* 8:106, 1977.

312. Walsh FB, Hoyt WK: *Clinical neuro-ophthalmology*, ed 3, Baltimore, 1969, Williams & Wilkins, p 1786.

313. Myoung CL, Heany LM, Jacobson RL, et al: Cerebrospinal fluid in cerebral hemorrhage and infarction, *Stroke* 6:638, 1975.

314. Kjellin KG, Soderstrom CE: Cerebral haemorrhages with atypical clinical patterns: A study of cerebral hematomas using CSF spectrophotometry and computerized transverse axial tomography ("EMI scanning"), *J Neurol Sci* 25:211, 1975.

315. Plum F, Posner JB: *The diagnosis of stupor and coma*, ed 3, Philadelphia, 1980, FA Davis.

316. Taveras JM, Wood EH: *Diagnostic neuroradiology*, vol 2, ed 2, Baltimore, 1976, Williams & Wilkins, p 1018.

317. Kowada M, Yamaguchi K, Matsuoka S, Ito Z: Extravasation of angiographic contrast material in hypertensive intracerebral hemorrhage, *J Neurosurg* 36:471, 1972.

318. Mizukami M, Araki G, Mihara H, et al: Arteriographically visualized extravasation in hypertensive intracerebral hemorrhage: Report of seven cases, *Stroke* 3:527, 1972.

319. Mizukami M, Araki G, Mihara H: Angiographic sign of good prognosis for hemiplegia in hypertensive intracerebral hemorrhage, *Neurology* 24:120, 1974.

320. Merritt HH: *A textbook of neurology*, ed 6, Philadelphia, 1979, Lea & Febiger, p 160.

321. Silliman S, McGill J, Booth R: Simultaneous bilateral hypertensive putaminal hemorrhages, *J Stroke Cerebrovasc Dis* 12:44, 2003.

322. Silverstein A: Intracranial hemorrhage in patients with bleeding tendencies, *Neurology* 11:310, 1961.

323. Gilles C, Brucher JM, Khoubesserian P, et al: Cerebral amyloid angiopathy as a cause of multiple intracerebral hemorrhages, *Neurology* 34:730, 1984.

324. Tapia JF, Kase CS, Sawyer RH, Mohr JP: Hypertensive putaminal hemorrhage presenting as pure motor hemiparesis, *Stroke* 14:505, 1983.

325. Kim JS, Lee JH, Lee MC: Small primary intracerebral hemorrhage: Clinical presentation of 28 cases, *Stroke* 25:1500, 1994.

326. Chung C, Caplan LR, Yamamoto Y, et al: Striatocapsular haemorrhage, *Brain* 123:1850, 2000.

327. Kim JS: Lenticulocapsular hemorrhages presenting as pure sensory stroke, *Eur Neurol* 42:128, 1999.

328. Jones HR, Baker RA, Kott HS: Hypertensive putaminal hemorrhage presenting with hemichorea, *Stroke* 16:130, 1985.

329. Altafullah I, Pascual-Leone A, Duvall K, et al: Putaminal hemorrhage accompanied by hemichorea-hemiballism, *Stroke* 27:1093, 1990.

330. Weisberg LA, Stazio A, Elliott D, et al: Putaminal hemorrhage: Clinical-computed tomographic correlations, *Neuroradiology* 32:200, 1990.

331. Mohr JP, Steinke W, Timsit SG, et al: The anterior choroidal artery does not supply the corona radiata and lateral ventricular wall, *Stroke* 22:1502, 1991.

332. D'Esposito M, Alexander MP: Subcortical aphasia: Distinct profiles following left putaminal hemorrhage, *Neurology* 45:38, 1995.

333. Weisberg LA, Elliott D, Shamsnia M: Massive putaminal-thalamic nontraumatic hemorrhage, *Comput Med Imaging Graph* 16:353, 1992.

334. Fuh JL, Wang SJ: Caudate hemorrhage: Clinical features, neuropsychological assessments and radiological findings, *Clin Neurol Neurosurg* 97:296, 1995.

335. Kumral E, Evyapan D, Balkir K: Acute caudate vascular lesions, *Stroke* 30:100, 1999.

336. Weisberg LA: Caudate hemorrhage, *Arch Neurol* 41:971, 1984.

337. Waga S, Fujimoto K, Okada M, et al: Caudate hemorrhage, *Neurosurgery* 18:445, 1986.

338. Steinke W, Tatemichi TK, Mohr JP, et al: Caudate hemorrhage with moyamoya-like vasculopathy from atherosclerotic disease, *Stroke* 23:1360, 1992.

339. Suzuki J, Kodama N: Moyamoya disease: A review, *Stroke* 14:104, 1983.

340. Stephen R, Stillwell D: *Arteries and veins of the human brain*, Springfield, Ill, 1969, Charles C Thomas.

341. Butler AB, Partian RA, Netsky MG: Primary intraventricular hemorrhage: A mild and remediable form, *Neurology* 22:675, 1972.

342. Beck DW, Menezes AH: Intracerebral hemorrhage in a patient with eclampsia, *JAMA* 246:1442, 1981.

343. Cambier J, Elghozi D, Strube E: Hémorragie de la tête du noyau caudé gauche, *Rev Neurol* 135:763, 1979.

344. Bertol V, Gracia-Naya M, Oliveros A, Gros B: Bilateral symmetric caudate hemorrhage, *Neurology* 41:1157, 1991.

345. Caplan LR: Caudate hemorrhage. In Kase CS, Caplan LR, editors: *Intracerebral hemorrhage*, Boston, 1994, Butterworth-Heinemann, p 329.

346. Mohr JP, Watters WC, Duncan GW: Thalamic hemorrhage and aphasia, *Brain Lang* 2:3, 1975.

347. Watson RT, Heilman KM: Thalamic neglect, *Neurology* 29:690, 1979.

348. Cambier J, Elghozi D, Strube E: Trois observations de lésions vasculaires du thalamus droit avec syndrome de l'hémisphere mineur: Discussion du concept de négligence thalamique, *Rev Neurol (Paris)* 136:105, 1980.

349. Schott B, Laurent B, Mauguiere F, et al: Négligence motrice par hématome thalamique droit, *Rev Neurol* 137:447, 1981.

350. Chung CS, Caplan LR, Han W, et al: Thalamic haemorrhage, *Brain* 119:1996, 1973.

351. Kumral E, Kocaer T, Ertubey NO, et al: Thalamic hemorrhage: A prospective study of 100 patients, *Stroke* 26:964, 1995.

352. Steinke W, Sacco R, Mohr JP, et al: Thalamic stroke: Presentation and prognosis of infarcts and hemorrhages, *Arch Neurol* 49:703, 1992.

353. Dromerick AX, Meschia JF, Kumar A, et al: Simultaneous bilateral thalamic hemorrhages following the administration of intravenous tissue plasminogen activator, *Arch Phys Med Rehab* 78:92, 1997.

354. Crum BA, Wijdicks EF: Thalamic hematoma from a ruptured posterior cerebral artery aneurysm, *Cerebrovasc Dis* 10:475, 2000.

355. Pozzati E: Thalamic cavernous malformations, *Surg Neurol* 53:30, 2000.

356. Barraquer-Bordas L, Illa I, Escartin A, et al: Thalamic hemorrhage: A study of 23 patients with a diagnosis by computed tomography, *Stroke* 12:524, 1981.

357. Waga S, Okada M, Yamamoto Y: Reversibility of Parinaud syndrome in thalamic hemorrhage, *Neurology (NY)* 29:407, 1979.

358. Keane JR: Transient opsoclonus with thalamic hemorrhage, *Arch Neurol* 37:423, 1980.

359. Keane JR: Contralateral gaze deviation with supratentorial hemorrhage: Three pathologically verified cases, *Arch Neurol* 32:119, 1975.

360. Denny-Brown D, Fischer EG: Physiological aspects of visual perception. II: The subcortical visual direction of behavior, *Arch Neurol* 33:228, 1976.

361. Pasik P, Pasik T, Bender MB: The pretectal syndrome in monkeys. I: Disturbances of gaze and body posture, *Brain* 92:521, 1969.

362. Christoff N: A clinicopathologic study of vertical eye movements, *Arch Neurol* 31:1, 1974.

363. Nashold BS, Seaber JH: Defects of ocular motility after stereotactic midbrain lesions in man, *Arch Ophthalmol* 88:245, 1972.

364. Christoff N, Anderson PJ, Bender MB: A clinicopathologic study of associated vertical eye movements, *Trans Am Neurol Assoc* 87:184, 1962.

365. Gilner LI, Avin B: A reversible ocular manifestation of thalamic hemorrhage: A case report, *Arch Neurol* 34:715, 1977.

366. Reynolds AF, Harris AB, Ojemann GA, et al: Aphasia and left thalamic hemorrhage, *J Neurosurg* 48:570, 1978.

367. Fisher CM: Some neuro-ophthalmological observations, *J Neurol Neurosurg Psychiatry* 30:383, 1967.

368. Pessin MS, Adelman LS, Prager RJ, et al: "Wrong-way eyes" in supratentorial hemorrhage, *Ann Neurol* 9:79, 1981.

369. Tijssen CC: Contralateral conjugate eye deviation in acute supratentorial lesions, *Stroke* 25:1516, 1994.

370. Alexander MP, LoVerme SR: Aphasia after left hemispheric intracerebral hemorrhage, *Neurology* 30:1193, 1980.

371. Heilman JM, Valenstein E: Frontal lobe neglect in man, *Neurology* 22:660, 1972.

372. Karussis D, Leker RR, Abramsky O: Cognitive dysfunction following thalamic stroke: A study of 16 cases and review of the literature, *J Neurol Sci* 172:25, 1999.

373. Liebson E: Anosognosia and mania associated with right thalamic haemorrhage, *J Neurol Neurosurg Psychiatry* 68:107, 2000.

374. Manabe Y, Kashibara K, Ota T, et al: Motor neglect following left thalamic hemorrhage: A case report, *J Neurol Sci* 171:69, 1999.

375. Dejerine J, Roussy G: Le syndrome thalamique, *Rev Neurol* 12:521, 1906.

376. Percheron SMJ: Les artères du thalamus humain, *Rev Neurol* 132:297, 1976.

377. Wilkins RH, Brody IA: The thalamic syndrome (Neurological Classics 18), *Arch Neurol* 20:559, 1969.

378. Fisher CM: Pure sensory stroke involving face, arm and leg, *Neurology* 15:76, 1965.

379. Abe K, Yorifuji S, Nishikawa Y: Pure sensory stroke resulting from thalamic haemorrhage, *Neuroradiology* 34:205, 1992.

380. Paciaroni M, Bogousslavsky J: Pure sensory syndromes in thalamic stroke, *Eur Neurol* 39:211, 1998.

381. Shintani S, Tsuruoka S, Shiigai T: Pure sensory stroke caused by a cerebral hemorrhage: Clinical-radiologic correlations in seven patients, *AJNR Am J Neuroradiol* 21:515, 2000.

382. Dobato JL, Villanueva JA, Gimenez-Roldan S: Sensory ataxic hemiparesis in thalamic hemorrhage, *Stroke* 21:1749, 1990.

383. Fisher CM: Ataxic hemiparesis: A pathologic study, *Arch Neurol* 35:126, 1978.

384. Mori S, Sadoshina S, Ibayashi S, et al: Impact of thalamic hematoma on six-month mortality and motor and cognitive functional outcome, *Stroke* 26:620, 2000.

385. Maeshima S, Truman G, Smith DS, et al: Functional outcome following thalamic haemorrhage: Relationship between motor and cognitive functions and ADL, *Disabil Rehabil* 11:459, 1997.

386. Masdeu JC, Rubino FA: Management of lobar intracerebral hemorrhage, medical or surgical, *Neurology* 34:381, 1984.

387. Weisberg LA: Subcortical lobar intracerebral hemorrhage: Clinical-computed tomographic correlations, *J Neurol Neurosurg Psychiatry* 48:1078, 1985.

388. Bogousslavsky J, Van Melle G, Regli F: The Lausanne Stroke Registry: Analysis of 1,000 consecutive patients with first stroke, *Stroke* 19:1083, 1988.

389. Kase CS: Lobar hemorrhage. In Kase CS, Caplan LR, editors: *Intracerebral hemorrhage*, Boston, 1994, Butterworth-Heinemann, p 363.

390. Faught E, Peters D, Bartolucci A, et al: Seizures after primary intracerebral hemorrhage, *Neurology* 39:1089, 1989.

391. Lipton RB, Berger AR, Lesser ML, et al: Lobar vs thalamic and basal ganglion hemorrhage: Clinical and radiographic features, *J Neurol* 234:86, 1987.

392. Sung C-Y, Chu N-S: Epileptic seizures in intracerebral hemorrhage, *J Neurol Neurosurg Psychiatry* 52:1273, 1989.

393. Arboix A, Comes E, Garcia-Eroles L, et al: Site of bleeding and early outcome in primary intracerebral hemorrhage, *Acta Neurol Scand* 105:282, 2002.

394. Passero S, Rocchi R, Rossi S, et al: Seizures after spontaneous supratentorial intracerebral hemorrhage, *Epilepsia* 43:1175, 2002.

395. Echlin FA, Arnett V, Zoll J: Paroxysmal high voltage discharges from isolated and partially isolated human and animal cerebral cortex, *EEG Clin Neurophysiol* 4:147, 1952.

396. Mohr JP, Pessin MS, Finkelstein S, et al: Broca aphasia: Pathologic and clinical aspects, *Neurology* 28:311, 1978.

397. Naeser MA, Hayward RW: The resolving stroke and aphasia: A case study with computerized tomography, *Arch Neurol* 36:233, 1979.

398. Yamada M, Itoh Y, Otomo E, et al: Subarachnoid haemorrhage in the elderly: A necropsy study of the association with cerebral amyloid angiopathy, *J Neurol Neurosurg Psychiatry* 56:543, 1993.

399. Miller JH, Wardlaw JM, Lammie GA: Intracerebral haemorrhage and cerebral amyloid angiopathy: CT features with pathological correlation, *Clin Radiol* 54:422, 1999.

400. Ohshima T, Endo T, Nukui H, et al: Cerebral amyloid angiopathy as a cause of subarachnoid hemorrhage, *Stroke* 21:480, 1990.

401. Tsushima Y, Tamura T, Unno Y, et al: Multifocal low-signal brain lesions on T2*-weighted gradient-echo imaging, *Neuroradiology* 42:499, 2000.

402. Knudsen KA, Rosand J, Karluk D, et al: Clinical diagnosis of cerebral amyloid angiopathy: Validation of the Boston criteria, *Neurology* 56:537, 2001.

403. Helweg-Larsen S, Sommer W, Strange P, et al: Prognosis for patients treated conservatively for spontaneous intracerebral hematomas, *Stroke* 15:1045, 1984.

404. Richardson A: Spontaneous intracerebral and cerebellar hemorrhage. In Russell RWR, editor: *Cerebral arterial disease*, New York, 1976, Churchill-Livingstone, p 210.

405. Steiner I, Gomori JM, Melded E: The prognostic value of the CT scan in conservatively treated patients with intracerebral hematoma, *Stroke* 15:279, 1984.

406. Sung CY, Chu NS: Late CT manifestations in spontaneous lobar hematoma, *J Comput Assist Tomogr* 25:938, 2001.

407. McKusick W, Richardson A, Taylor J: Primary intracerebral hemorrhage: A controlled trial of surgical and conservative treatment in 180 unsolicited cases, *Lancet* 2:221, 1961.

408. Crowell RM, Ojemann RG: Surgery for brain hemorrhage. In Moossy J, Reinmuth OM, editors: *Cerebrovascular diseases: Twelfth Research Conference*, Philadelphia, 1981, Lippincott-Raven, p 233.

409. Broderick JP, Adams HP, Barsan W, et al: Guidelines for the management of spontaneous intracerebral hemorrhage: A statement for healthcare professionals from a special writing group of the Stroke Council, American Heart Association, *Stroke* 30:905, 1999.

410. Flemming K, Wijdicks EFM, St. Louis EK, Li H: Predicting deterioration in patients with lobar haemorrhages, *J Neurol Neurosurg Psychiatry* 66:600, 1999.

411. Flemming KD, Wijdicks EF, Li H: Can we predict poor outcome at presentation in patients with lobar hemorrhage, *Cerebrovasc Dis* 11:183, 2001.

412. Mendelow AD, Gregson BA, Fernandes HM, et al: Early surgery versus initial conservative treatment in patients with spontaneous supratentorial intracerebral haematomas in the International Surgical Trial in INtracerebral Haemorrhage (STICH): A randomized trial, *Lancet* 365:387, 2005.

413. Little JR, Tubman DE, Ethier R: Cerebellar hemorrhage in adults: Diagnosis by computerized tomography, *J Neurosurg* 48:575, 1978.

414. Müller HR, Wüthrich R, Wiggli U, et al: The contribution of computerized axial tomography to the diagnosis of cerebellar and pontine hematomas, *Stroke* 6:467, 1975.

415. Freeman RE, Onofrio BM, Okazaki H, et al: Spontaneous intracerebellar hemorrhage, *Neurology* 23:84, 1973.

416. Hyland HH, Levy D: Spontaneous cerebellar hemorrhage, *Can Med Assoc J* 71:315, 1954.

417. Rey-Bellet J: Cerebellar hemorrhage: A clinicopathologic study, *Neurology* 10:217, 1960.

418. Richardson AE: Spontaneous cerebellar hemorrhage. In Vinken PJ, Bruyn GW, editors: *Handbook of clinical neurology*, Vol 12, Amsterdam, 1972, North-Holland Publishing, p 54.

419. Brennan RW, Bergland RM: Acute cerebellar hemorrhage: Analysis of clinical findings and outcome in 12 cases, *Neurology* 27:527, 1977.

420. McKissock W, Richardson A, Walsh L: Spontaneous cerebellar hemorrhage: A study of 34 consecutive cases treated surgically, *Brain* 83:1, 1960.

421. Norris JW, Eisen AA, Branch CL: Problems in cerebellar hemorrhage and infarction, *Neurology* 19:1043, 1969.

422. Fisher CM: The neurological examination of the comatose patient, *Acta Neurol Scand Suppl* 45:44, 1969.

423. Messert B, Leppik IE, Sato Y: Diplopia and involuntary eye closure in spontaneous cerebellar hemorrhage, *Stroke* 7:305, 1976.

424. Bosch EP, Kennedy SS, Aschenbrener CA: Ocular bobbing: The myth of its localizing value, *Neurology* 25:949, 1975.

425. Fisher CM: Ocular bobbing, *Arch Neurol* 11:543, 1964.

426. St. Louis EK, Wijdicks EF, Li H: Predicting neurologic deterioration in patients with cerebellar hematomas, *Neurology* 51:1364, 1998.

427. Brillman J: Acute hydrocephalus and death one month after nonsurgical treatment for acute cerebellar hemorrhage, *J Neurosurg* 50:374, 1979.

428. Yoshida S, Sasaki M, Oka H, et al: Acute hypertensive cerebellar hemorrhage with signs of lower brainstem compression, *Surg Neurol* 10:79, 1978.

429. Greenberg J, Skubick D, Shenkin H: Acute hydrocephalus in cerebellar infarct and hemorrhage, *Neurology (NY)* 29:409, 1979.

430. Heiman TD, Satya-Murti S: Benign cerebellar hemorrhages, *Ann Neurol* 3:366, 1978.

431. St. Louis EK, Wijdicks EF, Li H, et al: Predictors of poor outcome in patients with a spontaneous cerebellar hematoma, *Can J Neurol Sci* 27:32, 2000.

432. Kirollos RW, Tyagi AK, Ross SA, et al: Management of spontaneous cerebellar hematomas: A prospective treatment protocol, *Neurosurgery* 49:1378, 2001.

433. Roig C, Carvajal A, Illa I, et al: Hémorragies mésencéphaliques isolées, *Rev Neurol* 138:53, 1982.

434. Durward QJ, Barnett HJM, Barr HWK: Presentation and management of mesencephalic hematoma, *J Neurosurg* 56:123, 1982.

435. Morel-Maroger A, Metzger J, Bories J, et al: Les hématomes benins du tronc cérébral chez les hypertendus artériels, *Rev Neurol* 138:437, 1982.

436. Humphreys RP: Computerized tomographic definition of mesencephalic hematoma with evacuation through pedunculotomy, *J Neurosurg* 49:749, 1978.

437. LaTorre E, Delitala A, Sorano V: Hematoma of the quadrigeminal plate, *J Neurosurg* 49:610, 1978.

438. Scoville WB, Poppen JL: Intrapeduncular hemorrhage of the brain, *Arch Neurol Psychiatry* 61:688, 1949.

439. Galetta SL, Balcer IJ: Isolated fourth nerve palsy from midbrain hemorrhage, *J Neuroophthalmol* 18:204, 1998.

440. Isikay CT, Yucesan C, Yucemen N, et al: Isolated nuclear oculomotor nerve syndrome due to mesencephalic hematoma, *Acta Neurol Belg* 100:248, 2000.

441. Mizushima H, Seki T: Midbrain hemorrhage presenting with oculomotor nerve palsy: Case report, *Surg Neurol* 58:417, 2002.

442. Lee AG, Brown DG, Diaz PJ: Dorsal midbrain syndrome due to mesencephalic hemorrhage: Case report with serial imaging, *J Neuroophthalmol* 16:281, 1996.

443. Pego R, Martinez-Vazquez F, Branas F, et al: Hemorragia espontánea en la lamina cuadrigémina: Presentación de dos casos, *Rev Neurol* 25:1414, 1997.

444. Fang HCM, Foley JM: Hypertensive hemorrhages of the pons and cerebellum, *Arch Neurol Psychiatry* 72:638, 1954.

445. Caplan LR: Intracerebral hemorrhage. In Tyler HR, Dawson DM, editors: *Current neurology*, Vol II, Boston, 1979, Houghton Mifflin, p 185.

446. Kornyey S: Rapidly fatal pontile hemorrhage: Clinical and anatomic report, *Arch Neurol Psychiatry* 41:793, 1939.

447. Silverstein A: Primary pontile hemorrhage, *Confin Neurol* 29:33, 1967.

448. Silverstein A: Primary pontine hemorrhage. In Vinken PJ, Bruyn GW, editors: *Handbook of clinical neurology*, Vol 12, *Part II*, Amsterdam, 1972, North-Holland Publishing, p 37.

449. Jeong JH, Yoon SJ, Kang SJ, et al: Hypertensive pontine microhemorrhage, *Stroke* 33:925, 2002.

450. Dana C: Acute bulbar paralysis due to hemorrhage and softening of the pons and medulla, *Med Rec* 64:361, 1903.

451. Okudera T, Uemura K, Nakajima K, et al: Primary pontine hemorrhage: Correlations of pathologic features with postmortem microangiographic and vertebral angiography studies, *Mt Sinai J Med* 45:305, 1978.

452. Steegmann AT: Primary pontile hemorrhage, *J Nerv Ment Dis* 114:35, 1951.

453. Sharpe JA, Rosenberg MA, Hoyt WF, et al: Paralytic pontine exotropia: A sign of acute unilateral pontine gaze palsy and internuclear ophthalmoplegia, *Neurology* 24:1076, 1974.

454. Becker DH, Silverberg GD: Successful evacuation of an acute pontine hematoma, *Surg Neurol* 10:263, 1978.

455. Pierrott-Deseilligny C, Chain F, Serdaru M, et al: The "one-and-a-half" syndrome: Electro-oculographic analysis of five cases with deductions about the physiological mechanisms of lateral gaze, *Brain* 104:665, 1981.

456. Halsey JH, Ceballos R, Crosby EC: The supranuclear control of voluntary lateral gaze, *Neurology* 17:928, 1967.

457. Susac JO, Hoyt WF, Daroff RB, et al: Clinical spectrum of ocular bobbing, *J Neurol Neurosurg Psychiatry* 33:771, 1970.

458. Goto N, Kaneko M, Hosaka Y, et al: Primary pontine hemorrhage: Clinicopathologic correlations, *Stroke* 11:84, 1980.

459. Wijdicks EF, St. Louis E: Clinical profiles predictive of outcome in pontine hemorrhage, *Neurology* 49:1342, 1997.

460. Payne HA, Maravilla KR, Levinstone A, et al: Recovery from primary pontine hemorrhage, *Ann Neurol* 4:557, 1978.

461. O'Laoire SA, Crockard HA, Thomas DGT, et al: Brain-stem hematoma, *J Neurosurg* 56:222, 1982.

462. Zuccarello M, Iavicoli R, Pardatscher K, et al: Primary brain stem hematomas. Diagnosis and treatment, *Acta Neurochir* 54:45, 1980.

463. Gobernado JM, Fernandez de Molina AR, Gimeno A: Pure motor hemiplegia due to hemorrhage in the lower pons, *Arch Neurol* 37:393, 1980.

464. Schnapper RA: Pontine hemorrhage presenting as ataxic hemiparesis, *Stroke* 13:518, 1982.

465. Tuhrim S, Yang WC, Rubinowitz H, et al: Primary pontine hemorrhage and the dysarthria clumsy hand syndrome, *Neurology* 32:1027, 1982.

466. Freeman W, Ammerman HH, Stanley M: Syndromes of the pontile tegmentum, Foville's syndrome: Report of 3 cases, *Arch Neurol Psychiatry* 50:462, 1943.

467. Tyler HR, Johnson PC: Case records of the Massachusetts General Hospital (Case 36-1972), *N Engl J Med* 287:506, 1972.

468. Pullicino PM, Wong EH: Tonic downward and inward ocular deviation ipsilateral to pontine tegmental hemorrhage, *Cerebrovasc Dis* 10:327, 2000.

469. Lawrence WH, Lightfoote WE: Continuous vertical pendular eye movements after brainstem hemorrhage, *Neurology* 25:896, 1975.

470. Arseni C, Stanciu M: Primary hematomas of the brain stem, *Acta Neurochir* 28:323, 1973.

471. Kempe LG: Surgical removal of an intramedullary hematoma simulating Wallenberg's syndrome, *J Neurol Neurosurg Psychiatry* 27:78, 1964.

472. Mastaglia FL, Edis B, Kakulas BA: Medullary hemorrhage: A report of two cases, *J Neurol Neurosurg Psychiatry* 32:221, 1969.

473. Barinagarrementeria F, Cantú C: Primary medullary hemorrhage: Report of four cases and review of the literature, *Stroke* 25:1684, 1994.

474. Kumral E, Acarer A: Primary medullary hemorrhage with intractable hiccup, *J Neurol* 245:620, 1998.

475. Jung HH, Baumgartner RW, Hess K: Symptomatic secondary hemorrhagic transformation of ischemic Wallenberg's syndrome, *J Neurol* 247:463, 2000.

30 Aneurysmal Subarachnoid Hemorrhage

ERIC M. BERSHAD, JOSÉ I. SUAREZ

A woman, of forty years of age, and much given to drinking, was seiz'd with an apoplexy. From this she became paralytic in both sides, and was brought into the hospital at Padua, and there she soon died.... The vessels of the pia mater were so distended with blood, that the larger ones were almost black; and the smallest made a very beautiful appearance, as if injected with red wax.... [T]he trunk of that artery into which the vertebrals are conjoin'd, exhibited a small white elliptical spot.... I found it was not of that kind, which is generally us'd to be the beginning of an ossification, as I had thought; but somewhat soft in the parietes of the artery itself, and rather in the interior coat.

G. Morgagni, De sedibus et causis morborum (1761)[1]

Subarachnoid hemorrhage (SAH) refers to the extravasation of blood into the spaces filled with cerebrospinal fluid (CSF). In the absence of trauma, aneurysmal rupture is the most common cause of SAH. Often aneurysms remain silent until the cataclysmic rupture. Our understanding of the machinations underlying this condition has evolved; however, many issues remain unresolved. Despite advances in diagnosis and management, the mortality rate for SAH remains unacceptably high. The future holds promise, but there are obstacles to overcome.

Historical Aspects

Our concept of aneurysms began in ancient times. The Egyptian Papyrus of Ebers (c.1550 BC) contains an early description of an arterial aneurysm[2]; however, the first definite report of an intracranial aneurysm came later. Exactly when the first definite case report of SAH appeared in text is debated, although a vague description may have been referenced in Biblical writings.[3] Our modern understanding that the anatomic framework gives rise to intracranial aneurysms began in 1664 when Sir Christopher Wren, under the direction of Thomas Willis, illustrated the collateral arterial circulation at the base of the brain (circle of Willis).[4-6] In 1761, Morgagni[1] published *De sedibus et causis morborum (The Seats and Causes of Diseases)*, a collection of detailed clinicopathologic observations that may have included the earliest pathologically confirmed case of aneurysmal SAH. About 50 years later, in 1812, Cheyne[7] published *Cases of Apoplexy and Lethargy...*, which included an illustration of SAH presumably due to a ruptured aneurysm at the intracranial carotid artery bifurcation. In 1813, Blackall[8] reported a clinical case of aneurysmal SAH in *Observations on the Nature and Cure of Dropsies*, which vividly described the pathologic appearance of a top-of-the-basilar artery aneurysm as a "horse-bean." In 1859, William Gull[9] detailed a series of 62 cases of intracranial aneurysms that included thorough clinicopathologic descriptions. He astutely suggested that the presence of an acute severe headache should raise the suspicion of SAH; he also provided a possible description of delayed ischemic deficit related to vasospasm in a patient with a ruptured left middle cerebral artery aneurysm. The promulgation of lumbar puncture by Quincke[10] in 1891 paved the way for the routine premortem diagnosis of SAH. A major breakthrough came in 1927, when Moniz[11] first applied cerebral angiography to a living person to diagnose tumor; in 1933 he reported the successful visualization of an intracranial internal carotid aneurysm.[12] The successful clipping of an intracranial aneurysm by Dandy[13] in 1937 marked the beginning of an era in which active intervention for SAH superseded the nihilistic approach. The history of SAH continues with the advent of sophisticated neuroimaging techniques, multimodality brain monitoring, and endovascular therapy.

Epidemiology

Aneurysmal SAHs cause 2% to 7% of all strokes[14-17] but disproportionately account for 27% of stroke-related years of life lost before age 65.[18] The incidence of SAH varies substantially by region, ranging from 2 per 100,000 population per year in Beijing, China, up to 27 per 100,000 population per year in Japan.[19,20] Finland has a relatively high incidence of SAH, 22 per 100,000 population per year.[19] The worldwide aggregate incidence of SAH is 10.5 per 100,000 per year, which is about the same as the incidence in North America (United States and Canada).[21-23] The incidence of SAH has remained stable over approximately 40 years.[23,24] There is ethnic variability in the incidence of SAH, with a higher age-adjusted incidence among Mexican-Americans than in non-Hispanic whites.[16] The incidence of SAH increases with age. The mean age at presentation is 49 to 55 years.[14,19] There is a relative risk of SAH of 1.6:1 for women in comparison with men.[23,25] In North America, the relative risk of SAH is 2.1:1 for black in comparison with white persons.[26]

The prevalence of intracranial aneurysms in the general population is between 1% and 6% on the basis of autopsy studies, and 0.5% to 1% on the basis of angiographic data.[27] Of these, about 20% to 50% rupture during the person's lifetime.[28] About 12% to 45% of patients with aneurysmal SAH have multiple aneurysms.[29] The risk for development of a new (de novo) aneurysm after diagnosis of SAH is about 2% per year, according to results of a study using serial angiographic screenings.[30]

The case fatality rate for SAH has been gradually decreasing, by about 0.5% per year.[31] Between 1945 and 1974 in Rochester, Minnesota, the case fatality rate was 57%; it declined to 42% between 1974 and 1984.[32] The case fatality rate varies by region, with a 28-day age-adjusted mortality of 23% reported in Beijing, China, to 62% in former Yugoslavia.[19] Overall, approximately 10% to 20% of patients with SAH die before reaching the hospital, and about 25% die within 24 hours of the ictus.[14,31,33]

There are diurnal and seasonal variations in the occurrence of SAH.[20,34,35] In two Japanese studies, peaks of SAH occurred from 7 to 10 AM and from 5 to 8 PM, an effect attributed to circadian changes in blood pressure (BP).[20] The nadir diurnal occurrence was between 10 PM and 6 AM.[35] A seasonal variation in the incidence of SAH is not consistent in all studies.[20,35,36] A Japanese study found a greater predominance in spring than in summer for both sexes[20]; however, this pattern was not seen in another Japanese study.[35] A Danish study found a modest statistically significant increase in SAH hospitalization rates in the month of January over those in July.[36] Other factors that may influence SAH occurrence include changes in the ambient temperature, barometric pressure, and humidity.[34,37]

Risk Factors

Many potential risk factors for SAH have been studied, but only a few have been convincingly identified.[14,24,38-59] Risk factors are categorized as modifiable or nonmodifiable. The most important modifiable risk factors are cigarette smoking and hypertension; other modifiable risk factors for SAH include heavy alcohol use, cocaine abuse, caffeine and nicotine intake in pharmaceutical products, and use of nonsteroidal anti-inflammatory drugs, but these are less well established.[38,39,60] Contrary to traditional beliefs, oral contraceptive use, hypercholesterolemia, and exercise are probably not associated with an increased risk of SAH.[39,40]

Cigarette smoking is a robust modifiable risk factor for aneurysmal SAH.[38-41,43-53] In 1996, Teunissen and colleagues systematically reviewed studies evaluating risk factors for aneurysmal SAH.[40] Among two longitudinal and seven case-control studies that evaluated smoking as a possible risk factor,[41,43-50,61] the aggregate relative risk (RR) and odds ratio (OR) for SAH were 1.9 and 3.5, respectively, with smoking.[40] At least five subsequent retrospective studies found that active cigarette smoking was an independent risk factor for SAH.[38,39,51-53] Additionally, in one of these studies, previous smoking was also a potent independent risk factor for SAH, with an OR of 4.1.[38]

Hypertension is another robust modifiable risk factor for SAH.[38-41,51,53,54] In the review by Teunissen and colleagues[40] of seven case-control studies[44,45,47,48,50,61,62] and three longitudinal studies,[41,54,63] hypertension had an aggregate OR of 2.9 and an RR of 2.8. Furthermore, four subsequent retrospective studies demonstrated that hypertension was an independent risk factor for SAH.[38,39,51,53]

Heavy alcohol use is an inconsistently reported risk factor for SAH.[38-40,44,46,55-57] In the pooled analysis of SAH risk factors by Teunissen and colleagues,[40] which included two longitudinal series[55,56] and three case-control series,[44,46,57] heavy alcohol use (>150 g/day) was a statistically significant risk factor, with an RR of 4.7 and an OR of 1.5. In contrast, several other studies found that heavy alcohol use was not an independent predictor for SAH.[38,39] Broderick and associates[39] found that consumption of more than two alcoholic drinks per day was not an independent risk factor for SAH. Qureshi and coworkers[38] reported that alcohol use, defined as more than one alcoholic drink per day, was not an independent risk factor for SAH.[38]

Nonmodifiable risk factors for SAH include a family history of SAH in a first-degree relative, female sex, low educational achievement, low body mass index, and undetermined genetic factors.[14,24,39,41,58,59] Some known inherited conditions associated with SAH and/or intracranial aneurysms include adult dominant polycystic kidney disease (ADPKD), Ehlers-Danlos disease (type IV), alpha$_1$-antitrypsin deficiency, sickle cell disease, pseudoxanthoma elasticum, hereditary hemorrhagic telangiectasia, neurofibromatosis type I, tuberous sclerosis, fibromuscular dysplasia, and coarctation of the aorta.[14,24,42,64-68]

A family history of SAH in a close relative is an important nonmodifiable risk factor.[14,24,39,58,59] People with a first-degree relative with SAH have a relative risk of 3 to 7 for SAH in comparison with the general population[24]; however, having a second-degree relative with SAH does not significantly increase the risk over that of the general population.[69] A maternal history of SAH may portend higher risk than a paternal history.[58] Regarding the increased risk of SAH in patients with a family history of SAH, the clinical implications for screening are controversial. For example, a prospective observational study found that routine screening for aneurysms in first-degree relatives of patients with SAH did not translate into a hypothetical clinical benefit, owing to the anticipated postoperative disability that was expected to outweigh the reduction in mortality from the repair of asymptomatic aneurysms at low risk for rupture.[70]

Female gender is another important nonmodifiable risk factor for SAH. Women have 1.6 times the risk for SAH that men have, and the higher risk in women may increase further with advancing age.[71] The reasons for gender-related differences in SAH may be related to menstrual and hormonal influences.[14,23,25,62,72] An earlier age of menarche (<13 years old) and null gravidity are associated with significantly increased ORs of 3.2 and 4.2, respectively, for SAH.[72] Two studies found an increased risk of SAH with delayed age of initial parity.[73,74] Higher parity may reduce the risk of SAH.[75] Furthermore, a retrospective study reported a reduced risk of SAH in postmenopausal women taking hormone replacement therapy.[62]

Adult dominant polycystic kidney disease is a known risk factor for SAH.[76-79] Intracranial aneurysms are present in 5% to 40% of patients.[80] Patients with the disease who also have SAH tend to be younger, male, and have a higher proportion of middle cerebral artery aneurysms than the general population of patients with SAH.[81]

Causes of Subarachnoid Hemorrhage

Excluding trauma, rupture of a saccular (berry) aneurysm is the most common cause (85%) of SAH. Perimesencephalic hemorrhage (10%) is the next most common cause, followed by myriad uncommon etiologies including arteriovenous malformations (AVMs), intracranial arterial dissections, and others (5%) (Table 30-1).[24]

Perimesencephalic nonaneurysmal subarachnoid hemorrhage (PNSH) is a distinct form of nonaneurysmal SAH. The pathophysiology is not well known but may be associated with venous anomalies.[82,83] Clinically, patients present similarly to those with aneurysmal SAH; however, patients with PNSH are generally alert, without loss of consciousness at onset, and have no risk factors for aneurysms (i.e., hypertension and smoking). The standard CT definition of PNSH dictates that the blood is located mainly anterior to midbrain, in the interpeduncular cistern, or anterior to the pons, in the prepontine cistern, but may extend to the anterior ambient cistern, quadrigeminal cistern, or basal sylvian fissure. Also, there should be no involvement of the anterior hemispheric fissure, lateral sylvian fissure, or intraventricular hemorrhage (IVH).[84] Head CT is not sufficient by itself to diagnose PNSH because posterior circulation aneurysms may produce a similar pattern of hemorrhage. By definition, angiography reveals no aneurysm. Angiographic vasospasm is not uncommon; however, delayed cerebral ischemia (DCI) is rare. Some patients may experience hydrocephalus and may rarely require a permanent shunt.[85] The prognosis is usually excellent, and the risk of rebleeding is extremely low.[86]

TABLE 30-1 LESS COMMON CAUSES OF SPONTANEOUS SUBARACHNOID HEMORRHAGE

Category	Cause
Inflammatory	Vasculitis
Vascular	Perimesencephalic hemorrhage, cerebral arteriovenous malformation (AVM), intracranial arterial dissection,[370-372] carotid-cavernous fistula,[373] cerebral sinus venous thrombosis,[374] eclampsia, spinal AVM, spinal artery aneurysms,[375] moyamoya disease[376]*
Infectious	Mycotic aneurysms, gnathostomiasis (parasitic),[377] Lyme vasculitis[378]
Neoplastic	Pituitary apoplexy (adenoma), carcinomatous meningitis[379]
Hematologic	Coagulopathy, thrombocytopenia,[380] sickle cell disease
Drugs	Cocaine, amphetamines[379]
Other	Eclampsia[381]

*Mechanism thought to be rupture of transdural anastomotic vessels.[376]

Pathophysiology

The processes preceding catastrophic aneurysm rupture occur on a continuum that involves aneurysm formation, growth, and ultimate rupture. The dynamic interactions among inflammatory, hemodynamic, hormonal, and genetic contributors that drive this insidious process are gradually being elucidated.

Distribution and Types of Aneurysms

The saccular (berry) aneurysm is responsible for 85% of cases of aneurysmal SAH.[24] Less commonly, aneurysms may be fusiform or mycotic. Fusiform aneurysms are dilatations of the entire arterial circumference, usually related to atherosclerosis.[87] Mycotic (infectious) aneurysms are rare, may be saccular or fusiform, are usually associated with bacteremia, are typically seen in distal branches of the anterior circulation, and are found in the systemic arterial circulation. The best treatment for mycotic aneurysms is not well established but may involve antibiotics alone for aneurysms or adjunctive surgical or endovascular aneurysm repair.[88]

Intracranial aneurysms are usually solitary (70% to 75%) but may be multiple in some patients (25% to 50%).[89] The majority of saccular aneurysms arise from the circle of Willis and occur in the anterior circulation. The most common distribution for intracranial aneurysms includes the following arteries: anterior communicating (30%), posterior communicating (25%), middle cerebral (20%), internal carotid bifurcation (7.5%), and top of the basilar artery (7%).[90] Other possible locations for aneurysms are the ophthalmic, anterior choroidal, anterior cerebral, pericallosal, superior cerebellar, anterior inferior cerebellar, posterior inferior cerebellar, posterior cerebral, basilar, and cavernous internal carotid arteries.

Aneurysm Development

The origin of intracranial aneurysms stems from insidious and dynamic processes that slowly erode the structure of arterial wall. Traditionally, it was believed that congenital defects in the tunica media at arterial bifurcations gave rise to intracranial aneurysms; however, this hypothesis has been largely refuted.[91-93] First, because aneurysms form during life, it is likely that acquired factors rather than congenital abnormalities are implicated in the pathogenesis.[93,94] Next, the distribution of saccular aneurysms, predominantly in the anterior circulation, does not correlate well with the distribution of tunica media defects in the posterior circulation.[95] Also, tunica media defects may be present without evidence of aneurysms.[93] Additionally, pathologic specimens of aneurysms show a distinct pattern of sclerosis, ischemia, and degenerative changes, which suggests that atherosclerotic processes are involved.[96,97] Finally, the site of rupture of aneurysms on pathologic studies occurs distal to the supposed defects.[98]

During cerebral aneurysm pathogenesis, the arterial wall undergoes characteristic changes. Early on, hemodynamic factors such as hypertension result in endothelial cell injury as well as associated histopathologic findings

TABLE 30-2 CUMULATIVE (5-YEAR) RISK OF RUPTURE FOR UNRUPTURED SACCULAR ANEURYSMS

Size of Aneurysm (mm)	No History of SAH and Anterior Circulation Aneurysm	No History of SAH and Posterior Circulation or PCOM Aneurysm	History of SAH and Incidental Aneurysm
<7	0	2.5	1.5 anterior circulation; 3.5 posterior circulation (including PCOM)
7-12	2.6	14.5	n/a
13-24	14.5	18.4	n/a
>25	40	50	n/a

n/a, not available; PCOM, posterior communicating artery; SAH, subarachnoid hemorrhage.
Data derived from Wiebers DO, Whisnant JP, Huston J III, et al: Unruptured intracranial aneurysms: Natural history, clinical outcome, and risks of surgical and endovascular treatment. *Lancet* 362:103–110, 2003.

of balloon-like protrusions and crater-like concavities, cytoplasmic swelling, and subendothelial fibrin and cellular infiltration.[93] Other changes include degeneration of the arterial basement membrane and internal elastic lamina. Eventually, degeneration of the muscular tunica media occurs, possibly mediated by an apoptotic mechanism.[99] Hemodynamic stressors may occlude the vasa vasorum, resulting in smooth muscle ischemia. Alternatively, impaired diffusion of nutrients across a damaged internal elastic lamina and basement membrane may result in tunica media degeneration.[93]

Hemodynamic stress is considered a key mediator of aneurysm development.[92] Contributors to hemodynamic stress include hypertension, abnormal anatomy of the cerebral vasculature, and abnormal blood flow associated with certain conditions (i.e., arteriovenous malformations, sickle cell disease).[100-102] It is demonstrated in animal models that the combination of hypertension with unilateral carotid artery ligation consistently produces intracranial aneurysms.[100-102] Furthermore, a high prevalence of intracranial aneurysms is observed in patients with aplasia or hypoplasia of the internal carotid artery.[103] There is a growing awareness that hemodynamic conditions producing certain patterns of arterial wall shear stress result in degradation of the arterial wall.[104] Interestingly, it is areas of the arterial wall exposed to very low shear stress that are most prone to growth.[105]

In addition to hemodynamic factors, defects in arterial connective tissue structure (i.e., elastin and collagen) via either inherited or acquired conditions may predispose one to aneurysm development. Some evidence supporting this is the known association between certain diseases that affect connective tissue and aneurysms (i.e., collagen type III deficiency, alpha$_1$-antitrypsin).[106,107]

Inflammatory processes may also contribute to aneurysm development; however, it is unclear whether the inflammation is a primary cause of or a compensatory response to arterial wall stress. Chyatte and associates[108] found higher levels of complement, T lymphocytes, macrophages, monocytes, immunoglobulins, and vascular cell adhesion molecule-1 in the walls of unruptured aneurysms than in normal control vessels.

Cigarette smoking may induce a proteolytic state by increasing the ratio of plasma and arterial wall elastase levels to alpha$_1$-antitrypsin activity.[94] In rabbits, the application of topical elastase to the arterial wall resulted in saccular aneurysm formation, growth, and rupture.[109]

Hormonal factors such as estrogen are implicated in aneurysm development and SAH. Estrogen may exert beneficial effects on the cerebral blood vessels through mechanisms such as increased endothelial nitric oxide, mitochondrial production, and collagen strengthening.[71,110-112] Therefore, the decrease in estrogen levels in postmenopausal women may have an adverse effect on the vasculature and possibly increase the risk for SAH; however, this issue requires further study.

Aneurysm Rupture

The pathophysiology associated with aneurysm rupture is still being elucidated. Some clinical factors that may be useful to determine the risk of rupture of an unruptured aneurysm are the size and location of the aneurysm and a previous history of SAH (Table 30-2).[113]

Several investigators have evaluated the histology of saccular aneurysms to identify features that may be associated with rupture. Frösen and colleagues[114] evaluated the histology of 66 saccular aneurysms, both ruptured and unruptured, and found distinct patterns associated with ruptured aneurysms. Some of these were decellularization, apoptosis, matrix degeneration, loss of endothelialization, thrombus formation, and inflammatory infiltration.[114] Inflammatory cells consisted mainly of T lymphocytes and macrophages. Similarly, Kataoka and associates[115] found that ruptured aneurysms had significant inflammatory infiltration with macrophages and fragility of the wall compared to unruptured aneurysms.

Some anatomic features of the aneurysm may increase the risk of rupture; they include a smaller neck-to-body ratio and smaller caliber of associated draining arteries.[104]

There may be specific genetic factors predisposing an aneurysm to rupture. In one study, a specific polymorphism in the endothelial nitric oxide synthase gene was found significantly more often in patients with aneurysmal SAH than in community controls and patients with unruptured aneurysms.[116]

Clinical Presentation
Signs and Symptoms

The classic presentation of SAH is an acute and severe headache, often described as the "worst ever." The time to peak headache intensity is usually seconds.[24] However, occasionally the headache may be mild and may respond to over-the-counter analgesics.[117] Only a minority of patients have a warning "sentinel" headache days to weeks before an aneurysmal SAH, which probably represents a small aneurysmal leak.[118] Unfortunately, this history is usually obtained retrospectively, because the headache may be transient, and even if a head CT is performed during the headache, its findings will be negative about half the time.[119]

Syncope occurs in 50% of patients, a phenomenon that may be due to an abrupt rise in intracranial pressure (ICP), which exceeds the mean arterial pressure (MAP), thus resulting in a critically low cerebral perfusion pressure (CPP) and global cerebral ischemia. Seizures occur acutely in 6% to 16% of patients.[24,120,121]

Other common manifestations are nausea, vomiting, neck stiffness, photophobia, and phonophobia. Retinal or preretinal hemorrhages (Terson's syndrome) are seen on funduscopy in about 17% of patients, in relation to an acute rise in ICP; preretinal hemorrhages are associated with poor outcome.[122] Occasionally, meningeal signs are present owing to the chemical meningitis associated with SAH. A depressed level of consciousness (LOC) is very common and ranges from mild drowsiness to coma.

Focal neurologic deficits related to aneurysm rupture may include intracerebral hemorrhage (ICH), aneurysmal mass effect, and postictal paralysis after complex partial seizures. Classically, one may observe a third nerve palsy with pupillary dilation, which is related to extrinsic compression of the oculomotor nerve by a posterior communicating (PCOM) artery aneurysm. The pupil is characteristically large and poorly reactive to light owing to the interruption of the parasympathetic fibers traversing the outside of the oculomotor nerve. This syndrome may also be seen with posterior cerebral artery and superior cerebellar artery aneurysms. The finding of sixth nerve palsy may be a "false localizing sign," representing elevated ICP. Additionally, one may observe impaired upgaze, which is seen in association with hydrocephalus and is related to pressure on the dorsal midbrain vertical gaze centers. Other focal neurologic deficits may be related to anterior communicating (ACOM) artery or middle cerebral artery (MCA) aneurysms (Table 30-3).[14]

Acute cardiac abnormalities associated with SAH are discussed in more detail later in this chapter; however, several key points are addressed now. First, cardiac arrhythmias are very prevalent in aneurysmal SAH, occurring in up to 91% of patients, and may be life threatening.[123-125] Furthermore, electrocardiographic changes are very common, occurring in up to 100% of patients, and may even mimic acute myocardial infarction.[125] Some abnormalities include peaked P waves, a shortened PR interval, a prolonged QT interval, inverted T waves, prominent U waves, Q waves, and elevation or depression of the ST segment.[125]

TABLE 30-3 CLINICAL SYNDROMES RELATED TO SACCULAR ANEURYSMS

Location	Syndrome
Posterior communicating artery	Complete 3rd nerve palsy
Anterior communicating artery	Bilateral leg weakness, abulia
Middle cerebral artery	Contralateral hemiparesis, and aphasia or visuospatial defects
Internal carotid artery	Ophthalmoplegia, visual disturbances*
Basilar artery	Brainstem compression

*Ophthalmoplegia related to internal carotid artery aneurysms is due to cavernous sinus involvement. Related visual disturbances are due to either optic nerve or optic chiasm compression and manifest as unilateral visual loss or bitemporal hemianopia, respectively.

Misdiagnosis of Subarachnoid Hemorrhage

The clinical presentation of aneurysmal SAH is usually straightforward; however, in the community, initial misdiagnosis occurs in 23% to 51% of patients.[126] Occasionally patients present with seizure, acute confusional state, subdural hematoma, or head trauma, making the underlying diagnosis of aneurysmal SAH more elusive. A delayed diagnosis often has a disastrous outcome.[126,127] In one study, rebleeding occurred in 65% of patients who were initially misdiagnosed and was associated with high mortality.[128] Another study reported that of patients with an initial good clinical SAH grade, 91% had good or excellent outcome at 6 weeks when diagnosed correctly versus only 53% when the diagnosis was delayed.[127] The most common misdiagnoses are migraine headache and headache of unknown cause[126]; other misdiagnoses include meningitis, influenza, hypertensive crisis, myocardial infarction, arthritis, and psychiatric disease. The most common reasons for misdiagnoses of SAH are failure to obtain appropriate imaging study and misinterpretation of or failure to perform a lumbar puncture.[14]

Radiographic and Diagnostic Testing

The most appropriate initial diagnostic test for SAH is a non–contrast-enhanced head CT scan. The sensitivity of CT for acute SAH is very high initially but diminishes with increasing delay between the onset of symptoms and imaging. Newer CT scanners (third-generation or later) are reported to be 98% to 100% sensitive for detecting subarachnoid blood within 12 hours of onset of symptoms when compared with the "gold standard," lumbar puncture.[129-132] However, the sensitivity of CT drops to 93% at 24 hours and 50% at 7 days.[130] The accuracy of CT for SAH also depends on expert interpretation from a radiologist, because a preliminary reading by a nonexpert interpreter may be inaccurate.[133] Classically, the head CT reveals hyperintense signal in the basal subarachnoid cisterns. Other locations include the sylvian fissures, interhemispheric fissure, interpeduncular fossa, and suprasellar, ambient, and quadrigeminal cisterns.

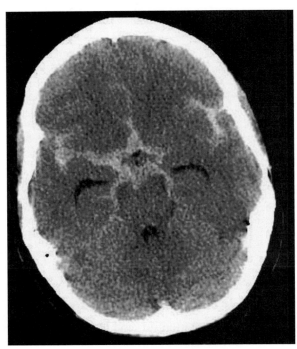

Figure 30-1 A non–contrast-enhanced head CT scan reveals extensive subarachnoid hemorrhage in the basal cisterns, sylvian fissures, and anterior interhemispheric fissure in a patient with a ruptured left posterior communicating artery aneurysm. There is also prominence of the temporal horns of the lateral ventricles, suggesting hydrocephalus.

There may also be associated intracerebral hemorrhage, intraventricular hemorrhage, subdural hematoma, cerebral edema, and hydrocephalus (Fig. 30-1). The pattern of blood seen on head CT scans may suggest a certain location of the underlying aneurysm; however, the accuracy of this approach is poor and thus has little diagnostic value.[29] The amount and location of blood on head CT scans remains one of the most important predictors of DCI (see Table 30-5).[134]

Lumbar puncture (LP) is considered the gold standard for detection of SAH. In patients with suspected SAH in whom head CT scan results are nondefinitive, it is absolutely essential to obtain an LP.[129] LP may be contraindicated in patients suspected to have focal mass lesions, elevated ICP, and herniation.[135] The presence of xanthochromia in the CSF strongly suggests SAH. In a retrospective study of patients with confirmed aneurysmal SAH (n = 111), xanthochromia was present in 100% of patients when the CSF was collected 12 hours to 2 weeks after onset of symptoms and analyzed by spectrophotometry.[136] Interestingly, xanthochromia was still present at 4 weeks after onset of symptoms in some (10 of 14) patients. Several hours after SAH, the lysing of red blood cells releases oxyhemoglobin, with subsequent formation of bilirubin, which has a yellowish appearance. This process may take up to 12 hours, so results of an LP performed too early after SAH may be falsely negative. One should evaluate CSF for xanthochromia with spectrophotometry rather than visual examination, which is not as sensitive. Most institutions rely on visual inspection of CSF. Other findings of

CSF analysis that are suggestive of but not definitive for the diagnosis of SAH include elevated protein, elevated D-dimer levels, presence of coagulation, crenated erythrocytes, and elevated opening pressure. It may be difficult to differentiate a "traumatic tap" from SAH. The finding of a serially decreasing red blood cell count from the first to the last CSF tube may suggest a traumatic tap, but because this decrement may also be seen with aneurysmal SAH, it is not definitive.[136,137] In contrast, xanthochromia is usually absent with a traumatic tap if the CSF is promptly analyzed.

MRI is not indicated as an initial diagnostic test for SAH; however, it may be useful if the head CT findings are negative, but results of the LP are abnormal. Mitchell and coworkers[138] found that gradient-echo T2-weighted MRI was 94% and 100% sensitive for detecting subarachnoid blood in the acute and subacute phases, respectively.[138] Additionally, Noguchi and associates[139,140] reported that the fluid-attenuated inversion recovery (FLAIR) MRI sequence detected SAH as well as non–contrast-enhanced head CT in the acute setting and better in the subacute to chronic phase.

The combination of normal CT and LP findings safely rules out SAH and thus should obviate cerebral angiography. In a prospective cohort study of patients with suspected SAH in whom CT and LP findings were negative, no SAH was observed in any patient during a 3-year follow-up.[141] Similarly, four other studies, one retrospective[142] and three prospective,[118,143,144] that evaluated patients with acute severe headache found no evidence of subsequent SAH or sudden death on long-term follow-up in patients with initially negative head CT and LP findings. Consequently, angiography is not routinely indicated in these patients, because the possibility of SAH is remote. Furthermore, the finding of a small incidental intracranial aneurysm does not imply that it has ruptured and may lead to unnecessary surgical or endovascular interventions that may result in perioperative morbidity and mortality.

Searching for the Aneurysm

After diagnosis of SAH, the next step is to promptly identify an aneurysm. Current practice dictates the early treatment of ruptured intracranial aneurysms. Delayed treatment of aneurysms increases the risk of rebleeding and may prohibit aggressive hemodynamic management of DCI.

Cerebral (Catheter) Angiography

Since its introduction in 1927 by Moniz,[12] cerebral angiography has remained the gold standard for diagnosis of intracranial aneurysms.[90,145] Advances in this technique have improved the diagnostic accuracy and decreased procedural morbidity. A "four-vessel" evaluation of the bilateral internal carotid arteries and vertebral arteries is necessary. The standard, digital subtraction angiography (DSA), may be supplemented by three-dimensional rotational angiography (3DRA) (Figs. 30-2 and 30-3). Van Rooij and colleagues[146] retrospectively reviewed the ability of this modality to detect aneurysms in the setting of a negative DSA result in patients with SAH. Remarkably,

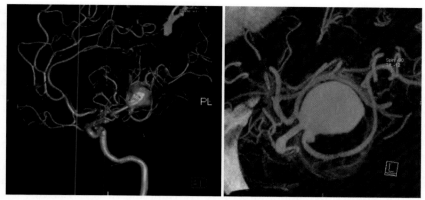

Figure 30-2 *Left,* Three-dimensional reconstruction angiogram (oblique anterolateral view) showing giant left middle cerebral artery bifurcation aneurysm, with several branches arising from aneurysm body. *Right,* CT angiogram of the same aneurysm (left lateral view).

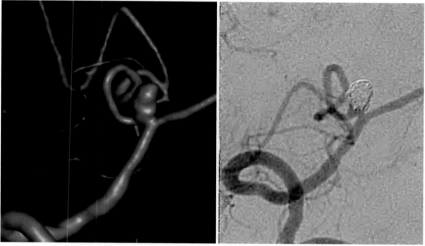

Figure 30-3 *Left,* Three-dimensional reconstruction angiogram showing a multilobed right posterior inferior cerebellar artery aneurysm. *Right,* Angiogram (AP right vertebral injection) showing coil occlusion of a posterior inferior cerebellar artery aneurysm.

three-dimensional rotational angiography revealed small (<5 mm) ruptured intracranial aneurysms in 18 of 23 (78%) of patients with negative DSA results; 16 of the 18 underwent subsequent treatment, either surgical (n = 7) or endovascular (n = 9).

Catheter angiography carries significant risks. Neurologic complications may include arterial dissection or rupture, ischemic stroke, and seizures. Nonneurologic complications include groin or retroperitoneal hematoma, contrast agent nephropathy, allergic reaction to contrast agent, and femoral artery dissection. With an experienced operator, there is about a 1.0% to 2.5% risk of neurologic complications, and 0.1% to 0.5% risk of permanent neurologic injury.[14,145,147,148] These complication rates apply to patients with various neurologic indications; patients who specifically have an angiogram for SAH may have different rates of complications. Interestingly, a study by Cloft and associates,[149] who reviewed the incidence of angiographic complications in patients with SAH, unruptured intracranial aneurysms, or arteriovenous malformations, found a combined rate of neurologic complications of 1.8%; however, the risk of permanent neurologic deficit was very low (0.07%).

CT Angiography

CT angiography (CTA) is emerging as an alternative diagnostic test for SAH; however, the diagnostic accuracy may be less than that of standard angiography.[14,150] The accuracy of CTA for detecting aneurysms varies widely in different studies. The sensitivity and specificity of CTA in comparison with those for DSA range from 77% to 100%, and 87% to 100%, respectively (see Fig. 30-2).[90,145,151-158]

Advantages of CTA include a quick procedural time, excellent anatomic rendering, and a low risk of complications. CTA reconstructed in 3D provides anatomically accurate relationships between the vascular structures and bone, which may be useful for surgical planning.[150,154] CTA poses less risk for iatrogenic complications than DSA because contrast agent is given intravenously for CTA, thus obviating the need for arterial manipulation. Interestingly, there are reported cases in which CTA revealed an aneurysm that was not seen with DSA.[159]

Some important limitations of CTA include a lower sensitivity for smaller aneurysms (<4 mm) and posterior circulation distribution aneurysms in comparison with DSA.[150,156] Furthermore, the large bolus of contrast agent needed for CTA may increase the risk of contrast-induced nephropathy, especially if performed in conjunction with DSA.[90]

Magnetic Resonance Angiography

Magnetic resonance angiography (MRA) is not appropriate to diagnose aneurysms in patients with suspected aneurysmal SAH. The sensitivity and specificity value for MRA for aneurysms in comparison with that for DSA ranges from 69% to 99%[90,145]; however, these studies were performed mostly in patients with unruptured aneurysms. The sensitivity for detecting small (<4 mm) aneurysms is poor. Some other limitations of MRA are the prolonged time required for scanning, susceptibility to motion artifact, and inability to be performed in patients who carry metallic objects such as pacemakers.

Angiographically "Negative" Subarachnoid Hemorrhage

In about 15% of patients with spontaneous SAH, results of the initial angiogram are negative; however, a second angiogram may reveal abnormalities in 2% to 24% of patients.[160] Thus, it is usual practice to obtain a second angiogram during initial hospitalization to exclude aneurysm and other vascular sources of SAH. The chance of finding an aneurysm is higher in patients in whom the initial CT scan showed a typical pattern for aneurysmal SAH than in patients in whom CT findings were negative but LP results positive.[161] Rarely, angiographically "negative" SAH may be due to spinal artery aneurysms or arteriovenous malformations; thus, MRI of the spinal cord should be considered.[162]

Grading Scales for Subarachnoid Hemorrhage

Numerous clinical and radiologic scales have been used to predict outcome after SAH.[163] Some of the clinical scales are Hunt and Hess,[164] Glasgow Coma Scale (GCS), World Federation of Neurological Surgeons (WFNS) scale,[165] and Prognosis on Admission of Aneurysmal Subarachnoid Hemorrhage (PAASH) scale (Table 30-4).[166] Radiologic grading scales include the Fisher scale,[167] modified Fisher scale,[134] and head CT grading scale (Table 30-5).

The Hunt and Hess scale is the most widely used clinical scale,[164] but its validity and reliability are suboptimal. The reason is the difficulty in grading subjective clinical symptoms and signs such as headache and level of consciousness.[24,163,168] Some newer scales (WFNS and PAASH) are more objective because they are largely based on the Glasgow Coma Scale (GCS), which is known to have good validity and reliability.[169-171] Recently, the

---

TABLE 30-4 CLINICAL GRADING SCALES FOR SUBARACHNOID HEMORRHAGE

Grade	Hunt and Hess Scale*	World Federation of Neurological Surgeons Scale	Prognosis on Admission of Aneurysmal Subarachnoid Hemorrhage Scale
1	Asymptomatic, mild headache, slight neck rigidity	GCS score 15	GCS score 15
2	Moderate to severe headache, neck rigidity, cranial nerve palsy	GCS score 13 or 14, without focal deficit	GCS score 11 to 14
3	Drowsiness, confusion, mild focal deficit	GCS score 13 or 14, with focal deficit	GCS score 8 to10
4	Stupor, moderate to severe hemiparesis	GCS score 7 to12	GCS score 4 to 7
5	Coma, decerebrate posturing	GCS score 3 to 6	GCS score 3

*Severe systemic conditions, including hypertension, diabetes mellitus, chronic obstructive pulmonary disease, coronary artery disease, and angiographically detected vasospasm, require advancing classification by one grade.
GCS, Glasgow Coma Scale.
Data from Hunt WE, Hess RM: Surgical risk as related to time of intervention in the repair of intracranial aneurysms. *J Neurosurg* 28:14-20, 1968; Report of World Federation of Neurological Surgeons Committee on a Universal Subarachnoid Hemorrhage Grading Scale. *J Neurosurg* 68:985-986, 1988; and Takagi K, Tamura A, Nakagomi T, et al: How should a subarachnoid hemorrhage grading scale be determined? A combinatorial approach based solely on the Glasgow Coma Scale. *J Neurosurg* 90: 680-687, 1999.

TABLE 30-5 HEAD CT GRADING SCALES FOR SUBARACHNOID HEMORRHAGE

Grade	Fisher Scale	Modified Fisher Scale
1	No visualization of blood	Diffuse thin SAH with no IVH
2	Diffuse thin layer <1 mm thick in vertical layers	Any IVH with thin or no visualized SAH
3	Localized clots and/or vertical layers <1 mm thick	Diffuse or localized thick SAH without IVH
4	Diffuse blood, but intraventricular or intracerebral clots	Diffuse or localized thick SAH with IVH

IVH, intraventricular hemorrhage; SAH, subarachnoid hemorrhage.
Data from Fisher CM, Kistler JP, Davis JM: Relation of cerebral vasospasm to subarachnoid hemorrhage visualized by computerized tomographic scanning. *Neurosurgery* 6:1-9, 1980; and Frontera JA, Claassen J, Schmidt JM, et al: Prediction of symptomatic vasospasm after subarachnoid hemorrhage: The modified Fisher scale. *Neurosurgery* 59: 21-27; discussion 21-27, 2006.

PAASH scale was compared with the WFNS scale, and the investigators in the study concluded that both scales had good ability to predict outcome; however, the PAASH scale performed even better than the WFNS scale owing to a more even distribution of outcome measures with ascending clinical grades.[172]

Radiologic scales have attempted to relate the amount of initial hemorrhage to the risk of DCI. In 1980, Fisher and coworkers[167] reported a scale that related the amount of SAH on initial head CT to subsequent risk of symptomatic vasospasm. The presence of thick SAH and vertical layering of blood in cisterns predicts the highest risk for development of symptomatic vasospasm; however, the Fisher scale has several limitations. First, the measurements used to determine blood thickness are based on printed CT images but have no relationship to true measurements. Second, an ascending grade does not correlate well with an increased risk of symptomatic vasospasm, because grade III rather than grade IV carries the highest risk. Third, ventricular blood is disregarded on the scale. Finally, the scale predicts DCI rather than long-term outcomes. A modified Fisher scale has been proposed that better accounts for ventricular blood and contains a more linear association between ascending grade and DCI.[134]

Management

Initial management of the patient with SAH begins with the stabilization of the airway, breathing, and circulation. Then attention turns to the institution of general supportive and neuroprotective measures, in anticipation of the known complications of SAH. Concurrently, one should make expeditious plans to secure the aneurysm (Table 30-6).

General Measures

Given the high likelihood of acute deterioration, one should manage patients with SAH in the intensive care unit (ICU). Admission to a specific neurologic ICU is preferable, because there is evidence that care of critically

TABLE 30-6 MANAGEMENT GUIDELINES AFTER SUBARACHNOID HEMORRHAGE

General measures	
Close monitoring of neurologic and hemodynamic status	Admit to intensive care unit (preferably neurologic unit)
Blood pressure	Avoid hypotension; keep blood pressure <160 mm Hg systolic before aneurysm secured, and <200 mm Hg once it is secured
Fluid management	Keep patient euvolemic with normal saline infusion (about 3 L daily)
Glucose	Sliding-scale insulin and/or intravenous insulin to keep glucose <140 mg/dL
Temperature	Acetaminophen 325-650 mg every 4-6 hours, and cooling devices as needed to keep temperature <37.5°C; identify fever source
Neuroprotection	Nimodipine 60 mg every 4 hours for 21 days
Seizure prophylaxis	Phenytoin 20 mg/kg load, then 100 mg IV every 8 hours for 3-7 days
Nutrition	Early feeding; place enteral feeding tube if swallowing inadequate
Stress ulcer prophylaxis	H_2 receptor antagonist, proton pump inhibitor, or sucralfate
Venous thromboembolism prophylaxis	Before aneurysm secured: sequential compression devices and elastic hose
	After aneurysm secured: enoxaparin 40 mg subcutaneously (SC) daily, or heparin 5000 units SC three times daily
Management of neurologic complications	
Rebleeding	Consider antifibrinolytics before aneurysm secured
	Early (<72 hours) securing of aneurysm: clipping or coiling
Hydrocephalus	External ventricular drainage
Seizures	If status epilepticus: lorazepam 0.1 mg/kg, and load phenytoin 20 mg/kg if not already done. Obtain electroencephalography immediately; identify etiology
Vasospasm	Screen with transcranial Doppler ultrasonography daily; confirm findings with angiography as clinically indicated
Delayed cerebral ischemia	Institute triple-H therapy; target central venous pressure to 8-12 mm Hg or pulmonary capillary wedge pressure to 12-16 mm Hg; consider intraarterial angioplasty/vasodilators
Management of systemic complications	
Cardiac dysfunction	β-blocker therapy if there is troponin elevation, narrow-complex tachyarrhythmias, or neurogenic stunned myocardium
Acute respiratory distress syndrome	Institute lung-protective ventilation with lower tidal volumes (6 mL/kg ideal body weight)
Infection/sepsis	Remove intravenous and bladder catheters promptly once not needed; handwashing; oral hygiene; early mobilization of patient; efficient weaning from ventilator
Electrolyte disturbance	Replete magnesium, potassium, phosphorus, and calcium as needed
Hyponatremia	Assess volume status to differentiate cerebral salt-wasting syndrome (CSWS) from syndrome of inappropriate antidiuretic hormone (secretion) (SIADH)
	If CSWS: aggressive fluid replacement with normal saline or hypertonic saline; consider oral sodium replacement; and fludrocortisone 0.1-0.2 mg orally twice daily if refractory
	If SIADH: fluid restriction, but carefully monitor central venous pressure to maintain euvolemia

ill neurologic patients by a neurointensive care team may enhance outcomes.[173,174]

Blood Pressure Management

The optimal BP target for patients with SAH is unknown and may vary among individuals or at different points during the disease course. Some of the factors that may influence BP management include the aneurysm status (secured or unsecured), presence of elevated ICP, integrity of the autoregulatory mechanism of cerebral vessels, and presence of vasospasm, DCI, or end-organ dysfunction.[175-177]

Cerebral autoregulation refers to the process of maintaining a constant cerebral blood flow (CBF) despite large fluctuations in CPP. Normally, CBF remains stable, with CPP values ranging from 50 to 150 mm Hg.[178] This process is due to modulation of cerebral arteriolar smooth muscle in response to changes in the CPP. The CPP is the difference between the MAP and the ICP. In patients with impaired cerebral autoregulation, the CBF becomes more closely linked to the MAP, and relatively small changes in the MAP may result in substantial changes in CBF. An increase or decrease in CBF beyond a certain threshold results in cerebral edema or cerebral ischemia, respectively. The autoregulatory mechanism may be impaired after SAH.[175,179] Thus, it is prudent to maintain CPP within a narrow range. Although not routinely used, several methods are available to check the integrity of the autoregulatory response. One can assess the mean CBF velocity change induced by changes in the MAP using transcranial Doppler (TCD) monitoring.[179] Jaeger and colleagues[175] evaluated changes in brain tissue oxygen pressure in response to changes in the CPP in patients with SAH. Those who had impaired autoregulation, defined as a significant change in brain tissue oxygenation for a given change in CPP, had a significantly higher incidence of delayed cerebral infarction.

Unsecured aneurysms are at risk for rebleeding; however, the literature has not conclusively identified hypertension as an independent predictor.[180,181] Nevertheless, the general consensus is that BP should be reduced to below 160 mm Hg in patients with unsecured aneurysms.[178] Care should be taken in the process, because excessive lowering may increase the risk of DCI in the setting of elevated ICP, vasospasm, or impaired cerebral autoregulation. In the American Heart Association/American Stroke Association (AHA/ASA) guidelines on SAH published in 2009, the recommendations regarding management of BP to prevent rebleeding are nonspecific, stating only, "blood pressure should be monitored and controlled to balance the risk of stroke, hypertension-related rebleeding, and maintenance of cerebral perfusion pressure."[182] Furthermore, intraoperatively induced hypotension is not advocated because of the possibility of harm from cerebral ischemia in patients who may have impaired cerebral autoregulation.

The presence of symptomatic vasospasm and DCI usually indicates a need to increase the BP to above the point at which symptoms resolve. The hypertensive component of triple-H therapy (hypertension, hypervolemia, and hemodilution; see later discussion) may require vasopressors to elevate the MAP above a certain threshold to improve the symptoms. The maximum BP target that is safe has not been well established, but generally the limit is a systolic BP of 200 to 220 mm Hg.[178]

The presence of end-organ dysfunction, such as hypertensive encephalopathy, aortic dissection, myocardial ischemia, pulmonary edema, or acute renal failure, may necessitate lowering the BP; however, there are no specific guidelines regarding this issue in patients with SAH. In patients with ischemic stroke, the usual goal is to reduce the BP by no more than 15% to avoid worsening ischemia.

In the case of symptomatic vasospasm and DCI, it may be necessary to induce hypertension as part of triple-H therapy. However, important systemic complications associated with induced hypertension include acute heart failure, myocardial ischemia, cardiac arrhythmias, and acute respiratory distress syndrome (ARDS). Some preferred choices for antihypertensive therapy are intravenous (IV) labetalol, esmolol, and nicardipine drip. Nitroprusside should be avoided because it can increase ICP.[14,178]

Fluid Management

The fluid management strategy in SAH depends on myriad factors, including the status of the aneurysm (secured or unsecured), and presence of vasospasm, DCI, cerebral edema, cerebral salt wasting, syndrome of inappropriate antidiuretic hormone (secretion) (SIADH), and diabetes insipidus. Although it is generally agreed that hypovolemia should be avoided, there are no solid data to determine whether euvolemia or hypervolemia should be the target of therapy. Euvolemia is achieved by keeping the central venous pressure (CVP) between 5 and 8 mm Hg with crystalloids or colloids. In patients with DCI, hypervolemia is achieved by targeting a central venous pressure between 8 and 12 mm Hg, or pulmonary capillary wedge pressure (PCWP) between 12 and 16 mm Hg.[14] In general, hypotonic fluids such as 0.45% saline, 5% dextrose in water (D_5W), and lactated Ringer's injection should be avoided because they may worsen cerebral edema.

Temperature Control

Fever is common in patients with SAH and is associated with a poor outcome.[183-185] Fever is associated with exacerbation of cerebral edema, elevated ICP, and vasospasm.[183,186-188] Infection is the most common reason for fever in patients with SAH; however, noninfectious etiologies, including venous thromboembolism, intraventricular hemorrhage, drug effect, and central fever, should be considered if results of the diagnostic work-up are unrevealing.[184] Some predictors of fever in patients with SAH include intraventricular hemorrhage and poor Hunt and Hess grade.[185]

Maintenance of normothermia can be achieved by antipyretic administration (i.e., acetaminophen), ice packs, water-circulating cooling blankets, adhesive surface cooling, or endovascular heat exchange catheters. The optimal method is unknown. Furthermore, despite retrospective data showing a strong association between fever and poor outcome,[183-185] there are no prospective data to support routine prophylaxis to maintain normothermia in patients with SAH.

Avoiding Hyperglycemia

Hyperglycemia is associated with poor outcome in aneurysmal patients with SAH.[189-192] In a retrospective study of 352 patients with SAH, Badjatia and colleagues[189] found that higher mean inpatient serum glucose levels were significantly associated with a longer ICU stay, symptomatic vasospasm, and poor neurologic outcome at hospital discharge. Additionally, Lanzino and associates[192] found that elevated admission and inpatient serum glucose values independently predicted increased mortality and worse neurologic outcome as measured on the Glasgow Outcome Scale (GOS).[192] In two large randomized controlled trials by Van den Berghe and coworkers,[193,194] intensive insulin therapy in critically ill patients to maintain blood glucose between 80 and 110 mg/dL reduced duration of both ICU and hospital stays, chance of renal failure, and duration of mechanical ventilation. In the first of the two studies, which enrolled patients in surgical ICUs, strict glucose control also reduced mortality[194]; however, this finding was not seen in the subsequent study of patients in medical ICUs.[193] A post hoc analysis of patients with acute brain injury who were enrolled in the first of these two randomized trials found that intensive insulin therapy was associated with fewer seizures, lower ICP, and better neurologic outcomes.[195] Currently, there are no large randomized trials specifically evaluating patients with SAH. A small pilot randomized trial (n = 78) of patients with SAH found that insulin therapy to maintain glucose between 80 and 120 mg/dL reduced infection rates (to 27%, vs. 42% in the control group; $P < .001$), but did not affect vasospasm, 6-month mortality, or neurologic outcome.[196]

In the absence of good-quality prospective data, the optimal target for blood glucose in SAH is uncertain. A reasonable goal is to keep blood glucose less than 140 mg/dL. Intravenous infusion of insulin may be necessary. One should be cautious to avoid hypoglycemia, which could potentially worsen outcome. Therefore, a well-designed insulin protocol with defined treatment for hypoglycemia may be helpful.

Nutrition

Acute brain injury induces a hypercatabolic state.[197] Early institution of nutrition is associated with enhanced outcomes in patients with traumatic brain injury[198-200]; however, there are currently no specific data evaluating early nutrition for patients with SAH. The enteral route is generally preferred, but total parenteral nutrition (TPN) may also be effective in brain-injured patients.[201]

Neuroprotective Agents

Myriad agents have been tested for neuroprotection in patients with aneurysmal SAH. Some of the agents tested include calcium antagonists (i.e., nimodipine, nicardipine, AT877),[202] aminosteroids (i.e., tirilazad), antioxidants (i.e., nicaraven and ebselen), and antiplatelet agents (i.e., aspirin, dipyridamole, nizofenone, ozagrel sodium, and OKY-46).[24] The only agent that has definitely improved outcome in randomized controlled trials is nimodipine.

Nimodipine and other calcium antagonists: A 2007 *Cochrane Database Systematic Review* evaluated 16 randomized trials of calcium antagonists in SAH involving 3361 patients.[202] The investigators found that oral nimodipine was associated with a significantly reduced relative risk (RR) of poor outcome (0.67; 95% [confidence interval] CI, 0.55–0.81) in comparison with controls. This beneficial effect was not seen for intravenous nimodipine or other calcium antagonists. The beneficial results were strongly influenced by the largest of the trials (n = 544), which randomly assigned patients to oral nimodipine 60 mg every 4 hours for 21 days or placebo.[203] Although generally safe, nimodipine has the potential to produce hypotension.[202]

Steroids: There is no evidence to support the routine use of steroids in patients with aneurysmal SAH. A 2005 *Cochrane Database Systematic Review* evaluated three randomized trials with 256 patients with aneurysmal SAH; however, because of the small number of patients, there was insufficient evidence to suggest either a beneficial or a harmful effect of steroids.[204] In a later study, Katayama and associates[205] found that prophylactic hydrocortisone for 10 days starting postoperatively in patients with aneurysmal SAH prevented hyponatremia and reduced the need for fluid supplementation; however, the patient outcomes were not significantly different from those in the placebo group.[205]

Statins: There has been interest in statins as possible neuroprotective agents in SAH. The physiologic rationale for using statins in SAH includes enhancement of nitric oxide production and reduction of free radical formation, which may attenuate vasospasm.[206,207] However, there is currently a paucity of evidence from randomized controlled trials to support the routine use of statins in patients with SAH. The available literature includes only small randomized pilot trials[179,208,209] or retrospective data.[210-213]

Although most of the available literature suggests that statins are safe and may possibly reduce vasospasm in patients with SAH, [179,209,212] some of the data do not support this finding.[211,214] There are three ongoing phase III randomized clinical trials to evaluate statins in aneurysmal SAH: the Simvastatin in Aneurysmal Subarachnoid Haemorrhage (STASH) trial, sponsored by Cambridge University Hospitals NHS foundation trust; the Simvastatin on Subarachnoid Hemorrhage-induced Vasospasm trial, sponsored by Brigham and Women's Hospital; and the Use of Simvastatin for the Prevention of Vasospasm in Aneurysmal Subarachnoid Hemorrhage trial, sponsored by the University of Illinois.[215]

Antiplatelets: DCI with subsequent infarction after aneurysmal SAH is a major source of long-term disability. Although the mechanism of infarction may be related to symptomatic vasospasm, thromboembolism may also be involved.[216] Previously, a systematic meta-analysis of the randomized data showed that antiplatelet drugs were beneficial in reducing delayed ischemia in patients with SAH.[217] In this analysis of 599 patients with SAH, antiplatelet agents significantly reduced the incidence of delayed ischemia (RR, 0.65; 95% CI, 0.47–0.89) but did not affect long-term outcome. Subsequently, Van den Bergh and colleagues[218] randomly assigned 161 patients to receive acetylsalicylic acid (aspirin), 100 mg, as suppository therapy or placebo for 14 days after aneurysmal

SAH. Unfortunately, the trial was stopped prematurely after an interim analysis suggested the futility of finding a statistically significant reduction in the primary endpoint, delayed ischemia. A 2007 *Cochrane Database Systematic Review* evaluated seven randomized trials involving 1385 patients with SAH. There was a trend toward better outcomes with antiplatelet drugs but a higher rate of intracranial hemorrhages; neither of these differences attained statistical significance.[219] In conclusion, there is currently no solid evidence to support the routine use of antiplatelet drugs after aneurysmal SAH.

Venous Thromboembolism Prophylaxis

Patients with SAH are at high risk for venous thromboembolism (VTE), either deep vein thrombosis or pulmonary embolism. The safety of anticoagulant use for prophylaxis of venous thromboembolism in patients with SAH is not well established. There is some indirect evidence from randomized trials that low-molecular-weight heparin may be relatively safe after the aneurysm has been secured. Siironen and coworkers[220] evaluated the efficacy of enoxaparin on mortality and neurologic outcome in patients with aneurysmal SAH. Although they were not specifically looking at venous thromboembolism in this trial, the researchers found that enoxaparin, 40 mg SC daily for 10 days, did not significantly increase bleeding complications or affect neurologic outcomes. In patients who have contraindications to anticoagulant prophylaxis, mechanical prophylaxis with sequential pneumatic compression devices and thigh-high elastic compression hose is advocated.[14,221]

Stress Ulcer Prophylaxis

Gastric stress ulcers are common in critically ill patients and are associated with worse outcome.[222] Important risk factors for stress ulcers include acute brain injury, mechanical ventilation, and coagulopathy. Measures that may help reduce the risk of ulcers include early feeding and administration of H_2 receptor antagonists (e.g., ranitidine, famotidine), proton pump inhibitors (PPIs) (e.g., pantoprazole, omeprazole), or sucralfate. Unfortunately, there are no randomized data to guide the optimal regimen in patients with SAH. Although H_2 receptor antagonists and proton pump inhibitors are effective at reducing stress ulcer formation, they also increase the risk of pneumonia. In a randomized trial, sucralfate did not raise gastric pH as much as ranitidine and was associated with a lower risk of "late-onset" pneumonia.[223] In fact, some randomized data from critically ill surgical patients raise the question of whether stress ulcer prophylaxis should be administered at all because of the low risk of clinically significant gastrointestinal bleeding and the increased risk of nosocomial pneumonia in this trial.[224]

Ventilator Management

Many patients with aneurysmal SAH require mechanical ventilation, and improper ventilator management increases patient mortality.[225,226] Some indications for mechanical ventilation in patients with SAH are respiratory failure due to impaired oxygenation or inadequate ventilation, elevated ICP, need for surgery, and inadequate airway protection.

The mode of ventilation is probably not important so long as the patient maintains good oxygenation and ventilation and does not receive excessive tidal volumes. The plateau pressure, as determined by a short end-inspiratory hold, should be less than 30 cm H_2O to help minimize the risk of ventilator-induced alveolar injury.[227] The patient should be made comfortable with ample sedation and analgesia.

The optimal target for oxygenation in patients with SAH is unknown. One must balance adequate brain oxygenation with the risk of oxygen toxicity. A 2004 *Cochrane Database Systematic Review* found that hyperbaric oxygen in patients with traumatic brain injury reduced mortality but did not improve neurologic outcome.[228] Hyperoxygenation may contribute to lung injury due to oxygen-mediated free radical formation.[229]

One should closely monitor carbon dioxide (Pco_2) levels in ventilated patients with SAH to avoid hypercarbia and excessive hypocarbia. The CBF increases linearly in response to changes in the Pco_2 level; an increase in Pco_2 can significantly increase the CBF and cerebral blood volume and lead to exacerbation of the ICP. In contrast, hyperventilation may do harm by reducing CBF and thus lowering the threshold for cerebral ischemia.

A critical concept in ventilator management is that patients should receive lower tidal volumes than traditionally used. There are compelling data from two randomized controlled trials demonstrating that traditional (high) tidal volumes (12 mL/kg) increase mortality over that seen with lower tidal volumes (6 mL/kg).[225,226] Although these studies were not specifically conducted in neurologic patients, it would be prudent to err on the side of lower tidal volumes, so long as the Pco_2 can be controlled. If the ICP is an issue, the respiratory rate can be set to a higher level to facilitate Pco_2 clearance. An important endpoint of lower tidal volume ventilation is the plateau pressure, which represents the alveolar pressure at end-inspiration; a high plateau pressure may facilitate ventilator-induced lung injury. The plateau pressure is easily checked with an end-inspiratory hold maneuver for 0.5 to 2 seconds at the end of inspiration.[225]

The application of positive end-expiratory pressure (PEEP) may reduce ventilator-induced lung injury by preventing alveolar derecruitment at end-expiration. Although there is a theoretical concern that positive end-expiratory pressure may increase the ICP by impairing venous return or lowering cardiac output, the data do not necessarily support this possibility.[230,231] Apuzzo and colleagues[230] found that application of positive end-expiratory pressure greater than 5 cm H_2O did slightly increase the ICP, but there was no associated reduction in the CPP. Furthermore, Huynh and associates[231] found that the higher levels of positive end-expiratory pressure (11 to 15 cm H_2O) were associated with reduced ICP and increased CPP in patients with severe brain injury.

Sedation and Analgesia

One should adequately control agitation and pain in the patient with SAH, because they may exacerbate hypertension and ICP and potentially increase the risk of aneurysmal rebleeding. However, one should start with low doses and carefully titrate upward to avoid oversedation, which will obscure neurologic findings.

The optimal agents are short acting and free of significant hemodynamic effects. For sedation, some reasonable choices include intermittent doses of lorazepam or midazolam, either orally or intravenously. In patients undergoing mechanical ventilation who require sedation, propofol or midazolam intravenous infusion is appropriate; both are easily titratable, although midazolam may require longer clearance time with prolonged use. Propofol characteristically lowers the BP, so supportive vasopressors may be needed.

Some initial analgesic choices include acetaminophen and codeine; however, these are usually inadequate.[232] Opiates such as morphine and fentanyl are usually needed but may lower the BP or contribute to delirium. Meperidine and tramadol are best avoided because they can trigger seizures. Diclofenac has antiplatelet effects and should be avoided. Continuous infusion of fentanyl is convenient for intubated patients; patient-controlled analgesia may be appropriate for awake and alert patients.

Nausea and vomiting may be problematic and can be controlled with ondansetron, which has minimal sedating effects. Alternatively, one can use metoclopramide, keeping in mind the potential for dystonic reactions.

Securing the Aneurysm: Surgical versus Endovascular Treatment

Early treatment of the aneurysm has largely replaced the traditional "wait and see" approach. The potential benefits of securing the aneurysm early include reducing the risk of rebleeding and allowing aggressive hemodynamic management. Unfortunately, there are a paucity of randomized data comparing approaches. In 2001, a *Cochrane Database Systematic Review* evaluated the literature and found only one randomized trial on the subject of timing of surgery for SAH.[233,234] The investigators concluded that patients who had early surgery had a trend toward better outcome (death or disability at 3 months) (95% CI, 0.13–1.02).[233,234] In 2002, de Gans and colleagues[235] performed a systematic review of the literature regarding the timing of aneurysm surgery; they included data from one randomized trial and 243 observational studies. They evaluated early (within 72 hours), intermediate (4 to 7 days), and late (>7 days) surgery. Although there were few randomized data to analyze, the investigators concluded that early or intermediate surgery was preferred to late surgery, especially for patients with good clinical grades. Neither of the systematic reviews included studies involving endovascular therapy, which has now become the preferred treatment modality for the majority of aneurysms.[236]

There is ongoing debate regarding the best modality to repair a given aneurysm. Some of the factors that are important to consider in choosing the best approach are aneurysm anatomy, patient characteristics, and institutional expertise (Table 30-7). The International Subarachnoid Hemorrhage Aneurysm Treatment Trial (ISAT) attempted to determine the optimal aneurysm therapy; however, many questions remain.[236] This was a European multicenter, randomized controlled trial of

TABLE 30-7 FACTORS THAT MAY INFLUENCE TYPE OF ANEURYSM TREATMENT

Factor	Surgery	Endo-vascular Treatment	Both
Wide neck to body ratio	×		
Giant aneurysm	×		
Mycotic aneurysm			×
Aneurysm feeds arterial branches			
Clinical equipoise		×	
Anterior circulation			×
Top-of-basilar aneurysm		×	
Fusiform aneurysm			×
MCA aneurysm	×		
Advanced age		×	
Poor clinical grade		×	
Multiple aneurysms		×	
High risk for surgery		×	
Patient preference		×	

2143 patients with aneurysmal SAH. The patients were randomly assigned to surgical clipping (n = 1070) or endovascular therapy (EVT) with coiling (n = 1073). The primary outcome was death or dependency at 1 year, as measured by the modified Rankin scale. EVT yielded a significantly lower rate of death or dependency than did surgical clipping (23.7% vs. 30.6%, respectively; P = .0019). The risk of early rebleeding was modestly higher in the EVT group.

There are some criticisms of the International Subarachnoid Hemorrhage Aneurysm Treatment Trial. First, prior to enrollment, there had to be agreement between the neurosurgeon and interventionalist that either treatment modality was acceptable for the given aneurysm. Consequently, a large number of patients were excluded from enrollment owing to the perception that one modality was superior. Second, the risk of early rebleeding (within 30 days) was found to be higher with EVT. In fact, a long-term follow-up study of patients enrolled in the trial revealed that retreatment of aneurysms after EVT was necessary in 17.4% of patients, compared with 3.8% in the surgically treated patients. The EVT retreatment occurred throughout the follow-up period and was more likely to be used in patients who were younger, had incomplete aneurysm occlusion, or had a wide aneurysm lumen. However, the long-term risk of rebleeding was rare and not significantly higher in the EVT group than in the surgically treated patients.[237] Even though a higher proportion of patients required retreatment after EVT, the benefit in outcome was maintained in comparison with that in surgically treated patients in long-term follow-up.[238] There is some evidence from a subgroup analysis of the International Subarachnoid Hemorrhage Aneurysm Treatment Trial data that elderly patients (age > 65 years; n = 243) may benefit more from EVT than from surgery. Although there was no significant benefit in independent outcome at 1 year with EVT (60.1% vs. 56.1% for surgery; P = ns), there was a significantly lower risk of epilepsy (0.7% vs. 12.9%, respectively; P < .001).[239]

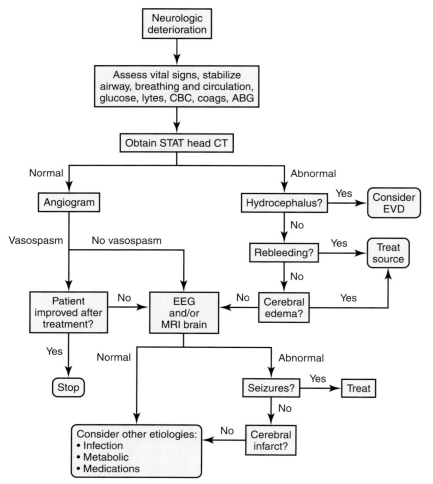

Figure 30-4   An approach to neurologic deterioration after SAH. ABG, arterial blood gas analysis; CBC, complete blood count; coags, coagulation studies; EEG, electroencephalography; EVD, external ventricular drain; lytes, electrolytes.

Neurologic Complications

One must remain vigilant to anticipate the myriad conditions that can lead to neurologic deterioration after SAH. A systematic approach can be helpful (Fig. 30-4). Some neurologic complications are aneurysmal rebleeding, hydrocephalus, seizures, vasospasm and DCI, and cerebral infarction (Table 30-8). Systemic complications may also contribute to apparent neurologic deterioration and are discussed later in the chapter (Table 30-9).

Aneurysmal Rebleeding

One of the most devastating early complications after SAH is aneurysmal rebleeding, which increases mortality up to 80%.[240] The risk of rebleeding peaks at 4% on the first day and is 1.5% per day for the next 2 weeks.[241] One study cites a risk of rebleeding of up to 17% on the first day after the ictus.[242] The cumulative risk of rebleeding is about 15% to 20% in the first 2 weeks[243] and about 50% by 6 months.[244] In a 2005 study of 573 patients, the cumulative short-term risk of rebleeding was found to be 6.9%, and most cases (72%) occurred within 72 hours.[181] Some patients may have rebleeding before seeking medical attention, so the true rate is unknown. Some known

TABLE 30-8   NEUROLOGIC COMPLICATIONS AFTER ANEURYSMAL SUBARACHNOID HEMORRHAGE

Etiology	Means of Diagnosis
Aneurysmal rebleeding	Head CT
Hydrocephalus	Head CT
Seizures: convulsive or non-convulsive	Electroencephalography
Delayed cerebral ischemia/symptomatic vasospasm	Transcranial Doppler ultrasonography, angiography, perfusion CT/MR
Ischemic stroke/intracerebral hemorrhage	Head CT, MRI of brain
Cerebral edema	Head CT, intracranial pressure monitoring

predictors of rebleeding are a history of sentinel headache, female gender, larger aneurysm size, higher Hunt and Hess clinical grade on admission, and time to surgery.[181,243,245,246] Some authorities speculate that placement of an external ventricular drain or lumbar puncture may increase the risk of rebleeding, but the literature does not support this proposition.[247,248]

TABLE 30-9 SYSTEMIC COMPLICATIONS ASSOCIATED WITH SUBARACHNOID HEMORRHAGE

Organ System	Complication(s)
Cardiac	Arrhythmias: sinus tachycardia, bradycardia, atrial flutter, atrial fibrillation, torsades de pointes, ventricular tachycardia, ventricular fibrillation
	Electrocardiographic abnormalities: T-wave inversion, peaked P waves, AV block, ST elevation or depression, QT prolongation, Q waves
	Neurogenic stunned myocardium
	Elevated cardiac enzymes
	Myocardial infarction
Pulmonary	Pneumonia: aspiration, nosocomial, ventilator-dependent
	Pulmonary edema
	Acute lung injury/acute respiratory distress syndrome
	Pulmonary embolism
	Pneumothorax
Infectious	Pneumonia, urinary tract infection, blood stream infection, sepsis, catheter-related infection, ventriculitis/meningitis
Hematologic	Thrombocytopenia
	Anemia
Endocrine	Cerebral salt-wasting syndrome
	Syndrome of inappropriate antidiuretic hormone secretion
	Hyperglycemia
	Central diabetes insipidus
	Adrenal insufficiency
Other	Deep venous thrombosis
	Gastrointestinal ulcers/bleeding
	Pressure ulcers
	Renal failure
	Allergic reaction
	Hepatic failure (rare)
	Electrolyte disturbances, especially hyponatremia, hypernatremia
	Systemic inflammatory response syndrome
	Fever

Clinically, rebleeding may manifest as an acute or worsening headache, decrease in the level of consciousness, loss of brainstem reflexes, posturing, respiratory arrest, or seizures.[120] Other manifestations include BP changes and elevated ICP. Rebleeding may manifest visually as an acute increase in external ventricular drainage or a change in the color of CSF from clear to red. One can confirm the diagnosis of rebleeding by urgent non–contrast-enhanced head CT. Definitive treatment of the aneurysm with EVT or surgical clipping markedly reduces the risk of rebleeding.

Before definitive treatment of the aneurysm, medical measures may help attenuate the risk of rebleeding. General measures, which are based mainly on common sense, include bed rest, maintaining a quiet and peaceful environment, treating pain, avoiding constipation, and controlling hypertension.[249] The literature is mixed about the effect of hypertension as a predictor of rebleeding.[180,181,250] The benefits of lowering BP may be offset by a higher risk of cerebral ischemia.[250]

Antifibrinolytic therapy with tranexamic acid or ε-aminocaproic acid (Amicar) reduces the risk of rebleeding but carries significant risks.[246] These agents inhibit plasminogen activation, which helps protect fibrin clots from degradation.[251] There is some evidence from randomized trials that short-term use of these agents (less than 72 hours) before definitive aneurysm treatment significantly reduces the risk of rebleeding without increasing the risk of ischemia[252]; however, it is uncertain whether long-term outcome is improved. A 2003 *Cochrane Database Systematic Review*, which included 1399 patients from 9 trials, concluded that antifibrinolytic agents reduced the risk of rebleeding (OR, 0.55; 95% CI, 0.42–0.71) but increased the risk of thromboembolism (OR, 1.39; 95% CI, 1.07–1.82) and did not improve neurologic outcome or mortality.[253] However, on the basis of the 2009 American Heart Association/American Stroke Association guidelines, a short course of antifibrinolytics before securing the aneurysm, or in patients deemed to be at low risk for vasospasm or in whom surgical delay is beneficial, is considered reasonable.[182] The usual dose of aminocaproic acid is a 5-g IV bolus, followed by an infusion of 1.5 g/hour for 24 to 48 hours.[14] A regimen for tranexamic acid is 1 g every 4 hours, with no bolus.[246] In addition to increasing the risk of ischemic stroke, other complications of antifibrinolytic therapy include venous thromboembolism, rhabdomyolysis, and acute renal failure.[246,254]

Hydrocephalus

The massive release of blood products into the CSF spaces may obstruct the ventricular system anywhere from the cerebral aqueduct to the arachnoid granulations and may lead to marked elevation in the ICP, resulting in herniation and brain death. Acute hydrocephalus occurs in about 20% of patients within 72 hours and is predicted by the demonstration of intraventricular blood rather than cisternal blood on head CT.[255] Acute hydrocephalus after SAH is associated with significantly increased mortality and neurologic impairment.[255,256]

The reasons underlying the association between acute hydrocephalus and worse outcome are unclear. One hypothesis is that lower CPP due to elevated ICP may increase the risk for cerebral ischemia; however, a 2007 study did not find a higher incidence of cerebral infarction in patients with SAH and acute hydrocephalus.[257]

The usual clinical findings in hydrocephalus include a progressively worsening level of consciousness and small, poorly reactive pupils in comatose patients.[255] Impaired upgaze due to dysfunction of the dorsal midbrain vertical gaze centers may be evident.[258] Diagnosis is made from non–contrast-enhanced head CT showing increased ventricular size. The "bicaudate index" provides an objective measurement of ventricular size on imaging studies; it is calculated by drawing a line between the maximum width of the lateral ventricles at the level of the caudate and dividing by the corresponding diameter of the line connecting the inner table of the skull at the same levels.[255,257] Hydrocephalus is present when the bicaudate index is greater than the 95% percentile adjusted for age (Table 30-10). Urgent external ventricular drainage may be life saving. A clinically dramatic response is often

TABLE 30-10 DIAGNOSIS OF HYDROCEPHALUS USING THE BICAUDATE INDEX

Age (yr)	95% Value of Bicaudate Index
<30	0.16
31-40	0.17
41-50	0.18
51-60	0.19
61-70	0.20
71-85	0.21

Data from Komotar RJ, Hahn DK, Kim GH, et al: The impact of microsurgical fenestration of the lamina terminalis on shunt-dependent hydrocephalus and vasospasm after aneurysmal subarachnoid hemorrhage. *Neurosurgery* 62:123-132; discussion 132-134, 2008; and Meese W, Kluge W, Grumme T et al: CT evaluation of the CSF spaces of healthy persons. *Neuroradiology* 19:131-136, 1980.

witnessed in comatose patients with SAH, who become alert and responsive shortly after placement of the external ventricular drain.

About 20% of patients with aneurysmal SAH require permanent shunting for chronic hydrocephalus.[259,260] The mechanism is not well determined but may be related to impairment of CSF absorption due to fibrosis of arachnoid villi in response to blood breakdown products and CSF inflammation.[261] Some retrospective data suggest that neurosurgical fenestration of the lamina terminalis to facilitate CSF drainage significantly reduces the occurrence of shunt dependence,[262,263] but other data do not support this finding.[260] A randomized controlled trial is needed to confirm the benefits of this approach.

Seizures

The incidence of seizures after aneurysmal SAH is 21% to 26%.[120,264] Furthermore, the presence of seizures at the onset of SAH is an independent risk factor for poor outcome.[265] Risk factors for seizures after SAH include poor-grade WFNS scale score on admission, thick cisternal blood clots, and aneurysmal rebleeding.[266,267] The efficacy of anticonvulsant prophylaxis of seizures after SAH is an area of controversy.[268] Traditionally, patients with SAH were started on anticonvulsants upon hospital admission and remained on the regimen for months to years. Later evidence suggests that long-term (>1 week) anticonvulsant prophylaxis may not be necessary and may even be harmful.[268-270] Anticonvulsant use is independently associated with worse outcome and may increase in-hospital complications.[269] Additionally, there is evidence that most seizures after SAH occur at the ictus rather than during hospitalization, the long-term risk of epilepsy is relatively low in survivors, and early prophylaxis does not prevent the long-term risk of epilepsy.[120,268,271] If anticonvulsant prophylaxis is used, there seems to be no benefit for an extended regimen. Chumnanvej and associates[270] retrospectively compared two different anticonvulsant regimens using phenytoin, evaluating seizure incidence and adverse effects. The traditional regimen consisted of phenytoin prophylaxis until hospital discharge, whereas the short regimen involved only 3 days of prophylaxis. The seizure incidences for the traditional and short prophylaxis regimens were not statistically different, 1.3% and 1.9%, respectively; however, the risk of hypersensitivity reaction was significantly higher in the traditional group (8.8% and 0.5%, respectively).[270] In survivors of SAH, the long-term risk of epilepsy is about 4% to 7%.[272-274]

Vasospasm, Delayed Cerebral Ischemia, and Infarction

One of the most feared complications after SAH is DCI and subsequent infarction, which is a source of major long-term disability. Although DCI is an anticipated complication, our treatment arsenal remains limited. One should understand an important distinction among radiologic vasospasm, symptomatic (clinical) vasospasm, and DCI. Radiologic evidence of vasospasm on angiography is found in about 66% of patients, whereas DCI occurs in about 32% to 46% of patients.[275,276] Symptomatic vasospasm is the most common cause of DCI; however, it has become clear that not all DCI is caused by vasospasm, as discussed later.[277]

The pathophysiology of DCI after SAH requires further elucidation. The instigating factor is thought to be related to extravasation of arterial blood, because the amount of subarachnoid blood in the basal subarachnoid cisterns correlates with the risk of DCI.[167,278] Second, the source of bleeding (i.e., arterial or venous) may be important. For example, it is known that the risk of vasospasm is exceedingly low after perimesencephalic hemorrhage, which may have a venous origin.[85] Oxyhemoglobin is implicated as the main trigger for vasospasm; however, this issue needs further confirmation.[279] Some of the subsequent mediators may be excess intracellular calcium,[280] free radical production,[281,282] neurogenic vascular dysfunction,[283] inflammatory infiltration of blood vessels,[284] and imbalances in vasoconstrictor and vasodilatory substances.[285]

DCI is usually related to vasospasm; however, attention has now turned to other etiologies, such as microthrombosis due to activation of the coagulation cascade and prolonged cortical spreading depression.[216,277,286,287] Stein and colleagues,[216] autopsying patients with SAH who died with or without DCI, found that patients with DCI had a much higher microclot burden, suggesting that thromboembolism played an important role in development of DCI in these patients. Interestingly, it was reported that patients with SAH who were undergoing aspirin therapy before aneurysmal rupture had a significantly lower risk of cerebral infarction.[288] Another interesting observation is that nimodipine, which improves outcome after SAH without affecting vasospasm, exerts fibrinolytic activity through a decrease in plasminogen-activator inhibitor-1 (PAI-1) levels.[289] Another potential cause for DCI that has gained attention is recurrent prolonged cortical spreading depression.[287] Dreier and associates[287] recorded spreading depolarization with electrocorticography in 18 patients with SAH who underwent surgical repair of an aneurysm. Recurrent spreading depolarizations were observed in 72% (n = 13) of cases and were closely correlated with subsequent DCI, with positive and negative predictive values of 86% and 100%, respectively.

The time course of vasospasm is usually predictable, with an onset beginning after 72 hours, a peak between days 6 to 8, and gradual resolution in 2 to 4 weeks.[14,290,291] It is unusual for vasospasm to begin within 72 hours after initial SAH.[292] Evidence of vasospasm may be observed on TCD ultrasonography up to 4 weeks after the ictus.[291]

Clinically, DCI may manifest subtly as worsening headache, confusion, decreasing level of consciousness, and eventual progression to a focal neurologic deficit.

The diagnosis of DCI is confirmed by urgently ruling out other causes of acute neurologic deterioration and demonstrating narrowing of the cerebral blood vessels on angiography (see Fig. 30-1). TCD monitoring is a useful noninvasive, bedside screening test for vasospasm. There is a good correlation between TCD evidence and angiographic demonstration of vasospasm. Vora and coworkers[293] demonstrated that mean CBF velocities less than 120 cm/sec and greater than or equal to 200 cm/sec had negative and positive predictive values of 94% and 87%, respectively, for demonstration of moderate to severe vasospasm on angiography; however, in most (57%) patients, CBF velocities were in the indeterminate range (120 to 199 cm/sec).[293] Other TCD measures that suggest vasospasm include an increase in flow velocity greater than 50 cm/sec in 24 hours and an elevated "Lindegaard" ratio. The Lindegaard ratio, which helps differentiate global hyperemia from vasospasm, is calculated as the ratio of the flow velocities in the middle cerebral artery and the ipsilateral *extracranial* internal carotid artery.[294] Ratios greater than 3 and greater than 6 are consistent with mild and severe vasospasm, respectively, whereas a ratio less than 3 in the setting of elevated blood flow velocities is consistent with global hyperemia, because the extracranial internal carotid artery does not have vasospasm but will increase with systemic hemodynamic factors. Although TCD evidence of vasospasm correlates well with angiographic demonstration of vasospasm, the sensitivity of TCD for DCI is less robust. Suarez and associates[295] found that the sensitivity of TCD evidence of vasospasm for detection of DCI was 73% for the anterior circulation; interestingly, angiography was only 80% sensitive.[295] This finding is consistent with the notion that there are other causes for DCI than strictly angiographic narrowing of the blood vessels. TCD has several limitations, including dependence on operator technique, patient-specific anatomic factors (i.e., abnormal bone window anatomy), and inability for insonation of distal arterial branches. Additionally, TCD blood flow velocities may be influenced by factors other than vasospasm, including BP, ICP, Pco_2, hematocrit, and patient age.[296] Furthermore, TCD is more accurate in the anterior circulation than in the posterior circulation. As such, different TCD criteria are proposed for assessing the posterior circulation.[297]

Perfusion CT of the head with or without CTA has shown promise for assessing the presence of symptomatic vasospasm.[298-301] Findings on perfusion CT that are consistent with DCI due to vasospasm include increases in cerebral blood volume, mean transit time, and time to peak and decreased CBF.[300,302]

Treatment of symptomatic vasospasm consists of medical and endovascular therapy. The cornerstone of medical management is triple-H therapy.[303] The hypertensive component of this therapy often requires a vasopressor such as phenylephrine, norepinephrine, or dopamine. Hypervolemia and hemodilution are achieved with aggressive crystalloid and colloid administration aimed at lowering hematocrit to about 30% to decrease blood viscosity. Endpoints of hypervolemia include targeting the central venous pressure to 8 to 12 mm Hg or pulmonary capillary wedge pressure to 14 to 18 mm Hg. Intermittent boluses of normal saline or human albumin may be necessary to achieve the desired hemodynamic endpoints.[304] Despite the widespread use of triple-H therapy, there are little prospective data supporting its efficacy. In 1982, Kassell and associates[303] retrospectively and prospectively evaluated a combination of volume expansion and induced hypertension in patients with SAH with angiographically confirmed symptomatic vasospasm. Of 58 patients, 43 had sustained improvement after the institution of triple-H therapy.[303] On the basis of findings in the largest retrospective series, symptoms referable to vasospasm improve with triple-H therapy in 60% to 74% of patients.[303,305] Potential complications of the approach include pulmonary edema, myocardial infarction, arrhythmias, acute respiratory distress syndrome, dilutional hyponatremia, and exacerbation of cerebral edema.[306] Additionally, there may be significant complications associated with the hemodynamic monitoring devices, either Swan-Ganz or central venous catheters, used to guide triple-H therapy. The Swan-Ganz catheter is no longer preferred because of its relative invasiveness; two large randomized controlled trials involving patients who either had acute lung injury or were high-risk surgical candidates showed no outcome benefit, but a higher complication rate was associated with pulmonary artery catheters than with central venous catheterization.[307,308]

Patients with DCI that is refractory to triple-H therapy may benefit from augmentation of cardiac output. Joseph and coworkers[309] found that CBF increased with dobutamine infusion independently of BP changes in patients with DCI. In patients with DCI who have heart failure or myocardial infarction and cannot tolerate triple-H therapy, some anecdotal reports describe improvement in symptoms with an intra-aortic balloon pump to augment CBF.[310,311]

Endovascular treatment for DCI is evolving, but large randomized trials of its use are lacking. EVT can be used alternatively or in conjunction with triple-H therapy. The two main approaches for EVT are intraarterial injection of vasodilators and/or transluminal balloon angioplasty.

Some IA vasodilators that have been used are papaverine, verapamil, nimodipine, and nicardipine.[312,313] Advantages of intraarterial vasodilators include immediate action and ability to alleviate distal arterial vasospasm; however, the effects of these agents are transient, and a second intervention may be necessary. Papaverine use has diminished owing to the observation that it may be neurotoxic.[314,315] Furthermore, intraarterial nicardipine may be longer acting than papaverine.[316] Although intraarterial vasodilators are generally safe, some possible complications of their use are hypotension, bradycardia, and elevation of ICP.[312,316]

Balloon angioplasty for DCI after SAH was first described in 1983 by Zubkov and associates,[317] who reported successful and prolonged response to treatment in 12 of 13 patients. A later pooled analysis of balloon angioplasty for DCI showed about a 60% response overall.[318] Clinical response is associated with increased CBF and decreased TCD-detected flow velocities.[318] Typically, balloon angioplasty involves gentle inflation of the balloon to successively larger volumes. A limitation of angioplasty is that the relatively large balloon size precludes dilation of smaller distal arteries. Possible complications of balloon angioplasty include those associated with angiography, such as arterial dissection, stroke, contrast allergy, and renal nephropathy, as well as catastrophic arterial rupture. After EVT, one can monitor blood flow velocities with TCD ultrasonography. A subsequent increase in TCD-detected flow velocities toward the level that previously produced symptoms can be used as a trigger for repeating EVT.

Cerebral Edema

The formation of cerebral edema after SAH occurs in 8% to 20% of patients and independently predicts poor outcome.[319,320] Cerebral edema may be present on admission or may develop subacutely. Predictors of acute cerebral edema include loss of consciousness at ictus and poor-grade Hunt and Hess scale value; late predictors include vasopressor use, large aneurysm size (>10 mm), and loss of consciousness at ictus.[320] Cerebral edema after SAH can be cytotoxic, vasogenic, hydrocephalic, or osmotic in origin. Cytotoxic edema may occur early, as a result of transient global cerebral ischemia due to the abrupt rise in ICP after aneurysmal rupture, or late, because of DCI. Hydrocephalic edema arises from impairment of CSF drainage and involves transependymal CSF flow. Vasogenic edema may occur from impairment of cerebral autoregulation, resulting in increased CBF and cerebral blood volume. Finally, osmotic edema may result from hyponatremia.[319]

Cerebral edema is reliably diagnosed from the presence of severe effacement of hemispheric sulci and basal cisterns, and blurring or finger-like extension of the gray-white matter junction at the level of the centrum semiovale.[320]

Medical Complications of Subarachnoid Hemorrhage

Multiorgan systemic disturbances are frequent after SAH and may be life threatening. Some of the medical complications are those seen in any critically ill patient receiving intensive care, and others are more specific to patients with SAH. Cardiac complications include neurogenic stunned myocardium, heart failure, myocardial infarction, and arrhythmias. Pulmonary complications include pneumonia, acute lung injury (ALI), acute respiratory distress syndrome, and pulmonary embolism. Endocrinologic disturbances include disorders of the hypothalamic-pituitary axis, cerebral salt wasting, and adrenal insufficiency. Infectious complications other than pneumonia include urinary tract infections, sepsis, and ventriculitis. Other medical complications are acute renal failure, electrolyte disturbances, deep venous thrombosis, gastrointestinal bleeding, and pressure ulcers.

Cardiac Complications

Cardiac dysfunction following SAH is common, occurring in 50% to 100% of patients, and includes arrhythmias, electrocardiographic abnormalities, neurogenic stunned myocardium, troponin elevation, heart failure, and myocardial infarction.[123-125,321] There may be genetic polymorphisms that predispose to development of cardiac dysfunction after SAH.[322]

Cardiac arrhythmias are frequent and range in severity from benign to life threatening.[124,323,324] Presence of serious arrhythmias occurs in about 4% of patients with SAH and independently predicts increased ICU length of stay, death, and poor neurologic outcome.[325] However, the cause of death in these patients is not usually related to the arrhythmia.[326]

Neurogenic stunned myocardium refers to acutely decreased left ventricular function that occurs shortly after aneurysmal rupture. On echocardiography, one observes a pattern of global or regional ventricular wall hypokinesis that is not usually referable to a distinct vascular territory.[327,328] Cardiac catheterization usually reveals normal-appearing coronary arteries.[329] Pathologic studies show a characteristic "contraction band necrosis."[330,331] The pathophysiology is thought to be related to sudden catecholamine surge. Ventricular function usually improves to normal spontaneously within a few weeks.[327,329]

Troponin elevation after SAH is also frequent. Multiple studies report that an elevated troponin-I value on admission is common after SAH and that it predicts cardiac dysfunction and poor outcome.[332-335] There is some evidence that β-blockade may have a beneficial effect on outcome in SAH; however, this possibility requires confirmation.[336,337]

Pulmonary edema is reported in about 29% of patients and may be related to both systolic and diastolic dysfunction after SAH.[338] The finding of elevated brain natriuretic peptide (BNP) after SAH may correlate with ventricular dysfunction and myocardial necrosis.[339]

Pulmonary Complications

Disturbances in pulmonary function may occur in SAH because of pulmonary edema, pneumonia, pulmonary embolism, and acute lung injury or acute respiratory distress syndrome. One study found abnormalities in oxygen exchange in 80% of patients with SAH and was associated with poor outcome.[340] Another study found that pulmonary dysfunction was associated with increased risk of DCI, thought to be due to the preclusion of aggressive hemodynamic therapy by tenuous lung function.[341]

Infection

Nosocomial infections are common after SAH. In a series of 573 consecutive patients with SAH, the following infections were identified: pneumonia (20%), urinary tract infection (13%), blood stream infection (8%), and meningitis or ventriculitis (5%).[342] In this study, pneumonia or blood stream infection independently predicted death or severe disability at 3 months.

Endocrine Disturbances

One should consider disorders of the hypothalamic-pituitary axis after SAH, which are likely underrecognized.[343-346] The most common hormonal abnormalities are deficiencies in growth hormone and adrenocorticotropic hormone. Acutely, patients may also have abnormalities in thyroid hormones that are compatible with euthyroid sick syndrome.[346] Deficiency in adrenocorticotropic hormone has direct clinical relevance because hypotension may increase the risk of DCI in the setting of vasospasm or elevated ICP. Similarly, central diabetes insipidus due to vasopressin deficiency has been described after clipping of anterior communicating artery aneurysms,[347,348] which could lead to rapid intravascular volume depletion and hypotension. Chronic endocrine disturbances occur in up to 55% of patients with SAH.[343,345,349] Patients with growth hormone deficiency after SAH may experience significant weight gain.[349]

Electrolyte Abnormalities

Abnormalities in serum electrolyte values are common after SAH and may be associated with poor outcome.[350-353] Thus, careful attention to electrolyte replacement is essential. Some of these disturbances are hyponatremia or hypernatremia, hypomagnesemia, hypokalemia, hypocalcemia, and hypophosphatemia.[350-355]

Hyponatremia should raise suspicion of cerebral salt-wasting syndrome (CSWS) or SIADH.[350,351] Hyponatremia may exacerbate cerebral edema and ICP. Hypernatremia may represent underlying central diabetes insipidus and is associated with a poor outcome.[351] Hypomagnesemia is associated with increased DCI.[352] Hypokalemia may contribute to life-threatening ventricular arrhythmias and prolongation of the QT interval.[124]

CSWS following neurologic injury was described as early as 1950[356] and has gradually gained widespread acceptance. Traditionally, hyponatremia after aneurysmal SAH was presumed to be due to SIADH; however, it has become clear that many cases of hyponatremia are due to renal sodium loss and have associated intravascular volume depletion. The differentiation of SIADH from CSWS is essential because the treatments vary markedly: SIADH requires fluid restriction, whereas CSWS requires aggressive volume replacement. Inappropriate fluid restriction in patients with CSWS may lead to dehydration and hypotension, which potentially increase the risk of DCI and cerebral infarction. The pathophysiology leading to CSWS is unclear. Berendes and associates[357] observed elevations of brain natriuretic peptide and depressed levels of aldosterone in patients with SAH with CSWS. Wijdicks and colleagues[358,359] observed elevations of both atrial natriuretic peptide (ANP) and brain natriuretic peptide above baseline in association with a negative fluid balance in patients with SAH.

The diagnosis of CSWS requires a determination of volume depletion. Volume depletion may be difficult to determine, and one should not rely on a single measure. The most accurate methods use radionuclide scanning with albumin or chromium-labeled red blood cells[360,361] but are expensive and not generally practical. Some bedside indicators of volume depletion include a central venous pressure less than 5 mm Hg, negative fluid balances, increased urine output, decreasing body weight, and low skin turgor. Laboratory tests are not generally useful to differentiate SIADH from CSWS. Treatment of CSWS involves aggressive volume and sodium replacement. Published regimens use various combinations of normal saline or hypertonic saline (3%) infusion, oral sodium replacement, and exogenous mineralocorticoids such as hydrocortisone and fludrocortisone.[362,363] Fludrocortisone is usually given at a dose of 0.1 mg daily up to 0.2 mg twice daily. Serious hypokalemia may result.[364] Treatment is gradually tapered over several weeks.

Outcomes

Despite advances in diagnosis and management of SAH, the outcome for most patients with aneurysmal SAH remains suboptimal. The case mortality rate is 40% to 50%; 10% to 20% of patients survive with severe disability, and 40% with independent function.[33] Some independent predictors of mortality and long-term disability include worse neurologic grade on admission, age, increasing systolic BP, fever, rebleeding, DCI and cerebral infarction, large aneurysm size (>10 mm), and elevated SAH Physiologic Derangement score.[185,365-368] The SAH Physiologic Derangement score combines a number of physiologic parameters—the arterioalveolar gradient and serum bicarbonate, glucose, and mean arterial pressure values—to create a score ranging from 0 to 8; a rising score strongly predicts neurologic disability and death. Patients with a score of 8 have a mortality approaching 80%, compared with about 10% for a score of 0.[365]

Long-term neurologic sequelae may be underrecognized. Hackett and coworkers,[369] interviewing 230 patients with SAH 1 year after onset, found that 46% reported impairment in cognitive function or mood.[369] The most common areas of impairment were memory (50%), mood (39%), speech (14%), and self-care (10%). Thus, quality of life after SAH may be impaired. Furthermore, there is about a 7% risk of epilepsy, which is associated with severe disability and reduced quality of life.[274]

REFERENCES

1. Morgagni G: *On the seats and causes of diseases investigated by anatomy,* London, 1761.
2. Haas LF: Papyrus of Ebers and Smith, *J Neurol Neurosurg Psychiatry* 67:578, 1999.
3. Pearce JM: Subarachnoid hemorrhage, *Semin Neurol* 26:148-150, 2006.
4. Pearce JM: The circle of Willis (1621-75), *J Neurol Neurosurg Psychiatry* 69:86, 2000.
5. Willis T: *Cerebri anatome: cui accessit nervorum descriptio et usus,* London, 1664, J Flesher.
6. Flamm ES: History of diagnosis and treatment of aneurysmal subarachnoid hemorrhage, *Neurosurg Clin N Am* 12:23-35, vii 2001.
7. Cheyne J: *Cases of apoplexy and lethargy: with observations upon the comatose diseases,* London, 1812, Thomas Underwood.
8. Blackall J: Observations on the nature and cure of dropsies, *London Quarterly Review* 428, 1813.
9. Gull W: Cases of aneurism of the cerebral vessels, *Guys Hospital Reports* 5:281-304, 1859.
10. Quincke H: *Verhandlungen des Congresses für Innere Medizin,* vol. 10, Wiesbaden, 1891, Zehnter Congress, pp 321-331.
11. Moniz E: L'encephalographie arterielle, son importance dans la localisation des tumerus cerebrales, *Rev Neurol (Paris)* 2, 1927.

12. Moniz E: Cerebral angiography. Its application in clinical practice and physiology, *Lancet* 225:1144-1147, 1933.

13. Dandy W: Intracranial aneurysm of the internal carotid artery cured by operation, *Ann Surg* 107:654-659, 1938.

14. Suarez JI, Tarr RW, Selman WR: Aneurysmal subarachnoid hemorrhage, *N Engl J Med* 354:387-396, 2006.

15. Sudlow CL, Warlow CP: Comparable studies of the incidence of stroke and its pathological types: Results from an international collaboration. International Stroke Incidence Collaboration, *Stroke* 28:491-499, 1997.

16. Rosamond W, Flegal K, Furie K, et al: Heart disease and stroke statistics—2008 update: A report from the American Heart Association Statistics Committee and Stroke Statistics Subcommittee, *Circulation* 117:e25-e146, 2008.

17. Feigin VL, Lawes CM, Bennett DA, et al: Stroke epidemiology: A review of population-based studies of incidence, prevalence, and case-fatality in the late 20th century, *Lancet Neurol* 2:43-53, 2003.

18. Johnston SC, Selvin S, Gress DR: The burden, trends, and demographics of mortality from subarachnoid hemorrhage, *Neurology* 50:1413-1418, 1998.

19. Ingall T, Asplund K, Mahonen M, et al: A multinational comparison of subarachnoid hemorrhage epidemiology in the WHO MONICA stroke study, *Stroke* 31:1054-1061, 2000.

20. Kozak N, Hayashi M: Trends in the incidence of subarachnoid hemorrhage in Akita Prefecture, Japan, *J Neurosurg* 106:234-238, 2007.

21. King JT Jr: Epidemiology of aneurysmal subarachnoid hemorrhage, *Neuroimaging Clin North Am* 7:659-668, 1997.

22. Ostbye T, Levy AR, Mayo NE: Hospitalization and case-fatality rates for subarachnoid hemorrhage in Canada from 1982 through 1991. The Canadian Collaborative Study Group of Stroke Hospitalizations, *Stroke* 28:793-798, 1997.

23. Linn FH, Rinkel GJ, Algra A, et al: Incidence of subarachnoid hemorrhage: Role of region, year, and rate of computed tomography: A meta-analysis, *Stroke* 27:625-629, 1996.

24. van Gijn J, Rinkel GJ: Subarachnoid haemorrhage: Diagnosis, causes and management, *Brain* 124:249-278, 2001.

25. Epidemiology of aneurysmal subarachnoid hemorrhage in Australia and New Zealand: Incidence and case fatality from the Australasian Cooperative Research on Subarachnoid Hemorrhage Study (ACROSS), *Stroke* 31:1843-1850, 2000.

26. Broderick JP, Brott T, Tomsick T, et al: The risk of subarachnoid and intracerebral hemorrhages in blacks as compared with whites, *N Engl J Med* 326:733-736, 1992.

27. Schievink WI: Intracranial aneurysms, *N Engl J Med* 336:28-40, 1997.

28. Brisman JL, Song JK, Newell DW: Cerebral aneurysms [see comment], *N Engl J Med* 355:928-939, 2006.

29. van der Jagt M, Hasan D, Bijvoet HW, et al: Validity of prediction of the site of ruptured intracranial aneurysms with CT, *Neurology* 52:34-39, 1999.

30. Juvela S, Porras M, Heiskanen O: Natural history of unruptured intracranial aneurysms: A long-term follow-up study, *J Neurosurg* 79:174-182, 1993.

31. Hop JW, Rinkel GJ, Algra A, et al: Case-fatality rates and functional outcome after subarachnoid hemorrhage: A systematic review, *Stroke* 28:660-664, 1997.

32. Ingall TJ, Whisnant JP, Wiebers DO, et al: Has there been a decline in subarachnoid hemorrhage mortality? *Stroke* 20:718-724, 1989.

33. Broderick JP, Brott TG, Duldner JE, et al: Initial and recurrent bleeding are the major causes of death following subarachnoid hemorrhage, *Stroke* 25:1342-1347, 1994.

34. Umemura K, Hirashima Y, Kurimoto M, et al: Involvement of meteorological factors and sex in the occurrence of subarachnoid hemorrhage in Japan, *Neurol Med Chir (Tokyo)* 48:101-107, 2008.

35. Inagawa T, Takechi A, Yahara K, et al: Primary intracerebral and aneurysmal subarachnoid hemorrhage in Izumo City, Japan. Part I: Incidence and seasonal and diurnal variations, *J Neurosurg* 93:958-966, 2000.

36. Fischer T, Johnsen SP, Pedersen L, et al: Seasonal variation in hospitalization and case fatality of subarachnoid hemorrhage—a nationwide Danish study on 9,367 patients, *Neuroepidemiology* 24:32-37, 2005.

37. Jehle D, Moscati R, Frye J, et al: The incidence of spontaneous subarachnoid hemorrhage with change in barometric pressure, *Am J Emerg Med* 12:90-91, 1994.

38. Qureshi AI, Suri MF, Yahia AM, et al: Risk factors for subarachnoid hemorrhage, *Neurosurgery* 49:607-612, discussion 612-613, 2001.

39. Broderick JP, Viscoli CM, Brott T, et al: Major risk factors for aneurysmal subarachnoid hemorrhage in the young are modifiable, *Stroke* 34:1375-1381, 2003.

40. Teunissen LL, Rinkel GJ, Algra A, et al: Risk factors for subarachnoid hemorrhage: A systematic review, *Stroke* 27:544-549, 1996.

41. Knekt P, Reunanen A, Aho K, et al: Risk factors for subarachnoid hemorrhage in a longitudinal population study, *J Clin Epidemiol* 44:933-939, 1991.

42. Schievink WI, Michels VV, Piepgras DG: Neurovascular manifestations of heritable connective tissue disorders: A review, *Stroke* 25:889-903, 1994.

43. Fogelholm R, Murros K: Cigarette smoking and subarachnoid haemorrhage: A population-based case-control study, *J Neurol Neurosurg Psychiatry* 50:78-80, 1987.

44. Juvela S, Hillbom M, Numminen H, et al: Cigarette smoking and alcohol consumption as risk factors for aneurysmal subarachnoid hemorrhage, *Stroke* 24:639-646, 1993.

45. Petitti DB, Wingerd J: Use of oral contraceptives, cigarette smoking, and risk of subarachnoid haemorrhage, *Lancet* 2(8083):234-235, 1978.

46. Longstreth WT Jr, Nelson LM, Koepsell TD, et al: Cigarette smoking, alcohol use, and subarachnoid hemorrhage, *Stroke* 23:1242-1249, 1992.

47. Canhao P, Pinto AN, Ferro H, et al: Smoking and aneurysmal subarachnoid haemorrhage: A case-control study, *J Cardiovasc Risk* 1:155-158, 1994.

48. Adamson J, Humphries SE, Ostergaard JR, et al: Are cerebral aneurysms atherosclerotic? *Stroke* 25:963-966, 1994.

49. Kawachi I, Colditz GA, Stampfer MJ, et al: Smoking cessation and decreased risk of stroke in women, *JAMA* 269:232-236, 1993.

50. Bonita R: Cigarette smoking, hypertension and the risk of subarachnoid hemorrhage: A population-based case-control study, *Stroke* 17:831-835, 1986.

51. Okamoto K, Horisawa R, Ohno Y: The relationships of gender, cigarette smoking, and hypertension with the risk of aneurysmal subarachnoid hemorrhage: A case-control study in Nagoya, Japan, *Ann Epidemiol* 15:744-748, 2005.

52. Jimenez-Yepes CM, Londono-Fernandez JL: Risk of aneurysmal subarachnoid hemorrhage: The role of confirmed hypertension, *Stroke* 39:1344-1346, 2008.

53. Kleinpeter G, Lehr S: Is hypertension a major risk factor in aneurysmal subarachnoid hemorrhage? *Wien Klin Wochenschr* 114:307-314, 2002.

54. Iso H, Jacobs DR Jr, Wentworth D, et al: Serum cholesterol levels and six-year mortality from stroke in 350,977 men screened for the multiple risk factor intervention trial, *N Engl J Med* 320:904-910, 1989.

55. Stampfer MJ, Colditz GA, Willett WC, et al: A prospective study of moderate alcohol consumption and the risk of coronary disease and stroke in women, *N Engl J Med* 319:267-273, 1988.

56. Donahue RP, Abbott RD, Reed DM, et al: Alcohol and hemorrhagic stroke. The Honolulu Heart Program, *JAMA* 255:2311-2314, 1986.

57. Gill JS, Shipley MJ, Tsementzis SA, et al: Alcohol consumption—a risk factor for hemorrhagic and non-hemorrhagic stroke, *Am J Med* 90:489-497, 1991.

58. Okamoto K, Horisawa R, Kawamura T, et al: Family history and risk of subarachnoid hemorrhage: A case-control study in Nagoya, Japan, *Stroke* 34:422-426, 2003.

59. Wang PS, Longstreth WT Jr, et al: Subarachnoid hemorrhage and family history: A population-based case-control study, *Arch Neurol* 52:202-204, 1995.

60. Juvela S: Nonsteroidal anti-inflammatory drugs as risk factors for spontaneous intracerebral hemorrhage and aneurysmal subarachnoid hemorrhage, *Stroke* 34:e34-e36, author reply e34-36, 2003.

61. Inman WH: Oral contraceptives and fatal subarachnoid haemorrhage, *Br Med J* 2:1468-1470, 1979.

62. Longstreth WT, Nelson LM, Koepsell TD, et al: Subarachnoid hemorrhage and hormonal factors in women: A population-based case-control study, *Ann Intern Med* 121:168-173, 1994.

63. Yano K, Reed DM, MacLean CJ: Serum cholesterol and hemorrhagic stroke in the Honolulu Heart Program, *Stroke* 20:1460-1465, 1989.

64. Yoshioka S, Kai Y, Uemura S, et al: [Ruptured cerebral aneurysm associated with coarctation of the aorta], *No To Shinkei* 42:1055-1060, 1990.

65. Putman CM, Chaloupka JC, Fulbright RK, et al: Exceptional multiplicity of cerebral arteriovenous malformations associated with hereditary hemorrhagic telangiectasia (Osler-Weber-Rendu syndrome), *AJNR Am J Neuroradiol* 17:1733-1742, 1996.

66. Schievink WI, Riedinger M, Maya MM: Frequency of incidental intracranial aneurysms in neurofibromatosis type 1, *Am J Med Genet* 134A:45-48, 2005.

67. Brill CB, Peyster RG, Hoover ED, et al: Giant intracranial aneurysm in a child with tuberous sclerosis: CT demonstration, *J Comput Assist Tomogr* 9:377-380, 1985.

68. Roman G, Fisher M, Perl DP, et al: Neurological manifestations of hereditary hemorrhagic telangiectasia (Rendu-Osler-Weber disease): Report of 2 cases and review of the literature, *Ann Neurol* 4:130-144, 1978.

69. Bromberg JE, Rinkel GJ, Algra A, et al: Subarachnoid haemorrhage in first and second degree relatives of patients with subarachnoid haemorrhage, *BMJ* 311:288-289, 1995.

70. Magnetic Resonance Angiography in Relatives of Patients with Subarachnoid Hemorrhage Study Group: Risks and benefits of screening for intracranial aneurysms in first-degree relatives of patients with sporadic subarachnoid hemorrhage, *N Engl J Med* 341:1344-1350, 1999.

71. Kongable GL, Lanzino G, Germanson TP, et al: Gender-related differences in aneurysmal subarachnoid hemorrhage, *J Neurosurg* 84:43-48, 1996.

72. Okamoto K, Horisawa R, Kawamura T, et al: Menstrual and reproductive factors for subarachnoid hemorrhage risk in women: A case-control study in Nagoya, Japan, *Stroke* 32:2841-2844, 2001.

73. Mhurchu CN, Anderson C, Jamrozik K, et al: Hormonal factors and risk of aneurysmal subarachnoid hemorrhage: An international population-based, case-control study, *Stroke* 32:606-612, 2001.

74. Yang CY, Chang CC, Kuo HW, et al: Parity and risk of death from subarachnoid hemorrhage in women: Evidence from a cohort in Taiwan, *Neurology* 67:514-515, 2006.

75. Gaist D, Pedersen L, Cnattingius S, et al: Parity and risk of subarachnoid hemorrhage in women: A nested case-control study based on national Swedish registries, *Stroke* 35:28-32, 2004.

76. Wakabayashi T, Fujita S, Ohbora Y, et al: Polycystic kidney disease and intracranial aneurysms: Early angiographic diagnosis and early operation for the unruptured aneurysm, *J Neurosurg* 58:488-491, 1983.

77. Oken BS: Intracranial aneurysms in polycystic kidney disease, *N Engl J Med* 309:927-928, 1983.

78. Chapman AB, Rubinstein D, Hughes R, et al: Intracranial aneurysms in autosomal dominant polycystic kidney disease, *N Engl J Med* 327:916-920, 1992.

79. van Dijk MA, Chang PC, Peters DJ, et al: Intracranial aneurysms in polycystic kidney disease linked to chromosome 4, *J Am Soc Nephrol* 6:1670-1673, 1995.

80. Yanaka K, Nagase S, Asakawa H, et al: Management of unruptured cerebral aneurysms in patients with polycystic kidney disease, *Surg Neurol* 62:538-545, discussion 545, 2004.

81. Gieteling EW, Rinkel GJ: Characteristics of intracranial aneurysms and subarachnoid haemorrhage in patients with polycystic kidney disease, *J Neurol* 250:418-423, 2003.

82. Watanabe A, Hirano K, Kamada M, et al: Perimesencephalic nonaneurysmal subarachnoid haemorrhage and variations in the veins, *Neuroradiology* 44:319-325, 2002.

83. Yamakawa H, Ohe N, Yano H, et al: Venous drainage patterns in perimesencephalic nonaneurysmal subarachnoid hemorrhage, *Clin Neurol Neurosurg* 110:587-591, 2008.

84. Rinkel GJ, Wijdicks EF, Vermeulen M, et al: Nonaneurysmal perimesencephalic subarachnoid hemorrhage: CT and MR patterns that differ from aneurysmal rupture, *AJNR Am J Neuroradiol* 12:829-834, 1991.

85. Rinkel GJ, Wijdicks EF, Vermeulen M, et al: The clinical course of perimesencephalic nonaneurysmal subarachnoid hemorrhage, *Ann Neurol* 29:463-468, 1991.

86. Greebe P, Rinkel GJ: Life expectancy after perimesencephalic subarachnoid hemorrhage, *Stroke* 38:1222-1224, 2007.

87. Findlay JM, Hao C, Emery D: Non-atherosclerotic fusiform cerebral aneurysms, *Can J Neurol Sci* 29:41-48, 2002.

88. Chun JY, Smith W, Halbach VV, et al: Current multimodality management of infectious intracranial aneurysms, *Neurosurgery* 48:1203-1213, discussion 1213-1214, 2001.

89. Rinne J, Hernesniemi J, Puranen M, et al: Multiple intracranial aneurysms in a defined population: Prospective angiographic and clinical study, *Neurosurgery* 35:803-808, 1994.

90. Brisman JL, Song JK, Newell DW: Cerebral aneurysms, *N Engl J Med* 355:928-939, 2006.

91. Stehbens WE: Heredity and the etiology of intracranial berry aneurysms, *Stroke* 27:2338-2340, 1996.

92. Stehbens WE: Etiology of intracranial berry aneurysms, *J Neurosurg* 70:823-831, 1989.

93. Inci S, Spetzler RF: Intracranial aneurysms and arterial hypertension: A review and hypothesis, *Surg Neurol* 53:530-540, discussion 540-542, 2000.

94. Juvela S, Poussa K, Porras M: Factors affecting formation and growth of intracranial aneurysms: A long-term follow-up study, *Stroke* 32:485-491, 2001.

95. Ferguson GG: The pathogenesis of intracranial saccular aneurysms, *Int Anesthesiol Clin* 20:19-24, 1982.

96. Krex D, Schackert HK, Schackert G: Genesis of cerebral aneurysms—an update, *Acta Neurochir (Wien)* 143:429-448, discussion 448-449, 2001.

97. Scanarini M, Mingrino S, Giordano R, et al: Histological and ultrastructural study of intracranial saccular aneurysmal wall, *Acta Neurochir (Wien)* 43:171-182, 1978.

98. Futami K, Yamashita J, Higashi S: Do cerebral aneurysms originate at the site of medial defects? Microscopic examinations of experimental aneurysms at the fenestration of the anterior cerebral artery in rats, *Surg Neurol* 50:141-146, 1998.

99. Kondo S, Hashimoto N, Kikuchi H, et al: Apoptosis of medial smooth muscle cells in the development of saccular cerebral aneurysms in rats, *Stroke* 29:181-188, discussion 189, 1998.

100. Nagata I, Handa H, Hashimoto N, et al: Experimentally induced cerebral aneurysms in rats: Part VI. Hypertension, *Surg Neurol* 14:477-479, 1980.

101. Hazama F, Hashimoto N: An animal model of cerebral aneurysms, *Neuropathol Appl Neurobiol* 13:77-90, 1987.

102. Kondo S, Hashimoto N, Kikuchi H, et al: Cerebral aneurysms arising at nonbranching sites: An experimental study, *Stroke* 28:398-403, discussion 403-404, 1997.

103. Zink WE, Komotar RJ, Meyers PM: Internal carotid aplasia/hypoplasia and intracranial saccular aneurysms: Series of three new cases and systematic review of the literature, *J Neuroimaging* 17:141-147, 2007.

104. Hassan T, Timofeev EV, Saito T, et al: A proposed parent vessel geometry-based categorization of saccular intracranial aneurysms: Computational flow dynamics analysis of the risk factors for lesion rupture, *J Neurosurg* 103:662-680, 2005.

105. Boussel L, Rayz V, McCulloch C, et al: Aneurysm growth occurs at region of low wall shear stress: Patient-specific correlation of hemodynamics and growth in a longitudinal study, *Stroke* 39:2997-3002, 2008.

106. van den Berg JS, Pals G, Arwert F, et al: Type III collagen deficiency in saccular intracranial aneurysms: Defect in gene regulation? *Stroke* 30:1628-1631, 1999.

107. Majamaa K, Myllyla VV: A disorder of collagen biosynthesis in patients with cerebral artery aneurysm, *Biochim Biophys Acta* 1225:48-52, 1993.

108. Chyatte D, Bruno G, Desai S, et al: Inflammation and intracranial aneurysms, *Neurosurgery* 45:1137-1146, 1999, discussion 1146-1147.

109. Miskolczi L, Guterman LR, Flaherty JD, et al: Saccular aneurysm induction by elastase digestion of the arterial wall: A new animal model, *Neurosurgery* 43:595-600, discussion 600-601, 1998.

110. McNeill AM, Zhang C, Stanczyk FZ, et al: Estrogen increases endothelial nitric oxide synthase via estrogen receptors in rat cerebral blood vessels: Effect preserved after concurrent treatment with medroxyprogesterone acetate or progesterone, *Stroke* 33:1685-1691, 2002.

111. Thomas T, Rhodin JA, Sutton ET, et al: Estrogen protects peripheral and cerebral blood vessels from toxicity of Alzheimer peptide amyloid-beta and inflammatory reaction, *J Submicrosc Cytol Pathol* 31:571-579, 1999.

112. Stirone C, Duckles SP, Krause DN, et al: Estrogen increases mitochondrial efficiency and reduces oxidative stress in cerebral blood vessels, *Mol Pharmacol* 68:959-965, 2005.

113. Wiebers DO, Whisnant JP, Huston J 3rd, et al: Unruptured intracranial aneurysms: Natural history, clinical outcome, and risks of surgical and endovascular treatment, *Lancet* 362:103-110, 2003.

114. Frösen J, Piippo A, Paetau A, et al: Remodeling of saccular cerebral artery aneurysm wall is associated with rupture: Histological analysis of 24 unruptured and 42 ruptured cases, *Stroke* 35:2287-2293, 2004.

115. Kataoka K, Taneda M, Asai T, et al: Structural fragility and inflammatory response of ruptured cerebral aneurysms: A comparative study between ruptured and unruptured cerebral aneurysms, *Stroke* 30:1396-1401, 1999.

116. Khurana VG, Meissner I, Meyer FB: Update on genetic evidence for rupture-prone compared with rupture-resistant intracranial saccular aneurysms, *Neurosurg Focus* 17:E7, 2004.

117. Weir B: Headaches from aneurysms, *Cephalalgia* 14:79-87, 1994.

118. Linn FH, Wijdicks EF, van der Graaf Y, et al: Prospective study of sentinel headache in aneurysmal subarachnoid haemorrhage, *Lancet* 344:590-593, 1994.

119. Leblanc R: The minor leak preceding subarachnoid hemorrhage, *J Neurosurg* 66:35-39, 1987.

120. Hart RG, Byer JA, Slaughter JR, et al: Occurrence and implications of seizures in subarachnoid hemorrhage due to ruptured intracranial aneurysms, *Neurosurgery* 8:417-421, 1981.

121. Pinto AN, Canhao P, Ferro JM: Seizures at the onset of subarachnoid haemorrhage, *J Neurol* 243:161-164, 1996.

122. Pfausler B, Belcl R, Metzler R, et al: Terson's syndrome in spontaneous subarachnoid hemorrhage: A prospective study in 60 consecutive patients, *J Neurosurg* 85:392-394, 1996.

123. Frontera JA, Parra A, Shimbo D, et al: Cardiac arrhythmias after subarachnoid hemorrhage: Risk factors and impact on outcome, *Cerebrovasc Dis* 26:71-78, 2008.

124. Andreoli A, di Pasquale G, Pinelli G, et al: Subarachnoid hemorrhage: Frequency and severity of cardiac arrhythmias. A survey of 70 cases studied in the acute phase, *Stroke* 18:558-564, 1987.

125. Sommargren CE: Electrocardiographic abnormalities in patients with subarachnoid hemorrhage, *Am J Crit Care* 11:48-56, 2002.

126. Edlow JA, Caplan LR: Avoiding pitfalls in the diagnosis of subarachnoid hemorrhage, *N Engl J Med* 342:29-36, 2000.

127. Mayer PL, Awad IA, Todor R, et al: Misdiagnosis of symptomatic cerebral aneurysm: Prevalence and correlation with outcome at four institutions, *Stroke* 27:1558-1563, 1996.

128. Neil-Dwyer G, Lang D: 'Brain attack'—aneurysmal subarachnoid haemorrhage: Death due to delayed diagnosis, *J R Coll Physicians Lond* 31:49-52, 1997.

129. van der Wee N, Rinkel GJ, Hasan D, et al: Detection of subarachnoid haemorrhage on early CT: Is lumbar puncture still needed after a negative scan? *J Neurol Neurosurg Psychiatry* 58:357-359, 1995.

130. Sames TA, Storrow AB, Finkelstein JA, et al: Sensitivity of new-generation computed tomography in subarachnoid hemorrhage, *Acad Emerg Med* 3:16-20, 1996.

131. Sidman R, Connolly E, Lemke T: Subarachnoid hemorrhage diagnosis: Lumbar puncture is still needed when the computed tomography scan is normal, *Acad Emerg Med* 3:827-831, 1996.

132. Boesiger BM, Shiber JR: Subarachnoid hemorrhage diagnosis by computed tomography and lumbar puncture: Are fifth generation CT scanners better at identifying subarachnoid hemorrhage? *J Emerg Med* 29:23-27, 2005.

133. Strub WM, Leach JL, Tomsick T, et al: Overnight preliminary head CT interpretations provided by residents: Locations of misidentified intracranial hemorrhage, *AJNR Am J Neuroradiol* 28:1679-1682, 2007.

134. Frontera JA, Claassen J, Schmidt JM, et al: Prediction of symptomatic vasospasm after subarachnoid hemorrhage: The modified Fisher scale, *Neurosurgery* 59:21-27, discussion 21-27, 2006.

135. Hillman J: Should computed tomography scanning replace lumbar puncture in the diagnostic process in suspected subarachnoid hemorrhage? *Surg Neurol* 26:547-550, 1986.

136. Vermeulen M, Hasan D, Blijenberg BG, et al: Xanthochromia after subarachnoid haemorrhage needs no revisitation, *J Neurol Neurosurg Psychiatry* 52:826-828, 1989.

137. Buruma OJ, Janson HL, Den Bergh FA, et al: Blood-stained cerebrospinal fluid: Traumatic puncture or haemorrhage? *J Neurol Neurosurg Psychiatry* 44:144-147, 1981.

138. Mitchell P, Wilkinson ID, Hoggard N, et al: Detection of subarachnoid haemorrhage with magnetic resonance imaging, *J Neurol Neurosurg Psychiatry* 70:205-211, 2001.

139. Noguchi K, Ogawa T, Inugami A, et al: Acute subarachnoid hemorrhage: MR imaging with fluid-attenuated inversion recovery pulse sequences, *Radiology* 196:773-777, 1995.

140. Noguchi K, Ogawa T, Seto H, et al: Subacute and chronic subarachnoid hemorrhage: Diagnosis with fluid-attenuated inversion-recovery MR imaging, *Radiology* 203:257-262, 1997.

141. Perry JJ, Spacek A, Forbes M, et al: Is the combination of negative computed tomography result and negative lumbar puncture result sufficient to rule out subarachnoid hemorrhage? *Ann Emerg Med* 51:707-713, 2008.

142. Wijdicks EF, Kerkhoff H, van Gijn J: Long-term follow-up of 71 patients with thunderclap headache mimicking subarachnoid haemorrhage, *Lancet* 2:68-70, 1988.

143. Markus HS: A prospective follow up of thunderclap headache mimicking subarachnoid haemorrhage, *J Neurol Neurosurg Psychiatry* 54:1117-1118, 1991.

144. Harling DW, Peatfield RC, Van Hille PT, et al: Thunderclap headache: Is it migraine? *Cephalalgia* 9:87-90, 1989.

145. Bederson JB, Awad IA, Wiebers DO, et al: Recommendations for the management of patients with unruptured intracranial aneurysms: A statement for healthcare professionals from the Stroke Council of the American Heart Association, *Stroke* 31:2742-2750, 2000.

146. van Rooij WJ, Peluso JP, Sluzewski M, et al: Additional value of 3D rotational angiography in angiographically negative aneurysmal subarachnoid hemorrhage: How negative is negative? *AJNR Am J Neuroradiol* 29:962-966, 2008.

147. Dion JE, Gates PC, Fox AJ, van Rooij WJ: Clinical events following neuroangiography: A prospective study, *Stroke* 18:997-1004, 1987.

148. Heiserman JE, Dean BL, Hodak JA, et al: Neurologic complications of cerebral angiography, *AJNR Am J Neuroradiol* 15:1401-1407, discussion 1408-1411, 1994.

149. Cloft HJ, Joseph GJ, Dion JE: Risk of cerebral angiography in patients with subarachnoid hemorrhage, cerebral aneurysm, and arteriovenous malformation: A meta-analysis, *Stroke* 30:317-320, 1999.

150. Anderson GB, Findlay JM, Steinke DE, et al: Experience with computed tomographic angiography for the detection of intracranial aneurysms in the setting of acute subarachnoid hemorrhage, *Neurosurgery* 41:522-527, discussion 527-528, 1997.

151. Uysal E, Yanbuloglu B, Erturk M, et al: Spiral CT angiography in diagnosis of cerebral aneurysms of cases with acute subarachnoid hemorrhage, *Diagn Interv Radiol* 11:77-82, 2005.

152. White PM, Wardlaw JM, Easton V: Can noninvasive imaging accurately depict intracranial aneurysms? A systematic review, *Radiology* 217:361-370, 2000.

153. White PM, Teasdale EM, Wardlaw JM, et al: Intracranial aneurysms: CT angiography and MR angiography for detection prospective blinded comparison in a large patient cohort, *Radiology* 219:739-749, 2001.

154. Harrison MJ, Johnson BA, Gardner GM, et al: Preliminary results on the management of unruptured intracranial aneurysms with magnetic resonance angiography and computed tomographic angiography, *Neurosurgery* 40:947-955, discussion 955-957, 1997.

155. Chappell ET, Moure FC, Good MC: Comparison of computed tomographic angiography with digital subtraction angiography in the diagnosis of cerebral aneurysms: A meta-analysis, *Neurosurgery* 52:624-631, discussion 630-631, 2003.

156. Dammert S, Krings T, Moller-Hartmann W, et al: Detection of intracranial aneurysms with multislice CT: Comparison with conventional angiography, *Neuroradiology* 46:427-434, 2004.

157. Agid R, Lee SK, Willinsky RA, et al: Acute subarachnoid hemorrhage: Using 64-slice multidetector CT angiography to "triage" patients' treatment, *Neuroradiology* 48:787-794, 2006.

158. Nijjar S, Patel B, McGinn G, et al: Computed tomographic angiography as the primary diagnostic study in spontaneous subarachnoid hemorrhage, *J Neuroimaging* 17:295-299, 2007.

159. Hashimoto H, Iida J, Hironaka Y, et al: Use of spiral computerized tomography angiography in patients with subarachnoid hemorrhage in whom subtraction angiography did not reveal cerebral aneurysms, *J Neurosurg* 92:278-283, 2000.

160. Schwartz TH, Solomon RA: Perimesencephalic nonaneurysmal subarachnoid hemorrhage: Review of the literature, *Neurosurgery* 39:433-440, discussion 440, 1996.

161. Little AS, Garrett M, Germain R, et al: Evaluation of patients with spontaneous subarachnoid hemorrhage and negative angiography, *Neurosurgery* 61:1139-1150, discussion 1150-1151, 2007.

162. Massand MG, Wallace RC, Gonzalez LF, et al: Subarachnoid hemorrhage due to isolated spinal artery aneurysm in four patients, *AJNR Am J Neuroradiol* 26:2415-2419, 2005.

163. Rosen DS, Macdonald RL: Subarachnoid hemorrhage grading scales: A systematic review, *Neurocrit Care* 2:110-118, 2005.

164. Hunt WE, Hess RM: Surgical risk as related to time of intervention in the repair of intracranial aneurysms, *J Neurosurg* 28:14-20, 1968.

165. Report of World Federation of Neurological Surgeons Committee on a universal subarachnoid hemorrhage grading scale, *J Neurosurg* 68:985-986, 1988.

166. Takagi K, Tamura A, Nakagomi T, et al: How should a subarachnoid hemorrhage grading scale be determined? A combinatorial approach based solely on the Glasgow Coma Scale, *J Neurosurg* 90:680-687, 1999.

167. Fisher CM, Kistler JP, Davis JM: Relation of cerebral vasospasm to subarachnoid hemorrhage visualized by computerized tomographic scanning, *Neurosurgery* 6:1-9, 1980.

168. Lindsay KW, Teasdale GM, Knill-Jones RP: Observer variability in assessing the clinical features of subarachnoid hemorrhage, *J Neurosurg* 58:57-62, 1983.

169. Braakman R, Avezaat CJ, Maas AI, Interobserver agreement in the assessment of the motor response of the Glasgow 'coma' scale, *Clin Neurol Neurosurg* 80:100-106, 1977.

170. Teasdale G, Jennett B: Assessment and prognosis of coma after head injury, *Acta Neurochir (Wien)* 34:45-55, 1976.

171. Jennett B, Teasdale G, Braakman R, et al: Predicting outcome in individual patients after severe head injury, *Lancet* 1:1031-1034, 1976.

172. van Heuven AW, Dorhout Mees SM, Algra A, Rinkel GJ: Validation of a prognostic subarachnoid hemorrhage grading scale derived directly from the Glasgow Coma Scale, *Stroke* 39:1347-1348, 2008.

173. Bershad EM, Feen ES, Hernandez OH, et al: Impact of a specialized neurointensive care team on outcomes of critically ill acute ischemic stroke patients, *Neurocrit Care*, 9:287-292, 2008.

174. Suarez JI, Zaidat OO, Suri MF, et al: Length of stay and mortality in neurocritically ill patients: Impact of a specialized neurocritical care team, *Crit Care Med* 32:2311-2317, 2004.

175. Jaeger M, Schuhmann MU, Soehle M, et al: Continuous monitoring of cerebrovascular autoregulation after subarachnoid hemorrhage by brain tissue oxygen pressure reactivity and its relation to delayed cerebral infarction, *Stroke* 38:981-986, 2007.

176. Handa Y, Hayashi M, Takeuchi H, et al: Time course of the impairment of cerebral autoregulation during chronic cerebral vasospasm after subarachnoid hemorrhage in primates, *J Neurosurg* 76:493-501, 1992.

177. Yamamoto S, Nishizawa S, Tsukada H, et al: Cerebral blood flow autoregulation following subarachnoid hemorrhage in rats: Chronic vasospasm shifts the upper and lower limits of the autoregulatory range toward higher blood pressures, *Brain Res* 782:194-201, 1998.

178. Mocco J, Rose JC, Komotar RJ, et al: Blood pressure management in patients with intracerebral and subarachnoid hemorrhage, *Neurosurg Clin North Am* 17(Suppl 1):25-40, 2006.

179. Tseng MY, Czosnyka M, Richards H, et al: Effects of acute treatment with pravastatin on cerebral vasospasm, autoregulation, and delayed ischemic deficits after aneurysmal subarachnoid hemorrhage: A phase II randomized placebo-controlled trial, *Stroke* 36:1627-1632, 2005.

180. Ohkuma H, Tsurutani H, Suzuki S: Incidence and significance of early aneurysmal rebleeding before neurosurgical or neurological management, *Stroke* 32:1176-1180, 2001.

181. Naidech AM, Janjua N, Kreiter KT, et al: Predictors and impact of aneurysm rebleeding after subarachnoid hemorrhage, *Arch Neurol* 62:410-416, 2005.

182. Bederson JB, Connolly ES Jr, Batjer HH, et al: Guidelines for the management of aneurysmal subarachnoid hemorrhage: A statement for healthcare professionals from a special writing group of the Stroke Council, American Heart Association, *Stroke* 40:994-1025, 2009.

183. Oliveira-Filho J, Ezzeddine MA, Segal AZ, et al: Fever in subarachnoid hemorrhage: Relationship to vasospasm and outcome, *Neurology* 56:1299-1304, 2001.

184. Commichau C, Scarmeas N, Mayer SA: Risk factors for fever in the neurologic intensive care unit, *Neurology* 60:837-841, 2003.

185. Fernandez A, Schmidt JM, Claassen J, et al: Fever after subarachnoid hemorrhage: Risk factors and impact on outcome, *Neurology* 68:1013-1019, 2007.

186. Clasen RA, Pandolfi S, Laing I, et al: Experimental study of relation of fever to cerebral edema, *J Neurosurg* 41:576-581, 1974.

187. Rossi S, Zanier ER, Mauri I, et al: Brain temperature, body core temperature, and intracranial pressure in acute cerebral damage, *J Neurol Neurosurg Psychiatry* 71:448-454, 2001.

188. Weir B, Disney L, Grace M, et al: Daily trends in white blood cell count and temperature after subarachnoid hemorrhage from aneurysm, *Neurosurgery* 25:161-165, 1989.

189. Badjatia N, Topcuoglu MA, Buonanno FS, et al: Relationship between hyperglycemia and symptomatic vasospasm after subarachnoid hemorrhage, *Crit Care Med* 33:1603-1609, quiz 1623, 2005.

190. Sato M, Nakano M, Asari J, et al: Admission blood glucose levels and early change of neurological grade in poor-grade patients with aneurysmal subarachnoid haemorrhage, *Acta Neurochir (Wien)* 148:623-636, discussion 626, 2006.

191. Alberti O, Becker R, Benes L, et al: Initial hyperglycemia as an indicator of severity of the ictus in poor-grade patients with spontaneous subarachnoid hemorrhage, *Clin Neurol Neurosurg* 102:78-83, 2000.

192. Lanzino G, Kassell NF, Germanson T, et al: Plasma glucose levels and outcome after aneurysmal subarachnoid hemorrhage, *J Neurosurg* 79:885-891, 1993.

193. van den Berghe G, Wilmer A, Hermans G, et al: Intensive insulin therapy in the medical ICU, *N Engl J Med* 354:449-461, 2006.

194. van den Berghe G, Wouters P, Weekers F, et al: Intensive insulin therapy in the critically ill patients, *N Engl J Med* 345:1359-1367, 2001.

195. van den Berghe G, Schoonheydt K, Becx P, et al: Insulin therapy protects the central and peripheral nervous system of intensive care patients, *Neurology* 64:1348-1353, 2005.

196. Bilotta F, Spinelli A, Giovannini F, et al: The effect of intensive insulin therapy on infection rate, vasospasm, neurologic outcome, and mortality in neurointensive care unit after intracranial aneurysm clipping in patients with acute subarachnoid hemorrhage: A randomized prospective pilot trial, *J Neurosurg Anesthesiol* 19:156-160, 2007.

197. Young B, Ott L, Yingling B, et al: Nutrition and brain injury, *J Neurotrauma* 9(Suppl 1):S375-S383, 1992.

198. Young B, Ott L, Twyman D, et al: The effect of nutritional support on outcome from severe head injury, *J Neurosurg* 67:668-676, 1987.

199. Hartl R, Gerber LM, Ni Q, et al: Effect of early nutrition on deaths due to severe traumatic brain injury, *J Neurosurg* 109:50-56, 2008.

200. Taylor SJ, Fettes SB, Jewkes C, et al: Prospective, randomized, controlled trial to determine the effect of early enhanced enteral nutrition on clinical outcome in mechanically ventilated patients suffering head injury, *Crit Care Med* 27:2525-2531, 1999.

201. Rapp RP, Young B, Twyman D, et al: The favorable effect of early parenteral feeding on survival in head-injured patients, *J Neurosurg* 58:906-912, 1983.

202. Dorhout Mees SM, Rinkel GJ, Feigin VL, et al: Calcium antagonists for aneurysmal subarachnoid haemorrhage, *Cochrane Database Syst Rev* (3) CD000277, 2007.

203. Pickard JD, Murray GD, Illingworth R, et al: Effect of oral nimodipine on cerebral infarction and outcome after subarachnoid haemorrhage: British Aneurysm Nimodipine Trial, *BMJ* 298:636-642, 1989.

204. Feigin VL, Anderson N, Rinkel GJ, et al: Corticosteroids for aneurysmal subarachnoid haemorrhage and primary intracerebral haemorrhage, *Cochrane Database Syst Rev* (3), CD004583, 2005.

205. Katayama Y, Haraoka J, Hirabayashi H, et al: A randomized controlled trial of hydrocortisone against hyponatremia in patients with aneurysmal subarachnoid hemorrhage, *Stroke* 38:2373-2375, 2007.

206. Trimble JL, Kockler DR: Statin treatment of cerebral vasospasm after aneurysmal subarachnoid hemorrhage, *Ann Pharmacother* 41:2019-2023, 2007.

207. McGirt MJ, Lynch JR, Parra A, et al: Simvastatin increases endothelial nitric oxide synthase and ameliorates cerebral vasospasm resulting from subarachnoid hemorrhage, *Stroke* 33:2950-2956, 2002.

208. Chou SH, Smith EE, Badjatia N, et al: A randomized, double-blind, placebo-controlled pilot study of simvastatin in aneurysmal subarachnoid hemorrhage, *Stroke* 9:2891-2893, 2008.

209. Lynch JR, Wang H, McGirt MJ, et al: Simvastatin reduces vasospasm after aneurysmal subarachnoid hemorrhage: Results of a pilot randomized clinical trial, *Stroke* 36:2024-2026, 2005.

210. Sillberg VA, Wells GA, Perry JJ: Do statins improve outcomes and reduce the incidence of vasospasm after aneurysmal subarachnoid hemorrhage: A meta-analysis, *Stroke* 79:380-386, 2008.

211. Kramer AH, Gurka MJ, Nathan B, et al: Statin use was not associated with less vasospasm or improved outcome after subarachnoid hemorrhage, *Neurosurgery* 62:422-427, discussion 427-430, 2008.

212. McGirt MJ, Blessing R, Alexander MJ, et al: Risk of cerebral vasospasm after subarachnoid hemorrhage reduced by statin therapy: A multivariate analysis of an institutional experience, *J Neurosurg* 105:671-674, 2006.

213. Parra A, Kreiter KT, Williams S, et al: Effect of prior statin use on functional outcome and delayed vasospasm after acute aneurysmal subarachnoid hemorrhage: A matched controlled cohort study, *Neurosurgery* 56:476-484, discussion 476-484, 2005.

214. Singhal AB, Topcuoglu MA, Dorer DJ, et al: SSRI and statin use increases the risk for vasospasm after subarachnoid hemorrhage, *Neurology* 64:1008-1013, 2005.

215. www.ClinicalTrials.gov, 2009, vol. 2009.

216. Stein SC, Browne KD, Chen XH, et al: Thromboembolism and delayed cerebral ischemia after subarachnoid hemorrhage: An autopsy study, *Neurosurgery* 59:781-787, discussion 787-788, 2006.

217. Dorhout Mees SM, Rinkel GJ, Hop JW, et al: Antiplatelet therapy in aneurysmal subarachnoid hemorrhage: A systematic review, *Stroke* 34:2285-2289, 2003.

218. van den Bergh WM, Algra A, Dorhout Mees SM, et al: Randomized controlled trial of acetylsalicylic acid in aneurysmal subarachnoid hemorrhage: The MASH Study, *Stroke* 37:2326-2330, 2006.

219. Dorhout Mees SM, van den Bergh WM, Algra A, et al: Antiplatelet therapy for aneurysmal subarachnoid haemorrhage, *Cochrane Database Syst Rev* (4), CD006184, 2007.

220. Siironen J, Juvela S, Varis J, et al: No effect of enoxaparin on outcome of aneurysmal subarachnoid hemorrhage: A randomized, double-blind, placebo-controlled clinical trial, *J Neurosurg* 99:953-959, 2003.

221. Black PM, Crowell RM, Abbott WM: External pneumatic calf compression reduces deep venous thrombosis in patients with ruptured intracranial aneurysms, *Neurosurgery* 18:25-28, 1986.

222. Stollman N, Metz DC: Pathophysiology and prophylaxis of stress ulcer in intensive care unit patients, *J Crit Care* 20:35-45, 2005.

223. Prod'hom G, Leuenberger P, Koerfer J, et al: Nosocomial pneumonia in mechanically ventilated patients receiving antacid, ranitidine, or sucralfate as prophylaxis for stress ulcer: A randomized controlled trial, *Ann Intern Med* 120:653-662, 1994.

224. Kantorova I, Svoboda P, Scheer P, et al: Stress ulcer prophylaxis in critically ill patients: A randomized controlled trial, *Hepatogastroenterology* 51:757-761, 2004.

225. Ventilation with lower tidal volumes as compared with traditional tidal volumes for acute lung injury and the acute respiratory distress syndrome. The Acute Respiratory Distress Syndrome Network, *N Engl J Med* 342:1301-1308, 2000.

226. Amato MB, Barbas CS, Medeiros DM, et al: Effect of a protective-ventilation strategy on mortality in the acute respiratory distress syndrome, *N Engl J Med* 338:347-354, 1998.

227. Hager DN, Krishnan JA, Hayden DL, et al: Tidal volume reduction in patients with acute lung injury when plateau pressures are not high, *Am J Respir Crit Care Med* 172:1241-1245, 2005.

228. Bennett MH, Trytko B, Jonker B: Hyperbaric oxygen therapy for the adjunctive treatment of traumatic brain injury, *Cochrane Database Syst Rev* (4), CD004609, 2004.

229. Lewis J, Veldhuizen R: Ventilation and oxygen: Just what the doctor ordered...unfortunately, *Crit Care Med* 32:2556-2557, 2004.

230. Apuzzo JL, Wiess MH, Petersons V, et al: Effect of positive end expiratory pressure ventilation on intracranial pressure in man, *J Neurosurg* 46:227-232, 1977.

231. Huynh T, Messer M, Sing RF, et al: Positive end-expiratory pressure alters intracranial and cerebral perfusion pressure in severe traumatic brain injury, *J Trauma* 53:488-492, discussion 492-493, 2002.

232. Roberts GC: Post-craniotomy analgesia: Current practices in British neurosurgical centres—a survey of post-craniotomy analgesic practices, *Eur J Anaesthesiol* 22:328-332, 2005.

233. Ohman J, Heiskanen O: Timing of operation for ruptured supratentorial aneurysms: A prospective randomized study, *J Neurosurg* 70:55-60, 1989.

234. Whitfield PC, Kirkpatrick PJ: Timing of surgery for aneurysmal subarachnoid haemorrhage, *Cochrane Database Syst Rev* (2), CD001697, 2001.

235. de Gans K, Nieuwkamp DJ, Rinkel GJ, et al: Timing of aneurysm surgery in subarachnoid hemorrhage: A systematic review of the literature, *Neurosurgery* 50:336-340, discussion 340-342, 2002.

236. Molyneux A, Kerr R, Stratton I, et al: International Subarachnoid Aneurysm Trial (ISAT) of neurosurgical clipping versus endovascular coiling in 2143 patients with ruptured intracranial aneurysms: A randomised trial, *Lancet* 360:1267-1274, 2002.

237. Campi A, Ramzi N, Molyneux AJ, et al: Retreatment of ruptured cerebral aneurysms in patients randomized by coiling or clipping in the International Subarachnoid Aneurysm Trial (ISAT), *Stroke* 38:1538-1544, 2007.

238. Molyneux AJ, Kerr RS, Yu LM, et al: International Subarachnoid Aneurysm Trial (ISAT) of neurosurgical clipping versus endovascular coiling in 2143 patients with ruptured intracranial aneurysms: A randomised comparison of effects on survival, dependency, seizures, rebleeding, subgroups, and aneurysm occlusion, *Lancet* 366:809-817, 2005.

239. Ryttlefors M, Enblad P, Kerr RS, et al: International Subarachnoid Aneurysm Trial of neurosurgical clipping versus endovascular coiling: Subgroup analysis of 278 elderly patients, *Stroke* 39:2720-2726, 2008.

240. Rosenorn J, Eskesen V, Schmidt K, et al: The risk of rebleeding from ruptured intracranial aneurysms, *J Neurosurg* 67:329-332, 1987.

241. Kassell NF, Torner JC: Aneurysmal rebleeding: A preliminary report from the Cooperative Aneurysm Study, *Neurosurgery* 13:479-481, 1983.

242. Fujii Y, Takeuchi S, Sasaki O, et al: Ultra-early rebleeding in spontaneous subarachnoid hemorrhage, *J Neurosurg* 84:35-42, 1996.

243. Torner JC, Kassell NF, Wallace RB, et al: Preoperative prognostic factors for rebleeding and survival in aneurysm patients receiving antifibrinolytic therapy: Report of the Cooperative Aneurysm Study, *Neurosurgery* 9:506-513, 1981.

244. Jane JA, Kassell NF, Torner JC, et al: The natural history of aneurysms and arteriovenous malformations, *J Neurosurg* 62:321-323, 1985.

245. Beck J, Raabe A, Szelenyi A, et al: Sentinel headache and the risk of rebleeding after aneurysmal subarachnoid hemorrhage, *Stroke* 37:2733-2737, 2006.

246. Chwajol M, Starke RM, Kim GH, et al: Antifibrinolytic therapy to prevent early rebleeding after subarachnoid hemorrhage, *Neurocrit Care* 8:418-426, 2008.

247. Hellingman CA, van den Bergh WM, Beijer IS, et al: Risk of rebleeding after treatment of acute hydrocephalus in patients with aneurysmal subarachnoid hemorrhage, *Stroke* 38:96-99, 2007.

248. Mehta V, Holness RO, Connolly K, et al: Acute hydrocephalus following aneurysmal subarachnoid hemorrhage, *Can J Neurol Sci* 23:40-45, 1996.

249. Lee K: Aneurysm precautions: A physiologic basis for minimizing rebleeding, *Heart Lung* 9:336-343, 1980.

250. Wijdicks EF, Vermeulen M, Murray GD, et al: The effects of treating hypertension following aneurysmal subarachnoid hemorrhage, *Clin Neurol Neurosurg* 92:111-117, 1990.

251. Burchiel KJ, Hoffman JM, Bakay RA: Quantitative determination of plasma fibrinolytic activity in patients with ruptured intracranial aneurysms who are receiving epsilon-aminocaproic acid: Relationship of possible complications of therapy to the degree of fibrinolytic inhibition, *Neurosurgery* 14:57-63, 1984.

252. Hillman J, Fridriksson S, Nilsson O, et al: Immediate administration of tranexamic acid and reduced incidence of early rebleeding after aneurysmal subarachnoid hemorrhage: A prospective randomized study, *J Neurosurg* 97:771-778, 2002.

253. Roos YB, Rinkel GJ, Vermeulen M, et al: Antifibrinolytic therapy for aneurysmal subarachnoid haemorrhage, *Cochrane Database Syst Rev* (3), CD001245, 2003.

254. Brown JA, Wollmann RL, Mullan S: Myopathy induced by epsilon-aminocaproic acid: Case report, *J Neurosurg* 57:130-134, 1982.

255. van Gijn J, Hijdra A, Wijdicks EF, et al: Acute hydrocephalus after aneurysmal subarachnoid hemorrhage, *J Neurosurg* 63:355-362, 1985.

256. Suarez-Rivera O: Acute hydrocephalus after subarachnoid hemorrhage, *Surg Neurol* 49:563-565, 1998.

257. Bakker AM, Dorhout Mees SM, Algra A, et al: Extent of acute hydrocephalus after aneurysmal subarachnoid hemorrhage as a risk factor for delayed cerebral infarction, *Stroke* 38:2496-2499, 2007.

258. Maramattom BV, Wijdicks EF: Dorsal mesencephalic syndrome and acute hydrocephalus after subarachnoid hemorrhage, *Neurocrit Care* 3:57-58, 2005.

259. Dorai Z, Hynan LS, Kopitnik TA, et al: Factors related to hydrocephalus after aneurysmal subarachnoid hemorrhage, *Neurosurgery* 52:763-769, discussion 769-771, 2003.

260. Komotar RJ, Hahn DK, Kim GH, et al: The impact of microsurgical fenestration of the lamina terminalis on shunt-dependent hydrocephalus and vasospasm after aneurysmal subarachnoid hemorrhage, *Neurosurgery* 62:123-132, discussion 132-134, 2008.

261. Massicotte EM, Del Bigio MR: Human arachnoid villi response to subarachnoid hemorrhage: Possible relationship to chronic hydrocephalus, *J Neurosurg* 91:80-84, 1999.

262. Tomasello F, d'Avella D, de Divitiis O: Does lamina terminalis fenestration reduce the incidence of chronic hydrocephalus after subarachnoid hemorrhage? *Neurosurgery* 45:827-831, discussion 831-832, 1999.

263. Komotar RJ, Olivi A, Rigamonti D, Tamargo RJ: Microsurgical fenestration of the lamina terminalis reduces the incidence of shunt-dependent hydrocephalus after aneurysmal subarachnoid hemorrhage, *Neurosurgery* 51:1403-1412, discussion 1412-1413, 2002.

264. Lin CL, Dumont AS, Lieu AS, et al: Characterization of perioperative seizures and epilepsy following aneurysmal subarachnoid hemorrhage, *J Neurosurg* 99:978-985, 2003.

265. Butzkueven H, Evans AH, Pitman A, et al: Onset seizures independently predict poor outcome after subarachnoid hemorrhage, *Neurology* 55:1315-1320, 2000.

266. Hasan D, Schonck RS, Avezaat CJ, et al: Epileptic seizures after subarachnoid hemorrhage, *Ann Neurol* 33:286-291, 1993.

267. Lin YJ, Chang WN, Chang HW, et al: Risk factors and outcome of seizures after spontaneous aneurysmal subarachnoid hemorrhage, *Eur J Neurol* 15:451-457, 2008.

268. Rhoney DH, Tipps LB, Murry KR, et al: Anticonvulsant prophylaxis and timing of seizures after aneurysmal subarachnoid hemorrhage, *Neurology* 55:258-265, 2000.

269. Rosengart AJ, Huo JD, Tolentino J, et al: Outcome in patients with subarachnoid hemorrhage treated with antiepileptic drugs, *J Neurosurg* 107:253-260, 2007.

270. Chumnanvej S, Dunn IF, Kim DH: Three-day phenytoin prophylaxis is adequate after subarachnoid hemorrhage, *Neurosurgery* 60:99-102, discussion 102-103, 2007.

271. Sundaram MB, Chow F: Seizures associated with spontaneous subarachnoid hemorrhage, *Can J Neurol Sci* 13:229-231, 1986.

272. Baker CJ, Prestigiacomo CJ, Solomon RA: Short-term perioperative anticonvulsant prophylaxis for the surgical treatment of low-risk patients with intracranial aneurysms, *Neurosurgery* 37:863-870, discussion 870-871, 1995.

273. Buczacki SJ, Kirkpatrick PJ, Seeley HM, et al: Late epilepsy following open surgery for aneurysmal subarachnoid haemorrhage, *J Neurol Neurosurg Psychiatry* 75:1620-1622, 2004.

274. Claassen J, Peery S, Kreiter KT, et al: Predictors and clinical impact of epilepsy after subarachnoid hemorrhage, *Neurology* 60:208-214, 2003.

275. Hijdra A, van Gijn J, Nagelkerke NJ, et al: Prediction of delayed cerebral ischemia, rebleeding, and outcome after aneurysmal subarachnoid hemorrhage, *Stroke* 19:1250-1256, 1988.

276. Solenski NJ, Haley EC Jr, Kassell NF, et al: Medical complications of aneurysmal subarachnoid hemorrhage: A report of the multicenter, cooperative aneurysm study. Participants of the Multicenter Cooperative Aneurysm Study, *Crit Care Med* 23:1007-1017, 1995.

277. Rabinstein AA, Friedman JA, Weigand SD, et al: Predictors of cerebral infarction in aneurysmal subarachnoid hemorrhage, *Stroke* 35:1862-1866, 2004.

278. Claassen J, Bernardini GL, Kreiter K, et al: Effect of cisternal and ventricular blood on risk of delayed cerebral ischemia after subarachnoid hemorrhage: The Fisher scale revisited, *Stroke* 32:2012-2020, 2001.

279. Macdonald RL, Weir BK: A review of hemoglobin and the pathogenesis of cerebral vasospasm, *Stroke* 22:971-982, 1991.

280. Tani E, Matsumoto T: Continuous elevation of intracellular Ca^{2+} is essential for the development of cerebral vasospasm, *Curr Vasc Pharmacol* 2:13-21, 2004.

281. Sano K, Asano T, Tanishima T, et al: Lipid peroxidation as a cause of cerebral vasospasm, *Neurol Res* 2:253-272, 1980.

282. Macdonald RL, Weir BK: Cerebral vasospasm and free radicals, *Free Radic Biol Med* 16:633-643, 1994.

283. Weir B, Macdonald RL, Stoodley M: Etiology of cerebral vasospasm, *Acta Neurochir Suppl* 72:27-46, 1999.

284. Dumont AS, Dumont RJ, Chow MM, et al: Cerebral vasospasm after subarachnoid hemorrhage: Putative role of inflammation, *Neurosurgery* 53:123-133, discussion 133-135, 2003.

285. Kolias AG, Sen J, Belli A: Pathogenesis of cerebral vasospasm following aneurysmal subarachnoid hemorrhage: Putative mechanisms and novel approaches, *J Neurosci Res* 87:1-11, 2008.

286. Vergouwen MD, Vermeulen M, Coert BA, et al: Microthrombosis after aneurysmal subarachnoid hemorrhage: An additional explanation for delayed cerebral ischemia, *J Cereb Blood Flow Metab* 28:1761-1770, 2008.

287. Dreier JP, Woitzik J, Fabricius M, et al: Delayed ischaemic neurological deficits after subarachnoid haemorrhage are associated with clusters of spreading depolarizations, *Brain* 129:3224-3237, 2006.

288. Juvela S: Aspirin and delayed cerebral ischemia after aneurysmal subarachnoid hemorrhage, *J Neurosurg* 82:945-952, 1995.

289. Roos YB, Levi M, Carroll TA, et al: Nimodipine increases fibrinolytic activity in patients with aneurysmal subarachnoid hemorrhage, *Stroke* 32:1860-1862, 2001.

290. Weir B, Grace M, Hansen J, et al: Time course of vasospasm in man, *J Neurosurg* 48:173-178, 1978.

291. Harders AG, Gilsbach JM: Time course of blood velocity changes related to vasospasm in the circle of Willis measured by transcranial Doppler ultrasound, *J Neurosurg* 66:718-728, 1987.

292. Kwak R, Niizuma H, Ohi T, et al: Angiographic study of cerebral vasospasm following rupture of intracranial aneurysms: Part I. Time of the appearance, *Surg Neurol* 11:257-262, 1979.

293. Vora YY, Suarez-Almazor M, Steinke DE, et al: Role of transcranial Doppler monitoring in the diagnosis of cerebral vasospasm after subarachnoid hemorrhage, *Neurosurgery* 44:1237-1247, discussion 1247-1248, 1999.

294. Alexandrov AV, Sloan MA, Wong LK, et al: Practice standards for transcranial Doppler ultrasound: part I—test performance, *J Neuroimaging* 17:11-18, 2007.

295. Suarez JI, Qureshi AI, Yahia AB, et al: Symptomatic vasospasm diagnosis after subarachnoid hemorrhage: Evaluation of transcranial Doppler ultrasound and cerebral angiography as related to compromised vascular distribution, *Crit Care Med* 30:1348-1355, 2002.

296. Sloan MA, Alexandrov AV, Tegeler CH, et al: Assessment: Transcranial Doppler ultrasonography: Report of the Therapeutics and Technology Assessment Subcommittee of the American Academy of Neurology, *Neurology* 62:1468-1481, 2004.

297. Sviri GE, Ghodke B, Britz GW, et al: Transcranial Doppler grading criteria for basilar artery vasospasm, *Neurosurgery* 59:360-366, discussion 360-366, 2006.

298. Binaghi S, Colleoni ML, Maeder P, et al: CT angiography and perfusion CT in cerebral vasospasm after subarachnoid hemorrhage, *AJNR Am J Neuroradiol* 28:750-758, 2007.

299. Laslo AM, Eastwood JD, Pakkiri P, et al: CT perfusion-derived mean transit time predicts early mortality and delayed vasospasm after experimental subarachnoid hemorrhage, *AJNR Am J Neuroradiol* 29:79-85, 2008.

300. van der Schaaf I, Wermer MJ, van der Graaf Y, et al: CT after subarachnoid hemorrhage: Relation of cerebral perfusion to delayed cerebral ischemia, *Neurology* 66:1533-1538, 2006.

301. Moftakhar R, Rowley HA, Turk A, et al: Utility of computed tomography perfusion in detection of cerebral vasospasm in patients with subarachnoid hemorrhage, *Neurosurg Focus* 21:E6, 2006.

302. Majoie CB, van Boven LJ, van de Beek D, et al: Perfusion CT to evaluate the effect of transluminal angioplasty on cerebral perfusion in the treatment of vasospasm after subarachnoid hemorrhage, *Neurocrit Care* 6:40-44, 2007.

303. Kassell NF, Peerless SJ, Durward QJ, et al: Treatment of ischemic deficits from vasospasm with intravascular volume expansion and induced arterial hypertension, *Neurosurgery* 11:337-343, 1982.

304. Suarez JI, Shannon L, Zaidat OO, et al: Effect of human albumin administration on clinical outcome and hospital cost in patients with subarachnoid hemorrhage, *J Neurosurg* 100:585-590, 2004.

305. Awad IA, Carter LP, Spetzler RF, et al: Clinical vasospasm after subarachnoid hemorrhage: Response to hypervolemic hemodilution and arterial hypertension, *Stroke* 18:365-372, 1987.

306. Lee KH, Lukovits T, Friedman JA: "Triple-H" therapy for cerebral vasospasm following subarachnoid hemorrhage, *Neurocrit Care* 4:68-76, 2006.

307. Sandham JD, Hull RD, Brant RF, et al: A randomized, controlled trial of the use of pulmonary-artery catheters in high-risk surgical patients, *N Engl J Med* 348:5-14, 2003.

308. Wheeler AP, Bernard GR, Thompson BT, et al: Pulmonary-artery versus central venous catheter to guide treatment of acute lung injury, *N Engl J Med* 354:2213-2224, 2006.

309. Joseph M, Ziadi S, Nates J, et al: Increases in cardiac output can reverse flow deficits from vasospasm independent of blood pressure: A study using xenon computed tomographic measurement of cerebral blood flow, *Neurosurgery* 53:1044-1051, discussion 1051-1052, 2003.

310. Rosen CL, Sekhar LN, Duong DH: Use of intra-aortic balloon pump counterpulsation for refractory symptomatic vasospasm, *Acta Neurochir (Wien)* 142:25-32, 2000.

311. Apostolides PJ, Greene KA, Zabramski JM, et al: Intra-aortic balloon pump counterpulsation in the management of concomitant cerebral vasospasm and cardiac failure after subarachnoid hemorrhage: Technical case report, *Neurosurgery* 38:1056-1059, discussion 1059-1060, 1996.

312. Sayama CM, Liu JK, Couldwell WT: Update on endovascular therapies for cerebral vasospasm induced by aneurysmal subarachnoid hemorrhage, *Neurosurg Focus* 21:E12, 2006.

313. Schuknecht B: Endovascular treatment of cerebral vasospasm following aneurysmal subarachnoid hemorrhage, *Acta Neurochir Suppl* 94:47-51, 2005.

314. Smith WS, Dowd CF, Johnston SC, et al: Neurotoxicity of intra-arterial papaverine preserved with chlorobutanol used for the treatment of cerebral vasospasm after aneurysmal subarachnoid hemorrhage, *Stroke* 35:2518-2522, 2004.

315. McAuliffe W, Townsend M, Eskridge JM, et al: Intracranial pressure changes induced during papaverine infusion for treatment of vasospasm, *J Neurosurg* 83:430-434, 1995.

316. Badjatia N, Topcuoglu MA, Pryor JC, et al: Preliminary experience with intra-arterial nicardipine as a treatment for cerebral vasospasm, *AJNR Am J Neuroradiol* 25:819-826, 2004.

317. Zubkov IuN, Nikiforov BM, Shustin VA: [1st attempt at dilating spastic cerebral arteries in the acute stage of rupture of arterial aneurysms], *Zh Vopr Neirokhir Im N N Burdenko* (6):17-23, 1983.

318. Hoh BL, Ogilvy CS: Endovascular treatment of cerebral vasospasm: Transluminal balloon angioplasty, intra-arterial papaverine, and intra-arterial nicardipine, *Neurosurg Clin North Am* 16:501-516, vi, 2005.

319. Mocco J, Prickett CS, Komotar RJ, et al: Potential mechanisms and clinical significance of global cerebral edema following aneurysmal subarachnoid hemorrhage, *Neurosurg Focus* 22:E7, 2007.

320. Claassen J, Carhuapoma JR, Kreiter KT, et al: Global cerebral edema after subarachnoid hemorrhage: Frequency, predictors, and impact on outcome, *Stroke* 33:1225-1232, 2002.

321. Urbaniak K, Merchant AI, Amin-Hanjani S, et al: Cardiac complications after aneurysmal subarachnoid hemorrhage, *Surg Neurol* 67:21-28, discussion 28-29, 2007.

322. Zaroff JG, Pawlikowska L, Miss JC, et al: Adrenoceptor polymorphisms and the risk of cardiac injury and dysfunction after subarachnoid hemorrhage, *Stroke* 37:1680-1685, 2006.

323. Di Pasquale G, Pinelli G, Andreoli A, et al: Holter detection of cardiac arrhythmias in intracranial subarachnoid hemorrhage, *Am J Cardiol* 59:596-600, 1987.

324. Estanol BV, Marin OS: Cardiac arrhythmias and sudden death in subarachnoid hemorrhage, *Stroke* 6:382-386, 1975.

325. Frontera JA, Parra A, Shimbo D, et al: Cardiac arrhythmias after subarachnoid hemorrhage: Risk factors and impact on outcome, *Cerebrovasc Dis* 26:71-78, 2008.

326. Zaroff JG, Rordorf GA, Newell JB, et al: Cardiac outcome in patients with subarachnoid hemorrhage and electrocardiographic abnormalities, *Neurosurgery* 44:34-39, 1999:discussion 39-40.

327. Kono T, Morita H, Kuroiwa T, et al: Left ventricular wall motion abnormalities in patients with subarachnoid hemorrhage: Neurogenic stunned myocardium, *J Am Coll Cardiol* 24:636-640, 1994.

328. Zaroff JG, Rordorf GA, Ogilvy CS, et al: Regional patterns of left ventricular systolic dysfunction after subarachnoid hemorrhage: Evidence for neurally mediated cardiac injury, *J Am Soc Echocardiogr* 13:774-779, 2000.

329. Mayer SA, Fink ME, Homma S, et al: Cardiac injury associated with neurogenic pulmonary edema following subarachnoid hemorrhage, *Neurology* 44:815-820, 1994.

330. Kitahara T, Masuda T, Soma K: [The etiology of sudden cardiopulmonary arrest in subarachnoid hemorrhage], *No Shinkei Geka* 21:781-786, 1993.

331. Wu DJ, Fujiwara H, Matsuda M, et al: Clinicopathological study of myocardial infarction with normal or nearly normal extracardiac coronary arteries: Quantitative analysis of contraction band necrosis, coagulation necrosis, hemorrhage, and infarct size, *Heart Vessels* 6:55-62, 1990.

332. Sandhu R, Aronow WS, Rajdev A, et al: Relation of cardiac troponin I levels with in-hospital mortality in patients with ischemic stroke, intracerebral hemorrhage, and subarachnoid hemorrhage, *Am J Cardiol* 102:632-634, 2008.

333. Ramappa P, Thatai D, Coplin W, et al: Cardiac troponin-I: A predictor of prognosis in subarachnoid hemorrhage, *Neurocrit Care* 8:398-403, 2008.

334. Naidech AM, Kreiter KT, Janjua N, et al: Cardiac troponin elevation, cardiovascular morbidity, and outcome after subarachnoid hemorrhage, *Circulation* 112:2851-2856, 2005.

335. Parekh N, Venkatesh B, Cross D, et al: Cardiac troponin I predicts myocardial dysfunction in aneurysmal subarachnoid hemorrhage, *J Am Coll Cardiol* 36:1328-1335, 2000.

336. Neil-Dwyer G, Cruickshank J, Stratton C: Beta-blockers, plasma total creatine kinase and creatine kinase myocardial isoenzyme, and the prognosis of subarachnoid hemorrhage, *Surg Neurol* 25:163-168, 1986.

337. Hamann G, Haass A, Schimrigk K: Beta-blockade in acute aneurysmal subarachnoid haemorrhage, *Acta Neurochir (Wien)* 121:119-122, 1993.

338. McLaughlin N, Bojanowski MW, Girard F, et al: Pulmonary edema and cardiac dysfunction following subarachnoid hemorrhage, *Can J Neurol Sci* 32:178-185, 2005.

339. Tung PP, Olmsted E, Kopelnik A, et al: Plasma B-type natriuretic peptide levels are associated with early cardiac dysfunction after subarachnoid hemorrhage, *Stroke* 36:1567-1569, 2005.

340. Vespa PM, Bleck TP: Neurogenic pulmonary edema and other mechanisms of impaired oxygenation after aneurysmal subarachnoid hemorrhage, *Neurocrit Care* 1:157-170, 2004.

341. Friedman JA, Pichelmann MA, Piepgras DG, et al: Pulmonary complications of aneurysmal subarachnoid hemorrhage, *Neurosurgery* 52:1025-1031, discussion 1031-1032, 2003.

342. Frontera JA, Fernandez A, Schmidt JM, et al: Impact of nosocomial infectious complications after subarachnoid hemorrhage, *Neurosurgery* 62:80-87, discussion 87, 2008.

343. Dimopoulou I, Kouyialis AT, Tzanella M, et al: High incidence of neuroendocrine dysfunction in long-term survivors of aneurysmal subarachnoid hemorrhage, *Stroke* 35:2884-2889, 2004.

344. Weant KA, Sasaki-Adams D, Dziedzic K, et al: Acute relative adrenal insufficiency after aneurysmal subarachnoid hemorrhage, *Neurosurgery* 63:645-649, 2008.

345. Schneider HJ, Kreitschmann-Andermahr I, Ghigo E, et al: Hypothalamopituitary dysfunction following traumatic brain injury and aneurysmal subarachnoid hemorrhage: A systematic review, *JAMA* 298:1429-1438, 2007.

346. Mangieri P, Suzuki K, Ferreira M, et al: Evaluation of pituitary and thyroid hormones in patients with subarachnoid hemorrhage due to ruptured intracranial aneurysm, *Arq Neuropsiquiatr* 61:14-19, 2003.

347. McIver B, Connacher A, Whittle I, et al: Adipsic hypothalamic diabetes insipidus after clipping of anterior communicating artery aneurysm, *BMJ* 303:1465-1467, 1991.

348. Nguyen BN, Yablon SA, Chen CY: Hypodipsic hypernatremia and diabetes insipidus following anterior communicating artery aneurysm clipping: Diagnostic and therapeutic challenges in the amnestic rehabilitation patient, *Brain Inj* 15:975-980, 2001.

349. Kreitschmann-Andermahr I, Hoff C, Saller B, et al: Prevalence of pituitary deficiency in patients after aneurysmal subarachnoid hemorrhage, *J Clin Endocrinol Metab* 89:4986-4992, 2004.

350. Kurokawa Y, Uede T, Ishiguro M, et al: Pathogenesis of hyponatremia following subarachnoid hemorrhage due to ruptured cerebral aneurysm, *Surg Neurol* 46:500-507, discussion 507-508, 1996.

351. Qureshi AI, Suri MF, Sung GY, et al: Prognostic significance of hypernatremia and hyponatremia among patients with aneurysmal subarachnoid hemorrhage, *Neurosurgery* 50:749-755, discussion 755-756, 2002.

352. van den Bergh WM, Algra A, van der Sprenkel JW, et al: Hypomagnesemia after aneurysmal subarachnoid hemorrhage, *Neurosurgery* 52:276-281,discussion 281-282, 2003.

353. Van de Water JM, Van den Bergh WM, Hoff RG, et al: Hypocalcaemia may reduce the beneficial effect of magnesium treatment in aneurysmal subarachnoid haemorrhage, *Magnes Res* 20:130-135, 2007.

354. Polderman KH, Bloemers FW, Peerdeman SM, et al: Hypomagnesemia and hypophosphatemia at admission in patients with severe head injury, *Crit Care Med* 28:2022-2025, 2000.

355. Fukui S, Katoh H, Tsuzuki N, et al: Multivariate analysis of risk factors for QT prolongation following subarachnoid hemorrhage, *Crit Care* 7:R7-R12, 2003.

356. Peters JP, Welt LG, Sims EA, et al: A salt-wasting syndrome associated with cerebral disease, *Trans Assoc Am Physicians* 63:57-64, 1950.

357. Berendes E, Walter M, Cullen P, et al: Secretion of brain natriuretic peptide in patients with aneurysmal subarachnoid haemorrhage, *Lancet* 349:245-249, 1997.

358. Wijdicks EF, Heublein DM, Burnett JC Jr: Increase and uncoupling of adrenomedullin from the natriuretic peptide system in aneurysmal subarachnoid hemorrhage, *J Neurosurg* 94:252-256, 2001.

359. Wijdicks EF, Schievink WI, Burnett JC Jr: Natriuretic peptide system and endothelin in aneurysmal subarachnoid hemorrhage, *J Neurosurg* 87:275-280, 1997.

360. Wijdicks EF, Vermeulen M, ten Haaf JA, et al: Volume depletion and natriuresis in patients with a ruptured intracranial aneurysm, *Ann Neurol* 18:211-216, 1985.

361. Betjes MG: Hyponatremia in acute brain disease: The cerebral salt wasting syndrome, *Eur J Intern Med* 13:9-14, 2002.

362. Sivakumar V, Rajshekhar V, Chandy MJ: Management of neurosurgical patients with hyponatremia and natriuresis, *Neurosurgery* 34:269-274, discussion 274, 1994.

363. Hasan D, Lindsay KW, Wijdicks EF, et al: Effect of fludrocortisone acetate in patients with subarachnoid hemorrhage, *Stroke* 20:1156-1161, 1989.

364. Taplin CE, Cowell CT, Silink M, et al: Fludrocortisone therapy in cerebral salt wasting, *Pediatrics* 118:e1904-e1908, 2006.

365. Claassen J, Vu A, Kreiter KT, et al: Effect of acute physiologic derangements on outcome after subarachnoid hemorrhage, *Crit Care Med* 32:832-838, 2004.

366. Roos EJ, Rinkel GJ, Velthuis BK, et al: The relation between aneurysm size and outcome in patients with subarachnoid hemorrhage, *Neurology* 54:2334-2336, 2000.

367. Qureshi AI, Suarez JI, Bhardwaj A, et al: Early predictors of outcome in patients receiving hypervolemic and hypertensive therapy for symptomatic vasospasm after subarachnoid hemorrhage, *Crit Care Med* 28:824-829, 2000.

368. Juvela S: Prehemorrhage risk factors for fatal intracranial aneurysm rupture, *Stroke* 34:1852-1857, 2003.

369. Hackett ML, Anderson CS: Health outcomes 1 year after subarachnoid hemorrhage: An international population-based study. The Australian Cooperative Research on Subarachnoid Hemorrhage Study Group, *Neurology* 55:658-662, 2000.

370. Thines L, Zairi F, Taschner C, et al: Subarachnoid hemorrhage from spontaneous dissection of the anterior cerebral artery, *Cerebrovasc Dis* 22:452-456, 2006.

371. Ogiichi T, Endo S, Onizuka K, et al: Non-aneurysmal subarachnoid hemorrhage associated with basilar artery dissection—autopsy case report, *(Tokyo) Neurol Med Chir* 37:612-615, 1997.

372. Nakatomi H, Nagata K, Kawamoto S, et al: Ruptured dissecting aneurysm as a cause of subarachnoid hemorrhage of unverified etiology, *Stroke* 28:1278-1282, 1997.

373. Hamani C, Andrade AF, Figueiredo EG, et al: Spontaneous subarachnoid hemorrhage as the primary manifestation of carotid cavernous fistulas: Case report, *Arq Neuropsiquiatr* 59:593-595, 2001.

374. Fountas KN, Faircloth LR, Hope T, et al: Spontaneous superior sagittal sinus thrombosis secondary to type II heparin-induced thrombocytopenia presenting as an acute subarachnoid hemorrhage, *J Clin Neurosci* 14:890-895, 2007.

375. Gonzalez LF, Zabramski JM, Tabrizi P, et al: Spontaneous spinal subarachnoid hemorrhage secondary to spinal aneurysms: Diagnosis and treatment paradigm, *Neurosurgery* 57:1127-1131, 2005:discussion 1127-1131.

376. Marushima A, Yanaka K, Matsuki T, et al: Subarachnoid hemorrhage not due to ruptured aneurysm in moyamoya disease, *J Clin Neurosci* 13:146-149, 2006.

377. Visudhiphan P, Chiemchanya S, Somburanasin R, et al: Causes of spontaneous subarachnoid hemorrhage in Thai infants and children: A study of 56 patients, *J Neurosurg* 53:185-187, 1980.

378. Jacobi C, Schwark C, Kress B, et al: Subarachnoid hemorrhage due to *Borrelia burgdorferi*-associated vasculitis, *Eur J Neurol* 13:536-538, 2006.

379. Biller J, Toffol GJ, Kassell NF, et al: Spontaneous subarachnoid hemorrhage in young adults, *Neurosurgery* 21:664-667, 1987.

380. Silvestrini M, Floris R, Tagliati M, et al: Spontaneous subarachnoid hemorrhage in an HIV patient, *Ital J Neurol Sci* 11:493-495, 1990.

381. Shah AK: Non-aneurysmal primary subarachnoid hemorrhage in pregnancy-induced hypertension and eclampsia, *Neurology* 61:117-120, 2003.

382. Meese W, Kluge W, Grumme T, et al: CT evaluation of the CSF spaces of healthy persons, *Neuroradiology* 19:131-136, 1980.

31 Arteriovenous Malformations and Other Vascular Anomalies

CHRISTIAN STAPF, J.P. MOHR, ANDREAS HARTMANN, HENNING MAST, ALEXANDER KHAW, JAE H. CHOI, JOHN PILE-SPELLMAN

Vascular malformations constitute an important cause of intracranial hemorrhage especially in younger patients. However, this group of pathologies is quite heterogeneous and comprises a large spectrum ranging from sporadic congenital lesions, such as brain arteriovenous malformations (AVMs), to genetically determined familial disorders that may progress over time, for example, familial cerebral cavernous malformations and hereditary hemorrhagic telangiectasia (Weber-Osler-Rendu disease).

In principle, vascular malformations may arise from any segment of the different functional units of the brain vasculature, including arteries, arterioles, capillaries, venules, and veins. This may be due to developmental derangement during the time of the vessel formation or may occur later in time because of external risk factors and genetic predisposition (Fig. 31-1). Many of these anomalies are associated with an increased risk of hemorrhage, because structural changes of the vascular wall lead to often progressive hemodynamic changes and lower resistance to intraluminal volume and pressure. However, the average risk of spontaneous hemorrhage appears to be rather low if the vascular malformation is diagnosed unruptured. Once hemorrhage has occurred all types are associated with higher bleeding rates.

Arteriovenous Malformations

History

The pathologic case material provides the earliest examples of what we call today a brain AVM. The 1846 publication by Viennese pathologist Rokitansky[1] may be the first to mention the existence of such lesions. He did not provide a detailed morphologic description of what he called "vascular brain tumors in pial tissue," but he was puzzled by the structural analogy between their "cavernous textures" and the "gaps, windows or canals in certain blastemas of the vascular system" that he had noted in embryonic tissue. This observation led him to the idea that a developmental derangement was the most likely underlying cause for this type of lesion. Half a century later, Carl Emmanuel, a pathologist working at Heidelberg University, published one of the first detailed histopathologic case studies.[2] He had already described "substantial enlargement of the microcirculatory pathways" reflecting the lack of a capillary bed in the angioma arteriale racemosum. Emmanuel's report is noteworthy because he appears to be the first researcher considering three possible causes of such lesions: congenital, secondary development from an innate telangiectasia, or a sequel to trauma. His landmark proposal drafted the three major etiologic concepts—embryologic derangement, dynamic development, and vascular trauma—upon which most future theories were built and further elaborated.[3]

Etiology

Growing insight into the embryology of the human cerebrovascular system during the first half of the 20th century fostered theories on the developmental basis of persistent cerebral arteriovenous (AV) shunts.[3-6] The introduction of cerebral angiography into clinical practice[7] offered the first in vivo opportunities for a better understanding of AVM angioarchitecture and its inherent flow pattern. Among the different types of intracerebral AV fistulas, vein of Galen aneurysmal malformations may actually constitute the only embryonic disorder (Table 31-1). The fistula links the choroidal artery system to a persistent ectatic median vein of the prosencephalon, which represents the embryonic precursor of the vein of Galen.[8,9]

Thanks to now routinely applied fetal ultrasound screening, an increasing number of vein of Galen aneurysmal malformations have been detected during gestation, and a few patients have been studied by prenatal MRI.[10,11] Information on comparable cases with an intrauterine diagnosis of a brain AVM, however, are lacking; none has as yet been reported from studies on routine fetal ultrasound evaluations, which are commonly performed between the 20th and 22nd gestational weeks.[12,13] Probably the youngest individual so far reported may be a preterm neonate (born at 32 weeks' gestation) who died during the second postnatal day from acute hemorrhage of an infratentorial AVM that was fed by the superior cerebellar artery.[14] The lack of observed cases in which a brain AVM was detected at earlier fetal stages hence challenges the widespread assumption that these lesions also arise from an embryonic disturbance at the time of the vessel formation.[15]

The vascular topography in many AVMs also argues against a genuine embryonic disorder. Brain AVMs

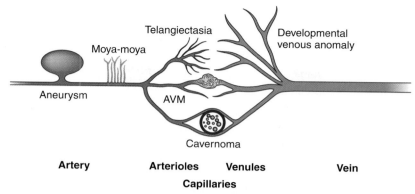

Figure 31-1 Vascular malformations and anomalies of the brain.

commonly affect distal arterial branches, and in roughly half the cases, the malformation is found in the border-zone region shared by the distal anterior, middle, and posterior cerebral arteries.[16] These "watershed areas" constitute anatomic remnants of the manifold artery-to-artery links that once covered the brain surface at its lissencephalic state. With the onset of cortical gyra-tion (29th gestational week), the original arterial mesh regresses, giving rise eventually to the defined arterial territories of the leptomeningeal arteries. In the dis-tal fields of these arterial territories, pial anastomoses between otherwise separated brain arteries persist, even though the number, size, and exact location of the lepto-meningeal anastomoses show numerous interindividual variations.[17-19] Their persistence may depend on the local composition of the extracellular matrix,[20] the formation of capillary basement membranes,[21,22] and the influence of angiogenetic factors on the course of the regression process.[23,24] This possibility suggests that the initial lesion may actually arise with a timely link to the for-mation of the arterial borderzones, that is, at some point after the 29th gestational week.[19,25] In one case report in which the interplay between cortical gyration and bor-derzone formation was disturbed by a primary migration

disorder such as schizencephaly, an AVM had developed at the site where the neural defect straddled the arterial borderzone territory.[26]

The relatively high rate of arterial aneurysms associ-ated with AVMs (up to 58% in two series)[27,28] has led to the notion of a similar underlying pathogenesis in AVMs and aneurysms,[29-31] thereby suggesting a structural or functional smooth muscle disorder in the context of AVM development. The formation of the arterial smooth muscle layer shows a spatiotemporal sequence, slowly progressing from proximal to distal arterial segments. In the human fetus, the first smooth muscle layer detected at proximal levels of the leptomeningeal arteries appears in the 16th gestational week, subsequently followed by the striatal (20th to 22nd gestational week), extrastria-tal medullary (term to first postnatal month), and corti-cal (6th to 9th month) arteries.[25] The time frame for this histologic maturation process coincides with the arterial borderzone development (29th gestational week to end of the 1st year of life). The idea of a primary smooth mus-cle defect at the level of the distal arterial branches may therefore provide a testable hypothesis for AVM develop-ment, especially in patients in whom the malformation is located in the arterial borderzone territory. On the basis

TABLE 31-1   DIFFERENTIAL DIAGNOSIS OF ARTERIOVENOUS (AV) MALFORMATIONS OF THE BRAIN: OTHER INTRACRANIAL AV FISTULAS

Entity*	Pathogenesis	Clinical Characteristics
Vein of Galen malformation[9,252]	Persistent dilated embryonic vein of the prosencephalon; posterior choroidal artery affected	Hemorrhage, congestive heart failure in neonates
Dural AV fistula[9]	Different types (congenital, traumatic, secondary to venous occlusion, etc.)	Arterial supply through meningeal arte-rial branches; high recurrence rate
Hereditary hemorrhagic telangiectasia (Rendu-Osler-Weber syndrome)[253]	Capillary regression leads to multiple small AV shunts in various tissues	Vascular abnormalities in nose, skin, lung, brain, and gastrointestinal tract
Encephalotrigeminal (Sturge-Weber syndrome)[254]	Phakomatosis	Neurocutaneous syndrome
Cerebro-retinal angiomatosis (von Hippel–Lindau disease)[254]	Phakomatosis	Neurocutaneous syndrome
Wyburn-Mason syndrome[255,256]	Phakomatosis	Neurocutaneous syndrome
Neovascular collateral vessels	Venous thrombosis or arterial occlusion may lead to focal angioneogenesis with false AV connections	Post-thrombotic syndrome, moyamoya disease, etc.
Traumatic AV fistulas	Traumatic disruption of adjacent arterial and venous vessel walls	Cavernous sinus fistula, etc.

*Superscript numbers indicate chapter references.

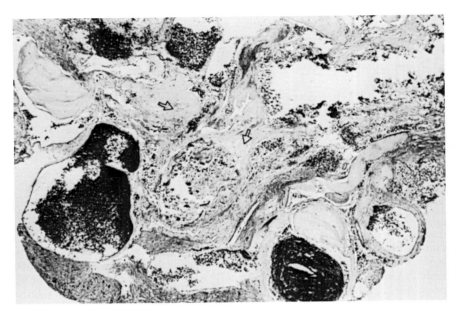

Figure 31-2 Photomicrograph of an arteriovenous malformation at low power, demonstrating areas of gliosis *(arrows)* between large thin-walled cavernous sinuses.

of theoretical vascular modeling, data from a study using the modeling now support the notion that a lack of local flow control at the distal arterial level may be the cause, rather than the result, of an AVM.[32]

The pathogenetic mechanisms leading to the lack of capillaries in the AVM nidus remain as yet unclear. The capillary density—that is, the number of capillaries in a given volume of brain tissue—remains stable after the fourth month of gestation, whereas the relative capillary volume in the cortex increases in a linear fashion from the end of the first trimester throughout infancy.[25,33] Any presumed capillary disease has as yet not found its morphologic correlate, and the morphology of endothelial cells in vessels within or adjacent to an AVM has been described as being normal.[34-40] A higher endothelial turnover in the AVM vasculature, however, may suggest the presence of active angiogenesis or ongoing vascular remodeling.[41]

Much effort is currently being devoted to defining the predisposing factors at the molecular level of the developing brain vasculature. Possible germline mutations affecting distinct angiogenetic pathways have been proposed to be the underlying cause of a variety of vascular malformations in the brain. As to AVMs, several candidate proteins are currently under investigation, including endothelial angiopoietin receptor Tie-2,[42-44] basic fibroblast growth factor (FGF-2),[45] nitric oxide synthase (NOS),[46] transforming growth factor-beta (TGF-β),[47,48] vascular endothelial growth factor (VEGF),[49] and endoglin.[50] Many of these proteins show mutual interactions,[43,47,51] commonly affect the signal pathways between the vascular endothelium and the smooth muscle layer of the arterial wall, but do not seem to affect the physiologic maturation process in the vessels involved. In fact, the basement membranes of AVM vessels have been shown to predominantly express laminin, a glycoprotein that is typically seen in mature (i.e., postembryonic) vessels.[22] Fibronectin, a histochemical marker for embryonic vessels, is barely detectable in AVMs,

suggesting that an AVM nidus consists of abnormal but not immature vessels.

Once the initial lesion has emerged, the permanent intraluminal stress arising from abnormal flow and pressure may lead to so-called secondary angiopathy, a nonreversible abnormal remodeling process in otherwise normal neighboring vessels.[9] Whether any of the suggested molecular factors may also play a role amid the biologic mechanisms that eventually lead to AVM growth, to secondary vascular changes, and to phenomena like spontaneous obliteration[52] and recurrence after successful therapy[53,54] has yet to be determined.

Morphology

An AVM resembles a tortuous agglomeration of abnormally dilated arteries and veins in the brain, commonly supplied through branches of one or more leptomeningeal arteries, and with drainage into deep veins, superficial veins, or both. In its core region or nidus, the AVM lacks a capillary bed, thereby allowing high-flow AV shunting through one or more fistulas.

Histologic evaluation of AVMs demonstrates that the walls of the large vascular components of the malformation are mostly devoid of elastic and significant muscular components (Fig. 31-2).[37,55] Within the malformation, the arteries show subendothelial thickening, medial hypertrophy, and, occasionally, thrombosis; the veins are thin walled and vary in size, with poorly developed muscular and elastic components. Corrosion preparations of AVMs injected with inert substances after removal of the brain at autopsy have shown that there is no normal cerebral tissue within the confines of an AVM (Fig. 31-3). The intense gliosis suggests that the neurons captivated within the margins of a malformation are probably nonfunctional (see Fig. 31-2). Presumably, cerebral function that should be located in the brain occupied by the malformation is displaced to the malformation's margins or even remote from it.[56,57]

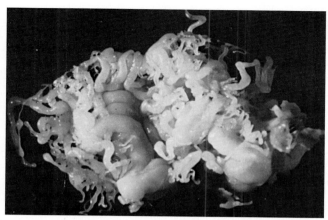

Figure 31-3 Corrosion specimen of an arteriovenous malformation obtained after the injection of acrylate into the malformation and dissolution of the soft tissue by potassium hydroxide. The specimen reveals the three-dimensional anatomy of the malformation and the configuration of the large venous sinusoids.

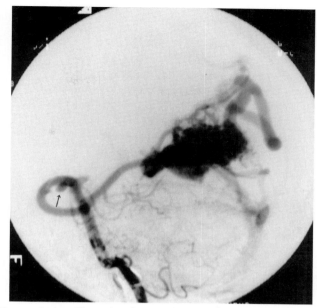

Figure 31-5 Flow-related arterial aneurysm *(arrow)* in a right occipital arteriovenous malformation fed by the ipsilateral posterior cerebral artery.

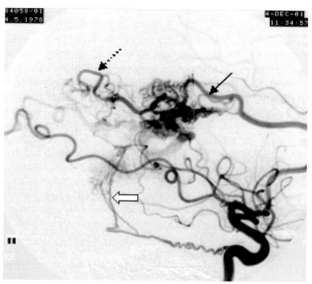

Figure 31-4 An "en passage" feeder vessel *(black arrow)* supplies the nidus, then continues to healthy brain tissue *(dotted arrow)*. Note the meningeal supply to a second nidus *(white arrow)*.

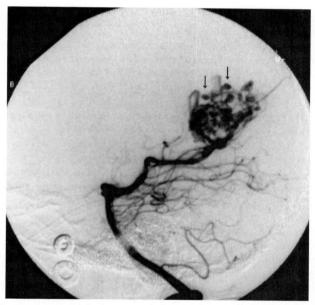

Figure 31-6 Multiple intranidal arterial aneurysms *(arrows)* in a right occipital arteriovenous malformation with feeders from the posterior cerebral artery.

Feeding arteries may supply the malformation directly via terminal branches or may continue "en passage," thereby supplying normal brain tissue distal to the AVM (Fig. 31-4). Arterial supply may arise from single arterial territories or may straddle the arterial borderzones, thereby recruiting feeding vessels from two or more adjacent arterial territories.[58] Deep arterial feeders originating from branches or main trunks of the major cerebral arteries in the lenticulostriate, choroidal, or thalamoperforating arteries may reach the AVM after passing through healthy brain tissue. In a few cases, feeding arteries may stenose or even occlude over time; in these instances, so-called moyamoya-type changes refer to any pattern of collateral small vessel recruitment due to proximal feeding artery stenosis or occlusion.

Concurrent arterial aneurysms are commonly defined as saccular dilatations of the lumen two or more times the width of the arterial vessel that carries the dilatation. Such arterial aneurysms may be located either on feeding arteries (so-called flow-related arterial aneurysms; Fig. 31-5), within the margins of the AVM nidus ("intranidal aneurysms"; Fig. 31-6), or on vessels unrelated to blood flow to the AVM.[59] The reported rates of concurrent aneurysms in patients with AVMs show large variations, ranging from 3%[60] to 58%.[61] Some of this variation may result from low interrater agreement.[62] Referral bias toward tertiary treatment centers may also influence the rate of detected aneurysms in the study cohort.[63] Finally, different study definitions of

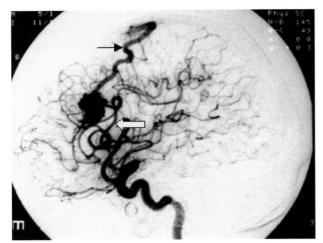

Figure 31-7 Angiogram of a compact arteriovenous malformation fed by branches of the middle cerebral artery *(white arrow)* and draining into a single superficial vein *(black arrow)*.

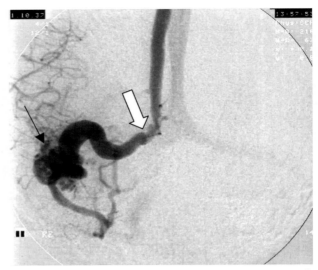

Figure 31-8 Arteriovenous malformation *(black arrow)* with a single large draining vein. Note the venous stenosis *(white arrow)*.

the term concurrent aneurysm may further contribute to variations in reported aneurysm rates. Therefore, there is now common agreement that infundibula, arterial ectasias (i.e., dilated feeding vessels), and intranidal aneurysmal dilatations seen during the venous phase of angiography are not to be diagnosed as arterial aneurysms.

The most common route of *venous AVM drainage* is toward the superficial veins of the brain directly or via collaterals to the major sinuses (Fig. 31-7). An alternative route is through deep venous channels that may reach the ependymal surface of the ventricular system and drain via the deep venous system. Variations of normal venous drainage anatomy may be found in up to 30% of all patients with AVM,[64,65] and adaptations of the venous system to compensate for the large blood volume leads to sometimes extensive collateral veins. In clinical AVM research, the overall venous drainage pattern is usually categorized as angiographically demonstrated drainage into the superficial cortical veins ("superficial venous drainage"), drainage into the deep venous system ("deep venous drainage") such as the internal cerebral veins, basal veins, and vein of Galen, and combined superficial and deep drainage. It is generally agreed that "in the posterior fossa, only cerebellar hemispheric veins that drain directly into the straight sinus, torcula Herophili, or transverse sinus are considered to be superficial."[66] Stenosis and thrombosis of venous drainage pathways have been described in prior observations.[67-69] For research purposes, "venous stenosis" is usually defined as a greater than twofold caliber narrowing of any draining vein outflow pathway seen in two angiographic views. Correspondingly, "venous ectasia" is usually recorded in cases with a greater than twofold caliber increase in any draining venous channel (Fig. 31-8).

Epidemiology

No population-based prevalence data on AVMs are currently available. Calculated estimates from hospital-based autopsy data may be unreliable, showing a wide range

from 5 to as many as 613 AVMs per 100,000 persons.[70-73] Given the patterns of case referral, it is no surprise that the larger series of cases of AVMs come mainly from surgical clinics. The low frequency of the disorder prevents all but a few interested physicians and surgeons from having any but a passing encounter with such cases. In one report of 100 patients evaluated angiographically for tandem lesions in a setting of high-grade carotid stenosis, two AVMs were found.[74]

Prior data from a large series in which more than 4000 volunteers were screened with brain MRI did not lead to the detection of any brain AVMs.[75,76] Assuming a hypothetical prevalence of 10 patients with AVMs per 100,000, brain MRI screening of 1 million people would be necessary to yield estimates with sufficiently narrow confidence intervals (CIs).[77]

Figure 31-9 summarizes available incidence rates for both AVM detection and associated intracranial hemorrhage (ICH). The age- and gender-adjusted incidence of ICH due to any type of intracranial vascular malformation is 0.82 per 100,000 (95% CI, 0.46-1.19) in a retrospective, population-based study conducted over 27 years in Olmsted County, Minnesota.[78,79] Of the 20 patients recorded, 17 (85%) had an underlying brain AVM. No separate incidence for AVM hemorrhage was calculated. In the Netherlands Antilles between 1980 and 1990, an annual incidence of 1.1 symptomatic AVMs per 100,000 people was described.[80] Of the 17 patients identified as having an AVM, 16 presented with ICH. In this fairly isolated and homogeneous population, however, an unusually high proportion of the patients with AVM (35%) had hereditary hemorrhagic telangiectasia (Rendu-Osler-Weber disease). Further, 25% of the patient cohort showed multiple brain AVMs, making it difficult to compare the findings with those in other populations. Finally, a mixed prospective and retrospective series from Linköping University, Sweden, estimated an AVM detection rate of 1.24 per 100,000 person-years (95% CI, 0.75-1.56).[81] The relatively high estimated incidence of AVM hemorrhage (0.87 per

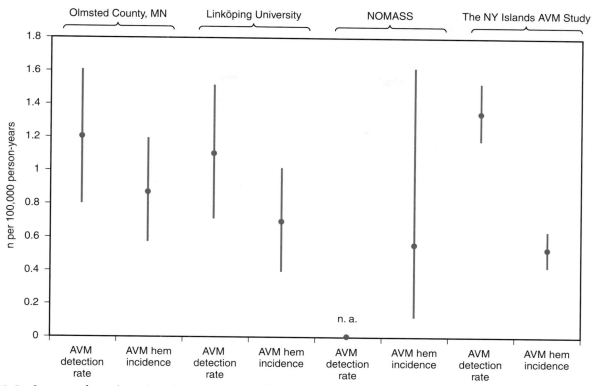

Figure 31-9 Synopsis of population-based arteriovenous malformation (AVM) detection rates and incidence of AVM hemorrhage. Average annual rates per 100,000 and 95% confidence limits are given on the basis of data from references 81, 82, 84, 86, and 166. hem, hemorrhage; n.a., not available; NOMASS, Northern Manhattan Stroke Study.

100,000 person-years; 95% CI, 0.57-1.19) may have been biased by patient referrals from outside the geographic study area. Incidence data derived from non–population-based studies have been shown to be highly variable, likely because of referral bias and under-ascertainment of AVM hemorrhage.

The New York Islands Study

The New York Islands AVM Hemorrhage Study is an ongoing prospective population-based survey determining the incidence of AVM hemorrhage and associated morbidity and mortality rates in a population defined by U.S. Post Office Zip Code boundaries. The New York islands—Manhattan Island, Staten Island, and Long Island (the last including the New York City boroughs of Brooklyn and Queens and the counties of Nassau and Suffolk)—contained a population of 9,429,541 persons according to the 2000 U.S. Census. Since March 15, 2000, all major New York Islands hospitals and their related hospital networks have cooperated prospectively to report weekly data on consecutive patients living in the study area with a diagnosis of brain AVM, and have included in their reports whether or not the patients had suffered AVM hemorrhage. Patients who are referred to these hospitals but live outside the Zip Code–defined study area are excluded from the study population.

As of June 14, 2002, 284 prospective patients with AVM were encountered, leading to a calculated prospective AVM detection rate of 1.34 per 100,000 person-years (95% CI, 1.18-1.49). Mean age among identified patients was 35 years (+/-18), and 49% were women.

Overall, 108 patients presented with a first-ever acute AVM hemorrhage; the currently estimated incidence of AVM hemorrhage in the New York Islands population is thus 0.51 per 100,000 person-years (95% CI, 0.41-0.61). The prevalence of AVM hemorrhage among detected cases (n = 144) was 0.68 per 100,000 person-years (95% CI, 0.57-0.79).[82]

Northern Manhattan Stroke Study

The Northern Manhattan Stroke Study (NOMASS) was a prospective, population-based, stroke incidence survey collecting data in a Zip Code–defined area in New York City that contained 136,623 white, black, and Hispanic residents older than 20 years, according to the 1990 U.S. Census. An active surveillance program was used to identify all hospitalized and nonhospitalized patients with first-ever (incident) stroke older than 20 years. All patients underwent CT, MRI, or both of the brain, and clinical data were systematically collected from their medical records.[83,84]

Data on all patients with incident ICH (i.e., any ICH or subarachnoid hemorrhage [SAH], with or without intraventricular blood) occurring between July 1, 1993, and June 30, 1997, were analyzed. Those suspected to have underlying AVMs underwent further studies, including cerebral angiography at the discretion of the treating physicians. The investigators did not include patients whose AVMs were identified before their strokes, nor those with ICH due to trauma, tumor, or any other type of intracranial vascular malformation (e.g., dural AV fistula, vein of Galen type malformation).

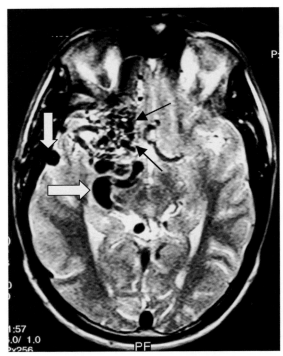

Figure 31-10 Large frontotemporal arteriovenous malformation *(black arrows)* with superficial and deep venous drainage *(white arrows)* and mass effect leading to midbrain compression.

Overall, first-ever ICH occurred in 207 patients during 546,492 person-years of observation, including 3 patients (1.4%) with an underlying brain AVM. The crude incidence rate for first-ever AVM hemorrhage in the adult population was 0.55 per 100,000 person-years (95% CI, 0.11–1.61).[85]

Genetics

The presumably congenital nature of AVMs might be expected to yield many cases with a family history, but the familial incidence appears to be quite rare.[86-90] Only seven families had been reported through 1990, involving 15 people in all. The mode of inheritance is uncertain. In contrast to the general male preponderance for AVMs reported in clinical surgical services, the sexes are equally represented in the scanty family history data, a feature that has been confirmed in the ongoing New York Islands study. With a greater awareness of the successes in surgery, greater effort is being made to diagnose the condition in the older population. In large modern centers, this effort at diagnosis has shifted the age of onset upward. Therefore, AVM is no longer to be considered a diagnosis mainly involving the young, even though most hemorrhages occur in younger patients. Dural and extracerebral AVMs are the only types thought to be usually acquired from trauma.

AVMs usually occur in isolation, unrelated to other disease states, but a few have been associated with the Rendu-Osler-Weber disease, most of them small.[91,92] In one large study, 31 of 136 patients from a hereditary hemorrhagic telangiectasia clinic were inferred from MRI findings to have cerebral AVMs.[92] Eighteen of these patients

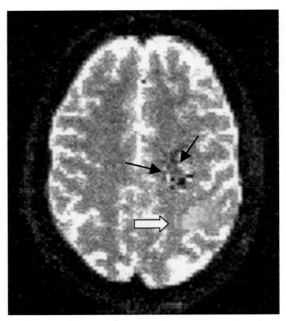

Figure 31-11 Functional magnetic resonance imaging study obtained as the patient performed finger-tapping shows brain activation *(white arrow)* in the vicinity of an arteriovenous malformation *(black arrows)* in slightly more posterior location than expected.

underwent angiogram; findings in all 18 were positive, and 7 had multiple (three or more) AVMs. The AVMs varied in size from 3 to 25 mm in maximal dimension. AVMs have also been described in the Wyburn-Mason syndrome.[93]

Diagnosis and Classification

Cerebral angiography represents the key imaging technique for adequate diagnosis, morphologic characterization (vascular supply and drainage, related aneurysms), and treatment planning for AVMs.[61,94] A meta-analysis has demonstrated that the risk of diagnostic angiography is significantly lower in patients with AVM (0.3%-0.8%) than in those evaluated for TIA or stroke (3.0%-3.7%).[95] Noninvasive conventional and functional MRI techniques are playing an increasing role in the interventional management because they facilitate localization of the nidus in relation to the brain (Fig. 31-10) and further identify functionally important brain areas adjacent to the nidus (Fig. 31-11).[96-98] Finally, based on flow velocity and resistance pattern, transcranial Doppler (TCD) ultrasonography (conventional B-mode, echo-enhanced, or color-coded TCD) has been demonstrated to be a noninvasive and cost-effective screening tool for both detection and follow-up evaluation of brain AVMs (Fig. 31-12).[99-101]

Despite proposals for a uniform terminology in clinical AVM research,[102] common international standards for diagnosing brain AVMs have not as yet been established.[62] Brain AVMs must be separated from other intracranial AV fistulas, which at times have similar morphologic features, because these lesions differ in terms of pathogenesis, natural course, and treatment strategies (Table 31-2). This nosologic heterogeneity in reported AVM series still confounds the literature and makes it difficult to compare

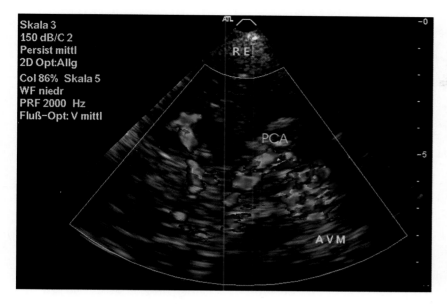

Figure 31-12 Transcranial color-coded duplex sonogram of a small midbrain arteriovenous malformation (AVM) mainly fed by the posterior cerebral artery (PCA).

different AVM study populations.[63,103] The ninth revision of the *International Classification of Diseases* (ICD-9)—still widely used in clinical and administrative practice—does not offer a separate code for brain AVMs, clustering them together with any other "congenital anomalies of cerebral vessels" such as cavernous malformations and unruptured arterial aneurysms.[104] The current ICD-10 codes provide an individual code for unruptured "arteriovenous malformations of cerebral vessels." Hemorrhage from the AVM, however, regardless of the bleeding location, is still classified among "other causes of SAH."[105]

Size

AVMs vary in size from tiny, so-called cryptic malformations (Fig. 31-13) to massive anomalies that encompass a number of cerebral lobes (Fig. 31-14). The arterial supply also varies enormously, from the extremes of all major cerebral, brainstem, or cerebellar arterial systems, to

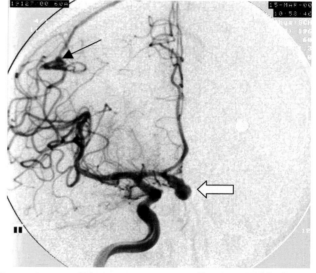

Figure 31-13 "Micro-arteriovenous malformation" *(black arrow)* and coincidental arterial aneurysm unrelated to the shunt flow *(white arrow)*.

TABLE 31-2 MULTIVARIATE LOGISTIC REGRESSION MODEL TESTING THE EFFECT OF DIFFERENT ANEURYSM TYPES ON INCIDENT HEMORRHAGE IN 463 PATIENTS WITH ARTERIOVENOUS MALFORMATION (AVM)

		95% Confidence	
	Odds Ratio	**Interval**	**P Value**
Feeding artery aneurysm	2.11	1.18–3.78	.012
Intranidal aneurysm	1.83	0.79–4.21	.158
Unrelated aneurysms	1.69	0.72–3.95	.228
Patient age	1.00	0.99–1.01	.923
Female gender	0.65	0.43–0.98	.042
AVM size*	0.94	0.93–0.96	?.0001
Deep venous drainage component	2.42	1.58–3.69	?.0001

*Maximum diameter in mm increments.

a single artery, to a single vein draining a fistula. The feeding arteries in the larger malformations frequently are abnormally enlarged and ectatic, reflecting the large loads they carry. Deep arterial feeders often feed the malformation as well. These deep vessels usually arise from branches or main trunks of the major cerebral arteries in the lenticulostriate, choroidal, or thalamoperforating arteries (Fig. 31-15) and reach the AVM after passing through healthy tissues. The venous drainage of AVMs eventually reaches recognizable venous channels, usually appearing abnormally distended because of the large volumes of blood flow through the shunt. The veins follow two basic routes, the more common being superficial drainage coursing over the cortex directly to the major sinuses or collateral venous channels that lead to the major sinuses. The other route is through deep venous

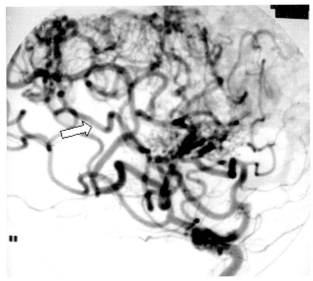

Figure 31-14 Large arteriovenous malformation with arterial supply throughout the hemisphere. Note the ectatic feeding arteries *(arrow)*.

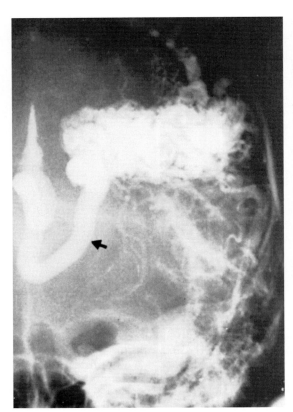

Figure 31-16 Cylinder-shaped arteriovenous malformation located in the frontal region and extending deep to the ventricle with a large vein draining to the ependyma *(arrow)*.

Location

No method has been generally agreed on for defining the epicenter of an AVM. The huge size of the arterial and venous channels may dwarf whatever fistula can be found, making it absurd to speak of a precise center of the malformation; some fistulas, however, are discrete enough to allow their determination as lobar, deep, and so forth. Careful volumetric studies suggest that there is no special predilection for AVMs in any part of the brain. The locations encountered seem simply to reflect the relative volume of the brain represented by a given region. The frontal lobe, occupying 30% of the brain volume, is shown to have 30% of the AVMs. The posterior fossa, at 12% of brain volume, has some 12% to 14% of the malformations.[106] When a center is said to be found, it is most often frontoparietal but can also be brainstem or cerebellar.[107] Location has not had a bearing on the tendency for hemorrhage, growth, regression, vascular complexity, or size. AVMs arising in the large lobes (e.g., frontal, occipital) seem to have about the same frequency of manifestation as headaches, seizures, and hemorrhage, the focal syndrome reflecting the brain region involved.[108]

AVMs are most commonly wedge-shaped with the apex of the wedge directed toward the ventricular system. However, these lesions may assume cylindrical or globoid forms in the white matter (Fig. 31-16). Among the hitherto less well-described locations are the brainstem,[109] choroidal artery territory,[110] anterior dura, and corpus callosum.[111] Fifty percent of AVMs appear to straddle

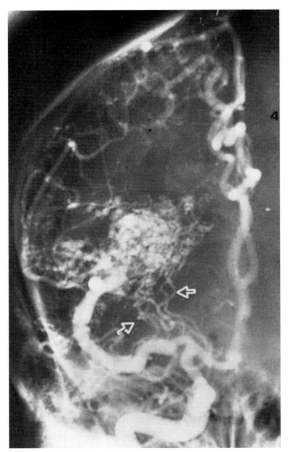

Figure 31-15 Example of a large arteriovenous malformation with a component of deep arterial feeders *(arrows)*.

channels that reach the ependymal surface of the ventricular system and drain via the deep venous system. In the larger lesions, there is often a dual venous network of drainage comprising both superficial and deep veins.

or are located near the arterial borderzone territories (Fig. 31-17).

Number

The vast majority of AVMs are single, but a growing proportion of patients have multiple AVMs (Fig. 31-18).[93,112] In one series of 203 patients, 19 (9%) had multiple AVMs.[93] When multiple, the lesions are usually small.

Clinical Syndromes

The vast majority of AVMs that become symptomatic manifest as hemorrhage.[79,113-117] Hemorrhage can be parenchymatous and subarachnoid. Unlike the hemorrhage in cerebral aneurysms, with which these lesions are often compared, the hemorrhage of AVMs into the subarachnoid

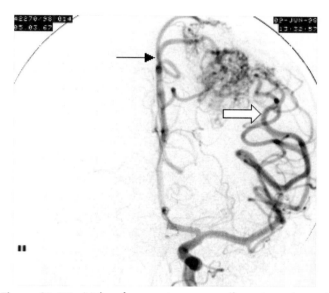

Figure 31-17 Nidus of an arteriovenous malformation is located in the borderzone between branches of the anterior cerebral artery *(black arrow)* and the middle cerebral artery *(white arrow)*.

space is generally confined to local subarachnoid spaces and does not spread widely into the large cisterns.

Risk of First Hemorrhage

The need for optimal treatment strategies for AVMs is driven by the risk of first hemorrhage, which is generally assumed to be 2% to 4% per year. For some subtypes, especially those smaller lesions deemed suitable for intervention, the risk may be as little as 1% per year,[83] and for those very large and complex, in the range of 3% to 6%.[99a] These recent reports show rates lower than those commonly quoted. Rates vary widely in reports from referral centers. They may stabilize over time.[63,99,118a] Preliminary prospective population-based estimates from the ongoing New York Islands AVM study suggest that about a third of all patients with AVM initially present with ICH.[119]

Factors Predisposing to Hemorrhage

Several studies have demonstrated an increased risk for hemorrhage in a setting of small AVM size, exclusive deep venous drainage,[120] and high intranidal pressures.[121] The impression that the smaller AVMs are more prone to hemorrhage has been held for many years,[115,122-126] being formed well before modern studies confirming this view, but has been superseded in modern studies by deep location and deep venous drainage. The role of deep venous drainage is a later discovery; a role for high intranidal pressures has long been suspected,[127] but modern microcatheter techniques were required before this suspicion could be confirmed.[128]

Clinical Syndromes Related to Hemorrhage

When acute bleeding occurs, the hematoma may expand within the AVM nidus, rupture into adjacent brain parenchyma, vent into the ventricular system and cause hemohydrocephalus, or spread into the subarachnoid space. Approximately half of the clinical presentations of AVMs are as ICH.[79,129-132] Although the malformation itself occupies space, it does not often manifest as a mass lesion in the absence of hemorrhage. In cases of stroke due to

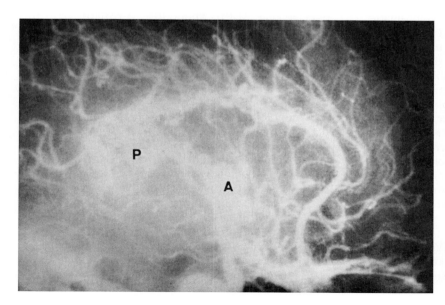

Figure 31-18 Tandem arteriovenous malformations involving the anterior third ventricle (A) and the roof structures of the posterior third ventricle (P). Even though the draining vein is common to these two malformations, they are distinct lesions.

causes other than AVM, the brain tissue was essentially healthy and normal before its disruption. Stroke from AVMs is different; the lesion is embedded in the brain, surrounded by healthy tissue, and its disordered vessels may draw circulation from healthy brain or provide blood to healthy brain distal to the malformation. The severity of neurologic deficit depends on the location and size of the hemorrhage.

Lesion Location

Lesion location plays a major role in clinical presentation. Those lesions located in polar regions of the brain with massive hemorrhage may cause little more than headache and nonfocal symptoms related to the mass effect and a rise in intracranial pressure. However, those lesions located in deep structures, such as the diencephalon, basal ganglion, or motor, sensory, and speech areas, may give rise to devastating neurologic deficits secondary to involvement of these areas. Because the hemorrhages are often subcortical and extend into the white matter, the fibers commonly separate without lasting impairment of function. Many patients with such lesions may make remarkable and often complete recovery from the initial hemorrhage even if it is massive. Unfortunately, some suffer fixed and sometimes catastrophic neurologic deficits after the initial hemorrhage, and these deficits remain for life.

The amount of subarachnoid blood varies, depending for the most part on two factors, the extent of the hemorrhage and the relationship of the AVM to large cisterns or to the ventricles. Many of the larger malformations project in a wedge-shaped fashion to the ventricle, where the dilated tortuous loops of veins may lie free without ependymal covering. This is a source of hemorrhage in such malformations and may lead to massive amounts of intraventricular blood with acute hydrocephalus and spread of the blood throughout the cerebrospinal fluid.

Settings for Rupture

The settings for the rupture include the familiar exertional states commonly encountered for other causes of hemorrhage. However, a few investigators have found no correlation with activity,[133] a point against advising asymptomatic patients to live a completely sedentary life. Pregnancy was once cautioned against and still remains a management conundrum[134]; however, the bleeding rate during pregnancy (0.031 patient-year) compares favorably with the risk in nonpregnant women (0.031 risk per patient-year),[135] indicating that pregnancy is not a greater risk for those without prior hemorrhage. Pregnancy, especially during the first trimester, was once believed to pose a greater risk of AVM hemorrhage, and some observers suggested cesarean section as a prudent measure to avoid complications during delivery.[135,136] There appears to be no greater hemorrhage risk for a woman during the various phases of pregnancy and, thus, no justification for abortion.

Underdiagnosis or Misdiagnosis

Both underdiagnosis and misdiagnosis of AVM are common. In some cases, the hemorrhagic onset of symptoms related to these lesions is not recognized by the patient or the treating physician. It may be passed off as a migraine type of headache or severe tension headache, or, when accompanied by a seizure, may be obscured. In a large series of patients with AVMs who underwent surgery, we have found approximately 15% with asymptomatic hemorrhages, identified from the finding of cystic encephalomalacia with pigmentation surrounding the site of hemorrhage; in all cases, a review of the clinical history showed no indication of previous hemorrhage. None of these hemorrhages was detected by CT scan or lumbar puncture and cerebrospinal fluid analysis. This significant incidence of clinically silent hemorrhage raises a question about the authenticity of statements that AVMs are dangerous only if they have previously hemorrhaged. Multiple hemorrhages associated with untreated AVMs are common.[137] However, the interval between these hemorrhages may be years or even decades.

Clinical Differences from Aneurysm Hemorrhage

Because hemorrhages from AVMs differ markedly from those of aneurysm and hypertension, it has long been believed that they should be easily differentiated from one another clinically. Although AVMs are buried in the brain, they are usually in continuity with the ventricle or cerebral surface. Thus, they can produce parenchymatous hemorrhage as well as SAH, intraventricular hemorrhage, or both. Because the lesions are arteriovenous, the hemorrhage is less violent than that from aneurysm and evolves over a longer period than the usual few seconds characteristic of aneurysmal rupture. Because the AVM hemorrhage arises in a malformation, it also has a less disruptive effect on cerebral function. Vasospasm, that discouraging accompaniment of ruptured aneurysms, is less prevalent with the SAH of an AVM because the hemorrhage is located away from the base of the brain and the volume of blood injected into the subarachnoid space is smaller.

Type of Syndromes

In our own experience, there are three distinct forms or syndromes of hemorrhage, as follows:
1. The AVM bleeds mainly into the ventricular system, producing hemocephalus rather than parenchymatous damage (Fig. 31-19). About 10% of patients have this clinical picture. An unrelenting course over minutes from the onset of headache to stupor is the typical presentation.
2. The hemorrhage affects the subarachnoid space in a fashion similar to that of a ruptured aneurysm, potentially including severe vasospasm (Fig. 31-20). About 10% of patients have this presentation, some on several occasions.
3. A deficit due to a parenchymatous hemorrhage occurs, followed by a satisfactory remission (Fig. 31-21). This condition is decidedly uncommon except in patients with lobar hemorrhage, whose diagnosis of hemorrhage is increasingly being documented by imaging, after which the lesions are not left alone to pursue their natural course.

Little information can be found in the literature to corroborate these syndromes. However, a few cases are described well enough to create a characteristic clinical picture of AVM rupture. Mackenzie[113] stated that "in most

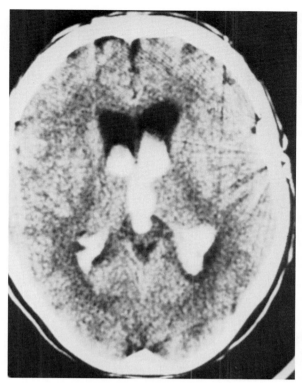

Figure 31-19 Massive intraventricular hemorrhage observed on CT after the rupture of a dural posterior fossa arteriovenous malformation.

cases there has been nothing remarkable about the history, the incident being simply one of sudden onset of severe headache, accompanied by neck stiffness, vomiting, and perhaps pyrexia." Deep hematomas in the basal ganglia have been described with the same smooth onset, hemiparesis, sensory disturbance, ocular motility disorders, and language and mental defects that are encountered in hypertensive hemorrhage.[138,139] Three such cases in the series reported by Wilson[140] were diagnosed only by surgical exploration, a finding that resurrects McCormick and Nofzinger's[141] long-standing contention that cryptic AVMs are more common than has been supposed. Data showing that AVMs cause as few as 10% of parenchymatous hematomas[139] may give some comfort to the physician faced with an etiologic diagnosis. Frequencies as high as 35% to 44% in other series[129] should promptly eliminate any complacency that an etiologic diagnosis can be made on clinical grounds alone.

Syndrome Severity and Clinical Course

The similarity of currently reported AVM hemorrhage incidence has prompted estimates of acute hemorrhage fatality or major morbidity from a variety of current databases. Prior reports have suggested the outcome can be benign. In the series described by Pia et al,[142] only 1 of 16 patients with hematomas 100 to 250 mL in size died, and 14 fully regained functional capacity. Four had slight to moderate hemiparesis, and 2 were asymptomatic. A few other reports have detailed patients who made remarkable functional improvements despite hemorrhage and extensive surgery. Garrido and Stein[138] described a

29-year-old man who had an extensive AVM fed by the lenticulostriate arteries. He experienced a hemorrhage with left hemiparesis, hemianopia, and memory impairment. After removal of this deep-seated lesion, the patient eventually improved enough to return to work.

Other, similar cases have been described in which deep hemorrhages and the causative AVM have been removed, with good results.[143] However, the outlook may not be as encouraging for all hematoma syndromes: Pertuiset et al[144] found that 19 of their patients with preoperative aphasia experienced no postoperative improvement. One might speculate that AVMs should have a better prognosis because some of the bleeding occurs into devitalized tissue. However, it may be premature to judge that such improvements are unique to hematomas from AVMs. Similar improvements have been shown with deep hypertensive hematomas if they are small, as noted by Hier and coworkers.[139] Ruff and Arbit[145] reported a single instance of acute minor motor aphasia precipitated by a hemorrhage from an AVM affecting the inferior frontal region of the dominant hemisphere. The clinical features and time course of improvement mimicked those documented in cases of infarction. As yet, no study has compared the outlook for hematomas of the same size from AVMs and other causes. In the limited experience with lobar hemorrhage[146] and caudate hemorrhage,[147] hemorrhages due to AVM had features identical to those attributed to other causes.

Our own post hoc analysis of 119 prospectively enrolled patients from the Columbia AVM databank showed 115 had a hemorrhage as the diagnostic event, and 27 of them suffered a second hemorrhage during follow-up; an additional 4 patients had other diagnostic symptoms but bled during follow-up.[148] The location of the incident bleeds was supratentorial in 99 (86%) patients. Of the 16 (14%) cases with infratentorial lesions, 4 (4%) were located in the brainstem, and 12 (10%) in the cerebellum. The type of initial and follow-up hemorrhage was identical in 23/27 patients (85%). Follow-up hemorrhages were similarly distributed: 29 (94%) supratentorial, and 2 (7%) infratentorial.

In 54 (47%; CI, 38%–56%) patients the incident hemorrhage resulted in no neurologic deficit, an additional 43 (37%; CI, 28%–46%) patients were independent in their daily activities (Rankin score 1). Fifteen (13%; CI, 7%–19%) patients were moderately disabled (Rankin score 2 or 3), and 3 (3%; CI, 0%–6%) were severely disabled (Rankin score 4). The mean Rankin score for the cases with incident hemorrhage was 0.76 (0.91), and for the cases with incident and follow-up hemorrhage the mean was 0.89 (1.09). The difference between the means of the two groups was not significant (0.13, 95% CI, −0.31–0.57). No patient had died during the observation period.

Parenchymal hemorrhages were most likely to result in a neurologic deficit (52%). Type and morbidity of hemorrhage during follow-up were similar to incident events. Twenty (74%) of 27 patients with both incident and follow-up hemorrhages were normal or independent (Rankin score 0 or 1). None of the patients with a hemorrhage during follow-up died during the observation period.

Hemorrhage from cerebral AVMs has proved to have a lower morbidity rate than hemorrhage from hypertension.[149] However, if AVMs have a better clinical outlook,

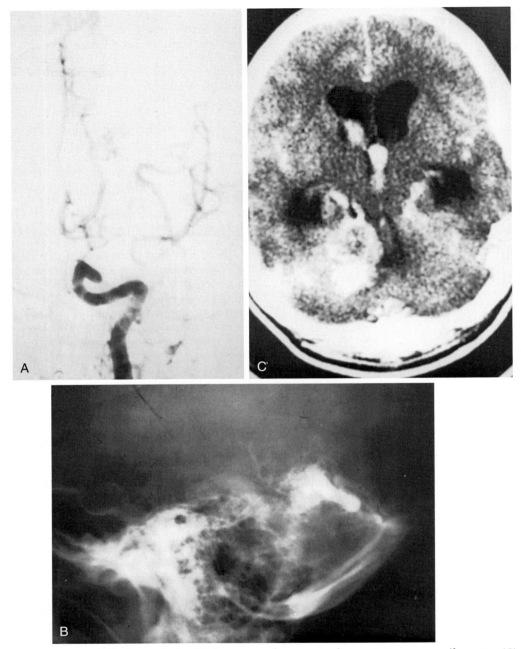

Figure 31-20 Intense vasospasm (A) observed after (B) the rupture of a posterior fossa arteriovenous malformation (C) with massive outpouring of blood into the basal cisterns and ventricles.

more effort to deal aggressively with such hematomas than is routinely the case in many institutions might be appropriate.

Risk of Rehemorrhage

Once hemorrhage has occurred, the risk of rehemorrhage is known to rise, but the extent and the timing of rehemorrhage are uncertain. In our own studies, an 18% annual rehemorrhage rate has been found in patients who already had bled.[150] Other studies report a wide variety of rates.[151] Graf et al[152] reviewed the records of 191 patients with AVMs, but the mean period of follow-up was relatively short (2 to 5 years). Nevertheless, they found a high rate of initial hemorrhage in the age group 11 to 35 years old, and the rate of rebleeding was about 2% a year. Smaller lesions were more prone to hemorrhage, and approximately 13% of the patients died as a result of the hemorrhage. It is generally accepted that approximately 15% of operated AVMs show evidence of prior but asymptomatic hemorrhage.[131]

Vasospasm

The rarity of vasospasm, symptomatic or merely an angiographic finding, has been a source of special commentary.[153,154] Although AVMs are generally said to be associated with a lower incidence of cerebral vasospasm

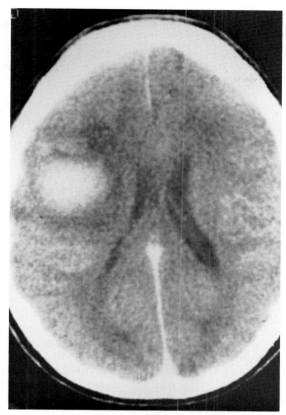

Figure 31-21 CT scan demonstrating parenchymatous hemorrhage after the rupture of a previously unsuspected arteriovenous malformation.

than cerebral aneurysms, this statement may be based on artifact, because AVMs (1) hemorrhage with less frequency into the large basal cisterns than aneurysms, (2) are less common than cerebral aneurysms, and (3) may be evaluated in the acute stage by arteriography, whereas spasm is generally seen on follow-up arteriography performed a few days after the SAH to evaluate the progress of a cerebral aneurysm or its readiness for surgery. The approach just described for vasospasm is not commonly the course of action taken with AVMs once they are identified. Anecdotal cases have certainly been observed in which delayed cerebral vasospasm has been intense after the rupture of an AVM; this spasm may go on to produce death or severe neurologic abnormalities (see Fig. 31-20). It is our impression that the incidence of cerebral vasospasm, in which the quantity of blood is sufficient within the entire subarachnoid space, is probably the same after rupture of a cerebral AVM as that after rupture of a cerebral aneurysm, but most AVMs do not rupture in ways that bring large amounts of blood into the basal cisterns. If present, vasospasm should be treated vigorously by whatever techniques are in current practice.

Aneurysms

Several retrospective studies suggested a higher risk of hemorrhage in patients with AVM and concurrent arterial aneurysms.[29,155-160] The retrospective actuarial analysis by Brown et al[161] demonstrated an increased annual risk of 7.0% for ICH in the setting of unruptured AVMs with

a concurrent arterial aneurysm (any coexisting saccular aneurysm seen on brain angiography) compared with a 1.7% per year risk for patients who have AVM without concurrent aneurysm. A few retrospective[162,163] and prospective[164,165] studies have found no independent effect of concurrent arterial aneurysms on the risk of ICH. The presence of such aneurysms, however, influences treatment decisions (i.e., surgical, endovascular, or radiation therapy) and acute patient management (i.e., invasive versus conservative care).

We undertook an analysis of our data to address these points. In a cross-sectional study, the 463 consecutive, prospectively enrolled patients from the Columbia AVM Databank were analyzed. Concurrent arterial aneurysms demonstrated on brain angiography were classified as (1) feeding artery aneurysms, (2) intranidal aneurysms, or (3) aneurysms unrelated to blood flow to the AVM. Clinical presentation (diagnostic event) was categorized as (1) ICH proven by imaging or (2) nonhemorrhagic presentation. Univariate and multivariate statistical models were applied to test the effect of age, gender, AVM size, venous drainage pattern, and the three different types of aneurysms on the risk of AVM hemorrhage at initial presentation.

ICH was the presenting symptom in 204 (44%) patients with AVM; 132 of them presented with ICH, 34 with intraventricular hemorrhage, and 29 with SAH. Because of missing data, the hemorrhage type was undefined in 9 patients. Of the 117 (25%) patients with concurrent arterial aneurysms, 93 had a single aneurysm type (54 had feeding artery aneurysms, 21 had intranidal aneurysms, and 18 had aneurysms unrelated to flow to the AVM). The remaining 24 patients showed more than one aneurysm type (10 with feeding artery and intranidal aneurysms, 10 with feeding artery and unrelated aneurysms, 1 with intranidal and unrelated aneurysms, and 3 with all three types of aneurysm).

Concurrent arterial aneurysms were significantly more common in patients presenting with AVM hemorrhage than in those with nonhemorrhagic AVM presentation ($P < .0001$). The difference remained significant ($P < .0001$) in a multivariate model controlling for age, gender, AVM size, and deep venous drainage (odds ratio 3.17; 95% CI, 1.91–5.28).

Feeding artery aneurysms were detected in 77 (17%) patients with AVM and were found significantly more often in those presenting with ICH than in those with nonhemorrhagic presentation (see Fig. 31-4). The difference remained significant in the multivariate model controlling for age, gender, AVM size, venous drainage pattern, and other concurrent aneurysm types (see Table 31-2). On the basis of these findings, the attributable risk of incident hemorrhage in feeding artery aneurysms for patients with AVM was estimated to be 6% (95% CI, 1%–11%). Feeding artery aneurysms were significantly more common among the 29 patients presenting with SAH (52%; n = 15) than in the 132 cases with intracerebral hemorrhage (17%; n = 23) or in the 34 patients with intraventricular hemorrhage (15%; n = 5; $P < .001$).

Intranidal aneurysms occurred in 35 (8%) patients with AVM. By univariate comparison, intranidal aneurysms were detected significantly more often in patients

TABLE 31-3 SEIZURE AS THE FIRST SIGN OF ARTERIOVENOUS MALFORMATION

Study (Year)*	No. of Cases	Cases with Seizure Presentation (%)				
		Total	Seizures Alone	Seizures plus Hemorrhage	Generalized Seizures	Focal Seizures
Stein and Wolpert (1980)[116,257]	121	43.8	36.8	7.4	—	—
Parkinson and Bachers (1980)[258]	100	67	—	—	—	—
Pertuiset et al (1979)[144]	162	37.6	25.3	12.3	41	59
Morello and Borghi (1973)[115]	154	35.0	20.1	14.9	—	—
Troupp et al (1970)[259]	138	26	—	—	—	—
Cooperative Study (1966)[129]	406	28	—	—	—	—
Paterson and McKissock (1956)[60]	110	46.4	—	—	—	—
Moody and Poppen (1970)[260]	105	50.5	40	10.5	55	45
Tönnis and Walter (1967)[261]	215	48.3	—	—	—	—
Krayenbühl and Yasargil (1959)[151]	608	41.2	—	—	—	—

*Superscript numbers indicate chapter references.

who presented with ICH (11%; n = 22) than in those without hemorrhagic presentation (5%; n = 13) (P = .023) (see Fig. 31-5). The effect of intranidal aneurysms on AVM hemorrhage, however, was not significant in the multivariate model controlling for age, gender, AVM size, venous drainage pattern, and the two other aneurysm types (see Table 31-2). No significant association was found for intranidal aneurysms with intracerebral hemorrhage (12%), intraventricular hemorrhage (15%), or SAH (3%) (P = .3) (see Table 31-2).

Thirty-two (7%) patients were found to have *arterial aneurysms unrelated to blood flow to the AVM*. No significant associations were found between unrelated arterial aneurysms and AVM hemorrhage at initial presentation or with ICH (7%), intraventricular hemorrhage (3%), or SAH (18%) (P = .2).

Our findings suggest that feeding artery aneurysms constitute an independent risk factor for hemorrhagic AVM presentation and may therefore be considered for surgical or endovascular treatment. However, a number of limitations should caution against final conclusions about treatment recommendations: Currently, population-based rates of death after AVM hemorrhage are unknown, and data from referral center patient cohorts may underestimate the overall frequency of AVM hemorrhage,[166] thereby leading to the possibility of a systematic error in this single-center analysis. Second, only 22% of our patients with incident ICH demonstrated aneurysms on an AVM feeding vessel, and only 52% of all patients presenting with SAH had a feeding artery aneurysm. Given the prevalence of feeding artery aneurysms in our sample, the attributable risk calculation suggests that only 6% of hemorrhages would have been prevented if all feeding artery aneurysms in the study sample had been eliminated.

Seizures

Seizures not caused by hemorrhage are the initial symptom in 16% to 53% of patients,[167] often alerting the physician to the presence of an AVM before it ruptures. Although seizure frequency has rarely been reported, the treatment response to antiepileptic medication is good.[168]

The available literature documents a remarkable variation in incidence of seizure (Table 31-3). The rate of seizure as a presenting feature of AVM varies from 28% (Cooperative Study) to 67%.[129] Reports vary too widely for one to consider that the severity,[169,170] ease of control with medication, and prognosis for hemorrhage are fully understood. The frequency of seizures correlates so poorly with AVM location that at present no specific relationships can be claimed. None was found in our series.

The *type of seizure* is often unreported. Several types of attacks labeled as seizures occur. The majority are partial or partial complex seizures, and the grand mal type is encountered in 27% to 35% of all seizures.[63,168] Some are typical focal epileptic seizures not associated with loss of consciousness. Others have been of the jacksonian type, with or without the loss of consciousness. Finally, several patients have experienced only a sudden loss of function, without tonic-clonic activity and without headache or loss of consciousness. Whether this last group has epilepsy per se is difficult to determine.[150] Ozer et al[171] were unable to distinguish focal AVM seizures from those of other causes in their 14 cases of seizure among 65 AVMs. Earlier opinions continue to influence clinical thinking but have been superseded by modern data. The most persistent opinion currently unsupported by data is the notion that there is more variation in type and frequency of attacks in AVM seizures than in cryptogenic or traumatic epilepsy.[113,172]

A small but separate literature exists for occipital AVMs, in which the seizures appear to have migrainous features,[173] including such complaints as "sudden dimming of everything in the right side of vision," "dimming of vision," and seeing "swirling spots of brightly colored lights," "red spots," or "frosted glass." In several cases, the visual complaints were followed by generalized seizure.

The *role of anatomic location* in seizure occurrence has received limited study, but suggestions have been made of a correlation of seizure with AVMs at the cortical surface. Turjman et al[177] found seizures associated with AVMs of the cerebral surface but not with deep AVMs. We did find an independent association of seizures at initial AVM presentation and a vascular borderzone location (odds ratio 2.2; 95% CI, 1.3-3.7).[176]

The incidence of seizures alone compared with *seizures in association with hemorrhage* varies widely. Hemorrhage occurred within 1 year in only 15% of

90 cases of seizure in the Cooperative Study.[129] Turjman et al[177] postulated a relationship between seizures and cortical AVMs and a history of hemorrhage.[178] Whether the character of the seizure differs when it is associated with hematoma is not certain.

Headache

Headache is the presenting symptom in 7% to 48% of patients with AVM.[167] In contrast to early assumptions,[179] the headache in AVM is of no distinctive type, frequency, persistence, or severity. Speculations about a pattern that distinguishes AVM headache from classic or common migraine or that recurrent unilateral headache reflects an underlying AVM have proved unfounded.[180] The former idea appears to have originated with Mackenzie,[113] who emphasized the tendency of the headaches to occur before the aura and for the aura to persist beyond the few minutes that typifies migraine, a finding not confirmed by others. Because headache is a common complaint in the population at large, it has been difficult to determine whether the headache associated with AVM is unique to the condition. That the character of the headache can be migrainous and have the classic aura is amply documented.[181,182]

Nevertheless, the notion that recurrent unilateral headache should arouse suspicion of an ipsilateral AVM is outmoded. It may have started with Northfield,[183] whose 1940 report stated that the headache "may affect only one side of the head, usually the side on which the angioma is situated." Very little evidence supports this claim. The yield for AVMs in evaluation for headache is low; in one study, only 0.2% of patients with normal neurologic findings who underwent neuroimaging for headache were diagnosed with an AVM.[184] Rates of response to pharmacologic headache treatment in patients with AVM have not been studied so far.

The postoperative disappearance of migraine headaches is not unusual and may occur after any type of operation. Disappearance of migraine after operation was a common feature of the early literature, which comprised mostly single case reports. The question raised now is whether all patients with migraine should be evaluated for an AVM. At the very least, CT with administration of a large bolus of contrast agent should be carried out in such patients. If anything suspicious is noted, then MRI should be performed.

Neurologic Deficit

Focal neurologic deficits without signs of underlying hemorrhage have been reported in 1% to 40% of patients with AVMs.[185] This wide range most likely reflects nonuniformity of definitions.[63] Slowly progressing neurologic deficits, which were once considered common,[186] are part of the presentation in only a few patients (4% to 8%). Progressing syndromes were thought to be due to "steal"—that is, cerebral artery hypotension leading to ischemia in brain tissue adjacent to the lesion caused by shunting of large blood volumes through the fistulas.[187,188] AVMs sometimes induce remarkable levels of arterial hypotension, but evidence for a causal link with symptoms is lacking.[185,189] Venous hypertension and mass effect of the nidus offer alternative explanations for progressing focal neurologic deficits.[190] Because AVMs occupy space, they may act like tumors, their bulk effect usually recognized by massive, distended draining veins, especially in the deep white matter.[190a] They may even hinder the circulation of cerebrospinal fluid, leading to hydrocephalus. Displacement of healthy brain tissue by the AVM sufficient to cause neurologic symptoms is rare.

Physiologic Studies

Physiologic evaluation of vascular malformations has centered on the study of AVMs.[191-195] Cerebral blood flow recordings indicate a varying degree of AV blood shunting within an AVM. The amount of shunting depends on the ratio of the feeding arteries to draining veins, the size of the lesion, and the number of shunts within the lesion. When arteriovenous shunting is great enough, left ventricular cardiac failure can occur, as has been seen in children with larger AVMs. Early intraoperative studies by Nornes and Grip[196] underscore the dynamic changes that occur in blood flow through these malformations during occlusion of the various nutrient arteries and with systemic changes of blood pressure and flow. The fall in pressures proceeds in an orderly manner from the parent artery through branches, leading finally to the AVM, where pressures may be quite low; by inference, pressures are also low in normal adjacent brain supplied by these branches.[197] Remarkably little difference is found between the shear forces in vessels involved by an AVM and those in healthy vessels.

Evidence is now clear that the large feeding arteries lack autoregulation.[198] Angiographic signs of disordered autoregulation after surgery include enlargement of an artery proximal to an AVM in the days after the malformation is occluded by either embolization or surgical ligation (Fig. 31-22). This postocclusion ectasia remains for days to weeks. Persistent ectasia leads to decreased flow and stasis in the arterial system proximal to the AVM,[128] indicating that obliteration of the shunt results in a global increase in blood flow.

In the postoperative state, arterial stasis, even vein thrombosis and venous infarction in the normal brain, has been described.[116,199] The pressure in the feeding arteries is initially high after surgery and may lead to hemorrhagic complications described by Spetzler et al[200] as "perfusion pressure breakthrough." The pressure and flow that drive the nutrient blood to an AVM are thought to be redirected to the normal circulation after the obliteration of an AVM. This rerouted blood pressures the local arteries beyond their capacities, resulting in edema and then hemorrhage in the area. Postoperative stasis, high arterial pressures, hemorrhagic complications, or a combination of these findings have been described by others as well.[107,128,201-204] Studies from our institution have indicated a shift of the autoregulation limits toward lower pressures, preserved responsiveness to CO_2, and pharmacologically induced vasodilatation in arteries adjacent to AVMs.[197,205]

Former assumptions of perfusion defects in the brain adjacent to an AVM have proved difficult to certify. In a study of 11 cases of hemispheral AVM, single-photon emission computed tomography (SPECT) was used to compare the regions of the AVM with a matching contralateral

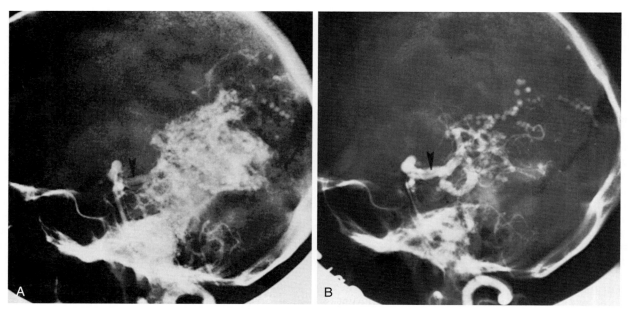

Figure 31-22 A, Large arteriovenous malformation (AVM) fed by a posterior cerebral artery *(arrowhead)*. B, Enlargement of the posterior cerebral artery *(arrowhead)* after successful embolic occlusion of portions of the AVM and feeding artery, with marked reduction of flow through the AVM but with enlargement of the feeding artery.

site before and after administration of acetazolamide. The defects in flow surrounding the AVM lesions were found to be related to the size of the AVM, not to any effects explained by local arterial pressure.[206] Preservation of cerebrovascular reserve was also evident, arguing against a specific defect in perfusion around an AVM such as that postulated for steal.

Other Vascular Malformations and Anomalies

Acquired Arteriovenous Fistulas

Some AV fistulas that appear on angiography to be AVMs actually constitute secondary lesions. Two major causes have been identified, trauma and venous thrombosis.

Trauma

Trauma to the brain surface from closed-head injury presumably may join or enlarge the existing AV shunts from their normal size of roughly 90 μm near the superior sagittal sinus and possibly in other sites. Once linked or enlarged, such fistulas would presumably lose their autoregulation and be subject to the same enlargement typical of any AV link. Patients with such lesions should have a history or should show evidence of prior head injury, and the injury should be confined to the brain surface. To date, no ready classification for these lesions has been developed.

Venous Thrombosis

Thrombosis of a large vein or sinus may create a high enough resistance to normal arterial flow to force creation of new pathways.[175,207,208] Angiography usually shows delayed filling of the carotid or vertebrobasilar arteries and those branches having access to a patent vein or sinus, such as the meningeal and other dural arteries,

which dilate and convolute in a manner seen in congenital AVMs. These shunts can develop in a fairly short time, possibly months. If sinus thrombosis occurs, a major hemorrhagic lesion may follow. There is still uncertainty about (1) whether the hypertrophied channels become independent of autoregulation or can be expected to subside if the venous obstruction is relieved is still unknown, (2) whether they have certain theoretical limits in size and extent or continue to develop until they hemorrhage, and (3) whether their proper treatment is ligation or neglect.

Dural Arteriovenous Fistulas

Dural arteriovenous fistulae (DAVFs) constitute AV shunts at the level of the meninges that are usually supplied by branches of the external carotid and/or vertebral artery (Fig. 31-23). Their venous channels usually empty into the major sinus, depending on the location of the AV shunt. They have an extracerebral location, may be congenital, but are mostly considered to develop secondary to physical or vascular trauma, in the setting of a sinus thrombosis. Often they present with pulse-synchronic bruits, headaches, and signs of increased intracranial pressure, but they may also cause progressive neurologic deficits and intracranial bleeding, including ICH. Those with direct or retrograde venous outflow into cerebral veins have been associated with hemorrhagic presentation or progressive neurologic symptoms at initial diagnosis, but no controlled longitudinal data exist on the actual longitudinal risk of these lesions. Nonetheless, the most widely used classification, as proposed by Cognard et al,[209] is mainly based on the venous outflow pattern as these characteristics may also impact on the endovascular treatment approach: In type I fistulas, meningeal branches shunt directly into a dural sinus without retrograde venous filling. Type II lesions are similar to type I but show venous reflux from the dural sinus into subarachnoid veins. Type

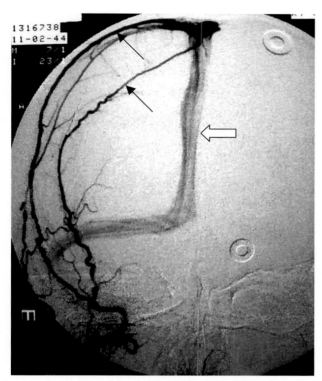

Figure 31-23 Dural fistula connecting branches of the external carotid artery *(black arrows)* with the superior sagittal sinus *(white arrow)*.

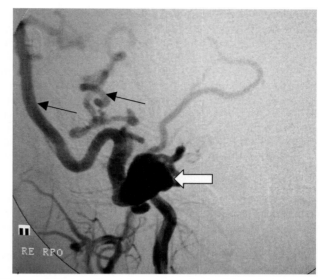

Figure 31-24 Carotid-cavernous fistula filling the cavernous sinus *(white arrow)* and draining through the intracranial venous system *(black arrows)*.

III fistulas connect directly to cortical veins. If the latter type shows venous ectasias, it is labeled type IV. The rare infratentorial type V lesions show retrograde venous drainage into the spinal venous system.[210]

A common presentation in a dural AV shunt is the carotid-cavernous fistula (Fig. 31-24). This subtype consists of mainly a single shunt (rarely several transdural feeders) which links the internal carotid artery during its passage through the cavernous sinus with a portion of the cavernous sinus. Although they often arise following trauma, they are also known to occur spontaneously, especially in the elderly. The classic symptom complex features an injected sclera of the affected eye, chemosis, ophthalmoplegia, a bruit, and, in severe cases, even loss of vision.[211]

Quite commonly, DAVFs are missed on standard CT, MRI, and MRA images, and their definite diagnosis is mainly based on diagnostic cerebral angiography after obligatory injection of the common carotid and vertebral arteries.

Most often, DAVFs are treated using an endovascular approach, either via the feeding artery system or via retrograde occlusion of the draining veins. Depending on the topographic location, direct embolization via transcranial puncture and neurosurgical occlusion of the venous draining system constitute alternative therapeutic strategies.

Vein of Galen Malformations

Vascular malformations that involve the vein of Galen region and that are characterized by venous dilatation of the great cerebral vein or its precursors have long been grouped together, regardless of vastly differing pathology. It was only in 1986 that Raybaud and Strother[8] described the dilated midline vein as the embryologic precursor of the vein of Galen, the median vein of the prosencephalon. The vein of Galen and the straight sinus form after the stage of the 50-mm embryo. Because the pallium is beginning to grow without established intrinsic vascularization between 21 to 23 mm (6 weeks' gestation) and 50 mm (11 weeks' gestation), the event leading to the defect must occur at the stage of the 21- to 23-mm embryo. There are fundamental differences between lesions in which the vein of Galen is absent (the malformation per se) and a situation in which a deep-seated AVM drains into a dilated vein of Galen. Prenatal diagnoses of the latter confirming true vein of Galen malformations further support their distinction from AVMs, for which in utero findings are yet missing.[10,11] Consequently, vein of Galen malformations become clinically manifest in neonates with cardiac failure due to high intracranial shunt flow, whereas infants present with macrocephaly or neurologic symptoms.[9] Vein of Galen malformations are usually not detected at later stages of life.

Telangiectasis

Telangiectases are uncommon anomalies composed of small clusters of capillary-like vessels located in the brainstem or cerebellum.[212] They are often deep and occasionally multiple. Their clinical significance is dubious. The telangiectases have long been considered curiosities for the pathologist to describe, with only rare clinical significance.[213] Although they frequently demonstrate small microhemorrhages on histologic examination, the hemorrhage does not appear to be large enough to create a clinical syndrome. In telangiectasia that manifests clinically, hemorrhage is the common mechanism, most often in the white matter of the brainstem, cerebellum, and diencephalic regions, their usual sites of occurrence. Rarely, the hemorrhages may be incapacitating or fatal, and postmortem examination may uncover the lesion as a thrombosed telangiectasia.

So-called familial hemorrhagic telangiectasia or Weber-Osler-Rendu syndrome is an autosomal dominant disorder associated with multiple "telangiectasias" elsewhere in the body, which actually constitute tiny vascular nodules with AV shunting.[214] Their number may increase during lifetime with the mostly affected organs being the mucosa, skin, and lungs. If located in the brain, these lesions may behave similar to sporadic AVMs and may cause spontaneous rupture with intracranial hemorrhage (see earlier).[215]

Cerebral Cavernous Malformations

Cerebral cavernous malformations (CCMs), or cavernomas, constitute abnormally enlarged postcapillary cavities without intervening brain parenchyma. They represent the only true venous malformation of the brain.

On the basis of autopsy data, prevalence estimates for CCMs in the general population range between 100 and 500 per 100,000. Women and men appear to be equally affected. The mean age at diagnosis spreads around age 30 in most later series, with an estimated annual detection rate of 0.56 per 100,000.[216] Because of their characteristic appearance on MRI (less so on CT), cavernous malformations are becoming more and more the subject of reports in the literature.[141,209,217-219] The proportion of familial cases ranges between 10% and 40% in most Western populations, but the highest frequency (50%) has been reported in Hispanic Americans, suggesting a genetic founder effect.[220] Patients harboring multiple CCMs or those with a familial CCM history have a high likelihood of carrying a genetic mutation.[88,221-223]

Generally, CCMs may occur anywhere, including the cortical surface, white matter pathways, basal ganglia, and deep in the brainstem. They rarely occupy a clinically significant amount of space in the brain but may be located in clinically important regions and are occasionally multiple. Although they are masses, they do not produce displacements commensurable with those of neoplasms. Their cavernous channels often show multiple areas of thrombosis and hemosiderin deposits as remnants of prior intracavernomatous (less often extracavernomatous) hemorrhage. Blood flow through these lesions is minimal, and therefore they are generally not seen on diagnostic angiograms.

In terms of imaging, CCMs may be recognized as round, slightly hyperdense lesions on noncontrast head CT, showing some ring enhancement after injection of contrast agent. In most cases, the diagnosis is easily established on brain MRI with a typical popcorn-shaped, mixed hyperintense and hypointense appearance and usually a hypointense perilesional signal on fluid-attenuated inversion recovery (FLAIR) and T2-weighted images. Gradient echo (T2*-weighted) imaging carries the highest sensitivity for the detection of CCM, revealing intralesional paramagnetic hemosiderin deposits as hypointense signals. Extracerebral manifestations may affect cranial nerves (rare, but most commonly the trigeminal, optic or oculomotor nerves), the spinal cord, the retina (in up to 5% of familial CCM cases), and the skin (visible as isolated hyperkeratotic cutaneous capillary venous malformations, so far described in cases with familial CCMs only).

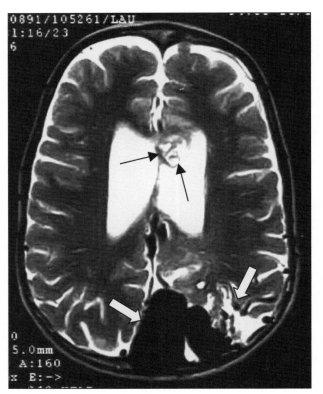

Figure 31-25 Cavernous malformation *(black arrows)* and large posterior arteriovenous malformation with ectatic draining veins *(white arrows)*.

Clinically, it is often difficult to determine a one-to-one relationship between lesion and symptoms. At initial diagnosis, the latter include epileptic seizures in 45% of cases, symptomatic hemorrhage in 30%, and headaches or other/unrelated symptoms leading to diagnostic imaging in 25%.[118,183,224-226] Overall, hemorrhage from cavernous malformations is not as common as hemorrhage from AVMs.[193,219,225,227] In patients in whom a CCM is found after MRI for chronic headache, it is very often difficult to determine a one-to-one relationship between lesion and symptoms.

Among patients with familial CCMs, 60% become symptomatic. The proportion of symptomatic patients among sporadic cases remains as yet unknown. Three different gene loci have been defined so far, all leading to autosomal dominant pattern of inheritance: *CCM1* or *KRIT1* is located on chromosome 7q and accounts for over 40% of familial cases (up to 70% in Hispanic Americans); *CCM2* or *MGC4607* is on chromosome 7p and can be found in roughly 30%; finally, *CCM3* or *PDCD10* has been mapped to chromosome 3q and is the underlying defect in 15%. Another 15% of familial cases show no mutation in the three loci, which is why at least one more gene defect can be suspected.[228,229] In some cases, an anomaly of endothelial growth factor has been identified (Fig. 31-25).[230]

In routine clinical practice, the diagnosis of CCMs should be stratified by patient history (symptomatic versus asymptomatic, family history), MRI data (anatomic location, single versus multiple CCMs, hemorrhagic versus nonhemorrhagic, with or without associated developmental venous anomaly), and genetic test results

TABLE 31-4 NEUROLOGIC CLASSIFICATION OF CEREBRAL CAVERNOUS MALFORMATION

	Parameter	
Clinical	Symptomatic Seizures Hemorrhage Headache	Asymptomatic
Family history	Positive Pedigree Pattern of inheritance	Negative
Imaging	MRI (T1-weighted ± contrast agent, T2-weighted or fluid-attenuated inversion recovery [FLAIR], T2*-weighted, or diffusion-weighted imaging)	
Number	Multiple anatomic locations	Single anatomic location
Size	Maximum cavernoma diameter	
Hemorrhage	Acute bleeding Extracavernomatous	Chronic hemosiderin Intralesional
Developmental venous anomaly	Present	Absent
Genetic testing	Positive: *CCM1 (KRIT1)* *CCM2 (MGC4607)* *CCM3 (PDCD10)*	Negative

(if performed). Ideally, the hemorrhage status is specified based on extracavernomatous versus intracavernomatous bleeding, and whether the MRI signal suggests acute blood or chronic hemosiderin deposits (Table 31-4).[231] In the early days of MRI in patients undergoing surgery for CCM, an initial morphologic classification based on their appearance on T1- and T2-weighted sequences was proposed, as follows: Type 1 cavernomas are hyperintense lesions indicating recent hemorrhage. Type 2 malformations are those most often seen in daily practice; they harbor mixed hyperintense and hypointense signals suggestive of mixed subacute and chronic hemorrhage signs or calcifications. Type 3 lesions are hypointense and mostly asymptomatic. Type 4 CCMs are also assumed to be asymptomatic and can be detected on gradient echo (T2*) imaging alone. The last group, however, may be difficult to differentiate from other causes of cerebral microbleeds, such as amyloid angiopathy, arteriosclerotic small vessel disease, CADASIL (cerebral autosomal dominant arteriopathy with subcortical infarcts and leukoencephalopathy), and vasculitis.[232]

On longitudinal patient follow-up, the number of CCMs may increase over time, especially in genetic CCM types. A given cavernoma may remain stable, increase in volume, or even regress.[233] The crude average hemorrhage risk of a cavernoma seems to be as low as 0.6% per year.[234] Factors favoring symptomatic hemorrhage include a history of prior cavernoma hemorrhage, strategic locations such as the brainstem and basal ganglia, and anticoagulation therapy.[235] Pregnancy as a risk factor for cavernoma hemorrhage remains controversial. No data exist on whether or not antiplatelet drugs or anticoagulation therapy modifies the risk of bleeding. Overall, even in genetically determined cases, the long-term prognosis is favorable, with 80% preserved long-term autonomy, but a less favorable outcome is seen in patients with brainstem CCM.[236]

If indicated, neurosurgical excision is the treatment of choice because outcome after stereotactic radiotherapy appears to have less favorable results.[237,239]

The decision for intervention is ideally based on a multidisciplinary discussion considering the overall profile of the patient (see Table 31-4). Surgery is generally limited to symptomatic CCMs associated with therapy-resistant epilepsy or progressive CCM enlargement, or after symptomatic CCM hemorrhage. If extralesional CCM bleeding has occurred, not only may surgical excision eliminate the risk of subsequent hemorrhage but also the risk of intervention itself may be lower because the surgical approach in the post acute phase is facilitated by the preexisting bleeding cavity. Owing to the progressive multiplication of lesions over time, surgical intervention is not generally recommended in patients with familial CCM. Resection of an associated developmental venous anomaly is contraindicated because its occlusion may lead to venous stasis, brain edema, and eventual hemorrhage.

Developmental Venous Anomalies

Developmental venous anomalies (DVAs) represent extreme variations of normal hemispheric white matter and tectal venous drainage. Formerly labeled with the now obsolete term "venous angioma," they constitute physiologic drainage pathways of normal brain tissue but have come under scrutiny because of the use of MRI (Fig. 31-26) and cerebral angiography. They are represented by a deep prominent vein that appears late on the venous phase of an arteriogram and is associated with a finger-like projection from the main vein resembling a broom or caput medusae. This appearance is characteristic on angiography, the lack of an arterial component in DVAs distinguishing them from AVMs. They are associated with cavernous malformations in more than 30% of cases[239] and often remain clinically asymptomatic. Their role in ischemic or hemorrhagic events may best be explained by secondary failure of efficient drainage of brain tissue due to insufficient autoregulation mechanisms or by undetected associated lesions, mostly cavernomas.[211] Their role in the physiologic drainage of normal brain tissue usually precludes any surgical or endovascular intervention.

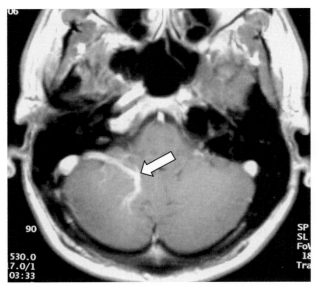

Figure 31-26 Developmental venous anomaly (DVA) of the cerebellum *(arrow)*.

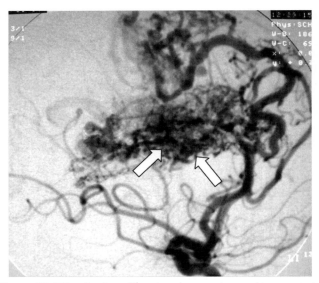

Figure 31-27 Angioproliferative changes *(arrows)* in an arteriovenous malformation resembling those found in moyamoya disease.

Moyamoya Disease

Moyamoya disease is an unusual form of chronic cerebrovascular occlusive disease with angiographic findings of bilateral stenosis or occlusion of the terminal portion of the internal carotid artery together with a vascular network at the base of the brain.[240] The Japanese word *moyamoya* has been translated as "hazy puff of smoke." The description arose from the initial angiographic appearance of this pathologic vascularization: The tiny size and large number of vessels imaged made the combination look like a cloud or a puff of smoke instead of single arteries. The numerous, dilated small vessels have also been termed "rete mirabile."[241]

Formerly described only in Japanese patients, moyamoya disease has now been found in other populations, although rarely. Annual incidence estimates of symptomatic moyamoya range between 0.06 per 100,000 in white patients and 0.54 per 100,000 in Japan, but seem to be almost twice as high in women and show two age distribution peaks, around 10 to 20 and 40 to 50 years.[240,242-245] Hereditary factors and ethnic origins may play a role in the occurrence or susceptibility to idiopathic moyamoya disease, as suggested by the occasional familial occurrence (12% in Japanese cases).[246] A secondary moyamoya syndrome may be seen in association with other congenital diseases, such as sickle cell anemia, von Recklinghausen's disease (neurofibromatosis type 1), and Down syndrome (trisomy 21).[247] However, the clinical manifestation and disease progression is not congenital and may also be seen as a secondary complication of early-onset intracranial atherosclerosis, autoimmune disease, vasculitis, meningitis, post-irradiation changes, cranial trauma, and brain neoplasm.[248,249]

In the vascular network of perforating arteries (the so-called moyamoya vessels), the following histologic changes can be observed: dilated vessels with a relatively thin wall, this type being more prominent in children, and thick-walled arteries showing luminal stenosis. With

hemodynamic stress or aging, the dilated arteries with attenuated walls may predispose to the formation of microaneurysms, the rupture of which is considered one of the mechanisms leading to parenchymatous hemorrhages in patients with moyamoya disease.

Clinically, ischemic and hemorrhagic symptoms are encountered. The ischemic type dominates in childhood, and transient ischemic attacks occur more often than infarctions, manifesting a variety of symptoms. The hemorrhagic type is more common in adult patients. Bleeding occurs, commonly in multiple and repetitive intervals, and massive bleeding, although infrequent, often leads to death.

Typical angiographic findings were considered indispensable to the diagnosis of moyamoya disease. As the quality of MRI and magnetic resonance angiography improved, however, the diagnosis was also made if either modality clearly demonstrated all the findings indicative of moyamoya. Moyamoya-type vascular changes have been observed in patients with AVMs (Fig. 31-27).[250] Whether the two entities are linked biologically or genetically, or whether the moyamoya-type vascular pathology observed in patients with AVMs merely results from hemodynamic changes associated with the AVM, remains unclear.

In advanced stages of moyamoya, some degree of early venous drainage may be seen on angiograms, suggesting AV shunting at the level of the neovessel network. On the other hand, moyamoya-type vascular changes have been observed on high-flow feeding arteries in brain AVMs. Whether the two entities are linked biologically, or whether the moyamoya-type vascular pathology observed in patients with AVM merely results from hemodynamic changes associated with the AVM remains as yet unclear. Some investigators envision a so-called high-flow angiopathy with the development of lesions to the intima in vessels feeding an AVM, the lesions building to the point of causing severe stenosis and occlusion of feeding arteries.[251] Another thesis is that the underlying process of severe stenosis known as moyamoya triggers sufficient vasodilatation in distal vessels as to cause AV links, which take on a life of their own and have the angiographic appearance of AVMs.

Ongoing Clinical Trials

Until recently, no randomized clinical trial has attempted to compare various forms of interventions with each other, nor with the "natural history" of AVMs discovered that had not bled. Evidence that rehemorrhage is common shortly after the first clinical hemorrhagic event prompted the initial well-intended assumptions that those discovered unbled should undergo attempts at eradication, this in hopes of being spared the unwelcome hemorrhage assumed to be likely in the future. Recent evidence suggests that the risk of hemorrhage may be far lower than the risk is when all forms of AVMs are lumped together.[83] Furthermore, many of the larger and more complex lesions with higher risk of hemorrhage are often considered too daunting to attempt eradication even after hemorrhage has occurred. Finally, hemorrhagic events from AVMs are clinically more mild than those from hypertension.[147a] All together, the rationale for intervention in those who have not bled can be argued as to have not having been established.[252] Based on these concerns, the National Institutes of Neurological Diseases and Stroke funded a clinical trial, A Randomized trial of Unruptured Brain Arteriovenous malformations (ARUBA) (1R01-NS51483, http://www.clinicaltrials.gov/ct/show/NCT00389181). This trial is limited to those unbled brain AVMs in which the lesion is deemed suitable for attempted eradication. It compares the outcomes from immediate prophylactic intervention against intervention that is deferred until hemorrhage occurs. The study period is for a minimum of 7 years following randomization. Both groups are treated medically for symptoms such as seizures or headache. To date, medical therapy is lacking to prevent hemorrhage. Organized in 2007, the trial remains under way as of the printing of this edition.[253]

REFERENCES

1. Rokitansky C: *Handbuch der allgemeinen pathologischen Anatomie*, Vienna, 1846, Braumüller & Seidel, pp 276-277.
2. Emmanuel C: Ein Fall von Angioma arteriale racemosum des Gehirns, *Deutsche Zeitschr Nervenheilk* 14:288-318, 1899.
3. Stapf C, Mohr JP, Mast H: History of concepts on the etiology of brain arteriovenous malformations, *Neurology* 58(Suppl 3):A342, 2002.
4. Mall FP: On the development of the blood-vessels of the brain in the human embryo, *Am J Anat* 4:1, 1905.
5. Evans HM: On the development of the aortae, cardinal and umbilical veins, and the other blood vessels of vertebrate embryos from capillaries, *Anat Rec* 3:498-519, 1909.
6. Streeter GL: The developmental alterations in the vascular system of the brain of the human embryo, *(Carnegie Inst Wash Pub 271.) Contrib Embryol* 8:5-38, 1918.
7. Moniz E: L'encéphalographie artérielle, son importance dans la localisation des tumeurs cérébrales, *Rev Neurol* 2:72-90, 1927.
8. Raybaud CA, Strother CM: Persisting abnormal embryonic vessels in intracranial arteriovenous malformations, *Acta Radiol Suppl* 369:136-138, 1986.
9. Lasjaunias P: *Vascular diseases in neonates, infants and children: Interventional neuroradiology management*, Berlin, 1997, Springer-Verlag.
10. Yuval Y, Lerner A, Lipitz S, et al: Prenatal diagnosis of vein of Galen aneurysmal malformation: Report of two cases with proposal for prognostic indices, *Prenat Diagn* 17:972-977, 1997.
11. Campi A, Scotti G, Filippi M, et al: Antenatal diagnosis of vein of Galen aneurysmal malformation: MR study of fetal brain and post-natal follow-up, *Neuroradiology* 38:87-90, 1996.
12. Pschyrembel W, Dudenhausen JW: *Praktische Geburtshilfe mit geburtshilflichen Operationen*, ed 17, Berlin, 1991, Walter de Gruyter.
13. Weaver DD, Brandt IK: *Catalog of prenatally diagnosed conditions*, ed 3, Baltimore, 1999, Johns Hopkins University Press.
14. Baird WF, Stitt DG: Arteriovenous aneurysm of the cerebellum in a premature infant, *Pediatrics* 24:455-457, 1959.
15. Padget DH: The development of the cranial arteries in the human embryo, *(Carnegie Inst Wash Pub 575.) Contrib Embryol* 32:205, 1948.
16. Stapf C, Mohr JP, Sciacca RR, et al: Incident hemorrhage risk of brain arteriovenous malformations located in the arterial border-zones, *Stroke* 31:2365-2368, 2000.
17. van den Bergh R, van der Eecken H: Anatomy and embryology of the cerebral circulation, *Prog Brain Res* 30:1, 1968.
18. Van den Bergh R, van der Eecken H: Anatomy and embryology of cerebral circulation, *Prog Brain Res* 30:1-25, 1968.
19. Van der Eecken HM, Fisher CM, Adams RD: The anatomy and functional significance of the meningeal arterial anastomoses of the human brain, *J Neuropathol Exp Neurol* 12:132-157, 1953.
20. Risau W, Lemmon V: Changes in the vascular extracellular matrix during embryonic vasculogenesis and angiogenesis, *Dev Biol* 125:441-450, 1988.
21. Bär T, Wolff JR: The formation of capillary basement membranes during internal vascularization of the rat's cerebral cortex, *Z Zellforsch* 133:231-248, 1972.
22. Krum JM, More NS, Rosenstein JM: Brain angiogenesis: Variations in vascular basement membrane glycoprotein immunoreactivity, *Exp Neurol* 111:152-165, 1991.
23. Bobik A, Campbell JH: Vascular derived growth factors: Cell biology, pathophysiology, and pharmacology, *Pharm Rev* 45:1-42, 1993.
24. Risau W: Angiogenetic factors, *Progr Growth Factor Res* 2:71-79, 1990.
25. Nelson MD, Gonzalez-Gomez I, Gilles FH: The search for human telencephalic ventriculofugal arteries, *AJNR Am J Neuroradiol* 12:215-222, 1991.
26. Hung PC, Wang HS, Yeh YS, et al: Coexistence of schizencephaly and intracranial arteriovenous malformation in an infant, *AJNR Am J Neuroradiol* 17:1921-1922, 1996.
27. Turjman F, Massoud TF, Viñuela F, et al: Correlation of the angioarchitectural features of cerebral arteriovenous malformations with clinical presentation of hemorrhage, *Neurosurgery* 37:856-862, 1995.
28. Meisel HJ, Mansmann U, Alvarez H, et al: Cerebral arteriovenous malformations and associated aneurysms: Analysis of 305 cases from a series of 662 patients, *Neurosurgery* 46:793-802, 2000.
29. Anderson RMCD, Blackwood W: The association of arteriovenous angioma and saccular aneurysm of arteries of the brain, *J Pathol Bacteriol* 77:101-110, 1959.
30. Voigt K, Beck U, Reinshagen G: A complex cerebral vascular malformation studied by angiography: Multiple aneurysms, angiomas and arterial ectasia, *Neuroradiology* 5:117-123, 1973.
31. Miyasaka K, Wolpert SM, Prager RJ: The association of cerebral aneurysms, infundibula, and intracranial arteriovenous malformations, *Stroke* 13:196-203, 1982.
32. Quick CM, Hashimoto T, Young WL: Lack of flow regulation may explain the development of arteriovenous malformations, *Neurol Res* 23:641-644, 2001.
33. Otto KB, Lierse W: Die Kappilarisierung verschiedener Teile des menschlichen Gehirns in der Fetalperiode und in den ersten Lebensjahren, *Acta Anat (Basel)* 77:25-36, 1970.
34. Laves W: Ein Fall von Angioma arteriali racemosum des Gehirnes im Bereiche der rechten Arter: Cerebri media, nebst einem Beitrag zur Frage der Entwicklung von Rankenangiomen im Gehirn, *Jahrb Psychiatr Neurol* 44:55, 1925.
35. Müller G: Zur Pathologie der arterio-venösen Rankenangiome des Gehirns, *Dtsch Z Nervenheilk* 172:361-376, 1954.
36. Kaplan HA, Aronson SM, Browder EJ: Vascular malformations of the brain: An anatomical study, *J Neurosurg* 18:635-830, 1961.
37. McCormick WF: The pathology of vascular ("arteriovenous") malformations, *J Neurosurg* 24:807-816, 1966.

38. Isoda K, Fukuda H, Takamura N, Hamamoto Y: Arteriovenous malformation of the brain: Histological study and micrometric measurement of abnormal vessels, *Acta Pathol Jpn* 31:883–893, 1981.

39. Challa VR, Moody DM, Brown WR: Vascular malformations of the central nervous system, *J Neuropathol Exp Neurol* 54:609–621, 1995.

40. Lamszus K, Schmidt NO, Ergün S, Westphal M: Isolation and culture of human neuromicrovascular endothelial cells for the study of angiogenesis in vitro, *J Neurosci Res* 55:370–381, 1999.

41. Hashimoto T, Mesa-Tejada R, Quick CM, et al: Evidence of increased endothelial cell turnover in brain arteriovenous malformations, *Neurosurgery* 49:124–131, 2001.

42. Gallione CJ, Pasyk KA, Boon LM, et al: A gene for familial venous malformations maps to chromosome 9p in a second large kindred, *J Med Genet* 32:197–199, 1995.

43. Hashimoto T, Lam T, Boudreau NJ, et al: Abnormal balance in the angiopoietin-Tie2 system in human brain arteriovenous malformations, *Circ Res* 89:111–113, 2001.

44. Vikkula M, Boon LM, Carraway KL, et al: Vascular dysmorphogenesis caused by an activating mutation in the receptor tyrosine kinase TIE2, *Cell* 87:1181–1190, 1996.

45. Rothbart D, Awad IA, Lee J, et al: Expression of angiogenic factors and structural proteins in central nervous system vascular malformations, *Neurosurgery* 38:915–924, 1996.

46. Hashimoto T, Emala CW, Joshi S, et al: Abnormal pattern of Tie-2 and vascular endothelial growth factor receptor expression in human cerebral arteriovenous malformations, *Neurosurgery* 47:910–918, 2000.

47. Hirschi KK, Rohovski SA, D'Amore PA: PDGF, TGF-beta, and heterotypic cell-cell interactions mediate endothelial cell-induced recruitment of 10T1/2 cells and their differentiation to a smooth muscle fate, *J Cell Biol* 141:805–814, 1998.

48. Malik G, Abdulrauf S, Yang XY, et al: Expression of transforming growth factor-beta complex in arteriovenous malformations, *Neurol Med Chir(Tokyo)* 38(Suppl):161–164, 1998.

49. Sonstein WJ, Kader A, Michelsen WJ, et al: Expression of vascular endothelial growth factor in pediatric and adult cerebral arteriovenous malformations: An immunocytochemical study, *J Neurosurg* 85:838–845, 1996.

50. Bourdeau A, Cymerman U, Paquet ME, et al: Endoglin expression is reduced in normal vessels but still detectable in arteriovenous malformations of patients with hereditary hemorrhagic telangiectasia type 1, *Am J Pathol* 156:911–923, 2000.

51. Blottner D: Nitric oxide and fibroblast growth factor in autonomic nervous system: Short- and long-term messengers in autonomic pathway and target organ control, *Prog Neurobiol* 51:423–438, 1997.

52. Abdulrauf SI, Malik GM, Awad IA: Spontaneous angiographic obliteration of cerebral arteriovenous malformations, *Neurosurgery* 44:280–287, 1999.

53. Kader A, Goodrich JT, Sonstein WJ, et al: Recurrent cerebral arteriovenous malformations after negative postoperative angiograms, *J Neurosurg* 85:14–18, 1996.

54. Robinson JR, Awad IA, Zhou P, et al: Expression of basement membrane and endothelial cell adhesion molecules in vascular malformations of the brain: Preliminary observations and working hypothesis, *Neurol Res* 17:49–58, 1995.

55. Yamada S, Liwnicz B, Lonser RR, Knierim D: Scanning electron microscopy of arteriovenous malformations, *Neurol Res* 21:541–544, 1999.

56. Burchiel KJ, Clarke H, Ojemann GA, et al: Use of stimulation mapping and corticography in the excision of arteriovenous malformations in sensorimotor and language-related neocortex, *Neurosurgery* 24:322–327, 1989.

57. Lazar RM, Marshall RS, Pile-Spellman J, et al: Interhemispheric transfer of language in patients with left frontal cerebral arteriovenous malformation 1, *Neuropsychologia* 38:1325–1332, 2000.

58. Stapf C, Mohr JP, Sciacca RR, et al: Incident hemorrhage risk of brain arteriovenous malformations located in the arterial borderzones, *Stroke* 31:2365–2368, 2000.

59. Stapf C, Mohr JP, Pile-Spellman J, et al: Concurrent arterial aneurysms in brain arteriovenous malformations with hemorrhagic presentation, *J Neurol Neurosurg Psychiatry* 73:294–298, 2002.

60. Paterson JH, McKissock W: A clinical survey of intracranial angiomas with special reference to their mode of progression and surgical treatment: A report of 110 cases, *Brain* 79:233, 1956.

61. Turjman F, Massoud TF, Vinuela F, et al: Aneurysms related to cerebral arteriovenous malformations: Superselective angiographic assessment in 58 patients, *AJNR Am J Neuroradiol* 15:1601–1605, 1994.

62. Stapf C, Hofmeister C, Mast H, et al: The feasibility of an Internet web-based, international study on brain arteriovenous malformations (The AVM World Study) [abstract], *Stroke* 31:322, 2000.

63. Hofmeister C, Stapf C, Hartmann A, et al: Demographic, morphological, and clinical characteristics of 1289 patients with brain arteriovenous malformation, *Stroke* 31:1307–1310, 2000.

64. Yasargil MG, editor: *Microneurosurgery*, New York, 1987, Thieme Medical.

65. Willinsky R, Lasjaunias P, terBrugge K, Pruvost P: Brain arteriovenous malformations: Analysis of the angio-architecture in relationship to hemorrhage (based on 152 patients explored and/or treated at the hospital de Bicetre between 1981 and 1986), *J Neuroradiol* 15:225–237, 1988.

66. Spetzler RF: Martin NA: A proposed grading system for arteriovenous malformations, *J Neurosurg* 65:476–483, 1986.

67. Nehls DG, Pittman HW: Spontaneous regression of arteriovenous malformations, *Neurosurgery* 11:776–780, 1982.

68. Willinsky R, Lasjaunias P, terBrugge K, Pruvost P: Brain arteriovenous malformations: Analysis of the angio-architecture in relationship to hemorrhage (based on 152 patients explored and/or treated at the hospital de Bicetre between 1981 and 1986), *J Neuroradiol* 15:225–237, 1988.

69. Morgan MK, Sekhon LH, Finfer S, Grinnell V: Delayed neurological deterioration following resection of arteriovenous malformations of the brain, *J Neurosurg* 90:695–701, 1999.

70. Courville CB: Intracranial tumors: Notes upon a series of three thousand verified cases with some current observations pertaining to their mortality, *Bull Los Angeles Neurol Soc* 32(Suppl 2):1–80, 1967.

71. Jellinger K: The morphology of centrally-situated angiomas. In Pia HW, Gleave JRW, Grote E, Zierski J, editors: *Cerebral angiomas: Advances in diagnosis and therapy*, New York, 1975, Springer-Verlag, pp 9–20.

72. Jellinger K: Vascular malformations of the central nervous system: A morphological overview, *Neurosurg Rev* 9:177–216, 1986.

73. Sarwar M, McCormick WF: Intracerebral venous angioma: Case report and review, *Arch Neurol* 35:323–325, 1978.

74. Griffiths PD, Worthy S, Gholkar A: Incidental intracranial pathology in patients investigated for carotid stenosis, *Neuroradiology* 38:25, 1996.

75. Yue NC, Longstreth WT Jr, Elster AD, et al: Clinically serious abnormalities found incidentally at MR imaging of the brain: Data from the Cardiovascular Health Study, *Radiology* 202:41–46, 1997.

76. Katzman GL, Dagher AP, Patronas NJ: Incidental findings on brain magnetic resonance imaging from 1000 asymptomatic volunteers, *JAMA* 282:36–39, 1999.

77. Berman MF, Sciacca RR, Pile-Spellman J, et al: The epidemiology of brain arteriovenous malformations, *Neurosurgery* 47:389–396, 2000.

78. Brown RD Jr, Wiebers DO, Torner JC, O'Fallon WM: Incidence and prevalence of intracranial vascular malformations in Olmsted County, Minnesota, 1965 to 1992, *Neurology* 46:949–952, 1996.

79. Brown RD Jr, Wiebers DO, Torner JC, O'Fallon WM: Frequency of intracranial hemorrhage as a presenting symptom and subtype analysis: A population-based study of intracranial vascular malformations in Olmsted Country, Minnesota, *J Neurosurg* 85:29–32, 1996.

80. Jessurun GA, Kamphuis DJ, van der Zande FH, Nossent JC: Cerebral arteriovenous malformations in The Netherlands Antilles: High prevalence of hereditary hemorrhagic telangiectasia-related single and multiple cerebral arteriovenous malformations, *Clin Neurol Neurosurg* 95:193–198, 1993.

81. Hillman J: Population-based analysis of arteriovenous malformation treatment, *J Neurosurg* 95:633–637, 2001.

82. Stapf C, Mast H, Sciacca R, et al: The New York Islands AVM Study: Design, study progress, and initial results, *Stroke* 34:E29-E33, 2003.

83. Stapf C, Mast H, Sciacca R, et al: Predictors of hemorrhage in patients with untreated brain arteriovenous malformations, *Neurology* 66:1350-1355, 2006.

84. Sacco RL, Boden-Albala B, Gan R, et al: Stroke incidence among white, black, and Hispanic residents of an urban community, *Am J Epidemiol* 147:259-268, 1998.

85. Stapf C, Labovitz DL, Sciacca RR, et al: Incidence of adult brain arteriovenous malformation hemorrhage in a prospective population-based stroke survey, *Cerebrovasc Dis* 13:43-46, 2002.

86. Barre RG, Suter CG, Rosenblum WI: Familial vascular malformation or chance occurrence? Case report of two affected family members, *Neurology* 28:98-100, 1978.

87. Boyd MC, Steinbok P, Paty DW: Familial arteriovenous malformations: Report of four cases in one family, *J Neurosurg* 62:597-599, 1985.

88. Dobyns WB, Michels VV, Groover RV, et al: Familial cavernous malformations of the central nervous system and retina, *Ann Neurol* 21:578-583, 1987.

89. Gerosa MA, Cappellotto P, Licata C, et al: Cerebral arteriovenous malformations in children (56 cases), *Childs Brain* 8:356-371, 1981.

90. Snead OC III, Acker JD, Morawetz R: Familial arteriovenous malformation, *Ann Neurol* 5:585-587, 1979.

91. Kadoya C, Momota Y, Ikegami Y, et al: Central nervous system arteriovenous malformations with hereditary hemorrhagic telangiectasia: Report of a family with three cases, *Surg Neurol* 42:234-239, 1994.

92. Putman CM, Chaloupka JC, Fulbright RK, et al: Exceptional multiplicity of cerebral arteriovenous malformations associated with hereditary hemorrhagic telangiectasia (Osler-Weber-Rendu syndrome), *AJNR Am J Neuroradiol* 17:1733-1742, 1996.

93. Willinsky RA, Lasjaunias P, terBrugge K, Burrows P: Multiple cerebral arteriovenous malformations (AVMs): Review of our experience from 203 patients with cerebral vascular lesions, *Neuroradiology* 32:207-210, 1990.

94. Meder JF, Nataf F, Delvat D, et al: [Radioanatomy of cerebral arteriovenous malformations], *Cancer Radiother* 2:173-179, 1998.

95. Cloft HJ, Joseph GJ, Dion JE: Risk of cerebral angiography in patients with subarachnoid hemorrhage, cerebral aneurysm, and arteriovenous malformation: a meta-analysis, *Stroke* 30:317-320, 1999.

96. Latchaw RE, Hu X, Ugurbil K, et al: Functional magnetic resonance imaging as a management tool for cerebral arteriovenous malformations, *Neurosurgery* 37:619-625, 1995.

97. Schlosser MJ, McCarthy G, Fulbright RK, et al: Cerebral vascular malformations adjacent to sensorimotor and visual cortex: Functional magnetic resonance imaging studies before and after therapeutic intervention, *Stroke* 28:1130-1137, 1997.

98. Zimmerman RS, Spetzler RF, Lee KS, et al: Cavernous malformations of the brain stem, *J Neurosurg* 75:32-39, 1991.

99. Mast H, Mohr JP, Thompson JL, et al: Transcranial Doppler ultrasonography in cerebral arteriovenous malformations: Diagnostic sensitivity and association of flow velocity with spontaneous hemorrhage and focal neurological deficit, *Stroke* 26:1024-1027, 1995.

99a. Laakso A, Dashti R, Juvela S, et al: Risk of hemorrhage in patients with untreated Spetzler-Martin grade IV and V arteriovenous malformations: A long-term follow-up study in 63 patients, *Neurosurgery* 2010 [Epub ahead of print].

100. Uggowitzer MM, Kugler C, Riccabona M, et al: Cerebral arteriovenous malformations: Diagnostic value of echo-enhanced transcranial Doppler sonography compared with angiography, *AJNR Am J Neuroradiol* 20:101-106, 1999.

101. Kilic T, Pamir MN, Budd S, et al: Grading and hemodynamic follow-up study of arteriovenous malformations with transcranial Doppler ultrasonography, *J Ultrasound Med* 17:729-738, 1998.

102. Reporting terminology for brain arteriovenous malformation clinical and radiographic features for use in clinical trials, *Stroke* 32:1430-1442, 2001.

103. Willinsky RA, Lasjaunias P, terBrugge K, Burrows P: Multiple cerebral arteriovenous malformations (AVMs): Review of our experience from 203 patients with cerebral vascular lesions, *Neuroradiology* 32:207-210, 1990.

104. U.S. Dept. of Health and Human Services, Public Health Service, Health Care Financing Administration. The International Classification of Diseases, 9th Revision, Clinical Modification: ICD-9. (Dept. of Health and Human Service Publication 91-1260.) 1991.

105. ICD-10: *International statistical classification of diseases and related health problems*, Geneva, 1992, World Health Organization.

106. Andoh T, Sakai N, Yamada H, et al: [Cerebellar AVM-clinical analysis of 14 cases], *No To Shinkei* 42:913-921, 1990.

107. Batjer HH, Devous MD Sr, Meyer YJ, et al: Cerebrovascular hemodynamics in arteriovenous malformation complicated by normal perfusion pressure breakthrough, *Neurosurgery* 22:503-509, 1988.

108. Kupersmith MJ, Vargas ME, Yashar A, et al: Occipital arteriovenous malformations: Visual disturbances and presentation, *Neurology* 46:953-957, 1996.

109. Symon L, Tacconi L, Mendoza N, Nakaji P: Arteriovenous malformations of the posterior fossa: A report on 28 cases and review of the literature, *Br J Neurosurg* 9:721-732, 1995.

110. Santoreneos S, Blumbergs PC, Jones NR: Choroid plexus arteriovenous malformations: A report of four pathologically proven cases and review of the literature, *Br J Neurosurg* 10:385-390, 1996.

111. Picard L, Miyachi S, Braun M, et al: Arteriovenous malformations of the corpus callosum: Radioanatomic study and effectiveness of intranidus embolization, *Neurol Med Chir (Tokyo)* 36:851-859, 1996.

112. Schlachter LB, Fleischer AS, Faria MA Jr, Tindall GT: Multifocal intracranial arteriovenous malformations, *Neurosurgery* 7:440-444, 1980.

113. Mackenzie I: The clinical presentation of cerebral angioma: A review of 50 cases, *Brain* 76:184, 1953.

114. Maspes PE, Marini G: Results of the surgical treatment of intracranial arteriovenous malformations, *Vasc Surg* 4:164-170, 1970.

115. Morello G, Borghi GP: Cerebral angiomas: A report of 154 personal cases and a comparison between the results of surgical excision and conservative management, *Acta Neurochir (Wien)* 28:135-155, 1973.

116. Stein BM, Wolpert SM: Arteriovenous malformations of the brain. I: Current concepts and treatment, *Arch Neurol* 37:1-5, 1980.

117. Trumpy JH, Eldevik P: Intracranial arteriovenous malformations: Conservative or surgical treatment? *Surg Neurol* 8:171-175, 1977.

118. Walter W: The influence of the type and localization of the angioma on the clinical syndrome. In Pia HW, Gleave JRW, Grote E, Zierski J, editors: *Cerebral angiomas: Advances in diagnosis and therapy*, New York, 1975, Springer-Verlag, p 271.

118a. Hernesniemi JA, Dashti R, Juvela S, et al: Natural history of brain arteriovenous malformations: A long-term follow-up study of risk of hemorrhage in 238 patients, *Neurosurgery* 63:823-829, 2008.

119. Stapf C, Mast H, Sciacca RR, et al: The New York Islands AVM Study: Detection rates for brain AVM and incident AVM hemorrhage, *Stroke* 32:368, 2001.

120. Marks MP, Lane B, Steinberg GK, Chang PJ: Hemorrhage in intracerebral arteriovenous malformations: Angiographic determinants, *Radiology* 176:807-813, 1990.

121. Duong DH, Young WL, Vang MC, et al: Feeding artery pressure and venous drainage pattern are primary determinants of hemorrhage from cerebral arteriovenous malformations, *Stroke* 29:1167-1176, 1998.

122. Crawford JV, Russell DS: Cryptic arteriovenous and venous hamartomas of the brain, *J Neurol Neurosurg Psychiatry* 19:1, 1956.

123. Dandy WE: Arteriovenous aneurysm of the brain, *Arch Surg (Chicago)* 17:190, 1928.

124. Forster DM, Steiner L, Hakanson S: Arteriovenous malformations of the brain: A long-term clinical study, *J Neurosurg* 37:562-570, 1972.

125. Fox JL: Embolization of an arteriovenous malformation of the brain stem, *Surg Neurol* 8:7, 1977.

126. Henderson WR, Gomez RD: Natural history of cerebral angiomas, *Br Med J* 4:571-574, 1967.

127. Kusske JA, Kelly WA: Embolization and reduction of the "steal" syndrome in cerebral arteriovenous malformations, *J Neurosurg* 40:313-321, 1974.

128. Young WL, Prohovnik I, Ornstein E, et al: The effect of arteriovenous malformation resection on cerebrovascular reactivity to carbon dioxide, *Neurosurgery* 27:257-266, 1990.

129. Troupp H, Marttila I, Halonen V: Arteriovenous malformations of the brain: Prognosis without operation, *Acta Neurochir* 22:125-128, 1970.

130. Höök OJ: Intracranial arteriovenous aneurysms: A follow-up study with particular attention to their growth, *Arch Neurol Psychiatry* 80:39, 1958.

131. Krayenbühl H, Siebenmann R: Small vascular malformations as a cause of primary intracerebral hemorrhage, *J Neurosurg* 22:7, 1965.

132. Mohr JP, Caplan LR, Melski JW, et al: The Harvard Cooperative Stroke Registry: A prospective registry, *Neurology* 28:754-762, 1978.

133. Paterson JH, McKissock W: A clinical survey of intracranial angiomas with special reference to their mode of progression and surgical treatment: A report of 110 cases, *Brain* 79:233, 1956.

134. Lanzino G, Jensen ME, Cappelletto B, Kassell NF: Arteriovenous malformations that rupture during pregnancy: A management dilemma, *Acta Neurochir (Wien)* 126:102-106, 1994.

135. Horton JC, Chambers WA, Lyons SL, et al: Pregnancy and the risk of hemorrhage from cerebral arteriovenous malformations, *Neurosurgery* 27:867-871, 1990.

136. Kelly DL Jr, Alexander E Jr, Davis CH Jr, Maynard DC: Intracranial arteriovenous malformations: Clinical review and evaluation of brain scans, *J Neurosurg* 31:422-428, 1969.

137. Guidetti B, Delitala A: Intracranial arteriovenous malformations: Conservative and surgical treatment, *J Neurosurg* 53:149-152, 1980.

138. Garrido E, Stein B: Removal of an arteriovenous malformation from the basal ganglion, *J Neurol Neurosurg Psychiatry* 41: 992-995, 1978.

139. Hier DB, Davis KR, Richardson EP Jr, Mohr JP: Hypertensive putaminal hemorrhage, *Ann Neurol* 1:152-159, 1977.

140. Wilson CDJ: Microsurgical treatment of intracranial vascular malformations, *J Neurosurg* 51:446, 1979.

141. McCormick WF, Nofzinger JD: "Cryptic" vascular malformations of the central nervous system, *J Neurosurg* 24:865-875, 1966.

142. Pia HW, Gleave JRW, Grote E, et al: *Cerebral angiomas: Advances in diagnosis and therapy*, New York, 1975, Springer-Verlag, p 285.

143. Hosobuchi Y, Fabricant J, Lyman J: Stereotactic heavy-particle irradiation of intracranial arteriovenous malformations, *Appl Neurophysiol* 50:248-252, 1987.

144. Pertuiset B, Sichez JP, Philippon J: Mortalité et morbidité après exérèse chirurgicale totale de 162 malformations artérioveneuses intracraniennes, *Rev Neurol* 135:319-329, 1979.

145. Ruff RM, Arbit E: Aphemia resulting from a left frontal hematoma, *Neurology* 31:353, 1981.

146. Kase CS, Williams JP, Wyatt DA, Mohr JP: Lobar intracerebral hematomas: Clinical and CT analysis of 22 cases, *Neurology* 32:1146-1150, 1982.

147. Stein R, Kase CS, Hier DB, et al: Caudate hemorrhage, *Neurology* 34:1549, 1984.

148. Hartmann A, Mast H, Mohr JP, et al: Morbidity of intracranial hemorrhage in patients with cerebral arteriovenous malformation, *Stroke* 29:931-934, 1998.

149. Choi JH, Mast H, Sciacca RR, et al: Clinical outcome after first and recurrent hemorrhage in patients with untreated brain arteriovenous malformation, *Stroke* 37:1243-1247, 2006 (Epub).

150. Mast H, Young WL, Koennecke HC, et al: Risk of spontaneous haemorrhage after diagnosis of cerebral arteriovenous malformation, *Lancet* 350:1065-1068, 1997.

151. Krayenbühl H, Yasargil G: *L'Aneurismo cerebral.* (Documenta Geigy, Series Chirurgica 4.) Basel, Geigy, 1959.

152. Graf CJ, Perret GE, Torner JC: Bleeding from cerebral arteriovenous malformations as part of their natural history, *J Neurosurg* 58:331-337, 1983.

153. Hayashi S, Arimoto T, Itakura T, et al: The association of intracranial aneurysms and arteriovenous malformation of the brain: Case report, *J Neurosurg* 55:971-975, 1981.

154. Lazar ML, Watts CC, Kilgore B, Clark K: Cerebral angiography during operation for intracranial aneurysms and arteriovenous malformations: Technical note, *J Neurosurg* 34:706-708, 1971.

155. Marks MP, Lane B, Steinberg GK, Chang PJ: Hemorrhage in intracerebral arteriovenous malformations: Angiographic determinants, *Radiology* 176:807-813, 1990.

156. Batjer HH, Devous MD Sr, Seibert GB, et al: Intracranial arteriovenous malformation: Relationships between clinical and radiographic factors and ipsilateral steal severity, *Neurosurgery* 23:322-328, 1988.

157. Lasjaunias P, Piske R, terBrugge K, Willinsky R: Cerebral arteriovenous malformations (C. AVM) and associated arterial aneurysms (AA). Analysis of 101 C. AVM cases, with 37 AA in 23 patients, *Acta Neurochir (Wien)* 91:29-36, 1988.

158. Turjman F, Massoud TF, Vinuela F, et al: Correlation of the angioarchitectural features of cerebral arteriovenous malformations with clinical presentation of hemorrhage, *Neurosurgery* 37:856-860, 1995.

159. Westphal M, Grzyska U: Clinical significance of pedicle aneurysms on feeding vessels, especially those located in infratentorial arteriovenous malformations, *J Neurosurg* 92:995-1001, 2000.

160. Redekop G, terBrugge K, Montanera W, Willinsky R: Arterial aneurysms associated with cerebral arteriovenous malformations: Classification, incidence, and risk of hemorrhage, *J Neurosurg* 89:539-546, 1998.

161. Brown RD Jr, Wiebers DO, Forbes GS: Unruptured intracranial aneurysms and arteriovenous malformations: Frequency of intracranial hemorrhage and relationship of lesions, *J Neurosurg* 73:859-863, 1990.

162. Langer DJ, Lasner TM, Hurst RW, et al: Hypertension, small size, and deep venous drainage are associated with risk of hemorrhagic presentation of cerebral arteriovenous malformations, *Neurosurgery* 42:481-486, 1998.

163. Nataf F, Meder JF, Roux FX, et al: Angioarchitecture associated with haemorrhage in cerebral arteriovenous malformations: A prognostic statistical model, *Neuroradiology* 39:52-58, 1997.

164. Mansmann U, Meisel J, Brock M, et al: Factors associated with intracranial hemorrhage in cases of cerebral arteriovenous malformation, *Neurosurgery* 46:272-279, 2000.

165. Stefani MA, Porter PJ, terBrugge KG, et al: Angioarchitectural factors present in brain arteriovenous malformations associated with hemorrhagic presentation, *Stroke* 33:920-924, 2002.

166. Brown RD Jr, Wiebers DO, Torner JC, O'Fallon WM: Incidence and prevalence of intracranial vascular malformations in Olmsted County, Minnesota, 1965 to 1992, *Neurology* 46:949-952, 1996.

167. Mast H, Mohr JP, Osipov A, et al: 'Steal' is an unestablished mechanism for the clinical presentation of cerebral arteriovenous malformations, *Stroke* 26:1215-1220, 1995.

168. Osipov A, Koennecke HC, Hartmann A, et al: Seizures in cerebral arteriovenous malformations: Type, clinical course, and medical management, *Interv Neuroradiol* 3:37-41, 1997.

169. Leblanc R, Feindel W, Ethier R: Epilepsy from cerebral arteriovenous malformations, *Can J Neurol Sci* 10:91-95, 1983.

170. Leblanc E, Meyer E, Zatorre R, et al: Functional PET scanning in the preoperative assessment of cerebral arteriovenous malformations, *Stereotact Funct Neurosurg* 65:60-64, 1995.

171. Ozer MN, Sencer W, Block J: A clinical study of cerebral vascular malformations: The significance of migraine, *J Mt Sinai Hosp* 31:403, 1964.

172. Olivecrona H, Ladenheim J: *Congenital arteriovenous aneurysms of the carotid and vertebral systems*, Berlin, 1957, Springer-Verlag.

173. Troost BT, Newton TH: Occipital lobe arteriovenous malformations: Clinical and radiologic features in 26 cases with comments on differentiation from migraine, *Arch Ophthalmol* 93:250-256, 1975.

174. Turjman F, Massoud TF, Sayre JW, et al: Epilepsy associated with cerebral arteriovenous malformations: A multivariate analysis of angioarchitectural characteristics, *AJNR Am J Neuroradiol* 16:345-350, 1995.

175. Graeb DA, Dolman CL: Radiological and pathological aspects of dural arteriovenous fistulas: Case report, *J Neurosurg* 64:962-967, 1986.

176. Stapf C, Mohr JP, Sciacca RR, et al: Incident hemorrhage risk of brain arteriovenous malformations located in the arterial borderzones, *Stroke* 31:2365-2368, 2000.

177. Turjman F, Massoud TF, Sayre JW, et al: Epilepsy associated with cerebral arteriovenous malformations: A multivariate analysis of angioarchitectural characteristics, *AJNR Am J Neuroradiol* 16:345-350, 1995.

178. Kilpatrick CJ, Davis SM, Tress BM, et al: Epileptic seizures in acute stroke, *Arch Neurol* 47:157-160, 1990.

179. Mackenzie I: The clinical presentation of cerebral angioma: A review of 50 cases, *Brain* 76:184, 1953.

180. Frishberg BM: Neuroimaging in presumed primary headache disorders, *Semin Neurol* 17:373–382, 1997.

181. Ennoksson P, Bynke H: Visual field defects in arteriovenous aneurysms of the brain, *Acta Ophthalmol* 36:586, 1958.

182. Lees F: The migrainous symptoms of cerebral angiomata, *J Neurol Neurosurg Psychiatry* 25:45, 1962.

183. Northfield DWC: Angiomatous malformations of the brain, *Guys Hosp Rep* 90:149, 1940.

184. Evans RW: Diagnostic testing for the evaluation of headaches, *Neurol Clin* 14:1, 1996.

185. Mast H, Mohr JP, Osipov A, et al: 'Steal' is an unestablished mechanism for the clinical presentation of cerebral arteriovenous malformations, *Stroke* 26:1215–1220, 1995.

186. Carter LP, Gumerlock MK: Steal and cerebral arteriovenous malformations, *Stroke* 26:2371–2372, 1995.

187. Carter LP, Gumerlock MK: Steal and cerebral arteriovenous malformations, *Stroke* 26:2371–2372, 1995.

188. Nornes H, Grip A: Hemodynamic aspects of cerebral arteriovenous malformations, *J Neurosurg* 53:456–464, 1980.

189. Young WL, Pile-Spellman J, Prohovnik I, et al: Evidence for adaptive autoregulatory displacement in hypotensive cortical territories adjacent to arteriovenous malformations. Columbia University AVM Study Project, *Neurosurgery* 34:601–610, 1994.

190. Miyasaka Y, Kurata A, Tanaka R, et al: Mass effect caused by clinically unruptured cerebral arteriovenous malformations, *Neurosurgery* 41:1060–1063, 1997.

190a. Choi JH, Mast H, Hartmann A, et al: Clinical and morphologic determinants of focal neurological deficits in patients with unruptured brain arteriovenous malformations, *J Neurol Sci* 287:126-130, 2009.

191. Feindel W, Yamamoto YL, Hodge CP: Red cerebral veins as an index of cerebral steal, *Scand J Clin Lab Invest Suppl*, 102: X:C, 1968.

192. Norlen G: Arteriovenous aneurysms of the brain: Report of ten cases of total removal of the lesion, *J Neurosurg* 6:475, 1949.

193. Numaguchi Y, Kitamura K, Fukui M, et al: Intracranial venous angiomas, *Surg Neurol* 18:193–202, 1982.

194. Shenkin HA, Spitz EB, Grant FC, Kety SS: Physiologic studies of arteriovenous anomalies of the brain, *J Neurosurg* 5:165, 1948.

195. Waltimo O: The relationship of size, density and localization of intracranial arteriovenous malformations to the type of initial symptom, *J Neurol Sci* 19:13–19, 1973.

196. Nornes H, Grip A: Hemodynamic aspects of cerebral arteriovenous malformations, *J Neurosurg* 53:456–464, 1980.

197. Fogarty-Mack P, Pile-Spellman J, Hacein-Bey L, et al: The effect of arteriovenous malformations on the distribution of intracerebral arterial pressures, *AJNR Am J Neuroradiol* 17:1443–1449, 1996.

198. Tarr RW, Johnson DW, Rutigliano M, et al: Use of acetazolamide-challenge xenon CT in the assessment of cerebral blood flow dynamics in patients with arteriovenous malformations, *AJNR Am J Neuroradiol* 11:441–448, 1990.

199. Spetzler RF, Wilson CB: Enlargement of an AVM documented by angiography: Case report, *J Neurosurg* 43:767, 1975.

200. Spetzler RF, Wilson CB, Weinstein P: Normal perfusion pressure breakthrough theory, *Clin Neurosurg* 25:651, 1978.

201. Kvam DA, Michelsen WJ, Quest DO: Intracerebral hemorrhage as a complication of artificial embolization, *Neurosurgery* 7:491–494, 1980.

202. Morgan MK, Johnston I, Besser M, Baines D: Cerebral arteriovenous malformations, steal, and the hypertensive breakthrough threshold: An experimental study in rats, *J Neurosurg* 66:563–567, 1987.

203. Mullan S, Brown FD, Patronas NJ: Hyperemic and ischemic problems of surgical treatment of arteriovenous malformations, *J Neurosurg* 51:757–764, 1979.

204. Muraszko K, Wang HH, Pelton G, Stein BM: A study of the reactivity of feeding vessels to arteriovenous malformations: Correlation with clinical outcome, *Neurosurgery* 26:190–199, 1990.

205. Young WL, Pile-Spellman J, Prohovnik I, et al: Evidence for adaptive autoregulatory displacement in hypotensive cortical territories adjacent to arteriovenous malformations. Columbia University AVM Study Project, *Neurosurgery* 34:601–610, 1994.

206. Hacein-Bey L, Nour R, Pile-Spellman J, et al: Adaptive changes of autoregulation in chronic cerebral hypotension with arteriovenous malformations: An acetazolamide-enhanced single-photon emission CT study, *AJNR Am J Neuroradiol* 16:1865–1874, 1995.

207. Lasjaunias P, Chiu M, ter Brugge K, et al: Neurological manifestations of intracranial dural arteriovenous malformations, *J Neurosurg* 64:724–730, 1986.

208. Svien HJ, McRae JA: Arteriovenous anomalies of the brain: Fate of patients not having definitive surgery, *J Neurosurg* 23:23–28, 1965.

209. Cognard C, Gobin YP, Pierot L, et al: Cerebral dural arteriovenous fistulas: Clinical and angiographic correlation with a revised classification of venous drainage, *Radiology* 194:671–680, 1995.

210. Al-Shahi R, Bhattacharya JJ, Currie DG, et al: Vascular Malformation Study Collaborators. Prospective, population-based detection of intracranial vascular malformations in adults: The Scottish Intracranial Vascular Malformation Study (SIVMS), *Stroke* 34:1163–1169, 2003.

211. Theaudin M, Saint-Maurice JP, Chapot R, et al: Diagnosis and treatment of dural carotid-cavernous fistulas: A consecutive series of 27 patients, *J Neurol Neurosurg Psychiatry* 78:174–179, 2007.

212. McCormick WF, Hardman JM, Boulter TR: Vascular malformations ("angiomas") of the brain, with special reference to those occurring in the posterior fossa, *J Neurosurg* 28:241–251, 1968.

213. Farrell DF, Forno LS: Symptomatic capillary telangiectasis of the brainstem without hemorrhage: Report of an unusual case, *Neurology* 20:341–346, 1970.

214. Johnson DW, Berg JN, Gallione CJ, et al: A second locus for hereditary hemorrhagic telangiectasia maps to chromosome 12, *Genome Res* 5:21–28, 1995.

215. Jessurun GA, Kamphuis DJ, van der Zande FH, Nossent JC: Cerebral arteriovenous malformations in The Netherlands Antilles. High prevalence of hereditary hemorrhagic telangiectasia-related single and multiple cerebral arteriovenous malformations, *Clin Neurol Neurosurg* 95:193–198, 1993.

216. Otten P, Pizzolato GP, Rilliet B, Berney J: [131 cases of cavernous angioma (cavernomas) of the CNS, discovered by retrospective analysis of 24,535 autopsies] 1, *Neurochirurgie* 35:31–82, 1989.

217. Hashim AS, Asakura T, Koichi U, et al: Angiographically occult arteriovenous malformations, *Surg Neurol* 23:431–439, 1985.

218. Tsitsopoulos P, Andrew J, Harrison MJ: Occult cerebral arteriovenous malformations, *J Neurol Neurosurg Psychiatry* 50:218–220, 1987.

219. Voigt K, Yasargil MG: Cerebral cavernous haemangiomas or cavernomas: Incidence, pathology, localization, diagnosis, clinical features and treatment. Review of the literature and report of an unusual case, *Neurochirurgia (Stuttg)* 19:59–68, 1976.

220. Labauge P, Denier C, Bergametti F, Tournier-Lasserve E: *Lancet Neurol* 6:237–244, 2007.

221. Rigamonti D, Spetzler RF, Medina M, et al: Cerebral venous malformations, *J Neurosurg* 73:560–564, 1990.

222. Kattapong VJ, Hart BL, Davis LE: Familial cerebral cavernous angiomas: Clinical and radiologic studies, *Neurology* 45:492–497, 1995.

223. Steiger HJ, Tew JM Jr: Hemorrhage and epilepsy in cryptic cerebrovascular malformations, *Arch Neurol* 41:722–724, 1984.

224. Fierstien SB, Pribram HW, Hieshima G: Angiography and computed tomography in the evaluation of cerebral venous malformations, *Neuroradiology* 17:137–148, 1979.

225. Giombini S, Morello G: Cavernous angiomas of the brain: Account of fourteen personal cases and review of the literature, *Acta Neurochir (Wien)* 40:61–82, 1978.

226. Pool JL, Potts DG: *Aneurysms and arteriovenous anomalies of the brain: Diagnosis and treatment*, New York, 1965, Harper & Row, p 463.

227. Saito Y, Kobayashi N: Cerebral venous angiomas: Clinical evaluation and possible etiology, *Radiology* 139:87–94, 1981.

228. Craig HD, Gunel M, Cepeda O, et al: Multilocus linkage identifies two new loci for a mendelian form of stroke, cerebral cavernous malformation, at 7p15-13 and 3q25.2-27, *Hum Mol Genet* 7:1851–1858, 1998.

229. Labauge P, Denier C, Bergametti F, Tournier-Lasserve E: *Lancet Neurol* 6:237–244, 2007.

230. Humphreys RP, Hoffman HJ, Drake JM, Rutka JT: Choices in the 1990s for the management of pediatric cerebral arteriovenous malformations, *Pediatr Neurosurg* 25:277–285, 1996.

231. Al-Shahi Salman R, Berg MJ, Morrison L, Awad IA: Hemorrhage from cavernous malformations of the brain: Definition and reporting standards, *Stroke* 40:3222–3230, 2008.

232. Viswanathan A, Chabriat H: Cerebral microhemorrhage, *Stroke* 37:550-555, 2006.

233. Clatterbuck RE, Moriarity JL, Elmaci I, Lee RR, Breiter SN, Rigamonti D: Dynamic nature of cavernous malformations: A prospective magnetic resonance imaging study with volumetric analysis, *J Neurosurgery* 93:981-986, 2000.

234. Labauge P, Brunerau L, Laberge S, Houtteville JP: Prospective follow-up of 33 asymptomatic patients with familial cerebral cavernous malformations, *Neurology* 57:1825-1828, 2001.

235. Lehnhardt FG, von Smekal U, Rückriem B, et al: Value of gradient-echo magnetic resonance imaging in the diagnosis of familial cerebral cavernous malformation, *Arch Neurol* 62:653-658, 2005.

236. Labauge P, Denier C, Bergametti F, Tournier-Lasserve E: Genetics of cavernous angiomas. *Lancet Neurol* 6:237-244, 2007.

237. Mathiesen T, Edner G, Kihlström L: Deep and brainstem cavernomas: A consecutive 8-year series, *J Neurosurgery* 99:31-37, 2003.

238. Pollock BE, Garces YI, Stafford SL, Foote RL, Schomberg PJ, Link MJ: Stereotactic radiosurgery for cavernous malformations, *J Neurosurg* 93:987-991, 2000.

239. Rabinov JD: Diagnostic imaging of angiographically occult vascular malformations 1, *Neurosurg Clin North Am* 10:419-432, 1999.

240. Masuda J, Ogata J, Yutani C: Smooth muscle cell proliferation and localization of macrophages and T cells in the occlusive intracranial major arteries in moyamoya disease, *Stroke* 24:1960-1967, 1993.

241. Nishimoto A, Takeuchi S: Abnormal cerebrovascular network related to the internal carotid arteries, *J Neurosurg* 29:255, 1968.

242. Goto Y, Yonekawa Y: Worldwide distribution of moyamoya disease, *Neurol Med Chir* 32:883-886, 1992.

243. Kuroda S, Ishikawa T, Houkin K, Nanba R, Hokari M, Iwasaki Y: Incidence and clinical features of disease progression in adult moyamoya disease, *Stroke* 36:2148-2153, 2005.

244. Uchino K, Johnston CS, Becker KJ, Tirschwell DL: Moyamoya disease in Washington State and California, *Neurology* 65:956-958, 2005.

245. Kuriyama S, Kusaka Y, Fujimura M, et al: Prevalence and clinico-epidemiological features of moyamoya disease in Japan. Findings from a nationwide epidemiological survey, *Stroke* 39:27-42, 2008.

246. Kuriyama S, Kusaka Y, Fujimura M, et al: Prevalence and clinicoepidemiological features of moyamoya disease in Japan. Findings from a nationwide epidemiological survey, *Stroke* 39:27-42, 2008.

247. Merkel KH, Ginsberg PL, Parker JC Jr, Post MJ: Cerebrovascular disease in sickle cell anemia: A clinical, pathological and radiological correlation, *Stroke* 9:45-52, 1978.

248. Ullrich NJ, Robertson R, Kinnamon DD, et al: Moyamoya following cranial irradiation for primary brain tumors in children, *Neurology* 68:932-938, 2007.

249. Fukui M, Members of the Research Committee on Spontaneous Occlusion of the Circle of Willis (Moyamoya Disease) of the Ministry of Health and Welfare, Japan. Guidelines for the diagnosis and treatment of spontaneous occlusion of the circle of Willis ('moyamoya' disease), *Clin Neurol Neurosurg* 99(Suppl 2):S238-S240, 1997.

250. Enam SA, Malik GM: Association of cerebral arteriovenous malformations and spontaneous occlusion of major feeding arteries: Clinical and therapeutic implications, *Neurosurgery* 45:1105-1111, 1999.

251. Pile-Spellman JM, Baker KF, Liszczak TM, et al: High-flow angiopathy: Cerebral blood vessel changes in experimental chronic arteriovenous fistula, *AJNR Am J Neuroradiol* 7:811-815, 1986.

252. Stapf C, Mohr JP, Choi JH, et al: Invasive treatment of unruptured brain arteriovenous malformations is experimental therapy, *Curr Opin Neurol* 19:63-68, 2006.

253. Mohr JP, Moskowitz AJ, Stapf C, et al: The ARUBA trial: Current status, future hopes, *Stroke* 241:e537-e540, 2010 (Epub).

32 Spinal Cord Ischemia

JOSHUA Z. WILLEY, HENRY J.M. BARNETT, J.P. MOHR

Spinal cord infarction, although rare, remains incompletely studied outside the cardiothoracic and vascular surgery literature. Its incidence is unknown, and no large epidemiologic study has been conducted. The increase in accidental production of cord infarct by modern cardiovascular surgery and the advances in imaging techniques, including computed tomography (CT) and magnetic resonance imaging (MRI), have led to more documentation.[1-3] One hopes that the better visualization of the spinal cord and improvements in the accurate localization, diagnosis, and management of vascular lesions may eventually improve its management.[4-6]

Historical Aspects

Blackwood,[7] reviewing the records of 3737 autopsies conducted over 50 years, found only five cases of spinal cord infarction. Surprisingly, no cases were due to atherosclerosis or hypertensive vascular disease. Slager and Webb,[8] however, found microinfarcts of the spinal cord in 3% of 200 consecutive autopsies performed in asymptomatic patients. Sandson and Friedman[9] described eight cases of spinal cord infarction, representing roughly 1.2% of all admissions for stroke in their center. Despite numerous well-documented case reports of spinal cord infarction, misconceptions still exist regarding its pathogenesis and clinical course.

Studies in animals reported in the distant past showed that aortic clamping led to paralysis. Clinically, paraparesis as a result of aortic obstruction was recognized at the end of the 19th century.[10] Bastian[11] in 1882 suggested that spinal cord softening may be the result of vascular occlusion; however, it was not until 1904 that Preobrashenski[12] described the syndrome of anterior spinal artery infarct.

Blood Supply to the Spinal Cord

The basic pattern of the arterial blood supply to the spinal cord consists of three longitudinal vessels that arise rostrally from the cervical region and descend as far as the conus medullaris, plus numerous feeder arteries and radicular vessels. Anastomoses between the descending and segmentally oriented vessels occur on the surface of the spinal cord, leading to the formation of a rich vascular plexus from which medullary vessels penetrate both white and gray matter. These vessels are end arteries and do not anastomose further.[2]

Longitudinal Arteries

There are three longitudinal arteries, the anterior spinal artery and the two posterior spinal arteries.

The *anterior spinal artery* forms rostrally from the union of the two anterior spinal branches of each vertebral artery at the level of the foramen magnum. From this site, it descends to the tip of the conus medullaris. It lies ventrally in relation to the anterior median sulcus (Fig. 32-1).[13,14] The caliber of the artery is largest in the lumbosacral region and smallest in the thoracic region, which has been considered a vulnerable zone for ischemia. The anterior spinal artery is reinforced by successive contributions of feeder arterial branches, which enter the artery in a caudal direction and supply the spinal cord below the point of entry. At the conus medullaris and along the filum terminale, the anterior spinal artery communicates through anastomotic branches with the posterior spinal arteries.[13,14]

The two *posterior spinal arteries* originate directly from the vertebral arteries (Fig. 32-2). Each vessel descends on the posterior surface of the spinal cord along the posterolateral sulcus. The arteries are commonly found to be discontinuous, and sometimes one artery moves across to supply the other side.[14] Throughout its course, each posterior spinal artery gives off branches that penetrate the cord to supply the posterior columns, dorsal gray matter, and superficial dorsal aspect of the lateral columns.

Radicular Tributary Arteries

Thirty-one pairs of radicular arteries penetrate the spinal canal through the intervertebral foramina. Usually seven or eight of these 62 radicular branches contribute to the vascularization of the spinal cord and define three major spinal arterial territories—cervicothoracic, midthoracic, and thoracolumbar.[5,15]

The *cervicothoracic* territory consists of the cervical spinal cord, its brachial plexus enlargement, and the first two or three thoracic segments. This territory is richly supplied by the anterior spinal artery arising from the intracranial vertebral arteries, the midcervical radicular branches of the vertebral artery, and the branches of the costocervical trunk. In the *midthoracic* territory, the radicular arteries supplying the middle and lower thoracic cord are less prominent.[16] This territory is usually supplied by a radicular branch arising at about the T7 level; it comprises the fourth to eighth segments of the thoracic cord.

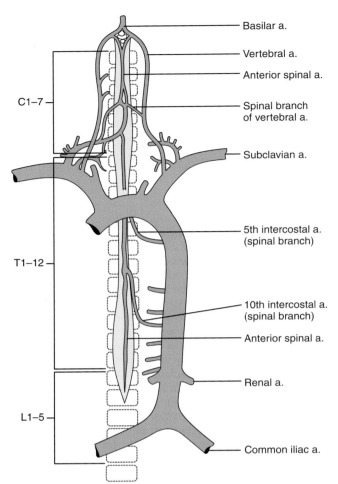

Figure 32-1 Extrinsic vascular supply of the spinal cord. Schematic representation of the anterior spinal artery. (Adapted from Gray H: Development and gross anatomy of the human body. In Clemente CD, editor: *Anatomy of the human body,* ed 30 (American ed), Philadelphia, 1984, Lea & Febiger; and Benavente OR, Barnett HJM: Spinal cord infarction. In Carter LP, Spetzler RF, editors: *Neurovascular surgery,* New York, 1995, McGraw-Hill, p 1229.)

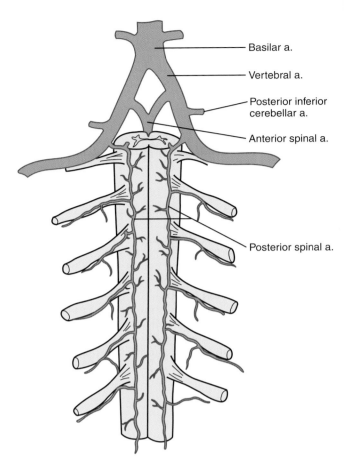

Figure 32-2 Extrinsic vascular supply of the spinal cord. Schematic representation of the posterior spinal arteries. (Adapted from Gray H: Development and gross anatomy of the human body. In Clemente CD, editor: *Anatomy of the human body,* ed 30 (American ed), Philadelphia, 1984, Lea & Febiger; and Benavente OR, Barnett HJM: Spinal cord infarction. In Carter LP, Spetzler RF, editors: *Neurovascular surgery,* New York, 1995, McGraw-Hill, p 1229.)

In addition to the lower thoracic segments, the *thoracolumbar* territory contains the lumbar enlargement, which relates to the lumbosacral plexus. This segment receives its blood supply from a single artery, called the artery of Adamkiewicz. Although the artery of Adamkiewicz is well-known by name, the site of origin varies widely from the left 9th, 10th, 11th, or 12th intercostal artery, and the artery itself varies considerably in size.[15] The artery of Adamkiewicz may be fed by collateral segmental arteries in the setting of chronic occlusive disease. These collaterals may have implications for the development of spinal cord infarction in the setting or aortic surgery. The collaterals may be visualized by magnetic resonance angiography.[17] This irregular augmentation of the anterior spinal artery system results in watershed areas that may be vulnerable to hypoperfusion, most marked in the thoracic area.[16] The radicular tributaries may be subdivided into two groups according to their origin. The first group consists of those derived from the subclavian artery; the second group is supplied directly from the aorta. At the level of the second thoracic spinal cord segment, the arterial supply changes from a subclavian supply to a direct aortic supply.[18]

Intrinsic Blood Supply of the Cord

When the radicular arteries reach the surface of the spinal cord, they form two distinct systems of intrinsic blood supply (Figs. 32-3 and 32-4). The first is the posterolateral and peripheral plexus formed by the two posterior spinal arteries, which are interconnected by anastomotic channels.[19] This plexus, a centripetal vascular territory, is formed by radial arteries directed inward as branches from the coronal arterial plexus surrounding the spinal cord. It supplies from one third to one half of the outer rim of the cord, including the lateral and ventral spinothalamic tracts. These radial arteries are longer in the posterior white columns than in the anterior and lateral columns. This difference in length could explain the size and localization of pathologic changes related to vascular disorders.[14]

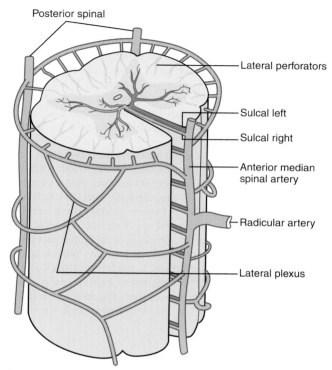

Figure 32-3 Intrinsic vascular supply of the cord. The central sulcal artery is supplied from the anterior median artery, and the lateral artery from the anterior and posterior spinal arteries, forming the vasa corona. (From Buchan AM, Barnett HJM: Infarction of the spinal cord. *J Neurosurg* 35:253, 1971.)

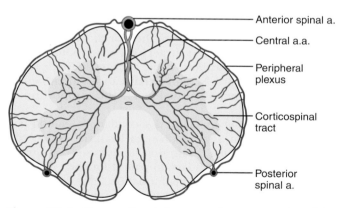

Figure 32-4 Cross-sectional diagrammatic representation of the territories of the anterior and posterior spinal arteries. (From Mawad ME, Rivera V, Crawford S, et al: Spinal cord ischemia after resection of the thoracoabdominal aortic aneurysms: MR findings in 24 patients. *AJNR Am J Neuroradiol* 155:987, 1990.)

The second arterial system to the spinal cord is a centrifugal system formed by the sulcal arteries, which arise from the anterior spinal artery and pass backward in the anterior medial sulcus. These arteries enter the gray commissure and, turning left or right, supply the gray matter and adjacent white matter. The corticospinal tract is nourished by both arterial systems.[14]

Both arterial systems are interconnected by a capillary anastomosis in the spinal cord. The number of sulcal arteries supplying each segment of the spinal cord varies

with the region of the cord. They are most numerous in the thoracolumbar segment and least numerous in the upper thoracic segment.[20]

Venous System

Two intrinsic venous systems and one extrinsic venous system drain the spinal cord.[15,19-22]

Intrinsic Venous System

The anterior median group (central veins) collects blood from both halves of the medial aspects of the anterior horns, anterior gray commissure, and white matter of the anterior funiculus. The central veins also drain adjacent levels above and below through intersegmental anastomoses. They commonly anastomose with other veins within the fissure. Finally, the central veins empty into the anterior median spinal vein.

The other group consists of radial veins that arise from capillaries near the periphery of the gray matter or from the white matter. They are radially oriented and directed outward toward the surface of the spinal cord, where they join the superficial plexus of veins surrounding the cord and form a venous vasa corona or corona plexus. These veins are more numerous in the white matter of the posterior and lateral funiculi, but they are also found in the anterior funiculus. The radial veins are more prominent at certain cervical and thoracic levels; they drain laterally from the gray matter of the lateral horns as well as posteriorly from the dorsal nucleus of Clarke.

Extrinsic Venous System

The extrinsic venous system is very conspicuous on the posterior aspect of the spinal cord and is especially prominent in the lumbosacral region. There is a rich anastomosis between the large venous trunks. The median posterior spinal vein descends in the region of the posterior median septum. This vessel drains blood from the posterior white columns and the end of the posterior horns.

The anterior spinal vein accompanies the anterior spinal artery and receives the sulcal veins. Both the anterior spinal veins and the median posterior spinal vein empty into the radicular veins, which accompany the anterior or posterior spinal roots. These radicular veins drain into the paravertebral and intervertebral plexuses, and then into the azygos and pelvic venous systems.[14] The absence of venous valves may allow infections in the abdominal cavity to spread to the spinal cord. Their absence also renders the spinal veins susceptible to Valsalva maneuvers, increasing the intraabdominal pressure.

Physiology of Spinal Cord Blood Flow

The regulation of spinal cord blood flow is similar to that of brain blood flow. The spinal cord blood vessels are affected by changes in P_{CO_2} and hypoxia. Hypercapnia increases blood flow. Autoregulation keeps the regional as well as the total spinal cord blood flow constant. As in the brain, the blood flow requirement and metabolic rate are high in the gray matter.[23,24]

The total cerebral blood flow of the human brain is 50 mL/min/100 g. Spinal cord flow varies, depending on the species and the area of cord studied.[24,25] In monkeys, total flow in cervical, upper trunk, and lumbar areas is 15, 10, and 20 mL/min/100 g, respectively.[25] The intrinsic blood supply of the cord is directly proportional to the area of gray matter, and this is most abundant in the thoracolumbar segment.[26] Consequently, this segment may be more vulnerable to hypoperfusion. In case series of spinal cord infarction, this location remains the most commonly involved, and the cervical cord is the second most commonly affected location in up to 25% of patients.[27]

Another important consideration is that the cord is contained within the spinal canal, which has fixed dimensions. Any changes in contents occur at the expense of cerebrospinal fluid (CSF), blood, or spinal tissue; a rise in intraspinal canal pressure causes a slowing of the spinal cord blood flow and consequent hypoxia.[18]

The blood flow of the spinal cord has a different pattern in the anterior and posterior systems. Flow in the anterior spinal artery is mainly caudal and unidirectional. Infarcts are most likely to be located in the anterior spinal artery distribution.[28] Flow in the posterior spinal arteries is bidirectional, caudal in the cervical and thoracic regions, and rostral in the lumbosacral region.[14]

Pathology of Spinal Cord Infarction

Spinal cord infarction results from interference with the circulation of the cord secondary to a generalized or localized reduction of blood flow. The locations of disease or obstruction that may lead to ischemia of the cord are the aorta, vertebral arteries, intercostal and lumbar arteries, radicular tributary arteries, anterior and posterior spinal arteries, small spinal vessels, and veins.[14] Heart disease leading to hypoperfusion and blood disorders may also interfere with the blood supply to the cord.[18]

The cellular events in spinal cord infarction are similar to those seen in cerebral infarction. An initial ischemic and inflammatory cascade is triggered,[29] including *N*-methyl-D-aspartate–mediated excitotoxic neuronal injury.[30] Subsequent cell death, delayed up to 2 days after the initial ischemic injury, occurs owing to apoptic cell death via activation of caspases. The delay up to 2 days after the initial injury may, in turn, be mediated after the failure of initial endogenous neuroprotective mechanisms.[31] The presence of heat shock proteins, which can be observed in a range of ischemic injuries, has been noted in CSF samples of patients undergoing aortic surgery with subsequent spinal cord stroke.[32] The presence of edema association with spinal cord infarction is mediated, in part, by varying expression of aquaporin-4.[33]

Depending on the intensity of tissue damage, the infarct can be complete or incomplete. In complete infarction, all cellular elements die. In incomplete infarction, some of the elements survive, especially blood vessels and, to a lesser extent, astrocytes. In addition, the damage can be only "cellular," being confined largely to neurons.

Initially, the infarcted area appears pale and swollen. In the central portion of the infarct, the neurons show ischemic changes (eosinophilic cytoplasm) (Fig. 32-5). The earliest change may be present after 6 hours. Astrocytes, oligodendroglial cells, and microglial cells, along with myelinated axons, disintegrate and give a granular appearance to the neuropil. These changes are followed by neovascularization, with endothelial hyperplasia and fragmentation of the tissue. In the next 2 to 3 weeks, the infarcted area is invaded by phagocytes. These cells liquefy the necrotic tissue, and cavitation occurs (Fig. 32-6). Finally, the astrocytes proliferate at the edges of the cavitation.[34] Because of the tight arrangement of the pathways in the cord, small infarcts are usually associated with more obvious symptoms and signs than similar lesions in the brain.[35]

Involvement of spinal cord blood vessels by atherosclerosis or thrombosis is uncommon, in contrast with the high frequency of similar vascular diseases in the cerebral vessels.[14,34,36] Perhaps this discrepancy can be explained by the fact that the blood pressure in the spinal arteries is lower than in other parts of the vascular system. This idea is supported by the occurrence of more frequent vascular disease in the spinal cords of patients with coarctation of the aorta, in which there is high blood pressure in the spinal cord system.[14] Postmortem examinations have traditionally been less thorough than the usually detailed pathologic surveillance of the cerebrum and its blood supply.

Etiology

Infarction of the spinal cord involving the territory supplied by the anterior spinal artery may result from interruption of the blood supply due to obstruction of the lumen of any vessel from the aorta to the intramedullary vasculature, from systemic hypoperfusion, or from a combination of the two (Table 32-1).[9] Syphilitic arteritis was the most common cause of spinal cord infarction in the prepenicillin era[9]; the next most common cause was atherosclerosis of the aorta, before aortic aneurysm reconstruction surgery grew in popularity. In small case series, cardiothoracic surgery is the leading cause of spinal cord ischemia that can be identified; a definite cause is not identified in a higher proportion of patients.[28,37,38]

Infarction of the spinal cord secondary to emboli has been described in association with bacterial endocarditis,[39,40] atrial myxoma,[41] mitral valve disease,[42] and paradoxical embolism secondary to patent foramen ovale or pulmonary arteriovenous malformation.[43,44]

Vertebral artery dissection has also been reported as a rare cause of spinal cord ischemia.[45] Fibrocartilaginous emboli (FCE) from herniated intervertebral disks are also a rare but well-recognized phenomenon causing spinal infarction. The mechanisms of FCE are poorly understood. Srigley et al[46] suggested that fragments of disk material are traumatically forced into bone marrow vertebral plexus and arterial channels. The patient usually experiences sudden onset of back or neck pain, which is followed by progressive and usually permanent spinal cord or brainstem dysfunction. A history of minor head or neck injury and a history of lifting a heavy load at the onset of symptoms is common. The infarction is typically central, with major involvement of the anterior and lateral horns. In more recent case series the cause of spinal cord ischemia is presumed to be FCE, based on the lack of available evidence for other causes.[47,48]

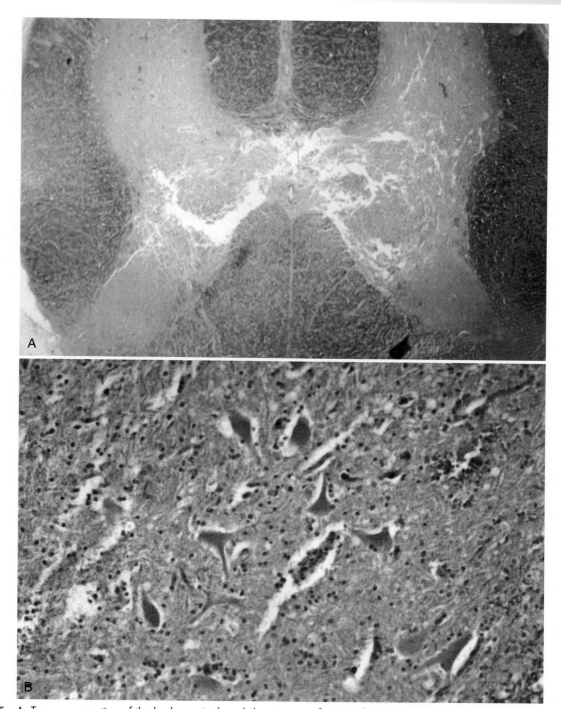

Figure 32-5   A, Transverse section of the lumbar spinal cord showing an infarct involving mainly the gray matter. Hematoxylin and eosin (H&E); magnification, × 1. B, Section from the anterior horn showing numerous ischemic neurons with dense eosinophilic cytoplasm. H&E; magnification, ×25. The patient had ischemic injury of the cord secondary to profound hypotension. (From Benavente OR, Barnett HJM: Spinal cord infarction. In Carter LP, Spetzler RF, editors: *Neurovascular surgery,* New York, 1995, McGraw-Hill, p 1229.)

The diagnosis of FCE is generally made at autopsy or during examination of surgical specimens, when emboli histologically identical to the fibrocartilage of the nucleus pulposus are identified in arteries, veins, or both, of the spinal circulation.[46,49] Tosi et al[50] reviewed 32 cases of histologically confirmed FCE and found a high incidence in young women (69%); a temporal relationship to significant trauma was present in only a minority of patients. In most of the cases (70%), embolization occurred in the cervical cord; in some, it extended to lower medullar and upper thoracic segments. Infarction was localized to the anterior spinal artery territory in most of the patients. The clinical course in this series showed some distinctive features. First, all patients had sudden onset of pain. Second, the

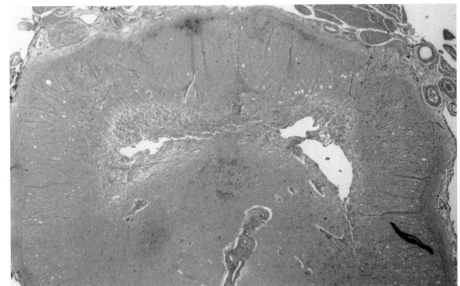

Figure 32-6 Thoracic spinal cord (transverse section) with a large infarct in the territory of the anterior spinal artery, with cavitation and vacuolation of the neuropil. Hematoxylin and eosin; magnification, ×1. The patient had a rupture of an aortic abdominal aneurysm. (From Benavente OR, Barnett HJM: Spinal cord infarction. In Carter LP, Spetzler RF, editors: *Neurovascular surgery,* New York, 1995, McGraw-Hill, p 1229.)

TABLE 32-1   CAUSES OF SPINAL CORD ISCHEMIA

Vasculitis
Polyarteritis nodosa[42]
Behçet's syndrome[157]
Giant cell arteritis[158]

Embolic causes
Atrial myxoma[41]
Mitral valve disease[42]
Bacterial endocarditis[39]
Patent foramen ovale[44]
Fibrocartilaginous emboli from herniated disks[46,50]

Systemic hypoperfusion
Cardiorespiratory arrest[63,65,159,160]
Traumatic rupture of aorta[161]
Dissection of aortic aneurysm[58,60,162]
Coarctation of aorta[50]

Iatrogenic causes
Thoracolumbar sympathectomy[66]
Surgical correction of scoliosis[67]
Cardiac catheterization[68]
Aortography[69]
Renal artery embolization[163]
Umbilical artery catheterization[164]
Vertebral angiography[52,70]
Aortic surgery[1,3]
Surgical repair of coarctation of aorta[85]
Retroperitoneal lymph node dissection[165]

Infectious causes
Syphilitic arteritis[8]
Mucormycosis[166]
Bacterial meningitis[167]

Miscellaneous causes
Sickle cell anemia[168]
Cocaine abuse[64]
Decompression sickness[169]
Antiphospholipid antibody syndrome[170]
Crohn's disease[171]
Cervical subluxation[172]
Atherosclerosis and thrombosis of aorta[105]

interval from onset of pain to maximal neurologic deficit ranged from 15 minutes to 48 hours; in cases of thrombotic infarction, neurologic deficits may appear first and, in most cases, manifest abruptly accompanied by pain. A third distinguishing feature of infarction secondary to thrombosis was that no patient with FCE showed significant improvement of neurologic deficit during the first 48 hours. Finally, evidence of cord swelling and increased T2 signal on MRI plus a collapsed intervertebral disk space at the appropriate level strongly suggested FCE.

Spinal cord ischemia associated with decompression sickness (caisson disease) has also been described. It results from circulating nitrogen bubbles that block small spinal arteries.[51] Primary thrombosis of the anterior spinal artery as a cause of spinal infarction has not been well-documented and is considered rare. Foo and Rossier,[52] reviewing 60 cases of anterior spinal artery syndrome, found seven patients in whom thrombosis of this vessel was the cause. In 24 others, no cause was found, and the thrombosis could not be considered primary.[52]

Dissection of an Aortic Aneurysm

Aortic aneurysm is a serious vascular disorder with a lifetime incidence of 2% to 6% and a 1-year mortality rate of 75% in untreated patients.[1] Neurologic complications of aortic aneurysms occur at different levels of the nervous system in the setting of rupture and are more likely to occur in the territory of the cerebral vasculature; spinal cord ischemia is present in a small minority of patients before surgery.[53] Aortic dissection is characterized by hemorrhage into the tunica media of the aorta, which separates the aortic wall into two layers. The dissection may extend up or down along the media, involving the innominate, carotid, or femoral arteries, narrowing the lumen of these arteries, and impairing blood flow. This condition is most commonly associated with arteriosclerosis, in which hypertension and aneurysmal dilatation of the aorta predispose to dissection.[56] Less often, dissecting aortic aneurysms occur in Marfan's syndrome, pregnancy, aortic stenosis, and hypothyroidism.[48] Dissecting aortic aneurysms can produce spinal cord ischemia when an important intercostal or lumbar artery is sheared or occluded at its origin. Hughes[48] reviewed the literature and found 11 cases of aortic dissection with spinal infarction confirmed by autopsy; the spinal damage was more extensive in some cases than in others. The dissection may involve one or several of the intercostal and lumbar arteries. The severity of impairment of blood flow determines the extent of spinal infarction. The other factor of importance is whether a large or small tributary artery is affected. In general, the midthoracic to lower thoracic cord is the region most often damaged because it is supplied by the intercostal arteries that are most frequently affected by aortic dissection.[36] If the artery of Adamkiewicz is involved, the area of maximal damage extends from the T10 to L1 levels. The midthoracic cord suffers the maximum insult because it is a watershed zone (T4 to T6) between the blood supply of the upper and lower parts of the cord.[51,57,58] The upper part of the cord, which is supplied from branches of the vertebral arteries, is rarely involved. The lumbosacral cord can be damaged if the dissection extends caudally. Necrosis involves gray matter and adjacent white matter, but the white matter at the periphery is sometimes spared. In severe cases, the total cross-section of the cord may be necrotic.[48] Acute onset of paraplegia or paraparesis with a thoracic sensory level can be a dramatic presentation in dissection of the aorta. Dissection is usually heralded by the sudden onset of severe pain in the chest or back or in both regions. However, a few cases of spinal cord infarction have been associated with painless dissecting aneurysms.[59] A review of the literature showed that, of 1805 patients with aortic dissection, 4.2% were seen with symptoms or signs of spinal cord damage.[60] Among patients with aortic aneurysms, those with thoracoabdominal dilatations tend to have a higher incidence of spinal cord infarction.[61]

Coarctation of the Aorta

Coarctation of the aorta is a congenital stenosis of the isthmus of the aorta. Coarctation has been divided into two types, infantile and adult. In the infantile type, a small segment of narrowing can occur before, at, or (most commonly) beyond the origin of the left subclavian artery. In the adult type, there is a vast anastomotic circulation between the arteries of the upper trunk and limbs and those beyond the stenosis in the lower trunk and legs. Arteries from the spinal cord form an important part of this anastomosis. Consequently, spinal complications occur in the adult type of coarctation.

The spinal cord can be also affected by ischemia secondary to hypotension. The caudal part of the cord is the most vulnerable because it is supplied by arteries originating from the aorta distal to the narrowed segment. Symptoms and signs of paresis and sensory and sphincter disturbances have been noted. These symptoms may sometimes be related to activity. In addition, the cord may be damaged as a result of hypertension in the anastomotic system. In this circumstance, the anterior spinal artery becomes enlarged and tortuous and compresses the spinal cord. However, the most common mechanism leading to cord damage is ischemia.[62]

Systemic Hypoperfusion

A profound and sustained drop in perfusion pressure may lead to an ischemic myelopathy involving primarily the watershed area of the midthoracic cord. Sandson and Friedman[9] reviewed 14 cases of spinal infarction secondary to hypoperfusion. All of the patients had paraplegia with areflexia and urinary dysfunction. In 13 patients, a sensory level was present in the thoracic region. Spinal cord infarction secondary to hypoperfusion occurs most often in the midthoracic region and predominately involves gray matter.[63,64] Azzarelli and Roessmann[65] studied 16 patients who had anoxic episodes (12 from cardiorespiratory arrest and four from pulmonary disease), concluding that the spinal cord was most vulnerable to hypoperfusion in the lumbosacral region. All of the lesions in this series were symmetrical and limited to the gray matter.

Iatrogenic Ischemia of the Spinal Cord

Because of the greater frequency of cardiovascular surgery and invasive diagnostic procedures, iatrogenic spinal cord infarction is encountered more frequently than before. Spinal cord ischemia has been associated with a number of surgical and diagnostic procedures, including thoracolumbar sympathectomy,[66] pneumonectomy,[51] and correction of scoliosis.[67] In these surgical procedures, ligation of an intercostal or lumbar artery probably causes spinal ischemia. Cardiac catheterization,[68] aortography,[69] vertebral angiography,[52,70] and spinal cord arteriography[71] have also been associated with cord infarction. Other procedures have been reported to be associated with spinal cord ischemia, notably epidural steroid injections in the treatment of back pain or spinal anesthesia.[72-75] Lumbar spine surgery with subsequent thoracic cord ischemia has been described as a consequence of microembolization,[76] while another group described a case of conus medullaris infarction after lumbar diskectomy from an occult dural arteriovenous fistula.[77] The treatment of spinal arteriovenous malformations and dural arteriovenous fistulas[78] has also been associated with spinal cord ischemia, although the actual risk of ischemic injury from the treatment is difficult to establish, as is whether the ischemia represents an arterial or venous thrombosis.

The replacement, by grafts, of segments of the thoracic or abdominal aorta and its transitory clamping continue to be associated with a low incidence of ischemic complications of the spinal cord.[79,80] The anterior spinal artery syndrome, the most common neurologic complication after aortic surgery, was first reported by Mehrez et al[81] in 1962. In another series, paraplegia associated with unruptured aortic aneurysm repair was present in 5% of 101 patients who underwent elective surgery.[3]

Crawford et al[1] also found that 6% of patients experienced permanent paraparesis or paraplegia after surgery, although more recent estimates place the risk closer to 3%.[82] Risk factors for the development of ischemic myelopathy include extent of the aneurysm (higher incidence of

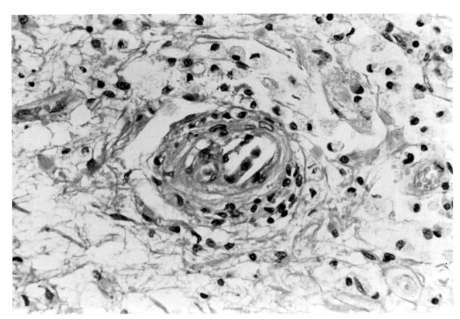

Figure 32-7 Obstruction of a small medullary artery within the spinal cord by atheromatous debris, including cholesterol clefts. The material came from a severely diseased thoracic aorta removed surgically after aneurysmal rupture. Many similar lesions, found at postmortem, caused this patient's total paraplegia at the T8 level.

paraplegia in large ruptured aneurysms with involvement of the entire descending aorta), the presence of previous dissection before surgery for an abdominal aortic aneurysm, the presence of prior cerebrovascular disease, and duration of clamping, which is longer in complicated operations.[1,82] Some researchers observe that the cord may be damaged during surgery as a result of ligation, resection, or embolization of the artery of Adamkiewicz[83] or, most commonly, because of sustained hypotension during clamping.[1] Others assert that the postoperative paraplegia is due in part to increased intracranial pressure and impairment of spinal blood perfusion during aortic cross-clamping.[84] Showers of atheromatous debris precipitated by the surgical handling of an ulcerated atherosclerotic plaque in the aorta may obstruct a number of intraspinal arterioles (Fig. 32-7).

Surgical repair of coarctation of the aorta also carries a risk of spinal cord injury, but the incidence of paraplegia after surgery is extremely low (0.4%). Curiously, neither the number of intercostal arteries involved during surgery nor the duration of clamping has been correlated with the incidence of spinal cord ischemia.[85]

Clinical Presentation of Spinal Cord Infarction

Spinal cord infarction has many similarities to cerebral infarction. In both, the clinical picture may be extremely diverse, depending on the vascular territory involved, the size of the lesion, its cause, and the status of the collateral circulation. The terms used to describe the pattern of duration of cerebrovascular disease can be applied to the spinal cord.

In patients of all ages in whom bilateral leg weakness or bilateral upper limb weakness simultaneously appear and any of the conditions exist as already described under the section on etiology (see Table 32-1), the clinician should be alerted to the possibility of spinal ischemia. In patients without these etiologic mechanisms present, particularly

in older patients, the sudden nearly simultaneous onset of bilateral symptoms and signs should arouse suspicion of spinal vascular disease. In the elderly with prominently calcified aortas, ischemia may result from an embolus of thrombotic or atheromatous material from an ulcerative lesion of a grossly diseased aorta. One of us (HJMB) has seen spinal cord ischemia precipitated by a sudden violent truncal twisting exertion in three such elderly subjects: once by a determinedly strenuous drive in golf, once in twisting from the front seat to pick a heavy object from the floor of the backseat of a car, and once after excessive twisting in a yoga program. If the neurologic manifestations are attributable to a specific arterial territory, the diagnosis is almost certain. Motor, sensory, and autonomic signs may be present. The findings may include paraparesis, tetraparesis, paraplegia, and loss of sphincter control, reflecting the level of the infarct, the vascular territory involved by the infarct, and the extension of the infarct.[35] If these signs remain for more than 24 hours, the event is referred to as a *complete infarct*. The same type of vascular event can be intermittent or less abrupt in onset, depending mainly on the underlying mechanism and on the presence of collateral circulation.

Transient ischemic attacks (TIAs) can theoretically involve the spinal cord. These focal neurologic deficits, which were previously defined by a duration of less than 24 hours, rarely precede spinal cord infarctions[18]; it is unclear to what degree the new definition of TIA, requiring no imaging evidence of acute infarction, will affect the prevalence of TIA.[86] Spinal TIAs are probably due to emboli arising from the heart or aorta, the site of ulcerative atherosclerotic disease, plus perhaps a combination of focal atherosclerotic stenosis and systemic hypotension.[16] It is surprising that TIAs of the spinal cord are not more frequently diagnosed because ulcerated atheromas and mural thrombi are common findings in the aortas of elderly patients.[35] Ischemic attacks may also occur in coarctation of the aorta due to the steal phenomenon.[87] Spinal TIAs have been reported in patients with spinal arteriovenous malformations (AVMs). The underlying mechanism is either the steal phenomenon, in which blood is shunted through a low-pressure AVM, or compression of the cord by the vascular malformation.[88]

The term *claudication of the cord* was introduced by Dejerine; it was thought to be a result of impaired blood flow secondary to arterial stenosis.[89] The term refers to transitory symptoms in the legs that are associated with exercise and that disappear with rest. Many of the early cases were attributed to syphilitic arteritis of the radicular arteries. Today, spinal AVMs are one of the most common causes of this syndrome.[88] Other reported causes are atherosclerosis and pronounced lumbar spondylosis or thoracic disk protrusion.[90,91] Intermittent spinal symptoms have also been described in patients with thoracolumbar spinal cord stenosis, in which the episodic neurologic dysfunction is presumably of vascular origin.[92,93]

The initial symptoms are heaviness in one or both legs that appears during activity and is relieved by rest. In addition, sensory symptoms, pain, or sphincter disturbances have been noted. When the patient is at rest, the neurologic examination generally discloses no significant abnormalities. After exercise, weakness of one or both legs and hyperreflexia and extensor plantar responses have been found.[38,91,94] Transient cord ischemia does not always preclude an infarction, but over long periods, a progressive reduction in exercise tolerance occurs, until a permanent deficit develops.[95]

The same pattern of presentation can be applied to claudication of the cauda equina. Intermittent claudication of the cauda equina, which is more common in males, is characterized by pain, numbness, and paresthesias with exercise and relief with rest. Symptoms begin in the lower back and buttocks and spread down the legs. Neurologic findings in a patient at rest are generally normal, but after exercise, minor motor and sensory disturbances may be found. The syndrome of cauda equina claudication has been associated with narrowing of the lumbar spinal canal,[96] disk protrusion, and achondroplasia.[97,98] Symptoms develop with actions or postures that involve extension of the lumbar spine. Relief occurs when the patient leans forward or squats. In a few patients, the precipitation of symptoms relates to exercise of the extremities, perhaps as a result of ischemia of cauda equina roots during exercise. It therefore seems that the syndrome of cauda equina claudication relates to exercise. It may be due to impaired blood flow through radicular arteries at points of constriction. Consequently, the blood supply cannot increase sufficiently during activity.[95,97,99]

In 1926, Foix and Alajouanine[100] described a syndrome of subacute or chronic progressive myelopathy. It was attributed to chronic ischemia of the spinal cord secondary to atherosclerosis, but this issue has been a subject of recurrent debate.[36] Many other conditions have been implicated in the cause of this entity. For instance, Clark and Cumming[101] reported a venous infarction of the spinal cord resulting in a subacute progressive myelopathy. The clinical picture consists of atrophy of the small muscles of the hands and hyperactive reflexes. Affected patients tend to have a history of hypertension and systemic atherosclerosis. The pathologic changes mainly involve the anterior horns and consist of small cavities or lacunes plus rarefaction of the neuropil. These types of changes have been observed principally in the lower cervical cord.

Familial cavernous angiomas, in which some members of a family are affected with spinal cord angiomas, have also been reported.[102]

Anterior Spinal Artery Syndrome

The territory supplied by the anterior spinal artery is the most common location of ischemic lesions of the spinal cord. Spiller[103] gave the first clinicopathologic description of anterior spinal artery syndrome in 1909. The underlying cause was syphilitic arteritis. Occlusion of this artery results in infarction of the anterior two thirds of the spinal cord. Involved structures are the anterior horns of the gray matter, the spinothalamic tracts, and the pyramidal tracts. The level of ischemia may be cervical, thoracic, or lumbosacral.[40,104]

Clinical Manifestations

Involvement of the vertebral arteries may produce infarction at the cervical level.[105] This syndrome is characterized by the sudden onset of radicular or diffuse neck pain followed by quadriparesis. Because of spinal shock, the paraplegia may remain flaccid for several days to weeks, and absence of reflexes is present. Disturbances in the control of vesical and rectal sphincters commonly occur. The sensory loss is marked and involves pain, temperature, pinprick, and light touch sensation below the segmental or dermatomal level of the lesion. However, proprioception, light touch, and vibration senses are almost always spared. Motor neuron signs may develop in the upper extremities, and spasticity of the legs, hyperreflexia, and extensor plantar responses may occur.[52,106] Proprioception and vibration sense may be affected with higher cervical lesions because of involvement of the medial lemniscus.[9]

Infarction of the spinal cord is most common at the thoracic level because of the presence of a watershed area in the midthoracic region.[9,14] The territory of the anterior spinal artery at this level can be infarcted by aortic or radicular artery disease. The typical thoracic infarction manifests as pain in the interscapular region followed by paraparesis or paraplegia sparing the arms, urinary and rectal incontinence or retention, and a sensory loss to pain and temperature that is most common at the T4 level. The initial spinal shock gives way to hypertonia, hyperreflexia, and extensor plantar responses below the level of the lesion.

Infarction of the lumbosacral region in the territory supplied by the anterior spinal artery may be caused by disease or obstruction of the radicular artery of Adamkiewicz. If the lesion is extensive, the patient is seen with a flaccid paraplegia due to damage of a large area of gray matter and, consequently, the motor neurons of the anterior horns. Autonomic dysfunction occurs; later, wasting of the legs associated with areflexia may be present.

Occlusion of a central sulcal artery produces small lesions in half of the spinal cord.[9,14,107] This disorder can manifest as an incomplete Brown-Séquard syndrome or as a suspended dissociated sensory loss consisting of impairment of pain and temperature sensation over the

TABLE 32-2 ANTERIOR SPINAL ARTERY SYNDROME

Back or neck pain of sudden onset
Rapidly progressive paraplegia
Flaccid paraplegia that soon becomes spastic
Areflexia at onset, which becomes hyperreflexic with extensor
   plantar response
Sensory level for pain and temperature
Preserved proprioception, light touch, and vibration sense
Urinary incontinence
Painful burning dysesthesias below the level of cord injury
   (during chronic phase)

TABLE 32-3 POSTERIOR SPINAL ARTERY SYNDROME

Sensory loss of proprioception, vibration, and light touch sensations; with sensory level
Preserved pain and temperature sensation, except at the level
   of the affected cord segment, where there is suspended
   global anesthesia
Motor function preserved
Loss of deep tendon and cutaneous reflexes at the level of the
   affected cord segment

segment affected by the infarct but with preserved sensation above and below the lesion. This is a rare phenomenon, attributed to embolic or thrombotic occlusion of the perforating branches of sulcal arteries, that produces a localized infarction and leaves the anterior spinal artery intact (Table 32-2).[10,108,109]

Posterior Spinal Artery Syndrome

Posterior spinal artery infarctions are less common than anterior infarctions, but they do occur.[39] The lesion mainly involves posterior columns and extends to the posterior horns. This syndrome manifests as a suspended pattern of total anesthesia at the affected level. The tendon and cutaneous reflexes for that specific spinal segment are abolished. Vibration and position senses are impaired below the affected level out of proportion to other sensory alterations. Paralysis, if present, is minimal and transient.[14] This syndrome has been described in association with atheromatous embolization,[110] intrathecal injection of phenol,[111] trauma, and syphilitic arteritis (Table 32-3).[40]

Venous Infarction

Venous infarction of the spinal cord is less common than arterial infarction, and most cases of venous infarction are diagnosed postmortem.[112] The most common causes of venous infarction in the spinal cord are vascular malformations of the spinal cord and acute compression by epidural processes such as hematomas and abscesses. Venous infarctions can be classified as hemorrhagic or nonhemorrhagic. The clinical features and the pathologic findings are remarkably constant. The hemorrhagic type has a sudden onset and severe pain in the back and sometimes in the legs and abdomen. Lower extremity weakness, producing a flaccid paraplegia or

quadriplegia, follows. The paralysis may be progressive over hours or days. Sensation is impaired in the legs and may involve the trunk or upper limbs, depending on the extent of the lesion. Bowel and bladder dysfunction invariably occurs.

The pathologic findings consist of a spinal cord disrupted by the hemorrhagic necrosis, which involves the central gray matter. This type of infarct tends to be more extensive in longitudinal and cross-sectional areas than anterior cord infarctions. The spinal veins are distended and obstructed. Hughes[112] reported seven cases of acute venous spinal cord infarction associated with acute thrombophlebitis; the most common underlying condition was systemic sepsis. Hemorrhagic venous infarction has also been associated with thrombophlebitis migrans, acute myelogenous leukemia, and tuberculosis.[113]

Nonhemorrhagic infarctions evolve slowly, with a clinical onset of as long as 1 year. Leg paralysis, sphincter dysfunction, and sensory loss without back pain are present. Survival time is longer than in hemorrhagic infarction. These types of infarctions are commonly associated with an underlying vascular malformation. This subacute neurologic syndrome, also called subacute necrotic myelitis, is attributed to intramedullary hypertension secondary to a spinal arteriovenous fistula.[112] The nonhemorrhagic infarctions tend to be at the T3 level or below; hemorrhagic infarctions have a more rostral location. Nonhemorrhagic infarctions have also been associated with polycythemia, thrombophlebitis, chronic meningitis, decompression sickness, and leg vein thrombosis and have been observed after sclerotherapy for esophageal varices.[113,114]

Differential Diagnosis

The differential diagnosis of spinal cord infarction is broad and includes all conditions that can manifest as an acute incomplete myelopathy or as early Guillain-Barré syndrome[115]: compressive lesions, spinal cord trauma, transverse myelitis, multiple sclerosis, intramedullary tumor, hematomyelia, and necrotizing myelitis.[9] An example of thoracic myelopathy complicating severe bacterial meningitis has also been reported.[116] In middle-aged or elderly patients with slowly progressive paraparesis, the diagnosis of vascular or arteriosclerotic myelopathy should be viewed with suspicion because many other diseases are more likely, including motor neuron disease, vitamin B_{12} deficiency, cervical spondylosis, and, less commonly, neoplasms, multiple sclerosis, and human T-cell leukemia-1 myelopathy. A single instance of angina-like presentation with midthoracic cord infarction has been reported.[117] Cervical manipulation may also be associated with cord infarction as well as the well-known brainstem and cerebellar infarction (Table 32-4).[118] A single instance of cord infarction associated with and assumed related to zolmitriptan therapy in a patient with migraine has been reported.[119]

Diagnostic Tests

A sudden neurologic deficit of spinal cord origin requires immediate investigation. Although ischemic disorders of the cord are uncommon, they must be diagnosed by

TABLE 32-4 DIFFERENTIAL DIAGNOSIS OF SPINAL CORD ISCHEMIA

Compressive myelopathy (tumor, epidural or subdural hematoma)
Traumatic myelopathy, including central cord syndrome
Disk herniation
Primary transverse myelitis
Transverse myelitis secondary to multiple sclerosis, Devic's syndrome, systemic lupus erythematosus
Acute necrotizing myelitis
Intramedullary spinal cord tumor
Arteriovenous malformation
Acute polyneuropathy
Guillain-Barré syndrome
Porphyria
Human immunodeficiency virus-related neuropathy (inflammatory demyelinating polyneuropathy)
Thallium

exclusion, and initial investigations must be designed to rule out a compressive myelopathy. The most important diagnostic aids in assessing vascular disease of the cord are CT, alone or with myelography, and MRI. CT and MRI have reduced the necessity of using plain radiographs, myelography, selective spinal angiography, and CSF analyses. A CT scan may show spinal cord swelling, but because of its poor spatial discrimination, CT has not contributed very much to diagnostic imaging of cord ischemia. Hemorrhagic infarctions are clearly visualized by CT. However, MRI produces more detailed and more useful images (Fig. 32-8).

MRI has become the method of choice for diagnosing spinal cord ischemia because it can reliably be used to exclude other causes of myelopathy, such as compressive lesions, intramedullary neoplasms, and cavitations. On MRI, the infarcted cord can have an increased diameter. Infarcts can be first seen on diffusion-weighted imaging (DWI) with high sensitivity within 8 hours of cord infarction.[120-122] Within 1 week after infarction the DWI changes will normalize, whereas T2 hyperintensity will become more prominent.[120] Once the blood–cord barrier becomes affected, enhancement of the ischemic or infarcted tissue can be seen after administration of gadolinium. In the subacute phase, high-intensity lesions are seen on T2-weighted images. A highly suggestive pattern for ischemia rather than another etiology of T2 hyperintensity in the spinal cord is intervetebral disk and vertebral body infarction in the adjacent level[123,124] and is particularly suggestive of aortic pathology.[125] There are instances of combined cord and cerebellar infarction with bilateral vertebral artery occlusion.[128] Sometimes the infarcts can be better visualized on contrast-enhanced T1-weighted MR images.[4-6,129,130] Fortuna et al[131] reviewed 61 cases of cord infarction diagnosed on MRI (T1-weighted images) during the early phase; they identified enlargement of the affected cord in about 50% and isodensity in most (70%) of the cases. On T2-weighted images, hyperintensity was noted in 90% of the cases. During later stages of cord infarction, T2-weighted images showed hyperintensity in most of the cases (86%).

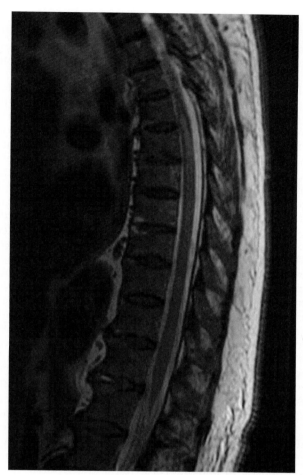

Figure 32-8 Sagittal T2-weighted magnetic resonance image of the thoracic cord shows an abnormal signal hyperintensity within the spinal cord (T4 to T6), without mass effect, consistent with cord infarction. (From Benavente OR, Barnett HJM: Spinal cord infarction. In Carter LP, Spetzler RF, editors: *Neurovascular surgery*, New York, 1995, McGraw-Hill, p 1229.)

The presence of concomitant hyperintensity of the vertebral body immediately below the spinal cord lesion on T2-weighted MR images is suggestive of cord ischemia. This finding has been observed in ischemia secondary to occlusion of the aorta and fibrocartilaginous emboli.[132] Although MRI is a highly sensitive tool for detecting infarction of the spinal cord, a definitive diagnosis is not always possible because the presence of other conditions, such as transverse myelitis, intramedullary tumors, and multiple sclerosis, cannot be entirely excluded. MRI should be routinely performed in every patient with a clinical picture suggestive of spinal cord infarction.

Treatment and Prognosis

No data are available regarding specific therapeutic regimens in patients who have had spinal cord ischemia or infarction. Multiple pharmacologic agents have been tested in animal models of spinal cord ischemia, including ketamine, carbamazepine, and inhibitors of the ischemic cascade; none have been tested prospectively yet in humans.[29,133-136] One case report points to the successful use of hyperbaric oxygen,[137] but this therapy remains completely unproven to date and has not been successful in cerebral infarction or other spinal cord injury mechanisms.[138]

Prevention of spinal cord ischemia during surgical treatment of aortic dissections remains the most active area of research. Endovascular procedures for aortic dissection appear to carry a lower risk of spinal cord ischemia in traumatic aortic injury.[139] Preventing prolonged and profound hypotension during aortic surgery is essential for reducing the incidence of perioperative cord ischemia. The use of bypass with distal perfusion remains one of the better studied methods for preventing spinal cord ischemia, and the use of surgical techniques to reattach ligated spinal arteries may not affect the risk of spinal cord ischemia. The most widely used and studied strategy for preventing postoperative spinal cord ischemia has been CSF shunting with the use of a lumbar drain under the premise that reducing CSF volume will improve spinal cord perfusion pressure. Case series from multiple sites have shown improved rates of spinal ischemia after the introduction of placement of a lumbar drain for CSF drainage in all patients compared with the historical experience before this protocol.[140] The combination of distal perfusion therapy and CSF drainage may be particularly effective in reducing the risk of spinal cord ischemia[82] and has, in some centers, virtually eliminated spinal cord ischemia.[141] The mode of CSF drainage remains controversial because excess CSF drainage may be associated with the development of subdural hematomas.[142,143] Lumbar CSF drainage may even be safe in patients receiving extracorporeal membrane oxygen.[144] The use of spinal somatosensory evoked potentials during surgery for a thoracoabdominal aneurysm has been shown to be a valuable guide in detecting whether the spinal cord is at risk, thereby allowing measures to be taken to prevent cord ischemia.[145,147] Motor evoked potentials, with demonstration of the presence of the artery of Adamkiewicz, may also help guide surgical treatment to minimize spinal cord ischemia.[148] In experimental animal models, selective hypothermia has proved to be efficacious in reducing paraplegia after prolonged aortic clamping, and increasingly, protocols using spinal fluid cooling after CSF diversion are being used and may be clinically effective.[149,150]

The combined use of elevating the mean arterial pressure, diverting CSF, and using hypothermia may account for much of the reduction in rates of spinal cord ischemia after surgical repairs.[151]

Correction of underlying pathogenic factors and modification of the usual risk factors, such as hypertension, heart disease, and diabetes mellitus, are important.[16] If the source is embolic, the use of anticoagulant or antiplatelet drugs should be considered.[18] Treatment is supportive, and special attention must be given to bowel and bladder function as well as to skin integrity. Bracken et al[152] have shown that methylprednisolone reduces the extent of disability after spinal cord trauma, so use of this agent immediately after establishment of a diagnosis of cord ischemia can be considered. There are no case series of spinal ischemia on which to rely.

The prognosis of spinal cord infarction is variable and depends on the extent of parenchymal damage and the cause. The prognosis seems to be worse in cases due to FCE.[50] Overall, about 24% of patients who have cord ischemia experience no improvement; the rest show some functional improvement, but only 20% have a good recovery with minimal disability.[38] Long-term outcome studies are isolated to small case series with variable follow-up times, in which authors have reported between 41% to 53% of patients gaining the ability to walk independently or with the help of a single assistive device.[27,28,37,153] The presence of chronic pain is a common and disabling feature for these patients over the long term.[27,154] The most significant predictor of recovery appears to be the severity of the initial impairment, although other associated factors have also included the initial presence of bladder dysfunction.[153,155,156]

REFERENCES

1. Crawford ES, Crawford JL, Safi HJ, et al: Thoracoabdominal aortic aneurysms: Preoperative and intraoperative factors determining immediate and long-term results of operations in 605 patients, *J Vasc Surg* 3:389, 1986.
2. Friedman SG, Moccio CG: Spinal cord ischemia following elective aortic reconstruction, *Ann Vasc Surg* 2:295, 1988.
3. Hollier LH, Symmonds JB, Pairolero PC, et al: Thoracoabdominal aortic aneurysm repair: Analysis of postoperative morbidity, *Arch Surg* 123:871, 1988.
4. Di Chiro G, Doppman JL, Dwyer AJ, et al: Tumors and arteriovenous malformations of the spinal cord: Assessment using MR, *Radiology* 156:689, 1985.
5. Mawad ME, Rivera V, Crawford S, et al: Spinal cord ischemia after resection of thoracoabdominal aortic aneurysms: MR findings in 24 patients, *AJNR Am J Neuroradiol* 155:987, 1990.
6. Nagashima C, Nagashima R, Morota N, Kobayashi S: Magnetic resonance imaging of human spinal cord infarction, *Surg Neurol* 35:368, 1991.
7. Blackwood W: Discussion on vascular disease of the spinal cord, *Proc R Soc Med* 51:543, 1958.
8. Slager UT, Webb AT: Pathologic findings in the spinal cord, *Arch Pathol* 96:388, 1973.
9. Sandson TA, Friedman JH: Spinal cord infarction: Report of 8 cases and review of the literature, *Medicine* 68:282, 1989.
10. Geldmacher DS, Nager BJ: Spinal cord vascular disease. In Bradley WG, Daroff RB, Fenichel GM, Marsden CD, editors: *Neurology in clinical practice*, vol 2, Bostons, 1991, Butterworth-Heinemann, p 983.
11. Bastian HC: Spinal cord softening. In Quain R, editor: *Dictionary for medicine*, London, 1882, Longmans Green, p 1479.
12. Preobrashenski PA: Syphilitic paraplegia with dissociated disturbance of sensation, *J Nevropatol i Psikhiatriia* 4:394–433, 1904.
13. Gray H: Developmental and gross anatomy of the central nervous system. In Clemente CD, editor: *Anatomy of the human body*, 30th ed. (American ed.) Philadelphia, 1984, Lea & Febiger, p 933.
14. Hughes JT: Vascular disorders of the spinal cord. In Vinken PJ, Bruyn GW, Klawans HL, editors: *Handbook of clinical neurology*, vol 55, Amsterdam, 1989, Elsevier, p 106.
15. Lozarthes G, Govaze A, Zadeh JO: Arterial vascularization of the spinal cord, *J Neurosurg* 35:253, 1971.
16. Satran R: Spinal cord infarction, *Stroke* 19:529, 1988.
17. Backes WH, Nijenhuis RJ, Mess WH, et al: Magnetic resonance angiography of collateral blood supply to spinal cord in thoracic and thoracoabdominal aortic aneurysm patients, *J Vasc Surg* 48:261–271, 2008.
18. Buchan AM, Barnett HJM: Infarction of the spinal cord. In Barnett HJM, Mohr JP, Stein BM, Yatsu FM, editors: *Stroke: Pathophysiology, diagnosis, and management*, ed 2, New York, 1986, Churchill Livingstone, p 709.
19. Gillilan LA: The arterial supply of the human spinal cord, *J Comp Neurol* 110:75–105, 1958.

20. Woollam DHM, Millen JW: The arterial supply of the spinal cord and its significance, *J Neurol Neurosurg Psychiatry* 18:97, 1955.

21. Gillilan LA: Veins of the spinal cord: Anatomic details; suggested clinical complications, *Neurology* 20:860, 1970.

22. Turnbull IM: Blood supply of the spinal cord. In Vinken PJ, Bruyn GN, editors: *Handbook of clinical neurology*, vol. 12, Amsterdam, 1972, Elsevier, p 478.

23. Marcus ML, Heistad DD, Ehrhardt JC, Abboud FM: Regulation of total and regional spinal cord blood flow, *Circ Res* 41:128, 1977.

24. Sandler AN, Tator CH: Regional spinal blood flow in primates, *J Neurosurg* 45:660–670, 1976.

25. Nystrom B, Stjernschantz J, Smedegard G: Regional spinal cord blood flow in the rabbit, cat and monkey, *Acta Neurol Scand* 70:307, 1984.

26. Such TH, Alexander L: Vascular system of the human spinal cord, *Arch Neurol Psychiatry* 41:660, 1939.

27. Masson C, Pruvo JP, Meder JF, et al: Spinal cord infarction: Clinical and magnetic resonance imaging findings and short term outcome, *J Neurol Neurosurg Psychiatry* 75:1431–1435, 2004.

28. Novy J, Carruzzo A, Maeder P, Bogousslavsky J: Spinal cord ischemia: Clinical and imaging patterns, pathogenesis, and outcomes in 27 patients, *Arch Neurol* 63:1113–1120, 2006.

29. Akuzawa S, Kazui T, Shi E, Yamashita K, Bashar AH, Terada H: Interleukin-1 receptor antagonist attenuates the severity of spinal cord ischemic injury in rabbits, *J Vasc Surg* 48:694–700, 2008.

30. Jellish WS, Zhang X, Langen KE, et al: Intrathecal magnesium sulfate administration at the time of experimental ischemia improves neurological functioning by reducing acute and delayed loss of motor neurons in the spinal cord, *Anesthesiology* 108:78–86, 2008.

31. Sakurai M, Nagata T, Abe K, et al: Survival and death-promoting events after transient spinal cord ischemia in rabbits: Induction of Akt and caspase 3 in motor neurons, *J Thorac Cardiovasc Surg* 125:370–377, 2003.

32. Hecker JG, Sundram H, Zou S, et al: Heat shock proteins HSP70 and HSP27 in the cerebral spinal fluid of patients undergoing thoracic aneurysm repair correlate with the probability of postoperative paralysis, *Cell Stress Chaperones* 13:435–446, 2008.

33. Xu WB, Gu YT, Wang YF, et al: Bradykinin preconditioning modulates aquaporin-4 expression after spinal cord ischemic injury in rats, *Brain Res* 1246:11–18, 2008.

34. Okazaki H: Cerebrovascular disease. In Okazaki H, editor: *Fundamentals of neuropathology*, ed 2, New York, 1989, Igaku-Shoin, p 27.

35. Moossy J: Vascular disease of the spinal cord. In Joynt RJ, editor: *Clinical neurology*, vol. 3, Philadelphia, 1991, Lippincott-Raven, p 1.

36. Jellinger K: Spinal cord arteriosclerosis and progressive vascular myelopathy, *J Neurol Neurosurg Psychiatry* 30:195, 1967.

37. Cheng MY, Lyu RK, Chang YJ, et al: Spinal cord infarction in Chinese patients. Clinical features, risk factors, imaging and prognosis, *Cerebrovasc Dis* 26:502–508, 2008.

38. Cheshire WP, Santos CC, Massey EW, Howard JF Jr: Spinal cord infarction: Etiology and outcome, *Neurology* 47:321–330, 1996.

39. Harrington AW: Embolism of the spinal cord, *Glasgow Med J* 103:28, 1925.

40. Hughes JT: Vascular disorders. In *Pathology of the spinal cord*, ed 2. (Major Problems in Pathology, Vol 6.) Philadelphia, 1978, WB Saunders, p 61.

41. Hirose G, Kosoegowa H, Takado M: Spinal cord ischemia and left atrial myxoma, *Arch Neurol* 24:228, 1971.

42. Whiteley AM, Hauw JJ, Escourolle R: A pathological survey of 41 cases of acute intrinsic spinal cord disease, *J Neurol Sci* 42:229, 1979.

43. Espinosa PS, Pettigrew LC, Berger JR: Hereditary hemorrhagic telangectasia and spinal cord infarct: Case report with a review of the neurological complications of HHT, *Clin Neurol Neurosurg* 110:484–491, 2008.

44. Mori S, Sadoshima S, Tagawa K, et al: Massive spinal cord infarction with multiple paradoxical embolism: A case report, *Angiology* 44:251–256, 1993.

45. Machnowska M, Moien-Afshari F, Voll C, Wiebe S: Partial anterior cervical cord infarction following vertebral artery dissection, *Can J Neurol Sci* 35:674–677, 2008.

46. Srigley JR, Lambert CD, Bilbao JM, Pritzker KPH: Spinal cord infarction secondary to intervertebral disc embolism, *Ann Neurol* 9:296, 1981.

47. Han JJ, Massagli TL, Jaffe KM: Fibrocartilaginous embolism—an uncommon cause of spinal cord infarction: A case report and review of the literature, *Arch Phys Med Rehabil* 85:153–157, 2004.

48. Raghavan A, Onikul E, Ryan MM, et al: Anterior spinal cord infarction owing to possible fibrocartilaginous embolism, *Pediatr Radiol* 34:503–506, 2004.

49. Case records of the Massachusetts General Hospital: Case 5, *N Engl J Med* 324:322, 1991.

50. Tosi L, Rigoli G, Beltramello A: Fibrocartilaginous embolism of the spinal cord: A clinical and pathogenetic reconsideration, *J Neurol Neurosurg Psychiatry* 60:55–60, 1996.

51. Henson RA, Parsons M: Ischaemic lesions of the spinal cord: An illustrated review, *Q J Med* 35:205, 1966.

52. Foo D, Rossier AB: Anterior spinal artery syndrome and its natural history, *Paraplegia* 21:1, 1983.

53. Gaul C, Dietrich W, Erbguth FJ: Neurological symptoms in aortic dissection: A challenge for neurologists, *Cerebrovasc Dis* 26:1–8, 2008.

54. Ross RT: Spinal cord infarction in disease and surgery of the aorta, *Can J Neurol Sci* 12:289, 1985.

55. Blanco M, Diez-Tejedor E, Larrea JL, Ramierez U: Neurologic complications of type I aortic dissection, *Acta Neurol Scand* 99:232, 1999.

56. Braunstein H: Pathogenesis of dissecting aneurysm, *Circulation* 28:1071, 1963.

57. Prendes JL: Neurovascular syndromes of aortic dissection, *Am Fam Physician* 23:175, 1981.

58. Waltimo O, Karli P: Aortic dissection and paraparesis, *Eur Neurol* 19:254, 1980.

59. Gerber O, Heyer EJ, Vieux U: Painless dissections of the aorta presenting as acute neurologic syndromes, *Stroke* 17:644, 1986.

60. Zull DN, Cydulka R: Acute paraplegia: A presenting manifestation of aortic dissection, *Am J Med* 84:765, 1988.

61. Lynch DR, Dawson TM, Raps EC, Galetta SL: Risk factors for the neurologic complications associated with aortic aneurysms, *Arch Neurol* 49:284, 1992.

62. Tyler HR, Clark OB: Neurological complications in patients with coarctation of aorta, *Neurology* 8:712, 1958.

63. Albert ML, Greer WER, Kantrowitz W: Paraplegia secondary to hypotension and cardiac arrest in a patient who has had previous thoracic surgery, *Neurology* 19:915, 1969.

64. Sawaya GR: Spinal cord infarction after cocaine use, *South Med J* 83:601, 1990.

65. Azzarelli B, Roessmann U: Diffuse "anoxic" myelopathy, *Neurology* 27:1049, 1977.

66. Hughes JT, Macintyre AG: Spinal cord infarction occurring during thoraco-lumbar sympathectomy, *J Neurol Neurosurg Psychiatry* 26:418, 1963.

67. MacEwen GD, Bunnell WP, Siram K: Acute neurological complications in the treatment of scoliosis, *J Bone Joint Surg* 57:404, 1975.

68. Blankenship JC: Spinal cord infarction resulting from cardiac catheterization, *Am J Med* 87:239, 1989.

69. Killen DA, Foster JH: Spinal cord injury as a complication of aortography, *Ann Surg* 152:211, 1960.

70. Lyon LW: Transfemoral vertebral angiography as cause of an anterior spinal artery syndrome, *J Neurosurg* 35:328, 1971.

71. Kieffer E, Fukui S, Chivas J, et al: Spinal cord arteriography: A safe adjunct before descending thoracic or thoracoabdominal aortic aneurysmectomy, *J Vasc Surg* 35:262, 2002.

72. LaFerlita BW: Postoperative paraplegia coincident with single shot spinal anaesthesia, *Anaesth Intensive Care* 35:605–607, 2007.

73. Lyders EM, Morris PP: A case of spinal cord infarction following lumbar transforaminal epidural steroid injection: MR imaging and angiographic findings, *AJNR Am J Neuroradiol* 30:1691, 2009.

74. Glaser SE, Falco F: Paraplegia following a thoracolumbar transforaminal epidural steroid injection, *Pain Physician* 8:309–314, 2005.

75. Muro K, O'Shaughnessy B, Ganju A: Infarction of the cervical spinal cord following multilevel transforaminal epidural steroid injection: Case report and review of the literature, *J Spinal Cord Med* 30:385–388, 2007.

76. Burbank SA, Vaccaro AR, Goins ML, et al: Thoracic paraparesis following an embolic vascular event during lumbar spinal surgery, *J Spinal Disord Tech* 19:68-72, 2006.

77. Stevens EA, Powers AK, Morris PP, Wilson JA: Occult dural arteriovenous fistula causing rapidly progressive conus medullaris syndrome and paraplegia after lumbar microdiscectomy, *Spine J* 9:e8-12, 2009.

78. Lee SH, Kim KT, Kim SM, Jo DJ: Extensive spinal cord infarction after surgical interruption of thoracolumbar dural arteriovenous fistula presenting with subarachnoid hemorrhage, *J Korean Neurosurg Soc* 46:60-64, 2009.

79. Kouchoukos NT, Masetti P, Rokkas CK, Murphy SF: Hypothermic cardiopulmonary bypass and circulatory arrest for operations on the descending thoracic and thoracoabdominal aorta, *Ann Thorac Surg* 74:S1885, 2002:discussion S1892.

80. Okita Y, Takamoto S, Ando M, et al: Repair for aneurysms of the entire descending thoracic aorta or thoracoabdominal aorta using a deep hypothermia, *Eur J Cardiothorac Surg* 12:120, 1997.

81. Mehrez IO, Nabseth DC, Hogan EL: Paraplegia following resection of abdominal aortic aneurysm, *Ann Surg* 156:890, 1962.

82. Estrera AL, Miller CC 3rd, Chen EP, et al: Descending thoracic aortic aneurysm repair: 12-year experience using distal aortic perfusion and cerebrospinal fluid drainage, *Ann Thorac Surg* 80:1290-1296, 2005:discussion 1296.

83. Reich MP: Paraplegia following resection of abdominal aortic aneurysm: Report of a case of atheromatous embolization to the anterior spinal artery, *Vasc Surg* 2:230-234, 1968.

84. Miyamoto K, Keno A, Wada T, Kimoto S: A new and simple method of preventing spinal cord damage following temporary occlusion of the thoracic aorta by draining the cerebrospinal fluid, *J Cardiovasc Surg* 16:188, 1960.

85. Brewer LA, Fosburg RG, Mulder GA, Verska JJ: Spinal cord complications following surgery for coarctation of the aorta, *J Thorac Cardiovasc Surg* 64:368, 1972.

86. Easton JD, Saver JL, Albers GW, et al: Definition and evaluation of transient ischemic attack: a scientific statement for healthcare professionals from the American Heart Association/American Stroke Association Stroke Council; Council on Cardiovascular Surgery and Anesthesia; Council on Cardiovascular Radiology and Intervention; Council on Cardiovascular Nursing; and the Interdisciplinary Council on Peripheral Vascular Disease. The American Academy of Neurology affirms the value of this statement as an educational tool for neurologists, *Stroke* 40:2276-2293, 2009.

87. Kendall BE, Andrew J: Neurogenic intermittent claudication associated with aortic steal from the anterior spinal artery complicating coarctation of the aorta, *J Neurosurg* 37:89, 1972.

88. Taylor JR, Van Allen MW: Vascular malformation of the cord with transient ischemic attacks, *J Neurosurg* 31:576, 1969.

89. Zulch KJ, Kurth-Schumacher R: The pathogenesis of "intermittent spinovascular insufficiency" ("spinal claudication of Dejerine") and other vascular syndromes of the spinal cord, *Vasc Surg* 4:116, 1970.

90. Bergmark G: Intermittent spinal claudication, *Acta Med Scand Suppl* 246:30, 1950.

91. Reichert FL, Rytand DA, Bruck EL: Arteriosclerosis of the lumbar segmental arteries producing ischemia of the spinal cord and consequent claudication of the thighs: A clinical syndrome with experimental confirmation, *Am J Med Sci* 187:794, 1934.

92. Neurogenic intermittent claudication [editorial], *BMJ* 1:662, 1969.

93. Wilson CB: Significance of the small lumbar spinal canal: Cauda equina compression syndromes due to spondylosis. III: Intermittent claudication, *J Neurosurg* 31:449, 1969.

94. Garcin R, Godlewski S, Rondot P: Etude clinique de medullopathies d'origine vasculaire, *Rev Neurol (Paris)* 106:558, 1962.

95. Aminoff MJ: Vascular disorders of the spinal cord. In Davidoff RA, editor: *Handbook of the spinal cord*, vol. 4, New York, 1987, Marcel Dekker, p 259.

96. Brish A, Lerner MA, Braham J: Intermittent claudication from compression of cauda equina by a narrowed spinal canal, *J Neurosurg* 21:207, 1964.

97. Blau JN, Logue K: Intermittent claudication of the cauda equina: An unusual syndrome resulting from central protrusion of a lumbar intervertebral disk, *Lancet* 277:1081, 1961.

98. Hancock DO, Phillips DG: Spinal compression in achondroplasia, *Paraplegia* 3:23, 1965.

99. Evans JG: Neurogenic intermittent claudication, *BMJ* 2:985, 1964.

100. Foix C, Alajouanine T: La myelite nécrotique subaige, *Rev Neurol* 36:601, 1926.

101. Clark CE, Cumming WJK: Subacute myelopathy caused by spinal venous infarction, *Postgrad Med J* 63:669, 1987.

102. Chen DH, Lipe HP, Qin Z, Bird TD: Cerebral cavernous malformation: Novel mutation in a Chinese family and evidence for heterogeneity, *J Neurol Sci* 196:91, 2002.

103. Spiller WG: Thrombosis of the cervical anterior median spinal artery: Syphilitic acute anterior poliomyelitis, *J Nerv Ment Dis* 36:601, 1909.

104. Hughes JT: The pathology of vascular disorders of the spinal cord, *Paraplegia* 2:207, 1965.

105. Hughes JT, Brownell B: Spinal cord ischemia due to arteriosclerosis, *Arch Neurol* 15:189, 1966.

106. Van Wieringen A: An unusual cause of occlusion of the anterior spinal artery, *Eur Neurol* 1:363, 1968.

107. Steegmann AT: Syndrome of the anterior spinal artery, *Neurology* 2:15, 1952.

108. Decroix JP, Ciaudo-Lacroix C, Lapresle J: Syndrome de Brown-Séquard du à un infarctus spinal, *Rev Neurol (Paris)* 140:585, 1984.

109. Paine RS, Byers RK: Transverse myelopathy in childhood, *Am J Dis Child* 85:151, 1953.

110. Perier O, Demanet JC, Henneaux J, Vincent AN: Existe-il un syndrome des artères spinales postérieures? À propos de deux observations anatomocliniques, *Rev Neurol* 103:396, 1960.

111. Hughes JT: Thrombosis of the posterior spinal arteries, *Neurology* 20:659, 1970.

112. Hughes JT: Venous infarction of the spinal cord, *Neurology* 21:794, 1971.

113. Kim RC, Smith HR, Henbest ML, Choi BH: Nonhemorrhagic venous infarction of the spinal cord, *Ann Neurol* 15:379, 1984.

114. Heller SL, Meyer JR, Russell EJ: Spinal cord venous infarction following endoscopy sclerotherapy for esophageal varices, *Neurology* 47:1081, 1996.

115. Hui AC, Wong KS, Fu M, Kay R: Ischaemic myelopathy presenting as Guillain-Barré syndrome, *Int J Clin Pract* 54:340, 2000.

116. Bhojo AK, Akhter N, Bakshi R, Wasay U: Thoracic myelopathy complicating acute meningococcal meningitis: MRI findings, *Am J Med Sci* 323:263, 2002.

117. Cheshire WP Jr: Spinal cord infarction mimicking angina pectoris, *Mayo Clin Proc* 75:1197, 2000.

118. Stevinson C, Honan W, Cooke B, Ernst E: Neurological complications of cervical spine manipulation, *J R Soc Med* 94:107, 2001.

119. Vijayan N, Peacock JH: Spinal cord infarction during use of zolmitriptan: A case report, *Headache* 40:57, 2000.

120. Kuker W, Weller M, Klose U, et al: Diffusion-weighted MRI of spinal cord infarction—high resolution imaging and time course of diffusion abnormality, *J Neurol* 251:818-824, 2004.

121. Loher TJ, Bassetti CL, Lovblad KO, et al: Diffusion-weighted MRI in acute spinal cord ischaemia, *Neuroradiology* 45:557-561, 2003.

122. Thurnher MM, Bammer R: Diffusion-weighted MR imaging (DWI) in spinal cord ischemia, *Neuroradiology* 48:795-801, 2006.

123. Amoiridis G, Ameridou I, Mavridis M: Intervertebral disk and vertebral body infarction as a confirmatory sign of spinal cord ischemia, *Neurology* 63:1755, 2004.

124. Bornke C, Schmid G, Szymanski S, Schols L: Vertebral body infarction indicating midthoracic spinal stroke, *Spinal Cord* 40:244-247, 2002.

125. Cheng MY, Lyu RK, Chang YJ, et al: Concomitant spinal cord and vertebral body infarction is highly associated with aortic pathology: A clinical and magnetic resonance imaging study, *J Neurol* 256:1418-1426, 2009.

126. Weidauer S, Dettmann E, Krakow K, Lanfermann H: [Diffusion-weighted MRI of spinal cord infarction. Description of two cases and review of the literature], *Nervenarzt* 73:999, 2002.

127. Stepper F, Lovblad KO: Anterior spinal artery stroke demonstrated by echo-planar DWI, *Eur Radiol* 11:2607, 2001.

128. Reich P, Muller-Schunk S, Leibetrau M, et al: Combined cerebellar and bilateral cervical posterior spinal artery stroke demonstrated on MRI, *Cerebrovasc Dis* 15:143, 2003.

129. Aichner F, Poewe W, Rogalsky W, et al: Magnetic resonance imaging in the diagnosis of spinal cord diseases, *J Neurol Neurosurg Psychiatry* 48:1220, 1985.
130. Elksnis SM, Hogg JP, Cunningham ME: MR imaging of spontaneous spinal cord infarction, *J Comput Assist Tomogr* 15:228, 1991.
131. Fortuna A, Ferrante L, Acqui M, Trillo G: Spinal cord ischemia diagnosed by MRI, *J Neuroradiol* 22:115–122, 1995.
132. Mikulis DJ, Ogilvy CS, McKee A, et al: Spinal cord infarction and fibrocartilaginous emboli, *AJNR Am J Neuroradiol* 13:155–160, 1992.
133. Hamaishi M, Orihashi K, Isaka M, et al: Low-dose edaravone injection into the clamped aorta prevents ischemic spinal cord injury, *Ann Vasc Surg* 23:128–135, 2009.
134. Seren M, Budak B, Turan N, et al: Collaborative therapy with nebivalol and L-NAME for spinal cord ischemia/reperfusion injury, *Ann Vasc Surg* 22:425–431, 2008.
135. Sirlak M, Eryilmaz S, Bahadir Inan M, et al: Effects of carbamazepine on spinal cord ischemia, *J Thorac Cardiovasc Surg* 136:1038–1043, 2008.
136. Yu QJ, Zhou QS, Huang HB, et al: Protective effect of ketamine on ischemic spinal cord injury in rabbits, *Ann Vasc Surg* 22:432–439, 2008.
137. Tofuku K, Koga H, Yamamoto T, Yone K, Komiya S: Spinal cord infarction following endoscopic variceal ligation, *Spinal Cord* 46:241–242, 2008.
138. New P: Inappropriate suggestion of benefit from hyperbaric oxygen for spinal cord injury, *Spinal Cord* 46:824, 2008.
139. Xenos ES, Abedi NN, Davenport DL, et al: Meta-analysis of endovascular vs open repair for traumatic descending thoracic aortic rupture, *J Vasc Surg* 48:1343–1351, 2008.
140. Cina CS, Abouzahr L, Arena GO, et al: Cerebrospinal fluid drainage to prevent paraplegia during thoracic and thoracoabdominal aortic aneurysm surgery: A systematic review and meta-analysis, *J Vasc Surg* 40:36–44, 2004.
141. Hnath JC, Mehta M, Taggert JB, et al: Strategies to improve spinal cord ischemia in endovascular thoracic aortic repair: Outcomes of a prospective cerebrospinal fluid drainage protocol, *J Vasc Surg* 48:836–840, 2008.
142. Wynn MM, Mell MW, Tefera G, Hoch JR, Acher CW: Complications of spinal fluid drainage in thoracoabdominal aortic aneurysm repair: A report of 486 patients treated from 1987 to 2008, *J Vasc Surg* 49:29–34, 2009:discussion 34-25.
143. Estrera AL, Sheinbaum R, Miller CC, et al: Cerebrospinal fluid drainage during thoracic aortic repair: Safety and current management, *Ann Thorac Surg* 88:9–15, 2009:discussion 15.
144. Cheung AT, Pochettino A, Guvakov DV, et al: Safety of lumbar drains in thoracic aortic operations performed with extracorporeal circulation, *Ann Thorac Surg* 76:1190–1196, 2003:discussion 1196-1197.
145. Shine TS, Harrison BA, De Ruyter ML, et al: Motor and somatosensory evoked potentials: Their role in predicting spinal cord ischemia in patients undergoing thoracoabdominal aortic aneurysm repair with regional lumbar epidural cooling, *Anesthesiology* 108:580–587, 2008.
146. Najibi S, Terramani TT, Weiss VJ, et al: Endoluminal versus open treatment of descending thoracic aortic aneurysms, *J Vasc Surg* 36:732, 2002.
147. Grabitz K, Sandmann W, Stuhmeier K, et al: The risk of ischemic spinal cord injury in patients undergoing graft replacement for thoracoabdominal aortic aneurysms, *J Vasc Surg* 23:230–240, 1996.
148. Ogino H, Sasaki H, Minatoya K, et al: Combined use of Adamkiewicz artery demonstration and motor-evoked potentials in descending and thoracoabdominal repair, *Ann Thorac Surg* 82:592–596, 2006.
149. Tabayashi K, Motoyoshi N, Saiki Y, et al: Efficacy of perfusion cooling of the epidural space and cerebrospinal fluid drainage during repair of extent I and II thoracoabdominal aneurysm, *J Cardiovasc Surg (Torino)* 49:749–755, 2008.
150. Wisselink W, Becker MO, Nguyen JH, et al: Protecting the ischemic spinal cord during aortic clamping: The influence of selective hypothermia and spinal cord perfusion pressure, *J Vasc Surg* 19:788–796, 1994.
151. Acher CW, Wynn M: A modern theory of paraplegia in the treatment of aneurysms of the thoracoabdominal aorta: An analysis of technique specific observed/expected ratios for paralysis, *J Vasc Surg* 49:1117–1124, 2009:discussion 1124.
152. Bracken MB, Shepard MJ, Holford TR, et al: Methylprednisolone administered for 24 or 48 hours, or 48 hours tirilazad mesylate, in the treatment of acute spinal cord injury: Results of the third National Acute Spinal Cord Injury randomized controlled trial, *JAMA* 277:1597, 1997.
153. Nedeltchev K, Loher TJ, Stepper F, et al: Long-term outcome of acute spinal cord ischemia syndrome, *Stroke* 35:560–565, 2004.
154. Pelser H, van Gijn J: Spinal infarction: A follow-up study, *Stroke* 24:896, 1993.
155. de Seze M, de Seze M, Joseph PA, et al: [Functional prognosis of paraplegia due to cord ischemia: A retrospective study of 23 patients], *Rev Neurol (Paris)* 159:1038–1045, 2003.
156. Salvador de la Barrera S, Barca-Buyo A, Montoto-Marques A, et al: Spinal cord infarction: Prognosis and recovery in a series of 36 patients, *Spinal Cord* 39:520–525, 2001.
157. Shakir RA, Sulaiman K, Kahn RA, Rudwan M: Neurological presentation of neuro-Behçet's syndrome: Clinical categories, *Eur Neurol* 30:249, 1990.
158. Gibb WRG, Urry PA, Lees AJ: Giant cell arteritis with spinal cord infarction and basilar artery thrombosis, *J Neurol Neurosurg Psychiatry* 48:945, 1985.
159. Imaizumi H, Ujike Y, Asai Y, et al: Spinal cord ischemia after cardiac arrest, *J Emerg Med* 12:789–793, 1994.
160. Rajan RK: Ischemic myelopathy following cardiac arrest, *Am Fam Physician* 29:221, 1984.
161. Keith WS: Traumatic infarction of the spinal cord, *Can J Neurol Sci* 1:124, 1974.
162. Thompson GB: Dissecting aortic aneurysm with infarction of the spinal cord, *Brain* 79:111, 1956.
163. Gang DL, Dole KB, Adelman LS: Spinal cord infarction following therapeutic renal artery embolization, *JAMA* 237:2841, 1977.
164. Lemke RP, Idiong N, Al-Saedi S, et al: Spinal cord infarct after arterial switch associated with an umbilical artery catheter, *Ann Thorac Surg* 62:1532, 1996.
165. Leibovitch I, Nash PA, Little JS, et al: Spinal cord ischemia after postchemotherapy retroperitoneal lymph node dissection for nonseminomatous germ cell cancer, *J Urol* 155:947, 1996.
166. von Pohle WR: Disseminated mucormycosis presenting with lower extremity weakness, *Eur Respir J* 9:1751, 1996.
167. Mathew P, Todd NV, Hadley DM, Adams JH: Spinal cord infarction following meningitis, *Br J Neurosurg* 7:701, 1993.
168. Rothman SM, Nelson JS: Spinal cord infarction in a patient with sickle cell anemia, *Neurology* 30:1072, 1980.
169. Rudar M, Urbanke A, Radonic M: Occlusion of the abdominal aorta with dysfunction of the spinal cord, *Ann Intern Med* 56:490, 1962.
170. Hasegawa M, Yamashita J, Yamashima T, et al: Spinal cord infarction associated with primary antiphospholipid syndrome in a young child, *J Neurosurg* 79:446, 1993.
171. Slot WB, Van Kasteel V, Coerkamp EG, et al: Severe thrombotic complications in a postpartum patient with active Crohn's disease resulting in ischemic spinal cord injury, *Dig Dis Sci* 40:1395, 1995.
172. Grinker RR, Guy CC: Sprain of cervical spine causing thrombosis of anterior spinal artery, *JAMA* 88:1140, 1927.

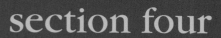

Specific Medical Diseases and Stroke

J. P. MOHR

For this, the fifth edition of *Stroke,* the authors in this section have updated their chapters and, in some cases, have written entirely new chapters on the aspects of a given disease that relate to stroke.

The topics chosen represent the major disease processes for which stroke is a prominent part of the clinical picture. Other diseases associated with stroke also exist, but the chosen list was considered to be the most important. Detailed description of the management of these diseases is deferred to the chapters on therapy.

The authors of some of the chapters in earlier editions have graciously added or even given way to new contributors.

Arterial Dissections and Fibromuscular Dysplasia

RICHARD M. ZWEIFLER, GERALD SILVERBOARD

Arterial Dissections
Epidemiology

Cervicocerebral arterial dissections account for approximately 2% of all ischemic strokes, but they are among the most important causes of stroke in young and middle-aged patients.[1-6] Most patients with dissection are between 30 and 50 years of age, with a mean age of approximately 40 years.[3,4] In patients younger than 45 years, arterial dissection is the second leading cause of stroke, accounting for 10% to 25% of ischemic strokes.[6-9] Although older studies reveal no overall gender predilection in adults, a 2006 study of 696 patients with spontaneous cervicocerebral dissection found a preponderance in males.[10] Females with arterial dissection are approximately 5 years younger at the time of dissection.[3,10] Childhood arterial dissections are unique in that they occur more commonly in boys.[11,12]

Population-based studies have reported the incidence of dissection as ranging from 2.6 to 2.9 cases per 100,000 per year.[2,3] The true incidence of cervicocerebral arterial dissection is likely higher than these estimates, however, because asymptomatic patients and patients with pain but no neurologic symptoms are underdiagnosed.[13] The annual incidence of cervical internal carotid artery (ICA) dissection was 3.5 per 100,000 in those older than 20 years in a Mayo Clinic series.[3] Seventy percent of cervical internal carotid dissections occur in patients between 35 and 50 years of age, with a mean age at presentation of 44 years; there is no sex predilection.[14] Patients with intracranial carotid dissection tend to be younger than those with cervical dissections. In a review of 59 reported cases of intracranial carotid dissection, the mean age at onset was 30 years, and there was a slight male predominance.[15] The annual incidence of spontaneous vertebral artery dissection is one third of ICA dissections,[5,16-18] with estimates of 1 to 1.5 per 100,000.[19] Extracranial vertebral artery dissection is more common, accounting for up to 15% of the reported cases of cervicocerebral dissection, whereas dissection of the intracranial vertebral artery is uncommon, accounting for approximately 5%.[20] The mean age at onset of intracranial vertebral dissection is the late 40s for isolated dissection and the late 30s for dissection with extension to the basilar artery.[21-24] In contrast to extracranial carotid and vertebral artery dissections, intracranial vertebral artery dissections are more common in men than in women.[21,25]

Pathology

Arterial dissections usually arise from an intimal tear that allows the development of an intramural hematoma (false lumen) (Figs. 33-1 and 33-2). In some patients, no communication between the true and false lumens can be demonstrated, suggesting that some dissections are the result of a primary intramedial hematoma. Furthermore, intimal disruption could occur as a result of rupture of a primary intramural hematoma into the intima. Although it is likely that the former mechanism is more common, both could occur.

The intramural hematoma is located within the layers of the tunica media but may be eccentric toward the intima (subintimal dissection) or adventitia (subadventitial dissection). Subintimal dissections are more likely to cause luminal stenosis, whereas subadventitial dissections may cause arterial dilatation (aneurysm). These aneurysms are often referred to as "false aneurysms" or "pseudoaneurysms," but they are true aneurysms because their walls contain blood vessel elements (i.e., media and adventitia)[19]; they are better termed "dissecting" aneurysms.[26,27] The absence of an external elastic lamina and a thin adventitia makes intracranial arteries prone to subadventitial dissection and subsequent subarachnoid hemorrhage (SAH). SAH is reported in about one fifth of intracranial ICA dissections and in more than half of intracranial vertebral artery dissections.[11,21,23,24,28-32]

Pathogenesis

The pathogenesis of most spontaneous arterial dissections is unknown. Dissections can be iatrogenic or due to severe trauma, in which cases the causes are obvious, but most occur spontaneously or are associated with antecedent trivial trauma. Precipitating events reported to antedate dissection include sudden head movement, coughing, vomiting, sneezing, chiropractic manipulation, performing yoga, painting a ceiling, vigorous nose blowing, sexual activity, anesthesia administration, resuscitation, and many types of sports activity.[33-49] Such activities may cause arterial injury due to mechanical stretching. A prospective study found that 81% of dissections were associated with some form of sudden neck movement.[36] Estimates of dissection risk following chiropractic manipulation vary widely with study methodology but range from 1 in 5.85 million manipulations[37] to as many as 1 in 20,000 manipulations.[50] One study found connective

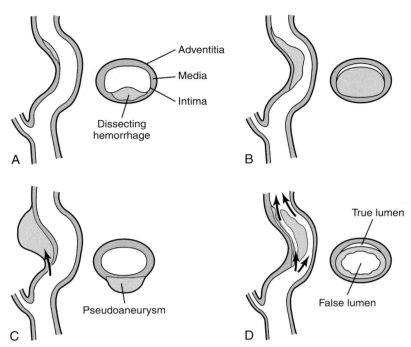

Figure 33-1 Anatomy of dissections. A, Lateral *(left)* and cross-sectional *(right)* schematic views of internal carotid artery demonstrate initial phase of intramedial and subintimal dissecting aneurysm; the three basic arterial layers (intima, media, and adventitia) are delineated. B, Comparable views of the progression of intramedial hemorrhage; the arterial lumen is reduced in size. C, Comparable views of an intramedial hemorrhage that dissects into the subadventitial rather than the subintimal plane, as in A and B; a large pseudoaneurysm results. D, Dissecting hemorrhage ruptures through the intima, establishing communication with the true lumen; recanalization may occur, enlarging the true or false lumen. (From Friedman AH, Day AL, Quisling RGJ, et al: Cervical carotid dissecting aneurysms. *Neurosurgery 7*:207, 1980.)

tissue disorders in one fourth of patients with cervical artery dissection after chiropractic manipulation.[51]

An underlying arteriopathy has been postulated to lead to structural instability of the arterial wall. Fibromuscular dysplasia (FMD) is found in approximately 15% to 20% of all patients with cervicocephalic dissection and is seen in more than half of those with bilateral carotid involvement.[3,52-57] From 1% to 5% of patients have an identifiable heritable connective tissue disorder,[58] such as Ehlers-Danlos syndrome type IV,[59-61] Marfan's syndrome,[54,55,62,63] autosomal dominant polycystic kidney disease,[55] osteogenesis imperfecta type I,[55] pseudoxanthoma elasticum,[55,64] type I collagen point mutation,[65] or alpha$_1$-antitrypsin deficiency.[66] Dissection has also been associated with other arteriopathies such as cystic medial necrosis[3,67] and moyamoya disease.[68-70] The associations with arterial redundancies (e.g., coils, kinks, and loops),[71,72] increased arterial distensibility,[73] widened aortic root,[74] and intracranial aneurysms[75,76] provide indirect evidence of an underlying arteriopathy.

Five percent of patients with spontaneous cervicocephalic dissection have at least one family member with a spontaneous dissection of the aorta or its main branches, including the vertebral and carotid arteries.[77] Atherosclerosis does not appear to be a risk factor.[27] Other reported risk factors for dissection are migraine,[78-80] recent infection,[81-83] pregnancy,[84,85] hyperhomocyst(e)inemia,[86,87] smoking,[27,88] hypertension,[27,89] and oral contraceptive use.[27] The possibility of an infectious etiology is supported by the reported seasonal variation of cervical artery dissection, with a 58% increase in frequency in the autumn.[56] Schievink and colleagues[90,91] have reported familial associations between dissection and multiple cutaneous lentigines and bicuspid aortic valves, suggesting an underlying neural crest defect.

Ultrastructural aberrations of dermal collagen fibrils and elastic fibers have been reported in 54% to 68% of patients with spontaneous cervical artery dissection in whom there is no clinical evidence of a known connective tissue disorder,[92-94] suggesting a molecular defect in the biosynthesis of the extracellular matrix.[95] Evidence of a generalized arteriopathy was reported by Volker and colleagues[96] in an ultrastructural study of superficial temporal artery specimens in patients with spontaneous cervicocephalic dissection. A study of skin biopsy specimens from healthy relatives of patients with dissection indicates a familial occurrence of connective tissue abnormalities.[97] No genetic mutation responsible for the majority of cases of cervical artery dissection has been identified.[93] Results of screening for mutations in the genes for type V procollagen (COL5A1),[98] type III collagen (COL3A1),[99,100] and tropoelastin (ELN)[101] have been negative.

Despite an association with many disorders (Table 33-1), the precise cause of cervicocephalic dissection remains unknown in most cases. The pathogenesis is likely multifactorial, with mechanical factors and underlying arteriopathy, possibly genetic or infectious, playing roles.

Sites of Dissection

Dissection of the extracranial carotid and vertebral arteries accounts for approximately 80% to 90% of all cervicocephalic dissections.[102,103] This disparity may be

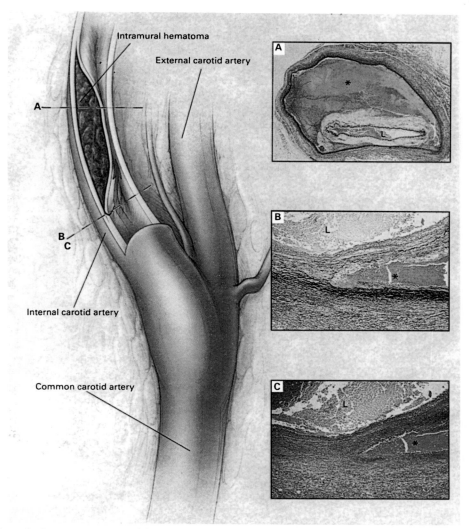

Figure 33-2 Pathologic findings in a 37-year-old woman with a dissection of the internal carotid artery. Photomicrographs of the right extracranial internal carotid artery (A through C) show a dissection within the outer layers of the tunica media, resulting in stenosis of the arterial lumen (L). The *dashed lines* on the left indicate the sites of the photomicrographs. A, The intramural hemorrhage (*) extends almost entirely around the artery (van Gieson stain, ×4). B and C, Higher-power views of the internal carotid artery at the point of dissection show fragmentation of elastic tissue (B; van Gieson stain, ×25), with the accumulation of pale ground-glass substance in the tunica media, indicated by the blue-staining mucopolysaccharides (C; Alcian blue, ×25). These changes are consistent with a diagnosis of cystic medial necrosis. (From Schievink WI: Spontaneous dissection of the carotid and vertebral arteries. *N Engl J Med* 344:898, 2001.)

explained by the greater mobility of the extracranial segments and the potential for injury by contact with bony structures such as the transverse processes of the upper cervical vertebrae and the styloid process (Fig. 33-3).[14] Extracranial ICA dissection typically occurs at least 2 cm distal to the bifurcation, near the C2-C3 vertebral level, and extends superiorly for a variable distance. It usually terminates before the artery enters the petrous bone, where mechanical support appears to limit further dissection in the majority of cases.[14] This location is distinct from that of atherosclerosis, which most commonly affects the ICA origin or the siphon. The vertebral artery is most mobile, and most susceptible to mechanical injury, at the C1-C2 level, as it leaves the transverse foramen of the axis and abruptly turns to enter the intracranial cavity (the V3 segment) (Fig. 33-4). The C1-C2 site is involved in one half to two thirds of all vertebral artery dissections and in 80% to 90% of rotation-related dissections.[17,104-107]

Intracranial arterial dissection is more common in children and adolescents than in adults, although intracranial dissection in children usually affects the anterior circulation, and intracranial posterior circulation dissection is more common in adults.[11] The most commonly involved intracranial sites are the supraclinoid segment of the ICA and the middle cerebral artery stem.[108,109] The most common site of intracranial vertebral artery dissection is the V4 segment at or near the origin of the posterior inferior cerebellar artery. At this level, the artery may be compressed during head maneuvers, the media and adventitia diminish in size and elastic components, and the external elastic lamina terminates. Approximately 20% of vertebral artery dissections involve both the extracranial and intracranial segments.[110]

TABLE 33-1 PREDISPOSING FACTORS FOR CERVICOCEPHALIC DISSECTION

Trauma
　Mild or trivial
　Major
　Iatrogenic
Arteriopathies
　Fibromuscular dysplasia
　Cystic medial necrosis
　Ehlers-Danlos syndrome type IV
　Marfan's syndrome
　Type I collagen point mutation
　Alpha$_1$-antitrypsin deficiency
　Osteogenesis imperfecta type I
　Pseudoxanthoma elasticum
　Autosomal-dominant polycystic kidney disease
　Moyamoya disease
　Redundancies (e.g., coils, kinks, and loops)
　Intracranial aneurysms
Migraine
Family history
Recent infection
Hyperhomocyst(e)inemia
Less well established
　Hypertension
　Pregnancy
　Smoking
　Oral contraceptives

Mechanisms of Ischemia

Cervicocephalic dissection can cause ischemic symptoms due to hemodynamic compromise secondary to luminal narrowing or occlusion, thromboembolism, or both. Several reports investigating the pattern of infarction in patients with carotid dissection indicate that most strokes are the result of distal embolization.[111-115] A high incidence of middle cerebral artery microemboli correlating with stroke symptoms has been found in patients with carotid artery dissection, further supporting a thromboembolic mechanism.[116]

Clinical Manifestations

Extracranial Carotid Artery Dissection

Local signs and symptoms: The major presenting features of extracranial carotid dissection are pain in the ipsilateral head, face, or neck associated with focal ischemic symptoms (cerebral or retinal). In about one third of cases, partial Horner's syndrome is present. Saver and Easton[20] summarized the clinical, radiologic, and prognostic features of 635 patients reported in the literature (Table 33-2).

Pain (in head, face, or neck) is the most common overall symptom, present in more than 80% of symptomatic cases, and is the initial presenting symptom in one half to two thirds of patients.[11,20,52,113,115,117-125]

Headache, present in 60% to 75% of patients, may precede other signs or symptoms by hours or weeks.[111,115,118,121,124,126] The pain is typically ipsilateral over the anterior head but may be more diffuse or bilateral, even with unilateral dissection.[79,124,127] Onset of headache is usually gradual, although sudden "thunderclap"

headache has been reported.[124,127] The headache is usually nonthrobbing and severe, and ipsilateral scalp tenderness may occur.[79,124,127] Unilateral neck pain is present in 20% to 30% of patients and may involve the anterior neck with radiation toward the ear, scalp, jaw, face, or pharynx.[111,115,124] Facial or orbital pain has been reported in more than 50% of cases.[124]

Ipsilateral partial oculosympathetic paresis (Horner's syndrome), present in approximately one third of patients, results from involvement of sympathetic fibers of the internal carotid plexus.[115,121,124] Ptosis and miosis are seen, but facial sweating remains intact (except for a focal area of the ipsilateral forehead) because the majority of sympathetic fibers supplying the face travel with the external carotid artery.[27]

Cranial nerve palsies have been reported in 12% of patients with spontaneous ICA dissection.[128] Lower cranial nerve palsies are most common and are found in approximately 5% to 10% of patients.[115,124,128] Figure 33-5 displays the anatomic relationship of the lower cranial nerves and the carotid artery. The most commonly affected cranial nerve is CN XII, followed in frequency by nerves IX, X, XI, and V.[124,128-134] The facial, oculomotor, abducens, and trochlear nerves may also be involved.[124,128,135] Dysgeusia is reported in about 10%.[124] Pulsatile tinnitus or a subjective bruit is reported in up to one fourth of patients, and an objective bruit may be heard in nearly one fifth.[52,64,124,136]

Ischemic signs and symptoms: Ischemic manifestations have been reported in 50% to 95% of patients,[115,118,124] although the highest rates were reported in older studies. At the time of the earlier reports, the diagnosis of dissection was typically suspected only in the presence of ischemic signs, and noninvasive diagnostic techniques were not available.[118] Most ischemic symptoms occur within 1 week of the onset of pain[118,124,126]; one study reported a median delay in the appearance of other symptoms of 4 days.[124] A 1998 case report describes a disabling stroke occurring 5 months after traumatic ICA dissection, although the patient did suffer a silent stroke at the time of the dissection.[137] Most infarctions are territorial (as opposed to borderzone), supporting an emboligenic etiology.[111-115] Transient ischemic attacks (TIAs) are common, being reported in about 50% of patients, and they are recurrent in half of the cases.[118] Of patients with stroke, approximately 75% report at least one preceding TIA.[118] Transient monocular blindness occurs in one fourth of cases.[124] Other ischemic ocular syndromes, such as central retinal artery occlusion and anterior ischemic optic neuropathy, are rare.[102,138,139]

Baumgartner and associates[115] have reported that dissections causing ischemic events are more often associated with occlusions and stenosis greater than 80%, and that dissections that do not cause ischemic events are more often associated with Horner's syndrome and lower cranial nerve palsies.

Intracranial Carotid and Middle Cerebral Artery Dissection

As noted previously, dissection of the intracranial ICA and its branches occurs in younger patients than extracranial dissection. A male preponderance has been

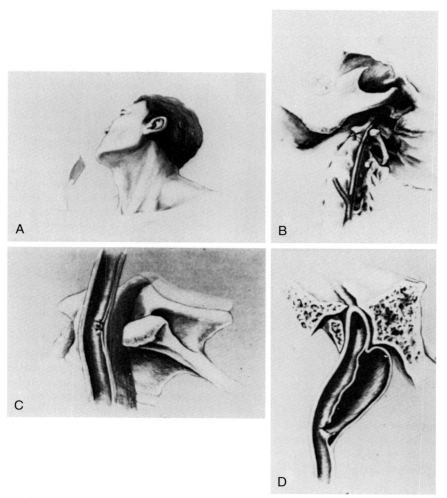

Figure 33-3 Presumed mechanism of carotid injury induced by neck rotation. A, Direction of hyperextension. B, Impingement of artery on the process of the vertebra. C, Intimal tear caused by impingement. D, Progression of intimal tear to dissection. (From Stringer WL, Kelly DLJ: Traumatic dissection of the extracranial internal carotid artery. *Neurosurgery* 6:123, 1980.)

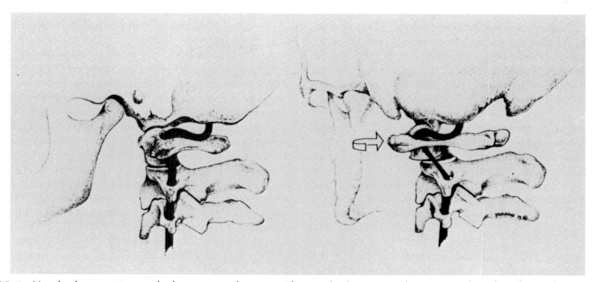

Figure 33-4 Vertebral artery injury with abrupt cervical rotation. The vertebral artery is subject to stretch and mechanical trauma between C1 and C2 when the neck is vigorously rotated and extended. (From Barnett HJM: Progress towards stroke prevention. *Neurology [NY]* 30:1212, 1980.)

TABLE 33-2 CLINICAL FEATURES OF EXTRACRANIAL CAROTID DISSECTION

No. of cases	635
Age	Mean 44.4 yr
	Range 4-74 yr
Sex	
Male	53%
Female	47%
Laterality	
Unilateral	86%
Left	60%
Right	40%
Bilateral	14%
*Major presenting complaint**	
Cerebral infarction	46%
Transient ischemic attack	30%
Neck or head pain	21%
Pulsatile tinnitus only	2%
Asymptomatic bruit only	2%
Associated features at diagnosis	
Symptoms	
Neck pain	20%
Headache	64%
Neck or head pain	67%
Tinnitus or subjective bruit	3%
Signs	
Partial Horner's syndrome	32%
Cervical bruit	18%
Linguinal paresis	6%
Early outcome	
Angiographic	
Normal or mildly stenotic vessel on follow-up imaging	70%
Clinical	
Neurologically normal	50%
Mild deficits only	21%
Moderate to severe deficits	25%
Death	4%

*Major presenting complaint leading to evaluation, not necessarily the initial symptom.
Data from references 11, 20, 117, 119, 120, 122, 123, 125, 191.

reported.[15] Severe unilateral headache is almost universally present, and ischemic symptoms typically occur with a much shorter delay (within minutes or hours) than in extracranial dissection. Seizures or syncope can be the presenting symptom, and half the patients have altered level of consciousness.[20] Three quarters of cases involve the supraclinoid ICA or the middle cerebral artery stem; the anterior cerebral artery is infrequently involved.[11,140] Although reported, bilateral dissections occur less commonly in the intracranial circulation than in the extracranial circulation.[70,109,141,142] SAH, resulting from subadventitial hematoma rupture through the external vessel wall, occurs in approximately 20% of cases.[15,109,143]

Extracranial Vertebral Artery Dissection

Saver and Easton[20] have previously summarized the clinical features and course of 174 cases of extracranial vertebral dissection from the literature (Table 33-3).

Local signs and symptoms: Headache occurs in one half to two thirds of patients with extracranial vertebral dissection and is typically ipsilateral and occipital.[20,106,110,124,144-146] The pain can be either throbbing or pressure-like.[124] Neck pain occurs in approximately half of patients and is typically gradual in onset.[20,106,110,124,144-147] The pain is usually unilateral but is bilateral in one third of cases.[124] Pulsatile tinnitus occurs less commonly with extracranial vertebral artery dissection than with extracranial ICA dissection.[110,136]

Ischemic signs and symptoms: The majority of patients with vertebral artery dissection have ischemic symptoms, although this fact may reflect an underdiagnosis of patients without ischemic manifestations. The median intervals between onsets of neck pain and headache and the development of ischemic symptoms are 2 weeks and 15 hours, respectively.[124] TIA has been reported to precede stroke in 13% of cases.[107] Lateral medullary signs and symptoms may be seen in isolation or in combination with other brainstem, posterior cerebral artery distribution, or upper cervical spinal cord findings.[14,52,107,124,148-152] Cervical radiculopathy (most commonly at C5-C6) has been reported, although it is unclear whether the etiology is ischemic or mechanical.[149,150]

Intracranial Vertebral and Basilar Artery Dissections

Intracranial vertebral artery dissection is distinguished clinically from extracranial dissection by the former's association with SAH. Coexistent SAH has been reported to occur in as many as one half to two thirds of adult cases,[21,23,24,28-32] but the association has not been reported in children.[11] Basilar artery dissections are rare. They may be isolated (primary) or associated with concomitant vertebral artery dissection. Clinical manifestations vary according to the extent of involvement. Primary basilar dissection typically manifests as rapidly progressive brainstem signs, although it can manifest as headache and more slowly developing focal signs or as a mass lesion due to intravascular hematoma.[25,29,109,110,143,153-178] Like other intracranial dissections, basilar artery dissections can manifest as SAH and dissecting aneurysm if the dissection plane is subadventitial or transmural.[29,109,143, 154,155, 159,163,164,172]

Diagnosis

When clinical presentation suggests cerebrovascular arterial dissection, whether spontaneous or traumatic in occurrence, an aggressive diagnostic approach is immediately warranted. The combination of MRI and MR angiography (MRA) are at present the most direct noninvasive modalities for confirmation of arterial dissection.[19, 179-186] In the traumatized patient in whom transport to an MRI unit may be an issue, carotid ultrasonography, transcranial Doppler (TCD) ultrasonography, or both can provide direct or indirect evidence of dissection.[187-193] Helical CT angiography (CTA) is also noninvasive and may be particularly advantageous in the traumatized patient with suspected arterial dissection.[194,195] Conventional angiography remains a mainstay in accurately defining the exact level and arterial territory of dissection and for imaging complications associated with dissection, such as pseudoaneurysm, double lumen, and presence of intraluminal or distal clot.[9,31,103,183,196] Neuroendovascular therapy,

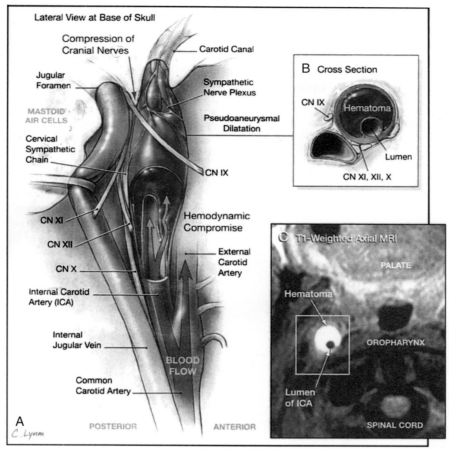

Figure 33-5 Anatomy of carotid artery dissection. A, Diagram demonstrating hematoma tracking into the vessel wall, resulting in a long segment of narrowing distal to the carotid artery bifurcation. B, Pseudoaneurysmal dilatation of the carotid artery at the base of the skull due to dissection may injure adjacent lower cranial nerves. C, T1-weighted axial magnetic resonance image of the upper neck. The hematoma in the wall of the internal carotid artery appears as a bright crescent around the residual vessel lumen (appearing as a dark flow void in the center of the vessel). CN, cranial nerve. (From Wityk RJ: Stroke in a healthy 46-year-old man. *JAMA* 285:2757, 2001.)

including balloon angioplasty and placement of stents and coils, is an option that may be performed in tandem with conventional angiography.

Ultrasonography

The combination of extracranial carotid B-mode imaging and carotid color-flow Doppler ultrasonography combined with TCD ultrasonography offers the most reliable systematic ultrasound investigation.[116,122,126,187-193,197] Extracranial vertebral artery dissection may also be diagnosed through a multimodal ultrasound approach.[197] Indirect rather than direct evidence of extracranial carotid artery dissection is often more prominent on ultrasound because extracranial carotid artery dissection typically occurs 2 cm or more distal to the carotid bulb, the latter being the more common site of atherosclerotic abnormalities.[20,188] Decrease or absence of flow velocities in the affected vessel, retrograde flow in supraorbital vessels, or bidirectional ICA flow suggests more distal obstruction or moderate- to high-grade stenosis resulting from dissection.[198] Direct ultrasound visualization of tapering of the ICA lumen may be achieved, as well as presence of true and false lumens with an intraluminal flap in 15% of cases (Figs. 33-6 and 33-7).[188,191]

Extracranial color-flow duplex ultrasonography has been effective in detecting abnormalities in extracranial vertebral artery dissection, similarly demonstrating indirect evidence of absence, reduction, or reversal of flow in the vertebral artery or, rarely, direct evidence of intimal hemorrhage.[189,190,197] The severity of stenosis and the presence of occlusion and site of dissection significantly affect the sensitivity and specificity of ultrasound in extracranial carotid and vertebral artery dissection.[188] Insonating the high cervical (retromandibular) region in extracranial carotid artery dissection and stepwise segmental insonation of the vertebral artery in extracranial vertebral artery dissection improve detection of suspected dissection.[20,188] TCD ultrasonography delineates flow abnormalities distal to vascular luminal narrowing or occlusion by dissection, including signs of carotid-carotid collateral cross-flow; artery-to-artery embolic middle cerebral artery stem occlusion is suggested when the middle cerebral artery signal is absent and the ipsilateral anterior cerebral and posterior cerebral artery velocities are increased.[20,193] Serial examinations of extracranial carotid and vertebral artery dissection for spontaneous or therapy-based recanalization with these ultrasound

TABLE 33-3 CLINICAL FEATURES OF EXTRACRANIAL VERTEBRAL DISSECTION

No. of cases	174
Age	Mean 38.9 yr
	Range 3-67 yr
Sex	
Male	43%
Female	57%
Laterality	
Unilateral	69%
Left	56%
Right	44%
Bilateral	31%
Clinical features at presentation *	
Cerebral infarction	75%
At onset	17%
Delayed	83%
Transient ischemic attack	25%
Neck pain	55%
Headache	53%
Head or neck pain	75%
Lateral medullary symptoms	33%
Associated conditions	
Hypertension	25%
Migraine	13%
Oral contraceptives (among women)	24%
Fibromuscular dysplasia	17%
Early outcome	
Angiographic	
Normal or mildly stenotic vessel on follow-up imaging	78%
Clinical	
Neurologically normal or mild deficits only	83%
Moderate to severe deficits	11%
Death	6%

*Major presenting complaint leading to evaluation, not necessarily the initial symptom.
Data from references 20, 144, 145, 146.

techniques allow outpatient monitoring and the use of clinical decision algorithms.[188-191,197,199]

Magnetic Resonance Imaging

MRI coupled with MRA currently offers sophisticated noninvasive imaging of cerebrovascular arterial dissection. Simultaneous definition of the brain and the major cervical and intracranial arteries is achieved with conventional T1- and T2-weighted and fluid attenuation inversion recovery (FLAIR) axial MRI with three-dimensional time-of-flight (TOF) MRA (Fig. 33-8). The typical abnormalities associated with dissection are most easily defined in extracranial carotid (Fig. 33-9) and vertebral artery dissection, whereas intracranial arterial dissection imaging often shows less specific abnormalities.[20] Characteristic imaging findings on MRI in extracranial carotid artery dissection include diminution or absence of signal flow void and a crescent sign, owing to narrowing of the vessel by intramural dissection of blood, which appears in a semilunar fashion as a spiraling periarterial rim of intramural hematoma in cross section on T1-weighted and fluid attenuation inversion recovery axial MR images (see Figs. 33-5C, 33-8, and 33-9).[19,20,179-186,200-203]

The intensity of the hematoma on T1- and T2-weighted images depends on the age of the dissection, because the hyperintense signal corresponds to intramural hematoma with methemoglobin signal intensity; in some dissections, all or part of the intramural hematoma appears hypointense on T2-weighted images as a result of acute clot deoxyhemoglobin or hemosiderin in the chronic type.[116] Subtle abnormalities also include (1) high signal intensity from the entire vessel, (2) significant compromise of the vessel lumen by adjoining tissue with abnormally increased signal, (3) enlargement of the vessel diameter, and (4) poor or no visualization of the vessel. Fat suppression techniques are important to differentiate small intramural hematomas from surrounding soft

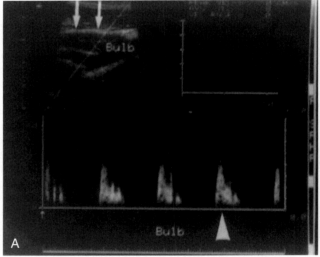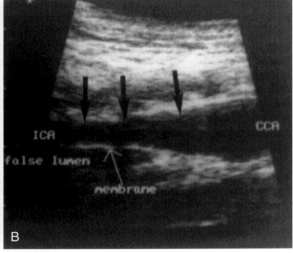

Figure 33-6 A, Duplex ultrasonogram demonstrates a patent bulb without atherosclerotic wall changes *(arrows)*. Doppler sample in the bulb demonstrates only short systolic flow signal without diastolic flow (stump flow) *(arrowhead)*. B, B-mode ultrasonogram of bulb and proximal internal carotid artery shows tapering luminal narrowing *(black arrows)* and a membrane *(white arrow)* separating true from false lumen. (From Sturzenegger M: Spontaneous internal carotid artery dissection: Early diagnosis and management in 44 patients. *J Neurol* 242:231, 1995.)

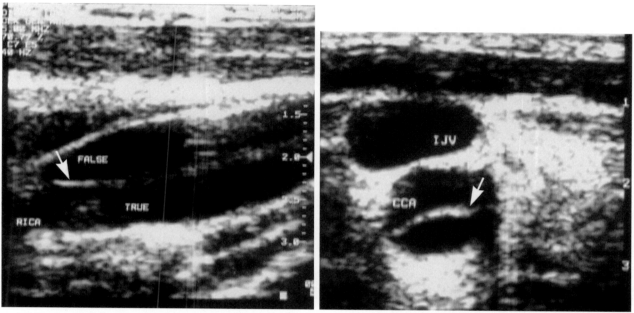

Figure 33-7 B-mode ultrasonography images of a carotid artery dissection demonstrating the true (TRUE) and false (FALSE) lumens separated by a membrane *(arrows)*. CCA, cervical carotid artery; IJV, internal jugular vein; RICA, right internal carotid artery. (Courtesy of Christine Miles, RVT.)

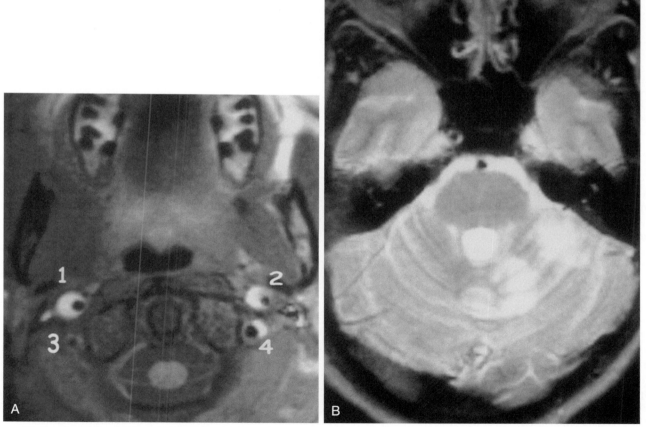

Figure 33-8 T1-weighted (A) and T2-weighted (B) axial MR images from a patient with vertigo and ataxia who was found to have a spontaneous four-vessel dissection. Note the crescents of methemoglobin in the walls of all the cerebral vessels. A, Dissection in the right internal carotid artery (1), left internal carotid artery (2), right vertebral artery (3), and left vertebral artery (4). The findings in the right vertebral artery (3) are subtle. B, Multiple cerebellar infarcts. (From Silverboard G, Tart R: Cerebrovascular arterial dissection in children and young adults. *Semin Pediatr Neurol* 7:278, 2000.)

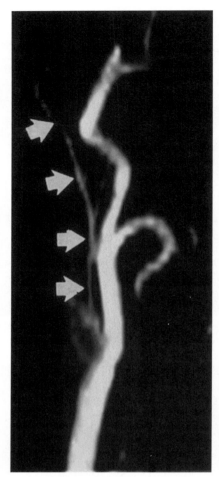

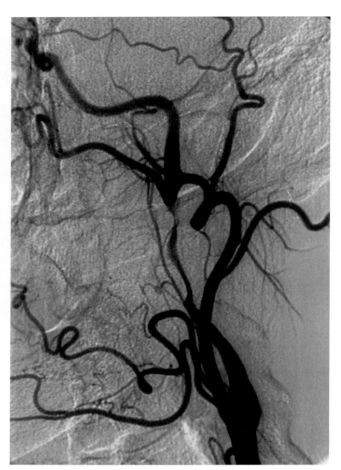

Figure 33-9 Lateral projection from an MR angiogram of a segmented cervical carotid artery, demonstrating complete occlusion of the high cervical portion of the internal carotid artery (arrows). This spontaneous dissection manifested as a minor stroke. The patient made a near-complete recovery with anticoagulation therapy. (From Silverboard G, Tart R: Cerebrovascular arterial dissection in children and young adults. *Semin Pediatr Neurol 7*:278, 2000.)

Figure 33-10 Digital subtraction angiogram (lateral view) showing irregular narrowing of the left internal carotid artery beginning approximately 3 cm distal to the bifurcation in a 38-year-old woman who presented with expressive aphasia and right hemiparesis. Note that the dissection terminates at the skull base, with a normal-appearing intracranial internal carotid artery.

tissues.[19] In the absence of significant luminal stenosis or compromise, MRI may detect carotid dissection missed by conventional angiography; however, MRI may fail to demonstrate mural hematoma even though associated vessel wall thickening is present. The pattern of stroke associated with extracranial carotid artery dissection is predominantly cortical (83%) and subcortical (60%) with the middle cerebral artery territory affected in 99%, the anterior cerebral artery territory in 4%, and the posterior cerebral artery territory in 3%, with borderzone infarcts in 5% of cases.[114,115] In extracranial carotid artery dissection, MRA in tandem with MRI constitutes the diagnostic study of choice, with sensitivity and specificity of 95% and 99%, respectively, for MRA and 84% and 99%, respectively, for MRI.[20,184] Dissecting aneurysms may be missed in the acute stage by three-dimensional time-of-flight MRA if the hematoma is isointense.[183]

Intracranial carotid arterial dissection produces less specific abnormalities on noninvasive studies, although MRI may demonstrate intramural hematoma.[20,204,205] The presence of SAH, occurring in one fifth of cases, is notable

and may clinically suggest dissection; however, cerebral angiography rather than MRI-MRA is the standard for diagnosis of intracranial carotid artery dissection.[20,31,103,110]

The extracranial vertebral artery distribution is the second most common site of dissection, typically at the C1-C2 site. Although unilateral extracranial vertebral artery dissection may go unrecognized owing to collateral flow by the uninvolved vertebral artery, bilateral vertebral artery dissection is well recognized. It may be associated with cerebellar, brainstem, or hemispheric infarction, which is demonstrated on routine MRI; concurrent carotid artery dissections may also occur.[20,110,206,207] The entire spectrum of MRI-MRA findings seen in extracranial carotid artery dissection may occur in extracranial vertebral artery dissection, although these two modalities are not as sensitive in extracranial vertebral artery dissection. One study reported sensitivity and specificity for MRI of 60% and 98% in extracranial carotid artery dissection and extracranial vertebral artery dissection, respectively, and 20% and 100%, respectively, for MRA.[184] Conventional angiography or CTA is warranted if MRI-MRA findings are nondiagnostic in spite of a high clinical index of suspicion for extracranial vertebral artery dissection.

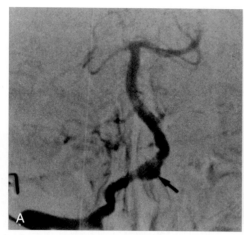
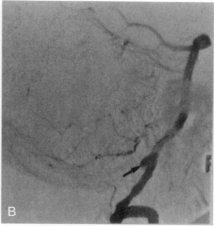

Figure 33-11   Vertebral angiography. A, Anteroposterior view showing right irregular aneurysm *(arrow)* with proximal narrowing. B, Lateral view. Aneurysm is more obvious *(arrow)*. (From Caplan LR, Baquis GD, Pessin MS, et al: Dissection of the intracranial vertebral artery. *Neurology* 38:868, 1988.)

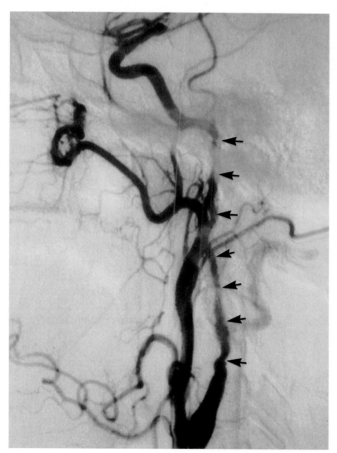

Figure 33-12   Lateral view from a digital subtraction angiogram showing the high cervical internal carotid artery. In this patient with fibromuscular dysplasia (more prominently seen on the opposite side; not shown), there is a long, irregular narrowing of the internal carotid artery. The dissection involves nearly the entire cervical portion of the internal carotid artery *(black arrows)*, starting just beyond the cervical bifurcation and ending in the petrous portion of the internal carotid artery with a normal carotid siphon. (From Silverboard G, Tart R: Cerebrovascular arterial dissection in children and young adults. *Semin Pediatr Neurol* 7:278, 2000.)

Intracranial vertebral artery dissection occurs at or near the origin of the posterior inferior cerebellar artery. Although the presentation is similar to that of extracranial vertebral artery dissection, with brainstem, cerebellar, or hemispheric infarction, intracranial vertebral artery dissection may be distinguished on the basis of its association with SAH.[20,21,23,24,28,29] MRI-MRA may demonstrate a crescent sign or may suggest a dissecting aneurysm, but angiography is warranted in most instances of intracranial vertebral or basilar artery dissection or suspected basilar artery embolization associated with vertebral artery dissection.

Angiography

Although the complementary use of MRI, MRA, CTA, and ultrasound is usually sufficient for the diagnosis of extracranial carotid artery dissection and some instances of extracranial vertebral artery dissection, angiography is the most definitive test for investigation of intracranial dissection as well as extracranial vertebral artery dissection. Angiography, although invasive, yields excellent delineation of abnormalities associated with dissection (Fig. 33-10), including intimal flaps, intraluminal clots, flame-shaped tapering occlusion, double lumen, vessel stenosis with string sign, and dissecting aneurysm formation. Double lumen and intimal flaps are the most specific angiographic findings in dissection. More often, angiographic features of intracranial dissection are not definitive but suggest dissection by demonstrating irregular or scalloped stenoses, a "string of beads," or complete vessel occlusion.[183] With intracranial dissection, angiography may delineate cerebral aneurysm from dissection causing SAH (Fig. 33-11). The finding at angiography of aneurysmal formation at a nonbifurcation location suggests dissection. Irregular narrowing of the affected artery may give a wavy ribbon appearance. The presence of FMD (Fig. 33-12) in 15% of cases may be associated with multivessel dissections.[208-210] Atherosclerotic disease should be suspected in lesions seen proximal to and within 2 cm of the carotid bifurcation.

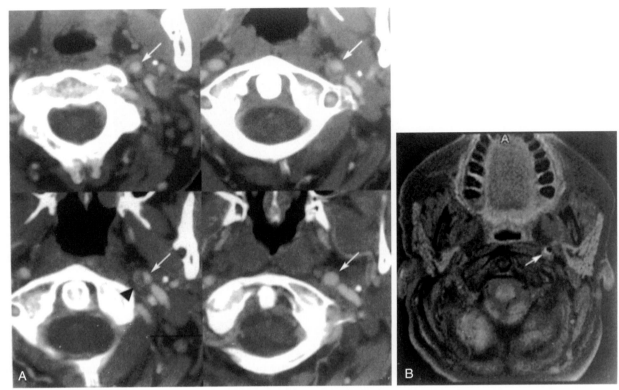

FIGURE 33-13 A, Axial multiplanar volume reconstruction CT angiograms obtained because of the possibility of acute carotid dissection shows that the caudal configuration of the internal carotid artery (ICA) is normal *(upper left, arrow)*. Moving rostrally in the neck *(upper right, lower left)*, the caliber of the ICA narrows *(arrows)*. A crescent-shaped intraluminal thrombus is visible *(lower left, arrowhead)*. Superior to the lesion *(lower right)*, the ICA is enlarged abnormally, suggesting a postdissection pseudoaneurysm *(arrow)*. B, The next day, a fat-saturated, T1-weighted axial MR image through the lesion shows a crescent-shaped area of abnormally high signal intensity *(arrow)* consistent with intramural thrombus related to the acute dissection. (From Fredenberg P, Forbes K, Toye L, et al: Assessment of cervical vascular injury with CT angiography. *BNI Q* 17:44, 2001.)

Computed Tomography

Advanced CT applications such as helical CTA may be particularly suited for investigation of dissection in traumatized patients (Fig. 33-13),[195] although CTA is gaining wider acceptance as a diagnostic option in nontraumatic dissection.[211] Traumatic effects depend on the extent and location of damage to the vessel wall. Dissection occurs more often in blunt than in penetrating trauma. CTA is rapid, allowing unstable patients to be imaged without compromising patient monitoring. Experience with CTA is limited, but in preliminary studies, it compares favorably with other diagnostic modalities, including catheter angiography.[195,211-213]

Treatment

Medical Therapy

Although treatment of extracranial cerebrovascular dissection is controversial and large controlled clinical trials are lacking, treatment is based on both empiric and clinical observations that most cerebral injuries, at least acutely, result from secondary thrombotic events, particularly artery-to-artery embolism.[20] Anticoagulation, with heparin given as immediate therapy in the symptomatic patient and warfarin given as subsequent therapy, has traditionally been the most commonly suggested therapy, with reassessment in the stable patient at 3 months by means of multimodal ultrasound studies, CTA, or MRI-MRA.[19,20,111,116,214] If imaging studies show that dissection has resolved, antiplatelet therapy may be warranted after discontinuation of warfarin; some investigators, however, would discontinue all therapies. If at 3 months reconstitution has not occurred and severe luminal irregularity or stenosis is noted, or if dissecting aneurysm persists, warfarin is continued for 3 months longer.[20]

Later data have prompted questions about the value of anticoagulation for cervicocephalic dissection. In a 2002 *Cochrane Review* on the use of antithrombotic drugs for carotid artery dissection, no evidence was found to support the routine use of anticoagulant or antiplatelet drugs for the treatment of extracranial carotid artery dissection.[215] A 2008 meta-analysis found no evidence of superiority of anticoagulants over antiplatelet agents.[216] The 2006 American Stroke Association (ASA) stroke prevention guidelines recommend that for patients with ischemic stroke or TIA and extracranial arterial dissection, use of warfarin for 3 to 6 months or use of antiplatelet agents is reasonable (class IIa, level of evidence B).[217] Engelter and colleagues[218] have proposed antiplatelet therapy for patients with a National Institutes of Health Stroke Scale score of 15 or higher, accompanying intracranial dissection, local compression syndromes without ischemic events, or concomitant diseases with increased bleeding risk. In patients with cervicocephalic dissection and (pseudo)occlusion of the dissected artery, high-intensity transient signals in transcranial ultrasound studies despite (dual) antiplatelets, multiple ischemic events in the same circulation, or free-floating thrombus, immediate anticoagulation is recommended. A prospective randomized controlled trial comparing anticoagulation with antiplatelet therapy in patients with cervicocephalic dissection is under way in Canada.

Historically, anticoagulation has typically been avoided in the presence of intracranial dissection because of the perceived increased risk of SAH. A published series of 81 patients with intracranial dissection suggests that anticoagulation may be safe in patients without associated aneurysm.[219] Other relative contraindications to anticoagulation are the presence of a large infarct with mass effect, hemorrhagic transformation of the infarcted arterial territory, and the presence of an intracranial aneurysm.[26]

Acute thrombolysis with tissue plasminogen activator (t-PA), given both intravenously and intraarterially through superselective arterial catheterization, has been administered safely after dissection-related stroke.[220-227] Increased intramural hemorrhage with exacerbation of dissection-related stenosis has not been reported. Experience with thrombolytic therapy after dissection is limited, however, with approximately 60 reported cases of carotid dissection and a handful of cases of vertebral dissection in the literature.[216]

Neuroendovascular Interventional Therapy

Neurovascular intervention is increasingly being employed in patients for whom medical therapy has failed and who have (1) persistent ischemic symptoms, (2) contraindications to anticoagulation, (3) surgically inaccessible lesions, (4) limited reserve due to involvement of other vessels, or (5) persistent or expanding dissecting aneurysm.[228] For both spontaneous and traumatic dissections, endovascular therapy in appropriate circumstances allows reestablishment of the true lumen by means of balloon angioplasty and stenting with either balloon-expandable or metallic self-expanding stents, resulting in the obliteration of the false lumen and restoration of hemodynamic flow in the true lumen and thereby reducing the risk of artery-to-artery embolism (Fig. 33-14).[26,30,170,228-247] Through the use of a covered stent or coil embolization placed through the interstices of the stent where necessary, obliteration of dissecting aneurysms in both the extracranial carotid and vertebral arteries may be accomplished (Fig. 33-15).[30,233,235,236,238,242,244,245,248] Endovascular therapy can reestablish hemodynamic flow in severely stenotic or totally occluded true lumens in select cases (Figs. 33-16 and 33-17); sequential reconstruction of the true lumen is accomplished by means of stents that provide gradual radial force, permitting apposition of the dissected segment to the vessel wall and thereby obliterating the false lumen and resolving the consequent loss of vascular continuity.[238,249] Extracranial and intracranial components of dissection can be addressed simultaneously if necessary.

When intracranial extension has occurred, endovascular techniques are also applicable and may be of particular benefit for balloon occlusion of intracranial dissection of the vertebral artery if temporary occlusion studies suggest adequate collateral blood flow. Long-term efficacy and endovascular therapy–related complications are still being assessed, although results of limited published series are promising.[220,248,250-253] Complications of endovascular intervention include retroperitoneal hemorrhage; vasospasm, which may be treated with angioplasty during the endovascular procedure; and the possibility of recurrent stenosis and distal embolism if there is large thrombus burden.[249] Because the risk of recurrent embolization is low and dissecting aneurysms do not usually rupture, stenting as an initial therapy is not warranted and should be reserved for cases in which medical therapy has failed.[26,215,249] When stenting is performed, antiplatelet agents are administered for at least 4 weeks to prevent stent occlusion.[249] There is a lack of prospective randomized data evaluating stenting for cervicocephalic dissection. Menon and colleagues[216] systematically reviewed the available literature, however, and reported a relatively low technical failure rate (5%) and a low perioperative complication rate (3.1%).

Surgical Therapy

With the advent of endovascular techniques, the need for surgical intervention as the treatment for symptomatic dissecting aneurysm or postdissection stenosis has decreased. Formerly, aneurysms accounted for 0.3% of extracranial ICA operations performed at the Cleveland Clinic[254] and 0.2% of those performed by the neurovascular surgical service at the Mayo Clinic.[249,255] Surgery is now reserved for patients who are symptomatic despite optimal medical therapy and who are not candidates for endovascular intervention.[26,249,256] Patients with impaired cerebral vasoreactivity who are at increased risk for stroke may need surgical revascularization.[26,257]

Surgical treatment consists of carotid ligation, aneurysmal resection with carotid reconstruction, and cervical-to-intracranial ICA bypass (supraclinoid or petrous ICA). Aneurysmal clipping is usually not an option because of the fusiform configuration usually found at surgery. Extracranial dissecting aneurysms rarely necessitate surgery; they often resolve spontaneously, particularly those that are not traumatic in origin.[249,258] Surgical excision of the symptomatic dissecting aneurysm with reconstruction of the ICA to eliminate the aneurysm and maintain the artery's hemodynamic flow may be accomplished with interposition of a saphenous vein graft or primary reanastomosis (Fig. 33-18).[26] Because the majority of carotid dissecting aneurysms occur in the distal carotid artery near the skull base, surgery may cause pharyngeal and superior laryngeal branch injuries of the vagus nerve and resultant, although usually transient, dysphonia or dysphagia.[26]

Carotid artery ligation, provided that adequate collateral flow is documented, has been performed. Complications include delayed ischemia due to embolization in the immediate postoperative period and potential long-term occurrence of cerebral ischemia or cerebral aneurysms.[26]

ACUTE CAROTID ARTERY DISSECTION

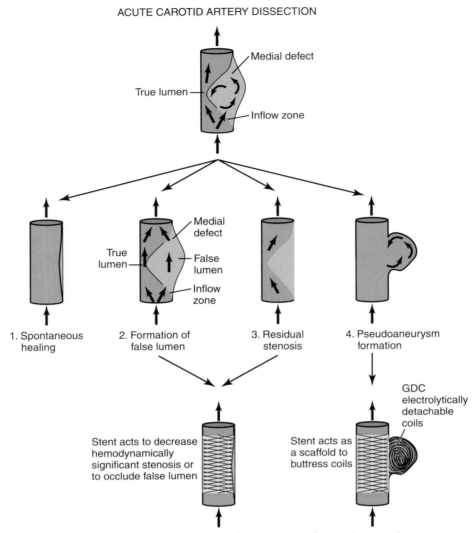

Figure 33-14   Simplified schematic illustration of the pathophysiologic process of carotid artery dissection proceeding from the acute stage to spontaneous healing (1), formation of false lumen (2), residual stenosis of varying degree or complete occlusion (3), or formation of a pseudoaneurysm (4). A stent is used in cases that have not responded to medical therapy, to relieve a hemodynamically significant stenosis, to occlude a false lumen, or to serve as a scaffold to enable coil embolization of a wide-necked pseudoaneurysm. GDC, Guglielmi detachable coil (Boston Scientific Corporation, Boston). *Arrows* indicate direction(s) of blood flow. (From Malek AM, Higashida RT, Phatouros CC, et al: Endovascular management of extracranial carotid artery dissection achieved using stent angiography. *AJNR Am J Neuroradiol* 21:1380, 2000.)

Because of the risk of recurrent dissection in another vessel, preservation of vessel integrity is a practical and potentially critical consideration. Schievink[26] favors cervical-to-intracranial ICA bypass using a saphenous vein graft between the cervical carotid artery and the petrous or supraclinoid portion of the ICA or, less often, the proximal middle cerebral artery.

Course and Prognosis

Although the clinical prognosis following extracranial carotid or vertebral dissection depends on the severity of the initial neurologic injury, in general it is quite good (Tables 33-2 to 33-4).[20] Complete or excellent recovery occurs in 75% to 85% of patients.[27,107,110,111,259] Mortality is less than 5%,[1,21] and significant neurologic deficits

persist in only 5% to 10% of patients.[27,110] Neurologic outcome is less favorable in patients with arterial occlusion,[138,260-262] traumatic dissections,[259] or intracranial dissection,[15,263] especially when it is associated with SAH.[29,148,219,264] For example, 50% of survivors of intracranial carotid artery dissection have major residual deficits.[12,15,263] The prognosis for basilar artery dissection is particularly poor, with mortality exceeding 60%.[265] The risk of recurrent stroke more than 2 weeks after the diagnosis of dissection is exceedingly low (0.4% per year), with the highest risk in the first year.[20] Persistent recurrent headache or neck pain is not uncommon and tends to occur more commonly in patients with traumatic dissections.[27,259,266]

Recurrent dissection in a previously involved artery is rare,[3-5,138,267,268] whereas the risk of recurrence in

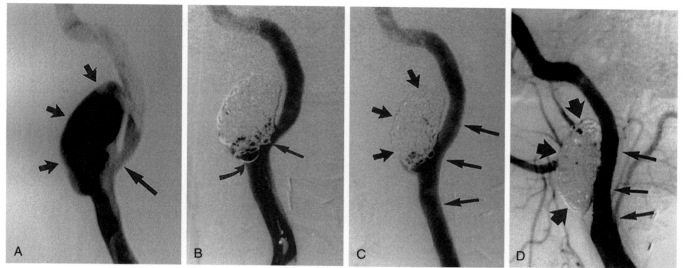

Figure 33-15 A 30-year-old woman with a left cervical internal carotid artery (ICA) pseudoaneurysm. A, Left internal carotid injection, lateral view, shows pseudoaneurysm *(short arrows)* and narrowed ICA *(long arrow)*. B, Left ICA angiogram after embolization with Guglielmi detachable coils shows the coils protruding into the parent artery *(arrows)*. C, Left ICA angiogram after embolization and stent placement shows the occluded pseudoaneurysm *(short arrows)* and the remodeled, stented carotid artery *(long arrows)*. D, At 6-month follow-up, a left common carotid angiogram shows total occlusion of the pseudoaneurysm *(short arrows)* and normal width and patency of the stented segment of the ICA *(long arrows)*. (From Klein GE, Szolar DH, Raith J, et al: Post-traumatic extracranial aneurysm of the internal carotid artery: Combined endovascular treatment with coils and stents. *AJNR Am J Neuroradiol* 18:1261, 1997.)

a previously uninvolved artery is low but not insignificant.[269] Schievink and colleagues[3] reported a 2% recurrence risk in the first month with a 1% annual risk thereafter, and other series have reported similar figures, with equal rates for carotid and vertebral dissections.[4,5,20] A 24-center study of 459 patients by Touze and associates[268] reported a stroke recurrence rate of only 0.3% per year, and a small study of 11 patients with triple or quadruple extracranial dissection reported no recurrence over 4 years.[270] In the Schievink series, risk declined with advancing age; the 10-year recurrence rate was 17% for patients younger than 45 years, and only 6% for patients older than 45 years (Fig. 33-19).[3] A family history of arterial dissection increased the risk of recurrence sixfold.[77] Presence of an underlying arteriopathy likewise increases the risk of recurrence.[4,5]

The angiographic prognosis of cervicocephalic dissection is favorable, although no correlation between angiographic and clinical prognoses has been found.[111,271] Angiographic stenoses improve or resolve in 80% to 90% of cases, with the rate of complete resolution averaging approximately 50% to 60% in published series.[27,110,111,180 182,196,259,271] Arterial occlusions recanalize in more than half of cases.[110,111,138,180,182,259] Complete resolution is seen in more than 20% of dissecting aneurysms,[110,179,182,196,259,272,273] and resolution or improvement is seen in approximately 50%.[110,179,182,196,259,271,273] Angiographic improvement occurs within the first 2 to 3 months after the dissection and is rare after 6 months.[19,20,111,126,138,185,188,214] Rupture of extracranial dissecting aneurysms is not commonly described; rather, thromboembolism from dissecting aneurysms or expansion of the aneurysm compressing adjacent structures merits continued monitoring.[11,179,249,272,274]

Fibromuscular Dysplasia
Epidemiology

Fibromuscular dysplasia (FMD) is an uncommon nonatheromatous, noninflammatory vasculopathy characterized by alternating fibrotic thickening and atrophy of the vessel wall. It affects women more commonly than men at a ratio of 2:1 and is more common in white persons.[275,276] Although commonly diagnosed in middle age (20 to 50 years), FMD can occur at any age. Population data regarding prevalence are lacking, although a single autopsy study reported histologically confirmed FMD of the internal carotid artery in 0.02% of 20,244 cases between 1968 and 1992.[275]

Pathology

FMD is classified based on the arterial layer that is primarily affected (intima, media, or adventitia). *Medial dysplasia*, the most common type, is further subdivided into three histologic types (medial fibroplasia, perimedial fibroplasia, and medial hyperplasia). Medial fibroplasia is the most common form (75% to 80%), leading to the classic "string of beads" appearance, in which the beads are larger than the normal vessel diameter. Perimedial fibroplasia accounts for less than 10% of FMD cases and occurs most commonly in girls between 5 and 15 years old. Histologically, there is extensive collagen deposition in the outer half of the media. Medial hyperplasia is rare and is characterized by smooth muscle cell hyperplasia without fibrosis. *Intimal fibroplasia*, which affects fewer than 10% of patients with FMD, is characterized by focal concentric stenosis, long smooth narrowing, or an arterial loop. The rarest form, *adventitial (periarterial)*

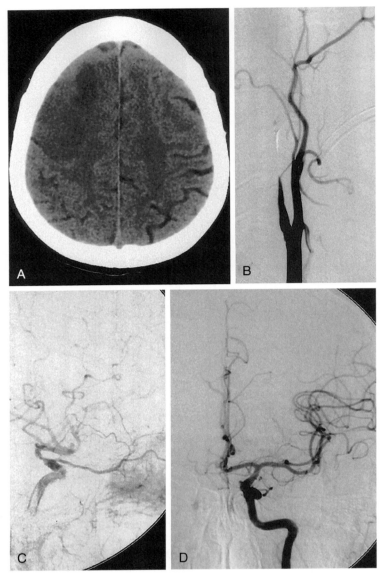

Figure 33-16 A 45-year-old woman noted to have left hemiparesis after diagnostic angiography. A, CT scan of the head shows evidence of a previous focal infarct as well as diffuse edema in the right posterior frontal lobe. B, Digital subtraction angiogram of the right common carotid artery reveals tapering of the right internal carotid artery (ICA) to a complete occlusion, with appearance consistent with dissection. C, Injection of the right external carotid artery shows retrograde collateral flow through the right ophthalmic artery, with filling of the cavernous segment of the right ICA. D, Injection of the left ICA shows no significant flow across the anterior communicating artery.

fibroplasia, is characterized by sharply localized, tubular areas of stenosis. Histologically, dense collagen replaces the fibrous tissue of the adventitia.

Pathogenesis

Although several risk factors have been identified (e.g., tobacco use and hypertension[277]), the etiology of FMD remains unknown. As with dissection, genetic factors likely play a role because FMD is more common in first-degree relatives of patients with renal artery FMD[278] and in individuals with the angiotensin-converting enzyme allele ACE-I.[279] Other associated conditions are Ehlers-Danlos syndrome (type IV) and alpha₁-antitripsin deficiency.[56,280-282] Additional hypotheses regarding pathogenesis have been

proposed, including ischemic, mechanical, toxic, hormonal, metabolic, and immunologic factors.[283-286] It remains most likely that the cause of FMD is multifactorial. Irrespective of the specific type and pathoetiology of FMD, the histopathologic changes are due to a fibroblast-like transformation of smooth muscle cells that allows them to produce extracellular matrix proteins, particularly collagen.[287]

Sites

FMD more commonly affects the extracranial vessels, with a predilection for the carotid artery.[288] Carotid involvement is typically bilateral[57,288] and adjacent to the C1-C2 interspace.[276,289] Vertebral involvement occurs in roughly 10% of cervicocephalic cases,[276,289] is typically

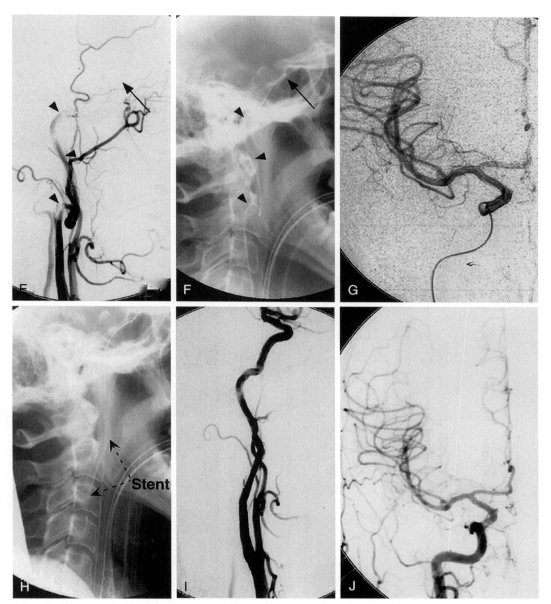

Figure 33-16, cont'd The treatment approach consisted of initial recanalization of the dissected right ICA, achieved by entering the true lumen with the use of a RAPIDTRANSIT Microcatheter (Codman & Shurtleff, Inc, Raynham, Mass) and Instinct-10 Microguidewire (E and F; *arrowheads*), which were advanced up to the cavernous portion of the right ICA (E and F; *arrow*). G, Superselective injection shows a patent right middle and anterior cerebral artery. H, An 8 mm × 2 cm WALLSTENT (Boston Scientific Corporation) was then deployed at the dissection site over a STABILIZER exchange Microguidewire (Cordis Corporation, Bridgewater, NJ) at the C2 level. The reconstitution of the lumen of the right ICA is shown by injection of the right common carotid artery (I), with resumption of intracranial perfusion (J). (From Malek AM, Higashida RT, Phatouros CC, et al: Endovascular management of extracranial carotid artery dissection achieved using stent angiography. *AJNR Am J Neuroradiol* 21:1380, 2000.)

randomly distributed,[288] and often coexists with carotid involvement.[289] Intracranial carotid or vertebral artery involvement occurs in up to 20% of cases and is typically limited to the intrapetrosal ICA or carotid siphon, although other vessels may be affected.[288,290,291]

Clinical Manifestations and Diagnosis

FMD is likely most often asymptomatic but may manifest as nonspecific symptoms (e.g., Horner's syndrome) or cause a stroke syndrome via hemodynamic compromise,[292,293] secondary thromboembolism,[288,294,295] or a direct complication (e.g., dissection,[3,53-55,262,296,297] aneurysm,[298] or arteriovenous fistula[299,300]).

The diagnosis of cervicocephalic FMD may be made in asymptomatic patients undergoing evaluation for another disorder or in patients with ischemic or nonischemic (e.g., bruit) symptoms. Imaging findings of cervicocephalic FMD typically fall into one of three categories. The most common is the typical string of beads appearance of alternating narrowing and dilation, most typically seen with the medial type (see Figs. 33-18 and 33-20). Unifocal

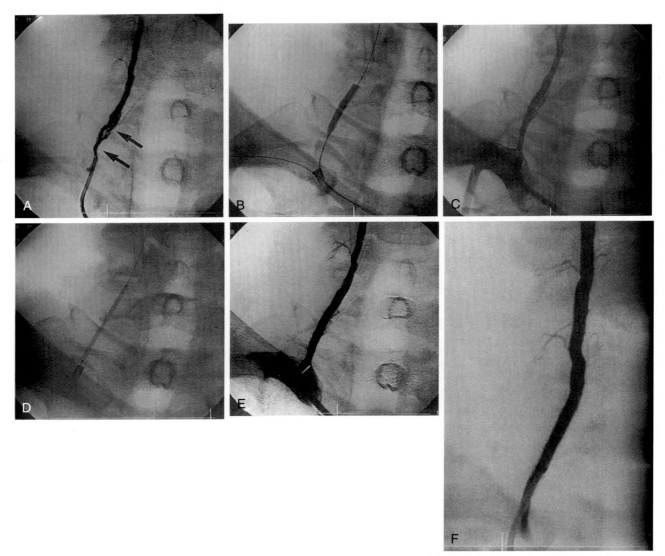

Figure 33-17 A, Traumatic dissection of proximal right vertebral artery in a 36-year-old man who suffered a brainstem infarction. After conservative treatment for 1 year, the vessel still appeared damaged, so endovascular therapy was offered. Note the multiple lumens *(arrows)* that force the interventionist to find the true lumen before inflating balloons and using stents. B, Once the true lumen is found, balloon angioplasty allows enlargement of this lumen in order to properly fit and deploy the stents. C, After predilation; note improvement of the true lumen, although further reconstruction of the vessel seems to be required. D, Balloon-expandable stent is properly positioned and deployed. E, Final result shows normalization of the true lumen of vessel with obliteration of false lumens. F, Six-month control follow-up angiogram shows preservation of the architecture of the vessel. (From Gomez CR, May AK, Terry JB, et al: Endovascular therapy of traumatic injuries of the extracranial cerebral arteries. *Crit Care Clin* 15:789, 1999.)

or multifocal tubular narrowing is less common and is not specific for any one histopathologic subtype. Finally, imaging may reveal less common associated phenomena such as diverticula, aneurysms, and arterial webs.

There are no published studies comparing different imaging techniques in the diagnosis of cervicocephalic FMD. Digital subtraction angiography has been long considered the gold standard, but noninvasive imaging techniques have been relied upon with increasing frequency. Duplex ultrasonography may reveal irregular patterns of stenosis suggestive of FMD[301] but is a nonspecific modality limited to evaluating the carotid bifurcation. MRA and CTA have become increasingly popular owing to their noninvasive characteristics and abilities

to image the complete cerebrovascular system. MRA artifact may mimic FMD[302]; when combined with MRI, MRA has the additional benefit of evaluation for associated ischemia.

Treatment

The prognosis of cervicocephalic FMD is typically fairly benign, and there are no prospective randomized controlled trials to guide therapy. Studies of stroke rates in patients with cervicocephalic FMD suffer from poor design but typically report low rates, even without therapy.[288,303-305] Corrin and associates,[304] for example, reported a recurrent stroke rate of 3.8% over 60 months.

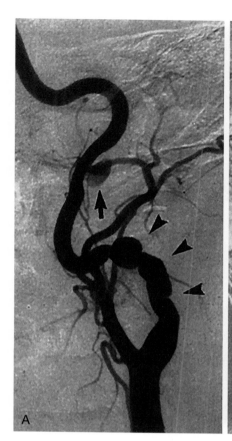
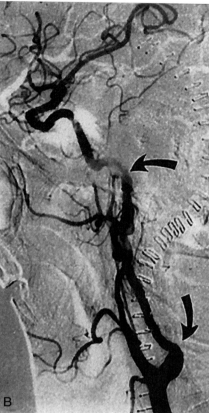

Figure 33-18 A, A lateral left common carotid angiogram reveals a spontaneous dissecting aneurysm *(arrow)* of the internal carotid artery and evidence of fibromuscular dysplasia *(arrowheads)*. B, A lateral left common carotid angiogram obtained after resection of the abnormal segment of artery and reconstruction with an interposition saphenous vein graft; *arrows* indicate the location of the anastomoses. (From Schievink WI: Spontaneous dissection of the carotid and vertebral arteries. *N Engl J Med* 344:898, 2001.)

TABLE 33-4   SURVEY OF LITERATURE ON OUTCOME OF MANAGEMENT IN 100 PATIENTS

Presenting Feature and Treatment*	Patients' Outcomes		
	Normal	**Minor Deficit†**	**Major Deficit or Death**
Major stroke (18 cases)			
No Rx or APT	0/13	1/13	12/13
Anticoagulation	1/4	2/4	1/4
Surgery	0	1/1	0
Single TIA or minor stroke (45 cases)			
No Rx or APT	15/17	2/17	0
Anticoagulation	14/16	1/16	1/16
Surgery	6/12	5/12	1/12
Multiple TIAs (15 cases)			
No Rx or APT	6/6	0	0
Anticoagulant	5/5	0	0
Surgery	3/4	1/4	0
Other (pain, tinnitus) (22 cases)			
No Rx or APT	18/20	1/20	1/20
Anticoagulation	2/2	0	0
Surgery	0	0	0
Total (in %)	70	14	16

*Major complaint on presentation to physician, not necessarily the initial symptom.
†Nondisabling deficit; residual Horner's syndrome considered normal.
APT, antiplatelet therapy; Rx, medical therapy; TIA, transient ischemic attack.
Data from 100 cases from English-language literature since 1975 on extracranial carotid artery dissection, in Hart RG, Easton JD: Dissections of cervical and cerebral arteries. *Neurol Clin* 1:155, 1993; plus references 88, 311, 312, 313, 314.

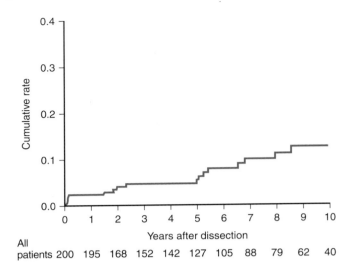

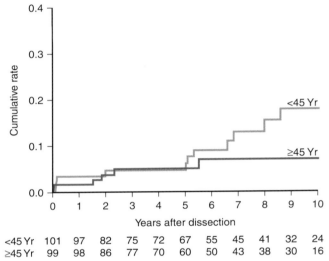

Figure 33-19 Cumulative rate of recurrent arterial dissection in all patients *(upper panel)* and according to age *(lower panel)*. The numbers shown below each panel are the numbers of patients at risk for recurrent dissection at each point. (From Schievink WI, Mokri B, O'Fallon M: Recurrent spontaneous cervical artery dissection. *N Engl J Med* 330:393, 1994.)

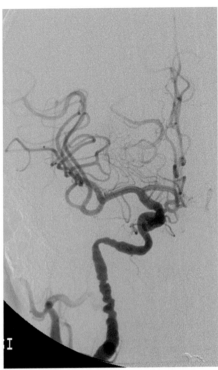

Figure 33-20 Digital subtraction angiogram of the carotid artery (lateral view) showing the typical string of beads pattern of alternating narrowing and dilation in fibromuscular dysplasia. (Image courtesy of John Agola, MD.)

For this reason, treatment should generally be conservative in nature, especially in asymptomatic patients.

For the majority of symptomatic FMD cases, initial medical therapy with antiplatelet agents or anticoagulants is recommended. In patients with cerebral aneurysms, antithrombotic therapy should be withheld until endovascular or surgical obliteration is achieved. For patients whose symptoms fail to respond to antithrombotic therapy, consideration of percutaneous transluminal angioplasty with or without endovascular stenting is appropriate, especially if there is hemodynamic compromise.[306,307] Surgical intervention is reserved for progressive clinical cases not amenable to endovascular therapy. Surgical procedures for FMD have included graduated internal dilatation, resection with end-to-side anastomosis or interposition graft, and extracranial-to-intracranial bypass in patients with hemodynamic compromise.[308-310]

REFERENCES

1. Chan MT, Nadareishvili ZG, Norris JW: Diagnostic strategies in young patients with ischemic stroke in Canada, *Can J Neurol Sci* 27:120, 2000.
2. Giroud M, Fayolle H, Andre N, et al: Incidence of internal carotid artery dissection in the community of Dijon, *J Neurol Neurosurg Psychiatry* 57:1443, 1994.
3. Schievink WI, Mokri B, O'Fallon M: Recurrent spontaneous cervical artery dissection, *N Engl J Med* 330:393, 1994.
4. Leys D, Moulin T, Stojkovic T, et al: Follow-up of patients with history of cervical artery dissection, *Cerebrovasc Dis* 4:43, 1995.
5. Bassetti C, Carruzzo A, Sturzenegger M, et al: Recurrence of cervical artery dissection: A prospective study of 81 patients, *Stroke* 27:1996, 1804.
6. Ducrocq X, Lacour JC, Debouverie M, et al: Accidents vasculaires cérébraux ischemiques du sujet jeune: Étude prospective de 296 patients ages 16 a 45 ans, *Rev Neurol (Paris)* 155:575, 1999.
7. Bogousslavsky J, Pierre P: Ischemic stroke in patients under age 45, *Neurol Clin* 10:113, 1992.
8. Gautier JC, Pradat-Diehl P, Loron P, et al: Accidents vasculaires cérébraux des sujets jeunes. Une etude de 133 patients age de 9 a 45 ans, *Rev Neurol (Paris)* 145:437, 1989.
9. Lisovoski F, Rousseaux P: Cerebral infarction in young people: A study of 148 patients with early cerebral angiography, *J Neurol Neurosurg Psychiatry* 54:576, 1991.
10. Arnold M, Kappeler L, Georgiadis D, et al: Gender differences in spontaneous cervical artery dissection, *Neurology* 67:1050, 2006.
11. Schievink WI, Mokri B, Jackers G: Spontaneous dissections of cervicocephalic arteries in childhood and adolescence, *Neurology* 44:1607, 1994.
12. Fullerton HJ, Johnston SC, Smith WS: Arterial dissection and stroke in children, *Neurology* 57:1155, 2001.
13. Leys D, Lucas C, Govert M, et al: Cervical artery dissections, *Eur Neurol* 37:3, 1997.
14. Hart RG, Easton JD: Dissections of cervical and cerebral arteries, *Neurol Clin* 1:155, 1983.

15. Bassetti C, Bogousslavsky J, Eskenasy-Cottier AC, et al: Spontaneous intracranial dissection in the anterior circulation, *Cerebrovasc Dis* 4:170, 1994.

16. Caplan LR, Zarins CK, Hemmat M: Spontaneous dissection of the extracranial vertebral arteries, *Stroke* 16:1030, 1996.

17. Hinse P, Thie A, Lachenmayer L: Dissection of the extracranial vertebral artery: Report of four cases and review of the literature, *J Neurol Neurosurg Psychiatry* 54:853, 1991.

18. Bertram M, Ringleb P, Fieback J, et al: Das spectrum neurologischer symptome bei dissektionen hirnversorgender Arterien, *Dtsch Med Wochenschr* 124:273, 1999.

19. Schievink WI: Spontaneous dissection of the carotid and vertebral arteries, *N Engl J Med* 344:898, 2001.

20. Saver JL, Easton JD. Dissections and trauma of cervicocerebral arteries. In Barnett HJM, Mohr JP, Stein BM, et al, editors: *Stroke: Pathophysiology, diagnosis, and management*, ed 3, New York, 1998, Churchill Livingstone, pp 769–786.

21. Caplan LR, Baquis GD, Pessin MS, et al: Dissection of the intracranial vertebral artery, *Neurology* 38:868, 1988.

22. Kawaguchi S, Sakaki T, Tsunoda S: Management of dissecting aneurysms of the posterior circulation, *Acta Neurochir (Wien)* 131:26, 1994.

23. Kitanaka C, Sasaki T, Eguchi T, et al: Intracranial vertebral artery dissections: Clinical, radiological features and surgical considerations, *Neurosurgery* 34:620, 1994.

24. Sasaki O, Ogawa H, Koike T, et al: A clinicopathologic study of dissecting aneurysms of the intracranial vertebral artery, *J Neurosurg* 75:874, 1991.

25. Bogousslavsky J: Dissections of the cerebral arteries—clinical effects, *Curr Opin Neurol Neurosurg* 1:63, 1988.

26. Schievink WI: The treatment of spontaneous carotid and vertebral artery dissections, *Curr Opin Cardiol* 15:318–321, 2000.

27. Mokri B, Sundt TM, Houser OW, et al: Spontaneous dissection of the cervical internal carotid artery, *Ann Neurol* 19:126, 1986.

28. Berger MS, Wilson CB: Intracranial dissecting aneurysms of the posterior circulation, *Neurosurgery* 61:882, 1984.

29. Friedman AH, Drake CG: Subarachnoid hemorrhage from intracranial dissecting aneurysm, *J Neurosurg* 60:325, 1984.

30. Halbach VV, Higashida R, Dowd CF, et al: Endovascular treatment of vertebral artery dissections and pseudoaneurysms, *J Neurosurg* 79:183, 1993.

31. Shimoji T, Bando K, Nakajima K, et al: Dissecting aneurysm of the vertebral artery: Report of seven cases and angiographic findings, *J Neurosurg* 61:1038, 1984.

32. Tsukahara T, Wada H, Satake K, et al: Proximal balloon occlusion for dissecting vertebral aneurysms accompanied by subarachnoid hemorrhage, *Neurosurgery* 36:914, 1995.

33. Beatty RA: Dissecting hematoma of the internal carotid artery following chiropractic manipulation, *J Trauma* 17:248, 1977.

34. Haldeman S, Kohlbeck F, McGregor M: Risk factors for vertebrobasilar artery dissection following cervical spine manipulation: A review of 60 cases, *Neurology* 46:A440, 1996.

35. Lee KP, Carlini WG, McCormick GF, et al: Neurologic complications following chiropractic manipulation: A survey of California neurologists, *Neurology* 45:1213, 1995.

36. Norria JW, Beletsky V, Nadareishvili ZG, et al: Sudden neck movement and cervical artery dissection, *CMAJ* 163:38, 2000.

37. Haldeman S, Carey P, Murray T, et al: Arterial dissections following cervical manipulation: The chiropractic experience, *CMAJ* 165:905, 2001.

38. Hufnagel A, Hammers A, Schonle PW, et al: Stroke following chiropractic manipulation of the cervical spine, *J Neurol* 246:683, 1999.

39. Mas J-L, Henin O, Bousser M-G, et al: Dissecting aneurysms of the vertebral artery and cervical manipulation: A case report with autopsy, *Neurology (NY)* 39:512, 1989.

40. Peters M, Bohl J, Thomke F, et al: Dissection of the internal carotid artery after chiropractic manipulation of the neck, *Neurology* 45:2284, 1995.

41. Rothwell DM, Bondy SJ, Williams JI: Chiropractic manipulation and stroke: A population-based case-control study, *Stroke* 32:1054, 2001.

42. Gould DB, Cunningham BS: Internal carotid artery dissection after remote surgery: Iatrogenic complications of anesthesia, *Stroke* 25:1276, 1994.

43. Schievink WI, Atkinson JLD, Bartleson JD, et al: Traumatic internal carotid dissections caused by blunt softball injuries, *Am J Emerg Med* 16:179, 1998.

44. Marks RL, Freed MM: Non-penetrating injuries of the neck in cerebrovascular accident, *Arch Neurol* 28:412, 1973.

45. Schneider RC, Gosch HH, Norell H, et al: Vascular insufficiency and differential distortion of the brain and spinal cord caused by cervical medullary football injuries, *J Neurosurg* 33:363, 1970.

46. Schneider RC: Serious and fatal neurosurgical football injuries, *Clin Neurosurg* 12:226, 1966.

47. Schneider RC, Gosch HH, Tareu JA, et al: Blood vessel trauma following head and neck injuries, *Clin Neurosurg* 19:312, 1972.

48. Ford FR: Syncope, vertigo, and disturbances of vision resulting from intermittent obstruction of the vertebral arteries due to deficit in the odontoid process and excessive mobility of the second cervical vertebrae, *Johns Hopkins Med J* 598:37–42, 1956.

49. Rogers L, Sweeney PJ: Stroke: A neurologic complication of wrestling, *Am J Sports Med* 7:352–354, 1979.

50. Vickers A, Zollman C: The manipulative therapies: Osteopathy and chiropractic, *BMJ* 319:1176, 1999.

51. Schievink WI, Mokri B, Piepgras DG, et al: Cervical artery dissections associated with chiropractic manipulation of the neck: The importance of pre-existing arterial disease and injury, *J Neurol* 243(Suppl 2):S92, 1996.

52. Fisher CM, Ojemann RG, Robertson GH: Spontaneous dissection of cervicocerebral arteries, *Can J Neurol Sci* 5:19, 1978.

53. Ringel SP, Harrison SH, Norenberg MD, et al: Fibromuscular dysplasia: Multiple "spontaneous" dissecting aneurysms of the major cervical arteries, *Ann Neurol* 1:301, 1977.

54. Schievink WI, Bjornsson J, Piepgras DG: Coexistence of fibromuscular dysplasia and cystic medial necrosis in a patient with Marfan's syndrome and bilateral carotid artery dissections, *Stroke* 25:2492–2496, 1994.

55. Schievink WI, Michels VV, et al: Neurovascular manifestations of heritable connective tissue disorders—a review, *Stroke* 25:889, 1994.

56. Schievink WI, Mokri B, Piepgras DG: Fibromuscular dysplasia of the internal carotid artery associated with alpha-1-antitrypsin deficiency, *Neurosurgery* 43:229, 1998.

57. Stanley JC, Fry WJ, Seeger JF, et al: Extracranial internal carotid and vertebral artery fibrodysplasia, *Arch Surg* 109:215, 1974.

58. Schievink WI, Wijdicks EFM, Michels VV, et al: Heritable connective tissue disorders in cervical artery dissections: A prospective study, *Neurology* 50:1166, 1998.

59. North KN, Whiteman DAH, Pepin MG, et al: Cerebrovascular complications in Ehlers-Danlos syndrome type IV, *Ann Neurol* 38:960, 1995.

60. Schievink WI, Limburg M, Dorthuys JE, et al: Cerebrovascular disease in Ehlers-Danlos syndrome type IV, *Stroke* 21:626, 1990.

61. Ulbricht D, Diederich NJ, Hermanns-Le T, et al: Cervical artery dissection: An atypical presentation with Ehlers-Danlos-like collagen pathology? *Neurology* 63:1708, 2004.

62. Austin MG, Schaefer RF: Marfan's syndrome, with unusual blood vessel manifestations, *Arch Pathol Lab Med* 64:205, 1957.

63. Youl BD, Coutellier A, Dubois B, et al: Three cases of spontaneous extracranial vertebral artery dissection, *Stroke* 21:618, 1990.

64. Mokri B, Sundt TM Jr, Houser OW: Spontaneous internal carotid dissection, hemicrania, and Horner's syndrome, *Arch Neurol* 36:677, 1979.

65. Mayer SA, Rubin BS, Starman BJ, et al: Spontaneous multivessel cervical artery dissection in a patient with a substitution of alanine for glycine (G13A) in the alpha 1 (I) chain of type I collagen, *Neurology* 47:552, 1996.

66. Schievink I, Prakash UBS, Piepgras DG, et al: α-Antitrypsin deficiency in intracranial aneurysms and cervical artery dissection, *Lancet* 343:452, 1994.

67. Brice JG, Crompton MR: Spontaneous dissecting aneurysms of the cervical internal carotid artery, *BMJ* 2:790, 1964.

68. Yuasa H, Tokito S, Izumi K, et al: Cerebrovascular moyamoya disease associated with an intracranial pseudoaneurysm, *J Neurosurg* 56:131, 1982.

69. Yamashita M, Tanaka K, Matsuo T, et al: Cerebral dissecting aneurysms in patients with moyamoya disease, *J Neurosurg* 58:120, 1983.

70. Adelman LS, Doe FD, Samat HB: Bilateral dissecting aneurysms of the internal carotid arteries, *Acta Neuropathol* 29:93, 1974.

71. Barbour PJ, Castaldo JE, Rae-Grant AD, et al: Internal carotid artery redundancy is significantly associated with dissection, *Stroke* 25:1201, 1994.

72. Ben Hamouda-M'Rad I, Biousse V, Bousser M-G, et al: Internal carotid artery redundancy is significantly associated with dissection, *Stroke* 26:1995, 1962.

73. Guillon B, Tzourio C, Biousse V, et al: Arterial wall properties in carotid artery dissection: An ultrasound study, *Neurology* 55:663, 2000.

74. Tzourio C, Cohen A, Lamisse N, et al: Aortic root dilatation in patients with spontaneous cervical artery dissection, *Circulation* 95:2351, 1997.

75. Schievink WI, Mokri B, Michels VV, et al: Familial association of intracranial aneurysms and cervical artery dissections, *Stroke* 22:1426–1430, 1991.

76. Schievink WI, Mokri B, Piepgras DG: Angiographic frequency of saccular intracranial aneurysms in patients with spontaneous cervical artery dissection, *J Neurosurg* 76:62–66, 1992.

77. Schievink WI, Mokri B, Piepgras DG, et al: Recurrent spontaneous arterial dissections: Risk in familial versus nonfamilial disease, *Stroke* 27:622, 1996.

78. D'Anglejean-Chatillon J, Ribeiro V, Mas JL, et al: Migraine—a risk factor for dissection of cervical arteries, *Headache* 29:560, 1989.

79. Fisher CM: The headache and pain of spontaneous carotid dissection, *Headache* 22:60, 1982.

80. Pezzini A, Grassi M, Del Zotto E, et al: Migraine mediates the influence of C677T MTHFR genotypes on ischemic stroke risk with a stroke-subtype effect, *Stroke* 38:3145, 2007.

81. Grau AJ, Brandt T, Forsting M, et al: Infection-associated cervical artery dissection: Three cases, *Stroke* 28:453, 1997.

82. Grau AJ, Brandt T, Buggle F, et al: Association of cervical artery dissection with recent infection, *Arch Neurol* 56:851, 1999.

83. Constantinescu CS: Association of varicella-zoster virus with cervical artery dissection in 2 cases [letter], *Arch Neurol* 57:427, 2000.

84. Wiebers DO, Mokri B: Internal carotid artery dissection after childbirth, *Stroke* 16:956, 1985.

85. Mas J-L, Bousser M-G, Corone P, et al: Dissecting aneurysm of the extracranial vertebral arteries and pregnancy, *Rev Neurol (Paris)* 143:761, 1987.

86. Gallai V, Caso V, Paciaroni M, et al: Mild hyperhomocyst(e)inemia: A possible risk factor for cervical artery dissection, *Stroke* 32:714, 2001.

87. Pezzini A, Del Zotto E, Archetti S, et al: Plasma homocysteine concentration, C677T *MTHFR* genotype, and 844ins68bp *CBS* genotype in young adults with spontaneous cervical artery dissection and atherothrombotic stroke, *Stroke* 33:664, 2002.

88. Mas J-L, Goeau C, Bousser M-G, et al: Spontaneous dissecting aneurysms of the internal carotid and vertebral arteries—two case reports, *Stroke* 16:125, 1985.

89. Mas JL, Bousser MG, Hasboun D, et al: Extracranial vertebral artery dissections: A review of 13 cases, *Stroke* 18:1037, 1987.

90. Schievink WI, Michels VV, Piepgras DG: A familial syndrome of arterial dissections with lentiginosis, *N Engl J Med* 332:579, 1995.

91. Schievink WI, Mokri B: Familial aorto-cervicocephalic arterial dissections and congenitally bicuspid aortic valve, *Stroke* 26:1995, 1935.

92. Brandt T, Hausser I, Orberk E, et al: Ultrastructural connective tissue abnormalities in patients with spontaneous cervicocerebral artery dissections, *Ann Neurol* 44:281, 1998.

93. Brandt T, Orberk E, Weber R, et al: Pathogenesis of cervical artery dissections: Association with connective tissue abnormalities, *Neurology* 57:24, 2001.

94. Dunac A, Blecic S, Jeangette S, et al: Stroke due to artery dissection: Role of collagen disease, *Cerebrovasc Dis* 8(Suppl 4):18, 1998.

95. Brandt T, Grond-Ginsbach C: Spontaneous cervical artery dissection: From risk factors toward pathogenesis [editorial], *Stroke* 33:657, 2002.

96. Volker W, Besselmann M, Dittrich R, et al: Generalized arteriopathy in patients with cervical artery dissection, *Neurology* 64:1508, 2005.

97. Grond-Ginsbach C, Weber R, Hausser I, et al: Familial connective tissue alterations in patients with spontaneous cervical artery dissections, *Cerebrovasc Dis* 10(Suppl 2):37, 2000.

98. Grond-Ginsbach C, Weber R, Haas J, et al: Mutations in the COL5A1 coding sequence are not common in patients with cervical artery dissections, *Stroke* 30:1887–1890, 1999.

99. Kiuvaniemi H, Prockop DJ, Wu Y, et al: Exclusion of mutations in the gene for type III collagen (COL3A1) as a common cause of intracranial aneurysms or cervical artery dissections: Results from sequence analysis of the coding sequences of type III collagen from 55 unrelated patients, *Neurology* 43:2652, 1993.

100. van den Berg JS, Limburg M, Kappelle LJ, et al: The role of type III collagen in spontaneous cervical arterial dissections, *Ann Neurol* 43:494, 1998.

101. Grond-Ginsbach C, Thomas-Feles C, Weber R, et al: Mutations in the tropoelastine gene (ELN) were not found in patients with spontaneous cervical artery dissection, *Stroke* 31:2000, 1935.

102. Guillon B, Levy C, Bousser MG: Internal carotid artery dissection: An update, *J Neurol Sci* 153:146, 1998.

103. Pelkonen O, Tikkakoski T, Leinonen S, et al: Intracranial arterial dissection, *Neuroradiology* 40:442, 1998.

104. Frisoni GB, Anzola GP: Vertebrobasilar ischemia after neck motion, *Stroke* 22:1452, 1991.

105. Josien E: Extracranial vertebral artery dissection: Nine cases, *J Neurol* 239:327, 1992.

106. Bin Saeed A, Shuaib A, Al-Sulaiti G, et al: Vertebral artery dissection: Warning symptoms, clinical features and prognosis in 26 patients, *Can J Neurol Sci* 27:292, 2000.

107. Arnold M, Bousser MG, Fahrni G, et al: Vertebral artery dissection: presenting findings and predictors of outcome, *Stroke* 37:2499, 2006.

108. Salari-Namin HR, Cohen SN: *Management of ischemic stroke*, New York, 2000, McGraw-Hill.

109. Manz HJ, Vester J, Laenstein B: Dissecting aneurysm of cerebral arteries in childhood and adolescence, *Virchows Arch* 384:325, 1979.

110. Mokri B, Houser OW, Sandock BA, et al: Spontaneous dissection of the vertebral arteries, *Neurology* 38:880, 1988.

111. Desfontaines P, Despland A: Dissection of the internal carotid artery: Aetiology, symptomatology, clinical and neurosonological follow-up and treatment in 60 consecutive cases, *Acta Neurol Psych Belg* 94:226, 1995.

112. Weiller C, Mullges W, Ringelstein EB, et al: Patterns of brain infarction in internal carotid artery dissections, *Neurosurg Rev* 14:111, 1991.

113. Steinke W, Schwartz A, Hennerici M: Topography of cerebral infarction associated with carotid artery dissection, *J Neurol* 243:323, 1996.

114. Lucas C, Moulin T, Deplanque D, et al: Stroke patterns of internal carotid artery dissection in 40 patients, *Stroke* 29:2646, 1998.

115. Baumgartner RW, Arnold M, Baumgartner I, et al: Carotid dissection with and without ischemic events: Local symptoms and cerebral artery findings, *Neurology* 57:827, 2001.

116. Srinivasan J, Newell DW, Sturzenegger M, et al: Transcranial Doppler in the evaluation of internal carotid artery dissection: Demonstration of a correlation between microemboli detected by transcranial Doppler and stroke: Usefulness of this technique for the evaluation of anticoagulation efficacy, *Stroke* 27:1226, 1996.

117. Ast G, Woimant F, Georges B, et al: Spontaneous dissection of the internal carotid artery in 68 patients, *Eur J Med* 2:466, 1993.

118. Biousse V, D'Anglejean-Chatillon J, Touboul P-J, et al: Time course of symptoms in extracranial carotid artery dissections, *Stroke* 26:235, 1995.

119. Cox LK, Bertorini T, Laster RE: Headaches due to spontaneous internal carotid artery dissection, *Headache* 31:12, 1991.

120. Early TF, Gregory RT, Wheeler JR, et al: Spontaneous carotid dissection: Duplex scanning in diagnosis and management, *J Vasc Surg* 14:391, 1991.

121. Mokri B: Spontaneous dissections of internal carotid arteries, *Neurologist* 3:104, 1997.

122. Mullges W, Ringelstein EB, Leibold M: Non-invasive diagnosis of internal carotid artery dissections, *J Neurol Neurosurg Psychiatry* 55:98, 1992.

123. Ramadan NM, Tietjen GE, Levine SR, et al: Scintillating scotomata associated with internal carotid artery dissection, *Neurology* 41:1084, 1991.

124. Silbert PL, Mokri B, Schievink WI: Headache and neck pain in spontaneous internal carotid and vertebral artery dissections, *Neurology* 45:1517, 1995.

125. Sue DE, Brant-Zawadzki MN, Chance J: Dissection of cranial arteries in the neck: Correlation of MRI and arteriography, *Neuroradiology* 34:273, 1992.

126. Sturzenegger M: Spontaneous internal carotid artery dissection: Early diagnosis and management in 44 patients, *J Neurol* 242:231, 1995.

127. Biousse V, D'Anglejean-Chatillon J, Touboul P-J, et al: Head pain in non-traumatic carotid artery dissections, *Cephalgia* 14:33, 1994.

128. Mokri B, Silbert PL, Schievink WI, et al: Cranial nerve palsy in spontaneous internal carotid and vertebral artery dissections, *Neurology* 46:356, 1996.

129. Francis KR, Williams DP, Troost BT: Facial numbness and dysesthesia: New features of carotid artery dissection, *Arch Neurol* 44:345, 1987.

130. Goodman JM, Zink WL, Cooper DF: Hemilingual paralysis caused by carotid artery dissection, *Arch Neurol* 40:653, 1983.

131. Guidetti D, Pisanello A, Giovanardi F, et al: Spontaneous carotid dissection presenting lower cranial nerve palsies, *J Neurol Sci* 184:203–207, 2001.

132. Panisset M, Eidelman BH: Multiple cranial neuropathy as a feature of internal carotid artery dissection, *Stroke* 21:141, 1990.

133. Sturzenegger M, Huber P: Cranial nerve palsies in spontaneous carotid artery dissection, *J Neurol Neurosurg Psychiatry* 56:1191, 1993.

134. Waespe W, Niesper J, Imhof H-G, et al: Lower cranial nerve palsies due to internal carotid dissection, *Stroke* 19:1561, 1988.

135. Gout O, Bonnaud I, Weill A, et al: Facial diplegia complicating a bilateral internal carotid artery dissection, *Stroke* 30:681, 1999.

136. Pelkonen O, Tikkakoski T, Luotonen J, et al: Pulsatile tinnitus as a symptom of cervicocephalic arterial dissection, *J Laryngol Otol* 118:193, 2006.

137. Martin PJ, Humphrey PRD: Disabling stroke arising five months after internal carotid artery dissection, *J Neurol Neurosurg Psychiatry* 65:136, 1998.

138. Bogousslavsky J, Despland PA, Regli F: Spontaneous carotid dissection with acute stroke, *Arch Neurol* 44:137, 1987.

139. Rao TH, Schneider LB, Patel M, et al: Central retinal artery occlusion from carotid dissection diagnosed by cervical computed tomography, *Stroke* 25:1271–1272, 1994.

140. Pozzati E, Galassi E, Godano U, et al: Regressing intracranial carotid occlusions in childhood, *Pediatr Neurosurg* 21:243, 1994.

141. Chang V, Rewcastle NB, Harwood-Nash DCF, et al: Bilateral dissecting aneurysms of the intracranial internal carotids in an 8-year-old boy, *Neurology (NY)* 25:573, 1975.

142. Nass R, Hays A, Chutorian A: Intracranial dissecting aneurysms in childhood, *Stroke* 13:204, 1982.

143. Adams HPJ, Aschenbrener CA, Kassell NF, et al: Intracranial hemorrhage produced by spontaneous dissecting intracranial aneurysm, *Arch Neurol* 39:773, 1982.

144. de Bray JM, Pennison-Besnier L, Dubas F, et al: Extracranial and intracranial vertebrobasilar dissections: Diagnosis and prognosis, *J Neurol Neurosurg Psychiatry* 63:46, 1977.

145. Provenzale JM, Morgenlander JC, Gress D: Spontaneous vertebral dissection: Clinical, conventional angiographic, CT, and MR findings, *J Comput Assist Tomogr* 20:185, 1996.

146. Takis C, Saver JL: *Cerebrovascular disease*, Philadelphia, 1997, Lippincott-Raven.

147. Chiras J, Marciano S, Vega Molina J, et al: Spontaneous dissecting aneurysm of the extracranial vertebral artery (20 cases), *Neuroradiology* 27:327, 1985.

148. Caplan LR, Zarins CK, Hemmati M: Spontaneous dissection of the extracranial vertebral arteries, *Stroke* 16:1030, 1985.

149. de Bray JM, Pennison-Besnier I, Giroud M: [Cervical deficit radiculopathy in 3 cases of vertebral artery dissection], *Rev Neurol (Paris)* 154:762, 1998.

150. Crum B, Mokri B, Fulgham J: Spinal manifestations of vertebral artery dissection, *Neurology* 55:304, 2000.

151. Weidauer S, Claus D, Gartenschlager M: Spinal sulcal artery syndrome due to spontaneous bilateral vertebral artery dissection, *J Neurol Neurosurg Psychiatry* 67:550, 1999.

152. Goldsmith P, Rowe D, Jager R, et al: Focal vertebral artery dissection causing Brown-Séquard's syndrome, *J Neurol Neurosurg Psychiatry* 64:415, 1998.

153. Adams HPJ, Aschenbrener CA, Kassell NF, et al: Intracranial hemorrhage produced by spontaneous dissecting aneurysms of the internal carotid arteries, *Acta Neuropathol* 29:93, 1974.

154. Alexander CB, Burger PC, Goree JA: Dissecting aneurysms of the basilar artery in two patients, *Stroke* 10:294, 1979.

155. Farrell MA, Gilbert JJ, Kaufmann JC: Fatal intracranial arterial dissection: Clinical pathological correlation, *J Neurol Neurosurg Psychiatry* 48:111, 1985.

156. Arunodaya GR, Vani S, Shankar SK, et al: Fibromuscular dysplasia with dissection of basilar artery presenting as "locked-in-syndrome," *Neurology* 48:1605, 1997.

157. Berkovic SF, Spokes RL, Anderson RM, et al: Basilar artery dissection, *J Neurol Neurosurg Psychiatry* 46:126, 1983.

158. Brihaye J, Retif J, Jeanmart L: Occlusion of the basilar artery in young patients, *Acta Neurochir* 24:143–156, 1971.

159. Woimant F, Spelle L: Spontaneous basilar artery dissection: Contribution of magnetic resonance imaging to diagnosis, *J Neurol Neurosurg Psychiatry* 58:540, 1995.

160. Campiche PR, Anzil AP, Zander E: Aneurysme dissequant de tronc basilaire, *Arch Suisse Neurol Neurochir Psychiatr* 104:209–223, 1969.

161. Crosato F, Terzian H: Gli aneurismi dissecanti intracranici, *Riv Pat Nerv Ment* 82:450–462, 1961.

162. Escourolle R, Gautier JC, Rosa A, et al: Aneurysme dissequant vertebrobasilaire, *Rev Neurol (Paris)* 128:95–104, 1973.

163. Hayman JA, Anderson RM: Dissecting aneurysm of the basilar artery, *Med J Aust* 2:360, 1966.

164. Hosoda K, Fujita S, Kawaguchi T, et al: Spontaneous dissecting aneurysms of the basilar artery presenting with subarachnoid hemorrhage, *J Neurosurg* 75:628, 1991.

165. Hyland HH: Thrombosis of intracranial arteries, *Arch Neurol Psychiatr* 30:342–356, 1933.

166. Kulla L, Deymeer F, Smith TW, et al: Intracranial dissecting and saccular aneurysms in polycystic kidney disease, *Arch Neurol* 39:776, 1983.

167. Nozicka A: Zerebrovaskulare erkrankungen bei jungen leuten bedingt durch dissezierendes aneurysma der basalen hirnarterien, *Hradec Kralove* 25:225–229, 1972.

168. Pasquier B, Couderc P, Pasquier D, et al: Hemodissection parietale obliterante ou anevrisme dissequant vertebro basilaire, *Sem Hop Paris* 52:2519–2527, 1976.

169. Pasquier B, N'Golet A, Pasquier D, et al: Vertebro-basilar dissecting aneurysm, *Sem Hop Paris* 55:487–488, 1979.

170. Perier O, Cauchie G, Demanet JC: Hematome intramural par dissection parietale (aneurysme dissequant) du tronc basilaire, *Acta Neurol Psych Belg* 64:1064–1074, 1964.

171. Perier O, Brihaye J, Dhaene R: Hemodissection parietale obliterante (anevrisme dissequant) de l'artere basilaire, *Acta Neurol Psych Belg* 66:123–141, 1966.

172. Pozzati E, Andreoli A, Padovani R, et al: Dissecting aneurysms of the basilar artery, *Neurosurgery* 36:254, 1995.

173. Redondo-Marco JA, Walb D: Zur frage des aneurysma dissecans am intrakraniellen gefabsystem, *Acta Neurochir* 16:278–290, 1969.

174. Scholefield BG: A case of aneurysm of the basilar artery, *Guys Hosp Rep* 74:485, 1924.

175. Sekino H, Nakamura N, Katoh Y, et al: Dissecting aneurysms of the vertebro-basilar system: Clinical and angiographic observations, *No Shinkei Geka* 9:125–133, 1981.

176. Takita K, Shirato H, Akasaka T, et al: Dissecting aneurysm of the vertebro-basilar artery, *No To Shinkei* 31:1211–1218, 1979.

177. Watson AJ: Dissecting aneurysm of arteries other than the aorta, *J Path Bact* 72:439–449, 1956.

178. Wolman L: Cerebral dissecting aneurysms, *Brain* 82:276–291, 1958.

179. Djouhri H, Guillon B, Brunereau L, et al: MR angiography for the long-term follow-up of dissecting aneurysms of the extracranial internal carotid artery, *Am J Roentgenol* 174:1137, 2000.

180. Kasner SE, Hankins LL, Bratina P, et al: Magnetic resonance angiography demonstrates vascular healing of carotid and vertebral artery dissections, *Stroke* 28:1997, 1993.

181. Kirsch EC, Kaim A, Engelter ST, et al: MR angiography in internal carotid artery dissection: Improvement of diagnosis by selective demonstration of the intramural hematoma, *Neuroradiology* 40:704, 1998.

182. Leclerc X, Lucas C, Godefroy O, et al: Preliminary experience using contrast-enhanced MRI angiography to assess vertebral artery structure for the follow-up of suspected dissection, *AJNR Am J Neuroradiol* 20:1482, 1999.

183. Provenzale JM: Dissection of the internal carotid and vertebral arteries: Imaging features, *ARJ Am J Roentgenol* 165:1099, 1995.

184. Levy C, Laissy JP, Raveau V, et al: Carotid and vertebral artery dissections: Three dimensional time-of-flight MR angiography and MR imaging versus conventional angiography, *Radiology* 190:97, 1994.

185. Jacobs A, Lanfermann H, Neveling M, et al: MRI and MRA-guided therapy of carotid and vertebral artery dissection, *J Neurol Sci* 39:329, 1997.

186. Mascalchi M, Bianchi MC, Mangiafico S, et al: MRI and MRI angiography of vertebral artery dissection, *Neuroradiology* 39:329, 1997.

187. de Bray JM, Lhoste P, Dubas F, et al: Ultrasonic features of extracranial carotid dissections: 47 cases studied by angiography, *J Ultrasound Med* 13:659, 1994.

188. Sturzenegger M, Mattle HP, Rivoir A, et al: Ultrasound findings in carotid artery dissection: Analysis of 43 patients, *Neurology* 45:691, 1995.

189. Hoffman M, Sacco RL, Chan S, et al: Noninvasive detection of vertebral artery dissection, *Stroke* 24:815, 1993.

190. Sturzenegger M, Mattle HP, Rivoir A, et al: Ultrasound findings in spontaneous extracranial vertebral artery dissection, *Stroke* 24:1993, 1910.

191. Steinke W, Rautenberg W, Schwartz A, et al: Noninvasive monitoring of internal carotid artery dissection, *Stroke* 25:998, 1994.

192. Hennerici M, Steinke W, Rautenberg W: High-resistance Doppler flow pattern in extracranial carotid dissection, *Arch Neurol* 46:670, 1989.

193. Baumgartner RW, Baumgartner I, Mattle HP, et al: Transcranial color-coded duplex sonography in the evaluation of collateral flow through the circle of Willis, *AJNR Am J Neuroradiol* 18:127, 1997.

194. Leclerc X, Godefroy O, Pruvo JP, et al: Computed tomographic angiography for the evaluation of carotid artery stenosis, *Stroke* 26:1577, 1995.

195. Fredenberg P, Forbes K, Toye L, et al: Assessment of cervical vascular injury with CT angiography, *BNI Q* 17:44, 2001.

196. Houser OW, Mokri B, Sundt TMJ, et al: Spontaneous cervical cephalic arterial dissection and its residuum: Angiographic spectrum, *AJNR Am J Neuroradiol* 5:27, 1984.

197. Lu C-J, Sun Y, Jeng J-S, et al: Imaging in the diagnosis and follow-up evaluation of vertebral artery dissection, *J Ultrasound Med* 19:263, 2000.

198. Alecu C, Fortrat JO, Ducrocq X, et al: Duplex scanning diagnosis of internal carotid artery dissections: A case control study, *Cerebrovasc Dis* 23:441, 2007.

199. Rothrock JF, Lim V, Press G, et al: Serial magnetic resonance and carotid duplex examinations in the management of carotid dissection, *Neurology (NY)* 39:686, 1989.

200. Provenzale JM, Barboriak DP, Taveras JM: Exercise-related dissection of craniocervical arteries: CT, MR, and angiographic findings, *J Comput Assist Tomogr* 19:268, 1995.

201. Scazzeri F, Mascalchi M, Calabrese R, et al: Case report: MRI and MR angiography of basilar artery dissection in a child, *Neuroradiology* 39:654, 1997.

202. Stapf C, Elkind SV, Mohr JP: Carotid artery dissection, *Annu Rev Med* 51:329, 2001.

203. Silverboard G, Tart R: Cerebrovascular arterial dissection in children and young adults, *Semin Pediatr Neurol* 7:278, 2000.

204. Brugieres P, Castrec-Carpo A, Heran F, et al: Magnetic resonance imaging in the exploration of dissection of the internal carotid artery, *J Neuroradiol* 16:1, 1989.

205. Gelbert F, Assouline E, Hodes JE, et al: MRI in spontaneous dissection of vertebral and carotid arteries, *Neuroradiology* 33:111, 1991.

206. Hart RG: Vertebral artery dissection, *Neurology (NY)* 38:987, 1988.

207. Quint DJ, Spickler EM: Magnetic resonance imaging demonstration of vertebral artery dissection: Report of 2 cases, *J Neurosurg* 72:964, 1990.

208. Osborn AG, Anderson RE: Angiographic spectrum of cervical and intracranial fibromuscular dysplasia, *Stroke* 8:617, 1997.

209. Chiu N, DeLong GR, Heinz ER: Intracranial fibromuscular dysplasia in a 5-year-old child, *Pediatr Neurol* 14:262, 1996.

210. Mokri B, Houser OW, Stanson AW: Multivessel cervicocephalic and visceral arterial dissections: Pathogenic role of primary arterial disease in cervicocephalic arterial dissections, *J Stroke Cerebrovasc Dis* 1:117, 1991.

211. Elijovich L, Kazmi K, Gauvrit J, et al: The emerging role of multidetector row CT angiography in the diagnosis of cervical arterial dissection: preliminary study, *Neuroradiology* 48:606, 2006.

212. Chen CJ, Tseng YC, Lee TH, et al: Multisection CT angiography compared with catheter angiography in diagnosing vertebral artery dissection, *AJNR Am J Neuroradiol* 25:769, 2004.

213. Vertinsky AT, Schwartz NE, Fischbein NJ, et al: Comparison of multidetector CT angiography and MR imaging of cervical arterial dissection, *AJNR Am J Neuroradiol* 29:1753, 2008.

214. Treiman GS, Treima RL, Foran RF, et al: Spontaneous dissection of the internal carotid artery: A nineteen-year clinical experience, *J Vasc Surg* 24:597, 1996.

215. Lyrer PA, Engelter ST: *Antithrombotic drugs for carotid artery dissection (Cochrane Review). The Cochrane Library Issue 1*, Oxford, 2002, Update Software.

216. Menon R, Kerry S, Norris JW, et al: Treatment of cervical arterial dissection: A systematic review and meta-analysis, *J Neurol Neurosurg Psychiatry* 79:1122, 2008.

217. Sacco RL, Adams R, Albers G, et al: Guidelines for prevention of stroke in patients with ischemic stroke or transient ischemic attack: a statement for healthcare professionals from the American Heart Association/American Stroke Association Council on Stroke: Co-Sponsored by the Council on Cardiovascular Radiology and Intervention: The American Academy of Neurology affirms the value of this guideline, *Stroke* 37:577, 2006.

218. Engelter ST, Brandt T, Debette S, et al: Antiplatelets versus anticoagulation in cervical artery dissection, *Stroke* 38:2605, 2007.

219. Metso TM, Metso AJ, Helenius J, et al: Prognosis and safety of anticoagulation in intracranial artery dissections in adults, *Stroke* 38:2007, 1837.

220. Price RF, Sellar R, Leung C, et al: Traumatic vertebral arterial dissection and vertebrobasilar arterial thrombosis successfully treated with endovascular thrombolysis and stenting, *AJNR Am J Neuroradiol* 19:1677, 1998.

221. Derex L, Nighoghossian N, Turjman F, et al: Intravenous tPA in acute ischemic stroke to internal carotid artery dissection, *Neurology* 54:2159, 2000.

222. Arnold M, Nedeltchev K, Sturzzenegger M, et al: Thrombolysis in patients with acute stroke caused by cervical artery dissection: Analysis of 9 patients and review of the literature, *Arch Neurol* 59:549, 2002.

223. Rudolf J, Neveling M, Grond M, et al: Stroke following internal carotid artery occlusion: A contraindication for intravenous thrombolysis, *Eur J Neurol* 6:51, 1999.

224. Sampognaro G, Turgut T, Connors JJ III, et al: Intra-arterial thrombolysis in a patient presenting with an ischemic stroke due to spontaneous internal carotid dissection, *Catheter Cardiovasc Interv* 48:312, 1999.

225. Ahmad HA, Gerraty RP, Davis SM, et al: Cervicocerebral artery dissections, *J Accid Emerg Med* 16:422, 1999.

226. Georgiadis D, Lanczik O, Schwab S, et al: IV thrombolysis in patients with acute stroke due to spontaneous carotid dissection, *Neurology* 64:1612, 2005.

227. Lavallee PC, Mazighi M, Saint-Maurice JP, et al: Stent-assisted endovascular thrombolysis versus intravenous thrombolysis in internal carotid artery dissection with tandem internal carotid and middle cerebral artery occlusion, *Stroke* 38:2270, 2007.

228. Gomez CR, May AK, Terry JB, et al: Endovascular therapy of traumatic injuries of the extracranial cerebral arteries, *Crit Care Clin* 15:789, 1999.

229. Bejjani GK, Monsein LH, Laird JR, et al: Treatment of symptomatic cervical carotid dissections with endovascular stents, *Neurosurgery* 44:755, 1999.

230. Yadav JS, Roubin GS, Iyer S, et al: Elective stenting of the extracranial carotid arteries, *Circulation* 95:376, 1997.

231. Malek AM, Higashida RT, Phatouros CC, et al: Endovascular management of extracranial carotid artery dissection achieved using stent angioplasty, *AJNR Am J Neuroradiol* 21:1380, 2000.

232. Hemphill JC III, Gress DR, Halbach VV: Endovascular therapy of traumatic injuries of the intracranial cerebral arteries, *Crit Care Clin* 15:811, 1999.

233. Manninen HI, Koivisto T, Saari T, et al: Dissecting aneurysms of all four cervicocranial arteries in fibromuscular dysplasia: Treatment with self-expanding endovascular stents, coil, embolization, and surgical ligation, *AJNR Am J Neuroradiol* 18:1216, 1997.

234. Dorros G, Cohn JM, Palmer LE: Stent deployment resolves a petrous carotid artery angioplasty dissection, *AJNR Am J Neuroradiol* 19:392, 1998.

235. Horowitz MB, Miller G III, Meyer Y, et al: Use of intravascular stents in treatment of internal carotid and extracranial vertebral artery pseudoaneurysms, *AJNR Am J Neuroradiol* 17:693, 1996.

236. Perez-Cruet MJ, Patwardhan RV, Mawad ME, et al: Treatment of dissecting pseudoaneurysm of the cervical internal carotid artery using a wall stent and detachable coils: Case report, *Neurosurgery* 40:622, 1997.

237. Lenthall RK, White BD, McConachie NS: Endovascular management of complete vertebral artery dissection presenting with subarachnoid hemorrhage, *Interv Neuroradiol* 5:161, 1999.

238. Siminonata F, Righi C, Scotti G: Post-traumatic dissecting aneurysm of extracranial internal carotid artery: Endovascular treatment with stenting, *Neuroradiology* 41:543, 1999.

239. Hurst RW, Haskal ZJ, Zager E, et al: Endovascular stent treatment of cervical internal carotid artery aneurysms with parent vessel preservation, *Surg Neurol* 40:313, 1998.

240. Singer RJ, Dake MD, Norbash A, et al: Covered stent placement for neurovascular disease, *AJNR Am J Neuroradiol* 18:507, 1996.

241. Hong MK, Satler LF, Gallino R, et al: Intravascular stenting as a definitive treatment of spontaneous carotid artery dissection, *Am J Cardiol* 79:538, 1997.

242. Matsuura JH, Rosenthall D, Jerius H, et al: Traumatic carotid artery dissection and pseudoaneurysm treated with endovascular coils and stent, *J Endovasc Surg* 4:339, 1997.

243. Mericle RA, Lanzino G, Wakhloo AK, et al: Stenting and secondary coiling of intracranial internal carotid artery aneurysm: technical case report, *Neurosurgery* 43:1229, 1998.

244. Klein GE, Szolar DH, Raith J, et al: Posttraumatic extracranial aneurysm of the internal carotid artery: Combined endovascular treatment with coils and stents, *AJNR Am J Neuroradiol* 18:1261–1264, 1997.

245. Miyachi S, Ishiguchi T, Taniguchi K, et al: Endovascular stenting of a traumatic dissecting aneurysm of the extracranial internal carotid artery—a case report, *Neurol Med Chir* 37:270, 1997.

246. Yamashita K, Okamoto S, Kim C, et al: Emergent treatment of iatrogenic dissection of the internal carotid artery with the Palmaz-Schatz stent—case report, *Neurol Med Chir* 37:336, 1997.

247. DeOcampo J, Brillman J, Levy DI: Stenting: A new approach to carotid dissection, *J Neuroimag* 7:187, 1997.

248. Scavee V, DeWispelaere JF, Mormont E, et al: Pseudoaneurysm of the internal carotid artery: Treatment with a covered stent, *Cardiovasc Interv Radiol* 24:283, 2001.

249. Schievink WI, Piepgras DG, McCaffrey TV, et al: Surgical treatment of extracranial internal carotid artery dissecting aneurysms, *Neurosurgery* 35:809, 1994.

250. Norris JW, Nadareishvili ZG, Rowe D, et al: Are the hazards of carotid stenting unacceptably high? *Neurology* 52(Suppl 2): A269, 1999.

251. Hobson RW II, Goldstein JE, Jamil Z, et al: Carotid restenosis: Operative and endovascular management, *J Vasc Surg* 29:228, 1999.

252. Vale FL, Fisher S III, Jordan WD Jr, et al: Carotid endarterectomy performed after progressive carotid stenosis following angioplasty and stent placement: Case report, *J Neurosurg* 87:940, 1997.

253. Coumans JV, Watson VE, Picken CA, et al: Saphenous vein interposition graft for recurrent carotid stenosis after prior endarterectomy and stent placement: Case report, *J Neurosurg* 90:567, 1999.

254. Painter TA, Hertzer NR, Beven EG, et al: Extracranial carotid aneurysms: Report of six cases and review of the literature, *J Vasc Surg* 2:312, 1985.

255. Sundt TM Jr, Pearson BW, Piepgras DG, et al: Surgical management of aneurysms of the distal extracranial internal carotid artery, *J Neurosurg* 64:169, 1986.

256. Coffin O, Maiza D, Galateau-Salle F, et al: Results of surgical management of internal carotid artery aneurysm by the cervical approach, *Ann Vasc Surg* 11:482, 1997.

257. Grubb RL, Derdeyn CP, Fritsch SM, et al: Importance of hemodynamic factors in the prognosis of symptomatic carotid occlusion, *JAMA* 280:1055, 1998.

258. Mokri B, Piepgras DG, Houser OW: Traumatic dissections of the extracranial internal carotid artery, *J Neurosurg* 68:189, 1988.

259. Mokri B: Traumatic and spontaneous extracranial internal carotid artery dissections, *J Neurol* 237:356, 1990.

260. Pozzati E, Giuliani G, Acciarri N, et al: Long-term follow-up of occlusive cervical carotid dissection, *Stroke* 21:528, 1990.

261. Milhaud K, de Freitas GR, van Melle G, et al: Occlusion due to carotid artery dissection, *Arch Neurol* 59:557, 2002.

262. Dziewas R, Konrad C, Drager B, et al: Cervical artery dissection: Clinical features, risk factors, therapy and outcome in 126 patients, *J Neurol* 250:1179, 2003.

263. de Bray JM, Pennison-Besnier I, Dubas F, et al: Extracranial and intracranial vertebrobasilar dissections: Diagnosis and prognosis, *J Neurol Neurosurg Psychiatry* 63:46, 1997.

264. Yamaura A, Ono J, Hirai S: Clinical picture of intracranial non-traumatic dissecting aneurysm, *Neuropathology* 1:85–90, 2000.

265. Saver JL, Easton JD, Hart RG: *Dissections and trauma of cervico-cerebral arteries*, New York, 1992, Churchill Livingstone.

266. Arboix A, Massons J, Oliveres M, et al: Analisis de 1,000 pacientes consecutivos con enfermedad cerebrovascular aguda: Registro de patologia cerebrovascular de L'Alianza-Hospital Central de Barcelona, *Med Clin (Barc)* 101:281, 1993.

267. Goldstein LB, Gray L, Hulette CM: Stroke due to recurrent ipsilateral carotid artery dissection in a young adult, *Stroke* 26:480–483, 1995.

268. Touze E, Gauvrit JY, Moulin T, et al: Risk of stroke and recurrent dissection after a cervical artery dissection: A multicenter study, *Neurology* 61:1347, 2003.

269. Dittrich R, Nassenstein I, Bachmann R, et al: Polyarterial clustered recurrence of cervical artery dissection seems to be the rule, *Neurology* 69:180, 2007.

270. Arnold M, De Marchis GM, Stapf C, et al: Triple and quadruple spontaneous cervical artery dissection: Presenting characteristics and long-term outcome, *J Neurol Neurosurg Psychiatry* 80:171–174, 2008.

271. Engelter ST, Lyrer PA, Kirsch EC, et al: Long-term follow-up after extracranial internal carotid artery dissection, *Eur Neurol* 44:199, 2000.

272. Guillon B, Brunereau L, Biousse V, et al: Long-term follow-up of aneurysms developed during extracranial internal carotid dissection, *Neurology* 53:117, 1999.

273. Touze E, Randoux B, Meary E, et al: Aneurysmal forms of cervical artery dissection: Associated factors and outcome, *Stroke* 32:418, 2001.

274. Benninger DH, Gandjour J, Georgiadis D, et al: Benign long-term outcome of conservatively treated cervical aneurysms due to carotid dissection, *Neurology* 69:486, 2007.

275. Schievink WI, Bjornsson J: Fibromuscular dysplasia of the internal carotid artery: A clinicopathological study, *Clin Neuropathol* 15:2, 1996.

276. Mettinger KL: Fibromuscular dysplasia and the brain II: Current concept of disease, *Stroke* 13:53, 1982.

277. Sang CN, Whelton PK, Hamper UM, et al: Etiologic factors in renovascular fibromuscular dysplasia: A case-control study, *Hypertension* 14:472, 1989.

278. Pannier-Moreau I, Grimbert P, Fiquet-Kempf B, et al: Possible familial origin of multifocal renal artery fibromuscular dysplasia, *J Hypertens* 15:1797, 1997.

279. Bofinger A, Hawley C, Fisher P, et al: Polymorphisms of the renin-angiotensin system in patients with multifocal renal arterial fibromuscular dysplasia, *J Hum Hypertens* 15:185, 2001.

280. Solder B, Streif W, Ellemunter H, et al: Fibromuscular dysplasia of the internal carotid artery in a child with alpha-1-antitrypsin deficiency, *Dev Med Child Neurol* 39:827, 1997.

281. Schievink WI, Bjornsson J, Parisi JE, et al: Arterial fibromuscular dysplasia associated with severe alpha 1-antitrypsin deficiency, *Mayo Clin Proc* 69:1040, 1994.

282. Schievink WI, Puumala MR, Meyer FB, et al: Giant intracranial aneurysm and fibromuscular dysplasia in an adolescent with alpha 1-antitrypsin deficiency, *J Neurosurg* 85:503, 1996.

283. Nakata Y, Shionoya S, Matsubara J, et al: An experimental study on the vascular lesions caused by disturbance of the vasa vasorum. 3: Influence of obstruction of the venous side of the vasa vasorum and the periaortic vein, *Jpn Circ J* 36:945, 1972.

284. Rothfield NJ: Fibromuscular arterial disease: Experimental studies, *Aust Radiol* 14:294, 1970.

285. Fievez M, Koerperich G, Dulieu J: Arterial fibromuscular dysplasia, *Ann Anat Pathol (Paris)* 20:357, 1975.

286. Paulson GW, Boesel CP, Evans WE: Fibromuscular dysplasia, *Arch Neurol* 35:287, 1978.

287. Bragin MA, Cherkasov AP: Morphogenesis of fibromuscular dysplasia of the renal arteries (an ultrastructural study), *Arkh Patol* 41:46, 1979.

288. So EL, Toole JF, Dalal P, et al: Cephalic fibromuscular dysplasia in 32 patients: Clinical findings and radiologic features, *Arch Neurol* 38:619, 1981.

289. Osborn AG, Anderson RE: Angiographic spectrum of cervical and intracranial fibromuscular dysplasia, *Stroke* 8:617, 1977.

290. Frens DB, Petajan JH, Anderson R: Fibromuscular dysplasia of the posterior cerebral artery: Report of a case and review of the literature, *Stroke* 5:161, 1974.

291. Hopkins LN, Budny JL: Fibromuscular dysplasia. In Wilkins RH, Rengachary SS, editors: *Neurosurgery*, New York, NY, 1985, McGraw Hill, pp 1293–1296.

292. Danza R, Baldizan J, Navarro T: Surgery of carotid kinking and fibromuscular dysplasia, *J Cardiovasc Surg* 24:628, 1983.

293. Rainer WG, Cramer GG, Newby JP, et al: Fibromuscular hyperplasia of the carotid artery causing positional cerebral ischemia, *Ann Surg* 167:444, 1968.

294. Balaji MR, DeWeese JA: Fibromuscular dysplasia of the internal carotid artery: Its occurrence with acute stroke and its surgical reversal, *Arch Surg* 115:984, 1980.

295. Morganlander JC, Goldstein LB: Recurrent transient ischemic attacks and stroke in association with an internal carotid artery web, *Stroke* 22:94, 1991.

296. Grotta JC, Ward RE, Flynn TC, et al: Spontaneous internal carotid artery dissection associated with fibromuscular dysplasia, *J Cardiovasc Surg* 23:512, 1982.

297. de Bray JM, Marc G, Pautot V, et al: Fibromuscular dysplasia may herald symptomatic recurrence of cervical artery dissection, *Cerebrovasc Dis* 23:448, 2007.

298. Kimura H, Hosoda K, Hara Y, et al: A very unusual case of fibromuscular dysplasia with multiple aneurysms of the vertebral artery and posterior inferior cerebellar artery, *J Neurosurg* 109:1108, 2008.

299. Hirai T, Korogi Y, Harada M, et al: Carotid-cavernous sinus fistula and aneurysmal rupture associated with fibromuscular dysplasia: A case report, *Acta Radiol* 37:49, 1996.

300. Reddy SV, Karnes WE, Earnest F 4th, et al: Spontaneous extracranial vertebral arteriovenous fistula with fibromuscular dysplasia: Case report, *J Neurosurg* 54:399, 1981.

301. Arning C, Grzyska U: Color Doppler imaging of cervicocephalic fibromuscular dysplasia, *Cardiovasc Ultrasound* 20:7, 2004.

302. Heiserman JE, Drayer BP, Fram EK, et al: MR angiography of cervical fibromuscular dysplasia, *AJNR Am J Neuroradiol* 13:1454, 1992.

303. Sandok BA: Fibromuscular dysplasia of the internal carotid artery, *Neurol Clin* 1:17-26, 1983.

304. Corrin LS, Sandok BA, Houser OW: Cerebral ischemic events in patients with carotid artery fibromuscular dysplasia, *Arch Neurol* 38:616, 1981.

305. Wells RP, Smith RR: Fibromuscular dysplasia of the internal carotid artery: A long term follow-up, *Neurosurgery* 10:39, 1982.

306. Wilms GE, Smits J, Baert AL, et al: Percutaneous transluminal angioplasty in fibromuscular dysplasia of the internal carotid artery: One year clinical and morphological follow-up, *Cardiovasc Interv Radiol* 8:20, 1985.

307. Curry TK, Messina LM: Fibromuscular dysplasia: When is intervention warranted? *Semin Vasc Surg* 16:190, 2003.

308. Chiche L, Bahnini A, Koskas F, et al: Occlusive fibromuscular disease of arteries supplying the brain: Results of surgical treatment, *Ann Vasc Surg* 11:496, 1997.

309. Collins GJ Jr, Rich NM, Clagett GP, et al: Fibromuscular dysplasia of the internal carotid arteries: Clinical experience and follow-up, *Ann Surg* 194:89, 1981.

310. Wesen CA, Elliott BM: Fibromuscular dysplasia of the carotid arteries, *Am J Surg* 151:448, 1986.

311. Benoit BG, Russell NA, Grimes JD, et al: Spontaneous dissection of carotid and vertebral arteries; Management considerations, *Can J Neurol Sci* 11:328, 1984.

312. Bogousslavsky J, Regli F, Despland A: Aneurysmes dissequants spontanes de l'artere carotide interne, *Rev Neurol (Paris)* 11:625, 1984.

313. Garcia-Merino JA, Gutierrez JA, Lopez-Lozano JJ: Double-lumen dissecting aneurysms of the internal carotid artery in fibromuscular dysplasia: A case report, *Stroke* 14:815, 1983.

314. Jackson MA, Hughes RC, Ward SC, et al: Headbanging and carotid dissection, *BMJ* 287:1262, 1983.

34 Collagen Vascular and Infectious Diseases

SACHIN AGARWAL, J.P. MOHR, MITCHELL S.V. ELKIND

Stroke is a relatively common complication of many inflammatory and collagen vascular diseases. Strokes in this setting are often ascribed to inflammation of arteries, although other mechanisms, including emboli and coagulation disturbances, play a prominent role. This chapter reviews the current clinical understanding of the inflammatory diseases that may be associated with stroke. The chapter concludes with some comments on the role of inflammation in atherosclerotic stroke.

Giant Cell Arteritis

Giant cell arteritis (GCA), also known as temporal arteritis, is an inflammatory disease affecting medium and large arteries throughout the body, including the aorta and most of its major branches.[1,2] Inflammation of the arteries of the head and neck is responsible for the major neurologic symptoms, prominent among them headache and vision loss, including monocular or binocular blindness. Stroke, although uncommon, is a well-documented and potentially fatal complication.

GCA is not rare. Reported age- and sex-adjusted incidence is 17 to 25 per 100,000 population among age group 50 years or older, and the incidence increases with age from 2.6 per 100,000 for those 50 to 59 years old to 44.6 per 100,000 for those older than 80 years.[3-5] There is a threefold higher incidence in women than in men.[3] Susceptibility is associated with northern European descent, and two thirds of those affected are women.[4,5] The incidence may be up to seven times higher among white than black persons, possibly in relation to the lower frequency of HLA-DR4 (D-related human leukocyte antigen) among the latter group.[6]

In GCA, the arterial wall is infiltrated with mononuclear cells (lymphocytes and plasma cells) and, to a lesser extent, eosinophils and neutrophils, predominantly in the media near the internal elastic lamina. Granulomas composed of multinucleated or foreign body giant cells are found along with the inflammatory cells but are not invariably present. The vessel may be necrotic in areas, especially in the media. Fibrinoid necrosis is usually not present.[7] Intimal proliferation and fibrosis may result in luminal narrowing and thrombosis.

There is evidence that GCA is a T-cell–dependent disease involving CD4+ T cells.[5] Moreover, T-cell activation in the nonlymphoid environment of the arterial wall requires activation of specialized antigen-presenting cells that release interferons and cytokines.[8] Later, activation of monocytes and macrophages is responsible for the systemic inflammatory syndrome in GCA and in polymyalgia rheumatica (PMR).[9] Resident cells of the arterial wall respond uniquely to the immune injury mediated by tissue-infiltrating cells.[10] The end result is an occlusive vasculopathy due to the rapid proliferation of the intima, or the formation of an aortic aneurysm due to destruction of the arterial wall.[5]

The etiology is unknown. Circulating immune complexes[11] and immunoglobulins[12] in the sera of patients with biopsy-proven GCA have been demonstrated. Several studies have demonstrated a higher frequency of certain histocompatibility antigens, including HLA-B8, HLA-DR4, and HLA-DRB1*04, among patients with GCA,[13] although others have not. Some genetic studies have demonstrated associations with polymorphisms in immune mediator genes, such as tumor necrosis factor (TNF) and intercellular adhesion molecule-1 (ICAM-1).[14,15] No infectious cause has been identified.

General Clinical Features

The most common presentation of GCA is headache.[16] It is usually constant, more commonly at night, and located predominantly in the temporal area, but it may radiate to the scalp, face, jaw, or occiput. Scalp tenderness is a frequent complaint, and many patients have swollen, nodular, or pulseless temporal arteries. Some patients have jaw claudication. Systemic symptoms include fever, weight loss, fatigue, and malaise. Many patients have arthralgias. Dementia, confusion, and psychiatric symptoms, such as depression, have been reported.[17]

Most patients with GCA have symptoms of PMR for weeks to months before headache, jaw claudication, or visual loss develops. Up to 44% of patients who present with PMR alone go on to have overt GCA, and 23% have serious ophthalmologic (sudden monocular or binocular blindness) or neurologic complications.[18] Patients with PMR are frequently found to have GCA on temporal artery biopsy. These findings support the notion that PMR and GCA are not two distinct nosologic entities but different manifestations of a common disease.

Visual loss is the most feared complication of GCA. Anterior ischemic optic neuropathy is the most common cause.[19] Posterior ischemic optic neuropathy and central retinal artery occlusion may also cause visual loss. Less often, the visual loss takes the form of homonymous hemianopia, even cortical blindness, as a result of posterior circulation infarction. Visual loss due to GCA rarely improves, despite treatment with corticosteroids.[19] Large series report visual loss in 40% to 50% of patients with GCA.[20]

Visual loss typically occurs suddenly, although 10% to 20% of patients experience transient loss of vision (transient monocular blindness) before fixed visual deficits develop.[20] Bilateral involvement occurs in 33% of patients. The disc is swollen and usually pale, flame hemorrhages may be seen, and disc atrophy subsequently develops. Afferent pupillary defects are common. Field defects are usually altitudinal and inferior, although inferior nasal defects, arcuate defects, and scotomas may be seen.[19]

Ophthalmoplegia, usually transient, occurs in 10% to 15% of patients, with cranial nerves III and VI being affected with equal frequency. Ophthalmoplegia in GCA is probably due to ischemic necrosis of extraocular muscles. GCA may also cause "orbital infarction syndrome," in which orbital pain, blindness, ophthalmoplegia, and anterior and posterior segment ischemia occur as a result of global orbital ischemia.[21]

Stroke is an uncommon complication of GCA. Studies from referral centers suggest that patients with GCA may be at higher risk for stroke during the active phase of the disease. Many strokes occur despite therapy with corticosteroids, sometimes within 2 weeks of initiation of treatment, and some have had stroke despite normalization of the erythrocyte sedimentation rate (ESR). Compared with the foci usually affected by atherosclerosis, GCA is more common in the brainstem and vertebral territories. Postmortem examinations usually document involvement of the extradural segments of the vessels only (Fig. 34-1),[22,23] although some have shown evidence of intradural involvement as well.[24-26]

Thrombotic occlusion due to arteritis in internal carotid arteries has also been described.[27] In each, the thrombus was found distal to the bifurcation. Sometimes the involved cavernous segments are completely occluded by thrombus, resulting in borderzone "distal field" infarction. Other patients have had artery-to-artery embolism with hemorrhagic infarction.[27]

Diagnosis

Diagnosis of GCA requires three of the following five criteria: age more than 50 years, new-onset localized headache, temporal artery tenderness or diminished pulse, ESR exceeding 50 mm/hr, and typical histologic findings on temporal artery biopsy.[28] Although the most common laboratory abnormality in patients with GCA is a markedly increased ESR, a normal ESR does not exclude the diagnosis.[29] An ESR higher than 50 mm/hr has a sensitivity of approximately 87%, but this parameter is normal in approximately 2% to 9% of biopsy-proven disease.[30] Elevated C-reactive protein (CRP) value appears to be a more sensitive indicator of disease. Simultaneous elevations of both ESR and CRP appear to provide the highest specificity (97%) for establishing the diagnosis.[31] Most patients have a mild to moderate normochromic or

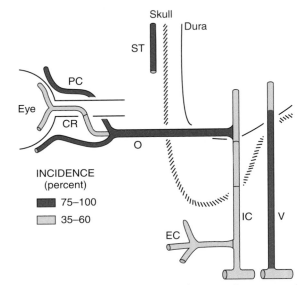

Figure 34-1 Pattern of involvement of giant cell arteritis in head and neck arteries. Note the high incidence of involvement of the vertebral artery (V), superior temporal artery (ST), ophthalmic artery (O), and posterior ciliary artery (PC). Intracranial arteries are rarely involved. CR, central retinal artery; EC, external carotid artery; IC, internal carotid artery. (From Wilkinson IMS, Russell RWR: Arteries of the head and neck in giant cell arteritis: A pathological study to show the pattern of arterial involvement. *Arch Neurol* 27:378, 1972.)

slightly hypochromic anemia. White blood cell counts are normal or moderately increased.

Temporal artery biopsy is the most specific diagnostic procedure. Biopsy is recommended for all patients in whom GCA is suspected. Bilateral temporal artery biopsy is recommended for highest sensitivity. In a retrospective study of 190 patients clinically diagnosed with GCA, biopsy findings were negative in 15.3%.[32] In one series of biopsy-proven cases, 86% were diagnosed through unilateral biopsy, and the remaining 14% only after biopsy of the other side.[33] A normal temporal artery biopsy does not exclude the diagnosis, however, because the disease may be segmental.[34] Other types of vasculitis may rarely cause inflammation of the temporal arteries and mimic the disease.[35,36] Complications of temporal artery biopsy are rare but include facial nerve injury, skin necrosis, eyebrow droop, and stroke.

Angiographic signs are uncommonly present, but the superficial temporal arteriogram may demonstrate areas of dilation and constriction along the length of the artery, and changes may also be seen in the internal carotid artery siphon segments. Angiographic abnormalities of intracranial arteries are rare and possibly represent cases of isolated granulomatous angiitis of the central nervous system (CNS). Color duplex ultrasonography has also been used in the diagnosis of GCA. In one study, a typical dark halo was seen around the lumen of the superficial temporal artery in 73% of patients, an abnormality that disappeared with treatment.[37] Fluorodeoxyglucose F-18 positron emission tomography may also show abnormal tracer uptake in the aorta and its branches in patients with GCA.[38] MRI of the brain may rarely show multifocal dural enhancement and temporalis muscle enhancement.[39]

Treatment and Prognosis

Once the diagnosis of GCA is suspected, steroid therapy should be started, and a temporal artery biopsy performed as soon as possible. Steroid therapy may be started before the biopsy. Some clinicians remain concerned that the initiation of steroid therapy may limit the diagnostic value of the temporal artery biopsy. An initial dosage of 40 to 60 mg/day of prednisone is recommended for the first month or until symptoms are controlled. Symptoms usually respond promptly to steroids, although visual loss and stroke may occur after initiation of treatment.

After clinical remission, steroid dose may be gradually tapered over 6 to 9 months to a maintenance dose of 7.5 to 10 mg prednisone daily.[40] Rapid tapering of the dosage may lead to relapse, including blindness. Steroids may be discontinued within 2 years because GCA often runs a self-limited course. Recurrence of symptoms or an increase in the ESR after initial control of the disease indicates relapse and should prompt resumption of higher doses of steroids. Relapse after withdrawal from steroids may not necessarily be accompanied by an increase in ESR, however. In one series, the mean duration of steroid therapy was 5.8 years, 12.8 years being the maximum.[41] The relapse rate after withdrawal of treatment was 47%; relapse occurred in 46% of the patients within 1 month and in 96% within 1 year after cessation of treatment. The relapse rate bore little relationship to the duration of treatment.[41] Alternate-day treatment regimens may be less effective than daily administration of steroids.[42] Some investigators advocate hospitalization and treatment with high-dose, pulsed intravenous administration of methylprednisolone for patients with acute visual loss.[43]

The role of steroid-sparing regimens in the treatment of GCA is not clear, but a small (n = 42) single-center, randomized trial has shown that combination therapy with methotrexate reduces the cumulative dose of prednisone taken while also diminishing the likelihood of relapse from 84% to 45%.[44] In contrast, a larger placebo-controlled trial involving 98 patients at 16 centers found that weekly methotrexate failed to lower the rate of relapse or the dose of corticosteroids.[45] There were some differences in the methodologies of the trials, including the protocol for steroid tapering, but the difference in outcomes is largely unexplained. The use of low- to medium-dose methotrexate for potential steroid-sparing effects is still unsettled. Newer agents such as infliximab are now being explored for GCA, even as monotherapy.[46]

GCA may cause death by stroke, myocardial infarction, or aortic rupture.[47] Epidemiologic studies and large clinical series, however, have not demonstrated shortened survival in patients with GCA.

Isolated Angiitis of the Central Nervous System

Primary (or granulomatous) angiitis of the CNS (PACNS) is an inflammatory arterial disease restricted to the cerebral circulation. Unlike GCA, PACNS occurs in patients of any age, is characterized by neurologic disease out of proportion to systemic illness, preferentially involves smaller arteries and veins, and often responds poorly to steroids alone. The diagnosis is difficult, and because it has often been made without pathologic confirmation, the true extent and characteristics of the disease are poorly understood.

Pathology

As in GCA, the pathologic process in PACNS is segmental. Any of the vessels of the brain and spinal cord may be involved, but most reports have noted a predilection for the small leptomeningeal vessels. The precapillary arterioles are most often affected, but some investigators have noted venular involvement.[48] Occasionally, the process may be quite focal, involving only one vessel or group of vessels, and the patient may present with a masslike lesion. The inflammatory infiltrate is composed of lymphocytes, plasma cells, granulomas with multinucleated giant cells, and, occasionally, neutrophils and eosinophils.[49] These infiltrates may involve any portion of the vessel wall. Some investigators have noted more inflammation in the intima and adventitia than the media.[48] Occasionally, thrombosis of larger intracranial arteries (internal carotid artery siphon, anterior cerebral, middle cerebral, posterior cerebral, and basilar arteries) is found.[50] Small aneurysms have also been reported.

The etiology of PACNS is unknown. Because many cases appear to be related to specific underlying infections or other illnesses, it is likely that this condition encompasses a spectrum of different diseases characterized by a vascular inflammatory reaction to a foreign antigen rather than a single nosologic entity. Other cases have been reported in association with Hodgkin's lymphoma, acquired immunodeficiency syndrome (AIDS),[51] primary intracerebral lymphoma, varicella encephalitis, leukemia, sarcoidosis, cerebral amyloid angiopathy, and varicella-zoster infection (Fig. 34-2).[52]

Clinical Features

The presentation of PACNS is heterogeneous and requires a high index of suspicion. Patients range widely in age from 3 to 96 years. The duration of illness is variable. Death may occur within days after presentation in some patients, whereas others have an indolent course lasting years.[53,54] Headache, nausea, vomiting, dementia, amnestic states, disorientation, confusion, somnolence, encephalopathy, or coma occurs early in the course of the disease in many patients. Multifocal neurologic symptoms and signs may develop in a stepwise, progressive fashion, with episodes of quantitative and qualitative worsening, usually occurring after variable periods of stabilization. Seizures are common. Ischemic or hemorrhagic stroke may occur.[50,55,56] Some patients have spinal cord involvement (either alone or in association with brain involvement), including progressive or acute myelopathy with incontinence and paraplegia.[57,58] Papilledema is common.

Systemic symptoms, such as fever and weight loss, are uncommon, distinguishing this entity from most rheumatologic conditions that can cause stroke, such as GCA and systemic lupus erythematosus. The ESR is usually not increased, and when abnormal, it is not as high as in GCA. Blood cell counts, electrolyte levels, and results of

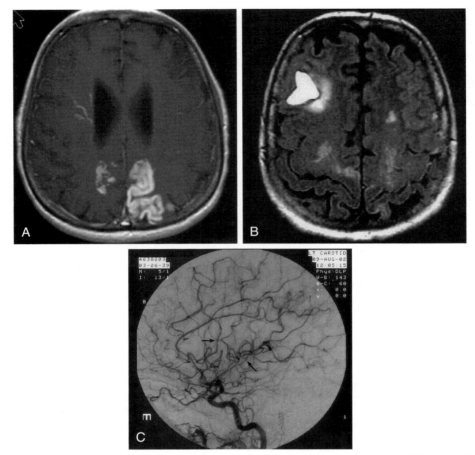

Figure 34-2 Cerebral vasculopathy associated with varicella zoster infection. A, Contrast-enhanced MR image of the brain, demonstrating enhancement of infarctions in bilateral occipital lobes. B, Fluid-attenuated inversion recovery (FLAIR) MR image showing increased signal in the right frontal lobe, a finding consistent with intracerebral hematoma. C, Cerebral angiogram. Note the beaded appearance of the middle cerebral and anterior cerebral artery branches *(arrows)*, a finding consistent with vasculitis.

serologic tests for collagen vascular disease are usually normal. The most consistent cerebrospinal fluid (CSF) abnormality is an increase in protein (frequently >100 mg/dL), although results of cerebrospinal fluid analysis may occasionally be normal. Increased immunoglobulin values are occasionally reported. Many patients have a moderate lymphocytic pleocytosis (usually <150 cells/mL), which thus manifests as a chronic meningitis.[59]

CT and MRI findings are heterogeneous and nonspecific. Cerebral angiographic results are usually abnormal, with alternating segments of concentric arterial narrowing and dilatation. However, cerebral angiographic findings may be normal, and abnormal constrictions found in vessels may also be due to a host of other causes, making reliance on angiography alone for the diagnosis problematic. Autopsy findings in visceral structures are usually normal but rarely may reveal small discrete foci of angiitis.[60] The most common neuropathologic finding is multiple small foci of infarction, followed by multiple foci of hemorrhage ("brain purpura," "petechiae"). Large infarcts and, less often, large confluent intraparenchymal hemorrhages may be present.[48,50,55,56] Occlusion of large or medium-sized vessels by thrombus is uncommon.[50,61] Subarachnoid blood and small aneurysms are rarely encountered.[55]

Retrospective studies have indicated that brain biopsy is the best test for the diagnosis of PACNS vasculitis[62,63] and is necessary to distinguish among tumor (especially lymphoma or intravascular malignant lymphomatosis), infection, and vasculitis (Fig. 34-3). Because PACNS has a predilection for leptomeningeal vessels, the procedure should include a leptomeningeal biopsy as well as a parenchymal biopsy. However, biopsy results have been negative in several subsequently autopsy-proven cases.[64]

Treatment

There is no standard treatment for isolated granulomatous angiitis of the CNS. Progression of the disease and death have frequently occurred despite treatment with high-dose steroids. Remissions have been reported with the use of prednisone, in some cases combined with cyclophosphamide.[65] Methotrexate has also been used as a steroid-sparing agent.[66]

A 2005 retrospective analysis among 12 patients found that small vessel PACNS relapsed in 30% of patients in the first 2 years despite treatment with prednisone and azathioprine.[67] The relapse continued at a similar rate through 6 years of follow-up, causing irreversible injury in half the patients with small vessel disease. In contrast,

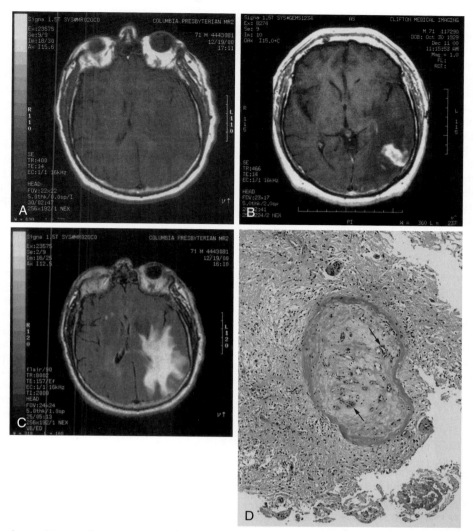

Figure 34-3   Cerebral vasculitis manifesting as a mass lesion. T1-weighted MR images before (A) and after (B) administration of contrast agent, showing the enhancement of a left temporoparietal mass lesion. C, T2-weighted MR image showing extensive edema around the lesion. D, Pathologic specimen from brain biopsy demonstrates an intraparenchymal blood vessel with chronic occlusive changes, mural fibrosis, and recanalization by small, thin-walled vessels *(arrows)*. The gray matter surrounding the blood vessel shows extensive gliosis and loss of neurons. Leukocytes, primarily lymphocytes, infiltrate the arterial adventitia and, to a lesser extent, the media, findings consistent with a chronic vasculitic process.

all patients with medium vessel PACNS were relapse-free during 6 years of follow-up, and all had discontinued low-dose prednisolone and azathioprine therapy by 24 months from presentation. Moreover, diagnosis of small vessel PACNS was more problematic than that of medium vessel disease, which caused angiographic abnormalities in all cases, with distinct, multiple vessel involvement.[67]

Takayasu's Arteritis

Takayasu's arteritis (pulseless disease, idiopathic aortitis) is a large vessel granulomatous arteritis that affects the aorta, its main branches, and, occasionally, the pulmonary artery. Although pathologic changes in the arteries are similar to those found in GCA, Takayasu's arteritis affects younger people, particularly women. Most cases have been reported from Asia, but the disease is found worldwide.[68] As in GCA, constitutional symptoms and increased

ESR are common in the acute phase. Symptoms such as arm claudication and syncope occur more frequently than retinal or cerebral ischemia. Brachial pressures and pulses are commonly asymmetrical, and there may be asymmetry between pressures in the arms and legs.

Cerebrovascular complications occur in patients with more advanced disease.[69] Cerebral infarction and retinal ischemia may occur subsequent to stenosis or occlusion of the extracranial carotid or vertebral arteries, but the intracranial arteries are rarely involved. It has been reported that delayed gadolinium-enhanced MRI is able to show evidence of delayed hyperenhancement in the aortic wall in patients with Takayasu's arteritis, which correlated with ESR and CRP values.[70,71] Fludeoxyglucose F 18 positron emission tomography can be a potent tool for the detection of metabolic activity in vasculitis because of increased uptake of the radiopharmaceutical in inflammatory cells in the vessel walls, including those of larger vessels such as the aorta, its main branches, and the femoral and pulmonary arteries.[72]

Treatment consists of corticosteroids, cytotoxic agents (cyclophosphamide), surgery, or a combination of these modalities. Cases of Takayasu's arteritis successfully treated with infliximab have been reported.[73-75] Combination therapy with minocycline, a matrix metalloproteinase inhibitor, and corticosteroids significantly decreased CRP, ESR, and disease activity score in association with a decrease in serum levels of metalloproteinases 3 and 9.[76]

Regression of carotid stenosis has been reported after administration of corticosteroids.[69] Various surgical reconstructive and bypass procedures have been used,[77-79] with apparent success in some patients, although postoperative anastomotic stenoses may occur. Some investigators advise delaying operation until after the inflammatory process can be controlled with corticosteroids,[68] but others have not found operating first to be problematic.[80] Some patients acquire unusual anastomotic vascular collateral patterns even without surgery.[81]

Polyarteritis Nodosa

Polyarteritis nodosa (PAN) is a necrotizing angiitis of the medium-sized to small muscular arteries throughout the body. The peripheral nervous system is more commonly involved than the CNS. The complications related to the CNS tend to occur late in the course of the disease, in the setting of renal failure, fever, and other systemic manifestations, and are not an independent predictor of death.[82] Diffuse or multifocal cerebral syndromes, such as headache, confusion, psychiatric syndromes, dementia, lymphocytic meningitis,[83] and generalized or focal seizures, are more common than stroke. Cerebral angiography may demonstrate multiple saccular aneurysms.[84] Autopsy demonstrates necrotizing vasculitis in large cerebral arteries, small meningeal arteries, or both.

Diagnostic studies in patients in whom PAN is suspected should include serologic tests for hepatitis B and C and antineutrophil cytoplasmic antibodies and may include visceral or cerebral angiography or biopsy of an organ system suspected of involvement. Treatment consists of corticosteroids and cyclophosphamide. In hepatitis B–associated PAN, combining an antiviral drug with plasma exchange facilitates seroconversion and prevents the development of long-term hepatic complications of hepatitis B infection.[85] Infantile PAN, a disease thought to be distinct from the adult form and possibly related to Kawasaki's disease, may cause stroke (infarction, aneurysmal subarachnoid hemorrhage) in children.[86]

Systemic Lupus Erythematosus

Reports on the neurologic manifestations of systemic lupus erythematosus (SLE) have long emphasized the high frequency of CNS complications, including stroke. Presence of neuropsychiatric disease (seizures and psychosis; cerebrovascular disease is not included) is considered one of the 13 cardinal manifestations of SLE recognized in the American College of Rheumatology (ACR) criteria for the disease.[87] Pathologic series have documented various cerebrovascular lesions, but findings in the brain and cerebral vessels at autopsy infrequently correlate with clinical syndromes.[88]

The proportion of patients with SLE in whom stroke develops is difficult to estimate. Stroke occurred one third as often as seizures and one fifth as often as psychiatric illness, perhaps justifying the American College of Rheumatology criteria. Other reports have documented clinical syndromes of cerebrovascular disease in 5.6% to 15%,[89,90] and about 6% of patients with SLE die of stroke.[91] Renal involvement, hypertension, and high titers of anti-DNA antibodies occur significantly more commonly in patients with SLE and stroke than in those with SLE without stroke.[90] Patients with SLE and cardiac valvular disease seem to have a high risk of stroke (87%).[89]

A prospective cohort study used the Framingham model to calculate the probability of cardiovascular events in patients with SLE. Such patients were found to have strikingly increased relative risks (RRs) of nonfatal myocardial infarction (RR = 10.1), death from cardiovascular disease (RR = 17), and stroke (RR = 7.9).[92] Increased prevalence of premature atherosclerosis in patients with SLE has been well established by autopsy series, although a 2006 study failed to show a strong association between SLE activity and duration with carotid plaque.[93]

Although *vasculitis* is frequently mentioned as an important cause of stroke in patients with SLE, documented vasculitic changes on postmortem examination are actually quite rare.[88,89] It has become increasingly recognized that cardiogenic brain embolism (with or without associated nonbacterial thrombotic endocarditis) is an important mechanism of stroke in patients with SLE. One study also found that microembolic signals detected on transcranial Doppler ultrasonography, possibly indicating embolic material, were more common in patients with SLE who had neuropsychiatric symptoms than in those who had no CNS symptoms, raising the possibility that microemboli may play an even broader role in SLE than previously suspected.[94] Documentation of cardiac sources of emboli in patients with SLE and stroke might prompt treatment with anticoagulants.

Thrombotic thrombocytopenic purpura (thrombocytopenia, microangiopathic hemolytic anemia, fever, renal failure, CNS signs) is another important but underdiagnosed mechanism of stroke in the terminal stages of SLE. Thrombotic thrombocytopenic purpura was documented in 14% in one of the necropsy series.[88]

Antiphospholipid antibodies, including antibodies and the lupus anticoagulant, are associated with cerebrovascular disease, systemic thrombotic events, spontaneous abortion, and thrombocytopenia.[15,101] These phenomena may be associated with antiphospholipid antibodies either in the setting of SLE or as a "primary" antiphospholipid syndrome (APS).[102] In one series,[90] lupus anticoagulant was detected in 38% and anticardiolipin antibodies in 43% of patients with SLE and stroke who were investigated for these abnormalities. The main therapy of antiphospholipid syndrome is long-term anticoagulation,[103] with the goal an International Normalized Ratio (INR) higher than 3.0.

Additional possible causes of infarction in patients with SLE are hypertension and hyperlipidemia, both of which are overrepresented among these patients.[104] Cerebral venous thrombosis is another uncommon but well-documented cerebrovascular complication in SLE. The mechanism of venous thrombosis may be multifactorial, including hypercoagulability due to lupus anticoagulant and anticardiolipin antibody.[105,106]

Wegener's Granulomatosis

Wegener's granulomatosis is a necrotizing granulomatous vasculitis involving the respiratory tract and other organ systems in association with glomerulonephritis. Nervous system complications include peripheral neuropathy and mononeuritis multiplex, CNS infection, local invasion by destructive granulomatous lesions causing cranial nerve palsies, and, rarely, CNS vasculitis.[107] Necrotizing granulomatous meningitis with leptomeningeal vasculitis may produce predominantly meningeal and encephalopathic syndromes or multiple cranial neuropathies, sometimes with prominent meningeal enhancement and confluent increased T2 signal abnormalities in white matter on brain MRI.[108,109] The presence of antineutrophil cytoplasmic antibodies facilitates diagnosis.[110] These antibodies have high specificity and sensitivity, and increases in their titer may indicate a relapse.[111] CNS complications may become less common with the advent of protocols combining cyclophosphamide and corticosteroids, which appear to be more effective than corticosteroids alone. A randomized, placebo-controlled trial evaluating etanercept for the maintenance of remission failed to show any efficacy, and there was a high rate of treatment-related complications, including solid cancers.[112] In this study, in addition to etanercept or placebo, patients received standard therapy including glucocorticoids plus cyclophosphamide or methotrexate.

Allergic Angiitis

Occasional reports of amaurosis fugax,[113] ischemic optic neuropathy,[113] subarachnoid hemorrhage,[114] and stroke-like syndromes[114] have been reported in patients with various forms of necrotizing "allergic" angiitis (Churg-Strauss syndrome).

Lymphomatoid Granulomatosis

Lymphomatoid granulomatosis is an "angiocentric and angiodestructive lymphoreticular proliferative and granulomatous disease" that primarily involves the lungs and may involve the CNS in approximately 20% of cases.[115] The disease may mimic Wegener's granulomatosis, and its progression to lymphoma has occurred. Clinical manifestations of CNS involvement usually consist of subacute, progressive syndromes of focal brain parenchymal or cranial nerve involvement that mimic neoplasm, encephalitis, or multiple sclerosis but rarely cerebrovascular disease.[116] Primary CNS involvement has been reported. Lymphomatoid granulomatosis involving the CNS and lungs has been successfully treated in one patient with rituximab monotherapy without any adverse effects; the patient stayed in remission for 18 months.[117]

Scleroderma

Only rarely does scleroderma (progressive systemic sclerosis) cause CNS problems directly.[118] Convulsions, stroke, and pathologic findings of arterial changes in the brains of patients with scleroderma may be the result of hypertension due to renal disease. Rarely, calcifications of cerebral vessels can be seen. Six percent of patients with scleroderma in one series had cerebrovascular disease, but the mechanisms involved were obscure.[118] Arteritis has only rarely been reported, and its relationship to the scleroderma may be coincidental.[119,120]

Rheumatoid Arthritis

CNS manifestations of rheumatoid arthritis are rare and tend to occur in the setting of long-established disease, with either clinical signs (fever, weight loss, active arthritis) or laboratory evidence (increase in rheumatoid factor titer or ESR) of disease activity. Rheumatoid meningitis ("pachymeningitis") has been reported as an asymptomatic finding at autopsy and may cause CNS symptoms and signs, including headache, visual loss, seizures, altered mental status, aphasia, memory loss, hemiparesis, and spinal cord compression.[121] Findings at autopsy include thickening and distention of the meninges with proteinaceous fluid. A large body of evidence supports the involvement of common proinflammatory cytokines in the development and progression of both rheumatoid arthritis and atherosclerosis. Proinflammatory cytokines such as interleukin-1, interleukin-6, and TNF-α produced within locally affected joints in rheumatoid arthritis may promote both traditional (e.g., dyslipidemia, insulin resistance) and nontraditional (e.g., oxidative stress) systemic cardiovascular risk factors.[122] The dura and leptomeninges demonstrate foci of inflammatory mononuclear cells and multinucleated giant cells.

CNS vasculitis, either isolated or in association with systemic rheumatoid vasculitis,[123] has been documented on rare occasions in patients with rheumatoid arthritis. Some of the patients in these cases also had pachymeningitis. One of the most feared neurologic complications of rheumatoid arthritis is compressive myelopathy secondary to C1-C2 vertebral subluxation, and a potential complication of C1-C2 subluxation is massive vertebrobasilar territory infarction due to vertebral artery thrombosis from pinching of the vertebral artery between the odontoid and rim of the foramen magnum or stretching of the vertebral arteries between the transverse foramina of the C1 and C2 vertebrae. Precipitation of vertebrobasilar ischemic symptoms has been associated with neck flexion, extension, and rotation in patients with C1-C2 subluxation.[124] In some, angiography has documented narrowing or occlusion of the vertebral arteries with these maneuvers.[124] Formation of vertebral artery pseudoaneurysms has also been reported.[125]

Sjögren's Syndrome

Sjögren's syndrome (xerostomia and keratoconjunctivitis sicca) may be diagnosed in conjunction with other collagen vascular diseases that have CNS complications. Primary Sjögren's syndrome is diagnosed when the disease is present without another collagen vascular disease. The frequency of CNS manifestations of primary Sjögren's syndrome is controversial because of the differences in populations studied and the difficulties of establishing the diagnosis and excluding other diseases. Multiple sclerosis–like,[126] stroke-like,[127] and dementing[127] syndromes have been reported. In one series, 7 of 87 patients (8%) with primary Sjögren's syndrome had CNS involvement, but most cases were not due to focal disease.[128] In another series, subcortical hyperintensities on MRI were seen in 51.3% of patients with the disease, compared with only 36.6% of age- and sex-matched controls.[129] Histopathologic documentation of the mechanisms involved is usually not available.

Sneddon's Syndrome

Livedo reticularis is a cutaneous condition characterized by a fixed, deep bluish red, reticulated pattern on the skin due to impaired superficial venous drainage of the skin. This cutaneous sign is found in several diseases, including PAN, SLE, rheumatoid arthritis, dermatomyositis, and cryoglobulinemia. Cerebrovascular disease in association with livedo reticularis is known as Sneddon's syndrome. Approximately 40% of patients have antiphospholipid antibodies,[130,131] and antiendothelial cell antibodies may also be seen.[132] Livedo reticularis usually precedes neurologic involvement but many manifest as stroke. The most common cerebrovascular manifestation in this syndrome is recurrent cerebral infarction.[133] Transient ischemic attacks, seizures, and dementia have been reported.[133] Dementia can be due to multiple small infarcts without overt acute clinical strokes,[134] but some patients appear to have dementia in the absence of infarction.[135] The mechanism of infarction is for the most part unknown.

Brain CT and MRI frequently document infarction involving the cortex or white matter.[136] Angiograms either are normal or demonstrate narrowing or occlusion of medium-sized arteries and their branches, sometimes with moya-moya-type collateral networks.[133,137] Cardiac valvular lesions may occur. Similar skin lesions and stroke have also been reported as due to atrial myxoma, suggesting that echocardiography to exclude cardiac lesions should be performed in patients with suspected Sneddon's syndrome.[138] Skin biopsies have usually demonstrated an occlusive, noninflammatory vasculopathy involving medium-sized arteries along with focal and segmental intimal hyperplasia due to fibroelastic proliferation or subendothelial cell proliferation.

Various antiplatelet and immunomodulatory agents, including steroids and azathioprine sodium, have not been effective in either antiphospholipid syndromes or Sneddon's syndrome.[139] Their failure and the reported success of warfarin may rationalize the use of anticoagulation. The use of warfarin may be further justified by the frequent presence of asymptomatic cardiac valvulopathy and the abundance of cerebral microemboli in patients with Sneddon's syndrome.[139]

Malignant Atrophic Papulosis

Malignant atrophic papulosis (Degos's disease, Köhlmeier-Degos disease) is a progressive vasculopathy that affects the skin, cerebral circulation, and other organ systems. The characteristic skin lesion consists of an umbilicated, raised papule with a white center. The appearance of cutaneous lesions usually precedes neurologic manifestations, sometimes by years. In some patients, however, neurologic manifestations may precede or accompany the development of cutaneous lesions.[140] Bowel infarction appears more common in young males, and perforations may occur.

Neurologic complications are varied and include transient ischemic attacks, stroke, progressive focal or multifocal deficits, and spinal cord involvement.[140] Angiographic findings are nonspecific, consisting of multiple branch occlusions and alternating segmental constriction and dilatation. Pathologic examination of brain vessels has documented a peculiar fibrous intimal proliferation between endothelium and internal elastic lamina, similar to vascular lesions in the skin,[140,141] and may be accompanied by thrombosis. The small meningeal arteries are frequently involved. Various therapies have been used, usually ineffectively, such as antiplatelet agents, anticoagulants, corticosteroids, and plasmapheresis.[142]

Behçet's Disease

Behçet's disease is a systemic inflammatory disorder with repeated exacerbations and remissions of symptoms. The diagnostic criteria require recurrent oral ulceration (at least three times in one 12-month period) as an essential symptom plus any two or more of the following symptoms or signs: genital ulceration, eye lesions (the iris is often involved in a distinct appearance), skin lesions, and a positive pathergy test result.[143] CNS involvement is more common in young male patients, age and sex being independent risk factors.[144] CNS complications usually occur in patients who have established cutaneous or ocular disease, but there are well-documented instances of neurologic presentation,[145] and some patients may have ocular and neurologic manifestations without oral or genital lesions.[146] Many patients present with a syndrome of aseptic meningitis or meningoencephalitis with fever and headache, with or without associated focal neurologic signs. There may be a fluctuating course with exacerbations and remissions that are atypical for cerebrovascular disease. Symptoms and signs of brainstem involvement and pseudobulbar palsy are frequently reported. Less often, neurologic presentations are sudden in onset and suggest stroke.[145] Some patients have presented with symptoms and signs of increased intracranial pressure, occasionally with minimal or no focal findings, due to angiographically documented cerebral venous sinus thrombosis.[147] Retinal ischemia and vasculitis have also been reported.[148]

Cerebrospinal fluid examination frequently demonstrates a moderate pleocytosis, predominantly lymphocytic, as well as an increased protein content, usually <100 mg/dL. Findings on MRI usually consist of increased signal intensity on T2-weighted images.[148,149] These lesions are usually found in the deep structures, including the brainstem, deep nuclei, and hypothalamus, and also in the hemispheric white matter, and they may enhance with the use of a contrast agent.[148,149] Unlike vascular lesions, these findings tend to resolve over time after treatment and frequently do not conform to a single arterial territory. These features, as well as leptomeningeal enhancement in some cases, might be more suggestive of an inflammatory process as opposed to vascular occlusion. Cerebral angiographic findings are usually normal.[150]

High-dose prednisone (20-100 mg/day orally) or pulse intravenous corticosteroid therapy (1 g/day of methylprednisolone for 3 days) is the mainstay of treatment and should be started immediately for the acute stage of CNS involvement, including increased intracranial pressure with headaches, aseptic meningitis, and meningoencephalitis.[151] After remission has been obtained, corticosteroids are tapered to 15 to 20 mg/day as maintenance. In most cases, however, corticosteroids are supplemented with cyclophosphamide, chlorambucil, azathioprine, or methotrexate.[151]

Cryoglobulinemia

There are rare reports of CNS complications in patients with mixed cryoglobulinemia. CNS manifestations include diffuse encephalopathic syndromes with focal signs, seizures, myelopathy, and, occasionally, ischemic stroke.[152] Mixed cryoglobulinemia is associated with a systemic vasculitis characterized by the deposition of circulating immune complexes in blood vessels. However, cryoglobulins are usually found in low concentrations and most patients have few or no clinical manifestations. Symptomatic disease occurs in less than 15% of patients.[153] Mixed cryoglobulinemia, especially type II, is regarded as the major causative factor of peripheral neuropathy and stroke syndromes in patients with hepatitis C virus infection.[153] Angiographic findings include narrowing of the major cerebral arteries with development of a moyamoya pattern of collateral vessels.[152] Mixed cryoglobulinemia may cause impairment of the vasa nervorum microcirculation by intravascular deposition of cryoglobulin leading to ischemia, and/or by necrotizing vasculitis from longstanding cryoglobulin precipitation, complement fixation, and rheumatoid factor activity.[154] The inflammatory infiltrate consists of lymphocytes and monocytes, but not polymorphonuclear monocytes.[154] Favorable outcome has been reported after treatment with corticosteroids, cyclophosphamide, and, in some cases, interferon.[155]

Retinocochleocerebral Vasculopathy (Susac's Syndrome)

Retinocochleocerebral vasculopathy, also known as Susac's syndrome, is a rare, perhaps underrecognized, condition that occurs almost exclusively in young women (85%) and is characterized by multiple microinfarcts affecting the brain, retina, and inner ear. Patients present with encephalopathy, visual loss, and hearing loss or tinnitus. The disease is often monophasic, but it may resolve slowly, and patients may suffer irreversible brain injury if the disease is well-established at presentation. Funduscopy reveals branch retinal artery occlusions. MRI shows multiple microinfarcts throughout the brain, but with a virtual pathognomonic predilection for the central callosum, at the distalmost territory of the penetrating vessels

supplying the corpus callosum (Fig. 34-4). Because of this involvement of the corpus callosum, the disorder may be mistaken for multiple sclerosis, but the location of lesions in the central corpus callosum, rather than peripherally as in multiple sclerosis, indicates a microvascular etiology. Cerebrospinal fluid examination may demonstrate a mild pleocytosis (predominantly lymphocytic) and increased protein content. The pathophysiology remains uncertain, although evidence now suggests that the condition is secondary to an autoimmune endotheliopathy affecting the microvasculature in the brain, eye, and ear. Anti-endothelial cell antibodies may be seen in some cases. Brain biopsies have shown swelling, necrosis, and sloughing of endothelium in capillaries and venules, fibrin deposition, and a minimally inflammatory deposition of complement within small vessels. The appearance is distinct from primary angiitis of the CNS, which manifests as marked inflammation, transmural inflammation of the vessel wall, and arterial necrosis.

Immunosuppressive therapy appears to be effective in preventing further deterioration in patients with Susac's syndrome. High-dose corticosteroid therapy is the mainstay, but additional agents, such as intravenous immunoglobulin, mycophenolate mofetil, and cyclophosphamide, are often necessary.[156] Rituximab is the newest agent to consider. Aspirin is a useful adjunct.

The Role of Inflammation in Atherosclerosis and Stroke

The role of inflammation in "garden variety" atherosclerosis and stroke has been well-established. According to a common theory of atherosclerosis, developed by Ross[157] and others, atherosclerosis is predominantly an inflammatory condition produced by a "response to injury" (Fig. 34-5). The role of inflammation in the atherosclerotic process can be divided into the following three phases: early development of atherosclerosis, progression of the atherosclerotic plaque, and acute plaque rupture (this event as yet of unclear significance for particle size embolized into the brain's arteries). Monocyte-derived macrophages and T lymphocytes have been found in human fatty streaks, the earliest stage of the disease process,[158-160] suggesting that immune processes may play an initiating or early role in the development of the lesion. Cytokines, including several interleukins, interferons, TNF, and several growth factors and colony-stimulating factors, have also been found within atheromatous lesions at all stages by means of various techniques.[161-165] As this process continues, there is an increase of inflammatory cells in the atheroma, which are recruited from the blood as well as undergoing multiplication within the lesion itself.[166-169] Endothelium-derived leukointegrins cause adherence of monocytes and T cells, particularly at branch points of arteries, where turbulence is prominent.[170-172] Changes in shear stress at these sites lead to upregulation of the genes responsible for the production of these molecules.[173-176] Animal studies confirm these data. Elevated levels of TNF-α and interleukin-1β increase monocyte recruitment into developing atherosclerotic lesions in mice.[177] Moreover, in knockout mice deficient in these adhesion molecules, atherosclerotic lesions are smaller despite lipid loading.[178]

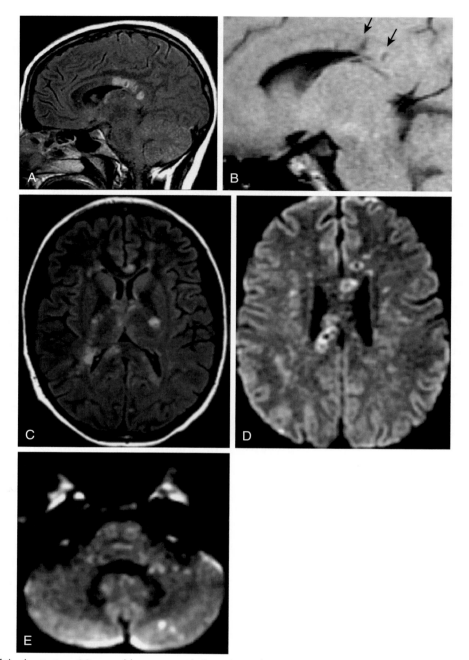

Figure 34-4 MRI of the brain in a 28-year-old woman with Susac's syndrome (retinocochleocerebral vasculopathy) who presented with encephalopathy, visual loss, and hearing loss during pregnancy. A, T2 fluid-attenuated inversion recovery (FLAIR) parasagittal image shows corpus callosal lesions, some with a ring of increased signal and a darker center. B, T1-weighted parasagittal image, similar cut, shows areas of T1 hypointensity *(arrows)* corresponding to the T2 bright lesions. C, T2-weighted FLAIR axial image shows additional lesions throughout the internal capsule and the genu, splenium, and tapetum of the corpus callosum. D, Diffusion-weighted (1000-b) axial image through the superior extent of the lateral ventricles shows several lesions with restricted diffusion through the central fibers of the corpus callosum, many with bright rings and dark centers. E, Diffusion-weighted (1000-b) axial image of the cerebellum and pons shows pinpoint lesions in the middle cerebellar peduncle and cerebellar cortex. (From Grinspan ZM, Willey JZ, Tullman MJ, et al: A 28-year-old pregnant woman with encephalopathy. *Neurology,* 73:e74-e79, 2009.)

Blockage of certain immunomodulatory molecules, such as CD40 ligand, which is expressed by macrophages, T cells, endothelium, and smooth muscle cells in atherosclerotic plaques, can reduce lesion formation.[179-182] Although this finding suggests that interference with inflammatory mechanisms could prevent the buildup of atherosclerotic lesions, the clinical implications remain uncertain in human beings.

Plaque rupture, the acute precipitant of approximately 50% of clinical events related to large vessel atherosclerosis, also involves inflammatory mechanisms. Rupture occurs at sites of the fibrous plaque where macrophages

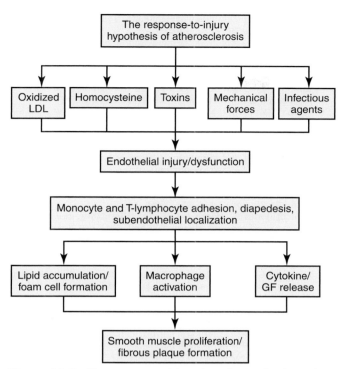

Figure 34-5 The response-to-injury hypothesis of atherosclerosis. GF, growth factor; LDL, low-density lipoprotein (cholesterol). (Adapted from Ross R: Atherosclerosis—an inflammatory disease. N Engl J Med 340:115, 1999.)

enter[183] and may be encouraged by destruction of the fibrous cap through upregulation and production of proteolytic enzymes, including metalloproteinases and collagenases derived from macrophages stimulated by activated T cells.[184] The profile of inflammatory cytokines in more advanced lesions, such as those taken from endarterectomy specimens, is predominantly a proinflammatory T-cell response.[185] Higher levels of macrophages and T cells[186] as well as of ICAM-1 and TNF-α [187,188] were found in endarterectomy specimens from patients with symptomatic carotid stenosis than in those with asymptomatic carotid stenosis. There can be great heterogeneity of inflammatory profiles within plaques, however.[189]

Of more direct interest to the clinician, epidemiologic studies have also generally shown that serologic evidence of inflammation is associated with atherosclerosis, coronary artery disease, and stroke. Leukocyte count is independently associated with carotid plaque cross-sectional thickness,[190] first ischemic stroke in healthy elderly individuals,[191] progression of carotid intima-media thickness,[192] and aortic arch atheroma[193] over time as well as with risk of atherosclerotic heart disease[194,195] and stroke,[196] even after adjustment of data for smoking. In a secondary analysis of a large clinical trial, short-term changes in leukocyte counts were found to result in a longer period of stroke risk.[197] It is not known whether this increase in leukocytes represented infection or some other proinflammatory phenomenon, but neutrophils appeared to be most closely associated with increased risk.

High-sensitivity CRP (hs-CRP) is probably the most-studied inflammatory marker in the prediction of stroke risk. There is some evidence that CRP gene polymorphisms are associated with plasma hs-CRP levels and stroke risk.[198] Hs-CRP predicts incident cerebrovascular events in several populations, and much of the early literature on this topic has been reviewed in a European consensus statement.[199] In the Women's Health Study, hs-CRP, interleukin-6, soluble ICAM-1, and serum amyloid A all predicted incident stroke among other cardiovascular events, but in multivariate models, hs-CRP was the only inflammatory marker that independently predicted risk.[200] Inclusion of hs-CRP improved the predictive ability of models over those containing lipid values and other risk factors alone.[200,201] In the Northern Manhattan Study, however, hs-CRP and serum amyloid A did not predict incident stroke, though they did predict incident myocardial infarction and death.[202] The mechanisms by which hs-CRP may be associated with stroke remain uncertain. Hs-CRP could be an "epiphenomenon," a marker of inflammation present in atherosclerosis but not directly responsible for it. Alternatively, there is evidence that CRP may play a more direct role. In vitro, for example, CRP stimulates release of cytokines and growth factors and also downregulates nitric oxide, a potent vasodilator.[203]

Some studies have suggested that hs-CRP also predicts prognosis after stroke, though most have been small, single-center studies and have assessed mortality rather than recurrent stroke.[199] In other studies, hs-CRP predicts progression of symptomatic intracranial atherosclerosis[204] and, if measured less than 3 hours after ischemic stroke onset and before treatment with thrombolysis, may be a measure of the probability of death after thrombolysis.[205] These data indicate that a simple blood test obtained at admission in patients with ischemic stroke probably has prognostic value. Its main disadvantage is that hs-CRP is nonspecific in origin, so acute increases in hs-CRP may occur in acute infection or other illness.

Several cellular adhesion molecules (CAMs) have been shown to play a major role in plaque initiation and development.[206,207] These molecules are expressed on the surfaces of vascular endothelial cells and leukocytes.[208] Soluble forms of CAMs, like E- and P-selectins, are thought to arise from shedding or proteolytic cleavage from endothelial cells and can serve as biomarkers in the circulation.[209] Murine models of targeted selectin gene disruption have clearly shown reduced leukocyte rolling and initial leukocyte adhesion to endothelium.[210] Moreover, higher levels of E-selectin have been found in patients with carotid artery atherosclerosis than in age- and sex-matched, normal controls.[211] Many inflammatory markers are associated with other risk factors, many of which are themselves associated with ischemic events.[212]

Inflammation may be associated not only with large vessel atherosclerosis, but also with cerebral small vessel disease. A polymorphism of the interleukin-6 gene that has been associated with increased inflammation has been found to be an independent risk factor for lacunar stroke.[213] In one study, patients with lacunar stroke and elevations of TNF-α and ICAM-1 were more likely to experience early neurologic deterioration and poor outcome at 3 months than patients without such elevations.[214]

There is also evidence from clinical trials that inflammatory markers may be used to determine optimal use and dose of statins. Studies have shown that statin therapy reduces hs-CRP[215,216] among healthy persons,[217] those with stable coronary disease,[218] and those with acute coronary syndrome.[219,220] The magnitude of the benefit associated with statin therapy correlated in part with the achieved hs-CRP level. In a secondary, but pre-specified, analysis of a large comparative statin trial in patients with acute coronary syndrome, lower event rates were found in patients in whom hs-CRP levels had been reduced to less than 2 mg/L, independent of lowering of the low-density lipoprotein cholesterol level.[221] The results also suggested an additive benefit of lowering both lipid and inflammatory measures. Of note, the benefit of lowering these markers was independent of the specific agent used, depending instead on the degree of success in lowering these parameters. Correlation of low-density lipoprotein cholesterol and hs-CRP levels was low, indicating measurement of independent phenomena. Similar results have been demonstrated with use of stroke as an outcome. Hs-CRP and other markers were measured and levels were related to stroke risk over time.[222] Of note, however, stroke risk was related to hs-CRP only in the placebo group, providing indirect evidence that statin treatment can reduce the risk associated with elevated hs-CRP.

A large randomized clinical trial among apparently healthy men and women with normal low-density lipoprotein cholesterol levels but elevated hs-CRP values who were randomly assigned to rosuvastatin therapy or placebo demonstrated a significant reduction in the incidence of major cardiovascular events, including stroke, with use of the agent.[223] This study has thus provided indirect evidence that statins are of benefit among patients with a marker of inflammation, although it may simply reflect a general benefit of statin therapy among all patients, with the greatest magnitude seen among those at higher risk.

The decision to measure hs-CRP or other markers in patients with stroke may be based on the U.S. Centers for Disease Control and Prevention/American Heart Association guidelines until further data are available. Because of the relative heterogeneity of causes of stroke in comparison with ischemic heart disease, these inflammatory marker measurements may prove to be especially useful in patients with stroke. No data yet demonstrate the validity of such an approach, however, and no current guidelines recommend measurement of inflammatory markers in patients with stroke or even provide appropriate levels to determine absolute risk. Thus, it remains to be proven how measuring these markers should affect secondary stroke prevention.

REFERENCES

1. Lie JT: Aortic and extracranial large vessel giant cell arteritis: A review of 72 cases with histopathologic documentation, *Semin Arthritis Rheum* 24:422, 1995.
2. Smith CA, Fidler WJ, Pinals RS: The epidemiology of giant cell arteritis: Report of a ten year study in Shelby County, Tennessee, *Arthritis Rheum* 26:1214, 1983.
3. Machado EBV, Michet CJ, Ballard DJ, et al: Trends in incidence and clinical presentation of temporal arteritis in Olmsted County, Minnesota, 1950-1985, *Arthritis Rheum* 31:745, 1988.
4. Hunder GG: Epidemiology of giant-cell arteritis, *Cleve Clin J Med* 69(Suppl 2):SII-79–SII-82, 2002.
5. Weyand CM, Goronzy JJ: Medium- and large-vessel vasculitis, *N Engl J Med* 349:160–169, 2003.
6. Love DC, Rapkin J, Lesser GR, et al: Temporal arteritis in blacks, *Ann Intern Med* 105:387, 1986.
7. Robbins SL, Cotran RS: Blood vessels. In *Pathological basis of disease*, ed 2, Philadelphia, 1979, WB Saunders, p 614.
8. Krupa WM, Dewan M, Jeon M-S, et al: Trapping of misdirected dendritic cells in the granulomatous lesions of giant cell arteritis, *Am J Pathol* 161:1815–1823, 2002.
9. Wagner AD, Goronzy JJ, Weyand CM: Functional profile of tissue-infiltrating and circulating CD68+ cells in giant cell arteritis: Evidence for two components of the disease, *J Clin Invest* 94:1134–1140, 1994.
10. Weyand CM, Goronzy JJ: Arterial wall injury in giant cell arteritis, *Arthritis Rheum* 42:844–853, 1999.
11. Park JR, Jones JG, Harkniss GD, et al: Circulating immune complexes in polymyalgia rheumatica and giant cell arteritis, *Ann Rheum Dis* 40:360, 1981.
12. Chess J, Albert DM, Bhan AK, et al: Serologic and immunopathologic findings in temporal arteritis, *Am J Ophthalmol* 96:283, 1983.
13. Gonzalez-Gay MA: Genetic epidemiology: Giant cell arteritis and polymyalgia rheumatica, *Arthritis Res* 3:154, 2001.
14. Mattey DL, Hajeer AH, Dababneh A, et al: Association of giant cell arteritis and polymyalgia rheumatica with different tumor necrosis factor microsatellite polymorphisms, *Arthritis Rheum* 43:1749, 2000.
15. Salvarani C, Casali B, Boiardi L, et al: Intercellular adhesion molecule 1 gene polymorphisms in polymyalgia rheumatica/giant cell arteritis: Association with disease risk and severity, *J Rheumatol* 27:1215, 2000.
16. Huston KA, Hunder GG: Giant cell (cranial) arteritis: A clinical review, *Am Heart J* 100:99, 1980.
17. Caselli RJ, Hunder GG, Whisnant JP: Neurologic disease in biopsy-proven giant cell (temporal) arteritis, *Neurology (NY)* 38:352, 1988.
18. Jones JG, Hazleman BL: Prognosis and management of polymyalgia rheumatica, *Ann Rheum Dis* 40:1, 1981.
19. Hayreh SS: Anterior ischemic optic neuropathy, *Arch Neurol* 38:675, 1981.
20. Russell RWR: Giant-cell arteritis: A review of 35 cases, *Q J Med* 28:471, 1959.
21. Borruat FX, Bogousslavsky J, Uffer S, et al: Orbital infarction syndrome, *Ophthalmology* 100:562, 1993.
22. Bogousslavsky J, Deruaz JP, Regli F: Bilateral obstruction of internal carotid artery from giant-cell arteritis and massive infarction limited to the vertebrobasilar area, *Eur Neurol* 24:57, 1985.
23. Collado A, Santamaria J, Ribalta T, et al: Giant-cell arteritis presenting with ipsilateral hemiplegia and lateral medullary syndrome, *Eur Neurol* 29:266, 1989.
24. Gibb WRG, Urry PA, Lees AJ: Giant cell arteritis with spinal cord infarction and basilar artery thrombosis, *J Neurol Neurosurg Psychiatry* 48:945, 1985.
25. Säve-Söderbergh J, Malmvall BO, Andersson R, et al: Giant cell arteritis as a cause of death: Report of nine cases, *JAMA* 255:493, 1986.
26. Thystrup J, Knudsen GM, Mogensen AM, et al: Atypical visual loss in giant cell arteritis, *Acta Ophthalmol (Copenh)* 72:759, 1994.
27. Butt Z, Cullen JF, Mutlukan E: Pattern of arterial involvement of the head, neck, and eyes in giant cell arteritis: Three case reports, *Br J Ophthalmol* 75:368, 1991.
28. Hunder GG, Bloch DA, Michel BA, et al: The American College of Rheumatology 1990 criteria for the classification of giant cell arteritis, *Arthritis Rheum* 33:1122, 1990.
29. Wong RL, Korn JH: Temporal arteritis without an elevated erythrocyte sedimentation rate: Case report and review of the literature, *Am J Med* 80:959, 1986.
30. Salvarani C, Hunder GG: Giant cell arteritis with low erythrocyte sedimentation rate: Frequency of occurrence in a population-based study, *Arthritis Rheum* 45:140–145, 2001.
31. Kyle V, Cawston TE, Hazleman BL: Erythrocyte sedimentation rate and C reactive protein in the assessment of polymyalgia rheumatica/giant cell arteritis on presentation and during follow up, *Ann Rheum Dis* 48:667–671, 1989.

32. Gonzalez-Gay MA, Garcia-Porrua C, Llorca J, et al: Biopsy-negative giant cell arteritis: Clinical spectrum and predictive factors for positive temporal artery biopsy, *Semin Arthritis Rheum* 30:249, 2001.

33. Hall S, Hunder GG: Is temporal artery biopsy prudent? *Mayo Clin Proc* 59:793, 1984.

34. Klein RG, Campbell RJ, Hunder GG, et al: Skip lesions in temporal arteritis, *Mayo Clin Proc* 51:504, 1976.

35. Hammoudeh M, Khan M: Cranial arteritis as the initial manifestation of malignant histiocytosis, *J Rheumatol* 9:443, 1982.

36. Morgan GJ Jr, Harris ED Jr: Non-giant cell temporal arteritis, *Arthritis Rheum* 21:362, 1978.

37. Schmidt WA, Kraft HE, Vorpahl K, et al: Color duplex ultrasonography in the diagnosis of temporal arteritis, *N Engl J Med* 337:1336, 1997.

38. Turlakow A, Yeung HW, Pui J, et al: Fludeoxyglucose positron emission tomography in the diagnosis of giant cell arteritis, *Arch Intern Med* 161:1003, 2001.

39. Joelsen E, Ruthrauff B, Ali F, et al: Multifocal dural enhancement associated with temporal arteritis, *Arch Neurol* 57:119, 2000.

40. Eberhardt RT, Dhadly M: Giant cell arteritis: Diagnosis, management, and cardiovascular implications, *Cardiol Rev* 15:55–61, 2007.

41. Andersson R, Malmvall BE, Bengtsson BA: Long-term corticosteroid treatment in giant cell arteritis, *Acta Med Scand* 220:465, 1986.

42. Hunder GG, Sheps SG, Allen GL, et al: Daily and alternate-day corticosteroid regimens in treatment of giant cell arteritis: Comparison in a prospective study, *Ann Intern Med* 82:613, 1975.

43. Rosenfeld SI, Kosmorsky GS, Klingele TG, et al: Treatment of temporal arteritis with ocular involvement, *Am J Med* 80:143, 1986.

44. Jover JA, Hernandez-Garcia C, Morado IC, et al: Combined treatment of giant-cell arteritis with methotrexate and prednisone: A randomized, double-blind, placebo-controlled trial, *Ann Intern Med* 134:106, 2001.

45. Hoffman G, Cid M, Hellmann D, et al: A multicenter, randomized, double-blind, placebo-controlled study of adjuvant methotrexate treatment for giant cell arteritis, *Arthritis Rheum* 46:1309–1318, 2002.

46. Uthman I, Kanj N, Atweh S: Infliximab as monotherapy in giant cell arteritis, *Clin Rheumatol* 25:109–110, 2006.

47. Lie JT: Aortic and extracranial large vessel giant cell arteritis: A review of 72 cases with histopathologic documentation, *Semin Arthritis Rheum* 24:422, 1995.

48. Budzilovich GN, Feigin I, Siegel H: Granulomatous angiitis of the nervous system, *Arch Pathol Lab Med* 76:250, 1963.

49. Cupps TR, Moore PM, Fauci AS: Isolated angiitis of the central nervous system, *Am J Med* 74:97, 1983.

50. Nagaratnam N, James WE: Isolated angiitis of the brain in a young female on the contraceptive pill, *Postgrad Med J* 63:1085, 1987.

51. Nogueras C, Sala M, Sasal M, et al: Recurrent stroke as a manifestation of primary angiitis of the central nervous system in a patient infected with human immunodeficiency virus, *Arch Neurol* 59:468, 2002.

52. Hayman M, Hendson G, Poskitt KJ, et al: Postvaricella angiopathy: Report of a case with pathologic correlation, *Pediatr Neurol* 24:387, 2001.

53. Berger JR, Romano J, Menkin M, et al: Benign focal cerebral vasculitis: Case report, *Neurology* 45:1731, 1995.

54. Johnson MD, Maciunas R, Creasy J, et al: Indolent granulomatous angiitis: Case report, *J Neurosurg* 81:472, 1994.

55. Biller J, Loftus CM, Moore SA, et al: Isolated central nervous system angiitis first presenting as spontaneous intracranial hemorrhage, *Neurosurgery* 20:310, 1987.

56. Koo EH, Massey EW: Granulomatous angiitis of the central nervous system: Protean manifestations and response to treatment, *J Neurol Neurosurg Psychiatry* 51:1126, 1988.

57. Caccamo DV, Garcia JH, Ho KL: Isolated granulomatous angiitis of the spinal cord, *Ann Neurol* 32:580, 1992.

58. Giovanini MA, Eskin TA, Mukherji SK, et al: Granulomatous angiitis of the spinal cord: A case report, *Neurosurgery* 34:540, 1994.

59. Anderson NE, Willoughby EW, Synek BJL: Leptomeningeal and brain biopsy in chronic meningitis, *Aust N Z J Med* 25:703, 1995.

60. Frayne JH, Gilligan BS, Essex WB: Granulomatous angiitis of the central nervous system, *Med J Aust* 145:410, 1986.

61. Marsden HB: Basilar artery thrombosis and giant cell arteritis [abstract], *Arch Dis Child* 49:75, 1974.

62. Alrawi A, Trobe JD, Blaivas M, Musch DC: Brain biopsy in primary angiitis of the central nervous system, *Neurology* 53:858, 1999.

63. Chu CT, Gray L, Goldstein LB, et al: Diagnosis of intracranial vasculitis: A multi-disciplinary approach, *J Neuropathol Exp Neurol* 58:30, 1998.

64. Younger DS, Hays AP, Brust JCM, et al: Granulomatous angiitis of the brain: An inflammatory reaction of diverse etiology, *Arch Neurol* 45:514, 1988.

65. Moore PM: Diagnosis and management of isolated angiitis of the central nervous system, *Neurology (NY)* 39:167, 1989.

66. Ebinger F, Mannhardt-Laakmann W, Zepp F: Cerebral vasculitis stabilised by methotrexate, *Eur J Pediatr* 159:712, 2000.

67. MacLaren K, Gillespie J, Shrestha S, et al: Primary angiitis of the central nervous system: Emerging variants, *Q J Med* 98:643–654, 2005.

68. Hall S, Barr W, Lie JT, et al: Takayasu arteritis: A study of 32 North American patients, *Medicine (Balt)* 64:89, 1985.

69. Ishikawa K, Yonekawa Y: Regression of carotid stenoses after corticosteroid therapy in occlusive thromboaortopathy (Takayasu's disease), *Stroke* 18:677, 1987.

70. Desai MY, Stone JH, Foo TKF, et al: Delayed contrast-enhanced MRI of the aortic wall in Takayasu's arteritis: Initial experience, *AJR Am J Roentgenol* 184:1427–1431, 2005.

71. Seko Y: Giant cell and Takayasu arteritis, *Curr Opin Rheumatol* 19:39–43, 2007.

72. Kobayashi Y, Ishii K, Oda K, et al: Aortic wall inflammation due to Takayasu arteritis imaged with ^{18}F-FDG PET coregistered with enhanced CT, *J Nucl Med* 46:917–922, 2005.

73. Uthman I, Kanj N, Atweh S: Infliximab as monotherapy in giant cell arteritis, *Clin Rheumatol* 25:109–110, 2005.

74. Rossa AD, Tavoni A, Merlini G, et al: Two Takayasu arteritis patients successfully treated with infliximab: A potential disease-modifying agent? *Rheumatology* 44:1074–1075, 2005.

75. Tanaka F, Kawakami A, Iwanaga N, et al: Infliximab is effective for Takayasu arteritis refractory to glucocorticoid and methotrexate, *Intern Med* 45:313–316, 2006.

76. Matsuyama A, Sakai N, Ishigami M, et al: Minocycline for the treatment of Takayasu arteritis, *Ann Intern Med* 143:394–395, 2005.

77. Friedrich H, Laas J, Walterbusch G, et al: Extra-intracranial bypass procedure with saphenous vein grafts, *Thorac Cardiovasc Surg* 34:57, 1986.

78. Giordano JM, Leavitt RY, Hoffman G, et al: Experience with surgical treatment of Takayasu's disease, *Surgery* 109:252, 1991.

79. Robbs JV, Human RR, Rajaruthnam P: Operative treatment of nonspecific aortoarteritis (Takayasu's arteritis), *J Vasc Surg* 3:605, 1986.

80. Shelhamer JH, Volkman DJ, Parrillo JE, et al: Takayasu's arteritis and its therapy, *Ann Intern Med* 103:121, 1985.

81. Masugata H, Yasuno M, Nishino M, et al: Takayasu's arteritis with collateral circulation from the right coronary artery to intracranial vessels: A case report, *Angiology* 43:448, 1992.

82. Guillevin L, Lhote F, Gayraud M, et al: Prognostic factors in polyarteritis nodosa and Churg-Strauss syndrome: A prospective study in 342 patients, *Medicine (Balt)* 75:17, 1996.

83. Harle JR, Disdier P, Ali Cherif A, et al: Démence curable et panartérite noueuse, *Rev Neurol (Paris)* 147:148, 1991.

84. Beattie DK, Hellier WP, Powell MP: Stroke-induced cardiovascular changes: A rare cause of death from polyarteritis nodosa, *Br J Neurosurg* 9:223, 1995.

85. Guillevin LC, Mahr A, Callard P, et al: The French Vasculitis Study Group: Hepatitis B virus-associated polyarteritis nodosa: Clinical characteristics, outcome, and impact of treatment in 115 patients, *Medicine* 84:5, 2005.

86. Engel DG, Gospe SM Jr, Tracy KA, et al: Fatal infantile polyarteritis nodosa with predominant central nervous system involvement, *Stroke* 26:699, 1995.

87. Tan EM, Cohen AS, Fries JF, et al: The 1982 revised criteria for the classification of systemic lupus erythematosus, *Arthritis Rheum* 25:1271, 1982.

88. Devinsky O, Petito CK, Alonso DR: Clinical and neuropathological findings in systemic lupus erythematosus: The role of vasculitis, heart emboli, and thrombotic thrombocytopenic purpura, *Ann Neurol* 23:380, 1988.

89. Futrell N, Millikan C: Frequency, etiology, and prevention of stroke in patients with systemic lupus erythematosus, *Stroke* 20:583, 1989.

90. Kitagawa Y, Gotoh F, Koto A, et al: Stroke in systemic lupus erythematosus, *Stroke* 21:1533, 1990.

91. Ward MM, Pyun E, Studenski S: Causes of death in systemic lupus erythematosus: Long-term follow-up of an inception cohort, *Arthritis Rheum* 38:1492, 1995.

92. Esdaile J, Abrahamowicz M, Grodzicky T, et al: Traditional risk factors fail to fully account for accelerated atherosclerosis in SLE, *Arthritis Rheum* 44:2331–2337, 2001.

93. Maksimowicz-McKinnon K, Magder LS, et al: Predictors of carotid atherosclerosis in systemic lupus erythematosus, *J Rheumatol* 33:2458–2463, 2006.

94. Kumral E, Evyapan D, Keser G, et al: Detection of microembolic signals in patients with neuropsychiatric lupus erythematosus, *Eur Neurol* 47:131, 2002.

95. Gharavi AE, Harris EN, Asherson RA, et al: Anticardiolipin antibodies: Isotype distribution and phospholipid specificity, *Ann Rheum Dis* 46:1, 1987.

96. Clinical and laboratory findings in patients with antiphospholipid antibodies and cerebral ischemia. The Antiphospholipid Antibodies in Stroke Study Group, *Stroke* 21:1268, 1990.

97. Briley DP, Coull BM, Goodnight SH Jr: Neurological disease associated with antiphospholipid antibodies, *Ann Neurol* 25:221, 1989.

98. Coull BM, Bourdette DN, Goodnight SH Jr, et al: Multiple cerebral infarctions and dementia associated with anticardiolipin antibodies, *Stroke* 18:1107, 1987.

99. Coull BM, Goodnight SH: Antiphospholipid antibodies, prethrombotic states, and stroke, *Stroke* 21:1370, 1990.

100. Gastineau DA, Kazmier FJ, Nichols WL, et al: Lupus anticoagulant: An analysis of the clinical and laboratory features of 219 cases, *Am J Hematol* 19:265, 1985.

101. Levine SR, Deegan MJ, Futrell N, et al: Cerebrovascular and neurologic disease associated with antiphospholipid antibodies: 48 cases, *Neurology (NY)* 40:1181, 1990.

102. Asherson RA, Khamashta MA, Ordi-Ros J, et al: The "primary" antiphospholipid syndrome: Major clinical and serological features, *Medicine (Balt)* 68:366, 1989.

103. Ruiz-Irastorza G, Khamashta MA, Hughes GR: Antiaggregant and anticoagulant therapy in systemic lupus erythematosus and Hughes' syndrome, *Lupus* 10:241–245, 2001.

104. Wierzbicki AS: Lipids, cardiovascular disease and atherosclerosis in systemic lupus erythematosus, *Lupus* 9:194, 2000.

105. Shiozawa Z, Yoshida M, Kobayashi K, et al: Superior sagittal sinus thrombosis and systemic lupus erythematosus, *Ann Neurol* 20:272, 1986.

106. Vidailhet M, Piett JC, Wechsler B, et al: Cerebral venous thrombosis in systemic lupus erythematosus, *Stroke* 21:1226, 1990.

107. Satoh J, Miyasaka N, Yamada T, et al: Extensive cerebral infarction due to involvement of both anterior cerebral arteries by Wegener's granulomatosis, *Ann Rheum Dis* 47:606, 1988.

108. Tishler S, Williamson T, Mirra SS, et al: Wegener granulomatosis with meningeal involvement, *AJNR Am J Neuroradiol* 14:1248, 1993.

109. Weinberger LM, Cohen ML, Remler BF, et al: Intracranial Wegener's granulomatosis, *Neurology* 43:1831–1834, 1993.

110. Specks U, Wheatley CL, McDonald TJ, et al: Anticytoplasmic autoantibodies in the diagnosis and follow-up of Wegener's granulomatosis, *Mayo Clin Proc* 64:28, 1989.

111. Nölle B, Specks U, Lüdemann J, et al: Anticytoplasmic autoantibodies: Their immunodiagnostic value in Wegener granulomatosis, *Ann Intern Med* 111:28, 1989.

112. Wegener's Granulomatosis Etanercept Trial (WGET) Research Group: Etanercept plus standard therapy for Wegener's granulomatosis, *N Engl J Med* 352:351–361, 2005.

113. Weinstein JM, Chui H, Lane S, et al: Churg-Strauss syndrome (allergic granulomatous angiitis): Neuro-ophthalmologic manifestations, *Arch Ophthalmol* 101:1217, 1983.

114. Chang Y, Kargas SA, Goates JJ, et al: Intraventricular and subarachnoid hemorrhage resulting from necrotizing vasculitis of the choroid plexus in a patient with Churg-Strauss syndrome, *Clin Neuropathol* 12:84, 1993.

115. Liebow AA, Carrington CRB, Friedman PJ: Lymphomatoid granulomatosis, *Hum Pathol* 3:457, 1972.

116. Hogan PJ, Greenberg MK, McCarty GE: Neurologic complications of lymphomatoid granulomatosis, *Neurology (NY)* 31:619, 1981.

117. Ishiura H, Morikawa M, Watanabe T, et al: Lymphomatoid granulomatosis involving central nervous system successfully treated with rituximab alone, *Arch Neurol* 65:662–665, 2008.

118. Averbuch-Heller L, Steiner I, Abramsky O: Neurologic manifestations of progressive systemic sclerosis, *Arch Neurol* 49:1292, 1992.

119. Whittaker R, Barnett A, Ryan P: Antiphospholipid syndrome in scleroderma, *J Rheumatol* 20:1598, 1993.

120. Lucivero V, Mezzapesa DM, Petruzzellis M, et al: Ischaemic stroke in progressive systemic sclerosis, *Neurol Sci* 25:230–233, 2004.

121. Bathon JM, Moreland LW, DiBartolomeo AG: Inflammatory central nervous system involvement in rheumatoid arthritis, *Semin Arthritis Rheum* 18:258, 1989.

122. Libby P: Role of inflammation in atherosclerosis associated with rheumatoid arthritis, *Am J Med* 121:S21–S31, 2008.

123. Singleton JD, West SG, Reddy VV, et al: Cerebral vasculitis complicating rheumatoid arthritis, *South Med J* 88:470, 1995.

124. Howell SJL, Molyneux AJ: Vertebrobasilar insufficiency in rheumatoid atlanto-axial subluxation: A case report with angiographic demonstration of left vertebral artery occlusion, *J Neurol* 235:189, 1988.

125. Fedele FA, Ho G Jr, Dorman BA: Pseudoaneurysm of the vertebral artery: A complication of rheumatoid cervical spine disease, *Arthritis Rheum* 29:136, 1986.

126. Alexander EL, Malinow K, Lejewski JE, et al: Primary Sjögren's syndrome with central nervous system disease mimicking multiple sclerosis, *Ann Intern Med* 104:323, 1986.

127. Caselli RJ, Scheithauer BW, Bowles CA, et al: The treatable dementia of Sjögren's syndrome, *Ann Neurol* 30:98, 1991.

128. Govoni M, Padovan M, Rizzo N, et al: CNS involvement in primary Sjögren's syndrome: Prevalence, clinical aspects, diagnostic assessment and therapeutic approach, *CNS Drugs* 15:597, 2001.

129. Escudero D, Latorre P, Codina M, et al: Central nervous system disease in Sjögren's syndrome, *Ann Intern Med* 146:239, 1995.

130. Tourbah A, Piette JC, Iba-Zizen MT, et al: The natural course of cerebral lesions in Sneddon syndrome, *Arch Neurol* 54:53, 1997.

131. Frances C, Papo T, Wechsler B, et al: Sneddon syndrome with or without antiphospholipid antibodies: A comparative study in 46 patients, *Medicine* 78:209, 1999.

132. Francés C, Le Tonquéze M, Salohzin KV, et al: Prevalence of anti-endothelial cell antibodies in patients with Sneddon's syndrome, *J Am Acad Dermatol* 33:64, 1995.

133. Rumpl E, Neuhofer J, Pallua A: Cerebrovascular lesions and livedo reticularis (Sneddon's syndrome): A progressive cerebrovascular disorder? *J Neurol* 231:324, 1985.

134. Wright RA, Kokmen E: Gradually progressive dementia without discrete cerebrovascular events in a patient with Sneddon's syndrome, *Mayo Clin Proc* 74:57, 1999.

135. Adair JC, Digre KB, Swanda RM, et al: Sneddon's syndrome: A cause of cognitive decline in young adults, *Neuropsychiatry Neuropsychol Behav Neurol* 14:197, 2001.

136. Stockhammer G, Felber SR, Zelger B, et al: Sneddon's syndrome: Diagnosis by skin biopsy and MRI in 17 patients, *Stroke* 24:685, 1993.

137. Boortz-Marx RL, Clark HB, Taylor S, et al: Sneddon's syndrome with granulomatous leptomeningeal infiltration, *Stroke* 26:492, 1995.

138. Weisshaar E, Claus G, Friedl A, et al: Atrial myxoma syndrome mimicking Ehrmann-Sneddon syndrome, *Dermatology* 195:404, 1997.

139. Aladdin Y, Hamadeh M, Butcher K: The Sneddon syndrome, *Arch Neurol* 65:834–835, 2008.

140. McFarland HR, Wood WG, Drowns BV, et al: Papulosis atrophicans maligna (Köhlmeier-Degos disease): A disseminated occlusive vasculopathy, *Ann Neurol* 3:388, 1978.

141. Burrow JN, Blumbergs PC, Iyer PV, et al: Köhlmeier-Degos disease: A multisystem vasculopathy with progressive cerebral infarction, *Aust N Z J Med* 21:49, 1991.

142. Shimazu S, Imai H, Kokubu S, et al: Long-term survival in malignant atrophic papulosis: A case report and review of the Japanese literature, *Nippon Geka Gakkai Zasshi* 89:1748, 1988.

143. International Study Group for Behçet's Disease: Criteria for diagnosis of Behçet's disease, *Lancet* 335:1078–1080, 1990.

144. Sakane T, Takeno M, Suzukin N, et al: Behçet's disease, *N Engl J Med* 341:1284–1291, 1999.
145. Iraguli VJ, Maravi E: Behçet syndrome presenting as cerebrovascular disease, *J Neurol Neurosurg Psychiatry* 49:838, 1986.
146. Lueck CJ, Pires M, McCartney AC, et al: Ocular and neurological Behçet's disease without orogenital ulceration? *J Neurol Neurosurg Psychiatry* 56:505, 1993.
147. Wechsler B, Vidailhet M, Piette JC, et al: Cerebral venous thrombosis in Behçet's disease: Clinical study and long-term follow-up of 25 cases, *Neurology* 42:614, 1992.
148. Al Kawi MZ, Bohlega S, Banna M: MRI findings in neuro-Behçet's disease, *Neurology* 41:405, 1991.
149. Morrissey SP, Miller DH, Hermaszewski R, et al: Magnetic resonance imaging of the central nervous system in Behçet's disease, *Eur Neurol* 33:287, 1993.
150. Zelenski JD, Capraro JA, Holden D, et al: Central nervous system vasculitis in Behçet's syndrome: Angiographic improvement after therapy with cytotoxic agents, *Arthritis Rheum* 32:217, 1989.
151. Evereklioglu C: Managing the symptoms of Behçet's disease, *Expert Opin Pharmacother* 5:317–328, 2004.
152. Petty GW, Duffy J, Huston J III: Cerebral ischemia in patients with hepatitis C virus infection and mixed cryoglobulinemia, *Mayo Clin Proc* 71:671, 1996.
153. Galossi A, Guarisco R, Bellis L, et al: Extrahepatic manifestations of chronic HCV infection, *J Gastrointest Liver Dis* 16:65–73, 2007.
154. Kanda T: Chronic hepatitis C infection and peripheral neuropathy: Is mixed cryoglobulinemia really important? *Intern Med* 42:377–378, 2003.
155. Acharya JN, Pacheco VH: Neurologic complications of hepatitis C, *Neurologist* 14:151–156, 2008.
156. Rennebohm RM, Egan RA, Susac JO: Treatment of Susac's syndrome, *Curr Treat Options Neurol* 10:67–74, 2008.
157. Ross R: Atherosclerosis: An inflammatory disease, *N Engl J Med* 340:115, 1999.
158. Munro JM, van der Walt JD, Munro CS, et al: An immunohistochemical analysis of human aortic fatty streaks, *Hum Pathol* 18:375, 1987.
159. Napoli C, D'Armiento FP, Mancini FP, et al: Fatty streak formation occurs in human fetal aortas and is greatly enhanced by maternal hypercholesterolemia: Intimal accumulation of low density lipoprotein and its oxidation precede monocyte recruitment into early atherosclerotic lesions, *J Clin Invest* 100:2680, 1997.
160. Stary HC, Chandler AB, Glagov S, et al: A definition of initial, fatty streak, and intermediate lesions of atherosclerosis: A report from the Committee on Vascular Lesions of the Council on Arteriosclerosis, American Heart Association, *Circulation* 89:2462, 1994.
161. Mazzone A, De Servi S, Ricevuti G, et al: Increased expression of neutrophil and monocyte adhesion molecules in unstable coronary artery disease, *Circulation* 88:358, 1993.
162. Galea J, Armstrong J, Gadsdon P, et al: Interleukin-1β in coronary arteries of patients with ischemic heart disease, *Arterioscler Thromb Vasc Biol* 16:1000, 1992.
163. Barath P, Fishbein MC, Cao J, et al: Detection and localization of tumor necrosis factor in human atheroma, *Am J Cardiol* 65:297, 1990.
164. van der Wal AC, Das PK, Bentz van de Berg D, et al: Atherosclerotic lesions in humans: In situ immunophenotypic analysis suggesting an immune-mediated response, *Lab Invest* 61:166, 1989.
165. Nilsson J: Cytokines and smooth muscle cells in atherosclerosis, *Cardiovasc Res* 27:1184, 1993.
166. Jonasson L, Holm J, Skalli O, et al: Regional accumulations of T cells, macrophages, and smooth muscle cells in the human atherosclerotic plaque, *Arteriosclerosis* 6:131, 1986.
167. Gown AM, Tsukada T, Ross R: Human atherosclerosis II: Immunocytochemical analysis of the cellular composition of human atherosclerotic lesions, *Am J Pathol* 125:191, 1986.
168. Libby P, Ross R: Cytokines and growth regulatory molecules. In Fuster V, Ross R, Topol EJ, editors: *Atherosclerosis and coronary artery disease* vol 1 Philadelphia, 1996, Lippincott-Raven, p 585.
169. Raines EW, Rosenfeld ME, Ross R: The role of macrophages. In Fuster V, Ross R, Topol EJ, editors: *Atherosclerosis and coronary artery disease,* vol 1, Philadelphia, 1996, Lippincott-Raven, p 539.

170. Chappell DC, Varner SE, Nerem RM, et al: Oscillatory shear stress stimulates adhesion molecule expression in cultured human endothelium, *Circ Res* 82:532, 1998.
171. Iiyama K, Hajra L, Iiyama M, et al: Patterns of vascular cell adhesion molecule-1 and intercellular adhesion molecule-1 expression in rabbit and mouse atherosclerotic lesions and at sites predisposed to lesion formation, *Circ Res* 85:199, 1999.
172. Tsuboi H, Ando J, Korenaga R, et al: Flow stimulates ICAM-1 expression time and shear stress dependently in cultured human endothelial cells, *Biochem Biophys Res Commun* 206:988, 1995.
173. Nagel T, Resnick N, Atkinson WJ, et al: Shear stress selectively upregulates intercellular adhesion molecule-1 expression in cultured human vascular endothelial cells, *J Clin Invest* 94:885, 1994.
174. Resnick N, Collins T, Atkinson W, et al: Platelet-derived growth factor B chain promoter contains a cis-acting fluid shear-stress-responsive element, *Proc Natl Acad Sci U S A* 90:4591, 1993.
175. Lin MC, Almus-Jacobs F, Chen HH, et al: Shear stress induction of the tissue factor gene, *J Clin Invest* 99:737, 1997.
176. Mondy JS, Lindner V, Miyashiro JK, et al: Platelet-derived growth factor ligand and receptor expression in response to altered blood flow in vivo, *Circ Res* 81:320, 1997.
177. Kim CJ, Khoo JC, Gillotte-Taylor K, et al: Polymerase chain reaction-based method for quantifying recruitment of monocytes to mouse atherosclerotic lesions in vivo: Enhancement by tumor necrosis factor alpha and interleukin-1beta, *Arterioscler Thromb Vasc Biol* 20:2000, 1976.
178. Hynes RO, Wagner DD: Genetic manipulation of vascular adhesion molecules in mice, *J Clin Invest* 98:2193, 1996.
179. Hollenbaugh D, Mischel-Petty N, Edwards CP, et al: Expression of functional CD40 by vascular endothelial cells, *J Exp Med* 182:33, 1995.
180. Mach F, Schonbeck U, Bonnefoy J-Y, et al: Activation of monocyte/macrophage functions related to acute atheroma complication by ligation of CD40: Induction of collagenase, stromelysin, and tissue factor, *Circulation* 96:396, 1997.
181. Schonbeck U, Mach F, Bonnefoy J-Y, et al: Ligation of CD40 activates interleukin 1(beta)-converting enzyme (capsase-1) activity in vascular smooth muscle and endothelial cells and promotes elaboration of active interleukin 1(beta), *J Biol Chem* 272:19569, 1997.
182. Mach F, Schonbeck U, Sukhova GK, et al: Reduction of atherosclerosis in mice by inhibition of CD40 signalling, *Nature* 394:200, 1998.
183. Lee RT, Libby P: The unstable atheroma, *Arterioscler Thromb Vasc Biol* 17:1859–1867, 1997.
184. Schonbeck U, Mach F, Sukhova GK, et al: Regulation of matrix metalloproteinase expression in human vascular smooth muscle cells by T lymphocytes: A role for CD40 signaling in plaque rupture? *Circ Res* 81:448, 1997.
185. Frostegard J, Ulfgren AK, Nyberg P, et al: Cytokine expression in advanced human atherosclerotic plaques: Dominance of pro-inflammatory (Th1) and macrophage-stimulating cytokines, *Atherosclerosis* 145:33, 1999.
186. Jander S, Sitzer M, Schumann R, et al: Inflammation in high-grade carotid stenosis: A possible role for macrophages and T cells in plaque destabilization, *Stroke* 29:1625, 1998.
187. DeGraba TJ, Siren AL, Penix L, et al: Increased endothelial expression of intercellular adhesion molecule-1 in symptomatic versus asymptomatic human carotid atherosclerotic plaque, *Stroke* 29:1405, 1998.
188. DeGraba TJ: Expression of inflammatory mediators and adhesion molecules in human atherosclerotic plaque, *Neurology* 49(Suppl 4):S15, 1997.
189. Falkenberg M, Bjornheden T, Oden A, et al: Heterogeneous distribution of macrophages, tumour necrosis factor alpha, tissue factor and fibrinolytic regulators in atherosclerotic vessels, *Eur J Vasc Endovasc Surg* 16:276, 1998.
190. Elkind MS, Cheng J, Boden-Albala B, et al: Elevated white blood cell count and carotid plaque thickness: The Northern Manhattan Stroke Study, *Stroke* 32:842, 2001.
191. Elkind MSV, Sciacca R, Boden-Albala B, et al: Relative elevation in leukocyte count predicts first cerebral infarction, *Neurology* 64:2121–2125, 2005.
192. Salonen R, Salonen JT: Progression of carotid atherosclerosis and its determinants: A population-based ultrasonography study, *Atherosclerosis* 81:33, 1990.

193. Sen S, Hinderliter A, Sen PK, et al: Association of leukocyte count with progression of aortic atheroma in stroke/transient ischemic attack patients, *Stroke* 38:2900-2905, 2007.
194. Yarnell JWG, Baker IA, Sweetnam PM, et al: Fibrinogen, viscosity, and white blood cell count are major risk factors for ischemic heart disease, *Circulation* 83:836, 1991.
195. Kannel WB, Anderson K, Wilson PW: White blood cell count and cardiovascular disease: Insights from the Framingham Study, *JAMA* 267:1253, 1992.
196. Grau AJ, Buggle F, Becher H, et al: The association of leukocyte count, fibrinogen and C-reactive protein with vascular risk factors and ischemic vascular diseases, *Thromb Res* 82:245, 1996.
197. Grau AJ, Boddy AW, Dukovic DA, et al: Leukocyte count as an independent predictor of recurrent ischemic events, *Stroke* 35:1147-1152, 2004.
198. Lange LA, Carlson CS, Hindorff LA, et al: Association of polymorphisms in the CRP gene with circulating C-reactive protein levels and cardiovascular events, *JAMA* 296:2703-2711, 2006.
199. Di Napoli M, Schwaninger M, Cappelli R, et al: Evaluation of C-reactive protein measurement for assessing the risk and prognosis in ischemic stroke: A statement for health care professionals from the CRP Pooling Project members, *Stroke* 36:1316-1329, 2005.
200. Ridker PM, Hennekens CH, Buring JE, Rifai N: C-reactive protein and other markers of inflammation in the prediction of cardiovascular disease in women, *N Engl J Med* 342:836-843, 2000.
201. Ridker PM, Buring JE, Rifai N, et al: Development and validation of improved algorithms for the assessment of global cardiovascular risk in women: The Reynolds Risk Score, *JAMA* 297:611-619, 2007.
202. Elkind MS, Luna JM, Moon YP, et al: High-sensitivity C-reactive protein predicts mortality but not stroke in a multi-ethnic cohort: The Northern Manhattan Study, *Neurology* 73:1300-1307, 2009.
203. Verma S, Szmitko PE, Yeh ETH: C-reactive protein: Structure affects function, *Circulation* 109:1914-1917, 2004.
204. Arenillas JF, Alvarez-Sabín J, Molina CA, et al: Progression of symptomatic intracranial large artery atherosclerosis is associated with a proinflammatory state and impaired fibrinolysis, *Stroke* 39:1456-1463, 2008.
205. Montaner J, Fernandez-Cadenas I, Molina CA, et al: Poststroke C-reactive protein is a powerful prognostic tool among candidates for thrombolysis, *Stroke* 37:1205-1210, 2006.
206. Carlos TM, Harlan JM: Leukocyte-endothelial adhesion molecules, *Blood* 84:2068-2101, 1994.
207. Frenette PS, Wagner DD: Insights into selectin function from knockout mice, *Thromb Haemost* 78:60-64, 1997.
208. O'Brien KD, McDonald TO, Chait A, et al: Neovascular expression of E-selectin, intercellular adhesion molecule-1, and vascular cell adhesion molecule-1 in human atherosclerosis and their relation to intimal leukocyte content, *Circulation* 93:672-682, 1996.
209. Pigott R, Dillon LP, Hemingway IH, et al: Soluble forms of E-selectin, ICAM-1 and VCAM-1 are present in the supernatants of cytokine activated cultured endothelial cells, *Biochem Biophys Res Commun* 187:584-589, 1992.
210. Price DT, Loscalzo J: Cellular adhesion molecules and atherogenesis, *Am J Med* 107:85-97, 1999.
211. Hwang SJ, Ballantyne CM, Sharrett AR, et al: Circulating adhesion molecules VCAM-1, ICAM-1, and E-selectin in carotid atherosclerosis and incident coronary heart disease cases: The Atherosclerosis Risk In Communities (ARIC) Study, *Circulation* 96:4219-4225, 1997.
212. Pearson TA, Mensah GA, Alexander RW, et al: Markers of inflammation and cardiovascular disease: Application to clinical and public health practice: A statement for healthcare professionals from the Centers for Disease Control and Prevention and the American Heart Association, *Circulation* 107:499-511, 2003.
213. Revilla M, Obach V, Cervera A, et al: A -174G/C polymorphism of the interleukin-6 gene in patients with lacunar infarction, *Neurosci Lett* 324:29-32, 2002.
214. Castellanos M, Castillo J, Garcia MM, et al: Inflammation-mediated damage in progressing lacunar infarctions: A potential therapeutic target, *Stroke* 33:982-987, 2002.
215. Ridker PM, Rifai N, Pfeffer MA, et al: Long-term effects of pravastatin on plasma concentration of C-reactive protein, *Circulation* 100:230-235, 1999.
216. Albert MA, Danielson E, Rifai N, et al: Effect of statin therapy on C-reactive protein levels: The Pravastatin Inflammation/CRP Evaluation (PRINCE), a randomized trial and cohort study, *JAMA* 286:64-70, 2001.
217. Ridker PM, Rifai N, Clearfield M, et al: Measurement of C-reactive protein for the targeting of statin therapy in the primary prevention of acute coronary events, *N Engl J Med* 344:1959-1965, 2001.
218. Ridker PM, Rifai N, Pfeffer MA, et al: Inflammation, pravastatin, and the risk of coronary events after myocardial infarction in patients with average cholesterol levels, *Circulation* 98:839-844, 1998.
219. Ridker PM, Cannon CP, Morrow D, et al: C-reactive protein levels and outcomes after statin therapy, *N Engl J Med* 352:20-28, 2005.
220. Morrow DA, de Lemos JA, Sabatine MS, et al: Clinical relevance of C-reactive protein during follow-up of patients with acute coronary syndromes in the Aggrastat-to-Zocor Trial, *Circulation* 114:228-281, 2006.
221. Ridker PM, Morrow DA, Rose LM, et al: Relative efficacy of atorvastatin 80 mg and pravastatin 40 mg in achieving the dual goals of low-density lipoprotein cholesterol <70 mg/dl and C-reactive protein <2 mg/l: An analysis of the PROVE-IT TIMI-22 trial, *J Am Coll Cardiol* 45:1644-1648, 2005.
222. Kinlay S, Schwartz GG, Olsson AG, et al: Inflammation, statin therapy, and risk of stroke after an acute coronary syndrome in the MIRACL study, *Arterioscler Thromb Vasc Biol* 28:142-147, 2008.
223. Everett BM, Glynn RJ, MacFadyen JG, et al: Rosuvastatin in the prevention of stroke among men and women with elevated levels of C-reactive protein: Justification for the use of statins in prevention: An intervention trial evaluating rosuvastatin (JUPITER), *Circulation* 121:143-150, 2010.

Moyamoya Disease

MASAHIRO YASAKA, JUNICHI MASUDA, JUN OGATA, TAKENORI YAMAGUCHI

Moyamoya disease is an unusual form of chronic cerebrovascular occlusive disease that is characterized by angiographic findings of bilateral stenosis or occlusion at the terminal portion of the internal carotid artery together with an abnormal vascular network at the base of the brain (Fig. 35-1).[1-6] The first report of a patient with this disease was published in 1957 by Takeuchi and Shimizu[7] with the diagnosis of "bilateral hypoplasia of the internal carotid arteries." This patient was a 29-year-old man who had been suffering from visual disturbance and hemiconvulsive seizures since the age of 10 years. Takeuchi and Shimizu[7] considered this arterial occlusion to be congenital hypoplasia that differed from the atherosclerotic lesion on the basis of the histologic examination of a branch of the external carotid artery. Since then, similar cases have been reported, mainly among the Japanese, and a variety of names have been applied to the condition—"cerebral juxta-basal telangiectasia" by Sano,[8] "cerebral arterial rete" by Handa and colleagues,[9] "rete mirabile" by Weidner and associates,[10] and "cerebral basal rete mirabile" by Nishimoto and Takeuchi.[11] The terms "spontaneous occlusion of the circle of Willis," used by Kudo,[12] and "moyamoya disease" are now commonly used in the literature. The term *moyamoya disease* was proposed by Suzuki and Takaku,[13] taken from the characteristic angiographic findings of an abnormal vascular network at the base of the brain; the Japanese word *moyamoya*, meaning "vague or hazy puff of smoke," describes its appearance.

Extensive investigations of patients with this characteristic angiographic finding have been conducted mainly by Japanese neurosurgeons over the past 50 years. As a result, the clinical entity of this disease and its concept have now been established. It is well known, for example, that progression of stenosis or occlusion of the intracranial major arteries, including the distal ends of the internal carotid arteries, is the primary lesion of this disease and that the abnormal vascular network (moyamoya vessels) at the base of the brain is their collateral supply, developed secondary to brain ischemia, although this finding on angiography characterizes the clinical category (see Fig. 35-1).[2,4-6,14] The guideline for the diagnosis of moyamoya disease was established and has been revised by the Research Committee on Spontaneous Occlusion of the Circle of Willis, organized by the Ministry of Health and Welfare, Japan (MHWJ), and the latest version (1997) was published not only in Japanese but also in English.[2,15] These publications help establish this disease as a clinical entity, and it is now known that moyamoya disease is widely distributed all over the world.[6,16,17] The epidemiology of moyamoya disease is discussed later.

Because the clinical features, radiologic findings, progress on etiology and pathogenesis, and pathologic findings have been sufficiently described in the previous edition of this textbook[6,18] and elsewhere,[4,14] we use the present chapter to add new knowledge on ultrasonography, MRI, and so on.

Guideline For Diagnosis

The guideline for the diagnosis of moyamoya disease has been developed by the MHWJ's Research Committee on Spontaneous Occlusion of the Circle of Willis (Tables 35-1 and 35-2).[2] It has been used not only for patient diagnosis but also for follow-up and further investigation into the etiology and pathogenesis of this unique and mysterious disorder.

Prior to 1995, the guideline stated that cerebral angiography is indispensable to diagnosis in all but the autopsied cases.[6] Because the quality of the images of MRI and MR angiography (MRA) has improved, the Research Committee conducted comparative studies to examine whether MRI and MRA could be substituted for conventional cerebral angiography.[6,19-21] They concluded in 1995 that the diagnosis of moyamoya disease can be made without conventional cerebral angiography if MRI and MRA clearly demonstrate all the findings that indicate moyamoya disease. The diagnostic criteria applied to the MRI and MRA were added as a supplemented reference in the revision (see Table 35-2).[2] The substitution of noninvasive imaging methods for invasive methods is helpful for patients, especially children.

This revision also contains the addition of autoimmune disorders to the list of disorders that should be excluded in any patient being evaluated for moyamoya disease, to avoid confusing this disease with other disorders in which vascular lesions resembling those of moyamoya disease can form.

Epidemiology

The incidence and prevalence of moyamoya disease in the Japanese have been surveyed by collaborative studies conducted by the research committees on the epidemiology of intractable diseases and on the spontaneous occlusion of the circle of Willis organized by the MHWJ in 1984, 1989, and 1994, and reported by Wakai and

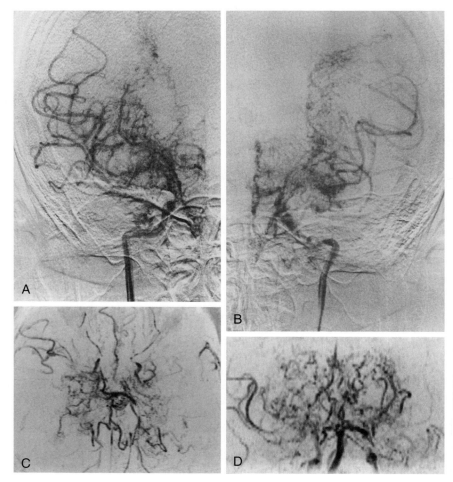

Figure 35-1 Conventional cerebral angiograms (A and B) and MR angiograms (C and D) in a 10-year-old boy with moyamoya disease. Anteroposterior views in conventional angiograms show (A) severe stenosis of the right middle cerebral artery (MCA) and (B) nearly complete occlusion of the left MCA. Well-developed basal moyamoya vessels are also seen. MR angiograms of this patient show findings similar to those observed on conventional angiograms: C, basal view; D, anteroposterior view. (From Houkin K, Aoki T, Takahashi A, et al: Diagnosis of moyamoya disease with magnetic resonance angiography. *Stroke* 25:2159, 1994.)

colleagues.[22] The estimated number of patients treated in Japan in 1994 was 3900 (95% confidence interval [CI], 3500–4400). The corresponding value surveyed in 1989 was 3300, but small hospitals (<200 beds) had not been included, so the 1994 figure was recalculated to exclude small hospitals and re-estimated as 3200. Therefore, the prevalence is considered unchanged from 1989 to 1994, and the annual prevalence and incidence are calculated to be 3.16 and 0.35 per 100,000 population, respectively. Female preponderance has been reported[6] and was also confirmed in the patient survey of 1994 by the finding of a female-to-male ratio of 1.8:1.[22] The largest peak in age distribution was observed in patients 10 to 14 years old, with a smaller peak in patients in their 40s. The age at onset was younger than 10 years in 47.8% of the patients (childhood moyamoya), although the disease had developed in some patients between the ages of 25 and 49 years (adult-type moyamoya) (Fig. 35-2).

Evidence of the familial occurrence of this disease has been accumulating in the medical literature.[4,6,23-25] According to the previously mentioned nationwide survey, family histories of moyamoya disease were found to be present in 10% of patients, and 13 pairs of monovular twins were registered as having the disease.[22] The contribution of hereditary factors to the occurrence of moyamoya disease is discussed later, in the section on etiology and pathogenesis.

Although regional predilection has never been reported within Japan, there are remarkable regional differences in the frequency of reported moyamoya worldwide.[6,16,17] After the report by Taveras in 1969,[26] reports of moyamoya disease have been growing among non-Japanese people, including white and black people, although it is rare in white patients.[17,27] None of the races has as high an incidence as the Japanese, but relatively large numbers of patients have been found in Korea[28,29] and China.[30,31]

Korean neurosurgeons performed the first nationwide cooperative survey of moyamoya disease in their country in 1988, and 289 patients were registered.[28] The reported clinical features of these patients, however, were different from those of Japanese patients. Therefore, it is important to examine whether this heterogeneity suggests racial and regional differences or whether it is related to any differences between the criteria used for diagnosis of moyamoya disease in the two countries. In 1995, the Japanese neurosurgeons Ikezaki and Fukui and their associates organized a collaborative study with Korean neurosurgeon Han and colleagues, analyzing the patients registered in Korea on the basis of questionnaires about the angiographic findings.[15,29,32] Because the guideline established by the MHWJ Research Committee was not strictly applied to the diagnosis of moyamoya disease in Korea, Ikezaki and Fukui reevaluated the registration records and divided the 451 registered Korean cases into definite (296), probable

TABLE 35-1 DIAGNOSTIC GUIDELINES FOR SPONTANEOUS OCCLUSION OF THE CIRCLE OF WILLIS (MOYAMOYA DISEASE)

(A) Cerebral angiography is indispensable for the diagnosis, and should present at least the following findings:
   1. Stenosis or occlusion at the terminal portion of the internal carotid artery and/or at the proximal portion of the anterior and/or middle cerebral arteries.
   2. Abnormal vascular networks seen in the vicinity of the occlusive or stenotic lesions in the arterial phase.
   3. These findings should present bilaterally.
(B) When magnetic resonance imaging (MRI) and magnetic resonance angiography (MRA) clearly demonstrate all the findings described below, conventional cerebral angiography is not mandatory:
   1. Stenosis or occlusion at the terminal portion of the internal carotid artery and at the proximal portion of the anterior and middle cerebral arteries on MRA.
   2. An abnormal vascular network in the basal ganglia on MRA. Note: An abnormal vascular network can be diagnosed when more than two apparent flow voids are seen in one side of the basal ganglia on MRI.
   3. B-1 and B-2 are seen bilaterally. (Refer to Image Diagnostic Guidelines by MRI and MRA [Table 35-2].)
(C) Because the etiology of this disease is unknown, cerebrovascular disease with the following basic diseases or conditions should thus be eliminated:
   1. Arteriosclerosis
   2. Autoimmune disease
   3. Meningitis
   4. Brain neoplasm
   5. Down syndrome
   6. Recklinghausen's disease
   7. Head trauma
   8. Irradiation to the head
   9. Others
(D) Instructive pathologic findings:
   1. Intimal thickening and the resulting stenosis or occlusion of the lumen are observed in and around the terminal portion of the internal carotid artery, usually on both sides. Lipid deposit is occasionally seen in thickened intima.
   2. Arteries constituting the circle of Willis such as the anterior and middle cerebral and posterior communicating arteries often show stenosis of varying degrees or occlusion associated with fibrocellular thickening of the intima, a waving of the internal elastic lamina, and an attenuation of the media.
   3. Numerous small vascular channels (perforators and anastomotic branches) are observed around the circle of Willis.
   4. Reticular conglomerates of small vessels are often seen in the pia mater.
Diagnosis: In reference to A-D mentioned above, the diagnostic criteria are classified as follows. Autopsy cases not undergoing cerebral angiography should be investigated separately while referring to D.
   1. Definite case: One that fulfills either A or B, and C.
In children, however, a case that fulfills A-1 and A-2 (or B-1 and B-2) on one side and with remarkable stenosis at the terminal portion of the internal carotid artery on the opposite side is also included.
   2. A probable case: One that fulfills A-1 and A-2 (or B-1 and B-2) and C (unilateral involvement).

From Fukui M: Guidelines for the diagnosis and treatment of spontaneous occlusion of the circle of Willis ("moyamoya" disease). Research Committee on Spontaneous Occlusion of the Circle of Willis (Moyamoya Disease) of the Ministry of Health and Welfare, Japan. *Clin Neurol Neurosurg* 99(Suppl 2):S238, 1997.

TABLE 35-2 IMAGE DIAGNOSTIC GUIDELINES FOR MOYAMOYA DISEASE BY MRI AND MRA

(A) When magnetic resonance imaging (MRI) and magnetic resonance angiography (MRA) clearly demonstrate all the findings described below, conventional cerebral angiography is not mandatory:
   1. Stenosis or occlusion at the terminal portion of the intracranial internal carotid artery and at the proximal portion of the anterior and middle cerebral arteries.
   2. An abnormal vascular network in the basal ganglia.
   3. A-1 and A-2 are seen bilaterally.
(B) Imaging methods and judgment.
   1. More than a 1.0 tesla magnetic field strength is recommended.
   2. There are no restrictions regarding MRA imaging methods.
   3. The imaging parameters, such as the magnetic field strength, the imaging methods, and the use of contrast medium, should be clearly documented.
   4. An abnormal vascular network can be diagnosed when more than two apparent flow voids are seen on one side of the basal ganglia on MRI.
   5. Either an over- or underestimation of the lesion could be made according to the imaging conditions. To avoid a false-positive diagnosis, only definite cases should thus be diagnosed on the MRI and MRA findings.
(C) Because similar vascular lesions secondary to other disorders are sometimes indistinguishable from this disease in adults, a diagnosis based on MRI and MRA without conventional angiography is thus only recommended in pediatric cases.

From Fukui M: Guidelines for the diagnosis and treatment of spontaneous occlusion of the circle of Willis ("moyamoya" disease). Research Committee on Spontaneous Occlusion of the Circle of Willis (Moyamoya Disease) of the Ministry of Health and Welfare, Japan. *Clin Neurol Neurosurg* 99(Suppl 2):S238, 1997.

(103), and unlikely (52) cases. Analysis of the definite cases showed that the clinical features of the Korean patients were quite similar to those of the Japanese patients.[15,32] The pattern of distribution for the age at onset showed the same two peaks (<10 years and 25 to 49 years) as that of the Japanese, although the adult population was 20% larger in the Korean sample than in the Japanese. There was a slight female predominance (ratio 1.3:1), and the incidence of hemorrhage was higher in females than in males. The incidence of brain infarction and hemorrhage was significantly higher, whereas the rates of transient ischemic attacks and seizures were lower in Korean than in Japanese subjects. The incidence of infarction in children and that of hemorrhage in both children and adults were also statistically higher in Koreans.

From these results, the higher incidence of hemorrhage and adult-type moyamoya are suggested to be the features of moyamoya disease in Korean patients, but the diagnostic criteria and the interpretation of the angiographic findings by neuroradiologists should be standardized in the two countries. Atherosclerotic cerebrovascular stenosis and occlusion should be excluded more carefully in the Korean patients before final conclusions are drawn. Such studies should be undertaken not only in Japan and Korea, but also in Western and other Asian countries for clarification of the racial significance and genetic background of this disease.

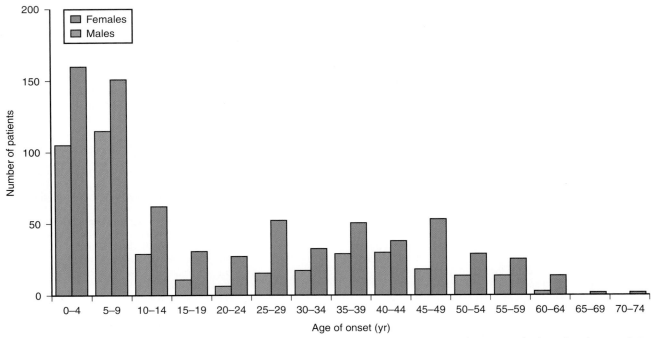

Figure 35-2 Distribution of age at onset and sex of patients with moyamoya disease. (From Wakai K, Tamakoshi A, Ikezaki K, et al: Epidemiological features of moyamoya disease in Japan: Findings from a nationwide survey. *Clin Neurol Neurosurg* 99[Suppl 2]:S1, 1997.)

Pathology

Pathologic observations of approximately 100 autopsy cases of moyamoya disease revealed various forms of cerebrovascular lesions in the brain, and their macroscopic and microscopic findings have been accumulated and described in the literature.[9,33-40] The lesion observed most commonly at autopsy is intracranial hemorrhage, which is a major cause of death for patients with moyamoya disease.[39] Massive parenchymatous hemorrhage (intracerebral hemorrhage) occurs frequently in the basal ganglia, thalamus, hypothalamus, cerebral peduncle, and midbrain, and often extends and ruptures to the intraventricular spaces.[39] Subarachnoid hemorrhage (SAH) also occurs, but primary SAH caused by rupture of aneurysms seems to be not so frequent as described previously, and many cases appear to be secondary extensions of parenchymatous hemorrhage.[6] In addition, old brain infarction and focal cortical atrophy of the brain are not uncommon findings and are often found in multiple.[39,40] Furthermore, the infarcts are mostly small and localized in the basal ganglia, internal capsule, thalamus, and subcortex. The large and arterial territorial infarcts[41] are rare in moyamoya disease, although occlusion of the intracranial major arteries is present. This finding may suggest the function of moyamoya vessels as a collateral pathway after arterial occlusion. The frequency and distribution of intracranial hemorrhage and infarction found at autopsy may not represent those of patients with moyamoya disease, and the pathologic specimens obtained from the circle of Willis and moyamoya vessels are biased by the unavoidable clinical modifications related to their deaths. Nevertheless, the histologic and immunohistochemical analyses of the postmortem materials have provided a significant amount of valuable information relating to the etiology and pathogenesis of lesion formation in this disease.

The Circle of Willis and the Major Branches

In the guideline for the diagnosis of moyamoya disease, the pathologic findings in the intracranial arteries from autopsied patients are included as an aid for diagnosis at autopsy of the disease in patients who did not undergo angiography during life (see Table 35-1).[2,3] The histologic appearance of the circle of Willis and the major branches of the patients with moyamoya disease is characteristic, but not peculiar to this disease.[35,36,40] Therefore, it is not always possible to diagnose moyamoya disease solely on the basis of pathologic findings.

On macroscopic observation, the circle of Willis and the major branches are tapered and narrowed entirely or partially with overgrown and dilated arteries branching from the circle of Willis (Fig. 35-3). The degree of tapering of arteries as well as the network formation of dilated arteries (moyamoya vessels) and their distributions vary from case to case. The distal ends of the internal carotid arteries are affected by severe narrowing or occlusion.

In conventional staining of specimens obtained from the circle of Willis or its major branches with lesion involvement, the arterial lumen is severely narrowed or occluded by fibrocellular intimal thickening (Figs. 35-4A and 35-5A).[35,36,38,40] The thickened intima appears to be in a laminated structure with duplication or triplication of internal elastic lamina and a wavy appearance. These features closely resemble the structure noted focally at arterial branching portions in normal controls, the so-called intimal cushion. The outer diameter of the affected artery

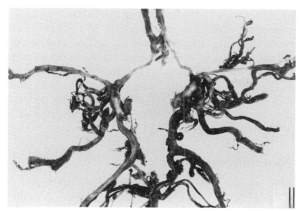

Figure 35-3 Macroscopic appearance of the circle of Willis in a 66-year-old woman with moyamoya disease at autopsy. Tapering of anterior and middle cerebral arteries can be seen bilaterally with network formation of dilated arteries (basal moyamoya vessels).

usually becomes smaller, and the underlying media are markedly attenuated. These histologic features are common to lesions at any site, although the extent of intimal thickenings and the distribution in the circle of Willis are variable in different patients.

Immunohistochemical staining of this lesion demonstrated that the thickened intima is composed mainly of smooth muscle cells (SMCs) (see Fig. 35-5B) that are phenotypically modulated from the contractile type to the synthetic.[38] With this immunohistochemical study, some of the SMCs in the intima were stained positively with the antibody for proliferating cell nuclear antigen (see Fig. 35-5C) and thereby were revealed to be proliferating. This evidence strongly suggests that SMC proliferation and phenotypic modulation contribute to the formation of fibrocellular intimal thickening in the circle of Willis in patients with moyamoya disease. Lipid deposition and lipid-containing macrophages (foam cells) have been

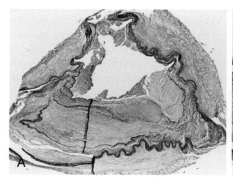
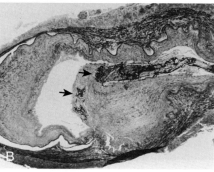

Figure 35-4 Microscopic appearance of the circle of Willis in patients with moyamoya disease at autopsy. A, Intracranial portion of right internal carotid artery of a 60-year-old woman (elastica van Gieson stain). B, Main trunk of the right middle cerebral artery of a 36-year-old man. *Arrows* indicate mural fibrin thrombi with its organization (Mallory's phosphotungstic acid-hematoxylin [PTAH] stain).

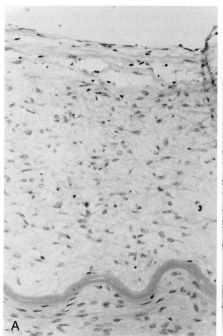
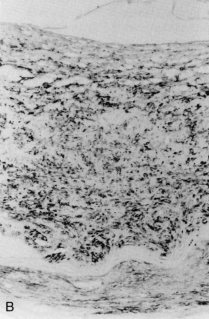
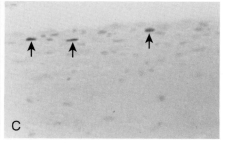

Figure 35-5 Microscopic appearance of the basilar artery of a 14-year-old girl with moyamoya disease at autopsy. A, H&E stain; B, immunohistochemical stain for muscle actin; C, staining for proliferating cell nuclear antigen (PCNA). *Arrows* in C indicate the nuclei stained positively for PCNA. (A and B from Masuda J, Ogata J, Yutani C: Smooth muscle cell proliferation and localization of macrophages and T-cells in the occlusive intracranial major arteries in moyamoya disease. *Stroke* 24:1960, 1993.)

found in some autopsy cases but are now considered features of atherosclerosis.[3]

Mural thrombi are often found in the stenotic lesions of the circle of Willis and the major branches (see Fig. 35-4*B*), but their frequency varies among reports.[35,36,38,42] Judging from their histologic features, the organization of such thrombi appears to contribute to the pathogenesis of fibrocellular intimal thickening, which is discussed in the section on etiology and pathogenesis.

Aneurysm formation, a relatively common finding in the circle of Willis in patients with moyamoya disease, and its pathology are summarized later.

Perforating Arteries (Moyamoya Vessels)

The vascular network at the base of the brain consists of dilated medium-sized or small muscular arteries branching off the circle of Willis, anterior choroidal arteries, intracranial portions of internal carotid arteries, and posterior cerebral arteries. These arteries form complex channels that usually connect to the distal portion of the anterior and middle cerebral arteries. Numerous small dilated and tortuous vessels originating from these channels enter into the base of the brain, corresponding to lenticulostriate and thalamoperforate arteries.

In microscopic observations, these perforating arteries in the brain parenchyma show various histologic changes. According to the morphometric analysis performed by Yamashita and colleagues,[39] the perforating arteries within the basal ganglia, thalamus, and internal capsule in patients with moyamoya disease can be divided into the following two groups: (1) a dilated artery with a relatively thin wall and (2) a thick-walled artery showing luminal stenosis. Dilatation of the arteries is more prominent in young patients than in adults. The majority of dilated arteries show fibrosis and marked attenuation of the media with occasional segmentation of the elastic lamina. With hemodynamic stress or aging, the dilated arteries with attenuated walls may predispose to focal protrusion (microaneurysm formation) of the arterial wall, and its rupture is considered one of the mechanisms leading to parenchymatous hemorrhage in patients with moyamoya disease (Fig. 35-6). The involvement by fibrinoid necrosis of the perforating arteries in the process of aneurysm formation has been shown in hypertensive parenchymatous hemorrhage but has never been confirmed pathologically in patients with moyamoya disease.

In contrast, the stenotic vessels are less common in young patients.[40] These vessels show concentric thickening of the intima with duplication of the elastic lamina and fibrosis of the tunica media (see Fig. 35-6). Partial dilatation with discontinuity of the elastic lamina and occluding thrombus formation with its organization and recanalization are occasionally found. The presence of these histologic changes in the perforating arteries indicates that the arterial obstructive changes in patients with moyamoya disease are not limited to the circle of Willis and their major branches.

Leptomeningeal Vessels

The leptomeningeal anastomoses among the three main cerebral arteries and transdural anastomoses from the external carotid arteries are commonly observed as an abnormal vascular network on cerebral angiograms in patients with moyamoya disease (so-called vault moyamoya).[4,14,43] Kono and associates[44] performed a histopathologic and morphometric study of the leptomeningeal vessels in autopsied brains with moyamoya disease and compared them with vessels from age-matched controls. These researchers clarified that such anastomoses are not newly formed vessels but merely dilated preexisting vessels in both arteries and veins. Attenuation or disruption of the internal elastic lamina is remarkable in patients with a short history of moyamoya disease, and fibrous intimal thickening is more prominent in patients with a longer history of the disease. These structural adaptations in the vascular walls of the leptomeningeal vessels suggest their participation in the collateral circulation at the cerebral cortical surfaces.

Aneurysm Formation

Intracranial aneurysms are frequently associated with moyamoya disease.[45-48] Such an association is far from coincidental because the frequency of aneurysms in patients with moyamoya disease is higher than in the general population. Intracranial aneurysms are of two types: major artery aneurysms (MAAs) developing from the circle of Willis, and peripheral artery aneurysms (PAAs) located on the moyamoya vessels, choroidal arteries, or any other peripheral arteries serving as collaterals.[45] SAH is caused by rupture of MAAs, whereas parenchymatous hemorrhage or intraventricular hemorrhage is caused by the rupture of PAAs in some cases.

MAAs are commonly found in the arterial complex of the anterior communicating artery–anterior cerebral artery in patients with unilateral moyamoya (probable cases) and in

Figure 35-6 Microscopic appearance of the perforating arteries of patients with moyamoya disease at autopsy. A, The artery in the right caudate nucleus of a 60-year-old woman with parenchymatous hemorrhage shows marked dilatation with rupture (elastica van Gieson stain). B, Some of the arteries in the left thalamus of a 39-year-old woman show luminal stenosis due to fibrous and edematous intimal thickening (hematoxylin & eosin stain).

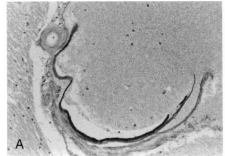
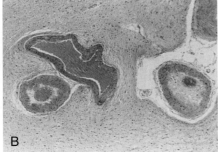

the basilar artery in patients with bilateral moyamoya (Fig. 35-7).[45] MAAs are fourfold higher in unilateral cases than in bilateral cases. Such anatomical distribution of MAAs could be explained if the aneurysms form as a result of increased blood flow through the relatively spared route of cerebral circulation as the stenotic process progresses. This increased blood flow exerts high pressure on the arterial wall, resulting in aneurysm formation in susceptible places such as branching sites. Histologically, the aneurysmal wall consists of endothelium with adventitial layers and a disappearance of internal elastic lamina and media, which is no different from the walls of saccular aneurysms commonly observed in SAH. Aneurysms formed by dissection of the intima from the media have also been reported in autopsy cases.[49,50]

PAAs are speculated to be responsible for parenchymatous hemorrhage. Two types of aneurysms are reported: saccular (true) aneurysms and pseudoaneurysms, consisting of fibrin and erythrocytes, that might be the result of rupture.[51] According to Herreman and coworkers,[45] the mean size of PAAs is half that of MAAs; PAAs may not be visualized angiographically in many cases. Thus, PAAs detected in angiography may represent only a subset of larger lesions. One third of angiographically visualized PAAs are reported to disappear spontaneously during the follow-up period; we have reported on the histology of a sclerosed PAA without rupture in an autopsy case[52] and suggested the pathologic processes by which the aneurysms disappear.

Extracranial Cervical Arteries and Systemic Arteries

The luminal stenosis due to fibrocellular intimal thickening has been described not only in intracranial arteries but also in extracranial arteries, including carotid arteries, renal arteries, pulmonary arteries, and coronary arteries,

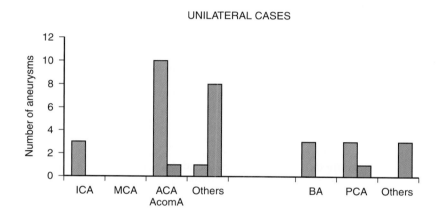

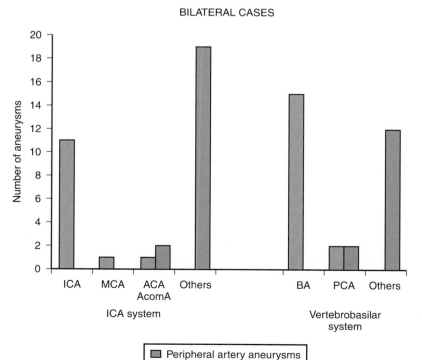

Figure 35-7 Locations of aneurysms in patients with moyamoya disease. ACA, anterior cerebral artery; AcomA, anterior communicating artery; BA, basilar artery; ICA, internal carotid artery; MCA, middle cerebral artery; PCA, posterior cerebral artery. (Data from Herreman F, Nathal E, Yasui N, et al: Intracranial aneurysm in moyamoya disease: Report of ten cases and review of the literature. *Cerebrovasc Dis* 4:329, 1994.)

in patients with moyamoya disease.[36,53] Yamashita and colleagues[54] reported the autopsy case of a 7-year-old Japanese girl with moyamoya disease associated with renovascular hypertension. The histologic study showed systemic involvement of concentric fibrocellular intimal thickening consisting of smooth muscle cells and elastic fibers in intracranial and extracranial carotid, coronary, and renal arteries; their histologic features were similar to those seen in fibromuscular dysplasia (FMD), intimal hyperplasia type. Several cases of renovascular hypertension associated with moyamoya disease have been reported in the literature,[55-57] many of which show the angiographic or pathologic appearance of FMD. Therefore, it is postulated that the systemic involvement of FMD or FMD-like vascular lesions is present in moyamoya disease, and hypertension may be a result of systemic involvement of the arterial lesions.

Ikeda measured the intimal thickness in various portions of the extracranial arteries of the autopsy cases with moyamoya disease and compared them with those in age- and sex-matched controls.[53] According to this study, the intimal thickening of the extracranial arteries is generally advanced in moyamoya disease compared with control cases, and mural thrombus formation and organization are also present in the extracranial arteries in moyamoya disease. Therefore, the intracranial lesion of moyamoya disease might be one of the manifestations of systemic illness, but no pathognomonic changes suggest any specific disease or etiologic factors of the illness; thus, the implications of these systemic changes are uncertain at present.

Etiology and Pathogenesis

There has been serious and continuing debate about whether moyamoya disease is acquired or congenital, and none of the proposed hypotheses for the pathogenesis of this disease has received general agreement.[3,4,6] Therefore, the cause remains unknown at present. Nevertheless, moyamoya disease is established as a clinical disease entity, and extensive clinical and pathologic studies have been conducted. As a result of this research, the following features are now generally accepted:

1. The progression of stenosis or occlusion of the circle of Willis and the major branches, including distal ends of the internal carotid arteries, is the primary finding in the disease.
2. An abnormal vascular network (moyamoya vessels) at the base of the brain consists of collateral vessels that have formed secondary to brain ischemia.
3. Clinical symptoms and signs are the manifestations of cerebrovascular events secondary to the previously described vascular lesions, including intracranial hemorrhage, infarct, and transient ischemic attacks (TIAs).
4. The major cellular components of the thickened intima formed in arteries of the circle of Willis and the major branches are smooth muscle cells. Migration and proliferation of smooth muscle cells in the intima, induced by unknown mechanisms, may lead to the intimal thickening in association with morphologic and biochemical alteration of extracellular matrix components including elastin, collagen, and other proteoglycans.

By contrast, the mechanisms responsible for inducing smooth muscle cell proliferation and migration in the arterial intima of patients with the disease are not yet identified. Furthermore, the reason that intimal thickening occurs in only limited arteries such as the circle of Willis is unknown. As previously mentioned, hereditary factors have long been suggested to play an important role in the etiology of moyamoya disease, as indicated by the high incidence among Japanese people,[16] occasional familial occurrence,[23] and association with some phenotypes of human leukocyte antigen (HLA)[58] or other congenital diseases, such as sickle cell anemia,[59] von Recklinghausen's disease,[60,61] and Down syndrome.[62,63] From results of a genetic study of patients in families with moyamoya disease, Fukuyama and associates[64,65] suggested a multifactorial mode of inheritance for the condition. Therefore, genetic linkage analysis of the pedigrees of patients with moyamoya disease of familial occurrence has been performed in several institutions and has demonstrated significant results. Inoue and coworkers[66,67] demonstrated a possible linkage between moyamoya disease and a region on chromosome 6 where the HLA gene is located. Ikeda and colleagues[68] performed the total genome search and found the possible linkage of markers located on chromosome 3p24.2-p26 in 16 families with moyamoya disease of familial occurrence. Yamauchi and associates,[69] performing a linkage analysis focused on chromosome 17, showed a possible linkage of chromosome 17q25 to familial moyamoya disease. Recently, chromosome 8q23 has been also suggested to have possible linkage to familial moyamoya disease.[70]

The extensive investigation focusing on the genes contained in or close to the candidate regions just described may yield clues for possible hypothesis explaining the pathogenesis of moyamoya disease.

Although hereditary factors may be involved in susceptibility to moyamoya disease, the majority of cases of the disease are sporadic, and the clinical manifestations and disease progression are not congenital. Through the accumulation of patient registrations and analysis of clinical data, acquired factors have been suggested in the occurrence and progression of moyamoya disease. Many hypotheses have been proposed; these include vasculitis with or without autoimmune mechanism,[13,14,71] infection (virus,[72] anaerobic bacteria such as *Propionibacterium acnes*[73]), thrombosis,[35,36,42] juvenile atherosclerosis,[35,36] cranial trauma,[74] abnormalities of sympathetic nerve endings,[69] and the postirradiation state.[75,76]

As noted in the discussion of pathology, microthrombi are frequently formed in the vasculature of patients with moyamoya disease.[35,36,38,42] Microthrombus appears to contribute to pathogenesis of the fibrocellular intimal thickening through its organization; this hypothesis explains the lamellated structure of the thickened intima of the lesions. If endothelial injury really occurs as the initiation of lesion formation, it is feasible to speculate that smooth muscle cell migration and proliferation in the intima are induced after injury. There has been substantial evidence that endothelial injury provokes phenotypic modulation and proliferation of smooth muscle cells and leads to neointima formation, not only in experimental animals[77-80] but also in patients with angioplasty restenosis.[80,81] In moyamoya disease, however, it is unclear to what extent this process is responsible for lesion formation. Furthermore, microthrombus is a nonspecific finding and reveals none of any specific etiologic factors in the endothelial injury.

None of the factors leading to endothelial injury has been identified in moyamoya disease. Ikeda and associates[82] detected loss of the endothelium covering the thickened intima in patients with moyamoya through the use of functional markers (thrombomodulin and von Willebrand factor). In relation to the hypotheses for the mechanisms of arterial injury, prothrombotic abnormalities, including inherited protein S deficiency and antiphospholipid antibodies, have been reported in some patients with moyamoya disease,[83,84] and chronic arteritis due to immunologic reactions may be implicated.[24,85] With cell type–specific immunohistochemistry, we previously demonstrated the presence of macrophages and T cells in the lesions, especially in the superficial layer of the thickened intima.[38] Such inflammatory cell infiltration observed in patients might, however, be a local reaction to microthrombi or a reflection of systemic inflammation or atherosclerotic changes unrelated to moyamoya disease. Therefore, it is not always easy to separate the histopathologic features of moyamoya disease from those of other pathologic changes, including atherosclerosis and various forms of arteritis.

In addition to the possible migration and proliferation of smooth muscle cells suggested in the genesis of intimal thickening and moyamoya vessel formation, many researchers have focused their attention on the growth factors and cytokines and their receptors, such as basic fibroblast growth factor (b-FGF),[86,87] platelet-derived growth factor (PDGF),[88] transforming growth factor-beta (TGF-β),[89] interleukin-1 (IL-1), prostaglandin E_2,[90] and hepatocyte growth factor (HGF).[91,92] Immunohistochemical staining[86,87] and measurements of these proteins in the cerebrospinal fluid[93,94] have been attempted in patients with moyamoya disease. These approaches may help introduce methods of molecular biology and vascular biology, which are now in rapid development in relation to the problem of angioplasty restenosis[79,81] and atherogenesis.[80] Genetic analysis and this work on candidate cytokines and their genes relevant to moyamoya disease may help identify the cause of the disorder.

Clinical Symptoms and Signs

Clinical symptoms and signs manifest as a result of the cerebrovascular events that occur in relation to pathologic changes in cerebral arteries in patients with moyamoya disease. Initial symptoms occur abruptly as attacks of cerebrovascular events including TIA, brain infarction, intracranial hemorrhage, and, occasionally, epileptic seizures. Some patients have shown no overt symptoms, and their disease was diagnosed from the angiography performed because of the familial occurrence of the disease.[19]

The MHWJ's Research Committee has defined four clinical types of moyamoya disease according to the initial symptoms and their frequencies in the registered patients accumulated until 1995,[95] as follows:

- Ischemic (63.4%)
- Hemorrhagic (21.6%)
- Epileptic (7.6%)
- Other (7.5%)

The ischemic type dominates in childhood moyamoya, representing 69% of cases in patients younger than 10 years; TIA occurs in 40% and infarction in 29% of patients manifesting a variety of symptoms, including motor paresis, disturbances of consciousness, speech disturbances, and sensory disturbances.[96] The course is sometimes repetitive and progressive and may result in cortical blindness, motor aphasia, or even a vegetative state within several years of onset. The ischemic symptoms (i.e., transient weakness and paresis) are provoked by some conditions involving hyperventilation, such as blowing to play wind instruments, blowing to cool something hot, and crying. They are considered to be induced by decreased cerebral blood flow (CBF) due to diminished Pa_{CO_2}. Ischemic deterioration is often precipitated by infection of the upper respiratory tract. Mental retardation and low IQ during the long follow-up are other important problems for children; this issue is further discussed in the section on disease progression and prognosis.

The hemorrhagic type is prevalent in adult patients, occurring in 66% of cases of the disease in adults, with a predominance of the hemorrhagic type in females.[96] Headache, disturbances of consciousness, and motor paresis are frequently encountered in the hemorrhagic type. Events triggering the bleeding are not identified, but hypertension and aging may be suggested as factors. Bleeding occurs often in multiple and repetitive intervals from several days to 10 years, and massive bleeding often leads to death.

Epilepsy was observed in about 5% of all patients, more than 80% of whom were children younger than 10 years.[96]

Laboratory Findings

Many groups have attempted to establish a diagnostic laboratory test for moyamoya disease, but none of the tests has proved successful. Some reports, however, showed fragments of data that provided valuable information concerning the etiology and pathogenesis of this disease. Infection by anaerobic bacteria such as *Propionibacterium acnes*,[73] cytomegalovirus, and Epstein-Barr virus,[72] for example, have been examined, with screening for specific antibodies and amplification of viral DNAs with polymerase chain reaction. The reported data suggest positive correlation with moyamoya disease.

Prothrombotic abnormalities have been reported not only in patients with moyamoya disease but also in children with cerebrovascular diseases. Deficiency of protein S and protein C have been reported in some patients with moyamoya disease.[83] Anticardiolipin antibody, an autoantibody against phosphatidyl-glycerol, itself a component of cell membrane phospholipid, showed higher percentages in patients with moyamoya disease than in controls.[84,85] These data suggest a possible connection between autoimmune mechanisms and moyamoya disease, because this antibody has been suggested to play an important role in arterial thrombus formation in brain infarction.[85,97]

Clinical Examination
Angiography

The fundamental angiographic finding in moyamoya disease is bilateral stenosis or occlusion at the intracranial portion of the internal carotid arteries together with a retiform arteriolar network (moyamoya vessels) at the base of the brain (see Figs. 35-1A and 35-1B). The stenotic or occlusive changes often extend along the arteries of the circle of Willis and their main branches. The vertebrobasilar system, however, has rarely been reported to be involved in this disease.[6,13,14] Formation of leptomeningeal collateral vessels, especially from the branches of the posterior cerebral artery, is frequently noted. Also usually present are transdural anastomoses via the ophthalmic artery, external carotid artery, and vertebral artery.

Suzuki and associates[13,14] divided the progression of moyamoya disease into the following six stages on the basis of angiographic findings, as follows: (1) narrowing of the carotid forks, (2) initial appearance of moyamoya vessels, (3) intensification of moyamoya vessels, (4) minimization of moyamoya vessels, (5) reduction of moyamoya vessels, and (6) disappearance of moyamoya vessels with collateral circulation only from the external carotid arteries. Kitamura and associates[4] confirmed these chronologic changes of angiographic findings in their followup patients; that is, as the narrowing of the main arteries advances, the moyamoya vessels increase in number, and they are later reduced when transdural anastomoses develop as disease progresses.

As noted previously, aneurysm formation is commonly seen in patients with moyamoya disease.

Computed Tomography

The features of moyamoya disease on computed tomography (CT) scans vary according to the clinical type. The most striking finding on conventional CT scans is high-density areas (HDAs) in the basal ganglia and thalamus, ventricular system, and subarachnoid spaces of the patients with the hemorrhagic type.[17,98] The HDAs resemble the topography of the hematoma in the internal type of hypertensive intracerebral hemorrhage.

In the ischemic type, CT scans reveal low-density areas (LDAs), which are relatively small and are usually confined to the cerebral cortex and subcortex, along with dilatation of cortical sulci and ventricles. Lacunar infarctions located in the basal ganglia and thalamus are sometimes seen in adults but are rare in children with the disease. Up to 40% of patients with the ischemic type, however, have no abnormalities on a conventional CT scan. Use of a contrast agent often visualizes tortuous and curvilinear vessels in the basal ganglia, which represent moyamoya vessels. The most proximal segments of the anterior and middle cerebral arteries are often poorly opacified.

Magnetic Resonance Imaging and Angiography

Because MRI and MRA are noninvasive techniques that can visualize various pathologic changes of the brain and the arterial tree, they have a big advantage over conventional angiography. MRI can demonstrate small subcortical lesions undetectable on CT. Brain infarctions in patients with moyamoya disease are usually small and located in the subcortex and are often multiple and bilateral. Brain atrophy and slight ventricular dilatation are also seen.[19-21,99] Stenotic or occlusive lesions at the distal ends of the internal carotid arteries can be demonstrated by MRA in most patients with this disease (see Figs. 35-1C and 35-1D). Apparent moyamoya vessels can be visualized as fine unusual vessels on MRA (see Figs. 35-1C and 35-1D) and also as a signal void on the MRI (Fig. 35-8), particularly in children. Small moyamoya vessels, however, are poorly visualized on both MRI and MRA, particularly in adults.

As described in the guideline for diagnosis of moyamoya disease, the MHWJ's Research Committee has concluded that this disease can be diagnosed without conventional angiography if MRI and MRA visualize the previously described findings bilaterally. To meet this agreement, the guideline was revised in 1995, and the diagnostic criteria on MRI and MRA were supplemented as shown in Table 35-2.[2] MRI and MRA have also shown to be useful imaging tools for postoperative assessment and

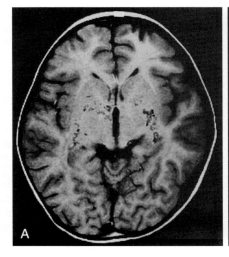
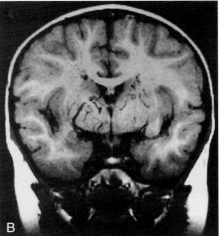

Figure 35-8 Typical MRI appearance of moyamoya vessels. A, Axial image reveals multiple signal voids in the basal ganglia. B, Coronal image shows well-developed basal moyamoya vessels in the bilateral basal ganglia. (From Houkin K, Aoki T, Takahashi A, et al: Diagnosis of moyamoya disease with magnetic resonance angiography. *Stroke* 25:2159, 1994.)

longitudinal follow-up of patients with moyamoya disease.[20,100,101] The prevention of rebleeding is important because the outcomes in patients with rebleeding were worse than in patients who did not rebleed (Fig. 35-9).[102] Kikuta et al investigated the incidence of asymptomatic microbleeds (MBs) in patients with moyamoya disease by using a 3-tesla magnetic resonance (MR) imaging unit. They found that the microbleeds were significantly more common in patients with moyamoya disease than in healthy individuals regardless of the disease type.[103] Future evaluation is necessary to elucidate whether microbleeds become a prediction factor of brain hemorrhage, and whether surgical revascularization prevents bleeding or not. The final results of the JAM trial are awaited.[104]

Ultrasonography

Because moyamoya disease is a type of systemic vascular disease, the extracranial internal and external carotid arteries, aorta, pulmonary artery, coronary artery, celiac trunk, and renal artery are reported to be involved, together with intracranial vessels.[18,105-107] Yang et al evaluated extracranial ICA by angiography in five patients with moyamoya disease and found stenotic lesion of the extracranial ICA in three (60%) of them.[106] The extracranial carotid artery is observed easily by conventional carotid ultrasonography, and its distal portion is also evaluated by transoral carotid ultrasonography (TOCU).[108-111] Takekawa et al performed carotid ultrasonography in a patient with moyamoya disease and found an increase in flow velocity at the external carotid artery functioning as a collateral pathway.[112] Yasaka et al investigated morphologic features of the extracranial ICA by conventional carotid ultrasonography and TOCU at 19 ICAs in 10 patients with moyamoya disease. He reported the presence of "champagne bottle neck sign" (diameter greatly reduced at the proximal portion of the ICA above the bulbus like a champagne bottle neck, so as to be less than half of that of the common carotid artery) in 14 ICAs (74%) and "diameter reversal sign" (diameter of the ICA is smaller than that of the external carotid artery) in 16 ICAs (84%) (Figs. 35-10 and 35-11).[113] They also demonstrated that the diameter of the extracranial distal ICA examined by TOCU in the same subjects was significantly smaller than that in the 28 ICAs of the 14 control subjects (2.4 ± 0.6 mm vs. 4.1 ± 0.5 mm, unpaired t-test, $P<0.0001$). The rapid internal diameter reduction at the proximal portion of the ICA, characterized by a "champagne bottle neck" or a "diameter reversal," seems an important morphologic feature of moyamoya disease and may be useful for early detection.[114]

Electroencephalography

Abnormal electroencephalographic (EEG) findings are more frequent in patients with childhood onset of the disease than in adults.[115] Such findings are related to permanent or transient ischemic changes due to a $Paco_2$ variation that is not specific for moyamoya disease.[4,6,14] Yoshii and Kudo summarized the EEG findings as follows: (1) diffuse and bilateral, abnormal, low-voltage or slow waves and spike waves, (2) "buildup" with the appearance of delta waves during hyperventilation, and (3) no effect on photic stimulation.[116]

Other Clinical Examinations

Because the symptoms of the ischemic type and epileptic type of moyamoya disease are caused by impairment of CBF due to arterial stenosis or occlusion, regional CBF and metabolic distribution have been measured by xenon inhalation and visualized with CT methods, including stable xenon-enhanced CT, dynamic CT, positron emission computed tomography (PET), and single-photon emission computed tomography (SPECT). Measurements of these physiologic and morphologic parameters have been useful for the follow-up of patients as well as evaluation of medical and surgical treatment and determination of prognosis.[117-123]

Disease Progression and Prognosis

In regard to disease progression and the prognosis for patients with moyamoya disease, there are remarkable differences between children and adults. In children, angiographic changes progress with time and sometimes rapidly,[124,125] and the formation of abnormal vascular networks at the base of the brain progresses from unilateral to bilateral during follow-up.[23,125,126] However, the prognosis for activities of daily life (ADLs) and life expectancy in children with moyamoya disease is generally fair, because irreversible ischemic and hemorrhagic complications are rarely encountered. More than 80% of such patients are in good health or in a state of independence, irrespective of treatment received. Nevertheless, many children are reported to be not well accommodated in social or school life because of poor intellectual ability, psychological impairment, and personality changes.[127-131] In general, the earlier the onset of the disease and the longer the period of suffering, the lower the mental function and quality of intelligence.

In adults, however, progression of angiographic changes is uncommon. Prognosis for ADLs and life expectancy, however, is poor because multiple and repetitive intracranial hemorrhages occur in many patients.

Treatment

The majority of patients with moyamoya (77%) have been treated surgically by any of the revascularization operations, whereas patients with mild or transient symptoms tend to be observed and given conservative treatment.[95] The surgical treatment is more effective than conservative treatment for the improvement in CBF, according to the physiologic parameters revealed by regional CBF measurement and PET studies, and is generally believed to have an advantage for a better prognosis.[1,117,132]

Medical Treatment

Vasodilators, antiplatelet agents, antifibrinolytic agents, and fibrinolytic agents are used in patients with moyamoya disease. Other medications, including anticonvulsants and steroids, are used in patients with the epileptic type and in patients with increased cranial pressure, respectively.[96,98]

Steroids are considered to be effective in certain cases, especially in patients with involuntary movements and during the active phase of recurrent ischemic or hemorrhagic attacks. This effect is presumed to be related to influences of steroids on edema, regional CBF, and vasculitis.

Antiplatelet agents, acetylsalicylic acid, and ticlopidine chloride may also be prescribed to prevent recurrence of ischemic attacks and thrombosis of the circle of Willis and the main branches, which is thought to play an important role in the progression of moyamoya disease. Other drugs, such as vasodilators, antifibrinolytics, and fibrinolytics, are occasionally used for similar purposes. The efficacy of these drugs in patients with moyamoya disease, however, has never been tested thoroughly in clinical trials.

Surgical Treatment

Surgical revascularizations are classified into the following three categories of surgical procedures: direct bypass surgery, indirect bypass surgery, and a combination of the two (Fig. 35-12).[1,133] Surgical revascularization has been performed to give additional collateral flow to the ischemic brain and thereby to improve regional CBF and prevent or minimize irreversible brain damage during follow-up. Also, collateral flow through the bypass is expected to have some effects in reducing hemodynamic stress on the moyamoya vessels and eventually to prevent the occurrence of hemorrhagic events. The evacuation of hematoma and ventricular drainage are performed in the acute stage of the hemorrhagic complication of moyamoya disease.

Superficial temporal artery–middle cerebral artery (STA-MCA) bypass is a direct revascularization surgery that was pioneered by Yasargil[134] and then applied to moyamoya disease by Karasawa and Kikuchi[135] and Reichmann and colleagues[136] independently. It is now generally accepted that this direct revascularization surgery seems to achieve a remarkable improvement in CBF and a better prognosis than conservative treatment.[117,137] This technique, however, requires skill in microvascular surgery, and it is not always possible to find a cortical branch suitable for anastomosis. Furthermore, careful intraoperative monitoring of blood pressure and $Paco_2$ is necessary; otherwise, there is a risk of perioperative ischemic complications.[118]

Indirect revascularizations are surgical procedures that aim to introduce external carotid flow into the internal carotid system via newly developed vascularization through the sutured tissues. Encephaloduroarteriosynangiosis (EDAS)[138] and encephalomyosynangiosis (EMS)[139] are the two representative procedures most commonly used in patients with moyamoya disease. Other operative methods, such as encephaloarteriosynangiosis (EAS), durapexy, and omentum transplantation,[140] also belong to this category. These operations can be performed in patients who do not have a cortical branch suitable for anastomoses, although revascularization is not always sufficient to give a collateral flow sufficient to prevent

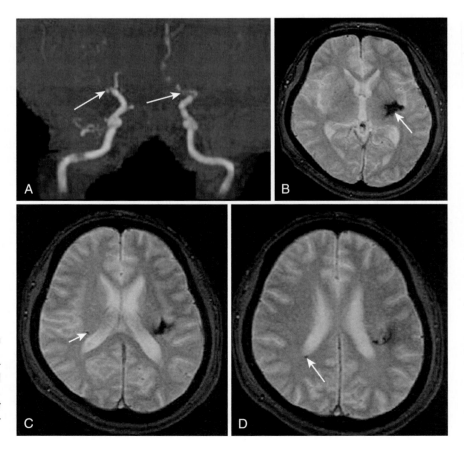

Figure 35-9 MR angiography and MRI in a 52-year-old patient with moyamoya disease. A, MR angiogram demonstrates occlusion or severe stenosis *(arrow)* at the bilateral distal portion of the internal carotid arteries. B to D, T2*-weighted MR images. B shows previous left putaminal hemorrhage *(arrow)*. C and D demonstrate multiple microbleeds *(arrows)*.

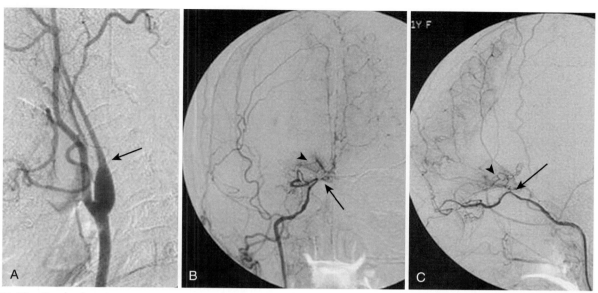

Figure 35-10 Cerebral angiograms in a patient with moyamoya disease. A, Reduction of the diameter of the internal carotid artery (ICA) at its proximal portion *(arrow)*. In the anteroposterior (B) and lateral (C) views, *arrows* indicate occlusion of the distal ICA, and *arrowheads* the vascular net at the basal brain. See also Fig. 35-11. (From Yasaka M, Ogata T, Yasumori K, et al: Bottle neck sign of the proximal portion of the internal carotid artery in moyamoya disease. *J Ultrasound Med* 25:1547-1552, 2006.)

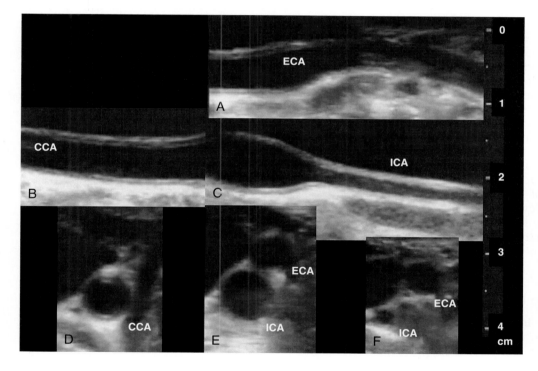

Figure 35-11 A to F, Conventional carotid ultrasonograms demonstrate signs of the "bottle neck" and "diameter reversal" in the same patient as shown in Fig. 35-10. CCA, common carotid artery; ECA, external carotid artery; ICA, internal carotid artery. (From Yasaka M, Ogata T, Yasumori K, et al: Bottle neck sign of the proximal portion of the internal carotid artery in moyamoya disease. *J Ultrasound Med* 25:1547-1552, 2006.)

ischemic symptoms. Therefore, the neurosurgeon often performs a *combination* of direct and indirect revascularization to obtain a better collateral flow.[137,141]

These surgical revascularizations are frequently performed in patients with the ischemic type of moyamoya disease (see Fig. 35-9), and the effect of surgery on improvement in regional CBF has been proved.[117,118,132,137,142] According to the follow-up study of registered patients who received surgery, surgical revascularization seems to be effective for the prevention of ischemic events and

for improvement in ADLs and intellectual activity, as long as the surgical procedure is chosen properly and performed successfully.[95,100,131,141] There is controversy as to whether the introduction of collateral flow by revascularization raises the risk of hemorrhagic events[1,143,144]; therefore, bypass surgery is not commonly performed in patients with the hemorrhagic type (see Fig. 35-9).[95,145] Rebleeding ratio has been reported to be lower in patients receiving bypass procedures, but the difference was not significant.[146,147] During the follow-up study after

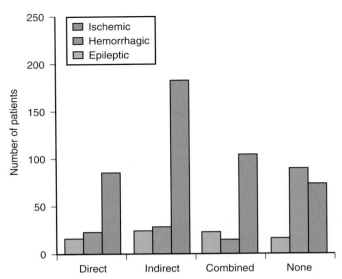

Figure 35-12 Selection of surgical revascularization procedure (x-axis) for patients with moyamoya disease according to type of initial attack. (Data from Fukui M, Kawano T: Follow-up study of registered cases in 1995. In Fukui M, editor: *Annual report [1995] by the Research Committee on Spontaneous Occlusion of the Circle of Willis [Moyamoya Disease]*. Ministry of Health and Welfare, Tokyo, 1996, p 12.)

surgery, however, moyamoya vessels actually diminished and often disappeared.[146] To evaluate the effect of bypass surgery on preventing recurrent bleeding, a prospective and randomized multicenter study, the Japan Adult Moyamoya (JAM) Trial, was initiated in January 2001.[148] This trial planned to register 160 patients from 23 hospitals in Japan and to allocate them randomly into two groups, direct bypass operation and nonoperation groups. Follow-up period was 5 years, and endpoints were recurrent brain hemorrhage, mortality, and morbidity.[104] The registration has been finished, and follow-up is ongoing.

The long-term effects of revascularization surgery on prognosis, including prevention of relapse of the hemorrhagic events and the improvement in ADLs and intelligence, have never been evaluated accurately, and the natural course of patients with moyamoya disease remains to be clarified.

Conclusion and Future Directions

As a result of the extensive investigation since the first report of this disease in 1957, moyamoya disease is now recognized as a true disease entity all over the world. Angiographic findings and pathophysiologic features of the disorder are well characterized, and the guidelines for diagnosis are also established, including the use of MRI and MRA.[2] Data concerning the epidemiology of the disease as well as the long-term effects of medical and surgical treatment on prognosis have been accumulating and need to be analyzed carefully and accurately.

In regard to the etiology and pathogenesis of this disease, great advances have been achieved, and such data are expected to provide important clues to solve the genesis of this mysterious disorder. Newer techniques, including molecular genetics, cell biology, and experimental

pathology, should be applied vigorously. The establishment of an experimental animal model of this disease will be extremely valuable.

REFERENCES

1. Fukui M: Current state of study on moyamoya disease in Japan, *Surg Neurol* 47:138, 1997.
2. Fukui M: Guidelines for the diagnosis and treatment of spontaneous occlusion of the circle of Willis ("moyamoya" disease). Research Committee on Spontaneous Occlusion of the Circle of Willis (Moyamoya Disease) of the Ministry of Health and Welfare, Japan, *Clin Neurol Neurosurg* 99(Suppl 2):S238, 1997.
3. Fukui M, Kono S, Sueishi K, et al: Moyamoya disease, *Neuropathology* 20(Suppl):S61, 2000.
4. Kitamura K, Fukui M, Oka K, et al: Moyamoya disease. In Toole JF, editor: *Handbook of clinical neurology*, Vol 11, Vascular diseases, Part III, Amsterdam, 1989, Elsevier, p p 293.
5. Masuda J, Ogata J, Yamaguchi T: Moyamoya disease. In Barnett HJM, Mohr JP, Stein BM, Yatsu FM, editors: *Stroke: Pathophysiology, diagnosis, and management*, ed 3, New York, 1998, Churchill Livingstone, p 815.
6. Yonekawa Y, Goto Y, Ogata N: Moyamoya disease: Diagnosis, treatment, and recent achievement. In Barnett HJM, Mohr JP, Stein BM, Yatsu FM, editors: *Stroke: Pathophysiology, diagnosis, and management*, ed 2, New York, 1992, Churchill Livingstone, p 721.
7. Takeuchi K, Shimizu K: Hypoplasia of the bilateral internal carotid arteries, *No To Shinkei* 9:37, 1957.
8. Sano K: Cerebral juxta-basal telangiectasia, *No To Shinkei* 17:748, 1965.
9. Handa H, Tani K, Kajikawa H, et al: Clinicopathological study on an adult case with cerebral arterial rete, *No To Shinkei* 21:181, 1969.
10. Weidner W, Hanafee W, Markham C: Intracranial collateral circulation via leptomeningeal and rete mirabile anastomosis, *Neurology* 15:39, 1965.
11. Nishimoto A, Takeuchi S: Abnormal cerebrovascular network related to the internal carotid arteries, *J Neurosurg* 29:255, 1968.
12. Kudo T: Spontaneous occlusion of the circle of Willis: A disease apparently confined to Japanese, *Neurology* 18:485, 1968.
13. Suzuki J, Takaku A: Cerebrovascular "moyamoya disease": A disease showing abnormal net-like vessels in base of brain, *Arch Neurol* 20:288, 1969.
14. Suzuki J, Kodama N: Moyamoya disease: A review, *Stroke* 14:104, 1983.
15. Ikezaki K, Han DH, Kawano T, et al: A clinical comparison of definite moyamoya disease between South Korea and Japan, *Stroke* 28:2513, 1997.
16. Goto Y, Yonekawa Y: Worldwide distribution of moyamoya disease, *Neurol Med Chir (Tokyo)* 32:883, 1992.
17. Yonekawa Y, Ogata N, Kaku Y, et al: Moyamoya disease in Europe, past and present status, *Clin Neurol Neurosurg* 99(Suppl 2):S58, 1997.
18. Masuda J, Ogata J, Yamaguchi T: Moyamoya Disease. In Mohr JP, Choi DW, Grotta JC, Weir B, Wolf PA, editors: *Stroke, Pathophysiology, diagnosis, and management*, ed 4, Philadelphia, 2004, Churchill Livingstone, pp 603–618.
19. Fukui M, Mizoguchi M, Matsushima T, et al: MR angiography in the families of moyamoya patients. In Fukui M, editor: *Annual report (1994) by research committee of spontaneous occlusion of the circle of Willis (moyamoya disease)*, Tokyo, 1995, Ministry of Health and Welfare, p 102.
20. Hasuo K, Mihara F, Matsushima T: MRI and MR angiography in moyamoya disease, *J Magn Reson Imaging* 8:762, 1998.
21. Houkin K, Aoki T, Takahashi A, et al: Diagnosis of moyamoya disease with magnetic resonance angiography, *Stroke* 25:2159, 1994.
22. Wakai K, Tamakoshi A, Ikezaki K, et al: Epidemiological features of moyamoya disease in Japan: Findings from a nationwide survey, *Clin Neurol Neurosurg* 99(Suppl 2):S1, 1997.
23. Kitahara T, Ariga N, Yamamura A, et al: Familial occurrence of moyamoya disease: Report of three Japanese families, *J Neurol Neurosurg Psychiatry* 42:208, 1979.
24. Kitahara T, Okumura K, Semba T, et al: Genetic and immunologic analysis of moyamoya disease, *J Neurol Neurosurg Psychiatry* 45:1048, 1982.

25. Yamada H, Nakamura S, Kageyama N: Moyamoya disease in mon-ovular twins: Case report, *J Neurosurg* 53:109, 1980.

26. Taveras JM: Multiple progressive intracranial arterial occlusion: A syndrome of children and young adults, *AJR Am J Roentgenol* 106:235, 1969.

27. Chiu D, Sheden P, Bratina P, et al: Clinical features of moyamoya disease in the United States, *Stroke* 29:1347, 1998.

28. Choi KS: Moyamoya disease in Korea: A cooperative study. In Suzuki J, editor: *Advances in surgery for cerebral stroke*, Tokyo, 1988, Springer-Verlag, p 107.

29. Han DH, Kwon OK, Byun BJ, et al: A co-operative study: Clinical characteristics of 334 Korean patients with moyamoya disease treated at neurosurgical institutes (1976-1994). The Korean Society for Cerebrovascular Disease, *Acta Neurochir (Wien)* 142:1263, 2000.

30. Hung CC, Tu YK, Su CF, et al: Epidemiological study of moyamoya disease in Taiwan, *Clin Neurol Neurosurg* 99(Suppl 2):S23, 1997.

31. Matsushima Y, Qian L, Aoyagi M: Comparison of moyamoya disease in Japan and moyamoya disease (or syndrome) in the People's Republic of China, *Clin Neurol Neurosurg* 99(Suppl 2):S19, 1997.

32. Ikezaki K, Han DH, Kawano T, et al: Epidemiological survey of moyamoya disease in Korea, *Clin Neurol Neurosurg* 99(Suppl 2):S6, 1997.

33. Hanakita J, Kondo A, Ishikawa J, et al: An autopsy case of moyamoya disease, *Neurol Surg* 10:531, 1982.

34. Hirayama A, Kowada M, Fukasawa H, et al: Cerebrovascular moyamoya disease: A case report and review of 12 autopsy cases in Japan, *No To Shinkei* 26:1215, 1974.

35. Hosoda Y, Ikeda E, Hirose S: Histopathological studies on spontaneous occlusion of the circle of Willis (cerebrovascular moyamoya disease), *Clin Neurol Neurosurg* 99(Suppl 2):S203, 1997.

36. Hosoda Y: Pathology of so-called "spontaneous occlusion of the circle of Willis," *Pathol Annu* 19:221, 1984.

37. Maki Y, Nakata Y: Autopsy of a case with an anomalous hemangioma of the internal carotid artery at the skull base, *No To Shinkei* 17:764, 1965.

38. Masuda J, Ogata J, Yutani C: Smooth muscle cell proliferation and localization of macrophages and T-cell in the occlusive intracranial major arteries in moyamoya disease, *Stroke* 24:1993, 1960.

39. Oka K, Yamashita M, Sadoshima S, et al: Cerebral hemorrhage in moyamoya disease at autopsy, *Virchows Arch* 392:247, 1981.

40. Yamashita M, Oka K, Tanaka K: Histopathology of the brain vascular network in moyamoya disease, *Stroke* 14:50, 1983.

41. Masuda J, Yutani C, Ogata J, et al: Atheromatous embolism in the brain: A clinicopathologic analysis of 15 autopsy cases, *Neurology* 44:1231, 1994.

42. Yamashita M, Oka K, Tanaka K: Cervico-cephalic arterial thrombi and thromboemboli in moyamoya disease: Possible correlation with progressive intimal thickening in the intracranial major arteries, *Stroke* 15:264, 1984.

43. Kodama N, Fujiwara S, Horie Y, et al: Transdural anastomosis in moyamoya disease: Vault moyamoya, *No Shinkei Geka* 8:729, 1980.

44. Kono S, Oka K, Sueishi K: Histopathologic and morphometric studies of leptomeningeal vessels in moyamoya disease, *Stroke* 21:1044, 1990.

45. Herreman F, Nathal E, Yasui N, et al: Intracranial aneurysm in moyamoya disease: Report of ten cases and review of the literature, *Cerebrovasc Dis* 4:329, 1994.

46. Kodama N, Suzuki J: Moyamoya disease associated with aneurysm, *J Neurosurg* 48:565, 1978.

47. Konishi Y, Kadowaki C, Hara M, et al: Aneurysms associated with moyamoya disease, *Neurosurgery* 16:484, 1985.

48. Nagamine Y, Takahashi S, Sonobe M: Multiple intracranial aneurysms associated with moyamoya disease: Case report, *J Neurosurg* 54:673, 1981.

49. Pilz P, Hartjes HJ: Fibromuscular dysplasia and multiple dissecting aneurysms of intracranial arteries. A further cause of moyamoya syndrome, *Stroke* 7:393, 1976.

50. Yamashita M, Tanaka K, Matsuo T, et al: Cerebral dissecting aneurysms in patients with moyamoya disease: Report of two cases, *J Neurosurg* 58:120, 1983.

51. Yuasa H, Tokito S, Izumi K, et al: Cerebrovascular moyamoya disease associated with an intracranial pseudoaneurysm: Case report, *J Neurosurg* 56:131, 1982.

52. Ogata J, Masuda J, Nishikawa M, et al: Sclerosed peripheral-artery aneurysm in moyamoya disease, *Cerebrovasc Dis* 6:248, 1996.

53. Ikeda E: Systemic vascular changes in spontaneous occlusion of the circle of Willis, *Stroke* 22:1358, 1991.

54. Yamashita M, Tanaka K, Kishikawa T, et al: Moyamoya disease associated with renovascular hypertension, *Hum Pathol* 15:191, 1984.

55. Godin M, Helias A, Tadie M, et al: Moyamoya syndrome and renal artery stenosis, *Kidney Int* 15:450, 1978.

56. Goldberg HJ: Moyamoya associated with peripheral vascular occlusive disease, *Arch Dis Child* 49:964, 1974.

57. Yamano T, Onouchi Z, Shimada M: Moyamoya disease and renal hypertension: A case probably caused by fibromuscular dysplasia, *Brain Dev* 6:184, 1974.

58. Aoyagi M, Ogami K, Matsushima Y, et al: Human leukocyte antigen in patients with moyamoya disease, *Stroke* 26:415, 1995.

59. Seeler RA, Royal JE, Powe L, et al: Moyamoya disease in children with sickle cell anemia and cerebrovascular occlusion, *J Pediatr* 93:808, 1978.

60. Erickson RP, Wooliscroft J, Allen RJ: Familial occurrence of intracranial arterial occlusive disease (moyamoya) in neurofibromatosis, *Clin Genet* 18:191, 1980.

61. Lamas E, Diez Lobato R, Cabello A, et al: Multiple intracranial arterial occlusions (moyamoya disease) in patients with neurofibromatosis: One case report with autopsy, *Acta Neurochir (Wien)* 45:133, 1978.

62. Mito T, Becker LE: Vascular dysplasia in Down syndrome: A possible relationship to moyamoya disease, *Brain Dev* 14:248, 1992.

63. Nagasaka T, Shiozawa Z, Kobayashi M, et al: Autopsy findings in Down's syndrome with cerebrovascular disorder, *Clin Neuropathol* 15:145, 1996.

64. Fukuyama Y, Kanai N, Osawa M: Clinical genetic analysis on moyamoya disease. In Yonekawa Y, editor: *Annual report (1991) by research committee on spontaneous occlusion of the circle of Willis*, Tokyo, 1992, Ministry of Health and Welfare, p 141.

65. Fukuyama Y, Sugahara N, Osawa M: A genetic study of idiopathic spontaneous multiple occlusion of the circle of Willis. In Yonekawa Y, editor: *Annual Report (1990) by research committee on spontaneous occlusion of the circle of Willis*, Tokyo, 1991, Ministry of Health and Welfare, p 139.

66. Inoue TK, Ikezaki K, Sasazuki T, et al: DNA typing of HLA in the patients with moyamoya disease, *Jpn J Hum Genet* 42:507, 1997.

67. Inoue TK, Ikezaki K, Sasazuki T, et al: Linkage analysis of moyamoya disease on chromosome 6, *J Child Neurol* 15:179, 2000.

68. Ikeda H, Sasaki T, Yoshimoto T, et al: Mapping of a familial moyamoya disease gene to chromosome 3p24.2-p26, *Am J Hum Genet* 64:533, 1999.

69. Yamauchi T, Tada M, Houkin K, et al: Linkage of familial moyamoya disease (spontaneous occlusion of the circle of Willis) to chromosome 17q25, *Stroke* 31:930, 2000.

70. Sakurai K, Horiuchi Y, Ikeda H, et al: A novel susceptibility locus for moyamoya disease on chromosome 8q23, *J Hum Genet* 49:278-281, 2004.

71. Kasai N, Fujiwara S, Kodama N, et al: The experimental study on causal genesis of moyamoya disease: Correlation with immunological reaction and sympathetic nerve influence for vascular changes, *No Shinkei Geka* 10:251, 1982.

72. Tanigawara T, Yamada H, Sasaki N, et al: Studies on cytomegalovirus and Epstein-Barr virus infection in moyamoya disease, *Clin Neurol Neurosurg* 99(Suppl 2):S225, 1997.

73. Yamada H, Deguchi K, Tanigawa T, et al: The relationship between moyamoya disease and bacterial infection, *Clin Neurol Neurosurg* 99(Suppl 2):S221, 1997.

74. Fernandes-Alvares E, Pineda M, Royo C, et al: Moyamoya disease caused by cranial trauma, *Brain Dev* 1:133, 1979.

75. Bitzer M, Topka H: Progressive cerebral occlusive disease after radiation therapy, *Stroke* 26:131, 1995.

76. Rajakulasingam K, Cerullo LJ, Raimondi AJ: Childhood moyamoya syndrome: Postradiation pathogenesis, *Childs Brain* 5:469, 1979.

77. Bai H-Z, Masuda J, Sawa Y, et al: Neointima formation after vascular stent implantation: Spatial and chronological distribution of smooth muscle cell proliferation and phenotypic modulation, *Arterioscler Thromb* 14:1994, 1846.

78. Masuda J, Tanaka K: A new model of cerebral arteriosclerosis induced by intimal injury using a silicone rubber cylinder in rabbits, *Lab Invest* 51:475, 1984.

79. Reidy MA, Fingerle J, Lindner V: Factors controlling the development of arterial lesions after injury, *Circulation* 86(Suppl III):1992, 1845.

80. Ross R: The pathogenesis of atherosclerosis: A perspective for the 1990s, *Nature* 362:801, 1993.

81. Casscells W: Migration of smooth muscle and endothelial cells: Critical events in restenosis, *Circulation* 86:723, 1992.

82. Ikeda E, Maruyama I, Hosoda Y: Expression of thrombomodulin in patients with spontaneous occlusion of the circle of Willis, *Stroke* 24:657, 1993.

83. Bonduel M, Hepner M, Sciuccati G, et al: Prothrombotic disorders in children with moyamoya syndrome, *Stroke* 32:1786, 2001.

84. Takanashi J, Sugita K, Miyazato S, et al: Antiphospholipid antibody syndrome in childhood strokes, *Pediatr Neurol* 13:323, 1995.

85. Hughes GRV: The antiphospholipid syndrome: Ten years on, *Lancet* 342:341, 1993.

86. Hoshimaru M, Takahashi JA, Kikuchi H, et al: Possible roles of basic fibroblast growth factor in the pathogenesis of moyamoya disease: An immunohistochemical study, *J Neurosurg* 75:267, 1991.

87. Suzui H, Hoshimaru M, Takahashi JA, et al: Immunohistochemical reactions for fibroblast growth factor receptor in arteries of patients with moyamoya disease, *Neurosurgery* 35:20, 1994.

88. Aoyagi M, Fukui N, Sakamoto H, et al: Altered cellular responses to serum mitogens, including platelet-derived growth factor, in cultured smooth muscle cells derived from arteries of patients with moyamoya disease, *J Cell Physiol* 147:191, 1991.

89. Hojo M, Hoshimaru M, Miyamoto S, et al: Role of transforming growth-β1 in the pathogenesis of moyamoya disease, *J Neurosurg* 89:623, 1998.

90. Yamamoto M, Aoyagi M, Fukai N, et al: Increase in prostaglandin E(2) production by interleukin-1β in arterial smooth muscle cells derived from patients with moyamoya disease, *Circ Res* 85:912, 1999.

91. Nanba R, Kuroda S, Ishikawa T, et al: Increased expression of hepatocyte growth factor in cerebrospinal fluid and intracranial artery in moyamoya disease, *Stroke* 35:2837-2842, 2004.

92. Kusaka N, Sugiu K, Tokunaga K, et al: Enhanced brain angiogenesis in chronic cerebral hypoperfusion after administration of plasmid human vascular endothelial growth factor in combination with indirect vasoreconstructive surgery, *J Neurosurg* 103:882-890, 2005.

93. Takahashi A, Sawamura Y, Houkin K, et al: The cerebrovascular fluid in patients in moyamoya disease contains a high level of basic fibroblast growth factor, *Neurosci Lett* 160:214, 1993.

94. Yoshimoto T, Houkin K, Takahashi A, et al: Angiogenic factors in moyamoya disease, *Stroke* 27:2160, 1996.

95. Fukui M, Kawano T: Follow-up study of registered cases in 1995. In Fukui M, editor: *Annual report (1995) by research committee on spontaneous occlusion of the circle of Willis (moyamoya disease)*, Tokyo, Japan, 1996, Ministry of Health and Welfare, p 12.

96. Handa H, Yonekawa Y, Goto Y, et al: Analysis of the filing data bank of 1500 cases of spontaneous occlusion of the circle of Willis and follow-up study of 200 cases for more than 5 years. In Handa H, editor: *Annual report (1984) by research committee on spontaneous occlusion of the circle of Willis*, Tokyo, Japan, 1985, Ministry of Health and Welfare, p 14.

97. Levine SR, Welch KMA: Cerebrovascular ischemia associated with lupus anticoagulant, *Stroke* 18:257, 1987.

98. Yamaguchi T, Tashiro M, Hasegawa Y: Collective analysis of the patients with spontaneous occlusion of the circle of Willis in Japan, registered from 1977 to 1982. In Gotoh F, editor: *Annual report (1982) by research committee on spontaneous occlusion of the circle of Willis (moyamoya disease)*, Tokyo, Japan, 1983, Ministry of Health and Welfare, p 15.

99. Yamada I, Suzuki S, Matsushima Y: Moyamoya disease: Comparison with MR angiography and MR imaging versus conventional angiography, *Radiology* 196:221, 1995.

100. Houkin K, Kuroda S, Nakayama N: Cerebral revascularization for moyamoya disease in children, *Neurosurg Clin N Am* 12:575, 2001.

101. Yamada I, Nakagawa T, Matsushima Y, et al: High-resolution turbo magnetic resonance angiography for diagnosis of moyamoya disease, *Stroke* 32:2001, 1825.

102. Morioka M, Hamada J, Todaka T, et al: High-risk age for rebleeding in patients with hemorrhagic moyamoya disease: long-term follow-up study, *Neurosurgery* 52:1049-1054, 2003.

103. Kikuta K, Takagi Y, Nozaki K, et al: Asymptomatic microbleeds in moyamoya disease: T2*-weighted gradient-echo magnetic resonance imaging study, *J Neurosurg* 102:470-475, 2005.

104. Miyamoto S: Ischemic cerebrovascular disease. Standardization of surgical treatment based on evidence. JAM (Japan Adult Moyamoya) trial group, *Jpn J Neurosurg* 15:326, 2006:(Abstract).

105. Kaczorowska M, Jozwiak S, Litwin M, et al: Moyamoya disease associated with stenosis of extracranial arteries: a case report and review of the literature, *Neurol Neurochir Pol* 39:242-246, 2005.

106. Yang SH, Li B, Wang CC, et al: Angiographic study of moyamoya disease and histological study in the external carotid artery system, *Clin Neurol Neurosurg* 99(Suppl 2):S61-S63, 1997.

107. Hoshimaru M, Kikuchi H: Involvement of the external carotid arteries in moyamoya disease: neuroradiological evaluation of 66 patients, *Neurosurgery* 31:398-400, 1992.

108. Yasaka M, Kimura K, Otsubo R, et al: Transoral carotid ultrasonography, *Stroke* 29:1383-1388, 1998.

109. Yakushiji Y, Yasaka M, Takada T, et al: Serial transoral carotid ultrasonographic findings in extracranial internal carotid artery dissection, *J Ultrasound Med* 24:877-880, 2005.

110. Kamouchi M, Kishikawa K, Okada Y, et al: Poststenotic flow and intracranial hemodynamics in patients with carotid stenosis: transoral carotid ultrasonography study, *AJNR Am J Neuroradiol* 26:76-81, 2005.

111. Kishikawa K, Kamouchi M, Okada Y, et al: Transoral carotid ultrasonography as a diagnostic aid in patients with severe carotid stenosis, *Cerebrovasc Dis* 17:106-110, 2004.

112. Takekawa H, Ebata A, Arai M, et al: Usefulness of carotid duplex ultrasonography in a patient with moyamoya disease, *No To Shinkei* 55:983-987, 2003.

113. Yasaka M, Ogata T, Yasumori K, Inoue T, Okada Y: Bottle Neck Sign of the Proximal Portion of the Internal Carotid Artery in Moyamoya Disease, *J Ultrasound Med* 25:1547-1552, 2006.

114. Yasuda C, Yakusiji Y, Eriguchi M, et al: Usefulness of carotid ultrasonography for the early detection of moyamoya disease, *Rinsho Shinkeigaku* 47:441-443, 2007.

115. Kodama N, Aoki Y, Hiraga H, et al: Electroencephalographic findings in children with moyamoya disease, *Arch Neurol* 36:16, 1979.

116. Yoshii N, Kudo T: Electroencephalographical study on occlusion of the Willis arterial ring, *Rinsho Shinkeigaku* 8:301, 1968.

117. Ikezaki K, Matsushima T, Kuwabara Y, et al: Cerebral circulation and oxygen metabolism in childhood moyamoya disease: A perioperative positron emission tomography study, *J Neurosurg* 81:843, 1994.

118. Iwama T, Hashimoto N, Yonekawa Y: The relevance of hemodynamic factors to perioperative ischemic complications in childhood moyamoya disease, *Neurosurgery* 38:1120, 1996.

119. Kuwabara Y, Ichiya Y, Otsuka M, et al: Cerebral hemodynamic changes in the child and adult with moyamoya disease, *Stroke* 21:272, 1990.

120. Kuwabara Y, Ichiya Y, Sasaki M, et al: Cerebral hemodynamics and metabolism in moyamoya disease-a positron emission tomography study, *Clin Neurol Neurosurg* 99(Suppl 2):S74, 1997.

121. Nariai T, Suzuki R, Hirakawa K, et al: Vascular reserve in chronic cerebral ischemia measured with acetazolamide challenge test: Comparison with positron emission tomography, *AJNR Am J Neuroradiol* 16:563, 1995.

122. Obara K, Fukuuchi Y, Kobari M, et al: Cerebral hemodynamics in patients with moyamoya disease and in patients with atherosclerotic occlusion of the major cerebral arterial trunks, *Clin Neurol Neurosurg* 99(Suppl 2):S86, 1997.

123. Taki W, Yonekawa Y, Kobayashi A, et al: Cerebral circulation and metabolism in adult's moyamoya disease-PET study, *Acta Neurochir (Wien)* 100:150, 1989.

124. Ezura M, Yoshimoto T, Fujiwara S, et al: Clinical and angiographic follow-up of childhood-onset moyamoya disease, *Childs Nerv Syst* 11:591, 1995.

125. Hirotsune N, Meguro T, Kawada S, et al: Long-term follow-up study of patients with unilateral moyamoya disease, *Clin Neurol Neurosurg* 99(Suppl 2):S178, 1997.

126. Kawano T, Fukui M, Hashimoto N, et al: Follow-up study of patients with "unilateral" moyamoya disease, *Neurol Med Chir (Tokyo)* 34:744, 1994.

127. Fukuyama Y, Mitsuishi Y, Umezu R: Intellectual prognosis of children with TIA type of spontaneous occlusion of the circle of Willis: With special reference to Wechsler's intelligence test and Benton's visual attention test. In Handa H, editor: *Annual report (1986) of research committee on spontaneous occlusion of the circle of Willis*, Tokyo, Japan, 1987, Ministry of Health and Welfare, p 43.

128. Imaizumi C, Imaizumi T, Osawa M, et al: Serial intelligence test scores in pediatric moyamoya disease, *Neuropediatrics* 30:294, 1999.

129. Imaizumi T, Hayashi K, Saito K, et al: Long-term outcomes of pediatric moyamoya disease monitored to adulthood, *Pediatr Neurol* 18:321, 1998.

130. Kurokawa T, Tomita S, Ueda K, et al: Prognosis of occlusive disease of circle of Willis (moyamoya disease) in children, *Pediatr Neurol* 12:288, 1969.

131. Matsushima Y, Aoyagi M, Nariai T, et al: Long-term intelligence outcome of post-encephalo-duro-arterio-synangiosis in childhood moyamoya patients, *Clin Neurol Neurosurg* 99(Suppl 2):S147, 1997.

132. Nakashima H, Meguro T, Kawada S, et al: Long-term results of surgically treated moyamoya disease, *Clin Neurol Neurosurg* 99(Suppl 2):S156, 1997.

133. Ueki K, Meyer JB: Moyamoya disease: The disorder and surgical treatment, *Mayo Clin Proc* 69:749, 1994.

134. Yasargil MG: *Microsurgery applied to neurosurgery*, Stuttgart, 1969, Thieme.

135. Karasawa J, Kikuchi H, Furuse S, et al: Treatment of moyamoya disease with STA-MCA anastomosis, *J Neurosurg* 49:679, 1978.

136. Reichmann O, Anderson RE, Roberts TC, et al: The treatment of intracranial occlusive cerebrovascular disease by STA-cortical MCA anastomosis. In Handa H, editor: *Microneurosurgery*, Tokyo, 1975, Igaku Shoin, p 31.

137. Matsushima T, Inoue T, Suzuki SO, et al: Surgical treatment of moyamoya disease in pediatric patients: Comparison between the results of indirect and direct revascularization procedures, *Neurosurgery* 31:401, 1992.

138. Matsushima Y, Inaba Y: Moyamoya disease in children and its surgical treatment: Introduction of a new surgical procedure and its follow-up angiograms, *Childs Brain* 11:155, 1984.

139. Karasawa J, Kikuchi H, Furuse S: A surgical treatment of moyamoya disease: Encephalomyosynangiosis, *Neurol Med Chir (Tokyo)* 17:29, 1977.

140. Karasawa J, Touhou H, Ohnishi H, et al: Cerebral revascularization using omental transplantation for childhood moyamoya disease, *J Neurosurg* 79:192, 1993.

141. Matsushima T, Inoue TK, Suzuki SO, et al: Surgical techniques and the results of a fronto-temporo-parietal combined indirect bypass procedure for children with moyamoya disease: A comparison with the results of encephalo-duro-arterio-synangiosis alone, *Clin Neurol Neurosurg* 99(Suppl 2):S123, 1997.

142. Shirane R, Yoshida Y, Takahashi T, et al: Assessment of encephalo-galeo-myo-synangiosis with dural pedicle insertion in childhood moyamoya disease: Characteristics of cerebral blood flow and oxygen metabolism, *Clin Neurol Neurosurg* 99(Suppl 2):S79, 1997.

143. Aoki N: Cerebrovascular bypass surgery for the treatment of moyamoya disease: Unsatisfactory outcome in the patients presenting with intracranial hemorrhage, *Surg Neurol* 40:372, 1993.

144. Srinivasan J, Britz GW, Newell DW: Cerebral revascularization for moyamoya disease in adults, *Neurosurg Clin N Am* 12:585, 2001.

145. Ikezaki K, Fukui M, Inamura T, et al: The current status of the treatment for hemorrhagic type moyamoya disease based on a 1995 nationwide survey in Japan, *Clin Neurol Neurosurg* 99(Suppl 2):S183, 1997.

146. Houkin K, Kamiyama H, Abe H, et al: Surgical therapy for adult moyamoya disease: Can surgical revascularization prevent the recurrence of intracerebral hemorrhage? *Stroke* 27:448, 1996.

147. Yoshida Y, Yoshimoto T, Shirane R, et al: Clinical course, surgical management, and long-term outcome of moyamoya patients with rebleeding after an episode of intracerebral hemorrhage: An extensive follow-up study, *Stroke* 30:2272, 1999.

148. Miyamoto S: Study on the management of moyamoya disease with hemorrhagic onset. In Yoshimoto T, editor: *Annual report (2000) by research committee on spontaneous occlusion of the circle of Willis*, Tokyo, Japan, 2001, Ministry of Health, Labor, and Welfare, p 61.

36 Migraine and Stroke

HANS C. DIENER, TOBIAS KURTH

Migraine is a chronic headache disorder with episodes of headache that are unilateral or bilateral in location, pulsating in quality, moderate to severe in intensity, and exacerbated by physical activity. Associated symptoms include nausea or vomiting, photophobia, and phonophobia. The prevalence of migraine is 12% to 18% in females and 6% to 8% in males.[1-4] The prevalence of migraine with aura (which includes familial hemiplegic migraine) is lower, around 4%, and about 25% of migraine patients have either migraine with aura or migraine both with and without aura.[5] Aura is a recurrent visual disorder manifesting in attacks of reversible focal neurologic symptoms that usually develops gradually over 5 to 20 minutes and lasts for less than 60 minutes. Various forms of migraine are recognized, generally classified according to the transient, though sometimes persistent, neurologic deficits that may precede, accompany, or outlast the headache phase. The most accepted current classification was published by the International Headache Society (IHS) in 2005 (Table 36-1).[6]

Migraine with aura of different types, retinal or ocular migraine, ophthalmoplegic migraine, familial hemiplegic migraine, and basilar artery migraine may mimic transient ischemic attack (TIA) or ischemic stroke may be associated with an increased stroke risk. Each may be transient, prolonged, or persistent.[7] When the aura symptoms of a migraine attack persist for more than 24 hours, *migraine-induced stroke* is suspected. The clinical features that often mimic stroke are described next.

Clinical Features

The most prevalent migraine syndromes include typical migraine headache without aura of neurologic deficit, and migraine headache associated with aura of neurologic deficit. Visual disturbances account for well over half the transient neurologic manifestations. Most frequently, these consist of positive phenomena such as stars, spark photopsia, complex geometric patterns, and fortification spectra. These positive phenomena may leave in their wake "negative" phenomena such as increasing scotoma and slowly developing hemianopia. The symptoms are characteristically slow in onset and slow in progression, although occasionally the onset is more abrupt, and a migraine headache may be confused with amaurosis fugax.[8] Visual symptoms sometimes progress to visual distortion or misperception, such as micropsia or dysmetropsia. The patterns of symptoms indicate the spread of neurologic dysfunction from the occipital cortex into the contiguous regions of the temporal or parietal lobes.[9-12] It is critical, in making the differential diagnosis from stroke, to establish that the neurologic deficit in aura crosses arterial territories. The second most common symptoms are somatosensory and characteristically hand and lower face (cheiro-oral) in distribution. Less frequently, the symptoms include aphasia, dysarthria, or clumsiness of one limb. Mostly, a slow, marchlike progression is characteristic.

Classification

The major problem that faces the clinician is a lack of consistency in the definition of migraine-related stroke in the studies conducted so far. Strict definition of terms is essential for future comprehensive epidemiologic or population-based studies. The following major questions arise:

- Does stroke occur in the course of the migraine attack, causing true migraine-induced cerebral infarction?
- Does migraine cause stroke because other risk factors for stroke are present to interact with the migraine-induced pathogenesis?
- Can stroke present as a migraine syndrome, that is, symptomatic migraine?

Some of the latest developments serve to clarify the association between migraine and stroke. The IHS classification has led to improved definitions of migraine and migraine-induced stroke in a more specific comprehensive manner.[13] New techniques of brain imaging have provided new insights into the relationship of the disorders through improvements in diagnosis.

Migrainous cerebral infarction (IHS 1.5.4) is described in the IHS classification as "one or more migrainous aura symptoms associated with an ischemic brain lesion in appropriate territory demonstrated by neuroimaging." Diagnostic criteria are as follows:

- The present attack in a patient with 1.2 *Migraine with aura* is typical of previous attacks except that one or more aura symptoms persists for more than 60 minutes.
- Neuroimaging demonstrates ischemic infarction in a relevant area.
- It is not attributed to another disorder.

Table 36-1 presents an extended classification of stroke in association with migraine or migraine-related stroke. Included in this classification is migrainous cerebral infarction.

TABLE 36-1   CLASSIFICATION OF MIGRAINE SUBTYPES

International Headache Society ICHD-II Code	World Health Organization ICD-10NA Code	Diagnosis (and Etiologic ICD-10 Code for Secondary Headache Disorders)
1.	[G43]	Migraine
1.1	[G43.0]	Migraine without aura
1.2	[G43.1]	Migraine with aura
1.2.1	[G43.10]	Typical aura with migraine headache
1.2.2	[G43.10]	Typical aura with nonmigraine headache
1.2.3	[G43.104]	Typical aura without headache
1.2.4	[G43.105]	Familial hemiplegic migraine
1.2.5	[G43.105]	Sporadic hemiplegic migraine
1.2.6	[G43.103]	Basilar-type migraine
1.3	[G43.82]	Childhood periodic syndromes that are commonly precursors of migraine
1.3.1	[G43.82]	Cyclical vomiting
1.3.2	[G43.820]	Abdominal migraine
1.3.3	[G43.821]	Benign paroxysmal vertigo of childhood
1.4	[G43.81]	Retinal migraine
1.5	[G43.3]	Complications of migraine
1.5.1	[G43.3]	Chronic migraine
1.5.2	[G43.2]	Status migrainosus
1.5.3	[G43.3]	Persistent aura without infarction
1.5.4	[G43.3]	Migrainous infarction
1.5.5	[G43.3] + [G40.x or G41.x]*	Migraine-triggered seizures
1.6	[G43.83]	Probable migraine
1.6.1	[G43.83]	Probable migraine without aura
1.6.2	[G43.83]	Probable migraine with aura
1.6.5	[G43.83]	Probable chronic migraine

*The additional code specifies the type of seizure.
ICD-10NA, *International Classification of Diseases, 10th revision: Neurological Adaptation;* ICHD-II, *International Classification of Headache Disorders,* 2nd ed.
Modified slightly from Headache Classification Subcommittee of the International Headache Society: The International Classification of Headache Disorders, 2nd edition. *Cephalalgia* 24(Suppl 1):1-160, 2004.

Migraine-Induced Stroke

Definition: See previous discussion.

The major problem with this definition is that the IHS classification does not permit the diagnosis of migraine-induced stroke in patients who have migraine without aura (see previous discussion). Perhaps, however, migraine without aura begins in "silent" brain areas and has the same pathogenesis as migraine with aura. This possibility is indicated by the blood flow measurements reported by Woods and colleagues,[9] who found a decrease of 30% to 40% in cerebral blood flow (CBF) in the occipital lobe in a woman during an episode of migraine without aura. Migraine-induced stroke might occur in patients without other vascular risk factors.

Coexisting Stroke and Migraine

Definition: A clearly defined clinical stroke syndrome must occur remotely in time from a typical attack of migraine.

Among young individuals, stroke is a rare event, whereas migraine is common. Clearly, the two conditions can coexist without migraine's being a contributive factor to stroke. When the two conditions coexist in the young, the true pathogenesis of stroke may be difficult to elucidate. A comorbidity of stroke risk in migraine sufferers

seems apparent from the case-control series reviewed later in this chapter, in which none of the strokes was directly induced by the migraine attack. This finding increases the clinical significance of coincident stroke and should serve to raise clinical consciousness of the need for stroke risk factor awareness in all migraine sufferers.

Stroke with Clinical Features of Migraine

Definition: A structural lesion unrelated to migraine pathogenesis that manifests as clinical features typical of migraine.

Symptomatic Cases

In symptomatic cases, established structural lesions of the central nervous system or cerebral vessels episodically cause symptoms typical of migraine with aura. Such cases should be termed "symptomatic migraine."[14] Cerebral arteriovenous malformations frequently masquerade as migraine with aura.[15] Migraine attacks associated with cerebral autosomal dominant arteriopathy with subcortical infarcts and leukoencephalopathy (CADASIL) also may be symptomatic of the membrane dysfunction associated with this disorder.[16-18] Subarachnoid hemorrhage, venous-sinus thrombosis, and viral meningitis can mimic migraine attacks with or without aura in patients who suffer from migraine or who have a family history of migraine.

Migraine Mimic

In this category, stroke due to acute and progressing structural disease is accompanied by headache and a constellation of progressive neurologic signs and symptoms indistinguishable from those of migraine. This might best be termed a migraine mimic.[19]

The diagnostic discrimination of a migraine mimic can be most difficult to define in patients with established migraine. Many of the cases described in the literature on the conceptual evolution of migraine-related stroke were likely migraine mimics, the diagnosis being hampered by limitation in investigative tools and uncertainty in the knowledge of migraine pathogenesis.

The issue of spontaneous carotid artery dissection is relevant because patients with migraine are at increased risk for dissections[20] and because the occurrence of a dissection as a typical migraine mimic has been reported.[21] Although the mechanism of pain production is not clearly understood, the occurrence of headache is an expected finding, present in 60% of patients[22] and greater in vertebral dissection, along with a variable incidence of ischemic complications, a combination that may mimic accompanied migraine. Fisher[23] analyzed 21 selected cases of angiographically documented cervical carotid dissection, observing that almost all patients (19 of 21) had ipsilateral pain in one or more regions of the head, including forehead, orbit, temple, retro-orbit, side of head, and frontal region. In addition, 12 patients had neck pain, usually in the upper neck and localized to a region including the mastoid, the upper carotid, behind or below the angle of the jaw, and along the sternocleidomastoid muscle. The pain was usually severe, often sudden in onset, described equally as steady or throbbing, and occasionally accompanied by alterations in ipsilateral scalp sensation. The duration ranged from several hours to 2 years, with most lasting no longer than 3 to 4 weeks. About three fourths of Fisher's patients experienced ischemic complications, and in half, the headache preceded the ischemic event by a few hours to 4 days. Other common diagnostic findings were Horner's syndrome, subjective bruit, dysgeusia, and visual scintillations.

Uncertain Classification

Complex or multiple factors: Many migraine-related strokes cannot be categorized with certainty.

Epidemiology

To date, many studies have evaluated the association between migraine and risk of stroke. The vast majority were retrospective studies,[24-35] followed by prospective studies,[36-41] a few cross-sectional studies,[42,43] and some studies using data from stroke registries.[44,45] Three retrospective case-control studies found increased risk of ischemic stroke among women younger than 45 years who reported a history of migraine with aura,[27,28,33] with risk estimates ranging from 3.8[28] to 8.4.[33] Two additional case-control studies found an increased risk for migraine sufferers with aura in both genders.[25,31] In only one case-control study, migraine without aura was associated with increased risk of ischemic stroke.[27] The association

between migraine and hemorrhagic stroke was evaluated in only one case-control study,[46] which found increased risk for those with a family history of migraine (odds ratio [OR] 2.30; 95% CI [CI], 1.35–3.90) and also suggested that there might be an increased risk among participants with migraine without aura (OR 1.84; 95% CI, 0.77–4.39). In another case-control study, the association between migraine and hemorrhagic stroke produced conflicting results, because the association was dependent on the control selection.[24] When the interaction between migraine and other risk factors for stroke was evaluated, the risk was more than tripled by smoking (OR 10)[27] and quadrupled by oral contraceptive use (ORs 14-17).[28,47] The combination of migraine, oral contraceptives, and smoking further increased the risk.

A meta-analysis of 11 case-control and three cohort studies published up to 2004 suggested that the risk of stroke is increased in individuals with migraine (pooled relative risk [RR] 2.16; 95% CI, 1.89–2.48). In this analysis, the risk was consistent among individuals who had migraine with aura (RR 2.27; 95% CI, 1.61–3.19) and migraine without aura (RR 1.83; 95% CI, 1.06–3.15) and was markedly increased for women taking oral contraceptives (RR 8.72; 95% CI, 5.05–15.05).[48]

Two large-scale prospective cohort studies and one population-based case-control study were published after the meta-analysis. The first used data from the Women's Health Study, which included more than 39,000 apparently healthy women 45 years or older.[36] This study found a 1.7-fold increased risk of ischemic stroke (RR 1.71; 95% CI, 1.11–2.66) for women who reported migraine with aura versus women without migraine. The associated risk was magnified in those women who were 45 to 55 years of age (RR 2.25; 95% CI, 1.30–3.91) and was not seen in the older age group. Migraine without aura was not associated with an increased risk of ischemic stroke.

The second prospective study used data from the Atherosclerosis Risk in Communities Study and included more than 12,000 men and women 55 years and older.[37] The study evaluated the migraine-stroke association in different time windows (i.e., retrospective and prospective). The only strict prospective evaluation (i.e., the migraine assessment preceded the stroke event) showed a 1.8-fold increased risk of ischemic stroke (RR 1.84; 95% CI, 0.89–3.82) in migraine sufferers with aura than in participants without migraine. The fact that the risk estimates did not reach statistical significance may be due to the specific migraine and aura classification used in the study. This study found no further effect modification by age, and the migraine-stroke association persisted after data were controlled for a large number of traditional stroke risk factors. The results of these prospective studies suggest that the migraine-stroke association may not be limited to individuals younger than 45.

The Stroke Prevention in Young Women Study matched 386 women age 15 to 49 years with first ischemic stroke with 614 age- and ethnicity-matched controls.[35] Subjects were classified as having no headache, probable migraine without visual symptoms, or probable migraine with visual symptoms. Compared with women without headache, those who reported probable migraine with visual symptoms had a 1.5-fold higher risk of ischemic stroke

(OR 1.5; 95% CI, 1.1–2.0), which was slightly attenuated after control for stroke risk factors. This risk further increased for women who reported a probable migraine frequency of at least 12 per year (OR 2.3; 95% CI, 1.5–3.5) and for those who had begun having migraines during the prior year (OR 6.7; 95% CI, 2.3–19.2). Women with probable migraine without visual symptoms were not at increased risk for ischemic stroke. When effect modification by smoking and oral contraceptive use was considered, the combination of smoking and oral contraceptive use increased the risk of ischemic stroke to sevenfold that in women without probable migraine. The risk in women who did smoke and use oral contraceptives was 10-fold that in women without probable migraine who did not smoke and who did not use oral contraceptives.[35]

Furthermore, migraine with aura is associated with silent brain infarcts, as reported by Kruit and colleagues.[43] In this study, randomly selected patients with migraine with aura (n = 161), patients with migraine without aura (n = 134), and controls (n = 140) who were frequency-matched to cases for age, sex, and place of residence were studied by means of MRI. The investigators found no significant difference between patients with migraine and controls in overall infarct prevalence (8.1% vs. 5.0%, respectively). However, patients with migraine had a higher prevalence of silent infarcts in the cerebellar region of the posterior circulation territory than did controls (5.4% vs. 0.7%, respectively; *P* = .02; adjusted OR, 7.1; 95% CI, 0.9–55). The adjusted OR was 13.7 (95% CI, 1.7–112) for patients with migraine with aura in comparison with that in controls. In patients with migraine with a frequency of attacks of one or more per month, the adjusted OR was 9.3 (95% CI, 1.1–76). The highest risk was in patients with migraine with aura who experienced one attack or more per month (OR, 15.8; 95% CI, 1.8–140).[43]

Because the absolute occurrence of ischemic stroke among migraine sufferers is a rare event, the absolute risks are considerably low. The estimated attributable risk from epidemiologic studies ranges from 18 to 40 additional ischemic stroke cases per 100,000 women per year.[36,48]

Potential Factors Increasing the Risk of Stroke among Patients with Migraine

Oral contraceptives are recognized to increase stroke risk in migraine sufferers and may cause coexisting stroke and migraine. In some instances, however, stroke occurs during the migraine attack, and the medication may have increased the risk of coagulopathy but may not have induced stroke in the absence of the migrainous process. The Collaborative Group for the Study of Stroke in Young Women used a case-control design to evaluate the risk of cerebrovascular disease in users of oral contraceptives.[24] The risk of cerebral thrombosis among women using oral contraceptives was 9.5 times greater than that among nonusers. The role of migraine was assessed in both users and nonusers of contraceptives. Among migraine sufferers not exposed to birth control pills, the risk of stroke was equivocal, depending on the control group used for comparison. The use of oral contraceptives in combination with migraine, however, increased the RR for thrombotic stroke from 2.0 to 5.9.

A study from Denmark found a multiplicative relationship between the risk of oral contraceptives and migraine.[30] A smaller French case-control study of women younger than 45 years found an increased risk for ischemic stroke among women who had migraine without aura (OR 3.0; 95% CI, 1.5–5.8). The risk was even greater in women suffering from migraine with aura (OR 6.2; 95% CI, 2.1–18.0).[27] There was a dose-effect relationship between risk of stroke and the dose of estrogen: The OR was 4.8 for pills containing 50 μg of estrogen, 2.7 for 30 to 40 μg, 1.7 for 20 μg, and 1 μg for progestogen. In none of these cases was the stroke induced by the migraine attack. Use of oral contraceptive in absence of migraine resulted in an OR of 3.5. The combination of oral contraceptive use and migraine resulted in an OR of 13.9 (95% CI, 5.5–35.1). A case control study from Italy in patients with TIA and stroke studied 308 patients aged 15 to 44 with either transient ischemic attack or stroke and 591 age- and sex-matched controls from seven university hospitals. A history of migraine was more frequent in patients than in controls, and none of the controls reported the combination of migraine and oral contraceptive use.[31] The latest data on this topic come from the Stroke Prevention in Young Women Study. In this study, the association between risk of stroke and probable migraine with aura was markedly increased in women who used oral contraceptives and smoked, but each factor individually only modestly increased the risk of stroke for women with probable migraine with aura.[35]

An interesting link had been described between migraine and cardiovascular risk factors. The Genetic Epidemiology of Migraine (GEM) study found that compared with controls, migraine sufferers are more likely to smoke and to have a parental history of early myocardial infarction. The study also found that migraine sufferers with aura are more likely to have an unfavorable cholesterol profile and an elevated blood pressure, to report a history of early-onset coronary heart disease or stroke, and to have a twofold greater risk of a high Framingham risk score–predicted 10-year risk of coronary heart disease even after adjustments for age were made.[49] Although, as mentioned previously, the risk of ischemic stroke is further increased for women with migraine with aura who smoke, newer data suggest that this association is limited to individuals without cardiovascular risk factors. For example, in the Stroke Prevention in Young Women Study, probable migraine with visual aura was associated with ischemic stroke only among women without hypertension, without diabetes, and without a history of myocardial infarction.[35] These results are complemented by data from the Women's Health Study.[50] The association between active migraine with aura and ischemic stroke was apparent only among women in the lowest Framingham risk score group. Interestingly, the association between migraine with aura and myocardial infarction in this cohort was apparent only among women with migraine with aura with high Framingham risk score. With regard to the individual components of the Framingham risk score, this diametric pattern of association was driven by a particularly increased risk of ischemic stroke among women with active migraine with aura who were young (45 to 49 years) and who had low total cholesterol values. In contrast, women with active migraine with aura who had high total cholesterol values had increased risk for myocardial infarction.[50]

Another interesting interrelationship exists among migraine, vascular disease, and the methylenetetrahydrofolate reductase (*MTHFR*) gene. The TT genotype of this polymorphism impairs enzyme activity, thus elevating homocysteine levels. Some studies have shown that carriers of the TT genotype are more likely to have migraine, in particular migraine with aura.[51] Although data from the Women's Health Study could not confirm this finding,[52] two studies have shown that women with migraine with aura who carry the TT polymorphism are at particular increased risk for ischemic stroke.[52,53]

Taking all these studies together, patients with migraine have an increased stroke risk, although the increase is small if one considers it in absolute numbers. The incidence of stroke caused directly by a migraine attack is low. Additional risk factors for stroke in migraine patients are migraine with aura, smoking, and oral contraceptive use, the last particularly if women also smoke. Further, there is evidence that with the exception of smoking, a low cardiovascular risk profile further increases the risk of stroke. In addition, specific genetic markers may also increase this risk. There is currently no strong evidence that migraine increases the risk of hemorrhagic stroke.

Neuroimaging

In a radiologic series of selected migrainous patients with or without focal neurologic deficits, the prevalence of CT scan abnormalities ranged from 34% to 71%. Cala and Mastaglia[54] reported a large series in which they examined 94 patients with a history of "recurrent migrainous headaches," of whom 6 showed evidence of cerebral infarction. Of these patients, 4 had fixed visual field defects with mesial occipital low densities. Of the 49 migrainous patients studied, 21 had evidence of low attenuation in the white matter, which was most extensive in the hemisphere on the side of the headache and contralateral to the sensory aura or signs.

Magnetic Resonance Imaging

The diagnosis of migraine-induced stroke has been greatly enhanced by the use of MRI. From the research viewpoint, great interest stemmed from observations of increased white matter lesions in approximately 30% of routinely studied migraine patients compared with healthy controls.[55] Lesions were found in the centrum semiovale and frontal white matter, in some cases extending to deeper structures in the region of the basal ganglia. In some series such findings were more prevalent in patients with the migraine subtypes associated with neurologic aura.[56] Not all case series found a greater incidence than controls, however. Another series found a higher incidence of white matter lesions in patients with migraine as well as in patients with tension-type headache.[57] The mechanisms of these changes remain to be determined. If relevant, they may represent small foci of ischemic infarction of obscure origin, or gliosis.

More important, two MRI studies found an increased prevalence of white matter lesions and silent brain infarcts in women with frequent migraine with aura.[43,58] Silent brain infarcts were preferentially observed in the occipital lobes and the posterior fossa. Whether these lesions are predictors of vascular dementia later in life or an increased risk of symptomatic brain infarcts is not yet known.

Positron Emission Tomography

Weiller and associates[59] found normal cortical blood flow during migraine attacks and after subcutaneous injection of 6 mg sumatriptan.

Headache of Vascular Disease

Not surprisingly, a major difficulty in differential diagnosis is that the symptom of head pain occurs in various forms of acute cerebrovascular disease, including ischemic stroke. The landmark experiments of Ray and Wolff[60] demonstrated that sensitivity to pressure, traction, and faradization occurred in the intracranial internal carotid artery, the first 1 to 2 cm of the middle cerebral artery stem, the first several centimeters of the anterior cerebral artery just beyond the A2 segment, and the first 1 to 2 cm of the vertebral, anterior, and posterior inferior cerebellar and pontine arteries. These sensitive structures, when electrically stimulated, provoke pain that is localized to specific areas of the scalp and face.

Fisher's[23,61] clinicopathologic observations extended these findings. A study of the headache syndromes due to ischemic cerebrovascular disease showed that most patients complained of the symptom at the onset of a persisting neurologic deficit, although in some cases headache was premonitory of or accompanied TIAs. The headache was usually not throbbing, often localized, and frequently lateralized ipsilateral to the presumed arterial occlusion; it was occasionally severe. Of special interest was the relatively high frequency of headache in posterior cerebral artery territory infarctions compared with that seen in carotid or basilar disease. Headache was the exception in lacunar strokes with pure motor or pure sensory syndromes, and no headaches occurred in any of the 58 patients with transient monocular blindness. Overall, the frequency of headache was 31% in carotid disease and 42% in vertebrobasilar disease. Mitsias and Ramadan[62] have extensively reviewed the literature on this topic up to 1997.

Drug-Induced Migraine–Related Stroke

Migraine-related stroke associated with ergot therapy is appropriately discussed in this category because it is impossible to confidently exclude an interaction of the drug with the migrainous process to induce stroke. Although rarely, ergot therapy even in therapeutic doses may produce focal and diffuse cerebral dysfunction. The peripheral vascular and central nervous system effects of ergot alkaloids in toxic doses have long been recognized, consisting of gangrene, seizures, encephalopathy, and coma. The mechanism responsible for diffuse cerebral dysfunction is not settled and may be the result of either a direct central nervous system toxic effect or severe cerebral vasoconstriction, although in therapeutic doses ergotamine usually has no effect on CBF. Scattered reports have appeared linking ergotamine use to focal disturbances in the ophthalmic and cerebral circulations, manifested as transient monocular blindness, bilateral papillitis, and sensorimotor deficits.[63-65] Epidemiologic studies show an increased stroke risk with the use of ergots but not of triptans.[66] Since the introduction of triptans, such as sumatriptan, there have also been scattered reports of strokelike events, but so far none that has been persuasive of primary involvement of the drug or can exclude its use in an event that mimics migraine. In most of the reported cases of stroke following injection of 6 mg sumatriptan, the time window between the injection and the stroke ranged from 5 to 329 days.[67] Only one case of sinus thrombosis was reported with the use of sumatriptan.[68] Another case report described spinal cord infarction after use of zolmitriptan.[69]

Angiography

The precipitation of migraine-like signs and symptoms during cerebral angiography is not uncommon and can potentially progress to stroke, although not all observers agree.[70] Angiography performed during migraine carries risk because of potential interaction with the migraine mechanism. Nevertheless, because arteriography can be complicated by stroke in all patients, the true pathogenesis of stroke cannot be attributed with certainty to migraine. In any case, in patients with migraine, CT or MR angiography should be performed when angiography is indicated.

Transient Focal Neurologic Events and Late-onset Migraine Accompaniments

Headache is not an invariable occurrence in migraine. Adding to the potential for diagnostic confusion is the occurrence of isolated migraine auras consisting of visual disturbances or focal deficits not accompanied by typical headache, often termed "migraine sine hemicrania." Charcot identified an incomplete form of ophthalmic migraine as "migraines ophtalmiques frustes" consisting only of "les troubles oculaires."

More controversial has been the entity of accompanied migraine without headache, originally described by Whitty.[71] Fisher[7,72] emphasized that the migrainous syndrome, despite the absence of headache, could be diagnosed on the basis of characteristic clinical features. Since then, painless transient and persistent migraine accompaniments have become more widely recognized.[73] The cause of late-onset migraine accompaniments has not been established. As the name of the syndrome suggests, the clinical features are essentially indistinguishable from those of migraine without headache. Brain imaging and cerebral arteriography do not reveal accountable structural lesions.

Hemorrhage

Cases of intracerebral hemorrhage due to migraine have been reported rarely and have been reviewed.[74] In our view, investigations have failed to establish true migraine-induced hemorrhage, most cases likely being symptomatic migraine or migraine mimics. Epidemiologic studies also failed to show an association between migraine and cerebral hemorrhage.[36] From the viewpoint of pathogenesis,

however, it is not unreasonable that ischemic softening of tissue during true migraine-induced cerebral infarction might become hemorrhagic, so dogmatism must be avoided. Experience with this entity in the context of the current IHS classification is awaited.

Retinal or Ocular Migraine

This group of disorders is designated as uncertain in classification because of limited clinical information; most clinical case reports or series were communicated prior to the development of contemporary, advanced neurologic investigation. Although transient homonymous scintillations or fortification scotoma are well-recognized cortical migrainous phenomena, monocular visual loss due to retinal involvement is less often a manifestation of migraine, although still a differential diagnostic point in the patient presenting with amaurosis fugax. Because both retinal and ciliary circulations may be affected, the term *ocular migraine* is preferred[75] and should be distinguished from the term *ophthalmic migraine*, which refers to any migrainous disturbance of vision, whether ocular or cortical.

Migraine that Mimics Stroke
Hemiplegic Migraine

Liveing,[76] in 1873, first described transient hemiparesis associated with a migraine attack. Whitty[77] classified the disorder into hemiplegic migraine with a family history of migraine with or without aura and familial hemiplegic migraine (FHM), in which attacks occur with stereotypical features in family members, often with severe and long-lasting hemiparesis or other persistent aura symptoms, and an autosomal dominant inheritance pattern.

The IHS classifies "hemiplegic migraine" under "migraine with typical aura" (IHS 1.2.1). FHM is classified as a subgroup of migraine with aura (IHS 1.2.4), and sporadic hemiplegic migraine as 1.2.5. The working definition for FHM includes the criteria for migraine with aura (1.2.1,1.2.2) with hemiplegic features that may be prolonged together with at least one first-degree relative with identical attacks. As noted previously, the overall prevalence of migraine with aura is around 4%; this figure includes hemiplegic migraine.

Hemiplegic migraine attacks are characterized by hemiparesis or hemiplegia. The arm and leg are involved in the majority of attacks, often combined with face and hand paresis. Less often, isolated facial and arm paresis occurs. The progression of the motor deficit is slow, with a spreading or marching quality. In most cases symptoms are accompanied by homolateral sensory disturbance, particularly cheiro-oral in distribution, again with a slowly spreading or marching quality. Infrequently, the hemiparesis may alternate from side to side, even during an attack.[78] Visual disturbance, which takes the form of hemianopic loss or typical visual aura, is common. Homolateral or contralateral localization of the visual disturbance is often obscure, however. When dysphasia occurs, it is more often expressive than receptive. The neurologic symptoms last 30 to 60 minutes and are followed by severe pulsating headache that is hemicranial or whole head in distribution. Nausea, vomiting, photophobia, and phonophobia are associated features. In severe cases, the aura can persist throughout the headache phase.

Manifestations of severe hemiplegic migraine attacks include fever, drowsiness, confusion, and coma, all of which can be prolonged from days to weeks.[78] Severe hemiplegic migraine may lead rarely to persistent minor neurologic deficit, in which the cumulative effect of repeated attacks progresses to profound multifocal neurologic deficit, even dementia.

FHM is characterized by the neurologic deficit described previously that is identical in at least one other first-degree relative. There is an autosomal dominant inheritance pattern of the disorder. Other neurologic deficits have been described in association with FHM. Most common is a syndrome of progressive cerebellar disturbance, dysarthria, nystagmus, and ataxia.[78] Retinitis pigmentosa, sensory neural deafness, tremor, dizziness, oculomotor disturbances with nystagmus, ataxia, and coma have also been described.[79,80] These neurologic deficits are present between attacks and are not part of the aura. Hemiplegic migraine attacks also may be part of other familial disorders affecting other systems, for example mitochondrial encephalomyopathy with lactic acidosis, and strokelike episodes syndrome (MELAS) and CADASIL.[18] Attacks of hemiplegic migraine are less likely to be stereotyped in family members with these conditions, however, because the migraine attack is probably "symptomatic" of the underlying brain disorder.

A breakthrough in establishing the cause of FHM was achieved during the clinical investigation of CADASIL.[81-83] This disease is characterized by recurring small deep infarcts, dementia, and leukoencephalopathy. Some patients also experience recurrent attacks of severe migraine-like headache with aura symptoms that include transient headache and hemiparesis. Joutel and coworkers[84,85] identified the gene locus on chromosome 19. Ophoff and colleagues[86] and Joutel and coworkers[87] have isolated, on chromosome 19p13.1, a gene encoding the alpha$_1$ subunit of a brain-specific voltage-gated P/Q type neuronal calcium channel (CACNL1A4) from patients with FHM. The third gene was identified by Dichgans and associates[88] on chromosome 2q24.

Several missense mutations were identified in the meantime.[89-91] The investigators also detected premature stop mutations predicted to disrupt the reading frame of CACNL1A4 in two unrelated patients with episodic ataxia type 2 (EA-2). Thus, FHM and episodic ataxia type 2 can be regarded as allelic channelopathies but of differing molecular mechanism, the former involving a gain-of-function variant of the Ca^{2+} channel subunit, and the latter a decrease in channel density. The results also indicate that different mutations in a single gene may cause phenotypic heterogeneity.[78,92]

Since this report, the same French group identified 10 different missense mutations in the *NOTCH3* genes of 14 unrelated families with CADASIL. The Notch genes are intimately involved in intercellular signaling during development. Proteins belonging to the Notch family are transmembrane receptors. Nine of the ten mutations either added or mutated a cysteine residue in one of the epidermal growth factor (EGF)–like repeats, which are to be found in the extracellular domain. It is likely that this mutation strongly affects protein conformation, although how it leads to CADASIL remains to be established. Possibly, however, membrane instability and abnormality of cell signaling could be the underlying basis of the migraine attacks in this disorder. The generalizability of the genetic findings in FHM, one of the rarest subtypes of migraine, to the more prevalent migraine subtypes also remains to be established. It must be noted that cases of nonfamilial hemiplegic migraine studied by Ophoff and colleagues[86] did not show mutations. Sometimes head trauma can lead to fatal brain edema in patients with FHM.[93]

Basilar Artery Migraine

The concept of basilar artery migraine (IHS 1.2.6) was first proposed by Bickerstaff.[94,95] The diagnostic criteria are those of migraine with aura, consisting of at least two of the following fully reversible symptoms, but no motor weakness: dysarthria, vertigo, tinnitus, hypacusia, diplopia, visual symptoms present simultaneously in both temporal and nasal fields of both eyes, ataxia, decreased level of consciousness, and simultaneously bilateral paresthesias.

Reviewing a personal series of 300 cases, Bickerstaff[95] noticed 34 patients whose attacks were usually heralded by visual disturbances—either complete visual loss or positive phenomena such as teichopsia so dazzling as to obscure the entire field of vision. Other basilar symptoms followed, including dizziness or vertigo; gait ataxia; dysarthria; tinnitus; bilateral acral, perioral, and lingual numbness; and paresthesias. These symptoms persisted for 2 to 60 minutes, ending abruptly, although the visual loss generally recovered more gradually. After the premonitory phase subsided, a severe throbbing occipital headache supervened and was accompanied by vomiting. The patients recovered completely, and between such attacks, many had episodes of classic migraine. Typically affected were adolescent girls. Attacks were usually infrequent and strongly related to menstruation. In Bickerstaff's series, all but 2 patients were younger than 23 years, and 26 of the 34 were girls. A clear-cut family history of migraine in close relatives was obtained in 82% of cases.

Lapkin and associates[96] encountered this entity in a younger population, reporting a group of 30 children with a mean age at onset of 7 years (range 7 months to 14 years). The duration of episodes ranged from minutes to many hours; one patient was symptomatic for nearly 3 days. Unlike in the adolescent cases previously described, the most common complaint was vertigo (73%), and visual disturbances occurred in 43% of cases. In children who were more severely affected, pyramidal tract dysfunction was observed as well as cranial nerve abnormalities, including internuclear ophthalmoplegia and facial nerve paresis. A family history of migraine was obtained in 86% of patients. During the follow-up period of 6 months to 3 years, none of the patients showed signs of progressive neurologic dysfunction, although one child was mentioned as having a permanent oculomotor nerve paralysis.

In the majority of cases of basilar migraine, the aura lasts between 5 and 60 minutes but can extend up to 3 days. Visual symptoms commonly occur first, predominantly in the temporal and nasal fields of vision. The visual disturbance may consist of blurred vision, teichopsia, scintillating scotoma, graying of vision, or total loss of vision. The features may start in one visual field and then spread to become bilateral. Bickerstaff pointed out that when vision is not completely obscured, diplopia might occur, usually as a sixth nerve weakness. Some form of diplopia may occur in up to 16% of cases.[97] Vertigo and gait ataxia are the next most common symptoms, each occurring in 63% of patients in one series.[97] The ataxia can be independent of vertigo. Tinnitus may accompany vertigo. Dysarthria is as common as ataxia and vertigo. Tingling and numbness, in the typical cheiro-oral spreading pattern seen in migraine with aura, occur in more than 60% of cases. This is usually bilateral and symmetric but may alternate sides with a hemidistribution. Occasionally, dysesthesias extend to the trunk. Bilateral motor weakness occurs in more than 50% of cases.

The syndrome of basilar artery migraine was later expanded to include alteration in consciousness. Bickerstaff[94] cited four cases of altered consciousness in detail and recorded a total of 8 of 32 patients with previously diagnosed basilar artery migraine. The onset of impaired consciousness occurred in the context of other basilar symptoms with a leisurely onset, not causing the patient to fall or incur self-injury, and was sometimes preceded by a dreamlike state. Ranging from drowsiness to stupor, the altered consciousness was akinetic and usually brief, lasting up to several minutes and not accompanied by rigidity, posturing, tongue biting, urinary incontinence, or changes in the respiratory pattern. As in the usual basilar artery migraine, a throbbing headache occurred on recovery. Laboratory investigations were generally unrevealing, with normal cerebrospinal fluid analysis and electroencephalography results. Lee and Lance[98] encountered seven patients with a similar syndrome of altered consciousness, using the term *migraine stupor*. Unlike the brief episodes observed by Bickerstaff,[94] the duration of stupor in their patients ranged from 2 hours to 5 days. Four patients showed aggressive and hysterical behavior during the attacks, leading to initial psychiatric diagnoses. Although impairment of consciousness in some form is common in basilar artery migraine, it progresses to stupor and prolonged coma. Other forms of altered consciousness are amnesia and syncope. Drop attacks are rare.

Headache occurs in almost all patients with basilar artery migraine. The headache has an occipital location in the majority and a throbbing, pounding quality and is accompanied by severe nausea and vomiting. It is unusual for the headache to be unilateral or localized to the more anterior parts of the cranium. Photophobia and phonophobia occur in one third to one half of patients. As with other forms of migraine, the symptoms may occur without headache, but usually in no more than 4% of cases.[97] Seizures have been observed in association with basilar migraine. Electroencephalographic changes without seizures, occurring with attacks of typical basilar artery migraine, also have been described. In all, electroencephalographic abnormalities are detected in less than one fifth of cases of basilar artery migraine and are mostly independent of any clinical manifestation of the disorder.

Permanent brainstem deficits as a result of basilar artery migraine have been reported rarely. None of Bickerstaff's cases had persisting neurologic disturbances; indeed, he stressed return to complete normality as a criterion for the diagnosis. Among the cases of migraine-associated stroke uncovered in the literature, only four of five have occurred in the vertebrobasilar territory, excluding the posterior cerebral artery. In Connor's presentation[99] of 18 cases of complicated migraine, 3 patients were considered to have lesions in the brainstem. In no instance did the transient episodes clearly resemble basilar artery migraine, as defined previously. Cerebral infarction specifically affecting the brainstem circulation territory understandably has been offered as evidence for a primary vascular cause of basilar migraine. Skinhoj and Paulson,[100] in studies performed during the migraine aura, found that angiographic findings were normal despite reduction of CBF, except for impaired filling in the top of the basilar artery.[100] Cerebral angiography can itself precipitate migraine aura, however, albeit after a time lag of hours. Nevertheless, the combination of the clinical features plus the arteriographic studies mentioned previously emphasizes a primary vascular alternative for the cause of basilar artery migraine. Cerebrovascular disease is the most serious disorder in the differential diagnosis of basilar artery migraine.

Ischemic stroke in the brainstem and posterior cortical regions, due to either cerebral embolism or thrombosis, manifests as a constellation of neurologic symptoms and signs of brainstem and posterior circulation defects accompanied in approximately one third of cases by headache. Basilar artery occlusive disease can, therefore, mimic basilar artery migraine. Another basilar artery migraine "mimic" for which migraine patients are at increased risk is vertebral artery dissection.

TIAs involving any part of the vertebrobasilar territory must figure largely in the differential diagnosis, particularly if basilar artery migraine occurs for the first time in later years of life. Certain familial disorders manifest as neurologic deficit in which attacks of hemiplegic or basilar migraine may be part of the symptom complex. This group includes CADASIL, MELAS, and variants of MELAS that are associated with seizures, particularly those occipital in origin.

Mechanisms

From the preceding review, it should be apparent that migraine can mimic cerebrovascular disorders, especially ischemic stroke, and stroke can mimic migraine. This fact poses diagnostic problems for the clinician that in most cases will be resolved. It is uncertain how much of the past literature on migraine-induced stroke described cerebrovascular disorders that were mistaken for migraine. This statement is made not to criticize these earlier reports but to recognize that they were communicated at a time when diagnostic tools were less well developed and that concepts of migraine mechanisms have changed. How a migraine attack can induce permanent neurologic deficit and brain damage remains to be determined. Perhaps even more intriguing is the question, what constitutes the comorbid increased risk for stroke between attacks? The latter is the most difficult to speculate on because although comorbid factors may be present (such as increased platelet aggregation), many are uncertain risk factors for stroke. Indeed, when definite risk factors for stroke are present in migraine sufferers, the stroke is attributed to this cause and not to migraine. On the basis of the epidemiologic data described, however, there must be stroke risk factors yet to be identified that are comorbid with migraine.

With regard to the mechanisms whereby stroke is induced during a migraine attack, information provides some limited understanding. The current literature on CBF has been reviewed. To summarize, spreading cortical depression of Leão may induce short-lived increases in CBF, followed by a more profound oligemia. Ischemic foci, however, may occasionally occur during attacks of migraine with aura. Possibly, SD is also associated with depolarization of intrinsic neurons that also supply intraparenchymal resistance microvessels, leading to constriction and a consequent flow reduction below the threshold for K^+ release from the neuron. Increased extracellular K^+ then might precipitate depolarization of contiguous cortical neurons. Alternatively, the decreased extracellular space and brain swelling that accompany spreading cortical depression and possibly migraine could increase microvascular resistance by mechanical compression. Thus, low flow in major intracerebral vessels may be due to increased downstream resistance, not major intracranial arterial vasospasm. Essentially, low CBF and sluggish flow in large intracerebral vessels during the aura of migraine, when combined with factors predisposing to coagulopathy, could lead, although rarely, to intravascular thrombosis and thus migraine-induced cerebral infarction. Release of vasoactive peptides and endothelin, activation of cytokines, and upregulation of adhesion molecules during the neurogenically mediated inflammatory response that may be responsible for headache also may induce intravascular thrombosis. This could explain why migraine-induced stroke usually respects intracranial arterial territories even though the aura involves more widespread brain regions. In addition, frequent aura, if due to spreading depression, could induce cytotoxic cell damage and gliosis based on glutamate release or excess intracellular calcium accumulation. This process could explain persistent neurologic deficit without evidence of ischemic infarction on the basis of selective neuronal necrosis. Increased extracellular K^+, which might precipitate rarely during episodes of migraine, probably relates to variability in the coagulation status, the degree of the neuronal and hemodynamic changes, and the interaction of each during the course of the migraine attack.

Migraine and Patent Foramen Ovale

Several studies have investigated a possible link between patent foramen ovale (PFO) and migraine. Del Sette and coworkers[101] compared 44 patients with migraine with aura, 73 patients younger than 50 years with focal cerebral ischemia, with 50 control individuals without cerebrovascular disease and migraine using transcranial Doppler ultrasonography. The prevalence of right-to-left shunt was significantly higher in patients with migraine

with aura (41%) and cerebral ischemia (35%) than in controls (8%). Anzola and colleagues[102] performed a case-control study in 113 consecutive patients with migraine with aura, 53 patients with migraine without aura, and 25 age-matched nonmigraine individuals. The prevalence of PFO was significantly higher in patients with migraine with aura (48%) than in patients with migraine without aura (23%) and controls (20%). Further studies confirmed by different methods (transcranial Doppler ultrasonography, transesophageal echocardiography) the relationship between PFO and migraine with aura.[103,104] There seems to be a much weaker association of PFO with migraine without aura and other headaches. A possible explanation might be that both conditions, migraine with aura and PFO, could be dominantly inherited and share a common genetic background.[105]

Coincident occurrence of two conditions, however, does not necessarily imply a causal relationship. Moreover, it is difficult to imagine how PFO would lead to a migraine attack with aura—a neural event in the occipital cortex caused by spreading depression. Even if small emboli arise from a PFO, they would travel preferentially into the anterior circulation rather than into the posterior cerebral artery.

Should PFOs be closed in patients with migraine? Even if we assume that there is a causal relationship between PFO and migraine, closure of PFO should then result in migraine improvement. To date, only one randomized and controlled prospective trial examining this issue has been performed, in the United Kingdom. The Migraine Intervention with STARFlex Technology (MIST) trial recruited patients with frequent migraine with aura that was refractory to preventive treatment (although topiramate and lamotrigine were not used).[106,107] The trial randomly assigned 147 patients to undergo either transcutaneous PFO closure with a STARFlex septal repair implant (NMT Medical, Boston) or a sham procedure. After 6 months, 135 patients had completed the trial. The primary endpoint, cure of migraine, was not significantly different between the two treatment groups. There was a trend for a reduction of migraine frequency in the operated group that was also not significant.[108] The procedure was associated with some serious adverse events—cardiac tamponade, pericardial effusion, retroperitoneal bleed, atrial fibrillation, and chest pain. Adverse events in the sham procedure group included incision site bleed, anemia, nosebleed, and a brainstem stroke.

In a retrospective study, 215 stroke patients with PFO were examined and underwent closure of PFO as a secondary prevention measure.[109] A year later, patients were asked about their migraine frequency before and after PFO closure to determine whether this intervention affected migraine attacks. Patients with a PFO and a history of stroke had higher migraine prevalence (22%) than the general population (10%). In patients with migraine with aura, percutaneous PFO closure reduced the frequency of migraine attacks by 54% (1.2 ± 0.8 vs. 0.6 ± 0.8 per month; $P = .001$) and in patients with migraine without aura by 62% (1.2 ± 0.7 vs. 0.4 ± 0.4 per month; $P = .006$). PFO closure did not have a statistically significant effect on headache frequency in patients with nonmigraine headaches. Several other retrospective studies found a similar relationship between PFO closure and migraine

TABLE 36-2   TREATMENT OF ACUTE MIGRAINE ATTACKS IN OTHERWISE HEALTHY PATIENTS AND IN PATIENTS WITH TRANSIENT ISCHEMIC ATTACK (TIA) OR STROKE AND PATIENTS AT RISK FOR STROKE*

Drug	Dose (mg)	Patients with Migraine without Vascular Risk	Patients with Migraine and with TIA or Stroke
Aspirin	500-1000	+++	+++
Paracetamol, acetaminophen	500-1000	++	++
Nonsteroidal anti-inflammatory drugs		+++	+++
Ergotamine oral	1-2	++	Contraindicated
α-Dihydroergocryptine, intravenous, subcutaneous (SC)		+++	Contraindicated
Sumatriptan	25-100 oral, 6 SC	+++	Contraindicated
Naratriptan	2.5	++	Contraindicated
Rizatriptan	10	+++	Contraindicated
Zolmitriptan	2.5	+++	Contraindicated
Eletriptan	20, 40, 80	+++	Contraindicated
Almotriptan	12.5	+++	Contraindicated
Frovatriptan	2.5	+	Contraindicated
Neuroleptics		+	+

*Number of plus signs indicates efficacy, from low (+) to high (+++), shown in clinical trials.

improvement.[110-115] However, with one exception, all of these studies had major limitations. First, even though migraine improves spontaneously with age, no study had a control group. Second, the high rate of placebo response can reduce the frequency of migraine by up to 70%. Third, after PFO closure, most patients received aspirin, which has a modest migraine prophylactic activity, at least in men.[116,117] Clopidogrel, given as an aspirin alternative, might also reduce migraine frequency.[118,119] Fourth, retrospective collection of headache data is highly unreliable; recall bias has a major influence on the results. Furthermore, the latest study observed that as many patients experience migraine improvement as experience new-onset migraine after PFO closure.[112]

Thus, to date, there is insufficient evidence to support the hypothesis that migraine frequency is improved by PFO closure. Additional properly conducted, prospective studies in patients with migraine that include control groups with other or no headaches are needed. These are under way in Europe and the United States. Until their results are known, PFO closure should not be used for the prophylaxis of migraine.

Stroke Prevention in Patients with Migraine

Most patients with TIA or stroke receive antiplatelet treatment. Aspirin lowers stroke risk[120] and has a weak preventive action in migraine.[117,121] Clopidogrel is more effective than aspirin in the prevention of the combined endpoint of stroke, myocardial infarction, and vascular death[122] and can be given to patients with migraine. In some patients clopidogrel might even improve migraine.[118] The combination of aspirin plus slow-release dipyridamole is more effective than aspirin in stroke prevention.[123] Dipyridamole may lead to headache in the first few days of intake. If it is tolerated over this period, the headache will improve. According to clinical experience, patients who used to suffer from migraine or patients from families with migraine get headache more often with dipyridamole than patients with no history of migraine. Titration of the dosage results

in a lower headache incidence and a lower rate of therapy dropout.[124] Anticoagulation poses no problem for patients with migraine. In patients with significant carotid stenosis angiography, carotid endarterectomy or stenting with angioplasty can induce migraine attacks in people who formerly had migraine or who still suffer from migraine.

Patients with hypertension and migraine should be treated with β-blockers that have shown efficacy in migraine prophylaxis, such as propranolol, metoprolol, bisoprolol, and atenolol.[125] Whether angiotensin-converting enzyme inhibitors such as lisinopril are effective in migraine prophylaxis is under debate.[126] Cholesterol-lowering drugs and antidiabetic treatment do not interfere with migraine or migraine treatment. Women with migraine with aura who suffer from additional diseases like hypertension, diabetes, and obesity and who are smoking should treat these risk factors and should be advised about the risk of oral contraceptives.[127,128]

Treatment of Migraine in Patients at Risk for Stroke or in Patients with Transient Ischemic Attack or Stroke

Migraine attack treatment with one of the triptans (almotriptan, eletriptan, frovatriptan, naratriptan, rizatriptan, sumatriptan, or zolmitriptan) is contraindicated in patients with TIA or stroke and in patients with multiple vascular risk factors (Table 36-2). The reason is that triptans have a vasoconstrictive action[129-131] and might result in a decrease of already decreased blood flow. For patients with vascular disease, calcitonin gene–related peptide (CGRP) antagonists are the drugs of choice in the future; these agents have no vasoconstrictive properties.[132] Ergot alkaloids are also contraindicated for the same reason.[131,133] Treatment of acute migraine attacks in patients at high risk for stroke is restricted to analgesic drugs. In some countries aspirin is available as an intravenous (IV) injection for the treatment of acute migraine attack; 1000 mg intravenous aspirin is inferior to 6 mg subcutaneous sumatriptan in terms of efficacy but is better tolerated.[134] Patients with frequent migraine attacks and vascular

TABLE 36-3 DRUGS FOR MIGRAINE PROPHYLAXIS IN OTHERWISE HEALTHY PATIENTS AND IN PATIENTS WITH TRANSIENT ISCHEMIC ATTACK (TIA) OR STROKE AND PATIENTS AT RISK FOR STROKE*

Drug	Dose (mg)	Patients with Migraine without Vascular Risk	Patients with Migraine and TIA or Stroke
Metoprolol	50-200	+++	+++
Propranolol	40-160	+++	+++
Bisoprolol	5-10	++	++
Flunarizine	5-10	+++	+++
Valproic acid	500-600	+++	+++
Gabapentin	2400	++	++
Topiramate	50-200	+++	+++
Pizotifen	1.5	+	Contraindicated
Methysergide	4-8	++	Contraindicated
Magnesium	500	+	+
α-Dihydroergocryptine	10	+	+
Aspirin	300	+	+

*Plus signs indicate efficacy, from low (+) to high (+++), shown in clinical trials.

disease should receive migraine prophylaxis (Table 36-3). Drugs of first choice are β-blockers.[125] They are effective and will also lower increased blood pressure. The later stroke trials indicate that lower blood pressure might even prevent vascular events in patients with normal blood pressure.[135] Flunarizine is not available in all countries but can be given to most patients with vascular disease.[136] The same is true for anticonvulsants.[137,138] Serotonin antagonists such as pizotifen and methysergide[139] are contraindicated in patients at risk for stroke. Aerobic exercise has migraine preventive action and lowers stroke risk.[140,141]

Patients who suffered cerebral or subarachnoid hemorrhage should not use acetylsalicylic acid to treat migraine attacks or nonsteroidal anti-inflammatory drugs (NSAIDs) for migraine prophylaxis. Triptans are contraindicated to treat headache after subarachnoidal hemorrhage. Valproic acid for migraine prophylaxis should be used only to control platelet count. The treatment of the acute phase of cerebral hemorrhage and subarachnoid hemorrhage is the same in patients with or without migraine.

Acknowledgments

HCD is supported by a grant from the German Ministry of Education and Science via the German Headache Consortium. TK is supported by NIH grants HL091880 and NS061836.

REFERENCES

1. Stewart WF, Lipton RB, Celentano DD, Reed ML: Prevalence of migraine headache in the United States: relation to age, race, income, and other sociodemographic factors, *JAMA* 267:64–69, 1992.
2. Lipton RB, Stewart WF: Epidemiology and comorbidity of migraine. In Goadsby PJ, Silberstein SD, editors: *Headache*, Boston, 1997, Butterworth-Heinemann, pp 75–97.
3. Stewart WF, Lipton RB, Celentano DD, Reed ML: Prevalence of migraine headache in the United States: Relation to age, income, race and other sociodemographic factors, *JAMA* 267:64–69, 1992.
4. Russel MB, Rasmussen BK, Thornvaldesen P, Olesen J: Prevalence and sex ratio of the subtypes of migraine, *Int J Epidemiol* 24:612–618, 1995.
5. Rasmussen BK, Olesen J: Migraine with aura and migraine without aura: An epidemiological study, *Cephalalgia* 12:221–228, 1992.
6. Headache Classification Subcommittee of the International Headache Society: The international classification of headache disorders, 2nd edition, *Cephalalgia* 24(Suppl 1):1–160, 2004.
7. Fisher CM: Late-life migraine accompaniments as a cause of unexplained transient ischemic attacks, *Can J Med Sci* 7:9, 1980.
8. Queiroz AP, Rapaport AM, Weeks RE, et al: Characteristics of migraine visual aura, *Headache* 37:137–141, 1997.
9. Woods RP, Iacoboni M, Mazziotta JC: Bilateral spreading cerebral hypoperfusion during spontaneous migraine headache, *N Engl J Med* 331:1689–1692, 1994.
10. Olesen J, Tfelt-Hansen P, Henriksen L, et al: Difference between cerebral blood flow reactions in classic and common migraine. In Rose FC, editor: *Advances in migraine research and therapy*, New York, 1982, Raven Press, pp 105–115.
11. Diener H: Positron emission tomography studies in headache, *Headache* 37:622–625, 1997.
12. Cutrer FM, Sorensen AG, Weisskopf RM, et al: Perfusion-weighted imaging defects during spontaneous migrainous aura, *Ann Neurol* 43:25–31, 1998.
13. Headache Classification Committee of the International Headache Society: Classification and diagnostic criteria for headache disorders, cranial neuralgias and facial pain, *Cephalalgia* 8(Suppl 7):1–93, 1988.
14. Olesen J, Friberg L, Olsen TS, et al: Ischaemia-induced (symptomatic) migraine attacks may be more frequent than migraine-induced ischaemic insults, *Brain* 116:187–202, 1993.
15. Silvestrini M, Cupini LM, Calabresi P, et al: Migraine with aura-like syndrome due to arteriovenous malformation: The clinical value of transcranial Doppler in early diagnosis, *Cephalalgia* 12:115–119, 1992.
16. Davous P: CADASIL: a review with proposed diagnostic criteria, *Eur J Neurol* 5:219–233, 1998.
17. Chabriat H, Vahedi K, Iba-Zizen MT, et al: Clinical spectrum of CADASIL: A study of 7 families, *Lancet* 346:934–939, 1995.
18. Dichgans M, Mayer M, Uttner I, et al: The phenotypic spectrum of CADASIL: Clinical findings in 102 cases, *Ann Neurol* 44:731–739, 1998.
19. Welch KM: Stroke and migraine–the spectrum of cause and effect, *Funct Neurol* 18(3):121–126, 2003.
20. Tzourio C, Benslamia L, Guillon B, et al: Migraine and the risk of cervical artery dissection: A case-control study, *Neurology* 59:435–437, 2002.
21. Ramadan NM, Tietjen GE, Levine SR, Welch KMA: Scintillating scotoma associated with internal carotid artery dissection, *Neurology* 41:1084–1087, 1991.
22. Sibert PL, Mokri B, Schievink WI: Headache and neck pain in spontaneous internal carotid and vertebral artery dissections, *Neurology* 45:1517–1522, 1995.
23. Fisher CM: The headache and pain of spontaneous carotid dissection, *Headache* 22:60, 1982.
24. Collaborative Group for the Study of Stroke in Young Women: Oral contraception and stroke in young women: Associated risk factors, *JAMA* 231:718–722, 1975.
25. Henrich JB, Horwitz RI: A controlled study of ischemic stroke risk in migraine patients, *J Clin Epidemiol* 42:773–780, 1989.
26. Tzourio C, Iglesias S, Hubert JB, et al: Migraine and risk of ischaemic stroke: A case-control study, *BMJ* 307:289–292, 1993.
27. Tzourio C, Tehindrazanarivelo A, Iglesias S, et al: Case-control study of migraine and risk of ischaemic stroke in young women, *BMJ* 310:830–833, 1995.
28. Chang CL, Donaghy M, Poulter N, World Health Organisation Collaborative Study of Cardiovascular Disease and Steroid Hormone Contraception: Migraine and stroke in young women: Case-control study, *BMJ* 318:13–18, 1999.
29. Marini C, Carolei A, Roberts R, et al: Focal cerebral ischemia in young adults: a collaborative case-control study. The National Research Council Study Group, *Neuroepidemiology* 12:70–81, 1993.

30. Lidegaard O: Oral contraceptivces, pregnancy and the risk of cerebral thromboembolism: the influence of diabetes, hypertension, migraine and previous thrombotic disease, *Br J Obstet Gynaecol* 102:153–159, 1995.

31. Carolei A, Marini C, DeMatteis G: History of migraine and risk of cerebral ischaemia in young adults, *Lancet* 347:1503–1506, 1996.

32. Haapaniemi H, Hillbom M, Juvela S: Lifestyle-associated risk factors for acute brain infarction among persons of working age, *Stroke* 28:26–30, 1997.

33. Donaghy M, Chang CL, Poulter N: on behalf of the European Collaborators of The World Health Organisation Collaborative Study of Cardiovascular Disease and Steroid Hormone Contraception. Duration, frequency, recency, and type of migraine and the risk of ischaemic stroke in women of childbearing age, *J Neurol Neurosurg Psychiatry* 73:747–750, 2002.

34. Schwaag S, Nabavi DG, Frese A, et al: The association between migraine and juvenile stroke: a case-control study, *Headache* 43:90–95, 2003.

35. MacClellan LR, Giles W, Cole J, et al: Probable migraine with visual aura and risk of ischemic stroke: The stroke prevention in young women study, *Stroke* 38:2438–2445, 2007.

36. Kurth T, Slomke MA, Kase CS, et al: Migraine, headache, and the risk of stroke in women: a prospective study, *Neurology* 64:1020–1026, 2005.

37. Stang PE, Carson AP, Rose KM, et al: Headache, cerebrovascular symptoms, and stroke: The Atherosclerosis Risk in Communities Study, *Neurology* 64:1573–1577, 2005.

38. Buring JE, Hebert P, Romero J, et al: Migraine and subsequent risk of stroke in the Physicians' Health Study, *Arch Neurol* 52:129–134, 1995.

39. Nightingale A, Farmer R: Ischemic stroke in young women: A nested case-control study using the UK General Practice Research Database, *Stroke* 35:1574–1578, 2004.

40. Hall G, Brown M, Mo J, MacRae K: Triptans in migraine: The risks of stroke, cardiovascular disease, and death in practice, *Neurology* 62:563–568, 2004.

41. Velentgas P, Cole JA, Mo J, et al: Severe vascular events in migraine patients, *Headache* 44:642–651, 2004.

42. Merikangas KR, Fenton BT, Cheng SH, et al: Association between migraine and stroke in a large-scale epidemiological study of the United States, *Arch Neurol* 54:362–368, 1997.

43. Kruit M, van Buchem M, Hofman P, et al: Migraine as a risk factor for subclinical brain lesions, *JAMA* 291:427–434, 2004.

44. Sochurkova D, Moreau T, Lemesle M, et al: Migraine history and migraine-induced stroke in the Dijon stroke registry, *Neuroepidemiology* 18:85–91, 1999.

45. Milhaud D, Bogousslavsky J, van Melle G, Liot P: Ischemic stroke and active migraine, *Neurology* 57:1805–1811, 2001.

46. Chang CL, Donaghy M, Poulter N: Migraine and stroke in young women: case-control study. The World Health Organisation Collaborative Study of Cardiovascular Disease and Steroid Hormone Contraception, *BMJ* 318:13–18, 1999.

47. Tzourio C, Tehindrazanarivelo A, Iglesias S, et al: Case-control study of migraine and risk of ischaemic stroke in young women, *BMJ* 310:830–833, 1995.

48. Etminan M, Takkouche B, Isorna FC, Samii A: Risk of ischaemic stroke in people with migraine: Systematic review and meta-analysis of observational studies, *BMJ* 330:63–65, 2005.

49. Scher AI, Terwindt GM, Picavet HS, et al: Cardiovascular risk factors and migraine: the GEM population based study, *Neurology* 64:614–620, 2005.

50. Kurth T, Schürks M, Logroscino G, et al: Migraine, vascular risk, and cardiovascular events in women: Prospective cohort study, *BMJ* 337:a636, 2008.

51. Scher AI, Terwindt GM, Verschuren WM, et al: Migraine and MTHFR C677T genotype in a population-based sample, *Ann Neurol* 59:372–375, 2006.

52. Schurks M, Zee RY, Buring JE, Kurth T: Interrelationships among the MTHFR 677C>T polymorphism, migraine, and cardiovascular disease, *Neurology* 71:505–513, 2008.

53. Pezzini A, Grassi M, Del Zotto E, et al: Migraine mediates the influence of C677T MTHFR genotypes on ischemic stroke risk with a stroke subtype effect, *Stroke* 38:3145–3151, 2007.

54. Cala LA, Mastaglia FL: Computerized axial tomography findings in patients with migrainous headaches, *BMJ* 2:149–150, 1976.

55. Igarashi H, Sakai F, Kan S, et al: Magnetic resonance imaging of the brain in patients with migraine, *Cephalalgia* 11:69–74, 1991.

56. Fazekas F, Koch M, Schmidt R, et al: The prevalence of cerebral damage varies with migraine type: A MRI study, *Headache* 32:287–291, 1992.

57. De Benedittis G, Lorenzetti A, Sina C, et al: Magnetic resonance imaging in migraine and tension type headache, *Headache* 35:264–268, 1995.

58. Kruit MC, Launer LJ, Ferrari MD, van Buchem MA: Brain stem and cerebellar hyperintense lesions in migraine, *Stroke* 37:1109–1112, 2006.

59. Weiller C, May A, Limmroth V, et al: Brain stem activation in spontaneous human migraine attacks, *Nature Med* 1:658–660, 1995.

60. Ray BS, Wolff HG: Experimental studies on headache: Pain-sensitive structures of the head and their significance in headache, *Arch Surg* 41:813–856, 1940.

61. Fisher CM: Headache in cerebrovascular disease. In Vinken PJ, Bruyn GW, editors: *Handbook of clinical neurology*, Amsterdam, 1968, Elsevier, pp 124–126.

62. Mitsias P, Ramadan NM: Headache in ischemic cerebrovascular disease. Part I: clinical features, *Cephalalgia* 12:269–274, 1992.

63. Brohult J, Forsberg O, Hellstrom R: Multiple arterial thrombosis after oral contraceptives and ergotamine, *Acta Med Scand* 181:453, 1967.

64. Merkhoff GC, Poter JM: Ergot intoxication: Historical review and description, *Ann Surg* 180:773, 1974.

65. Senter HJ, Liebermann AN: Cerebral manifestations of ergotism. Report of a case and review of the literature, *Stroke* 7:88–92, 1976.

66. Wammes-van der Heijden EA, Rahimtoola H, Leufkens HG, et al: Risk of ischemic complications related to the intensity of triptan and ergotamine use, *Neurology* 67:1128–1134, 2006.

67. Fox AW: Comparative tolerability of oral 5-HT 1B/1D agonists, *Headache* 40:521–527, 2000.

68. Cavazos JE, Carees JB, Chilukuri VR: Sumatriptan-induced stroke in sagittal sinus thrombosis, *Lancet* 343:1105–1106, 1994.

69. Vijayan N, Peacock JH: Spinal cord infarction during use of zolmitriptan: A case report, *Headache* 40:57–60, 2000.

70. Shuaib A, Hachinski C: Migraine and the risks from angiography, *Arch Neurol* 45:911–912, 1988.

71. Whitty CWM: Migraine without headache, *Lancet* 2(7510):283, 1967.

72. Fisher CM: Migraine accompaniments versus arteriosclerotic ischemia, *Trans Am Neuol Assoc* 93:211, 1968.

73. Wijman CA, Wolf PA, Kase CS, et al: Migrainous visual accompaniments are not rare in late life: The Framingham Study, *Stroke* 29:1539–1543, 1998.

74. Caplan L: Intracerebral hemorrhage revisited, *Neurology* 38:624, 1988.

75. Corbett JJ: Neuro-ophthalmic complications of migraine and cluster headaches, *Neurol Clin* 1:973–995, 1983.

76. Liveing E: *On megrim, sick-headache, and some allied disorders: a contribution to the pathology of nerve-storms*, London, 1873, J & A Churchill.

77. Whittey CWM: Familial hemiplegic migraine, *J Neurol Neurosurg Psychiatry* 16:172, 1953.

78. Ducros A, Denier C, Joutel A, et al: The clinical spectrum of familial hemiplegic migraine associated with mutations in a neuronal calcium channel, *N Engl J Med* 345:17–24, 2001.

79. Elliott MA, Peroutka SJ, Welch S, May EF: Familial hemiplegic migraine, nystagmus, and cerebellar atrophy, *Ann Neurol* 39:100–106, 1996.

80. Vahedi K, Denier C, Ducros A, et al: CACNA1A gene de novo mutation causing hemiplegic migraine, coma and cerebellar atrophy, *Neurology* 55:1040–1042, 2000.

81. Hutchinson M, Oriordan J, Javed M, et al: Familial hemiplegic migraine and autosomal dominant arteriopathy with leukoencephalopathy (CADASIL), *Ann Neurol* 38:817–824, 1995.

82. Chabriat H, Vahedi K, Iba-Zizen MT, et al: Clinical spectrum of CADASIL: A study of 7 families, *Lancet* 346:934–939, 1995.

83. Chabriat H, Tournier-Lasserve E, Vahedi K, et al: Autosomal dominant migraine with MRI white-matter abnormalities mapping to the CADASIL locus, *Neurology* 45:1086–1091, 1995.

84. Joutel A, Corpechet C, Ducros A, et al: Notch3 mutations in CADASIL, a hereditary adult-onset condition causing stroke and dementia, *Nature* 383:707–710, 1996.

85. Joutel A, Corpechot C, Vayssière C, et al: Characterization of Notch3 mutations in CADASIL patients, *Neurology* 48:1729-1730, 1997.

86. Ophoff RA, Terwindt GM, Vergouwe MN, et al: Familial hemiplegic migraine and episodic ataxia type-2 are caused by mutations in the Ca²⁺ channel gene CACNLA4, *Cell* 87:543-552, 1996.

87. Joutel A, Bousser M, Biouse V, et al: A gene for familial hemiplegic migraine maps to chromosome 19, *Nat Genet* 5:40-45, 1993.

88. Dichgans M, Freilinger T, Eckstein G, et al: Mutation in the neuronal voltage-gated sodium channel SCN1A in familial hemiplegic migraine, *Lancet* 366:371-377, 2005.

89. Terwindt GM, Ophoff RA, Haan J, et al: Variable clinical expression of mutations in the P/Q-type calcium channel gene in familial hemiplegic migraine, *Neurology* 50:1105-1110, 1998.

90. Terwindt GM, Ophoff RA, Haan J, et al: Familial hemiplegic migraine: a clinical comparison of families linked and unlinked to chromosome 19, *Cephalalgia* 16:153-155, 1996.

91. Carrera P, Piatti M, Stenirri S, et al: Genetic heterogeneity in Italian families with familial hemiplegic migraine, *Neurology* 53:26-32, 1999.

92. Battistini S, Stenirri S, Piatti M, et al: A new CACNA1A gene mutation in acetazolamide-responsive familial hemiplegic migraine and ataxia, *Neurology* 53:38-43, 1999.

93. Kors EE, Terwindt GM, Vermeulen FLMG, et al: Delayed cerebral edema and fatal coma after minor head trauma: role of CACNA1A calcium channel subunit gene and relationship with familial hemiplegic migraine, *Ann Neurol* 49:753-760, 2001.

94. Bickerstaff ER: The basilar artery and migraine epilepsy syndrome, *Proc R Soc Med* 55:167, 1962.

95. Bickerstaff ER: Basilar artery migraine, *Lancet* 1(7211):15, 1961.

96. Lapkin ML, French JH, Golden GS: The EEG in childhood basilar artery migraine, *Neurology* 27:580, 1977.

97. Sturzenegger MH, Meienberg O: Basilar artery migraine: a follow-up study of 82 cases, *Headache* 25:408, 1985.

98. Lee CH, Lance JW: Migraine stupor, *Headache* 17:32, 1977.

99. Connor RCR: Complicated migraine. A study of permanent neurological and visual defects caused by migraine, *Lancet* 2(7265):1072-1075, 1962.

100. Skinhoj E, Paulson OB: Regional cerebral blood flow in the internal carotid artery distribution during migraine, *BMJ* 3:569-570, 1969.

101. Del Sette M, Angeli S, Leandri M, et al: Migraine with aura and right-to-left shunt on transcranial Doppler: a case-control study, *Cerebrovasc Dis* 8:327-330, 1998.

102. Anzola GP, Magoni M, Guindani M, et al: Potential source of cerebral embolism in migraine with aura: a transcranial Doppler study, *Neurology* 52:1622-1625, 1999.

103. Schwerzmann M, Nedeltchev K, Lagger F, et al: Prevalence and size of directly detected patent foramen ovale in migraine with aura, *Neurology* 65:1415-1418, 2005.

104. Carod-Artal FJ, da Silveira Ribeiro L, Braga H, et al: Prevalence of patent foramen ovale in migraine patients with and without aura compared with stroke patients. A transcranial Doppler study, *Cephalalgia* 26:934-939, 2006.

105. Wilmshurst PT, Pearson MJ, Nightingale S, et al: Inheritance of persistent foramen ovale and atrial septal defects and the relationship to familial migraine with aura, *Heart* 90:1245-1247, 2004.

106. Lampl C, Bonelli S, Ransmayr G: Efficacy of topiramate in migraine aura prophylaxis: preliminary results of 12 patients, *Headache* 44:174-177, 2004.

107. Lampl C, Katsarava Z, Diener HC, Limmroth V: Lamotrigine reduces migraine aura and migraine attacks in patients with migraine with aura, *J Neurol Neurosurg Psychiatry* 76:1730-1732, 2005.

108. Dowson A, Mullen MJ, Peatfield R, et al: Migraine Intervention with STARFlex Technology (MIST) trial: a prospective, multicenter, double-blind, sham-controlled trial to evaluate the effectiveness of patent foramen ovale closure with STARFlex septal repair implant to resolve refractory migraine headache, *Circulation* 117:1397-1404, 2008.

109. Schwerzmann M, Wiher S, Nedeltchev K, et al: Percutaneous closure of patent foramen ovale reduces the frequency of migraine attacks, *Neurology* 62:1399-1401, 2004.

110. Post M, Thijs V, Herroelen L, Budts W: Closure of a patent foramen ovale is associated with a decrease in prevalence of migraine, *Neurology* 62:1439-1440, 2004.

111. Wilmshurst PT, Nightingale S, Walsh KP, Morrison WL: Effect on migraine of closure of cardiac right-to-left shunts to prevent recurrence of decompression illness or stroke or for haemodynamic reasons, *Lancet* 356(9242):1648-1651, 2000.

112. Mortelmans K, Post M, Thijs V, et al: The influence of percutaneous atrial septal defect closure on the occurrence of migraine, *Eur Heart J* 26:1533-1537, 2005.

113. Reisman M, Christofferson RD, Jesurum J, et al: Migraine headache relief after transcatheter closure of patent foramen ovale, *J Am Coll Cardiol* 45:493-495, 2005.

114. Azarbal B, Tobis J, Suh W, et al: Association of interatrial shunts and migraine headaches: impact of transcatheter closure, *J Am Coll Cardiol* 45:489-492, 2005.

115. Anzola GP, Frisoni GB, Morandi E, et al: Shunt-associated migraine responds favorably to atrial septal repair: a case-control study, *Stroke* 37:430-434, 2006.

116. Buring JE, Peto R, Hennekens CH, et al: Low-dose aspirin for migraine prophylaxis, *JAMA* 264:1711-1713, 1990.

117. Diener HC, Hartung E, Chrubasik J, et al: A comparative study of acetylsalicylic acid and metoprolol for the prophylactic treatment of migraine. A randomised, controlled, double-blind, parallel group phase III study, *Cephalalgia* 21:140-144, 2001.

118. Wilmshurst PT, Nightingale S, Walsh KP, Morrison WL: Clopidogrel reduces migraine with aura after transcatheter closure of persistent foramen ovale and atrial septal defects, *Heart* 91:1173-1175, 2005.

119. Sharifi M, Burks J: Efficacy of clopidogrel in the treatment of post-ASD closure migraines, *Catheter Cardiovasc Interv* 63:255, 2004.

120. Antiplatelet Trialists Collaboration: Collaborative overview of randomised trials of antiplatelet therapy. I: Prevention of death, myocardial infarction, and stroke by prolonged antiplatelet therapy in various categories of patients, *BMJ* 308:81-106, 1994.

121. Bensenor IM, Cook NR, Lee I-M, et al: Low-dose aspirin for migraine prophylaxis in women, *Cephalalgia* 21:175-183, 2001.

122. CAPRIE Steering Committee: A randomised, blinded, trial of clopidogrel versus aspirin in patients at risk of ischaemic events (CAPRIE), *Lancet* 348:1329-1339, 1996.

123. Diener HC, Cuhna L, Forbes C, et al: European Stroke Prevention Study 2: Dipyridamole and acetylsalicylic acid in the secondary prevention of stroke, *J Neurol Sci* 143:1-13, 1996.

124. Chang YJ, Ryu SJ, Lee TH: Dose titration to reduce dipyridamole-related headache, *Cerebrovasc Dis* 22:258-262, 2006.

125. Silberstein SD, for the US Headache Consortium. Practice parameter: evidence-based guidelines for migraine headache (an evidence-based review). Report of the Quality Standards Subcommitee of the American Academy of Neurology, *Neurology* 55:754-763, 2000.

126. Schrader H, Stovner LJ, Helde G, et al: Prophylactic treatment of migraine with angiotensin converting enzyme inhibitor (lisinopril): randomised, placebo-controlled, crossover trial, *BMJ* 322:19-22, 2001.

127. Bousser M-G: Migraine, female hormones, and stroke, *Cephalalgia* 19:75-79, 1999.

128. MacGregor A: Gynaecological aspects of migraine, *Rev Contemp Pharmacother* 11:75-90, 2000.

129. Jansen I, Edvinson L, Mortensens A, Olesen J: Sumatriptan is a potent vasoconstrictor in human dural arteries via a 5-HT1-like receptor, *Cephalalgia* 12:202-205, 1992.

130. Longmore J, Hargreaves RJ, Boulanger CM, et al: Comparison ot the vasoconstrictor properties of the 5-HT1D-receptor agonists rizatriptan (MK-462) and sumatriptan in human isolated coronary artery: outcome of two independent studies using different experimental protocols, *Funct Neurol* 12:3-9, 1997.

131. Saxena PR, den Boer MO, Ferrari MD: The pharmacology of anti-migrainous drugs, *Clin Neuropharm* 15:375A-376A, 1992.

132. Olesen J, Diener H, Husstedt IW, et al: Calcitonin gene-related peptide (CGRP) receptor antagonist BIBN4096BS is effective in the treatment of migraine attacks, *N Engl J Med* 350:1104-1110, 2004.

133. Saxena VK, De Deyn PP: Ergotamine: its use in the treatment of migraine and its complications, *Acta Neurol Napoli* 14:140-146, 1992.

134. Diener HC, for the ASASUMAMIG Study Group: Efficacy and safety of intravenous acetylsalicylic acid lysinate compared to subcutaneous sumatriptan and parenteral placebo in the acute treatment of migraine. A double-blind, double-dummy, randomized, multicenter, parallel group study, *Cephalalgia* 19:581-588, 1999.

135. Hansson L, Zanchetti A, Carruthers SG, et al: Effects of intensive blood-pressure lowering and low-dose aspirin in patients with hypertension: principal results of the Hypertension Optimal Treatment (HOT) randomised trial, *Lancet* 351:1755–1762, 1998.

136. Diener HC, Peters C, Rudizo M, et al: Ergotamine, flunarizine and sumatriptan do not change cerebral blood flow velocity in normal subjects and migraineurs, *J Neurol* 238:245–250, 1991.

137. Mathew NT, Rapoport A, Saper J, et al: Efficacy of gabapentin in migraine prophylaxis, *Headache* 41:119–128, 2001.

138. Klapper J, on behalf of the Divalproex Sodium in Migraine Prophylaxis Study Group: Divalproex sodium in migraine prophylaxis: a dose-controlled study, *Cephalalgia* 17:103–108, 1997.

139. Silberstein SD: Methysergide, *Cephalalgia* 18:421–435, 1998.

140. Sacco RL, Gan R, Boden-Albala B, et al: Leisure-time physical activity and ischemic stroke risk - The Northern Manhattan Stroke Study, *Stroke* 29:380–387, 1998.

141. Wannamethee G, Shaper AG: Physical activity and stroke in British middle aged men, *BMJ* 304:597–601, 1992.

37 Hypertensive Encephalopathy

CATHERINE LAMY, JEAN-LOUIS MAS

The term *hypertensive encephalopathy* was introduced by Oppenheimer and Fishberg[1] in 1928 to designate a constellation of neurologic symptoms that punctuated the course of severe hypertension. Hypertensive encephalopathy is currently defined as an acute syndrome characterized by elevated blood pressure associated with rapidly progressive signs and symptoms, including headache, seizures, altered mental status, visual disturbances, and other focal or diffuse neurologic signs.[1-3] Neuroimaging typically reveals a reversible vasogenic edema involving parietooccipital regions in a relatively symmetrical pattern.[4-7] Its pathogenesis is still incompletely understood, although it seems to be related to breakthrough of autoregulation and to endothelial dysfunction, leading to cerebral edema.[6,8,9] Recognition is important to avoid unnecessary evaluation and orient treatment toward prompt control of blood pressure.

Pathogenesis

The brain is protected from extremes of blood pressure by an autoregulation system that ensures constant perfusion over a wide range of systemic pressures (Fig. 37-1). Under normal circumstances, brain vessels possess intrinsic vascular tone. In response to systemic hypotension, cerebral arterioles dilate to maintain adequate perfusion, whereas vessels constrict in response to high pressure.[7,10] The basic mechanism of autoregulation of cerebral blood flow is still controversial. The autoregulatory vessel caliber changes are most likely mediated by an interplay between myogenic and metabolic mechanisms. The endothelium plays a central role in blood pressure homeostasis by secreting relaxing factors such as nitric oxide and vasoconstriction factors (thromboxane A_2 and endothelin). In normotensive individuals, cerebral blood flow remains unchanged between mean blood pressures of approximately 60 mm Hg and 150 mm Hg.[8,11,12] At pressures above the upper limit of autoregulation, hypertensive encephalopathy may occur. Conversely, when cerebral perfusion pressure decreases below the lower limit of autoregulation, cerebral blood flow decreases and cerebral ischemia occurs. There may be differences between individuals in the degree of hypertension that can give rise to autoregulatory dysfunction leading to encephalopathy as well as differences within a single person over time, depending on comorbid factors. The degree of hypertension required to induce encephalopathy depends on the baseline pressure.[10] Rapidly developing, fluctuating, or intermittent hypertension carries a particular risk for hypertensive encephalopathy. Long-standing hypertension causes a shift of the cerebral blood flow curve to the right, presumably owing to structural changes (vascular hypertrophy and inward remodeling) and diminished responsiveness of resistance vessels. Therefore, sudden elevations to relatively higher blood pressures are required to produce hypertensive encephalopathy in a patient with chronic hypertension than in a normotensive person.[10] In children and young adults, the curve may shift to the left, leaving them more at risk for the development of hypertensive encephalopathy.[2]

Over the previous century, two theories were advanced to explain the pathogenesis of hypertensive encephalopathy. The earlier theory postulated that hypertensive encephalopathy results from intense cerebral autoregulatory vasoconstriction in response to acute hypertension, resulting in decreased cerebral blood flow, ischemia, and subsequent edema involving mainly the borderzone arterial regions.[2,8] The direct observation of alternating constriction and dilatation during episodes of acute rise in blood pressure in hypertensive rats' pial vessels seemed to confirm this hypothesis.[2]

The current popular theory implicates forced vasodilatation of cerebral vessels (autoregulation breakthrough) rather than vasoconstriction as the major component of hypertensive encephalopathy that results in the extravasation of fluid into the interstitium, termed vasogenic edema. In fact, patterns of cerebral blood flow with acute hypertension may be complex with both low-flow and high-flow areas coexisting in adjacent cortical regions. The concept of breakthrough of autoregulation has been initially characterized as a passive phenomenon, as the autoregulatory capacity of vessels is exceeded and the vessels dilate passively. Later evidence suggests that breakthrough of autoregulation may be an active process initiated by calcium-dependent potassium channels. This process generates reactive oxygen species and an active increase in permeability of the blood-brain barrier as well as an increase in vesicular transport, rather than disruption of tight junctions.[13] Abnormalities in vasoactive factors released by the endothelium may contribute to the pathophysiology of hypertensive encephalopathy. Ultimately, loss of endothelial fibrinolytic activity, activation of coagulation and platelets, and degranulation of damaged endothelium may promote further inflammation, thrombosis, and vasoconstriction.[12]

The preferential distribution of white matter lesions in posterior brain regions is recognized but not fully understood. One likely explanation involves the regional

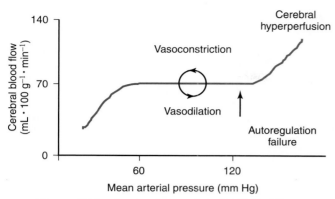

Figure 37-1 Autoregulation of cerebral blood flow.

heterogeneity of the sympathetic innervation.[14] It is known that anterior cerebral circulation is richly innervated by sympathetic nerves from the superior cervical ganglion, in contrast to the vertebrobasilar vessels, which are relatively devoid of sympathetic innervation.[15] It is possible that sympathetically mediated vasoconstriction protects the anterior circulation from overperfusion in acute hypertension.[14]

Pathologic Features

The neuropathologic findings of hypertensive encephalopathy as shown in autopsy studies[16,17] consist of varying degrees of vascular alterations (fibrinoid necrosis of arterioles, thrombosis of arterioles and capillaries), and of parenchymal lesions (microinfarcts, petechial hemorrhages, cerebral edema). Ring hemorrhage around a thrombosed precapillary constitutes the classic microscopic lesion. If hypertensive encephalopathy develops in a patient with long-standing hypertension, a variety of additional hypertensive cerebrovascular changes may be found, including medial atrophy, hyperplasia, hyalinization, and microaneurysms.

The lesions are most often multiple and bilateral, being most prominent in the deep white matter and at the gray-white junction in the watershed and posterior areas; the brainstem is usually severely affected.[16] They may also be present in the basal ganglia, diencephalon, and cerebral cortex. Their extent and severity vary but are generally correlated with the severity of neurologic manifestations and blood pressure, especially during the terminal stage. Brain swelling, occasionally sufficient to cause herniation of cerebellar tonsils through the foramen magnum, has been documented. The vascular changes are not confined to the brain and may also affect the eyes (retinal hemorrhages, papilledema), kidneys (fibrinoid arteriolar lesions of glomeruli), and other organs.[16] These findings, however, may not be representative of those in surviving patients, instead representing the extreme of a spectrum of abnormalities. A brain biopsy performed in one patient with hypertensive encephalopathy has been reported to demonstrate white matter edema with no evidence of vessel wall damage or infarction, consistent with MRI findings of vasogenic edema; the patient made a full neurologic recovery, and follow-up MRI revealed complete resolution of lesions.[18]

Clinical Features

The classic clinical manifestations of hypertensive encephalopathy include severe headache, nausea and vomiting, mental abnormalities including confusion and diminished spontaneity, and speech, seizures, and visual disturbances.[2,3,5,6,16]

Alterations in consciousness range in severity from mild somnolence to frank confusion, stupor, or coma in extreme cases. Temporary restlessness and agitation may alternate with lethargy. The mental functions are slowed; memory and the ability to concentrate are impaired, although severe amnesia is unusual. Abnormalities of visual perception are nearly always detectable. Patients often report blurred vision. Hemianopia, visual neglect, visual hallucinations,[19] and frank cortical blindness may occur. Papilledema may be present with flame-shaped retinal hemorrhages and exudates,[2] but normal ocular fundus findings do not exclude a diagnosis of hypertensive encephalopathy. The tendon reflexes are often brisk, and some patients have weakness and incoordination. Occasionally, focal neurologic signs may be noted.

The onset is usually subacute, with symptoms developing over 24 to 48 hours, but may be heralded by a seizure.[20] The electroencephalogram may show focal sharp waves, slowing, or normal findings.[6] Examination of the cerebrospinal fluid in patients with hypertensive encephalopathy has revealed elevated pressure,[3] mild pleocytosis, and elevated protein concentration.[2]

The clinical presentation of hypertensive encephalopathy is often nonspecific.[6] The differential diagnosis includes various neurologic conditions, such as stroke, venous thrombosis, and encephalitis, all of which can mimic hypertensive encephalopathy, and transient elevations of blood pressure may be the consequence of cerebral lesions. Therefore, patients with hypertension and altered neurologic status represent a difficult diagnosis problem, and hypertensive encephalopathy should remain a diagnosis of exclusion.

Neuroradiologic Features

The most characteristic imaging pattern in hypertensive encephalopathy is the presence of edema involving the white matter of the posterior portions of both cerebral hemispheres, especially the parietooccipital regions (Fig. 37-2), in a relatively symmetric pattern.[4-7] The calcarine and paramedian occipital lobe structures are usually spared, a feature that could help distinguish hypertensive encephalopathy from bilateral infarction in the posterior cerebral artery territory.[4] The involvement of other posterior structures, such as the cerebellum and brainstem, is common. Isolated or predominant posterior fossa lesions (Fig. 37-3) are more scarce.[21,22] In some rare cases, the posterior fossa lesions are severe enough to cause hydrocephalus.[23] Spinal cord involvement has been reported.[24] Although the abnormalities affect primarily the subcortical white matter, the cortex and the basal ganglia may also be involved. A tendency for the milder cases to have a greater involvement of gray than white matter has been reported, suggesting that the edema may originate in the cortex.[25] Imaging findings that may be regarded as

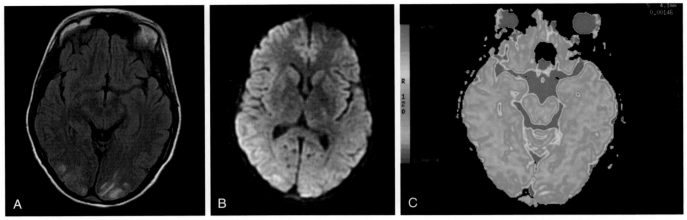

Figure 37-2 Eclampsia in a 28-year-old woman, who had severe headaches, generalized seizures, and blurred vision, and complete clinical recovery after delivery. A, Axial fluid-attenuated inversion recovery (FLAIR) MR image showing bilateral high signal in the occipital regions. B, Diffusion-weighted MR image with normal signal in the occipital regions. C, ADC (apparent diffusion coefficient) MRI map showing increased ADC in the posterior regions.

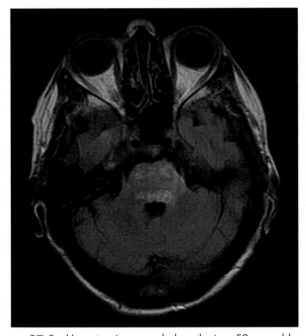

Figure 37-3 Hypertensive encephalopathy in a 52-year-old man. The patient presented with headache, nausea, and unsteady gait. He was drowsy and dysarthric. His blood pressure was 230 mm Hg systolic/150 mm Hg diastolic. This axial fluid-attenuated inversion recovery (FLAIR) MR image shows an extensive increased signal in the brainstem. After blood pressure was controlled, neurologic symptoms improved over days. MRI control 7 weeks later showed complete resolution of abnormalities.

atypical, such as significant anterior involvement, hemorrhagic lesions, signal enhancement due to disruption of the blood-brain barrier, and unilateral lesions are possible.[6,26-29]

The abnormalities are often apparent on CT scan but are best depicted by MRI.[28,29] The most commonly observed abnormalities on MRI are punctate or confluent areas of increased foci on proton density and T2-weighted images. Fluid-attenuated inversion recovery (FLAIR)

sequences improve the ability to detect subtle peripheral lesions and have showed cortical lesions to be more common than previously thought.[25] Gradient-echo imaging may reveal petechial hemorrhages.[29] Large parenchymal hemorrhages have been described in severe cases.[28,29]

In most patients who undergo follow-up CT or MRI, these striking findings usually regress after appropriate therapy, suggesting transient edema rather than true infarction.[4-6] When typical clinical risk factors are not present, follow-up MRI may be key in the diagnosis. However, initial differentiation between reversible and permanent parenchymal lesions cannot be made on the basis of conventional MRI or CT. Recurrent episodes of hypertensive encephalopathy have been occasionally reported.[30]

Diffusion-weighted MRI sequences show increased apparent diffusion coefficient (ADC) in the involved brain regions consistent with vasogenic edema in the majority of cases (see Fig. 37-2), with a predominant watershed distribution.[31-35] These areas with increased ADC values may appear hyperintense, hypointense, or isointense on diffusion-weighted imaging (DWI), depending on the amount of the "T2 shine-through" effect. Interpretation of diffusion-weighted MR images alone, without the benefit of quantitative diffusion information, may underestimate the extension of lesions.[33,36]

ADC values provide a wealth of prognostic information. Lesions with high ADC values are most often reversible, whereas those with decreased ADC values usually progress to true infarction.[6,33,36-38] The extent of signal changes on T2-weighted MRI and DWI and of ADC values seem to correlate well with patient outcome and can help guide more aggressive treatment in more severely affected patients.

Both single-photon emission CT[7] and perfusion-weighted MRI[39] have shown preserved or increased perfusion to edematous portions of the brain in patients with hypertensive encephalopathy. These data support the hypothesis that the condition begins with hyperperfusion, resulting in failure of autoregulation and breakthrough accumulation of vasogenic edema. Further perfusion-weighted imaging is needed to clarify the precise evolution of lesions in hypertensive encephalopathy.

Diffuse vasoconstriction, focal vasoconstriction, vasodilatation, and even string of beads appearance, consistent with vasospasm, have been demonstrated at catheter or MR angiography in patients with eclampsia and preeclampsia.[40-42] Results of follow-up MRA demonstrated reversibility of this vasculopathy.[7] These imaging features are close to those of reversible cerebral vasoconstriction syndrome,[43] which has been associated with various conditions such as postpartum state and exposure to various vasoactive substances.

Causes

Hypertensive encephalopathy occurs as a result of a sudden, sustained rise in blood pressure, from any cause, sufficient to exceed the upper limit of cerebral blood flow autoregulation. As would be predicted from the physiology of autoregulation (see earlier discussion), the degree of hypertension required to precipitate encephalopathy depends on the premorbid pressure. Previously normotensive individuals can show signs of encephalopathy at blood pressures as low as 160 mm Hg systolic, 100 mm Hg diastolic (160/100 mm Hg).[12] The condition may occur at any age but is most common in the second to fourth decades of life.

Antihypertensive treatment has markedly reduced the incidence of hypertensive encephalopathy in individuals with known hypertension. However, abrupt elevations of blood pressure (characteristically above 220/110 mm Hg) in patients with chronic hypertension who are receiving either no treatment or insufficient treatment or in patients whose treatment has been discontinued may cause hypertensive encephalopathy. Acute or chronic renal disease (acute glomerular nephropathy, renal artery stenosis, renal infarction, renal failure) is one of the most common causes of hypertensive encephalopathy.[12] Whether the greater tendency toward development of hypertensive encephalopathy in patients with renal hypertension than in those with essential hypertension is related to increased circulating permeability factors or to endothelial damage remains to be determined.

Eclampsia is usually considered a form of hypertensive encephalopathy on the basis of similarities in clinical, radiologic, and pathologic features.[17,44,45] The fluid accumulation often observed during pregnancy may accentuate the tendency for brain edema to develop. However, there is not always a good correlation between symptoms and signs of eclampsia and level of blood pressure.[46] Several findings suggest that vascular endothelial damage may play a role in preeclampsia/eclampsia.[46,47] Preeclampsia/eclampsia is a multisystem disorder characterized by abnormal vascular response to placentation that is associated with increased systemic vascular resistance, enhanced platelet aggregation, activation of the coagulation system, and endothelial cell dysfunction.[48] The increase in peripheral resistance and blood pressure may be mediated, at least in part, by a substantial increase in sympathetic vasoconstrictor activity, as suggested by a study that used intraneural recordings of sympathetic nerve activity in skeletal muscle nerve fascicles of women

with preeclampsia.[49] The precise mechanism underlying the increased sympathetic nerve activity remains, however, to be determined. Endothelial damage is thought to be due to the secretion of trophoblastic cytotoxic factors originating from a poorly perfused fetoplacental unit. Generalized endothelial dysfunction may lead to (1) increased sensitivity to normally circulating pressor agents and impaired synthesis of vasoactive compounds, which may result in vasospasm and reduced organ perfusion, (2) platelet activation with transitory platelet-rich microvascular occlusion, (3) activation of the coagulation cascade, and (4) loss of fluid from the intravascular compartment.[50]

Other clinical situations associated with hypertensive encephalopathy include vasculitis (systemic lupus erythematosus, polyarteritis nodosa); endocrine disorders (pheochromocytoma, primary aldosteronism); porphyria; thermal injury; scorpion envenomation; cocaine or amphetamine abuse; and use of over-the-counter stimulants (phenylpropanolamine hydrochloride, ephedrine, pseudoephedrine, caffeine).[5,6,12,51] Hypertensive encephalopathy may also occur in previously normotensive patients after bilateral carotid endarterectomy, in association with carotid baroreceptor failure syndrome.[52]

Hinchey and colleagues[4] reported on 15 patients with a reversible syndrome of headache, altered mental status, seizures, and visual loss, associated with posterior white matter changes on neuroimaging, that they termed reversible posterior leukoencephalopathy syndrome. Of the 15 patients, 7 were receiving immunosuppressive therapy (cyclosporine or tacrolimus) after transplantation or as treatment for aplastic anemia, 1 was receiving interferon-alpha for melanoma, 3 had eclampsia, and 4 had hypertensive encephalopathy. Most of the patients had an abrupt increase in blood pressure, but 3 of 15 were normotensive. Because MRI has shown that lesions can occur in both gray and white matter, a new name, *posterior reversible encephalopathy syndrome* (PRES), was coined.[6,25,51] This clinicoradiologic syndrome has been subsequently described in children[53] and has been recognized in a growing number of medical conditions, including disorders such as myeloproliferative disorders, human immunodeficiency virus (HIV) infection, thrombotic thrombocytopenic purpura, and hemolytic-uremic syndrome; treatment with erythropoietin, granulocyte-stimulating factor, intravenous immunoglobulin, interleukin, immunosuppressant agents such as cisplatin, cytarabine, and vincristine, cyclosporine, tacrolimus, gemcitabine, and tiazofurin; antiangiogenic therapies; blood transfusion; and exposure to contrast media.[5,6,51] Although most of the patients had some degree of hypertension, blood pressure levels were usually lower than those typically encountered with pure hypertensive encephalopathy.

Failure of the autoregulatory capabilities of the cerebral vessels, itself resulting from various mechanisms, including hypertension and endothelial dysfunction, may represent a common pathophysiologic mechanism leading to this syndrome. Immunosuppressive drugs can damage the blood-brain barrier by various means: direct toxic effects on the vascular endothelium, endothelial dysfunction secondary to the vascular endothelial growth factor (VEGF) inhibition, vasoconstriction caused by release of endothelin, and increases in thromboxane and prostacyclin causing microthrombi.[4,51] The additional role of seizures has been suggested.[4,51,54] Seizures can result in elevations of blood pressure, regional hyperperfusion breakdown of the blood-brain barrier, and vasogenic edema. Infection, shock, or severe metabolic abnormalities (e.g., hyponatremia, hypomagnesemia, hypercalcemia, renal or hepatic dysfunction) may also be contributing factors.[4,6,51] Hypertension may therefore be the sole cause leading to PRES or may act as a contributing factor.

Treatment

Hypertensive encephalopathy is regarded as a hypertensive emergency, which is defined as any situation that requires immediate blood pressure reduction (not necessarily to normal ranges) to prevent or limit target organ damage. As there have been no large clinical trials, treatment of hypertensive encephalopathy is dictated by consensus.[12]

Most experts recommend that mean arterial blood pressure should not be lowered by more than 20% during the first hour, with a target diastolic blood pressure of 100 to 110 mm Hg.[55] If possible, patients should be admitted to an intensive care unit, and the blood pressure lowered under constant monitoring. Intravenous administration of antihypertensive drugs is generally preferred. Excessive drops in pressure must be avoided, particularly in the elderly patient and the patient with preexisting hypertension, because they may precipitate renal, cerebral, or coronary ischemia. Although not evidence-based, the use of anticonvulsants in patients with hypertensive encephalopathy who are having seizures is reasonable.[12,55]

Suitable agents in the management of hypertensive encephalopathy must satisfy a number of criteria, as follows: are usable by intravenous injection, have rapid onset of action, and are easily titrated with a short half-life allowing more flexible use. The drugs proposed include nicardipine, urapidil, labetalol, and sodium nitroprusside.[12,55,56] There is insufficient evidence from randomized controlled trials to determine which drug or drug class is most effective in reducing mortality and morbidity.[57]

Nicardipine is a second-generation calcium channel antagonist. It is an arterial vasodilator with no negative inotropic activity. The onset of action of intravenous nicardipine is 5 to 15 minutes from administration, with a duration of action of 4 to 6 hours. Nicardipine has been demonstrated to increase coronary blood flow with favorable effect on myocardial oxygen balance. As a result of its rapid onset of action, its ease of use (dosage independent of body weight), and its demonstrated efficacy, nicardipine has become the first-line treatment for hypertensive emergencies.[55,56]

Labetalol has both α-blocking and β-blocking activity, with a recognized value in the majority of hypertensive emergencies except for acute heart failure. The β-blocking effect of labetalol is about a fifth that of propranolol. The hypotensive effect of labetalol begins within 2 to 5 minutes, reaching a peak at 5 to 15 minutes after administration and lasting for about 2 to 4 hours. It has the advantage of maintaining cardiac output and cerebral and coronary blood flow, and it is associated with good clinical safety, provided that the usual contraindications to β-blockers are observed. Adverse effects include nausea, vomiting, and flushing. Bradycardia, heart block, bronchospasm, and heart failure can also complicate its use.[12,55,56]

Urapidil is a peripheral A1 postsynaptic receptor antagonist as well as a central 5-hydroxytryptamine 1A receptor agonist. Its vasodilatory action is not accompanied by reflex tachycardia or any significant modification of the renin-angiotensin system. Urapidil decreases both cardiac preload and afterload and also induces selective pulmonary and renal vasodilatation. It has a good safety profile; its single contraindication is aortic stenosis.[55] Sodium nitroprusside is a short-acting arterial and venous dilatator that induces a simultaneous reduction in cardiac preload and afterload, making it useful in the treatment of hypertensive crises accompanied by heart failure. It should be given only by continuous intravenous infusion (0.25-2 µg/kg/min). However, several of the following factors limit its use. First, by increasing intracranial pressure, nitroprusside decreases the cerebral flow rate. Second, it is common for blood pressure to be unintentionally below a safe target level during treatment. Third, nitroprusside promotes baroreflex activation, causing tachycardia that can exacerbate acute coronary syndromes and heart failure. Other complications include cyanate or thiocyanate toxicity when the drug is given for a long period (days), especially in patients with hepatic or renal dysfunction. Finally, nitroprusside infusion requires intra-arterial monitoring of blood pressure, which may not otherwise be required. It is now less widely used as first-line treatment because of its adverse effects and the availability of other drugs that are easier to use.[12,55,56]

Other parenteral drugs used for hypertensive emergencies include fenoldopam, a selective postsynaptic dopamine-1 receptor agonist. Reported side effects of fenoldopam include headache, flushing, and increased intraocular pressure. Enalaprilat is an angiotensin-converting enzyme inhibitor available for intravenous administration. Its onset of action is delayed for 15 minutes, and it does not reach peak effect for about 1 hour. The relative slow onset limits its use in hypertensive encephalopathy. In addition, angiotensin-converting enzyme inhibitors should be used cautiously in patients who are hypovolemic or in those with underlying renal artery stenosis, because these drugs can lead to precipitous falls in blood pressure. Intravenous hydralazine is a commonly administered arteriolar vasodilator that is effective for hypertensive emergencies associated with pregnancies. The most common adverse effect of hydralazine administration is unpredictable hypotension.[58] Phentolamine, clonidine, and diazoxide are no longer part of the treatment of hypertensive emergencies.

Oral therapy should be instituted before parenteral agents are discontinued.

The management of hypertensive encephalopathy also includes early recognition and removal of exacerbating factors such as immunosuppressive drugs.[4] Delivery is the ultimate cure for eclampsia. If convulsions have occurred, parenteral magnesium sulfate is the treatment of choice.[59] The role of prophylactic magnesium sulfate in preeclampsia is less clear. There is also long-standing experience with several suitable antihypertensive drugs. The parenteral antihypertensive drugs most commonly used during pregnancy are labetalol, nicardipine, hydralazine, and urapidil.[55,58,60] Angiotensin-converting enzyme inhibitors and angiotensin receptor antagonists are contraindicated in pregnancy because of unacceptable fetal side effects.

REFERENCES

1. Oppenheimer BS, Fishberg AM: Hypertensive encephalopathy, *Arch Intern Med* 41:264-278, 1928.
2. Dinsdale HB: Hypertensive encephalopathy, *Stroke* 13:717-719, 1982.
3. Healton EB, Brust JC, Feinfeld DA, et al: Hypertensive encephalopathy and the neurologic manifestations of malignant hypertension, *Neurology* 32:127-132, 1982.
4. Hinchey J, Chaves C, Appignani B, et al: A reversible posterior leucoencephalopathy syndrome, *N Engl J Med* 334:494-500, 1996.
5. Lamy C, Oppenheim C, Meder JF, et al: Neuroimaging in posterior reversible encephalopathy syndrome, *J Neuroimaging* 14:89-96, 2004.
6. Lee VH, Wijdicks EF, Manno EM, et al: Clinical spectrum of reversible posterior leukoencephalopathy syndrome, *Arch Neurol* 65:205-210, 2008.
7. Schwartz RB, Jones KM, Kalina P, et al: Hypertensive encephalopathy: Findings on CT, MR imaging and SPECT imaging in 14 cases, *AJR Am J Roentgenol* 159:379-383, 1992.
8. Bartynski WS: Posterior reversible encephalopathy syndrome, part 2: Controversies surrounding pathophysiology of vasogenic edema, *AJNR Am J Neuroradiol* 29:1043-1049, 2008.
9. Hinchey JA: Reversible posterior leukoencephalopathy syndrome: What have we learned in the last 10 years? *Arch Neurol* 65:175-176, 2008.
10. Strandgaard S, Paulson OB: Cerebral autoregulation, *Stroke* 15:415, 1984.
11. Slama M, Modeliar SS: Hypertension in the intensive care unit, *Curr Opin Cardiol* 21:279-287, 2006.
12. Vaughan CJ, Delanty N: Hypertensive emergencies, *Lancet* 356:411-417, 2000.
13. Heistad DD: What's new in the cerebral microcirculation? *Microcirculation* 8:365-375, 2001.
14. Beausang-Linder M, Bill A: Cerebral circulation in acute arterial hypertension: Protective effect of sympathetic nervous activity, *Acta Physiol Scand* 111:193-199, 1981.
15. Bill A, Linder J: Sympathetic control of cerebral blood flow in acute arterial hypertension, *Acta Physiol Scand* 96:114-121, 1976.
16. Chester EM, Agamanolis DP, Banker BQ, et al: Hypertensive encephalopathy: A clinicopathologic study of 20 cases, *Neurology* 28:928-939, 1978.
17. Richards A, Graham D, Bullock R: Clinicopathological study of neurological complications due to hypertensive disorders of pregnancy, *J Neurol Neurosurg Psychiatry* 51:416-421, 1988.
18. Schiff D, Lopes MB: Neuropathological correlates of reversible posterior leukoencephalopathy, *Neurocrit Care* 2:303-305, 2005.
19. Tallaksen CM, Kerty E, Bakke S: Visual hallucinations in a case of reversible hypertension-induced brain oedema, *Eur J Neurol* 5:615-618, 1998.
20. Bakshi R, Bates V, Mechtler L, et al: Occipital seizures as the major clinical manifestation of reversible posterior leukoencephalopathy syndrome: Magnetic resonance imaging findings, *Epilepsia* 39:296-299, 1998.
21. Casey SO, Truwit CL: Pontine reversible edema: A newly recognized imaging variant of hypertensive encephalopathy? *AJNR Am J Neuroradiol* 21:243-245, 2000.
22. Sèze JD, Mastain B, Stojkovic T, et al: Unusual MR findings of the brainstem in arterial hypertension, *AJNR Am J Neuroradiol* 21:391-394, 2000.
23. Wang MC, Escott EJ, Breeze RE: Posterior fossa swelling hydrocephalus resulting from hypertensive encephalopathy: Case report and review of the literature, *Neurosurgery* 44:1325-1327, 1999.
24. Milia A, Moller J, Pilia G, et al: Spinal cord involvement during hypertensive encephalopathy: Clinical and radiological findings, *J Neurol* 255:142-143, 2008.
25. Casey SO, Sampaio RC, Michel E, et al: Posterior reversible encephalopathy syndrome: Utility of fluid-attenuated inversion recovery MR imaging in the detection of cortical and subcortical lesions, *AJNR Am J Neuroradiol* 21:1199-1206, 2000.
26. Bartynski WS, Boardman JF: Distinct imaging patterns and lesion distribution in posterior reversible encephalopathy syndrome, *AJNR Am J Neuroradiol* 28:1320-1327, 2007.
27. McKinney AM, Short J, Truwit CL, et al: Posterior reversible encephalopathy syndrome: Incidence of atypical regions of involvement and imaging findings, *AJR Am J Roentgenol* 189:904-912, 2007.
28. Schwartz RB, Bravo SM, Klufas RA, et al: Cyclosporine neurotoxicity and its relationship to hypertensive encephalopathy: CT and MR findings in 16 cases, *AJR Am J Roentgenol* 165:627-631, 1995.
29. Weingarten K, Barbut D, Filippi C, et al: Acute hypertensive encephalopathy: Findings on spin-echo and gradient-echo MR imaging, *AJR Am J Roentgenol* 162:665-670, 1994.
30. Kanazawa M, Sanpei K, Kasuga K: Recurrent hypertensive brainstem encephalopathy, *J Neurol Neurosurg Psychiatry* 76:888-890, 2005.
31. Coley SC, Porter DA, Calamante F, et al: Quantitative MR diffusion mapping and cyclosporine induced neurotoxicity, *AJNR Am J Neuroradiol* 20:1507-1510, 1999.
32. Engelter ST, Provenzale JM, Petrella JR: Assessment of vasogenic edema in eclampsia using diffusion imaging, *Neuroradiology* 42:818-820, 2000.
33. Provenzale JM, Petrella JR, Cruz LCH, et al: Quantitative assessment of diffusion abnormalities in posterior reversible encephalopathy syndrome, *AJNR Am J Neuroradiol* 22:1455-1461, 2001.
34. Schaefer PW, Buonanno FS, Gonzales RG, et al: Diffusion-weighted imaging discriminates between cytotoxic and vasogenic edema in a patient with eclampsia, *Stroke* 28:1082-1085, 1997.
35. Schwartz RB, Mulkern RV, Gudbjartsson H, et al: Diffusion-weighted MR imaging in hypertensive encephalopathy: Clues to pathogenesis, *AJNR Am J Neuroradiol* 19:859-862, 1998.
36. Covarrubias DJ, Luetmer PH, Campeau NG: Posterior reversible encephalopathy syndrome: Prognostic utility of quantitative diffusion-weighted MR images, *AJNR Am J Neuroradiol* 23:1038-1048, 2002.
37. Ay H, Buonanno F, Schaefer P, et al: Posterior leukoencephalopathy without severe hypertension: Utility of diffusion-weighted MRI, *Neurology* 51:1369-1376, 1998.
38. Koch S, Rabinstein A, Falcone S, et al: Diffusion-weighted imaging shows cytotoxic and vasogenic edema in eclampsia, *AJNR Am J Neuroradiol* 22:1068-1070, 2001.
39. Jones BV, Egelhoff JC, Patterson RJ: Hypertensive encephalopathy in children, *Am J Neuroradiol* 18:101-106, 1997.
40. Bartynski WS, Boardman JF: Catheter angiography, MR angiography, and MR perfusion in posterior reversible encephalopathy syndrome, *AJNR Am J Neuroradiol* 29:447-455, 2008.
41. Trommer B, Homer D, Mikhael M: Cerebral vasospasm and eclampsia, *Stroke* 19:326-329, 1988.
42. Tsukimori K, Ochi H, Yumoto Y, et al: Reversible posterior encephalopathy syndrome followed by MR angiography-documented cerebral vasospasm in preeclampsia-eclampsia: Report of 2 cases, *Cerebrovasc Dis* 25:377-380, 2008.
43. Ducros A, Boukobza M, Porcher R, et al: The clinical and radiological spectrum of reversible cerebral vasoconstriction syndrome: A prospective series of 67 patients, *Brain* 130:3091-3101, 2007.
44. Digre KB, Varner MW, Osborn AG, et al: Cranial magnetic resonance imaging in severe preeclampsia vs eclampsia, *Arch Neurol* 50:399-406, 1993.
45. Manfredi M, Beltramello A, Bongiovanni LG, et al: Eclamptic encephalopathy: Imaging and pathogenetic considerations, *Acta Neurol Scand* 96:277-282, 1997.
46. Schwartz RB, Feske SK, Polak JF, et al: Preeclampsia-eclampsia: Clinical and neuroradiographic correlates and insights into the pathogenesis of hypertensive encephalopathy, *Radiology* 217:371-376, 2000.
47. Mas JL, Lamy C: Severe preeclampsia/eclampsia: Hypertensive encephalopathy of pregnancy? *Cerebrovasc Dis* 8:53-58, 1998.
48. Sibai B, Dekker G, Kupferminc M: Pre-eclampsia, *Lancet* 365:785-799, 2005.
49. Schobel HP, Fischer T, Heuszer K, et al: Preeclampsia—a state of sympathetic overactivity, *N Engl J Med* 335:1480-1485, 1996.
50. Roberts JM, Redman CWG: Pre-eclampsia: More than pregnancy-induced hypertension, *Lancet* 34:1447-1450, 1993.

51. Bartynski WS: Posterior reversible encephalopathy syndrome, part 1: Fundamental imaging and clinical features, *AJNR Am J Neuroradiol* 29:1036-1042, 2008.

52. Ille O, Woimant F, Pruna A, et al: Hypertensive encephalopathy after bilateral endarterectomy, *Stroke* 26:488-491, 1995.

53. Pavlakis SG, Frank Y, Chusid R: Hypertensive encephalopathy, reversible occipitoparietal encephalopathy or reversible posterior leukoencephalopathy: Three names for an old syndrome, *J Child Neurol* 14:277-281, 1999.

54. Obeid T, Shami A, Karsou S: The role of seizures in reversible posterior leukoencephalopathy, *Seizure* 13:277-281, 2004.

55. Slama M, Modeliar SS: Hypertension in the intensive care unit, *Curr Opin Cardiol* 21:279-287, 2006.

56. Varon J: Treatment of acute severe hypertension: current and newer agents, *Drugs* 68:283-297, 2008.

57. Perez MI, Musini VM: Pharmacological interventions for hypertensive emergencies: A Cochrane Systematic Review, *J Hum Hypertens* 22:596-607, 2008.

58. McCoy S, Baldwin K: Pharmacotherapeutic options for the treatment of preeclampsia, *Am J Health Syst Pharm* 66:337-344, 2009.

59. Duley L, Gulmezoglu AM, Henderson-Smart DJ: Magnesium sulphate and other anticonvulsants for women with pre-eclampsia, *Cochrane Database Syst Rev* (2):CD000025, 2003.

60. Sibai B, Dekker G, Kupferminc M: Pre-eclampsia, *Lancet* 365:785-799, 2005.

38 Atherosclerotic Disease of the Proximal Aorta

MARCO R. DI TULLIO, SHUNICHI HOMMA

The presence of atherosclerotic plaques in the aorta is a risk factor for ischemic stroke. The proximal portion of the aorta, where the origin of blood vessels that supply the brain is located, may be the site of origin of cerebral embolism, providing an explanation for cerebral ischemic events otherwise considered of unknown etiology. This chapter reviews the principal studies on the association of aortic plaques and ischemic stroke and the related diagnostic and therapeutic issues.

Frequency of Aortic Plaques in the General Population

The atherosclerotic process in the aorta develops throughout life but becomes especially evident after the fourth decade, and the prevalence and number of atherosclerotic lesions increase continuously thereafter. In the Stroke Prevention: Assessment of Risk in a Community (SPARC) study,[1] the prevalence of "simple" (plaques <4 mm in thickness, without ulceration or mobile debris) or "complex" (plaques ≥4 mm or with complex features) atherosclerotic lesions was evaluated by transesophageal echocardiography (TEE) in 588 volunteers older than 44 years. Overall, aortic atherosclerosis of any degree and complex atherosclerosis in any segment of the aorta were present in 51.3% and 7.6% of subjects, respectively. Atherosclerosis of any degree was identified in the ascending aorta in 8.4%, the aortic arch in 31.0%, and the descending aorta in 44.9% of subjects; corresponding figures for complex atherosclerosis were 0.2%, 2.2%, and 6.0%. Atherosclerosis of any degree in any aortic segment was found to increase from approximately 17% in the group 45 to 54 years old to more than 80% in subjects older than 75 years. Complex atherosclerosis was virtually absent in the younger subgroup but was seen in more than 20% of patients older than 75 years. In a TEE study from Australia on healthy volunteers older than 59 years, the prevalence of simple plaques in the aortic arch was 22%, and that of complicated plaques (≥5 mm or with an irregular, ulcerated surface) was 4%.[2]

The prevalence of aortic atherosclerosis in the general population may depend on the characteristics, and especially the risk factor distribution, of the sample studied. In the triethnic study group of the Aortic Plaque and Risk of Ischemic Stroke (APRIS) study, TEE showed the prevalence of aortic arch atherosclerosis of any degree in 209 stroke-free volunteers older than 55 years from northern Manhattan to be 62.2%, and that of large (≥4 mm) arch plaques 23.9%.[3] These figures, which are much higher than those in the other studies, were obtained in patients with a greater burden of atherosclerotic risk factors. The APRIS study group had higher frequencies of diabetes (23.0% vs. 8.9%), hypertension (69.4% vs. 55.2%), and both past and current smoking history (60.3% vs. 39.0% and 16.1% vs. 8.2%, respectively) than the SPARC subjects.

Aortic Plaques and Ischemic Stroke
Pathology Studies

The first report of a strong association between aortic arch plaques and ischemic stroke came from a large autopsy case-control study conducted in France by Amarenco and colleagues and published in 1992.[4] The researchers showed a much greater frequency of ulcerated aortic plaques in elderly patients who had died from a stroke than in patients who had died from other neurologic diseases (26% vs. 5%; age-adjusted odds ratio [OR] 4.0; 95% confidence interval [CI], 2.1-7.8). Importantly, the highest frequency of ulcerated plaques was observed in patients with unexplained (cryptogenic) stroke (61% vs. 28%; adjusted OR 5.7; 95% CI, 2.4-3.6), thus providing a potential pathogenic mechanism for the stroke. The lack of association between ulcerated plaques and presence of significant carotid artery stenosis and atrial fibrillation, two other important sources for brain embolism, suggested an independent role of aortic plaques in the stroke risk. Among patients with ulcerated plaques, only 3% were younger than 60 years, suggesting that ulcerated plaques could be a new potential stroke risk factor exclusively in elderly subjects.

In a 1996 necropsy study, Khatibzadeh and coworkers[5] found evidence of arterial embolization in 40 of 120 unselected patients (33%). Complicated aortic arch plaques were significantly associated with arterial embolism (OR, 5.8; 95% CI, 1.1-31.7), independent of and with a similar strength to the associations of severe ipsilateral carotid artery disease and atrial fibrillation with arterial embolism.

In Vivo Studies—Transesophageal Echocardiography

TEE, the most sensitive and most widely used technique for examining the proximal portion of the aorta, has allowed the study of the association between aortic plaques and

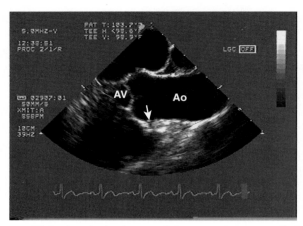

Figure 38-1 Longitudinal view of the ascending aorta (Ao) by transesophageal echocardiography. The entire ascending aorta is visualized from the aortic valve (AV) to the initial curvature of the aortic arch. The takeoff of the right coronary artery is visible *(arrow).*

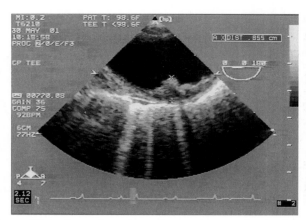

Figure 38-3 Protruding atherosclerotic plaque in the distal aortic arch. Measurement of plaque thickness, perpendicular to the major axis of the aortic lumen, is shown. Plaque thickness (0.855 cm) is displayed in the upper right corner.

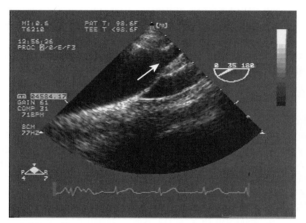

Figure 38-2 Transesophageal echocardiography visualization of the midportion to distal portion of the aortic arch. The takeoff of the left subclavian artery is visible *(arrow).*

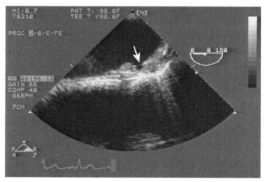

Figure 38-4 Complex plaque in the distal aortic arch. A large ulceration *(arrow)* is visible.

ischemic stroke in vivo. The proximity of the esophagus to the aorta and the absence of interposed structures allow the use of high-frequency ultrasound transducers, providing high-resolution images of the vessel. In the search for aortic plaques as the potential cause of ischemic stroke, the portion of aorta proximal to the takeoff of the left subclavian artery is the focus of the examination. Although the existence of retrograde diastolic flow has been demonstrated in the aorta,[6,7] its occurrence is probably an infrequent mechanism for embolization to the brain. Therefore, plaques that are located more distally in the aorta are an unlikely cause of stroke. The initial portion of the aorta can be accurately visualized by TEE from the aortic valve level to the initial curvature of the arch (Fig. 38-1). The midportion and distal portions of the aortic arch are also visible in all patients (Fig. 38-2). A small portion of the vessel (proximal arch) cannot be visualized owing to the interposition of the trachea and is therefore a "blind spot" in the examination, although the introduction of multiplane transducers has allowed for a more complete visualization of the vessel in most patients. It is possible to make an

accurate TEE assessment for the presence of plaques and their thickness (Fig. 38-3), as well as for the presence of ulcerations (Fig. 38-4) or superimposed thrombus (Figs. 38-5 to 38-7). TEE has been shown to be highly sensitive and specific in the detection of aortic plaques.[8,9] Its diagnostic accuracy for presence of thrombus is also high (sensitivity 91%, specificity 90%).[9] However, the sensitivity of TEE for detecting small ulcerations of the plaque surface, which may carry an additional risk for further embolic events,[2,10,11] has been described as less than optimal (approximately 75%).[6,7] The reproducibility of TEE measurements of aortic plaque thickness has been shown to be very good, with agreement of 84% to 88% for the diagnosis of large ($\geq$4 mm) plaque.[12]

TEE is a safe, although semi-invasive, diagnostic test. Major complications are uncommon and due mainly to unsuspected preexisting esophageal disease. In a European series of more than 10,000 patients,[13] one death was observed. In an additional 2.7% of patients, the test could not be performed because of unsuccessful intubation (1.9%) or patient intolerance (0.8%). Similar results were obtained in a study from the Mayo Clinic involving 15,381 consecutive patients, with two deaths

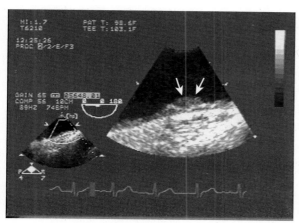

Figure 38-5 Enlarged view of a plaque in the midportion of the aortic arch. Hypoechoic material suggestive of thrombus *(arrows)* appears superimposed on the brightly echogenic plaque.

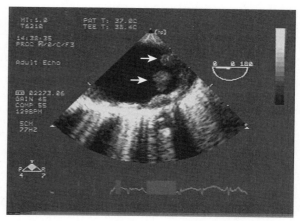

Figure 38-7 Complex atherosclerotic plaque of the distal aortic arch. Two large thrombi *(arrows)* are visible.

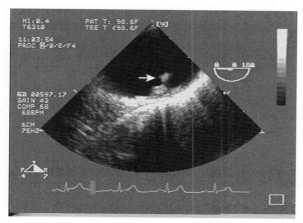

Figure 38-6 Complex plaque in the midportion of the aortic arch. A large pedunculated portion can be seen *(arrow)*, which was highly mobile in real-time imaging.

(0.01%) and a 1.7% overall incidence of complications.[14] In another series of 901 patients, intubation was unsuccessful in 1.2% of cases, there were no deaths, and a low incidence (0.6%) of major complications was observed.[15] Our experience in patients with stroke has shown no higher frequency of patient discomfort, unsuccessful intubation, or significant complications.[16] Moreover, the test can be safely performed even in patients of very advanced age.[17]

Case-Control Studies

Tunick and colleagues[18] first reported a higher frequency of aortic plaques 5 mm or thicker in 122 patients referred for TEE with a history of arterial embolism than in 122 age- and sex-matched patients with other cardiologic diagnoses (27% vs. 9%; OR, 3.2; 95% CI, 1.6-6.5). This retrospective study, in which data were not adjusted for other potential embolic sources, was followed by other case-control studies that focused on the risk of ischemic stroke associated with TEE-detected aortic arch plaques. The principal studies in this category are summarized in Table 38-1. Amarenco and colleagues[19] studied 250 patients

with acute ischemic stroke older than 60 years and 250 controls. They found that arch plaques between 1 and 3.9 mm in thickness were associated with stroke after adjustment for conventional stroke risk factors (adjusted OR, 4.4) but that a sharp increase in risk was present for plaques 4 mm or thicker (adjusted OR, 9.1; 95% CI, 3.3-25.2). Also, only the stroke risk associated with plaques 4 mm or thicker was independent of the presence of carotid stenosis and atrial fibrillation.[19] The investigators speculated that the sharp increase in risk observed for larger plaques might depend on the more frequent presence of superimposed thrombus, which would be included in the measurement of plaque thickness, and to a more frequent presence of mobile components, a circumstance also observed in other studies.[20] In this study, plaques 4 mm or thicker were also significantly more frequent in patients with cryptogenic stroke than in patients with stroke of determined origin (28.2% vs. 8.1%; OR, 4.7; 95% CI, 2.2-10.1).

Similar results, except for the association with cryptogenic stroke, were obtained in an Australian study by Jones and coworkers,[2] who studied 215 patients with stroke and 202 healthy volunteers older than 59 years (see Table 38-1). In that study, plaques 5 mm or more in thickness or with ulcerated or mobile components were associated with a much greater stroke risk (adjusted OR, 7.1; 95% CI, 2.7-18.4) than smaller, smooth plaques (adjusted OR, 2.3; 95% CI, 1.2-4.2). However, the frequency of large or complex plaques was similar in patients with cryptogenic stroke (20%) and in patients with stroke of determined origin (23%).

In 106 patients with stroke older than 40 years and 114 age- and gender-matched controls, we found an increased risk of stroke associated with aortic plaques 5 or more mm in thickness (adjusted OR, 2.6; 95% CI, 1.1-5.9).[10] The risk was entirely due to the subgroup of patients older than 59 years, whereas the prevalence of large plaques was very low (3%) both in patients with stroke and in controls younger than that age cutoff (see Table 38-1), underscoring that large aortic plaques appear to represent a relevant clinical entity only in the elderly.

TABLE 38-1 ASSOCIATION BETWEEN PROXIMAL AORTIC PLAQUES AND ISCHEMIC STROKE: TRANSESOPHAGEAL ECHOCARDIOGRAPHIC CASE-CONTROL STUDIES

Study (Reference No.)	Cases/Controls (N)	Age (Years)	Type of Atheroma	Controls (%)	Patients with Stroke (%)	Adjusted Odds Ratio* (95% CI)
Amarenco et al[19]	250/250	≥60	1-3.9 mm	22	46	4.4 (2.8–6.8)
			≥4 mm	2	14	9.1 (3.3–25.2)
Jones et al[2]	215/202	≥60	<5 mm, smooth	22	33	2.3 (1.2–4.2)
			≥5 mm, complex	4	22	7.1 (2.7–18.4)
Di Tullio et al[10]	106/114	≥40	≥5 mm	13	26	2.6 (1.1–5.9)
	30/36	<60		3	3	1.2 (0.7–20.2)
	76/78	≥60		18	36	2.4 (1.1–5.7)
Di Tullio et al[22]	255/209	≥55	≥4 mm	24	49	2.4 (1.3–4.6)

*Adjusted for conventional stroke risk factors (also see text).
CI, confidence interval.

TABLE 38-2 RECURRENCE RATE OF EMBOLIC EVENTS AND STROKE IN PATIENTS WITH AND WITHOUT PROXIMAL AORTIC PLAQUES: TRANSESOPHAGEAL ECHOCARDIOGRAPHIC PROSPECTIVE STUDIES

Study (Reference No.)	Aortic Plaque Present/Aortic Plaque Absent (N)	Follow-up (Months)	Type of Plaque	Aortic Plaque Absent (%)	Aortic Plaque Present (%)	Adjusted* Relative Risk (95% CI)
Tunick et al[23]	42/42	14	≥4 mm	7	33	4.3 (1.2–15.0)
Mitusch et al[24]	47/136	16	≥5 mm/mobile vs. <5 mm	4.1/yr	13.7/yr	4.3 (1.5–12.0)
FAPS[25]†	331	24-48	≥4mm	2.8/yr	11.9/yr	3.8 (1.8–7.8)
				5.9/yr	26.0/yr	3.5 (2.1–5.9)
Tanaka et al[26]	42/42	14	≥4mm	7	33	4.3 (1.2–15.0)
Fujimoto et al[27]	42/42	14	≥4 mm	7	33	4.3 (1.2–15.0)

*Adjusted for conventional stroke risk factors (also see text).
†Only study conducted on patients with ischemic stroke. Data in first row refer to recurrence rate of stroke; data in second row refer to recurrence rate of all embolic events.

Using epiaortic ultrasonography instead of TEE, Davila-Roman and associates[21] studied the prevalence of aortic plaques in 1200 subjects older than 49 years undergoing cardiac surgery, 158 of whom had experienced a previous embolic event.[21] The researchers found plaques 3 mm or thicker in 26.6% of patients with a previous cerebrovascular event and in 18.1% of those without it. Aortic plaques, arterial hypertension, atrial fibrillation, and carotid artery stenosis were independently associated with neurologic events in that study.

In a later study, we reported similar results in 255 patients with stroke and in 209 age-, gender-, and race/ethnicity-matched controls from the APRIS study. Large aortic arch plaques (≥4 mm) were again found to be associated with an increased stroke risk after adjustment for other stroke risk factors (adjusted OR, 2.4; 95% CI, 1.3–4.6; see Table 38-1).[22] Complex plaque morphology and coexisting hypercoagulability increased the stroke risk, as discussed later in the chapter.

Prospective Studies

Investigators have also prospectively confirmed the role of aortic arch plaques as a risk factor for peripheral and cerebral embolization, by following up patients who had a first stroke or other embolic event and comparing the embolic recurrence rate in patients with and without proximal aortic plaques (Table 38-2). After a mean follow-up of 14 months, Tunick and colleagues[23] noted a significantly greater incidence of cerebral or peripheral embolic events in 42 patients with protruding aortic atheromas than in control subjects matched for age, gender, and hypertension status (33% vs. 7%; relative risk [RR], 4.3; 95% CI, 1.2–15.0). Similar results were reported by Mitusch and associates[24] in a group of 47 patients with large or mobile arch plaques compared with 136 patients with small or no atheroma. In that study, recurrence rate of embolic events was 13.7% per year in patients with plaques that were either 5 mm or more in thickness or mobile, and 4.1% per year in patients with plaques less than 5 mm thick (RR, 4.3; 95% CI, 1.5–12.0). In a French multicenter study of 331 patients with stroke 60 years or older,[25] arch plaques 4 mm or more in thickness were associated with an almost four-fold increase in risk of recurrent stroke, after data were adjusted for the presence of carotid stenosis, atrial fibrillation, peripheral artery disease, and other conventional risk factors (see Table 38-2). In the subgroup with large plaques, the recurrence rate was highest in patients whose index stroke was cryptogenic (16.4/100 person-years). In that study, the incidence of all vascular events was also significantly greater in patients with large plaques (RR, 3.5; see Table 38-2). The increased risk of recurrent stroke related to large arch plaques was confirmed in two later prospective studies. In 236 patients with ischemic stroke, Tanaka and colleagues[26] observed an increased risk of recurrent stroke or myocardial infarction in patients with arch plaques ≥3.5 mm (see Table 38-2). Fujimoto and coworkers[27] followed up 283 patients with embolic stroke and no significant occlusive lesion in cerebral arteries for a mean 3.4 years. Patients who experienced a recurrent stroke (32, or 11.3%) had significantly higher prevalence of arch plaques ≥4 mm (41% vs. 22%) and of plaque extension to the cephalic branches (63% vs. 39%; see Table 38-2).

In a report from the SPARC study,[1] the importance of the association between aortic atherosclerosis and cerebrovascular events has been questioned. In 581 community-derived subjects who underwent TEE in that study, large (≥4 mm), ulcerated, or mobile plaques were associated with a history of coronary artery disease (OR, 2.35; 95% CI, 1.1–5.0) but not with a history of ischemic stroke (OR, 1.37; 95% CI, 0.44–4.3), leading the investigators of the study to question the importance of aortic plaques as a risk factor for stroke in the community. The inclusion in that study of younger subjects (45 years was the age cutoff for inclusion in the study) may have diluted the strength of the association observed between aortic plaques and stroke. Also, the prevalence of severe plaques in the proximal aorta was low (2.4%). However, we reported similar findings from the follow-up of the control group of the APRIS study (age >54 years), in which the presence of large aortic arch plaques was not associated with stroke and vascular events (hazard ratio [HR], 1.05; 95% CI, 0.37–3.03).[3] These observations suggest that the risk of stroke from arch plaques incidentally detected in otherwise healthy subjects may be lower than that generally reported in the literature, which was obtained in subjects who had previous stroke or peripheral embolic events or were referred for TEE because of another coexisting condition.

Plaque Morphology and Stroke Risk

The role of aortic plaques as a risk factor for stroke has been established mainly on the basis of the thickness of the plaque, with either 4 mm or 5 mm chosen as the threshold for increased risk. It is unclear, however, whether plaque thickness is directly related to the stroke mechanism or is rather a marker of diffuse atherosclerosis, which may in fact be responsible for the increased stroke risk. We have demonstrated that differences exist in the plaque-related stroke risk between genders.[28] In our study, aortic plaques 4 mm or thicker were significantly more frequent in men than in women (31.5% vs. 20.3%; P = .025), and were associated with ischemic stroke in both men (adjusted OR, 6.0; 95% CI, 2.1–16.8) and women (adjusted OR, 3.2; 95% CI, 1.2–8.8), after adjustment for other established stroke risk factors. Plaques 3 to 3.9 mm in thickness, however, were significantly associated with stroke in women (adjusted OR, 4.8; 95% CI, 1.7–15.0) but not in men (adjusted OR, 0.8; 95% CI, 0.2–3.0). This observation suggests that plaque thickness, instead of identifying the actual culprit lesion for the stroke, may

be a marker of diffuse atherosclerosis, including intracranial atherosclerosis, or of other conditions that may differ between genders and are possibly related to the stroke mechanism.[25] In any case, plaque progression, defined as increase in thickness over time, has been shown to be associated with a higher incidence of vascular events. In 117 patients with stroke or transient ischemic attack, those who showed plaque progression over 1 year were significantly more likely to experience a vascular event (stroke, transient ischemic attack, myocardial infarction, or death) over a median follow-up of 1.7 years than those with no plaque progression (51% vs. 11%; P < .0001).[29]

The complex morphology of a plaque appears to be more directly related to the stroke mechanism. As mentioned earlier, morphologic features of the plaque, such as ulceration and mobility, have been linked with an increased stroke risk,[1,5,8-11,20] especially in the case of cryptogenic stroke. Stone and associatees[11] showed a significantly greater frequency of ulcerated plaques in 23 patients with cryptogenic stroke than in 26 patients with stroke of determined origin (39% vs. 8%; P < .001). In our experience in 152 elderly patients with stroke and 152 age-matched controls,[20] ulcerated or mobile plaques were found to be a much stronger risk factor for stroke than large but noncomplex plaques (Table 38-3). Our study confirmed that plaques 4 mm or thicker were indeed associated with an increased stroke risk (adjusted OR, 4.3; 95% CI, 2.1–8.7); however, when these large plaques were divided on the basis of the presence or absence of ulceration (defined as a discrete indentation of at least 2 mm in width and depth) or mobile components, the stroke risk associated with those complex feature was exceedingly high (adjusted OR, 17.1), whereas large but noncomplex plaques carried only a modest increase in risk (adjusted OR, 2.4; see Table 38-3). This difference remained even after patients with other conditions possibly related to stroke, such as atrial fibrillation, carotid stenosis of 60% or greater, and intracranial atherosclerosis, were excluded from the analysis. Cohen and coworkers[30] studied the impact of plaque morphology (ulceration, hypoechoic components, or calcification) on the risk of recurrent vascular events in a prospective study of 334 patients with stroke older than 60 years and followed up for 2 to 4 years. In patients with plaques 4 mm or greater, the presence of ulcerations or hypoechoic components was not found to increase the risk of vascular events. However, the absence of calcification was associated with the strongest increase in risk (adjusted RR, 10.3; 95% CI, 4.2–25.2), and the presence of calcification was found to decrease the risk of subsequent events (adjusted RR, 1.2; 95% CI, 0.6 to 2.1), possibly signaling a more stable lesion.

These observations suggest that although the thickness of the plaque represents the most readily available marker of the risk of embolization associated with arch aortic plaques, the plaque's morphologic features strongly affect the embolic potential of the lesion, possibly opening the field to new therapeutic approaches in individual patients. It should be remembered that whenever TEE identifies a protruding mobile component on a plaque, that component represents thrombus superimposed on atherosclerotic material and usually occurs on ulcerated plaques. This observation has been confirmed by several

TABLE 38-3 EFFECT OF AORTIC PLAQUE MORPHOLOGY ON THE RISK OF ISCHEMIC STROKE

	Patients with Stroke (N = 152)		Control Subjects (N = 152)		Unadjusted Odds Ratio* (95% CI)	Adjusted Odds Ratio* (95% CI)
	N	%	N	%		
No plaque	28	18.4	55	36.2	—	—
Small plaque (<4 mm)†	56	36.8	68	44.7	1.6 (0.9–2.9)	1.9 (1.0–3.6)
Large plaque (≥4 mm)	68	44.8	29	19.1	4.6 (2.5–8.6)	4.3 (2.1–8.7)
Noncomplex plaque	34	22.4	25	16.5	2.7 (1.3–5.3)	2.4 (1.1–5.1)
Complex plaque	34	22.4	4	2.6	16.7 (5.4–51.8)	17.1 (5.1–57.3)
Ulcerated	24	15.8	3	2.0	15.7 (4.4–56.7)	15.8 (4.1–61.4)
Mobile	10	6.6	1	0.7	19.6 (2.4–161.3)	21.3 (2.4–193.2)

*Adjusted for age, gender, arterial hypertension, diabetes mellitus, and hypercholesterolemia.
†No complex forms were present among small plaques.
CI, confidence interval.

studies that have correlated the TEE findings with data derived from the histopathologic examination of the aorta.[4,5,24,25,31,32] Mobile components superimposed on an aortic plaque are infrequently seen in elderly patients with stroke, at a rate ranging from 1.6% to 8.7% in different studies (Table 38-4).[2,8,11,19,20,22,33,34] When present, however, they represent a very strong risk factor for brain embolization. In our study, mobile components superimposed on a plaque were present in 6.6% of elderly patients with stroke and were associated with a more than 20-fold increase in the risk of stroke, after adjustment of data for other conventional stroke risk factors (see Table 38-4).[20] Occasionally, mobile thrombi without severe atherosclerotic changes can be seen in the aortic arch of patients younger than 60 years who present with an embolic event (23 cases out of 27,855 TEE examinations in a multicenter cardiology study).[35] These thrombi, which usually have an insertion site on small atherosclerotic plaques, appear to represent a rare variant of atherosclerotic disease associated with embolic events in younger patients.[35]

The potential for embolism to the brain of large plaques, and even more of complex plaques, has been confirmed with transcranial Doppler ultrasonographic monitoring. With this technique, continuous monitoring of the blood flow into the middle cerebral arteries is obtained. Monitoring can be done simultaneously on the arteries of both sides and maintained for prolonged periods. The passage of small particles in the area interrogated by the ultrasound beam produces a characteristic high-intensity transient signal (HITS) (Fig. 38-8), the identification of which can be made more accurate through the application of appropriate filters. Using this technique over 30 minutes in 46 patients with acute ischemic stroke, Rundek and colleagues[36] showed the presence of HITS in a much larger proportion of patients with stroke and plaques 4 mm or thicker than in patients with small or no plaques, even in the absence of other TEE-detected possible embolic sources (70% vs. 18%; $P = .007$). Moreover, all patients with large and complex plaques were found to have HITS, compared with 39% of patients with large but noncomplex plaques ($P = .005$). Similar results about the association

TABLE 38-4 PREVALENCE OF MOBILE THROMBI SUPERIMPOSED ON PROXIMAL AORTIC PLAQUES IN PATIENTS WITH ISCHEMIC STROKE

Study	Patients (N)	Mobile Thrombi	
		N	%
Toyoda et al[8]	62	3	4.8
Nihoyannopoulos et al[33]	152	3	2.0
Jones et al[2]	202	11	5.4
Amarenco et al[19]			
Unselected	250	7	2.8
Cryptogenic	78	6	7.7
Stone et al[11]			
Unselected	49	2	4.1
Cryptogenic	23	2	8.7
Di Tullio et al[20]	152	10	6.6
Ueno et al[34]	167	12	7.2
Di Tullio et al[22]	255	4	1.6

between plaques 4 mm or thicker and HITS were obtained in patients with cryptogenic stroke in a study by Castellanos and associates,[37] in which data on plaque complexity were not reported.

In summary, aortic plaque thickness of 4 mm or greater has been shown to be associated with increased risk of stroke and remains a useful tool for risk stratification, although part of the risk may come from superimposed thrombus included in the measurement of plaque thickness. Plaque thickness is also a marker of diffuse atherosclerosis, which may also play an important role in the stroke mechanism. The presence of complex morphologic features of a plaque, and especially of mobile components, appears more directly related to stroke mechanism in individual patients. Overall, the incidence of recurrent embolic events in patients with large or mobile aortic plaques has been estimated to be more than 14% per year, underscoring the need for effective secondary prevention strategies.[38]

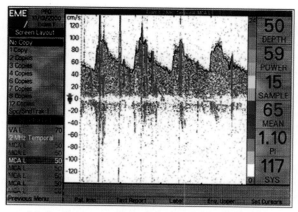

Figure 38-8 Transcranial Doppler examination of the middle cerebral artery. High-intensity transient signals (HITSs) are visualized as vertical high-amplitude signals with narrow spectrum superimposed on the normal blood flow.

Natural History of Aortic Plaques

The natural history of atherosclerotic plaques in the proximal aorta has not been extensively studied. From the information available, however, it appears that plaque size and morphology are important in determining the evolution of a plaque over time. Montgomery and colleagues[39] followed 30 patients who were found to have aortic atherosclerosis (12 with plaque thickness <5 mm, 8 with plaque thickness <5 mm, and 10 with mobile components) on initial TEE. A second TEE examination was then performed at 12 months. Although no significant changes were seen in subjects with smaller plaques, new mobile lesions had developed in 4 of 8 patients with plaques of 5 mm or greater. In patients who had mobile lesions at the time of the initial study, such lesions had resolved in 70% of cases, but new mobile lesions were observed in another 70%. Overall, although 20 of 30 patients (67%) had no change in the degree of atherosclerosis, substantial changes had occurred in the plaque morphology. In another study on 78 patients with stroke or transient ischemic attack, plaque progression over 9 months was observed in 37% of cases and was more frequent in the arch than in other aortic segments.[40] Using transthoracic echocardiographic examination of the aortic arch from a suprasternal window, Geraci and Weinberger[41] studied the plaque progression in 89 patients followed for up to 18 months (mean 7.7 months). Although plaques less than 4 mm thick at baseline showed changes in thickness in only 23% of cases, plaques 4 mm or thicker showed changes in thickness, upward or downward, in 52% of cases. It therefore appears that large aortic plaques are extremely dynamic lesions whose appearance may change considerably over a relatively short period.

Aortic Plaques in Patients with Stroke of Different Race or Ethnicity

Most studies on the association between atherosclerotic plaques in the proximal portion of the aorta and ischemic stroke have been conducted in white populations.

Some information, however, is available for black and Hispanic patients that allows a comparison of plaque frequencies, which is important in the light of the different prevalence of risk factors for atherosclerosis in different race and ethnic groups. In a retrospective study of 1553 patients with ischemic stroke (889 white, 664 black), Gupta and colleagues[42] found a higher prevalence of aortic plaques in white than in black patients in the ascending aorta (14.7% vs. 11.1%; $P = .04$), aortic arch (67.7% vs. 62.2%; $P = .03$), and descending aorta (58.4% vs. 50.3%; $P = .002$). The plaque burden (sum of maximum plaque thickness at the three aortic locations) was also significantly higher in white patients (4.97 mm vs. 4.28 mm; $P = .007$); prevalences of plaques 4 mm or thicker (25.9% vs. 18.7%; $P < .001$) and of complex plaques—defined as protruding, ulcerated, mobile, or calcified regardless of plaque thickness (26.3% vs. 19.0%; $P < .001$)—were also greater in white patients, but *only* in the aortic arch. These findings were observed despite a higher prevalence of arterial hypertension and diabetes mellitus in black patients and cannot therefore be explained by differences in conventional stroke risk factor distribution. In our case-control study in patients with ischemic stroke older than 59 years from the triethnic community of northern Manhattan, plaques 4 mm or thicker had similar frequencies in white, black, and Hispanic subjects (24.1%, 20.0%, and 22.5%, respectively).[20] However, complex plaques were twice as frequent in white subjects than in black and Hispanic subjects (32.3%, 15.6%, and 16.3%, respectively). Complex plaques were associated with a strong increase in stroke risk in all three race-ethnic subgroups. As in the Gupta study,[42] the frequency of arterial hypertension and diabetes mellitus in our study was significantly lower in white subjects than in the other two race-ethnic subgroups, and that of hypercholesterolemia was significantly lower in white subjects than in black subjects. The prevalence of plaques 4 mm or thicker in the overall study population (44.8%) was much higher in our study than in the similar study from France (14.4%)[19] and also higher than the frequency of plaques that were either 5 mm or thicker or complex in the similar study from Australia (22%).[2] Therefore, even though the stroke risks associated with large or complex plaques appeared similar in the three studies, the attributable risk of stroke from proximal aortic plaques may be greater in the population of the United States, underscoring the need for effective preventive measures and risk factor reduction.

Factors Associated with Aortic Plaques in Patients with Stroke

Although differences in traditional risk factors for stroke and atherosclerosis alone do not seem to explain racial and ethnic differences in frequency of aortic plaques, some of these risk factors are indeed associated with the presence of these plaques. Age is the strongest and universally accepted predictor of aortic atherosclerosis.[1,2,4,5,10,19-21,43,44] Cigarette smoking has consistently been shown to be associated with aortic atherosclerosis[2,19,21,43,44] and is the most important modifiable risk factor for the development of aortic plaques. Arterial hypertension has also been shown to be associated with proximal aortic atherosclerosis,[4,44] especially in the case of ulcerated lesions.[4] In the SPARC study, systolic and pulse pressure variables (office and ambulatory), but no diastolic variables, were associated with atherosclerosis and complex atherosclerosis in the aorta after adjustments for age and smoking history.[44] The association between diabetes mellitus and aortic atherosclerosis has been supported in some studies,[2] and negated in others,[43,44] at least after adjustment for other risk factors.[43] Hypercholesterolemia has been found to be associated with aortic atherosclerosis in some studies,[21,43,45] and treatment with 3-hydroxy-3-methylglutaryl coenzyme A (HMG-CoA) reductase inhibitors (statins) has been shown to induce regression of aortic atherosclerotic lesions in humans.[46-48]

Variables besides traditional risk factors have been identified that are associated with aortic atherosclerosis and are possibly cofactors in increasing the embolic risk associated with aortic plaques. As mentioned earlier, the embolic potential of aortic plaque is related at least in part to the presence of superimposed thrombus. It is therefore conceivable that the coexistence of a hypercoagulable state in a patient with aortic arch plaque may increase the likelihood of superimposed thrombus formation, further enhancing the embolic potential of the lesion. Procoagulant properties have been demonstrated in atherosclerotic aortas; increased tissue factor expression and activity have been observed in the atherosclerotic intima that may lead to thrombus formation as the result of its exposure to the flowing blood.[49] Among coagulation factors, an increased fibrinogen level has been shown to be a risk factor for cardiovascular disease and ischemic stroke[50,51] and to be associated with degree of carotid stenosis,[52-54] abdominal aortic atheromas,[52] and peripheral atherosclerotic disease.[55,56] Atherogenic effects of fibrinogen have been described and possibly result from its interactions with some lipoproteins. In fact, fibrinogen has been shown to modulate the atherogenic effects of lipoprotein(a) [Lp(a)][57] and to increase the risk of severe carotid atherosclerosis and stroke in patients with low levels of high-density-lipoprotein cholesterol.[58] The association between fibrinogen and carotid artery disease has been shown to be particularly strong in the elderly.[59] Moreover, interracial differences have been reported in the levels of fibrinogen, with black subjects having higher levels than white subjects[60] and both groups having higher levels than Asian subjects.[61] Fibrinogen has also been shown to be independently associated with aortic atherosclerosis in a group of 148 patients who underwent TEE for valvular heart disease.[43] In that study, there was a relation between fibrinogen levels and severities of both aortic atherosclerosis and coronary artery disease.

Plasma homocysteine has also been found to be independently associated with aortic atherosclerosis diagnosed by TEE. In 82 cardiac patients, Tribouilloy and coworkers[62] found, in a multivariate analysis including usual risk factors for atherosclerosis, that age, male gender, and low-density-lipoprotein (LDL) cholesterol and homocysteine levels were the only factors independently associated with severity of aortic atherosclerosis. These findings suggest that homocysteine may be a marker of atherosclerotic lesion in large arterial vessels. Homocysteine was also shown to be independently associated with aortic arch atheroma progression over a period of 9 months in a group of 78 patients with stroke or transient ischemic attack, whereas no conventional risk factor for atherosclerosis was shown to have similar independent effect. Endothelial dysfunction causing plaque progression and a hypercoagulable state resulting in thrombus deposition were invoked as possible mechanisms for the finding.[40]

As mentioned earlier, the presence of a hypercoagulable state in patients with large aortic plaques could increase the embolic potential. In the APRIS study, prothrombin fragment 1.2 (F1.2), an indicator of thrombin generation, was associated with large plaques in patients with stroke ($P = .02$) but not in control subjects. Over a mean follow-up of 55.1 ± 37.2 months, patients with stroke who had large plaques and F1.2 levels over the median value had significantly higher risk of recurrent stroke and death than those with large plaques but lower F1.2 levels (230/1000 person-years vs. 85/1000 person-years; $P = .05$).[22] This observation indicates that in patients presenting with acute ischemic stroke, large aortic plaques are associated with blood hypercoagulability (as indicated by F1.2 level), suggesting a role for coagulation activation in the stroke mechanism.

The embolic potential of an aortic atheroma is also related to its lipid content. Cholesterol crystal emboli have been documented pathologically in peripheral arteries of patients in whom large atheromas are seen on TEE.[63-65] In addition to the association of total and LDL cholesterol with aortic plaques, mentioned earlier, Lp(a) has been shown to be an independent marker of aortic atherosclerosis.[66] Lp(a) is a complex between LDL and apoprotein(a). In spite of the close structural resemblance between LDL and Lp(a), these particles have very different metabolic properties. Serum Lp(a) levels are under strong genetic influence and are determined mainly by the synthetic rate of apoprotein(a), a protein with a striking similarity to plasminogen. This homology to plasminogen has prompted the speculation that Lp(a) may be an important risk factor for both atherosclerosis and thrombosis. It has been suggested that the atherogenic activity of Lp(a) might result from its inhibiting effect on plasminogen activation, with consequent decrease in plasmin formation. This in turn reduces the activation of transforming growth factor-β, a potent inhibitor of smooth muscle cell proliferation.[67] In addition, Lp(a) has been detected in atherosclerotic plaques, where it combines with fibrin and attenuates the clearance of this protein, promoting atherogenesis and vascular dysfunction.[68]

In summary, some lipid and coagulation abnormalities are associated with proximal aortic atherosclerosis; such abnormalities may be of importance in the progression of the atherosclerotic plaque and are possibly implicated as cofactors in determining the plaque's embolic potential. The study and consequent better understanding of the relation between lipid metabolism, coagulation, and proximal aortic atherosclerosis might provide indications for preventive and therapeutic measures in patients with proximal aortic plaques.

Proximal Aortic Plaques and Carotid Artery Disease

The relation between proximal aortic plaques and carotid artery disease, another important risk factor for ischemic stroke, has been investigated in several studies. In the autopsy study by Amarenco and colleagues,[4] ulcerated aortic plaques were as frequent in patients with carotid stenosis greater than 75% than in patients without it. In the case-control TEE study by Amarenco and associates,[19] no correlation was observed between aortic plaques 4 mm or thicker and carotid stenosis greater than 70%. We observed that the frequency of carotid stenosis greater than 60% rose with increasing aortic plaque thickness[10]; however, the positive predictive value of carotid stenosis greater than 60% for arch plaque 5 mm or thicker was only 16%, suggesting that although a general correlation exists between aortic and carotid atherosclerosis, one condition cannot be predicted on the basis of the other in individual patients. Jones and coworkers[2] obtained similar results, reporting a positive predictive value of carotid disease for aortic plaque of 57%. In a later study, Kallikazaros and colleagues[69] reported, in a group of 62 patients with cardiac disease, that presence of carotid plaque had good positive predictive value (83%) and acceptable sensitivity (75%) and specificity (74%) for presence of aortic plaque, but lower negative predictive value (63%). In summary, a general correlation exists between carotid atherosclerosis and aortic atherosclerosis, but one cannot be reliably predicted from the presence of the other, with the possible exception of patients with cardiac disease, in whom the relation appears to be closer.[69]

Proximal Aortic Plaques and Coronary Artery Disease

The relation between aortic atherosclerosis and coronary artery disease has been extensively studied. In a TEE study of 61 patients who had previously undergone coronary angiography, Fazio and associates[70] found atherosclerotic plaques in the thoracic aorta in 37 of 41 patients (90%) with obstructive coronary disease (defined as ≥50% left main coronary artery stenosis or ≥70% stenosis in the left anterior descending, circumflex, or right coronary arteries), but in only 2 of 20 patients (10%) with no or nonobstructive coronary disease. In that study, the presence of aortic plaque on TEE had 90% sensitivity and 90% specificity for obstructive coronary artery disease. In 153 consecutive patients undergoing coronary angiography and TEE, Khoury and colleagues[71] detected plaques in the aorta of 90 of 97 patients (93%), in comparison with 12 of 55 patients (22%) with normal coronary arteries. The aortic arch had evidence of plaque in 80% of patients with coronary stenosis greater than 50%. In the SPARC study,[1] aortic plaques were independently associated with history of myocardial infarction and coronary bypass surgery. In the population-based Rotterdam Coronary Calcification Study,[72] coronary calcification, assessed in 2013 subjects by electron-beam CT, showed a graded association with aortic calcification, considered a marker of atherosclerosis. In that study, the association was stronger than that between coronary calcification and carotid disease.

Therefore, a strong association between aortic atherosclerosis and coronary artery disease has been widely documented. However, the strength of this association appears slightly lower in elderly patients. In the study by Khoury and colleagues,[71] the specificity of the presence of aortic plaques for the diagnosis of coronary artery disease was found to be decreased in patients older than 63 years in comparison with younger patients (64% vs. 90%, respectively). In another study of 84 patients with cardiac disease,[73] the presence of aortic plaques failed to predict significant coronary artery disease in patients older than 69 years, but it was a strong predictor in younger patients.

Aortic Plaques and Atheroembolism

Besides being the site of origin of thromboembolism to the brain and the peripheral circulation, the atherosclerotic aorta can also give origin to atheroembolic phenomena, in which cholesterol crystal emboli are sent to various segments of the arterial circulation. Atheroembolism is generally characterized by small embolic particles that lodge in small arterioles (<200 μm in diameter)[74] and may occur spontaneously or following vascular surgery, arteriography, or anticoagulation.[75,76] The clinical consequences of atheroembolism are variable, depending on the location of the target organ and the number and frequency of embolic episodes. Therefore, atheroembolism has a wide spectrum of clinical presentations, from clinically silent episodes recognized only during diagnostic procedures[77-79] to complex clinical pictures characterized by multiple organ involvement (brain, retina, kidneys, gastrointestinal tract, lower limbs).[80,81] The simultaneous or consecutive involvement of different body segments may, in fact, greatly facilitate a correct diagnosis in cases of subtle or subacute clinical presentation.

Older age appears to be the strongest risk factor for atheroembolism from an aortic source. All 16 patients with atheroembolism reported by Gore and Collins[80] were older than 60 years. In that study, 12 of 13 autopsied patients had evidence of embolism to multiple sites. Older age and aortic atherosclerosis have a major impact on the risk of atheroembolism following cardiac surgery, as discussed in the next section.

Proximal Aortic Plaques and Cardiac Surgery

Aortic atherosclerosis is widely recognized as a strong risk factor for atheroembolic events, especially stroke, after cardiac surgery. As the mean age of the general population increases and indications for cardiac surgery in the elderly expand, an ever-increasing number of elderly subjects undergo open heart surgery, raising the number of subjects at high risk for atheroembolic events. Blauth and colleagues,[82] studying the autopsies of 221 subjects who had undergone cardiac surgery, identified embolic disease in 69 (31%), which was atheroembolic in nature in more than two thirds of cases. The brain was the most common target organ (16%), followed by spleen (11%), kidney (10%), and pancreas (7%). Atheroembolism was multiple in 63% of subjects and was more common after coronary artery procedures than after valvular procedures (26% vs. 9%; $P = .008$). Atheroembolic events occurred in 37% of patients with severe atherosclerosis of the ascending aorta but in only 2% of patients without significant aortic disease ($P < .0001$), and 96% of patients who had evidence of atheroemboli had severe atherosclerosis of the ascending aorta. In that study, there was a strong relationship between age, severe aortic atherosclerosis, and atheroembolism.

The consequences of atheroembolism during or after cardiac surgery may be devastating. In a 2003 autopsy study, death was directly attributed to the embolic event (intraoperative cardiac failure due to coronary embolization in 3, massive stroke in 2, and extensive gastrointestinal embolization in 1) in 6 of 29 patients (21%) who had evidence of atheroemboli.[83] Proximal aortic atherosclerosis is also associated with the severity of postoperative neurologic complications. In a multicenter prospective study on adverse cerebral outcomes after coronary bypass surgery in 2108 patients from 24 U.S. institutions, the most severe complications (focal injury, or stupor or coma at discharge) were predicted by proximal aortic atherosclerosis, history of neurologic disease, and older age.[84] In 921 consecutive patients undergoing cardiac surgery in another study, the incidence of postoperative stroke was 8.7% in patients with atherosclerotic disease of the ascending aorta and 1.8% in patients without it ($P < .0001$).[85] Logistic regression indicated that aortic atherosclerosis was the strongest predictor of perioperative stroke. In yet another study, aortic atherosclerosis was shown to be a predictor of both early (immediately after surgery) and delayed (after initial uneventful recovery) stroke in 2972 patients undergoing cardiac surgery.[86] In that study, 82% of early strokes and 71% of delayed strokes occurred in patients 65 years of age or older.

The increased risk of stroke during coronary artery bypass in patients with proximal aortic plaques has been related to the effects of cannulation of the aorta to establish extracorporeal circulation. Ura and colleagues[87] performed epiaortic echocardiography before cannulation and after decannulation in 472 patients undergoing cardiac surgery with extracorporeal circulation. In 16 patients (3.4%), these investigators found a new lesion in the intima of the ascending aorta after decannulation. In 10 of 16 patients (63%), the new lesions were severe, with mobile components or disruption of the intimal layer. Three patients in this group had a postoperative stroke. Thickness of the plaque near the site of aortic manipulation was associated with the development of a new lesion. The frequency of new lesion was 33.3% with plaque thickness 4 mm or greater, 11.8% with plaque thickness 3 to 4 mm, and only 0.8% with plaque thickness less than 3 mm. It has been suggested that the incidence of perioperative stroke and vascular events in patients with severe proximal aortic atherosclerosis can be reduced by modifications in surgical approach. Trehan and associates[88] performed TEE in 3660 patients scheduled for coronary artery bypass surgery and found proximal aortic atheromas with mobile components in 104 (2.84%). In those patients, these researchers modified the surgical approach, the most frequent change being off-pump surgery (88 of 104 patients). The incidences of stroke and vascular events at 1 week after surgery were 0.96% and 1.92%, respectively, and there were no embolic events in the 88 patients who had undergone off-pump surgery. Therefore, preoperative TEE evaluation of the proximal aorta and evolution in surgical techniques may decrease the incidence of stroke associated with coronary artery bypass surgery.

Proximal Aortic Plaques and Cardiac Catheterization

There is a high risk of embolism to the brain when severe proximal atherosclerosis is present in subjects undergoing catheter-based diagnostic or therapeutic procedures involving the aortic arch. Because a TEE examination of the aorta is not usually performed before intraaortic procedures, the presence of aortic plaques is not known to the operator, a circumstance that increases the risk of embolic events after the procedure, especially in elderly patients. The awareness of the presence of aortic plaques, and the consequent modification of the catheterization technique, can be of great importance in reducing the risk of embolic sequelae. Karalis and associates[89] performed cardiac catheterization via the usual femoral approach in 59 patients with aortic atherosclerosis and in 71 control patients. The incidence of embolic events was 17% in patients with aortic atherosclerosis and 3% in controls ($P = .01$). No embolic events occurred in 11 patients with aortic atherosclerosis in whom a brachial approach instead of a femoral approach was used. It is therefore evident that the identification of subjects at high risk for atheroembolism (elderly, with history of prior embolic events or evidence of atherosclerosis in other body segments, or with multiple risk factors for atherosclerosis) can be invaluable in identifying the patients who should be referred for TEE before intraaortic procedures and could drastically reduce the incidence of embolic complications.

Obviously, the same consideration just discussed for diagnostic cardiac catheterization applies to therapeutic procedures involving the aorta. Keeley and Grines[90] evaluated the frequency of aortic debris retrieval during placement of guiding catheters in 1000 consecutive patients undergoing percutaneous revascularization procedures. In more than 50% of cases, guiding catheter placement was associated with scraping of debris from the aorta. The investigators underscored the fact that great attention to allowing debris to exit the back of the catheter was essential to prevent the injection of atheromatous debris into the bloodstream. Karalis and associates[89] also compared the results of intraaortic balloon pump placement in 10 patients with aortic atherosclerosis and in 12 patients without it. An embolic event related to the procedure was observed in 5 patients (50%) in the former group, and in none in the latter ($P = .02$). The researchers concluded that when aortic debris is detected, and especially when mobile components are identified, performing brachial rather than femoral catheterization and avoiding placement of an intraaortic balloon pump may reduce the risk of embolism.

Treatment of Proximal Aortic Plaques

Although the role of proximal aortic plaques as a risk factor for cerebral and peripheral embolism has become increasingly evident in the past decade, the best treatment options to reduce the risk of a first or recurrent embolic event in patients with aortic plaque are not yet clearly defined. Several preventive and therapeutic possibilities have been suggested and are reviewed in this section.

Systemic Anticoagulation

Because most embolic events associated with large or complex proximal aortic plaques are thought to be thromboembolic in origin, systemic anticoagulation has been suggested as an option to reduce their incidence in patients with this type of plaque. Dressler and colleagues[91] reported on the frequency of recurrent vascular events in 31 subjects presenting with a systemic embolic event and a mobile aortic plaque on TEE, according to the use of warfarin. Treatment was not randomized, and although 79% of patients (11 of 14) with medium or large mobile components received warfarin, only 53% (9 of 17) of those with small mobile components (diameter ≤1mm) did. Overall, 45% of patients not receiving warfarin had a vascular event over a mean follow-up of approximately 10 months, compared with 5% of those receiving warfarin. Corresponding figures for stroke were 27% and 0%, respectively. Annual incidence of stroke in the group not receiving warfarin was 32%. The investigators concluded that warfarin was protective against recurrent embolic events in patients with mobile plaques and that the dimension of the mobile component should not be used to assess the need for anticoagulation. Prospective results from the Stroke Prevention in Atrial Fibrillation (SPAF) study[92] showed significant reduction of the rate of embolic events in patients with protruding atheromas treated with adjusted-dose warfarin (international normalized ratio [INR], 2 to 3) in comparison with patients treated with low-intensity warfarin (INR, 1.2 to 1.5) plus aspirin (325 mg/day). Overall, patients with complex aortic plaques had a fourfold higher stroke incidence than patients without plaques, and adjusted-dose warfarin decreased the risk by 75% (P = .005). Of course, all patients in that study had nonvalvular atrial fibrillation, precluding the direct extrapolation of the results to the general population.

Although the use of oral anticoagulation in patients with mobile plaques appears logical and is supported by the aforementioned studies, its use in patients with large but nonmobile lesions is more controversial. In 50 patients with atheromas 4 mm or larger but without mobile components followed for 22 ± 10 months, Ferrari and coworkers[93] found a substantial incidence of stroke in patients treated with aspirin or ticlopidine (5/23, or 21.7%), compared with no stroke in 27 patients treated with warfarin (P = .01). This study was small, however, and the treatment was not randomized. In 2009, we reported on the incidence of recurrent stroke and death in 516 patients with acute ischemic stroke treated with aspirin or warfarin as part of the Patent Foramen Ovale in Cryptogenic Stroke Study (PICSS). Over a follow-up of 2 years, large plaques (≥4 mm) remained associated with an increased risk of events (adjusted HR, 2.12, 95% CI, 1.04–4.32), especially those with complex morphology (HR, 2.55, 95%CI, 1.10–5.89). The risk was highest among patients with cryptogenic stroke, both for large plaques (HR, 6.42, 95% CI, 1.62–25.46) and for large complex plaques (HR, 9.50, 95% CI, 1.92–47.10).[94] Therefore, medical treatment with warfarin or aspirin did not seem to affect the significance of the association between large arch plaques and recurrent events. Although event rates tended to be lower in the warfarin group than in the aspirin group (2-year event rate in patients with large plaques, 23.0% and 30.2%, respectively; P = .21), the difference between the two treatments was not statistically significant.[95] Further studies with larger patient populations are needed to evaluate the possibility of differences in efficacy between warfarin and aspirin or other antiplatelet agents in specific patient subgroups, such as patients with cryptogenic stroke.

The safety of systemic anticoagulation in patients with aortic plaques has traditionally been questioned,[96] because anticoagulation might induce bleeding within the plaque, with consequent ulceration and risk of embolization. Moreover, anticoagulation might remove the thrombin coating from ulcerated atheromas and therefore facilitate microembolization of cholesterol crystals.[97,98] Atheroembolism is a real clinical entity, and its sequelae[73-80] and association with anticoagulation[75,76] in patients with aortic atherosclerosis have been discussed earlier in the chapter. However, its incidence after systemic anticoagulation appears to be rather low. In the SPAF study,[99] adjusted-dose treatment with warfarin (INR, 2 to 3) was associated with an incidence of cholesterol embolization of 0.7% per year.

Antiplatelet Medications

As mentioned earlier, antiplatelet therapy with aspirin or ticlopidine has been reported to be less protective against recurrent embolic events than warfarin therapy in patients with large or complex plaques,[91-93] but this has been seen generally in small studies without treatment randomization. The only data from a randomized study come from PICSS[94] and are summarized earlier, in the section on systemic anticoagulation. The combination of aspirin and clopidogrel is being tested against warfarin in patients with large plaques.[100] More data are therefore needed to assess the role of antiplatelet agents in the prevention of aortic plaque–related embolic events, their relative efficacy in comparison with warfarin, and the identification of patients for whom either treatment is suitable.

Thrombolysis

Thrombolysis has occasionally been used to treat large mobile plaques with seemingly very high embolic potential.[101] The high risk of major hemorrhagic complications, especially in elderly patients, and the questionable advantages of thrombolysis over anticoagulation make it an unlikely therapeutic choice in patients with mobile plaques, so thrombolysis should be reserved for selected cases. Like systemic anticoagulation, thrombolysis has also been associated with atheroembolic complications in patients with aortic atherosclerosis,[102] although the incidence of this complication is probably rather low.[103]

Statins

The use of statins to prevent embolic events in patients with large or complex aortic plaques appears to have a powerful rationale, because statins may induce plaque stabilization through the reduction of the lipid content, with consequent reduced frequency of ulceration and superimposed thrombus formation. As mentioned earlier, statins have been shown to induce plaque regression in humans.[46-48] To date, no randomized trial has assessed the efficacy of statins for this indication. The only available data come from Tunick and colleagues,[104] who retrospectively identified 519 patients with severe thoracic aortic plaques and determined the incidence of embolic events according to treatment status (statins, warfarin, or antiplatelet medications). Treatment was not randomized, and patients taking each class of medication were matched with patients of similar age and embolic risk profile not taking that medication. Over an average follow-up of 34 ± 26 months, embolic events occurred in 111 patients (21%). In multivariate analysis, statin treatment was found to be independently protective against recurring events ($P = .0001$). In the matched analysis, the relative risk reduction was 59%. No protective effect was found for warfarin or antiplatelet medication. Although with the limitations of the retrospective nonrandomized design, this study represents preliminary evidence of the efficacy of statins in preventing embolic events in patients with severe aortic plaques, which deserves confirmation in randomized prospective studies.

Surgery

Aortic endarterectomy has been proposed as a preventive measure in patients with large mobile plaques in the proximal aorta at impending risk for embolism, especially when cardiac surgery is performed. However, the surgical procedure on the aorta in itself carries a high risk, especially for the potential to dislodge parts of the mobile component of the plaque and precipitate an embolic event. Stern and colleagues[105] performed intraoperative TEE in 3404 patients undergoing heart surgery, finding complex plaques (≥5 mm, or mobile) in 268 (8%). Arch endarterectomy was performed in 43 patients in an attempt to prevent intraoperative stroke. The intraoperative stroke rate in the 268 patients was high (15.3%), as was mortality (14.9%). On multivariate analysis, age and arch endarterectomy were found to be independently associated with intraoperative stroke. The OR for stroke of arch endarterectomy was 3.6 ($P = .01$). Therefore, the use of arch endarterectomy should be carefully considered only in very selected cases.

Resection and graft replacement of a severely atherosclerotic segment of ascending aorta were performed by Rokkas and Kouchoukos and associates[106] in 81 patients (mean age 71 years) undergoing coronary bypass surgery. In that study, the 30-day mortality was 8.6% (7 patients). Perioperative strokes occurred in 4 patients (4.9%), and transient neurologic deficits in 2 (2.5%). During the follow-up, only one stroke occurred 4 months after the procedure. However, 3-year survival was only 40%, with mortality being secondary mainly to complications from generalized atherosclerosis. In 17 patients who underwent graft replacement of the ascending aorta for severe atherosclerosis during elective coronary bypass grafting, King and colleagues[107] reported a hospital mortality of 23.5%, compared with only 2.3% in 89 patients who underwent replacement for ascending thoracic aortic aneurysm ($P = .006$). Cerebrovascular event rates were 17.6% and 3.4%, respectively ($P = .05$). Nonfatal postoperative complications were observed in 53% of the patients with atherosclerosis, compared with 20% of controls ($P = .01$).

From the cumulative evidence presented, surgical procedures on a severe atherosclerotic proximal aorta are associated with substantial morbidity and mortality and should be reserved for carefully selected cases.

Future Directions

The most important advancements in the field of proximal aortic plaques and ischemic stroke will likely come from the results of randomized clinical trials to test preventive and therapeutic options in patients with proximal aortic atherosclerosis. However, as the general population ages, the number of subjects with atherosclerotic disease will increase, and the identification of subjects at high risk for embolic events to target for primary prevention measures will become more and more important. Better, easier, and noninvasive ways to identify high-risk aortic plaques will be needed. This need may entail both a more accurate assessment of plaque morphology and attempts to identify plaques that are more likely to rupture and give origin to embolic events (vulnerable plaques).

Newer Imaging Modalities

As mentioned earlier, the assessment of stroke risk in patients with proximal aortic plaques has been based on plaque thickness and morphology. The measure of plaque thickness, although very helpful for risk stratification, is a monodimensional measurement of a three-dimensional lesion and may therefore not convey all the information about the plaque embolic potential in individual subjects. Also, plaque thickness and morphology characteristics are usually evaluated by TEE, a semi-invasive technique that does not lend itself to be a screening tool in asymptomatic elderly subjects. Transthoracic echocardiography from a suprasternal or supraclavicular approach would be a much easier and more widely applicable technique, provided that questions on its sensitivity in comparison with TEE, especially for identification of complex plaque morphology, can be addressed. Real-time three-dimensional echocardiographic equipment has become available that with further technical refinements might prove very useful in the noninvasive evaluation of the aortic arch. Figure 38-9 displays an example of an ulcerated plaque in the distal portion of the aortic arch visualized by TEE, commonly available transthoracic echocardiography, and real-time three-dimensional echocardiography. The advantages of the three-dimensional technique over the traditional transthoracic image in displaying the real extension of the

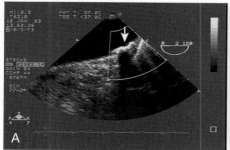
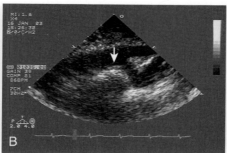
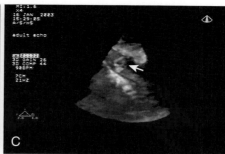

Figure 38-9 A, Transesophageal echocardiography visualization of a calcified plaque in the distal aortic arch. A large ulceration *(arrow)* is shown. B, Same plaque as in A, visualized from the suprasternal transthoracic approach. No definite ulceration is visible. C, Transthoracic three-dimensional imaging of the same plaque. Rotation of the transducer plane has allowed a better visualization of the plaque, and the entire area of ulceration *(arrow)* is now visible.

plaque and the characteristics of its ulceration are apparent; the three-dimensional technique allows a representation of the plaque characteristics that appears at least as good as that obtained by TEE. Further technical refinements, including transducers with smaller footprints to better fit into the suprasternal notch, and studies assessing the accuracy of the new technique in comparison with TEE are needed to evaluate the potential and applicability of this new technique.

Noninvasive techniques besides echocardiography have been shown to have excellent accuracy for the detection of proximal aortic plaques. MRI has been shown to correlate well with TEE for aortic plaque determination[108] and to accurately quantify the fibrotic and lipidic components of the plaque in animal models.[109] Compared with TEE, dual-helical CT has shown sensitivity of 87%, specificity of 82%, and overall accuracy of 84% for the detection of aortic plaques.[110]

A combination of different techniques, such as positron emission tomography (PET) and MRI, has been successfully applied to the imaging of plaques in the aortic arch (Fig. 38-10).

Identification of the Vulnerable (High-Risk) Plaque

The noninvasive identification of the vulnerable plaque, or a plaque that is at higher risk for rupture and consequent superimposed thrombus formation, would be of great importance in trying to prevent embolic sequelae. As discussed before, MRI has shown potential for identifying fibrotic and lipidic components of a plaque.[109] Contrast agents have been introduced that may enhance this capability. Superparamagnetic iron oxide has been found to localize to aortic atherosclerotic plaques in animal models, allowing the detection of iron-laden macrophages in the aortic subendothelium[111] and therefore possibly providing a new noninvasive modality for imaging of inflammatory aortic plaques. Contrast agents have been developed that target activated matrix metalloproteinases, enzymes that have been implicated in the propensity of a plaque to rupture.[112] Positron emission tomography with fludeoxyglucose F 18 is a promising tool for visualizing inflammation in an atherosclerotic plaque and has been shown to be able to visualize statin-induced reduction in the degree of inflammation.[113] Further development of these techniques may improve our ability to identify those plaques that are more likely to become sources of cerebral embolization.

Summary

Large and complex plaques in the proximal portion of the thoracic aorta have been established as a risk factor for ischemic stroke, especially cryptogenic, and other arterial embolic events in patients older than 60 years. The frequency of embolic events, both spontaneous and precipitated by diagnostic or therapeutic procedures on the aorta, has been defined. Progress has been made in aortic plaque imaging and in the understanding of morphologic characteristics and associated factors that affect the plaque-related embolic risk. Initial therapeutic data have been obtained, although further investigation remains to be done in that regard. Further advancement is expected to come from improved techniques for the identification of high-risk plaques and from randomized treatment trials aimed at reducing the risk of embolic events associated with severe proximal aortic atherosclerosis.

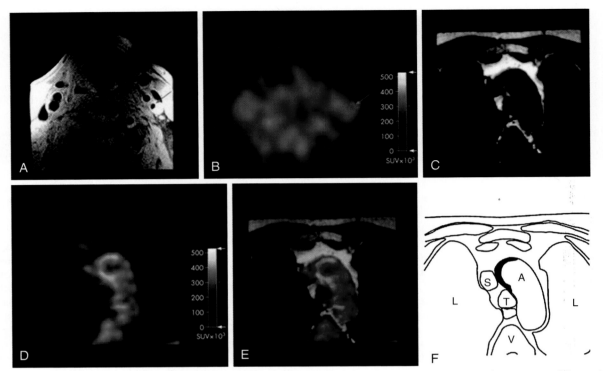

Figure 38-10   Co-registered axial fluorodeoxyglucose F-18 (FDG) positron emission tomography scan and MR image of the neck (A and B) and chest (C to E), showing minimal tracer uptake in the ipsilateral carotid artery *(arrow)* and high uptake into an eccentric plaque in the arch of the aorta. F, Schematic of chest MR images, showing the aortic arch (A) with plaque, lungs (L), superior vena cava (S), trachea (T), and vertebral body (V). (Reprinted with permission from Moustafa RR, Azquierdo D, Weissberg PL, et al: Neurological picture: Identifying aortic plaque inflammation as a potential cause of stroke. *J Neurol Neurosurg Psychiatry* 79:236, 2008. © BMJ Publishing Group Ltd.)

REFERENCES

1. Agmon Y, Khandheria BK, Meissner I, et al: Relation of coronary artery disease and cerebrovascular disease with atherosclerosis of the thoracic aorta in the general population, *Am J Cardiol* 89:262–267, 2002.
2. Jones EF, Kalman JM, Calafiore P, et al: Proximal aortic atheroma:An independent risk factor for cerebral ischemia, *Stroke* 26:218–224, 1995.
3. Russo C, Jin Z, Rundek T, et al: Atherosclerotic disease of the proximal aorta and the risk of vascular events in a population-based cohort: The Aortic Plaques and Risk of Ischemic Stroke (APRIS) study, *Stroke* 40:2313–2318, 2009.
4. Amarenco P, Duyckaerts C, Tzourio C, et al: The prevalence of ulcerated plaques in the aortic arch in patients with stroke, *N Engl J Med* 326:221–225, 1992.
5. Khatibzadeh M, Mitusch R, Stierle U, et al: Aortic atherosclerotic plaques as a source of systemic embolism, *J Am Coll Cardiol* 27:664–669, 1996.
6. Tenenbaum A, Motro M, Feinberg MS, et al: Retrograde flow in the thoracic aorta in patients with systemic emboli: A transesophageal echocardiographic evaluation of mobile plaque motion, *Chest* 118:1703–1708, 2000.
7. Harloff A, Strecker C, Frydrychowicz AP, et al: Plaques in the descending aorta: A new risk factor for stroke: Visualization of potential embolization pathways by 4D MRI, *J Magn Reson Imaging* 26:1651–1655, 2007.
8. Toyoda K, Yasaka M, Nagata S, et al: Aortogenic embolic stroke: A transesophageal echocardiographic approach, *Stroke* 23:1056–1061, 1992.
9. Vaduganathan P, Ewton A, Nagueh SF, et al: Pathologic correlates of aortic plaques, thrombi and mobile "aortic debris" imaged in vivo with transesophageal echocardiography, *J Am Coll Cardiol* 30:357–363, 1997.
10. Di Tullio MR, Sacco RL, Gersony D, et al: Aortic atheromas and acute ischemic stroke: A transesophageal echocardiographic study in an ethnically mixed population, *Neurology* 46:1560–1566, 1996.
11. Stone DA, Hawke MW, LaMonte M, et al: Ulcerated atherosclerotic plaques in the thoracic aorta are associated with cryptogenic stroke: A multiplane transesophageal echocardiographic study, *Am Heart J* 130:105–108, 1995.
12. Weber A, Jones EF, Zavala JA, et al: Intraobserver and interobserver variability of transesophageal echocardiography in aortic arch atheroma measurement, *J Am Soc Echocardiogr* 21:129–133, 2008.
13. Daniel WG, Erbel R, Kasper W, et al: Safety of transesophageal echocardiography: A multicenter survey of 10,419 examinations, *Circulation* 83:817–821, 1991.
14. Oh JK, Seward JB, Tajik AJ: *Transesophageal echocardiography: The echo manual*, ed 2, 1999, Lippincott Williams & Wilkins, pp 23–36.
15. Chee TS, Quek SS, Ding ZP, et al: Clinical utility, safety, acceptability and complications of transoesophageal echocardiography (TEE) in 901 patients, *Singapore Med J* 36:479–483, 1995.
16. Weslow RG, Di Tullio MR: Sacco RL: Safety and tolerability of transesophageal echocardiography in stroke patients, *Cerebrovasc Dis* 5:243, 1995.
17. Zabalgoitia M, Gandhi DK, Evans J, et al: Transesophageal echocardiography in the awake elderly patient: Its role in the clinical decision-making process, *Am Heart J* 120:1147–1153, 1990.
18. Tunick PA, Perez JL, Kronzon I: Protruding atheromas in the thoracic aorta and systemic embolization, *Ann Intern Med* 115:423–427, 1991.

19. Amarenco P, Cohen A, Tzourio C, et al: Atherosclerotic disease of the aortic arch and the risk of ischemic stroke, *N Engl J Med* 331:1474-1479, 1994.

20. Di Tullio MR, Sacco RL, Savoia MT, et al: Aortic atheroma morphology and the risk of ischemic stroke in a multiethnic population, *Am Heart J* 139:329-336, 2000.

21. Davila-Roman VG, Barzilai B, Wareing TH, et al: Atherosclerosis of the ascending aorta: Prevalence and role as an independent predictor of cerebrovascular events in cardiac patients, *Stroke* 25:2010-2016, 1994.

22. Di Tullio MR, Homma S, Jin Z, et al: Aortic atherosclerosis, hypercoagulability and stroke: The Aortic Plaques and Risk of Ischemic Stroke (APRIS) Study, *J Am Coll Cardiol* 52:855-861, 2008.

23. Tunick PA, Rosenzweig BP, Katz ES, et al: High risk for vascular events in patients with protruding aortic atheromas: A prospective study, *J Am Coll Cardiol* 23:1085-1090, 1994.

24. Mitusch R, Doherty C, Wucherpfennig H, et al: Vascular events during follow-up in patients with aortic arch atherosclerosis, *Stroke* 28:36-39, 1997.

25. Atherosclerotic disease of the aortic arch as a risk factor for recurrent ischemic stroke: The French Study of Aortic Plaques in Stroke Group, *N Engl J Med* 334:1216-1221, 1996.

26. Tanaka M, Yasaka M, Nagano K, et al: Moderate atheroma of the aortic arch and the risk of stroke, *Cerebrovasc Dis* 21:26-31, 2006.

27. Fujimoto S, Yasaka M, Otsubo R, et al: Aortic arch atherosclerotic lesions and the recurrence of ischemic stroke, *Stroke* 35:1426-1429, 2004.

28. Di Tullio MR, Sacco RL, Savoia MT, et al: Gender differences in the risk of ischemic stroke associated with aortic atheromas, *Stroke* 31:2623-2627, 2000.

29. Sen S, Hinderliter A, Sen PK, et al: Aortic arch atheroma progression and recurrent vascular events in patients with stroke or transient ischemic attack, *Circulation* 116:928-935, 2007.

30. Cohen A, Tzourio C, Bertrand B, et al: Aortic plaque morphology and vascular events: A follow-up study in patients with ischemic stroke. FAPS Investigators. French Study of Aortic Plaques in Stroke, *Circulation* 96:3838-3841, 1997.

31. Tunick PA, Culliford AT, Lamparello PJ, et al: Atheromatosis of the aortic arch as an occult source of multiple systemic emboli, *Ann Intern Med* 114:391-392, 1991.

32. Tunick PA, Lackner H, Katz ES, et al: Multiple emboli from a large aortic arch thrombus in a patient with thrombotic diathesis, *Am Heart J* 124:239-241, 1992.

33. Nihoyannopoulos P, Joshi J, Athanasopoulos G, et al: Detection of atherosclerotic lesions in the aorta by transesophageal echocardiography, *Am J Cardiol* 71:1208-1212, 1993.

34. Ueno Y, Kimura K, Iguchi Y, et al: Mobile aortic plaques are a cause of multiple brain infarcts seen on diffusion-weighted imaging, *Stroke* 38:2470-2476, 2007.

35. Laperche T, Laurian C, Roudaut R, et al: Mobile thromboses of the aortic arch without aortic debris: A transesophageal echocardiographic finding associated with unexplained arterial embolism: The Filiale Echocardiographie de la Societe Francaise de Cardiologie, *Circulation* 96:288-294, 1997.

36. Rundek T, Di Tullio MR, Sciacca RR, et al: Association between large aortic arch atheromas and high-intensity transient signals in elderly stroke patients, *Stroke* 30:2683-2686, 1999.

37. Castellanos M, Serena J, Segura T, et al: Atherosclerotic aortic arch plaques in cryptogenic stroke: A microembolic signal monitoring study, *Eur Neurol* 45:145-150, 2001.

38. Zavala JA, Amarenco P, Davis SM, et al: Aortic arch atheroma, *Int J Stroke* 1:74-80, 2006.

39. Montgomery DH, Ververis JJ, McGorisk G, et al: Natural history of severe atheromatous disease of the thoracic aorta: A transesophageal echocardiographic study, *J Am Coll Cardiol* 27:95-101, 1996.

40. Sen S, Oppenheimer SM, Lima J, et al: Risk factors for progression of aortic atheroma in stroke and transient ischemic attack patients, *Stroke* 33:930-935, 2002.

41. Geraci A, Weinberger J: Natural history of aortic arch atherosclerotic plaque, *Neurology* 54:749-751, 2000.

42. Gupta V, Nanda NC, Yesilbursa D, et al: Racial differences in thoracic aorta atherosclerosis among ischemic stroke patients, *Stroke* 34:408-412, 2003.

43. Tribouilloy C, Peltier M, Colas L, et al: Fibrinogen is an independent marker for thoracic aortic atherosclerosis, *Am J Cardiol* 81:321-326, 1998.

44. Agmon Y, Khandheria BK, Meissner I, et al: Independent association of high blood pressure and aortic atherosclerosis: A population-based study, *Circulation* 102:2087-2093, 2000.

45. Di Tullio MR, Savoia MT, Sacco RL: Aortic arch atheromas and ischemic stroke in patients of different race-ethnicity, *Neurology* 46:A441, 1996.

46. Pitsavos CE, Aggeli KI, Barbetseas JD, et al: Effects of pravastatin on thoracic aortic atherosclerosis in patients with heterozygous familial hypercholesterolemia, *Am J Cardiol* 82:1484-1488, 1998.

47. Corti R, Fayad ZA, Fuster V, et al: Effects of lipid-lowering by simvastatin on human atherosclerotic lesions: A longitudinal study by high-resolution, noninvasive magnetic resonance imaging, *Circulation* 104:249-252, 2001.

48. Corti R, Fuster V, Fayad ZA, et al: Lipid lowering by simvastatin induces regression of human atherosclerotic lesions: Two years' follow-up by high-resolution noninvasive magnetic resonance imaging, *Circulation* 106:2884-2887, 2002.

49. Sueishi K, Ichikawa K, Nakagawa K, et al: Procoagulant properties of atherosclerotic aortas, *Ann N Y Acad Sci* 748:185-192, 1995.

50. Qizilbash N: Fibrinogen and cerebrovascular disease, *Eur Heart J* 16(Suppl A):42-45, 1995.

51. Kannel WB, D'Agostino RB, Belanger AJ: Update on fibrinogen as a cardiovascular risk factor, *Ann Epidemiol* 2:457-466, 1992.

52. Levenson J, Giral P, Razavian M, et al: Fibrinogen and silent atherosclerosis in subjects with cardiovascular risk factors, *Arterioscler Thromb Vasc Biol* 15:1263-1268, 1995.

53. Heinrich J, Schulte H, Schonfeld R, et al: Association of variables of coagulation, fibrinolysis and acute-phase with atherosclerosis in coronary and peripheral arteries and those arteries supplying the brain, *Thromb Haemost* 73:374-379, 1995.

54. Agewall S, Wikstrand J, Suurkula M, Tengborn L, Fagerberg B: Carotid artery wall morphology, haemostatic factors and cardiovascular disease. An ultrasound study in men at high and low risk for atherosclerotic disease, *Blood Coagul Fibrinolysis* 5:895-904, 1994.

55. Smith FB, Lowe GD, Fowkes FG, Rumley A, Rumley AG, Donnan PT, Housley E: Smoking, haemostatic factors and lipid peroxides in a population case control study of peripheral arterial disease, *Atherosclerosis* 102:155-162, 1993.

56. Lassila R, Peltonen S, Lepantalo M, et al: Severity of peripheral atherosclerosis is associated with fibrinogen and degradation of cross-linked fibrin, *Arterioscler Thromb* 13:1738-1742, 1993.

57. Willeit J, Kiechl S, Santer P, Oberhollenzer F, Egger G, Jarosch E, Mair A: Lipoprotein(a) and asymptomatic carotid artery disease: Evidence of a prominent role in the evolution of advanced carotid plaques: The Bruneck Study, *Stroke* 26:1582-1587, 1995.

58. Szirmai IG, Kamondi A, Magyar H, Juhasz C: Relation of laboratory and clinical variables to the grade of carotid atherosclerosis, *Stroke* 24:1811-1816, 1993.

59. Willeit J, Kiechl S: Prevalence and risk factors of asymptomatic extracranial carotid artery atherosclerosis. A population-based study, *Arterioscler Thromb* 13:661-668, 1993.

60. Folsom AR, Wu KK, Conlan MG, et al: Distributions of hemostatic variables in blacks and whites: Population reference values from the Atherosclerosis Risk in Communities (ARIC) Study, *Ethn Dis* 2:35-46, 1992.

61. Iso H, Folsom AR, Sato S, Wu KK, Shimamoto T, Koike K, Iida M, Komachi Y: Plasma fibrinogen and its correlates in Japanese and US population samples, *Arterioscler Thromb* 13:783-790, 1993.

62. Tribouilloy CM, Peltier M, Iannetta Peltier MC, Trojette F, Andrejak M, Lesbre JP: Plasma homocysteine and severity of thoracic aortic atherosclerosis, *Chest* 118:1685-1689, 2000.

63. Katz ES, Tunick PA, Kronzon I: Observations of coronary flow augmentation and balloon function during intraaortic balloon counterpulsation using transesophageal echocardiography, *Am J Cardiol* 69:1635-1639, 1992.

64. Coy KM, Maurer G, Goodman D, Siegel RJ: Transesophageal echocardiographic detection of aortic atheromatosis may provide clues to occult renal dysfunction in the elderly, *Am Heart J* 123:1684-1686, 1992.

65. Koppang JR, Nanda NC, Coghlan C, Sanyal R: Histologically confirmed cholesterol atheroemboli with identification of the source by transesophageal echocardiography, *Echocardiography* 9:379-383, 1992.

66. Peltier M, Iannetta Peltier MC, Sarano ME, Lesbre JP, Colas JL, Tribouilloy CM: Elevated serum lipoprotein(a) level is an independent marker of severity of thoracic aortic atherosclerosis, *Chest* 121:1589-1594, 2002.

67. Bartens W, Wanner C: Lipoprotein(a): New insights into an atherogenic lipoprotein, *Clin Invest* 72:558-567, 1994.

68. Rabbani LE, Loscalzo J: Recent observations on the role of hemostatic determinants in the development of the atherothrombotic plaque, *Atherosclerosis* 105:1-7, 1994.

69. Kallikazaros IE, Tsioufis CP, Stefanadis CI, et al: Closed relation between carotid and ascending aortic atherosclerosis in cardiac patients, *Circulation* 102:III263-III268, 2000.

70. Fazio GP, Redberg RF, Winslow T, Schiller NB: Transesophageal echocardiographically detected atherosclerotic aortic plaque is a marker for coronary artery disease, *J Am Coll Cardiol* 21:144-150, 1993.

71. Khoury Z, Gottlieb S, Stern S, Keren A: Frequency and distribution of atherosclerotic plaques in the thoracic aorta as determined by transesophageal echocardiography in patients with coronary artery disease, *Am J Cardiol* 79:23-27, 1997.

72. Oei HH, Vliegenthart R, Hak AE, et al: The association between coronary calcification assessed by electron beam computed tomography and measures of extracoronary atherosclerosis: the Rotterdam Coronary Calcification Study, *J Am Coll Cardiol* 39:1745-1751, 2002.

73. Matsumura Y, Takata J, Yabe T, et al: Atherosclerotic aortic plaque detected by transesophageal echocardiography: Its significance and limitation as a marker for coronary artery disease in the elderly, *Chest* 112:81-86, 1997.

74. Soloway HB, Aronson SM: Atheromatous emboli to central nervous system: Report of 16 cases, *Arch Neurol* 11:657-667, 1964.

75. Ben-Horin S, Bardan E, Barshack I, et al: Cholesterol crystal embolization to the digestive system: Characterization of a common, yet overlooked presentation of atheroembolism, *Am J Gastroenterol* 98:1471-1479, 2003.

76. Theriault J, Agharazzi M, Dumont M, et al: Atheroembolic renal failure requiring dialysis: Potential for renal recovery: A review of 43 cases, *Nephron Clin Pract* 94:c11-c18, 2003.

77. Bruno A, Russell PW, Jones WL, et al: Concomitants of asymptomatic retinal cholesterol emboli, *Stroke* 23:900-902, 1992.

78. Bruno A, Jones WL, Austin JK, et al: Vascular outcome in men with asymptomatic retinal cholesterol emboli: A cohort study, *Ann Intern Med* 122:249-253, 1995.

79. Mouradian M, Wijman CA, Tomasian D, et al: Echocardiographic findings of patients with retinal ischemia or embolism, *J Neuroimaging* 12:219-223, 2002.

80. Gore I, Collins DP: Spontaneous atheromatous embolization: Review of the literature and a report of 16 additional cases, *Am J Clin Pathol* 33:416-426, 1960.

81. Hauben M, Norwich J, Shapiro E, et al: Multiple cholesterol emboli syndrome—six cases identified through the spontaneous reporting system, *Angiology* 46:779-784, 1995.

82. Blauth CI, Cosgrove DM, Webb BW, et al: Atheroembolism from the ascending aorta: An emerging problem in cardiac surgery, *J Thorac Cardiovasc Surg* 103:1104-1111, 1992.

83. Doty JR, Wilentz RE, Salazar JD, et al: Atheroembolism in cardiac surgery, *Ann Thorac Surg* 75:1221-1226, 2003.

84. Roach GW, Kanchuger M, Mangano CM, et al: Adverse cerebral outcomes after coronary bypass surgery: Multicenter Study of Perioperative Ischemia Research Group and the Ischemia Research and Education Foundation Investigators, *N Engl J Med* 335:1857-1863, 1996.

85. van der Linden LJ, Hadjinikolaou L, Bergman P, Lindblom D: Postoperative stroke in cardiac surgery is related to the location and extent of atherosclerotic disease in the ascending aorta, *J Am Coll Cardiol* 38:131-135, 2001.

86. Hogue CW Jr, Murphy SF, Schechtman KB, Davila-Roman VG: Risk factors for early or delayed stroke after cardiac surgery, *Circulation* 100:642-647, 1999.

87. Ura M, Sakata R, Nakayama Y, Goto T: Ultrasonographic demonstration of manipulation-related aortic injuries after cardiac surgery, *J Am Coll Cardiol* 35:1303-1310, 2000.

88. Trehan N, Mishra M, Kasliwal RR, Mishra A: Reduced neurological injury during CABG in patients with mobile aortic atheromas: A five-year follow-up study, *Ann Thorac Surg* 70:1558-1564, 2000.

89. Karalis DG, Quinn V, Victor MF, et al: Risk of catheter-related emboli in patients with atherosclerotic debris in the thoracic aorta, *Am Heart J* 131:1149-1155, 1996.

90. Keeley EC, Grines CL: Scraping of aortic debris by coronary guiding catheters: A prospective evaluation of 1,000 cases, *J Am Coll Cardiol* 32:1861-1865, 1998.

91. Dressler FA, Craig WR, Castello R, Labovitz AJ: Mobile aortic atheroma and systemic emboli: Efficacy of anticoagulation and influence of plaque morphology on recurrent stroke, *J Am Coll Cardiol* 31:134-138, 1998.

92. Transesophageal echocardiographic correlates of thromboembolism in high-risk patients with nonvalvular atrial fibrillation: The Stroke Prevention in Atrial Fibrillation Investigators Committee on Echocardiography, *Ann Intern Med* 128:639-647, 1998.

93. Ferrari E, Vidal R, Chevallier T, Baudouy M: Atherosclerosis of the thoracic aorta and aortic debris as a marker of poor prognosis: Benefit of oral anticoagulants, *J Am Coll Cardiol* 33:1317-1322, 1999.

94. Di Tullio MR, Russo C, Jin Z, et al: Aortic arch plaques and risk of recurrent stroke and death, *Circulation* 119:2376-2382, 2009.

95. Russo C, Di Tullio MR, Jin Z, et al: Warfarin vs. aspirin for prevention of recurrent stroke and death in patients with large aortic arch plaques, *J Am Coll Cardiol [abstract]*, 51 (10):A318, 2008.

96. Moldveen-Geronimus M, Merriam JC Jr: Cholesterol embolization: From pathological curiosity to clinical entity, *Circulation* 35:946-953, 1967.

97. Hollier LH, Kazmier FJ, Ochsner J, et al: "Shaggy" aorta syndrome with atheromatous embolization to visceral vessels, *Ann Vasc Surg* 5:439-444, 1991.

98. Hilton TC, Menke D, Blackshear JL: Variable effect of anticoagulation in the treatment of severe protruding atherosclerotic aortic debris, *Am Heart J* 127:1645-1647, 1994.

99. Blackshear JL, Zabalgoitia M, Pennock G, et al: Warfarin safety and efficacy in patients with thoracic aortic plaque and atrial fibrillation. SPAF TEE Investigators. Stroke Prevention and Atrial Fibrillation. Transesophageal echocardiography, *Am J Cardiol* 83:453-455, 1999:A9.

100. Donnan GA, Davis SM, Jones EF, Amarenco P: Aortic source of brain embolism, *Curr Treat Options Cardiovasc Med* 5:211-219, 2003.

101. Hausmann D, Gulba D, Bargheer K, et al: Successful thrombolysis of an aortic-arch thrombus in a patient after mesenteric embolism, *N Engl J Med* 327:500-501, 1992.

102. Geraets DR, Hoehns JD, Burke TG, Grover-McKay M: Thrombolytic-associated cholesterol emboli syndrome: Case report and literature review, *Pharmacotherapy* 15:441-450, 1995.

103. Aggarwal K, Tjahja IE: Atheroembolic disease following administration of tissue plasminogen activator (TPA), *Clin Cardiol* 19:906-908, 1996.

104. Tunick PA, Nayar AC, Goodkin GM, et al: Effect of treatment on the incidence of stroke and other emboli in 519 patients with severe thoracic aortic plaque, *Am J Cardiol* 90:1320-1325, 2002.

105. Stern A, Tunick PA, Culliford AT, et al: Protruding aortic arch atheromas: risk of stroke during heart surgery with and without aortic arch endarterectomy, *Am Heart J* 138:746-752, 1999.

106. Rokkas CK, Kouchoukos NT: Surgical management of the severely atherosclerotic ascending aorta during cardiac operations, *Semin Thorac Cardiovasc Surg* 10:240-246, 1998.

107. King RC, Kanithanon RC, Shockey KS, et al: Replacing the atherosclerotic ascending aorta is a high-risk procedure, *Ann Thorac Surg* 66:396-401, 1998.

108. Fayad ZA, Nahar T, Fallon JT, et al: In vivo magnetic resonance evaluation of atherosclerotic plaques in the human thoracic aorta: A comparison with transesophageal echocardiography, *Circulation* 101:2503-2509, 2000.

109. Helft G, Worthley SG, Fuster V, Zaman AG, Schechter C, Osende JI, Rodriguez OJ, Fayad ZA, Fallon JT, Badimon JJ: Atherosclerotic aortic component quantification by noninvasive magnetic resonance imaging: An in vivo study in rabbits, *J Am Coll Cardiol* 37:1149-1154, 2001.

110. Tenenbaum A, Garniek A, Shemesh J, et al: Dual-helical CT for detecting aortic atheromas as a source of stroke: Comparison with transesophageal echocardiography, *Radiology* 208:153–158, 1998.

111. Litovsky S, Madjid M, Zarrabi A, et al: Superparamagnetic iron oxide-based method for quantifying recruitment of monocytes to mouse atherosclerotic lesions in vivo: Enhancement by tissue necrosis factor-alpha, interleukin-1beta, and interferon-gamma, *Circulation* 107:1545–1549, 2003.

112. Lancelot E, Amirbekian V, Brigger I, et al: Evaluation of matrix metalloproteinases in atherosclerosis using a novel noninvasive imaging approach, *Arterioscler Thromb Vasc Biol* 28:425–432, 2008.

113. Tahara N, Kai H, Ishibashi M, et al: Simvastatin attenuates plaque inflammation: Evaluation by fluorodeoxyglucose positron emission tomography, *J Am Coll Cardiol* 48:1825–1831, 2006.

39 CADASIL: Cerebral Autosomal Dominant Arteriopathy with Subcortical Infarcts and Leukoencephalopathy

HUGUES CHABRIAT, ANNE JOUTEL, ELISABETH TOURNIER-LASSERVE, MARIE-GERMAINE BOUSSER

CADASIL (cerebral autosomal dominant arteriopathy with subcortical infarcts and leukoencephalopathy)[1] is an inherited small artery disease of midadulthood that was identified through the use of clinical, magnetic resonance imaging (MRI), pathologic, and genetic tools in the 1990s.[2,3] The disease is due to mutations of the *NOTCH3* gene on chromosome 19,[4] which lead to an accumulation of the ectodomain of this receptor within the vascular wall. CADASIL is responsible for subcortical ischemic events and leads progressively to dementia with pseudobulbar palsy. The disease was first reported in European families. Today, CADASIL has been diagnosed in European, American, African, and Asiatic pedigrees and reported on all continents. The disease remains probably largely underdiagnosed.

History

In 1955, Van Bogaert[5] reported two sisters belonging to a family originating from Belgium who had a "subcortical encephalopathy of Binswanger's type of rapid course" with onset during midadulthood. Their clinical presentation included dementia, gait disturbances, pseudobulbar palsy, seizures, and focal neurologic deficits. Two other sisters had died at age 36 and 43 years after a progressive dementia. The father had a stroke at age 51 and died after a myocardial infarct. The pathologic examination revealed widespread areas of white matter rarefaction in the brain associated with multiple small infarcts, mainly located in the white matter and basal ganglia.[5]

In 1977, Sourander and Walinder[6,7] called "hereditary multi-infarct dementia" a familial condition observed in a Swedish pedigree and characterized by dementia associated with pseudobulbar palsy occurring 10 to 15 years after recurrent strokelike episode. Age at onset was between 29 and 38 years, and age at death varied from 30 to 53 years. These researchers reported brain lesions identical to those observed by Van Bogaert in three cases also caused by small vessel disease in the brain. The walls of the small arteries were thickened, causing a reduction of their lumens. Atherosclerosis of basal arteries was found in only one family

member. In the pedigree, the condition followed an autosomal dominant pattern of transmission. The disease was only recently distinguished from CADASIL.[8]

Up to 1993, several families having diseases close in presentation to the cases already described were reported, with the use of numerous terms and eponyms for their condition—chronic familial vascular encephalopathy,[9] familiäre zerebrale Arteriosklerose,[10] familiäre zerebrale Gefäßerkrankung,[11] démence sous-corticale familiale avec leucoencéphalopathie artériopathique,[12] familial disorder with subcortical ischemic strokes, dementia and leukoencephalopathy,[13] and slowly progressive familial dementia with recurrent strokes and white matter hypodensities on computed tomography (CT) scan.[14]

In 1976, we saw a 50-year-old patient with a clinical history of recurrent lacunar infarcts who presented with a large and widespread hypodensity of the white matter on CT scan. He had no vascular risk factors, in particular, no hypertension. Ten years later, his daughter came to see us for a long history of attacks of migraine with aura and transient ischemic attacks and for a recent minor stroke. CT and MRI showed lesions in the white matter identical to those observed in her father. These two observations were the basis of an extensive clinical, MRI, and genetic study of the whole family, which was a very large one originating from the western part of France called Loire-Atlantique. The data were first presented as "recurrent strokes in a family with diffuse white matter and muscular lipidosis—a new mitochondrial cytopathy?"[2] then as "autosomal dominant syndrome with strokelike episodes and leukoencephalopathy,"[15] and later as "autosomal dominant leukoencephalopathy and subcortical ischemic strokes."[2] Because of the confusion raised by all these different names, we proposed the acronym CADASIL (cerebral autosomal dominant arteriopathy with subcortical infarcts and leukoencephalopathy) in 1993 to designate this disease and highlight its main characteristics.[2] After genetic analysis in the large family from Loire-Atlantique, the affected gene was located on chromosome 19 in the same year.[1] In 1996, various mutations of the *NOTCH3* gene were found to be responsible for the disease. Since then, CADASIL has been recognized in hundreds of families on all continents. Genetic testing is now currently used for diagnosis. The gene identification was also crucial to better understanding of the pathophysiology of the disease and for the development of transgenic mouse models of the disease.[16]

Clinical Presentation

The earliest clinical manifestations of CADASIL are attacks of migraine with aura. Despite their frequency, which is four times that in the general population,[17,18] these manifestations are inconstant, observed in only 20% to 30% of symptomatic subjects. Migraine with aura is five times more frequent in patients with CADASIL than in the general population, in contrast to migraine without aura, which has the same frequency as in the general population. When present, migraine with aura is usually the first symptom, with an average onset at age 30 years (range 6 to 48 years), occurring 10 years earlier in women.[19] An early age was found to be correlated in only one study with a high serum homocysteine level.[20] Most frequently, attacks are typical, with visual or sensory aura symptoms lasting 20 to 30 minutes, followed by a headache lasting a few hours; 50% of the patients, however, have atypical attacks, with basilar, hemiplegic, or prolonged aura, and a few patients have very severe attacks, with confusion, fever, meningitis, or coma.[19,21-23] The frequency of attacks is highly variable, and trigger factors are the usual ones identified for migraine.[19] Migraine with aura may be the prominent symptom of CADASIL in some families. The frequency of migraine attacks can also differ largely among affected subjects, from one attack in a lifetime to several attacks per month.[19]

Stroke is the most frequent clinical manifestation of the disease. About two thirds of symptomatic subjects have had transient ischemic attacks or a completed stroke.[24] These events occur at a mean age of 41 ± 9 years (extreme limits from 20 to 65 years).[17,18,24] Two thirds of them are classic lacunar syndromes: pure motor stroke, ataxic hemiparesis, pure sensory stroke, sensory motor stroke. Other focal neurologic deficits of abrupt onset are less frequently observed: dysarthria either isolated or associated with motor or sensory deficit, monoparesis, paresthesias of one limb, isolated ataxia, nonfluent aphasia, and hemianopia.[17] The onset of the neurologic deficit can be progressive over several hours. Some neurologic deficits occur suddenly and are associated with headache. When they are transient, they can mimic attacks of migraine with aura. Ischemic events usually occur in the absence of vascular risk factors. However, they are also observed in some patients with one or several vascular risk factors, most frequently in tobacco users or hypertensive subjects. The influence of such factors on the clinical and MRI phenotype remains unknown.[4,18]

About 20% of patients with CADASIL have a history of severe episodes of mood disturbances. The frequency is again widely variable among families.[17,25] A few patients have a severe depression of the melancholic type, sometimes alternating with typical manic episodes.[17,18,21,26] The location of ischemic lesions in basal ganglia or in frontal white matter may play a key role in their occurrence.[27,28] Apathy characterized by a lack of motivation associated with a reduction in voluntary behavior has recently been recognized as a major clinical manifestation present in about 40% of patients, independent of depression.[29]

Dementia is the second most common clinical manifestation of CADASIL. It is reported in one third of symptomatic patients. The location of cerebral lesions explains the "subcortical" aspect of the cognitive deficit. The neuropsychological deficit of this syndrome with a progressive or stepwise course is mainly responsible for attention deficit, apathy, and memory impairment.[12,17,30] Aphasia, apraxia, and agnosia are rare or observed only at the end stage of the disease.[12,14] The cognitive deficit is often subtle, particularly at the onset of the disease, and can be detected with a battery of neuropsychological testing. Tests of executive functions can detect the earliest cognitive alterations before age 35 years.[31] The cognitive decline can occur either suddenly, stepwise, or progressively in the total absence of ischemic events, mimicking a degenerative dementia.[17,21] The frequency and severity of cognitive decline can vary among different members of a given family. The variable location and severity of cerebral tissue damage might play a key role. In a positron emission tomography study of two affected brothers, one demented and the other asymptomatic, a severe cortical metabolic depression was found in the demented subject, who only had infarcts within basal ganglia and thalamus.

Furthermore, we recently observed that the severity of white matter microstructural damage is strongly related to the clinical status in CADASIL.[32] This observation agrees with the correlations observed between the clinical status and the load of infarctions within the white matter[33] and with atrophy.[34] Therefore, the degree of tissue destruction or neuronal loss is crucial to the cognitive status of CADASIL patients. When dementia is present at a mean age of 60 years, it is observed in the absence of any other clinical manifestations in only 10% of cases. Dementia is always associated with pyramidal signs, pseudobulbar palsy, gait difficulties, urinary incontinence, or a combination of these conditions.[35] The cognitive and functional decline is usually progressive. The patient becomes bedridden and often dies after pulmonary complications of swallowing difficulties. Baudrimont and colleagues[2] reported that one patient with CADASIL died after the occurrence of a deep cerebral hematoma. Dementia is present in 90% of cases before death, which occurs at a median age of 64 years in men and 69 years in women.[18]

Other neurologic manifestations have occasionally been reported in CADASIL. Focal or generalized seizures have been observed in 6% to 10% of cases.[17,18] Deafness of acute or rapid onset has been observed in several cases.[15] The lack of cranial nerve palsy, spinal cord disease, and symptoms of muscular origin is noteworthy in CADASIL. The cause of the radiculopathy reported in one case by Ragno and associates[26] has not been determined.

Finally, the natural history of the disease is summarized in Figure 39-1. CADASIL starts between 20 and 30 years in one fifth of the patients as attacks of migraine with aura. Ischemic manifestations, observed in two thirds of the patients, occur mainly during the fourth and fifth decades. Executive dysfunction and apathy are frequent clinical manifestations after the age of stroke onset. They are sometimes associated with severe mood disturbances.

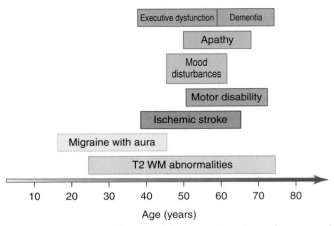

Figure 39-1 Natural history of the main clinical manifestations of CADASIL (cerebral autosomal dominant arteriopathy with subcortical infarcts and leukoencephalopathy). T2 WM, abnormalities in white matter as seen on T2-weighted MRI. (Modified from Chabriat H, Joutel A, Dichgans M, et al: CADASIL. *Lancet Neurol* 8:643-653,2009.)

Dementia mainly occurs during the sixth decade and is nearly constant before death.

Neuroimaging

MRI is crucial for the diagnosis of CADASIL. The findings are always abnormal in symptomatic subjects.[2,17,35] In addition, the signal abnormalities can be detected during a presymptomatic period of variable duration. MRI signal abnormalities are observed as early as 20 years of age. After age 35, all subjects having the affected gene have an abnormal MRI.[3,36] The frequency of asymptomatic subjects with abnormal MRI findings decreases progressively with aging among the gene carriers and becomes very low after 60 years.

T1-weighted MR images show punctiform or nodular hypointense signals in basal ganglia and white matter. T2-weighted images show hyperintensities in the regions often associated with widespread areas of increased signal in the white matter.[31] The severity of MRI signal abnormalities is variable. These lesions dramatically increase with age in affected patients. In subjects younger than 40 years, hyperintensities on T2-weighted images are usually punctuate or nodular with a symmetrical distribution and predominate in periventricular areas and in the centrum semiovale. Later in life, white matter lesions are diffuse and can involve the whole of white matter, including the U fibers under the cortex. The frequency of signal abnormalities in the external capsule (two thirds of cases) and in the anterior part of the temporal lobes is noteworthy.[37] Brainstem lesions are observed mainly in the pons.[32] The medulla is usually spared. Cortical or cerebellar lesions are exceptional. They have been observed in only two patients older than 60 years. CT can reveal the white matter and basal ganglia lesions but is much less sensitive than MRI.[38]

Other MRI findings include dilated perivascular spaces with typical "état criblé" in some cases[39] and microbleeds detected on gradient-echo images in 25% to 69% of subjects[40,41] related to age, glycosylated hemoglobin content, and blood pressure values.[42]

Findings of cerebral angiography performed in 14 patients belonging to seven affected families were normal except in one patient, in whom a detectable narrowing of small arteries was seen.[17] Weller and coworkers[43] reported a worsening of the neurologic status in two patients with CADASIL after angiography, the findings of which were normal, with a possible vasospasm in one patient. One patient had a severe headache, vomiting, confusion, somnolence, and a grand mal seizure that resolved within several hours.[43] Dichgans and associates[44] later confirmed the high frequency of neurologic complications after angiography in patients with CADASIL. Ultrasound studies and echocardiography findings are usually normal, although a high frequency of patent foramen ovale (47%) has been reported in an Italian series.[45] Cerebrospinal fluid examination findings are usually normal, although oligoclonal bands with pleiocytosis have been reported.[38] An isolated increase in complement factor B has been reported in three patients with CADASIL.[46] Electromyographic findings are essentially normal. A monoclonal immunoglobulin was detected in the sera of a few isolated cases.[15]

Pathology

Macroscopic examination of the brain shows a diffuse myelin pallor and rarefaction of the hemispheric white matter sparing the U fibers.[2,47] Lesions predominate in the periventricular areas and centrum semiovale. They are associated with lacunar infarcts located in the white matter and basal ganglia (lentiform nucleus, thalamus, caudate) (Fig. 39-2).[47,48] The most severe hemispheric lesions are the most profound.[2,12] In the brainstem, the lesions are more marked in the pons and are similar to the pontine rarefaction of myelin of ischemic origin described by Pullicino and colleagues.[49] Microscopic investigations showed that the wall of cerebral and leptomeningeal arterioles is thickened with a significant reduction of the lumen.[2] Such abnormalities can also be detected by leptomeningeal biopsy.[50] Some inconstant features are similar to those reported in patients with hypertensive encephalopathy: duplication and splitting of internal elastic lamina, adventitial hyalinosis and fibrosis, and hypertrophy of the media.[51] However, a distinctive feature is the presence of a granular material within the media and extending into the adventitia. The periodic acid-Schiff (PAS)–positive staining response suggested the presence of glycoproteins; results of staining for amyloid substance and elastin are negative.[2,48,52,53] Immunohistochemistry does not support the presence of immunoglobulins. By contrast, the endothelium of the vessels is usually spared. Sometimes, the smooth muscle cells are not detectable and have been replaced by collagen fibers.[51] On electron microscopy, the smooth muscle cells appear swollen and often degenerated, some with multiple nuclei. A granular, electron-dense, osmiophilic material has been seen within the media.[47] This material consists of granules about 10 to 15 nm in diameter.[51] It is localized close to the cell membrane of the smooth muscle cells, where it appears very dense. The smooth muscle cells are separated by large amounts of the unidentified material. In a single case, these vascular abnormalities were found to be associated with typical lesions of Alzheimer's disease.[54]

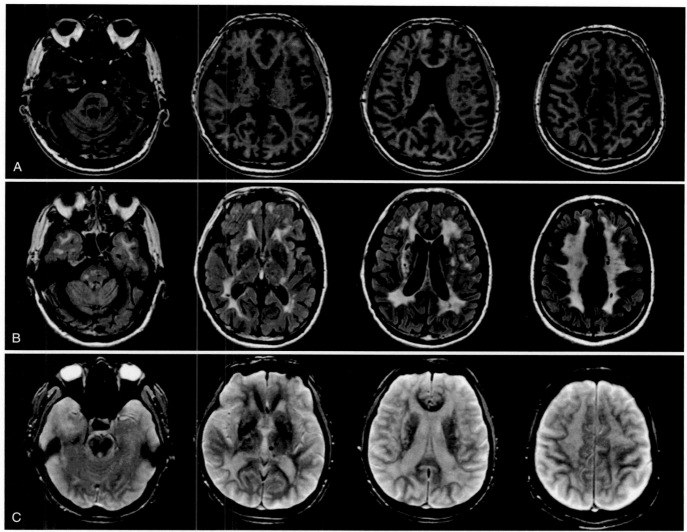

Figure 39-2 MRI aspects of CADASIL (cerebral autosomal dominant arteriopathy with subcortical infarcts and leukoencephalopathy) in a 61-year-old patient with a history of stroke, gait difficulties, and cognitive complaints. A, T1-weighted MR images showing lacunar infarcts located in the brainstem (pons), thalamus, and lentiform nuclei. B, On fluid-attenuated inversion recovery (FLAIR) images, the small deep infarcts are detected in association with diffuse and confluent white matter hyperintensities involving the anterior part of the temporal lobes. C, On T2*-weighted or gradient-echo images, microbleeds are visible as small hypointense foci in the thalamus and brainstem. (Modified from Chabriat H, Joutel A, Dichgans M, et al: CADASIL. *Lancet Neurol* 8:643-653, 2009.)

Ruchoux and associates[48,55,56] made the crucial observation that the vascular abnormalities observed in the brain were also detectable in other organs. The granular and osmiophilic material surrounding the smooth muscle cells as seen with electron microscopy is also present in the media of arteries located in the spleen, liver, kidneys, muscle, and skin and also in the wall of carotid and aortic arteries.[48,55] These vascular lesions can also be detected by nerve biopsy.[57] The presence of this material in the skin vessels allows one to confirm the diagnosis of CADASIL in difficult cases by means of punch skin biopsies,[58] although the sensitivity and specificity of this method have not yet been completely established.[48,55,59] Skin biopsy immunostaining with a Notch3 monoclonal antibody revealing the accumulation of Notch3 protein in the vessel wall is also another diagnostic tool of high sensitivity (85% to 95%) and specificity (95% to 100%).[60,61]

Genetics

The clinical penetrance of the disease is related to age and is close to 100% after age 50 years. The penetrance based on MRI features reaches 100% at age 35 years. In the absence of a positive familial history, the diagnosis of CADASIL should not be ruled out, because of the possibility of de novo mutations of the *NOTCH3* gene.[62]

CADASIL is caused by stereotyped mutations of the *NOTCH3* gene. This gene is a 2321–amino acid protein; it is a transmembrane receptor with an extracellular domain containing 34 EGF (epidermal growth factor) repeats (including 6 cysteine residues) and 3 Lin repeats associated with an intracellular and a transmembrane domains. The stereotyped missense mutations responsible for the disease are within epidermal growth factor–like (EGF-like) repeats and only located in the extracellular domain of the Notch3 protein. In 70% of cases, they are located within exons 3 and 4, which encode the first five EGF domains. All mutations in CADASIL lead to an uneven number of cysteine residues and presumably alter the function of the receptor.

The Notch3 protein is expressed exclusively in vascular smooth muscle cells.[63] The protein undergoes a proteolytic cleavage leading to an extracellular and a transmembrane fragment. After cleavage, these two fragments form a heterodimer at the cell surface. The ectodomain of the Notch3 receptor accumulates within the vessel walls of affected subjects. This accumulation is found near but not within the characteristic granular osmiophilic material seen on electron microscopy. It is observed in all vascular smooth muscle cells and in pericytes within all organs (brain, heart, muscles, lungs, skin). An abnormal clearance of the Notch3 ectodomain from the smooth muscle cell surface is presumed to cause this accumulation.[63]

The identification of the gene for CADASIL was a crucial step in developing a molecular diagnostic test that is now currently used for the diagnosis of the disease. More than 95% of mutations in the *NOTCH3* gene are missense mutations. Others are small in-frame deletions or splice-site mutations.[64-68] Remarkably, all mutations lead to an odd number of cysteine residues within a given epidermal growth factor repeats.[52,65,69-73] De novo mutations have been reported, but their exact frequency is unknown.[62,74] Two homozygous patients have so far been described.[75,76] Genetic testing is the gold standard for the diagnosis of CADASIL. Screening of the 23 exons encoding the 34 EGF repeats has 100% specificity when it detects a mutation leading to an odd number of cysteine residues within an EGFR. Its sensitivity is also close to 100%.[70,72,77]

Diagnosis

CADASIL should be considered in any patient with transient ischemic attacks or strokes, severe mood disorders, or attacks of migraine with aura or dementia in whom MRI discloses widespread signal abnormalities in the subcortical white matter and basal ganglia. This association should prompt a genealogic study of the family, including all first- and second-degree relatives. Clinical or neuroimaging data, or both, obtained from these sources are crucial to confirm the hereditary origin of the disease. The diagnosis can be confirmed by genetic testing with or without skin biopsy (see previous discussion).

The clinical and MRI presentation of CADASIL is very close to that of Binswanger's disease (BD), although the two conditions differ on the following three points: Unlike CADASIL, Binswanger's disease occurs most often in hypertensive patients, is not associated with migraine with aura, and is not recognized as an autosomal dominant condition. However, it should be noted that the familial character has not been systematically evaluated in most cases of Binswanger's disease and that, conversely, sporadic mutations of the *NOTCH3* gene are possible.[62] On MRI, involvement of the external capsule and anterior white matter of temporal lobes appears more frequent and severe in CADASIL, a feature useful for differential diagnosis. Some causes of vascular leukoencephalopathies are

easy to recognize. Amyloid angiopathies of hereditary origin can manifest as ischemic strokes and MRI white matter signal abnormalities but are essentially characterized by recurrent lobar cerebral hemorrhages and the presence of amyloid deposits within the wall of brain vessels.[78,79]

The "familial young-onset arteriosclerotic leukoencephalopathy" reported in Japanese pedigrees is an autosomal recessive condition also called CARASIL (cerebral autosomal recessive arteriopathy with subcortical infarcts and leukoencephalopathy), associated with alopecia and skeletal abnormalities secondary to a thickening of the intima of small cerebral vessels. It is caused by mutations of the HtrA serine protease 1 (*HTRA1*) gene that repress signaling by transforming growth factor-β family members.[80,81] The hereditary leukoencephalopathy described by Lossos and associates,[82] a disorder with increased skin collagen content, leads to a progressive dementia and is associated with palmoplantar keratoderma.[82] CADASIL, particularly at onset, can be difficult to differentiate from multiple sclerosis. The autosomal dominant pattern of transmission of the disease, the absence of optic nerve and spinal cord involvement, and the symmetrical distribution of white matter signal abnormalities often associated with basal ganglia infarcts on MRI are the most helpful signs of the disease.[64] Also, adrenoleukodystrophy, an X-linked metabolic disorder with accumulation of very-long-chain fatty acids, can be observed in adults but, unlike CADASIL, does not involve basal ganglia; the cerebral disease is progressive and associated with spinal cord and peripheral nerve demyelination.

Other ischemic small vessel diseases with clinical and MRI presentations close to that observed in CADASIL and autosomal dominant transmission but distinct from CADASIL have been identified.[83]

Conclusion

CADASIL is a systemic genetic disease of vascular smooth muscle cells. Genetic and pathologic research now suggests that the accumulation of the ectodomain of the Notch3 protein is associated with the severe ultrastructural alterations of the arteriolar wall observed in this disease. Other data suggest that the arteriolar wall changes may result in cerebral hypoperfusion leading to the progressive accumulation of tissue lesions. These lesions predominate in the most vulnerable cerebral areas possibly because of the distinctive angioarchitecture of the brain. Finally, both the variable severity of the tissue destruction within the white matter and basal ganglia and their different locations might be important sources of the variability in clinical severity seen in the members of a given family.

Not only is the research performed in CADASIL crucial to determining the best target for future prevention of the disease, but it is also important for a better understanding of the pathophysiology of small artery diseases. CADASIL can be regarded as a unique model to investigate the determinants of vascular dementia, the clinical correlates of ischemic white matter lesions, and the natural history of tissue damage in small vessel disease. Furthermore, the identification of the *Notch3* gene is a major step in the dismantling of the group of cerebral vascular disorders associated with leukoaraiosis.

REFERENCES

1. Tournier-Lasserve E, Joutel A, Melki J, et al: Cerebral autosomal dominant arteriopathy with subcortical infarcts and leukoencephalopathy maps to chromosome 19q12, *Nat Genet* 3:256-259, 1993.
2. Baudrimont M, Dubas F, Joutel A, et al: Autosomal dominant leukoencephalopathy and subcortical ischemic stroke. A clinicopathological study, *Stroke* 24:122-125, 1993.
3. Joutel A, Corpechot C, Ducros A, et al: Notch3 mutations in CADASIL, a hereditary adult-onset condition causing stroke and dementia, *Nature* 383:707-710, 1996.
4. Chabriat H, Joutel A, Vahedi K, et al: [CADASIL (cerebral autosomal dominant arteriopathy with subcortical infarcts and leukoencephalopathy)], *J Mal Vasc* 21:277-282, 1996.
5. Van Bogaert L: Encephalopathie sous-corticale progressive (Binswanger) à évolution rapide chez deux soeurs, *Med Hellen* 961-972, 1955.
6. Sourander P, Walinder J: Hereditary multi-infarct dementia. Morphological and clinical studies of a new disease, *Acta Neuropathol (Berl)* 39:247-254, 1977.
7. Sourander P, Walinder J: Hereditary multi-infarct dementia, *Lancet* 1(8019):1015, 1977.
8. Low WC, Junna M, Borjesson-Hanson A, et al: Hereditary multi-infarct dementia of the Swedish type is a novel disorder different from NOTCH3 causing CADASIL, *Brain* 130:357-367, 2007.
9. Stevens DL, Hewlett RH, Brownell B: Chronic familial vascular encephalopathy, *Lancet* 1:1364-1365, 1977.
10. Gerhard: Familiäre zerebrale Arteriosklerose, *Zbl Allgemein Pathol Bd* 163, 1980.
11. Colmant H: Familiäre zerebrale Gefäberkrankung, *Zbl Allgemein Pathologie Bd* (1/2):124, 1980:163.
12. Davous P, Fallet-Bianco C: [Familial subcortical dementia with arteriopathic leukoencephalopathy. A clinico-pathological case], *Rev Neurol (Paris)* 147:376-384, 1991.
13. Mas JL, Dilouya A, De Recondo J: A familial disorder with subcortical ischemic strokes, dementia and leukoencephalopathy, *Neurology* 42:1015-1019, 1992.
14. Salvi F, Michelucci R, Plasmati R, et al: Slowly progressive familial dementia with recurrent strokes and white matter hypodensities on CT scan, *Ital J Neurol Sci* 13:135-140, 1992.
15. Tournier-Lasserve E, Iba-Zizen MT, Romero N, Bousser MG: Autosomal dominant syndrome with strokelike episodes and leukoencephalopathy, *Stroke* 22:1297-1302, 1991.
16. Ruchoux MM, Domenga V, Brulin P, et al: Transgenic mice expressing mutant Notch3 develop vascular alterations characteristic of cerebral autosomal dominant arteriopathy with subcortical infarcts and leukoencephalopathy, *Am J Pathol* 162:329-342, 2003.
17. Chabriat H, Vahedi K, Iba-Zizen MT, et al: Clinical spectrum of CADASIL: A study of 7 families. Cerebral autosomal dominant arteriopathy with subcortical infarcts and leukoencephalopathy, *Lancet* 346:934-939, 1995.
18. Dichgans M, Mayer M, Uttner I, et al: The phenotypic spectrum of CADASIL: Clinical findings in 102 cases, *Ann Neurol* 44:731-739, 1998.
19. Vahedi K, Chabriat H, Levy C, et al: Migraine with aura and brain magnetic resonance imaging abnormalities in patients with CADASIL, *Arch Neurol* 61:1237-1240, 2004.
20. Singhal S, Bevan S, Barrick T, et al: The influence of genetic and cardiovascular risk factors on the CADASIL phenotype, *Brain* 127:2031-2038, 2004.
21. Verin M, Rolland Y, Landgraf F, et al: New phenotype of the cerebral autosomal dominant arteriopathy mapped to chromosome 19: Migraine as the prominent clinical feature, *J Neurol Neurosurg Psychiatry* 59:579-585, 1995.
22. Schon F, Martin RJ, Prevett M, et al: "CADASIL coma": An underdiagnosed acute encephalopathy, *J Neurol Neurosurg Psychiatry* 74:249-252, 2003.
23. Requena I, Indakoetxea B, Lema C, et al: [Coma associated with migraine], *Rev Neurol* 29:1048-1051, 1999.
24. Desmond DW, Moroney JT, Lynch T, et al: The natural history of CADASIL: A pooled analysis of previously published cases, *Stroke* 30:1230-1233, 1999.
25. Chabriat H, Tournier-Lasserve E, Vahedi K, et al: Autosomal dominant migraine with MRI white-matter abnormalities mapping to the CADASIL locus, *Neurology* 45:1086-1091, 1995.
26. Ragno M, Tournier-Lasserve E, Fiori MG, et al: An Italian kindred with cerebral autosomal dominant arteriopathy with subcortical infarcts and leukoencephalopathy (CADASIL), *Ann Neurol* 38:231-236, 1995.
27. Bhatia K, Marsden C: The behavioural and motor consequences of focal lesions of the basal ganglia in man, *Brain* 117:859-876, 1994.
28. Aylward ED, Roberts-Willie JV, Barta PE, et al: Basal ganglia volume and white matter hyperintensities in patients with bipolar disorder, *Am J Psychiatry* 5:687-693, 1994.
29. Reyes S, Viswanathan A, Godin O, et al: Apathy: A major symptom in CADASIL, *Neurology* 72:905-910, 2009.
30. Davous P, Bequet D: [CADASIL—a new model for subcortical dementia], *Rev Neurol (Paris)* 151:634-639, 1995.
31. Chabriat H, Levy C, Taillia H, et al: Patterns of MRI lesions in CADASIL, *Neurology* 51:452-457, 1998.
32. Chabriat H, Mrissa R, Levy C, et al: Brain stem MRI signal abnormalities in CADASIL, *Stroke* 30:457-459, 1999.
33. Viswanathan A, Gschwendtner A, Guichard JP, et al: Lacunar lesions are independently associated with disability and cognitive impairment in CADASIL, *Neurology* 69:172-179, 2007.
34. Viswanathan A, Godin O, Jouvent E, et al: Impact of MRI markers in subcortical vascular dementia: A multi-modal analysis in CADASIL, *Neurobiol Aging* 31:1629-1636, 2010.
35. Bousser MG, Tournier-Lasserve E: Summary of the proceedings of the First International Workshop on CADASIL. Paris, May 19-21, 1993. *Stroke* 25:704-707, 1994.
36. Chabriat H, Bousser MG, Pappata S: Cerebral autosomal dominant arteriopathy with subcortical infarcts and leukoencephalopathy: A positron emission tomography study in two affected family members, *Stroke* 26:1729-1730, 1995.
37. van Den Boom R, Lesnik Oberstein SA, van Duinen SG, et al: Subcortical lacunar lesions: an MR imaging finding in patients with cerebral autosomal dominant arteriopathy with subcortical infarcts and leukoencephalopathy, *Radiology* 224:791-796, 2002.
38. Chabriat H, Joutel A, Vahedi K, et al: [CADASIL. Cerebral autosomal dominant arteriopathy with subcortical infarcts and leukoencephalopathy], *Rev Neurol (Paris)* 153:376-385, 1997.
39. Cumurciuc R, Guichard JP, Reizine D, et al: Dilation of Virchow-Robin spaces in CADASIL, *Eur J Neurol* 13:187-190, 2006.
40. Lesnik Oberstein SA, van den Boom R, van Buchem MA, et al: Cerebral microbleeds in CADASIL, *Neurology* 57:1066-1070, 2001.
41. Dichgans M, Holtmannspotter M, Herzog J, et al: Cerebral microbleeds in CADASIL: A gradient-echo magnetic resonance imaging and autopsy study, *Stroke* 33:67-71, 2002.
42. Viswanathan A, Guichard JP, Gschwendtner A, et al: Blood pressure and haemoglobin A1c are associated with microhaemorrhage in CADASIL: A two-centre cohort study, *Brain* 129:2375-2383, 2006.
43. Weller M, Petersen D, Dichgans J: Cerebral angiography complications link CADASIL to familial hemiplegic migraine, *Neurology* 46:844, 1996.
44. Dichgans M, Petersen D: Angiographic complications in CADASIL, *Lancet* 349:776-777, 1997.
45. Zicari E, Tassi R, Stromillo ML, et al: Right-to-left shunt in CADASIL patients: Prevalence and correlation with clinical and MRI findings, *Stroke* 39:2155-2157, 2008.
46. Unlu M, de Lange RP, de Silva R, et al: Detection of complement factor B in the cerebrospinal fluid of patients with cerebral autosomal dominant arteriopathy with subcortical infarcts and leukoencephalopathy disease using two-dimensional gel electrophoresis and mass spectrometry, *Neurosci Lett* 282:149-152, 2000.
47. Gutierrez-Molina M, Caminero Rodriguez A, Martinez Garcia C, et al: Small arterial granular degeneration in familial Binswanger's syndrome, *Acta Neuropathol (Berl)* 87:98-105, 1994.
48. Ruchoux MM, Guerouaou D, Vandenhaute B, et al: Systemic vascular smooth muscle cell impairment in cerebral autosomal dominant arteriopathy with subcortical infarcts and leukoencephalopathy, *Acta Neuropathol (Berl)* 89:500-512, 1995.
49. Pullicino P, Ostow P, Miller L, et al: Pontine ischemic rarefaction, *Ann Neurol* 37:460-466, 1995.
50. Lammie GA, Rakshi J, Rossor MN, et al: Cerebral autosomal dominant arteriopathy with subcortical infarcts and leukoencephalopathy (CADASIL)—confirmation by cerebral biopsy in 2 cases, *Clin Neuropathol* 14:201-206, 1995.

51. Zhang WW, Ma KC, Andersen O, et al: The microvascular changes in cases of hereditary multi-infarct disease of the brain, *Acta Neuropathol (Berl)* 87:317-324, 1994.

52. Joutel A, Corpechot C, Ducros A, et al: Notch3 mutations in cerebral autosomal dominant arteriopathy with subcortical infarcts and leukoencephalopathy (CADASIL), a mendelian condition causing stroke and vascular dementia, *Ann N Y Acad Sci* 826:213-217, 1997.

53. Ruchoux MM, Maurage CA: CADASIL: Cerebral autosomal dominant arteriopathy with subcortical infarcts and leukoencephalopathy, *J Neuropathol Exp Neurol* 56:947-964, 1997.

54. Gray F, Robert F, Labrecque R, et al: Autosomal dominant arteriopathic leuko-encephalopathy and Alzheimer's disease, *Neuropathol Appl Neurobiol* 20:22-30, 1994.

55. Ruchoux MM, Chabriat H, Bousser MG, et al: Presence of ultrastructural arterial lesions in muscle and skin vessels of patients with CADASIL, *Stroke* 25:2291-2292, 1994.

56. Lucas C, Pasquier F, Leys D, et al: [CADASIL: A new familial disease responsible for cerebral infarction and dementia], *Rev Med Interne* 16:290-292, 1995.

57. Schroder JM, Sellhaus B, Jorg J: Identification of the characteristic vascular changes in a sural nerve biopsy of a case with cerebral autosomal dominant arteriopathy with subcortical infarcts and leukoencephalopathy (CADASIL), *Acta Neuropathol (Berl)* 89:116-121, 1995.

58. Furby A, Vahedi K, Force M, et al: Differential diagnosis of a vascular leukoencephalopathy within a CADASIL family: Use of skin biopsy electron microscopy study and direct genotypic screening, *J Neurol* 245:734-740, 1998.

59. Sabbadini G, Francia A, Calandriello L, et al: Cerebral autosomal dominant arteriopathy with subcortical infarcts and leucoencephalopathy (CADASIL). Clinical, neuroimaging, pathological and genetic study of a large Italian family, *Brain* 118(Pt 1):207-215, 1995.

60. Joutel A, Favrole P, Labauge P, et al: Skin biopsy immunostaining with a Notch3 monoclonal antibody for CADASIL diagnosis, *Lancet* 358:2049-2051, 2001.

61. Lesnik Oberstein SA, van Duinen SG, van den Boom R, et al: Evaluation of diagnostic NOTCH3 immunostaining in CADASIL, *Acta Neuropathol (Berl)* 106:107-111, 2003.

62. Joutel A, Dodick DD, Parisi JE, et al: De novo mutation in the Notch3 gene causing CADASIL, *Ann Neurol* 47:388-391, 2000.

63. Joutel A, Andreux F, Gaulis S, et al: The ectodomain of the Notch3 receptor accumulates within the cerebrovasculature of CADASIL patients, *J Clin Invest* 105:597-605, 2000.

64. Auer DP, Putz B, Gossl C, et al: Differential lesion patterns in CADASIL and sporadic subcortical arteriosclerotic encephalopathy: MR imaging study with statistical parametric group comparison, *Radiology* 218:443-451, 2001.

65. Dichgans M, Ludwig H, Muller-Hocker J, et al: Small in-frame deletions and missense mutations in CADASIL: 3D models predict misfolding of Notch3 EGF-like repeat domains, *Eur J Hum Genet* 8:280-285, 2000.

66. Dotti MT, De Stefano N, Bianchi S, et al: A novel NOTCH3 frameshift deletion and mitochondrial abnormalities in a patient with CADASIL, *Arch Neurol* 61:942-945, 2004.

67. Chabriat H, Joutel A, Vahedi K, et al: [CADASIL (cerebral autosomal dominant arteriopathy with subcortical infarcts and leukoencephalopathy): clinical features and neuroimaging], *Bull Acad Natl Med* 184:1523-1531, discussion 1531-1523, 2000.

68. Holtmannspotter M, Peters N, Opherk C, et al: Diffusion magnetic resonance histograms as a surrogate marker and predictor of disease progression in CADASIL: A two-year follow-up study, *Stroke* 36:2559-2565, 2005.

69. Bianchi S, Dotti MT, Federico A: Physiology and pathology of notch signalling system, *J Cell Physiol* 207:300-308, 2006.

70. Joutel A, Vahedi K, Corpechot C, et al: Strong clustering and stereotyped nature of Notch3 mutations in CADASIL patients, *Lancet* 350:1511-1515, 1997.

71. Joutel A, Chabriat H, Vahedi K, et al: Splice site mutation causing a seven amino acid Notch3 in-frame deletion in CADASIL, *Neurology* 54:1874-1875, 2000.

72. Peters N, Opherk C, Bergmann T, et al: Spectrum of mutations in biopsy-proven CADASIL: Implications for diagnostic strategies, *Arch Neurol* 62:1091-1094, 2005.

73. Dichgans M, Herzog J, Gasser T: NOTCH3 mutation involving three cysteine residues in a family with typical CADASIL, *Neurology* 57:1714-1717, 2001.

74. Coto E, Menendez M, Navarro R, et al: A new de novo Notch3 mutation causing CADASIL, *Eur J Neurol* 13:628-631, 2006.

75. Tuominen S, Juvonen V, Amberla K, et al: Phenotype of a homozygous CADASIL patient in comparison to 9 age-matched heterozygous patients with the same R133C Notch3 mutation, *Stroke* 32:1767-1774, 2001.

76. Liem MK, Lesnik Oberstein SA, Vollebregt MJ, et al: Homozygosity for a NOTCH3 mutation in a 65-year-old CADASIL patient with mild symptoms: A family report, *J Neurol* 255:1978-1980, 2008.

77. Monet M, Domenga V, Lemaire B, et al: The archetypal R90C CADASIL-NOTCH3 mutation retains NOTCH3 function in vivo, *Hum Mol Genet* 16:982-992, 2007.

78. Greenberg SM, Vonsattel JP, Stakes JW, et al: The clinical spectrum of cerebral amyloid angiopathy: Presentations without lobar hemorrhage, *Neurology* 43:2073-2079, 1993.

79. Greenberg SM, Vonsattel JP: Diagnosis of cerebral amyloid angiopathy. Sensitivity and specificity of cortical biopsy, *Stroke* 28:1418-1422, 1997.

80. Razvi SS, Bone I: Single gene disorders causing ischaemic stroke, *J Neurol* 253:685-700, 2006.

81. Fukutake T, Hirayama K: Familial young-onset arteriosclerotic leukoencephalopathy with alopecia and lumbago without arterial hypertension, *Eur Neurol* 35:69-79, 1995.

82. Lossos A, Cooperman H, Soffer D, et al: Hereditary leukoencephalopathy and palmoplantar keratoderma: A new disorder with increased skin collagen content, *Neurology* 45:331-337, 1995.

83. Verreault S, Joutel A, Riant F, et al: A novel hereditary small vessel disease of the brain, *Ann Neurol* 59:353-357, 2006.

Reversible Cerebral Vasoconstriction Syndromes

ANEESH B. SINGHAL, ANNE DUCROS

Reversible cerebral vasoconstriction syndromes are a group of conditions characterized by reversible multifocal narrowing of the cerebral arteries, typically associated with recurrent sudden, severe (thunderclap) headaches and often complicated by ischemic or hemorrhagic strokes.[1,2] A typical case is illustrated in Figure 40-1. Over the past 60 years, this enigmatic reversible angiographic phenomenon has been reported under a variety of names and eponyms, each reflecting the associated clinical setting (Table 40-1) or the presumed pathophysiology—for example, migrainous "vasospasm" or "angiitis"[3,4]; thunderclap headache with reversible vasospasm[5-7]; postpartum cerebral angiopathy, angiitis, or vasospasm[8]; drug-induced cerebral arteritis or angiopathy[9,10]; Call's or Call-Fleming syndrome[11,12]; central nervous system (CNS) pseudovasculitis[13]; and benign angiopathy of the central nervous system.[14] Only recently has it become apparent that patients with reversible cerebral arterial narrowing have similar clinical, laboratory, imaging, and prognostic features regardless of the associated underlying condition(s).[15-17] The descriptive term *reversible cerebral vasoconstriction syndrome* (RCVS) has been proposed to facilitate the recognition and management of this group of disorders.[1]

History, Evolution, and Associated Conditions

Stroke was historically attributed to cerebral "vasospasm" for centuries. However, from the 1950s onward, the work of C.M. Fisher and others enumerated pathologic causes of stroke, such as carotid atherosclerosis, lipohyalinosis, and cardioembolism. As a result, "vasospasm" disappeared from the stroke lexicon except in the setting of aneurysmal subarachnoid hemorrhage. Ironically, Dr. Fisher himself was later instrumental in bringing to world attention the phenomenon of reversible segmental cerebral vasoconstriction. In the early 1970s, he described unusual cases of postpartum women with transient neurologic dysfunction associated with reversible cerebral arterial irregularities.[18] One patient was discussed at the first Sâlpetrière Hospital stroke conference in Paris[19]; at the second conference, Rascol and associates[20] presented four similar cases, and the entity became known as "postpartum angiopathy." Over the next decade, similar cases were documented in association with such diverse conditions as pregnancy,[9] migraine,[4,21,22] vasoconstrictive

drugs and medications,[9,10] neurosurgical procedures,[23] hypercalcemia,[24] and even unruptured saccular aneurysms.[5] In 1987, Marie Fleming presented the cases of two patients with transient cerebral arterial narrowing at the Boston Stroke Society meeting held at Massachusetts General Hospital. Dr. Fisher promptly recognized the similarity between her cases and others previously reported, and in a collaborative effort reported on 19 patients.[11] Thereafter, some investigators referred to this syndrome as Call's or Call-Fleming syndrome,[25-27] but the use of variable terminology persisted.

Meanwhile, this syndrome was probably being misinterpreted as primary angiitis primary angiitis of the central nervous system (PACNS), an inflammatory condition affecting brain arteries, because of overlapping angiographic as well as clinical features such as headache, seizures, and stroke.[28-30] Calabrese and colleagues[14] recognized that these patients did not exhibit the typical progressive course of PACNS; instead, their angiographic abnormalities reversed promptly and clinical resolution occurred within weeks, even without immunosuppressive therapy. These researchers suspected that the patients had a transient or mild form of PACNS and proposed the term "benign angiopathy of the central nervous system" (BACNS).[14] Calabrese's group subsequently analyzed the clinical characteristics and long-term outcomes of BACNS and concluded that it is consistent with RCVS.[31,32]

Over the past few years, it has become apparent that the same clinicoangiographic syndrome has been reported separately by stroke neurologists, headache specialists, obstetricians, internists, and rheumatologists, each in turn imparting their own biases to nomenclature, theories of pathogenesis, and clinical approach. The proposal and adoption of the broad term RCVS, along with provisional diagnostic criteria (Table 40-2), have encouraged retrospective and prospective studies that have helped characterize the syndrome.[1,2,33-35] The now-routine use of relatively noninvasive angiographic techniques, such as computed tomography angiography (CTA) and magnetic resonance angiography (MRA), combined with the widespread use of illicit drugs such as ecstasy and cocaine and of serotonergic and sympathomimetic medications, makes it likely that vascular neurologists and other specialists will encounter an increasing number of patients with RCVS.

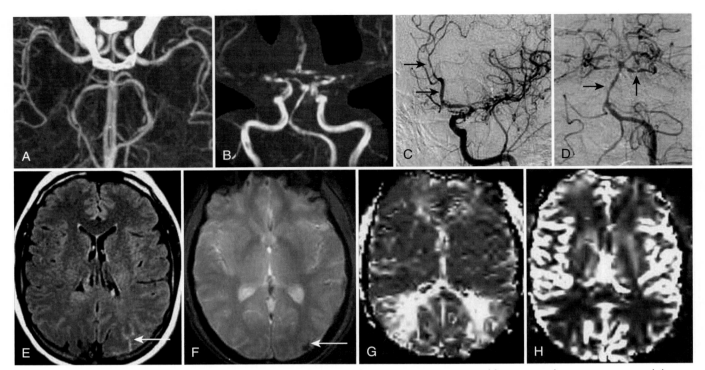

Figure 40-1 Typical case of reversible cerebral vasoconstriction syndrome (RCVS). A 44-year-old woman with prior migraine and depression experienced a sudden, excruciating (thunderclap) headache while exercising. The headache did not resemble her prior migraines and resolved over 30 minutes. Over the next week, 3 more thunderclap headaches occurred. Blood pressure and neurologic findings were normal. CT angiogram (A), MR angiogram (B), and digital subtraction angiogram (C and D) show segmental narrowing and dilatation of multiple intracerebral arteries. Note the abnormal dilatation followed by abrupt narrowing of the anterior cerebral artery (*arrows,* C), the basilar artery (*horizontal arrow,* D) and the superior cerebellar artery (*vertical arrow,* D). This "sausage on a string" appearance is characteristic of RCVS. Brain MRI showed sulcal hyperintensity in the left occipital lobe on axial fluid-attenuated inversion recovery (FLAIR) images (*arrow,* E), and corresponding sulcal hypointensity on gradient-echo images (*arrow,* F), consistent with cortical surface subarachnoid hemorrhage. Perfusion-weighted MRI showed abnormally increased mean transit time (G) and reduced cerebral blood flow (H) in the "watershed" regions of the bilateral middle and posterior cerebral arteries; fortunately these regions did not progress to infarction. Cerebrospinal fluid examination findings were normal. Results of extensive tests for vasculitis were negative. She was treated with nimodipine. Over the next 2 weeks, her headaches resolved, and follow-up brain imaging showed resolution of the subarachnoid blood and vascular abnormalities.

Demographics and Clinical Features

Once considered rare, RCVS is being reported with increasing frequency, presumably as a result of the widespread use of relatively noninvasive imaging tests such as CT and MRA as well as greater awareness of the syndrome. Cases have been documented from numerous countries including France, the United States, Mexico, Canada, Spain, South Africa, China, India, Japan, and Australia. RCVS appears to affect individuals of all races. Most patients are young adults in the age range of 25 to 50 years, with a mean age of approximately 42 years.[2,34] Children can be affected.[36] There is an impressive female preponderance (2:1 to 10:1, depending on the case series), even after cases related to pregnancy have been accounted for.

The onset is typically dramatic with a sudden "worst ever" headache that reaches its peak intensity within seconds, often referred to as a "thunderclap headache."[5,37] Screaming, agitation, confusion, and collapse due to the extreme severity of the pain are common. Many patients report trigger factors, such as orgasm, physical exertion, acute stressful or emotional situations, straining, coughing, sneezing, bathing, and swimming. The syndrome is known to occur in certain clinical settings (see Table 40-1). More than 80% of patients experience thunderclap headaches, and the rest have subacute or less severe headaches; the absence of headache at onset is exceptional. The location of the headache could be occipital, vertex, or diffuse. It is usually throbbing and accompanied by nausea, emesis, or photosensitivity, but patients with migraines clearly identify the thunderclap headaches as different from their usual headaches. Severe pain usually subsides within 1 to 2 hours, although 50% to 75% of patients report mild baseline headache between acute exacerbations. Thunderclap headaches recur frequently over the ensuing 1 to 3 weeks, with an average of four recurrences; however, the intensity and frequency diminish over time. Headache remains the only symptom in one half to three fourths of patients.

The frequency of other neurologic signs and symptoms varies according to the method of case ascertainment.[1,2,33-35] Generalized tonic-clonic seizures are reported in 0 to 21% of patients at the time of presentation; however, recurrent seizures are rare. Focal neurologic deficits from ischemic stroke or parenchymal hematoma are reported in 9% to 63%, the frequency being higher in inpatient series. Visual deficits are common,

TABLE 40-1   CONDITIONS ASSOCIATED WITH REVERSIBLE CEREBRAL VASOCONSTRICTION SYNDROME

Idiopathic	No identifiable precipitating factor Associated with headache disorders (migraine, primary thunderclap headache,* benign exertional headache, benign sexual headache, and primary cough headache)
Exposure to medications, drugs, and blood products	Phenylpropanolamine, pseudoephedrine, amphetamine derivatives,* methergine, bromocriptine, ergotamine tartrate, sumatriptan,* isometheptene, oral contraceptives, lisuride, licorice, selective serotonin reuptake inhibitors (SSRIs),* cocaine, ecstasy, marijuana,* lysergic acid diethylamide (LSD), tacrolimus (FK-506), cyclophosphamide,* erythropoietin,* intravenous immune globulin (IVIG),* red blood cell transfusion*
Pregnancy and puerperium	Early puerperium, late pregnancy, eclampsia,* preeclampsia,* delayed postpartum eclampsia*
Miscellaneous conditions	Hypercalcemia, porphyria,* pheochromocytoma, bronchial carcinoid tumor, unruptured saccular cerebral aneurysm, head trauma, spinal subdural hematoma, postcarotid endarterectomy,* neurosurgical procedures, cervical arterial dissection

*Also associated with the reversible posterior leukoencephalopathy syndrome.

TABLE 40-2   SUMMARY OF CRITICAL ELEMENTS FOR THE DIAGNOSIS OF REVERSIBLE CEREBRAL VASOCONSTRICTION SYNDROMES

1. Transfemoral angiography or indirect (CT or MR) angiography documenting segmental cerebral artery vasoconstriction.
2. No evidence for aneurysmal subarachnoid hemorrhage.
3. Normal or near-normal cerebrospinal fluid analysis results (total protein content < 80 mg/dL, white blood cell count <10/mm^3, normal glucose content).
4. Severe, acute headache, with or without additional neurologic signs and symptoms.
5. The diagnosis cannot be confirmed until reversibility of the angiographic abnormalities is documented within 12 weeks after onset or, if death occurs before the follow-up studies are completed, autopsy rules out conditions such as vasculitis, intracranial atherosclerosis, and aneurysmal subarachnoid hemorrhage, which can also manifest as headache and stroke.

Modified from Calabrese LH, Dodick DW, Schwedt TJ, et al: Narrative review: Reversible cerebral vasoconstriction syndromes. *Ann Intern Med* 146:34-44, 2007.

including scotomas, blurring, hemianopia, and cortical blindness (full or partial Balint's syndrome). Hemiplegia, tremor, ataxia, and aphasia have also been reported. Some patients demonstrate acute transient deficits consistent with transient ischemic attacks, and others have subacute and recurrent positive visual or sensory symptoms mimicking the aura of migraine. Most patients have brisk tendon reflexes. Blood pressure can be normal or elevated from the pain, the disease itself, or the associated condition (e.g., eclampsia). Over the next few weeks, most patients show gradual resolution of visual and other focal neurologic signs or symptoms. Few are left with minor or moderate permanent deficits. Less than 5% experience progressive cerebral arterial vasoconstriction culminating in massive strokes, brain edema, severe morbidity, or death.[38-40]

Laboratory Findings

Blood counts, erythrocyte sedimentation rate, serum electrolyte levels, and liver and renal function test results are usually normal. Tests for rheumatoid factor, antinuclear and antinuclear cytoplasmic antibodies, Lyme disease antibodies, and urine vanillylmandelic acid and 5-hydroxyindoleacetic acid are useful to rule out vasculitis and evaluate for vasoactive tumors (e.g., pheochromocytoma, carcinoid) that have been associated with RCVS. Serum and urine toxicology screens, in addition to a careful medication history, are important to uncover exposure to vasoactive drugs and medications. Cerebrospinal fluid examination findings are normal (protein level less than 60 mg/dL, fewer than 5 white blood cells per mm^3) in more than 85% of patients[34]; minor

abnormalities can result from ischemic or hemorrhagic strokes. There is no role for brain biopsy or temporal artery biopsy other than to rule out cerebral vasculitis when the diagnosis of RCVS cannot be secured within the clinical context, including presentation and associated conditions (see Tables 40-1 and 40-2) and brain imaging and angiographic findings. Distinguishing RCVS from cerebral vasculitis can be challenging and is discussed further later (see "Differential Diagnosis"). Brain and temporal artery biopsies as well as full autopsy in patients who died from progressive vasoconstriction have shown normal arterial histology.[21,27,39] However, in some cases, the interpretation of pathologic samples can be difficult because prolonged severe vasoconstriction can itself induce secondary inflammation.[41]

Brain Imaging

Patients with RCVS typically present to the emergency department for evaluation of thunderclap headaches and appropriately undergo urgent brain and vascular imaging to rule out secondary causes. Between 30% and 70% of patients ultimately diagnosed with RCVS show no parenchymal lesion on initial head CT or brain MRI, despite having widespread vasoconstriction on concomitant cerebral angiography.[2,34,42-44] Brain scans remain normal in 15% of cases reported from inhospital settings; this number is much higher in emergency department case series. The wide variability in the frequency of abnormal brain imaging findings reflects the wide clinical spectrum, which ranges from isolated headache and normal brain imaging findings (more common), to the more pernicious course with multiple strokes, seizures, and permanent neurologic impairment.

Abnormal brain imaging findings can consist of a variety of lesions, either initially or on follow-up studies (Fig. 40-2). Ischemic stroke is the most frequent lesion, followed by cortical surface (nonaneurysmal) subarachnoid hemorrhage, parenchymal hemorrhage, and reversible

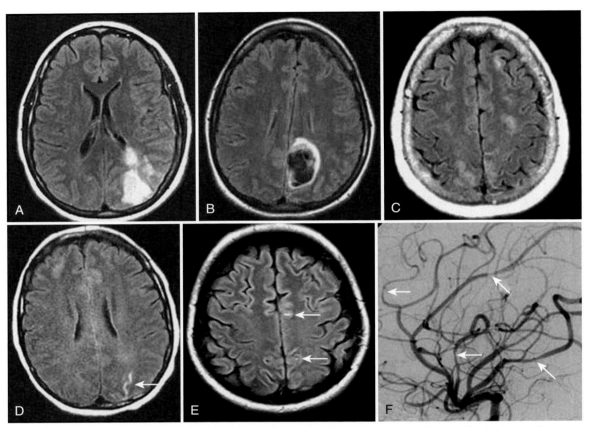

Figure 40-2　Brain MRI findings in reversible cerebral vasoconstriction syndrome (RCVS). A to E, Axial fluid-attenuated inversion recovery (FLAIR) images show the typical brain imaging abnormalities in RCVS, including an ischemic stroke in the watershed distribution of the left middle and posterior cerebral artery (A), parenchymal brain hemorrhage (B), reversible hyperintense lesions (brain edema) in subcortical regions (C), nonaneurysmal cortical surface subarachnoid hemorrhage *(arrow)* overlying the left hemisphere (D), and dilated cortical surface vessels *(arrows)* overlying the left hemisphere (E). However, it is important to note that in many patients with RCVS, no parenchymal lesion is seen on brain MRI. F, Digital subtraction angiogram from a patient with RCVS shows the typical segmental narrowing ("sausaging") of multiple cerebral arteries that usually reverse within weeks. (From Calabrese LH, Singhal AB: Primary angiitis of the central nervous system (PACNS) and reversible cerebral vasoconstriction syndromes (RCVS). In Stone JH, editor: *A clinician's pearls and myths in rheumatology,* New York, 2010, Springer.)

brain edema.[2,34,42-44] Any combination of lesions can be present. Infarcts are often bilateral and symmetrical and located in arterial "watershed" regions of the cerebral hemispheres. Cerebellar infarcts are also common. Smaller infarcts typically abut the cortical-subcortical junction, and larger infarcts are often wedge shaped. Perfusion-weighted MRI may show areas of hypoperfusion. Cortical surface hemorrhages are typically minor, restricted to a few sulcal spaces.[45-47] Single as well as multiple lobar hemorrhages can occur. Subdural hemorrhage has been reported.[48] It appears that hemorrhages are more common in women and are more frequently associated with medication or drug exposure. Interestingly, some patients with negative initial imaging findings go on to have lobar hemorrhage after their second or third headache exacerbation, reflecting the dynamic nature of this condition. Fluid-attenuated inversion recovery (FLAIR) MRI may show dot or linear hyperintensities within sulcal spaces, which are distinct from subarachnoid hemorrhage and reflect slow flow within dilated surface vessels.[49] The presence of reversible brain edema, in a distribution similar to that in the reversible posterior

leukoencephalopathy syndrome, suggests an overlapping pathophysiology between these syndromes.[47]

The diagnosis of RCVS can be considered only after documentation of the presence of cerebral vasoconstriction with transfemoral, CT, or MR angiography. Findings of the first angiogram can be normal if it is performed within 3 to 5 days after symptom onset. In one study, 21% of patients with RCVS had normal findings on initial MRA, and 9% had normal findings on both MRA and transcranial Doppler ultrasonography.[2] The rate of diagnosis can be increased by repeating the angiographic study after a few days; however, the value of repeat testing is limited by the usually benign nature of this condition. Angiographic abnormalities are dynamic, with different segments (usually the more proximal segments) becoming affected over time. Angiography often reveals arterial dissection and unruptured saccular aneurysms,[5,50,51] and in some patients the vasoconstriction can affect the extracranial internal carotid or vertebral artery.[52] Patients with typical clinical features have been diagnosed on the basis of elevated blood flow velocities on transcranial Doppler ultrasonography.[53] This noninvasive bedside tool has usefulness in monitoring the progression of vasoconstriction,[33] although there is little correlation between ultrasonographic and angiographic findings, and most investigators prefer angiographic studies to establish resolution and confirm the diagnosis. The time course of vasoconstriction is variable, but most patients show resolution within 3 months.

Prospective case series have highlighted the characteristic temporal pattern and relationship of clinical features and arterial abnormalities.[2] Thunderclap headaches recur frequently over the first week, with the last attack occurring an average of 7 to 8 days after onset.[2] Mild baseline headaches may then persist in 70% of patients, lasting a mean of 22 days[2,33]; some patients have chronic headaches. Brain hemorrhage and brain edema are early complications, occurring during the first week, whereas ischemic complications occur significantly later, at the end of the second week.[2] Ischemic complications may thus occur when the headaches have improved or even resolved.

Differential Diagnosis

RCVS is easily recognized from the features outlined in Table 40-2. Most patients report severe thunderclap headaches and have benign cerebrospinal fluid findings, characteristic brain imaging features, and vascular abnormalities that resolve over a few weeks. Individually, however, the clinical and imaging features carry a wide range of differential diagnoses.

Thunderclap headaches can signify a variety of ominous conditions, including aneurysmal subarachnoid hemorrhage, parenchymal hemorrhage, cerebral artery dissection, and cerebral venous sinus thrombosis.[37] These conditions are easily excluded with appropriate brain imaging. Patients with negative initial brain scan results are often subjected to a second imaging procedure to exclude these secondary conditions; however, the presence of three or four recurrent thunderclap headaches points to a diagnosis of RCVS. If imaging findings are negative and the patient does not prove to have vasoconstriction, primary headache disorders such as primary thunderclap headache, primary exertional headache, and orgasmic headache are usually considered.[54] In one study, 39% of patients presenting with thunderclap headache and normal brain MRI findings proved to have vasoconstriction on MRA, and those with and without vasoconstriction had similar clinical features, suggesting that RCVS and primary thunderclap headache belong to the same spectrum of disorders.[43]

Migraine is another consideration because a prior history of migraine is frequently elicited and because abnormal cerebral angiographic results have been documented in migraine.[55,56] Although there may be some overlap, RCVS appears distinct from migraine because unlike migraine it rarely (if ever) recurs, the nature of the headache is dissimilar, and the angiographic abnormalities persist for several weeks. Nevertheless, attribution of the severe headache and even the stroke to migraine is a common problem, frequently leading to inappropriate treatment with antimigraine agents such as sumatriptan, which can exacerbate vasoconstriction and stroke.[27,57]

Brain imaging demonstration of infarction or hemorrhage might raise consideration of the broad range of etiologies for stroke in young adults. The presence of thunderclap headache and cerebral vasoconstriction appropriately raises initial concern for a ruptured brain aneurysm. The presence of cortical surface subarachnoid hemorrhage (which occurs in up to 22% of patients with RCVS) adds to the diagnostic dilemma.[45,46] However it should be noted that in patients with aneurysmal subarachnoid hemorrhage, cerebral "vasospasm" can be evident within hours and then reappears days or a week or so later. It is restricted to the artery surrounded by blood rather than affecting multiple distant arteries, and cerebral angiography does not reveal the alternating segments of arterial dilatation that give RCVS the characteristic "sausage on a string" appearance. Moreover, subarachnoid hemorrhage from ruptured aneurysms is usually deep-seated, for example, in the sylvian fissure, rather than restricted to a few cortical sulci as in RCVS.

Cerebral angiographic abnormalities can raise suspicion for cerebral arteriopathies such as intracranial atherosclerosis, infectious arteritis, vasculitis, and fibromuscular dysplasia. Detailed medical history and laboratory testing usually help distinguish these conditions from RCVS. The one condition that historically has been difficult to exclude is PACNS, because features such as headache, focal deficits, stroke, seizures, and angiographic irregularities are common to both conditions. An understandable presumptive diagnosis of "vasculitis" based on angiographic features alone may lead to the risks of brain biopsy and to the adverse effects of long-term immunosuppressive therapy. Delays of several days before such steps are taken should help distinguish RCVS, in which the initial clinical syndrome is typically more stable and even improving, from PACNS, in which clinical status may be worsening. Dramatic clinical presentations with explosive headaches, normal cerebrospinal fluid findings, and normal brain imaging strongly favor a diagnosis of RCVS. Furthermore, in patients with RCVS, there is often a history of associated cofactors to provide clues to the diagnosis, such as a temporal relationship with childbirth or incriminating drug exposure (see Table 40-1). Imaging clues that strongly favor a diagnosis of RCVS in the appropriate clinical setting are the absence of brain lesions on initial imaging and the presence of cortical surface subarachnoid hemorrhages, lobar hemorrhage, symmetrical "watershed" territory infarctions (usually high parietal), and bilateral edematous lesions.[34,42,44] Angiographic findings of smooth concentric narrowing and dilatation affecting multiple medium-sized intracerebral arteries and their branches ("string of beads" or "sausage on a string" appearance) is characteristic for RCVS, whereas "notched," irregular, and eccentric narrowing, presumably due to arterial inflammation, predicts PACNS.[35] Though rare exceptions exist,[58] the reversibility over days to weeks is the feature that best distinguishes this disorder from PACNS and other arteriopathies. The anxiety of awaiting for reversal affects even the most experienced clinical teams.

Etiology and Pathophysiology

The etiology of the prolonged but reversible vasoconstriction, and the relationship between acute headache and vasoconstriction, is not known. Altered cerebral arterial tone due to abnormal vascular receptor activity or sensitivity appears critical; it may result from either a spontaneous or evoked central vascular discharge or a variety of exogenous or endogenous factors, including vasoconstrictive drugs and medications, female reproductive hormones, hypercalcemia, and others (see Table 40-1). The anatomic basis to explain both the vasoconstriction and the headache may be the dense innervation of cerebral blood vessels with sensory afferents from the first division of the trigeminal nerve and dorsal root of C2. At the molecular level, it is reasonable to postulate a role for the numerous immunologic and biochemical factors known to be involved in vasospasm associated with aneurysmal subarachnoid hemorrhage (catecholamines, endothelin-1, serotonin, nitric oxide, prostaglandins).[59] Serotonin is believed to play a central role in RCVS, on the basis of the association of the syndrome with serotonin-enhancing medications and tumors.[25,27,57] Some authorities have speculated that the vasoconstriction is related to transient vasculitis, but findings of histologic studies do not support a role for inflammation.[39]

Management

In the absence of controlled trials, management is guided by observational data and expert opinion. For patients who present with thunderclap headache but have not undergone vascular imaging, empiric therapy is not justified. Once cerebral vasoconstriction has been documented, however, treatment can be considered. It is important to note that RCVS is usually self-limited, with clinical and angiographic resolution occurring spontaneously within a few weeks. Therefore simple observation alone is reasonable, especially in patients who show no signs of clinical progression. Calcium channel blockers such as nimodipine and verapamil,[26] brief courses of glucocorticoids,[60] magnesium sulfate,[61] serotonin antagonists, and even dantrolene[62] have been administered in an effort to relieve the vasoconstriction. Data from two prospective case series suggest that nimodipine does not affect the time course of cerebral vasoconstriction.[2,33] However, nimodipine might relieve the number and intensity of headaches, and it has documented effects on the smaller vasculature not easily imaged by angiography. These agents can be discontinued after resolution of symptoms or angiographic abnormalities. Balloon angioplasty and direct intraarterial administration of nicardipine, papaverine, milrinone, and nimodipine have been used with variable success.[63-65] These interventions carry a high risk of reperfusion injury and should be reserved for patients exhibiting clear signs of clinical progression.[39] Unfortunately, no known clinical or imaging features reliably predict disease progression.

Patients with severe angiographic abnormalities are often admitted to the intensive care unit for neurologic monitoring and blood pressure management. The goals of blood pressure control need careful consideration. Theoretically, pharmacologically induced hypertension can induce further cerebral vasoconstriction or result in brain hemorrhage, and in the setting of cerebral vasoconstriction, even mild hypotension can trigger ischemic stroke.[66] Acute seizures may warrant treatment; however, long-term seizure prophylaxis is probably unnecessary.

It is logical to avoid further exposure to any potential precipitating factors, such as marijuana, cocaine, exercise stimulants, and amphetamines. The pain of RCVS-associated headache is extreme and frequently warrants round-the-clock use of opioid analgesics. Sumatriptan and the ergot derivatives are contraindicated because of their vasoconstrictive actions.[27,57] Patients should be counseled to avoid physical exertion, the Valsalva maneuver, and other known triggers of recurrent headaches for a few weeks. Usual stroke preventive medications, such as antiplatelets, anticoagulants, and cholesterol-lowering agents, are probably not indicated.

Outcome and Prognosis

Most patients with RCVS have complete resolution of headaches and angiographic abnormalities within days to weeks. Less than 15% to 20% of patients are left with residual deficits from stroke. Progressive vasoconstriction resulting in progressive symptoms[63] or death[38-40] can occur in rare cases. It should be noted that "reversibility" in the term RCVS refers to the dynamic and reversible nature of vasoconstriction; clinical deficits from brain damage might persist, and the vasoconstriction (particularly if severe and prolonged) may not fully reverse in some patients. Recurrence of an "episode" of RCVS is extremely rare.[67] Some patients go on to have intractable chronic migraine-like headaches or depression.

REFERENCES

1. Calabrese LH, Dodick DW, Schwedt TJ, Singhal AB: Narrative review: Reversible cerebral vasoconstriction syndromes, *Ann Intern Med* 146:34–44, 2007.
2. Ducros A, Boukobza M, Porcher R, et al: The clinical and radiological spectrum of reversible cerebral vasoconstriction syndrome. A prospective series of 67 patients, *Brain* 130:3091–3101, 2007.
3. Serdaru M, Chiras J, Cujas M, Lhermitte F: Isolated benign cerebral vasculitis or migrainous vasospasm? *J Neurol Neurosurg Psychiatry* 47:73–76, 1984.
4. Jackson M, Lennox G, Jaspan T, Jefferson D: Migraine angiitis precipitated by sex headache and leading to watershed infarction, *Cephalalgia* 13:427–430, 1993.
5. Day JW, Raskin NH: Thunderclap headache: Symptom of unruptured cerebral aneurysm, *Lancet* 2:1247–1248, 1986.
6. Slivka A, Philbrook B: Clinical and angiographic features of thunderclap headache, *Headache* 35:1–6, 1995.
7. Dodick DW, Brown RD Jr, Britton JW, Huston J III: Nonaneurysmal thunderclap headache with diffuse, multifocal, segmental, and reversible vasospasm, *Cephalalgia* 19:118–123, 1999.
8. Bogousslavsky J, Despland PA, Regli F, Dubuis PY: Postpartum cerebral angiopathy: Reversible vasoconstriction assessed by transcranial Doppler ultrasounds, *Eur Neurol* 29:102–105, 1989.
9. Henry PY, Larre P, Aupy M, et al: Reversible cerebral arteriopathy associated with the administration of ergot derivatives, *Cephalalgia* 4:171–178, 1984.
10. Raroque HG Jr, Tesfa G, Purdy P: Postpartum cerebral angiopathy. Is there a role for sympathomimetic drugs? *Stroke* 24:2108–2110, 1993.
11. Call GK, Fleming MC, Sealfon S, et al: Reversible cerebral segmental vasoconstriction, *Stroke* 19:1159–1170, 1988.
12. Singhal AB, Caviness VS, Begleiter AF, et al: Cerebral vasoconstriction and stroke after use of serotonergic drugs [see comment], *Neurology* 58:130–133, 2002.
13. Razavi M, Bendixen B, Maley JE, et al: CNS pseudovasculitis in a patient with pheochromocytoma, *Neurology* 52:1088–1090, 1999.
14. Calabrese LH, Gragg LA, Furlan AJ: Benign angiopathy: A distinct subset of angiographically defined primary angiitis of the central nervous system, *J Rheumatol* 20:2046–2050, 1993.
15. Singhal AB: Cerebral vasoconstriction syndromes, *Top Stroke Rehabil* 11:1–6, 2004.

16. Singhal AB: Cerebral vasoconstriction without subarachnoid blood: Associated conditions, clinical and neuroimaging characteristics, *Ann Neurol* S59-S60, 2002.

17. Singhal AB, Bernstein RA: Postpartum angiopathy and other cerebral vasoconstriction syndromes, *Neurocrit Care* 3:91-97, 2005.

18. Fisher CM: Cerebral ischemia—less familiar types (review), *Clin Neurosurg* 18:267-336, 1971.

19. Millikan CH: Accidents vasculaires cerebraux chez les femmes agees de 15 a 45 ans. In Castaigne P, Gautier J-C, editors: *Maladies vasculaires cerebrales I: Conference de la Salpetriere, 1975, Hospital de la Salpetriere,* Paris, 1975, J-B Balliere, pp 77-84.

20. Rascol A, Guiraud B, Manelfe C, Clanet M: Accidents vasculaires cerebraux de la grossesse et du post partum. In *II Conference de la Salpetriere sue les maladies vasculaires cerebrales; 1979, Hospital de la Salpetriere,* Paris, 1979, JB Balliere, pp 84-127.

21. Serdaru M, Chiras J, Cujas M, Lhermitte F: Isolated benign cerebral vasculitis or migrainous vasospasm? *J Neurol Neurosurg Psychiatry* 47:73-76, 1984.

22. Case records of the Massachusetts General Hospital: Weekly clinicopathological exercises. Case 35-1985. Abrupt onset of headache followed by rapidly progressive encephalopathy in a 30-year-old woman, *N Engl J Med* 313:566-575, 1985.

23. Suwanwela C, Suwanwela N: Intracranial arterial narrowing and spasm in acute head injury, *J Neurosurg* 36:314-323, 1972.

24. Yarnell PR, Caplan LR: Basilar artery narrowing and hyperparathyroidism: Illustrative case, *Stroke* 17:1022-1024, 1986.

25. Noskin O, Jafarimojarrad E, Libman RB, Nelson JL: Diffuse cerebral vasoconstriction (Call-Fleming syndrome) and stroke associated with antidepressants, *Neurology* 67:159-160, 2006.

26. Nowak DA, Rodiek SO, Henneken S, et al: Reversible segmental cerebral vasoconstriction (Call-Fleming syndrome): Are calcium channel inhibitors a potential treatment option? *Cephalalgia* 23:218-222, 2003.

27. Singhal AB, Caviness VS, Begleiter AF, et al: Cerebral vasoconstriction and stroke after use of serotonergic drugs, *Neurology* 58:130-133, 2002.

28. Snyder BD, McClelland RR: Isolated benign cerebral vasculitis, *Arch Neurol* 35:612-614, 1978.

29. Bettoni L, Juvarra G, Bortone E, Lechi A: Isolated benign cerebral vasculitis. Case report and review, *Acta Neurol Belg* 84:161-173, 1984.

30. van Calenbergh F, van den Bergh V, Wilms G: Benign isolated arteritis of the central nervous system, *Clin Neurol Neurosurg* 88:267-273, 1986.

31. Hajj-Ali RA, Furlan A, Abou-Chebel A, Calabrese LH: Benign angiopathy of the central nervous system: Cohort of 16 patients with clinical course and long-term followup, *Arthritis Rheum* 47:662-669, 2002.

32. Hajj-Ali RA, Calabrese LH: Central nervous system vasculitis, *Curr Opin Rheumatol* 21:10-18, 2009.

33. Chen SP, Fuh JL, Chang FC, et al: Transcranial color Doppler study for reversible cerebral vasoconstriction syndromes, *Ann Neurol* 63:751-757, 2008.

34. Singhal AB, Hajj-Ali R, Calabrese LH: Reversible cerebral vasoconstriction syndrome: Two-center experience of 139 cases, *J Neuro Sci* 285(Suppl 1):S100-S101, 2009.

35. Fok JW, Nogueira RG, Singhal AB: *Cerebral angiographic features can distinguish reversible cerebral vasoconstriction syndromes from primary angiitis of the CNS,* Bangkok, 2009, Paper presented at 19th World Congress of Neurology.

36. Kirton A, Diggle J, Hu W, Wirrell E: A pediatric case of reversible segmental cerebral vasoconstriction, *Can J Neurol Sci* 33:250-253, 2006.

37. Schwedt TJ, Matharu MS, Dodick DW: Thunderclap headache, *Lancet Neurol* 5:621-631, 2006.

38. Buckle RM, Du Boulay G, Smith B: Death due to cerebral vasospasm, *J Neurol Neurosurg Psychiatry* 27:440-444, 1964.

39. Singhal AB, Kimberly WT, Schaefer PW, Hedley-Whyte ET: Case records of the Massachusetts General Hospital. Case 8-2009. A 36-year-old woman with headache, hypertension, and seizure 2 weeks post partum, *N Engl J Med* 360:1126-1137, 2009.

40. Williams TL, Lukovits TG, Harris BT, Harker Rhodes C: A fatal case of postpartum cerebral angiopathy with literature review, *Arch Gynecol Obstet* 275:67-77, 2007.

41. Calado S, Vale-Santos J, Lima C, Viana-Baptista M: Postpartum cerebral angiopathy: Vasospasm, vasculitis or both? *Cerebrovasc Dis* 18:340-341, 2004.

42. Singhal AB, Topcuoglu MA, Caviness VS, Koroshetz WJ: Call-Fleming syndrome versus isolated cerebral vasculitis: MRI lesion patterns, *Stroke* 34:264, 2003.

43. Chen SP, Fuh JL, Lirng JF, et al: Recurrent primary thunderclap headache and benign CNS angiopathy: Spectra of the same disorder? *Neurology* 67:2164-2169, 2006.

44. Singhal AB: Brain hemorrhages in reversible cerebral vasoconstriction syndromes (RCVS), *Neurology* 68:A221-A222, 2007.

45. Edlow BL, Kasner SE, Hurst RW, et al: Reversible cerebral vasoconstriction syndrome associated with subarachnoid hemorrhage, *Neurocrit Care* 7:203-210, 2007.

46. Moustafa RR, Allen CM, Baron JC: Call-Fleming syndrome associated with subarachnoid haemorrhage: Three new cases, *J Neurol Neurosurg Psychiatry* 79:602-605, 2008.

47. Singhal AB: Postpartum angiopathy with reversible posterior leukoencephalopathy, *Arch Neurol* 61:411-416, 2004.

48. Santos E, Zhang Y, Wilkins A, et al: Reversible cerebral vasoconstriction syndrome presenting with haemorrhage, *J Neurol Sci* 276:189-192, 2009.

49. Iancu-Gontard D, Oppenheim C, Touze E, et al: Evaluation of hyperintense vessels on FLAIR MRI for the diagnosis of multiple intracerebral arterial stenoses, *Stroke* 34:1886-1891, 2003.

50. Arnold M, Camus-Jacqmin M, Stapf C, et al: Postpartum cervicocephalic artery dissection, *Stroke* 39:2377-2379, 2008.

51. Singhal AB: Thunderclap headache, reversible cerebral arterial vasoconstriction, and unruptured aneurysms, *J Neurol Neurosurg Psychiatry* 73:96, author reply 97, 2002.

52. Rothrock JF, Walicke P, Swenson MR, et al: Migrainous stroke, *Arch Neurol* 45:63-67, 1988.

53. Bogousslavsky J, Despland PA, Regli F, Dubuis PY: Postpartum cerebral angiopathy: Reversible vasoconstriction assessed by transcranial Doppler ultrasounds, *Eur Neurol* 29:102-105, 1989.

54. The International Classification of Headache Disorders, ed 2. *Cephalalgia* 2004;24(Suppl 1):9-160.

55. Masuzawa T, Shinoda S, Furuse M, et al: Cerebral angiographic changes on serial examination of a patient with migraine, *Neuroradiology* 24:277-281, 1983.

56. Sanin LC, Mathew NT: Severe diffuse intracranial vasospasm as a cause of extensive migrainous cerebral infarction [see comment], *Cephalalgia* 13:289-292, 1993.

57. Meschia JF, Malkoff MD, Biller J: Reversible segmental cerebral arterial vasospasm and cerebral infarction: Possible association with excessive use of sumatriptan and Midrin, *Arch Neurol* 55:712-714, 1998.

58. Calado S, Vale-Santos J, Lima C, Viana-Baptista M: Postpartum cerebral angiopathy: Vasospasm, vasculitis or both? *Cerebrovasc Dis* 18:340-341, 2004.

59. Dietrich HH, Dacey RG Jr: Molecular keys to the problems of cerebral vasospasm, *Neurosurgery* 46:517-530, 2000.

60. Hajj-Ali RA, Furlan A, Abou-Chebel A, Calabrese LH: Benign angiopathy of the central nervous system: Cohort of 16 patients with clinical course and long-term followup, *Arthritis Rheum* 47:662-669, 2002.

61. Singhal AB: Postpartum angiopathy with reversible posterior leukoencephalopathy, *Arch Neurol* 61:411-416, 2004.

62. Muehlschlegel S, Rordorf G, Bodock M, Sims JR: Dantrolene mediates vasorelaxation in cerebral vasoconstriction: A case series, *Neurocrit Care* 10:116-121, 2009.

63. Ringer AJ, Qureshi AI, Kim SH, et al: Angioplasty for cerebral vasospasm from eclampsia, *Surg Neurol* 56:373-378, discussion 378-379, 2001.

64. Song JK, Fisher S, Seifert TD, et al: Postpartum cerebral angiopathy: Atypical features and treatment with intracranial balloon angioplasty, *Neuroradiology* 46:1022-1026, 2004.

65. Bouchard M, Verreault S, Gariepy JL, Dupre N: Intra-arterial milrinone for reversible cerebral vasoconstriction syndrome, *Headache* 49:142-145, 2009.

66. Rosenbloom MH, Singhal AB: CT angiography and diffusion-perfusion MR imaging in a patient with ipsilateral reversible cerebral vasoconstriction after carotid endarterectomy, *AJNR Am J Neuroradiol* 28:920-922, 2007.

67. Ursell MR, Marras CL, Farb R, et al: Recurrent intracranial hemorrhage due to postpartum cerebral angiopathy: Implications for management, *Stroke* 29:1995-1998, 1998.

41 Coagulation Abnormalities in Stroke

BRUCE M. COULL, KENDRA DRAKE

emostasis is a complex, highly evolved system involving intricate chemical interactions among soluble clotting factors, blood elements, and vascular tissues all working in concert to stop bleeding when blood vessels are damaged. Coagulation per se is the component of hemostasis that involves the transformation of liquid blood to a solid clot. Practically all ischemic strokes involve activation of hemostasis, sometimes under pathologic circumstances, whereas a variety of impairments in clotting factors and platelet function sometimes contribute to intracranial bleeding. The formation of a thrombus within an artery is a frequent consequence of vascular endothelial injury, such as happens with rupture of an atherosclerotic plaque or from relative stasis of blood in the auricle of the fibrillating left atrium. Abnormalities in hemostasis that predispose to thrombotic events are referred to as either a "hypercoagulable state" or a "thrombophilia," whereas conditions in which thrombotic events are more prevalent, such as diabetes mellitus, are considered to be a *prothrombotic state;* however, these terms are frequently interchanged. A detailed understanding of the hypercoagulable state hones the mechanistic diagnosis of stroke and may also help define treatment. Some measures of hemostatic function show promise as biomarkers for monitoring the risk of stroke.

Pathogenesis of Thrombosis

Vascular Injury

Hemostasis is a complex system of reactions that are normally held in check by a dynamic interplay between the normal blood vessel endothelial surface and certain regulatory plasma proteins that prevent activation of platelets and the prothrombin pathway.[1] The circulating regulatory plasma proteins include protein C, protein S, antithrombin III (ATIII), tissue factor pathway inhibitor (TFPI), and protein Z.[2,3] On the vascular endothelium, a key protein, thrombomodulin, promotes the activation of protein C. The combination of activated protein C with another natural anticoagulant, protein S, results in a complex that can rapidly inactivate activated coagulation factors Va and VIIIa, thereby suppressing thrombin activation (see, for example, Fig. 41-1). Protein S is found in the plasma as both an active (free) and an inactive (C4b-binding protein) form. A member of the coagulation cascade, protein Z, along with protein Z–related protease inhibitor, directly degrades factor Xa.

The vascular endothelium forms another key element in the regulation of hemostasis by expressing a number of regulatory molecules on the endothelial surface. Among these are thrombomodulin and the glycosaminoglycan, heparin, which by binding ATIII, greatly amplifies the ATIII functional ability to rapidly neutralize thrombin and other activated prothrombotic serine proteases, including factors Xa and IXa.[4,5] Healthy vascular endothelium also inhibits platelet adhesion and aggregation by several mechanisms. When the endothelium is stimulated by local injury, inflammation, or other thrombogenic processes, prostacyclin (PGI$_2$) is released. PGI$_2$ causes vasodilatation and inhibits platelet plug formation. Vascular endothelium also synthesizes and releases nitric oxide, a potent vasodilator and inhibitor of platelet activation.[6,7] Furthermore, if a clot does begin to form, the vascular endothelium promotes local fibrinolysis via the synthesis and release of tissue plasminogen activator (t-PA).

Although usually a barrier against thrombosis, the normal vascular endothelium becomes a strongly prothrombotic surface when injured.[6] Mediators of inflammation such as interleukin-1, tumor necrosis factor, and immune complexes can induce the endothelium to express tissue factor and other such substances, expose binding sites for clotting factors, and downregulate thrombomodulin expression.[5] With severe injury, endothelial cells may be lost from the vascular surface altogether, thereby exposing thrombogenic subendothelial tissues, as happens with rupture of an atheromatous plaque.[8,9] The brain vascular endothelium also appears to vary in its effectiveness as a barrier against thrombosis because the expression of thrombomodulin within the cerebral circulation varies regionally and is limited in amount compared with systemic vessels.[10-12]

Factor V Leiden, Antithrombin III, Protein C, Protein S, and Protein Z Deficiencies; Prothrombin G20210A Polymorphism; and von Willebrand Factor

Hereditary Deficiencies

Genetic modifications that affect function or concentration of the regulatory coagulation proteins in the hemostatic pathways are associated with an increased risk of

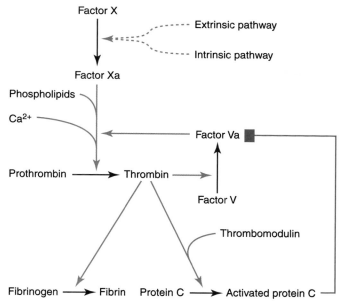

Figure 41-1 Regulation of factor V activity by thrombin and activated protein C. Thrombin activates protein C, which degrades factor V. Factor V Leiden is resistant to inactivation by protein C, which leads to a hypercoagulable state. (Adapted from Hamedani AG, Cole JW, Mitchell BD, et al: Meta-analysis of factor V Leiden and ischemic stroke in young adults: The importance of case ascertainment. *Stroke* 41:1599-1603, 2010.)

stroke. As a general rule the risk is similar for both ischemic stroke and myocardial infarction (MI) in adults, but there are some exceptions. Abnormalities in proteins S, C, and ATIII are associated most strongly with stroke in neonates and young children.[13] Their role in adult stroke is less certain, but recent studies suggest importance in selected populations. For example, the Atherosclerosis Risk in Communities Study (ARIC), reported a direct inverse relationship between protein C levels and the risk of ischemic stroke but not MI across the entire cohort.[14] An unsuspected finding was that the increased risk of stroke was not confined only to individuals with the abnormal low levels but correlated across the entire population in a manner similar to population studies of hypertension.

The presence of factor V Leiden,[15] activated protein C (APC) resistance,[16] and the prothrombin G20210A gene mutation[17] and low levels of protein Z have all been associated with increased risk of stroke.[18] APCR, caused by a mutation in factor V (factor V Leiden), which renders factor Va unable to be cleaved by APC, is by far the most common inherited defect associated with venous thrombosis. This mechanism and the related role of thrombin activation and protein C are summarized in Figure 41-1. In white populations, the factor V Leiden defect is present in 5% to 7% of the normal population and accounts for more than 95% of the total APC resistance. The factor V Leiden mutation appears in 20% of individuals with a first episode of deep venous thrombosis and in 60% of individuals with recurrent venous thromboses due to hypercoagulable states.

Although APC resistance due to factor V Leiden has a well-recognized association with cerebral venous

thrombosis,[15] the relationship to arterial stroke in adults is less certain; currently, the strongest evidence suggests a role in children with stroke.[19] In adult populations such as in the Physicians' Health Study, the presence of factor V Leiden did not increase the risk of stroke or MI,[20] and similar results have been found in some case-control studies[21]; however, in one large study, factor V Leiden was significantly more common in patients with large infarcts (13.6%; $P < 0.025$; confidence interval [CI], 1.16–4.34) than in the stroke-free control subjects (6.5%).[22] Furthermore, a meta-analysis of 18 case-control studies in adults, both young and those older than 50 years, with stroke found inconsistent results with such a heterogeneous mixture of subjects. Among unselected individuals with ischemic stroke, the odds ratio for factor V Leiden was 1.40 (P = NS), whereas the odds ratio associating stroke with factor V Leiden was statistically significant at 2.73 (P = 0.003) when individuals who were likely to have a prothrombotic state were specified.[23]

In adults with stroke, the association between inherited deficiencies in protein C, protein S, and ATIII and *arterial* thrombosis is less convincing.[24,25] Case-control and cohort studies provide inconsistent results: some show a positive relationship to stroke while others show a negative relationship. Such discrepancies reflect differences in the selection of subjects to be tested. In a prospective case-control study that initially enrolled subjects with acute MI, it was found on follow-up that individuals with low levels of protein C and/or antithrombin, even if in the low normal range, tended to have an increased risk of recurrent cardiovascular events including stroke.[26] Similarly, a reduced protein C level measured at the time of acute stroke has been correlated with a poor clinical outcome.

An increased risk of stroke is also reported with elevated levels of von Willebrand factor (vWF), factor VIIIc, and plasma fibrinogen.[27,28] Unlike the other regulatory proteins that interact with normal vascular endothelial function, vWF comes into play when endothelium is damaged and the factor interacts with platelet activation. The levels of vWF are influenced by inflammation, genetic influences (e.g., ABO blood groups), and a metalloprotease, "A Disintegrin And Metalloprotease with ThromboSpondin motif (ADAMTS13)."[28] When coupled with inflammation, high levels of vWF triple the relative risk of stroke compared with individuals with low vWF levels. Lip et al[29] found that constantly elevated vWF levels in persons with chronic atrial fibrillation were associated with an increased likelihood of cardioembolic-related stroke. From a clinical perspective many of these studies emphasize the importance of the role of inflammation as a critical influence on levels and function. When considering the results of measurements obtained during the early phase of stroke, one must keep in mind that levels of these substances can be affected by the extent of the early inflammatory phase response. For example, one study reported that low protein S levels were common in patients hospitalized for any reason,[30] which makes the role of this substance in stroke much more difficult to establish.

A single mutation in the 3′-untranslated region of the prothrombin gene resulting in a G-to-A (glycine-to-alanine) substitution has been associated with familial thrombophilia.[17] Prothrombin, or factor II, is the precursor of thrombin. A vitamin K–dependent zymogen, this protein is produced by the liver and has a central role in the conversion of fibrinogen to fibrin. Prothrombin also has inhibitory functions that limit the hemostasis process (see Fig. 41-1). Thrombin also has regulatory functions that are important in the pathogenesis of atherosclerosis, such as initiating platelet aggregation and endothelial activation.

Factor II G20210A occurs in about 2.5% of the general population and in 6% of patients with a family history of venous thrombosis.[31] This mutation is seen almost exclusively in white persons; in the presence of traditional vascular risk factors, the addition of factor II G20210A has a synergistic effect on the risk of MI, but results are conflicting.[17] Few studies have investigated the role of factor II G20210A in stroke. A case-control study of consecutive patients with stroke or transient ischemic attack (TIA) found no difference in prevalence of the prothrombin mutation between the patients and control subjects.[21] Another study of 72 young patients with stroke and without traditional vascular risk factors found an increased prevalence in patients compared with control subjects (9.7% of patients had heterozygous mutations versus 2.5% of control subjects; 2.8% of patients had homozygous mutations versus 0% of control subjects).[14] The stroke risk associated with the heterozygous mutation was increased 3.8-fold, either mutation was increased 5.5-fold, and the homozygous mutation was increased 208-fold. From a clinical perspective more studies are needed to clarify the role of this mutation in stroke from either a diagnostic or therapeutic perspective.

Acquired Deficiencies

Acquired deficiencies of ATIII and proteins C and S are associated with a prothrombotic state and thereby to brain infarction in a variety of special clinical settings, as listed in Table 41-1.

Reductions of the anticoagulant proteins have been found in perioperative settings in women who are pregnant or taking oral contraceptives and in patients with malignancies, hepatic failure, or nephrotic syndrome. Short-term fluctuations of anticoagulant protein levels can also follow plasmapheresis and hemodialysis. In a patient with any of the foregoing conditions who experiences TIA, stroke, or amaurosis fugax, careful evaluation may uncover one of these prothrombotic states.

Laboratory Investigation

Genetic tests are available for factor V Leiden and the prothrombin G20210A polymorphism.[32] For deficiencies of protein C, protein S, and ATIII, the underlying defect may be attributable to several different mutations, and DNA testing is not practical. In general, in situations for which genetic tests are unavailable (or their results would be negative in the case of acquired deficiencies), functional or activity-based assays should be used. Ten percent of defects are in the functional aspect of the molecule and would be missed with antigen assays.[32]

For protein C, functional assays are based on measurement of the anticoagulant activity of APC against the natural substrates, factors VIIIa and Va, or measurement of

TABLE 41-1 ACQUIRED DEFICIENCIES OF ANTITHROMBIN III AND PROTEINS C AND S

Consumption coagulopathy
Disseminated intravascular coagulation (shock, sepsis)
Surgery
Preeclampsia
Liver dysfunction
Acute hepatic failure
Cirrhosis
Renal disease
Nephrotic syndrome
Hemolytic-uremic syndrome
Malignancies
Leukemia (acute promyelocytic leukemia)
Malnutrition or gastrointestinal loss
Vascular reconstruction (diabetes, age)
Protein-calorie deprivation
Inflammatory bowel disease
Various medicines (i.e., warfarin)
Estrogens-progestins
Heparin
L-Asparaginase
Other
Vasculitis (? systemic lupus erythematosus)
Infection—neutropenia
Hemodialysis
Plasmapheresis

the amidolytic activity against small synthetic substrates. The former should be the test of choice because it better mimics in vivo conditions.[32] These tests are commercially available, but their results may be affected by conditions such as APC resistance and high concentrations of factor VIII and may be difficult to interpret.[33,34] These problems can be avoided through the use of amidolytic assays with snake venom as the activator. APC resistance can be assessed in plasma with activated partial thromboplastin time (aPTT)-based methods.[35] These are simple, inexpensive, and sensitive to the APC resistance syndrome as well as to factor V Leiden.[32] For protein S, a functional assay should be theoretically superior to antigen measurement; however, available functional assays are based on the APC cofactor activity of protein S and are not very specific. The distribution of protein S in the plasma is 60% of the whole protein bound to C4b-binding protein, and 40% is free and active as APC cofactor.[36] The most common defect in protein S is a normal total protein S level but decreased levels of free protein S.[37] Thus, if one assays only the total protein S level, many cases of protein S defect will be missed. In a study of protein S deficiency established by genetic testing in a large kindred, levels of free protein S distinguished carriers from noncarriers much better than levels of the whole protein, suggesting that it may not be necessary to measure both free and total protein S.[38] The measurement of ATIII antigen is not adequate for screening patients because many patients with dysfunctional AT deficiency have normal antigen levels and they would not be diagnosed by ATIII antigen determination.[32] The two types of functional assays for ATIII deficiency are progressive inhibitory activity (performed without heparin) and heparin cofactor activity. Both may be performed with either thrombin or factor

Xa as the target enzyme. The assay using heparin cofactor activity is able to detect all clinically relevant cases of ATIII deficiency. Factor Xa is probably a better target enzyme than thrombin because factor Xa is not affected by the presence of the other main plasma inhibitor of thrombin, heparin cofactor II.[39]

Activation of Hemostasis and Fibrin Formation

Many methods are available to measure both activation and breakdown products of coagulation and fibrinolysis.[40,41] Among these is the activation peptide ($F_{1.2}$), which is cleaved from prothrombin by factor Xa to form thrombin. Although the circulating plasma levels of $F_{1.2}$ reflect ongoing activation of hemostasis, routine measures of $F_{1.2}$ have not found clinical utility. The conversion of fibrinogen to a cross-linked fibrin clot is a complex multistep process that is mediated by thrombin. In the first step, thrombin cleaves fibrinopeptides A and B to form circulating fibrin monomers. The circulating fibrin monomer is then covalently cross-linked by thrombin-activated factor XIII. When the fibrin clot is lysed via fibrinolysis, specific breakdown products form; they include either nonspecific fibrin(ogen) degradation products or D-dimer that is specific to fibrin degradation.[42-44]

During the early phase of ischemic stroke, the intense activation of coagulation produces elevations of hemostatic markers, including prothrombin activation fragment $F_{1.2}$, fibrinopeptide A, and thrombin–antithrombin complex.[29,45-50]

These elevations decline slowly but may persist for weeks to months.[45,48] Some studies have found persistent elevation of these markers in patients after stroke compared with control subjects.[50-52] One possible conclusion from these data is that there is an underlying prothrombotic state in patients with cerebrovascular disease. High levels of hemostatic markers have been found in patients with atrial fibrillation.[53-57] Levels of these markers are reduced by anticoagulation[58-61] and have been reported to decline after cardioversion.[62]

In the Edinburgh Artery Study, after adjustment for traditional vascular risk factors, several hemostatic factors were found to be associated with stroke and MI: plasma fibrinogen level, t-PA antigen, and fibrin–D-dimer. This study also found that, in older men and women, the presence of increased coagulation activity and disturbed fibrinolysis predicted future vascular events.[63] A later study confirmed these results and also found that levels of C-reactive protein, D-dimer, and fibrinogen after an initial ischemic stroke were predictive of a new stroke.[64]

Fibrinogen itself is a strong independent risk factor for MI and stroke.[3,63,65-71] Fibrinogen levels increase after stroke,[72] and fibrinogen elevations are associated with an increased risk of further cardiovascular events in stroke survivors.[72,73] Patients with infection-associated stroke have higher levels of fibrinogen after stroke than those without a recent infection.[74] Possible mechanisms for the higher risk of stroke include activation of hemostasis, increased blood viscosity, a reflection of underlying inflammation, and decreased cerebral blood flow.[68,75] Fibrinogen also plays a critical role in platelet activation through binding to platelet glycoprotein IIb–IIIa

membrane receptors,[76] which might be another mechanism favoring thrombosis.

Fibrinolysis

Homeostasis depends on the balance between clot formation and clot degradation, or *fibrinolysis*. Depression of fibrinolytic activity can tip the balance toward thrombosis. The fibrinolytic system is equilibrated between t-PA and its primary inhibitor, plasminogen activator inhibitor type 1 (PAI-1). Either reductions of t-PA or elevations of PAI-1 can inhibit fibrinolysis and predispose to thrombosis. Both of these mechanisms have been suggested as operating in venous thrombosis[77] but have not been comprehensively studied in stroke. Several rare inherited conditions are associated with depressed fibrinolysis, however, including plasminogen deficiency, qualitative plasminogen abnormalities, plasminogen activator deficiency, elevation of PAI-1, dysfibrinogenemia, and factor XII/pre-kallikrein deficiency.[78-84] These disorders usually manifest as venous thrombosis, but cases of arterial thrombosis including stroke have been described.

Fibrinolytic degradation products such as cross-linked D-dimer are increased after stroke,[45,49,51,85,86] and their levels are correlated with infarct size, stroke severity, and subsequent mortality.[48] Weak levels of D-dimer occur later than peak levels of fibrin markers, which suggests a relative excess of fibrin formation over fibrin(ogen)olysis in the early phase of stroke. Functional assays have shown a reduction in the extent that fibrinolytic activity can be stimulated after stroke.[87,88] Although elevations of both t-PA antigen and PAI-1 antigen have been observed after stroke,[50,89-91] the elevations of t-PA antigen do not necessarily indicate greater plasma fibrinolytic activity because much of the t-PA antigen may be bound to PAI-1 antigen. Prospective population studies have demonstrated the seemingly paradoxic finding that elevations of t-PA antigen are associated with a greater risk of MI and stroke.[17,92,93] Elevations of t-PA antigen are also associated with the severity of carotid atherosclerosis.[94] Elevations of t-PA antigen do not necessarily denote increased fibrinolytic activity but instead may indicate an ongoing response to atherosclerosis and thrombosis and greater clot formation rather than a more effective fibrinolytic response. Furthermore, like the increase in PGI_2 seen in patients with atherosclerosis, t-PA antigen elevation may merely be a marker for ongoing endothelial damage.[95] These markers may eventually provide additional information for identifying patients at a high risk of stroke.

Lipoprotein (a)—or Lp(a)—can inhibit fibrinolysis in vitro and may have a similarly important effect in vivo, and elevated levels of Lp(a) increase the risk of stroke and MI.[96] Lp(a) has substantial homology to plasminogen, the precursor to plasmin.[97] Lp(a) also stimulates the release of PAI-1 from endothelial cells and effectively competes with plasminogen for binding either to fibrin or to the surface of vascular endothelial cells, inhibiting fibrinolysis.[98,99] Lp(a) levels have been found to be high in selected populations with cerebrovascular disease, and most but not all studies have shown Lp(a) elevation to be a potent risk factor for stroke, especially in young patients.[100-105] However, Lp(a) levels do not appear to be associated with stroke characteristics, recurrence, or prognosis.[98,99] Unfortunately, there is no established treatment for increased Lp(a) levels, and management consists of aggressively controlling other risk factors, especially lowering the low-density lipoprotein (LDL) cholesterol level to less than 100 mg/dL.

Platelet Adhesion, Activation, and Aggregation

Platelet activation is related to cerebral ischemia, both as a potential cause of stroke and as a result of platelet exposure to the ischemic brain.[106] Atherothrombosis occurs when the vessel wall is damaged, for example, by rupture of an atherosclerotic plaque, exposing collagen fibers and subendothelial matrix proteins.[107] The first process in thrombosis is the adhesion of platelets to subendothelial matrix proteins, with activation of adhered platelets and stimulation of a large number of other platelets to form a platelet aggregate. Other coagulation proteins assemble on this aggregate and ultimately lead to thrombosis and possibly vessel occlusion.[108] Platelet activation, under certain conditions, can cause thrombus formation even in the absence of vessel wall injury; examples are thrombosis in disseminated coagulopathy and platelet activation as a stroke mechanism in some people with antiphospholipid antibodies.[106] Some conditions, such as cerebrovascular disease and MI, have been associated with a long-term increase in platelet activation, as evidenced by elevated serum levels of platelet release proteins[45,46,85,109-111] and by urinary metabolites of thromboxane.[112,113] There is some evidence that platelet activation occurs in ischemic brain tissue and continues for some time after the initial event. Using a primate focal ischemia model, Del Zoppo et al[114] have provided evidence that platelet activation occurs in the ischemic brain area. Whether the risk of stroke in people with persistent platelet activation is increased, however, is not clear.

Patients with myeloproliferative disease (MPD), including polycythemia rubra vera (PV) and essential thrombocythemia (ET), have increases in platelet reactivity and platelet counts as well as large, dysfunctional platelets, which are strongly associated with stroke.[115-117] Thrombosis occurs more frequently in PV and ET than in acute myelocytic leukemia or chronic granulocytic leukemia and is a major cause of morbidity and mortality in patients with these myeloproliferative disorders. Up to 40% of patients with PV or ET experience a thrombotic episode, and the incidence of thrombosis could be as high as 75% per year. Arterial occlusions are more common than venous events,[117-122] and stroke is often the presenting feature of both PV and ET. At the time of diagnosis, 25% of patients with myeloproliferative syndromes manifest atherosclerosis, and 50% of patients have evidence of carotid intimal thickening. Increasing age, elevated hematocrit level, and treatment with phlebotomy in PV all predispose to thromboembolism. Importantly, the magnitude of the elevation of the platelet count does not correlate with the risk of thrombosis. In one study, the average platelet count at the time of stroke was 600,000 cells/mm,[3] but two thirds of patients had counts lower than 400,000 cells/mm.[3] In the absence of MPD, secondary thrombocytosis is an occasional but much less common cause of stroke.[123,124]

Antiplatelet therapy, usually with aspirin, is recommended for treatment of patients with cerebral, coronary artery, or peripheral vascular thrombosis.[125] Aspirin irreversibly inhibits platelet cyclooxygenase through acetylation and attenuates thromboxane A_2, a potent stimulator of platelet activation.[106] Dipyridamole inhibits platelet activation through inhibition of platelet phosphodiesterase activity, ultimately blocking calcium-mediated platelet activation.[126] Ticlopidine and clopidogrel inhibit the excitatory receptor P2Y1, thereby blocking adenosine diphosphate–induced platelet aggregation.[127] Platelet inhibitors also usually suppress the platelet hyperreactivity associated with MPD and can prolong the usually shortened mean platelet survival time.[128] As well as its antithrombotic effects, aspirin may inhibit platelet secretion of vascular growth factors and inflammatory cytokines, thereby reducing chronic vascular damage. In addition to pharmacologic antithrombotic measures, lowering of elevated platelet counts should be considered in patients with MPD and a history of thrombosis. Hydroxyurea (e.g., 1 g daily to start) has been shown in a randomized trial to prevent thrombotic complications in patients with essential thrombocytosis.[128,129] A platelet count of 250,000 to 450,000 cells/mm[3] is an appropriate target. The use of anagrelide to lower platelet counts should be considered for cases refractory to hydroxyurea or for patients unable to tolerate the drug.[128]

Heparin-Induced Thrombocytopenia

Heparin-induced thrombocytopenia (HIT) is a potentially serious consequence of heparin administration. The syndrome happens when antibodies, usually immunoglobulin G (IgG), are produced that bind the heparin-platelet factor 4 (PF4) complex.[130,131] The antibody binding causes further platelet activation that produces more PF4 release, thereby propagating the cycle. Although platelets are consumed and the counts fall, the syndrome is characterized by vascular occlusive events rather than bleeding. HIT occurs 6 to 10 days after heparin exposure and is associated with a significant thrombocytopenia and a high risk of thrombotic events, including stroke.[130-135] The incidence of HIT is 1% to 5%. The risk is higher with higher doses of heparin but has been described after very low doses such as those used for intravenous line flushes.[136-139] HIT provides some insight into how immune mechanisms promote thrombosis.[131,140] The interaction between heparin and PF4 leads to platelet activation, endothelial damage, and thrombosis.[141] The HIT-related antibodies are usually IgG antibodies that bind to a complex of heparin and PF4.[142] HIT antibodies may also bind to heparan on the surface of endothelial cells and stimulate the production of tissue factor on the endothelial cell surface.[143] Heparin–PF4 complexes bind to Fc gamma RII A receptors (CD32) and induce platelet activation associated with more release of PF4, leading to a propagation of the HIT process. An elevation of circulating adhesion molecules (selectins) has also been observed in HIT.[144] Platelet–neutrophil complexes are mediated by P-selectin, which is also important in leukocyte adhesion. This finding supports a role for inflammation in the underlying pathophysiology of HIT. Platelet activation leads to release of platelet microparticles, triggering an activation of the coagulation system.[144]

A 14-year retrospective review found that in patients diagnosed with isolated HIT the 30-day risk of thrombosis was 53%.[138] Most thromboses were venous. Although platelet counts in HIT may fall to as low as 20,000 cells/mm,[3] hemorrhagic complications are uncommon. HIT is often seen in postoperative settings, perhaps because of the combined influence of surgery-induced inflammation and heparin exposure. Atkinson et al[133] have emphasized the relationship between HIT and ischemic stroke after carotid endarterectomy. Becker and Miller,[130] reviewing data on 29 patients with HIT II-related stroke from the literature, found that few patients had previous cerebrovascular disease and that most patients either died (25%) or were left disabled after their strokes. HIT has also been associated with cerebral venous thrombosis.[145] Other risk factors for the development of HIT II are diabetes, neoplasm, heart failure, infection, antiphospholipid antibodies, and trauma.[141] The diagnosis of HIT is based on a combination of clinical findings and demonstration of heparin-dependent antiplatelet antibodies.[138,146,147]

Prevention of HIT is the best management strategy, and platelet counts should be closely monitored in patients undergoing heparin therapy. Once HIT is recognized, heparin should be promptly discontinued; thrombosis risk is high in these patients, however, so some antithrombotic treatment must be given.[148] Because low-molecular-weight heparin will cross-react with antiheparin antibodies, this agent cannot be used for anticoagulation in patients with HIT.[137] Currently, heparinoids and recombinant hirudins are appropriate treatments in patients with HIT.[149-151] Thrombin inhibitors may also have a role. Many patients need long-term anticoagulation with warfarin; however, this therapy cannot be initiated until platelet counts have normalized because the severe drop in protein C in HIT contraindicates early treatment with warfarin.[149,151]

Antiphospholipid Antibodies

Although not recognized as such at the time, the first test utilizing a partial antiphospholipid (aPL) antibody assay was developed in 1906 by Wassermann and colleagues as a serologic test for syphilis.[152,153] Consisting of a heterogeneous group of immunoglobulins, aPLs are directed against anionic phospholipids, phospholipid–protein complexes, or phospholipid binding proteins.[152-154] aPL antibodies are produced in a variety of clinical situations and are associated with a hypercoagulable state characterized primarily by thrombosis, thrombocytopenia, and fetal loss. In the 1950s it was noted that some patients with systemic lupus erythematosus (SLE) often had prolonged aPTTs and false-positive results on Venereal Disease Research Laboratory (VDRL) tests[155] but experienced thrombotic episodes despite the elevation of the aPTT. Among these thrombotic events are a variety of cerebrovascular manifestations.

Bowie et al[156] first described the association of aPLs and thrombosis in 1963. In a 1972 review, Feinstein and Rapaport[157] called this phenomenon the *lupus anticoagulant* because of the occurrence in persons with SLE.

Harris et al,[158] recognizing that cardiolipin is a major component of the VDRL test, developed and popularized the anticardiolipin (aCL) antibody test in 1983.

The lupus anticoagulant (LA) test is a functional assay characterized by prolongation of phospholipid-dependent coagulation, whereas aCL antibodies are identified by immunoassay and target molecular variants of cardiolipin to measure antibody concentration and binding avidity.[152,159,160] Positive results of either test have been independently associated with thrombosis, and their combined presence and repeated positivity amplify the risk of thrombotic complications.[161,162] The preponderance of evidence, however, indicates that the LA test is more specific for patients at risk of thromboembolic events.[159,160] In contrast, the aCL antibody test is a more sensitive assay but is nonspecific, and positive results could also be found in various other individuals, such as those taking certain medications, those with malignancies or infectious diseases, and even in some healthy individuals.[152,159,161] Other aPL-related antibodies such as antiphosphatidylserine, phosphatidylethanolamine, and phosphatidylinositol have been less frequently studied, and their significance is still emerging.[163-165]

In 1990, three groups independently recognized that aPL antibodies were not directed against phospholipids alone but rather against a complex of plasma glycoprotein β_2 glycoprotein I (β_2GPI) and phospholipid. The cationic plasma glycoprotein β_2GPI, or apolipoprotein H, was noted to be an antigenic target that identifies most but not all aPL antibodies.[160,165,166] Data suggest that endothelial cells have cell surface receptors that attract and bind to β_2GPI, which in turn can attract aPL antibodies, which can lead to endothelial cell activation, increased secretion of proinflammatory cytokines, release of tissue factor, and subsequent initiation of the coagulation cascade.[153,165] One of the most promising aspects of the discovery of β_2GPI as a target antigen for aPL is that β_2GPI, a minor natural anticoagulant, competes in vitro for available phospholipid surface area needed for assembly of the prothrombinase complex, thereby inhibiting prothrombinase activity. It is thought that only autoimmune aPL antibodies react in vivo with β_2GPI after binding to phospholipids; therefore, immunoassays for β_2GPI have been added to the revised criteria for definite antiphospholipid syndrome (APS).[159,160,167] In some studies, the presence of β_2GPI antibodies rivals the presence of other aPL antibody markers in identifying patients with the highest risk of thrombosis.[168]

The Sapporo diagnostic criteria for APS were revised in 2006 and include the clinical criteria of either vascular thrombosis or pregnancy morbidity as well as the laboratory criteria of aCL antibody, LA, or anti-β_2GPI antibody on at least two occasions at least 6 weeks apart (Table 41-2).[167] Antibodies to other negatively charged phospholipids (e.g., phosphatidylserine and phosphatidylethanolamine) are also associated with these and other clinical manifestations; however, with an evidence-based medicine approach, there are insufficient data for these antibodies to be included in a rigorous classification system. Other clinical manifestations that have been associated with aPLs are livedo reticularis, optic changes, primary adrenal insufficiency, and a variety of neurologic

TABLE 41-2 REVISED SAPPORO CLASSIFICATION CRITERIA FOR THE ANTIPHOSPHOLIPID SYNDROME

Antiphospholipid antibody syndrome (APS) is present if at least one of the following clinical criteria and one of the laboratory criteria are met:

Clinical criteria
1. Vascular thrombosis—One or more clinical episodes of arterial, venous, or small vessel thrombosis, in any tissue or organ
2. Pregnancy and morbidity
   a. One or more unexplained deaths of a morphologically normal fetus at or beyond the tenth week of gestation
   b. One or more premature births of a morphologically normal neonate before the 34th week of gestation
   c. Three or more unexplained consecutive spontaneous abortions before the 10th week of gestation

Laboratory criteria
1. Lupus anticoagulant (LA) present in plasma, on two or more occasions at least 12 weeks apart
2. Anticardiolipin (aCL) antibody of IgG and/or IgM isotype present in medium or high titer on two or more occasions at least 12 weeks apart
3. Anti-β_2 glycoprotein-I antibody of IgG and/or IgM isotype present on two or more occasions at least 12 weeks apart

Adapted from Miyakis S, Lockshin MD, Atsumi T, et al: International consensus statement on an update of the classification criteria for definite antiphospholipid syndrome (APS). *J Thromb Haemost* 4:295-306, 2006.

symptoms including movement disorders, epilepsy, and dementia.[154,169-172] Once again, the strength of the association between these clinical manifestations and the presence of aPLs is not strong enough for them to be included as diagnostic features.

Individuals with APS but without SLE or other rheumatologic or autoimmune disorders have primary APS (PAPS). Those with APS along with SLE or other collagen vascular diseases have secondary APS.[152,160,173] However, the recent consensus statement on APS advises against using the term *secondary* APS because most of these individuals have SLE and documenting the coexistence of SLE (or another disease) is more advantageous for classification.[167] Turiel et al[173] found that the main independent risk factors for vascular complications in PAPS patients were previous thrombosis and high IgG aCL titers (>40 GPL units). However, in those with APS and SLE, aPLs impart an increased risk of thrombosis that is at least equal to and may be greater than that observed in PAPS.[174,175] Cerebrovascular ischemia associated with APS generally occurs at a younger age; however, in the absence of clinical complications, the presence of aPLs does not indicate APS, and the role in predicting thrombotic events is controversial.[168,173] The prevalence of aPLs in healthy adults rises with age and is estimated to be as high as 12% to 50% in healthy elders, depending on the test used for detection.[153]

One of the largest studies to evaluate the natural history and risk factors for recurrent thrombosis in patients with aPLs comes from the Italian Registry of 360 patients studied prospectively for 4 years.[176] Inclusion criteria were presence of aPLs and availability of the subject for follow-up. aPL assays were performed clinically for a thrombotic event, a coagulation abnormality suggesting the presence of LA, or a disease known to be associated with APS. Treatment was at the discretion of the physician. Over the 4-year period, 34 patients had thrombotic events, including 10 strokes and six TIAs. Risk factors for thrombosis in this cohort included an aCL antibody titer greater than 40 GPL units and either a prior thrombotic event or SLE. Other studies have also evaluated the association of APS with recurrent stroke.[58,176,177-180] Some[176,178-182] but not all[162,177,183] have suggested an association with recurrent thrombosis. Most of these studies are small to medium-sized case series, however, and their results thus cannot be considered conclusive. It is crucial to know whether APS raises the risk of recurrent stroke.

Many case-control studies have shown an association between different types of aPL antibodies and initial stroke,[184-191] but some have not.[192-195] The methodologic differences among studies, such as the type of aPL studied, sample size, and study population, could explain these discrepant results. It is interesting, however, that many of the larger studies found an association between aPLs and incident stroke, whereas the association with recurrent stroke is weaker. The explanation is not clear but may be related to the higher importance of other stroke risk factors in the risk of recurrent stroke, which overshadow the recurrent stroke risk contributed by aPLs.[182]

Few prospective studies have examined the association between aPL and either an initial stroke or MI. However, patients included in these studies would not meet current criteria for APS as these studies were limited to performance of aCL antibody testing performed on only one occasion.[196,197] The first prospective association between aCL and stroke was reported by Brey et al[185] in a study of the association between aCL and stroke and MI in men enrolled in the Honolulu Heart Program over 20 years. Only the presence of β_2GPI-dependent aCL IgG antibodies was significantly associated with incident ischemic stroke and MI. However, this association was attenuated during the last 5 years of follow-up. The risk factor-adjusted relative odds for men with the presence versus the absence of β_2GPI-dependent aCL of the IgG class was 2.2 at 15 years.

The clinical presentation of stroke and TIA associated with aPLs does not have particular distinguishing features. Both large and small cerebral arterial occlusions in the anterior and posterior circulations as well as venous occlusions are all reported to occur. Although deep lacunar infarctions and isolated white matter signal-enhancing lesions are detected on magnetic resonance imaging (MRI) and large brain infarctions occur, most strokes are relatively small and involve the cortex and subjacent white matter.[58] No single mechanism for stroke associated with aPLs has been established, but a few pathologic reports have demonstrated nonspecific microvascular platelet–fibrin plugs, which suggest possible thrombosis in situ. However, cardiac valvular lesions, predominantly left-sided and mitral, often accompany APS and could also be responsible for these lesions.[162,166,198]

Mechanisms underlying the aPL-associated vascular events, in the absence of SLE, are probably multifactorial and include associations of strokes with valvular disease,[162,166] cerebral microemboli,[185,199] thrombosis and endothelial hyperplasia,[153,200,201] antibodies to brain endothelium,[202,203] and adhesion molecule expression.[204] Some aPLs interfere with the vascular endothelial anticoagulant functions, whereas others directly activate endothelial thrombogenic mechanisms. Membranes of circulating white blood cells and platelets have also been implicated as a target for prothrombotic binding of aPLs. The thrombogenicity of aPLs may stem from their targeting of prothrombin on damaged membrane surfaces and their interference with the APC pathway. aPLs can interfere with thrombomodulin-induced protein C activation and also with protein S cofactor function for protein C. The importance of platelet activation in the process is supported by analysis of brain tissue removed from patients with aPL-related stroke, in which small arteries and microvessels are occluded by platelet–fibrin plugs. Single-photon emission computed tomography[205,206] and MRI spectroscopy[207] studies show diffuse damage that is compatible with many of these mechanisms. It is likely that the mechanism underlying the aPL-associated stroke in a given patient may affect the treatment response. Animal models of stroke in APS exist but are complex and therefore not yet suitable for evaluating therapy.[202,208] There have been reports of strokes in animals immunized with β_2GPI, but they seem to occur late in the disease and affect only a few animals.[209]

The thorough evaluation of patients in whom aPL is suspected often requires multiple testing procedures because, unfortunately, no one test can adequately screen a patient for aPLs.[210] An effective initial screen is a sensitive aPTT test and the aCL assay. If results of these evaluations are negative but clinical suspicion remains high, then the following tests should be performed: (1) kaolin clotting time, (2) dilute Russell viper venom time (dRVVT), and (3) lupus inhibitor screen (different aPTT reagents). One caveat about aPL testing is that levels of aPLs may fall during thrombotic events, so tests may have to be repeated when the patient reaches a steady state. It cannot be stressed enough that all patients with suspected aPL-associated clinical manifestations should also be carefully evaluated for other potential causes.

Secondary stroke prevention treatments such as platelet antiaggregant and anticoagulant therapy have been used in both APS and in cerebrovascular disease associated with aPL immunoreactivity. The largest study of recurrent stroke was performed by the prospective Antiphospholipid Antibody in Stroke Study (APASS) group. The APASS group, in collaboration with the Warfarin-Aspirin for Recurrent Stroke Study (WARSS) group, completed the first prospective study of the role of aPLs in recurrent ischemic stroke.[162] This controlled and blinded study initiated in 1993 compared the risk of recurrent stroke and other thromboembolic disease over a 2-year follow-up period in patients with ischemic stroke who were randomly assigned to receive either aspirin therapy (325 mg/day) or warfarin therapy (target international normalized ratio [INR] range, 1.4 to 2.8). A single aPL determination was performed in each patient at study entry. The rates of recurrent stroke were not found to be statistically different between treatment groups, and there were no differences in major bleeding complication rates.[162]

Therefore, it appears that in patients who test positive for aPLs at the time of ischemic stroke, including those with low titers of aCL and/or IgA aCL, and who do not have either atrial fibrillation or high-grade carotid stenosis, aspirin therapy is equivalent to warfarin therapy (INR of approximately 2.2) in both efficacy and major bleeding complication rate. Both the aspirin dose and INR value utilized for this study were based on current treatment recommendations for secondary prevention of ischemic stroke in patients without aPLs at the time the study was undertaken over 15 years ago. It is important to note that the analyses that are currently available from the WARSS or APASS data do not address the issue of whether meeting the proposed criteria for the diagnosis of definite APS is an important factor in stroke recurrence or therapeutic response.

It is possible yet unproven that higher doses of warfarin are superior for prevention of recurrence in aPL-associated ischemic stroke. Khamashta et al,[211] in a highly selected cohort that was studied retrospectively, found that high-dose anticoagulant therapy is associated with better outcomes. However, this potential benefit must be weighed against the considerably high hemorrhagic complication rate reported in that study. Further, the patients in the study did not undergo further aPL testing and would not fulfill current criteria for APS. Crowther et al[181] more recently performed a randomized double-blind trial of 114 patients followed up for 2.7 years. Recurrent thrombosis including MI, deep venous thrombosis, pulmonary embolism, and stroke, occurred in 3.4% (2/58) of those patients assigned to moderate-intensity warfarin (average INR, 2.3) and in 10.7% (6/56) of those assigned to receive high-intensity warfarin (average INR, 3.3). In addition, 22.4% (13/58) of the moderate-intensity group and 37.5% (21/56) of the high-intensity group discontinued warfarin prematurely because of either thrombosis while receiving therapy or complications; however, there was no difference in bleeding rates between the two groups. These results suggest that high-intensity warfarin therapy with an INR of 3.1 to 4.0 is not more efficacious than moderate-intensity warfarin with an INR of 2.0 to 3.0 for prevention of recurrent thrombosis in patients with aPL antibodies. Thus, whether either moderate-intensity or high-intensity warfarin therapy can prevent recurrent stroke or other thrombotic episodes remains an open question. It is possible that subgroups of patients with different risks of recurrence will be identified in the coming years. With the current level of knowledge, however, patients with previous arterial thrombosis and persistent medium-high titers of aCL, LA, or both seem to be at the highest risk of recurrent events. Currently, there is no evidence to support the use of any specific treatment strategies for primary prevention of aPL-associated ischemic stroke.[182]

Although it is possible to suppress LA with prednisone, this treatment, except as indicated for coexisting SLE or other connective tissue diseases, has not been effective for prevention of vascular events.[212] For a few patients who experience the catastrophic variant of APS that resembles disseminated intravascular coagulation, the combination of corticosteroids with plasmapheresis and/or intravenous immunoglobulin and possibly immunosuppression has been effective for short-term management.[213-215]

Sneddon's Syndrome

Sneddon's syndrome is an uncommon condition characterized by ischemic stroke and widespread livedo reticularis in the absence of other systemic diseases. Approximately three of four individuals with Sneddon's syndrome have increased levels of aPLs.[216,217] Besides livedo reticularis, some patients with the syndrome experience Raynaud's phenomenon and acrocyanosis. Sneddon's syndrome typically affects young adults and is more common in women than in men and has been linked to tobacco use. Skin biopsies, which are particularly useful for diagnosing aPL-seronegative individuals, show focal epidermal ulceration with chronic inflammatory infiltrates in the dermis, without evidence of vasculitis.[218] Neurologic symptoms associated with Sneddon's syndrome include headaches, vertigo, TIA, retinal artery occlusion, ischemic stroke, and mental deterioration and vascular dementia, presumably from recurrent stroke.[217] However, the presence of aPLs in individuals with Sneddon's syndrome indicates a worse prognosis.[216] Individuals with Sneddon's syndrome are typically younger and have fewer stroke risk factors than most persons with stroke, except that migraine-like headaches and hypertension are common in these individuals. Some individuals with Sneddon's syndrome experience progressive cognitive deterioration leading to dementia, despite having only minor or minimal clinical stroke-like episodes. Such progressive decline can happen even in persons receiving antithrombotic therapy. This clinical course epitomizes the observations of Sneddon[219] and Rebello et al,[220] who emphasized that stroke in affected individuals often leaves little neurologic deficit but the subjects gradually became demented nonetheless. Unfortunately, except for the possible relationship to high aCL levels and the presence of LA and livedo reticularis, no specific laboratory or clinical finding predicts who will likely develop Sneddon's. Many individuals with Sneddon's syndrome eventually experience complex partial seizures.

What sets Sneddon's apart from other forms of aPL syndromes is not understood. It has been hypothesized that endothelial dysfunction and cell detachment with perivascular inflammation in small arterioles are the initiating events, which are followed by occlusion of the vascular lumen by mononuclear cells, erythrocytes, and fibrin, which leads to a cellular and fibrotic plug. It has yet to be determined whether the vascular occlusive events of Sneddon's syndrome reflect primary endothelial cell dysfunction or an unusual arteriosclerotic-like condition of young adults or result from recurrent thrombotic events in the setting of a hypercoagulable state or possibly from a combination of these conditions.[216]

Homocystinuria and Homocystinemia

The 20-fold or higher increases in plasma homocysteine, homocystine, cysteine–homocysteine, and related mixed disulfides (together termed *homocyst(e)ine* [Hcy]) that typify homocystinuria produce premature atherosclerosis that is frequently complicated by early stroke or other large arterial occlusions.[221] Homocystinuria is a metabolic consequence of one of several inborn errors of metabolism that impair cystathionine β-synthase (CBS) and several other enzyme systems important for methionine metabolism (Fig. 41-2). These are autosomal recessive traits, and persons homozygous for CBS deficiency often develop premature atherosclerosis and thromboembolic complications, including stroke, by age 30 years.[222] The classic phenotype of homocystinuria includes ocular, vascular, skeletal, and nervous system abnormalities. Affected individuals may have a marfanoid habitus, with arm spans greater than body height, setting-sun lenticular

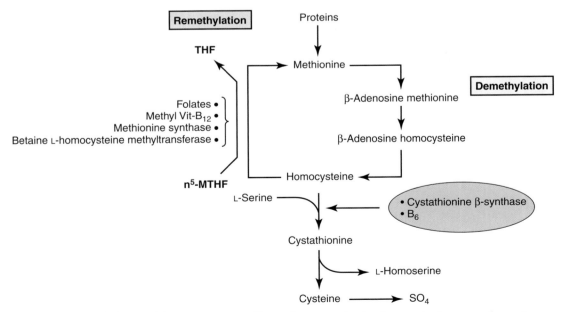

Figure 41-2 Methionine metabolism and homocysteinemia. Plasma homocysteine levels may rise because of genetic or acquired metabolic deficiencies in pathways of methionine metabolism. The principal causes are dysfunction of the cystathionine β-synthase enzyme system for cysteine metabolism and dysfunction of remethylation of the tetrahydrofolate (THF) pathway, and these may occur with folate or vitamin B_{12} deficiencies. See text for details. B_6, vitamin B_6; B_{12}, vitamin B_{12}; n^5-MTHF, methyltetrahydrofolate.

dislocations, and cognitive impairment. A malar flush and livedo reticularis are sometimes present, but the phenotypic expression varies considerably; some individuals with homocystinuria exhibit none of these characteristics. About 0.3% to 1.5% of the general population may be heterozygous for CBS deficiency, and the estimated incidence of homocystinuria is approximately 1 in 332,000 live births.[222] In obligate heterozygotes, CBS activity is reduced by 50%, but whether these individuals are at increased risk of stroke is not known.

In contrast to homocystinuria, modest elevations in plasma Hcy levels and related metabolites are now recognized as independent risk factors for ischemic stroke and related forms of atherosclerotic vascular disease.[196,223-228] As many as 30% of subjects with ischemic stroke have plasma levels of Hcy approximately 1.5 times higher than levels measured in healthy individuals of similar age and same sex.[229-231] Elevated plasma Hcy levels are also observed in subjects with silent strokes, white matter hyperintensities, and persons with brain atrophy.[210,232-234] Hcy levels are lower in premenopausal women than in men of similar age, but levels increase with age; after menopause, gender differences disappear altogether. Clarke et al[235] found plasma Hcy levels to be inversely related to red cell folate and serum vitamin B_2 levels, and there is a direct relationship between plasma Hcy levels and decreasing renal function and hyperuricemia. However, the association of high plasma Hcy levels with other stroke risk factors, such as hypertension and diabetes mellitus, is weak, and the current consensus is that an elevated plasma Hcy level is an independent risk factor for stroke.[226,236] Malinow et al[237] found that modest rises in levels of Hcy (>10.5 mmol/L) in asymptomatic adults increased the odds of carotid intimal thickening more than threefold compared with subjects whose plasma Hcy levels were less than 5.88 mmol/L.

Elderly subjects with plasma Hcy levels of 14 to 16 mmol/L have a relative risk of stroke of approximately 2.8 compared with subjects with levels lower than 10 mmol/L. In the Rotterdam study, the risk of stroke and MI rose in direct relationship with the total homocysteine level.[225] The Framingham study also found nonfasting total Hcy levels to be an independent risk factor for incident stroke in the elderly.[210] On the basis of these findings, the attributable risk of stroke due to such modest increases in Hcy could be very significant because of the high prevalence of this mild Hcy elevation.

Dietary folate deficiency raises Hcy levels, and before 1996, almost 90% of Americans did not ingest the minimum 400 μg/day of folate. The U.S. Food and Drug Administration published a regulation that, starting in 1998, all enriched-flour breads, rice, pasta, cornmeal, and other cereal grain products would be required to contain 140 μg of folic acid per 100 g of flour. The goal of this policy was to increase folic acid intake among women of child-bearing potential and reduce the risk of neural tube defects in their children. Since that time, studies evaluating the effect of vitamin supplementation have shown only a modest further reduction in Hcy levels. Thus, the effect of what was once suspected to be a major health problem and potential stroke risk factor may have been lessened by a change in public health policy.[238]

Besides genetic predispositions, many individuals are at risk of hyperhomocysteinemia because of acquired defects in methionine metabolism. As shown in Figure 41-2, decreased CBS activity and reduced remethylation of Hcy may produce hyperhomocysteinemia via abnormalities in folate-, cobalamin-, or betaine-dependent metabolic pathways. Data from case-control studies of healthy subjects as well as subjects with vascular disease indicate that an inverse relationship exists between plasma levels of folate and vitamin B_{12} and plasma concentrations of Hcy.

A mutation in methylenetetrahydrofolate reductase (MTHFR) in the folate pathway has been correlated with an increase in plasma Hcy levels and may possibly be a risk factor for cardiovascular disease.[239] The common thermolabile MTHFR variant results from a C-to-T point mutation at nucleotide C677T (changing alanine to valine), which significantly reduces the enzyme's basal activity.[240] This mutation is prevalent in the population: the frequency of heterozygotes is 40% to 50% and that of homozygotes is 5% to 15% in several populations. The presence of the mutation is associated with elevated plasma Hcy levels and possibly an increase in the rate of MI.[241,242] Studies on the C677T mutation as a risk factor for MIs and other vascular disease have given variable results. Kluijtmans et al[242] reported an odds ratio of 3:1 for premature MI with the C677T mutation in a select group of patients. Gallagher et al[241] also reported a higher risk in both heterozygotes and homozygotes for the C677T mutation. However, other studies have not shown an association between C677T and MI and other vascular diseases.[243] Data are currently lacking for support of this mutation as a risk factor for stroke.

Numerous studies indicate that homocystinemia promotes the development of premature atherosclerosis, and the vascular pathology of large arteries from subjects with homocystinemia demonstrates features typical of atherosclerosis, such as fibrous intimal plaques, medial fibrosis, and disruption of the internal elastic membranes.[244] Accumulation of lipids is less conspicuous in affected arteries, and despite the documentation of premature atherosclerosis, the vascular occlusive events appear to be disproportionate to the severity of arterial disease. Converging lines of evidence from experimental studies have demonstrated that Hcy damages vascular endothelial cells and interferes with the regulatory functions of endothelial cells in coagulation and nitric oxide generation.[245,246]

Probably all young persons with unexplained stroke and especially those with premature atherosclerosis should undergo plasma Hcy measurement.[227] A single plasma determination is probably an effective screen, but some researchers have advocated giving a methionine load beforehand, as doing so might increase the number of subjects testing positive by up to 30%. If an Hcy elevation is detected, first-degree relatives of the patient should also be tested. Because hyperhomocysteinemia is not limited to young people, elderly patients with stroke and TIA due to atherosclerosis should be considered for Hcy testing if an obvious cause for the atherosclerosis is lacking. As indicated in Figure 41-2, when an elevation of Hcy is detected, serum folate and vitamin B_{12} levels should also be measured. Establishing the presence of hyperhomocysteinemia has clinical utility because, even in the absence of low serum folate or B_{12} levels, plasma homocysteine may be lowered with dietary supplements of folic acid, biotin, and vitamins B_{12} and B_6.[227,237]

Sickle Cell Disease

A critical single-point mutation that causes the substitution of valine for glutamic acid in the hemoglobin β chain underlies sickle cell anemia (SSA) and its consequent disease, sickle cell disease (SCD). Biochemically, when exposed to acidotic or hypoxemic environments, the hydrophobic valine residue polymerizes, resulting in a gel that changes red cell morphology.[247] The extremely rigid, sickled erythrocyte produces a tremendous increase in blood viscosity that contributes to red blood cell sludging in the microcirculation during sickle crises. Even in the absence of crisis, SSA can cause a progressive occlusive systemic vasculopathy leading to SCD involving many organs, including the brain. This untoward result happens in approximately 30% of individuals with SSA, which suggests that other factors buffer the effects of the HbSS gene. Individuals with SCD are at increased risk of vascular occlusive events, often recurrent, including catastrophic stroke, as well as infarctions of the kidney, lung, bone, skin, and eye. Symptoms usually begin in early childhood, but occasionally, persons with SSA may live into early or middle adulthood before manifesting adverse effects.

The prevalence of sickle trait (HbSA) in black Americans is estimated at about 8.5%; hemoglobin HbSS occurs in up to 0.16%, and the variant HbSC occurs in 0.21%. SCD occurs in approximately 1 in 500 black births in the United States,[247a] and the incidence of cerebrovascular disease is 10 times greater in blacks with SCD than in those without SCD.[248] Roughly 11% of those with SCD develop clinically overt stroke by age 20,[248-250] which peaks at age 10 but increases to 24% overt stroke by age 45.[251] The highest incidence of stroke occurs between the ages of 2 and 9 years, and a second peak occurs after age 20[251,252]; unfortunately, up to two thirds of individuals with first stroke experience recurrent infarcts.[253] Typically, infarctions include both deep brain and cortical structures, but brainstem, spinal cord, and retinal infarctions as well as dural sinus thrombosis are reported. Pavlakis et al[254] have emphasized the occurrence of watershed or borderzone infarctions, particularly in territories of the middle cerebral artery. They speculate that a combination of occlusive arteriopathy and perfusion failure produces watershed strokes. Silent infarcts (evidence of ischemic injury by imaging in the absence of clinical history of stroke but with possible associated cognitive impairment) are also relatively common and increase with age; their overall incidence is 17% to 22%.[248,249,255,256] Silent infarcts are also a strong independent risk factor for overt stroke in this population. The Cooperative Study of Sickle Cell Disease (CSSCD) found a 14-fold increase in the stroke rate in patients with silent infarction on brain MRI compared with those with normal brain MRI findings.[257]

The susceptibility to ischemic stroke in persons with SCD appears to involve genes outside the beta-globin locus, especially genes that affect immune regulation and inflammation.[249,256] Particular HLA phenotypes of interest include DPB1*0401 (susceptible to stroke) and BPB1*1701 (protective).[256] Transforming growth factor-beta pathway genes, AGT microsatellite alleles, the SELP gene, and SNPs in VCAM-1, IL4R, and ADRB2 are all associated with increased risk of stroke in SCD, but further study is needed.[249,252,258-262] It also appears that excess alpha genes may be a risk factor for stroke in SCD, whereas alpha gene deletion (alpha thalassemia) is protective.[263]

Other risk factors for stroke in patients with SCD are anemia with persistent hemoglobin levels below 7 g/dL, recent or recurrent episodes of chest pain, increased leukocyte count, elevated blood pressure, and the moyamoya phenomenon on brain imaging.[249,253,256,264-266] Parvovirus B19-induced aplasia has also been associated with stroke occurring coincident with the infection, possibly secondary to severely lowered hemoglobin, but the reason for this observation is unclear.[251,267] Chronic hemoglobin desaturation could increase the risk of stroke by perturbing endothelial function and limiting oxygen delivery to the brain. Children with SCD who demonstrate decreased daytime SpO_2 (2% to 3% absolute difference), which declines over time, appear to be at increased risk of stroke.[268] A useful clinical marker is high middle cerebral artery blood flow velocities, as evidenced by transcranial Doppler (TCD) ultrasonography. Abnormal TCD velocities greater than 200 cm/s were identified in 5% to 10% of children with SCD and confer a 10% annual risk for developing primary stroke in children.[269] TCD velocities in adults with SCD are lower than in children but are still elevated compared with adult control subjects.[248,270]

As SCD develops, sickled cells adhere to endothelium, contributing to a cascade of acute inflammatory cells and clotting factors resulting in a nidus for thrombus formation and a relative deficiency of nitric oxide that reduces the compensatory vasodilatation and contributes to endothelial expression of cell adhesion molecules and activation of hemostatic pathways, including activation of platelets.[247,271] There is progressive segmental narrowing of the distal internal carotid artery, portions of the circle of Willis, and proximal branches of the major intracranial arteries. Pathologically, this large vessel arteriopathy demonstrates intimal proliferation and an increase in fibroblasts and smooth muscle cells within the arterial wall. This process is schematized in Figure 41-3. The progressive nature of this occlusive arteriopathy is evidenced by the development of the moyamoya phenomenon in 20% to 40% of individuals who have had an overt stroke. In addition to disease in large arteries, sickled cells can plug the microcirculation and cerebral veins.[252]

Besides brain infarctions, these alterations of arterial, capillary, and venous circulation increase the risk of intracerebral hemorrhage (ICH). Although the prevalence of ischemic stroke outnumbers that of ICH, ICH occurs more often in adults between the ages of 20 and 30 years.[247] ICH in SCD can result either from medial necrosis of cerebral arterioles with subsequent vascular rupture or from venous thrombosis that happens with elevated blood viscosity and sludging. The combination of increased cerebral mean arterial blood flow velocities, increased cerebral blood flow, and intracerebral blood volume, which are only partially explained by the underlying anemia, probably contributes to the predisposition to ICH.[272]

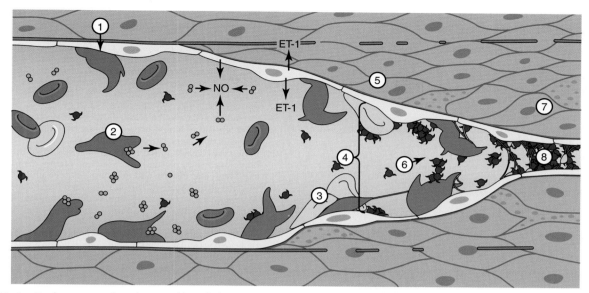

Figure 41-3 Occlusive vasculopathy in sickle cell disease. The sickle erythrocyte adheres to vascular endothelium (1), undergoes hemolysis (2), thereby producing a proinflammatory state with leukocyte adhesion and platelet activation at the vessel wall (3,4,5). These events promote endothelin release and antagonize the effects of nitric oxide (NO) on vascular tone and promote smooth muscle proliferation leading to a progressive occlusive vasculopathy. (Adapted from Switzer JA, Hess DC, Nichols FT, et al: Pathophysiology and treatment of stroke in sickle-cell disease: Present and future. *Lancet Neurol* 5:501-512, 2006.)

Although some asymptomatic persons with SSA may tolerate HbSS of up to 50%, the mainstay of treatment for SCD is repeated exchange transfusion to maintain the concentration of HbSS at less than 30%. Transfusion provides benefit by correcting low oxygen carrying capacity and improving microvascular perfusion by decreasing the proportion of sickled red cells as well as intravascular hemolysis.[273] The Stroke Prevention Trial in Sickle Cell Anemia (STOP) evaluated the role of repeated red cell transfusion in children with increased stroke risk and abnormal TCD and showed a decreased incidence of stroke from 10% per year to less than 1% per year[269,273-275] in children maintained with transfusions. Therefore, children with sickle cell disease should have regular screening TCD and undergo transfusion for confirmed TCD velocities greater than 200 cm/s.[269,275] Pegelow et al[276] also showed that transfusion therapy reduced recurrent silent lesions. Transfusion therapy should be maintained over the long term because discontinuation results in a high rate of reversion to abnormal blood flow velocities on TCD and stroke.[273,274] However, the optimal duration of therapy remains undefined. Scothorn et al[277] report that, in the 2-year period after an initial stroke, patients with SCD are particularly vulnerable to development of a second stroke but that, after 2 years, those with an antecedent or concurrent medical event at the time of initial stroke have a much lower recurrent stroke risk.

Hematopoietic stem-cell transplantation (HSCT) is the only curative treatment available for SCD and might be more effective than transfusion, specifically for prevention of cerebrovascular disease, but its use has been limited by transplant-related morbidity and mortality. The timing of bone marrow transplantation is controversial. One would like to perform HSCT before end-stage organ damage occurs yet limit this therapy to patients destined to experience these complications. Therefore, it is generally reserved for those with severe disease, even though those with less severe disease have better outcomes.[278]

Hydroxyurea has decreased the incidence of sickle cell crisis in adults and children with severe disease by increasing hematocrit, inhibiting erythrocyte sickling by increasing HbF, reducing red cell adhesion, and decreasing lactate dehydrogenase and total bilirubin concentrations.[279] It has been shown to provide similar protection as compared with long-term transfusion for decreased TCD velocity and stroke, but the long-term side effects are not known.[250,279] Inhaled nitric oxide and sodium nitrate have also been proposed as potential treatments for SCD because they increase vasodilatation; however, further investigations are needed.[271]

Screening of Patients with Stroke for Coagulopathies

Besides the usual routine clinical tests for coagulation, the majority of individuals with stroke and TIA do not require an extensive evaluation to look for abnormalities in the hemostatic system or to diagnose a hypercoagulable state.[280,281] The yield of screening is likely to be highest in those who are young, in those with repeated unexplained strokes, and in those with a prior history of thrombosis (particularly venous thrombosis). Patients with unexplained cerebral venous thrombosis (i.e., cortical vein or sagittal sinus thrombosis) should be investigated for hypercoagulable conditions, especially APC resistance. Patients with livedo reticularis and left heart valvular abnormalities and women with a history of spontaneous abortion should be screened for aPL antibodies. Hemoglobin electrophoresis should be considered in young black patients. A suggested approach is summarized in Tables 41-2 and 41-3.

TABLE 41-3 LABORATORY SCREENING TESTS FOR COAGULOPATHIES IN SELECTED PATIENTS

Protein C, protein S, and antithrombin III measurements by functional assay

Free protein S antigen measurement

Anticardiolipin antibody assay by enzyme-linked immunosorbent assay (ELISA)

Functional assay for lupus anticoagulant

Hemoglobin electrophoresis (especially in black people)

Homocyst(e)ine measurement

Lipoprotein(a) measurement

Either factor V Leiden by polymerase chain reaction or functional assay for activated protein C resistance

Thrombin time for dysfibrinogenemia

REFERENCES

1. Levy JH, Dutton RP, Hemphill JC III, et al: Multidisciplinary approach to the challenge of hemostasis, *Anesth Analg* 110: 354-364, 2010.
2. Esmon CT: Molecular events that control the protein C anticoagulant pathway, *Thromb Haemost* 70:29, 1993.
3. Vasse M: Protein Z, a protein seeking a pathology, *Thromb Haemost* 100:548-556, 2008.
4. Bombeli T, Meuller M, Haeberli A: Anticoagulant properties of the vascular endothelium, *Thromb Haemost* 77:408, 1997.
5. Wu KK, Thiagarajan P: Role of endothelium in thrombosis and hemostasis, *Annu Rev Med* 47:315, 1996.
6. Félétou M, Vanhoutte PM: Endothelial dysfunction: A multifaceted disorder (The Wiggers Award Lecture), *Am J Physiol Heart Circ Physiol* 291:H985-H1002, 2006.
7. Galley HF, Webster NR: Physiology of the endothelium, *Br J Anaesth* 93:105-113, 2004.
8. Breitenstein A, Tanner FC, Lüscher TF: Tissue factor and cardiovascular disease: Quo vadis? *Circ J* 74:3-12, 2010.
9. Jennings LK: Mechanisms of platelet activation: need for new strategies to protect against platelet-mediated atherothrombosis, *Thromb Haemost* 102:248-257, 2009.
10. Boffa MC: Thrombomodulin in human brain microvasculature [letter], *Lupus* 4:165, 1995.
11. Tran ND, Wong VL, Schreiber SS, et al: Regulation of brain capillary endothelial thrombomodulin mRNA expression, *Stroke* 27:2304, 1996.
12. Kwaan HC, Samama MM: The significance of endothelial heterogeneity in thrombosis and hemostasis, *Semin Thromb Hemost* 36:286-300, 2010.
13. Kenet G, Lütkhoff LK, Albisetti M, et al: Impact of thrombophilia on risk of arterial ischemic stroke or cerebral sinovenous thrombosis in neonates and children: A systematic review and meta-analysis of observational studies, *Circulation* 121:1838-1847, 2010.
14. Folsom AR, Ohira T, Yamagishi K, et al: Low protein C and incidence of ischemic stroke and coronary heart disease: The Atherosclerosis Risk in Communities (ARIC) Study, *J Thromb Haemost* 7:1774-1778, 2009.
15. Laugesaar R, Kahre T, Kolk A, et al: Factor V Leiden and prothrombin 20210G>A [corrected] mutation and paediatric ischaemic stroke: A case-control study and two meta-analyses.[Erratum appears in Acta Paediatr 2010 Jul;99(7):1112], *Acta Paediatr* 99:1168-1174, 2010.
16. Press RD, Liu XY, Beamer N, et al: Ischemic stroke in the elderly—role of the common factor V mutation causing resistance to activated protein C, *Stroke* 27:44, 1996.
17. Bentley P, Peck G, Smeeth L, et al: Causal relationship of susceptibility genes to ischemic stroke: Comparison to ischemic heart disease and biochemical determinants, *PLoS ONE* 5(2):e9136, 2010.
18. Staton J, Sayer M, Hankey GJ, et al: Protein Z gene polymorphisms, protein Z concentrations, and ischemic stroke, *Stroke* 36:1123-1127, 2005.
19. Herak DC, Antolic MR, Krleza JL, et al: Inherited prothrombotic risk factors in children with stroke, transient ischemic attack, or migraine, *Pediatrics* 123:e653-e660, 2009.
20. Ridker PM, Vaughan DE, Stampfer MJ, et al: Endogenous tissue-type plasminogen activator and risk of myocardial infarction, *Lancet* 341:1165, 1993.
21. Moskau S, Smolka K, Semmler A, et al: Common genetic coagulation variants are not associated with ischemic stroke in a case-control study, *Neurol Res* 32:519-522, 2010.
22. Szolnoki Z, Somogyvari F, Kondacs A, et al: Evaluation of the roles of the Leiden V mutation and ACE I/D polymorphism in subtypes of ischemic stroke, *J Neurol* 248:756, 2001.
23. Hamedani AG, Cole JW, Mitchell BD, et al: Meta-analysis of factor V Leiden and ischemic stroke in young adults: The importance of case ascertainment, *Stroke* 41:1599-1603, 2010.
24. Reiner AP, Carty CL, Jenny NS, et al: PROC, PROCR and PROS1 polymorphisms, plasma anticoagulant phenotypes, and risk of cardiovascular disease and mortality in older adults: The Cardiovascular Health Study, *J Thromb Haemost* 6:1625-1632, 2008.
25. de Moerloose P, Boehlen F: Inherited thrombophilia in arterial disease: A selective review, *Semin Hematol* 44:106-113, 2007.
26. Pelkonen KM, Wartiovaara-Kautto U, Nieminen MS, et al: Low normal level of protein C or of antithrombin increases risk for recurrent cardiovascular events, *Blood Coagul Fibrinolysis* 16:275-280, 2005.
27. Wieberdink RG, van Schie MC, Koudstaal PJ, et al: High von Willebrand factor levels increase the risk of stroke: The Rotterdam study, *Stroke* 41:2151-2156, 2010.
28. Bongers TN, de Maat MPM, vaan Goor M-LPJ, et al: High von Willebrand factor levels increase the risk of first ischemic stroke. Influence of ADAMTS13, inflammation, and genetic variability, *Stroke* 37:2672-2677, 2006.
29. Lip GY, Lane D, Van Walraven C, et al: Additive role of plasma von Willebrand factor levels to clinical factors for risk stratification of patients with atrial fibrillation. [Erratum appears in Stroke 37:2444, 2006], *Stroke* 37:2294-2300, 2006.
30. Mayer SA, Sacco RL, Hurlet-Jensen A, et al: Free protein S deficiency in acute ischemic stroke: A case-control study, *Stroke* 24:224, 1993.
31. Poort SR, Rosendaal FR, Reitsma PH, et al: A common genetic variation in the 3′-untranslated region of the prothrombin gene is associated with elevated plasma prothrombin levels and an increase in venous thrombosis, *Blood* 88:3698, 1996.
32. Tripodi A, Mannucci PM: Laboratory investigation of thrombophilia, *Clin Chem* 47:1597, 2001.
33. De Moerloose P, Reber G, Bouviar CA: Spuriously low levels of protein C with Protac activation clotting assay [letter], *Thromb Haemost* 59:543, 1988.
34. Faioni EM, Franchi F, Asti D, et al: Resistance to activated protein C mimicking dysfunctional protein C: Diagnostic approach, *Blood Coagul Fibrinolysis* 7:349, 1996.
35. Jorquera JI, Montoro JM, Fernandez MA, et al: Modified test for activated protein C resistance [letter], *Lancet* 344:1162, 1994.
36. Dahlback B: The protein C anticoagulant system: Inherited defects as basis for venous thrombosis, *Thromb Res* 77:1, 1995.
37. Comp PC, Doray D, Patton D, et al: An abnormal distribution of protein S occurs in functional protein S deficiency, *Blood* 67:504, 1986.
38. Simmonds RE, Ireland H, Lane DA, et al: Clarification of the risk for venous thrombosis associated with hereditary protein S deficiency by investigation of a large kindred with a characterized gene defect, *Ann Intern Med* 128:8, 1998.
39. Demers C, Henderson P, Blajchman MA, et al: An antithrombin III assay based on factor Xa inhibition provides a more reliable test to identify congenital antithrombin III deficiency than an assay based on thrombin inhibition, *Thromb Haemost* 69:231, 1993.
40. Leroy-Matheron C, Lamare M, Levent M, et al: Markers of coagulation activation in inherited protein S deficiency, *Thromb Res* 67:607, 1992.
41. Paramo JA: Prothrombin fragments in cardiovascular disease, *Adv Clin Chem* 51:1-23, 2010.
42. Alkjaersig N, Fletcher A: Catabolism and excretion of fibrinopeptide A, *Blood* 60:148, 1982.
43. Nossel H: Relative proteolysis of the fibrinen Bβ chain by thrombin and plasmin as a determinant of thrombosis, *Nature* 291:165, 1981.
44. Owen J, Kvam D, Nossel H, et al: Thrombin and plasmin activity and platelet activation in the development of venous thrombosis, *Blood* 60:476, 1983.
45. Feinberg WM, Bruck DC, Ring ME, et al: Hemostatic markers in acute stroke, *Stroke* 20:592, 1989.

46. Feinberg WM, Erickson LP, Bruck D, et al: Hemostatic markers in acute ischemic stroke: Association with stroke type, severity, and outcome, *Stroke* 27:1296, 1996.

47. Jones SL, Close CF, Mattock MB, et al: Plasma lipid and coagulation factor concentrations in insulin dependent diabetics with microalbuminuria, *BMJ* 298:487, 1989.

48. Takano K, Yamaguchi T, Kato H, et al: Activation of coagulation in acute cardioembolic stroke, *Stroke* 22:12, 1991.

49. Takano K, Yamaguchi T, Uchida K: Markers of a hypercoagulable state following acute ischemic stroke, *Stroke* 23:194, 1992.

50. Tohgi H, Takahahi H, Chiba K, et al: Coagulation-fibrinolysis system in poststroke patients receiving antiplatelet medication, *Stroke* 24:801, 1993.

51. Tohgi H, Kawashima M, Taa K, et al: Coagulation-fibrinolysis abnormalities in acute and chronic phases of cerebral thrombosis and embolism, *Stroke* 21:1663, 1990.

52. Yamazaki M, Uchiyama S, Maruyama S: Alterations of haemostatic markers in various subtypes and phases of stroke, *Blood Coagul Fibrinolysis* 4:707, 1993.

53. Asakura H, Hifumi S, Jokaji H, et al: Prothrombin fragment F 1+2 and thrombin-antithrombin complex are useful markers of the hypercoagulable state in atrial fibrillation, *Blood Coagul Fibrinolysis* 3:469, 1992.

54. Carter AM, Catto AJ, Grant PJ: Association of the alpha-fibrinogen Thr312Ala polymorphism with poststroke mortality in subjects with atrial fibrillation, *Circulation* 9:2423, 1999.

55. Feinberg WM, Bruck DC, Pearce LA: Intravascular coagulation in patients with atrial fibrillation [abstract], *Neurology (NY)* 41:298, 1991.

56. Gustafsson C, Blomback M, Britton M, et al: Coagulation factors and the increased risk of stroke in nonvalvular atrial fibrillation, *Stroke* 21:47, 1990.

57. Kumagai K, Fukunami M, Ohmori M, et al: Increased intravascular clotting in patients with chronic atrial fibrillation, *J Am Coll Cardiol* 16:377, 1990.

58. Clinical and laboratory findings in patients with antiphospholipid antibodies and cerebral ischemia. Antiphospholipid Antibody in Stroke Study Group (APASS), *Stroke* 21:1268, 1990.

59. Feinberg WM, Cornell ES, Nightingale SD, et al: Relationship between prothrombin activation fragment $F_{1.2}$ and international normalized ratio (INR) in patients with atrial fibrillation, *Stroke* 28:1101, 1997.

60. Kistler JP, Singer DE, Millenson MM, et al: Effect of low-intensity warfarin anticoagulation on level of activity of the hemostatic system in patients with atrial fibrillation, *Stroke* 24:1360, 1993.

61. Lip GYH, Lip PL, Zarafis J, et al: Fibrin D-dimer and β-thromboglobulin as markers of thrombogenesis and platelet activation in atrial fibrillation: Effects of introducing ultra-low-dose warfarin and aspirin, *Circulation* 94:425, 1996.

62. Lip GY: Fibrinogen and cardiovascular disorders, *Q J Med* 88:155, 1995.

63. Smith FB, Lee AJ, Fowkes FGR, et al: Hemostatic factors as predictors of ischemic heart disease and stroke in the Edinburgh artery study, *Arterioscler Thromb Vasc Biol* 17:3321, 1997.

64. Di Napoli M, Papa F: for the Villa Pini Stroke Data Bank Investigators: Inflammation, hemostatic markers, and antithrombotic agents in relation to long-term risk of new cardiovascular events in first-ever ischemic stroke patients, *Stroke* 33:1763, 2002.

65. Cook NS, Ubben D: Fibrinogen as a major risk factor in cardiovascular disease, *Trends Pharmacol Sci* 11:444, 1990.

66. Ernst E, Resch KL: Fibrinogen as a cardiovascular risk factor: A meta-analysis and review of the literature, *Ann Intern Med* 118:956, 1993.

67. Kannel WB, Wolf PA, Castelli WP, et al: Fibrinogen and risk of cardiovascular disease: The Framingham study, *JAMA* 258:1183, 1987.

68. Lowe GD, Lee AJ, Rumley A, et al: Blood viscosity and risk of cardiovascular events: The Edinburgh Artery Study, *Br J Haematol* 96:168, 1997.

69. Qizilbash N: Fibrinogen and cerebrovascular disease, *Eur Heart J* 16(Suppl A):42, 1995.

70. Wilhelmsen L, Svardsudd K, Korsan-Bengtsen K: Fibrinogen as a risk factor for stroke and myocardial infarction, *N Engl J Med* 311:50, 1984.

71. Yarnell JWG, Baker IA, Sweetnam PM, et al: Fibrinogen, viscosity, and white blood cell count are major risk factors for ischemic heart disease, *Circulation* 83:836, 1991.

72. Coull B, Beamer N, de Garmo P, et al: Chronic blood hyperviscosity in subjects with acute stroke, transient ischemic attack, and risk factors for stroke, *Stroke* 22:162, 1991.

73. Resch KL, Ernst E, Matrai A, et al: Fibrinogen and viscosity as risk factors for subsequent cardiovascular events in stroke survivors, *Ann Intern Med* 117:371, 1992.

74. Ameriso SF, Wong VLY, Quismorio FP, et al: Immunohematologic characteristics of infection-associated cerebral infarction, *Stroke* 22:1004, 1991.

75. Ernst E: Fibrinogen as a cardiovascular risk factor: Interrelationship with infections and inflammation, *Eur Heart J* 14(Suppl K):82, 1993.

76. Cahill M, Mistry R, Barnett DB: The human platelet fibrinogen receptor: clinical and therapeutic significance, *Br J Clin Pharmacol* 33:3, 1992.

77. Juhan-Vague I, Valdier J, Alessi M, et al: Deficient t-PA release and elevated PA inhibitor levels in patients with spontaneous or recurrent deep venous thrombosis, *Thromb Haemost* 57:67, 1987.

78. Berdeaux D, Marlar R: Report of an American family with elevated PAI-1 as a cause of multiple thromboses responsive to prednisone [abstract], *Thromb Haemost* 65:1044, 1991.

79. Dolan G, Greaves M, Cooper P, et al: Thrombovascular disease and familial plasminogen deficiency: A report of three kindred, *Br J Haematol* 70:417, 1988.

80. Francis R: Clinical disorders of fibrinolysis: A critical review, *Blut* 59:1, 1989.

81. Furlan A, Lucas F, Craciun R, et al: Stroke in a young adult with familial plasminogen disorder, *Stroke* 22:1598, 1991.

82. Hart RG, Kanter MC: Hematologic disorders and ischemic stroke: A selective review, *Stroke* 21:1111, 1990.

83. Jorgenson M, Bonnevie-Nielsen V: Increased concentration of the fast-acting plasminogen activator inhibitor in plasma associated with familial venous thrombosis, *Br J Haematol* 65:175, 1987.

84. Nagayama T, Shinohara Y, Nagayama M, et al: Congenitally abnormal plasminogen in juvenile ischemic cerebrovascular disease, *Stroke* 24:2104, 1993.

85. Feinberg WM, Bruck DC: Time course of platelet activation following acute ischemic stroke, *J Stroke Cerebrovasc Dis* 1:124, 1991.

86. Fisher M, Francis R: Altered coagulation in cerebral ischemia: Platelet, thrombin, and plasmin activity, *Arch Neurol* 47:1075, 1990.

87. Glueck C, Rorick M, Scherler M, et al: Hypofibrinolytic and atherogenic risk factors for stroke, *J Lab Clin Med* 125:319, 1995.

88. Kempter B, Peinemann A, Biniasch O, et al: Decreased fibrinolytic stimulation by short-term venous occlusion test in patients with cerebrovascular disease, *Thromb Res* 79:363, 1995.

89. Brockman MJ, Schwendemann G, Stief TW: Plasminogen activator inhibitor in acute stroke, *Mol Chem Neuropathol* 14:143, 1991.

90. Lindgren A, Lindoff C, Norrving B, et al: Tissue plasminogen activator and plasminogen activator inhibitor-1 in stroke patients, *Stroke* 27:1066, 1996.

91. Margaglione M, Di Minno G, Grandone E, et al: Abnormally high circulation levels of tissue plasminogen activator and plasminogen activator inhibitor-1 in patients with a history of ischemic stroke, *Arterioscler Thromb Vasc Biol* 14:1741, 1994.

92. de Bono D: Significance of raised plasma concentrations of tissue-type plasminogen activator and plasminogen activator inhibitor in patients at risk from ischaemic heart disease, *Br Heart J* 71:504, 1994.

93. Ridker PM: Plasma concentration of endogenous tissue plasminogen activator and the occurrence of future cardiovascular events, *J Thromb Thrombolysis* 1:35, 1994.

94. Salomaa V, Stinson V, Kark JD, et al: Association of fibrinolytic parameters with early atherosclerosis: The ARIC Study. Atherosclerosis Risk in Communities Study, *Circulation* 91:284, 1995.

95. Oates JA, FitzGerald GA, Branch RA, et al: Clinical implications of prostaglandin and thromboxane A_2 formation, *N Engl J Med* 319:689, 1988.

96. Scott J: Lipoprotein (a): Thrombogenesis linked to atherosclerosis at last? *Nature* 341:22, 1989.

97. McLean JW, Tomlinson JE, Kuang WJ, et al: cDNA sequence of human apolipoprotein (a) is homologous to plasminogen, *Nature* 330:132, 1987.

98. Etingin OR, Hajjar DP, Hajjar KA, et al: Lipoprotein (a) regulates plasminogen activator inhibitor-1 expression in endothelial cells: A potential mechanism in thrombogenesis, *J Biol Chem* 266:2459, 1991.

99. Hajjar KA, Gavish D, Breslow JL, et al: Lipoprotein (a) modulation of endothelial cell surface fibrinolysis and its potential role in atherosclerosis, *Nature* 339:303, 1989.

100. Franceschini G, Cofrancesco E, Safa O, et al: Association of lipoprotein (a) with atherothrombotic events and fibrinolytic variables: A case-control study, *Thromb Res* 78:227, 1995.

101. Jürgens F, Költringer P: Lipoprotein (a) in ischemic cerebrovascular disease: A new approach to the assessment of stroke, *Neurology (NY)* 37:513, 1987.

102. Lassila R, Manninen V: Hypofibrinolysis and increased lipoprotein (a) coincide in stroke, *J Lab Clin Med* 125:301, 1995.

103. Schreiner PJ, Chambless LE, Brown SA, et al: Lipoprotein (a) as a correlate of stroke and transient ischemic attack prevalence in a biracial cohort: The ARIC study, *Ann Epidemiol* 4:351, 1994.

104. Shintani S, Kikuchi S, Hamaguchi H, et al: High serum lipoprotein (a) is an independent risk factor for cerebral infarction, *Stroke* 24:965, 1993.

105. Zenker G, Költringer P, Boné G, et al: Lipoprotein (a) as a strong indicator for cerebrovascular disease, *Stroke* 17:942, 1986.

106. Del Zoppo GL: The role of platelets in ischemic stroke, *Neurology* 51(Suppl 3):S9, 1998.

107. Hennerici MG: The unstable plaque, *Cerebrovascular Diseases* 17(Suppl 3):17, 2004.

108. Fitzgerald DJ: Vascular biology of thrombosis, *Neurology* 57(Suppl 2):S1, 2001.

109. Fisher M, Levine PH, Fullerton A, et al: Marker proteins of platelet activation in patients with cerebrovascular disease, *Stroke* 39:692, 1982.

110. Shah AB, Beamer N, Coull BM: Enhanced in vivo platelet activation in subtypes of ischemic stroke, *Stroke* 16:643, 1985.

111. Taomoto K, Asada M, Kanazaua Y, et al: Usefulness of the measurement of plasma-thromboglobulin (beta-TG) in cerebrovascular disease, *Stroke* 14:518, 1983.

112. Koudstall P, Ciabattoni G, van Gijn J, et al: Increased thromboxane biosynthesis in patients with acute cerebral ischemia, *Stroke* 24:219, 1993.

113. Van Kooten F, Ciabattoni G, Patrono C, et al: Evidence for episodic platelet activation in acute ischemic stroke, *Stroke* 25:278, 1994.

114. Del Zoppo GL, Copeland BR, Harker LA, et al: Experimental acute thrombotic stroke in baboons, *Stroke* 17:1254, 1986.

115. Arboix A, Besses C, Acin P, et al: Ischemic stroke as first manifestation of essential thrombocythemia: Report of six cases, *Stroke* 26:1463, 1995.

116. Jabaily J, Iland HJ, Laszlo J, et al: Neurologic manifestations of essential thrombocythemia, *Ann Intern Med* 99:513, 1983.

117. Alvarez-Larran A, Cervantes F, Bellosillo B, et al: Essential thrombocythemia in young individuals: Frequency and risk factors for vascular events and evolution to myelofibrosis in 126 patients, *Leukemia* 21:1218, 2007.

118. De Stefano V, Za T, Rossi E, et al: Recurrent thrombosis in patients with polycythemia vera and essential thrombocythemia: Incidence, risk factors, and effect of treatments, *Haematologica* 93:372, 2008.

119. Johnson M, Gernsheimer T, Johansen K: Essential thrombocytosis: Underemphasized cause of large-vessel thrombosis, *J Vasc Surg* 22:443, 1995.

120. Murphy S, Peterson P, Iland H, et al: Experience of the Polycythemia Vera Study Group with essential thrombocythemia: A final report on diagnostic criteria, survival, and leukemic transition by treatment, *Semin Hematol* 34:29, 1997.

121. Riuniti O, Barbui T, Finazzi G, et al: Polycythemia vera: The natural history of 1213 patients followed for 20 years, *Ann Intern Med* 123:656, 1995.

122. Vadher BD, Machin SJ, Patterson KG, et al: Life-threatening thrombotic and haemorrhagic problems associated with silent myeloproliferative disorders, *Br J Haematol* 85:213, 1993.

123. Williams B, Morton C: Cerebral vascular accident in a patient with reactive thrombocytosis: A rare cause of stroke, *Am J Med Sci* 336:279, 2008.

124. Saxena VK, Brands C, Crols R, et al: Multiple cerebral infarctions in a young patient with secondary thrombocythemia, *Acta Neurol* 15:297, 1993.

125. Albers GW, Amarenco P, Easton JD, et al: American College of Chest Physicians: Antithrombotic and thrombolytic therapy for ischemic stroke: American College of Chest Physicians Evidence-Based Clinical Practice Guidelines (8th Edition), *Chest* 133(Suppl 6):630S, 2008.

126. Hervey PS, Goa KL: Extended-release dipyridamole/aspirin, *Drugs* 58:469, 1999.

127. Quinn MJ, Fitzgerald DJ: Ticlopidine and clopidogrel, *Circulation* 100:1667, 1999.

128. Van Genderen PJJ, Mulder PGH, Waleboer M, et al: Prevention and treatment of thrombotic complications in essential thrombocythaemia: Efficacy and safety of aspirin, *Br J Haematol* 97:179, 1997.

129. Harrisnon CN, Campbell PJ, Buck G, et al: Hydroxyurea compared with anagerlide in high-risk essential thrombocythemia, *N Engl J Med* 353:33, 2005.

130. Becker PS, Miller VT: Heparin-induced thrombocytopenia, *Stroke* 20:1449, 1989.

131. Otis SA: Zehnder JL. Heparin-induced thrombocytopenia: Current status and diagnostic challenges, *Am J Hematol* 85:700–706, 2010.

132. Ansell J, Deykin D: Heparin-induced thrombocytopenia and recurrent thromboembolism, *Am J Hematol* 8:325, 1980.

133. Atkinson JL, Sundt TM Jr, Kazmier FJ, et al: Heparin-induced thrombocytopenia and thrombosis in ischemic stroke, *Mayo Clin Proc* 63:353, 1988.

134. Bell WR: Heparin-associated thrombocytopenia and thrombosis, *J Lab Clin Med* 111:600, 1988.

135. King DJ, Keltron JG: Heparin-associated thrombocytopenia, *Ann Intern Med* 100:535, 1984.

136. Fabris F, Ahmad S, Cella G, et al: Pathophysiology of heparin-induced thrombocytopenia: Clinical and diagnostic implications: A review, *Arch Pathol Lab Med* 124:1657, 2000.

137. Fabris F, Luzzatto G, Stefani PM, et al: Heparin-induced thrombocytopenia, *Haematologica* 85:72, 2000.

138. Warkentin TE, Kelton JG: Heparin and platelets, *Hematol Oncol Clin North Am* 4:243, 1990.

139. Warkentin TE, Levine MN, Hirsh J, et al: Heparin-induced thrombocytopenia in patients treated with low-molecular-weight heparin or unfractionated heparin, *N Engl J Med* 332:1330, 1995.

140. Aster R: Heparin-induced thrombocytopenia: Understanding improves but questions remain, *J Lab Clin Med* 127:418, 1996.

141. Goor Y, Goor O, Eldor A: Heparin-induced thrombocytopenia with thrombotic sequelae: A review, *Autoimmun Rev* 1:183, 2002.

142. Horsewood P, Warkentin TE, Hayward CP, et al: The epitope specificity of heparin-induced thrombocytopenia, *Br J Haematol* 95:161, 1996.

143. Cines DB, Tomasaki A, Tannenbaum S: Immune endothelial cell injury in heparin-associated thrombocytopenia, *N Engl J Med* 316:581, 1987.

144. Walenga JM, Jeske WP, Messmore HS: Mechanisms of venous and arterial thrombosis in heparin-induced thrombocytopenia, *J Thromb Thrombolysis* 10(Suppl):S13, 2000.

145. Kyritsis AP, Williams EC, Schutta HS: Cerebral venous thrombosis due to heparin-induced thrombocytopenia, *Stroke* 21:1503, 1990.

146. Spencer FA: Heparin-induced thrombocytopenia: Patient profiles and clinical manifestations, *J Thromb Thrombolysis* 10(Suppl):S21, 2000.

147. Warkentin TE: Heparin-induced thrombocytopenia: A clinicopathological syndrome, *Thromb Haemost* 82:439, 1999.

148. Wallis DE, Workman DL, Lewis BE, et al: Failure of heparin cessation as treatment for heparin-induced thrombocytopenia, *Am J Med* 106:629, 1999.

149. Greinacher A: Treatment of heparin-induced thrombocytopenia, *Thromb Haemost* 82:457, 1999.

150. Lewis BE, Walenga JM, Wallis DE: Anticoagulation with Novastan (argatroban) in patients with heparin-induced thrombocytopenia, and heparin-induced thrombocytopenia and thrombosis syndrome, *Semin Thromb Hemost* 23:197, 1997.

151. Lubenow N, Greinacher A: Management of patients with heparin-induced thrombocytopenia: Focus on recombinant hirudin, *J Thromb Thrombolysis* 10(Suppl):S47, 2000.

152. Lim W, Crowther MA, Eikelboom JW: Management of antiphospholipid antibody syndrome: A systematic review, *JAMA* 295:1050–1057, 2006.

153. Janardhan V, Wolf PA, Kase CS, et al: Anticardiolipin antibodies and risk of ischemic stroke and transient ischemic attack: The Framingham cohort and offspring study, *Stroke* 35:736–741, 2004.

154. Lim W, Crowther MA: Antiphospholipid antibodies: A critical review of the literature, *Curr Opin Hematol* 14:494–499, 2007.

155. Arnout J, Vermylen J: Lupus anticoagulants: Mechanistic and diagnostic considerations. In Khamashta MA, editor: *Hughes syndrome: Antiphospholipid syndrome*, London, 2000, Springer-Verlag, p 225.

156. Bowie WEJ, Thompson JH, Pasacuzzi CA, et al: Thrombosis in systemic lupus erythematosus despite circulating anticoagulants, *J Clin Invest* 62:416, 1963.

157. Feinstein DI, Rapaport SI: Acquired inhibitors of blood coagulation, *Prog Hemost Thromb* 1:75, 1972.

158. Harris EN, Boey ML, Mackworth-Young CG, et al: Anticardiolipin antibodies: Detection by radioimmunoassay and association with thrombosis in systemic lupus erythematosus, *Lancet* 2:1211, 1983.

159. Caso V, Parnetti L, Panarelli P, et al: Selection of thrombogenetic antiphospholipid antibodies in cerebrovascular disease patients, *J Neurol* 250:593-597, 2003.

160. Galli M, Luciani D, Bertolini G, et al: Lupus anticoagulants are stronger risk factors for thrombosis than anticardiolipin antibodies in the antiphospholipid syndrome: A systematic review of the literature, *Blood* 101:1827-1832, 2003.

161. Ruiz-Irastorza G, Hunt BJ, Khamashta MA: A systematic review of secondary thromboprophylaxis in patients with antiphospholipid antibodies, *Arthritis Rheum* 57:1487-1495, 2007.

162. Levine SR, Brey RL, Tilley BC, et al: Antiphospholipid antibodies and subsequent thrombo-occlusive events in patients with ischemic stroke, *JAMA* 35:736-741, 2004.

163. Gonzales-Portillo F, McIntyre JA, Wagenknecht DR, et al: Spectrum of antiphospholipid antibodies (aPL) in patients with cerebrovascular disease, *J Stroke Cerebrovasc Dis* 10:222-226, 2001.

164. Okuma H, Kitagawa Y, Takagi S, et al: Prevalence rates of antiphospholipid antibodies in ischemic stroke patients, *Intern Med* 45:1017-1018, 2006.

165. Nojima J, Kuratsune H, Suehisa E, et al: Strong correlation between the prevalence of cerebral infarction and the presence of anti-cardiolipin/beta2-glycoprotein I and antiphosphatidylserine/prothrombin antibodies: Co-existence of these antibodies enhances ADP-induced platelet activation in vitro, *Thromb Haemost* 91:967-976, 2004.

166. Brey RL: Antiphospholipid antibodies in young adults with stroke, *J Thromb Thrombolysis* 20:105-112, 2005.

167. Miyakis S, Lockshin MD, Atsumi T, et al: International consensus statement on an update of the classification criteria for definite antiphospholipid syndrome (APS), *J Thromb Haemost* 4: 295-306, 2006.

168. Ali HY, Abdullah ZA: Anti-beta(2)-glycoprotein I autoantibody expression as a potential biomarker for strokes in patients with anti-phospholipid syndrome, *J Immunotoxicol* 5:173-177, 2008.

169. Suvajac G, Stojanovich L, Milenkovich S: Ocular manifestations in antiphospholipid syndrome, *Autoimmun Rev* 6:409-414, 2007.

170. Espinosa G, Cervera R, Font J, et al: Adrenal involvement in the antiphospholipid syndrome, *Lupus* 12:569-572, 2003.

171. Arnson Y, Shoenfeld Y, Alon E, et al: The antiphospholipid syndrome as a neurological disease, *Semin Arthritis Rheum* 40: 97-108, 2010.

172. Cavera R, Piette J-C, Font J, et al: Antiphospholipid syndrome. Clinical and immunologic manifestations and patterns of disease expression in a cohort of 1000 patients, *Arthritis Rheum* 46:1019-1027, 2002.

173. Turiel M, Sarzi-Puttini P, Peretti R, et al: Thrombotic risk factors in primary antiphospholipid syndrome: A 5-year prospective study, *Stroke* 36:1490-1494, 2005.

174. Horbach DA, Oort EV, Donders RC, et al: Lupus anticoagulant is the strongest risk factor for both venous and arterial thrombosis in patients with systemic lupus erythematosus: Comparison between different assays for the detection of antiphospholipid antibodies, *Thromb Haemost* 76:916, 1996.

175. Goldstein R, Moulds JM, Smith CD, et al: MHC studies of the primary antiphospholipid antibody syndrome and of antiphospholipid antibodies in systemic lupus erythematosus, *J Rheum* 23:1173, 1996.

176. Finazzi G, Brancaccio V, Moia M, et al: Natural history and risk factors for thrombosis in 360 patients with antiphospholipid antibodies: A four-year prospective study from the Italian registry, *Am J Med* 100:530, 1996.

177. Antiphospholipid Antibody in Stroke Study (APASS) Group: Anticardiolipin antibodies and the risk of recurrent thromboocclusive events and death, *Neurology* 48:91, 1997.

178. Levine SR, Salowich-Palm L, Sawaya KL, et al: IgG anticardiolipin antibody titer > 40 GPL and the risk of subsequent thromboocclusive events and death: A prospective cohort study, *Stroke* 28:1660, 1997.

179. Ruiz Irastorza G, Khamashta MA, Hunt BJ, et al: Bleeding and recurrent thrombosis in definite antiphospholipid syndrome: Analysis of a series of 66 patients treated with oral anticoagulation to a target international normalized ratio of 3.5, *Arch Intern Med* 162:1164, 2002.

180. Verro P, Levine SR, Tietjen GE: Cerebrovascular ischemic events with high positive anticardiolipin antibodies, *Stroke* 29:2245, 1998.

181. Crowther MA, Ginsberg JS, Julian J, et al: A comparison of two intensities of warfarin for the prevention of recurrent thrombosis in patients with the antiphospholipid antibody syndrome, *N Engl J Med* 349:1133-1138, 2003.

182. Brey RL: Management of the neurological manifestations of APS—what do the trials tell us? *Thromb Res* 114:489-499, 2004.

183. van Goor MP, Alblas CL, Leebeek FW, et al: Do antiphospholipid antibodies increase the long-term risk of thrombotic complications in young patients with a recent TIA or ischemic stroke?, *Acta Neurol Scand* 109:410-415, 2004.

184. Locht H, Wiik A: IgG and IgM isotypes of anti-cardiolipin and anti-beta2-glycoprotein I antibodies reflect different forms of recent thrombo-embolic events, *Clin Rheumatol* 25:246-250, 2006.

185. Brey RL, Abbott RD, Sharp DS, et al: Beta-2-glycoprotein 1dependent (B2GP1-dep) anticardiolipin antibodies are an independent risk factor for ischemic stroke in the Honolulu Heart Cohort, *Stroke* 32:1701-1706, 2001.

186. Brey RL, Stallworth CL, McGlasson DL, et al: Antiphospholipid antibodies and stroke in young women, *Stroke* 33:2396, 2002.

187. Nagaraja D, Christopher R, Manjari T: Anticardiolipin antibodies in ischemic stroke in the young: Indian experience, *J Neurol Sci* 150:137, 1997.

188. Tuhrim S, Rand JH, Wu X, et al: Antiphosphatidylserine antibodies are independently associated with ischemic stroke, *Neurology* 53:1523-1527, 1999.

189. Tuhrim S, Rand JH, Wu XX, et al: Elevated anticardiolipin antibody titer is an independent risk factor for stroke in a multiethnic population independent of isotype or degree of positivity, *Stroke* 30:1561-1565, 1999.

190. Toschi V, Motta A, et al: High prevalence of antiphosphatidylinositol antibodies in young patients with cerebral ischemia of undetermined cause, *Stroke* 29:1759-1764, 1998.

191. Zielinska J, Rygiewicz D, Wierzchowska E, et al: Anticardiolipin antibodies are an independent risk factor for ischemic stroke, *Neurol Res* 21:653-657, 1999.

192. Metz LM, Edworthy S, Mydlarski R, et al: The frequency of phospholipid antibodies in an unselected stroke population, *Can J Neurol Sci* 25:64, 1998.

193. Tanne D, D'Olhaberriague L, Schultz LR, et al: Anticardiolipin antibodies and their associations with cerebrovascular risk factors, *Neurology* 52:1368-1373, 1999.

194. Ahmed E, Stegmayr B, Trifunovic J, et al: Anticardiolipin antibodies are not an independent risk factor for stroke. An incident case-referent study nested within the MONICA and Vasterbotten cohort project, *Stroke* 31:1289-1293, 2000.

195. Blohorn A, Guegan-Massardier E, Triquenot Y, et al: Antiphospholipid antibodies in the acute phase of cerebral ischemia in young adults: A descriptive study of 139 patients, *Cerebrovasc Dis* 13:156-162, 2002.

196. Ridker PM, Manson JE, Buring JE, et al: Homocysteine and risk of cardiovascular disease among postmenopausal women, *JAMA* 281:1817, 1999.

197. Wu R, Nityanand S, Berglund L, et al: Antibodies against cardiolipin and oxidatively modified LDL in 50-year-old men predict myocardial infarction, *Arterioscler Thromb Vasc Biol* 17:3159, 1997.

198. Turiel M, Muzzupappa S, Gottardi B, et al: Evaluation of cardiac abnormalities and embolic sources in primary antiphospholipid syndrome by transesophageal echocardiography, *Lupus* 9: 406-412, 2000.

199. Rademacher J, Sohngen D, Specker C, et al: Cerebral microembolism: A disease marker for ischemic cerebrovascular events in the antiphospholipid syndrome of systemic lupus erythematosus? *Acta Neurol Scand* 99:356, 1999.

200. Chen WH, Kao YF, Lan MY, et al: The increase of blood anticardiolipin antibody depends on the underlying etiology in cerebral ischemia, *Clin Appl Thromb Hemost* 12:69-76, 2006.
201. Shoenfeld Y, Ziporen L: Lessons from experimental APS models, *Lupus* 7(Suppl 2):S158, 1998.
202. Katzav A, Shoenfeld Y, Chapman J: The pathogenesis of neural injury in animal models of the antiphospholipid syndrome, *Clin Rev Allergy Immunol* 38:196-200, 2010.
203. Lanir N, Zilberman M, Yron I, et al: Reactivity patterns of antiphospholipid antibodies and endothelial cells: Effect of antiendothelial antibodies on cell migration, *J Lab Clin Med* 131:548, 1998.
204. Kaplanski G, Cacoub P, Farnarier C, et al: Increased soluble vascular cell adhesion molecule 1 concentrations in patients with primary or systemic lupus erythematosus-related antiphospholipid syndrome: Correlations with the severity of thrombosis, *Arthritis Rheum* 43:55, 2000.
205. Hilker R, Thiel A, Geisen C, et al: Cerebral blood flow and glucose metabolism in multi-infarct dementia related to primary antiphospholipid antibody syndrome, *Lupus* 9:311, 2000.
206. Kao CH, Lan JL, Hsieh JF, et al: Evaluation of regional cerebral blood flow with ^{99m}Tc-HMPAO in primary antiphospholipid antibody syndrome, *J Nucl Med* 40:1446, 1999.
207. Sabet A, Sibbitt WL, Stidley CA, et al: Neurometabolite markers of cerebral injury in the antiphospholipid antibody syndrome of systemic lupus erythematosus, *Stroke* 29:2254, 1998.
208. Nowacki P, Ronin-Walknowska E, Ossowicka-Stepinska J: Central nervous system involvement in pregnant rabbits with experimental model of antiphospholipid syndrome, *Folia Neuropathol* 36:38, 1998.
209. Garcia CO, Kanbour-Shakir A, Tang H, et al: Induction of experimental antiphospholipid syndrome in PL/J mice following immunization with beta 2 GPI, *Am J Reprod Immunol* 37:118, 1997.
210. Bostom AG, Selhub J, Jacques PF, et al: Power shortage: Clinical trials testing the "homocysteine hypothesis" against a background of folic acid-fortified cereal grain flour, *Ann Intern Med* 135:133, 2001.
211. Khamashta MA, Cuadrado MJ, Mujic F, et al: The management of thrombosis in the antiphospholipid-antibody syndrome, *N Engl J Med* 332:993, 1995.
212. Julkunen H, Hedman C, Kauppi M: Thrombolysis for acute ischemic stroke in the primary antiphospholipid syndrome, *J Rheumatol* 24:181, 1997.
213. Bucciarelli S, Erkan D, Espinosa G, et al: Catastrophic antiphospholipid syndrome: Treatment, prognosis, and the risk of relapse, *Clin Rev Allergy Immunol* 36:80-84, 2009.
214. Uthman I, Shamseddine A, Taher A: The role of therapeutic plasma exchange in the catastrophic antiphospholipid syndrome, *Transfus Apher Sci* 33:11-17, 2005.
215. Ioannou Y, Lambrianides A, Cambridge G, et al: B cell depletion therapy for patients with systemic lupus erythematosus results in a significant drop in anticardiolipin antibody titres, *Ann Rheum Dis* 67:246-425, 2008.
216. Ayoub N, Esposita G, Barete S, et al: Protein Z deficiency in antiphospholipid-negative Sneddon's syndrome, *Stroke* 35:1329-1332, 2004.
217. Boesch SM, Plorer AL, Auer AJ, et al: The natural course of Sneddon syndrome: Clinical and magnetic resonance imaging findings in a prospective six year observation study, *J Neurol Neurosurg Psychiatry* 74:542-544, 2003.
218. Levine SR, Langer SL, Albers JW, et al: Sneddon's syndrome: An antiphospholipid antibody syndrome? *Neurology (NY)* 38:798, 1998.
219. Sneddon IB: Cerebrovascular lesions and livedo reticularis, *Br J Dermatol* 77:180, 1965.
220. Rebello M, Val JF, Garijo F, et al: Livedo reticularis and cerebrovascular lesions (Sneddon's syndrome), *Brain* 106:965, 1983.
221. Skovby F, Gaustadnes M, Mudd SH: A revisit to the natural history of homocystinuria due to cystathionine beta-synthase deficiency, *Mol Genet Metab* 99:1-3, 2010.
222. Testai FD: Gorelick PB: Inherited metabolic disorders and stroke part 2: Homocystinuria, organic acidurias, and urea cycle disorders, *Arch Neurol* 67:148-153, 2010.
223. Graham IM, Daly LE, Refsum HM, et al: Plasma homocysteine as a risk factor for vascular disease, *JAMA* 277:1775, 1997.
224. Bostom AG, Rosenberg IH, Silbershatz H, et al: Nonfasting plasma total homocysteine levels and stroke incidence in elderly persons: The Framingham Study, *Ann Intern Med* 131:352, 1999.
225. Bots ML, Launer LJ, Lindemans J, et al: Homocysteine and short-term risk of myocardial infarction and stroke in the elderly: The Rotterdam Study, *Arch Intern Med* 159:38, 1999.
226. Boushey CJ, Beresford SAA, Omenn GS, et al: A quantitative assessment of plasma homocysteine as a risk factor for vascular disease—probable benefits of increasing folic acid intakes, *JAMA* 274:1049, 1995.
227. Fortin IJ, Genest J Jr: Measurement of homocyst(e)ine in the prediction of atherosclerosis, *Clin Biochem* 28:155, 1995.
228. Hogeveen M, Blom HJ, Van Amerongen M, et al: Hyperhomocysteinemia as a risk factor for ischemic and hemorrhagic stroke in newborn infants, *J Pediatr* 141:429, 2002.
229. Boers GHJ, Smals AGH, Trijbels FJM, et al: Heterozygosity for homocystinuria in premature peripheral and cerebral occlusive arterial disease, *N Engl J Med* 313:709, 1985.
230. Brattstrom LE, Israelsson B, Jeppson J-O, et al: Folic acid: An innocuous means to reduce plasma homocysteine, *Scand J Clin Lab Invest* 48:215, 1988.
231. Coull BM, Malinow MR, Beamer N, et al: Elevated plasma homocyst(e)ine concentration as a possible independent risk factor for stroke, *Stroke* 21:572, 1990.
232. Longstreth WT Jr, Katz R, Olson J, et al: Plasma total homocysteine levels and cranial magnetic resonance imaging findings in elderly persons: The Cardiovascular Health Study, *Arch Neurol* 61:67-72, 2004.
233. Wright CB, Paik MC, Brown TR, et al: Total homocysteine is associated with white matter hyperintensity volume: The Northern Manhattan Study, *Stroke* 36:1207-1211, 2005.
234. Seshadri S, Wolf PA, Beiser AS, et al: Association of plasma total homocysteine levels with subclinical brain injury: Cerebral volumes, white matter hyperintensity, and silent brain infarcts on volumetric magnetic resonance imaging in the Framingham Offspring Study, *Arch Neurol* 65:642-649, 2008.
235. Clarke R, Daly L, Robinson K, et al: Hyperhomocysteinemia: An independent risk factor for vascular disease, *N Engl J Med* 324:1149, 1991.
236. Perry IJ, Refsum H, Morris RW, et al: Prospective study of serum total homocysteine concentration and risk of stroke in middle-aged British men, *Lancet* 346:1395, 1995.
237. Malinow MR, Nieto FJ, Szklo M, et al: Carotid artery intimal-medial wall thickening and plasma homocyst(e)ine in asymptomatic adults: The Atherosclerosis Risk in Communities Study, *Circulation* 87:1107, 1993.
238. Bouillanne O, Millaire A, De Groote P, et al: Prevalence and clinical significance of antiphospholipid antibodies in heart valve disease: A case-control study, *Am Heart J* 132:790, 1996.
239. Kang SS, Passen EL, Ruggie N, et al: Thermolabile defect of methylenetetrahydrofolate reductase in coronary artery disease, *Circulation* 88:1463, 1993.
240. Frost P, Blom HJ, Milos R, et al: A candidate genetic risk factor for vascular disease: A common mutation in methylenetetrahydrofolate reductase [letter], *Nat Genet* 10:111, 1995.
241. Gallagher PM, Meleady R, Shields DC, et al: Homocysteine and risk of premature coronary heart disease: Evidence for a common gene mutation, *Circulation* 94:2154, 1996.
242. Kluijtmans LAJ, Van den Heuvel LPWJ, Boers GHJ, et al: Molecular genetic analysis of mild hyperhomocysteinemia: A common mutation in the methylenetetrahydrofolate reductase gene is a genetic risk factor for cardiovascular disease, *Am J Hum Genet* 58:35, 1996.
243. DeLoughery TG, Evans A, Sadeghi A, et al: Common mutation in methylenetetrahydrofolate reductase—correlation with homocysteine metabolism and late-onset vascular disease, *Circulation* 94:3074, 1996.
244. McCully KS: Vascular pathology of homocysteinemia: implications for the pathogenesis of atherosclerosis, *Am J Pathol* 56:111, 1969.
245. Harpel PC, Zhang X, Borth W: Homocysteine and hemostasis: Pathogenic mechanisms predisposing to thrombosis, *J Nutr* 126(Suppl 4):1285S, 1996.
246. Upchurch GR Jr, Welch GN, Loscalzo J: Homocysteine, EDRF, and endothelial function, *J Nutr* 126(Suppl 4):1290S, 1996.
247. Prengler M, Pavlakis SG, Prohovnik I, et al: Sickle cell disease: The neurological complications, *Ann Neurology* 51:543-552, 2002.
247a. Wahl S, Quirolo KC: Current issues in blood transfusion for sickle cell disease, *Curr Opin Pediatr* 21:15-21, 2009.

248. Sampaio SG, Vicari P, Figueiredo MS, et al: Brain magnetic resonance imaging abnormalities in adult patients with sickle cell disease. Correlation with transcranial Doppler findings, *Stroke* 40:2408-2412, 2009.
249. Hoppe C, Klitz W, Cheng S, et al: Gene interactions and stroke risk in children with sickle cell anemia, *Blood* 103:2391-2396, 2004.
250. Sumoza A, de Bisotti R, Sumoza D, et al: Hydroxyurea (HU) for prevention of recurrent stroke in sickle cell anemia (SCA), *Am J Hematol* 71:161-165, 2002.
251. Wong WY, Powars DR: Overt and incomplete (silent) cerebral infarction in sickle cell anemia: Diagnosis and management, *Neuroimaging Clin N Am* 17:269-280, 2007.
252. Switzer JA, Hess DC, Nichols FT, et al: Pathophysiology and treatment of stroke in sickle-cell disease: Present and future, *Lancet Neurol* 5:501-512, 2006.
253. Dobson SR, Holden KR, Nietert PJ, et al: Moyamoya syndrome in childhood sickle cell disease: A predictive factor for recurrent cerebrovascular events, *Blood* 99:3144-3150, 2002.
254. Pavlakis SG, Bello J, Prohovnik I, et al: Brain infarction in sickle cell anemia: magnetic resonance imaging correlates, *Ann Neurol* 23:125, 1988.
255. Steen RG, Emudianughe T, Hankins GM, et al: Brain imaging findings in pediatric patients with sickle cell disease, *Radiology* 228(1):216-225, 2003.
256. Hoppe C, Klitz W, Noble J, et al: Distinct HLA associations by stroke subtype in children with sickle cell anemia, *Blood* 101:2865-2869, 2003.
257. Miller ST, Macklin EA, Pegelow CH, et al: Silent infarction as a risk factor for overt stroke in children with sickle cell anemia: A report from the Cooperative Study of Sickle Cell Disease, *J Pediatr* 139:385, 2001.
258. Sebastiani P, Ramoni MF, Nolan V, et al: Genetic dissection and prognostic modeling of overt stroke in sickle cell anemia, *Nat Genet* 37:435-440, 2005.
259. Hayward P: Genetic model predicts stroke in sickle-cell disease, *Lancet Neurol* 4:277, 2005.
260. Taylor JGVI, Tang DC, Savage SA, et al: Variants in the VCAM1 gene and risk for symptomatic stroke in sickle cell disease, *Blood* 100:4303-4309, 2002.
261. Romana M, Diara JP, Doumbo L, et al: Angiotensinogen gene associated polymorphisms and risk of stroke in sickle cell anemia: Additional data supporting an association, *Am J Hematol* 76:310-311, 2004.
262. Tang DC, Prauner R, Lui W, et al: Polymorphisms within the angiotensinogen gene (GT-repeat) and the risk of stroke in pediatric patients with sickle cell disease: A case-control study, *Am J Hematol* 68:164-169, 2001.
263. Sarnaik SA, Ballas SK: Molecular characteristics of pediatric patients with sickle cell anemia and stroke, *Am J Hematol* 67:179-182, 2001.
264. Miller ST, Sleeper LA, Pegelow CH, et al: Prediction of adverse outcomes in children with sickle cell disease, *N Engl J Med* 342:83-89, 2000.
265. Kratovil T, Bulas D, Driscoll MC, et al: Hydroxyurea therapy lowers TCD velocities in children with sickle cell disease, *Pediatr Blood Cancer* 47:894-900, 2006.
266. Strouse JJ, Holbert ML, DeBaun MR, et al: Primary hemorrhagic stroke in children with sickle cell disease is associated with recent transfusion and use of corticosteroids, *Pediatrics* 118:1916-1924, 2006.
267. Wierenga KJ, Serjeant BE, Serjeant GR: Cerebrovascular complications and parvovirus infection in homozygous sickle cell disease, *J Pediatr* 139:438-442, 2001.
268. Quinn CT, Sargent JW: Daytime steady-state haemoglobin desaturation is a risk factor for overt stroke in children with sickle cell anaemia, *Br J Haematol* 140:336-339, 2008.
269. Adams RJ, McKie VC, Hsu L, et al: Prevention of a first stroke by transfusions in children with sickle cell anemia and abnormal results on transcranial Doppler ultrasonography, *N Engl J Med* 339:5-11, 1998.
270. Valadi N, Silva GS, Bowman LS, et al: Transcranial Doppler ultrasonography in adults with sickle cell disease, *Neurology* 67:572-574, 2006.
271. Kato GJ, Gladwin MT: Evolution of novel small-molecule therapeutics targeting sickle cell vasculopathy, *JAMA* 300:2638-2646, 2008.
272. Adams RJ, Ohene-Frempong K, Wang W: Sickle cell and the brain, *Hematology Am Soc Hematol Educ Program* 31-46:2001.
273. Adams RJ, Brambilla D: Optimizing Primary Stroke Prevention in Sickle Cell Anemia (STOP 2) Trial Investigators: Discontinuing prophylactic transfusions used to prevent stroke in sickle cell disease, *N Engl J Med* 353:2769-2778, 2005.
274. Brousse V, Hertz-Pannier L, Consigny Y, et al: Does regular blood transfusion prevent progression of cerebrovascular lesions in children with sickle cell disease? *Ann Hematol* 88:785-788, 2009.
275. Lee MT, Piomelli S, Granger S, et al: Stroke Prevention Trial in Sickle Cell Anemia (STOP): Extended follow-up and final results, *Blood* 108:847-852, 2006.
276. Pegelow CH, Wang W, Granger S, et al: Silent infarcts in children with sickle cell anemia and abnormal cerebral artery velocity, *Arch Neurol* 58:2017-2021, 2001.
277. Scothorn D, Price C, Schwartz D, et al: Risk of recurrent stroke in children with sickle cell disease receiving blood transfusion therapy for at least five years after initial stroke, *J Pediatr* 140:348, 2002.
278. Bhatia M, Walters MC: Hematopoietic cell transplantation for thalassemia and sickle cell disease: Past, present and future, *Bone Marrow Transplant* 41:109-117, 2008.
279. Zimmerman SA, Schultz WH, Burgett S, et al: Hydroxyurea therapy lowers transcranial Doppler flow velocities in children with sickle cell anemia, *Blood* 110:1043-1047, 2007.
280. Bushnell C, Goldstein LB: Screening for hypercoagulable syndromes following stroke, *Curr Atheroscler Rep* 5:291-298, 2003.
281. Rahemtullah A, Van Cott EM: Hypercoagulation testing in ischemic stroke, *Arch Pathol Lab Med* 131:890-901, 2007.

Stroke and Substance Abuse

JOHN C.M. BRUST

Drug dependence is "a state of psychic or physical dependence, or both, on a drug, arising in a person following administration of that drug on a periodic or continuous basis."[1] Drug abuse, on the other hand, refers to the perception that recreational use of a substance is harmful, regardless of whether the substance is taken continuously, periodically, or infrequently, and regardless of whether it is legally available. When alcohol and tobacco are included, millions of Americans are substance abusers, and many of them are at increased risk of stroke, either occlusive or hemorrhagic.[2-4] Mechanisms vary, including a higher incidence of atherosclerotic infarction in alcohol drinkers, cerebral complications of endocarditis common in parenteral drug abusers, and vasculitides affecting users of particular substances.

Opiates

The most commonly abused opiate drug is heroin (diacetylmorphine), which is administered by injection or, especially since the advent of the AIDS epidemic, by snorting or smoking. Stroke affects heroin users by diverse mechanisms. Injectors are at risk of infectious endocarditis, especially with *Staphylococcus aureus* and *Candida*,[5-8] affecting the mitral, aortic, and tricuspid valves with equal frequency[9] and often causing cerebral emboli.

Stroke associated with endocarditis can be occlusive or hemorrhagic. Infarction follows embolic vessel occlusion or, less often, bacterial or fungal meningitis. Cerebral or subarachnoid hemorrhage usually occurs after rupture of a septic (mycotic) aneurysm.[10,11] Unlike saccular (berry) aneurysms, septic aneurysms are more likely to manifest with subtle or insidiously progressive neurologic or systemic symptoms (e.g., headache, fever, syncope, hemiparesis, aphasia) than with a sudden onset suggesting subarachnoid hemorrhage; also, cerebrospinal fluid (CSF) white cell pleocytosis may occur in asymptomatic patients with endocarditis days before mycotic aneurysm ruptures.[12] The infrequency with which mycotic aneurysms spontaneously disappear during antimicrobial therapy, the high mortality associated with their rupture, and the relative ease (compared with saccular aneurysms) of their surgical removal support the view that cerebral angiography should be performed in patients with endocarditis who have either unexplained neurologic symptoms or abnormal CSF findings and that once found, most mycotic aneurysms should be promptly excised.[12] Mycotic aneurysms in heroin users have also occurred on the carotid and subclavian arteries.[13,14] Heroin users

are at risk of hemorrhagic stroke secondary to hepatitis, liver failure, and deranged clotting or secondary to heroin nephropathy with uremia or malignant hypertension.

In one report, nine heroin addicts had stroke unassociated with endocarditis.[15] In three, ranging in age from 41 to 45 years, the relation of stroke to heroin was uncertain: one patient, while using heroin, had an intracerebral hemorrhage in the presence of probable heroin nephropathy and malignant hypertension; another, who was normotensive, had a basal ganglia hemorrhage 3 days after beginning methadone detoxification; the third, who was mildly hypertensive, had a probable capsular infarct 6 weeks after starting methadone maintenance. In the other six patients, ages 25 to 38 years, heroin appeared to be more directly causal. Four of the patients, all of whom were normotensive, had probable cerebral infarcts in association with loss of consciousness after intravenous injection of heroin. Cerebral angiographic results were normal in one of the patients but in another showed stenosis of the internal carotid artery at the siphon and of the proximal anterior cerebral artery, plus occlusion of the middle cerebral artery; the changes suggested primary vessel disease more than emboli. Cerebral infarction occurred in the two remaining patients who were using heroin at the time, although the strokes were not related to overdose and did not follow recent injections. In one of these patients, who was normotensive, cerebral angiography suggested widespread small vessel constrictions consistent with arteritis. None of these patients was using oral contraceptives or had other illnesses that would predispose to stroke. Consistent with hypersensitivity, one patient had 10% eosinophilia, serum hypergammaglobulinemia, and a positive direct Coombs test result, and another had an erythrocyte sedimentation rate (ESR) of 94 mm/h and positive latex fixation titers. Except for cocaine in one patient (whose stroke followed an acute reaction to heroin), these nine patients were using no other drugs.

Other reports of stroke in heroin abusers include that of a 19-year-old man who had taken heroin intravenously weekly for a year and had used lysergic acid diethylamide (LSD) intermittently; he experienced sudden global aphasia, and cerebral angiography suggested diffuse angiitis.[16] A 21-year-old woman demonstrated hemiparesis 2 weeks after starting daily heroin use and 6 hours after an intravenous injection.[17] Symptoms began with vomiting, headache, sweating, and shortness of breath, suggesting anaphylaxis, and cerebral angiography showed narrowing and irregularity of the distal internal carotid artery, suggesting arteritis. Eosinophilia and the fact that her husband had shared her heroin were consistent with hypersensitivity to heroin or to an adulterant. A normotensive 20-year-old man who had used heroin occasionally for 2 years took his first intravenous injection in 8 months and experienced sudden left homonymous hemianopia and incoordination; cerebral angiography showed "beading" of the right posterior cerebral artery.[18] Acute severe cerebellar ataxia followed intraarterial injection of heroin in another patient.[19]

Other heroin-associated infarcts resulted in aphasia and cortical blindness.[20,21] Ischemic stroke has also occurred after heroin sniffing[22]; in one such case, involving a 34-year-old man, cerebral angiographic results were normal.[23] A young man had an intracerebral hemorrhage within minutes of intravenous injection of heroin.[24] Opiate withdrawal symptoms and cerebral infarction were reported in two newborns whose mothers had used codeine during pregnancy.[25]

Heroin could cause stroke by a number of possible mechanisms.[15,26] After heroin overdose, hypoventilation and hypotension can produce permanent brain damage with bilateral cerebral leukoencephalopathy.[27] Hemiplegia has appeared on awakening from naloxone-responsive coma[15,28]; overdoses have also caused spastic quadriparesis, dementia, deafness, seizures, dystonia, and ballism.[29,30] Delayed postanoxic encephalopathy also occurs.[31] Bilateral globus pallidus infarction is commonly observed at autopsy in heroin users,[32,33] and hemichorea was present in a patient with heroin stroke.[15] A 17-year-old boy developed respiratory failure and shock while snorting heroin; on regaining consciousness he was cognitively impaired, and magnetic resonance imaging (MRI) revealed globus pallidus infarction.[34] In some cases an awkward position of the neck during overdose coma might have kinked the carotid artery and further decreased cerebral perfusion.[28] MRI revealed bilateral borderzone infarction in a young man who developed seizures and left hemiparesis three days after injecting heroin. Hypotension was never evident, however, and angiography showed reversible bilateral segmental narrowing of the supraclinoid internal carotid, middle cerebral, and anterior cerebral arteries.[35]

Direct toxic injury from either heroin or an adulterant is another possibility. Heroin is often mixed with quinine and lactose or mannitol; other reported adulterants include talc, starch, curry powder, abrasive cleanser, caffeine, and strychnine.[26] Quinine caused amblyopia in a heroin addict[36] and might contribute to acute adverse reactions with pulmonary edema or sudden death after parenteral injection.[37] There is no evidence, however, linking quinine to stroke.

Embolization of foreign material to the brain has not been observed in parenteral heroin users (even though the jugular vein is commonly used, with occasional accidental arterial injection) but has been documented at autopsy in abusers of other opiates.[38,39] Probably because of restricted heroin supply, pentazocine (Talwin) and tripelennamine (Pyribenzamine) ("Ts and Blues") were widely abused in Chicago and other Midwestern cities during the 1970s. Oral tablets were crushed, suspended in water, passed through cotton or a cigarette filter, and injected intravenously, and cerebral infarcts and hemorrhages occurred in users.[40] Common at autopsy was pulmonary arteriolar occlusion by microcrystalline cellulose or particulate magnesium silicate (talc), which had been used to bind pentazocine and tripelennamine. Such microemboli also reached the brain, especially when multiple lung emboli produced pulmonary hypertension and opened "functional pulmonary arteriovenous shunts." "Beaded arteries" were seen at cerebral angiography in "Ts and Blues" stroke patients, consistent with emboli, vasculitis, or both.[26]

Talc microemboli were also found at autopsy in the liver, spleen, and central nervous system of a parenteral paregoric abuser.[41] A young man who several times a day injected pulverized unfiltered meperidine tablets intravenously had occasional seizures after injection and then experienced difficulty with concentration, impaired memory, and visual blurring; fundal hemorrhages and areas of arterial occlusion were seen, and his symptoms improved with abstinence.[42]

Posterior cerebral artery occlusion followed intravenous injection of a melted hydromorphone (Dilaudid) suppository; the authors speculated that the mechanism was paradoxic fat embolism of the product's cocoa butter content.[43]

Some heroin strokes follow the first injection after weeks or months of abstinence, and laboratory findings further suggest an immunologic cause. Heroin nephropathy may be immunologically mediated[44]; the C3 component of complement is reduced in patients with heroin pulmonary edema; and heroin addicts frequently have hypergammaglobulinemia[45] (including elevated IgM independent of IgG and IgA levels[46-48]), circulating immune complexes,[41] antibodies to smooth muscle and lymphocyte membranes,[46] false-positive serologic tests,[45] and lymph node hypertrophy.[26] Opium, morphine, codeine, and meperidine, moreover, have caused urticaria, angioneurotic edema, and anaphylaxis.[49] Whether the offending antigen is the opiate or a contaminant is unclear, but morphine binding by gamma globulin is reported in addicts[50] and experimental animals.[51]

Relevant to heroin stroke and its possible mechanisms is heroin myelopathy. Acute paraparesis, sensory loss, and urinary retention occur shortly after injection, frequently after a period of abstinence.[52-56] In some, symptoms are present on awakening from coma. Proprioception and vibratory sense are often preserved relative to loss of spinothalamic sensory modalities, which suggests infarction in the territory of the anterior spinal artery,[57] and in a patient with bilateral pallidal infarction, there was also MRI evidence of spinal cord borderzone infarction.[33] Several hours after snorting heroin, a man awoke with flaccid paralysis of the legs and urinary retention; MRI showed midthoracic transverse myelitis.[58] Autopsy in one patient showed necrosis "confined almost entirely" to the upper thoracic spinal cord gray matter and in another demonstrated additional involvement of the anterior aspect of the posterior columns and a pyramidal tract in the lower thoracic cord.[53] If these lesions were cord infarcts, their possible causes, as with cerebral stroke in heroin users, include "borderzone" infarction during a period of coma, hypoventilation, and hypotension, as well as hypersensitivity reaction. Consistent with the latter, one young man, remaining conscious, had several episodes of numbness and weakness of both legs for a few minutes after injection.[54] Eleven days after injection an adolescent demonstrated a rash on the chest and feet and 6 days later became paraplegic after a second injection.[55] Cord biopsy in another patient showed vasculitis affecting mainly small arteries and arterioles, with "double refractile fragments" in inflamed tissue, including vessel walls.[59] (Such foreign particles are also seen in the skin of heroin addicts.[60]) A patient at Harlem Hospital had heroin injected into a vessel over his midthoracic spine and within 30 minutes experienced paraparesis and then urinary retention and sensory loss below that level. Myelographic findings were normal. Regardless of whether the vessel injected was arterial or venous, the common intercostal origins of the posterior cutaneous and spinal arteries or veins would have allowed injected material direct access to the spinal cord; it remains uncertain, however, whether the damage was direct toxicity, hypersensitivity, or embolism of foreign material.

A man using intravenous heroin for the first time in 2 years became comatose and apneic; after he received an opiate antagonist, quadriplegia, anarthria, dysphagia, and sensory loss consistent with a ventral pontine lesion developed over several hours.[61] Recovery was partial, and whether the lesion was vascular was not determined.

Amphetamine and Related Agents

Although their manufacture was greatly reduced after the 1972 Controlled Substances Act, amphetamine and similar psychostimulants are still produced in huge quantities. During the 1990s methamphetamine became the fastest growing illegal drug in North America and parts of Europe. Swallowed, injected, snorted, or smoked, it is often taken with heroin, and samples contain a variety of pharmacologically active and inactive adulterants.[2] Strokes common to any parenteral drug abuse are encountered. There are also strokes that may be unique to these agents.

Acutely amphetamine can cause excitement, hypertension, and a rectal temperature exceeding 109°F, followed by coma, vascular collapse, and death; at autopsy, diffuse cerebral edema and petechiae are seen, without large infarcts or hematomas.[62-64] In dogs or rabbits[65-67] given lethal doses of amphetamine, severe hyperpyrexia, myocardial fiber necrosis, and neuronal degeneration in the cerebral cortex and cerebellum were seen. Curare prevented the fever and the fatal course, which suggests that the hyperpyrexia was secondary to muscle hyperactivity and that death was secondary to heat stroke. Fever may have also contributed to similar brain pathologic findings in cats receiving long-term methamphetamine over 2 weeks, although, in that study, neuronal catecholamine depletion was suspected as the primary cause.[68]

Significant brain hemorrhage was not present in these experimental animals but has been found, along with focal neurologic signs, in animal and human cases of heat stroke,[69] often with severe clotting abnormalities, including decreased prothrombin activity, thrombocytopenia, hypofibrinogenemia, and fibrinolysis.[70] However, hyperpyrexia and disturbed clotting have not been described in patients with intracranial hemorrhage after amphetamine/methamphetamine use.

Reports of amphetamine use in the literature include more than 40 patients, ages 16 to 60 years.[71] Oral, intravenous, nasal, and inhalational routes of administration have been reported. Most were chronic users, but in several patients, stroke followed a first exposure. The dose was usually unknown, but in one case was as low as 80 mg. Except for one instance each of diethylpropion and pseudoephedrine, all the reported patients took amphetamine or methamphetamine; seven also took methylphenidate, LSD, dimethoxymethylamphetamine ("STP"), cocaine, heroin, or barbiturates. Severe headaches usually occurred within minutes of drug use. Blood pressure was elevated in the majority of patients in whom it was recorded, and diastolic pressure were as high as 120 mm Hg in five. Eight patients died, usually soon after admission. Computed tomography (CT) variably showed intracerebral hemorrhage (frequently lobar) or subarachnoid hemorrhage. In some patients, angiography revealed irregular narrowing (beading) of distal cerebral arteries, suggesting (but not pathognomonic for) vasculitis; some of these patients had taken the drug only orally. Vasculitic changes were present at autopsy in three patients (including one whose angiogram showed only an avascular mass). In another patient, a cerebral vascular malformation was seen on both angiography and CT.

Thus, some of these amphetamine/methamphetamine-induced intracranial hemorrhages seem to have been secondary to acute hypertension, some to cerebral vasculitis, and some to a combination of the two; however, in others neither feature was apparent. A case report described cerebral vasculitis at autopsy after methamphetamine-associated intracerebral hemorrhage.[100] Another autopsy report of methamphetamine-associated intracerebral hemorrhage found no evidence of vasculitis.[99] Although acute hypertension secondary to amphetamine could be causal, it might have been a transient result of the stroke in some patients. Conversely, in other patients, fleeting blood pressure elevations could have been missed.

Amphetamine/methamphetamine-associated ischemic strokes have been less frequently reported.[102] In one case a Brown-Séquard syndrome followed an attempt to inject methamphetamine into a jugular vein.[105] Ischemic stroke occurred in a young man after intranasal use of amphetamine combined with caffeine.[106] Cerebral vasculitis and brain infarction were found at autopsy in a man who had been using intravenous methamphetamine for nearly a decade.[107] Right occipital lobe infarction occurred in a woman 3 months after last injecting methamphetamine; magnetic resonance angiography showed segmental narrowing of the right posterior cerebral artery, which was still present 4 months later.[108] Two young women had carotid artery dissection and middle cerebral artery territory infarction after methamphetamine use.[109]

Two epidemiologic studies addressed the association of amphetamine/methamphetamine and stroke. In a population-based case-control study of women aged 15 to 44 years, amphetamine/methamphetamine was a risk factor for combined hemorrhagic and ischemic stroke (odds ratio, 3.8).[110] Some women in that study used both cocaine and amphetamine/methamphetamine, and drug use was based on self-report at a later interview; claims did not always match what was recorded in the medical record, including positive results on urine drug screening. Hospitalized control subjects, moreover, did not undergo drug screening, and if they were even less likely than case patients to report drug use, the risk of stroke might be exaggerated. A case-control study using a cross-sectional design based on more than 3 million patients discharged from Texas hospitals over a 3-year period found that amphetamine/methamphetamine increased the risk of hemorrhagic stroke (odds ratio, 4.95) but not ischemic stroke; amphetamine/methamphetamine also increased the risk of death after hemorrhagic stroke (odds ratio, 2.63).[111]

Amphetamine-induced cerebral vasculitis appears to be of more than one type. Necrotizing angiitis, sometimes affecting the nervous system, occurred in 14 Los Angeles abusers of multiple drugs, including amphetamine, methamphetamine, barbiturates, chlordiazepoxide, diazepam, marijuana, hydroxyzine, LSD, heroin, meperidine, mescaline, oxycodone, oxymorphone, dimethoxymethylamphetamine, and strychnine.[112] All but two patients used intravenous methamphetamine, and one used it exclusively. Five patients were asymptomatic; in the others, symptoms included fever, weight loss, malaise, weakness, skin rash, pneumonitis, pulmonary edema, hematuria, proteinuria, renal failure, abdominal pain, pancreatitis, gastrointestinal hemorrhage, arthralgia, myalgia, peripheral neuropathy, anemia, leukocytosis, and hemolysis. One patient had renal failure, severe hypertension, papilledema, retinal detachment, "progressive encephalopathy," and, at autopsy, vasculitis affecting pontine arterioles. Another, who had demonstrated "mental obtundation" and hypertension, at autopsy showed "recent and resolving cerebral and pontine infarction," "marked cerebellar hemorrhage," and vasculitis in the cerebrum, cerebellum, and brainstem. Vessel lesions consisted initially of fibrinoid necrosis of the media and intima, with infiltration by neutrophils, eosinophils, lymphocytes, and histiocytes; later, there was destruction of muscular and elastic components, replacement by collagen, and often "a nodular (nodose) bulge with nearly aneurysmal dilatation."

The authors considered these lesions, which affected only muscular arteries and arterioles, typical for polyarteritis nodosa and distinguished them from hypersensitivity angiitis, which involves small arteries, capillaries, and venules. They further noted that more than one drug or adulterant could have caused these lesions and that, in contrast to polyarteritis nodosa, the lesions observed in these patients were not associated with the presence of hepatitis antigen.[113,114]

Although such brain lesions have been found pathologically in amphetamine/methamphetamine abusers,[82,102] in some, cerebral arteritis has been presumed on the basis of cerebral angiography,[71,72,76,86,96,115-117] and sometimes the relation to amphetamine abuse has been tenuous. In a report of three young men who experienced ischemic strokes in association with intranasal methamphetamine, cerebral angiography revealed supraclinoid beading of the internal carotid artery in one, occlusion of the internal carotid artery near its origin in another, and

supraclinoid occlusion of the internal carotid artery in the third.[118] In another report, thalamic infarction followed intranasal methamphetamine use, but angiography was not performed.[119]

A radiographic study of 19 young drug abusers, most taking intravenous methamphetamine and hospitalized for coma or stroke, revealed widespread segmental constrictions of large and medium-sized cerebral arteries and stenosis or occlusion of many penetrating arterioles (beading).

Such a finding could reflect either multiple emboli, vasculitis, or spontaneous segmental vasoconstriction.[115] The same researchers then gave rhesus monkeys intravenous methamphetamine, 1.5 mg/kg (considered the lower limit of dosage for most abusers), and performed serial cerebral angiograms for 2 weeks.[120] Several animals studied 10 minutes after receiving the drugs showed an irregularly decreased caliber of small cerebral vessels; a return to normal was seen at 24 hours. In others, these changes occurred in both small and large vessels and persisted for the 2-week period; in one animal, the changes actually worsened with time. Clinically, the animals had hypertension and behavioral changes. Postmortem examination at 2 weeks revealed subarachnoid hemorrhage in some animals, with numerous brain petechial hemorrhages, infarcts, edema, microaneurysms, and perivascular white blood cell cuffing. In a later study, monkeys received intravenous methamphetamine three times weekly.[121] After either a month or a year, serial angiograms showed occlusions and slow blood flow in small cerebral arteries, and autopsy revealed attenuated and fragmented brain arterioles and capillaries, microaneurysms, dilated venules, petechiae, neuronal loss, and gliosis. Talc crystals were present in capillaries (the drug was given as crushed methamphetamine tablets); however, arguing against the notion that such particles play a critical role in the vasculitis was the finding that in the animals receiving crushed placebo tablets containing all ingredients except methamphetamine, vasculitis was minimal or absent.

In rats receiving 2 weeks of intravenous methamphetamine, electron microscopy showed that brain capillaries had abnormal "budding" from the luminal walls of endothelial cells and vesicles within the endothelial cell cytoplasm.[121] These changes affected vessels smaller than 100 μm and would therefore be missed on angiography. (The vulnerability of small vessels might be related to their separate innervation; large cerebral vessels are innervated by the peripheral sympathetic nervous system, but nerve terminals on smaller arteries appear to be from central noradrenergic neurons.[122])

Angiographic and histologic changes also occurred in rats and monkeys receiving methylphenidate (Ritalin).[121]

These lesions are different from those of polyarteritis nodosa, in which elastic arteries, capillaries, and veins are spared. Whether the lesions in methamphetamine users are the result of direct toxicity or hypersensitivity is unclear, nor can the possibility be excluded that the early angiographic findings are secondary to subarachnoid hemorrhage (although beading of distal pial arteries in subarachnoid hemorrhage is rare).[72] In an adolescent amphetamine abuser with mononeuritis multiplex, sural nerve biopsy showed apparent hypersensitivity angiitis of medium and small muscular arteries, arterioles, venules, and veins, with fibrinoid necrosis and infiltration by polymorphonuclear leukocytes, lymphocytes, eosinophils, and plasma cells.[123] The central nervous system, however, was clinically unaffected.

A study using single-photon emission CT (SPECT) found reduced cerebral blood flow in the cingulate cortex of both long-term and short-term abstinent methamphetamine users.[124]

In mice, pretreatment with methamphetamine exacerbated damage after middle cerebral artery ligation.[125]

Phenylpropanolamine (PPA), a drug similar to but less potent than amphetamine, was marketed, sometimes with ephedrine or caffeine, in over-the-counter decongestants and diet pills, as well as in drugs made deliberately to resemble amphetamine ("look-alike pills").[126,127] Acute hypertension, severe headache, psychiatric symptoms, seizures, and hemorrhagic stroke have occurred in users.[127-137]

A case reported as "cerebral arteritis" in a PPA user was based simply on angiographic beading.[138] PPA with caffeine, from a commercial diet preparation, produced subarachnoid hemorrhage in rats receiving it intraperitoneally at three to six times the recommended dose.[133]

In 2000, a case-control study involving 43 U.S. hospitals found that appetite suppressants containing PPA increase the risk of subarachnoid or intracerebral hemorrhage in women (odds ratio, 16.58). No men in that study used PPA-containing diet pills, but a trend toward higher hemorrhagic stroke risk was observed in men and women using PPA-containing cough and cold remedies. The greater risk associated with diet pills was attributed to higher daily doses.[139] That year, the U.S. Food and Drug Administration (FDA) ordered products containing PPA to be withdrawn from the market.[140]

A subsequent report from Mexico described 16 patients with ischemic or hemorrhagic stroke occurring within 24 hours of ingesting decongestants containing PPA.[141,142] A Korean case-control study found PPA contained in cold remedies to be a risk factor for hemorrhagic stroke, both intracerebral (odds ratio, 1.68) and subarachnoid (odds ratio, 3.96).[143]

Ephedrine and pseudoephedrine are present in over-the-counter decongestants and bronchodilators. Complications of these agents include headache, tachyarrhythmia, hypertensive emergency, and hemorrhagic and occlusive stroke.[144-150] A young man who had previously used "speed" and LSD had a subarachnoid hemorrhage within an hour of ingesting pills that turned out to be ephedrine.[151] Cerebral angiographic results were initially normal, but angiography performed a week later showed beading and branch occlusions suggesting arteritis; a biopsy from grossly normal skin showed periluminal deposits of IgM and the C3 component of complement in dermal vessels, consistent with circulating immune complexes.

Multiple hemorrhagic cerebral infarcts and cerebrovascular beading occurred in a woman who received ephedrine intravenously for emergency treatment of hypotension.[152]

Rupture of a cerebral vascular malformation occurred in a man who had used pseudoephedrine daily for more than a year.[153] Thunderclap headache and bilateral severe cerebral vasoconstriction in the absence of subarachnoid hemorrhage (Call-Fleming syndrome) occurred in a woman soon after taking pseudoephedrine and dextromethorphan.[154]

Dietary supplements containing ephedra alkaloids (ma huang) are popular in the United States for energy enhancement and weight reduction. Cardiotoxicity (including sudden death) and ischemic and hemorrhagic strokes were reported in users.[155-161] A review of 140 adverse events associated with ephedra use revealed stroke in 10 people and seizures in seven.[159] These products often contain caffeine, which, as an adenosine receptor antagonist, probably aggravates ephedra's vasoconstrictor and pressor actions.

A case-control study found a nonsignificant trend toward hemorrhagic stroke and the use of ephedra-containing products, and in 2003 they were banned by the U.S. FDA.[162]

Other amphetamine-like drugs promoted as diet pills and anecdotally associated with stroke include phentermine, phendimetrazine,[163] diethylpropion,[80] and fenfluramine.[164,165] A cohort study found that dexfenfluramine, fenfluramine, and phentermine increased the risk of stroke (odds ratio, 2.4), but confidence intervals were wide.[166] After reports of valvular heart disease in users, fenfluramine and dexfenfluramine were removed from the U.S. market.[167]

3,4-Methylenedioxymethamphetamine (MDMA, "ecstasy") and 3,4-methylenedioxyethamphetamine (MDEA) are "designer drugs" with both amphetamine-like and hallucinogen-like properties.[2] Adolescents and young adults often ingest ecstasy tablets while dancing frenetically at "rave" parties, and reported complications, sometimes fatal, include ischemic and hemorrhagic stroke.[168-178] An 18-year-old boy had a rupture of a middle cerebral artery saccular aneurysm while using ecstasy.[179] A 25-year-old woman who abused both MDMA and cocaine developed basilar artery occlusion.[180] Three days after taking MDMA orally a 26-year-old woman developed a pure amnestic syndrome that was still present a year later; bilateral globus pallidus hyperintensities on MRI were interpreted as ischemic injury, and the authors speculated that serotonin-induced vasospasm within the hippocampi caused the amnesia.[181]

A young woman who injected crushed methylphenidate tablets into her jugular veins experienced immediate right hemiplegia after a left injection and, 2 months later, left hemiplegia after a right injection; presumably she inadvertently injected into her carotid arteries.[182]

Intraretinal talc microemboli have been seen in the fundi of intravenous methylphenidate abusers.[38,183] In some there were retinal vascular and choroidal abnormalities, neovascularization, and vitreous hemorrhage,[183] and in one abuser, who had not had a clinical stroke, talc and cornstarch emboli were also present in arterioles, capillaries, and veins of the brain and lung.[38] Infarction of the medial medulla in a young woman occurred a few minutes after intravenous injection of methylphenidate; at autopsy there was systemic granulomatosis due to talc and talc deposits in small vessels around the medullary infarct.[39]

As with amphetamine/methamphetamine, cerebral "vasculitis" has been presumed without pathologic confirmation in a number of reports of methylphenidate-associated stroke.[184] A 12-year-old boy taking methylphenidate in prescribed dosage had an ischemic stroke, and cerebral angiography showed cerebral arterial irregularities and occlusions.[185] Ischemic stroke with similar angiographic changes affected an 8-year-old boy taking methylphenidate therapeutically.[186]

Mycotic subclavian and carotid aneurysms have been reported after inadvertent intraarterial injection of phentermine.[187]

Death has followed parenteral[188] or oral[189] abuse of propylhexedrine from nasal decongestant inhalers; stroke has not yet been reported in such patients, and the cause of death has been uncertain.

Cerebral and retinal infarcts were reported in chronic intranasal abusers of sprays and drops containing the sympathomimetics oxymetazoline and phenoxazoline.[190,191]

Intracerebral hemorrhage occurred in a young man after intravenous self-administration of epinephrine.[192] A normotensive 73-year-old man had a thalamic hemorrhage after repeated heavy use of an epinephrine inhaler.[193]

Cocaine

Before the 1980s cocaine hydrochloride was usually sniffed or, less often, injected. The emergence of smokable alkaloidal "crack" cocaine allowed much larger doses and more prolonged intoxication than with intranasal (and unsmokable) cocaine hydrochloride. An epidemic of crack cocaine use ensued, and with it a flood of reports describing medical complications, including stroke.[194]

Parenteral cocaine users are at risk of stroke related to infection, including endocarditis, AIDS, and hepatitis. They also experience strokes caused directly by the drug itself, whether taken intranasally, intravenously, or intramuscularly or smoked as crack.[195,196] The first report of a cocaine-related stroke appeared in 1977; a middle-aged, mildly hypertensive man injected cocaine intramuscularly after drinking a bottle of wine and an hour later abruptly experienced aphasia and right hemiparesis; CSF findings were normal, and cerebral angiography was refused.[197] The same year, fatal rupture of a cerebral saccular aneurysm occurred in a young man sniffing cocaine.[198] Further cases were not reported until the mid-1980s, but by 2002, more than 600 cases of cocaine-related stroke had been described, about half occlusive and half hemorrhagic.[39,199-277]

Ischemic strokes have included transient ischemic attacks and infarction of cerebrum, thalamus, brainstem, spinal cord, retina, and peripheral oculomotor nerve.[212,233,278-286]

Infarction has occurred in newborns whose mothers used cocaine shortly before delivery[205] and in pregnant women.[195,212,233,278] Pontomesencephalic infarction in a cocaine sniffer was associated with extensive destruction of osteocartilaginous structures of the nose, sinuses, and palate.[276] Bilateral hippocampal infarction followed cocaine-induced cardiac arrest.[277] In some cases, cerebral infarction was attributed to vasculitis on the basis

of angiographic findings[228]; such changes, however, could represent either cocaine-induced cerebral vasoconstriction or vasospasm after undiagnosed subarachnoid hemorrhage.[287] Autopsies usually show histologically normal cerebral vessels,[195,236,247] although in five cases, mild cerebral vasculitis was observed at biopsy or autopsy.[203,216,233,245] In these cases, cerebral angiographic findings were normal. Conversely, in a man with multiple cerebral infarcts diagnosed both clinically and on MRI, angiography showed "multifocal areas of segmental stenosis and dilatation," yet brain biopsy revealed no evidence of vasculitis.[241] A young crack smoker had middle cerebral artery branch occlusion, cardiomyopathy, and a left atrial thrombus.[252] A 20-year-old with no other risk factors had superior cerebellar artery occlusion 6 months after the last use of cocaine, which raises the possibility of delayed effects.[288]

In a 27-year-old occasional cocaine sniffer with "heaviness and paresthesias" in the legs and occasional "forgetfulness," MRI revealed multiple periventricular white matter lesions.[270] A young man who had used cocaine "regularly" for 10 years demonstrated progressively impaired cognition; CT revealed patchy areas consistent with infarction, and cerebral angiography showed marked stenosis of the internal carotid and middle cerebral arteries with moyamoya-like collateral vessels.[286] A young woman who had been using crack for 12 years experienced mental deterioration progressing to mutism over several weeks; CT showed diffuse cerebral atrophy, but SPECT showed more focal reductions in perfusion.[289]

MRI studies in asymptomatic long-term cocaine users found abnormal cerebral white matter signals consistent with "subclinical vascular events."[290] In a study of 32 cocaine-dependent subjects, cerebral white matter hyperintensities on MRI were significantly more frequent among cocaine users than among heroin users (odds ratio, 2.54) or normal control subjects (odds ratio, 2.90).[291]

A population-based study of young adults found that cocaine conferred significant risk of "early retinal vascular abnormalities."[292]

Intracerebral or subarachnoid hemorrhage has occurred during or within hours of cocaine use or has shown a less clear temporal relationship.[247,293-295] In some instances there has been other substance use, especially ethanol. Parenchymal hemorrhages have been located in the cerebrum, brainstem, and cerebellum.[247,272,281,282,285,296,297]

Also described are superior saggital sinus thrombosis with hemorrhagic venous infarction, mycotic aneurysm rupture, dural arteriovenous fistula, spontaneous spinal epidural hematoma, and bleeding into embolic infarction or glioma.[271,281,298,299] Nearly half the patients with cocaine-associated intracranial hemorrhage who underwent angiography had saccular aneurysms or vascular malformations.

Of 150 consecutive patients with subarachnoid hemorrhage, 17 had used cocaine within 72 hours, and mortality and morbidity rates were worse among the cocaine users, perhaps because of drug-aggravated vasospasm.[262] In another study, 27 of 440 patients with ruptured aneurysms had used cocaine within 72 hours, and although vasospasm was more likely among the cocaine users, there was no difference in clinical outcome.[300] Cerebral hemorrhages have occurred in newborns and postpartum women.[195,224,242]

Autopsies on patients with cocaine-induced intracranial hemorrhage have revealed histologically normal cerebral vessels.[218,293]

A case-control study from Atlanta failed to find any association between crack use and stroke.[301] This unexpected finding was probably related to lack of information regarding acute crack use in more than half of the subjects and controls as well as the fact that nearly half of the controls with information available had used crack, many acutely, raising the possibility that crack users are more likely than nonusers to be hospitalized for a variety of reasons. A population-based study of 10,085 young adults identified 33 with nonfatal stroke and concluded that cocaine use was not a risk factor.[302] In that study the diagnosis of stroke was based on physician report and "lifetime cocaine use" (i.e., use not necessarily associated temporarily with the stroke) was based on patient report.

A case-control study of women aged 15 to 44 years found that cocaine use was a strong risk factor for stroke (odds ratio, 13.9).[110] A case-control study of men and women aged 18 to 49 years found that cocaine use within 3 days was a strong risk factor for subarachnoid hemorrhage (odds ratio, 24.97).[303]

The mechanisms of cocaine-related stroke are diverse. Striking, if one considers that cocaine and amphetamine have similar actions and effects, is the high frequency of underlying aneurysm or vascular malformation in hemorrhagic strokes in cocaine users compared with amphetamine users and, conversely, the frequency of vasculitis in amphetamine users compared with cocaine users.[304] Cocaine hydrochloride is more often associated with hemorrhagic than occlusive stroke, whereas hemorrhagic and occlusive strokes occur with roughly equal frequency in crack users; however, the rising prevalence of stroke since the appearance of crack is probably attributable to wider use and higher dosage rather than to a peculiarity of crack itself.[305]

Coronary artery vasoconstriction has been documented during cardiac catheterization, and cocaine-induced myocardial infarction, cardiac arrhythmia, and cardiomyopathy carry a risk of embolic stroke.[306] More significant, however, is cocaine's effects on systemic and cerebral circulation. By blocking reuptake of norepinephrine from sympathetic nerve endings (and probably also by affecting calcium flux and serotonin reuptake), cocaine is a vasoconstrictor both systemically and intracranially.[307-311] Acute hypertension can result, leading to intracranial hemorrhage, especially in subjects with underlying aneurysms or vascular malformations.[247] Cerebral vasoconstriction probably causes occlusive stroke, and it is possibly significant that cocaine metabolites, which in some long-term users are detectable in urine for weeks, also cause cerebral vasospasm.[312,313] In healthy young cocaine users, intravenous cocaine caused dose-related cerebral vasoconstriction (as detected by magnetic resonance angiography),[314] and Doppler ultrasonography revealed increased cerebrovascular resistance that persisted for at least 1 month during abstinence.[315] In women, cocaine-induced cerebral vasospasm is hormonally influenced, occurring during the luteal phase of

the menstrual cycle but not during the follicular phase.[316] The situation is complex, however, because cerebral and peripheral vessels frequently respond differently to similar stimuli. Whereas intraluminal cocaine constricted cat and rat pial vessels in vitro, topical cocaine dilated pial vessels in living rats[307,312,317] and intravenous cocaine produced both vasoconstriction and vasodilatation of cerebral vessels in rabbits.[318,319] In swine, cocaine given intravenously caused carotid artery constriction, but there was no response in vitro, which suggests that at least in that species the vasoconstriction effect was indirect, through "release of humoral and/or neural vasoactive substances."[320] Other animal studies show either a central or a peripheral mechanism of action for cocaine-induced vasocontriction.[321,322] Cocaine-induced cerebral vasospasm was reportedly most prominent in brain areas rich in dopamine (which has vasoconstrictor effects on intracortical vessels), and the vasospasm was blocked by dihydropyridine calcium channel antagonists.[323] In rabbits cocaine-induced cerebral vasospasm was dependent on endothelin-1 release.[324] Cultured canine vascular smooth muscle cells underwent apoptosis when exposed to cocaine.[325]

Active cocaine users have increased platelet aggregation to adenosine diphosphate, and the abnormality improves with abstinence.[326] In vitro studies with platelets are conflicting. Cocaine reportedly enhanced the response of platelets to arachidonic acid, thereby promoting aggregation.[327] It also, however, directly inhibited fibrinogen binding to activated platelets and caused dissociation of preformed platelet aggregates.[328] In rabbits, repeated cocaine injections caused arteriosclerotic aortopathy.[329] In a cocaine user with symptoms of coronary artery disease, protein C and antithrombin III levels were depleted but returned to normal, with clearing of symptoms, when use of the drug was discontinued.[330] In long-term cocaine users, immediate administration of cocaine caused erythrocytosis and increased levels of von Willebrand factor.[331]

Ethanol reportedly enhances cocaine toxicity; in the presence of ethanol, cocaine is metabolized to cocaethylene, which, perhaps even more powerfully than cocaine itself, binds to the synaptic dopamine transporter and blocks reuptake.[332] Cocaine and ethanol synergistically depress myocardial contraction,[333] and a study using SPECT found that cerebral perfusion was reduced to a greater degree in subjects who abused both cocaine and ethanol than in those who abused cocaine alone.[334]

Human studies using control subjects suggest that long-term cocaine use produces subtle cognitive impairment,[335-338] but unlike methamphetamine, cocaine does not produce morphologic damage at dopaminergic or serotonergic nerve endings.[339,340] Studies with positron emission tomography (PET) and SPECT in long-term cocaine users found irregularly decreased blood flow in the cerebral cortex; in some of these subjects, CT or MRI findings were normal, and in some (but not all), PET and SPECT abnormalities were associated with deficits on psychometric testing.[341-346]

How cocaine affects the fetus is controversial. Perinatal and neonatal strokes—both occlusive and hemorrhagic— may be underrecognized in newborns exposed to cocaine in utero.[263,347] Cerebral blood flow studies during the first few days of life in cocaine-exposed neonates are consistent with persisting vasoconstriction.[348] Some investigators speculate that cocaine-induced vasospasm during the first trimester is responsible for CNS malformations (including encephalocele, holoprosencephaly, and hypoplastic cerebellum).[223] Others have doubted such causality.[349] Adolescents exposed to cocaine in utero had significantly reduced global cerebral blood flow compared with control subjects.[350]

Phencyclidine

Phencyclidine (PCP, "angel dust") became a widely abused U.S. street drug in the 1970s; it can be smoked, eaten, or injected. Large doses cause psychosis, myoclonus, nystagmus, seizures, coma, and sometimes fatal respiratory and circulatory collapse.[351] Hypertension can occur both early and late during intoxication[351-353] and may be related to enhancement of the action of catecholamines and serotonin.[354] However, contractile responses of isolated basilar and middle cerebral arteries to PCP were not prevented or reversed by methysergide, phentolamine, atropine, diphenhydramine, or indomethacin, which raises the possibility of PCP receptors on cerebral blood vessels.[355]

A 13-year-old boy became comatose after taking PCP; admission blood pressure was normal, and he became more alert. Three days later, however, his condition deteriorated, and his blood pressure was 220/130 mm Hg. Autopsy revealed an intracerebral hemorrhage.[353] The urine of a 6-year-old boy who became unresponsive with seizures and right hemiparesis was found to contain PCP; CT demonstrated left parietooccipital lucency and vessel enhancement, suggesting a vascular malformation. He recovered, and cerebral angiography was not performed.[352] A young man collapsed after smoking PCP; his blood pressure was 180/100 mm Hg, and autopsy showed subarachnoid hemorrhage without parenchymal hematoma.[356] A 17-year-old boy with PCP in his blood died after perforation of the ventral surface of the basilar artery.[357] A 44-year-old diabetic, hypertensive man had two episodes of amaurosis fugax a few hours after smoking PCP; his carotid arteries were angiographically normal, and symptoms did not recur during abstinence.[358] Hypertensive encephalopathy followed PCP ingestion in a young woman with systemic lupus erythematosus and a history of migraine.[359]

Lysergic Acid Diethylamide

In high doses, LSD causes severe hypertension, obtundation, and convulsions.[2] In vitro spasm of cerebral vessel strips immersed in LSD-containing solution was prevented or reversed by methysergide.[355] After ingesting four LSD capsules, a 14-year-old boy experienced seizures and, 4 days later, left hemiplegia; carotid angiography showed progressive narrowing of the internal carotid artery from its origin to the siphon, with occlusion at its bifurcation.[360]

A young woman demonstrated sudden left hemiplegia a day after oral ingestion of LSD; angiography showed marked constriction of the internal carotid artery at the siphon; 9 days later, the vessel was occluded at that level.[361]

A 19-year-old with acute aphasia and cerebral angiographic findings consistent with arteritis had used both LSD and heroin, but the time relationship of either drug to the stroke was not stated.[16] Another patient with angiographic evidence of vasculitis had used both LSD and "diet pills."[115]

Marijuana

Marijuana is the most widely used illicit drug in the United States. Reports of marijuana-related stroke are few, however, and not all are convincing.[362] Two young men had only conjugate deviation of the eyes for days or weeks after marijuana use,[363,364] and another young man awoke with dysarthria and hemiparesis the morning after smoking marijuana.[365] In none of these patients was imaging performed. Two young men, both hypertensive cigarette smokers, experienced hemiparesis during marijuana smoking, and CT showed cerebral infarction.[366] Reports describe transient ischemic attacks during marijuana smoking, in some cases followed by infarction.[367-372] Several cases involve cerebellar infarction in teenagers[373,374]; in one of these, the infarct included the territories of the posterior inferior, anterior inferior, and superior cerebellar arteries while entirely sparing the brainstem.[373] Occipital lobe infarction occurred 15 minutes after smoking cannabis in a young man who had smoked several joints per week for many years.[375] A 36-year-old man with no stroke risk factors and negative results on work-up had three cerebral infarcts 1 and 1½ years apart, each time immediately after smoking hashish.[376] In some cases marijuana smoking was accompanied by heavy ethanol consumption. In one of these, MR angiography demonstrated vasospastic narrowing of branches of the left middle and anterior cerebral arteries.[377] Other reports describe cerebral infarction during an episode of coital headache,[378] in an adolescent heterozygous for factor V Leiden mutation,[379] and in a 27-year-old man receiving cisplatin chemotherapy.[380]

A single report of intracerebral hemorrhage in a cannabis user involved a young woman who took daily buprenorphine for heroin addiction and who had smoked several joints daily for over a decade. After the appearance of headache, she continued to smoke cannabis; although her neurologic examination was normal, CT showed a temporal lobe hemorrhage and angiography revealed diffuse cerebral arterial narrowing.[381]

A hospital-based case-control study failed to identify marijuana use as an independent risk factor for stroke.[382]

Proposed mechanisms for alleged marijuana-induced stroke include systemic hypotension (not documented) and cerebral vasospasm. Endocannabinoid receptors are present on sympathetic nerve terminals on systemic and cerebral vessels, and they have vasorelaxant actions both endothelium-independent and dependent.[383,384] Human volunteers receiving infusions of Δ-9-tetrahydrocannibinol (THC, the psychoactive compound in cannabis) developed symptomatic postural hypotension, and transcranial Doppler sonography showed marked reductions in cerebral blood velocity.[385] In another study of volunteers, infusion of THC increased cerebral blood flow in several regions of the cerebral cortex.[386] In both heavy and moderate marijuana users, abstinent for a month, transcranial Doppler sonography demonstrated increased pulsatility index, a measure of cerebrovascular resistance.[387] Cerebral blood volume was increased in marijuana smokers within 36 hours of last use.[388]

Marijuana smoking has been associated with paroxysmal atrial fibrillation and myocardial infarction.[389-391]

In rats, THC has vasoconstrictor action on systemic vessels.[392]

Barbiturates

Usually abused orally, barbiturates and other sedatives and tranquilizers can cause cerebral infarction with overdose and diffusely decreased brain perfusion, but neither occlusive nor hemorrhagic stroke has otherwise been reported. A 20-year-old man taking a combination of secobarbital and strychnine ("M and Ms") orally became comatose with right hemiplegia, and cerebral angiography showed widespread segmental vascular irregularity consistent with arteritis; he had been taking other drugs as well for at least 10 years.[116] Cerebral vasculitis was also found in four other barbiturate abusers; two also abused chlorpromazine, one took other unidentified drugs, and the fourth apparently used only barbiturates, but whether orally or parenterally was not revealed.[115] In monkeys receiving dissolved secobarbital capsules, 1.5 mg/kg intravenously three times a week for 1 year, cerebral angiography showed narrowing of small arteries. Histologic examination found scattered talc crystals in brain capillaries, without cellular reaction; one animal had a frontal lobe microinfarct.[116]

Inhalants

Inhalation of vapors to achieve euphoric intoxication is common in the United States, especially among children. Substances include aerosols, enamels, paint thinners, lighter fluid, cleaning fluid, glues, cements, gasoline, and anesthetics. Death results from violence, accidents, suffocation, aspiration, or cardiac arrhythmia. A 12-year-old who sniffed glue developed hemiplegia, and cerebral angiography showed occlusion of the middle cerebral artery; a proposed mechanism was vasospasm caused by trichloroethylene sensitization of vessel receptors to circulating catecholamines.[393] Radioisotope brain scanning in a boy with status epilepticus after toluene sniffing showed several wedge-shaped areas of increased uptake in both cerebral hemispheres, consistent with infarcts.[394] A 43-year-old man had an aneurysmal subarachnoid hemorrhage while watching a pornographic movie and inhaling amyl nitrite.[395]

Alcohol

Coronary artery disease and myocardial infarction are less prevalent in people who drink moderate amounts of alcohol than in abstainers.[396,397] Heavy drinkers have an increased risk of coronary artery disease, however, resulting in an increased risk of cardioembolic stroke

secondary to cardiac wall hypokinesia or arrhythmia. Alcohol intoxication and withdrawal are also directly associated with cardiac arrhythmia ("holiday heart"),[398] and thromboembolism is a prominent feature of alcoholic cardiomyopathy.[202] A large body of literature has addressed whether short-term or long-term alcohol use is a risk factor for stroke, independent of its cardiac effects or other risk factors.[399-403]

Retrospective studies, most notably from Finland, found an association between recent heavy alcohol use and both ischemic and hemorrhagic strokes.[404-407] The Finnish studies, however, used population prevalence data as a control, and other similarly designed analyses found either no such association[408] or an association only with intracerebral hemorrhage.[409] One study found that the association between alcohol intoxication and stroke disappeared when data were corrected for cigarette smoking.[410,411] The Finnish investigators, reporting that among young adults more strokes occurred during weekends and holidays than expected, observed a stronger association in young women than in young men, which suggests factors other than simply ethanol.

Numerous case-control and cohort studies have addressed the relationship of stroke to chronic alcohol use.[412,438] Contradictory findings are not surprising because studies have differed in endpoints chosen (e.g., total stroke, ischemic stroke, hemorrhagic stroke, or stroke mortality), amount and duration of alcohol consumption, correction for other risk factors (especially hypertension and smoking), ethnicity and socioeconomics of populations being studied, and selection of control subjects. Drinkers tend to be overrepresented among hospitalized control subjects, which leads to the impression that alcohol is protective against stroke; they tend to be underrepresented among community control subjects identified by a questionnaire, which leads to the impression that alcohol is a risk factor for stroke.[439]

Among cohort studies, the Yugoslavia Cardiovascular Disease Study found increased stroke mortality among drinkers, and although the association was especially strong for people with hypertension, it persisted with adjustment for blood pressure.[440,441] A reduced risk was found for modest drinkers. In the Honolulu Heart Study, heavy drinkers had a higher risk of hemorrhagic stroke independent of other risk factors, including hypertension and smoking.[442-445] There was no comparable risk for ischemic stroke. The Framingham Study described lower than expected stroke incidence among "moderate" drinkers and higher rates in both heavy drinkers and nondrinkers.[446] In the Nurses' Health Study, independent of smoking and hypertension, there was an inverse association between modest alcohol intake (fewer than two drinks daily) and ischemic stroke and a positive association at higher intakes; subarachnoid hemorrhage was associated with both low and high alcohol intakes.[447] In the Lausanne Stroke Registry, the severity of internal carotid artery stenosis inversely correlated with "light-to-moderate" alcohol intake; there were too few patients to assess heavy intake.[448] The Japanese Hisayama Study found that heavy drinking conferred higher risk of cerebral hemorrhage in persons with hypertension, whereas light alcohol consumption reduced the risk of cerebral infarction.[449] Four other Japanese studies found either a positive association between stroke mortality and alcohol intake,[450,451] independent associations between alcohol and hemorrhagic but not ischemic stroke,[452] no association between alcohol and ischemic stroke,[453] or a reduced risk of ischemic stroke among mild-to-moderate drinkers and increased risk among heavy drinkers.[454]

A 1989 review of 62 epidemiologic studies concluded that ethnicity played a role in the disparate results.[455] Among white people, moderate doses of alcohol seemed to protect against ischemic stroke, whereas higher doses increased risk. (This pattern is similar to that for alcohol and coronary artery disease.) Among the Japanese, little association seemed to exist between alcohol and ischemic stroke. In both populations, all doses of alcohol seemed to increase the risk of both intracerebral and subarachnoid hemorrhage.

An Australian case-control study found that low doses of ethanol (less than 20 g/day) were protective against "all strokes, all ischemic strokes, and primary intracerebral hemorrhage."[456] A British case-control study found that the protective effect of "light or moderate" drinking compared with nondrinking disappeared when data were corrected for exercise and obesity.[457] In an Italian case-control study, the role of alcohol as a risk factor for stroke "was practically lost" after correction for previous strokes, hypertension, diabetes, obesity, and hyperlipidemia.[412,458] A study from Denmark found that moderate wine drinking reduced the likelihood of stroke, moderate drinking of "spirits" increased the likelihood, and moderate drinking of beer had no effect in either direction.[459] Another Danish study found a decreased risk of stroke (ischemic, hemorrhagic, or not specified) in wine drinkers but not in beer or liquor drinkers.[460]

A Finnish study found that recent heavy drinking increased the risk of embolic stroke in patients with a source of thrombus in the heart or large cerebral vessels.[461] Another Finnish study found a higher risk for hemorrhagic stroke in binge-drinking young adults.[462]

In the Northern Manhattan Stroke Study, "moderate" ethanol intake (two drinks daily) protected against ischemic stroke. Protection was questionable for three to five drinks daily, and seven or more drinks increased the risk. There was no difference in benefit or risk between young and older subjects, between men and women, among white, black, and Hispanic people, or among drinkers of wine, beer, and liquor.[463] In the U.S. Physicians' Health Study, the risk of ischemic stroke was significantly lower in subjects who had more than one drink weekly than in those who drank less. There was no difference in risk reduction between those who had one drink weekly and those who had one or more drinks daily.[464]

In the Framingham Study, when results were stratified according to age, ethanol intake reduced the risk of ischemic stroke only in subjects ages 60 to 69 years, and when results were stratified according to type of beverage, only wine was protective.[465] Remote but not current drinking of 12 or more grams of ethanol daily increased the risk of ischemic stroke in men but not in women; these subjects were older and more often used tobacco.[466]

In the Cardiovascular Health Study the relative risks of ischemic stroke were 0.85, 0.75, 1.06, and 1.03 for 1, 1 to 6, 7 to 13, and 14 or more drinks per week.[467] There were lower risks among drinkers than abstainers in apoE4-negative subjects but higher risks among drinkers than abstainers in apoE4-positive subjects. The apoE4 allele is associated with lower levels of high-density lipoprotein (HDL) and increased risk of vascular disease.[468] In another report from the Cardiovascular Health Study, red wine was associated with risk reduction in a dose-dependent manner, but other beverages were not.[469]

In a prospective study of more than 60,000 Chinese men, alcohol consumption increased the risk of both ischemic and hemorrhagic stroke in a dose-related fashion.[436] In neither stroke subtype could a protective or J-shaped relationship be found, which was consistent with other studies of Asian subjects.[470]

In 2003 a meta-analysis of 19 cohort studies and 16 case-control studies over a period of 2 decades found that compared with abstention, consumption of 12 to 24 g of ethanol per day reduced the risk of ischemic stroke (relative risk, 0.72) but not of hemorrhagic stroke. Consumption of more than 60 g per day increased the risk of both ischemic stroke (relative risk, 1.69) and hemorrhagic stroke (relative risk, 2.18). Thus, as with myocardial infarction (and with the possible exception of East Asians), a J-shaped association appears to exist for ethanol consumption and risk of ischemic stroke, whereas a more linear association exists for ethanol consumption and risk of hemorrhagic stroke.[471]

Studies with duplex ultrasonography and angiography have shown that heavy ethanol consumption raises the risk of carotid artery atherosclerosis, whereas low ethanol intake has a beneficial effect.[472,473] Similarly, a study using CT found that one to five drinks daily reduced the risk of leukoaraiosis in patients with stroke, whereas heavier alcohol consumption increased the risk.[474] The Japanese Hisayama study found alcohol to be an independent risk factor for "vascular dementia."[475] The U.S. Cardiovascular Health Study found a "U-shaped" relationship between alcohol consumption and MRI white matter abnormalities; one to seven drinks per week was most protective.[476] Other studies describe a similar relationship between moderate ethanol consumption and improved cognitive performance; the degree to which such benefit is related to alcohol's effects on cerebral circulation is uncertain.[477-482] In the Rotterdam Study, alcohol was especially effective in reducing the risk of "vascular dementia."[483]

In 2006 the American Heart Association recommended that men limit their alcohol intake to no more than two drinks per day and that women should limit their intake to no more than one drink per day. One drink was considered either 12 ounces of beer, 4 ounces of wine, or 1.5 ounces of 80-proof spirits.[484]

As with coronary artery disease, several mechanisms might explain the association between alcohol and stroke.[485] Alcohol raises blood pressure in the short and long term,[440,442,486-496] perhaps related to increased adrenergic activity and to increased blood levels of cortisol, renin, aldosterone, and vasopressin.[497] Corticotropin-releasing hormone is sympathoexcitatory when administered centrally; in healthy subjects, dexamethasone blocked the increased sympathetic discharge and the increased blood pressure induced by intravenous ethanol.[498] The decline in systolic blood pressure seen during the first week after a stroke is greater in heavy drinkers than in light drinkers or abstainers,[499] and with abstinence, blood pressure may become normal.[500] Perhaps related to its protective effects, alcohol lowers blood levels of low-density lipoproteins (LDLs) and elevates levels of HDLs.[501-504]

Alcohol seems preferentially to protect large vessels from atherosclerosis, perhaps accounting for ethnic differences in patterns of protection or risk.[505] The relationship is uncertain, however, because alcohol may not raise blood levels of the more protective HDL-2 subfraction.[506,507] In the Northern Manhattan Stroke Study, the protective effect of moderate alcohol consumption on stroke risk was independent of the HDL cholesterol level.[463] In the Framingham Study, among men with the apoE2 allele, LDL cholesterol was lower in drinkers than in nondrinkers; among those with the apoE4 allele, LDL cholesterol was higher in drinkers.[508] In the Cardiovascular Health Study alcohol intake was associated with decreased total LDL particles, decreased levels of small LDL, HDL, and very-low-density lipoprotein particles, and higher levels of large LDL and medium- and large-sized HDL particles.[509]

Although heavy alcohol consumption is associated with elevated blood glucose levels, mild-to-moderate drinking lowers the risk of developing type 2 diabetes mellitus.[397,510,511]

Alcohol immediately decreases fibrinolytic activity, increases factor VIII level, increases platelet reactivity to adenosine diphosphate (ADP), and shortens bleeding time.[512-517] Ethanol raises endogenous tissue plasminogen activator,[518] reduces plasma fibrinogen levels,[519] increases levels of prostacyclin,[520,521] decreases platelet function,[480,522-526] and stimulates release of endothelin from endothelial cells.[527] In long-term alcoholics, diminished levels of clotting factors, excessive fibrinolysis, and platelet abnormalities appear to be secondary to liver disease.[497,528]

During or after ethanol withdrawal, "rebound thrombocytosis" and platelet hyperaggregability are observed.[529,530] In rats this rebound followed withdrawal from ethanol or white wine but not from red wine.[531] Human subjects with alcoholism undergoing withdrawal had decreased platelet response to activators[532] and decreased levels of tissue-type plasminogen activator inhibitor.[533]

Nondrinkers and heavy drinkers have higher blood levels of C-reactive protein than moderate drinkers, which is an observation relevant to the probable role of inflammation in atherosclerosis.[534]

Acute alcohol intoxication is accompanied by cerebral vasodilation[535] and blood–brain barrier leakage of albumin,[536] perhaps contributing to the severity of traumatic intracerebral hemorrhage during drinking.[537] Increased cerebral blood flow is also observed during alcohol withdrawal.[538] Compared with nondrinkers, subjects consuming less than one drink per week had increased global cerebral blood flow, whereas in those consuming more than 15 drinks per week cerebral blood flow was decreased.[539] Alcohol-related hemoconcentration may contribute to reduced cerebral blood flow.[497]

In vitro studies involving a variety of mammals show ethanol to be a potent vasoconstrictor of basilar and middle cerebral artery segments.[540] In living rats, ethanol caused vasoconstriction of cerebral arterioles[541] and blocked the vasodilation produced by hypoxia and hypercapnea,[542] acetylcholine, histamine, and ADP but not the vasodilation produced by nitroglycerin or the vasoconstriction produced by a thromboxane analogue.[543] In cultured canine vascular smooth muscle cells, ethanol exposure caused depletion of intracellular magnesium ion.[544] Such an effect could lead to calcium ion overloading, causing both hypertension and cerebral vasoconstriction, and, indeed, pretreatment of animals with magnesium ion prevents ethanol-induced strokes.[545-547]

Hyperhomocysteinemia is a risk factor for both myocardial ischemia and ischemic stroke, and alcoholics often have elevated blood homocysteine levels secondary to deficiency of folate, pyridoxine, or cobalamin.[548]

Studies suggesting a special protective benefit of wine, especially red wine, have led to speculation that the responsible constituents might be free radical scavengers in the form of polyphenols and flavonoids, which, by reducing oxidative damage to LDLs, might reduce atherogenesis.[549-554] Ethanol itself, however, is pro-oxidant.[555]

Tobacco

Epidemiologic studies show smoking to be a major risk factor for coronary artery and peripheral vascular diseases.[556-560] Although a few reports have found no such relationship or have demonstrated only insignificant trends toward higher risk of stroke among smokers,[561-564] most case-control and cohort studies show that smoking does raise the risk of both ischemic and hemorrhagic stroke.[3,303,411,423,435,565-590] In women smokers, the risk of ischemic and hemorrhagic stroke is enhanced in those taking oral contraceptives.[591-595] In a prospective cohort study of middle-aged women, smoking increased stroke risk in a dose-dependent fashion; for those smoking 25 or more cigarettes daily, the relative risk for all stroke was 3.7 and for subarachnoid hemorrhage was 9.8, independent of other risk factors including oral contraceptives, hypertension, and alcohol.[596] In a study of ischemic stroke in young women, the odds ratio comparing smokers with never smokers was 2.2 for 1 to 10 cigarettes per day, 2.5 for 11 to 20, 4.3 for 21 to 39, and 9.1 for 40 or more.[597] In another report, smoking in hypertensive men and women carried a 15-fold risk for subarachnoid hemorrhage and was a greater risk than hypertension itself.[566] In another study, the treatment of hypertension reduced stroke incidence in nonsmokers but not in smokers.[598] Tobacco smoking, hypertension, and high blood cholesterol levels appear to interact synergistically as stroke risk factors.[599] Patients with ischemic stroke who smoke tend to be younger than those who do not.[600]

In the Honolulu Heart Program, stroke risk was independent of coronary artery disease.[601] The Framingham Study found smoking to be a risk factor for subarachnoid hemorrhage and, independent of age and hypertension, for both ischemic and hemorrhagic stroke; this risk was dose-dependent and disappeared when smoking ceased.[602,603] Other researchers have confirmed reduction of stroke risk with cessation of smoking,[577,583,604] but a small long-term excess risk persists.[605] Smoking is a risk factor for central retinal artery occlusion as well as for aortic plaque formation.[606,607]

Smokers were not overrepresented among 624 consecutive patients with nonarteritic ischemic optic neuropathy.[608] Among smokers, the risk of stroke mortality is reduced in those who smoke cigarettes with lower tar yield.[609] On the other hand, stroke was reported after application of a nicotine patch.[610] Several studies found that passive as well as active smoking increased stroke risk,[605,611-614] although a meta-analysis of 16 such studies concluded that a causal relationship was "only suggestive."[615]

A study from Sweden found that although smokeless tobacco (oral snuff) did not increase the risk of stroke, it did increase the risk of fatal stroke.[616]

A study from the United Kingdom estimated that an intensive smoking reduction program (as had been adopted but then abandoned in California) would prevent 455 strokes during the year 2000 and 11,304 strokes by 2010.[617]

A European study, noting a decrease in stroke prevalence in Western Europe but a rise in Eastern Europe, attributed the difference to the higher prevalence of tobacco use in Eastern Europe.[618] A study from China estimated that (1) in 1990, 600,000 Chinese deaths (500,000 in men) were attributable to tobacco, (2) by 2000, this figure would rise to 800,000, and (3) of all Chinese males currently younger than 30 years of age, one third would die prematurely as a consequence of smoking and that 5% to 8% of their deaths would be caused by stroke.[619]

Several possible mechanisms could underlie tobacco's association with risk of stroke.[620] Smoking aggravates atherosclerosis. In a study of identical twins who were discordant for smoking, carotid plaques were significantly more prominent in the smokers, and in other reports, smoking correlated in dose-related fashion with severity of extracranial carotid atherosclerosis.[448,621-623]

In the Atherosclerosis Risk in Communities Study, current cigarette smoking was associated with a 50% increase in the progression over 3 years of carotid artery atherosclerosis compared with nonsmoking; past smoking was associated with a 25% increase, and passive exposure to environmental smoke was associated with a 20% increase.[624] Smoking one cigarette causes transient increases in arterial wall stiffness that increase the likelihood of plaque formation.[625] The reduction in stroke risk with cessation of smoking, however, argues against the possibility that such large vessel atherosclerosis is paramount.[493,626-628] Carbon monoxide in cigarette smoke reduces blood's oxygen-carrying capacity, and nicotine constricts coronary arteries.[629,630] Coronary artery constriction and the greater myocardial oxygen demand induced by cocaine are exacerbated by concomitant tobacco smoking.[631] In animals, nicotine damages endothelium, and increased numbers of circulating endothelial cells are found in smokers.[632,633] A German study found that neonates and children during the first month of life who were exposed to environmental tobacco smoke already demonstrated endothelial cell damage.[634] In mice with long-term exposure to nicotine, aortic walls

exhibited subendothelial edema and swelling of endothelial cells and mitochondria.[633] Bovine endothelial cells exposed to nicotine demonstrated giant cell formation and cellular vacuolization.[635] Cigarette smoking produces superoxide anions, reduces production and availability of nitric oxide, and increases production and release of endothelin.[636]

Smoking immediately raises blood pressure, systolic more than diastolic.[637,638] Whether smoking is a risk factor for chronic hypertension is less clear,[639] although it does accelerate the progression of chronic hypertension to malignant hypertension.[640,641] Smokers become tachycardic, and atrial fibrillation has been observed after chewing nicotine gum.[629]

Smoking activates the coagulant pathway, increases platelet reactivity, and inhibits prostacyclin formation.[626,642-647] It raises blood fibrinogen levels, which is a linkage noted in several stroke studies, and polycythemia secondary to smoking increases blood viscosity.[646] In cultures of human brain endothelial cells, nicotine increased production of plasminogen activator inhibitor-1 (PAI-1).[647]

In rats, nicotine-induced depletion of tissue plasminogen activator was associated with enhanced focal ischemic brain injury.[648] Increased plasma levels of PAI-1 are found in smokers.[649,650] The increased risk of subarachnoid hemorrhage in smokers has been blamed on greater elastolytic activity in the serum.[651] Smokers who receive intravenous thrombolysis for either acute myocardial infarction or acute ischemic stroke have a better early outcome than nonsmokers.[652] A proposed mechanism is that increased circulating levels of fibrinogen induced by smoking makes thrombolysis more effective.[653]

The relative contributions of nicotine, tars, and the gaseous constituents of cigarette smoke to cardiovascular disease are uncertain.[654] Transdermal or oral nicotine produces plasma levels of platelet activation products (platelet factor 4 and β-thromboglobulin) and von Willebrand factor that are intermediate between those of smokers and nonsmokers.[655]

Although stroke was reported after application of a nicotine patch,[610] a meta-analysis of 35 clinical trials involving the transdermal nicotine patch found no excess incidence of myocardial infarction or stroke.[656] Effects of tobacco smoke and nicotine on cerebral blood flow are complex because nicotine has both direct and indirect effects on cerebral vessels themselves as well as on neuronal nicotinic receptors, and both carbon dioxide and nitric oxide are vasodilators. In volunteers, several puffs on a lighted cigarette during a 5-minute period increased middle cerebral artery flow velocity in all subjects; onset and offset were detected within a few seconds of starting and stopping smoking. The effect was independent of CO_2 autoregulation, and in fact, smoking suppressed CO_2-induced vasodilation by 56% in men (but by only 5% in women).[657]

In rats, inhalation of tobacco smoke caused brief constriction of pial arterioles followed by dilation; nicotine infusion caused only vasodilation. The vasodilation was considered the result of sympathetic activation; the vasoconstriction was considered partially the result of thromboxane A_2 induced by other constituents in cigarette smoke.[658] In lenticulostriate arterioles of rats with long-term exposure to nicotine, calcium channels were upregulated and calcium-activated potassium channels were downregulated; the effect was considered the result of decreased bioavailability of endogenous nitric oxide.[659] Nicotine-induced vasodilation of porcine basilar arteries denuded of endothelium was abolished by the nitric oxide synthase inhibitor N-nitro-L-arginine; nicotine was considered to act on nicotinic receptors on presynaptic adrenergic nerve terminals, releasing norepinephrine, which in turn releases nitric oxide from neighboring nitric-oxidergic nerves.[660] In rats, a vasodilator area in the medulla is excited by both hypoxia and microinjections of nicotine.[661]

A possible role for inflammation in tobacco's effects on vessels and coagulation factors is suggested by an increased risk of stroke among young female smokers carrying single nucleotide polymorphisms for particular mediators of inflammation.[662]

Progressive multifocal symptoms were observed in four young women who smoked and used oral contraceptives. Cerebral angiography demonstrated moyamoya vessels, and abnormal study results included elevated ESR, presence of antinuclear antibodies, and elevated CSF IgG. Disease progression ceased with discontinuation of oral contraceptives and reduction in smoking.[663] In another series of 39 patients with moyamoya disease, the use of tobacco and oral contraceptives was also overrepresented.[664]

An elderly man had syncopal spells whenever he stood up after smoking a cigarette; the spells ceased when he stopped smoking. SPECT showed decreased cerebral perfusion "in the posterior circulation structures" after this patient smoked a cigarette or chewed nicotine gum.[665]

REFERENCES

1. Eddy NB, Halbach H, Isbell H, Seevers MH: Drug dependence: Its significance and characteristics, *Bull World Health Organ* 32:721, 1965.
2. Brust JCM: *Neurological aspects of substance abuse*, ed 2, Newton, MA, 2004, Butterworth-Heinemann.
3. Kokkinos J, Levine SR: Stroke, *Neurol Clin* 11:577, 1993.
4. Patel AN: Self-inflicted strokes, *Ann Intern Med* 76:823, 1972.
5. Banks T, Fletcher R, Ali N: Infective endocarditis in heroin addicts, *Am J Med* 55:444, 1973.
6. Buttner A, Mall G, Penning R, et al: The neuropathology of heroin abuse, *Forensic Sci Int* 113:435, 2000.
7. Borne J, Riascos R, Cuellar H, et al: Neuroimaging in drug and substance abuse. Part II: Opioids and solvents, *Top Magn Reson Imaging* 16:239, 2005.
8. Tuazon CU, Sheagren JN: Staphylococcal endocarditis in parenteral drug abusers: Source of the organism, *Ann Intern Med* 82:788, 1975.
9. Hubbell G, Cheitlin MD, Rapaport E: Presentation, management, and follow-up evaluation of infective endocarditis in drug addicts, *Am Heart J* 102:85, 1981.
10. Amine AB: Neurosurgical complications of heroin addiction: Brain abscess and mycotic aneurysm, *Surg Neurol* 7:385, 1977.
11. Gilroy J, Andaya L, Thomas VJ: Intracranial mycotic aneurysms and subacute bacterial endocarditis in heroin addiction, *Neurology* 23:1193, 1973.
12. Brust JCM, Dickinson PCT, Hughes JEO, Holtzman RNN: The diagnosis and treatment of cerebral mycotic aneurysms, *Ann Neurol* 27:238, 1990.
13. Ledgerwood AM, Lucas CE: Mycotic aneurysm of the carotid artery, *Arch Surg* 109:496, 1974.
14. Ho K, Rassekh Z: Mycotic aneurysm of the right subclavian artery: A complication of heroin addiction, *Chest* 74:116, 1978.
15. Brust JCM, Richter RW: Stroke associated with addiction to heroin, *J Neurol Neurosurg Psychiatry* 39:194, 1976.
16. Lignelli GJ, Buchheit WA: Angiitis in drug abusers, *N Engl J Med* 284:112, 1971.
17. Woods BT, Strewler GJ: Hemiparesis occurring six hours after intravenous heroin injection, *Neurology* 22:863, 1972.
18. King J, Richards M, Tress B: Cerebral arteritis associated with heroin abuse, *Med J Aust* 2:444, 1978.
19. Celius EG: Neurologic complications in heroin abuse: Illustrated by two unusual cases, *Tidsskr Nor Laegeforen* 117:356, 1997.
20. Kortikale Blindheit nach Heroin intoxication. Nuklearmedizin 2:N16, 2000.
21. Munoz Casares FC, Serrano Castro P, Linan Lopez M, et al: Sudden aphasia in a young woman, *Rev Clin Esp* 199:325, 1999.
22. Bartolomei F, Nicoli F, Swiader L, Gastaut JL: Accident vasculaire cérébral ischémique après prise nasale d'héroïne: Une nouvelle observation, *Presse Med* 21:983, 1992.
23. Herskowitz A, Gross E: Cerebral infarction associated with heroin sniffing, *South Med J* 66:778, 1973.
24. Knoblauch AL, Buchholz M, Koller MG, Kistler H: Hemiplegie nach Injektion von Heroin, *Schweiz Med Wochenschr* 113:402, 1983.
25. Reynolds EW, Riel-Romero RMS, Bada HS: Neonatal abstinence syndrome and cerebral infarction following maternal codeine use during pregnancy, *Clin Pediatr* 46:639, 2007.
26. Caplan LR, Hier DB, Banks G: Stroke and drug abuse, *Stroke* 13:869, 1982.
27. Ginsberg MD, Hedley-Whyte ET, Richardson EP: Hypoxic-ischemic leukoencephalopathy in man, *Arch Neurol* 33:5, 1976.
28. Jensen R, Olsen TS, Winther BB: Severe non-occlusive ischemic stroke in young heroin addicts, *Acta Neurol Scand* 81:354, 1990.
29. Shoser BG, Groden C: Subacute onset of oculogyric crisis and generalized dystonia following intranasal administration of heroin, *Addiction* 94:431, 1999.
30. Vila N, Chamorro A: Ballistic movements due to ischemic infarcts after intravenous heroin overdose: Report of two cases, *Clin Neurol Neurosurg* 99:259, 1997.
31. Protass LM: Delayed postanoxic encephalopathy after heroin use, *Ann Intern Med* 74:738, 1971.
32. Anderson SN, Skullerud K: Hypoxic/ischemic brain damage, especially pallidal lesions, in heroin addicts, *Forensic Sci Int* 102:51, 1999.
33. Niehaus L, Roricht S, Meyer BU, Sander B: Nuclear magnetic resonance tomography detection of heroin-associated CNS lesions, *Aktuelle Radiol* 7:309, 1997.
34. Zuckerman GB, Ruiz DC, Keller IA, et al: Neurologic complications following intranasal administration of heroin in an adolescent, *Ann Pharmacother* 30:778, 1996.
35. Niehaus L, Meyer B-U: Bilateral borderzone brain infarctions in association with heroin abuse, *J Neurol Sci* 160:180, 1998.
36. Brust JCM, Richter RW: Quinine amblyopia related to heroin addiction, *Ann Intern Med* 74:84, 1971.
37. Levine LH, Hirsch CS, White LW: Quinine cardiotoxicity: A mechanism for sudden death in narcotic addicts, *J Forensic Sci* 18:167, 1973.
38. Atlee W: Talc and cornstarch emboli in eyes of drug abusers, *JAMA* 219:49, 1972.
39. Mizutami T, Lewis R, Gonatas N: Medial medullary syndrome in a drug abuser, *Arch Neurol* 37:425, 1980.
40. Caplan LR, Thomas C, Banks G: Central nervous system complications of addiction to "T's and Blues," *Neurology* 32:623, 1982.
41. Butz WC: Disseminated magnesium and silicate associated with paregoric addiction, *J Forensic Sci* 15:581, 1970.
42. Lee J, Sapira JD: Retinal and cerebral microembolization of talc in a drug abuser, *Am J Med Sci* 265:75, 1973.
43. Biter S, Gomez CR: Stroke following injection of a melted suppository, *Stroke* 24:741, 1993.
44. Cunningham EE, Brentjens JR, Zielezny MA, et al: Heroin nephropathy: A clinicopathologic and epidemiologic study, *Am J Med* 68:47, 1980.
45. Becker C: Medical complications of drug abuse, *Adv Intern Med* 24:183, 1979.
46. Husby G, Pierce PE, Williams RL: Smooth muscle antibody in heroin addicts, *Ann Intern Med* 83:801, 1975.

47. Nickerson DS, Williams RL, Boxmeyer M, et al: Increased opsonic capacity of serum in chronic heroin addiction, *Ann Intern Med* 72:671, 1970.

48. Ortona L, Laghi V, Cauda R: Immune function in heroin addicts, *N Engl J Med* 300:45, 1979.

49. Schoenfeld MR: Acute allergic reactions to morphine, codeine, meperidine hydrochloride, and opium alkaloids, *N Y State J Med* 60:2591, 1960.

50. Ryan JJ, Parker CW, Williams RL: Gamma-globulin binding of morphine in heroin addicts, *J Lab Clin Med* 80:155, 1972.

51. Ringle DA, Herndon BL: In vitro morphine binding by sera from morphine-treated rabbits, *J Immunol* 109:174, 1972.

52. Lee MC, Randa DC, Gold LH: Transverse myelopathy following the use of heroin, *Minn Med* 59:82, 1976.

53. Pearson J, Richter RW, Baden MM, et al: Transverse myelopathy as an illustration of the neurologic and neuropathologic features of heroin addiction, *Hum Pathol* 3:109, 1972.

54. Richter RW, Rosenberg RN: Transverse myelitis associated with heroin addiction, *JAMA* 206:1255, 1968.

55. Schein PS, Yessayun L, Mayman CI: Acute transverse myelitis associated with intravenous opium, *Neurology* 21:101, 1971.

56. Sahni V, Garg D, Garg S, et al: Unusual complications of heroin abuse: transverse myelitis, rhabdomyolysis, compartment syndrome, and ARF, *Clin Toxicol* 46:153, 2008.

57. Henson RA, Parsons M: Ischemic lesions of the spinal cord: An illustrated review, *Q J Med* 36:205, 1967.

58. McCreary M, Emerman C, Hanna J, Simon J: Acute myelopathy following intranasal insufflation of heroin: A case report, *Neurology* 55:316, 2000.

59. Judice DJ, LeBlanc HJ, McGarry PA: Spinal cord vasculitis presenting as spinal cord tumor in a heroin addict, *J Neurosurg* 48:131, 1978.

60. Hirsch CS: Dermatopathology of narcotic addiction, *Hum Pathol* 3:37, 1972.

61. Hall JH, Karp HR: Acute progressive ventral pontine disease in heroin abuse, *Neurology* 23:6, 1973.

62. Jordan SC, Hampson F: Amphetamine poisoning associated with hyperpyrexia, *Br Med J* 2:844, 1960.

63. Lewis E: Hyperpyrexia with antidepressant drugs, *Br Med J* 2:1671, 1965.

64. Zalis EG, Parmley LF: Fatal amphetamine poisoning, *Arch Intern Med* 112:822, 1963.

65. Zalis EG, Lundberg GD, Knutson RA: The pathophysiology of acute amphetamine poisoning with pathologic correlation, *J Pharmacol Exp Ther* 158:115, 1967.

66. Kasirsky G, Zaidi IH, Tansy MF: LD50 and pathologic effects of acute and chronic administration of methamphetamine HCl in rabbits, *Res Commun Chem Pathol Pharmacol* 3:215, 1972.

67. Zalis EG, Kaplan G, Lundberg GD, Knutson RA: Acute lethality of the amphetamines in dogs and its antagonism with curare, *Proc Soc Exp Biol Med* 18:557, 1965.

68. Escalante OD, Ellinwood EH: Central nervous system cytopathological changes in cats with chronic methedrine intoxication, *Brain Res* 21:151, 1970.

69. Clowes GHA, O'Donnell TF: Heat stroke, *N Engl J Med* 291:564, 1974.

70. Shibolet S, Coll R, Gilat T, Sohar E: Heatstroke: Its clinical picture and mechanism in 36 cases, *Q J Med* 36:525, 1967.

71. Cahill DW, Knipp H, Mosser J: Intracranial hemorrhage with amphetamine abuse, *Neurology* 31:1058, 1981.

72. Chynn KY: Acute subarachnoid hemorrhage, *JAMA* 233:55, 1973.

73. Coroner's Report: Amphetamine overdose kills boy, *Pharm J* 198:172, 1967.

74. Delaney P, Estes M: Intracranial hemorrhage with amphetamine abuse, *Neurology* 30:1125, 1980.

75. D'Souza T, Shraberg D: Intracranial hemorrhage associated with amphetamine use, *Neurology* 31:922, 1981.

76. Edwards K: Hemorrhagic complications of cerebral arteritis, *Arch Neurol* 34:549, 1977.

77. Gericke OL: Suicide by ingestion of amphetamine sulfate, *JAMA* 128:1098, 1945.

78. Goodman SJ, Becker DP: Intracranial hemorrhage associated with amphetamine abuse, *JAMA* 212:480, 1970.

79. Hall CD, Blanton DE, Scatliff JH, Morris CE: Speed kills: Fatality from the self administration of methamphetamine intravenously, *South Med J* 66:650, 1973.

80. Harrington H, Heller HA, Dawson D, et al: Intracerebral hemorrhage and oral amphetamine, *Arch Neurol* 40:503, 1983.

81. Kane FJ, Keeler MH, Reifler CB: Neurological crisis following methamphetamine, *JAMA* 210:556, 1969.

82. Kessler JT, Jortner BS, Adapon BD: Cerebral vasculitis in a drug abuser, *J Clin Psychiatry* 39:559, 1978.

83. Lloyd JTA, Walker DRH: Death after combined dexamphetamine and phenylzine, *Br Med J* 2:168, 1965.

84. LoVerme S: Complications of amphetamine abuse. In Culebras A, editor: *Clini-Pearls* Vol 2, No 8. Syracuse, NY, Creative Medical Publications, 1979, p 5.

85. Lukes SA: Intracerebral hemorrhage from an arteriovenous malformation after amphetamine injection, *Arch Neurol* 40:60, 1983.

86. Margolis MT, Newton TH: Methamphetamine ("speed") arteritis, *Neuroradiology* 2:179, 1971.

87. Matick H, Anderson D, Brumlik J: Cerebral vasculitis associated with oral amphetamine overdose, *Arch Neurol* 40:253, 1983.

88. Olsen ER: Intracranial hemorrhage and amphetamine usage, *Angiology* 28:464, 1977.

89. Poteliakhoff A, Roughton BC: Two cases of amphetamine poisoning, *Br Med J* 1:26, 1956.

90. Shukla D: Intracranial hemorrhage associated with amphetamine use, *Neurology* 32:917, 1982.

91. Tibbetts JC, Hinck VC: Conservative management of a hematoma in the fourth ventricle, *Surg Neurol* 1:253, 1973.

92. Weiss SR, Raskind R, Morganstern NL, et al: Intracerebral and subarachnoid hemorrhage following use of methamphetamine ("speed"), *Int Surg* 53:123, 1970.

93. Yarnell PR: "Speed" headache and hematoma, *Headache* 17:69, 1977.

94. Yatsu FM, Wesson DR, Smith DE: Amphetamine abuse. In Richter RW, editor: *Medical aspects of drug abuse*, Hagerstown, Md, 1975, Harper & Row, p 50.

95. Yen DJ, Wang SJ, Ju TH, et al: Stroke associated with methamphetamine inhalation, *Eur Neurol* 34:16, 1994.

96. Yu YJ, Cooper DR, Wellenstein DE, Block B: Cerebral angiitis and intracerebral hemorrhage associated with methamphetamine abuse: Case report, *J Neurosurg* 58:109, 1983.

97. Delaney P: Intracranial hemorrhage associated with amphetamine use, *Neurology* 31:923, 1981.

98. Chen H-J, Liang C-L, Lu K, et al: Rapidly growing internal carotid artery aneurysm after amphetamine abuse. Case Report, *Am J Forensic Med Pathol* 24:32, 2003.

99. McGee SM, McGee DN, McGee MB: Spontaneous intracerebral hemorrhage related to methamphetamine abuse. Autopsy findings and clinical correlation, *Am J Forensic Med Pathol* 25:334, 2004.

100. Shibata S, Mari K, Sekine I, et al: Subarachnoid and intracerebral hemorrhage associated with necrotizing angiitis due to methamphetamine abuse: an autopsy case, *Neurol Med Chir (Tokyo)* 31:49, 1991.

101. Chaudhuri C, Salahudeen AK: Massive intracerebral hemorrhage in an amphetamine addict, *Am J Med Sci* 317:350, 1999.

102. Perez JA, Arsura EL, Strategos S: Methamphetamine-related stroke: four cases, *J Emerg Med* 17:469, 1999.

103. Miranda J, O'Neill D: Stroke associated with amphetamine use, *Ir Med J* 95:281, 2002.

104. Schuff A, Skopp G, Pedalund I, et al: Cerebral hemorrhage after the consumption of amphetamine, *Arch Kriminol* 216:36, 2005.

105. Huang W, Ralph J, Marco E, et al: Incomplete Brown-Séquard syndrome after methamphetamine injection into the neck, *Neurology* 60:2015, 2003.

106. Lambrecht GL, Malbrain ML, Chew SL, et al: Intranasal caffeine and amphetamine causing stroke, *Acta Neurol Belg* 93:146, 1993.

107. Bostwick DG: Amphetamine induced cerebral vasculitis, *Hum Pathol* 12:1031, 1981.

108. Miller MA, Coon TP: Delayed ischemic stroke associated with methamphetamine use, *J Emerg Med* 31:305, 2006.

109. McIntosh A, Hungs M, Kostanian V, et al: Carotid artery dissection and middle cerebral artery stroke following methamphetamine use, *Neurology* 67:2259, 2006.

110. Petitti DB, Sidney S, Quesenberry C, et al: Stroke and cocaine or amphetamine use, *Epidemiology* 9:596, 1998.
111. Westover AN, McBride S, Haley RW: Stroke in young adults who abuse amphetamines or cocaine. A population-based study of hospitalized patients, *Arch Gen Psychiatry* 64:495, 2007.
112. Citron BP, Halpern M, McCarron M, et al: Necrotizing angiitis associated with drug abuse, *N Engl J Med* 283:1003, 1970.
113. Gocke DJ, Christian CL: Angiitis in drug abusers, *N Engl J Med* 284:112, 1971.
114. Citron BP, Peters RL: Angiitis in drug abusers, *N Engl J Med* 284:111, 1971.
115. Rumbaugh CL, Bergeron RT, Fang HCH, McCormick R: Cerebral angiographic changes in the drug abuse patient, *Radiology* 101:335, 1971.
116. Rumbaugh CL, Fang HCH: The effects of drug abuse on the brain, *Med Times* 108:37S, 1980.
117. DeSilva DA, Wang MC, Lee MP, et al: Amphetamine-associated ischemic stroke: Clinical presentation and proposed pathogenesis, *J Stroke Cerebrovasc Dis* 16:185, 2007.
118. Rothrock JF, Rubenstein R, Lyden PD: Ischemic stroke associated with methamphetamine inhalation, *Neurology* 38:589, 1988.
119. Sachdeva K, Woodward KG: Caudal thalamic infarction following intranasal methamphetamine use, *Neurology* 39:305, 1989.
120. Rumbaugh CL, Bergeron T, Scanlon RL, et al: Cerebral vascular changes secondary to amphetamine abuse in the experimental animal, *Radiology* 101:345, 1971.
121. Rumbaugh CL, Fang HCH, Higgins RE, et al: Cerebral microvascular injury in experimental drug abuse, *Invest Radiol* 11:282, 1976.
122. Hartman BK, Zide D, Udenfriend A: The use of dopamine beta-hydroxylase as a marker for the central noradrenergic nervous system in rat brain, *Proc Natl Acad Sci U S A* 69:2722, 1972.
123. Stafford CR, Bogdanoff BM, Green L, Spector HB: Mononeuropathy multiplex as a complication of amphetamine angiitis, *Neurology* 25:570, 1975.
124. Hwang J, Lyoo IK, Kim SJ, et al: Decreased cerebral blood flow of the right anterior cingulate cortex in long-term and short-term abstinent methamphetamine users, *Drug Alcohol Depend* 82:177, 2006.
125. Wang Y, Haysahi T, Chang C-F, et al: Methamphetamine potentiates ischemia/reperfusion insults after transient middle cerebral artery ligation, *Stroke* 32:775, 2001.
126. Blum A: Phenylpropanolamine: An over-the-counter amphetamine? *JAMA* 245:1346, 1981.
127. Mueller SM: Neurologic complications of phenylpropanolamine use, *Neurology* 33:650, 1983.
128. Bernstein E, Diskant B: Phenylpropanolamine: A potentially hazardous drug, *Ann Emerg Med* 11:315, 1982.
129. Forman HP, Levin S, Stewart B, et al: Cerebral vasculitis and hemorrhage in an adolescent taking diet pills containing phenylpropanolamine: Case report and review of the literature, *Pediatrics* 83:737, 1989.
130. Kane FJ, Greene BQ: Psychotic episodes associated with the use of common proprietary decongestants, *Am J Psychiatry* 123:484, 1966.
131. King J: Hypertension and cerebral hemorrhage after trimolets ingestion, *Med J Aust* 2:258, 1979.
132. Lovejoy FH: Stroke and phenylpropanolamine, *Pediatr Alert* 12:45, 1981.
133. Mueller SM, Ertel PJ: Subarachnoid hemorrhage associated with over-the-counter diet medications, *Stroke* 14:16, 1983.
134. Mueller SM, Solow EB: Seizures associated with a new combination "pick-me-up" pill, *Ann Neurol* 11:322, 1982.
135. Ostern S, Dodson WH: Hypertension following Ornade ingestion, *JAMA* 194:472, 1965.
136. Schaffer CB, Pauli MW: Psychotic reaction caused by proprietary oral diet agents, *Am J Psychiatry* 137:1256, 1980.
137. Wharton BK: Nasal decongestants and paranoid psychosis, *Br J Psychiatry* 117:429, 1970.
138. Ryu SJ, Lin SK: Cerebral arteritis associated with oral use of phenylpropanolamine: Report of a case, *J Formos Med Assoc* 94:53, 1995.
139. Kernan WN, Viscdi CM, Brass LM, et al: Phenylpropanolamine and the risk of hemorrhagic stroke, *N Engl J Med* 343:1826, 2000.
140. Fleming GA: The FDA, regulation, and the risk of stroke, *N Engl J Med* 343:1886, 2000.
141. Cantu C, Arauz A, Murillo-Bonilla LM, et al: Stroke associated with sympathomimetics contained in over-the-counter cough and cold drugs, *Stroke* 34:1667, 2003.
142. Brust JCM: Over-the-counter cold remedies and stroke, *Stroke* 34:1673, 2003.
143. Yoon B-W, Park BJ, Bae HJ, et al: Phenylpropanolamine contained in cold remedies and risk of hemorrhagic stroke, *Neurology* 68:146, 2007.
144. Bruno A, Nolte KB, Chapin J: Stroke associated with ephedrine use, *Neurology* 43:1313, 1993.
145. Garcia-Albea E: Subarachnoid hemorrhage and nasal vasoconstrictor abuse, *J Neurol Neurosurg Psychiatry* 46:875, 1983.
146. Loizou LA, Hamilton JG, Tsementzis SA: Intracranial hemorrhage in association with pseudoephedrine overdose, *J Neurol Neurosurg Psychiatry* 45:471, 1982.
147. Mariani PJ: Pseudoephedrine-induced hypertensive emergency: Treatment with labetalol, *Am J Emerg Med* 4:141, 1986.
148. Pentel P: Toxicity of over-the-counter stimulants, *JAMA* 252:1898–1903, 1984.
149. Stoessl AJ, Young G, Feasby TE: Intracerebral hemorrhage and angiographic beading following ingestion of catecholaminergics, *Stroke* 16:734, 1985.
150. Kurth T: Over-the-counter cough and cold medication use and risk for hemorrhagic stroke, *Neurology* 61:724, 2003.
151. Wooten MR, Khangure MS, Murphy MJ: Intracerebral hemorrhage and vasculitis related to ephedrine abuse, *Ann Neurol* 13:337, 1983.
152. Mourand I, Ducrocq X, Lacour JC, et al: Acute reversible cerebral arteritis associated with parenteral ephedrine use, *Cerebrovasc Dis* 9:355, 1999.
153. Baker SK, Silva JE, Lam KK: Pseudoephedrine-induced hemorrhage associated with a cerebral vascular malformation, *Can J Neurol Sci* 32:248, 2005.
154. Singhal AB, Caviness VS, Begleiter AF, et al: Cerebral vasoconstriction and stroke after use of serotonergic drugs, *Neurology* 58:130, 2002.
155. Adverse events associated with ephedrine-containing products-Texas, December 1993-September 1995, *JAMA* 276:1711, 1996.
156. Josefson D: Herbal stimulant causes U.S. deaths, *BMJ* 312:1378, 1996.
157. Theoharides TC: Sudden death of a healthy college student related to ephedrine toxicity from a ma huang-containing drink, *J Clin Psychopharmacol* 17:437, 1997.
158. Vahedi K, Domingo V, Amarenco R, Bousser MG: Ischemic stroke in a sportsman who consumed MaHuang extract and creatine monohydrate for body building, *J Neurol Neurosurg Psychiatry* 68:112, 2000.
159. Haller CA, Benowitz NL: Adverse cardiovascular and central nervous system events associated with dietary supplements containing ephedra alkaloids, *N Engl J Med* 343:1833, 2000.
160. Shekelle PG, Hardy ML, Morton SC, et al: Efficacy and safety of ephedra and ephedrine for weight loss and athletic performance. A meta-analysis, *JAMA* 289:1537, 2003.
161. Karch SB: Use of ephedra-containing products and risk for hemorrhagic stroke, *Neurology* 61:724, 2003.
162. Morgenstern MD, Viscoli CM, Kernan WN, et al: Use of ephedra-containing products and risk for hemorrhagic stroke, *Neurology* 60:132, 2003.
163. Kokkinos J, Levine SR: Possible association of ischemic stroke with phentermine, *Stroke* 24:310, 1993.
164. Wen PY, Feske SK, Teoh SK, Steig PE: Cerebral hemorrhage in a patient taking fenfluramine and phentermine for obesity, *Neurology* 49:632, 1997.
165. Schwitler J, Agosti R, Ott P, et al: Small infarctions of cochlear, retinal, and encephalic tissue in young women, *Stroke* 23:903, 1992.
166. Darby LE, Myers MW, Jick H: Use of dexfenfluramine, fenfluramine, and phentermine and the risk of stroke, *Br J Clin Pharmacol* 47:565, 1999.
167. Gardin JM, Schumacher D, Constantine G, et al: Valvular abnormalities and cardiovascular status following exposure to dexfenfluramine or phentermine/fenfluramine, *JAMA* 283:1703, 2000.
168. Schifano F, Oyefeso A, Webb L, et al: Review of deaths related to taking ecstasy, England and Wales, 1997-2000, *BMJ* 326:80, 2003.

169. McEvoy AW, Kitchen ND, Thomas DG: Intracerebral hemorrhage and drug abuse in young adults, *Br J Neurosurg* 14:449, 2000.

170. Hanyu S, Ikeguchi K, Imai H, et al: Cerebral infarction association with 3,4-methylenedioxymethamphetamine ("Ecstasy") abuse, *Eur Neurol* 35:173, 1995.

171. McCann U, Slate SO, Ricuarte GA: Adverse reaction with 3, 4-methylenedioxymethamphetamine (MDMA, ecstasy), *Drug Saf* 15:107, 1996.

172. Harris DP, DeSilva R: "Ecstasy" and intracerebral hemorrhage, *Scott Med J* 37:150, 1992.

173. Gledhill JA, Moore DF, Bell D, et al: Subarachnoid hemorrhage associated with MDMA abuse, *J Neurol Neurosurg Psychiatry* 56:1036, 1993.

174. Hughes JC, McCabe M, Evans RJ: Intracranial haemorrhage associated with ingestion of "ecstasy," *Arch Emerg Med* 10:372, 1993.

175. Schlaeppi M, Price A, de Torrente A: Hemorrhagie cerebrale et "ecstasy," *Schweiz Rundsch Med Prax* 88:568, 1999.

176. Jacks AS, Hykin PJ: Retinal hemorrhage caused by "ecstasy," *Br J Ophthalmol* 82:842, 1998.

177. Manchanda S, Connolly MJ: Cerebral infarction in association with Ecstasy abuse, *Postgrad Med J* 69:874, 1993.

178. Reneman L, Habraken JB, Majoie CB, et al: MDMA ("Ecstasy") and its association with cerebrovascular accidents: Preliminary findings, *Am J Neuroradiol* 21:1001, 2000.

179. Auer J, Berent R, Weber T, et al: Subarachnoid hemorrhage with "Ecstasy" abuse in a young adult, *Neurol Sci* 23:199, 2002.

180. Vallée JH, Crozier S, Guillerin R, et al: Acute basilar artery occlusion treated by thromboaspiration in a cocaine and ecstasy abuser, *Neurology* 61:839, 2003.

181. Spatt J, Glawar B, Mamoli B: A pure amnestic syndrome after MDMA ("ecstasy") ingestion, *J Neurol Neurosurg Psychiatry* 62:418, 1997.

182. Chillar RK, Jackson AL: Reversible hemiplegia after presumed intracarotid injection of Ritalin, *N Engl J Med* 304:1305, 1981.

183. Tse DT, Ober RR: Talc retinopathy, *Am J Ophthalmol* 90:624, 1980.

184. Thomalla G, Kucinski T, Weiller C, et al: Cerebral vasculitis following oral methylphenidate intake in an adult: A case report, *World J Biol Psychiatry* 7:56, 2006.

185. Trugman JM: Cerebral arteritis and oral methylphenidate, *Lancet* 1:584, 1988.

186. Schteinschnaider A, Plaghos LL, Garbugino S, et al: Cerebral arteritis following methylphenidate use, *J Child Neurol* 15:265, 2000.

187. Hamer R, Phelp D: Inadvertent intra-arterial injection of phentermine: A complication of drug abuse, *Ann Emerg Med* 10:148, 1981.

188. Anderson RJ, Garza H, Garriott JC, Dimaio V: Intravenous propylhexedrine (Benzedrex) abuse and sudden death, *Am J Med* 67:15, 1979.

189. Riddick L, Reisch R: Oral overdose of propylhexedrine, *J Forensic Sci* 26:834, 1981.

190. Margaral LE, Sanborn GE, Donoso LA, et al: Branch retinal artery occlusion after excessive use of nasal spray, *Ann Ophthalmol* 17:500, 1985.

191. Montalban J, Ibanez L, Rodriguez C, et al: Cerebral infarction after excessive use of nasal decongestants, *J Neurol Neurosurg Psychiatry* 52:541, 1989.

192. Delodovici ML, Cavaletti G, Crespi V, et al: Intracerebral hemorrhage following intravenous administration of epinephrine, *Riv Neurol* 59:64, 1989.

193. Cartwright MS, Reynolds PS: Intracerebral hemorrhage associated with over-the-counter inhaled epinephrine, *Cerebrovasc Dis* 19:415, 2005.

194. Kaku DA, Lowenstein DH: Emergence of recreational drug abuse as a major risk factor for stroke in young adults, *Ann Intern Med* 113:821, 1990.

195. Levine SR, Brust JCM, Futrell N, et al: Cerebrovascular complications of the use of the "crack" form of alkaloidal cocaine, *N Engl J Med* 323:699, 1990.

196. Koch S, Sacco RL: Cocaine-associated stroke: some new insights? *Nat Clin Pract Neurol* 4:579, 2008.

197. Brust JCM, Richter RW: Stroke associated with cocaine abuse? *N Y State J Med* 77:1473, 1977.

198. Lundberg GD, Garriott JC, Reynolds PC, et al: Cocaine-related death, *J Forensic Sci* 22:402, 1977.

199. Mittleman RE, Wetli CV: Cocaine and sudden "natural" death, *J Forensic Sci* 32:11, 1987.

200. Altes-Capella J, Cabezudo-Artero JM, Forteza-Rei J: Complications of cocaine abuse, *Ann Intern Med* 107:940, 1987.

201. Baquero M, Alfaro A: Progressive bleeding in spontaneous thalamic hemorrhage, *Neurologia* 9:364, 1994.

202. Caplan LR, Hier DB, DeCruz I: Cerebral embolism in the Michael Reese Stroke Registry, *Stroke* 14:530, 1983.

203. Case records of the Massachusetts General Hospital: Weekly clinicopathological exercises. Case 27-1993: A 32-year-old man with the sudden onset of a right-sided headache and left hemiplegia and hemianesthesia, *N Engl J Med* 329:117, 1993.

204. Chadan N, Thierry A, Sautreaux JL, et al: Rupture aneurysmale et toxicomanie á la cocaine, *Neurochirurgie* 37:403, 1990.

205. Chasnoff IJ, Bussey ME, Savich R, Stack CM: Perinatal cerebral infarction and maternal cocaine use, *J Pediatr* 108:456, 1986.

206. Cregler LL, Mark H: Medical complications of cocaine abuse, *N Engl J Med* 315:1495, 1986.

207. Cregler LL, Mark H: Relation of stroke to cocaine abuse, *NY State J Med* 87:128, 1987.

208. Daras M, Tuchman AJ, Koppel BS, et al: Neurovascular complications of cocaine, *Acta Neurol Scand* 90:124, 1994.

209. Daras M, Tuchman AJ, Marks S: Central nervous system infarction related to cocaine abuse, *Stroke* 22:1320, 1991.

210. DeBroucker T, Verstichel P, Cambier J, De-Truchis P: Accidents neurologiqes après prise de cocaine, *Presse Med* 18:541, 1989.

211. Derby LE, Myers MW, Jick H: Use of dexfenfluramine, fenfluramine and phentermine and the risk of stroke, *Br J Clin Pharmacol* 47:565, 1999.

212. Devenyi P, Schneiderman JF, Devenyi RG, Lawby L: Cocaine-induced central retinal artery occlusion, *CMAJ* 138:129, 1988.

213. Devore RA, Tucker HM: Dysphagia and dysarthria as a result of cocaine abuse, *Otolaryngol Head Neck Surg* 98:174, 1988.

214. Dominguez R, Vila-Coro AA, Slopis JM, Bohan TP: Brain and ocular abnormalities in infants with in utero exposure to cocaine and other street drugs, *Am J Dis Child* 145:688, 1991.

215. Engstrand BC, Daras M, Tuchman AJ, et al: Cocaine-related ischemic stroke, *Neurology* 39(Suppl 1):186, 1989.

216. Fredericks RK, Lefkowitz DS, Challa VER, Troost BT: Cerebral vasculitis associated with cocaine abuse, *Stroke* 22:1437, 1991.

217. Golbe LI, Merkin MD: Cerebral infarction in a user of free-base cocaine ("crack"), *Neurology* 36:1602, 1986.

218. Green R, Kelly KM, Gabrielson T, et al: Multiple intracerebral hemorrhages after smoking "crack" cocaine, *Stroke* 21:957, 1990.

219. Guidotti M, Zanasi S: Cocaine use and cerebrovascular disease: Two cases of ischemic stroke in young adults, *Ital J Neurol Sci* 11:153, 1990.

220. Hall JAS: Cocaine-induced stroke: First Jamaican case, *J Neurol Sci* 98:347, 1990.

221. Hamer JJ, Kamphuis DJ, Rico RE: Cerebral hemorrhages and infarcts following use of cocaine, *Ned Tijdschr Geneeskd* 135:333, 1991.

222. Harruff RC, Phillips AM, Fernandez GS: Cocaine-related deaths in Memphis and Shelby County: Ten-year history, 1980-1989, *J Tenn Med Assoc* 84:66, 1991.

223. Heier LA, Carpanzano CR, Mast J, et al: Maternal cocaine abuse: The spectrum of radiologic abnormalities in the neonatal CNS, *AJR* 157:1105, 1991.

224. Henderson CE, Torbey M: Rupture of intracranial aneurysm associated with cocaine use during pregnancy, *Am J Perinatol* 5:142, 1988.

225. Hoyme HE, Jones KL, Dixon SD, et al: Prenatal cocaine exposure and fetal vascular disruption, *Pediatrics* 85:743, 1990.

226. Jacobs IG, Roszler MH, Kelly JK, et al: Cocaine abuse: Neurovascular complications, *Radiology* 170:223, 1989.

227. Kaku DA, Lowenstein DH: Recreational drug use: A growing risk factor for stroke in young people, *Neurology* 39(Suppl 1):16, 1989.

228. Kaye BR, Fainstat M: Cerebral vasculitis associated with cocaine abuse, *JAMA* 258:2104, 1987.

229. Klonoff DC, Andrews BT, Obana WG: Stroke associated with cocaine use, *Arch Neurol* 46:989, 1989.

230. Konzen JP, Levine SR, Charbel FT, Garcia JH: The mechanisms of alkaloidal cocaine-related stroke, *Neurology* 42(Suppl 3):249, 1992.

231. Koppel BS, Kaunitz AM, Daras M, et al: Cocaine-associated stroke during pregnancy, *Ann Neurol* 32:239, 1992.

232. Kramer LD, Locke GE, Ogunyemi A, Nelson L: Neonatal cocaine-related seizures, *J Child Neurol* 5:60, 1990.

233. Krendel DA, Ditter SM, Frankel MR, Ross WK: Biopsy-proven cerebral vasculitis associated with cocaine abuse, *Neurology* 40:1092, 1990.

234. Lehman LB: Intracerebral hemorrhage after intranasal cocaine use, *Hosp Physician* 7:69, 1987.

235. Levine SR, Washington JM, Jefferson MF, et al: "Crack" cocaine-associated stroke, *Neurology* 37:1849–1853, 1987.

236. Levine SR, Welch KM: Cocaine and stroke, *Stroke* 19:779, 1988.

237. Libman RB, Masters SR, de Paola A, Mohr JP: Transient monocular blindness associated with cocaine abuse, *Neurology* 43:228, 1993.

238. Lichtenfield PJ, Rubin DB, Feldman RS: Subarachnoid hemorrhage precipitated by cocaine snorting, *Arch Neurol* 41:223, 1984.

239. Lowenstein DH, Massa SM, Rowbotham MC, et al: Acute neurologic and psychiatric complications associated with cocaine abuse, *Am J Med* 83:841, 1987.

240. Mangiardi JR, Daras M, Geller ME, et al: Cocaine-related intracranial hemorrhage: Report of nine cases and reviews, *Acta Neurol Scand* 77:177, 1988.

241. Martin K, Rogers T, Kavanaugh A: Central nervous system angiopathy associated with cocaine abuse, *J Rheumatol* 22:780, 1995.

242. Mercado A, Johnson G, Calver D, Sokol RJ: Cocaine, pregnancy, and postpartum intracerebral hemorrhage, *Obstet Gynecol* 73:467, 1989.

243. Meza I, Estrad CA, Montalvo JA, et al: Cerebral infarction associated with cocaine use, *Henry Ford Hosp Med J* 37:50, 1989.

244. Moore PM, Peterson PL: Nonhemorrhagic cerebrovascular complications of cocaine abuse, *Neurology* 39(Suppl 1):302, 1989.

245. Morrow PL, McQuillen JB: Cerebral vasculitis associated with cocaine abuse, *J Forensic Sci* 38:732, 1993.

246. Nalls G, Disher A, Darabagi J, et al: Subcortical cerebral hemorrhages associated with cocaine abuse: CT and MR findings, *J Comput Assist Tomogr* 13:1, 1989.

247. Nolte KB, Brass LM, Fletterick CF: Intracranial hemorrhage associated with cocaine abuse: A prospective autopsy study, *Neurology* 46:1291, 1996.

248. Nolte KB, Gelman BB: Intracerebral hemorrhage associated with cocaine abuse, *Arch Pathol Lab Med* 113:812, 1989.

249. Nwosu CM, Nwabueze AC, Ikeh VO: Stroke at the prime of life: A study of Nigerian Africans between the ages of 16 and 45 years, *East Afr Med J* 69:384, 1992.

250. Peterson PL, Moore PM: Hemorrhagic cerebrovascular complications of crack cocaine abuse, *Neurology* 39(Suppl 1):302, 1989.

251. Peterson PL, Roszler M, Jacobs I, Wilner HI: Neurovascular complications of cocaine abuse, *J Neuropsychiatry Clin Neurosci* 3:143–149, 1991.

252. Petty GW, Brust JCM, Tatemichi TK, Barr ML: Embolic stroke after smoking "crack" cocaine, *Stroke* 21:1632, 1990.

253. Qureshi AI, Safdar K, Patel M, et al: Stroke in young black patients: Risk factors, subtypes, and prognosis, *Stroke* 26:1995, 1995.

254. Ramadan J, Levine SR, Welch KMA: Pontine hemorrhage following "crack" cocaine use, *Neurology* 41:946, 1991.

255. Reeves RR, McWilliams ME, Fitzgerald MJ: Cocaine-induced ischemic cerebral infarction mistaken for a psychiatric syndrome, *South Med J* 88:352, 1995.

256. Rogers JN, Henry TE, Jones AM, et al: Cocaine-related deaths in Pima Country, Arizona, 1982-1984, *J Forensic Sci* 31:1404, 1986.

257. Rowbotham MC: Neurologic aspects of cocaine abuse, *West J Med* 149:442, 1988.

258. Rowley HA, Lowenstein DH, Rowbotham MC, Simon RP: Thalamomesencephalic strokes after cocaine abuse, *Neurology* 39:428, 1989.

259. Sauer CM: Recurrent embolic stroke and cocaine-related cardiomyopathy, *Stroke* 22:1203, 1991.

260. Schwartz ICA, Cohen JA: Subarachnoid hemorrhage precipitated by cocaine snorting, *Arch Neurol* 41:705, 1984.

261. Seaman ME: Acute cocaine abuse associated with cerebral infarction, *Ann Emerg Med* 19:34, 1990.

262. Simpson RK, Fischer DK, Narayan RK, et al: Intravenous cocaine abuse and subarachnoid hemorrhage: Effect on outcome, *Br J Neurosurg* 4:27, 1990.

263. Singer LT, Yamashita TS, Hawkins S, et al: Increased incidence of intraventricular hemorrhage and developmental delay in cocaine-exposed, very low birth weight infants, *J Pediatr* 124:765, 1994.

264. Sloan MA, Kittner SJ, Rigamonti D, Price TR: Occurrence of stroke associated with use/abuse of drugs, *Neurology* 41:1358, 1991.

265. Sloan MA, Mattioni TA: Concurrent myocardial and cerebral infarctions after intranasal cocaine use, *Stroke* 23:427, 1992.

266. Spires MC, Gordon EF, Choudhuri M, et al: Intracranial hemorrhage in a neonate following prenatal cocaine exposure, *Pediatr Neurol* 5:324, 1989.

267. Tardiff K, Gross E, Wu J, et al: Analysis of cocaine-positive fatalities, *J Forensic Sci* 34:53, 1989.

268. Toler KA, Anderson B: Stroke in an intravenous drug user secondary to the lupus anticoagulant, *Stroke* 19:274, 1988.

269. Vivancos F, Diez-Tejedor E, Martinez N, et al: Stroke due to abuse of cocaine, *J Neurol* 24(Suppl 1):S39, 1994.

270. Weingarten KO: Cerebral vasculitis associated with cocaine abuse or subarachnoid hemorrhage? *JAMA* 259:1658, 1988.

271. Wojak JC, Flamm ES: Intracranial hemorrhage and cocaine use, *Stroke* 18:712, 1987.

272. Fessler RD, Esshaki CM, Stankewitz RC, et al: The neurovascular complications of cocaine, *Surg Neurol* 47:339, 1997.

273. Hoebert M, Houben MP, Jansen BP, et al: Cerebral infarction after cocaine use, *Ned Tijdschr Geneeskd* 150:2789, 2006.

274. Schreiber AL, Formal CS: Spinal cord infarction secondary to cocaine use, *Am J Phys Med Rehabil* 86:158, 2007.

275. Anand S, Chodorowski Z, Wisniewski M, et al: A cocaine-associated quadriplegia and motor aphasia after first use of cocaine, *Przegl Lek* 64:316, 2007.

276. Zandio Amorena B, Erro Aguire ME, Cabada T, et al: Cocaine-induced brain stem stroke associated to cranial midline destructive lesions, *Neurologia* 23:55, 2008.

277. Bolouri MR, Small GA: Neuroimaging of hypoxia and cocaine-induced hippocampal stroke, *J Neuroimaging* 14:290, 2004.

278. Mody CK, Miller BL, McIntyre HB, et al: Neurologic complications of cocaine abuse, *Neurology* 38:1189, 1988.

279. DiLazzaro V, Restuccia D, Oliviero A, et al: Ischemic myelopathy associated with cocaine: Clinical, neurophysiological, and neuroradiological features, *J Neurol Neurosurg Psychiatry* 63:531, 1997.

280. Migita DS, Devereaux MW, Tomsak RL: Cocaine and pupillary-sparing oculomotor paresis, *Neurology* 49:1466, 1997.

281. Brown E, Prajer J, Lee HY, Ramsey RG: CNS complications of cocaine abuse: Prevalence, pathophysiology, and neuroradiology, *AJR Am J Roentgenol* 159:137, 1992.

282. Mena I, Giombetti RJ, Miller BL, et al: Cerebral blood flow changes with acute cocaine intoxications: Clinical correlations with SPECT, CT, and MRI, *NIDA Res Monogr* 138:161, 1994.

283. Sawaya GR, Kaminski MJ: Spinal cord infarction after cocaine use, *South Med J* 83:601, 1990.

284. Strupp M, Hamann GF, Brandt T: Combined amphetamine and cocaine abuse caused mesencephalic ischemia in a 16-year-old boy—due to vasospasm? *Eur Neurol* 43:181, 2000.

285. Tolat D, O'Dell WO, Golamco-Estrella SP, Avella H: Cocaine-associated stroke: Three cases and rehabilitation considerations, *Brain Inj* 14:383, 2000.

286. Storen EC, Wijdicks EFM, Crum BA, Schultz G: Moyamoya-like vasculopathy from cocaine dependency, *AJNR Am J Neuroradiol* 21:1008, 2000.

287. Levine SR, Brust JCM, Welch KMA: Cerebral vasculitis associated with cocaine abuse or subarachnoid hemorrhage, *JAMA* 259:1648, 1988.

288. Deringer PM, Hamilton LL, Whelan MA: A stroke associated with cocaine use, *Arch Neurol* 47:502, 1990.

289. LaMonica G, Donatelli A, Katz JL: A case of mutism subsequent to cocaine abuse, *J Subst Abuse Treat* 17:109, 1999.

290. Bartzokis G, Beckson M, Hance DB, et al: Magnetic resonance imaging evidence of "silent" cerebrovascular toxicity in cocaine dependence, *Biol Psychiatry* 45:1203, 1999.

291. Streeter LIK, Ahn KH, Lee HK, et al: White matter hyperintensities in subjects with cocaine and opiate dependence and healthy comparison subjects, *Psychiatry Res* 131:135, 2004.

292. Leung IY, Lais S, Ren S, et al: Early retinal vascular abnormalities in African-American cocaine users, *Am J Ophthalmol* 146:612, 2008.

293. Aggarwal SK, Williams V, Levine SR, et al: Cocaine-associated intracranial hemorrhage: Absence of vasculitis in 14 cases, *Neurology* 46:1741, 1996.

294. Davis GG, Swalwell CI: The incidence of acute cocaine or methamphetamine intoxication in deaths due to ruptured cerebral (berry) aneurysms, *J Forensic Sci* 41:626, 1996.

295. Kibayashi K, Mastri AR, Hirsch CS: Cocaine-induced intracerebral hemorrhage: Analysis of predisposing factors and mechanisms causing hemorrhagic strokes, *Hum Pathol* 26:659, 1996.

296. Egido-Herrero JA, Gonzalez JL: Pontine hemorrhage after abuse of cocaine, *Rev Neurol* 25:137, 1997.

297. Oyesiku NM, Colohan AR, Barrow DL, Reisner A: Cocaine-induced aneurysmal rupture: An emergent factor in the natural history of intracranial aneurysms, *Neurosurgery* 32:518, 1993.

298. Samkoff LM, Daras M, Kleiman A, Koppell BS: Spontaneous spinal epidural hematoma: Another neurologic complication of cocaine? *Arch Neurol* 53:819, 1996.

299. Keller TM, Chappell ET: Spontaneous acute epidural hematoma precipitated by cocaine abuse: Case report, *Surg Neurol* 47:12, 1997.

300. Conway JE, Tamargo RJ: Cocaine use is an independent risk factor for cerebral vasospasm after aneurysmal subarachnoid hemorrhage, *Stroke* 32:2338, 2001.

301. Qureshi AI, Akbar MS, Czander E, et al: Crack cocaine use and stroke in young patients, *Neurology* 48:341, 1997.

302. Qureshi AI, Suri FK, Guterman LR, et al: Cocaine use and the likelihood of non-fatal myocardial infarction and stroke. Data from the Third National Health and Nutrition Examination Survey, *Circulation* 103:502, 2001.

303. Broderick JP, Viscoli CM, Brott T, et al: Major risk factors for aneurysmal subarachnoid hemorrhage in the young are modifiable, *Stroke* 34:1375, 2003.

304. Brust JCM: Vasculitis owing to substance abuse, *Neurol Clin* 15:945, 1997.

305. Levine SR, Brust JCM, Futrell N, et al: A comparative study of the cerebrovascular complications of cocaine: Alkaloidal vs. hydrochloride, *Neurology* 41:1173, 1991.

306. Frishman WH, Del Vecchio A: Cardiovascular manifestations of substance abuse: Part 1: Cocaine, *Heart Dis* 5:187, 2003.

307. Huang QF, Gebrewold A, Altura BT, Altura BM: Cocaine-induced cerebral vascular damage can be ameliorated by Mg^{2+} in rat brain, *Neurosci Lett* 109:113, 1990.

308. Isner JM, Chokshi SK: Cocaine and vasospasm, *N Engl J Med* 321:1604, 1989.

309. Konzen JP, Levine SR, Garcia JH: Vasospasm and thrombus formation as possible mechanisms of stroke related to alkaloidal cocaine, *Stroke* 26:1114, 1995.

310. Zhang X, Schrott LM, Sparber SB: Evidence for a serotonin-mediated effect of cocaine causing vasoconstriction and herniated umbilici in chicken embryos, *Pharmacol Biochem Behav* 59:585, 1998.

311. Treadwell SD, Robinson TG: Cocaine use and stroke, *Postgrad Med J* 83:389, 2007.

312. Powers RH, Madden JA: Vasoconstrictive effects of cocaine, metabolites and structural analogs on rat cerebral arteries, *FASEB J* 4:A1095, 1990.

313. Weiss RD, Gawin FH: Protracted elimination of cocaine metabolites in long-term, high-dose cocaine abusers, *Am J Med* 85:879, 1988.

314. Kaufman MJ, Levin JM, Ross MH, et al: Cocaine-induced cerebral vasoconstriction detected in humans with magnetic resonance angiography, *JAMA* 279:376, 1998.

315. Herning RI, King DE, Better WE, Cadet JL: Neurovascular deficits in cocaine abusers, *Neuropsychopharmacology* 21:110, 1999.

316. Kaufman MJ, Levin JM, Maas LC, et al: Cocaine-induced cerebral vasoconstriction differs as a function of sex and menstrual cycle phase, *Biol Psychiatry* 49:774, 2001.

317. Dohi S, Jones D, Hudak ML, Traystman RJ: Effects of cocaine on pial arterioles in cats, *Stroke* 21:1710, 1990.

318. Diaz-Tejedor E, Tejada J, Munoz J: Cerebral arterial changes following cocaine IV administration: An angiographic study in rabbits, *J Neurol* 239(Suppl 2):S38, 1992.

319. Wang A-M, Suojanen JN, Colucci VM: Cocaine- and methamphetamine-induced acute cerebral vasospasm: An angiographic study in rabbits, *Am J Neuroradiol* 11:1141, 1990.

320. Nunez BD, Miao L, Ross JN, et al: Effects of cocaine on carotid vascular reactivity in swine after balloon vascular injury, *Stroke* 25:631, 1994.

321. Mo W, Arruda JA, Dunea G, Singh AK: Cocaine-induced hypertension: Role of the peripheral nervous system, *Pharmacol Res* 40:139, 1999.

322. Vongpatanasin W, Monsour Y, Chavoshon B, et al: Cocaine stimulates the human cardiovascular system via a central mechanism of action, *Circulation* 100:497, 1999.

323. Johnson BA, Devous MD, Ruiz P, et al: Treatment advances for cocaine-induced ischemic stroke: Focus on dihydropyridine class calcium channel antagonists, *Am J Psychiatry* 158:1191, 2001.

324. Yoon SH, Zuccarello M, Rapoport RM: Acute cocaine induces endothelin-1 constriction of rabbit basilar artery, *Endothelium* 14:137, 2007.

325. Su J, Li J, Li W, et al: Cocaine induces apoptosis in vascular muscle cells: potential roles in strokes and brain damage, *Eur J Pharmacol* 482:61, 2003.

326. Kosten TR, Tucker K, Gottschalk PC, et al: Platelet abnormalities associated with cerebral perfusion defects in cocaine dependence, *Biol Psychiatry* 55:91, 2004.

327. Togna G, Tempesta E, Togna AR, et al: Platelet responsiveness and biosynthesis of thromboxane and prostacyclin in response to in vitro cocaine treatment, *Haemostasis* 15:100, 1985.

328. Jennings LK, White MM, Sauer CM, et al: Cocaine-induced platelet defects, *Stroke* 24:1352, 1993.

329. Langner RO, Bement CL, Perry LE: Arteriosclerotic toxicity of cocaine, *NIDA Res Monogr* 88:325, 1988.

330. Chokshi SK, Moore R, Pandian NG, Isner JM: Reversible cardiomyopathy associated with cocaine intoxication, *Ann Intern Med* 111:1039, 1989.

331. Siegel AJ, Sholar MB, Mendelson JH, et al: Cocaine-induced erythrocytosis and increase in von Willebrand factor: Evidence for drug-related blood doping and prothrombotic effects, *Arch Intern Med* 159:1999, 1925.

332. Randell T: Cocaine, alcohol mix in body to form even longer lasting, more lethal drug, *JAMA* 267:1043, 1992.

333. Wilson LD, Henning RJ, Suttheimer C, et al: Cocaethylene causes dose-dependent reductions in cardiac function in anesthetized dogs, *J Cardiovasc Pharmacol* 26:965, 1995.

334. Gottschalk PC, Kosten TR: Cerebral perfusion defects in combined cocaine and alcohol dependence, *Drug Alcohol Depend* 68:95, 2002.

335. O'Malley S, Adamse M, Heaton RK, Gawin FH: Neuropsychological impairment in chronic cocaine abusers, *Am J Drug Alcohol Abuse* 18:131, 1992.

336. Weinrieb RM, O'Brien CP: Persistent cognitive deficits attributed to substance abuse, *Neurol Clin* 11:663, 1993.

337. Bolla KI, Rothman R, Cadet JL: Dose-related neurobehavioral effects of chronic cocaine use, *J Neuropsychiatry Clin Neurosci* 11:361, 1999.

338. Smelson DA, Roy A, Santana S, Engelhart C: Neuropsychological deficits in withdrawn cocaine-dependent males, *Am J Drug Alcohol Abuse* 25:377, 1999.

339. Davidson C, Gow AJ, Lee TH, et al: Methamphetamine neurotoxicity: Necrotic and apoptotic mechanisms and relevance to human abuse and treatment, *Brain Res Rev* 36:1, 2001.

340. Seiden LS, Kleven MS: Lack of toxic effects of cocaine on dopamine and serotonin neurons in the rat brain, *NIDA Res Monogr* 88:276, 1988.

341. Holman BL, Carvalho PA, Mendelson J, et al: Brain perfusion is abnormal in cocaine-dependent polydrug users: A study using technetium-99m-HMPAO and ASPECT, *J Nucl Med* 32:1206, 1991.

342. Strickland TL, Stein R: Cocaine-induced cerebrovascular impairment: Challenges to neuropsychological assessment, *Neuropsychol Rev* 5:69, 1995.

343. Tumeh SS, Nagel JS, English RJ, et al: Cerebral abnormalities in cocaine abusers: Demonstration by SPECT perfusion brain scintigraphy, *Radiology* 176:821, 1990.

344. Volkow ND, Fowler JS, Wolf AP, Gillespie A: Metabolic studies of drugs of abuse. In Harris L, editor: *Problems of drug dependence*, 1990. (NIDA Research Monograph 105.) Washington DC, US Department of Health and Human Services, 1991, p 47.

345. Tucker KA, Potenza MN, Beauvais JE, et al: Perfusion abnormalities and decision making in cocaine dependence, *Biol Psychiatry* 56:527, 2004.

346. Bolla K, Ernst M, Kiehl K, et al: Prefrontal cortical dysfunction in abstinent cocaine abusers, *J Neuropsychiatry Clin Neurosci* 16:456, 2004.

347. Dixon SD, Bejar R: Echoencephalographic findings in neonates associated with maternal cocaine and methamphetamine use: Incidence and clinical correlates, *J Pediatr* 115:770, 1989.

348. King TA, Perlman JM, Laptook AR, et al: Neurologic manifestations of in utero cocaine exposure in near-term and term infants, *Pediatrics* 96:259, 1995.

349. Volpe BJ: Effect of cocaine use on the fetus, *N Engl J Med* 327:399, 1992.

350. Rao H, Wang J, Gianetta J, et al: Altered resting cerebral blood flow in adolescents with in utero cocaine exposure revealed by perfusion functional MRI, *Pediatrics* 120:e1245, 2007.

351. McCarron MM, Schultze BW, Thompson GA, et al: Acute phencyclidine intoxication: Incidence of clinical findings in 1000 cases, *Ann Emerg Med* 10:237, 1981.

352. Crosley CJ, Binet EF: Cerebrovascular complications in phencyclidine intoxication, *J Pediatr* 94:316, 1979.

353. Eastman JW, Cohen SN: Hypertensive crisis and death associated with phencyclidine poisoning, *JAMA* 231:1270, 1975.

354. Illett KF, Jarrott B, O'Donnell SR, et al: Mechanism of cardiovascular actions of 1-(1-phenylcyclohexyl) piperidine hydrochloride (phencyclidine), *Br J Pharmacol Chemother* 28:73, 1966.

355. Altura B, Altura BM: Phencyclidine, lysergic acid diethylamide, and mescaline: Cerebral artery spasms and hallucinogenic activity, *Science* 212:1051, 1981.

356. Besson HA: Intracranial hemorrhage associated with phencyclidine abuse, *JAMA* 248:585, 1982.

357. Boyko OB, Burger PC, Heinz ER: Pathological and radiological correlation of subarachnoid hemorrhage in phencyclidine abuse: Case report, *J Neurosurg* 67:446, 1987.

358. Ubogu EE: Amaurosis fugax associated with phencyclidine inhalation, *Eur Neurol* 46:98, 2001.

359. Burns RS, Lerner SE: The effects of phencyclidine in man: A review. In Domino EF, editor: *PCP (Phencyclidine): Historical and current perspectives*, Ann Arbor, Mich, 1981, NPP Books, p 449.

360. Sobel J, Espinas OE, Friedman SA: Carotid artery obstruction following LSD capsule ingestion, *Arch Intern Med* 127:290, 1971.

361. Lieberman AN, Bloom W, Kishore PS, Lin JP: Carotid artery occlusion following ingestion of LSD, *Stroke* 5:213, 1974.

362. Moussouttas M: Cannabis use and cerebrovascular disease, *Neurologist* 10:47, 2004.

363. Barrett CP, Braithwaite RA, Teale JD: Unusual case of tetrahydrocannabinol intoxication confirmed by radioimmunoassay, *Br Med J* 2:166, 1977.

364. Mohan H, Sood GC: Conjugate deviation of the eyes after cannabis intoxication, *Br J Ophthalmol* 48:160, 1964.

365. Cooles P, Michaud R: Stroke after heavy cannabis smoking, *Postgrad Med J* 63:511, 1987.

366. Zachariah SB: Stroke after heavy marijuana smoking, *Stroke* 22:406, 1991.

367. Dis A, Gomis M, Rodriguez-Campello A, et al: Factors associated with a high risk of stroke recurrence in patients with transient ischemic attack or minor stroke, *Stroke* 39:1717, 2008.

368. Barnes D, Palace J, O'Brien MD: Stroke following marijuana smoking, *Stroke* 9:1381, 1992.

369. Lawson TM, Rees A: Stroke and transient ischemic attacks in association with substance abuse in a young man, *Postgrad Med J* 72:692, 1996.

370. McCarron MO, Thomas AM: Cannabis and alcohol in stroke, *Postgrad Med J* 73:448, 1997.

371. Mousak A, Agathos P, Kerezoudi E, et al: Transient ischemic attack in heavy cannabis smokers—how "safe" is it? *Eur Neurol* 44:42, 2000.

372. Haubrich C, Diehl R, Dönges M, et al: Recurrent transient ischemic attacks in a cannabis smoker, *J Neurol* 252:369, 2005.

373. White D, Martin D, Geller T, et al: Stroke associated with marijuana abuse, *Pediatr Neurosurg* 32:92, 2000.

374. Geller T, Loftis L, Brink DS: Cerebellar infarction in adolescent males associated with acute marijuana use, *Pediatrics* 113:e365, 2004.

375. Finsterer J, Christian P, Wolfgang K: Occipital stroke shortly after cannabis consumption, *Clin Neurol Neurosurg* 106:305, 2004.

376. Mateo I, Pinedo A, Gomez-Beldarrain M, et al: Recurrent stroke associated with cannabis use, *J Neurol Neurosurg Psychiatry* 76:435, 2005.

377. Mesec A, Rot V, Grad A: Cerebrovascular disease associated with marijuana abuse: a case report, *Cerebrovasc Dis* 11:284, 2001.

378. Alvaro LC, Irondo I, Villaverde FJ: Sexual headache and stroke in a heavy cannabis smoker, *Headache* 42:224, 2002.

379. Marinella MA: Stroke after marijuana smoking in a teenager with factor V Leiden mutation, *South Med Assoc J* 94:1217, 2001.

380. Russmann S, Winkler A, Lövblad KO, et al: Lethal ischemic stroke after cisplatin-based chemotherapy for testicular carcinoma and cannabis inhalation, *Eur Neurol* 48:178, 2002.

381. Renard D, Gaillard N: Brain hemorrhage and cerebral vasospasm associated with chronic use of cannabis and buprenorphine, *Cerebrovasc Dis* 25:282, 2008.

382. Sloan MA, Duh S-H, Mayder LS, et al: Marijuana and the risk of stroke, *Stroke* 30:57, 2000.

383. Randall MD, Kendall DA: Endocannabinoids: a new class of vasoactive substances, *Trends Pharmacol Sci* 19:55, 1998.

384. Hillard CJ: Endocannabinoids and vascular function, *J Pharmacol Exp Ther* 294:27, 2000.

385. Matthew RJ, Wilson WH, Davis R: Postural syncope after marijuana: A transcranial Doppler study of the hemodynamics, *Pharmacol Biochem Behav* 75:309, 2003.

386. Matthew RJ, Wilson WH, Turkington TG, et al: Time course of tetrahydrocannabinol-induced changes in regional cerebral blood flow measured with positron emission tomography, *Psychiatry Res* 116:173, 2002.

387. Herning RI, Better WE, Tate K, et al: Cerebrovascular perfusion in marijuana users during a month of monitored abstinence, *Neurology* 64:488, 2005.

388. Sneider JT, Pope HG, Silveri MM, et al: Altered regional blood volume in chronic cannabis smokers, *Exp Clin Psychopharmacol* 14:422, 2006.

389. Kosier DA, Filipiak KJ, Stolarz P, et al: Paroxysmal atrial fibrillation following marijuana intoxication: A two-case report of possible association, *Int J Cardiol* 78:183, 2001.

390. Mittleman MA, Lewis RA, Maclure M, et al: Triggering myocardial infarction by marijuana, *Circulation* 103:2805, 2001.

391. Jones RT: Cardiovascular system effects of marijuana, *J Clin Pharmacol* 42:58S, 2002.

392. Adams MD, Earnhardt JT, Dewcy WL, Harris LS: Vasoconstrictor actions of delta-8- and delta-9-tetrahydrocannabinol in the rat, *J Pharmacol Exp Ther* 196:649, 1976.

393. Parker MJ, Tarlow MJ, Milne-Anderson J: Glue sniffing and cerebral infarction, *Arch Dis Child* 59:675, 1984.

394. Lamont CM, Adams FG: Glue-sniffing as a cause of a positive radioisotope brain scan, *Eur J Nucl Med* 7:387, 1982.

395. Nudelman RW, Saleman M: Blue movie, *JAMA* 257:3230, 1987.

396. Mukamal KJ, Chung H, Jenny NS, et al: Alcohol consumption and the risk of coronary heart disease in older adults: The Cardiovascular Health Study, *J Am Geriatr Soc* 54:30, 2006.

397. Klatsky AL: Alcohol, cardiovascular disease and diabetes mellitus, *Pharmacol Res* 55:237, 2007.

398. Thornton JR: Atrial fibrillation in healthy non-alcoholic people after an alcoholic binge, *Lancet* 2:1013, 1984.

399. Katsuki S, Omae T: Stroke prone profiles in the Japanese. In Engel A, Larsson T, editors: *First Thule International Symposium on Stroke*, Stockholm, 1966, Nordiska Bokhandein, 1967, p 215.

400. Klassen AC, Loewenson RB, Resch JA: Cerebral atherosclerosis in selected chronic disease states, *Atherosclerosis* 18:321, 1973.

401. Lee K: Alcoholism and cerebral thrombosis in the young, *Acta Neurol Scand* 59:270, 1979.

402. Okada H, Horibe H, Yoshiyuki O, et al: A prospective study of cerebrovascular disease in Japanese rural communities, Akabane and Asahi. Part 1: evaluation of risk factors in the occurrence of cerebral hemorrhage and thrombosis, *Stroke* 7:599–607, 1976.

403. Ramanova MV, Romanov NS: Cerebral circulation disturbance in patients with chronic alcoholism, *Sov Med* 7:148, 1978.

404. Hillbom M, Kaste M: Does ethanol intoxication promote brain infarction in young adults? *Lancet* 2:1181, 1978.

405. Hillbom M, Kaste M: Ethanol intoxication: A risk factor for ischemic brain infarction in adolescents and young adults, *Stroke* 12:422, 1981.

406. Hillbom M, Kaste M: Alcohol intoxication: A risk factor for primary subarachnoid hemorrhage, *Neurology* 32:706, 1982.

407. Hillbom M, Kaste M: Ethanol intoxication: A risk factor for ischemic brain infarction, *Stroke* 14:694, 1983.

408. Hilton-Jones O, Warlow CP: The cause of stroke in the young, *J Neurol* 232:137, 1985.

409. Moorthy G, Price TR, Tuhrim S, et al: Relationship between recent alcohol intake and stroke type? The NINCDS Stroke Data Bank, *Stroke* 17:141, 1986.

410. Gorelick PB, Rodin MB, Langenberg P, et al: Is acute alcohol ingestion a risk factor for ischemic stroke? Results of a controlled study in middle-aged and elderly stroke patients at three urban medical centers, *Stroke* 18:359, 1987.

411. Gorelick PB, Rodin MB, Langenberg P, et al: Weekly alcohol consumption, cigarette smoking, and the risk of ischemic stroke: Results of a case-control study at three urban medical centers in Chicago, Illinois, *Neurology* 39:339, 1989.

412. Beghi E, Bogliun G, Cosso P, et al: Stroke and alcohol intake in a hospital population: A case-control study, *Stroke* 26:1691, 1995.

413. Boysen G, Nyboe J, Appleyard M, et al: Stroke incidence and risk factors for stroke in Copenhagen, Denmark, *Stroke* 19:1345, 1988.

414. Cullen K, Stenhouse NS, Wearne KL: Alcohol and mortality in the Busselton study, *Int J Epidemiol* 11:67, 1982.

415. Fuchs CS, Stampfer MJ, Colditz GA, et al: Alcohol consumption and mortality among women, *N Engl J Med* 332:1245, 1995.

416. Goldberg RJ, Burchfiel CM, Benfante R, et al: Lifestyle and biologic factors associated with atherosclerotic disease in middle-aged men: 20-year findings from the Honolulu Heart Program, *Arch Intern Med* 155:686, 1995.

417. Gordon T, Doyle JT: Drinking and mortality: The Albany Study, *Am J Epidemiol* 125:263, 1987.

418. Hansagi H, Romelsjo A, Gerhardsson de Verdier M, et al: Alcohol consumption and stroke mortality: 20 year follow-up of 15,077 men and women, *Stroke* 26:1768, 1995.

419. Herman B, Schmintz PIM, Leyten ACM, et al: Multivariate logistic analysis of risk factors for stroke in Tilburg, the Netherlands, *Am J Epidemiol* 118:514, 1983.

420. Khaw AL, Barrett-Connor E: Dietary potassium and stroke-associated mortality: A 12-year prospective study, *N Engl J Med* 316:235, 1987.

421. Kiechl S, Willeit J, Egger G, et al: Alcohol consumption and carotid atherosclerosis: Evidence of dose-dependent atherogenic and antiatherogenic effects. Results from the Bruneck Study, *Stroke* 25:1593, 1994.

422. Klatsky AL, Friedman GD, Siegelaub AB: Alcohol and mortality: A ten-year Kaiser-Permanente experience, *Ann Intern Med* 95:139, 1981.

423. Lee TK, Huang ZS, Ng SK, et al: Impact of alcohol consumption and cigarette smoking on stroke among the elderly in Taiwan, *Stroke* 26:790, 1995.

424. Oleckno WA: The risk of stroke in young adults: An analysis of the contribution of cigarette smoking and alcohol consumption, *Public Health* 102:45, 1988.

425. Paganini-Hill A, Ross RK, Henderson BE: Post-menopausal oestrogen treatment and stroke: A prospective study, *BMJ* 297:519, 1988.

426. Palomaki H, Kaste M: Regular light-to-moderate intake of alcohol and the risk of ischemic stroke: Is there a beneficial effect? *Stroke* 24:1993, 1828.

427. Peacock PB, Riley CP, Lampton TD, et al: The Birmingham stroke, epidemiology, and rehabilitation study. In Stewart G, editor: *Trends in epidemiology: Applications to health service research and training*, Springfield, Ill, 1972, Charles C Thomas, p 231.

428. Rodgers H, Aitken PD, French JM, et al: Alcohol and stroke: A case control study of drinking habits past and present, *Stroke* 24:1473, 1993.

429. Sasaki S, Zhang XH, Kesteloot H: Dietary sodium, potassium, saturated fat, alcohol, and stroke mortality, *Stroke* 26:783, 1995.

430. Semenciw RM, Morrison MI, Mao Y, et al: Major risk factors for cardiovascular disease mortality in adults: Results from the Nutrition Canada Survey Study, *Int J Epidemiol* 17:317, 1988.

431. Stemmermann GN, Hayashi T, Resch JA, et al: Risk factors related to ischemic and hemorrhagic cerebrovascular disease at autopsy: The Honolulu Heart Study, *Stroke* 15:23, 1984.

432. Taylor JR, Combs-Orme T: Alcohol and strokes in young adults, *Am J Psychiatry* 142:116, 1985.

433. Athyros VG, Liberopoulos EN, Mikhailidis DP, et al: Association of drinking pattern and alcohol beverage type with the prevalence of metabolic syndrome, diabetes, coronary heart disease, stroke, and peripheral arterial disease in a Mediterranean cohort, *Angiology* 58:689, 2008.

434. Feigin VL, Rinkel GJ, Lowes CM, et al: Risk factors for subarachnoid hemorrhage: An updated systematic review of epidemiological studies, *Stroke* 36:2773, 2005.

435. Lu M, Ye W, Adami HO, et al: Stroke incidence in women under 60 years of age related to alcohol intake and smoking habit, *Cerebrovasc Dis* 25:517, 2008.

436. Bazzano LA, Gu D, Reynolds K, et al: Alcohol consumption and risk for stroke among Chinese men, *Ann Neurol* 62:569, 2007.

437. Ariesen MJ, Claus SP, Rinkel GJE, et al: Risk factors for intracerebral hemorrhage in the general population: A systematic review, *Stroke* 34:2060, 2003.

438. Sturgeon JD, Folsom AR, Longstreth WT, et al: Risk factors for intracerebral hemorrhage in a pooled prospective study, *Stroke* 38:2718, 2007.

439. Ben-Shlomo Y, Markowe H, Shipley M, Marmot MG: Stroke risk from alcohol consumption using different control groups, *Stroke* 23:1093, 1992.

440. Kozararevic D, McGee D, Vojvodic N, et al: Frequency of alcohol consumption and morbidity and mortality: The Yugoslavia Cardiovascular Disease Study, *Lancet* 1(8169):613, 1980.

441. Kozarevic DJ, Vodvodic N, Gordon T, et al: Drinking habits and death: The Yugoslavia Cardiovascular Disease Study, *Int J Epidemiol* 12:145, 1983.

442. Blackwelder WC, Yano K, Rhoads GC, et al: Alcohol and mortality: The Honolulu Heart Study, *Am J Med* 68:164, 1980.

443. Donahue RP, Abbott RD, Reed DM, Yano K: Alcohol and hemorrhagic stroke: The Honolulu Heart Study, *JAMA* 255:2311, 1986.

444. Kagan A, Popper JS, Rhoads GG, Yano K: Dietary and other risk factors for stroke in Hawaiian Japanese men, *Stroke* 16:390, 1985.

445. Takeya Y, Popper JS, Shimizu Y, et al: Epidemiologic studies of coronary heart disease and stroke in Japanese men living in Japan, Hawaii, and California: Incidence of stroke in Japan and Hawaii, *Stroke* 15:15, 1984.

446. Wolf PA, D'Agostino RB, Odell P, et al: Alcohol consumption as a risk factor for stroke: The Framingham Study, *Ann Neurol* 24:177, 1988.

447. Stamfer MJ, Coditz GA, Willett WC, et al: A prospective study of moderate alcohol consumption and the risk of coronary disease and stroke in women, *N Engl J Med* 319:267, 1988.

448. Bogousslavsky J, Van Melle G, Despland PA, Regli F: Alcohol consumption and carotid atherosclerosis in the Lausanne Stroke Registry, *Stroke* 21:715, 1990.

449. Kiyohara Y, Kato I, Iwamoto H, et al: The impact of alcohol and hypertension on stroke incidence in a general Japanese population. The Hisayama Study, *Stroke* 26:368, 1995.

450. Kono S, Ikeda M, Ogata M, et al: The relationship between alcohol and mortality among Japanese physicians, *Int J Epidemiol* 12:437, 1983.

451. Kono S, Ikeda M, Tokudome S, et al: Alcohol and mortality: A cohort study of male Japanese physicians, *Int J Epidemiol* 15:527, 1986.

452. Tanaka H, Ueda Y, Hayashi M, et al: Risk factors for cerebral hemorrhage and cerebral infarction in a Japanese rural community, *Stroke* 13:62, 1982.

453. Tanaka H, Hayaski M, Date C, et al: Epidemiologic studies of stroke in Shibata, a Japanese provincial city: Preliminary report on risk factors for cerebral infarction, *Stroke* 16:773, 1985.

454. Iso H, Kitamara A, Shimamoto T, et al: Alcohol intake and the risk of cardiovascular disease in middle-aged Japanese men, *Stroke* 26:767, 1995.

455. Camargo CA: Moderate alcohol consumption and stroke: The epidemiologic evidence, *Stroke* 20:1611, 1989.

456. Jamrozik K, Broadhurst RJ, Anderson CS, Stewart-Wynne EG: The role of lifestyle factors in the etiology of stroke: A population-based case-control study in Perth, Western Australia, *Stroke* 25:51, 1994.

457. Shinton R, Sagar G, Beevers G: The relation of alcohol consumption to cardiovascular risk factors and stroke: The West Birmingham Stroke Project, *J Neurol Neurosurg Psychiatry* 56:458, 1993.

458. Beghi E, Bogliun G, Cosso P, et al: Cerebrovascular disorders and alcohol intake: Preliminary results of a case-control study, *Ital J Neurol Sci* 13:209, 1992.

459. Gronback M, Deis A, Sorensen TI, et al: Mortality associated with moderate intakes of wine, beer, or spirits, *BMJ* 10:1165, 1995.

460. Truelson T, Gronbaek M, Schnohr P, Boysen G: Intake of beer, wine, and spirits and risk of stroke: The Copenhagen City Heart Study, *Stroke* 29:2467, 1998.

461. Hillbom M, Numminen H, Juvela S: Recent heavy drinking of alcohol and embolic stroke, *Stroke* 30:2307, 1999.

462. Juvela S, Hillbom M, Palomäki H: Risk factors for spontaneous intracerebral hemorrhage, *Stroke* 26:1558, 1995.

463. Sacco RL, Elkind M, Baden-Albala B, et al: The protective effect of moderate alcohol consumption on ischemic stroke, *JAMA* 281:53, 1999.

464. Berger K, Ajani UA, Case CS, et al: Light-to-moderate alcohol and the risk of stroke among U.S. male physicians, *N Engl J Med* 341:1557, 1999.

465. Djoussé L, Ellison RC, Beiser A, et al: Alcohol consumption and risk of ischemic stroke: The Framingham Study, *Stroke* 33:907, 2002.

466. Dulli DA: Alcohol, ischemic stroke, and lessons from a negative study, *Stroke* 33:890, 2002.

467. Mukamal KJ, Chung H, Jenny NS, et al: Alcohol use and risk of ischemic stroke among older adults: The Cardiovascular Health Study, *Stroke* 36:2005, 1830.

468. Klatsky AL: Alcohol and stroke. An epidemiological labyrinth, *Stroke* 36:2005, 1835.

469. Mukamal KJ, Ascherio A, Mittleman MA, et al: Alcohol and risk for ischemic stroke in men: the role of drinking patterns and usual beverage, *Ann Intern Med* 142:11, 2005.

470. Sacco RL: Alcohol and stroke risk: an elusive dose-response relationship, *Ann Neurol* 62:551, 2007.

471. Reynolds K, Lewis LB, Nolan JDL: Alcohol consumption and risk of stroke. A meta-analysis, *JAMA* 289:579, 2003.

472. Palomaki H, Kaste M, Raininko R, et al: Risk factors for cervical atherosclerosis in patients with transient ischemic attack or minor ischemic stroke, *Stroke* 24:970, 1993.

473. Schminke V, Luedemann J, Berger K, et al: Association between alcohol consumption and subclinical carotid atherosclerosis. The Study of Health in Pomerania, *Stroke* 36:1746, 2005.

474. Jorgensen HS, Nakagama H, Raaschou HO, Olsen TS: Leukoaraiosis in stroke patients: The Copenhagen Stroke Study, *Stroke* 26:588, 1995.

475. Yoshitake T, Kiyohara Y, Kato I, et al: Incidence and risk factors of vascular dementia and Alzheimer's disease in a defined elderly Japanese population: The Hisayama Study, *Neurology* 45:1161, 1995.

476. Mukamal KJ, Longstreth WT, Mittleman MA, et al: Alcohol consumption and subclinical findings on magnetic resonance imaging of the brain in older adults: The Cardiovascular Health Study, *Stroke* 32:939, 2001.

477. Elias PK, Elias MF, D'Agostino RB, et al: Alcohol consumption and cognitive performance, *Am J Epidemiol* 150:580, 1999.

478. DeCarli C, Miller BL, Swan GE, et al: Cerebrovascular and brain morphologic correlates of mild cognitive impairment in the National Heart, Lung, and Blood Institute Twin Study, *Arch Neurol* 58:43, 2001.

479. Herbert LE, Scherr PA, Beckett LA, et al: Relation of smoking and low-to-moderate alcohol consumption to change in cognitive function: A longitudinal study in a defined community of older persons, *Am J Epidemiol* 137:881, 1993.

480. Hendrie HC, Gao S, Hall KS, et al: The relationship between alcohol consumption, cognitive performance, and daily functioning in an urban sample of older black Americans, *J Am Geriatr Soc* 44:1158, 1996.

481. Dufovil C, Ducimetierre P, Alperovitch A: Sex differences in the association between alcohol consumption and cognitive performance: EVA Study Group, *Am J Epidemiol* 146:405, 1997.

482. Lemeshow S, Letenneur L, Dartigues JF, et al: Illustration of analysis taking into account complex survey considerations: The association between wine consumption and dementia in the PAQUID Study, *Am J Epidemiol* 148:298, 1998.

483. Ruitenberg A, van Swieten JC, Witteman JCM, et al: Alcohol consumption and the risk of dementia: The Rotterdam Study, *Lancet* 359:281, 2002.

484. Lichtenstein A, Appel L, Brands M, et al: Nutrition Committee. AHA Science Advisory: Diet and Lifestyle Recommendations Revision 2006: a science advisory for healthcare professionals from the Nutrition Committee, *Circulation* 114:82, 2006.

485. Hillbom M, Numminen H: Alcohol and stroke: Pathophysiologic mechanisms, *Neuroepidemiology* 17:281, 1998.

486. Beilin LJ: Alcohol and hypertension, *Clin Exp Pharmacol Physiol* 22:185, 1995.

487. Brackett DJ, Gauvin DV, Lerner MR, et al: Dose- and time-dependent cardiovascular responses induced by ethanol, *J Pharmacol Exp Ther* 268:78, 1994.

488. Janssens E, Mounier-Vehier F, Hamon M, Leys D: Small subcortical infarcts and primary subcortical hemorrhages may have different risk factors, *J Neurol* 242:425, 1995.

489. Lip GY, Beevers DG: Alcohol, hypertension, coronary disease, and stroke, *Clin Exp Pharmacol Physiol* 22:189, 1995.

490. MacMahon S: Alcohol consumption and hypertension, *Hypertension* 9:111, 1987.

491. MacMahon SW, Norton RN: Alcohol and hypertension: Implications for prevention and treatment, *Ann Intern Med* 105:124, 1986.

492. Russell M, Cooper ML, Frone M, et al: Drinking patterns and blood pressure, *Am J Epidemiol* 128:917, 1988.

493. Tell GS, Rutan GH, Kronmal RA, et al: Correlates of blood pressure in community-dwelling older adults: The Cardiovascular Health Study, *Hypertension* 23:59, 1994.

494. Fuchs FD, Chambless LE, Whelton PK, et al: Alcohol consumption and the incidence of hypertension: The Atherosclerosis Risk in Communities Study, *Hypertension* 37:1242, 2001.

495. Cushman WC: Alcohol consumption and hypertension, *J Clin Hypertension* 3:166, 2001.

496. Okubo Y, Miyamoto T, Suwazano Y, et al: Alcohol consumption and blood pressure in Japanese men, *Alcohol* 23:149, 2001.

497. Gorelick PB: Alcohol and stroke, *Stroke* 18:268, 1987.

498. Randin D, Vollenweider P, Tappy L, et al: Suppression of alcohol-induced hypertension by dexamethasone, *N Engl J Med* 332:1733, 1995.

499. Harper G, Castleden CM, Potter JF: Factors affecting changes in blood pressure after acute stroke, *Stroke* 25:1726, 1994.

500. Longstreth WT, Koepsell TD, Yerby MS, van Belle G: Risk factors for subarachnoid hemorrhage, *Stroke* 16:377, 1985.

501. Baranoa E, Lieber CS: Alcohol and lipids, *Recent Dev Alcohol* 14:97, 1998.

502. Camargo CA, Williams PT, Vranizan KM, et al: The effect of moderate alcohol intake on serum apolipoproteins A-I and A-II: A controlled study, *JAMA* 253:2854, 1985.

503. Haskell WJ, Camargo C, Williams PT, et al: The effect of cessation and resumption of moderate alcohol intake on serum high-density lipoprotein subfractions: A controlled study, *N Engl J Med* 310:805, 1984.

504. Van Tol A, Hendriks HD: Moderate alcohol consumption: Effects on lipids and cardiovascular disease risk, *Curr Opin Lipidol* 12:19, 2001.

505. Reed DM, Resch JA, Hayashi T, et al: A prospective study of cerebral artery atherosclerosis, *Stroke* 19:820, 1988.

506. Avogaro P, Cazzolato G, Belussi F, Bittolo Bon G: Altered apoprotein composition of HDL-2 and HDL-3 in chronic alcoholics, *Artery* 10:317, 1982.

507. Gorelick PB: The status of alcohol as a risk factor for stroke, *Stroke* 20:1607, 1989.

508. Corella D, Tucker K, Lahoz C, et al: Alcohol drinking determines the effect of the APOE locus on LDL-cholesterol concentrations in men: The Framingham Offspring Study, *Am J Clin Nutr* 73:736, 2001.

509. Mukamal KJ, Mackey RH, Kuller LH, et al: Alcohol consumption and lipoprotein subclasses in older adults, *J Clin Endocrinol Metab* 92:2559, 2007.

510. O'Keefe JH, Bybee KA, Lavie CJ: Alcohol and cardiovascular health. The razor-sharp double-edged sword, *J Am Coll Cardiol* 50:1009, 2007.

511. Koppes LL, Dekker JM, Hendriks HF, et al: Moderate alcohol consumption lowers the risk of type 2 diabetes: A meta-analysis of prospective observational studies, *Diabetes Care* 28:719, 2005.

512. Hillbom M, Kangasaho M, Kaste M, et al: Acute ethanol ingestion increases platelet reactivity: Is there a relationship to stroke? *Stroke* 16:19, 1985.

513. Hillbom M, Kaste M, Rasi V: Can ethanol intoxication affect hemocoagulation to increase the risk of brain infarction in young adults? *Neurology* 33:381, 1983.

514. Lang WE: Ethyl alcohol enhances plasminogen activator secretion by endothelial cells, *JAMA* 250:772, 1983.

515. Lee K, Nielsen JD, Zeeberg I, Gormsen J: Platelet aggregation and fibrinolytic activity in young alcoholics, *Acta Neurol Scand* 62:287, 1980.

516. Meade TW, Chakrabarti R, Haines AP, et al: Characteristics affecting fibrinolytic activity and plasma fibrinogen concentrations, *Br Med J* 1:153, 1979.

517. Numminen A, Syrjälä M, Benthin G, et al: The effect of acute ingestion of a large dose of alcohol on the hemostatic system and its circadian variation, *Stroke* 31:1269, 2000.

518. Ricker PM, Vaughn DE, Stampfer MJ, et al: Association of moderate alcohol consumption and plasma concentration of endogenous tissue-type plasminogen activator, *JAMA* 272:929, 1994.

519. DiMinno G, Mancini M: Drugs affecting plasma fibrinogen levels, *Cardiovasc Drugs Ther* 6:25, 1992.

520. Jakubowski JA, Vaillancourt R, Deykin D: Interaction of ethanol, prostacyclin, and aspirin in determining human platelet reactivity in vitro, *Arteriosclerosis* 8:436, 1988.

521. Landolfi R, Steiner M: Ethanol raises prostacyclin in vivo and in vitro, *Blood* 64:679, 1984.

522. Fenn CG, Littleton JM: Inhibition of platelet aggregation by ethanol: The role of plasma and platelet membrane lipids, *Br J Pharmacol* 73:305P, 1981.

523. Kangasaho M, Hillbom M, Kaste M, Vapaatalo H: Effects of ethanol intoxication and hangover on plasma levels of thromboxane B2 and 6-keto-prostaglandin F1 alpha symbol and on thromboxane B2 formation by platelets in man, *Thromb Haemost* 48:232, 1982.

524. Quintana RP, Lasslo A, Dugdale ML, et al: Effects of ethanol and of other factors on ADP-induced aggregation of human blood platelets in vitro, *Thromb Res* 20:405, 1980.

525. Torres Duarte AP, Gong QS, Young J, et al: Inhibition of platelet aggregation in whole blood by alcohol, *Thromb Res* 78:107, 1995.

526. LaCoste L, Hung J, Lam JY: Acute and delayed antithrombotic effects of alcohol in humans, *Am J Cardiol* 87:82, 2001.

527. Tsaji S, Kawano S, Michida T, et al: Ethanol stimulates immunoreactive endothelin-1 and -2 release from cultured human umbilical vein endothelial cells, *Alcohol Clin Exp Res* 16:347, 1992.

528. Fujii Y, Takeuchi S, Tanaka R, et al: Liver dysfunction in spontaneous intracerebral hemorrhage, *Neurosurgery* 35:592, 1994.

529. Haselager EM, Vreeken J: Rebound thrombocytosis after alcohol abuse: A possible factor in the pathogenesis of thromboembolic disease, *Lancet* 1(8015):774, 1977.

530. Hutton RA, Fink FR, Wilson DT, Marjot DH: Platelet hyperaggregability during alcohol withdrawal, *Clin Lab Haematol* 3:223, 1981.

531. Ruf JC, Berger JL, Renaud S: Platelet rebound effect of alcohol withdrawal and wine drinking in rats: Relation to tannins and lipid peroxidation, *Arterioscler Thromb Vasc Biol* 15:140, 1995.

532. Neiman J, Rand ML, Jakowec DM, Packham MA: Platelet responses to platelet-activating factor are inhibited in alcoholics undergoing alcohol withdrawal, *Thromb Res* 56:399, 1989.

533. Delahousse B, Maillot F, Gabriel I, et al: Increased plasma fibrinolysis and tissue-type plasminogen activator/tissue-type plasminogen activator inhibitor ratios after ethanol withdrawal in chronic alcoholics, *Blood Coagul Fibrinolysis* 12:59, 2001.

534. Imhof A, Froehlich M, Brenner H, et al: Effect of ethanol consumption on systemic markers of inflammation, *Lancet* 357:763, 2001.

535. McQueen JD, Sklar FK, Posey JB: Autoregulation of cerebral blood flow during alcohol infusion, *J Stud Alcohol* 39:1477, 1978.

536. Persson LI, Rosengren LE, Johansson BB, Hansson HA: Blood-brain barrier dysfunction to peroxidase after air embolism, aggravated by acute ethanol intoxication, *J Neurol Sci* 42:65, 1979.

537. Flamm ES, Demopoulos HB, Seligman ML, et al: Ethanol potentiation of central nervous system trauma, *J Neurosurg* 46:328, 1977.

538. Hemmingsen R, Barry DL, Hertz MM, Klinken L: Cerebral blood flow and oxygen consumption during ethanol withdrawal in the rat, *Brain Res* 173:259, 1979.

539. Christie IC, Price J, Edwards L, et al: Alcohol consumption and cerebral blood flow among older adults, *Alcohol* 42:269, 2008.

540. Zhang A, Altura BT, Altura BM: Ethanol-induced contraction of cerebral arteries in diverse mammals and its mechanism of action, *Eur J Pharmacol* 248:229, 1993.

541. Gordon EL, Nguyen TS, Ngai AC, Winn HR: Differential effects of alcohols on intracerebral arterioles: ethanol alone causes vasoconstriction, *J Cereb Blood Flow Metab* 15:532, 1995.

542. Sun H, Zhao H, Sharpe M, et al: Effect of chronic alcohol consumption on brain damage following transient focal ischemia, *Brain Res* 73:2008, 1994.

543. Mayhan WG: Responses of cerebral arterioles during chronic ethanol exposure, *Am J Physiol* 262:H787, 1992.

544. Altura BM, Zhang A, Cheng TP, Altura BT: Ethanol promotes rapid depletion of intracellular free Mg in cerebral vascular smooth muscle cells: Possible relation to alcohol-induced behavioral and stroke-like effects, *Alcohol* 10:563, 1993.

545. Altura BM, Altura BT: Association of alcohol in brain injury, headaches, and stroke with brain tissue and serum levels of ionized magnesium: A review of recent findings and mechanisms of action, *Alcohol* 19:119, 1999.

546. Altura BM, Altura BT: Role of magnesium and calcium in alcohol-induced hypertension and strokes as probed by in vivo television microscopy, digital image microscopy, optical spectroscopy, ^{31}P-NMR spectroscopy and a unique magnesium ion-selective electrode, *Alcohol Clin Exp Res* 18:1057, 1994.

547. Altura BM, Gebrewold A, Altura BT, Gupta RK: Role of brain [Mg^{2+}] in alcohol-induced hemorrhagic stroke in a rat model: A ^{31}P-NMR in vivo study, *Alcohol* 12:131, 1995.

548. Cravo ML, Camilo ME: Hyperhomocysteinemia in chronic alcoholism: Relations to folic acid and vitamins B6 and B12 status, *Nutrition* 19:296, 2000.

549. Bell JR, Donovan JL, Wong R, et al: (+)-Catechin in human plasma after a single serving of reconstituted red wine, *Am J Clin Nutr* 71:103, 2000.

550. German JB, Walzam RK: The health benefits of wine, *Annu Rev Nutr* 20:561, 2000.

551. Malarcher AM, Giles WH, Croft JB, et al: Alcohol intake, type of beverage, and the risk of cerebral infarction in young women, *Stroke* 32:77, 2001.

552. Wollin SD, Jones PJ: Alcohol, red wine, and cardiovascular disease, *J Nutr* 131:1401, 2001.

553. Corder R, Mullen W, Khan NQ, et al: Red wine procyanidins and vascular health, *Nature* 444:566, 2006.

554. Saremi A, Arora R: The cardiovascular implications of alcohol and red wine, *Am J Ther* 15:265, 2008.

555. Puddey IB, Croft KD: Alcohol, stroke, and coronary heart disease: Are there anti-oxidants and pro-oxidants in alcoholic beverages that might influence the development of atherosclerotic cardiovascular disease? *Neuroepidemiology* 18:292, 1999.

556. Aronow WS, Kaplan NM: Smoking. In Kaplan NM, Stamler J, editors: *Prevention of coronary heart disease*, Philadelphia, 1983, WB Saunders, p 50.

557. Doll R, Hill AB: Mortality of British doctors in relation to smoking: Observations on coronary thrombosis, *Natl Cancer Inst Monogr* 19:205, 1966.

558. Kannel WB, D'Agostino RB, Belanger AL: Fibrinogen, cigarette smoking, and risk of cardiovascular disease: Insights from the Framingham Study, *Am Heart J* 113:1006, 1987.

559. Palmer JR, Rosenberg: Shapiro S: "Low yield" cigarettes and the risk of nonfatal myocardial infarction in women, *N Engl J Med* 320:1569, 1989.

560. Kroger K, Buss C, Govern M, et al: Risk factors in young patients with peripheral atherosclerosis, *Int Angiol* 19:206, 2000.

561. Davanipour Z, Sobel E, Alter M, et al: Stroke/transient ischemic attack in the Lehigh Valley: Evaluation of smoking as a risk factor, *Ann Neurol* 24:130, 1988.

562. Herman B, Leyten ACM, van Luuk JH, et al: An evaluation of risk factors for stroke in a Dutch community, *Stroke* 13:334, 1982.

563. Kannel WB, Dawber TR, Cohen ME, et al: Vascular disease of the brain-epidemiologic aspects. The Framingham Study, *Am J Public Health* 55:1355, 1965.

564. Nilsson S, Cartensen JM, Perhagen G: Mortality among male and female smokers in Sweden: A 33 year follow up, *J Epidemiol Community Health* 55:825, 2001.

565. Bloch C, Richard JL: Risk factors for atherosclerotic diseases in the Prospective Parisian Study. I: Comparison with foreign studies, *Rev Epidemiol Sante Publique* 33:108, 1985.

566. Bonita R: Cigarette smoking, hypertension, and the risk of subarachnoid hemorrhage: A population-based case-control study, *Stroke* 17:831, 1986.

567. Bonita R, Scragg R, Stewart A, et al: Cigarette smoking and risk of premature stroke in men and women, *BMJ* 293:6, 1986.

568. Candelise L, Bianchi F, Galligoni F, et al: Italian multicenter study on cerebral ischemic attacks. III: Influence of age and risk factors on cerebral atherosclerosis, *Stroke* 15:379, 1984.

569. U.S. Department of Health and Human Services: The health consequences of smoking: Nicotine addiction: A report of the Surgeon General. (DHHS Publication No [CDC] 88-8406.) Washington, DC, US Government Printing Office, 1988.

570. Doll R, Gray R, Hafner B, et al: Mortality in relation to smoking: Twenty-two years' observations on female British doctors, *Br Med J* 1:967, 1980.

571. Hammond EC: Smoking in relation to mortality and morbidity: Finding in the first 34 months of follow-up in a prospective study started in 1959, *J Natl Cancer Inst* 32:1161, 1964.

572. Hammond EC: Smoking in relation to death rates of one million men and women, *Natl Cancer Inst Monogr* 19:127, 1966.

573. Harmsen P, Rosengren A, Tsipogianni A, Wilhelmsen L: Risk factors for stroke in middle-aged men in Göteborg, Sweden, *Stroke* 21:223, 1990.

574. Herrschaft H: Prophylaxe zerbraler Durchblutungsstörungen, *Fortschr Neurol Psychiatr* 53:337, 1985.

575. Juvela S, Hillbom M, Numminen H, Koskinen P: Cigarette smoking and alcohol consumption as risk factors for aneurysmal subarachnoid hemorrhage, *Stroke* 24:639, 1993.

576. Kahn HA: The Dorn study of smoking and mortality among US veterans: Report on 81/2 years of observations, *Natl Cancer Inst Monogr* 19:1, 1966.

577. Koch A, Reuther R, Boos R, et al: Risikofactoren bei cerebralen Durchblutungesstörungen, *Verh Dtsch Ges Inn Med* 83:1773, 1977.

578. Kurtzke JF: *Epidemiology of cerebrovascular disease*, New York, 1969, Springer-Verlag.

579. Love BB, Biller J, Jones MP, et al: Cigarette smoking: A risk factor for cerebral infarction in young adults, *Arch Neurol* 47:693, 1990.

580. Molgaard CA, Bartok A, Peddercord KM, et al: The association between cerebrovascular disease and smoking: A case-control study, *Neuroepidemiology* 5:88, 1986.

581. Paffenbarger RS Jr, Wing AL: Chronic disease in former college students. XI: Early precursors of nonfatal stroke, *Am J Epidemiol* 94:524, 1971.

582. Paffenbarger RS Jr, Wing A: Characteristics in youth predisposing to fatal stroke in later years, *Lancet* 1(7493):753, 1967.

583. Rogot E: Smoking and general mortality among US veterans, 1954-1969. Bethesda Md, National Heart and Lung Institute, 1974.

584. Salonen JT, Puska P, Tuomilehto J, et al: Relation of blood pressure, serum lipids, and smoking to the risk of cerebral stroke: A longitudinal study in eastern Finland, *Stroke* 13:327, 1982.

585. Shinton R, Beevers G: Meta-analysis of relation between cigarette smoking and stroke, *BMJ* 298:789, 1989.

586. Tuomilehto J, Bonita R, Stewart A, et al: Hypertension, cigarette smoking, and the decline in stroke incidence in eastern Finland, *Stroke* 22:7, 1991.

587. Benson RT, Sacco RL: Stroke prevention: Hypertension, diabetes, tobacco, and lipids, *Neurol Clin* 18:309, 2000.

588. Kissela BM, Saverbeck L, Woo D, et al: Subarachnoid hemorrhage: A preventable disease with a heritable component, *Stroke* 33:1321, 2002.

589. Anderson CS, Feigin V, Bennett D, et al: Active and passive smoking and the risk of subarachnoid hemorrhage: an international population-based case-control study, *Stroke* 35:633, 2004.

590. Koshinen LO, Blomstedt PC: Smoking and non-smoking tobacco as risk factors in subarachnoid hemorrhage, *Acta Neurol Scand* 114:33, 2006.

591. Collaborative Group for the Study of Stroke in Young Women: Oral contraception and increased risk of cerebral ischemia or thrombosis, *N Engl J Med* 288:871, 1973.

592. Frederiksen H, Ravenholt RT: Thromboembolism, oral contraceptives, and cigarettes, *Public Health Rep* 85:197, 1970.

593. Goldbaum GM, Kendrick JS, Hogelin GC, Gentry EM: The relative impact of smoking and oral contraceptive use on women in the United States, *JAMA* 258:1339, 1987.

594. Petitti DB, Wingerd J: Use of oral contraceptives, cigarette smoking, and risk of subarachnoid hemorrhage, *Lancet* 2(8083):234, 1978.

595. Royal College of General Practitioners: *Oral contraceptives and health*, London, 1974, Pitman.

596. Colditz GA, Bonita R, Stampfer MJ, et al: Cigarette smoking and risk of stroke in middle-aged women, *N Engl J Med* 318:937, 1988.

597. Bhat VM, Cole JW, Sorkin JD, et al: Dose-response relationship between cigarette smoking and risk of ischemic stroke in young women, *Stroke* 39:2439, 2008.

598. Medical Research Council Working Party: MRC trial of treatment of mild hypertension: Principal results, *BMJ* 291:97, 1985.

599. Pandey MR: Tobacco smoking and hypertension, *J Indian Med Assoc* 97:367, 1999.

600. Christensen HK, Guasorra AD, Boysen G: Ischemic stroke occurs among younger smokers, *Ugeskr Laeger* 163:7057, 2001.

601. Abbott RD, Reed DM, Yano K: Risk of stroke in male cigarette smokers, *N Engl J Med* 315:717, 1986.

602. Sacco RL, Wolf PA, Bharucha NE, et al: Subarachnoid and intracerebral hemorrhage: Natural history, prognosis, and precursive factors in the Framingham Study, *Neurology* 34:847, 1984.

603. Wolf PA, D'Agostino RB, Kannel WB, et al: Cigarette smoking as a risk factor for stroke: The Framingham Study, *JAMA* 259:1025, 1988.

604. Wannamethee SG, Shaper AG, Whincup PH, Walker M: Smoking cessation and the risk of stroke in middle-aged men, *JAMA* 274:155, 1995.

605. Taylor BV, Oudit GY, Kalman PG, Liu P: Clinical and pathophysiological effects of active and passive smoking on the cardiovascular system, *Can J Cardiol* 14:1129, 1998.

606. Blackshear JL, Pearce LA, Hart RG, et al: Aortic plaque in atrial fibrillation: Prevalence, predictors, and thromboembolic implications, *Stroke* 30:834, 1999.

607. Framme C, Spiegel D, Roider J, et al: Central retinal artery occlusion: Importance of selective intra-arterial fibrinolysis, *Ophthalmologe* 98:725, 2001.

608. Hayreh SS, Jonas JB, Zimmerman MB: Nonarteritic ischemic optic neuropathy and tobacco smoking, *Ophthalmology* 114:804, 2007.

609. Tang JL, Morris JK, Wald NJ, et al: Mortality in relation to tar yield of cigarettes: A prospective study of four cohorts, *BMJ* 311:1530, 1995.

610. Pierce JR: Stroke following application of a nicotine patch, *Ann Pharmacol* 28:402, 1994.

611. Bonita R, Duncan J, Truelsen T, et al: Passive smoking as well as active smoking increases the risk of acute stroke, *Tob Control* 8:156, 1999.

612. Heuschmann PU, Heidrich J, Wellmann J, et al: Stroke mortality and morbidity attributable to passive smoking in Germany, *Eur J Cardiovasc Prev Rehabil* 14:793, 2007.

613. He Y, Lam TH, Jiang B, et al: Passive smoking and risk of peripheral arterial disease and ischemic stroke in Chinese women who never smoked, *Circulation* 118:1535, 2008.

614. Garcia-Nunez C, Saez J, Garcia-Nunez JM, et al: Passive smoking as a cerebrovascular risk factor, *Rev Neurol* 45:577, 2007.

615. Lea PN, Forey BA: Environmental tobacco smoke exposure and risk of stroke in nonsmokers: a review of meta-analysis, *Stroke Cerebrovasc Dis* 15:190, 2006.

616. Hergens MP, Lambe M, Pershagen G, et al: Smokeless tobacco and the risk of stroke, *Epidemiology* 19:794, 2008.

617. Naidoo B, Stevens W, McPherson K: Modelling the short term consequences of smoking cessation in England on the hospitalization rates for acute myocardial infarction and stroke, *Tob Control* 9:397, 2000.

618. La Vecchia C, Levi F, Lucchini F, Negri E: Trends in mortality from major diseases in Europe, 1980-1993, *Eur J Epidemiol* 14:1, 1998.

619. Liu BQ, Peto R, Chen ZM, et al: Emerging tobacco hazards in China. 1: Retrospective proportional mortality study of one million deaths, *BMJ* 317:1411, 1998.

620. Hawkins BT, Brown RC, Davis TP: Smoking and ischemic stroke: A role for nicotine? *Trends Pharmacol Sci* 23:8, 2002.

621. Haapanen A, Koskenvuo M, Kaprio J, et al: Carotid arteriosclerosis in identical twins discordant for cigarette smoking, *Circulation* 80:10, 1989.

622. Whisnant JP, Homer D, Ingall TJ, et al: Duration of cigarette smoking is the strongest predictor of severe extracranial carotid atherosclerosis, *Stroke* 21:707, 1990.

623. Mast H, Thompson JLP, Lin I-F, et al: Cigarette smoking as a determinant of high-grade carotid artery stenosis in Hispanic, black and white patients with stroke or transient ischemic attack, *Stroke* 29:908, 1998.

624. Howard G, Wagenknecht LE, Burke GL, et al: Cigarette smoking and progression of atherosclerosis: The Atherosclerosis Risk in Communities (ARIC) Study, *JAMA* 279:119, 1998.

625. Kool MJ, Hoeks AP, Struijker Boudier HA, et al: Short and long-term effects of smoking on arterial wall properties in habitual smokers, *J Am Coll Cardiol* 22:1993, 1881.

626. Murchison LE, Fyfe T: Effects of cigarette smoking on serum lipids, blood glucose, and platelet adhesiveness, *Lancet* 2(7456):182, 1966.

627. Rogers RL, Meyer JS, Shaw TG, et al: Cigarette smoking decreases cerebral blood flow suggesting increased risk for stroke, *JAMA* 250:2796, 1983.

628. Kaufman DJ, Roman MJ, Devereux RB, et al: Prevalence of smoking and its relationship with carotid atherosclerosis in Alaskan Eskimos of the Norton Sound region: the GOCADAN study, *Nicotine Tob Res* 10:483, 2008.

629. Benowitz NL: Pharmacologic aspects of cigarette smoking and nicotine addiction, *N Engl J Med* 319:1318, 1988.

630. Maouad J, Fernandez F, Barrillon A, et al: Diffuse or segmental narrowing (spasm) of coronary arteries during smoking demonstrated on angiography, *Am J Cardiol* 53:354, 1984.

631. Moliterno DJ, Willard JE, Lange RA, et al: Coronary vasoconstriction induced by cocaine, cigarette smoking, or both, *N Engl J Med* 330:454, 1994.

632. Davis JW, Shelton L, Eigenberg DA, et al: Effects of tobacco and non-tobacco cigarette smoking on endothelium and platelets, *Clin Pharmacol Ther* 37:529, 1985.

633. Zimmerman M, McGreachie J: The effect of nicotine on aortic endothelium: A quantitative ultrastructural study, *Atherosclerosis* 63:33, 1987.

634. Haustein KO: Health consequences of passive smoking, *Wien Med Wochenschr* 150:233, 2000.

635. Talloss JH, Booyse FM: Effects of various agents and physical damage on giant cell formation in bovine aortic endothelial cell cultures, *Microvasc Res* 16:51, 1978.

636. Rhaman MM, Laher I: Structural and functional alteration of blood vessels caused by cigarette smoking: an overview of molecular mechanisms, *Curr Vasc Pharmacol* 5:276, 2007.

637. Pardell H, Amario P, Hernandez R: Pathogenesis and epidemiology of arterial hypertension, *Drugs* 56(Suppl 2):1, 1998.

638. Green MS, Jucha E, Luz Y: Blood pressure in smokers and non-smokers: Epidemiologic findings, *Am Heart J* 111:932, 1986.

639. Isles C, Brown JJ, Cumming AM, et al: Excess smoking in malignant phase hypertension, *Br Med J* 1:579, 1979.

640. Mehta MC, Jain AC, Billie M: Combined effects of alcohol and nicotine on cardiovascular performance in a canine model, *J Cardiovasc Pharmacol* 31:930, 1998.

641. Belch JJ, McArdle BM, Burns P, et al: The effects of acute smoking on platelet behavior, fibrinolysis, and haemorheology in habitual smokers, *Thromb Haemost* 51:6, 1984.

642. Nadler JL, Velasso JS, Horton R: Cigarette smoking inhibits prostacyclin formation, *Lancet* 1(8336):1248, 1983.

643. Seiss W, Lorenz R, Roth P, Weber PC: Plasma catecholamines, platelet aggregation and associated thromboxane formation after physical exercise, smoking, or norepinephrine infusion, *Circulation* 66:44, 1982.

644. Miller GJ, Bauer KA, Cooper JA, Rosenberg RD: Activation of the coagulant pathway in cigarette smokers, *Thromb Haemost* 79:549, 1998.

645. Nair S, Kulkarni S, Camoens NM, et al: Changes in platelet glycoprotein receptors after smoking—a flow cytometric study, *Platelets* 12:20, 2001.

646. Schwarcz TH, Hogan LA, Endean ED, et al: Thromboembolic complications of polycythemia: Polycythemia vera versus smokers' polycythemia, *J Vasc Surg* 17:518, 1993.

647. Zidovetski R, Chen P, Fisher M, Hofman FM: Nicotine increases plasminogen activator inhibitor-1 production by human brain endothelial cells via protein kinase C-associated pathway, *Stroke* 30:651, 1999.

648. Wang L, Kittaka M, Sun N, et al: Chronic nicotine treatment enhances focal ischemic brain injury and depletes free pool of brain microvascular tissue plasminogen activator in rats, *J Cereb Blood Flow Metab* 17:136, 1997.

649. Margaglione M, Capucci G, d'Addedda M, et al: PAI-1 plasma levels in the general population without evidence of atherosclerosis: Relation to environmental and genetic determinants, *Arterioscler Thromb Vasc Biol* 18:562, 1998.

650. Simpson AJ, Gray RS, Moore NR, Booth NA: The effects of chronic smoking on the fibrinolytic potential of plasma and platelets, *Br J Haematol* 97:208, 1997.

651. Fogelholm R: Cigarette smoking and subarachnoid hemorrhage: A population-based case-control study, *J Neurol Neurosurg Psychiatry* 50:78, 1987.

652. Orbiagele B, Saver JL: The smoking–thrombolysis paradox and acute ischemic stroke, *Neurology* 65:293, 2005.

653. Levine SR: Smoke without fire: The complex effects of cigarette smoking on thrombolytic therapy for acute ischemic stroke, *Neurology* 65:183, 2005.

654. Benowitz NL: The role of nicotine in smoking-related cardiovascular disease, *Prev Med* 26:412, 1997.

655. Blann AD, Steele C, McCollum CN: The influence of smoking and of oral and transdermal nicotine on blood pressure, and haematology and coagulation indices, *Thromb Haemost* 78:1093, 1997.

656. Greenland S, Satterfield MH, Lanes SF: A meta-analysis to assess the incidence of adverse effects associated with the transdermal nicotine patch, *Drug Saf* 18:297, 1998.

657. Domino EF, Minoshima S, Guthrie S, et al: Nicotine effects on regional cerebral blood flow in awake, resting tobacco users, *Synapse* 38:313, 2000.

658. Iida M, Iida H, Dohi S, et al: Mechanisms underlying cerebrovascular effects of cigarette smoking in rats in vivo, *Stroke* 29:1656, 1998.

659. Gerzanich V, Zhang F, West GA, Simard JM: Chronic nicotine alters NO signaling of Ca (2^+) channels in cerebral arterioles, *Circ Res* 88:359, 2001.

660. Zhang W, Edvinsson L, Lee TJ: Mechanism of nicotine-induced relaxation in the porcine basilar artery, *J Pharmacol Exp Ther* 284:790, 1998.

661. Golanov EV, Ruggiero DA, Reis DJ: A brainstem area mediating cerebrovascular and EEG responses to hypoxic excitation of rostral ventrolateral medulla in rat, *J Physiol* 529:413, 2000.

662. Cole JW, Brown DW, Giles WH, et al: Ischemic stroke risk, smoking, and the genetics of inflammation in a biracial population: The Stroke Prevention in Young Women Study, *Thromb J* 6:11, 2008.

663. Levine SR, Fagan SC, Floberg J, et al: Moya-moya, oral contraceptives, and cigarette use, *Ann Neurol* 24:155, 1988.

664. Peerless SJ: Risk factors of moyamoya disease in Canada and the USA, *Clin Neurol Neurosurg* 99(Suppl 2):S45, 1997.

665. Fukada H, Kitani M, Omodani H: ^{99}mTc-HMPAO brain SPECT imaging in a case of repeated syncopal episodes associated with smoking, *Stroke* 28:1461, 1997.

43 Cardiac Diseases

DAVID M. GREER, SHUNICHI HOMMA, KAREN L. FURIE

Embolism is the major mechanism of stroke in the United States, accounting for 60% of all ischemic strokes.[1] Up to 25% of these embolic strokes have a readily identifiable specific cardioembolic cause, atrial fibrillation (AF).[1] AF affects 9% of men aged 65 years and older.[2-4] In addition, approximately 25% to 30% of strokes in the young (younger than 45 years) can be attributed to cardiac embolism.[5,6] Table 43-1 estimates the prevalence of various cardiac conditions in embolic ischemia and infarction.[7] The economic toll of embolic strokes in the United States amounts to $39 billion annually in both direct and indirect health care costs.[8-10]

In comparison with that after other subtypes of stroke, the prognosis after a cardioembolic stroke is poor.[11] There is a 6.5% risk of recurrence within 7 days, and the in-hospital mortality rate is 27.3%.[11] The 5-year mortality rate for cardioembolic stroke has been reported as high as 80%.[12]

Clinical Features of Cardioembolic Transient Ischemic Attack or Stroke

Cardioembolism as a proven cause of stroke can be inferred as the diagnosis and distinguished from other stroke subtypes on the basis of (1) *absence* of a large artery stenosis or occlusion in the vessel supplying the ischemic territory, (2) a clinical syndrome or radiographic appearance *inconsistent* with a small vessel (lacunar) stroke, (3) *absence* of unusual precipitants of stroke (i.e., vasculitis), and (4) *absence* of an atheroma of the aortic arch larger than 4 mm. Up to 18% of patients with presumed lacunar syndromes concomitantly have high-risk factors for cardioembolism.[13,14]

Clinical features of cardioembolic stroke are summarized in Table 43-2. The onset of symptoms due to cardioembolism is usually sudden, and repetitive stereotyped transient ischemic attacks (TIAs), associated most commonly with low flow due to large vessel atherosclerotic disease, are unusual in embolic stroke. Less than a third of patients experience transient ischemic symptoms before the stroke.[15-18] The size of the emboli partially determines which vessels are affected. Small emboli can cause symptoms of retinal ischemia.[19-23] In a balloon catheter model of embolism, the majority of emboli were found to occlude the middle cerebral artery or one of its branches; the next most commonly affected vessel was the basilar artery and its branches, and then the anterior cerebral artery.[24] The size and composition of the embolus vary according to the underlying cardiac disorder (Table 43-3).

Valvular lesions may result in the embolization of calcified particles.

Atrial myxomas can cause tumor emboli. In nonbacterial thrombotic endocarditis (NBTE), platelets are the main component of the embolic material, whereas emboli from left ventricular aneurysms contain mainly fibrinous material.[25]

The sudden onset of symptoms, observed in 25% to 82% of possible cardioembolic strokes, has low specificity, inasmuch as the onset is sudden in 66% of strokes from other mechanisms.[15,16] Sudden onset and loss of consciousness are also insensitive for determining that symptoms are due to embolism.[15,11,26] In 1967, Fisher and Pearlman[27] described "non-sudden" cerebral embolism with stuttering progression, which they attributed to vacillating flow around an embolus lodged in the intracranial circulation. Seizures related to acute stroke are more common in patients with cardiac embolism.[28] There may be fluctuations in symptoms as the embolus lyses and fragments move downstream.[29] In addition, early clinical improvement or recovery may be due either to the recruitment of collateral sources of blood flow or to distal migration of the embolus.

Patients at high risk for cardioembolism are more likely to have large infarcts (half a lobe or larger) that involve both deep and superficial structures and are visible on initial head CT (Fig. 43-1).[18,26,30,31] Strokes caused by cardioembolism from AF commonly lead to a significant neurologic disability.[32] A pattern of multiple infarctions involving multiple vascular territories is distinctive for cardioembolism.[18,32-34] Cerebral or cerebellar surface branch occlusion by an embolus may lead to focal infarctions causing specific syndromes of focal motor deficits, isolated aphasia, hemiataxia, or hemianopia.[18,35,36] Posterior cerebral artery territory infarcts, in particular, are commonly caused by cardiac embolism.[37,38] Embolic

TABLE 43-1 CARDIAC CONDITIONS ASSOCIATED WITH CEREBRAL EMBOLI

Source	Percentage of All Cardiogenic Emboli
Nonvalvular atrial fibrillation	45
Acute myocardial infarction	15
Ventricular aneurysm	10
Rheumatic heart disease	10
Prosthetic cardiac valve	10
Other	10

TABLE 43-2 CLINICAL CHARACTERISTICS OF CARDIOEMBOLIC STROKE

Clinical features	Neurologic history and findings
	Sudden onset
	Isolated focal deficit
	Seizure at onset
	Loss of consciousness at onset
	Peak of deficit at onset
	Involvement of more than one vascular territory
	Evidence of systemic embolization
Neuroimaging findings	Multiple infarcts in more than one vascular territory
	Deep and superficial infarctions
	Hemorrhagic conversion
	Absence of large artery stenosis or occlusion in parent vessels
	Rapid recanalization of intracranial vessels on transcranial Doppler ultrasonography

TABLE 43-3 CHARACTERISTICS OF EMBOLI BY SOURCE

Source	Type	Size
Atrial fibrillation	Fibrin	Large
Left ventricular thrombus	Fibrin	Large
Myxoma	Myxomatous	Small or large
Infective endocarditis	Septic debris	Small or large
Degenerative valvular disease	Calcium	Small

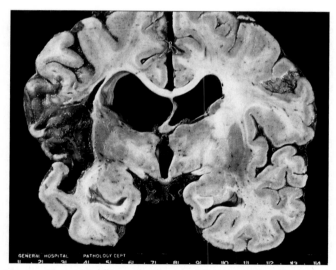

Figure 43-1 Middle cerebral artery (MCA) territory infarction. A complete MCA territory infarction due to stem occlusion is common in embolic stroke. (From Rosenberg R, editor: *Atlas of clinical neurology*, Philadelphia, 1998, Current Medicine.)

strokes are believed to be more prone to hemorrhagic conversion, a complication detected on follow-up CT in approximately 20% of cardioembolic strokes.[39] Hemorrhagic conversion occurs when there is spontaneous lysis of the thrombus with reperfusion into infarcted tissue.

Between 30% and 60% of patients with ischemic stroke have a possible source of cardiac embolism.[25,40] It is important to recognize, however, that the detection of a potential cardiac source of embolism depends, to a large extent, on the thoroughness of the evaluation. For example, one study demonstrated that 15% of potential embolic sources were detected only after cardiac monitoring and two-dimensional (2D) transthoracic echocardiography.[41] In addition, ascribing a stroke to a definite cardioembolic cause can be difficult because of a coexistent mechanism involving a potential noncardiac source of embolus (e.g., large vessel atherosclerosis in approximately 30% of cases). [18,25,42-45]

Diagnostic Studies

A thorough cardiac assessment of patients with stroke is necessary for accurate diagnosis of the mechanism of cerebral ischemia and to help establish prognosis. A standard 12-lead electrocardiogram (ECG) can identify patients who are in sustained AF and can detect acute myocardial ischemia; however, a 24- to 48-hour portable cardiac monitor is essential to detect paroxysmal AF, and the result is not always positive despite numerous such studies in the same patient.[42] More extended cardiac monitoring may be more sensitive to the detection of AF, and in a patient in whom the index of suspicion is high, this testing should be considered.[46,47] A clinical history of angina pectoris or abnormal electrocardiography findings (e.g., anterior wall myocardial infarction [MI], left ventricular hypertrophy, or inverted T waves) have associated hazard ratios of 1.6 to 3.2 for nonfatal MI or cardiac death in patients with TIA or minor stroke.[48]

Transthoracic echocardiography (TTE) is an essential part of the embolic evaluation. M-mode and two-dimensional echocardiography can define the cardiac chambers, valves, and left ventricular function. The use of agitated saline allows for detection of an intracardiac shunt, such as a patent foramen ovale (PFO). The proper detection of a shunt with this procedure requires an adequate Valsalva maneuver, with crossing of the bubble from the right atrium to the left atrium seen upon release of the Valsalva maneuver after two to four cardiac cycles. The more delayed appearance of bubbles is suggestive of a pulmonary source of shunting, such as a pulmonary arteriovenous malformation (AVM). TTE may be insensitive for masses and thrombi in the left atrium and upon the mitral valve, requiring further studies (see later).[49,50]

Transesophageal echocardiography (TEE) is more sensitive in detecting abnormalities in the left atrium and appendage, atrial septum, mitral valve, and aortic arch.[51-53] The cost-effectiveness of performing TEE in all patients with stroke remains controversial.[54,55] This evaluation is recommended for patients with a suspected embolic stroke in whom cardiac monitoring and TTE findings are unremarkable and in young patients with stroke. It actually may be less sensitive for the detection of PFO with agitated saline, because patients who are sedated for the procedure are less able to perform an adequate Valsalva maneuver.

Embolus detection by *transcranial Doppler* (TCD) ultrasonography can be used to identify microemboli present in a variety of potential cardiac sources (AF, infectious endocarditis, cardiomyopathy, aortic stenosis, mitral stenosis, and PFO).[56] The frequency of high-intensity transient signals (HITS) did not appear to vary according to echocardiographic diagnosis in one study, but another demonstrated a higher rate (33%) of microembolization in patients with high-risk sources of embolism (e.g., prosthetic valves) than in patients with other, lower-risk cardiac conditions (e.g., AF [15%]).[56,57]

Approach to Management

Once the clinical presentation, radiographic appearance, and vascular and cardiac evaluations suggest or confirm cardioembolism as the definitive source for the stroke or TIA, the focus shifts to management, mainly the question whether to use anticoagulant or antiplatelet therapy. Table 43-4 summarizes potential cardiac conditions according to the strength of indication for anticoagulation. Although the early period after stroke appears to be the highest risk period for recurrent embolization, it is also the period of greater risk of hemorrhagic conversion. One study examining the utility of immediate anticoagulation for a stroke due to any presumed mechanism but occurring in a patient with AF did not demonstrate a benefit of anticoagulation in the first 2 weeks.[58] Still, in patients at higher risk for embolism, such as those with mechanical prosthetic valves or left ventricular thrombi, immediate anticoagulation should be considered.[59]

For long-term prevention of stroke, AF is the only condition for which warfarin has been shown to be superior to aspirin.[59] Still, anticoagulation is often used in situations with the potential for recurrent embolization. In the Warfarin Aspirin Recurrent Stroke Study (WARSS), warfarin was weakly (absolute risk reduction, 9%) superior to aspirin therapy in patients in whom an embolic stroke was suspected but there was no evidence of a definite cardiac source; this difference was not statistically significant, however.[60] Currently, there are no data specifically comparing aspirin with other antiplatelet agents for the prevention of cardioembolic stroke.

Specific Cardiac Conditions Causing Cerebral Embolism

The numerous structural and functional cardiac conditions associated with transient cerebral symptoms and infarction are described here in greater detail (see Table 43-1). Although cardiac testing can reveal a potential source, the neurologist must determine whether the symptoms, physical findings, and results of neuroimaging support the causal relationship. This determination includes analyzing whether the caliber of occluded vessel correlates with the expected embolus size.

Structural Cardiac Defects

Cardiomyopathy

The reported annual stroke rates (1.3% to 3.5% per year) that were derived from cardiac trials likely underestimate the actual risk of stroke.[7,61-65] The risk of stroke is

TABLE 43-4 CLASSIFICATION OF CARDIOEMBOLIC CEREBRAL ISCHEMIC EVENTS

Definite cardioembolism:
  Antithrombotic therapy considered the standard of practice:
    Left ventricular thrombus
    Left atrial thrombus
    Recent transmural anterior myocardial infarction
    Rheumatic valvular disease
    Mechanical prosthetic valve
    Atrial fibrillation
  Antithrombotic therapy may be of value:
    Nonbacterial thrombotic endocarditis
  Antithrombotic therapy contraindicated:
    Bacterial endocarditis
    Atrial myxoma
Possible cardioembolism:
  Mitral annular calcification
  Mitral valve prolapse
  Cardiomyopathy
  Patent foramen ovale
  Atrial flutter
  Sick sinus syndrome
  Valve strands
  Left atrial spontaneous echo contrast seen on
    transesophageal echocardiogram

inversely related to the ejection fraction (EF), with as much as a 58% increase in thromboembolic events for every 10% decrease in EF, but not to the functional classification (New York Heart Association [NYHA] Functional Class).[64,66] There is a fourfold risk of stroke in patients who are 50 to 59 years old and have congestive heart failure.[4,67] The rate of stroke in patients with nonischemic dilated cardiomyopathy is approximately 1.5% to 3.5%.[62,68] In patients with cardiomyopathy, AF is often a complicating factor that further raises the risk of stroke. Other factors include decreased apical flow and a possible intracardiac hypercoagulable state. Patients with CHF have been found to have increased sympathetic activity, which may lead to increased platelet activation as well as increased levels of β-thyroid–binding globulin, D dimer, von Willebrand factor, fibrinopeptide A, thrombin-antithrombin complexes, β-thromboglobulin, and P-selectin; they also have impaired vascular endothelial function, which impairs the release of nitric oxide, further contributing to platelet adhesion. In the Survival and Ventricular Enlargement (SAVE) study, patients with EF values of 29% to 35% (mean 32%) had a stroke rate of 0.8% per year; the rate in patients with EF values of 28% or less (mean 23%) was 2.5% per year.[64] The Warfarin and Antiplatelet Therapy in Chronic Heart Failure (WATCH) trial was a prospective, three-arm randomized trial comparing warfarin (international normalized ration [INR] goal 2.0 to 3.0), aspirin (162 mg/day), and clopidogrel (75 mg/day) in patients with an EF ≤30% and NYHA class II to IV. The study was stopped early at 1587 patients after poor enrollment rates and without showing a significant difference between the treatment arms, although there was a suggestion of a benefit for warfarin in reducing nonfatal stroke and hospitalization, as secondary endpoints were analyzed.[69] Compared with placebo,

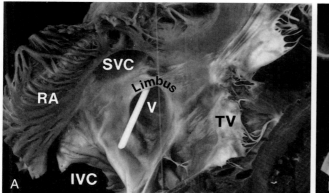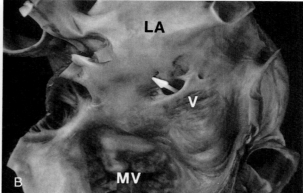

Figure 43-2 Patent foramen ovale, shown in autopsy specimen. A, Right atrial (RA) view shows a probe in the foramen ovale, between limbus and valve (V) of fossa ovalis. B, Left atrial (LA) view shows the probe exiting through the ostium secundum, the prominent fenestration in the valve. Normally, when left atrial pressure exceeds right atrial pressure, the valve of the fossa ovalis is impressed against the limbus and closes the foramen ovale. IVC, inferior vena cava; MV, mitral valve; SVC, superior vena cava; TV, tricuspid valve. (From Hagen PT, Scholz DG, Edwards WD: Incidence and size of patent foramen ovale during the first 10 decades of life: An autopsy study of 965 normal hearts. *Mayo Clin Proc* 59:17, 1984.)

warfarin has been shown to significantly reduce the risk of stroke by 40% to 55% in patients with ischemic and nonischemic cardiomyopathy.[70,71] However, the Sixty Plus Reinfarction Study failed to show a significant risk reduction in stroke using an INR value as high as 2.7 to 4.5.[72] A study comparing the efficacy of warfarin and aspirin for the prevention of stroke in patients with low EF is currently under way.[63]

Acute Myocardial Infarction

Within 2 to 4 weeks of acute MI, 2.5% of patients suffer a stroke.[73,74] Stroke is more common with anterior wall MI (4% to 12% of cases) than with inferior wall MI (1%) and usually occurs within the first 2 weeks.[73,74] Left ventricular thrombus develops in approximately 40% of patients with an anterior wall MI and can be detected with TTE. The thrombus usually develops in the first 2 weeks, coinciding with the period of highest risk for embolic stroke.[73-75] However, there have been reports of development of a left ventricular thrombus as a late complication of anterior wall MI, and patients with low EF due to MI have a cumulative stroke risk of 8.1% after 5 years.[64,76] Despite the absence of clinical trial data, clinicians commonly choose to administer anticoagulation immediately and then maintain it for at least 3 to 6 months in patients in whom left ventricular thrombus is detected. The thrombus may resolve with anticoagulant therapy or may persist for several months. Intravenous tissue-type plasminogen activator (t-PA) has been used safely in patients with acute ischemic stroke and left ventricular thrombus.[77] After MI, warfarin alone for INR 2.1 or in combination with aspirin at 75 mg daily resulted in fewer reinfarctions, thromboembolic events, and deaths compared with aspirin at 16 mg daily alone. However, the warfarin-treated patients had a fourfold higher risk for major hemorrhage.[78]

Patent Foramen Ovale

Paradoxic embolism, or crossing of a venous thrombus into the arterial system, can occur in a patient with a PFO (Fig. 43-2).[79] The resultant right-to-left shunt may appear

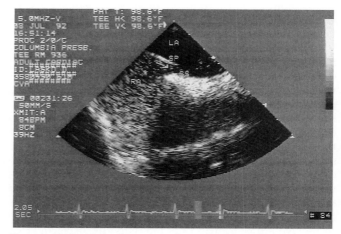

Figure 43-3 Vertical transesophageal echocardiographic view of fossa ovalis area demonstrating the passage of microbubbles through the patent foramen ovale (arrow) from right atrium (RA) into left atrium (LA). Separation of septum primum (SP) from septum secundum (SS) is clearly visualized. (From Homma S, DiTullio MR, Sacco RL: Patent foramen ovale and ischemic stroke. In Barnett HJM, et al, editors: *Stroke: Pathophysiology, diagnosis, and management,* ed 3, New York, 1998, Churchill Livingstone.)

only in the setting of elevated right heart pressures, as occurs with a Valsalva maneuver or with pulmonary hypertension (Fig. 43-3). PFO is common in the general population (20% to 25%),[80] so care should be taken to establish a causal relationship of PFO with cerebral ischemic symptoms before PFO-specific treatment is initiated for secondary prevention of stroke.[79,81]

Strokes in association with PFO occur commonly in the pial convexity branches, as expected, but also in the basilar artery distribution.[82,83] Thrombus is believed to emanate from either a leg or pelvic vein. The latter should not be overlooked in the search for venous thrombus in the patient with a PFO and cerebral ischemic symptoms. In addition, there is conjecture that microthrombi can form within the PFO itself, particularly when there is a coexistent atrial septal aneurysm.[84]

In a study reported by Mas et al.,[85] the risk of recurrent stroke after 4 years of follow-up was 2.3% in patients with PFO alone (95% confidence interval [CI], 0.3%–4.3%), 15.2% among patients with both patent foramen ovale and atrial septal aneurysm (95% CI, 1.8%–28.6%), and 4.2% in patients with neither (95% CI, 1.8%–6.6%). These investigators found no recurrent strokes in patients with atrial septal aneurysms alone. The principal author continues to emphasize uncertainties in risk factors and management.[86] A later report described a high prevalence of PFO in older patients with cryptogenic stroke, but methodologic issues obscure the significance of the findings.[87]

Larger defects (>2 mm) with a higher degree of shunting, as measured by the number of microbubbles crossing into the left atrium, have been associated with cryptogenic embolism.[82,88] Whether the mean diameter of a PFO affects the risk of embolism remains unsettled. One study showed significantly larger diameters in patients with stroke or TIA than in control subjects. In that study, a PFO more than 4 mm in diameter was associated with a higher risk of TIAs (odds ratio [OR], 3.4; 95% CI, 1.0–11; $P = .04$), ischemic strokes (OR, 12; 95% CI, 3.3–44; $P = .0001$), and multiple strokes (OR, 27; 95% CI, 4.7–160; $P = .0002$).[89] Others have shown no clear relationship,[90] including a large Spanish study showing no relationship with PFO size and stroke event rates, even including patients whose shunts were considered "massive."[91] In the PFO in the Cryptogenic Stroke Study, there was no difference in rates of recurrent stroke or death between those with PFO (14.8%) and those without (15.4%) in the entire population or the subset with a cryptogenic mechanism (14.3% versus 12.7%). Neither PFO size nor the association of an atrial septal aneurysm increased the risk of stroke or death. These patients were randomized as part of the Warfarin Aspirin Recurrent Stroke Study (WARSS) to receive either aspirin (325 mg daily) or warfarin (INR 1.4 to 2.8) for 2 years. Treatment did not affect time to primary endpoints in patients with PFO.[92]

TEE is more sensitive than TTE with contrast agent in detecting a PFO.[93] However, TTE is risk free, and positive findings may eliminate the need for additional invasive testing.[94] Two-dimensional TEE measurement of PFO size may be more accurate than the traditionally used contrast agent technique.[95] Patients with cerebral ischemic symptoms and a PFO should undergo noninvasive studies of the legs to rule out deep vein thrombosis, and a pelvic vein MR venogram (MRV) or CT venogram (CTV) should be considered.[94]

It remains unclear whether warfarin is superior to aspirin for stroke prevention after an initial cerebral ischemic event. Current clinical trial data argue against anticoagulation for asymptomatic individuals with PFO. Transcatheter closure of PFO is available; however, according to one series, there remains a risk of persistent shunting after such treatment in up to 20% of patients. After transcatheter closure, the annual risk of stroke or TIA has been reported to remain 3.2% per year.[96] This persistent risk may be explained in part by alternative mechanisms of stroke. Later studies have investigated the safety and efficacy of different devices used for transcatheter closure; however, these are mostly case series and non-randomized studies.[97-101] Furthermore, radiofrequency ablation of atrial fibrillation is possible at the time of transcatheter PFO closure.[102] A controversy exists concerning nickel allergy for some devices containing nickel, which may trigger a local allergic reaction.[103]

Additional studies are needed to identify patients most likely to benefit from transcatheter closure of PFO and to improve performance of the devices used for the procedure. Concerns for safety,[104] reports of delayed-onset atrial fibrillation,[105] and uncertainty about the need for closure have led to a call for[106] and presence of ongoing clinical trials comparing best medical therapy with closure. Two randomized studies are ongoing to address the benefit of catheter-based closure versus medical management, CLOSURE 1 and RESPECT (www.stroketrials.org). Results for the CLOSURE trial are anticipated in October 2010.

Left Atrial Myxoma

An embolic event occurs in up to 3% to 50% of patients with atrial myxoma. Atrial myxoma is the most common primary cardiac tumor but is found in only 75 out of 1 million autopsies. Multiple events have been reported, some separated in time by months to years. The friability of the tumor lends itself to embolism of tumor fragments (Fig. 43-4).[107,108] Myxomas can be detected on TTE or TEE. The treatment is surgical resection.

Spontaneous Echo Contrast

Spontaneous echo contrast (SEC), a marker of disordered flow and hemostatic activation in the left atrium, is often seen on TEE in patients with AF.[55,109,110] SEC is associated with a higher risk of thromboembolism in mitral valve disorders.[111,112] Numerous studies have established an association between SEC and intracardiac thrombus formation, but SEC has not been shown to be an independent risk factor for embolic stroke.[111-114]

Mitral Valve Strands

Lambl's excrescences, or mitral valve strands, are filamentous processes on the ventricular surface of the aortic valve or the atrial surface of the mitral valve; they are detectable on TEE. Histologically, the strands are composed of endothelialized connective tissue. One study found that mitral valve strands were more common in patients with a history of recent cerebral ischemic events (6.3%) than in control subjects who had neither (0.3%). In young patients in whom cardioembolic stroke was suspected, 16% were found to have mitral valve strands, often without another identifiable cardiac source.[115] Other retrospective studies have shown that mitral valve strands are found more commonly in younger patients and in patients with a recent embolic event (10.6% to 53%) than in patients referred because of findings on TEE performed for other reasons (2.3% to 15%).[116-118]

Dysrhythmias

Atrial Fibrillation

Thrombi in AF arise from the left atrium and atrial appendage. The combination of rheumatic heart disease (RHD) and AF carries a stroke risk 17 times that in

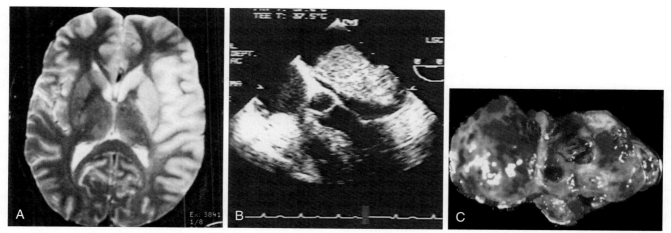

Figure 43-4 *A,* T2-weighted MR image of the brain in a patient with left middle cerebral artery territory infarction due to atrial myxoma embolization. *B,* Echocardiogram showing a large atrial myxoma above the mitral valve during systole. *C,* Pathologic specimen showing a gelatinous atrial myxoma with numerous cysts. (From Rosenberg R, editor: *Atlas of clinical neurology,* Philadelphia, 1998, Current Medicine.)

normal controls (who have neither AF nor RHD).[3] Of all the definite or possible mechanisms of cardioembolic stroke, AF has been the most extensively studied.[119-125] It is the most common cause of embolic stroke, accounting for 25% to 30% of all embolic strokes.[7] AF is the only cardioembolic source of stroke that has been subjected to randomized clinical trials evaluating the efficacy of antithrombotic and antiplatelet therapies for stroke prevention.[125] The rate of AF-related stroke rises with age.[3,4] Younger patients with AF who are free of cardiac disease, diabetes, and hypertension have an extremely low rate of stroke (1.3% per 15 years).[119, 126] Beginning at age 65 years, however, the annual risk of stroke is 3% to 5% per year; the risk increases to 10% per year or higher by age 80 years, with women predominating.[4] The age-related risk is independent of other major risk factors (diabetes, hypertension, previous stroke, and congestive heart failure).[119] Multiple grading schemes are available for quantifying the risk of stroke in patients with nonvalvular atrial fibrillation. These consistently find a prior stroke or TIA to be the highest risk for another event, but otherwise may give variable rates of prediction based on other risk factors.[127]

The five aforementioned randomized primary and secondary prevention trials have demonstrated the efficacy and safety of warfarin in preventing AF-related stroke.[119-125] Pooled data from these trials demonstrated a 68% reduction in ischemic stroke (95% CI, 50%-79%) and an intracerebral hemorrhage rate of less than 1% per year. The data for aspirin suggest a much more modest effect. One European study randomly assigned patients with stroke or TIA with AF to aspirin (300 mg daily) versus placebo, and found a nonsignificant 16% relative risk reduction.[128] The Stroke Prevention in Atrial Fibrillation (SPAF) III study suggested that patients with low-risk AF (without prior stroke/TIA, hypertension, low EF, or advanced age and female sex) may be treated as safely with aspirin as with warfarin, the rates of thromboembolism also being similar.[122] The Atrial Fibrillation Clopidogrel Trial with Irbesartan for Prevention of Vascular Events (ACTIVE) randomly divided patients with AF and

at least one stroke risk factor to receive either warfarin or the combination of aspirin (75-100 mg daily) and clopidogrel (75 mg daily). The trial was terminated early because of a lack of comparative efficacy in preventing embolic events in the aspirin plus clopidogrel arm, even though the agents caused equivalent rates of hemorrhage (INR goal, 2-3).[129] Even in patients with AF who cannot take warfarin, the combination of aspirin and clopidogrel was not found to be superior to aspirin alone in a subgroup analysis of the Clopidogrel for High Atherothrombotic Risk and Ischemic Stabilization, Management and Avoidance (CHARISMA) randomized trial.[130] The ACTIVE A study found, in patients with AF who could not take warfarin and who were randomly assigned to either the combination of aspirin and clopidogrel or aspirin alone, ischemic events were significantly prevented, but at a cost of relatively the same number of major hemorrhagic events.[131]

Oral anticoagulation for secondary stroke prevention in patients with AF is associated with a small but definite risk of hemorrhage, particularly intracerebral hemorrhage, which is more common in elderly patients (>75 years).[119] Despite the increased risk of intracerebral hemorrhage in patients aged older than 85 years, there continues to be a benefit of anticoagulation for AF, and care should be taken to ensure that these patients' INR values stay within the target range, because higher values significantly increase the risk.[132]

Independent risk factors associated with a higher risk of stroke include age older than 65 years, previous history of stroke or TIA, hypertension, and diabetes mellitus. Impaired left ventricular function was identified as an additional risk factor in the SPAF study population. In a pooled analysis of seven separate studies conducted by the SPAF study investigators, AF with a prior stroke or TIA carried the strongest risk for future stroke, an estimated rate of 6% to 9% per year.[133] Despite these findings, only 30% to 60% of patients with AF receive appropriate anticoagulation therapy.[134] Long-term oral anticoagulation with a goal INR of 2.0 to 3.0 is recommended for patients with AF and a recent stroke or TIA.[135]

An alternative approach in the future may include complete isolation of the left atrial appendage, perhaps obviating the need for anticoagulation. Because the vast majority (estimated at 90%) of thrombi in AF form in the left atrial appendage, mechanical isolation of this compartment is an attractive theoretical approach. Preliminary studies have lent some credence to this notion, and a randomized trial is ongoing.[136]

TTE findings can also be factored into risk stratification. Moderate to severe impairment of left ventricular function is associated with a 2.5-fold greater risk of stroke. A left atrial anteroposterior diameter greater than 2.5 cm/ m² was also found to be a predictor of cerebral embolism. In the SPAF study, 26% of patients had no clinical risk factor and normal TTE findings. These patients had a low risk of stroke (<1% per year). Approximately one third of patients considered at low risk according to clinical criteria are reclassified as having a high risk on the basis of echocardiographic findings.[137-140]

TEE has greater sensitivity for detecting abnormalities in the left atrium. SEC, reduced left atrial appendage emptying, and left atrial thrombus are markers of higher stroke risk. In addition, TEE is better able to visualize aortic plaque.[141,142] In patients with high-risk clinical factors, the presence of any left atrial abnormality or an aortic arch atheroma shown to be larger than 4 mm on TEE was found to raise the risk of stroke by as much as 20% per year.[143]

The use of anticoagulation for acute cardioembolic stroke due to AF is controversial. There is a significant risk of hemorrhagic conversion of the acute infarction (1.7% to 4.4%), particularly with larger strokes.[144-147] Conversely, the risk of recurrent embolism ranges from 0.1% to 1.3% in the first 2 weeks.[58,148,149] There are meager data supporting the use of anticoagulation in the acute setting, but they derive mostly from nonblinded studies and small case series.[150,151] A study of immediate therapy in patients with AF and ischemic stroke appeared to show no benefit of anticoagulation over antiplatelet therapy[58]; patients randomly assigned within 30 hours of stroke onset to receive dalteparin (100 IU/kg subcutaneously [SC] twice daily) or aspirin (160 mg daily) had a higher rate of stroke recurrence or progression, death, or symptomatic intracerebral hemorrhage (24.6% vs. 16.9%; $P = 0.048$) and of extracerebral hemorrhages (5.8% vs. 1.8%; $P = .028$). Major limitations of this study were that a significant proportion of the strokes in this study were characterized as lacunar, suggesting that the mechanism of stroke may not have been cardioembolic, and higher risk patients may not have been enrolled in this trial, as it was left to the treating physicians' discretion.

Sick Sinus Syndrome

Sick sinus syndrome (SSS), also referred to as tachycardia-bradycardia syndrome, is more common in older patients and is often attributed to ischemia, degeneration, or neuromuscular disease. Patients may experience atrial flutter and AF as part of this syndrome.[152] SSS has been associated with a higher risk of stroke; systemic embolism occurs in 16% of patients with SSS, in comparison with only 1.9% of patients with complete heart block.[153,154] The treatment of choice is surgical insertion of an atrial on-demand pacemaker.[155] Antithrombotic therapy has not been directly compared with antiplatelet therapy in this population, although clearly, in patients with paroxysmal AF, warfarin is recommended. An atrial pacemaker, of course, does not prevent the occurrence of AF, and thus antithrombotic therapy is still warranted.

Atrial Flutter

Atrial flutter is an unstable rhythm that belies underlying atrial disease and commonly degenerates into AF. In a study examining a large Medicare database, the stroke risk in patients with atrial flutter (relative risk [RR], 1.41) was determined to be higher than in a control group but lower than in patients with AF (RR, 1.64). Patients with atrial flutter who subsequently experienced an episode of AF had a higher risk of stroke (RR, 1.56) than patients with atrial flutter who never had a subsequent episode of AF (RR, 1.11).[156] Left atrial appendage velocities are similar in patients with AF and patients with AF-flutter (an intermediate form with elements of both AF and atrial flutter); thus, the risk of left atrial thrombus formation should be comparable in the two conditions.[157]

Largely because of the risk of intermittent AF in patients with atrial flutter, it is appropriate to consider anticoagulation in patients who present with atrial flutter and coexistent cardiac disease that predisposes to left atrial thrombus.[148]

Valvular Disease

Mitral Annular Calcification

Mitral annular calcification (MAC) has been associated with a higher risk of ischemic stroke.[158-160] This disorder is associated with aging, ischemic heart disease, and cardiac arrhythmias. Because patients with MAC are also at risk of stroke by other mechanisms, it is unclear whether there is a causal relationship (i.e., that thrombus calcific debris embolizes from the degenerated valve) or merely whether mitral annulus calcification is a marker of systemic atherosclerosis and intrinsic cardiac dysfunction.

Prosthetic Valves

The rate of embolism in patients with mechanical prosthetic valves who are receiving anticoagulation approximates that of patients with bioprosthetic valves who are not, approximately 3% to 4% annually for mitral valves and 1.3% to 3.2% for aortic valves.[161-163] It is recommended that patients with bioprosthetic valves undergo anticoagulation either for the first 3 months or on a long-term basis if there is evidence of AF, left atrial thrombus, or previous emboli.[164] Adding aspirin to warfarin therapy in patients with mechanical valves and high-risk bioprosthetic valves is superior to warfarin alone in reducing rates of vascular mortality and systemic embolism (1.9% per year versus 8.5% per year, respectively) without a significant increase in major bleeding complications.[165]

Mitral Stenosis

Mitral stenosis, often related to rheumatic heart disease, is associated with left atrial thrombus in 15% to 17% of cases in autopsy series (Fig. 43-5).[166,167] The annual rate of

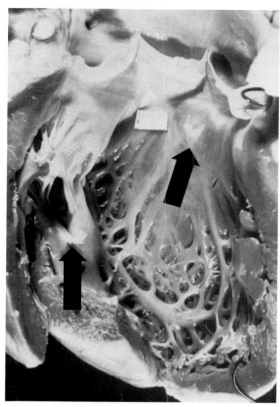

Figure 43-5 Pathologic specimen showing mitral stenosis resulting from rheumatic heart disease with "jet lesions" *(arrows)* on the wall of the left ventricle. (From Hinchey JA, Furlan AJ, Barnett HJM: Cardiogenic brain embolism: Incidence, varieties, and treatment. In Barnett HJM, editors: *Stroke: Pathophysiology, diagnosis, and management,* ed 3, New York, Churchill Livingstone, 1998.)

stroke is approximately 2% in patients with mitral stenosis, and recurrent embolism is common. Warfarin should be considered when there is a strong suspicion of coexistent AF.[168]

Infective Endocarditis

Stroke occurs in 15% to 20% of patients with infective endocarditis, usually within the first 48 hours (Fig. 43-6). Appropriate antibiotic therapy dramatically reduces the risk of stroke, and late embolism occurs in less than 5% of cases.[168,169] An elevated erythrocyte sedimentation rate in the setting of cerebral ischemic symptoms and fever or a new heart murmur should trigger a diagnostic evaluation including serial blood cultures, a transthoracic echocardiogram, and, if a high level of suspicion remains, TEE. Neurologic complications of infective endocarditis, including ischemic and hemorrhagic infarctions, toxic encephalopathy, arteritis, meningitis, and subarachnoid hemorrhage, contribute to the high mortality rate (15% to 20%) associated with this condition despite antibiotic therapy.[170,171] Infective endocarditis can be complicated by mycotic aneurysms, which can rupture, causing subarachnoid hemorrhage. Mycotic aneurysms can be differentiated from berry aneurysms on the basis of their location in the distal cerebral vasculature (third or fourth branch from the circle of Willis). When subarachnoid hemorrhage occurs in this setting, it is more superficial and is not generally complicated by vasospasm. The presence of strokes or hemorrhages, even if small, poses a challenge in this population, because definitive therapy often requires surgical valve replacement. This procedure requires large doses of anticoagulation, so it should be delayed if possible in the acute setting to let the lesions heal. It is commonly

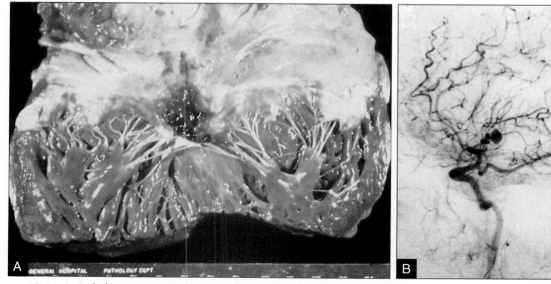

Figure 43-6 A, Pathologic specimen showing a large hemorrhagic vegetation. B, Left common carotid angiogram showing an aneurysm of a proximal branch of the left middle cerebral artery. (From Rosenberg R, editor: *Atlas of clinical neurology,* Philadelphia, 1998, Current Medicine.)

recommended to wait a minimum of 2 weeks after an ischemic or hemorrhagic cerebral event and longer if possible (4 to 6 weeks).

The most common organisms causing native valve endocarditis are streptococci, staphylococci, and enterococci. More rarely, other species of bacteria, fungi, spirochetes, and rickettsiae can infect valves.[172] Echocardiography has not been shown to be useful in predicting risk of embolism, and early antibiotic therapy is still the mainstay of treatment.[170,173] The risk of subarachnoid hemorrhage is considered by many authorities to represent a contraindication to the use of anticoagulation in infectious endocarditis. Noninvasive MR arteriography or CT angiography have largely replaced conventional transfemoral angiography in screening for mycotic aneurysms.[174]

Nonbacterial Thrombotic Endocarditis

Also known as marantic endocarditis, NBTE is associated with malignancy, often in combination with Trousseau's syndrome (Fig. 43-7).[175] The clinical manifestation may be one of focal deficits referable to one or more vascular territories, or a nonfocal encephalopathy.[176] NBTE should be suspected in all cases of stroke in patients with an underlying malignancy and is best diagnosed with echocardiography, either TEE or TTE.[175] Some clinicians recommend anticoagulation to prevent recurrent embolism, especially in a patient with a coexistent hypercoagulable state; however, the efficacy of anticoagulation in this setting has not been proven.

Libman-Sacks endocarditis represents an atypical form of NBTE associated with systemic lupus erythematosus.[177-179] It is often associated with an antiphospholipid antibody–mediated systemic hypercoagulable state. There are no proven treatment strategies for Libman-Sacks endocarditis and the antiphospholipid antibody syndrome.[178] Although anticoagulation is often used, particularly in patients with transient ischemic symptoms or stroke, the target INR range is debated.

Other Valvular Disorders

Mitral regurgitation is associated with a higher risk of stroke, largely because of coexistent AF in the majority of cases.[180,181] *Aortic stenosis* can also cause stroke, mainly through embolization of calcific material.[182] One case-control study demonstrated that *mitral valve prolapse* is considerably less common among young patients with stroke or transient ischemic symptoms than previously reported, yielding a crude OR of 0.70 in patients with mitral valve prolapse in relation to controls (95% CI, 0.15–2.80; $P = 0.80$); after adjustment for age and sex, the OR was found to be 0.59 (95% CI, 0.12–2.50; $P = 0.62$).[183] *Mitral valve papillary fibroelastoma* is a rare tumor detectable on echocardiography that can result in stroke and requires surgical resection.[184-186]

Cardiac Procedures

Coronary Artery Bypass Surgery–Related Embolism

Approximately 3% to 6% of patients undergoing coronary artery bypass grafting or valve replacement surgery experience a perioperative stroke.[187,188] The mechanism of stroke may be cardioembolism, low flow (distal field or watershed hypotensive ischemia), or artery-to-artery emboli from the aortic arch.[189] Most delayed strokes are due to postoperative AF, particularly in the setting of low

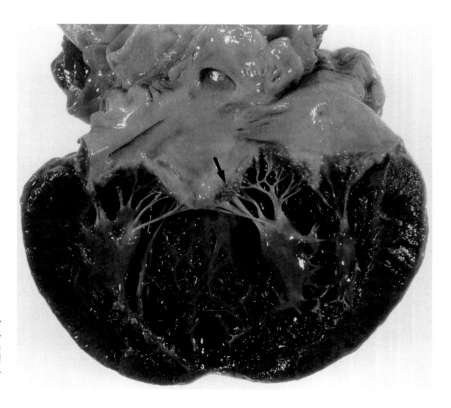

Figure 43-7 Mitral valve vegetations of nonbacterial thrombotic endocarditis *(arrow).* (From Rogers LR, Cho ES, Kempin S, Posner JB: Cerebral infarction from nonbacterial thrombotic endocarditis: Clinical and pathological study including the effects of anticoagulation. *Am J Med* 83:746, 1987.)

EF.[187,190] Clinical factors such as age more than 75 years, recent MI or unstable angina, history of previous stroke, carotid artery disease, hypertension, diabetes, previous coronary artery surgery, postoperative AF, low EF, and history of pulmonary or renal insufficiency are associated with higher risk of stroke.[187,191,192] Diffusion-weighted MRI is more sensitive than CT for visualizing these acute infarcts, which are often multiple and may manifest as encephalopathy.[193] There appears to be a posterior circulation predominance to the pattern of infarction after coronary artery bypass grafting.[194]

Cardiac Catheterization

Cardiac catheterization can result in ischemic stroke, usually embolic. The embolus may occur secondary to an artery-to-artery cause from the disruption of atherosclerotic plaque in the aorta or to cardiac injury during the procedure. The risk of stroke has been found to be significantly associated with the severity of coronary artery disease (OR, 1.96) and the duration of fluoroscopy (OR, 1.65). Diffusion-weighted MRI was shown to be sensitive for detecting multiple silent infarcts and small vessel infarcts.[195] Hypertension, age more than 60 years, peripheral vascular disease, emergency performance of the procedure, and angioplasty raise the risk of catheterization-related thromboembolic complications.[196]

Cardiac Embolism and the Hemostatic System

Atrial fibrillation, a model for embolic stroke, has been linked to alterations in the hemostatic system.[197-202] Local hemostatic factors in the endocardium are likely responsible for the development of left atrial thrombi.[203] As in other vascular beds, the regulation of this signaling is under genetic control, although a variety of external stimuli modulate the expression. In patients with AF, the level of prothrombin fragment F1+2, a byproduct of the conversion of prothrombin to thrombin and thus a measure of thrombin generation, increases with age in parallel with the rate of stroke.[204] The overwhelming majority of patients experience a dramatic reduction in stroke risk with warfarin, which correlates well with a reduction in the level of activity of the hemostatic system. In addition, aspirin has little effect on F1+2, corresponding to its relative lack of efficacy in stroke prevention in patients with AF.

Other studies have confirmed that levels of prothrombotic factor are increased in AF (factor VIII, fibrinogen, thrombin-antithrombin complex), as are levels of those involved in fibrinolysis (tissue plasminogen activator, D dimer).[107-202] Von Willebrand factor levels are a marker of endothelial damage associated with AF as well.[201,202] Platelet activation has been shown to play a role in AF. Elevations in platelet factor 4, β-thromboglobulin, and P-selectin have been demonstrated in patients with AF.[197,201] This increased hemostatic activity is not unique to AF and suggests a common mechanism of stroke among other cardiac conditions associated with risk of embolism—left ventricular aneurysm,[205] mitral stenosis,[206] and heart failure.[207]

Therefore, it appears that aberrant flow in the heart secondary to structural disease may result in endothelial disruption, triggering local thrombus formation. The stability of the thrombus is mediated by the integrity of fibrin cross linking. The genetic control regulating the interaction between the endothelium and the coagulation system may, in part, explain why some high-risk patients remain free of embolic events. These genetic influences may also be at play in cases of high-risk patients who experience emboli while undergoing therapeutic anticoagulation. The interaction between the endocardial surface and the coagulation system requires additional study.

REFERENCES

1. Sacco RL, Ellenberg JH, Mohr JP, et al: Infarcts of undetermined cause: The NINCDS Stroke Data Bank, *Ann Neurol* 25:382-390, 1989.
2. Kannel WB, Wolf PA, Benjamin EJ, et al: Prevalence, incidence, prognosis, and predisposing conditions for atrial fibrillation: Population-based estimates, *Am J Cardiol* 82:2N-9N, 1998.
3. Wolf PA, Dawber TR, Thomas HE Jr, et al: Epidemiologic assessment of chronic atrial fibrillation and risk of stroke: The Framingham study, *Neurology* 28:973-977, 1978.
4. Wolf PA, Abbott RD, Kannel WB: Atrial fibrillation: A major contributor to stroke in the elderly. The Framingham Study, *Arch Intern Med* 147:1561-1564, 1987.
5. Kittner SJ, Stern BJ, Wozniak M, et al: Cerebral infarction in young adults: The Baltimore-Washington Cooperative Young Stroke Study, *Neurology* 50:890-894, 1998.
6. Adams HP Jr, Butler MJ, Biller J, et al: Nonhemorrhagic cerebral infarction in young adults, *Arch Neurol* 4:793-796, 1986.
7. Cardiogenic brain embolism: Cerebral Embolism Task Force, *Arch Neurol* 43:71-84, 1986.
8. American Heart Association: *Heart and stroke facts: Statistical supplement*, Dallas, 2008, American Heart Association.
9. Diringer MN, Edwards DF, Mattson DT, et al: Predictors of acute hospital costs for treatment of ischemic stroke in an academic center, *Stroke* 30:724-728, 1999.
10. Lloyd-Jones D, Adams R, Carnethon M, et al: Heart Disease and Stroke Statistics—2009 Update: A report from the American Heart Association Statistics Committee and Stroke Statistics Committee, *Circulation* 119:e21-e181, 2009.
11. Arboix A, Vericat MC, Pujades R, et al: Cardioembolic infarction in the Sagrat Cor-Alianza Hospital of Barcelona Stroke Registry, *Acta Neurol Scand* 96:407-412, 1997.
12. Petty GW, Brown RD Jr, Whisnant JP, et al: Ischemic stroke subtypes: A population-based study of functional outcome, survival, and recurrence, *Stroke* 31:1062-1068, 2000.
13. Horowitz DR, Tuhrim S, Weinberger JM, Rudolph SH: Mechanisms in lacunar infarction, *Stroke* 23:325-327, 1992.
14. Staaf G, Samuelsson M, Lindgren A, et al: Sensorimotor stroke: Clinical features, MRI findings, and cardiac and vascular concomitants in 32 patients, *Acta Neurol Scand* 97:93-98, 1998.
15. Ramirez-Lassepas M, Cipolle RJ, Bjork RJ, et al: Can embolic stroke be diagnosed on the basis of neurologic clinical criteria? *Arch Neurol* 44:87-89, 1987.
16. Caplan LR, Hier DB, D'Cruz I: Cerebral embolism in the Michael Reese Stroke Registry, *Stroke* 14:530-536, 1983.
17. Foulkes MA, Wolf PA, Price TR, et al: The Stroke Data Bank: Design, methods, and baseline characteristics, *Stroke* 19:547-554, 1988.
18. Bogousslavsky J, Cachin C, Regli F, et al: Cardiac sources of embolism and cerebral infarction-clinical consequences and vascular concomitants: The Lausanne Stroke Registry, *Neurology* 41:855-859, 1991.
19. Appen RE, Wray SH, Cogan DG: Central retinal artery occlusion, *Am J Ophthalmol* 79:374-381, 1975.
20. Babikian VL, Wijman CA, Hyde C, et al: Cerebral microembolism and early recurrent cerebral or retinal ischemic events, *Stroke* 28:1314-1318, 1997.
21. Hankey GJ, Slattery JM, Warlow CP: Prognosis and prognostic factors of retinal infarction: A prospective cohort study, *BMJ* 302:499-504, 1991.
22. Babikian VL, Hyde C, Pochay V, et al: Clinical correlates of high-intensity transient signals detected on transcranial Doppler sonography in patients with cerebrovascular disease, *Stroke* 25:1570-1573, 1994.

23. Murkin JM: Etiology and incidence of brain dysfunction after cardiac surgery, *J Cardiothorac Vasc Anesth* 13(Suppl 1):12-77, 1999.

24. Gacs G, Merei FT, Bodosi M: Balloon catheter as a model of cerebral emboli in humans, *Stroke* 13:39-42, 1982.

25. Cardiogenic brain embolism: The second report of the Cerebral Embolism Task Force, *Arch Neurol* 46:727-743, 1989.

26. Timsit SG, Sacco RL, Mohr JP, et al: Brain infarction severity differs according to cardiac or arterial embolic source, *Neurology* 43:728-733, 1993.

27. Fisher CM, Pearlman A: The nonsudden onset of cerebral embolism, *Neurology* 17:1025-1032, 1967.

28. Kraus JA, Berlit P: Cerebral embolism and epileptic seizures: The role of the embolic source, *Acta Neurol Scand* 97:154-159, 1998.

29. Minematsu K, Yamaguchi T, Omae T: 'Spectacular shrinking deficit': Rapid recovery from a major hemispheric syndrome by migration of an embolus, *Neurology* 42:157-162, 1992.

30. Kittner SJ, Sharkness CM, Sloan MA: Features on initial computed tomography scan of infarcts with a cardiac source of embolism in the NINDS Stroke Data Bank, *Stroke* 23:1748-1751, 1992.

31. Ringelstein EB, Koschorke S, Holling A, et al: Computed tomographic patterns of proven embolic brain infarctions, *Ann Neurol* 26:759-765, 1989.

32. Jørgensen HS, Nakayama H, Reith J, et al: Acute stroke with atrial fibrillation: The Copenhagen Stroke Study, *Stroke* 27:1765-1769, 1996.

33. Bogousslavsky J, Bernasconi A, Kumral E: Acute multiple infarction involving the anterior circulation, *Arch Neurol* 53:50-57, 1996.

34. Bogousslavsky J, Van Melle G, Regli F, et al: Pathogenesis of anterior circulation stroke in patients with nonvalvular atrial fibrillation: The Lausanne Stroke Registry, *Neurology* 40:1046-1050, 1990.

35. Horowitz DR, Tuhrim S: Stroke mechanisms and clinical presentation in large subcortical infarctions, *Neurology* 49:1538-1541, 1997.

36. Bogousslavsky J, Van Melle G, Regli F: Middle cerebral artery pial territory infarcts: A study of the Lausanne Stroke Registry, *Ann Neurol* 25:555-560, 1989.

37. Yamamoto Y, Georgiadis AL, Chang HM, Caplan LR: Posterior cerebral artery territory infarcts in the New England Medical Center Posterior Circulation Registry, *Arch Neurol* 56:824-832, 1999.

38. Pessin MS, Lathi ES, Cohen MB, et al: Clinical features and mechanism of occipital infarction, *Ann Neurol* 21:290-299, 1987.

39. Hart RG, Easton JD: Hemorrhagic infarcts, *Stroke* 17:586-589, 1986.

40. Mast H, Thompson JL, Voller H, et al: Cardiac sources of embolism in patients with pial artery infarcts and lacunar lesions, *Stroke* 25:776-781, 1994.

41. Rem JA, Hachinski VC, Boughner DR, et al: Value of cardiac monitoring and echocardiography in TIA and stroke patients, *Stroke* 16:950-956, 1985.

42. Jabaudon D, Sztajzel J, Sievert K, et al: Usefulness of ambulatory 7-day ECG monitoring for the detection of atrial fibrillation and flutter after acute stroke and transient ischemic attack, *Stroke* 35:1647-1651, 2004.

43. Tayal AH, Tian M, Kelly KM, et al: Atrial fibrillation detected by mobile cardiac outpatient telemetry in cryptogenic TIA or stroke, *Neurology* 71:1696-1701, 2008.

44. Bogousslavsky J, Hachinski VC, Boughner DR, et al: Cardiac and arterial lesions in carotid transient ischemic attacks, *Arch Neurol* 43:223-228, 1986.

45. Moncayo J, Devuyst G, Van Melle G, Bogousslavsky J: Coexisting causes of ischemic stroke, *Arch Neurol* 57:1139-1144, 2000.

46. Hornig CR, Haberbosch W, Lammers C, et al: Specific cardiological evaluation after focal cerebral ischemia, *Acta Neurol Scand* 93:297-302, 1996.

47. Bogousslavsky J, Regli F, Maeder P, et al: The etiology of posterior circulation infarcts: A prospective study using magnetic resonance imaging and magnetic resonance angiography, *Neurology* 43:1528-1533, 1993.

48. Pop GA, Koudstaal PJ, Meeder HJ, et al: Predictive value of clinical history and electrocardiogram in patients with transient ischemic attack or minor ischemic stroke for subsequent cardiac and cerebral ischemic events. The Dutch TIA Trial Study Group, *Arch Neurol* 51:333-341, 1994.

49. Popp RL: Echocardiography (2), *N Engl J Med* 323:165-172, 1990.

50. Popp RL: Echocardiography (1), *N Engl J Med* 323:101-109, 1990.

51. Pop G, Sutherland GR, Koudstaal PJ, et al: Transesophageal echocardiography in the detection of intracardiac embolic sources in patients with transient ischemic attacks, *Stroke* 21:560-565, 1990.

52. Hata JS, Ayres RW, Biller J, et al: Impact of transesophageal echocardiography on the anticoagulation management of patients admitted with focal cerebral ischemia, *Am J Cardiol* 72:707-710, 1993.

53. Pearson AC, Labovitz AJ, Tatineni S, et al: Superiority of transesophageal echocardiography in detecting cardiac source of embolism in patients with cerebral ischemia of uncertain etiology, *J Am Coll Cardiol* 17:66-72, 1991.

54. Warner MF, Momah KI: Routine transesophageal echocardiography for cerebral ischemia: Is it really necessary? *Arch Intern Med* 156:1719-1723, 1996.

55. McNamara RL, Lima JA, Whelton PK, et al: Echocardiographic identification of cardiovascular sources of emboli to guide clinical management of stroke: A cost-effectiveness analysis, *Ann Intern Med* 127:775-787, 1997.

56. Sliwka U, Job FP, Wissuwa D, et al: Occurrence of transcranial Doppler high-intensity transient signals in patients with potential cardiac sources of embolism: A prospective study, *Stroke* 26:2067-2070, 1995.

57. Tong DC, Bolger A, Albers GW: Incidence of transcranial Doppler-detected cerebral microemboli in patients referred for echocardiography, *Stroke* 25:2138-2141, 1995.

58. Berge E, Abdelnoor M, Nakstad PH, et al: Low molecular-weight heparin versus aspirin in patients with acute ischaemic stroke and atrial fibrillation: A double-blind randomised study. HAEST Study Group. Heparin in Acute Embolic Stroke Trial, *Lancet* 200;355:1205-1210.

59. del Zoppo GJ: Antithrombotic treatments in acute ischemic stroke, *Curr Opin Hematol* 7:309-315, 2000.

60. Mohr JP, Thompson JL, Lazar RM, et al: A comparison of warfarin and aspirin for the prevention of recurrent ischemic stroke, *N Engl J Med* 345:1444-1451, 2001.

61. Katz SD, Marantz PR, Biasucci L, et al: Low incidence of stroke in ambulatory patients with heart failure: A prospective study, *Am Heart J* 126:141-146, 1993.

62. Fuster V, Gersh BJ, Guiliani ER, et al: The natural history of idiopathic dilated cardiomyopathy, *Am J Cardiol* 47:525-531, 1981.

63. Pullicino PM, Halperin JL, Thompson JL: Stroke in patients with heart failure and reduced left ventricular ejection fraction, *Neurology* 54:288-294, 2000.

64. Loh E, Sutton MS, Wun CC, et al: Ventricular dysfunction and the risk of stroke after myocardial infarction, *N Engl J Med* 336:251-257, 1997.

65. Cleland JG: Anticoagulant and antiplatelet therapy in heart failure, *Curr Opin Cardiol* 12:276-287, 1997.

66. Dries DL, Rosenberg YD, Waclawiw MA, et al: Ejection fraction and risk of thromboembolic events in patients with systolic dysfunction and sinus rhythm: Evidence for gender differences in the studies of left ventricular dysfunction trials, *J Am Coll Cardiol* 29:1074-1080, 1997.

67. Kannel WB, Wolf PA, Verter J: Manifestations of coronary disease predisposing to stroke. The Framingham study, *JAMA* 250:2942-2946, 1983.

68. Segal JP, Stapleton JF, McClellan JR, et al: Idiopathic cardiomyopathy: Clinical features, prognosis and therapy, *Curr Probl Cardiol* 3:1-48, 1978.

69. Massie BM, Collins JF, Ammon SE, et al: Randomized trial of warfarin, aspirin and clopidogrel in patients with chronic heart failure: The Warfarin and Antiplatelet therapy in Chronic Heart Failure (WATCH) trial, *Circulation* 119:1559-1561, 2009.

70. Effect of long-term oral anticoagulant treatment on mortality and cardiovascular morbidity after myocardial infarction: Anticoagulants in the Secondary Prevention of Events in Coronary Thrombosis (ASPECT) Research Group, *Lancet* 343:499-503, 1994.

71. Smith P, Arnesen H, Holme I: The effect of warfarin on mortality and reinfarction after myocardial infarction, *N Engl J Med* 323:147-152, 1990.

72. A double-blind trial to assess long-term oral anticoagulant therapy in elderly patients after myocardial infarction. Report of the Sixty Plus Reinfarction Study Research Group, *Lancet* 2:989-994, 1980.

73. Komrad MS, Coffee CE, Coffee KS, et al: Myocardial infarction and stroke, *Neurology* 34:1403-1409, 1984.

74. Puletti M, Cusmano E, Testa MG, et al: Incidence of systemic thromboembolic lesions in acute myocardial infarction, *Clin Cardiol* 9:331-333, 1986.

75. Asinger RW, Mikell FL, Elsperger J, et al: Incidence of left-ventricular thrombosis after acute transmural myocardial infarction: Serial evaluation by two-dimensional echocardiography, *N Engl J Med* 305:297-302, 1981.

76. Stratton JR, Resnick AD: Increased embolic risk in patients with left ventricular thrombi, *Circulation* 75:1004-1011, 1987.

77. Derex L, Nighoghossian N, Perinetti M, et al: Thrombolytic therapy in acute ischemic stroke patients with cardiac thrombus, *Neurology* 57:2122-2125, 2001.

78. Hurlen M, Abdelnoor M, Smith P, et al: Warfarin, aspirin, or both after myocardial infarction, *N Engl J Med* 347:969-974, 2002.

79. Sacco RL, Homma S, Di Tullio MR: Patent foramen ovale: A new risk factor for ischemic stroke, *Heart Dis Stroke* 2:235-241, 1993.

80. Lechat P, Mas JL, Lescault G, et al: Prevalence of patent foramen ovale in patients with stroke, *N Engl J Med* 318:1148-1152, 1988.

81. Di Tullio M, Sacco RL, Gopal A, et al: Patent foramen ovale as a risk factor for cryptogenic stroke, *Ann Intern Med* 117:461-465, 1992.

82. Steiner MM, Di Tullio MR, Rundek T, et al: Patent foramen ovale size and embolic brain imaging findings among patients with ischemic stroke, *Stroke* 29:944-948, 1998.

83. Barinagarrementeria F, Amaya LE, Cantu C: Causes and mechanisms of cerebellar infarction in young patients, *Stroke* 28:2400-2404, 1997.

84. Hanna JP, Sun JP, Furlan AJ, et al: Patent foramen ovale and brain infarct: Echocardiographic predictors, recurrence, and prevention, *Stroke* 25:782-786, 1994.

85. Mas JL, Arquizan C, Lamy C, et al: Recurrent cerebrovascular events associated with patent foramen ovale, atrial septal aneurysm, or both, *N Engl J Med* 345:1740-1746, 2001.

86. Mas JL: Patent foramen ovale and stroke: Still a controversial issue, *Rev Med Interne* 30:737-740, 2009.

87. Handke M, Harloff A, Olschewski M, et al: Patent foramen ovale and cryptogenic stroke in older patients, *N Engl J Med* 357:2262-2268, 2007.

88. Homma S, Di Tullio MR, Sacco RL, et al: Characteristics of patent foramen ovale associated with cryptogenic stroke: A biplane transesophageal echocardiographic study, *Stroke* 25:582-586, 1994.

89. Schuchlenz HW, Weihs W, Horner S, Quehenberger F: The association between the diameter of a patent foramen ovale and the risk of embolic cerebrovascular events, *Am J Med* 109:456-462, 2000.

90. Kutty S, Brown K, Qureshi AM, Latson LA: Maximal potential patent foramen diameter does not correlate with the type or frequency of the neurologic event prior to closure, *Cardiology* 113:111-115, 2009.

91. Serena J, Marti-Fàbregas J, Santamarina E, et al: CODICIA, Right-to-Left Shunt in Cryptogenic Stroke Study; Stroke Project of the Cerebrovascular Diseases Study Group, Spanish Society of Neurology: Recurrent stroke and massive right-to-left shunt: Results from the prospective Spanish multicenter (CODICIA) study, *Stroke* 39:3131-3136, 2008.

92. Homma S, Sacco RL, Di Tullio MR, et al: Effect of medical treatment in stroke patients with patent foramen ovale: Patent foramen ovale in Cryptogenic Stroke Study, *Circulation* 105:2625-2631, 2002.

93. Hausmann D, Mügge A, Becht I, Daniel WG: Diagnosis of patent foramen ovale by transesophageal echocardiography and association with cerebral and peripheral embolic events, *Am J Cardiol* 70:668-672, 1992.

94. Lethen H, Flachskampf FA, Schneider R, et al: Frequency of deep vein thrombosis in patients with patent foramen ovale and ischemic stroke or transient ischemic attack, *Am J Cardiol* 80:1066-1069, 1997.

95. Schuchlenz HW, Weihs W, Beitzke A, et al: Transesophageal echocardiography for quantifying size of patent foramen ovale in patients with cryptogenic cerebrovascular events, *Stroke* 33:293-296, 2002.

96. Hung J, Landzberg MJ, Jenkins KJ, et al: Closure of patent foramen ovale for paradoxical emboli: Intermediate-term risk of recurrent neurological events following transcatheter device placement, *J Am Coll Cardiol* 35:1311-1316, 2000.

97. Krizanic F, Sievert J, Pfeiffer D, et al: Clinical evaluation of a novel occluder device (Occlutech) for percutaneous transcather closure of patent foramen ovale (PFO), *Clin Res Cardiol* 97:872-877, 2008.

98. Taaffe M, Fischer E, Baranowski A, et al: Comparison of three patent foramen ovale closure devices in a randomized trial (Amplatzer versus CardioSEAL-STARflex versus Helex occluder), *Am J Cardiol* 101:1353-1358, 2008.

99. Luermans JG, Post MC, Schrader R, et al: Outcome after percutaneous closure of a patent foramen ovale using the Intrasept device: a multi-centre study, *Catheter Cardiovasc Interv* 71:822-828, 2008.

100. Mullen MJ, Hildick-Smith D, De Giovanni JV, et al: BioSTAR Evaluation Study (BEST): A prospective, multicenter, phase I clinical trial to evaluate the feasibility, efficacy, and safety of the BioSTAR bioabsorbable septal repair implant for the closure of atrial-level shunts, *Circulation* 114:1962-1967, 2006.

101. Buscheck F, Sievert H, Kleber F, et al: Patent foramen ovale using the Premere device: The results of the CLOSEUP trial, *J Interv Cardiol* 19:328-333, 2006.

102. Lakkireddy D, Rangisetty U, Prasad S, et al: Intracardiac echo-guided radiofrequency catheter ablation of atrial fibrillation in patients with atrial septal defect or patent foramen ovale repair: A feasibility, safety, and efficacy study, *J Cardiovasc Electrophysiol* 19:1143-1144, 2008.

103. Reddy BT, Patel JB, Powell DL, et al: Interatrial shunt closure devices in patients with nickel allergy, *Catheter Cardiovasc Interv* 74:647-651, 2009.

104. Mohr JP, Homma S: Patent cardiac foramen ovale: stroke risk and closure, *Ann Intern Med* 139:787-788, 2003.

105. Staubach S, Steinberg DH, Zimmermann W, et al: New onset atrial fibrillation after patent foramen ovale closure, *Catheter Cardiovasc Interv* 74:889-895, 2009.

106. O'Gara PT, Messe SR, Tuzcu EM, et al: American Heart Association; American Stroke Association; American College of Cardiology Foundation: Percutaneous device closure of patent foramen ovale for secondary stroke prevention: A call for completion of randomized clinical trials. A science advisory from the American Heart Association/American Stroke Association and the American College of Cardiology Foundation, *J Am Coll Cardiol* 53:2014-2018, 2009.

107. Sandok BA, von Estorff I, Giuliani ER: CNS embolism due to atrial myxoma: Clinical features and diagnosis, *Arch Neurol* 37:485-488, 1980.

108. Roeltgen DP, Weimer GR, Patterson LF: Delayed neurologic complications of left atrial myxoma, *Neurology* 31:8-13, 1981.

109. Zotz RJ, Müller M, Genth-Zotz S, et al: Spontaneous echo contrast caused by platelet and leukocyte aggregates? *Stroke* 32:1127-1133, 2001.

110. Peverill RE, Graham R, Gelman J, et al: Haematologic determinants of left atrial spontaneous echo contrast in mitral stenosis, *Int J Cardiol* 81:235-242, 2001.

111. Castello R, Pearson AC, Labovitz AJ: Prevalence and clinical implications of atrial spontaneous contrast in patients undergoing transesophageal echocardiography, *Am J Cardiol* 65:1149-1153, 1990.

112. Daniel WG, Nellessen U, Schröder E, et al: Left atrial spontaneous echo contrast in mitral valve disease: An indicator for an increased thromboembolic risk, *J Am Coll Cardiol* 11:1204-1211, 1988.

113. Castello R, Pearson AC, Fagan L, et al: Spontaneous echocardiographic contrast in the descending aorta, *Am Heart J* 120:915-919, 1990.

114. Comess KA, DeRook FA, Beach KW, et al: Transesophageal echocardiography and carotid ultrasound in patients with cerebral ischemia: Prevalence of findings and recurrent stroke risk, *J Am Coll Cardiol* 23:1598-1603, 1994.

115. Tice FD, Slivka AP, Walz ET, et al: Mitral valve strands in patients with focal cerebral ischemia, *Stroke* 27:1183-1186, 1996.

116. Freedberg RS, Goodkin GM, Perez JL, et al: Valve strands are strongly associated with systemic embolization: A transesophageal echocardiographic study, *J Am Coll Cardiol* 26:1709-1712, 1995.

117. Orsinelli DA, Pearson AC: Detection of prosthetic valve strands by transesophageal echocardiography: Clinical significance in patients with suspected cardiac source of embolism, *J Am Coll Cardiol* 26:1713-1718, 1995.

118. Roberts JK, Omarali I, Di Tullio MR, et al: Valvular strands and cerebral ischemia: Effect of demographics and strand characteristics, *Stroke* 28:2185-2188, 1997.

119. Risk factors for stroke and efficacy of antithrombotic therapy in atrial fibrillation: Analysis of pooled data from five randomized controlled trials, *Arch Intern Med* 154:1449-1457, 1994.

120. Warfarin versus aspirin for prevention of thromboembolism in atrial fibrillation: Stroke Prevention in Atrial Fibrillation II Study, *Lancet* 343:687-691, 1994.

121. Adjusted-dose warfarin versus low-intensity, fixed-dose warfarin plus aspirin for high-risk patients with atrial fibrillation: Stroke Prevention in Atrial Fibrillation III randomised clinical trial, *Lancet* 348:633-638, 1996.

122. Patients with nonvalvular atrial fibrillation at low risk of stroke during treatment with aspirin: Stroke Prevention in Atrial Fibrillation III Study. The SPAF III Writing Committee for the Stroke Prevention in Atrial Fibrillation Investigators, *JAMA* 279:1273-1277, 1998.

123. The effect of low-dose warfarin on the risk of stroke in patients with nonrheumatic atrial fibrillation: The Boston Area Anticoagulation Trial for Atrial Fibrillation Investigators, *N Engl J Med* 323:1505-1511, 1990.

124. Stroke Prevention in Atrial Fibrillation Study: Final results, *Circulation* 84:527-539, 1991.

125. Secondary prevention in non-rheumatic atrial fibrillation after transient ischaemic attack or minor stroke. EAFT (European Atrial Fibrillation Trial) Study Group, *Lancet* 342:1255-1262, 1993.

126. Nabavi DG, Allroggen A, Reinecke H, et al: Absence of circulating microemboli in patients with lone atrial fibrillation, *Neurol Res* 21:566-568, 1999.

127. Stroke Risk in Atrial Fibrillation Working Group: Comparison of 12 risk stratification schemes to predict stroke in patients with nonvalvular atrial fibrillation, *Stroke* 39:1901-1910, 2008.

128. EAFT (European Atrial Fibrillation Trial) Study Group: Secondary prevention in non-rheumatic atrial fibrillation after transient ischemic attack or minor stroke, *Lancet* 342:1255-1262, 1993.

129. Connolly S, Pogue J, Hart R, et al: Clopidogrel plus aspirin versus oral anticoagulation for atrial fibrillation in the Atrial fibrillation Clopidogrel Trial with Irbesartan for prevention of Vascular Events (ACTIVE W): A randomized controlled trial, *Lancet* 367:1903-1912, 2006.

130. Hart RG, Bhatt DL, Hacke W, et al: Clopidogrel and aspirin versus aspirin alone for the prevention of stroke in patients with a history of atrial fibrillation: subgroup analysis of the CHARISMA randomized trial, *Cerebrovasc Dis* 25:344-347, 2008.

131. ACTIVE Investigators, Connolly SJ, Pogue J, et al: Effect of clopidogrel added to aspirin in patients with atrial fibrillation, *N Engl J Med* 360:2066-2078, 2009.

132. Fang MC, Chang Y, Hylek EM, et al: Advanced age, anticoagulation intensity, and risk for intracranial hemorrhage among patients taking warfarin for atrial fibrillation, *Ann Intern Med* 141:745-752, 2004.

133. The Stroke Risk in Atrial Fibrillation Working Group: Independent predictors of stroke in patients with atrial fibrillation, *Neurology* 69:546-554, 2007.

134. Albers GW, Bittar N, Young L, et al: Clinical characteristics and management of acute stroke in patients with atrial fibrillation admitted to US university hospitals, *Neurology* 48:1598-1604, 1997.

135. Albers GW, Amarenco P, Easton JD, et al: Antithrombotic and Thrombolytic Therapy for Ischemic Stroke. American College of Chest Physicians Evidence-Based Clinical Practice Guidelines (8th Edition), *Chest* 133:630S-669S, 2008.

136. Sick PB, Schuler G, Hauptmann KE, et al: Initial worldwide experience with the WATCHMAN left atrial appendage system for stroke prevention in atrial fibrillation, *J Am Coll Cardiol* 49:1490-1495, 2007.

137. Asinger RW: Role of transthoracic echocardiography in atrial fibrillation, *Echocardiography* 17:357-364, 2000.

138. Egeblad H, Andersen K, Hartiala J, et al: Role of echocardiography in systemic arterial embolism: A review with recommendations, *Scand Cardiovasc J* 32:323-342, 1998.

139. Predictors of thromboembolism in atrial fibrillation. II: Echocardiographic features of patients at risk. The Stroke Prevention in Atrial Fibrillation Investigators, *Ann Intern Med* 116:6-12, 1992.

140. Echocardiographic predictors of stroke in patients with atrial fibrillation: A prospective study of 1066 patients from 3 clinical trials, *Arch Intern Med* 158:1316-1320, 1998.

141. Abe Y, Asakura T, Gotou J, et al: Prediction of embolism in atrial fibrillation: Classification of left atrial thrombi by transesophageal echocardiography, *Jpn Circ J* 64:411-415, 2000.

142. Fagan SM, Chan KL: Transesophageal echocardiography risk factors for stroke in nonvalvular atrial fibrillation, *Echocardiography* 17:365-372, 2000.

143. Transesophageal echocardiographic correlates of thromboembolism in high-risk patients with nonvalvular atrial fibrillation: The Stroke Prevention in Atrial Fibrillation Investigators Committee on Echocardiography, *Ann Intern Med* 128:639-647, 1998.

144. Babikian VL, Kase CS, Pessin MS, et al: Intracerebral hemorrhage in stroke patients anticoagulated with heparin, *Stroke* 20:1500-1503, 1989.

145. Rothrock JF, Dittrich HC, McAllen S, et al: Acute anticoagulation following cardioembolic stroke, *Stroke* 20:730-734, 1989.

146. Bogousslavsky J, Regli F: Anticoagulant-induced intracerebral bleeding in brain ischemia: Evaluation in 200 patients with TIAs, emboli from the heart, and progressing stroke, *Acta Neurol Scand* 71:464-471, 1985.

147. Lodder J, van der Lugt PJ: Evaluation of the risk of immediate anticoagulant treatment in patients with embolic stroke of cardiac origin, *Stroke* 14:42-46, 1983.

148. Stoddard MF: Risk of thromboembolism in acute atrial fibrillation or atrial flutter, *Echocardiography* 17:393-405, 2000.

149. Sacco RL, Foulkes MA, Mohr JP, et al: Determinants of early recurrence of cerebral infarction: The Stroke Data Bank, *Stroke* 20:983-989, 1989.

150. Cerebral Embolism Study Group: Immediate anticoagulation of embolic stroke: A randomized trial, *Stroke* 14:668-676, 1983.

151. Chamorro A, Vila N, Ascaso C, et al: Heparin in acute stroke with atrial fibrillation: Clinical relevance of very early treatment, *Arch Neurol* 56:1098-1102, 1999.

152. Rubenstein JJ, Schulman CL, Yurchak PM, et al: Clinical spectrum of the sick sinus syndrome, *Circulation* 46:5-13, 1972.

153. Fairfax AJ, Lambert CD, Leatham A: Systemic embolism in chronic sinoatrial disorder, *N Engl J Med* 295:190-192, 1976.

154. Fairfax AJ, Lambert CD: Neurological aspects of sinoatrial heart block, *J Neurol Neurosurg Psychiatry* 39:576-580, 1976.

155. Santini M, Alexidou G, Ansalone G, et al: Relation of prognosis in sick sinus syndrome to age, conduction defects and modes of permanent cardiac pacing, *Am J Cardiol* 65:729-735, 1990.

156. Biblo LA, Yuan Z, Quan KJ, et al: Risk of stroke in patients with atrial flutter, *Am J Cardiol* 87:346-349, 2001.

157. Santiago D, Warshofsky M, Li Mandri G, et al: Left atrial appendage function and thrombus formation in atrial fibrillation-flutter: A transesophageal echocardiographic study, *J Am Coll Cardiol* 24:159-164, 1994.

158. Nair CK, Thomson W, Ryschon K, et al: Long-term follow-up of patients with echocardiographically detected mitral annular calcium and comparison with age- and sex-matched control subjects, *Am J Cardiol* 63:465-470, 1989.

159. Nishide M, Irino T, Gotoh M, et al: Cardiac abnormalities in ischemic cerebrovascular disease studied by two-dimensional echocardiography, *Stroke* 14:541-545, 1983.

160. de Bono DP, Warlow CP: Mitral-annulus calcification and cerebral or retinal ischaemia, *Lancet* 2:383-385, 1979.

161. Chesebro JH, Adams PC, Fuster V: Antithrombotic therapy in patients with valvular heart disease and prosthetic heart valves, *J Am Coll Cardiol* 8(Suppl B):41B-56B, 1986.

162. Kuntze CE, Ebels T, Eijgelaar A, et al: Rates of thromboembolism with three different mechanical heart valve prostheses: Randomised study, *Lancet* 1:514-517, 1989.

163. Kuntze CE, Blackstone EH, Ebels T: Thromboembolism and mechanical heart valves: A randomized study revisited, *Ann Thorac Surg* 66:101-117, 1998.

164. Olesen KH, Rygg IH, Wennevold A, et al: Long-term follow-up in 185 patients after mitral valve replacement with the Lillehei-Kaster prosthesis: Overall results and prosthesis-related complications, *Eur Heart J* 8:680-688, 1987.

165. Turpie AG, Gent M, Laupacis A, et al: A comparison of aspirin with placebo in patients treated with warfarin after heart-valve replacement, *N Engl J Med* 329:524-529, 1993.

166. Coulshed N, Epstein EJ, McKendrick CS, et al: Systemic embolism in mitral valve disease, *Br Heart J* 32:26-34, 1970.

167. Szekely P: Systemic embolism and anticoagulant prophylaxis in rheumatic heart disease, *BMJ* 1:1209-1212, 1964.

168. Szekely P: Rheumatic heart disease in three decades (1942-1971), *Singapore Med J* 14:417-419, 1973.

169. Salgado AV, Furlan AJ, Keys TF, et al: Neurologic complications of endocarditis: A 12-year experience, *Neurology* 39:173-178, 1989.

170. Hart RG, Foster JW, Luther MF, Kanter MC: Stroke in infective endocarditis, *Stroke* 21:695-700, 1990.

171. Pruitt AA, Rubin RH, Karchmer AW, Duncan GW: Neurologic complications of bacterial endocarditis, *Medicine (Baltimore)* 57:329-342, 1978.

172. Karchmer AW: Infective endocarditis. In Braunwald E, Fauci AS, Kasper DL, et al: *Harrison's principles of internal medicine*, ed 15, New York, 2001, McGraw-Hill.

173. Buda AJ, Zotz RJ, LeMire MS, et al: Prognostic significance of vegetations detected by two-dimensional echocardiography in infective endocarditis, *Am Heart J* 112:1291-1296, 1986.

174. Salgado AV, Furlan AJ, Keys TF: Mycotic aneurysm, subarachnoid hemorrhage, and indications for cerebral angiography in infective endocarditis, *Stroke* 18:1057-1060, 1987.

175. Lopez JA, Ross RS, Fishbein MC, Siegel RJ: Nonbacterial thrombotic endocarditis: A review, *Am Heart J* 113:773-784, 1987.

176. Rogers LR, Cho ES, Kempin S, Posner JB: Cerebral infarction from non-bacterial thrombotic endocarditis: Clinical and pathological study including the effects of anticoagulation, *Am J Med* 83:746-756, 1987.

177. Lopez JA, Fishbein MC, Siegel RJ: Echocardiographic features of nonbacterial thrombotic endocarditis, *Am J Cardiol* 59:478-480, 1987.

178. Futrell N, Millikan C: Frequency, etiology, and prevention of stroke in patients with systemic lupus erythematosus, *Stroke* 20:583-591, 1989.

179. Gorelick PB, Rusinowitz MS, Tiku M, et al: Embolic stroke complicating systemic lupus erythematosus, *Arch Neurol* 42:813-815, 1985.

180. Pomerance A: Cardiac pathology and systolic murmurs in the elderly, *Br Heart J* 30:687-689, 1968.

181. Pomerance A: Cardiac pathology in the aged, *Geriatrics* 23:101-104, 1968.

182. Kapila A, Hart R: Calcific cerebral emboli and aortic stenosis: Detection of computed tomography, *Stroke* 17:619-621, 1986.

183. Gilon D, Buonanno FS, Joffe MM, et al: Lack of evidence of an association between mitral-valve prolapse and stroke in young patients, *N Engl J Med* 341:8-13, 1999.

184. Cesena FH, Pereira AN, Dallan LA, et al: Papillary fibroelastoma of the mitral valve 12 years after mitral valve commissurotomy, *South Med J* 92:1023-1028, 1999.

185. Muir KW, McNeish I, Grosset DG, et al: Visualization of cardiac emboli from mitral valve papillary fibroelastoma, *Stroke* 27:1133-1134, 1996.

186. Kasarskis EJ, O'Connor W, Earle G: Embolic stroke from cardiac papillary fibroelastomas, *Stroke* 19:1171-1173, 1988.

187. Roach GW, Kanchuger M, Mangano CM, et al: Adverse cerebral outcomes after coronary bypass surgery. Multicenter Study of Perioperative Ischemia Research Group and the Ischemia Research and Education Foundation Investigators, *N Engl J Med* 335:1857-1863, 1996.

188. Barbut D, Caplan LR: Brain complications of cardiac surgery, *Curr Probl Cardiol* 22:449-480, 1997.

189. Salazar JD, Wityk RJ, Grega MA, et al: Stroke after cardiac surgery: Short- and long-term outcomes, *Ann Thorac Surg* 72:1195-1201, 2001.

190. Hogue CW Jr, Murphy SF, Schechtman KB, et al: Risk factors for early or delayed stroke after cardiac surgery, *Circulation* 100:642-647, 1999.

191. Newman MF, Wolman R, Kanchuger M, et al: Multicenter preoperative stroke risk index for patients undergoing coronary artery bypass graft surgery. Multicenter Study of Perioperative Ischemia (McSPI) Research Group, *Circulation* 94(Suppl):II74-II80, 1996.

192. Stamou SC, Corso PJ: Coronary revascularization without cardiopulmonary bypass in high-risk patients: A route to the future, *Ann Thorac Surg* 71:1056-1061, 2001.

193. Wityk RJ, Goldsborough MA, Hillis A, et al: Diffusion- and perfusion-weighted brain magnetic resonance imaging in patients with neurologic complications after cardiac surgery, *Arch Neurol* 58:571-576, 2001.

194. Barbut D, Grassineau D, Lis E, et al: Posterior distribution of infarcts in strokes related to cardiac operations, *Ann Thorac Surg* 65:1656-1659, 1998.

195. Segal AZ, Abernathy WB, Palacios IF, et al: Stroke as a complication of cardiac catheterization: Risk factors and clinical features, *Neurology* 56:975-977, 2001.

196. Jackson JL, Meyer GS, Pettit T: Complications from cardiac catheterization: Analysis of a military database, *Mil Med* 165:298-301, 2000.

197. Lip GY, Lip PL, Zarifis J, et al: Fibrin D-dimer and beta-thromboglobulin as markers of thrombogenesis and platelet activation in atrial fibrillation: Effects of introducing ultra-low-dose warfarin and aspirin, *Circulation* 94:425-431, 1996.

198. Lip GY, Lowe GD, Rumley A, Dunn FG: Fibrinogen and fibrin D-dimer levels in paroxysmal atrial fibrillation: Evidence for intermediate elevated levels of intravascular thrombogenesis, *Am Heart J* 131:724-730, 1996.

199. Lip GY, Rumley A, Dunn FG, et al: Plasma fibrinogen and fibrin D-dimer in patients with atrial fibrillation: Effects of cardioversion to sinus rhythm, *Int J Cardiol* 51:245-251, 1995.

200. Lip GY, Lowe GD, Rumley A, et al: Increased markers of thrombogenesis in chronic atrial fibrillation: Effects of warfarin treatment, *Br Heart J* 73:527-533, 1995.

201. Gustafsson C, Blombäck M, Britton M, et al: Coagulation factors and the increased risk of stroke in nonvalvular atrial fibrillation, *Stroke* 21:47-51, 1990.

202. Mitusch R, Siemens HJ, Garbe M, et al: Detection of a hypercoagulable state in nonvalvular atrial fibrillation and the effect of anticoagulant therapy, *Thromb Haemost* 75:219-223, 1996.

203. Rosenberg RD, Aird WC: Vascular-bed-specific hemostasis and hypercoagulable states, *N Engl J Med* 340:1555-1564, 1999.

204. Kistler JP, Singer DE, Millenson MM, et al: Effect of low-intensity warfarin anticoagulation on level of activity of the hemostatic system in patients with atrial fibrillation. BAATAF Investigators, *Stroke* 24:1360-1365, 1993.

205. Lip GY, Lowe GD, Metcalfe MJ, et al: Effects of warfarin therapy on plasma fibrinogen, von Willebrand factor, and fibrin D-dimer in left ventricular dysfunction secondary to coronary artery disease with and without aneurysms, *Am J Cardiol* 76:453-458, 1995.

206. Yamamoto K, Ikeda U, Seino Y, et al: Coagulation activity is increased in the left atrium of patients with mitral stenosis, *J Am Coll Cardiol* 25:107-112, 1995.

207. Jafri SM, Ozawa T, Mammen E, et al: Platelet function, thrombin and fibrinolytic activity in patients with heart failure, *Eur Heart J* 14:205-212, 1993.

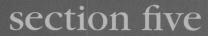

Diagnostic Studies

RÜDIGER VON KUMMER

The chapters in this section cover the main imaging modalities used for the assessment of the pathology and pathophysiology of stroke.

The chapter authors have focused their efforts on the indications for the use of each individual method, have provided enough description of the techniques to set the scientific background, but have minimized the broader issues of diagnosis and treatment for the individual stroke subtypes. The main emphasis of each chapter is on the findings in various settings of stroke.

A few of the methods have expanded enormously and with them some changes in authorship. Leading among the expanded topics are magnetic resonance imaging and angiography, which has become a field in itself. Similar expanding consideration applies to duplex extracranial and transcranial Doppler insonation and B-mode imaging. Positron emission tomography and single-photon emission computed tomography have such limited use in clinical practice that they have been dropped from the chapter list.

44 Ultrasonography

STEPHEN MEAIRS, MICHAEL HENNERICI, J.P. MOHR

The continuous development of noninvasive ultrasound techniques has resulted in a variety of diagnostic applications for assessment of cerebrovascular diseases. In this chapter, we discuss the clinical merits and limitations of ultrasound for evaluation of both acute and advanced atherosclerotic disease. We outline approaches for identification of stroke etiology and summarize how neurosonology is used for the monitoring of stroke patients. We also address recent developments in both qualitative and quantitative assessment of cerebral perfusion as well as ultrasonographic techniques for molecular imaging. Finally, we discuss ultrasound technologies for the therapy of stroke, including sonothrombolysis, drug delivery to the brain, gene therapy, and stimulation of angiogenesis.

Ultrasound Technology

Doppler Ultrasonography

Ultrasonographic Doppler techniques are commonly used for examining the intracranial and extracranial arteries supplying the brain. Interpretation of Doppler signals is based on analysis of the audio signals and of the frequency spectrum. The *Doppler effect* is named after Christian Doppler, who in 1842 described the change in frequency of light emitted by moving objects. This effect is familiar to anyone who has stood in one place and listened to a source of sound passing by. The sound rises in pitch as the source approaches the listener and then equally drops off as the source moves away after passing. In clinical applications, this effect is known as the *Doppler frequency shift*, which is the difference between emitted and received ultrasonography frequency, and is proportional to the velocity of moving blood cells.

Continuous-wave (CW) Doppler systems use two transducers, one of which emits while the other receives ultrasound continuously (Fig. 44-1). Although this simple system is easily applicable for the detection of a broad range of alterations in flow velocity, including the high blood flow velocities associated with severe stenosis, it provides only limited information about the topographic origin of the ultrasound-reflecting source. In contrast, pulsed-wave (PW) Doppler systems, in which ultrasound is both emitted from and received by a single piezoelectric crystal in the transducer, can provide a depth estimate of the site being insonated (Fig. 44-2). This feature, along with information on the direction of the Doppler frequency shift, is used in transcranial PW Doppler ultrasonography to locate and differentiate intracranial cerebral arteries. Although CW and PW Doppler techniques are simple, inexpensive screening procedures for detection of stenoses and occlusions in the extracranial arteries, they have been largely replaced by more sophisticated ultrasonographic techniques offering real-time display of the vessel walls and lumen combined with color-coded visualization of blood flow (Fig. 44-3). Transcranial PW Doppler, however, still plays a significant role in the transcranial investigation of cerebrovascular disease.

Imaging Techniques

A number of complementary ultrasonographic techniques are available for the evaluation of the intracranial and extracranial arteries and for the visualization of the brain parenchyma. These are complemented by approaches utilizing the nonlinear behavior of ultrasound contrast agents (UCAs).

B-mode scanning displays the morphologic features of normal and diseased vessels. Because the extracranial carotid and vertebral arteries lie near the skin, linear-array transducers are commonly used at ultrasound frequencies of 7.0 to 12.0 MHz. A number of transcranial imaging applications for assessment of structural alterations in the brain have emerged. The brain must be imaged through the temporal bone window, so these applications usually employ 2.0-MHz phased or curved-array transducers.

Duplex ultrasonography combines integrated PW Doppler spectrum analysis and B-mode scanning. In addition to providing information about the presence and morphology of arterial lesions, the B-mode image serves as a guide for the placement of the PW Doppler sample volume (Fig. 44-4). Distinct criteria of the Doppler spectrum analysis (see later) are then used to evaluate hemodynamics and to categorize carotid artery stenoses. The common carotid artery (CCA), internal carotid artery (ICA), and external carotid artery (ECA) are usually characterized by a relatively distinct Doppler frequency spectrum, which allows their identification on insonation with a PW Doppler system. The emission frequency of the integrated PW Doppler system ranges between 4 and 7 MHz.

Color Doppler flow imaging (CDFI) preserves the advantages of duplex ultrasonography and superimposes color-coded blood flow patterns on the gray-scale B-mode image.[1-3] With the use of a defined color scale, the direction and the average mean velocity of moving blood cells within the sample volume at a given point in time are encoded. Generation of color signals is based on

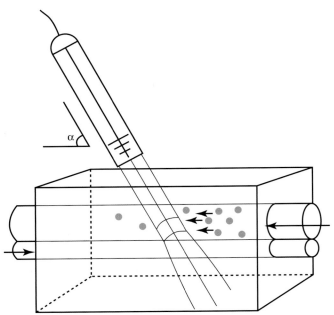

Figure 44-1 Continuous-wave Doppler ultrasonography uses a single piezo crystal for both transmitting and receiving ultrasound signals. (From Hennerici M, Rautenberg W, Steinke W: Ultrasonography. In Mohr JP, Gautier J-C, editors: *Guide to clinical neurology,* St. Louis, 1995, Churchill Livingstone, p 185.)

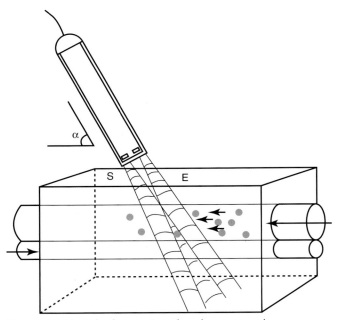

Figure 44-2 Pulsed-wave Doppler ultrasonography uses separate piezo crystals, one of which emits (E) and the other receives (S) ultrasound waves. This allows location of the sample volume. (From Hennerici M, Rautenberg W, Steinke W: Ultrasonography. In Mohr JP, Gautier J-C, editors: *Guide to clinical neurology,* St. Louis, 1995, Churchill Livingstone, p 185.)

the detection of frequency and phase shifts by means of a multigate transducer. The technique of autocorrelation is used to obtain a real-time visualization of color-coded hemodynamics.

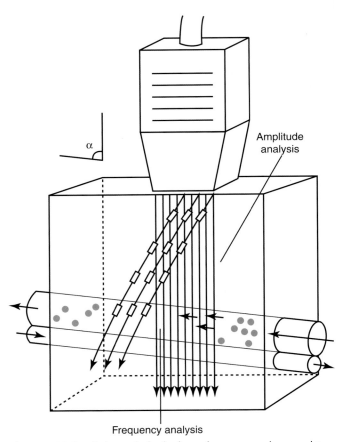

Figure 44-3 Color-coded duplex ultrasonography combines B-mode echotomography and flow velocity signals for structural and hemodynamic analysis. (From Hennerici M, Rautenberg W, Steinke W: Ultrasonography. In Mohr JP, Gautier J-C, editors: *Guide to clinical neurology,* St. Louis, 1995, Churchill Livingstone, p 185.)

Power Doppler imaging (PDI) displays the amplitude of Doppler signals. Color and brightness of the signals are related to the number of blood cells producing the Doppler shift. PDI is more sensitive for detection of blood flow than CDFI (Table 44-1). The reason is that PDI is less angle-dependent than CDFI, thus allowing better display of curving or tortuous vessels. Reliance on Doppler amplitude means that there is no aliasing, which appears when an analog signal is sampled at a frequency that is lower than half of its maximum frequency. The lack of aliasing of signal improves the display of vessel wall disease in areas of turbulent flow. Moreover, more of the dynamic range of the Doppler signal can be used in PDI to improve sensitivity. PDI is a valuable technique for displaying plaque surface structure (Fig. 44-5).

Real-time compound imaging is a modality that enhances ultrasonographic visualization and characterization of carotid artery plaques.[4,5] This technique acquires ultrasound beams, which are steered off-axis from the orthogonal beams used in conventional ultrasonography. The number of frames and steering angles varies, depending on the transducer characteristics. Frames acquired from sufficiently different angles contain independent random speckle patterns, which are averaged to reduce speckle and improve tissue differentiation.

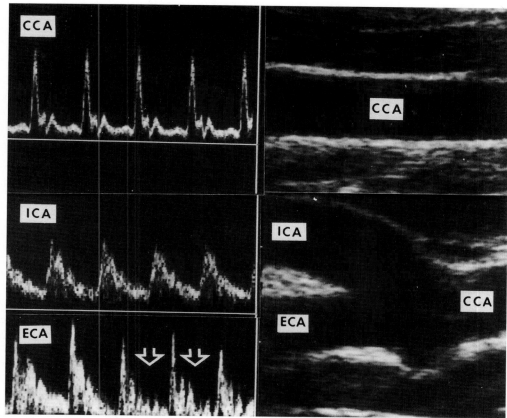

Figure 44-4 Duplex system analysis of a normal carotid artery. Doppler frequency spectra *(left)* and B-mode echotomograms *(right)* of the common carotid artery (CCA) and the bifurcation with internal carotid artery (ICA) and external carotid artery (ECA). High systolic flow and low diastolic flow and transmitted oscillation *(open arrows)* in the ECA from tapping of the superficial temporal artery. Flow in the ICA is high in diastole, reflecting a low-resistance pattern. The Doppler waveform in the CCA reflects the two vascular beds it supplies, but it is dominated by the low-resistance flow to the brain.

TABLE 44-1 TECHNICAL DIFFERENCES BETWEEN COLOR DOPPLER FLOW IMAGING (CDFI) AND POWER DOPPLER IMAGING (PDI)

	CDFI	PDI
Physical principle	Frequency and phase shift	Echo amplitude
Color-coded information	Mean velocity and direction	Density of blood cells
Hemodynamic information	Display in real time	None
Angle dependence of color display	Present	Absent
Aliasing phenomenon	Above Nyquist limit	Absent
	Good definition of plaque surface	Improved display of high-grade stenoses
Intravascular color contrast		Improved visualization in calcified plaques
Motion artifacts	Rare	Frequent

Three-dimensional (3D) ultrasonography can be used for both qualitative and quantitative analysis of plaques in the carotid artery. Surface features of carotid plaques can be clearly demonstrated by 3D ultrasonography. In some cases, the use of this modality may lead to a diagnosis not obtainable with other imaging techniques.[6] One method of 3D ultrasonography image acquisition involves the use of position and orientation measurement (POM) devices capable of tracking scanheads in six degrees of freedom (6-DOF).[7-10] This approach allows "freehand" scanning to collect image data from different perspectives and potentially offers the ability to maximize tissue information that is not readily available from one imaging plane alone (Fig. 44-6). Methods for enhanced reconstruction and visualization of 6-DOF ultrasonography data have been developed.[11]

Monitoring Early Atherosclerosis

Intima–Media Thickness

Pignoli et al[12] were the first to characterize a "double-line" pattern of the normal carotid artery wall with B-mode ultrasonography. They described the first echogenic line on the far wall as representing the lumen–intima interface

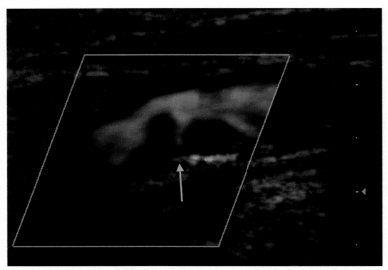

Figure 44-5   Deep plaque ulceration *(arrow)* in the left internal carotid artery as depicted by power Doppler imaging. The plaque is practically anechoic, typical of lipid-filled plaques.

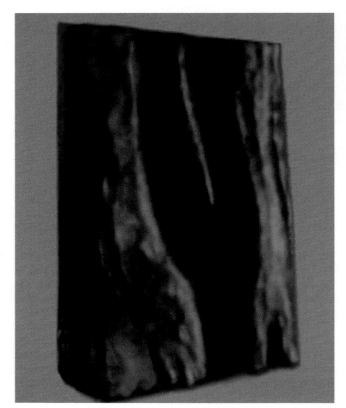

Figure 44-6   Volume rendering of the three-dimensional ultrasound reconstruction of the carotid artery. Data were acquired with a position and orientation device that tracks the transducer during freehand scanning.

and the second line as corresponding to the media–adventitia interface. Significantly, they demonstrated that the distance between these two echogenic lines correlated highly with measurements of intima–media thickness (IMT) in tissue specimens from common carotid arteries. This initial report on measurement of IMT with

B-mode scanning was later validated in vitro[13] and was shown to enable good intraobserver and interobserver reproducibility.[14]

Many studies have used high-resolution ultrasonography to establish associations between common carotid IMT, cardiovascular risk factors, and the prevalence of cardiovascular disease (CVD). The growing importance of common carotid IMT is reflected by its use as a surrogate endpoint.

IMT Sampling

Because the focal location of sites of reactive intimal thickening and initial plaque development in the carotid arteries is related to geometric transitions, the selection of precise regions for measurement of IMT is important (Fig 44-7). Any single examination by ultrasonography may not identify the site of maximal intimal thickening. Therefore, IMT examinations over a range of incident angles and axial locations are necessary. Several IMT sampling protocols have been introduced. Some use IMT measurements of the CCA, where the double-line pattern is easier to visualize. Others include IMT at the carotid bifurcation and at the ICA. Some studies have calculated IMT means obtained from both normal and abnormal walls.[15,16] The use of these aggregate measurements has been shown to improve reliability.[17] The type of IMT sampling used—combined measurements at different sites, measurements only at the CCA, and mean or maximum wall thickness—may largely depend on the research question and on the relative emphasis accorded to confirmed atherosclerotic lesions.[18]

Serial Measurements of IMT

A major source of error in the longitudinal assessment of IMT is the difficulty of retrieving the same echographic view of the vessel. Although the mean IMT might be regarded as a reproducible variable by which to evaluate differences between populations exposed to diverse risk

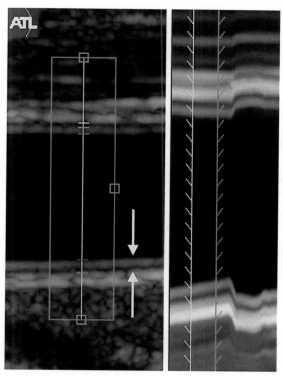

Figure 44-7 Intima-medial thickness (IMT) measurements can be performed for a defined segment of the cardiac cycle with the use of automated systems. *Left,* The green region of interest specifies the area in which IMT (as shown with *white arrows*) is measured. *Right,* A user-defined specification of the segment of the cardiac cycle (diastole) in the M-mode display of arterial diameter over time.

factors, evolutionary or therapy-induced changes in the individual may be better monitored in defined carotid sectors. External reference points have been proposed to improve reproducibility.[19]

Quality Control

Sources of potential variability in IMT measurements associated with both image acquisition (sonographers) and interpretation (readers) have led to development of quality control procedures in many laboratories. These procedures include periodic expert review by trained neurologists or neuroradiologists, replicate baseline readings to identify outliers, standard films to check against reader variability and drift, second readings for data verification, use of standardized ultrasound equipment, and appropriate blinding of sonographers and technicians to clinical status or treatment assignment.

Pathophysiologic Correlates

Although an increased IMT is generally considered to reflect early atherosclerotic plaque formation, this consideration may not always be true. Intimal hyperplasia and intimal fibrocellular hypertrophy are two types of non-atherosclerotic intimal reactions associated with local modifications of flow and mural tension that are likely to represent adaptive or self-limiting compensatory changes. Intimal fibrocellular hypertrophy, a layered widening of

both smooth muscle cells and matrix fibers, can be quite extensive in a particular arterial segment and is not necessarily of uniform width. Early atherosclerotic lesions, on the other hand, are characterized by a focal eccentric accumulation of lipid in the intima, in the extracellular matrix interstices, and in smooth muscle cells and macrophages. These early lesions do not project into the vessel lumen or modify the surface contour, and endothelial cells are anatomically intact. Superimpositions of intimal fibrocellular hypertrophy, intimal hyperplasia, and atherosclerosis are common. IMT, as measured by B-mode scanning, is a heterogeneous entity reflecting normal ageing and atherosclerosis, the differentiation of which is limited and possible, to some extent, only from subsequent follow-up studies.

Clinical Studies of IMT

Eight large prospective studies of the relationship between the degree of carotid IMT (CIMT) and the risk of CVD have been performed. The results have demonstrated that increased CIMT is significantly associated with risk for myocardial infarction, stroke, coronary heart disease, death, or a combination of these.[20-28] An additional study with more than 13,000 participants had similar results.[29] In several investigations, the adjusted relative risks associated with the greatest degrees of wall thickness were sufficiently high that they would be expected to improve clinical risk prediction in appropriately selected patients.[20-22,24,25]

Identifying Early Carotid Plaque

Observational studies have likewise demonstrated the predictive power of the presence of carotid plaque.[25-27,29-34] In these studies, the relative risks associated with plaque were similar to or slightly higher than those observed with increased CIMT. In one study, the presence of carotid plaque significantly improved the area under the receiver operating characteristic curve for prediction of all-cause mortality even after risk factors and use of medications were considered.[34] There was not a uniform definition of carotid plaque in these studies.[35] Most investigations identified plaque as focal widening relative to adjacent segments with protrusion into the lumen and/or having a minimum wall thickness.[35] A report from the American Society of Echocardiography (ASE) and the Society of Vascular Medicine and Biology defined nonobstructive plaque as the presence of focal thickening at least 50% greater than that of the surrounding vessel wall.[36] A precise definition of plaque was provided by the Mannheim CIMT Consensus, which agreed that plaque should be defined as a focal structure that encroaches into the arterial lumen at least 0.5 mm, is 50% of the surrounding IMT, or demonstrates a thickness of greater than or equal to 1.5 mm.[37,38] This definition has been adopted by the ASE in their last updated consensus statement on assessment of subclinical vascular disease.[39]

The ASE consensus recommends that the clinical usefulness of CIMT measurement and plaque detection is related to the patient's pretest CVD risk, which is altered by the relative risk based on the test results. Measuring

CIMT and identifying carotid plaque by ultrasound are most useful for refining CVD risk assessment in patients at intermediate CVD risk (Framingham Risk Scores [FRS], 6% to 20% without established coronary heart disease, peripheral arterial disease, cerebrovascular disease, diabetes mellitus, or abdominal aortic aneurysm). Patients with the following clinical circumstances also might be considered for CIMT measurement and carotid plaque detection: (1) family history of premature CVD in a first-degree relative (men <55 years old, women <65 years old); (2) individuals younger than 60 years old with severe abnormalities in a single risk factor (e.g., genetic dyslipidemia) who otherwise would not be candidates for pharmacotherapy; or (3) women younger than 60 years old with at least two CVD risk factors. This test can be considered if the level of aggressiveness of preventive therapies is uncertain and additional information about the burden of subclinical vascular disease or future CVD risk is needed. Imaging should not be performed in patients with established atherosclerotic vascular disease or if the results would not be expected to alter therapy. Strict attention to quality control in image acquisition, measurement, interpretation, and reporting is necessary for implementation of this technique in clinical practice. Serial studies of CIMT to address progression or regression are not recommended for use in clinical practice.[39]

Endothelium-Dependent Flow-Mediated Vasodilation

Endothelial dysfunction may be evaluated with high-frequency ultrasonographic imaging of the brachial artery to assess endothelium-dependent flow-mediated dilation (FMD) of blood vessels.[40] The technique provokes the release of nitric oxide, resulting in vasodilation, which serves as an index of vasomotor function. Ischemia-induced hyperemia in the distal forearm is usually used as a stimulus to produce a twofold to fivefold increase in brachial blood flow.[41,42] Standard techniques involve scanning of the artery and measuring its diameter during three conditions: at baseline, during reactive hyperemia (induced by inflation for a period of 5 minutes and then deflation of a sphygmomanometer cuff around the limb distal to the scanned part of the artery), and finally after administration. A detailed description of ultrasonographic assessment of FMD with guidelines for research application of this technique has been published by the International Brachial Artery Reactivity Task Force.[43]

Ultrasonographic studies of FMD have demonstrated an abnormal endothelium-dependent vasodilation in subjects with coronary artery disease (CAD).[44] Patients with CAD had lower FMD than control subjects, and this difference was statistically significant after smokers were excluded. Not only is brachial artery reactivity impaired in patients with CAD, but the impairment is also related to the extent and severity of CAD.[45] Hypercholesterolemia is associated with abnormal FMD in children and in adults, and significant correlations exist between levels of low-density lipoprotein and Lp(a) lipoprotein and endothelium-dependent vasodilation.[40,46]

Active cigarette smoking has been shown to be associated with endothelial dysfunction in otherwise healthy teenagers and young adults in a dose-dependent manner,[47] as is passive smoking.[48,49] More recently, obesity has been shown to be significantly associated with endothelial dysfunction.[50] These studies also demonstrate the potential reversibility of endothelial dysfunction: after smoking cessation or prolonged withdrawal from environmental tobacco smoke exposure, some improvement of endothelial function may be observed.

Assessment of Advanced Atherosclerotic Disease

Insonation of the ophthalmic artery can be used as an indirect test for detection of significant carotid artery stenosis.[51-54] This periorbital technique rapidly provides information about the existence of collateral pathways. In the presence of severe stenosis or occlusion of the ICA, retrograde blood supply from the ECA via the ophthalmic anastomosis can be easily detected with CW Doppler ultrasonography. However, with sufficient collateralization from the contralateral carotid artery or the vertebrobasilar systems, orthograde perfusion of the ophthalmic artery may occur. Accordingly, this indirect test fails to detect even hemodynamically significant ipsilateral carotid obstruction in up to 20% of patients. Thus, although detection of retrograde perfusion in the ophthalmic artery is a strong indicator of severe disease within the ipsilateral extracranial carotid system, finding normal perfusion of the ophthalmic branches cannot exclude severe carotid stenosis or occlusion.

Doppler ultrasonography can detect various degrees of extracranial carotid obstruction. According to the distribution of abnormal blood flow patterns measured within, proximal to, or distal to a narrowed arterial segment, this technique provides data on the extent, site, and severity of lesions of more than 40% lumen narrowing. In such lesions, the sensitivity (92% to 100%) and specificity (93% to 100%) of various Doppler techniques have been shown to be similar to those of arteriography.[55,56] Special transducers can be used to assess distal extracranial lesions of the ICA, such as carotid dissections,[57] fibromuscular dysplasia, and atypically located atherosclerosis.

Grading Carotid Artery Stenosis

Recommendations[58] for the interpretation of maximum Doppler shift velocities (Table 44-2), systolic velocity ratios, and residual area to quantify ICA stenosis are summarized here.

Mild stenosis (40% to 60% of lumen diameter) is characterized by a local increase of peak and mean flow velocities. Systolic peak velocities range above 120 cm/s (4-MHz probe).

Moderate stenosis (60% to 80%) shows a distortion of normal pulsatile flow in addition to a local increase of peak and mean frequencies. Typically, systolic flow decelerations are found in the poststenotic segment. The systolic peak velocity ranges from 120 to 240 cm/s.

Severe stenosis (more than 80% as estimated by Doppler studies) produces markedly increased peak flow

TABLE 44-2 CRITERIA FOR THE CLASSIFICATION OF INTERNAL CAROTID ARTERY STENOSIS BY PULSED-WAVE DOPPLER SONOGRAPHY

Diameter Stenosis (%)	Peak Systolic Frequency (kHz)	Peak Systolic Velocity (cm/s)	End-Diastolic Frequency (kHz)	End-Diastolic Velocity (cm/s)
40-60	>4.0	>120	<1.3	<40
61-80	>4.0	>120	>1.3	>40
81-90	>8.0	>240	>3.3	>100

velocities exceeding 240 cm/s and occasionally reaching more than 600 cm/s (Fig. 44-8). In addition, prestenotic and poststenotic blood flow velocities are significantly lower than those in the contralateral, unaffected carotid artery. Retrograde flow in the ophthalmic artery may occur.

Subtotal stenosis (more than 95%) is characterized by variable, usually low peak flow velocities, which decrease once a stenosis becomes pseudoocclusive. This condition is difficult to separate from complete occlusion and may be misdiagnosed.

ICA occlusion is characterized by the absence of any signal along the cervical course of the ICA. Frequently, a low-velocity Doppler signal with a predominant reversed signal component and absence of diastolic flow can be recorded at the presumed origin of the ICA (stump flow). Blood flow velocity in the CCA is reduced, and frequently, retrograde perfusion of the ophthalmic artery occurs. The diagnosis of carotid occlusion by B-mode ultrasound alone is not reliable because the residual vascular lumen frequently cannot be visualized adequately in complicated, heterogeneous, partially calcified high-grade

obstructions. In acute thrombotic occlusion, echo-lucent material fills the vascular lumen, which can hardly be differentiated on gray scale from blood flow in a patent ICA. CW Doppler and duplex ultrasonography techniques have a significantly higher accuracy for the diagnosis of ICA occlusion; however, differentiation of this entity from a subtotal stenosis is sometimes difficult. The PW Doppler spectrum and color signals in ICA occlusion typically demonstrate a marked reduction of the systolic and diastolic blood flow velocity in the CCA and an internalized ECA with high diastolic flow velocity, indicating collateral supply via the ophthalmic artery. Color-coded intravascular Doppler signals are absent in the occluded ICA; however, blue-coded flow reversal in the residual stump at the bifurcation (stump flow) may occur. The capacity of modern CDFI and PDI instruments to detect very slow blood flow velocities has markedly improved the sensitivity for the diagnosis of a subtotal ICA stenosis and pseudoocclusion.

CCA occlusion is a relatively rare condition that can be diagnosed reliably by conventional duplex ultrasonography and CDFI.[59,60] It is important to assess whether the

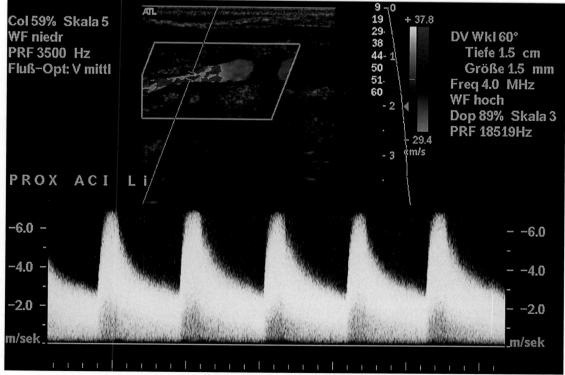

Figure 44-8 The Doppler spectrum identifies a high-grade stenosis of the carotid artery with maximum peak velocity exceeding 600 cm/s, causing left hemispheric stroke. Color Doppler flow imaging demonstrates a mosaic pattern indicating high-flow velocity and mixed turbulence.

ICA distal to the CCA occlusion is patent because patency of this area is a prerequisite for surgical intervention.[61-64] CDFI typically displays blue-coded signals in the ECA because of reversed flow direction and orthograde filling of the ICA in the absence of Doppler signals in the CCA.

Severe intracranial obstructions within the carotid siphon or the middle cerebral artery (MCA) may lead to dampened spectra in the ipsilateral extracranial carotid artery. In addition, alterations of flow direction and signal frequency may occur in the ophthalmic artery, depending on the site and severity of the lesion. Intracranial arteriovenous malformations (AVMs) and shunts may lead to increased flow velocities in the ipsilateral proximal vessel segments. Such findings on extracranial Doppler examination should therefore prompt an appropriate evaluation for suspected intracranial AVM.

The combination of B-mode imaging and PW Doppler ultrasonography in duplex instruments considerably improves the accuracy of the noninvasive diagnosis and grading of carotid stenosis. The degree of stenosis can be estimated from distinct variables in the Doppler frequency spectrum. However, instead of Doppler shift frequencies, equivalent flow-velocity values can be obtained after correction of the Doppler insonation angle according to the flow direction in the vessel segment. In CDFI, three sources of information are available for the classification of carotid stenosis: the Doppler frequency spectrum, measurement of the residual vessel lumen, and characteristic color-flow patterns.

Doppler frequency spectrum. Assessment of the Doppler spectrum is important because it can often be recorded even when plaque calcification prevents adequate visualization of both color-flow patterns and the residual vessel lumen. Variables from the Doppler spectrum such as the peak systolic frequency or velocity[65-67] (see Table 44-2) agree well with angiography for grading of carotid stenosis.

Measurement of residual vessel lumen. The methodologic limitations of measurements of residual vessel lumen with B-mode imaging are well documented.[68-70] With the use of sequential longitudinal and transverse sections, both CDFI and PDI allow more reliable assessment of plaque configuration and relative obstruction by contrasting the intravascular surface.[71-75] If a concentric stenosis is assumed, the percentage area reduction in cross-sections is higher than the relative diameter. There is good correlation between transverse lumen reduction on CDFI and diameter reduction on corresponding angiograms of carotid stenosis.[75,76] Measurement of local diameter and area reduction in carotid stenosis can be performed more reliably by PDI than by CDFI because of better visualization of the residual stenotic lumen by the former technique.[77,78]

The volumetric potential of 3D ultrasonography has important clinical implications in serial follow-up studies for observing the progression or regression of stenotic lesions and for evaluating the outcome of interventional procedures such as endarterectomy and stent placement.[79] The use of advanced imaging systems for acquisition and offline analysis of electrocardiography-gated, axial B-mode scans allows reliable quantification of carotid artery plaques.[80] In comparison with other techniques for the quantification of atherosclerotic lesions, 3D ultrasound angiography offers a precise quantitative method for prospective, clinical studies of atherosclerosis.[81]

Color Doppler flow patterns. Color Doppler flow patterns can provide complementary information for establishing the severity of carotid artery stenosis. Mild stenosis is associated with a relatively long segment of decreased color saturation with an absence of or minimal poststenotic turbulence.[3] In moderate obstructions, the decreased color saturation is more circumscribed, and flow velocity remains high during diastole. Poststenotic flow is turbulent, and flow reversal occurs frequently (Fig. 44-9). Severe stenosis is characterized by a mosaic pattern indicating high flow velocity and mixed turbulence.[82] A short segment of maximal color fading or aliasing with severe poststenotic turbulence and flow reversal provides further evidence for severe stenosis.[3]

Vertebral Artery Stenosis

Examination of the extracranial vertebral artery with ultrasonography is limited to its origin from the subclavian artery, its proximal pretransverse segment, short intertransverse segments between the third and sixth cervical vertebrae, and the atlas loop. Although PW Doppler criteria for vertebral artery stenosis are similar to those used for diagnosis of carotid artery stenosis and have been defined by several duplex studies, detection and classification of stenosis or occlusion in the vertebral arteries are more difficult than in the carotid arteries.[83-85] One reason for this difficulty is that variations in arterial caliber are common in vertebral arteries. In addition, numerous collateral pathways of the vertebral system can permit orthograde flow to the basilar artery even in the presence of vertebral occlusion. These features make examination of the vertebral artery at several locations

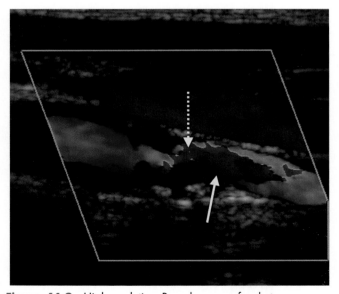

Figure 44-9 High-resolution B-mode scan of a heterogeneous, asymptomatic plaque in the right internal carotid artery. The display is facilitated with color Doppler flow imaging, showing a 70% stenosis with turbulent flow *(dotted arrow)*. The plaque is weakly echogenic at the surface with calcifications near the arterial wall. The *blue area* represents flow reversal *(white arrow)*.

mandatory. CDFI allows noninvasive quantification of flow in the vertebral artery system in more than 95% of all patients[86] and facilitates identification of the proximal segment and ostium, the predominant location of extracranial vertebral stenosis, as well as identification of the atlas loop.[87,88] Using this technique, investigators have documented normal flow velocities of the vertebral artery origin (V0 segment), the pretransverse segment (V1), and the intertransverse (V2) segment.[89]

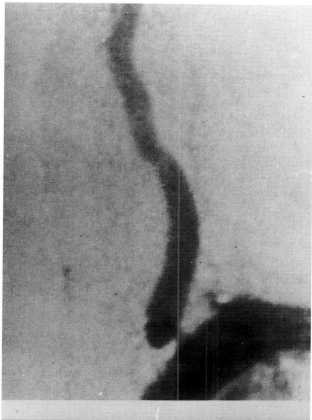

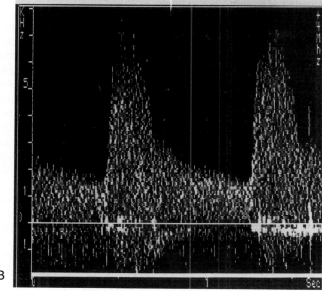

Figure 44-10 Tight stenosis at the origin of the vertebral artery. A, Angiogram; B, Doppler spectra.

Correct interpretation of Doppler results in a vertebral artery requires knowledge of Doppler variables from both the contralateral vertebral artery and the carotid system. For example, an increase in the systolic or diastolic velocity profile of the proximal vertebral artery, although suggestive of stenosis, can also occur as a compensatory response to a variety of conditions of the contralateral vertebral artery, such as hypoplasia, aplasia, stenosis, occlusion, and severe obstruction of the carotid system.

The predominant site of extracranial vertebral artery stenosis is the ostium of the subclavian artery (Fig. 44-10). The atlas loop (V3) and intracranial (V4) segment are involved less commonly, and stenoses in the intertransverse segments are rare. A peak systolic frequency exceeding 4 kHz assessed by means of the integrated PW Doppler system indicates a relevant vertebral stenosis. Features of color-coded Doppler signals correspond to those of carotid stenosis. As luminal narrowing is greater, decreased color saturation becomes more circumscribed, and turbulence, as well as poststenotic flow reversal, becomes more severe. Hemodynamically significant obstruction of the intracranial vertebral artery produces a high-resistance Doppler waveform with a resistivity index exceeding 0.80.[88] However, the Doppler spectrum may be normal if flow to the ipsilateral posterior inferior cerebellar artery is preserved. In acute proximal vertebral artery occlusion, PW Doppler spectra cannot be recorded, and color Doppler signals are absent in the pretransverse and intertransverse segments. However, demonstration of the vascular lumen differentiates this condition from vertebral hypoplasia, which is defined in pathoanatomic studies as a decrease in vascular lumen diameter to less than 2 mm.[90]

Plaque Morphology

Because of its noninvasive nature, real-time capabilities, and general availability, ultrasonography has been the most extensively utilized imaging technique for the study of carotid plaque morphology. High-resolution B-mode imaging alone, and in conjunction with color Doppler flow and PDI techniques, has been used to define variables for identification of symptomatic or vulnerable plaques. The variables have included echogenicity, surface structure, and ulcerations of the plaques.

Carotid artery plaques of homogeneous, moderate-intensity echogenicity consist mainly of fibrotic tissue.[91,92] Such plaques rarely show ulceration, perhaps accounting for the lack of a significant correlation between homogeneous echogenicity and the occurrence of focal cerebral ischemia. Heterogeneous plaques, by comparison, represent matrix deposition, cholesterol accumulation, necrosis, calcification, and intraplaque hemorrhage.[91-93] Several studies have demonstrated that high-resolution B-mode scanning can characterize echomorphologic features of carotid plaques (Fig. 44-11) that correlate with histopathologic criteria.[94] Although echolucent areas within the plaque may represent thrombotic material or hemorrhage, lipid accumulation may have similar echogenicity.[95] Plaque calcification causes acoustic shadowing. Depending on the location of the plaque and on the extent of calcification, acoustic shadowing can be a major obstacle to adequate ultrasonographic visualization.

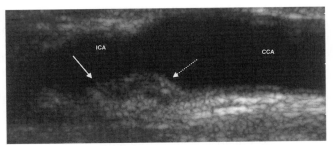

Figure 44-11 B-mode scan (using a 8- to 13-MHz, dynamic-range, linear transducer) of heterogeneous plaque *(arrows)* of the internal carotid artery (ICA) at the level of the carotid bifurcation. The fibrous cap displays stronger echoes on the proximal plaque surface *(broken arrow)* than on its more distal surface *(solid arrow)*, where thinning of the cap is evident. The plaque displays a relatively smooth surface structure protruding into the lumen of the ICA. Beneath the plaque surface is an area of weaker echoes, corresponding to lipid accumulation. CCA, Common carotid artery.

Initial studies of plaque echogenicity with B-mode ultrasonography reported an association between heterogeneous plaques and the occurrence of cerebrovascular events.[96-100] Support for this association was provided by several investigations of endarterectomy specimens that suggested a correlation between intraplaque hemorrhage and transient ischemic attacks (TIAs) and stroke.[101-104] Later studies, however, were unable to confirm these observations.[105-107]

Whether differences in plaque echogenicity can distinguish between symptomatic and asymptomatic plaques continues to be a debatable subject. Later ultrasonographic studies have renewed the notion that heterogeneous carotid plaques are more often associated with intraplaque hemorrhage and neurologic events and have concluded that evaluation of plaque morphology may be helpful in selecting patients for carotid endarterectomy.[108-110] Other researchers argue that lipid-rich plaques are more prone to rupture and suggest that an association between intraplaque hemorrhage and a high lipid content as revealed by B-mode scanning may support this theory.[111] These findings have been negated by yet other research groups who find little correlation between plaque morphology and histologic specimens.[112] A definitive study on the significance of heterogeneous plaque structure found no differences in volume of intraplaque hemorrhage, lipid core, necrotic core, or plaque calcification in patients with highly stenotic carotid lesions undergoing endarterectomy, regardless of preoperative symptom status.[113]

Attempts to characterize plaque surface structure with B-mode scanning have been disappointing. Although a relatively good differentiation between smooth, irregular, and ulcerative plaque surfaces has been obtained for postmortem carotid artery specimens,[92] the accuracy of in vivo findings in comparison with findings at carotid endarterectomy has been considerably poorer.[65,94,112,114] Commonly used variables for identification of plaque ulceration have been surface defects showing a depth and length of 2 mm or more with a well-defined base in the recess. B-mode imaging using these criteria has failed to provide a satisfactory diagnostic yield for ulcerative plaques, with a sensitivity of only 47%.[94] Other groups have been unable to distinguish between the presence and absence of intimal ulcerations with B-mode scans.[115] Diagnostic sensitivity for detection of plaque ulceration with ultrasonography is affected by the severity of carotid stenosis, increasing to 77% in plaques associated with 50% or less stenosis.[94]

Whether plaque surface irregularities or ulcerations are useful variables for defining patients at risk of carotid embolism remains unclear. Advocates of a pathophysiologic relationship maintain that ulcerations represent fertile ground for potential thrombosis and consequent embolic events. This contention is supported by studies demonstrating an association between angiographically defined ulcerations and an increased risk of stroke in medically treated symptomatic patients.[116] In spite of the poor sensitivity and specificity of arteriography for detection of plaque ulceration,[94] it should be remembered that many ulcers are smooth and thick, containing no thrombus at all[117] for putative plaque embolism. Moreover, pathologic studies have shown that, in asymptomatic carotid plaques with stenosis exceeding 60%, there is a higher frequency of plaque hemorrhages, ulcerations, and mural thrombi as well as of numerous healed ulcerations and organized thrombi.[118] Likewise, comparisons of symptomatic with asymptomatic large and stenotic carotid endarterectomy plaques have revealed a high incidence of complex plaque structure and complications in each.[105,119] There appears, therefore, to be little difference in plaque constituents or plaque surface structure between specimens from symptomatic and asymptomatic patients. These findings suggest that a simple description of plaque structure or an identification of plaque ulceration as depicted in current clinical imaging techniques—ultrasonography, magnetic resonance imaging (MRI) and angiography—may be inadequate for predicting the vulnerability of carotid plaques. This viewpoint is in line with recent recommendations from the American Society of Echocardiography and the Society of Vascular Medicine and Biology.[39]

Plaque Motion

Experimental work has suggested that analysis of plaque motion—that is, translational plaque movements coincident with those of arterial walls, plaque rotations, and local, plaque-specific deformations—may provide new insights into plaque modeling as well as into mechanisms of plaque rupture with subsequent embolism. Plaque surface movement may be attributable to deformations resulting from propagation of multiple local internal tears in the plaque. Theoretically, identification of local variations in surface deformability might provide information on the relative vulnerability of a plaque to fissuring or rupture.

Four-dimensional (4D) ultrasonography has been used to acquire temporal 3D ultrasonography data on carotid artery plaques. Motion detection algorithms were used to determine apparent velocity fields of the plaque surface. This technique allowed characterization of plaque motion patterns in patients with symptomatic and asymptomatic carotid artery disease.[120] Asymptomatic plaques showed a homogeneous orientation and magnitude of computed surface velocity vectors, coincident with arterial wall movement. Symptomatic plaques, however, demonstrated evidence of plaque deformation, irrespective of arterial wall movements. Other groups have reported similar findings.[121,122] Indeed, the variables of maximal surface velocity and maximal relative surface velocity were significantly lower in asymptomatic plaques, suggesting more homogeneous motion patterns. Clustering using fuzzy c-means correctly classified 74% of plaques based on texture features only and 79% of plaques based on motion features only.[123] Classification performance reached 84% when a combination of motion and texture features was used. Enhanced block-matching algorithms for characterization of plaque motion have been described and compared with motion detection using optical flow.[124] Studies are lacking, however, showing that detection of altered plaque motion can identify patients at risk.

Imaging of Plaque Angiogenesis

The presence of newly generated blood vessels within atherosclerotic lesions has been recognized for more than 70 years,[125] but only recently has the in vivo evaluation of angiogenesis received attention for its possible role in assessing the vulnerability of atheroma. Histologic studies have, indeed, shown that microvessels are not usually present in the normal human intimal layers and that the intima becomes vascularized only with the development of the atherosclerotic process and when its layer grows in thickness.[126] Angiogenesis and microvessels observed in coronary atheromas in histologic studies have proved to be strongly associated with unstable angina and myocardial infarction. Direct visualization of the adventitial vasa vasorum and plaque neovascularization is now possible with contrast-enhanced ultrasound imaging.[127-131] Microbubbles can be readily visualized in the fibrous tissue of carotid plaques that histologically correspond to newly generated vessels,[128] thus confirming that plaques undergo angiogenesis that could be related to progression and remodeling. Larger studies are needed to clarify the prognostic value of plaque vascularization and to evaluate the role of this new application for monitoring therapies aimed at plaque remodeling. First pilot study results suggest that this approach could be useful for identification of carotid plaque instability.[132]

Nonatherosclerotic Vascular Disease

Carotid Artery Dissection

Ultrasonography is useful for diagnosis of carotid artery dissection, a cause of transient or permanent neurologic deficits, particularly in young patients. ICA dissection usually occurs spontaneously and results in a typical syndrome of focal cerebral deficits, headache, neck pain, ipsilateral cranial nerve palsy (ninth and twelfth), and ipsilateral Horner's syndrome.

Various patterns can be observed in carotid dissection. CDFI can show marked flow reversal at the origin of the ICA in systole and the absence of or minimal blood flow in diastole, which is a pattern that corresponds to a high-resistance bidirectional Doppler signal.[133] B-mode scans can demonstrate a tapered lumen and occasionally a floating intimal flap.[134] Narrowing of the true lumen by the false lumen thrombus can be associated with a low-velocity Doppler waveform. The direction of flow in a patent false lumen can vary from being forward to being reversed or bidirectional. The flow dynamics in carotid dissections are complex and depend primarily on the presence of thrombus within the false lumen, the entry and exit flaps if the false lumen is patent, the motion of the flap wall, and the extent of the dissection.[135] In some patients, the only finding may be a retromandibular high-velocity signal associated with a distal stenosis of the cervical carotid artery.[136]

Follow-up examinations of carotid dissections demonstrate gradual normalization of the Doppler spectrum, which indicates recanalization of the ICA within a few weeks to months in more than two thirds of patients.[137] Carotid aneurysms can occur as complications of ICA dissections. Their follow-up with angiography and MR angiography (MRA) or MRI can be complemented with ultrasonography because of development of broad-band transducers with improved axial resolution and depth penetration.[57]

Vertebral Artery Dissection

Vertebral artery dissection is one of the most common causes of brainstem strokes in young patients.[138,139] It manifests as neck pain, occipital headache, and signs and symptoms of brainstem or cerebellar ischemia in about 90% of patients and commonly leaves a permanent deficit.[140-142] The role of ultrasonography in diagnosis of this condition remains uncertain. There is no pathognomonic ultrasonographic finding for vertebral artery dissection if the lesion affects the V2 through V4 segments. Examination of the atlas loop can reveal absence of flow signals, low bidirectional flow signals, or low poststenotic flow signals.[143] In dissections of the V1 segment, the stenotic segment can be visualized, whereas absence of flow in the intertransverse segments should similarly raise the question of vertebral dissection. Further findings can include a localized increase in the diameter of the artery with hemodynamic signs of stenosis or occlusion at the same level, decreased pulsatility, and the presence of intravascular echogenicity in the enlarged segment.[144,145] Occasionally, the specific finding of an intramural hematoma is found.[146]

A recent study assessed the sensitivity of ultrasound as compared with MRI of the neck and MRA for the detection of cervical artery dissection in 52 patients.[147] Two dissections affecting the internal carotid artery (n = 2; 8%) and two dissections of the vertebral artery (n = 2; 8%) had normal initial ultrasound findings. Thus, the sensitivity of ultrasound in detecting cervical artery dissection is high; it is approximately 92% for both vascular territories. However, intramural hematomas may be missed either when they are located outside the arterial segments directly visible by ultrasound or if they are too small to cause hemodynamically significant stenosis.[147] Ultrasound provides reliable follow-up of vertebral artery dissection in all patients seen with stenosis or occlusion but does not allow for detection of pseudoaneurysms of the vertebral artery.[148]

Transcranial Doppler (TCD) can be helpful in determining the length of dissection.[149] In one study, combined use of extracranial and TCD and duplex ultrasonography methods was found to improve the diagnostic yield of detection of vertebral artery dissection. Consideration of any abnormal ultrasonographic finding resulted in a diagnostic yield of 86%, whereas reliance on definite abnormal findings (i.e., absence of flow signal, severely reduced flow velocities, absence of diastolic flow, bidirectional flow, or stenosis signal) resulted in a diagnostic yield of only 64%.[143] Similar results were obtained in another study, in which ultrasonographic abnormalities (i.e., high-resistance signal, occlusion, and bilateral retrograde flow) were found in eight of 10 vertebral artery dissections.[150] Detection of abnormal flow patterns in the vertebral artery in cases of suspected dissection may guide further diagnostic imaging procedures and therapeutic measures. However, because unremarkable ultrasound findings do not exclude the diagnosis of vertebral dissection, further workup in these cases is mandatory.

Inflammatory Disease of the Carotid Arteries

In patients with Takayasu arteritis, increased IMT relative to that in control subjects has been reported.[151] IMT was diffusely thickened (bilaterally in 79% of the patients), whereas only rarely did the carotid artery show localized IMT thickening. Altogether, abnormal ultrasound findings were noted in 83% of the CCAs, whereas only 39% of the CCAs showed angiographically detectable alterations. CCA involvement with sparing of the internal and external carotid arteries is frequent in Takayasu arteritis.[152] The involved CCA shows diffuse or circumferential thickening of the vessel wall, which is significantly thicker in active than in inactive lesions, whereas hyperechogenicity has been observed in both active and inactive disease.[152]

Transcranial Doppler in the Evaluation of Stroke

TCD uses high-energy bidirectional pulsed Doppler, typically at a low frequency of 2 MHz, for intracranial vascular examination via transtemporal, transorbital, and transnuchal bone windows (Fig. 44-12). Applications for TCD in stroke imaging include detection of intracranial stenosis and occlusion, evaluation of intracranial collateral circulations, detection of vasospasm in subarachnoid hemorrhage (SAH), and assessment of cerebral autoregulation. TCD monitoring techniques are available for detection of high-intensity transient signals suggestive of microembolism and for surveillance of intracranial hemodynamics during stroke therapy. The introduction of transcranial CDFI has led to greater accuracy in vessel identification. Reports on the merits of transcranial CDFI for detection of cerebral aneurysms, evaluation of AVMs, and characterization of vessel morphology are now available.

Technological advances have enhanced the capabilities of TCD. They include transcranial PDI, contrast-enhanced CDFI, 3D transcranial PDI, and contrast harmonic perfusion imaging.

With conventional TCD, intracranial basal arteries are identified from flow direction, depth of the Doppler sample volume, and probe position (Table 44-3). Because flow velocities of intracranial vessels are known to vary

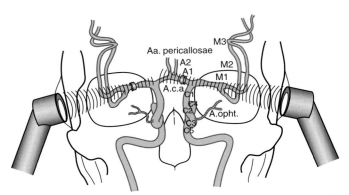

Figure 44-12 Schematic illustration of the position of the sample volume inside the skull, using the transtemporal approach. Aa. pericallosae, Pericallosal arteries; A.c.a., anterior communicating artery; A. opht., ophthalmic artery; C1 through C5, segments of the internal carotid artery; M1, M2, and M3, segments of the middle cerebral artery.

with age and sex,[153] hematocrit value,[154] and end-tidal partial pressure of carbon dioxide, a standardized TCD examination procedure is mandatory.[155] Normal values for flow velocities in the basal cerebral arteries have been determined in several studies (Table 44-4).[55,156-161] Optimal performance and correct interpretation of TCD studies require knowledge of both the clinical setting and the results of extracranial ultrasonographic examinations.

Transcranial CDFI facilitates identification of basal cerebral arteries.[162] Although conventional TCD assumes

TABLE 44-3 TRANSCRANIAL DOPPLER CRITERIA FOR THE IDENTIFICATION OF BASAL INTRACRANIAL VESSELS USING THE TRANSTEMPORAL, TRANSORBITAL, AND NUCHAL APPROACHES

Vessel	Probe	Depth (mm)	Flow Direction
Transtemporal approach			
MCA	Medial	30-65	Toward probe
ACA	Medial	55-80	Away from probe
ICA	Caudal	55-75	Toward probe
PCA, P1	Posterior	55-80	Toward probe
PCA, P2	Posterior	55-75	Away from probe
Transorbital approach			
Ophthalmic artery		30-60	Toward probe
ICA, C4, C5		60-80	Toward probe
ICA, C2, C3		60-80	Away from probe
Nuchal approach			
VA		50-100	Away from probe
BA		75-120	Away from probe

ACA, Anterior cerebral artery; BA, basilar artery; ICA, internal carotid artery; MCA, middle cerebral artery; PCA, posterior cerebral artery; VA, vertebral artery.

TABLE 44-4 NORMAL VALUES OF TRANSCRANIAL DOPPLER EXAMINATION

Vessel	Age Group (yr)	Systolic Peak Velocity (cm/s)	Mean Velocity (cm/s)	Diastolic Velocity (cm/s)
MCA (50 mm)	<40	94.5 ± 13.6	58.4 ± 8.4	45.6 ± 6.6
	40-60	91.0 ± 16.9*	57.7 ± 11.5*	44.3 ± 9.5*
	>60	78.1 ± 15.0†	44.7 ± 11.1†	31.9 ± 9.1*
ACA (70 mm)	<40	76.4 ± 16.9	47.3 ± 13.6	36.0 ± 9.0
	40-60	86.4 ± 20.1	53.1 ± 10.5	41.1 ± 7.4†
	>60	73.3 ± 20.3	45.3 ± 13.5	34.2 ± 8.8†
PCA (60 mm)	<40	53.2 ± 11.3	34.3 ± 7.8	25.9 ± 6.5
	40-60	60.1 ± 20.6	36.6 ± 9.8	28.7 ± 7.5†
	>60	51.0 ± 11.9	29.9 ± 9.3	22.0 ± 6.9†
VA/BA (75 mm)	<40	56.3 ± 7.8	34.9 ± 7.8	27.0 ± 5.3
	40-60	59.5 ± 17.0	36.4 ± 11.7	29.2 ± 8.4†
	>60	50.9 ± 18.7	30.5 ± 12.4	21.2 ± 9.2†
Pulsatility index (all age groups)				
MCA		0.92 ± 0.25		
ACA		0.8 ± 0.16		
PCA		0.88 ± 0.21		

ACA, Anterior cerebral artery; BA, basilar artery; MCA, middle cerebral artery; PCA, posterior cerebral artery; VA, vertebral artery.
*$P < 0.02$.
†$P < 0.05$.

a 0-degree Doppler angle for the calculation of flow velocities, transcranial CDFI allows correction for the Doppler insonation angle. The magnitude of the angle of insonation and the effect on flow velocity estimates in intracranial vessels have been determined through visually controlled measurements of the Doppler insonation angle made by color-flow imaging; angle-corrected peak systolic flow velocities were 3% to 30% higher than uncorrected velocity readings obtained with conventional Doppler ultrasonography.[163] Similar findings were reported in another study; in 14.5% of subjects, the angle-corrected velocity was 25% to 50% higher, and in 10.8%, it was more than 50% higher than the uncorrected velocity readings.[164] Although transcranial CDFI is considered by many to be the ultrasonic method of choice for evaluation of the intracranial circulation, there are no data on the failure rate of transcranial CDFI in a large group of patients. There are no prospective data on the ability of transcranial CDFI to detect intracranial stenosis in a large group of patients.

Intracranial Stenosis and Occlusion

Significant narrowing of intracranial arteries results in localized increases in mean and peak flow velocities, turbulence and reversed flow phenomena, and reduction of prestenotic or poststenotic flow velocities.[165-167] Stenosis that narrows the lumen by more than 50% can be reliably detected in arterial segments with anatomically favorable insonation angles such as the M1 segment of the MCA and the P1 segment of the posterior cerebral artery (PCA).

A reliable diagnosis of occlusion in the M1 segment can be made only when unequivocal evidence of blood flow in the ipsilateral anterior cerebral artery (ACA) or PCA can be obtained, thus differentiating this condition from high ultrasound attenuation and poor echo window insonation. Further findings supporting MCA occlusion are dampened spectra in segments proximal to the

occlusion, reversed flow direction in distal MCA branches, and abnormally elevated flow velocities in the ipsilateral ACA.[168] In one series of 467 patients, the sensitivity for the detection of MCA occlusion by TCD was 79% and the specificity was 100%.[169] Contrast-enhanced transcranial CDFI may be more accurate than TCD in demonstrating occlusions of the MCA[170] and is particularly useful in cases of inadequate bone windows.[171] A multicenter study has demonstrated that transcranial CFDI is a feasible, fast, and valid noninvasive bedside method for evaluating the MCA in an acute stroke setting, particularly when contrast enhancement is applied.[172]

TCD examinations of the vertebrobasilar arteries are less reliable than those of the anterior circulation. The junction of the basilar artery is difficult to define by TCD criteria alone, and investigation of the entire course of the basilar artery, which is usually limited by excessive insonation depth with poor signal-to-noise ratio,[173] can be achieved in only 30% of patients. As in the anterior circulation, partial obstructions are easier to detect than total occlusion. Using intraarterial digital subtraction angiography (DSA) as a standard reference, two groups of investigators have found that TCD demonstrated sensitivities of 74% to 87% and specificities of 80% to 86% for detection of large vessel occlusive disease of the intracranial vertebrobasilar system.[174,175] Best results, however, are obtained when TCD is used in combination with cerebral angiography[173] or MRA.[176] Unfortunately, TCD detection of basilar artery occlusion is poor, with a sensitivity of only 36%.[177] This fact is of major clinical importance in the evaluation of patients suspected of having acute basilar artery thrombosis.

Three-dimensional ultrasonographic imaging of the intracranial vessels allows a comprehensive visualization of the basal arteries and circle of Willis. Details not appreciated on 2D images alone are shown well with this technique. In particular, the origin of small arteries perpendicular or diagonal to the scanning plane can be easily identified with 3D ultrasonography. Contrast-enhanced 3D PDI may allow superior demonstration of intracerebral vascular disease and increase operator diagnostic confidence.[178] Measurement of 3D transcranial images can be a difficult task because the appearance of surface reconstructions of intracranial arteries can be significantly affected by the quality of the acquired images, the accuracy of the spatial registration, the reconstruction algorithm used, and the selection of isosurface variables. Moreover, there can be significant distortion of the ultrasound beam when it traverses the temporal bone window, leading to unpredictable results in some cases.[179] Nevertheless, first reports on the characterization of intracranial stenosis with 3D PDI have been encouraging.[180] Further work is needed to validate the ability of 3D ultrasonography to provide accurate data for quantitative assessment of the intracranial arteries and to establish variables for standardization of this technique.

Assessment of Intracranial Collateralization

The presence of intracranial collateralization in patients with stenosis or occlusion of the extracranial carotid arteries can be investigated with conventional TCD. Findings compatible with the presence of collateral flow over the anterior communicating artery include retrograde flow in the ipsilateral ACA, increased peak and mean velocities in both ACAs, increased velocities and low-frequency signals in the midline indicating functional stenosis of the anterior communicating artery, and decreased MCA velocity during compression of the contralateral CCA. Collateralization from the posterior circulation is suggested by increased velocities in the ipsilateral P1 segment of the PCA or in the basilar artery as well as by low-frequency signals in the posterior communicating artery. Leptomeningeal anastomosis, although more difficult to assess, may be associated with increased velocities in the proximal and distal segments of the PCA and with retrograde flow signals in distal MCA branches. TCD can also detect retrograde flow in the ophthalmic artery, which is another avenue for collateralization.

Flow velocities in the MCA distal to significant stenosis and occlusion vary with regard to the efficacy of intracranial collateralization. Although reduced MCA velocities and pulsatility indexes have been found ipsilateral to symptomatic carotid occlusion,[181,182] normal peak and mean velocities indicating adequate collateralization have been reported in asymptomatic patients.[183]

Microembolic Signal Detection

TCD can be used to detect microembolic signals (MES) entering the cerebral circulation. This technique, first reported over two decades ago,[184] may identify patients who are at increased risk of stroke during interventional investigations and carotid surgery.[185] The methodology of MES detection consists of fixing a Doppler probe with a frequency of approximately 2 MHz over the temporal bone and adjusting its position, orientation, and the Doppler sample volume depth to obtain a good signal from blood flow within the ipsilateral MCA. Because a microembolus has different acoustic properties from those of the blood in which it is traveling, there is a transient increase in the back-scattered ultrasonic power as it passes through the Doppler sample volume (high-intensity transient signals, or HITS); therefore, careful monitoring of the Doppler signal provides a means of classification and artifact rejection (Fig. 44-13). HITS corresponding to both gaseous and solid microembolic materials have been detected during angiography,[186,187] carotid angioplasty,[188] open heart surgery,[189,190] and carotid endarterectomy[191,192] as well as in patients with TIAs or stroke,[193-196] asymptomatic carotid stenosis,[197] heart valve prosthesis,[198,199] and intracranial arterial disease.[200]

Definition of High-Intensity Transient Signals

HITS are usually visualized in the fast Fourier transform (FFT). In 1995, using this signal analysis approach, a consensus committee[201] proposed the following three criteria for defining HITS: (1) duration is less than 300 ms, (2) exceeds the background by at least 3 dB, and (3) is unidirectional within the Doppler velocity spectrum. HITS detection can be performed by insonation of any of the three major vessels of the circle of Willis, although monitoring of the carotid arteries[202] and the jugular veins[203] has also been reported. In most cases, the main stem of the MCA is insonated with a 2-MHz probe via the temporal bone window. Sophisticated multigate techniques have been developed that interrogate two sample volumes along a vessel to enable better differentiation between artifacts and moving particles (Fig. 44-14).

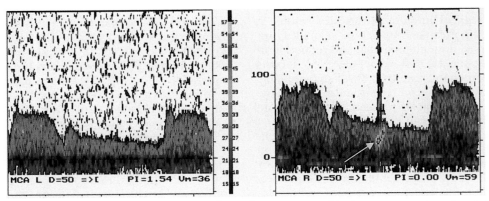

Figure 44-13 Two images showing simultaneous transcranial Doppler monitoring of high-intensity transient signals (HITS) in the left and right middle cerebral arteries (MCAs). Note the HITS *(arrow)* occurring in the right MCA, presumably of microembolic origin.

Differentiation

To date, most studies of embolic signals have relied on trained human observers to identify candidate events and to distinguish between true embolic signals and signals due to other mechanisms. Indeed, the detection of HITS shows a high interobserver agreement,[204-206] with kappa values in the range of 0.95. The technique is very time-consuming, however, and there are a number of drawbacks associated with HITS monitoring, in terms of both cost and reliability.

If the technique is to become widely accepted in clinical practice, some form of automatic recognition will become mandatory. A number of attempts have been made to provide commercial automated systems, but none has been independently shown to be able to discriminate between artifacts and signals due to microemboli.[207] Such systems must also be capable of distinguishing between signals from emboli of different types because the clinical consequences of microemboli, although currently unclear, are expected to vary greatly; for example, patients with prosthetic heart valves can show more than 40,000 HITS per day or more than 1 million HITS per month without any neurologic or neuropsychological sequelae. Signal analysis techniques, such as simultaneous insonation with two frequencies (e.g., 1 and 2 MHz),[208] nonlinear forecasting,[209] recognition of specific postembolic spectral patterns,[210] and the application of the narrow band hypothesis[211] have been introduced to illuminate specific properties of HITS. Applications for automatic online microembolic signal detection with the use of a multifrequency Doppler instrument[212,213] and a rule-based expert system[214] have given favorable results, which suggests that such approaches may well provide the necessary basis for automatic MES detection systems in the future.

Localizing the Source of Embolism in Patients with Stroke

Data on the frequency of HITS suggestive of microemboli from the heart or from the proximal arteries of the intracranial circulation have been variable.[215,216] In patients with heart valve prostheses, thousands of clinically silent events can be recorded, whereas in patients with symptomatic carotid stenoses, HITS are relatively rare events. It appears that emboli of cardiac and carotid origin may have different ultrasonic characteristics, which are probably related to composition and size.[217] The clinical relevance of these features, however, is unclear.

After the report of HITS detection during carotid endarterectomy,[218] similar signals that occurred spontaneously were recognized in patients with symptomatic carotid artery disease.[193,195,197] Because the MES disappeared after carotid endarterectomy,[194,219,220] it was assumed that the atherosclerotic carotid plaque had been the source of the signals. In an unselected group of patients with stroke examined within 1 month of cerebral infarction, however, the prevalence of ipsilateral MES in the largest series published was approximately 10%.[221] If the interval after the acute event is shorter, the prevalence of MES may increase. In another study, monitoring with TCD within 2 days after admission showed that approximately 25% of an unselected group of patients had MES.[222] Patients with a carotid stenosis of at least 40% have been reported to have significantly more MES (39%) than those without a carotid stenosis (18%). Similarly, the prevalence of MES in a comparable group of patients was reported to approach 50% when monitoring was performed immediately after admission and 1 and 2 days thereafter.[223] Of the studied group, 44% of patients had a carotid stenosis or occlusion, and 62% of these patients were MES positive.

Apart from the role of the timing of examination in determining the likelihood of MES detection in symptomatic carotid artery disease,[219,224,225] the severity of carotid stenosis may correlate with the number of measured MES; that is, the more severe the narrowing, the more MES are detected.[223,226,227] Interestingly, complete carotid occlusion has been found to be associated with a high MES count.[227] Contrary to the preceding discussion on the doubtful relevance of plaque ulcerations in pathoanatomic studies, other studies maintain that there is a relationship between preoperative MES count and carotid plaque ulceration.[228] Similarly, HITS monitored in the MCAs of patients with carotid stenosis have been

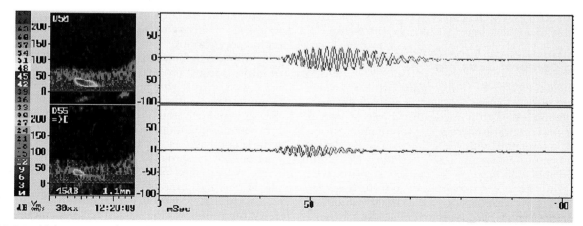

Figure 44-14 Multigate Doppler technique for improved identification of microemboli. Here the middle cerebral artery is insonated simultaneously at two locations. The delay in time between the appearance of high-intensity signals at the two gates is strong evidence for a microembolic particle. (An artifact would appear simultaneously at both gates.)

reported to correlate with the appearance of ipsilateral plaque ulceration.[229]

There is some evidence that HITS detected during the dissection phase of carotid endarterectomy may correlate with clinically silent infarctions demonstrated with MRI.[191] Moreover, in a few cases, a relationship between persistent particulate embolization in the immediate postoperative period and both incipient carotid artery thrombosis and the development of major neurologic deficits has been observed.[192] In carotid angioplasty, embolization at the time of intervention is very common but usually asymptomatic. Late embolization, occurring in a minority of patients, may account for the small but significant risk of delayed stroke.[188]

Carotid dissections can cause neurologic deficits by either hemodynamic or embolic mechanisms. Because anticoagulants are often used in this setting to prevent neurologic deterioration and stroke recurrence, it would be valuable to differentiate between the two mechanisms. HITS detection would seem an ideal technique for this purpose. Reports on the relationship between MES and the clinical or imaging features of carotid dissection, however, have been conflicting. One study of patients with carotid dissections reported that the detection of HITS had no clinical significance,[230] but another investigation found that MES occurrence on serial TCD monitoring sessions was associated with an increased risk of early ischemic recurrence.[231] Further studies are necessary to settle this issue.

HITS occur predominantly in patients with large vessel territory stroke patterns and persisting deficits, most likely due to artery-to-artery or cardiogenic embolism.[221] In contrast, patients with small vessel disease are only occasionally seen with HITS. Thus, the detection of HITS may support the classification of the individual pathogenesis of cerebral ischemia, particularly when multiple risk constellations for stroke coexist. Moreover, detection of recurrent microembolic events by TCD monitoring can provide useful guidance for pathophysiologically oriented treatment of patients with stroke.[221] Microembolism can also occur in giant cell arteritis[232] and may be related to disease activity in systemic lupus erythematosus with antiphospholipid syndrome.[233] HITS are also significantly associated with large aortic arch atheromas in elderly patients with stroke, which is an observation supporting the causal role of aortic atheromas in ischemic stroke.[234]

Predicting Cerebral Ischemia

Microemboli detected by TCD in patients with stroke may be associated with a higher prevalence of prior cerebrovascular ischemia,[224,227] thus suggesting a role of MES as a risk factor for cerebral ischemia. Asymptomatic carotid stenoses are associated with MES but to a much lesser extent than symptomatic stenoses.[220,226,235,236] Detection of asymptomatic embolization in carotid stenosis with TCD monitoring, however, may predict short-term ipsilateral stroke risk. This supports the use of the technique to identify patients at high risk of recurrent stroke for therapeutic interventions and as a surrogate marker to evaluate antithrombotic medication.[237] Studies addressing early recurrent ischemic events after stroke or TIA in patients

with a carotid stenosis[238,239] have found the presence of MES to be a predictor for early ischemic recurrence.

Interventional Trials Using MES Detection

In patients with recent symptomatic carotid stenosis, combination therapy with clopidogrel and aspirin was shown to be more effective than aspirin alone in reducing asymptomatic embolization.[240] Similar results were obtained in the Clopidogrel plus Aspirin for Infarction Reduction (CLAIR) trial. Patients with acute ischemic stroke or TIA who had symptomatic large artery stenosis in the cerebral or carotid arteries and in whom microembolic signals were present on transcranial Doppler were randomly assigned within 7 days of symptom onset to receive clopidogrel plus aspirin or aspirin alone for 7 days. Results of this trial demonstrated that combination therapy with clopidogrel and aspirin is more effective than aspirin alone in reducing microembolic signals in patients with predominantly intracranial symptomatic stenosis.[241]

Future Aspects of Microembolic Signal Detection

In the majority of cases in which HITS are detected, whether these phenomena are associated with an increased risk of functional or morphologic brain damage remains unclear.[225] This problem has been compounded by the wide variety of variables used by different investigators for MES detection. The International Consensus Group on Microembolus Detection reported guidelines for the proper use of microembolism detection by TCD in clinical practice and scientific investigations.[207] They suggested that technical instruments (i.e., ultrasound device, transducer size and type, FFT size, FFT length, FFT overlap, and high-pass filter settings), methodology (i.e., identification of arteries insonated, insonation depth, detection threshold, scale settings, axial extension of sample volume, and recording time), and methods for analysis and interpretation (i.e., algorithms for signal intensity measurement, standardization of interobserver and intraobserver variability, and comparison of semiautomatic embolus detection algorithms) should be reported and validated in each laboratory to establish the required sensitivity and specificity for clinical use and scientific application.

If embolus detection is to realize its full potential, both in clinical trials and in routine monitoring situations, it is necessary to derive automatic methods of processing Doppler data so that vast amounts of information can be speedily and accurately evaluated. As novel applications for dynamic quantitative evaluation of cerebral perfusion with second-generation ultrasonography contrast agents emerge,[242,243] approaches using systems that can automatically analyze multiple gaseous particles may prove beneficial. Such techniques could be applied, for example, to discriminate embolus material through the use of targeted microbubbles that attach to solid emboli and hence establish their characteristics from the bubble signatures. Indeed, first results of using abciximab immunobubbles for detection of solid emboli seem promising.[244]

The cardiac conditions producing MES are heterogeneous; therefore, the prevalence of MES is highly variable. The data from patients after myocardial infarction, endocarditis, patent foramen ovale (PFO), mitral valve prolapse, dilatative cardiomyopathy, and intracardiac thrombus are promising, but only small patient cohorts have been investigated by means of TCD in these categories.[245] MES in atrial fibrillation, or derived from athero-aortic plaques, have been investigated more intensively, but again, larger cohorts need to be explored to draw firm conclusions. In all cardiac diseases there is a lack of large prospective studies that would allow reliable correlation of MES with clinical events.[245] Compared with knowledge about carotid artery disease, the current knowledge about the impact of cardiogenic MES on the patient's risk is sparse. This should encourage clinical research in this promising field.

Dolichoectatic Arteries and Intracranial Vasculopathies

Noninvasive diagnosis of intracranial dolichoectatic arteries,[246] a cause of TIAs or stroke,[247] can be achieved with TCD in combination with computed tomography (CT) or MRI. The dramatic reduction in peak and mean flow velocities that is often observed in these patients suggests a thromboembolic mechanism of ischemia in slow flow territories. TCD is also sensitive and specific for the detection of arterial vasculopathy in sickle cell disease[248,249] and has been used for assessment of reversible multisegmental narrowing of cerebral arteries in postpartum cerebral angiopathy.[250]

Detection of Right-to-Left Cardiac Shunts

Paradoxic embolism through a PFO is a known cause of embolic strokes and TIAs in patients with stroke of uncertain etiology. TCD monitoring of the basal intracranial vessels during intravenous injection of appropriate contrast media that does not normally pass through the lungs can be used for the detection of right-to-left shunts through documentation of microbubbles reaching the brain.[251-253] TCD findings correlate well with those of transesophageal echocardiography when a standardized procedure including the Valsalva maneuver is used.[254] In some patients, TCD studies can identify microbubbles in the absence of PFO, thus suggesting pulmonary shunting. Careful CT assessment of the thorax can identify such abnormal pathways, which sometimes require interventional treatment.

Contrast TCD performed with galactose suspension (Echovist), but not with saline, has 100% sensitivity for identification of a cardiac right-to-left shunt that has been proven by transesophageal echocardiography (TEE).[255] The sensitivity of diagnosing PFO with both TCD and TEE may be higher with injection of contrast media into the femoral vein than into the antecubital vein.[256] This difference may be related to different inflow patterns to the right atrium because inferior vena caval flow is directed to the right atrial septum and superior vena caval flow to the tricuspid valve. The timing of the Valsalva maneuver, the dose of the contrast medium, and the patient's posture during the examination are further factors influencing detection of PFO.[257,258]

Echocontrast Studies in Stroke Diagnosis

The ability of intravenous contrast media to increase the echogenicity of flowing blood has been known for some time.[259] However, only recently has there been an increasing demand for the use of echo-enhancing agents in assessment of cerebrovascular disease. Common applications employing contrast agents are TCD studies in patients with severe hyperostosis of the skull, quantification of internal carotid stenosis in the presence of calcification, differentiation between internal carotid occlusion and pseudoocclusion, assessment of intracranial aneurysms and AVMs, and investigation of the basilar and intracranial vertebral arteries.

Commercially available contrast agents consist of microbubbles with average diameters from 3 to 6 μm in concentrations typically on the order of 10^8 microbubbles per milliliter. The microbubbles are normally stabilized against dissolution by surfactants, phospholipids, or a surface layer of partially denatured albumin. Current contrast agents can enhance the ultrasound signal by 10 to 30 dB,[260] thus enabling the detection of flow in deeper and smaller vessels.

The first generation of ultrasonography contrast agents consisted of air-filled microbubbles. However, because of the low concentration of air gases in the systemic circulation, the air contained inside these agents quickly diffuses out of the microbubbles after injection into the body.[261] The type of gas inside the bubble determines the dwell time in the circulation[262] and can also affect the backscattered signal in both linear and nonlinear regimens.[263] Thus, a second generation of ultrasonic agents was developed and consists of microbubbles containing less soluble gases, such as perfluorocarbons and sulfur hexafluoride.

Echogenic liposomes are similar in terms of their chemical composition to phospholipid-coated microbubbles but consist of phospholipid bilayers encapsulating a mixture of liquid and gas. This type of agent also offers enhanced stability compared with gas microbubbles and is particularly attractive for drug delivery applications, as larger quantities of either aqueous or nonaqueous material can be encapsulated. Because of their lower gas content compared with microbubble agents, higher doses of echogenic liposomes (i.e., particles per unit volume) are required to obtain equivalent levels of contrast enhancement during imaging and specific pulse regimens are required to initiate drug release.

Carotid Artery Stenosis

Clinical studies with echo contrast agents have claimed to be effective in improving diagnostic confidence in patients with carotid artery stenosis. Contrast enhancement reduces operator variability, improves ultrasonographic image quality, and aids in distinguishing between pseudoocclusions and true occlusions.[264] Although first reports on the use of ultrasonic contrast media to investigate carotid arteries suggested a significant improvement in characterization and quantification of severe internal carotid stenosis,[265,266] further studies demonstrated that unenhanced PDI provides the same diagnostic yield as the combined approach for assessment of carotid artery pseudoocclusion.[266] As the analysis of the data from the European Carotid Surgery Trial has shown that patients with subtotal ICA stenosis do not benefit from carotid endarterectomy,[267] the clinical importance of distinguishing between pseudoocclusions and true occlusions with ultrasonography has diminished. In this context, the use of echo contrast agents for detection of carotid artery pseudoocclusion is not justified.

Insufficient Transcranial Bone Windows

In TCD, insonation through the temporal bone window is often impaired by an insufficient signal-to-noise ratio, especially in elderly patients. Echo contrast agents have been shown to yield conclusive TCD findings in most patients in whom ultrasonography penetration is insufficient. Most studies have been performed with the galactose-based microbubble agent Levovist. Depending on the concentration of Levovist, the average maximal TCD signal enhancement is approximately 12.0 ± 5.4 dB for 300 mg/mL.[268] Albunex has likewise been shown to improve the quality of TCD examinations through better visualization of the ICA, the MCA, and the circle of Willis,[269] although the relatively short duration of the contrast enhancement is a limiting factor.

Contrast agents have also been shown to enhance diagnoses by transcranial CDFI in patients with poor tissue penetration in whom imaging of vessels would otherwise be inadequate.[270] Other studies have confirmed these initial findings in patients whose basal arteries could not be assessed adequately with transcranial CDFI. After administration of Levovist, more than 85% of examinations of the MCA, the ACA, the P1 and P2 segments of the PCA, and the supraclinoid portion of the ICA siphon were satisfactory.[271] Moreover, the use of intravenous contrast material often enables the entire circle of Willis to be evaluated from a single temporal-bone acoustic window in both PDI and CDFI.[272] Contrast agents have also been used to enable intracranial insonation through lateral and paramedian frontal bone windows, thus offering a further approach to study the circle of Willis, the venous midline vasculature, and the frontal parenchyma.[273] The technical success rate of 3D transcranial PDI investigations has also been improved with contrast agents.[274]

There is good evidence that echo contrast agents are valuable in TCD examinations of patients with acute cerebrovascular disease. In an investigation of patients seen with ischemic strokes and TIAs who had insufficient temporal bone windows, results of contrast-enhanced transcranial CDFI studies in 66% of patients were conclusive.[275] These findings have been confirmed by a similar study of patients with acute stroke in whom investigations performed without contrast enhancement were inadequate.[276]

The quality of transtemporal precontrast enhancement scans is strongly predictive of the potential diagnostic benefit that is to be expected from application of an intravenous contrast agent. In patients whose intracranial structures are not visible in B-mode imaging and whose vessel segments are not depicted with CDFI, there is little chance that the use of a contrast agent will provide diagnostic confidence.[277] This has also been shown in patients with acute cerebral ischemia. In one study, the identification of any cerebral artery before contrast enhancement provided an overall accuracy of 97% in predicting that an investigation with contrast agent would be conclusive, whereas in patients in whom vessel identification was not possible before the use of contrast enhancement, there were no conclusive contrast studies.[275]

Intracranial Vertebral and Basilar Arteries

Examinations of the intracranial vertebral arteries and the basilar artery are also facilitated with echo contrast agents. The use of an echo contrast agent for insonation through the foramen magnum during color-coded duplex ultrasonography can increase the depth at which vessels can be identified[278] and can improve the number of pathologic findings not seen in unenhanced scans by about 20%.[279] Moreover, echo contrast enhancement of the vertebral and basilar arteries may significantly improve diagnostic accuracy. This is particularly true in cases of acute basilar artery occlusion because the detection rate of basilar artery flow for contrast-enhanced transcranial CDFI is more than 98%, as opposed to 76% without contrast agent.[280] Some evidence suggests that PDI may be just as effective as contrast-enhanced transcranial CDFI in visualizing the vertebrobasilar system.[281]

Intracranial Aneurysms

Contrast-enhanced transcranial CDFI and contrast-enhanced PDI (CE PDI) employing Levovist have been used to detect and measure the size of intracranial aneurysms.[282] Although CE PDI missed four of 36 angiographically verified aneurysms in one study, measurements of aneurysm size correlated well with angiographic findings. Other ultrasonographic studies have suggested that aneurysm dimensions may vary with intracranial pressure (ICP), in that they are larger and less pulsatile at low ICP and smaller but more pulsatile at high ICP.[283] Intraoperative transcranial CDFI allows characterization and localization of aneurysms,[284] as well as identification of vessels potentially threatened by clipping,[285] whereas intraoperative microvascular Doppler ultrasonography has been shown to be an effective alternative to intraoperative angiography for assessment of vessel patency in aneurysm surgery.[286] An important remaining question is whether, in cases of acute SAH, TCD is capable of detecting not only the bleeding aneurysm but also other asymptomatic aneurysms that may require neurosurgical intervention.

Arteriovenous Malformations

Transcranial CE PDI with Levovist has also been used to evaluate AVMs.[287] In one study, CE PDI identified all angiographically confirmed AVMs in patients with adequate temporal bone windows. Although this technique slightly underestimated AVM size, it consistently showed feeding arteries. Coincidental blood supply from another intracranial or extracranial vessel, however, was missed by CE PDI in all cases. In another study, transcranial color-coded duplex sonography allowed visualization of 42 of 54 AVMs, for a sensitivity of 77.8%.[288] Blood flow imaging, a 2D ultrasound modality that offers angle-independent visualization of flow, has been used to discern between feeding arteries and draining veins during surgery for AVMs.[289]

Venous Thrombosis

TCD methods can also be used to evaluate the basal cerebral veins, which can be identified on the basis of their anatomic relation to specific arteries.[290] As in other applications, power- and frequency-based color-coded duplex ultrasonography aids in the assessment of cerebral veins and sinuses.[291] Standardized protocols for intracranial venous examinations and reference data for clinical applications have been described.[292]

Evidence suggests that TCD can detect and monitor intracranial venous hemodynamics and collateral pathways in patients with confirmed cerebral venous thrombosis (CVT).[293,294] Transcranial CDFI evaluation of venous drainage patterns in acute CVT has shown that both initially normal venous flow and normalization of initially diseased venous flow within 90 days of CVT are related to a favorable outcome.[295] Transcranial CDFI appears to enable a more reliable evaluation of the major deep cerebral veins and posterior fossa sinuses in cases of sinus thrombosis. The anterior and middle portions of the superior sagittal sinus and cortical veins, however, cannot be assessed by this means.[296] Here, increased venous blood flow velocity can be used as indirect evidence of a CVT. Superior evaluation of transverse sinus thrombosis can be obtained with the use of echo contrast agents[297] (see later). Further prospective studies are needed to establish the sensitivity and specificity of neurosonologic techniques for diagnosis and monitoring of intracranial venous thrombosis.

Ultrasound Monitoring in Acute Stroke

Monitoring of Thrombolysis

Recanalization time as determined in vitro is an important measure of thrombolysis when a clot is exposed to tissue-type plasminogen activator (t-PA) (Fig. 44-15). This time is usually given as the time of complete clot dissolution with washout to the distal vasculature and the veins. In human strokes, complete recanalization correlates with clinical recovery, as predicted from animal models. Recanalization, however, is a process that often begins many minutes before restoration of cerebral blood flow because t-PA binding and activity on the clot surface are proportional to the area exposed to blood flow. Once recanalization starts, the clot softens and partially dissolves. As a result, residual flow improves, which allows more t-PA to bind with fibrinogen sites. This process facilitates clot lysis and continually improves residual flow until the clot breaks up under the pressure of arterial blood pulsations.

Recanalization time may be an important clinical variable indicating thrombolysis. Although prolonged clot dissolution delays complete recanalization and may be associated with a longer duration of cerebral ischemia, a sudden increase in blood flow may disrupt the blood-brain barrier and lead to edema or hemorrhage. Alexandrov et al[298] have addressed this issue using real-time ultrasonography monitoring of residual flow signals during thrombolysis with t-PA in patients with occlusion of the MCA or basilar artery. These researchers classified recanalization as sudden (abrupt appearance of a normal or stenotic low-resistance signal), stepwise (flow improvement over 1 to 29 minutes), or slow (≥30 minutes to improvement). The results showed that recanalization began at a median of 17 minutes and was completed at 35

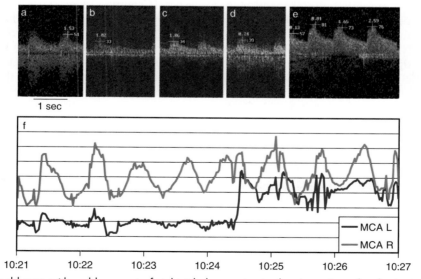

Figure 44-15 A 63-year-old man with sudden onset of right-sided sensorimotor hemiparesis and aphasia at 8:30 AM. A, Transcranial Doppler ultrasonography shows a minimal signal in the left middle cerebral artery (MCA). B and C, Cerebral blood flow velocity decreases further. D, An improvement in signal intensity is detected at 10:24 AM, signifying the onset of recanalization. E, The signal abruptly changes to a normal waveform in less than 1 second. F, Recanalization starts within minutes of administration of a bolus of tissue-type plasminogen activator and is complete within seconds, leading to complete recanalization of the distal M1 segment of the MCA.

minutes after bolus administration of t-PA, with a mean duration of recanalization of 23 ± 16 minutes. Complete recanalization occurred considerably faster (median, 10 minutes) than partial recanalization (median, 30 minutes). Importantly, rapid arterial recanalization was associated with better short-term improvement, whereas slow flow improvement and dampened flow signals were less favorable prognostic signs. These findings, by providing valuable information on temporal patterns of recanalization, may assist in identification of patients who need additional pharmacologic or interventional treatment.

Recently, an international consensus on grading intracranial flow obstruction (COGIF score) with transcranial color-coded Doppler was proposed (Table 44-5).[299] The COGIF score can be applied for both baseline evaluation and assessment of recanalization during follow-up. The major grades of the COGIF score comprise vessel occlusion (grade 1), partial recanalization (grades 2 and 3), and established perfusion (grade 4).

Grade 1: MCA main stem occlusion. The main diagnostic criterion of the occlusion of the M1 segment is the absence of a color Doppler flow signal and its Doppler spectrum in the location of the proximal MCA segment. Because the absence of Doppler signals may be a consequence of an insufficient acoustic bone window, a reliable diagnosis of arterial occlusion requires sufficient visibility of the other arteries (ACA A1-segment, C1-segment of intracranial ICA) or veins (deep middle cerebral vein) of the anterior circulation or visibility of the contralateral anterior circulation.

Grades 2-3: Low-flow phenomena in the M1 segment of the MCA may be found as a result of a partial recanalization of the M1 segment or the carotid T, an upstream carotid obstruction, or a downstream obstruction (i.e., distal main stem or MCA branch occlusions). Upstream or downstream obstruction must be differentiated from partial recanalization of the M1.

Grade 4: Different Doppler patterns are integrated, including normal flow (4a), stenotic flow (4b), and high-flow velocities in hyperperfusion (4c). All patterns indicate established perfusion.

Detection of MES by TCD at the site of arterial obstruction can indicate clot dissolution. Alexandrov et al[300] detected clusters of MES distal to a high-grade M1 stenosis before spontaneous clinical recovery; they also documented minimal MCA flow signals followed by MES,

increased velocities, and normal flow signals over a period of 2 minutes preceding complete recanalization.[300] Further studies are needed to establish the role of MES detection in monitoring of thrombolytic therapy.

Monitoring of Midline Shift

Transcranial color-coded duplex ultrasonography is a noninvasive, easily reproducible, and reliable method for monitoring midline dislocation of the third ventricle in patients with stroke.[301] It is well suited for monitoring the space-occupying effect of both supratentorial and infratentorial strokes during treatment in critical care and stroke units.[302] The technique can also be used to facilitate the identification of patients who are unlikely to survive without decompressive craniectomy.[303] Studies confirm that TCD is a reliable noninvasive method for serially monitoring patients with large MCA infarctions, showing that the degree of midline shift correlates significantly with ICP measurements.[304]

Assessment of Vasospasm

TCD has become a standard examination procedure for detection, quantification, and follow-up of vasospasms after SAH.[159,305,306] Vasospasms generally occur on the fourth day after SAH, and peak flow velocities can be observed between the 11th and 18th days. Normalization of flow velocities occurs within the third or fourth week after SAH. A rapid increase of velocities 4 to 8 days after SAH is associated with a higher risk of ischemic stroke.

Although early reports claimed that TCD results mirror the extent of obstruction commonly demonstrated in angiograms of stroke-prone patients after SAH, other observations have questioned a simple focal narrowing of the arterial lumen, analogous to that in atherosclerotic disease, as the cause of altered Doppler flow patterns after SAH. The pathophysiology of subarachnoid vasospasm is complex. Elevated ICP may lead to an increase in vasomotor resistance of capillary and arteriolar vessels with consequent dampening of the Doppler flow velocity in major proximal arteries. This may result in false-negative Doppler results despite angiographically demonstrable vasospasm. Moreover, local flow turbulences may be found despite normal angiographic findings if peripheral vasomotor dysregulation and large vessel vasoconstriction occur subsequent to SAH.

Importantly, TCD findings in patients with SAH are greatly influenced by changing therapeutic concepts. Only 28% of patients treated with calcium channel blockers have a significant increase in flow velocities before the onset of delayed ischemic stroke, which suggests that vasospasm may occur in more distal arterial segments inaccessible to TCD insonation.[307] TCD is further limited in patients with SAH by its relatively poor diagnostic accuracy in the ACA territory, a common site of aneurysms.[308]

Increased Intracranial Pressure

TCD can be useful in monitoring ICP in patients with bleeding diatheses and other contraindications to invasive ICP monitoring. Simultaneous recordings of Doppler

TABLE 44-5 CONSENSUS ON GRADING INTRACRANIAL FLOW (COGIF) OBSTRUCTION SCORE

COGIF Score	Transcranial Color Doppler Flow Pattern
1	No flow
2	Low flow velocities without diastolic flow
3	Low flow velocities with diastolic flow
4	Established perfusion (a) Flow velocities equal to contralateral side (b) High focal flow velocities (stenosis) (c) High segmental flow velocities (hyperperfusion)

signals from the basal cerebral arteries, systemic blood pressure, and ICP with epidural devices have shown that a progressive reduction in diastolic and systolic velocities can occur with increasing ICP. Moreover, various patterns of flow alterations have been demonstrated in different regions of the brain, indicating the existence of varying pressure gradients inside the skull.[309] When the ICP rises above diastolic blood pressure, Doppler signals from the basal cerebral arteries are severely altered. Mild or moderate increases in ICP, however, can be compensated for by an increase in the systemic blood pressure, thus resulting in normal TCD findings. Measurements of the absolute ICP value cannot be performed with this method, but changes in TCD findings parallel changes in ICP value, if a constant arterial CO_2 content and a constant level of distal vasoconstriction is assumed. Thus, at least under certain conditions, a quantitative estimation of the ICP could be made on the basis of consistent relationships between flow velocity variables recorded from intracranial arteries and continuous but noninvasive arterial blood pressure measurement. Schmidt et al[310] supported this concept and showed that a mathematical model could predict ICP modulations from shapes of arterial blood flow and pulse noninvasively. These preliminary findings suggest that TCD may prove useful in evaluating strategies to improve cerebral autoregulation as well as in the optimal management of ICP control.

Functional Studies

The introduction of bilateral continuous TCD monitoring has resulted in the development of a variety of sophisticated applications as supplementary tools to positron emission tomography (PET) and functional MRI studies. They include evaluation of functional recovery after stroke.

Changes in cerebral perfusion during motor activity in patients with stroke who have early recovery of motor function may be monitored with TCD.[311,312] Increased flow velocities in both the contralateral and ipsilateral MCAs during motor tasks have been demonstrated, suggesting that areas of the healthy hemisphere can be activated soon after a focal ischemic injury and can contribute to the positive evolution of a functional deficit. This phenomenon of contralateral recovery from activation is not transient because it is evident months after stroke onset. In patients with Broca aphasia after ischemic stroke, a similar increase in MCA flow velocities has been detected after successful speech therapy, providing additional support for contralateral hemispheric involvement in functional recovery after stroke.[313]

Ultrasonographic Brain Perfusion Imaging

Because perfusion imaging may detect ischemic lesions earlier than CT and may distinguish the stroke subtype and severity of cerebral ischemia, there is growing interest in the use of perfusion imaging to predict recovery, differentiate stroke pathogenesis, and monitor therapy. Advanced contrast-specific ultrasound imaging technologies now allow assessment of brain perfusion in stroke patients.

Contrast-Specific Imaging Techniques

Contrast Harmonic Imaging

Contrast harmonic imaging (CHI) is based on the nonlinear emission of harmonics by resonant microbubbles pulsating in an ultrasound field. The emission at twice the driving frequency, termed the *second harmonic*, can be detected and separated from the fundamental frequency. The advantage of the harmonic over the fundamental frequency is that microbubbles of contrast agent resonate with harmonic frequencies, whereas adjacent tissues do so very little. In this way, CHI may enhance the signal-to-noise ratio and the ability of B-mode scanners to differentiate bubbles in the tissue vascular space from the echogenic surrounding avascular tissue.

Pulse-Inversion Contrast Harmonic Imaging

Pulse-inversion CHI (PICHI) is a technique that minimizes some of the shortcomings of CHI. It uses a two-pulse sequence with an 180-degree phase difference to cancel the effect of transmitted second harmonics on the received signal.[314] In PICHI two pulses are transmitted down each ray line, instead of only a single pulse as is done with conventional harmonic or fundamental imaging. The first is a normal pulse, and the second is an inverted replica of the first so that wherever there was a positive pressure on the first pulse there is an equal negative pressure on the second. Any linear target that responds equally to positive and negative pressures will reflect back to the transducer equal but opposite echoes. These are then added and all stationary linear targets cancel, as shown in Figure 44-16.

Microbubbles respond differently to positive and negative pressures and do not reflect identical inverted waveforms. Figure 44-17 illustrates the effect that inverting one of the pulses has on nonlinear components generated by microbubbles. When the responses are added together the fundamental component cancels and the second harmonic components add constructively. PICHI preserves axial resolution and avoids harmonic frequency overlaps, thus providing improved ultrasonographic visualization of adult brain tissue.[243]

Power Modulation

An alternative to changing the phase of each successive pulse that is transmitted is to change the amplitude of successive pulses in a group. This technique is referred to as *power modulation (PM) imaging*. PM detects the

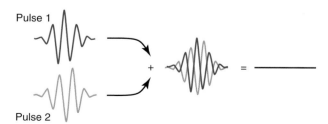

Figure 44-16 By adding two consecutive bubble echoes from inverted pulses, pulse inversion cancels fundamental echoes without filtering.

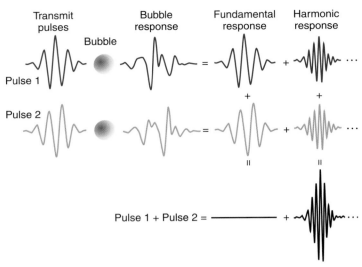

Figure 44-17 Pulse-inversion harmonic imaging signal processing.

differential nonlinear response generated from two different excitations. In PM, a low-amplitude pulse is transmitted to estimate the linear response of a target volume. Then a slightly higher amplitude pulse is transmitted to elicit a nonlinear response from the target volume. On reception, the lower amplitude signal is rescaled by the factor between transmitted pulses and is then subtracted. The resulting difference at the fundamental frequency represents energy that has "leaked out" of the second pulse into the higher harmonics (Fig. 44-18).

Power Modulated Pulse-Inversion Imaging

Pulse inversion can also be combined with power modulation imaging (PMPI). In this case, both the phase and amplitude are altered between pulses. The pulses are again scaled on reception but are then added. The main difference between PM and PMPI is the fact that PMPI produces a slightly higher second harmonic component than does PM, which is still slightly lower than pulse inversion. Often much of the difference seen between these pulsing sequences is not necessarily due to the method itself as much as the choice of other variables used during the optimization process, such as where the receiver filters are placed with respect to the fundamental or harmonic. The nonlinear fundamental is more sensitive but has worse resolution because of its lower frequency. Because of the attenuation and distortion in the skull, sensitivity is generally the most important consideration in transcranial contrast imaging, which makes the nonlinear fundamental in either PM or PMPI the dominant component.

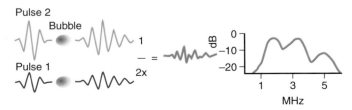

Figure 44-18 Power modulation signal processing.

High Mechanical Index Perfusion Studies

Most studies on assessment of cerebral perfusion after UCA injection have applied high mechanical index (MI) ultrasound imaging, regardless of the technique used for contrast-specific imaging. The MI, originally defined to predict the onset of cavitation in fluids, is a measure of acoustic output and also describes the likelihood of microbubble disruption. Until recently there was no alternative to high MI imaging because lower acoustic outputs were unable to detect microbubbles in the brain. Therefore, because bubbles are destroyed in the microcirculation with high MI imaging, a triggered pulsing sequence is implemented to allow for replenishment of new bubbles in the ultrasound scan plane. Accordingly, most early studies of cerebral perfusion were performed with triggered harmonic gray-scale imaging techniques (i.e., conventional, PM, or PMPI) analyzing the bolus kinetics in healthy subjects to determine the best method for detection of UCA in the cerebral microcirculation.[315-328] In some experiments, fundamental color duplex technologies based on the power Doppler mode and contrast agent destruction were used (e.g., contrast burst imaging and time variance imaging).

Low Mechanical Index Perfusion Imaging

Recently low-MI real-time perfusion techniques have been introduced that allow the detection of UCA in the cerebral microcirculation with little or no bubble destruction as compared with the high-MI imaging (Fig. 44-19). Because of minimal contrast-agent bubble destruction, a high frame rate can be applied, which leads to a better time resolution of bolus kinetics (Fig. 44-20). Low-MI imaging of contrast agent also avoids the shadowing effect, a significant problem associated with high-MI imaging. As previously noted, high-MI imaging destroys microbubbles in brain tissue. Because of the high acoustic intensities that are emitted by bursting bubbles, bubbles that are "behind" the emitting bubbles (further away from the ultrasound transducer) are "shadowed" by

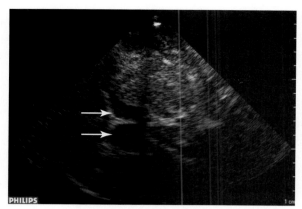

Figure 44-19 Real-time display of brain perfusion with low mechanical index perfusion imaging of the brain on a Philips IU22 platform with the use of a 1- to 5-MHz dynamic pulsed array transducer. The contrast agent is delivered to the capillaries, which are then depicted with contrast-specific ultrasound as a homogeneous contrast enhancement in brain tissue. For anatomic reference, the *arrows* show the well-delineated frontal horns of the lateral ventricles.

this effect and thus obscured from data analysis. Thus, areas of tissue that are shadowed may not be available for analysis of tissue perfusion. The problem of shadowing is basically eliminated with low-MI imaging because bubbles are not destroyed with such low acoustic pressures. Moreover, the technique can obtain multiplanar real-time images of brain perfusion.[329] This is a significant breakthrough for ultrasound perfusion imaging because previous approaches were confined to a single image plane and therefore limited in their assessment of the extents of brain infarction and low perfusion states. The disadvantage of this new low-MI technique, however, is the limited investigation depth due to the low MI used. Successful perfusion imaging of the contralateral hemisphere has not yet been demonstrated with this technique.

Bolus, Destruction, and Refill Kinetics

After UCA bolus injection, time intensity curves (TICs) with contrast wash-in and washout phases can be generated with the use of contrast-specific imaging and can be further analyzed. Different variables of these curves can be extracted (Fig. 44-21), such as the time to peak intensity (TPI), the peak intensity (PI), the mean transit time (MTT), the peak width, full width at 90% of the maximum intensity, full width at half the maximum intensity (FWHM), the area under the curve (AUC), the positive gradient (PG, defined as PI/TPI), and the peak signal increase (PSI). These parameters can then be displayed as parametric images.[330]

Several studies have shown that such variables may be suitable for assessment of the perfusion state, particularly the analysis of local time-intensity curves in prespecified region of interest[331] or the visual interpretation of parametric images.[330,332-335] MRI and PET studies in acute stroke patients have demonstrated the diagnostic value of TPI maps for differentiation between unaffected parenchyma, penumbra, and ischemic core area.[336] Similar

results have been achieved with ultrasound perfusion techniques.

Destruction kinetics involves destruction of contrast agent microbubbles at a constant frame rate with the use of a high MI. After contrast bolus injection, microbubbles are destroyed with a series of high-energy pulses. Local perfusion status is analyzed in selected regions of interest by destruction curves and acoustic intensity differences obtained before and after microbubble destruction.[337,338] There are three mathematical models for analyzing the diminution curve: a linear, a simple exponential, and a complex exponential (contrast burst depletion imaging; CODIM) model.[318,323,338,339] Figure 44-22 provides an example of the use of microbubble destruction imaging (MDI) to assess cerebral perfusion in a patient with a high-grade carotid stenosis.

High-MI ultrasound pulses lead to microbubble destruction within the field of insonation. If a constant concentration of contrast agent is delivered to brain tissue with a constant UCA infusion rate, then after destruction with high-MI ultrasound, new microbubbles will enter this field with a certain velocity, will travel a determined distance, and will fill a certain tissue volume depending on blood velocity. The intensity of the echo response signal is directly related to the contrast agent concentration in the tissue; therefore, the blood flow assessment is based on monitoring the intensity of the echo response signal of the insonated volume after bubble destruction. Low-MI ultrasound imaging can be used to monitor microbubble replenishment in real time (Fig. 44-23) after the application of destruction pulses at high MI. The behavior of the refill kinetics can be assessed with an exponential curve fit.[340] The parameters of this exponential curve are related to cerebral blood flow: blood flow velocity is directly related to the rate constant β, the fractional vascular volume is related to the plateau echo enhancement (A), and the product of both (A × β) is associated with blood flow.[242]

Safety of Ultrasound Perfusion Imaging

The commercially available UCAs Levovist, Optison, and SonoVue have been shown to have contrast-enhancing properties in human brain perfusion imaging. No severe adverse events have been documented in numerous volunteer studies published on brain perfusion analysis using these contrast agents, which have included hundreds of patients.

One study investigated the integrity of the blood–brain barrier (BBB) in humans after bubble destruction of Levovist and Optison with transcranial color-coded sonography.[341] MRI examinations with gadolinium (Gd-MRI) were performed during both early and late phases after insonation. Ultrasound transmission power levels were kept within diagnostic limits and resembled standard settings in brain perfusion studies. Using a triple dose of gadolinium to increase sensitivity and considering the potential time dependence of BBB changes, the authors showed that insonation of Levovist and Optison did not lead to any detectable difference in T1 signal intensities in two defined brain regions in Gd-MRI. Moreover, they found no signs of focal signal enhancement or focal brain damage. In another study on patients with small-vessel

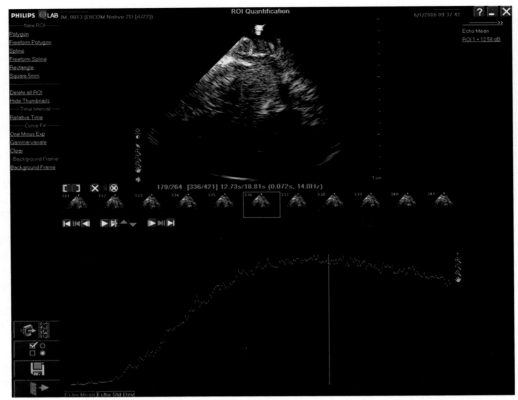

Figure 44-20 Real-time acoustic intensity curve of the contrast agent SonoVue after bolus injection on a Philips IU22 platform with the use of a 1- to 5-MHz dynamic pulsed array transducer. A very low mechanical index of 0.017 is used, which is then attenuated about 90% by the skull bone before entering the brain. A *region of interest* has been drawn in the upper image to determine where mean acoustic intensity will be measured. The *smaller images in the middle* of the figure are the individual image frames at 14 Hz. The *red curve* displays the mean acoustic intensity of contrast bolus arrival from the region of interest for a total of 264 frames during 18.81 seconds.

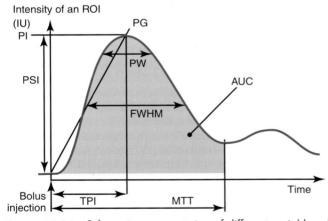

Figure 44-21 Schematic representation of different variables of the time-intensity curve available for perfusion assessment. AUC, Area under the curve; FWHM, full width at half the maximum intensity; IU, intensity units (linear scale); MTT, mean transit time; PG, positive gradient; PI, peak intensity; PSI, peak signal increase; PW, peak width; ROI, region of interest; TPI, time-to-peak intensity.

disease and intact BBB, standard contrast-enhanced ultrasound perfusion imaging did not lead to MRI-detectable BBB changes.[342] These studies provide further evidence of the safety of both UCAs themselves and the exposure levels of current ultrasonic equipment used for transcranial investigations.

Brain Perfusion Imaging in Acute Ischemic Stroke Patients

UCA *bolus kinetics* were analyzed in most perfusion imaging studies in acute ischemic stroke. Different nonlinear imaging modalities (harmonic imaging, PM, and pulse inversion imaging) with high-MI triggering and different contrast agents (Levovist, Optison, and SonoVue) were used.[243,331,333,335,337,343-350] In one study, stroke MRI with diffusion-weighted imaging (DWI) and perfusion maps were used to validate the threshold of PI reduction and TTP delay for the diagnosis of a diffusion or perfusion impairment.[344] The results of this study showed that an area with isolated contrast influx delay in areas without impaired water diffusion could be separated from healthy tissue with parameters of the wash-in kinetics. For a peak signal with more than one third of the amplitude of the healthy tissue and a delay of more than 4 seconds, isolated TTP prolongation without DWI abnormalities could be suspected.

Ultrasound perfusion imaging can be performed as an emergency diagnostic procedure within a few minutes before starting thrombolytic therapy.[351] Beside contrast bolus kinetics, *diminution kinetics* after bolus injection of SonoVue was evaluated in the early phase of ischemic stroke (<24 hours) and compared with perfusion MRI.[337] This study showed the diagnostic potential of this fast imaging technique to obtain information on regions of reduced perfusion in the early phase of ischemic stroke.

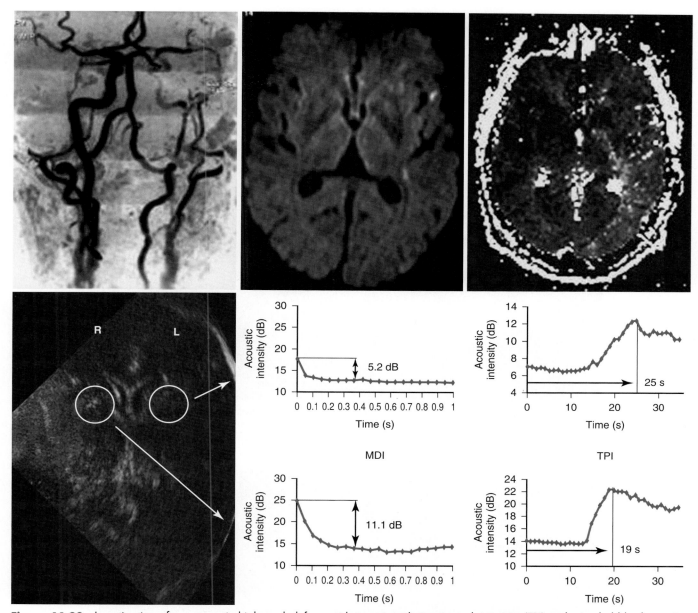

Figure 44-22 Investigation of symptomatic high-grade left carotid stenosis with time-to-peak intensity (TPI) and microbubble destruction imaging (MDI) using SonoVue. The *upper magnetic resonance (MR) images* demonstrate the high-grade stenosis with MR angiography *(left)*, left hemispheric diffusion-weighted image (DWI) lesions *(middle)*, and perfusion deficit in left hemisphere with perfusion-weighted imaging *(right)*. For TPI, triggered imaging was used (frame rate 1 Hz) to measure time to maximum acoustic intensity. For destruction imaging, repetitive sequences of high-energy pulses at high frame rate (14 Hz) resulting in complete microbubble destruction were applied. Analysis of TPI and MDI were undertaken in both hemispheres in the territory of the middle cerebral arteries *(circles)*. Note both prolonged TPI and decreased destruction intensities in left hemisphere.

Because individual microbubbles can now be depicted flowing through small vessels in the brain with low-MI imaging, it is possible to track these bubbles and map perfusion over time. Dynamic microvascular microbubble maps provide excellent demarcation of MCA infarctions (Fig. 44-24) and provide impressive displays of low-velocity tissue microbubble refill after destruction with high-MI imaging.[342] In brain regions showing delayed contrast bolus arrival on perfusion-weighted MRI, ultrasound shows decreased or absent microbubble refill kinetics.

Stroke Therapy with Ultrasound

Sonothrombolysis

Mounting evidence from in vitro experiments and animal studies indicates that application of ultrasound as an adjunct to thrombolytic therapy offers a promising approach for improving recanalization of occluded intracerebral vessels. Ultrasound together with microbubbles can further enhance the adjunct effect of sonothrombolysis and may even be applied as a new approach for clot

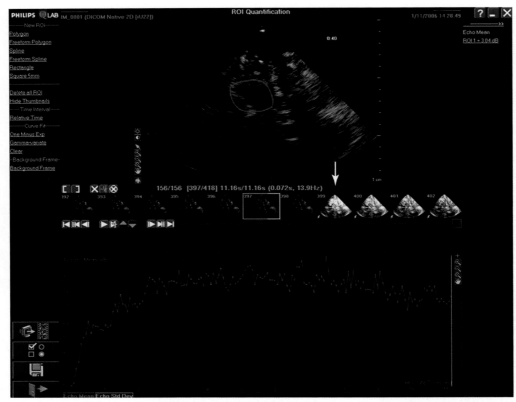

Figure 44-23 Real-time acoustic intensity curve of the contrast agent SonoVue demonstrating refill after bubble destruction with transient high mechanical index imaging. Mean acoustic intensity is measured in the *region of interest* in the upper image. The *smaller images in the middle of the figure* are the individual image frames at 14 Hz. The *arrow* shows the first of a series of high mechanical index images for microbubble destruction.

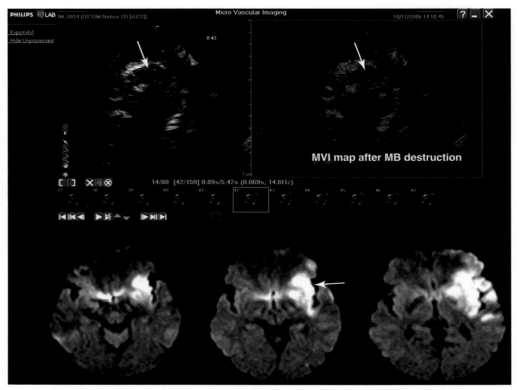

Figure 44-24 Microvascular map of left MCA infarction *(arrows)* characterized by absent or diminished contrast agent. The excellent infarction demarcation compares well with MRI diffusion-weighted imaging *(bottom images)*. MB, Microbubble; MCA, middle cerebral artery; MRI, magnetic resonance imaging; MVI, microvascular imaging.

lysis without thrombolytic drugs.[352] Further possibilities are specific targeting of thrombus with microbubbles, as well as local drug delivery with ultrasound-sensitive liposomes.

Ultrasound-Enhanced t-PA Thrombolysis

The potential for high-frequency ultrasound to dissolve intraarterial thrombi was first reported by Sobbe et al in 1974.[353] In these experiments, a 26.5-kHz ultrasound transducer was used to recanalize thrombosed iliofemoral arteries in dogs with minimal complications. Further studies using catheter-based or transcutaneous ultrasound focused on the ability of ultrasound to enhance the effect of fibrinolytic agents in recanalizing acutely thrombosed arteries.[354-360]

In vitro studies have shown various levels of thrombolytic improvement averaging 30% to 40% and have required 1 to 3 hours of insonation to achieve the effect.[361] Frequencies from 20 kHz to 2 MHz have provided thrombolytic activity, and lower frequencies have penetrated the skull more efficiently than higher frequencies. Several animal studies also show positive results in various vascular beds, including coronary arteries. Living animal systems are much more complex and can show the effect of the animal's endogenous t-PA in ischemia. This can produce positive effects with very small amounts of ultrasound. Intensity levels of 0.6 W/cm^2 to 2.0 W/cm^2 have proven therapeutic without evidence of safety issues.[362]

Clinical Studies of Ultrasound-Enhanced Thrombolysis

The Combined Lysis of Thrombus in Brain Ischemia Using Transcranial Ultrasound and Systemic tPA (CLOTBUST) study[363] was a multicenter randomized clinical trial of 126 patients who had acute ischemic stroke due to occlusion of the MCA. All patients were treated with intravenous t-PA within 3 hours after the onset of symptoms. Target patients received 2-MHz, PW transcranial Doppler monitoring for a duration of 2 hours, as well as t-PA. A complete reperfusion or dramatic clinical recovery was observed in 49% of the patients in the target group (t-PA + US) and in only 30% of the control group. No secondary effects linked with ultrasound exposure were identified. Similar findings were found in a pilot study showing a higher grade of recanalization after 1 hour with ultrasound combined with t-PA.[364]

Some have questioned the therapeutic efficacy of commercial TCD devices for treatment of ischemic stroke because of the high attenuation of ultrasound by temporal bone.[365] Experimental studies[366] were not conclusive when they attempted to show that such low acoustic pressures through the human skull are unable to produce a thrombolytic effect, but recent simulations of the CLOTBUST study confirm that acoustic pressures were operative, which are lower than literature values reported as effective for ultrasound thrombolysis.[367] However, as noted above, it is likely that very low acoustic pressures can have biological effects in vivo, perhaps through acceleration of clot lysis with endogenous t-PA.

The Transcranial Low-Frequency Ultrasound-Mediated Thrombolysis in Brain Ischemia (TRUMBI) trial was stopped prematurely because of the occurrence of a higher number of intracerebral hemorrhages after t-PA treatment combined with transcranial sonication at 300 kHz.[368] Unlike the CLOTBUST study, rigorous MRI monitoring was performed in all patients and not just in those in whom control imaging after thrombolysis was warranted clinically. This led to detection of MRI evidence of hemorrhage in 93% of the target patients and in 42% of the control patients in TRUMBI. Among these hemorrhages, all were classified as hemorrhagic transformation in the t-PA–only group versus 61% in the t-PA plus ultrasound group. Five hemorrhages in the target group were symptomatic hemorrhages, possibly linked to ultrasound exposure.

The reason for hemorrhages in the TRUMBI trial is unclear. Indeed, experimental animal work in rats[369] was unable to demonstrate harmful secondary effects of ultrasound with the use of the TRUMBI variables. One study suggested that hemorrhages in TRUMBI were related to abnormal permeability of the human BBB that was induced by wide-field low-frequency insonation.[370] Wang et al hypothesize that, in TRUMBI, a pulse length of 765 mm combined with a very wide beam can cause overlap many times as the wave runs its course back and forth across the brain, reflecting off the skull. Therefore, the instantaneous intensity of ultrasound in the brain tissue may multiply constructively at some localized sites of brain tissue, resulting in MIs that are larger than the maximum limit set by the US Food and Drug Administration (FDA).[371] However, a recent simulation demonstrated that acoustic pressures in TRUMBI were indeed only slightly above the inertial cavitation threshold.[367] Nevertheless, standing waves were postulated, which resolved after small alterations of the ultrasound variables. These results suggest that fine tuning of sonothrombolysis variables with sophisticated simulation software could help to improve the safety of this promising adjunct therapy.

Microbubble-Enhanced Thrombolysis with t-PA

Numerous studies have shown significant amplification of lysis with the addition of microbubbles to the combination of thrombolytic drugs and ultrasound.[372-376] Although the therapeutic mechanism is not fully understood, it probably involves both stable and inertial cavitation modes. The microbubble lowers the threshold for thrombolysis by providing a preexisting bubble that can easily be made to cavitate by ultrasound. Stable cavitation can produce microstreaming in the area and dramatically enlarge the bubble momentarily. This will cause localized mechanical stress on adjacent clots. The surface of the clot will erode, and penetration and numerous microscopic holes inside the clot have even been demonstrated.[377] Microstreaming also leads to a dramatic increase in delivery of thrombolytic drug to the clot.[378] More energy delivered to the microbubble can lead to inertial cavitation, which ends with violent disruption of the bubble. This can produce microjets that are also effective in eroding clots.[379] However, recent data suggest that stable cavitation is more effective than inertial cavitation in clot lysis.[380] Pressure waves interact with bubbles, which causes expansion and contraction. This can lead to "pumping" of energy from the traveling wave, "focusing" and reemitting it locally, sometimes at other, perhaps better frequencies.

Improved clinical thrombolysis with microbubbles in combination with ultrasound and thrombolytic drugs shows great promise, but the optimal techniques, indications, and contraindications have not yet been well-defined. Moreover, optimal microbubble dosage, delivery, required thrombolytic drug dosage, and optimal ultrasound characteristics all remain uncertain.[372-376] Microbubbles that have been used for thrombolysis include lipid, albumin, or galactose spheres ranging in size from 0.5 micron to about 5 microns surrounding a gas or air bubble. Commercially available Definity and Optison are FDA approved in the United States for endocardial border imaging, and Levovist and SonoVue are available in Europe. However, none are approved for thrombolysis.

Clinical Studies of Microbubble-Enhanced Thrombolysis

The first clinical use of microbubbles in acute stroke was performed with Levovist added to standard t-PA therapy augmented with continuous TCD.[381] Outcomes were improved to a 55% sustained recanalization rate compared with 41% with the use of t-PA and continuous TCD and 24% with t-PA alone. Clinical improvement was improved by more than 4 points on the National Institutes of Health Stroke Scale in 55% compared with 41% with t-PA and continuous TCD and 31% with t-PA alone. No increased symptomatic intracranial hemorrhage was encountered. Further pilot studies have likewise provided evidence for enhancement of thrombolysis with ultrasound and microbubbles in MCA stroke[382] and basilar artery occlusion.[383]

Clot Lysis with Ultrasound and Microbubbles without Thrombolytic Drugs

In vitro and in vivo thrombolysis without thrombolytic drugs has been readily accomplished with microbubbles and ultrasound.[374,375,380,384-389] In vitro examples show a predominately mechanical effect of the bubble encountering the clot and eroding it when activated by ultrasound.[374,380,384] In vivo examples are more complex, in that interactions include endothelial factors triggered by local ischemia, as well as an endogeneous t-PA effect originating from the ischemic vessel wall.[375,385-389]

Early success of microbubble thrombolysis without a thrombolytic drug was shown by Birnbaum et al in 1998 using a rabbit iliac artery model and a small amount of clot.[375] Later evidence included two studies of thrombosed canine dialysis grafts using two types of albumin microbubbles by Culp.[385,386] Investigations in the rete mirabilis of pigs showed that it was possible to deliver adequate ultrasound to the center of a human scale head and still achieve the therapeutic effect of ultrasound augmentation of lysis when only microbubbles were used as a thrombolytic agent.[387] A subsequent study[388] used albumin microbubbles tagged with the GPIIb/IIIa inhibitor, eptifibatide, to promote accumulation of the bubbles at the clot with enhanced sonothrombolysis. In another investigation microbubbles targeted to human platelets (immunobubbles) were developed with the use of abciximab, an antibody fragment specific for the GPIIb/IIIa receptor expressed by activated platelets. The immunobubbles were shown to improve visualization of human clots both in vitro and in an in vivo model of acute arterial thrombotic occlusion, thus demonstrating the feasibility of using a therapeutic agent for selective targeting in vascular imaging.[390] Recently, a specific advantage of targeted abciximab immunobubbles for enhancing sonothrombolysis has been demonstrated.[391]

Only a few reports have addressed safety issues of treatment with ultrasound and microbubbles in animal models. The results have consistently documented a lack of detrimental features in both ischemic[392] and hemorrhagic models.[393]

Emerging Applications

Molecular Imaging

Molecular imaging can be defined as the characterization and measurement of biological processes at the cellular and molecular level by means of remote imaging detectors. Goals of molecular imaging include noninvasive detection of disease with the use of disease-associated molecular signatures, in vivo delineation of complex molecular mechanisms of disease, and detection of gene expression. Targeted ultrasound techniques combine ultrasound imaging technology with specific contrast agents for the assessment of molecular or genetic signatures of disease. Because of the high echogenicity of UCAs in comparison with tissue or plasma, the echo from a single microbubble can be detected with ultrasonographic imaging techniques. This means that the system is sensitive to a volume on the order of 0.004 picoliters,[394] thus offering a high level of resolution.

Addition of targeted ligands to microbubbles opens new avenues for the identification of vascular occlusion or areas of vascular injury. Adhesion molecules such as the integrin $\alpha_v\beta_3$, intercellular adhesion molecule-1 (ICAM-1), and fibrinogen receptor GPIIb/IIIa are overexpressed in regions of angiogenesis, inflammation, and thrombus, respectively. These molecular signatures can be used to localize UCAs through the use of complementary receptor ligands. This approach has been demonstrated for imaging of angiogenesis with the use of microbubbles targeted to α_v-integrins.[395] Likewise, lipid-based perfluorobutane-filled microbubbles have been synthesized with various densities of anti–ICAM-1 monoclonal antibodies conjugated to the bubble shell to investigate early stages of atherosclerosis.[396] Targeted microbubbles directed to the GPIIb/IIIa receptor of activated platelets have also been developed for visualization of thrombus,[390,397,398] and leukocyte-targeted microbubbles can be used to characterize the severity of postischemic myocardial inflammation[399] and to identify inflamed plaques.[400]

Contrast ultrasound perfusion imaging and molecular imaging with microbubbles targeted to activated neutrophils, α_5-integrins, or vascular cell adhesion molecule (VCAM-1) have been performed in murine models of vasculogenesis and hind-limb ischemia produced by arterial occlusion in wild-type or monocyte chemotactic protein-1-deficient mice.[401] On targeted imaging, signal enhancement from α_5-integrins and VCAM-1 coincided with the earliest appearance of regional blood flow. Targeted imaging demonstrated early signal enhancement for neutrophils, monocyte α_5-integrin, and VCAM-1 at day 2 when blood flow was very low.[401] Thus, different components of the inflammatory response that participate in vascular development and remodeling can be assessed separately with ultrasound molecular imaging.

Recent data show that noninvasive ultrasound molecular imaging of endothelial activation can detect the lesion-prone vascular phenotype before the appearance of obstructive atherosclerotic lesions.[402] This approach was demonstrated in mice deficient for the low-density lipoprotein receptor and the Apobec-1 editing peptide (DKO mice) as an age-dependent model of atherosclerosis. Ultrasound molecular imaging of the proximal thoracic aorta with contrast agents targeted to P-selectin and VCAM-1 showed selective signal enhancement for DKO mice, while en face microscopy demonstrated preferential attachment of targeted microbubbles to regions of lesion formation.

Ultrasound molecular imaging can detect important intravascular events that participate in cardiovascular and cerebrovascular diseases including inflammatory responses, angiogenesis, and thrombus formation. The potential clinical role of this technology will be contingent on further refinement of targeted microbubble chemistry and studies that indicate that the unique diagnostic information from molecular imaging can positively affect patient care.[403]

Opening the Blood–Brain Barrier

The BBB is a significant obstacle for delivery of both small molecules and macromolecular agents. Indeed, potential therapeutic substances, which cannot be applied in the presence of an intact BBB, are neuropeptides, proteins, and chemotherapeutic agents. Likewise, large molecules such as monoclonal antibodies, recombinant proteins, antisense, or gene therapeutics do not cross the BBB.

There is a good deal of evidence showing that ultrasound can be used to permeate blood–tissue barriers. Large molecules and genes can cross the plasma membrane of cultured cells after application of acoustic energy.[404] Indeed, electron microscopy has revealed ultrasound-induced membrane porosity in both in vitro and in vivo experiments.[405] High-intensity focused ultrasound has been shown to allow selective and nondestructive disruption of the BBB in rats.[406] If microbubbles are introduced to the blood stream before focused ultrasound exposure, the BBB can be transiently opened at the ultrasound focus without acute neuronal damage.[407] Thus, the introduction of cavitation nuclei into the blood stream can confine the ultrasound effects to the vasculature and reduce the intensity needed to produce BBB opening. This can diminish the risk of tissue damage and make the technique more easily applied through the intact skull. In most studies, the confirmation of BBB disruption has been obtained with MR contrast imaging at targeted locations[407-409] or with postmortem histologic examination.[406,410]

Targeted delivery of antibodies to the brain has been accomplished with focused ultrasound. Dopamine D_4 receptor–targeting antibody was injected intravenously and shown to recognize antigen in the murine brain after disruption of the BBB with ultrasound.[408] Likewise, doxorubicin, a chemotherapeutic drug that does not cross the BBB, has been administered to the brain with the use of ultrasound and microbubbles.[411] Different levels of doxorubicin in the brain were achieved through alteration of the microbubble concentration. These results are encouraging and provide an important framework for future studies aimed at local disruption of the BBB for delivery of macromolecular agents to the brain.

Several avenues of transcapillary passage after ultrasound sonication have been identified. These included transcytosis, passage through endothelial cell cytoplasmic openings, opening of tight junctions, and free passage through injured endothelium.[412] One study investigated the integrity of the tight junctions (TJs) in rat brain microvessels after BBB disruption by ultrasound bursts (1.5-MHz) in combination with Optison.[413] BBB disruption, as evidenced by leakage of intravenously administered horseradish peroxidise (HRP) and lanthanum chloride, was paralleled by the apparent disintegration of the TJ complexes and the redistribution and loss of the immunosignals for occludin, claudin-5, and ZO-1. At 6 and 24 hours after sonication, no HRP or lanthanum leakage was observed, and the barrier function of the TJs, as indicated by the localization and density of immunosignals, appeared to be completely restored. The results of these studies demonstrate that the effect of ultrasound on TJs is very transient, lasting less than 4 hours.

Although much effort has been undertaken to demonstrate the safety of BBB opening with ultrasound and microbubbles, further work is needed to elucidate the molecular effects of this application. Recent data demonstrate that at the upper thresholds of acoustic pressure for safe BBB opening a reorganization of gap-junctional plaques in both neurons and astrocytes may occur.[414] This is important because gap junctions allow transfer of information between adjacent cells and are responsible for tissue homeostasis. Likewise, there is evidence that focused ultrasound-induced opening of the BBB in the presence of UCAs can lead to increased ubiquitinylation of proteins in neuronal cells,[415] which indicates that brain molecular stress pathways are affected by this treatment.

Ultrasound-Enhanced Gene Therapy

Ultrasound may be a valuable tool in gene therapy by virtue of its ability to enhance transgene expression through a process termed *sonoporation*. Simple exposure to ultrasound has been shown to enhance transgene expression in vascular cells by up to tenfold after naked DNA transfection. Likewise, transfection studies performed with the use of marker genes that do not exert a fluorescent protein demonstrated that ultrasound consistently increased gene expression in cell lines such as HeLa, NIH t-3, and COS-1 cells.[416] The enhancement of transfection occurred at levels of ultrasound of about 0.5 W/cm² and a duration of exposure of only about 15 seconds and did not appreciably heat the cells or adversely affect their survival. Similar results on the effect of ultrasound on gene expression have been obtained in cell cultures during liposomal transfection experiments.[417] Cultured neuronal cell types that are effectively sonoporated include chick retinal neurons, chick dorsal forebrain, chick optic tectum, PC12 cells, rat cerebellar neurons, and mouse hippocampal neurons. Depending on the type of cell and conditions of sonoporation, the transfection efficacy has been as high as 20%.[418] In the presence of microbubbles, a synergistic effect for sonoporation is attained, and cavitation is a likely mechanism. This new technology holds the promise of delivering genes more selectively than other methods and less invasively than direct injection.

The capacity of ultrasound-targeted microbubble destruction to deliver angiogenic genes, improve perfusion, and recruit progenitor cells after a myocardial infarction in mice was recently evaluated.[419] The physiologic impact of VEGF and SCF gene delivery was confirmed by increased myocardial recruitment of VEGF receptor 2– and SCF receptor–expressing cells. Consequently, capillary and arteriolar density (factor VIII and alpha-smooth muscle actin staining), myocardial perfusion, and cardiac function were all enhanced in recipients of VEGF or SCF. These results proved promising opportunities for influencing angiogenesis and recruiting progenitor cells after cerebral infarction.

Targeted Drug Delivery with Ultrasound

Microbubbles not only are used to enhance the effects of ultrasound on gene expression but also may be employed as carriers of gene therapeutic agents.[416,420] There are a number of ways to entrap different drugs with microbubbles. One technique is to incorporate them into the membrane- or wall-forming materials that stabilize microbubbles. Charged drugs can be stabilized in or onto the surfaces of microbubbles by virtue of electrostatic interactions. In this way, cationic lipid-coated microbubbles can bind DNA, which is a polyanion and binds avidly to cationic (positively charged) microbubbles. Drugs can also be incorporated into the interior of microbubbles (gas-filled microspheres). Another way to entrap drugs in microbubbles is to create a layer of oil (e.g., triacetin) to stabilize the outer surface of the bubble. Hydrophobic drugs can then be incorporated into the oil layer. Regardless of the technique used to incorporate the drugs, they are released when ultrasound energy cavitates the microbubble. These methods for making drug-carrying microbubbles are most applicable to drugs that are highly active. This is the case for gene-based drugs, in which the amount of gene injected is usually on the order of micrograms or milligrams. Therefore, large volumes of bubbles are not required to deliver highly active drugs such as gene-based ones.

A number of studies have shown that entrapment of t-PA into liposomes provides a selective targeting so that the efficacy of fibrinolytic agents is improved.[421-425] Moreover, ultrasound may be used to target liposomal drug delivery. Mechanisms of enhancement include acoustic cavitational effects and acoustic radiation force.[426] Novel developments include the combination of nanotechnology with microbubbles for drug delivery, which may have implications for thrombolysis.[427,428]

Combined ultrasound-sensitive thrombolytic drug delivery combined with specific targeting is highly attractive. Targeting of clot-dissolving therapeutics has the potential to decrease the frequency of complications while simultaneously increasing treatment effectiveness. This is achieved by concentrating the available drug at the desired site and permitting a lower systemic dose. A fibrin-specific, liquid perfluorocarbon nanoparticle that is surface modified to deliver the plasminogen activator streptokinase has been developed and shows such characteristics.[429] Effective concentrations of targeted streptokinase were orders of magnitude lower than equivalently efficacious levels of free drug. As little as 1% surface targeting of streptokinase nanoparticles produced significant decreases in clot volumes in 1 hour.[429]

REFERENCES

1. Merritt CR: Doppler color flow imaging, *J Clin Ultrasound* 15:591–597, 1987.
2. Middleton WD, Foley WD, Lawson TL: Color-flow Doppler imaging of carotid artery abnormalities, *Am J Roentgenol* 150:419–425, 1988.
3. Steinke W, Kloetzsch C, Hennerici M: Carotid artery disease assessed by color Doppler flow imaging: Correlation with standard Doppler sonography and angiography, *AJNR Am J Neuroradiol* 11:259–266, 1990.
4. Jespersen SK, Wilhjelm JE, Sillesen H: In vitro spatial compound scanning for improved visualization of atherosclerosis, *Ultrasound Med Biol* 26:1357–1362, 2000.
5. Kofoed SC, Gronholdt ML, Wilhjelm JE, et al: Real-time spatial compound imaging improves reproducibility in the evaluation of atherosclerotic carotid plaques, *Ultrasound Med Biol* 27:1311–1317, 2001.
6. Meairs S, Timpe L, Beyer J, et al: Acute aphasia and hemiplegia during karate training, *Lancet* 356:40, 2000.
7. Detmer PR, Baschein G, Hodges TC, et al: 3D ultrasonic image feature localization based on magnetic scanhead tracking: In vitro calibration and validation, *Ultrasound Med Biol* 20:923–936, 1994.
8. Hodges TC, Detmer PR, Burns DH, et al: Ultrasonic three-dimensional reconstruction: In vitro and in vivo volume and area measurement, *Ultrasound Med Biol* 20:719–729, 1994.
9. Leotta DF, Detmer PR, Martin RW: Performance of a miniature magnetic position sensor for three-dimensional ultrasound imaging, *Ultrasound Med Biol* 23:597–609, 1997.
10. Barry CD, Allott CP, John NW, et al: Three-dimensional freehand ultrasound: Image reconstruction and volume analysis, *Ultrasound Med Biol* 23:1209–1224, 1997.
11. Meairs S, Beyer J, Hennerici M: Reconstruction and visualization of irregularly sampled three- and four-dimensional ultrasound data for cerebrovascular applications, *Ultrasound Med Biol* 26:263–272, 2000.
12. Pignoli P, Tremoli E, Poli A, et al: Intimal plus medial thickness of the arterial wall: A direct measurement with ultrasound imaging, *Circulation* 74:1399–1406, 1986.
13. Wong M, Edelstein J, Wollman J, et al: Ultrasonic-pathological comparison of the human arterial wall. Verification of intima-media thickness, *Arterioscler Thromb* 13:482–486, 1993.
14. Riley WA, Barnes RW, Applegate WB, et al: Reproducibility of non-invasive ultrasonic measurement of carotid atherosclerosis. The Asymptomatic Carotid Artery Plaque Study, *Stroke* 23:1062–1068, 1992.
15. Zanchetti A, Bond MG, Hennig M, et al: Calcium antagonist lacidipine slows down progression of asymptomatic carotid atherosclerosis: Principal results of the European Lacidipine Study on Atherosclerosis (ELSA), a randomized, double-blind, long-term trial, *Circulation* 106:2422–2427, 2002.
16. Folsom AR, Eckfeldt JH, Weitzman S, et al: Relation of carotid artery wall thickness to diabetes mellitus, fasting glucose and insulin, body size, and physical activity. Atherosclerosis Risk in Communities (ARIC) Study Investigators, *Stroke* 25:66–73, 1994.
17. Furberg CD, Borhani NO, Byington RP, et al: Calcium antagonists and atherosclerosis. The Multicenter Isradipine/Diuretic Atherosclerosis Study, *Am J Hypertens* 6:24S–29S, 1993.

18. Crouse JR: Sources of arterial wall thickness measurement variability. In Touboul PJ, editor: *Intima media thickness and atherosclerosis: Predicting the risk?* New York, 1997, Parthenon, pp 59–68.

19. Baldassarre D, Werba JP, Tremoli E, et al: Common carotid intima-media thickness measurement. A method to improve accuracy and precision, *Stroke* 25:1588–1592, 1994.

20. Chambless LE, Heiss G, Folsom AR, et al: Association of coronary heart disease incidence with carotid arterial wall thickness and major risk factors: The Atherosclerosis Risk in Communities (ARIC) Study, 1987-1993, *Am J Epidemiol* 146:483–494, 1997.

21. O'Leary DH, Polak JF, Kronmal RA, et al: Carotid-artery intima and media thickness as a risk factor for myocardial infarction and stroke in older adults. Cardiovascular Health Study Collaborative Research Group, *N Engl J Med* 340:14–22, 1999.

22. Chambless LE, Folsom AR, Clegg LX, et al: Carotid wall thickness is predictive of incident clinical stroke: The Atherosclerosis Risk in Communities (ARIC) study, *Am J Epidemiol* 151:478–487, 2000.

23. Lorenz MW, von Kegler S, Steinmetz H, et al: Carotid intima-media thickening indicates a higher vascular risk across a wide age range: Prospective data from the Carotid Atherosclerosis Progression Study (CAPS), *Stroke* 37:87–92, 2006.

24. Salonen JT, Salonen R: Ultrasound B-mode imaging in observational studies of atherosclerotic progression, *Circulation* 87:II56–II65, 1993.

25. Kitamura A, Iso H, Imano H, et al: Carotid intima-media thickness and plaque characteristics as a risk factor for stroke in Japanese elderly men, *Stroke* 35:2788–2794, 2004.

26. Rosvall M, Janzon L, Berglund G, et al: Incident coronary events and case fatality in relation to common carotid intima-media thickness, *J Intern Med* 257:430–437, 2005.

27. van der Meer IM, Bots ML, Hofman A, et al: Predictive value of noninvasive measures of atherosclerosis for incident myocardial infarction: The Rotterdam Study, *Circulation* 109:1089–1094, 2004.

28. Lorenz MW, Markus HS, Bots ML, et al: Prediction of clinical cardiovascular events with carotid intima-media thickness: a systematic review and meta-analysis, *Circulation* 115:459–467, 2007.

29. Belcaro G, Nicolaides AN, Ramaswami G, et al: Carotid and femoral ultrasound morphology screening and cardiovascular events in low risk subjects: A 10-year follow-up study (the CAFES-CAVE study 1), *Atherosclerosis* 156:379–387, 2001.

30. Hunt KJ, Evans GW, Folsom AR, et al: Acoustic shadowing on B-mode ultrasound of the carotid artery predicts ischemic stroke: the Atherosclerosis Risk in Communities (ARIC) study, *Stroke* 32:1120–1126, 2001.

31. Prabhakaran S, Rundek T, Ramas R, et al: Carotid plaque surface irregularity predicts ischemic stroke: The northern Manhattan study, *Stroke* 37:2696–2701, 2006.

32. Prabhakaran S, Singh R, Zhou X, et al: Presence of calcified carotid plaque predicts vascular events: The Northern Manhattan Study, *Atherosclerosis* 195:e197–e201, 2007.

33. Spence JD, Eliasziw M, DiCicco M, et al: Carotid plaque area: A tool for targeting and evaluating vascular preventive therapy, *Stroke* 33:2916–2922, 2002.

34. Stork S, van den Beld AW, von Schacky C, et al: Carotid artery plaque burden, stiffness, and mortality risk in elderly men: A prospective, population-based cohort study, *Circulation* 110:344–348, 2004.

35. Wyman RA, Mays ME, McBride PE, et al: Ultrasound-detected carotid plaque as a predictor of cardiovascular events, *Vasc Med* 11:123–130, 2006.

36. Roman MJ, Naqvi TZ, Gardin JM, et al: Clinical application of noninvasive vascular ultrasound in cardiovascular risk stratification: A report from the American Society of Echocardiography and the Society of Vascular Medicine and Biology, *J Am Soc Echocardiogr* 19:943–954, 2006.

37. Touboul PJ, Hennerici MG, Meairs S, et al: Mannheim intima-media thickness consensus, *Cerebrovasc Dis* 18:346–349, 2004.

38. Touboul PJ, Hennerici MG, Meairs S, et al: Mannheim carotid intima-media thickness consensus (2004-2006). An update on behalf of the Advisory Board of the 3rd and 4th Watching the Risk Symposium, 13th and 15th European Stroke Conferences, Mannheim, Germany, 2004, and Brussels, Belgium, 2006, *Cerebrovasc Dis* 23:75–80, 2007.

39. Stein JH, Korcarz CE, Hurst RT, et al: Use of carotid ultrasound to identify subclinical vascular disease and evaluate cardiovascular disease risk: a consensus statement from the American Society of Echocardiography Carotid Intima-Media Thickness Task Force. Endorsed by the Society for Vascular Medicine, *J Am Soc Echocardiogr* 21:93–111, 2008.

40. Celermajer DS, Sorensen KE, Gooch VM, et al: Non-invasive detection of endothelial dysfunction in children and adults at risk of atherosclerosis, *Lancet* 340:1111–1115, 1992.

41. Corretti MC, Plotnick GD, Vogel RA: Technical aspects of evaluating brachial artery vasodilatation using high-frequency ultrasound, *Am J Physiol* 268:H1397–H1404, 1995.

42. Uehata A, Lieberman EH, Gerhard MD, et al: Noninvasive assessment of endothelium-dependent flow-mediated dilation of the brachial artery, *Vasc Med* 2:87–92, 1997.

43. Corretti MC, Anderson TJ, Benjamin EJ, et al: Guidelines for the ultrasound assessment of endothelial-dependent flow-mediated vasodilation of the brachial artery: A report of the International Brachial Artery Reactivity Task Force, *J Am Coll Cardiol* 39:257–265, 2002.

44. Corretti MC, Plotnick GD, Vogel RA: Correlation of cold pressor and flow-mediated brachial artery diameter responses with the presence of coronary artery disease, *Am J Cardiol* 75:783–787, 1995.

45. Neunteufl T, Katzenschlager R, Hassan A, et al: Systemic endothelial dysfunction is related to the extent and severity of coronary artery disease, *Atherosclerosis* 129:111–118, 1997.

46. Arcaro G, Zenere BM, Travia D, et al: Non-invasive detection of early endothelial dysfunction in hypercholesterolaemic subjects, *Atherosclerosis* 114:247–254, 1995.

47. Celermajer DS, Sorensen KE, Georgakopoulos D, et al: Cigarette smoking is associated with dose-related and potentially reversible impairment of endothelium-dependent dilation in healthy young adults, *Circulation* 88:2149–2155, 1993.

48. Celermajer DS, Adams MR, Clarkson P, et al: Passive smoking and impaired endothelium-dependent arterial dilatation in healthy young adults, *N Engl J Med* 334:150–154, 1996.

49. Thomas GN, Chook P, Yip TW, et al: Smoking without exception adversely affects vascular structure and function in apparently healthy Chinese: Implications in global atherosclerosis prevention, *Int J Cardiol* 128:172–177, 2008.

50. Woo KS, Chook P, Yu CW, et al: Overweight in children is associated with arterial endothelial dysfunction and intima-media thickening, *Int J Obes Relat Metab Disord* 28:852–857, 2004.

51. Maroon JC, Pieroni DW, Campbell RL: Ophthalmosonometry: An ultrasonic method for assessing carotid blood flow, *J Neurosurg* 30:238–246, 1969.

52. Melis-Kisman E, Mol JMF: L'application de l'effet Doppler à l'exploration cérébrovasculaire - Rapport préliminaire, *Rev Neurol (Paris)* 122:470–472, 1970.

53. Müller HR: Direktionelle Dopplersonographie der A. frontalis medialis, *EEG EMG Z Elektroenzephalogr Elektromyogr Verwandte Geb* 2:816–823, 1971.

54. LoGerfo FW, Mason GR: Directional Doppler studies of supraorbital artery flow in internal carotid stenosis and occlusion, *Surgery* 76:723–728, 1974.

55. Büdingen HJ, von Reutern GM: *Ultraschalldiagnostik der hirnversorgenden arterien*, Stuttgart, 1994, Thieme.

56. Hennerici M, Neuerburg-Heusler D: *Vascular diagnosis with ultrasound*, Stuttgart - New York, 1998, Thieme.

57. Meairs S, Hennerici M: Long-term follow-up of aneurysms developed during extracranial internal carotid artery dissection, *Neurology* 54:2190, 2000.

58. De Bray JM, Glatt B: Quantification of atheromatous stenosis in the extracranial internal carotid artery, *Cerebrovasc Dis* 5:414–426, 1995.

59. Levine SR, Welch KM: Common carotid artery occlusion, *Neurology* 39:178–186, 1989.

60. Zbornikova V, Lassvik C: Common carotid artery occlusion: Haemodynamic features, *Cerebrovasc Dis* 1:136–141, 1991.

61. Belkin M, Mackey WC, Pessin MS, et al: Common carotid artery occlusion with patent internal and external carotid arteries: Diagnosis and surgical management, *J Vasc Surg* 17:1019–1028, 1993.

62. Dashefsky SM, Cooperberg PL, Harrison PB, et al: Total occlusion of the common carotid artery with patent internal carotid artery. Identification with color flow Doppler imaging, *J Ultrasound Med* 10:417–421, 1991.

63. Riles TS, Imparato AM, Posner MP, et al: Common carotid occlusion, *Ann Surg* 199:363-366, 1984.
64. Steinke W, Rautenberg W, Sliwka U, et al: Common carotid artery occlusion: Clinical significance of a patent internal carotid artery, *Neurol Sci* 20:140, 1993.
65. Robinson ML, Sacks D, Perlmutter GS, et al: Diagnostic criteria for carotid duplex sonography, *AJR Am J Roentgenol* 151:1045-1049, 1988.
66. Taylor DC, Strandness DE Jr: Carotid artery duplex scanning, *J Clin Ultrasound* 15:635-644, 1987.
67. Zwiebel WJ, Knighton R: Duplex examination of the carotid arteries, *Semin Ultrasound CT MRI* 11:97-135, 1990.
68. Comerota AJ, Cranley A, Cook S: Real-time B-mode imaging in diagnosis of cerebrovascular disease, *Surgery* 89:718-729, 1981.
69. Ricotta JJ, Bryan FA, Bond MG, et al: Multicenter validation study of real-time (B-mode) ultrasound, arteriography, and pathologic examination, *J Vasc Surg* 6:512-520, 1987.
70. Zwiebel WJ, Austin CW, Sackett JF, et al: Correlation of high-resolution, B-mode and continuous-wave Doppler sonography with arteriography in the diagnosis of carotid stenosis, *Radiology* 149:523-532, 1983.
71. Sliwka U, Rother J, Steinke W, et al: [The value of duplex sonography in cerebral ischemia] Die bedeutung der duplexsonographie bei zerebralen ischamien, *Bildgebung* 58:182-191, 1991.
72. Erickson SJ, Mewissen MW, Foley WD, et al: Stenosis of the internal carotid artery: Assessment using color Doppler imaging compared with angiography, *AJR Am J Roentgenol* 152:1299-1305, 1989.
73. Middleton WD, Foley WD, Lawson TL: Flow reversal in the normal carotid bifurcation: Color Doppler flow imaging analysis, *Radiology* 167:207-210, 1988.
74. Steinke W, Kloetzsch C, Hennerici M: Variability of flow patterns in the normal carotid bifurcation, *Atherosclerosis* 84:121-127, 1990.
75. Steinke W, Hennerici M, Rautenberg W, et al: Symptomatic and asymptomatic high-grade carotid stenoses in Doppler color-flow imaging, *Neurology* 42:131-138, 1992.
76. Sitzer M, Fuerst G, Fischer H, et al: Between-method correlations in quantifying internal carotid stenosis, *Stroke* 24:1513-1518, 1993.
77. Steinke W, Meairs S, Ries S, et al: Sonographic assessment of carotid artery stenosis: Comparison of power Doppler imaging and color Doppler flow imaging, *Stroke* 27:91-94, 1996.
78. Griewing B, Morgenstern C, Driesner F, et al: Cerebrovascular disease assessed by color-flow and power Doppler ultrasonography: Comparison with digital subtraction angiography in internal carotid artery stenosis, *Stroke* 27:95-100, 1996.
79. Yao J, van Sambeek MR, Dall'Agata A, et al: Three-dimensional ultrasound study of carotid arteries before and after endarterectomy; analysis of stenotic lesions and surgical impact on the vessel, *Stroke* 29:2026-2031, 1998.
80. Delcker A, Diener HC: Quantification of atherosclerotic plaques in carotid arteries by three-dimensional ultrasound, *Br J Radiol* 67:672-678, 1994.
81. Griewing B, Schminke U, Morgenstern C, et al: Three-dimensional ultrasound angiography (power mode) for the quantification of carotid artery atherosclerosis, *J Neuroimaging* 7:40-45, 1997.
82. Hallam MJ, Reid JM, Cooperberg PL: Color-flow Doppler and conventional duplex scanning of the carotid bifurcation: Prospective, double-blind, correlative study, *AJR Am J Roentgenol* 152:1101-1105, 1989.
83. Ackerstaff RG, Hoeneveld H, Slowikowski JM, et al: Ultrasonic duplex scanning in atherosclerotic disease of the innominate, subclavian and vertebral arteries: A comparative study with angiography, *Ultrasound Med Biol* 10:409-418, 1984.
84. Bendick PJ, Jackson VP: Evaluation of the vertebral arteries with duplex sonography, *J Vasc Surg* 3:523-530, 1986.
85. Davis PC, Nilsen B, Braun IF, et al: A prospective comparison of duplex scanning vs angiography of the vertebral arteries, *Am J Neuroradiol* 7:1059-1064, 1986.
86. Bendick PJ, Glover JL: Hemodynamic evaluation of vertebral arteries by duplex ultrasound, *Surg Clin North Am* 70:235-244, 1990.
87. Bartels E: [Color-coded Doppler sonography of the vertebral arteries. Comparison with conventional duplex sonography] Farbkodierte Dopplersonographie der vertebralarterien. Vergleich mit der konventionellen duplexsonographie, *Ultraschall Med* 13:59-66, 1992.
88. Trattnig S, Schwaighofer B, Hubsch P, et al: Color-coded Doppler sonography of vertebral arteries, *J Ultrasound Med* 10:221-226, 1991.
89. Kuhl V, Tettenborn B, Eicke BM, et al: Color-coded duplex ultrasonography of the origin of the vertebral artery: Normal values of flow velocities, *J Neuroimaging* 10:17-21, 2000.
90. Fisher CM, Gore I, Okabe N, et al: Atherosclerosis of the carotid and vertebral arteries - extracranial and intracranial, *J Neuropathol Exp Neurol* 24:455-476, 1965.
91. Goes E, Janssens W, Maillet B, et al: Tissue characterization of atheromatous plaques: Correlation between ultrasound image and histological findings, *J Clin Ultrasound* 18:611-617, 1990.
92. Hennerici M, Reifschneider G, Trockel U, et al: Detection of early atherosclerotic lesions by duplex scanning of the carotid artery, *J Clin Ultrasound* 12:455-464, 1984.
93. Wolverson MK, Bashiti HM, Peterson GJ: Ultrasonic tissue characterisation of atheromatous plaques using high resolution real time scanner, *Ultrasound Med Biol* 9:599-609, 1983.
94. Comerota AJ, Katz ML, White JV, et al: The preoperative diagnosis of the ulcerated carotid atheroma, *J Vasc Surg* 11:505-510, 1990.
95. Bock RW, Lusby RJ: Carotid plaque morphology and interpretation of the echolucent lesion. In Labs KH, Jäger KA, Fitzgerald DE, Woodcock JP, Neuerburg-Heusler D, editors: *Diagnostic vascular imaging*, London, 1992, Arnold, pp 225-236.
96. Bluth EI, Kay D, Merritt CRB, et al: Sonographic characterization of carotid plaque: Detection of hemorrhage, *AJR Am J Roentgenol* 146:1061-1065, 1986.
97. Langsfeld M, Gray Weale AC, Lusby RJ: The role of plaque morphology and diameter reduction in the development of new symptoms in asymptomatic carotid arteries, *J Vasc Surg* 9:548-557, 1989.
98. O'Donnell TF, Erdoes L, Mackay WC, et al: Correlation of B-mode ultrasound imaging and arteriography with pathologic findings at carotid endarterectomy, *Arch Surg* 120:443-449, 1985.
99. Sterpetti AV, Schultz RD, Feldhaus RJ, et al: Ultrasonographic features of carotid plaque and the risk of subsequent neurologic deficits, *Surgery* 104:652-660, 1988.
100. Aldoori MI, Baird R: Duplex scanning and plaque histology in cerebral ischaemia, *Eur J Vasc Surg* 1:159-164, 1987.
101. Imparato AM, Riles TS, Gostein F: The carotid bifurcation plaque: Pathologic findings associated with cerebral ischemia, *Stroke* 10:238-245, 1979.
102. Fisher M, Blumenfeld AM, Smith TW: The importance of carotid artery plaque disruption and hemorrhage, *Arch Neurol* 44:1086-1089, 1987.
103. Imparato AM, Riles TS, Mintzer R, et al: The importance of hemorrhage in the relationship between gross morphologic characteristics and cerebral symptoms in 376 carotid artery plaques, *Ann Surg* 197:195-203, 1983.
104. Lusby RJ, Ferrell LD, Ehrenfeld WK, et al: Carotid plaque hemorrhage. Its role in production of cerebral ischemia, *Arch Surg* 117:1479-1488, 1982.
105. Bassiouny HS, Davis H, Massawa N, et al: Critical carotid stenoses: Morphologic and chemical similarity between symptomatic and asymptomatic plaques, *J Vasc Surg* 9:202-212, 1989.
106. Leen EJ, Feeley TM, Colgan MP, et al: "Haemorrhagic" carotid plaque does not contain haemorrhage, *Eur J Vasc Surg* 4:123-128, 1990.
107. Lennihan L, Kupsky WJ, Mohr JP, et al: Lack of association between carotid plaque hematoma and ischemic cerebral symptoms, *Stroke* 18:879-881, 1987.
108. AbuRahma AF, Kyer PD, Robinson PA, et al: The correlation of ultrasonic carotid plaque morphology and carotid plaque hemorrhage: Clinical implications, *Surgery* 124:721-726, 1998.
109. Park AE, McCarthy WJ, Pearce WH, et al: Carotid plaque morphology correlates with presenting symptomatology, *J Vasc Surg* 27:872-878, 1998.
110. Golledge J, Cuming R, Ellis M, et al: Carotid plaque characteristics and presenting symptom, *Br J Surg* 84:1697-1701, 1997.
111. Nielsen TG, Laursen H, Gronholdt ML, et al: Histopathological features of in situ vein bypass stenoses, *Eur J Vasc Endovasc Surg* 14:492-498, 1997.
112. Droste DW, Karl M, Bohle RM, et al: Comparison of ultrasonic and histopathological features of carotid artery stenosis, *Neurol Res* 19:380-384, 1997.
113. Hatsukami TS, Ferguson MS, Beach KW, et al: Carotid plaque morphology and clinical events, *Stroke* 28:95-100, 1997.

114. Widder B, Paulat K, Hackspacher J, et al: Morphological characterization of carotid artery stenoses by ultrasound duplex scanning, *Ultrasound Med Biol* 16:349-354, 1990.

115. Bluth EI, McVay LVI, Merritt CR, et al: The identification of ulcerative plaque with high resolution duplex carotid scanning, *J Ultrasound Med* 7:73-76, 1988.

116. Eliasziw M, Strifler JY, Fox AJ, et al: Significance of plaque ulceration in symptomatic patients with high-grade carotid stenosis, *Stroke* 25:304-308, 1994.

117. Fischer CM, Ojemann RJ: A clinico-pathologic study of carotid endarterectomy plaques, *Rev Neurol* 142:573, 1986.

118. Svindland A, Torvik A: Atherosclerotic carotid disease in asymptomatic individuals: An histological study of 53 cases, *Acta Neurol Scand* 78:506-517, 1988.

119. Glagov S, Bassiouny HS, Giddens DP, et al: Intimal thickening: morphogenesis, functional significance and detection, *J Vasc Invest* 1:1-14, 1995.

120. Meairs S, Hennerici M: Four-dimensional ultrasonographic characterization of plaque surface motion in patients with symptomatic and asymptomatic carotid artery stenosis, *Stroke* 30:1807-1813, 1999.

121. Lenzi GL, Vicenzini E: The ruler is dead: An analysis of carotid plaque motion, *Cerebrovasc Dis* 23:121-125, 2007.

122. Bang J, Dahl T, Bruinsma A, et al: A new method for analysis of motion of carotid plaques from RF ultrasound images, *Ultrasound Med Biol* 29:967-976, 2003.

123. Stoitsis J, Golemati S, Nikita KS, et al: Characterization of carotid atherosclerosis based on motion and texture features and clustering using fuzzy c-means, *Conf Proc IEEE Eng Med Biol Soc* 2:1407-1410, 2004.

124. Stoitsis J, Golemati S, Dimopoulos A, et al: Analysis and quantification of arterial wall motion from B-mode ultrasound images: Comparison of block-matching and optical flow, *Conf Proc IEEE Eng Med Biol Soc* 5:4469-4472, 2005.

125. Paterson JC: Capillary rupture with intimal haemorrhage as the causative factor in coronary thrombosis, *Arch Pathol* :474-487, 1938.

126. Geiringer E: Intimal vascularisation and atherosclerosis. Histologic characteristics of carotid atherosclerotid plaque, *J Pathol Bacteriol* 63:201-211, 1951.

127. Feinstein SB: Contrast ultrasound imaging of the carotid artery vasa vasorum and atherosclerotic plaque neovascularization, *J Am Coll Cardiol* 48:236-243, 2006.

128. Vicenzini E, Giannoni MF, Puccinelli F, et al: Detection of carotid adventitial vasa vasorum and plaque vascularization with ultrasound cadence contrast pulse sequencing technique and echocontrast agent, *Stroke* 38:2841-2843, 2007.

129. Shah F, Balan P, Weinberg M, et al: Contrast-enhanced ultrasound imaging of atherosclerotic carotid plaque neovascularization: A new surrogate marker of atherosclerosis? *Vasc Med* 12:291-297, 2007.

130. Purushothaman KR, Sanz J, Zias E, et al: Atherosclerosis neovascularization and imaging, *Curr Mol Med* 6:549-556, 2006.

131. Huang PT, Huang FG, Zou CP, et al: Contrast-enhanced sonographic characteristics of neovascularization in carotid atherosclerotic plaques, *J Clin Ultrasound* 36:346-351, 2008.

132. Giannoni MF, Vicenzini E, Citone M, et al: Contrast carotid ultrasound for the detection of unstable plaques with neoangiogenesis: A pilot study, *Eur J Vasc Endovasc Surg* 37:722-727, 2009.

133. Hennerici M, Steinke W, Rautenberg W: High-resistance Doppler flow pattern in extracranial carotid dissection, *Arch Neurol* 46:670-672, 1989.

134. Steinke W, Rautenberg W, Schwartz A, et al: Ultrasonographic diagnosis and monitoring of cervicocephalic arterial dissection, *Cerebrovasc Dis* 2:195, 1992.

135. Sidhu PS, Jonker ND, Khaw KT, et al: Spontaneous dissections of the internal carotid artery: Appearances on colour Doppler ultrasound, *Br J Radiol* 70:50-57, 1997.

136. Sturzenegger M, Mattle HP, Rivoir A, et al: Ultrasound findings in carotid artery dissection: Analysis of 43 patients, *Neurology* 45:691-698, 1995.

137. Steinke W, Rautenberg W, Schwartz A, et al: Noninvasive monitoring of internal carotid artery dissection, *Stroke* 25:998-1005, 1994.

138. Caplan LR, Zarins CK, Hemmatti M: Spontaneous dissection of the extracranial vertebral arteries, *Stroke* 16:1030-1038, 1985.

139. Hart RG: Vertebral artery dissection, *Neurology* 38:987-989, 1988.

140. Greselle JF, Zenteno M, Kien P, et al: Spontaneous dissection of the vertebro-basilar system. A study of 18 cases (15 patients), *J Neuroradiol* 14:115-123, 1987.

141. Josien E: Extracranial vertebral artery dissection: Nine cases, *J Neurol* 239:327-330, 1992.

142. Mokri B, Houser OW, Sandok BA, et al: Spontaneous dissections of the vertebral arteries, *Neurology* 38:880-885, 1988.

143. Sturzenegger M, Mattle HP, Rivoir A, et al: Ultrasound findings in spontaneous extracranial vertebral artery dissection, *Stroke* 24:1910-1921, 1993.

144. Touboul PJ, Mas JL, Bousser MG, et al: Duplex scanning in extracranial vertebral artery dissection, *Stroke* 19:116-121, 1988.

145. Bartels E, Flügel KA: Evaluation of extracranial vertebral artery dissection with duplex color-flow imaging, *Stroke* 27:290-295, 1996.

146. Lu CJ, Sun Y, Jeng JS, et al: Imaging in the diagnosis and follow-up evaluation of vertebral artery dissection, *J Ultrasound Med* 19:263-270, 2000.

147. Nebelsieck J, Sengelhoff C, Nassenstein I, et al: Sensitivity of neurovascular ultrasound for the detection of spontaneous cervical artery dissection, *J Clin Neurosci* 16:79-82, 2009.

148. Wessels T, Mosso M, Krings T, et al: Extracranial and intracranial vertebral artery dissection: Long-term clinical and duplex sonographic follow-up, *J Clin Ultrasound* 36:472-479, 2008.

149. De Bray JM, Missoum A, Dubas F, et al: [Doppler transcranial ultrasonography in carotid and vertebral dissections: 36 cases involving angiography] Le Doppler transcranien dans les dissections carotidiennes et vertebrales: Etude de 36 cas arteriographies, *J Mal Vasc* 19:35-40, 1994.

150. Hoffmann M, Sacco RL, Chan S, et al: Noninvasive detection of vertebral artery dissection, *Stroke* 24:815-819, 1993.

151. Maeda H, Handa N, Matsumoto M, et al: Carotid lesions detected by B-mode ultrasonography in Takayasu's arteritis: "Macaroni sign" as an indicator of the disease, *Ultrasound Med Biol* 17:695-701, 1991.

152. Park SH, Chung JW, Lee JW, et al: Carotid artery involvement in Takayasu's arteritis: Evaluation of the activity by ultrasonography, *J Ultrasound Med* 20:371-378, 2001.

153. Ackerstaff RG, Keunen RW, van Pelt W, et al: Influence of biological factors on changes in mean cerebral blood flow velocity in normal ageing: A transcranial Doppler study, *Neurol Res* 12:187-191, 1990.

154. Brass LM, Pavlakis SG, DeVivo D, et al: Transcranial Doppler measurements of the middle cerebral artery. Effect of hematocrit, *Stroke* 19:1466-1469, 1988.

155. Gomez CR, Brass LM, Tegeler CH, et al: The transcranial Doppler standardization project, *J Neuroimaging* 3:190-192, 1993.

156. Aaslid R, Markwalder TM, Nornes H: Noninvasive transcranial Doppler ultrasound recording of flow velocity in basal arteries, *J Neurosurg* 57:769-774, 1982.

157. Arnolds BJ, von Reutern GM: Transcranial Doppler sonography. Examination technique and normal reference values, *Ultraschall Med* 12:115-123, 1987.

158. Büdingen HJ, Staudacher T: Die identifizierung der arteria basilaris mit der transkraniellen Dopplersonographie, *Ultraschall Med* 8:95-101, 1987.

159. Harders A: *Neurosurgical applications of transcranial Doppler sonography*, Vienna, 1986, Springer.

160. Hennerici M, Rautenberg W, Sitzer G, et al: Transcranial Doppler ultrasound for the assessment of intracranial arterial flow velocity: Part 1. Examination technique and normal values, *Surg Neurol* 27:439-448, 1987.

161. Lindegaard KF, Bakke SJ, Grolimund P, et al: Assessment of intracranial hemodynamics in carotid artery disease by transcranial Doppler ultrasound, *J Neurosurg* 63:890-898, 1985.

162. Bogdahn U, Becker G, Winkler J, et al: Transcranial color-coded real-time sonography in adults, *Stroke* 21:1680-1688, 1990.

163. Bartels E, Flugel KA: Quantitative measurements of blood flow velocity in basal cerebral arteries with transcranial duplex color-flow imaging. A comparative study with conventional transcranial Doppler sonography, *J Neuroimaging* 4:77-81, 1994.

164. Eicke BM, Tegeler CH, Dalley G, et al: Angle correction in transcranial Doppler sonography, *J Neuroimaging* 4:29-33, 1994.

165. Hennerici M, Rautenberg W, Schwartz A: Transcranial Doppler ultrasound for the assessment of intracranial arterial flow velocity: Part 2. Evaluation of intracranial arterial disease, *Surg Neurol* 27:523-532, 1987.

166. Lindegaard KF, Bakke SJ, Aaslid R, et al: Doppler diagnosis of intracranial arterial occlusive disorders, *J Neurol Neurosurg Psychiatry* 49:510-518, 1986.

167. Spencer MP, Whisler D: Transorbital Doppler diagnosis of intracranial arterial stenosis, *Stroke* 17:916-921, 1986.

168. Mattle H, Grolimund P, Huber P, et al: Transcranial Doppler sonographic findings in middle cerebral artery disease, *Arch Neurol* 45:289-295, 1988.

169. Rautenberg W, Schwartz A, Mull M, et al: Noninvasive detection of intracranial stenoses and occlusions, *Stroke* 21:149, 1990.

170. Goertler M, Kross R, Baeumer M, et al: Diagnostic impact and prognostic relevance of early contrast-enhanced transcranial color-coded duplex sonography in acute stroke, *Stroke* 29:955-962, 1998.

171. Postert T, Braun B, Federlein J, et al: Diagnosis and monitoring of middle cerebral artery occlusion with contrast-enhanced transcranial color-coded real-time sonography in patients with inadequate acoustic bone windows, *Ultrasound Med Biol* 24:333-340, 1998.

172. Gerriets T, Goertler M, Stolz E, et al: Feasibility and validity of transcranial duplex sonography in patients with acute stroke, *J Neurol Neurosurg Psychiatry* 73:17-20, 2002.

173. Mull M, Aulich A, Hennerici M: Transcranial Doppler ultrasonography versus arteriography for assessment of the vertebrobasilar circulation, *J Clin Ultrasound* 18:539-549, 1990.

174. Cher LM, Chambers BR, Smidt V: Comparison of transcranial Doppler with DSA in vertebrobasilar ischaemia, *Clin Exp Neurol* 29:143-148, 1992.

175. Tettenborn B, Estol C, DeWitt LD, et al: Accuracy of transcranial Doppler in the vertebrobasilar circulation, *J Neurol* 237:159, 1990.

176. Röther J, Wentz KU, Rautenberg W, et al: Magnetic resonance angiography in vertebrobasilar ischemia, *Stroke* 24:1310-1315, 1993.

177. Meairs S, Steinke W, Mohr JP, Hennerici M: Ultrasound imaging and Doppler sonography. In Barnett HJM, Mohr JP, Stein BM, Yatsu F, editors: *Stroke: Pathophysiology, diagnosis and management*, ed 3, New York, 1998, Churchhill Livingstone, pp 207-326.

178. Postert T, Braun B, Pfundtner N, et al: Echo contrast-enhanced three-dimensional power Doppler of intracranial arteries, *Ultrasound Med Biol* 24:953-962, 1998.

179. Deverson S, Evans DH, Bouch DC: The effects of temporal bone on transcranial Doppler ultrasound beam shape, *Ultrasound Med Biol* 26:239-244, 2000.

180. Klotzsch C, Bozzato A, Lammers G, et al: Contrast-enhanced three-dimensional transcranial color-coded sonography of intracranial stenoses, *AJNR Am J Neuroradiol* 23:208-212, 2002.

181. Schneider PA, Rossman ME, Bernstein EF, et al: Effect of internal carotid artery occlusion on intracranial hemodynamics. Transcranial Doppler evaluation and clinical correlation, *Stroke* 19:589-593, 1988.

182. Schneider PA, Rossman ME, Torem S, et al: Transcranial Doppler in the management of extracranial cerebrovascular disease: Implications in diagnosis and monitoring, *J Vasc Surg* 7:223-231, 1988.

183. Rautenberg W, Hennerici M: Intracranial hemodynamic measurements in patients with severe asymptomatic extracranial carotid disease, *Cerebrovasc Dis* 1:216-222, 1991.

184. Padayachee TS, Gosling RG, Bishop CC, et al: Monitoring middle cerebral artery blood velocity during carotid endarterectomy, *Br J Surg* 73:98-100, 1986.

185. Naylor AR: Transcranial Doppler monitoring during carotid endarterectomy. In Hennerici M, Meairs S, editors: *Cerebrovascular ultrasound: Theory, practice and future developments*, Cambridge, 2001, Cambridge University Press, pp 317-323.

186. Rautenberg W, Schwartz A, Hennerici M: Transkranielle dopplersonographic während der zerebralen angiographie. In Widder B, editor: *Transkranielle Dopplersonographie bei zerebrovaskulären erkrankungen*, Berlin, 1987, Springer, pp 144-148.

187. Markus HS, Loh A, Isrrael D, et al: Microscopic air embolism during cerebral angiography and strategies for avoidance, *Lancet* 341:784-787, 1993.

188. Markus HS, Clifton A, Buckenham T, et al: Carotid angioplasty. Detection of embolic signals during and after the procedure, *Stroke* 25:2403-2406, 1994.

189. Ries F, Eicke M: Auswirkungen der extrakorporalen zirkulation auf die intrazerebrale hämodynamik: Erklärung postoperativer neuropsychiatrischer komplikationen. In Widder B, editor: *Transkranielle Doppler-sonographie bei zerebrovaskulären erkrankungen*, Berlin, 1987, Springer, pp 100-110.

190. Bunegin L, Wahl D, Albin MS: Detection and volume estimation of embolic air in the middle cerebral artery using transcranial Doppler sonography, *Stroke* 25:593-600, 1994.

191. Jansen C, Ramos LM, van Heesewijk JP, et al: Impact of microembolism and hemodynamic changes in the brain during carotid endarterectomy, *Stroke* 25:992-997, 1994.

192. Gaunt ME, Martin PJ, Smith JL, et al: Clinical relevance of intraoperative embolization detected by transcranial Doppler ultrasonography during carotid endarterectomy: A prospective study of 100 patients, *Br J Surg* 81:1435-1439, 1994.

193. Siebler M, Sitzer M, Steinmetz H: Detection of intracranial emboli in patients with symptomatic extracranial carotid artery disease, *Stroke* 23:1652-1654, 1992.

194. Siebler M, Sitzer M, Rose G, et al: Silent cerebral embolism caused by neurologically symptomatic high-grade carotid stenosis. Event rates before and after carotid endarterectomy, *Brain* 116:1005-1015, 1993.

195. Grosset DG, Georgiadis D, Abdullah I, et al: Doppler emboli signals vary according to stroke subtype, *Stroke* 25:382-384, 1994.

196. Georgiadis D, Grosset DG, Quin RO, et al: Detection of intracranial emboli in patients with carotid disease, *Eur J Vasc Surg* 8:309-314, 1994.

197. Markus HS, Droste DW, Brown MM: Detection of asymptomatic cerebral embolic signals with Doppler ultrasound, *Lancet* 343:1011-1012, 1994.

198. Grosset DG, Cowburn P, Georgiadis D, et al: Ultrasound detection of cerebral emboli in patients with prosthetic heart valves, *J Heart Valve Dis* 3:128-132, 1994.

199. Georgiadis D, Mallinson A, Grosset DG, et al: Coagulation activity and emboli counts in patients with prosthetic cardiac valves, *Stroke* 25:1211-1214, 1994.

200. Diehl RR, Sliwka U, Rautenberg W, et al: Evidence for embolization from a posterior cerebral artery thrombus by transcranial Doppler monitoring, *Stroke* 24:606-608, 1993.

201. Consensus Committee of the Ninth International Cerebral Hemodynamics Symposium: Basic identification criteria of Doppler microembolic signals, *Stroke* 26:1123, 1995.

202. Georgiadis D, Baumgartner RW, Karatschai R, et al: Further evidence of gaseous embolic material in patients with artificial heart valves, *J Thorac Cardiovasc Surg* 115:808-810, 1998.

203. Valdueza JM, Harms L, Doepp F, et al: Venous microembolic signals detected in patients with cerebral sinus thrombosis, *Stroke* 28:1607-1609, 1997.

204. Georgiadis D, Kaps M, Siebler M, et al: Variability of Doppler microembolic signal counts in patients with prosthetic cardiac valves, *Stroke* 26:439-443, 1995.

205. Markus H, Bland JM, Rose G, et al: How good is intercenter agreement in the identification of embolic signals in carotid artery disease? *Stroke* 27:1249-1252, 1996.

206. Van Zuilen EV, Mess WH, Jansen C, et al: Automatic embolus detection compared with human experts. A Doppler ultrasound study, *Stroke* 27:1840-1843, 1996.

207. Ringelstein EB, Droste DW, Babikian VL, et al: Consensus on microembolus detection by TCD. International Consensus Group on Microembolus Detection, *Stroke* 29:725-729, 1998.

208. Georgiadis D, Wenzel A, Zerkowski HR, et al: Influence of transducer frequency on Doppler microemboli signals in an in vivo model, *Neurol Res* 20:198-200, 1998.

209. Keunen RW, Stam CJ, Tavy DL, et al: Preliminary report of detecting microembolic signals in transcranial Doppler time series with nonlinear forecasting, *Stroke* 29:1638-1643, 1998.

210. Ries F, Tiemann K, Pohl C, et al: High-resolution emboli detection and differentiation by characteristic postembolic spectral patterns, *Stroke* 29:668-672, 1998.

211. Roy E, Abraham P, Montresor S, et al: The narrow band hypothesis: An interesting approach for high-intensity transient signals (HITS) detection, *Ultrasound Med Biol* 24:375–382, 1998.

212. Russell D, Brucher R: Online automatic discrimination between solid and gaseous cerebral microemboli with the first multifrequency transcranial Doppler, *Stroke* 33:1975–1980, 2002.

213. Brucher R, Russell D: Automatic online embolus detection and artifact rejection with the first multifrequency transcranial Doppler, *Stroke* 33:1969–1974, 2002.

214. Fan L, Evans DH, Naylor AR: Automated embolus identification using a rule-based expert system, *Ultrasound Med Biol* 27:1065–1077, 2001.

215. International workshop on cerebral embolism, *Cerebrovasc Dis* 5:67–158, 1995.

216. Rautenberg W, Ries S, Bäzner H, et al: Emboli detection by TCD monitoring, *Can J Neurol Sci* 20:138–139, 1993.

217. Grosset DG, Georgiadis D, Kelman AW, et al: Quantification of ultrasound emboli signals in patients with cardiac and carotid disease, *Stroke* 24:1922–1924, 1993.

218. Spencer MP, Thomas GI, Nicholls SC, et al: Detection of middle cerebral artery emboli during carotid endarterectomy using transcranial Doppler ultrasonography, *Stroke* 21:415–423, 1990.

219. Van Zuilen EV, Moll FL, Vermeulen FE, et al: Detection of cerebral microemboli by means of transcranial Doppler monitoring before and after carotid endarterectomy, *Stroke* 26:210–213, 1995.

220. Markus HS, Thomson ND, Brown MM: Asymptomatic cerebral embolic signals in symptomatic and asymptomatic carotid artery disease, *Brain* 118:1005–1011, 1995.

221. Daffertshofer M, Ries S, Schminke U, et al: High-intensity transient signals in patients with cerebral ischemia, *Stroke* 27:1844–1849, 1996.

222. Koennecke HC, Mast H, Trocio SH Jr, et al: Frequency and determinants of microembolic signals on transcranial Doppler in unselected patients with acute carotid territory ischemia. A prospective study, *Cerebrovasc Dis* 8:107–112, 1998.

223. Sliwka U, Lingnau A, Stohlmann WD, et al: Prevalence and time course of microembolic signals in patients with acute stroke. A prospective study [published errata appear in Stroke 1997 Sep;28(9):1847 and 1999 Jan;30(1):192], *Stroke* 28:358–363, 1997.

224. Tong DC, Albers GW: Transcranial Doppler-detected microemboli in patients with acute stroke, *Stroke* 26:1588–1592, 1995.

225. Forteza AM, Babikian VL, Hyde C, et al: Effect of time and cerebrovascular symptoms of the prevalence of microembolic signals in patients with cervical carotid stenosis, *Stroke* 27:687–690, 1996.

226. Wijman CA, Babikian VL, Matjucha IC, et al: Cerebral microembolism in patients with retinal ischemia, *Stroke* 29:1139–1143, 1998.

227. Eicke BM, von Lorentz J, Paulus W: Embolus detection in different degrees of carotid disease, *Neurol Res* 17:181–184, 1995.

228. Sitzer M, Muller W, Siebler M, et al: Plaque ulceration and lumen thrombus are the main sources of cerebral microemboli in high-grade internal carotid artery stenosis, *Stroke* 26:1231–1233, 1995.

229. Valton L, Larrue V, Arrue P, et al: Asymptomatic cerebral embolic signals in patients with carotid stenosis. Correlation with appearance of plaque ulceration on angiography, *Stroke* 26:813–815, 1995.

230. Oliveira V, Batista P, Soares F, et al: HITS in internal carotid dissections, *Cerebrovasc Dis* 11:330–334, 2001.

231. Molina CA, Alvarez-Sabin J, Schonewille W, et al: Cerebral microembolism in acute spontaneous internal carotid artery dissection, *Neurology* 55:1738–1740, 2000.

232. Schauble B, Wijman CA, Koleini B, et al: Ophthalmic artery microembolism in giant cell arteritis, *J Neuroophthalmol* 20:273–275, 2000.

233. Fukuchi K, Kusuoka H, Watanabe Y, et al: Correlation of sequential MR images of microsphere-induced cerebral ischemia with histologic changes in rats, *Invest Radiol* 34:698–703, 1999.

234. Rundek T, Di Tullio MR, Sciacca RR, et al: Association between large aortic arch atheromas and high-intensity transient signals in elderly stroke patients, *Stroke* 30:2683–2686, 1999.

235. Siebler M, Kleinschmidt A, Sitzer M, et al: Cerebral microembolism in symptomatic and asymptomatic high-grade internal carotid artery stenosis, *Neurology* 44:615–618, 1994.

236. Babikian VL, Hyde C, Pochay V, et al: Clinical correlates of high-intensity transient signals detected on transcranial Doppler sonography in patients with cerebrovascular disease, *Stroke* 25:1570–1573, 1994.

237. Markus HS, MacKinnon A: Asymptomatic embolization detected by Doppler ultrasound predicts stroke risk in symptomatic carotid artery stenosis, *Stroke* 36:971–975, 2005.

238. Valton L, Larrue V, le Traon AP, et al: Microembolic signals and risk of early recurrence in patients with stroke or transient ischemic attack, *Stroke* 29:2125–2128, 1998.

239. Babikian VL, Wijman CA, Hyde C, et al: Cerebral microembolism and early recurrent cerebral or retinal ischemic events, *Stroke* 28:1314–1318, 1997.

240. Markus HS, Droste DW, Kaps M, et al: Dual antiplatelet therapy with clopidogrel and aspirin in symptomatic carotid stenosis evaluated using Doppler embolic signal detection: The Clopidogrel and Aspirin for Reduction of Emboli in Symptomatic Carotid Stenosis (CARESS) trial, *Circulation* 111:2233–2240, 2005.

241. Wong KS, Chen C, Fu J, et al: Clopidogrel plus aspirin versus aspirin alone for reducing embolisation in patients with acute symptomatic cerebral or carotid artery stenosis (CLAIR study): A randomised, open-label, blinded-endpoint trial, *Lancet Neurol* 9:489–497, 2010.

242. Wei K, Jayaweera AR, Firoozan S, et al: Quantification of myocardial blood flow with ultrasound-induced destruction of microbubbles administered as a constant venous infusion, *Circulation* 97:473–483, 1998.

243. Meairs S, Daffertshofer M, Neff W, et al: Pulse-inversion contrast harmonic imaging: Ultrasonographic assessment of cerebral perfusion, *Lancet* 355:550–551, 2000.

244. Martin MJ, Chung EM, Goodall AH, et al: Enhanced detection of thromboemboli with the use of targeted microbubbles, *Stroke* 38:2726–2732, 2007.

245. Dittrich R, Ringelstein EB: Occurrence and clinical impact of microembolic signals (MES) in patients with chronic cardiac diseases and atheroaortic plaques–a systematic review, *Curr Vasc Pharmacol* 6:329–334, 2008.

246. Schwartz A, Rautenberg W, Hennerici M: Dolichoectatic intracranial arteries: Review of selected aspects, *Cerebrovasc Dis* 3:273–279, 1993.

247. Rautenberg W, Aulich A, Röther J, et al: Stroke and dolichoectatic intracranial arteries, *Neurol Res* 14:201–203, 1992.

248. Adams RJ, Nichols FT, Aaslid R, et al: Cerebral vessel stenosis in sickle cell disease: Criteria for detection by transcranial Doppler, *Am J Pediatr Hematol Oncol* 12:277–282, 1990.

249. Adams RJ, Nichols FT, Figueroa R, et al: Transcranial Doppler correlation with cerebral angiography in sickle cell disease, *Stroke* 23:1073–1077, 1992.

250. Bogousslavsky J, Despland PA, Regli F, et al: Postpartum cerebral angiopathy: Reversible vasoconstriction assessed by transcranial Doppler ultrasounds, *Eur Neurol* 29:102–105, 1989.

251. Chimowitz MI, Nemec JJ, Marwick TH, et al: Transcranial Doppler ultrasound identifies patients with right- to-left cardiac or pulmonary shunts, *Neurology* 41:1902–1904, 1991.

252. Di Tullio M, Sacco RL, Venketasubramanian N, et al: Comparison of diagnostic techniques for the detection of a patent foramen ovale in stroke patients, *Stroke* 24:1020–1024, 1993.

253. Itoh T, Matsumoto M, Handa N, et al: Paradoxical embolism as a cause of ischemic stroke of uncertain etiology. A transcranial Doppler sonographic study, *Stroke* 25:771–775, 1994.

254. Jauss M, Kaps M, Keberle M, et al: A comparison of transesophageal echocardiography and transcranial Doppler sonography with contrast medium for detection of patent foramen ovale, *Stroke* 25:1265–1267, 1994.

255. Droste DW, Lakemeier S, Wichter T, et al: Optimizing the technique of contrast transcranial Doppler ultrasound in the detection of right-to-left shunts, *Stroke* 33:2211–2216, 2002.

256. Hamann GF, Schatzer KD, Frohlig G, et al: Femoral injection of echo contrast medium may increase the sensitivity of testing for a patent foramen ovale, *Neurology* 50:1423–1428, 1998.

257. Schwarze JJ, Sander D, Kukla C, et al: Methodological parameters influence the detection of right-to-left shunts by contrast transcranial Doppler ultrasonography, *Stroke* 30:1234–1239, 1999.

258. Droste DW, Jekentaite R, Stypmann J, et al: Contrast transcranial Doppler ultrasound in the detection of right-to-left shunts: Comparison of Echovist-200 and Echovist-300, timing of the Valsalva maneuver, and general recommendations for the performance of the test, *Cerebrovasc Dis* 13:235–241, 2002.

259. Ophir J, Parker KJ: Contrast agents in diagnostic ultrasound, *Ultrasound Med Biol* 15:319–333, 1989.

260. Burns PN: Overview of echo-enhanced vascular ultrasound imaging for clinical diagnosis in neurosonology, *J Neuroimaging* 7(Suppl 1):S2-14, 1997.

261. Van Liew HD, Raychaudhuri S: Stabilized bubbles in the body: Pressure-radius relationships and the limits to stabilization, *J Appl Physiol* 82:2045-2053, 1997.

262. Kabalnov A, Bradley J, Flaim S, et al: Dissolution of multicomponent microbubbles in the bloodstream: 2, Experiment, *Ultrasound Med Biol* 24:751-760, 1998.

263. Chang PH, Shung KK, Levene HB: Quantitative measurements of second harmonic Doppler using ultrasound contrast agents, *Ultrasound Med Biol* 22:1205-1214, 1996.

264. Strandness DE, Eikelboom BC: Carotid artery stenosis–where do we go from here? *Eur J Ultrasound* 7(Suppl 3):S17-S26, 1998.

265. Sitzer M, Furst G, Siebler M, et al: Usefulness of an intravenous contrast medium in the characterization of high-grade internal carotid stenosis with color Doppler-assisted duplex imaging, *Stroke* 25:385-389, 1994.

266. Sitzer M, Rose G, Furst G, et al: Characteristics and clinical value of an intravenous echo-enhancement agent in evaluation of high-grade internal carotid stenosis, *J Neuroimaging* 7(Suppl 1):S22-S25, 1997.

267. Rothwell PM, Gutnikov SA, Warlow CP: Reanalysis of the final results of the European Carotid Surgery Trial, *Stroke* 34:514-523, 2003.

268. Ries F, Honisch C, Lambertz M, et al: A transpulmonary contrast medium enhances the transcranial Doppler signal in humans, *Stroke* 24:1903-1909, 1993.

269. Haggag KJ, Russell D, Brucher R, et al: Contrast enhanced pulsed Doppler and colour-coded duplex studies of the cranial vasculature, *Eur J Neurol* 6:443-448, 1999.

270. Otis S, Rush M, Boyajian R: Contrast-enhanced transcranial imaging. Results of an American phase-two study, *Stroke* 26:203-209, 1995.

271. Gerriets T, Seidel G, Fiss I, et al: Contrast-enhanced transcranial color-coded duplex sonography: Efficiency and validity, *Neurology* 52:1133-1137, 1999.

272. Murphy KJ, Bude RO, Dickinson LD, et al: Use of intravenous contrast material in transcranial sonography, *Acad Radiol* 4:577-582, 1997.

273. Stolz E, Kaps M, Kern A, et al: Frontal bone windows for transcranial color-coded duplex sonography, *Stroke* 30:814-820, 1999.

274. Delcker A, Turowski B: Diagnostic value of three-dimensional transcranial contrast duplex sonography, *J Neuroimaging* 7:139-144, 1997.

275. Baumgartner RW, Arnold M, Gonner F, et al: Contrast-enhanced transcranial color-coded duplex sonography in ischemic cerebrovascular disease, *Stroke* 28:2473-2478, 1997.

276. Nabavi DG, Droste DW, Kemeny V, et al: Potential and limitations of echocontrast-enhanced ultrasonography in acute stroke patients: A pilot study, *Stroke* 29:949-954, 1998.

277. Nabavi DG, Droste DW, Schulte-Altedorneburg G, et al: Diagnostic benefit of echocontrast enhancement for the insufficient transtemporal bone window, *J Neuroimaging* 9:102-107, 1999.

278. Iglseder B, Huemer M, Staffen W, et al: Imaging the basilar artery by contrast-enhanced color-coded ultrasound, *J Neuroimaging* 10:195-199, 2000.

279. Droste DW, Nabavi DG, Kemeny V, et al: Echocontrast enhanced transcranial colour-coded duplex offers improved visualization of the vertebrobasilar system, *Acta Neurol Scand* 98:193-199, 1998.

280. Koga M, Kimura K, Minematsu K, et al: Relationship between findings of conventional and contrast-enhanced transcranial color-coded real-time sonography and angiography in patients with basilar artery occlusion, *AJNR Am J Neuroradiol* 23:568-571, 2002.

281. Postert T, Meves S, Bornke C, et al: Power Doppler compared to color-coded duplex sonography in the assessment of the basal cerebral circulation, *J Neuroimaging* 7:221-226, 1997.

282. Griewing B, Motsch L, Piek J, et al: Transcranial power mode Doppler duplex sonography of intracranial aneurysms, *J Neuroimaging* 8:155-158, 1998.

283. Wardlaw JM, Cannon J, Statham PF: Does the size of intracranial aneurysms change with intracranial pressure? Observations based on color "power" transcranial Doppler ultrasound, *J Neurosurg* 88:846-850, 1998.

284. Woydt M, Greiner K, Perez J, et al: Intraoperative color duplex sonography of basal arteries during aneurysm surgery, *J Neuroimaging* 7:203-207, 1997.

285. Mursch K, Schaake T, Markakis E: Using transcranial duplex sonography for monitoring vessel patency during surgery for intracranial aneurysms, *J Neuroimaging* 7:164-170, 1997.

286. Bailes JE, Tantuwaya LS, Fukushima T, et al: Intraoperative microvascular Doppler sonography in aneurysm surgery, *Neurosurgery* 40:965-970, 1997.

287. Uggowitzer MM, Kugler C, Riccabona M, et al: Cerebral arteriovenous malformations: Diagnostic value of echo-enhanced transcranial Doppler sonography compared with angiography, *AJNR Am J Neuroradiol* 20:101-106, 1999.

288. Bartels E: Evaluation of arteriovenous malformations (AVMs) with transcranial color-coded duplex sonography: Does the location of an AVM influence its sonographic detection? *J Ultrasound Med* 24:1511-1517, 2005.

289. Lindseth F, Lovstakken L, Rygh OM, et al: Blood flow imaging: An angle-independent ultrasound modality for intraoperative assessment of flow dynamics in neurovascular surgery, *Neurosurgery* 65:149-157, 2009.

290. Valdueza JM, Schmierer K, Mehraein S, et al: Assessment of normal flow velocity in basal cerebral veins. A transcranial Doppler ultrasound study, *Stroke* 27:1221-1225, 1996.

291. Baumgartner RW, Gonner F, Arnold M, et al: Transtemporal power- and frequency-based color-coded duplex sonography of cerebral veins and sinuses, *AJNR Am J Neuroradiol* 18:1771-1781, 1997.

292. Stolz E, Kaps M, Kern A, et al: Transcranial color-coded duplex sonography of intracranial veins and sinuses in adults. Reference data from 130 volunteers, *Stroke* 30:1070-1075, 1999.

293. Valdueza JM, Hoffmann O, Weih M, et al: Monitoring of venous hemodynamics in patients with cerebral venous thrombosis by transcranial Doppler ultrasound, *Arch Neurol* 56:229-234, 1999.

294. Canhao P, Batista P, Ferro JM: Venous transcranial Doppler in acute dural sinus thrombosis, *J Neurol* 245:276-279, 1998.

295. Stolz E, Gerriets T, Bodeker RH, et al: Intracranial venous hemodynamics is a factor related to a favorable outcome in cerebral venous thrombosis, *Stroke* 33:1645-1650, 2002.

296. Stolz E, Kaps M, Dorndorf W: Assessment of intracranial venous hemodynamics in normal individuals and patients with cerebral venous thrombosis, *Stroke* 30:70-75, 1999.

297. Ries S, Steinke W, Neff KW, et al: Echocontrast-enhanced transcranial color-coded sonography for the diagnosis of transverse sinus venous thrombosis, *Stroke* 28:696-700, 1997.

298. Alexandrov AV, Burgin WS, Demchuk AM, et al: Speed of intracranial clot lysis with intravenous tissue plasminogen activator therapy: Sonographic classification and short-term improvement, *Circulation* 103:2897-2902, 2001.

299. Nedelmann M, Stolz E, Gerriets T, et al: Consensus recommendations for transcranial color-coded duplex sonography for the assessment of intracranial arteries in clinical trials on acute stroke, *Stroke* 40:3238-3244, 2009.

300. Alexandrov AV, Demchuk AM, Felberg RA, et al: Intracranial clot dissolution is associated with embolic signals on transcranial Doppler, *J Neuroimaging* 10:27-32, 2000.

301. Stolz E, Gerriets T, Fiss I, et al: Comparison of transcranial color-coded duplex sonography and cranial CT measurements for determining third ventricle midline shift in space-occupying stroke, *AJNR Am J Neuroradiol* 20:1567-1571, 1999.

302. Bertram M, Khoja W, Ringleb P, et al: Transcranial colour-coded sonography for the bedside evaluation of mass effect after stroke, *Eur J Neurol* 7:639-646, 2000.

303. Gerriets T, Stolz E, Konig S, et al: Sonographic monitoring of midline shift in space-occupying stroke: An early outcome predictor, *Stroke* 32:442-447, 2001.

304. Horstmann S, Koziol JA, Martinez-Torres F, et al: Sonographic monitoring of mass effect in stroke patients treated with hypothermia. Correlation with intracranial pressure and matrix metalloproteinase 2 and 9 expression, *J Neurol Sci* 276:75-78, 2009.

305. Aaslid R, Huber P, Nornes H: Evaluation of cerebrovascular spasm with transcranial Doppler ultrasound, *J Neurosurg* 60:37-41, 1984.

306. Seiler RW, Grolimund P, Aaslid R, et al: Cerebral vasospasm evaluated by transcranial ultrasound correlated with clinical grade and CT-visualized subarachnoid hemorrhage, *J Neurosurg* 64:594-600, 1986.

307. Laumer R, Steinmeier R, Gönner R, et al: Cerebral hemodynamics in subarachnoid hemorrhage evaluated by transcranial Doppler sonography, *Neurosurgery* 31:1-9, 1993.

308. Lennihan L, Petty GW, Fink E, et al: Transcranial Doppler detection of anterior cerebral vasospasm, *J Neurol Neurosurg Psychiatry* 56:906-909, 1993.

309. Hassler W, Steinmetz H, Gawlowski J: Transcranial Doppler ultrasonography in raised intracranial pressure and in intracranial circulatory arrest, *J Neurosurg* 68:745-751, 1988.

310. Schmidt B, Klingelhofer J, Schwarze JJ, et al: Noninvasive prediction of intracranial pressure curves using transcranial Doppler ultrasonography and blood pressure curves, *Stroke* 28:2465-2472, 1997.

311. Silvestrini M, Cupini LM, Placidi F, et al: Bilateral hemispheric activation in the early recovery of motor function after stroke, *Stroke* 29:1305-1310, 1998.

312. Caramia MD, Palmieri MG, Giacomini P, et al: Ipsilateral activation of the unaffected motor cortex in patients with hemiparetic stroke, *Clin Neurophysiol* 111:1990-1996, 2000.

313. Silvestrini M, Troisi E, Matteis M, et al: Correlations of flow velocity changes during mental activity and recovery from aphasia in ischemic stroke, *Neurology* 50:191-195, 1998.

314. Krishnan S, O'Donnell M: Transmit aperture processing for nonlinear contrast agent imaging, *Ultrason Imaging* 18:77-105, 1996.

315. Seidel G, Greis C, Sonne J, et al: Harmonic grey scale imaging of the human brain, *J Neuroimaging* 9:171-174, 1999.

316. Postert T, Muhs A, Meves S, et al: Transient response harmonic imaging: An ultrasound technique related to brain perfusion, *Stroke* 29:1901-1907, 1998.

317. Eyding J, Krogias C, Wilkening W, et al: Parameters of cerebral perfusion in phase-inversion harmonic imaging (PIHI) ultrasound examinations, *Ultrasound Biol* 29:1379-1385, 2003.

318. Eyding J, Wilkening W, Reckhardt M, et al: Contrast burst depletion imaging (CODIM): A new imaging procedure and analysis method for semiquantitative ultrasonic perfusion imaging, *Stroke* 34:77-83, 2003.

319. Eyding J, Wilkening W, Krogias C, et al: Validation of the depletion kinetic in semiquantitative ultrasonographic cerebral perfusion imaging using 2 different techniques of data acquisition, *J Ultrasound Med* 23:1035-1040, 2004.

320. Harrer JU, Klotzsch C: Second harmonic imaging of the human brain: The practicability of coronal insonation planes and alternative perfusion parameters, *Stroke* 33:1530-1535, 2002.

321. Krogias C, Postert T, Meves S, et al: Semiquantitative analysis of ultrasonic cerebral perfusion imaging, *Ultrasound Med Biol* 31:1007-1012, 2005.

322. Meves SH, Wilkening W, Thies T, et al: Comparison between echo contrast agent-specific imaging modes and perfusion-weighted magnetic resonance imaging for the assessment of brain perfusion, *Stroke* 33:2433-2437, 2002.

323. Meyer K, Seidel G: Transcranial contrast diminution imaging of the human brain: A pilot study in healthy volunteers, *Ultrasound Med Biol* 28:1433-1437, 2002.

324. Pohl C, Tiemann K, Schlosser T, et al: Stimulated acoustic emission detected by transcranial color Doppler ultrasound: A contrast-specific phenomenon useful for the detection of cerebral tissue perfusion, *Stroke* 31:1661-1666, 2000.

325. Postert T, Hoppe P, Federlein J, et al: Contrast agent specific imaging modes for the ultrasonic assessment of parenchymal cerebral echo contrast enhancement, *J Cereb Blood Flow Metab* 20:1709-1716, 2000.

326. Seidel G, Algermissen C, Christoph A, et al: Visualization of brain perfusion with harmonic gray scale and power Doppler technology: An animal pilot study, *Stroke* 31:1728-1734, 2000.

327. Seidel G, Meyer K, Metzler V, et al: Human cerebral perfusion analysis with ultrasound contrast agent constant infusion: A pilot study on healthy volunteers, *Ultrasound Med Biol* 28:183-189, 2002.

328. Wiesmann M, Seidel G: Ultrasound perfusion imaging of the human brain, *Stroke* 31:2421-2425, 2000.

329. Kern R, Perren F, Kreisel S, et al: Multi-planar transcranial ultrasound imaging: Standards, landmarks and correlation with magnetic resonance imaging, *Ultrasound Med Biol* 31:311-315, 2005.

330. Wiesmann M, Meyer K, Albers T, et al: Parametric perfusion imaging with contrast-enhanced ultrasound in acute ischemic stroke, *Stroke* 35:508-513, 2004.

331. Federlein J, Postert T, Meves S, et al: Ultrasonic evaluation of pathological brain perfusion in acute stroke using second harmonic imaging, *J Neurol Neurosurg Psychiatry* 69:616-622, 2000.

332. Eyding J, Krogias C, Schollhammer M, et al: Contrast-enhanced ultrasonic parametric perfusion imaging detects dysfunctional tissue at risk in acute MCA stroke, *J Cereb Blood Flow Metab* 26:576-582, 2006.

333. Eyding J, Nolte-Martin A, Krogias C, et al: Changes of contrast-specific ultrasonic cerebral perfusion patterns in the course of stroke; reliability of region-wise and parametric imaging analysis, *Ultrasound Med Biol* 33:329-334, 2007.

334. Holscher T, Wilkening W, Draganski B, et al: Transcranial ultrasound brain perfusion assessment with a contrast agent-specific imaging mode: Results of a two-center trial, *Stroke* 36:2283-2285, 2005.

335. Seidel G, Meyer-Wiethe K, Berdien G, et al: Ultrasound perfusion imaging in acute middle cerebral artery infarction predicts outcome, *Stroke* 35:1107-1111, 2004.

336. Sobesky J, Zaro WO, Lehnhardt FG, et al: Which time-to-peak threshold best identifies penumbral flow? A comparison of perfusion-weighted magnetic resonance imaging and positron emission tomography in acute ischemic stroke, *Stroke* 35:2843-2847, 2004.

337. Kern R, Perren F, Schoeneberger K, et al: Ultrasound microbubble destruction imaging in acute middle cerebral artery stroke, *Stroke* 35:1665-1670, 2004.

338. Meyer-Wiethe K, Cangur H, Seidel GU: Comparison of different mathematical models to analyze diminution kinetics of ultrasound contrast enhancement in a flow phantom, *Ultrasound Med Biol* 31:93-98, 2005.

339. Lucidarme O, Kono Y, Corbeil J, et al: Validation of ultrasound contrast destruction imaging for flow quantification, *Ultrasound Med Biol* 29:1697-1704, 2003.

340. Meairs S: Contrast-enhanced ultrasound perfusion imaging in acute stroke patients, *Eur Neurol* 59(Suppl 1):17-26, 2008.

341. Schlachetzki F, Holscher T, Koch HJ, et al: Observation on the integrity of the blood-brain barrier after microbubble destruction by diagnostic transcranial color-coded sonography, *J Ultrasound Med* 21:419-429, 2002.

342. Jungehulsing GJ, Brunecker P, Nolte CH, et al: Diagnostic transcranial ultrasound perfusion-imaging at 2.5 MHz does not affect the blood-brain barrier, *Ultrasound Med Biol* 34:147-150, 2008.

343. Eyding J, Krogias C, Wilkening W, et al: Detection of cerebral perfusion abnormalities in acute stroke using phase inversion harmonic imaging (PIHI): Preliminary results, *J Neurol Neurosurg Psychiatry* 75:926-929, 2004.

344. Meyer-Wiethe K, Cangur H, Schindler A, et al: Ultrasound perfusion imaging: Determination of thresholds for the identification of critically disturbed perfusion in acute ischemic stroke: A pilot study, *Ultrasound Med Biol* 33:851-856, 2007.

345. Meyer K, Wiesmann M, Albers T, et al: Harmonic imaging in acute stroke: Detection of a cerebral perfusion deficit with ultrasound and perfusion MRI, *J Neuroimaging* 13:166-168, 2003.

346. Postert T, Federlein J, Weber S, et al: Second harmonic imaging in acute middle cerebral artery infarction. Preliminary results, *Stroke* 30:1702-1706, 1999.

347. Schlachetzki F, Hoelscher T, Dorenbeck U, et al: Sonographic parenchymal and brain perfusion imaging: Preliminary results in four patients following decompressive surgery for malignant middle cerebral artery infarct, *Ultrasound Med Biol* 27:21-31, 2001.

348. Seidel G, Albers T, Meyer K, et al: Perfusion harmonic imaging in acute middle cerebral artery infarction, *Ultrasound Med Biol* 29:1245-1251, 2003.

349. Shiogai T, Takayasu N, Mizuno T, et al: Comparison of transcranial brain tissue perfusion images between ultraharmonic, second harmonic, and power harmonic imaging, *Stroke* 35:687-693, 2004.

350. Stolz E, Allendorfer J, Jauss M, et al: Sonographic harmonic grey scale imaging of brain perfusion: Scope of a new method demonstrated in selected cases, *Ultraschall Med* 23:320-324, 2002.

351. Niesen W, Marouf W, Weiller C, et al: Transcranial perfusion sonography preceding thrombolysis: Perfusion deficit correlates with clinical as well as vascular status, *Cerebrovasc Dis* 25:27, 2008.

352. Meairs S, Culp W: Microbubbles for thrombolysis of acute ischemic stroke, *Cerebrovasc Dis* 27(Suppl 2):55-65, 2009.

353. Sobbe A, Stumpff U, Trubestein G, et al: [Thrombolysis by ultrasound (author's transl)], *Klin Wochenschr* 52:1117-1121, 1974.

354. Harpaz D, Chen X, Francis CW, et al: Ultrasound accelerates urokinase-induced thrombolysis and reperfusion, *Am Heart J* 127:1211-1219, 1994.

355. Rosenschein U, Gaul G, Erbel R, et al: Percutaneous transluminal therapy of occluded saphenous vein grafts: Can the challenge be met with ultrasound thrombolysis? *Circulation* 99:26-29, 1999.

356. Luo H, Birnbaum Y, Fishbein MC, et al: Enhancement of thrombolysis in vivo without skin and soft tissue damage by transcutaneous ultrasound, *Thromb Res* 89:171-177, 1998.

357. Riggs PN, Francis CW, Bartos SR, et al: Ultrasound enhancement of rabbit femoral artery thrombolysis, *Cardiovasc Surg* 5:201-207, 1997.

358. Hamm CW, Steffen W, Terres W, et al: Intravascular therapeutic ultrasound thrombolysis in acute myocardial infarctions, *Am J Cardiol* 80:200-204, 1997.

359. Rosenschein U, Roth A, Rassin T, et al: Analysis of coronary ultrasound thrombolysis endpoints in acute myocardial infarction (ACUTE trial). Results of the feasibility phase, *Circulation* 95:1411-1416, 1997.

360. Yock PG, Fitzgerald PJ: Catheter-based ultrasound thrombolysis, *Circulation* 95:1360-1362, 1997.

361. Daffertshofer M, Hennerici M: Ultrasound in the treatment of ischaemic stroke, *Lancet Neurol* 2:283-290, 2003.

362. Daffertshofer M, Fatar M: Therapeutic ultrasound in ischemic stroke treatment: Experimental evidence, *Eur J Ultrasound* 16:121-130, 2002.

363. Alexandrov AV, Molina CA, Grotta JC, et al: Ultrasound-enhanced systemic thrombolysis for acute ischemic stroke, *N Engl J Med* 351:2170-2178, 2004.

364. Eggers J, Koch B, Meyer K, et al: Effect of ultrasound on thrombolysis of middle cerebral artery occlusion, *Ann Neurol* 53:797-800, 2003.

365. Pfaffenberger S, Devcic-Kuhar B, Kollmann C, et al: Can a commercial diagnostic ultrasound device accelerate thrombolysis? An in vitro skull model, *Stroke* 36:124-128, 2005.

366. Meairs S, Dempfle CE: In vitro models for assessing transcranial ultrasound-enhanced thrombolysis, *Stroke* 36:929-930, 2005.

367. Baron C, Aubry J-F, Tanter M, et al: Simulation of intracranial acoustic fields in clinical trials of sonothrombolysis, *Ultrasound Med Biol* 35:1148-1158, 2009.

368. Daffertshofer M, Gass A, Ringleb P, et al: Transcranial low-frequency ultrasound-mediated thrombolysis in brain ischemia: Increased risk of hemorrhage with combined ultrasound and tissue plasminogen activator: Results of a phase ii clinical trial, *Stroke* 36:1441-1446, 2005.

369. Daffertshofer M, Huang Z, Fatar M, et al: Efficacy of sonothrombolysis in a rat model of embolic ischemic stroke, *Neurosci Lett* 361:115-119, 2004.

370. Reinhard M, Hetzel A, Kruger S, et al: Blood-brain barrier disruption by low-frequency ultrasound, *Stroke* 37:1546-1548, 2006.

371. Wang Z, Moehring MA, Voie AH, et al: In vitro evaluation of dual mode ultrasonic thrombolysis method for transcranial application with an occlusive thrombosis model, *Ultrasound Med Biol* 34:96-102, 2008.

372. Tachibana K, Tachibana S: Albumin microbubble echo-contrast material as an enhancer for ultrasound accelerated thrombolysis, *Circulation* 92:1148-1150, 1995.

373. Porter TR, LeVeen RF, Fox R, et al: Thrombolytic enhancement with perfluorocarbon-exposed sonicated dextrose albumin microbubbles, *Am Heart J* 132:964-968, 1996.

374. Cintas P, Nguyen F, Boneu B, et al: Enhancement of enzymatic fibrinolysis with 2-MHz ultrasound and microbubbles, *J Thromb Haemost* 2:1163-1166, 2004.

375. Birnbaum Y, Luo H, Nagai T, et al: Noninvasive in vivo clot dissolution without a thrombolytic drug: Recanalization of thrombosed iliofemoral arteries by transcutaneous ultrasound combined with intravenous infusion of microbubbles, *Circulation* 97:130-134, 1998.

376. Tsivgoulis G, Alexandrov AV: Ultrasound-enhanced thrombolysis in acute ischemic stroke: Potential, failures, and safety, *Neurotherapeutics* 4:420-427, 2007.

377. Everbach EC, Francis CW: Cavitational mechanisms in ultrasound-accelerated thrombolysis at 1 MHz, *Ultrasound Med Biol* 26:1153-1160, 2000.

378. Datta S, Coussios CC, Ammi AY, et al: Ultrasound-enhanced thrombolysis using Definity as a cavitation nucleation agent, *Ultrasound Med Biol* 34:1421-1433, 2008.

379. Miller MW, Miller DL, Brayman AA: A review of in vitro bioeffects of inertial ultrasonic cavitation from a mechanistic perspective, *Ultrasound Med Biol* 22:1131-1154, 1996.

380. Datta S, Coussios CC, McAdory LE, et al: Correlation of cavitation with ultrasound enhancement of thrombolysis, *Ultrasound Med Biol* 32:1257-1267, 2006.

381. Molina CA, Ribo M, Rubiera M, et al: Microbubble administration accelerates clot lysis during continuous 2-MHz ultrasound monitoring in stroke patients treated with intravenous tissue plasminogen activator, *Stroke* 37:425-429, 2006.

382. Perren F, Loulidi J, Poglia D, et al: Microbubble potentiated transcranial duplex ultrasound enhances IV thrombolysis in acute stroke, *J Thromb Thrombolysis* 25:219-223, 2008.

383. Pagola J, Ribo M, Alvarez-Sabin J, et al: Timing of recanalization after microbubble-enhanced intravenous thrombolysis in basilar artery occlusion, *Stroke* 38:2931-2934, 2007.

384. Porter TR, Kricsfeld D, Lof J, et al: Effectiveness of transcranial and transthoracic ultrasound and microbubbles in dissolving intravascular thrombi, *J Ultrasound Med* 20:1313-1325, 2001.

385. Culp WC, Porter TR, Xie F, et al: Microbubble potentiated ultrasound as a method of declotting thrombosed dialysis grafts: Experimental study in dogs, *Cardiovasc Intervent Radiol* 24:407-412, 2001.

386. Culp WC, Porter TR, McCowan TC, et al: Microbubble-augmented ultrasound declotting of thrombosed arteriovenous dialysis grafts in dogs, *J Vasc Interv Radiol* 14:343-347, 2003.

387. Culp WC, Erdem E, Roberson PK, et al: Microbubble potentiated ultrasound as a method of stroke therapy in a pig model: Preliminary findings, *J Vasc Interv Radiol* 14:1433-1436, 2003.

388. Culp WC, Porter TR, Lowery J, et al: Intracranial clot lysis with intravenous microbubbles and transcranial ultrasound in swine, *Stroke* 35:2407-2411, 2004.

389. Xie F, Tsutsui JM, Lof J, et al: Effectiveness of lipid microbubbles and ultrasound in declotting thrombosis, *Ultrasound Med Biol* 31:979-985, 2005.

390. Alonso A, Della Martina A, Stroick M, et al: Molecular imaging of human thrombus with novel abciximab immunobubbles and ultrasound, *Stroke* 38:1508-1514, 2007.

391. Alonso A, Dempfle CE, Della MA, et al: In vivo clot lysis of human thrombus with intravenous abciximab immunobubbles and ultrasound, *Thromb Res* 124:70-74, 2009.

392. Fatar M, Stroick M, Griebe M, et al: Effect of combined ultrasound and microbubbles treatment in an experimental model of cerebral ischemia, *Ultrasound Med Biol* 34:1414-1420, 2008.

393. Stroick M, Alonso A, Fatar M, et al: Effects of simultaneous application of ultrasound and microbubbles on intracerebral hemorrhage in an animal model, *Ultrasound Med Biol* 32:1377-1382, 2006.

394. Dayton PA, Ferrara KW: Targeted imaging using ultrasound, *J Magn Reson Imaging* 16:362-377, 2002.

395. Leong-Poi H, Christiansen J, Klibanov AL, et al: Noninvasive assessment of angiogenesis by ultrasound and microbubbles targeted to alpha(v)-integrins, *Circulation* 107:455-460, 2003.

396. Weller GE, Villanueva FS, Klibanov AL, et al: Modulating targeted adhesion of an ultrasound contrast agent to dysfunctional endothelium, *Ann Biomed Eng* 30:1012-1019, 2002.

397. Schumann PA, Christiansen JP, Quigley RM, et al: Targeted-microbubble binding selectively to GPIIb IIIa receptors of platelet thrombi, *Invest Radiol* 37:587-593, 2002.

398. Tardy I, Pochon S, Theraulaz M, et al: In vivo ultrasound imaging of thrombi using a target-specific contrast agent, *Acad Radiol* 9(Suppl 2):S294-S296, 2002.

399. Christiansen JP, Leong-Poi H, Klibanov AL, et al: Noninvasive imaging of myocardial reperfusion injury using leukocyte-targeted contrast echocardiography, *Circulation* 105:1764-1767, 2002.

400. Lindner JR: Detection of inflamed plaques with contrast ultrasound, *Am J Cardiol* 90:32L-35L, 2002.

401. Behm CZ, Kaufmann BA, Carr C, et al: Molecular imaging of endothelial vascular cell adhesion molecule-1 expression and inflammatory cell recruitment during vasculogenesis and ischemia-mediated arteriogenesis, *Circulation* 117:2902-2911, 2008.

402. Kaufmann BA, Carr CL, Belcik JT, et al: Molecular imaging of the initial inflammatory response in atherosclerosis: Implications for early detection of disease, *Arterioscler Thromb Vasc Biol* 30:54–59, 2010.

403. Piedra M, Allroggen A, Lindner JR: Molecular imaging with targeted contrast ultrasound, *Cerebrovasc Dis* 27(Suppl 2):66–74, 2009.

404. Taniyama Y, Tachibana K, Hiraoka K, et al: Local delivery of plasmid DNA into rat carotid artery using ultrasound, *Circulation* 105:1233–1239, 2002.

405. Ogawa K, Tachibana K, Uchida T, et al: High-resolution scanning electron microscopic evaluation of cell-membrane porosity by ultrasound, *Med Electron Microsc* 34:249–253, 2001.

406. Mesiwala AH, Farrell L, Wenzel HJ, et al: High-intensity focused ultrasound selectively disrupts the blood-brain barrier in vivo, *Ultrasound Med Biol* 28:389–400, 2002.

407. Hynynen K, McDannold N, Vykhodtseva N, et al: Noninvasive MR imaging-guided focal opening of the blood-brain barrier in rabbits, *Radiology* 220:640–646, 2001.

408. Kinoshita M, McDannold N, Jolesz FA, et al: Targeted delivery of antibodies through the blood-brain barrier by MRI-guided focused ultrasound, *Biochem Biophys Res Commun* 340:1085–1090, 2006.

409. McDannold N, Vykhodtseva N, Hynynen K: Targeted disruption of the blood-brain barrier with focused ultrasound: Association with cavitation activity, *Phys Med Biol* 51:793–807, 2006.

410. McDannold N, Vykhodtseva N, Raymond S, et al: MRI-guided targeted blood-brain barrier disruption with focused ultrasound: Histological findings in rabbits, *Ultrasound Med Biol* 31:1527–1537, 2005.

411. Treat LH, McDannold N, Vykhodtseva N, et al: Targeted delivery of doxorubicin to the rat brain at therapeutic levels using MRI-guided focused ultrasound, *Int J Cancer* 121:901–907, 2007.

412. Sheikov N, McDannold N, Vykhodtseva N, et al: Cellular mechanisms of the blood-brain barrier opening induced by ultrasound in presence of microbubbles, *Ultrasound Med Biol* 30:979–989, 2004.

413. Sheikov N, McDannold N, Sharma S, et al: Effect of focused ultrasound applied with an ultrasound contrast agent on the tight junctional integrity of the brain microvascular endothelium, *Ultrasound Med Biol* 34:1093–1104, 2008.

414. Alonso A, Reinz E, Jenne JW, et al: Reorganization of gap junctions after focused ultrasound blood–brain barrier opening in the rat brain, *J Cereb Blood Flow Metab* 30:1394–1402, 2010.

415. Alonso A, Reinz E, Fatar M, et al: Neurons but not glial cells overexpress ubiquitin in the rat brain following focused ultrasound-induced opening of the blood-brain barrier, *Neuroscience* 169:116–124, 2010.

416. Unger EC, Hersh E, Vannan M, et al: Local drug and gene delivery through microbubbles, *Prog Cardiovasc Dis* 44:45–54, 2001.

417. Unger EC, McCreery TP, Sweitzer RH: Ultrasound enhances gene expression of liposomal transfection, *Invest Radiol* 32:723–727, 1997.

418. Fischer AJ, Stanke JJ, Omar G, et al: Ultrasound-mediated gene transfer into neuronal cells, *J Biotechnol* 122:393–411, 2006.

419. Fujii H, Sun Z, Li SH, et al: Ultrasound-targeted gene delivery induces angiogenesis after a myocardial infarction in mice, *JACC Cardiovasc Imaging* 2:869–879, 2009.

420. Shohet RV, Chen S, Zhou YT, et al: Echocardiographic destruction of albumin microbubbles directs gene delivery to the myocardium, *Circulation* 101:2554–2556, 2000.

421. Nguyen PD, O'Rear EA, Johnson AE, et al: Thrombolysis using liposomal-encapsulated streptokinase: An in vitro study, *Proc Soc Exp Biol Med* 192:261–269, 1989.

422. Heeremans JL, Prevost R, Bekkers ME, et al: Thrombolytic treatment with tissue-type plasminogen activator (t-PA) containing liposomes in rabbits: A comparison with free t-PA, *Thromb Haemost* 73:488–494, 1995.

423. Perkins WR, Vaughan DE, Plavin SR, et al: Streptokinase entrapment in interdigitation-fusion liposomes improves thrombolysis in an experimental rabbit model, *Thromb Haemost* 77:1174–1178, 1997.

424. Leach JK, O'Rear EA, Patterson E, et al: Accelerated thrombolysis in a rabbit model of carotid artery thrombosis with liposome-encapsulated and microencapsulated streptokinase, *Thromb Haemost* 90:64–70, 2003.

425. Wang SS, Chou NK, Chung TW: The t-PA-encapsulated PLGA nanoparticles shelled with CS or CS-GRGD alter both permeation through and dissolving patterns of blood clots compared with t-PA solution: An in vitro thrombolysis study, *J Biomed Mater Res A* 91:753–761, 2009.

426. Xi X, Yang F, Chen D, et al: A targeting drug-delivery model via interactions among cells and liposomes under ultrasonic excitation, *Phys Med Biol* 53:3251–3265, 2008.

427. Vandenbroucke RE, Lentacker I, Demeester J, et al: Ultrasound assisted siRNA delivery using PEG-siPlex loaded microbubbles, *J Control Release* 126:265–273, 2008.

428. Lentacker I, Vandenbroucke RE, Lucas B, et al: New strategies for nucleic acid delivery to conquer cellular and nuclear membranes, *J Control Release* 132:279–288, 2008.

429. Marsh JN, Senpan A, Hu G, et al: Fibrin-targeted perfluorocarbon nanoparticles for targeted thrombolysis, *Nanomedicine (Lond)* 2:533–543, 2007.

45

Computed Tomography–Based Evaluation of Cerebrovascular Disease

IMANUEL DZIALOWSKI, VOLKER PUETZ, RÜDIGER VON KUMMER

This chapter studies the clinical efficacy of computed tomography (CT) in patients with acute ischemic or hemorrhagic stroke. We will discuss noncontrast CT (NCT) as well as CT angiography (CTA) and CT perfusion imaging (CTP) for acute stroke. Because of the differing prognosis between anterior and posterior circulation ischemic strokes, we will separately discuss CT imaging for these. In theory, CT, like magnetic resonance imaging (MRI), can be clinically effective in patients with acute stroke on five different levels: (1) technical capacity, (2) diagnostic accuracy, (3) diagnostic impact, (4) therapeutic impact, and (5) patient outcome or prognostic impact.[1]

We will focus on the use of CT in the acute stroke setting. Whenever applicable, we will compare CT with MRI—the other important acute stroke imaging modality discussed in a separate chapter.

Noncontrast CT
Feasibility and Technical Capacity

A potential advantage of CT over MRI is its wide availability and excellent feasibility.[2] Even with older generation scanners a plain CT scan can be performed within minutes. Performing a CTA or CTP requires a spiral CT scanner, the application of contrast media, and processing afterward. Each examination will usually only require an extra 5 minutes' scan time. Recently, CT scanners with up to 320 detector rows that cover a tissue volume of 16 cm thickness have become available.[3] These scanners can examine the whole brain in less than 1 second and can repeatedly image the entire cerebral circulation, allowing time-resolved images of the brain vessels and whole brain CTP.

Detection of Infarct Core

Acute brain ischemia below the cerebral blood flow (CBF) threshold of 20 to 30 mL/100 g/min leads to loss of neurologic function, cell membrane dysfunction with cellular edema (so-called cytotoxic edema), and subsequent shrinkage of the extracellular space. This type of edema is potentially reversible and can be visualized by MRI with diffusion-weighted imaging (DWI). Acute severe brain ischemia with CBF values below 10 mL/100 g/min causes

immediate net water uptake into gray matter.[4,5] This so-called ionic edema[6] characterizes brain tissue destined for tissue necrosis, even with early reperfusion.[7] Only this net uptake of water into brain tissue causes a decrease in x-ray attenuation on CT.[4] The decrease in x-ray attenuation is linearly and indirectly correlated to the amount of water uptake. A 1% increase in tissue water causes a decrease of approximately 2 Hounsfield units (HU) in x-ray attenuation that can be detected by the human eye.[8] CT is thus a very specific method for depicting irreversible brain infarction.[9]

Early Signs of Infarction on NCT

Early changes visible on head CT during ischemia are often summarized as "early ischemic changes" (EIC). We should, however, distinguish between at least three different kinds of EIC with different pathophysiologic and diagnostic relevance:

1. Reduced x-ray attenuation of gray matter is the common cause of CT signs such as "loss of the insular or cortical ribbon," "obscuration of the lentiform nucleus," reduction in gray matter–white matter contrast, or "hypodensity." These phenomena are all consequences of ionic cerebral edema and thus represent ischemic damage (infarction) on CT (Fig. 45-1B).

2. Isolated brain tissue swelling without reduced x-ray attenuation (Fig. 45-2): this phenomenon has been extensively studied recently and is likely caused by compensatory vasodilation with an increase of cerebral blood volume (CBV).[10-12] It seems to represent tissue at risk of infarction that might be salvaged with reperfusion (ischemic penumbra). It can be observed in 10% to 20% of ischemic brain regions.[10] The presence of isolated cortical swelling on CT—even if very extensive—should NOT keep stroke neurologists from attempting urgent recanalization but should rather be taken as a challenge. It is therefore a mistake to call brain tissue swelling per se an "early CT sign of infarction" and to lump this phenomenon together with ischemic x-ray hypoattenuation.

3. The hyperdense artery sign is highly specific for the presence of an intraarterial thrombus,[13] but its detection depends on the thrombus' hematocrit value, which

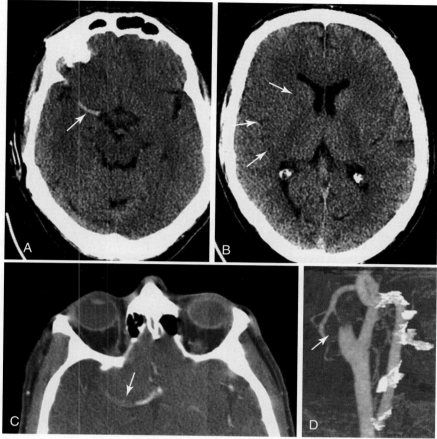

Figure 45-1   Acute middle cerebral artery (MCA) infarction in a patient with occlusion of the internal carotid artery (ICA) and MCA. A, Hyperdense MCA sign *(arrow)* on baseline noncontrast CT (NCT) scan. B, NCT with hypoattenuation of the right lentiform nucleus, head of caudate nucleus, and insula *(arrows)*. C, Intracranial CT angiography (CTA) source image showing right proximal MCA occlusion *(arrow)*. D, Extracranial CTA maximal intensity projection of the right common carotid artery, external carotid artery, and ICA showing proximal ICA occlusion.

determines its x-ray attenuation.[14] The term *EIC* should not be used for this sign because arterial obstruction by an intraluminal thrombus can be fully compensated for by collateral flow. An arterial obstruction is not a "sign" of brain ischemia but may cause brain ischemia (see Fig. 45-1A).

Diagnostic Accuracy

In the first 6 hours after ischemic stroke, two of three stroke patients will develop ionic edema that can be detected by NCT.[15] Poor sensitivity of NCT is often blamed for the fact that ischemic (i.e., ionic) edema cannot be diagnosed early in each and every patient with ischemic stroke. However, stroke symptoms occur at CBF reduction to 20 to 30 mL/100 g/min, which is well above the accepted threshold for occurrence of ionic edema. We can thus assume that around one third of ischemic stroke patients have not yet developed relevant ionic edema (i.e., no irreversible damage) and may have an excellent prognosis if reperfusion is achieved. X-ray hypoattenuation on early NCT, however, is subtle and hard to detect without training (see Fig. 45-1B). Interrater reliability for ischemic tissue hypoattenuation varies between a kappa value of 0.4 and 0.6.[16] The "sensitivity" of NCT for evidence of infarction on follow-up imaging varies between 20% and

87% depending on image quality, experience, and training.[15] Using systematic scores like the Alberta Stroke Program Early CT Score (ASPECTS) facilitates detection of x-ray hypoattenuation and improves reliability and sensitivity.[17] Once a hypoattenuating area has been detected, it is highly predictive of subsequent infarction.[9]

Diagnostic Impact

The diagnostic impact of stroke imaging refers to the proportion of patients in whom the specific diagnosis of stroke type relies on imaging. NCT has a huge diagnostic impact simply by differentiating ischemic from hemorrhagic stroke, enabling a specific therapy like thrombolysis to be administered. In addition, the extent of hypoattenuation on NCT is an important positive predictor of thrombolysis-induced brain hemorrhage, which is the most feared complication of thrombolysis.[18-20] MR DWI is highly sensitive for ischemic brain tissue, even above the CBF level of the penumbra and indicates brain tissue at high risk, if not already irreversibly injured, whereas hypoattenuation on NCT depicts irreversible tissue damage with high specificity. The detection of areas with high signal intensity on DWI may allow assessment of the pattern of affected brain territories and the cause

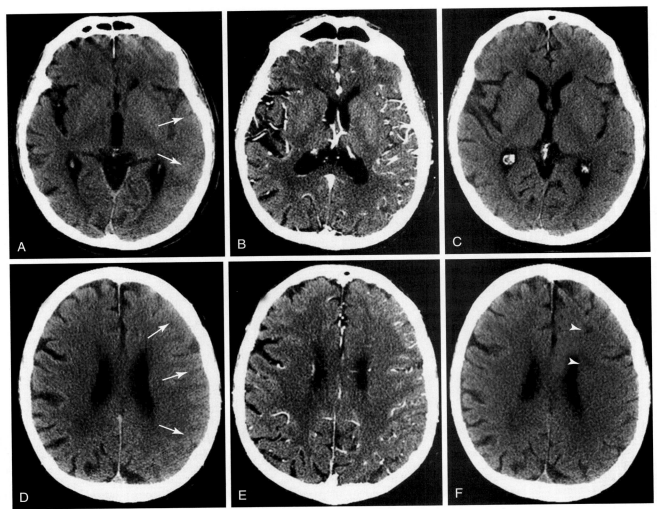

Figure 45-2 A 79-year-old man seen with acute aphasia and right-sided hemiplegia. Baseline noncontrast CT (NCT) shows hemispheric cortical swelling *(arrows)* without hypoattenuation (A, D). CT angiography demonstrates dilated cortical vessels in these regions (B, E). The patient had marked spontaneous clinical improvement. Follow-up NCT (C, F) 3 days later revealed minor infarcts in the internal borderzone *(arrowheads)* and regressive cortical swelling.

of stroke early on and signals an increased risk of stroke in patients with transient ischemic attacks (TIAs).[21]

Therapeutic Impact

In acute ischemic stroke, thrombolysis with intravenous (IV) recombinant tissue plasminogen activator (rt-PA) within 3 hours of stroke onset can increase the proportion of nondisabled patients by an absolute 13%.[22] The therapeutic time window of 3 hours may be extended in the future because treatment with IV rt-PA has recently shown a beneficial effect, that is, between 3 and 4.5 hours from symptom onset with an absolute effect size for improved functional outcome of 7%.[23] The National Institute of Neurological Disorders and Stroke (NINDS) rt-PA Study Group was able to prove benefit for thrombolysis simply by using NCT to identify ischemic stroke patients. The European Cooperative Acute Stroke Study (ECASS) investigators used NCT to additionally exclude patients with extended ischemic edema.[24] These studies show that NCT is sufficient to identify a group of

patients in whom IV thrombolytics have a moderate beneficial effect within 4.5 hours of symptom onset. Interestingly, none of the completed, large, phase III trials of IV thrombolysis selected patients on the basis of a visible arterial occlusion—the target pathology for immediate recanalizing therapies—and did not check for recanalization by treatment. Only the Prolyse in Acute Cerebral Thromboembolism (PROACT) studies investigated the therapeutic impact of thrombolysis in patients selected by angiographically proven middle cerebral artery (MCA) occlusion and slight edema on NCT.[25,26] Intraarterial infusion of prourokinase within 6 hours of symptom onset achieved an absolute effect size of 15%.

Prognostic Impact

The impact of CT on the functional outcome of stroke patients is the most important level of clinical efficacy. As shown above, NCT enables thrombolysis in ischemic stroke patients and thereby reduces long-term disability. Moreover, the information on the extent of x-ray hypoattenuation on NCT is prognostically relevant. There is good evidence that patients with extended hypoattenuation (infarction) on NCT have a poorer natural history and less chance to benefit from thrombolysis.[18,20,27]

In summary, brain tissue imaging by NCT ignores the changes above the CBF threshold of irreversible injury, with the exception of brain tissue swelling without hypoattenuation due to compensatory vasodilation. NCT has a rather low sensitivity for identifying brain ischemia but a high specificity for identifying irreversible ischemic injury. One may conclude that mainly patients who have small volumes of hypoattenuating brain tissue on NCT but severe symptoms will benefit from reperfusion therapy. In fact, several studies have demonstrated that the response to thrombolytic therapy is associated with the extent of hypoattenuation on early CT.[20]

CTA
Feasibility and Technical Capacity

The advent of "helical" or "spiral" acquisition has enabled CT scanners to acquire data very rapidly. With this technique, data acquisition occurs continuously while the gantry table moves the patient through the gantry, so a volume of interest can be scanned in a relatively short time.

A CTA study of the neck and head requires about 5 minutes' examination time and the application of contrast media. Usually, an IV bolus of about 100 mL of an iodinated, nonionic and isoosmolar or low osmolar contrast agent is given, and image acquisition will be initiated when the contrast reaches the aortic arch or common carotid artery. In our experience, feasibility of CTA is excellent and images are diagnostic in almost every patient. Immediately after data acquisition, CTA source images can be viewed, and large vessel occlusions can be diagnosed instantaneously (see Fig. 45-1C). Within a few minutes, 3D reformats can be generated, enabling detection of peripheral vessel and other abnormalities (see Fig. 45-1D).

The utility of CTA is tremendous, and it has already replaced conventional catheter angiography in many situations. Recent technical development enables CTA with time-resolution (4D-CTA) and digital subtraction of the bone.

Diagnostic Accuracy

Intracranial Disease

The need for rapid decision making makes CTA an ideal technique in the detection of large vessel intracranial arterial stenosis or occlusion (see Fig. 45-1). For intracranial atherosclerotic stenosis, noninvasive imaging modalities should identify lesions with high sensitivity and specificity as compared with the gold standard of digital subtraction angiography (DSA). In the prospective Stroke Outcomes and Neuroimaging of Intracranial Atherosclerosis (SONIA) Trial, both transcranial Doppler (TCD) ultrasound and magnetic resonance angiography (MRA) noninvasively identified 50% to 99% of intracranial large vessel stenoses with a substantial negative predictive value of about 90%.[28] However, the positive predictive value (PPV) was only 36% for TCD and 59% for MRA. Thus the authors concluded that abnormal findings on TCD or MRA require a confirmatory test such as angiography to reliably identify stenosis.

Compared with MRA, CTA has increased sensitivity (70% versus 98%, respectively) and PPV (65% versus 93%, respectively) for revealing intracranial arterial stenosis.[29] Similar results were found in a recent study, where the sensitivity of CTA to detect 50% or greater intracranial stenosis was 97.1% and the specificity was 99.5%.[30] Thus, CTA seems sufficient to detect or rule out significant intracranial atherosclerotic stenosis. We have recently used CTA to detect intracranial nonocclusive thrombi (iNOT; Fig. 45-3) in patients seen with acute ischemic stroke and TIAs.[31] These thrombi seem to be rare (2.7% of patients in our study) but indicate stroke patients with increased risk of clinical deterioration during the hospital course.

CTA also has excellent accuracy in detecting intracranial arterial occlusion. Lev et al[32] studied 44 consecutive patients with acute ischemic stroke who underwent CTA of the circle of Willis within 6 hours of onset of symptoms. A total of 572 vessels was evaluated, and angiographic correlation was available for 224 of these vessels. Sensitivity and specificity of CTA were both 98%, and accuracy was 99%. The mean time for CTA reconstruction was 15 minutes. The results of Lev et al have been confirmed by a study by Nguyen-Huynh et al,[30] in which

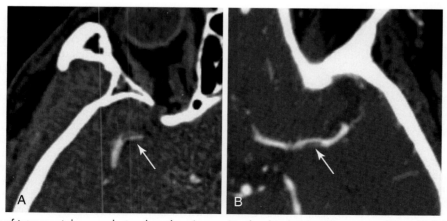

Figure 45-3 Example of intracranial nonocclusive thrombus (arrows) in the distal right M1 segment (A) and left M1 segment (B).

both the sensitivity and specificity of CTA to detect large artery intracranial occlusion were 100%.

As an additional prognostic factor and for the purpose of immediate treatment decisions, the intracranial thrombus extent can be estimated with CTA. Patients' prognoses and responses to therapy can be judged by a 10-point clot burden score (CBS; Fig. 45-4). CBS is a simple measure of the location and extent of intracranial thrombus.[33] Patients with a higher thrombus burden (i.e., lower CBS scores) had higher baseline Institutes of Health Stroke Scale (NIHSS) scores and more extended infarctions compared with patients with less thrombus burden. Moreover, CBS was an independent predictor of independent functional outcomes and death in this study. These results have been confirmed in a recent study by Tan et al.[34] Their study also demonstrated a correlation of CBS with the perfusion defects on CTP maps and CTA source images and confirmed the hypothesis that a higher thrombus burden is associated with lower recanalization rates with IV thrombolysis.[34,35]

In summary, CTA is an ideal tool for the rapid and accurate detection of intracranial stenosis and occlusion of major intracranial arteries and may help to differentiate patients who will benefit from specific recanalization techniques.

Extracranial Carotid Artery Disease

Cerebral angiography has been the diagnostic procedure of choice for the quantification of extracranial carotid artery stenosis. Although generally safe, angiography is still associated with a 0.5% to 5% rate of stroke as a complication when used in routine clinical practice.[36,37] With the advent of ultrafast helical CT imaging, the complication is avoided, and CTA is being used with increasing frequency in the diagnosis of extracranial carotid artery disease. An example of severe right internal carotid stenosis is depicted in Fig. 45-5A, on conventional arteriography, and in Fig. 45-5B, on CTA (axial cuts).

Several studies to date have reported excellent agreement between conventional catheter cerebral angiography and CTA. In a comparative study of CTA, conventional angiography, and MRA, a strong correlation was found between CTA and angiography ($r = 0.987$; $P < 0.0001$) in 128 carotid bifurcations in 64 patients.[38] CTA has the additional benefit of providing precise information regarding the surrounding vascular and bony anatomy, including arterial wall calcification that is not depicted by DSA or MRA.

In a prospective study, 40 patients (80 carotid arteries) underwent evaluation by CTA, digital DSA, and Doppler ultrasonography.[39] The overall correlation between Doppler ultrasonography and DSA was less robust ($r = 0.808$) than that between CTA and DSA ($r = 0.92$); CTA provided superb correlation in the detection of mild stenosis (0% to 29%), stenosis greater than 50%, and carotid occlusion and had sensitivities and specificities exceeding 0.90. CTA performed less well in the detection of 70% to 99% stenosis and had a sensitivity of 0.73 (axial source images) and a PPV of only 0.62 (negative predictive value, 0.95). The relatively poorer degree of discrimination on CTA in this study between moderate (50% to 69%) and severe (70% to 99%) stenosis is an important limiting factor to consider in the use of this technology. It is hoped that further prospective data acquisition with simultaneous 320-slice technology will shed additional light on this issue.

Detection of Infarct Core

In addition to providing information on the vessel status, CTA may also predict the fate of ischemic brain parenchyma; that is, it improves early detection of ischemic infarction.[40] Viewing the CTA source images at a low contrast and window level (e.g., 40/40 HU) downstream to a large vessel occlusion, CTA will show an area of diminished tissue contrast enhancement (Figs. 45-6 and 45-7). This area likely represents severely hypoperfused brain tissue that will be irreversibly damaged without reperfusion. In comparison with NCT, the sensitivity and accuracy in prediction of final infarct extension can be improved.[41,42] CTA source images closely correlated to MR DWI sequences.[43]

Diagnostic Impact

The diagnostic impact of CTA is probably still underestimated. Within minutes, CTA reliably diagnoses arterial occlusions and stenoses from the aortic arch to the distal intracranial arterial segments. Compared with MRI, CTA is sensitive for calcified plaques and can thus elucidate the underlying stroke etiology in many cases. It was already shown that patients with MCA occlusion have a lesser chance to benefit from IV thrombolytics if the ipsilateral carotid is obstructed.[44] A systematic study of arterial pathology with CTA may enable more specific treatments of arterial occlusions. In addition, CTA can distinguish patients seen with seizures and postictal paresis (Todd's paralysis) from those with true ischemic hemiparesis and early seizures by demonstrating arterial occlusion.[45]

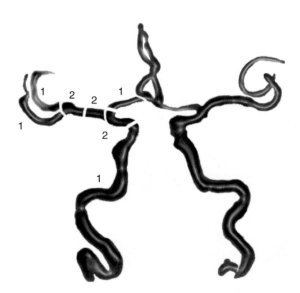

Figure 45-4 A 10-point clot burden score (CBS): 1 or 2 points each (as indicated) are subtracted for absent contrast opacification on CT angiography in the infraclinoid internal carotid artery (ICA) (1), supraclinoid ICA (2), proximal M1 segment (2), distal M1 segment (2), M2 branches (1 each) and A1 segment (1). The CBS score applies only to the symptomatic hemisphere.

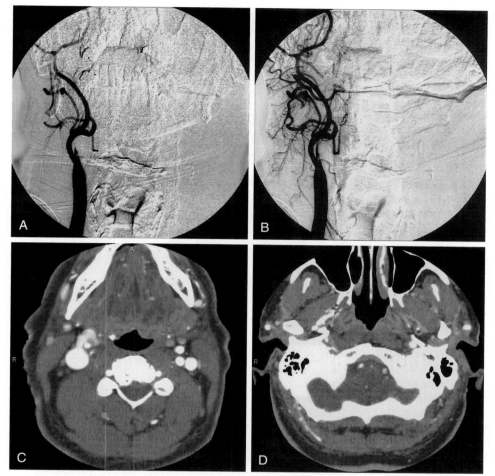

Figure 45-5 Conventional angiographic depiction (A, B) of right internal carotid artery occlusion in a patient seen with an acute ischemic right middle cerebral artery distribution infarction. CT angiography source images (C, D) confirm right ICA occlusion *(arrow)*.

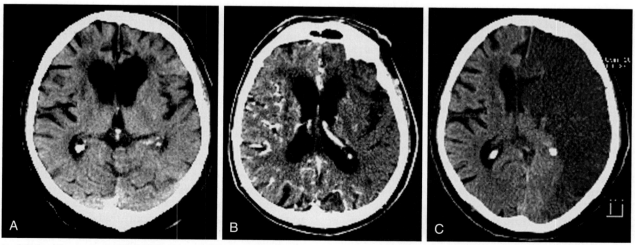

Figure 45-6 Noncontrast CT (NCT) (A) and CT angiography (CTA) source images (B) of a patient 1 hour after acute aphasia and right hemiparesis. NCT shows subtle hypoattenuation of left basal ganglia, insula, and anterior cerebral artery (ACA) territory. CTA clearly shows contrast hypoattenuation in the complete middle cerebral artery and ACA territory caused by an internal carotid artery occlusion. Follow- up CT (C) shows the resulting infarction.

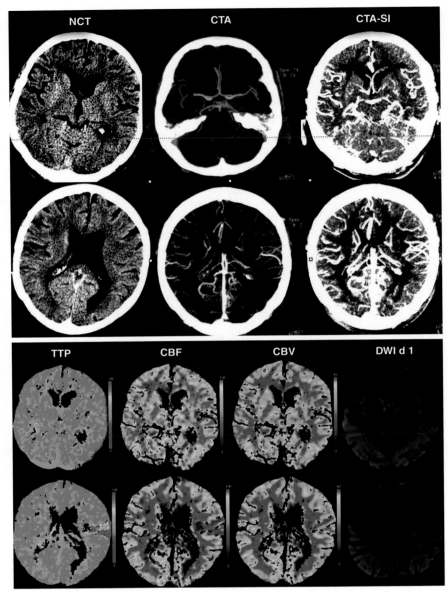

Figure 45-7 Noncontrast CT (NCT), CT angiography (CTA), and CT perfusion imaging (CTA-SI) of an 82-year-old patient 2 hours after aphasia and mild right hemiparesis. NCT and CTA results are normal without evidence of intracranial arterial occlusion *(upper two rows)*. Time-to-peak (TTP) and cerebral blood flow (CBF) parameter maps reveal hypoperfusion in the left insula and corona radiata without reduction of cerebral blood volume (CBV, *lower two rows*). After thrombolysis with recombinant tissue plasminogen activator (rt-PA), follow-up MRI-diffusion-weighted imaging (DWI) shows a tiny infarction in the left insula.

Therapeutic Impact

The usefulness of CTA for therapeutic decision making has not yet been prospectively studied. There is evidence from secondary analyses of randomized trials that patients with a small core of infarction on NCT (or possibly CTA source images) and an intracranial large vessel occlusion on CTA might be ideal candidates for recanalization, even beyond the accepted time window.[46] This hypothesis is currently being studied in at least two large, randomized controlled trials.[47]

Many centers use CTA to select acute ischemic stroke patients for intraarterial interventions. The PROACT II study demonstrated that patients with an MCA occlusion benefit from intraarterial thrombolysis up to 6 hours after onset.[25] Another approach for patients with known intracranial occlusions is the intravenous–intraarterial bridging concept. The Interventional Management of Stroke III trial currently investigates whether this strategy is superior to standard IV thrombolysis.[47] Potentially, patients with proximal arterial occlusion (e.g., carotid T occlusion) and/or large thrombus burden may benefit from additional intraarterial therapy, whereas patients with minor thrombus burden (e.g., MCA M2 branch occlusion) may have no additional benefit. Estimation of thrombus burden with a CBS could be a simple and readily available tool to help in deciding whether a patient will benefit from aggressive treatment paradigms.

CTA might also be useful for excluding patients without visible arterial occlusion from thrombolysis. Angiographic studies have shown that no arterial occlusion can be detected in one third of patients seen within 6 hours of onset.[48] A systematic comparison of the efficacy of thrombolysis in acute ischemic stroke patients with arterial occlusion versus those without arterial occlusion, however, has not yet been performed.

CT Perfusion Imaging
Technical Capacity and Feasibility

With the development of helical CT scanning technology, it is now possible to track a bolus of IV contrast material as it passes through the brain. The measurement technique for CBF has its theoretical basis in the central volume principle,[49] which relates CBF (mL/100g/min), CBV (mL/100 g), and mean transit time (MTT; seconds) by the following equation:

$$CBF = \frac{CBV}{MTT}$$

It is assumed that a linear relationship exists between the CT enhancement and the concentration of contrast material within brain tissue and arteries. After IV administration of a bolus of iodinated contrast agent, measurements are made of the arterial enhancement curve, $C_a(t)$, the supplying artery, and the tissue enhancement curve, $Q(t)$, for a region of the central parenchyma. For the calculation of MTT, a mathematical process of deconvolution is applied to the functions $C_a(t)$ and $Q(t)$ to determine an impulse function, $R(t)$, which would be the theoretical tissue enhancement curve obtained from a rapidly injected bolus of contrast material. The MTT is calculated from the following formula:

$$MTT = \frac{\text{area underneath } R(t)}{\text{height of } R(t) \text{ plateau}}$$

CBV is calculated from $Q(t)$ and $C_a(t)$, the two parameters measured directly during the CTP study:

$$CBV = \frac{\text{area underneath } Q(t)}{\text{area underneath } C_a(t)}$$

Although this technique is rapidly evolving, difficulties remain and include patient motion artifacts, partial averaging effects, effects of drawing regions of interest (ROIs) directly over arterial vessels, and the proper selection of the arterial input vessel to yield the most accurate results. Another still significant limitation is the incomplete coverage of the volume of brain tissue scanned during contrast passage. Depending on the CT manufacturer, only about 2 to 4 cm (craniocaudal extension) of brain tissue can be covered. This volume is usually placed at the level of the basal ganglia so that perfusion of all major supratentorial vascular territories can be captured. New-generation CT scanners with up to 320 detector rows will provide whole-brain perfusion images.

Attempts at quantitative validation of this technology in humans through comparison with other techniques, such as xenon-CT, are ongoing.[50,51]

Diagnostic Accuracy

CTP parameter maps improve diagnostic accuracy for tissue at risk and irreversibly damaged brain tissue.[42,50,52,53] For example, Lin et al studied 28 patients with multimodal CT seen with territorial infarction within 3 hours of symptom onset and assessed 280 ASPECTS regions for a relative CBV reduction. They found a 91% sensitivity and 100% specificity for predicting a DWI lesion on follow-up imaging.[52] Parsons et al[42] showed that CBV best predicts final infarct extent in patients with major reperfusion, whereas CBF and MTT were the best predictor of final infarct size in patients without reperfusion. In some patients with MCA branch or other distal intracranial occlusions not recognized on CTA, time-to-peak (TTP) or MTT parameter maps are helpful in identifying the presence and site of occlusion (Fig. 45-7).

Diagnostic Impact

CTP facilitates and improves identification of the infarct core and has the potential to identify tissue at risk. Acute multimodal CT imaging is limited in detecting small ischemic lesions. In patients with normal NCT, CTA, and CTP findings but persistent neurologic deficit, immediate MR DWI will usually show one or multiple small ischemic lesions, for example, in the brainstem or one that is bihemispheric. In patients without a DWI lesion an ischemic cause becomes very unlikely.

Therapeutic and Prognostic Impact

The therapeutic impact of CTP is still unclear. Acute stroke patients presenting within 4 to 5 hours of symptom onset should not be excluded from thrombolysis on the grounds of CTP imaging findings. In patients presenting beyond the accepted time window for thrombolysis, CTP might help to identify the tissue at risk, thereby facilitating decision making on late recanalization strategies.

Similar to NCT, CTP is prognostically relevant because it identifies the core of infarction. Patients with an extensive CBV lesion have reduced chances of achieving an independent functional outcome.[42,54]

Limitations of a Multimodal CT Protocol

Before initiation of a multimodal CT examination, the following contraindications should be kept in mind: known renal insufficiency, contrast media allergy, hyperthyroidism, medication with the oral antidiabetic metformin, and pregnancy. Because acute ischemic stroke with the option of thrombolysis is an emergency, waiting for laboratory results such as serum creatinine level should not delay the performance of CT. The risk of developing relevant radiocontrast media nephropathy in acute stroke patients seems to be reasonably low (<0.5%).[55,56] In patients taking metformin, the serum creatinine level should be checked at baseline and up to 3 days after the examination so that metformin accumulation with subsequent lactate acidosis is avoided.

Depending on the CT manufacturer, data on the effective radiation dose varies between 5 and 10 mSv. A relevant individual risk of radiation-induced intracranial neoplasm seems only to exist in children.[57] Because of the rapidly increasing frequency of CT examinations, however, there is a cumulative risk that should not be neglected.

Posterior Circulation CT Imaging
Ischemic Stroke

About 20% of cerebrovascular ischemic events involve the posterior circulation.[58] Clinical signs and symptoms are frequently less specific compared with anterior circulation stroke. Isolated transient loss-of-consciousness or dizziness can be misattributed to vertebrobasilar ischemia, whereas many cases of true vertebrobasilar ischemia remain undiagnosed.[59] However, similar to anterior circulation stroke, early diagnosis is crucial for initiating systemic thrombolysis or mechanical revascularization procedures. The relevance of acute brain imaging with CT is to reliably rule out intracranial hemorrhaging and to identify patients with basilar artery occlusion. Latter patients have a devastating prognosis: nearly 80% die or are severely disabled if treated conservatively.[60]

The sensitivity of DWI for identifying final infarction is better than NCT in posterior circulation ischemia.[61] This is relevant in differentiating cerebral ischemic events from other disease entities with similar clinical symptomatology (e.g., basilar migraine or vestibular neuritis). The reliability of CT to detect hypodensity in the posterior circulation is limited by bony and beam hardening artifacts in the posterior fossa. Newer-generation CT scanners with helical scan techniques seem to diminish this limitation[62] but have not been analyzed systematically. The sensitivity for detection of a final infarct in the posterior circulation is improved with CTA source images compared with NCT (Fig. 45-8).[63] Studies comparing the sensitivity of CTA source images with MR DWI have not been performed.

A hyperdense basilar artery sign[64] (see Fig. 45-8) and a hyperdense posterior cerebral artery sign[65] specifically indicate occlusion of these arteries. By application of CTA, vertebrobasilar occlusion can be diagnosed with high sensitivity and specificity.[32] In the study by Lev et al, the diagnostic accuracy of CTA was 96% for vertebral artery occlusion and 100% for basilar artery occlusion. Thus, in a patient with patency of the basilar artery on CTA, the diagnosis of symptomatic basilar artery occlusion can be excluded. In contrast, evidence of basilar artery occlusion on CTA should immediately prompt recanalization strategies. In patients with clinically suspected posterior circulation ischemia, both basilar artery occlusion and vertebral artery occlusion on CTA are predictors of increased risk of mortality and poorer functional outcome.[66]

In contrast to anterior circulation stroke, posterior circulation stroke currently has limited imaging-based selection criteria for identifying patients who may benefit from thrombolysis. Multimodal CT and MRI have only been analyzed in smaller patient series. Demonstration of small DWI lesions or a diffusion–perfusion mismatch have been proposed for identifying patients with basilar artery occlusion who may potentially benefit from thrombolysis.[24,67] A TTP delay in the posterior cerebral artery territory on CTP parameter maps indicates vertebrobasilar

occlusion.[68] The therapeutic and prognostic implications of these techniques for patients with posterior circulation strokes need to be studied.

Quantification of CTA source image hypoattenuation in the posterior circulation with a systematic score, the posterior circulation Acute Stroke Prognosis Early CT Score, identified patients with basilar artery occlusion who were unlikely to have a favorable functional outcome despite recanalization of the basilar artery.[63] In a similar study, CTA source image hypoattenuation in the mesencephalon and pons indicated patients with basilar artery occlusion and poor functional outcomes.[69] Both studies demonstrate that CTA source image hypoattenuation can identify areas with ischemic changes in the posterior circulation, including the brainstem. Moreover, this information has prognostic relevance in patients with basilar artery occlusion. However, these findings need to be validated prospectively and should not currently influence immediate treatment decision making in patients with posterior circulation strokes, particularly for those with basilar artery occlusion.

NCT and CTA in Acute Hemorrhagic Stroke

NCT is the imaging modality of choice in the diagnosis of acute intracerebral hemorrhage. It seems to easily detect the hyperdense (60 to 80 HU) appearance of a fresh blood clot. Studies on the reliability and validity of this finding have not, however, been performed. The conditions under which intracerebral blood is not hyperdense on CT are not well studied. Low hematocrit levels and impairment of clotting may be possible conditions. CT is as sensitive and specific as MRI in detecting acute intracranial hemorrhage. CT is less sensitive in detecting subacute or old intracerebral hematomas.[70] The location of intracerebral hematoma is key in determining etiology. A deep (or basal ganglia) intracerebral hemorrhage is usually hyperdense, as are thalamic, pontine, or cerebellar locations. Lobar hematomas may be caused by sinus thrombosis, arteriovenous malformations, brain tumors, or coagulation disorders, including therapeutic anticoagulation.

The utility of CTA after NCT has shown intracerebral hemorrhage is tremendous and might replace catheter angiography in the future. Cerebral aneurysms can be diagnosed accurately down to a diameter of 2 mm.[71] Similarly, arteriovenous malformations and venous thrombosis can be diagnosed in many cases.

Approximately 30% of acute hemorrhagic stroke patients show evidence of hematoma growth within the first hours after onset.[72] This increase in hematoma size is a key factor in predicting a poor prognosis for the disease. When CTA source images are used, it is possible to predict hematoma growth early on. The so-called spot sign characterizes a leak of contrast media that is clearly hyperdense in relation to the surrounding hematoma. Wada et al[73] found the spot sign in 13 of 39 patients (33%) with acute intracerebral hemorrhage within the first 3 hours. The presence of the spot sign was significantly correlated with a poor functional outcome. Several studies are currently testing the predictive value of this sign, and further studies are planned to investigate whether patients with a positive spot sign will respond to factor VIIa therapy.

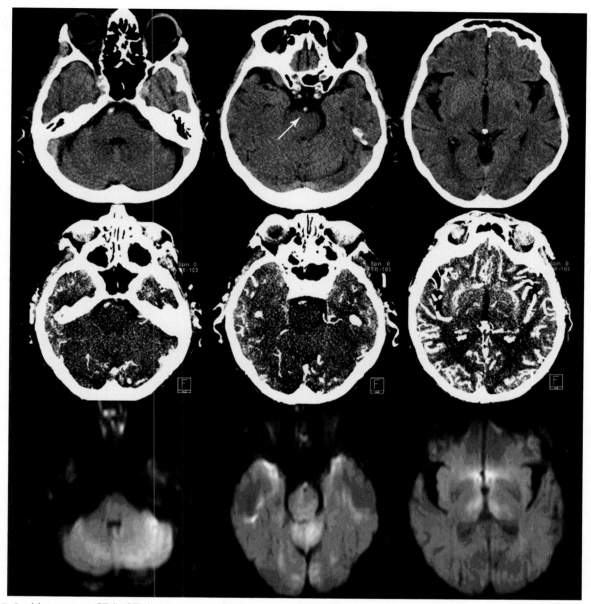

Figure 45-8 Noncontrast CT (NCT) *(upper row)* and CT angiography (CTA) source images *(middle row)* of a patient with acute basilar artery occlusion 3.5 hours and 4.5 hours after symptom onset, respectively. NCT demonstrates hyperdense basilar artery sign *(arrow)* but does not reveal early ischemic changes. CTA source images demonstrate hypoattenuation in all posterior circulation territories (posterior circulation Acute Stroke Prognosis Early CT Score [pc-ASPECTS] = 0). The patient was treated with systemic thrombolysis with alteplase. Diffusion-weighted MRI *(lower row)* performed after thrombolysis (6.5 hours after symptom onset) demonstrates lesions in the same territories (pc-ASPECTS = 0). (Images courtesy of the Seaman Family MR Research Centre, University of Calgary, Canada.)

Acknowledgment

We would like to acknowledge Charles A. Jungreis and Steven Goldstein for their work on the previous edition of this chapter.

REFERENCES

1. Kent DL, Larson EB: Disease, level of impact, and quality of research methods. Three dimensions of clinical efficacy assessment applied to magnetic resonance imaging, *Invest Radiol* 27:245-254, 1992.
2. Hand PJ, Wardlaw JM, Rowat AM, et al: Magnetic resonance brain imaging in patients with acute stroke: Feasibility and patient related difficulties, *J Neurol Neurosurg Psychiatry* 76:1525-1527, 2005.
3. Murayama K, Katada K, Nakane M, et al: Whole-brain perfusion CT performed with a prototype 256-detector row CT system: Initial experience, *Radiology* 250:202-211, 2009.
4. Schuier FJ, Hossmann KA: Experimental brain infarcts in cats. II. Ischemic brain edema, *Stroke* 11:593-601, 1980.
5. Todd NV, Picozzi P, Crockard HA, et al: Reperfusion after cerebral ischemia: Influence of duration of ischemia, *Stroke* 17:460-466, 1986.
6. Simard JM, Kent TA, Chen M, et al: Brain oedema in focal ischaemia: Molecular pathophysiology and theoretical implications, *Lancet Neurol* 6:258-268, 2007.
7. Dzialowski I, Klotz E, Goericke S, et al: Ischemic brain tissue water content: CT monitoring during middle cerebral artery occlusion and reperfusion in rats, *Radiology* 243:720-726, 2007.

8. Dzialowski I, Weber J, Doerfler A, et al: Brain tissue water uptake after middle cerebral artery occlusion assessed with CT, *J Neuroimaging* 14:42-48, 2004.

9. von Kummer R, Bourquain H, Bastianello S, et al: Early prediction of irreversible brain damage after ischemic stroke at CT, *Radiology* 219:95-100, 2001.

10. Na DG, Kim EY, Ryoo JW, et al: CT sign of brain swelling without concomitant parenchymal hypoattenuation: Comparison with diffusion- and perfusion-weighted MR imaging, *Radiology* 235:948-992, 2005.

11. Parsons MW, Pepper EM, Bateman GA, et al: Identification of the penumbra and infarct core on hyperacute noncontrast and perfusion CT, *Neurology* 68:730-736, 2007.

12. Butcher KS, Lee SB, Parsons MW, et al: Differential prognosis of isolated cortical swelling and hypoattenuation on CT in acute stroke, *Stroke* 38:941-947, 2007.

13. von Kummer R, Meyding-Lamade U, Forsting M, et al: Sensitivity and prognostic value of early CT in occlusion of the middle cerebral artery trunk, *AJNR Am J Neuroradiol* 15:9-15, 1994:discussion 16-18.

14. Kirchhof K, Welzel T, Mecke C, et al: Differentiation of white, mixed, and red thrombi: Value of CT in estimation of the prognosis of thrombolysis phantom study, *Radiology* 228:126-130, 2003.

15. Wardlaw JM, Mielke O: Early signs of brain infarction at CT: Observer reliability and outcome after thrombolytic treatment—systematic review, *Radiology* 235:444-453, 2005.

16. Marks MP, Holmgren EB, Fox AJ, et al: Evaluation of early computed tomographic findings in acute ischemic stroke, *Stroke* 30:389-392, 1999.

17. Barber PA, Demchuk AM, Zhang J, et al: Validity and reliability of a quantitative computed tomography score in predicting outcome of hyperacute stroke before thrombolytic therapy, *Lancet* 355:1670-1674, 2000.

18. Dzialowski I, Hill MD, Coutts SB, et al: Extent of early ischemic changes on computed tomography (CT) before thrombolysis: Prognostic value of the Alberta Stroke Program Early CT Score in ECASS II, *Stroke* 37:973-978, 2006.

19. Lansberg MG, Albers GW, Wijman CA: Symptomatic intracerebral hemorrhage following thrombolytic therapy for acute ischemic stroke: A review of the risk factors, *Cerebrovasc Dis* 24:1-10, 2007.

20. von Kummer R, Allen KL, Holle R, et al: Acute stroke: Usefulness of early CT findings before thrombolytic therapy, *Radiology* 205:327-333, 1997.

21. Coutts SB, Simon JE, Eliasziw M, et al: Triaging transient ischemic attack and minor stroke patients using acute magnetic resonance imaging, *Ann Neurol* 57:848-854, 2005.

22. Tissue plasminogen activator for acute ischemic stroke: The National Institute of Neurological Disorders and Stroke rt-Pa Stroke Study Group, *N Engl J Med* 333:1581-1587, 1995.

23. Hacke W, Kaste M, Bluhmki E, et al: Thrombolysis with alteplase 3 to 4.5 hours after acute ischemic stroke, *N Engl J Med* 359:1317-1329, 2008.

24. Ostrem JL, Saver JL, Alger JR, et al: Acute basilar artery occlusion: Diffusion-perfusion MRI characterization of tissue salvage in patients receiving intra-arterial stroke therapies, *Stroke* 35:e30-e34, 2004.

25. Furlan A, Higashida R, Wechsler L, et al: Intra-arterial prourokinase for acute ischemic stroke. The PROACT II Study: A randomized controlled trial. Prolyse in acute cerebral thromboembolism, *JAMA* 282:2003-2011, 1999.

26. del Zoppo GJ, Higashida RT, Furlan AJ, et al: PROACT: A phase II randomized trial of recombinant pro-urokinase by direct arterial delivery in acute middle cerebral artery stroke. PROACT investigators. Prolyse in acute cerebral thromboembolism, *Stroke* 29:4-11, 1998.

27. Hill MD, Buchan AM: Thrombolysis for acute ischemic stroke: Results of the Canadian Alteplase For Stroke Effectiveness Study, *CMAJ* 172:1307-1312, 2005.

28. Feldmann E, Wilterdink JL, Kosinski A, et al: The stroke outcomes and neuroimaging of intracranial atherosclerosis (SONIA) trial, *Neurology* 68:2099-2106, 2007.

29. Bash S, Villablanca JP, Jahan R, et al: Intracranial vascular stenosis and occlusive disease: Evaluation with CT angiography, MR angiography, and digital subtraction angiography, *AJNR Am J Neuroradiol* 26:1012-1021, 2005.

30. Nguyen-Huynh MN, Wintermark M, English J, et al: How accurate is CT angiography in evaluating intracranial atherosclerotic disease? *Stroke* 39:1184-1188, 2008.

31. Puetz V, Dzialowski I, Coutts SB, et al: Frequency and clinical course of stroke and transient ischemic attack patients with intracranial nonocclusive thrombus on computed tomographic angiography, *Stroke* 40:193-199, 2009.

32. Lev MH, Farkas J, Rodriguez VR, et al: CT angiography in the rapid triage of patients with hyperacute stroke to intraarterial thrombolysis: Accuracy in the detection of large vessel thrombus, *J Comput Assist Tomogr* 25:520-528, 2001.

33. Puetz V, Dzialowski I, Hill MD, et al: Intracranial thrombus extent predicts clinical outcome, final infarct size and hemorrhagic transformation in ischemic stroke: The clot burden score, *Int J Stroke* 3:230-236, 2008.

34. Tan IY, Demchuk AM, Hopyan J, et al: CT angiography clot burden score and collateral score: Correlation with clinical and radiologic outcomes in acute middle cerebral artery infarct, *AJNR Am J Neuroradiol* 30:525-531, 2009.

35. Lee KY, Han SW, Kim SH, et al: Early recanalization after intravenous administration of recombinant tissue plasminogen activator as assessed by pre- and post-thrombolytic angiography in acute ischemic stroke patients, *Stroke* 38:192-193, 2007.

36. Mamourian A, Drayer BP: Clinically silent infarcts shown by MR after cerebral angiography, *AJNR Am J Neuroradiol* 11:1084, 1990.

37. Johnston DC, Chapman KM, Goldstein LB: Low rate of complications of cerebral angiography in routine clinical practice, *Neurology* 57:2012-2014, 2001.

38. Sameshima T, Futami S, Morita Y, et al: Clinical usefulness of and problems with three-dimensional CT angiography for the evaluation of arteriosclerotic stenosis of the carotid artery: Comparison with conventional angiography, MRA, and ultrasound sonography, *Surg Neurol* 51:301-308, 1999:discussion 308-309.

39. Anderson GB, Ashforth R, Steinke DE, et al: CT angiography for the detection and characterization of carotid artery bifurcation disease, *Stroke* 31:2168-2174, 2000.

40. Ezzeddine MA, Lev MH, McDonald CT, et al: CT angiography with whole brain perfused blood volume imaging: Added clinical value in the assessment of acute stroke, *Stroke* 33:959-966, 2002.

41. Coutts SB, Lev MH, Eliasziw M, et al: Aspects on CTA source images versus unenhanced CT: Added value in predicting final infarct extent and clinical outcome, *Stroke* 35:2472-2476, 2004.

42. Parsons MW, Pepper EM, Chan V, et al: Perfusion computed tomography: Prediction of final infarct extent and stroke outcome, *Ann Neurol* 58:672-679, 2005.

43. Schramm P, Schellinger PD, Klotz E, et al: Comparison of perfusion computed tomography and computed tomography angiography source images with perfusion-weighted imaging and diffusion-weighted imaging in patients with acute stroke of less than 6 hours' duration, *Stroke* 35:1652-1658, 2004.

44. Rubiera M, Ribo M, Delgado-Mederos R, et al: Tandem internal carotid artery/middle cerebral artery occlusion: An independent predictor of poor outcome after systemic thrombolysis, *Stroke* 37:2301-2305, 2006.

45. Sylaja PN, Dzialowski I, Krol A, et al: Role of CT angiography in thrombolysis decision-making for patients with presumed seizure at stroke onset, *Stroke* 37:915-917, 2006.

46. Hill MD, Rowley HA, Adler F, et al: Selection of acute ischemic stroke patients for intra-arterial thrombolysis with pro-urokinase by using ASPECTS, *Stroke* 34:1925-1931, 2003.

47. Khatri P, Hill MD, Palesch YY, et al: Methodology of the interventional management of stroke III trial, *Int J Stroke* 3:130-137, 2008.

48. Kassem-Moussa H, Graffagnino C: Nonocclusion and spontaneous recanalization rates in acute ischemic stroke: A review of cerebral angiography studies, *Arch Neurol* 59:1870-1873, 2002.

49. Meier P, Zierler KL: On the theory of the indicator-dilution method for measurement of blood flow and volume, *J Appl Physiol* 6:731-744, 1954.

50. Murphy BD, Fox AJ, Lee DH, et al: Identification of penumbra and infarct in acute ischemic stroke using computed tomography perfusion-derived blood flow and blood volume measurements, *Stroke* 37:1771-1777, 2006.

51. Wintermark M, Thiran JP, Maeder P, et al: Simultaneous measurement of regional cerebral blood flow by perfusion CT and stable xenon CT: A validation study, *AJNR Am J Neuroradiol* 22:905-914, 2001.

52. Lin K, Rapalino O, Law M, et al: Accuracy of the Alberta Stroke Program Early CT Score during the first 3 hours of middle cerebral artery stroke: Comparison of noncontrast CT, CT angiography source images, and CT perfusion, *AJNR Am J Neuroradiol* 29: 931–936, 2008.

53. Tan JC, Dillon WP, Liu S, et al: Systematic comparison of perfusion-CT and CT-angiography in acute stroke patients, *Ann Neurol* 61:533–543, 2007.

54. Gasparotti R, Grassi M, Mardighian D, et al: Perfusion CT in patients with acute ischemic stroke treated with intra-arterial thrombolysis: Predictive value of infarct core size on clinical outcome, *AJNR Am J Neuroradiol* 30:722–727, 2009.

55. Krol AL, Dzialowski I, Roy J, et al: Incidence of radiocontrast nephropathy in patients undergoing acute stroke computed tomography angiography, *Stroke* 38:2364–2366, 2007.

56. Josephson SA, Dillon WP, Smith WS: Incidence of contrast nephropathy from cerebral CT angiography and CT perfusion imaging, *Neurology* 64:1805–1806, 2005.

57. Brenner DJ, Hall EJ: Computed tomography—an increasing source of radiation exposure, *N Engl J Med* 357:2277–2284, 2007.

58. Savitz SI, Caplan LR: Vertebrobasilar disease, *N Engl J Med* 352:2618–2626, 2005.

59. Ferro JM, Pinto AN, Falcao I, et al: Diagnosis of stroke by the non-neurologist. A validation study, *Stroke* 29:1106–1109, 1998.

60. Schonewille WJ, Algra A, Serena J, et al: Outcome in patients with basilar artery occlusion treated conventionally, *J Neurol Neurosurg Psychiatry* 76:1238–1241, 2005.

61. Muir KW, Buchan A, von Kummer R, et al: Imaging of acute stroke, *Lancet Neurol* 5:755–768, 2006.

62. Schulte-Altedorneburg G, Bruckmann H: [Imaging techniques in diagnosis of brainstem infarction], *Nervenarzt* 77:731–743, 2006:quiz 744.

63. Puetz V, Sylaja PN, Coutts SB, et al: Extent of hypoattenuation on CT angiography source images predicts functional outcome in patients with basilar artery occlusion, *Stroke* 39:2485–2490, 2008.

64. Vonofakos D, Marcu H, Hacker H: CT diagnosis of basilar artery occlusion, *AJNR Am J Neuroradiol* 4:525–528, 1983.

65. Krings T, Noelchen D, Mull M, et al: The hyperdense posterior cerebral artery sign: A computed tomography marker of acute ischemia in the posterior cerebral artery territory, *Stroke* 37:399–403, 2006.

66. Sylaja PN, Puetz V, Dzialowski I, et al: Prognostic value of CT angiography in patients with suspected vertebrobasilar ischemia, *J Neuroimaging* 18:46–49, 2008.

67. Renard D, Landragin N, Robinson A, et al: MRI-based score for acute basilar artery thrombosis, *Cerebrovasc Dis* 25:511–516, 2008.

68. Nagahori T, Hirashima Y, Umemura K, et al: Supratentorial dynamic computed tomography for the diagnosis of vertebrobasilar ischemic stroke, *Neurol Med Chir (Tokyo)* 44:105–110, 2004:discussion 110–101.

69. Schaefer PW, Yoo AJ, Bell D, et al: CT angiography-source image hypoattenuation predicts clinical outcome in posterior circulation strokes treated with intra-arterial therapy, *Stroke* 39:3107–3109, 2008.

70. Kidwell CS, Chalela JA, Saver JL, et al: Comparison of MRI and CT for detection of acute intracerebral hemorrhage, *JAMA* 292: 1823–1830, 2004.

71. Chen W, Wang J, Xin W, et al: Accuracy of 16-row multislice computed tomographic angiography for assessment of small cerebral aneurysms, *Neurosurgery* 62:113–121, 2008:discussion 121–112.

72. Brott T, Broderick J, Kothari R, et al: Early hemorrhage growth in patients with intracerebral hemorrhage, *Stroke* 28:1–5, 1997.

73. Wada R, Aviv RI, Fox AJ, et al: CT angiography "spot sign" predicts hematoma expansion in acute intracerebral hemorrhage, *Stroke* 38:1257–1262, 2007.

46

Magnetic Resonance Imaging of Cerebrovascular Diseases

STEVEN WARACH, ALISON E. BAIRD, KRISHNA A. DANI, MAX WINTERMARK, CHELSEA S. KIDWELL

Nuclear magnetic resonance techniques were first employed in the 1940s, and the first images were obtained in the 1970s. In the 1980s structural MRI emerged as a clinically useful diagnostic modality for stroke and other neurologic disorders.[1-5] In the detection of ischemic stroke lesions MRI is more sensitive than CT, particularly for small infarcts and in sites such as the cerebellum and brainstem and deep white matter.[6-8] In the investigation of ischemic stroke, conventional structural MRI techniques, such as T1-weighted imaging (T1WI), T2-weighted imaging (T2WI), and fluid-attenuated inversion recovery (FLAIR) imaging, begin to reliably detect ischemic parenchymal changes beyond the first 12 to 24 hours after onset. These methods can be combined with MR angiography (MRA) to noninvasively assess the intracranial and extracranial vasculature. However, within the critical first 3 to 6 hours, the period of greatest therapeutic opportunity, these methods do not adequately assess the extent and severity of ischemic changes.

The 1990s witnessed the development of reliable imaging of ischemic events within the first 6 hours from onset. Diffusion-weighted imaging (DWI) sequences have been developed that are sensitive to the self-diffusion of water and early ischemic changes,[9,10] as have contrast-based perfusion-sensitive techniques that delineate hemodynamic changes.[11,12] These techniques were recognized for their potential clinical utility in the early detection and investigation of patients with stroke.[13,14] That initial optimism began to bear fruit as further technical developments, most notably echoplanar imaging (EPI),[15] made diffusion and perfusion MRI feasible in routine clinical practice. The detection of hyperacute intraparenchymal hemorrhagic stroke by susceptibility-weighted MRI also has been established as comparable to CT. In combination with MRA, the multimodal stroke MRI examination opened the door for the detection of the site, age, extent, mechanism, and tissue viability of acute stroke lesions in a single imaging study. A number of potential clinical applications have emerged that could allow therapeutic and clinical decisions to be based on the physiologic state of the tissue in addition to clinical assessment. Stroke MRI is applied as a multimodal examination to evaluate the stroke patient for arterial pathology, hemodynamic changes, hyperacute parenchymal injury, subacute and chronic infarct, and evidence of acute or chronic hemorrhage (Fig. 46-1). Beyond its role as an aid in routine clinical diagnosis, the most promising applications of current MRI methodology are as a patient selection tool for experimental and interventional therapies and as a biomarker of therapeutic response in clinical trials.

In this review, we describe the applications of structural and functional MR techniques in cerebrovascular diseases. First, the relevant technologic and methodologic aspects are discussed, then the pathophysiologic considerations and background, followed by the potential clinical applications. Broader applications of MRI to specific cerebrovascular topics are illustrated in the other chapters in this book. A fuller treatment of the technical topics discussed in this chapter may be found elsewhere.[16,17]

General Principles and Basic Pulse Sequences

Routine MR imaging is based on the interaction of radio waves with atomic nuclei (most commonly protons or hydrogen nuclei) in tissue. Hydrogen is present in nearly all of the organs of the body. Protons have a net magnetic moment such that when they are placed in a magnetic field they align with the magnetic field and can be excited by radiofrequency (RF) pulses. Water and fat protons are the most extensively imaged nuclei. Other nuclei can be imaged, such as phosphorus, sodium, and fluorine, but these are much less abundant than hydrogen and have no current clinical application to stroke.

In MRI the patient is placed in a strong magnetic field. In general, this main magnetic field is always on, so safety precautions around the MRI scanner are essential even when a scan is not being performed. The strength of the magnetic field depends on the specific scanner. In practice, most of the current clinical MRI is performed at 1.5 Tesla (1.5 T), but lower and higher field strength scanners are also in use. Over the past decade clinical 3.0-T MRI has become commonplace. The next decade may see 7.0-T MRI become a product for routine clinical use.[18] In general, for brain and cerebrovascular imaging, higher field strengths give greater signal-to-noise ratio, which is advantageous for reducing scanning time and improving spatial resolution. To acquire images, RF pulses are

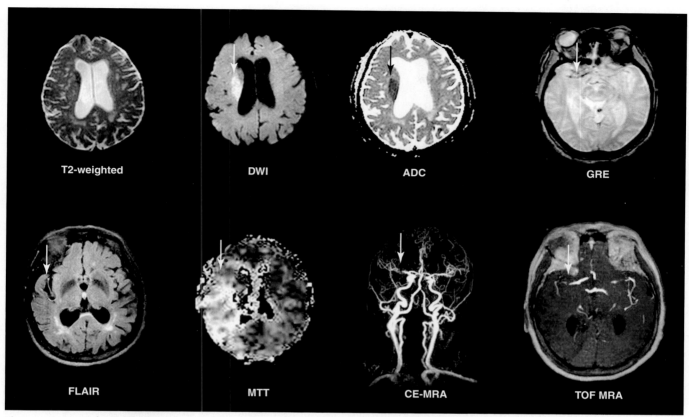

| T2-weighted | DWI | ADC | GRE |

| FLAIR | MTT | CE-MRA | TOF MRA |

Figure 46-1 Multimodal MRI of acute stroke. *Arrows* point to the sequence-specific acute cerebrovascular pathology. T2-weighted image from the b0 images of the diffusion-weighted imaging (DWI) sequence appears normal. DWI image shows acute ischemic injury as a region of relative hyperintensity. The apparent diffusion coefficient (ADC) is reduced, as is characteristic of hyperacute stroke. The gradient recalled echo (GRE) image illustrates the susceptibility blooming of an acute thrombus *(arrow)*. Fluid-attenuated inversion recovery (FLAIR) image shows hyperintense middle cerebral artery (MCA) distal to the occlusion. The mean transit time (MTT) map of the perfusion-weighted image illustrates delayed perfusion in the right MCA territory. The contrast-enhanced (CE) and time-of-flight (TOF) MR angiograms identify the site of occlusion in the right MCA.

applied at the Larmor frequency of hydrogen, the proton's resonant spin frequency. The energy from the RF pulses is absorbed and then released until the tissue being scanned has reemitted the energy absorbed and undergone relaxation. The *echo time* (TE) is the time the machine waits after the applied RF pulse to receive the RF echo from the patient. The *repetition time* (TR) is the time between RF pulses. The energy released occurs over a short time according to two relaxation constants, known as T1 (longitudinal relaxation constant) and T2 (transverse relaxation constant). Varying the TE and TR enables images of different contrast to be obtained, depending on which of the constants is dominant in the tissue. Spatial localization of the signal source from the tissue is achieved by the superimposition of brief gradient magnetic field pulses.

Conventional Pulse Sequences

Conventional MRI pulse sequences include T2WI, T1WI, proton density imaging (PDI), and FLAIR imaging. These are of most value in the evaluation of subacute and chronic stroke. The conventional sequences are based on two families of sequences termed spin echo (or fast spin echo) and gradient echo. In the former, the energy is refocused with the use of a series of RF pulses, whereas

the latter uses a reversal of the magnetic field gradient to refocus the energy. The gradient echo sequences are most useful for MR angiography and hemorrhage detection.

T1-weighted images: T1-weighted images are based on the longitudinal relaxation of spins. They are generated primarily from sequences of short TE and short TR; the shorter the TE and TR, the more T1-weighted the image is. On T1WI, the cerebrospinal fluid (CSF) has low signal intensity, whereas fat has high signal intensity. Gray matter appears less intense (darker) than white matter. Ischemic infarcts appear hypointense on T1WI. The T1WI is not an essential part of the multimodal stroke MRI examination but is valuable in specific cases: axial fat-suppressed T1WI of neck soft tissue can identify the intramural thrombus of an arterial dissection.[19]

T2-weighted images: T2-weighted images are based on the transverse relaxation of spins. They are generated from sequences of long TE and long TR. On T2WI, the CSF signal is hyperintense, whereas fat has almost no signal. Gray matter appears less intense (darker) than white matter. Ischemic lesions also appear hyperintense and may be difficult to distinguish from normal CSF spaces, a potential problem for smaller lesions.

Proton density images: Proton density images are generated with long TR and short TE, and the CSF and fat are

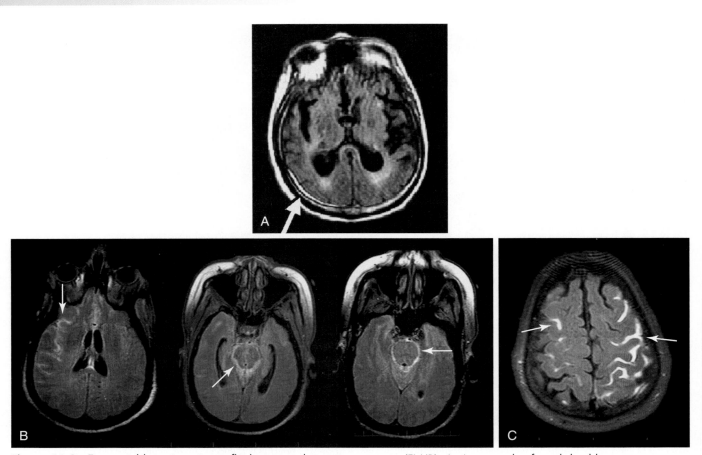

Figure 46-2 Extra-axial hyperintensity on fluid-attenuated inversion recovery (FLAIR). A, An example of a subdural hematoma seen on fluid-attenuated inversion recovery image (FLAIR) *(arrow)*, with clear contrast between the hyperintensity of the blood and the background tissue. This small subdural hematoma was not seen on CT. B, FLAIR images from a 47-year-old man with a subarachnoid hemorrhage. Blood appears hyperintense in the subarachnoid space at multiple levels. C, FLAIR images showing gadolinium enhancement of cerebrospinal fluid in hemispheric sulci *(arrows)* after intravenous tissue-type plasminogen activator (t-PA) treatment. This is the hyperintense acute reperfusion marker (HARM) sign, which indicates early blood-brain barrier disruption in stroke and is associated with reperfusion and increased risk of hemorrhagic transformation. The HARM sign is more likely to be seen following thrombolytic therapy. The main imaging differential is blood, which can be ruled out by gradient recalled echo MRI or CT.

of similar signal intensity. One advantage of PDI is that lesions appear hyperintense relative to CSF, although in practice PDI has been supplanted by FLAIR imaging.

Fluid-attenuated inversion recovery images: On fluid-attenuated inversion recovery (FLAIR) images, an additional RF pulse (inversion pulse) is applied with the purpose of nulling signal from the CSF. As applied in routine practice, on T2-weighted FLAIR imaging the CSF signal is nearly fully suppressed and appears dark as in T1WI, but the lesions appear bright, as in T2WI, allowing better visualization of cortical lesions and periventricular lesions. In practice, FLAIR imaging is used in place of PDI and is often used in preference to T2WI, although FLAIR acquisition times are somewhat longer. Some radiologists prefer both FLAIR imaging and T2WI for the comprehensive head MRI examination, because of the diagnostic advantages of the latter for noncerebrovascular pathologies. Unique features of FLAIR sequences for acute stroke imaging include hyperintensity of extraaxial blood (e.g., subarachnoid hemorrhage [SAH],[20] subdural hematoma, Fig. 46-2A and B) and delayed gadolinium enhancement of intrasulcal CSF,

indicative of early blood-brain barrier disruption (Fig. 46-2C).[21] FLAIR imaging may also depict hyperintense arterial signal indicative of very slow flow associated with acute occlusions or severe stenosis (Fig. 46-3).[22,23] A disadvantage of FLAIR imaging is its high sensitivity to pulsation artifacts of CSF that may suggest SAH.

Advanced Stroke MRI

MRI provides valuable information in the emergency acute stroke evaluation, supplementing the anatomical information obtained from conventional sequences. These protocols include DWI, perfusion MRI (MRP), MRA, and gradient recalled echo (GRE) imaging. EPI became a clinical application essential to diffusion and perfusion imaging, because its short acquisition time minimizes the effects of motion due to either head movement or physiologic brain pulsations. These sequences allow a multimodal evaluation of the patient with acute stroke by imaging tissue injury, perfusion, and the vasculature within the short period feasible for an acute stroke evaluation.

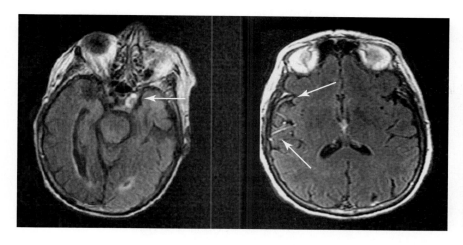

Figure 46-3 Fluid-attenuated inversion recovery (FLAIR) hyperintense vessel sign. *Left,* Hyperintense vessel sign on FLAIR imaging in a patient with a 2-hour-old occlusion of the left internal carotid artery *(arrow).* Note the normal flow void (hypointensity) of the contralateral carotid artery. *Right,* Hyperintense vessel *(arrows)* sign in branches of the right middle cerebral artery territory distal to an occlusion, indicating slow flow in a patient with penumbral flow in that territory.

Diffusion-weighted imaging: DWI has transformed the diagnosis of ischemic stroke in its earliest stage, from reliance on a mostly clinical inference about the presence, localization, and size of an ischemic lesion, to imaging confirmation of the infarct. This technique is the only brain imaging method to reliably demonstrate ischemic parenchymal impact within the first minutes to hours after onset, well before changes are detectable on CT and T2WI or FLAIR MR images (Figs. 46-1 and 46-4). DWI detects the self-diffusion of water, which is the mobility of water molecules among other water molecules (brownian motion).[9,24] With use of single-shot EPI, whole-brain DWI of stroke can be obtained in a scanning time as little as 2 seconds[25]; in current practice, however, multiple DWI acquisitions are obtained and combined for greater signal-to-noise ratio. The typical DWI pulse sequence actually acquires two sets of images, one with and the other without diffusion weighting. An EPI T2WI sequence is set without diffusion weighting. A bipolar pair of diffusion-sensitizing magnetic field gradient pulses to the T2WI pulse sequence cause a dephasing and then rephasing of the spinning protons in water molecules.[24] Where there has been net displacement of a water molecule (i.e., protons) between application of the two diffusion gradient pulses (on the order of tens of milliseconds), there is a net dephasing and subsequent signal loss in the resulting image. The more the water has moved, the greater the signal loss, so that signal intensity is reduced everywhere but relatively less where water movement is restricted. CSF appears very dark, normal brain appears intermediate, and ischemic brain, where parenchymal diffusion is reduced, appears relatively bright.

DWI is quantitative in that it both measures a physiologic parameter—the apparent diffusion coefficient (ADC) of water in mm²/sec—and can define the acute ischemic lesion volume, which can be used to study ischemic pathophysiology in vivo. The ADC is calculated from the reduction in signal intensity that occurs with diffusion weighting. Thus a DWI pulse sequence usually contains at least two sets of images, one without diffusion weighting, a T2WI, and one with high diffusion weighting. The strength of diffusion weighting is described by a set of pulse sequence features called the b-value, so these two sets of images may be referred to as b0, indicating the T2WI without diffusion weighting, and the b1000, referring to the most commonly used b-value in practice.

Diffusion measurements also contain geometric information, primarily axonal orientation, because DWI acquires its information in one direction at a time. This anisotropy results in higher signal perpendicular to fiber tracts and lower signal parallel to them. For routine stroke imaging, it is preferable to minimize anisotropy by effectively averaging the diffusion measurements across three orthogonal directions, reducing the hyperintensity not due to ischemia, a potential confounding factor for small ischemic lesion in white matter tracts. These averaged images are often referred to as *isotropic DWI.* Diffusion tensor imaging (DTI)[26,27] is a type of DWI that, rather than eliminate anisotropy, uses this information to determine the direction and integrity of degenerated white matter tracts and its impact on stroke recovery.[28,29]

In acute cerebral ischemia, the ischemic lesion appears hyperintense (bright) on DWI and hypointense (dark) on an ADC map (see Figs. 46-1 and 46-4). This appearance reflects cytotoxic edema and a reduction in the volume and increased tortuosity of the extracellular space. As the ischemic lesion evolves through the phases of cytotoxic edema, ionic edema, vasogenic edema, tissue necrosis, and cavitation, the ADC normalizes and then becomes elevated in the chronic phase of stroke. This feature makes it possible to distinguish old ischemic lesions from new by calculation of the ADC value. As a rule of thumb, DWI hyperintensity without T2WI or FLAIR changes must imply reduced ADC and can be taken as evidence of acute ischemic impact. A combination of DWI with FLAIR in a single pulse sequence eliminates partial volume effects of CSF in the brain parenchyma and increases lesion contrast,[30,31] but this method is not in common practice because it lengthens acquisition times and reduces the signal-to-noise ratio. Signal hyperintensity on DWI can persist during later stages of stroke (the "T2 shine-through" effect) and cannot by itself be evidence of acute ischemic stroke. In addition, nonischemic pathologies may be associated with DWI hyperintensity.[32] For these reasons, in patients with suspected ischemic stroke, DWI should always be interpreted with T2WI and FLAIR and ideally with a calculation of the ADC.

Perfusion imaging: Brain perfusion, defined in the broadest sense as some aspect of cerebral circulation,

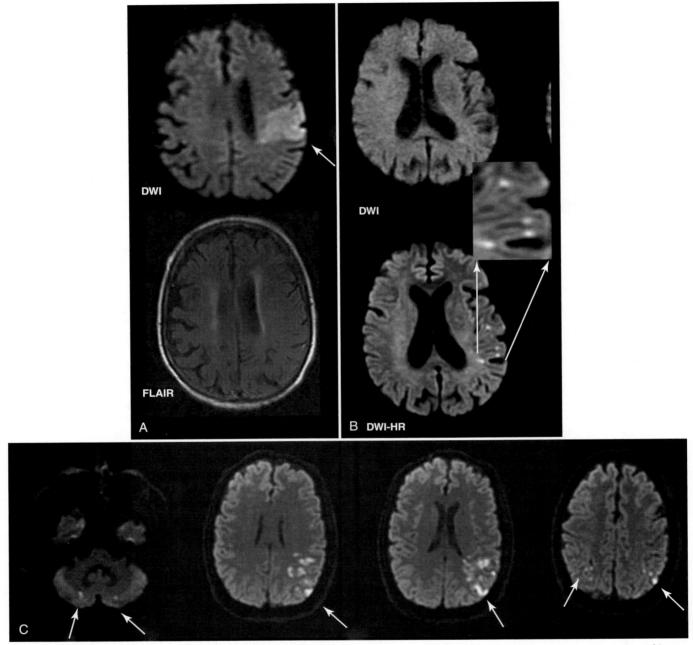

Figure 46-4 Detection of hyperacute ischemic stroke with diffusion-weighted imaging (DWI). A, The characteristic MRI pattern of hyperacute ischemic stroke, which is DWI positive *(arrow)* and fluid-attenuated inversion recovery (FLAIR) negative. B, High-resolution DWI (DWI-HR) may reveal punctate acute ischemic lesions not seen on the more typical lower-resolution DWI. The use of DWI-HR may further reduce the probability of false-negative DWI in stroke. C, Acute ischemic lesions *(arrows)* in multiple arterial territories suggestive of cardioembolic mechanism.

may be studied by various MRI strategies. Two MRI methods, one requiring the injection of contrast agent and the other not, have been used to study abnormal perfusion in human stroke (mainly ischemic) (Fig. 46-5). The first strategy, which is the standard method in clinical practice, is dynamic susceptibility contrast (DSC) imaging, involves a bolus injection of gadolinium and the rapid acquisition of a series of susceptibility-weighted or T2*-weighted images repeated every 1 to 2 seconds through an entire brain volume.[11,12] The intravascular passage of

gadolinium in sufficiently high concentration distorts the local magnetic field owing to magnetic susceptibility effects, causing dephasing of spins in brain tissue adjacent to the blood vessels and therefore results in signal loss. The amount of signal loss over time in a series of rapidly acquired images has been shown to be proportional to cerebral blood volume (CBV) in healthy brain tissue. The time it takes for the change in signal intensity to reach a maximum is the time to peak (TTP) and is related to the mean transit time (MTT) of an idealized bolus of contrast

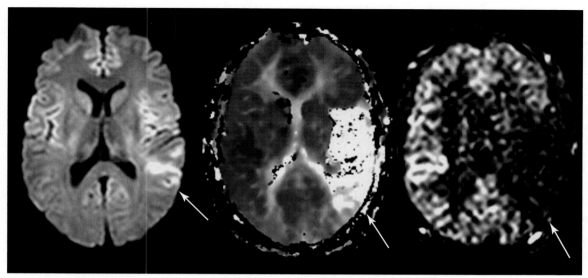

Figure 46-5 MR perfusion imaging. A, Acute ischemic changes in left middle cerebral artery territory on diffusion-weighted imaging (DWI). B, Larger region of ischemia on perfusion mean transit time (MTT) map using the standard dynamic susceptibility contrast (DSC) method. C, MR perfusion without gadolinium is acquired using arterial spin labeling (ASL), showing a comparable perfusion defect on this relative cerebral blood flow map obtained 1 hour 40 minutes after stroke onset. *Arrows* point to regions of abnormality.

agent. Because cerebral blood flow (CBF) in these intravascular models equals the ratio CBV/MTT, information about cerebral blood flow can potentially be inferred with this technique. In patients with acute stroke, qualitative perfusion maps of the relative MTT (rMTT), relative CBF, and relative CBV can be generated, permitting visualization of perfusion defects in acute infarcts, tissue reperfusion occurring after recanalization of blood vessels, and hyperperfusion of subacute infarcts. Postprocessing of the MRP images occurs within minutes of image acquisition at the scanner and so the images are rapidly available to the treating physician. The optimal and accurate quantification of these and other perfusion parameters is an area of intense investigation,[33-39] but in clinical practice, the MRP source images and scanner-generated perfusion maps are sufficient to determine the presence or absence of acute focal ischemia. For cases in which patient head movement during MRP acquisition renders the maps inadequate for diagnosis, assessment of the individual source MRP images is required, because these EPI source images are virtually unaffected by patient motion.

Because of the recognized toxicity of gadolinium-based contrast agents in patients with renal failure, there has been increased interest in MR perfusion methods that do not require contrast agent administration. The second MR perfusion strategy involves arterial spin labeling (ASL) methods, which use RF inversion pulses to magnetically label spins in the arterial supply to brain regions, using arterial water as an endogenous diffusible tracer.[40-43] It can be applied either as pulsed,[44,45] as continuous labeling,[46] or as a combination of both. In ischemic stroke, ASL appears to give comparable diagnostic information to that from the gadolinium bolus tracking methods (see Fig. 46-5),[47] although the reduced signal-to-noise ratio requires averaging of multiple acquisitions, requiring significantly longer acquisition times, and thus is more vulnerable to motion artifacts. However, the

more straightforward quantitative measurement of tissue perfusion with ASL[48,49] is an advantage of this methodology over the bolus tracking method. Innovations have now permitted multiple brain slices to be imaged with ASL,[50] and we predict that ASL perfusion methods will soon become available for routine imaging on most MRI scanners.

Magnetic resonance angiography: In cerebrovascular diagnosis, MRA with contrast-enhanced (CE) or time-of-flight (TOF) methods are the standard approaches. In CE-MRA, a rapid MR acquisition is timed to a bolus injection of contrast agent over a large field of view, permitting routine imaging of the vasculature from the aortic arch through to the branches of the circle of Willis (see Fig. 46-1). The vascular anatomy is outlined by the blood containing the contrast agent.

In TOF MRA, no contrast agent injection is required, and the vascular signal depends on direction and velocity of blood flowing into the plane of imaging. The magnetization of protons in stationary tissue occurs through saturation by repeated low-flip-angle RF pulses, whereas protons in the vessels flowing into the tissue remain unsaturated and appear relatively bright. The data are then postprocessed for an angiographic reconstruction. In practice, inspection of the source images is often necessary to evaluate subtle or ambiguous findings, and most scanners permit scrolling through a reformatted slab of source MRA images for this purpose (see Fig. 46-1). For imaging of the arteries of the circle of Willis, three-dimensional rather than two-dimensional TOF MRA is the most common method of MRA in clinical practice, since it gives superior spatial resolution and is less prone to signal loss from turbulent flow at sites of stenoses. For MRA of the neck arteries, two-dimensional MRA is added because it is more sensitive to detection of slower flow.

Limitations of TOF MRA are its tendency to overestimate the degree of stenosis (particularly when there is slow or turbulent flow or calcifications) and its insensitivity to collateral sources of flow. Its advantages include greater spatial resolution than CE-MRA for the intracranial circulation and its application to the imaging of the cerebral venous system (MR venography). TOF is an alternative for patients unable to receive gadolinium-based contrast agents. Notwithstanding its tendency to overestimate the degree of stenosis, MRA rivals CT angiography and conventional angiography for the detection of arterial stenoses, occlusions, and dissections.[51-54] The sensitivity of MRA to detect aneurysm after SAH is estimated to be 69% to 100%, with a specificity of 75% to 100%.[55] The sensitivity for smaller aneurysms is less.[56]

Susceptibility-Weighted Imaging

Susceptibility-weighted imaging (SWI) refers to a family of MRI sequences in which the tissue contrast is based on magnetic susceptibility differences between different tissue types. Magnetic susceptibility is the property of matter that distorts an applied magnetic field. Although often a source of artifacts at the interface of differing tissue types or in the presence of metal, this principle can be used to make pulse sequences sensitive to hemorrhage, to functional changes in blood oxygenation, and to hemodynamic parameters. The conventional GRE pulse sequence (commonly called T2*-weighted images) is sensitive to the susceptibility effects of paramagnetic molecules such as gadolinium-containing contrast agents as well as deoxyhemoglobin and other hemoglobin breakdown products that are present during all stages of intracranial hemorrhage. Single-shot EPI has intrinsic susceptibility weighting, and EPI using a GRE technique, as in MRP, is the most sensitive of all to susceptibility effects in routine clinical practice. A specific variation of GRE, termed simply SWI, measures phase differences and may be more sensitive than conventional GRE in the detection of acute hemorrhage, chronic microbleeds, and cerebral veins.[57-59]

Spectroscopy

Magnetic resonance spectroscopy (MRS) allows the noninvasive in vivo assessment of brain chemistry by measuring resonances from important metabolites. Clinical studies of MRS have been performed predominantly on ^{1}H nuclei (proton MRS), for which there is a relatively favorable signal-to-noise ratio compared with MRS of other nuclei. Although data collection from single voxels (single voxel spectroscopy) is more straightforward, differences between tissue compartments following stroke are more easily appreciated with chemical shift imaging (CSI). In CSI, spectra from multiple voxels within a grid corresponding to one or more slices are displayed. Typically metabolite peaks are presented as a spectrum in the "frequency domain" on a scale expressed in parts per million (ppm), which conventionally runs from right to left. CSI data can also be displayed as a color-coded "map" overlying a structural image, but it should be stressed that analysis of individual spectra is mandatory. Although a large number of metabolites can be detected, particularly in those studies using a short TE, stroke studies have focused on metabolites with large peaks

TABLE 46-1 MRI SEQUENCES IN ACUTE STROKE

Sequence	Primary Diagnostic Use in Cerebrovascular Disease
Diffusion-weighted imaging (DWI)	Hyperacute acute ischemic lesions Distinguish old lesions from new by apparent diffusion coefficient (ADC) imaging
T2-weighted imaging (T2WI)	Subacute and chronic ischemic lesions Rule out noncerebrovascular pathology
Fluid-attenuated inversion recovery (FLAIR)	Subacute and chronic ischemic lesions Rule out noncerebrovascular pathology Hyperintense vessel sign Blood-brain barrier breakdown
Gradient recalled echo (GRE)	Acute intracranial hemorrhage Hemorrhagic transformation Microbleeds Intravascular thrombus
MR angiography (MRA)	Acute arterial occlusion Other arterial lesions: stenosis, dissection, aneurysm MR venogram for sinus and cerebral venous thrombosis
Perfusion-weighted imaging (PWI)	Focal hemodynamic defect Diffusion-perfusion mismatch as marker of ischemic penumbra

including *N*-acetyl-L-aspartate (NAA) at 2.01 ppm, lactate at 1.33 ppm, and, to a lesser extent, choline at 3.22 ppm and creatine at 3.03 ppm. Values of metabolite peaks can be expressed in relative terms, for example, as a ratio to another metabolite within the same voxel, or to the same metabolite in a voxel in the contralateral hemisphere. Absolute concentrations may be derived by using the signal from water as an internal reference[60] or, less commonly, by using a reference solution placed in the scanner external to the patient.

Stroke MRI Examination

The objective of multimodal MRI of acute stroke, also referred to as the stroke MRI examination, is to obtain diagnostic information about the acute parenchymal injury, subacute or chronic infarct, arterial pathology, tissue perfusion, and presence of hemorrhage. The full multimodal MR sequences listed in Table 46-1 can be acquired within 15 to 20 minutes of scanning. Approximately, 10% to 15% of patients suspected of acute stroke may not have MRI because of contraindications. All patients must be screened by MRI personnel for safety related to metal or electronic devices. Updated online resources relating to MRI safety are available (e.g., <www.mrisafety.com>). In 2006, a link between gadolinium-based contrast agents and nephrogenic systemic fibrosis (NSF), a potentially debilitating fibrosing disease of the skin and viscera occurring in patients with chronic kidney disease, was recognized. Readers are referred to European and North American guidelines for specific management recommendations.[61,62] In general, caution is recommended (i.e., use only agents without reports of associated NSF and the lowest possible dose, and obtain patient's consent) when the glomerular filtration rate (GFR) is between 30 and 60 mL/min/1.73 m^2 in the patient with chronic kidney disease, but local hospital policies may differ. Gadolinium should not be used when the GFR is less than 30 mL/min/1.73 m² or if the patient is dialysis dependent. Estimated GFR based on serum creatinine is used to screen patients undergoing MRI for this risk.

Transient Ischemic Attacks

Standard MRI

Conventional MRI (e.g., T1WI) is more sensitive than standard CT in identifying both new and preexisting ischemic lesions in patients with transient ischemic attacks (TIAs) (employing the classic definition of TIA as a focal neurologic deficit of vascular etiology that resolves within 24 hours). In various studies, standard MRI sequences have shown evidence of at least one infarct somewhere in the cerebrum in 46% to 81% of patients with TIA.[63,64] Some of these infarcts are in locations that could have accounted for the deficits observed during the TIA. Among patients meeting clinical criteria for TIA, 31% to 39% demonstrate neuroanatomically relevant infarcts on conventional MRI.[63,65] It is difficult with both conventional MRI and CT to determine what proportion of these appropriately localized infarcts occurred at the time of the index TIA and what proportion existed prior to the presenting event.

The earliest report of MRI findings in patients with TIA came from Awad et al.[66] This group studied 22 patients with both MRI and CT. They found that 77% of patients had focal ischemic changes on MRI compared with 32% on CT. However, the majority of lesions did not correlate with symptomatology. Fazekas et al[63] reported the results of conventional MRI in 62 patients with hemispheric TIAs. Forty-five of these patients also underwent contrast-enhanced studies. The researchers found that 81% of their cohort had MRI evidence of focal ischemic injury, and that 31% demonstrated evidence of an acute TIA-associated infarct. The majority of infarcts identified as acute (68%) were less than 1.5 cm in diameter, and 58% were purely cortical. Thirty-seven percent of the acute infarcts were multiple in nature. Contrast enhancement occurred in five of the 45 patients studied and in two of

these patients was essential to the delineation of the acute lesion. Evidence of infarction in these patients was associated with a higher frequency of a history of vascular or cardiac disorders.

Additional insight regarding lesion location and clinical characteristics of patients with TIA-associated lesions on conventional MRI comes from two other studies. In their report of 64 patients with carotid territory TIAs studied with MRI, Kimura et al[65] found that 16 of 41 patients demonstrated contrast enhancement. The majority of contrast-enhancing lesions were cortical (81%). Aphasia or confusional state, hypertension, and presence of an emboligenic cardiac or arterial source were more frequently observed in patients with enhancement. The higher rate of contrast enhancement in this study than in the report by Fazekas et al[63] may be related to differences in patient characteristics and timing of the MRI studies. Bhadelia et al[64] studied 100 patients with TIA from the Cardiovascular Health Study imaged with standard MRI sequences.[64] Brain infarcts were demonstrated in 46% of the patients with TIA, compared with 28% of patients without a history of TIA. In stepwise logistic regression analysis, diastolic blood pressure and internal carotid intima-media thickness were predictive of infarction on MRI. These investigators also found an increased frequency of cortical infarcts and multiple infarcts in the patients with TIA.[64]

Advanced MR Techniques: Diffusion-Weighted Imaging, Perfusion MRI

MRI techniques of diffusion weighting and perfusion permit greater visualization of the dynamic tissue response to acute ischemia and have afforded new insights into the pathophysiology of TIA (Fig. 46-6). Numerous series show convergent results regarding the frequency of DWI positivity among patients with TIA.[67-74] In a pooled analysis of 19 studies, the aggregate rate of DWI positivity was 39%, with frequency ranging from 25% to 67%.[75]

Several studies have demonstrated that DWI positivity is associated with specific clinical characteristics, including longer symptom duration, motor deficits, aphasia, and

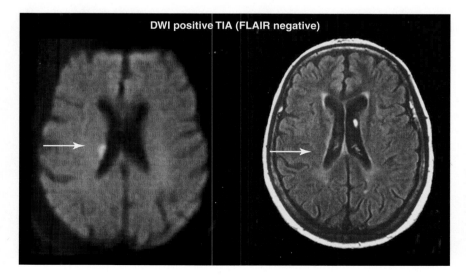

DWI positive TIA (FLAIR negative)

Figure 46-6 Diffusion-weighted imaging (DWI) of a transient ischemic attack (TIA). MRI findings in a 63-year-old man with a 30-minute episode of left arm weakness, imaged 4 hours after resolution. *Left,* DWI sequence shows right periventricular white matter lesion *(arrow)* not apparent on the fluid-attenuated inversion recovery (FLAIR) sequence *(right, arrow).*

large vessel occlusion demonstrated on MRA.[67,76,77] In a multicenter analysis of 808 patients, presence of motor symptoms, longer duration of TIA, and MRI within 24 hours of resolution of symptoms were univariate predictors of DWI positivity.[78] DWI positivity was more frequent in patients who underwent MRI within 24 hours of symptom resolution than in those imaged later than 24 hours (37.1% versus 29.8%, respectively; odds ratio [OR], 1.39; 95% confidence interval [CI], 1.00–1.93).

The sensitivity and specificity of DWI offers unique precision in characterizing the vascular and anatomic localization of ischemic TIA lesions. This information provides important insights into the underlying etiologic mechanism. In the series reported by Kidwell et al,[67] DWI results altered the attending physician's opinion regarding vascular localization, anatomic localization, and probable TIA mechanism in approximately a third of patients per category. Another study conducted by Schulz et al[78a] looked at the utility of DWI in patients presenting late with subacute TIA and studied 136 patients with TIAs a median 17 days after symptom onset. These investigators found that DWI showed a high signal lesion in 13% of these patients. For patients who had one or multiple lesions on T2WI, DWI helped clarify whether the lesions were related to a recent ischemic event in 31% of this group. Compared with T2WI alone, DWI provided additional information in 13% of TIAs, such as clarification of clinical diagnosis or vascular territory.

Several studies have assessed the follow-up imaging characteristics of patients with positive and negative results on DWI. In the series by Kidwell at el,[67] only five of nine patients (56%) undergoing follow-up imaging demonstrated a subsequent infarct in the region corresponding to the original DWI abnormality (Fig. 46-7). In a study of 33 "DWI-positive" patients with TIA, Oppenheim et al[79] found that 26 (79.6%) had a subsequent infarct on follow-up imaging. Conversely, Sylaja et al,[80] exploring the characteristics of "DWI-negative" patients with TIA, found that patients with brainstem location ischemia or lacunar syndromes were most likely to have a negative initial DWI result and a positive follow-up imaging result.

Of particular importance are studies demonstrating that DWI positivity has important prognostic implications. Specifically, these studies have shown that patients with TIA who have abnormalities on DWI scans have a higher risk of recurrent ischemic events than those without such abnormalities.[73,77,81] Purroy et al[77] performed MRI within 7 days of symptom onset in 83 patients with classic TIA. New vascular events were seen in 19.3% of cases and were associated with symptom duration of more than 1 hour and a DWI abnormality. Vascular events occurred in 40% of patients with both of these features.

Another study evaluated the ABCD score for stratifying risk in patients with classic TIA assessed on DWI.[82] The predictive value of a DWI lesion was higher than the other predictors examined (even after adjustment for the

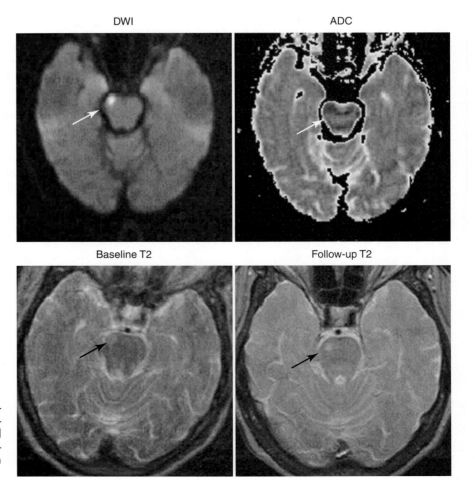

DWI   ADC

Baseline T2   Follow-up T2

Figure 46-7 Follow-up imaging demonstrates a subsequent infarct in the region corresponding to the original diffusion-weighted imaging (DWI) abnormality in transient ischemic attack (TIA). ADC, apparent diffusion coefficient.

ABCD score) for a variety of subsequent risks, including stroke or death within 90 days. Another study, conducted by Calvet et al,[73] sought to combine the predictive ability of the ABCD score with the predictive value of DWI and TIA etiology; they followed up 343 patients with TIA (339 of whom underwent DWI) for 3 months subsequent to TIA. ABCD score and positive DWI result were found to be associated with increased 7-day and 3-month risks of stroke.

Several reports have now provided new insights into the role of perfusion imaging findings in patients with clinical TIAs. These studies have demonstrated that MRP provides additive value to DWI and in some cases is more sensitive than DWI in detecting acute ischemic changes in some patients with TIA. Because MRP is able to detect regions of relative hypoperfusion that do not reach the threshold of tissue bioenergetic compromise required to cause a lesion on DWI, a greater number of patients with modest degrees of ischemia may be detected with this technique.

Mlynash et al[72] assessed the value of combined DWI and MRP in patients with suspected hemispheric TIA. Imaging was performed within 48 hours of stroke onset, and lesions were correlated with suspected clinical localization and baseline characteristics. Although 33% of patients had a lesion on MRP and 35% of patients had a lesion on DWI, the combined yield of DWI plus MRP was 51%. In a similar study, Krol et al[83] found that 21 of 62 patients with TIA (33.9%) had evidence of a perfusion abnormality as defined by rMTT delay. This group found no relationship between the presence of a perfusion abnormality and the patient's clinical outcome.

In summary, DWI and MRP play important roles in the diagnosis of TIA and provide vital prognostic information that can guide management. Patients with TIA who have DWI lesions, especially multiple lesions, are at higher risk of recurrent ischemic events. These studies can also assist with stroke localization and understanding of the mechanism of the stroke. Moreover, taken as a whole, these neuroimaging studies suggest a need to reexamine the utility and accuracy of the current time-based definition of TIA. Accumulating evidence suggests that any time cutoff for TIA is inaccurate in reflecting end-organ injury. Accordingly, efforts are under way to redefine TIAs using a tissue-based definition that takes into account the fundamental physiologic processes indexed by imaging or other laboratory measures, rather than a strict time limit.[75]

Ischemic Stroke

Potential early MRI findings in patients with acute stroke are summarized in Table 46-2. Within the first few hours of ischemia, standard MRI sequences (T1WI, T2WI, and FLAIR) are relatively insensitive to ischemia, showing abnormalities in less than 50% of cases.[84] The earliest changes, seen as increased signal on T2WI and FLAIR sequences, are due to a net increase in overall tissue water content, a process which takes several hours to develop to levels visible on MR. These changes are rarely seen prior to 6 hours from onset and by 12 to 24 hours can be readily appreciated. Although the majority of ischemic lesions are evident on both CT and conventional MRI by

TABLE 46-2 EARLY MRI FINDINGS IN ACUTE ISCHEMIC STROKE

Hyperintensity on diffusion-weighted imaging, with minimal or no changes on T2-weighted imaging (T2WI) or fluid-attenuated inversion recovery (FLAIR) imaging
Hypointensity on apparent diffusion coefficient (ADC) imaging
Hypointense ("blooming") artery sign of acute intravascular thrombus on gradient recalled echo (GRE) imaging
Arterial occlusion on MR angiography
Absence of arterial flow-void, indicative of occlusion, on T2WI or FLAIR imaging
Hyperintense vessel sign, indicative of slow or collateral flow, on FLAIR imaging
Focal reduction or absence of contrast on dynamic perfusion source images
Focal reduction or absence of perfusion on perfusion parameter maps

24 hours, standard MRI is superior to CT in identifying lesions earlier as well as lesions that are smaller or in the posterior fossa.[6,7] Conventional MR sequences are sensitive to patient motion, degrading image quality. Whereas ischemic parenchymal changes are not apparent on conventional sequences in the first few hours, intravascular signs of acute stroke may be apparent: absence of arterial flow void on T2WI, intravascular hyperintensity on FLAIR (see Figs. 46-1 and 46-3)[22,85,86] and the hypointense intravascular sign due to acute thrombus on GRE sequences (Figs. 46-1 and 46-8).[87,88]

DWI allows visualization of regions of ischemia within minutes of symptom onset.[89] Decreased water diffusion associated with cytotoxic edema causes an increased (bright) signal on DWI sequences, which can be quantitatively measured on the ADC maps, where darker areas represent decreased diffusion. The increase in signal on DWI may persist for several weeks or longer partially owing to a T2 effect. The average ADC, however, remains reduced for only 4 to 7 days then returns to normal or supranormal levels within 7 to 10 days from ischemia onset.[30,90,91] Although the average ADC generally follows this pattern, studies have now clearly demonstrated that marked heterogeneity of the ADC value can occur within the ischemic lesion, even in the hyperacute time window.[92]

DWI has a high degree of sensitivity (88% to 100%) and specificity (95% to 100%) for acute ischemia, even at very early time points.[93-96] In the study by Ay et al,[93] of 782 consecutive patients presenting with stroke-like deficits, DWI had positive results in 765, and negative results in 27, including 10 patients with nonstroke etiologies for their deficits and 10 patients with reversible deficits. Studies performed in the acute stroke setting have consistently demonstrated marked superiority in accuracy of diagnosis of ischemic change for DWI (95% to 100%) over that for CT (42% to 75%) or standard MRI sequences such as FLAIR (46%).[97-100] A study comparing DWI lesions with pathologically confirmed infarction at autopsy also demonstrated an overall accuracy of 95%.[101] Occasionally, DWI hyperintensities may be seen in a number of other cerebral disorders, including status epilepticus, tumors, infections, and Creutzfeldt-Jakob disease.

A prospective, blinded comparison of DWI with noncontrast CT in a consecutive series of 356 patients referred for emergency assessment of suspected acute

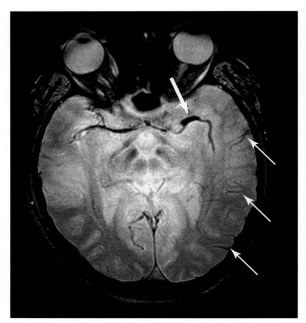

Figure 46-8 The blooming hypointensity of an acute arterial thrombus on gradient recalled echo (GRE) MRI *(large arrow)*. The *small arrows* point to dilated veins commonly seen on GRE within the penumbral region, as defined on diffusion-perfusion mismatch (not shown).

stroke proved the superiority of DWI in a broad, representative sample.[102] The sensitivity of DWI for ischemic acute stroke ranged from 73% (within 3 hours after the event) to 92% (more than 12 hours). By contrast, the sensitivity of CT at these times was 12% and 16%, respectively. The specificity of MRI for stroke detection was 92% (at 3 hours) and 97% (more than 12 hours).[102] The superiority of DWI over CT was observed regardless of clinical severity or time from stroke onset to scan. A 2010 practice guideline of the American Academy of Neurology recommended that DWI should be performed for the most accurate diagnosis of acute ischemic stroke.[103]

Despite the high sensitivity of DWI, clinicians must recognize that false-negative results might occur with this technique: The reported rate of false-negative results with DWI in the previously described study was 17% (versus 84% for CT) for the entire sample and 27% (versus 88% for CT) within the first 3 hours.[102] Mild or small infarcts, early imaging, and brainstem location are factors associated with false-negative scans, and the false-negative rate is higher when patients have two or more of these factors than when individuals have one or none.[80,102] Other studies have also reported sensitivity of DWI for the diagnosis of acute ischemic stroke is higher than that of CT (39% to 75%) or FLAIR (46%).[100,104]

Information on the natural history of diffusion imaging lesion growth comes from several clinical trials and case series. Warach et al[105] analyzed serial imaging studies from patients enrolled in the placebo arm of a neuroprotective trial and demonstrated that the natural history of diffusion lesions is to grow over time during the acute and subacute periods.[105] Ischemic lesions follow a relatively consistent pattern of growth during the first 3

days, followed by subsequent decrease in size to days 5 to 7.[106-109]

Numerous studies have shown that initial diffusion lesion volume correlates well both with final infarct volume and neurologic and functional outcomes in patients with stroke, suggesting that DWI can provide important early prognostic information.[108,110-116] Building on this data, Baird et al[117] demonstrated the combination of clinical and DWI factors provided better prediction of stroke recovery than any factor alone.

Although these correlations have been repeatedly demonstrated in anterior circulation ischemia, several small case series have suggested that acute DWI lesion volumes correlate poorly with clinical measures in the posterior circulation, because small strategic brainstem infarcts can lead to devastating clinical syndromes and large cerebellar infarcts may cause minimal symptomatology.[118]

An increasing number of studies have provided data demonstrating the clinical utility of DWI in current practice.[119,120] Diffusion-weighted imaging allows early identification of lesion size, neuroanatomic site, and vascular territory involved. A distinctive advantage of DWI is its ability to distinguish acute from chronic ischemia, allowing new lesions to be identified in patients even when they are near or within areas of prior ischemic injury.[121,122] Another important insight into stroke pathophysiology offered by DWI is the frequent visualization of multiple acute lesions in different vascular territories in patients who have only one clinically symptomatic acute insult, providing evidence of an embolic stroke mechanism.

Perfusion imaging employing the bolus contrast passage method is playing an ever more important role in the initial evaluation and treatment of the patient with acute stroke. Perfusion measures that can be derived from this technique include MTT, relative CBV (rCBV), time to peak measures, and relative CBF (rCBF). Quantitative measures of cerebral tissue perfusion may be calculated using an arterial input function.[34,37,123,124] Controversy persists regarding the best perfusion measure and the ability to obtain reliable quantitative perfusion measures in the acute stroke setting.

Both DWI and T2WI have allowed the detection of many silent or previously undetected small cortical and cerebellar infarcts. Further, on DWI, it has been more recognized that there are frequently multiple acute infarcts and that new ischemic lesions can occur over time. In the study by Baird et al,[125] multiple acute lesions were seen in 17% of patients. These lesions were attributed to multiple emboli. They occurred in both anterior and posterior circulations or in both cerebral hemispheres in 3% to 5% of patients, suggesting that there was a proximal source of embolism. Otherwise the lesions were seen in the vascular territories of one hemisphere and attributed to multiple emboli or to the breakup of an embolus.

Multiple DWI lesions of different ages are associated with early recurrence of stroke and a high risk of future ischemic events.[126] Multiple acute DWI lesions predict early recurrent strokes: In a study of patients with stroke who underwent imaging within 6 hours of onset, 34% of individuals had additional lesions when reimaged 1 week later, and in almost 50% of these patients, the new lesions were outside the area of perfusion abnormality at baseline.[127] Patients with multiple DWI lesions or large artery disease are more likely to have recurrent lesions than stroke patients with single lesions on DWI[127] for up to 90 days, but greatest risk is during the first month after the initial stroke.[128]

DWI lesions can help identify stroke etiology, because certain lesion patterns are associated with specific stroke subtypes.[129] Single cortical-subcortical lesions, multiple lesions in the anterior and posterior circulation, and multiple lesions in multiple cerebral territories are associated with cardioembolism.[125,129] Multiple lesions in the unilateral anterior circulation, and small scattered lesions in one vascular territory, particularly in a watershed distribution, are related to large artery atherosclerosis.[129,130] These imaging patterns, together with information obtained from other MRI sequences, such as MRA, might help in the selection of the most appropriate measures for secondary prevention of stroke.

In general, acute ischemic stroke shows no signs on FLAIR imaging in the first 6 hours from onset, with areas of hyperintensity evolving thereafter. In patients with unwitnessed onset of stroke, including individuals whose deficits are present on awakening, a DWI lesion without a matching hyperintensity on FLAIR imaging suggests that the stroke occurred within 6 hours. Studies to evaluate the use of MRI in this setting to select for patients for treatment are ongoing.[131-134]

Because CSF signal is suppressed on FLAIR imaging, it is a very sensitive to detect blood or gadolinium-based contrast agents in the CSF and can, therefore, readily identify SAH and subdural hemorrhage. Early blood-brain barrier disruption in stroke appears as delayed gadolinium enhancement of hemispheric sulci on FLAIR sequences (see Fig. 46-2).[21] Such enhancement—termed hyperintense acute reperfusion marker, or HARM—is associated with reperfusion, thrombolytic therapy, an increase in the risk of hemorrhagic transformation, and an increase in plasma matrix metalloproteinase-9.[21,135-137]

In patients with acute ischemic stroke, portions of the intracranial arterial tree can appear hyperintense on FLAIR imaging (see Fig. 46-3). This hyperintense vessel sign is indicative of slow blood flow distal to the site of acute arterial obstruction. This slowdown in blood flow is attributable to anterograde flow through an incomplete occlusion, or flow via leptomeningeal collaterals, and is associated with large diffusion-perfusion mismatch, but is not predictive of response to thrombolytic therapy.[22,23,138,139]

Subacute infarcts are characterized by varying amounts of vasogenic edema and sometimes hemorrhagic transformation of the infarct. Vasogenic edema is maximum between 1 and 6 days but persists to varying degrees for 3 or 4 weeks. The T2-weighted and FLAIR images show signal hyperintensity in the area of infarction. On T1WI the area of infarction appears hypointense. After the administration of gadolinium, there is usually enhancement of the lesion on T1WI or of the blood vessels within the ischemic lesion, indicating slow flow in the area of infarction. In acute or subacute stroke, gadolinium enhancement occurs in regions of blood-brain barrier breakdown. The typical sequence of enhancement of the infarct is that enhancement is uncommon in the first 6 days, is most common between 7 and 30 days and disappears after that but can persist for up to 6 weeks.[140] Two patterns of enhancement have been seen, a slowly progressive form that follows the T2WI changes and then an early form of enhancement which may be associated with better outcome. Occasionally a fogging effect may be seen in this phase or in the acute phase that is postulated to be due to developing hemorrhagic infarction.

On DWI, the ischemic lesion may be isointense (phase of pseudodnormalization) or, less frequently, hyperintense, as in the acute phase. Over time, as the ischemic lesion evolves through the phases of cytotoxic edema, vasogenic edema, and tissue necrosis and cavitation, the ADC normalizes (termed "pseudonormalization") and then becomes elevated in the chronic phase of stroke. This feature makes it possible to distinguish old ischemic lesions from new by calculating the ADC.

In the chronic stage of stroke the edema that was present in the subacute phase has resolved. At very late time points there may be atrophy and cavity formation. On T2-weighted and FLAIR imaging, infarcts appear hyperintense. On T1WI, infarcts are hypointense and no longer have contrast enhancement. On DWI there is the T2 shine-through pattern and the ADC is elevated.

Wallerian degeneration may be seen as a secondary phenomenon in the white matter tracts. Kuhn et al[141] showed the wallerian degeneration after cerebral infarction on sequential MRI.

Incidental focal hyperintensities in the subcortical white matter demonstrated by T2-weighted or FLAIR images are both a common feature in patients undergoing brain MRI for cerebrovascular or other indications and indicative of chronic microvascular disease. Awad et al[142-145] found these to be associated with advanced age, history of hypertension, and pathologic changes such as arteriosclerosis, dilated perivascular spaces, and vascular ectasia, and to be indications of chronic cerebrovascular disease.[142-145] These incidental or silent white matter hyperintensities have also been studied extensively by Fazekas et al,[146-151] who confirmed their association with risk factors for cerebrovascular disease. These associations were most strong with age but also with reduced white matter CBF, history of hypertension, diabetes, or cardiac disease, elevated fibrinogen values, and reduced levels of total cholesterol and α-tocopherol. These white matter lesions may progress in number and frequency but their clinical significance in the asymptomatic patient for cognitive decline or risk of stroke independent of the other coexisting stroke risk factors is uncertain.

Tissue Metabolite Changes in Infarction

The expected changes in the major metabolites following stroke have been broadly characterized with respect to the infarct core. Although the physiologic role of *NAA* is not clear, it has been considered to be a marker of neuronal integrity[152] on the basis of its predominantly neuronal localization.[153] NAA values have consistently been shown to fall after stroke,[154-160] with greater decreases in the center than in the periphery of the lesion.[157,161] Continuing decreases are seen throughout the first 2 weeks after stroke,[160] and levels remain chronically low or absent.

Lactate levels are raised within the infarct and manifest as a "doublet" peak at 1.33 ppm, projecting above and below the baseline at long and intermediate TEs, respectively. Lactate production results from anaerobic glycolysis and is generally considered to be undetectable in the healthy brain. However, later studies have suggested that low levels of lactate may be detectable in a proportion of older healthy volunteers[162] and in the hemisphere contralateral to stroke lesions.[160] Animal studies of both ex vivo[163] and in vivo MRS[161] suggest lactate is present within minutes of ischemia and continues to increase over hours, particularly in the center of the ischemic lesion. Reperfusion after focal ischemia precipitates a gradual decrease in lactate over days[161,164] but a decline in lactate is also seen in permanent MCA occlusion models.[161] Clinical studies are consistent with these findings, with high levels of lactate detected in patients imaged in the hyperacute phase,[165,166] which subsequently fall within the first week[155,156] and are undetectable after 2 weeks.[157,160] Measurements after a number of months have shown a second rise in lactate levels,[160] consistent with the presence of inflammatory infiltrate.

The *creatine* peak is influenced by both creatine and phosphocreatine and therefore can be considered to be a marker of energy stores. Reductions in this peak are also seen after stroke,[154,155,157,159] but are less dramatic than for NAA.[156] Changes in the *choline* peak, which represents total choline levels and is a marker of cell membrane turnover, have been more variably reported, with levels after stroke shown to be decreased,[154,159] unchanged,[157] or increased.[155] Although decreases may represent cell loss, it has been postulated that increases may represent myelin damage in infarct regions with a significant proportion of white matter.[158] The finding that MRS can reveal substantial metabolic heterogeneity in tissues demonstrating only small differences in ADC value[165] suggests a potential value for MRS in addition to conventional sequences for the description of the functional status of tissue. The possibility of using MRS to refine the MR definition of "tissue at risk" remains interesting. It has been hypothesized that tissue with a raised lactate but normal NAA levels may indicate metabolically compromised yet intact neurons, and therefore the ischemic penumbra (Fig. 46-9).[158]

Animal studies consistently show the presence of lactate at the earliest imaged time points.[161,167]

NAA levels demonstrate an early reduction with as much as 20% within an hour[161] and 50% within 6 hours.[167] In human studies little data are collected during the hyperacute phase of stroke. However, one study demonstrated that the MRP-DWI mismatch region matched the region of normal NAA and raised lactate,[165] whereas another study showed that in the "mismatch" area lactate values were less, and those of NAA greater, compared with measurements from the lesion on DWI.[166] Values in individual subjects are likely to be influenced by the degree and duration of ischemia and the nature of collateral circulation. Determination of the metabolite thresholds that define the penumbra, including how much of a reduction in NAA is acceptable, must be prospectively tested in a large cohort of subjects imaged using CSI during the hyperacute phase of stroke.

MRS studies also have the potential to provide markers of the efficacy of therapy, either in clinical practice or in trials. Such markers may include the measurement of brain temperature in different tissue compartments,[168,169] assessment of the interplay between ischemia and redox status,[170] or, theoretically, even the demonstration that certain drugs have actually reached the target tissues. In addition, MRS studies have shown that metabolite changes in the hemisphere ipsilateral to stenosis of an internal carotid artery include a reduction of NAA, an increase in choline, and sometimes an increase in lactate.[171,172] Such changes can be reversed with carotid endarterectomy, particularly in patients who do not have lactate in the lesion prior to surgery,[171] and in those in whom the postoperative CBV is demonstrably improved.[173] MRS may also aid evaluation of prognosis after stroke, with measurements of lactate-to-choline ratios[174] or changes in NAA[175] correlated with clinical outcome.

MRS has a number of important limitations. First, even under ideal conditions, signal-to-noise ratio is limited by the low concentration of brain metabolites relative to water. Second, movement of patients during scanning not only may distort spectra and introduce confounding signal from scalp lipid but also may displace the head from

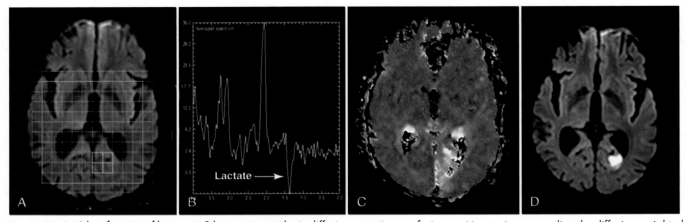

Figure 46-9 Identification of lactate in 2-hour acute stroke in diffusion-negative, perfusion-positive region, preceding the diffusion-weighted imaging (DWI) lesion. A, Baseline DWI with magnetic resonance spectroscopy (MRS) grid overlaid. B, MRS abscissa from highlighted voxels in A, which shows the presence of lactate *(arrow)*. C, Baseline lesion on mean transit time (MTT) map. D, Follow-up DWI demonstrating lesion in region on early lactate peak.

TABLE 46-3   APPEARANCE OF HEMORRHAGE ON VARIOUS MRI SEQUENCES

Stage	T1-Weighted	T2-Weighted	Fluid-Attenuated Inversion Recovery	Gradient Recalled Echo or T2*
Hyperacute (<12 h)	Isointense or mildly hyperintense	Hyperintense	Hyperintense	Hypointense rim
Acute (12 h to 2 days)	Isointense or hypointense	Hypointense	Hypointense	Hypointense rim gradually progressing centrally
Early subacute (2-7 days)	Hyperintense	Hypointense	Hypointense	Hypointense
Late subacute (8 days to 1 month)	Hyperintense	Hyperintense	Hyperintense	Hypointense
Chronic (>1 month to years)	Isointense or hypointense	Hypointense	Hypointense	Slitlike hyperintense or isointense core surrounded by a hypointense rim

its original position, thereby limiting the spatial sensitivity of the technique. Finally, interpretation of metabolite ratios requires an appreciation that all major metabolites may change after stroke and with aging.[176]

In summary, MRS provides an opportunity to study brain biochemistry in vivo after stroke. This technique may potentially image the ischemic penumbra, provide prognostic information, and may offer additional imaging endpoints in clinical trials. However, every effort must be made to reduce likely sources of artifact and error.

Hemorrhage

Although CT has traditionally been considered the gold standard for the assessment of hemorrhage, advances in MRI techniques have provided both improved diagnostic capabilities for detection of intracranial hemorrhage and better understanding of the underlying pathophysiology, etiology, and prognosis of these disorders.

The appearance of blood on various MRI sequences depends on the stage of evolution of the blood breakdown products (Table 46-3).[177] The hemoglobin that is present in freshly extravasated blood exists primarily in the form of oxyhemoglobin, which is nonparamagnetic. However, conversion of intracellular oxyhemoglobin to deoxyhemoglobin likely begins at the periphery of the hematoma almost immediately. Deoxyhemoglobin contains four unpaired electrons, making it highly paramagnetic. Around day 2 or 3, deoxyhemoglobin is converted to methemoglobin, which initially is formed intracellularly then becomes extracellular as the red blood cells lyse. Around day 7, macrophages and phagocytes begin transforming the methemoglobin to hemosiderin and ferritin.

Conventional T1- and T2-weighted MRI sequences are highly sensitive for the detection of subacute and chronic blood, but they are less sensitive to parenchymal hemorrhage less than 6 hours old. Studies now suggest that hyperacute parenchymal blood can be accurately detected using GRE/T2* sequences or EPI SWI.[178-180] Echoplanar T2*-weighted imaging can be performed with a very low acquisition time (seconds), representing a significant advantage in patients with acute intracranial hemorrhage who are unable to cooperate or lie still for extended periods of time.

The hallmark of hyperacute hemorrhage on these sequences is a rim of hypointense signal surrounding an isointense core (Fig. 46-10). Subsequently, in the acute

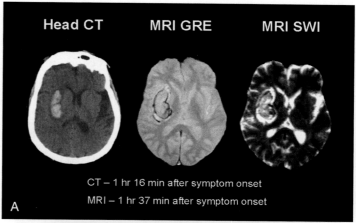

Head CT   MRI GRE   MRI SWI

CT – 1 hr 16 min after symptom onset
MRI – 1 hr 37 min after symptom onset

A

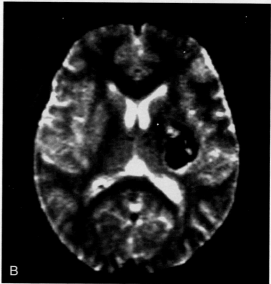

B

Figure 46-10 A, An example of an acute intraparenchymal hematoma, less than 2 hours from onset, on CT as well as gradient recalled echo (GRE) MRI and MRI using echoplanar imaging (EPI) and susceptibility weighted imaging (SWI). Note on MRI the appearance of a heterogenous central hypointense periphery of the hematoma, surrounded by the hyperintense rim of edema. B, In a hematoma at a later point, approximately 3 hours from onset in this figure, hypointensity predominates.

and subacute stages, the hematoma becomes diffusely hypointense, and in the chronic stage, the hematoma appears as a slitlike signal with a hyperintense or isointense core with a rim of hypointensity.

Several large multicenter prospective studies have demonstrated that these MRI sequences are as reliable as CT in the identification of acute blood.[102,181,182] In some cases, MRI detects hemorrhages that are not evident on CT.[181,183] These findings have allowed MRI to be employed as the sole imaging modality to evaluate patients with acute stroke at capable centers. However, up to 20% of patients with acute stroke may not tolerate or may have contraindications to MRI.[184]

Intraparenchymal Hemorrhage

The most frequent underlying etiologies of adult primary intracerebral hemorrhage (ICH) are hypertension and cerebral amyloid angiopathy (CAA), and MRI findings can often assist in making this determination. Primary ICH associated with hypertension most often occurs in deep brain structures (e.g., putamen, thalamus, cerebellum, and pons). In contrast, primary ICH occurring in lobar regions,

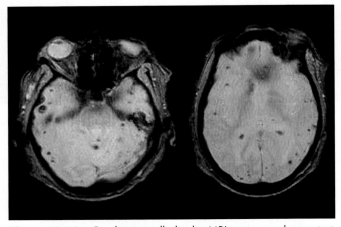

Figure 46-11 Gradient recalled echo MRI sequence demonstrating multiple scattered old microbleeds (punctate hypointensities) from a patient with cerebral amyloid angiopathy.

particularly in the elderly, is most commonly related to CAA but may also be associated with hypertension.[185] CAA-related hemorrhage is frequently characterized by a distinct pattern of lobar microbleeds (see later).

MRI is superior to CT in identifying underlying structural lesions that are less frequent causes of parenchymal ICH (e.g., arteriovenous malformations, tumors) and in quantifying the amount and extent of perihematomal edema. A contrast study is indicated in patients without a clear underlying etiology or in hemorrhages occurring in unusual locations.[186]

MRI techniques have provided new insights into the underlying pathophysiology of ICH, specifically the role of ongoing secondary neuronal injury in the perihematomal region. A number of studies (but not all) have demonstrated perihematomal regions of hypoperfusion, or bioenergetic compromise, or both.[187,188] These MRI studies have suggested that approximately one third of patients imaged in the acute phase may have reduced perihematomal ADC values.[187,189,190] Further studies have characterized the evolving time course, with ADC values being low within the first day and then gradually elevated, likely reflecting the evolution of perihematomal edema.

In aggregate, these studies suggest that there may be a subset of patients with a rim of perihematomal hypoperfusion and possibly ischemia in the hyperacute phase. It is likely that this region rapidly disappears in the subacute phase as edema and inflammation evolve.[188,191] The development of edema and toxicity from blood breakdown products are the most significant contributors to ongoing perihematomal injury. MRI studies thus have the potential to monitor the impact of these findings on recovery and in the future may be used as surrogate outcome markers for studies of putative interventions.[192,193]

Microbleeds

GRE or T2* sequences have the ability to detect clinically silent prior microbleeds, not visualized on CT (Figs. 46-11 and 46-12). Microbleeds are usually defined as punctate, homogeneous, rounded, hypointense parenchymal lesions less than 5 to 10 mm in size. A number of studies have demonstrated that the pathologic correlate of

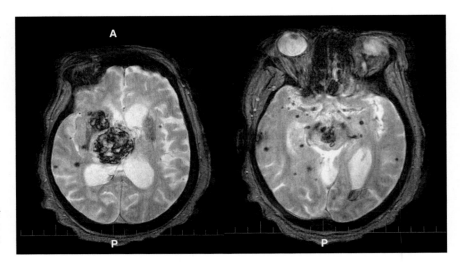

Figure 46-12 Example of GRE from a patient with ICH attributable to hypertensive disease, in whom microbleeds are most commonly found in deep and infratentorial regions.

GRE-visualized microbleeds is a region with hemosiderin-laden macrophages that occur adjacent to small vessels. These findings are indicative of previous extravasation of blood at the vessel wall.[194]

MRI evidence of microbleeds is seen in 38% to 80% of patients with primary ICH, in 21% to 26% of patients with ischemic stroke, and in 5% to 6% of asymptomatic or healthy elderly individuals.[195-197] Hypertension, CAA, advancing age, and, much less commonly, cerebral autosomal dominant arteriopathy with silent infarcts and leukoaraiosis (CADASIL) have been identified as the most important risk factors for microbleeds.[198-201]

A growing body of evidence indicates that microbleeds represent a marker of a bleeding-prone angiopathy.[202-204] Several case reports and small series suggested that patients with microbleeds may be at increased risk for development of hemorrhage following antithrombotic or thrombolytic therapies. In contrast, two large series did not show an increased risk of hemorrhage in patients treated with intravenous tissue plasminogen activator (t-PA).[205,206] However, in both of these studies, very few patients were included who had a large microbleed burden, thus representing a potentially biased sample. The risk of hemorrhage in patients with a large number of microbleeds (more than 5) remains unanswered.

The pattern of microbleed topography can provide insights into the underlying risk factors and etiology, particularly in patients with primary ICH. It has been shown that microbleeds are a common occurrence in patients with CAA and most frequently are found in lobar regions (see Fig. 46-11).[198] A pattern of multiple lobar microbleeds in the setting of a lobar ICH is highly suggestive of CAA as the underlying etiology. In contrast, in patients with ICH attributable to hypertensive disease, microbleeds are most commonly found in deep and infratentorial regions, although it is likely that hypertension may also contribute to lobar located microbleeds (see Fig. 46-12).[201]

A growing number of studies indicate that the presence of microbleeds and the overall microbleed burden have important prognostic significance. One study demonstrated that the total number of microbleeds predicts risk of future symptomatic hemorrhage in patients with probable CAA.[207] In addition, new microbleeds demonstrated on repeat MRI were found to also predict increased risk of future symptomatic ICH. Moreover, microbleed burden and rate of accumulation were found to predict cognitive decline and poor neurologic or functional outcome in this population.[207]

The presence and lesion burden of microbleeds appear to also be a significant prognostic factor in hypertensive hemorrhage and ischemic stroke. For example, several studies have shown a correlation between microbleeds and new vascular events.[199,208,209] In addition, Kwa et al[197] found that microbleeds were significantly associated with leukoaraiosis. Finally, some studies have also suggested that there may be racial and ethnic differences in the frequency of microbleeds.[210] Copenhaver et al[210] found that microbleeds were more prevalent in black patients with primary ICH (74%) than in whites (42%) (*P* = .005).[210] In this study, after data were adjusted for age, hypertension, and alcohol use, race was an independent predictor of microbleeds.

Hemorrhagic Transformation

Hemorrhagic transformation (HT) of an ischemic infarction is a common occurrence, visualized in up to 42% of patients in pathologic series. Numerous studies have demonstrated that hemorrhagic transformation is much more frequent in cardioembolic strokes, with estimates ranging from 30% to 74% in CT studies. The frequency of HT is also significantly increased in patients treated with thrombolytic or mechanical revascularization therapies, with rates of asymptomatic HT ranging from 10.6% to 67.8% in IV thrombolytic trials and 57% in the second Prolyse in Acute Cerebral Thromboembolism (PROACT II) trial of intraarterial pro-urokinase.[210a]

The MRI evolution of blood breakdown products is similar to that seen with primary ICH (see Table 46-3). However, gradient echo sequences may demonstrate regions of petechial hemorrhage not visualized with CT or standard MR sequences. Prospective studies, employing serial MRI with gradient echo sequences, are required to clarify the frequency of these findings in various stroke subtypes and their role in antithrombotic treatment decisions. The most commonly used radiologic classification system for rating the type and severity of hemorrhagic transformation was developed for head CT scans and divides hemorrhage into two major categories, hemorrhagic infarct (HI) and parenchymal hematoma (PH), each with two subcategories based on severity. However, it is important to note that the application of this classification system to MRI has not been systematically assessed and compared with CT. Thus, the prognostic significance of these categories is unclear for MRI.

MRI information can, however, assist in distinguishing hemorrhagic transformation of an ischemic infarct from a primary hematoma. Most hemorrhagic transformations are smaller than the field of the ischemic infarct as seen on DWI. Primary hematomas also tend to have rounder edges and often have a greater amount of surrounding edema than would be seen in an ischemic stroke. Finally, hematomas frequently do not respect vascular territories.

A growing number of studies have evaluated the clinical and radiologic (including MRI) predictors of HT in the setting of thrombolytic therapy. Contrast agent extravasation has been identified as an important marker of blood-brain barrier disruption and therefore a predictor of HT.[21,211,212] Also, a growing number of MRI studies have identified additional imaging characteristics predictive of HT. Several of these studies have suggested that a large baseline DWI lesion, low ADC values, or both are also independent predictors of subsequent symptomatic hemorrhage.[213-215] These findings provide potential imaging biomarkers for testing of treatments designed to minimize risk of blood-brain barrier opening and subsequent hemorrhagic transformation.

Subarachnoid Hemorrhage

Later studies have explored the clinical utility of MRI sequences in patients with subarachnoid hemorrhage (SAH). Although standard spin-echo sequences are relatively insensitive to subarachnoid blood, newer sequences, including FLAIR and gradient echo T2* imaging, have been shown to have modest sensitivity, particularly in the subacute phase when the CT result is often negative.[216-218] Subarachnoid blood appears as a region of high signal intensity relative to normal CSF on FLAIR sequences and as a region of hypointensity on gradient echo images. Overall, studies have suggested that FLAIR imaging is as sensitive as CT for acute SAH, but compared with the findings at lumbar puncture, the findings on FLAIR imaging are not definitive in excluding acute SAH.[217,219-221]

Evaluation of patients with SAH and vasospasm is an emerging role for multimodal MRI. Several reports have demonstrated that patients with vasospasm secondary to aneurysmal SAH demonstrate a high rate of DWI lesions, often indicative of silent ischemia.[222,223] In studies employing perfusion imaging, these ischemic lesions were associated with regions of hemodynamic compromise and angiographic evidence of vessel vasospasm.[224-226] Later studies have employed combined diffusion and perfusion imaging to characterize the pathophysiology and evolution of ischemia due to vasospasm.[227,228]

Subdural and Epidural Hematomas

Subdural hematomas appear as crescent-shaped lesions adjacent to the brain parenchyma. The MRI appearance depends on the age of the hematoma and the sequences acquired. In the acute stage, subdural hemorrhages appear as hyperintense on FLAIR and T2-weighted sequences. On GRE sequences, they may be isointense or hypointense in the acute stage, on the basis of the stage of blood breakdown products. In the subacute stage, they appear hypointense. In the chronic stage, subdural hematomas appear as either isointense or mixed signals, depending on the degree of blood reabsorption.

Epidural hematomas appear as lentiform (biconvex) extraaxial lesions adjacent to the brain parenchyma. The displaced dura appears as a thin line of low signal intensity between the brain and hematoma. Rapid enlargement may lead to significant midline shift, often associated with herniation. MRI signal intensities usually follow the previously described temporal evolution of intraparenchymal ICH.

Vascular Pathology

MRA rivals conventional angiography and CT angiography for the detection of arterial stenoses and occlusions,[51-54,229] although there is a tendency of MRA, especially TOF, to overestimate the degree of stenosis because of dephasing of protons caused by turbulent flow or calcifications at the site of the stenosis. Also the smaller intracranial vessels are not well visualized with MRA. A normal screening MRA is reliable to exclude hemodynamically significant stenoses. False-positive results can arise when the degree of carotid stenosis is overestimated or when the carotid artery is kinked or changes direction abruptly, in the distal carotid artery as it enters the carotid canal, owing to susceptibility artifact between vessel and bone, and in the presence of surgical clips. A false-positive occlusion on MRA is usually deducible by the reconstitution of flow distal to the point of signal loss. Sensitivity and specificity for carotid occlusion have been found to be 100% for most

studies. In general, if MRA shows no stenosis or a stenosis of less than 70%, no further evaluation is necessary. If MRA shows a stenosis of 70% or more, duplex ultrasonography should be performed. If results of the two studies agree, no further evaluation is suggested,[230,231] and appropriate management can be provided. If MRA and duplex ultrasonography do not agree, then further evaluation with conventional angiography is recommended. The most promising new approach is contrast-enhanced MRA of the carotid arteries, in which a more rapid MR acquisition is timed to a bolus injection of contrast agent over a larger field of view in less than 1 minute and compares favorably to conventional angiography for the diagnosis of carotid stenosis.[232-235] The accuracy of this contrast-enhanced MRA technique for the detection of vascular disease of vertebral artery origins and the aortic arch is being investigated.

The diagnosis of dissection of the internal carotid or vertebral artery can be made with MRI and MRA.[236-239] Findings suggestive of dissection on MRI are increased signal from parts of or the entire vessel wall on axial T1-weighted images (with fat suppression) consistent with hematoma (Fig. 46-13), a border of increased signal surrounding the lumen with luminal narrowing, poor or absence of visualization of the vessel, or significant compromise of the vessel lumen by adjacent abnormally increased signal tissue. If a false lumen with an intimal flap is present, it is best appreciated on the T2WI. Vessel abnormalities such as narrowings, aneurysmal dilatation, and a second lumen may be demonstrable by MRA. When a TOF technique is used, MRA may show a normal or simply widened outer contour of the vessel at the site of dissection. This is caused by the addition of signal from the vessel wall due to methemoglobin in the hematoma, and by the high-flow lumen. False-negative MRI/MRA assessments for dissection occur, and CT angiography is recommended if there is a high degree of clinical suspicion and the MR results are negative.

MRA has a sensitivity of 92% to 95% for the detection of intracranial aneurysms.[240,241] The sensitivity of MRA to detect aneurysm after SAH is 69% to 100%, with a specificity of 75% to 100%.[55] The sensitivity of this technique for the detection of small aneurysms is lower.[56] Lesions

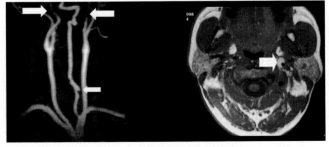

Figure 46-13 MR images from a 48-year-old man with dissections *(arrows)* of bilateral carotid and vertebral arteries. *Left,* Power-injector contrast-enhanced neck MR angiogram shows an intimal flap in the left vertebral artery as well as progressive tapering of the distal internal carotid arteries. *Right,* A T1-weighted axial MR image through the internal carotid artery illustrates the pathognomonic crescent sign of dissection. In this image, the blood within the vessel wall of the right internal carotid artery appears hyperintense.

as small as 2 to 3 mm in diameter have been shown by MRA, and the technique has occasionally demonstrated small aneurysms missed on conventional angiography.[242] However, aneurysms smaller than 5 mm may be missed with MRA. Slow flow and turbulence within small aneurysms may interfere with their detection in up to 27% of cases, leading to limitation in study interpretation.[243] These problems can be partially overcome by using intravenous contrast media. Small aneurysms may be difficult to differentiate from vessel loops because, unlike with conventional angiography, there is no increase in signal at the point of vessel overlap with use of an MIP (maximum intensity projection) algorithm. The use of MRA as a screening test for the detection of aneurysms is controversial.[244,245] If aneurysm size is the only factor, the insensitivity to small aneurysms may not be of clinical consequence. The accuracy of MRA in detecting small aneurysms is likely to improve as techniques are further refined.

A newer application of vascular imaging with MRI is high spatial resolution multimodal imaging of the carotid plaque to identify the various components, such as lipid deposits, fibrous caps, calcium, and thrombus.[246-248] Although not yet a routine practice, high-resolution carotid plaque imaging appears promising as a way to document decreased lipid content and plaque stabilization following lipid-lowering therapy[249] and to identify a ruptured fibrous cap associated with a recent history of TIA or stroke.[248]

Cerebral Venous Thrombosis

Although diagnosis of cerebral venous thrombosis remains a diagnostically challenging entity, advances in MRI have substantially aided in the ability of physicians to perform a rapid, noninvasive, and comprehensive neuroimaging evaluation. Moreover, MRI has provided further insight into the underlying differences in the pathophysiologic processes involved in venous versus arterial infarction. In cerebral venous thrombosis, breakdown of the blood-brain barrier combined with venous congestion leads to a unique combination of coexistent vasogenic and cytotoxic edema, which in turn often leads to frank infarction, hemorrhage, or both. MRI studies are able to visualize venous congestion, venous infarction, and hemorrhage.

Venous hypertension may produce cytotoxic edema, vasogenic edema, or a combination of the two. These changes can be visualized as hyperintensity on T2-weighted or FLAIR images. If venous hypertension is mild, no signal abnormalities may occur. In patients with superior sagittal sinus thromboses, parasagittal lesions are common and may be bilateral. Transverse sinus thrombosis frequently causes posterior temporal lobe lesions, whereas thrombosis of the deep sinus system often causes bithalamic lesions. With contrast agent administration, there may be lesion enhancement in a tumor-like pattern. Hemorrhagic transformation of venous infarction occurs frequently and has the typical MR appearance of hemorrhage based on the stage of the blood breakdown product (see earlier discussion of hemorrhage).

Vessel occlusion is usually well demonstrated by MR venography (MRV) (Fig. 46-14), making angiography unnecessary in the majority of cases. MRV has been accepted as the procedure of choice in the diagnosis of sagittal sinus thrombosis.[250,251] It is particularly valuable because the clinical diagnosis of sinus venous thrombosis is often occult because of a wide spectrum of clinical presentation and a highly variable clinical presentation. Direct findings of cerebral thrombosis by MRV include lack of typical high flow signal from a sinus and direct visualization of thrombus on individual frames of the 2D slices. These must be distinguished from an aplastic or hypoplastic sinus and from the appearance of a sinus after recanalization. Thrombosed veins and/or sinuses may also be visualized on axial gradient echo T2*-weighted sequences with greater conspicuity than standard T1- and T2-weighted scans.[252,253] One group reported that the sensitivity of T2*WI and T1WI sequences to detect clot in the sinuses or veins was estimated at 90% and 71%, respectively, between days 1 and 3.[254] Of note, T2*SWI detected 97% of thrombosed cortical veins, even in the absence of visible occlusion on MRV.

Studies now suggest that the majority of cases can be initially diagnosed by a combination of MRI studies, including T1WI, T2WI, DWI, GRE, FLAIR, MRA, and MRV, and that MRI provides a useful means for follow-up.[255,256] Several reports have begun to elucidate the diffusion-perfusion MR characteristics of venous sinus thrombosis. Abnormal DWI signal intensity may be associated with

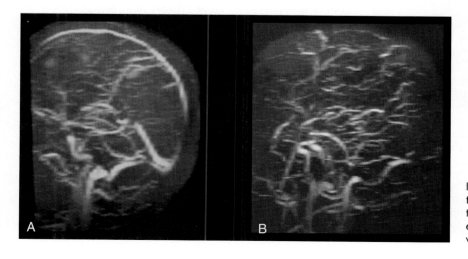

Figure 46-14 A, Normal MR venogram of the brain. B, Straight sinus thrombosis. Note the lack of flow signal in the straight sinus, lateral sinus, vein of Galen, and internal cerebral veins.

low ADC values indicative of cytotoxic edema, high ADC values indicative of vasogenic edema, or mixed values indicative of a combination of both vasogenic and cytotoxic edema.[250,257,258] Consequently, MR lesions caused by venous thrombosis are more frequently reversible than those due to arterial ischemia, because of the reversibility of vasogenic edema. Several groups have also demonstrated perfusion imaging abnormalities, including increased MTT[259] and increased CBV.[260]

MRI-Guided Acute Stroke Therapy

A full clinical multimodal stroke MRI study for acute stroke is feasible even within a 3-hour thrombolysis time window, and the additional diagnostic information obtained with MRI could result in more appropriate application of thrombolytic therapy and better cost-effectiveness.[261-266] Several large stroke centers rely on MRI to screen patients for thrombolytic and other interventional treatments.[267] The mismatch between volumes of DWI and MRP lesions can be used to approximate the ischemic penumbra.[106,268,269] Some of the DWI lesion is potentially reversible, and some of the peripheral region of the perfusion abnormality does not progress to infarction (Fig. 46-15). The Echoplanar Imaging Thrombolytic Evaluation Trial (EPITHET) as well as the Diffusion and Perfusion Imaging Evaluation for Understanding Stroke Evolution (DEFUSE), Desmoteplase in Acute Ischemic Stroke (DIAS), and Dose Escalation of Desmoteplase for Acute Ischemic Stroke (DEDAS) studies showed that patients with a DWI-MRP mismatch could benefit from acute thrombolytic therapy.[270-273] The DEFUSE study involved patients treated with intravenous alteplase 3 to 6 hours after onset of symptoms. These patients were not selected on the basis of the DWI-MRP mismatch; however, early reperfusion in patients with a mismatch

(an MRP lesion of at least 10 mL in size and at least 20% larger than a DWI lesion) was associated with a favorable clinical outcome, and the benefit of treatment was even greater in individuals with a target mismatch profile: with the mismatch pattern but excluding a malignant profile, that is, neither DWI nor MRP lesion exceeding 100 mL. Patients without a mismatch did not benefit from reperfusion.[270] In the EPITHET, treatment with intravenous alteplase led to attenuation of infarct volume growth in patients with a mismatch.[271] The trials of desmoteplase (DIAS and DEDAS) enrolled patients in whom a DWI-MRP mismatch was found 3 to 9 hours from onset of symptoms and were the only studies to use outcome on MRI as a selection criterion in a randomized controlled manner for late thrombolysis. The DIAS and DEDAS studies showed a positive dose-response relationship for desmoteplase on early reperfusion and found that beneficial clinical effects were seen in patients treated with desmoteplase.[272,273] DIAS-2, a phase 3 study, did not confirm the clinical benefit of desmoteplase, although the reason for this result is not well understood.[274] Results of these late thrombolysis trials are encouraging, but much work remains to fully develop the role of the diffusion-perfusion mismatch in selecting patients for thrombolysis.[275]

The role of MRI in acute stroke management is an area of intense research. The results from MRI-based clinical trials are helping to refine the mismatch concept, and penumbral imaging is a promising tool that will help us identify individuals who might benefit from thrombolysis beyond the current therapeutic window.[270-274,276]

Multimodality MRI may have a valuable role in the prediction of tissue outcome, which could help identify the tissue destined to become infarcted at the earliest times after stroke onset. The combination of DWI and perfusion imaging allows the identification of four ischemic patterns. In approximately 70% of patients studied within 24 hours of symptom onset, there is a "perfusion-diffusion mismatch," in which the area of DWI abnormality is surrounded by a larger area of hypoperfusion, most commonly measured by the rMTT perfusion map. It has been proposed that this tissue that is hypoperfused but has a normal DWI signal may be the tissue that is ischemic but not yet irreversibly injured and that is at risk for infarct progression. In other patients, the DWI lesion is larger than the perfusion lesion in approximately 10% (presumed partial or total reperfusion) of cases, and in 10% to 15%, the DWI and perfusion lesions are of equivalent size (likely little viable tissue, operationally defined as a completed infarct).

Several studies have demonstrated that baseline MR perfusion lesion volumes correlate well with final infarct volume as well as neurologic and functional outcomes and, in fact, correlate somewhat better than the baseline diffusion lesion volumes.[111,113,116,277] It is speculated that the stronger association is explained by the fact that the perfusion lesion volume identifies all tissue at risk of infarction if vessel recanalization does not occur. Several groups have reported that CBV measures provide the greatest accuracy in predicting final infarct size and clinical outcome.[278-281]

Diffusion/perfusion MR studies have begun to elucidate the evolution of ischemic lesions in humans. It

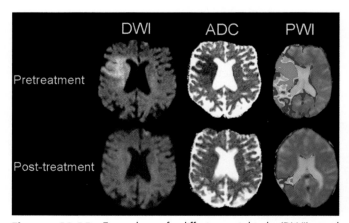

Figure 46-15 Examples of diffusion-weighted (DWI) and perfusion-weighted (PWI) imaging from a patient treated with intraarterial thrombolytic therapy for a right middle cerebral artery occlusion. *Top row* shows pretreatment images, and *bottom row,* early post-treatment images. Perfusion images are in the form of color-coded maps of the time to peak of the residue function (Tmax) with *red* indicating greatest delay. Following vessel recanalization, there is complete reversal of initial DWI and apparent diffusion coefficient (ADC) abnormalities and almost complete reversal of the initial perfusion lesion.

has been suggested that early MRI can characterize the ischemic penumbra as regions of perfusion but not diffusion abnormality (diffusion-perfusion mismatch) (see Figs. 46-1 and 46-15). These are regions in which blood flow is reduced but in which tissue bioenergetic failure, as evidenced by cytotoxic edema, has not yet developed. This hypothesis is supported by studies demonstrating that the natural history of diffusion MRI abnormalities is to grow over time as noted previously, particularly in patients imaged early after symptom onset.[105,106,109,282] An important finding that arose from combined diffusion-perfusion studies was that a substantial number of patients still have regions of mismatch up to 24 hours or longer after symptom onset, even though the frequency of patients with mismatch gradually decreases over time since onset.[282,283]

Serial MRI studies performed in patients with mismatch have confirmed that infarct growth occurs primarily in patients with large regions of mismatch,[106,108,113,279,284] suggesting gradual failure of the ischemic penumbra within the region of mismatch as it is incorporated into the infarct core. Schellinger et al,[285] studying patients with mismatch and evidence of a vessel occlusion at baseline, found that patients with subsequent early recanalization had substantially smaller final infarct lesions than those without recanalization and better clinical outcome.[285]

Although mismatch may provide a simple and practical means of identifying the penumbra in acute stroke, it is important to note that prior animal studies and later case series in humans undergoing thrombolytic therapy have shown that diffusion abnormalities can be partially reversed with early reperfusion.[286-288] These data suggest that early after ischemia onset, the penumbra likely includes not only regions of diffusion-perfusion mismatch but also portions of the region of diffusion abnormality (see Fig. 46-15).

Efforts have been under way to identify thresholds distinguishing tissue that will proceed to infarction from salvageable penumbral tissue. Several groups have found that relative ADC values could reliably differentiate regions that would proceed to infarction from those that would not within the initial hypoperfused region.[289] These findings are in accord with those of Schlaug et al,[268] who found ADC values of 56.4% of normal in the core, and values of 91.3% in the penumbra. However, these findings apply generally to untreated patients or patients in whom early recanalization does not occur. In patients with early vessel recanalization, ADC decreases may not reliably indicate tissue infarction independent of the duration and severity of ischemia.[290] Thresholds for infarct progression, malignant middle cerebral artery infarct, and risk of hemorrhagic transformation may be identified with quantitative diffusion or perfusion MRI,[202,291-299] but these thresholds are not absolute thresholds; rather, they depend on the technique of measurement and analysis, the time from onset, the therapeutic intervention, and interactions with other physiologic and clinical variables.[300]

Several prior studies have delineated perfusion thresholds that distinguish benign oligemia from ischemic penumbral tissue by determining values that predicted final infarct size in patients not being treated with thrombolysis, in whom the infarct grows to consume the entire penumbra to the benign oligemia border.[294,297,301,302]

A large number of studies have analyzed early MRI characteristics in patients with untreated stroke to identify predictors of final infarct volume. These natural history studies generally provide predictive models of tissue outcome, assuming that early recanalization does not occur in most patients. Schlaug et al[268] used a logistic regression model to differentiate regions of ultimate infarction and noninfarction on the basis of baseline perfusion measures to operationally define the ischemic penumbra. Other groups have employed generalized linear model algorithms, multiparametric ISODATA (Iterative Self-Organizing Data Analysis) techniques, and other automated strategies to predict final tissue status. All of these approaches have demonstrated good overall accuracy.[296,301,303]

Several groups have reported that an altered evolution of infarction can be visualized on serial diffusion and perfusion imaging studies in patients undergoing intravenous thrombolytic therapy. Inhibition of lesion growth has been clearly demonstrated in patients experiencing reperfusion in comparison with patients with persistent perfusion deficits or vessel occlusions.[304,305] In addition, several groups have found regions of higher ADC values within the initial ischemic field on follow-up imaging in patients undergoing reperfusion within 36 hours of onset than in patients not undergoing reperfusion, suggesting tissue salvage.[306,307] Further compelling data come from Parsons et al,[174] who compared MRI signatures in patients treated with intravenous t-PA within 6 hours of onset and a group of matched controls. These investigators found a significant decrease in the amount of mismatch tissue proceeding to infarction as well as less infarct expansion in the thrombolysis-treated group.

These studies suggest that it is feasible and potentially advantageous to use diffusion-perfusion MRI to select patients for thrombolytic therapy, employing MRI to characterize the degree of perfusion impairment and amount of remaining salvageable tissue. Efforts are under way to identify specific MRI signatures and criteria to distinguish regions of reversible and irreversible infarction. Kidwell et al[286] used automated image registration techniques to analyze diffusion-perfusion MRI data from patients treated with intra-arterial thrombolytic therapy. Stepwise discriminant analysis was performed using baseline ADC, MTT, rCBV, and rCBF values to identify tissue that was labeled as infarction or normal at day 7. In this preliminary model, baseline diffusion-perfusion MRI variables distinguished ultimate tissue infarction from noninfarction to a high degree. There is also a growing body of data suggesting that baseline MRI characteristics may be used to predict risk of hemorrhagic transformation.[202,299] Further characterization of the MRI signatures of penumbra, core infarction, and hemorrhage risk may allow extension of the time window for treatment beyond current standards and improve safety by enabling treatment decisions to be based on individual patient pathophysiology rather than rigid time windows.

In addition to demonstrating lesion evolution through infarct growth in patients with mismatch and a persistent vessel occlusion, serial multimodal MRI studies have provided important additional insights into the evolving pathophysiology of human ischemia, particularly in patients undergoing vessel recanalization. The phenomenon of postischemic hyperperfusion has been demonstrated in approximately half of patients undergoing successful vessel recanalization with intraarterial thrombolysis.[308] In addition, late secondary ischemic injury, visualized on DWI and ADC maps, has now been demonstrated in humans, as in animal models, following vessel recanalization.[202] These findings may become important targets for neuroprotective therapy in the future.

DWI lesion volume correlates with acute stroke severity as measured by the National Institutes of Health Stroke Scale (NIHSS) score.[111] Further, DWI lesion size, clinical stroke severity, and a number of other clinical factors each provide prognostic information in ischemic stroke. Baird et al[117] reported that the combination of clinical factors (NIHSS score and time in hours from onset to MRI scanning) and DWI factors (DWI lesion volume) allowed improved prediction of stroke recovery as early as 3 to 6 hours after onset of symptoms. The findings were externally validated in an independent series of patients with high sensitivity and specificity. The investigators developed a three-item scale for the early prediction of stroke recovery, a total score of 5 to 7 indicating a high likelihood of recovery.[117]

REFERENCES

1. Bydder GM, Steiner RE, Young IR, Hall AS, Thomas DJ, Marshall J, Pallis CA, Legg NJ: Clinical NMR imaging of the brain: 140 cases, *AJR Am J Roentgenol* 139:215–236, 1982.
2. Brant-Zawadzki M, Davis PL, Crooks LE, Mills CM, Norman D, Newton TH, Sheldon P, Kaufman L: NMR demonstration of cerebral abnormalities: Comparison with CT, *AJR Am J Roentgenol* 140:847–854, 1983.
3. Buonanno FS, Kistler JP, DeWitt LD, Pykett IL, Brady TJ: Proton (1H) nuclear magnetic resonance (NMR) imaging in stroke syndromes, *Neurol Clin* 1:243–262, 1983.
4. Bydder GM, Steiner RE, Thomas DJ, Marshall J, Gilderdale DJ, Young IR: Nuclear magnetic resonance imaging of the posterior fossa: 50 cases, *Clin Radiol* 34:173–188, 1983.
5. Ramadan NM, Deveshwar R, Levine SR: Magnetic resonance and clinical cerebrovascular disease. An update, *Stroke* 20:1279–1283, 1989.
6. Bryan RN, Levy LM, Whitlow WD, Killian JM, Preziosi TJ, Rosario JA: Diagnosis of acute cerebral infarction: Comparison of CT and MR imaging, *AJNR Am J Neuroradiol* 12:611–620, 1991.
7. Yuh WT, Crain MR, Loes DJ, Greene GM, Ryals TJ, Sato Y: MR imaging of cerebral ischemia: Findings in the first 24 hours, *AJNR Am J Neuroradiol* 12:621–629, 1991.
8. Amarenco P, Kase CS, Rosengart A, Pessin MS, Bousser MG, Caplan LR: Very small (border zone) cerebellar infarcts. Distribution, causes, mechanisms and clinical features, *Brain* 116:161–186, 1993.
9. Le Bihan D, Breton E, Lallemand D, Grenier P, Cabanis E, Laval-Jeantet M: MR imaging of intravoxel incoherent motions: Application to diffusion and perfusion in neurologic disorders, *Radiology* 161:401–407, 1986.
10. Moseley ME, Cohen Y, Mintorovitch J, et al: Early detection of regional cerebral ischemia in cats: Comparison of diffusion- and T2-weighted MRI and spectroscopy, *Magn Reson Med* 14:330–346, 1990.
11. Belliveau JW, Rosen BR, Kantor HL, et al: Functional cerebral imaging by susceptibility-contrast NMR, *Magn Reson Med* 14:538–546, 1990.
12. Rosen BR, Belliveau JW, Buchbinder BR, et al: Contrast agents and cerebral hemodynamics, *Magn Reson Med* 19:285–292, 1991.
13. Warach S, Chien D, Li W, Ronthal M, Edelman RR: Fast magnetic resonance diffusion-weighted imaging of acute human stroke, *Neurology* 42:1717–1723, 1992.
14. Warach S, Li W, Ronthal M, Edelman RR: Acute cerebral ischemia: Evaluation with dynamic contrast-enhanced MR imaging and MR angiography, *Radiology* 182:41–47, 1992.
15. Stehling MK, Turner R, Mansfield P: Echo-planar imaging: Magnetic resonance imaging in a fraction of a second, *Science* 254:43–50, 1991.
16. Edelman R, Hesselink J, Zlatkin M, Crues J, editors: *Clinical magnetic resonance imaging*, ed 3, Philadelphia, PA, 2006, Elsevier.
17. Davis S, Fisher M, Warach S, editors: *Magnetic resonance imaging in stroke*, Cambridge, UK, 2003, Cambridge University Press.
18. Duyn JH: Study of brain anatomy with high-field MRI: Recent progress. *Magn Reson Imaging*
19. Shah GV, Quint DJ, Trobe JD: Magnetic resonance imaging of suspected cervicocranial arterial dissections, *J Neuroophthalmol* 24:315–318, 2004.
20. Noguchi K, Ogawa T, Inugami A, Toyoshima H, Okudera T, Uemura K: MR of acute subarachnoid hemorrhage: A preliminary report of fluid-attenuated inversion-recovery pulse sequences, *AJNR Am J Neuroradiol* 15:1940–1943, 1994.
21. Latour LL, Kang DW, Ezzeddine MA, Chalela JA, Warach S: Early blood-brain barrier disruption in human focal brain ischemia, *Ann Neurol* 56:468–477, 2004.
22. Toyoda K, Ida M, Fukuda K: Fluid-attenuated inversion recovery intraarterial signal: An early sign of hyperacute cerebral ischemia, *AJNR Am J Neuroradiol* 22:1021–1029, 2001.
23. Kamran S, Bates V, Bakshi R, Wright P, Kinkel W, Miletich R: Significance of hyperintense vessels on FLAIR MRI in acute stroke, *Neurology* 55:265–269, 2000.
24. Moseley ME, Kucharczyk J, Mintorovitch J, et al: Diffusion-weighted MR imaging of acute stroke: Correlation with T2-weighted and magnetic susceptibility-enhanced MR imaging in cats, *AJNR Am J Neuroradiol* 11:423–429, 1990.
25. Warach S, Gaa J, Siewert B, Wielopolski P, Edelman RR: Acute human stroke studied by whole brain echo planar diffusion-weighted magnetic resonance imaging, *Ann Neurol* 37:231–241, 1995.
26. Basser PJ, Mattiello J, LeBihan D: Estimation of the effective self-diffusion tensor from the NMR spin echo, *J Magn Reson B* 103:247–254, 1994.
27. Pierpaoli C, Jezzard P, Basser PJ, Barnett A, Di Chiro G: Diffusion tensor MR imaging of the human brain, *Radiology* 201:637–648, 1996.
28. Liang Z, Zeng J, Zhang C, Liu S, Ling X, Wang F, Ling L, Hou Q, Xing S, Pei Z: Progression of pathological changes in the middle cerebellar peduncle by diffusion tensor imaging correlates with lesser motor gains after pontine infarction, *Neurorehabil Neural Repair* 23:692–698, 2009.
29. Nelles M, Gieseke J, Flacke S, et al: Diffusion tensor pyramidal tractography in patients with anterior choroidal artery infarcts, *AJNR Am J Neuroradiol* 29:488–493, 2008.
30. Lansberg MG, Thijs VN, O'Brien MW, et al: Evolution of apparent diffusion coefficient, diffusion-weighted, and T2-weighted signal intensity of acute stroke, *AJNR Am J Neuroradiol* 22:637–644, 2001.
31. Latour LL, Warach S: Cerebral spinal fluid contamination of the measurement of the apparent diffusion coefficient of water in acute stroke, *Magn Reson Med* 48:478–486, 2002.
32. Schaefer PW: Diffusion-weighted imaging as a problem-solving tool in the evaluation of patients with acute strokelike syndromes, *Top Magn Reson Imaging* 11:300–309, 2000.
33. Rempp KA, Brix G, Wenz F, Becker CR, Guckel F, Lorenz WJ: Quantification of regional cerebral blood flow and volume with dynamic susceptibility contrast-enhanced MR imaging, *Radiology* 193:637–641, 1994.
34. Smith AM, Grandin CB, Duprez T, Mataigne F, Cosnard G: Whole brain quantitative CBF, CBV, and MTT measurements using MRI bolus tracking: Implementation and application to data acquired from hyperacute stroke patients, *J Magn Reson Imaging* 12:400–410, 2000.
35. Smith AM, Grandin CB, Duprez T, Mataigne F, Cosnard G: Whole brain quantitative CBF and CBV measurements using MRI bolus tracking: Comparison of methodologies, *Magn Reson Med* 43:559–564, 2000.
36. Ostergaard L, Sorensen AG, Kwong KK, et al: High resolution measurement of cerebral blood flow using intravascular tracer bolus passages. Part II: Experimental comparison and preliminary results, *Magn Reson Med* 36:726–736, 1996.

37. Ostergaard L, Johannsen P, Host-Poulsen P, et al: Cerebral blood flow measurements by magnetic resonance imaging bolus tracking: Comparison with [(15)O]H2O positron emission tomography in humans, *J Cereb Blood Flow Metab* 18:935–940, 1998.

38. Calamante F, Christensen S, Desmond PM, Ostergaard L, Davis SM, Connelly A: The physiological significance of the time-to-maximum (Tmax) parameter in perfusion MRI, *Stroke* 41:1169–1174, 2010.

39. Christensen S, Mouridsen K, Wu O, et al: Comparison of 10 perfusion MRI parameters in 97 sub-6-hour stroke patients using voxel-based receiver operating characteristics analysis, *Stroke* 40:2055–2061, 2009.

40. Roberts DA, Detre JA, Bolinger L, Insko EK, Leigh JS Jr: Quantitative magnetic resonance imaging of human brain perfusion at 1.5 T using steady-state inversion of arterial water, *Proc Natl Acad Sci U S A* 91:33–37, 1994.

41. Wells JA, Lythgoe MF, Choy M, Gadian DG, Ordidge RJ, Thomas DL: Characterizing the origin of the arterial spin labelling signal in MRI using a multiecho acquisition approach, *J Cereb Blood Flow Metab* 29:1836–1845, 2009.

42. Hendrikse J, Petersen ET, van Laar PJ, Golay X: Cerebral border zones between distal end branches of intracranial arteries: MR imaging, *Radiology* 246:572–580, 2008.

43. van Laar PJ, van der Grond J, Hendrikse J: Brain perfusion territory imaging: Methods and clinical applications of selective arterial spin-labeling MR imaging, *Radiology* 246:354–364, 2008.

44. Kim SG, Tsekos NV, Ashe J: Multi-slice perfusion-based functional MRI using the FAIR technique: Comparison of CBF and BOLD effects, *NMR Biomed* 10:191–196, 1997.

45. Edelman RR, Siewert B, Darby DG, et al : Qualitative mapping of cerebral blood flow and functional localization with echo-planar MR imaging and signal targeting with alternating radio frequency, *Radiology* 192:513–520, 1994.

46. Detre JA, Alsop DC: Perfusion magnetic resonance imaging with continuous arterial spin labeling: Methods and clinical applications in the central nervous system, *Eur J Radiol* 30:115–124, 1999.

47. Siewert B, Schlaug G, Edelman RR, Warach S: Comparison of EPISTAR and T2*-weighted gadolinium-enhanced perfusion imaging in patients with acute cerebral ischemia, *Neurology* 48:673–679, 1997.

48. Buxton RB, Frank LR, Wong EC, Siewert B, Warach S, Edelman RR: A general kinetic model for quantitative perfusion imaging with arterial spin labeling, *Magn Reson Med* 40:383–396, 1998.

49. Wong EC, Buxton RB, Frank LR: Quantitative perfusion imaging using arterial spin labeling, *Neuroimaging Clin North Am* 9:333–342, 1999.

50. Alsop DC, Detre JA: Multisection cerebral blood flow MR imaging with continuous arterial spin labeling, *Radiology* 208:410–416, 1998.

51. Debrey SM, Yu H, Lynch JK, et al: Diagnostic accuracy of magnetic resonance angiography for internal carotid artery disease: A systematic review and meta-analysis, *Stroke* 39:2237–2248, 2008.

52. Raghavan P, Mukherjee S, Gaughen J, Phillips CD: Magnetic resonance angiography of the extracranial carotid system, *Top Magn Reson Imaging* 19:241–249, 2008.

53. Babiarz LS, Romero JM, Murphy EK, et al: Contrast-enhanced MR angiography is not more accurate than unenhanced 2D time-of-flight MR angiography for determining > or = 70% internal carotid artery stenosis, *AJNR Am J Neuroradiol* 30:761–768, 2009.

54. Provenzale JM, Sarikaya B: Comparison of test performance characteristics of MRI, MR angiography, and CT angiography in the diagnosis of carotid and vertebral artery dissection: A review of the medical literature, *AJR Am J Roentgenol* 193:1167–1174, 2009.

55. Wardlaw JM, White PM: The detection and management of unruptured intracranial aneurysms, *Brain* 123:205–221, 2000.

56. Korogi Y, Takahashi M, Mabuchi N, et al: Intracranial aneurysms: Diagnostic accuracy of MR angiography with evaluation of maximum intensity projection and source images, *Radiology* 199:199–207, 1996.

57. Greer DM, Koroshetz WJ, Cullen S, et al: Magnetic resonance imaging improves detection of intracerebral hemorrhage over computed tomography after intra-arterial thrombolysis, *Stroke* 35:491–495, 2004.

58. Mittal S, Wu Z, Neelavalli J, Haacke EM: Susceptibility-weighted imaging: Technical aspects and clinical applications, part 2, *AJNR Am J Neuroradiol* 30:232–252, 2009.

59. Haacke EM, Mittal S, Wu Z, et al: Susceptibility-weighted imaging: Technical aspects and clinical applications, part 1, *AJNR Am J Neuroradiol* 30:19–30, 2009.

60. Barker PB, Soher BJ, Blackband SJ, et al: Quantitation of proton NMR spectra of the human brain using tissue water as an internal concentration reference, *NMR in Biomedicine* 6:89–94, 1993.

61. Leiner T, Kucharczyk W: NSF prevention in clinical practice: Summary of recommendations and guidelines in the United States, Canada, and Europe, *J Magn Reson Imaging* 30:1357–1363, 2009.

62. Thomsen HS: How to avoid nephrogenic systemic fibrosis: Current guidelines in Europe and the United States, *Radiol Clin North Am* 47:871–875, 2009:vii.

63. Fazekas F, Fazekas G, Schmidt R, et al: Magnetic resonance imaging correlates of transient cerebral ischemic attacks, *Stroke* 27:607–611, 1996.

64. Bhadelia RA, Anderson M, Polak JF, et al: Prevalence and associations of MRI-demonstrated brain infarcts in elderly subjects with a history of transient ischemic attack. The Cardiovascular Health Study, *Stroke* 30:383–388, 1999.

65. Kimura K, Minematsu K, Wada K, et al: Lesions visualized by contrast-enhanced magnetic resonance imaging in transient ischemic attacks, *J Neurol Sci* 173:103–108, 2000.

66. Awad I, Modic M, Little JR, et al: Focal parenchymal lesions in transient ischemic attacks: Correlation of computed tomography and magnetic resonance imaging, *Stroke* 17:399–403, 1986.

67. Kidwell CS, Alger JR, Di Salle F, et al: Diffusion MRI in patients with transient ischemic attacks, *Stroke* 30:1174–1180, 1999.

68. Engelter ST, Provenzale JM, Petrella JR, Alberts MJ: Diffusion MR imaging and transient ischemic attacks, *Stroke* 30:2762–2763, 1999.

69. Ay H, Buonanno FS, Schaefer PW, et al: Clinical and diffusion-weighted imaging characteristics of an identifiable subset of TIA patients with acute infarction [abstract], *Stroke* 30:235A, 1999.

70. Takayama H, Mihara B, Kobayashi M, et al: [Usefulness of diffusion-weighted MRI in the diagnosis of transient ischemic attacks], *No To Shinkei* 52:919–923, 2000.

71. Bisschops RHC, Kappelle LJ, Mali W, van der Grond J: Hemodynamic and metabolic changes in transient ischemic attack patients, *Stroke* 33:110–115, 2001.

72. Mlynash M, Olivot JM, Tong DC, et al: Yield of combined perfusion and diffusion MR imaging in hemispheric TIA, *Neurology* 72:1127–1133, 2009.

73. Calvet D, Touze E, Oppenheim C, Turc G, Meder JF, Mas JL: DWI lesions and TIA etiology improve the prediction of stroke after TIA, *Stroke* 40:187–192, 2009.

74. Boulanger JM, Coutts SB, Eliasziw M, Subramaniam S, Scott J, Demchuk AM: Diffusion-weighted imaging-negative patients with transient ischemic attack are at risk of recurrent transient events, *Stroke* 38:2367–2369, 2007.

75. Easton JD, Saver JL, Albers GW, et al: Definition and evaluation of transient ischemic attack. A scientific statement for healthcare professionals from the American Heart Association/American Stroke Association Stroke Council; Council on Cardiovascular Surgery and Anesthesia; Council on Cardiovascular Radiology and Intervention; Council on Cardiovascular Nursing; and the Interdisciplinary Council on Peripheral Vascular Disease, *Stroke* 40:2276–2293, 2009.

76. Crisostomo RA, Garcia MM, Tong DC: Detection of diffusion-weighted MRI abnormalities in patients with transient ischemic attack: Correlation with clinical characteristics, *Stroke* 34:932–937, 2003.

77. Purroy F, Montaner J, Rovira A, et al: Higher risk of further vascular events among transient ischemic attack patients with diffusion-weighted imaging acute ischemic lesions, *Stroke* 35:2313–2319, 2004.

78. Shah SH, Saver JL, Kidwell CS, et al: A multicenter pooled, patient-level data analysis of diffusion-weighted MRI in TIA patients, *Stroke*:38, 2007.

78a. Schulz UG, Briley D, Meagher T, et al: Diffusion-weighted MRI in 300 patients presenting late with subacute transient ischemic attack or minor stroke, *Stroke* 35(11):2459–2465, 2004.

79. Oppenheim C, Lamy C, Touze E, et al: Do transient ischemic attacks with diffusion-weighted imaging abnormalities correspond to brain infarctions? *AJNR Am J Neuroradiol* 27:1782–1787, 2006.

80. Sylaja PN, Coutts SB, Krol A, et al: When to expect negative diffusion-weighted images in stroke and transient ischemic attack, *Stroke* 39:1898–1900, 2008.

81. Prabhakaran S, Chong JY, Sacco RL: Impact of abnormal diffusion-weighted imaging results on short-term outcome following transient ischemic attack, *Arch Neurol* 64:1105–1109, 2007.

82. Cucchiara BL, Messe SR, Taylor RA, et al: Is the ABCD score useful for risk stratification of patients with acute transient ischemic attack? *Stroke* 37:1710–1714, 2006.

83. Krol AL, Coutts SB, Simon JE, et al: Perfusion MRI abnormalities in speech or motor transient ischemic attack patients, *Stroke* 36:2487–2489, 2005.

84. Mohr JP, Biller J, Hilal SK, et al: Magnetic resonance versus computed tomographic imaging in acute stroke, *Stroke* 26:807–812, 1995.

85. Maeda M, Yamamoto T, Daimon S, et al: Arterial hyperintensity on fast fluid-attenuated inversion recovery images: A subtle finding for hyperacute stroke undetected by diffusion-weighted MR imaging, *AJNR Am J Neuroradiol* 22:632–636, 2001.

86. Koga M, Kimura K, Minematsu K, Yamaguchi T: Hyperintense MCA branch sign on FLAIR-MRI, *J Clin Neurosci* 9:187–189, 2002.

87. Flacke S, Urbach H, Keller E, et al: Middle cerebral artery (MCA) susceptibility sign at susceptibility-based perfusion MR imaging: Clinical importance and comparison with hyperdense MCA sign at CT, *Radiology* 215:476–482, 2000.

88. Chalela JA, Haymore JB, Ezzeddine MA, et al: The hypointense MCA sign, *Neurology* 58:1470, 2002.

89. Baird AE, Warach S: Magnetic resonance imaging of acute stroke, *J Cereb Blood Flow Metab* 18:583–609, 1998.

90. Schlaug G, Siewert B, Benfield A, et al: Time course of the apparent diffusion coefficient (ADC) abnormality in human stroke, *Neurology* 49:113–119, 1997.

91. Fiebach JB, Jansen O, Schellinger PD, et al: Serial analysis of the apparent diffusion coefficient time course in human stroke, *Neuroradiology* 44:294–298, 2002.

92. Nagesh V, Welch KM, Windham JP, et al: Time course of ADCw changes in ischemic stroke: Beyond the human eye! *Stroke* 29:1778–1782, 1998.

93. Ay H, Buonanno FS, Rordorf G, et al: Normal diffusion-weighted MRI during stroke-like deficits, *Neurology* 52:1784–1792, 1999.

94. Lovblad KO, Laubach HJ, Baird AE, et al: Clinical experience with diffusion-weighted MR in patients with acute stroke, *AJNR Am J Neuroradiol* 19:1061–1066, 1998.

95. van Everdingen KJ, van der Grond J, Kappelle LJ, et al: Diffusion-weighted magnetic resonance imaging in acute stroke, *Stroke* 29:1783–1790, 1998.

96. Gonzalez RG, Schaefer PW, Buonanno FS, et al: Diffusion-weighted MR imaging: Diagnostic accuracy in patients imaged within 6 hours of stroke symptom onset, *Radiology* 210:155–162, 1999.

97. Mullins ME, Schaefer PW, Sorensen AG, et al: CT and conventional and diffusion-weighted MR imaging in acute stroke: Study in 691 patients at presentation to the emergency department, *Radiology* 224:353–360, 2002.

98. Perkins CJ, Kahya E, Roque CT, et al: Fluid-attenuated inversion recovery and diffusion- and perfusion-weighted MRI abnormalities in 117 consecutive patients with stroke symptoms, *Stroke* 32:2774–2781, 2001.

99. Lansberg MG, Norbash AM, Marks MP, et al: Advantages of adding diffusion-weighted magnetic resonance imaging to conventional magnetic resonance imaging for evaluating acute stroke, *Arch Neurol* 57:1311–1316, 2000.

100. Barber PA, Darby DG, Desmond PM, et al: Identification of major ischemic change. Diffusion-weighted imaging versus computed tomography, *Stroke* 30:2059–2065, 1999.

101. Kelly PJ, Hedley-Whyte ET, Primavera J, et al: Diffusion MRI in ischemic stroke compared to pathologically verified infarction, *Neurology* 56:914–920, 2001.

102. Chalela JA, Kidwell CS, Nentwich LM, et al: Magnetic resonance imaging and computed tomography in emergency assessment of patients with suspected acute stroke: A prospective comparison, *Lancet* 369:293–298, 2007.

103. Schellinger PD, Bryan RN, Caplan LR, et al: Evidence-based guideline: The role of diffusion and perfusion MRI for the diagnosis of acute ischemic stroke: Report of the Therapeutics and Technology Assessment Subcommittee of the American Academy of Neurology, *Neurology* 75:177–185, 2010.

104. Lansberg MG, Albers GW, Beaulieu C, Marks MP: Comparison of diffusion-weighted MRI and CT in acute stroke, *Neurology* 54:1557–1561, 2000.

105. Warach S, Pettigrew LC, Dashe JF, et al: Effect of citicoline on ischemic lesions as measured by diffusion-weighted magnetic resonance imaging. Citicoline 010 Investigators, *Ann Neurol* 48:713–722, 2000.

106. Baird AE, Benfield A, Schlaug G, et al: Enlargement of human cerebral ischemic lesion volumes measured by diffusion-weighted magnetic resonance imaging, *Ann Neurol* 41:581–589, 1997.

107. Lansberg MG, O'Brien MW, Tong DC, et al: Evolution of cerebral infarct volume assessed by diffusion-weighted magnetic resonance imaging, *Arch Neurol* 58:613–617, 2001.

108. Beaulieu C, de Crespigny A, Tong DC, et al: Longitudinal magnetic resonance imaging study of perfusion and diffusion in stroke: Evolution of lesion volume and correlation with clinical outcome, *Ann Neurol* 46:568–578, 1999.

109. Schwamm LH, Koroshetz WJ, Sorensen AG, et al: Time course of lesion development in patients with acute stroke: Serial diffusion- and hemodynamic-weighted magnetic resonance imaging, *Stroke* 29:2268–2276, 1998.

110. Warach S, Dashe JF, Edelman RR: Clinical outcome in ischemic stroke predicted by early diffusion-weighted and perfusion magnetic resonance imaging: A preliminary analysis, *J Cereb Blood Flow Metab* 16:53–59, 1996.

111. Lovblad KO, Baird AE, Schlaug G, et al: Ischemic lesion volumes in acute stroke by diffusion-weighted magnetic resonance imaging correlate with clinical outcome, *Ann Neurol* 42:164–170, 1997.

112. Tong DC, Yenari MA, Albers GW, OB M, et al: Correlation of perfusion- and diffusion-weighted MRI with NIHSS score in acute (<6.5 hour) ischemic stroke, *Neurology* 50:864–870, 1998.

113. Barber PA, Darby DG, Desmond PM, et al: Prediction of stroke outcome with echoplanar perfusion- and diffusion-weighted MRI, *Neurology* 51:418–426, 1998.

114. Thijs VN, Adami A, Neumann-Haefelin T, Clinical and radiological correlates of reduced cerebral blood flow measured using magnetic resonance imaging, *Arch Neurol* 59:233–238, 2002.

115. Thijs VN, Lansberg MG, Beaulieu C, et al: Is early ischemic lesion volume on diffusion-weighted imaging an independent predictor of stroke outcome? A multivariable analysis, *Stroke* 31:2597–2602, 2000.

116. Baird AE, Lovblad KO, Dashe JF, et al: Clinical correlations of diffusion and perfusion lesion volumes in acute ischemic stroke, *Cerebrovasc Dis* 10:441–448, 2000.

117. Baird AE, Dambrosia J, Janket S, et al: A three-item scale for the early prediction of stroke recovery, *Lancet* 357:2095–2099, 2001.

118. Linfante I, Llinas RH, Schlaug G, et al: Diffusion-weighted imaging and National Institutes of Health Stroke Scale in the acute phase of posterior-circulation stroke, *Arch Neurol* 58:621–628, 2001.

119. Lutsep HL, Albers GW, DeCrespigny A, et al: Clinical utility of diffusion-weighted magnetic resonance imaging in the assessment of ischemic stroke, *Ann Neurol* 41:574–580, 1997.

120. Lee LJ, Kidwell CS, Alger J, et al: Impact on stroke subtype diagnosis of early diffusion-weighted magnetic resonance imaging and magnetic resonance angiography, *Stroke* 31:1081–1089, 2000.

121. Fitzek C, Tintera J, Muller-Forell W, et al: Differentiation of recent and old cerebral infarcts by diffusion-weighted MRI, *Neuroradiology* 40:778–782, 1998.

122. Schonewille WJ, Tuhrim S, Singer MB, Atlas SW: Diffusion-weighted MRI in acute lacunar syndromes. A clinical-radiological correlation study, *Stroke* 30:2066–2069, 1999.

123. Ostergaard L, Sorensen AG, Kwong KK, et al: High resolution measurement of cerebral blood flow using intravascular tracer bolus passages. Part II: Experimental comparison and preliminary results, *Magn Reson Med* 36:726–736, 1996.

124. Ostergaard L, Weisskoff RM, Chesler DA, et al: High resolution measurement of cerebral blood flow using intravascular tracer bolus passages. Part I: Mathematical approach and statistical analysis, *Magn Reson Med* 36:715–725, 1996.

125. Baird AE, Lovblad KO, Schlaug G, et al: Multiple acute stroke syndrome: Marker of embolic disease? *Neurology* 54:674-678, 2000.
126. Sylaja PN, Coutts SB, Subramaniam S, et al: Acute ischemic lesions of varying ages predict risk of ischemic events in stroke/TIA patients, *Neurology* 68:415-419, 2007.
127. Kang DW, Latour LL, Chalela JA, et al: Early ischemic lesion recurrence within a week after acute ischemic stroke, *Ann Neurol* 54:66-74, 2003.
128. Kang DW, Latour LL, Chalela JA, et al: Early and late recurrence of ischemic lesion on MRI: Evidence for a prolonged stroke-prone state?, *Neurology* 63:2261-2265, 2004.
129. Kang DW, Chalela JA, Ezzeddine MA, Warach S: Association of ischemic lesion patterns on early diffusion-weighted imaging with TOAST stroke subtypes, *Arch Neurol* 60:1730-1734, 2003.
130. Chaves CJ, Silver B, Schlaug G, et al: Diffusion- and perfusion-weighted MRI patterns in borderzone infarcts, *Stroke* 31:1090-1096, 2000.
131. Cho AH, Sohn SI, Han MK, et al: Safety and efficacy of MRI-based thrombolysis in unclear-onset stroke. A preliminary report, *Cerebrovasc Dis* 25:572-579, 2008.
132. Ebinger M, Galinovic I, Rozanski M, et al: Fluid-attenuated inversion recovery evolution within 12 hours from stroke onset: A reliable tissue clock?, *Stroke* 41:250-255, 2010.
133. Song SS, Ritter CH, Ku KD, et al: The upper time limit of DWI positive—FLAIR negative MRI in witnessed-onset acute ischemic strokes is less than 6 hours: Implications for the design of wake-up stroke treatment trials, *Stroke* 41:e48, 2010.
134. Thomalla G, Rossbach P, Rosenkranz M, et al: Negative fluid-attenuated inversion recovery imaging identifies acute ischemic stroke at 3 hours or less, *Ann Neurol* 65:724-732, 2009.
135. Kidwell CS, Latour L, Saver JL, et al: Thrombolytic toxicity: Blood brain barrier disruption in human ischemic stroke, *Cerebrovasc Dis* 25:338-343, 2008.
136. Warach S, Latour LL: Evidence of reperfusion injury, exacerbated by thrombolytic therapy, in human focal brain ischemia using a novel imaging marker of early blood-brain barrier disruption, *Stroke* 35(Suppl 1):2659-2661, 2004.
137. Barr TL, Latour LL, Lee KY, et al: Blood-brain barrier disruption in humans is independently associated with increased matrix metalloproteinase-9, *Stroke* 41:e123-128, 2010.
138. Schellinger PD, Chalela JA, Kang DW, et al: Diagnostic and prognostic value of early MR Imaging vessel signs in hyperacute stroke patients imaged <3 hours and treated with recombinant tissue plasminogen activator, *AJNR Am J Neuroradiol* 26:618-624, 2005.
139. Lee KY, Latour LL, Luby M, et al: Distal hyperintense vessels on FLAIR: An MRI marker for collateral circulation in acute stroke?, *Neurology* 72:1134-1139, 2009.
140. Crain MR, Yuh WT, Greene GM, et al: Cerebral ischemia: Evaluation with contrast-enhanced MR imaging, *AJNR Am J Neuroradiol* 12:631-639, 1991.
141. Kuhn MJ, Mikulis DJ, Ayoub DM, et al: Wallerian degeneration after cerebral infarction: Evaluation with sequential MR imaging, *Radiology* 172:179-182, 1989.
142. Awad IA, Johnson PC, Spetzler RF, Hodak JA: Incidental subcortical lesions identified on magnetic resonance imaging in the elderly. II. Postmortem pathological correlations, *Stroke* 17:1090-1097, 1986.
143. Awad IA, Spetzler RF, Hodak JA, et al: Incidental subcortical lesions identified on magnetic resonance imaging in the elderly. I. Correlation with age and cerebrovascular risk factors, *Stroke* 17:1084-1089, 1986.
144. Awad IA, Spetzler RF, Hodak JA, et al: Incidental lesions noted on magnetic resonance imaging of the brain: Prevalence and clinical significance in various age groups, *Neurosurgery* 20:222-227, 1987.
145. Awad IA, Masaryk T, Magdinec M: Pathogenesis of subcortical hyperintense lesions on magnetic resonance imaging of the brain. Observations in patients undergoing controlled therapeutic internal carotid artery occlusion, *Stroke* 24:1339-1346, 1993.
146. Fazekas F, Kleinert R, Offenbacher H, et al: The morphologic correlate of incidental punctate white matter hyperintensities on MR images, *AJNR Am J Neuroradiol* 12:915-921, 1991.
147. Schmidt R, Fazekas F, Kleinert G, et al: Magnetic resonance imaging signal hyperintensities in the deep and subcortical white matter. A comparative study between stroke patients and normal volunteers, *Arch Neurol* 49:825-827, 1992.
148. Schmidt R, Fazekas F, Hayn M, et al: Risk factors for microangiopathy-related cerebral damage in the Austrian stroke prevention study, *J Neurol Sci* 152:15-21, 1997.
149. Schmidt R, Schmidt H, Fazekas F, et al: Apolipoprotein E polymorphism and silent microangiopathy-related cerebral damage. Results of the Austrian Stroke Prevention Study, *Stroke* 28:951-956, 1997.
150. Schmidt R, Fazekas F, Kapeller P, et al: MRI white matter hyperintensities: Three-year follow-up of the Austrian Stroke Prevention Study, *Neurology* 53:132-139, 1999.
151. Fazekas F, Niederkorn K, Schmidt R, et al: White matter signal abnormalities in normal individuals: Correlation with carotid ultrasonography, cerebral blood flow measurements, and cerebrovascular risk factors, *Stroke* 19:1285-1288, 1988.
152. Saunders DE: MR spectroscopy in stroke, *Br Med Bull* 56:334-345, 2000.
153. Simmons ML, Frondoza CG, Coyle JT: Immunocytochemical localization of *N*-acetyl-aspartate with monoclonal antibodies, *Neuroscience* 45:37-45, 1991.
154. Duijn JH, Matson GB, Maudsley AA, et al: Human brain infarction: Proton MR spectroscopy, *Radiology* 183:711-718, 1992.
155. Saunders DE, Howe FA, van den Boogaart A, et al: Continuing ischemic damage after acute middle cerebral artery infarction in humans demonstrated by short-echo proton spectroscopy, *Stroke* 26:1007-1013, 1995.
156. Graham GD, Blamire AM, Rothman DL, et al: Early temporal variation of cerebral metabolites after human stroke. A proton magnetic resonance spectroscopy study, *Stroke* 24:1891-1896, 1993.
157. Gideon P, Henriksen O, Sperling B, et al: Early time course of *N*-acetylaspartate, creatine and phosphocreatine, and compounds containing choline in the brain after acute stroke. A proton magnetic resonance spectroscopy study, *Stroke* 23:1566-1572, 1992.
158. Gillard JH, Barker PB, van Zijl PC, et al: Proton MR spectroscopy in acute middle cerebral artery stroke, *AJNR Am J Neuroradiol* 17:873-886, 1996.
159. Wardlaw JM, Marshall I, Wild J, et al: Studies of acute ischemic stroke with proton magnetic resonance spectroscopy: Relation between time from onset, neurological deficit, metabolite abnormalities in the infarct, blood flow, and clinical outcome, *Stroke* 29:1618-1624, 1998.
160. Munoz Maniega S, Cvoro V, Chappell FM, et al: Changes in NAA and Lactate following ischemic stroke. A serial MR spectroscopic imaging study, *Neurology* 71:7, 2008.
161. Higuchi T, Fernandez EJ, Maudsley AA, et al: Mapping of lactate and *N*-acetyl-l-aspartate predicts infarction during acute focal ischemia: In vivo 1H magnetic resonance spectroscopy in rats, *Neurosurgery* 38:121-129, 1996:discussion 129-130.
162. Sijens PE, den Heijer T, de Leeuw FE, et al: MR spectroscopy detection of lactate and lipid signals in the brains of healthy elderly people, *Euro Rad* 11:1495-1501, 2001.
163. Peeling J, Wong D, Sutherland GR: Nuclear magnetic resonance study of regional metabolism after forebrain ischemia in rats, *Stroke* 20:633-640, 1989.
164. Allen K, Busza AL, Crockard HA, et al: Acute cerebral ischaemia: Concurrent changes in cerebral blood flow, energy metabolites, pH, and lactate measured with hydrogen clearance and 31P and 1H nuclear magnetic resonance spectroscopy. III. Changes following ischaemia, *J Cereb Blood Flow Meta* 8:816-821, 1988.
165. Nicoli F, Lefur Y, Denis B, et al: Metabolic counterpart of decreased apparent diffusion coefficient during hyperacute ischemic stroke: A brain proton magnetic resonance spectroscopic imaging study, *Stroke* 34:e82-87, 2003.
166. Singhal AB, Ratai E, Benner T, et al: Magnetic resonance spectroscopy study of oxygen therapy in ischemic stroke, *Stroke* 38:2851, 2007.
167. Monsein LH, Mathews VP, Barker PB, et al: Irreversible regional cerebral ischemia: Serial MR imaging and proton MR spectroscopy in a nonhuman primate model, *AJNR Am J Neuroradiol* 14:963-970, 1993.
168. Karaszewski B, Wardlaw JM, Marshall I, et al: Measurement of brain temperature with magnetic resonance spectroscopy in acute ischemic stroke, *Ann Neurol* 60:438-446, 2006.

169. Marshall I, Karaszewski B, Wardlaw JM, et al: Measurement of regional brain temperature using proton spectroscopic imaging: Validation and application to acute ischemic stroke, *Magn Reson Imaging* 24:699-706, 2006.

170. An L, Latour L, Dani K, Warach S: Simultaneous measurement of glutathione and other metabolites in stroke patients by j-difference spectroscopy, *Proc Intl Soc Mag Reson Med* 17:379, 2009.

171. van der Grond J, Balm R, Klijn CJ, et al: Cerebral metabolism of patients with stenosis of the internal carotid artery before and after endarterectomy, *J Cereb Blood Flow Metab* 16:320-326, 1996.

172. Tsuchida C, Kimura H, Sadato N, et al: Evaluation of brain metabolism in steno-occlusive carotid artery disease by proton MR spectroscopy: A correlative study with oxygen metabolism by PET. [see comment], *J Nucl Med* 41:1357-1362, 2000.

173. Kim GE, Lee JH, Cho YP, Kim ST: Metabolic changes in the ischemic penumbra after carotid endarterectomy in stroke patients by localized in vivo proton magnetic resonance spectroscopy (1H-MRS), *Cardiovasc Surg* 9:345-355, 2001.

174. Parsons MW, Li T, Barber PA, et al: Combined H MR spectroscopy and diffusion-weighted MRI improves the prediction of stroke outcome, *Neurology* 55:498-505, 2000.

175. Federico F, Simone IL, Conte C, et al: Prognostic significance of metabolic changes detected by proton magnetic resonance spectroscopy in ischaemic stroke, *J Neurol* 243:241-247, 1996.

176. Haga KK, Khor YP, Farrall A, Wardlaw JM: A systematic review of brain metabolite changes, measured with 1H magnetic resonance spectroscopy, in healthy aging, *Neurobiol Aging* 30:353-363, 2009.

177. Kidwell CS, Wintermark M: Imaging of intracranial haemorrhage, *Lancet Neurol* 7:256-267, 2008.

178. Patel MR, Edelman RR, Warach S: Detection of hyperacute primary intraparenchymal hemorrhage by magnetic resonance imaging, *Stroke* 27:2321-2324, 1996.

179. Linfante I, Llinas RH, Caplan LR, Warach S: MRI features of intracerebral hemorrhage within 2 hours from symptom onset, *Stroke* 30:2263-2267, 1999.

180. Schellinger PD, Jansen O, Fiebach JB, et al: A standardized MRI stroke protocol: Comparison with CT in hyperacute intracerebral hemorrhage, *Stroke* 30:765-768, 1999.

181. Kidwell CS, Chalela JA, Saver JL, et al: Comparison of MRI and CT for detection of acute intracerebral hemorrhage, *JAMA* 292: 1823-1830, 2004.

182. Fiebach JB, Schellinger PD, Jansen O, et al: diffusion-weighted: MR imaging in randomized order: Diffusion-weighted imaging results in higher accuracy and lower interrater variability in the diagnosis of hyperacute ischemic stroke, *Stroke* 33:2206-2210, 2002.

183. Packard AS, Kase CS, Aly AS, Barest GD: Computed tomography-negative" intracerebral hemorrhage: Case report and implications for management, *Arch Neurol* 60:1156-1159, 2003.

184. Singer OC, Sitzer M, du Mesnil de Rochemont R, Neumann-Haefelin T: Practical limitations of acute stroke MRI due to patient-related problems, *Neurology* 62:1848-1849, 2004.

185. Lang EW, Ren Ya Z, Preul C, et al: Stroke pattern interpretation: The variability of hypertensive versus amyloid angiopathy hemorrhage, *Cerebrovasc Dis* 12:121-130, 2001.

186. Broderick J, Connolly S, Feldmann E, et al: Guidelines for the management of spontaneous intracerebral hemorrhage in adults: 2007 update: A guideline from the American Heart Association/American Stroke Association Stroke Council, High Blood Pressure Research Council, and the Quality of Care and Outcomes in Research Interdisciplinary Working Group, *Stroke* 38:2001-2023, 2007.

187. Kidwell CS, Saver JL, Mattiello J, et al: Diffusion-perfusion MR evaluation of perihematomal injury in hyperacute intracerebral hemorrhage, *Neurology* 57:1611-1617, 2001.

188. Butcher KS, Baird T, MacGregor L, et al: Perihematomal edema in primary intracerebral hemorrhage is plasma derived, *Stroke* 35:1879-1885, 2004.

189. Forbes KP, Pipe JG, Heiserman JE: Diffusion-weighted imaging provides support for secondary neuronal damage from intraparenchymal hematoma, *Neuroradiology* 45:363-367, 2003.

190. Pascual AM, Lopez-Mut JV, Benlloch V, et al: Perfusion-weighted magnetic resonance imaging in acute intracerebral hemorrhage at baseline and during the 1st and 2nd week: A longitudinal study, *Cerebrovasc Dis* 23:6-13, 2007.

191. Herweh C, Juttler E, Schellinger PD, et al: Evidence against a perihemorrhagic penumbra provided by perfusion computed tomography, *Stroke* 38:2941-2947, 2007.

192. Siddique MS, Fernandes HM, Wooldridge TD, et al: Reversible ischemia around intracerebral hemorrhage: A single-photon emission computerized tomography study, *J Neurosurg* 96:736-741, 2002.

193. Murakami M, Fujioka S, Oyama T, et al: Serial changes in the regional cerebral blood flow of patients with hypertensive intracerebral hemorrhage—long-term follow-up SPECT study, *J Neurosurg Sci* 49:117-124, 2005.

194. Fazekas F, Kleinert R, Roob G, et al: Histopathologic analysis of foci of signal loss on gradient-echo T2*-weighted MR images in patients with spontaneous intracerebral hemorrhage: Evidence of microangiopathy-related microbleeds, *AJNR Am J Neuroradiol* 20:637-642, 1999.

195. Roob G, Lechner A, Schmidt R, et al: Frequency and location of microbleeds in patients with primary intracerebral hemorrhage, *Stroke* 31:2665-2669, 2000.

196. Roob G, Schmidt R, Kapeller P, et al: MRI evidence of past cerebral microbleeds in a healthy elderly population, *Neurology* 52:991-994, 1999.

197. Kwa VI, Franke CL, Verbeeten B Jr, Stam J: Silent intracerebral microhemorrhages in patients with ischemic stroke. Amsterdam Vascular Medicine Group, *Ann Neurol* 44:372-377, 1998.

198. Greenberg SM, Briggs ME, Hyman BT, et al: Apolipoprotein E epsilon 4 is associated with the presence and earlier onset of hemorrhage in cerebral amyloid angiopathy, *Stroke* 27:1333-1337, 1996.

199. Tsushima Y, Aoki J, Endo K: Brain microhemorrhages detected on T2*-weighted gradient-echo MR images, *AJNR Am J Neuroradiol* 24:88-96, 2003.

200. Dichgans M, Holtmannspotter M, Herzog J, et al: Cerebral microbleeds in CADASIL: A gradient-echo magnetic resonance imaging and autopsy study, *Stroke* 33:67-71, 2002.

201. Kinoshita T, Okudera T, Tamura H, et al: Assessment of lacunar hemorrhage associated with hypertensive stroke by echo-planar gradient-echo T2*-weighted MRI, *Stroke* 31:1646-1650, 2000.

202. Kidwell CS, Saver JL, Villablanca JP, et al: Magnetic resonance imaging detection of microbleeds before thrombolysis: An emerging application, *Stroke* 33:95-98, 2002.

203. Wong KS, Chan YL, Liu JY, et al: Asymptomatic microbleeds as a risk factor for aspirin-associated intracerebral hemorrhages, *Neurology* 60:511-513, 2003.

204. Chalela JA, Kang DW, Warach S: Multiple cerebral microbleeds: MRI marker of a diffuse hemorrhage-prone state, *J Neuroimaging* 14:54-57, 2004.

205. Kakuda W, Thijs VN, Lansberg MG, et al: Clinical importance of microbleeds in patients receiving IV thrombolysis, *Neurology* 65:1175-1178, 2005.

206. Fiehler J, Albers GW, Boulanger JM, et al: Bleeding risk analysis in stroke imaging before thromboLysis (BRASIL): Pooled analysis of T2*-weighted magnetic resonance imaging data from 570 patients, *Stroke* 38:2738-2744, 2007.

207. Greenberg SM, Eng JA, Ning M, et al: Hemorrhage burden predicts recurrent intracerebral hemorrhage after lobar hemorrhage, *Stroke* 35:1415-1420, 2004.

208. Boulanger JM, Coutts SB, Eliasziw M, et al: Cerebral microhemorrhages predict new disabling or fatal strokes in patients with acute ischemic stroke or transient ischemic attack, *Stroke* 37:911-914, 2006.

209. Imaizumi T, Horita Y, Hashimoto Y, et al: Dotlike hemosiderin spots on T2*-weighted magnetic resonance imaging as a predictor of stroke recurrence: A prospective study, *J Neurosurg* 101:915-920, 2004.

210. Copenhaver BR, Hsia AW, Merino JG, et al: Racial differences in microbleed prevalence in primary intracerebral hemorrhage, *Neurology* 71:1176-1182, 2008.

210a. Furlan A, Higashida R, Wechsler L, et al: Intra-arterial prourokinase for acute ischemic stroke. The PROACT II study: A randomized controlled trail. Prolyse in Acute Cerebral Thromboembolism, *JAMA* 282(21):2003-2011, 1999.

211. Lin K, Kazmi KS, Law M, et al: Measuring elevated microvascular permeability and predicting hemorrhagic transformation in acute ischemic stroke using first-pass dynamic perfusion CT imaging, *AJNR Am J Neuroradiol* 28:1292-1298, 2007.

212. Bang OY, Buck BH, Saver JL, et al: Prediction of hemorrhagic transformation after recanalization therapy using T2*-permeability magnetic resonance imaging, *Ann Neurol* 62:170-176, 2007.

213. Lansberg MG, Thijs VN, Bammer R, et al: Risk factors of symptomatic intracerebral hemorrhage after tPA therapy for acute stroke, *Stroke* 38:2275-2278, 2007.

214. Singer OC, Humpich MC, Fiehler J, et al: Risk for symptomatic intracerebral hemorrhage after thrombolysis assessed by diffusion-weighted magnetic resonance imaging, *Ann Neurol*, 2007.

215. Selim M, Fink JN, Kumar S, et al: Predictors of hemorrhagic transformation after intravenous recombinant tissue plasminogen activator: Prognostic value of the initial apparent diffusion coefficient and diffusion-weighted lesion volume, *Stroke* 33:2047-2052, 2002.

216. Singer MB, Atlas SW, Drayer BP: Subarachnoid space disease: Diagnosis with fluid-attenuated inversion-recovery MR imaging and comparison with gadolinium-enhanced spin-echo MR imaging—blinded reader study, *Radiology* 208:417-422, 1998.

217. Mitchell P, Wilkinson ID, Hoggard N, et al: Detection of subarachnoid haemorrhage with magnetic resonance imaging, *J Neurol Neurosurg Psychiatry* 70:205-211, 2001.

218. Wiesmann M, Mayer TE, Yousry I, et al: Detection of hyperacute subarachnoid hemorrhage of the brain by using magnetic resonance imaging, *J Neurosurg* 96:684-689, 2002.

219. Mohamed M, Heasly DC, Yagmurlu B, Yousem DM: Fluid-attenuated inversion recovery MR imaging and subarachnoid hemorrhage: Not a panacea, *AJNR Am J Neuroradiol* 25:545-550, 2004.

220. Noguchi K, Seto H, Kamisaki Y, et al: Comparison of fluid-attenuated inversion-recovery MR imaging with CT in a simulated model of acute subarachnoid hemorrhage, *AJNR Am J Neuroradiol* 21:923-927, 2000.

221. Woodcock RJ Jr, Short J, Do HM, et al: Imaging of acute subarachnoid hemorrhage with a fluid-attenuated inversion recovery sequence in an animal model: Comparison with non-contrast-enhanced CT, *AJNR Am J Neuroradiol* 22:1698-1703, 2001.

222. Condette-Auliac S, Bracard S, Anxionnat R, et al: Vasospasm after subarachnoid hemorrhage: Interest in diffusion-weighted MR imaging, *Stroke* 32:1818-1824, 2001.

223. Hadeishi H, Suzuki A, Yasui N, et al: Diffusion-weighted magnetic resonance imaging in patients with subarachnoid hemorrhage, *Neurosurgery* 50:741-747, 2002:discussion 747-748.

224. Rordorf G, Koroshetz WJ, Copen WA, et al: Diffusion- and perfusion-weighted imaging in vasospasm after subarachnoid hemorrhage, *Stroke* 30:599-605, 1999.

225. Shimoda M, Takeuchi M, Tominaga J, et al: Asymptomatic versus symptomatic infarcts from vasospasm in patients with subarachnoid hemorrhage: Serial magnetic resonance imaging, *Neurosurgery* 49:1341-1348, 2001:discussion 1348-1350.

226. Griffiths PD, Wilkinson ID, Mitchell P, et al: Multimodality MR imaging depiction of hemodynamic changes and cerebral ischemia in subarachnoid hemorrhage, *AJNR Am J Neuroradiol* 22:1690-1697, 2001.

227. Hattingen E, Blasel S, Dettmann E, et al: Perfusion-weighted MRI to evaluate cerebral autoregulation in aneurysmal subarachnoid haemorrhage, *Neuroradiology* 50:929-938, 2008.

228. Weidauer S, Lanfermann H, Raabe A, et al: Impairment of cerebral perfusion and infarct patterns attributable to vasospasm after aneurysmal subarachnoid hemorrhage: A prospective MRI and DSA study, *Stroke* 38:1831-1836, 2007.

229. Siewert B, Patel MR, Warach S: Magnetic resonance angiography, *Neurologist* 1:167-184, 1995.

230. Anderson CM, Saloner D, Lee RE, et al: Assessment of carotid artery stenosis by MR angiography: Comparison with x-ray angiography and color-coded Doppler ultrasound, *AJNR Am J Neuroradiol* 13:989-1003, 1992:discussion 1005-1008.

231. Long A, Lepoutre A, Corbillon E, Branchereau A: Critical review of non- or minimally invasive methods (duplex ultrasonography, MR- and CT-angiography) for evaluating stenosis of the proximal internal carotid artery, *Eur J Vasc Endovasc Surg* 24:43-52, 2002.

232. Huston J 3rd, Fain SB, Wald JT, et al: Carotid artery: Elliptic centric contrast-enhanced MR angiography compared with conventional angiography, *Radiology* 218:138-143, 2001.

233. Sundgren PC, Sunden P, Lindgren A, et al: Carotid artery stenosis: Contrast-enhanced MR angiography with two different scan times compared with digital subtraction angiography, *Neuroradiology* 44:592-599, 2002.

234. Remonda L, Senn P, Barth A, et al: Contrast-enhanced 3D MR angiography of the carotid artery: Comparison with conventional digital subtraction angiography, *AJNR Am J Neuroradiol* 23:213-219, 2002.

235. Randoux B, Marro B, Koskas F, et al: Carotid artery stenosis: Prospective comparison of CT, three-dimensional gadolinium-enhanced MR, and conventional angiography, *Radiology* 220:179-185, 2001.

236. Sue DE, Brant-Zawadzki MN, Chance J: Dissection of cranial arteries in the neck: Correlation of MRI and arteriography, *Neuroradiology* 34:273-278, 1992.

237. Provenzale JM, Barboriak DP, Taveras JM: Exercise-related dissection of craniocervical arteries: CT, MR, and angiographic findings, *J Comput Assist Tomogr* 19:268-276, 1995.

238. Rother J, Schwartz A, Rautenberg W, Hennerici M: Magnetic resonance angiography of spontaneous vertebral artery dissection suspected on Doppler ultrasonography, *J Neurol* 242:430-436, 1995.

239. Stringaris K, Liberopoulos K, Giaka E, et al: Three-dimensional time-of-flight MR angiography and MR imaging versus conventional angiography in carotid artery dissections, *Int Angiol* 15:20-25, 1996.

240. Ross JS, Masaryk TJ, Modic MT, et al: Intracranial aneurysms: Evaluation by MR angiography, *AJNR Am J Neuroradiol* 11:449-455, 1990.

241. Huston J 3rd, Nichols DA, Luetmer PH, et al: Blinded prospective evaluation of sensitivity of MR angiography to known intracranial aneurysms: Importance of aneurysm size, *AJNR Am J Neuroradiol* 15:1607-1614, 1994.

242. Curnes JT, Shogry ME, Clark DC, Elsner HJ: MR angiographic demonstration of an intracranial aneurysm not seen on conventional angiography, *AJNR Am J Neuroradiol* 14:971-973, 1993.

243. Schuierer G, Huk WJ, Laub G: Magnetic resonance angiography of intracranial aneurysms: Comparison with intra-arterial digital subtraction angiography, *Neuroradiology* 35:50-54, 1992.

244. Ronkainen A, Puranen MI, Hernesniemi JA, et al: Intracranial aneurysms: MR angiographic screening in 400 asymptomatic individuals with increased familial risk, *Radiology* 195:35-40, 1995.

245. Raaymakers TW, Buys PC, Verbeeten B Jr, et al: MR angiography as a screening tool for intracranial aneurysms: Feasibility, test characteristics, and interobserver agreement, *AJR Am J Roentgenol* 173:1469-1475, 1999.

246. Fayad ZA, Fuster V: Clinical imaging of the high-risk or vulnerable atherosclerotic plaque, *Circ Res* 89:305-316, 2001.

247. Yuan C, Mitsumori LM, Beach KW, Maravilla KR: Carotid atherosclerotic plaque: Noninvasive MR characterization and identification of vulnerable lesions, *Radiology* 221:285-299, 2001.

248. Yuan C, Zhang SX, Polissar NL, et al: Identification of fibrous cap rupture with magnetic resonance imaging is highly associated with recent transient ischemic attack or stroke, *Circulation* 105:181-185, 2002.

249. Zhao XQ, Yuan C, Hatsukami TS, et al: Effects of prolonged intensive lipid-lowering therapy on the characteristics of carotid atherosclerotic plaques in vivo by MRI: A case-control study, *Arterioscler Thromb Vasc Biol* 21:1623-1629, 2001.

250. Chu K, Kang DW, Yoon BW, Roh JK: Diffusion-weighted magnetic resonance in cerebral venous thrombosis, *Arch Neurol* 58:1569-1576, 2001.

251. Yuh WT, Simonson TM, Wang AM, et al: Venous sinus occlusive disease: MR findings, *AJNR Am J Neuroradiol* 15:309-316, 1994.

252. Idbaih A, Boukobza M, Crassard I, et al: MRI of clot in cerebral venous thrombosis: High diagnostic value of susceptibility-weighted images, *Stroke* 37:991-995, 2006.

253. Selim M, Fink J, Linfante I, et al: Diagnosis of cerebral venous thrombosis with echo-planar T2*-weighted magnetic resonance imaging, *Arch Neurol* 59:1021-1026, 2002.

254. Santhosh K, Kesavadas C, Thomas B, et al: Susceptibility weighted imaging: A new tool in magnetic resonance imaging of stroke, *Clin Radiol* 64:74-83, 2009.

255. Lafitte F, Boukobza M, Guichard JP, et al: MRI and MRA for diagnosis and follow-up of cerebral venous thrombosis (CVT), *Clin Radiol* 52:672-679, 1997.

256. Bousser MG, Ferro JM: Cerebral venous thrombosis: An update, *Lancet Neurol* 6:162-170, 2007.

257. Lovblad KO, Bassetti C, Schneider J, et al: Diffusion-weighted mr in cerebral venous thrombosis, *Cerebrovasc Dis* 11:169-176, 2001.

258. Ducreux D, Oppenheim C, Vandamme X, et al: Diffusion-weighted imaging patterns of brain damage associated with cerebral venous thrombosis, *AJNR Am J Neuroradiol* 22:261-268, 2001.

259. Doege CA, Tavakolian R, Kerskens CM, et al: Perfusion and diffusion magnetic resonance imaging in human cerebral venous thrombosis, *J Neurol* 248:564-571, 2001.

260. Keller E, Flacke S, Urbach H, Schild HH: Diffusion- and perfusion-weighted magnetic resonance imaging in deep cerebral venous thrombosis, *Stroke* 30:1144-1146, 1999.

261. Kang DW, Chalela JA, Dunn W, Warach S: MRI screening before standard tissue plasminogen activator therapy is feasible and safe, *Stroke* 36:1939-1943, 2005.

262. Schellinger PD, Jansen O, Fiebach JB, et al: Feasibility and practicality of MR imaging of stroke in the management of hyperacute cerebral ischemia, *AJNR Am J Neuroradiol* 21:1184-1189, 2000.

263. Kohrmann M, Juttler E, Fiebach JB, et al: MRI versus CT-based thrombolysis treatment within and beyond the 3 h time window after stroke onset: A cohort study, *Lancet Neurol* 5:661-667, 2006.

264. Schellinger PD, Thomalla G, Fiehler J, et al: MRI-based and CT-based thrombolytic therapy in acute stroke within and beyond established time windows: An analysis of 1210 patients, *Stroke* 38:2640-2645, 2007.

265. Earnshaw SR, Jackson D, Farkouh R, Schwamm L: Cost-effectiveness of patient selection using penumbral-based MRI for intravenous thrombolysis, *Stroke* 40:1710-1720, 2009.

266. Solling C, Hjort N, Ashkanian M, et al: Safety and efficacy of MRI-based selection for recombinant tissue plasminogen activator treatment: Responder analysis of outcome in the 3-hour time window, *Cerebrovasc Dis* 27:223-229, 2009.

267. Hjort N, Butcher K, Davis SM, et al: Magnetic resonance imaging criteria for thrombolysis in acute cerebral infarct, *Stroke* 36:388-397, 2005.

268. Schlaug G, Benfield A, Baird AE, et al: The ischemic penumbra: Operationally defined by diffusion and perfusion MRI, *Neurology* 53:1528-1537, 1999.

269. Warach S: Thrombolysis in stroke beyond three hours: Targeting patients with diffusion and perfusion MRI, *Ann Neurol* 51:11-13, 2002.

270. Albers GW, Thijs VN, Wechsler L, et al: Magnetic resonance imaging profiles predict clinical response to early reperfusion: The diffusion and perfusion imaging evaluation for understanding stroke evolution (DEFUSE) study, *Ann Neurol* 60:508-517, 2006.

271. Davis SM, Donnan GA, Parsons MW, et al: Effects of alteplase beyond 3 h after stroke in the Echoplanar Imaging Thrombolytic Evaluation Trial (EPITHET): A placebo-controlled randomised trial, *Lancet Neurol* 7:299-309, 2008.

272. Hacke W, Albers G, Al-Rawi Y, et al: The Desmoteplase in Acute Ischemic Stroke Trial (DIAS): A phase II MRI-based 9-hour window acute stroke thrombolysis trial with intravenous desmoteplase, *Stroke* 36:66-73, 2005.

273. Furlan AJ, Eyding D, Albers GW, et al: Dose Escalation of Desmoteplase for Acute Ischemic Stroke (DEDAS): Evidence of safety and efficacy 3 to 9 hours after stroke onset, *Stroke* 37:1227-1231, 2006.

274. Hacke W, Furlan AJ, Al-Rawi Y, et al: Intravenous desmoteplase in patients with acute ischaemic stroke selected by MRI perfusion-diffusion weighted imaging or perfusion CT (DIAS-2): A prospective, randomised, double-blind, placebo-controlled study, *Lancet Neurol* 8:141-150, 2009.

275. Donnan GA, Baron JC, Ma H, Davis SM: Penumbral selection of patients for trials of acute stroke therapy, *Lancet Neurol* 8:261-269, 2009.

276. Merino JG, Latour LL, An L, et al: Reperfusion half-life: A novel pharmacodynamic measure of thrombolytic activity, *Stroke* 39:2148-2150, 2008.

277. Tong DC, Yenari MA, Albers GW, et al: Correlation of perfusion- and diffusion-weighted MRI with NIHSS score in acute (<6.5 hour) ischemic stroke, *Neurology* 50:864-870, 1998.

278. Kluytmans M, van Everdingen KJ, Kappelle LJ, et al: Prognostic value of perfusion- and diffusion-weighted MR imaging in first 3 days of stroke, *Eur Radiol* 10:1434-1441, 2000.

279. Sorensen AG, Copen WA, Ostergaard L, et al: Hyperacute stroke: Simultaneous measurement of relative cerebral blood volume, relative cerebral blood flow, and mean tissue transit time, *Radiology* 210:519-527, 1999.

280. Ueda T, Yuh WT, Maley JE, et al: Outcome of acute ischemic lesions evaluated by diffusion and perfusion MR imaging, *AJNR Am J Neuroradiol* 20:983-989, 1999.

281. Karonen JO, Liu Y, Vanninen RL, et al: Combined perfusion- and diffusion-weighted MR imaging in acute ischemic stroke during the 1st week: A longitudinal study, *Radiology* 217:886-894, 2000.

282. Neumann-Haefelin T, Wittsack HJ, Wenserski F, et al: Diffusion- and perfusion-weighted MRI. The DWI/PWI mismatch region in acute stroke, *Stroke* 30:1591-1597, 1999.

283. Darby DG, Barber PA, Gerraty RP, et al: Pathophysiological topography of acute ischemia by combined diffusion-weighted and perfusion MRI, *Stroke* 30:2043-2052, 1999.

284. Karonen JO, Vanninen RL, Liu Y, et al: Combined diffusion and perfusion MRI with correlation to single-photon emission CT in acute ischemic stroke. Ischemic penumbra predicts infarct growth, *Stroke* 30:1583-1590, 1999.

285. Schellinger PD, Fiebach JB, Jansen O, et al: Stroke magnetic resonance imaging within 6 hours after onset of hyperacute cerebral ischemia, *Ann Neurol* 49:460-469, 2001.

286. Kidwell CS, Saver JL, Mattiello J, et al: Thrombolytic reversal of acute human cerebral ischemic injury shown by diffusion/perfusion magnetic resonance imaging, *Ann Neurol* 47:462-469, 2000.

287. Lutsep HL, Nesbit GM, Berger RM, Coshow WR: Does reversal of ischemia on diffusion-weighted imaging reflect higher apparent diffusion coefficient values? *J Neuroimaging* 11:313-316, 2001.

288. Uno M, Harada M, Okada T, Nagahiro S: Diffusion-weighted and perfusion-weighted magnetic resonance imaging to monitor acute intra-arterial thrombolysis, *J Stroke Cerebrovasc Dis* 9:113-120, 2000.

289. Desmond PM, Lovell AC, Rawlinson AA, et al: The value of apparent diffusion coefficient maps in early cerebral ischemia, *AJNR Am J Neuroradiol* 22:1260-1267, 2001.

290. Fiehler J, Foth M, Kucinski T, et al: Severe ADC decreases do not predict irreversible tissue damage in humans, *Stroke* 33:79-86, 2002.

291. Oppenheim C, Samson Y, Manai R, et al: Prediction of malignant middle cerebral artery infarction by diffusion-weighted imaging, *Stroke* 31:2175-2181, 2000.

292. Oppenheim C, Grandin C, Samson Y, et al: Is there an apparent diffusion coefficient threshold in predicting tissue viability in hyperacute stroke? *Stroke* 32:2486-2491, 2001.

293. Oppenheim C, Samson Y, Dormont D, et al: DWI prediction of symptomatic hemorrhagic transformation in acute MCA infarct, *J Neuroradiol* 29:6-13, 2002.

294. Grandin CB, Duprez TP, Smith AM, et al: Which MR-derived perfusion parameters are the best predictors of infarct growth in hyperacute stroke? Comparative study between relative and quantitative measurements, *Radiology* 223:361-370, 2002.

295. Rohl L, Sakoh M, Simonsen CZ, et al: Time evolution of cerebral perfusion and apparent diffusion coefficient measured by magnetic resonance imaging in a porcine stroke model, *J Magn Reson Imaging* 15:123-129, 2002.

296. Wu O, Koroshetz WJ, Ostergaard L, et al: Predicting tissue outcome in acute human cerebral ischemia using combined diffusion- and perfusion-weighted MR imaging, *Stroke* 32:933-942, 2001.

297. Thijs VN, Adami A, Neumann-Haefelin T, et al: Relationship between severity of MR perfusion deficit and DWI lesion evolution, *Neurology* 57:1205-1211, 2001.

298. Fiehler J, Knab R, Reichenbach JR, et al: Apparent diffusion coefficient decreases and magnetic resonance imaging perfusion parameters are associated in ischemic tissue of acute stroke patients, *J Cereb Blood Flow Metab* 21:577-584, 2001.

299. Tong DC, Adami A, Moseley ME, Marks MP: Prediction of hemorrhagic transformation following acute stroke: Role of diffusion- and perfusion-weighted magnetic resonance imaging, *Arch Neurol* 58:587-593, 2001.

300. Warach S: Tissue viability thresholds in acute stroke: The 4-factor model, *Stroke* 32:2460-2461, 2001.

301. Rose SE, Chalk JB, Griffin MP, et al: MRI based diffusion and perfusion predictive model to estimate stroke evolution, *Magn Reson Imaging* 19:1043-1053, 2001.

302. Liu Y, Karonen JO, Vanninen RL, et al: Cerebral hemodynamics in human acute ischemic stroke: A study with diffusion- and perfusion-weighted magnetic resonance imaging and SPECT, *J Cereb Blood Flow Metab* 20:910-920, 2000.

303. Jacobs MA, Mitsias P, Soltanian-Zadeh H, et al: Multiparametric MRI tissue characterization in clinical stroke with correlation to clinical outcome: Part 2, *Stroke* 32:950-957, 2001.

304. Jansen O, Schellinger P, Fiebach J, et al: Early recanalisation in acute ischaemic stroke saves tissue at risk defined by MRI, *Lancet* 353:2036–2037, 1999.

305. Schellinger PD, Jansen O, Fiebach JB, et al: Monitoring intravenousrecombinanttissueplasminogenactivatorthrombolysisforacute ischemic stroke with diffusion and perfusion MRI, *Stroke* 31:1318–1328, 2000.

306. Marks MP, Tong DC, Beaulieu C, et al: Evaluation of early reperfusion and i.v. tPA therapy using diffusion- and perfusion-weighted MRI, *Neurology* 52:1792–1798, 1999.

307. Taleb M, Lovblad KO, El-Koussy M, et al: Reperfusion demonstrated by apparent diffusion coefficient mapping after local intra-arterial thrombolysis for ischaemic stroke, *Neuroradiology* 43:591–594, 2001.

308. Kidwell CS, Saver JL, Mattiello J, et al: Diffusion-perfusion MRI characterization of post-recanalization hyperperfusion in humans, *Neurology* 57:2015–2021, 2001.

47 Cerebral Angiography

RONALD J. SATTENBERG, JEFFREY L. SAVER, Y. PIERRE GOBIN, DAVID S. LIEBESKIND

After Egas Moniz invented cerebral angiography in 1927, it became the method of choice for the diagnosis of brain lesions[1,2] until the development of computed tomography (CT) and later magnetic resonance imaging (MRI) limited the indication for catheter angiography to visualization of cerebral vessels. CT angiography (CTA) and magnetic resonance angiography (MRA) have demonstrated excellent performance in noninvasively imaging large cervicocerebral vessels, further reducing the need for invasive angiography. Other noninvasive imaging techniques such as duplex ultrasonography and transcranial Doppler ultrasonography provide hemodynamic information that further limits the indications for cerebral angiography. Because of its ability to show the smallest vascular lesions and detail, however, cerebral angiography is still the gold standard for imaging the cervicocerebral vasculature and related flow. Moreover, the dramatic expansion of percutaneous treatments for ischemic and hemorrhagic cerebrovascular disease has brought a resurgence in catheter angiography as a necessary prelude and guide to endovascular interventions.

Technique

Cerebral angiography is increasingly performed by a diverse range of specialists, and this diversity has prompted the publication of qualification requirements for diagnostic and interventional procedures.[3] With miniaturization and other advances in catheter technology and the development of nonionic contrast agents, cerebral angiography is now usually a straightforward procedure that takes 30 to 60 minutes to complete. Cerebral angiography is painless and can generally be performed with the use of local anesthesia administered at the groin and no or mild sedation. General anesthesia is required only in patients unable to cooperate or in children. With the use of a closure device[4] such as a collagen plug or percutaneous arterial suture for hemostasis, patients may be ambulatory within 1 hour after the procedure is completed, and anticoagulation need not be halted before the procedure. However, closure devices are only used in a select population of patients. Without closure devices, the patient can usually ambulate within 6 to 8 hours.

Vascular access is most often obtained via the common femoral artery and rarely via the brachial or axillary artery. After arterial puncture, an arterial sheath is placed into the artery. A *sheath* is a short catheter with a diaphragm at its exterior end that allows the passage and manipulation of additional smaller catheters without damaging the femoral artery. Catheterization of the aortic arch and further selective catheterizations are performed with the combined use of a catheter and a guidewire. A plethora of catheters and guidewires are available. Selection of the catheters and guidewires used in a particular patient is based on the patient's vascular anatomy, the diagnostic question to be answered by the procedure, and the preferences of the operator. A hockey stick–shaped catheter and a guidewire with a simple 45-degree curve are commonly used, both with hydrophilic coating. For difficult anatomy, other catheter shapes are available. The catheter is continuously flushed with heparinized saline to prevent thrombus formation.

The precise vessels catheterized depend on the indication for the procedure. Sometimes catheterizing only one vessel is all that is required, for instance, for immediate follow-up evaluation after aneurysm clipping. At other times, the bilateral vertebral arteries, bilateral external and internal carotid arteries, and bilateral common carotid arteries all must be catheterized. In many instances, catheterization and angiography of the aortic arch and three to four vessels are necessary. The injection variables employed may alter contrast bolus delivery and have considerable effects on the opacification of downstream arteries, parenchyma, and veins.[5] Standardized technique is therefore important for comparison of angiographic results.

At the very end of the procedure, the common femoral artery sheath is removed, and manual compression is applied at the access site until hemostasis is obtained. Arteriotomy closing devices are now routinely used. These are essentially tools that percutaneously place a suture into or a plug at the puncture site to obtain immediate hemostasis. The indications for the use of a percutaneous closure device vary among institutions. One common approach is not to use these devices for routine angiography, but to reserve their application in patients who are undergoing anticoagulation, who are being treated with thrombolytics, or who have coagulation deficits from other causes.

Risks

The risk of cerebral angiography has declined over the years. Increasing procedural safety is due to many factors, including nonionic contrast agents, new catheters and guidewires that have safer designs and are made of less thrombogenic materials, and digital subtraction angiography.[6,7]

The risks of cerebral angiography are related to patient age and medical condition, the number of catheter exchanges, the total time for the procedure, and the load of contrast agent.[6,8] Contrast-induced neurotoxicity may elicit neurologic symptoms.[9] Headaches or even transient encephalopathy during angiography have also been documented, although the underlying factors that trigger such events remain unclear.[10-12] Interestingly, some data suggest that the performance of cerebral angiography may directly affect the tone of the vasculature, and vasodilation is the condition most often noted.[13] Increased use of angiography as part of therapeutic interventions and introduction of novel acquisition techniques that may increase radiation exposure also warrant consideration in the future.[14] Cerebral angiography is more risky in the elderly and in patients with particular conditions that predispose to thrombus formation on the catheter (hypercoagulable states) and to vessel dissection and rupture (e.g., Marfan's disease). In the setting of acute ischemic stroke, it has also been suggested that microcatheter injections may predispose to hemorrhagic transformation.[15]

Many studies have been performed to quantify the risks of cerebral angiography.[16] Hankey et al[17] reviewed several series and found the general risk for permanent neurologic sequelae after cerebral angiography to be 1%. The mortality rate was less than 0.1%. The overall risk for a neurologic complication was about 4%.[17] In a prospective study by Dion et al,[6] of 1002 cerebral angiography procedures, the rate of permanent neurologic deficit was 0.1% and that of transient deficits was 1.2%. Other studies cite a persistent neurologic deficit rate of 0.3% to 0.5% and a total neurologic complication rate of 0.5% to 2%.[7] The most recent data suggest angiography complication rates that may be exceedingly low.[16,18,19] Kaufmann et al[16] reported neurologic complications in 2.63%, including 0.14% with strokes and permanent disability, and a mortality rate of 0.06% in a consecutive series of 19,826 procedures. Fifi et al[18] reported a complication rate of 0.30% across 3636 diagnostic cerebral angiograms over a 6-year period. Recent studies have also considered operator training or specialty as a factor in complication rates.[20]

Among the potential neurologic complications of cerebral angiography are embolic events and vascular dissections. Transcranial Doppler ultrasonography studies monitoring for microembolic events during diagnostic angiography have shown that although nonpathogenic air emboli introduced at the time of contrast injection are common, formed element emboli are uncommon.[21] Symptomatic air embolism during angiography may occur in 0.08% of procedures.[22] Carotid or vertebral artery dissections secondary to catheterization depend on operator experience and are less frequent (0.4%) with the newer, safer catheter designs. Although neurologically symptomatic complications from cerebral angiography are rare, clinically silent "complications," diagnosed on diffusion-weighted MRI, are more common, being found in 26% of diagnostic angiography procedures.[23] Covert MRI diffusion lesions are associated with the presence of multiple vascular risk factors, greater difficulty in probing vessels, amount of contrast medium needed, longer fluoroscopy time, and the use of multiple catheters.[23]

One particular concern of cerebral angiography in the setting of recently ruptured cerebral aneurysms is the risk of precipitating rebleeding by injecting contrast agent with an increased pressure head. This risk is extremely low. In a meta-analysis of 415 patients with acute subarachnoid hemorrhage, Cloft et al[24] found no cases of rebleeding during angiography.

Nonneurologic complications consist of local complications (i.e., hematoma, pseudoaneurysm, and infection), renal failure, contrast agent allergies, and arterial occlusions. Contrast or even heparin during angiography may also cause transient reductions in serum calcium values, possibly due to chelation.[25] In a cooperative study among leading interventional radiologic societies, nonneurologic major complication rates were as follows: renal failure, 0% to 0.15%; arterial occlusion requiring surgical intervention, 0% to 0.4%; arteriovenous fistula or pseudoaneurysm, 0.01% to 0.22%; and hematoma requiring transfusion or evacuation, 0.26% to 1.5%.[8] Recent use of percutaneous closure devices has demonstrated low rates of complications, although the use of concomitant antithrombotic agents may increase events.[4]

When an allergy to iodine contrast medium is known before procedure initiation, premedication with steroids and antihistamines is usually sufficient to prevent any adverse reactions. In patients with previous severe allergy such as shock, in whom iodine is contraindicated even with premedication, gadolinium-based contrast agents, which are radiopaque as well as paramagnetic, may be used.

Angiographic Cerebral Vasculature: Normal Anatomy

To recognize and understand vascular disease, one must first be acquainted with the normal angioarchitecture of the cerebrovascular system and its variants. The three phases of an angiographic imaging sequence—arterial, capillary, and venous—are shown in Figures 47-1 to 47-3. Each phase has its particular sensitivity for the different pathologic entities. One should be able to recognize common variants, such as persistent fetal anomalies, vascular fenestrations (Fig. 47-4), and collateral pathways.

Indications
Intracranial Hemorrhage

Intracranial hemorrhage may be epidural, subdural, subarachnoid, or intraparenchymal.

Epidural hemorrhage is usually secondary to head trauma. The vessels coursing in the epidural space, most notably the middle meningeal artery, are torn, and arterial bleeding results. These hemorrhages are often associated with skull fractures. Because epidural hemorrhages are usually of traumatic origin, correlation with the clinical history as well as noninvasive imaging almost invariably identifies the cause, obviating the need for angiographic evaluation.

Subdural hemorrhage (SDH) is secondary to bleeding from the cortical bridging veins that drain into the superior sagittal sinus or other dural sinuses. The characteristic angiographic appearance is a lentiform avascular

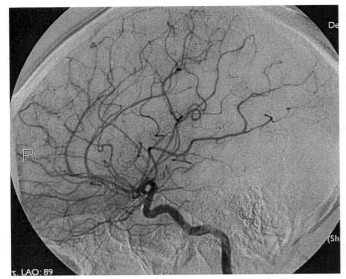

Figure 47-1 Internal carotid artery injection, lateral projection, arterial phase. The arteries are primarily opacified during this phase.

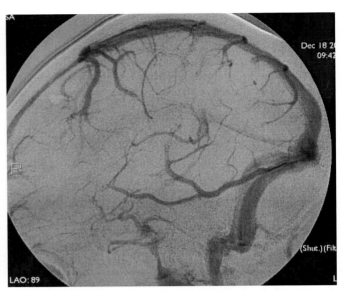

Figure 47-3 Internal carotid artery injection, lateral projection, venous phase. The veins are primarily opacified during this phase.

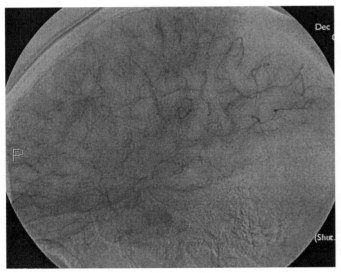

Figure 47-2 Internal carotid artery injection, lateral projection, capillary phase. No significant arterial or venous opacification is noted during this phase.

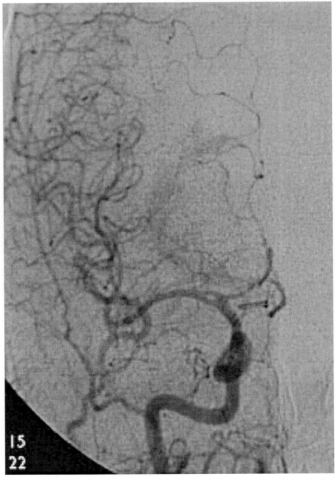

Figure 47-4 Common carotid artery injection, anteroposterior projection. Note the "filling defect" in the M1 segment, just at the carotid bifurcation. This is a fenestration.

collection outlined by displaced cortical vessels. The cortical bridging veins are vulnerable to venous hypertension or tearing in the subdural space secondary to trauma. Venous hypertension can be caused by a variety of reasons, including sinus thrombosis and dural arteriovenous fistulas (Fig. 47-5). Uncommonly, a subdural hematoma may result when an intracerebral aneurysm that previously hemorrhaged creates adhesions that direct subsequent hemorrhaging into the subdural compartment. In this situation, an intraparenchymal focus of hemorrhage is also often present, detection of which should raise the suspicion for aneurysmal bleeding. In a subdural hemorrhage, if a dural arteriovenous fistula or aneurysm is suspected, cerebral angiography should be performed.

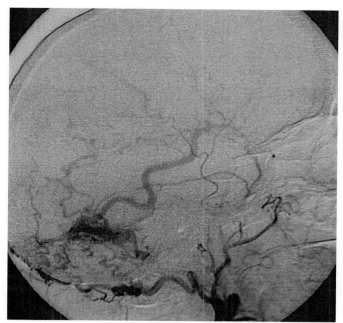

Figure 47-5 External carotid artery injection, lateral projection. There is arterial and early venous opacification with contrast simultaneously. The dural fistula is also opacified.

However, if trauma or significant brain parenchyma atrophy is present in an older patient, angiography should be reserved.

Subarachnoid hemorrhage (SAH) has an incidence of 6 to 8 per 100,000 person-years, and studies suggest that 2% to 6% of the population have an intracranial aneurysm. In 85% of SAHs, the cause is a ruptured aneurysm, usually a berry aneurysm. Among the other causes of SAH are trauma (in which case a parenchyma focus of contusion or hemorrhage is often seen on imaging), intraparenchymal hemorrhage extending into the ventricular system, cerebral or cervical arteriovenous malformation (AVMs) or fistula, venous thrombosis, mycotic aneurysm, nonaneurysmal perimesencephalic hemorrhage, vasculitis, and dissections; some SAHs are cryptogenic.

In less than 5% of AVMs that bleed, the hemorrhage is confined to the subarachnoid space, and no intraparenchymal blood is present. Generally, if the findings of angiography performed in the early phase of a nontraumatic SAH are normal, the procedure should be repeated after 1 week. There are several explanations why an aneurysm may not be detected on angiography; among these are parenchymal hematoma compressing the aneurysm; thrombus in the aneurysm, its neck, or both; perianeurysmal vasospasm; and suboptimal views of the region harboring the aneurysm. The diagnostic yield of a second cerebral angiogram in eight different series was 17%.[26] If findings on the second angiogram are also normal, a third angiographic procedure performed several months later can be of benefit. In one series, aneurysm was detected by a third angiogram in 1 of 14 patients.[26] For a patient in whom a CT scan shows a truly perimesencephalic hemorrhage pattern, the probability that cerebral angiography will reveal a vertebrobasilar aneurysm is 4%.[27] Thus, the diagnosis of perimesencephalic hemorrhage

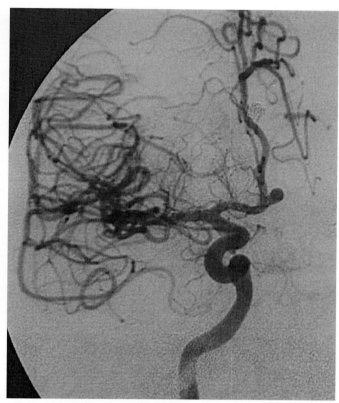

Figure 47-6 Right internal carotid artery injection, frontal projection, demonstrates an anterior communicating artery aneurysm. The aneurysm dome points superomedially.

requires normal findings on a cerebral angiogram. In a truly perimesencephalic pattern of SAH, a second angiographic procedure is not necessary if findings of the first angiogram are normal.[28]

Berry or sacciform aneurysms are the most prevalent intracranial aneurysms. They are localized mostly in the anterior circulation (90%) as follows: anterior communicating artery, 40%; middle cerebral artery bifurcation, 30%; intracranial internal carotid artery, 20%; and posterior circulation, 10%. Other cerebral aneurysms are fusiform, traumatic (pseudoaneurysm), mycotic, or dissecting. A selection of aneurysms is illustrated in Figures. 47-6 to 47-18. Cerebral aneurysms have been associated with autosomal dominant polycystic kidney disease and Marfan's syndrome.

Angiography should evaluate the location of the aneurysm, size of the neck and dome (dome–neck ratio), morphology, and relationship to the parent vessel and should show whether the aneurysm incorporates the origin of other vessels. Multiple aneurysms are found in 20% of aneurysmal SAHs, and it may be difficult to identify which aneurysm bled and should be treated first. Three important features indicating the causative aneurysm are (1) the location of the aneurysm in relation to the SAH, (2) the aneurysm shape, because a ruptured aneurysm may be lobulated or have a teat, and (3) the aneurysm size. Active extravasation of contrast material from an aneurysm at the time of angiography is exceptional and indicates intraprocedural rupture. Three-dimensional rotational angiography

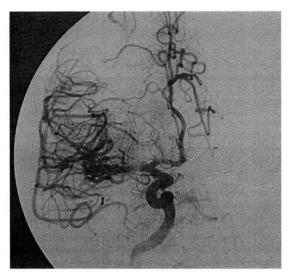

Figure 47-7 Right internal carotid artery injection, anteroposterior projection, after embolization. The anterior communicating artery aneurysm seen previously is no longer opacifying.

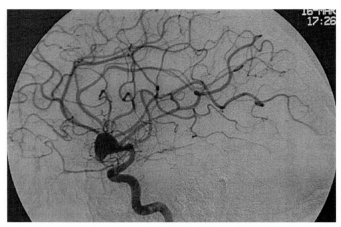

Figure 47-9 Internal carotid artery injection, lateral projection, arterial phase, demonstrating a large anterior communicating artery aneurysm.

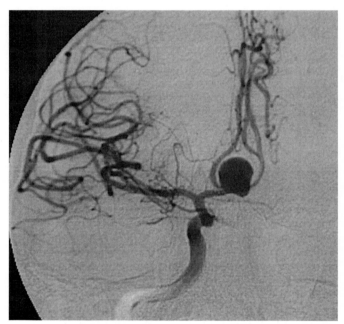

Figure 47-8 Right internal carotid artery injection, frontal view, arterial phase, demonstrating a large anterior communicating artery aneurysm. Notice how the A2 segments of the anterior cerebral artery are splayed by the aneurysm.

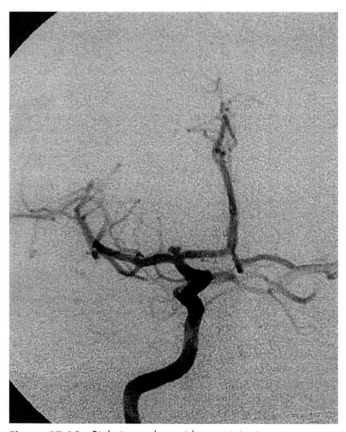

Figure 47-10 Right internal carotid artery injection, anteroposterior projection, arterial phase, demonstrating a carotid bifurcation aneurysm. The aneurysm is bilobed and irregular in contour.

may be more sensitive for aneurysm detection[29-31] yet may still result in a 4.2% rate of angiogram-negative SAH.[32] Angiography may also be used for later assessment of arterial status after definitive treatment of an aneurysm, and evidence shows very low complication rates.[33]

Intraparenchymal hemorrhage can be secondary to a variety of pathologic entities, including hypertension (80%), amyloid angiopathy, trauma, hemorrhagic transformation of ischemic stroke, arterial dissection, tumor, sinus thrombosis, AVM, cavernous hemangioma, and saccular aneurysm. About 20% of hemorrhages due to

intracranial aneurysms have an intraparenchymal component, especially if a mycotic aneurysm is the cause. If an AVM is suspected on MRI or CT, angiography is required to characterize the lesion, its venous drainage, arterial feeding arteries (feeders), and nidus. The characteristic angiographic appearance of an AVM consists of enlarged arterial feeders, a nidus, and early draining veins (Figs. 47-19 to 47-22).

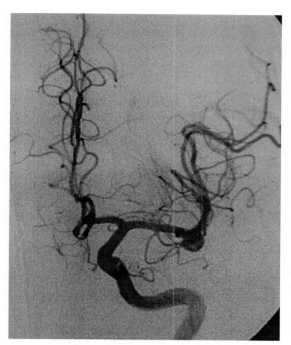

Figure 47-11 Left internal carotid artery injection, frontal projection, arterial phase, demonstrating a middle cerebral artery aneurysm. The aneurysm dome is pointing inferiorly.

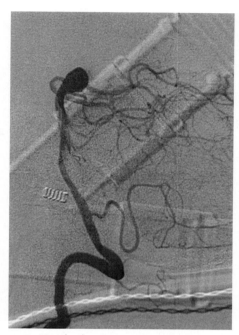

Figure 47-13 Vertebral artery injection, lateral projection, arterial phase, demonstrating a basilar tip aneurysm.

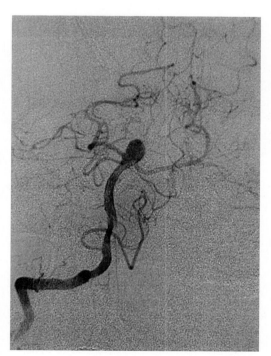

Figure 47-12 Right vertebral artery injection, frontal projection, arterial phase, demonstrating a basilar tip aneurysm.

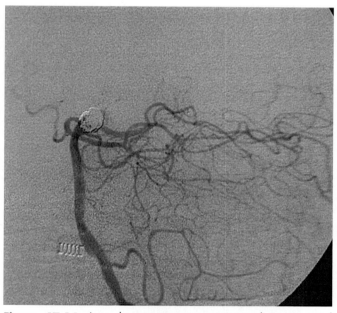

Figure 47-14 Lateral projection, posterior circulation, arterial phase. Status: postembolization; the basilar tip aneurysm is no longer opacifying.

The association of AVMs and aneurysms on the arterial feeders is well-known and is secondary to the high-flow state through the AVM (Figs. 47-21 and 47-22). Furthermore, selection of optimal treatment modalities for AVMs requires knowledge of the detailed angioarchitecture of the lesion. For example, the presence of a lenticulostriate arterial supply to the nidus makes surgery more difficult (see Fig. 47-22).

In general, angiography is indicated in the evaluation of intracranial hemorrhage in (1) any patient younger than 70 years with a lobar hemorrhage and (2) any patient of any age with a deep hemorrhage who does not have a history of hypertension or CT or MRI evidence of small vessel arteriopathy.

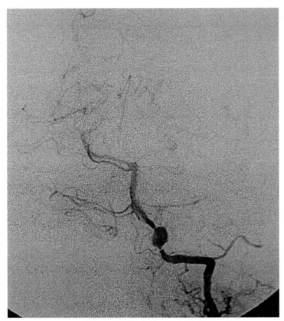

Figure 47-15 Vertebral artery injection, frontal projection, demonstrating a vertebrobasilar aneurysm. Notice how the contrast column rapidly narrows and there is significantly decreased opacification of the vasculature distal to the aneurysm. This is consistent with a dissecting aneurysm.

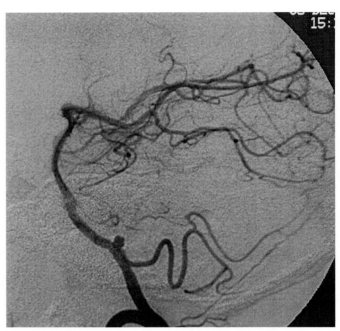

Figure 47-17 Vertebral artery injection, lateral projection, arterial phase, demonstrating a posterior inferior cerebellar artery (PICA) aneurysm.

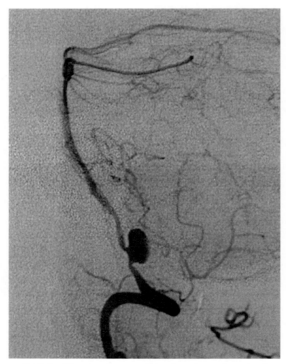

Figure 47-16 Vertebral artery injection, lateral projection, arterial phase, demonstrating a dissecting vertebrobasilar aneurysm.

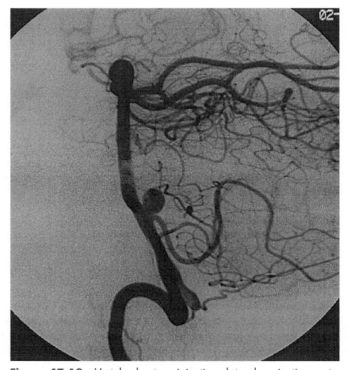

Figure 47-18 Vertebral artery injection, lateral projection, arterial phase, demonstrating both a basilar tip aneurysm and a posterior inferior cerebellar artery aneurysm.

Ischemia

Cerebral Infarction and Transient Ischemic Attack

Cerebral angiography remains a mainstay in the evaluation of cerebral ischemia in the young (e.g., <45 years), in whom the potential causes are diverse and include entities often best characterized on angiographic studies, including vasculitis and dissection. Pediatric neuroendovascular procedures are being performed with increasing frequency, for various indications.[34] Even when detailed imaging features of ischemia are evident

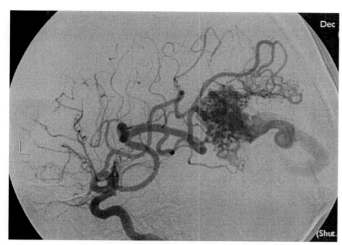

Figure 47-19 Internal carotid artery injection, lateral projection, arterial phase, demonstrating early venous opacification, as well as a nidus, consistent with an arteriovenous malformation.

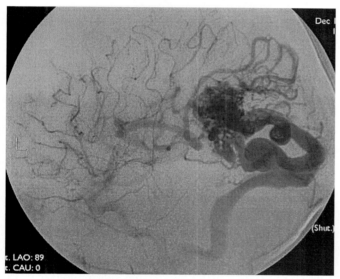

Figure 47-20 Internal carotid artery injection, lateral projection, venous phase, demonstrating the venous phase of an arteriovenous malformation. Note the enlarged vein draining the arteriovenous malformation nidus.

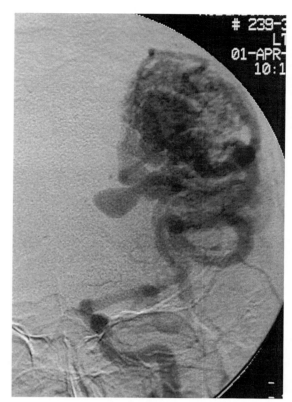

Figure 47-21 Left internal carotid artery injection, anteroposterior projection, arterial phase, demonstrating an enlarged middle cerebral artery vasculature feeding an arteriovenous malformation with an aneurysm whose dome points inferomedially.

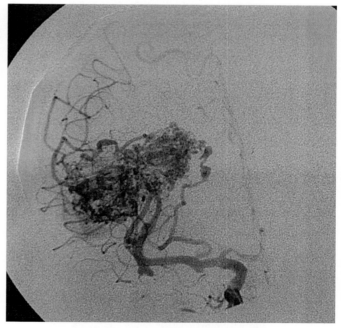

Figure 47-22 Right internal carotid artery injection, frontal projection, arterial phase, demonstrating an arteriovenous malformation being opacified by middle cerebral arterial vessels, as well as a lenticulostriate artery originating from the M1 segment of the middle cerebral artery.

on multimodal CT or MRI, angiography may still provide further information.[35,36]

Angiography remains fundamentally important in the evaluation of cervical carotid atherosclerosis. The decision whether to proceed with carotid endarterectomy or carotid stenting depends on the extent of stenosis at the carotid bifurcation. In general, patients with symptomatic carotid disease benefit from surgical intervention if the severity of stenosis on angiography is 50% to 99%, whereas those with asymptomatic stenosis derive a modest benefit from surgery if the severity of stenosis is 60% to 99%. The common noninvasive imaging modalities, carotid duplex ultrasonography, CTA, and MRA, are generally quite good, but each has intrinsic as well as operator- and reader-dependent limitations. When two noninvasive tests provide congruent results regarding

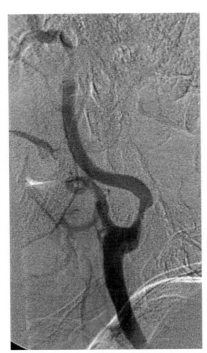

Figure 47-23 Common carotid artery injection, lateral projection, arterial phase, demonstrates an internal carotid artery stenosis just distal to the bifurcation.

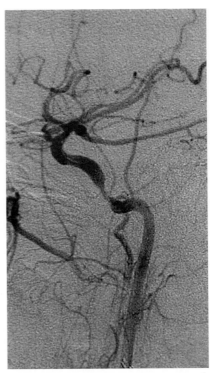

Figure 47-25 Common carotid artery injection, lateral projection, arterial phase, demonstrating a stenosis in the petrous segment of the internal carotid artery. Note that there is also opacification of some of the external carotid artery vasculature.

the severity of stenosis, a decision for or against surgery may be made with confidence. If noninvasive test results disagree, however, catheter angiography is desirable for definitively characterizing the lesion.

Although both modalities can assess the severity of an internal carotid artery stenosis well, an important advantage of cerebral angiography over standard carotid duplex ultrasonography is that the evaluation of the morphology of a plaque is better accomplished by catheter angiography (Figs. 47-23 and 47-24). Plaque morphology can be very important because, even if stenosis is not severe, an ulcerated plaque can be the cause of transient ischemic attacks (TIAs) and similarly may be the harbinger of a stroke. Arterial wall imaging with CT or MRI may be another option in the future.

Intracranial atherosclerotic stenosis is one cause of cerebral infarction and TIAs (Figs. 47-25 and 47-26). For middle cerebral artery atherosclerotic stenosis, a stroke rate of up to 10% annually has been reported. The Warfarin-Aspirin Symptomatic Intracranial Disease (WASID) trial demonstrated that aspirin may be as effective as anticoagulation in this disorder.[37] Particular risk factors, such as severe degree of luminal arterial stenosis, have also been noted and indicate a high risk of recurrent ischemia.[38] Accurate determination of luminal stenosis with angiography is therefore important in risk assessment. The intracranial vasculature can be assessed with CTA, MRA, and transcranial Doppler ultrasonography to some extent; however, these intracranial vessels are smaller in diameter than the internal carotid artery, and the sensitivity and specificity of noninvasive studies for

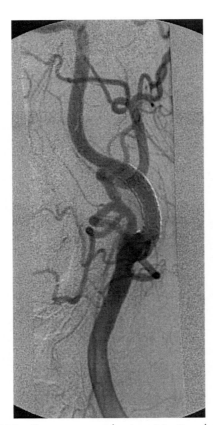

Figure 47-24 Common carotid artery injection, lateral projection, arterial phase, demonstrating internal carotid artery status after angioplasty and stent placement. The stenotic segment is no longer present.

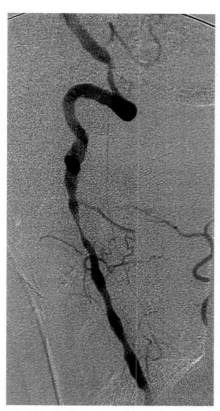

Figure 47-26   Vertebral artery injection, lateral projection, arterial phase. Note the tandem stenoses.

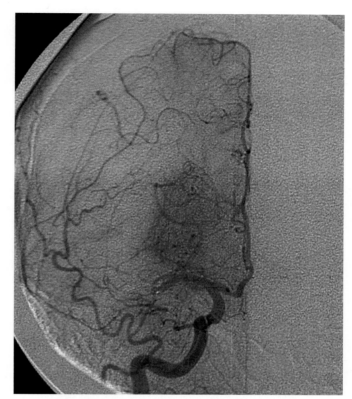

Figure 47-27   Right internal carotid artery injection, frontal projection, demonstrating an abrupt M1 segment "cutoff."

detecting and characterizing intracranial stenoses are not yet as well documented as for cervical stenoses. In fact, the Stroke Outcomes and Neuroimaging of Intracranial Atherosclerosis (SONIA) trial showed prominent discordance in noninvasive angiographic detection rates.[39] Quantifying the severity of intracranial stenosis at angiography requires a different measurement technique from that used for extracranial stenosis—that established by the North American Symptomatic Carotid Endarterectomy Trial (NASCET). Intracranial vessels tend to taper distal to stenoses, leading to possible underestimation of the extent of narrowing if the NASCET method were employed. A standardized measure has been introduced for intracranial stenoses, where percent stenosis = [(1 − (D(stenosis)/D(normal)))] × 100, where D(stenosis) = the diameter of the artery at the site of the most severe stenosis and D(normal) = the diameter of the proximal normal artery.[40]

Acute Ischemia

In approximately 80% of acute ischemic strokes, early angiography demonstrates a large artery occlusion, either embolic (from arterial origin or cardioembolic) or due to in situ atherothrombosis. Cerebral angiography is indicated as an emergency procedure if intraarterial thrombolysis or mechanical thrombectomy is being considered. In the last several years, mechanical devices for clot retrieval and aspiration have been cleared by the United States Food and Drug Administration for restoration of cerebral arterial patency in the setting of acute ischemic

stroke.[41-45] More recent efforts have expanded revascularization techniques to possibly include stenting of intracranial arteries to restore patency.[46-48]

The cerebral angiographic findings in acute ischemic stroke are varied. One finding is the abrupt cutoff of a vessel (Figs. 47-27 to 47-33). If an embolus is the cause, a meniscus sign may be seen. The clot burden or volume of thrombus may also be assessed at angiography, facilitating the planning of revascularization approaches.[49] Another finding is a relatively bare area seen in the capillary phase of the examination (this is perhaps the most sensitive angiographic sign of ischemia). Collateralization should be assessed in acute strokes because the presence of collateral vessels indicates that the hypoperfused region has some blood supply, so irreversible injury may not occur for some time. Collateralization can take the following forms: (1) flow through the circle of Willis (i.e., anterior communicating artery and posterior communicating artery); (2) flow from the external carotid artery through the ophthalmic artery and then to the internal carotid artery, and (3) leptomeningeal collateral flow. In the subacute phase, hours to weeks after ischemic strokes, "luxury perfusion" (hyperperfusion visualized as increased contrast radiodensity) may be seen.

The recent increase in endovascular therapies for revascularization as a treatment for acute ischemic stroke has led to increased investigation of serial angiographic changes that may accompany revascularization of an occluded cerebral artery. Recanalization and re-occlusion may be readily illustrated at angiography.[50] The role of

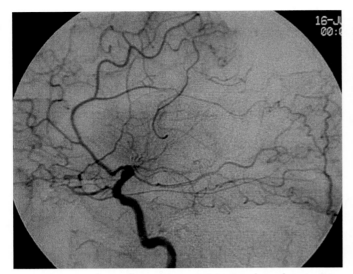

Figure 47-28 Internal carotid artery injection, lateral projection, demonstrating the absence of opacification of the middle cerebral artery vasculature.

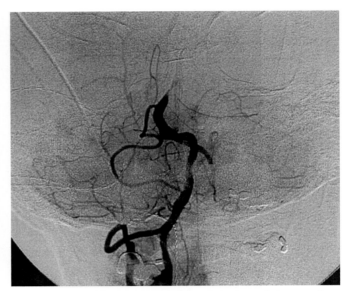

Figure 47-30 This anteroposterior projection of the vertebrobasilar artery demonstrates occlusion of the basilar artery. Notice the parenchymal blush.

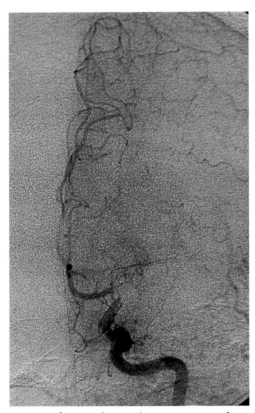

Figure 47-29 Left internal carotid artery injection, frontal projection, demonstrates significant occlusion at the top of the internal carotid artery at its bifurcation. Note that some opacification of the left anterior cerebral artery vasculature is seen.

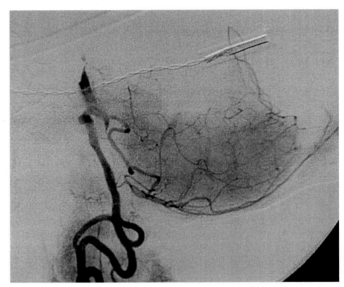

Figure 47-31 Vertebral artery injection, lateral projection, demonstrating an abrupt "cutoff" of the basilar artery opacification.

collateral circulation as a key facet of ischemic pathophysiology[51,52] and pivotal determinant of recanalization has been underscored by angiographic analyses in this setting. Revascularization after thrombolysis or thrombectomy has also been the focus of intense investigation as the distinction between recanalization, or restoration of proximal arterial patency, and reperfusion of the downstream territory has become apparent.[53] The use of specific angiographic scales, as well as the inherent advantages or disadvantages of each tool, has become an important area of research because such features of revascularization may have different implications on the neurologic outcome of the stroke patient. Consideration of serial angiographic details, including features of collateral flow, arterial patency, and downstream territorial perfusion, with the use of validated scales and methodology[54] will be important in linking the technical success of endovascular devices with treatment outcomes in clinical trials,[42,44] future registries, and routine clinical practice.

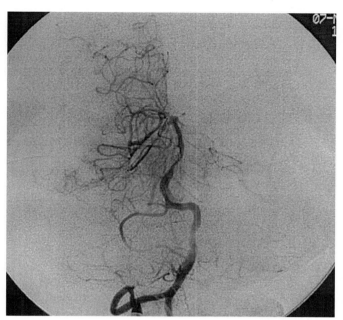

Figure 47-32 Vertebral artery injection, anteroposterior projection, after thrombolysis, demonstrates opacification of the entire basilar artery and the posterior cerebral artery vasculature.

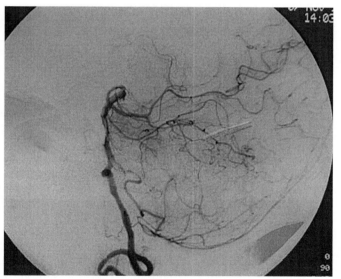

Figure 47-33 Vertebral artery injection, lateral projection, demonstrating basilar artery status after thrombolysis with opacification of the entire basilar artery as well as posterior cerebral artery opacification.

Arteriovenous Malformations

An *arteriovenous malformation* is an abnormal connection between arteries and veins without an intervening capillary, producing a high-flow state with arteriovenous shunting of blood (see Figs. 47-19 to 47-22). These lesions can be associated with headaches, seizures, and other neurologic symptoms. Hemorrhages may be due to nidus vessel rupture, to rupture of an associated aneurysm, or to venous congestion. Associated aneurysms may be in the nidus or on a feeding artery, so-called flow-related

aneurysms (see Figs. 47-21 and 47-22). This diagnosis is often made or at least suspected on MRI, MRA, or CTA. Although time-resolved noninvasive angiographic techniques have been refined,[55] cerebral angiography remains necessary for adequately characterizing the arterial feeders and venous drainage and its dynamics, as well as for searching for associated aneurysms.

Treatment is based on the characteristics of the AVM and whether it involves neurologically eloquent territory. Among the treatment modalities are endovascular embolization, surgery, and stereotactic radiation surgery. Often, a combination of two or three therapies is required (see Chapter 65).

Cervicocephalic Artery Dissection

Cervicocephalic arterial dissection has many possible causes, including trauma, fibromuscular dysplasia, and other vasculopathies. Dissection can manifest as ischemic stroke and, less often, SAH. The diagnosis of dissection can often be made on MRI, MRA, or CTA. In particular, nonenhanced axial T1-weighted, fat-saturated MR images are sensitive for subacute dissection because the blood in the vessel wall appears as high-signal intensity, contrasting with the flow void in the vessel lumen. Characteristic of dissection on angiography is tapering or narrowing of the vessel, in some cases to a string, or even total occlusion; in other cases, a flap may be visualized. Dissecting aneurysms may also be seen (see Figs. 47-15 and 47-16). Affected patients are most often managed medically. However, in case of progressing ischemia, an endovascular procedure involving angioplasty and stenting may be beneficial.

Vasculitis

Intracranial vasculitis is suspected when multiple cerebral infarcts are detected in different vascular territories. There are many causes of intracranial vasculitis, both autoimmune and infectious. CT and especially MRI can strongly suggest the diagnosis in conjunction with the clinical history, but a cerebral angiogram is generally required for confirmation. The angiographic findings in intracranial vasculitis range from normal to demonstration of focal concentric narrowings, most prominent in the more distal vasculature. This appearance may mimic the vasospasm of SAH, but the clinical history distinguishes the two entities. Cerebral angiography is important in confirming the diagnosis of vasculitis before a patient is subjected to long-term corticosteroid and cytotoxic therapies with their potential side effects. In rare cases, angiography may be unrevealing because of vasculitic changes primarily situated at more diminutive vessel calibers.[56]

Another benefit of cerebral angiography in suspected vasculitis is that the external carotid artery can be injected as part of the procedure so that a superficial temporal artery biopsy can be planned, if it is indicated to aid in diagnosis.

Takayasu's arteritis involves the proximal segments of the supra-aortic arteries. Its angiographic appearance is shown in Figure 47-34.

Fibromuscular Dysplasia

Fibromuscular dysplasia is a vasculopathy of medium-sized arteries, with a prevalence of 0.5% to 0.7%.[57,58] This entity affects the cervical and intracranial vasculature.

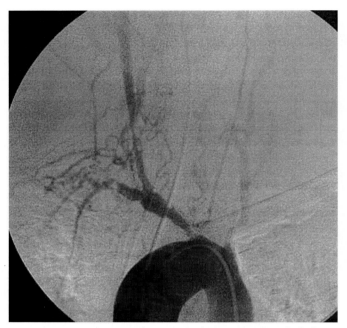

Figure 47-34   Aortic arch injection demonstrating multiple large vessel tandem stenoses in Takayasu's arteritis. Notice how poorly the arch vessels are opacifying secondary to stenoses at vessel origins.

Most lesions occur at the C1-C2 level and spare the proximal aspect of the supra-aortic arteries.[57] The diagnosis is often made incidentally on cerebral angiography performed for diagnosis of intracranial aneurysm or dissection, both of which are often associated with fibromuscular dysplasia. The characteristic angiographic finding is alternation of dilated and stenosed regions to give a "string of beads" appearance or, alternatively, a long tubular stenosis.

Moyamoya Syndrome

Moyamoya disease is a condition named for its cerebral angiographic appearance—*moya moya* is the Japanese word for "puff of smoke." The cloudlike collateral networks of vessels in moyamoya disease are multiple small channels formed in response to the chronic occlusive vasculopathy affecting large arteries at the base of the brain, mainly the distal internal carotid artery (see Chapter 35). Moyamoya disease can produce both ischemic and hemorrhagic strokes; cerebral infarcts predominate in children, and hemorrhagic and ischemic events are relatively equally common in adults. Among the pathologic concomitants of this disease are aneurysms and AVMs, which were detected in 11% of patients reported by Chiu et al.[59] Moyamoya syndrome has recently been characterized in reports from Europe and North America, offering insight on this rare disorder.[60,61]

The diagnosis of moyamoya disease may be suspected from MRI or MRA findings. Cerebral angiography is required, however, for confirmation, precise anatomic depiction, and study of the external carotid circulation to guide revascularization therapy. The angiographic findings consist of bilateral stenotic occlusive disease in the intracranial internal carotid artery with thin multiple

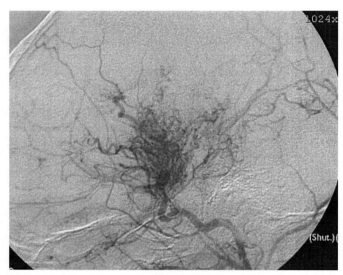

Figure 47-35   Internal carotid artery injection, lateral projection, demonstrating absence of the normal vasculature and a "puff of smoke" appearance to the distribution of opacification.

collateral vessels (Fig. 47-35). The angiographic changes occur idiopathically in moyamoya disease but also in response to stenosing vasculopathy from diverse identified causes (moyamoya syndrome), including radiation vasculopathy, Down's syndrome, and early-onset intracranial atherosclerosis.

Cerebral Arterial Vasospasm

Arterial vasospasm of the intracranial arteries after SAH has an associated 15% to 20% risk of mortality (see Chapter 40).[62] Vasospasm is most common between 3 and 10 days after SAH. It is the principal cause of death and disability once the aneurysm has been secured by clipping or coiling. The diagnosis of vasospasm is generally suspected from clinical findings as well as transcranial Doppler ultrasonography, but confirmation usually requires a cerebral angiogram. Admission angiographic cerebral circulation time may be used to predict subsequent angiographic vasospasm after aneurysmal SAH.[63] Patients with symptomatic vasospasm despite adequate medical management, including hypertensive–hypervolemic therapy, are usually candidates for urgent cerebral angiography and angioplasty (balloon and/or chemical). In a patient with vasospasm, angiography shows narrowing of the vessels in a single or multiple regions. Spasm in the proximal intracranial arteries may be amenable to balloon angioplasty, and more distal spasm may be treated with intraarterial injection of papaverine or nicardipine.[64]

Cerebral Venous Thrombosis

Cerebral venous thrombosis refers to the occlusion of the cerebral veins or sinuses by thrombus (see Chapter 28). The superior sagittal sinus is affected in 72% of cases, and the lateral sinuses are affected in 70%.[65] Multiple predisposing factors are associated with cerebral venous thrombosis, and a predisposing factor is identified in as many as 80% of cases.[65] Among these factors are intracranial infection, sepsis, brain surgery, tumor, hormonal causes, puerperium, oral contraceptives, hypercoagulable states, and dehydration. The clinical scenario is often one of slow progression of symptoms. Initial symptoms are generally nonspecific. A headache is the most common presenting symptom. Additional common symptoms are papilledema, vomiting, seizures, and focal neurologic deficits. CT or MRI findings often suggest the diagnosis.

The angiographic appearance of cerebral venous thrombosis is characteristically seen in the venous phase of the imaging sequence. There is no (or little) opacification of the thrombosed sinus. A long arterial injection as well as a long imaging time must be used so as to give the venous system an adequate chance to opacify. Anteroposterior (AP), lateral, and oblique views should be obtained. Oblique imaging is very valuable because often the entire sinus cannot be shown on the lateral view, and the anterior and posterior aspects of the sinus overlap on a true AP view. Imaging of superior sagittal sinus thrombosis is shown in Figure 47-36.

Anticoagulation is usually the first treatment attempted for cerebral venous thrombosis. If the patient's symptoms progress or there is no improvement over time, local catheter-guided pharmacologic or mechanical thrombolysis can be considered.

Brain Death

The diagnosis of brain death rarely requires a cerebral angiogram. The use of an invasive test for the diagnosis of brain death is regarded as problematic in some countries. If confirmatory laboratory tests are needed to supplement clinical findings, a diagnosis can be established with the use of nuclear medicine, electrophysiology, transcranial Doppler ultrasonography, and other noninvasive methods. Multimodal CT, including CTA and CT perfusion,

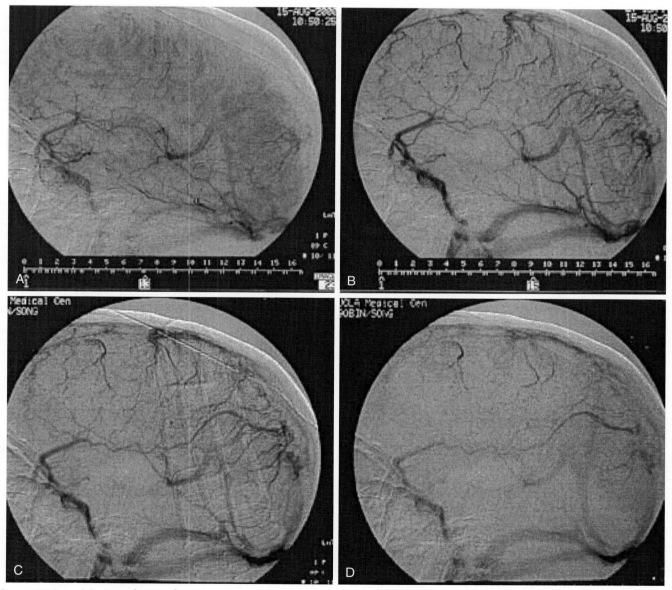

Figure 47-36 A-D, Lateral view of entire venous phase demonstrating no significant opacification of the superior sagittal sinus. (Images are a sequence of the "venous phase"—A being earlier than D.)

has recently been studied and holds promise as a potential rapid alternative for diagnosis of brain death.[66-69] For brain death to be diagnosed on cerebral angiography, there should be no contrast opacification of intracranial vessels after injection of contrast agent into the brachiocephalic vasculature. The shutdown of the entire cerebral circulation reflects increased intracranial pressure due to brain swelling.

REFERENCES

1. Wolpert SM: Neuroradiology classics, *AJNR Am J Neuroradiol* 20:1752-1753, 1999.
2. Rosenbaum AE, Eldevik OP, Mani JR, et al: In re: Amundsen P. Cerebral angiography via the femoral artery with particular reference to cerebrovascular disease. *Acta Neurol Scand* 1967; (Suppl 31):115, *AJNR Am J Neuroradiol* 22:584-589, 2001.
3. Qureshi AI, Abou-Chebl A, Jovin TG: Qualification requirements for performing neurointerventional procedures: A Report of the Practice Guidelines Committee of the American Society of Neuroimaging and the Society of Vascular and Interventional Neurology, *J Neuroimaging* 18:433-447, 2008.
4. Geyik S, Yavuz K, Akgoz A, et al: The safety and efficacy of the Angio-Seal closure device in diagnostic and interventional neuroangiography setting: A single-center experience with 1,443 closures, *Neuroradiology* 49:739-746, 2007.
5. Ahmed AS, Deuerling-Zheng Y, Strother CM, et al: Impact of intraarterial injection parameters on arterial, capillary, and venous time-concentration curves in a canine model, *AJNR Am J Neuroradiol* 30:1337-1341, 2009.
6. Dion JE, Gates PC, Fox AJ, Barnett HJ, Blom RJ: Clinical events following neuroangiography: A prospective study, *Stroke* 18: 997-1004, 1987.
7. Leffers AM, Wagner A: Neurologic complications of cerebral angiography. A retrospective study of complication rate and patient risk factors, *Acta Radiol* 41:204-210, 2000.
8. Quality improvement guidelines for adult diagnostic neuroangiography: Cooperative study between the ASNR, ASITN, and the SCVIR. American Society of Neuroradiology. American Society of Interventional and Therapeutic Neuroradiology. Society of Cardiovascular and Interventional Radiology, *AJNR Am J Neuroradiol* 21:146-150, 2000.
9. Frontera JA, Pile-Spellman J, Mohr JP: Contrast-induced neurotoxicity and selective cortical injury, *Cerebrovasc Dis* 24:148-151, 2007.
10. Gil-Gouveia R, Fernandes Sousa R, Lopes L, Campos J, Pavao Martins I: Headaches during angiography and endovascular procedures, *J Neurol* 254:591-596, 2007.
11. Gil-Gouveia RS, Sousa RF, Lopes L, et al: Post-angiography headaches, *J Headache Pain* 9:327-330, 2008.
12. Guimaraens L, Vivas E, Fonnegra A, et al: Transient encephalopathy from angiographic contrast: a rare complication in neurointerventional procedures, *Cardiovasc Intervent Radiol* 33:383-388, 2010.
13. Kochanowicz J, Lewszuk A, Kordecki K, et al: Diagnostic cerebral angiography affects the tonus of the major cerebral arteries, *Med Sci Monit* 13(Suppl 1):55-58, 2007.
14. Bridcut RR, Murphy E, Workman A, et al: Patient dose from 3D rotational neurovascular studies, *Br J Radiol* 80:362-366, 2007.
15. Khatri P, Broderick JP, Khoury JC, et al: Microcatheter contrast injections during intra-arterial thrombolysis may increase intracranial hemorrhage risk, *Stroke* 39:3283-3287, 2008.
16. Kaufmann TJ, Huston J 3rd, Mandrekar JN, et al: Complications of diagnostic cerebral angiography: evaluation of 19,826 consecutive patients, *Radiology* 243:812-819, 2007.
17. Hankey GJ, Warlow CP, Sellar RJ: Cerebral angiographic risk in mild cerebrovascular disease, *Stroke* 21:209-222, 1990.
18. Fifi JT, Meyers PM, Lavine SD, et al: Complications of modern diagnostic cerebral angiography in an academic medical center, *J Vasc Interv Radiol* 20:442-447, 2009.
19. Thiex R, Norbash AM, Frerichs KU: The safety of dedicated-team catheter-based diagnostic cerebral angiography in the era of advanced noninvasive imaging, *AJNR Am J Neuroradiol* 31: 230-234, 2010.
20. Hussain SI, Wolfe TJ, Lynch JR, et al: Diagnostic cerebral angiography: The interventional neurology perspective, *J Neuroimaging* 20:251-254, 2010.
21. Gerraty RP, Bowser DN, Infeld B, et al: Microemboli during carotid angiography. Association with stroke risk factors or subsequent magnetic resonance imaging changes? *Stroke* 27:1543-1547, 1996.
22. Gupta R, Vora N, Thomas A, et al: Symptomatic cerebral air embolism during neuro-angiographic procedures: Incidence and problem avoidance, *Neurocrit Care* 7:241-246, 2007.
23. Bendszus M, Koltzenburg M, Burger R, et al: Silent embolism in diagnostic cerebral angiography and neurointerventional procedures: A prospective study, *Lancet* 354:1594-1597, 1999.
24. Cloft HJ, Joseph GJ, Dion JE: Risk of cerebral angiography in patients with subarachnoid hemorrhage, cerebral aneurysm, and arteriovenous malformation: A meta-analysis, *Stroke* 30:317-320, 1999.
25. Hassan AE, Hussain MS, Chowdhury F, et al: Changes in serum calcium levels associated with catheter-based cerebral angiography, *J Neuroimaging* 17:336-338, 2007.
26. van Gijn J, Rinkel GJ: Subarachnoid haemorrhage: Diagnosis, causes and management, *Brain* 124:249-278, 2001.
27. Ruigrok YM, Rinkel GJ, Buskens E, et al: Perimesencephalic hemorrhage and CT angiography: A decision analysis, *Stroke* 31:2976-2983, 2000.
28. Huttner HB, Hartmann M, Kohrmann M, et al: Repeated digital subtraction angiography after perimesencephalic subarachnoid hemorrhage? *J Neuroradiol* 33:87-89, 2006.
29. Pedicelli A, Rollo M, Di Lella GM, et al: 3D rotational angiography for the diagnosis and preoperative assessment of intracranial aneurysms: Preliminary experience, *Radiol Med* 112:895-905, 2007.
30. van Rooij WJ, Peluso JP, Sluzewski M, Beute GN: Additional value of 3D rotational angiography in angiographically negative aneurysmal subarachnoid hemorrhage: How negative is negative? *AJNR Am J Neuroradiol* 29:962-966, 2008.
31. van Rooij WJ, Sprengers ME, de Gast AN, et al: 3D rotational angiography: The new gold standard in the detection of additional intracranial aneurysms, *AJNR Am J Neuroradiol* 29:976-979, 2008.
32. Ishihara H, Kato S, Akimura T, et al: Angiogram-negative subarachnoid hemorrhage in the era of three dimensional rotational angiography, *J Clin Neurosci* 14:252-255, 2007.
33. Ringer AJ, Lanzino G, Veznedaroglu E, et al: Does angiographic surveillance pose a risk in the management of coiled intracranial aneurysms? A multicenter study of 2243 patients, *Neurosurgery* 63:845-849, 2008:discussion 849.
34. Wolfe TJ, Hussain SI, Lynch JR, et al: Pediatric cerebral angiography: Analysis of utilization and findings, *Pediatr Neurol* 40:98-101, 2009.
35. Liebeskind DS: Location, location, location: Angiography discerns early MR imaging vessel signs due to proximal arterial occlusion and distal collateral flow, *AJNR Am J Neuroradiol* 26:2432-2433, 2005.
36. Sanossian N, Saver JL, Alger JR, et al: Angiography reveals that fluid-attenuated inversion recovery vascular hyperintensities are due to slow flow, not thrombus, *AJNR Am J Neuroradiol* 30:564-568, 2009.
37. Chimowitz MI, Lynn MJ, Howlett-Smith H, et al: Comparison of warfarin and aspirin for symptomatic intracranial arterial stenosis, *N Engl J Med* 352:1305-1316, 2005.
38. Kasner SE, Lynn MJ, Chimowitz MI, et al: Warfarin vs aspirin for symptomatic intracranial stenosis: Subgroup analyses from WASID, *Neurology* 67:1275-1278, 2006.
39. Feldmann E, Wilterdink JL, Kosinski A, et al: The Stroke Outcomes and Neuroimaging of Intracranial Atherosclerosis (SONIA) trial, *Neurology* 68:2099-2106, 2007.
40. Samuels OB, Joseph GJ, Lynn MJ, et al: A standardized method for measuring intracranial arterial stenosis, *AJNR Am J Neuroradiol* 21:643-646, 2000.
41. Gobin YP, Starkman S, Duckwiler GR, et al: MERCI 1: A phase 1 study of mechanical embolus removal in cerebral ischemia, *Stroke* 35:2848-2854, 2004.
42. Smith WS, Sung G, Saver J, et al: Mechanical thrombectomy for acute ischemic stroke: Final results of the Multi MERCI trial, *Stroke* 39:1205-1212, 2008.

43. Smith WS, Sung G, Starkman S, et al: Safety and efficacy of mechanical embolectomy in acute ischemic stroke: Results of the MERCI trial, *Stroke* 36:1432-1438, 2005.

44. The Penumbra Pivotal Stroke Trial: safety and effectiveness of a new generation of mechanical devices for clot removal in intracranial large vessel occlusive disease, *Stroke* 40:2761-2768, 2009.

45. Bose A, Henkes H, Alfke K, et al: The Penumbra System: a mechanical device for the treatment of acute stroke due to thromboembolism, *AJNR Am J Neuroradiol* 29:1409-1413, 2008.

46. Brekenfeld C, Schroth G, Mattle HP, et al: Stent placement in acute cerebral artery occlusion: Use of a self-expandable intracranial stent for acute stroke treatment, *Stroke* 40:847-852, 2009.

47. Levy EI, Mehta R, Gupta R, et al: Self-expanding stents for recanalization of acute cerebrovascular occlusions, *AJNR Am J Neuroradiol* 28:816-822, 2007.

48. Levy EI, Siddiqui AH, Crumlish A, et al: First Food and Drug Administration-approved prospective trial of primary intracranial stenting for acute stroke: SARIS (stent-assisted recanalization in acute ischemic stroke), *Stroke* 40:3552-3556, 2009.

49. Qureshi AI, Alkawi A, Hussein HM, Divani AA: Angiographic analysis of intravascular thrombus volume in patients with acute ischemic stroke, *J Endovasc Ther* 14:475-482, 2007.

50. Qureshi AI, Hussein HM, Abdelmoula M, et al: Subacute recanalization and reocclusion in patients with acute ischemic stroke following endovascular treatment, *Neurocrit Care* 10:195-203, 2009.

51. Liebeskind DS: Collateral circulation, *Stroke* 34:2279-2284, 2003.

52. Liebeskind DS: Collaterals in acute stroke: Beyond the clot, *Neuroimaging Clin N Am* 15:553-573, 2005.

53. Tomsick T: Timi, TIBI, TICI: I came, I saw, I got confused, *AJNR Am J Neuroradiol* 28:382-384, 2007.

54. Higashida RT, Furlan AJ, Roberts H, et al: Trial design and reporting standards for intra-arterial cerebral thrombolysis for acute ischemic stroke, *Stroke* 34:e109-e137, 2003.

55. Eddleman CS, Jeong HJ, Hurley MC, et al: 4D radial acquisition contrast-enhanced MR angiography and intracranial arteriovenous malformations: Quickly approaching digital subtraction angiography, *Stroke* 40:2749-2753, 2009.

56. Salvarani C, Brown RD Jr, Calamia KT, et al: Angiography-negative primary central nervous system vasculitis: A syndrome involving small cerebral vessels, *Medicine (Baltimore)* 87:264-271, 2008.

57. Kubis N, Von Langsdorff D, Petitjean C, et al: Thrombotic carotid megabulb: Fibromuscular dysplasia, septae, and ischemic stroke, *Neurology* 52:883-886, 1999.

58. Finsterer J, Strassegger J, Haymerle A, Hagmuller G: Bilateral stenting of symptomatic and asymptomatic internal carotid artery stenosis due to fibromuscular dysplasia, *J Neurol Neurosurg Psychiatry* 69:683-686, 2000.

59. Chiu D, Shedden P, Bratina P, Grotta JC: Clinical features of moyamoya disease in the United States, *Stroke* 29:1347-1351, 1998.

60. Kraemer M, Heienbrok W, Berlit P: Moyamoya disease in Europeans, *Stroke* 39:3193-3200, 2008.

61. Hallemeier CL, Rich KM, Grubb RL Jr, et al: Clinical features and outcome in North American adults with moyamoya phenomenon, *Stroke* 37:1490-1496, 2006.

62. Lysakowski C, Walder B, Costanza MC, Tramer MR: Transcranial Doppler versus angiography in patients with vasospasm due to a ruptured cerebral aneurysm: A systematic review, *Stroke* 32:2292-2298, 2001.

63. Udoetuk JD, Stiefel MF, Hurst RW, et al: Admission angiographic cerebral circulation time may predict subsequent angiographic vasospasm after aneurysmal subarachnoid hemorrhage, *Neurosurgery* 61:1152-1159, 2007:discussion 1159-1161.

64. Linfante I, Delgado-Mederos R, Andreone V, et al: Angiographic and hemodynamic effect of high concentration of intra-arterial nicardipine in cerebral vasospasm, *Neurosurgery* 63:1080-1086, 2008:discussion 1086-1087.

65. Allroggen H, Abbott RJ: Cerebral venous sinus thrombosis, *Postgrad Med J* 76:12-15, 2000.

66. Escudero D, Otero J, Marques L, et al: Diagnosing brain death by CT perfusion and multislice CT angiography, *Neurocrit Care* 11:261-271, 2009.

67. Frampas E, Videcoq M, de Kerviler E, et al: CT angiography for brain death diagnosis, *AJNR Am J Neuroradiol* 30:1566-1570, 2009.

68. Greer DM, Strozyk D, Schwamm LH: False positive CT angiography in brain death, *Neurocrit Care* 11:272-275, 2009.

69. Quesnel C, Fulgencio JP, Adrie C, et al: Limitations of computed tomographic angiography in the diagnosis of brain death, *Intensive Care Med* 33:2129-2135, 2007.

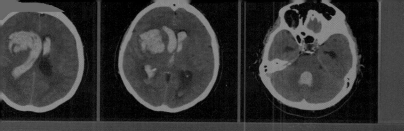

Therapy

PART A: MEDICAL THERAPY

JAMES C. GROTTA

The treatment of acute stroke begins with prehospital management, before the neurologist is even involved, including the extremely important contribution of emergency medicine. The various aspects of thrombolysis, both intravenous and intraarterial, are covered in detail, including a review of thrombolytic agents, clinical trial data pertaining to benefits and risks, community experience, guidelines, and, finally, practical tips.

Specialized care in stroke units and intensive care units is addressed with emphasis on the effectiveness and components of each. Details of good ICU care are reviewed with attention to correcting disturbed physiology and treatment of specific stroke syndromes. The possibility of reversing the pathologic cascade of injury at the cellular level is followed by a detailed review of neuroprotective agents, with an eye on how to finally establish the utility of such therapy.

Treatment of specific stroke conditions (e.g., dissection and venous thrombosis) is covered with an emphasis on what is known and where new information is needed, as well as selection of patients for surgical intervention. The emerging scientific inquiry and evidence surrounding stroke rehabilitation, which is discussed in detail, will provide much valuable new information, including measurement of outcome, treatment of stroke complications during recovery, and various rehabilitation techniques. A new chapter on cell-based treatment has been added to cover the exciting area of "restorative therapy."

The topic of secondary prevention begins with a detailed review of platelet physiology in stroke, the mechanism of various antiplatelet agents and choices among them based on clinical trial data, and new antiplatelet strategies. Cardioembolic stroke and its prevention is then covered in detail, as is treatment to modify important risk factors such as blood pressure and cholesterol and the selection of patients for carotid intervention.

The section concludes with an enlightening review of all aspects of conducting clinical research studies in stroke prevention and treatment. Principles of data analysis are covered, and the section finishes by discussing the roles of the U.S. Federal Drug Administration, Institutional Research Boards, and informed consent.

PART B: INTERVENTIONAL THERAPY

RÜDIGER VON KUMMER

This new section covers the interventional therapy of ischemic and hemorrhagic stroke and interventional prophylactic approaches to treating arterial diseases and vascular malformations associated with a risk for brain ischemia or intracranial hemorrhage. It begins with an extended overview, including discussion of the latest trials on carotid artery stenting. Sections on intraarterial thrombolysis, mechanical recanalization, and dural arteriovenous malformations have been thoroughly revised. New chapters on the treatment of intracranial aneurysms and vascular malformations of the brain have been added. Interventional therapy of stroke patients is a rapidly growing field that now requires its own section.

PART C: SURGICAL THERAPY

MARC R. MAYBERG

The application of surgical therapies to *completed* stroke, whether ischemic or hemorrhagic, has been relatively limited, with a few exceptions. Thus, most surgical treatments have been directed toward *preventing* ischemic stroke or intracranial hemorrhage in patients at risk. This may be changing with the emergence of new therapies based on new technologies. With the evolution of cerebrovascular devices and techniques has come a cycle of innovation, enthusiasm for novel treatment, and tempered application based on scientific data. In the past, exciting new surgical therapies, which seemed

logical and successfully modified cerebrovascular physiology (e.g., extracranial-intracranial bypass for ischemia), subsequently proved ineffective and were discarded. Existing standards of practice in cerebrovascular surgery, such as carotid endarterectomy, were questioned and subsequently verified by well-designed clinical trials. This cycle of change in surgical treatment for stroke has continued, as reflected in this section.

Surgical therapy includes a variety of topics: the genetic basis for cerebral aneurysms and arteriovenous malformations (genomic insights into the pathogenesis of these disorders will likely lead to better measures to identify individuals at risk and diagnose these lesions prior to hemorrhagic events); the rapidly accumulating data on treatment of spontaneous intracerebral and intraventricular hemorrhage (recent large prospective randomized clinical trials are defining the role of surgery in these disorders and delineating clinical features related to history and outcomes); carotid endarterectomy as a measure to prevent stroke (exciting new data from the first prospective randomized direct comparison between microsurgical and endovascular treatment is presented, as well as a large body of data from prior trails for endarterectomy versus medical therapy); the microsurgical treatment of cerebral aneurysms (in addition to considerations regarding patient selection, surgical approach and technique, these chapters review the comparison of open microsurgical treatment to endovascular therapy and specific indications for each treatment); and microsurgical and radiosurgical therapy for arteriovenous malformations of the brain and spinal cord. The genetics, natural history, and optimal treatment of cavernous malformations is also summarized.

New technologies have emerged to identify subsets of patients who might benefit from extracranial-intracranial bypass. In addition, there has been a growing interest in decompressive craniectomy for large hemispheric cerebral infarction. Similarly, the emergent treatment of cerebellar hemorrhage and infarction is often lifesaving and is associated with excellent outcomes.

These chapters describe a dynamic period in the treatment of stroke, wherein practitioners from multiple specialties are using a better understanding of the pathophysiology and natural history of cerebrovascular disorders to apply advanced technologies to the treatment of stroke.

48 Prehospital and Emergency Department Care of the Patient with Acute Stroke

OPEOLU ADEOYE, ARTHUR PANCIOLI

Optimal care of patients with acute stroke depends on rapid recognition of symptoms by the patient or bystanders in the prehospital setting, activation of emergency medical services (EMS), and transport to a hospital capable of delivering state-of-the art acute stroke care 24 hours a day. Table 48-1 highlights current recommendations for the rapid evaluation of stroke patients. After EMS notification or self-arrival in the emergency department (ED) by the stroke patient, any breakdown in the rapid sequence of events necessary to deliver optimal care could adversely impact patient outcomes. This chapter addresses the roles that prehospital care providers and ED teams play in the evaluation and management of patients with acute stroke.

The EMS community and ED team play important roles in the evaluation and management of patients with acute stroke. In 2004, the American Heart Association/American Stroke Association (AHA/ASA) convened a taskforce on the development of stroke systems. That taskforce determined that the approach to care in many systems across the United States was fragmented and that this uneven approach may contribute to stroke morbidity and mortality.[1] The taskforce identified the prehospital and ED phases of care as key components within stroke care. Subsequently, an ASA expert panel was convened and issued specific recommendations for optimizing prehospital care of the stroke patient within the larger system of stroke care[2]:

1. Stroke systems should require appropriate processes that ensure rapid access to EMS for acute stroke patients.
2. EMS responders should use protocols, tools, and training that meet current ASA/AHA guidelines for stroke care.
3. Prehospital providers, emergency physicians, and stroke experts should collaborate in the development of EMS training, assessment, treatment, and transportation protocols for stroke patients.
4. Patients should be transported to the nearest stroke center for evaluation and care if a stroke center is located within a reasonable transport distance and transport time.

This last point should be particularly emphasized as it may have implications for regional practices, whereby, as in the case of trauma victims and trauma centers, a closer hospital may be bypassed so that a stroke patient may be better served, evaluated, and treated at a certified stroke center; it may also entail crossing state lines. Given the time-sensitive nature of acute stroke treatment, preexisting systems should facilitate the appropriate prehospital and ED care of stroke patients. One example of a systematic approach improving care is seen in an Australian prospective cohort study that used historical controls; implementation of a prehospital stroke triage protocol that included bypass of non-stroke center hospitals improved thrombolytic administration among stroke patients from 4.7% before the intervention to 21.4% after the intervention.[3]

The Course of Events for the Acute Stroke Patient

Speed and efficiency of initial management, diagnosis, and communication are significant components of the contribution to acute stroke care provided by prehospital and ED teams. An analysis of the course of events that transpires between the onset of a patient's symptoms and the delivery of definitive therapies is warranted. The major components in the evaluation and treatment process of patients with acute stroke can be divided into prehospital and ED phases, as follows.

TABLE 48-1 GUIDELINES FOR RAPID EVALUATION OF THE PATIENT WITH ACUTE STROKE

Period Measured	Optimal Time (min)
From ED arrival to emergency physician evaluation	10
From ED arrival to CT scan	25
From ED arrival to CT scan interpretation	50
From ED arrival to initiation of therapy (80% compliance)*	60

*Target should be compliance with these guidelines in at least 80% of cases.
CT, Computed tomography; ED, emergency department.

Prehospital Components

1. Recognition of stroke symptoms by the patient or family members
2. First contact with medical care (for example, phoning 911 in the United States)
3. Dispatch of appropriate level of prehospital care providers
4. Prehospital evaluation, management, and transport
5. Prehospital identification of stroke
6. Prehospital notification of pending ED arrival

Emergency Department

1. ED triage
2. ED evaluation and management
3. Divergence of pathway according to whether stroke is ischemic or hemorrhagic
4. Disposition of patient from the ED

The single largest component of the delay between symptom onset and definitive therapy exists between symptom onset and arrival at the ED. In a population-based study conducted in the Greater Cincinnati/Northern Kentucky region in 1999, only 26% of stroke patients arrived in the ED in less than 3 hours after symptom onset; only an additional 9% arrived from 3 to 8 hours after onset.[4] Thus, it is clear that the prehospital times must be decreased if the number of patients eligible for immediate therapy is to be improved.

Recognition of Stroke Symptoms by the Patient or Family Members

Possibly the largest component in the prehospital delay is failure of the patient or family members to recognize stroke symptoms and act accordingly. In recognition of this, the AHA recently issued a statement that summarizes the issues relating to delayed presentation in acute stroke and offered some suggestions for further study regarding approaches for minimizing prehospital delay.[5] Factors that have been shown to be associated with delay in arrival at the ED are as follows[6-13]:

- The patient (or family member) initially phones the primary care physician instead of the local emergency service phone number.
- The patient lives alone.
- Stroke begins while the patient is asleep.
- Symptoms appear while the patient is at home versus at work.
- The stroke is mild rather than severe.

In addition, stroke often damages the areas of the brain that control either the patient's perception of a problem or the patient's ability to communicate. In a population-based study in Corpus Christi, Texas, only 4.3% of stroke patients who utilized EMS activated EMS themselves.[14] However, the major reasons for time-to-treatment delay appear to be the lack of recognition of stroke signs and symptoms and the lack of a proper response. In another survey conducted in greater Cincinnati, Ohio, only 37% of patients with stroke, their family members, or both knew at the onset of the patient's stroke that the symptoms were due to a stroke.[15] Of the 163 patients, 62 (38%) did not know a single warning symptom of stroke and another 45 (28%) could identify only one symptom.

The lack of knowledge of the warning signs of and risk factors in stroke was quantified in a large telephone survey in the greater Cincinnati, Ohio, area in 1995.[16] That survey assessed the level of stroke knowledge within a population whose demographics matched those of patients with acute stroke. Using open-ended questions, the researchers in this study found that only 57% of the respondents were able to name even one warning sign of stroke. Similarly, only 68% could name even one risk factor for stroke. Persons older than 75 years were significantly less likely to be able to name one stroke warning sign or one risk factor than younger persons. Another survey was performed in 2000 within the same community and with the identical methodology to both reassess the level of stroke knowledge and look for incremental change in the overall level of stroke knowledge in the public.[17] The researchers found an increase in the public knowledge of stroke warning signs, in that 70% of respondents in the 2000 survey were able to name at least one stroke warning sign. Although this survey population had a slightly higher number of respondents who described themselves as having at least "some college," which may account for the increase in knowledge of stroke warning signs, there was no change in the percentage of respondents who could name one risk factor.

Unfortunately, therefore, a significant portion of the general public still has minimal knowledge and understanding of stroke warning signs and risk factors. Inadequate public awareness of the importance of stroke symptoms may lead to a significant delay in presentation of stroke victims for treatment. Such a relationship was noted in a multicenter study in Sweden. In the prospective study of factors influencing the time from onset of stroke or transient ischemic attack (TIA) to hospital arrival, both a lack of awareness of the need to seek medical attention and the failure to use direct ambulance transport were found to increase the prehospital delay.[18]

First Contact with Medical Care

The EMS system is the point of first medical contact for about half of people having acute stroke.[6,7,10] Although the symptomatology and presentation of many acute strokes are dramatic enough to lead patients or bystanders toward prompt action, less dramatic presentations often lead to significant delay. A French study has previously demonstrated that initially contacting the general practitioner or primary care physician (PCP) was associated with less likelihood of EMS use by stroke patients.[13] A recent survey presenting case vignettes to 395 PCPs in Germany found that working as a general practitioner (odds ratio [OR], 0.3; 95% confidence interval [CI], 0.2 to 0.6) and practice location outside a metropolitan area ($P = 0.002$) independently decreased the probability of admitting suspected stroke patients as a medical emergency when first contact to PCPs was by phone.[19]

Unfortunately, any action other than the immediate activation of the EMS system via 911 or equivalent will lead to significant delays in treatment. The Second Delay in Accessing Stroke Healthcare study (DASH II) was a prospective multicenter study that enrolled 617 patients with suspected stroke.[20] EMS use was found to be associated with decreased prehospital and in-hospital delays to care. Patients who used EMS had a median prehospital delay time of 2.85 hours compared with 4.03 hours for those who did not use EMS ($P = 0.002$). Those who used EMS had significantly shorter times from symptom onset to arrival, time to seeing an emergency physician, time to computed tomography (CT) scan, and time to being seen by a neurologist.[20] In another study, use of the EMS system shortened time to arrival as well as time to treatment in patients with acute stroke. Patients arriving by ambulance were more likely to arrive earlier (OR for arrival within 3 hours, 3.7) than individuals arriving via other modes of transport and were more likely to be seen by a physician within 15 minutes of arrival (OR, 2.3).[21] Thus, it is clear that the use of the EMS system is one critical link in reducing delay to ED arrival for patients with acute stroke.

Dispatch of Appropriate Level of Prehospital Providers

Once the EMS-911 system is activated, EMS dispatchers gather initial information and dispatch prehospital care providers. Thus, the first triage by any form of medical provider occurs on receipt of the 911 call. However, in one study, dispatchers without specific training in stroke could identify only 52% of verified cases of stroke. Ambulance units were dispatched to the scene for preliminary diagnosis other than stroke in 48% of cases.[22]

In a retrospective review of San Francisco dispatcher performance for acute stroke or TIA calls, dispatchers were able to identify cases as "cerebrovascular accidents" only 31% of the time.[23] In the majority of cases in this study (59%), ambulances were dispatched at lower priority than they would have been for an identified stroke. Surprisingly, 51% of callers to 911 used the word *stroke* to describe their emergency, but only 48% of the patients for whom *stroke* was used in the 911 call were categorized by dispatchers as having cerebrovascular accidents.[23]

This decision about the level of prehospital provider to dispatch to a possible stroke victim is relatively important. One study indicated that advanced life support (ALS) transport might be better suited to the evaluation and transport of potential stroke victims. In that study, up to 29% of patients with acute ischemic stroke required prehospital interventions for treatable medical conditions, including compromised airway and cardiac instability. The patients transported by basic life support units arrived at the hospital earlier (40 ± 1 minutes) than those transported by ALS units staffed by paramedics (45 ± 1 minutes; $P = .004$). However, patients transported by ALS units were seen by a physician sooner after arrival at the ED (10 ± 2 minutes) than those who arrived via basic life support units (20 ± 4 minutes; $P = .02$). Thus, although the transport times were similar, the level of care for patients transported by ALS teams was higher. In that community, stroke is treated as a level I emergency equivalent to trauma and myocardial infarction.[24] Not all local EMS networks treat stroke as a level I emergency.[1,2]

As already mentioned, a recent AHA/ASA expert panel recommended that prehospital providers, emergency physicians, and stroke experts should collaborate in the development of EMS training, assessment, treatment, and transportation protocols for stroke.[2] This should facilitate education of local providers and appropriate-level dispatch for possible stroke cases.

Prehospital Evaluation and Management

On identification of a potential stroke victim, prehospital care providers must begin stabilization of the patient and measures aimed toward diagnosis (Table 48-2). An assessment of the patient's airway, breathing, and circulation (ABCs) with measurement of vital signs and pulse oximetry must be performed, and abnormalities must be addressed. The initial assessment should proceed with application of a cardiac monitor, measurement of the patient's serum glucose level, initiation of intravenous (IV) access, and application of supplemental oxygen. Notably, these measures should be performed during transport of the patient and, unless resuscitative measures are required, should not delay transport.

One critical component of the prehospital care provider's assessment is to attempt to establish the exact time of onset of the patient's symptoms and to elicit the history of relevant events surrounding the episode, such as trauma, seizure activity, or migraine headache. Prehospital care providers have shown great creativity in eliciting key elements of the patient's history to help establish time of onset.

In addition to stabilization and establishing time of onset, prehospital care providers should pay specific attention to the management of blood pressure, fluid status, and glucose level. Interventions to lower blood pressure should not be attempted in the prehospital setting. The differentiation between acute hemorrhagic and acute ischemic stroke requires neurologic imaging and determines the aggressiveness of blood pressure management once the patient is in the ED. Thus, elevations of blood pressure should not be treated before the patient's arrival in the ED.

The prehospital administration of IV fluids to the patient with stroke should also be approached with caution. Dextrose-containing fluids, such as 5% dextrose in water, should be administered only to patients with

TABLE 48-2 GUIDELINES FOR PREHOSPITAL MANAGEMENT OF STROKE

Do...	Do Not...
Determine time of onset	Give large amounts of IV fluids
Assess with Prehospital Stroke Scale	Give dextrose without evidence of hypoglycemia
Give supplemental oxygen	Reduce blood pressure with vasoactive agents
Attach cardiac monitor	Delay transport
Establish IV access	
Measure blood glucose level	
Perform ABCs (ensure airway, breathing, and circulation)	
Treat hypotension	
Give nothing by mouth (NPO)	
Alert emergency department	
Ensure rapid transport	

documented hypoglycemia. For resuscitation needs, isotonic crystalloid is the fluid of choice and should be given as needed to appropriately treat the patient with stroke and associated shock.[25]

Hypoglycemia is a potential stroke mimic that must be ruled out or treated. Ideally, hypoglycemia can be diagnosed in the prehospital setting by paramedics and other ALS providers. If hypoglycemia is documented and symptoms of stroke are present, administration of 50% dextrose in water is appropriate. Intramuscular glucagon may be given instead of dextrose if there is difficulty obtaining venous access. The severity of the patient's symptoms, the time of glucose administration, and subsequent changes in the patient's clinical status must be documented by the EMS provider. Administration of glucose to a patient with suspected stroke but without documented hypoglycemia should be avoided because elevations of the serum glucose level have been associated with worse outcomes after ischemic stroke.[26-28]

Prehospital Identification of Stroke

Ideally, prehospital providers should be well versed in acute stroke recognition and should quickly initiate protocols for acute stroke.[29] Two tools, the Los Angeles Prehospital Stroke Screen (LAPSS) and the Cincinnati Prehospital Stroke Scale (CPSS), have emerged for use by prehospital care providers to allow for early stroke recognition and communication with hospital-based teams.

The LAPSS was created to be a stroke recognition tool specifically for prehospital care personnel (Fig. 48-1).[30] It is a one-page instrument that takes less than 3 minutes to perform. The LAPSS consists of four history items, three physical examination items, and a serum glucose test. In a prospective validation study of the LAPSS, paramedics identified acute stroke victims with a sensitivity of 91% and a specificity of 97%.[31]

The CPSS is a three-item neurologic examination that was developed to assist prehospital care providers in identifying patients with stroke who may be candidates for thrombolysis (Table 48-3). The CPSS was derived via the selection of the three most sensitive and specific components of the National Institutes of Health Stroke Scale (NIHSS)[32]—facial palsy, arm weakness, and speech abnormality. When performed by a trained physician, this scale has been shown to be effective in identifying such patients. The CPSS can be taught in approximately 10 minutes and performed in less than 1 minute.

The CPSS has also been shown to identify potential stroke victims accurately when performed by prehospital care providers.[33] Correlation for the total score (number of abnormal items) between prehospital care providers and physicians was excellent. The CPSS is valid in identifying patients with stroke (sensitivity, 66%; specificity, 87%), especially anterior circulation stroke (sensitivity, 88%). In the evaluation study, presence of a single abnormality on the CPSS identified all patients with anterior circulation stroke who would have been candidates for thrombolytic therapy. The addition of a test for ataxia to the CPSS would have identified six of the 10 patients with posterior circulation stroke who were not identified

in this study. However, ataxia is one of the most poorly reproducible items on the NIHSS and is not included in the CPSS.

Both the LAPSS and the CPSS have been widely utilized in and are accepted tools for the EMS community. The LAPSS has greater overall sensitivity but requires slightly more time to perform. The CPSS is rapidly taught and performed but has a lower sensitivity for posterior circulation stroke.

Prehospital Notification of Pending Emergency Department Arrival

The use of EMS or advance hospital notification by EMS providers has been associated with decreased arrival to CT times in the ED and increased likelihood of treatment with thrombolytics.[34-37] Thus, to help diminish the time from symptom onset to definitive therapy for a patient with stroke, prehospital care providers can facilitate rapid delivery of therapy via an advance notification call to the patient's destination hospital. Armed with tools such as the LAPSS or CPSS, prehospital care providers can, with very good accuracy, make a presumptive diagnosis of acute stroke and set an ED or "stroke team" into motion via advance notification.

Organizations designed to improve stroke care have formally recognized the importance of EMS in systems such as "stroke centers." In a recommendation for the establishment of primary stroke centers, Alberts et al[38] state, "It is vital that the EMS system be integrated with the stroke center. The stroke center should be able to communicate effectively with EMS personnel in the out-of-hospital setting during transportation of a patient experiencing an acute stroke. The ED should be able to efficiently receive and triage patients with stroke arriving via EMS. The stroke center staff should support and participate in educational activities involving EMS personnel." The community of prehospital care providers and the physician leaders in this field are committed to continuous improvement in stroke care and explicitly endorse ongoing efforts to include EMS in the continuum of acute stroke care.[20] To this end, it should be reemphasized that appropriate prehospital stroke triage entails EMS personnel taking the patient to the closest hospital best equipped to fully evaluate and treat the patient's stroke, independent of all other considerations.

Emergency Department Time Delays

Delays in the ED are another barrier to the optimal triage and treatment of patients with acute stroke. Table 48-1 lists the recommendations of the National Institute of Neurological Diseases and Stroke (NINDS)-sponsored National Symposium on Rapid Identification and Treatment of Acute Stroke for time intervals from symptom onset to ED arrival for a patient with suspected stroke.[39]

This conference also provided a recommended algorithm for triage and the evaluation of patients with stroke in the ED. Triage of patients, which is based on stroke severity, available resources, and time from symptom onset, is one way to focus resources appropriately. For example, the patient with a mild or moderate stroke and

Los Angeles Prehospital Stroke Screen (LAPSS)

1. Patient Name: ____________ Last ____________ First
2. Information History from:
   [ ] Patient
   [ ] Family Member ____________ Name ____________ Phone
   [ ] Other
3. Last known time patient was at baseline or deficit free and awake: Military Time: ________ Date: ________

SCREENING CRITERIA:

	Yes	Unknown	No
4. Age > 45	[ ]	[ ]	[ ]
5. History of seizures or epilepsy **absent**	[ ]	[ ]	[ ]
6. Symptom duration **less than** 24 hours	[ ]	[ ]	[ ]
7. At baseline, patient is **not** wheelchair bound or bedridden	[ ]	[ ]	[ ]

	Yes	No
8. Blood glucose between 60 and 400:	[ ]	[ ]

9. Exam: **LOOK FOR OBVIOUS ASYMMETRY**

	Normal	**Right**	**Left**
Facial Smile/Grimace:	_	_ Droop	_ Droop
Grip:	_	_ Weak Grip _ No Grip	_ Weak Grip _ No Grip
Arm Strength	_	_ Drifts Down _ Falls Rapidly	_ Drifts Down _ Falls Rapidly

	Yes	No
Based on exam, patient has **only unilateral** (and not bilateral) weakness:	[ ]	[ ]
10. **Items 4,5,6,7,8,9 all YES's (or unknown) LAPSS screening criteria met:**	[ ]	[ ]

11. If LAPSS criteria for stroke met, call receiving hospital with a "code stroke"; if not, then return to the Appropriate Treatment Protocol. (Note: the patient may still be experiencing a stroke even if LAPSS criteria are not met.)

Figure 48-1 The Los Angeles Prehospital Stroke Screen. (From Kidwell CS, Saver JL, Schubert GB, et al: Design and retrospective analysis of the Los Angeles Prehospital Stroke Screen [LAPSS]. *Prehosp Emerg Care* 2:267-273, 1998.)

stable neurologic deficit who presents more than 6 hours after symptom onset should be evaluated promptly, but it is more urgent to treat a patient who is a potential candidate for a thrombolytic agent within a very small time window (e.g., 3 hours).

Opportunities for physicians to intervene exist only for a limited time regardless of whether a patient is having an ischemic or a hemorrhagic stroke. Delays in patient arrival and delivery of care can significantly affect a patient's potential for a good outcome. Each previously presented element in the course of events for the patient with acute stroke is discussed here.

Until the patient is stabilized and imaging is performed, the care of a patient with acute stroke should be kept on a course aimed at early intervention. Directing acute stroke care toward a rapid, aggressive path of intervention requires a "paradigm shift" from the approach used in the recent past. This shift is similar to the changes in practice mentality for acute myocardial infarction (AMI) that first occurred with the availability of thrombolytic agents and then again with the advent of percutaneous intervention. A comparison of therapy for acute ischemic stroke with that of AMI is illustrative of the impediments to this paradigm shift.

TABLE 48-3 THE CINCINNATI PREHOSPITAL STROKE SCALE*

Facial Droop	Have patient smile or show teeth
Normal	Both sides move equally
Abnormal	One side does not move as well
Arm Drift	Patient closes eyes and holds both arms out
Normal	Both sides move equally
Abnormal	One side does not move as well
Speech	Have patient say "you can't teach an old dog new tricks."
Normal	Patient uses correct words without slurring
Abnormal	Slurs words, uses inappropriate words, or is unable to speak

*Any one or more abnormal findings is suggestive of acute stroke.

Despite reports that almost half the patients with ischemic stroke arrive at an ED within 3 hours of symptom onset, only 3.6% of more than 17,000 patients with potential stroke documented in the two NINDS studies were eligible for treatment (alteplase or placebo) within this time.[40] In contrast, approximately 33% of eligible patients with AMI, according to the National Registry for Myocardial Infarction II, are currently treated with a thrombolytic agent (26%) or alternative reperfusion methods (7%), such as invasive cardiac catheterization or angioplasty.[41]

Currently, the major difference is the perception among physicians and hospitals that myocardial infarction is a medical emergency but stroke is not. For example, in the NINDS study, the goal for time from patient arrival at the ED to treatment was 55 minutes.[40] In contrast, current guidelines for myocardial infarction recommend 30 minutes from arrival to treatment.[42]

To optimize the chance of successful treatment, management protocols for patients with stroke similar to those for patients with AMI or trauma must be designed. In patients with acute stroke, the average time in eight hospitals in Houston, Texas, from arrival in the ED to evaluation by a physician was 28 minutes; for patients brought to Greater Cincinnati hospitals, the elapsed time was 10 minutes for those who arrived by ALS units, and 20 minutes for patients brought by basic life support units. Times from patient arrival in an ED to performance of a CT scan were 100 minutes in Houston and either 47 minutes (ALS unit transport) or 69 minutes (basic life support unit transport) in greater Cincinnati. In Houston, the availability of a designated "stroke team" shortened the time from arrival to examination by a physician by 13 minutes and to CT by 63 minutes.[24,43] The results of these studies illustrate areas where delays currently occur in the evaluation of patients with stroke in the ED and the important effect that stroke teams can have in improving early evaluation and treatment.

Emergency Department Triage

Triage is derived from the French term *trier*, which means to sort or prioritize. This seemingly simple act of setting the patient's priority level via triage is one of the most important aspects of the ED management of an acute stroke. Like the decision a patient or family member makes about whether to call 911, the triage nurse's assignment of a patient with stroke to the critical care arena within an ED rather than to a "noncritical" bed entirely changes the dynamic of the patient's evaluation and treatment. Hospital-based systems seeking to improve the speed and efficiency of evaluation for patients with stroke must involve the ED nursing staff in the effort and must provide education to enable ED triage nurses to assign patients with acute stroke to receive the highest priority of care. It is also useful to give the ED nursing staff clear, concise guidelines for the triage of such patients. Similarly, having a well-understood and easily activated "acute stroke care pathway" with ED orders and a template for documentation can dramatically improve the management of acute stroke.[44,45]

Emergency Department Evaluation and Management

The patient with a possible acute stroke must immediately be stabilized. The ABC assessment is primary. Simultaneously, the diagnostic evaluation must be initiated.

Airway

Airway compromise and the need for intubation may have multiple causes. They include diminished level of consciousness and inability to protect the airway, impairment of oropharyngeal mobility and sensation, and loss of protective reflexes due to ischemic or compressive brainstem dysfunction. Intubation and mechanical ventilation are the primary mechanism for airway protection in the ED setting.

The decision to intubate a patient is based on answering the following three fundamental clinical questions:

1. Is there a failure of airway maintenance or protection?
2. Is there a failure of ventilation or oxygenation?
3. What is the anticipated clinical course?

A common clinical error in airway assessment and management occurs when a patient is found to be "breathing on his or her own." Although they may be breathing, patients with stroke may be at serious risk of aspiration, at which point airway protection should be considered. If a patient cannot adequately maintain oxygen saturation despite supplemental oxygen or cannot properly eliminate carbon dioxide, mechanical ventilation is required. Finally, patients whose status can be expected to deteriorate or who require prolonged procedures such as angiography should be considered for early intubation under controlled circumstances.[46]

Before sedation and intubation, the emergency physician should take a few moments to perform as complete a neurologic examination as is safe for the patient. Once sedation and intubation are achieved, a significant component of the diagnostic and prognostic data is compromised because baseline neurologic data can no longer be obtained. It is therefore critical to record baseline neurologic status before these interventions.

If a patient requires intubation, rapid sequence intubation should be performed (Table 48-4). This process begins with careful preparation of all necessary equipment and medication so as to provide as controlled an environment as possible. During intubation, careful consideration must be given to avoiding raising the intracranial pressure (ICP).

TABLE 48-4 RAPID SEQUENCE INTUBATION

Preparation
Preoxygenation
Pretreatment:
  Lidocaine 1.5 mg/kg IV
  Vecuronium 0.01 mg/kg IV
  Fentanyl 3 µg/kg (over 1 minute)
Paralysis with induction:
  Etomidate 0.3 mg/kg IV
  Succinylcholine 1.5 mg/kg IV
Placement—confirm tube placement
Postintubation management

Adapted from Walls R, editor: *Manual of emergency airway management*, Philadelphia, 2000, Lippincott Williams & Wilkins.

The patient should be thoroughly preoxygenated and then should receive a sedative-induction agent. Etomidate and thiopental are commonly used as induction agents for rapid sequence intubation. Etomidate, an ultra-short-acting nonbarbiturate hypnotic, is a superb induction agent; it is given in a dose of 0.3 mg/kg IV. Etomidate causes very little alteration in hemodynamics and therefore has gained considerable favor in the induction of critically ill patients. Thiopental is a short-acting barbiturate that has been used for many years as an induction agent. It should be used only in hypertensive patients, if at all, because of its propensity for reducing systolic blood pressure, an effect that may be detrimental to the patient with acute stroke.

Additional premedication should include IV lidocaine (1.5 mg/kg), which is given for its purported ability to blunt the hemodynamic response and possibly blunt the rise in ICP that is associated with laryngoscopy. Blunting the hemodynamic response is necessary because of the rich sensory innervation of the supraglottic larynx. The use of the laryngoscope results in significant sympathetic activity and a marked catecholamine discharge. If autoregulation is impaired, the hemodynamic response may result in an increase in ICP. Ideally, the lidocaine should be given at least 3 minutes before intubation. In addition, opiates can be used to decrease the sympathetic response. Fentanyl, given in a dose of 3 µg/kg, can be used as an adjunct to block the potential hemodynamic response and the potential rise in ICP due to laryngoscopy.[47]

A defasciculating dose of a nondepolarizing neuromuscular blocking agent should also be part of the premedication before laryngoscopy; an example is vecuronium, 0.01 mg/kg IV. Such an agent is given to blunt the rise in ICP that can occur in relation to the fasciculations that result from the use of a depolarizing neuromuscular blocking agent. Ideally, this dose is given 3 minutes before the use of a depolarizing neuromuscular blocking agent. Neuromuscular blockade should be achieved with a short-acting agent, such as succinylcholine, in a dose of 1.5 to 2 mg/kg IV. Prolonged paralysis is undesirable because of the loss of clinical signs and symptoms. Sedation must be maintained after intubation, however, to avoid agitation and elevation of ICP.

The ED team must be constantly aware that any patient with an altered level of consciousness may have suffered trauma. A careful examination for evidence of injury is required. Cervical spine immobilization is required for all traumatized patients with altered level of consciousness.

Breathing

Once the airway has been addressed, the patient's respiratory status must be assessed. Patients may also have significant comorbidity, such as congestive heart failure, chronic obstructive pulmonary disease, or cancer. Oxygen delivery and oxygenation should be optimized. Patients commonly receive supplemental oxygen therapy, although there is no literature currently supporting the routine use of supplemental oxygen in patients with stroke but without hypoxia.[25,48] Because up to a third of patients with stroke experience pneumonia within 1 month of the stroke, aspiration pneumonia prevention must begin in the ED. Elevation of the head to 30 degrees, careful pulmonary toilet, and strict avoidance of any oral intake until a formal swallowing evaluation has been performed are imperative.

Circulation

Once a patient has been determined to be capable of protecting the airway or the airway has been secured and adequate ventilation and oxygenation have been established, attention is turned to the cardiovascular status. This assessment should address hypertension, hypotension, and electrocardiographic (ECG) abnormalities.

Hypertension

Hypertension is extremely common in patients with acute stroke and should be treated cautiously, if at all.[25,49,50] The management of hypertension depends on the cause of the stroke.[51] Hypertension in patients with presumed aneurysmal subarachnoid hemorrhage (SAH) or other vascular anomalies, in which the hypertension may actually be detrimental, should be treated more aggressively. Patients with acute ischemic stroke, unless dramatically hypertensive, should be treated conservatively. If it is deemed critical to alter a patient's blood pressure, the following principles should guide the choice of agents and approach to the ED management of hypertension. First, short-acting, titratable agents should be used; examples are labetalol, nicardipine, and esmolol. Second, physicians should start with very low doses and titrate the dosage according to desired parameters. Third, physicians should avoid agents that may be harmful; diuretics should be avoided except in the setting of acute and compromising heart failure. Oral medications and unpredictable medications, such as sublingual nifedipine, should be avoided. Also, using more than one medication with different mechanisms of action in the acute setting may be particularly dangerous. The combination of two antihypertensive agents may have a summary effect significantly greater than the presumed individual effects of the two medications at their standard dosing. Finally, the goal should be a relatively slow and modest reduction in blood pressure to avoid a significant diminution in perfusion. For this reason, sodium nitroprusside should be avoided.[51]

The lack of prospective controlled trials to support a specific target range for the safe treatment of blood pressure in acute stroke leaves the physician wanting.[25] Commonly used guidelines advocate using titratable short-acting vasoactive medications when systolic pressure exceeds 220 mm Hg or diastolic blood pressure exceeds 120 mm/mc (the so-called hypertensive emergency). Systolic blood pressure lower than 220, or diastolic blood pressure lower than 120, can be treated with either careful observation or medications such as intravenous labetalol with careful dosage titration. The AHA guidelines recommend that the blood pressure not exceed 185 mm Hg systolic or 110 mm/mc diastolic at the time of initiation of IV thrombolytics.[25] The use of aggressive agents such as nitroprusside to lower the blood pressure into the "treatable range" is not advisable. Simple bedside maneuvers such as elevation of the head of the bed may help control hypertension by improving cerebral venous drainage.[25,51]

Hypotension

Hypotension can decrease cerebral perfusion pressure and subsequently lead to a significant extension of an area of cerebral infarction. During an acute stroke, perfusion of ischemic areas is directly related to the mean arterial pressure. Hypotension should be evaluated and aggressively treated. As an initial intervention, putting the patient's head down flat can increase blood pressure and cerebral perfusion and can sometimes result in clinical improvement. In addition, hypotension can be treated with IV fluids, inotropic agents, or vasopressors as necessary to maintain perfusion and prevent extension of an infarct. Physicians must search for a cause for a patient's relative hypotension. The emergency physician must be constantly vigilant for other diseases, such as AMI, gastrointestinal bleeding, occult trauma, aortic dissection, and sepsis.

Electrocardiographic Abnormalities

An evaluation of the patient's cardiac rhythm and an ECG are imperative. Cardiac rhythm can be significantly affected by acute stroke or may be the underlying cause of a patient's acute stroke. Cardiac rhythm disturbances such as atrial fibrillation are a significant risk factor for ischemic stroke. Similarly, acute or subacute myocardial infarction can precipitate either cardiovascular compromise leading to cerebral hypoperfusion or thrombus presenting as cerebrovascular embolism. Finally, acute dissection of the thoracic aorta may involve the carotid and/or vertebral arteries. Patients who have hemodynamic compromise or chest pain at the time of presentation with acute stroke should be evaluated for potential AMI or thoracic aortic dissection. In addition, patients who are mute or who have significant difficulty communicating should be even more aggressively screened for these possibilities. A baseline ECG and a chest radiograph should be considered. Conversely, cardiac rhythm and function can be affected by acute stroke. Hemispheric ischemic strokes that involve the insula and both SAH and intracerebral hemorrhage (ICH) can affect cardiac rhythm. ECG changes such as T-wave inversion occur in 50% to 75% of patients with acute stroke.[52]

Other Issues

Issues that must be addressed in the ED in addition to stabilization of the airway, breathing, and circulation include hyperglycemia, hyperpyrexia, seizures, and emesis.

Hyperglycemia

Patients with hyperglycemia at the time of the acute stroke have worse outcomes.[27] In the NINDS rt-PA Stroke Trial, a higher admission blood glucose level was associated with lower odds of desirable clinical outcome and a greater likelihood of a symptomatic ICH, regardless of recombinant tissue plasminogen activator (rt-PA) treatment.[26] Elevated glucose levels in patients with stroke may be partly due to a stress response. An alternative, speculative hypothesis is that elevated glucose levels may worsen brain injury, in part through the anaerobic metabolism of glucose in ischemic tissues with production of lactic acid. If this hypothesis is true, residual blood flow to the ischemic area would appear to be necessary for glucose-mediated injury. Glucose levels are not related to outcomes after lacunar infarcts.[28] For this reason, IV fluids should not include glucose, and patients with hyperglycemia should be treated with insulin to achieve euglycemia. The Glucose Insulin in Stroke Trial (GIST-UK) randomly assigned ischemic and hemorrhagic stroke patients seen within 24 hours of symptom onset who had elevated blood glucose levels at admission to aggressive glucose control versus standard therapy. Unfortunately, the trial was stopped because of slow enrollment, and fewer than half of the 2355 patients it would have taken to detect a 6% mortality difference were ultimately enrolled.[53] In the recently published Glucose Regulation in Acute Stroke Patients (GRASP) pilot trial, 72 ischemic stroke patients were randomized to tight glucose control (goal, 70 to 110 mg/dL), loose control (goal, 70 to 200 mg/dL), or control usual care (goal, 70 to 300 mg/dL). The feasibility and safety of two insulin infusion protocol targets were assessed.[54] The insulin infusion protocol was found to be safe and feasible. However, the study was not powered to detect a functional outcome benefit, and a phase 3 trial is in the planning stages.[54] Thus, while hyperglycemia should be avoided, it remains unclear whether aggressive early glucose reduction would be beneficial in the setting of acute stroke.

Hyperpyrexia

Temperature control is also important. Elevations in brain temperature have been shown to worsen cerebral ischemia and are associated with increases in stroke severity, infarct size, and mortality rates, as well as worse outcomes.[55,56] In a study of 390 patients with acute ischemic stroke, each temperature increase of 1°C raised the risk of poor outcome by a factor of 2.2.[57] Elevations in temperature have the greatest effect in the first 24 hours after stroke. Hyperthermia is easy to underestimate because brain temperature is higher than core body temperature and varies within regions of the brain.[58] Trials of hypothermia in patients who have experienced cardiac arrest have had encouraging results[59,60]; results of studies of the use of induced hypothermia in acute ischemic stroke have also been encouraging but are not definitive.[61] At this time, fever of any degree, even mild hyperthermia, should be treated with antipyretics (acetaminophen), and its cause should be investigated.

Seizures

Seizures can be a serious complication of acute stroke. They occur in approximately 5% of patients with acute ischemic stroke and may be related to involvement of the cerebral cortex or to very large strokes. The incidence of seizures in patients with ICH is approximately 25%. Seizures occur most commonly in patients with lobar hemorrhages or hemorrhages that extend into the cortex.[62] Seizures or seizure-like episodes occur in approximately 25% of patients with acute SAH.

Acute seizures are managed with benzodiazepines; if unsuccessful, these agents should be followed with barbiturates. Patients with acute stroke and seizure should receive a loading dose of fosphenytoin or phenytoin as soon as possible after the initiation of seizure activity. The principal advantage of fosphenytoin is that, unlike phenytoin, it can be dissolved in water. Fosphenytoin does not cause tissue necrosis if the patient has extravasation from an IV site, and it can be given intramuscularly. Both phenytoin and fosphenytoin can cause hypotension. The only significant detraction from the use of fosphenytoin is that it is significantly more expensive than phenytoin. Divalproex sodium (Depakote), a commonly used anticonvulsant, should be avoided in the setting of ICH because this agent has an antiplatelet effect, which may be deleterious in hemorrhagic stroke. In the setting of acute ischemic stroke, phenytoin should be administered after a seizure, but no evidence exists to support its prophylactic use.[25] Continuous electroencephalographic monitoring should be considered in comatose patients or in those with a poor neurologic examination unexplained by the primary stroke, as nonconvulsive seizures may be responsible for poor responsiveness. A careful examination by the emergency physician should be undertaken to ensure that poor responsiveness is not due to neurologic posturing that may indicate worsening of a mass lesion or progression of mass effect.

Emesis

Emesis is relatively common in acute hemorrhagic stroke and, because it may increase ICP, may be deleterious. Thus, throughout the ED phase of the patient's care, emesis should be avoided or controlled. Phenothiazine antiemetics such as promethazine (Phenergan) are usually adequate but do carry the theoretical burden of decreasing a patient's seizure threshold and causing sedation. The newer antiemetic agents known as the 5-hydroxytryptamine receptor antagonists (also known as the serotonin antagonists) are superior inhibitors of nausea and vomiting; they neither decrease the seizure threshold nor cause sedation. The prototype agent in this class is ondansetron. The use of serotonin antagonists should be considered early in acute stroke if emesis occurs and is especially important for hemorrhagic stroke.

Diagnostic Studies

Basic diagnostic studies should be included in the initial evaluation of patients with acute stroke. The AHA recommends an ECG, chest radiograph, complete blood count, platelet count, and measurements of partial thromboplastin time, prothrombin time, serum electrolyte levels, and serum glucose level.[25] Other laboratory studies (such as cardiac enzymes) should be ordered as indicated.

Divergence of Pathways Based on Ischemic Versus Hemorrhagic Stroke

Once the initial stabilization and evaluation of a patient with stroke have been accomplished, laboratory and imaging data will lead to a divergence of potential pathways for treatment. First, the clinician is charged with ruling out stroke mimics while proceeding on the course toward rapid institution of stroke management. Second, although there is significant overlap in presentation, the management of acute ischemic stroke differs considerably from that of acute ICH and SAH.

Stroke Mimics

A number of stroke mimics may be encountered in an ED. The most common are hypoglycemia, seizure with postictal paralysis, migraine headaches, a lesion in the brain, systemic infection, trauma, positional vertigo, and metabolic derangements.[63] Because rapid stroke evaluation is labor intensive and costly and because the definitive therapies may carry significant risk, stroke mimics must be ruled out as early as possible in the ED.

Ischemic Stroke

Management

Currently, the optimal therapy for an appropriately selected patient with acute ischemic stroke is the initiation of thrombolysis. The ED's role in the treatment of ischemic stroke with thrombolytics is highly system dependent. The patient with undifferentiated stroke must be kept on the "fast track" toward therapy until either (1) the patient is deemed an appropriate candidate and therapy is offered or (2) the patient is clearly excluded from thrombolytic intervention because of well-defined exclusion criteria.

A number of procedures can ensure that appropriate candidates are considered for therapy in the ED. First, the consistent and reinforced use of the NIHSS confirms and quantifies the extent of the stroke, facilitates discussions about risks and benefits, improves communication among colleagues, and allows for accurate reassessment of progress. Second, a stroke team whose role and availability are clearly defined has been shown to be one of the essential elements in optimizing rapid stroke treatment. Ideally, ED faculty would be members of this team.[37] Third, an agreed-on clinical pathway should be developed and implemented by the institution along with emergency physicians and nurses, the stroke team, laboratory services, radiology services, and hospital administration; this pathway should be initiated in the ED.

The ED team can also provide a significant service to the patient with acute stroke by considering the possibility of and ruling out concomitant cardiovascular diseases such as AMI and dissection of a thoracic aortic aneurysm. Both of these entities can precipitate an acute ischemic stroke, and both involve medical–surgical management issues that must be addressed. Diagnostic modalities, such as a CT scan of the chest with an IV contrast agent, may be required if a thoracic aortic dissection is suspected on either clinical or radiologic grounds.

Each hospital should develop a treatment plan for patients with acute stroke that reflects its abilities and limitations.[37] Hospitals without brain imaging facilities should never treat patients with a thrombolytic agent. Hospitals with easy access to brain imaging facilities, radiologic expertise, and an experienced physician should be able to treat appropriately identified patients with IV alteplase. However, in a hospital without an active intensive care unit or neurosurgical expertise, it is probably best that patients treated with alteplase be transferred immediately after treatment has begun to a hospital with these capabilities.

Telemedicine will likely play an increasingly important role in the treatment of patients with stroke in rural hospitals. In a recent prospective, randomized study, stroke experts at a hub site evaluated patients seen at four spoke sites either by telephone or by telemedicine. One hundred and eleven patients were randomly assigned to telemedicine, and 111 were randomly assigned to telephone. The primary outcome was whether the decision to give thrombolytics was correct, as determined by expert adjudication. Thrombolytic therapy was given in 28% of the telemedicine group and in 23% of the telephone group ($P = 0.43$). Treatment decisions were more likely to be correct in the telemedicine group compared with the telephone group (OR, 10.9; 95% CI, 2.7 to 44.6; $P = 0.0009$), and the hub consultant made correct decisions more frequently with telemedicine than with the telephone (OR, 7.2; 95 CI, 2.1 to 24.6; $P = 0.0009$).[64] This study provides the strongest evidence to date of the feasibility of appropriate thrombolytic therapy through the use of telemedicine and is thus very encouraging. Limitations included not determining whether telemedicine, in fact, increased the use of thrombolytics for stroke at the remote sites and a longer duration of time from call to decision to treat in the telemedicine arm. Future studies will likely focus on whether telemedicine increases the use of thrombolytics for stroke in remote locations and whether outcomes are improved for patients initially seen at centers without on-site stroke experts.

Prevention of Complications

The ED team may initiate critical preventive measures in the care of patients with acute stroke. Ideally, the measures would be initiated via the predefined stroke treatment pathway. They include not giving the patient anything by mouth, initiating a consultation for a formal swallowing study, and beginning prophylaxis against deep venous thrombosis in patients not receiving thrombolytics. Because urosepsis is a significant risk, use of Foley catheters should be avoided whenever possible.[65] Finally, it cannot be overemphasized that the initiation of a stroke treatment pathway in the ED will help ensure complete and consistent care throughout a patient's hospitalization.

Special Consideration: Transient Ischemic Attacks

TIAs have been previously defined as "temporary focal brain or retinal deficits caused by vascular disease that clear completely in less than 24 hours."[66] Neurovascular experts have now defined the TIA as "a brief episode of

neurologic dysfunction caused by focal brain ischemia, with clinical symptoms typically lasting less than 1 hour and without evidence of accompanying infarction on brain imaging."[67] This newer definition should help clinicians avoid labeling mild strokes as TIAs.

TIAs are common and represent a significant warning of ischemic stroke.[68] On the basis of estimates of stroke incidence, approximately 300,000 TIAs occur each year in the United States.[69,70] In one study, one in 15 individuals older than 65 years reported a history of TIA.[71] Labeled by some clinicians as "unstable angina of the brain," this disease and its significance are becoming increasingly well understood.

Identification of TIAs in the ED is a complex and difficult task. TIAs often manifest as vague complaints that can be difficult to discern, especially in the patient without a classic medical history for the disease. Another problem is the fact that, in the majority of cases of true TIA, the symptoms have abated by the time the patient is evaluated by an emergency physician. In addition, the differential diagnosis of TIAs is extensive; it includes syncope, seizure and/or Todd's paralysis, hypoglycemia, complicated migraines, multiple sclerosis, neuromuscular disorders, SAH, Bell's palsy, neoplasm, hemorrhagic stroke, functional disorders, and vertigo. These factors combine to make the identification of TIAs difficult. It is important for the ED physician to realize that a TIA is the final common pathway of a number of disease processes and is not necessarily an entity unto itself. For that reason, the history and physical examination are of paramount importance in the diagnosis of the source of the TIA. Careful questioning of paramedics, family, friends, and other possible witnesses is usually required.

The role of the ED in the care of the patient with a suspected TIA has three primary components. The first is identification of the possibility of TIA and initiation of a rapid and aggressive evaluation to look for causes, which is a process aimed at reducing stroke risk. The second is prevention of ischemic stroke via the institution of antiplatelet or antithrombotic agents. Third is the disposition of the patient, with a strong emphasis on admission to the hospital so that monitoring and completion of the evaluation can be facilitated. Nonrandomized studies suggest that urgent preventive intervention may reduce subsequent stroke risk in patients with TIAs.[72,73]

Hemorrhagic Stroke

Intracerebral Hemorrhage

ED management for patients with ICH consists of standard resuscitative techniques such as airway management and hemodynamic monitoring for stability. Blood pressure control is a primary directive of the emergency physician for patients with dramatic hypertension in the setting of ICH. This therapy should be thought of as an attempt to reduce the pressure driving the continuation of intracerebral bleeding.[51]

The exact parameters for blood pressure control remain widely controversial: some researchers advocate significant blood pressure drops, while other, more conservative practitioners advocate mean arterial pressure drops of 20%. The most promising study of blood pressure management in ICH to date was the Intensive Blood Pressure Reduction in Acute Cerebral Hemorrhage (INTERACT) pilot study.[74] Four hundred and four patients with spontaneous ICH who presented within 6 hours of symptom onset and were hypertensive on arrival (systolic blood pressure, 150 to 200 mm Hg) were randomly assigned to early intensive blood pressure lowering (target systolic blood pressure, 140 mm Hg; n = 203) or standard guideline-based blood pressure management (target systolic blood pressure, 180 mm Hg; n = 201). The primary efficacy end point was proportional change in hematoma volume at 24 hours. From randomization to 1 hour, mean systolic blood pressure was 153 mm Hg in the intensive group and 167 mm Hg in the guideline group (difference, 13.3 mm Hg; 95% CI, 8.9 to 17.6 mm Hg; $P < 0.0001$); from 1 to 24 hours, systolic blood pressure was 146 mm Hg in the intensive group and 157 mm Hg in the guideline group (10.8 mm Hg; 95% CI, 7.7 to 13.9 mm Hg; $P < 0.0001$). Mean proportional hematoma growth was 36.3% in the guideline group and 13.7% in the intensive group (difference, 22.6%; 95% CI, 0.6 to 44.5%; $P = 0.04$) at 24 hours. The authors concluded that early intensive blood pressure reduction is clinically feasible, well-tolerated, and seems to reduce hematoma growth in ICH.[74] Further studies are warranted to confirm these findings. The most recent AHA guidelines recommend consideration of aggressive blood pressure reduction if systolic blood pressure is more than 200 or mean arterial pressure is more than 150; a target blood pressure of 160/90 is suggested if systolic blood pressure is greater than 180 or mean arterial pressure is greater than 130 but increased ICP is not suspected.[75]

Because nitroprusside, verapamil, and hydralazine are all cerebral vasodilators, these agents may be suboptimal and should be avoided in the setting of presumed increased intracerebral pressure associated with intracerebral hematomas. Additional choices for blood pressure control in the setting of ICH are labetalol, nicardipine, and esmolol.[51] Management of elevated ICP may be initiated in the ED. In the setting of an acute herniation syndrome, hyperventilation can be instituted. This measure immediately lowers cerebral blood flow and thereby decreases ICP. Hyperventilation should not be instituted for patients other than those with impending herniation syndrome, however, because of a theoretical concern that the perihematoma regions will suffer significant ischemia due to the decrease in intracerebral blood flow. Hypertonic saline and mannitol can also be used but should be reserved for the patient with herniation syndrome or with a hematoma so large that herniation can be expected.

The ED team must remain vigilant for rapid changes in the neurologic status of patients with ICH. For many years, it was believed that ICH occurred over a brief time and that growth in hemorrhage volume was arrested very shortly after ictus. Brott et al,[76] however, found that substantial growth in the volume of hematomas occurred in 26% of patients within the first hour after baseline CT. In addition, growth occurred in 12% of patients between 1 hour and 20 hours after baseline CT. Thus, 38% of patients had substantial growth (greater than one third of the volume) in the first 20 hours after baseline CT scanning. These results reveal a significant potential for a decline in a patient's neurologic status while the patient remains in the ED, and the treatment team must maintain a constant watch to be able to respond appropriately to such a change. Patients who are seen early, those with prior antiplatelet use, and those with large baseline ICHs or any intraventricular hemorrhage on the initial CT are particularly susceptible to hematoma expansion.[77] Unfortunately, no proven treatments exist for hematoma expansion. The most promising study to date was the Recombinant Activated Factor VII (rFVIIa) for Acute Intracerebral Hemorrhage trial.[78] In this randomized controlled trial, Mayer et al randomly assigned 399 ICH patients to treatment with rFVIIa or placebo within 4 hours of symptom onset. Treatment with rFVIIa demonstrated an absolute reduction in death and severe disability of 15% compared with results achieved with placebo. Corresponding to this clinical benefit, there was a significant decrease in hemorrhage expansion with rFVIIa compared with results achieved with placebo, as demonstrated on CT scanning. Also, compared with placebo, a small increase in frequency of thromboembolic adverse events ($P = 0.12$) was observed. Unfortunately, in the subsequent phase III Efficacy and Safety of Recombinant Activated Factor VII for Acute Intracerebral Hemorrhage (FAST) trial,[79] no mortality or functional outcome difference was observed between the 841 patients randomly assigned to placebo or rFVIIa, despite successful reduction of hematoma growth. Before publication of the FAST trial results, the AHA guidelines issued a class IIb recommendation for use of rFVIIa but suggested its use be limited to clinical trial settings only.[75]

A potential role of the ED physician in consultation with neurologists and neurosurgeons is to provide prognostic information to families. The prognosis of ICH is quite poor, in that the mortality rate can be up to 50% within 30 days; half of the deaths occur in the first 48 hours.[80] Clinical indicators that can be used to aid in determining the prognosis of patients with ICH include the volume of hemorrhage, the level of consciousness on arrival at the ED, and the presence or absence of intraventricular extension.[81,82]

Volume of ICH has been estimated by Lisk et al[82] and Kothari et al.[83] The formula for an ellipsoid is as follows:

$$1/3 \times \pi \times (ABC)/2$$

where A, B, and C are the three dimensions of an ellipsoid that approximates the ICH.

This formula can be simplified by acknowledging that π is approximately 3 and then reducing the formula to $ABC/2$. For the bedside $ABC/2$ method, the CT slice with the largest area of hemorrhage is identified. The largest diameter (A) of the hemorrhage on this slice is measured. The largest diameter 90 degrees to A on the same slice is measured next (B). Finally, the number of slices on which any amount of hemorrhage is seen multiplied by the slice thickness is calculated as the third dimension (C). Multiplying A, B, and C together and dividing by 2 will give the approximate volume of the ICH. This method has been shown to be extremely accurate compared with computer modeling of the ICH volume.[83]

Although these prediction rules are reasonably reliable in terms of predicting ICH mortality, questions have been raised about the potential for overly aggressive early withdrawal of care. In fact, withdrawal of care was found to be the most common cause of death in a series of 1421 ICH patients.[84] Thus, the current AHA guidelines recommend aggressive therapy for the majority of ICH patients for a period of 24 hours to avoid the self-fulfilling prophesy of declaring a patient has a poor prognosis, then committing the patient to that prognosis through early care withdrawal.[75]

Special Consideration: Anticoagulant-Associated Intracerebral Hemorrhage

In ICH patients with coagulopathy due to concomitant medical conditions or medications, specific therapies are available depending on the primary process. Recent estimates suggest that one in every five cases of ICH occur in patients receiving warfarin.[85,86] In these patients, current options for correcting the coagulopathy include administration of vitamin K, fresh frozen plasma (FFP), prothrombin complex concentrates (PCC), and rFVIIa. Vitamin K should be administered because it addresses the effects of warfarin, but its onset of activity is far beyond the early time window when it would have an impact on limiting hematoma expansion. Some concerns are frequently raised about anaphylactic reactions after IV administration of vitamin K. The emergency physician and others caring for patients with life-threatening bleeding receiving anticoagulation should be aware that a retrospective analysis of the experience at the Mayo Clinic over 5 years found the incidence of anaphylactoid reaction from IV vitamin K to be three in 10,000 administrations, similar to that for *all* penicillins.[87] Thus, vitamin K may be as safely administered as other medications that are routinely used in medical practice. A slow infusion over an hour may be preferred to a bolus infusion. Patients with elevated international normalized ratio (INR, >1.3) due to warfarin should also be treated promptly with FFP. Time to initiation of FFP infusion has been found to be highly predictive of normalization of INR at 24 hours in warfarin-associated hemorrhages.[88] ICH patients receiving anticoagulation have a higher mortality rate than patients not receiving anticoagulation, and higher INR levels in patients receiving anticoagulation have been associated with worse outcomes.[89] Given the life-threatening impact of anticoagulant-associated ICH, 10 to 12 mL/kg of FFP should be rapidly administered to correct the coagulopathy.

Hospitals without the ability to care for patients with warfarin-associated ICH should administer both vitamin K and FFP before the transfer of patients to tertiary care centers, if possible. Delaying this critical intervention may allow for further hematoma expansion and the associated worse outcomes. PCCs require much smaller volume infusions than FFP and are thought to act more rapidly in reversing anticoagulation from warfarin than FFP and, as such, may result in less hematoma expansion in the setting of ICH.[90-92] However, these products also have an increased risk of thromboembolic events ranging from superficial thrombophlebitis to deep venous thromboses, pulmonary emboli, or disseminated intravascular coagulation.[91,92] Thus, larger clinical trials are required before PCCs may be recommended for routine use in warfarin-associated ICH.

The use of rFVIIa for warfarin-associated ICH has been suggested. In a study of seven patients with warfarin-associated ICH, 15 to 90 µg/kg of rFVIIa was given in addition to standard therapy (FFP and vitamin K).[93] Rapid normalization of INR occurred, but rebound increased INR developed, and full doses of FFP and vitamin K were still required. The rebound phenomenon presumably occurred as a result of the short half-life of rFVIIa (2.6 hours). Another study compared 13 patients with warfarin-associated ICH treated with rFVIIa plus vitamin K and FFP to 15 patients treated with vitamin K and FFP alone.[94] A fourfold faster decrease in INR was found in the rFVIIa treated group compared with the standard therapy group. Although rFVIIa may be a potential therapy for warfarin-associated ICH, larger prospective studies are needed.

Patients who develop an ICH while receiving heparin therapy should be treated promptly with protamine sulfate to reverse the effects of heparinization. For every 100 units of continuous heparin infusion per hour, 1 mg of protamine may be given. The same dose may be administered to patients who received a bolus of heparin. Patients receiving antiplatelet therapies may be more difficult to treat because of the long half-life of some agents. In addition to platelet administration, desmopressin (DDAVP) may be given to improve platelet function and aggregation in the setting of these agents. Patients with underlying coagulopathies due to comorbidities such as liver disease, essential thrombocytopenia, hemophilia, and von Willebrand's disease should be treated with the appropriate replacement product, which addresses the underlying condition. Failure to initiate these therapies specifically aimed at limiting hematoma expansion may expose patients to further bleeding and clinical deterioration.

Subarachnoid Hemorrhage

The most critical issue in the ED management of acute SAH is making the diagnosis. The diagnosis is not difficult in the setting of catastrophic SAH; nevertheless, hidden within the myriad patients with headaches who are seen at an ED are those few individuals with SAH whose symptoms are limited to a headache. Such patients have the best prognosis if the diagnosis is made but also the greatest likelihood that the diagnosis will be missed.

Patients with acute cephalgia account for approximately 1.2% of the more than 100 million ED encounters per year in the United States.[95] On the basis of this statistic, more than 1 million patients per year seen at an ED are evaluated for acute headaches. Buried within that group are approximately 30,000 patients with aneurysmal SAH, of whom only 48% are seen with symptoms that would lead to their assignment to Hunt and Hess category 1 or 2.[96] Thus, patients with aneurysmal SAH who are assigned to Hunt and Hess category 1 or 2 at presentation represent approximately 1% of ED headache evaluations. It is exactly those patients in whom great vigilance is required to maximize their potential for a favorable outcome.

In the ED, the diagnosis is based on clinical suspicion followed by a non–contrast-enhanced head CT scanning; if CT does not yield a diagnosis, lumbar puncture is performed. There has been a debate in the emergency medicine literature regarding the need to perform lumbar puncture in all patients to rule out SAH if findings on head CT scanning performed with a third- or fourth-generation scanner are negative for SAH.[97-99] It is likely that the latest generation CT scanners are extremely sensitive for detection of SAH (reportedly 93.1% to 97.5% sensitive for scans obtained within 24 hours of ictus); they are, unfortunately, not 100% sensitive.[100,101] Thus, the standard evaluation for patients with the sudden onset of a severe (often termed *thunderclap*) headache remains imaging, followed by lumbar puncture when imaging findings are normal.

Specific ED management of patients with nontraumatic SAH revolves around the basics of resuscitation and stabilization as well as management of the frequent complications of acute SAH. First, consultation with a neurosurgeon is required as soon as this diagnosis is made. Second, as with any potentially critically ill ED patient, the ED physician must begin with the ABCs of treatment. Patients with SAH frequently are seen with or progress to obtundation. Endotracheal intubation of obtunded patients protects them from aspiration caused by depressed airway protective reflexes and allows for hyperventilation, if required.

Management of hypertension in the acute phase of SAH remains somewhat controversial. Recommendations have advocated blood pressure control for patients with significantly elevated blood pressure. Some experts have recommended antihypertensive agents for a systolic blood pressure greater than 150 mm Hg.[102] Others have advocated keeping the mean arterial pressure (MAP) below 120 mm Hg; mean blood pressure is calculated from diastolic blood pressure (DBP) and systolic blood pressure (SBP) as follows[103]:

$$MAP = DBP + 1/3(SBP - DBP)$$

When medications are required for blood pressure control, the clinician should use only agents that can be titrated rapidly. Patients receiving vasoactive agents require invasive arterial line monitoring because labile blood pressure is common in acute SAH.[51]

Pulmonary Edema, Cardiac Events, Electrocardiography, Dysrhythmias

Left ventricular dysfunction occurs in an estimated 22% of SAH patients[104] and is predicted by elevations in cardiac troponin I and abnormal ECG findings. Although reversible, this left ventricular dysfunction predisposes a sizeable proportion of SAH patients to pulmonary edema, hypotension, and cardiac arrhythmias. The mechanisms responsible for these derangements in SAH are poorly understood, but it is postulated to be due to increased ICP resulting in a catecholamine surge. ED treatment measures should prevent further complications. The ED team should monitor cardiac activity, oximetry, automated blood pressure measurements, and end-tidal carbon dioxide and should avoid excessive or inadequate hyperventilation. The head of the patient's bed should be elevated to 30 degrees so that intracranial venous drainage can occur.

If the patient manifests evidence of herniation, a number of interventions should be started. The patient should receive osmotic agents, such as mannitol or hypertonic saline, and hyperventilation should be initiated or maintained.

Disposition from the Emergency Department

Patients with hemorrhagic stroke or large ischemic stroke and all patients receiving rt-PA for an acute ischemic stroke should be admitted to a dedicated neuroscience intensive care unit, if available, or the stroke care unit or general intensive care unit. Of note, special attention should be given to patients with posterior circulation strokes; they may benefit from a high level of monitoring. Patients with smaller ischemic strokes who are deemed unlikely to be at risk of clinically significant cerebral edema would ideally be assigned to a monitored bed in a dedicated stroke unit. Because dedicated stroke units do not exist in many facilities, predesignated monitored beds should be assigned to where the acute stroke care pathway is well understood. Hospitals without the required capabilities should have a prearranged transfer agreement with a facility that can meet these requirements. It is rare for a patient with stroke to be discharged from the ED to other than an inpatient bed.

One area of considerable importance to the ED team is disposition of the patient with a suspected TIA. The disposition of the patient with a neurologic emergency such as TIA should be no different from that of any other patient with critical status and is in many ways analogous to that of the patient with unstable angina. Nonetheless, patients with neurologic emergencies commonly are not admitted and do not receive the urgent evaluation that data suggest they need to prevent recurrence or evolution of their medical problems. The disposition of an ED patient with a suspected TIA requires great care. TIAs represent a significant warning of potentially impending stroke.

When considering disposition of such a patient, the emergency physician must keep in mind the short-term prognosis after a suspected TIA. In an early incidence study from Rochester, Minnesota, investigators found a 10% incidence of ischemic stroke in the 3 months after a TIA.[105] In a study of 1707 patients evaluated for TIA in EDs, 10.5% experienced a stroke within 90 days of diagnosis, 2.6% were hospitalized for cardiac events, and 1.4% died of causes other than stroke.[106] This risk of stroke was more than 50 times that expected in a cohort of similar age.[68,69] Half of the strokes occurred within 2 days of the TIAs.[106] A recent cross-sectional study of mostly community hospitals across 11 states in the United States found that 53% of patients with TIAs were admitted to the hospital.[107] Another study over a 10-year period found that 54% of patients with TIAs were admitted from the ED and the admission rate did not change over the 10 years. The strongest predictors of hospital admission were location in the northeast region of the United States and the performance of a head CT in the ED.[108]

Nonrandomized studies suggest that urgent preventive intervention may reduce subsequent stroke risk in patients with TIAs.[71,72] Thus, the emergency physician should initiate the evaluation of a TIA patient beyond a baseline CT, when possible. The physician should also initiate or advance the patient's antiplatelet therapy. Then, the patient's care can be turned over to a primary care provider or neurologist for continuation of the observation and completion of the necessary evaluation.

The basis for admission is the rapid evaluation of these TIA patients for the cause of disease. While recently published risk stratification scores such as the ABCD[2] score hold promise in terms of deriving a tool that may guide emergency physicians in identifying high-risk patients,[109] it should be noted that all patients seen in the ED in the derivation and validation cohorts were admitted to the hospital. Other patients were seen in outpatient settings. Thus, the ED TIA patient population likely represents a high-risk group that warrants more aggressive evaluation and intervention. One possible solution for these patients is an observation unit with clinical protocols for diagnostic testing (e.g., carotid duplex ultrasonography and echocardiography) and rapid disposition with risk factor modification and follow-up. These protocols have yet to be implemented on a national scale but do hold promise for the treatment of TIA and other diseases.

It is critical that the emergency physician consider the literature that highlights the significant potential morbidity that TIA heralds. It is becoming clear that initial therapeutic intervention, thorough evaluation, initial testing, and admission with subsequent testing must be undertaken to prevent devastating harm to this group of patients. Because half of TIA patients are discharged home from the ED, this change is truly a paradigm shift for many practitioners and consultants.[107,108]

Conclusion

The care of a patient with an acute stroke should exist as a continuum from access to prehospital care through definitive therapies. Prehospital care providers are critical players in the pursuit of optimal care for acute stroke. As the point of first medical contact for many stroke victims, they serve as the first opportunity for identification of stroke and for the initiation of the cascade of events that must occur to optimize a patient's chance for recovery. The prehospital arena has been shown to be a part of a patient's care in which the greatest delays between symptom onset and definitive therapy occur. It is within this arena that symptom recognition and a decision to act based on symptom recognition make the difference between potential eligibility for acute therapy and automatic exclusion based on time. The fact that "all care begins prehospital" for the patient with acute stroke must not be lost on researchers and treating physicians. Improvements in public education, prehospital care provider education, protocol development, triage and communication, and destination selection can mean the difference between the implementation of advanced therapies and a lost opportunity.

The ED is the next critical point in the care of a patient with stroke. In the ED, stabilization and a carefully coordinated evaluation, in concert with appropriate subspecialists, optimizes the patient's chance to receive the most appropriate definitive therapy in the shortest time. This process involves significant preplanning with the establishment of clear delineation of responsibilities and a well-designed stroke care pathway. Thus, a major focus in the initial management of acute ischemic stroke revolves around well-orchestrated coordination of patient care to ensure that physician evaluation and diagnostic testing are performed very quickly. During this "golden hour of stroke," however, there remain multiple patient care issues for the clinician.[110]

Such system building, with the emphasis on prehospital and ED teams, represents a new paradigm in acute stroke care and will serve to create opportunities for patients to receive optimal therapies in an efficient manner.

REFERENCES

1. Schwamm LH, Pancioli A, Acker JE 3rd, et al: Recommendations for the establishment of stroke systems of care: recommendations from the American Stroke Association's Task Force on the Development of Stroke Systems, *Circulation* 111:1078-1091, 2005.
2. Acker JE 3rd, Pancioli AM, Crocco TJ, et al: Implementation strategies for emergency medical services within stroke systems of care: a policy statement from the American Heart Association/American Stroke Association Expert Panel on Emergency Medical Services Systems and the Stroke Council, *Stroke* 38:3097-3115, 2007.
3. Quain DA, Parsons MW, Loudfoot AR, et al: Improving access to acute stroke therapies: A controlled trial of organised pre-hospital and emergency care, *Med J Aust* 189:429-433, 2008.
4. Kleindorfer DO, Broderick JP, Khoury J, et al: Emergency department arrival times after acute ischemic stroke during the 1990s, *Neurocrit Care* 7:31-35, 2007.
5. Moser DK, Kimble LP, Alberts MJ, et al: Reducing delay in seeking treatment by patients with acute coronary syndrome and stroke, *Circulation* 114:168-182, 2006.
6. Barsan W, Brott T, Broderick J, et al: Time of hospital presentation in patients with acute ischemic stroke, *Arch Intern Med* 153:2558-2561, 1993.
7. Adeoye O, Lindsell C, Broderick J, et al: Emergency medical services use by stroke patients: A population based study, *Am J Emerg Med* 27:141-145, 2009.
8. Anderson N, Broad J, Bonita R: Delays in hospital admission and investigation in acute stroke, *BMJ* 311:162, 1995.
9. Fogelholm R, Murros K, Rissanen A, et al: Factors delaying hospital admission after acute stroke, *Stroke* 27:398-400, 1996.
10. Rosamond DW, Gorton RA, Hinn AR, et al: Rapid response to stroke symptoms: The delay in accessing stroke healthcare (DASH) study, *Acad Emerg Med* 5:45-51, 1998.
11. Ferro J, Melo T, Oliveria V, et al: An analysis of the admission delay of acute strokes, *Cerebrovasc Dis* 4:71-75, 1994.
12. Jorgensen H, Nakauama H, Reith J, et al: Factors delaying hospital admission in acute stroke, *Neurology* 47:383-387, 1996.
13. Derex L, Adeleine P, Nighoghossian N: Factors influencing early admission in a French stroke unit, *Stroke* 33:153-159, 2002.
14. Wein TH, Staub L, Felberg R, et al: Activation of emergency medical services for acute stroke in a nonurban population: The T.L.L. Temple Foundation Stroke Project, *Stroke* 31:1925-1928, 2000.
15. Kothari R, Sauerbeck L, Jauch E, et al: Patients' awareness of stroke signs, symptoms, and risk factors, *Stroke* 28:1871-1875, 1997.
16. Pancioli A, Broderick J, Kothari R, et al: Public perception of stroke warning signs and potential risk factors, *JAMA* 279:1288-1292, 1998.
17. Schneider A, Pancioli A, Khoury J, et al: Trends in community knowledge of the warning signs and risk factors for stroke, *JAMA* 289:343-346, 2003.
18. Webster P, Radberg J, Lundgren B: Factors associated with delayed admission to hospital and in-hospital delays in acute stroke and TIA: A prospective, multicenter study, *Stroke* 30:40-48, 1999.
19. Roebers S, Wagner M, Ritter MA, et al: Attitudes and current practice of primary care physicians in acute stroke management, *Stroke* 38:1298-1303, 2007.
20. Schroeder EB, Rosamond WD, Morris DL, et al: Determinants of use of emergency medical services in a population with stroke symptoms: The Second Delay in Accessing Stroke Healthcare (DASH II) Study, *Stroke* 31:2591-2596, 2000.

21. Lacy C, Suh D-C, Bueno M, et al: Delay in presentation and evaluation for acute stroke. Stroke Time Registry for Outcomes Knowledge and Epidemiology (STROKE), *Stroke* 32:63–69, 2001.

22. Kothari R, Barsan WG, Brott T, et al: Frequency and accuracy of prehospital diagnosis of acute stroke, *Stroke* 26:937–941, 1995.

23. Porteous G, Corry M, Smith W: Emergency medical services dispatcher identification of stroke and transient ischemic attack, *Prehosp Emerg Care* 3:211–216, 1999.

24. Kothari R, Barsan WG, Brott T, et al: Frequency and accuracy of prehospital diagnosis of acute stroke. *Stroke* 26(6):937–941, 1995.

25. Adams H, del Zoppo G, Alberts MJ, et al: Guidelines for the early management of adults with acute ischemic stroke: A guideline from the American Heart Association/American Stroke Association, *Stroke* 38:1655–1711, 2007.

26. Bruno A, Levine SR, Frankel M, et al: Relation between admission glucose level and outcome in the NINDS rt-PA Stroke Trial, *Stroke* 59:669–674, 2002.

27. Wass C, Lanier W: Glucose modulation of ischemic brain injury: Review and clinical recommendations, *Mayo Clin Proc* 71:801–812, 1996.

28. Bruno A, Biller J, Adams HP Jr, et al: Acute blood glucose level and outcome from ischemic stroke, *Neurology* 52:280–284, 1999.

29. Zachariah B, Van Cott C, Dunford J: Dispatch life support and the acute stroke patient: Making the right call. In Marler J, Winters-Jones P, Emr M, editors: *Proceedings of a National Symposium on Rapid Identification and Treatment of Acute Stroke*, Bethesda, Md, 1997, The National Institute of Neurological Disorders and Stroke, pp 29–33.

30. Kidwell CS, Saver JL, Schubert GB, et al: Design and retrospective analysis of the Los Angeles Prehospital Stroke Screen (LAPSS), *Prehosp Emerg Care* 2:267–273, 1998.

31. Kidwell CS, Starkman S, Eckstein M, et al: Identifying stroke in the fields. Prospective validation of the Los Angeles Prehospital Stroke Screen (LAPSS), *Stroke* 31:71–76, 2000.

32. Kothari R, Hall K, Brott T, et al: Early stroke recognition: Developing an out-of-hospital NIH Stroke Scale, *Acad Emerg Med* 4:986–990, 1997.

33. Kothari R, Pancioli A, Liu T, et al: Cincinnati Prehospital Stroke Scale: Reproducibility and validity, *Ann Emerg Med* 33:373–378, 1999.

34. Abdullah AR, Smith EE, Biddinger PD, et al: Advance hospital notification by EMS in acute stroke is associated with shorter door-to-computed tomography time and increased likelihood of administration of tissue-plasminogen activator, *Prehosp Emerg Care* 12:426–431, 2008.

35. California acute stroke pilot registry (CASPR) investigators: Prioritizing interventions to improve rates of thrombolysis for ischemic stroke, *Neurology* 64:654–659, 2005.

36. Rossnagel K, Jungehulsing GJ, Nolte CH, et al: Out-of-hospital delays in patients with acute stroke, *Ann Emerg Med* 44:476–483, 2004.

37. Sahni R: Acute stroke: Implications for prehospital care. National Association of EMS Physicians Standards and Clinical Practice Committee, *Prehosp Emerg Care* 4:270–272, 2000.

38. Alberts MJ, Hademenos G, Latchaw RE, et al: Recommendations for the establishment of primary stroke centers, *JAMA* 283:3102–3109, 2000.

39. Bock B: Response system for patients presenting with acute ischemic stroke. In Marler J, Winters-Jones P, Emr M, editors: *Proceedings of a National Symposium on Rapid Identification and Treatment of Acute Stroke*, Bethesda, Md, 1997, The National Institute of Neurological Disorders and Stroke, pp 55–57.

40. Anonymous: Tissue plasminogen activator for acute ischemia stroke. The National Institute of Neurological Disorders and Stroke rt-PA Stroke Study Group, *N Engl J Med* 333:1581–1587, 1995.

41. National Registry of Myocardial Infarction II (NRMI II). Quarterly Data Report, 1996: *Ohio Data (September)*, San Francisco, 1996, Genentech.

42. Emergency department: Rapid identification and treatment of patients with acute myocardial infarction. National Heart Attack Alert Program Coordinating Committee, 60 Minutes To Treatment Working Group, *Ann Emerg Med* 23:311–329, 1994.

43. Bratina P, Greenberg L, Pasteur W, et al: Current emergency department management of stroke in Houston, TX, *Stroke* 26:409–414, 1995.

44. Baraff L, Lee TJ, Kader S, et al: Effect of a practice guideline on the process of emergency department care of falls in elder patients, *Acad Emerg Med* 6:1216–1223, 1999.

45. Bonnono C, Criddle LM, Lutsep H, et al: Emergi-paths and stroke teams: An emergency department approach to acute ischemic stroke, *J Neurosci Nurs* 32:298–305, 2000.

46. Walls R: The decision to intubate. In Walls R, editor: *Manual of Emergency Airway Management*, Philadelphia, 2000, Lippincott Williams & Wilkins, pp 3–7.

47. Walls R, Murphy M: Increased intracranial pressure. In Walls R, editor: *Manual of Emergency Airway Management*, Philadelphia, 2000, Lippincott Williams & Wilkins, pp 159–163.

48. Pancioli AM, Bullard MJ, Grulee ME, et al: Supplemental oxygen use in ischemic stroke patients: Does utilization correspond to need for oxygen therapy? *Arch Intern Med* 162:49–52, 2002.

49. Lisk D, Grotta JC, Lamki LM, et al: Should hypertension be treated after acute stroke? A randomized controlled trial using single photon emission computed tomography, *Arch Neurol* 50:855–862, 1993.

50. Powers W: Acute hypertension after stroke: The scientific basis for treatment decisions, *Neurology* 43:461–467, 1993.

51. Pancioli AM: Hypertension management in neurologic emergencies, *Ann Emerg Med* 51(3S):524–527, 2008.

52. Dimant J, Grob D: Electrocardiographic changes and myocardial damage in patients with acute cerebrovascular accidents, *Stroke* 8:448–455, 1977.

53. Gray CS, Hildreth AJ, Sandercock PA, et al: Glucose-potassium-insulin infusions in the management of post-stroke hyperglycaemia: The UK Glucose Insulin in Stroke Trial (GIST-UK), *Lancet Neurol* 6:397–406, 2007.

54. Johnston KC, Hall CE, Kissela BM, et al: GRASP Investigators. Glucose Regulation in Acute Stroke Patients (GRASP) trial: A randomized pilot trial. *Stroke* 40(12):3804–3809, 2009. Epub Oct 15 2009.

55. Azzimondi G, Bassein L, Nonino F, et al: Fever in acute stroke worsens prognosis. A prospective study, *Stroke* 26:2040–2043, 1995.

56. Hajat C, Hajat S, Sharma P: Effects of post-stroke pyrexia on stroke outcome: A meta-analysis of studies in patients, *Stroke* 31:410–414, 2000.

57. Reith J, Jorgensen H, Pedersen PM, et al: Body temperature in acute stroke: Relation to stroke severity, infarct size, mortality, and outcome, *Lancet* 347:422–425, 1996.

58. Schwab S, Spranger M, Aschoff A, et al: Brain temperature monitoring and modulation in patients with severe MCA infarction, *Neurology* 48:762–767, 1997.

59. Bernard S, Gray TW, Buist MD, et al: Treatment of comatose survivors of out-of-hospital cardiac arrest with induced hypothermia, *N Engl J Med* 346:557–563, 2002.

60. The Hypothermia After Cardiac Arrest Study Group: Mild therapeutic hypothermia to improve the neurologic outcome after cardiac arrest, *N Engl J Med* 346:549–556, 2002.

61. Schwab S, Georgiadis D, Berrouschot J, et al: Feasibility and safety of moderate hypothermia after massive hemispheric infarction, *Stroke* 32:2033–2035, 2001.

62. Vespa PM, O'Phelan K, Shah M, et al: Acute seizures after intracerebral hemorrhage: A factor in progressive midline shift and outcome, *Neurology* 60:1441–1446, 2003.

63. Libman R, Wirkowski E, Alvir J, et al: Conditions that mimic stroke in the emergency department: Implications for acute stroke trials, *Arch Neurol* 52:1119–1122, 1995.

64. Meyer BC, Raman R, Hemmen T, et al: Efficacy of site-independent telemedicine in the STRokE DOC trial: A randomised, blinded, prospective study, *Lancet Neurol* 7:787–795, 2008.

65. Roth EJ, Lovell L, Harvey RL, et al: Incidence of and risk factors for medical complications during stroke rehabilitation, *Stroke* 32:523–529, 2001.

66. The Study Group on TIA Criteria and Detection: XI. Transient focal cerebral ischemia: Epidemiologic and clinical aspects, *Stroke* 5:277–284, 1974.

67. Albers GW, Caplan LR, Easter JD, et al: Transient ischemic attack—proposal for a new definition, *N Engl J Med* 347:1713–1716, 2002.

68. Brown RJ, Petty GW, O'Fallon WM, et al: Incidence of transient ischemic attack in Rochester, Minnesota, 1985-1989, *Stroke* 29:2109–2113, 1998.

69. Broderick J, Brott T, Kothari R, et al: The Greater Cincinnati/Northern Kentucky Stroke Study: Preliminary first-ever total incidence rates of stroke among blacks, *Stroke* 29:415-421, 1998.

70. Williams G, Jiang JG, Matchar DB, et al: Incidence and occurrence of total (first-ever and recurrent) stroke, *Stroke* 30:2523-2528, 1999.

71. Rothwell PM, Giles MF, Chandratheva A, et al: Early use of Existing Preventive Strategies for Stroke (EXPRESS) study, *Lancet* 370:1432-1442, 2007.

72. Lavallee PC, Meseguer E, Abboud H, et al: A transient ischaemic attack clinic with round-the-clock access (SOS-TIA): Feasibility and effects, *Lancet Neurol* 6:953-960, 2007.

73. National Stroke Association: *TIA/Mini Strokes: Public Knowledge and Experience—Roper Starch Worldwide Survey. Roper Starch Worldwide*, Englewood, Colo, 2000, National Stroke Association, pp 55.

74. Anderson CS, Huang Y, Wang JG, et al: Intensive blood pressure reduction in acute cerebral hemorrhage trial (INTERACT): A randomised pilot trial, *Lancet Neurol* 7:391-399, 2008.

75. Broderick J, Connolly S, Feldmann E, et al: Guidelines for the management of spontaneous intracerebral hemorrhage in adults: 2007 update: A guideline from the American Heart Association/American Stroke Association Stroke Council, *Stroke* 38:2001-2023, 2007.

76. Brott T, Broderick J, Kothari R, et al: Early hemorrhage growth in patients with intracerebral hemorrhage, *Stroke* 28:1-5, 1997.

77. Broderick JP, Diringer MN, Hill MD, et al: Determinants of intracerebral hemorrhage growth: an exploratory analysis, *Stroke* 38:1072-1075, 2007.

78. Mayer SA, Brun NC, Begtrup K, et al: Recombinant activated factor VII for acute intracerebral hemorrhage, *N Engl J Med* 352:777-785, 2005.

79. Mayer SA, Brun NC, Begtrup K, et al: Efficacy and safety of recombinant activated factor VII for acute intracerebral hemorrhage, *N Engl J Med* 358:2127-2137, 2008.

80. Hemphill JC 3rd, Bonovich DC, Besmertis L, et al: The ICH score: a simple, reliable grading scale for intracerebral hemorrhage, *Stroke* 32:891-897, 2001.

81. Broderick J, Brott T, Duldner J, et al: Volume of intracerebral hemorrhage: A powerful and easy-to-use predictor of 30-day mortality, *Stroke* 24:987-993, 1993.

82. Lisk D, Pasteur W, Rhoades H, et al: Early presentation of hemispheric intracerebral hemorrhage: Prediction of outcome and guidelines for treatment allocation, *Neurology* 44:133-139, 1994.

83. Kothari R, Brott T, Broderick J, et al: The ABCs of measuring intracerebral hemorrhage volume, *Stroke* 27:1304-1305, 1996.

84. Zurasky JA, Aiyagari V, Zazulia AR, et al: Early mortality following spontaneous intracerebral hemorrhage, *Neurology* 64:725-727, 2005.

85. Hart RG, Tonarelli SB, Pearce LA: Avoiding central nervous system bleeding during antithrombotic therapy: Recent data and ideas, *Stroke* 36:1588-1593, 2005.

86. Flaherty ML, Kissela B, Woo D, et al: The increasing incidence of anticoagulant-associated intracerebral hemorrhage, *Neurology* 68:116-121, 2007.

87. Reigert-Johnson DL, Volcheck GW: The incidence of anaphylaxis following intravenous phytonadione (vitamin K_1): a 5-year retrospective review, *Ann Allergy Asthma Immunol* 89:400-406, 2002.

88. Goldstein JN, Thomas SH, Frontiero V, et al: Timing of fresh frozen plasma administration and rapid correction of coagulopathy in warfarin-related intracerebral hemorrhage, *Stroke* 37:151-155, 2006.

89. Rosand J, Eckman MH, Knudsen KA, et al: The effect of warfarin and intensity of anticoagulation on outcome after intracerebral hemorrhage, *Arch Intern Med* 164:880-884, 2004.

90. Huttner HB, Schellinger PD, Hartmann M, et al: Hematoma growth and outcome in treated neurocritical care patients with intracerebral hemorrhage related to oral anticoagulant therapy: Comparison of acute treatment strategies using vitamin K, fresh frozen plasma, and prothrombin complex concentrates, *Stroke* 37:1465-1470, 2006.

91. Makris M, Greaves M, Phillips WS, et al: Emergency oral anticoagulant reversal: The relative efficacy of infusions of fresh frozen plasma and clotting factor concentrate on correction of the coagulopathy, *Thromb Haemost* 77:477-480, 1997.

92. Lankiewicz MW, Hays J, Friedman KD, et al: Urgent reversal of warfarin with prothrombin complex concentrate, *J Thromb Haemost* 4:967-970, 2006.

93. Freeman WD, Brott TG, Barrett KM, et al: Recombinant factor VIIa for rapid reversal of warfarin anticoagulation in acute intracranial hemorrhage, *Mayo Clin Proc* 79:1495-1500, 2004.

94. Brody DL, Aiyagari V, Shackleford AM, Diringer MN: Use of recombinant factor VIIa in patients with warfarin-associated intracranial hemorrhage, *Neurocrit Care* 2:263-267, 2005.

95. Morgenstern L, Huber JC, Luna-Gonzales H, et al: Headache in the emergency department, *Headache* 41:537-541, 2001.

96. Whisnant JP, Sacco SE, O'Fallon WF, et al: Referral bias in aneurysmal subarachnoid hemorrhage, *J Neurosurg* 78:726-732, 1993.

97. Sidman R, Connolly E, Lemke T: Subarachnoid hemorrhage diagnosis: Lumbar puncture is still needed when the computed tomography scan is normal, *Acad Emerg Med* 3:827-831, 1996.

98. Edlow JA, Wyer PC: How good is a negative cranial computed tomographic scan result in excluding subarachnoid hemorrhage?, *Ann Emerg Med* 36:507-517, 2000.

99. Prosser RL Jr, Edlow JA, Wyer PC: Feedback: Computed tomography for subarachnoid hemorrhage, *Ann Emerg Med* 37:679-680, 2001.

100. Sames TA, Storrow AB, Finkelstein JA, et al: Sensitivity of new-generation computed tomography in subarachnoid hemorrhage, *Acad Emerg Med* 3:16-20, 1996.

101. Morgenstern LB, Luna-Gonzales H, Huber JC, et al: Worst headache and subarachnoid hemorrhage: Prospective, modern computed tomography and spinal fluid analysis, *Ann Emerg Med* 32:297-304, 1998.

102. Bernardini GL, DeShaies RM: Critical care of intracerebral and subarachnoid hemorrhage, *Curr Neurol Neurosci Rep* 1:568-576, 2001.

103. Biller J, Godersky JC, Adams HP Jr: Management of aneurysmal subarachnoid hemorrhage, *Stroke* 19:1300, 1988.

104. Naidech AM, Kreiter KT, Janjua N, et al: Cardiac troponin elevation, cardiovascular morbidity, and outcome after subarachnoid hemorrhage, *Circulation* 112:2851-2856, 2005.

105. Whisnant J, Matsumoto N, Elveback L: Transient cerebral ischemic attacks in a community—Rochester, Minnesota, 1955 through 1969, *Mayo Clin Proc* 48:194-198, 1973.

106. Johnston S, Gress DR, Browner WS, et al: Short-term prognosis after emergency-department diagnosis of transient ischemic attack, *JAMA* 284:2901-2906, 2000.

107. Coben JH, Owens PL, Steiner CA, Crocco TJ: Hospital and demographic influences on the disposition of transient ischemic attack, *Acad Emerg Med* 15:171-176, 2008.

108. Edlow JA, Kim S, Pelletier AJ, et al: National study on emergency department visits for transient ischemic attack, 1992-2001, *Acad Emerg Med* 13:666-672, 2006.

109. Johnston SC, Rothwell PM, Nguyen-Huynh MN, et al: Validation and refinement of scores to predict very early stroke risk after transient ischaemic attack, *Lancet* 369:283-292, 2007.

110. Thurman J, Jauch EC: Emergency department management of acute ischemic stroke, *Emerg Med Clin North Am* 20:609-630, 2002.

Intravenous Thrombolysis

WENDY BROWN, LAMA AL-KHOURY, GILDA TAFRESHI, PATRICK D. LYDEN

Thrombolysis offers the simplest and most direct treatment for thrombotic disorders, including ischemic strokes. Plasminogen activators produce clinical improvement in patients with coronary artery thrombosis, peripheral vascular disease, venous thrombosis, pulmonary embolism, and acute ischemic stroke. According to the pivotal National Institutes of Neurological Disorders and Stroke (NINDS) study, intravenous (IV) tissue plasminogen activator (t-PA) improved the clinical outcome of all types of ischemic stroke (i.e., large artery, embolic, and small vessel or lacunar strokes) if treatment began within 3 hours of the onset of symptoms.[1] Consequently, the U.S. Food and Drug Administration (FDA) approved recombinant t-PA (rt-PA) for the treatment of acute ischemic strokes within 3 hours of onset, excluding all patients with intracranial hemorrhage (ICH).

To date, other IV agents have proved useful, but none is yet approved by the FDA for treatment of ischemic stroke. In this chapter we review the historical background of thrombolytic therapy in preclinical and clinical trials, summarize the different agents in previous as well as current use, and discuss the management protocol for thrombolytic treatment in patients with stroke.

Thrombosis and Thrombolysis

Thrombosis involves the processes of endothelial injury, platelet adherence and aggregation, and thrombin generation. Thrombin plays a major role in clot formation; it is responsible for cleaving fibrinogen to fibrin, which forms the clot matrix. Thrombin also activates factor XIII, which accomplishes interfibrin cross-linking.[2] Figure 49-1 illustrates the coagulation cascade.[3] In a process involving platelet membrane receptors and phospholipids, thrombin is generated locally by the extrinsic and intrinsic pathways. Factors V and XIII interact with specific platelet membrane phospholipids to facilitate activation of factor X to factor Xa and the conversion of prothrombin to thrombin on the platelet surface. Platelet-bound thrombin-modified factor V (factor Va) serves as a high-affinity platelet receptor for factor Xa, which accelerates the rate of thrombin generation. The relative platelet–fibrin composition of a specific thrombus depends on regional blood flow or shear stress. At arterial flow rates, thrombi are predominantly platelet rich, whereas at lower venous flow rates, activation of coagulation predominates. The efficacy of thrombolysis perhaps depends on the relative fibrin content and fibrin cross-linking, the latter possibly determined by the age of the thrombus. Theoretically, therefore, plasminogen

activators may act less well on fibrin-poor clots, but such distinctions have not been observed clinically.

In addition to both endothelial cell-derived antithrombotic characteristics and circulating anticoagulants (activated protein C and protein S), thrombus growth is limited by the endogenous thrombolytic system, in which plasmin plays a central role. One effect of endogenous thrombolysis is continuous remodeling of the thrombus. This effect results from the preferential conversion of plasminogen to plasmin on the thrombus surface, where fibrin binds t-PA in proximity to its substrate plasminogen, accelerating plasmin formation. Plasminogen activation may also occur on cells that express plasminogen receptors and produce plasminogen activators, such as endothelial and polymorphonuclear cells. If sufficient quantities of plasminogen activators are produced or administered, plasminogen can be activated in plasma, where it cleaves circulating fibrinogen and fibrin to produce fibrin split products.

The naturally circulating plasminogen activators, t-PA and single chain urokinase-type PA (scu-PA), catalyze plasmin formation from plasminogen. In the circulation, plasmin rapidly binds to its inhibitor, α_2-antiplasmin, and is inactivated. Endogenous fibrinolysis is modulated by several inhibitors of plasmin and plasminogen activators. The half-life of plasmin in the circulation is estimated to be approximately 0.1 second. α_2-Antiplasmin is the primary inhibitor of fibrinolysis through plasmin inhibition by binding to excessive plasmin. Thrombospondin interferes with the t-PA–mediated, fibrin-associated activation of plasminogen. Contact activation inhibitors and C1 inhibitor have indirect effects on thrombolysis.

A competitive inhibitor of plasminogen is histidine-rich glycoprotein (HRG). In addition to inhibitors of plasmin, there are specific plasminogen activator inhibitors that decrease the activity of t-PA, scu-PA, and urokinase (UK) plasminogen activator (u-PA). Both plasma t-PA and u-PA are inhibited by plasminogen activator inhibitor-1 (PAI-1), which is derived from platelets and endothelial cells. The potential risk for thrombosis reflects the relative concentrations of circulating PAI-1 and the endogenous plasminogen activators t-PA and u-PA. In addition, other plasminogen activator inhibitors are derived from different tissues. Within the thrombus, however, plasmin is protected from this inhibitor and t-PA is also relatively protected from circulating plasma inhibitors. This is why plasmin and t-PA can achieve their fibrinolytic effect better within the clot than in serum and also why clot lysis can be achieved with a relatively low risk of bleeding

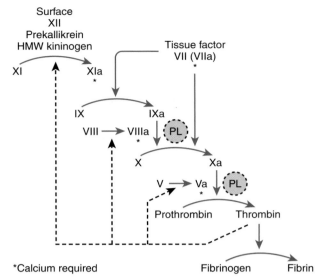

Surface
XII
Prekallikrein
HMW kininogen

Tissue factor
VII (VIIa)
*

Figure 49-1 Coagulation cascade. The different factors of the coagulation system are portrayed. The cascade culminates in the conversion of prothrombin to thrombin. The *dashed lines* show the autocatalytic action of thrombin. PL, Phospholipids. (From Douglas S: Coagulation history. *Br J Haematol* 107:22-32, 1999.)

when these agents are used. Plasminogen activation is enhanced further by the complex formed by t-PA, fibrin, and plasminogen. The complex increases the clot-selective fibrinolytic activity of t-PA. Fibrinolysis occurs predominantly within the thrombus and at its surface. Lysis of thrombus is augmented by contributions from local blood flow.[2] During thrombus consolidation, plasminogen bound to fibrin and to platelets allows local release of plasmin. Within the circulation, plasmin cleaves the fibrinogen to different fragments, which incorporate into the fibrin and cause destabilization of its network, therefore allowing further degradation.[2]

All thrombolytic agents in current use are obligate plasminogen activators that act on fibrin and thrombin. Current thrombolytic agents are either endogenous plasminogen activators, which are involved in physiologic fibrinolysis, or exogenous plasminogen activators, which are not.[2]

Endogenous Plasminogen Activators

Tissue-Type Plasminogen Activator

Tissue-type plasminogen activator is a single-chain, 70-kilodalton (kDa), glycosylated serine protease. It has four domains: finger or F domain, growth factor or E domain, two kringle regions (K1 and K2), and a serine protease domain. The COOH-terminal serine protease domain has the active site for the cleavage of plasminogen. The two kringle domains of t-PA (Fig. 49-2) are similar to the kringle domains on plasminogen. The finger domain residues and the K2 domain residues are responsible for fibrin affinity. The single t-PA chain is converted to the double-chain t-PA form by plasmin cleavage of the arginine (position 275)–isoleucine (position 276) bond. Both the single- and double-chain forms are enzymatically active and have fibrin-selective properties. The

plasma half-life of the single- and double-chain forms is 3 to 8 minutes. Tissue-type plasminogen is secreted by endothelial cells, neurons, astrocytes, and microglia. It is cleared by the liver. It is considered to be fibrin dependent because of favorable activation of plasminogen in association with fibrin. Exercise and certain vasoactive substances, such as desmopressin, raise t-PA levels. Heparin and heparan sulfate increase t-PA activity.[2] Recombinant DNA techniques are used to produce rt-PA for commercial use in both single-chain (alteplase) and double-chain (dulteplase) forms. Figure 49-2 illustrates the amino acid sequence of t-PA.[4]

Urokinase

Urokinase plasminogen activator and its precursor scu-PA, or pro-UK, are glycoproteins. Urokinase is synthesized by endothelial, renal, and malignant cells. The single-chain pro-UK possesses fibrin-selective plasmin-generating activity. Pro-UK has been synthesized by recombinant techniques to be used as an exogenous agent. Removal of the amino acid lysine at position 158 from scu-PA by plasmin produces the high molecular weight (HMW) double-chain u-PA (54 kDa) linked by the disulfide bridge; further cleavage produces the low molecular weight (LMW) u-PA (31 kDa). Both LMW and HMW forms are enzymatically active. HMW u-PA activates plasminogen to plasmin directly. The half-life of the two forms is 9 to 12 minutes.[2] Pro-UK has been studied in patients with stroke but has not been approved for clinical use.

Novel Plasminogen Activators

Different mutant forms of t-PA and u-PA have been developed through alteration of the original amino acid sequences by point mutations and deletions. These changes alter the specificity and stability of the molecules. A good example is TNK-t-PA (tenecteplase), a mutant form of t-PA with delayed clearance and a longer half-life than t-PA. In patients with myocardial infarction (MI), TNK has a half-life of 17 ± 7 minutes, as compared with 3.5 ± 1.4 minutes for alteplase.[5] TNK has higher fibrin selectivity and greater resistance to plasminogen-activator inhibitor with enhanced lytic activity on the thrombus and induces earlier reperfusion than t-PA. The name TNK is derived from the fact that the molecule is produced through alteration of the amino acid sequence at the T, N, and K domains of t-PA, as portrayed in Figure 49-3, resulting in the improved characteristics already described.[6]

TNK was shown to be effective for the treatment of coronary thrombosis. The Assessment of the Safety and Efficacy of New Thrombolytic Trial–study 1 (ASSENT-1) evaluated the safety of TNK in 3325 patients with MI. The ICH rates were 0.7% with the 30-mg dose and 0.6% with the 40-mg dose of TNK, which are similar to rates for t-PA in previous MI trials. The rate of serious bleeding complications requiring transfusions was 1.4% for TNK compared with 7% for t-PA (statistically significant difference with the lesser bleeding rates in the TNK group).[7] In ASSENT-2, 16,949 patients with acute MI were assigned to receive either a single-bolus dose of TNK or a 30-minute infusion of t-PA. All patients also received heparin

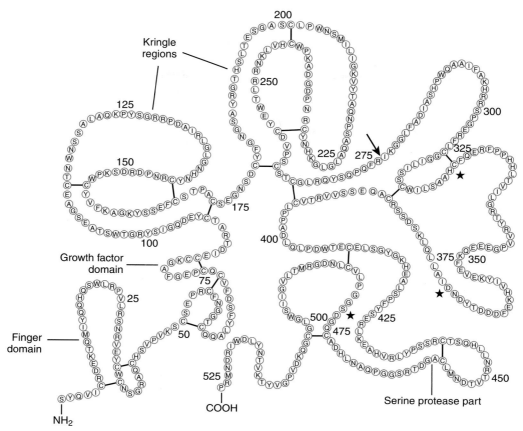

Figure 49-2 Schematic representation of the amino acid sequence of t-PA. The amino acids are represented by their letter symbols. *Black bars* indicate the disulfide bonds. The active site residues histidine-322, asparagine-371, and serine-478 are indicated with an *asterisk*. The *arrow* indicates the plasmin cleavage site for conversion of single-chain to double chain t-PA. (From Collen D: Fibrin-selective thrombolytic therapy for acute myocardial infarction. *Circulation* 93:857-865, 1996.)

and aspirin. The ICH rates were statistically similar in the two groups (0.93% in the TNK group and 0.94% in the t-PA group). There was a slightly but statistically significantly lower rate of major bleeding requiring transfusion with TNK (4.25% for the TNK group versus 5.49% for the t-PA group; $P = 0.0003$). The ASSENT-2 investigators concluded that TNK, which has higher fibrin specificity than t-PA and can be given as a single bolus, is associated with a lesser overall systemic bleeding rate but a similar ICH rate when given to patients with acute MI.[8]

After these successes with coronary thrombosis, it was natural to pursue an indication for cerebral thrombosis. A dose-finding study showed safety in acute stroke patients treated with TNK. Twenty-five patients were enrolled into each tier, and the study included four TNK dose tiers. Patients were followed up at 24 hours, at discharge, and at 3 months. Symptomatic ICHs within 36 hours of treatment did not occur in the first two tiers, but *asymptomatic* ICH occurred in 8% and 32% in the first two tiers, respectively. Clinical systemic bleeding that did not require treatment occurred in 16% and 40% in the first two tiers, respectively.[9] Two hemorrhages occurred at the highest dose tier after 13 patients were enrolled, prompting a halt to the trial.[9] A phase 2 study of the best two doses of TNK was organized and funded, but unfortunately the FDA imposed an additional two tiers. As a

result, enrollment in the trial proceeded poorly, and it was abandoned after several years. Thus, although TNK appears to be more effective than rt-PA and to have fewer complications, conclusive evidence of this remains lacking.

Microplasmin

A recombinant form of human microplasminogen has recently been investigated. Whereas t-PA is a specific proteolytic enzyme that converts the inactive proenzyme plasminogen to plasmin, microplasmin is a truncated form of plasmin, which, in recent years, has been tested in rodent models of ischemic stroke for safety and neuroprotective properties. It has been shown that in mice with inactivation of genes encoding α_2-antiplasmin, this inactivation significantly reduced infarct size after ischemia, which suggests that there may be some neuroprotective properties inherent in the molecule.[10] Microplasmin reacts with α_2-antiplasmin and neutralizes it. Microplasmin was tested in two rabbit clot embolic stroke models, both small and large, with escalating weight-based dosing. Microplasmin improved behavioral rating scores 60 minutes after embolization without increasing hemorrhagic conversion.[11] There have been no human studies up to now; however, this seems to be a promising new agent for further study.

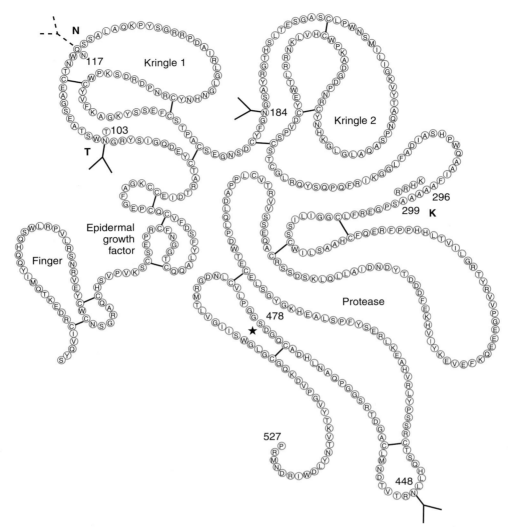

Figure 49-3 The structure of the mutant form of t-PA called TNK-t-PA. This name is given to this compound because of substitution at the T site (asparagine for threonine at position 103), N site (glutamine for asparagine at position 117), and K site (replacing one lysine, one histidine, and two arginines with four alanines at positions 296 through 299) of the original t-PA molecule. The t-PA and TNK structures have the following domains: finger domain, epidermal growth factor domain, the two kringle structures, as well as the serine protease domain. Glycosylation sites are marked by a Y. The *star* marks the serine site where plasminogen activation occurs. There are *short lines* that show the bridging between the different loops of the molecule. The amino acid substitutions enhance the selectivity and increase the half-life of the molecule, as fully explained in the text. (From Benedict CR, Refino CF, Keyt BA, et al: New variant of human tissue plasminogen activator [TPA] with enhanced efficacy and a lower incidence of bleeding compared with recombinant human TPA. *Circulation* 92:3032-3040, 1995.)

Exogenous Plasminogen Activators

Exogenous plasminogen activators are produced or extracted from nonhuman sources. Pharmacologic quantities of endogenous plasminogen activators produced by recombinant techniques, such as rt-PA, or produced through different mutations in the original physiologic plasminogen activator molecules, such as TNK, have already been discussed.

Streptokinase

Streptokinase (SK) is a single-chain polypeptide derived from group C β-hemolytic streptococci. SK combines with plasminogen, and the complex activates circulating plasminogen to plasmin and undergoes conversion to SK–plasmin itself. This complex is not inhibited by α_2–antiplasmin, but SK activity can be eliminated by the presence of SK-neutralizing antibodies produced after previous infection with streptococci. The kinetics of SK elimination are complex, consisting of an initial half-life of 4 minutes and a second half-life of 30 minutes.[2]

Anisoylated Plasminogen-Streptokinase Activator Complex

Anisoylated plasminogen-streptokinase activator complex (APSAC) consists of plasminogen and SK bound noncovalently. Its fibrin selectivity originates from its plasminogen-mediated fibrin-binding properties. In the presence of fibrin, SK allows formation of plasmin within the complex, after activation of the acyl-protected active site of plasminogen.[2]

The half-life of APSAC is 70 minutes, which is longer than that of t-PA. APSAC has been studied in patients with cardiac disease. In a double-blind study, 382 patients with acute MI were randomly assigned to receive APSAC, or t-PA, or a combination of both. The patency of the infarct-related artery at 1 hour and at 90 minutes and complete reperfusion rates were highest in the t-PA group. The rate of "unsatisfactory outcome," a composite of clinical endpoints assessed through hospital discharge, was lowest for the t-PA group, although the difference was not statistically significant. The mortality rate at 6 weeks was lowest in the t-PA group (2.2% with t-PA, 8.8% with APSAC, and 7.2% with the combination treatment; P value for t-PA versus APSAC was 0.02, and that for t-PA versus combination therapy was 0.06).[12]

Both APSAC and SK can be used in the thrombolytic treatment of acute MI. However, their longer half-lives, the production of anti-SK antibodies to the two agents, and the higher frequency of hypotension and allergic reactions (side effects) compared with t-PA give t-PA the priority as a thrombolytic agent. All three agents have been approved for use in treatment of acute MI.[13] APSAC has not yet been studied in patients with stroke.

Plasminogen Activators Derived from Saliva of *Desmodus rotundus*

The recombinant plasminogen activators that are identical to the ones derived from the saliva of the vampire bat (*Desmodus rotundus*) include an alpha form that is more fibrin dependent than t-PA. Its half-life is also longer than that of t-PA. Experimental studies have shown that the recombinant alpha-1 form and the bat plasminogen activator may be superior to t-PA in sustaining recanalization and may cause less fibrinogenolysis.[14,15] The Desmoteplase in Acute Ischemic Stroke Study (DIAS) was a dose-finding randomized, phase 2 trial designed to evaluate the safety and efficacy of IV desmoteplase.[16] This study selected patients between 3 and 9 hours after stroke onset based on mismatch of perfusion-weighted/diffusion-weighted MRI. Eligible patients had a National Institutes of Health Stroke Scale (NIHSS) score between 4 and 20 and MRI evidence of perfusion/diffusion mismatch. The perfusion/diffusion mismatch is considered to be reflective of the "ischemic penumbra," which is potentially salvageable tissue. Fixed doses of desmoteplase were evaluated, but the evaluation was terminated early due to the excessive rate of symptomatic ICH, defined as a four-point or more worsening of the NIHSS with CT-confirmed ICH. Subsequently, the lower weight-adjusted doses were investigated in 57 patients. A significantly higher rate of reperfusion was observed with desmoteplase compared with placebo (P = 0.0012). Early reperfusion was found to correlate favorably with clinical outcome assessed by the NIHSS, modified Rankin scale, and Barthel Index (BI) at 90 days (P = 0.0028).

The Dose Escalation of Desmoteplase in Acute Stroke (DEDAS) study accompanied the DIAS study to further define the safety and efficacy of IV desmoteplase in patients with perfusion/diffusion mismatch 3 to 9 hours after stroke onset.[17] DEDAS was a randomized, placebo-controlled, body weight–adjusted dose-escalation study. Included were patients with an NIHSS score of 4 through 20 with a perfusion/diffusion mismatch on MRI. The primary safety end point was symptomatic ICH defined as in the DIAS study. The study randomly assigned 37 patients:

14 received an IV bolus of 90 µg/kg of desmoteplase over 1 to 2 minutes, and 15 received 125 µg/kg. As was seen in the DIAS trial, reperfusion was found to correlate with a good clinical outcome at 90 days compared with those without reperfusion (P = 0.003). Also, no symptomatic ICHs were observed.

Subsequently, DIAS 2, a prospective, randomized, double-blind, placebo-controlled study was completed to confirm the results of the DIAS/DEDAS studies and to further evaluate the safety and efficacy of desmoteplase.[18] Patients were included if they had an NIHSS score between 4 and 24 and onset of symptoms within 3 to 9 hours, as well as a perfusion/diffusion mismatch on MRI of 20%. Perfusion CT was also allowed depending on site experience. There was no statistically significant difference in clinical outcome between the 90 µg/kg or 125 µg/kg of desmoteplase or placebo. Symptomatic ICH, defined as in DIAS, was observed in 4% of patients in the desmoteplase groups. Questions have been raised, however, regarding the reproducibility of the perfusion studies in DIAS 2, which allowed site investigators to use an "eyeball" method (i.e., nonquantitative) measurement of mismatch. Post-hoc data analysis suggested that there may have been important overestimation and underestimation of mismatch in DIAS 2 (personal communication, Greg Albers, MD). Desmoteplase will be studied again in DIAS 3 and DIAS 4, trials organized to find a positive effect of desmoteplase on clinical outcomes without the use of mismatch selection criteria from imaging. Instead, patients will be selected if imaging documents a large artery occlusion and the absence of large areas of infarcted brain (hypodensity on CT imaging).

Staphylokinase

Staphylokinase (STK) is a polypeptide derived from *Staphylococcus aureus*. It combines with plasminogen irreversibly and activates free plasminogen. The complex plasmin–STK has relative fibrin specificity because, in the absence of fibrin, this complex is inhibited by α_2-antiplasmin. Recombinant STK has been used in experimental models of acute MI[2] but not in models of stroke.

Ancrod

Ancrod is a purified fraction of venom from the Malaysian pit viper (*Calloselasma rhodostoma*) and induces rapid defibrinogenation in humans by splitting fibrinopeptide A from fibrinogen.[19] This agent has been the target for acute ischemic stroke since the 1980s.[20,21] Ancrod is given as a continuous infusion for up to 72 hours, and fibrinogen levels are checked before treatment and at designated intervals during and after treatment to determine the activity. Ancrod's effects on plasma fibrinogen levels can be measured. The dosing strategy is to maintain a target fibrinogen level throughout the 5 to 7 days of dosing.[22]

The North American Stroke Treatment with Ancrod Trial (STAT) was a randomized clinical trial that enrolled patients within 3 hours of stroke onset with pretreatment blood pressures maintained at 185 mm Hg systolic/105 mm Hg diastolic or less.[23] The patients received IV ancrod or placebo continuously for 72 hours, then intermittently for 2 days so that a target fibrinogen level could be obtained, which was based on their pretreatment fibrinogen level. This study was found to increase the proportion of patients with ischemic stroke who had a favorable functional status, as measured by a BI score of 95 or greater at 90 days. This study showed significant efficacy ($P = 0.041$), and similar mortality rates were seen between ancrod treatment and placebo. Significantly more asymptomatic ICHs were also found in the ancrod group than in the placebo group at rates similar to those found in the NINDS t-PA trial. Following this study was the European Stroke Treatment with Ancrod Trial (ESTAT), which administered treatment within 6 hours of acute stroke onset.[24] ESTAT was a randomized, double-blind placebo-controlled, phase 3 trial of 1222 patients randomly assigned to ancrod or placebo. Unlike the STAT study, treatment was started within 6 hours of symptom onset and blood pressure was allowed to be 220/120 mm Hg or less. As in the STAT study, pretreatment fibrinogen levels were measured, and infusions were adjusted to maintain a prespecified target fibrinogen range. The time to treatment was more than 3 hours in 43% of the ancrod-treated group and in 42% of the placebo-treated group. Functional outcome at 3 months, as measured by a BI score greater than 95 or return to prestroke values, was similar in the ancrod and placebo groups. Symptomatic ICH occurred significantly more often in patients given ancrod compared with those given placebo ($P = 0.007$).

A pivotal phase 3 trial was organized to confirm whether ancrod significantly altered the outcome after stroke in a large cohort of patients. The dose was carefully titrated to fibrinogen. Unfortunately, the trial was halted after an interim analysis for futility, which suggests that ancrod does not benefit patients with acute stroke.

Preclinical Studies of Thrombolysis for Acute Stroke

Considerable preclinical development showed that thrombolysis might be an effective stroke therapy. After recombinant technology was developed to produce large quantities of t-PA, animal studies could be conducted to show that t-PA, administered immediately after experimental embolic occlusion, caused reperfusion with significantly less neurologic damage. This development

helped overcome the negative experience of early human use that accumulated before modern imaging techniques.

As early as 1963, Meyer et al[25] studied embolic stroke models in cats and monkeys and administered IV or intraarterial bovine or human plasmin; this treatment resulted in clot lysis without higher rates of hemorrhagic infarction.[25]

In 1983, del Zoppo et al[26] demonstrated in baboons that after 3 hours of reversible balloon inflation compressing the middle cerebral artery (MCA), intracarotid administration of UK improved neurologic function and reduced infarct size without an increase in the rate of ICH detectable by CT. In 1985, Zivin et al[27] documented that t-PA could substantially improve neurologic function after embolization with artificially made clots. These studies together strongly suggested that thrombolysis, by restoring blood flow soon after stroke onset, could prevent neurologic deficits.

Preclinical trials also yielded insights into the potential risks of thrombolysis. In 1986, del Zoppo et al[28] studied t-PA–induced hemorrhagic transformation of ischemic baboon brains within 3.5 hours of MCA occlusion followed by 30 minutes of reperfusion. There was no significant difference in incidence or volume of infarct-related hemorrhage between any of the t-PA groups and the control group. In 1987, Slivka and Pulsinelli[29] investigated the hemorrhagic potential of both t-PA and SK given 24 hours after experimental strokes in rabbits as well as that of SK given 1 hour after experimental stroke. These investigators found that the thrombolytic agents increased the risk of ICH unless they were given early after the insult.[29] In 1989, Lyden et al[30] found no difference in the frequency of hemorrhagic transformation in the ischemic brains of rabbits whether t-PA was administered 10 minutes, 8 hours, or even 24 hours after cerebral embolism. In 1991, Clark et al[31] demonstrated that aspirin and t-PA act synergistically to cause intracranial bleeding in the rabbit embolism model.

To learn whether hemorrhagic risk was associated with thrombolytic agents in general or with a particular agent specifically, Lyden et al[32] compared t-PA, SK, and saline given after embolic stroke in rabbits. SK, but not t-PA, was associated with a significant increase in ICH rate and size. Table 49-1 demonstrates those results.[32] It should

TABLE 49-1 RATES OF INTRACRANIAL HEMORRHAGE AND THROMBOLYSIS IN RABBITS WITH EMBOLIC STROKES AFTER ADMINISTRATION OF T-PA AS COMPARED WITH STREPTOKINASE AND SALINE*

Treatment	Dose	Time (min)	n	Hemorrhage No.	Hemorrhage %	Thrombolysis No.	Thrombolysis %
Saline		†	48	12	25	17	35
t-PA	3 mg/kg	90	16	5	31	9	56
t-PA	5 mg/kg	90	22	3	14	15	68
t-PA	10 mg/kg	90	11	4	36	10	91†
SK	30,000 units/kg	5	11	6	55	5	45
SK	30,000 units/kg	90	17	11	65‡	14	82†
SK	30,000 units/kg	300	12	10	83‡	10	83†

*Results of t-PA treatment at 5 minutes and 4, 8, and 24 hours are contained in references 2 and 3.
†Saline-treated control rabbits were treated 5, 90, or 300 minutes after embolization.
‡$p < 0.05$ different from saline by chi-squared test.
ICH, Intracranial hemorrhage; SK, streptokinase; Time, time after embolization that treatment was initiated; t-PA, tissue-type plasminogen activator.
From Lyden PD, Madden KP, Clark WA, et al: Comparison of cerebral hemorrhage rates following tissue plasminogen activator or streptokinase treatment for embolic strokes in rabbits. *Stroke* 21:981-983, 1990.

be noted that there was no clear dose-response effect for hemorrhages, and the doses used were comparable to the those used for cardiac disease in humans. Only the rabbits in which t-PA achieved thrombolysis had twice the frequency of ICH than those given placebo,[32] which suggests that reperfusion might be the basis for the higher rate of hemorrhagic transformation.

In summary, preclinical studies suggested that t-PA had reliably opened cerebral arteries in embolic experimental models. Considerable benefit was achieved if thrombolysis occurred early after occlusion onset. Hemorrhages occurred after thrombolysis and seemed to be related to the particular agent used, and SK carried a greater risk than t-PA.

Clinical Studies of Thrombolysis for Acute Stroke

The clinical development of thrombolysis for stroke proceeded logically from preclinical testing. Early experiments benefited from preclinical data and emphasized several factors: agent, dose, timing, and concomitant management. We review first human-use studies that documented thrombolysis in humans after administration of thrombolytic agents.

Dose-ranging studies yielded important data about the dose of t-PA to use in pivotal trials; the efficacy of the agents seemed to be counterbalanced by hemorrhages at higher doses. Large placebo-controlled trials confirmed the efficacy and hazards of these agents as well as observations from preclinical studies that SK was more hazardous. Finally, after regulatory approval of t-PA for treatment of acute stroke, open-label studies confirmed the findings of the definitive trials and showed that IV thrombolysis is feasible and efficacious in a variety of settings. Data from experimental cerebral ischemia studies pointed to the need to treat acute stroke within a few hours, and this observation also proved true in human trials.

Feasibility Studies

Results of early attempts to achieve thrombolysis for acute ischemic stroke were discouraging, especially in studies conducted without the benefit of brain CT to exclude hemorrhage; in these preliminary trials, patients were enrolled within significantly longer time windows than currently approved. In 1965, Meyer et al[33] studied 73 patients with acute progressive strokes; the treatment group received SK plus anticoagulation, and the control group received anticoagulation only. There was a higher incidence of death in the treatment group, and better clinical improvement in the control group.[33]

In 1976, Fletcher et al[34] studied 31 patients with acute ischemic stroke who were treated with one of three different doses of IV UK; treatment was given within 36 hours of symptom onset. The study concluded that UK could be administered to patients in doses that achieve substantial thrombolysis without producing other than mild coagulation deficits; this study could not address the efficacy of the treatment, however, because the number of patients was too low. The mortality rate was 16%, and there was no placebo group for comparison. On the basis

of these two studies, which were widely discussed, IV thrombolysis for stroke was abandoned pending better agents and better selection procedures.

After the efficacy and safety of t-PA were proved in animal models, thrombolysis was pursued again in acute clinical stroke trials. In 1992, del Zoppo et al[35] studied 139 patients with acute ischemic stroke who received different doses of IV t-PA within 8 hours of stroke onset. An angiogram confirmed occlusion of an extracranial or intracranial arterial cerebral blood supply in all patients. Exclusion criteria included a minor deficit, a transient ischemic attack (TIA), a clinically large stroke with a combination of hemiplegia, impaired consciousness, and forced gaze deviation, blood pressure higher than 200 mm Hg systolic, 120 mm Hg diastolic, and radiologic (CT) evidence of bleeding or radiologic evidence of significant mass effect or midline shift. Patients with early CT hypoattenuation changes were not excluded from the study. Primary endpoints were angiographic recanalization and ICH with neurologic deterioration. This landmark study reestablished the clinical promise of thrombolysis; 40% of all patients experienced recanalization of occluded arteries. Intriguingly, there was no relation between dose and recanalization, but patients with distal (i.e., smaller) clots showed higher recanalization rates. The frequency of all hemorrhages was 30.8%, although symptomatic hemorrhages occurred in 9.6% of all patients. The mortality rate during hospitalization was 12.5%. There was no increase in hemorrhages with doses comparable to those used to achieve coronary reperfusion, although it could not be assumed that the safe and effective dose for acute coronary events would be the perfect dose for acute stroke treatment. Therefore, the effective and safe dose for stroke treatment was yet to be determined.

In 1992, the first in a series of government-sponsored trials appeared. In a dose-finding trial sponsored by the NINDS, 74 patients with acute ischemic stroke received escalating doses of t-PA (0.35 to 1.08 mg/kg) within the time window of 90 minutes. Intracranial hematomas did not occur in any of the 58 patients who received doses of 0.85 mg/kg or less. Intracranial hematomas occurred with higher doses. Hemorrhages associated with neurologic deterioration (symptomatic hemorrhages) occurred in three of the 74 patients, although such hemorrhages did not occur at t-PA doses of less than 0.95 mg/kg. Major improvement, manifesting as a significant improvement in the NIHSS score, occurred at 2 hours in 30% of the patients and at 24 hours in 46% of patients. Major neurologic improvement was not related to the dose of t-PA. The investigators concluded that the highest safe dose of t-PA was probably less than 0.95 mg/kg, but it is important to keep in mind that this conclusion was based on only three symptomatic hemorrhages occurring in a total experience of 74 patients. The distinct possibility remains that a higher dose could, in fact, prove to be safe and more efficacious.[36]

In 1992, Haley et al[37] studied 20 patients with acute ischemic stroke in another dose-escalating trial in which t-PA treatment was given between 91 and 180 minutes after stroke onset. The risks of symptomatic ICH were 10% overall and 17% with the two higher dosage levels (the three doses used were 0.6 mg/kg, 0.85 mg/kg, and

0.95 mg/kg). Three patients (15%) improved by 4 points on the NIHSS at 24 hours.[37]

Mori et al[38] conducted a trial in Japan in which either 6 million or 12 million units of IV t-PA or placebo was administered within 6 hours of stroke onset. Using angiograms before and after thrombolysis, these investigators confirmed that t-PA increased the rate of MCA recanalization. Of considerable importance is the fact that functional outcome measured by the BI score was also significantly improved by thrombolysis. Like the del Zoppo trial, this trial established unequivocally that IV thrombolytics could open occluded cerebral vessels. Further, and perhaps even more important, the trial results suggested that angiographic confirmation of cerebral vessel occlusion might not be essential before IV thrombolysis.[38]

In 1993, in the "bridging trial," a forerunner of the definitive NINDS study, Haley et al[39] studied 27 patients who received 0.85 mg/kg of IV t-PA or placebo within 3 hours of stroke onset. This was a randomized, double-blinded, placebo-controlled study. Despite the small sample size, there was suggestion of early neurologic improvement (at 24 hours) in the patients treated with t-PA. In the treatment arm in which therapy was given up to 90 minutes after stroke onset, six of the 10 patients who received t-PA improved by 4 or more points on the NIHSS, compared with one of the 10 patients given placebo. In the treatment arm in which therapy was given between 91 and 180 minutes after stroke onset, two patients in the t-PA group and two patients from the placebo subgroups improved by 4 or more points on the NIHSS at 24 hours.[39] The results of the bridging trial anticipated those of the larger NINDS study in a surprising number of respects. Nevertheless, large, rigorous, placebo-controlled, randomized trials were needed to confirm any beneficial effects afforded by IV thrombolytic agents.

Large, Randomized, Multicenter, Placebo-Controlled Trials

ECASS

Published in 1995, the European Cooperative Acute Stroke Study (ECASS) included 620 patients treated with 1.1 mg/kg of IV t-PA or placebo within 6 hours of stroke onset.[40] The trial showed no significant efficacy in the intent-to-treat primary analysis. On exclusion of patients with protocol violations (109 patients, 17.4%), a target population of 511 patients was selected for further analysis. Protocol violations consisted of inclusion of patients with large strokes (i.e., hypodensity of greater than one third of the MCA territory on CT), concurrent use of anticoagulants or volume expanders, detection of hemorrhage on baseline CT, uncontrolled hypertension, and lack of complete follow-up. The first hypothesis in this study was that there would be a 15-point difference in the BI between the two groups in the study, favoring the t-PA treatment group. The second hypothesis was that there would be a difference on the modified Rankin Scale (mRS) score in favor of the t-PA group.

In the target population, there was a 1-point difference in the mRS score between the two groups (P = 0.035) in favor of the t-PA group. There was no statistically significant difference in ICH rates between the groups, but there

was an increase in frequency of large parenchymal hemorrhages in the t-PA group and an increase in frequency of hemorrhagic infarcts in the placebo group. There was no statistically significant difference in mortality rates at 30 days.[40] Although ECASS failed to show a benefit (the hypothesis was not proved), subsequent analyses showed a significant treatment effect. In particular, on post hoc reanalysis of ECASS with the use of NINDS global endpoint statistics, a statistically significant treatment effect was detected in the intent-to-treat group. This finding suggests that ECASS might have shown a beneficial effect of thrombolytic agents in stroke even though one cannot definitely reach that conclusion from a post hoc analysis.[41] Furthermore, when the patients treated within 3 hours were examined separately (38 given placebo, 49 given t-PA), a nonstatistically significant treatment effect (Fig. 49-4A) was demonstrated by the same statistical analysis methods used in the NINDS study (global odds ratio [OR],

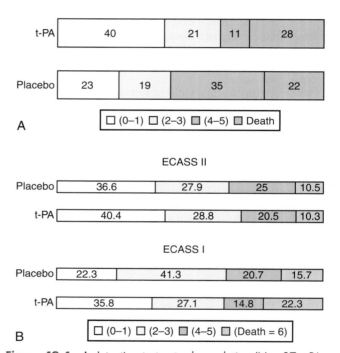

Figure 49-4 A, Intention to treat subpopulation (N = 87, t-PA = 49, placebo = 38) in the ECASS-I patients who received treatment within 3 hours, using the same analysis method implemented previously in NINDS: global odds ratio is 2.3 (0.9, 5.3), P = 0.07. The results are not statistically significant because of the small number of patients within 3 hours. B, Patient outcome by modified Rankin scale (mRS) in ECASS-I and ECASS-II. Both ECASS-I and ECASS-II were positive for the endpoint of mRS ≤ 2 (no disability to slight disability). Each *bar* shows the percent of patients with that grade. Grade 0: asymptomatic patients. Grade 1: no significant disability despite symptoms; patient is able to carry out all usual activities and duties. Grade 2: slight disability; the patient is unable to carry out all previous activities but able to look after his or her affairs without assistance. Grade 3: moderate disability with the requirement of some help but with preservation of the ability to walk without assistance. Grade 4: moderately severe disability with inability to walk without assistance and inability to attend to one's own bodily needs without assistance. Grade 5: severe disability; the patient is bedridden, incontinent, and requires constant nursing care and attention. Grade 6 is death.

2.3; $P = 0.07$).[42] The ECASS post hoc analyses suggested that an independent 3-hour trial might show a benefit for thrombolytic agents.

The NINDS Studies

In December 1995, the NINDS study was published; it was a randomized, placebo-controlled, multicenter trial that showed the efficacy of t-PA in treating acute ischemic strokes within 3 hours of onset.[1] This NINDS study differed from ECASS in several respects besides the dose of t-PA and time to treatment. Most importantly, NINDS protocol required that the blood pressure had to be controlled to below 185 mm Hg systolic, 95 mm Hg diastolic. Table 49-2 summarizes the inclusion and exclusion criteria of the NINDS study.

The NINDS study had two parts with identical protocol but different endpoints. Part 1 tested whether t-PA showed clinical activity, as indicated by a statistically significant difference on the primary endpoint, chosen arbitrarily to be either an improvement of 4 or more points on the NIHSS or complete resolution of the neurologic deficit within 24 hours. Part 2 used a global test statistic to assess clinical outcome after 3 months, based on scores on the BI, mRS, Glasgow Outcome Scale (GOS), and NIHSS. Part 1 enrolled 291 patients (144 in the t-PA group and 147 in the placebo group), and part 2 enrolled 333 patients (168 patients in the t-PA group and 165 patients in the placebo group). In part 1, on the primary endpoint, the number of patients improving by 4 or more points on the NIHSS at 24 hours was 67 (47%) in the t-PA group and 57 (39%) in the placebo group (not statistically significant, with a P value of 0.21).[1] Subsequent analysis showed that any other cutoff improvement in the 24-hour NIHSS score, such as 5 or more points, would have yielded a statistically significant difference between the two groups (Fig. 49-5).[43]

In part 2 of the NINDS, benefit was observed on all four primary efficacy measures (i.e., NIHSS, BI, mRS, and GOS scores) at 3 months from onset of stroke. Figure 49-6 demonstrates the increase in proportion of patients with good clinical outcomes in the t-PA group compared with the placebo group as measured by these scales. Patients treated with t-PA were 30% to 50% more likely to have minimal or no disability at 3 months, depending on the outcome measure. For example, the percentage of patients with an mRS score of 1 or less at 3 months was 39% in the t-PA group versus 26% in the placebo group (statistically significant difference in favor of t-PA). Symptomatic ICH occurred in 6.4% of patients who received treatment but only in 0.6% of patients who received placebo. Mortality rates at 3 months were not statistically different between the two groups, being 17% in the t-PA group and 21% in the placebo group.[1] Thus, despite an increased risk of hemorrhage, the mortality rate was not affected, and IV t-PA provided considerable benefit and improved outcomes, as depicted in Figure 49-7. Furthermore, the NINDS data analysis showed that t-PA treatment resulted in a more favorable outcome regardless of the subtype of stroke (small-vessel, large-vessel, or cardioembolic stroke) diagnosed at baseline.[1]

Further subgroup analysis of the NINDS data showed that the only variables independently associated with

TABLE 49-2 INCLUSION AND EXCLUSION CRITERIA OF THE NINDS STUDY*

Inclusion criteria of NINDS
Ischemic stroke of defined onset <3 hours
Deficit measurable on NIHSS
Baseline CT of the brain without evidence of hemorrhage

Exclusion criteria of NINDS
A prior stroke within the last 3 months PTP
Major surgery within the last 14 days PTP
Serious head trauma within the last 3 months PTP
History of ICH
Systolic BP >185 mm Hg or diastolic BP >110 mm Hg or if aggressive treatment was required to lower the BP to below these limits
Rapidly improving or minor symptoms
Symptoms suggestive of SAH
Gastrointestinal bleeding or urinary tract hemorrhage within 3 weeks PTP
Arterial puncture at a noncompressible site within the last 7 days PTP
Seizure at the onset of symptoms
Anticoagulants or heparin within 48 hours before stroke onset or elevated PTT or elevated PT >15 sec
Platelet count <100,000/mL
Blood glucose <50 mg/dL or above 400 mg/dL

*Tissue Plasminogen Activator for Acute Ischemic Stroke.
BP, Blood pressure; CT, computed tomography; ICH, intracranial hemorrhage; NIHSS, National Institutes of Health Stroke Scale; NINDS, National Institute of Neurological Disorders and Stroke; PT, prothrombin time; PTP, prior to presentation; PTT, partial thromboplastin time; SAH, subarachnoid hemorrhage.
Tissue plasminogen activator for acute ischemic stroke. The National Institute of Neurological Disorders and Stroke rt-PA Stroke Study Group. *N Engl J Med* 333:1581-1587, 1995.

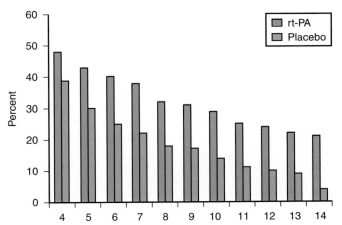

Figure 49-5 The percentage of patients within each improvement category of National Institutes of Health Stroke Scale (NIHSS) at 24 hours in Part 1 of National Institute of Neurological and Communicable Diseases and Stroke (NINDS) study. The improvement in NIHSS score at 24 hours was significantly better in the t-PA treated group as compared with placebo ($P < 0.05$) in each of the categories of improvement in the NIHSS score, except for a drop of NIHSS of ≥4 points (chosen as the primary endpoint of Part I of NINDS). Therefore, had the primary endpoint been chosen to be a drop in NIHSS at 24 hours ≥ any number other than 4, Part 1 would have shown a statistically significant benefit of t-PA at 24 hours.

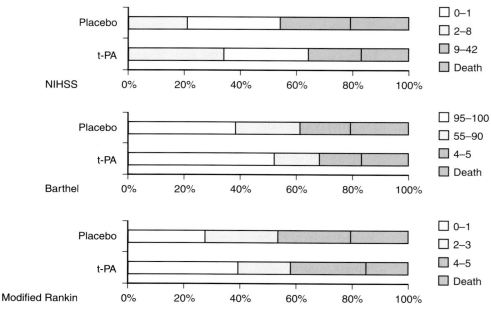

Figure 49-6   Statistically significant improvement on all primary outcome measures at 3 months in National Institute of Neurological and Communicable Diseases and Stroke (NINDS) study, Part 2. National Institutes of Health Stroke Scale (NIHSS), Barthel Index, and modified Rankin Scale (mRS) at 3 months are depicted here, and there is a statistically significant improvement in the t-PA treated patients as compared with placebo in each of these categories as well as in the Glasgow Outcome Scale (GOS), which is not shown here.

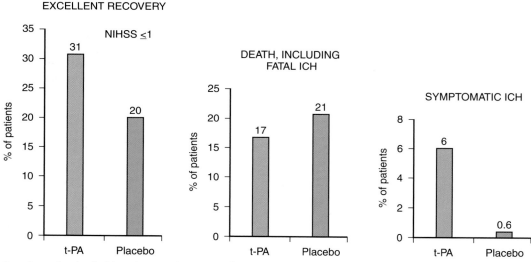

Figure 49-7   Benefit and risk of t-PA in National Institute of Neurological and Communicable Diseases and Stroke (NINDS) for Acute Stroke Trial: Benefit from t-PA is shown as a statistically significant higher percent of patients with National Institutes of Health Stroke Scale (NIHSS) score of 0–1 in the t-PA group as compared with placebo. Risk is depicted as a statistically significant increase in symptomatic intracranial hemorrhage (ICH) at 36 hours that is attributable to t-PA treatment. Despite that risk, there is no significant difference in mortality between the t-PA and placebo groups at 3 months.

an increased risk of symptomatic ICH in the t-PA-treated patients were the baseline severity of the stroke as measured by the NIHSS, brain edema defined by hypodensity on baseline CT, and mass effect on baseline CT (before treatment).[44] These factors did not interact with treatment, however, which suggests that such factors might not be predictive in excluding patients from treatment.

Subsequent prespecified analyses of the NINDS database with the use of a global statistical method showed

sustained, statistically significant benefit at 6-month and 1-year follow-up points: the OR values for a favorable outcome in the t-PA group compared with the placebo group were 1.7 with a 95% confidence interval of 1.3 to 2.3 at 6 months and 1.7 with a 95% confidence interval of 1.2 to 2.3 at 1 year.[45] At 1 year, the range of absolute increase in the percentage of patients with a favorable outcome was 11% to 13%, and the range of relative increase in the percentage of patients with a favorable outcome was 32%

to 46% for the three outcome scales (mRS, BI, and GOS). Patients treated with t-PA were at least 30% more likely to be independent at 1 year than those given placebo. Importantly, favorable outcomes were not accompanied by an increase in severe disability or mortality. The proportion of patients surviving between 3 months and 12 months after stroke was consistently higher in the t-PA group than in the placebo group. However, there was no statistically significant difference in mortality at 6 months and 1 year. After adjustment for those variables, treatment with t-PA still offered better outcomes.

As was the case for the 3-month follow-up data, there was no evidence of interaction between the subtype of stroke at baseline and treatment, meaning that all stroke subtypes (large-vessel, small-vessel, and embolic) benefitted from t-PA. Moreover, there was no significant difference in the incidence of recurrent stroke between the t-PA and placebo groups at 1 year.[45] Furthermore, another analysis of the NINDS data addressed finding the binary measures that predicted effectiveness of t-PA during the first 3 months. Measures using NIHSS and mRS scores of 1 or less were the most sensitive discriminators of effectiveness of t-PA in the NINDS study. The best measure was NIHSS score of 2 or less at 24 hours. High-quality analysis of the volume of brain infarction as measured by CT was not as sensitive in detecting a treatment effect as the clinical scale measures.[46]

ECASS II

ECASS II was a multicenter double-blind, randomized trial of 800 patients with acute stroke who received either 0.9 mg/kg t-PA (409 patients) or placebo (391 patients) within 6 hours of stroke onset.[47] Exclusion criteria were similar to those for the NINDS, with the addition of evidence of early infarction changes on CT greater than one third of the MCA territory, coma or stupor, and hemiplegia with fixed eye deviation. The use of anticoagulants and antiplatelet agents was prohibited for the first 24 hours after random assignment of patients to treatment.

There were 72 protocol violations (17%), 34 in the t-PA group and 38 in the placebo group; the majority resulted from failure to abide by the CT criteria. There was no statistically significant difference in the proportion of favorable outcomes (mRS score 0 to 1 at day 90) between the two groups; favorable outcomes occurred in 40.3% of the t-PA group and in 36.6% of the placebo group ($P \geq 0.05$). A post hoc analysis of the 90-day mRS score, classifying each patient as either functionally independent (mRS score, ≤ 2) or dependent (mRS score, >2), found a statistically significant difference between the two groups in favor of t-PA (54.3% in the t-PA group versus 46.0% in the placebo group with an 8.3% absolute difference; $P = 0.024$). The incidence of symptomatic ICH was higher in the t-PA group (8.8%) than in the placebo group (3.4%).[47] Figure 49-4B shows the mRS scores for the t-PA and placebo groups at 90 days in both ECASS-1 and ECASS-2.

Streptokinase Trials

Three clinical trials attempted to investigate the benefits and risks of SK treatment in acute stroke. These trials were all terminated prematurely because of complications. The Multicentre Acute Stroke Trial in Europe (MAST-E) was a double-blind, placebo-controlled, randomized study of SK published in 1996.[48] Patients with acute MCA strokes presenting within 6 hours of onset received either 1.5 million units of IV SK or placebo. There was no difference in the primary outcome measures (death and severe disability and mRS score ≥ 3 at 6 months after treatment). In-hospital death and symptomatic ICH occurred more often in the SK group. The use of anticoagulants or antiplatelet agents was allowed: 65% of patients given SK and 75% of patients given placebo received heparin concomitantly with thrombolysis, and 20% of patients in each group also received aspirin. At 6 months, the mortality rate was higher in the SK group ($P = 0.06$). There was a trend toward less severe disability with SK and a significantly shorter rehabilitation or nursing home stay ($P = 0.003$). This study found no evident benefit from SK treatment.[48]

The Multicentre Acute Stroke Trial in Italy (MAST-I), published in 1995,[49] was a randomized controlled trial that studied patients who received IV SK, SK plus aspirin, aspirin alone, or placebo within 6 hours of stroke onset. Anticoagulants were to be avoided in this trial, except for limited doses of subcutaneous heparin for prophylaxis of deep venous thrombosis. There was no proved benefit in any therapy group. Symptomatic hemorrhages were more common in the SK groups than in the placebo and aspirin-only groups. Aspirin plus SK therapy was associated with a statistically significant increase in early mortality compared with placebo.[49]

In the Australian Streptokinase (ASK) study,[50] 340 patients were randomly assigned to receive either placebo or SK intravenously within 4 hours of stroke onset. The study had to be suspended because of poorer outcomes in the SK group. There was no relationship between the dose of SK and the risk of hemorrhage. The hematoma rate was 9.6% in the SK group and 0% in the placebo group for patients who received treatment within 3 hours of stroke onset. The SK group had higher mortality, worse clinical outcome, and increased ICH rates. Hypotension was an adverse event that occurred in the SK-treated patients. Subsequent analysis comparing the 70 patients treated within 3 hours and the 270 patients treated after 3 hours of stroke onset found that earlier treatment was associated with better outcomes than was later treatment.[51]

A further multivariate meta-analysis of all patients from previous SK studies (MAST-E, MAST-I, ASK, and others) showed that concomitant use of aspirin increased the mortality in SK-treated patients (17% without aspirin versus 91% with aspirin treatment, $P = 0.005$).[52] There remains clinical uncertainty, therefore, whether SK might have shown benefit if tested with the same protocol as used in the NINDS rt-PA trial. This issue remains unsolved.

The ATLANTIS Study

The Alteplase Thrombolysis for Acute Noninterventional Therapy in Ischemic Stroke (ATLANTIS) study, published in 1999, was a double-blind, randomized trial evaluating the efficacy and safety of treatment with 0.9 mg/kg of IV t-PA in patients with acute ischemic strokes within 6 hours of stroke onset (part A).[53] After an interim safety analysis, the treatment window was changed to 5 hours (part B)[54] because of concerns about safety in patients treated between 5 and 6 hours of onset. The trial ended prematurely in 1998 on the basis of analysis that the treatment was unlikely to be beneficial. In the final analysis of part B, the median time to treatment was 4.5 hours; a minority of patients received treatment within 3 hours. There was no difference in the primary endpoint, that is, in the percentage of patients with an NIHSS score of ≤1 at 90 days. The symptomatic ICH rate, however, was greater in the t-PA group.

Albers et al[55] retrospectively evaluated data for the ATLANTIS patients who had received t-PA or placebo within the 3-hour time window. The primary endpoint was the percentage of patients who had complete recovery, as determined by an NIHSS score of ≤1 at 90 days after treatment. The total number of patients was 61: 38 in the placebo arm and 23 in the t-PA arm. The patients receiving t-PA were significantly more likely to have a favorable outcome, defined as an NIHSS score of ≤1 ($P = 0.01$); 60.9% of the t-PA group had an NIHSS score of ≤1 at 3 months versus only 26.3% in the placebo group, with an absolute difference of 34.6% (OR, 4.4; $P < 0.01$). The symptomatic ICH rate was 13% in the t-PA group versus 0% in the placebo group (statistically significant difference; $P = 0.05$). There was a trend toward higher mortality in the t-PA group that did not reach statistical significance.[55]

Pooled Analysis of NINDS, ECASS II, and ATLANTIS

Despite its proven effectiveness in treating acute ischemic strokes, alteplase is still only given to a minority of patients with acute ischemic strokes, primarily because of the short time window in which it is currently being used.[56] In 2004, the investigators of the ATLANTIS, ECASS II, and NINDS studies performed a pooled analysis of six randomized controlled trials of alteplase given up to 6 hours to determine the effect of time to treatment on functional outcome.[57] A total of 2775 patients were included from the NINDS trials,[1] the ECASS trials[40,47] and the ATLANTIS trials.[53,54] The median onset to treatment was 243 minutes. The study confirmed a clear association between time to treatment and meaningful recovery. As the time interval to treatment increased, the odds of a favorable outcome (defined as an mRS of <2) decreased ($P < 0.005$). The odds ratios were 2.8 (95% confidence interval, 1.8 to 4.5) for 0 to 90 minutes, 1.6 (1.1 to 2.2) for 91 to 180 minutes, 1.4 (1.1 to 1.9) for 180 to 270 minutes, and 1.2 (0.9 to 1.5) for 271 to 360 minutes. Symptomatic ICH occurred in 5.9% of patients treated with alteplase compared with 1.1% of placebo-treated patients ($P < 0.0001$). An association was found between ICH and treatment with alteplase as well as age but not with time to treatment. The hazard ratio for death adjusted for baseline NIHSS was not significantly different from 1.0 for patients treated within 270 minutes but exceeded 1.0 for patients treated from 271 to 360 minutes (1.0; 1.02 to 2.07).[56] The results of this study confirmed a strong association between time to treatment with alteplase and treatment efficacy, but it also suggested a potential benefit beyond 3 hours. The most important finding in the pooled analysis, however, was a confirmation that the odds of favorable outcome declined with every minute delay from symptom onset.

SITS-MOST

The Safe Implementation of Thrombolysis in Stroke-Monitoring Study (SITS-MOST) was a prospective, multicenter, observational study that was initiated as a requirement of the approval of alteplase by the European Medicines Agency (EMEA) in 2002.[58] The purpose of the trial was to confirm the safety of alteplase when given within 3 hours in routine clinical practice. Participating centers had to have routine monitoring and comprehensive care for all stroke patients. Safety and functional outcomes were compared with pooled results from the NINDS, ECASS I and II, and the ATLANTIS trials for patients treated within 3 hours. Between 2002 and 2006, 6483 patients received alteplase. At 7 days, the rate of symptomatic hemorrhage was 7.3% (468/6438) compared with 8.6% (40/465) in the pooled randomized analysis. In the SITS-MOST, 54.8% of patients had good functional outcomes (defined as an mRS of 0 to 2) compared with 49% in the pooled analysis.[58] While SITS-MOST confirmed the safety of alteplase in routine clinical practice, it should be noted that the study did not include patients older than 80 years or with an NIHSS score of 25 or higher.

Additional analysis of SITS-MOST data suggested that new centers, that is, those that began thrombolytic programs for the first time, could deliver thrombolytic therapy as safely as more experienced centers. This finding, although counterintuitive, suggests that centers without active programs can design and initiate teams to deliver thrombolytic therapy to stroke patients with good safety and efficacy.[58]

SITS-ISTR

The SITS (Safe Implementation of Treatments in Stroke) is an interactive database of unselected patients treated with thrombolysis for acute strokes in more than 700 clinical centers in 35 countries. The SITS-ISTR study was a retrospective study of 664 patients registered with the SITS-ISTR between 2002 and 2007 who were treated with alteplase between 3 and 4.5 hours after symptom onset.[59] The rates of functional independence (defined as an mRS of 0 to 2) and symptomatic ICH were compared with patients registered in the SITS-ISTR who were treated within 3 hours. Differences between the treatment groups suggested a possible selection bias because patients treated between 3 and 4.5 hours were younger (65 years compared with 68 years, $P < 0.0001$), had a lower median NIHSS score (11 versus 12, $P < 0.0001$), and were more likely to be treated in experienced stroke centers. There was no difference between groups in rate of functional independence (58% versus 56.3%) or symptomatic ICH (2.2% versus 1.6%). The authors concluded that alteplase can be safely given at 4 to 4.5 hours but acknowledged the need for a randomized controlled study to confirm their findings.

ECASS III

In 2002, the EMEA approved alteplase with two requirements. The first request was for the implementation of an observational study, which resulted in the SITS-MOST study. The second was for a randomized trial in which the time window was extended beyond 3 hours.

The ECASS III trial was a randomized controlled, double-blind trial of 821 patients with acute ischemic stroke who received either 0.9 mg/kg of alteplase (418) intravenously or placebo (403) at 3 to 4.5 hours after symptom onset.[60] Patients with a history of diabetes and a previous stroke and an NIHSS score of more than 25 were excluded. Treatment groups were generally well-matched, but patients treated beyond 3 hours had a significantly higher mean NIHSS compared with the alteplase group (11.6 versus 10.7, $P = 0.03$). The average time to treatment was 3 hours and 59 minutes in the alteplase group and 3 hours and 58 minutes in the placebo group. Of the patients in the alteplase group, 52% had a favorable outcome (defined as an mRS of ≤ 1) compared with 45.2% in the placebo group ($P < 0.04$). The difference remained significant even after adjustment for the baseline NIHSS score (OR, 1.42; 95% confidence interval, 1.02 to 1.98, $P = 0.04$). The rate of symptomatic ICH was 2.4% in the alteplase group compared with 0.3% in the placebo group ($P = 0.008$).

Some critics argue that the use of the mRS changed significantly between the ECASS II and the ECASS III trials and that the unusually high response rate in the placebo group reflects this secular trend. Others, however, noted the fact that the ECASS III resembled the NINDS trial in important respects—other than the age and severity limits—and that the statistically significant result confirms the original NINDS trial of rt-PA for acute stroke.[61]

On the basis of this study, the European Stroke Organization modified its guidelines to include patients with symptom onset up to 4.5 hours,[62] and other countries are expected to follow. The critical point, however, is that increasing the time window for thrombolysis should increase the number of acute strokes that can be treated with alteplase, not provide a reason to delay treatment. While the ECASS III study shows that alteplase is still effective when given after 3 hours, early treatment is essential because its benefit is time dependent.[57,61]

Community Experience of Thrombolysis for Acute Stroke

On the basis of the results of the two NINDS studies and the post hoc analysis of the ECASS trials, the FDA approved t-PA as treatment for acute ischemic stroke in June 1996. Almost immediately, critics suggested that somehow the trials had been conducted only in specialized stroke centers and therefore the results could not be generalized to the larger stroke population. Despite the fact that the NINDS study included more patients randomly assigned for treatment at community medical centers than in academic centers, a need existed to demonstrate efficacy in community experience. Several such observational studies have now appeared, and the results nearly uniformly confirm those of the ECASS and NINDS studies. If the NINDS protocol is not followed, however, lower response rates and higher hemorrhage rates can be observed. Table 49-3 summarizes the majority of the observational studies to date.

In 1998, Chiu et al[63] published the first *Houston* community experience, which evaluated 30 patients with

acute ischemic stroke who were treated with IV t-PA between December 1995 and December 1996 at a dose of 0.9 mg/kg. The rate of symptomatic ICH was 7%, and the rate of fatal ICH was 3%. On follow-up in December 1996, 37% of patients had recovered to fully independent function (BI, 95 to 100), and 30% of patients had no disability (mRS score, 0 to 1). The 3-month mortality rate was 20% (compared with 17% in the corresponding NINDS group). Three patients were treated outside the 3-hour window. This study concluded that t-PA therapy is a feasible, safe, and effective treatment for acute ischemic stroke in one academic and three community medical centers. There was no difference in any outcome or safety measure between the two types of medical centers.[63]

In 1998, Grond et al[64] published the *Cologne* community experience, in which 100 patients (22% of 453 patients with a presumed diagnosis of stroke) received t-PA; 26 were treated within 90 minutes of stroke onset. The average time from emergency department (ED) arrival to treatment (door-to-needle time) was 48 minutes, and the average arrival time from stroke onset was 78 minutes. At 3 months after t-PA therapy, 53% of patients had recovered with fully independent function (BI, 95 to 100), 40% had no disability (mRS score, 0 to 1), and 42% had an NIHSS score of 0 to 1. Symptomatic ICH occurred in 5%, fatal ICH occurred in 1%, and total ICH occurred in 11%. The mortality rate was 12%. The investigators concluded that thrombolysis was effectively applied in acute stroke treatment with acceptable efforts and that the outcome and complication rates were comparable to those of the NINDS studies.

In 1999, the *Oregon* experience was published.[65] Thirty-three patients with acute ischemic stroke received t-PA within 3 hours of stroke onset. The exclusion criteria were the same as those for the NINDS study, with the addition of excluding patients with ischemic changes of more than one third of the MCA territory on CT. The mean baseline NIHSS score was 16.6, as compared with 14 in the NINDS study. The percentage of patients achieving full or almost full recovery at 3 months, as measured by an mRS score of 0 to 1, was 36.4%, compared with 39% in the NINDS study. Symptomatic ICH occurred in 9.1%, compared with 6.4% in the NINDS trial, and occurred in patients with severe strokes (NIHSS score, ≥ 20). The mortality rate was 18.2% (6.1% secondary to ICH) versus 17% (3% secondary to ICH) in the NINDS study. The Oregon study results were compared with the NINDS study results, and t-PA was found to be a feasible and efficacious treatment.[65]

The initial *Cleveland* community experience with t-PA was published in 2000.[66] It showed more hemorrhages and fewer "responders" than the NINDS study. The objective was to estimate the rate of t-PA use in the community, the outcomes of t-PA treatment, and the incidence of ICH. The study was a chart review that enrolled patients from 29 hospitals in the metropolitan areas of Cleveland, Ohio. An attempt was made to collect all cases prospectively, but most of the cases were actually reviewed in retrospect. Of 3948 patients with acute ischemic strokes seen between 1997 and 1998, 17% were admitted within 3 hours of onset. The median NIHSS score was 12. Only 1.8% received t-PA treatment. Symptomatic hemorrhage

TABLE 49-3 SUMMARY OF THE INTRAVENOUS T-PA STUDIES IN STROKE

Year	Series	N (t-PA)	t-PA mg/kg	S. ICH	T. ICH	Outcome
1992	NINDS (<90 min)[36]	74	0.35-1.08	4%	—	46%[a]
1992	Haley et al (90-180 min)[37]	20	0.6-0.95	10%	—	15%[b]
1992	Mori et al, 6 h[38]	31 (19)	*PH*	*HI*	*T.ICH*	*mean HSS[c]*
		20 MIU	*11%*	*56%*	*67%*	*−9 (±18.6)*
		30 MIU	*10%*	*30%*	*40%*	*−20.3 (±19.4)*
		Pl.	*8%*	*33%*	*42%*	*−29.7(±27.7)*
1993	Bridging Trial, 3 h[39]	27 (14)	0.85	0% for t-PA <90 min	—	57% t-PA 15% Pl.[d]
1995	ECASS, 6 h[40]	620 (313)	1.1	—	43% t-PA Pl. 37%	35.7% t-PA 29.3% Pl.[e]
1995	NINDS, 3 h[1]	624 (312)	0.9	6.4% 0.6% Pl.	—	39% t-PA 26% Pl.(ss)[f]
1997	ECASS-II 6 h[47]	800 (409)	0.9	8.8% t-PA 3.4% Pl.	—	40.3% t-PA 36.6% Pl.[g]
1997	ECASS-II Post hoc[47]	—	—	—	—	54.3% t-PA 46% Pl. (ss)[h]
1998	Houston, 3 h[63]	30	0.9	7%	10%	30%[i]
1998	Cologne, 3 h[64]	100	0.9	5%	11%	40%[j]
1998	Lyon, 7 h[74]	100	0.8		7%	45%[k]
1999	Oregon, 3 h[65]	33	0.9	9.1%		36.4%[l]
1999 (1991-1993)	ATLANTIS-A (6 h)[53]	142 (71)	0.9	11% t-PA 0% Pl.	—	40% t-PA 21% Pl.[m]
1999 (1993-1998)	ATLANTIS-B (3-5 h)[54]	547 (272)	0.9	7% t-PA 1.1% Pl.	—	34% t-PA 32% Pl.[n]
2000	Cleveland, 3 h[66]	70	0.9	15.7%	—	Increased death[o]
2000	STARS, 3 h[68]	389	0.9	3.3%	11.5%	35%[p]
2000	Vancouver, 3 h[69]	46	0.9	2.2% (36 h)	—	43%[q]
2001	Berlin, 3 h[71]	75	0.9	—	2.7%	40%[r]
2001	Calgary, 3 h[70]	84	0.9	7.1%	—	54%[s]
2001	Houston, 3 h[72]	269	0.9	5.6%[t]	—	—
2002	ATLANTIS<3 h[55]	61 (23)	0.9	13% t-PA 0% Pl.	—	t-PA 60.9% Pl. 26.3%[u]
2002	CASES, 3 h[73]	1099	0.9	4.6%	—	46%[v]
In press	Lyon, 7 h[76]	200	0.8	5.5%		35%[w]

ATLANTIS, Alteplase Thrombolysis for Acute Noninterventional Therapy in Ischemic Stroke Study; ATLANTIS-A, ATLANTIS Part A; ATLANTIS-B, ATLANTIS Part B; CASES, Canadian Activase for Stroke Effectiveness Study; ECASS, European Cooperative Acute Stroke Study; h, hour; HI, hemorrhagic infarct; HSS, hemispheric stroke scale at day 30 (mean from baseline); min, minute; mRS, modified Rankin Scale; NIH, National Institutes of Health; NIHSS, National Institutes of Health Stroke Scale; NINDS, National Institute of Neurological Diseases and Stroke; N(t-PA), total number of patients (patients who received t-PA); PH, parenchymal hematoma; Pl., placebo; S. ICH, symptomatic intracerebral hemorrhage; ss, statistically significant; STARS, Standard Treatment with Alteplase to Reverse Stroke trial; T. ICH, total intracerebral hemorrhage; t-PA, tissue-type plasminogen activator. Superscript numbers indicate chapter references.

[a]NIHSS improvement ≥4 at 24 h.
[b]As in (a).
[c]Every 500,000 MIU of t-PA corresponds to 1 mg. HSS ranges from 0 to 100.
[d]As in (a). ICH was 0% for the group who received t-PA within 90 min from onset.
[e]Identical median mRS = 3 for t-PA and the placebo group; 35.7% of t-PA patients with mRS ≤2 versus 29.3% in the placebo group (intention-to-treat analysis).
[f]Percent of patients with mRS ≤1 at 3 months in the t-PA and placebo groups; ss, statistically significant difference (better in t-PA group).
[g]mRS ≤1 at 90 days. No statistically significant difference between t-PA and placebo.
[h]Statistically significant difference between t-PA and placebo groups for mRS ≤2.
[i]mRS ≤1 on follow-up in Dec. 1996 of all 30 patients. Enrollment was between Dec. 1995-Dec. 1996.
[j]mRS ≤1 at 3 months.
[k]mRS ≤1 at day 90.
[l]mRS ≤1 at 3 months.
[m]NIHSS ≤1 at 90 days.
[n]NIHSS ≤1 at 90 days.
[o]Increased protocol violations and deaths. Only 1.8% were treated with t-PA.
[p]mRS ≤1 at 30 days.
[q]mRS ≤1 at 13 months.
[r]mRS ≤1 at 3 months.
[s]mRS ≤2 at 3 months.
[t]Mean baseline NIHSS 14.4(±6.1). At 24 hours mean NIHSS 10(±8). Mean discharge NIHSS 7(±7).
[u]NIHSS ≤1 at 90 days. Post-hoc analysis of the ATLANTIS patients who received t-PA within 3 hours from onset.
[v]Independent (mRS ≤2) at 90 days.
[w]mRS ≤1 at 3 months.

occurred in 15.7% of the patients given t-PA, but 50% of the cases with t-PA treatment had protocol violations. Deviations from the protocol included use of antiplatelet agents or anticoagulants within 24 hours of treatment with t-PA, treatment beyond the 3-hour window, and deviation from the blood pressure guidelines. The in-hospital mortality rate and the length of hospital stay were significantly higher in the t-PA group.

The differences between the initial Cleveland community survey and all others probably are due in part to differences in methodology. In this trial, nurse abstractors attempted to find cases after the fact; a case ascertainment bias toward difficult cases with memorable adverse outcomes would be hard to avoid. In other series, cases of stroke were collected prospectively by the stroke team physicians.

The Cleveland group published a second report of the Cleveland community experience with IV t-PA.[67] This was a retrospective chart review of all patients with ischemic stroke who presented to the Cleveland Clinic Health System between June 2000 and June 2001. A stroke quality improvement (SQI) program had been implemented before that, starting in 1999. The SQI included very frequent review of acute stroke data, performance monitoring, implementation of stroke protocol in the ED, a 24-hour stroke beeper, and medical education about acute stroke management and IV t-PA use. The results showed that IV t-PA was given in 18.8% of patients who arrived within the 3-hour time window. Protocol deviations occurred in 19.1% of those patients who received t-PA; symptomatic ICH occurred in 6.4%, which is a rate that is comparable with that in the NINDS study. The authors concluded that IV t-PA could be given safely to appropriate patients with stroke at the community hospital level.[67]

In summary, the higher rate of protocol violations in the initial Cleveland community experience had led to the higher frequency of adverse events. Moreover, after extensive education and retraining, the symptomatic ICH rate and protocol violations declined in Cleveland.

The results of the *STARS* (Standard Treatment with Alteplase to Reverse Stroke) study were published in March 2000; Albers et al[68] looked at 389 consecutive patients with stroke enrolled between February 1997 and December 1998 from different academic and community hospitals in the United States. Those patients were seen with acute ischemic stroke within 3 hours of onset. The median NIHSS score was 13. Protocol violations occurred in 127 patients (32.6%). The violations were anticoagulant use, treatment outside the recommended period, and nonadherence to blood pressure guidelines. The measure of recovery was mRS score at 30 days after t-PA treatment; the mRS score was ≤1 in 35% of patients and ≤2 (independence) in 43% of patients. Symptomatic ICH occurred in 3.3% of patients, and asymptomatic ICH occurred in 8.2%. This study showed favorable clinical outcomes with t-PA treatment and a relatively low rate of symptomatic hemorrhage, comparable with that of the NINDS studies.[68]

In December 2000, the *Vancouver* study was published. Chapman et al[69] studied 46 consecutive patients with ischemic stroke (combined retrospective and prospective study) who received t-PA within the 3-hour time window. The NINDS inclusion and exclusion criteria were applied. Symptomatic ICH at 36 hours occurred in 2.2% of patients. At 13-months' follow-up, 22% of patients were dead (similar to NINDS results); 43% of patients had a favorable outcome, consisting of an mRS score of 0 to 1, and 48% had a BI of 95 to 100.[69]

In April 2001, Barber et al[70] published the *Calgary* experience, in which 2165 consecutive patients with acute stroke in Calgary, Canada, treated between October 1996 and December 1999 were studied. Of these patients, 1168 (53.9%) were given a diagnosis of ischemic stroke. Hemorrhagic stroke was diagnosed in 31.8%, and TIAs were diagnosed in 13.9%. Of the 1168 patients with ischemic stroke, 73.1% were excluded from the study because of delayed presentation. Causes for delay included uncertain time of onset (24.2%), waiting to see whether the deficit would improve (29%), transfer from another hospital (8.9%), and poor accessibility to the treating hospital (patient's home a long distance from the treating hospital or transfer of patients from an outlying hospital) (5.7%). Of the 1168 patients with ischemic stroke, 314 patients (27%) were admitted to the hospital within 3 hours of onset, and 84 of the 314 (26.7%) received IV t-PA. Exclusion of the rest of the patients seen within the 3-hour window was due to different reasons: 13.1% had mild strokes, 18.2% showed clinical improvement, 13.6% had other protocol exclusions, 8.9% experienced ED referral delay, and 8.3% had significant morbidity. At 3 months, 54% of the patients included in the study had an mRS score ≤ 2. The symptomatic ICH rate was 7.1%. Only 4.7% of all patients seen during the study period were treated with t-PA; the majority of t-PA treatment exclusions were related to a delay in presentation. Of those patients whose strokes were considered too mild to be treated or who showed rapid improvement, 32% either remained dependent on hospital discharge or died during hospital admission. This finding implied that a third of the patients who were excluded because of minimal deficits or dramatic improvement had poor outcomes, which raises the question of whether such patients should also be treated.

In May 2001, the *Berlin* study was published.[71] Cases of acute ischemic stroke were collected over 2 years; only 75 of the patients, or 9.4%, received IV t-PA. The median baseline NIHSS score was 13 ± 6. Average time for initiation of thrombolysis was 144 minutes from onset; 17% of patients were treated after 3 hours of onset. Cerebral hemorrhages occurred in 2.7%. The outcome at 3 months was good (mRS score, 0 to 1) in 40%, moderate (mRS score, 2 to 3) in 32%, and poor (mRS score, 4 to 5) in 13%. The mortality rate was 15%. It was noticed in this study that, over time, the median door-to-CT time and door-to-needle time shortened and the number of patients treated per month increased from two to four. The investigators, Koennecke et al,[71] concluded that IV t-PA is safe and efficacious and that the performance of the stroke team and the number of patients enrolled can improve with time.

In an article published in December 2001, Grotta et al[72] described their own *Houston* community experience with t-PA treatment in patients with acute ischemic stroke between January 1996 and June 2000. The design was a prospective inception cohort registry of patients seen by the stroke team at the University of Texas–Houston Medical School and three community hospitals in addition to a retrospective medical record review of all patients treated with t-PA within the same 4-year period. A total of 269 patients were treated, representing 15% of all patients who were seen with acute ischemic stroke during the study period. The mean door-to-needle time was 70 minutes, and 28% of patients were treated within 2 hours of onset. The symptomatic ICH rate was 4.5%. Protocol violations occurred in 13% of all treated patients, and patients with protocol violations had an ICH rate of 15%. The mean NIHSS score was 14.4 ± 6.1 before treatment, 10 ± 8 at 24 hours, and 7 ± 7 on discharge. The in-hospital mortality rate was 15%. These investigators concluded that IV t-PA could be given in up to 15% of patients with acute ischemic stroke with a low risk of intracerebral bleeding; they also concluded that successful experience with such treatment depends not only on the experience and organization of the treating team but also on following the treatment protocol.[72]

In May 2002, the final results of the Canadian Activase for Stroke Effectiveness Study (CASES) were published.[73] A total of 1099 stroke patients who were treated with IV t-PA were enrolled between February 1999 and June 2001. The median baseline NIHSS score was 15 (range, 2 to 40). On follow-up evaluation at 90 days after the stroke, 30% of those patients had minimal or no residual neurologic deficit, and 46% were independent (mRS, 0 to 2). The ICH rate was 4.6%. Protocol violations occurred in 15%. Predictors of outcome were baseline NIHSS, baseline ASPECT score (evaluates the radiologic changes of stroke on brain CT), patient age, atrial fibrillation, and the patient's baseline serum sugar level. Predictors of ICH were mean arterial blood pressure as well as baseline serum glucose level. The CASES group concluded that IV alteplase (Activase) is safe and efficacious in Canada.[73]

The *Lyon* trial was a phase 2 trial of thrombolysis using a protocol that was very different from that of the NINDS study: The t-PA dose was 0.8 mg/kg; 10% of the dose was given as an IV bolus, and the remaining 90% was given as IV drip over 1 hour after that.[74] The time window for t-PA administration was 7 hours after stroke; the majority of patients received the t-PA within 3 to 6 hours. Heparin or LMW heparin was also given. The initial results of the first 100 patients were published in 1998[74]: at 90 days, 45% of the patients had good results (mRS score, 0 to 1), 18% had a moderate outcome (mRS score, 2 to 3), and 31% of patients had serious neurologic outcomes (mRS score, 4 to 5). Of the 11 patients treated within 6 to 7 hours of stroke onset, 45% had good results. Death occurred in 6% of the patients, two of whom had intracerebral hematoma after having received IV heparin within the first 24 hours. The intracerebral hematoma rate was 7%. The results of the Lyon trial were updated in an abstract published in 2002.[75] The rate of good outcome (mRS score, ≤1) at 5 years was 37.4%. The mortality rate was 23.9%. Further later data analysis available to us evaluated a total of 200 patients in the Lyon trial.[76] The rate of good outcomes (mRS score, 0 and 1) was 35% at 3 months. The rate of parenchymal anatomic hematoma within 7 days was 9%, and that of symptomatic hematomas was 5.5%. Mortality at 3 months occurred in 11.5%. Independent predictive factors of poor outcomes appeared to be structured hypodensity on Day 1 CT, hyperdense MCA sign, internal carotid thrombosis, gray–white matter indistinction, no IV heparin within 24 hours or after 24 hours, the use of LMW heparin, and the use of mannitol.

Guidelines for Intravenous Thrombolysis in Acute Stroke

Given the relationship between adverse events and protocol violations, it is important to understand the NINDS protocol for the use of t-PA in acute stroke. The study was originally intended to be a phase 2B confirmatory dose-finding and safety study, not a definitive phase 3 protocol, but because it proved efficacy, no further phase 3 trial was pursued. Therefore, the protocol contains some idiosyncrasies that were never intended to be included in the FDA package insert.

Treatment Protocol

Patients should be seen within the 3-hour window of stroke onset.[77] Thrombolysis should not be implemented unless (1) the stroke diagnosis is established by a physician with expertise in stroke and (2) brain CT is assessed by a physician with expertise in reading this imaging study. A total dose of 0.9 mg/kg of recombinant t-PA is given, not to exceed a maximal dose of 90 mg. The first 10% of the dose is given as an IV bolus, and the rest of the dose (90%) is given as an IV drip over the following hour. A list of inclusion and exclusion criteria is used to determine whether a patient should be given t-PA. These criteria were defined by the NINDS study (see Table 49-2) and were adopted nearly verbatim by the FDA, even though they were not intended for clinical use.[77] At this time, it is important to follow these guidelines, but the physician's judgment is required in individual cases.

Expedited Treatment Protocol

Although studies are now beginning to show that alteplase may be safely given beyond the 3-hour window, the chance of a favorable outcome diminishes with time; thus treatment should still be rendered as soon as possible. In 2006, Sattin et al[78] demonstrated that alteplase could be safely given using an expedited protocol with a benchmark onset-to-treatment time of less than 2 hours. This protocol avoids delays pending coagulation studies or platelet count, unless clinically indicated, and allows no delays pending a formal CT interpretation by a radiologist. Between July 2003 and June 2005, 781 patients were evaluated for acute stroke with the use of this protocol, and 103 patients (13.2%) received t-PA. Of those patients treated with alteplase, 49 (47.6%) were treated within 2 hours of symptom onset. The overall rate of symptomatic hemorrhage in the group treated in less than 2 hours was two of 49 (4.1%), which was not significantly different from the rate of 6.4% in the NINDS trial ($P = 0.42$) or from the group treated between 2 and 3 hours, who had a rate of two of 54 (3.7%). While this study demonstrated that an expedited protocol is feasible and appears safe, it reflects the experience in only one institution; thus its generalization to other centers cannot be made.

Although it is important to follow the guidelines, a physician's judgment is required in individual cases, especially in those cases in which the safety of thrombolysis is not known. Many physicians may also decide to administer alteplase in extreme situations in which the benefits seem to outweigh the risks, despite a contraindication. As experience with alteplase increases, it is likely that there will be more circumstances in which patients are deliberately or inadvertently given alteplase in "off-label" situations. In 2007, Aleu et al[79] performed a literature review that identified 273 patients who received off-labeled IV or intraarterial t-PA for acute ischemic stroke. Hemorrhagic complications occurred in a total of 36 patients; 19 of 273 patients (6.95%) had a symptomatic ICH and 17 of 273 (6.22%) had extracranial hemorrhages.

Patients are excluded for any of the exclusion criteria; we consider some of the more important criteria in the following discussion.

Use of Oral Anticoagulants, Prothrombin Time Longer than 15 Seconds, or International Normalized Ratio 1.7 or Greater

This criterion is obviously needed to exclude patients receiving anticoagulation therapy. In the original trial,[1] any patient was excluded who had consumed any oral warfarin (Coumadin) in the previous day, no matter what the prothrombin time might be at the time of the stroke. The final package insert was written in such a way, however, as to allow thrombolysis even if the patient has taken warfarin recently; the criterion is only that the international normalized ratio (INR) be less than 1.7. The physician confronted with this situation must use judgment and must proceed thoughtfully; however, generally, we recommend thrombolytic treatment if the INR is below the stated limit even if the patient has taken warfarin before the stroke occurred. In routine practice, physicians *should not wait* for INR results before beginning the rt-PA bolus, unless some clinical clue suggests that the patient may have below-normal coagulation status.

Use of Heparin in the Last 24 Hours with a Prolonged Partial Thromboplastin Time

This is an absolute contraindication, given the potential risk of hemorrhaging. We are aware of anecdotal cases in which heparin was reversed with protamine, and t-PA was given after the partial thromboplastin time was recorded as normal. Because this approach has never been studied for safety, we cannot recommend it and do not use it routinely in our own practice. We are also aware of many cases in which reocclusion occurs after successful thrombolysis; preliminary data using serial transcranial ultrasonography has indicated that the reocclusion rate may be as high as 27%.[80] Certainly, after coronary thrombolysis, heparin is required to maintain vessel patency. We believe that further study on this point is warranted.

Platelet Count Less than 100,000 cells/mm³

The limit of 100,000 cells/mm³ for the platelet count is arbitrary and was chosen by the NINDS investigators on the basis of limited review of literature and consultation with hematologists. No one knows, however, how many functioning platelets are needed to protect a patient from hemorrhaging during thrombolysis. The physician should exercise caution and judgment; in some situations, it may be wise to treat a patient with a platelet count below the limit.

Prior Stroke within the Last 3 Months

The time limit on prior stroke was set somewhat arbitrarily at 3 months, and no mention is made of severity. For example, does a minor motor lacune with signs lasting 3 days and resolving completely contraindicate thrombolytic therapy for 3 months? The physician must use considerable judgment in individual cases and consider the following questions:

- How mild was the prior stroke?
- Did it resolve completely or partially?
- How long ago was the prior stroke?
- What is the potential for bleeding into the prior stroke if thrombolysis is used today?

There may be situations in which the benefit of treating the current stroke outweighs the risk due to recent, resolved minor stroke.

Head Trauma within the Last 3 Months

The considerations applying to this exclusion criterion are similar to those mentioned for prior stroke. The guidelines do not mention severity. The critical question for the clinician is as follows: how likely is the previous head trauma to predispose the patient to bleeding if thrombolysis is given now? The benefit of thrombolysis for the current event may outweigh the potential risks of bleeding after minor head trauma in the previous 3 months.

Major Surgery within the Last 14 Days

This contraindication is generally absolute, although we often consult with the surgeon who performed the surgery before making the decision. Often the devastation of the current stroke outweighs any harm that could be caused by rebleeding at the operative site. An individual exception to this exclusion rule could be considered in rare cases after careful consideration and discussion with the patient or family or both regarding the risks of hemorrhage.

Pretreatment Systolic Blood Pressure Greater than 185 mm Hg or Diastolic Blood Pressure Greater than 110 mm Hg

This exclusion criterion is absolute. If gentle antihypertensive therapy, such as 10 to 20 mg of IV labetalol, or an infusion of 5 mg/h nicardipine does not bring the blood pressure under the limits, no thrombolytic agents should be used. Hypertension at the time of thrombolysis has been shown to predict hemorrhagic transformation. On the other hand, the careful physician should be aware that most patients with stroke have elevated blood pressure on arrival at the ED. The first blood pressure values obtained by paramedics or the triage nurse must not be used to exclude the patient from t-PA therapy. The patient should be allowed to acclimate to the ED for a few minutes; often, the blood pressure declines spontaneously. The patient who exhibits persistent hypertension despite the passage of time and gentle antihypertensive therapy should always be excluded from t-PA treatment.

Rapidly Improving Neurologic Signs

This exclusion criteria causes considerable discomfort for most physicians because stroke symptoms wax and wane over the first few hours. To qualify as rapidly improving, the symptoms must improve monotonically and dramatically. Patients whose deficits oscillate from severe to mild or who show only slight improvement should be treated. Generally, patients with TIA have complete resolution of symptoms within 1 or 2 hours. Patients who show only slight improvement over the first hour should be treated. The risk of ICH associated with thrombolytic treatment in a patient with TIA appears to be extremely low.[81] In an observational study by Odzemir et al,[82] 13 patients with marked clinical fluctuations defined as an increase or decrease on the NIHSS of 4 points were treated with alteplase. Only one patient had an asymptomatic hemorrhage, and all patients had a favorable functional outcome.

Isolated Mild Neurologic Deficits

Patients with isolated mild neurologic deficits, such as isolated ataxia, isolated hemisensory loss, or isolated dysarthria, tend to recover completely with little residual effect. This criterion assumes a careful neurologic examination and a search for symptoms that could easily be overlooked, such as quadrantanopsia, hemispatial neglect, and mild expressive aphasia. The only patients who should be excluded from t-PA therapy are those with pure sensory or isolated ataxic symptoms. Also, individual judgment must be used; an isolated, mild expressive aphasia could end the career of a patient who speaks for a living. We routinely consider treating mild aphasia if the patient works in an occupation such as teaching, television broadcasting, or therapy. Likewise, an isolated hemianopsia could end some careers, such as truck or taxi driving, and treatment could be considered. Mild symptoms other than pure dysarthria or sensory deficit are associated with adverse outcomes. As mentioned earlier, of the patients studied by Barber et al[70] whose deficits were considered mild or were rapidly improving, 32% were dependent at hospital discharge or died during hospital admission. Therefore, unless the symptoms are truly isolated to a purely sensory deficit or dysarthria, the patient should be treated. This study was confirmed by Smith et al[83]: of all stroke patients arriving at one institution within 3 hours, 34% were not given thrombolytic therapy because of mild deficits; of these, 27% had poor functional outcomes.

Prior or Current Intracerebral Hemorrhage

This contraindication is relative: if the patient has ever had an ICH, thrombolysis should not be used if the cause was such that thrombolytic therapy is likely to promote rebleeding. Individual exceptions may be considered if the bleeding was due to some nonrecurring condition, such as remote history of posttraumatic subdural hematoma that is proven to be resolved.

Blood Glucose Level Less than 50 mg/dL or Greater than 400 mg/dL

Hypoglycemia should be treated with glucose replacement; the deficit will most likely resolve, but if it does not, then thrombolysis could be considered. Hypoglycemia mimics stroke in 1.7% of cases.[84] On the other hand, incidental hypoglycemia could accompany a stroke and should not exclude the patient from therapy if the neurologic deficit persists despite blood glucose correction. Hyperglycemia is associated with increased hemorrhage risk and very low rates of successful outcome. Again, if insulin therapy brings the glucose value down to an acceptable level, it would theoretically be permissible to treat with t-PA. This approach has not been studied, however, and cannot be recommended in routine practice.

Seizure at the Onset of Stroke

The purpose of this exclusion is to ensure that post-ictal paralysis is not mistaken for stroke. In actual practice, some patients with stroke do suffer tonic or clonic jerks, which witnesses may report to paramedics or the physicians as seizures. Generally, post-ictal paralysis occurs in a patient with a known seizure disorder who has a typical tonic-clonic convulsion. Physicians must sort out from witnesses what actually occurred and whether the movements were tonic–clonic. There is probably little risk, however, in giving a thrombolytic to a patient with no stroke and post-ictal paralysis; one could argue for erring on the side of treatment, reasoning that failure to treat the patient with true ischemic stroke could result in much greater harm.

Gastrointestinal or Genitourinary Bleeding

Excluding patients with gastrointestinal or genitourinary bleeding from thrombolytic therapy is necessary because thrombolysis could activate bleeding from sources in the gastrointestinal or genitourinary tract. On the other hand, many patients consider blood loss inconsequential compared with the devastating effects of stroke. It is important to consider the nature of the bleeding, how recently it occurred, and how difficult it might be to control if it were to recur. Women with active menstruation and menometrorrhagia have been successfully and safely treated with t-PA for acute stroke, after consultation with the gynecologist, because an urgent uterine artery embolization or ligation could easily be performed to halt uncontrollable bleeding.[85] Giving such therapy to a patient with colonic polyposis or diverticulosis, however, could result in bleeding that would be far less easily controlled. Considerable physician judgment is required in this setting, and full discussion with the patient or family or both about the potential risks and benefits is essential.

Recent Myocardial Infarction

This is an absolute contraindication because of the possibility of pericardial rupture and tamponade. No specific time limit is specified, but *recent* is generally considered to be on the order of weeks. As with other exclusion criteria, one must consider the size of the myocardial infarct, the treatment given, and the current status of the patient in assessing the potential risk of cardiac rupture in a specific case.

Additional Treatment Considerations

Thrombolytic treatment should not be given unless ancillary care and the facility to handle bleeding complications are present, best provided in an intensive care unit setting. We are aware of many stroke units and "step-down" care units that are perfectly appropriate for monitoring patients after thrombolysis. Vital signs and neurologic examinations (neuro-checks) are required for monitoring the patient for blood loss (causing hypotension), hypertension above the posttreatment limits, neurologic deterioration (suggesting hemorrhage or reocclusion), and other complications of stroke.

Risks and benefits of thrombolytic treatment should be explained to the family, and consent should be obtained. Consent can be waived if the patient is not fit to give it and no family member is available. We recommend, however, that if any deviation from the protocol is contemplated, full consent from the family be obtained before it is initiated.

Early Computed Tomography Findings Are Not Contraindications to Treatment

In 1997, von Kummer et al[86] analyzed the ECASS data and concluded that the clinical severity of stroke could be associated with hemorrhagic infarction and that the risk of hemorrhagic infarction might be increased when early CT changes indicating hypoattenuation and mass effect are detected. It was clear that hemorrhaging and death occurred more frequently in patients with early ischemic changes constituting more than one third of the MCA territory. They also concluded that rising age and treatment with t-PA were related to the risk of increased parenchymal hemorrhaging. However, the analysis was post hoc and therefore should have served to generate hypotheses, not guide patient care. Furthermore, the finding was not statistically significant, even in the first report. Unfortunately, the logical caveats expressed by these investigators in their report went unheeded, and the result has been widely applied as a common reason not to treat patients who would otherwise qualify.

In a retrospective analysis, the NINDS group looked at early ischemic changes (EICs) on baseline CT scans and tried to correlate them with outcome, CT lesion volume at 3 months, development of symptomatic ICH, and negative or positive interaction with t-PA treatment.[87] The EICs based on von Kummer's original report were (1) loss of distinction between gray matter and white matter, (2) hypodensity or hypoattenuation on baseline CT, or (3) compression of cerebrospinal fluid spaces (sulcal effacement). The hyperdense MCA sign was not included. Overall, EICs were present in 35% of the patients given placebo and in 28% of the patients given t-PA (similar in the two groups; $P = 0.09$). There was a strong association between stroke severity as measured by the NIHSS and the incidence of EICs; after correction for the NIHSS variable, however, there was no proven interaction between t-PA treatment and EIC. In other words, there was no higher risk associated with t-PA treatment when EICs were present on baseline CT. The patients given t-PA seemed to have a better outcome regardless of whether they had EICs. The findings are summarized in Figure 49-8. The

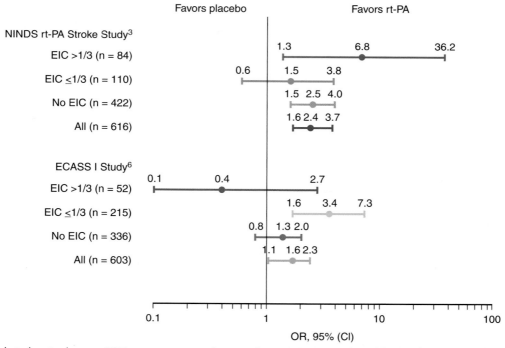

Figure 49-8 Early ischemic changes (EIC) are not contraindications for t-PA treatment. The odds ratio from ECASS for patients with EIC of more than one third of the middle cerebral artery vascular territory shows that there was no statistical difference in bad outcome between the t-PA and placebo groups in the presence of these early ischemic changes but that there was benefit with t-PA treatment in the NINDS for Acute Stroke Trial even in the presence of these early ischemic changes. (From Patel S, Levine S, Tilley B, et al: Lack of clinical significance of early ischemic changes on computed tomography in acute stroke. *JAMA* 286:2830-2838, 2001.)

investigators in this study concluded that the presence of EICs should not be contraindications in the decision for t-PA treatment if the patient otherwise meets eligibility criteria. They also commented that the analysis of the ECASS data and conclusions about EICs prohibiting treatment should have been established after correction for the variable of stroke severity. Gilligan et al[88] published similar results arising from the reanalysis of the ASK trial in 2002. The authors found that predictors of major hemorrhage were SK treatment and elevated systolic blood pressure before treatment (>165 mm Hg); however, EICs less than one third or more than one third of MCA territory were not associated with major hemorrhaging.

In an attempt to reconcile the two positions and the contradiction between the analyses of the two studies (ECASS and NINDS), we may argue that the implication of ischemic changes in more than one third of the MCA territory on early CT might be different beyond 3 hours (ECASS) than they would be within 3 hours (NINDS). In the latter case, a substantial portion of the remaining two thirds of the MCA territory might be hypoperfused but still salvageable if lysis of the clot is successful, which might result in a clinical benefit to offset the risk of bleeding. Beyond 3 hours, however, a smaller ischemic area might still be penumbral and have less of a hypothetical volumetric mismatch between the hypoperfused area and the irreversibly injured area.

It appears, therefore, that the CT findings should be used with caution in selecting patients for thrombolytic therapy. Certainly, a hemorrhage contraindicates therapy. Areas of marked hypodensity, suggesting that the stroke is more than 3 hours old, should give the physician pause. Mild EIC such as sulcal effacement, loss of gray–white matter distinction, or loss of the so-called insular ribbon sign, no matter how large a portion of the MCA territory is involved, should not necessarily contraindicate therapy if the patient otherwise qualifies for treatment. Presence of the so-called hyperdense MCA sign, or hyperdense dot sign,[89] should not be regarded as a contraindication to therapy either, although the prospects for a good outcome are very low in this setting, regardless of the type of treatment. Figure 49-9 demonstrates the CT of a 40-year-old man with the different CT signs mentioned and EICs at baseline and 24 hours after thrombolysis.

Considerable research is ongoing to find imaging variables that may guide selection of treatment. It is probably true that many patients with remaining salvageable brain tissue are deprived of useful treatment if physicians strictly adhere to the 3-hour time limit. Similarly, it is clear that many patients do not have salvageable brain tissue even earlier than 3 hours after stroke onset. There remains a need for a truly reliable, rapid, and widely available imaging method that will indicate when brain tissue becomes irretrievably damaged. Many techniques, such as magnetic resonance imaging (MRI) diffusion and perfusion techniques, have been proposed and are under intense evaluation. To date, however, no imaging modality has proved better for selection of patients for particular therapies than existing published clinical criteria.

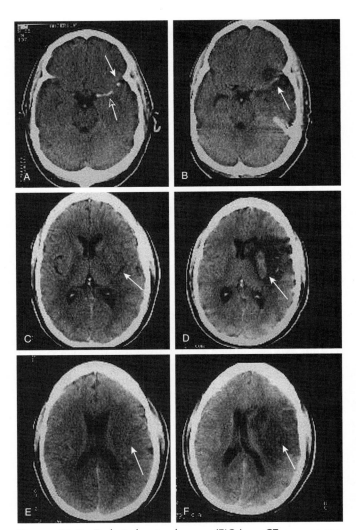

Figure 49-9 Early ischemic changes (EICs) on CT are not contraindications for thrombolysis. This is the brain CT of a 40-year-old man with acute left hemispheric stroke on presentation (A, C, and E) and 48 hours after thrombolysis (B, D, and F). A, A linear hyperdense middle cerebral artery (MCA) sign *(open head white arrow)* and a hyperdense dot MCA sign *(closed head white arrow)*, on presentation. B, The hyperdense MCA sign 48 hours later. C, Portrays loss of the left insular ribbon as one of the early ischemic changes. D, Portrays an island of relative hyperdensity within the stroke bed that might be either hemorrhagic transformation or an island of spared nonischemic brain tissue within the ischemic bed at 24 hours after thrombolysis. E, Portrays ischemic-related hypodense changes in the MCA territory on presentation. F, Portrays progression of the hypodense ischemic changes at 48 hours.

Effect of Time to Thrombolytic Treatment

Thrombolytic therapy should be administered within 3 hours from time of onset, as discussed before, but a 2000 analysis of the NINDS study data showed that the benefit of treatment was higher when t-PA was given earlier in this time window.[90] This analysis showed that patients treated within 90 minutes of stroke onset had greater odds of improvement at 24 hours and a higher favorable 3-month outcome than patients treated between 91 and 180 minutes after onset. The time of treatment within

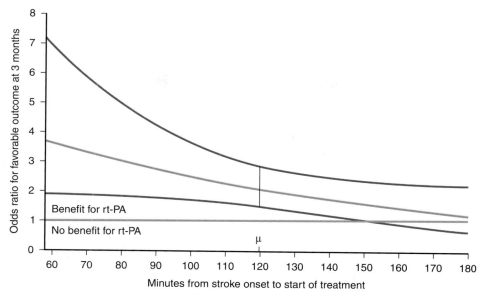

Figure 49-10   Time to treatment effect: This figure shows that t-PA benefit disappears as the time from onset to t-PA treatment approaches 3 hours. (From Marler J, Tilley B, Lu M, et al: Early stroke treatment associated with better outcome: The NINDS rt-PA Stroke Study. *Neurology* 55:1649-1655, 2000.)

3 hours had no effect on the ICH rate.[90] Therefore, the earliest possible treatment is recommended, not for fear of ICH but because of decreased benefit with later treatment. Figure 49-10 shows that the OR for a favorable outcome approaches 1 as the time to treatment approaches 3 hours (the benefit of t-PA is greater than that of placebo if the OR is greater than 1, as depicted in the graph).[90]

Generalized Efficacy of t-Pa for Acute Stroke

A post hoc analysis of the NINDS data was conducted to try to establish whether any factors might have had negative interactions with t-PA treatment or, in other words, to identify any pretreatment patient information that significantly affected the patient's response to t-PA treatment.[91] The investigators included 27 baseline variables to check for possible interaction with t-PA treatment. These variables were age, race, sex, cigarette smoking, alcohol abuse, diabetes mellitus, hypertension, baseline NIHSS score, percentage of correct t-PA dose received, history of atherosclerosis, history of atrial fibrillation, history of other cardiac disease, prior stroke, aspirin administration, baseline stroke subtype, early CT findings, presence or absence of thrombus, weight, admission and baseline mean arterial blood pressure, admission and baseline systolic as well as admission and baseline diastolic blood pressure, centers of treatment, time from stroke onset to treatment, and admission temperature. This analysis also tested interactions among these factors and among confounding variables. Independent of t-PA therapy, outcome was related to age by deficit or age by NIHSS score, diabetes, age by blood pressure interaction, and early CT findings. These factors and their interactions altered the patient's long-term outcome but did not alter the likelihood of a favorable response to t-PA treatment; the efficacy of t-PA as shown by the NINDS data were generalized to all subgroups. The investigators concluded that treatment

for patients with acute stroke should be selected according to the NINDS guidelines and that further subselection is not supported.[91]

Recanalization and Arterial Reocclusion after t-Pa Treatment

Early studies by del Zoppo et al[35] and Mori et al,[38] as described earlier, showed that IV t-PA could recanalize the cerebral vessels on angiograms. Further data have been published to support their conclusions. In 2002, Alexandrov et al[92] published the results of a series of 60 consecutively treated patients with occlusion of the M1 or M2 segment of the MCA who received t-PA (bolus followed by IV infusion) and were monitored by transcranial Doppler ultrasonography for 2 hours after t-PA treatment. The median prebolus NIHSS score was 16, and the median time to administration of the bolus was 120 minutes; 58% of patients received the t-PA within the first 2 hours. Recanalization was complete in 30% (18 patients), partial in 48% (29 patients), and null in 22% (13 patients). Early reocclusion occurred in 34% of patients given t-PA who experienced any initial recanalization, accounting for two thirds of deteriorations after improvement. Note that reocclusion occurred more often in patients with earlier and partial recanalization, along with secondary neurologic deterioration and higher in-hospital mortality. Nevertheless, patients with reocclusion had better long-term outcomes than patients without any early recanalization.[92]

Management During and After Thrombolytic Treatment[77]

As mentioned before, the patient should be admitted to a skilled care unit, such as an intensive care unit or a stroke care unit that provides close observation, careful cardiovascular monitoring, and frequent neurologic evaluations. Blood pressure should be monitored and controlled carefully during the treatment and the following 24 hours. An excessively high blood pressure might predispose the patient to bleeding intracranially, whereas low blood pressure might worsen cerebral ischemia. According to American Heart Association recommendations, blood pressure should be monitored every 15 minutes for 2 hours from the start of t-PA infusion, then every 30 minutes for 6 hours, then every 60 minutes over the rest of the 24 hours after initiation of t-PA treatment.[77]

The protocol for blood pressure treatment after thrombolysis is listed in Table 49-4. Recommended drugs listed in the table were selected because of their rapid onset of action and their predictable effects with a low potential for overshooting.[93] Note that in the NINDS study, these medications were used, in addition to other medications such as IV nicardipine, hydralazine, sublingual nifedipine, and sustained-release or topical nitroglycerin.[94] Furthermore, although abrupt substantial declines in mean arterial pressure have been shown to reduce cerebral flow, the threshold below which it is unsafe to lower mean arterial pressure is unknown. The blood pressure eligibility criteria that were applied are similar to those used in the t-PA dose-finding trial. The blood pressure management algorithm was used because of the low incidence of symptomatic hemorrhaging in the pilot study and recognition of the potential link between high blood pressure and ICH.[36,37]

Post hoc analyses of data from the NINDS study have shown that, after randomization but not before, blood pressure treatment was associated with a less favorable 3-month outcome in the t-PA group. However, because of the nonrandomized use of antihypertensive therapy and the many post hoc comparisons leading to statistical errors, the significance of this observation was unclear, and the importance of controlling blood pressure after thrombolysis still holds because of the possible association of ICH with high blood pressure.[94]

Central lines and arterial puncture should be restricted in the first 24 hours after thrombolytic treatment. However, the physician should be aware that the serum half-life of t-PA is very short, and after 20 minutes, there is very little systemic thrombolytic activity. Therefore, if clinical circumstances require a central line or triple-lumen catheter for monitoring of cardiopulmonary pressures, such a line could be safely established an hour or more after thrombolysis was complete. Urinary tract instrumentation (placement of a Foley catheter) should be avoided during infusion of t-PA and at least 30 minutes after the infusion ends. Placement of a nasogastric tube should be avoided during the first 24 hours after initiation of treatment; as with central lines and arterial puncture, we routinely insert this catheter earlier if required by patient circumstances.[77]

For 36 hours after thrombolysis, hemorrhagic complications of t-PA are the major worry; these can be intracranial or extracranial hemorrhages. If bleeding is suspected, then a blood specimen is collected for measurement of hemoglobin level, hematocrit, partial thromboplastin time, prothrombin time, INR, platelet count, and fibrinogen level. Blood should be typed and cross-matched when the need for transfusion arises. Arterial or venous sites should be compressed if they are the bleeding source.

TABLE 49-4 EMERGENCY MANAGEMENT OF ARTERIAL HYPERTENSION FOR PATIENTS RECEIVING THROMBOLYTIC TREATMENT FOR ACUTE ISCHEMIC STROKE

Indication that patient is eligible for treatment with intravenous rt-PA or other acute reperfusion intervention.
Blood pressure level
 Systolic >185 mm Hg or diastolic >110 mm Hg
  Labetalol 10 to 20 mg IV over 1 to 2 minutes, may repeat ×1; or
  Nitropaste 1 to 2 inches; or
  Nicardipine infusion, 5 mg/h, titrate up by 0.25 mg/h at 5- to 15-minute intervals, maximum dose 15 mg/h; when desired blood pressure attained, reduce to 3 mg/h
 If blood pressure does not decline and remains >185/110 mm Hg, do not administer rt-PA.
Management of blood pressure during and after treatment with rt-PA or other acute reperfusion intervention.
 Monitor blood pressure every 15 minutes during treatment and then for another 2 hours, then every 30 minutes for 6 hours, and then every hour for 16 hours.
Blood pressure level
 Systolic 180 to 230 mm Hg or diastolic 105 to 120 mm Hg
  Labetalol 10 mg IV over 1 to 2 minutes, may repeat every 10 to 20 minutes, maximum dose of 300 mg; or
  Labetalol 10 mg IV followed by an infusion at 2 to 8 mg/min
 Systolic >230 mm Hg or diastolic 121 to 140 mm Hg
  Labetalol 10 mg IV over 1 to 2 minutes, may repeat every 10 to 20 minutes, maximum dose of 300 mg; or
  Labetalol 10 mg IV followed by an infusion at 2 to 8 mg/min; or
  Nicardipine infusion, 5 mg/h, titrate up to desired effect by increasing 2.5 mg/h every 5 minutes to maximum of 15 mg/h
 If blood pressure not controlled, consider sodium nitroprusside.

From Adams HP Jr, del Zoppo G, Alberts M, et al: Guidelines for the early management of adults with ischemic stroke. *Stroke* 38: 1655-1711, 2007.

If major life-threatening bleeding occurs, including ICH, gastrointestinal bleeding, and retroperitoneal bleeding, thrombolytic treatment should be stopped if it is still going. Urgent CT of the brain should be obtained for suspected ICH.[77] Neurosurgical consultation for possible surgical intervention should also be obtained. Surgery should not be performed, however, unless the fibrinolytic state is corrected; such a correction usually requires both cryoprecipitate and fresh frozen plasma to overcome clotting factor deficiencies induced by the t-PA. The presence of immediate neurosurgical treatment, however, is not a mandatory element of using rt-PA for acute ischemic stroke because the efficacy of early surgery has never been established.

For major extracranial hemorrhages, the appropriate emergency imaging techniques should be performed, along with surgical consultations and interventions when appropriate. For 24 hours after IV t-PA treatment, patients should not receive aspirin, heparin, warfarin, or other antithrombotic or antiplatelet drugs.[77] As mentioned elsewhere, however, reocclusion may be a considerable problem after thrombolysis, and we are concerned that further studies of postthrombolytic anticoagulation are lacking.

Predictors of Good Outcome with Thrombolytic Treatment

In a 2001 article, Demchuk et al[95] analyzed data collected from 1205 patients treated in different centers in Germany, the United States, and Canada with IV t-PA as per NINDS protocol. A good outcome was defined as an mRS score of 0 to 1, and a poor outcome was an mRS score greater than 1. The independent predictors of good outcome in patients treated with IV t-PA, in relative order of decreasing magnitude, were milder baseline stroke severity, no history of diabetes mellitus, normal CT scan result, normal pretreatment blood glucose level, and normal pretreatment blood pressure. Confounding was observed among the variables: history of diabetes, CT scan appearance, baseline serum glucose level, and blood pressure (baseline mean arterial pressure), suggesting important relationships among these variables. Symptomatic ICH was associated with a poor outcome. The known risk factors for poor outcome in untreated patients, such as age and stroke mechanism, were not associated with outcome in this cohort study.

Risks of Thrombolysis

Plasminogen activators raise the risk of ICH by altering the framework of the platelet plug and by changing vascular permeability as well as the integrity of the vascular basal lamina at the site of injury; the latter two effects contribute to dissolution of the blood–brain barrier. Therefore, there is an increased risk of brain edema and ICH.[2] As mentioned before, subgroup analysis of the NINDS data showed that the only variables that were independently associated with an increased risk of symptomatic ICH were baseline stroke severity as measured by NIHSS, the amount of edema defined by acute hypodensity, and mass effect on CT before treatment (baseline CT).[96] Table 49-3 summarizes the rates of ICH with t-PA in the various clinical studies.

Reperfusion injury is another hypothetical risk. It has been shown that reperfusion is associated with a secondary wave of glutamate and other neurotransmitter release, which results in calcium influx and excitotoxicity. Restoration of blood flow might allow synthesis of damaging proteins and other cytokines as well as a supply of oxygen to ischemic areas, providing a substrate for peroxidation of lipids and formation of free radicals. Moreover, thrombolysis might allow the clot to break and cause secondary embolization to a distal vascular distribution.

Cost-Effectiveness of Thrombolysis

The cost-effectiveness of t-PA was demonstrated in 1998, in a study that used certain assumptions about stroke costs and outcomes based on data from the literature and from the NINDS study. Even though it shortened the stay at the hospital, t-PA therapy increased the hospital cost by $15,000 per patient for each additional patient who was discharged home rather than to a nursing home or in-patient rehabilitation center. On the other hand, t-PA reduced the costs of nursing home care and rehabilitation. The overall effect on both acute and long-term care costs (90% certainty) to the health care system is a net decrease of more than $4,000,000 for every 1000 patients treated.[97] These results have been confirmed in other trials.[98,99]

Combination Treatment

Combining thrombolysis with other treatment regimens has not proved to be beneficial so far in clinical studies. Previous studies have combined anticoagulants with fibrinolysis. In the MAST-E study,[48] 65% of the patients received SK and 75% of the placebo group also received heparin. There was no evidence of statistically significant benefit, and the study was terminated early because of increased ICH in the SK group. It is recommended that no anticoagulants be given within 24 hours of t-PA treatment. Previous studies have shown that SK with antiplatelet treatment (aspirin) is associated with a higher risk of ICH compared with SK alone or aspirin alone (MAST-I).[49] Clinical studies have not tested t-PA in combination with aspirin. Experimental models, however, have shown that t-PA with heparin is safe and did not increase the rate of ICH.[18] A small group of patients (n = 30) received a combination of t-PA and heparin in a feasibility study described by von Kummer et al[100]; these researchers concluded that when the combination treatment was given within 6 hours of stroke onset, the incidence of fatal ICH occurred in 9% of patients, whereas asymptomatic hemorrhagic infarction occurred in 28%. Reperfusion occurred in 34% of patients 90 minutes after initiation of thrombolysis and in 53% within 12 to 24 hours of thrombolysis initiation. Good clinical outcomes correlated with reperfusion ($P <$ 0.05). Future randomized controlled studies are needed to determine whether this or other antithrombotic strategies combined with IV t-PA are better than thrombolysis alone, weighing the benefits and risks involved.

Neuroprotective agents in combination with thrombolysis have been tested in experimental models and in clinical studies. Studies showed benefit in animals receiving neuroprotective agents within a short time window after the cerebrovascular occlusion. In 1991, Zivin and Mazzarella[101] used MK-801, a glutamate antagonist, followed by thrombolysis with t-PA and proved that such a combination was more effective than t-PA alone in reducing neurologic damage after stroke. MK-801 had no effect when used alone in the same stroke model. In 1999, Zhang et al[102] showed that combining anti-CD18 antibodies, which prevent adhesion of white blood cells to the endothelium, with thrombolysis prolonged the effective time window of thrombolysis from 2 hours to 4 hours. Anti-CD18 antibodies alone had no effect. Neuroprotective agents can reduce the side effects of thrombolysis because they enhance the integrity of the vascular endothelium and protect ischemic brain tissue from the hypothetical reperfusion injury discussed earlier. These results were not mirrored in clinical studies, most probably because these agents were given at a prolonged time from the onset of stroke.

Several clinical studies combined thrombolysis with neuroprotective agents. However, the two latest studies have failed to show benefit. In October 2001, Grotta[103] published the results of a study in which patients received IV t-PA alone or t-PA plus the neuroprotective agent lubeluzole. This agent works via inhibition of the glutamate-activated nitrous oxide pathway. Eighty-nine patients were randomly assigned to various treatments, but the study was terminated prematurely because another larger study using lubeluzole alone showed no benefit for such monotherapy. Note that lubeluzole was given before the end of the 1-hour t-PA drip (less than 4 hours from onset). There was no difference between the two treatment groups in the primary outcome measures: BI, mortality, ICH, and serious adverse events. This study showed that such a combination treatment is safe and feasible.

In October 2001, Lyden et al[104] reported the results of a randomized study in which t-PA was given within 3 hours of stroke onset with or without clomethiazole administered within 12 hours of stroke onset. There was no significant difference between the two groups in the primary end points, serious adverse events, and mortality at 3 months. This trial proved that such a combination was feasible and safe. There was no benefit in outcome as measured by BI, mRS, and NIHSS, with the combination treatment as compared with the t-PA group alone. However, there was benefit from the combination treatment in patients with total anterior circulation strokes, as well as decreased ICH on CT at 24 hours, even though the clomethiazole plus t-PA group had a higher frequency of edema and early ischemic changes on baseline CT. Future studies combining neuroprotective agents with thrombolysis should be pursued, keeping in mind that the neuroprotective agent should be administered earlier, and maybe earlier than the thrombolytic treatment, in light of animal models that show benefit only with very early administration of neuroprotective agents.

Hypothermia in combination with thrombolysis is under investigation. Future studies will evaluate whether hypothermia might prolong the time window of thrombolysis so that benefit might be achieved from t-PA given in combination with induced hypothermia even later than 3 hours after stroke onset.[105] Initial experience shows that hypothermia can be combined safely with thrombolysis; pivotal trials are being organized.[105,106]

Intraarterial thrombolysis in combination with IV thrombolysis is discussed in Chapter 62.

Conclusion

Thrombolysis with the use of IV t-PA is safe and improves the outcome of patients with stroke, despite a higher risk of ICH (but no increased risk of mortality). The emphasis should be on (1) treating the patient as early as possible, (2) excluding ICH on CT before treatment, and (3) controlling hypertension before and after treatment. A specialized unit setting is ideal for monitoring the patient. Treatment with anticoagulants and antiplatelet agents are forbidden within the first 24 hours after thrombolysis,

according to the NINDS protocol. Newer generation thrombolytic agents are currently under study for acute stroke treatment and, because they are more clot-selective, may show a greater rate of lysis with a lower risk of bleeding. It is hoped that future clinical studies using combination treatments of IV thrombolysis with intraarterial lytics or mechanical clot disruption, antithrombotic therapy, or neuroprotective agents within a short time window might build on the positive results obtained so far with t-PA.

REFERENCES

1. Tissue plasminogen activator for acute ischemic stroke: NINDS rt-PA Stroke Study Group, *N Engl J Med* 333:1581–1587, 1995.
2. Lyden PD: *Thrombolytic Therapy for Stroke*, ed 2, Totowa, NJ, 2005, Humana Press.
3. Douglas S: Coagulation history, *Br J Haematol* 107:22–32, 1999.
4. Collen D: Fibrin-selective thrombolytic therapy for acute myocardial infarction, *Circulation* 93:857–865, 1996.
5. Verstraete M: Third generation thrombolytic drugs, *Am J Med* 109:52–58, 2000.
6. Benedict CR, Refino CJ, et al: New variant of human tissue plasminogen activator (tPA) with enhanced efficacy and a lower incidence of bleeding compared with recombinant human tPA, *Circulation* 92:3032–3040, 1995.
7. Van de Werf F, Cannon C, Luyten A, et al: Safety assessment of single-bolus administration of TNK tissue-plasminogen activator in acute myocardial infarction: The ASSENT-1 trial, *Am Heart J* 137:786–791, 2000.
8. Van de Werf F, Barron HV, Armstrong P, et al: Incidence and predictors of bleeding events after fibrinolytic therapy with fibrin-specific agents, *Eur Heart J* 22:2253–2261, 2001.
9. Haley EC, Lyden PD, Hemmen TM, et al: A pilot dose-escalation safety study of tenecteplase in acute ischemic stroke, *Stroke* 36:607–612, 2005.
10. Suzuki Y, Chen F, Ni Y, et al: Microplasmin reduces ischemic brain damage and improves neurological function in a rat stroke model monitored with MRI, *Stroke* 35:2402–2406, 2004.
11. Lapchak PA, Arauju DM, Pakola S, et al: Microplasmin, a novel thrombolytic that improves behavioral outcome after embolic strokes in rabbits, *Stroke* 33:2279–2284, 2002.
12. Cannon CP: Comparison of front-loaded recombinant tissue-type plasminogen activator, anistreplase and combination thrombolytic therapy for acute myocardial infarction: Results of the Thrombolysis in Myocardial Infarction (TIMI) 4 trial, *J Am Coll Cardiol* 24:1602–1610, 1994.
13. Cairns J, Fuster V, Gore J, Kennedy JW: Coronary thrombolysis, *Cardiopulm Crit Care J* 108:401S–423S, 1995.
14. Witt W, Baldus B, Bringmann P, Cashion L, et al: Thrombolytic properties of *Desmodus rotundus* (vampire bat) salivary plasminogen activator in experimental pulmonary embolism in rats, *Blood* 79:1213–1217, 1992.
15. Mellott MJ, Stabilito II, Holahan MA, et al: Vampire bat salivary plasminogen activation in a canine model of arterial thrombosis, *Arterioscler Thromb* 12:212–221, 1992.
16. Hacke W, Albers GW, Al-Rawi Y, et al: The Desmoteplase in Acute Ischemic Stroke Trial (DIAS): A phase II MRI-based 9-Hour window acute stroke thrombolysis trial with intravenous desmoteplase, *Stroke* 36:66–73, 2005.
17. Furlan AJ, Albers GW, Al-Rawi Y, et al: Dose Escalation of Desmoteplase for Acute Ischemic Stroke (DEDAS): Evidence of safety and efficacy 3 to 9 hours after stroke onset, *Stroke* 37:1227–1231, 2006.
18. Hacke W, Furlan AJ, Al-Rawi Y, et al: Intravenous desmoteplase in patients with acute ischaemic stroke selected by MRI perfusion-diffusion weighted imaging or perfusion CT (DIAS-2): A prospective, randomised, double-blind, placebo-controlled study, *Stroke* 8:141–150, 2009.
19. Bell W, Pitney W, Oakley L, et al: Therapeutic defibrination in the treatment of thrombotic disease, *Lancet* 1:490–493, 1968.
20. Hossman V, Heiss WD, Beweymeyer H, Wiedemann G: Controlled trial of ancrod in acute ischemic stroke, *Arch Neurol* 40:803–808, 1983.

21. Olinger CP, Brott TG, Barsan WG, et al: Use of ancrod in acute or progressing ischemic cerebral infarction, *Ann Emerg Med* 17:1208-1209, 1983.

22. Levy DE, Trammel J, Wasiewski WW, et al: Ancrod for acute ischemic stroke: a new dosing regimen derived from analysis of prior ancrod stroke studies, *J Stroke Cerebrovasc Dis* 18:23-27, 2009.

23. Sherman DG, Atkinson RP, Chippendale T, et al: Intravenous ancrod for treatment of acute ischemic stroke: The STAT study: a randomized controlled trial. Stroke Treatment with Ancrod Trial, *JAMA* 283:2395-2403, 2000.

24. Hennerici MG, Kay R, Bogousslavsky J, et al: Intravenous ancrod for acute ischaemic stroke in the European Stroke Treatment with Ancrod Trial: A randomised controlled trial, *Lancet* 368:1871-1878, 2006.

25. Meyer JS, Gilroy J, Barnhart ME, et al: Therapeutic thrombolysis in cerebral thromboembolism. In Siekert W, Whisnant JGS, editors: *Cerebral Vascular Diseases*, Philadelphia, 1963, Grune & Stratton, pp 160-175.

26. del Zoppo G, Copeland BR, Waltz TA, et al: The beneficial effect of intracarotid urokinase on acute stroke in a baboon model, *Stroke* 17:638-643, 1986.

27. Zivin JA, Fisher M, DeGirolami U, et al: Tissue plasminogen activator reduces neurological damage after cerebral embolism, *Science* 230:1289-1292, 1985.

28. del Zoppo G, Copeland BR, Harker LA, et al: Experimental acute thrombotic stroke in baboons, *Stroke* 17:1254-1265, 1986.

29. Slivka A, Pulsinelli WA: Hemorrhagic complications of thrombolytic therapy in experimental stroke, *Stroke* 18:1148-1156, 1987.

30. Lyden PD, Zivin JA, Clark WA, et al: Tissue plasminogen activator mediated thrombolysis of cerebral emboli and its effect on hemorrhagic infarction in rabbits, *Neurology* 39:703-708, 1989.

31. Clark WM, Madden KP, Lyden PD, Zivin JA: Cerebral hemorrhagic risk of aspirin or heparin therapy with thrombolytic treatment in rabbits, *Stroke* 22:872-876, 1991.

32. Lyden PD, Madden KP, Clark WA, et al: Comparison of cerebral hemorrhage rates following tissue plasminogen activator or streptokinase treatment for embolic stroke in rabbits, *Stroke* 21:981-983, 1990.

33. Meyer JS, Gilroy J, Barnhart ME, Johnson JF: Therapeutic thrombolysis in cerebral thromboembolism: Randomized evaluation of intravenous streptokinase. In Millikan CH, Siekert RG, Whisnant JP, editors: *Cerebral Vascular Diseases Fourth Princeton Conference*, New York, 1965, Grune & Stratton, pp 200-213.

34. Fletcher AP, Alkjaersig N, Lewis M, et al: A pilot study of urokinase therapy in cerebral infarction, *Stroke* 7:135-142, 1976.

35. del Zoppo G, Poeck K, Pessin MS, et al: Recombinant tissue plasminogen activator in acute thrombotic and embolic stroke, *Ann Neurol* 32:78-86, 1992.

36. Brott TG, Haley EC Jr, Levy DE, et al: Urgent therapy for stroke. Part I: Pilot study of tissue plasminogen activator administered within 90 minutes, *Stroke* 23:632-640, 1992.

37. Haley EC Jr, Levy DE, Brott TG, et al: Urgent therapy for stroke. Part II: Pilot study of tissue plasminogen activator administered 91-180 minutes from onset, *Stroke* 23:641-645, 1992.

38. Mori E, Yoneda Y, Tabuchi M, et al: Intravenous recombinant tissue plasminogen activator in acute carotid artery territory stroke, *Neurology* 42:976-982, 1992.

39. Haley EC, Brott TG, Sheppard GL, et al: Pilot randomized trial of tissue plasminogen activator in acute ischemic stroke, *Stroke* 24:1000-1004, 1993.

40. Hacke W, Kaste M, Fieschi C, et al: Intravenous thrombolysis with recombinant tissue plasminogen activator for acute hemispheric stroke: The European Cooperative Acute Stroke Study (ECASS), *JAMA* 274:1017-1025, 1995.

41. Hacke W, Bluhmki E, Steiner T, et al: Dichotomized efficacy end points and global end-point analysis applied to the ECASS intention-to-treat data set, *Stroke* 29:2073-2075, 1998.

42. Steiner T, Bluhmki E, Kaste M, et al: The ECASS 3-hour cohort, *Cerebrovasc Dis* 8:198-203, 1998.

43. Haley EC Jr, Lewandowski C, Tilley BC, et al: Myths regarding the NINDS rt-PA stroke trial: Setting the record straight. NINDS rt-PA Stroke Study Group, *Ann Emerg Med* 30:676-682, 1997.

44. Intracerebral hemorrhage after intravenous t-PA therapy for ischemic stroke: NINDS rt-PA Stroke Study Group, *Stroke* 28:2109-2118, 1997.

45. Kwiatkowski TG, Libman R, Frankel M, et al: Effects of tissue plasminogen activator for acute ischemic stroke at one year, *N Engl J Med* 340:1781-1787, 1999.

46. Broderick JP, Lu M, Kothari R, et al: Finding the most powerful measures of the effectiveness of tissue plasminogen activator in the NINDS tPA stroke trial, *Stroke* 31:2335-2341, 2000.

47. Hacke W, Kaste M, Fieschi C, et al: Randomised double-blind placebo-controlled trial of thrombolytic therapy with intravenous alteplase in acute ischaemic stroke (ECASS II), *Lancet* 352:1245-1251, 1998.

48. Multicenter Acute Stroke Trial—Europe Study Group (MAST-E): Thrombolytic therapy with streptokinase in acute ischemic stroke, *N Engl J Med* 335:145-150, 1996.

49. Randomised controlled trial of streptokinase, aspirin, and combination of both in treatment of acute ischaemic stroke: Multicentre Acute Stroke Trial-Italy (MAST-I) Group, *Lancet* 346:1509-1514, 1995.

50. Donnan GA, Davis SM, Chambers BR, et al: Streptokinase for acute ischemic stroke with relationship to time of administration: Australian Streptokinase (ASK) Trial Study Group, *JAMA* 276:961-966, 1996.

51. Donnan GA, Davis SM, Chambers BR, et al: ASK Trial: Unfavourable outcome if treated more than three hours after onset [abstract], *Cerebrovasc Dis* 5:225-273, 1995.

52. Cornu C, Boutitie F, Candelise L, et al: Streptokinase in acute ischemic stroke: An individual patient data meta-analysis: The Thrombolysis in Acute Stroke Pooling Project, *Stroke* 31:1555-1560, 2000.

53. Clark WM, Albers GW, Madden KP, et al: The rtPA (alteplase) 0-6 hour acute stroke trial, part A (A027g): Results of a double-blind, placebo-controlled, multicenter study, *Stroke* 31:811-816, 2000.

54. Clark W, Wissman S, Albers GW, et al: Recombinant tissue-type plasminogen activator (alteplase) for ischemic stroke 3 to 5 hours after symptom onset, *JAMA* 282:2019-2024, 1999.

55. Albers GW, Clark W, Madden K, Hamilton S: ATLANTIS Trial: Results for patients treated within 3 hours of stroke onset, *Stroke* 33:493-496, 2002.

56. Albers GW, Olivet JM: Intravenous alteplase for ischaemic stroke, *Lancet* 369:249-250, 2007.

57. Hacke W, Donnan G, Fieschii C, et al: Association of outcome with early stroke treatment: Pooled analysis of Atlantis, ECASS, and the NINDS rt-PA stroke trials, *Lancet* 363, 768-764:2004.

58. Wahlgren N, Ahmed N, Davalos A, et al: Thrombolysis with alteplase for acute ischemic stroke in the Safe Implementation of Thrombolysis in Stroke-Monitoring Study (SITS-MOST): An observational study, *Lancet* 369:275-282, 2007.

59. Wahlgren N, Ahmed N, Davalos A, et al: Thrombolysis with alteplase 3-4.5 h after acute ischaemic stroke (SITS-ISTR): An observational study, *Lancet* 372:1303-1309, 2008.

60. Hacke W, Kaste M, Bluhmki E, et al: Thrombolysis with alteplase 3 to 4.5 hours after acute ischemic stroke, *N Engl J Med* 359:1317-1329, 2008.

61. Lyden PD: Thrombolytic therapy for acute stroke—not a moment to lose, *N Engl J Med* 359:1393-1395, 2008.

62. http: www.eso-stroke.org/pdf/ESO%20Guidelines_update_Jan_2009.pdf, Accessed March 31, 2009.

63. Chiu D, Krieger D, Villar-Cordova C, et al: Intravenous tissue plasminogen activator for acute ischemic stroke feasibility, safety, and efficacy in the first year of clinical practice, *Stroke* 29:18-22, 1998.

64. Grond M, Stenzel C, Schmulling S, et al: Early intravenous thrombolysis for acute ischemic stroke in a community based approach, *Stroke* 29:1544-1549, 1998.

65. Egan R, Lutsep HL, Clark WM, et al: Open label tissue plasminogen activator for stroke: The Oregon experience, *J Stroke Cerebrovasc Dis* 8:287-290, 1999.

66. Katzan I, Furlan A, Lloyd L, et al: Use of tissue-type plasminogen activator for acute ischemic stroke: The Cleveland area experience, *JAMA* 283:1151-1158, 2000.

67. Katzen IMM, Hammer MDM, Furlan AJM: Quality improvement and tissue-type plasminogen activator for acute stroke. A Cleveland update, *Stroke* 34:799-800, 2003.

68. Albers GW, Bates V, Clark W, et al: Intravenous tissue-type plasminogen activator for treatment of acute stroke: The Standard Treatment with Alteplase to Reverse Stroke (STARS) study, *JAMA* 283:1145-1150, 2000.

69. Chapman KM, Woolfenden AR, Graeb D, et al: Intravenous tissue plasminogen activator for acute ischemic stroke, *Stroke* 31:2920-2924, 2000.

70. Barber PA, Zhang J, Demchuk A, et al: Why are stroke patients excluded from TPA therapy? *Neurology* 56:1015-1020, 2001.

71. Koennecke HC, Nohr R, Leistner S, Marx P: Intravenous tPA for ischemic stroke team: Performance over time, safety and efficacy in a single center-2-year experience, *Stroke* 32:1074-1078, 2001.

72. Grotta J, Burgin WS, El-Mitwalli A, et al: Intravenous tissue-type plasminogen activator therapy for ischemic stroke, *Arch Neurol* 58:2009-2013, 2001.

73. Hill MD, Buchan AM: Canadian Activase for Stroke Effectiveness Study (CASES), *Can J Neurol Sci* 28:232-238, 2001.

74. Trouillas P, Nighoghossian N, Derex L, et al: Thrombolysis with intravenous rtPA in a series of 100 cases of acute carotid territory stroke. Determination of etiological, topographic, and radiological outcome factors, *Stroke* 29:2529-2540, 1998.

75. Trouillas P, Nighoghossian N, Derex L, Honnorat J: Prognosis at 5 years of acute cerebral infarcts of the carotid territory treated by intravenous rtPA: Data from the Lyon thrombolysis registry, *Stroke* 33:395, 2002.

76. Trouillas P, Nighoghossian N, Derex L, et al: Final results of the Lyon rtPA protocol (200 cases): Effect of intravenous rtPA within 7 hours without radiological and clinical exclusions in carotid territory acute cerebral infarcts [Letter], *Stroke* 34:284, 2003.

77. Adams HP Jr, del Zoppo G, Alberts M, et al: Guidelines for the early management of adults with ischemic stroke, *Stroke* 38:1655-1711, 2007.

78. Sattin JA, Olson SE, Liu L, et al: An expedited code stroke protocol is feasible and safe, *Stroke* 37:2935-2939, 2006.

79. Aleu A, Mellado P, Lichy C, et al: Hemorrhagic complications after off-label thrombolysis for ischemic stroke, *Stroke* 38:417-422, 2007.

80. Grotta J, Alexandrov AV: Early arterial re-occlusion in patients treated with 0.9 mg/kg IV TPA [abstract], *Stroke* 33:354, 2002.

81. Lyden P, Lu M, Kwiatkowski TG, et al: Thrombolysis in patients with transient neurologic deficits, *Neurology* 57:2125-2128, 2001.

82. Ozdemir O, Beletsky O, Chan R, et al: Thrombolysis in patients with marked clinical fluctuations in neurologic status due to cerebral ischemia, *Arch Neurol* 65:1041-1043, 2008.

83. Smith EE, Abdullah Petkovska I, et al: Poor outcomes in patients who do not receive intravenous tissue plasminogen activator because of mild or improving ischemic stroke, *Stroke* 36:2497-2499, 2005.

84. Hemmen TM, Meyer BC, McClean TL, Lyden PD: Identification of nonischemic stroke mimics among 411 code strokes at the University of California, San Diego, stroke center, *J Stroke Cerebrovasc Dis* 17:23-25, 2008.

85. Wein TH, Hickenbottom SL, Morgenstern B, et al: Safety of tissue plasminogen activator for acute stroke in menstruating women, *Stroke* 33:2506-2508, 2002.

86. von Kummer R, Allen KL, Holle R, et al: Acute stroke: Usefulness of early CT findings before thrombolytic therapy, *Radiology* 205:327-333, 1997.

87. Patel S, Levine S, Tilley B, et al: Lack of clinical significance of early ischemic changes on computed tomography in acute stroke, *JAMA* 286:2830-2838, 2001.

88. Gilligan A, Markus R, Read S, et al: Baseline blood pressure but not early computed tomography changes predicts major hemorrhage after streptokinase in acute ischemic stroke, *Stroke* 33:2236-2242, 2002.

89. Barber P, Demchuk A, Hudon ME, et al: Hyperdense sylvian fissure MCA "dot" sign, *Stroke* 32:84-88, 2001.

90. Marler JR, Tilley BC, Lu M, et al: Early stroke treatment associated with better outcome: The NINDS rt-PA stroke study, *Neurology* 55:1649-1655, 2000.

91. Generalized efficacy of t-PA for acute stroke: NINDS rt-PA Stroke Study Group, *Stroke* 28:2119-2125, 1997.

92. Alexandrov AV, Grotta JC: Arterial reocclusion in stroke patients treated with intravenous tissue plasminogen activator, *Neurology* 59:862-867, 2002.

93. Brott TG, MacCarthy EP: Antihypertensive therapy in stroke. In Fisher M, editor: *Medical therapy of acute stroke*, New York, 1989, Marcel Dekker, pp 117-141.

94. Brott T, Lu M, Kothari R, et al: Hypertension and its treatment in the NINDS rt-PA stroke trial, *Stroke* 29:1504-1509, 1998.

95. Demchuk AM, Tanne D, Hill MD, et al: Predictors of good outcome after intravenous tPA for acute ischemic stroke, *Neurology* 57:474-480, 2001.

96. The NINDS: t-PA Stroke Study Group: Intracerebral hemorrhage after intravenous t-PA therapy for ischemic stroke, *Stroke* 28:2109-2118, 1997.

97. Fagen SC, Morgenstern LB, Petitta A, et al: Cost-effectiveness of tissue plasminogen activator for acute ischemic stroke, *Neurology* 50:883-890, 1998.

98. Demaerschalk BM, Yip TR: Economic benefit of increasing utilization of intravenous tissue plasminogen activator for acute ischemic stroke in the United States, *Stroke* 37:943-944, 2006.

99. Sandercock P, Berge E, Dennis M, e al: Cost-effectiveness of thrombolysis with recombinant tissue plasminogen activator for acute ischemic stroke assessed by a model based on UK NHS costs, *Stroke* 35:1490-1497, 2004.

100. von Kummer R, Hacke W: Safety and efficacy of intravenous tissue plasminogen activator and heparin in acute middle cerebral artery stroke, *Stroke* 23:646-652, 1992.

101. Zivin J, Mazzarella V: Tissue plasminogen activator plus glutamate antagonist improves outcome after embolic stroke, *Arch Neurol* 48:1235-1238, 1991.

102. Zhang RL, Zhang ZG, Chopp M: Increased therapeutic efficacy with rt-PA and anti-CD18 antibody treatment of stroke in the rat, *Neurology* 52:273-279, 1999.

103. Grotta J: Combination therapy stroke trial, *Cerebrovasc Dis* 12:258-263, 2001.

104. Lyden P, Jacoby M, Schim J, et al: The Clomethiazole Acute Stroke Study in tissue-type plasminogen activator-treated stroke (CLASS-T): Final results, *Neurology* 57:1199-1205, 2001.

105. Guluma KZ, Hemmen TM, Olson SE, et al: A trial of therapeutic hypothermia via endovascular approach in awake patients with acute ischemic stroke: Methodology, *Acad Emerg Med* 13:820-827, 2006.

106. Hemmen TM, Lyden PD: Induced hypothermia for acute stroke, *Stroke* 37:794-799, 2007.

50 Antithrombotic Therapy for Treatment of Acute Ischemic Stroke

HAROLD P. ADAMS, JR., PATRICIA H. DAVIS

Because most ischemic strokes are secondary to arterial thromboembolism, antithrombotic agents (i.e., anticoagulants and antiplatelet agents) are a mainstay of medical treatment to prevent ischemic stroke. The utility of these medications in long-term management to prevent stroke or recurrent stroke is well established.[1-3] Oral anticoagulants are of confirmed usefulness in the prevention of cardioembolic stroke among patients with high-risk heart diseases, including most patients with atrial fibrillation.[3,4] Antiplatelet agents are the standard medical therapy for lowering the risk of stroke among patients with arterial diseases, including those patients with either intracranial or extracranial atherosclerosis.[2] Because of their established efficacy in long-term care and because most strokes are secondary to formation of clots, there continues to be considerable interest in the emergency use of either anticoagulant or antiplatelet agents in the setting of acute stroke. Antithrombotic agents, especially heparin, often are prescribed by clinicians.[5,6] With the exception of aspirin and clopidogrel, these medications are given parenterally, usually intravenously or subcutaneously (Table 50-1). These agents may be used as the primary intervention or as an adjunct to other measures aimed at restoring perfusion to the brain. The rationale for these medications includes halting the propagation of an intraarterial thrombus, forestalling early recurrent embolization, and maintaining collateral flow to the area of ischemia. In addition, their adjunctive use after mechanical or pharmacologic thrombolysis centers on preventing rethrombosis or reocclusion after recanalization. In particular, intravenously administered antiplatelet agents are given in conjunction with emergency angioplasty and stenting. Antithrombotic agents also are a potential therapy for those patients with stroke who are bedridden and have an increased risk of deep vein thrombosis (DVT) and pulmonary embolism, which add to the morbidity and potential mortality of the neurologic event. The antithrombotic medications are used both to prevent and to treat these thromboembolic events. However, physicians are uncertain about which patients to emergently treat with antithrombotic medications and when to start these medications. Fortuitously, the results of several clinical trials performed in the past 15 years have provided data to guide clinicians on the use of antithrombotic agents in the management of patients with ischemic stroke. These results have been used to formulate recommendations included in the guidelines for treatment of acute ischemic stroke.[7,8] Several reviews have also discussed the role of antithrombotic therapy in ischemic stroke.[3,9,10]

Pharmacology

Heparin, Low-Molecular-Weight Heparins, and Danaparoid

The glycosaminoglycans *heparin*, *low-molecular-weight (LMW) heparins*, or *danaparoid* have been used for more than 60 years. They continue to be used widely for treatment of patients with acute ischemic stroke. Heparin is a mixture of glycosaminoglycans that is usually obtained from porcine or bovine sources. Its molecular weight ranges from 5000 to 30,000 daltons (d).[11] Recently, a form of heparin that can be given orally has been developed.[12] The formulation facilitates transport of the drug across the gastrointestinal epithelium.[13] However, heparin usually is given either subcutaneously or intravenously. Because of the high risk of local bleeding at the injection site, heparin is not given intramuscularly. The antithrombotic effects of heparin are immediate if it is given intravenously in a bolus dose followed by a continuous intravenous infusion. A lag of several hours in achieving antithrombotic responses follows subcutaneous administration, and as a result, therapeutic levels may not be reached for 24 hours.

Heparin binds to plasma proteins, platelet-derived proteins, and endothelial cells. Differences in levels of those proteins might explain variations in clinical responses to heparin among patients. Heparin binds to and alters the conformation of antithrombin, which in turn increases the ability of antithrombin to inactivate thrombin, activated factor X (factor Xa), and activated factor IX (factor IXa). Heparin binds to the amino terminus of the molecule site of antithrombin, which leads to a conformational change in the antithrombin. This change increases the ability of antithrombin to inactivate thrombin by a ratio of 1000 to 4000 times. Heparin does not directly affect either thrombin or factor Xa already incorporated in a formed thrombus; thus, it does not have thrombolytic effects.[14] The ratio of inhibition of activated thrombin to factor Xa is 1:1. Heparin also prevents fibrin formation through its inhibition of thrombin-induced activation of platelets and factors V and VIII. It does not affect factor Xa already bound to platelets. Heparin also inactivates

TABLE 50-1 ANTITHROMBOTIC AGENTS THAT MAY BE USED IN THE MANAGEMENT OF PATIENTS WITH ACUTE ISCHEMIC STROKE

Anticoagulants
  Glycosaminoglycans
    Heparin
    Low-molecular-weight heparins
    Danaparoid
  Direct thrombin inhibitors
    Argatroban
  Antithrombin
  Protein C
Antiplatelet agents
  Aspirin
  Clopidogrel
  Glycoprotein IIb/IIIa receptor blockers
    Abciximab
    Eptifibatide (Integrilin)

TABLE 50-2 WEIGHT-BASED REGIMEN FOR ADMINISTRATION OF UNFRACTIONATED HEPARIN

Initial dosage regimen
80 units/kg intravenous bolus
Followed by 18 units/kg/h
Check aPTT in 6 h

Adjustment of dosage
aPTT level of <35 s (approximately 1.2 × control)
  Administer another 50 units/kg bolus
  Increase infusion to 22 units/kg/h (increase 4 units/h)
aPTT level of 35 to 45 s (approximately 1.2 to 1.5 × control)
  Administer another 40 units/kg bolus
  Increase infusion to 20 units/kg/h (increase 2 units/h)
aPTT level of 46 to 70 s (approximately 1.5 to 2.3 × control)
  Continue infusion at 18 units/kg/h
aPTT level of 71 to 90 s (approximately 2.3 to 3 × control)
  Decrease infusion to 16 units/kg/h (decrease 2 units/h)
aPTT level of >90 s (approximately 3 × control)
  Halt infusion for 1 h
  Restart infusion at 16 units/kg/h
  Decrease infusion to 15 units/kg/h (decrease 3 units/h)

aPTT, activated partial thromboplastin time.

thrombin through heparin cofactor II, which is an action that occurs at high concentrations and is independent from its effects on antithrombin. In addition, the high-molecular-weight components of heparin can alter endothelial modulation of clotting factors and interact with platelet factor IV. The binding of heparin to von Willebrand factor also affects platelet function.[11,15,16]

Heparin also binds to macrophages and endothelial cells. This binding, which is saturable, relates to the rapid clearance of heparin from the circulation, and this effect may explain variations in responses among patients. In addition, an individual patient's response may change over time. Some of the differences in responses may occur for no obvious reason. Heparin has a narrow therapeutic window; differences between safe but effective doses and dangerous levels are small.[14] There is a strong association between the risk of serious bleeding and increases in the dose of heparin. Some patients are relatively resistant to the actions of heparin (heparin resistance). This response may be secondary to a deficiency of antithrombin or to an elevation of heparin-binding proteins, including fibrinogen, factor VIII, or platelet factor 4.[17] Heparin does not cross the placenta.

The activated partial thromboplastin time (aPTT) is the most widely used test to monitor the biologic (antithrombotic) effects of heparin. This test measures responses to heparin-induced inhibition of thrombin, factor Xa, and factor IXa. The optimal level of anticoagulation is uncertain but is assumed to be approximately 1.5 times control values. The aPTT test has a number of serious limitations. Variability in reagents between institutions may lead to spurious aPTT results.[15] Patients with the lupus anticoagulant–antiphospholipid antibody syndrome often have falsely elevated aPTT values; in this situation, monitoring heparin therapy with this test may be problematic. Alternative ways to assess heparin's activity include measuring inhibition of factor Xa or measuring heparin levels via neutralization with protamine sulfate. However, the usual therapeutic level of heparin that achieves inhibition of factor Xa to 0.3 to 0.7 U/mL.[15,18] These tests are not widely available and may be more difficult to perform than measurements of aPTT.

Most high-risk patients receive 5000 units of heparin twice a day for prevention of DVT. A different regimen is often given to patients with acute thrombotic events. The usual daily dose is approximately 24,000 to 30,000 units to maintain a therapeutic antithrombotic effect. Traditionally, a bolus of heparin (usually 5000 units) is given to start treatment; thereafter, heparin is given as a continuous intravenous infusion, often in an hourly dose of 1000 units. Initially, the aPTT value is markedly prolonged, so follow-up assessments are usually delayed until 6 hours after the initiation of therapy. Depending on the results, the infusion may be increased or decreased in increments of 100 U/h, and the aPTT is reassessed in 6 hours. This approach, although time-honored, has a number of limitations. It does not account for the marked variations in responses among patients. Some patients have excessive anticoagulation with an increased risk of bleeding, whereas others receive insufficient anticoagulation with a resultant loss of efficacy. The patient's weight is an important variable that affects biologic responses to heparin. As a result, weight-based nomograms are now used to administer heparin.[17,19-21] Current guidelines now recommend a nomogram, such as that included in Table 50-2, for initiation of heparin treatment and subsequent adjustments in doses in response to levels of anticoagulation.[7]

Heparin also has subtle anti-inflammatory actions that may differ from its effects on coagulation factors.[22-24] In addition, heparin may have effects on major neurotransmitters of the brain. The interactions of these effects and the potential utility of heparin for treatment of patients with acute brain ischemia are not obvious.

Because of the many limitations of unfractionated (traditional) heparin, other parenterally administered, rapidly acting anticoagulants have been developed.[25,26] The leading alternatives are the LMW heparins and danaparoid. Potential advantages include a long period of antithrombotic action and a predictable dose-antithrombotic effect. These medications have a weak effect on thrombin and selective antithrombotic actions on factor Xa. These agents are also of biologic origin and are largely created by the chemical or enzymatic depolarization of unfractionated heparin. The LMW heparins weigh approximately 1000 to 10,000 d. The reduction into low-weight compounds leads to lessened binding to platelets, proteins, endothelial cells, and macrophages. These effects probably explain the longer duration of effect and the relatively predictable responses to the use of the LMW heparins.

The LMW heparins and danaparoid have a reduced effect on thrombin function compared with unfractionated heparin but more selective inhibition of factor Xa. The ratio for thrombin and factor Xa is approximately 1:2 to 1:4. Because these agents do not affect thrombin activity except in very high concentrations, assessment of the responses by the use of the aPTT is unreliable. Rather, measuring inhibition of factor Xa tests the antithrombotic effects of these medications. The desired levels are 0.3 to 0.7 U/mL. However, the reliability of laboratory measurements of antifactor Xa activity is uncertain. Because these agents are excreted renally, the level of anticoagulation may be high among patients with renal failure.[16] Clinical trials have demonstrated that neonates and infants need a relatively higher dose of the LMW heparins than do older children or adults to achieve targeted levels for inhibition of factor Xa.[27]

Although the LMW heparins and danaparoid may be given intravenously, most clinical studies have focused on subcutaneously administered regimens, particularly in the scenario of preventing DVT. Usually, patients receive an injection twice daily. Although the dosage of these agents usually is not adjusted to the patient's weight, a weight-based nomogram may also be appropriate. The responses to specific LMW heparins generally are similar, but the specific pharmacologic effects differ; thus, these agents should be evaluated individually. In particular, the ratio of antithrombin activity to antifactor Xa activity varies among the several compounds. As a result, data about the efficacy and safety of one LMW heparin may not be automatically applicable to another agent.

Other Anticoagulants

Because of the lag between the initiation of therapy with vitamin K antagonists and an antithrombotic response, these agents are not used as an intervention for treatment of acute ischemic stroke. Most of these agents are given orally, although warfarin is available in a parenteral formulation. In addition, these medications may have an initial and transient prothrombotic effect through their initial inhibition of the actions of proteins C and S, which limit their applicability.

Direct thrombin inhibitors may affect unbound thrombin and produce a more reliable antithrombotic effect than unfractionated heparin. These agents also do not affect platelet function. *Hirudin*, originally derived from the salivary gland of the medicinal leech, now is available with the use of recombinant technology (*lepirudin*).[28,29] It is a potent and irreversible inhibitor of thrombin function. The anticoagulant activity of hirudin is monitored by the aPTT. Antihirudin antibodies may develop within 5 days of treatment in 40% to 70% of patients treated with lepirudin. These antibodies may increase drug potency. Hirudin and lepirudin have been used in the treatment

of patients with unstable heart disease, but they have not been used to treat patients with stroke.[30] *Bivalirudin (hirulog)* is another direct thrombin inhibitor that has been used to treat patients with unstable heart disease.

Argatroban is a selective thrombin inhibitor that competitively acts at the active site of thrombin; it has an immediate antithrombotic effect.[31,32] Argatroban has a short half-life (approximately 50 minutes); thus, anticoagulation may be initiated or terminated more rapidly than with either unfractionated heparin or the LMW heparins. It also is monitored by the aPTT. In experimental stroke models, it has been administered successfully with tissue plasminogen activator (t-PA).[33] *Ximelagatran* is a direct thrombin inhibitor that was tested in the long-term prophylaxis against thromboembolism among patients with atrial fibrillation, but it had significant hepatotoxicity.[34] *Dabigatran* is another direct thrombin inhibitor that was as effective as warfarin in preventing thromboembolism with less risk of bleeding when administered at a lower dose. At a higher dose, it was more effective than warfarin in preventing stroke and systemic embolism but had a similar rate of bleeding.[35]

In addition, direct or indirect inhibition of activated factors VII, IX, or X is a potential intervention.[28] These agents include *idraparinux, rivaroxaban, apixaban,* and *edoxaban*.[36] Rivaroxaban was effective in preventing venous thromboembolism after major orthopedic surgery in four phase 3 trials.[36] There are double-blind trials testing three Xa inhibitors for stroke prevention in atrial fibrillation; these are ARISTOTLE (apixaban), ROCKET-AF (rivaroxaban) and ENGAGE-AF TIMI 48 (edoxaban).[37] Activated protein C is produced by the complex of thrombin and thrombomodulin. It inhibits activated factors V and VIII. Several agents, including activated protein C concentrates, are being developed.[28] Thus, it is likely that several new anticoagulants may be available in the future.

Antiplatelet Agents

Aspirin irreversibly blocks the cyclooxygenase (COX) activity of prostaglandin (PG) H synthase 1 (COX-1) and 2 (COX-2) by acetylation of a serine residue of the COX channel.[38-40] Aspirin's actions on platelet COX-1 are approximately 170-fold more potent than on monocyte COX-2.[41] It produces a permanent defect of thromboxane A_2–dependent platelet function that induces platelet aggregation and causes vasoconstriction. Aspirin also alters endothelial production of prostacyclin, an agent that inhibits platelet aggregation and induces vasoconstriction. The potentially prothrombotic effects of prostacyclin inhibition appear to be less relevant clinically because the endothelial cells may regenerate new COX unlike the anuclear platelet, in which COX inhibition is irreversible.[42]

The antithrombotic actions of aspirin occur over a broad range of doses. Because the effects of endothelial production of prostacyclin may be dose-related, lower doses of aspirin may be more effective in preventing thrombosis than larger doses. Aspirin is readily absorbed, so peak plasma levels are reached within 30 to 40 minutes.[43] Enteric coating of the tablet does delay absorption. A single dose of 100 mg of aspirin has an almost immediate effect on platelet aggregation.[42] These effects mean that aspirin might be useful in the setting of acute ischemic stroke. Lower doses of aspirin (<100 mg) may take longer than 24 hours to achieve maximal suppression of COX. Subsequently, lower daily doses are able to maintain the antiplatelet effects. Thus, the minimum initial dose of aspirin appears to be at least 160 mg; that is the dose used in the Chinese Acute Stroke Trial.[44] Other potential antiplatelet actions may be the result of platelet activation by neutrophils, which is mediated by nitric oxide, and enhancement of the production of nitric oxide by endothelial cells.[41,45] The utility of aspirin as a neuroprotective agent for use in acute stroke is not established, but there is evidence that strokes may be less severe among patients who have previously used aspirin.[46-48] There have been concerns that patients may develop resistance to aspirin and that higher doses of the medication may be needed to achieve antiplatelet effects.[49-51]

Dipyridamole blocks the actions of phosphodiesterase and is an action that in turn limits the reuptake of adenosine in the platelets.[52] This agent also prolongs platelet survival and produces vasodilation.[53] The interval from initiation of treatment with dipyridamole to the achievement of antiplatelet effects is not established. Presumably there is some lag; as a result, the medication probably will not be used to treat acute ischemic stroke, although in combination with aspirin, it is effective in preventing recurrent stroke.[54]

The thienopyridines, *ticlopidine, clopidogrel, prasugrel, ticagrelor,* and *cangrelor,* inhibit platelet aggregation induced by adenosine diphosphate by blocking the platelet receptor P2Y12, which interacts with fibrinogen.[39,55,56] The ability of clopidogrel to limit platelet aggregation occurs in a dose-dependent manner. The inhibition of platelet function starts within 2 hours of a 300-mg loading dose of clopidogrel and is irreversible.[57,58] Clopidogrel is a prodrug that requires a two-step activation process by the cytochrome P-450 (CYP) isoenzymes. Inhibition of these enzymes, particularly CYP2C19, by other drugs such as fluoxetine or by competition for the catalytic site on CYP2C19 by proton pump inhibitors can lead to interindividual variability in platelet aggregation.[59,60] There are also genetic variations that affect the antiplatelet response to clopidogrel. Carriers of specific alleles of CYP2C19 and CYP3A4 had less response to clopidogrel and a higher risk of recurrent vascular events after myocardial infarction (MI).[61,62] The clinical usefulness of genotyping patients to select the appropriate antiplatelet agent or to adjust the dose is unproven.[63,64] Prasugrel has a tenfold to 100-fold greater inhibition of platelet aggregation than either clopidogrel or ticlopidine. Prasugrel also has more rapid effects on platelet function than clopidogrel and produces irreversible inhibition. It is also a prodrug but requires only one-step activation by CYP enzymes and is not affected by genetic variability of these isoenzymes. Prasugrel was approved by the U.S. Food and Drug Administration in 2009 for the treatment of patients with acute myocardial ischemia because there was a significant reduction in ischemic events when it was compared with clopidogrel.[65] The effects of these medications dissipate over several days after their use is stopped.[66] Ticagrelor, unlike clopidogrel and prasugrel, binds reversibly to the P2Y12 receptor and has a half-life of 7 to 8 hours. It is not a prodrug, has a rapid onset of action, and is more potent than clopidogrel. It is more effective than clopidogrel in patients with acute coronary syndromes in preventing vascular death, MI, or stroke.[67] Cangrelor is an intravenous adenosine triphosphate analogue that reversibly binds to the P2Y12 platelet receptor. It has a half-life of 3 to 6 minutes, and the antiplatelet effect is gone within 60 minutes after the infusion is stopped. The use of periprocedural cangrelor in the CHAMPION trial was not more effective than placebo in reducing death, MI, or revascularization at 48 hours.[68] Because its rapid onset and offset of action are important assets, further trials are recommended.[69]

The glycoprotein (integrin) IIb/IIIa receptor antagonists are potent blockers of platelet aggregation by affecting the binding of fibrinogen to the platelets.[70-74] These agents do not affect platelet adhesion, but they do limit formation of a clot.[75,76] Their pharmacologic effects vary.[73,77] *Abciximab* is a monoclonal chimeric murine-human antibody that blocks the receptor.[78] A bolus dose of abciximab may block more than 80% of the platelet receptors and maintain antiplatelet effects for several hours.[52,79] With blockade of more than 90% of the platelet receptors, bleeding time is prolonged. Platelet function is inhibited within 2 hours of administration of a bolus dose. Gradual recovery of platelet function develops over the next 12 hours. An infusion of abciximab also maintains the antiplatelet effects during subsequent hours. The usual loading dose of abciximab is 0.25 mg/kg, and the maintenance infusion is 0.125 mcg/kg/min (maximum, 10 mcg/min). The antiplatelet effects of abciximab are potentiated by the concomitant administration of aspirin.[78] Abciximab also may have some effect on the formation of thrombin. Abciximab in conjunction with other antithrombotic medications has been used to treat patients with acute coronary artery disease, including those having emergency mechanical interventions.[80,81]

Tirofiban is a nonpeptide derivative of tyrosine. It selectively and rapidly blocks the glycoprotein IIb/IIIa receptor.[52] Marked inhibition of platelet aggregation and prolongation of the bleeding time occur within 5 minutes of the start of an intravenous infusion of the medication. The effects begin to disappear within 1.5 hours after the infusion is halted.[52] Tirofiban is used to treat acute coronary artery occlusion.[77,82,83]

Eptifibatide is a heptapeptide that has high affinity and specificity for the glycoprotein IIb/IIIa receptor.[52] It also affects integrin-mediated binding of the smooth muscle cells to thrombospondin and prothrombin.[84] After administration of a bolus dose followed by an intravenous infusion, platelet aggregation is diminished markedly within 1 hour.[85] Eptifibatide also affects thrombin generation and markedly prolongs the bleeding time. The bleeding time rapidly normalizes after halting the infusion of eptifibatide. The agent is used to treat patients with acute coronary artery occlusions.[86-88] The usual dose is 180 mcg/kg (maximum, 22.6 mg) over 1 to 2 minutes followed by a continuous infusion of 2 mcg/kg/min (maximum dose, 15 mg/h).

Thrombin mediates platelet activation via an interaction with the protease-activated receptor 1 (PAR-1) on the platelet. SCH 530348 is a competitive and selective inhibitor of the PAR-1 receptor without affecting the production of fibrin by thrombin. The (TRA 2°P)-TIMI 50 trial is a double-blind, placebo-controlled trial testing the addition of SCH 530348 compared with placebo to standard therapy in patients with MI, peripheral vascular disease, or stroke. The endpoints are cardiovascular death, MI, stroke, or coronary revascularization.[89]

Safety of Emergency Antithrombotic Treatment for Patients with Acute Ischemic Stroke

Physicians are concerned about the safety of emergency administration of antithrombotic medications in the treatment of patients with acute ischemic stroke. Intracranial hemorrhage, including hemorrhagic transformation of the infarction, is the major complication of any therapy aimed at restoring or improving perfusion to the brain. The risks for major bleeding after treatment of stroke are highlighted by the trials of thrombolytic therapy, several of which were halted prematurely because of bleeding complications.[90-94] Besides symptomatic hemorrhagic transformation of the infarction or other intracranial hemorrhage, bleeding complications also may occur in other locations in the body. In addition, some of the antithrombotic agents also may be associated with nonhemorrhagic complications. Recent clinical trials provide data about the safety of these agents when patients with recent ischemic stroke are treated.

Heparin

While unfractionated heparin has been used extensively for treatment of patients with acute ischemic stroke, information about its associated risk of bleeding is relatively limited. Early studies, performed in the 1960s, provided little data about bleeding complications.[95-99] Bleeding was not a major problem in the trial conducted by Duke et al.[100] The Cerebral Embolism Study Group did not report bleeding complications related to heparin among 45 patients with presumed stroke usually due to cardioembolism.[101-103] In another report, the same group linked the risk of hemorrhage to the severity of the brain injury.[104] Although asymptomatic hemorrhagic transformation (detection of bleeding on brain imaging but without neurologic worsening) is commonly observed after embolic stroke affecting the cerebral hemisphere, Japanese investigators found a higher risk of symptomatic hemorrhage among patients treated with heparin.[105] Slivka and Levy reviewed their experience with heparin administered to 69 patients with progressing stroke; two patients had neurologic worsening secondary to intracerebral hemorrhage.[106] In 2008, Sandercock et al found that heparin is associated with an increased risk of bleeding.[107]

Data on the safety of heparin are shown in Table 50-3. Camerlingo et al administered heparin within 3 hours of onset of stroke to 208 patients, 13 of whom had symptomatic hemorrhages.[108] A Spanish study involved heparin administered to 83 patients within 72 hours of cardioembolic stroke.[108a] Eight patients had hemorrhages, and six of these died. Two doses of subcutaneously administered heparin were tested in the International Stroke

Trial. Intracranial bleeding was diagnosed in 16 of 2429 patients (0.7%) given the lower dose and in 43 of 2426 patients (1.8%) receiving the higher dose.[109] In a subgroup of patients with atrial fibrillation, the rates of hemorrhage were 1.3% and 2.8% for the lower and higher doses of heparin.[110] Van den Berg et al reported major hemorrhagic complications in 0.8% of 664 patients who received heparin for treatment of acute ischemic stroke.[111] An Italian trial tested intravenous heparin administered within 3 hours of onset of stroke and subsequently adjusted to maintain an aPTT of 2 to 2.5 times the control.[108] Symptomatic intracranial hemorrhages occurred in 6.2% of patients given heparin compared with 1.4% of the patients receiving placebo ($P = 0.008$). Major extracranial hemorrhage also was more common in the heparin-treated group (2.9% versus 1.4%). Petty et al calculated that the risk of bleeding with heparin was 0.3 per 100 person-days.[112] The risk of bleeding with heparin is generally associated with the level of anticoagulation and the dose of medication. In addition, the likelihood of bleeding complications of heparin is higher in women, in people older than 70 years, and in those with renal failure.[113,114] Heparin also has been given in conjunction with thrombolytic agents. Studies of intraarterially administered prourokinase involved the use of heparin as a concomitant therapy.[115-117] The risk of bleeding approached 10% and was increased with the larger of the two doses of heparin. On the other hand, two studies did not report a higher risk of bleeding complications when heparin was administered after the use of alteplase.[118,119]

Nonneurologic hemorrhages also may complicate heparin. One study of heparin for evolving stroke reported that 10 of 69 patients had bleeding complications; most were nonneurologic.[106] In the International Stroke Trial, extracranial hemorrhage was diagnosed in 33 of 2426 patients (1.4%) given the higher dose of heparin and in 10 of 2429 patients (0.4%) receiving low-dose heparin.[109] The most common locations for serious bleeding are the gastrointestinal tract, urinary system, retroperitoneal space, and joints. These hemorrhages may lead to major morbidity or increased rates of mortality. Minor hemorrhages, which may necessitate cessation of heparin treatment, include microscopic hematuria, epistaxis, bruising, and minor rectal bleeding.

Heparin should be discontinued if a patient experiences severe bleeding. Protamine sulfate also may be administered. The calculated dosage of protamine is based on the assumption that heparin has a half-life of approximately 60 minutes and that the dosage of the antidote corresponds to the amount of heparin given in the previous 90 minutes.[15] Approximately 1 mg of protamine sulfate can negate the effects of 100 units of heparin. Intravenous protamine sulfate should be infused slowly (over at least 10 minutes) because it can induce hypotension. Anaphylaxis may also complicate administration of protamine.[15]

Osteoporosis may complicate long-term administration of heparin, but this potential complication should not be a major issue during short-term therapy. A transient prothrombotic state may follow the sudden termination of heparin. The frequency and the importance of this phenomenon are not clear. However, one study

TABLE 50-3 RATES OF SYMPTOMATIC INTRACRANIAL HEMORRHAGE AND SERIOUS EXTRACRANIAL HEMORRHAGE WITH ANTITHROMBOTIC TREATMENT OF ACUTE ISCHEMIC STROKE

Trial	Agent	Intracranial Hemorrhage		Extracranial Hemorrhage	
		N	%	N	%
Unfractionated heparin					
Chamorro[108a]	Heparin	8/83	9.6	—	
Camerlingo[177]	Heparin	2/45	4.4	0/45	0
IST	LD heparin	16/2429	0.7	10/2429	0.4
	HD heparin	43/2426	1.8	33/2426	1.4
Camerlingo[108]	Heparin	13/208	6.2	6/208	2.9
RAPID	Heparin	2/32	6.3	—	
LMW heparins or danaparoid					
FISS	LD nadroparin	0/100	0	4/100	4.0
	HD nadroparin	0/101	0	6/101	5.9
TOAST	Danaparoid	19/638	2.9	25/638	3.9
FISS-bis	LD nadroparin	10/271	3.7	—	
	HD nadroparin	15/245	6.1	—	
HAEST	Dalteparin	6/224	2.7	13/224	5.8
TOPAS	Certoparin	2/99	2.0	1/99	1.0
	Certoparin	1/102	0.9	0	0
	Certoparin	2/103	1.9	0	0
	Certoparin	4/100	4.0	5/100	5.0
TAIST	LD tinzaparin	3/507	0.6	2/507	0.4
	HD tinzaparin	7/486	1.4	4/486	0.8
Wong[136]	Nadroparin	1/180	0.5	25/180	14.0
Antiplatelet agents					
MAST	Aspirin	3/153	1.9	—	
IST	Aspirin	87/9720	0.9	109/9720	1.1
CAST	Aspirin	115/10,335	1.1	86/10,335	0.8
HAEST	Aspirin	4/225	1.8	4/225	1.8
TAIST	Aspirin	1/491	0.2	2/491	0.4
Wong	Aspirin	5/173	2.8	10/173	5.7
Abciximab	Abciximab	0/54	0	0/54	0
AbESTT	Abciximab	8/195	4.1	3/195	1.5
AbESTT-II	Abciximab	23/397	5.8	24/394	6.1

Abciximab, Abciximab in Ischemic Stroke Study; AbESTT, Abciximab Emergent Stroke Treatment Trial; CAST, Chinese Acute Stroke Trial; FISS, Fraxiparin in Stroke Study; HAEST, Heparin in Acute Embolic Stroke Trial; IST, International Stroke Trial; LD, low-dose; HD, high-dose; LMW, low-molecular-weight; MAST, Multicentre Acute Stroke Trial—Italy; RAPID, Rapid Anticoagulation Prevents Ischemic Damage study; TAIST, Tinzaparin in Acute Ischemic Stroke; TOAST, Trial of Org 10172 in Acute Stroke Treatment; TOPAS, Therapy of Patients with Acute Stroke.

found recurrent ischemic events after the cessation of heparin.[120]

Thrombocytopenia is a potential complication of treatment with heparin. A modest decline in platelet count may appear in up to 80% of patients who receive heparin for more than 3 days.[121] Ramirez-Lassepas et al found a greater than 40% decline in platelet count among 21 of 137 patients with stroke who were treated with heparin. These declines were asymptomatic.[122] A more severe, autoimmune-mediated thrombocytopenia may complicate the use of heparin.[121,123-125] Because heparin is a foreign protein, abnormal IgG or IgM antibodies may be found in many patients receiving heparin.[126] This finding usually appears 5 to 15 days after heparin is started. Prior use of heparin may sensitize a patient, and a second exposure may induce a severe thrombocytopenia within hours.[121,127] The autoimmune reaction is not related to the dose of heparin. The diagnosis of heparin-induced thrombocytopenia (HIT) is based on an unexplained drop in the platelet count of at least 50% or skin lesions at sites of heparin injection and the presence of HIT antibodies. The

secondary white clot syndrome may lead to myocardial or cerebral ischemia.[128,129] The neurologic complications may mimic those of thrombotic thrombocytopenia purpura. Because of the considerable risk of thrombocytopenia, patients receiving heparin should have their platelet counts checked every 2 to 3 days. Heparin should be stopped if a decline in platelet count is detected. Patients with HIT with thrombosis should be treated with hirudin or argatroban.[130,131]

Low-Molecular-Weight Heparins and Danaparoid

Bleeding is also the most likely potential complication of treatment with an LMW heparin or danaparoid. Because of a more predictable dose–response relationship, the risk of bleeding appears to be less with these agents than with unfractionated heparin. Clinical studies have confirmed a better safety profile with these agents than that for heparin.[16] The long duration of their pharmacologic actions is a potential disadvantage if serious bleeding does happen.

Clotting factors may be administered to a patient with serious bleeding after the administration of an LMW heparin, but the effectiveness of this therapy is uncertain. Protamine sulfate is not an effective antidote.

The safety of these agents in patients with acute ischemic stroke has been evaluated in several clinical trials (see Table 50-3). Most of the trials have tested subcutaneous administration. A trial performed in Hong Kong found no increase in the risk of intracranial or extracranial hemorrhage with the administration of nadroparin.[132] However, a second trial of nadroparin found a significantly increased risk of serious bleeding.[24] Symptomatic bleeding was diagnosed in 2.8% of 250 patients given placebo, in 3.7% of 271 patients receiving a low dose of nadroparin, and in 6.1% of 245 patients receiving a higher dose of the agent. In a study comparing aspirin or dalteparin in patients with atrial fibrillation and recent stroke, symptomatic intracranial hemorrhage was diagnosed in 2.7% of the patients given the LMW heparin and in 1.8% of patients receiving aspirin.[133] Extracranial hemorrhage also was more common among the patients treated with dalteparin. A German trial tested four doses of certoparin; the risks of symptomatic intracranial or extracranial bleeding were the greatest among the group that received the highest dose of the medication.[134] In a trial that tested two doses of tinzaparin in comparison with aspirin, the risks for symptomatic intracranial hemorrhage were 0.2% for aspirin, 0.6% for low-dose tinzaparin, and 1.4% for the highest dose of tinzaparin.[135] This trial did not find that medication-related extracranial bleeding was a problem. Wong et al[136] compared the utility of aspirin or a LMW heparin, nadroparin, in patients with recent stroke associated with large artery occlusive disease. The rates of hemorrhagic transformation of the infarction and severe adverse events were similar in both treatment groups.

One trial tested the intravenous administration of danaparoid in treatment of patients with acute ischemic stroke.[137] The medication was given with a bolus followed by a continuous intravenous infusion, and subsequent treatment was adjusted according to levels of inhibition of factor Xa. Enrollment of patients with more than a moderately severe stroke (as indicated by a National Institutes of Health Stroke Scale [NIHSS] score of 15 or greater) was halted because of an unacceptably high rate of symptomatic intracranial hemorrhage. Overall, symptomatic hemorrhage occurred in 6 of 628 patients given placebo (0.9%) and in 19 of 638 patients treated with danaparoid (2.9%). Extracranial hemorrhage also was significantly increased with danaparoid. A meta-analysis of the randomized trials of anticoagulants among patients with cardioembolism concluded that early administration of anticoagulants is associated with a significant increase in the risk of symptomatic intracranial bleeding (2.5% versus 0.7%; odds ratio, 2.89; 95% confidence interval, 1.19 to 7.01).[138]

A Finnish trial tested enoxaparin or unfractionated heparin in preventing venous thromboembolic events among patients with lower limb paralysis.[139] Fewer patients had hemorrhagic transformation of the infarction with enoxaparin (13.2%) than with unfractionated heparin (18.9%). A recent clinical trial compared the utility of enoxaparin or unfractionated heparin in preventing DVT after stroke.[140] The trial, which involved enrollment within 48 hours after stroke, did not assess the ability of the two anticoagulants to improve the neurologic outcome. Symptomatic intracranial hemorrhage or extracranial bleeding was diagnosed in 11 of 666 patients given enoxaparin and in 6 of 669 patients given heparin; most of the difference was due to a higher rate of extracranial bleeding with enoxaparin (7 versus 0). Another clinical trial compared the utility of certoparin, an LMW heparin, or unfractionated heparin in preventing venous thromboembolic complications among patients treated within 24 hours of stroke.[141] The rates of major bleeding complications were similar in the two treatment groups: 1.1% with certoparin and 1.8% with heparin. Burak et al[142] administered enoxaparin to eight children with acute ischemic stroke; no bleeding complications were noted. An Indian study administered nadroparin and aspirin to 20 patients with acute ischemic stroke; no difference in the rate of bleeding was noted when compared with 20 patients who received only aspirin.[143] A systematic review that compared aspirin or LMW heparin after stroke found that the anticoagulant was associated with a significant increase in major extracranial hemorrhage.[144] Among patients treated within 24 hours, symptomatic intracranial hemorrhage was significantly more common among patients treated with heparin.

Thrombocytopenia is a potential complication of treatment with the LMW heparins and danaparoid, but the risk of this complication is lower than with unfractionated heparin.[125,145] Because of the potential for cross-reactivity, patients who have experienced autoimmune heparin-associated thrombocytopenia probably should not receive the LMW heparins. Danaparoid is no longer available for administration.

Other Antithrombotic Agents

The other rapidly acting antithrombotic agents have not been extensively tested in the setting of acute ischemic stroke. Antithrombin was administered to 20 patients with cardioembolic stroke, and two hemorrhages were diagnosed.[146] LaMonte et al[32] performed a multicenter trial that enrolled 171 patients within 12 hours of stroke; two different doses of argatroban were tested. The primary outcome of this safety trial was symptomatic intracranial hemorrhage; it occurred in 5.1% of 59 subjects treated with the larger dose of argatroban, 3.4% of 58 subjects in the lower dose group, and in none of the 52 subjects in the control group. Argatroban, carefully adjusted to prolong the aPTT 1.75 times control levels, has also been administered as an adjunct to standard full-dose t-PA to 20 patients with middle cerebral artery occlusions as part of an ongoing safety study. Symptomatic intracranial hemorrhages were diagnosed in two, and one death occurred.[147,148] Some of the other agents, such as hirudin, have been tested in situations other than stroke, and the risk of bleeding was relatively high.[30]

Antiplatelet Agents

The safety of administration of aspirin within 48 hours of onset of stroke was explored in two large trials, and the medication was compared with LMW heparin in other clinical trials.[44,109,133,135,136] It also has been evaluated as an adjunct to intravenous thrombolytic therapy. One trial found that early administration of aspirin was relatively safe, but when it was added to streptokinase, the risk of intracranial hemorrhage was very high.[94] In the Chinese Acute Stroke Trial, bleeding events developed in 115 of 10,335 patients (1.1%) who received aspirin within 48 hours of onset of stroke.[44] In the International Stroke Trial, hemorrhages were reported in 87 of the 9720 patients treated with aspirin (0.9%).[109] The risk was lower among those patients who received aspirin without concomitant heparin; only 26 of 4858 patients had bleeding (0.5%). Two trials comparing aspirin or LMW heparin reported less bleeding with aspirin, but a more recent trial did not find any difference in hemorrhagic complications.[133,135] While the likelihood of serious intracranial bleeding is relatively low with aspirin, there is some associated risk from the early use of the medication after stroke. In addition, serious extracranial bleeding, particularly gastrointestinal hemorrhage, may complicate the use of aspirin.

Clopidogrel is administered as a monotherapy or in conjunction with aspirin and other antithrombotic agents in a variety of clinical settings. It has been given to patients with recent transient ischemic attacks (TIAs), but it has not been used as an acute intervention for treatment of acute ischemic stroke. Kennedy et al administered clopidogrel (300-mg loading dose followed by 75 mg daily) or placebo in addition to aspirin to patients with recent TIA or minor ischemic stroke; two of 198 patients receiving aspirin and clopidogrel had intracranial hemorrhage compared with no cases of bleeding among 194 patients treated with aspirin alone.[149] In a pilot study of 40 patients treated within 36 hours of onset of TIA or minor ischemic stroke with 300 mg clopidogrel and 325 mg of aspirin, the risk of intracerebral hemorrhage was low.[150] Two trials of the longer-term administration of the combination of aspirin and clopidogrel in comparison with monotherapy with either aspirin or clopidogrel alone found higher rates of bleeding with the combination.[151,152] The MATCH trial enrolled only patients with ischemic cerebrovascular disease.[151] In the ACTIVE-A trial, patients with atrial fibrillation received either the combination of aspirin and clopidogrel with an associated 2.0% per year risk of major bleeding or aspirin alone with a 1.3% per year risk ($P < 0.001$).[153] Because of the success of early administration of the combination of clopidogrel (loading dose) and aspirin in patients with myocardial ischemia, a similar strategy could be tested in acute ischemic stroke; an important issue will be safety. Similarly, further evidence about the safety of clopidogrel in the first hours after stroke is needed because the medication may be used as an adjunct for those patients receiving mechanical interventions to restore perfusion.

The greater potency of platelet inhibition of prasugrel and ticagrelor compared with clopidogrel is associated with a higher risk of serious bleeding. In a trial of patients with acute coronary syndromes, those with a history of TIA or stroke had a risk of intracranial hemorrhage of 2.3% for prasugrel versus 0% for clopidogrel ($P = 0.02$).[154] Similarly, the use of ticagrelor is associated with a higher risk of hemorrhagic stroke than with clopidogrel; thus it is recommended that both these drugs should be avoided in patients with cerebrovascular disease.[155] Ticagrelor also caused dyspnea, bradyarrhythmias, and increased serum levels of uric acid and creatinine. Cangrelor was associated with an excess of groin hematomas when used during percutaneous coronary interventions but not other forms of major bleeding, and bleeding was not increased in patients with a history of cerebrovascular disease.[68]

The parenterally administered glycoprotein IIb/IIIa receptor blockers have been given alone and in conjunction with thrombolytic agents in patients with acute ischemic stroke. The experience is greatest with abciximab, which has been tested in a series of clinical trials. A dose escalation study of abciximab reported no hemorrhages among 54 subjects; no dosage relationship was found.[156] A dose confirmation study reported seven cases of symptomatic hemorrhage among 195 subjects administered abciximab compared with two cases in 199 subjects treated with placebo.[157] Asymptomatic hemorrhages detected by CT were more common among the group treated with placebo than among persons treated with abciximab. Other serious bleeding was reported in three subjects in the abciximab group and in two in the placebo group. An international trial testing abciximab given within 6 hours after stroke was halted prematurely after 808 patients were enrolled; symptomatic intracranial hemorrhages were more common among those treated with abciximab than among those assigned to receive placebo.[158] A subgroup of patients treated within 3 hours of awakening with a stroke had a high rate of bleeding with abciximab. Mitsias et al tested abciximab in a series of patients with acute hemispheric cerebral infarction; few bleeding events were diagnosed.[159,160] In a series of 24 patients with neurologic deterioration after a subcortical infarct, infusion of eptifibatide was not associated with any intracerebral hemorrhages.[161] Mandava et al administered the combination of abciximab and heparin to 35 patients with stroke; one case of symptomatic and four cases of asymptomatic hemorrhage were reported.[162] Qureshi et al reported one symptomatic intracranial hemorrhage among 20 patients receiving abciximab in addition to reteplase.[163] The same group reported two asymptomatic hemorrhages among 20 patients who were treated with eptifibatide and reteplase.[164] Five patients were treated with half-dose abciximab and thrombolytic therapy; one intracranial hemorrhage was diagnosed.[165] In a study evaluating the utility of abciximab, intraarterial t-PA, and mechanical interventions in 47 patients with acute occlusions in the vertebrobasilar circulation, 3% had symptomatic intracranial hemorrhage.[166] Glycoprotein IIb/IIIa receptor blockers were given as an adjunct to pharmacologic and mechanical intraarterial thrombolysis; three of 21 patients had asymptomatic hemorrhagic transformation of the infarction detected on imaging. Twenty-one patients received intravenously administered tirofiban followed by intraarterial urokinase and mechanical thrombolysis; intracranial hemorrhages were diagnosed in five cases (three of these were fatal).[167] In the ReoPro and Retavase to treat Acute Stroke study (ROSIE/ROSIE-CT), an open-label dose-escalation study, the safety of abciximab combined with a thrombolytic agent is being tested.[168] In the Combination Anti-platelet and Anti-coagulant Treatment after Lysis of Ischemic Stroke trial (CATALIST), the safety of adding eptifibatide to aspirin, tinzaparin, and standard intravenous t-PA therapy will be tested.[169]

In the dose-escalation and safety CLEAR trial, eptifibatide was given in combination with low-dose intravenous t-PA within 3 hours after the onset of acute ischemic stroke and compared with standard-dose intravenous t-PA. When the 69 patients given combination therapy were compared with the 25 patients given standard-dose intravenous t-PA, no difference was seen in the symptomatic intracranial hemorrhage rate.[170] A phase 2 trial to test this combination, the CLEAR-ER trial, is currently enrolling patients.[171] Based on a systemic review, Ciccone et al concluded that the glycoprotein IIb/IIIa receptor blockers were associated with nonsignificant increases in symptomatic intracranial hemorrhages or major extracranial hemorrhages.[172]

Conclusions

Clinical trials confirm that both anticoagulants and antiplatelet agents are associated with a modest but significant risk of serious bleeding complications. The likelihood for either major extracranial or symptomatic intracranial hemorrhage appears to be greatest with unfractionated heparin, the LMW heparins, argatroban, and danaparoid. Bleeding side effects also appear to be greater with the glycoprotein IIb/IIIa receptor blockers than with aspirin. Information about clopidogrel is too limited to make any firm conclusions about its safety, and the other thienopyridines have not been tested in stroke patients.

Although the risk of bleeding is relatively low with anticoagulants, it is high enough to mandate that strong evidence for efficacy is needed to justify their use. The LMW heparins do not appear to be either more dangerous or safer than unfractionated heparin. The risk of serious bleeding complications increases with the dose of unfractionated heparin or LMW heparin. No data correlate the risk of bleeding with either subcutaneous or intravenous administration of heparin or LMW heparins. The use of a bolus dose to start anticoagulation does not seem to be particularly dangerous, despite common admonitions against this practice. The likelihood of hemorrhage with heparin or LMW heparins is associated with the severity of neurologic impairments or the size of stroke on the initial brain imaging study. Anticoagulants probably cannot be given with a reasonable level of safety to patients with findings of multilobar infarction. Patients with more severe strokes (NIHSS score >15) and those with a large area of hypodensity on CT probably should not be treated with either unfractionated heparin or one of the LMW heparins.

Starting aspirin within 48 hours after stroke is accompanied by a relatively low rate of symptomatic bleeding. The other antiplatelet agents appear to confer a sufficiently high risk of serious bleeding complications that strong evidence for efficacy is needed to justify their use. The safety of a combination of either an anticoagulant or antiplatelet agent with a thrombolytic agent has not been established. At present, current guidelines recommend delaying the start of these medications until at least 24 hours after intravenous treatment with t-PA.[7]

Besides intracranial bleeding, physicians should be alert to nonneurologic hemorrhagic complications after the use of an anticoagulant or antiplatelet agent. Patients with active bleeding or other illnesses that are associated with a high chance of serious bleeding (e.g., recent surgery or recent trauma) may be well-served by not receiving these medications. Agent-specific issues such as thrombocytopenia also should be kept in mind when antithrombotic medications are administered to patients with acute ischemic stroke.

Efficacy of Treatment of Acute Ischemic Stroke

There has been considerable uncertainty about the efficacy of antithrombotic agents in improving outcomes after acute ischemic stroke. Unless there is strong evidence of efficacy, these medications, which may be associated with serious neurologic or medical complications, should not be administered. Meta-analyses have shown that heparin and the LMW heparins are effective in lowering the risk of DVT after stroke.[173] However, most physicians are not prescribing antithrombotic medications in the setting of acute ischemic stroke with the primary goal of preventing DVT and pulmonary embolism. The primary goal has been to limit brain injury and improve neurologic outcome by halting neurologic worsening and preventing early recurrent thromboembolism. Some subgroups of patients with stroke, such as those with cardioembolism, large artery atherosclerosis, or arterial dissection have been preferentially treated with urgent anticoagulation. Although these medications are prescribed widely, strong clinical data on their efficacy are limited.[107,174,175]

Unfractionated Heparin

Several small studies of heparin were performed before the development of modern brain imaging studies.[95,97-99,176] In general, these studies' results suggested that emergency administration of heparin was potentially effective. Still, major methodologic problems weaken these data. Two studies included randomized assignment, but the numbers of enrolled subjects were too few to produce definitive results.[97,98] Three other studies used historical controls for comparisons.[95,99,176] In the 1980s, a randomized, placebo-controlled trial tested the potential utility of intravenously administered heparin.[100] Approximately 200 subjects, with stable neurologic deficits, were enrolled but most did not receive treatment until more than 24 hours after onset of stroke. Not surprisingly, no net benefit from treatment was noted.

In a series of studies, the Cerebral Embolism Study Group tested the potential utility of heparin.[101-104] These studies showed a trend toward a lower rate of recurrent embolization. The investigators also estimated that the risk of early recurrent stroke may be as high as 12%.[101] On the basis of a retrospective review of 44 patients with embolic stroke, heparin was estimated to halve the risk of early recurrent stroke. However, the meta-analysis performed by Sandercock et al[173] could not confirm the efficacy of heparin for improving outcomes after stroke or lowering the risk of recurrent embolization.

In a study that included initiating treatment within 5 hours of onset of stroke to 45 patients, improvement was noted in 23.[177] In an uncontrolled study, Dahl et al administered heparin to 52 patients with progressing stroke, and neurologic worsening stopped in 38; 11 patients experienced neurologic worsening despite heparin therapy.[178] Haley et al found no benefit from heparin when it was administered to 36 patients with progressing stroke.[179] Chamorro et al gave heparin to 231 patients with recent embolic stroke and noted recurrent events in 5 patients.[179a] In a historical control study, Rödén-Jüllig and Britton compared outcomes among 314 patients not receiving heparin with those in 907 patients treated with anticoagulants.[180] Progression of neurologic deficits was noted in 28% of patients who did not receive heparin and in 21% of those who did, and the investigators concluded that heparin did not improve outcomes or halt neurologic worsening. Another trial reported that recurrent strokes occurred in 2.4% of 664 patients who received heparin for treatment of acute ischemic stroke.[111]

In a very large trial that enrolled approximately 20,000 participants, investigators of the International Stroke Trial tested two doses of subcutaneously administered heparin against placebo (Tables 50-3 through 50-6).[109] Within 48 hours of onset of stroke, subjects were assigned treatment with either 5000 units (low dose) or 12,500 units (high dose) of heparin twice a day. Some subjects also received aspirin. The trial does have weaknesses in design. For a sizable number of patients enrolled in the trial, baseline brain imaging studies were not performed beforehand to exclude primary hemorrhages. Thus, some subjects with de novo hemorrhage might have been treated. Both the treating physicians and the subjects were aware of the treatment allocation; this information may have biased the physicians' and subjects' reporting of adverse experiences. No monitoring of the level of anticoagulation and no adjustment of doses of heparin were included. As a result, some subjects may have received excessive doses of heparin that could raise the odds of major bleeding complications, whereas other subjects might have received insufficient doses of heparin; thus, the effectiveness of therapy may have been lost. The trial demonstrated a modest decline in the frequency of recurrent stroke within the first 14 days with the use of heparin. No reduction in mortality or an improvement in the rate of favorable outcomes was seen. As a result, the trial found no net benefit from treatment with heparin. No net benefit from treatment with

TABLE 50-4 RATES OF EARLY RECURRENT STROKE AFTER ANTITHROMBOTIC THERAPY FOR ACUTE ISCHEMIC STROKE

| Trial | Agent | Treatment | | Comparison Group | | |
		N	%	Type	N	%
Unfractionated heparin						
IST	LD heparin	78/2429	1.6	Control	214/4859	2.2
	HD heparin	86/2426	1.8			
IST—AF	Heparin	44/1557	2.8	Control	79/1612	4.9
LMW heparins and danaparoid						
FISS	LD nadroparin	2/101	1.9	Placebo	5/105	4.7
	HD nadroparin	1/102	1			
TOAST	Danaparoid	7/638	1.1	Placebo	7/628	1.1
TOAST—CE	Danaparoid	0/143	0	Placebo	2/123	1.6
HAEST	Dalteparin	19/224	8.5	Aspirin	17/225	7.5
TOPAS	Certoparin	3/99	3.0			
	Certoparin	3/102	2.9			
	Certoparin	4/103	3.9			
	Certoparin	3/100	3.0			
TAIST	LD tinzaparin	24/507	4.7	Aspirin	15/491	3.1
	HD tinzaparin	16/486	3.3			
TAIST—CE	Tinzaparin	4/256	1.6	Aspirin	2/112	1.8
Wong[136]	Nadroparin	8/180	4.0	Aspirin	8/173	5.0
Antiplatelet agents						
MAST	Aspirin	1/153	0.6	Control	0/156	0
IST	Aspirin	275/9719	2.8	Control	368/9714	3.8
CAST	Aspirin	220/10,335	2.1	Placebo	258/10,320	2.5
HAEST	Aspirin	17/225	7.5	Dalteparin	19/224	8.5
TAIST	Aspirin	15/491	3.2	Tinzaparin	40/993	4.0
Wong	Aspirin	8/173	5.0	Nadroparin	8/180	4.0
Abciximab	Abciximab	1/54	2.0	Placebo	1/20	5.0
AbESTT	Abciximab	7/195	3.9	Placebo	8/199	3.9
AbESTT-II	Abciximab	12/403	2.9	Placebo	7/398	1.7

Abciximab, Abciximab in Ischemic Stroke Study; AbESTT, Abciximab Emergent Stroke Treatment Trial; AF, atrial fibrillation; CAST, Chinese Acute Stroke Trial; CE, cardioembolic; FISS, Fraxiparin in Stroke Study; HAEST, Heparin in Acute Embolic Stroke Trial; IST, International Stroke Trial; LD, low-dose; HD, high-dose; LMW, low-molecular-weight; MAST, Multicentre Acute Stroke Trial—Italy; TAIST, Tinzaparin in Acute Ischemic Stroke; TOAST, Trial of Org 10172 in Acute Stroke Treatment; TOPAS, Therapy of Patients with Acute Stroke.

heparin was also noted among the subgroup of patients who had atrial fibrillation.

Despite the publication of the results of the International Stroke Trial, interest persisted in the potential usefulness of heparin for treatment of patients with recent stroke. Additional clinical trials have been reported. In a small multicenter clinical trial, Chamorro et al tested intravenously administered heparin with adjustments in dosage in response to aPTT.[181] The trial was halted prematurely when only 67 subjects were enrolled because of slow enrollment. Not surprisingly, outcomes between the two treatment groups were not different. In a single-center, placebo-controlled study, Camerlingo et al enrolled 418 subjects in a clinical trial that tested intravenous heparin administered within 3 hours of onset of stroke.[108a] Favorable outcomes were found in 81 of 208 subjects given heparin and in 60 of 210 subjects in the control group.

Low-Molecular-Weight Heparins and Danaparoid

Several trials tested subcutaneously administered LMW heparins (see Tables 50-3 through 50-6). Two dosages of nadroparin (4100 anti-factor Xa units daily or 4100 anti-factor Xa units twice daily) were tested in a placebo-controlled trial performed by Kay et al.[132,182] Medications were started within 48 hours of stroke and continued for 10 days. No monitoring of the level of anticoagulation or adjustment of doses was performed. Recurrent strokes occurred more frequently in the subjects receiving placebo than in either group that received nadroparin. At

an assessment performed 6 months after stroke, excellent outcomes were significantly more common among the subjects who received the larger dose of nadroparin than among those who received placebo. However, no differences in favor of nadroparin were found at the end of the early treatment period or at 3 months. The reason for the differences in responses at 3 months and 6 months is not clear. A second trial of nadroparin tested two doses of nadroparin against placebo. A weight-based treatment regimen was used; the lower dose was 85 anti-factor Xa units/day, and the large dose was doubled. The medications were administered within 24 hours of onset of stroke, but no monitoring or dose adjustments were included. No improvement in outcomes was noted.[183]

A Norwegian trial tested dalteparin or aspirin in preventing early recurrent stroke or improving outcomes among patients with atrial fibrillation who had strokes.[133] The arrhythmia was used as a surrogate for the diagnosis of cardioembolic stroke. Dalteparin was given subcutaneously for 10 days, and no monitoring of anticoagulation or adjustment of the dose was performed. Recurrent strokes occurred in 8.5% of 224 subjects treated with dalteparin and in 7.5% of 225 subjects receiving aspirin. No differences in the rates of favorable outcomes were found between the two treatment groups. German investigators evaluated four doses of subcutaneously administered certoparin (3000 U/day, 3000 U/twice a day, 5000 U/twice a day, or 8000 U/twice a day) in a study that enrolled approximately 400 subjects.[134] Therapy was initiated within 12 hours of stroke. Levels of anticoagulation were not monitored, and adjustments in the doses were not made during the 12 to 16 days of treatment. No

TABLE 50-5   RATES OF NEUROLOGIC WORSENING AFTER TREATMENT OF ACUTE ISCHEMIC STROKE

| Trial | Agent | Treatment | | Comparison Group | | |
		N	%	Type	N	%
Unfractionated heparin						
Rödén-Jüllig[180]	Heparin		30	Control		33
RAPID	Heparin	8/32	25	Aspirin	7/35	20
LMW heparins and danaparoid						
TOAST	Danaparoid	63/635	10	Placebo	62/633	9.9
HAEST	Dalteparin	24/224	10.7	Aspirin	17/225	7.6
TAIST	LD tinzaparin	55/508	11.4	Aspirin	58/491	11.9
	HD tinzaparin	58/486	11.9			
Wong[136]	Nadroparin	10/180	6	Aspirin	8/173	5
Antiplatelet agents						
MAST	Aspirin	18/153	11.8	Control	21/156	13.4
IST	Aspirin	567/4858	11.7	Control	604/4859	12.4
CAST	Aspirin	545/10,335	5.3	Placebo	614/10,320	5.9
HAEST	Aspirin	17/225	7.6	Dalteparin	24/224	10.7
TAIST	Aspirin	58/491	11.9	Tinzaparin	116/993	11.7
RAPID	Aspirin	7/35	20.0	Heparin	8/32	25.0
Wong[136]	Aspirin	8/173	5.0	Nadroparin	10/180	6.0
Abciximab	Abciximab	6/54	11.0	Placebo	3/20	15.0
AbESTT	Abciximab	14/195	7.1	Placebo	24/199	12.0
AbESTT-II	Abciximab	35/403	8.6	Placebo	45/398	11.3

Abciximab, Abciximab in Ischemic Stroke Study; AbESTT, Abciximab Emergent Stroke Treatment Trial; AF, atrial fibrillation; CAST, Chinese Acute Stroke Trial; CE, cardioembolic; FISS, Fraxiparin in Stroke Study; HAEST, Heparin in Acute Embolic Stroke Trial; HD, high-dose; IST, International Stroke Trial; LD, low-dose; LMW, low-molecular-weight; MAST, Multicentre Acute Stroke Trial—Italy; TAIST, Tinzaparin in Acute Ischemic Stroke; TOAST, Trial of Org 10172 in Acute Stroke Treatment; TOPAS, Therapy of Patients with Acute Stroke.

TABLE 50-6 RATES OF FAVORABLE OUTCOMES AFTER ANTITHROMBOTIC TREATMENT OF ACUTE ISCHEMIC STROKE

Trial	Agent	Treatment		Comparison Group		
		N	%	Type	N	%
Unfractionated heparin						
IST	LD heparin	1776/4860	36.5	Control	3852/9718	36.9
	HD heparin	1802/4856	37.1			
Camerlingo[108]	Heparin	81/208	38.9	Control	60/210	28.6
RAPID	Heparin	13/32	40.6	Aspirin	19/35	54.3
LMW heparins and danaparoid						
FISS	LD nadroparin	48/101	47.5	Placebo	37/105	35.2
	HD nadroparin	57/102	55.8			
TOAST	Danaparoid	482/641	75.2	Placebo	467/634	73.6
FISS-bis	LD nadroparin	155/271	57.2	Placebo	142/250	56.8
	HD nadroparin	145/245	59.2			
HAEST	Dalteparin	76/224	33.9	Aspirin	79/225	35.1
TOPAS	Certoparin	37/96	38.5			
	Certoparin	38/97	39.2			
	Certoparin	36/98	36.7			
	Certoparin	42/96	43.7			
TAIST	LD tinzaparin	188/507	38.3	Aspirin	206/491	42.5
	HD tinzaparin	181/486	38.4			
Wong[136]	Nadroparin	131/180	72.7	Aspirin	119/173	68.9
Antiplatelet agents						
MAST	Aspirin	59/153	38.6	Control	50/156	32.1
IST	Aspirin	1860/4858	38.3	Control	1795/4859	36.9
CAST	Aspirin	7182/10335	69.5	Placebo	7054/10321	68.3
HAEST	Aspirin	79/225	35.1	Dalteparin	76/224	33.9
TAIST	Aspirin	206/491	42.5	Tinzaparin	369/993	38.3
Wong	Aspirin	119/173	68.9	Nadroparin	131/180	72.7
Abciximab	Abciximab	24/54	44.0	Placebo	8/20	40.0
AbESTT	Abciximab	97/200	48.5	Placebo	80/200	40.0
AbESTT-II	Abciximab	154/403	38.2	Placebo	167/398	41.9

Abciximab, Abciximab in Ischemic Stroke Study; AbESTT, Abciximab Emergent Stroke Treatment Trial; CAST, Chinese Acute Stroke Trial; FISS, Fraxiparin in Stroke Study; HAEST, Heparin in Acute Embolic Stroke Trial; HD, high-dose; IST, International Stroke Trial; LD, low-dose; LMW, low-molecular-weight; MAST, Multicentre Acute Stroke Trial—Italy; RAPID, Rapid Anticoagulation Prevents Ischemic Damage study; TAIST, Tinzaparin in Acute Ischemic Stroke; TOAST, Trial of Org 10172 in Acute Stroke Treatment; TOPAS, Therapy of Patients with Acute Stroke.

differences in the rates of recurrent stroke or favorable outcomes were seen among the groups. In a three-arm treatment trial, two doses of tinzaparin (100 anti-factor Xa U/kg or 175 anti-factor Xa U/kg) were compared with aspirin (300 mg/day).[135] The doses of tinzaparin were not adjusted to the level of anticoagulation. Treatment was started within 48 hours of stroke. No reduction in mortality or improvement in the rate of favorable outcome was seen with either dose of tinzaparin. The presumed cause of stroke did not affect responses to treatment.

Intravenously administered danaparoid was compared with placebo in a randomized trial that enrolled approximately 1300 subjects.[137] Patients were enrolled within 24 hours of onset of stroke. Treatment was initiated with a bolus dose and maintained with a continuous infusion for 7 days. Infusion rates were adjusted in response to levels of inhibition of factor Xa. A weight-based regimen also was used. No differences were noted between the two treatment groups in the rates of neurologic worsening or early recurrent stroke. No reduction in the rate of early recurrent embolism among those patients with presumed cardioembolic stroke was noted between the two treatment groups. Although a trend in favor of treatment with danaparoid was detected during the first 7 days, no

difference in outcomes was found at 3 months. Patients with stroke secondary to large artery atherosclerosis (primarily stenosis or occlusion of the internal carotid artery) seemed to benefit from treatment.[184] This response was not replicated in the trial of tinzaparin described previously.[135] In a meta-analysis of the trials of LMW heparins and danaparoid, Bath et al could not establish efficacy of these agents in any group of patients with acute ischemic stroke.[185]

Subsequently, Wong et al tested nadroparin (3800 anti-factor Xa U twice daily) or aspirin (160 mg daily) in 603 subjects.[136] Enrollment was within 48 hours of onset of stroke; 353 subjects had evidence of large artery occlusive disease demonstrated by vascular imaging. Almost all the subjects had primarily intracranial stenoses. Favorable outcomes were similar in the two treatment groups. Another trial looked at the utility of early anticoagulation in treatment of patients with atrial fibrillation as identified by clinical variables or laboratory findings of D-dimer, prothrombin fragments (1 + 2), soluble fibrin monomer, or C-reactive protein. Dalteparin (100 U/kg twice a day) or aspirin (160 mg/day) was administered, and outcomes at 3 months were compared. No improvement in outcomes with administration of dalteparin was found.[186] A small study from India reported that the addition of nadroparin to aspirin reduced mortality and morbidity rates from stroke at 4 weeks.[143] Based on a database search that identified eight children, Burak et al concluded that enoxaparin could be an effective alternative to unfractionated heparin in children.[142]

In a meta-analysis of the trials testing unfractionated heparin or LMW heparins in patients with cardioembolic stroke, Paciaroni et al found that the medications were associated with a nonsignificant reduction in recurrent stroke within 7 to 14 days (3.0% versus 4.9%; odds ratio, 0.68, 95% confidence interval [CI], 0.44 to 1.06; $P = 0.09$). No major difference in disability or death at follow-up was seen (73.5% versus 73.8%; odds ratio, 1.01, 95% CI, 0.82 to 1.24; $P = 0.9$).[138]

Other Antithrombotic Agents

Yasaka et al administered antithrombin to patients and noted no recurrent stroke events.[146] A pilot study of argatroban enrolled 171 subjects treated within 12 hours after onset of stroke.[32] Argatroban was given in a bolus (100 μg/kg) and followed by an intravenous infusion at 3 μg/kg/min (n = 59) or 1 μg/kg/min (n = 58). Target aPTTs were 2.25 times the control for the higher dose and 1.75 times the control for the lower dose. Fifty-four subjects received placebo. No differences in outcomes, including mortality rate, were noted. Low-dose argatroban carefully titrated to prolong the aPTT at 1.75 times control values combined with standard full-dose intravenous t-PA is being tested in a pilot study. In the first reported cohort of 15 subjects, recanalization was complete in six cases and partial in four others.[147] Reocclusion of the previous patent artery occurred in three subjects. Additional research on argatroban and other antithrombotic agents is ongoing.

Antiplatelet Agents

Aspirin has been examined in several clinical trials (see Tables 50-3 through 50-6).[187] Aspirin often has been the reference agent for trials testing LMW heparins. In general, aspirin was as effective as the anticoagulant in preventing recurrent stroke, in achieving favorable outcomes, and in preventing mortality.

In one trial, the rate of favorable outcomes improved when aspirin was administered alone or in combination with streptokinase.[94] Recurrent stroke was observed in only one of 153 patients given aspirin alone. A multicenter trial comparing intravenous t-PA combined with aspirin compared with thrombolytic therapy alone has started.[188] In the International Stroke Trial, aspirin (300 mg daily) was given alone to 4858 subjects and in conjunction with heparin to another 4861 subjects.[109] Recurrent stroke was diagnosed in 156 (3.2%) of the subjects who received only aspirin and in 119 (2.4%) of the subjects who were given both aspirin and heparin. The reduction in recurrent events was statistically significant. The rates of recurrent stroke among patients treated with aspirin alone and with heparin, in comparison with the rates in those not taking aspirin, are shown in Table 50-5. The rates of death or disability were modestly reduced in patients who were treated with either aspirin or the combination of heparin and aspirin, but the differences were not significant. In the randomized Chinese Acute Stroke Trial, which enrolled more than 20,000 subjects, aspirin (160 mg/day) was compared with placebo.[44] Therapy was started within 48 hours of stroke and continued for 28 days. The long interval from onset of stroke and the long treatment period are sources of concern; in particular, the long treatment period during which the control group received placebo overlaps with the time that many physicians would consider that long-term stroke preventive medications should have been started. Aspirin reduced the risk of recurrent stroke: rates of stroke were 2.1% (220/10,335) in the aspirin group and 2.5% (258/10,320) in the placebo group. The trial found a modest decline in mortality and disability with aspirin (30.5% versus 31.6% for placebo). The investigators of the CAST and International Stroke Trials had prespecified an analysis of combined data; the results found a significant reduction in the prevention of recurrent strokes (7 per 1000), and a benefit was seen in all subgroups of patients for improving outcomes.

A small Swedish placebo-controlled, randomized, double-blind trial tested the usefulness of aspirin (325 mg/day) in preventing progressing stroke.[189] Patients who had taken an antiplatelet agent within 72 hours before the stroke were excluded. The medication was started within 48 hours of stroke. At 5 days, progression of neurologic impairments was found in 15.9% of the 220 subjects treated with aspirin and in 16.7% of the subjects assigned placebo. No differences in outcomes were found.

The FASTER trial enrolled 392 patients with TIA or minor stroke, and all patients received aspirin in addition to either a 300-mg loading dose of clopidogrel or placebo and simvastatin versus placebo in a factorial design. The trial was stopped early because of difficulty recruiting patients due to the widespread use of statins, but the risk of recurrent stroke within 90 days was 7.1% in the clopidogrel group and 10.8% on placebo (risk ratio, 0.7; 95% CI, 0.3 to 1.2).[149] A larger trial (Platelet-Oriented Inhibition in New TIA and minor ischemic stroke [POINT] trial) is testing a loading dose of 600 mg of clopidogrel versus placebo in addition to aspirin in patients with minor stroke or high-risk TIA.[190]

Small anecdotal studies reported on the responses to glycoprotein IIb/IIIa receptor blockers in patients with ischemic cerebrovascular disease, including the use of these medications as an adjunct to angioplasty and stenting.[33,160,163,165,191-194] These medications have been given as a monotherapy or in conjunction with thrombolytic agents or anticoagulants.[195] Eckert et al found that the addition of abciximab to t-PA and endovascular interventions was associated with improved degrees of recanalization and neurologic outcomes.[166] Another study used low-pressure angioplasty supplemented in some cases with eptifibatide.[196] They concluded that the regimen was successful in achieving recanalization and in preventing reocclusion. Qureshi et al found that eptifibatide within 24 hours of treatment with thrombolytic therapy may help prevent subsequent neurologic worsening.[164] An uncontrolled study looked at abciximab for treatment of acute ischemic stroke.[159] The agent was started 3 to 24 hours after the onset of stroke, and the patients were monitored clinically and with diffusion-weighted magnetic resonance imaging scans. Average improvement of NIHSS scores was 4 points, and seven of 26 subjects showed decreases in the area of ischemia on follow-up scans.

A pilot dose-escalation study of abciximab found that the medication might improve outcomes among patients treated within 24 hours of stroke.[156] A second dose-confirmation, randomized, double-blinded, placebo-controlled study tested the efficacy of abciximab when started within 6 hours of onset of stroke.[157] Abciximab was given in a 0.25 mg/kg bolus followed by a 12-hour infusion of 0.125 μg/kg/min (maximum, 10 μg/min). The trial, which enrolled 400 patients, showed a nonsignificant shift in favorable outcomes at 3 months (odds ratio, 1.20; 95% CI, 0.84 to 1.70; $P = 0.33$). The benefit was strongest among patients treated within 5 hours of onset of stroke. The results of this trial prompted the Abciximab in Emergent Stroke Treatment Trial-II, which enrolled subjects into three groups: those enrolled within 5 hours of stroke onset, 5 to 6 hours after stroke, or within 3 hours of awakening with a stroke.[158] The trial was halted prematurely when an interim analysis did not demonstrate a favorable risk–benefit ratio. A small trial of tirofiban compared with aspirin within 6 hours of the onset of acute ischemic stroke was halted early because of no difference between the two groups.[197]

Conclusions

Preventing Early Recurrent Stroke

The data from clinical trials provide conflicting evidence as to whether early administration of antithrombotic agents is effective in lowering the risk of early recurrent stroke. On the basis of the information collected from several of the larger trials, the risk of early recurrent stroke is much lower than was assumed previously.[44,109,137] A reasonable estimate is that approximately 2% of patients have recurrent stroke within 1 week of the stroke. By 2 weeks, the rate probably increases to between 3% and 4%. Although the risk of recurrent stroke is higher in patients with presumed cardioembolic stroke, the rates are approximately 2% to 8% in the first 7 to 14 days.[109,110,133,137] However, although the risk of early recurrent stroke is not high, the likelihood of a poorer neurologic outcome after a second event is considerable. Initiation of therapy to prevent this complication is important. Other crucial issues are (1) when to start therapies to prevent recurrent stroke, (2) whether to maintain anticoagulation on a long-term basis, and (3) selection of the best agent for the individual patient.

Because the overall risk of early recurrent embolization is relatively low, demonstration of the efficacy of emergency anticoagulation in lessening that risk will be difficult. Some trials have not specifically evaluated the utility of anticoagulants in preventing early recurrent stroke, and others have not demonstrated that unfractionated heparin, LMW heparins, or danaparoid are effective. At present, early anticoagulation has not been established as efficacious in preventing early recurrent stroke, including presumed cardioembolic stroke. There has been no subgroup of stroke patients identified who have been judged as having a very high risk of recurrent stroke and who might benefit from emergency anticoagulation.

Results of the large trials of aspirin are somewhat conflicting. Although aspirin lowered the risk of early recurrences, the benefit from aspirin was reduced when the aggregate of hemorrhagic and ischemic stroke was evaluated.[44,109] In trials of LMW heparin, aspirin was administered as the control medication. In the trial conducted by Berge et al, the rate of recurrent embolic stroke among patients with atrial fibrillation was slightly lower among the patients treated with aspirin than among those receiving dalteparin.[133] Overall, the results suggest that aspirin, started within 48 hours of stroke, may produce a modest reduction in the risk of early recurrent stroke. Thus, starting aspirin within 48 hours of the event is a reasonable treatment option for most patients with ischemic stroke.[7] The decision to start aspirin should be influenced by other therapies administered in the early period. Aspirin should not be started in lieu of other effective treatments for acute stroke, such as t-PA. Aspirin should not be started sooner than 24 hours after the administration of t-PA.[7] No other antiplatelet agent has been shown to be effective in reducing the likelihood of recurrent stroke within the first days after a stroke.

Halting Neurologic Worsening

Neurologic worsening (stroke-in-evolution) is associated with a greater likelihood of poor outcomes; thus, preventing this deterioration should be a primary focus of acute stroke care.[198] As a result, antithrombotic agents often are prescribed to patients who are judged to be at risk of neurologic decline. Prediction of those patients who will deteriorate cannot be made with certainty.[198,199] Some patients might be diagnosed through direct observation of stroke-in-evolution. Others may be judged as having a high risk of neurologic worsening on the basis of clinical findings. Neurologic decline seems to be more common with strokes in the vertebrobasilar circulation than in the carotid circulation.[200] Patients with multilobar or large brainstem strokes are at high risk of neurologic worsening. Unfortunately, these patients also have a high risk for hemorrhagic complications that lead to neurologic decline. The risk of hemorrhagic complications is increased by both anticoagulants and antiplatelet agents. In addition, neurologic worsening may be secondary to a number of medical or neurologic complications of stroke that are not ameliorated by antithrombotic medications. Severe brain edema, hydrocephalus, increased intracranial pressure, seizures, electrolyte disturbances, and infections are potential causes of neurologic decline.[201-204] None of these conditions may be successfully treated with antithrombotic agents.

Clinical trials that have examined the impact of anticoagulants or antiplatelet agents on halting neurologic worsening have reported neutral results.[44,109,133,135-137,157, 158,180,181] Overall, the trials report that the frequency of neurologic deterioration within the first 7 to 10 days after stroke was approximately 10% regardless of whether the patient received antithrombotic therapy. These disappointing results are those reported by uncontrolled trials in which anticoagulants were administered to patients with presumed stroke-in-evolution. Overall, the data suggest that the effect of antithrombotic therapy in halting neurologic deterioration after stroke is likely to be small.

Improving Neurologic Outcomes

Overall, the data from the clinical trials of unfractionated heparin, LMW heparins, and danaparoid are similar. The trials do not show a net long-term benefit from initiation of anticoagulant therapy within the first 12 to 48 hours after stroke.[24,109,134-137,181] A small Italian trial of heparin given within 3 hours of onset of stroke showed borderline efficacy.[108a] Still, the general trend is that emergency anticoagulation does not lessen disability or mortality rates after stroke. Although there are real differences among the individual trials, probably reflecting the nature of the populations enrolled in the studies, the results of the trials generally are similar. There is no evidence that anticoagulants are more effective in any subgroup of patients, including those with cardioembolic events or large artery atherosclerosis. The success with unfractionated heparin is not better or worse than that achieved with the LMW heparins. The likelihood of a therapeutic response does not seem to be influenced by the mode of administration, the use of a bolus dose to start treatment, or the level of anticoagulation. The data about argatroban are too limited to determine whether it is effective.

Most of the information about the utility of antiplatelet agents comes from two large trials testing aspirin.[44,109] Although there are marked differences in the rates of favorable outcomes between the two trials, the aggregate data suggest that starting aspirin within 48 hours of onset of stroke is associated with a modest improvement in the rate of favorable outcomes. Several of the trials of anticoagulants included aspirin as part of the control management; these studies show that aspirin is at least equal to the anticoagulants.[133,135,136] No data about the utility of clopidogrel are available. The data from recent trials testing the parenterally administered glycoprotein IIb/IIIa receptor blockers are mixed.[157,158] Preliminary studies of abciximab suggested that the agent might be effective, but the recent international trial did not demonstrate any benefit in improving neurologic outcomes. Unless the data from ongoing or future trials of emergency administration of antiplatelet agents provide positive results, the present evidence suggests that these medications do not improve outcomes.

Prevention of Deep Vein Thrombosis

DVT and pulmonary embolism are important causes of morbidity and mortality after stroke.[201,205] Bedridden patients with a paralyzed lower extremity have the greatest risk of these complications. In this group, the rate of DVT is estimated to be approximately 25% to 50%.[68,206,207] Pulmonary embolism accounts for approximately 5% to 25% of deaths after stroke, and most of these vascular events occur more than 1 week after stroke.[207-209] Institution of measures to prevent DVT is a quality indicator for inpatient management of patients with recent stroke. Several measures, including early mobilization, can prevent DVT.[210]

Antithrombotic agents are the principal medical therapy for prevention or treatment of DVT. Kelly et al concluded that the short-term administration of low-dose unfractionated heparin did not have a sustained benefit in forestalling venous thromboembolic disease.[208,209] However, other studies have concluded that early administration of antithrombotic agents, including heparin and LMW heparins, to patients with stroke is effective.[173] Some studies found that the LMW compounds are superior to heparin.[140,211,212] During the last few years, additional data have demonstrated the utility of anticoagulants in preventing DVT and pulmonary embolism. A large international trial compared unfractionated heparin and enoxaparin in 1762 subjects with recent ischemic stroke and found no difference in risk of bleeding but a lower rate of venous thromboembolism in the enoxaparin group.[140,213] Current guidelines recommend anticoagulants for the prevention of DVT after stroke.[7]

Besides preventing DVT, anticoagulants have been shown to be effective in preventing pulmonary embolism among high-risk bedridden patients with recent stroke. Guidelines recommend parenteral administration of anticoagulants to lessen the likelihood of pulmonary embolism in high-risk patients.[7] Still, it is reasonable to withhold anticoagulants in some patients at high risk of hemorrhagic transformation such as those with multilobar infarctions.

Aspirin provides some protection against DVT and pulmonary embolism. It is an alternative to treatment with anticoagulants.[214] Antithrombotic stockings and external pneumatic calf compression devices also reduce the risk of DVT and pulmonary embolism for a patient who cannot receive anticoagulants.[215] Placement of a filter in the inferior vena cava (Greenfield filter) can also be used to prevent pulmonary embolism in patients who cannot receive antithrombotic agents. Intravenous infusions of heparin are prescribed to patients with pulmonary embolism.

Other Indications

With the initiation of therapy, warfarin lowers the levels of the antithrombotic factors, proteins C and S, before its effects on prothrombin are detected. Thus, a transient hypercoagulable state might occur during the first days of starting warfarin. The complication of a prothrombotic state with secondary ischemic events is most commonly detected among patients who have an inherited or acquired deficiency of protein C or protein S. Because of the concern about this risk, many physicians prescribe a brief course of heparin or an LMW heparin during the initiation of treatment with warfarin. The utility of this strategy is not known. An alternative approach is to start with low doses of warfarin so that inhibition of both the prothrombotic and antithrombotic clotting factors occurs at approximately the same time.

Parenteral anticoagulants may also be started in a manner similar to that used for starting antithrombotic therapy to prevent recurrent ischemic events in high-risk patients with cardiogenic embolism. Either heparin or LMW heparins may be administered until the desired international normalized ratio (INR) is achieved with warfarin. In this situation, treatment with the parenteral anticoagulants should be considered as a transitional step toward long-term treatment and not part of the immediate management of the stroke. However, there may be increased risk of bleeding with this strategy. In a retrospective review of 204 patients with cardioembolic stroke, those who were treated with warfarin and bridged with heparin or enoxaparin had an increased risk of serious bleeding compared with those treated with warfarin without bridging.[216] The timing of initiation of anticoagulation after an infarction has not been established. Current guidelines recommend that these agents not be started within 24 hours after treatment with t-PA.

Anticoagulation has been recommended for treatment of patients with stroke secondary to extracranial arterial dissection. There is a concern about intracranial bleeding with anticoagulants given to patients with intracranial arterial dissections because subarachnoid hemorrhage is a known complication of the arterial lesion. A Cochrane review in 2003 and a meta-analysis in 2008 that included more than 700 patients did not show any difference in efficacy or complications between antiplatelet and anticoagulant therapy in preventing stroke, TIA, or death.[217,218] A nonrandomized study of 298 consecutive patients with spontaneous dissection of the cervical carotid artery also showed no difference in efficacy.[219] At 3 months, the recurrent event rate of ischemic stroke was low: 0.3%. The Cervical Artery Dissection in Stroke Study (CADISS) is a randomized controlled trial in which antiplatelet therapy is being compared with anticoagulation with heparin followed by warfarin in patients with cervical artery dissection. A feasibility phase of 250 subjects is being conducted to determine the necessary sample size and to see if an adequate number of patients can be recruited.[220]

Patients with acute ischemic heart disease often receive anticoagulants, antiplatelet agents, or both as part of the treatment regimen to limit the cardiac injury. These agents are administered as adjuncts to pharmacologic or mechanical thrombolysis. A similar strategy may be important in treating acute brain ischemia. There are cases of arterial reocclusion with neurologic worsening after successful recanalization with the administration of intravenous t-PA. Concomitant administration of an anticoagulant or antiplatelet agent might limit the occurrence of reocclusion. The concern is whether the addition of the antithrombotic medications would increase the risk of serious intracranial bleeding. One trial of streptokinase and aspirin reported a very high rate of hemorrhage. Other small studies suggest that antithrombotic medications may be administered with a reasonable degree of safety in this situation. Still, considerable research is needed to determine whether adjunctive antithrombotic therapy is safe and effective.

Current Status of Antithrombotic Therapy

The many clinical trials performed in the last 10 to 15 years provide little support for the emergency administration of a rapidly acting anticoagulant for treatment of a patient with an acute ischemic stroke. These medications are associated with a small but statistically significant risk of intracranial hemorrhage or other serious bleeding. The risk of hemorrhage is less than that attributed to emergency administration of thrombolytic medications, but the anticoagulants have not been found to improve

neurologic outcomes, halt neurologic worsening, or forestall early recurrent stroke. Because of the lack of efficacy, the use of medications that have real risk is problematic. Although emergency anticoagulation has not been established as efficacious, many physicians continue to prescribe these medications, often in the setting of neurologic decline or a presumed high risk of recurrent stroke. These medications are also administered to patients who cannot be treated with t-PA. In this situation, the physician should recognize that the value of emergency anticoagulation is not confirmed.

If anticoagulants are to be prescribed for the treatment of acute ischemic stroke, several steps should be taken to increase the safety of their use. These medications should not be prescribed until the presence of a primary brain hemorrhage has been excluded on a brain imaging study. If the medications are to be started 24 hours after treatment with t-PA, a brain imaging study should be performed to exclude bleeding before starting the anticoagulants. Anticoagulation should be delayed several days if a brain imaging study shows a multilobar infarction, hemorrhagic transformation of the infarction, or if the patient has severe neurologic impairments. Monitoring both the level of anticoagulation to avoid an overdose and the platelet count to detect secondary thrombocytopenia should be done to lower the risk of serious complications. Determining the most likely cause of stroke and starting long-term stroke prophylactic therapies (either oral anticoagulants or antiplatelet agents) could limit the exposure to heparin.

Early administration of aspirin modestly reduces the frequency of recurrent events and improves outcomes. Aspirin's utility in the emergency management of stroke (within the first hours) is not clear. The use of aspirin should not be regarded as equal to thrombolytic therapy in improving outcomes after stroke. Still, starting aspirin within the first 48 hours after stroke seems prudent. Starting antiplatelet agents could eliminate the need for anticoagulants. There appear to be no particular limitations for starting aspirin with regard to the severity of stroke as determined by clinical and brain imaging findings. Aspirin should not be given within 24 hours after treatment with t-PA. Currently, the glycoprotein IIb/IIIa receptor blockers should not be prescribed to patients with ischemic stroke. Further research on the utility of antiplatelet agents is under way.

Future of Antithrombotic Therapy

Investigators in the future may wish to reevaluate the utility of rapidly acting anticoagulants or antiplatelet agents in patients with acute ischemic stroke. Some recommendations for future trials would include (1) a modern clinical trial design including blinding of treatment allocation, (2) presumably intravenous administration of the agent to rapidly achieve biological responses, (3) monitoring of the level of anticoagulation so that adjustments could be made to avoid both overdosage and underdosage (the monitoring would need to be done in such a way as to keep the treatment allocations unknown to the investigators), and (4) careful selection of subjects based on the primary goal of treatment.

The future role of antiplatelet agents and anticoagulants in the management of patients with acute ischemic stroke might be as a component in multimodality therapy. An approach similar to that employed in cardiology may be applicable to acute stroke. The adjunctive use of antithrombotic medications may maintain the efficacy of pharmacologic or mechanical thrombolysis. The use of these medications might lower the risk of bleeding because the dose of the thrombolytic agents may be reduced. Several preliminary studies have evaluated the combination of thrombolysis and antithrombotic agents; while the results are promising, considerable additional research is needed. Hopefully, future clinical trials will test the safety and efficacy of multimodality thrombolytic and antithrombotic therapy for treatment of patients with acute ischemic stroke.

REFERENCES

1. Adams RJ, Albers G, Alberts MJ, et al: Update to the AHA/ASA recommendations for the prevention of stroke in patients with stroke and transient ischemic attack, *Stroke* 39:1647-1652, 2008.
2. Sacco RL, Adams R, Albers G, et al: Guidelines for prevention of stroke in patients with ischemic stroke or transient ischemic attack: a statement for healthcare professionals from the American Heart Association/American Stroke Association Council on Stroke: Co-sponsored by the Council on Cardiovascular Radiology and Intervention: the American Academy of Neurology affirms the value of this guideline, *Circulation* 113:e409-e449, 2006.
3. Albers GW, Amarenco P, Easton JD, et al: Antithrombotic and thrombolytic therapy for ischemic stroke, *Chest* 133:630S-669S, 2008.
4. Hart RG, Pearce LA, Aguilar MI: Meta-analysis: Antithrombotic therapy to prevent stroke in patients who have nonvalvular atrial fibrillation, *Ann Intern Med* 146:857-867, 2007.
5. Burgin WS, Staub L, Chan W, et al: Acute stroke care in non-urban emergency departments, *Neurology* 57:2006-2012, 2001.
6. Schmidt WP, Heuschmann P, Taeger D, Henningsen H: Determinants of IV heparin treatment in patients with ischemic stroke, *Neurology* 63:2407-2409, 2004.
7. Adams HP Jr, del Zoppo G, Alberts MJ, et al: Guidelines for the early management of adults with ischemic stroke: a guideline from the American Heart Association/American Stroke Association Stroke Council, Clinical Cardiology Council, Cardiovascular Radiology and Intervention Council, and the Atherosclerotic Peripheral Vascular Disease and Quality of Care Outcomes in Research Interdisciplinary Working Groups: The American Academy of Neurology affirms the value of this guideline as an educational tool for neurologists, *Stroke* 38:1655-1711, 2007.
8. del Zoppo GJ, Saver JL, Jauch EC, Adams HP Jr: on behalf of the American Heart Association Stroke Council. Expansion of the time window for treatment of acute ischemic stroke with intravenous tissue plasminogen activator: A Science Advisory from the American Heart Association/American Stroke Association, *Stroke* 40:2945-2948, 2009.
9. Novakovic R, Toth G, Purdy PD: Review of current and emerging therapies in acute ischemic stroke, *J Neurointerv Surg* 1:13-26, 2009.
10. Hankey GJ, Eikelboom JW: Antithrombotic drugs for patients with ischaemic stroke and transient ischaemic attack to prevent recurrent major vascular events, *Lancet Neurol* 9:273-284, 2010.
11. Hirsh J, Bauer KA, Donati MB, et al: Parenteral anticoagulants, *Chest* 133:141S-159S, 2008.
12. Mousa SA, Zhang F, Aljada A, et al: Pharmacokinetics and pharmacodynamics of oral heparin solid dosage form in healthy human subjects, *J Clin Pharmacol* 47:1508-1520, 2007.
13. Arbit E, Goldberg M, Gomez-Orellana I, Majuru S: Oral heparin: Status review, *Thromb J* 4:6, 2006.
14. Fareed J, Callas D, Hoppensteadt DA, et al: Antithrombin agents as anticoagulants and antithrombotics. Implications in drug development, *Med Clin North Am* 82:569-586, 1998.
15. Hirsh J, Anand SS, Halperin JL, Fuster V: Guide to anticoagulant therapy: Heparin, *Circulation* 103:2994-3018, 2001.
16. Hirsh J, Warkentin TE, Shaughnessy SG, et al: Heparin and low-molecular-weight heparin. Mechanisms of action, pharmacokinetics, dosing, monitoring, efficacy, and safety, *Chest* 119:64S-94S, 2001.
17. Hirsh J, Warkentin TE, Raschke R, et al: Heparin and low-molecular-weight heparin: mechanisms of action, pharmacokinetics, dosing considerations, monitoring, efficacy, and safety, *Chest* 114:489S-510S, 1998.
18. Hirsh J, Dalen JE, Anderson DR, et al: Oral anticoagulants: mechanism of action, clinical effectiveness, and optimal therapeutic range, *Chest* 114:445S-469S, 1998.
19. Becker RC, Ansell J: Antithrombotic therapy. An abbreviated reference for clinicians, *Arch Intern Med* 155:149-161, 1995.
20. Raschke RA, Reilly BM, Guidry JR, et al: The weight-based heparin dosing nomogram compared with a "standard care" nomogram. A randomized controlled trial, *Ann Intern Med* 119:874-881, 1993.
21. Raschke R, Hirsh J, Guidry JR: Suboptimal monitoring and dosing of unfractionated heparin in comparative studies with low-molecular-weight heparin, *Ann Intern Med* 138:720-723, 2003.
22. Chamorro A: Immediate anticoagulation in acute focal brain ischemia revisited: Gathering the evidence, *Stroke* 32:577-578, 2001.
23. Chamorro A: Role of inflammation in stroke and atherothrombosis, *Cerebrovasc Dis* 17(Suppl 3):1-5, 2004.
24. Chamorro A: Heparin in acute ischemic stroke: the case for a new clinical trial, *Cerebrovasc Dis* 9(Suppl 3):16-23, 1999.
25. Hirsh J, Weitz JI: New antithrombotic agents, *Lancet* 353:1431-1436, 1999.
26. Hirsh J, O'Donnell M, Eikelboom JW: Beyond unfractionated heparin and warfarin: Current and future advances, *Circulation* 116:552-560, 2007.
27. Nowak-Gottl U, Bidlingmaier C, Krumpel A, Kenet G: Pharmacokinetics, efficacy, and safety of LMWHs in venous thrombosis and stroke in neonates, infants and children, *Br J Pharmacol* 153:1120-1127, 2008.
28. Weitz JI, Hirsh J: New anticoagulant drugs, *Chest* 119:95S-107S, 2001.
29. Hirsh J: New anticoagulants, *Am Heart J* 142:S3-S8, 2001.
30. Topol EJ, Fuster V, Harrington RA, et al: Recombinant hirudin for unstable angina pectoris. A multicenter, randomized angiographic trial, *Circulation* 89:1557-1566, 1994.
31. LaMonte M: Argatroban in thrombotic stroke, *Pathophysiol Haemost Thromb* 32(Suppl 3):39-45, 2002.
32. LaMonte MP, Nash ML, Wang DZ, et al: Argatroban anticoagulation in patients with acute ischemic stroke (ARGIS-1). A randomized, placebo-controlled safety study, *Stroke* 35:1677-1682, 2004.
33. Morris DC, Zhang L, Zhang ZG, et al: Extension of the therapeutic window for recombinant tissue plasminogen activator with argatroban in a rat model of embolic stroke, *Stroke* 32:2635-2640, 2001.
34. Akins PT, Feldman HA, Zoble RG, et al: Secondary stroke prevention with ximelagatran versus warfarin in patients with atrial fibrillation: Pooled analysis of SPORTIF III and V clinical trials, *Stroke* 38:874-880, 2007.
35. Connolly SJ, Ezekowitz MD, Yusuf S, et al: Dabigatran versus warfarin in patients with atrial fibrillation, *N Engl J Med* 361:1139-1151, 2009.
36. Garcia D, Libby E, Crowther MA: The new oral anticoagulants, *Blood* 115:15-20, 2010.
37. Verheugt FWA: Novel oral anticoagulants to prevent stroke in atrial fibrillation, *Nat Rev Cardiol* 7:149-154, 2010.
38. Roth GJ, Calverley DC: Aspirin, platelets, and thrombosis: Theory and practice, *Blood* 83:885-898, 1994.
39. Harker LA, Fuster V: Pharmacology of platelet inhibitors, *J Am Coll Cardiol* 8:21B-32B, 1986.
40. Alberts MJ, Bergman DL, Molner E, et al: Antiplatelet effect of aspirin in patients with cerebrovascular disease, *Stroke* 35:175-178, 2004.
41. Awtry EH, Loscalzo J: Aspirin, *Circulation* 101:1206-1218, 2000.
42. Burch JW, Stanford N, Majerus PW: Inhibition of platelet prostaglandin synthetase by oral aspirin, *J Clin Invest* 61:314-319, 1978.
43. Patrono C, Baigent C, Hirsh J, Roth G: Antiplatelet drugs, *Chest* 133:199S-233S, 2008.

44. CAST (Chinese Acute Stroke Trial) Collaborative Group: CAST: Randomised placebo-controlled trial of early aspirin use in 20,000 patients with acute ischaemic stroke, *Lancet* 349:1641-1649, 1997.

45. Nagamatsu Y, Tsujioka Y, Hashimoto M, et al: The differential effects of aspirin on platelets, leucocytes and vascular endothelium in an in vivo model of thrombus formation, *Clin Lab Haematol* 21:33-40, 1999.

46. Grotta JC, Lemak NA, Gary H, et al: Does platelet antiaggregant therapy lessen the severity of stroke? *Neurology* 35:632-636, 1985.

47. Kalra L, Perez I, Smithard DG, Sulch D: Does prior use of aspirin affect outcome in ischemic stroke? *Am J Med* 108:205-209, 2000.

48. Wilterdink JL, Bendixen B, Adams HP Jr, et al: Effect of prior aspirin use on stroke severity in the Trial of Org 10172 in Acute Stroke Treatment (TOAST), *Stroke* 32:2836-2840, 2001.

49. Macchi L, Sorel N, Christiaens L: Aspirin resistance; definitions, mechanisms, prevalence, and clinical resistance, *Curr Pharm Des* 12:251-258, 2006.

50. Helgason CM, Bolin KM, Hoff JA, et al: Development of aspirin resistance in persons with previous ischemic stroke, *Stroke* 25:2331-2336, 1994.

51. Grundmann K, Jaschonek K, Kleine B, et al: Aspirin non-responder status in patients with recurrent cerebral ischemic attacks, *J Neurol* 250:63-66, 2003.

52. Patrono C, Coller B, Dalen JE, et al: Platelet-active drugs, *Chest* 119:39S-63S, 2001.

53. Rivey MP, Alexander MR, Taylor JW: Dipyridamole: A critical evaluation, *Drug Intell Clin Pharm* 18:869-880, 1984.

54. Sacco RL, Diener HC, Yusuf S, et al: Aspirin and extended-release dipyridamole versus clopidogrel for recurrent stroke, *N Engl J Med* 359:1238-1251, 2008.

55. Patrono C, Coller B, Dalen JE, et al: Platelet-active drugs: The relationships among dose, effectiveness, and side effects, *Chest* 114:470S-488S, 1998.

56. Quinn MJ, Fitzgerald DJ: Ticlopidine and clopidogrel, *Circulation* 100:1667-1672, 1999.

57. Helft G, Osende JI, Worthley SG, et al: Acute antithrombotic effect of a front-loaded regimen of clopidogrel in patients with atherosclerosis on aspirin, *Arterioscler Thromb Vasc Biol* 20:2316-2321, 2000.

58. Pache J, Kastrati A, Mehilli J, et al: Clopidogrel therapy in patients undergoing coronary stenting: Value of a high-loading-dose regimen, *Catheter Cardiovasc Interv* 55:436-441, 2002.

59. Ho PM, Maddox TM, Wang L, et al: Risk of adverse outcomes associated with concomitant use of clopidogrel and proton pump inhibitors following acute coronary syndrome, *JAMA* 301:937-944, 2009.

60. Liu T: Drug interaction between clopidogrel and proton pump inhibitors, *Pharmacotherapy* 30:275-289, 2010.

61. Freedman JE, Hylek EM: Clopidogrel, genetics, and drug responsiveness, *N Engl J Med* 360:411-413, 2009.

62. Shuldiner AR, O'Connell JR, Bliden KP, et al: Association of cytochrome P450 2C19 genotype with the antiplatelet effect and clinical efficacy of clopidogrel therapy, *JAMA* 302:849-857, 2009.

63. Roden DM, Stein CM: Clopidogrel and the concept of high-risk pharmacokinetics, *Circulation* 119:2127-2130, 2009.

64. Bhatt DL: Tailoring antiplatelet therapy based on pharmacogenomics: How well do the data fit? *JAMA* 302:896-897, 2009.

65. Wiviott SD, Braunwald E, McCabe CH, et al: Prasugrel versus clopidogrel in patients with acute coronary syndromes, *N Engl J Med* 357:2001-2015, 2007.

66. Weber AA, Braun M, Hohlfeld T, et al: Recovery of platelet function after discontinuation of clopidogrel treatment in healthy volunteers, *Br J Clin Pharmacol* 52:333-336, 2001.

67. Wallentin L, Becker RC, Budaj A, et al: Ticagrelor versus clopidogrel in patients with acute coronary syndromes, *N Engl J Med* 361:1045-1057, 2009.

68. Bhatt DL, Lincoff AM, Gibson CM, et al: Intravenous platelet blockade with cangrelor during PCI, *N Engl J Med* 361:2330-2341, 2009.

69. Kastrati A, Ndrepepa G: Cangrelor—a champion lost in translation? *N Engl J Med* 361:2382-2384, 2009.

70. Quinn M, Fitzgerald DJ: Long-term administration of glycoprotein IIb/IIIa antagonists, *Am Heart J* 135:S113-S118, 2006.

71. Coller BS, Anderson K, Weisman HF: New antiplatelet agents: platelet GPIIb/IIIa antagonists, *Thromb Haemost* 74:302-308, 1995.

72. Theroux P: Oral inhibitors of platelet membrane receptor glycoprotein IIb/IIIa in clinical cardiology: Issues and opportunities, *Am Heart J* 135:S107-S112, 2006.

73. Dickfeld T, Ruf A, Pogatsa-Murray G, et al: Differential antiplatelet effects of various glycoprotein IIb-IIIa antagonists, *Thromb Res* 101:53-64, 2001.

74. Gawaz M, Ruf A, Neumann F, et al: Effect of glycoprotein IIb-IIIA receptor antagonism on platelet membrane glycoproteins after coronary stent placement, *Thromb Haemost* 80:994-1001, 2010.

75. Proimos G: Platelet aggregation inhibition with glycoprotein IIb-IIIa inhibitors, *J Thromb Thrombolysis* 11:99-110, 2001.

76. Frelinger AL III, Furman MI, Krueger LA, Barnard MR, Michelson AD: Dissociation of glycoprotein IIb/IIIa antagonists from platelets does not result in fibrinogen binding or platelet aggregation, *Circulation* 104:1374-1379, 2001.

77. Bhatt DL, Topol EJ: Current role of platelet glycoprotein IIb/IIIa inhibitors in acute coronary syndromes, *JAMA* 284:1549-1558, 2000.

78. Schneider DJ, Baumann PQ, Holmes MB, et al: Time and dose dependent augmentation of inhibitory effects of abciximab by aspirin, *Thromb Haemost* 85:309-313, 2001.

79. Tcheng JE, Ellis SG, George BS, et al: Pharmacodynamics of chimeric glycoprotein IIb/IIIa integrin antiplatelet antibody Fab 7E3 in high-risk coronary angioplasty, *Circulation* 90:1757-1764, 1994.

80. Schomig A, Kastrati A, Dirschinger J, et al: Coronary stenting plus platelet glycoprotein IIb/IIIa blockade compared with tissue plasminogen activator in acute myocardial infarction. Stent versus Thrombolysis for Occluded Coronary Arteries in Patients with Acute Myocardial Infarction Study Investigators, *N Engl J Med* 343:385-391, 2000.

81. Kastrati A, Mehilli J, Neumann FJ, et al: Abciximab in patients with acute coronary syndromes undergoing percutaneous coronary intervention after clopidogrel pretreatment: The ISAR-REACT 2 Randomized Trial, *JAMA* 295:1531-1538, 2006.

82. Vernon SM: Glycoprotein IIb/IIIa antagonists and low-molecular weight heparin in acute coronary syndromes, *Cardiol Clin* 19:235-252, 2000.

83. Topol EJ, Moliterno DJ, Herrmann HC, et al: Comparison of two platelet glycoprotein IIb/IIIa inhibitors, tirofiban and abciximab, for the prevention of ischemic events with percutaneous coronary revascularization, *N Engl J Med* 344:1888-1894, 2001.

84. Lele M, Sajid M, Wajih N, Stouffer GA: Eptifibatide and 7E3, but not tirofiban, inhibit alpha(v)beta(3) integrin-mediated binding of smooth muscle cells to thrombospondin and prothrombin, *Circulation* 104:582-587, 2001.

85. Gilchrist IC, O'Shea JC, Kosoglou T, et al: Pharmacodynamics and pharmacokinetics of higher-dose, double-bolus eptifibatide in percutaneous coronary intervention, *Circulation* 104:406-411, 2001.

86. O'Shea JC, Hafley GE, Greenberg S, et al: Platelet glycoprotein IIb/IIIa integrin blockade with eptifibatide in coronary stent intervention: the ESPRIT trial: a randomized controlled trial, *JAMA* 285:2468-2473, 2001.

87. Marso SP, Bhatt DL, Roe MT, et al: Enhanced efficacy of eptifibatide administration in patients with acute coronary syndrome requiring in-hospital coronary artery bypass grafting. PURSUIT Investigators, *Circulation* 102:2952-2958, 2000.

88. Lincoff AM, Califf RM, Van de Werf F, et al: Mortality at 1 year with combination platelet glycoprotein IIb/IIIa inhibition and reduced-dose fibrinolytic therapy vs conventional fibrinolytic therapy for acute myocardial infarction. GUSTO V randomized trial, *JAMA* 288:2130-2135, 2002.

89. Morrow DA, Scirica BM, Fox KAA, et al: Evaluation of a novel antiplatelet agent for secondary prevention in patients with a history of atherosclerotic disease: Design and rationale for the Thrombin-Receptor Antagonist in Secondary Prevention of Atherothrombotic Ischemic Events (TRA 2°P)-TIMI 50 trial, *Am Heart J* 158:335-341, 2009.

90. Donnan GA, Davis SM, Chambers BR, et al: Streptokinase for acute ischemic stroke with relationship to time of administration: Australian Streptokinase (ASK) Trial Study Group, *JAMA* 276:961-966, 1996.

91. Hommel M, Boissel JP, Cornu C, et al: Termination of trial of streptokinase in severe acute ischaemic stroke. MAST Study Group, *Lancet* 345:578-579, 1995.

92. The National Institute of Neurological Disorders and Stroke rt-PA Stroke Study Group: Tissue plasminogen activator for acute ischemic stroke, *N Engl J Med* 333:1581-1587, 1995.

93. Multicenter Acute Stroke Trial—Europe Study Group: Thrombolytic therapy with streptokinase in acute ischemic stroke, *N Engl J Med* 335:145-150, 1996.

94. Multicentre Acute Stroke Trial—Italy (MAST-I) Group: Randomised controlled trial of streptokinase, aspirin, and combination of both in treatment of acute ischaemic stroke, *Lancet* 346:1509-1514, 1995.

95. Millikan CH: Therapeutic agents—current status. Anticoagulant therapy in cerebrovascular disease. In Siekert RD, Whisnant JP, editors: *Cerebral vascular disease, fourth conference*, New York, 1965, Grune and Stratton, pp 181-184.

96. Millikan CH, McDowell FH: Treatment of progressing stroke, *Stroke* 12:397-409, 1981.

97. Baker RN, Broward JA, Fong HC, et al: Anticoagulant therapy in cerebral infarction. Report on cooperative study, *Neurology* 12:823-835, 1962.

98. Carter AB: Anticoagulation treatment in progressing stroke, *Br Med J* 2:70-73, 1961.

99. Fisher CM: Anticoagulant therapy in cerebral thrombosis and cerebral embolism. A national cooperative study, interim report, *Neurology* 11:119-131, 1961.

100. Duke RJ, Bloch RF, Turpie AG, et al: Intravenous heparin for the prevention of stroke progression in acute partial stable stroke, *Ann Intern Med* 105:825-828, 1986.

101. Cerebral Embolism Study Group: Immediate anticoagulation and embolic stroke. A randomized trial, *Stroke* 14:668-676, 1983.

102. Cerebral Embolism Study Group: Immediate anticoagulation of embolic stroke: Brain hemorrhage and management options, *Stroke* 15:779-789, 1984.

103. Cerebral Embolism Study Group: Cardioembolic stroke, early anticoagulation, and brain hemorrhage, *Arch Intern Med* 147:636-640, 1987.

104. Cerebral Embolism Task Force: Cardiogenic brain embolism, *Arch Neurol* 43:71-84, 1986.

105. Okada Y, Yamaguchi T, Minematsu K, et al: Hemorrhagic transformation in cerebral embolism, *Stroke* 20:598-603, 1989.

106. Slivka A, Levy D: Natural history of progressive ischemic stroke in a population treated with heparin, *Stroke* 21:1657-1662, 1990.

107. Sandercock P, Counsell C, Kamal A: Anticoagulants for acute ischemic stroke, *Cochrane Database Syst Rev Oct* 8(4):CD000024, 2008.

108. Camerlingo M, Salvi P, Belloni G, et al: Intravenous heparin started within the first 3 hours after onset of symptoms as a treatment for acute nonlacunar hemispheric cerebral infarctions, *Stroke* 36:2415-2420, 2005.

108a. Chamorro A, Vila N, Saiz A, et al: Early anticoagulation after large embolic infarction. A safety study, *Neurology*, 45:861-865, 1995.

109. International Stroke Trial Collaborative Group. The International Stroke Trial (IST): A randomised trial of aspirin, subcutaneous heparin, both, or neither among 19,435 patients with acute ischaemic stroke, *Lancet* 349:1569-1581, 1997.

110. Saxena R, Lewis S, Berge E, et al: Risk of early death and recurrent stroke and effect of heparin in 3169 patients with acute ischemic stroke and atrial fibrillation in the International Stroke Trial, *Stroke* 32:2333-2337, 2001.

111. van den Berg E, Lohmann N, Friedburg D, Rabe F: Report of general temporary anticoagulation in the treatment of acute cerebral and retinal ischaemia, *Vasa* 26:222-227, 1997.

112. Petty GW, Brown RD Jr, Whisnant JP, et al: Frequency of major complications of aspirin, warfarin, and intravenous heparin for secondary stroke prevention, *Ann Intern Med* 130:14-22, 1999.

113. Levine M, Raskob GE, Landefeld CS, Hirsch J: Hemorrhagic complications of anticoagulant treatment, *Chest* 108:276S-290S, 1995.

114. Levine MN, Raskob G, Landefeld S, Kearon C: Hemorrhagic complications of anticoagulant treatment, *Chest* 114:511S-523S, 1998.

115. Furlan AJ, Higashida R, Wechsler L, Schultz G: PROACT II Investigators. PROACT II. Recombinant prourokinase (r-ProUK) in acute cerebral thromboembolism. Initial trial results, *Stroke* 30:234, 1999.

116. del Zoppo GJ, Higashida RT, Furlan AJ: PROACT: A phase II randomized trial of recombinant pro-urokinase by direct arterial delivery in acute middle cerebral artery stroke. PROACT Investigators. Prolyse in Acute Cerebral Thromboembolism, *Stroke* 29:4-11, 1998.

117. Furlan A, Higashida R, Wechsler L, et al: Intra-arterial prourokinase for acute ischemic stroke. The PROACT II Study: A randomized controlled trial, *JAMA* 282:2003-2011, 1999.

118. Grond M, Rudolf J, Neveling M, et al: Risk of immediate heparin after rt-PA therapy in acute ischemic stroke, *Cerebrovasc Dis* 7:318-323, 1997.

119. Trouillas P, Nighoghossian N, Derex L, et al: Thrombolysis with intravenous rtPA in a series of 100 cases of acute carotid territory stroke: Determination of etiological, topographic, and radiological outcome factors, *Stroke* 29:2529-2540, 1998.

120. Slivka A, Levy DE, Lapinski RH: Risk associated with heparin withdrawal in ischaemic cerebrovascular disease, *J Neurol Neurosurg Psychiatry* 52:1332-1336, 1989.

121. Horne MK, Alkins BR: Platelet binding of IgG from patients with heparin induced thrombocytopenia, *J Lab Clin Med* 127:435-442, 1996.

122. Ramirez-Lassepas M, Cipolle RJ, Rodvold KA, et al: Heparin induced thrombocytopenia in patients with cerebrovascular ischemic disease, *Neurology* 34:736-740, 1986.

123. Atkinson JL, Sundt TMJ, Kazmier FJ, et al: Heparin-induced thrombocytopenia and thrombosis in ischemic stroke, *Mayo Clin Proc* 63:353-361, 1988.

124. Becker PS, Miller VT: Heparin-induced thrombocytopenia, *Stroke* 20:1449-1459, 1989.

125. Kappers-Klunne MC, Boon DM, Hop WC, et al: Heparin-induced thrombocytopenia and thrombosis: A prospective analysis of the incidence in patients with heart and cerebrovascular diseases, *Br J Haematol* 96:442-446, 1997.

126. Greinacher A, Potzsch B, Amiral J, et al: Heparin-associated thrombocytopenia: Isolation of the antibody and characterization of a multimolecular PF4-heparin complex as the major antigen, *Thromb Haemost* 71:247-251, 1994.

127. Gupta AK, Kovacs MJ, Sauder DN: Heparin-induced thrombocytopenia, *Ann Pharmacother* 32:55-59, 1998.

128. Boon DM, Michiels JJ, Tanghe HL, Kappers-Klunne MC: Heparin-induced thrombocytopenia with multiple cerebral infarctions simulating thrombotic thrombocytopenic purpura. A case report, *Angiology* 47:407-411, 1996.

129. Warkentin TE, Bernstein RA: Delayed-onset heparin-induced thrombocytopenia and cerebral thrombosis after a single administration of unfractionated heparin, *N Engl J Med* 348:1067-1069, 2003.

130. Kanagasabay RR, Unsworth-White MJ, Robinson G, et al: Cardiopulmonary bypass with danaparoid sodium and ancrod in heparin-induced thrombocytopenia, *Ann Thorac Surg* 66:567-569, 1998.

131. Lewis BE, Walenga JM, Wallis DE: Anticoagulation with Novastan (argatroban) in patients with heparin-induced thrombocytopenia and heparin-induced thrombocytopenia and thrombosis syndrome, *Semin Thromb Hemost* 23:197-202, 1997.

132. Kay R, Wong KS, Yu YL, et al: Low-molecular-weight heparin for the treatment of acute ischemic stroke, *N Engl J Med* 333:1588-1593, 1995.

133. Berge E, Abdelnoor M, Nakstad PH, Sandset PM: on behalf of the HAEST Study Group. Low-molecular-weight heparin versus aspirin in patients with acute ischaemic stroke and atrial fibrillation: A double-blind randomised study, *Lancet* 355:1205-1210, 2000.

134. Diener HC, Ringelstein EB, von Kummer R, et al: Treatment of acute ischemic stroke with the low-molecular-weight heparin certoparin, *Stroke* 32:22-29, 2001.

135. Bath PM, Lindenstrom E, Boysen G, et al: Tinzaparin in acute ischaemic stroke (TAIST): A randomised aspirin-controlled trial, *Lancet* 358:683-684, 2001.

136. Wong KS, Chen C, Ng PW, et al: Low-molecular-weight heparin compared with aspirin for the treatment of acute ischaemic stroke in Asian patients with large artery occlusive disease: A randomised study, *Lancet* 6:407-413, 2007.

137. The Publications Committee for the Trial of ORG 10172 in Acute Stroke Treatment (TOAST) Investigators. Low-molecular-weight heparinoid, ORG 10172 (danaparoid), and outcome after acute ischemic stroke: A randomized controlled trial, *JAMA* 279:1265–1272, 1998.

138. Paciaroni M, Agnelli G, Micheli S, Caso V: Efficacy and safety of anticoagulant treatment in acute cardioembolic stroke: A meta-analysis of randomized controlled trials, *Stroke* 38:423–430, 2007.

139. Hillbom M, Erila T, Sotaniemi K, et al: Enoxaparin vs heparin for prevention of deep-vein thrombosis in acute ischaemic stroke: A randomized, double-blind study, *Acta Neurol Scand* 106:84–92, 2002.

140. Sherman DG, Albers GW, Bladin C, et al: The efficacy and safety of enoxaparin versus unfractionated heparin for the prevention of venous thromboembolism after acute ischaemic stroke (PREVAIL Study): An open-label randomised comparison, *Lancet* 369:1347–1355, 2007.

141. Diener HC, Ringelstein EB, von Kummer R, et al: Prophylaxis of thrombotic and embolic events in acute ischemic stroke with the low-molecular-weight heparin certoparin: Results of the PROTECT Trial, *Stroke* 37:139–144, 2006.

142. Burak CR, Bowen MD, Barron TF: The use of enoxaparin in children with acute, nonhemorrhagic ischemic stroke, *Pediatr Neurol* 29:295–298, 2003.

143. Sarma GR, Roy AK: Nadroparin plus aspirin versus aspirin alone in the treatment of acute ischemic stroke, *Neurol India* 51:208–210, 2003.

144. Bath P: Anticoagulants and antiplatelet agents in acute ischaemic stroke, *Lancet Neurol* 1:405, 2002.

145. Warkentin TE, Levine MN, Hirsh J, et al: Heparin-induced thrombocytopenia in patients treated with low-molecular-weight heparin or unfractionated heparin, *N Engl J Med* 332:1330–1335, 1995.

146. Yasaka M, Yamaguchi T, Moriyasu H, et al: Antithrombin III and low-dose heparin in acute cardioembolic stroke, *Cerebrovasc Dis* 5:35–42, 1995.

147. Sugg RM, Pary JK, Uchino K, et al: Argatroban tPA stroke study: Study design and results in the first treated cohort, *Arch Neurol* 63:1057–1062, 2006.

148. Barreto AD, Grotta JC: The Argatroban and tPA Stroke Study, *Prog Neurothera Neuropsychopharm* 3:35–47, 2008.

149. Kennedy J, Hill MD, Ryckborst KJ, et al: Fast assessment of stroke and transient ischaemic attack to prevent early recurrence (FASTER): A randomised controlled pilot trial, *Lancet Neurol* 6:961–969, 2007.

150. Meyer DM, Albright KC, Allison TA, Grotta JC: LOAD: A pilot study of the safety of loading of aspirin and clopidogrel in acute ischemic stroke and transient ischemic attack, *J Stroke Cerebrovasc Dis* 17:26–29, 2001.

151. Diener HC, Bogousslavsky J, Brass LM, et al: Aspirin and clopidogrel compared with clopidogrel alone after recent ischaemic stroke or transient ischaemic attack in high-risk patients (MATCH): Randomised, double-blind, placebo-controlled trial, *Lancet* 364:331–337, 2004.

152. Bhatt DL, Fox KAA, Hacke W, et al: Clopidogrel and aspirin versus aspirin alone for the prevention of atherothrombotic events, *N Engl J Med* 354:1706–1717, 2006.

153. Connolly SJ, Pogue J, Hart RG, et al: Effect of clopidogrel added to aspirin in patients with atrial fibrillation, *N Engl J Med* 360:2066–2078, 2009.

154. Bhatt DL: Intensifying platelet inhibition—navigating between scylla and charybdis, *N Engl J Med* 357:2078–2081, 2007.

155. Schomig A: Ticagrelor—is there need for a new player in the antiplatelet-therapy field? *N Engl J Med* 361:1108–1111, 2009.

156. The Abciximab in Ischemic Stroke Investigators: Abciximab in acute ischemic stroke: A randomized, double-blind, placebo-controlled, dose-escalation study, *Stroke* 31:601–609, 2000.

157. Abciximab Emergent Stroke Treatment Trial (AbESTT) Investigators: Emergency administration of abciximab for treatment of patients with acute ischemic stroke: Results of a randomized phase 2 trial, *Stroke* 36:880–890, 2005.

158. Adams HP Jr, Effron MB, Torner J, et al: Emergency administration of abciximab for treatment of patients with acute ischemic stroke results of an international phase III trial, *Stroke* 39:87–99, 2008.

159. Mitsias PD, Lu M, Morris D, et al: Treatment of acute supratentorial ischemic stroke with abciximab is safe and may result in early neurological improvement. A preliminary report, *Cerebrovasc Dis* 18:249–250, 2004.

160. Mitsias PD, Lu M, Silver B, et al: MRI-guided, open trial of abciximab for ischemic stroke within a 3- to 24-hour window, *Neurology* 65:612–615, 2005.

161. Martin-Schild S, Shaltoni H, Abraham AT, et al: Safety of eptifibatide for subcortical stroke progression, *Cerebrovasc Dis* 28:595–600, 2009.

162. Mandava P, Thiagarajan P, Kent TA: Glycoprotein IIb/IIIa antagonists in acute ischaemic stroke: Current status and future directions, *Drugs* 68:1019–1028, 2008.

163. Qureshi AI, Harris-Lane P, Kirmani JF, et al: Intra-arterial reteplase and intravenous abciximab in patients with acute ischemic stroke: An open-label, dose-ranging, phase I study, *Neurosurgery* 59:789–797, 2006.

164. Qureshi AI, Hussein HM, Janjua N, et al: Postprocedural intravenous eptifibatide following intraarterial reteplase in patients with acute ischemic stroke, *J Neuroimaging* 18:50–55, 2008.

165. Morris DC, Silver B, Mitsias P, et al: Treatment of acute stroke with recombinant tissue plasminogen activator and abciximab, *Acad Emerg Med* 10:1396–1399, 2003.

166. Eckert B, Koch C, Thomalla G, et al: Aggressive therapy with intravenous abciximab and intra-arterial rtPA and additional PTA/stenting improves clinical outcome in acute vertebrobasilar occlusion: combined local fibrinolysis and intravenous abciximab in acute vertebrobasilar stroke treatment (FAST): Results of a multicenter study, *Stroke* 36:1160–1165, 2005.

167. Mangiafico S, Cellerini M, Nencini P, et al: Intravenous tirofiban with intra-arterial urokinase and mechanical thrombolysis in stroke: Preliminary experience in 11 cases, *Stroke* 36:2154–2158, 2005.

168. ReoPro and retavase to treat acute stroke. http://www.clinicaltrials.gov/ct2/show/NCT00046293?term=ReoPro&rank=4. Accessed Feb. 1, 2010.

169. Combination Anti-platelet and Anti-Coagulant Treatment After Lysis of ischemic Stroke Trial (CATALIST). http://www.clinicaltrials.gov/ct2/show/NCT00061373?term=CATALIST&rank=1. Accessed Feb. 1, 2010.

170. Pancioli AM, Broderick J, Brott T, et al: The combined approach to lysis utilizing eptifibatide and rt-PA in acute ischemic stroke: The CLEAR Stroke Trial, *Stroke* 39:3268–3276, 2008.

171. Study of the combination therapy of RT-PA and eptifibatide to treat acute ischemic stroke (CLEAR-ER). http://www.clinicaltrials.gov/ct2/show/NCT00894803?term=CLEAR-ER&rank=1. Accessed Feb. 1, 2010.

172. Ciccone A, Abraha I, Santilli I: Glycoprotein IIb-IIIa inhibitors for acute ischemic stroke, *Stroke* 38:1113–1114, 2007.

173. Sandercock PA, van den Belt AG, Lindley RI, Slattery J: Antithrombotic therapy in acute ischaemic stroke: An overview of the completed randomised trials, *J Neurol Neurosurg Psychiatry* 56:17–25, 1993.

174. Adams HP Jr: Emergent use of anticoagulation for treatment of patients with ischemic stroke, *Stroke* 33:856–861, 2002.

175. Coull BM, Williams LS, Goldstein LB, et al: Anticoagulants and antiplatelet agents in acute ischemic stroke. Report of the Joint Stroke Guideline Development Committee of the American Academy of Neurology and the American Stroke Association (a division of the American Heart Association), *Neurology* 59:13–22, 2002.

176. Gentling E, Barnett HJM, Fields WS, et al: Cerebral ischemia. The role of thrombosis and antithrombotic therapy, *Stroke* 8:150–175, 1977.

177. Camerlingo M, Casto L, Ferraro F, et al: Immediate anticoagulation with heparin for first-ever ischemic stroke in the carotid artery territories observed within 5 hours of onset, *Arch Neurol* 51:462–467, 1994.

178. Dahl T, Sandset PM, Abildgaard U: Heparin treatment in 52 patients with progressive ischemic stroke, *Cerebrovasc Dis* 4:101–105, 1994.

179. Haley E Jr, Kassell N, Torner J: Failure of heparin to prevent progression in progressing ischemic infarction, *Stroke* 19:10–14, 1988.

179a. Chamorro A, Vila N, Ascaso C, Blanc R: Heparin in acute stroke with atrial fibrillation. Clinical relevance of very early treatment, *Arch Neurol* 56:1098–1102, 1999.

180. Rödén-Jüllig A, Britton M: Effectiveness of heparin treatment for progressing ischaemic stroke: Before and after study, *J Intern Med* 248:287-291, 2000.

181. Chamorro A, Busse O, Obach V, et al: The Rapid Anticoagulation Prevents Ischemic Damage Study in Acute Stroke—final results from the writing committee, *Cerebrovasc Dis* 19:402-404, 2006.

182. Kay R, Wong KS, Woo J: Pilot study of low-molecular-weight heparin in the treatment of acute ischemic stroke, *Stroke* 25:684-685, 1994.

183. Hommel M: Fraxiparin in ischemic stroke study (FISS-bis), *Cerebrovasc Dis* 8:19, 1998.

184. Adams HP Jr, Bendixen BH, Leira E, et al: Treatment of ischemic stroke in patients with occlusion or stenosis of the internal carotid artery, *Neurology* 53:122-125, 1999.

185. Bath PM, Iddenden R, Bath FJ: Low-molecular-weight heparins and heparinoids in acute ischemic stroke. A meta-analysis of randomized controlled trials, *Stroke* 31:1770-1778, 2000.

186. O'Donnell MJ, Berge E, Sandset PM: Are there patients with acute ischemic stroke and atrial fibrillation that benefit from low-molecular-weight heparin? *Stroke* 37:452-455, 2006.

187. Antithrombotic Trialists' Collaboration: Collaborative meta-analysis of randomised trials of antiplatelet therapy for prevention of death, myocardial infarction, and stroke in high risk patients, *BMJ* 324:71-86, 2002.

188. Zinkstok S, Vermeulen M, Stam J, de Haan R, Roos Y: Antiplatelet therapy in combination with rt-PA thrombolysis in ischemic stroke (ARTIS): Rationale and design of a randomized controlled trial, *Cerebrovasc Dis* 29:79-81, 2009.

189. Rödén-Jüllig A, Britton M, Malmkvist K, Leijd B: Aspirin in the prevention of progressing stroke: A randomized controlled study, *J Intern Med* 254:584-590, 2003.

190. Platelet-Oriented Inhibition in New TIA and Minor Ischemic Stroke (POINT) Trial. http://www.clinicaltrials.gov/ct2/show/NCT00991029?term=POINT&rank=1. Accessed Feb. 1, 2010.

191. Qureshi AI, Suri FK, Khan J, et al: Abciximab as an adjunct to high-risk carotid or vertebrobasilar angioplasty: Preliminary experience, *Neurosurgery* 46:1316-1325, 2000.

192. Lee KY, Heo JH, Lee SI, Yoon WB: Rescue treatment with abciximab in acute ischemic stroke, *Neurology* 56:1585-1587, 2001.

193. Ho DS, Wang Y, Chui M, et al: Intracarotid abciximab injection to abort impending ischemic stroke during carotid angioplasty, *Cerebrovasc Dis* 11:300-304, 2001.

194. Mandava P, Lick SD, Kent TA, et al: Initial safety experience of abciximab and heparin for acute ischemic stroke, *Cerebrovasc Dis* 19:276-278, 2005.

195. Del Pace S, Scheggi V: Acute ischaemic stroke treated with combined intra-arterial thrombolysis and intravenous tirofiban despite oral anticoagulant therapy at an international normalised ratio > or = 2.0, *Intern Emerg Med* 1:250-252, 2006.

196. Nogueira RG, Schwamm LH, Buonanna FS, et al: Low-pressure balloon angioplasty with adjuvant pharmacological therapy in patients with acute ischemic stroke caused by intracranial arterial occlusions, *Neuroradiology* 50:331-340, 2008.

197. Torgano T, Zeccz B, Monzani V, et al: Effect of intravenous tirofiban and aspirin in reducing short-term and long-term neurologic deficit in patients with ischemic stroke; a double-blind randomized trial, *Cerebrovasc Dis* 29:275-281, 2010.

198. Rödén-Jüllig A: Progressing stroke, Epidemiology. *Cerebrovasc Dis* 7(Suppl 5):2-5, 1997.

199. Tai H, Uchiyama S, Ohara K, et al: Deteriorating ischemic stroke in 4 clinical categories classified by the Oxfordshire Community Stroke Project, *Stroke* 31:2049-2054, 2000.

200. Yamamoto H, Bogousslavsky J, Van Melle G: Different predictors of neurological worsening in different causes of stroke, *Arch Neurol* 55:481-486, 1998.

201. van der Worp HB, Kappelle LJ: Complications of acute ischaemic stroke, *Cerebrovasc Dis* 8:124-132, 1998.

202. Davalos A, Castillo J: Potential mechanisms of worsening, *Cerebrovasc Dis* 7(Suppl 5):19-24, 1997.

203. Davalos A, Toni D, Iweins F, et al: Neurological deterioration in acute ischemic stroke: Potential predictors and associated factors in the European Cooperative Acute Stroke Study (ECASS), *Stroke* 30:2631-2636, 1999.

204. Davalos A, Cendra E, Teruel J, et al: Deteriorating ischemic stroke: Risk factors and prognosis, *Neurology* 40:1865-1869, 1990.

205. Wijdicks EF, Scott JP: Pulmonary embolism associated with acute stroke, *Mayo Clin Proc* 72:297-300, 1997.

206. Warlow C, Ogston D, Douglas AS: Deep vein thrombosis in the legs after stroke, *BMJ* 1:1178-1188, 1976.

207. Oppenheimer S, Hachinski V: Complications of acute stroke, *Lancet* 339:721-727, 1992.

208. Kelly J, Rudd A, Lewis R, Hunt BJ: Venous thromboembolism after acute stroke, *Stroke* 32:262-267, 2001.

209. Kelly J, Rudd A, Lewis RR, et al: Venous thromboembolism after acute ischemic stroke. A prospective study using magnetic resonance direct thrombus imaging, *Stroke* 35:2320-2325, 2004.

210. Langhorne P: Measures to improve recovery in the acute phase of stroke, *Cerebrovasc Dis* 9(Suppl 5):2-5, 1999.

211. Gould MK, Dembitzer AD, Sanders GD, Garber AM: Low-molecular-weight heparins compared with unfractionated heparin for treatment of acute deep venous thrombosis. A cost-effectiveness analysis, *Ann Intern Med* 130:789-799, 1999.

212. Koopman MM, Buller HR: Low-molecular-weight heparins in the treatment of venous thromboembolism, *Ann Intern Med* 128:1037-1039, 1998.

213. Sherman DG, Soltes S, Samuel R, Chibedi-Deroche D: Enoxaparin versus unfractionated heparin in the prevention of venous thromboembolism after acute ischemic stroke: Rationale, design, and methods of an open-label, randomized, parallel-group multicenter trial, *J Stroke Cerebrovasc Dis* 14:95-101, 2005.

214. Pulmonary Embolism Prevention (PEP) Trial Collaborative Group: Prevention of pulmonary embolism and deep vein thrombosis with low dose aspirin: Pulmonary Embolism Prevention (PEP) trial, *Lancet* 355:1295-1302, 2000.

215. Kamran SI, Downey D, Ruff RL: Pneumatic sequential compression reduces the risk of deep vein thrombosis in stroke patients, *Neurology* 50:1683-1688, 1998.

216. Hallevi H, Albright KC, Martin-Schild S, et al: Anticoagulation after cardioembolic stroke: To bridge or not to bridge? *Arch Neurol* 65:1169-1173, 2008.

217. Menon R, Kerry S, Norris JW, Markus HS: Treatment of cervical artery dissection: A systematic review and meta-analysis, *J Neurol Neurosurg Psychiatry* 79:1122-1127, 2008.

218. Lyrer P, Engelter S: Antithrombotic drugs for carotid artery dissection, *Cochrane Database System Rev 3*, CD000255, 2003.

219. Georgiadis D, Arnold M, von Buedingen HC, et al: Aspirin vs anticoagulation in carotid artery dissection: A study of 298 patients, *Neurology* 72:1810-1815, 2009.

220. The CADISS: Trial Investigators. Antiplatelet therapy vs. anticoagulation in cervical artery dissection: rationale and design of the Cervical Artery Dissection in Stroke Study (CADISS), *Int J Stroke* 2:292-296, 2007.

51 General Stroke Management and Stroke Units

MARKKU KASTE, RISTO O. ROINE

Only thrombolytic therapy and stroke unit care have been shown to improve the outcome of stroke. Intravenous (IV) and intraarterial delivery of thrombolysis were discussed in Chapters 49 and 62. This chapter characterizes stroke unit care, including all aspects of general stroke management that can optimally be delivered in stroke units. There is strong evidence that treatment of patients with ischemic stroke in stroke units significantly results in lower rates of death, dependency, and the need for institutional care than treatment in general medical wards (level I evidence). The acute stroke unit is a key element in the critical care pathway and the chain of recovery of a patient with stroke after emergency care in the emergency department.[1]

Short History of Stroke Units

The first stroke units were established in North America in the 1960s. They were modeled after coronary care units but failed to have any effect on mortality or morbidity.[2-4] In the 1970s rehabilitation stroke units were created and involved multidisciplinary teams and staff education, but their effects were not evaluated critically.[5] Nonintensive care acute stroke units supplemented by early mobilization and rehabilitation were created in the 1970s and 1980s in North America,[6,7] the United Kingdom,[8] and Scandinavia.[9-11] At first they focused on diagnosis, prevention of complications, education of staff, and research but soon also included early rehabilitation, involvement of family, and multidisciplinary teamwork. Two studies verified that organized stroke care could improve the recovery of the patient with a stroke.[8,11]

The findings of two studies, demonstrating better functional outcome for patients treated in stroke units than for those treated in general medical wards, led to a number of randomized trials, the majority of which were carried out in the United Kingdom and Scandinavian countries.[10-24] Langhorne et al,[25] the first to perform a meta-analysis on the results of these trials, showed that stroke unit care saves lives. The Stroke Unit Trialists' Collaboration then verified these results and demonstrated that organized care in stroke units also reduced the rates of death or institutional care and death or dependency.[26]

Stroke Unit Design

The observed benefits are apparent for a wide variety of stroke services, including stroke centers, acute stroke units, combined acute and rehabilitation stroke units, rehabilitation stroke units admitting patients after a delay of 1 or 2 weeks, and mobile stroke teams.[27]

A *stroke center* consists of a comprehensive stroke service that offers the infrastructure to bring patients as quickly as possible to the stroke center. It provides immediate diagnosis and treatment, as well as early rehabilitation, and refers patients to the appropriate further treatment, rehabilitation, and secondary prevention. A stroke center offers not only acute stroke unit services but also 24-hour availability of laboratory, neuroradiologic, and ultrasonographic diagnostic services and neurosurgical and cardiologic services (Table 51-1).[28] Stroke centers need a large catchment area, and most often, they are a part of a large teaching hospital located in a metropolitan area.

Stroke units provide a disease-specific service in a geographically defined area of a hospital ward and are exclusively dedicated to the management of patients with stroke. Such units can be organized in a variety of medical departments: neurology, internal medicine, geriatric medicine, and rehabilitation medicine. The most distinctive features are a coordinated multidisciplinary team, specialization (i.e., medical and nursing expertise in stroke and rehabilitation), educational programs for the staff, and involvement of caregivers. These basic principles of the Scandinavian model for a combined acute-rehabilitation stroke unit have been scientifically evaluated in Umeå, Sweden, Trondheim, Norway, and Helsinki, Finland.[11,19,22] Germany has established national guidelines for stroke units. According to the German guidelines, stroke units are divided into different levels according to equipment and staff, but they should all have computed tomography (CT) scanning and diagnostic ultrasonography available 24 hours a day.[29,30]

Although there is an agreement that stroke units are dedicated exclusively to stroke patients, not much evidence-based data exist about the components that should be present in different types of stroke units.[30-33] In a recent survey among European stroke experts the levels of care were defined.[34] According to experts, all facilities

TABLE 51-1 REQUIREMENTS FOR ACUTE STROKE UNITS

Minimum requirements for stroke centers

Written protocols for diagnostic and treatment guidelines and operational procedures for medical and nursing staff

Availability of CT 24 hours a day

Availability of blood tests 24 hours a day, including immediate availability of coagulation parameters

Availability of neurosonographic investigations 24 hours a day (color-coded duplex ultrasonography of extracranial vessels and transcranial Doppler ultrasonography of intracranial vessels)

Continuous or frequent monitoring of blood pressure, levels of blood gases and blood glucose, and body temperature

Continuous ECG monitoring and availability of ECG within 24 hours

Close cooperation of neurologists, internists, neuroradiologists, and neurosurgeons in evaluation and treatment

Trained nursing staff specialized in acute care of stroke

Early rehabilitation, including physical therapy, speech therapy, neuropsychology, and occupational therapy

Established network of rehabilitation facilities

Additional facilities recommended in acute stroke units

Diffusion and perfusion MRI and MRA

CT angiography and perfusion CT

Transesophageal echocardiography

Cerebral angiography

CT, Computed tomography; ECG, electrocardiography; MRA, magnetic resonance angiography; MRI, magnetic resonance imaging.
Modified from Kaste M, Skyhoj Olsen T, Orgogozo J-M, et al for the European Stroke Initiative (EUSI) Executive Committee: Organization of stroke care: Education, stroke units and rehabilitation. *Cerebrovasc Dis* 10(Suppl 3):1-11, 2000.

considered necessary should be available in comprehensive stroke centers (CSC) (Table 51-2),[34] and research and teaching should also be important parts of the activity. In primary stroke centers (PSC) all stroke patients should receive the highest level of care except for a few specific investigations or treatments requiring resources and expertise available only in a few hospitals (see Table 51-2).[34] The third level should include the minimum level of care considered necessary by the experts for any hospital ward (AHW) treating stroke patients (see Table 51-2).[34] The eight components considered absolutely necessary by more than 75% of experts for both CSCs and PSCs were a multidisciplinary team, stroke-trained nurses, brain CT available 24 hours a day 7 days a week (24/7), CT priority for stroke patients, extracranial Doppler sonography, automated electrocardiographic monitoring, IV recombinant tissue plasminogen activator (rt-PA) protocol available 24/7, and an in-house emergency department. Eleven other components in the fields of vascular surgery, neurosurgery, interventional radiology, and clinical research were considered to be necessary in CSCs by more than 75% of the experts. Only eight components—brain CT 24/7, CT priority for stroke patients, in-house emergency department with dedicated staff, stroke care map for patient admission, stroke pathway, prevention program, and collaboration with outside rehabilitation center—were considered important for AHW but not absolutely necessary by more than 50% of the experts.[34] This classification is close to that of the Brain Attack Coalition and the

German and Swiss models, although it does not closely relate to stroke units included in the Cochrane systematic review.[33,35-38]

Mixed assessment-rehabilitation units, which, in essence, are generic disability services, have an interest and expertise in the assessment and rehabilitation of disabling illnesses but do not exclusively manage patients with stroke. These units often combine acute admission with a period of rehabilitation, whereas delayed admission units admit patients after at least 1 week. The results of the Stroke Unit Trialists' Collaboration demonstrated that both such types of units can positively influence outcomes for patients with stroke (Table 51-3).[30-39] Obviously, such units do not fulfill the modern concept of acute stroke unit care, targeted at preventing early complications like aspiration.[39]

All the different models of stroke unit care incorporate specialist multidisciplinary team care coordinated through weekly meetings. The mixtures of staff available are similar in organized stroke unit settings and conventional care settings, consisting of medical nurses, physiotherapy staff, occupational therapists, speech therapists, and social workers.[33] The main difference is in the practice and organization of care. Stroke unit care most often includes a coordinated multidisciplinary team, staffing by people with an interest in stroke, staff education programs, routine provision of information to patients and caregivers, and involvement of caregivers as well as technical and human resources for delivering stroke unit care (see Table 51-1).[28] All members of the team must know the principles of good medical care and early rehabilitation and how to deliver it. The specialized rehabilitation personnel in conventional care settings usually work only during ordinary working hours, whereas in stroke units, the patients are treated 24 hours a day. Accordingly, all members of the staff in stroke units must be capable of participating in all activities of acute stroke care and rehabilitation. Mobile stroke teams have not been able to reduce death, dependency, or need for institutional care compared with conventional care in general medical wards.[40] Although not proven, it is possible that skilled nursing staff available 24 hours a day in a geographically defined area in the early stage of stroke is necessary for prevention of early complications.

Effectiveness of Stroke Unit Care

Most randomized trials of stroke unit care have involved a relatively small number of patients and, accordingly, have not been able to verify differences in hard endpoints, such as case-fatality rates. A meta-analysis of those trials have verified, however, that patients receiving stroke unit care are more likely to survive, return home, and regain physical independence. Furthermore, secondary complications of stroke are less common in patients receiving stroke unit care.[39] Table 51-4 summarizes the differences between stroke unit care and conventional care.[39] Analysis of recent Cochrane systematic reviews revealed that stroke unit care is able to reduce stroke progression/recurrence, infections, complications, and bedsores.[41] In the United Kingdom, stroke unit care has been shown to

TABLE 51-2 COMPONENTS CONSIDERED ESSENTIAL* FOR STROKE CARE

CSC
Stroke-trained physician (24/7)
Interventional neuroradiologist on call
Neurosurgeon on call
Multidisciplinary team
CEA vascular surgeon
Stroke-trained nurses
Emergency department staff
Physician expert in carotid ultrasonology
Physician expert in echocardiography
Social worker
Physician trained in rehabilitation
Speech therapy start within 2 days
Physiotherapy start within 2 days
Brain CT scan 24/7
CT priority for stroke patients
MRI (T_1-, T_2-, T_2^*- weighted, FLAIR) 24/7
Diffusion-weighted MRI
Extracranial Doppler sonography 24/7
Extracranial duplex sonography 24/7
TCD 24/7
CT angiography 24/7
Magnetic resonance angiography 24/7
Transfemoral cerebral angiography 24/7
Transthoracic echocardiography
Transesophageal echocardiography
Automated ECG monitoring (bedside)
Automated monitoring of pulse oximetry
Automated monitoring of BP
Automated monitoring of breathing
Monitoring of temperature
Intravenous rt-PA protocols 24/7
Intraarterial thrombolysis 24/7
Respiratory support
Surgery for hematoma
Carotid surgery
Angioplasty and stenting
Hemicraniectomy
Ventricular drainage
Surgery for hematoma
Emergency department (in-house)
Stroke outpatient clinic
Multidisciplinary ICU
Inpatient rehabilitation (in-house)
Outpatient rehabilitation available
Collaboration with outside rehabilitation center
Anticoagulation clinic
Stroke faculty
Stroke care map for patient admission
Stroke database
Intravenous rt-PA protocols
Community stroke awareness program
Prevention program
Stroke pathways

Clinical research
Research grants
Drug research
Stroke clinical fellowship
Stroke study coordinator
Stroke research unit

PSC
Neurologist on call
Neurologist on staff
Stroke-trained physician (24/7)
Diagnostic radiologist on call
Multidisciplinary team
Stroke-trained nurses
Emergency department staff
Physician expert in carotid ultrasonology
Social worker
Speech therapy start within 2 days
Physiotherapy start within 2 days
Brain CT scan 24/7
CT priority for stroke patients
Extracranial Doppler sonography
Extracranial duplex sonography
Transthoracic echocardiography
Transesophageal echocardiography
Automated ECG monitoring at bedside
Automated monitoring of pulse oximetry
Automated monitoring of blood pressure
Automated monitoring of breathing
Monitoring of temperature
Intravenous rt-PA protocols 24/7
Emergency department (in-house)
Stroke outpatient clinic
Multidisciplinary ICU
Inpatient rehabilitation (in-house)
Outpatient rehabilitation available
Collaboration with outside rehabilitation center
Stroke care map for patient admission
Intravenous rt-PA protocols
Community stroke awareness program
Prevention program
Stroke pathways

AHW
Emergency department staff
Brain CT scan 24/7
CT priority for stroke patients
Emergency department (in-house)
Collaboration with outside rehabilitation center
Stroke care map for patient admission
Prevention program
Stroke pathways

*Considered absolutely necessary by more than 50% of the experts.
AHW, Any hospital ward; BP, blood pressure; CEA, carotid endarterectomy; CSC, comprehensive stroke center; CT, computed tomography; ECG, electrocardiographic; FLAIR, fluid-attenuated inversion recovery; ICU, intensive care unit; MRI, magnetic resonance imaging; PSC, primary stroke center; rt-PA, recombinant tissue plasminogen activator; TCD, transcranial Doppler.
From Leys D, Ringelstein EB, Kaste M, Hacke W; European Stroke Initiative Executive Committee: The main components of stroke unit care: Results of a European expert survey. *Cerebrovasc Dis* 23:344-352, 2007.

TABLE 51-3   STROKE UNIT CARE VERSUS CONVENTIONAL CARE: OUTCOME AT THE END OF FOLLOW-UP

Outcome	Stroke Unit (n/N)	Control (n/N)	Stroke Units Better*
Death	340/1626	417/1623	0.81 (0.68, 0.96)
Death or institutional care	640/1597	755/1600	0.75 (0.65, 0.87)
Death or dependency	843/1409	944/1421	0.71 (0.60, 0.84)

*Expressed as odds ratio (95% confidence interval fixed).
Modified from Langhorne P, Dennis M: *Stroke units: an evidence-based approach*, London, 1998, BMJ Books.

TABLE 51-4   CHARACTERISTICS OF STROKE UNIT CARE AND CONVENTIONAL CARE

Characteristic(s)	Stroke Unit Care	Conventional Care
Coordination of rehabilitation		
Multidisciplinary team and weekly meetings	All	Some
Caregivers routinely involved	Most	Some
Specialization of staff		
Physicians interested in stroke	Most	Some
Physicians interested in rehabilitation	Most	Some
Nurses interested in stroke	Most	Some
Nurses interested in rehabilitation	Most	Some
Education, training, and research		
Regular staff training	Most	Some
Routine information provision to caregivers	Most	Some
Participation in stroke trials	Some	Some
Comprehensiveness of rehabilitation input		
All who need it receive physical and occupational therapy	Most	Some
Earlier start of physical and occupational therapy	Most	Some
Protocol for medical investigations and treatment	Some	None
Intensity of Input		
Enhanced nurse-to-patient ratio	Some	Some
More intensive physical and occupational therapy	Some	Some

Modified from Langhorne P, Dennis M: *Stroke units: an evidence-based approach*, London, 1998, BMJ Books.

be more effective than either stroke team or domiciliary management of stroke.[42]

With the advent of new invasive therapeutic modalities, such as hypothermia and hemicraniectomy in malignant middle cerebral artery (MCA) infarction, the need for intensive stroke care has reemerged, although this approach has not been tested in randomized controlled trials.[43]

Who Benefits?

Subgroup analyses of randomized trials revealed that all patients, regardless of age, sex, and severity of stroke, benefit from stroke unit care (Table 51-5).[39] The only exceptions are patients admitted in a coma, whose high case-fatality rate is not affected by stroke unit care.

The numbers are relatively small but suggest that elderly patients and patients with severe stroke benefit most. Young patients and patients with mild strokes have better outcomes regardless of where they receive care.

Patients with mild strokes do not gain benefit from stroke unit care in terms of increased chance of survival, but more survivors of mild stroke are independent in their daily lives. Approximately 25 mild strokes need to be treated for stroke unit care to result in one more independent survivor (number of patients needed to be treated to make statistical difference [NNT] = 25). For patients with moderate stroke, the NNT is 17 for one more survivor and 33 for one more independent survivor. For patients with severe stroke, the NNT is 17 for one more survivor but 100 for one more independent survivor. Because of the small numbers, these figures are imprecise, and the 95% confidence interval (CI) includes the possibility of no benefit. However, the results suggest that there is no firm reason to exclude patients from stroke unit care on the basis of gender, age, or stroke severity.

Stroke unit care seems to be beneficial in all types of settings. In systematic review, the mean reduction in the proportion of patients dead or institutionalized at late follow-up was 26% in geriatric medicine stroke units, 28% in general medicine stroke units, 28% in neurologic stroke units, and 33% in rehabilitation medicine stroke units.[33]

Are There Long-Term Benefits of Stroke Unit Care?

Both of the two trials of stroke unit care with a 5-year follow-up demonstrate that the odds ratios (ORs) for adverse outcomes continue to favor stroke unit care.[44-46] The ORs are for death, 0.63 (0.45, 0.89); for death or institutional care, 0.62 (0.43, 0.89); and for death or dependency, 0.59 (0.38, 0.92). The first study extended the follow-up to 10 years after stroke and found a similar pattern of results. The ORs in this study are for death, 0.46 (0.23, 0.91); for death or institutional care, 0.40 (0.18, 0.86); and for death or dependency, 0.62 (0.26, 1.46).[47]

TABLE 51-5 ORGANIZED STROKE UNIT CARE VERSUS CONVENTIONAL CARE: DEATH OR INSTITUTIONAL CARE AT THE END OF FOLLOW-UP

	Stroke Unit (n/N)	Control (n/N)	Stroke Units Better* (Risk of Death or Institutional Care)	
			OR	95 CI Fixed
Sex				
Female	172/418	193/384	0.77	(0.60, 0.98)
Male	120/366	158/364	0.66	(0.51, 0.85)
Age				
<75 years	241/839	273/796	0.77	(0.63, 0.94)
≥75 years	202/398	290/7422	0.69	(0.56, 0.85)
Severity				
Mild	36/287	47/273	0.95	(0.66, 1.36)
Moderate	279/649	317/627	0.70	(0.58, 0.84)
Severe	179/229	199/232	0.55	(0.38, 0.81)

*Expressed as odds ratio (OR) (95% confidence interval [CI] fixed).
Modified from Langhorne P, Dennis M: *Stroke units: an evidence-based approach*, London, 1998, BMJ Books.

Availability of Stroke Unit Care

The first Pan-European Consensus Meeting on Stroke Management, jointly organized by the World Health Organization (WHO) Regional Office for Europe and the European Stroke Council, recommended that stroke units should be established on a large scale throughout Europe so that by the year 2005 all patients in Europe with acute stroke should have access to care in specialized stroke units or from stroke teams.[48] This ambitious goal was not reached, but in Sweden the majority of stroke patients (up to 80%) are already treated in stroke units, according to the Swedish national quality assessment register for stroke care, Riks-Stroke.[49] This also applies in Germany. The Norwegian Board of Health has recommended that all hospitals treating stroke patients should have stroke units. In Germany, stroke patients are treated nationwide in stroke units, and according to the German Stroke Data Bank, the results are equally as good as those published by the Stroke Unit Trialists' Collaboration in 1997.[50]

The second Pan-European Consensus Meeting on Stroke Management, jointly organized by the WHO Regional Office for Europe, International Stroke Society, and the European Stroke Council, stated that all stroke patients should have access to a continuum of care from organized stroke units in the acute stage to appropriate rehabilitation and secondary prevention by 2015.[51] The random survey of European hospitals admitting stroke patients revealed that only 13.5% of stroke patients are treated in CSCs and PSCs, 44.1% are treated in AHWs, and 42.3% of acute stroke patients are admitted to hospitals that do not have the minimum facilities for acute stroke care as specified by the European Stroke Organisation (ESO). Only in Finland, Luxembourg, Sweden, and the Netherlands did most hospitals of the survey have appropriate level of care.[52] Accordingly, in Europe there is still a long way to go until the goals specified in the Helsingborg Declaration of 2006 are met.

TABLE 51-6 MAIN GOALS OF STROKE CARE IN AN ACUTE STROKE UNIT

Maintenance of vital functions
Recanalization of the occluded cerebral artery
Treatment of unstable cerebral ischemia and prevention of progressing stroke
Prevention and treatment of infarct edema
Prevention of acute medical complications
Prevention of recurrent stroke
Early rehabilitation

General Stroke Management

A general recommendation of the ESO is that all patients with stroke should be treated in specialized stroke units.[28] The acute stroke unit is the third step in the critical pathway for stroke, after prehospital emergency care and care in the emergency department (see Chapter 48). The main goals of stroke care at a stroke unit are shown in Table 51-6. Optimally, all stroke patients and even high-risk TIA patients should be admitted to a stroke unit as an emergency. Prevention of recurrent stroke and early rehabilitation are important aspects of stroke management in stroke units, thoroughly reviewed in Chapters 56 and 58. Secondary prevention should start as early as possible or on admission to the stroke unit at the latest. It is recommended that aspirin should be given after ischemic stroke if thrombolysis is not administered or 24 hours after thrombolysis. Selection of treatment should be based on the most likely cause of the stroke and all risk factors of the patient, and it is vital that both a secondary prevention strategy and a rehabilitation plan is developed before the patient is discharged from the stroke unit.

Vital Functions

The clinical condition of the patient with acute stroke should be stabilized in the emergency department, before arrival at the acute stroke unit. For a patient in whom airway, breathing, or cardiovascular function (the ABCs) is compromised, intensive care facilities are used until the clinical situation is stable. The exceptions are patients in whom the prognosis is obviously poor, a fatal course is inevitable, or there are other reasons to withhold aggressive therapies. In other words, the patient should be stabilized in the emergency department before the next step of the critical pathway—transfer to the acute stroke unit—is taken.

The decision where to treat the patient depends on local resources and the level of care and monitoring at the stroke unit; some stroke units do have intensive care facilities, such as continuous arterial blood pressure (BP) monitoring, central venous catheters, mechanical ventilators, and continuous positive airway pressure (CPAP) ventilation. The vital functions of a patient with stroke are stable if (1) the patient has a secure airway and ventilatory function, (2) BP is not extremely high or low, (3) the cardiac rhythm is hemodynamically sufficient, and (4) unstable coronary ischemia is not present. Endotracheal intubation is indicated for patients with reduced consciousness, and controlled ventilation is needed for patients with spontaneous hypoventilation.

The patient with acute stroke, even the one with milder symptoms or with stable vital functions, must be recognized as an urgently ill medical patient.[53,54] Even transitory, rapidly resolving, or fluctuating symptoms may be associated with complete acute occlusion of the internal carotid artery (ICA) or even occlusion of the MCA trunk in patients with excellent collateral circulation. If the artery is not recanalized, the situation is likely to lead to embolic complications of the progressing thrombus and to worsening of the patient's clinical status. In some cases, hemodynamic ischemia may accentuate the symptoms, if the patient is dehydrated, hypotensive, or is immediately mobilized without knowledge of the state of recanalization.

Recanalization

The first goal of the emergency medical services (EMS) personnel during the hyperacute stage at the scene and again in the emergency department is to define whether the patient is a candidate for thrombolytic therapy. IV and intraarterial thrombolysis as well as mechanical thrombectomy are extensively covered in other chapters and therefore are not touched on here (see Chapters 49, 61, and 62).

Even if the patient is not a candidate for thrombolysis, the next step is to rapidly evaluate whether the occluded cerebral artery has already been recanalized.[55] Fortunately, several methods are readily available in most stroke centers. The intraluminal thrombus is often visible as a hyperdensity on the initial CT scan, showing as the characteristic dense media sign but also as the dense posterior, anterior, or basilar artery sign.[56] In borderline cases, the CT diagnosis can be difficult, and persistent arterial occlusion can be suspected only because of calcified atherosclerotic arteries. If the dense artery sign matches the perfusion defect in perfusion CT images, the artery has not recanalized.[57,58] CT angiography, if available, will answer this question. Magnetic resonance angiography

(MRA) is also sensitive but is more time-consuming and is not always readily available to diagnose lack of blood flow in the artery. The same holds true for single-photon emission computed tomography (SPECT) using fluorodeoxyglucose (FDG) or hexamethyl-propyleneamine-oxime (HM-PAO) and for positron emission tomography (PET) using FDG.

The dynamic recanalization process calls for more feasible methods that can be repeated at the bedside or used in continuous monitoring mode. Transcranial Doppler (TCD) ultrasonography is a dynamic monitoring method available at the bedside; it is based on blood flow velocity measurement using Doppler ultrasonography (see Chapter 44). The demonstration of recanalization with TCD ultrasonography is very straightforward, and the method can be used to follow the recanalization process as it is actually taking place.[59] Typical recanalization patterns of the MCA with repeated TCD ultrasonography measurements have been reported in patients.[60] A new thrombolysis in brain ischemia (TIBI) classification, analogous to the angiographic thrombolysis in myocardial ischemia (TIMI) classification to measure residual flow and recanalization of cardiac vessels, has been developed for noninvasive monitoring of intracranial vessel residual flow signals with TCD ultrasonography. TIBI classification as determined by emergency TCD ultrasonography correlated with initial stroke severity, clinical recovery, and mortality in patients with stroke who were treated with IV t-PA, and a flow-grade improvement has been found to correlate with clinical improvement.[60,61]

Unstable Cerebral Ischemia and Progressing Stroke

The unstable phase of cerebral ischemia generally extends up to the point that recanalization is complete and, in some cases, beyond, depending on the status of the cerebrovascular tree and the overall cardiopulmonary condition of the patient. The unstable phase is characterized by both persisting arterial occlusion and fluctuating symptoms due to reduced perfusion or embolization of the thrombus that may or may not be accentuated if the BP falls or as the patient is mobilized.[62]

Progressing stroke is an old concept, originated before the era of modern imaging technology. Development of the penumbral area into infarction has been demonstrated by several perfusion methods, including perfusion-weighted imaging (PWI), which is based on magnetic resonance imaging (MRI). Deterioration of the clinical condition of the patient has many potential reasons; however, only a few are directly related to the thrombus itself.[63] Because of the heterogeneous nature of progressing stroke, it should not be used for research or clinical decision making unless the diagnosis is based on recanalization, mismatched patterns on diffusion-weighted imaging (DWI) and PWI, or both. Treatment of progressing symptoms can be successful only if the pathophysiologic mechanism or multiple mechanisms behind the deterioration have been clarified. The main reasons for progressing stroke include most of the acute complications, which can be prevented in well-organized stroke unit care and, if they do occur, can be treated (Table 51-7).

TABLE 51-7 REASONS FOR DETERIORATION IN ACUTE ISCHEMIC STROKE

Systemic causes
Dehydration
Arterial hypotension
Extreme degrees of arterial hypertension
Increased body temperature, fever
Hyperglycemia
Hypoventilation, CO_2 retention
Hypoxia
Aspiration and pneumonia
Sepsis, infection
Pulmonary embolism
Myocardial ischemia
Cardiac arrhythmias
Congestive heart failure
Neurogenic pulmonary edema
Hypoglycemia
Epileptic seizure activity
Hyponatremia and other disturbances
    of electrolyte balance
Overhydration
Thiamine deficiency
Organic delirium
Psychiatric factors

Causes related to arterial occlusion or cerebral infarct
Reembolization
Progressing thrombosis
Reocclusion
Infarct edema
Increased intracranial pressure and reduced perfusion pressure
Compartmental brain herniation
Hemorrhagic transformation
Decreasing collateral flow
Reduced perfusion due to multiple stenosing arterial lesions
Extension of the infarct core
Extension of the penumbral area

Prevention and Treatment of Infarct Edema and Elevated Intracranial Pressure

Patients with large hemispheric strokes, defined as exceeding 50% of the MCA territory, are at risk of development of cerebral edema that could produce mass effect and may lead to herniation. The clinical picture is that of a progressive decline in level of consciousness, sighing, and vomiting, followed by decorticate or decerebrate posturing and pupillary dilation as the herniation proceeds. Intracranial pressure (ICP) is not usually elevated during the early phase of herniation, but there may be a gradient between the hemispheres that can be observed even noninvasively by TCD ultrasonography. Direct monitoring of ICP is generally not recommended but is being used in some intensive stroke care units.[64] Increased ICP is covered in more detail in Chapter 52. Close monitoring of neurologic status and serial CT scans are the diagnostic method of choice for guiding interventions.

Ischemic brain edema occurs during the first 24 to 48 hours after ischemic infarcts. In younger patients, brain edema with elevated ICP may become a major complication, possibly leading to herniation and death.[65] Such patients usually show a rapid decline in consciousness and demonstrate the signs of herniation 2 to 4 days after

onset of symptoms. The outcome is fatal in the majority of patients: the mortality rate is about 80% for standard treatment.[66,67]

According to historical studies, acute massive brain swelling with subsequent transtentorial herniation after MCA infarction is found in 13% of autopsied patients with stroke, and raised ICP due to edema is common.[67,68] The time course of edema formation after stroke has been studied in patients more than 50 years ago.[69] Brain edema involving the gray and white matter surrounding the infarcted tissue could be seen within 24 hours, reached its maximum on days 3 to 5, and then subsided completely within 2 weeks. A malignant MCA infarct has been defined as a space-occupying infarct of at least the total MCA territory, with signs of an increasing space-occupying effect on serial CT scans with a midline shift of more than 10 mm at the septum pellucidum level (see Chapters 52 and 78).[66,70] Such an infarct is commonly caused by an embolic occlusion of either the distal ICA or the proximal MCA trunk. The outcome is often fatal, and a mortality rate of up to 80% has been reported for standard care.[65,66]

Based on a pooled analysis of smaller studies, hemicraniectomy is now the treatment of choice and level I class A recommendation for the patient with malignant MCA infarct.[53]

Development of clinically significant edema in the infarct area and especially the transformation into malignant MCA infarct can often be predicted on clinical grounds as well as through the use of DWI or other perfusion methods, and several studies have addressed this question.[67,71-75] A lesion found on DWI that exceeds 145 cm^3 has been demonstrated to be highly predictive of a malignant course with 100% sensitivity and 94% specificity, although with wide confidence intervals.[72]

Hemorrhagic transformation of the infarct is often asymptomatic but can be a factor in the unfavorable course of a large infarct. Therefore efforts to prevent hemorrhagic transformation seem justified.[76-80] However, after thrombolytic therapy, hemorrhagic transformation signifies recanalization and is generally not associated with clinical deterioration. Basic management of elevated ICP after stroke usually consists of (1) placement of the patient in a semi-sitting position with elevation of the head and upper trunk to approximately 30 degrees, (2) avoidance of noxious stimuli, (3) pain relief, and (4) a low normal body temperature (36°C to 37°C). Because the head-up position may also lead to a decrease in mean arterial BP (MAP), the head position should be individualized and adjusted so that cerebral perfusion pressure (CPP) (MAP − ICP) can be optimized. Osmotherapy with 10% glycerol (250 mL of 10% glycerol over 60 minutes every 6 hours) or 15% mannitol (100 to 200 mL every 4 to 6 hours) is usually given intravenously at the first sign of space-occupying edema.[81] The effect of glycerol may last somewhat longer than that of mannitol and may be less commonly associated with a rebound increase in ICP. Hypertonic saline (up to 5% or more) has been used for the same purpose and has often been reported to be more effective than mannitol.[82] Hypotonic and glucose-containing solutions are avoided, and a slightly negative fluid balance can be a target. One must keep in mind, however, that, especially in the early phase of an infarct, dehydration is known to be detrimental. Dexamethasone and other corticosteroids are useless and are relatively contraindicated.

A short-acting barbiturate such as thiopental given as a bolus results in rapid reduction in ICP but may be harmful if there is a significant drop in MAP and CPP. Propofol (10 mg/mL as a continuous infusion of 10 to 30 mL/h) is commonly used for sedation of patients receiving mechanical ventilation, but its effects on the ICP have not been well studied. In case of severe compromise of cerebral perfusion by rising ICP, the fastest way to restore intracranial circulation is volume loading with induction of hypertension by vasopressors. If the ICP is being directly measured, the CPP should be kept above 70 mm Hg. Alternatively, TCD ultrasonography may be used to ensure sufficient blood flow velocity and perfusion pressure, although absolute values are not available. During vasoactive treatment, continuous or intermittent monitoring of MCA blood flow by TCD ultrasonography may also be used to exclude significant arterial spasm due to higher doses of vasopressors.

Only a few studies have addressed conservative treatment of infarct edema. Hypertonic saline with hydroxyethyl starch and glycerol have been reported to improve early mortality rates for malignant MCA infarct.[81,82] A systematic review of the use of glycerol in ischemic stroke found a significant 35% OR reduction (95% CI, 3% to 56%) in the early mortality rate, although only 601 patients were included in the meta-analysis.[80] A single study of 173 patients that was both randomized and double-blinded showed a 60% reduction in the early mortality rate during the first week of IV glycerol therapy.[82] Thus, there is at least some evidence that glycerol may be helpful, but it has not been properly tested in the setting of malignant MCA infarct or in patients with infarct edema. Ten percent saline rapidly and effectively decreases ICP but may lead to cardiovascular compromise or osmotic injury, especially in the presence of hyponatremia; therefore it is not recommended for general use.[81,83]

According to a recent pooled analysis of smaller randomized trials, hemicraniectomy (discussed in Chapters 52 and 78) effectively improves the outcome in malignant MCA stroke and is currently recommended by the ESO guidelines.[53,84]

Prevention of Acute Medical Complications

General Stroke Care

In addition to recanalization of the occluded vessel, there are other almost as urgent goals in the early management of stroke. Basically, the outcome of the patient depends heavily on the appearance of imminent medical complications involving different organ systems (e.g., cardiopulmonary system, gastrointestinal system, kidneys, skin, muscles, and peripheral and central nervous systems), fluid balance, coagulation, fibrinolysis, and nutritional and other disturbances of homeostasis (see Table 51-7). The subtype of stroke according to the Trial of Org 10172 in Acute Stroke Treatment (TOAST) classification is important, even for assessment of risk of recurrence and mortality, and affects secondary preventive strategies that should be initiated immediately.[85] Adequate treatment

and preservation of vital functions constitute the basis of all therapeutic measures in acute stroke, even those outside the stroke unit environment. The consensus is that management of general medical problems is the basis for stroke treatment.[53,54,86-89]

Fluid and Electrolyte Balance

Almost all patients with stroke are somewhat dehydrated on admission, which is a condition that has been found to correlate with a less favorable outcome.[90] Several reasons may account for dehydration after acute stroke—swallowing, communication, and cognitive problems as well as immobility, infection, diuretic therapy, hyperthermia, and restlessness—and preexisting dehydration, from whatever cause, may have had an acute prothrombotic effect that resulted in thromboembolic stroke. Patients who have lain for hours or even days after stroke before being found and brought for treatment represent a subgroup of patients with stroke who are at very high risk of worsening and death. These patients commonly have multiple medical complications on admission, such as severe dehydration, decubitus ulcer, aspiration pneumonia, urinary tract infection, rhabdomyolysis, renal insufficiency, and, possibly, imminent multiorgan failure. Although the issue has not been explicitly studied, a common observation in the stroke unit is that such patients have the worst overall prognosis.

In the prehospital care setting, one of the first things to be done for a patient with stroke is to establish an IV line with Ringer's solution or physiologic saline; rehydration will continue at the stroke unit. IV fluid therapy is virtually always needed, and no patient with stroke should be deprived of it during the early phase. The fluid balance during the first 24 hours after stroke should be more or less positive, depending on the level of dehydration on admission, which can be assessed by measurement of hematocrit and osmolality. Because both volume depletion and volume overloading should be avoided, the fluid balance of a patient with acute stroke must be closely monitored, especially during the unstable phase.

Sometimes more complex electrolyte disturbances ensue, as seen in such cases with low intake of salt or, very rarely, preexisting syndrome of inappropriate antidiuretic hormone (SIADH). It is our impression that the occurrence of SIADH is very exceptional after stroke and that hyponatremia and volume depletion are usually caused by the cerebral salt wasting (CSW) syndrome, which can be confused with SIADH. In these cases, the conventional recommendation to restrict fluids so that hyponatremia can be corrected carries a risk and may even prove fatal; instead, volume loading and sodium loading must be performed. As a rule, fluid restriction is virtually never indicated in acute stroke. In very severe stroke with compression or destruction of the hypothalamus, lack of antidiuretic hormone may lead to diabetes insipidus, which must be treated with vasopressin.

Cardiovascular Management

Cardiac arrhythmias and myocardial ischemia secondary to stroke are very common. Significant alterations in the ST segments and the T waves on an electrocardiogram (ECG) may appear in the early phase, representing true myocardial ischemia, sometimes in the absence of coronary disease.[91,92] Cardiac enzymes may be elevated in stroke, more commonly in severe stroke, including stroke due to intracerebral or subarachnoid hemorrhage.[93] The routine treatment for this phenomenon, which depends mainly on excess circulating catecholamines, is beta-blocker or α and beta-blocker therapy. Beta-blockers are routinely administered to protect the myocardium, especially in more severe stroke. One must, however, abide by any preexisting and acute contraindications to this therapeutic modality, such as bronchoconstriction, congestive heart failure, severe bradycardia, and disturbances of atrioventricular or intraventricular conduction (i.e., prolonged PQ or QT interval).

An initial ECG should be performed in every stroke patient followed by continuous ECG monitoring, which is recommended for the majority of patients, especially for patients with cardiac symptoms or hemodynamic instability. A continuously recording automated ECG monitoring and analyzing system is likely to improve the diagnostics of significant arrhythmias, such as atrial fibrillation. Cardiac enzyme levels are routinely monitored for 24 hours or for several days in unstable patients. Etiologic studies, including echocardiography and invasive cardiologic evaluation, are an essential part of the diagnostic work-up for many patients with stroke. Readily available cardiologic consultations are a must for an acute stroke unit.

Blood Pressure Management

A transient elevation of arterial BP is the rule at the onset of stroke, occurring in 80% of patients with acute stroke.[94,95] This elevation has been viewed as a beneficial physiologic response to ischemia that does not need to be treated under most circumstances.[96] It has been attributed to a number of factors, such as catecholamine secretion in response to stress, neuroendocrine factors, alcohol, and topographic presentation of the infarct.[97-104] The BP usually declines during the first few days.[103-108] Although the general recommendation has been not to treat a moderate elevation in BP during the first few days, the issue is not entirely settled.[107] It is suggested that sudden lowering of the BP in the acute stage of occlusive stroke may either reduce the CPP in the ischemic portion of the brain or provoke an ischemic steal, especially with the use of vasodilators such as calcium entry blockers.[106,109-112] Deficient autoregulation of cerebral blood flow (CBF) and watershed infarctions associated with critical internal carotid stenosis or occlusion may be accentuated after hypotensive therapy or acetazolamide administration, which is a possibility that should also be kept in mind for amaurosis fugax due to unilateral carotid stenosis.[105,110]

The natural course of BP in the early phase of various subtypes of stroke is not very well known, but the elevation in BP is usually seen to decline spontaneously within a week after stroke without the use of intervening medications.[95] Chamorro et al[107,113] conducted an observational study of 24-hour BP recordings in patients with strokes of various types and in hospital control subjects, immediately after presentation to the hospital and 7 days after admission. These researchers observed a lower incidence of brain edema in patients who received antihypertensive treatment during the early phase of stroke than in those who did not, even when the MAP on admission was significantly higher in the former group. Complete recovery was more common in patients with edema who were treated with moderate BP reduction.[113] It has been suggested that poststroke hypertension could be deleterious, facilitating edema formation in the ischemic tissue. Pharmacologic elevation of BP as a therapeutic intervention has been studied, but the results are not conclusive.[114] This mode of therapy is used in intensive stroke units as a rescue therapy in emergent situations when increasing ICP leads to rapid reduction of CPP. Invasive hemodynamic monitoring and intensive care facilities are needed for this therapy.

An increase in BP is a protective physiologic mechanism, and deficient autoregulation in the acute stage may lead to a severely reduced perfusion pressure in case of a sudden drop in BP. Some exceptions to this rule are acute congestive heart failure due to severe hypertension, hypertensive encephalopathy, subarachnoid hemorrhage, immediate or progressing hypertensive or anticoagulant-induced intracranial hemorrhage, hyperperfusion syndrome after carotid endarterectomy, myocardial ischemia, dissection of the thoracic or abdominal aorta, and the use of thrombolytic therapy.

According to the current recommendations of the American Heart Association (AHA) and the ESO, BP values exceeding 220 mm Hg systolic, 130 mm Hg diastolic (220/130 mm Hg) should be treated actively even on admission.[53,54] The decision to treat also depends on the previous BP level as well as on the use of anticoagulants or thrombolytic therapy, during and after which BP readings of 180/100 mm Hg should not be exceeded. No recommendations currently exist on how to deal with BP in the setting of expansive infarct edema with or without increased ICP.

We use TCD ultrasonography to assess intracranial hemodynamics on an individual basis to optimize BP level according to the actual cardiopulmonary status of the patient. On the basis of current evidence, there is no need to revise existing recommendations. There may be a shift toward somewhat lower BP levels, but more aggressive lowering of BP may necessitate monitoring of intracranial hemodynamics.

Impressive progress has been made in the secondary prevention of stroke with antihypertensive treatment, although the topic is not within the scope of this chapter. Secondary prevention studies generally do not answer questions about how and when antihypertensive therapy should be used during the early phase of stroke. However, a beneficial effect on long-term outcome has been convincingly demonstrated for diuretics, beta-blockers, and two angiotensin-converting enzyme (ACE) inhibitors, which also makes them a logical choice in acute care. ACE inhibitors carry less risk of accentuating cerebral ischemia and have been reported to protect the brain from the ischemia associated with BP reduction.

Vasodilators typically cause a severe ischemic steal phenomenon and should be avoided, except when strongly indicated as, for example, in myocardial ischemia. The drugs of choice for emergency IV antihypertensive treatment are (1) labetalol in IV boluses of 10 mg, which can be repeated as necessary, or as a continuous infusion at 30 to 60 mg/h and (2) enalapril in repeated boluses of 1 mg every 15 to 30 minutes. Nicardipine can be used with a starting dose of 2 to 5 mg/h as a continuous infusion (or nimodipine, 1 to 2 mg/h); one must keep in mind, however, that calcium entry blockers can lead to steal of blood flow from ischemic to healthy regions of the brain and that the effect of a sharp drop in BP can be harmful. The use of peroral nifedipine is discouraged by most treatment guidelines, including those of the American Stroke Association. In resistant cases, sodium nitroprusside can be considered, although this agent carries the risk of severe compromise of cerebral perfusion with a sudden drop of BP, reflex tachycardia, and myocardial ischemia. Either IV nimodipine or IV nitroglycerin effectively treats elevated BP when there is a special indication, such as subarachnoid hemorrhage or myocardial ischemia, for the use of either of these drugs.

There is some evidence for a deleterious effect of BP reduction on stroke. A word of caution about the use of dihydropyridine derivatives to lower the BP is therefore appropriate. The Intravenous Nimodipine West European Stroke Trial (INWEST) found a correlation between nimodipine-induced reduction in BP and an unfavorable outcome of acute stroke.[115] Diastolic but not systolic BP reduction was associated with neurologic worsening after the IV administration of high-dose nimodipine for acute stroke.[109] It is unclear whether this negative effect was mediated through deficient autoregulation or reduced myocardial perfusion, which has a correlation to the diastolic BP. Nimodipine is highly effective in subarachnoid hemorrhage and is sometimes used for vasculitis, postpartum angiography, or cerebrovascular spasm of unknown cause, although there are no controlled studies to support this use. Oral nifedipine is contraindicated as emergency antihypertensive treatment in stroke according to most published guidelines, mainly because of the possibility of severe steal from ischemic regions and an uncontrolled drop in BP.[53,54]

Respiratory Function and Prevention of Pulmonary Complications

In acute ischemic stroke, early changes in ventilatory drive and early respiratory disturbances due to reduced consciousness are rare. However, patients with complete MCA infarct, large supratentorial hemorrhage, or brainstem stroke may have early ventilatory problems. Patients with severe stroke are continuously monitored with pulse oximetry, and supplemental oxygen should be used in the emergency and unstable phases, until stabilization of recanalization and later on, if needed, according to pulse oximetry and arterial blood gas values or if signs of myocardial ischemia develop. Usually, 2 to 4 L/min administered via nasal tube are sufficient, but mask ventilation may be needed to deliver more oxygen. Temporary CPAP ventilation is sometimes necessary for refractory pulmonary edema. CPAP can also be used for severe obstructive sleep apnea, which is commonly diagnosed in acute stroke patients, and is also known to be an important risk factor for stroke, most likely mediated by its cardiovascular effects.

The adequacy of ventilation must be ensured as part of any routine check of vital functions. Hypoxia must be excluded by oxygen saturation and with arterial blood gas measurement, if appropriate. Hypoventilation must be excluded, especially in patients with even slightly decreased consciousness in case of aspiration pneumonia. The combination of hypoxia, hypoventilation, and low CPP is the worst case scenario.

If intubation is indicated, it should be preplanned and performed by an experienced anesthesiologist because CBF can be compromised during the procedure; such compromise may also provoke unwanted autonomic reflexes and BP changes, thereby precipitating intracranial shifts or bleeding. The following findings are sufficient indications for intubation:

- Unconsciousness (Glasgow Coma Scale [GCS] score < 8)
- Inability to swallow or clear secretions from the mouth
- Absence of cough and gag reflexes
- Severe stridor

A patient with stroke should undergo intubation only if the possibility for independent recovery is present; that is, intubation should not be used only to prolong the terminal phase. Some patients clearly benefit from ventilator treatment, and independent recovery is possible.[116,117]

Chest radiographs show that most patients with acute stroke have at least slight pulmonary congestion or even pulmonary edema. The presence of either finding does not necessarily indicate volume overloading or even congestive heart failure; the condition may be neurogenic and related to a burst of catecholamines. Neurogenic or catecholamine-induced edema often responds well to IV labetalol, especially in cases of extreme degrees of arterial hypertension. Slight pulmonary edema in a patient with acute stroke is generally not treated by fluid restriction or diuretics, unless the edema is severe or oxygenation is compromised.

One of the most important risks in the early phase after stroke is aspiration pneumonia. Bacterial pneumonia accounts for 15% to 25% of stroke-related deaths. The majority of the pneumonias are caused by aspiration.[118] Aspiration is commonly found in patients with reduced consciousness as well as in patients with impaired gag reflexes or swallowing disturbances, which occur after conditions besides brainstem stroke. All patients who have severe stroke, who are initially unconscious or vomiting, or who lay for hours after stroke before being found and brought for treatment are assumed to have aspirated, implicating the need for antibiotics covering both the aerobic and anaerobic pathogens of aspiration pneumonia. It is not a good idea to wait for distinct signs of pneumonia because the delay may worsen the outcome, and aspiration pneumonia is one of the most common medical complications of stroke and also has the highest impact on survival.[119-122]

Nasogastric feeding may be helpful in the prevention of aspiration pneumonia, although it does not completely abolish the risk. Other reasons for pneumonia are poor cough (hypostatic pneumonia) and immobilization. Frequent changes of the patient's position in bed and pulmonary physical therapy may prevent this type of pneumonia.

Immobilization and Mobilization

Any patient with stroke should be mobilized as soon as considered safe. However, this is not an automatic routine, and the permission to mobilize the patient must be given by the treating physician. There are a number of situations in which mobilization is believed to carry a risk, although this is another area lacking evidence-based data.

Unstable cerebral ischemia, like unstable coronary ischemia, should be a contraindication for mobilization. Normally, the unstable phase ends as the vessel becomes recanalized, either spontaneously or as a result of thrombolytic therapy. Thrombolysis is followed by immobilization for 24 hours. Hemodynamic ischemia is typically enhanced by orthostatic hypotension. Volume depletion must, of course, be corrected before the patient is allowed to stand up. Intracerebral bleeding is progressive in a high proportion (up to 70%) of patients with intracranial hemorrhage, who should be immobilized for 24 hours or as long as progression is considered possible. Unstable cardiopulmonary status, coronary ischemia, and pulmonary embolism are typical contraindications to mobilization of a stroke patient, but respiratory insufficiency is usually not because the ventilatory function commonly improves with sitting and upright positions.

Mobilization takes place in a controlled fashion, meaning that both vital functions and neurologic symptoms are monitored during the process, and possible sensorimotor or cognitive deficits are taken into account to protect the patient.

Urinary Tract Infection

Urinary tract infection is one of the most common medical complications of acute cerebral infarction. Urinary retention is common in the early phase after stroke. The majority of hospital-acquired urinary tract infections are associated with the use of indwelling catheters. A bladder catheter is usually needed, however, to ensure correct fluid balance and to follow diuresis hour by hour. Intermittent catheterization is not always feasible in the setting of severe stroke and incontinence, which may contribute to decubitus ulcer. Suprapubic catheters are considered to carry a lower risk of infection. Acidification may reduce the risk of infection, whereas intermittent catheterization has not been shown to do so. Once urinary infection is seen, appropriate antibiotics should be started. However, prophylactic antibiotics are not recommended.

Pulmonary Embolism and Deep Venous Thrombosis

Pulmonary embolism is one of the most common causes of death in patients with ischemic cerebral infarction, even in patients who otherwise would have had an excellent recovery from the stroke.[119-122] The risk of deep venous thrombosis and pulmonary embolism can be reduced by early mobilization and by the use of subcutaneous heparin or low-molecular-weight heparin.[123]

However, this effect seems to be counterbalanced by an increase in the rate of hemorrhagic complications.[124] Nevertheless, prophylaxis with subcutaneous low-dose heparin, 5000 IU every 12 hours, is recommended for bedridden patients with stroke until mobilization, as recommended by the ESO and American Stroke Association guidelines.[53,54] Tachypnea, pain, and oxygen desaturation may be signs of pulmonary embolism or pneumonia. The lower extremities should be examined daily to detect signs of deep venous thrombosis, which can be excluded by venous ultrasonography. Physical therapy and the use of support or pump stockings are suggested as an alternative to low-molecular-weight heparin.

Decubitus Ulcer

Frequent turning of immobilized patients is essential for prevention of decubitus ulcers. The skin of the incontinent patient must be kept dry. For patients at particularly high risk, an air- or fluid-filled oscillating decubitus mattress system should be used. If the decubitus ulcer does not respond to conservative treatment, antibiotic therapy for several days may be justified, before definitive surgical débridement.

Seizures

Partial (focal) or secondary generalized epileptic seizures may occur in the early phase of ischemic stroke. Lorazepam (1 to 4 mg IV) or diazepam (5 to 10 mg IV) followed by IV fosphenytoin loading when necessary is a common choice for the treatment of seizures. Carbamazepine, levetiracetam, or lamotrigine can also be used. Monitoring with electroencephalography (EEG) may be useful in some cases, but routine EEG monitoring is not recommended.

Delirium, Depression, and Psychiatric Problems

Acute organic delirium is common and must be recognized and treated promptly because of the high morbidity and mortality rates associated with it. Heavy use of alcohol, malnutrition, and infection are known predisposing factors, but delirium may also develop in previously healthy patients. IV lorazepam in bolus doses of 1 to 2 mg can be administered and haloperidol, when needed, can be added in cases of severe restlessness, agitation, aggressiveness, and psychotic behavior. Parenteral thiamine substitution is started on admission for all patients at risk of delirium.

Treatment of depression is not within the scope of this discussion (see Chapter 56). Approximately one third of patients with stroke have moderate to severe depression in the early period after stroke. Citalopram lacks pharmacologic interactions and has been shown to be useful in the treatment of poststroke depression.[125] Recently, escitalopram was shown to be effective in reducing the occurrence of depression in acute stroke patients in a randomized trial.[126] The general attitude in the stroke unit is often the best way to combat depression, but both antidepressive and anxiolytic medications must be used when indicated. A psychiatric consultation is rarely needed during the early phase, except for a severe exacerbation of a preexisting psychiatric disorder.

Special Aspects

Body Temperature and Induced Hypothermia

Body temperature is commonly elevated to above 37.5°C in the early phase of stroke.[127-130] It may be a marker of stroke severity, may reflect infectious complications, or may be an independent prognostic factor adversely affecting morbidity and mortality. In experimental ischemia models, temperature is the main determinant of infarct size in both focal and global cerebral ischemia, and even postischemic hypothermia is neuroprotective.[131-134] There is now compelling evidence that even mild hyperthermia has a clear-cut, clinically significant deleterious effect in acute stroke and may lead to expanding infarct, edema, hemorrhage, and increased ICP.[128,130,131,135,136] A landmark work by Reith et al[130] is the largest retrospective study showing that admission body temperature is highly correlated with initial stroke severity and infarct size as well as with poor outcome and mortality. These researchers found that the relative risk of poor outcome increased by a factor of 2.2 per each 1°C rise in body temperature. Furthermore, this relationship was independent of stroke severity, and the presence of infection was not independently predictive of poor outcome. The relationship between body temperature and outcome could be demonstrated even in mild stroke.[130]

The significance of elevated body temperature in stroke was probably first suggested in 1976 by Hindfelt[137] in a retrospective series of patients, although the beneficial effect of cool ambient temperature was anecdotally mentioned and even emphasized as a treatment modality in a Finnish home physician book more than 100 years ago.[138] Fever was confirmed as an independent predictor of unfavorable outcome in the 1990s.[128] As a result, interest in lowering body temperature of patients with acute stroke grew. Several pilot studies on hypothermia have been published, but pivotal multicenter studies are still lacking. External cooling pads or blankets or endovascular cooling catheters to decrease body temperature to between 32°C and 33°C have been used for at least 24 hours or up to 3 days after the onset of stroke.[139] However, prolonged hypothermia may be deleterious because the rate of infectious complications is believed to rise rapidly after the first day or so. In most hypothermia studies, relaxed general anesthesia was found to be necessary, except for one study favoring very mild hypothermia of 35°C to 36°C in conscious, lightly sedated patients who were given meperidine to control shivering. In nonintensive stroke units external cooling devices are usually preferred, but in neurocritical care units endovascular cooling is also an option.

Hypothermia is a promising approach to combat worsening edema and rising ICP.[136,140] This measure has been reported to markedly lower elevated ICP, although it has a distinct rebound effect unless the hypothermia is tapered very slowly. So far, these approaches are not applicable to the majority of patients with stroke and should probably be reserved for patients with malignant MCA infarcts only until there is evidence from randomized controlled trials that the therapy is safe and effective. However, if very mild hypothermia in awake patients, applicable in ordinary stroke units, proves safe and effective, it is likely to have a major impact on stroke care.[141] Even now, many stroke units combat fever aggressively, and routine administration of propacetamol or acetaminophen is common; for acetaminophen, a mean reduction of 0.4°C for 24 hours compared with placebo has been demonstrated.[142]

Mild hypothermia with brain temperatures between 33°C and 35°C was demonstrated to be safe and to reduce both mortality and ICP in a small number of patients with malignant MCA infarct.[143] Randomized controlled trials have demonstrated that therapeutic hypothermia is safe and effective after cardiac arrest and is increasingly used in most countries according to current treatment guidelines.[144-147] Even though the results of large-scale interventional studies in stroke are still awaited, normothermia or perhaps mild hypothermia in selected cases should have a high priority in the acute care of stroke.

Blood Glucose and Hyperglycemia

A substantial proportion (up to 50%) of patients with acute stroke are hyperglycemic on admission. Hyperglycemia has various effects that lead to increased infarct size and hemorrhagic transformation in experimental reperfusion models.[148] The mechanism of action of hyperglycemia is believed to be the endothelial expression of adhesion factors, promotion of vasospasm, production of reactive oxygen species, and upregulation of nuclear factor kappa-B (NF-κB) by oxidating products of glycosylation, leading to inflammation and metabolic tissue injury related to a high lactate level and low pH.[149]

An elevated blood glucose level leads to a 12-fold increase in the rate of hemorrhagic complications with intraarterial thrombolysis, as reported by the second Prolyse in Acute Cerebral Thromboembolism Trial (PROACT II) investigators.[150] There is some evidence that hyperglycemia may also enhance hemorrhagic transformation in patients, as it does in experimental reperfusion models.

Admission hyperglycemia is associated with increased infarct size.[151] The strong and consistent association between admission hyperglycemia and poor prognosis after stroke observed in nondiabetic patients suggests that glucose level is an important risk factor for morbidity and mortality after stroke.[152] After ischemic stroke, even a mildly elevated admission blood glucose level of 110 to 126 mg/dL (6.1 to 7.0 mmol/L) was associated with an increased risk of 30-day mortality in nondiabetic patients only (relative risk, 3.28; 95% CI, 2.32 to 4.64). In nondiabetic stroke survivors, mild acute hyperglycemia seems to be associated with in-hospital mortality and a higher risk of poor functional recovery.[152]

Elevated blood glucose levels are known to be a marker for poor outcome in ischemic stroke, subarachnoid hemorrhage, brain trauma, and global ischemia caused by cardiac arrest and are known to enhance edema in experimental ischemia models. Very strict blood glucose control (80 to 110 mg/dL [4.4 to 6.1 mmol/L]) has significantly reduced the early mortality rate of patients admitted to a surgical intensive care unit by 42% (95% CI, 22% to 62%).[153]

What are the clinical implications of these data? Based on experimental data and the association of hyperglycemia and poor outcome, it has been recommended that no glucose-containing solutions be given to patients with stroke, especially during the first few days and even longer if the situation remains unstable or there is threatening edema or hemorrhagic transformation. Blood glucose levels exceeding 144 mg/dL (8 mmol/L) are to be treated with small doses of rapidly acting subcutaneous insulin or, in resistant cases, IV insulin infusion.[53,54] In several stroke guidelines, the cutoff value has been 180 mg/dL (10 mmol/L). There has been a shift toward lower values, but treatment levels lower than 144 mg/dL (8 mmol/L) may be possible only in the intensive care setting.[153] The UK Glucose Insulin in Stroke Trial (GIST-UK) failed to show any benefit from insulin treatment of elevated blood glucose levels in acute stroke.[154] Nevertheless, control of the blood glucose level, especially during the early phase of stroke, is another top priority, probably equal in importance to the control of body temperature.

Conclusions

Stroke unit care is highly evidence-based medicine (especially in stroke units without intensive care facilities, mixed assessment/rehabilitation stroke units, or rehabilitation stroke units). Only one trial supports the effectiveness of a mobile stroke team[14]; accordingly, there is not enough data to reliably estimate the effectiveness of the mobile stroke team model. Such a team provides good service for delivering thrombolysis in a metropolitan area, but it does not have the advantages of ordinary stroke unit care in a geographically defined area provided by highly motivated multidisciplinary staff, the effectiveness of which has been verified.[39] Stroke unit care is cost-effective and reduces the likelihood of death, disability, and the need for institutional care.[39,155-161] These benefits are not restricted to any special group of patients. All stroke patients, regardless of age, sex, or severity of stroke, benefit from stroke unit care. The beneficial effect is long-standing for up to 5 to 10 years.[44]

The Pan-European Consensus Meeting on Stroke Management, organized by the WHO Regional Office for Europe together with the European Stroke Council, recommended in 1995 that all patients with acute stroke have easy access to stroke unit care by the year 2005.[48] The recommendations of the ESO, on behalf of the European Stroke Council, the European Neurological Society, and the European Federation of Neurological Societies, state that acute stroke care should take place in stroke units.[87,162] Recommendations of the Advisory Working Group on Stroke Center Identification Options of the AHA aim to improve the capacity of hospitals to provide organized care to stroke patients.[163] Dedicated stroke unit care is already in large-scale practice, especially in Germany and the Scandinavian countries, experience from which demonstrates that the results of the meta-analysis of the Stroke Unit Trialists' Collaboration can be achieved on a population level.[49,50]

REFERENCES

1. Committee on Acute Cardiac Care, Council on Clinical Cardiology, American Heart Association: Critical pathways: A review, *Circulation* 101:461-465, 2000.
2. Kennedy FB, Pozen TJ, Gableman EH, et al: Stroke intensive care—an appraisal, *Am Heart J* 80:188-196, 1970.
3. Drake WE, Hamilton MJ, Carlsson M, et al: Acute stroke management and patient outcome: The value of neurovascular care units (NCU), *Stroke* 4:933-945, 1973.
4. Pitner SE, Mance CJ: An evaluation of stroke intensive care: Results in a municipal hospital, *Stroke* 4:737-741, 1973.
5. Isaacs B: Five years' experience of a stroke unit, *Health Bull* 35:94-98, 1977.
6. McCann C, Cuthbertson RA: Comparison of two systems for stroke rehabilitation in a general hospital, *J Am Geriatr Soc* 24:211-216, 1976.
7. Feigenson JS, Gitlow HS, Greenberg SD: The disability oriented rehabilitation unit—a major factor influencing stroke outcome, *Stroke* 10:5-8, 1979.
8. Garraway WM, Akhtar AJ, Hockey L, Prescott RJ: Management of acute stroke in the elderly: Preliminary results of a controlled trial, *BMJ* 280:1040-1044, 1980.
9. Von Arbin M, Britton M, de Faire U, et al: A study of stroke patients treated in a non-intensive stroke unit or in general medical wards, *Acta Med Scand* 208:81-85, 1980.
10. Hamarin E: Early activation after stroke: Does it make a difference? *Scand J Rehabil Med* 14:101-109, 1982.
11. Strand T, Asplund K, Eriksson S, et al: A non-intensive stroke unit reduces functional disability and the need for long term hospitalization, *Stroke* 16:29-34, 1985.
12. Feldman DJ, Lee PR, Unterecker J, et al: A comparison of functionally orientated medical care and formal rehabilitation in the management of patients with hemiplegia due to cerebrovascular disease, *J Chron Dis* 15:297-310, 1962.
13. Gordon EE, Kohn KH: Evaluation of rehabilitation methods in the hemiplegic patient, *J Chron Dis* 19:3-16, 1966.
14. Wood-Dauphinee S, Shapiro S, Bass E: A randomized trial of team care following stroke, *Stroke* 15:864-872, 1984.
15. Garraway WM, Alchtar AJ, Hockey L, Prescott RJ: Management of acute stroke in the elderly: Follow-up of a controlled trial, *BMJ* 281:827-829, 1980.
16. Fagerberg B, Blomstrand C: Do stroke units save lives? *Lancet* 342:992, 1993.
17. Hankey G, Deleo D, Stewart-Wynne EG: Acute hospital care for stroke patients: A randomized trial, *Cerebrovasc Dis* 5:228, 1995.
18. Ilmavirta M: Stroke unit and outcome of brain infarction [Dissertation]. Tampere, Finland, Acta Universitatis Tampereisis, series A 410, 1994.
19. Indredavik B, Bakke F, Haheim LL, Holme I: Benefit of stroke unit: A randomised controlled trial, *Stroke* 22:1026-1031, 1991.
20. Juby LC, Lincoln NB, Berman P: The effect of a stroke rehabilitation unit on functional and psychological outcome: A randomised controlled trial, *Cerebrovasc Dis* 6:106-110, 1996.
21. Kalra L, Dale P, Crome P: Improving stroke rehabilitation: A controlled study, *Stroke* 24:1462-1467, 1993.
22. Kaste M, Palomäki H, Sarna S: Where and how should elderly stroke patients be treated? A randomized trial, *Stroke* 26:249-253, 1995.
23. Sivenius J, Pyörälä K, Heinonen OP, et al: The significance of intensity of rehabilitation after stroke: A controlled trial, *Stroke* 16:928-931, 1985.
24. Stevens RS, Ambler NR, Warren MD: A randomized controlled trial of a stroke rehabilitation ward, *Age Ageing* 13:65-75, 1984.
25. Langhorne P, Williams BO, Gilchrist W, Howie K: Do stroke units save lives? *Lancet* 342:395-398, 1993.
26. Stroke Unit Trialists' Collaboration: Collaborative systematic review of the randomised trials of organised in-patient (stroke unit) care after stroke, *BMJ* 314:1151-1159, 1997.
27. Langhorne P, Duncan P: Does the organisation of postacute stroke care really matter? *Stroke* 32:268-274, 2001.
28. Kaste M, Skyhoj Olsen T, Orgogozo J-M, et al: for the EUSI Executive Committee. Organization of stroke care: Education, stroke units and rehabilitation. European Stroke Initiative (EUSI), *Cerebrovasc Dis* 10(Suppl 3):1-11, 2000.
29. Diener HC: Future organisation of stroke service: A model for acute stroke management. In Wahlgren NG, Magnus von Arbin M, editors: *Update on Stroke Therapy 1998-1999*, Stockholm, 1999, pp 173-180.
30. Ringelstein EB, Berlit P, Busse O, et al: Konzepte der überregionalen und regionalen Schlaganfallversorgung in Deutschland, *Akt Neurol* 27:101-104, 2000.
31. Hacke W, Kaste M, Bogousslavsky J, et al: European Stroke Initiative Recommendations for Stroke Management—Update 2003, *Cerebrovasc Dis* 16:311-337, 2003.

32. Berlit P, Busse O, Diener H, et al für die Kommission 1.06: Empfehlungen für die Einrichtung von Schlaganfallspe-zialstationen ('Stroke Units'), *Nervenarzt* 69:180-185, 1998.

33. Stroke Unit Trialists' Collaboration: How do stroke units improve patient outcomes? A collaborative systematic review of the randomized trials, *Stroke* 28:2139-2144, 1997.

34. Leys D, Ringelstein EB, Kaste M, Hacke W: European Stroke Initiative Executive Committee. The main components of stroke unit care: results of a European expert survey, *Cerebrovasc Dis* 23:344-352, 2007.

35. Ringelstein E, Busse O, Grond M: 'Time is brain. Competence is brain.' Die Weiterentwicklung des Stroke-Unit-Konzeptes in Europa, *Nervenarzt* 76:1024-1027, 2005.

36. Engelter S, Lyrer P: Stroke units in der Schweiz: Bedarfanalyse, Richtlinien und Anforderungsp-rofil, *Schweiz Med Forum* 4:200-2003, 2004.

37. Alberts MJ, Latchaw RE, Selman WR, et al: Recommendations for comprehensive stroke centers: A consensus statement from the Brain Attack Coalition, *Stroke* 36:1597-1616, 2005.

38. Stroke Unit Trialists' Collaboration: Organised inpatient (stroke unit) care for stroke, *Cochrane Database Syst Rev* 4:CD000197, 2007.

39. Langhorne P, Dennis M: *Stroke units: an evidence-based approach*, London, 1998, BMJ Books.

40. Langhorne P, Dey P, Woodman M, et al: Is stroke unit care portable? A systematic review of the clinical trials, *Age Ageing* 34:324-330, 2005.

41. Govan L, Langhorne P, Weir CJ: Stroke Unit Trialists Collaboration. Does the prevention of complications explain the survival benefit of organized inpatient (stroke unit) care? Further analysis of a systematic review, *Stroke* 38:2536-2540, 2007.

42. Kalra L, Evans A, Perez I, et al: Alternative strategies for stroke care: A prospective randomised controlled study of stroke unit, stroke team, and domiciliary management of stroke, *Lancet* 356:894-899, 2000.

43. Hacke W, Schwab S, de Georgia M: Intensive care of acute stroke, *Cerebrovasc Dis* 4:385-392, 1994.

44. Indredavik B, Slordahl SA, Bakke F, et al: Stroke unit treatment: Long-term effects, *Stroke* 28:1861-1866, 1997.

45. Indredavik B, Bakke F, Slordahl SA, et al: Stroke unit treatment improves long-term quality of life: A randomized controlled trial, *Stroke* 29:895-899, 1998.

46. Lincoln NB, Husbands S, Trescoli C, et al: Five year follow up of a randomised controlled trial of a stroke rehabilitation unit, *BMJ* 320:549, 2000.

47. Indredavik B, Bakke F, Slordahl SA, et al: Stroke unit treatment: 10-year follow-up, *Stroke* 30:1524-1527, 1999.

48. Aboderin I, Venables G: Stroke management in Europe. Pan-European Consensus Meeting on Stroke Management, *J Intern Med* 240:173-180, 1996.

49. Riks-Stroke—a Swedish national quality register for stroke care, *Cerebrovasc Dis* 15(Suppl 1):5-7, 2003.

50. Kostanalyse der Schlaganfall-Behandlung in Deutschland: Eine Auswertung der Schlaganfall-Datenbank der Stiftung Deutsche Schlaganfall-Hilfe, *Ak Neurol* 29:181-190, 2002.

51. Kjellström T, Norrving B, Shatchkute A: Helsingborg Declaration 2006 on European stroke strategies, *Cerebrovasc Dis* 23:231-241, 2007.

52. Leys D, Ringelstein EB, Kaste M, Hacke W: Executive Committee of the European Stroke Initiative. Facilities available in European hospitals treating stroke patients, *Stroke* 38:2985-2991, 2007.

53. European Stroke Organisation (ESO) Executive Committee; ESO Writing Committee. Guidelines for management of ischaemic stroke and transient ischaemic attack 2008, *Cerebrovasc Dis* 25(5):457-507, 2008.

54. Adams HP, Brott T, Crowell RM, et al: Guidelines for the management of patients with acute ischemic stroke, *Stroke* 25:1901-1904, 1994.

55. Von Kummer R, Holle R, Rosin L, et al: Does arterial recanalization improve outcome in carotid territory stroke? *Stroke* 26:581-587, 1995.

56. Leys D, Pruvo JP, Godefroy O, et al: Prevalence and significance of hyperdense middle cerebral artery in acute stroke, *Stroke* 23:317-324, 1992.

57. Mayer TE, Hamann GF, Baranczyk J, et al: Dynamic CT perfusion imaging of acute stroke, *Am J Neuroradiol* 21:1441-1449, 2000.

58. Wolpert SM, Brückmann H, Greenlee R, et al: Neuroradiologic evaluation of patients with acute stroke treated with recombinant tissue plasminogen activator. The rt-PA Acute Stroke Study Group, *AJNR Am J Neuroradiol* 14:3-13, 1993.

59. Kaps M, Link A: Transcranial sonographic monitoring during thrombolytic therapy, *AJNR Am J Neuroradiol* 19:758-760, 1998.

60. Demchuk AM, Burgin WS, Christou I, et al: Thrombolysis in brain ischemia (TIBI) Transcranial Doppler flow grades predict clinical severity, early recovery, and mortality in patients treated with intravenous tissue plasminogen activator, *Stroke* 32:89-93, 2001.

61. Burgin SW, Malkoff M, Felberg RA, et al: Transcranial Doppler ultrasound criteria for recanalization after thrombolysis for middle cerebral artery stroke, *Stroke* 31:1128-1132, 2000.

62. Alexandrov AV, Felberg RA, Demchuk AM, et al: Deterioration following spontaneous improvement: Sonographic findings in patients with acutely resolving symptoms of cerebral ischemia, *Stroke* 31:915-919, 2000.

63. Jansen O, Schellinger P, Fiebach J, et al: Early recanalisation in acute ischaemic stroke saves tissue at risk defined by MRI, *Lancet* 353:2036-2037, 1999.

64. Schwab S, Aschoff A, Spranger M, et al: The value of intracranial pressure monitoring in acute hemispheric stroke, *Neurology* 47:393-398, 1996.

65. Hacke W, Schwab S, Horn M, et al: "Malignant" middle cerebral artery territory infarction: Clinical course and prognostic signs, *Arch Neurol* 53:309-315, 1996.

66. Rieke K, Schwab S, Krieger D, et al: Decompressive surgery in space occupying hemispheric infarction: Results of an open, prospective study, *Crit Care Med* 23:1576-1587, 1995.

67. Krieger DW, Demchuk AM, Kasner SE, et al: Early clinical and radiological predictors of fatal brain swelling in ischemic stroke, *Stroke* 30:287-292, 1999.

68. Ng LK, Nimmanniyta J: Massive cerebral infarction with severe brain swelling: a clinicopathological study, *Stroke* 1(3):158-163, 1970.

69. Shaw CM, Alvord EC, Berry GR: Swelling of the brain following ischemic infarction with arterial occlusion, *Arch Neurol* 1:161-177, 1959.

70. Schwab S, Steiner T, Aschoff A, et al: Early hemicraniectomy in patients with complete middle cerebral artery infarction, *Stroke* 29:1888-1893, 1998.

71. Steiger HJ: Outcome of acute supratentorial cerebral infarction in patients under 60: Development of a prognostic grading system, *Acta Neurochir (Wien)* 111:73-79, 1991.

72. Oppenheim C, Samai Y, Manai R, et al: Prediction of malignant middle cerebral artery infarction by diffusion-weighted imaging, *Stroke* 31:2175-2181, 2000.

73. Alexandrov AV, Black SE, Ehrlich LE, et al: Simple visual analysis of brain perfusion on HMPAO SPECT predicts early outcome in acute stroke, *Stroke* 27:1537-1542, 1996.

74. Berrouschot J, Barthel H, von Kummer R, et al: 99m-Technetium-ethyl-cysteinate-dimer single-photon emission CT can predict fatal ischemic brain edema, *Stroke* 29:2556-2562, 1998.

75. Andrefsky JA, Sila CA, Steiner CP, et al: Prediction of life-threatening brain swelling from large supratentorial hemispheric infarction comparing ellipsoid volume estimation (EVE) to computer assisted 3-D volumetric analysis (CAVA) within 48 hours of stroke onset, *Neurology* 52:101, 1999.

76. Berger C, Fiorelli M, Steiner T, et al: Hemorrhagic transformation of ischemic brain tissue asymptomatic or symptomatic? *Stroke* 32:1330-1335, 2001.

77. Molina CA, Montaner J, Abilleira S, et al: Timing of spontaneous recanalization and risk of hemorrhagic transformation in acute cardioembolic stroke, *Stroke* 32:1079-1084, 2001.

78. Morfis L, Schwartz RS, Poulos R, Howes LG: Blood pressure changes in acute cerebral infarction and hemorrhage, *Stroke* 28:1401-1405, 1997.

79. Broderick JP, Hagen T, Brott T, Tomsick T: Hyperglycemia and hemorrhagic transformation of cerebral infarcts, *Stroke* 26:484-487, 1995.

80. Righetti E, Celani MG, Cantisani T, et al: Glycerol for acute stroke (Cochrane Review). In *The Cochrane Library,* Issue 2. Oxford, 2004, Update Software.

81. Bayer AJ, Pathy MS, Newcombe R: Double-blind randomised trial of intravenous glycerol in acute stroke, *Lancet* 329:405-408, 1987.

82. Schwarz S, Schwab S, Bertram M, et al: Effects of hypertonic saline hydroxyethyl starch solution and mannitol in patients with increased intracranial pressure after stroke, *Stroke* 29:1550-1555, 1998.

83. Schwarz S, Georgiadis D, Aschoff A, Schwab S: Effects of hypertonic (10%) saline in patients with raised intracranial pressure after stroke, *Stroke* 33:136-140, 2002.

84. Vahedi K, Hofmeijer J, Juettler E, et al: for DECIMAL, DESTINY, and HAMLET investigators. Early decompressive surgery in malignant infarction of the middle cerebral artery: A pooled analysis of three randomised controlled trials, *Lancet Neurol* 6(3):215-222, 2007.

85. Kolominsky-Rabas PL, Weber M, Gefeller O, et al: Epidemiology of ischemic stroke subtypes according to TOAST criteria: Incidence, recurrence, and long-term survival in ischemic stroke subtypes: A population-based study, *Stroke* 32:2735-2740, 2001.

86. Recommendations on stroke prevention, diagnosis, and therapy. Report of the WHO Task Force on Stroke and Other Cerebrovascular Disorders, *Stroke* 20:1407-1431, 1989.

87. Hacke W, Kaste M, Olsen TS, et al: European Stroke Initiative recommendations for stroke management, *Cerebrovasc Dis* 10:335-351, 2000.

88. The European Ad Hoc Consensus Group: European strategies for early intervention in stroke, *Cerebrovasc Dis* 6:315-324, 1996.

89. Optimizing intensive care in stroke: A European perspective. A report of an Ad Hoc Consensus Group meeting, *Cerebrovasc Dis* 7:113-128, 1997.

90. Bhalla A, Sankaralingam S, Dundas R, et al: Influence of raised plasma osmolarity on clinical outcome after acute stroke, *Stroke* 31:2043-2048, 2000.

91. Norris JW, Hachinski VC, Myers MG, et al: Serum cardiac enzymes in stroke, *Stroke* 10:548-553, 1979.

92. Norris J: Effects of cerebrovascular lesions on the heart, *Neurol Clin* 1:87-101, 1983.

93. Kaste M, Somer H, Konttinen A: Heart type creatine kinase isoenzyme (CK MB) in acute cerebral disorders, *Br Heart J* 40:802-805, 1978.

94. Yatsu FM, Zivin J: Hypertension in acute ischemic strokes: Not to treat, *Arch Neurol* 42:999-1000, 1985.

95. Lavin P: Management of hypertension in patients with acute stroke, *Arch Intern Med* 146:66-68, 1986.

96. Waltz AG: Effect of blood pressure on blood flow in ischemic and in non-ischemic cerebral cortex, *Neurology* 18:613-621, 1968.

97. Ito A, Omae T, Katsuki S: Acute changes in blood pressure following vascular diseases in the brain stem, *Stroke* 4:80-84, 1973.

98. Carlberg B, Asplund K, Hägg E: High blood pressure in acute stroke: Is it white coat hypertension? *J Intern Med* 228:291-292, 1990.

99. Carlberg B, Asplund K, Hägg E: Course of blood pressure in different subsets of patients after acute stroke, *Cerebrovasc Dis* 1:281-287, 1991.

100. Carlberg B, Asplund K, Hägg E: Factors influencing admission blood pressure levels in patients with acute stroke, *Stroke* 22:527-530, 1991.

101. Olsson T, Marklund N, Gustafson Y, Nasman B: Abnormalities at different levels of the hypothalamic-pituitary-adrenocortical axis early after stroke, *Stroke* 23:1573-1576, 1992.

102. Myers MG, Norris JW, Hachinski VC, Sole MJ: Plasma norepinephrine in stroke, *Stroke* 12:200-203, 1981.

103. Jansen PAF, Schulte BPM, Poels EFJ, Gribnau FWJ: Course of blood pressure after cerebral infarction and transient ischemic attack, *Clin Neurol Neurosurg* 89:243-246, 1987.

104. Harper G, Castleden CM, Potter JF: Factors affecting changes in blood pressure after acute stroke, *Stroke* 25:1726-1729, 1994.

105. Wallace JD, Levy LL: Blood pressure after stroke, *JAMA* 246:2177-2180, 1981.

106. Britton M, Carlsson A, Faire UD: Blood pressure course in patients with acute stroke and matched controls, *Stroke* 17:861-864, 1986.

107. Chamorro A, Vila N, Ascaso C, et al: Blood pressure and functional recovery in acute ischemic stroke, *Stroke* 29:1850-1853, 1998.

108. Oppenheimer S, Hachinski V: Complications of acute stroke, *Lancet* 339:721-724, 1992.

109. Ahmed N, Näsman P, Wahlgren NG: Effect of intravenous nimodipine on blood pressure and outcome after acute stroke, *Stroke* 31:1250-1255, 2000.

110. Graham DI: Ischemic brain following emergency blood pressure lowering in hypertensive patients, *Acta Med Scand* 678(Suppl):61-69, 1982.

111. Power WJ: Acute hypertension after stroke: The scientific basis for treatment decisions, *Neurology* 43:461-467, 1993.

112. Jörgensen HS, Nakayama H, Raaschou HO, Olsen TS: Effect of blood pressure and diabetes on stroke in progression, *Lancet* 344:156-159, 1994.

113. Chamorro A: Blood pressure in acute ischemic stroke and functional recovery. In Wahlgren NG, editor: *Update on stroke therapy 2001-2002*, Stockholm, 2001, Repro Print AB, pp 193-203.

114. Rordorf G, Cramer SC, Efird JT, et al: Pharmacological elevation of blood pressure in acute stroke: Clinical effects and safety, *Stroke* 28:2133-2138, 1997.

115. Wahlgren NG, MacMahon DG, De Keyser J, et al: The Intravenous Nimodipine West European Trial (INWEST) of nimodipine in the treatment of acute ischemic stroke, *Cerebrovasc Dis* 4:204-210, 1994.

116. Grotta J, Pasteur W, Khwaja G, et al: Elective intubation for neurologic deterioration after stroke, *Neurology* 45:640-644, 1995.

117. Berrouschot J, Rössler A, Köster J, Schneider D: Mechanical ventilation in patients with hemispheric ischemic stroke, *Crit Care Med* 28:2956-2961, 2000.

118. Horner J, Massey E, Riski J, et al: Aspiration following stroke: Clinical correlates and outcome, *Neurology* 38:1359-1362, 1988.

119. Davenport RJ, Dennis MS, Wellwood I, Warlow CP: Complications after acute stroke, *Stroke* 27:415-420, 1996.

120. Langhorne P, Stott DJ, Robertson L, et al: Medical complications after stroke: A multicenter study, *Stroke* 31:1223-1229, 2000.

121. Roth EJ, Lovell L, Harvey RL, et al: Incidence of and risk factors for medical complications during stroke rehabilitation, *Stroke* 32:523-529, 2001.

122. Johnston KC, Li JY, Lyden PD, et al: Medical and neurological complications of ischemic stroke: Experience from the RANTTAS trial. RANTTAS Investigators, *Stroke* 29:447-453, 1998.

123. Kelly J, Rudd A, Lewis R, Hunt BJ: Venous thromboembolism after acute stroke, *Stroke* 32:262-267, 2001.

124. International Stroke Trial (IST): A randomised trial of aspirin, subcutaneous heparin, both, or neither among 19,435 patients with acute ischaemic stroke. International Stroke Trial Collaborative Group, *Lancet* 349:1569-1581, 1997.

125. Andersen G, Vestergaard K, Lauritzen L: Effective treatment of post-stroke depression with the selective serotonin reuptake inhibitor citalopram, *Stroke* 25:1099-1104, 1994.

126. Robinson RG, Jorge RE, Moser DJ, et al: Escitalopram and problem-solving therapy for prevention of poststroke depression: a randomized controlled trial, *JAMA* 299(20):2391-2400, 2008.

127. Christensen H, Boysen G, Christensen E: Body temperature in acute stroke, *Cerebrovasc Dis* 10(Suppl 2):101, 2000.

128. Castillo J, Martinez F, Leira R, et al: Mortality and morbidity of acute cerebral infarction related to temperature and basal analytic parameters, *Cerebrovasc Dis* 4:56-71, 1994.

129. Castillo J, Davalos T, Marrugat J, Noya M: Timing for fever-related brain damage in acute ischemic stroke, *Stroke* 29:2455-2460, 1998.

130. Reith J, Jörgensen HS, Pedersen PM, et al: Body temperature in acute stroke: Relation to stroke severity, infarct size, mortality, and outcome, *Lancet* 347:422-425, 1996.

131. Busto R, Globus MY, Dietrich WD, et al: Effects of mild hypothermia on ischemia-induced release of neurotransmitters and free fatty acids in rat brain, *Stroke* 20:904-910, 1989.

132. Yamamoto H, Hong SC, Soleau S, et al: Mild postischemic hypothermia limits cerebral injury following transient focal ischemia in rat neocortex, *Brain Res* 718:207-211, 1996.

133. Shimizu T, Naritomi H, Kakud W, et al: Mild hypothermia is effective for the treatment of acute embolic stroke if induced within 24 hours after onset but not in the later phase, *J Cereb Blood Flow Metab* 17:42, 1997.

134. Kawai N, Okauchi M, Morisaki K, Nagao S: Effects of delayed intraischemic and postischemic hypothermia on a focal model of transient cerebral ischemia in rats, *Stroke* 31:1982-1989, 2000.

135. Maher J, Hachinski V: Hypothermia as a potential treatment for cerebral ischemia, *Cerebrovasc Brain Metab Rev* 5:277-300, 1993.

136. Ginsberg MD, Busto R: Combating hyperthermia in acute stroke: A significant clinical concern, *Stroke* 29:529-534, 1998.

137. Hindfelt B: The prognostic significance of subfebrility and fever in ischaemic cerebral infarction, *Acta Neurol Scand* 53:72-79, 1976.

138. Wistrand AT: Kotilääkäri [English translation: Home Physician]. Helsinki, Sampo, 1901.

139. Georgiadis D, Schwarz S, Kollmar R, Schwab S: Endovascular cooling for moderate hypothermia in patients with acute stroke: First results of a novel approach, *Stroke* 32:2550-2553, 2001.

140. Ginsberg MD, Sternau LL, Globus MY, et al: Therapeutic modulation of brain temperature: Relevance to ischemic brain injury, *Cerebrovasc Brain Metab Rev* 4:189-225, 1992.

141. Kammersgaard LP, Rasmussen BH, Jorgensen HS, et al: Feasibility and safety of inducing modest hypothermia in awake patients with acute stroke through surface cooling: A case-control study, *Stroke* 31:2251-2256, 2000.

142. Kasner SE, Wein T, Piriyawat P, et al: Acetaminophen for altering body temperature in acute stroke: A randomized clinical trial, *Stroke* 33:130-135, 2002.

143. Schwab S, Schwarz S, Spranger M, et al: Moderate hypothermia in the treatment of patients with severe middle cerebral artery infarction, *Stroke* 29:2461-2466, 1998.

144. Marion DW, Penrod LE, Kelsey SF, et al: Treatment of traumatic brain injury with moderate hypothermia, *N Engl J Med* 336:540-546, 1997.

145. Clifton GL, Miller ER, Choi SC, et al: Lack of effect of induction of hypothermia after acute brain injury, *N Engl J Med* 344:556-563, 2001.

146. Zeiner A, Holzer M, Behringer W, et al: Mild resuscitative hypothermia to improve neurological outcome after cardiac arrest: A clinical feasibility trial. Hypothermia After Cardiac Arrest (HACA) Study Group, *Stroke* 31:86-94, 2000.

147. Mild therapeutic hypothermia after cardiac arrest, *N Engl J Med* 346:549-556, 2002.

148. Kawai N, Keep RF, Betz AL, Dietrich WD: Hyperglycemia and the vascular effects of cerebral ischemia, *Stroke* 28:149-154, 1997.

149. Kent TA, Soukup VM, Fabian RH: Heterogeneity affecting outcome from acute stroke therapy: Making reperfusion worse, *Stroke* 32:2318-2327, 2001.

150. Kase CS, Furlan AJ, Wechsler LR, et al: Symptomatic intracranial hemorrhage after intraarterial thrombolysis with recombinant prourokinase in acute ischemic stroke: The PROACT II Study, *Neurology* 54(Suppl 3):A260-A261, 2000.

151. Toni D, De Michele M, Fiorelli M, et al: Influence of hyperglycemia on infarct size and clinical outcome of acute ischemic stroke patients with intracranial arterial occlusion, *J Neurol Sci* 123:129-133, 1994.

152. Capes SE, Hunt D, Malmberg K, et al: Stress hyperglycemia and prognosis of stroke in nondiabetic and diabetic patients: A systematic overview, *Stroke* 32:2426-2432, 2001.

153. Van Den Berghe G, Wouters P, Weekers F, et al: Intensive insulin therapy in critically ill patients, *N Engl J Med* 345:1359-1367, 2001.

154. Gray CS, Hildreth AJ, Sandercock PA, et al: Glucose-potassium-insulin infusions in the management of post-stroke hyperglycaemia: the UK Glucose Insulin in Stroke Trial (GIST-UK), *Lancet Neurol* 6:397-406, 2007.

155. Gladman JRF: Stroke units: Are they cost effective? *Br J Hosp Med* 47:91-93, 1992.

156. Jörgensen HS, Nakayama H, Raaschou HO, et al: The effect of stroke units: Reductions in mortality, discharge rate to nursing home, length of hospital stay, and cost: A community-based study, *Stroke* 26:1178-1182, 1995.

157. Jörgensen HS, Nakayama H, Raaschou HO, Skyhöj Olsen T: Acute stroke care and rehabilitation: An analysis of direct cost and its clinical and social determinants. The Copenhagen Stroke Study, *Stroke* 28:1138-1141, 1997.

158. Ronnig OM, Guldvog B: Stroke units versus general medical wards. I: Twelve and 18 month survival, a randomised controlled trial, *Stroke* 29:58-62, 1998.

159. Caro JJ, Huybrechts KF, Duchesne I: Management patterns and costs of acute ischemic stroke: An international study. Stroke Economic Analysis Group, *Stroke* 31:582-590, 2000.

160. Claesson L, Gosman-Hedström G, Johannesson M, et al: Resource utilization and costs of stroke unit care integrated in a care continuum: A 1-year controlled, prospective, randomized study in elderly patients. The Göteborg 701 Stroke Study, *Stroke* 31:2569-2577, 2000.

161. Fagerberg B, Claesson L, Gosman-Hedström G, Blomstrand C: Effect of acute stroke unit care integrated in a care continuum vs conventional treatment: A randomized 1-year study of elderly patients. The Göteborg 701 Stroke Study, *Stroke* 31:2578-2584, 2000.

162. Brainin M: Neurological acute stroke care: The role of European neurology. European Federation of Neurological Societies Task Force, *Eur J Neurol* 4:435-441, 1997.

163. Adams R, Acker J, Alberts M, et al: Recommendations for improving the quality of care through stroke centers and systems: An examination of stroke center identification options from the Advisory Working Group on Stroke Center Identification Options of the American Stroke Association, *Stroke* 33:326, 2002.

52 Critical Care of the Patient with Acute Stroke

JENNIFER DIEDLER, MAREK SYKORA, WERNER HACKE

Initial clinical assessment of patients with severe stroke should concentrate on the following issues:
1. Vital functions (pulmonary function, heart rate, blood pressure).
2. Neurologic symptoms; severity of neurologic deficit based on validated stroke scales.
3. Time of symptom onset and potential eligibility for specific treatment options.
4. Blood sampling for electrolytes, full blood count, and coagulation studies.

One should always bear in mind that most emergency measures depend on the cause of the stroke (ischemic versus hemorrhagic). Thus, it is vital that appropriate neuroimaging studies not be unnecessarily delayed. Additionally, caution is warranted to avoid measures that have the potential to interfere with further treatment options (for example, insertion of a central venous line in a patient eligible for thrombolysis).

General Principles of Neurologic Critical Care
Ancillary Tests

Diagnostic studies and their indications in stroke patients are discussed in detail elsewhere in this book (see Chapters 44 to 47). As a general rule, the need for further diagnostics has to be weighed carefully against the potential risk that in-house transportations bear for the critically ill. These procedures usually require disconnection from the ventilator to a transportable ventilator or other ventilator suitable for use in MRI scanners, which may not be tolerated easily by patients with severe pulmonary dysfunction. Moreover, monitoring is not as good as on the intensive care unit (ICU), and the options for intervention during critical situations may be limited. Before transportation of a critically ill patient, one should always question the therapeutic consequences that are likely to be drawn from the results. If there are no consequences, one should not perform the procedure. Diagnostic procedures that do not require transportation of the patient should be preferred. Optimal neuromonitoring, as will described later in the chapter, may help reduce the need for imaging.

If a diagnostic or therapeutic procedure requiring transportation of the patient cannot be avoided, careful preparation is obligatory. The physician has to decide about the medications that may be discontinued and the adequate monitoring that must be taken along; catheters need to be fixed properly; extraventricular drainage should be closed during transportation to avoid overdrainage. Emergency medication should be taken along, and long waits in the imaging suite for the actual imaging procedure should be avoided. Deeper sedation frequently becomes necessary for transportation and to allow acquisition of diagnostic studies of acceptable quality. One should bear in mind, however, that the clinical evaluation of the patient may be markedly limited thereafter; short-acting sedatives should be preferred. All patients with severe stroke must be accompanied by a physician or trained physician-extender during all diagnostic procedures.

Clinical Examinations

Every neurointensive care patient should undergo a complete clinical examination at least three times per day. Because of analgosedation, the neurologic examination frequently is restricted to evaluation of pupillary and brainstem reflexes, motor reaction upon painful stimuli, reflex status, and pathologic reflexes. Particularly, signs of raised intracranial pressure (ICP) and transtentorial herniation, such as sequential loss of brainstem reflexes, have to be recognized immediately. New motor deficits or pathologic reflexes may indicate enlargement of infarction or vasospasm in patients with subarachnoid hemorrhage (SAH). Changes in ventilator settings, such as the need to switch from assisted ventilation to fully controlled mechanical ventilation under stable levels of sedation, may indicate loss of brainstem function. Auscultation of heart and lung, palpation and auscultation of the abdomen, and careful inspection of the patient (edema, signs of dehydration, skin lesions, wounds) complete the clinical examination. Additionally, ventilator settings, blood gas analyses, laboratory parameters, temperature, urinary excretion, and central venous pressure (CVP) have to be reviewed regularly by the attending physicians.

Pulmonary Function and Mechanical Ventilation

Maintenance of adequate oxygenation is essential in patients with acute stroke, and hypoxia could be deleterious for the ischemic penumbra. Avoidance of hypercapnia is of equal importance, as it potentially leads to

TABLE 52-1   INDICATIONS FOR MECHANICAL VENTILATION

$Po_2 < 70$ mm Hg despite O_2 administration via nasal probe or facial mask
$Pco_2 > 60$ mm Hg (except for patients with chronic obstructive airway disease and chronically elevated CO_2)
Vital capacity < 500-600 mL
Clinical signs of respiratory failure (tachypnea, use of accessory muscles)
Severe respiratory acidosis
Airway protection (gag and swallowing reflexes absent, level of consciousness decreased)

vasodilation in the cerebral arterioles supplying healthy brain tissue, thereby reducing blood supply to the lesion site, where cerebral vessels are already maximally dilated under resting conditions. Transcutaneous evaluation of oxygen saturation constitutes the minimal requirement for monitoring of pulmonary function. Mechanical ventilation should be initiated when Pao_2 values drop below 60 to 70 mm Hg, $Paco_2$ values exceed 50 to 60 mm Hg, or both. Other clinical signs of respiratory failure are tachypnea exceeding 35 breaths per minute, dyspnea with use of accessory muscles, and respiratory acidosis (Table 52-1).

Respiratory failure in patients with acute stroke is mostly associated with aspiration pneumonia, impaired central respiratory drive, or neurogenic pulmonary edema (NPE). During the course of the disease, however, respiratory function can be compromised by the development of various pathologic conditions, including atelectasis or pneumonia due to immobilization, decreased level of consciousness, epileptic seizures, and critical illness polyneuropathy. Additionally, patients with severe stroke undergo mechanical ventilation for performance of diagnostic or therapeutic interventions or airway protection when gag reflex is absent or reduced. The percentage of unselected patients with stroke who undergo mechanical ventilation has been reported as 10%.[1] Significant differences in rate of mechanical ventilation have been found to be related to the cause of stroke; Mayer et al[1] reported that 5% of patients with ischemic stroke, 26% of patients with intracerebral hemorrhage (ICH), and 47% of patients with subarachnoid hemorrhage (SAH) underwent mechanical ventilation, whereas Gujjar et al[2] found rates of 6% for ischemic stroke and 30% for ICH.

As the prognosis of patients with acute stroke undergoing mechanical ventilation in the past has been rather poor (mortality rates between 49% and 93%) the identification of clinical predictors of adverse outcome is crucial.[2-5] A Glasgow Coma Scale (GCS) score less than 10 was found to predict mortality in most studies. Other factors were older age, absence of brainstem reflexes, intubation because of respiratory failure, and bradycardia.[1,2,5,6] These data can obviously provide no guidelines for individual patients. Still, it is important to bear them in mind, particularly when one is discussing the issue of mechanical ventilation with a patient's family.

Orotracheal intubation is the approach of first choice because it enables the use of larger-diameter tubes, avoids the tube contamination that occurs during passage of oronasal tubes, and is associated with a lower prevalence of maxillary sinusitis.[7,8] Any drugs used before intubation should preferably be short-acting. We recommend sufentanil (0.3 to 1.0 mg/kg), followed by etomidate (0.3 to 0.5 mg/kg) or propofol (1.5 to 3 mg/kg) in combination with a nondepolarizing neuromuscular blocking agent such as rocuronium (0.9 to 1 mg/kg), given in rapid sequence, to avoid long-term influence on the hemodynamic situation. Continuous infusion of sedatives and analgesics is warranted for the duration of mechanical ventilation. Further details on sedation and analgesia are given in the next section of this chapter.

Ventilator settings should be adjusted to provide a Pao_2 of 80 to 100 mm Hg, a $Paco_2$ between 38 and 42 mm Hg and a pH between 7.35 and 7.45. Pressure- or volume-controlled ventilation modes can be applied. Inspiration-to-expiration (I:E) ratio can initially be set at 1:2, and positive end-expiratory pressure (PEEP) at 5 to 8 cm H_2O. For volume-controlled ventilation, tidal volume can initially be set at 6 to 8 mL/kg, inspiratory flow at 30 L/min, and frequency at 10 to 15 breaths/min. For pressure-controlled ventilation, initial setting could be 12 to 14 cm H_2O above PEEP. End-inspiratory pressures should not exceed 30 to 35 cm H_2O. Ventilation parameters have to be adjusted regularly, according to blood gas values. Preexisting pulmonary disorders such as chronic obstructive pulmonary disease (COPD), pneumonia, or the development of acute respiratory distress syndrome (ARDS) may require more invasive ventilator settings. Lung-protective strategies include the "baby-lung concept," which involves use of low tidal volume, low inspiratory pressure, and high PEEP levels.[9]

Theoretically, higher PEEP levels result in higher intrathoracic pressure and reduced venous return and thereby may promote an increase in ICP. Moreover, the PEEP could affect cerebral perfusion pressure (CPP) by lowering mean arterial pressure (MAP). In a 2005 study in patients with SAH, stepwise elevation of PEEP to 20 cm H_2O (14.7 mm Hg) resulted in an increase in cerebrospinal fluid (CSF) and a significant decrease of MAP and regional cerebral blood flow (CBF).[10] However, reduction of CBF depended on MAP changes as a result of disturbed cerebrovascular autoregulation, and normalization of MAP restored regional CBF to baseline values. Likewise, PEEP levels up to 12 mm Hg have not been found to increase ICP in patients with acute stroke.[11] Equally, it was shown that alterations of the I:E ratio from 1:2 to 1:1 do not influence ICP or CPP and could therefore be readily applied in patients with acute stroke.[12] In summary, PEEP application seems to be safe, provided that MAP is maintained. However, monitoring of MAP, ICP, and CPP is desirable.

Orotracheal or nasotracheal intubation is potentially associated with the risk of laryngeal or tracheal stenosis and phonation disability. Whited[13] described a 2% incidence of laryngeal stenosis in patients who had been intubated fewer than 6 days; the incidence rose to approximately 5% in patients intubated for 6 to 11 days. These findings were not confirmed in later studies. Colice et al[14] described mucosal ulceration and varying severity of laryngeal edema in 94% of patients intubated longer than 4 days; these changes were mostly reversible, and duration of intubation did not influence the incidence of laryngeal lesions. Dunham and LaMonica[15] observed no differences in incidence of laryngeal complications whether patients underwent early or late tracheostomy.

In addition to reducing the risk of the complications just described, tracheostomy is associated with several advantages over orotracheal or nasotracheal intubation. They include patient comfort, a more secure airway, improved suctioning, reduced need for analgosedation, and faster weaning from mechanical ventilation—all of which result in a shorter stay in the ICU. A study by Scales et al[16] in mechanically ventilated patients in the ICU found that early tracheostomy (≤10 days) was associated with a modest survival benefit. Weaning from mechanical ventilation took place more quickly in the early tracheostomy group. Each additional delay of tracheotomy of 1 day was associated with increased mortality with a number-needed-to-treat of 71 to save one life per week of delay. In contrast, a systematic review and meta-analysis comparing early with late tracheostomy in trauma patients found no difference in days of mechanical ventilation, length of ICU stay, and frequency of pneumonia except for patients with severe brain injury.[17] It thus appears that especially brain-injured patients who are not likely to be weaned from mechanical ventilation within 10 days would profit from early tracheostomy; identification of such patients is not always straightforward, however. Qureshi et al[18] examined 69 mechanically ventilated patients with infratentorial lesions; unsuccessful weaning was found to be associated with a GCS score lower than 7 as well as brainstem deficits.[18] Huttner et al[19] investigated predictive factors for tracheostomy after supratentorial ICH and found that patients with low GCS scores due to large hematomas and complicating hydrocephalus who were suffering from COPD were at highest risk for an extended period of ventilation.

In conclusion, we perform early tracheostomy in patients who are likely to require ventilatory support for more than 10 days or who are without a functioning gag reflex and require tracheostomy for airway protection.

Sedation and Analgesia

Patients treated in the ICU are exposed to various stress factors, including anxiety, unfamiliar auditory and visual stimuli, awareness of severe illness, and sleep disturbances. Medical conditions such as pain, respiratory insufficiency, cardiovascular impairment, and sepsis constitute further stress factors; the same is true for several treatment options, particularly mechanical ventilation. Inadequate sedation and analgesia can cause combativeness syndrome, which results in a higher metabolic rate and greater oxygen consumption, potentially further endangering the ischemic penumbra. Furthermore, mechanical ventilation is greatly compromised, or even impossible, with inadequate sedation. Sedation is a major issue in intracranial hypertension, because coughing or straining raises ICP.

A variety of drugs are available for sedation of patients in ICU. For a list of drugs, dosages, and potential side effects, see Table 52-2.

Benzodiazepines probably are the most frequently administered drugs for long-term sedation. They vary in their potency, onset of duration and action, distribution, and metabolism including presence or absence of active metabolites. Patient-specific factors such as age, prior alcohol abuse, and concomitant drug therapy affect the intensity and duration of benzodiazepine activity. Especially older patients exhibit a slower clearance of benzodiazepines. Accumulation of benzodiazepines and their active metabolites, especially under continuous infusion, may produce prolonged oversedation. Moreover, tolerance may occur within hours to several days of therapy, and escalating doses have been reported. Midazolam is a benzodiazepine with a rapid onset and short duration with single doses (elimination half-time 1.5 to 2.5 hours). However, accumulation and prolonged sedative effects are commonly observed after long-term sedation with midazolam, especially in the elderly, in obese patients, and in patients with low albumin levels or renal insufficiency. Yet the use of the benzodiazepine antagonist flumazenil is problematic after prolonged therapy because of the risk of inducing withdrawal syndromes.

Propofol is an intravenous, general anesthetic agent with rapid onset and short duration of sedation, even after longer infusion. Common adverse effects include severe hypotension and bradycardia. Prolonged administration of high doses of propofol have been associated with lactic acidosis and hypertriglyceridemia, because the agent is available in a phospholipid emulsion (1.1 kcal/mL). Propofol has safely been used in neuroanesthesia and has been shown to reduce elevated ICP in patients with traumatic brain injury.[20]

Studies comparing the effects of propofol and midazolam have reported a reliable, safe, and controllable sedation for both agents.[21-25] The main observed differences were (1) a higher incidence of arterial hypotension in patients receiving propofol and (2) a faster recovery in patients treated with propofol, also resulting in faster weaning. The use of midazolam infusion for treatment of refractory status epilepticus is well established; case reports suggest that propofol also possesses therapeutic potential for patients with this condition.[26] Additionally, initial comparisons have described no differences in antiepileptic properties between the two agents.[27]

Ketamine has strong analgetic effects and induces a dissociative anesthesia. Because of its psychomimetic effect—inducing nightmares and hallucinations—it should preferably be combined with other sedative agents. Ketamine possesses sympathomimetic properties leading to higher cardiac output and bronchodilation. The use of ketamine in patients in neurologic ICUs for its putative effect on ICP has been debated. However, studies now suggest that it can be administered safely in the patient with elevated ICP if the patient is under sedation (propofol or midazolam) and $Paco_2$ is maintained by controlled mechanical ventilation.[28,29]

Clonidine as a central α-agonist can be recommended for light sedation, as add-on therapy to reduce dose requirements of sedatives, and to treat drug withdrawal syndromes in the ICU. Side effects include bradycardia and hypotension.

Treatment of conditions with potential to aggravate the patient, in particular inadequate analgesia, is an important measure that may reduce the amount of sedation required. The same is true for nonmedical measures,

TABLE 52-2 SEDATIVES COMMONLY USED IN PATIENTS TREATED IN INTENSIVE CARE UNITS

Drug	Dose	Onset of Action	Duration of Action	Comments
Adrenergic inhibitors				
Labetalol	20-80 mg bolus every 10 min, up to 300 mg; 0.5-2.0 mg/min infusion	5-10 min	3-6 h	Indicated in ischemic and hemorrhagic stroke; contraindicated in acute heart failure
Esmolol	250-500 μg/kg/min bolus then 50-100 μg/kg/min infusion	1-2 min	10-30 min	Indicated in stroke and aortic dissection; contraindicated in bradycardia, atrioventricular block, heart failure, and bronchospasm
Urapidil	1.25-2.5 mg bolus; 5-40 mg/h infusion	3-5 min	4-6 h	Indicated in most hypertensive emergencies including stroke; avoid in coronary ischemia
Vasodilators				
Nitroprusside*	0.2-10 μg/kg/min as infusion	within seconds	2-5 min	Indicated in most hypertensive emergencies, including stroke, when diastolic blood pressure >140 mm Hg; contraindicated in high intracranial pressure
Nicardipine	5-15 mg/h infusion	5-10 min	0.5-4 h	Indicated in stroke; contraindicated in acute heart failure, coronary ischemia, and aortic stenosis
Enalaprilat	1.25-5 mg every 6 h	15-30 min	6-12 h	Indicated in acute left ventricular failure; avoid in acute myocardial infarction and hypotension
Hydralazine	10-20 mg bolus	10-20 min	1-4 h	Indicated in eclampsia; avoid in tachycardia and coronary ischemia
Fenoldopam	0.1-0.3 μg/kg/min infusion	<5 min	30 min	Indicated in most hypertensive emergencies, including stroke; avoid in glaucoma, tachycardia, and portal hypertension
Diuretic				
Furosemide	20-40 mg bolus	2-5 min	2-3 h	Avoid in hypokalemia, eclampsia, and pheochromocytoma

Adapted from Steiner T, Kaste M, Forsting M, et al: Recommendations for the management of intracranial haemorrhage - part I: Spontaneous intracerebral haemorrhage. The European Stroke Initiative Writing Committee and the Writing Committee for the EUSI Executive Committee. *Cerebrovasc Dis* 22:294-316, 2006.

such as communicating with and reassuring the patient and tempering psychological problems.

It must be stressed that sedation is never a substitute for adequate analgesia. Almost every patient in an ICU experiences pain at some point; the treatment of choice depends on the cause and severity of the pain. Nonopioid agents (paracetamol, salicylate, or nonsteroidal agents such as indomethacin, ibuprofen, and diclofenac) may be adequate in some cases. Still, most patients require opioids for satisfactory pain control.

Three members of this group are being routinely applied: fentanyl, sufentanil, and the ultra-short-acting remifentanil. Fentanyl possesses an approximately 100 to 150 times higher analgesic potency than morphine. The maximal effect is already reached 4 to 5 minutes after intravenous infusion. Fentanyl accumulates in fatty tissue and has an elimination half-time of 219 minutes. Its redistribution can cause significant rebound effects after its discontinuation, and even respiratory depression. Fentanyl is applied as a continuous intravenous infusion, at doses ranging between 0.05 and 0.3 mg/h, usually combined with midazolam or propofol.

Sufentanil (not available on the U.S. market) has an analgesic potency approximately 1000 times higher than that of morphine. Its context-sensitive half-life is significantly shorter than that of fentanyl during continuous infusion (elimination half-time 64 minutes), making it the agent of choice in many neurologic ICUs. Moreover, it is reported to provide better patient comfort with less respiratory depression than fentanyl.[30] Sufentanil has an additional sedative effect, which reduces the required dose of sedatives. It is applied as continuous intravenous infusion at rates of 0.5 to 0.75 μg/kg/h.

Remifentanil (not available on the U.S. market) is an ultra-short-acting opioid that is increasingly used today in neuroanesthesia and neurointensive care. It has the shortest elimination half-time, the smallest volume of distribution, and the highest clearance rate of all opioids. Its context-sensitive half-life remains stable even after long-term continuous infusion (elimination half-time, 6 to 14 minutes). These characteristics make remifentanil highly attractive for patients in neurologic ICUs, in whom regular clinical evaluation of the neurologic status is desirable. Analgesia-based sedation with remifentanil has been found to permit significantly faster and more predictable awakening for neurologic assessment.[31,32]

Although later studies have shown that sufentanil did not lead to respiratory depression in spontaneously breathing ICU patients when adequate levels of analgesia and sedation were maintained,[33] we apply high-potency opioids very cautiously in awake, spontaneously breathing patients. Alternatives may be less potent agents, such as piritramid (3.75 to 15 mg intravenously [IV]) and tramadol (50 to 100 mg IV [not available on the U.S. market]).

A frequent complication in long-term treatment with opioids is gastrointestinal hypomotility leading to pharmacologically induced subileus. Prophylactic application of laxative agents may be considered. Although good cardiovascular properties are reported with use of fentanyl and sufentanil, hypotension and bradycardia may occur, especially when large doses are rapidly administered intravenously. Studies of the effects of remifentanil on ICP have suggested that infusion of the drug usually decreases ICP with minimal changes in CPP.[32] However, the exact effects of sufentanil, fentanyl, and remifentanil on cerebral hemodynamics remain uncertain.[34-37]

Although patients with acute brain injury, edema, and elevated ICP may require deeper sedation levels (see later discussion on treatment of elevated ICP), the need for sedation should be reevaluated daily, and sedation levels should be assessed regularly. Commonly used scores for assessment of sedation levels include the Ramsay sedation scale (RSS) and the Sedation-Agitation Scale (SAS). Although not designed for patients receiving neurologic intensive care, these scales generally can be applied to patients with brain injury, keeping in mind that brain injury such as aphasia or hemiparesis may impede adequate reaction.

Fluid and Electrolyte Balance

Fluid and electrolyte disturbances are common findings in ICU patients. They may be due to (1) sympathetic responses to ischemic or hemorrhagic neuronal injury, (2) unbalanced fluid and electrolyte substitution (calculation of daily fluid requirement; see Table 52-3), (3) unbalanced nutritional regimen, or (4) administration of diuretics and other drugs (particularly osmotherapeutics). Sympathetic nervous system stimulation reduces renal blood flow, thus activating the renin-angiotensin system and increasing the secretion of aldosterone, an effect that in turn causes sodium retention and kaliuresis. Antidiuretic hormone (ADH) secretion may also be affected by central nervous system lesions, resulting in sodium and water retention and decreased urine output (syndrome of inappropriate antidiuretic hormone secretion [SIADH]) or in diabetes insipidus. Finally, release of brain-derived natriuretic peptide (BNP) has been associated with cerebral salt wasting syndrome (CSWS; see later).

Fluid disturbances can be assessed by (1) clinical observation, (2) evaluation of fluid intake and output, (3) measurement of CVP via a central venous line or pulse contour continuous cardiac output monitoring, and (4) measurements of serum osmolarity, urine osmolarity, and serum sodium concentration. Sodium, the main electrolyte of the extracellular fluid, accounts for more than 90% of its osmolarity. There is a close relationship between sodium and water shifts. Sodium concentrations and the hydration state of the patient provide the required information for diagnosis and the treatment of fluid imbalances. Isotonic volume depletion is the most common abnormality encountered. The treatment of

TABLE 52-3 ASSESSMENT OF DAILY FLUID REQUIREMENT

Basal requirement	30 mL per kg body weight
+ Urinary output	Urine volume over last 24 hours
+ Stool water	Approximately 100 mL/day (more in diarrhea)
+ Insensible loss	Approximately 800 mL/day (spontaneously breathing patient)
	Approximately 400 mL/day (mechanically ventilated patient)
	Fever correction: add 500 mL per 1°C > 37°C

choice is enteral or IV administration of isotonic fluids. Careful fluid balancing and monitoring of the CVP are warranted to allow determination of the amount of fluids needed. In patients with concomitant left ventricular failure, chest radiograph, echocardiography, or pulse contour continuous cardiac output analysis should be used to avoid potentially deleterious fluid overload.

For hypernatremic or hyponatremic states, the therapeutic regimen depends on the hydration state of the patient. Hyponatremia is the most common electrolyte disturbance in the neurologic ICU. Rapidly developing and severe hyponatremia (serum sodium level 110 mmol/L) may lead to generalized seizures, coma, and brain edema. The differential diagnosis includes SIADH and CSWS. The correct and early diagnosis is important, because the recommended fluid management is exactly opposite in the two conditions. Although SIADH is caused by excessive secretion of ADH leading to water retention, hypervolemia, and secondary diuresis and natriuresis, CSWS is associated with the release of brain natriuretic factor, resulting in diuresis, natriuresis, and concomitant hypovolemia. Therefore, treatment of SIADH is based on water restriction, but treatment of CSWS requires fluid and sodium administration. Differential diagnosis of both syndromes requires correct estimation of hydration state, measurement of urine volume, serum, and urine osmolality and the ratio of both, and urine sodium concentration. However, whether the two syndromes are separate entities or rather different manifestations of a common pathophysiologic origin remains controversial. Some studies claim that hyponatremia more frequently should be attributed to CSWS than to SIADH,[38-40] and other studies entirely doubt the concept of CSWS.[41,42]

In the setting of a central diabetes insipidus, subcutaneous (SC) or IV administration of 2 to 5 units of aqueous vasopressin or 1 to 5 µg of its analog, desmopressin (DDAVP), effectively reduces water diuresis. Further details concerning fluid management are provided in textbooks of clinical medicine.

Nutrition

Nutrition in hospitalized patients with acute stroke is an often overlooked, although significant issue. Davalos et al[43] reported protein-energy malnutrition in 16.3% of 104 patients admitted with acute stroke, and in 26.4% and 35% of the same population after the first and second weeks in hospital, respectively; additionally, malnutrition was identified as an independent predictor of poor outcome. Similar results were reported by Gariballa et al[44]; they assessed 96 patients with acute stroke upon admission and after 2 weeks, and 51 of them again at 4 weeks. They found that nutritional status deteriorated significantly during the study period. Serum albumin concentrations showed a significant association with infective complications and were an independent predictor of death at 3 months. Davalos et al[43] postulated a hypercatabolic state due to stress reaction or a neuroendocrine response to injury that modified the carbohydrate metabolism as possible explanation for the observed malnutrition. The demonstrated prognostic significance of malnutrition in patient outcome highlights the importance of an adequate caloric and protein supply in patients with acute stroke. Rough estimates for basal energy expenditure (BEE) are 25 kcal/kg/day for adults between 20 and 30 years, 22.5 kcal/kg/day for adults between 30 and 70 years, and 20 kcal/kg/day for those older than 70 years. A closer estimation is provided by the formula of Harris and Benedict, as follows:

$$BEE \ (men) = 66.5 + (13.75 \times weight \ in \ kg) + (5 \times height \ in \ cm) - (6.8 \times age \ in \ years)$$

$$BEE \ (women) = 655 + (9.6 \times weight \ in \ kg) + (1.8 \times height \ in \ cm) - (4.7 \times age \ in \ years)$$

For nutritional support of the critically ill, partly contradictory guidelines exist,[45-47] because there is little evidence from randomized controlled trials on the issue. Consideration of some basic pathophysiologic mechanisms may be helpful to guide therapy. Typically, different metabolic stages can be distinguished during critical illness. An initial phase of reduced metabolism that has been found predominantly in trauma patients is followed by a catabolic stage. In this stage, acute-phase proteins are synthesized and regulation of metabolism underlies stress hormones such as epinephrine, cortisol, and glucagon. Metabolism thereby becomes detached from substrate intake; independently from the external supply of glucose, gluconeogenesis in the liver is triggered, and cells of organs such as the muscle develop insulin resistance in order to ensure substrate supply to the brain. This phase is then followed by an anabolic stage with a high energy expenditure that, in contrast to the previous phase, is reactive to external energy supply.

A meta-analysis has shown that parenteral hyperalimentation may increase complication and mortality rates in critically ill patients.[48] An uncontrolled observational study of ICU patients found that moderate caloric intake (33% to 65% of recommended caloric intake target of 25 kcal/kg/day, or approximately 9 to 18 kcal/kg per day) was associated with better outcomes than higher levels of caloric intake.[49] Other studies have provided evidence for the negative effect of hyperglycemia on survival of critically ill patients.[50] However, the fact that energy expenditure and reactivity to external supply of substrates vary during the different phases of critical illness renders the use of fixed formulas problematic. Current guidelines state that substituted energy during acute critical illness should not exceed 25 to 30 kcal/kg/day, and in the acute phase 15 to 20 kcal/kg/day are sufficient. Afterwards, energy supply should be augmented slowly to ≈1.2 times (≈1.5 times for patients with malnutrition) of the actual energy turnover. Therefore, nutritional concepts may constantly change during the intensive care stay; in contrast, during acute sepsis, hyperalimentation and hyperglycemia should be avoided, and a patient who is to be weaned from the respirator should be provided with an adequate energy supply. It is important to note, that although hyperalimentation may be harmful, nutritional support offering an adequate caloric input should not be delayed in patients receiving critical care. Delaying initiation of nutritional support exposes the patients to energy deficits that cannot be compensated later on. Essential amino acids, fatty acids, and vitamins are already included in standard parenteral and enteral feeding preparations. Protein requirements in critically ill patients may be higher (1.2 to 1.5 g per kg body weight) than in nonstressed, healthy persons (0.8 g per kg body weight).

It has been suggested that enteral rather than parenteral nutrition should be pursued in the ICU. If possible, oral feeding should be allowed. However, supplemental nutritional support is required in most patients treated in a neurocritical care unit because of depressed levels of consciousness, impaired swallowing function, or mechanical ventilation. For nutritional support, enteral nutrition with a nasogastric tube is the approach of first choice. Patients who are bound to require long-term enteral nutritional support may be considered for percutaneous endoscopic gastrostomy (PEG), which is better tolerated and causes fewer local complications. The enteral route has several advantages, including simpler application, lower risk of infection, utilization of the normal physiologic functions of digestion and absorption, maintenance of the intestinal mucosa, and lower cost. Intestinal function and motility must be regularly monitored (bowel sounds, aspiration of gastric residuals) and, if necessary, supported by a stimulant such as metoclopramide. Gastric retention enhances the risk of regurgitation and pulmonary aspiration. If motility is still not restored, postpyloric feeding (endoscopically placed nasoduodenal or nasojejunal probe) or parenteral nutrition should be considered. Another common complication of enteral feeding is diarrhea, which occurs as a result of the hyperosmolar electrolyte solutions or of quick buildup of enteral feeding after an extended period of fasting or parenteral nutrition.

Additional parenteral nutrition is indicated when enteral feeding does not cover nutritional requirements. A peripheral venous line is adequate for short-term parenteral nutrition, provided that the osmolarity of the infused solutions does not exceed approximately 1000 mOsm/kg. Long-term parenteral nutrition, meeting the patients' full caloric and protein requirements without giving an excess fluid volume, requires hyperosmolar formulas of up to 1800 mOsm/kg. These are very irritating to the venous endothelium and thus must be administered via central venous lines (see earlier discussion). Complications of parenteral feeding thereby include the risks associated with the necessity of a central catheter.

Nutritional support should be carefully monitored. This includes assessment of blood glucose levels at least every 4 hours, daily assessment of blood urea (daily increase < 30 mg/dL), and measurement of triglyceride levels at least twice per week (<400 mg/dL). Hyperglycemia often requires continuous insulin infusion. In case insulin requirements exceed 6 IE per hour, external glucose supply should be lowered. Further monitoring of nutritional therapy includes regular assessment of albumin, electrolytes, phosphate, and liver enzymes. Liver function abnormalities, with mild to moderate elevations of serum liver enzyme activity and bilirubin, are also very common but usually benign and self-limiting.

Blood Pressure Control

A variety of drugs can be used for treatment of acute arterial hypertension. Continuous infusion of intravenous drugs with a short half-time provides optimal therapeutic control. Modes of action and potential influence on ICP and CBF of the intravenous antihypertensive agents most commonly used in intensive care are described in this section. Specific aspects of managing blood pressure according to cause of stroke and individual findings are covered later in the chapter.

Peripheral Vasodilators

Vasodilators cause relaxation of arterial and venous smooth muscle cells. This effect is accompanied by baroreceptor-mediated tachycardia. These agents are also active in the cerebral vasculature, increasing CBF and ICP. In patients with acute stroke, cerebral vessels supplying the affected brain region are already maximally dilated. Thus, use of vasodilators can result in vasodilation of the vessels supplying unaffected brain regions, causing a redistribution of CBF (steal phenomenon) and potentially aggravating ischemic injury. Although this pathophysiologic concept has not been demonstrated in clinical studies, most institutions refrain from using vasodilators in patients with acute stroke.

The most commonly used vasodilators are nitroprusside, nitroglycerin, and hydralazine. Nitroprusside and nitroglycerin, which have a fast onset and short duration of action, should be administered as continuous intravenous infusions. The main limitation of nitroprusside is the risk of cyanide intoxication, particularly in association with doses exceeding 18 μg/kg/h or used longer than 48 to 72 hours. Nitroglycerin has been shown to dilate large cerebral arteries.[51] Rogers et al[52] demonstrated significant ICP increases in association with the decrease in arterial blood pressure in a cat model. Cottrell et al[53] reported similar findings in five anesthetized patients. Thus, the use of nitroglycerin is not indicated in patients with intracranial hypertension. Hydralazine has a slower onset of action, although its effect after intravenous bolus administration lasts for approximately 4 hours. Like nitroprusside and nitroglycerin, hydralazine is best administered as a continuous intravenous infusion. Studies on head-injured patients showed that hydralazine administration is associated with increases in ICP.[54,55] To date, no clinical studies have examined the effect of hydralazine in patients with acute stroke.

Adrenergic Agents

Urapidil (not available on the U.S. market) is an α_1-receptor antagonist that has both a peripheral effect and a central effect. Owing to its central effect, administration of urapidil is not associated with tachycardia. Animal studies demonstrated that urapidil does not influence ICP when applied as a continuous intravenous infusion.[56,57] Results of its bolus administration were not unanimous; one study described an ICP increase in cats with experimental cerebral cold lesions,[57] and the other described no ICP effects in dogs with intracranial hypertension.[56] Still, loss of cerebral autoregulation and significant decrease in CPP were reported.[58] A clinical study in eight patients undergoing craniotomy for intracerebral tumor showed that the decrease in systemic arterial blood pressure due to urapidil does not influence ICP.[59]

Clonidine stimulates α_2-adrenergic inhibitory neurons in the medulla, thus reducing sympathetic nervous system outflow. This reduction leads to decreases in arterial blood pressure, heart rate, and cardiac output. Clonidine also has sedative and analgesic properties.[60,61] It can be administered orally, subcutaneously, and as an IV infusion. Acute withdrawal results in rebound hypertension. The effects of clonidine on CBF remain unclear. Greene et al[62] used clonidine in 13 patients with severe hypertension. Goal blood pressure was reached in 12 patients; a significant increase in CBF (>10%) occurred in 5 patients, and a significant decrease in 4. The magnitude of CBF changes depended on the initial values, patients with initially low CBF experiencing an increase and those with initially high CBF a decrease. Asgeirsson et al[63] found no effect of clonidine on CBF and ICP in six severely head-injured patients. Kanawati et al[64] observed a significant reduction in CBF after administration of clonidine; because this effect could not be reproduced with use of a structural analogue of clonidine that does not cross the blood-brain barrier, these investigators suggested that the CBF response to clonidine is mediated by central mechanisms rather than by alterations in CPP. Favre et al[65] observed significant changes in MAP and CPP in 12 patients who received clonidine during the preinduction period while ICP remained unchanged. Ter Minassian et al[66] also observed significant decreases in MAP and CPP after intravenous administration of clonidine; in contrast to the previous study, they found that clonidine also resulted in a transient increase in ICP in three subjects.[66] Thus, although thoroughly studied, the effects of clonidine on CBF remain unclear. The effect of clonidine on the cerebrovascular CO_2 response is also a matter of debate, with two studies reporting a reduced response,[65,67] and another an increased response.[68]

Propranolol is a nonselective β-antagonist. Its administration results in decreases in blood pressure, heart rate, and cardiac output. No effect of propranolol on ICP was observed after oral administration in patients with intracerebral hemorrhage[69] or in patients with head injury.[59] Equally, no effect on CBF was noted in 31 hypertensive patients after long-term propranolol therapy.[70] Because this agent can be administered only orally or by slow IV injection, it cannot be used for long-term control of hypertension in the ICU.

Labetalol is a mixed α- and β-antagonist. It can lower MAP by reducing systemic vascular resistance while preventing reflex tachycardia through the additional β-blockade. Labetalol can be administered as a continuous intravenous infusion, a feature that augments its applicability in ICU. This agent appears to have no effect on ICP in experimental studies using animal models[71,72] or in clinical studies in hypertensive patients.[73] Orlowski et al[74] observed a slight but statistically significant greater ICP reduction in patients treated with nitroprusside alone than in patients treated either with labetalol or with a combination of labetalol and nitroprusside. As with other agents in this category, studies examining the effectiveness of labetalol in patients with acute stroke are lacking.

Calcium Channel Blockers

Calcium channel blockers cause vasodilation (more pronounced in arteries than in veins) and decrease in heart rate, myocardial contractility, and conduction at the atrioventricular node. These effects can lead to myocardial depression, atrioventricular block, bradycardia, heart failure, and even cardiac arrest. Nifedipine and nicardipine are the most commonly used calcium channel blockers.

Nifedipine was shown to produce a discrete but statistically significant elevation in ICP when given intravenously to cats with normal baseline ICP; this increase, however, was larger in the presence of intracranial hypertension.[75] Similar results were reported by Anger et al[76] in a further animal study; Wusten et al[77] observed significant increase in ICP after administration of nifedipine but found that administration of urapidil did not influence ICP. Likewise Tateishi et al[78] reported a significant ICP increase, ranging from 1 to 10 mm Hg, in 10 patients with head trauma or cerebrovascular disease. Bertel et al[79] compared oral nifedipine with placebo in 25 hypertensive patients who did not have intracranial disease. These researchers observed significant reductions in MAP with nifedipine; however, in this study, nifedipine administration resulted in CBF elevation in four of five patients in whom CBF was evaluated. Current stroke guidelines do not recommend the sublingual administration of nifedipine because of a prolonged effect and the potential of a precipitous decline in blood pressure.[80]

Nicardipine is a potent vasodilator that also affects cerebral blood vessels. Its effect on CBF remains unclear. Sakabe et al[81] observed significant postischemic rises in CBF in both nicardipine-treated and control animals; CBF significantly decreased in the control group but remained unchanged in the nicardipine-treated group. Kittaka et al[82] observed no CBF changes with administration of nicardipine after an ischemic insult in rats; in contrast, in an animal model without intracranial disease, Tanaka et al[83] saw CBF increases after administration of the agent. Interestingly, Sakabe et al[81] observed no improvement in neurologic outcome in treated animals, but Kittaka et al[82] reported significant decreases in neuron-specific enolase and in infarction and edema volume, which were associated with an improved neurologic outcome, with treatment. After topical application of nicardipine during extracranial-to-intracranial bypass procedures, Gaab et al[84] observed a marked dilation in the small cortical arteries; a nicardipine infusion, however, was associated

with an increase in cerebral P_{O_2}. Akopov et al[85] could demonstrate no consistent pattern in regional (r) global CBF changes in 75 hypertensive patients with symptoms of chronic ischemic cerebrovascular disorders. Abe et al,[86] however, reported a moderate increase in local CBF after administration of nicardipine.

Halpern et al[87] compared the efficacy and safety of intravenous nicardipine and sodium nitroprusside in the treatment of postoperative hypertension. In that study involving 137 patients, intravenous nicardipine controlled hypertension more rapidly than sodium nitroprusside (14 ± 1 minutes versus 30 ± 3.5 minutes, respectively) and the total number of dose changes required was lower with nicardipine. Other studies came to similar results.[88,89]

Lisk et al[90] examined the effect of nicardipine, captopril, or clonidine in hypertensive patients with acute ischemic stroke (treated within 72 hours of onset). Nicardipine administration resulted in the most marked drop in MAP. A total of four patients demonstrated a MAP decrease greater than 16%, which was associated with sustained or decreased CBF. Three of these four patients were treated with nicardipine. Administration of nicardipine also appears to increase ICP; Nishikawa et al[91] observed significant rises in CSF pressure (approximately 5 mm Hg) with administration of nicardipine, which were associated with significant decreases in MAP and CPP, in 17 patients without intracranial disease. Interestingly, this effect was not influenced by the dose administered (0.1 to 0.3 mg/kg).

Angiotensin-Converting Enzyme Inhibitors

Various angiotensin-converting enzyme (ACE) inhibitors have been developed. Of those, enalapril is the only agent currently available for intravenous administration and therefore also the one relevant for use in neurocritical care units. Enalapril apparently has no effect on CBF in patients without intracranial disease or in patients with a unilateral stenosis of the internal carotid artery greater than 70%.[92,93] Kobayashi et al[94] observed a mean 8% CBF increase in patients with chronic cerebral infarction given enalapril. These findings, together with its insignificant side effects, suggest that enalapril is an attractive alternative for treatment of arterial hypertension in patients with acute stroke. An important contraindication is stenosis of the renal artery. A dose of 1.25 mg is administered intravenously over 5 minutes; continuous application is possible, but a total dose of 10 mg/day should not be exceeded.

Maintenance or Elevation of Arterial Blood Pressure

Maintenance of adequate cerebral perfusion is essential for patients with acute brain injury. Patients with arterial hypotension should initially be assessed clinically, and underlying conditions (for example, arrhythmia or hypovolemia) treated accordingly, before catecholamines are administered. One should note that cardiac failure due to acute myocardial ischemia is a common cause of acute hypotension that should be excluded before other measures are initiated. Other frequent causes of severe hypotension include hypovolemia, sepsis, and iatrogenically induced hypotension due to sedation or excessive application of antihypertensive agents. Crystalloid or colloid fluids should be applied and fluid homeostasis maintained through precise evaluation of fluid intake and output. The target value of CVP lies between 8 and 12 cm H_2O. In prolonged, severe hypotonia, pulse contour continuous cardiac output monitoring may provide useful parameters to guide cardiocirculatory treatment. Catecholamines are administered after adequate optimization of volume status in order to enhance cardiac output and optimize systemic peripheral resistance. All catecholamines augment cardiac oxygen consumption and are arrhythmogenic. No studies have yet compared the efficacy or side effects of various catecholamines in patients with acute stroke, so no definitive recommendations are possible. Norepinephrine is a strong vasopressor and the drug of choice for augmenting peripheral systemic resistance, for example, during septic shock. Dobutamine is administered to enhance cardiac output. Epinephrine is the catecholamine of choice for cardiovascular resuscitation. Specific therapeutic concepts utilizing induced arterial hypertension are discussed later.

Invasive Monitoring Procedures

Central Venous Line

Venous access can be achieved by catheterizing a peripheral vein. Although several veins can be used, one must bear in mind that antecubital veins are not appropriate in awake and mobile patients because of discomfort and the risk of thrombosis; risk of thrombosis also prohibits the use of pedal veins, except in immobile bedridden patients. Central venous lines should be used (1) if no peripheral venous access can be obtained, (2) for administration of drugs that irritate peripheral veins or can cause tissue necrosis after extravasation, and (3) in unstable patients requiring several intravenous lines for drug administration.

The femoral, internal jugular, external jugular, and subclavian veins can be used for central venous access. Each approach has its own advantages and disadvantages. It is important to note that cannulation of the internal jugular vein should be avoided in patients with, or in danger of potential development of, intracranial hypertension, because of possible impairment of cerebral venous drainage. Puncture of the internal carotid artery may occur, but the incidence of pneumothorax is quite low. Cannulation of the subclavian vein bears an increased risk of pneumothorax; on the other hand, this vein does not collapse and can therefore be used in cases of shock or hypovolemia. Although cannulation of the femoral vein is relatively easy, this approach should be used only as a last resort, mainly because of the risk of infection. The position of all central venous lines, except for those inserted in the femoral vein, should be verified on a chest radiograph before they are used.

Pulse Contour Analysis

Pulse contour analysis has replaced the use of pulmonary artery catheters for monitoring of cardiac output in many intensive care units. It has the advantage of being less invasive than the pulmonary artery catheter, diminishing the risk of severe complications; in patients who already

have a central line, the system requires only an additional central artery catheter. The PiCCO (pulse contour cardiac output system, Pulsion Medical Systems AG, Munich) uses transpulmonary thermodilution and pulse contour analysis to calculate cardiac output, stroke volume variation, intrathoracic blood volume, and extravascular lung water. Thereby, cardiac function can be monitored continuously and volume status can be better estimated than from the use of the unreliable CVP alone. There are first reports on the use of pulse contour analysis to direct hypertensive and hypervolemic therapy in patients with vasospasm,[95] and more studies are to follow. A valuable, completely noninvasive alternative for hemodynamic monitoring is transthoracic echocardiography.

Invasive Monitoring of Arterial Blood Pressure

The main indications for peripheral arterial cannulation are continuous direct blood pressure measurement and access for blood sampling, particularly in patients whose peripheral veins are inadequate for repeated blood sampling. The radial artery is most commonly used. The pulse of the ulnar artery should be confirmed as palpable before cannulation of the radial artery is attempted. Alternatively, evaluation of the ulnar artery can be performed with Doppler ultrasonography.

Invasive Monitoring of Intracranial Pressure

ICP monitoring is essential in patients at risk for ICP increase during the course of their disease, particularly comatose or sedated patients, in whom clinical assessment is not feasible. ICP monitoring reduces the need for neuroradiologic examinations and allows evaluation of the effectiveness of diverse therapeutic approaches. From ICP and MAP, CPP is calculated as follows:

$$CPP = MAP - ICP$$

ICP monitoring is routinely performed unilaterally; tissue shifts in the contralateral hemisphere are therefore detected with a certain temporal latency. The exact effects of this issue on the clinical relevance of ICP monitoring have not yet been systematically studied. Still, in our experience in patients undergoing bilateral ICP monitoring, the role of this latency is minor, because initial pressure gradients rapidly resolve. Furthermore, ICP transducers are mostly inserted in the affected hemisphere, so that ICP increases are readily recognized. Currently, monitoring can be performed with intraventricular, intraparenchymatous, or epidural catheters as well as subarachnoid bolts.

Intraventricular catheters (IVCs) possess the highest accuracy and still are the reference standard for ICP monitoring. First introduced in 1953, they continue to constitute an attractive option for ICP monitoring, because they also allow CSF drainage. An IVC is mostly introduced through a skin incision and bur-hole over the posterior frontal lobe of the nondominant hemisphere, and forwarded for 5 to 8 cm, or until CSF is encountered. A three-way stopcock allows CSF drainage. The amount of CSF drained can be regulated by adjustment of the height of the reservoir. The external acoustic meatus usually serves as reference point for estimating reservoir height. Simultaneous performance of ICP monitoring and CSF drainage is a common mistake; the ICP measured under these conditions equals the atmospheric pressure. Thus, drainage must be temporarily interrupted to achieve an accurate measurement. The accuracy of the measured ICP can be compromised by accumulation of blood clots, debris, or air in the lumen of an IVC.

The major complication of IVCs is infection, the actual incidence of which varies widely among the different studies (0% to 22%),[96-98] probably largely because of the various definitions for ventriculostomy-related infections. One large series has been reported by Bota et al,[98] who analyzed clinical, laboratory, and microbiologic data from 638 critically ill patients in whom an external ventriculostomy catheter was placed; incidence rate of ventriculitis was 9%. This figure is in line with data from a review by Lozier et al,[99] who found an 8.8% incidence of positive CSF culture results. These investigators proposed definition criteria for five categories of CSF infections in patients who underwent ventriculostomy, ranging from contamination, through colonization, suspected infection, and ventriculostomy-related infection to ventriculitis. According to these criteria, diagnosis of ventriculostomy-related infection requires progressively declining glucose CSF level, increasing CSF protein level and pleocytosis, and at least one positive CSF culture result without clinical symptoms other than fever. Patients with ventriculitis should additionally have clinical signs of meningitis, including nuchal rigidity. However, the value of CSF glucose, CSF protein, and standard laboratory parameters, such as peripheral leukocyte count, has been doubted by other researchers.[100,101] New approaches include assessment of intrathecal interleukin-6 levels but need to be evaluated in larger patient series.[102]

Several factors in the risk of IVC-associated infection remain unclear; they are (1) the potential influence of the duration of intraventricular catheterization and (2) the usefulness of prophylactic antibiotic treatment. In a prospective study of 172 consecutive neurosurgical patients, Mayhall et al[97] identified ventricular catheterization for longer than 5 days as a risk factor for infection (ventriculitis or meningitis). Previous ventriculostomy, however, did not raise the risk of infection in subsequent procedures. These researchers thus concluded that an IVC should remain in place for up to 5 days, after which the catheter should be removed and re-inserted at a different site. These results were challenged by Holloway et al,[96] who did not observe significant differences in infection rates between patients in whom catheters were replaced prior to 5 days and those whose catheters remained in place for longer periods; these results suggest that catheter exchange is not beneficial.[96] In this context, it must be noted that even the association between duration of IVC and infection still is not unequivocally documented and remains a matter of debate. In their review, Lozier et al[99] found that extended duration of ventriculostomy is correlated with an increasing risk for infections during the first 10 days of catheterization. Likewise, Bota et al[98] reported a peak in infection risk at day 9, followed by a rapid decrease after day 10. Other risk factors for ventriculostomy-related infections were intraventricular

hemorrhage (IVH), SAH, cranial fracture with CSF leak systemic infections, and catheter irrigation.[99]

Prophylactic use of antibiotics was reported as beneficial by some investigators,[103,104] but not by others.[105,106] According to a 1999 survey, 72% of centers do use antibiotics (mainly cephalosporins and semisynthetic penicillins) in patients with IVCs.[106] This issue remains unclear and should be addressed in a randomized controlled trial. We currently do not use prophylactic antibiotic treatment.

Friedman and Vries[107] reported that percutaneous tunneling of the IVC reduces the infection rate; they encountered no infections after 100 consecutive procedures in 66 patients, with a mean drainage duration of 6.2 days.[107] This finding was later confirmed by Khanna et al,[108] who reported no infection during the first 16 days after IVC insertion in a series of 100 consecutive procedures; the overall infection incidence in their patients was quite low (4% for an average IVC duration of 18.3 days).

Parenchymal or subdural bleeding along the insertion site constitutes a further complication of IVC. Its incidence, however, is negligibly low.

Prior to removal of the IVC, it is vital to acquire some information about the CSF absorption. For this purpose, catheter drainage should be discontinued for 24 hours, and ICP values closely monitored. Provided that ICP values do not rise by more than 15 to 20 mm Hg during this period, removal of the catheter can be regarded as safe. The quantity of drained CSF is a further indicator for the patency of CSF absorption and the necessity of external drainage; CSF drainage less than 250 mL/day with the reservoir hanging 20 cm above the external acoustic meatus indicates an adequate CSF absorption.

ICP monitoring with an *epidural catheter* is the least invasive approach, in which bleeding complications or infections are extremely rare. Unfortunately, this method is also the most vulnerable to artifacts, and the results are therefore not reproducible. Kosteljanetz et al[109] examined the efficacy of epidural catheters in 35 neurosurgical patients. Satisfactory catheter function was noted in approximately two thirds of cases. In 7 patients, ICP was simultaneously monitored with IVCs and epidural catheters; differences in measured ICP values of up to 25 mm Hg were noted. The researchers thus concluded that epidural catheters do not constitute an appropriate method for ICP monitoring. Bruder et al[110] reported similar findings; they observed no agreement between epidural and intraparenchymatous ICP values.

ICP measurement with a catheter-tip *intraparenchymal microtransducer* is a popular alternative to the ventricular catheter. Parenchymal ICP probes are likely to cause less damage to brain tissue and are associated with low infection rates. On the other hand, problems regarding zero drift and robustness have been reported in various laboratory and clinical studies.[111-115] The three different techniques of pressure transduction are fiberoptic, piezoelectric, and pneumatic.

Fiberoptic systems are based on a device sensing changes in light reflection off a pressure-sensitive diaphragm. They have been shown to have a relatively good zero drift and sensitivity stability. Good long-term zero drift properties are crucial: Although devices provide an electrical calibration for calibration of external monitors, their recordings cannot be corrected for inherent zero drift of the catheter once it is placed, their pressure output being dependent on zero drift of the sensor. Piezoelectric systems based on silicon chips seem to be more robust than fiberoptic transducers.[116] The Spiegelberg ICP monitoring system (Spiegelberg AG, Hamburg) is an example of a special pneumatic catheter-transducer system. ICP is measured by a catheter that has an air-pouch balloon situated at its top. The pressure within the internal air pouch balloon is equivalent to the surrounding pressure and is transduced by an external strain-gauge transducer. This design allows an automatic in vivo zeroing of the ICP system.

The current guidelines for brain trauma state that in the current state of technology, the ventricular catheter connected to an external strain gauge is the most accurate, lowest cost, and most reliable method of monitoring ICP. ICP transduction via fiberoptic or catheter-tip micro-strain-gauge devices placed in ventricular catheters provide similar benefits but at higher costs. Other devices such as subarachnoid, subdural, and epidural monitors are less accurate.

Multimodality brain monitoring: The rationale for multimodality monitoring in large ischemic stroke is the protection of healthy brain tissue adjacent to the infarcted area or in the contralateral hemisphere that may become affected by the expanding brain edema. In patients with intracranial hemorrhage, brain monitoring is applied to allow recognition of secondary brain injury caused by rebleeding or by the space-occupying effects of the hematoma and the surrounding edema or to detect vasospasm in SAH. Thus, the main goals of multimodality brain monitoring are (1) to detect deterioration before irreversible secondary brain injury develops,[117-122] (2) to monitor the effect of therapeutic measures,[123-125] and (3) to predict outcome.[126,127] The benefit of extensive brain monitoring in terms of clinical outcome has yet to be determined. In an early series, ICP monitoring in patients with malignant middle cerebral artery (MCA) infarction predicted clinical outcome but was not helpful in guiding long-term treatment of increased ICP.[128] Moreover, the authors stated that in most cases, clinical signs of herniation preceded ICP increase. However, all patients in the series were treated conservatively and in none did elevation of ICP trigger decompressive surgery. With the advent and evaluation of new therapeutic strategies, brain monitoring becomes increasingly meaningful. Multimodality brain monitoring in addition to ICP and CPP includes measurement of brain tissue oxygen pressure (Ptio$_2$), cerebral microdialysis, measurement of CBF, and eventually continuous electroencephalographic (EEG) monitoring.

Brain tissue partial pressure of oxygen (Ptio$_2$) is measured by a microprobe that is usually placed within the frontal white matter or the region of interest, such as the penumbra of an infarct or adjacent to a hematoma. Depending on the catheter, measurements of brain temperature, pH, tissue partial pressure of oxygen and carbon dioxide, and ICP can be made simultaneously. The measured tissue surface is approximately 17 mm^2. The measured values depend on localization of the catheter: Oxygen levels are highest in areas with dense populations of neurons, such as the cortex, and lowest in the white matter. Most of the experience so far with this method has been gained in patients with traumatic brain injury or SAH. However, we routinely use Ptio$_2$ monitoring for the indications previously listed as supplements to ICP and CPP measurements. Normal values are 20 mm Hg in white matter and 35 to 45 mm Hg in gray matter.

Cerebral microdialysis likewise requires the placement of a small catheter ($\approx$0.65 mm diameter) within the brain tissue. It allows analysis of various substances derived from the extracellular space in brain tissue, such as glucose and its metabolites lactate and pyruvate, the neurotransmitter glutamate, and glycerol, which is set free from membrane phospholipids during neuronal cell decay. Additionally, post hoc analyses using high-performance liquid chromatography can be performed. Under aerobic conditions, glucose is metabolized to pyruvate and adenosine triphosphate; in contrast, during hypoxia, the end product will be lactate instead. Thus, the lactate-to-pyruvate ratio is a sensitive indicator of lack of oxygen or ischemia. Another sensitive parameter to detect ischemia is glutamate, moderately high levels indicating ischemia in a reversible state and excessively high levels and a concomitant increase in glycerol indicating an irreversible loss of neurons. These changes in the extracellular milieu often precede elevations of ICP or manifestation of new neurologic deficits.

CBF can be estimated by a variety of techniques, including transcranial Doppler (TCD) ultrasonography, xenon-CT, single-photon emission CT (SPECT), oxygen-15 positron emission tomography (PET), perfusion CT, and perfusion-weighted MRI. Except for TCD, these methods do not offer the possibility of continuous monitoring. Placement of a thermal diffusion probe offers the possibility for continuously assessing regional cerebral perfusion on the basis of the tissue's ability to dissipate heat. Other systems measure ICP and changes in CBF by means of laser Doppler flowmetry.

Continuous EEG (cEEG) monitoring in the ICU setting usually was used to detect (nonconvulsive) seizures, to monitor burst suppression during barbiturate therapy, to assess levels of sedation, or to predict outcome.[129] With the advent of digital EEG and quantitative EEG analysis, EEG monitoring has become more user-friendly. Reports have now shown the value of cEEG monitoring and quantitative EEG analysis to predict vasospasm in patients with SAH.[130,131]

Treatment of Raised Intracranial Pressure

The main goal of ICP treatment is to minimize or, if possible, eliminate secondary ischemic insults and mechanical damage caused by shifts and local compression of brain tissue. The focus has hereby changed from the initially proposed regimen, which was purely ICP-oriented, to a regimen aiming at maintaining CPP. Sustained CPP drops can result in hypoperfusion of ischemic brain regions, because the supplying arterioles are maximally dilated and cerebral autoregulation is impaired (Figs. 52-1 and 52-2).

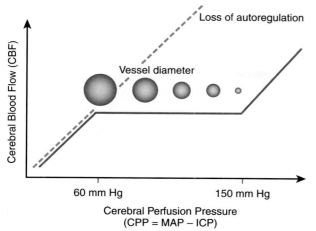

Figure 52-1 Autoregulation of cerebral blood flow (CBF). The cerebral vascular bed is capable of maintaining a constant CBF from a mean arterial blood pressure of 60 to 150 mm Hg. This phenomenon of "autoregulation" is achieved through either a reduction (vasodilation) or an increase (vasoconstriction) of arterial resistances when the cerebral perfusion pressure (CPP) decreases or increases. If the autoregulation is impaired *(dotted line)*, the CBF passively changes with the CPP. ICP, intracranial pressure.

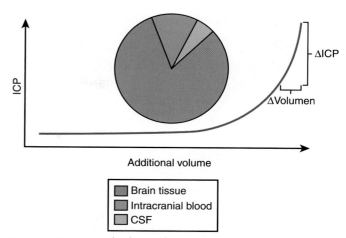

Figure 52-2 Cerebral compliance. An increase of edematous brain tissue requires a compensatory decrease of the other two physiologic compartments contained in the skull, intravascular blood and cerebrospinal fluid (CSF). After the failure of these very limited compensatory mechanisms, the ICP rapidly rises, and even a small increase in the intracranial volume (Δvolumen) may substantially raise the intracranial pressure (ΔICP). However, in this situation, even a small reduction in brain edema can dramatically lower the ICP.

Basic Measures

Although the optimal blood pressure in patients with intracranial hypertension remains unknown, it is important to avoid sustained hypotensive episodes encompassing the risk of further ischemic brain injury, especially in patients with disturbed autoregulation. We usually maintain CPP above 60 to 70 mm Hg. In patients with traumatic brain injury, Steiner et al[132] used continuous assessment of autoregulatory parameters in order to calculate optimal CPP. In a cohort of 114 head-injured patients, these researchers could show that outcome at 6 months correlated with the difference between CPP and CPP_{opt}. However, data on optimal CPP levels and their association with outcome in stroke patients are lacking.

Avoidance of hypovolemia is the simplest way to maintain blood pressure; in patients with a central line, CVP should be kept above 8 mm Hg. Crystalloid solutions, colloid solutions, and blood products can be used, in the order given. In patients with decreased peripheral resistance, vasopressors can be necessary; dopamine and epinephrine are the drugs of first choice. Dobutamine is the drug of choice when arterial hypotension is presumed to be caused by decreased cardiac output.

Keeping the patient's head elevated 15 to 30 degrees increases cerebral venous and CSF outflow, and could thus contribute to an ICP reduction. On the other hand, such a position compromises venous return to the heart, possibly decreasing arterial pressure. Ropper et al[133] examined the influence of body position on ICP in 19 patients in ICU; ICP was lowest when the head was raised to 60 degrees in 10 patients and with the head horizontal in 2 patients; ICP remained unchanged in both positions in 5 patients. Rosner and Coley[134] examined the effect of various head positions (0 to 50 degrees, in steps of 10 degrees) on ICP and CPP. An average ICP decrease of 1 mm Hg was noted for each step but was associated

with a reduction in CPP of 2 to 3 mm Hg. CPP was not beneficially affected by any degree of head elevation and was maximal in the horizontal position. Feldman et al[135] observed no significant changes in CPP with elevation of the patient's head from horizontal to 30 degrees, and ICP was significantly reduced. Similar results were reported by Meixensberger et al,[136] who also found that brain tissue oxygen pressure remained unaffected by the body position. Moraine et al,[137] however, observed no ICP changes when the patient's head was elevated from horizontal to 30 degrees; ICP values did drop, however, when the head was further elevated to 45 degrees. At the same time, CBF gradually decreased with head elevation from horizontal to 45 degrees, a change that these investigators attributed mainly to changes in arteriovenous pressure gradients.

It must be noted that all of the studies just summarized examined patients with severe head injury. In a study in 18 patients with acute stroke, ICP, MAP, and CPP values were compared when head position was changed from horizontal to 30 degrees of elevation. A mild but statistically significant reduction in ICP was evident; it was accompanied by a reduction in MAP of a much higher magnitude, so this maneuver mildly reduced ICP at the expense of a CPP reduction.[138] Likewise, Ropper et al[133] observed different behaviors of the monitored parameters among the patients studied. We thus suggest that optimal head positioning be decided on an individual basis, rather than the routine positioning of all patients with 30-degree head elevation as is currently practiced in most ICUs.

Specific Treatment

Osmotherapeutic agents are hypertonic solutions of low molecular weight that increase serum osmolarity, thus creating an osmotic gradient between blood and brain tissue.

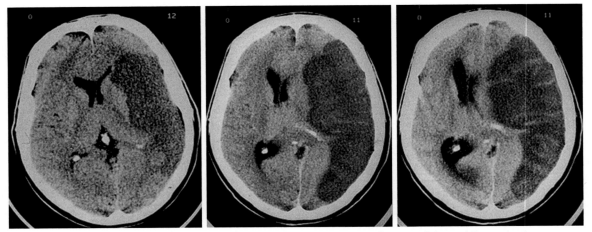

Figure 52-3 *Left to right,* Course of edema formation in complete infarction of the middle cerebral artery.

An intact blood-brain barrier is essential for this osmotic gradient. Migration of osmotic substances through the damaged blood-brain barrier can reverse the osmotic gradient and aggravate brain edema (rebound effect). This result was demonstrated by Kaufmann and Cardoso[139] in 23 cats with a cortical cold injury and vasogenic edema, and by Garcia-Sola et al[140] in a goat model in which inflation of an epidural balloon was used to produce intracranial hypertension. Furthermore, volume reduction is more pronounced in the healthy hemisphere; this could potentially increase the pressure gradient between the two hemispheres and facilitate displacement and herniation of brain tissue. It must be noted, however, that such an increase in the pressure gradient constitutes a pathophysiologic model, which has not been substantiated in any animal or clinical studies. The few available data in humans are inconsistent.[141-143]

Mannitol is the most commonly used osmotherapeutic agent. In addition to drawing water from interstitial and intercellular spaces, this agent may improve rheologic properties of blood. Initially, mannitol leads to an increased intravascular volume, resulting in reduction of hematocrit and higher MAP levels. Provided that autoregulation is intact, a concomitant increase in CPP leads to cerebral vasoconstriction, which is followed by reduction of cerebral blood volume and finally of ICP.

The effectiveness of mannitol was demonstrated in several studies examining patients with head injury.[144-146] Pollay et al[147] also described a synergistic effect of mannitol and furosemide in reducing ICP, related to preferential excretion of water through the renal distal tubule, which sustains the osmotic gradient, and potentially also to reduced production of CSF. Although a large body of animal studies has investigated the effects of mannitol on cerebral ischemia and edema formation (Fig. 52-3), few clinical trials have investigated the use of mannitol in patients with stroke. Most experimental studies found beneficial effects of mannitol on edema formation, lowering of ICP, and infarct volume.[148,149] However, enhanced brain swelling and midline shift after repetitive doses of mannitol have been reported.[139] Bereczki et al[150] analyzed the case-fatality rate with respect to mannitol treatment in 805 patients with stroke. These investigators could not

find any association between mannitol use and better prognosis at 30 days and 1 year after stroke. Depending on the factors included in the logistic regression models, mannitol either did not have a significant effect on the case-fatality rate or was associated with an adverse outcome.

In their Cochrane Database analysis, Bereczki et al[150,151] evaluated the evidence for the effectiveness of mannitol in patients with acute ischemic and hemorrhagic stroke. These researchers identified a total of three randomized studies comparing the effect of mannitol with placebo or open control in patients with ischemic stroke or nontraumatic intracerebral hemorrhage. On the basis of three trials (involving 21 and 128 patients with ICH, and 77 patients with ischemic stroke), neither beneficial nor harmful effects could be proved. Thus, the use of mannitol in patients with acute stroke is based solely on the results of experimental studies or of studies in patients with head trauma.

However, these trials were not designed to investigate efficacy of reducing edema formation in malignant, space-occupying ischemic stroke. In this special setting, some case series have described effective lowering of ICP with the use of mannitol. In 10 of 14 episodes, single doses of 40 g mannitol in eight patients with hemispheric stroke and massive brain edema did effectively lower elevated ICP for up to 4 hours.[152] Likewise, in another observational study, mannitol effectively reduced ICP in association with a concomitant increase in CPP and brain tissue oxygen pressure in the ipsilateral and contralateral hemispheres.[153] Effects on long-term outcome have not been investigated, but the data suggest that mannitol can be efficiently employed to manage an acute ICP crisis and to bridge the time until further interventions such as hemicraniectomy can be initiated.

The sugar glycerol is another frequently used osmotic agent. Theoretically, the risk of a rebound phenomenon is lower than with mannitol, because glycerol can be metabolized by the brain. As with mannitol, the occurrence of a rebound phenomenon remains controversial.[154] Biestro et al[155] compared the effectiveness of mannitol and glycerol for decreasing ICP, using a modified therapeutic intensity level to compare the two approaches. Although both agents were effective at reducing ICP, the duration of this effect was longer for glycerol, leading these investigators to suggest that glycerol is best used as basic treatment and that a bolus of mannitol should be applied to counteract sudden increases in ICP. A 2004 Cochrane Database review identified 10 randomized studies involving a total of 482 mannitol-treated patients in comparison with 463 control patients.[156] Despite a small favorable effect of glycerol treatment on short-term survival, results have to be interpreted cautiously owing to the relatively small number of patients and the fact that most of the trials were performed in the pre-CT era. Moreover, there was no evidence of benefit in long-term survival or functional outcome. Focusing on intensive care treatment, it has to be noted that in only a few patients was stroke confirmed by CT and in only one study were clinical signs of brain edema used as inclusion criterion. There is no randomized clinical trial addressing the effect of glycerol on outcome in patients with massive brain edema secondary to hemispheric infarction.

Theoretically, 40% sorbital solutions can be applied as well. However, they have two major drawbacks: (1) they are metabolized through the liver, and thus cannot be used in patients with liver dysfunction, and (2) they are contraindicated in patients with fructose intolerance. For this reason, we refrain from their routine use.

The effectiveness of hypertonic saline solutions in the treatment of intracranial hypertension after head trauma has been documented in several studies.[157,158] Gemma et al[159] observed a comparable ICP decrease after the administration of 7.5% hypertonic saline or 20% mannitol in 50 patients during elective supratentorial procedures. In a similar study, Schwarz et al[152] compared the effects of a combination of hypertonic saline–hydroxyethyl starch (HS-HES) with those of mannitol; both substances were effective in reducing ICP. In contrast, Qureshi et al[160] reported a favorable trend toward ICP reduction after infusion of 3% saline in acetate in patients with head trauma (n = 8) or postoperative edema (n = 6), but not in patients with nontraumatic intracranial hemorrhage (n = 8) or ischemic stroke (n = 6). This result could not be reproduced, however, in a later study conducted in our department that examined the effect of hypertonic saline in eight patients with stroke and increased ICP, in whom the standard mannitol treatment showed no effect; treatment with 75 mL of 10% saline over 15 minutes resulted in an ICP reduction in all cases. Maximal ICP decrease (mean, 9.9 mm Hg) was observed 20 minutes after the end of the infusion. No side effects were noted.[161] Thus, few studies have examined the effectiveness of hypertonic saline in patients with acute stroke, and the results, as described previously, were not unanimous. The optimum concentration of hypertonic saline remains controversial; multiple concentrations ranging from 3% to 23.4% have been tested with different application schedules in patients with traumatic brain injury.[162] Severe side effects of hypertonic saline solutions include severe hypernatremia, congestive heart failure, and pulmonary edema.

Given the results already summarized, no evidence-based recommendation can be made on the use of osmotic agents in stroke. Regardless of the therapeutic regimen, it is vital to monitor serum electrolyte levels and osmolarity closely (at least twice daily) while osmotic agents are used. We initially use mannitol (100 mL of a 20% mannitol solution) for control of intracranial hypertension. This is given as bolus infusion (over 15 minutes), preferably through a central line. Because the half-life of mannitol is short (approximately 1 hour), several administrations (4 to 6 per day) are necessary. In predisposed patients, a cumulative dose of 300 g may already be nephrotoxic and may induce tubular necrosis. Therefore, mannitol accumulation in the serum has to be monitored. This can be done by simultaneous calculation and measurement of serum osmolality.[163] Usually, the two values should be identical. If mannitol accumulates, an osmolar gap occurs, with serum osmolality exceeding the calculated osmolality. We aim for a target serum osmolarity of 320 mOsm/L, avoiding higher values in an effort to minimize the risk of acute tubular necrosis and because of the previously cited risk of rebound effect. We often combine mannitol with furosemide in an attempt to increase the osmotic gradient. If mannitol therapy is not sufficient for ICP control, we use HS-HES, a hypertonic saline, or both.

Tromethamine (Tham) has been shown to decrease ICP in animal models.[164] It acts by entering the CSF compartment, reducing cerebral acidosis, and causing vasoconstriction, thus reducing ICP. A prospective randomized clinical trial in 149 patients with severe head injury who received either Tham or placebo for 5 days demonstrated that the use of Tham was associated with (1) a significantly lower incidence of ICP values exceeding 20 mm Hg during the first two treatment days and (2) a significantly lower number of patients with barbiturate coma requiring treatment.[165] Nevertheless, no difference in outcome between the two groups was observed at 3, 6, or 12 months.

Tham should always be infused via a central line, because extravasation leads to severe tissue necrosis. Initially, the effectiveness of the agent should be assessed by infusion of 1 mmol/kg in 100 mL of 5% glucose over 45 minutes. Continuous Tham infusion should be initiated only if the first application leads to an ICP reduction by approximately 10 to 15 mm Hg. The dose is adapted so as to achieve and then maintain blood pH between 7.5 and 7.55.

Hyperventilation results in reduction in $Paco_2$, which causes vasoconstriction, thus reducing CBF, cerebral blood volume, and, subsequently, ICP. This effect usually occurs within minutes of initiation of hyperventilation. It must be noted that metabolic autoregulation is not intact in ischemic brain regions, where brain arterioles are maximally dilated. Vasoconstriction is therefore limited to vessels supplying unaffected brain tissue, a feature that could theoretically lead to redistribution of CBF (reverse steal phenomenon). Michenfelder and Milde,[166] examining the effect of hypocapnia in a primate model of acute ischemic stroke, found no differences in mortality or level of neurologic function with use of hyperventilation, although they did note a tendency toward smaller infarct volumes. The applicability of hyperventilation is limited by the following major factors: (1) cerebral vasoconstriction can result in cerebral ischemia and (2) the induced elevation of CSF pH is compensated by the choroid plexus within hours, in contrast to the much slower compensation of blood pH, which can require several days. This latter finding implies that the effect of hyperventilation lasts for only a few hours, after which cerebral vessels regain their normal diameter. Termination of hyperventilation at this stage results in an increase of Pa_{CO_2} in both blood and CSF, which in turn causes cerebral vasodilation, potentially leading to a rebound effect on ICP. In a randomized trial, Muizelaar et al[167] examined the effects of hyperventilation alone, hyperventilation plus Tham, and normoventilation (control) in 113 patients with severe head injury, who were divided into two subgroups according to the initial motor score.[167] These investigators observed a significantly worse outcome at 3 and 6 months after injury in patients with severe motor scores who were treated with hyperventilation alone. They also demonstrated that hyperventilation alone, in contrast to hyperventilation plus Tham, could not sustain CSF alkalinization. A variety of clinical studies on head injury have suggested that hyperventilation has deleterious effects on cerebral oxygenation[168,169] and metabolism.[170]

Hyperventilation is a treatment option for short interventions, to counteract sudden ICP elevations. Under these conditions, the risk of rebound is minimal. Hyperventilation is easily induced through an approximate 10% increase in tidal volume, a target arterial P_{CO_2} level being 30 to 35 mm Hg. However, with regard to the large body of evidence indicating possible deleterious effects of hyperventilation on cerebral oxygenation, metabolism, and blood flow, and the lack of any beneficial effect on outcome, long-term hyperventilation cannot be recommended in patients with stroke.[171]

The main effects of *barbiturates* are decreases in cerebral metabolism and CBF; the mechanism of these changes is unclear, although an enhancement of the binding of gamma-aminobutyric acid (GABA) to its receptor and a direct effect on vascular tone have been postulated.[172] The effect of barbiturates on ICP appears to be less uniform than that of other agents. ICP reductions were observed in 11 of 15 patients with nontraumatic lesions by Woodcock et al[173]; in 14 of 21 patients with neurosurgical trauma by Lee et al[174]; in 50 of 60 patients with acute ischemic stroke by Schwab et al[175]; and in 57 of 67 patients with severe head injuries by Cormio et al,[176] who found that ICP values were reduced but remained higher than 20 mm Hg in 27 of 67 patients. Schwartz et al[177] found no differences in efficacy between barbiturate coma and mannitol in reducing ICP in 95 patients with head injury. Only 5 of 60 (8%) patients treated with barbiturates survived in the study reported by Schwab et al.[175] Sustained ICP control was achieved only in the 5 survivors. It must be noted, however, that barbiturates were mostly used as the last line of treatment, after failure of other treatment options; thus, outcome in some patients treated with barbiturates may already have been predetermined by the extent of brain lesions. In another series involving 21 patients with elevated ICP after large MCA infarction, ICP was temporarily decreased in every case by barbiturate treatment, but this effect was associated with reductions in cerebral oxygen pressure and CPP.[153]

Because of several potential and partially severe side effects of barbiturate coma (marked arterial hypotension, myocardial damage, electrolyte disturbances, impairment of liver function, predisposition to infection), this treatment should be used only as a therapy of last choice, accompanied by invasive monitoring of arterial blood pressure and frequent evaluations of serum electrolyte and liver enzyme levels. Barbiturates should be infused slowly over a separate venous line. Thiopental is the barbiturate used most in neurocritical care unit. It is advisable to apply a bolus injection of 100 mg of thiopental initially and to proceed with further applications only if a marked ICP reduction is observed. The barbiturate effect is monitored on the basis of the appearance of a burst-suppression pattern on EEG. Serum levels of barbiturates are not reliable.

Qizilbash et al[178] have reviewed the use of *corticosteroids* for acute stroke. Seven trials involving 453 patients were chosen for analysis; the follow-up period varied between 1 and 12 months, and only one study utilized CT to exclude hemorrhagic stroke.[178] The reviewers concluded that corticosteroid treatment did not influence mortality at 1 year or improve functional outcome in survivors. Reported adverse effects included gastrointestinal hemorrhage, infection, and hyperglycemia. A clinical study of corticosteroid therapy in 93 patients with supratentorial intracranial hemorrhage found no evidence of a beneficial effect, and the rates of complications already mentioned were significantly increased.[179] Obviously, the possibility that inclusion of patients with hemorrhagic infarcts may have influenced the results of early studies cannot be ruled out. Thus, it is possible that a subgroup of patients with ischemic stroke (particularly those with large infarcts and vasogenic edema) could potentially benefit from corticosteroid treatment. At the same time, the adverse effects observed in these early trials discourage the conduct of further research in this area.

As early as 1901, Kocher suggested performing decompressive surgery (*hemicraniectomy*) in order to alleviate intracranial hypertension.[180] Decompressive surgery is based on purely mechanical considerations. The vector of brain extension is reverted into the newly created compensatory spaces so as to relieve the pressure on the midline structures. The rationale of removing a part of the neurocranium is simply to create space for the expanding brain. This maneuver ideally normalizes the ICP and reduces ventricular compression and midline shift. CBF can also be restored, thus increasing tissue oxygen supply. In this way, secondary damage to the surrounding healthy tissue may be avoided.

Most studies on decompressive surgery have been performed in the context of malignant infarction of the MCA and traumatic brain injury. Occasionally, hemicraniectomy was carried out in patients with venous sinus thrombosis, SAH, or brain infections. Several animal stroke models provide evidence that decompressive surgery improves cerebral perfusion and reduces the volume of infarction.[181-183] Likewise, in animal models of traumatic brain injury, it could be shown that decompression significantly reduced secondary brain damage.[184] Although there is a large body of evidence that decompressive surgery effectively lowers ICP and probably mortality,[185,186] there is still intense debate as to whether it also improves outcome. The applicability of this approach in various stroke syndromes is discussed later in the chapter.

Normal body temperature is 37° C, with a significant diurnal variation of ±0.6° C. Body core temperature can be measured at varying sites; the shell temperatures are measured sublingual, axillary, or cutaneous. Core temperatures reflect tympanic membrane, esophageal, rectal, bladder, and intravasal temperature measurements. *Hypothermia* is defined as mild (>33° C), moderate (29 to 33° C), or deep (<29° C).

With drop of core body temperature, the systemic oxygen demand lessens. Correspondingly, decreases in carbon dioxide production, plasma potassium levels, and carbohydrate metabolism are observed. Several studies have demonstrated a neuroprotective effect of moderate hypothermia in animal models of focal cerebral ischemia.[187-189] Potential underlying neuroprotective mechanisms include decrease in excitatory amino acid levels,[190,191] stabilization of the blood-brain barrier and cell membranes,[192,193] and a downregulation of cerebral metabolism.[194] Additionally, alteration of CBF during hypothermia may contribute to its neuroprotective effects.[194]

Deep hypothermia has routinely been used during open heart surgery and also occasionally for cerebral protection during neurosurgical operations. Although initial clinical studies in patients with brain injury suggested a potential clinical benefit of moderate hypothermia,[195,196] these results could not be confirmed in a later multicenter trial.[197] Yet, moderate hypothermia appears to improve outcomes in patients with coma after resuscitation from out-of-hospital cardiac arrest.[198,199] Application of moderate hypothermia for ischemic stroke is detailed later in this chapter.

Antiepileptic therapy: Reported frequencies for epileptic seizures in acute stroke range from 2% to 23%, depending on study design, diagnostic criteria, duration of follow-up, study population, and the extent of monitoring. Incidence seems to be higher in hemorrhagic stroke.[200] In ICH, lobar location and small hemorrhages seem to be associated with the occurrence of seizures within 24 hours after ictus.[201] Seizures are usually partial, and secondary generalization may occur. Later reports have focused on the occurrence of nonconvulsive seizures. Vespa et al[200] performed continuous EEG monitoring of 109 patients with acute ischemic or hemorrhagic stroke. Electroencephalographic seizures occurred in 28% of patients with ICH, compared with 6% of patients with ischemic stroke. The risk for recurrent seizures after stroke in the acute phase is unclear, estimates ranging from 20% to 80%.[80] History of alcohol abuse increased the risk of status epilepticus in patients with ICH.[201] Data from MRI studies suggest that prolonged seizures may be associated with formation of cerebral edema, which could potentially increase ICP.[179-182] The same holds true for seizure-related cerebral vasodilation, and increases in oxygen and substrate demand can aggravate cerebral ischemia. In the study by Vespa et al,[200] posthemorrhagic nonconvulsive seizures were associated with a significant increase in midline shift.

Few data are available on the utility of prophylactic application of antiepileptic drugs after stroke. Prophylactic administration of antiepileptic drugs is therefore not recommended in current guidelines for the management of ischemic or hemorrhagic stroke. An exception may be in patients with lobar hemorrhages.[202] In a small prospective study, prophylactic use of antiepileptic treatment in patients with lobar hemorrhage led to a reduction in seizures.[201] We administer antiepileptics only in patients who experience seizures. Epileptic seizures should be treated initially with intravenous benzodiazepines, followed by phenytoin (18 to 20 mg/kg) if the first agents are unsuccessful. In the case of refractory status epilepticus, please refer to current guidelines, for example, those provided by the European Federation of Neurological Societies (http://www.efns.org).

Prevention of Deep Vein Thrombosis and Pulmonary Embolism

Early in-hospital mortality in patients with acute stroke has been attributed not only to neurologic deterioration caused by brain edema, recurrent ischemia, or hemorrhage growth but also to secondary medical complications such as aspiration pneumonia, cardiac complication, sepsis, and pulmonary embolism.[203-205] The incidence of pulmonary embolism after acute stroke shows a large variation among studies.[206] Incidences between 0% and 46% in postmortem studies have been reported. A study by Widjicks et al[207] found that pulmonary embolism was associated with sudden death in 50% of cases; in the other cases, clinical diagnosis was based on the occurrence of sudden dyspnea, pleuritic pain, or tachycardia. Studies applying MR direct thrombus imaging have reported high incidences of deep vein thrombosis (DVT) (17.7%) in patients with hemiplegic stroke treated with aspirin and compression stockings.[208]

The risk of DVT and pulmonary embolism can be reduced by hydration and early mobilization, although the latter is not an option for many ICU patients. Compression stockings have been found effective in surgical patients, but their efficacy after stroke remains unproven.[209] Studies in patients with ischemic stroke have shown that administration of low-molecular-weight heparin (LMWH) reduced the incidence of DVT and pulmonary embolism without increasing the risk of intracerebral hemorrhage.[206,210,211] Current guidelines therefore recommend the use of low-dose subcutaneous heparin or LMWHs for patients with ischemic stroke at high risk for DVT or pulmonary embolism.[80,212]

Because of the fear of trigger rebleeding in patients with hemorrhagic stroke, thromboembolism prophylaxis is frequently withheld during the first days after ICH or administered at half of the normal dose in patients at high risk for CVT. The intermittent use of pneumatic compression devices has recently been recommended.[202,213] However, in a small randomized trial, Boeer et al have compared early with late application of low-dose subcutaneous heparin in patients with hemorrhagic stroke. The group of patients in whom prophylaxis was started on the second day after ICH onset had significant lower rate of pulmonary embolism than patients in whom treatment was initiated on days 4 and 10 after ictus. No overall increase in rebleeding was observed in any of the groups. Therefore, it has been recommended that in neurologically stable patients, low-dose heparin can be started on the second day after onset of ICH.[214] Other guidelines recommend starting after day 3 or 4.[202] Monitoring of partial thromboplastin time or anti–factor Xa level has been recommended.

A special issue arises in patients receiving vasopressors. A small study has investigated bioavailability of subcutaneous LMWH in ICU patients undergoing vasopressor therapy. The vasopressor group had lower plasma concentrations of factor Xa activity than ICU patients not receiving vasopressors and postoperative controls and might therefore be insufficiently protected from venous thromboembolism. This finding could be caused by impaired perfusion of subcutaneous tissue due to pharmacologically induced adrenergic vasoconstriction. These results suggest that ICU patients receiving vasopressors may need a different mode of administration to attain adequate thrombosis prophylaxis.[215]

Management of Blood Glucose

Post-stroke hyperglycemia is a common finding and occurs in 43% to 68% of patients.[216] Several large clinical trials have found an association between post-stroke hyperglycemia and higher mortality and poor functional outcome.[216-219] Suggested mechanisms include tissue acidosis secondary to anaerobic glycolysis, lactic acidosis, and free radical production.[220,221] Other investigators argue that hyperglycemia may be part of a stroke-related stress response and may reflect the seriousness of the event itself.[222]

Furthermore, in a study involving critically ill surgical patients, van den Berghe et al[50] had shown that intensive insulin therapy in order to keep blood glucose levels between 80 and 110 mg/dL lowered in-hospital mortality from 10.9% to 7.2%.[50] This was achieved mostly by reducing deaths from multiorgan failure with a proven septic focus. However, in a follow-up study by the same group in medical ICU patients, intensive insulin therapy had no beneficial effects on survival rates but was associated with fivefold to sixfold increase in hypoglycemic events.[223] Despite these conflicting results, intensive insulin therapy had been widely advocated, especially in patients with severe sepsis.[224] This procedure has now been challenged by the results of a large trial on intensive insulin therapy in severe sepsis.[225] The trial had to be stopped prematurely for safety reasons. The rate of severe hypoglycemia was higher in the intensive insulin therapy group than in the conventional insulin therapy group (17.0% versus 4.1%), as was the rate of serious adverse events (10.9% versus 5.2%).

Likewise, the largest randomized trial so far of blood glucose management in patients with stroke found no difference in mortality or functional outcome rates between patients with mild-to-moderate glucose elevations (median 137 mg/dL) that were not treated with insulin and patients receiving intensive insulin therapy targeted to achieve blood glucose levels between 72 and 126 mg/dL.[226] Therefore, current guidelines do not recommend the routine use of insulin infusion in patients with stroke and moderate hyperglycemia, referring to the common practice to treat blood glucose levels higher than 180 mg/dL.[212] The new guidelines for glucose management in critically ill septic patients recommend maintaining blood glucose levels below 150 mg/dL.[227]

Temperature Management

In experimental stroke, hyperthermia was associated with increased infarct size and poor outcome.[228,229] A retrospective study of patients with supratentorial ICH found a high incidence of fever, especially in patients with ventricular hemorrhage. The duration of fever was associated with poor outcome and appeared to be an independent prognostic factor.[230] Research in experimental cerebral ischemia revealed a variety of possible mechanisms by which hyperthermia contributes to worse outcome. These include enhanced release of neurotransmitters, exaggerated production of oxygen radicals, more extensive breakdown of the blood-brain barrier, increased numbers of potentially damaging ischemic depolarizations in the focal ischemic penumbra and impaired recovery of energy metabolism, enhanced inhibition of protein kinases, and worsening of cytoskeletal proteolysis.[231] The basic pathophysiologic principles probably also apply to patients with ICH. A raise in body temperature should prompt a search for an infectious focus, and treatment should aim to maintain body temperature below 37.5° C. A frequently used agent is acetaminophen or paracetamol; external cooling with cooling blankets may work well. Some centers employ an intravenous cooling catheter to keep body temperature at the desired level. The theoretical benefits of hypothermia were discussed previously.

Specific Treatment of Various Stroke Syndromes
Acute Large Middle Cerebral Artery Stroke

The clinical course of severe infarction of the MCA (malignant MCA syndrome) or of infarction of the MCA plus the anterior cerebral artery (ACA), the posterior cerebral artery (PCA), or both that is treated with medical therapy alone follows a predictable pattern in most patients.[232,233] Within the first few hours after onset of symptoms, patients with large supratentorial infarcts are typically fully awake, although some may show mild drowsiness. Bilateral motor signs, coma, posturing, and pupillary abnormalities are usually not observed in the very early phase of large supratentorial infarcts. Neurologic deterioration occurs during the first 24 hours in most patients with large supratentorial infarcts, corresponding to the development of brain edema. Such patients lose consciousness to varying degrees from drowsiness to coma. Pupillary enlargement and loss of pupillary reactivity—initially occurring only on the side of the infarction and later bilaterally—nausea, vomiting, posturing, and abnormal breathing patterns are signs of secondary brainstem dysfunction due to impending herniation. If ICP is being monitored, it is typically only moderately elevated (≈20 mm Hg), at the onset of deterioration. ICP values subsequently rise over the next 24 to 48 hours. Elevated ICP is a reliable prognostic sign, and an ICP exceeding 30 mm Hg is usually associated with a fatal course.[128]

Most patients demonstrating neurologic deterioration within the first few hours after stroke onset eventually die. Various predictors for deterioration and poor clinical outcome have been identified. Regarding vascular disease, distal internal carotid artery (ICA) occlusion almost uniformly indicates fatal outcome. Proximal occlusion of the MCA stem is also an unfavorable radiologic finding, typically leading to a complete MCA infarction, including the basal ganglia, which are often spared in patients with a more distal MCA occlusion. It seems plausible that the extent of the infarcted area closely correlates with mortality. Complete MCA plus ACA infarcts and infarcts involving the complete hemisphere are usually lethal. Rapid onset of neurologic deterioration with loss of consciousness during the first 6 hours indicates an aggressive course of the disease and is associated with a high mortality.[232] The extent of brain edema depends largely on the size and location of the infarct but also shows substantial individual variability. As a general rule, young and middle-aged patients have less compensation capacity for space-occupying intracranial lesions than older patients with cerebral atrophy.

A large hemispheric infarct must be recognized in the emergency department as a life-threatening condition that requires prompt and massive intervention. After stabilization of the airway, breathing, and circulation, the initial diagnostic evaluation and transfer of the patient to a neurocritical care unit should not be delayed. If indicated, early reperfusion therapies can be initiated in the emergency department. Venous access, continuous monitoring of blood pressure, electrocardiography (ECG), and pulse oxygenation are part of routine intensive care measures. Continuous ECG monitoring is especially important because neurogenic cardiac arrhythmias are commonly observed, particularly in patients with large infarcts of the right hemisphere. Although respiratory problems are uncommon upon presentation, their frequency sharply rises within the first 24 hours, reflecting increasing brain edema and brainstem dysfunction. Most patients with large infarcts require ventilatory support. To achieve sufficient cerebral oxygenation, oxygen should be insufflated via a face mask to achieve arterial P_{O_2} values greater than 90 mm Hg. Indications for intubation and mechanical ventilation were discussed earlier.

Hemicraniectomy

For a long time, only nonrandomized studies, retrospective case series, and a Cochrane Database review employing heterogeneous inclusion criteria had suggested that decompressive surgery may be beneficial in malignant MCA infarction (Fig. 52-4).[234-237] The results of a pooled analysis of three randomized controlled trials of early decompressive surgery in malignant media infarction have now been published.[238] All trials had defined basically similar inclusion criteria, and for the pooled analysis, the following inclusion criteria were applied: age between 18 and 60 years; clinical deficits assessed by National Institutes of Health Stroke Scale (NIHSS) greater than 15 and decrease in the level of consciousness to a score of 1 or more on item 1a of the NIHSS; and CT signs of an infarct of at least 50% of the MCA territory or infarct volume greater than 145 cm³ on diffusion-weighted MRI (DWI); and inclusion within 45 hours after onset of symptoms (i.e., 48 hours to treatment). In total, data from 93 patients were included from the three trials: 51 were randomly allocated to undergo surgery and 42 to receive conservative treatment. The primary outcome measure was the score on the modified Rankin scale (mRS) at 1 year dichotomized between favorable (0-4) and unfavorable (5 and death) outcome. Secondary outcome measures were mortality at 1 year and a dichotomization of the mRS score between 0 to 3 and 4 to death. The distribution of the mRS score at 1 year differed significantly between the two groups: more patients in the surgery group had an mRS score ≤ 4 (75% versus 24%; $P < .0001$) or ≤ 3 (43% versus 21%; $P < .014$). Likewise, mortality at 1 year was significantly different: 78% of patients who underwent surgery versus 29% in the conservative group survived ($P < .0001$). The number needed to treat (NNT) was 2 for survival with an mRS score ≤ 4, 4 for survival with an mRS score ≤ 3, and 2 for survival irrespective of functional outcome. Hence, the investigators concluded that decompressive surgery undertaken within 48 hours of stroke onset reduces mortality and increases

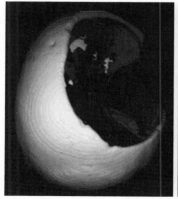
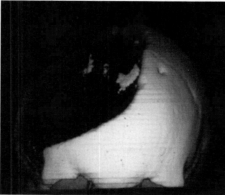
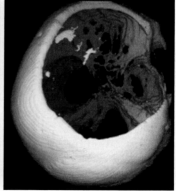

FIGURE 52-4 Three-dimensional CT reconstruction of decompressive surgery after space-occupying infarction of the middle cerebral artery. Note the extension of the bone flap.

the number of patients with a favorable functional outcome. On the basis of the data from the pooled analysis, the probability of surviving in a condition of being permanently dependent on the assistance of others (mRS score 4) increases more than tenfold, whereas the probability of survival with an mRS score ≤ 3 doubles. Yet, the risk of severe disability (mRS score 5) was not increased. However, the criticism was raised that a mRS score of 4 already implies that the patient will be unable to walk and will persistently be dependent on the assistance of others, whereas the end result of the best medical treatment is either death or survival with a high probability of a favorable outcome (defined as mRS ≤ 3, 75% of patients who survived under best medical care).[239] Information about quality of life of survivors is therefore essential in order to resolve these issues. Studies on quality of life following decompressive surgery for malignant media infarction have produced divergent results. Some found an acceptable to good functional outcome,[240-246] but others obtained less promising results,[247-249] particularly in older patients. Moreover, standard outcome measures such as Barthel Index (BI), Glasgow Outcome Scale, and mRS, with their emphasis on motor abilities, may not account for all remaining deficits, and cognitive impairments and communication skills are considered to be particularly crucial for determining quality of life. A study by Kastrau et al[244] assessed recovery from aphasia in patients with infarction of the dominant hemisphere. They found significant improvements in aphasic symptoms in 13 of 14 patients during a mean observation period of 470 days.[244] At the same time, data about quality of life of patients after conservative treatment are scarce. One study involving 62 patients found a mean BI of 32 for patients receiving conservative treatment, a BI of 33 for patients who underwent hemicraniectomy within 24 hours, and a BI of 27 for those who had late (>24 hours) hemicraniectomy after a minimum follow-up period of 1.5 years.[242] Another study found no significant difference in the BI at 3 months between survivors undergoing hemicraniectomy and those receiving conservative treatment.[250]

The surgical technique commonly used consists of removal of a bone flap with a diameter of 12 cm (including the frontal, parietal, temporal, and parts of the occipital squamae). The dura is initially fixed at the edge of the craniotomy, to prevent epidural bleeding, and subsequently opened. An adjusted, biconvex dural patch made of lyophilized cadaver dura or homologous temporal fascia is then placed into the incision. Although the size varies, dural patches 15 to 20 cm in length and 2.5 to 3.5 cm in width are generally used.

The ideal timing for decompressive surgery remains a matter of discussion; because the clinical course in patients with massive cerebral infarction (more than two thirds of the MCA territory) is highly predictable, it does not appear reasonable to wait for the appearance of clinical deterioration before performing surgery. One must also take into account that several hours may pass between the decision for surgery and its performance and that the procedure itself requires approximately 3 hours. Thus, the patient may be unnecessarily exposed to the risk of mesencephalic ischemia, which greatly worsens clinical status and outcome. We advocate surgery within 24 hours of symptom onset for any patient with (1) neuroradiologic signs of massive MCA infarction and (2) deterioration of clinical status since admission. We occasionally refrain from awaiting even this initial clinical deterioration in patients with complete MCA infarction. We also refrain from applying a rigid age limit for decompressive surgery, tending to rely on the health and social condition of each patient prior to the ischemic infarct. For patients with infarctions of the dominant hemisphere, we discuss prognosis—and particularly, probable residual deficit—with the family, in an attempt to assess the patient's viewpoint about disabled survival.

In summary, on the basis of the currently available data, it seems reasonable to state that decompressive surgery in malignant MCA infarction decreases mortality and there is good evidence that it does so without increasing the number of severely disabled survivors. Remaining questions concern quality of life, the optimal timing of surgery, and whether there should be an age limit. However, because the decision for surgery should always be made on an individual basis for each patient, it seems fair to also consider patients older than 60 years for hemicraniectomy, depending on their premorbid status.

Moderate Hypothermia

As already discussed previously in this chapter, hypothermia (1) theoretically offers neuroprotective effects and (2) may help control ICP. Because patients with acute stroke were rarely treated with hypothermia within the first 12 hours after symptom onset, neuroprotection has barely been considered an issue in case studies on hypothermia in ischemic stroke. Those studies have rather focused on the effect of hypothermia on reduction of brain edema and control of ICP.

The first clinical trial on the effect of moderate hypothermia (33° C) in patients with severe MCA infarction was reported by Schwab et al[251] in 1998. Hypothermia was induced at a mean of 14 hours after symptom onset and maintained for 72 hours. Mortality was only 44%, and survivors had a favorable outcome, with a mean BI of 70, even though all patients had met the criteria for diagnosis of a "malignant" MCA infarction. Although hypothermia significantly reduced ICP, a secondary rise in ICP, occasionally exceeding initial ICP levels and requiring additional treatment with osmotherapeutics, was observed upon rewarming. The rewarming period constitutes a critical phase, because metabolic needs potentially outstrip oxygen delivery. This ICP rebound after rewarming might be due to a hypermetabolic response after induced hypothermia, which has already been described after cardiopulmonary bypass surgery. Schwab et al[252] reported similar results in a multicenter observational study of 50 prospective patients with cerebral infarction involving at least the complete MCA territory who were treated with moderate hypothermia (33° C). Overall mortality was 38%; 8% of patients died during hypothermia, and 30% during rewarming owing to uncontrollable ICP increase. Neurologic outcomes were expressed as a score of 28 on the NIHSS and a score of 2.9 on the mRS at 4 weeks and at 3 months after stroke, respectively. Krieger et al[253] reported initial results in 10 patients with acute ischemic stroke (NIHSS score 19.8 ± 3.3) who were treated with moderate hypothermia (32° C) after thrombolysis.[253] Mortality was 33%, and the mean mRS score at 3 months was 3.1 ± 2.3.

Hypothermia affects virtually every organ system. Ventricular ectopy and fibrillation limit the extent of hypothermia, but this effect is known to occur only at temperatures below 30° C. Pneumonia was the only severe side effect of moderate hypothermia in the first study reported by Schwab et al.[251] The complications of moderate hypothermia most commonly described in the later multicenter trial were thrombocytopenia (70%), bradycardia (62%), and pneumonia (48%).[252] Four patients (8%) died during hypothermia, because of severe coagulopathy, cardiac failure, or uncontrollable intracranial hypertension. Complications in the 10 patients studied by Krieger et al[253] were bradycardia (n = 5), ventricular ectopy (n = 3), hypotension (n = 3), melena (n = 2), fever after rewarming (n = 3), and infection (n = 4). Also, 4 patients with chronic atrial fibrillation experienced a rapid ventricular rate, and 3 patients had myocardial infarctions during hypothermia.

Initially, surface cooling with cooling blankets, alcohol applied to exposed skin, or application of ice bags to groin, axilla, and neck were used to induce hypothermia. This approach, however, requires intensive effort from the medical and nursing staff for induction as well as maintenance of the target temperature. A novel technique using endovascular cooling has now been described.[254] It uses a central line with a single infusion lumen (e.g., ICY, Alsius Corporation, Irvine, Calif, or Celsius Control System by Innercool Therapies, San Diego, Calif) and one further lumen that ends in three balloons, sized 8 mm, 5 mm, and 5 mm in diameter, located at the distal end of the catheter. The balloons are perfused with a sterile solution of normal saline via a closed-loop tubing system. The tubing is connected to a mobile temperature management device placed at the patient's bedside. The device consists of a water bath with adjustable temperature; a pump circulates the saline solution through the water bath. The catheter is inserted into the femoral vein and advanced to the inferior vena cava. Initial results of this approach were promising, as target temperature was reached after 3 ± 1 hours (range, 2 to 4.5 h) and deviations from the target temperature were minimal (>0.2° C or >0.3° C during 21% or 10% of the time, respectively).[254] However, the advantages of this approach over surface cooling have not been evaluated in large-scale studies.

Taking into account the results of the pooled analysis of three randomized controlled trials on hemicraniectomy and the available evidence for hypothermia, in patients with large MCA infarction, surgical decompression has now to be considered as the therapy of first choice for those younger than 60 years, regardless of the affected hemisphere.

This consideration is in line with the results of the only study that has compared effectiveness of decompressive surgery and hypothermia in controlling intracranial hypertension and reducing mortality. In this study, a total of 36 patients with severe acute ischemic stroke were treated with hemicraniectomy (n = 17) or moderate hypothermia (n = 19). Age, baseline NIHSS score, sex, cranial CT findings, level of consciousness, and time to treatment were similar in the two groups. Mortality was 12% for the hemicraniectomy group and 47% for the moderate hypothermia group; 1 patient treated with moderate hypothermia died of treatment complication (sepsis), and 3 of ICP crises that occurred during rewarming. The researchers concluded that in patients with acute ischemic stroke, hemicraniectomy is associated with lower rates of both mortality and complications than moderate hypothermia.[255]

New clinical applications for hypothermia may therefore focus on the early neuroprotective effect rather than the potential to decrease brain edema and ICP. As mentioned previously, the studies so far conducted on hypothermia in ischemic stroke did not focus on neuroprotection. Promising data derive from two studies in patients after cardiac arrest.[198,199] The positive results of these studies led to inclusion of hypothermia in current guidelines for resuscitation. However, limiting factors for large-scale clinical application of early hypothermia for neuroprotection in acute ischemic stroke include the question about the required depth of hypothermia and thereby its feasibility in awake patients. Until now hypothermia has been restricted to intubated and sedated patients. The use of hypothermia in ischemic stroke remains experimental, and no evidence-based recommendation can currently be given.

Blood Pressure Management

Blood pressure management is a critical issue in the treatment of acute stroke. Both hypertension and hypotension can be associated with poor outcome after stroke.[256] Theoretical reasons to lower blood pressure in the acute phase are decreasing the risk of severe hemorrhagic transformation, especially after thrombolysis, to prevent further cardiovascular damage and eventually to diminish the formation of brain edema. On the other hand, it is feared that aggressive reduction of blood pressure may negatively affect cerebral perfusion, especially in the penumbra, and thereby enlarge ischemic damage of the brain. Furthermore, it has to be kept in mind that in a majority of patients, blood pressure spontaneously declines during the first hours after stroke. The additional effect of sedative medication may enhance this effect in ICU patients.

A systematic review of blood pressure management in acute stroke has failed to provide evidence that active management of blood pressure influences patient outcomes.[257] In the absence of conclusive, evidence-based data, current guidelines recommend cautious initiation of treatment when systolic or diastolic blood pressure exceeds 220 mm Hg or 120 mm Hg, respectively, or in the presence of other medical factors that may require lowering of blood pressure, such as cardiac insufficiency and pulmonary edema.[80,212] Lower thresholds apply for patients after intravenous or intraarterial thrombolysis. Special caution is required in patients with hemodynamic causes of stroke. No specific antihypertensive agent can be recommended (see previous discussion). However, intravenous application should be preferred for better controllability. The use of sublingual administration of nifedipine is discouraged because of the potential for a prolonged and precipitous effect. Larger studies on blood pressure management in ischemic stroke are currently ongoing.[258]

On the basis of experimental data, induced hypertension to increase CBF in potentially salvageable tissue seems attractive based on experimental data.[259] In a preliminary report, Rordorf et al[259a] observed an improvement of the NIHSS score in 7 of 13 patients with acute stroke during phenylephrine infusion and were able to establish a blood pressure threshold for this improvement in 6 patients. Hillis et al[260] performed serial DWI and perfusion-weighted MRI (PWI) studies before and during the period of induced hypertension. After 3 days, patients who were treated with induced hypertension showed an improvement in neurologic status, no further change in DWI lesion volume and a reduction of PWI abnormality. Finally, Schwarz et al[260a] examined the influence of sudden increases in MAP, which were induced by norepinephrine, during 47 monitoring sessions in 19 patients with severe ischemic stroke. These investigators noted a slight increase in ICP, accompanied by significant increases in CPP and in mean flow velocity of the MCA supplying the affected hemisphere. No hemorrhagic complications or other side effects were observed. However, those data are preliminary, and evaluation through further studies is therefore warranted before elevation of blood pressure is implemented in clinical routine.

Acute Basilar Artery Occlusion

Occlusion of the basilar artery is cause of the most desolate strokes and associated with a grave prognosis; early studies reported a mortality rate of up to 90%.[261-263] Without treatment the chances for survival or independent outcome are negligible. Survival depends mainly on immediate recanalization.[264] The clinical presentation consists of sudden onset of severe motor and bulbar symptoms, such as tetraplegia, ophthalmoplegia, and dysarthria, combined with reduced consciousness. A gradual or stuttering course may occur as well.

A 2006 meta-analysis compared intravenous thrombolysis (IVT) (n = 76) with intraarterial thrombolysis (IAT) (n = 344) for basilar artery occlusion.[265] Although IAT using recombinant tissue-type plasminogen activator (rt-PA) was associated with a significantly higher recanalization rate (65%) than IVT (53%), survival rates were equal (76% and 78%, respectively). A total of 24% of patients receiving IAT and 22% receiving IVT had good outcomes. Without recanalization, the likelihood of good outcome was close to zero (2%). The researchers thus draw two main conclusions: (1) the route of drug delivery does not make a difference in clinical outcome and (2) the chances of recanalization, without which a favorable outcome seems impossible, were slightly higher after IAT. Therefore, centers that have 24-hour interventional neuroradiology should employ IAT. Moreover, the intraarterial approach offers mechanical options like percutaneous transluminal angioplasty (PTA), stenting, and catheter devices for thrombus extraction.[266] However, centers without interventional neuroradiology availability should not delay treatment but immediately start IVT.

Eckert et al[267] compared the combined approach employing intravenous application of the platelet GP IIb/IIIa antagonist abciximab, intraarterial recombinant tissue-type plasminogen activator (rt-PA), and additional PTA/stenting with a historical control group that was treated with intraarterial rt-PA monotherapy.[267] The combined therapy showed a trend toward better neurologic outcome (34% versus 17%) and a significantly lower mortality rate (38% versus 68%). The rationale for applying antiplatelet agents and/or immediate PTA/stenting is to prevent reocclusion. Reocclusion rates of 17% have been reported during IAT.[268] Reocclusion may be a reason why in the meta-analysis discussed previously, there was no significant benefit of IAT in survival rates despite significantly higher recanalization rates.

There is no established time window for recanalization therapy in basilar artery occlusion; however, aggressive treatment more than 12 hours after onset of symptoms or in patients already presenting with complete loss of brainstem reflexes seems not to be justified.

Our routine emergency protocol for patients with reduced consciousness and suspected acute basilar occlusion includes immediate CT with CT angiography. If CT angiography confirms the clinical diagnosis, a bridging IVT therapy with rt-PA is started in combination with intravenous application of the platelet GP IIb/IIIa antagonist tirofiban; the patient is immediately transferred to angiography for IAT with rt-PA. Owing to reduction of consciousness, most patients have already been intubated and mechanically ventilated in the emergency department. Patients who are still awake are intubated for the angiography procedure; short-acting sedatives such as propofol and remifentanil should be preferred for immediate neurologic assessment following the procedure in order to estimate prognosis. Postangiography radiologic assessment includes CT or MRI to exclude intracerebral hemorrhage. All patients with acute basilar artery occlusion are transferred to the ICU.

Cerebellar Infarction

Cerebellar infarction accounts for 1.9% to 10.5% of cases in clinicopathologic series of patients with cerebral infarctions. Neurologic deterioration occurs as a result of a growing mass effect of the infarcted cerebellum in the posterior fossa. Therefore, patients with signs of increased pressure in the posterior fossa on cranial CT should be carefully monitored in a neurocritical care unit. One must always bear in mind that deterioration in such a patient can occur within minutes, although the clinical condition prior to this point can appear stable or even to be improving. Although there seems to be a maximum of deterioration of consciousness around the third day within ictus,[269] deterioration can occur any time within the first 2 weeks after onset of a cerebellar infarct and may be later than that in supratentorial stroke, indicating the need for prolonged monitoring in conservatively treated patients with cerebellar infarcts.

No controlled study has yet assessed the efficacy of decompressive surgery for cerebellar infarctions. Nevertheless, this is an important issue, because increasing mass effect of the infarcted cerebellum in the posterior fossa can lead to clinical deterioration and brainstem compression. Identifying patients with cerebellar infarctions who are bound to experience intracranial hypertension is not always straightforward; prognostic factors include underlying size of the infarction, hemorrhagic transformation, and poor collateral blood flow. One must keep in mind that neurologic deterioration can also be caused by occlusive hydrocephalus or progression of concurrent brainstem infarction. Close clinical monitoring and frequent CT scanning to estimate the severity of obstructive hydrocephalus are mandatory. In patients with fast decline of consciousness, decompressive surgery of the posterior fossa—with or without removal of infarcted cerebellar tissue—is significantly better than ventriculostomy.[270,271] Ventriculostomy alone may be a temporary measure, but great care must be taken in such a procedure because it may promote ascending herniation. We do not use this approach in patients with additional basilar artery thrombosis and large brainstem infarcts.

Because it is often difficult to clearly distinguish the mechanisms leading to further clinical deterioration, testing of somatosensory evoked potentials (SSEPs) and brainstem auditory evoked potentials (BAEPs) provide further information for treatment decisions. Patients with normal BAEP and SSEP results are usually treated with osmotherapeutics. Prolonged interpeak latencies in BAEPs and altered amplitudes in SSEPs may indicate the need for decompressive surgery. Ventriculostomy is the treatment of choice in patients with CT findings indicating hydrocephalus alone.

Spontaneous Intracerebral Hemorrhage

ICH accounts for 10% to 17% of all strokes.[214] In retrospective studies, mortality within the first month was between 35% and 52%; only 20% of patients regained functional independence by 6 months. Volume of ICH, GCS score on admission, age more than 80 years, infratentorial origin of ICH, and presence of intraventricular blood have been identified as independent predictors of 30-day mortality.[272] However, implementation of do-not-resuscitate orders in patients with ICH may have led to self-fulfilling prophecies and to a pessimistic overestimation of prognosis in ICH. Of importance, it has been shown that treatment within specialized neurologic intensive care units can decrease the mortality rate to 28% to 38%, compared with 25% to 83% for patients treated in general intensive care units.[273] Moreover, there has been a large increase in clinical trials of ICH, providing hope for new and effective treatments for patients with ICH. Because more than half of patients with ICH require intubation and mechanical ventilation,[2] the neurointensivist must know these options to be able to make meaningful therapeutic decisions in time.

Three pathophysiologic concepts are considered of high importance for intensive care treatment of patients with ICH and have been the target of later studies. First, ICH is a dynamic process; in about one third of patients, substantial hematoma enlargement occurs within the first 24 hours[274] and is visualized in up to 70% of patients in whom CT is performed within 3 hours after onset of symptoms.[275] Although it remains unclear whether this enlargement is due to rebleeding or continuous bleeding, hemorrhage growth has been shown to be an independent determinant of mortality and functional outcome after ICH.[275] Each 1-mL growth of hematoma has been associated with a 7% increase in risk of death or disability.[275,276] Thus, attenuation of hematoma growth is a major therapeutic strategy. Second, a low-density region develops frequently surrounding the hematoma. Thrombin and several serum proteins were suggested to trigger an inflammatory reaction in the perihematomal zone.[277-279] Additionally, Sansing et al[280] have proposed that interaction of thrombin with factors released from activated platelets at the site of hemorrhage increases vascular permeability, thereby contributing to the development of edema. Parallel to ICH enlargement, perihematomal edema seems to grow during the first 24 hours.[281] Furthermore, significant, delayed edema growth can occur up to 2 weeks after ictus. The prognostic and pathophysiologic significance of brain edema in ICH remains controversial. Edema volume has not been independently associated with worse outcome but was associated with increased mass effect and neurologic deterioration in one study.[282] On the other hand, another group has found an association between early edema size relative to hemorrhage volume and good outcome.[283] Also, 36% to 50% of patients with ICH have additional IVH. Intraventricular blood volume was found to be significantly associated with mortality at 30 days; concomitant hydrocephalus was identified as an independent predictor of early mortality.[284]

Therapeutic strategies for ICH therefore must first target cessation of hematoma enlargement and prevention of deleterious consequences of mass effect evoked by the hemorrhage itself and the surrounding edema. Development of hydrocephalus has to be monitored, and adequate measures such as placement of an extraventricular drain must be taken in time.

Medical Treatment

Considering aforementioned prognostic significance, hematoma expansion seems an ideal therapeutic target. Thus the use of hemostatic agents has been tried in ICH and SAH with various agents, including tranexamic acid, ε-aminocaproic acid, and aprotinin, with disappointing results. *Recombinant activated factor VII* (rFVIIa) was originally developed for patients with hemophilia, in whom it was applied to stop intracerebral bleeding. It acts locally at the sites of tissue injury and vascular wall disruption by binding to tissue factor. It thus generates small amounts of thrombin sufficient to activate platelets. At higher doses, rFVIIa directly activates factor X on the surfaces of activated platelets, leading to a thrombin burst and acceleration of coagulation. Following two small prospective, randomized dose-escalating phase 2a trials, a larger phase 2 trial was performed involving 399 patients with spontaneous ICH. Patients were randomly assigned to treatment with 40, 80, or 160 µg/kg rFVIIa within 4 hours of ictus. Compared with placebo, treatment with rFVIIa limited hematoma expansion, decreased mortality, and improved 3-month clinical outcome; a 5% increase in arterial thromboembolic events was found within the group receiving the highest dose. The results lead to initiation of a larger phase 3 trial[285] that included 841 patients within 3 hours of ICH onset; patients with a GCS score less than 5 were excluded: 268 patients were randomly assigned to placebo, 276 patients to receive 20 µg/kg rFVIIa, and 297 patients to receive 80 µg/kg rFVIIa within 4 hours of stroke. At 24 hours, treatment with 80 µg/kg significantly reduced hemorrhage growth in comparison with placebo (26% versus 11%), corresponding to a moderate but statistically significant reduction of 3.8 mL in the volume of growth compared with placebo. Total final lesion volumes at 72 hours were similar in the three groups. There were no significant differences in survival or functional outcome among the three groups. The overall frequency of thromboembolic serious adverse events was similar in the three groups; however, arterial events were significantly more frequent in the 80-µg rFVIIA group than in the placebo group. The investigators point out imbalances between groups, with a higher rate of intraventricular extension in the treatment group; moreover, they attribute the disappointing results mainly to the fact that the placebo group had much more favorable outcome than the placebo group of the previous phase 2a trial (mortality 19% versus 29%; mRS score 5 and 6, 24% versus 45%). However, other studies on neuroprotective treatment in ICH found comparably low mortality rates.[286,287] Thus, outcomes of ICH may have improved because of advances in neurointensive care. Other investigators have pointed out that special subgroups need to be defined who may benefit from different treatments. For example, rFVIIa treatment within an earlier time window may prove beneficial for outcome. However, of 8886 patients screened, only 841 were eligible for the phase 3 rFVIIa study. Ultra-early treatment will require a high level of logistics in primary care of patients with ICH.

Blood Pressure Management

Severe hypertension is commonly observed in patients with acute ICH. On the basis of the available evidence, no general conclusion can be drawn about the optimal blood pressure management in patients with hemorrhagic stroke. Current guidelines recommend maintaining systolic blood pressure lower than 180 mm Hg and diastolic blood pressure lower than 105 mm Hg. MAP should not exceed 130 to 120 mm Hg.[202,214] Importance was placed on selecting a target blood pressure on the basis of individual patient factors, such as baseline blood pressure, history of hypertension, presumed cause of hemorrhage, age, and elevated ICP.

Two main pathophysiologic considerations have to be weighed against each other. The rationale for lowering blood pressure is to avoid hemorrhagic expansion, which is especially important for hemorrhages caused by aneurysms or arteriovenous malformations. On the other hand, aggressive lowering of blood pressure bears the theoretical risk of inducing ischemia in the edematous region adjacent to the hemorrhage.

Studies underlining and mitigating the importance of both principles have been published so far. However, little prospective evidence has been available to clearly support a specific blood pressure threshold. Several questions remain unresolved:

- Does hypertension promote hemorrhage growth? Or is it rather a bystander effect of hematoma enlargement? Does reduction of blood pressure result in better patient outcome?

- Is autoregulation impaired in ICH? If so, does overaggressive treatment of blood pressure decrease CPP and thereby worsen brain injury and finally patient outcome? What are the mechanisms involved?

A randomized pilot trial has investigated the relation between blood pressure and hemorrhage growth[276]; results from this trial will probably be considered in future guidelines. Patients with spontaneous ICH were included within 6 hours of onset and randomly assigned to early intensive lowering of blood pressure with a target systolic blood pressure of 140 mm Hg (n = 203) or guideline-based management (n = 201) with a target systolic blood pressure of 180 mm Hg. Mean baseline hematoma volumes were 14.2 mL and 12.7 mL, respectively. Mean blood pressure in the first hour was 153 mm Hg in the intensive group versus 167 mm Hg in the guideline group. Within the first 24 hours, blood pressure values were 146 mm Hg and 157 mm Hg, respectively. At 24 hours, mean proportional hematoma growth was 36.3% in the guideline group versus 13.7 % in the intensive group. The mean absolute difference in hematoma volume between both groups was 1.7 mL at 24 hours (compared with ≈4 mL difference between treatment and control groups in the rFVIIa studies). The effect of aggressive blood pressure lowering on clinically meaningful outcomes such as death and disability remains to be investigated. Although Davis et al[275] could show that for each 10% increase in hematoma growth, there was a 5% increase in hazard of death and a 16% greater likelihood of worsening by 1 point on the mRS, attenuation of hematoma growth may not translate into clinical outcome, as was found in the latest rFVIIa study.[285]

Although prospective studies in animals and humans have challenged the concept of major ischemia in the perihematomal edema,[71,288] human MRI and single-photon emission CT data indicate the existence of a rim of tissue at risk for secondary ischemia in large hematomas with elevated ICP.[289,290] Yet, later MRI and CT studies again have dispelled this concept.[291,292] Few data are available to date with respect to autoregulation in ICH. In a human positron emission tomography study, Powers et al[288] found that reduction in MAP by 15% (mean 142 ± 10 to 119 ± 11 mm Hg) did not result in CBF reduction. In an earlier single-photon emission CT study, Kuwata et al[293] reported that autoregulation in the perihematomal zone seemed to be preserved in the acute phase; however, global CBF significantly dropped in both hemispheres after reducing MAP was reduced by more than 20%. It may be relevant to consider that patients with stroke frequently suffer from chronic hypertension and their brain autoregulatory curve may be shifted to the right. Although CBF remains constant for MAP levels between 50 and 120 mm Hg in normal individuals, patients with chronic hypertension can be at risk for critical hypoperfusion at MAP levels that would be tolerated by normal individuals. The same holds true for patients with elevated ICP. Mainly on the basis of data from patients with traumatic brain injury and one study in patients with ICH, current guidelines recommend a preservation of a CPP higher than 60 mm Hg.[294,295] However, as discussed previously, further research is to be done in the field with respect to studies claiming that optimal CPP may differ among patients and should be determined by autoregulatory parameters.[132]

Appropriate agents for blood pressure management were discussed earlier.

Coagulation and Reversal of Anticoagulation

Early assessment and correction of the coagulation status of a patient with ICH are particularly important, because this parameter may affect both the progression of cerebral bleeding and the incidence of early rebleeding. A therapeutic dilemma arises in patients with anticoagulant-associated ICH and an underlying condition associated with a high risk of recurrent embolism. Between 0.3% and 0.6% of patients undergoing warfarin anticoagulation suffer ICH, risk factors for which include age, intensity of anticoagulation, and leukoaraiosis. However, the annual risk of 5% to 10% for a thromboembolic complication without anticoagulation in patients with prosthetic valves can be translated as a 2-week risk of 0.2% to 0.4%, which should be weighed against a rather high risk of early rebleeding.[214,296]

Patients with a prolonged activated partial thromboplastin time because of heparin therapy should be treated with protamine sulfate, 1 mg/100 IU of heparin, adjusted to the time since last heparin use (30-60 minutes, 0.5-0.75 mg/IU; 60-120 minutes, 0.375-0.5 mg/IU; >120 minutes, 0.25-0.375 mg/IU[202]). The total dose should not exceed 50 mg, and the infusion rate should be less than 5 mg/min; eventually prothrombin complex concentrates (PCCs) or fresh frozen plasma (FFP) may be added. LMWHs are increasingly employed for anticoagulation in clinical practice. However, there is no uniformly effective or specific antidote to reverse bleeding complications. Protamine sulfate only partially antagonizes the anticoagulant effects of LMWHs. PCCs have proved more efficient.[297] A prolonged prothrombin time due to phenprocoumon or warfarin therapy should be reversed with intravenous PCC, FFP, or both. Dosages and composition of factors of PCC largely vary among products, and details should be obtained from the manufacturer. For FFP, the following approximation can be applied: 10 mL/kg will reduce an INR of 4.2 to 2.4, an INR of 3.0 to 2.1, or an INR of 2.4 to 1.8; reducing an INR of 4.2 to 1.4 would therefore require 40 mL/kg.[214] Treatment must be combined with vitamin K₁ (1-2 × 5-10 mg IV), because the half-lives of phenprocoumon (7 days) and warfarin (24 hours) exceed those of vitamin K–dependent factors. Currently, there are no randomized clinical trials comparing PCC with FFP. The use of FFP may require infusion of relatively large volumes of plasma. The necessary time for infusion may allow hematoma enlargement and can lead to volume overload, at worst provoking heart failure. Moreover, concentration of factors varies among batches, making the degree of effectiveness somewhat unpredictable.[202] PCCs can correct coagulopathy faster when administered in smaller volumes, at the price of a higher risk for thromboembolic complications. Repeated measurements of coagulation status are necessary; INR should be reevaluated 15 minutes after application of PCC. Some reports also suggest the off-label use of rFVIIa to normalize INR in warfarin-associated hemorrhage.[298-300] However,

concerns have been raised, given the potentially larger risk of thromboembolic complications in subjects already prone to embolism.

Re-initiation of anticoagulation primarily concerns patients with a high risk of cardiogenic embolism associated with mechanical heart valves or atrial fibrillation. Current guidelines have summarized the available data as follows: In 114 patients from three clinical series, antagonizing anticoagulation with FFP and discontinuation of warfarin for a mean of 7 to 10 days was associated with embolism in 5% of patients. Rebleeding upon re-institution of anticoagulation between days 7 and 10 occurred in 1 patient (0.8%). Seven additional clinical series involving 78 patients used PCC for reversal of anticoagulation, resulting in 5% of thromboembolic events; hematoma expansion occurred in 6%.[202] These limited data suggest that reversal of anticoagulation with FFP or PCC seems to be safe in patients with high risk for cardioembolic events; re-initiation of warfarin appears to be safe within the first 7 to 14 days.

Symptomatic ICH is one of the most severe complications of thrombolytic therapy. According to American Heart Association guidelines,[202] currently recommended options include infusion of platelets (6 to 8 U) and cryoprecipitate containing factor VIII. However, these guidelines are not evidence-based; we routinely use ε-aminocaproic acid (5 g over 15 to 30 min) and cryoprecipitate for ICH associated with thrombolytic therapy.

Surgery

ICH comprises a heterogeneous group of pathologic conditions. Thus, the underlying origin and the location of hemorrhage as well as the neurologic status on presentation have to be carefully considered in the decision for or against surgical treatment. With respect to surgery, one classically distinguishes between supratentorial and infratentorial ICHs. Another important question is the presence or absence of intraventricular extension and concomitant hydrocephalus. In the following we summarize surgical approaches for "spontaneous" supratentorial and infratentorial nonaneurysmal ICH, the treatment of hydrocephalus and IVH. The neurointensivist frequently and urgently is confronted with these therapeutic decisions. Special considerations regarding ICH caused by arteriovenous malformation or cavernous angiomas are discussed in another chapter.

The rationale for *clot evacuation in supratentorial ICH* consists in alleviation of pressure exerted by the hematoma on the surrounding tissue. Large hemorrhages may result in elevated ICP, eventually followed by midline shift, brainstem compression, and herniation; smaller hematomas may compromise perfusion in the surrounding tissue and thereby promote secondary brain injury. The evidence for a zone of hypoperfusion surrounding the hematoma has been discussed previously. Experimental studies have shown that removal of the mass lesion improved perfusion in the surrounding brain tissue.[301,302] The three main questions with regard to surgery in supratentorial ICH are in whom, how, and when to operate.

Despite completion of a large, multicenter randomized trial, the indication for surgery in supratentorial ICH

TABLE 52-4 SUMMARY OF SURGICAL TRIALS FOR SPONTANEOUS INTRACRANIAL HEMORRHAGE

Study or Subcategory	Treatment (n/N)	Control (n/N)	Peto OR 95% CI	Weight (%)	Peto OR (95% CI)
McKissock et al, 1961	58/80	46/91		9.83	1.81 (1.01–3.27)
Auer et al, 1989	21/50	46/91		5.54	0.32 (0.15–0.71)
Juvela et al, 1989	12/26	10/26		2.88	1.36 (*0.46–4.05)
Batjer et al, 1990	4/8	11/13		0.94	0.20 (0.03–1.33)
Chen et al, 1992	15/64	11/63		4.64	1.44 (0.61–3.40)
Morgenstern et al, 1998	3/17	4/17		1.27	0.71 (0.14–3.63)
Zuccarello et al, 2000	2/9	3/11		0.87	0.77 (0.11–5.62)
Cheng et al, 2001	26/266	34/234		11.73	0.64 (0.37–1.09)
Teernstra et al, 2003	20/36	20/34		3.87	0.88 (0.34–2.25)
Hosseini et al, 2003	3/20	9/17		1.84	0.19 (0.05–0.72)
Hattori et al, 2004	9/121	20/121		5.70	0.42 (0.209–0.92)
Mendelow et al, 2005	173/477	189/505		50.88	0.95 (0.73–1.23)
Total (95% CI)	1183	1182		100.00	0.85 (0.71–1.02)

Total events: 346 treatment, 392 control
Test for heterogeneity: $\chi^2 = 26.29$, df = 11 ($P = .006$), F = 58.2%
Test for overall effect: Z = 1.73 ($P = .08$)

0.1 0.2 0.5 1 2 5 10
Favors treatment   Favors control

CI, confidence interval; OR, odds ratio.
Adapted from Steiner T, Kaste M, Forsting M, et al: Recommendations for the management of intracranial haemorrhage - part I: Spontaneous intracerebral haemorrhage. The European Stroke Initiative Writing Committee and the Writing Committee for the EUSI Executive Committee. *Cerebrovasc Dis* 22:294-316, 2006.

itself, the optimal technique, and best timing are still uncertain. The results of a meta-analysis of 12 prospective RCTs on surgery in supratentorial ICH are summarized in Table 52-4. The largest trial so far has been the International Surgical Trial in Intracerebral Hemorrhage (STICH) which was published in 2005.[303] This trial involved 1033 patients from 83 centers, 503 of whom were randomly assigned to early surgery and 530 to initial best conservative treatment (later evacuation was allowed if necessary and took place in about a quarter of patients) on the basis of the "uncertainty principle." Patients were eligible for inclusion if they had spontaneous, supratentorial ICH with onset of symptoms within 72 hours and the responsible neurosurgeon was uncertain about the benefit of either—medical or surgical—treatment. Patients with a GCS score less than 5 and clots smaller than 2 cm were preferentially excluded. Upon inclusion, hematoma evacuation by the method of choice of the responsible neurosurgeon had to be undertaken within 24 hours. Primary outcome measures were mortality and disability at 6 months as measured by the extended Glasgow Outcome Scale (GOS), using a parallel-group trial design that divided patients into good and poor prognosis groups with differing definitions of favorable outcome. In the intention-to-treat analysis, no significant difference regarding favorable outcome between the surgical (26% favorable outcome) and conservative (24% favorable outcome) groups was found. Surgery within 96 hours was associated with a statistically insignificant absolute benefit of 2.3% in 6-month outcome. The same statistically insignificant trend in favor of surgery was found for the

other outcome parameters—mortality, mRS score, and BI. Thus, early surgery offered no benefit over initial conservative treatment. However, a subgroup analysis identified that patients with superficial, lobar hematomas (1 cm or less from cortical surface) and those with GCS scores of 9 to 12 were more likely to benefit from surgery, but the difference did not reach statistical significance. In contrast, of patients presenting in coma with initial GCS score ≤ 8, nearly all had unfavorable outcomes; early surgery even raised the relative risk for poor outcome by 8%, suggesting that surgery is probably harmful in this subgroup of patients.

These results need to be interpreted with respect to those of the previous randomized trials. Taking the available evidence into account, current treatment strategies largely depend on (1) hemorrhage size and location and (2) clinical impairment and course of neurologic symptoms. Table 52-5 summarizes our current procedure regarding surgical or nonsurgical treatment in special subgroups of patients.

Other approaches apart from standard craniotomy—chosen by the majority of surgeons in the STICH trial—comprise stereotactic or endoscopic aspiration of hematomas and thrombolytic therapy of intracerebral or intraventricular blood clots. These techniques offer promise (Auer 1989, Zuccarello 1999) but have not yet been validated in randomized clinical trials.

As for indication and surgical technique, the question about the ideal timing of intervention remains unresolved. Despite promising results from an early report[304] on clot extraction of putaminial hemorrhages

TABLE 52-5 RECOMMENDATIONS FOR SURGICAL OR NONSURGICAL TREATMENT OF INTRACEREBRAL HEMORRHAGE (ICH)

Location of ICH	Clinical and/or CT Features	Treatment
Putamen	Alert, small ICH (<30 mL)	Nonsurgical
	Comatose, large ICH (>60 mL)	Nonsurgical
	Drowsy, intermediate ICH (30-60 mL)	Consider evacuation
Caudate	Alert or drowsy, with intraventricular hemorrhage and hydrocephalus	Consider ventriculostomy
Thalamus	Drowsy or lethargic, with blood in the 3rd ventricle and hydrocephalus	Consider ventriculostomy
Lobar white matter	Drowsy or lethargic, with intermediate ICH (20-60 mL), progressive decline in level of consciousness	Consider evacuation
Pons, midbrain, medulla	—	Nonsurgical
Cerebellum	Noncomatose, with ICH >3 cm in diameter, and/or hydrocephalus, and/or effacement of quadrigeminal cistern	Evacuation recommended, preceded by ventriculostomy if status is actively deteriorating

within 7 hours of ictus, a subsequent single-center randomized trial provided evidence for an increased of risk of rebleeding in 4 of 11 patients who underwent ultra-early surgery, less than 4 hours after ictus. Results in the same study were better for patients operated in the 12-hour time frame.[305] Mortality rate in these patients was 18%, compared with 29% in the conservative arm. However, this finding did not translate into improved functional outcome. In another small study, patients randomly allocated to surgery underwent clot evacuation during the first 9 hours after symptom onset. No difference in outcome and mortality from medical treatment was found.[306] In the STICH trial, the average time from the onset of symptoms to surgery was 30 hours, and only 16% of patients were treated within 12 hours. In summary, no clear evidence indicates that ultra-early surgery improves functional outcome. In contrast, delayed evacuation by craniotomy seems to offer little benefit, even more so in comatose patients with deep hemorrhage.

Corresponding to the uncertainty about the pathophysiologic role of brain edema in ICH, only little evidence has been published about *decompressive surgery (hemicraniectomy) for supratentorial ICH*. Murthy et al[307] report on 12 patients with supratentorial hypertensive ICH who underwent hematoma evacuation and decompressive hemicraniectomy. Of 11 surviving patients, 6 had a good functional outcome (mRS score ≤3) at a mean follow-up time of 17 months. In another small study on clot evacuation in patients with primary supratentorial hemorrhage, in 15 patients in whom progression of brain swelling was anticipated, decompressive craniectomy was performed after clot removal. The combination of decompressive craniectomy and hematoma evacuation showed promising results in a subgroup of severely compromised patients.[308]

Unlike with supratentorial hematomas, the indication for surgery in *cerebellar hematomas* is undisputed, despite the complete lack of prospective trials. A class I recommendation of the current American Heart Association guidelines states that patients with cerebellar hemorrhage larger than 3 cm and neurologic deterioration or brainstem compression and/or hydrocephalus from

ventricular obstruction should undergo surgical removal of the hemorrhage as soon as possible.[202] This recommendation is based on nonrandomized series of patients reporting good outcomes for surgically treated patients with cerebellar hemorrhages larger than 3 cm, hydrocephalus, or brainstem compression. Medical management of patients with smaller hemorrhages without signs of brainstem compression as decrease in vigilance seems to be justified.[309,310]

No recommendation can be made for surgical evacuation of brainstem hematomas, because the tissue destruction caused by the initial bleeding precludes any benefit. Anecdotal reports of successful surgical treatment of hematomas located in the vicinity of the fourth ventricle constitute neurosurgical rarities.

Intraventricular Hemorrhage and Hydrocephalus

One differentiates between primary and secondary intraventricular hemorrhage. Primary IVH constitutes a distinct entity; it originates from intraventricular structure such as the choroid plexus. Symptoms are similar to those of SAH (severe headache of acute onset, neck stiffness, depressed level of consciousness), although motor deficit usually is either absent or minimal. Prognosis is more benign than that of secondary IVH.[311] Secondary IVH occurs in up to 40% of all patients with ICH and in up to 20% of all patients with SAH. There is strong evidence that IVH contributes to mortality after cerebral hemorrhage. Retrospective studies identified the presence and amount of intraventricular blood, time to clearance of the ventricles, and development of hydrocephalus as independent predictors of poor outcome.[284,312] Hydrocephalus due to IVH develops via two different pathomechanisms. In the acute phase, obstruction of the third and fourth ventricles results in obstructive hydrocephalus. Later, malresorptive hydrocephalus may occur owing to loss of function of pacchionian granulations. Typically, decline in the level of consciousness is the major symptom of a developing hydrocephalus.

External ventricular drainage (EVD) is the treatment of choice that lowers the ICP immediately. Typically, the

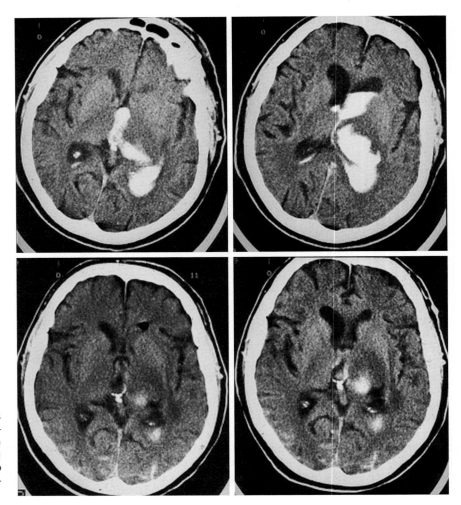

Figure 52-5 Intraventricular thrombolysis after basal ganglia hemorrhage with intraventricular bleeding. Time course of therapy with recombinant tissue-plasminogen activator (rt-PA) for thrombolysis of intraventricular blood. *Top row*, before treatment; *bottom row*, after treatment.

EVD is placed ipsilateral to the hemorrhage. In case of occlusion of the foramina of Monro, bilateral placement of EVDs may become necessary. The drainage has to be continued until the ventricular clot has dissolved, and CSF circulation normalized. Although a lifesaving procedure, placement of a ventricular drainage does not affect the clot resolution or the incidence of communicating hydrocephalus. Therefore, IVT was proposed as an effective measure to hasten the resolution of the intraventricular blood clot, reduce the duration of extraventricular drainage, decrease the severity and incidence of communicating hydrocephalus, and lower IVH-associated mortality. Clinical experience with this approach has grown over the last years.[313-315] The use of urokinase or streptokinase has been widely replaced by administration of rt-PA, dosages varying between 4 and 20 mg.[316] At the moment, one prospective study on intraventricular thrombolysis with rt-PA is ongoing (at www.clearivh.com). This study was preceded by two randomized pilot dose-finding studies employing 1 mg rt-PA every 8 hours until clearing of the third and fourth ventricles or a cumulative dose of 8 mg. The results have not been published so far, but the preliminary data seem promising. Complications that may counteract the advantages of IVT are secondary hemorrhage and EVD infection. Therefore, vascular malformations should be ruled out with either CT angiography or conventional angiography before intraventricular lysis is initiated (Fig. 52-5).

A promising approach to shorten the need for EVD is placement of a lumbar drainage. In a retrospective series including 55 patients with ICH, Huttner et al[317] investigated the effect of placement of lumbar drainage on duration of need for an EVD. Placement of lumbar drainage was performed in patients with persistent hydrocephalus after complete clearing of the third and fourth ventricles. In these cases, a communication between the inner and outer CSF spaces was assumed, and lumbar drainage was performed with clamped EVD. EVD was reopened only when ICP increased. As soon as clamping of the EVD was tolerated for at least 24 hours without an increase in ICP and no enlargement of the ventricles was observed on the CT scan, the EVD was removed. After that, the lumbar drainage was clamped every other day and hydrocephalus was monitored by CT scan. If no hydrocephalus recurred, the lumbar drainage was removed. After five futile attempts to clamp the lumbar drainage, a ventriculoperitoneal shunt was placed. In this small series, placement of a lumbar drainage shortened the duration of required EVD, and the frequency of a ventriculoperitoneal shunt was reduced. The investigators do not report an increased risk for axial herniation or infection.

Subarachnoid Hemorrhage

SAH from the rupture of an intracranial aneurysm is often devastating and accounts for approximately one fourth of all cerebrovascular deaths. Despite great advances in the surgical, endovascular, and intensive care management of patients with aneurysmal SAH, the morbidity and mortality of this disease remain unacceptably high. Only about half of patients admitted to qualified neurocritical care centers with the diagnosis of aneurysmal SAH have a good clinical outcome.[318] Many patients die of the initial bleed or further complications associated with the disease, the most detrimental complications being early rebleeding and vasospasm. Of the survivors, about 50% are left disabled and dependent on the help of others.[319] Because SAH is treatable and even curable at particular stages, management decisions are critical. As the loss of functional independence is a common consequence of aneurysmal bleeding despite surgical clipping or endovascular therapy of the aneurysm, the best medical management may complement efforts to improve outcome.

General Management

The basic goal of intensive care management in acute SAH is to avoid or treat such serious complications as early rebleeding, vasospasm, elevation of ICP through intraparenchymal or subdural hematoma, acute hydrocephalus, and brain swelling. The general ICU management of patients with SAH basically does not differ from that of other patients with stroke. However, there are some special aspects to consider. Positive fluid balance with at least 3000 mL preferably of isotonic crystalloids should be kept to reduce the risk of vasospasm and hyponatremia. Hypotension increases the risk of vasospasm, and delayed ischemia should therefore be avoided.[320] Until the aneurysm is secured, the MAP should not exceed 60 to 90 mm Hg. Systolic blood pressures higher than 160 mm Hg may be associated with increased risk of rerupture of the aneurysm.[321] Because cerebral autoregulation is impaired in SAH, systolic blood pressure values up to 200 mm Hg should be tolerated after the aneurysm is secured, in order to lower the risk of cerebral infarction.[322] Only extreme hypertensive blood pressure values (>200 mm Hg) should be treated with antihypertensives such as urapidil, beta-blockers, clonidine, and angiotensin-converting enzyme inhibitors. In addition, nimodipine or nicardipine may be advantageously used in this setting. In the acute phase, activities that may lead to elevation of blood pressure or ICP should strongly be avoided. Suctioning, transports, and positioning should be accompanied by additive sedation. Effective analgesia is imperative, and mild sedation may be necessary in agitated patients. Stool softeners are prescribed, particularly in patients receiving opioids. Prophylaxis of DVT is provided by stockings or pneumatic compression devices. Low-dose heparin or LMWH should be used in all patients with proposed longer immobilization. Patients requiring catecholamine pressure support should receive preferably low-dose heparin intravenously. However, the potential risks of prophylactic low-dose heparin or LMWH has not been sufficiently studied in patients with SAH.

Nevertheless, in neurosurgical studies including also patients with SAH, low-dose heparin or LMWH was not associated with rebleeding events.[323,324] After endovascular treatment with coils, full-dose heparinization (activated partial thromboplastin time [aPTT] 1.5 to 2×) for 24 hours is needed. Subsequently, antiplatelet therapy (ASA 100 mg) can be started for 6 months. This measure has been found to reduce the rate of ischemic complications following endovascular treatment of aneurysm.[325] If a stent was used for the positioning of the coils, dual-antiplatelet therapy (ASA + clopidogrel) is indicated for 6 months. Prophylactic anticonvulsive treatment is not indicated. Anticonvulsants should be administered individually in high-risk patients or in patients with positive history of seizures.

Fever, a common complication in SAH, is known to negatively affect outcome.[326] Body temperature higher than 38.0° C should be therefore aggressively treated with acetaminophen, paracetamol, or cooling blankets. When temperature is refractory to all therapy, normothermia or hypothermia may be induced as a neuroprotective measure.[327] Hyperglycemia after SAH relates to delayed ischemia and poor outcome and represents another important therapeutic target.[328,329] However, intensive insulin regimens should be applied with caution because insulin-related decrease in cerebral glucose and elevation of anaerobic metabolites have been observed even with normoglycemia or hyperglycemia.[330,331] Nosocomial infection as pneumonia and blood stream infections after SAH are independently associated with poor outcome, so infection control should be applied vigorously.[332]

Rebleeding

In the first few hours after the initial bleed, more than 10% of all patients demonstrate clinical deterioration, suggesting that rebleeding has occurred.[333,334] The mortality rate following rebleeding in patients with SAH is approximately 50%.[335] To date, there is no method for identifying the patients with a higher risk for rebleeding. The probability of rebleeding is about 4% the first day after the bleed and about 1.5% per day thereafter.[336] Overall, the incidence of rebleeding is reportedly 20% in the first 2 weeks and 50% within the first 6 months after the initial bleed.[318,337] After this time, the risk gradually decreases to a level of 3% per year. Several predisposing factors for rebleeding have been identified. They are female gender, early admission after SAH, poor neurologic grade, poor general medical condition, and systolic blood pressure greater than 160 mm Hg.[336]

Antifibrinolytics

Clot formation and tissue damage stimulate fibrinolytic activity in the CSF, thus raising the risk of rebleeding; this observation constituted the rationale for the use of antifibrinolytic drugs. Aminocaproic acid and tranexamic acid were used. A randomized placebo-controlled trial, a nonrandomized trial, and other reports assessing the efficacy of antifibrinolytic therapy showed a significantly lower incidence of rebleeding. However, mortality was not altered with this kind of therapy, which was associated with a higher incidence of ischemic stroke.[338,339]

Important side effects of antifibrinolytic therapy were a greater tendency for bleeding after discontinuation of therapy, diuresis, diarrhea, abdominal discomfort, nausea, and dizziness.[340]

A Cochrane Library review showed no benefit of antifibrinolytics in patients with aneurysmal SAH,[341] but a few later studies are indicating that early, short-term therapy may be effective and safe.[342]

Acute Hydrocephalus

Symptomatic obstructive hydrocephalus occurs in 15% to 20% of patients with SAH.[343] A characteristic history consists of gradual obtundation after a lucid interval of a few hours. Insertion of an external ventricular catheter results in significant improvement within 1 or 2 days, even if it may carry a higher risk of rebleeding. The improvement can be explained by an abrupt decrease of ICP due to CSF drainage. Clinically, a slowly developing hydrocephalus can be assumed in a patient who demonstrates vertical gaze palsy, decline of cognitive functions, and progressive lethargy. Ventriculostomy is especially recommended in patients with Hunt and Hess grades IV or V[344] and may precede the treatment of ruptured aneurysm. A depression in level of consciousness indicates the need for CT scanning. If hydrocephalus is present, ventriculomegaly will be evident. It is best discerned through comparison of the current CT scan with earlier scans. In this situation, an external ventricular shunt is indicated. In patients with large amounts of intraventricular blood, intraventricular fibrinolysis therapy with low doses of rt-PA (2 mg every 12 hours for 3 days) may improve clinical outcome, even though this observation needs confirmation in randomized clinical trials.[315] There is an association of shunt-dependent hydrocephalus with Hunt and Hess grade on admission, incidence of repeated SAH, anterior communicating artery (ACoA) aneurysm, and IVH.[345,346] Lumbar drainage may represent an effective option if an extraventricular drain is needed longer and may be associated with reduction of cerebral vasospasm.[317,347,348]

Vasospasm

Up to 25% of patients with a ruptured aneurysm experience delayed cerebral ischemia, mainly between day 5 and day 14 after the initial bleeding.[335,349] Ischemia is the prominent cause of death and disability after SAH. The total amount of subarachnoid blood is a strong risk factor, but its distribution does not predict the site of ischemia.[350] Thus, vasospasm occurs more commonly in patients with a poor Hunt and Hess grade SAH. The time course of vasospasm is consistent with an immune-mediated response, and later observations suggest that immunologic processes, including activation of the complement system, may be involved. Contraction of the arterial smooth muscle and morphologic changes in the vessel wall and along its endothelial surface occur in response to injury.[351] Studies examining the various components of blood for their potential to produce vasospasm have been reported.[349,351] Many of these components can cause vasospasm, although no single spasmogen has been identified. Other potential contributors to vasospasm are mechanical wall disruption, inflammation, and free radical formation. The clinical presentation of vasospasm is a gradual

process, although it can also be abrupt on rare occasions or insidious with minor transient changes. Patients may complain of increased headache or may manifest meningism, seizures, decreased consciousness, or new focal neurologic deficits. A new deficit can range from a minor paresis to hemiplegia, aphasia, or behavioral change.[352]

The detection of vasospasm is possible with TCD ultrasonography, which demonstrates increased blood flow velocity due to arterial narrowing in the basal cerebral arteries. However, there is uncertainty about the diagnostic specificity of TCD ultrasonography. Only flow velocities greater than 120 to 200 cm/s are highly predictive for the diagnosis of vasospasm.[353] The sensitivity and specificity of TCD ultrasonography in diagnosing vasospasm in comparison with angiography were reported to be adequate in the MCA, but not in the ACA or PCA. Comparison of TCD ultrasonographic findings with regional CBF measurements[354,355] indicates that the sensitivity and specificity of the modality may be inadequate to guide major medical decisions, although it may still be useful as a noninvasive screening tool. TCD ultrasonographic signs of vasospasm are listed in Table 52-6. However, cerebral angiography is the gold standard for the diagnosis of vasospasm and can be both diagnostic and therapeutic. Novel modalities like DWI, DWI/PWI mismatch, single-photon emission CT, perfusion CT, perfusion MRI, and xenon CT in detecting and quantifying vasospasm are under research.[356-359] In contrast to TCD ultrasonography, these methods depict the cerebral perfusion and possibly the tissue at risk and may become increasingly helpful in therapeutic decision making.

Treatment with hypervolemia, hemodilution, and induced hypertension therapy, also called *triple-H therapy*, aims to increase CBF and improve microcirculation by raising systolic blood pressure and cardiac output.[360] In the first larger patient series, reported by Kassell et al,[361] the combination of induced hypertension and volume expansion reversed neurologic deficits in 43 of 58 patients. It is hypothesized that a defect in cerebral autoregulation renders the perfusion of the brain passively dependent on systolic blood pressure. Triple-H therapy is indicated when severe vasospasm is found on TCD ultrasonography or a patient demonstrates progressive neurologic deterioration.

Hypervolemia is induced by infusion of isotonic saline or plasma expanders, aiming at a CVP of 10 to 14 mm

TABLE 52-6 FINDINGS OF TRANSCRANIAL DOPPLER ULTRASONOGRAPHY THAT INDICATE VASOSPASM

Intensity-weighted mean velocity	>3 kHz (120 cm/s) = borderline >4 kHz (160 cm/s) = significant >5 kHz (200 cm/s) = critical
Maximum systolic velocity	>4 kHz (160 cm/s) = relevant >7.5 kHz (300 cm/s) = critical
MCA/ICA index	>3.0
Velocity increase during the first 6 days	>50%/day or >1 kHz (40 cm/s)/day
Pulsatility of signals	Pulsatility index >1.0 Resistance index >0.6

MCA/ICA index, mean carotid artery flow velocity divided by internal carotid artery mean flow velocity.

Hg. If no clinical improvement is achieved, the additional use of vasopressors, such as dobutamine, dopamine, and norepinephrine, should be considered for induced hypertension. Continuous infusion is titrated to achieve a mean increase in arterial blood pressure to 20 to 30 mm Hg above the baseline value, with systolic blood pressure values up to 180 mm Hg. MAP values of 90 to 130 mm Hg and CPP values of 80 to 120 mm Hg should be the targets. Sometimes systolic blood pressure as high as 240 mm Hg is required to achieve adequate CPP. Although catecholamine-based vasopressor therapy is reported to occasionally reverse neurologic deficits, the cerebrovascular and metabolic effects of such agents in this situation are unclear. When catecholamines cross the blood-brain barrier, which is disrupted with vasospasm,[362] they have been reported to produce hypermetabolism and hyperemia in animals. Concomitant infusion of albumin and other fluids also leads to decreases in hematocrit value and blood viscosity. Animal studies have shown that the optimal hematocrit is 33%, because the oxygen-carrying capacity of the blood is not compromised.[363] This concept has been applied to clinical care in determining the endpoint for hemodilution therapy.[364] However, hemodilution remains a controversial component of triple-H therapy, because one study showed that patients with SAH who have higher admission hemoglobin concentration and higher mean hemoglobin value had better outcomes.[365] It seems that certain components of triple-H therapy are more effective than others in reversing delayed ischemia. Hypertension and normovolemia have been reported to improve cerebral oxygenation more effectively and with less complication than hypervolemia/hemodilution.[366,367]

Although the benefit of triple-H therapy has not yet been proven by randomized studies, the rate of permanent ischemic deficits seems to be lower than expected. Triple-H therapy is used either prophylactically or in the phase of reversible neurologic deficit with impending ischemia but without complete infarction.[352,368] However, controversy exists regarding its prophylactic versus therapeutic application.[369] Prophylactic effect of triple-H therapy to prevent vasospasm could not be shown.[370] Some evidence suggests that if infarction is present, triple-H therapy may cause further deterioration.[371] Also, pulmonary and cerebral edema, cardiac dysregulation due to volume overload, myocardial infarction, and the risk of rebleeding seem to be more common with this treatment. The overall incidence of systemic complications associated with triple-H therapy is 7% to 17% for pulmonary edema, 2% for myocardial infarction, 3% to 35% for dilutional hyponatremia, and 3% for coagulopathy.[372,373] Thus, triple-H therapy should be terminated in stepwise fashion as soon as delayed ischemic neurologic deficit resolves. Swan-Ganz catheters may be useful for a better guidance of triple-H therapy. Less invasive pulse contour continuous cardiac output monitoring can be also used effectively to achieve therapeutic targets.[95]

The use of *calcium channel blockers* is based on the assumption that they can reduce the frequency of vasospasm by inhibiting the calcium influx in the smooth muscle cells of the vasculature. Other factors may be preservation of oxidative metabolism, cell membrane stabilization, and microrheologic effects.[374] Nimodipine

or nicardipine is the drug of choice. Nimodipine, which is more commonly used, significantly reduces delayed cerebral ischemia and improves outcome.[375,376] A systematic review of all randomized trials of calcium antagonist therapy in SAH showed a significant reduction in the frequency of poor outcome.[377,378] On the basis of these data, it is generally recommended that all patients with SAH receive nimodipine, 60 mg enterally every 4 to 6 hours or, in Europe, as an initial IV formula (1 mg/h for 1 to 2 hours, followed by continuous infusion of 1 to 6 mg/h); later, oral nimodipine (60 mg, 4-6 times per day) may be given for 2 to 3 weeks after SAH. Side effects include pulmonary right-to-left shunt and hypotension, which affects the coronary blood flow and the digestive tract muscles.

Tirilazad, a potent in vitro inhibitor of free radical–mediated lipid peroxidation, has been studied in several trials.[379-381] The only beneficial effect on outcome was seen in a subgroup of men who were treated with a dosage of 6 mg/kg/day.[379]

Another interesting therapeutic option is the use of *antiplatelet agents* such as aspirin, because several studies have demonstrated an activation of platelets within the first 3 days after SAH. Retrospective data suggest that patients who used salicylates before a hemorrhage had a significantly lower risk for delayed ischemia. Data from a pilot study suggest that this treatment is safe and feasible.[382] In a meta-analysis, antiplatelet drugs were shown to significantly reduce the risk of delayed ischemia with no increase in ICH.[383]

Positive results for the use of magnesium in animal SAH studies have been duplicated in a phase 2 study investigating the effect of 64 mmol magnesium per day in 238 patients with SAH, which showed reduction in delayed ischemia and increase in good outcome at 3 months.[384] These encouraging results should be confirmed in a phase 3 trial that is under way.[385]

The previous use or the initiation of acute *statin therapy* may be effective in reducing vasospasm.[386-388] It is proposed that statins have neuroprotective properties related to the induction of the nitric oxide synthase pathway and immunomodulatory effects. However, the evidence in SAH is limited to small studies. One meta-analysis has shown that statins may significantly reduce the incidence of vasospasm, delayed ischemic deficit, and also mortality.[389]

Endothelin, a potent vasoconstrictor, has been implicated in the pathogenesis of vasospasm. A phase 2a study with clazosentan, an *endothelin receptor A antagonist*, in 34 patients with SAH reported significant reduction of the incidence and severity of vasospasm.[390] Most recently, results from Clazosentan to Overcome Neurological Ischemia and Infarction Occurring After Subarachnoid Hemorrhage (CONSCIOUS-1), a larger trial with clazosentan in 413 patients with SAH, have been published. Clazosentan significantly decreased moderate to severe angiographic vasospasm and showed a trend for reduction in vasospasm-related morbidity and mortality, albeit not significant.[391]

Nicardipine prolonged-release implants are placed to the subarachnoid space preoperatively. However, the evidence supporting their use is still very scarce. In a prospective randomized phase 2a study with 32 patients with SAH, such implants significantly reduced the incidence of angiographic vasospasm, delayed ischemia, and reduced mortality.[392]

The evidence for neuroprotective effects of *hypothermia* is persuasive. Induced mild hypothermia may have some benefit in patients with poor clinical grade who have refractory vasospasms and severe brain edema. Some centers routinely use hypothermia in the early postoperative phase in such patients. However, until now, no evidence on this issue has been published. Mild intraoperative cooling has not been shown to have any benefit in patients with SAH and good clinical grade.[393] In animal experiments, hypothermia reduces hypoperfusion and metabolic alterations in the acute phase of SAH[394] and may represent an option in refractory vasospasm.

Invasive approaches for the treatment of vasospasm include endovascular techniques such as balloon angioplasty, intra-arterial administration of papaverine, and a combination thereof.

Papaverine is an alkaloid compound and a powerful vasodilator. It acts directly on the smooth muscle cells of the arterial wall by transendothelial absorption. *Intraarterial papaverine infusion* is often associated with vasospasm in distal vessels.[395-397] Papaverine may be administered in patients with severe vasospasm who cannot be treated with angioplasty.[398] However, papaverine can transiently produce signs of neurologic deterioration during infusion, depending on the vascular territory infused, such as hemiparesis, seizures, pupillary changes, unconsciousness, increased ICP, and cardiovascular collapse.[399] Doses of approximately 300 mg may be intraarterially infused for 20 minutes to 1 hour. On angiography, notable changes in diameter are observed in 50% of patients, whereas clinical improvement is often less impressive (occurring in about one in four patients). The vasodilatory effect of papaverine is significantly reduced when vasospasm is present for several days and secondary histologic changes of the vessel have already occurred.[400]

Multiple complications and short-lasting effect of papaverine have led to the growing use of *other vasodilators*. In small series, intraarterial nimodipine, nicardipine, verapamil, and milrinone have been tested. Intraarterial nimodipine in a selected patient group resulted in reduction of angiographic vasospasm and increase in cerebral perfusion.[401] Similarly, milrinone infused intra-arterially was effective and safe for reversal of vasospasm after SAH.[402] Recently, intraventricular nicardipine has been used in therapy of refractory vasospasm.[403] However, evidence from controlled studies is still lacking.

When neurologic manifestations of delayed cerebral ischemia due to vasospasm cannot be reversed by medical therapy, balloon catheters may be used to dilate the narrowed arteries. Transluminal *angioplasty* has been shown to effectively reverse angiographic signs of vasospasm of proximal accessible vessels in 75% of cases refractory to conventional treatment with triple-H therapy.[404] The carotid artery, vertebral artery, proximal MCA, and the entire basilar artery can be treated with transluminal angioplasty, whereas this technique does not seem safe to perform beyond the proximal portion of the anterior, middle, and posterior cerebral arteries.[405,406] Results in patients with delayed ischemia who underwent angioplasty for vasospasm were very encouraging.[404,406,407] Delayed treatment as a salvage procedure seems to be less successful. Generally speaking, angioplasty is reserved for patients who have already undergone surgery or endovascular closure of the aneurysm. Obvious complications include rupture of an unclipped aneurysm, vessel rupture, arterial dissection, and vessel occlusion. *Vessel stenting* might be an option for the therapy of massive narrowing of the proximal portions of the three basal cerebral arteries.

Intracisternal fibrinolysis aims to decrease the incidence of symptomatic vasospasm by injection of rt-PA in the basal cistern. Several studies showed that this therapy might decrease vasospasm but does not affect outcome after 3 months.[315,408,409] IVH occurs in up to 20% of patients with SAH. There is strong evidence that IVH contributes to mortality after cerebral hemorrhage or SAH.[410,411] Routine clinical management consists of an external ventricular drainage, which lowers the ICP immediately, but the drainage must be continued until the ventricular clot has dissolved and CSF circulation has normalized. Clotted blood often blocks the drain, necessitating its removal and insertion of a second catheter. Prolonged drainage, however, increases the risk of infection, with higher rates of ventriculitis after the first week of intraventricular catheter placement. The drainage itself prevents acute hydrocephalus but does not affect resolution of the clot or incidence of communicating hydrocephalus. IVT was therefore proposed as an effective measure to hasten the resolution of the intraventricular blood clot, reduce the duration of extraventricular drainage, decrease the extent and incidence of communicating hydrocephalus, and thereby lower the death rate associated with IVH.

Clinical experience with this approach has grown over the last 15 years. However, a wide variety of dosages and substances (urokinase or rt-PA) have been used. To perform intraventricular thrombolysis in patients with a large amount of intraventricular blood after ICH, we use 1 mg rt-PA every 8 hours. A multicenter phase 2 trial (CLEAR-IVH)[412] of intraventricular rt-PA in patients with intraventricular blood after ICH has been presented most recently with astonishing reduction of mortality to 17% versus 65% in the placebo arm (XVIII European Stroke Conference, Nice, 2008).[413] Before the initiation of thrombolysis, vascular malformations and aneurysms must be ruled out with either CTA or conventional angiography.

Decompressive *hemicraniectomy* can improve outcome in patients with severe cerebral edema due to SAH. In small series of SAH patients with intractable brain edema, hemicraniectomy has been shown to improve survival and outcome and represents a useful adjunct modality for management of refractory intracranial hypertension in patients with poor-grade SAH. Patients with progressive brain edema without radiologic signs of infarction and those with hematoma probably benefit most.[414,415]

Extracranial Complications

A variety of extracranial complications arise as direct consequences of the SAH. They include abnormalities in cardiovascular, pulmonary, endocrine, and electrolyte homeostasis. Many of these abnormalities can be attributed to a post-SAH "hyperadrenergic state"—for example, myocardial infarction and cardiac dysrhythmia. Acute pulmonary edema can also result from massive sympathetic discharge. Other complications are gastrointestinal hemorrhage after stress ulcer following SAH.

Serum catecholamine levels rise dramatically after SAH; there seems to be a connection between the peak of vasospasm after SAH and symptom development corresponding to serum catecholamine levels.[416,417] Systemic hypertension can often be seen after SAH and is most likely related to elevations in catecholamine and renin levels secondary to the bleeding.[418] Other causes of hypertension are increased ICP, seizures, pain, agitation, and vasospasm. Severe arterial hypertension is associated with a higher rate of rebleeding, a higher incidence of vasospasm, and death.[419]

Cardiac arrhythmia and electrocardiographic changes are common problems in many patients after SAH. Arrhythmia can sometimes be severe and life-threatening, whereas ECG changes have a broad variety of patterns, some of which indicate myocardial ischemia. Morphologic changes in the ventricular wall consistent with myocardial ischemia have been observed after poor Hunt and Hess grade SAH. Neurogenic pulmonary edema is another rare complication of SAH.

Fluid and sodium imbalance represent a manifestation of hypothalamic dysfunction after SAH, which occurs in about one third of patients. Both hypovolemia and hyponatremia are common.[420,421] The clinical picture can be consistent with the syndrome of inappropriate antidiuretic hormone secretion (SIADH).[38] In addition, the kidney may be unable to retain sodium, an inability consistent with observed rises in atrial natriuretic factor, constituting CSWS.[422]

Invasive Neuromonitoring

Clear guidelines for instituting multimodal monitoring in patients with SAH have not yet been established. ICP monitoring may provide data for appropriate treatment of elevated ICP. However, ICP monitoring to evaluate CPP may not reflect the needs of the individual patient if it is the only method used. There is evidence that the continuous measurement of the partial oxygen pressure of brain ($PtiO_2$) may represent an important alternative in the monitoring of patients with SAH, especially those who are at risk for vasospasm and delayed cerebral ischemia.[119-121] Several experimental and clinical studies have shown that the continuous measurement of the $PbrO_2$ significantly reflects changes in blood oxygenation, ventilation, ICP, and CPP. Additionally, as described previously in this chapter, cerebral microdialysis[122,423] and measurement of regional CBF[424] may be helpful to monitor the clinical course and provide guidance for further therapeutic decisions. Prospective trials of multimodality brain monitoring–guided treatment protocols are needed to demonstrate impact on clinical outcomes.

REFERENCES

1. Mayer SA, Copeland D, Bernardini GL, et al: Cost and outcome of mechanical ventilation for life-threatening stroke, *Stroke* 31:2346-2353, 2000.
2. Gujjar AR, Deibert E, Manno EM, et al: Mechanical ventilation for ischemic stroke and intracerebral hemorrhage: Indications, timing, and outcome, *Neurology* 51:447-541, 1998.
3. Grotta J, Pasteur W, Khwaja G, et al: Elective intubation for neurologic deterioration after stroke, *Neurology* 45:640-644, 1995.
4. Bushnell CD, Phillips-Bute BG, Laskowitz DT, et al: Survival and outcome after endotracheal intubation for acute stroke, *Neurology* 52:1374-1381, 1999.
5. Steiner T, Mendoza G, De Georgia M, et al: Prognosis of stroke patients requiring mechanical ventilation in a neurological critical care unit, *Stroke* 28:711-715, 1997.
6. Burtin P, Bollaert PE, Feldmann L, et al: Prognosis of stroke patients undergoing mechanical ventilation, *Intensive Care Med* 20:32-36, 1994.
7. Holzapfel L, Chevret S, Madinier G, et al: Influence of long-term oro- or nasotracheal intubation on nosocomial maxillary sinusitis and pneumonia: Results of a prospective, randomized, clinical trial, *Crit Care Med* 21:1132-1138, 1993.
8. Salord F, Gaussorgues P, Marti-Flich J, et al: Nosocomial maxillary sinusitis during mechanical ventilation: A prospective comparison of orotracheal versus the nasotracheal route for intubation, *Intensive Care Med* 16:390-393, 1990.
9. Kirkpatrick AW, Meade MO, Mustard RA, et al: Strategies of invasive ventilatory support in ARDS, *Shock* 6(Suppl 1):S17-S22, 1996.
10. Muench E, Bauhuf C, Roth H, et al: Effects of positive end-expiratory pressure on regional cerebral blood flow, intracranial pressure, and brain tissue oxygenation, *Crit Care Med* 33:2367-2372, 2005.
11. Georgiadis D, Schwarz S, Baumgartner RW, et al: Influence of positive end-expiratory pressure on intracranial pressure and cerebral perfusion pressure in patients with acute stroke, *Stroke* 32:2088-2092, 2001.
12. Georgiadis D, Schwarz S, Kollmar R, et al: Influence of inspiration: Expiration ratio on intracranial and cerebral perfusion pressure in acute stroke patients, *Intensive Care Med* 28:1089-1093, 2002.
13. Whited RE: A prospective study of laryngotracheal sequelae in long-term intubation, *Laryngoscope* 94:367-377, 1984.
14. Colice GL, Stukel TA, Dain B: Laryngeal complications of prolonged intubation, *Chest* 96:877-884, 1989.
15. Dunham CM, LaMonica C: Prolonged tracheal intubation in the trauma patient, *J Trauma* 24:120-124, 1984.
16. Scales DC, Thiruchelvam D, Kiss A, et al: The effect of tracheostomy timing during critical illness on long-term survival, *Crit Care Med* 36:2547-2557, 2008.
17. Dunham CM, Ransom KJ: Assessment of early tracheostomy in trauma patients: a systematic review and meta-analysis, *Am Surg* 72:276-281, 2006.
18. Qureshi AI, Suarez JI, Parekh PD, et al: Prediction and timing of tracheostomy in patients with infratentorial lesions requiring mechanical ventilatory support, *Crit Care Med* 28:1383-1387, 2000.
19. Huttner HB, Kohrmann M, Berger C, et al: Predictive factors for tracheostomy in neurocritical care patients with spontaneous supratentorial hemorrhage, *Cerebrovasc Dis* 21:159-165, 2006.
20. Kelly DF, Goodale DB, Williams J, et al: Propofol in the treatment of moderate and severe head injury: a randomized, prospective double-blinded pilot trial, *J Neurosurg* 90:1042-1052, 1999.
21. Aitkenhead AR, Pepperman ML, Willatts SM, et al: Comparison of propofol and midazolam for sedation in critically ill patients, *Lancet* 2:704-709, 1989.
22. Barrientos-Vega R, Mar Sanchez-Soria M, Morales-Garcia C, et al: Prolonged sedation of critically ill patients with midazolam or propofol: Impact on weaning and costs, *Crit Care Med* 25:33-40, 1997.
23. Chamorro C, de Latorre FJ, Montero A, et al: Comparative study of propofol versus midazolam in the sedation of critically ill patients: Results of a prospective, randomized, multicenter trial, *Crit Care Med* 24:932-939, 1996.
24. Shafer A: Complications of sedation with midazolam in the intensive care unit and a comparison with other sedative regimens, *Crit Care Med* 26:947-956, 1998.

25. Weinbroum AA, Halpern P, Rudick V, et al: Midazolam versus propofol for long-term sedation in the ICU: A randomized prospective comparison, *Intensive Care Med* 23:1258-1263, 1997.

26. Stecker MM, Kramer TH, Raps EC, et al: Treatment of refractory status epilepticus with propofol: Clinical and pharmacokinetic findings, *Epilepsia* 39:18-26, 1998.

27. Prasad A, Worrall BB, Bertram EH, et al: Propofol and midazolam in the treatment of refractory status epilepticus, *Epilepsia* 42:380-386, 2001.

28. Bourgoin A, Albanese J, Wereszczynski N, et al: Safety of sedation with ketamine in severe head injury patients: Comparison with sufentanil, *Crit Care Med* 31:711-717, 2003.

29. Albanese J, Arnaud S, Rey M, et al: Ketamine decreases intracranial pressure and electroencephalographic activity in traumatic brain injury patients during propofol sedation, *Anesthesiology* 87:1328-1334, 1997.

30. Bailey PL, Streisand JB, East KA, et al: Differences in magnitude and duration of opioid-induced respiratory depression and analgesia with fentanyl and sufentanil, *Anesth Analg* 70:8-15, 1990.

31. Karabinis A, Mandragos K, Stergiopoulos S, et al: Safety and efficacy of analgesia-based sedation with remifentanil versus standard hypnotic-based regimens in intensive care unit patients with brain injuries: A randomised, controlled trial (ISRCTN50308308), *Crit Care* 8:R268-R280, 2004.

32. Tipps LB, Coplin WM, Murry KR, et al: Safety and feasibility of continuous infusion of remifentanil in the neurosurgical intensive care unit, *Neurosurgery* 46:596-601, 2000:discussion 601-602.

33. Prause A, Wappler F, Scholz J, et al: Respiratory depression under long-term sedation with sufentanil, midazolam and clonidine has no clinical significance, *Intensive Care Med* 26:1454-1461, 2000.

34. Fodale V, Schifilliti D, Pratico C, et al: Remifentanil and the brain, *Acta Anaesthesiol Scand* 52:319-326, 2008.

35. Hanel F, Werner C, von Knobelsdorff G, et al: The effects of fentanyl and sufentanil on cerebral hemodynamics, *J Neurosurg Anesthesiol* 9:223-227, 1997.

36. Trindle MR, Dodson BA, Rampil IJ: Effects of fentanyl versus sufentanil in equianesthetic doses on middle cerebral artery blood flow velocity, *Anesthesiology* 78:454-460, 1993.

37. Werner C, Kochs E, Bause H, et al: Effects of sufentanil on cerebral hemodynamics and intracranial pressure in patients with brain injury, *Anesthesiology* 83:721-726, 1995.

38. Nelson PB, Seif SM, Maroon JC, et al: Hyponatremia in intracranial disease: Perhaps not the syndrome of inappropriate secretion of antidiuretic hormone (SIADH), *J Neurosurg* 55:938-941, 1981.

39. Wijdicks EF, Vermeulen M, ten Haaf JA, et al: Volume depletion and natriuresis in patients with a ruptured intracranial aneurysm, *Ann Neurol* 18:211-216, 1985.

40. Sivakumar V, Rajshekhar V, Chandy MJ: Management of neurosurgical patients with hyponatremia and natriuresis, *Neurosurgery* 34:269-274, 1994:discussion 274.

41. Brimioulle S, Orellana-Jimenez C, Aminian A, et al: Hyponatremia in neurological patients: cerebral salt wasting versus inappropriate antidiuretic hormone secretion, *Intensive Care Med* 34:125-131, 2008.

42. Oh MS, Carroll HJ: Cerebral salt-wasting syndrome. We need better proof of its existence, *Nephron* 82:110-114, 1999.

43. Davalos A, Ricart W, Gonzalez-Huix F, et al: Effect of malnutrition after acute stroke on clinical outcome, *Stroke* 27:1028-1032, 1996.

44. Gariballa SE, Parker SG, Taub N, et al: Influence of nutritional status on clinical outcome after acute stroke, *Am J Clin Nutr* 68:275-281, 1998.

45. Kreymann KG: Early nutrition support in critical care: A European perspective, *Curr Opin Clin Nutr Metab Care* 11:156-159, 2008.

46. Kreymann KG, Berger MM, Deutz NE, et al: ESPEN Guidelines on Enteral Nutrition: Intensive care, *Clin Nutr* 25:210-223, 2006.

47. Heyland DK, Dhaliwal R, Drover JW, et al: Canadian clinical practice guidelines for nutrition support in mechanically ventilated, critically ill adult patients, *JPEN J Parenter Enteral Nutr* 27:355-373, 2003.

48. Heyland DK, MacDonald S, Keefe L, et al: Total parenteral nutrition in the critically ill patient: a meta-analysis, *JAMA* 280:2013-2019, 1998.

49. Krishnan JA, Parce PB, Martinez A, et al: Caloric intake in medical ICU patients: consistency of care with guidelines and relationship to clinical outcomes, *Chest* 124:297-305, 2003.

50. van den Berghe G, Wouters P, Weekers F, et al: Intensive insulin therapy in the critically ill patients, *N Engl J Med* 345:1359-1367, 2001.

51. Kistler JP, Vielma JD, Davis KR, et al: Effects of nitroglycerin on the diameter of intracranial and extracranial arteries in monkeys, *Arch Neurol* 39:631-634, 1982.

52. Rogers MC, Hamburger C, Owen K, et al: Intracranial pressure in the cat during nitroglycerin-induced hypotension, *Anesthesiology* 51:227-229, 1979.

53. Cottrell JE, Gupta B, Rappaport H, et al: Intracranial pressure during nitroglycerin-induced hypotension, *J Neurosurg* 53:309-311, 1980.

54. Robertson CS, Clifton GL, Taylor AA, et al: Treatment of hypertension associated with head injury, *J Neurosurg* 59:455-460, 1983.

55. Skinhoj E, Overgaard J: Effect of dihydralazine on intracranial pressure in patients with severe brain damage, *Acta Med Scand Suppl* 678:83-87, 1983.

56. Puchstein C, Van Aken H, Anger C, et al: Influence of urapidil on intracranial pressure and intracranial compliance in dogs, *Br J Anaesth* 55:443-448, 1983.

57. Seifert V, Hussein S, Stolke D, et al: Modification of intracranial pressure by urapidil following experimental cold lesions in the cat, *Anasth Intensivther Notfallmed* 21:218-222, 1986.

58. Van Aken H, Puchstein C, Anger C, et al: The influence of urapidil, a new antihypertensive agent, on cerebral perfusion pressure in dogs with and without intracranial hypertension, *Intensive Care Med* 9:123-126, 1983.

59. Anger C, van Aken H, Feldhaus P, et al: Permeation of the blood-brain barrier by urapidil and its influence on intracranial pressure in man in the presence of compromised intracranial dynamics, *J Hypertens Suppl* 6:S63-S64, 1988.

60. Bernard JM, Kick O, Bonnet F: Comparison of intravenous and epidural clonidine for postoperative patient-controlled analgesia, *Anesth Analg* 81:706-712, 1995.

61. Hall JE, Uhrich TD, Ebert TJ: Sedative, analgesic and cognitive effects of clonidine infusions in humans, *Br J Anaesth* 86:5-11, 2001.

62. Greene CS, Gretler DD, Cervenka K, et al: Cerebral blood flow during the acute therapy of severe hypertension with oral clonidine, *Am J Emerg Med* 8:293-296, 1990.

63. Asgeirsson B, Grande PO, Nordstrom CH, et al: Effects of hypotensive treatment with alpha 2-agonist and beta 1-antagonist on cerebral haemodynamics in severely head injured patients, *Acta Anaesthesiol Scand* 39:347-351, 1995.

64. Kanawati IS, Yaksh TL, Anderson RE, et al: Effects of clonidine on cerebral blood flow and the response to arterial CO_2, *J Cereb Blood Flow Metab* 6:358-365, 1986.

65. Favre JB, Gardaz JP, Ravussin P: Effect of clonidine on ICP and on the hemodynamic responses to nociceptive stimuli in patients with brain tumors, *J Neurosurg Anesthesiol* 7:159-167, 1995.

66. ter Minassian A, Beydon L, Decq P, et al: Changes in cerebral hemodynamics after a single dose of clonidine in severely head-injured patients, *Anesth Analg* 84:127-132, 1997.

67. Maekawa T, Cho S, Fukusaki M, et al: Effects of clonidine on human middle cerebral artery flow velocity and cerebrovascular CO_2 response during sevoflurane anesthesia, *J Neurosurg Anesthesiol* 11:173-177, 1999.

68. Lee HW, Caldwell JE, Dodson B, et al: The effect of clonidine on cerebral blood flow velocity, carbon dioxide cerebral vasoreactivity, and response to increased arterial pressure in human volunteers, *Anesthesiology* 87:553-558, 1997.

69. Feibel JH, Baldwin CA, Joynt RJ: Catecholamine-associated refractory hypertension following acute intracranial hemorrhage: Control with propranolol, *Ann Neurol* 9:340-343, 1981.

70. Globus M, Keren A, Eldad M, et al: The effect of chronic propranolol therapy on regional cerebral blood flow in hypertensive patients, *Stroke* 14:964-967, 1983.

71. Qureshi AI, Wilson DA, Hanley DF, et al: Pharmacologic reduction of mean arterial pressure does not adversely affect regional cerebral blood flow and intracranial pressure in experimental intracerebral hemorrhage, *Crit Care Med* 27:965-971, 1999.

72. Van Aken H, Puchstein C, Schweppe ML, et al: Effect of labetalol on intracranial pressure in dogs with and without intracranial hypertension, *Acta Anaesthesiol Scand* 26:615-619, 1982.

73. Griffith DN, James IM, Newbury PA, et al: The effect of beta-adrenergic receptor blocking drugs on cerebral blood flow, *Br J Clin Pharmacol* 7:491-494, 1979.

74. Orlowski JP, Shiesley D, Vidt DG, et al: Labetalol to control blood pressure after cerebrovascular surgery, *Crit Care Med* 16:765-768, 1988.

75. Griffin JP, Cottrell JE, Hartung J, et al: Intracranial pressure during nifedipine-induced hypotension, *Anesth Analg* 62:1078-1080, 1983.

76. Anger C, Wusten R, Woulters P, et al: The behavior of intracranial pressure and intracranial compliance in nifedipine-induced hypotension, *Anasth Intensivther Notfallmed* 23:303-308, 1988.

77. Wusten R, Hemelrijck J, Mattheussen M, et al: Effect of nifedipine and urapidil on autoregulation of cerebral circulation in the presence of an intracranial space occupying lesion, *Anasth Intensivther Notfallmed* 25:140-145, 1990.

78. Tateishi A, Sano T, Takeshita H, et al: Effects of nifedipine on intracranial pressure in neurosurgical patients with arterial hypertension, *J Neurosurg* 69:213-215, 1988.

79. Bertel O, Conen D, Radu EW, et al: Nifedipine in hypertensive emergencies, *Br Med J (Clin Res Ed)* 286:19-21, 1983.

80. Adams HP Jr, del Zoppo G, Alberts MJ, et al: Guidelines for the early management of adults with ischemic stroke, *Circulation* 115:e478-e534, 2007.

81. Sakabe T, Nagai I, Ishikawa T, et al: Nicardipine increases cerebral blood flow but does not improve neurologic recovery in a canine model of complete cerebral ischemia, *J Cereb Blood Flow Metab* 6:684-690, 1986.

82. Kittaka M, Giannotta SL, Zelman V, et al: Attenuation of brain injury and reduction of neuron-specific enolase by nicardipine in systemic circulation following focal ischemia and reperfusion in a rat model, *J Neurosurg* 87:731-737, 1997.

83. Takata Y, Yoshizumi T, Ito Y, et al: Comparison of withdrawing antihypertensive therapy between diuretics and angiotensin converting enzyme inhibitors in essential hypertensives, *Am Heart J* 124:1574-1580, 1992.

84. Gaab MR, Czech T, Korn A: Intracranial effects of nicardipine, *Br J Clin Pharmacol* 20(Suppl 1):67S-74S, 1985.

85. Akopov SE, Simonian NA, Kazarian AV: Effects of nifedipine and nicardipine on regional cerebral blood flow distribution in patients with arterial hypertension, *Methods Find Exp Clin Pharmacol* 18:685-692, 1996.

86. Abe K, Iwanaga H, Inada E: Effect of nicardipine and diltiazem on internal carotid artery blood flow velocity and local cerebral blood flow during cerebral aneurysm surgery for subarachnoid hemorrhage, *J Clin Anesth* 6:99-105, 1994.

87. Halpern NA, Goldberg M, Neely C, et al: Postoperative hypertension: A multicenter, prospective, randomized comparison between intravenous nicardipine and sodium nitroprusside, *Crit Care Med* 20:1637-1643, 1992.

88. Neutel JM, Smith DH, Wallin D, et al: A comparison of intravenous nicardipine and sodium nitroprusside in the immediate treatment of severe hypertension, *Am J Hypertens* 7:623-628, 1994.

89. Dorman T, Thompson DA, Breslow MJ, et al: Nicardipine versus nitroprusside for breakthrough hypertension following carotid endarterectomy, *J Clin Anesth* 13:16-19, 2001.

90. Lisk DR, Grotta JC, Lamki LM, et al: Should hypertension be treated after acute stroke? A randomized controlled trial using single photon emission computed tomography, *Arch Neurol* 50:855-862, 1993.

91. Nishikawa T, Omote K, Namiki A, et al: The effects of nicardipine on cerebrospinal fluid pressure in humans, *Anesth Analg* 65:507-510, 1986.

92. Fagan SC, Robert S, Ewing JR, et al: Cerebral blood flow changes with enalapril, *Pharmacotherapy* 12:319-323, 1992.

93. Patel RV, Ramadan NM, Levine SR, et al: Effects of ramipril and enalapril on cerebral blood flow in elderly patients with asymptomatic carotid artery occlusive disease, *J Cardiovasc Pharmacol* 28:48-52, 1996.

94. Kobayashi S, Yamaguchi S, Okada K, et al: The effect of enalapril maleate on cerebral blood flow in chronic cerebral infarction, *Angiology* 43:378-388, 1992.

95. Segal E, Greenlee JD, Hata SJ, et al: Monitoring intravascular volumes to direct hypertensive, hypervolemic therapy in a patient with vasospasm, *J Neurosurg Anesthesiol* 16:296-298, 2004.

96. Holloway KL, Barnes T, Choi S, et al: Ventriculostomy infections: the effect of monitoring duration and catheter exchange in 584 patients, *J Neurosurg* 85:419-424, 1996.

97. Mayhall CG, Archer NH, Lamb VA, et al: Ventriculostomy-related infections. A prospective epidemiologic study, *N Engl J Med* 310:553-559, 1984.

98. Bota DP, Lefranc F, Vilallobos HR, et al: Ventriculostomy-related infections in critically ill patients: a 6-year experience, *J Neurosurg* 103:468-472, 2005.

99. Lozier AP, Sciacca RR, Romagnoli MF, et al: Ventriculostomy-related infections: A critical review of the literature, *Neurosurgery* 51:170-181, 2002:discussion 181-182.

100. Pfisterer W, Muhlbauer M, Czech T, et al: Early diagnosis of external ventricular drainage infection: results of a prospective study, *J Neurol Neurosurg Psychiatry* 74:929-932, 2003.

101. Schade RP, Schinkel J, Roelandse FW, et al: Lack of value of routine analysis of cerebrospinal fluid for prediction and diagnosis of external drainage-related bacterial meningitis, *J Neurosurg* 104:101-108, 2006.

102. Schoch B, Regel JP, Nierhaus A, et al: Predictive value of intrathecal interleukin-6 for ventriculostomy-related Infection, *Zentralbl Neurochir* 69:80-86, 2008.

103. Poon WS, Ng S, Wai S: CSF antibiotic prophylaxis for neurosurgical patients with ventriculostomy: A randomised study, *Acta Neurochir Suppl* 71:146-148, 1998.

104. Wyler AR, Kelly WA: Use of antibiotics with external ventriculostomies, *J Neurosurg* 37:185-187, 1972.

105. Aucoin PJ, Kotilainen HR, Gantz NM, et al: Intracranial pressure monitors. Epidemiologic study of risk factors and infections, *Am J Med* 80:369-376, 1986.

106. Prabhu VC, Kaufman HH, Voelker JL, et al: Prophylactic antibiotics with intracranial pressure monitors and external ventricular drains: A review of the evidence, *Surg Neurol* 52:226-236, 1999:discussion 236-237.

107. Friedman WA, Vries JK: Percutaneous tunnel ventriculostomy. Summary of 100 procedures, *J Neurosurg* 53:662-665, 1980.

108. Khanna RK, Rosenblum ML, Rock JP, et al: Prolonged external ventricular drainage with percutaneous long-tunnel ventriculostomies, *J Neurosurg* 83, 1995:79179-4.

109. Kosteljanetz M, Borgesen SE, Stjernholm P, et al: Clinical evaluation of a simple epidural pressure sensor, *Acta Neurochir (Wien)* 83:108-111, 1986.

110. Bruder N, N'Zoghe P, Graziani N, et al: A comparison of extradural and intraparenchymatous intracranial pressures in head injured patients, *Intensive Care Med* 21:850-852, 1995.

111. Citerio G, Piper I, Cormio M, et al: Bench test assessment of the new Raumedic Neurovent-P ICP sensor: A technical report by the BrainIT group, *Acta Neurochir (Wien)* 146:1221-1226, 2004.

112. Munch E, Weigel R, Schmiedek P, et al: The Camino intracranial pressure device in clinical practice: Reliability, handling characteristics and complications, *Acta Neurochir (Wien)* 140:1113-1119, 1998:discussion 1119-1120.

113. Schurer L, Munch E, Piepgras A, et al: Assessment of the CAMINO intracranial pressure device in clinical practice, *Acta Neurochir Suppl* 70:296-298, 1997.

114. Piper I, Barnes A, Smith D, et al: The Camino intracranial pressure sensor: is it optimal technology? An internal audit with a review of current intracranial pressure monitoring technologies, *Neurosurgery* 49:1158-1164, 2001:discussion 1164-1165.

115. Signorini DF, Shad A, Piper IR, et al: A clinical evaluation of the Codman MicroSensor for intracranial pressure monitoring, *Br J Neurosurg* 12:223-227, 1998.

116. Bavetta S, Norris JS, Wyatt M, et al: Prospective study of zero drift in fiberoptic pressure monitors used in clinical practice, *J Neurosurg* 86:927-930, 1997.

117. Berger C, Annecke A, Aschoff A, et al: Neurochemical monitoring of fatal middle cerebral artery infarction, *Stroke* 30:460-463, 1999.

118. Berger C, Dohmen C, Maurer MH, et al: Cerebral microdialysis in stroke, *Nervenarzt* 75:113-123, 2004.

119. Charbel FT, Du X, Hoffman WE, et al: Brain tissue PO(2), PCO(2), and pH during cerebral vasospasm, *Surg Neurol* 54:432-437, 2000:discussion 438.

120. Kiening KL, Unterberg AW, Bardt TF, et al: Monitoring of cerebral oxygenation in patients with severe head injuries: Brain tissue PO2 versus jugular vein oxygen saturation, *J Neurosurg* 85:751-757, 1996.

121. Rose JC, Neill TA, Hemphill JC 3rd: Continuous monitoring of the microcirculation in neurocritical care: An update on brain tissue oxygenation, *Curr Opin Crit Care* 12:97-102, 2006.

122. Skjoth-Rasmussen J, Schulz M, Kristensen SR, et al: Delayed neurological deficits detected by an ischemic pattern in the extracellular cerebral metabolites in patients with aneurysmal subarachnoid hemorrhage, *J Neurosurg* 100:8-15, 2004.

123. Berger C, Kiening K, Schwab S: Neurochemical monitoring of therapeutic effects in large human MCA infarction, *Neurocrit Care* 9:352-356, 2008.

124. Berger C, Sakowitz OW, Kiening KL, et al: Neurochemical monitoring of glycerol therapy in patients with ischemic brain edema, *Stroke* 36:e4-e6, 2005.

125. Berger C, Stauder A, Xia F, et al: Neuroprotection and glutamate attenuation by acetylsalicylic acid in temporary but not in permanent cerebral ischemia, *Exp Neurol* 210:543-548, 2008.

126. Dohmen C, Bosche B, Graf R, et al: Identification and clinical impact of impaired cerebrovascular autoregulation in patients with malignant middle cerebral artery infarction, *Stroke* 38:56-61, 2007.

127. Dohmen C, Bosche B, Graf R, et al: Prediction of malignant course in MCA infarction by PET and microdialysis, *Stroke* 34:2152-2158, 2003.

128. Schwab S, Aschoff A, Spranger M, et al: The value of intracranial pressure monitoring in acute hemispheric stroke, *Neurology* 47:393-398, 1996.

129. Claassen J, Mayer SA: Continuous electroencephalographic monitoring in neurocritical care, *Curr Neurol Neurosci Rep* 2:534-540, 2002.

130. Claassen J, Hirsch LJ, Kreiter KT, et al: Quantitative continuous EEG for detecting delayed cerebral ischemia in patients with poor-grade subarachnoid hemorrhage, *Clin Neurophysiol* 115:2699-2710, 2004.

131. Claassen J, Mayer SA, Hirsch LJ: Continuous EEG monitoring in patients with subarachnoid hemorrhage, *J Clin Neurophysiol* 22:92-98, 2005.

132. Steiner LA, Czosnyka M, Piechnik SK, et al: Continuous monitoring of cerebrovascular pressure reactivity allows determination of optimal cerebral perfusion pressure in patients with traumatic brain injury, *Crit Care Med* 30:733-738, 2002.

133. Ropper AH, O'Rourke D, Kennedy SK: Head position, intracranial pressure, and compliance, *Neurology* 32:1288-1291, 1982.

134. Rosner MJ, Coley IB: Cerebral perfusion pressure, intracranial pressure, and head elevation, *J Neurosurg* 65:636-641, 1986.

135. Feldman Z, Kanter MJ, Robertson CS: Effect of head elevation on intracranial pressure, cerebral perfusion pressure, and cerebral blood flow in head-injured patients, *J Neurosurg* 76:207-211, 1992.

136. Meixensberger J, Baunach S, Amschler J, et al: Influence of body position on tissue-pO2, cerebral perfusion pressure and intracranial pressure in patients with acute brain injury, *Neurol Res* 19:249-253, 1997.

137. Moraine JJ, Berre J, Melot C: Is cerebral perfusion pressure a major determinant of cerebral blood flow during head elevation in comatose patients with severe intracranial lesions? *J Neurosurg* 92:606-614, 2000.

138. Schwarz S, Georgiadis D, Aschoff A, et al: Effects of body position on intracranial pressure and cerebral perfusion in patients with large hemispheric stroke, *Stroke* 33:497-501, 2002.

139. Kaufmann AM, Cardoso ER: Aggravation of vasogenic cerebral edema by multiple-dose mannitol, *J Neurosurg* 77:584-589, 1992.

140. Garcia-Sola R, Pulido P, Capilla P: The immediate and long-term effects of mannitol and glycerol. A comparative experimental study, *Acta Neurochir (Wien)* 109:114-121, 1991.

141. Carhuapoma JR, Qureshi AI, Bhardwaj A, et al: Interhemispheric intracranial pressure gradients in massive cerebral infarction, *J Neurosurg Anesthesiol* 14:299-303, 2002.

142. Manno EM, Adams RE, Derdeyn CP, et al: The effects of mannitol on cerebral edema after large hemispheric cerebral infarct, *Neurology* 52:583-587, 1999.

143. Videen TO, Zazulia AR, Manno EM, et al: Mannitol bolus preferentially shrinks non-infarcted brain in patients with ischemic stroke, *Neurology* 57:2120-2122, 2001.

144. Muizelaar JP, Lutz HA 3rd, Becker DP: Effect of mannitol on ICP and CBF and correlation with pressure autoregulation in severely head-injured patients, *J Neurosurg* 61:700-706, 1984.

145. Mendelow AD, Teasdale GM, Russell T, et al: Effect of mannitol on cerebral blood flow and cerebral perfusion pressure in human head injury, *J Neurosurg* 63:43-48, 1985.

146. Kirkpatrick PJ, Smielewski P, Piechnik S, et al: Early effects of mannitol in patients with head injuries assessed using bedside multimodality monitoring, *Neurosurgery* 39:714-720, 1996:discussion 720-721.

147. Pollay M, Fullenwider C, Roberts PA, et al: Effect of mannitol and furosemide on blood-brain osmotic gradient and intracranial pressure, *J Neurosurg* 59:945-950, 1983.

148. Karibe H, Zarow GJ, Weinstein PR: Use of mild intraischemic hypothermia versus mannitol to reduce infarct size after temporary middle cerebral artery occlusion in rats, *J Neurosurg* 83:93-98, 1995.

149. Paczynski RP, He YY, Diringer MN, et al: Multiple-dose mannitol reduces brain water content in a rat model of cortical infarction, *Stroke* 28:1437-1443, 1997:discussion 1444.

150. Bereczki D, Fekete I, Prado GF, et al: Mannitol for acute stroke, *Cochrane Database Syst Rev* (3):CD001153, 2007.

151. Bereczki D, Liu M, do Prado GF, et al: Mannitol for acute stroke, *Stroke* 39:512, 2008.

152. Schwarz S, Schwab S, Bertram M, et al: Effects of hypertonic saline hydroxyethyl starch solution and mannitol in patients with increased intracranial pressure after stroke, *Stroke* 29:1550-1555, 1998.

153. Steiner T, Pilz J, Schellinger P, et al: Multimodal online monitoring in middle cerebral artery territory stroke, *Stroke* 32:2500-2506, 2001.

154. Steiner T, Ringleb P, Hacke W: Treatment options for large hemispheric stroke, *Neurology* 57:S61-S68, 2001.

155. Biestro A, Alberti R, Galli R, et al: Osmotherapy for increased intracranial pressure: Comparison between mannitol and glycerol, *Acta Neurochir (Wien)* 139:725-732, 1997:discussion 732-733.

156. Righetti E, Celani MG, Cantisani T, et al: Glycerol for acute stroke, *Cochrane Database Syst Rev* (2):CD000096, 2004.

157. Gunnar W, Jonasson O, Merlotti G, et al: Head injury and hemorrhagic shock: Studies of the blood brain barrier and intracranial pressure after resuscitation with normal saline solution, 3% saline solution, and dextran-40, *Surgery* 103:398-407, 1988.

158. Hartl R, Medary MB, Ruge M, et al: Hypertonic/hyperoncotic saline attenuates microcirculatory disturbances after traumatic brain injury, *J Trauma* 42:S41-S47, 1997.

159. Gemma M, Cozzi S, Tommasino C, et al: 7.5% hypertonic saline versus 20% mannitol during elective neurosurgical supratentorial procedures, *J Neurosurg Anesthesiol* 9:329-334, 1997.

160. Qureshi AI, Suarez JI: Use of hypertonic saline solutions in treatment of cerebral edema and intracranial hypertension, *Crit Care Med* 28:3301-3313, 2000.

161. Schwarz S, Georgiadis D, Aschoff A, et al: Effects of hypertonic (10%) saline in patients with raised intracranial pressure after stroke, *Stroke* 33:136-140, 2002.

162. Ogden AT, Mayer SA, Connolly ES Jr: Hyperosmolar agents in neurosurgical practice: The evolving role of hypertonic saline, *Neurosurgery* 57:207-215, 2005:discussion 207-215.

163. Dorman HR, Sondheimer JH, Cadnapaphornchai P: Mannitol-induced acute renal failure, *Medicine (Baltimore)* 69:153-159, 1990.

164. Gaab MR, Seegers K, Smedema RJ, et al: A comparative analysis of THAM (Tris-buffer) in traumatic brain oedema, *Acta Neurochir Suppl (Wien)* 51:320-323, 1990.

165. Wolf AL, Levi L, Marmarou A, et al: Effect of THAM upon outcome in severe head injury: A randomized prospective clinical trial, *J Neurosurg* 78:54-59, 1993.

166. Michenfelder JD, Milde JH: Failure of prolonged hypocapnia, hypothermia, or hypertension to favorably alter acute stroke in primates, *Stroke* 8:87-91, 1977.

167. Muizelaar JP, Marmarou A, Ward JD, et al: Adverse effects of prolonged hyperventilation in patients with severe head injury: A randomized clinical trial, *J Neurosurg* 75:731-739, 1991.

168. Imberti R, Bellinzona G, Langer M: Cerebral tissue PO_2 and $SjvO_2$ changes during moderate hyperventilation in patients with severe traumatic brain injury, *J Neurosurg* 96:97-102, 2002.

169. Imberti R, Ciceri M, Bellinzona G, et al: The use of hyperventilation in the treatment of plateau waves in two patients with severe traumatic brain injury: Contrasting effects on cerebral oxygenation, *J Neurosurg Anesthesiol* 12:124-127, 2000.

170. Marion DW, Puccio A, Wisniewski SR, et al: Effect of hyperventilation on extracellular concentrations of glutamate, lactate, pyruvate, and local cerebral blood flow in patients with severe traumatic brain injury, *Crit Care Med* 30:2619-2625, 2002.

171. Bardutzky J, Schwab S: Antiedema therapy in ischemic stroke, *Stroke* 38:3084-3094, 2007.

172. Olsen RW: GABA-benzodiazepine-barbiturate receptor interactions, *J Neurochem* 37:1-13, 1981.

173. Woodcock J, Ropper AH, Kennedy SK: High dose barbiturates in non-traumatic brain swelling: ICP reduction and effect on outcome, *Stroke* 13:785-787, 1982.

174. Lee MW, Deppe SA, Sipperly ME, et al: The efficacy of barbiturate coma in the management of uncontrolled intracranial hypertension following neurosurgical trauma, *J Neurotrauma* 11:325-331, 1994.

175. Schwab S, Spranger M, Schwarz S, et al: Barbiturate coma in severe hemispheric stroke: Useful or obsolete? *Neurology* 48:1608-1613, 1997.

176. Cormio M, Gopinath SP, Valadka A, et al: Cerebral hemodynamic effects of pentobarbital coma in head-injured patients, *J Neurotrauma* 16:927-936, 1999.

177. Schwartz ML, Tator CH, Rowed DW, et al: The University of Toronto head injury treatment study: A prospective, randomized comparison of pentobarbital and mannitol, *Can J Neurol Sci* 11:434-440, 1984.

178. Qizilbash N, Lewington SL, Lopez-Arrieta JM: Corticosteroids for acute ischaemic stroke, *Cochrane Database Syst Rev* (2):CD000064, 2002.

179. Poungvarin N, Bhoopat W, Viriyavejakul A, et al: Effects of dexamethasone in primary supratentorial intracerebral hemorrhage, *N Engl J Med* 316:1229-1233, 1987.

180. Kocher T, Hirnerschütterung, Hirndruck und chirurgische Eingriffe bei Hirnkrankheiten. Wien Hölder, 1901.

181. Doerfler A, Engelhorn T, Heiland S, et al: Perfusion- and diffusion-weighted magnetic resonance imaging for monitoring decompressive craniectomy in animals with experimental hemispheric stroke, *J Neurosurg* 96:933-940, 2002.

182. Doerfler A, Forsting M, Reith W, et al: Decompressive craniectomy in a rat model of "malignant" cerebral hemispheric stroke: experimental support for an aggressive therapeutic approach, *J Neurosurg* 85:853-859, 1996.

183. Forsting M, Reith W, Schabitz WR, et al: Decompressive craniectomy for cerebral infarction. An experimental study in rats, *Stroke* 26:259-264, 1995.

184. Zweckberger K, Stoffel M, Baethmann A, et al: Effect of decompression craniotomy on increase of contusion volume and functional outcome after controlled cortical impact in mice, *J Neurotrauma* 20:1307-1314, 2003.

185. Yoo DS, Kim DS, Cho KS, et al: Ventricular pressure monitoring during bilateral decompression with dural expansion, *J Neurosurg* 91:953-959, 1999.

186. Jaeger M, Soehle M, Meixensberger J: Improvement of brain tissue oxygen and intracranial pressure during and after surgical decompression for diffuse brain oedema and space occupying infarction, *Acta Neurochir Suppl* 95:117-118, 2005.

187. Colbourne F, Corbett D, Zhao Z, et al: Prolonged but delayed postischemic hypothermia: A long-term outcome study in the rat middle cerebral artery occlusion model, *J Cereb Blood Flow Metab* 20:1702-1708, 2000.

188. Corbett D, Hamilton M, Colbourne F: Persistent neuroprotection with prolonged postischemic hypothermia in adult rats subjected to transient middle cerebral artery occlusion, *Exp Neurol* 163:200-206, 2000.

189. Huh PW, Belayev L, Zhao W, et al: Comparative neuroprotective efficacy of prolonged moderate intraischemic and postischemic hypothermia in focal cerebral ischemia, *J Neurosurg* 92:91-99, 2000.

190. Nakashima K, Todd MM: Effects of hypothermia on the rate of excitatory amino acid release after ischemic depolarization, *Stroke* 27:913-918, 1996.

191. Winfree CJ, Baker CJ, Connolly ES Jr, et al: Mild hypothermia reduces penumbral glutamate levels in the rat permanent focal cerebral ischemia model, *Neurosurgery* 38:1216-1222, 1996.

192. Dietrich WD, Busto R, Halley M, et al: The importance of brain temperature in alterations of the blood-brain barrier following cerebral ischemia, *J Neuropathol Exp Neurol* 49:486-497, 1990.

193. Karibe H, Zarow GJ, Graham SH, et al: Mild intraischemic hypothermia reduces postischemic hyperperfusion, delayed postischemic hypoperfusion, blood-brain barrier disruption, brain edema, and neuronal damage volume after temporary focal cerebral ischemia in rats, *J Cereb Blood Flow Metab* 14:620-627, 1994.

194. Krafft P, Frietsch T, Lenz C, et al: Mild and moderate hypothermia (alpha-stat) do not impair the coupling between local cerebral blood flow and metabolism in rats, *Stroke* 31:1393-1400, 2000:discussion 1401.

195. Clifton GL, Allen S, Barrodale P, et al: A phase II study of moderate hypothermia in severe brain injury, *J Neurotrauma* 10:263-271, 1993:discussion 273.

196. Marion DW, Obrist WD, Carlier PM, et al: The use of moderate therapeutic hypothermia for patients with severe head injuries: A preliminary report, *J Neurosurg* 79:354-362, 1993.

197. Clifton GL, Miller ER, Choi SC, et al: Lack of effect of induction of hypothermia after acute brain injury, *N Engl J Med* 344:556-563, 2001.

198. The Hypothermia after Cardiac Arrest Study Group: Mild therapeutic hypothermia to improve the neurologic outcome after cardiac arrest, *N Engl J Med* 346:549-556, 2002.

199. Bernard SA, Gray TW, Buist MD, et al: Treatment of comatose survivors of out-of-hospital cardiac arrest with induced hypothermia, *N Engl J Med* 346:557-563, 2002.

200. Vespa PM, O'Phelan K, Shah M, et al: Acute seizures after intracerebral hemorrhage: A factor in progressive midline shift and outcome, *Neurology* 60:1441-1446, 2003.

201. Passero S, Rocchi R, Rossi S, et al: Seizures after spontaneous supratentorial intracerebral hemorrhage, *Epilepsia* 43:1175-1180, 2002.

202. Broderick J, Connolly S, Feldmann E, et al: Guidelines for the management of spontaneous intracerebral hemorrhage in adults: 2007 update: a guideline from the American Heart Association/American Stroke Association Stroke Council, High Blood Pressure Research Council, and the Quality of Care and Outcomes in Research Interdisciplinary Working Group, *Circulation* 116:e391-e413, 2007.

203. Johnston KC, Li JY, Lyden PD, et al: Medical and neurological complications of ischemic stroke: Experience from the RANTTAS trial. RANTTAS Investigators, *Stroke* 29:447-453, 1998.

204. Weimar C, Roth MP, Zillessen G, et al: Complications following acute ischemic stroke, *Eur Neurol* 48:133-140, 2002.

205. Langhorne P, Stott DJ, Robertson L, et al: Medical complications after stroke: A multicenter study, *Stroke* 31:1223-1229, 2000.

206. Kamphuisen PW, Agnelli G, Sebastianelli M: Prevention of venous thromboembolism after acute ischemic stroke, *J Thromb Haemost* 3:1187-1194, 2005.

207. Wijdicks EF, Scott JP: Pulmonary embolism associated with acute stroke, *Mayo Clin Proc* 72:297-300, 1997.

208. Kelly J, Rudd A, Lewis RR, et al: Venous thromboembolism after acute ischemic stroke: a prospective study using magnetic resonance direct thrombus imaging, *Stroke* 35:2320-2325, 2004.

209. Mazzone C, Chiodo GF, Sandercock P, et al: Physical methods for preventing deep vein thrombosis in stroke, *Cochrane Database Syst Rev* (4):CD001922, 2004.

210. Diener HC, Ringelstein EB, von Kummer R, et al: Prophylaxis of thrombotic and embolic events in acute ischemic stroke with the low-molecular-weight heparin certoparin: Results of the PROTECT Trial, *Stroke* 37:139-144, 2006.

211. Sherman DG, Albers GW, Bladin C, et al: The efficacy and safety of enoxaparin versus unfractionated heparin for the prevention of venous thromboembolism after acute ischaemic stroke (PREVAIL Study): An open-label randomised comparison, *Lancet* 369:1347-1355, 2007.

212. European Stroke Organization Executive Committee: Guidelines for management of ischaemic stroke and transient ischaemic attack 2008, *Cerebrovasc Dis* 25:457-507, 2008.

213. Albers GW, Amarenco P, Easton JD, et al: Antithrombotic and thrombolytic therapy for ischemic stroke: The Seventh ACCP Conference on Antithrombotic and Thrombolytic Therapy, *Chest* 126:483S-512S, 2004.

214. Steiner T, Kaste M, Forsting M, et al: Recommendations for the management of intracranial haemorrhage—part I: Spontaneous intracerebral haemorrhage. The European Stroke Initiative Writing Committee and the Writing Committee for the EUSI Executive Committee, *Cerebrovasc Dis* 22:294-316, 2006.

215. Dorffler-Melly J, de Jonge E, Pont AC, et al: Bioavailability of subcutaneous low-molecular-weight heparin to patients on vasopressors, *Lancet* 359:849-850, 2002.

216. Capes SE, Hunt D, Malmberg K, et al: Stress hyperglycemia and prognosis of stroke in nondiabetic and diabetic patients: A systematic overview, *Stroke* 32:2426-2432, 2001.

217. Scott JF, Robinson GM, French JM, et al: Prevalence of admission hyperglycaemia across clinical subtypes of acute stroke, *Lancet* 353:376-377, 1999.

218. Oppenheimer SM, Hoffbrand BI, Oswald GA, et al: Diabetes mellitus and early mortality from stroke, *Br Med J (Clin Res Ed)* 291:1014-1015, 1985.

219. Weir CJ, Murray GD, Dyker AG, et al: Is hyperglycaemia an independent predictor of poor outcome after acute stroke? Results of a long-term follow up study, *BMJ* 314:1303-1306, 1997.

220. Lindsberg PJ, Roine RO: Hyperglycemia in acute stroke, *Stroke* 35:363-364, 2004.

221. Parsons MW, Barber PA, Desmond PM, et al: Acute hyperglycemia adversely affects stroke outcome: A magnetic resonance imaging and spectroscopy study, *Ann Neurol* 52:20-28, 2002.

222. Candelise L, Landi G, Orazio EN, et al: Prognostic significance of hyperglycemia in acute stroke, *Arch Neurol* 42:661-663, 1985.

223. Van den Berghe G, Wilmer A, Hermans G, et al: Intensive insulin therapy in the medical ICU, *N Engl J Med* 354:449-461, 2006.

224. Dellinger RP, Carlet JM, Masur H, et al: Surviving Sepsis Campaign guidelines for management of severe sepsis and septic shock, *Crit Care Med* 32:858-873, 2004.

225. Brunkhorst FM, Engel C, Bloos F, et al: Intensive insulin therapy and pentastarch resuscitation in severe sepsis, *N Engl J Med* 358:125-139, 2008.

226. Gray CS, Hildreth AJ, Sandercock PA, et al: Glucose-potassium-insulin infusions in the management of post-stroke hyperglycaemia: The UK Glucose Insulin in Stroke Trial (GIST-UK), *Lancet Neurol* 6:397-406, 2007.

227. Dellinger RP, Levy MM, Carlet JM, et al: Surviving Sepsis Campaign: International guidelines for management of severe sepsis and septic shock, *Crit Care Med* 2008(36):296-327, 2008.

228. Fukuda H, Kitani M, Takahashi K: Body temperature correlates with functional outcome and the lesion size of cerebral infarction, *Acta Neurol Scand* 100:385-390, 1999.

229. Takagi K: Body temperature in acute stroke, *Stroke* 33:2154-2155, 2002:author reply 2154-2155.

230. Schwarz S, Hafner K, Aschoff A, et al: Incidence and prognostic significance of fever following intracerebral hemorrhage, *Neurology* 54:354-361, 2000.

231. Ginsberg MD, Busto R: Combating hyperthermia in acute stroke: A significant clinical concern, *Stroke* 29:529-534, 1998.

232. Hacke W, Schwab S, Horn M, et al: 'Malignant' middle cerebral artery territory infarction: Clinical course and prognostic signs, *Arch Neurol* 53:309-315, 1996.

233. Berrouschot J, Sterker M, Bettin S, et al: Mortality of space-occupying ('malignant') middle cerebral artery infarction under conservative intensive care, *Intensive Care Med* 24:620-623, 1998.

234. Schwab S, Steiner T, Aschoff A, et al: Early hemicraniectomy in patients with complete middle cerebral artery infarction, *Stroke* 29:1888-1893, 1998.

235. Gupta R, Connolly ES, Mayer S, et al: Hemicraniectomy for massive middle cerebral artery territory infarction: A systematic review, *Stroke* 35:539-543, 2004.

236. Rieke K, Schwab S, Krieger D, et al: Decompressive surgery in space-occupying hemispheric infarction: Results of an open, prospective trial, *Crit Care Med* 23:1576-1587, 1995.

237. Morley NC, Berge E, Cruz-Flores S, et al: Surgical decompression for cerebral oedema in acute ischemic stroke, *Cochrane Database Syst Rev* (3):CD003435, 2002.

238. Vahedi K, Hofmeijer J, Juettler E, et al: Early decompressive surgery in malignant infarction of the middle cerebral artery: A pooled analysis of three randomised controlled trials, *Lancet Neurol* 6:215-222, 2007.

239. Puetz V, Campos CR, Eliasziw M, et al: Assessing the benefits of hemicraniectomy: What is a favourable outcome? *Lancet Neurol* 6:580, 2007.

240. Pillai A, Menon SK, Kumar S, et al: Decompressive hemicraniectomy in malignant middle cerebral artery infarction: An analysis of long-term outcome and factors in patient selection, *J Neurosurg* 106:59-65, 2007.

241. Chen CC, Cho DY, Tsai SC: Outcome of and prognostic factors for decompressive hemicraniectomy in malignant middle cerebral artery infarction, *J Clin Neurosci* 14:317-321, 2007.

242. Wang KW, Chang WN, Ho JT, et al: Factors predictive of fatality in massive middle cerebral artery territory infarction and clinical experience of decompressive hemicraniectomy, *Eur J Neurol* 13:765-771, 2006.

243. Harscher S, Reichart R, Terborg C, et al: Outcome after decompressive craniectomy in patients with severe ischemic stroke, *Acta Neurochir (Wien)* 148:31-37, 2006:discussion 37.

244. Kastrau F, Wolter M, Huber W, et al: Recovery from aphasia after hemicraniectomy for infarction of the speech-dominant hemisphere, *Stroke* 36:825-829, 2005.

245. Curry WT Jr, Sethi MK, Ogilvy CS, et al: Factors associated with outcome after hemicraniectomy for large middle cerebral artery territory infarction, *Neurosurgery* 56:681-692, 2005:discussion 681-692.

246. Woertgen C, Erban P, Rothoerl RD, et al: Quality of life after decompressive craniectomy in patients suffering from supratentorial brain ischemia, *Acta Neurochir (Wien)* 146:691-695, 2004.

247. Uhl E, Kreth FW, Elias B, et al: Outcome and prognostic factors of hemicraniectomy for space occupying cerebral infarction, *J Neurol Neurosurg Psychiatry* 75:270-274, 2004.

248. Foerch C, Lang JM, Krause J, et al: Functional impairment, disability, and quality of life outcome after decompressive hemicraniectomy in malignant middle cerebral artery infarction, *J Neurosurg* 101:248-254, 2004.

249. Holtkamp M, Buchheim K, Unterberg A, et al: Hemicraniectomy in elderly patients with space occupying media infarction: improved survival but poor functional outcome, *J Neurol Neurosurg Psychiatry* 70:226-228, 2001.

250. Mori K, Aoki A, Yamamoto T, et al: Aggressive decompressive surgery in patients with massive hemispheric embolic cerebral infarction associated with severe brain swelling, *Acta Neurochir (Wien)* 143:483-491, 2001:discussion 491-492.

251. Schwab S, Schwarz S, Spranger M, et al: Moderate hypothermia in the treatment of patients with severe middle cerebral artery infarction, *Stroke* 29:2461-2466, 1998.

252. Schwab S, Georgiadis D, Berrouschot J, et al: Feasibility and safety of moderate hypothermia after massive hemispheric infarction, *Stroke* 32:2033-2035, 2001.

253. Krieger DW, De Georgia MA, Abou-Chebl A, et al: Cooling for acute ischemic brain damage (Cool AID): An open pilot study of induced hypothermia in acute ischemic stroke, *Stroke* 32:1847-1854, 2001.

254. Georgiadis D, Schwarz S, Kollmar R, et al: Endovascular cooling for moderate hypothermia in patients with acute stroke: First results of a novel approach, *Stroke* 32:2550-2553, 2001.

255. Georgiadis D, Schwarz S, Aschoff A, et al: Hemicraniectomy and moderate hypothermia in patients with severe ischemic stroke, *Stroke* 33:1584-1588, 2002.

256. Castillo J, Leira R, Garcia MM, et al: Blood pressure decrease during the acute phase of ischemic stroke is associated with brain injury and poor stroke outcome, *Stroke* 35:520-526, 2004.

257. Interventions for deliberately altering blood pressure in acute stroke, *Cochrane Database Syst Rev* (2):CD000039, 2001.

258. Potter J, Robinson T, Ford G, et al: CHHIPS (Controlling Hypertension and Hypotension Immediately Post-Stroke) Pilot Trial: Rationale and design, *J Hypertens* 23:649-655, 2005.

259. Astrup J, Siesjo BK, Symon L: Thresholds in cerebral ischemia—the ischemic penumbra, *Stroke* 12:723-725, 1981.

259a. Rordorf G, Koroshetz WJ, Ezzeddine MA, et al: A pilot study of drug-induced hypertension for treatment of acute stroke, *Neurology* 56(9):1210-1213, 2001.

260. Hillis AE, Ulatowski JA, Barker PB, et al: A pilot randomized trial of induced blood pressure elevation: Effects on function and focal perfusion in acute and subacute stroke, *Cerebrovasc Dis* 16:236-246, 2003.

260a. Schwarz S, Georgiadis D, Aschoff A, Schwab S: Effects of hypertension on intracranial pressure and flow velocities of the middle cerebral arteries in patients with large hemispheric stroke, *Stroke* 33:998-1004, 2002.

261. Archer CR, Horenstein S: Basilar artery occlusion: Clinical and radiological correlation, *Stroke* 8:383-390, 1977.

262. Castaigne P, Lhermitte F, Gautier JC, et al: Arterial occlusions in the vertebro-basilar system. A study of 44 patients with post-mortem data, *Brain* 96:133-154, 1973.

263. Fields WS, Ratinov G, Weibel J, et al: Survival following basilar artery occlusion, *Arch Neurol* 15:463-471, 1966.

264. Hacke W, Zeumer H, Ferbert A, et al: Intra-arterial thrombolytic therapy improves outcome in patients with acute vertebrobasilar occlusive disease, *Stroke* 19:1216-1222, 1988.

265. Lindsberg PJ, Mattle HP: Therapy of basilar artery occlusion: A systematic analysis comparing intra-arterial and intravenous thrombolysis, *Stroke* 37:922-928, 2006.

266. Gobin YP, Starkman S, Duckwiler GR, et al: MERCI 1: A phase 1 study of Mechanical Embolus Removal in Cerebral Ischemia, *Stroke* 35:2848-2854, 2004.

267. Eckert B, Koch C, Thomalla G, et al: Aggressive therapy with intravenous abciximab and intra-arterial rtPA and additional PTA/stenting improves clinical outcome in acute vertebrobasilar occlusion: combined local fibrinolysis and intravenous abciximab in acute vertebrobasilar stroke treatment (FAST): Results of a multicenter study, *Stroke* 36:1160-1165, 2005.

268. Qureshi AI, Siddiqui AM, Kim SH, et al: Reocclusion of recanalized arteries during intra-arterial thrombolysis for acute ischemic stroke, *AJNR Am J Neuroradiol* 25:322-328, 2004.

269. Jauss M, Krieger D, Hornig C, et al: Surgical and medical management of patients with massive cerebellar infarctions: Results of the German-Austrian Cerebellar Infarction Study, *J Neurol* 246:257-264, 1999.

270. Chen HJ, Lee TC, Wei CP: Treatment of cerebellar infarction by decompressive suboccipital craniectomy, *Stroke* 23:957-961, 1992.

271. Heros RC: Surgical treatment of cerebellar infarction, *Stroke* 23:937-938, 1992.

272. Hemphill JC 3rd, Bonovich DC, Besmertis L, et al: The ICH score: A simple, reliable grading scale for intracerebral hemorrhage, *Stroke* 32:891-897, 2001.

273. Diringer MN, Edwards DF: Admission to a neurologic/neurosurgical intensive care unit is associated with reduced mortality rate after intracerebral hemorrhage, *Crit Care Med* 29:635-640, 2001.

274. Brott T, Broderick J, Kothari R, et al: Early hemorrhage growth in patients with intracerebral hemorrhage, *Stroke* 28:1-5, 1997.

275. Davis SM, Broderick J, Hennerici M, et al: Hematoma growth is a determinant of mortality and poor outcome after intracerebral hemorrhage, *Neurology* 66:1175-1181, 2006.

276. Anderson CS, Huang Y, Wang JG, et al: Intensive blood pressure reduction in acute cerebral haemorrhage trial (INTERACT): A randomised pilot trial, *Lancet Neurol* 7:391-399, 2008.

277. Lee KR, Colon GP, Betz AL, et al: Edema from intracerebral hemorrhage: The role of thrombin, *J Neurosurg* 84:91-96, 1996.

278. Castillo J, Davalos A, Alvarez-Sabin J, et al: Molecular signatures of brain injury after intracerebral hemorrhage, *Neurology* 58:624-629, 2002.

279. Abilleira S, Montaner J, Molina CA, et al: Matrix metalloproteinase-9 concentration after spontaneous intracerebral hemorrhage, *J Neurosurg* 99:65-70, 2003.

280. Sansing LH, Kaznatcheeva EA, Perkins CJ, et al: Edema after intracerebral hemorrhage: Correlations with coagulation parameters and treatment, *J Neurosurg* 98:985-992, 2003.

281. Gebel JM Jr, Jauch EC, Brott TG, et al: Natural history of perihematomal edema in patients with hyperacute spontaneous intracerebral hemorrhage, *Stroke* 33:2631-2635, 2002.

282. Zazulia AR, Diringer MN, Derdeyn CP, et al: Progression of mass effect after intracerebral hemorrhage, *Stroke* 30:1167-1173, 1999.

283. Gebel JM Jr, Jauch EC, Brott TG, et al: Relative edema volume is a predictor of outcome in patients with hyperacute spontaneous intracerebral hemorrhage, *Stroke* 33:2636-2641, 2002.

284. Diringer MN, Edwards DF, Zazulia AR: Hydrocephalus: a previously unrecognized predictor of poor outcome from supratentorial intracerebral hemorrhage, *Stroke* 29:1352-1357, 1998.

285. Mayer SA, Brun NC, Begtrup K, et al: Efficacy and safety of recombinant activated factor VII for acute intracerebral hemorrhage, *N Engl J Med* 358:2127-2137, 2008.

286. Lyden PD, Shuaib A, Lees KR, et al: Safety and tolerability of NXY-059 for acute intracerebral hemorrhage: The CHANT Trial, *Stroke* 38:2262-2269, 2007.

287. Haley EC Jr, Thompson JL, Levin B, et al: Gavestinel does not improve outcome after acute intracerebral hemorrhage: An analysis from the GAIN International and GAIN Americas studies, *Stroke* 36:1006-1010, 2005.

288. Powers WJ, Zazulia AR, Videen TO, et al: Autoregulation of cerebral blood flow surrounding acute (6 to 22 hours) intracerebral hemorrhage, *Neurology* 57:18-24, 2001.

289. Kidwell CS, Saver JL, Mattiello J, et al: Diffusion-perfusion MR evaluation of perihematomal injury in hyperacute intracerebral hemorrhage, *Neurology* 57:1611-1617, 2001.

290. Sills C, Villar-Cordova C, Pasteur W, et al: Demonstration of hypoperfusion surrounding intracerebral hematoma in humans, *J Stroke Cerebrovasc Dis* 6:17-24, 1996.

291. Schellinger PD, Fiebach JB, Hoffmann K, et al: Stroke MRI in intracerebral hemorrhage: Is there a perihemorrhagic penumbra? *Stroke* 34:1674-1679, 2003.

292. Herweh C, Juttler E, Schellinger PD, et al: Evidence against a perihemorrhagic penumbra provided by perfusion computed tomography, *Stroke* 38:2941-2947, 2007.

293. Kuwata N, Kuroda K, Funayama M, et al: Dysautoregulation in patients with hypertensive intracerebral hemorrhage. A SPECT study, *Neurosurg Rev* 18:237-245, 1995.

294. Fernandes HM, Siddique S, Banister K, et al: Continuous monitoring of ICP and CPP following ICH and its relationship to clinical, radiological and surgical parameters, *Acta Neurochir Suppl* 76:463-466, 2000.

295. Robertson CS, Valadka AB, Hannay HJ, et al: Prevention of secondary ischemic insults after severe head injury, *Crit Care Med* 27:2086-2095, 1999.

296. Flibotte JJ, Hagan N, O'Donnell J, et al: Warfarin, hematoma expansion, and outcome of intracerebral hemorrhage, *Neurology* 63:1059-1064, 2004.

297. Firozvi K, Deveras RA, Kessler CM: Reversal of low-molecular-weight heparin-induced bleeding in patients with pre-existing hypercoagulable states with human recombinant activated factor VII concentrate, *Am J Hematol* 81:582-589, 2006.

298. Deveras RA, Kessler CM: Reversal of warfarin-induced excessive anticoagulation with recombinant human factor VIIa concentrate, *Ann Intern Med* 137:884-888, 2002.

299. Brody DL, Aiyagari V, Shackleford AM, et al: Use of recombinant factor VIIa in patients with warfarin-associated intracranial hemorrhage, *Neurocrit Care* 2:263-267, 2005.

300. Freeman WD, Brott TG, Barrett KM, et al: Recombinant factor VIIa for rapid reversal of warfarin anticoagulation in acute intracranial hemorrhage, *Mayo Clin Proc* 79:1495-1500, 2004.

301. Nehls DG, Mendelow DA, Graham DI, et al: Experimental intracerebral hemorrhage: Early removal of a spontaneous mass lesion improves late outcome, *Neurosurgery* 27:674-682, 1990:discussion 682.

302. Kingman TA, Mendelow AD, Graham DI, et al: Experimental intracerebral mass: Time-related effects on local cerebral blood flow, *J Neurosurg* 67:732-738, 1987.

303. Mendelow AD, Gregson BA, Fernandes HM, et al: Early surgery versus initial conservative treatment in patients with spontaneous supratentorial intracerebral haematomas in the International Surgical Trial in Intracerebral Haemorrhage (STICH): a randomised trial, *Lancet* 365:387-397, 2005.

304. Kaneko M, Tanaka K, Shimada T, et al: Long-term evaluation of ultra-early operation for hypertensive intracerebral hemorrhage in 100 cases, *J Neurosurg* 58:838-842, 1983.

305. Morgenstern LB, Demchuk AM, Kim DH, et al: Rebleeding leads to poor outcome in ultra-early craniotomy for intracerebral hemorrhage, *Neurology* 56:1294-1299, 2001.

306. Zuccarello M, Brott T, Derex L, et al: Early surgical treatment for supratentorial intracerebral hemorrhage: A randomized feasibility study, *Stroke* 30:1833-1839, 1999.

307. Murthy JM, Chowdary GV, Murthy TV, et al: Decompressive craniectomy with clot evacuation in large hemispheric hypertensive intracerebral hemorrhage, *Neurocrit Care* 2:258-262, 2005.

308. Maira G, Anile C, Colosimo C, et al: Surgical treatment of primary supratentorial intracerebral hemorrhage in stuporous and comatose patients, *Neurol Res* 24:54-60, 2002.

309. van Loon J, Van Calenbergh F, Goffin J, et al: Controversies in the management of spontaneous cerebellar haemorrhage. A consecutive series of 49 cases and review of the literature, *Acta Neurochir (Wien)* 122:187-193, 1993.

310. Da Pian R, Bazzan A, Pasqualin A: Surgical versus medical treatment of spontaneous posterior fossa haematomas: A cooperative study on 205 cases, *Neurol Res* 6:145-151, 1984.

311. Butler AB, Partain RA, Netsky MG: Primary intraventricular hemorrhage. A mild and remediable form, *Neurology* 22:675-687, 1972.

312. Tuhrim S, Horowitz DR, Sacher M, et al: Volume of ventricular blood is an important determinant of outcome in supratentorial intracerebral hemorrhage, *Crit Care Med* 27:617-621, 1999.

313. Naff NJ, Hanley DF, Keyl PM, et al: Intraventricular thrombolysis speeds blood clot resolution: Results of a pilot, prospective, randomized, double-blind, controlled trial, *Neurosurgery* 54:577-583, 2004:discussion 583-584.

314. Lee MW, Pang KY, Ho WW, et al: Outcome analysis of intraventricular thrombolytic therapy for intraventricular haemorrhage, *Hong Kong Med J* 9:335-340, 2003.

315. Nieuwkamp DJ, de Gans K, Rinkel GJ, et al: Treatment and outcome of severe intraventricular extension in patients with subarachnoid or intracerebral hemorrhage: A systematic review of the literature, *J Neurol* 247:117-321, 2000.

316. Huttner HB, Staykov D, Bardutzky J, et al: Treatment of intraventricular hemorrhage and hydrocephalus, *Nervenarzt* 79:1369-1370, 2008.

317. Huttner HB, Nagel S, Tognoni E, et al: Intracerebral hemorrhage with severe ventricular involvement: Lumbar drainage for communicating hydrocephalus, *Stroke* 38:183-187, 2007.

318. Kassell NF, Torner JC, Jane JA, et al: The International Cooperative Study on the Timing of Aneurysm Surgery. Part 2: Surgical results, *J Neurosurg* 73:37-47, 1990.

319. Hop JW, Rinkel GJ, Algra A, et al: Quality of life in patients and partners after aneurysmal subarachnoid hemorrhage, *Stroke* 29:798-804, 1998.

320. Handa Y, Kubota T, Tsuchida A, et al: Effect of systemic hypotension on cerebral energy metabolism during chronic cerebral vasospasm in primates, *J Neurosurg* 78:112-119, 1993.

321. Ohkuma H, Tsurutani H, Suzuki S: Incidence and significance of early aneurysmal rebleeding before neurosurgical or neurological management, *Stroke* 32:1176-1180, 2001.

322. van Gijn J, Rinkel GJ: Subarachnoid haemorrhage: Diagnosis, causes and management, *Brain* 124:249-278, 2001.

323. Nurmohamed MT, van Riel AM, Henkens CM, et al: Low molecular weight heparin and compression stockings in the prevention of venous thromboembolism in neurosurgery, *Thromb Haemost* 75:233-238, 1996.

324. Iorio A, Agnelli G: Low-molecular-weight and unfractionated heparin for prevention of venous thromboembolism in neurosurgery: A meta-analysis, *Arch Intern Med* 160:2327-2332, 2000.

325. Brooks NP, Turk AS, Niemann DB, et al: Frequency of thromboembolic events associated with endovascular aneurysm treatment: Retrospective case series, *J Neurosurg* 108:1095-1100, 2008.

326. Fernandez A, Schmidt JM, Claassen J, et al: Fever after subarachnoid hemorrhage: risk factors and impact on outcome, *Neurology* 68:1013-1019, 2007.

327. Badjatia N, O'Donnell J, Baker JR, et al: Achieving normothermia in patients with febrile subarachnoid hemorrhage: Feasibility and safety of a novel intravascular cooling catheter, *Neurocrit Care* 1:145-156, 2004.

328. Frontera JA, Fernandez A, Claassen J, et al: Hyperglycemia after SAH: Predictors, associated complications, and impact on outcome, *Stroke* 37:199-203, 2006.

329. Badjatia N, Topcuoglu MA, Buonanno FS, et al: Relationship between hyperglycemia and symptomatic vasospasm after subarachnoid hemorrhage, *Crit Care Med* 33:1603-1609, 2005.

330. Schlenk F, Graetz D, Nagel A, et al: Insulin-related decrease in cerebral glucose despite normoglycemia in aneurysmal subarachnoid hemorrhage, *Crit Care* 12:R9, 2008.

331. Kerner A, Schlenk F, Sakowitz O, et al: Impact of hyperglycemia on neurological deficits and extracellular glucose levels in aneurysmal subarachnoid hemorrhage patients, *Neurol Res* 29:647-653, 2007.

332. Frontera JA, Fernandez A, Schmidt JM, et al: Impact of nosocomial infectious complications after subarachnoid hemorrhage, *Neurosurgery* 62:80-87, 2008:discussion 87.

333. Kassell NF, Torner JC: Aneurysmal rebleeding: A preliminary report from the Cooperative Aneurysm Study, *Neurosurgery* 13:479-481, 1983.

334. Fujii Y, Takeuchi S, Sasaki O, et al: Ultra-early rebleeding in spontaneous subarachnoid hemorrhage, *J Neurosurg* 84:35-42, 1996.

335. Biller J, Godersky JC, Adams HP Jr: Management of aneurysmal subarachnoid hemorrhage, *Stroke* 19:1300-1305, 1988.

336. Torner JC, Kassell NF, Wallace RB, et al: Preoperative prognostic factors for rebleeding and survival in aneurysm patients receiving antifibrinolytic therapy: Report of the Cooperative Aneurysm Study, *Neurosurgery* 9:506-513, 1981.

337. Ojemann RG: Management of the unruptured intracranial aneurysm, *N Engl J Med* 304:725-726, 1981.

338. Vermeulen M, Lindsay KW, Murray GD, et al: Antifibrinolytic treatment in subarachnoid hemorrhage, *N Engl J Med* 311:432-437, 1984.

339. Roos Y: Antifibrinolytic treatment in subarachnoid hemorrhage: A randomized placebo-controlled trial. STAR Study Group, *Neurology* 54:77-82, 2000.

340. Glick R, Green D, Ts'ao C, et al: High dose epsilon-aminocaproic acid prolongs the bleeding time and increases rebleeding and intraoperative hemorrhage in patients with subarachnoid hemorrhage, *Neurosurgery* 9:398-401, 1981.

341. Roos YB, Rinkel GJ, Vermeulen M, et al: Antifibrinolytic therapy for aneurysmal subarachnoid haemorrhage, *Cochrane Database Syst Rev* (2):CD001245, 2000.

342. Starke RM, Kim GH, Fernandez A, et al: Impact of a protocol for acute antifibrinolytic therapy on aneurysm rebleeding after subarachnoid hemorrhage, *Stroke* 39:2617-2621, 2008.

343. van Gijn J, Hijdra A, Wijdicks EF, et al: Acute hydrocephalus after aneurysmal subarachnoid hemorrhage, *J Neurosurg* 63:355-362, 1985.

344. Bailes JE, Spetzler RF, Hadley MN, et al: Management, morbidity and mortality of poor-grade aneurysm patients, *J Neurosurg* 72:559-566, 1990.

345. Gruber A, Reinprecht A, Bavinzski G, et al: Chronic shunt-dependent hydrocephalus after early surgical and early endovascular treatment of ruptured intracranial aneurysms, *Neurosurgery* 44:503-509, 1999:discussion 509-512.

346. Kosteljanetz M: CSF dynamics in patients with subarachnoid and/or intraventricular hemorrhage, *J Neurosurg* 60:940-946, 1984.

347. Hasan D, Lindsay KW, Vermeulen M: Treatment of acute hydrocephalus after subarachnoid hemorrhage with serial lumbar puncture, *Stroke* 22:190-194, 1991.

348. Klimo P Jr, Kestle JR, MacDonald JD, et al: Marked reduction of cerebral vasospasm with lumbar drainage of cerebrospinal fluid after subarachnoid hemorrhage, *J Neurosurg* 100:215-224, 2004.

349. Treggiari-Venzi MM, Suter PM, Romand JA: Review of medical prevention of vasospasm after aneurysmal subarachnoid hemorrhage: A problem of neurointensive care, *Neurosurgery* 48:249-261, 2001:discussion 261-262.

350. Shimoda M, Oda S, Tsugane R, et al: Prognostic factors in delayed ischaemic deficit with vasospasm in patients undergoing early aneurysm surgery, *Br J Neurosurg* 11:210-215, 1997.

351. Wilkins RH: Cerebral vasospasm, *Crit Rev Neurobiol* 6:51-77, 1990.

352. Heros RC, Zervas NT, Varsos V: Cerebral vasospasm after subarachnoid hemorrhage: An update, *Ann Neurol* 14:599-608, 1983.

353. Vora YY, Suarez-Almazor M, Steinke DE, et al: Role of transcranial Doppler monitoring in the diagnosis of cerebral vasospasm after subarachnoid hemorrhage, *Neurosurgery* 44:1237-1247, 1999:discussion 1247-1248.

354. Laumer R, Steinmeier R, Gonner F, et al: Cerebral hemodynamics in subarachnoid hemorrhage evaluated by transcranial Doppler sonography. Part 1. Reliability of flow velocities in clinical management, *Neurosurgery* 33:1-8, 1993:discussion 8-9.

355. Steinmeier R, Laumer R, Bondar I, et al: Cerebral hemodynamics in subarachnoid hemorrhage evaluated by transcranial Doppler sonography. Part 2. Pulsatility indices: Normal reference values and characteristics in subarachnoid hemorrhage, *Neurosurgery* 33:10–18, 1993:discussion 18–19.

356. Ohtonari T, Kakinuma K, Kito T, et al: Diffusion-perfusion mismatch in symptomatic vasospasm after subarachnoid hemorrhage, *Neurol Med Chir (Tokyo)* 48:331–336, 2008:discussion 336.

357. Sviri GE, Mesiwala AH, Lewis DH, et al: Dynamic perfusion computerized tomography in cerebral vasospasm following aneurysmal subarachnoid hemorrhage: A comparison with technetium-99m-labeled ethyl cysteinate dimer-single-photon emission computerized tomography, *J Neurosurg* 104:404–410, 2006.

358. Yonas H, Gur D, Claassen D, et al: Stable xenon-enhanced CT measurement of cerebral blood flow in reversible focal ischemia in baboons, *J Neurosurg* 73:266–273, 1990.

359. Hattingen E, Blasel S, Dettmann E, et al: Perfusion-weighted MRI to evaluate cerebral autoregulation in aneurysmal subarachnoid haemorrhage, *Neuroradiology* 50:919–938, 2008.

360. Origitano TC, Wascher TM, Reichman OH, et al: Sustained increased cerebral blood flow with prophylactic hypertensive hypervolemic hemodilution ("triple-H" therapy) after subarachnoid hemorrhage, *Neurosurgery* 27:729–739, 1990:discussion 739–740.

361. Kassell NF, Peerless SJ, Durward QJ, et al: Treatment of ischemic deficits from vasospasm with intravascular volume expansion and induced arterial hypertension, *Neurosurgery* 11:337–343, 1982.

362. Germano A, d'Avella D, Imperatore C, et al: Time-course of blood-brain barrier permeability changes after experimental subarachnoid haemorrhage, *Acta Neurochir (Wien)* 142:575–580, 2000:discussion 580–581.

363. Wood JH, Kee DB Jr: Hemorheology of the cerebral circulation in stroke, *Stroke* 16:765–772, 1985.

364. Awad IA, Carter LP, Spetzler RF, et al: Clinical vasospasm after subarachnoid hemorrhage: Response to hypervolemic hemodilution and arterial hypertension, *Stroke* 18:365–372, 1987.

365. Naidech AM, Drescher J, Ault ML, et al: Higher hemoglobin is associated with less cerebral infarction, poor outcome, and death after subarachnoid hemorrhage, *Neurosurgery* 59:775–779, 2006:discussion 779–780.

366. Muench E, Horn P, Bauhuf C, et al: Effects of hypervolemia and hypertension on regional cerebral blood flow, intracranial pressure, and brain tissue oxygenation after subarachnoid hemorrhage, *Crit Care Med* 35:1844–1851, 2007:quiz 1852.

367. Raabe A, Beck J, Keller M, et al: Relative importance of hypertension compared with hypervolemia for increasing cerebral oxygenation in patients with cerebral vasospasm after subarachnoid hemorrhage, *J Neurosurg* 103:974–981, 2005.

368. Solomon RA, Fink ME, Lennihan L: Prophylactic volume expansion therapy for the prevention of delayed cerebral ischemia after early aneurysm surgery. Results of a preliminary trial, *Arch Neurol* 45:325–332, 1988.

369. Lee KH, Lukovits T, Friedman JA: "Triple-H" therapy for cerebral vasospasm following subarachnoid hemorrhage, *Neurocrit Care* 4:68–76, 2006.

370. Treggiari MM, Walder B, Suter PM, et al: Systematic review of the prevention of delayed ischemic neurological deficits with hypertension, hypervolemia, and hemodilution therapy following subarachnoid hemorrhage, *J Neurosurg* 98:978–984, 2003.

371. Shimoda M, Oda S, Tsugane R, et al: Intracranial complications of hypervolemic therapy in patients with a delayed ischemic deficit attributed to vasospasm, *J Neurosurg* 78:423–429, 1993.

372. Buckland MR, Batjer HH, Giesecke AH: Anesthesia for cerebral aneurysm surgery: Use of induced hypertension in patients with symptomatic vasospasm, *Anesthesiology* 69:116–119, 1988.

373. Hasan D, Wijdicks EF, Vermeulen M: Hyponatremia is associated with cerebral ischemia in patients with aneurysmal subarachnoid hemorrhage, *Ann Neurol* 27:106–108, 1990.

374. Siesjo BK: Cellular calcium metabolism, seizures, and ischemia, *Mayo Clin Proc* 61:299–302, 1986.

375. Hongo K, Kobayashi S: Calcium antagonists for the treatment of vasospasm following subarachnoid haemorrhage, *Neurol Res* 15:218–224, 1993.

376. Barker FG 2nd, Ogilvy CS: Efficacy of prophylactic nimodipine for delayed ischemic deficit after subarachnoid hemorrhage: A meta-analysis, *J Neurosurg* 84:405–414, 1996.

377. Feigin VL, Rinkel GJ, Algra A, et al: Calcium antagonists for aneurysmal subarachnoid haemorrhage, *Cochrane Database Syst Rev* (3):CD000277, 2000.

378. Dorhout Mees SM, Rinkel GJ, Feigin VL, et al: Calcium antagonists for aneurysmal subarachnoid haemorrhage, *Cochrane Database Syst Rev* (3):CD000277, 2007.

379. Kassell NF, Haley EC Jr, Apperson-Hansen C, et al: Randomized, double-blind, vehicle-controlled trial of tirilazad mesylate in patients with aneurysmal subarachnoid hemorrhage: A cooperative study in Europe, Australia, and New Zealand, *J Neurosurg* 84:221–228, 1996.

380. Haley EC Jr, Kassell NF, Apperson-Hansen C, et al: A randomized, double-blind, vehicle-controlled trial of tirilazad mesylate in patients with aneurysmal subarachnoid hemorrhage: A cooperative study in North America, *J Neurosurg* 86:467–474, 1997.

381. Lanzino G, Kassell NF, Dorsch NW, et al: Double-blind, randomized, vehicle-controlled study of high-dose tirilazad mesylate in women with aneurysmal subarachnoid hemorrhage. Part I. A cooperative study in Europe, Australia, New Zealand, and South Africa, *J Neurosurg* 90:1011–1017, 1999.

382. Hop JW, Rinkel GJ, Algra A, et al: Randomized pilot trial of postoperative aspirin in subarachnoid hemorrhage, *Neurology* 54:872–878, 2000.

383. Dorhout Mees SM, Rinkel GJ, Hop JW, et al: Antiplatelet therapy in aneurysmal subarachnoid hemorrhage: A systematic review, *Stroke* 34:2285–2289, 2003.

384. van den Bergh WM, Algra A, van Kooten F, et al: Magnesium sulfate in aneurysmal subarachnoid hemorrhage: A randomized controlled trial, *Stroke* 36:1011–1015, 2005.

385. Dorhout Mees S.M: Magnesium in aneurysmal subarachnoid hemorrhage (MASH II) phase III clinical trial. MASH-II study group, *Int J Stroke* 3:63–65, 2008.

386. Parra A, Kreiter KT, Williams S, et al: Effect of prior statin use on functional outcome and delayed vasospasm after acute aneurysmal subarachnoid hemorrhage: A matched controlled cohort study, *Neurosurgery* 56:476–484, 2005:discussion 476–484.

387. Tseng MY, Czosnyka M, Richards H, et al: Effects of acute treatment with pravastatin on cerebral vasospasm, autoregulation, and delayed ischemic deficits after aneurysmal subarachnoid hemorrhage: a phase II randomized placebo-controlled trial, *Stroke* 36:1627–1632, 2005.

388. Lynch JR, Wang H, McGirt MJ, et al: Simvastatin reduces vasospasm after aneurysmal subarachnoid hemorrhage: Results of a pilot randomized clinical trial, *Stroke* 36:2024–2026, 2005.

389. Sillberg VA, Wells GA, Perry JJ: Do statins improve outcomes and reduce the incidence of vasospasm after aneurysmal subarachnoid hemorrhage. A Meta-Analysis, *Stroke* 39:2622–2626, 2008.

390. Vajkoczy P, Meyer B, Weidauer S, et al: Clazosentan (AXV-034343), a selective endothelin A receptor antagonist, in the prevention of cerebral vasospasm following severe aneurysmal subarachnoid hemorrhage: results of a randomized, double-blind, placebo-controlled, multicenter phase IIa study, *J Neurosurg* 103:9–17, 2005.

391. Macdonald RL, Kassell NF, Mayer S, et al: Clazosentan to Overcome Neurological Ischemia and Infarction Occurring After Subarachnoid Hemorrhage (CONSCIOUS-1). Randomized, double-blind, placebo-controlled phase 2 dose-finding trial, *Stroke* 39:3015–3021, 2008.

392. Barth M, Capelle HH, Weidauer S, et al: Effect of nicardipine prolonged-release implants on cerebral vasospasm and clinical outcome after severe aneurysmal subarachnoid hemorrhage: A prospective, randomized, double-blind phase IIa study, *Stroke* 38:330–336, 2007.

393. Todd MM, Hindman BJ, Clarke WR, et al: Mild intraoperative hypothermia during surgery for intracranial aneurysm, *N Engl J Med* 352:135–145, 2005.

394. Schubert GA, Poli S, Mendelowitsch A, et al: Hypothermia reduces early hypoperfusion and metabolic alterations during the acute phase of massive subarachnoid hemorrhage: A laser-Doppler-flowmetry and microdialysis study in rats, *J Neurotrauma* 25:539–548, 2008.

395. Elliott JP, Newell DW, Lam DJ, et al: Comparison of balloon angioplasty and papaverine infusion for the treatment of vasospasm following aneurysmal subarachnoid hemorrhage, *J Neurosurg* 88:277-284, 1998.

396. Clouston JE, Numaguchi Y, Zoarski GH, et al: Intraarterial papaverine infusion for cerebral vasospasm after subarachnoid hemorrhage, *AJNR Am J Neuroradiol* 16:27-38, 1995.

397. Tsurushima H, Hyodo A, Yoshii Y: Papaverine and vasospasm, *J Neurosurg* 92:509-511, 2000.

398. Kaku Y, Yonekawa Y, Tsukahara T, et al: Superselective intra-arterial infusion of papaverine for the treatment of cerebral vasospasm after subarachnoid hemorrhage, *J Neurosurg* 77:842-847, 1992.

399. Tsurushima H, Kamezaki T, Nagatomo Y, et al: Complications associated with intraarterial administration of papaverine for vasospasm following subarachnoid hemorrhage—two case reports, *Neurol Med Chir (Tokyo)* 40:112-115, 2000.

400. Kassell NF, Helm G, Simmons N, et al: Treatment of cerebral vasospasm with intra-arterial papaverine, *J Neurosurg* 77:848-852, 1992.

401. Hanggi D, Turowski B, Beseoglu K, et al: Intra-arterial nimodipine for severe cerebral vasospasm after aneurysmal subarachnoid hemorrhage: Influence on clinical course and cerebral perfusion, *AJNR Am J Neuroradiol* 29:1053-1060, 2008.

402. Fraticelli AT, Cholley BP, Losser MR, et al: Milrinone for the treatment of cerebral vasospasm after aneurysmal subarachnoid hemorrhage, *Stroke* 39:893-898, 2008.

403. Goodson K, Lapointe M, Monroe T, et al: Intraventricular nicardipine for refractory cerebral vasospasm after subarachnoid hemorrhage, *Neurocrit Care* 8:247-252, 2008.

404. Newell DW, Eskridge J, Mayberg M, et al: Endovascular treatment of intracranial aneurysms and cerebral vasospasm, *Clin Neurosurg* 39:348-360, 1992.

405. Higashida RT, Halbach VV, Cahan LD, et al: Transluminal angioplasty for treatment of intracranial arterial vasospasm, *J Neurosurg* 71:648-653, 1989.

406. Eskridge JM, McAuliffe W, Song JK, et al: Balloon angioplasty for the treatment of vasospasm: Results of first 50 cases, *Neurosurgery* 42:510-516, 1998:discussion 516-517.

407. Polin RS, Coenen VA, Hansen CA, et al: Efficacy of transluminal angioplasty for the management of symptomatic cerebral vasospasm following aneurysmal subarachnoid hemorrhage, *J Neurosurg* 92:284-290, 2000.

408. Findlay JM, Weir BK, Kassell NF, et al: Intracisternal recombinant tissue plasminogen activator after aneurysmal subarachnoid hemorrhage, *J Neurosurg* 75:181-188, 1991.

409. Rohde V, Schaller C, Hassler WE: Intraventricular recombinant tissue plasminogen activator for lysis of intraventricular haemorrhage, *J Neurol Neurosurg Psychiatry* 58:447-451, 1995.

410. Mayfrank L, Hutter BO, Kohorst Y, et al: Influence of intraventricular hemorrhage on outcome after rupture of intracranial aneurysm, *Neurosurg Rev* 24:185-191, 2001.

411. Steiner T, Diringer MN, Schneider D, et al: Dynamics of intraventricular hemorrhage in patients with spontaneous intracerebral hemorrhage: Risk factors, clinical impact, and effect of hemostatic therapy with recombinant activated factor VII, *Neurosurgery* 59:767-773, 2006:discussion 773-774.

412. CLEAR-IVH Study home page. http://biosgroup-johnshopkins medicine.health.officelive.com/background.aspx.

413. Report of the 17th European Stroke Conference, May 13-16, Nice, France, 2008.

412. Schirmer CM, Hoit DA, Malek AM: Decompressive hemicraniectomy for the treatment of intractable intracranial hypertension after aneurysmal subarachnoid hemorrhage, *Stroke* 38:987-992, 2007.

413. Buschmann U, Yonekawa Y, Fortunati M, et al: Decompressive hemicraniectomy in patients with subarachnoid hemorrhage and intractable intracranial hypertension, *Acta Neurochir (Wien)* 149:59-65, 2007.

414. Minegishi A, Ishizaki T, Yoshida Y, et al: Plasma monoaminergic metabolites and catecholamines in subarachnoid hemorrhage. Clinical implications, *Arch Neurol* 44:423-428, 1987.

415. Staub F, Graf R, Gabel P, et al: Multiple interstitial substances measured by microdialysis in patients with subarachnoid hemorrhage, *Neurosurgery* 47:1106-1115, 2000:discussion 1115-1116.

416. Wijdicks EF, Vermeulen M, van Gijn J: Hyponatraemia and volume status in aneurysmal subarachnoid haemorrhage, *Acta Neurochir Suppl (Wien)* 47:111-113, 1990.

417. Disney L, Weir B, Grace M, et al: Trends in blood pressure, osmolality and electrolytes after subarachnoid hemorrhage from aneurysms, *Can J Neurol Sci* 16:299-304, 1989.

418. Kurokawa Y, Uede T, Ishiguro M, et al: Pathogenesis of hyponatremia following subarachnoid hemorrhage due to ruptured cerebral aneurysm, *Surg Neurol* 46:500-507, 1996:discussion 507-508.

419. Diringer M, Ladenson PW, Stern BJ, et al: Plasma atrial natriuretic factor and subarachnoid hemorrhage, *Stroke* 19:1119-1124, 1988.

420. Harrigan MR: Cerebral salt wasting syndrome: A review, *Neurosurgery* 38:152-160, 1996.

421. Sarrafzadeh AS, Sakowitz OW, Kiening KL, et al: Bedside microdialysis: A tool to monitor cerebral metabolism in subarachnoid hemorrhage patients? *Crit Care Med* 30:1062-1070, 2002.

422. Vajkoczy P, Horn P, Thome C, et al: Regional cerebral blood flow monitoring in the diagnosis of delayed ischemia following aneurysmal subarachnoid hemorrhage, *J Neurosurg* 98:1227-1234, 2003.

Pharmacologic Modification of Acute Cerebral Ischemia

NICOLE R. GONZALES, JAMES C. GROTTA

Pharmacologic therapy of acute ischemic stroke promises the opportunity to reduce brain injury and hence disability in a large proportion of patients with stroke. Treatments are needed that can be proven effective for important clinical outcomes in well-designed clinical trials. Optimally, these treatments should be low in morbidity, cost, and complexity so that they can be quickly and widely used in emergency settings of variable sophistication, as are common in the care of most patients with stroke worldwide.

Background: Preclinical and Clinical Cytoprotection

The Definition and Role of Cytoprotection

Pharmacologic therapy of ischemic stroke can be split into broad groups on the basis of the sequence and location of physiologic events thought to occur on occlusion of a cerebral artery, although as in most complex biological systems, these events overlap both temporally and spatially. Since the previous edition of this chapter was written, an additional aspect of ischemic injury has emerged: ischemic preconditioning, in which a noxious stimulus given below the threshold of damage can induce protection when a subsequent deleterious event occurs. The mechanisms of ischemic preconditioning are currently the focus of ongoing study, and important mediators include Toll-like receptors (TLRs)[1] and astrocyte-mediated mechanisms.[2] There is mounting evidence that the genomic response to the ischemic cascade can be reprogrammed,[1] thus introducing the concept of prophylactic ischemic stroke therapy in high-risk patients (e.g., those undergoing endovascular and surgical procedures with periprocedural risk of ischemic stroke).

The next group of therapies targets the events occurring within the artery lumen by reversing the arterial occlusion and restoring perfusion to damaged brain tissue. The prototypes of such therapy are thrombolytics, fibrinolytics, and anticoagulants. Reversing arterial occlusion has been the area of greatest clinical success to date in stroke treatment. Other therapies targeting later events will probably have much less impact on outcome than fast removal of the offending arterial occlusion, and it is even possible that further improvement in treatment cannot be achieved unless it is also accompanied by reperfusion of the damaged tissue. Much can be learned from the preclinical and

clinical development of these "reperfusion" drugs, and the lessons will be brought into this chapter. However, such therapy is discussed in detail in other chapters and so is not specifically addressed further here.

A third, broad category of pharmacotherapy for stroke targets the consequences of arterial occlusion on the blood vessel wall, neuron, glia, and neuronal environment. Although often labeled *neuroprotection,* this approach to therapy actually has a wide variety of targets, many of which are nonneuronal, so a more appropriate term would be *cytoprotection*. Common to this approach is the effort to improve outcome by preventing progression to cellular death of tissue initially damaged by the ischemic event. Although unlikely to salvage irreversibly damaged cells, such therapies may "modify" the biologic perturbations induced at the cellular level in brain tissue whose fate still hangs in the balance. This type of pharmacotherapy is the subject of the present chapter.

A final category of stroke pharmacotherapy aims to augment recovery of brain function by targeting events during the restorative phase occurring after tissue damage is complete. This therapy is the subject of another chapter.

The concept of cytoprotection relies on the principle that delayed cellular injury occurs after ischemia. Neurons suffer irreversible damage after only a few minutes of complete cessation of blood flow. Such a condition might exist during cardiac arrest. In most instances of acute focal brain ischemia, however, if a state of zero blood flow occurs, it would only be in the core of the ischemic region. The larger surrounding penumbral area receives reduced blood flow, which causes loss of normal function that may lead to permanent cellular damage if uncorrected but allows for recovery if blood flow is restored by either clot lysis or collateral flow.

Because ischemia is clearly a process and not an instantaneous event, there is potential both for modifying the process after the clinical ictus and for altering the final outcome. It is equally apparent from experimental models that if cytoprotective treatments are to succeed, they must be instituted within a few minutes after the onset of ischemia. Previous clinical trials may have failed because such treatment was delayed and was therefore unlikely to render a benefit.

The concept of cytoprotection is not new in the clinical domain. It has been known for years that hypothermia reduces ischemic neuronal injury. Accidental hypothermia can protect a drowning victim from otherwise fatal hypoxic-ischemic brain damage. Animal models of both global and focal ischemia confirm the beneficial effects of hypothermia. The benefit of hypothermia in treating global cerebral ischemic injury after cardiac arrest has also been dramatically demonstrated in humans. The importance of this result cannot be overemphasized because it is the first proof that experimental brain cytoprotection, which can be demonstrated so readily in the laboratory, can be translated into human benefit. The mechanism of action of hypothermia is uncertain but probably is related to effects on multiple cytotoxic events that occur after ischemia.

Targets of Cytoprotection: The Ischemic Cascade

A major accomplishment of in vivo and in vitro model systems of cerebral ischemia is an understanding of the *ischemic cascade*. The details of the physiologic events that constitute the brain's response to injury and this cascade are discussed in detail in other chapters. Each step of this cascade might be a potential target for therapeutic intervention. Several variables exist that may affect the pathobiology of the ischemic cascade and, consequently, the severity of injury; the most important are the depth of blood flow reduction, its duration before reperfusion occurs, its distribution (i.e., global or focal), comorbidities (e.g., diabetes or hypertension), and the adequacy of reperfusion, if one assumes that reperfusion occurs. However, many of the events that have been described seem to follow in a fairly predictable order.[3-7]

First, there is reduction of blood flow, followed rapidly by ion channel dysregulation, depletion of intracellular energy stores, membrane depolarization, inhibition of protein synthesis, and calcium overloading. These processes are accompanied by an initial increase in both oxygen extraction and glucose metabolism, as well as lactic acidosis. Membrane depolarization causes opening of voltage-operated calcium channels, allowing disruption of tightly regulated neuronal calcium homeostasis. Glutamate is released from metabolic and synaptic stores and, in the presence of glycine, activates the *N*-methyl-D-aspartate (NMDA) ionotropic glutamate receptor. The immediate consequence is increased sodium permeability and cellular swelling (cytotoxic edema), but the more damaging event is further elevation of intracellular calcium through the NMDA-associated ion channel. Further perturbations in ion flux occur as a result of glutamate's effect on α-amino-3-hydroxy-5-methyl-4-isoxazole propionic acid (AMPA) and metabotropic receptors. Documented increases in other neurotransmitters, such as γ-aminobutyric acid (GABA), dopamine, and norepinephrine, may also be damaging. More recently, the sulfonylurea receptor 1 (SUR 1)–regulated nonselective cation–adenosine triphosphate (NCCa-ATP) channel and acid-sensing ion channel 1a have been implicated in the pathogenesis of ischemic injury.

Increased intracellular calcium activates a large number of damaging enzymatic pathways. Calcium (through calmodulin) activates protein kinases such as CaM kinase II and protein kinase C, which may imbalance neuronal homeostasis by causing protein phosphorylation. Other pivotal enzyme systems activated by calcium are (1) the proteases, such as calpain, which causes cytoskeletal proteolysis, as well as activation of programmed cell death, for example, via mitochondrial release of apoptosis-inducing factor (AIF); (2) lipases, such as phospholipase A, which leads to production of arachidonic acid and free radical formation, and phospholipase C, which via generation of inositol 1,4,5-trisphosphate (IP3) results in release of intracellular calcium stores, and (3) nitric oxide synthase (NOS), which increases nitric acid (NO) and consequently the potent pro-oxidative peroxynitrites. The consequences of free radical production and these enzyme perturbations are widespread and include damage to proteins, lipids, and DNA; disruption of neuronal (and endothelial) membrane and cytoskeletal integrity; and disruption of nuclear and mitochondrial function, leading to irreversible brain tissue damage. Damaged mitochondria release various factors (e.g., cytochrome c, Smac, AIF, or endonuclease G) involved in programmed cell death. The best characterized, cytochrome c, represents a key step in assembly of the apoptosome and activation of caspase-9 during the initial stages of apoptosis.

Increased gene expression in ischemic regions, including those induced by spreading depolarization initiated by ischemia, could have damaging consequences. Adhesion molecules, such as intercellular adhesion molecule-1 (ICAM-1), P- and E-selectins, and integrins (e.g., CD18), enable interaction of white blood cells with vascular endothelium and extravasation, which leads to parenchymal cell damage, production of blood–brain barrier damage, and obstruction of the microcirculation, resulting in "no reflow." Growth factors such as nerve growth factor (NGF) and basic fibroblast growth factor (bFGF) may result in further increased production of NO. This NO-cGMP-PKG mechanism may have a prosurvival component. Cytokines such as tumor necrosis factor-α (TNFα) and interleukin-1β (IL-1β) activate their respective receptors and transcription factors, such as nuclear factor kappa B (NFκB), which in turn promote and perpetuate the proinflammatory response and may also set in motion the activity of various caspases. The consequence of these nuclear pathways is alteration in DNA structure and function leading to delayed cellular death (apoptosis). Additionally, there is growing evidence that TLR signaling plays an important role in aggravating stroke-mediated brain injury.

The biology of the recovery phase after ischemic injury is less well understood but is the subject of intensive investigation. Many of the same events that are triggered by interruption of blood flow probably also stimulate the recovery process at later stages. First, local and hematogenous inflammatory cells may remove damaged or destroyed tissue. Theoretically, this removal may help provide a suitable environment for developing new neuronal connections, neurogenesis, and in-growth of progenitor cells. There is evidence that glutamate release (mainly via NMDA receptor), NO-cGMP-PKG activation, and various calcium-activated enzymes such as CaM-kinase II, metalloproteinase-9, and numerous growth factors act in concert to stimulate production of new dendritic connections between surviving cells, axonogenesis, and stimulation of nascent progenitor cells.

Preclinical Stroke Models

The development of reproducible, relatively simple animal models mimicking cerebral ischemia in humans subsequently led to numerous preclinical studies testing the efficacy of cytoprotective therapies that targeted each of the steps of the ischemic cascade. Rodents have been most commonly used for these studies. Although the general nature of the cerebral damage produced by ischemia is the same among species, the severity and other features may differ not only between species but also among various strains and within strains, depending on age, gender, and size. To maintain reproducibility of results of such studies, investigators must pay careful attention to the choice of anesthetic as well as to physiologic variables, such as brain temperature, oxygenation, blood flow, and acid-base balance. These variables must be carefully controlled both during and after ischemia. The standardization of physiologic variables is an important difference between animal stroke models and human stroke, the latter being characterized by great variability in severity and other phenotypic features. Broadly, the models can be divided into those of global forebrain ischemia, which reflect the type of cerebral injury incurred with cardiac arrest, and those of unilateral carotid and/or middle cerebral artery (MCA) occlusion, similar to what occurs with ischemic stroke in humans. Many permutations of these models exist.

Global ischemia is usually produced through permanent occlusion of the vertebral arteries and temporary occlusion of the carotid arteries bilaterally, often in association with some degree of induced hypotension to produce total cessation of flow. This goal is difficult to achieve because of the rich muscular collateral network present in most species. Flow is usually restored by reversal of the carotid occlusion and hypotension, which is similar to what occurs with resuscitation after cardiac arrest. The resultant morphologic injury to the cortex, striatum, and hippocampus develops in a predictable and delayed manner and correlates both spatially and temporally with pathologic changes seen after cardiac arrest in humans. In particular, damage to the CA1 sector of the hippocampus has proven to be easily quantitated and correlates with testable and measurable changes in memory.[8-10]

Models of focal ischemia may involve either permanent or reversible unilateral occlusion of the MCA or carotid artery (or both), sometimes coupled with hypotension or contralateral occlusion of the carotid artery to reduce collateral flow.[11-14] Occlusions have been produced by ligation or other external means, by endovascular obstruction by injected clots or suture material, or by thrombosis induced by local activation of coagulation. All models are characterized by geographically measurable damage to cortex and usually striatum of varying severity according to strain of species, duration and depth of ischemia, and location of arterial occlusion. Such injury can also be measured by a number of behavioral tests of motor and proprioceptive function.

Preclinical Testing of Cytoprotective Therapies

The disturbing reality is that despite the substantial positive effect of cytoprotective drugs in animal stroke models—except for hypothermia after cardiac arrest—results of all clinical trials of this approach to stroke treatment have been neutral (no effect) or negative (harmful). Before we discuss this conundrum, we deal with several general themes that have proved useful in achieving positive results with cytoprotective therapies in preclinical models. Careful attention to these issues will be important in achieving positive results with neuroprotective drugs, either in the laboratory or at the bedside.

The Need for Careful Physiologic Monitoring

Core temperature, blood glucose concentration, pH, oxygenation, blood pressure, and cerebral blood flow and collateral circulation all have important effects on outcome after ischemia. If these variables are not controlled in the laboratory, variability in stroke severity occurs and consistent results are not detected. For instance, if cerebral blood flow is not monitored during an experiment in which the MCA is occluded, animals in two comparison treatment groups may have different levels of ischemic insult; thus differences in outcome may be due to these imbalances rather than to the therapy that is being tested. Minor differences in the location or number of vessels occluded or in the level of blood pressure can have major effects on the depth and distribution of cerebral hypoperfusion. As another example, some drugs, such as the glutamate antagonists, can lower brain temperature. Unless this effect is monitored, positive results occurring from the neuroprotective properties of hypothermia may be attributed to the drug instead.

Penumbra as Target

Because cytoprotective therapies are aimed at interrupting the ischemic cascade in tissue that is not yet dead, most logically they should be tested in animal models of focal cerebral ischemia in which there is a relatively extensive ischemic penumbra. *Penumbra* can be operationally defined as tissue that has been exposed to a reduction in perfusion shy of the threshold leading to immediate destruction but that would not survive without reperfusion or cytoprotective intervention.[3,4] Such regions of "penumbral level" hypoperfusion are most often seen in MCA occlusion models with rather extensive cortical involvement and in which the damage is of a moderate nature, more typical of reversible occlusion models. Penumbra is also time-related; it gradually disappears over minutes to hours after arterial occlusion to become incorporated into the irreversibly damaged "core," or areas that spontaneously improve their perfusion and function ("benign oligemia"). It is likely that both in the laboratory and at the bedside, strokes with extensive penumbral tissue are the most likely to respond to cytoprotection and vice versa; that is, strokes with irreversible damage are the least likely. The current challenge is reliable determination of penumbra. The hope is that the ischemic penumbra can be imaged as a surrogate marker of reversible versus irreversible injury. So far, this surrogate marker remains elusive.

Reperfusion Injury

There is considerable debate regarding whether reperfusion itself has damaging effects. Certainly, if there is disruption of the blood–brain barrier, reperfusion can be associated with cerebral edema and hemorrhage. However, even in the absence of such gross abnormalities, reperfusion after a period of occlusion long enough to produce cellular injury may result in increased production of free radicals, gene expression, and inflammatory events that may augment cellular damage. Experimental evidence has shown greater histologic damage, particularly in cortex, after temporary MCA occlusion lasting 3 hours than in permanent MCA occlusion.[15,16] Many cytoprotective drugs are especially effective in animal models of reperfusion that incorporate some element of reperfusion injury. The effort to understand the effect of neuroprotective therapies on reperfusion injury deserves greater attention.

Downstream Targets

Prophylactic treatment with cytoprotective drugs may be possible in some cases (i.e., before high-risk surgical procedures), but in most patients, these drugs are started at some point after the onset of the stroke. Many of the initial events in the ischemic cascade, such as release of glutamate and increase in intracellular calcium, occur almost instantaneously, and their effect might not be dampened by a cytoprotective agent even if it is started as early as 1 or 2 hours after the onset of ischemia. This has been reflected in the relatively brief 30- to 60-minute maximal time window of therapeutic efficacy of these drugs in laboratory models and in the failure of clinical trials to show benefit when these drugs were started as late as 6 to 24 hours after stroke onset. Later events in the cascade, such as production of NO and free radicals, inflammatory cytokines, transcription factors, and caspases may be more effectively targeted by postischemic cytoprotective therapies. These events represent the final pathways to cellular death, and their treatment has led to robust protection in animal stroke models.

Multimodality Therapy

An understanding of the ischemic cascade has enabled us to design cytoprotective therapy aimed at each of these steps. This has led to the emerging concept that multimodality therapy may be necessary to maximize a therapeutic attack on acute ischemic stroke. A therapy targeting only one of these processes is unlikely to result in a therapeutic "home run." A multimodality approach to neuroprotection will probably be more effective clinically than the use of a single agent. The negative or neutral results of clinical trials of drugs targeting specific neurotransmitter pathways (see later), despite their efficacy in animal models, suggest that, to detect a signal of clinical efficacy, we need a more potent intervention that might be achieved only by simultaneously targeting multiple pathways. However, such clinical studies will be complex and more difficult to design and carry out. The dosing, benefit, and interactions of the various candidate combinations must be worked out in animal models before this approach can be taken at the bedside.

Combinations of reperfusion and neuroprotective strategies have been shown to be effective in several laboratories. Uematsu et al.[17] found that the neuronal calcium signal increased after MCA occlusion in rats and that the increase was not attenuated by reperfusion. The noncompetitive NMDA ion channel blocker MK-801 administered during ischemia was able to attenuate intracellular calcium and increase the amount of neuronal salvage over that achieved only by reperfusion. Zivin and Mazzarella[18] reported a positive effect of the thrombolytic tissue plasminogen activator (t-PA) in a rabbit autologous clot embolism model. MK-801 had no beneficial effect by itself in this model, but when added to t-PA, this agent was able to increase efficacy by approximately 33% over that achieved by t-PA alone. In a later study, the same investigators found anti-ICAM-1 to have an additive effect on t-PA,[19] and other laboratories have found other cytoprotective drugs that improve outcome over that achieved by t-PA alone.

Combinations of various cytoprotective therapies are also more effective than the use of one alone. Uematsu et al.[17] found that the addition of the dihydropyridine, voltage-operated calcium channel antagonist nimodipine to MK-801 augmented the beneficial effect on both calcium and neuronal necrosis. Hypothermia has been combined with pharmacologic cytoprotective agents to provide additional benefit. In some cases, drug combinations may be effective even though the individual components used alone have little or no effect.

Early Pharmacologic Intervention May Influence Functional Recovery

As we have learned more about the biology of neurologic recovery after stroke (covered in other chapters), it has become apparent that brain plasticity and functional recovery depend on the contributions of synaptogenesis, dendritic arborization, trophic factors, and progenitor cells. The timing and amount of these reparative processes may be influenced by neurotransmitter function, inflammation, and gene expression that all occur earlier and that may be the targets of neuroprotective pharmacotherapy. For example, one could envision that an antiglutamatergic drug given soon after stroke to reduce necrosis might also have the unwanted negative effect of inhibiting synaptogenesis, which also depends to some extent on glutamatergic function.

The outcome in rodent stroke models used to test neuroprotective drugs is usually measured by histologic quantification of infarct volume within the first few days after stroke onset. These measures may miss an additional positive effect of the drug on recovery or an inhibitory effect on reparative processes. Evaluation of behavioral outcome during the weeks after stroke may provide a more accurate picture of the effect of a neuroprotective agent on the complex interaction of acute injury and delayed recovery.

Relevance of Animal Models

Much has been written about the failure of benefit in clinical trials of neuroprotective drugs despite the positive results of the same drugs in animal models.[20,21] Such discordance has raised the question of whether the animal models of stroke, particularly rodent models, reflect what is occurring in human stroke. Indeed, the juvenile lissencephalic rodent brain used in most laboratory studies may not respond to ischemic injury or to a neuroprotective drug the same way as an elderly gyrencephalic human brain. However, data correlating thresholds of both the depth and duration of perfusion needed to produce irreversible damage have been similar in rodents and humans,[22,23] such that the positive results of thrombolytic trials in patients with stroke were predicted by data from animal models. Similarly, the success of hypothermia after cardiac arrest in humans was predicted by the benefit seen with a similar protocol after global forebrain ischemia in rodents.[24-26] Therefore, although biological differences between rodent and human brain certainly exist, it is likely that the discrepancy between results of clinical and laboratory testing of neuroprotective drugs rests more on differences between the way we have tested drugs in the laboratory and how we have designed the clinical trials to test them at the bedside.

This principle has been demonstrated in a review of preclinical neuroprotection studies that compared the experimental efficacy of interventions that have been taken forward to clinical trials with that of drugs that have only been tested in the laboratory.[27] There was no evidence that drugs used clinically were more effective experimentally than those tested only in animal models. The results of this review highlight the importance of the quality of trial design in the preclinical stages of development because it provides the foundation for translational clinical trials. Even the most well-designed clinical trials are doomed to failure if the premise on which they are based is not solid.

Stroke Therapy Academic Industry Roundtables (STAIR) are consensus conferences on translational stroke research and have addressed how to reconcile our laboratory and clinical studies to achieve successful translation of laboratory results.[21,28,29] Some of the conferences' recommendations for making our laboratory studies more reliable were as follows:

1. Evaluate most drugs in both permanent and transient models of ischemia.
2. Provide an adequate dose–response curve.
3. Determine the therapeutic index between efficacy and toxicity; a narrow index would indicate less clinical utility.
4. Explore the time window of benefit.
5. Perform studies with blinded assessment of outcome and with careful monitoring of potentially confounding physiologic variables.
6. Measure outcome both histologically and functionally and both immediately and at later points.
7. Ensure that preclinical studies follow the intent-to-treat model of clinical trials—animals should not be excluded from the analysis just because they are "data outliers" and so on.
8. Before proceeding to clinical trials, a drug should be seen to have positive results consistently in multiple laboratories and with multiple models. Comparison of magnitude of benefit with positive controls may be useful for determining relative efficacy.
9. Test novel first-in-class drugs in gyrencephalic species.

In the following discussion, we describe some of the important things we need to do in the future design of clinical trials to achieve the success realized in the laboratory.

Important Issues to Clarify in Design of Future Clinical Trials

Standardization of Stroke

Along with time to treatment, the biggest discrepancy between laboratory and clinical trials has been in the area of standardized stroke physiology, severity, type, location,

perfusion, and reversibility. We have already emphasized that controlling physiologic variables is important in detecting a therapeutic effect in laboratory stroke models. This control is more difficult to achieve in patients who have a wide variety of underlying illness such as pulmonary disease (hypoxia), cardiac disease (hypotension, reduced cardiac output), diabetes (elevated blood glucose and lactate levels), advanced age and associated atherosclerosis (reduced collateral circulation), and infection (fever). Distribution of such underlying conditions that are known to influence outcome must be balanced among the treatment groups in any clinical trial.

The single most important determinant of stroke outcome is stroke severity, as reflected in the clinical deficit.[30] This deficit can be quantitated with various stroke scales. It is critical that the distribution and level of stroke severity be comparable in the treatment groups of any stroke trial. Most patients with very minor deficits recover spontaneously, and those with very severe deficits often do not survive. Patients at these extremes of the clinical spectrum therefore only provide "noise" in the analysis because their data are least likely to show a difference between an effective treatment and the control group. Most trials now use the baseline stroke scale to exclude patients with the most minor or severe strokes and to ensure that the treated groups are well balanced in the critical variable of stroke severity. However, there is debate about what the thresholds should be. Most investigators would agree that patients with National Institute of Health Stroke Scale (NIHSS) scores lower than 5 usually will recover spontaneously and might be excluded from clinical trials. However, some of these patients with "mild" strokes do show deterioration, and excluding them may eliminate a subset of patients who could substantially benefit from treatment. Because the NIHSS scores are higher (worse) in patients with left hemisphere strokes,[31] the upper cutoff may differ in patients with left and right hemisphere lesions. Studies have shown that death due to cerebral swelling begins to occur more frequently with NIHSS scores of 15 to 20 for right hemisphere and 20 to 25 for left hemisphere lesions.

In addition to stroke severity, strokes might be standardized on the basis of type or location of stroke and presence of penumbra. This would best be achieved by imaging the infarct immediately and accepting into the trial only patients with lesions in certain locations (e.g., cortical or subcortical), depending on the optimal target tissue identified in laboratory and exploratory phase 2 studies.

The presence of reversible damage, or penumbra, is likely to be even more important than location. Numerous studies have attempted to define the imaging signature of penumbral tissue.[32-39] From a practical standpoint, the most progress has been made with magnetic resonance imaging (MRI), although recent progress in computed tomographic (CT) physiologic imaging may provide accurate and more widely applicable information. A complete discussion of MRI and CT in acute stroke is beyond the scope of this chapter and is addressed in another chapter. However, most investigators agree that the existence of a volumetric "mismatch" between the area of severely decreased perfusion (indicating tissue at risk of infarction) and a smaller area of very low diffusion of water (diffusion-weighted imaging [DWI]) on MRI or very low cerebral blood volume (CBV) on CT (both indicating irreversibly damaged tissue) is operationally the best indicator that penumbra still exists. This mismatch is seen in almost all patients imaged within the first 2 to 3 hours after stroke onset but may also be seen to a lesser extent as long as 6 to 8 hours after stroke. Perhaps relying on the presence of this mismatch rather than on an arbitrary stopwatch would better help select patients for cytoprotective clinical trials. A final advantage of using imaging to identify and standardize the selection of patients with stroke is that the DWI or CBV abnormality might provide a baseline index of stroke extent that might be compared with the final infarct volume to determine whether the therapeutic intervention has been successful in preventing any growth of the infarct after admission.[40] To date, however, the appropriate imaging thresholds for distinguishing either penumbra from benign oligemia or irreversibly from reversibly injured core tissue are still uncertain and under intense investigation.

Such issues of stroke standardization and selection of the optimal set of patients for a pivotal efficacy trial should be worked out in multiphasic phase 2 studies before embarking on a large phase 3 efficacy trial.

Sample Size

As will become apparent in the discussion of the individual clinical trials that have been conducted, most have been insufficiently powered to detect small clinical benefits. If one considers that t-PA given within 3 hours of stroke onset produced an absolute difference of 12% to 15% in good outcome in a trial of roughly 300 patients,[41] then a trial of a cytoprotective drug, which would most likely produce substantially less effect than t-PA, would have to be much larger to reach significance. Later efficacy trials, such as the Glycine Antagonist (gavestinel) in Neuroprotection (GAIN International) study,[42] the Intravenous Magnesium Efficacy in Acute Stroke trial (IMAGES),[43] and Stroke—Acute Ischemic NXY Treatment (SAINT)[44] were powered to detect a 5% difference in outcome, which is a treatment effect that is more realistic to expect. A good example of what can be expected in effect size in a cytoprotective trial is the experience with citicoline, in which a significant treatment effect of 5% was seen in a meta-analysis of 1652 patients.[45]

Unfortunately, the sample size cannot be determined from pilot studies. It would seem prudent, therefore, to be conservative and to plan to enroll a large number of patients into the efficacy trial. If, by some chance, the drug is particularly effective and fewer patients are needed to prove efficacy, this fact will become apparent to the Data Safety and Monitoring Committee during the trial, and the trial could be terminated early (for efficacy) because it would become unethical to continue to randomly assign patients to the untreated arm. However, the failure of trials to date has discouraged investment in such large, expensive studies.

Time

Perhaps the biggest deficiency of clinical trials to date has been the substantial delay in starting treatment compared with animal studies. The calcium antagonist and glutamate antagonist trials are excellent examples (see later). In the laboratory, these drugs work only if started within an hour or so of the onset of ischemia, presumably because they are targeting events that occur immediately on the interruption of blood flow. The clinical trials testing these compounds, however, enrolled patients 6 to 12 hours after stroke onset. There are many reasons for designing trials to allow delayed therapy; mainly, they include the difficulty in accruing large numbers of patients into trials within 1 to 3 hours of onset and marketing pressures dictating that treating so few patients would not be profitable. However, these are practical and not biological reasons, and our negative experiences to date tell us that we must pay more attention to the biology of the disease to be successful. The clinical trial, therefore, should reflect the time window determined in preclinical studies.

It is possible to treat patients more rapidly after stroke onset, as evidenced by the successful National Institute of Neurological Diseases and Stroke (NINDS) t-PA trial (treatment given within 90 to 180 minutes)[41] and later studies temporally linking use of t-PA within 3 hours and random assignment to therapy with the cytoprotective agent.[46] Even more aggressive have been efforts to train paramedics to recognize stroke with sufficient accuracy to allow field administration of the first dose of the cytoprotective drug.[47]

Coupling Cytoprotection with Reperfusion

Besides the practical issue of delivering drug faster, there are other theoretical advantages of coupling cytoprotection with the use of t-PA or other reperfusion strategies. Logically, it would allow greater penetration of the cytoprotective agent into the target tissue than if the arterial occlusion remained untreated. Furthermore, as already discussed, one of the consequences of reperfusion might be a second wave of pathologic events leading to "reperfusion injury" that might be advantageously targeted by the cytoprotective agent.

Dose

It will become apparent in the discussion to follow that several cytoprotective drugs have been taken through clinical trial progression from phase 1 to large phase 3 efficacy trials even though side effects limited the doses that were given so that blood levels of drug analogous to those that had been protective in animals were never achieved in humans. Often, patients with stroke do not tolerate drugs that have sedative, behavioral, or cardiovascular side effects. It is critical that careful phase 2 trials determine both the maximal tolerated dose of drug in patients with stroke and the likelihood that the dose will have an adequate effect.

More Sensitive Outcome Measures

Animal stroke models most often rely on histologic outcome, whereas clinical trials in humans are based on functional performance. Which measure is more sensitive? More important, which is more important to patients? Clearly, patients are more interested in what they can do functionally regardless of what an MR image or CT scan shows. Fortunately, analyses from the NINDS trial suggest that clinical endpoints are just as sensitive as infarct volume endpoints, at least as measured by CT.[48] Furthermore, in animal models that incorporate both histologic and behavioral outcomes, the two have been shown to correlate very closely. Therefore, it appears there is little reason to abandon functional outcome measures in clinical trials. However, if we could find a stroke volume endpoint that proves to be more sensitive than functional measures, this endpoint might be used in phase 2 trials as a "surrogate" to determine whether functional success would be likely in a larger efficacy trial. As mentioned, MRI may provide such a surrogate by determining the effect of a therapy on the growth of infarct volume from baseline DWI to later T2-weighted measurements.[40]

Another question concerns the best functional outcome measure to use. This issue is still uncertain because no one measurement reflects the total clinical condition of the patient. Clearly, any scale that is used to measure outcome must be validated as reflecting a true deficit in function, its entire range and distribution in patients with stroke must be understood, and its reliability with repeated measurements and among different examiners must be established. What is the best scale to measure stroke outcome? Is it a measure of the neurologic findings (e.g., NIHSS), the amount of disability (e.g., modified Rankin Scale [mRS]), the functional independence (e.g., Barthel Index [BI]), or the quality of life (e.g., EuroQOL).[49,50] Fortunately, these measures generally correlate with one another, but which of them is the most valid, reliable, and sensitive needs to be determined.

Even when that issue has been determined, questions arise as to how to measure effect. Should the effect of a drug be evaluated along the entire spectrum of the scale, or should the scale be dichotomized into good and bad outcomes? The latter is often necessary because the distribution of patients with stroke is not normally distributed on most scales. However, the dichotomy leaves out important data in the middle ranges of stroke outcome. Furthermore, is it better to use a single scale or multiple scales? The NINDS study used a global outcome statistic that incorporated data from several clinical scales simultaneously into one odds ratio for good versus poor outcome.[51] A disadvantage of this approach is that it requires dichotomization of the scales that are used. Further work must be done to obtain the most information from our scales so that their sensitivity in detecting a meaningful difference between treatment groups can be increased.

More Potent Therapies Are Needed

As previously discussed, it appears that greater efficacy can be achieved in animal models by targeting events that occur "downstream" in the ischemic cascade and by multimodality and combination therapies that target multiple steps simultaneously. Clinical trials are starting to test these approaches. However, such clinical trials pose several theoretical and practical problems. Many of the drugs targeting downstream events such as growth factors do not readily cross the blood–brain barrier. Furthermore, although inflammation and apoptosis may have negative effects, these processes may also have a positive reparative role, as we have pointed out.

In the case of combination therapies, the traditional approach has been that each component must be tested separately and the combination must be more effective than the sum of the components. However, this approach would require a multiple-armed trial of huge numbers of patients, which is impractical if urgent therapy were also part of the protocol. One could argue that, because most single drugs that are approved by the U.S. Food and Drug Administration (FDA) do not have a unique mechanism of action but instead have multiple effects, testing of drug combinations should be allowed without requiring testing of their individual components, particularly in a disease for which so few therapeutic options exist and clinical trials are so difficult to perform. These difficult issues must be addressed. One way or the other, the complex issues of how to dose the various components of the combination and how to deal with their interactions and side effects need to be worked out in careful phase 2 studies before larger efficacy trials are initiated.

Clinical Cytoprotective Therapy Trials

To date, many cytoprotective drugs have reached the stage of pivotal phase 3 efficacy trials in patients with acute stroke (Table 53-1). Unfortunately, throughout the neuroprotective literature, the phrase "failure to demonstrate efficacy" is a common thread in the many trials with neutral or negative results despite the largely encouraging results yielded by preclinical studies. The reasons for this discrepancy are multiple and have been discussed in the preceding paragraphs. Many of the later trials have addressed deficiencies of the previous ones with more rigorous trial design, including more specific patient selection criteria (ensuring homogeneity of stroke location and severity), stratified randomization algorithms (time-to-treat), narrowed therapeutic window, and pharmacokinetic monitoring. Current trials have also incorporated biological surrogate markers of toxicity and outcome, such as serum drug levels and neuroimaging. Lastly, multimodal therapies and coupled cytoprotection–reperfusion strategies are being investigated to optimize tissue salvage. Recently completed phase 1 and 2 trials and ongoing cytoprotective clinical trials are listed in Tables 53-2 and 53-3, respectively.

In the remainder of this chapter, we focus on individual therapeutic strategies, emphasizing what has been learned from these trials in terms of both trial design and the biological effect (or lack thereof) of these agents.

Calcium Antagonists

The first practical pharmacologic agents to be clinically evaluated for cytoprotection in stroke were the calcium channel antagonists. There are several classes of calcium channels that play a role in brain ischemia. The presynaptic voltage-activated N-type calcium channels are largely restricted to neurons and regulate neurotransmitter release. The ubiquitous voltage-gated L-type calcium channels trigger excitation–contraction coupling in smooth muscle and regulate vasomotor tone. These L-type calcium channels are sensitive to the dihydropyridine compounds, of which nimodipine and nicardipine are examples. Calcium influx through NMDA receptor–mediated channels is both ligand- and voltage-dependent. Other classes of calcium channels have distinct activation or inactivation

TABLE 53-1 PAST AND CURRENT CYTOPROTECTIVE CLINICAL TRIALS

Drug	Phase	Latest Extent of Time Window (h)	Adequate Power*	Adequate Dose	Dose-Limiting Adverse Effects	Results	N
Calcium antagonists							
Nimodipine	3	6-48	+	?	Hypotension	Neutral	
Nicardipine	2	12		?	Hypotension	Neutral	
Glutamate antagonists							
Selfotel	3	6-12	+	No	Neuropsychological	Negative	
Dextrorphan	2	48		Yes	Neuropsychological	Neutral	
Aptiganel (Cerestat)	3	6-24	+	Yes	Hypertension	Negative	
AR-R15696AR	2	12		Yes	Neuropsychological	Neutral	
Magnesium							
IMAGES	3	12	+	Yes	No	Neutral	2589
FAST-MAG	3†	2		Yes	No	?	
AMPA antagonists							
YM872	2b	3-6	+	?	?	Neutral	
ZK200775	2	24		?	Sedation	Negative	
Indirect glutamate modulators							
Eliprodil	3	?	?	?	?	Negative	
Gavestinel	3	6	+	Yes	No	Neutral	
Sipatrigine	2	12		?	Neuropsychological	Negative	
Fosphenytoin	2/3	4	+	?	No	Neutral	
BMS-204352	3	6	+	?	No	Neutral	
Lifarizine	2	?		?	Hypotension	Neutral	
Lubeluzole	3	4-8	+	No	Cardiac	Neutral	
Other neurotransmitter modulators							
Trazodone	2	?	?	?	?	Neutral	
Repinotan	3	6	+	Yes	?	Negative	660
ONO-2506	2/3	6	+	?	?	?	
Opioid antagonists							
Naloxone	2	8-60		?	No	Neutral	
Nalmefene	3	6	+	?	No	Neutral	
GABA agonists							
Clomethiazole	3	12	+	Yes	Sedation	Neutral	
Diazepam	3	12	+	?	?	Neutral	880
Free radical scavengers							
Tirilazad	3	6	+	?	No	Negative	
Ebselen	3	48	+	?	?	?	394
NXY-059	3	6	+	Yes	No	Neutral	3195
Anti-inflammatory agents							
Enlimomab	3	6	+	Yes	Fever	Negative	
LeukArrest	3	12		?	?	Neutral	
FK-506	2†	12		?	?	?	
Steroids	2	48		?	Infection	Negative	
Membrane stabilizers, trophic factor							
GM1	3	72	+	?	No	Neutral	
Cerebrolysin	2	12-24		?	No	Positive trend	
Citicoline	3†	24	+	?	No	Positive pooled analysis	
Albumin	3†	5		Yes		?	
EPO	3	6		?	?	?	522
bFGF	2/3	6	+	?	Hypotension	Negative	
Hypothermia	1	5-24		Yes	Pneumonia, arrhythmia, hypotension	?	50
Caffeinol	2	4		Yes	No	?	20

TABLE 53-1 PAST AND CURRENT CYTOPROTECTIVE CLINICAL TRIALS—CONT'D

Drug	Phase	Latest Extent of Time Window (h)	Adequate Power*	Adequate Dose	Dose-Limiting Adverse Effects	Results	N
Oxygen							
DCLHb	2	18		?	Hypertensive nephropathy	Negative	
HBO	2/3†	24		?	?	Neutral	

*Relevant only to phase 2b or 3 efficacy trial.
†Currently enrolling.
AMPA, α-amino-3-hydroxy-5-methyl-4-isoxazole proprionic acid; bFGF, basic fibroblast growth factor; DCLHb, diaspirin-cross-linked hemoglobin; EPO, erythropoietin; FAST-MAG, Field Administration of Stroke Therapy—Magnesium Trial; GABA, γ-aminobutyric acid; GM1, genetic marker (monosialo-ganglioside); HBO, hyperbaric oxygen; IMAGES, Intravenous Magnesium Efficacy in Acute Stroke study.

TABLE 53-2 RECENTLY COMPLETED PHASE 1 AND 2 CLINICAL TRIALS

Treatment	Phase	Treatment Window (h)	Result
Albumin (ALIAS)	1	18	Ongoing phase 3 trial of human serum albumin (2 g/kg IV) compared with placebo within 5 h of stroke onset
Carbamylated erythropoietin (CEPO)	1	12-48	Ongoing follow-up study further evaluating safety and pharmacokinetics
Interferon beta-1a	1	24	Unknown
Granulocyte colony-stimulating factor (G-CSF)	2	12	Ongoing multinational, multicenter, randomized, double-blind, placebo-controlled phase 2 trial
Caffeinol/hypothermia	2	4	Uncertain
Endovascular cooling (ICTUS-L)	1	6	Planned prospective, multisite phase 2/3 pivotal efficacy trial of thrombolysis combined with hypothermia in awake patients with moderately severe middle cerebral artery distribution strokes
Lovastatin (NeuSTART)	1	24	Follow-up study planned

ALIAS, Albumin in Acute Stroke Trial; CEPO, Safety Study of Carbamylated Erythropoietin to Treat Patients With Acute Ischemic Stroke; ICTUS-L, Intra-vascular Cooling in the Treatment of Stroke—Longer tPA Window Trial; NeuSTART, The Neuroprotection with Statin Therapy for Acute Recovery Trial.

TABLE 53-3 ONGOING CYTOPROTECTIVE CLINICAL TRIALS

Drug	Phase	Latest Extent of Time Window (h)	Current Enrollment	Planned N
Minocycline	1/2	6	40	60
G-CSF (AXIS 2)	2	5	?	350
Magnesium (FAST-MAG)	3	2	814	1298
Citicoline	3	24	900	2600
Albumin (ALIAS-Part 2)	3	5	26	1100
Erythropoietin	3	6	?	?

ALIAS-Part 2, Albumin in Acute Stroke Trial; AXIS 2, AX200 for the Treatment of Ischemic Stroke; FAST-MAG, Field Administration of Stroke Therapy–Magnesium Trial; G-CSF, granulocyte colony-stimulating factor.

characteristics or resemble L-type channels but are insensitive to dihydropyridines. Many calcium channel antagonists have been reported to preferentially antagonize the cerebral vascular smooth muscle and have a high affinity for calcium channels in the inactivated state, such as those found in the depolarized environment of the ischemic penumbra.[52] This selective interaction may be beneficial for the neuroprotectant potential of these agents.

The calcium channel antagonist that has undergone the most extensive investigation in stroke is *nimodipine*. The cytoprotective effect of nimodipine results from its ability to block calcium influx and prevent the excessive accumulation of intracellular calcium that initiates the final common pathway to cell death. Nimodipine has been studied in experimental models of cerebral ischemia[53] and in clinical trials of subarachnoid hemorrhage, head injury, and cardiac arrest, as well as acute focal ischemia.[53,54]

Oral nimodipine has been investigated in ischemic stroke in at least 29 randomized placebo-controlled trials. These studies enrolled patients with treatment time windows ranging from 12 to 48 hours, used nimodipine doses between 60 and 240 mg/day, and treated patients for periods of 14 to 28 days. A few of the earlier studies found a significant difference in mortality and neurologic function in favor of nimodipine therapy[55-59]; however, subsequent larger studies and a later meta-analysis failed to replicate this benefit.[53,60] Several studies have actually shown a better outcome in the placebo-treated patients, which is a finding attributed to hypotension induced by both oral and intravenous (IV) administration of the drug.[61-63]

The most extensive meta-analysis of 22 calcium antagonist trials, studying more than 6800 patients, did not demonstrate any beneficial effect of treatment, even in subgroups receiving early treatment (within 12 hours of stroke onset) (Fig. 53-1).[53] In addition, meta-analysis limited to the "good-quality" trials showed a statistically significant negative effect of calcium antagonists. A similar analysis of "poor-" and "moderate-quality" trials found that calcium antagonists exerted no effect on outcome. In fact, the results of this meta-analysis prompted the premature termination of the Very Early Nimodipine Use in Stroke (VENUS) trial, which was designed to determine the efficacy of nimodipine administered within 6 hours of stroke onset.[64] The interim analysis of 454 patients showed no effect of nimodipine; within the ischemic stroke subgroup, however, an increase in poor outcome at 3 months was found in the nimodipine-treated patients (relative risk [RR], 1.4; 95% confidence interval [CI], 1.0–2.1).

Another dihydropyridine calcium channel antagonist, *nicardipine*, has been tested in a pilot stroke study.[65] Hypotension was a common and dose-related side effect that could potentially negate the overall benefit of treatment.

In summary, given the weight of the evidence, calcium antagonists cannot be considered generally effective in improving the outcome of ischemic stroke and may even cause a worsened outcome. The lack of effect, or the presence of detrimental effect, may be due to the hypotension caused by blocking of the vascular smooth muscle cells.

Blockade of L-type calcium channels in the setting of maximal vasodilation and impaired autoregulation within the ischemic region may cause relative hypotension and a steal phenomenon with shunting of blood flow to nonischemic regions, thereby further decreasing perfusion to the penumbra.[66] Another plausible explanation for the failure of calcium antagonists to show efficacy is that neurotransmitter release is a proximal event in the excitotoxic cascade with immediate effects; therefore, any delay in administration of the drug precludes its theoretical efficacy in preventing cell necrosis. Delayed or prolonged use of L-type calcium antagonists may actually induce apoptotic cell death because modest increases in calcium inhibit apoptosis.[67] This mechanism may overcome other protective actions of these agents. Ultraearly antagonism of other receptor subtypes, such as the N-type, may be more beneficial in penumbral preservation through inhibition of neurotransmitter release without undesired hypotension. Such agents have demonstrated cytoprotection in animal models, but they have not been extensively studied in humans because of poor blood–brain barrier permeability of these peptides.[68] We discuss methods to improve drug delivery at the end of the chapter. Lastly, critical review of these studies highlights the importance of beginning treatment as quickly as possible, that is, within a few hours of injury as opposed to the 24- or 48-hour treatment window allowed in some studies. The importance of adequate sample size necessary to demonstrate modest benefit is also underscored.[69]

Glutamate Antagonists

NMDA receptor antagonists were the first class of therapeutic agents for acute stroke to proceed from development in the laboratory to testing in humans that employed modern

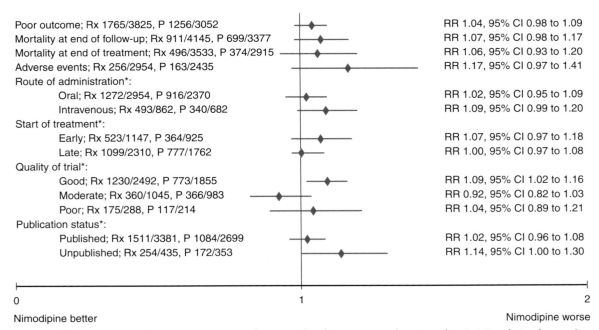

Poor outcome; Rx 1765/3825, P 1256/3052	RR 1.04, 95% CI 0.98 to 1.09
Mortality at end of follow-up; Rx 911/4145, P 699/3377	RR 1.07, 95% CI 0.98 to 1.17
Mortality at end of treatment; Rx 496/3533, P 374/2915	RR 1.06, 95% CI 0.93 to 1.20
Adverse events; Rx 256/2954, P 163/2435	RR 1.17, 95% CI 0.97 to 1.41
Route of administration*:	
Oral; Rx 1272/2954, P 916/2370	RR 1.02, 95% CI 0.95 to 1.09
Intravenous; Rx 493/862, P 340/682	RR 1.09, 95% CI 0.99 to 1.20
Start of treatment*:	
Early; Rx 523/1147, P 364/925	RR 1.07, 95% CI 0.97 to 1.18
Late; Rx 1099/2310, P 777/1762	RR 1.00, 95% CI 0.97 to 1.08
Quality of trial*:	
Good; Rx 1230/2492, P 773/1855	RR 1.09, 95% CI 1.02 to 1.16
Moderate; Rx 360/1045, P 366/983	RR 0.92, 95% CI 0.82 to 1.03
Poor; Rx 175/288, P 117/214	RR 1.04, 95% CI 0.89 to 1.21
Publication status*:	
Published; Rx 1511/3381, P 1084/2699	RR 1.02, 95% CI 0.96 to 1.08
Unpublished; Rx 254/435, P 172/353	RR 1.14, 95% CI 1.00 to 1.30

0   1   2

Nimodipine better   Nimodipine worse

Figure 53-1 Results from meta-analyses comparing nimodipine to placebo in acute ischemic stroke. 0, Nimodipine better; 2, nimodipine worse; CI, confidence intervals; P, placebo group; RR, relative risk; Rx, treatment group; *, assessment of analyses indicated poor outcome. (Adapted from Horn J, Limburg M: Calcium antagonists for ischemic stroke: A systematic review. *Stroke* 32:570, 2001.)

principles of clinical trial design, of which the most important was relatively early treatment. The potential utility of NMDA antagonists in stroke was first recognized when it was observed that a hypoxic or ischemic insult results in elevation of brain levels of the excitatory neurotransmitter glutamate. The excitotoxic theory of ischemic brain injury implicates glutamate as a pivotal mediator of cell death via ligand-gated receptors (NMDA and AMPA receptors), as reviewed previously. The NMDA receptor is a complex ligand-gated ion channel that requires activation by glutamate and glycine as well as concomitant membrane depolarization to overcome a voltage-dependent block by magnesium ions.

The complex structure of the NMDA receptor provides multiple sites for therapeutic inhibition. Competitive NMDA antagonists bind directly to the glutamate site of the NMDA receptor to inhibit the action of glutamate. Noncompetitive antagonists block the NMDA-associated ion channel in a use-dependent manner. Other sites on the NMDA receptor susceptible to antagonism are the glycine site and the polyamine site. Prototypes of these competitive and noncompetitive NMDA antagonists have been studied in phase 3 clinical trials for the treatment of stroke.

CGS19755 (selfotel) is a competitive NMDA receptor antagonist that limits neuronal damage in animal stroke models.[70-72] Phase 2 studies of selfotel revealed that the dosing regimen was limited by dose-related adverse neuropsychiatric adverse events including hallucinations, agitation, confusion, dysarthria, ataxia, delirium, paranoia, and somnolence. A dose of 1.5 mg/kg was settled on for phase 3 trials, which did not achieve the plasma concentrations that were found to be neuroprotective in animal models. Phase 3 parallel studies in the United States and Europe were suspended after 31% of planned enrollment had been accomplished, however, because of an unfavorable efficacy-to-toxicity ratio.[73] The proportion of patients with neurologic progression or decreased arousal was higher in the selfotel group, as were both 8- and 30-day mortality rates. There was no difference between selfotel and placebo in the primary endpoint of functional independence, even when stroke subtype subgroup analysis was performed.

We may conclude from these trials that selfotel is not efficacious as a cytoprotectant and may potentially exert a neurotoxic effect in patients with severe stroke. The selfotel trials exhibit an important principle of cytoprotectant failure—the narrow therapeutic index. Animal models determined that a plasma selfotel level of 40 μg/mL was cytoprotective. However, the highest tolerated level in human patients with stroke was only half of this target cytoprotective concentration (21 μg/mL), and even these "subtherapeutic" levels produced marked neurologic and psychiatric effects.[74]

The noncompetitive NMDA antagonist *dextrorphan* was also evaluated in a pilot study within 48 hours of hemispheric cerebral infarction.[75] As with selfotel, adverse effects of dextrorphan occurred in a dose-dependent fashion: nystagmus, somnolence, nausea, vomiting, and hypotension at the highest loading doses. During the maintenance infusion, the most common side effects were agitation, confusion, hallucinations, and hypertension. There were no differences in the outcome between patients receiving placebo and those receiving low-, medium-, or high-dose dextrorphan. Unlike with selfotel, the plasma concentrations of dextrorphan achieved were comparable to the cytoprotective level determined in cell culture and animal models. At present, no further clinical trials of dextrorphan are in progress.

A multicenter placebo-controlled, double-blind, randomized trial of the noncompetitive NMDA antagonist CNS1102 (aptiganel, *Cerestat*) was then conducted to evaluate the safety and tolerability of escalating doses (3, 4.5, 6, and 7.5 mg) of aptiganel and to determine the pharmacokinetic properties of the drug.[76] Forty-six patients with ischemic carotid artery territory stroke (NIHSS score, 4 to 20) were enrolled within 24 hours of symptom onset. The dose regimen that was adopted (4.5-mg bolus followed by 0.75 mg/h infusion) successfully achieved the target cytoprotective plasma concentration (>10 ng/mL), which had been identified in animal studies. This dose was associated with moderately increased systolic blood pressure (≈30 mm Hg), which responded to antihypertensive agents, and adverse neurologic experiences (mild sedation and confusion) that patients easily tolerated. However, no suggestion of treatment effect was found in this study.

On the basis of these results, a nested phase 2–phase 3 study was performed to compare low-dose (3-mg bolus then 0.5 mg/h; total 9 mg) and high-dose (5-mg bolus then 0.75 mg/h; total 14 mg) aptiganel regimens with placebo.[77] Patients with clinical diagnoses of ischemic stroke were randomly assigned to one of three treatment arms within 6 hours of symptom onset. There were no criteria for stroke severity or syndrome, and no stratified randomization procedure was used to enforce recruitment of patients within a 3-hour window. Phase 3 enrollment was terminated early when analysis of the phase 2 data revealed an increase in mortality within the aptiganel cohort. Analysis of available phase 3 data (628 patients) showed no difference in 90-day outcome, as measured by mRS, among the three groups. The difference in 90-day mortality was not significant, but mortality at 120 days was marginally increased in the high-dose group. On the basis of this evidence, aptiganel is not efficacious when given within 6 hours of onset of stroke and may be harmful at higher doses.

Phase 2 studies have been conducted to study the safety and tolerability of a novel low-affinity, use-dependent NMDA antagonist, *AR-R15696AR*. The 2002 trial demonstrated that a dosing regimen capable of achieving cytoprotective concentrations produced a significant excess of side effects compared with placebo, including nausea, vomiting, fever, agitation, dizziness, and hallucinations.[78] No positive treatment effect on BI or NIHSS score was observed at 1 month. As with other NMDA antagonists, the unfavorable efficacy-to-toxicity ratio has halted further investigation of this agent.[78]

Magnesium (Mg^{2+}) is theoretically an ideal neuroprotectant because of its diverse mechanisms of action, low cost, ease of administration, wide therapeutic index, good blood–brain barrier permeability, and established safety profile. Mg^{2+} ions endogenously function as a physiologic voltage-dependent block of the NMDA receptor ion channel and inhibitor of ischemia-induced glutamate release.[79] In addition to these antiexcitotoxic actions,

Mg^{2+} antagonizes voltage-gated calcium (Ca^{2+}) channels of all types, promotes vasodilation, enhances mitochondrial buffering of calcium overloading, prevents depletion of ATP, and inhibits the inflammatory response and calcium-mediated activation of intracellular enzymes.[79-81] Preclinical models show that magnesium sulfate ($MgSO_4$) consistently reduces infarct volume: a dose–response relationship is demonstrated within easily achieved serum levels (1.49 mmol/L).[82] Postischemic $MgSO_4$ treatment given 6 hours after embolization significantly reduces infarct volume by 48% compared with placebo.[82] This model mimics clinical reality, in which patients present for treatment hours after the onset of ischemia. However, as with previous agents, the benefit of Mg^{2+} has been shown only in some laboratories in some models.

The theoretical benefit of Mg^{2+} is augmented by the finding that up to 80% of patients with stroke have significantly decreased serum ionized Mg^{2+} levels, and 15% show an elevated ionized Ca^{2+}/Mg^{2+} ratio, which is a state promoting increased vascular tone.[83] Low cerebrospinal fluid Mg^{2+} levels have been associated with significantly larger cortical infarcts and greater likelihood of persistent neurologic deficit, whereas high cerebrospinal fluid Mg^{2+} levels are significantly correlated with neurologic improvement from baseline findings and smaller deficit at follow-up for patients with cortical or subcortical infarct.[84] These findings suggest that relative magnesium deficiency may play a role in the pathophysiology of ischemia and that magnesium treatment may have therapeutic utility.

Several pilot studies have already demonstrated the safety and tolerability of IV Mg^{2+} in patients with acute ischemic stroke.[80,85] Administration of $MgSO_4$ as a loading dose (8 to 16 mmol) followed by a 24-hour continuous infusion (65 mmol) has been studied in more than 3000 patients with stroke treated within 48 hours, in whom there were no significant adverse events. The majority of these studies have not revealed the significant hypotension or hyperglycemia that was experienced in some preclinical evaluations of $MgCl$.[86] The majority of reported adverse events was the expected complications of the initial stroke and did not differ from those reported in patients given placebo. A dose optimization study identified a dose (16 mmol bolus, 24-hour continuous infusion of 65 mmol) capable of achieving the minimum neuroprotective serum levels in all patients while producing no adverse events.[85] A systematic review of four phase 2 clinical trials disclosed a nonsignificant, 8% absolute reduction in the combined endpoint of death or functional dependence.[43]

The IMAGES Study Group conducted a large phase 3 trial of $MgSO_4$ administered within 12 hours of onset designed to detect a 5.5% absolute difference in death or dependence.[87] A total of 2589 patients were randomly assigned within 12 hours of acute stroke to receive either $MgSO_4$ intravenously or placebo. The primary outcome was a global endpoint statistic expressed as the common odds ratio for death or disability at day 90. The efficacy dataset included 2386 patients. The primary outcome was not improved by magnesium (odds ratio [OR], 0.95; 95% CI, 0.80–1.13, $P = 0.59$). Planned subgroup analyses showed benefit of magnesium in noncortical strokes ($P = 0.011$); however, greater benefit had been expected in the cortical group.

One of the greatest impediments to translating experimental efficacy to a clinical reality is the delay in administration of potentially cytoprotective therapies. Ongoing trials of magnesium administration have been designed to specifically address this issue. The Field Administration of Stroke Therapy—Magnesium (FAST-MAG) pilot study was an open-label evaluation of the safety and feasibility of paramedic-initiated magnesium therapy to patients with stroke identified in the field by the Los Angeles Prehospital Stroke Screen (LAPSS).[47] The average time to treatment was only 29 minutes from symptom onset, which is the shortest onset-to-treatment interval reported to date. More than two thirds of patients had a good functional outcome.

A phase 3 multicenter, randomized, placebo-controlled trial is enrolling patients to evaluate the efficacy of field-administered, hyperacute Mg^{2+} therapy (given within 2 hours of stroke onset). Because patients are identified by the paramedics before neuroimaging, both ischemic and hemorrhagic strokes will be included. Analyses will be based on time-to-treatment stratification, and the primary endpoint is the shift in the distribution of functional outcomes on the mRS–global disability, assessed at 90 days.[88] As of August 2009, 814 patients (of 1298 planned) have been enrolled. The median interval from "last known well" to the start of the study agent is 46 minutes. Treatment was initiated within 1 hour of onset in 72% and between 1 to 2 hours in 26%. Median pretreatment stroke severity on the Los Angeles Motor Scale (LAMS) is 4. Adjudicated final diagnoses are acute cerebral ischemia in 73%, intracerebral hemorrhage in 24%, and stroke mimic in 3% (Saver, personal communication).

In summary, although preclinical studies of competitive and noncompetitive NMDA antagonists suggest that they can effectively protect penumbral regions, results of clinical studies have thus far been disappointing. Trial design, lacking forced time-to-treatment stratification and patient selection criteria for stroke homogeneity, may have contributed to these results. As with calcium antagonists, achieving neuroprotection by blocking glutamate-induced damage means interrupting events that are triggered almost immediately after the onset of ischemia; thus the time to treatment from onset must be brief. This small time window, seen in all animal studies, was ignored in all clinical trials of these drugs except for the FAST-MAG trial.

Even more important, the negative clinical results with NMDA antagonists may be attributed to the dose-limiting phencyclidine-like side effects, which prevent achievement of therapeutic drug levels in brain tissue. An understanding of the clinically apparent neurotoxicity of NMDA antagonists involves a condition described as "NMDA receptor hypofunction." NMDA antagonists have been shown to induce large vacuoles within the adult rodent brain that may signify irreversible damage.[89,90] Molecular experiments have demonstrated that an indirect complex network disturbance is responsible for the NMDA receptor hypofunction. Blockade of NMDA receptors on subcortical inhibitory neurons leads to disinhibition of glutamatergic and cholinergic cortical projections.[91] This disinhibited state, coupled with simultaneous stimulation of non-NMDA glutamate receptors, may lead to enhanced neurotoxicity. Concurrent administration of GABAergic or α-adrenergic agents appears to diminish the excitotoxic damage.[92] Finally, a model of immature rodents demonstrates that administration of NMDA antagonists during the period of synaptogenesis triggers diffuse apoptotic degeneration throughout the brain.[93]

These complex interactions indicate the potential problems with using drugs that target specific neurotransmitter function. Attempts have been made to develop strategies inhibiting glutamate-induced damage while avoiding the toxicity profile of direct NMDA receptor antagonism. Several agents with such properties have been tested in phase 2 and 3 trials, including polyamine site blockers, glycine antagonists, AMPA receptor antagonists, presynaptic glutamate release inhibitors, ion channel blockers, and GABA agonists. These agents are discussed individually in the following sections.

Agents Acting Indirectly on Glutamate

Eliprodil, an antagonist of the polyamine site of the NMDA receptor, has been evaluated in phase 2 and phase 3 trials involving patients with acute stroke. However, the data remain unpublished, and further investigation has stopped because of an unsatisfactory risk–benefit ratio.[94]

GV150526 (gavestinel) is a novel glycine site antagonist at the NMDA receptor complex. It exhibits neuroprotective effects in experimental stroke models at established plasma levels (10 to 30 µg/mL) with a paucity of toxicity and an extended time window (6 hours).[95] Gavestinel has no known antiplatelet or anticoagulant effects. Therefore, Bordi et al.[95] believed that this compound could be safely administered before performance and interpretation of neuroimaging so that treatment delays could be avoided.

Multiple smaller clinical trials have demonstrated the safety of gavestinel.[96-98] Subsequently, two large phase 3 randomized, placebo-controlled, double-blind trials failed to demonstrate the efficacy of gavestinel despite statistical power adequate to detect even small differences. The GAIN Americas trial randomly assigned 1367 patients to treatment or placebo within 6 hours of stroke onset, and concomitant treatment with IV t-PA was allowed in eligible patients.[99] Patients were stratified at randomization by age (younger or older than 75 years) and initial stroke severity (NIHSS score, 2 to 5, 6 to 13, or >13). Patients were well-matched for baseline characteristics. Mean NIHSS score was 12, and median time to treatment was 5.2 hours. No statistically significant difference in mortality rate or 3-month outcome measures (BI, mRS, or NIHSS score) was found between the gavestinel and placebo groups.

As previously described, the GAIN International trial recruited 1804 patients within 6 hours of stroke onset and used the same dosing regimen and stratified randomization schema as the GAIN Americas trial.[42] The primary efficacy measure, survival combined with 3-month BI, was analyzed only in the ischemic stroke population (721 patients given gavestinel; 734 given placebo). Secondary endpoints were BI (at 7 days and 1 month), NIHSS score (at 7 days, 1 and 3 months), mRS (at 1 and 3 months), death within 3 months, and global statistical test of combined neurologic status (NIHSS 1 or less, BI score 95 or more, mRS 1 or less) at 3 months. In comparison with placebo, gavestinel had no effect on primary or secondary outcome measures when baseline NIHSS score and age were included as covariates

in proportional odds models. Minor adverse events (transient increase in liver function values and phlebitis) were seen more commonly in the gavestinel group, but no significant differences were found in rates of serious adverse events.

The neutral results of the large gavestinel trials are disconcerting for several reasons. First, the clinical testing closely mimicked the experimental models that had exhibited neuroprotection even after 6 hours of ischemia. Second, these trials incorporated an adequate number of patients to exclude a clinically significant benefit of gavestinel, which is a point that has been used to criticize previous trials. Third, these trials appropriately stratified patients according to baseline stroke severity and age, which are factors that may otherwise cause imbalances within treatment and placebo groups, thereby confounding results. Fourth, "supratherapeutic" levels of the neuroprotective agent were achieved with only minimal and tolerable side effects. Therefore, unlike with other modulators of glutamate activity, doses of gavestinel were not limited by intolerability of "therapeutic" doses.

The reason for the neutral results for gavestinel clinical trials remains to be identified. It is possible that the time window to effectively antagonize glutamate is simply less than 6 hours and that the neuroprotective benefit of infarct size reduction in animals does not translate into improved functional outcome measured in clinical trials. Just as likely, however, is that expectations for gavestinel were overinflated because only positive preclinical results were published (it is common for negative results in animal studies to go unreported). Mild beneficial effects were seen only in carefully standardized stroke models that do not reflect the heterogeneity of patients with stroke, in whom more robust efficacy would be needed to achieve clinical significance.

Blockade of glutamate-activated AMPA receptors represents another target of cytoprotection with several advantages over NMDA receptor antagonism. AMPA receptors are colocalized with NMDA receptors on cortical neurons but are also present on oligodendrocytes in the white matter.[100] These receptors are more permeable to sodium and mediate fast synaptic transmission and depolarization, thereby facilitating activation of NMDA receptors. Favorable attributes of AMPA antagonism include potential preservation of both cortical and subcortical regions as well as reduction of secondary activation of NMDA receptor and voltage-gated calcium channels. One promising AMPA antagonist, *YM872*, exhibits high-affinity competitive activity at the AMPA receptor as well as low affinity for the NMDA receptor, the glycine site on the NMDA receptor, and the kainite receptor. In animal models, this agent has demonstrated reduction of infarct volume comparable with that seen with NMDA receptor antagonists.[101] A phase 1 clinical trial showed that a 24-hour infusion of 1.25 mg/kg/h was tolerated in elderly volunteers, although central nervous system side effects limited the use of higher doses and longer infusion times.[102]

Enrollment was terminated prematurely in two concurrent YM872 clinical trials, the AMPA Receptor Antagonist Treatment in Ischemic Stroke (ARTIST) trials, on the basis of an interim futility analysis. These multicenter, randomized, double-blind, placebo-controlled trials were designed to "fill in the gaps" left by past neuroprotection trials: combination of reperfusion and neuroprotection strategies and the use of a biological marker of efficacy. The ARTIST+ trial compared the efficacy of YM872 plus t-PA with that of placebo plus t-PA. Preclinical data have demonstrated that coadministration of t-PA and YM872 within 2 hours of stroke imparts a higher level of cytoprotection than either agent alone.[103] Patients with acute hemispheric ischemic stroke and a moderate to severe deficit (NIHSS score, 7 to 23; level of consciousness [LOC] score, 0 to 1) treated with standard protocol t-PA were eligible. The planned enrollment was 600 patients, and more than 400 patients were enrolled. YM872 administration was started before the end of t-PA infusion and continued for 24 hours. Primary efficacy-outcome measures included neurologic function and disability scales.

The second trial, ARTIST MRI, evaluated the safety and potential efficacy of YM872 administered to patients with stroke within 6 hours of onset and used MRI as a surrogate marker of outcome. Baseline ischemic lesion volume on DWI was compared with final lesion volume on T2-weighted imaging with fluid-attenuated inversion recovery (FLAIR) to detect the effect of YM872 on lesion growth. The abandonment of these very well-designed trials is disappointing. Further investigation of YM872 is not planned at this time.

Another approach to the biological monitoring of neurotherapeutics is highlighted in a stroke trial investigating another AMPA antagonist, *ZK200775*.[104] This dose-finding trial utilized serum concentrations of S-100B and neuron-specific enolase as peripheral markers of glial and neuronal injury, respectively. The study found a significant worsening in the mean NIHSS score 48 hours after the start of treatment in the highest dose group (525 mg/48 hours). This neurologic deterioration was associated with a higher than expected elevation in serum S-100B levels in a multiple regression analysis controlling for stroke severity. There was no significant increase in neuron-specific enolase. Although these data suggest glial rather than neuronal damage, the oligodendrocytes are critical for neuronal homeostasis, and glial damage may contribute to neuronal dysfunction. These results provide corroborative evidence of the potential toxicity of glutamate antagonists suggested by the clinically apparent dose-related toxicity observed in previous trials. Such markers may be useful surrogate markers of cytoprotection and toxicity in future trials.

Inhibitors of glutamate release are a heterogeneous group of agents, including anticonvulsants and antidepressants. The proposed mechanism of action for these drugs is ion channel blockade.

The antiepileptic drug *lamotrigine* inhibits glutamate release and has shown beneficial effects in a rodent model of focal cerebral ischemia when administered immediately after ischemia.[105] However, a 2-hour delay of treatment produced no effect on infarct volume or neurologic outcome in two models.[105,106] To our knowledge, no clinical stroke trials of lamotrigine have been performed because the preclinical efficacy of immediate drug administration cannot be replicated in patients with stroke. Similarly, a derivative of lamotrigine, *sipatrigine (BW619C89)*, is a use-dependent sodium channel antagonist that inhibits presynaptic glutamate release. It has been shown to decrease glutamate release during ischemia[107]; like lamotrigine, however, sipatrigine reduced infarct volume only when administered at the onset of ischemia.[108] This agent has been evaluated in phase 2 clinical trials in patients within 12 hours of stroke onset.[109] As with selfotel, continuous infusion of sipatrigine produced intolerable neuropsychiatric effects (e.g., sedation, agitation, confusion, hallucinations, and visual disturbances) while showing no trend of improving outcomes in a small cohort of 27 patients. A subsequent two-part trial evaluating the maximum tolerated dose and efficacy of sipatrigine was halted early by the trial sponsor, and further clinical development of the drug for stroke has ceased.[110]

Preclinical studies have shown that *phenytoin* can reduce neuronal injury, possibly by inhibiting the spread of electrical depolarization in penumbral regions, thereby reducing postischemic glutamate release. Fosphenytoin, an aqueous-soluble rapidly injectable prodrug of phenytoin, is another sodium channel blocker. A multicenter combined phase 2–3 evaluation of IV fosphenytoin within 4 hours of acute stroke was terminated prematurely after interim analysis of 462 enrolled patients showed no difference between placebo and fosphenytoin in any of the functional or disability outcomes.[110]

A novel calcium-sensitive, maxi-K potassium channel opener, *BMS-204352 (MaxiPost)*, causes neuronal hyperpolarization, decreased calcium influx, and glutamate release.[111] Phase 1 and 2a studies revealed no safety concerns. However, a phase 3 trial, the Potassium-Channel Opening Stroke Trial (POST) of 1978 patients with moderate to severe cortical strokes (NIHSS score, 6 to 20) treated within 6 hours of onset failed to show any significant beneficial effect compared with placebo.[110]

The pilot study of another ion channel blocker, *lifarizine*, also suggested reduced mortality rates and improved outcomes, but because the drug causes hypotension, further clinical testing is not planned.[112]

Lubeluzole is a novel benzothiazole compound that has emerged as a neuroprotective agent in animal models of focal ischemia.[113-115] In some laboratories, lubeluzole has reduced infarct volume and improved neurologic outcome in animal models even when administered up to 6 hours after infarct induction.[113] Lubeluzole administered 1 hour after photochemically induced infarct attenuated the growth and density of ischemic damage in the periphery of infarct, the presumed penumbra, as measured by serial DWI with apparent diffusion coefficient (ADC) mapping.[115] There are several putative mechanisms by which lubeluzole protects the penumbral region in these models. First, lubeluzole normalizes neuronal activity in the peri-infarct region by inhibiting glutamate release possibly via blockade of non–L-type calcium channels.[116] Additionally, blockade of sodium channels and taurine release by lubeluzole suggests that it may reduce osmoregulatory stress in the peri-infarct zone.[117] Finally, lubeluzole downregulates the glutamate-induced NOS pathway and diminishes NO-related neurotoxicity.[118]

A phase 2 placebo-controlled clinical trial of lubeluzole in acute ischemic stroke suggested that the agent lowers mortality and disability rates in some patients.[119] Subjects with acute ischemic stroke in the MCA territory were treated within 6 hours of onset of symptoms. Prolongation of the QT interval on electrocardiography was observed at plasma drug concentrations of 100 ng/mL or greater in the phase 1 study but was not confirmed in this trial. The low-dose lubeluzole group experienced no excess of cardiac arrhythmias compared with the placebo group, although there was a higher incidence of ventricular fibrillation in the high-dose lubeluzole group. The overall mortality rate was 6% for the low-dose regimen, 18% for placebo, and 35% for the high-dose regimen. The trial was terminated prematurely when a multivariate logistic regression analysis found this significant imbalance in 28-day mortality favoring treatment with the low-dose regimen. The excess mortality in the high-dose group was partially due to imbalanced randomization of subjects: this group had more severe strokes. When multivariate regression analysis accounted for stroke severity, high-dose treatment had no effect on mortality. BI scores tended to be higher in the low-dose lubeluzole group, but no significant differences in efficacy measures were found among the groups.

On the basis of the results of this pilot study, subsequent phase 3 randomized, multicenter, double-blind, placebo-controlled trials adopted the low-dose regimen to test the efficacy of lubeluzole in patients with acute ischemic stroke. However, it is essential to note that the low-dose regimen produced a mean plasma concentration (61 ± 22 ng/mL) that is below the minimal neuroprotective level established in animals (100 ng/mL).[120]

Three large-scale, multicenter, double-blind, placebo-controlled, randomized, phase 3 trials of low-dose lubeluzole in patients with stroke have produced conflicting results. The European and Australian trial randomly assigned 725 patients to treatment within 6 hours of onset and demonstrated similar overall mortality rates, rates of adverse events, and clinical outcomes in all placebo- and lubeluzole-treated patients.[121] However, an unplanned post hoc analysis found that lubeluzole treatment decreased mortality among patients with mild to moderate stroke as measured by the Clinical Global Impression rating. The North American trial involved 721 patients treated within 6 hours of onset of moderate to severe hemispheric stroke (NIHSS score, >7).[122] The mean time to treatment was 4.7 hours. The primary outcome measure, mortality at 12 weeks, was not significantly different between groups; however, the extent of functional recovery (BI score) and disability (mRS) at 3 months significantly favored lubeluzole over placebo after the data were controlled for appropriate covariates. The odds of favorable outcome were 38% higher with lubeluzole according to the global test statistic. This study also confirmed the safety of the low-dose regimen, reporting no significant differences in cardiac-related complications or adverse events.

The third trial evaluating the efficacy of low-dose lubeluzole randomly assigned to treatment a total of 1786 patients who were stratified according to time to treatment (0 to 6 hours and 6 to 8 hours).[123] During the trial, a target stroke population (core stroke group) was defined on the basis of results of a meta-analysis identifying patients who might benefit from treatment. The core stroke group consisted of patients with ischemic stroke, excluding patients 75 years or older with severe strokes, who were treated within 6 hours. Only the core stroke group was used in the primary efficacy analyses. Lubeluzole had no significant effect on mortality or 12-week functional status in the core stroke group. Similar neutral results were found in the nontarget population, including all patients treated within 6 to 8 hours of onset and patients 75 years or older with severe stroke. The most commonly reported adverse experiences were fever, constipation, and headache. Lubeluzole-treated patients experienced more cardiac events, including atrial fibrillation and QT interval prolongation, but this higher rate was not associated with increased mortality.

Finally, lubeluzole was the first potentially neuroprotective agent to be evaluated in a dedicated combination trial with t-PA. Patients who qualified for and received IV t-PA within 3 hours of symptom onset were randomly allocated 1:1 to receive either lubeluzole or placebo.[46] The lubeluzole infusion was started before the end of the 1-hour t-PA infusion. Eighty-nine patients were enrolled before the trial was terminated early because of negative results of the previously described concurrent lubeluzole phase 3 trial.[123] In the enrolled patients (45% of the planned population), t-PA and the study drug were administered at a mean of 2.5 and 3.2 hours from symptom onset, respectively. There were no significant differences in rates of death, intracerebral hemorrhage, or serious adverse events or in functional outcomes (BI) between the lubeluzole and placebo groups. These results demonstrate the safety and feasibility of linking ultraearly neuroprotection with thrombolysis; however, the premature stoppage of enrollment led to a study with insufficient power to detect efficacy.

A systematic review of five randomized trials, involving a total of 3510 patients, found no evidence that lubeluzole given at any dose reduced the odds of death or dependency at the end of follow-up (OR, 1.03; 95% CI, 0.91–1.19).[124] At any given dose, however, lubeluzole was associated with a significant excess of cardiac conduction disorders.

There are several reasons that the lubeluzole trials may have failed to show efficacy. As with many other agents, the time from stroke onset to drug administration is most likely too long to meaningfully inhibit glutamate release and action. Although an extended 6-hour time window for efficacious treatment has been reported, other animal models have failed to replicate the efficacy of lubeluzole initiated more than 30 minutes after ischemia. The discrepancy in results between the North American and European trials may be in part due to time to drug initiation. In the North American trial, the mean interval was 4.7 hours. Although a similar mean is not reported by the European trial, more than 80% of patients were treated after 4 hours, which may potentially have led to lessened efficacy. Also, dose-limiting side effects, primarily cardiac, led to a narrow therapeutic index with resultant serum drug levels below the minimum neuroprotective level reported in animal studies. Although the combination trial of lubeluzole and t-PA required treatment within 4 hours, its early termination yielded a small sample size and a study with insufficient power to detect efficacy.

Other Neurotransmitter Modulators

Serotonin agonists may exert cytoprotection via several actions at presynaptic and postsynaptic 5-hydroxytryptamine-1A (5-HT_{1A}) receptors. Primarily, activation of this receptor causes neuronal membrane hyperpolarization by opening G protein–coupled potassium channels.[125] Activation of presynaptic serotonin receptors may lead to a reduction in glutamate release.[126] Lastly, these agents may inhibit apoptosis.[127]

One small trial of 49 patients with acute stroke failed to show greater efficacy of a serotonin reuptake inhibitor, *trazodone*, on mortality or neurologic deficit compared with placebo.[128] The neuroprotective efficacy, safety, and tolerability of *repinotan (BAY x 3702)*, a serotonin agonist of the 5-HT$_{1A}$ subtype, were also tested. This drug produced a 55% reduction of infarct volume in experimental models of permanent focal ischemia. A phase 2 trial of repinotan identified 1.25 mg/day given for 3 days as a dose that is well-tolerated by patients with stroke and may improve neurologic outcome at 3 months.[129] The results of a double-blind, placebo-controlled phase 3 efficacy trial comparing repinotan to placebo in patients with moderate to severe stroke (NIHSS scores, 8 to 23) within 6 hours of symptom onset have been submitted for publication. The study had negative results.[110]

ONO-2506 is a novel neurotransmitter modulator. Its proposed mechanism of action is modulation of glutamate transporter uptake capacity and expression of GABA receptors.[130] A safety and efficacy study of ONO-2506, which recruited patients with stroke within 6 hours of onset of a radiographically confirmed cortical infarct, was terminated; however, details have not been published.[110]

The endogenous opioids act at the kappa (κ) opioid receptor as excitatory neurotransmitters and potentiators of ischemic injury. Opiate receptor antagonists have exhibited cytoprotective activity in preclinical focal and global models of ischemia.[131-133] Several small trials of *naloxone* have not conclusively shown efficacy in acute ischemic stroke.[134-138] The equivocal results are likely due to insufficient power of these small studies to detect small but significant treatment effects. Also, naloxone is relatively nonspecific for the kappa receptor.

In a phase 2a trial, *nalmefene* (0.1 mg/kg), an opiate antagonist that has relatively pure activity at the kappa receptor, was administered within 6 hours of stroke onset and was found to be tolerable and possibly efficacious.[139] A subsequent phase 2b dose-comparison trial established that nalmefene doses up to 60 mg are safe in patients with stroke. Although no overall treatment effect was observed, a subgroup analysis suggested that nalmefene may confer a beneficial effect in young patients (<70 years old).[140]

On the basis of phase 2 data, a phase 3 trial was designed to study the safety and efficacy of 60 mg of nalmefene.[141] A total of 368 patients were randomly assigned to undergo treatment within 6 hours of stroke onset. The study found no significant treatment effect on 3-month outcome with any of the planned analyses, including secondary analyses in young patients and thrombolytic-treated patients.

There are several potential explanations for the negative results of the opioid antagonist trials. As with other upstream modulators of excitotoxicity, delayed treatment may not confer neuroprotection because the pivotal steps in the cascade have already occurred by the time of treatment. Also, the trial design did not enforce recruitment of adequate numbers of patients to the subgroups most likely to derive benefit (e.g., young patients, patients with moderate to severe deficits, and patients eligible for thrombolytic treatment), which resulted in insufficient power. Last, no pharmacokinetic studies were performed, so the adequacy of dosage is unknown.

Enhancement of GABA-induced inhibition may be a useful target of cytoprotection. *Clomethiazole* is a GABA agonist that theoretically prevents damage due to excessive excitatory neurotransmitters by enhancing inhibition at the GABA$_A$ receptor level.[142] Activation of the GABA receptor increases chloride conductance and membrane hyperpolarization, thereby depressing neuronal depolarization and excitability.[143] Clomethiazole has been shown to exhibit neuroprotection in several focal ischemia models.[144,145]

A dose-escalation trial demonstrated an acceptable safety profile in patients with acute stroke with a dose that produced plasma concentration levels comparable to that which provided neuroprotection in preclinical studies.[146]

The Clomethiazole Acute Stroke Study (CLASS) evaluated clomethiazole in a randomized, placebo-controlled fashion in patients with hemispheric ischemic stroke with a moderate to severe deficit who were treated within 12 hours of onset.[147] Efficacy analysis of 1353 patients revealed a nonsignificant 1.2% difference favoring clomethiazole in achievement of functional independence as assessed by BI. Sedation, the most common adverse event, led to withdrawal of treatment in 15.6% of patients. Subgroup analyses found a significant beneficial effect of clomethiazole in two overlapping groups: patients with severe baseline neurologic deficit and those classified as having a total anterior circulation stroke. An interaction between stroke syndrome classification and treatment was identified. In patients with total anterior circulation strokes, 40.8% of clomethiazole-treated patients reached relative functional independence compared with 29.8% of placebo-treated patients, which suggests that patients with the largest strokes may have a larger penumbra that may be salvaged by cytoprotective therapy.

The Clomethiazole Acute Stroke Study in Ischemic Stroke (CLASS-I) was designed to test the hypothesis generated by the previous CLASS trial, which was that clomethiazole is effective in patients with large ischemic anterior circulation strokes.[148] Patients with ischemic stroke who showed evidence of higher cortical dysfunction plus visual field and motor deficits were randomly assigned within 12 hours of onset to receive either placebo or clomethiazole. There was no evidence of drug efficacy on any of the outcome variables, including NIHSS score, BI, mRS, and 30-day lesion volume.

The absence of treatment effect occurred despite adequate trial design, appropriate patient selection, and adequate plasma drug concentrations. As with other trials, the lack of efficacy is most likely due to either the prolonged treatment time window or the inadequate prediction of human pharmacokinetics based on rodent data.

A large randomized controlled international trial evaluated the effect of *diazepam*, a benzodiapine with established GABAergic activity, within 12 hours of stroke onset.[149] This trial randomly assigned 880 patients, within 12 hours of acute stroke, to 10 mg diazepam followed by 10-mg tablets twice daily for 3 days or placebo. There was no statistical difference in the primary outcome measure (mRS <3 at 3 months) between groups.

In summary, a large number of drugs that target glutamate and other neurotransmitter functions have shown efficacy in preclinical studies but not in clinical trials. A major factor has been side effects that limit dose, but even in studies that have achieved therapeutic dose ranges and that have been sufficiently powered, such as the GAIN and CLASS trials, results have been neutral or negative. There is a recurrent theme in preclinical studies of benefit being seen when treatment is administered very early after ischemia. In subsequent clinical trials, however, a much larger treatment window was allowed. Currently, the best remaining hope for this strategy is with ongoing trials of magnesium (FAST-MAG), which has employed a very rapid time to treatment.

Free Radical Scavengers, Adhesion Molecule Blockers, Steroids, and Other Anti-Inflammatory Strategies

Other strategies of neuroprotection attack later stages of the ischemic cascade. NO synthesis is induced by stimulation of glutamate receptors, and NO in turn has a number of complex actions relevant to ischemia and cell injury. Endothelium-derived NO causes vasodilatation beneficial to ischemic brain, but neuronal NO generates oxygen free radicals that are toxic to cells. In animal models of stroke, NOS inhibitors have complex effects befitting the dual role of NO in cerebral ischemia. The usefulness of NO modulation in stroke will likely hinge on the ability to favorably manipulate the beneficial and deleterious effects of NO.

Reactive oxygen intermediates play a role in ischemic tissue damage and represent another target for cytoprotection. Free radical scavengers affect a late stage of the ischemic process. *Tirilazad mesylate* is a 21-aminosteroid free radical scavenger and potent membrane lipid peroxidation inhibitor that has shown neuroprotective promise in focal ischemia and subarachnoid hemorrhage models.[150,151] This agent protects the microvascular endothelium and maintains intact blood–brain barrier and cerebral autoregulatory mechanisms. Unfortunately, its penetration into the brain parenchyma is limited, possibly leading to unsatisfactory efficacy in stroke, as demonstrated by clinical trials to date.[152] However, a new group of antioxidants, pyrrolopyrimidines, with significantly improved blood–brain barrier penetrance, have demonstrated successful neuroprotection in focal ischemia with a postischemic treatment window of 4 hours.[152]

A sequential dose-escalation trial determined that tirilazad doses of up to 6 mg/kg/day for 3 days are safe and well tolerated when administered within 6 hours of acute stroke.[153] A phase 3 randomized trial of tirilazad therapy started within 6 hours of stroke onset was terminated prematurely after a preplanned interim analysis of 660 patients determined the futility of continued enrollment.[154] No statistically significant difference was found in the proportion of patients demonstrating a favorable outcome because of tirilazad treatment administered at a median of 4.3 hours. The lack of drug efficacy in this trial was in part ascribed to inadequate dosing, especially in women, and a second tirilazad trial was designed using higher dosing regimens.[155] This trial was discontinued prematurely after safety concerns were raised in a concurrent European

trial, despite trends toward reduced rates of mortality and dependence in both men and women. A systematic review of six randomized controlled trials involving more than 1700 patients included previously unpublished data from two large European trials with negative results.[156] This review found that tirilazad actually increases rates of death and disability by one fifth.

Whether tirilazad not only exhibits a lack of neuroprotection but may also induce worsening within specific populations of patients with stroke is still unclear. Potential reasons for these conclusions include controversial results of preclinical studies,[157] delay in drug administration (>75% of patients were treated >3 hours after stroke onset), thrombophlebitis causing a systemic inflammatory state, and inadequate blood–brain barrier permeability. Finally, it is possible that generation of free radicals plays a positive role in the recovery of patients with stroke.

Ebselen is another type (selenoorganic) of antioxidant that potentially inhibits lipid peroxidation through multiple mechanisms. These mechanisms include inhibition of lipoxygenase within the arachidonate cascade, blocked production of superoxide anions by activated leukocytes,[158] inhibition of inducible NOS,[159] and glutathione-like inhibition of membrane lipid peroxidation.[160] In animal ischemia models, pretreatment and concurrent treatment with ebselen have led to reduction in infarct size and a decrease in cerebral edema.[161]

A single randomized efficacy trial has shown that early treatment with ebselen improved outcome after acute ischemic stroke.[162] Ebselen was administered orally to patients within 48 hours of ischemic stroke onset (mean time to treatment, 29.7 hours). There was no statistically significant difference in mortality. Intention-to-treat analysis demonstrated that ebselen therapy achieved a significantly better outcome at 1 month, but only a trend to improvement was observed at 3 months. Although the ebselen group contained slightly more patients with mild impairment than the placebo group, the difference was not significant, and the efficacy of ebselen was also demonstrated in patients with moderate to severe deficits. Ebselen treatment given within 24 hours significantly improved the likelihood of good recovery on the Glasgow Outcome Scale compared with placebo (42% versus 22%; $P = 0.038$), whereas treatment after 24 hours led to no significant differences between the groups. The ebselen-treated patients were marginally more likely to report adverse events, but the incidence was not significantly different from that in the placebo group. On the basis of the results of this adequately powered trial, ebselen is believed to be safe and possibly efficacious. A multicenter phase 3 ebselen trial was completed in 2002 with a total of 394 patients; however, the results have not been reported.[110]

Free radicals are produced during ischemia and reperfusion and contribute to the neuronal injury after stroke. Edaravone (MCI-186) is a free radical scavenger whose mechanism of neuroprotection includes inhibition of endothelial cell injury, delayed neuronal death, and prevention of edema after ischemia.[163,164] Preclinical study demonstrated that even when administered 6 hours after onset of ischemia, edaravone significantly reduced infarct volume and improved neurologic deficit. In addition, edaravone reduced microglial activation, iNOS expression, and nitrotyrosine formation at a later period. These results indicate that edaravone may exert an early neuroprotective effect through early free radicals scavenging and a late anti-inflammatory effect; the results also suggest that edaravone may expand the therapeutic window in stroke patients.[165] A Japanese multicenter randomized clinical trial of edaravone was published in 2003. Patients were randomly assigned to edaravone or placebo within 72 hours after symptom onset. A significant improvement in functional outcome on the mRS at 3 months was noted in the edaravone group ($P = 0.0382$).[166] Edaravone has been approved in Japan since 2001 as a neuroprotective agent for treatment of acute cerebral infarct within 24 hours after symptom onset.[164] A phase 2 randomized controlled safety study is currently recruiting patients with acute ischemic stroke within 24 hours of symptom onset. This study will assess the safety, tolerability and local tolerance of MCI-186. Secondary outcome measures include pharmacokinetics and neurologic outcome.[167]

Several nitrone free radical-trapping agents (spin-trap agents) have demonstrated neuroprotection in rodent models of both transient and permanent focal ischemia.[168,169] NXY-059 (disodium 4-((tert-butylimino) methyl) benzene-1,3-disulfonate N-oxide) is a novel nitrone-based compound that has free radical-trapping properties. Despite its greater water solubility, NXY-059 has shown greater efficacy in reduction of infarct size and improvement in neurologic outcome than the free radical-trapping agent PBN (α-phenyl-N-tert-butyl nitrone) when given at equimolar doses.[170] The neuroprotective efficacy of NXY-059 is retained even when the agent is given up to 5 hours after onset of ischemia.[170] In a primate model of permanent focal ischemia, NXY-059 significantly decreased neurologic disability and reduced infarct volume in both cortical and subcortical regions.[171] Pharmacokinetic studies show that NXY-059 produces dose-dependent neuroprotection at unbound plasma concentrations of 30 to 80 μmol/L.[169]

The SAINT I study[172] was a randomized, double-blind, placebo-controlled trial involving 1722 patients with acute ischemic stroke who were randomly assigned to receive a 72-hour infusion of placebo or IV NXY-059 within 6 hours after the onset of the stroke. The primary outcome was disability at 90 days, as measured according to scores on mRS for disability. All patients received standard of care, including IV rt-PA, when indicated.

Approximately 96% of the patients assigned to NXY-059 achieved plasma concentrations of NXY-059 greater than 150 μmol/L. Analysis for the primary outcome was positive. Among the 1699 subjects included in the efficacy analysis, NXY-059 significantly improved the overall distribution of scores on the mRS compared with placebo ($P = 0.038$). The OR for improvement across all categories of the scale was 1.20 (95% CI, 1.01–1.42). Rates of adverse events and mortality were similar in the two groups. Although the effect on disability was moderate, it was believed to be consistent with a neuroprotective action. Additional support for the suggestion that NXY-059 was neuroprotective was a biological signal from post hoc analysis, which revealed that treatment with NXY-059 significantly reduced the incidence of intracranial hemorrhage among patients in whom alteplase was also used.[173]

As expected, these findings generated much excitement, and confirmation of these results was planned in SAINT II. Based on the results of SAINT I, the SAINT II protocol was modified to include an increase in the sample size from 1700 to 3200 patients, which would provide at least 80% power to detect an OR of 1.2 (across all cutoff points of the mRS), which was seen in SAINT I. In addition, a revised approach to analysis of the NIHSS score and a prospective analysis of intracerebral hemorrhage were planned.[44] The efficacy analysis was based on 3195 patients (1588 in the NXY-059 group and 1607 in the placebo group). Prognostic factors were well-balanced between the treatment groups. Mortality and adverse event rates were similar in the two groups. The distribution of scores on the mRS did not differ between the NXY-059 and placebo groups ($P = 0.33$; OR, 0.94; 95% CI, 0.83–1.06). Analysis of categorized scores on the mRS confirmed the lack of benefit: the OR for trichotomization into mRS scores of 0 to 1 versus 2 to 3 versus 4 to 6 was 0.92 (95% CI, 0.80–1.06). There was no evidence of efficacy for any of the secondary endpoints. Alteplase was administered to 44% of patients in both groups; however, there was no difference in the frequency of symptomatic or asymptomatic hemorrhage between treatment groups. The authors concluded that NXY-059 is ineffective for the treatment of acute ischemic stroke within 6 hours after the onset of symptoms. Lastly, a pooled analysis of the SAINT trials confirmed neutral results, not only in the overall population but also in important prespecified subgroups, such as those treated early after stroke or those who were offered alteplase.[174]

The SAINT II investigators considered whether the conflicting results of the two trials might be related to the higher rate of alteplase use in SAINT II. However, no evidence of an interaction between alteplase use and the effect of NXY-059 was found in either trial.[44] Although NXY-059 was tested rigorously in the preclinical setting relative to other neuroprotective agents, in retrospect, investigators identified red flags in the preclinical stages including lack of benefit across animal models and concerns with timing of administration.[175] The results from SAINT II are disappointing, but they highlight many opportunities for improvement in both preclinical testing of neuroprotective agents and in clinical trial design.

Complex inflammatory processes mediate ischemic- and reperfusion-related brain injury, representing an ideal downstream target for cytoprotection. Modulation of cytokines, inflammatory-related enzymes (NOS), endothelial leukocyte interactions, leukocyte activation, and gene transcription factors has been investigated in experimental models and a few clinical trials.

Various models of focal ischemia have demonstrated greater expression of leukocyte-endothelial adhesion molecules,[176,177] and the absence of adhesion molecules in knockout mice significantly reduces infarct size.[178,179] Antiadhesion molecule strategies have shown efficacy only in models of transient ischemia, which supports the belief that neuroprotection imparts significant benefit only if coupled with reperfusion.[180,181] Furthermore, animal studies have demonstrated that a combination of t-PA and antiadhesion molecule therapy (antibodies to either intracellular adhesion molecule 1[182] or CD18) significantly reduces infarct volume and neurologic deficit score more than either agent alone, even when administered up to 4 hours after induction of ischemia.[14,183]

Although there is contradictory evidence for upregulation of inflammatory adhesion molecules in patients with ischemic stroke, the majority of studies demonstrate elevations in circulating adhesion molecules (soluble [s] ICAM-1, soluble vascular cell adhesion molecule-1 (VCAM-1), sP-selectin, and sE-selectin).[184-186] Elevated ICAM-1 expression has been observed on microvessels within infarcts in patients surviving 15 hours to 6 days after stroke.[187]

Enlimomab is a murine monoclonal anti-ICAM-1 antibody that has undergone phase 3 testing in patients with stroke. A phase 3 trial compared the efficacy of enlimomab with placebo in 625 patients with ischemic stroke who received treatment within 6 hours of symptom onset.[188] The target serum drug level was achieved in 96.6% of patients after the first dose, and adequate trough levels were maintained throughout the duration of treatment. Enlimomab treatment was associated with worse disability and greater mortality rates than was placebo. This negative treatment effect was evident by day 5 of treatment and was confirmed with adjustments for age and stroke severity. The hazard of death averaged over the first 90 days was 43% higher in enlimomab-treated patients than in placebo-treated patients.

There are several possible explanations for the negative effect of enlimomab. First, enlimomab is a different type of antibody from that used in experimental models. Murine anti-ICAM antibody may have led to upregulation of endogenous adhesion molecules and precipitated a paradoxic inflammatory response. It has been shown that all enlimomab-treated patients develop anti-mouse antibodies.[189] An experimental model was subsequently designed to mimic the clinical trial that had negative results. First, administration of this murine antibody to rats was shown to lead to production of host humoral responses against the protein, consisting of the activation of complement, neutrophils, and the microvascular system.[190] Second, no preclinical model delayed treatment for 6 hours or administered the drug for 5 consecutive days as in the clinical trial. Most important, animal studies showed no treatment benefit in permanent ischemia models. Only a minority of patients (4% to 24%) had spontaneous reperfusion; hence most enrolled patients were not comparable with transient ischemia models, which were associated with treatment benefit. Therefore, the rational approach to future immunomodulatory therapies would be development of a humanized anti-adhesion molecule strategy with a revised (shorter) dosage regimen coupled with thrombolysis.

To this end, a humanized immunoglobulin (Ig) G1 antibody against human CD18 (*Hu23F2G* or rovelizumab, *LeukArrest*) was developed to block leukocyte infiltration while avoiding the complications of enlimomab due to sensitization. A phase 3 trial enrolled patients within 12 hours of stroke onset, allowed concomitant use of t-PA, and employed a reduced frequency of dosing schema compared with enlimomab: The three groups received either a single dose at enrollment, the first dose at enrollment and a second dose 60 hours later, or placebo. The phase 3 trial of rovelizumab was terminated after interim futility analysis determined that treatment was unlikely to confer significant benefit if the trial were continued. To date, the data from this trial remain unpublished.

The immunomodulator, interferon-β (IFN-β), has been evaluated in a small number of preclinical trials. Its well-known side effect profile in patients with multiple sclerosis provides the opportunity to move forward more quickly in clinical trials of acute stroke. While the exact mechanism by which IFN-β provides neuroprotection is not clear, potential mechanisms include a reduction in neutrophil infiltration, decreased blood–brain barrier disruption,[191] and promotion of cell survival factors possibly mediated by NF-κB activation.[192] The preclinical data in acute ischemic stroke, however, is limited and conflicting. One study utilizing a transient model of ischemia demonstrated a reduction in infarct volume 1 day after stroke when IFN-β was administered even as long as 6 hours after symptom onset.[193] Similar results have been seen in a rabbit model of subcortical stroke.[194] One recent study has been reported in which IFN-β failed to demonstrate neuroprotection both in histologic and functional measures.[195] A randomized controlled dose-escalation phase 1 trial of IFN-β1a administered within 24 hours of symptom onset was recently completed.[110] Five dose cohorts of five patients (4:1 active:placebo) were studied at 11 μg, 22 μg, 44 μg, 66 μg, and 88 μg administered daily for 7 days. The results have not yet been published.

Leukocyte activation is another event in the inflammatory process that may be interrupted. A recombinant protein inhibitor of CD11b/CD18 receptor (*UK-279276*) blocks neutrophil activation and has shown neuroprotection in animal models of focal ischemia.[196] The Acute Stroke Therapy by Inhibition of Neutrophils (ASTIN) study was an adaptive phase 2 dose-response finding, proof-of-concept study to establish whether UK-279276 improves recovery in acute ischemic stroke. The investigators utilized a Bayesian sequential design with real-time efficacy data capture and continuous reassessment of the dose response using a double-blind, randomized, adaptive allocation to 1 of 15 doses (dose range, 10 to 120 mg) or placebo and early termination for efficacy or futility. The primary endpoint was change from baseline to day 90 on the Scandinavian Stroke Scale. Nine hundred sixty-six acute stroke patients (887 ischemic, 204 cotreated with IV t-PA) were treated within 6 hours of symptom onset. There was no treatment effect for UK-279276, and the trial was stopped early for futility. The authors concluded that UK-279276 was well-tolerated and without serious side effects but that it did not improve recovery in patients with acute ischemic stroke. The adaptive design facilitated early termination for futility.[197]

Promising new strategies are developing to target other "downstream" events of the ischemic–excitotoxic cascade: the calcium-dependent enzymatic reactions mediating necrotic and apoptotic cell death. Theoretically, because these processes occur "later" in the cascade, the therapeutic time window may be longer. Several important enzymes have been characterized as potential targets of neuroprotection. Calpain, a ubiquitous protease, mediates cell death via cleavage of structural and regulatory proteins. Caspase-3 is another protease that cleaves homeostatic proteins and may execute apoptosis.[198] Stress-activated mitogen-activated protein kinase (MAPK) is an enzyme that has been linked to inflammatory cytokine production and apoptosis.[199] Inhibition of these enzymes may be effective in preserving the structural integrity of neurons.

Multiple experimental models have demonstrated the efficacy of calpain, caspase, and protein kinase inhibitors in reducing infarct volume when used up to 6 hours after onset of ischemia.[200-203] The inability of these large protein compounds to cross the blood–brain barrier, however, has thus far limited clinical development, although novel strategies are being developed to enhance delivery of neurotherapeutics to the brain.

Minocycline has demonstrated protective effects in hypoxic-ischemic, focal, and global ischemia models.[204,205] Minocycline, a semisynthetic second-generation drug of the tetracycline group, is a safe and readily available compound that exerts anti-inflammatory effects such as inhibition of microglial activation[206] and production of other inflammatory mediators.[205] Furthermore, minocycline may inhibit the activity of matrix metalloproteinases (MMPs) and diminish permeability of the blood–brain barrier. An additional putative protective action of minocycline is inhibition of caspase, inducible NOS (iNOS), and p38 MAPK.[207] The neuroprotective efficacy of minocycline has been demonstrated in animal models even when delayed up to 4 hours,[205] has been shown to be as neuroprotective as hypothermia,[208] and may extend the t-PA treatment time window in ischemic stroke models.[209] Minocycline appears to be an ideal neuroprotective candidate on the basis of its established safety profile, good central nervous system penetration, wide availability, and inexpensive cost. Interestingly, the possibility of a gender-related response to treatment, with no reduction in infarct size in female rodents, was recently reported[210] and highlights an important trial design aspect that may need to be taken into account in future studies.

The results of an open-label, evaluator-blinded study that included 152 patients was recently reported.[211] Minocycline at a dosage of 200 mg was administered orally for 5 days within 6 to 24 hours after onset of stroke. The primary outcome measure was change in NIHSS score from baseline to day 90 in the minocycline group compared with placebo. Seventy-four patients received minocycline, and 77 received placebo. NIHSS, mRS, and BI scores were all significantly improved in minocycline-treated patients. Rates of adverse events and hemorrhagic transformation did not differ by treatment group. The trial did have some limitations, including the pseudorandomized design and open-label treatment. In addition, the placebo group did unusually poorly in this particular trial. Nonetheless, these findings support the preclinical data, which suggested a potential benefit of minocycline in acute ischemic stroke.

There are currently two ongoing clinical trials of minocycline in patients with acute ischemic stroke. The first is a Pilot Study of Treatment With Intravenous Enoxaparin and/or Oral Minocycline to Limit Infarct Size After Ischemic Stroke.[212] The study is a randomized, single-blind (outcomes assessor), parallel assignment, efficacy study. Patients will be assigned to one of three treatment groups: enoxaparin IV, or oral minocycline 200 mg, or both enoxaparin IV and oral minocycline 200 mg. The primary outcome measure is an index of salvaged ischemic penumbra and final infarct volume based on quantitative volumetric analyses of pretreatment and posttreatment perfusion-weighted and diffusion-weighted brain MRI within approximately 7 days of stroke onset. The study began in April 2009 and has a planned enrollment of 64 patients. The second trial, Minocycline to Improve Neurologic Outcome (MINO),[213] is designed to determine which of four different IV doses (between 3 and 10 mg/kg) of minocycline is safe and tolerated in patients with acute ischemic stroke; the result will be carried forward in future treatment trials. As of February 2009, 40 of 60 planned patients have been enrolled, and no significant infusion reactions have occurred.[214]

Tacrolimus (FK506) has been widely used for prevention of transplant organ rejection and has been investigated as a potential neuroprotectant because of its immunosuppressive properties. Tacrolimus suppresses the calcium-dependent signal transduction pathway that promotes proliferation of helper T cells by inhibition of calcineurin.[215] Apoptotic cell death is also attenuated by tacrolimus.[216] Multiple animal models demonstrate the neuroprotective effects of this agent through both histologic and radiographic evidence of reduction in infarct volume.[46,217-220]

A new formulation of this agent, FK506 Lipid Complex-Gilead (FK506 LCG), has been developed for the acute stroke indication. Preliminary studies demonstrated a dose-dependent hypothermia and increase in blood pressure in animals and a transient increase in blood pressure and heart rate in humans. Overall, this compound was well-tolerated, and a randomized, double-blind, placebo-controlled, dose-escalation study is planned to determine the safety, tolerability, and pharmacokinetics of FK506 LCG in patients with stroke.

Corticosteroids theoretically may interrupt the inflammatory cascade that occurs during stroke. Experimental data suggest that corticosteroids activate endothelial NOS activity via a nontranscriptional pathway, thereby augmenting regional cerebral blood flow and reducing infarct volume.[221] Although corticosteroids substantially reduce stroke size in experimental models, trials using various routes of administration, dosage, and duration of treatment with *dexamethasone* have failed to demonstrate a beneficial effect of steroids.[222,223] Steroids do, however, raise rates of infection and hyperglycemic complications. A systematic review of published randomized trials comparing steroids with placebo in treatment given within 48 hours of onset concluded that there is insufficient evidence to justify corticosteroid use after ischemic stroke.[224] In this review, data from 453 patients within seven trials revealed that treatment did not reduce rates of mortality or improve outcome. The substantial delay from stroke onset to drug administration is a possible culprit in the negative results. Additionally, the detrimental side effects of corticosteroids may be mediated by the transcriptional genomic activities of steroids, thereby limiting their clinical utility.[221] Therefore, novel compounds that selectively activate nontranscriptional glucocorticoid receptor activity may provide neuroprotection without the deleterious effects.[225] Such compounds are under development.

A growing interest in studying the pleiotropic effects of the 3-hydroxy-3-methylglutaryl coenzyme A (HMG CoA) reductase inhibitors ("*statins*") has uncovered a potential neuroprotective effect. A murine focal ischemia model demonstrated that long-term (14 to 28 days) or prophylactic treatment with mevastatin upregulates endothelial

NOS, reduces infarct size, and improves neurologic deficit in a dose- and time-dependent manner independent of serum cholesterol levels.[226] Other preclinical models utilizing different statins have also demonstrated attenuation of the size of the infarct[227,228] and improvement in functional outcome.[229] Meta-analyses of clinical statin trials support a clinical benefit in humans through lowering of stroke risk by approximately 30%.[230] The possible mechanisms of neuroprotection include improved endothelial function, increased endothelial NOS activity, antioxidant effects, promotion of neovascularization, and anti-inflammatory properties.

The Neuroprotection with Statin Therapy for Acute Recovery Trial (NeuSTART) is the first clinical trial evaluating the use of lovastatin in the early stage of stroke.[231] NeuSTART is a multicenter phase 1b dose-escalation and dose-finding study in which 33 patients with acute ischemic stroke will be administered lovastatin in increasing doses from 1 to 10 mg/kg daily for 3 days beginning within 24 hours after symptom onset. The primary safety outcome will be the occurrence of myotoxicity or hepatotoxicity. The study is designed to determine the highest dose of lovastatin that can be administered with less than 10% risk of toxicity.

Human serum albumin is a multifunctional protein with neuroprotective properties in experimental models of focal ischemia even when administered up to 4 hours after induction of reversible ischemia.[232] Several mechanisms have been speculated for its neuroprotective capacity, including inhibition of lipid peroxidation (antioxidant), maintenance of microvascular integrity, inhibition of endothelial cell apoptosis,[233] hemodilution, and mobilization of the free fatty acids required for restoration of damaged neurons.[234] Although nonalbumin hemodilution trials have not demonstrated a benefit, these were designed to test efficacy of hemodilution, not cytoprotection per se.

The Albumin in Acute Stroke (ALIAS) Pilot Trial was a phase 1, dose-escalation study designed to evaluate the safety and tolerability of increasing doses of albumin in patients with acute ischemic stroke.[235] Eighty-two subjects (mean age, 65 years) received albumin almost 8 hours after stroke onset. Forty-two patients also received standard-of-care IV t-PA. Age-related plasma brain natriuretic peptide levels increased at 24 hours after albumin administration but did not predict cardiac adverse events. The only albumin-related adverse event was mild or moderate pulmonary edema, which occurred in 13% of subjects and was readily managed with diuretics. In the t-PA–treated subgroup, symptomatic intracranial hemorrhage occurred in one of 42 subjects. In terms of functional outcome, the probability of good outcome (mRS 0 to 1 or NIHSS score 0 to 1 at 3 months) at the highest three albumin doses was 81% greater than in the lower dose tiers (RR, 1.81; 95% CI, 1.11–2.94). The t-PA–treated subjects who received higher doses of albumin were three times more likely to achieve a good outcome than subjects receiving lower dose albumin, which suggests a positive synergistic effect between albumin and t-PA.[235]

These promising preliminary results have led to a multicenter, randomized, placebo-controlled efficacy trial of albumin in acute ischemic stroke—the ALIAS-Part 2 Trial, which began enrollment in 2006. ALIAS-Part 2 is a phase 3 trial in which human serum albumin, at a dose of 2 g/kg, administered IV over 2 hours will be compared with placebo isovolumic normal saline in patients with acute ischemic stroke. The major change in ALIAS-Part 2 is that infusion of the study drug begins *within 5 hours* of stroke onset. Patients are treated according to the best standard of care including concurrent treatment with IV or intraarterial thrombolysis, when appropriate. The primary outcome will be determined at 3 months. The primary hypothesis is that if the composite outcome of an mRS of 0 to 1 or NIHSS score of 0 to 1 at 3 months (or both) is used, then the proportion of patients with improved outcomes will be greater by 10% or more in the active treatment group. The trial is estimated to conclude in 2011, with an estimated enrollment of 1100 patients.[110] In addition to the primary outcome measure, the ALIAS-Part 2 Trial will also examine whether albumin therapy does in fact reduce symptomatic intracerebral hemorrhage after t-PA.

The peroxisome proliferator activated receptor-gamma (PPARγ) is a member of the nuclear receptor superfamily, which controls glucose and lipid metabolism. In addition, PPARγ has been shown to be involved in systemic and vascular processes such as cellular differentiation,[201] inflammation,[236,237] and atherosclerosis.[238-240] In animal studies, the use of the PPARγ agonists in ischemic stroke models decreases infarct volume and is associated with improved neurologic outcomes in treated animals compared with controls. Their beneficial effects may be due to the repression of inflammatory mediators,[241,242] inhibition of NF-κB,[243] upregulation of antioxidant enzymes including catalase and superoxide dismutase,[242,244,245] and release of growth factors.[246] The promise of these agents is their potential to influence multiple molecular mechanisms.[247] These findings are consistent across different central nervous system models of disease. The clinically relevant PPARγ agonists are the thiazolidinediones (TZDs), pioglitazone, and rosiglitazone, which are FDA approved for the treatment of type 2 diabetes. There is currently an ongoing study of pioglitazone for secondary stroke prevention, the Insulin Resistance Intervention after Stroke Trial (IRIS); however, to our knowledge, there are no clinical studies evaluating the TZDs for treatment of acute ischemic stroke.

Membrane "Stabilizers" and Trophic Factors

SUR1, while best known for its role in the formation of K_ATP channels, has recently been associated with a nonselective cation channel, the NC(Ca-ATP) channel, in ischemic astrocytes, which is regulated by SUR1. NC(Ca-ATP) is opened by depletion of ATP and, when opened, leads to cytotoxic edema and cell necrosis.[248] This channel is upregulated in neurons, astrocytes, and capillary endothelial cells after central nervous system ischemia or injury. Blocking this channel by SUR1 inhibitors results in improvement in neurologic function in rodent models of ischemic stroke.[248] Moreover, the SUR1 antagonist, glibenclamide, has been shown to have a significant benefit across multiple ischemic stroke models with a large window for treatment opportunity (4 to 6 hours after ischemic insult).[249]

Retrospective clinical evaluation of the sulfonylureas for stroke has demonstrated interesting results. One study reviewed medical records of diabetic patients with stroke who were hospitalized within 24 hours of symptom onset. This cohort included 33 patients who were taking a sulfonylurea at the time of admission through discharge and 28 patients who served as control subjects. The primary outcome of major neurologic improvement was reached by 36% of patients in the treatment group and by 7% in the control group ($P = 0.007$).[250] This outcome appeared to be most beneficial in patients with nonlacunar stroke. In a different publication, the same group also reported that the initial presentation of stroke in diabetic patients may also be less severe for those who are taking sulfonylureas compared with other hyperglycemic treatments.[251] While there are no clinical trials of SUR1 inhibitors registered at this time, plans for phase 1 and 2 trials are in progress. Two doses will be used, and the emphasis will be on patients with NIHSS scores of 6 to 15 who have evidence of vascular occlusion. The treatment window will extend to 6 hours.[252]

The monosialoganglioside *GM-1* is thought to limit excitotoxicity and facilitate nerve repair and regrowth. In a study of 792 patients with acute stroke, there was a nonsignificant trend toward greater recovery in patients treated for 3 weeks with GM-1 than in those given placebo.[253] Post hoc analysis showed a statistically significant difference in neurologic outcome favoring GM-1 in the subgroup of patients treated within 4 hours. There was no difference in mortality rates, and the drug had no significant side effects. A Cochrane meta-analysis reported that there is not enough evidence to conclude that gangliosides are beneficial in acute stroke. In addition, caution was warranted due to sporadic cases of Guillain-Barré syndrome after ganglioside therapy.[254]

Cerebrolysin is a compound consisting of free amino acids and biologically active small peptides that are products of the enzymatic breakdown of lipid free brain products. Experimental models have demonstrated neuroprotection, although the mechanism of action is unclear.[255] Several small European trials have suggested that cerebrolysin administered as a continuous infusion (20 to 50 mL/day) for 20 days results in better motor function and global function than placebo.[256] Larger clinical trials would be required to confirm neuroprotection and determine the pharmacokinetics–pharmacodynamics of this peptide.

Energy failure and activation of phospholipases during ischemia lead to breakdown of cellular membranes and, ultimately, to neuronal death. *Cytidine-5'-diphosphocholine* (*citicoline*), is the rate-limiting intermediate in the biosynthesis of phosphatidylcholine, is incorporated into the membrane of injured neurons, and may prevent membrane breakdown into free radical–generating lipid byproducts. Citicoline has exhibited a neuroprotective effect in a variety of central nervous system injury models, including focal ischemia.[257] However, the neuroprotective capacity is modest and is lost if treatment is started beyond 3 hours after onset of injury.[258] Despite the extensive work performed with experimental models, the exact mechanism of action of citicoline remains elusive. However, it is believed to be due to increased phosphatidylcholine synthesis and inhibition of phospholipase A_2 within the injured brain. During ischemia, the choline supply is limited, and membrane phospholipids are hydrolyzed to provide a source of choline for neurotransmitter synthesis. This autocannibalism ultimately leads to death of cholinergic neurons.[258] Additionally, there is evidence that citicoline reduces expression of procaspases and other proteins involved in apoptotic cell death after focal ischemia.[259]

Pharmacokinetic–pharmacodynamic studies show that orally administered citicoline is nearly completely absorbed, blood levels peak at 6 hours, and the brain uptakes citicoline metabolites as early as 30 minutes after dosing.[260] Although bioavailability is the same with oral and IV administration, brain uptake is approximately four times higher with the IV route (0.5% oral dose versus 2% IV dose). Encapsulation of citicoline within liposomes may increase brain availability to 23% of the administered dose.

A randomized dose-response trial in 259 patients found a significant difference in functional outcome (BI and mRS), neurologic function (NIHSS), and cognitive function (Mini-Mental State Examination) favoring oral citicoline.[261] Both 500 mg and 2000 mg citicoline had significant effects on favorable outcome at 3 months (BI) after adjustment for initial stroke severity. There were no deaths and no dose-related serious adverse events, with the exception of mild dizziness experienced at 2000 mg/day. A subsequent phase 3 U.S. trial randomly assigned 394 patients with acute ischemic stroke to receive placebo or citicoline (500 mg by mouth daily) starting within 24 hours of stroke onset and continuing for 6 weeks. Patients with moderate to severe strokes (NIHSS score > 4) within the MCA territory were included.[262] An imbalance of stroke severity occurred: significantly more patients with NIHSS scores less than 8 were assigned to the placebo group. There was no statistical difference in planned secondary analyses, and the primary efficacy analysis was rendered unreliable because of the nonproportional distribution of patient BI scores. Post hoc analyses revealed that, in the subgroup of patients with baseline NIHSS scores higher than 7, citicoline-treated patients were significantly more likely to achieve a full recovery (placebo, 21%; citicoline, 33%; $P = 0.05$). No difference between treatment arms was seen in patients with NIHSS scores of 7 or less.

Partly on the basis of this subgroup analysis, another large phase 3 trial was conducted to evaluate the efficacy of higher dose citicoline (2000 mg/day) administered within 24 hours of onset to patients with baseline NIHSS scores higher than 7.[263] There was no difference between citicoline- and placebo-treated patients in the planned primary outcome, defined as improvement in NIHSS score of more than 7 points from the baseline value. However, post hoc analyses found a significant positive effect of treatment on recovery and on a global test of multiple outcomes. The neutral results of this trial are likely due to the chosen primary endpoint, which may not be reflective of recovery.

An important trial evaluating the effect of citicoline on MRI-demonstrated lesion volume showed the potential utility of neuroimaging as a surrogate marker of neuroprotective efficacy.[40] One hundred patients who had baseline NIHSS scores higher than 4 and who were seen with an abnormality on DWI within 24 hours of stroke onset were randomly assigned to receive either placebo or citicoline (500 mg/day) for 6 weeks. Follow-up MRI was performed at 12 weeks. At 12 weeks, the ischemic lesion volume had expanded by 180% in the placebo group compared with 34% in the citicoline group. Baseline predictors of change in lesion size included volume of perfusion deficit, baseline NIHSS score, initial DWI volume, arterial lesion on magnetic resonance angiography, and elapsed time from onset (≤12 hours versus >12 hours). A significant association was found between reduction of lesion volume and improvement of NIHSS score by 7 points or more.

Finally, IV citicoline at various doses (750 to 1000 mg/day) and treatment durations (10 to 30 days) has been evaluated in several non-U.S. trials, all of which showed significant improvements in recovery. A small pilot study comparing the efficacy of citicoline (1000 mg/day for 30 days) with that of placebo found that 71% of citicoline-treated patients improved from baseline compared with only 31% of placebo-treated patients.[264] The largest trial involved 272 patients randomly assigned to receive either citicoline (1000 mg/day for 14 days) or placebo. In this trial, a 26% relative difference on a global improvement rating scale favoring citicoline treatment over placebo was demonstrated.[265]

A meta-analysis of seven controlled clinical stroke trials showed that citicoline treatment was associated with significant reductions in rates of long-term death or disability.[266] A later pooled analysis of oral citicoline clinical trials in acute ischemic stroke sought to determine the effects of citicoline on neurologic recovery.[45] Individual patient data were extracted from four trials and pooled into a solitary database. Of 1652 total patients, 1372 fulfilled the inclusion criteria (583 placebo, 789 citicoline). Three-month recovery (composite NIHSS score <1, mRS score <1, BI value >95) was achieved in 25.2% of citicoline-treated patients compared with 20.2% of placebo-treated patients (Table 53-4). The largest difference in recovery was seen in patients treated with the highest dose (2000 mg) of citicoline. An international randomized multicenter placebo-controlled study began enrollment in 2006 to confirm the efficacy findings noted in the pooled analysis.[167] The study has enrolled 900 of a planned 2600 patients[110] who are randomly assigned within 24 hours of symptom onset to either placebo or citicoline (1 g/12 hour IV) during 3 days followed by 6 weeks of oral treatment. The primary outcome measure is total recovery at 3 months, based on a global test analysis including the NIHSS, mRS, and BI.

Finally, the combination of citicoline and IV thrombolysis has been shown to significantly reduce infarct volume compared with either treatment alone in a rat embolic stroke model, although this treatment combination has not yet been tested in humans.[267] Given the positive results of the meta-analyses just described, clinical evaluation of the combination of citicoline and t-PA appears to be the logical next step.

Estrogen exerts a multifaceted modulation of neurons, and various injury models have demonstrated the neuroprotection imparted by this hormone.[268,269] Although the exact neuroprotective mechanism has not been determined, there are many candidate actions. They include induction of antiapoptotic Bcl-2 proteins,[270] complex interactions with neurotrophins, activation of the cyclic adenosine monophosphate (cAMP)–protein kinase A–cAMP response element binding protein (CREB) pathway (antiapoptotic), attenuation of glutamate receptor activation, and decreasing intracellular calcium.[271] Clinical and epidemiologic data indirectly support the neuroprotective role of estrogen in the finding that premenopausal women have fewer strokes and that tamoxifen (an estrogen receptor antagonist) increases stroke risk.[272,273] No acute neuroprotection trials have been conducted in human patients with stroke.

TABLE 53-4 META-ANALYSES OF CITICOLINE STUDIES INTENT-TO-TREAT SET: GEE-ESTIMATED PROBABILITIES OF GLOBAL RECOVERY AFTER 12 WEEKS OF FOLLOW-UP

	Citicoline, %	Placebo, %	OR	95% CI	P
Citicoline vs placebo (4 trials, 1372 patients)	25.2	20.2	1.33	1.10-1.62	0.0034
Doses					
Citicoline 500 mg vs placebo					
Study 001a[261]	27.7	11.4	2.98	1.25-7.02	0.0129
Study 007[262]	24.2	16.6	1.61	0.93-2.78	0.089
Study 010[40]	17.1	24	0.65	0.28-1.48	0.3078
Overall	20.8	15.7	1.42	0.96-2.093	0.0782
Citicoline 1000 mg vs placebo					
Study 001a[261]	9.1	10.7	0.84	0.35-2.15	0.7096
Citicoline 2000 mg vs placebo					
Study 001a[261]	25.19	9.8	3.098	1.18-8.12	0.0214
Study 018[263]	28.47	23.25	1.314	1.0-1.65	0.0183
Overall	27.9	21.9	1.38	1.10-1.72	0.0043

*Superscript numbers indicate chapter references.
CI, Confidence interval; GEE, generalized estimating equation; OR, odds ratio.
From Davalos A, Castillo J, Alvarez-Sabin J, et al: Oral citicoline in acute ischemic stroke: An individual patient data pooling analysis of clinical trials. *Stroke* 33:2850, 2002.

Erythropoietin (EPO) is a mediator of the physiologic response to hypoxia via activation of the EPO receptor, a member of the cytokine receptor superfamily. Both astrocytes and neurons produce EPO in response to hypoxia, and this glycoprotein has been demonstrated to cross the blood–brain barrier.[274] The overall result of EPO receptor activation is cell proliferation, inhibition of apoptosis, and erythroblast differentiation.[275] EPO may also provide antioxidant activity and resistance to glutamate toxicity.[276,277] A focal ischemia model demonstrated that intraperitoneal epoetin alfa administered 6 hours after ischemia provided 50% protection, and this protection occurs via an antiapoptotic mechanism.[278,279] An initial safety and subsequent proof-of-concept study showed that intravenously administered EPO is safe and able to enter the brain in patients with stroke. In addition, treatment with EPO was associated with an improvement in clinical outcomes at 1 month.[280] A phase 3 randomized controlled trial that enrolled 522 patients within 6 hours of symptom onset was recently completed. This study evaluated the effect of a 3-day high-dose, IV EPO treatment on functional outcome (BI) at 90 days. The results have not yet been published.[110] Because of the potential of EPO to stimulate production of red blood cells and to promote blood coagulation, a modified version of EPO, Lu AA24493 or carbamylated erythropoietin (CEPO), has been developed and studied in a phase 1 trial. A subsequent study further evaluating safety and pharmacokinetics is currently ongoing.[281] The latter two trials have initiated treatment between 12 and 48 hours after symptom onset.

Trophic factors are emerging as potential cytoprotective agents, although their role may be more important in the recovery phase. *bFGF* (*trafermin [Fiblast]*) is a polypeptide that is trophic for brain neurons, glia, and endothelial cells and may prevent downregulation of antiapoptotic proteins such as Bcl-2.[282] Animal studies have shown that bFGF is effective in reducing infarct volume in acute ischemia models and in promoting synaptogenesis and functional recovery.[283,284] Additionally, synergistic protective effects have been observed for the combination of bFGF with either citicoline or caspase inhibitors.[285,286]

A double-blind, placebo-controlled clinical trial compared two doses of bFGF (5 mg or 10 mg) with placebo.[287] Patients with acute, moderate to severe stroke (NIHSS score >6) were randomly assigned within 6 hours of onset to receive a single 24-hour infusion of either bFGF or placebo. An interim efficacy analysis predicted only a nominal chance of significant benefit, and the trial was terminated after enrollment of 286 of the 900 patients planned. A nonsignificant trend for favorable outcome was seen in the low-dose group, whereas a nonsignificant disadvantage was seen in the high-dose group. Post hoc analysis further suggested efficacy of the low-dose regimen. Dose-dependent adverse events included leukocytosis and relative hypotension. An unpublished, multicenter, controlled phase 2/3 trial of bFGF was halted after interim analysis revealed a significant higher mortality rate in patients treated with this agent.

The poor penetration of the blood–brain barrier by bFGF necessitates high systemic doses, and peripheral side effects may offset the therapeutic effect. Conjugation of bFGF to a blood–brain barrier drug-delivery vector (OX26-SA) has demonstrated neuroprotection at a lower, systemically administered dosage in a rodent model.[288]

Other trophic factors, such as platelet-derived growth factor, insulin-derived growth factor, and glial cell line-derived neurotrophic factor, have also shown promise in neuroprotective models, possibly through angiogenic mechanisms.[289-291] They have not been studied in humans.

Granulocyte colony-stimulating factor (G-CSF) is a colony-stimulating factor hormone. It is a glycoprotein, growth factor, or cytokine produced by a number of different tissues to stimulate the bone marrow to produce granulocytes and stem cells. In acute stroke, G-CSF has been shown to be neuroprotective, antiapoptotic, and anti-inflammatory. In chronic stroke, G-CSF improves neurologic function weeks after stroke, induces neurogenesis, and enhances plasticity and stem cell mobilization from bone marrow. A phase 2 randomized, double-blind, placebo-controlled trial evaluating the safety and tolerability of AX 200 (G-CSF) compared with placebo in patients with acute stroke within 12 hours of symptom onset was completed in 2007. Patients with MCA infarct confirmed by MRI were randomly assigned on a 1:2 basis to receive either placebo or one of four different escalating doses of AX 200 (30, 90, 135, 180 µg/kg total) as an IV infusion.[110] A total of 44 patients were recruited. Thromboembolic complications (stroke and heart attack) were similar between G-CSF and placebo (7/30 versus 4/14, respectively) and serious adverse events were evenly distributed between groups.[292] Based on these findings, AXIS 2 (AX200 for the Treatment of Ischemic Stroke—A Multinational, Multicenter, Randomized, Double-blind, Placebo-Controlled phase 2 trial) has recently begun recruiting patients (NCT00927836).[293] The dose under evaluation is 135 µg/kg. The primary outcome measure is improvement on mRS relative to placebo-treated patients at 90 days. Enrollment of 350 patients is planned.[293]

Many of the novel neuroprotectants, especially trophic factors and anti-inflammatory agents, exist as peptides unable to cross the blood–brain barrier. Animal models have demonstrated enhancement of delivery and neuroprotection when protein agents are conjugated to a delivery vector. Such enhanced delivery mechanisms include (1) reformulation of the neurotherapeutic protein by conjugation and biotinylation and (2) creation of a fusion protein linked to transduction domains. Enhanced drug delivery systems have several benefits. First, obviously, they may enable delivery of neurotherapeutic agents that otherwise do not have access to the brain. Second, neuroprotection may be achieved at lower systemic doses, thereby allowing administration of agents that previously had dose-limiting side effects. Last, conjugation of an agent to blood–brain barrier delivery vectors may decrease its distribution to peripheral organs. Experimental models have already demonstrated these benefits. Bcl-XL, an antiapoptotic peptide member of the *Bcl-2* protooncogene family, has successfully been fused to the HIV TAT protein, has penetrated the blood–brain barrier after systemic administration, and has imparted neuroprotection.[294]

Hypothermia

The neuroprotective action of mild to moderate (29°C to 35°C) systemic hypothermia has been demonstrated in numerous animal models of global and focal cerebral ischemia.[295-304] The many hypothesized mechanisms for this protection include restoration of neurotransmitter balance,[305,306] reduction in cerebral metabolism,[307] preservation of the blood–brain barrier,[302] inhibition of apoptosis,[302,308] and attenuation of the inflammatory response.[309,310] Perhaps the consistent and robust benefit of hypothermia in multiple laboratories and animal models is due to the fact that it works through multiple pathways, all conspiring to have a greater effect than more precisely targeted therapies. Many of the clinically relevant questions regarding hypothermia have been addressed with varying degrees of success in animal studies: optimal mechanism of induction, target temperature, therapeutic time window, duration of treatment, rewarming, safety, reduction of shivering threshold, and persistence of benefit.

Several general principles have emerged from the extensive work investigating the cerebroprotective effects of hypothermia.[301] First, hypothermia applied during the ischemic period (intraischemic) is more protective than hypothermia applied after reperfusion (postischemic). Second, the efficacy of postischemic hypothermia depends on the interval between onset of ischemia and induction of hypothermia, achievement of target temperature, and duration of treatment. Third, hypothermia is more efficacious for global ischemia–reperfusion than for focal ischemia and more efficacious for transient focal ischemia than for permanent focal ischemia, which suggests that hypothermia may be most beneficial when coupled with thrombolysis and recanalization.

Hypothermia after cardiac arrest has been investigated with the use of surface cooling techniques.[24,25,311,312] Two large trials have conclusively established the neuroprotective effects and safety of hypothermia after cardiac arrest.[24,25] These studies are the first proof of the principle that neuroprotection can be realized in humans. The median time to achieve the target temperature from return of spontaneous circulation was 8 hours with surface cooling. Neurologic outcomes were significantly better in patients treated with hypothermia than in control subjects in both trials. The efficacy demonstrated, despite relatively long times to achieve the target temperature, is consistent with animal studies after global forebrain ischemia, which showed that such delayed therapy can be beneficial if it is continued for 12 to 24 hours.[26]

In the clinical treatment of stroke with hypothermia, rapid induction, precise temperature control, and ease of administration are critical requirements for the therapy. Cooling can be initiated through surface (skin) cooling or endovascular methods, such as catheter-based systems or IV infusions of chilled fluids. Surface cooling using previous technologies may induce hypothermia slowly and can overshoot the target temperature.[313] More recent versions of surface cooling units may approach the cooling power of endovascular methods with greater control. Endovascular cooling via specialized IV catheters may be a more efficient means of inducing and maintaining hypothermia and may possibly enhance the efficacy of neuroprotection. Endovascular cooling devices have been shown to reliably induce hypothermia, maintain the target temperature, and provide stable rewarming without rebound temperature elevation such as that seen with surface cooling.[314,315]

Several early studies have looked at the safety and feasibility of hypothermia in patients with ischemic stroke.[314,316-320]

However, the majority of these studies have focused on salvage hypothermic management of elevated intracranial pressure in patients with malignant MCA territory infarcts rather than as a stand-alone neuroprotective modality. These early studies have utilized surface cooling methods to achieve significant depths of hypothermia requiring sedation and neuromuscular blockade to enable patient tolerance of cooling. In one series of 50 consecutive patients with large MCA infarcts and severe deficits (mean NIHSS score, 25) who did not receive thrombolysis, hypothermia was initiated at a mean 22 ± 9 hours from symptom onset with surface cooling in ventilated, sedated, and paralyzed patients.[318] The mean time to reach the target temperature (32°C to 33°C) was 6.5 hours, and the mean duration of hypothermia was 17 hours. Hypothermia in this study population was effective in management of elevated intracranial pressure but was also associated with significant adverse effects (e.g., pneumonia, arrhythmias, and hypotension).

Data are accumulating to support the beneficial effect and safety of mild (34°C to 35°C) hypothermia in comparison with the moderate-to-severe hypothermia that is often accompanied by increased systemic adverse effects.[302,321,322] The duration of hypothermia has been studied over a variety of maintenance periods from 1 to 72 hours, and substantial protection has been shown even at the shortest duration of 1 hour.[323] The Cooling for Acute Ischemic Brain Damage (COOL-AID) study group completed two clinical trials of hypothermia in acute ischemic stroke in patients with severe MCA infarcts. The first study used surface cooling,[314] and the second used endovascular cooling.[324] Hypothermia (target, 31°C to 33°C) was achieved with surface cooling within 5 hours after onset (after IV t-PA) or within 8 hours (after endovascular thrombolysis). Both trials demonstrated feasibility but were not powered to answer questions regarding safety and efficacy.

A case-control study reported by Kammersgaard et al.[317] illustrated the feasibility of moderate hypothermia administered to awake patients within 12 hours of stroke onset. Hypothermia was initiated on admission with surface cooling to achieve 35.5°C and was maintained for 6 hours. Pethidine (meperidine) was effectively used to reduce shivering in all patients. These data support the feasibility of using mild hypothermia to treat awake patients with stroke without the inherent risks of intubation, sedation, and paralysis.

The Intravascular Cooling in the Treatment of Stroke-Longer t-PA Window (ICTuS-L) was a phase 1 trial originally designed to establish the safety of endovascular cooling combined with t-PA. In addition, by enrolling patients treated with t-PA from 3 to 6 hours after onset, extension of the therapeutic time window for thrombolysis using hypothermia would also be evaluated. There were a total of six treatment groups: patients who were seen within 3 hours received t-PA with or without hypothermia (groups 1 and 2) and patients who were seen within 3 to 6 hours of symptom onset randomly assigned to hypothermia plus t-PA, hypothermia alone, t-PA alone, or no treatment assignment (standard of care) comprised groups 3 through 6. ICTuS-L utilized an aggressive antishivering regimen, including buspirone and meperidine. ICTuS-L began in 2003; however, in 2008 both SITS-ISTR and ECASS 3 showed that IV thrombolysis was effective in patients treated between 3 and 4.5 hours after symptom onset. At this point, the investigators elected to close the ICTuS-L study early for analysis. As of December 2008, 59 patients were enrolled in ICTuS-L: 28 patients were randomly assigned to hypothermia and 30 patients were randomly assigned to normothermia. Overall, the rate of serious adverse events between those who received t-PA and those who did not were equivalent. Pneumonia occurred more frequently in the hypothermia patients than in the normothermia patients (7/28 versus 2/30, $P < 0.05$). This led to a change in the protocol to decrease the risk of development of pneumonia. The rates of intracranial hemorrhage, including both asymptomatic and symptomatic, were comparable in the two groups at 48 hours (33% hypothermia, 25% normothermia). There appeared to be no other safety concerns besides pneumonia, specifically, no increased risk of deep vein thrombosis due to the endovascular catheter; no liver, renal or hematologic concerns; and no coagulopathy.

The ICTuS-L trial confirmed that hypothermia, using an endovascular catheter, can be safely combined with thrombolytic therapy and that an aggressive antishivering protocol is feasible in awake stroke patients. ICTuS 2/3 is a planned prospective, multisite phase 2/3 pivotal efficacy trial of thrombolysis combined with hypothermia in awake patients with moderately severe MCA distribution strokes. This trial will investigate the clinical efficacy of hypothermia, further delineate safety in combination with thrombolysis, and confirm that the changes to the treatment protocol successfully limit the occurrence of pneumonia. The target population in phase 2 will include 450 assessable patients and in phase 3 will include 1600 assessable patients diagnosed with acute ischemic stroke. IV infusion of cooled saline will be added to the hypothermia protocol and will be followed by catheter placement for endovascular hypothermia therapy as soon as possible. Patients will receive hypothermia therapy to 33°C for 24 hours followed by 12 hours of controlled rewarming to 36.5°C (normothermia). Each subject will be followed up for 90 days after the onset of their stroke.

Hypothermia remains one of the most potent neuroprotective agents yet studied. The use of a treatment protocol that obviates the need for intubation makes this early treatment more relevant for practical clinical use. Future studies will investigate the effect of hypothermia on clinical outcome, the safety of combination with thrombolysis, and the potential for utilization with other neuroprotective modalities as discussed next.

Caffeinol

A novel combination of caffeine and ethanol (*caffeinol*) has demonstrated more robust neuroprotection than many other experimental and clinically relevant agents tested in the laboratory.[325] When used individually, caffeine had no effect, and ethanol actually increased infarct volume. The protective mechanism of the combination remains largely unknown but may be due to the synergistic effect of caffeine and ethanol on the excitatory–inhibitory balance between neurotransmitter systems and is currently being investigated with microdialysis studies. Adenosine and NMDA receptor antagonism and GABA enhancement are hypothesized to be mechanistically involved in this neurochemical action. Despite the unknown mechanism of action, animal studies have demonstrated a significant 83% reduction in infarct volume with the early administration of the combination of caffeine, 10 mg/kg, and 5% ethanol (0.325 g/kg), given intravenously over 120 minutes in rats subjected to experimental transient focal cerebral ischemia. Significant benefit was seen with treatment given up to 3 hours after stroke but was ineffective with permanent ischemia, in animals pretreated with ethanol, and in largely subcortical strokes.[326,327] Extensive work has shown that combining IV t-PA with caffeinol imparts no greater risk of intracranial hemorrhage in vivo and no reduction of t-PA fibrinolytic activity in vitro.[328]

An open-label, dose-escalation pilot study of caffeine and ethanol in patients with acute ischemic stroke identified the optimal dose resulting in plasma levels comparable with those producing therapeutic effect in animals (caffeine, 5 to 10 μg/mL; ethanol, 30 to 50 mg/dL) and that is clinically tolerated by patients without any significant adverse effects.[329]

Combining caffeinol with hypothermia to 35°C conferred greater neuroprotection in a transient focal ischemia model than either caffeinol or hypothermia alone. In this model, hypothermia was started 60 minutes after the onset of ischemia and continued for 240 minutes. A second clinical trial designed to establish the feasibility and safety of administering both caffeinol and mild systemic hypothermia to patients with acute ischemic stroke who had been treated with IV t-PA within 5 hours of symptom onset has recently been completed.[330] Twenty patients with acute ischemic stroke were treated with caffeinol (8 to 9 mg/kg caffeine + 0.4 g/kg IV ethanol over 2 hours, started within 4 hours after symptom onset) and hypothermia (started within 5 hours of symptom onset and continued for 24 hours (target temperature, 33°C to 35°C) followed by 12 hours of rewarming). IV t-PA was given to eligible patients. Meperidine and buspirone were used to suppress shivering. All patients received caffeinol, and most reached target blood levels. Cooling was attempted in 18 patients via endovascular (n = 8) or surface (n = 10) approaches. Two patients were not cooled because of catheter or machine failure. Thirteen patients reached the target temperature; average time from symptom onset was 9 hours and 43 minutes. The cooling protocol was revised to optimize the chances of reaching the target temperature. The biggest obstacle to cooling in awake patients was shivering, which required an aggressive antishivering protocol. Three patients died: one from symptomatic hemorrhage, one from malignant cerebral edema, and one from unrelated medical complications. No adverse events were attributed to caffeinol. At this point, the details of feasibility have been identified, and a prospective placebo-controlled randomized study is needed to further assess safety and to test the efficacy of caffeinol, hypothermia, or both.

Blood Substitutes and Oxygen Delivery

Compounds derived from human hemoglobin have a dual property: they may be neuroprotective through improvement in tissue oxygenation and may also augment perfusion because of their low viscosity. Several cell-free hemoglobin solutions are under clinical evaluation, but development has been cautious because of concerns about potential allergic and infectious complications as well as nephrotoxicity. The agent that went farthest in clinical development is *diaspirin–cross-linked hemoglobin (DCLHb)*, human hemoglobin derived from banked red blood cells, heat treated, and cross-linked to diaspirin to prevent dissociation. Its oxygen affinity is similar to that of blood. Probably because hemoglobin binds endothelial NO, it has a slight pressor effect. Studies in animal stroke models have consistently shown better perfusion of ischemic regions and reduction in infarct size.[331-334] The drug may be particularly effective in maintaining flow and oxygenation in the core of the infarct, thereby maintaining it in a "penumbral" state until definitive reperfusion by spontaneous or therapeutic thrombolysis occurs. In one study, DCLHb was able to double the length of time MCA occlusion could be withstood before ischemic damage appeared.[334]

A multicenter, randomized, single-blind phase 2 safety and dose-finding trial randomly assigned 85 patients to receive either DCLHb or saline.[335] Patients who had acute ischemic stroke in the anterior circulation and were identified within 18 hours of onset of symptoms were enrolled. DCLHb caused a rapid rise in mean arterial blood pressure. The pressor effect was not accompanied by complications or excessive need for antihypertensive treatment. Multivariate logistic regression analysis showed that a severe stroke at baseline and treatment with DCLHb (OR, 4.0; CI, 1.4–12.0) were independent predictors of worse outcome (mRS, 3 to 6) at 3 months. More serious adverse events and deaths occurred in DCLHb-treated patients than in control patients.

Normobaric hyperoxia (NBO) confers cortical protection when administered within 30 minutes of ischemia in rodents.[336] Practically, NBO therapy is easier to deliver than hyperbaric oxygen (HBO) therapy. Because of its simplicity, low cost, and safety, NBO may be initiated by first responders in the field. A phase 2 randomized controlled trial has recently been conducted to compare the safety and efficacy of treating acute ischemic stroke patients with NBO (within 9 hours of symptom onset) to standard medical treatment. This trial also assessed the therapeutic potential of NBO in extending the time window for administering thrombolytics.[110] Results are not yet available.

HBO treatment presumably increases oxygen delivery to the ischemic penumbra, thereby prolonging the functional activity of this potentially salvageable tissue. Administration of 100% oxygen at greater than atmospheric ambient pressure increases the amount of oxygen physically dissolved in blood. Other postulated protective actions are inhibition of neutrophil sequestration[337] and reduction of peri-infarct glucose, glutamate, and pyruvate levels.[338] Although the majority of animal models demonstrate a beneficial effect of HBO therapy on outcome and infarct volume,[339-343] others do not,[344-346] and controversy prevails regarding the neuroprotective potential of this modality in both clinical and experimental focal ischemia. Increased free radical generation and lipid peroxidation is a theoretical risk of HBO therapy that may counteract its neuroprotective mechanisms of action. A study of HBO delivery at 3 atm in a rodent model of focal ischemia demonstrated neuroprotection without alteration of lipid peroxidation.[343]

Human experience with ischemic stroke and HBO treatment yields similar conflicting results.[347,348] A double-blind pilot study compared the safety and efficacy of HBO

therapy and hyperbaric air (HBA) given to patients within 24 hours of onset of ischemic stroke.[348] A total of 34 patients were exposed to 40 minutes of hyperbaric treatment (17 HBO, 17 HBA) at 1.5 atm for 10 dives total. The mean Orgogozo neurologic assessment score at 1 year was significantly better in the HBO therapy than HBA therapy group, but no statistical difference was found in either the mRS scores or the net difference between pretreatment and posttreatment scores. This study concluded that HBO treatment was safe and possibly efficacious.

Conclusion

Encouraging signals have been detected in human studies of both hypothermia after cardiac arrest and citicoline for ischemic stroke, suggesting that clinically meaningful cytoprotection after stroke may still be achievable despite 10 years of trials of various agents that have largely failed to demonstrate it. An ongoing large trial of prehospital administered magnesium is nearing completion. If results of this trial are also negative, it should be determined once and for all that delayed treatment with drugs targeting single "upstream" events will not succeed. Phase 1 and 2 trials are now being designed to reflect the lessons learned from earlier trials. These lessons include (1) ultraearly treatment (FAST-MAG study); (2) targeting "downstream" events (e.g., trophic factors, EPO, albumin), which may be more amenable to postischemic treatment; and (3) combining agents that together have high potency by targeting multiple pathways (e.g., caffeinol, hypothermia, and t-PA). It is hoped that one or more of these approaches or some even more efficacious approach to cytoprotection will prove effective. Before valuable resources are committed to more large phase 3 studies, however, (1) any agent that seems promising should first show robust benefit in careful and thorough preclinical testing in multiple laboratories and models with clinically realistic treatment delay and (2) carefully conducted phase 1 and 2 trials should demonstrate that neuroprotective doses of the agent can be achieved in patients with stroke without unacceptable toxicity.

REFERENCES

1. Marsh BJ, Williams-Karnesky RL, Stenzel-Poore MP: Toll-like receptor signaling in endogenous neuroprotection and stroke, *Neuroscience* 158(3):1007-1020, 2009.
2. Trendelenburg G, Dirnagl U: Neuroprotective role of astrocytes in cerebral ischemia: focus on ischemic preconditioning, *Glia* 50(4):307-320, 2005.
3. Hossmann KA: Viability thresholds and the penumbra of focal ischemia, *Ann Neurol* 36(4):557-565, 1994.
4. Ginsberg M: Neuroprotection in brain ischemia: An update, *Neuroscientist* 1(95):164, 1995.
5. DeGraba TJ, Ostrow PT, Strong RA, et al: The temporal relation of calcium-calmodulin binding and neuronal damage after global ischemia, *Stroke* 23:876, 1992.
6. Bredesen DE: Neural apoptosis, *Ann Neurol* 38(6):839-851, 1995.
7. Sharp FR, Lu A, Tang Y, et al: Multiple molecular penumbras after focal cerebral ischemia, *J Cereb Blood Flow Metab* 20:1011, 2000.
8. Pulsinelli WA, Brierley JB: A new model of bilateral hemispheric ischemia in the unanesthetized rat, *Stroke* 10(3):267-272, 1979.
9. Pulsinelli WA, Brierley JB, Plum F: Temporal profile of neuronal damage in a model of transient forebrain ischemia, *Ann Neurol* 11(5):491-498, 1982.
10. Volpe BT, Pulsinelli WA, Tribuna J, et al: Behavioral performance of rats following transient forebrain ischemia, *Stroke* 15(3):558-562, 1984.

11. Chen ST, Hsu CY, Hogan EL, et al: A model of focal ischemic stroke in rats: Reproducible extensive cortical infarction, *Stroke* 17:738, 1986.

12. Brint S, Jacewicz M, Kiessling M, et al: Focal brain ischemia in rat: Method for reproducible neocortical infarction using tandem occlusion of the distal middle cerebral and ipsilateral common carotid arteries, *J Cereb Blood Flow Metab* 8:474, 1988.

13. Buchan A, Xue D, Slivka A: A new model of temporary focal neocortical ischemia in the rat, *Stroke* 23:273, 1992.

14. Zhang RL, Zhang ZG, Chopp M: Increased therapeutic efficacy with rt-PA and anti-CD18 antibody treatment of stroke in the rat, *Neurology* 52:273, 1999.

15. Yang GY, Betz AL: Reperfusion-induced injury to the blood-brain barrier after middle cerebral artery occlusion in rats, *Stroke* 25(8):1658-1664, 1994:discussion 1664-1655.

16. Aronowski J, Strong R, Grotta JC: Reperfusion injury: Demonstration of brain damage produced by reperfusion after transient focal ischemia in rats, *J Cereb Blood Flow Metab* 17(10):1048-1056, 1997.

17. Uematsu D, Araki N, Greenberg J, et al: Combined therapy with MK-801 and nimodipine for protection of ischemic brain damage, *Neurology* 41:88, 1991.

18. Zivin J, Mazzarella V: Tissue plasminogen activator plus glutamate antagonist improves outcome after embolic stroke, *Arch Neurol* 48:1235, 1991.

19. Bowes M, Rothlein R, Fagan S, et al: Monoclonal antibodies preventing leukocyte activation reduce experimental neurologic injury and enhance efficacy of thrombolytic therapy, *Neurology* 45:815, 1995.

20. Grotta JC: The current status of neuronal protective therapy: Why have all neuronal protective drugs worked in animals but none so far in stroke patients? *Cerebrovasc Dis* 4:115, 1994.

21. Fisher M, Ratan R: New perspectives on developing acute stroke therapy, *Ann Neurol* 53:10, 2003.

22. Jones TH, Morawetz RB, Crowell RM, et al: Thresholds of focal cerebral ischemia in awake monkeys, *J Neurosurg* 54:773, 1981.

23. Kaplan B, Brint S, Tanabe J, et al: Temporal thresholds for neocortical infarction in rats subjected to reversible focal cerebral ischemia, *Stroke* 22:1032, 1991.

24. Bernard SA, Gray TW, Buist MD, et al: Treatment of comatose survivors of out-of-hospital cardiac arrest with induced hypothermia, *N Engl J Med* 346:557, 2002.

25. The Hypothermia after Cardiac Arrest Study Group: Mild therapeutic hypothermia to improve the neurologic outcome after cardiac arrest, *N Engl J Med* 346(8):549-556, 2002.

26. Colbourne F, Li H, Buchan AM: Indefatigable CA1 sector neuroprotection with mild hypothermia induced 6 hours after severe forebrain ischemia in rats, *J Cereb Blood Flow Metab* 19:742, 1999.

27. O'Collins VE, Macleod MR, Donnan GA, et al: 1,026 experimental treatments in acute stroke, *Ann Neurol* 59(3):467-477, 2006.

28. Recommendations for standards regarding preclinical neuroprotective and restorative drug development, *Stroke* 30(12):2752-2758, 1999.

29. STAIR-II Recommendations for clinical trial evaluation of acute stroke therapies, *Stroke* 32(7):1598-1606, 2001.

30. Adams HP, Davis PH, Leira EC, et al: Baseline NIH Stroke Scale score strongly predicts outcome after stroke, *Neurology* 53:126, 1999.

31. Woo D, Broderick J, Kothari R, et al: Does the National Institutes of Health Stroke Scale favor left hemisphere strokes? *Stroke* 30:2355, 1999.

32. Heiss WD, Graf R, Lottgen J, et al: Repeat positron emission tomographic studies in transient middle cerebral artery occlusion in cats: Residual perfusion and efficacy of postischemic reperfusion, *J Cereb Blood Flow Metab* 17:388, 1997.

33. Baron JC: Mapping the ischaemic penumbra with PET: implications for acute stroke treatment, *Cerebrovasc Dis* 9(4):193-201, 1999.

34. Marchal G, Beaudouin V, Rioux P, et al: Prolonged persistence of substantial volumes of potentially viable brain tissue after stroke: A correlative PET-CT study with voxel-based data analysis, *Stroke* 27:599, 1996.

35. Neumann-Haeflin T, Moseley ME, Albers GW: New magnetic resonance imaging methods for cerebrovascular disease: Emerging clinical applications, *Ann Neurol* 31:559, 2000.

36. Schellinger PD, Fieback JB, Jansen O, et al: Stroke magnetic resonance imaging within 6 hours after onset of hyperacute cerebral ischemia, *Ann Neurol* 49:460, 2001.

37. Schlaug G, Benfield A, Baird AE, et al: The ischemic penumbra: operationally defined by diffusion perfusion MRI, *Neurology* 53:1528, 1999.

38. Li F, Silva MD, Liu KF, et al: Secondary decline in apparent diffusion coefficient and neurological outcome after a short period of focal brain ischemia in rats, *Ann Neurol* 48:236, 2000.

39. Kidwell CS, Saver JL, Mattiello J, et al: Thrombolytic reversal of acute human cerebral ischemic injury shown by diffusion/perfusion magnetic resonance imaging, *Ann Neurol* 47:462, 2000.

40. Warach S, Pettigrew LC, Dashe JF, et al: Effect of citicoline on ischemic lesions as measured by diffusion-weighted magnetic resonance imaging. Citicoline 010 Investigators, *Ann Neurol* 48(5):713-722, 2000.

41. Tissue plasminogen activator for acute ischemic stroke: The National Institute of Neurological Disorders and Stroke rt-PA Stroke Study Group, *N Engl J Med* 333(24):1581-1587, 1995.

42. Lees KR, Asplund K, Carolei A, et al: Glycine antagonist (gavestinel) in neuroprotection (GAIN International) in patients with acute stroke: A randomised controlled trial. GAIN International Investigators, *Lancet* 355(9219):1949-1954, 2000.

43. Muir KW: Magnesium for neuroprotection in ischaemic stroke: rationale for use and evidence of effectiveness, *CNS Drugs* 15(12):921-930, 2001.

44. Shuaib A, Lees KR, Lyden P, et al: NXY-059 for the treatment of acute ischemic stroke, *N Engl J Med* 357(6):562-571, 2007.

45. Davalos A, Castillo J, Alvarez-Sabin J, et al: Oral citicoline in acute ischemic stroke: An individual patient data pooling analysis of clinical trials, *Stroke* 33(12):2850-2857, 2002.

46. McCarter JF, McGregor AL, Jones PA, et al: FK 506 protects brain tissue in animal models of stroke, *Transplant Proc* 33(3):2390-2392, 2001.

47. Saver JL, Kidwell CS, Leary M, et al: The Field Administration of Stroke Therapy-Magnesium: A study of prehospital neuroprotective therapy. Abstract presented at the Ongoing Clinical Trials Session, Fort Lauderdale, Fla, 2001, 26th International Stroke Conference.

48. Effect of intravenous recombinant tissue plasminogen activator on ischemic stroke lesion size measured by computed tomography: NINDS; The National Institute of Neurological Disorders and Stroke (NINDS) rt-PA Stroke Study Group, *Stroke* 31(12):2912-2919, 2000.

49. Hantson L: Neurologic scales in the assessment of stroke. In Grotta J, Miller L, Buchan AM, editors: *Ischemic stroke: Recent advances in understanding and therapy*, Southbourough, Mass, 1995, International Business Communications.

50. Duncan PW, Lai SM, Bode RK, et al: Stroke impact scale-16, *Neurology* 60:291, 2003.

51. Tilley BC, Marler J, Geller NL, et al: Use of a global test for multiple outcomes in stroke trials with application to the National Institute of Neurological Disorders and Stroke t-PA Stroke Trial, *Stroke* 27(11):2136-2142, 1996.

52. Bean BP: Nitrendipine block of cardiac calcium channels: High-affinity binding to the inactivated state, *Proc Natl Acad Sci U S A* 81(20):6388-6392, 1984.

53. Horn J, de Haan RJ, Vermeulen M, et al: Nimodipine in animal model experiments of focal cerebral ischemia: a systematic review, *Stroke* 32(10):2433-2438, 2001.

54. Grotta JC: Clinical aspects of the use of calcium antagonists in cerebrovascular disease, *Clin Neuropharmacol* 14(5):373-390, 1991.

55. Gelmers HJ: The effects of nimodipine on the clinical course of patients with acute ischemic stroke, *Acta Neurol Scand* 69(4):232-239, 1984.

56. Gelmers HJ, Gorter K, de Weerdt CJ, et al: A controlled trial of nimodipine in acute ischemic stroke, *N Engl J Med* 318(4):203-207, 1988.

57. Paci A, Ottaviano P, Trenta A, et al: Nimodipine in acute ischemic stroke: a double-blind controlled study, *Acta Neurol Scand* 80(4):282-286, 1989.

58. Gelmers HJ, Hennerici M: Effect of nimodipine on acute ischemic stroke. Pooled results from five randomized trials, *Stroke* 21(12 Suppl):IV81-84, 1990.

59. Nag D, Garg RK, Varma M: A randomized double-blind controlled study of nimodipine in acute cerebral ischemic stroke, *Indian J Physiol Pharmacol* 42(4):555-558, 1998.

60. Clinical trial of nimodipine in acute ischemic stroke: The American Nimodipine Study Group, *Stroke* 23(1):3-8, 1992.

61. Wahlgren N, MacMahon D, De Keyser J, et al: Intravenous Nimodipine West European Stroke Trial (INWEST) of nimodipine in the treatment of acute ischemic stroke. The INWEST Study Group, *Cerebrovasc Dis* 4:204, 1994.

62. Kaste M, Fogelholm R, Erila T, et al: A randomized, double-blind, placebo-controlled trial of nimodipine in acute ischemic hemispheric stroke, *Stroke* 25(7):1348-1353, 1994.

63. Ahmed N, Nasman P, Wahlgren NG: Effect of intravenous nimodipine on blood pressure and outcome after acute stroke, *Stroke* 31(6):1250-1255, 2000.

64. Horn J, de Haan RJ, Vermeulen M, et al: Very Early Nimodipine Use in Stroke (VENUS): a randomized, double-blind, placebo-controlled trial, *Stroke* 32(2):461-465, 2001.

65. Rosenbaum D, Zabramski J, Frey J, et al: Early treatment of ischemic stroke with a calcium antagonist, *Stroke* 22(4):437-441, 1991.

66. Kobayashi T, Mori Y: Ca2+ channel antagonists and neuroprotection from cerebral ischemia, *Eur J Pharmacol* 363(1):1-15, 1998.

67. Koh JY, Cotman CW: Programmed cell death: Its possible contribution to neurotoxicity mediated by calcium channel antagonists, *Brain Res* 587(2):233-240, 1992.

68. Buchan AM, Gertler SZ, Li H, et al: A selective N-type Ca(2+)-channel blocker prevents CA1 injury 24 h following severe forebrain ischemia and reduces infarction following focal ischemia, *J Cereb Blood Flow Metab* 14(6):903-910, 1994.

69. Ginsberg MD: Neuroprotection for ischemic stroke: Past, present and future, *Neuropharmacology* 55(3):363-389, 2008.

70. Grotta JC, Picone CM, Ostrow PT, et al: CGS-19755, a competitive NMDA receptor antagonist, reduces calcium-calmodulin binding and improves outcome after global cerebral ischemia, *Ann Neurol* 27(6):612-619, 1990.

71. Simon R, Shiraishi K: N-methyl-D-aspartate antagonist reduces stroke size and regional glucose metabolism, *Ann Neurol* 27(6):606-611, 1990.

72. Simmonds J, Sailer T, Moyer J: The effects of CGS-19755 in rat focal cerebral ischemia produced by tandem ipsilateral common carotid artery and middle cerebral artery occlusion, *Abstr Soc Neurosci* 19:1647, 1993.

73. Davis SM, Lees KR, Albers GW, et al: Selfotel in acute ischemic stroke: Possible neurotoxic effects of an NMDA antagonist, *Stroke* 31(2):347-354, 2000.

74. Steinberg GK, Perez-Pinzon MA, Maier CM, et al: CGS-19755: Correlation of in vitro neuroprotection, protection against experimental ischemia and CSF levels in cerebrovascular surgery patients [abstract]. In Proceedings of the 5th International Symposium on Pharmacology of Cerebral Ischemia, July 20-22, 1994.

75. Albers GW, Atkinson RP, Kelley RE, et al: Safety, tolerability, and pharmacokinetics of the N-methyl-D-aspartate antagonist dextrorphan in patients with acute stroke. Dextrorphan Study Group, *Stroke* 26(2):254-258, 1995.

76. Dyker AG, Edwards KR, Fayad PB, et al: Safety and tolerability study of aptiganel hydrochloride in patients with an acute ischemic stroke, *Stroke* 30(10):2038-2042, 1999.

77. Albers GW, Goldstein LB, Hall D, et al: Aptiganel hydrochloride in acute ischemic stroke: A randomized controlled trial, *JAMA* 286(21):2673-2682, 2001.

78. Diener HC, Al Khedr A, Busse O, et al: Treatment of acute ischaemic stroke with the low-affinity, use-dependent NMDA antagonist AR-R15896AR. A safety and tolerability study, *J Neurol* 249(5):561-568, 2002.

79. Muir KW: Magnesium in stroke treatment, *Postgrad Med J* 78(925):641-645, 2002.

80. Muir KW, Lees KR: A randomized, double-blind, placebo-controlled pilot trial of intravenous magnesium sulfate in acute stroke, *Stroke* 26(7):1183-1188, 1995.

81. Weglicki WB, Phillips TM: Pathobiology of magnesium deficiency: A cytokine/neurogenic inflammation hypothesis, *Am J Physiol* 263(3 Pt 2):R734-737, 1992.

82. Yang Y, Li Q, Ahmad F, et al: Survival and histological evaluation of therapeutic window of post-ischemia treatment with magnesium sulfate in embolic stroke model of rat, *Neurosci Lett* 285(2):119-122, 2000.

83. Altura BT, Memon ZI, Zhang A, et al: Low levels of serum ionized magnesium are found in patients early after stroke which result in rapid elevation in cytosolic free calcium and spasm in cerebral vascular muscle cells, *Neurosci Lett* 230(1):37-40, 1997.

84. Lampl Y, Geva D, Gilad R, et al: Cerebrospinal fluid magnesium level as a prognostic factor in ischaemic stroke, *J Neurol* 245(9):584-588, 1998.

85. Muir KW, Lees KR: Dose optimization of intravenous magnesium sulfate after acute stroke, *Stroke* 29(5):918-923, 1998.

86. Izumi Y, Roussel S, Pinard E, et al: Reduction of infarct volume by magnesium after middle cerebral artery occlusion in rats, *J Cereb Blood Flow Metab* 11(6):1025-1030, 1991.

87. Muir KW, Lees KR, Ford I, et al: Magnesium for acute stroke (Intravenous Magnesium Efficacy in Stroke Trial): randomised controlled trial, *Lancet* 363(9407):439-445, 2004.

88. Saver JL, Kidwell CS, Hamilton S, et al: The field administration of stroke therapy—magnesium. abstract presented at the ongoing clinical trials session, San Antonio, Tex, February 7-9, 2002, 27th International Stroke Conference.

89. Olney JW, Labruyere J, Price MT: Pathological changes induced in cerebrocortical neurons by phencyclidine and related drugs, *Science* 244(4910):1360-1362, 1989.

90. Horvath ZC, Czopf J, Buzsaki G: MK-801-induced neuronal damage in rats, *Brain Res* 753(2):181-195, 1997.

91. Farber NB, Kim SH, Dikranian K, et al: Receptor mechanisms and circuitry underlying NMDA antagonist neurotoxicity, *Mol Psychiatry* 7(1):32-43, 2002.

92. Kim SH, Price MT, Olney JW, et al: Excessive cerebrocortical release of acetylcholine induced by NMDA antagonists is reduced by GABAergic and alpha2-adrenergic agonists, *Mol Psychiatry* 4(4):344-352, 1999.

93. Olney JW, Wozniak DF, Jevtovic-Todorovic V, et al: Drug-induced apoptotic neurodegeneration in the developing brain, *Brain Pathol* 12(4):488-498, 2002.

94. Lees KR: Cerestat and other NMDA antagonists in ischemic stroke, *Neurology* 49(5 Suppl 4):S66-69, 1997.

95. Bordi F, Pietra C, Ziviani L, et al: The glycine antagonist GV150526 protects somatosensory evoked potentials and reduces the infarct area in the MCAo model of focal ischemia in the rat, *Exp Neurol* 145(2 Pt 1):425-433, 1997.

96. Dyker AG, Lees KR: Safety and tolerability of GV150526 (a glycine site antagonist at the N-methyl-D-aspartate receptor) in patients with acute stroke, *Stroke* 30(5):986-992, 1999.

97. Phase II studies of the glycine antagonist GV150526 in acute stroke: The North American experience. The North American Glycine Antagonist in Neuroprotection (GAIN) Investigators, *Stroke* 31(2):358-365, 2000.

98. Lees KR, Lavelle JF, Cunha L, et al: Glycine antagonist (GV150526) in acute stroke: A multicentre, double-blind placebo-controlled phase II trial, *Cerebrovasc Dis* 11(1):20-29, 2001.

99. Sacco RL, DeRosa JT, Haley EC Jr, et al: Glycine antagonist in neuroprotection for patients with acute stroke: GAIN Americas: A randomized controlled trial, *JAMA* 285(13):1719-1728, 2001.

100. Akins PT, Atkinson RP: Glutamate AMPA receptor antagonist treatment for ischaemic stroke, *Curr Med Res Opin* (18 Suppl 2):s9-13, 2002.

101. Kawasaki-Yatsugi S, Ichiki C, Yatsugi S, et al: Neuroprotective effects of an AMPA receptor antagonist YM872 in a rat transient middle cerebral artery occlusion model, *Neuropharmacology* 39(2):211-217, 2000.

102. Van Hoogdalem E, de Vos R, Hefting NR, et al: Clinical experience with YM872, a novel AMPA receptor antagonist for acute ischemic stroke [abstract], *Stroke* 30:264, 1999.

103. Suzuki M, Sasamata M, Miyata K: Neuroprotective effects of YM872 coadministered with t-PA in a rat embolic stroke model, *Brain Res* 959(1):169-172, 2002.

104. Elting JW, Sulter GA, Kaste M, et al: AMPA antagonist ZK(200775 in patients with acute ischemic stroke: Possible glial cell toxicity detected by monitoring of S-100B serum levels, *Stroke* 33:2813, 2002.

105. Smith SE, Meldrum BS: Cerebroprotective effect of lamotrigine after focal ischemia in rats, *Stroke* 26(1):117-121, 1995:discussion 121-112.

106. Traystman RJ, Klaus JA, DeVries AC, et al: Anticonvulsant lamotrigine administered on reperfusion fails to improve experimental stroke outcomes, *Stroke* 32(3):783-787, 2001.

107. Leach MJ, Swan JH, Eisenthal D, et al: BW619C89, a glutamate release inhibitor, protects against focal cerebral ischemic damage, *Stroke* 24(7):1063-1067, 1993.

108. Kawaguchi K, Graham SH: Neuroprotective effects of the glutamate release inhibitor 619C89 in temporary middle cerebral artery occlusion, *Brain Res* 749:131, 1991.

109. Muir KW, Holzapfel L, Lees KR: Phase II clinical trial of sipatrigine (619C89) by continuous infusion in acute stroke, *Cerebrovasc Dis* 10(6):431-436, 2000.

110. The Internet Stroke Center, Stroke Trials Registry: www.strokecenter.org. Accessed August 1, 2009.

111. Gribkoff VK, Starrett JE Jr, Dworetzky SI: The pharmacology and molecular biology of large-conductance calcium-activated (BK) potassium channels, *Adv Pharmacol* 37:319-348, 1997.

112. Squire IB, Lees KR, Pryse-Phillips W, et al: Efficacy and tolerability of lifarizine in acute ischemic stroke. A pilot study. Lifarizine Study Group, *Ann N Y Acad Sci* 765:317-318, 1995.

113. De Ryck M, Keersmaekers R, Clincke G, et al: Lubeluzole, a novel benzothiazole, protects neurologic function after cerebral thrombotic stroke in rats: An apparent stereospecific effect [abstract], *Abstr Soc Neurosci* 20:185, 1994.

114. Aronowski J, Strong R, Grotta JC: Treatment of experimental focal ischemia in rats with lubeluzole, *Neuropharmacology* 35(6):689-693, 1996.

115. De Ryck M, Verhoye M, Van der Linden AM: Diffusion-weighted MRI of infarct growth in a rat photochemical stroke model: Effect of lubeluzole, *Neuropharmacology* 39(4):691-702, 2000.

116. Hernandez-Guijo JM, Gandia L, de Pascual R, et al: Differential effects of the neuroprotectant lubeluzole on bovine and mouse chromaffin cell calcium channel subtypes, *Br J Pharmacol* 122(2):275-285, 1997.

117. Scheller DK, De Ryck M, Kolb J, et al: Lubeluzole blocks increases in extracellular glutamate and taurine in the peri-infarct zone in rats, *Eur J Pharmacol* 338(3):243-251, 1997.

118. Lesage AS, Peeters L, Leysen JE: Lubeluzole, a novel long-term neuroprotectant, inhibits the glutamate-activated nitric oxide synthase pathway, *J Pharmacol Exp Ther* 279(2):759-766, 1996.

119. Diener HC, Hacke W, Hennerici M, et al: Lubeluzole in acute ischemic stroke. A double-blind, placebo-controlled phase II trial. Lubeluzole International Study Group, *Stroke* 27(1):76-81, 1996.

120. De Ryck M, Keersmaekers R, Duytschaever H, et al: Lubeluzole protects sensorimotor function and reduces infarct size in a photochemical stroke model in rats, *J Pharmacol Exp Ther* 279(2):748-758, 1996.

121. Diener HC: Multinational randomised controlled trial of lubeluzole in acute ischaemic stroke. European and Australian Lubeluzole Ischaemic Stroke Study Group, *Cerebrovasc Dis* 8(3):172-181, 1998.

122. Grotta J: Lubeluzole treatment of acute ischemic stroke. The US and Canadian Lubeluzole Ischemic Stroke Study Group, *Stroke* 28(12):2338-2346, 1997.

123. Diener HC, Cortens M, Ford G, et al: Lubeluzole in acute ischemic stroke treatment: A double-blind study with an 8-hour inclusion window comparing a 10-mg daily dose of lubeluzole with placebo, *Stroke* 31(11):2543-2551, 2000.

124. Gandolfo C, Sandercock P, Conti M: Lubeluzole for acute ischaemic stroke, *Cochrane Database Syst Rev* 1:CD001924, 2002.

125. Davies MF, Deisz RA, Prince DA, et al: Two distinct effects of 5-hydroxytryptamine on single cortical neurons, *Brain Res* 423(1-2):347-352, 1987.

126. Matsuyama S, Nei K, Tanaka C: Regulation of glutamate release via NMDA and 5-HT1A receptors in guinea pig dentate gyrus, *Brain Res* 728(2):175-180, 1996.

127. Schaper C, Zhu Y, Kouklei M, et al: Stimulation of 5-HT(1A) receptors reduces apoptosis after transient forebrain ischemia in the rat, *Brain Res* 883(1):41-50, 2000.

128. Ramirez-Lessepas M, Patrick BK, Snyder BD, et al: Failure of central nervous system serotonin blockage to influence outcome in acute cerebral infarction. A double blind randomized trial, *Stroke* 17(5):953-956, 1986.

129. Teal P, Silver FL, Simard D: The BRAINS study: Safety, tolerability, and dose-finding of repinotan in acute stroke, *Can J Neurol Sci* 32(1):61-67, 2005.

130. Pettigrew LC, Kasner SE, Albers GW, et al: Safety and tolerability of arundic acid in acute ischemic stroke, *J Neurol Sci* 251(1-2):50-56, 2006.

131. Hariri RJ, Supra EL, Roberts JP, et al: Effect of naloxone on cerebral perfusion and cardiac performance during experimental cerebral ischemia, *J Neurosurg* 64(5):780-786, 1986.

132. Namba S, Nishigaki S, Fujiwara N, et al: Opiate-antagonist reversal of neurological deficits—experimental and clinical studies, *Jpn J Psychiatry Neurol* 40(1):61-79, 1986.

133. Baskin DS, Kuroda H, Hosobuchi Y, et al: Treatment of stroke with opiate antagonists—effects of exogenous antagonists and dynorphin 1-13, *Neuropeptides* 5(4-6):307-310, 1985.

134. Fallis RJ, Fisher M, Lobo RA: A double blind trial of naloxone in the treatment of acute stroke, *Stroke* 15(4):627-629, 1984.

135. Jabaily J, Davis JN: Naloxone administration to patients with acute stroke, *Stroke* 15(1):36-39, 1984.

136. Adams HP Jr, Olinger CP, Barsan WG, et al: A dose-escalation study of large doses of naloxone for treatment of patients with acute cerebral ischemia, *Stroke* 17(3):404-409, 1986.

137. Olinger CP, Adams HP Jr, Brott TG, et al: High-dose intravenous naloxone for the treatment of acute ischemic stroke, *Stroke* 21(5):721-725, 1990.

138. Federico F, Lucivero V, Lamberti P, et al: A double blind randomized pilot trial of naloxone in the treatment of acute ischemic stroke, *Ital J Neurol Sci* 12(6):557-563, 1991.

139. Clark WM, Coull BM, Karukin M, et al: Randomized trial of Cervene, a kappa receptor-selective opioid antagonist, in acute ischemic stroke, *J Stroke Cerebrovasc Dis* 6(1):35-40, 1996.

140. Clark W, Ertag W, Orecchio E, et al: Cervene in acute ischemic stroke: Results of a double-blind, placebo-controlled, dose-comparison study, *J Stroke Cerebrovasc Dis* 8(4):224-230, 1999.

141. Clark WM, Raps EC, Tong DC, et al: Cervene (nalmefene) in acute ischemic stroke: Final results of a phase III efficacy study. The Cervene Stroke Study Investigators, *Stroke* 31(6):1234-1239, 2000.

142. Green AR, Hainsworth AH, Jackson DM: GABA potentiation: A logical pharmacological approach for the treatment of acute ischaemic stroke, *Neuropharmacology* 39(9):1483-1494, 2000.

143. Moody EJ, Skolnick P: Chlormethiazole: Neurochemical actions at the gamma-aminobutyric acid receptor complex, *Eur J Pharmacol* 164(1):153-158, 1989.

144. Cross AJ, Jones JA, Baldwin HA, et al: Neuroprotective activity of chlormethiazole following transient forebrain ischaemia in the gerbil, *Br J Pharmacol* 104(2):406-411, 1991.

145. Marshall JW, Cross AJ, Ridley RM: Functional benefit from clomethiazole treatment after focal cerebral ischemia in a nonhuman primate species, *Exp Neurol* 156(1):121-129, 1999.

146. Wester P, Strand T, Wahlgren NG, et al: An open study of clomethiazole in patients with acute cerebral infarction, *Cerebrovasc Dis* 8(3):188-190, 1998.

147. Wahlgren NG, Ranasinha KW, Rosolacci T, et al: Clomethiazole Acute Stroke Study (CLASS): Results of a randomized, controlled trial of clomethiazole versus placebo in 1360 acute stroke patients, *Stroke* 30(1):21-28, 1999.

148. Lyden P, Shuaib A, Ng K, et al: Clomethiazole Acute Stroke Study in ischemic stroke (CLASS-I): Final results, *Stroke* 33(1):122-128, 2002.

149. Lodder J, van Raak L, Hilton A, et al: Diazepam to improve acute stroke outcome: Results of the early GABA-ergic activation study in stroke trial. A randomized double-blind placebo-controlled trial, *Cerebrovasc Dis* 21(1-2):120-127, 2006.

150. Hall ED, Pazara KE, Braughler JM: 21-Aminosteroid lipid peroxidation inhibitor U74006F protects against cerebral ischemia in gerbils, *Stroke* 19(8):997-1002, 1988.

151. Zuccarello M, Marsch JT, Schmitt G, et al: Effect of the 21-aminosteroid U-74006F on cerebral vasospasm following subarachnoid hemorrhage, *J Neurosurg* 71(1):98-104, 1989.

152. Hall ED, Andrus PK, Smith SL, et al: Neuroprotective efficacy of microvascularly-localized versus brain-penetrating antioxidants, *Acta Neurochir Suppl* 66:107-113, 1996.

153. Safety study of tirilazad mesylate in patients with acute ischemic stroke (STIPAS), *Stroke* 25(2):418-423, 1994.

154. A randomized trial of tirilazad mesylate in patients with acute stroke (RANTTAS): The RANTTAS Investigators, *Stroke* 27(9):1453-1458, 1996.
155. Haley EC Jr: High-dose tirilazad for acute stroke (RANTTAS II). RANTTAS II Investigators, *Stroke* 29(6):1256-1257, 1998.
156. Tirilazad mesylate in acute ischemic stroke: A systematic review. Tirilazad International Steering Committee, *Stroke* 31(9): 2257-2265, 2000.
157. Beck T, Bielenberg GW: Failure of the lipid peroxidation inhibitor U74006F to improve neurological outcome after transient forebrain ischemia in the rat, *Brain Res* 532:336, 1990.
158. Ichikawa S, Omura K, Katayama T, et al: Inhibition of superoxide anion production in guinea pig polymorphonuclear leukocytes by a seleno-organic compound, ebselen, *J Pharmacobiodyn* 10(10):595-597, 1987.
159. Hattori R, Inoue R, Sase K, et al: Preferential inhibition of inducible nitric oxide synthase by ebselen, *Eur J Pharmacol* 267(2): R1-2, 1994.
160. Maiorino M, Roveri A, Coassin M, et al: Kinetic mechanism and substrate specificity of glutathione peroxidase activity of ebselen (PZ51), *Biochem Pharmacol* 37(11):2267-2271, 1988.
161. Takasago T, Peters EE, Graham DI, et al: Neuroprotective efficacy of ebselen, an anti-oxidant with anti-inflammatory actions, in a rodent model of permanent middle cerebral artery occlusion, *Br J Pharmacol* 122(6):1251-1256, 1997.
162. Yamaguchi T, Sano K, Takakura K, et al: Ebselen in acute ischemic stroke: A placebo-controlled, double-blind clinical trial. Ebselen Study Group, *Stroke* 29(1):12-17, 1998.
163. Watanabe T, Yuki S, Egawa M, et al: Protective effects of MCI-186 on cerebral ischemia: Possible involvement of free radical scavenging and antioxidant actions, *J Pharmacol Exp Ther* 268(3):1597-1604, 1994.
164. Yoshida H, Yanai H, Namiki Y, et al: Neuroprotective effects of edaravone: A novel free radical scavenger in cerebrovascular injury, *CNS Drug Rev* 12(1):9-20, 2006.
165. Zhang N, Komine-Kobayashi M, Tanaka R, et al: Edaravone reduces early accumulation of oxidative products and sequential inflammatory responses after transient focal ischemia in mice brain, *Stroke* 36(10):2220-2225, 2005.
166. Edaravone Acute Infarction Study Group: Effect of a novel free radical scavenger, edaravone (MCI-186), on acute brain infarction. Randomized, placebo-controlled, double-blind study at multicenters, *Cerebrovasc Dis* 15(3):222-229, 2003.
167. Safety and pharmacokinetics of MCI-186 in subjects with acute ischemic stroke: http://clinicaltrials.gov. Accessed August 1, 2009.
168. Zhao Z, Cheng M, Maples KR, et al: NXY-059, a novel free radical trapping compound, reduces cortical infarction after permanent focal cerebral ischemia in the rat, *Brain Res* 909:46, 2001.
169. Sydserff SG, Borelli AR, Green AR, et al: Effect of NXY-059 on infarct volume after transient or permanent middle cerebral artery occlusion in the rat; studies on dose, plasma concentration and therapeutic time window, *Br J Pharmacol* 135(1):103-112, 2002.
170. Kuroda S, Tsuchidate R, Smith ML, et al: Neuroprotective effects of a novel nitrone, NXY-059, after transient focal cerebral ischemia in the rat, *J Cereb Blood Flow Metab* 19(7):778-787, 1999.
171. Marshall JW, Duffin KJ, Green AR, et al: NXY-059, a free radical-trapping agent, substantially lessens the functional disability resulting from cerebral ischemia in a primate species, *Stroke* 32(1):190-198, 2001.
172. Lees KR, Zivin JA, Ashwood T, et al: NXY-059 for acute ischemic stroke, *N Engl J Med* 354(6):588-600, 2006.
173. Lees KR, Davalos A, Davis SM, et al: Additional outcomes and subgroup analyses of NXY-059 for acute ischemic stroke in the SAINT I trial, *Stroke* 37(12):2970-2978, 2006.
174. Diener HC, Lees KR, Lyden P, et al: NXY-059 for the treatment of acute stroke: pooled analysis of the SAINT I and II Trials, *Stroke* 39(6):1751-1758, 2008.
175. Savitz SI, Schabitz WR: A critique of SAINT II: Wishful thinking, dashed hopes, and the future of neuroprotection for acute stroke, *Stroke* 39(4):1389-1391, 2008.
176. Okada Y, Copeland BR, Mori E, et al: P-selectin and intercellular adhesion molecule-1 expression after focal brain ischemia and reperfusion, *Stroke* 25(1):202-211, 1994.

177. Zhang RL, Chopp M, Zaloga C, et al: The temporal profiles of ICAM-1 protein and mRNA expression after transient MCA occlusion in the rat, *Brain Res* 682:182, 1995.
178. Soriano SG, Coxon A, Wang YF, et al: Mice deficient in Mac-1 (CD11b/CD18) are less susceptible to cerebral ischemia/reperfusion injury, *Stroke* 30(1):134-139, 1999.
179. Kitagawa K, Matsumoto M, Mabuchi T, et al: Deficiency of intercellular adhesion molecule 1 attenuates microcirculatory disturbance and infarction size in focal cerebral ischemia, *J Cereb Blood Flow Metab* 18(12):1336-1345, 1998.
180. Clark WM, Madden KP, Rothlein R, et al: Reduction of central nervous system ischemic injury in rabbits using leukocyte adhesion antibody treatment, *Stroke* 22(7):877-883, 1991.
181. Zhang RL, Chopp M, Jiang N, et al: Anti-intercellular adhesion molecule-1 antibody reduces ischemic cell damage after transient but not permanent middle cerebral artery occlusion in the Wistar rat, *Stroke* 26(8):1438-1442, 1995:discussion 1443.
182. Enlimomab Acute Stroke Trial Investigators: Use of anti-CAM-1 therapy in ischemic stroke: Results of the Enlimomab Acute Stroke Trial. *Neurology* 57:1428-1434, 2001.
183. Zhang RL, Zhang ZG, Chopp M, et al: Thrombolysis with tissue plasminogen activator alters adhesion molecule expression in the ischemic rat brain, *Stroke* 30:624, 1999.
184. Fassbender K, Mossner R, Motsch L, et al: Circulating selectin- and immunoglobulin-type adhesion molecules in acute ischemic stroke, *Stroke* 26(8):1361-1364, 1995.
185. Bitsch A, Klene W, Murtada L, et al: A longitudinal prospective study of soluble adhesion molecules in acute stroke, *Stroke* 29:2129, 1998.
186. Frijns CJ, Kappelle LJ, van Gijn J, et al: Soluble adhesion molecules reflect endothelial cell activation in ischemic stroke and in carotid atherosclerosis, *Stroke* 28(11):2214-2218, 1997.
187. Lindsberg PJ, Carpen O, Paetau A, et al: Endothelial ICAM-1 expression associated with inflammatory cell response in human ischemic stroke, *Circulation* 94(5):939-945, 1996.
188. Use of anti-ICAM-1 therapy in ischemic stroke: Results of the Enlimomab Acute Stroke Trial, *Neurology* 57(8):1428-1434, 2001.
189. Schneider D, Berrouschot J, Brandt T, et al: Safety, pharmacokinetics and biological activity of enlimomab (anti-ICAM-1 antibody): An open-label, dose escalation study in patients hospitalized for acute stroke, *Eur Neurol* 40(2):78-83, 1998.
190. Furuya K, Takeda H, Azhar S, et al: Examination of several potential mechanisms for the negative outcome in a clinical stroke trial of enlimomab, a murine anti-human intercellular adhesion molecule-1 antibody: A bedside-to-bench study, *Stroke* 32(11): 2665-2674, 2001.
191. Veldhuis WB, Floris S, van der Meide PH, et al: Interferon-beta prevents cytokine-induced neutrophil infiltration and attenuates blood-brain barrier disruption, *J Cereb Blood Flow Metab* 23(9):1060-1069, 2003.
192. Yang CH, Murti A, Pfeffer SR, et al: Interferon alpha/beta promotes cell survival by activating nuclear factor kappa B through phosphatidylinositol 3-kinase and Akt, *J Biol Chem* 276(17): 13756-13761, 2001.
193. Veldhuis WB, Derksen JW, Floris S, et al: Interferon-beta blocks infiltration of inflammatory cells and reduces infarct volume after ischemic stroke in the rat, *J Cereb Blood Flow Metab* 23(9):1029-1039, 2003.
194. Liu H, Xin L, Chan BP, et al: Interferon-beta administration confers a beneficial outcome in a rabbit model of thromboembolic cerebral ischemia, *Neurosci Lett* 327(2):146-148, 2002.
195. Maier CM, Yu F, Nishi T, et al: Interferon-beta fails to protect in a model of transient focal ischemia, *Stroke* 37(4):1116-1119, 2006.
196. Jiang N, Chopp M, Chahwala S: Neutrophil inhibitory factor treatment of focal cerebral ischemia in the rat, *Brain Res* 788(1-2): 25-34, 1998.
197. Krams M, Lees KR, Hacke W, et al: Acute Stroke Therapy by Inhibition of Neutrophils (ASTIN): An adaptive dose-response study of UK-279,276 in acute ischemic stroke, *Stroke* 34(11):2543-2548, 2003.
198. Manabat C, Han BH, Wendland M, et al: Reperfusion differentially induces caspase-3 activation in ischemic core and penumbra after stroke in immature brain, *Stroke* 34(1):207-213, 2003.
199. Robertson GS, Crocker SJ, Nicholson DW, et al: Neuroprotection by the inhibition of apoptosis, *Brain Pathol* 10(2):283-292, 2000.

200. Satoh S, Ikegaki I, Suzuki Y, et al: Neuroprotective properties of a protein kinase inhibitor against ischaemia-induced neuronal damage in rats and gerbils, *Br J Pharmacol* 118(7):1592-1596, 1996.

201. Wang KK, Nath R, Posner A, et al: An alpha-mercaptoacrylic acid derivative is a selective nonpeptide cell-permeable calpain inhibitor and is neuroprotective, *Proc Natl Acad Sci U S A* 93(13):6687-6692, 1996.

202. Barone FC, Irving EA, Ray AM, et al: SB 239063, a second-generation p38 mitogen-activated protein kinase inhibitor, reduces brain injury and neurological deficits in cerebral focal ischemia, *J Pharmacol Exp Ther* 296:312, 2001.

203. Markgraf CG, Velayo NL, Johnson MP, et al: Six-hour window of opportunity for calpain inhibition in focal cerebral ischemia in rats, *Stroke* 29(1):152-158, 1998.

204. Yrjanheikki J, Keinanen R, Pellikka M, et al: Tetracyclines inhibit microglial activation and are neuroprotective in global brain ischemia, *Proc Natl Acad Sci U S A* 95:15769, 1998.

205. Yrjanheikki J, Tikka T, Keinanen R, et al: A tetracycline derivative, minocycline, reduces inflammation and protects against focal cerebral ischemia with a wide therapeutic window, *Proc Natl Acad Sci U S A* 96:13496, 1999.

206. Yenari MA, Xu L, Tang XN, et al: Microglia potentiate damage to blood-brain barrier constituents: Improvement by minocycline in vivo and in vitro, *Stroke* 37(4):1087-1093, 2006.

207. Wang CX, Yang T, Noor R, et al: Delayed minocycline but not delayed mild hypothermia protects against embolic stroke, *BMC Neurol* 2:2, 2002.

208. Nagel S, Su Y, Horstmann S, et al: Minocycline and hypothermia for reperfusion injury after focal cerebral ischemia in the rat: Effects on BBB breakdown and MMP expression in the acute and subacute phase, *Brain Res* 1188:198-206, 2008.

209. Murata Y, Rosell A, Scannevin RH, et al: Extension of the thrombolytic time window with minocycline in experimental stroke, *Stroke* 39(12):3372-3377, 2008.

210. Li J, McCullough LD: Sex differences in minocycline-induced neuroprotection after experimental stroke, *J Cereb Blood Flow Metab* 29(4):670-674, 2009.

211. Lampl Y, Boaz M, Gilad R, et al: Minocycline treatment in acute stroke: An open-label, evaluator-blinded study, *Neurology* 69(14):1404-1410, 2007.

212. Jonas S: Pilot study of treatment with intravenous enoxaparin and/or oral minocycline to limit infarct size after ischemic stroke: http://clinicaltrials.gov. Accessed August 1, 2009.

213. Fagan SC, Waller JL, Fenwick TN, et al: Minocycline to improve neurologic outcome in stroke (MINOS): A dose-finding study, *Stroke* 41:2283-2287, 2010.

214. Hess D: Between bench and bedside: challenges in the translation of high-impact targets into clinical trials: minocycline, San Diego, Calif, 2009, International Stroke Conference.

215. Asai A, Qiu J, Narita Y, et al: High level calcineurin activity predisposes neuronal cells to apoptosis, *J Biol Chem* 274:34450, 1999.

216. Herr I, Martin-Villalba A, Kurz E, et al: FK506 prevents stroke-induced generation of ceramide and apoptosis signaling, *Brain Res* 826(2):210-219, 1999.

217. Bochelen D, Rudin M, Sauter A: Calcineurin inhibitors FK506 and SDZ ASM 981 alleviate the outcome of focal cerebral ischemic/reperfusion injury, *J Pharmacol Exp Ther* 288(2):653-659, 1999.

218. Ebisu T, Katsuta K, Fujikawa A, et al: Early and delayed neuroprotective effects of FK506 on experimental focal ischemia quantitatively assessed by diffusion-weighted MRI, *Magn Reson Imaging* 19(2):153-160, 2001.

219. Arii T, Kamiya T, Arii K, et al: Neuroprotective effect of immunosuppressant FK506 in transient focal ischemia in rat: Therapeutic time window for FK506 in transient focal ischemia, *Neurol Res* 23(7):755-760, 2001.

220. Takamatsu H, Tsukada H, Noda A, et al: FK506 attenuates early ischemic neuronal death in a monkey model of stroke, *J Nucl Med* 42(12):1833-1840, 2001.

221. Limbourg FP, Huang Z, Plumier JC, et al: Rapid nontranscriptional activation of endothelial nitric oxide synthase mediates increased cerebral blood flow and stroke protection by corticosteroids, *J Clin Invest* 110(11):1729-1738, 2002.

222. Mulley G, Wilcox RG, Mitchell JR: Dexamethasone in acute stroke, *Br Med J* 2(6143):994-996, 1978.

223. Norris JW, Hachinski VC: High dose steroid treatment in cerebral infarction, *Br Med J (Clin Res Ed)* 292(6512):21-23, 1986.

224. Qizilbash N, Lewington SL, Lopez-Arrieta JM: Corticosteroids for acute ischaemic stroke, *Cochrane Database Syst Rev* 2:CD000064, 2000.

225. Vayssiere BM, Dupont S, Choquart A, et al: Synthetic glucocorticoids that dissociate transactivation and AP-1 transrepression exhibit antiinflammatory activity in vivo, *Mol Endocrinol* 11(9):1245-1255, 1997.

226. Amin-Hanjani S, Stagliano NE, Yamada M, et al: Mevastatin, an HMG-CoA reductase inhibitor, reduces stroke damage and upregulates endothelial nitric oxide synthase in mice, *Stroke* 32(4):980-986, 2001.

227. Laufs U, Gertz K, Dirnagl U, et al: Rosuvastatin, a new HMG-CoA reductase inhibitor, upregulates endothelial nitric oxide synthase and protects from ischemic stroke in mice, *Brain Res* 942(1-2):23-30, 2002.

228. Sironi L, Cimino M, Guerrini U, et al: Treatment with statins after induction of focal ischemia in rats reduces the extent of brain damage, *Arterioscler Thromb Vasc Biol* 23(2):322-327, 2003.

229. Balduini W, De Angelis V, Mazzoni E, et al: Simvastatin protects against long-lasting behavioral and morphological consequences of neonatal hypoxic/ischemic brain injury, *Stroke* 32(9):2185-2191, 2001.

230. Blauw GJ, Lagaay AM, Smelt AHM, et al: Stroke, statins, and cholesterol: A meta-analysis of randomized, placebo-controlled, double-blind trials with HMG-CoA reductase inhibitors, *Stroke* 28:946, 1997.

231. Elkind MS, Sacco RL, MacArthur RB, et al: The Neuroprotection with Statin Therapy for Acute Recovery Trial (NeuSTART): An adaptive design phase I dose-escalation study of high-dose lovastatin in acute ischemic stroke, *Int J Stroke* 3(3):210-218, 2008.

232. Belayev L, Liu Y, Zhao W, et al: Human albumin therapy of acute ischemic stroke: Marked neuroprotective efficacy at moderate doses and with a broad therapeutic window, *Stroke* 32(2):553-560, 2001.

233. Zoellner H, Hofler M, Beckmann R, et al: Serum albumin is a specific inhibitor of apoptosis in human endothelial cells, *J Cell Sci* 109(Pt 10):2571-2580, 1996.

234. Rodriguez de Turco EB, Belayev L, Liu Y, et al: Systemic fatty acid responses to transient focal cerebral ischemia: Influence of neuroprotectant therapy with human albumin, *J Neurochem* 83(3):515-524, 2002.

235. Ginsberg MD, Hill MD, Palesch YY, et al: The ALIAS Pilot Trial: A dose-escalation and safety study of albumin therapy for acute ischemic stroke—I: Physiological responses and safety results, *Stroke* 37(8):2100-2106, 2006.

236. Bishop-Bailey D: Peroxisome proliferator-activated receptors in the cardiovascular system, *Br J Pharmacol* 129(5):823-834, 2000.

237. Blanquart C, Barbier O, Fruchart JC, et al: Peroxisome proliferator-activated receptors: Regulation of transcriptional activities and roles in inflammation, *J Steroid Biochem Mol Biol* 85(2-5):267-273, 2003.

238. Ailhaud G: Cell surface receptors, nuclear receptors and ligands that regulate adipose tissue development, *Clin Chim Acta* 286(1-2):181-190, 1999.

239. Duez H, Fruchart JC, Staels B: PPARs in inflammation, atherosclerosis and thrombosis, *J Cardiovasc Risk* 8(4):187-194, 2001.

240. Francis GA, Annicotte JS, Auwerx J: PPAR agonists in the treatment of atherosclerosis, *Curr Opin Pharmacol* 3(2):186-191, 2003.

241. Sundararajan S, Gamboa JL, Victor NA, et al: Peroxisome proliferator-activated receptor-gamma ligands reduce inflammation and infarction size in transient focal ischemia, *Neuroscience* 130(3):685-696, 2005.

242. Hwang J, Kleinhenz DJ, Lassegue B, et al: Peroxisome proliferator-activated receptor-gamma ligands regulate endothelial membrane superoxide production, *Am J Physiol Cell Physiol* 288(4):C899-905, 2005.

243. Chung SW, Kang BY, Kim SH, et al: Oxidized low density lipoprotein inhibits interleukin-12 production in lipopolysaccharide-activated mouse macrophages via direct interactions between peroxisome proliferator-activated receptor-gamma and nuclear factor-kappa B, *J Biol Chem* 275(42):32681-32687, 2000.

244. Zhao X, Zhang Y, Strong R, et al: 15d-Prostaglandin J2 activates peroxisome proliferator-activated receptor-gamma, promotes expression of catalase, and reduces inflammation, behavioral dysfunction, and neuronal loss after intracerebral hemorrhage in rats, *J Cereb Blood Flow Metab* 26(6):811–820, 2006.

245. Shimazu T, Inoue I, Araki N, et al: A peroxisome proliferator-activated receptor-gamma agonist reduces infarct size in transient but not in permanent ischemia, *Stroke* 36(2):353–359, 2005.

246. Giannini S, Serio M, Galli A: Pleiotropic effects of thiazolidinediones: Taking a look beyond antidiabetic activity, *J Endocrinol Invest* 27(10):982–991, 2004.

247. Vemuganti R: Therapeutic potential of PPAR gamma activation in stroke, *PPAR Res* 2008:1–9, 2008.

248. Simard JM, Chen M, Tarasov KV, et al: Newly expressed SUR1-regulated NC(Ca-ATP) channel mediates cerebral edema after ischemic stroke, *Nat Med* 12(4):433–440, 2006.

249. Simard JM, Yurovsky V, Tsymbalyuk N, et al: Protective effect of delayed treatment with low-dose glibenclamide in three models of ischemic stroke, *Stroke* 40(2):604–609, 2009.

250. Kunte H, Schmidt S, Eliasziw M, et al: Sulfonylureas improve outcome in patients with type 2 diabetes and acute ischemic stroke, *Stroke* 38(9):2526–2530, 2007.

251. Simard JM, Woo SK, Bhatta S, et al: Drugs acting on SUR1 to treat CNS ischemia and trauma, *Curr Opin Pharmacol* 8(1):42–49, 2008.

252. Simard JM: Between bench and bedside: Challenges in the translation of high-impact targets into clinical trials: NS-Ca-ATP channels, San Diego, Calif, 2009, International Stroke Conference.

253. Lenzi GL, Grigoletto F, Gent M, et al: Early treatment of stroke with monosialoganglioside GM-1. Efficacy and safety results of the Early Stroke Trial, *Stroke* 25(8):1552–1558, 1994.

254. Candelise L, Ciccone A: Gangliosides for acute ischaemic stroke, *Cochrane Database Syst Rev* 4:CD000094, 2001.

255. Schwab M, Antonow-Schlorke I, Zwiener U, et al: Brain-derived peptides reduce the size of cerebral infarction and loss of MAP2 immunoreactivity after focal ischemia in rats, *J Neural Transm Suppl* 53:299–311, 1998.

256. Ladurner F: Neuroprotection in acute ischaemic stroke [abstract], *Stroke* 32:323, 2001.

257. Rao AM, Hatcher JF, Dempsey RJ: CDP-choline: Neuroprotection in transient forebrain ischemia of gerbils, *J Neurosci Res* 58:697, 1999.

258. Adibhatla RM, Hatcher JF, Dempsey RJ: Citicoline: Neuroprotective mechanisms in cerebral ischemia, *J Neurochem* 80:12, 2002.

259. Krupinski J, Ferrer I, Barrachina M, et al: CDP-choline reduces pro-caspase and cleaved caspase-3 expression, nuclear DNA fragmentation, and specific PARP-cleaved products of caspase activation following middle cerebral artery occlusion in the rat, *Neuropharmacology* 42(6):846–854, 2002.

260. Galletti P, De Rosa M, Cotticelli MG, et al: Biochemical rationale for the use of CDPcholine in traumatic brain injury: Pharmacokinetics of the orally administered drug, *J Neurol Sci* (103 Suppl):S19–25, 1991.

261. Clark WM, Warach SJ, Pettigrew LC, et al: A randomized dose-response trial of citicoline in acute ischemic stroke patients. Citicoline Stroke Study Group, *Neurology* 49(3):671–678, 1997.

262. Clark WM, Williams BJ, Selzer KA, et al: A randomized efficacy trial of citicoline in patients with acute ischemic stroke, *Stroke* 30(12):2592–2597, 1999.

263. Clark WM, Wechsler LR, Sabounjian LA, et al: A phase III randomized efficacy trial of 2000 mg citicoline in acute ischemic stroke patients, *Neurology* 57(9):1595–1602, 2001.

264. Corso EA, Arena M, Ventimiglia A, et al: [CDP choline in cerebral vasculopathy: Clinical evaluation and instrumental semeiology], *Clin Ter* 102(4):379–386, 1982.

265. Tazaki Y, Sakai F, Otomo E, et al: Treatment of acute cerebral infarction with a choline precursor in a multicenter double-blind placebo-controlled study, *Stroke* 19(2):211–216, 1988.

266. Saver J, Wilterdink J: Choline precursors in acute and subacute stroke: A meta-analysis, *Stroke* 32:1598, 2002.

267. Andersen M, Overgaard K, Meden P, et al: Effects of citicoline combined with thrombolytic therapy in a rat embolic stroke model, *Stroke* 30:1464, 1999.

268. Toung TJ, Traystman RJ, Hurn PD: Estrogen-mediated neuroprotection after experimental stroke in male rats, *Stroke* 29(8):1666–1670, 1998.

269. Simpkins JW, Rajakumar G, Zhang YQ, et al: Estrogens may reduce mortality and ischemic damage caused by middle cerebral artery occlusion in the female rat, *J Neurosurg* 87(5):724–730, 1997.

270. Dubal DB, Shughrue PJ, Wilson ME, et al: Estradiol modulates bcl-2 in cerebral ischemia: A potential role for estrogen receptors, *J Neurosci* 19(15):6385–6393, 1999.

271. Green PS, Simpkins JW: Neuroprotective effects of estrogens: Potential mechanisms of action, *Int J Dev Neurosci* 8:347, 2000.

272. Paganini-Hill A, Ross RK, Henderson BE: Postmenopausal oestrogen treatment and stroke: a prospective study, *BMJ* 297(6647):519–522, 1988.

273. Gail MH, Costantino JP, Bryant J, et al: Weighing the risks and benefits of tamoxifen treatment for preventing breast cancer, *J Natl Cancer Inst* 91(21):1829–1846, 1999.

274. Pardridge WM: Drug delivery to the brain, *J Cereb Blood Flow Metab* 17(7):713–731, 1997.

275. Siren AL, Ehrenreich H: Erythropoietin—a novel concept for neuroprotection, *Eur Arch Psychiatry Clin Neurosci* 251(4):179–184, 2001.

276. Sakanaka M, Wen TC, Matsuda S, et al: In vivo evidence that erythropoietin protects neurons from ischemic damage, *Proc Natl Acad Sci U S A* 95(8):4635–4640, 1998.

277. Morishita E, Masuda S, Nagao M, et al: Erythropoietin receptor is expressed in rat hippocampal and cerebral cortical neurons, and erythropoietin prevents in vitro glutamate-induced neuronal death, *Neuroscience* 76(1):105–116, 1997.

278. Brines ML, Ghezzi P, Keenan S, et al: Erythropoietin crosses the blood-brain barrier to protect against experimental brain injury, *Proc Natl Acad Sci U S A* 97:10526, 2000.

279. Siren AL, Fratelli M, Brines M, et al: Erythropoietin prevents neuronal apoptosis after cerebral ischemia and metabolic stress, *Proc Natl Acad Sci U S A* 98(7):4044–4049, 2001.

280. Ehrenreich H, Hasselblatt M, Dembowski C, et al: Erythropoietin therapy for acute stroke is both safe and beneficial, *Mol Med* 8(8):495–505, 2002.

281. Safety and pharmacokinetic study of carbamylated erythropoietin (CEPO) to treat patients with acute ischemic stroke: http://www.clinicaltrials.gov. Accessed August 2009.

282. Ay I, Sugimori H, Finklestein SP: Intravenous basic fibroblast growth factor (bFGF) decreases DNA fragmentation and prevents downregulation of Bcl-2 expression in the ischemic brain following middle cerebral artery occlusion in rats, *Brain Res Mol Brain Res* 87(1):71–80, 2001.

283. Kawamata T, Dietrich WD, Schallert T, et al: Intracisternal basic fibroblast growth factor enhances functional recovery and upregulates the expression of a molecular marker of neuronal sprouting following focal cerebral infarction, *Proc Natl Acad Sci U S A* 94(15):8179–8184, 1997.

284. Li Q, Stephenson D: Postischemic administration of basic fibroblast growth factor improves sensorimotor function and reduces infarct size following permanent focal cerebral ischemia in the rat, *Exp Neurol* 177:531, 2002.

285. Schabitz WR, Li F, Irie K, et al: Synergistic effects of a combination of low-dose basic fibroblast growth factor and citicoline after temporary experimental focal ischemia, *Stroke* 30(2):427–431, 1999:discussion 431–422.

286. Ma J, Qiu J, Hirt L, et al: Synergistic protective effect of caspase inhibitors and bFGF against brain injury induced by transient focal ischaemia, *Br J Pharmacol* 133(3):345–350, 2001.

287. Bogousslavsky J, Victor SJ, Salinas EO, et al: Fiblast (trafermin) in acute stroke: Results of the European-Australian phase II/III safety and efficacy trial, *Cerebrovasc Dis* 14(3-4):239–251, 2002.

288. Song BW, Vinters HV, Wu D, et al: Enhanced neuroprotective effects of basic fibroblast growth factor in regional brain ischemia after conjugation to a blood-brain barrier delivery vector, *J Pharmacol Exp Ther* 301(2):605–610, 2002.

289. Krupinski J, Issa R, Bujny T, et al: A putative role for platelet-derived growth factor in angiogenesis and neuroprotection after ischemic stroke in humans, *Stroke* 28(3):564–573, 1997.

290. Semkova I, Krieglstein J: Neuroprotection mediated via neurotrophic factors and induction of neurotrophic factors, *Brain Res Brain Res Rev* 30(2):176–188, 1999.

291. Wang Y, Chang CF, Morales M, et al: Protective effects of glial cell line-derived neurotrophic factor in ischemic brain injury, *Ann N Y Acad Sci* 962:423-437, 2002.

292. Schabitz W: Between bench and bedside: Challenges in the translation of high-impact targets into clinical trials: G-CSF, San Diego, Calif, 2009, International Stroke Conference.

293. AXIS 2: AX200 for the Treatment of Ischemic Stroke (AXIS-2): http://www.clinicaltrials.gov. Accessed July 5, 2009.

294. Kilic E, Dietz GP, Hermann DM, et al: Intravenous TAT-Bcl-Xl is protective after middle cerebral artery occlusion in mice, *Ann Neurol* 52(5):617-622, 2002.

295. Busto R, Dietrich WD, Globus MYT, et al: Small differences in intraischemic brain temperature critically determine the extent of ischemic neuronal injury, *J Cereb Blood Flow Metab* 7:729, 1987.

296. Buchan A, Pulsinelli WA: Hypothermia but not N-methyl-D-aspartate antagonist MK-801 attenuates neuronal damage in gerbils subjected to transient global ischemia, *J Neurosci* 10:311, 1990.

297. Minamisawa H, Nordstrom CH, Smith ML, et al: The influence of mild body and brain hypothermia on ischemic brain damage, *J Cereb Blood Flow Metab* 10(3):365-374, 1990.

298. Coimbra C, Wieloch T: Hypothermia ameliorates neuronal survival when induced 2 hours after ischaemia in the rat, *Acta Physiol Scand* 146(4):543-544, 1992.

299. Meden P, Overgaard K, Pedersen H, et al: The influence of body temperature on infarct volume and thrombolytic therapy in a rat embolic stroke model, *Brain Res* 647(1):131-138, 1994.

300. Corbett D, Nurse S, Colbourne F: Hypothermic neuroprotection. A global ischemia study using 18- to 20-month-old gerbils, *Stroke* 28(11):2238-2242, 1997:discussion 2243.

301. Barone FC, Feuerstein GZ, White RF: Brain cooling during transient focal ischemia provides complete neuroprotection, *Neurosci Biobehav Rev* 21:31, 1997.

302. Maier CM, Ahern K, Cheng ML, et al: Optimal depth and duration of mild hypothermia in a focal model of transient cerebral ischemia: Effects on neurologic outcome, infarct size, apoptosis, and inflammation, *Stroke* 29(10):2171-2180, 1998.

303. Corbett D, Hamilton M, Colbourne F: Persistent neuroprotection with prolonged postischemic hypothermia in adult rats subjected to transient middle cerebral artery occlusion, *Exp Neurol* 163(1):200-206, 2000.

304. Kawai N, Okauchi M, Morisaki K, et al: Effects of delayed intraischemic and postischemic hypothermia on a focal model of transient cerebral ischemia in rats, *Stroke* 31(8):1982-1989, 2000:discussion 1989.

305. Nakashima K, Todd MM: Effects of hypothermia on the rate of excitatory amino acid release after ischemic depolarization, *Stroke* 27(5):913-918, 1996.

306. Koizumi H, Fujisawa H, Ito H, et al: Effects of mild hypothermia on cerebral blood flow—independent changes in cortical extracellular levels of amino acids following contusion trauma in the rat, *Brain Res* 747(2):304-312, 1997.

307. Sick TJ, Xu G, Perez-Pinzon MA: Mild hypothermia improves recovery of cortical extracellular potassium ion activity and excitability after middle cerebral artery occlusion in the rat, *Stroke* 30(11):2416-2421, 1999:discussion 2422.

308. Babu PP, Yoshida Y, Su M, et al: Immunohistochemical expression of Bcl-2, Bax and cytochrome c following focal cerebral ischemia and effect of hypothermia in rat, *Neurosci Lett* 291:196, 2000.

309. Ishikawa M, Sekizuka E, Sato S, et al: Effects of moderate hypothermia on leukocyte-endothelium interaction in the rat pial microvasculature after transient middle cerebral artery occlusion, *Stroke* 30(8):1679-1686, 1999.

310. Inamasu J, Suga S, Sato S, et al: Post-ischemic hypothermia delayed neutrophil accumulation and microglial activation following transient focal cerebral ischemia in rats, *J Neuroimmunol* 109:66, 2000.

311. Zeiner A, Holzer M, Sterz F, et al: Mild resuscitative hypothermia to improve neurological outcome after cardiac arrest. A clinical feasibility trial. Hypothermia After Cardiac Arrest (HACA) Study Group, *Stroke* 31(1):86-94, 2000.

312. Felberg RA, Krieger DW, Chuang R, et al: Hypothermia after cardiac arrest: Feasibility and safety of an external cooling protocol, *Circulation* 104(15):1799-1804, 2001.

313. Abou-Chebl A, DeGeorgia MA, Andrefsky JC, et al: Technical refinements and drawbacks of a surface cooling technique for the treatment of severe acute ischemic stroke, *Neurocrit Care* 1(2):131-143, 2004.

314. Krieger DW, De Georgia MA, Abou-Chebl A, et al: Cooling for Acute Ischemic Brain Damage (COOL AID): an open pilot study of induced hypothermia in acute ischemic stroke, *Stroke* 32(8):1847-1854, 2001.

315. Hemmen TM, Lyden PD: Induced hypothermia for acute stroke, *Stroke* 38(Suppl 2):794-799, 2007.

316. Schwab S, Schwarz S, Spranger M, et al: Moderate hypothermia in the treatment of patients with severe middle cerebral artery infarction, *Stroke* 29(12):2461-2466, 1998.

317. Kammersgaard LP, Rasmussen BH, Jorgensen HS, et al: Feasibility and safety of inducing modest hypothermia in awake patients with acute stroke through surface cooling: A case-control study: The Copenhagen Stroke Study, *Stroke* 31(9):2251-2256, 2000.

318. Schwab S, Georgiadis D, Berrouschot J, et al: Feasibility and safety of moderate hypothermia after massive hemispheric infarction, *Stroke* 32(9):2033-2035, 2001.

319. Steiner T, Friede T, Aschoff A, et al: Effect and feasibility of controlled rewarming after moderate hypothermia in stroke patients with malignant infarction of the middle cerebral artery, *Stroke* 32(12):2833-2835, 2001.

320. Georgiadis D, Schwarz S, Kollmar R, et al: Endovascular cooling for moderate hypothermia in patients with acute stroke: First results of a novel approach, *Stroke* 32(11):2550-2553, 2001.

321. Krieger DW, Yenari MA: Therapeutic hypothermia for acute ischemic stroke: What do laboratory studies teach us? *Stroke* 35(6):1482-1489, 2004.

322. Ehrlich MP, McCullough JN, Zhang N, et al: Effect of hypothermia on cerebral blood flow and metabolism in the pig, *Ann Thorac Surg* 73(1):191-197, 2002.

323. Zhang RL, Chopp M, Chen H, et al: Postischemic (1 hour) hypothermia significantly reduces ischemic cell damage in rats subjected to 2 hours of middle cerebral artery occlusion, *Stroke* 24(8):1235-1240, 1993.

324. De Georgia MA, Krieger DW, Abou-Chebl A, et al: Cooling for Acute Ischemic Brain Damage (COOL AID): A feasibility trial of endovascular cooling, *Neurology* 63(2):312-317, 2004.

325. Strong R, Grotta JC, Aronowski J: Combination of low dose ethanol and caffeine protects brain from damage produced by focal ischemia in rats, *Neuropharmacology* 39(3):515-522, 2000.

326. Belayev L, Khoutorova L, Zhang Y, et al: Caffeinol confers cortical but not subcortical neuroprotection after transient focal cerebral ischemia in rats, *Brain Res* 1008(2):278-283, 2004.

327. Lapchak PA, Song D, Wei J, et al: Pharmacology of caffeinol in embolized rabbits: Clinical rating scores and intracerebral hemorrhage incidence, *Exp Neurol* 188(2):286-291, 2004.

328. Aronowski J, Strong R, Shirzadi A, et al: Ethanol plus caffeine (caffeinol) for treatment of ischemic stroke: Preclinical experience, *Stroke* 34(5):1246-1251, 2003.

329. Piriyawat P, Labiche LA, Burgin WS, et al: Pilot dose-escalation study of caffeine plus ethanol (caffeinol) in acute ischemic stroke, *Stroke* 34(5):1242-1245, 2003.

330. Martin-Schild S, Hallevi H, Shaltoni H, et al: Combined neuroprotective modalities coupled with thrombolysis in acute ischemic stroke: A pilot study of caffeinol and mild hypothermia, *J Stroke Cerebrovasc Dis* 18(2):86-96, 2009.

331. Bowes M, Burhop K, Zivin JA: Diaspirin cross-linked hemoglobin improves neurological outcome following reversible but not irreversible CNS ischemia in rabbits, *Stroke* 25:2253, 1994.

332. Cole DJ, Schell RM, Przybelski RJ, et al: Focal cerebral ischemia in rats: Effect of hemodilution with alpha-alpha cross-linked hemoglobin on CBF, *J Cereb Blood Flow Metab* 12(6):971-976, 1992.

333. Cole DJ, Schell RM, Drummond JC, et al: Focal cerebral ischemia in rats. Effect of hypervolemic hemodilution with diaspirin cross-linked hemoglobin versus albumin on brain injury and edema, *Anesthesiology* 78(2):335-342, 1993.

334. Grotta J, Aronowski J: DCLHb for focal ischemia and reperfusion, *Cerebrovasc Dis* 6:189, 1996.

335. Saxena R, Wijnhoud AD, Carton H, et al: Controlled safety study of a hemoglobin-based oxygen carrier, DCLHb, in acute ischemic stroke, *Stroke* 30(5):993-996, 1999.

336. Singhal AB, Dijkhuizen RM, Rosen BR, et al: Normobaric hyperoxia reduces MRI diffusion abnormalities and infarct size in experimental stroke, *Neurology* 58(6):945-952, 2002.
337. Atochin DN, Fisher D, Demchenko IT, et al: Neutrophil sequestration and the effect of hyperbaric oxygen in a rat model of temporary middle cerebral artery occlusion, *Undersea Hyperb Med* 27:185, 2000.
338. Badr AE, Yin W, Mychaskiw G, et al: Effect of hyperbaric oxygen on striatal metabolites: A microdialysis study in awake freely moving rats after MCA occlusion, *Brain Res* 916:85, 2001.
339. Burt J, Kapp JP, Smith RR: Hyperbaric oxygen and cerebral infarction in the gerbil, *Surg Neurol* 28:265, 1987.
340. Weinstein PR, Anderson GG, Telles DA: Results of hyperbaric oxygen therapy during temporary middle cerebral artery occlusion in unanesthetized cats, *Neurosurgery* 20(4):518-524, 1987.
341. Veltkamp R, Warner DS, Domoki F, et al: Hyperbaric oxygen decreases infarct size and behavioral deficit after transient focal cerebral ischemia in rats, *Brain Res* 853(1):68-73, 2000.
342. Chang C, Niu KC, Hoffer BJ, et al: Hyperbaric oxygen therapy for treatment of postischemic stroke in adult rats, *Exp Neurol* 166:298, 2000.
343. Sunami K, Takeda Y, Hashimoto M, et al: Hyperbaric oxygen reduces infarct volume in rats by increasing oxygen supply to the ischemic periphery, *Crit Care Med* 28(8):2831-2836, 2000.
344. Jacobson I, Lawson DD: The effect of hyperbaric oxygen on experimental cerebral infarction in the dog: With preliminary correlations of cerebral blood flow at 2 atmospheres of oxygen, *J Neurosurg* 20:849-859, 1963.
345. Roos JA, Jackson-Friedman C, Lyden P: Effects of hyperbaric oxygen on neurologic outcome for cerebral ischemia in rats, *Acad Emerg Med* 5(1):18-24, 1998.
346. Hjelde A, Hjelstuen M, Haraldseth O, et al: Hyperbaric oxygen and neutrophil accumulation/tissue damage during permanent focal cerebral ischaemia in rats, *Eur J Appl Physiol* 86(5):401-405, 2002.
347. Anderson DC, Bottini AG, Jagiella WM, et al: A pilot study of hyperbaric oxygen in the treatment of human stroke, *Stroke* 22:1137, 1991.
348. Nighoghossian N, Trouillas P, Adeleine P, et al: Hyperbaric oxygen in the treatment of acute ischemic stroke. A double-blind pilot study, *Stroke* 26(8):1369-1372, 1995.

54

Treatment of "Other" Stroke Etiologies

SCOTT E. KASNER, BRETT L. CUCCHIARA

The relatively uncommon or "other determined causes" of stroke often require therapeutic approaches that are distinct from the strategies employed for the more typical atherothromboembolic, cardioembolic, and small vessel occlusive strokes. These unusual stroke etiologies are myriad but can be broadly classified as vascular, hematologic, and miscellaneous diseases (Tables 54-1 through 54-3). The clinical manifestations, pathophysiology, and diagnostic considerations for these disorders are discussed elsewhere in this text, while this chapter will address the unique issues of treatment of those disorders for which specific therapies have been proposed. Because of the relative rarity of these stroke etiologies, most of the putative treatments have not been subjected to randomized clinical trials and are supported by limited data from observational or descriptive studies.

Vascular Disorders

The extracranial and intracranial arteries are susceptible to a diverse set of nonatherosclerotic disorders that may cause stroke (see Table 54-1). In young stroke victims, these nonatherosclerotic vasculopathies are particularly overrepresented, accounting for approximately 20% to 30% of strokes.[1-6] These disorders can be further classified as inflammatory and noninflammatory.

Noninflammatory Vasculopathies

Arterial Dissection

Dissection of the internal carotid artery and vertebral artery may occur as a result of significant head and neck trauma but may also occur spontaneously or after a trivial injury. A number of underlying connective tissue disorders appear to be risk factors for spontaneous dissection, including fibromuscular dysplasia (FMD), Marfan's syndrome, Ehlers-Danlos syndrome (type IV), osteogenesis imperfecta, and other genetic conditions in which collagen is abnormally formed.[7-11] At present, none of these underlying conditions are amenable to treatment.

Ischemic stroke may result from either extracranial or intracranial dissection. However, intracranial dissection may also produce subarachnoid hemorrhage and will be discussed separately later in this chapter. The clinical manifestations of extracranial carotid and vertebral artery dissection are distinct, but their treatment appears to be identical.

In the first 3 hours after the onset of acute ischemic stroke, thrombolytic therapy must be considered,[12] regardless of whether dissection is suggested by the patient's history or examination. Intravenous tissue plasminogen activator (t-PA) is contraindicated in patients with a known history of recent major systemic trauma, but spontaneous dissection is not easily diagnosed during the critical time window. There is a theoretical risk of causing increased hemorrhage into the vessel wall.[13] However, there have been no reports to substantiate the theoretical risk. To the contrary, two case series, involving 11 and 33 patients, respectively, found no dissection-specific complications related to intravenous t-PA and demonstrated outcomes with t-PA comparable to patients with more typical stroke causes.[14,15] In the time window between 4.5 and 8 hours after symptom onset, intravenous t-PA is no longer a viable option, but intraarterial thrombolysis is a potential treatment[16] that has been used successfully for stroke due to dissection.[17-21] In these cases, the catheter tip is placed in the distal thrombus beyond the site of the dissection, thus minimizing the exposure of the torn intima to the thrombolytic agent. Emergent endovascular therapy using angioplasty and stenting with or without thrombolysis has also been reported in cases with high-risk large vessel occlusions or demonstrable penumbral tissue defined by diffusion/perfusion magnetic resonance imaging (MRI) and fluctuating or progressive symptoms despite anticoagulation.[22-25]

The optimal strategy for prevention of stroke in patients with arterial dissection is controversial. Options include anticoagulation, antiplatelet therapy, angioplasty with or without stenting, surgery, or conservative observation without specific medical or surgical therapy. As stroke related to dissection may be a result of thromboembolism or hemodynamic compromise, treatment should be directed at the mechanism by which the dissection caused the stroke. Thromboembolism seems to be the dominant mechanism,[26] and microembolic signals are detectable with transcranial Doppler (TCD) monitoring in about half of patients.[27] Historically, early anticoagulation with heparin or low-molecular-weight heparin has been widely recommended at the time of diagnosis,[28-31] particularly because the risk of stroke appears to be greatest in the first few days after the initial vascular injury.[32-34] As with thrombolysis, it has been proposed that immediate anticoagulation of an acute dissection could cause

TABLE 54-1   UNUSUAL VASCULOPATHIES

Noninflammatory vasculopathies
Dissection
Fibromuscular dysplasia
Vasospasm after subarachnoid hemorrhage
Reversible cerebral vasoconstriction syndromes
Radiation-induced vasculopathy
Moyamoya disease
Hereditary disorders
  Homocystinuria, Fabry disease, CADASIL

Inflammatory vasculopathies
Isolated angiitis of the central nervous system
Temporal (giant cell) arteritis
Collagen vascular diseases
  Polyarteritis nodosa, Churg-Strauss angiitis, systemic lupus
  erythematosus, Wegener's granulomatosis, Henoch-
  Schönlein purpura, rheumatoid arthritis, cryoglobulinemia,
  Takayasu disease
Infectious arteriopathy
  Syphilis, tuberculosis, bacterial and fungal infections,
  varicella-zoster virus, human immunodeficiency virus
Toxin-related arteriopathy
  Amphetamines, cocaine, phenylpropanolamine, LSD, heroin
Neoplasm-related arteriopathy

CADASIL, cerebral autosomal dominant arteriopathy with subcortical infarcts and leukoencephalopathy; LSD, lysergic acid diethylamide.

TABLE 54-2   HEMATOLOGIC CAUSES OF STROKE

Disorders of coagulation
Hereditary disorders
  Factor V Leiden mutation, prothrombin G20210A mutation,
  protein C deficiency, protein S deficiency, antithrombin III
  deficiency, other factor deficiencies
Acquired disorders
  Disseminated intravascular coagulation
  Antiphospholipid antibody syndrome
  Factor excess, deficiency, or dysfunction
    Dysfibrinogenemia, nephrotic syndrome, liver disease,
    pregnancy, paroxysmal nocturnal hemoglobinuria,
    iatrogenic causes

Red cell disorders
Hemoglobinopathies
  Sickle cell disease, hemoglobin SC disease
Polycythemia rubra vera

Platelet disorders
Essential thrombocytosis
Sticky platelet syndrome

TABLE 54-3   MISCELLANEOUS UNUSUAL CAUSES OF STROKE

Migraine-related stroke
Mitochondrial encephalopathy, lactic acidosis, and strokelike
  episodes (MELAS)
Atypical embolism
  Fat embolism, tumor embolism, air embolism, cholesterol
  embolism
Cerebral venous thrombosis

artery dissection in 34 case series similarly showed no difference in subsequent stroke risk (1.9% antiplatelet versus 2.0% anticoagulant) or death.[36] However, these pooled analyses included both retrospective and prospective studies, most involving fewer than 20 patients. Such studies are highly prone to publication bias because small groups of patients with dissection who fare well without subsequent events are unlikely to be reported. Therefore, the pooled analyses may overestimate the risk of recurrent stroke. In a retrospective cohort of 432 patients from 24 centers with carotid or vertebral dissection, the 1-year incidence of subsequent stroke was only 0.3%.[37] In a prospective cohort study of 298 patients from two centers with carotid dissections followed up for 3 months, only one patient had a stroke (on day 3 of anticoagulation), which yielded a 3-month incidence of only 0.3% (95% confidence interval [CI], 0%–1.9%), and the incidence of major bleeding with anticoagulation was 2%.[38] The risk of stroke in these two cohort studies was lower than in the pooled analyses, which supports the idea of publication bias in that meta-analysis; however, the data from both cohort studies are also limited given their nonrandomized nature. If the low risk is confirmed in future studies, then it would seem unlikely that aggressive treatment with anticoagulation would be beneficial. At the present time, antithrombotic therapy with either antiplatelet or anticoagulant therapy is reasonable.

Dissections usually heal over time, and patients are commonly given antithrombotic therapy for at least 3 months. The 3-month duration of therapy is arbitrary, and some authors suggest that imaging studies be repeated to confirm recanalization of the dissected vessel before a change in therapy.[13,33,39] Patients with complete vascular healing can probably be treated with antiplatelet therapy or no therapy. Similarly, patients with complete and persistent occlusions or irregularity also appear to be at low risk and prolonged anticoagulation is not necessary. A dissecting aneurysm (often erroneously referred to as a *pseudoaneurysm*) may occur in 5% to 40% of patients with dissection.[30,40-45] These have been thought to represent a potential source of thromboembolism and to pose a risk of arterial rupture. Consequently, aggressive treatments such as ligation of the parent artery, bypass procedures, and stenting have been advocated.[46-51] However, long-term observational data have demonstrated a very low risk of complications related to these aneurysms, arguing against aggressive intervention. The three case series that have been reported included a total of 89 patients with 109 aneurysms, and average follow-up has ranged from 3 to 6.5 years. No cases of aneurysm rupture were identified, and there were only three recurrent cerebral

worsening hemorrhage into the vessel wall, but this has never been proven to occur. No controlled clinical trials have addressed the issue of antithrombotic therapy for dissection, but there are numerous published case series and two meta-analyses of these series comparing anticoagulant and antiplatelet therapy. A Cochrane systematic review of 327 patients with carotid dissection spanning 26 case series found no difference in death or disability nor recurrent stroke (anticoagulation, 1.7%; antiplatelet, 3.8%; no therapy, 3.3%).[35] Another systematic review involving 762 patients with either carotid or vertebral ischemic events, none of which was clearly related to the aneurysm.[45,52,53] Most of these patients were treated with either early anticoagulation for a few months followed by long-term antiplatelet therapy or antiplatelet therapy alone.

Most ischemic strokes due to dissection are a result of early thromboembolic phenomena, but a minority appear to be due to hemodynamic compromise.[54,55] The prognosis may be worse in these cases, and revascularization procedures such as stenting or surgery have occasionally been proposed in this setting, although prospective studies do not currently exist.[54,56,57] Routine treatment of clinically asymptomatic persistent stenosis after dissection is probably not warranted given that the procedural risk seems to outweigh the long-term risk of stroke with medical management.[58]

Intracranial dissection may result in either ischemic stroke or subarachnoid hemorrhage. In the setting of subarachnoid hemorrhage, anticoagulation is contraindicated, and patients should be medically managed similar to patients with aneurysmal subarachnoid hemorrhage. In the setting of ischemic stroke, the same treatment principles likely apply as for extracranial dissection, but this has not been studied. Caution and vigilance is certainly warranted because hemorrhage may be catastrophic. It has been proposed that intracranial dissections that cause ischemia could be treated with surgical extracranial-to-intracranial arterial bypass[13] so that anticoagulation can be avoided, but again data regarding this approach are completely lacking. At least one case of immediate extracranial-to-intracranial arterial bypass surgery after intraarterial thrombolysis in a patient with intracranial carotid dissection has been reported.[59]

Some dissections are believed to occur without producing any symptoms and therefore are presumed to remain completely unrecognized. Therefore, it is possible that some dissections have a benign prognosis and do not require therapy. Unfortunately, there is no reliable method to identify these low-risk patients at present, and observation without therapy cannot be recommended.

Patients who have had cervicocerebral arterial dissections should probably avoid activities that may cause sudden rotation or extension of the neck. However, no real data exist to define the limits of activity for these patients. There is no apparent reason to manage their physical therapy differently during rehabilitation after stroke because of the dissection.

Fibromuscular Dysplasia

FMD is a noninflammatory arteriopathy that predominantly affects the extracranial cephalic, renal, splanchnic, and iliac arteries. About one third of patients with FMD also harbor intracranial berry aneurysms. FMD is frequently an incidental finding on conventional angiography but is occasionally associated with stroke. When FMD is implicated as a cause of ischemic stroke, it is usually by way of a poorly characterized predisposition toward arterial dissection, although local atherosclerosis and local in situ thrombosis have been described.[60-67] Hypertension is extremely common in patients with FMD and must be aggressively controlled so that the development of cardiovascular and cerebrovascular atherosclerotic disease can

be prevented. A thorough evaluation of the renal arteries is indicated for identification of FMD causing renal artery stenosis and secondary hypertension, which may be effectively treated with renal artery angioplasty in many cases.[68]

Immediate treatment of stroke attributed to FMD has not been reported. As with dissection, FMD is often not diagnosed in the hyperacute period. There is no current evidence to suggest a differential response to thrombolytic therapy in patients with FMD.

Prevention of stroke and treatment of FMD are largely unknown because there is a paucity of information about its natural history, although it is often believed to be benign. In a series of 79 patients with FMD, only one elderly patient had a stroke in the territory of the affected artery, and it occurred 18 years after the initial diagnosis.[64] Two other elderly patients had strokes in regions that were unrelated to the affected vessel, about 4 and 11 years after diagnosis. All three of these patients were not receiving treatment, and no strokes or transient ischemic attacks occurred among patients treated with antithrombotic medications. Thus, even without therapy, the risk of stroke related to FMD appears to be relatively low and may be particularly minimal in younger patients in whom FMD is an often incidental finding. Nevertheless, antithrombotic strategies should be considered because they appear to further ameliorate the risk, most importantly among patients with FMD and stroke without an alternative etiology. In most cases, antiplatelet therapy is generally preferable to anticoagulation because the annual risk of stroke (approximately 1% to 2%) appears to be less than the bleeding risk attributable to anticoagulation.[69-71] Anticoagulation with warfarin should be carefully considered as a short-term therapy for patients with dissections (as already described).

Surgical and endovascular treatment has been advocated for patients with FMD causing symptomatic focal carotid artery stenosis. Because FMD is often associated with atherosclerosis, patients with accessible symptomatic carotid artery stenosis that appears atherosclerotic should probably be managed as if the FMD were an incidental anomaly.[72] In the absence of concomitant atherosclerosis, surgical intraluminal dilatation of the FMD-related stenosis has been attempted with mixed results.[60,65,73-78] Perioperative morbidity is estimated at 3% to 6% and may negate any potential benefit compared with medical therapy alone or no therapy at all. Angioplasty and/or stenting of FMD has also been successfully performed in a number of cases and is increasingly used, although the efficacy of this approach in stroke prevention has not been formally assessed.[79-87] Surgical considerations for FMD-associated intracranial aneurysms are likely to be similar to those for all intracranial aneurysms.

Vasospasm after Subarachnoid Hemorrhage

Among survivors of aneurysmal subarachnoid hemorrhage, symptomatic vasospasm is a leading cause of morbidity and mortality. Although vasospasm resembles a dynamic constrictive process, there is evidence that it is largely a proliferative arteriopathy. Compromise of the vascular lumen may lead to impaired cerebral autoregulation

TABLE 54-4 DRUGS ASSOCIATED WITH REVERSIBLE CEREBRAL VASOCONSTRICTION SYNDROME

Sympathomimetic drugs
Phenylpropanolamine, pseudoephedrine, amphetamine and amphetamine derivatives, cocaine, ephedra-containing herbal supplements, isometheptene

Serotonergic drugs
Serotonin selective reuptake inhibitors, sumatriptan, ergotamine

Miscellaneous
Bromocriptine, lisuride, tacrolimus, cyclophosphamide, erythropoietin, intravenous immune globulin

and ultimately to ischemia. This nonatherosclerotic vasculopathy and its treatment are discussed extensively elsewhere in this text and will not be reiterated here.

Reversible Cerebral Vasoconstriction Syndromes

Reversible cerebral vasoconstriction syndrome (RCVS) encompasses several interrelated disorders associated with dysregulation of cerebral vascular tone, leading to vasoconstriction of medium and large arteries.[88] RCVS has been previously known by other names, including benign angiopathy of the central nervous system and Call-Fleming syndrome. Patients often present with thunderclap headaches, and subarachnoid hemorrhage, intracerebral hemorrhage, or ischemic stroke may occur. A number of vasoactive drugs have been identified as possible precipitants of RCVS (Table 54-4).[89-99] A detailed history with attention to these agents should be taken, and their use, if present, should be permanently discontinued. Rarely, RCVS occurs secondary to underlying conditions, including pheochromocytoma, carcinoid tumors, hypercalcemia, porphyria, or after vascular or neurosurgical procedures.[88] Such conditions should be identified and specific treatment implemented, as appropriate.

Optimal treatment for RCVS is uncertain given the lack of any controlled therapeutic trials. Spontaneous recovery without intervention has been reported.[91,98,100] Treatment with calcium channel blockers, particularly nimodipine and verapamil, has been proposed based on anecdotal evidence and the possibly comparable role of calcium channel blockers in treating vasospasm after aneurysmal subarachnoid hemorrhage.[100-103] If they are used, care should be taken in patients with extensive segmental vascular narrowing so that decreased cerebral perfusion and subsequent ischemia are avoided. A short course of high-dose steroids has also been suggested as a possible therapy based on efficacy in experimentally induced vasoconstriction.[100,104] Magnesium sulfate is often used in patients with RCVS in the postpartum period given parallels with the central nervous system involvement seen with eclampsia.[105]

Follow-up imaging to confirm resolution of vasoconstriction is generally warranted so that the duration of treatment can be determined. TCD may be used as a noninvasive modality for monitoring and follow-up and is particularly useful if elevated blood flow velocities are present initially.[106-108]

Radiation-Induced Vasculopathy

Radiotherapy for cancers of the head and neck often leads to delayed toxicity to the nervous system. Cerebral necrosis is the predominant result, but vascular endothelial damage is believed to be a critical component of its pathogenesis.[109,110] In addition, larger vessels are often affected by fibrosis and accelerated atherosclerosis at atypical locations.[111-114] The extracranial carotid and vertebral arteries, intracranial vessels of the circle of Willis, and the microvasculature may all be affected, depending on the field and dose of radiation. Microvascular disease tends to be particularly insidious and progressive. Anticoagulation with heparin and warfarin was reported to be beneficial in a small series of patients with radiation-induced nervous system disease.[109] Longer term treatment for small vessel disease has not been assessed, and neither has the role of antiplatelet therapy. For large vessel disease, angioplasty with or without stenting and carotid endarterectomy have been reported to be viable treatment options for some patients.[115-120] The endovascular approach may be preferable for radiation-induced carotid disease because local scarring and soft tissue injury from radiation often makes the surgical field for endarterectomy less manageable. For patients with radiation-induced intracranial disease, encephaloduroarteriomyosynangiosis combined with superficial temporal artery to middle cerebral artery (STA-MCA) bypass has been reported.[121]

Moyamoya Disease

Moyamoya disease is a rare idiopathic arteriopathy in which there is progressive stenosis and occlusion of the terminal portions of the internal carotid arteries and formation of an anomalous vascular network at the base of the brain. A similar vascular pattern may occur with systemic diseases, including severe atherosclerosis, hemoglobinopathies, prothrombotic disorders, radiation therapy, head trauma, and inflammatory or infectious diseases, and is often labeled as *quasimoyamoya* or *moyamoya syndrome* rather than moyamoya disease.[122,123] Patients with moyamoya disease are prone to ischemic stroke, intracerebral hemorrhage, and aneurysm formation with subsequent subarachnoid hemorrhage. Ischemic complications tend to predominate in children, while hemorrhage is more typical of moyamoya in adults, but this pattern is not constant. Epilepsy is also common in moyamoya, occurring in about 5% of all patients[124,125] and usually relates to the underlying cerebrovascular disease. Medical and surgical treatments exist for moyamoya disease, but their rigorous assessment has been limited by the rarity of the disease. Management of concurrent vascular risk factors, such as hypertension or smoking, is recommended so that additional vascular injury is prevented. Further, in quasimoyamoya, treatment should target the underlying disorder when possible.

Ischemic stroke in moyamoya should initially be treated with supportive measures as with other ischemic strokes. Hyperacute therapy with intravenous t-PA has not been assessed in this setting, and discretion with this approach is advised because of the propensity for intracerebral hemorrhage in moyamoya. Antiplatelet therapies are frequently used to prevent recurrent cerebral thromboembolic events, in both the short and long term, although this approach has not been formally evaluated in this population. Further, there is no specific information about the choice of antiplatelet agent, although dipyridamole has a vasodilatory effect that is conjectured to offer a potential but untested benefit. Anticoagulation with warfarin has also not been studied, but because of the risk of intracerebral hemorrhage, it should probably be used with caution in moyamoya.

Other vasodilators, calcium channel antagonists in particular, are believed to improve transient ischemic symptoms in moyamoya and may also offer modest prevention against stroke. Corticosteroids are also believed to be useful in some patients, notably when there is evidence of cerebral edema or vascular inflammation. However, there are considerable data that argue against the use of steroids for more typical causes of ischemic stroke[126-130] that make this approach somewhat dubious. Further, inflammation does not appear to play a major role in the pathophysiology of moyamoya, which, again, argues against the empiric use of steroids.

Medical management of intracerebral hemorrhage due to moyamoya is similar to that due to the more common causes and is again principally supportive. As with hypertensive hemorrhage, surgical evacuation is controversial[131,132] and may offer limited benefit because the intraparenchymal hemorrhages of moyamoya tend to be deep. Management of subarachnoid hemorrhage due to rupture of a moyamoya-related aneurysm is also similar to the management of more generic aneurysms. However, the surgical issues are quite distinct because the abnormal network of moyamoya vessels is extremely susceptible to manipulation. Moreover, the aneurysms tend to be in unusual locations or in the posterior circulation, thereby complicating the approach. Endovascular techniques have limited utility in dealing with aneurysms of the anterior circulation because the occlusion of the terminal internal carotid artery renders them inaccessible. Vasospasm after subarachnoid hemorrhage may contribute substantially to morbidity and mortality in moyamoya, particularly because cerebral perfusion is already impaired. Early detection of vasospasm is therefore critical, yet noninvasive diagnosis with TCD ultrasonography may be unreliable because of the obliteration of the major intracranial cerebral vessels. When suspected, the diagnosis of vasospasm should be pursued with angiography and aggressively treated as already outlined, although the utility of hypervolemic–hypertension–hemodilution therapy or nimodipine in this setting is unknown.

There are some patients with moyamoya for whom the disease is relatively benign, limited to mild, transient symptoms, and conservative medical therapy may suffice.[133] However, in the majority of patients, these medical therapies offer very limited efficacy, and more aggressive surgical therapies should be considered. Occasionally, moyamoya is discovered incidentally in asymptomatic patients. A small observational study of 40 such patients in Japan found a 3.2% annual stroke risk among 34 nonsurgically treated patients, and no subsequent stroke among six surgically treated patients, which suggests a possible benefit for aggressive surgical therapies even in patients without symptoms.[134]

Surgical revascularization procedures have two key goals: (1) improving regional cerebral blood flow so that ischemic complications are prevented, and (2) alleviating the pressure and/or flow through deep moyamoya collateral vessels, thus reducing the risk of hemorrhage. Direct bypass (such as STA-MCA anastomosis), indirect bypass (such as encephaloduroarteriosynangiosis and encephaloduroarteriomyosynangiosis), or a combination of both have been described as effective treatments in a number of series and small uncontrolled studies,[135-143] but their roles have never been studied in a randomized clinical trial. A single case report of successful angioplasty for early moyamoya has been published.[144] These surgical techniques and their proposed importance in moyamoya are described in detail elsewhere in this text.

Hyperhomocyst(e)inemia and Homocystinuria

Elevated levels of the amino acid homocyst(e)ine appear to cause endothelial injury and proliferation of vascular smooth muscle cells, thereby leading to premature atherosclerosis.[145,146] In addition, homocyst(e)ine may interfere with endogenous anticoagulant mechanisms, resulting in a prothrombotic state.[147,148] Homocyst(e)ine levels can be reduced with folic acid, pyridoxine (vitamin B_6), and cyanocobalamin (vitamin B_{12}) supplementation.

Homocystinuria is a rare autosomal recessive disease caused by a genetic deficiency of cystathionine synthase. This defect leads to high blood levels of homocysteine and excretion of homocysteine in the urine and is associated with a number of clinical symptoms including vascular disease and thromboembolic events. Most patients develop clinical symptoms during early childhood, although vascular events often occur in early adulthood. Treatment is aimed at normalizing homocysteine levels through vitamin B_6, B_{12}, and folate supplementation. For patients who do not respond to vitamin supplementation, a methionine-restricted, cystine-supplemented diet is added to vitamin therapy. Betaine has also been used as an adjunctive therapy.[149] A multicenter observational study demonstrated a substantial reduction in vascular events in patients with homocystinuria treated with aggressive homocysteine-lowering therapy compared with historical control subjects.[150]

In contrast to the specific situation of homocystinuria, the role of vitamin supplementation in patients with modest hyperhomocyst(e)inemia and vascular disease is much less clear. While hyperhomocyst(e)inemia appears to be independently associated with risk of ischemic stroke, it is uncertain whether this is a cause or effect of vascular disease.[143,144] Controlled trials of homocysteine-lowering therapy have shown some beneficial effects on surrogate indicators of vascular function; however, these indicators may not directly correlate with clinical vascular events.[149,150] Two large randomized trials assessed the role of vitamin therapy in preventing recurrent vascular events following stroke: the Vitamins in Stroke Prevention

(VISP) study and the Vitamins to Prevent Stroke Study (VITATOPS). The VISP trial randomized 3680 patients with stroke to either high-dose (daily doses of 25 mg B_6, 0.4 mg B_{12}, 2.5 mg folic acid) or low-dose (200 mg B_6, 6 mg B_{12}, 20 mg folic acid) vitamin supplementation.[151] There was a mean reduction in homocysteine levels of 2 mmol/L, but no benefit was seen on any vascular endpoint. A subgroup analysis of the VISP trial focused on the patients theoretically most likely to benefit from treatment.[152] In this analysis, patients with low and very high B_{12} levels at baseline were excluded in an attempt to eliminate patients with B_{12} malabsorption (low levels) and those receiving B_{12} supplementation outside of the study (very high levels). In the remaining 2155 patients, a 21% relative reduction in the composite endpoint of stroke, coronary event, or death was demonstrated ($p = 0.05$) with high-dose compared to low-dose vitamin supplementation.

VITATOPS randomized 8164 patients with stroke TIA to either placebo or vitamin supplementation (daily doses of 25 mg B_6, 500 mg B_{12}, 2 mg folic acid).[153] Over a median follow-up period of 3.4 years, the primary endpoint of stroke, MI, or vascular death occurred in 15.1% of patients in the vitamin arm compared to 16.6% in the placebo arm (RR 0.91; 95% CI, 0.82-1.00, $p = 0.05$). Vitamin therapy was associated with modest reductions in stroke and vascular death, but not myocardial infarction. No adverse events were seen with vitamin therapy. Other randomized trials have assessed vitamin therapy in patients with known coronary artery disease or other vascular disease but have not focused specifically on patients with prior stroke. These trials have uniformly failed to show benefit to homocysteine lowering therapy.[154-156] Based on the totality of the current data, it remains uncertain whether vitamin supplementation for prevention of recurrent vascular events in patients with stroke and elevated homocysteine is beneficial (outside the specific context of homocystinuria).

Fabry Disease

Fabry disease is a rare X-linked inherited deficiency of the lysosomal enzyme alpha-galactosidase, which causes lipid deposition in the vascular endothelium and results in progressive vasculopathy of the brain, heart, skin, and kidneys.[159] Angiokeratoma on the trunk are often the only early sign, but cerebral arteriopathy usually becomes clinically evident in young men by the fourth decade and occasionally in older women.[160] The intracranial vertebrobasilar system is often dolichoectatic and may be the proximate source of ischemic stroke, although cardiogenic embolism and progressive small vessel occlusive disease with deep infarctions are also observed.[159,161,162] In young stroke victims, Fabry disease may be underdiagnosed. In a German cohort of 721 patients aged 18 to 55 with cryptogenic stroke, the Fabry mutation was found in 4.9% of men and in 2.4% of women.[163]

Antiplatelet agents are believed to be useful in preventing ischemic events related to existing vascular disease,[163] but the disease itself was untreatable and the prognosis was quite poor until recombinant alpha-galactosidase A became available as an intravenous infusion. In a randomized controlled trial of 58 patients with Fabry disease, alpha-galactosidase was given intravenously at a

dose of 1 mg/kg every other week for 20 weeks.[164] Only 31% of patients in the treated group developed new microvascular endothelial lipid deposits after 20 weeks compared with 100% of the patients in the placebo group ($P < 0.001$). In addition, after 6 months of open-label therapy provided to all subjects, all patients in the former placebo group and 98% of patients in the former recombinant alpha-galactosidase A group had clearance of microvascular endothelial deposits. Because alpha-galactosidase A replacement therapy effectively clears endothelial deposits from affected organs in patients with Fabry disease, it should presumably arrest the disease process and should therefore be instituted promptly after the diagnosis is established. Subsequent trials demonstrated clinical improvements in kidney function, but the impact on cardiac function has been inconsistent.[165-168] Enzyme replacement therapy has been shown to have a favorable effect on cerebral blood flow, but the risk of stroke appears substantial despite therapy.[169,170] Higher enzyme doses may be needed for stroke prevention, and this is an area of active research.[171] The major adverse effects of recombinant alpha-galactosidase A infusions are fever and rigors, which may occur in 25% to 50% of treated patients, but may be minimized with slow infusion rates and premedication with acetaminophen and hydroxyzine.

Inflammatory Vasculopathies

Cerebrovascular disease may rarely occur as a result of derangement of cell-mediated and antibody-mediated immune responses. The vasculitides are a heterogeneous group of disorders in which inflammation of the blood vessels causes vascular narrowing, occlusion, or necrosis, which may result in cerebral ischemia, infarction, or hemorrhage.[172] Vasculitis may be a primary process (isolated angiitis of the central nervous system) or may occur secondary to an identifiable systemic inflammatory disorder, infection, toxin, or neoplasm. Immunosuppression appears to be the key element of treatment (Table 54-5).

Isolated Angiitis of the Central Nervous System

Isolated angiitis of the central nervous system (IACNS) affects only the brain and spinal cord, and there is a complete absence of any systemic manifestation of the disease. Symptoms of IACNS may include headache, seizure, stroke, and multifocal encephalopathy. In the early descriptions of this disease, the prognosis was uniformly poor, but immunotherapy may alter the course of the disease. Clinical and angiographic improvement has been attributed to corticosteroids and cyclophosphamide, but because of the profound rarity of IACNS, randomized clinical trials have not been performed. In a review of the literature and description of eight additional cases, Calabrese and Mallek[173] observed that nearly all untreated patients died or were persistently dependent, whereas four of 13 treated with steroids and 10 of 13 treated with both steroids and cyclophosphamide improved. In a series of 101 patients from the Mayo Clinic, 34 of 42 patients (81%) treated initially with prednisone alone had a favorable response compared with 38 of 47 patients (81%) treated

TABLE 54-5 IMMUNOSUPPRESSIVE DRUGS USED IN THE TREATMENT OF INFLAMMATORY VASCULOPATHIES

Drug	Indications	Dosing Regimen	Adverse Effects
Prednisone or methylprednisolone	IACNS GCA CVD-related ? Infection-related ? Toxin-related ? Neoplasm-related	*Induction:* 0.5-2 mg/kg/day orally or: up to 1000 mg/day IV for acute or severe cases *Taper:* as tolerated over 3-12 months *Maintenance:* 5-10 mg/day orally	Infections, cushingoid features, adrenal insufficiency, behavioral/mood changes, osteopenia, diabetes mellitus, many others
Cyclophosphamide	IACNS CVD-related	*Induction:* 1-2 mg/kg/day orally or: 750 mg/m^2 BSA IV monthly for acute, severe cases *Taper:* as tolerated over 3-12 months *Maintenance:* lowest dose without recurrent symptoms; consider switch to azathioprine	Bone marrow suppression, infections, malignancy, nausea/vomiting, alopecia, hemorrhagic cystitis, diarrhea, rash
Azathioprine*	IACNS GCA CVD-related	*Induction:* not used as induction therapy *Maintenance:* start 1 mg/kg/day orally; increase by 0.5 mg/kg/day every 4 weeks to max. 2.5 mg/kg/day	Bone marrow suppression, infections, hepatotoxicity, nausea/vomiting, diarrhea
Methotrexate†	GCA CVD-related	*Induction and maintenance:* 10 mg/day orally	Bone marrow suppression, hepatotoxicity, nephrotoxicity, nausea/vomiting, fatigue, fever/chills

*Used as an alternative to cyclophosphamide.
†Used in conjunction with corticosteroids.
BSA, Body surface area; CVD, collagen vascular disorder; GCA, giant cell (temporal) arteritis; IACNS, isolated angiitis of the central nervous system; IV, intravenous.

with cyclophosphamide (most of whom also received treatment with steroids).[174] The median duration of treatment was approximately 10 months with both steroids and cyclophosphamide. Relapse leading to a change in therapy occurred in 26 of 101 patients (26%). In contrast, others[175,176] have found that corticosteroids alone offered a transient effect at best and that combination therapy with cyclophosphamide was required for a clinical benefit. The appropriate dosage for both medications is unclear and varies among centers. For induction therapy, prednisone or prednisolone 1 to 2 mg/kg per day is recommended at the time of diagnosis; tapering should occur over 3 to 12 months to a minimal dose of 5 to 10 mg/day. Some centers initiate steroid treatment with intravenous pulse steroids, such as methylprednisolone 1 g daily for 1 to 6 days.[174] Cyclophosphamide should be started at 1 to 2 mg/kg per day, but more aggressive treatment with intravenous cyclophosphamide may be useful for patients with more acute or severe symptoms, in the form of either 3 to 6 monthly pulses of 750 mg/m^2 body surface area or 15 mg/kg.[172,177] Patients may be followed up with serial neurologic examination, neuropsychiatric testing, cerebrospinal fluid examination, and/or MRI at 3- to 6-month intervals. Serial angiography is seldom necessary. If remission or stabilization occurs, then cyclophosphamide may be gradually weaned over several months and replaced with the better tolerated azathioprine 2 mg/kg per day as maintenance therapy in some cases,[172] although the role of this agent is untested. These therapeutic regimens have only been evaluated for relatively brief terms of a few years, and their longer term efficacy has not been described. Longer term therapy seems to be required for patients who relapse. One study

of 12 patients found a high relapse rate in patients with predominantly small vessel involvement, whereas no patients with middle sized vessel involvement relapsed, which suggests that patients with small vessel vasculitis may require longer term or more aggressive treatment.[178] Titration of medication doses is somewhat empiric in response to each individual patient's clinical response. Patients taking cyclophosphamide or azathioprine require careful monitoring of the leukocyte count for evidence of bone marrow suppression. In addition, oral fluid intake must be increased so that the risk of hemorrhagic cystitis is minimized. Antiemetics may be needed to manage nausea, particularly with intravenous pulse cyclophosphamide. Finally, patients must be monitored and treated for steroid-induced diabetes mellitus while taking steroids.

Other immunomodulatory approaches, including other chemotherapeutic agents, plasma exchange, and intravenous immunoglobulin, have not been studied in IACNS beyond individual case reports. Similarly, the role of antithrombotic medication in IACNS has not been evaluated.

Temporal (Giant Cell) Arteritis

Temporal (giant cell) arteritis is a systemic inflammatory vasculopathy that should be considered in any stroke patient older than 50 years.[179] Treatment decisions are often necessary before confirmation of the diagnosis. If the clinical features (described elsewhere) are present, the erythrocyte sedimentation rate (ESR) is elevated, or both, a unilateral temporal artery biopsy should be performed. Corticosteroids, the mainstay of therapy, can be initiated before the biopsy and will not affect the results if performed within approximately 10 to 14 days.[179,180] For patients seen with acute visual loss, immediate treatment with high-dose (up to 1000 mg daily) intravenous methylprednisolone for 3 to 5 days has been advocated by some authors,[181,182] although others have suggested that intravenous steroid pulses offer no benefit compared with oral therapy but carry greater expense and risk.[183,184] Chevalet et al performed a randomized clinical trial of 164 patients with uncomplicated temporal arteritis comparing three dosing regimens: 240 mg intravenous pulse of methylprednisolone (IVMP) followed by 0.7 mg/kg/day oral prednisone (group 1), or 0.7 mg/kg/day oral prednisone without an IV pulse (group 2), or 240 mg IVMP followed by 0.5 mg/kg/day oral prednisone (group 3).[185] Steroid doses were then tapered starting 6 months after therapy. At 1 year, there were no significant differences among the three groups with regard to clinical symptoms, laboratory parameters, or steroid-related side effects. In contrast, Mazlumzadeh et al performed a randomized clinical trial in 27 patients with temporal arteritis comparing a 3-day course of IVMP (15 mg/kg per day) to placebo. All patients were also treated with 40 mg/day of prednisone. Patients randomly assigned to IVMP were able to taper steroids more rapidly and had a higher frequency of sustained remission after stopping steroid treatment.[186] Further, Chan et al performed a retrospective cohort study of 100 patients with acute visual loss due to giant cell arteritis and found that there was an increased likelihood of improved vision in the group treated with intravenous steroids (40%) compared with those who received oral steroids (13%).[187] Based on these data, the role of intravenous steroids remains somewhat uncertain, and some authors recommend using high-dose intravenous steroids only for those patients whose clinical condition progresses in the face of oral steroids.[188,189]

Regardless of whether intravenous steroids are used, maintenance therapy with daily oral prednisone, starting at 40 to 80 mg daily (0.5 to 1.0 mg/kg),[190] should be initiated; eventual gradual tapering should then occur. The goal of maintenance therapy is to prevent subsequent ischemic events, and the taper should likely be adjusted according to the patient's clinical response, ESR, and C-reactive protein level. There is great controversy over the duration of therapy and the rapidity of the taper. However, in a cohort study involving 90 patients, the timing of cessation of therapy had no effect on the risk of recurrent symptoms.[191] A reasonable approach is treatment for 4 weeks until clinical signs and symptoms have resolved and the ESR and C-reactive protein level have normalized, then reduction of the steroid dose gradually every 1 to 2 weeks by 10% or less of the total daily dose.[192] If symptoms recur or there is an increase in ESR or C-reactive protein level during the taper, the prednisone dose should be increased by 20 to 40 mg/day for 2 to 3 weeks, then the taper can be resumed. Careful attention should be given to steroid side effects such as diabetes, hypertension, osteoporosis, avascular necrosis of the hip, cataracts, and gastrointestinal bleeding. Calcium (1000 to 1500 mg/day) and vitamin D (800 IU/day) supplementation is recommended.[192] Bisphosphonates may be appropriate for patients with reduced bone mineral density. In the setting of concurrent aspirin therapy, the use of a proton pump inhibitor to protect gastric mucosa should be considered.

Experience with other immunosuppressive agents for temporal arteritis is limited. Methotrexate has been studied in three randomized controlled trials, and an individual patient data meta-analysis of the 161 patients in these trials has been published.[193] All patients were treated with steroids initially. Adjunctive methotrexate significantly lowered the risk of first relapse ($P = 0.04$) and second relapse ($P = 0.02$). The estimated numbers needed to treat were 3.6 to prevent a first relapse and 4.7 to prevent a second relapse. The overall incidence of adverse events, including typical steroid side effects, did not differ between the methotrexate and placebo arms. It therefore appears reasonable to consider the use of adjunctive methotrexate to reduce the risk of relapse, but it does not appear that methotrexate is effective at reducing the incidence of steroid side effects. Azathioprine was shown to reduce the required dose of corticosteroids in a randomized trial involving 31 patients with temporal arteritis and/or polymyalgia rheumatica.[194] Based on these limited data, the role of azathioprine remains poorly defined, but it may be reasonable to consider if a steroid-sparing agent is required and methotrexate is not tolerated. Cyclosporine A offered no benefit over steroids alone in a small open trial.[195] The tumor necrosis factor-alpha inhibitor infliximab has been tested in a randomized trial of 44 patients with temporal arteritis and was found to be ineffective and associated with a higher rate of infection.[196]

In patients with stroke related to temporal arteritis, it seems logical to use antiplatelet therapy to reduce the risk of recurrent vascular events, although this has not been subject to randomized trials. Two small observational studies do support a significant reduction in ischemic events in patients with temporal arteritis treated with antithrombotic therapy.[197,198]

Cerebral Vasculitis Related to Collagen Vascular Disorders

Systemic vasculitides include polyarteritis nodosa, Sjögren's disease, Churg-Strauss angiitis, Wegener's granulomatosis, Henoch-Schönlein purpura, cryoglobulinemia, systemic lupus erythematosus, scleroderma, and rheumatoid arthritis, each of which is characterized by the pattern of involvement of other organ systems.[199-211] Neurologic involvement is variable in each of these disorders and is typically less prominent than the other features but may be the initial manifestation in some cases. Further, neurologic symptoms, when present, are rarely due to cerebral vasculitis or cerebritis but are rather more frequently related to cardiac emboli (such as nonbacterial thrombotic endocarditis), hypercoagulable states (such as antiphospholipid antibody syndrome), or atherosclerosis (as a result of renovascular hypertension or steroid-induced diabetes mellitus).[212,213] Treatment of the cerebral component is, in general, dictated by the treatment of the systemic disease and often includes corticosteroids and other immunosuppressant agents.[199,214] When the diagnosis of concomitant cerebral vasculitis exists and persists despite treatment of the systemic process, then more aggressive treatment, such as that for

IACNS, may be warranted, but again, data to support this approach are lacking.

Cerebral Vasculitis Related to Infection

Among the secondary causes of vasculitis, infectious etiologies include meningovascular syphilis, tuberculous meningitis, other bacterial (*Streptococcus pneumoniae, Neisseria*) meningitis, fungal (*Aspergillus, Candida, Coccidioides, Cryptococcus, Histoplasma,* and *Mucor*) meningoencephalitides, neurocysticercosis, varicella-zoster virus (VZV) encephalitis, human immunodeficiency virus (HIV), and hepatitis C virus.[215-248] Specifically directed antimicrobial therapy is advisable for each of these disorders and may improve the vasculopathic angiographic findings,[221] although this approach may not necessarily improve the clinical course.[249,250] Immunosuppressive regimens are often used in patients with persisting vasculopathy,[221,249,251] although the efficacy of this approach is unproven. The role of antiplatelet agents, anticoagulation, and thrombolysis in infection-related vasculopathy is also uncertain, and caution is advised because there may be a necrotizing component of the vasculitis as well as dysfunction of the blood–brain barrier, thereby increasing the risk of intracerebral hemorrhage.[252]

Cerebral Vasculitis Related to Toxins

Toxins implicated in cerebral vasculitis include cocaine, amphetamines, heroin, lysergic acid diethylamide (LSD), and inhaled volatile solvents (glue sniffing), although these may result in a process more like vasospasm after subarachnoid hemorrhage than a true inflammatory vasculitis.[253-258] Other sympathomimetic agents, including ephedrine and phenylpropanolamine, may have similar effects.[259-261] In the setting of acute ischemic stroke associated with drug use (cocaine, in particular), there is evidence to suggest that a combination of vasospasm and superimposed thrombosis may occur.[262] In such cases, thrombolysis may be a reasonable therapeutic option in the first few hours, whereas antiplatelet therapy may be appropriate later in the course.[263]

No specific therapy has been shown to improve the vasculopathy, but the offending agent should certainly be removed.[258] Patients should be closely monitored and treated for symptoms of drug withdrawal. As many abusers of illicit drugs also abuse alcohol, a low threshold should exist for initiating benzodiazepines for symptoms or signs of alcohol withdrawal.

Ideal therapy for ongoing vasculitis among users of methamphetamine has not been identified, in part because the pathogenesis of the vasculitis is unclear. Steroid therapy has been used in some patients on a short-term basis, but there is little evidence to suggest this is beneficial.[258] Calcium channel blockers have been advocated for the treatment of cocaine users with vasospasm/vasculitis, but no formal data exist regarding efficacy.

Long-term secondary stroke prevention strategies should include cessation of the identified abused drug. Antiplatelet therapy is probably indicated for patients with ischemic stroke, although there are limited data specifically applicable to stroke in the setting of drug abuse.

Cerebral Vasculitis Related to Neoplasms

Arteriopathies may rarely complicate the course of systemic neoplasms. The small and middle-sized intracranial arteries may be affected by carcinomatous or lymphomatous meningitis, as well as intravascular lymphomatosis. The prognosis is quite poor in these cases. Steroids, palliative chemotherapy, and radiation therapy may offer some transient benefit for the inflammatory vasculopathy, although in some cases this approach led to acute worsening of symptoms.[264-267]

Hematologic Disorders

Ischemic stroke may be associated with a number of hereditary and acquired prothrombotic states, including abnormalities of red cell or platelet function, coagulation factors, or endogenous fibrinolysis (see Table 54-2). These disorders are uncommon, but are overrepresented among young stroke victims and should be considered when no alternative etiology is identified.[1-4]

Prothrombotic Disorders

Disorders of the Coagulation System

The factor V Leiden, prothrombin G20210A, and methylenetetrahydrofolate reductase (MTHFR) C677T gene mutations have been associated with a hypercoagulable state, particularly with regard to venous thrombosis. Meta-analysis of published studies suggests that the relationship between these genetic variants and arterial events such as ischemic stroke is relatively modest but possibly stronger in younger patients.[268,269] Stroke is also associated with inherited deficiencies of protein C, protein S, and antithrombin III, which are far less common but are probably associated with a higher risk of recurrent thrombotic events; acquired deficiencies may also occur because these factors may be depleted in nephrotic syndrome, hepatic disease, and pregnancy. Prothrombotic tendencies are also found in association with oral contraceptive use, systemic inflammatory disorders, and malignancies. Hyperhomocyst(e)inemia may also predispose to thrombosis, as already described.

In the hyperacute setting of ischemic stroke, these underlying inherited or acquired disorders may not be recognized, and patients may be treated with standard thrombolytic or antithrombotic therapy.[270] Chronic anticoagulation is often recommended for secondary prevention among stroke survivors with a confirmed prothrombotic state, although this remains controversial and guidelines suggest that either antiplatelet or anticoagulant therapy may be considered.[271,272] Those rare patients with known protein C or protein S deficiencies should not be initially treated with warfarin unless heparin is given concurrently because there is a small risk of inducing a transient hypercoagulable state.[273] Given the modest association of the factor V, prothrombin G20210A, and MTHFR C677T gene mutations with arterial events, it is probably reasonable to use antiplatelet therapy for secondary stroke prevention in these patients unless multiple thrombotic events have occurred.

Antiphospholipid Antibody Syndrome

Antiphospholipid antibodies (aPLs) may occur with systemic disorders or may occur in isolation; they appear to be an independent risk factor for both arterial and venous thromboembolism in some but not all studies, as their presence may be confounded by other disorders or medications.[274-283] The mechanism by which aPLs may lead to thrombosis is uncertain, but they appear to interfere with endogenous anticoagulants, protein C, and platelet homeostasis. Moreover, aPLs are relatively common, occurring in up to 10% of the normal population,[284,285] which suggests that not all patients with this laboratory abnormality require specific treatment. In most asymptomatic patients with aPLs, there is no well-defined role for primary prevention. However, asymptomatic patients with systemic lupus erythematosus and aPLs appear to be at very high risk of thromboembolic events[286] and should perhaps receive prophylactic treatment, although this issue has not been directly studied. Finally, a distinction should be made between the mere presence of aPLs and the aPL syndrome, which is characterized by the occurrence of thromboembolic events and medium- to high-titer aPLs or a positive lupus anticoagulant on two separate measurements at least 6 weeks apart.[287]

In the acute setting, t-PA has been used for stroke due to aPL syndrome.[270] However, assessment of the eligibility of such patients for thrombolysis may be obscured if the partial thromboplastin time (PTT) is spuriously elevated owing to the presence of aPL. Elevated PTT is an exclusion criterion for the use of intravenous t-PA but only if the patient has received heparin or has a known predisposition for bleeding (such as a factor deficiency).[288] This is not the case with aPL, so patients with falsely elevated PTTs due to aPL should still be considered candidates for thrombolysis. Anti–t-PA antibodies have been identified in patients with aPL syndrome[289] that may theoretically attenuate the potential effect of thrombolysis, but this has not been evaluated.

Preventative strategies for patients who have had stroke or other thromboembolic events include antithrombotic and immunomodulatory therapies. The prospective Antiphospholipid Antibody Stroke Study (APASS) specifically addressed the role of aPL in a large population of patients with noncardioembolic stroke as part of the Warfarin versus Aspirin for Recurrent Stroke Study (WARSS).[290] In APASS, 1770 patients had testing for aPL before the initiation of antithrombotic therapy, and 41% were classified as aPL positive.[291] During 2 years of follow-up, there was no difference in the incidence of thromboocclusive events between patients with and without aPL. Further, there was no difference in the risk of these events between those treated with warfarin or aspirin. Several important limitations of this study should be noted. First, patients enrolled in WARSS/APASS were, for the most part, older (mean age, 62 years) with typical atherosclerotic risk factors and mostly lacunar strokes. Second, aPLs were measured on only a single occasion; therefore it is unknown what proportion of patients would have met criteria for aPL syndrome. Third, the vast majority of aPL-positive patients had low- to medium-titer antibodies (only 0.2% of patients had high-titer positive

IgG anticardiolipin antibodies). The results of APASS do emphasize that older patients with typical atherosclerotic risk factors, a single thrombotic event, and positive aPL at a single measurement should be managed with antiplatelet therapy alone. These findings probably should not be extrapolated, however, to patients who meet criteria for aPL syndrome.

In a retrospective study of 147 patients with aPL syndrome, recurrent thromboembolic events occurred in 101 patients during a median follow-up period of 6 years.[292] The relative risk of recurrence was dramatically and significantly lower in patients treated with warfarin to maintain the international normalized ratio (INR) ≥ 3.0 (relative risk, 0.05; 95% CI, 0.01–0.16) compared with those treated with aspirin or with lower levels of anticoagulation. Corticosteroids, azathioprine, and cyclophosphamide had no significant effect on thrombotic events in this study. Similarly, a later study with 61 patients followed up for a median of 77 months showed that warfarin significantly reduced the risk of recurrence by about 75% when the prothrombin ratio (patient versus control) was maintained between 1.5 and 2.0.[293] Aspirin was no better than observation without treatment. Immunosuppressive regimens again had no preventative effect, and prednisone in particular appeared to increase the risk of thrombotic episodes. More recently, two randomized controlled trials enrolling 114 and 109 patients, respectively, compared high-intensity warfarin (goal INR, 3.0 to 4.0 to 4.5) to moderate intensity warfarin (goal INR, 2.0 to 3.0) in aPL syndrome.[294,295] Both studies found no benefit and more bleeding complications with higher intensity warfarin. On the basis of these data, it is recommended that patients with aPL syndrome who are treated with warfarin should have a goal INR of 2.0 to 3.0.

Catastrophic antiphospholipid antibody syndrome refers to the rare but dramatic occurrence of thrombotic events involving multiple organ systems over a short period of time (generally < 7 days) in patients with aPLs. This condition is associated with a poor prognosis, and aggressive treatment is required. Given the rarity of the condition, treatment recommendations are based entirely on clinical experience.[296] Intravenous heparin should be started immediately and administered for 7 to 10 days before conversion to oral anticoagulation. High-dose steroids are recommended to attenuate cytokine release from widespread tissue necrosis. Plasmapheresis and/or intravenous immunoglobulin is used in an attempt to modulate the pathogenic aPLs. If progression occurs despite these interventions, then more aggressive immunosuppresion with cyclophosphamide or rituximab should be considered.

Disseminated Intravascular Coagulation

Disseminated intravascular coagulation (DIC) is caused by disequilibrium of the coagulation system that usually occurs in the context of malignancy, sepsis, surgical/obstetric complications, or trauma. Fibrin and platelet thrombi form in the microcirculation and obstruct tissue perfusion.[297] Simultaneously, free platelets are depleted and fibrin degradation products are formed, which results in a systemic lytic state. Both ischemic stroke and intracerebral hemorrhage may occur in DIC.[297-299]

Treatment should be directed primarily toward correcting the underlying or precipitating disorder, if possible. When ischemic thromboembolic events are the prevailing process, anticoagulation with heparin or low-molecular-weight heparin is generally advised to prevent additional events, but this is controversial.[300-302] Thrombolysis is likely contraindicated in patients with ischemic stroke due to DIC because of low platelet counts, depleted coagulation factors, and the increased risk of hemorrhage, although this remains speculative given the lack of clinical data.

After the acute thrombotic event, if the underlying disorder cannot be treated, long-term prophylactic therapy should be considered for chronic DIC. Chronic DIC does not typically respond well to oral anticoagulation with warfarin, so parenteral heparin or low-molecular-weight heparin is preferred.[300,301]

When intracerebral or systemic hemorrhage is the predominant event, bleeding should be controlled by replacement of depleted clotting factors and platelets. Antithrombotic therapy should be avoided. In some patients with DIC and bleeding refractory to conventional therapy, recombinant factor VIIa has been suggested as a possible additional therapeutic option.[303]

Sickle Cell Disease

Sickle cell disease rarely has stroke as its presenting symptom, but stroke may occur in 10% to 20% of patients with the disorder.[304,305] Sickle trait alone may also be rarely associated with stroke, particularly in the setting of severe dehydration or hypoxia. Sickle cell disease causes a progressive nonatherosclerotic large vessel arteriopathy that, in the extreme, may evolve into a quasimoyamoya pattern.[306,307] Increased blood viscosity during a sickle crisis may impair perfusion, and infarction may also occur owing to direct occlusion of the microvasculature by cellular aggregates. The coexisting anemia may cause compensatory arteriolar vasodilatation and increase cerebral blood flow, which may, in turn, increase the risk of intracerebral hemorrhage.[308]

Early treatment of stroke due to sickle cell disease consists of emergent simple blood transfusion or exchange transfusion to reduce the proportion of sickle hemoglobin (HbS) to less than 30%, although this approach is based on consensus rather than evidence.[309] Generic supportive measures are indicated in the acute setting, aiming for normovolemia, normothermia, and normoglycemia. Thrombolytic therapy for acute ischemic stroke may be associated with an increased risk of intracerebral hemorrhage; however, formal studies to evaluate this have not been performed, and there is no definite reason to withhold this treatment option from patients who otherwise meet standard eligibility criteria.[309] At least one case report of successful thrombolysis for cerebral venous sinus thrombosis in sickle cell disease has been reported.[310]

Transfusion therapy is better characterized as a strategy for prevention of stroke in sickle cell disease. The Stroke Prevention Trial in Sickle Cell Anemia (STOP) was a randomized clinical trial that tested whether long-term transfusion therapy could reduce the risk of stroke in 130 high-risk children with the disease.[311] Participants were identified as being at high risk if TCD ultrasonography revealed velocities exceeding 200 cm/s in the intracranial internal carotid artery or the middle cerebral artery. Transfusions were performed to maintain the HbS concentration at less than 30% of the total hemoglobin. Only one of 63 children treated with transfusion therapy developed a stroke compared with 11 of 67 who received standard care ($P < 0.001$). The study was terminated prematurely because of the overwhelming benefit: a 92% reduction in the risk of stroke. Transfusion is strongly recommended as first-line, primary prevention in children at high risk based on this study and may be advisable as secondary prevention in children and adults who have already had cerebrovascular events. The optimal concentration of HbS for long-term secondary prevention is controversial, ranging from 30% to 60%.[312-314] The optimal duration of transfusion therapy was assessed in the Optimizing Stroke Prevention in Sickle Cell Anemia (STOP 2) trial.[315] This trial enrolled 79 patients with sickle cell disease, no history of stroke, and elevated TCD velocities who had undergone at least 30 months of transfusion therapy with normalization of their TCD velocities. Patients were randomly assigned to continued transfusion therapy versus discontinuation of transfusion therapy. In the 41 patients who stopped transfusion therapy, 14 developed recurrent high-risk TCD velocities and two experienced a stroke. The 38 patients who continued transfusion therapy had neither of these endpoints.

As short-term or prophylactic therapy, transfusions can be performed as either simple transfusions or exchange transfusions. Simple transfusions are straightforward transfusions of packed red blood cells to reduce the relative proportion of HbS. The number of required units of blood is based on the patient's pretransfusion levels of HbS and total hematocrit and an estimate of the total circulating blood volume. The short-term risks of simple transfusion are volume overloading and hyperviscosity; therefore it is most suited for patients who are already severely anemic, volume depleted, or both. Exchange transfusions allow for reduction in the HbS level without increasing the hematocrit level. This can be performed manually or automatically with the use of apheresis equipment, and both approaches involve removal of about 2 units (about one liter) of blood with replacement of about 4 units of packed red blood cells and normal saline, depending on the initial HbS level and the patient's size. Over the long-term, exchange transfusions may be better tolerated than simple transfusions and pose a lower risk of iron toxicity but are more expensive and require exposure to more units of blood. Blood-borne infections are infrequent, but their risk increases with chronic transfusion therapy. With either approach, transfusions are also associated with alloimmunization, but this may be minimized with the use of red blood cells that are phenotypically matched for specific antigens (Kell blood group and Rh antigens C and E).[316] In a retrospective review of patients treated with transfusion therapy for secondary stroke prevention, eight of 14 (57%) of those treated with initial simple transfusion had recurrent strokes compared with eight of 38 (21%) of those treated with exchange transfusion.[317] These data must be interpreted cautiously given the nonrandomized nature of the observations.

Hydroxyurea is a chemotherapeutic agent that appears to increase the concentration of fetal hemoglobin and improve red blood cell survival.[318] It has also been shown to increase cerebral oxygenation as measured by near-infrared spectroscopy.[319] Several studies have shown that treatment with hydroxyurea lowers TCD flow velocities, suggesting a possible benefit in stroke prevention.[320-322] In a double-blind clinical trial, 299 patients with frequent painful sickle crises (without a history of stroke) were randomly assigned to receive either hydroxyurea or placebo and were followed up for a mean of 21 months.[323] Hydroxyurea was given at an initial dose of 15 mg/kg per day and increased by 5 mg/kg per day every 12 weeks, unless bone marrow suppression (neutrophil count, <2000/mm^3; platelet count, <80,000/mm^3; or hemoglobin, <4.5 g/dL) occurred. If marrow depression occurred, treatment was stopped until blood counts recovered and was then resumed at a lower dose. The maximum dose in the study was 35 mg/kg per day. Painful crises occurred at a median rate of 2.5 times per year in treated patients compared with 4.5 times per year among those given placebo (P < 0.001). Time between crises was also extended by hydroxyurea therapy. The study was too small to address the effect of treatment on the risk of stroke, although the findings are encouraging because the mechanism by which painful crises occur is likely similar to the pathogenesis of stroke. One small prospective study in 35 children with a history of stroke suggested that hydroxyurea plus phlebotomy might be as similarly effective as chronic transfusion therapy and iron chelation for long-term recurrent stroke prevention.[324] A multicenter trial comparing these two strategies for secondary stroke prevention plans to randomize 130 patients and began enrollment in 2006.[325] The major side effect of hydroxyurea is reversible, dose-related bone marrow suppression.

Quasimoyamoya disease resulting from sickle cell disease should presumably be managed in a manner similar to that for true moyamoya disease, as already described.[326-329] Bone marrow or hematopoietic stem cell transplantation may be considered for patients with high-risk sickle cell disease and may reduce the risk of recurrent stroke, although this remains controversial.[330,331]

Other strategies undergoing investigation in clinical trials include the use of overnight continuous positive airway pressure to prevent nocturnal oxygen desaturation, which has been associated with an increased risk of stroke, and the use of aspirin for stroke prevention.[332] Additionally, an ongoing randomized trial is investigating the role of transfusion therapy in patients with sickle cell disease and clinically silent cerebral infarction with normal TCD velocities.[332]

Miscellaneous Disorders

Migraine-Related Stroke

Epidemiologic evidence demonstrates that patients with migraines, particularly migraine with aura, have an increased risk of stroke.[333] However, the mechanism by which migraine is linked to stroke remains uncertain. Migraine is associated with a slowly spreading wave of cortical depolarization, which may cause a transient increase in cerebral blood flow followed by a period of relative hypoperfusion.[334,335] Migraine is also associated with abnormalities of platelet, coagulation, and endothelial function that may contribute to an increased risk of stroke.[336-340] In some patients, angiography has demonstrated evidence of an arteriopathy similar to vasospasm.[341-343] Further, mitochondrial abnormalities have been detected in some patients with migraine-induced stroke.[344] Finally, there appears to be an increased prevalence of patent foramen ovale in patients with migraine, which suggests the possibility that microembolism may link migraine and stroke in some patients.[345]

Early treatment specific for migraine-induced stroke has not been formally evaluated. Further, because migraine-related stroke is largely a diagnosis of exclusion, characterization in the early period before decisions are made about treatment is probably not feasible. Therefore, given mechanistic data suggesting coagulation and platelet activation in migraine, it seems reasonable to use thrombolytic and antithrombotic medications as would be used in stroke due to more typical causes.

Vasodilator agents have been administered to patients with migraine-related stroke and suspected or documented angiographic anomalies, although the efficacy of these agents is uncertain. Theoretically, migraine-related stroke might be treated immediately by inducing cerebral vasodilation to increase cerebral blood flow and/or inhibit the propagation of cortical spreading depressions. This may be accomplished with inhalation of 10% CO_2, isoproterenol, or nitrates, as these maneuvers may abolish the aura of migraine.[346-348] However, hypotension, confusion, and worsening headache as side effects of these treatments likely outweigh their unproven benefits. Calcium channel antagonists have also been used for this purpose, including intravenous nicardipine or oral nimodipine in a manner similar to that for vasospasm after subarachnoid hemorrhage, although there is little support from the literature.[348] Cerebral vasoconstrictive medications used for abortive migraine therapy, including ergots and triptans, should be avoided because of the concern that they may further reduce cerebral blood flow to the ischemic territory or precipitate a recurrent event.[342,343,349,350]

Long-term prevention of stroke recurrence in migraine-related stroke should probably include antiplatelet therapy, although, again, this has not been formally tested. Oral calcium channel antagonists including verapamil or amlodipine are widely used on the basis of theoretically preventing future vasoconstrictive episodes; again, however, evidence for this approach is lacking. Smoking cessation and aggressive treatment of traditional vascular risk factors are warranted in all patients with migraine, particularly those who have experienced stroke. Furthermore, given epidemiologic evidence suggesting a roughly eightfold increase in stroke risk in patients with migraine taking oral contraceptive agents, these should be discontinued after migraine-related stroke and alternative contraceptive strategies employed.[333,351]

Mitochondrial Encephalopathy, Lactic Acidosis, and Strokelike Episodes

Inherited abnormalities in the mitochondrial respiratory chain complexes may lead to the syndrome of mitochondrial encephalopathy, lactic acidosis, and strokelike episodes (MELAS). Stroke is usually attributed to a metabolic disturbance rather than a vascular mechanism, although there may be altered function of the smooth muscle cells in the microvasculature.[352] Several mutations have been identified in this syndrome, and no specific therapy is available to replace the abnormal gene product.[353,354] Supportive care includes the removal of offending systemic conditions and medications, such as hypoxemia, acidosis, infection, or barbiturates, if present. Administration of agents that alter mitochondrial metabolism has been used to limit the production of excess lactic acid. The drug used most often, coenzyme Q10 at a dose of 150 mg daily, has been shown to reduce abnormally elevated ratios of lactate:pyruvate,[355] although its clinical effect is uncertain. Moreover, there appears to be tremendous variability among patients with MELAS in their biochemical response to coenzyme Q that likely determines whether they will show any response to this intervention.[356] Fortunately, coenzyme Q is extremely well-tolerated and has no significant side effects, such that empiric use is sensible in patients with MELAS. Sodium dichloroacetate also appears to reduce lactate and pyruvate, and early reports suggested a possible clinical benefit.[357] However, a small randomized controlled trial involving 30 patients comparing dichloroacetate to placebo demonstrated unacceptable peripheral nerve toxicity associated with this agent without evidence of clinical benefit.[358] Several reports have suggested a role for l-arginine in the treatment of patients with MELAS, in that it may improve endothelial dysfunction and tissue perfusion.[359-361] In one study of 24 patients with MELAS, intravenous infusion of l-arginine seemed to attenuate the neurologic symptoms occurring during acute strokelike episodes, and long-term oral L-arginine supplementation appeared to decrease the frequency and severity of subsequent episodes.[362] Given the lack of a comparator placebo group, these observations must be interpreted cautiously. Other agents that have been reported in isolated case reports to be potentially beneficial include idebenone, vitamins K_3 (menadiol sodium diphosphate) and C, riboflavin, niacin, thiamine, and pyridoxine.[356,363-365]

Cerebral Venous Thrombosis

Cerebral venous thrombosis (CVT) is a rare but important cause of stroke for which specific therapy is available. Etiologic treatment is a principal consideration. CVT related to an infectious etiology, seen most commonly in children with otitis, sinusitis, tonsillitis, or pharyngitis, requires early administration of appropriate antibiotics. In adults, most cases are not related to infection, but systemic processes often are implicated.[366] A number of infrequent but potentially treatable causes of CVT include severe dehydration, malignancy, myeloproliferative disorders, hypercoagulable states, and inflammatory bowel disease, all of which require treatment of the systemic disorder for maximal treatment of the CVT and prevention of recurrent events. Many adult cases are associated with pregnancy and the puerperium and are more readily treated after the delivery of the child. Oral contraceptive agents have also been implicated as risk factors and should be discontinued.[351,367,368] The cause remains unknown in about 20% of cases.[369]

Symptomatic management of CVT should include attention to the treatment of seizures, metabolic derangements, cerebral edema, and elevated intracranial pressure, as dictated by the clinical situation. Seizures usually respond to standard anticonvulsant agents. Cerebral edema may be medically treated with mannitol, glycerol, acetazolamide, dextran, barbiturates, or corticosteroids, although there is considerable debate about the relative advantages of each.[369-371] Osmotherapy with mannitol or glycerol in repeated boluses may be particularly useful in dealing with abrupt elevations of intracranial pressure, particularly while more specific thrombolytic or antithrombotic medications are being initiated. Acetazolamide tends to be most useful in patients with relatively mild symptoms but is unlikely to offer great benefit in patients with severe cerebral edema. Corticosteroids have no proven role in CVT and may increase the risk of systemic infection. Barbiturates are problematic because they obscure the neurologic examination and may cause significant hypotension. In very severe cases, consideration may be given to lumbar puncture, shunting, or surgical decompression.[366] Decompressive craniectomy has been reported in cases with clinical signs of impending or active herniation, and some patients have had surprisingly good outcomes at long-term follow-up.[372,373] These invasive approaches may, however, limit the use of antithrombotic or thrombolytic treatments that are more likely to relieve the venous hypertension and the resultant cerebral edema. On the other hand, in one series of four patients undergoing decompressive craniectomy, half-dose heparin was restarted 12 hours postoperatively and full-dose heparin was resumed at 24 hours without bleeding complications.[373]

Therapeutic options for dealing with the thrombosis itself include anticoagulation, pharmacologic thrombolysis, mechanical devices for clot removal, or conservative observation. The role of anticoagulation in the treatment of CVT is rooted in a long history of controversy. Anticoagulation prevents further thrombus formation, thereby preventing the development of venous infarctions, both bland and hemorrhagic. However, in patients with hemorrhagic venous infarction due to CVT, anticoagulation may pose a risk of increased intracerebral bleeding. Some authors favor anticoagulation with heparin only in patients without radiologic and cerebrospinal fluid evidence of hemorrhage, while others favor a more aggressive stance and recommend heparin even in patients with documented hemorrhagic infarctions. CVT is one of the few uncommon causes of stroke that has been subjected to randomized controlled clinical trials. Einhaupl et al[374] planned to study 60 patients with CVT, randomly assigning them to receive either intravenous heparin (adjusted to a PTT of 80 to 100 seconds) or placebo saline infusion. The study was halted prematurely after only 20 patients were enrolled because of the dramatic and statistically significant benefit of heparin. At 3 months after treatment, eight of the 10 heparin-treated patients had complete recovery, and the remaining two had slight residual deficits. In contrast, only one patient in the placebo group had complete recovery, six had residual deficits, and three died ($P < 0.01$). Moreover, the benefit of heparin was demonstrable after only 3 days of treatment.

Einhaupl et al also performed a retrospective analysis to evaluate the role of heparin in CVT with hemorrhagic venous infarction and found that, of 43 patients, the mortality rates were 15% among patients treated with heparin and 69% among those not treated with heparin. A clinical trial of nadroparin, a low-molecular-weight heparin, was performed in 60 patients with CVT. The results were less dramatic than with unfractionated heparin, with a nonsignificant reduction in poor outcomes: 13% of the treated group and 21% in the placebo group. There were no new symptomatic intracerebral hemorrhages associated with nadroparin.[375] It is unclear whether there is a real difference in the efficacy of unfractionated and low-molecular-weight heparins or if the difference between these two studies reflects the relatively small size of both. Nevertheless, these two randomized trials taken together suggest a 15.5% (95% CI, -6% to 37%) reduction in death or dependence with anticoagulant treatment, although the sample size remained too small to draw a definitive conclusion.[375] Based on these results, acute anticoagulation is recommended for the majority of patients with CVT, even in the presence of hemorrhagic infarction. Reflecting this, in the International Study on Cerebral Vein and Dural Sinus Thrombosis (ISCVT), a multicenter, prospective, observational study, more than 80% of patients were treated with immediate anticoagulation.[376]

Thrombolysis offers the possibility of a more aggressive intervention than heparin, but its role remains poorly defined. Intravenous thrombolytic therapy for CVT has been reported to be of value in a few case series, but data are limited.[377,378] Local infusion of urokinase or t-PA into dural sinus thrombosis has been more widely used, although no controlled trials have been published.[379] In most reported series of local thrombolysis, relatively low doses of thrombolytic agent are administered (t-PA, 1 to 2 mg/h) as a continuous infusion. Mechanical thrombolysis, in particular with the use of rheolytic thrombectomy (Angiojet catheter), has been increasingly reported, typically in conjunction with pharmacologic thrombolysis.[380-385] Most series have also treated patients concurrently with intravenous heparin as already described. In a nonrandomized comparison of 40 patients with superior sagittal sinus thrombosis, 16 of 20 patients (80%) treated with local urokinase returned to normal compared with only 9 of 20 (45%) treated with heparin (P = 0.019), even though patients in the thrombolysis group had more severe deficits before treatment.[386] A systematic review of 72 studies reporting 169 patients treated with pharmacologic thrombolysis, including roughly 30% with hemorrhagic infarcts, found a relatively low rate of bleeding complications (5% intracerebral hemorrhage with neurologic deterioration, 2% extracranial hemorrhage requiring transfusion), and good outcomes were achieved in most patients. However, a prospective case series of 20 patients treated with pharmacologic and mechanical thrombolysis, 70% of whom had hemorrhagic infarction, found a much higher risk of symptomatic hemorrhage (25%), raising the possibility of publication bias in prior case reports.[387] Until a randomized clinical trial is performed and given the apparent efficacy of heparin in most cases, thrombolytic therapy should probably be reserved for patients who decline despite adequate anticoagulation

or patients who rapidly deteriorate owing to extensive thrombosis in multiple venous sinuses; it may also possibly be reserved for patients with thrombosis of the deep venous system, given the worse prognosis associated with this location.[376,388,389]

After early treatment with intravenous heparin and/or thrombolytics, oral anticoagulation with warfarin is typically used for ongoing therapy, although the ideal duration of therapy has not been established. Many authors recommend warfarin empirically for 1 to 3 months,[369] whereas others use MRI and MR venography to determine whether flow is reestablished before discontinuing therapy. Prolonged anticoagulation therapy may be required for refractory cases or for patients with an underlying prothrombotic state.[390] In women with CVT related to pregnancy or the puerperium, many experts advocate prophylactic anticoagulation during future pregnancies.[369] If the CVT developed during a prior pregnancy, then subcutaneous low molecular weight heparin is often recommended during the next pregnancy and for up to 8 weeks postpartum. If the prior CVT was a puerperal event, then anticoagulation is solely used for 4 to 8 weeks after delivery.

REFERENCES

1. Adams HP Jr, Butler MJ, Biller J, Toffol GJ: Nonhemorrhagic cerebral infarction in young adults, *Arch Neurol* 43:793-796, 1986.
2. Adams HP Jr, Kappelle LJ, Biller J, et al: Ischemic stroke in young adults. Experience in 329 patients enrolled in the Iowa Registry of Stroke in young adults, *Arch Neurol* 52:491-495, 1995.
3. Bogousslavsky J, Pierre P: Ischemic stroke in patients under age 45, *Neurol Clin* 10:113-124, 1992.
4. Carolei A, Marini C, Ferranti E, et al: A prospective study of cerebral ischemia in the young. Analysis of pathogenic determinants. The National Research Council Study Group, *Stroke* 24:362-367, 1993.
5. Knoflach M, Furtner M, Mair A, et al: [Juvenile stroke—results from the Austrian Stroke Registry.], *Wien Med Wochenschr* 158:453-457, 2008.
6. Leys D, Bandu L, Henon H, et al: Clinical outcome in 287 consecutive young adults (15 to 45 years) with ischemic stroke, *Neurology* 59:26-33, 2002.
7. Brandt T, Hausser I, Orberk E, et al: Ultrastructural connective tissue abnormalities in patients with spontaneous cervicocerebral artery dissections, *Ann Neurol* 44:281-285, 1998.
8. Mayer SA, Rubin BS, Starman BJ, Byers PH: Spontaneous multivessel cervical artery dissection in a patient with a substitution of alanine for glycine (g13a) in the alpha 1 (I) chain of type I collagen, *Neurology* 47:552-556, 1996.
9. van den Berg JS, Limburg M, Kappelle LJ, et al: The role of type III collagen in spontaneous cervical arterial dissections, *Ann Neurol* 43:494-498, 1998.
10. Brandt T, Morcher M, Hausser I: Association of cervical artery dissection with connective tissue abnormalities in skin and arteries, *Front Neurol Neurosci* 20:16-29, 2005.
11. Volker W, Ringelstein EB, Dittrich R, et al: Morphometric analysis of collagen fibrils in skin of patients with spontaneous cervical artery dissection, *J Neurol Neurosurg Psychiatry* 79:1007-1012, 2008.
12. The National Institute of Neurological Disorders and Stroke rt-PA Stroke Study Group: Tissue plasminogen activator for acute ischemic stroke, *N Engl J Med* 333:1581-1587, 1995.
13. Saver JL, Easton JD: Dissections and trauma of cervicocerebral arteries. In Barnett HJM, Mohr JP, Stein BM, Yatsu FM, editors: *Stroke: Pathophysiology, diagnosis, and management*, New York, 1998, Churchill Livingstone, pp 769-786.
14. Derex L, Nighoghossian N, Turjman F, et al: Intravenous t-PA in acute ischemic stroke related to internal carotid artery dissection, *Neurology* 54:2159-2161, 2000.

15. Georgiadis D, Lanczik O, Schwab S, et al: IV thrombolysis in patients with acute stroke due to spontaneous carotid dissection, *Neurology* 64:1612-1614, 2005.

16. Furlan A, Higashida R, Wechsler L, et al: Intra-arterial prourokinase for acute ischemic stroke. The PROACT II Study: A randomized controlled trial, *JAMA* 282:2003-2011, 1999.

17. Sampognaro G, Turgut T, Conners JJ 3rd, et al: Intra-arterial thrombolysis in a patient presenting with an ischemic stroke due to spontaneous internal carotid artery dissection, *Catheter Cardiovasc Interv* 48:312-315, 1999.

18. Price RF, Sellar R, Leung C, et al: Traumatic vertebral arterial dissection and vertebrobasilar arterial thrombosis successfully treated with endovascular thrombolysis and stenting, *AJNR: Am J Neuroradiol* 19:1677-1680, 1998.

19. Gomez CR, May AK, Terry JB, et al: Endovascular therapy of traumatic injuries of the extracranial cerebral arteries, *Crit Care Clin* 15:789-809, 1999.

20. Arnold M, Nedeltchev K, Sturzenegger M, et al: Thrombolysis in patients with acute stroke caused by cervical artery dissection: Analysis of 9 patients and review of the literature, *Arch Neurol* 59:549-553, 2002.

21. Cerrato P, Berardino M, Bottacchi E, et al: Vertebral artery dissection complicated by basilar artery occlusion successfully treated with intra-arterial thrombolysis: Three case reports, *Neurol Sci* 29:51-55, 2008.

22. Cohen JE, Leker RR, Gotkine M, et al: Emergent stenting to treat patients with carotid artery dissection: Clinically and radiologically directed therapeutic decision making, *Stroke* 34:e254-257, 2003.

23. Lavallee PC, Mazighi M, Saint-Maurice J-P, et al: Stent-assisted endovascular thrombolysis versus intravenous thrombolysis in internal carotid artery dissection with tandem internal carotid and middle cerebral artery occlusion, *Stroke* 38:2270-2274, 2007.

24. Abboud H, Houdart E, Meseguer E, Amarenco P: Stent assisted endovascular thrombolysis of internal carotid artery dissection, *J Neurol Neurosurg Psychiatry* 76:292-293, 2005.

25. Cohen JE, Gomori JM, Grigoriadis S, et al: Intra-arterial thrombolysis and stent placement for traumatic carotid dissection with subsequent stroke: A combined, simultaneous endovascular approach, *J Neurol Sci* 269:172-175, 2008.

26. Mokri B: Cervicocephalic arterial dissections. In Bogousslavsky J, Caplan LR, editors: *Uncommon causes of stroke*, Cambridge, 2001, Cambridge University Press, pp 211-229.

27. Molina CA, Alvarez-Sabin J, Schonewille W, et al: Cerebral microembolism in acute spontaneous internal carotid artery dissection, *Neurology* 55:1738-1740, 2000.

28. Leys D, Lucas C, Gobert M, et al: Cervical artery dissections, *Eur Neurol* 37:3-12, 1997.

29. Hart RG, Easton JD: Dissections of cervical and cerebral arteries, *Neurol Clin* 1:155-182, 1983.

30. Sturzenegger M: Spontaneous internal carotid artery dissection: Early diagnosis and management in 44 patients, *J Neurol* 242:231-238, 1995.

31. Hill MD, Hwa G, Perry JR: Extracranial cervical artery dissection, *Stroke* 31:799, 2000.

32. Lucas C, Moulin T, Deplanque D, et al: Stroke patterns of internal carotid artery dissection in 40 patients, *Stroke* 29:2646-2648, 1998.

33. Kasner SE, Hankins LL, Bratina P, et al: Magnetic resonance angiography demonstrates vascular healing of carotid and vertebral artery dissections, *Stroke* 28:1993-1997, 1997.

34. Biousse V, D'Anglejan-Chatillon J, Touboul P-J, et al: Time course of symptoms in extracranial carotid artery dissections. A series of 80 patients, *Stroke* 36:235-239, 1995.

35. Lyrer P, Engelter S: Antithrombotic drugs for carotid artery dissection, *Cochrane Database Syst Rev* 3:CD000255, 2003.

36. Menon R, Kerry S, Norris JW, Markus HS: Treatment of cervical artery dissection: A systematic review and meta-analysis, *J Neurol Neurosurg Psychiatry* 79:1122-1127, 2008.

37. Touze E, Gauvrit J-Y, Moulin T, et al: Risk of stroke and recurrent dissection after a cervical artery dissection: A multicenter study, *Neurology* 61:1347-1351, 2003.

38. Georgiadis D, Arnold M, von Buedingen HC, et al: Aspirin versus anticoagulation in carotid artery dissection: A study of 298 patients, *Neurology* 72:1810-1815, 2009.

39. Jacobs A, Lanfermann H, Szelies B, et al: MRI- and MRA-guided therapy of carotid and vertebral artery dissections (abstract), *Cerebrovasc Dis* 6(Suppl 2):80, 1996.

40. Mokri B, Sundt TM, Houser OW, Piepgras DG: Spontaneous dissection of the cervical internal carotid artery, *Ann Neurol* 19:126-138, 1986.

41. Levy C, Laissy JP, Raveau V, et al: Carotid and vertebral artery dissections: Three-dimensional time-of-flight MR angiography and MR imaging versus conventional angiography, *Radiology* 190:97-103, 1994.

42. Mokri B: Traumatic and spontaneous extracranial internal carotid artery dissections, *J Neurol* 237:356-361, 1990.

43. Houser OW, Mokri B, Sundt TM, et al: Spontaneous cervical cephalic arterial dissection and its residuum: Angiographic spectrum, *AJNR Am J Neuroradiol* 5:27-34, 1983.

44. Leclerc X, Godefroy O, Salhi A, et al: Helical CT for the diagnosis of extracranial internal carotid artery dissection, *Stroke* 27:461-466, 1996.

45. Benninger DH, Gandjour J, Georgiadis D, et al: Benign long-term outcome of conservatively treated cervical aneurysms due to carotid dissection, *Neurology* 69:486-487, 2007.

46. Perez-Cruet MJ, Patwardhan RV, Mawad ME, Rose JE: Treatment of dissecting pseudoaneurysm of the cervical internal carotid artery using a wall stent and detachable coils: Case report, *Neurosurgery* 40:622-625, 1997:discussion 625-626.

47. Candon E, Marty-Ane C, Pieuchot P, Frerebeau P: Cervical-to-petrous internal carotid artery saphenous vein in situ bypass for the treatment of a high cervical dissecting aneurysm: Technical case report, *Neurosurgery* 39:863-866, 1996.

48. Treiman GS, Treiman RL, Foran RF, et al: Spontaneous dissection of the internal carotid artery: A nineteen-year clinical experience, *J Vasc Surg* 24:597-605, 1996:discussion 605-597.

49. Schievink WI, Piepgras DG, McCaffrey TV, Mokri B: Surgical treatment of extracranial internal carotid artery dissecting aneurysms, *Neurosurgery* 35:809-815, 1994:discussion 815-806.

50. Morgan MK, Sekhon LH: Extracranial-intracranial saphenous vein bypass for carotid or vertebral artery dissections: A report of six cases, *J Neurosurg* 80:237-246, 1994.

51. Chiche L, Praquin B, Koskas F, Kieffer E: Spontaneous dissection of the extracranial vertebral artery: Indications and long-term outcome of surgical treatment, *Ann Vasc Surg* 19:5-10, 2005.

52. Guillon B, Brunereau L, Biousse V, et al: Long-term follow-up of aneurysms developed during extracranial internal carotid artery dissection, *Neurology* 53:117-122, 1999.

53. Touze E, Randoux B, Meary E, et al: Aneurysmal forms of cervical artery dissection: Associated factors and outcome, *Stroke* 32:418-423, 2001.

54. Mokri B: Spontaneous dissections of internal carotid arteries, *Neurologist* 3:104-119, 1997.

55. Bogousslavsky J, Despland P-A, Regli F: Spontaneous carotid dissection with acute stroke, *Arch Neurol* 44:137-140, 1987.

56. DeOcampo J, Brillman J, Levy DI: Stenting: A new approach to carotid dissection, *J Neuroimaging* 7:187-190, 1997.

57. Malek AM, Higashida RT, Phatouros CC, et al: Endovascular management of extracranial carotid artery dissection achieved using stent angioplasty, *AJNR Am J Neuroradiol* 21:1280-1292, 2000.

58. Muller BT, Luther B, Hort W, et al: Surgical treatment of 50 carotid dissections: Indications and results, *J Vasc Surg* 31:980-988, 2000.

59. Ogiwara H, Maeda K, Hara T, et al: Spontaneous intracranial internal carotid artery dissection treated by intra-arterial thrombolysis and superficial temporal artery-middle cerebral artery anastomosis in the acute stage—case report, *Neurol Med Chir (Tokyo)* 45:148-151, 2005.

60. Collins GJ Jr, Rich NM, Clagett GP, et al: Fibromuscular dysplasia of the internal carotid arteries. Clinical experience and follow-up, *Ann Surg* 194:89-96, 1981.

61. Vles JS, Hendriks JJ, Lodder J, Janevski B: Multiple vertebro-basilar infarctions from fibromuscular dysplasia related dissecting aneurysm of the vertebral artery in a child, *Neuropediatrics* 21:104-105, 1990.

62. Perez-Higueras A, Alvarez-Ruiz F, Martinez-Bermejo A, et al: Cerebellar infarction from fibromuscular dysplasia and dissecting aneurysm of the vertebral artery. Report of a child, *Stroke* 19:521-524, 1988.

63. Dufour JJ, Lavigne F, Plante R, Caouette H: Pulsatile tinnitus and fibromuscular dysplasia of the internal carotid, *J Otolaryngol* 14:293-295, 1985.

64. Corrin LS, Sandok BA, Houser OW: Cerebral ischemic events in patients with carotid artery fibromuscular dysplasia, *Arch Neurol* 38:616-618, 1981.

65. Wesen CA, Elliott BM: Fibromuscular dysplasia of the carotid arteries, *Am J Surg* 151:448-451, 1986.

66. Mettinger KL, Ericson K: Fibromuscular dysplasia and the brain. I. Observations on angiographic, clinical and genetic characteristics, *Stroke* 13:46-52, 1982.

67. Mettinger KL: Fibromuscular dysplasia and the brain. II. Current concept of the disease, *Stroke* 13:53-58, 1982.

68. Slovut DP, Olin JW: Fibromuscular dysplasia, *N Engl J Med* 350:1862-1871, 2004.

69. The Stroke Prevention in Atrial Fibrillation Investigators: Bleeding during antithrombotic therapy in patients with atrial fibrillation, *Arch Intern Med* 156:409-416, 1996.

70. Evans A, Kalra L: Are the results of randomized controlled trials on anticoagulation in patients with atrial fibrillation generalizable to clinical practice? *Arch Intern Med* 161:1443-1447, 2001.

71. Evans A, Perez I, Yu G, Kalra L: Secondary stroke prevention in atrial fibrillation: Lessons from clinical practice, *Stroke* 31:2106-2111, 2000.

72. Hooshmand H, Boykin ME, Vines FS, Lee HM: Fibromuscular dysplasia of the extracranial internal carotid arteries associated with an ulcerative plaque, *Stroke* 3:67-70, 1972.

73. Effeney DJ, Ehrenfeld WK, Stoney RJ, et al: Why operate on carotid fibromuscular dysplasia? *Arch Surg* 115:1261-1265, 1980.

74. Effeney DJ, Ehrenfeld WK, Stoney RJ, Wylie EJ: Fibromuscular dysplasia of the internal carotid artery, *World J Surg* 3:179-186, 1979.

75. Stewart MT, Moritz MW, Smith RB 3rd, et al: The natural history of carotid fibromuscular dysplasia, *J Vasc Surg* 3:305-310, 1986.

76. Smith DC, Smith LL, Hasso AN: Fibromuscular dysplasia of the internal carotid artery treated by operative transluminal balloon angioplasty, *Radiology* 155:645-648, 1985.

77. Smith LL, Smith DC, Killeen JD, et al: Operative balloon angioplasty in the treatment of internal carotid artery fibromuscular dysplasia, *J Vasc Surg* 6:482-487, 1987.

78. Van Damme H, Sakalihasan N, Limet R: Fibromuscular dysplasia of the internal carotid artery. Personal experience with 13 cases and literature review, *Acta Chir Belg* 99:163-168, 1999.

79. van den Hoven RW, Mali WP, Theodorides T: Transluminal dilatation of the internal carotid artery in fibromuscular dysplasia—a case history, *Angiology* 39:272-275, 1988.

80. Jooma R, Bradshaw JR, Griffith HB: Intimal dissection following percutaneous transluminal carotid angioplasty for fibromuscular dysplasia, *Neuroradiology* 27:181-182, 1985.

81. Wilms GE, Smits J, Baert AL, et al: Percutaneous transluminal angioplasty in fibromuscular dysplasia of the internal carotid artery: One year clinical and morphological follow-up, *Cardiovasc Intervent Radiol* 8:20-23, 1985.

82. Dublin AB, Baltaxe HA, Cobb CA 3rd: Percutaneous transluminal carotid angioplasty and detachable balloon embolization in fibromuscular dysplasia, *AJNR: Am J Neuroradiol* 5:646-648, 1984.

83. Belan A, Vesela M, Vanek I, et al: Percutaneous transluminal angioplasty of fibromuscular dysplasia of the internal carotid artery, *Cardiovasc Intervent Radiol* 5:79-81, 1982.

84. Hasso AN, Bird CR, Zinke DE, Thompson JR: Fibromuscular dysplasia of the internal carotid artery: Percutaneous transluminal angioplasty, *AJR Am J Roentgenol* 136:955-960, 1981.

85. Balaji MR, DeWeese JA: Fibromuscular dysplasia of the internal carotid artery: Its occurrence with acute stroke and its surgical reversal, *Arch Surg* 115:984-986, 1980.

86. Finsterer J, Strassegger J, Haymerle A, et al: Bilateral stenting of symptomatic and asymptomatic internal carotid artery stenosis due to fibromuscular dysplasia, *J Neurol Neurosurg Psychiatry* 69:683-686, 2000.

87. Takigami M, Baba T, Saitou K: [Percutaneous transluminal angioplasty in fibromuscular dysplasia of the internal carotid artery: Case report], *No Shinkei Geka* 30:301-306, 2002.

88. Calabrese LH, Dodick DW, Schwedt TJ, Singhal AB: Narrative review: Reversible cerebral vasoconstriction syndromes, *Ann Intern Med* 146:34-44, 2007.

89. Ichiki M, Watanabe O, Okamoto Y, et al: [A case of reversible cerebral vasoconstriction syndrome (RCVS) triggered by a Chinese herbal medicine], *Rinsho Shinkeigaku* 48:267-270, 2008.

90. Noskin O, Jafarimojarrad E, Libman RB, Nelson JL: Diffuse cerebral vasoconstriction (Call-Fleming syndrome) and stroke associated with antidepressants, *Neurology* 67:159-160, 2006.

91. Singhal AB, Bernstein RA: Postpartum angiopathy and other cerebral vasoconstriction syndromes, *Neurocrit Care* 3:91-97, 2005.

92. Janssens E, Hommel M, Mounier-Vehier F, et al: Postpartum cerebral angiopathy possibly due to bromocriptine therapy, *Stroke* 26:128-130, 1995.

93. Levine SR, Washington JM, Jefferson MF, et al: "Crack" cocaine-associated stroke, *Neurology* 37:1849-1853, 1987.

94. Merkel PA, Koroshetz WJ, Irizarry MC, et al: Cocaine-associated cerebral vasculitis, *Semin Arthritis Rheum* 25:172-183, 1995.

95. Henry PY, Larre P, Aupy M, et al: Reversible cerebral arteriopathy associated with the administration of ergot derivatives, *Cephalalgia* 4:171-178, 1984.

96. Le Coz P, Woimant F, Rougemont D, et al: [Benign cerebral angiopathies and phenylpropanolamine], *Rev Neurol (Paris)* 144:295-300, 1988.

97. Raroque HG Jr, Tesfa G, Purdy P: Postpartum cerebral angiopathy. Is there a role for sympathomimetic drugs? *Stroke* 24:2108-2110, 1993.

98. Singhal AB, Caviness VS, Begleiter AF, et al: Cerebral vasoconstriction and stroke after use of serotonergic drugs, *Neurology* 58:130-133, 2002.

99. Nighoghossian N, Derex L, Trouillas P: Multiple intracerebral hemorrhages and vasospasm following antimigrainous drug abuse, *Headache* 38:478-480, 1998.

100. Hajj-Ali RA, Furlan A, Abou-Chebel A, et al: Benign angiopathy of the central nervous system: Cohort of 16 patients with clinical course and long-term follow up, *Arthritis Rheum* 47:662-669, 2002.

101. Nowak DA, Rodiek SO, Henneken S, et al: Reversible segmental cerebral vasoconstriction (Call-Fleming syndrome): Are calcium channel inhibitors a potential treatment option? *Cephalalgia* 23:218-222, 2003.

102. Dodick DW: Reversible segmental cerebral vasoconstriction (Call-Fleming syndrome): The role of calcium antagonists, *Cephalalgia* 23:163-165, 2003.

103. Lu SR, Liao YC, Fuh JL, et al: Nimodipine for treatment of primary thunderclap headache, *Neurology* 62:1414-1416, 2004.

104. Chen D, Nishizawa S, Yokota N, et al: High-dose methylprednisolone prevents vasospasm after subarachnoid hemorrhage through inhibition of protein kinase c activation, *Neurol Res* 24:215-222, 2002.

105. Singhal AB: Postpartum angiopathy with reversible posterior leukoencephalopathy, *Arch Neurol* 61:411-416, 2004.

106. Rubiera del Fueyo M, Molina Cateriano CA, Arenillas Lara JF, et al: [Reversible segmental cerebral vasoconstriction: The value of duplex transcranial Doppler in its diagnosis and follow up], *Rev Neurol* 38:530-533, 2004.

107. Chen SP, Fuh JL, Chang FC, et al: Transcranial color Doppler study for reversible cerebral vasoconstriction syndromes, *Ann Neurol* 63:751-757, 2008.

108. Bogousslavsky J, Despland PA, Regli F, et al: Postpartum cerebral angiopathy: Reversible vasoconstriction assessed by transcranial Doppler ultrasounds, *Eur Neurol* 29:102-105, 1989.

109. Glantz MJ, Burger PC, Friedman AH, et al: Treatment of radiation-induced nervous system injury with heparin and warfarin, *Neurology* 44:2020-2027, 1994.

110. Jellinger K, Sturm KW: Delayed radiation myelopathy in man. Report of twelve necropsy cases, *J Neurol Sci* 14:389-408, 1971.

111. Mitchell WG, Fishman LS, Miller JH, et al: Stroke as a late sequela of cranial irradiation for childhood brain tumors, *J Child Neurol* 6:128-133, 1991.

112. Peterson DI, Alfonso F, Geslani B: Cerebral infarction due to radiation accelerated arteriosclerosis, *Bull Clin Neurosci* 52:43-46, 1987.

113. Nardelli E, Fiaschi A, Ferrari G: Delayed cerebrovascular consequences of radiation to the neck. A clinicopathologic study of a case, *Arch Neurol* 35:538-540, 1978.

114. Conomy JP, Kellermeyer RW: Delayed cerebrovascular consequences of therapeutic radiation. A clinicopathologic study of a stroke associated with radiation-related carotid arteriopathy, *Cancer* 36:1702-1708, 1975.

115. Andros G, Schneider PA, Harris RW, et al: Management of arterial occlusive disease following radiation therapy, *Cardiovasc Surg* 4:135-142, 1996.

116. Carmody BJ, Arora S, Avena R, et al: Accelerated carotid artery disease after high-dose head and neck radiotherapy: Is there a role for routine carotid duplex surveillance? *J Vasc Surg* 30:1045-1051, 1999.

117. Kashyap VS, Moore WS, Quinones-Baldrich WJ: Carotid artery repair for radiation-associated atherosclerosis is a safe and durable procedure, *J Vasc Surg* 29:90-96, 1999:discussion 97-99.

118. Brown MM: Surgery, angioplasty, and interventional neuroradiology, *Curr Opin Neurol Neurosurg* 6:66-73, 1993.

119. Cohen JE, Rajz G, Lylyk P, et al: Protected stent-assisted angioplasty in radiation-induced carotid artery stenosis, *Neurol Res* 27(Suppl 1):S69-72, 2005.

120. Harrod-Kim P, Kadkhodayan Y, Derdeyn CP, et al: Outcomes of carotid angioplasty and stenting for radiation-associated stenosis, *AJNR Am J Neuroradiol* 26:1781-1788, 2005.

121. Ishikawa T, Houkin K, Yoshimoto T, Abe H: Vasoreconstructive surgery for radiation-induced vasculopathy in childhood, *Surg Neurol* 48:620-626, 1997.

122. Suzuki J: *Moyamoya disease*, Berlin, 1986, Springer-Verlag.

123. Bonduel M, Hepner M, Sciuccati G, et al: Prothrombotic disorders in children with moyamoya syndrome, *Stroke* 32:1786-1792, 2001.

124. Imaizumi T, Hayashi K, Saito K, et al: Long-term outcomes of pediatric moyamoya disease monitored to adulthood, *Pediatr Neurol* 18:321-325, 1998.

125. Nakase H, Ohnishi H, Touho H, et al: Clinical study of epileptic type moyamoya disease in children, *Jpn J Psychiatry Neurol* 46:419-420, 1992.

126. Norris JW: Steroid therapy in acute cerebral infarction, *Arch Neurol* 33:69-71, 1976.

127. Norris JW, Hachinski VC: High dose steroid treatment in cerebral infarction, *BMJ* 292:21-23, 1986.

128. Patten BM, Mendell J, Bruun B, et al: Double-blind study of the effects of dexamethasone on acute stroke, *Neurology* 22:377-383, 1972.

129. Bauer RB, Tellez H: Dexamethasone as treatment in cerebrovascular disease: 2. A controlled study in acute cerebral infarction, *Stroke* 4:547-555, 1973.

130. Qizilbash N, Lewington SL, Lopez-Arrieta JM: Corticosteroids for acute ischaemic stroke, *Cochrane Database Syst Rev* 2:CD000064, 2002.

131. Morgenstern LB, Frankowski RF, Shedden P, et al: Surgical treatment for intracerebral hemorrhage (STICH): A single-center, randomized clinical trial, *Neurology* 51:1359-1363, 1998.

132. Morgenstern LB, Demchuk AM, Kim DH, et al: Rebleeding leads to poor outcome in ultra-early craniotomy for intracerebral hemorrhage, *Neurology* 56:1294-1299, 2001.

133. Fukui M, Kawano T: Follow-up study of registered cases in 1995. In Fukui M, editor: *Annual report (1995) by research committee on spontaneous occlusion of the circle of Willis*, Toyko, 1996, Ministry of Health and Welfare.

134. Kuroda S, Hashimoto N, Yoshimoto T, et al: Radiological findings, clinical course, and outcome in asymptomatic moyamoya disease: Results of multicenter survey in Japan, *Stroke* 38:1430-1435, 2007.

135. Houkin K, Ishikawa T, Yoshimoto T, et al: Direct and indirect revascularization for moyamoya disease: Surgical techniques and peri-operative complications, *Clin Neurol Neurosurg* 99:S142-145, 1997.

136. Srinivasan J, Britz GW, Newell DW: Cerebral revascularization for moyamoya disease in adults, *Neurosurg Clin N Am* 12:585-594, 2001:ix.

137. Houkin K, Kuroda S, Nakayama N: Cerebral revascularization for moyamoya disease in children, *Neurosurg Clin N Am* 12:575-584, 2001:ix.

138. Irikura K, Miyasaka Y, Kurata A, et al: The effect of encephalomyo-synangiosis on abnormal collateral vessels in childhood moyamoya disease, *Neurol Res* 22:341-346, 2000.

139. Kawaguchi S, Okuno S, Sakaki T: Effect of direct arterial bypass on the prevention of future stroke in patients with the hemorrhagic variety of moyamoya disease, *J Neurosurg* 93:397-401, 2000.

140. Houkin K, Kuroda S, Ishikawa T, et al: Neovascularization (angiogenesis) after revascularization in moyamoya disease. Which technique is most useful for moyamoya disease? *Acta Neurochir (Wien)* 142:269-276, 2000.

141. Morimoto M, Iwama T, Hashimoto N, et al: Efficacy of direct revascularization in adult moyamoya disease: Haemodynamic evaluation by positron emission tomography, *Acta Neurochir (Wien)* 141:377-384, 1999.

142. Golby AJ, Marks MP, Thompson RC, et al: Direct and combined revascularization in pediatric moyamoya disease, *Neurosurgery* 45:50-58, 1999:discussion 58-60.

143. Matsushima T, Inoue T, Katsuta T, et al: An indirect revascularization method in the surgical treatment of moyamoya disease—various kinds of indirect procedures and a multiple combined indirect procedure, *Neurol Med Chir(Tokyo)* 38:297-302, 1998.

144. Rodriguez GJ, Kirmani JF, Ezzeddine MA, et al: Primary percutaneous transluminal angioplasty for early moyamoya disease, *J Neuroimaging* 17:48-53, 2007.

145. Lentz SR: Does homocysteine promote atherosclerosis? *Arterioscler Thromb Vasc Biol* 21:1385-1386, 2001.

146. Hankey GJ, Eikelboom JW: Homocysteine and stroke, *Curr Opin Neurol* 14:95-102, 2001.

147. Lentz SR: Mechanisms of thrombosis in hyperhomocysteinemia, *Curr Opin Hematol* 5:343-349, 1998.

148. Lentz SR, Sadler JE: Inhibition of thrombomodulin surface expression and protein C activation by the thrombogenic agent homocysteine, *J Clin Invest* 88:1906-1914, 1991.

149. Yap S: Classical homocystinuria: Vascular risk and its prevention, *J Inherit Metab Dis* 26:259-265, 2003.

150. Yap S, Boers GH, Wilcken B, et al: Vascular outcome in patients with homocystinuria due to cystathionine beta-synthase deficiency treated chronically: A multicenter observational study, *Arterioscler Thromb Vasc Biol* 21:2080-2085, 2001.

151. Fallon UB, Elwood P, Ben-Shlomo Y, et al: Homocysteine and ischaemic stroke in men: The Caerphilly Study, *J Epidemiol Community Health* 55:91-96, 2001.

152. Hackam DG, Peterson JC, Spence JD: What level of plasma homocyst(e)ine should be treated? Effects of vitamin therapy on progression of carotid atherosclerosis in patients with homocyst(e)ine levels above and below 14 micromol/l, *Am J Hypertens* 13:105-110, 2000.

153. The VITATOPS Trial Study Group: B vitamins in patients with recent transient ischemic attack or stroke in the vitamins to prevent stroke (VITATOPS) trial: A randomised, double-blind, parallel, placebo-controlled trial, *Lancet Neurol* 9:855-865, 2010.

154. Spence JD, Bang H, Chambless LE, et al: Vitamin intervention for stroke prevention trial: An efficacy analysis, *Stroke* 36:2404-2409, 2005.

155. Hankey GJ, Algra A, Chen C, et al: VITATOPS, the Vitamins To Prevent Stroke Trial: Rationale and design of a randomised trial of B-vitamin therapy in patients with recent transient ischaemic attack or stroke (nct00097669) (isrctn74743444), *Int J Stroke* 2:144-150, 2007.

156. Ebbing M, Bleie O, Ueland PM, et al: Mortality and cardiovascular events in patients treated with homocysteine-lowering B vitamins after coronary angiography: A randomized controlled trial, *JAMA* 300:795-804, 2008.

157. Bonaa KH, Njolstad I, Ueland PM, et al: Homocysteine lowering and cardiovascular events after acute myocardial infarction, *N Engl J Med* 354:1578-1588, 2006.

158. The Heart Outcomes Prevention Evaluation I: Homocysteine lowering with folic acid and b vitamins in vascular disease, *N Engl J Med* 354:1567-1577, 2006.

159. Utsumi K, Yamamoto N, Kase R, et al: High incidence of thrombosis in Fabry's disease, *Intern Med* 36:327-329, 1997.

160. Ashley GA, Shabbeer J, Yasuda M, et al: Fabry disease: Twenty novel alpha-galactosidase A mutations causing the classical phenotype, *J Hum Genet* 46:192-196, 2001.

161. Castro LH, Monteiro ML, Barbosa ER, et al: Fabry's disease in a female carrier with bilateral thalamic infarcts: A case report and a family study, *Rev Paul Med* 112:649-653, 1994.

162. Frustaci A, Chimenti C, Ricci R, et al: Improvement in cardiac function in the cardiac variant of Fabry's disease with galactose-infusion therapy, *N Engl J Med* 345:25-32, 2001.

163. Rolfs A, Bottcher T, Zschiesche M, et al: Prevalence of Fabry disease in patients with cryptogenic stroke: A prospective study, *Lancet* 366:1794-1796, 2005.

164. Eng CM, Guffon N, Wilcox WR, et al: Safety and efficacy of recombinant human alpha-galactosidase A—replacement therapy in Fabry's disease, *N Engl J Med* 345:9-16, 2001.

165. Banikazemi M, Bultas J, Waldek S, et al: Agalsidase-beta therapy for advanced Fabry disease: A randomized trial, *Ann Intern Med* 146:77-86, 2007.

166. Bierer G, Balfe D, Wilcox WR, et al: Improvement in serial cardiopulmonary exercise testing following enzyme replacement therapy in Fabry disease, *J Inherit Metab Dis* 29:572-579, 2006.

167. Germain DP, Waldek S, Banikazemi M, et al: Sustained, long-term renal stabilization after 54 months of agalsidase beta therapy in patients with Fabry disease, *J Am Soc Nephrol* 18:1547-1557, 2007.

168. Beer M, Weidemann F, Breunig F, et al: Impact of enzyme replacement therapy on cardiac morphology and function and late enhancement in Fabry's cardiomyopathy, *Am J Cardiol* 97:1515-1518, 2006.

169. Moore DF, Scott LT, Gladwin MT, et al: Regional cerebral hyperperfusion and nitric oxide pathway dysregulation in Fabry disease: Reversal by enzyme replacement therapy, *Circulation* 104:1506-1512, 2001.

170. Wilcox WR, Banikazemi M, Guffon N, et al: Long-term safety and efficacy of enzyme replacement therapy for Fabry disease, *Am J Hum Genet* 75:65-74, 2004.

171. Germain DP: Fabry disease: The need to stratify patient populations to better understand the outcome of enzyme replacement therapy, *Clin Ther* 29(Suppl A):S17-18, 2007.

172. Ferro JM: Vasculitis of the central nervous system, *J Neurol* 245:766-776, 1998.

173. Calabrese LH, Mallek JA: Primary angiitis of the central nervous system. Report of 8 new cases, review of the literature, and proposal for diagnostic criteria, *Medicine* 67:20-39, 1988.

174. Salvarani C, Brown RD Jr, Calamia KT, et al: Primary central nervous system vasculitis: Analysis of 101 patients, *Ann Neurol* 62:442-451, 2007.

175. Moore PM: Diagnosis and management of isolated angiitis of the central nervous system, *Neurology* 39:167-173, 1989.

176. Woolfenden AR, Tong DC, Marks MP, et al: Angiographically defined primary angiitis of the CNS: Is it really benign? *Neurology* 51:183-188, 1998.

177. Barron TF, Ostrov BE, Zimmerman RA, et al: Isolated angiitis of the CNS: Treatment with pulse cyclophosphamide, *Pediatr Neurol* 9:73-75, 1992.

178. MacLaren K, Gillespie J, Shrestha S, et al: Primary angiitis of the central nervous system: Emerging variants, *QJM* 98:643-654, 2005.

179. Lee AG, Brazis PW: Temporal arteritis: A clinical approach, *J Am Geriatr Soc* 47:1364-1370, 1999.

180. Guevara RA, Newman NJ, Grossniklaus HE: Positive temporal artery biopsy 6 months after prednisone treatment, *Arch Ophthalmol* 116:1252-1253, 1998.

181. Swannell AJ: Polymyalgia rheumatica and temporal arteritis: Diagnosis and management, *BMJ* 314:1329-1332, 1997.

182. Sailler L, Carreiro M, Ollier S, et al: [Non-complicated Horton's disease: Initial treatment with methylprednisolone 500 mg/day bolus for three days followed by 20 mg/day prednisone-equivalent. Evaluation of 15 patients], *Rev Med Interne* 22:1032-1038, 2001.

183. Cornblath WT, Eggenberger ER: Progressive visual loss from giant cell arteritis despite high-dose intravenous methylprednisolone, *Ophthalmology* 104:854-858, 1997.

184. Hayreh SS, Zimmerman B: Management of giant cell arteritis. Our 27-year clinical study: New light on old controversies, *Ophthalmologica* 217:239-259, 2003.

185. Chevalet P, Barrier JH, Pottier P, et al: A randomized, multicenter, controlled trial using intravenous pulses of methylprednisolone in the initial treatment of simple forms of giant cell arteritis: A one year followup study of 164 patients, *J Rheumatol* 27:1484-1491, 2000.

186. Mazlumzadeh M, Hunder GG, Easley KA, et al: Treatment of giant cell arteritis using induction therapy with high-dose glucocorticoids: A double-blind, placebo-controlled, randomized prospective clinical trial, *Arthritis Rheum* 54:3310-3318, 2006.

187. Chan CC, Paine M, O'Day J: Steroid management in giant cell arteritis, *Br J Ophthalmol* 85:1061-1064, 2001.

188. Staunton H, Stafford F, Leader M, et al: Deterioration of giant cell arteritis with corticosteroid therapy, *Arch Neurol* 57:581-584, 2000.

189. Kupersmith MJ, Langer R, Mitnick H, et al: Visual performance in giant cell arteritis (temporal arteritis) after 1 year of therapy, *Br J Ophthalmol* 83:796-801, 1999.

190. Nesher G, Rubinow A, Sonnenblick M: Efficacy and adverse effects of different corticosteroid dose regimens in temporal arteritis: A retrospective study, *Clin Exp Rheumatol* 15:303-306, 1997.

191. Andersson R, Malmvall BE, Bengtsson BA: Long-term corticosteroid treatment in giant cell arteritis, *Acta Med Scand* 220:465-469, 1986.

192. Salvarani C, Cantini F, Hunder GG: Polymyalgia rheumatica and giant-cell arteritis, *Lancet* 372:234-245, 2008.

193. Mahr AD, Jover JA, Spiera RF, et al: Adjunctive methotrexate for treatment of giant cell arteritis: An individual patient data meta-analysis, *Arthritis Rheum* 56:2789-2797, 2007.

194. De Silva M, Hazleman BL: Azathioprine in giant cell arteritis/polymyalgia rheumatica: A double-blind study, *Ann Rheum Dis* 45:136-138, 1986.

195. Schaufelberger C, Andersson R, Nordborg E: No additive effect of cyclosporin A compared with glucocorticoid treatment alone in giant cell arteritis: Results of an open, controlled, randomized study, *Br J Rheumatol* 37:464-465, 1998.

196. Hoffman GS, Cid MC, Rendt-Zagar KE, et al: Infliximab for maintenance of glucocorticosteroid-induced remission of giant cell arteritis: A randomized trial, *Ann Intern Med* 146:621-630, 2007.

197. Lee MS, Smith SD, Galor A, et al: Antiplatelet and anticoagulant therapy in patients with giant cell arteritis, *Arthritis Rheum* 54:3306-3309, 2006.

198. Nesher G, Berkun Y, Mates M, et al: Low-dose aspirin and prevention of cranial ischemic complications in giant cell arteritis, *Arthritis Rheum* 50:1332-1337, 2004.

199. Moore PM, Calabrese LH: Neurologic manifestations of systemic vasculitides, *Semin Neurol* 14:300-306, 1994.

200. Montaner J, Dominguez J, Molina C, et al: [Stroke and scleroderma. Cerebral Raynaud?], *Neurologia* 16:236-237, 2001.

201. Reichart MD, Bogousslavsky J, Janzer RC: Early lacunar strokes complicating polyarteritis nodosa: Thrombotic microangiopathy, *Neurology* 54:883-889, 2000.

202. Murphy JM, Gomez-Anson B, Gillard JH, et al: Wegener granulomatosis: MR imaging findings in brain and meninges, *Radiology* 213:794-799, 1999.

203. Savitz JM, Young MA, Ratan RR: Basilar artery occlusion in a young patient with Wegener's granulomatosis, *Stroke* 25:214-216, 1994.

204. Chatzis A, Giannopoulos N, Baharakakis S, et al: Unusual cause of a stroke in a patient with seronegative rheumatoid arthritis, *Cardiovasc Surg* 7:659-660, 1999.

205. Nagahiro S, Mantani A, Yamada K, et al: Multiple cerebral arterial occlusions in a young patient with Sjogren's syndrome: Case report, *Neurosurgery* 38:592-595, 1996:discussion 595.

206. Bragoni M, Di Piero V, Priori R, et al: Sjogren's syndrome presenting as ischemic stroke, *Stroke* 25:2276-2279, 1994.

207. Ohno T, Matsuda I, Furukawa H, et al: Recovery from rheumatoid cerebral vasculitis by low-dose methotrexate, *Intern Med* 33:615-620, 1994.

208. Gururaj AK, Chand RP, Chuah SP: Cerebral infarction in juvenile rheumatoid arthritis, *Clin Neurol Neurosurg* 90:261-263, 1988.

209. Doll NJ, Salvaggio JE: Stroke and gangrene: Complications of therapeutic plasma exchange therapy, *Clin Exp Dial Apheresis* 5:415-421, 1981.

210. Serena M, Biscaro R, Moretto G, et al: Peripheral and central nervous system involvement in essential mixed cryoglobulinemia: A case report, *Clin Neuropathol* 10:177-180, 1991.

211. Escudero D, Latorre P, Codina M, et al: Central nervous system disease in Sjogren's syndrome, *Ann Med Interne (Paris)* 146:239-242, 1995.

212. Futrell N, Schultz LR, Millikan C: Central nervous system disease in patients with systemic lupus erythematosus, *Neurology* 42:1649-1657, 1992.

213. Futrell N, Millikan C: Frequency, etiology, and prevention of stroke in patients with systemic lupus erythematosus, *Stroke* 20:583-591, 1989.

214. Jayne D: Evidence-based treatment of systemic vasculitis, *Rheumatology* 39:585-595, 2000.

215. Brightbill TC, Ihmeidan IH, Post MJ, et al: Neurosyphilis in HIV-positive and HIV-negative patients: Neuroimaging findings, *AJNR: Am J Neuroradiol* 16:703-711, 1995.

216. Ries S, Schminke U, Fassbender K, et al: Cerebrovascular involvement in the acute phase of bacterial meningitis, *J Neurol* 244:51-55, 1997.

217. Zalduondo FM, Provenzale JM, Hulette C, et al: Meningitis, vasculitis, and cerebritis caused by CNS histoplasmosis: Radiologic-pathologic correlation, *AJR Am J Roentgenol* 166:194-196, 1996.

218. Hsu SS, Kim HS: Meningococcal meningitis presenting as stroke in an afebrile adult, *Ann Emerg Med* 32:620-623, 1998.

219. Oschmann P, Dorndorf W, Hornig C, et al: Stages and syndromes of neuroborreliosis, *J Neurol* 245:262-272, 1998.

220. Qureshi AI, Janssen RS, Karon JM, et al: Human immunodeficiency virus infection and stroke in young patients, *Arch Neurol* 54:1150-1153, 1997.

221. Berkefeld J, Enzensberger W, Lanfermann H: MRI in human immunodeficiency virus-associated cerebral vasculitis, *Neuroradiology* 42:526-528, 2000.

222. Picard O, Brunereau L, Pelosse B, et al: Cerebral infarction associated with vasculitis due to varicella zoster virus in patients infected with the human immunodeficiency virus, *Biomed Pharmacother* 51:449-454, 1997.

223. Sarazin L, Duong H, Bourgouin PM, et al: Herpes zoster vasculitis: Demonstration by MR angiography, *J Comput Assist Tomogr* 19:624-627, 1995.

224. Gjerstad L, Nyberg-Hansen R, Bjorland O, et al: Herpes zoster ophthalmicus with cerebral angiitis and reduced cerebral blood flow, *Acta Neurol Scand* 74:460-466, 1986.

225. MacKenzie RA, Forbes GS, Karnes WE: Angiographic findings in herpes zoster arteritis, *Ann Neurol* 10:458-464, 1981.

226. Yankner BA, Skolnik PR, Shoukimas GM, et al: Cerebral granulomatous angiitis associated with isolation of human T-lymphotropic virus type III from the central nervous system, *Ann Neurol* 20:362-364, 1986.

227. Kalita J, Bansal R, Ayagiri A, et al: Midbrain infarction: A rare presentation of cryptococcal meningitis, *Clin Neurol Neurosurg* 101:23-25, 1999.

228. Vernino S, Wijdicks EF, McGough PF: Coma in fulminant pneumococcal meningitis: New MRI observations, *Neurology* 51:1200-1202, 1998.

229. Grimes DA, Lach B, Bourque PR: Vasculitic basilar artery thrombosis in chronic *Candida albicans* meningitis, *Can J Neurol Sci* 25:76-78, 1998.

230. Barinagarrementeria F, Cantu C: Frequency of cerebral arteritis in subarachnoid cysticercosis: An angiographic study, *Stroke* 29:123-125, 1998.

231. Bonawitz C, Castillo M, Mukherji SK: Comparison of CT and MR features with clinical outcome in patients with Rocky Mountain spotted fever, *AJNR: Am J Neuroradiol* 18:459-464, 1997.

232. Huang LT: *Salmonella* meningitis complicated by brain infarctions, *Clin Infect Dis* 22:194-195, 1996.

233. Rojas-Echeverri LA, Soto-Hernandez JL, Garza S, et al: Predictive value of digital subtraction angiography in patients with tuberculous meningitis, *Neuroradiology* 38:20-24, 1996.

234. Weststrate W, Hijdra A, de Gans J: Brain infarcts in adults with bacterial meningitis, *Lancet* 347:399, 1996.

235. Azuma T, Matsubara T, Shima Y, et al: Neurosteroids in cerebrospinal fluid in neurologic disorders, *J Neurol Sci* 120:87-92, 1993.

236. Hsieh FY, Chia LG, Shen WC: Locations of cerebral infarctions in tuberculous meningitis, *Neuroradiology* 34:197-199, 1992.

237. Kerr L, Filloux FM: Cerebral infarction as a remote complication of childhood *Haemophilus influenzae* meningitis, *West J Med* 157:179-182, 1992.

238. Gallagher PG, Ball WS: Cerebral infarctions due to CNS infection with, *Enterobacter sakazakii, Pediatr Radiol* 21:135-136, 1991.

239. Goel A, Pandya SK, Satoskar AR: Whither short-course chemotherapy for tuberculous meningitis? *Neurosurgery* 27:418-421, 1990.

240. Floret D, Delmas MC, Cochat P: Cerebellar infarction as a complication of pneumococcus meningitis, *Pediatr Infect Dis J* 8:57-58, 1989.

241. Yu YL, Woo E, Chan FL, et al: Cerebral infarction in cryptococcal meningitis, *Clin Exp Neurol* 26:193-197, 1989.

242. Barinagarrementeria F, Del Brutto OH: Neurocysticercosis and pure motor hemiparesis, *Stroke* 19:1156-1158, 1988.

243. Johns DR, Tierney M, Parker SW: Pure motor hemiplegia due to meningovascular neurosyphilis, *Arch Neurol* 44:1062-1065, 1987.

244. Freedman MS, Macdonald RD: Herpes zoster ophthalmicus with delayed cerebral infarction and meningoencephalitis, *Can J Neurol Sci* 14:312-314, 1987.

245. Walterspiel JN: *Kingella kingae* meningitis with bilateral infarcts of the basal ganglia, *Infection* 11:307-309, 1983.

246. Snyder RD, Stovring J, Cushing AH, et al: Cerebral infarction in childhood bacterial meningitis, *J Neurol Neurosurg Psychiatry* 44:581-585, 1981.

247. de Carvalho CA, Allen JN, Zafranis A, et al: Coccidioidal meningitis complicated by cerebral arteritis and infarction, *Hum Pathol* 11:293-296, 1980.

248. Casato M, Saadoun D, Marchetti A, et al: Central nervous system involvement in hepatitis C virus cryoglobulinemia vasculitis: A multicenter case-control study using magnetic resonance imaging and neuropsychological tests, *J Rheumatol* 32:484-488, 2005.

249. Melanson M, Chalk C, Georgevich L, et al: Varicella-zoster virus DNA in CSF and arteries in delayed contralateral hemiplegia: Evidence for viral invasion of cerebral arteries, *Neurology* 47:569-570, 1996.

250. Pagnoux C, Cohen P, Guillevin L: Vasculitides secondary to infections, *Clin Exp Rheumatol* 24:S71-81, 2006.

251. Taylor CL, Varma A, Herwadkar A, et al: Successful reversal of threatening carotid artery occlusion in HIV-associated non-aneurysmal vasculitis, *Int J STD AIDS* 19:141-142, 2008.

252. Reynard CA, Calain P, Pizzolato GP, et al: Severe acute myocardial infarction during a staphylococcal septicemia with meningoencephalitis. A possible contraindication to thrombolytic treatment, *Intensive Care Med* 18:247-249, 1992.

253. Meadows R, Verghese A: Medical complications of glue sniffing, *South Med J* 89:455-462, 1996.

254. Petitti DB, Sidney S, Quesenberry C, et al: Stroke and cocaine or amphetamine use, *Epidemiology* 9:596-600, 1998.

255. Sloan MA, Kittner SJ, Feeser BR, et al: Illicit drug-associated ischemic stroke in the Baltimore-Washington Young Stroke Study, *Neurology* 50:1688-1693, 1998.

256. Aggarwal SK, Williams V, Levine SR, et al: Cocaine-associated intracranial hemorrhage: Absence of vasculitis in 14 cases, *Neurology* 46:1741-1743, 1996.

257. Brust JC: Vasculitis owing to substance abuse, *Neurol Clin* 15:945-957, 1997.

258. Calabrese LH, Duna GF: Drug-induced vasculitis, *Curr Opin Rheumatol* 8:34-40, 1996.

259. Mourand I, Ducrocq X, Lacour JC, et al: Acute reversible cerebral arteritis associated with parenteral ephedrine use, *Cerebrovasc Dis* 9:355-357, 1999.

260. Kernan WN, Viscoli CM, Brass LM, et al: Phenylpropanolamine and the risk of hemorrhagic stroke, *N Engl J Med* 343:1826-1832, 2000.

261. Bruno A, Nolte KB, Chapin J: Stroke associated with ephedrine use, *Neurology* 43:1313-1316, 1993.

262. Konzen JP, Levine SR, Garcia JH: Vasospasm and thrombus formation as possible mechanisms of stroke related to alkaloidal cocaine, *Stroke* 26:1114-1118, 1995.

263. Bendixen BH, Cucchiara B, Kasner SE: Stroke associated with drug abuse. In Gilman S, editor: *Medlink neurology (CD-ROM, updated every 4 months),* San Diego, Calif, 2001, Medlink.

264. Gutmann DH, Cantor CR, Piacente GJ, et al: Cerebral vasculopathy and infarction in a woman with carcinomatous meningitis, *J Neurooncol* 9:183-185, 1990.

265. Kastenbauer S, Wiesmann M, Pfister HW: Cerebral vasculopathy and multiple infarctions in a woman with carcinomatous meningitis while on treatment with intrathecal methotrexate, *J Neurooncol* 48:41-45, 2000.

266. Klein P, Haley EC, Wooten GF, et al: Focal cerebral infarctions associated with perivascular tumor infiltrates in carcinomatous leptomeningeal metastases, *Arch Neurol* 46:1149-1152, 1989.

267. Calamia KT, Miller A, Shuster EA, et al: Intravascular lymphomatosis. A report of ten patients with central nervous system involvement and a review of the disease process, *Adv Exp Med Biol* 455:249-265, 1999.

268. Casas JP, Hingorani AD, Bautista LE, et al: Meta-analysis of genetic studies in ischemic stroke: Thirty-two genes involving approximately 18,000 cases and 58,000 controls, *Arch Neurol* 61:1652–1661, 2004.

269. Kim RJ, Becker RC: Association between factor V Leiden, prothrombin G20210A, and methylenetetrahydrofolate reductase C677T mutations and events of the arterial circulatory system: A meta-analysis of published studies, *Am Heart J* 146:948–957, 2003.

270. Julkunen H, Hedman C, Kauppi M: Thrombolysis for acute ischemic stroke in the primary antiphospholipid syndrome, *J Rheumatol* 24:181–183, 1997.

271. Coull BM, Skaff PT: Disorders of coagulation. In Bogousslavsky J, Caplan L, editors: *Uncommon causes of stroke*, Cambridge, 2001, Cambridge University Press, pp 86–95.

272. Sacco RL, Adams R, Albers G, et al: Guidelines for prevention of stroke in patients with ischemic stroke or transient ischemic attack: A statement for healthcare professionals from the American Heart Association/American Stroke Association Council on Stroke: Co-sponsored by the Council on Cardiovascular Radiology and Intervention: The American Academy of Neurology affirms the value of this guideline, *Stroke* 37:577–617, 2006.

273. Sallah S, Abdallah JM, Gagnon GA: Recurrent warfarin-induced skin necrosis in kindreds with protein S deficiency, *Haemostasis* 28:25–30, 1998.

274. Ginsburg KS, Liang MH, Newcomer L, et al: Anticardiolipin antibodies and the risk for ischemic stroke and venous thrombosis, *Ann Intern Med* 117:997–1002, 1992.

275. Ahmed E, Stegmayr B, Trifunovic J, et al: Anticardiolipin antibodies are not an independent risk factor for stroke: An incident case-referent study nested within the Monica And Vasterbotten Cohort Project, *Stroke* 31:1289–1293, 2000.

276. Brey RL, Abbott RD, Curb JD, et al: Beta(2)-glycoprotein 1-dependent anticardiolipin antibodies and risk of ischemic stroke and myocardial infarction: The Honolulu Heart Program, *Stroke* 32:1701–1706, 2001.

277. Daif AK: Anticardiolipin antibodies as an independent risk factor for stroke in young Saudis, *Funct Neurol* 13:285–289, 1998.

278. Kenet G, Sadetzki S, Murad H, et al: Factor V Leiden and antiphospholipid antibodies are significant risk factors for ischemic stroke in children, *Stroke* 31:1283–1288, 2000.

279. Levine SR, Salowich-Palm L, Sawaya KL, et al: IgG anticardiolipin antibody titer > 40 GPL and the risk of subsequent thrombo-occlusive events and death. A prospective cohort study, *Stroke* 28:1660–1665, 1997.

280. Metz LM, Edworthy S, Mydlarski R, et al: The frequency of phospholipid antibodies in an unselected stroke population, *Can J Neurol Sci* 25:64–69, 1998.

281. Muir KW, Squire IB, Alwan W, et al: Anticardiolipin antibodies in an unselected stroke population, *Lancet* 344:452–456, 1994.

282. Tuhrim S, Rand JH, Wu XX, et al: Elevated anticardiolipin antibody titer is a stroke risk factor in a multiethnic population independent of isotype or degree of positivity, *Stroke* 30:1561–1565, 1999.

283. Zielinska J, Ryglewicz D, Wierzchowska E, et al: Anticardiolipin antibodies are an independent risk factor for ischemic stroke, *Neurol Res* 21:653–657, 1999.

284. Coull BM, Levine SR, Brey RL: The role of antiphospholipid antibodies in stroke, *Neurol Clin* 10:125–143, 1992.

285. Vila P, Hernandez MC, Lopez-Fernandez MF, et al: Prevalence, follow-up and clinical significance of the anticardiolipin antibodies in normal subjects, *Thromb Haemost* 72:209–213, 1994.

286. Love PE, Santoro SA: Antiphospholipid antibodies: Anticardiolipin and the lupus anticoagulant in systemic lupus erythematosus (SLE) and in non-SLE disorders. Prevalence and clinical significance, *Ann Intern Med* 112:682–698, 1990.

287. Wilson WA, Gharavi AE, Koike T, et al: International consensus statement on preliminary classification criteria for definite antiphospholipid syndrome: Report of an international workshop, *Arthritis Rheum* 42:1309–1311, 1999.

288. The NINDS rt-PA Stroke Study Group: Intracerebral hemorrhage after intravenous t-PA therapy for ischemic stroke, *Stroke* 28:2109–2118, 1997.

289. Cugno M, Dominguez M, Cabibbe M, et al: Antibodies to tissue-type plasminogen activator in plasma from patients with primary antiphospholipid syndrome, *Br J Haematol* 108:871–875, 2000.

290. Mohr JP, Thompson JLP, Lazar RM, et al: A comparison of warfarin and aspirin for the prevention of recurrent ischemic stroke, *N Engl J Med* 345:1444–1451, 2001.

291. APASS Investigators: Antiphospholipid antibodies and subsequent thrombo-occlusive events in patients with ischemic stroke, *JAMA* 291:576–584, 2004.

292. Khamashta MA, Cuadrado MJ, Mujic F, et al: The management of thrombosis in the antiphospholipid-antibody syndrome, *N Engl J Med* 332:993–997, 1995.

293. Krnic-Barrie S, O'Connor CR, Looney SW, et al: A retrospective review of 61 patients with antiphospholipid syndrome. Analysis of factors influencing recurrent thrombosis, *Arch Intern Med* 157:2101–2108, 1997.

294. Crowther MA, Ginsberg JS, Julian J, et al: A comparison of two intensities of warfarin for the prevention of recurrent thrombosis in patients with the antiphospholipid antibody syndrome, *N Engl J Med* 349:1133–1138, 2003.

295. Finazzi G, Marchioli R, Brancaccio V, et al: A randomized clinical trial of high-intensity warfarin vs. conventional antithrombotic therapy for the prevention of recurrent thrombosis in patients with the antiphospholipid syndrome (WAPS), *J Thromb Haemost* 3:848–853, 2005.

296. Asherson RA, Cervera R, de Groot PG, et al: Catastrophic antiphospholipid syndrome: International consensus statement on classification criteria and treatment guidelines, *Lupus* 12:530–534, 2003.

297. Bowie EJ, Owen CA: The clinical pathology of intravascular coagulation, *Bibl Haematol* 49:217–224, 1983.

298. Graus F, Rogers LR, Posner JB: Cerebrovascular complications in patients with cancer, *Medicine* 64:16–35, 1985.

299. Schwartzman RJ, Hill JB: Neurologic complications of disseminated intravascular coagulation, *Neurology* 32:791–797, 1982.

300. de Jonge E, Levi M, Stoutenbeek CP, et al: Current drug treatment strategies for disseminated intravascular coagulation, *Drugs* 55:767–777, 1998.

301. Handin RI: Coagulation disorders. In Braunwald E, Isselbacher KJ, Petersdorf RG, et al: *Harrison's principles of internal medicine*, New York, 1988, McGraw-Hill, pp 1475–1480.

302. Levi M: Disseminated intravascular coagulation, *Crit Care Med* 35:2191–2195, 2007.

303. Franchini M, Manzato F, Salvagno GL, et al: Potential role of recombinant activated factor VII for the treatment of severe bleeding associated with disseminated intravascular coagulation: A systematic review, *Blood Coagul Fibrinolysis* 18:589–593, 2007.

304. Earley CJ, Kittner SJ, Feeser BR, et al: Stroke in children and sickle-cell disease: Baltimore-Washington Cooperative Young Stroke Study, *Neurology* 51:169–176, 1998.

305. Ohene-Frempong K, Weiner SJ, Sleeper LA, et al: Cerebrovascular accidents in sickle cell disease: Rates and risk factors, *Blood* 91:288–294, 1998.

306. Jeffries BF, Lipper MH, Kishore PR: Major intracerebral arterial involvement in sickle cell disease, *Surg Neurol* 14:291–295, 1980.

307. Gerald B, Sebes JI, Langston JW: Cerebral infarction secondary to sickle cell disease: Arteriographic findings, *AJR Am J Roentgenol* 134:1209–1212, 1980.

308. Prohovnik I, Pavlakis SG, Piomelli S, et al: Cerebral hyperemia, stroke, and transfusion in sickle cell disease, *Neurology* 39:344–348, 1989.

309. Adams RJ: Stroke prevention and treatment in sickle cell disease, *Arch Neurol* 58:565–568, 2001.

310. Sidani CA, Ballourah W, El Dassouki M, et al: Venous sinus thrombosis leading to stroke in a patient with sickle cell disease on hydroxyurea and high hemoglobin levels: Treatment with thrombolysis, *Am J Hematol* 83:818–820, 2008.

311. Adams RJ, McKie VC, Hsu L, et al: Prevention of a first stroke by transfusions in children with sickle cell anemia and abnormal results on transcranial Doppler ultrasonography, *N Engl J Med* 339:5–11, 1998.

312. Cohen AR, Martin MB, Silber JH, et al: A modified transfusion program for prevention of stroke in sickle cell disease, *Blood* 79:1657–1661, 1992.

313. Miller ST, Jensen D, Rao SP: Less intensive long-term transfusion therapy for sickle cell anemia and cerebrovascular accident, *J Pediatr* 120:54–57, 1992.

314. Adams RJ, McKie VC, Brambilla D, et al: Stroke prevention trial in sickle cell anemia, *Control Clin Trials* 19:110–129, 1998.

315. Adams RJ, Brambilla D: Discontinuing prophylactic transfusions used to prevent stroke in sickle cell disease, *N Engl J Med* 353:2769-2778, 2005.

316. Vichinsky EP, Luban NL, Wright E, et al: Prospective RBC phenotype matching in a stroke-prevention trial in sickle cell anemia: A multicenter transfusion trial, *Transfusion* 41:1086-1092, 2001.

317. Hulbert ML, Scothorn DJ, Panepinto JA, et al: Exchange blood transfusion compared with simple transfusion for first overt stroke is associated with a lower risk of subsequent stroke: A retrospective cohort study of 137 children with sickle cell anemia, *J Pediatr* 149:710-712, 2006.

318. Ballas SK, Marcolina MJ, Dover GJ, et al: Erythropoietic activity in patients with sickle cell anaemia before and after treatment with hydroxyurea, *Br J Haematol* 105:491-496, 1999.

319. Tavakkoli F, Nahavandi M, Wyche MQ, et al: Effects of hydroxyurea treatment on cerebral oxygenation in adult patients with sickle cell disease: An open-label pilot study, *Clin Ther* 27:1083-1088, 2005.

320. Zimmerman SA, Schultz WH, Burgett S, et al: Hydroxyurea therapy lowers transcranial Doppler flow velocities in children with sickle cell anemia, *Blood* 110:1043-1047, 2007.

321. Gulbis B, Haberman D, Dufour D, et al: Hydroxyurea for sickle cell disease in children and for prevention of cerebrovascular events: The Belgian experience, *Blood* 105:2685-2690, 2005.

322. Kratovil T, Bulas D, Driscoll MC, et al: Hydroxyurea therapy lowers TCD velocities in children with sickle cell disease, *Pediatr Blood Cancer* 47:894-900, 2006.

323. Charache S, Terrin ML, Moore RD, et al: Effect of hydroxyurea on the frequency of painful crises in sickle cell anemia, *N Engl J Med* 332:1317-1322, 1995.

324. Ware RE, Zimmerman SA, Sylvestre PB, et al: Prevention of secondary stroke and resolution of transfusional iron overload in children with sickle cell anemia using hydroxyurea and phlebotomy, *J Pediatr* 145:346-352, 2004.

325. Wang WC: The pathophysiology, prevention, and treatment of stroke in sickle cell disease, *Curr Opin Hematol* 14:191-197, 2007.

326. Merkel KH, Ginsberg PL, Parker JC Jr, et al: Cerebrovascular disease in sickle cell anemia: A clinical, pathological and radiological correlation, *Stroke* 9:45-52, 1978.

327. Garza-Mercado R: Pseudomoyamoya in sickle cell anemia, *Surg Neurol* 18:425-431, 1982.

328. Chiu D, Shedden P, Bratina P, et al: Clinical features of moyamoya disease in the United States, *Stroke* 29:1347-1351, 1998.

329. Hankinson TC, Bohman LE, Heyer G, et al: Surgical treatment of moyamoya syndrome in patients with sickle cell anemia: Outcome following encephaloduroarteriosynangiosis, *J Neurosurg Pediatr* 1:211-216, 2008.

330. Walters MC, Storb R, Patience M, et al: Impact of bone marrow transplantation for symptomatic sickle cell disease: An interim report. Multicenter investigation of bone marrow transplantation for sickle cell disease, *Blood* 95:1918-1924, 2000.

331. Woodard P, Helton KJ, Khan RB, et al: Brain parenchymal damage after haematopoietic stem cell transplantation for severe sickle cell disease, *Br J Haematol* 129:550-552, 2005.

332. Kirkham FJ, Lerner NB, Noetzel M, et al: Trials in sickle cell disease, *Pediatr Neurol* 34:450-458, 2006.

333. Etminan M, Takkouche B, Isorna FC, et al: Risk of ischaemic stroke in people with migraine: Systematic review and meta-analysis of observational studies, *BMJ* 330:63, 2005.

334. Lauritzen M: Spreading depression and migraine, *Pathol Biol (Paris)* 40:332-337, 1992.

335. Olesen J: Cerebral blood flow in migraine with aura, *Pathol Biol (Paris)* 40:318-324, 1992.

336. Broderick JP, Swanson JW: Migraine-related strokes. Clinical profile and prognosis in 20 patients, *Arch Neurol* 44:868-871, 1987.

337. Hering-Hanit R, Friedman Z, Schlesinger I, et al: Evidence for activation of the coagulation system in migraine with aura, *Cephalalgia* 21:137-139, 2001.

338. Lassen LH, Ashina M, Christiansen I, et al: Nitric oxide synthase inhibition in migraine, *Lancet* 349:401-402, 1997.

339. Zeller JA, Frahm K, Baron R, et al: Platelet-leukocyte interaction and platelet activation in migraine: A link to ischemic stroke? *J Neurol Neurosurg Psychiatry* 75:984-987, 2004.

340. Tietjen GE, Al-Qasmi MM, Athanas K, et al: Increased von Willebrand factor in migraine, *Neurology* 57:334-336, 2001.

341. Spierings EL: Angiographic changes suggestive of vasospasm in migraine complicated by stroke, *Headache* 30:727-728, 1990.

342. Meschia JF, Malkoff MD, Biller J: Reversible segmental cerebral arterial vasospasm and cerebral infarction: Possible association with excessive use of sumatriptan and midrin, *Arch Neurol* 55:712-714, 1998.

343. Sanin LC, Mathew NT: Severe diffuse intracranial vasospasm as a cause of extensive migrainous cerebral infarction, *Cephalalgia* 13:289-292, 1993.

344. Ojaimi J, Katsabanis S, Bower S, et al: Mitochondrial DNA in stroke and migraine with aura, *Cerebrovasc Dis* 8:102-106, 1998.

345. Schwerzmann M, Nedeltchev K, Meier B: Patent foramen ovale closure: A new therapy for migraine, *Catheter Cardiovasc Interv* 69:277-284, 2007.

346. Alvarez WC: The present day treatment of migraine, *Mayo Clin Proc* 9:22, 1934.

347. Kupersmith MJ, Hass WK, Chase NE: Isoproterenol treatment of visual symptoms in migraine, *Stroke* 37:484-486, 1987.

348. Silberstein SD, Saper JR, Freitag FG: Migraine: Diagnosis and treatment. In Silberstein SD, Lipton RB, Dalessio DJ, editors: *Wolff's headache and other head pain*, Oxford, 2001, Oxford University Press, pp 121-237.

349. Jayamaha JE, Street MK: Fatal cerebellar infarction in a migraine sufferer whilst receiving sumatriptan, *Intensive Care Med* 21:82-83, 1995.

350. Lindboe CF, Dahl T, Rostad B: Fatal stroke in migraine: A case report with autopsy findings, *Cephalalgia* 9:277-280, 1989.

351. Gillum LA, Mamidipudi SK, Johnston SC: Ischemic stroke risk with oral contraceptives: A meta-analysis, *JAMA* 284:72-78, 2000.

352. Ohama E, Ohara S, Ikuta F, et al: Mitochondrial angiopathy in cerebral blood vessels of mitochondrial encephalomyopathy, *Acta Neuropathol* 74:226-233, 1987.

353. Hirano M, Pavlakis SG: Mitochondrial myopathy, encephalopathy, lactic acidosis, and strokelike episodes (MELAS): Current concepts, *J Child Neurol* 9:4-13, 1994.

354. DiMauro S, Moraes CT: Mitochondrial encephalomyopathies, *Arch Neurol* 50:1197-1208, 1993.

355. Chan A, Reichmann H, Kogel A, et al: Metabolic changes in patients with mitochondrial myopathies and effects of coenzyme Q10 therapy, *J Neurol* 245:681-685, 1998.

356. Matthews PM, Ford B, Dandurand RJ, et al: Coenzyme q10 with multiple vitamins is generally ineffective in treatment of mitochondrial disease, *Neurology* 43:884-890, 1993.

357. Kimura S, Ohtuki N, Nezu A, et al: Clinical and radiologic improvements in mitochondrial encephalomyelopathy following sodium dichloroacetate therapy, *Brain Dev* 19:535-540, 1997.

358. Kaufmann P, Engelstad K, Wei Y, et al: Dichloroacetate causes toxic neuropathy in MELAS: A randomized, controlled clinical trial, *Neurology* 66:324-330, 2006.

359. Koga Y, Ishibashi M, Ueki I, et al: Effects of l-arginine on the acute phase of strokes in three patients with MELAS, *Neurology* 58:827-828, 2002.

360. Kubota M, Sakakihara Y, Mori M, et al: Beneficial effect of l-arginine for stroke-like episode in MELAS, *Brain Dev* 26:481-483, 2004:discussion 480.

361. Koga Y, Akita Y, Junko N, et al: Endothelial dysfunction in MELAS improved by l-arginine supplementation, *Neurology* 66:1766-1769, 2006.

362. Koga Y, Akita Y, Nishioka J, et al: L-Arginine improves the symptoms of strokelike episodes in MELAS, *Neurology* 64:710-712, 2005.

363. Napolitano A, Salvetti S, Vista M, et al: Long-term treatment with idebenone and riboflavin in a patient with MELAS, *Neurol Sci* 21:S981-982, 2000.

364. Argov Z, Bank WJ, Maris J, et al: Treatment of mitochondrial myopathy due to complex III deficiency with vitamins K3 and C: A 31P-NMR follow-up study, *Ann Neurol* 19:598-602, 1986.

365. DiMauro S, Hirano M, Schon EA: Mitochondrial encephalomyopathies: Therapeutic approaches, *Neurol Sci* 21:S901-908, 2000.

366. Bousser M-G, Chiras J, Bories J, et al: Cerebral venous thrombosis—a review of 38 cases, *Stroke* 16(2):199-213, 1985.

367. Martinelli I, Sacchi E, Landi G, et al: High risk of cerebral-vein thrombosis in carriers of a prothrombin-gene mutation and in users of oral contraceptives, *N Engl J Med* 338:1793-1797, 1998.

368. de Bruijn SF, Stam J, Vandenbroucke JP: Increased risk of cerebral venous sinus thrombosis with third-generation oral contraceptives. Cerebral venous sinus thrombosis study group, *Lancet* 351:1404, 1998.

369. Bousser M-G, Ross Russell R: *Cerebral venous thrombosis*, London, 1997, WB Saunders Co.

370. Maruishi M, Kato H, Nawashiro H, et al: Successful treatment of increased intracranial pressure by barbiturate therapy in a patient with severe sinus thrombosis after failure of osmotic therapy. A case report, *Acta Neurochir (Wien)* 120:88-91, 1993.

371. Goldberg AL, Rosenbaum AE, Wang H, et al: Computed tomography of dural sinus thrombosis, *J Comput Assist Tomogr* 10:16-20, 1986.

372. Stefini R, Latronico N, Cornali C, et al: Emergent decompressive craniectomy in patients with fixed dilated pupils due to cerebral venous and dural sinus thrombosis: Report of three cases, *Neurosurgery* 45:626-629, 1999:discussion 629-630.

373. Keller E, Pangalu A, Fandino J, et al: Decompressive craniectomy in severe cerebral venous and dural sinus thrombosis, *Acta Neurochir Suppl* 94:177-183, 2005.

374. Einhaupl KM, Villringer A, Meister W, et al: Heparin treatment in sinus venous thrombosis, *Lancet* 338:597-600, 1991.

375. de Bruijn SFTM, Stam J, for the Cerebral Venous Sinus Thrombosis Study Group: Randomized, placebo-controlled trial of anticoagulant treatment with low-molecular-weight heparin for cerebral sinus thrombosis, *Stroke* 30:484-488, 1999.

376. Ferro JM, Canhao P, Stam J, et al: Prognosis of cerebral vein and dural sinus thrombosis: Results of the International Study on Cerebral Vein and Dural Sinus Thrombosis (ISCVT), *Stroke* 35:664-670, 2004.

377. Castaigne P, Laplane D, Bousser MP: Superior sagittal sinus thrombosis, *Arch Neurol* 34:788-789, 1977.

378. DiRocco C, Iannelli A, Leone G, et al: Heparin-urokinase treatment in aseptic dural sinus thrombosis, *Arch Neurol* 38:431-435, 1981.

379. Canhao P, Falcao F, Ferro JM: Thrombolytics for cerebral sinus thrombosis: A systematic review, *Cerebrovasc Dis* 15:159-166, 2003.

380. Agner C, Deshaies EM, Bernardini GL, et al: Coronary Angiojet catheterization for the management of dural venous sinus thrombosis. Technical note, *J Neurosurg* 103:368-371, 2005.

381. Zhang A, Collinson RL, Hurst RW, et al: Rheolytic thrombectomy for cerebral sinus thrombosis, *Neurocrit Care* 9:17-26, 2008.

382. Curtin KR, Shaibani A, Resnick SA, et al: Rheolytic catheter thrombectomy, balloon angioplasty, and direct recombinant tissue plasminogen activator thrombolysis of dural sinus thrombosis with preexisting hemorrhagic infarctions, *AJNR Am J Neuroradiol* 25:1807-1811, 2004.

383. Chow K, Gobin YP, Saver J, et al: Endovascular treatment of duralsinusthrombosiswithrheolyticthrombectomyandintra-arterial thrombolysis, *Stroke* 31:1420-1425, 2000.

384. Kirsch J, Rasmussen PA, Masaryk TJ, et al: Adjunctive rheolytic thrombectomy for central venous sinus thrombosis: Technical case report, *Neurosurgery* 60:E577-578, 2007:discussion E578.

385. Opatowsky MJ, Morris PP, Regan JD, et al: Rapid thrombectomy of superior sagittal sinus and transverse sinus thrombosis with a rheolytic catheter device, *AJNR Am J Neuroradiol* 20:414-417, 1999.

386. Wasay M, Bakshi R, Kojan S, et al: Nonrandomized comparison of localurokinasethrombolysisversussystemicheparinanticoagulation for superior sagittal sinus thrombosis, *Stroke* 32:2310-2317, 2001.

387. Stam J, Majoie CBLM, van Delden OM, et al: Endovascular thrombectomy and thrombolysis for severe cerebral sinus thrombosis: A prospective study, *Stroke* 39:1487-1490, 2008.

388. Bousser M-G: Cerebral venous thrombosis: Nothing, heparin, or local thrombolysis? *Stroke* 30:481-483, 1999.

389. Kasner SE, Gurian JH, Grotta JC: Urokinase treatment of sagittal sinus thrombosis with venous hemorrhagic infarction, *J Stroke Cerebrovasc Dis* 7:421-425, 1998.

390. Ferro JM, Canhao P: Acute treatment of cerebral venous and dural sinus thrombosis, *Curr Treat Options Neurol* 10:126-137, 2008.

55

Medical Therapy of Intracerebral and Intraventricular Hemorrhage

LEWIS B. MORGENSTERN, DARIN B. ZAHURANEC

Blood frightens people. Although acute hemorrhage is white rather than red on a CT scan, it usually prompts an emergency department physician to rapidly call a tertiary referral center to transfer the patient. The physician accepting the call at the referral center is frequently left wondering what the referral center can do for the patient that the local community hospital cannot. The good news is that although we still have no "magic bullet" to treat intracerebral and intraventricular hemorrhage, aggressive therapy is likely to reduce mortality and improve outcome. Surgery remains controversial, and many therapies can be provided at any hospital with a good intensive care unit and neurologic or neurosurgical expertise.

In this chapter, we discuss medical therapy of spontaneous intracerebral hemorrhage (ICH) and intraventricular hemorrhage (IVH) in adults. Epidemiology, clinical presentation, imaging, and surgical treatment are covered elsewhere in this book. Care for ICH or IVH begins in the community with prompt recognition, transport, and triage of the patient with acute stroke. In the emergency department, after a *stat* head CT scan determines that a spontaneous cerebral hemorrhage has occurred and a search for the cause begins, therapy commences with blood pressure control and assessment of cerebral edema. A watchful eye for hydrocephalus and intensive care unit (ICU) complications is critical. Early feeding and rehabilitation are important.

We begin with emergency department management of the patient with acute ICH or IVH and follow it with a discussion of the utility of specialized wards for patients with ICH or IVH and the importance of aggressive medical therapies. We then consider edema, hydrocephalus, and ventricular drainage procedures; instillation of "lytics" is considered in this section. Next we discuss rebleeding and the steps to prevent this serious complication. Brief consideration is given to the circumstances special to warfarin-related cerebral hemorrhage. Finally, we deal with patient selection for surgical interventions and the predictors of outcome. Primary IVH is rare.[1] One study found that primary IVH accounted for only 3% of all cases of IVH.[2] We therefore discuss ICH and IVH as one entity.

Emergency Department Management

Table 55-1 reviews the steps in the care of patients with ICH or IVH. Initial concerns should focus on the ABCs of emergency therapy. The patient who has brainstem injury or in whom aspiration or trauma is associated with the cerebral bleed may have compromise of airway or breathing. These complications are treated with airway management (with adequate cervical spine protection for those in whom trauma is suspected) and intubation, as discussed later. Patients who have been immobile for long periods before they are brought to the emergency department may have rhabdomyolysis and renal failure; these possibilities should be kept in mind.[3]

The Importance of Aggressive Medical Therapies
Stroke Units and Intensive Care Units

Patients with ICH or IVH should be cared for in specialized units where personnel are familiar with both intensive care procedures and neurologic injury. At the minimum, this statement implies training of nurses to perform neurologic examinations and to promptly recognize deterioration so that rescue therapies can be instituted to halt worsening. The evidence in support of providing care in specialized hospital areas comes from the data on stroke units[4-6] and specific studies on the role of stroke units in caring for patients with ICH. Ronning et al[7] randomly assigned 121 patients with ICH to care in an acute stroke unit or a general medical ward. Thirty-day mortality rate in the stroke unit patients was 39%, compared with 63% in the general medical ward group. No difference between the groups was found for the proportions of patients discharged home and patients requiring placement in long-term facilities.

The decision to assign patients to a neurologic ICU rather than a general ICU is also supported by a study that examined outcome in 1038 patients with ICH in 43 ICUs in the United States.[8] Those who were *not* in a neurologic ICU had a higher odds ratio (OR) for mortality, of 3.4 (95% confidence interval [CI], 1.7–7.6). Patients in the ICUs that had a full-time intensivist on staff had a lower mortality rate (OR, 0.39; 95% CI, 0.2–0.7). For a more detailed description of stroke critical care please see Chapter 52.

Fever

Stroke units not only provide rescue treatment for patients with worsening neurologic signs but also give prophylaxis against complications and avoid conditions that are toxic

TABLE 55-1 EMERGENCY DEPARTMENT CONSIDERATIONS FOR SUSPECTED INTRACEREBRAL HEMORRHAGE (ICH)

1. Secure airway, breathing, and circulation.
2. Check for history of recent head trauma, hypertension, tumor, arteriovenous malformation (AVM), aneurysm, clotting disorder, or chemotherapy
3. Order *stat* head CT scan.
4. Collect and send specimens for complete blood count, prothrombin time, partial thromboplastin time, chemistry panel, and urine drug screen.
5. Insert intravenous and Foley bladder catheters.
6. If CT confirms ICH and increased ICP is not suspected: Reduce blood pressure slowly by no more than 15%-20% to mean arterial pressure of 110 mm Hg if possible.
7. Obtain neurologic and neurosurgical consultations.
8. Suspect aneurysm or AVM if CT shows subarachnoid hemorrhage or hemorrhage in an atypical location or if the patient is not known to have hypertension.
9. Watch the patient closely for signs of deterioration; repeat CT if deterioration occurs.
10. Invoke intracranial pressure protocol if Glasgow Coma Scale score is less than 14.
11. Treat fever and hyperglycemia or hypoglycemia.

TABLE 55-2 REPRESENTATIVE STANDARD ORDERS FOR PATIENTS ADMITTED TO AN INTENSIVE CARE UNIT OR STROKE UNIT WITH CEREBRAL HEMORRHAGE

Admit to Intensive Care Unit/Stroke Unit
Diagnosis: intracerebral hemorrhage
Condition: critical
Vital signs: q1h with neurologic checks and pulse oximetry
Activity: bed rest; have patient up with therapists after 24 hours if stable
Call physician if: temp >38.0° C (obtain chest x-ray, urinalysis and urine culture, blood culture × 2, and give acetaminophen, 1g q6h, and cooling blanket to keep temp <38.0°C); mean arterial blood pressure >120 mm Hg; finger-stick glucose q6h, call if glucose >150 or <70 mg/dL for sliding scale; pulse <60, >120 bpm; respirations <8, >24 min; change in National Institutes of Health Stroke Scale score of ≥2 points
Diet: NPO until cleared by speech pathologist
Allergies: ?
Lab tests: electrolytes, blood chemistry, blood counts including platelets, coagulation profile
IV fluids: normal saline at 80 mL/hour
Pneumatic compression stockings; may add heparin 5000 U SC q8-12 hours after 1-4 days
Ventilator settings as needed
Histamine (H_2) blocker

to damaged neurons. Representative standard orders are shown in Table 55-2. Fever is an independent predictor of poor outcome in ICH.[9] No studies have been performed to document that lowering body temperature improves outcome, but there is good evidence that patients with stroke do worse if they have fever.[10,11] In patients with elevated temperatures, an infectious source should be sought assiduously. Prompt use of acetaminophen and of mechanical cooling devices (blankets) is advocated.

Hyperglycemia

Elevated serum glucose concentration is associated with poor outcome in ICH.[12] Efforts to control glucose with an insulin drip have not proved useful to date.[13] A high serum glucose level may also predispose to ICH after intravenous administration of recombinant tissue-type plasminogen activator (rt-PA) for acute ischemic stroke.[14] Ensuring metabolic homeostasis by striving for normal glucose levels through adequate replacement of fluid volume is desirable.

Hypertension

Blood pressure management of the patient with acute ICH or IVH remains controversial, but a consensus is emerging.[3] Although lowering the blood pressure in acute hemorrhage holds the theoretical promise of preventing rebleeding, many researchers have worried that perihematomal ischemia may be worsened. Evidence now suggests that this concern is a moot point. Experimental laboratory data in dogs first showed that lowering mean arterial pressure (MAP) within normal limits of cerebral autoregulation did not detrimentally affect regional cerebral blood flow or intracranial pressure (ICP).[15] Positron emission tomography (PET) also fails to demonstrate tissue hypoxia surrounding cerebral hematomas in humans.[16] Powers et al[17] performed a controlled trial of

blood pressure reduction in acute patients with ICH and measured perihematomal and global cerebral blood flow; neither declined.

A pilot trial of blood pressure reduction in human intracerebral hemorrhage has been reported.[18] The Intensive Blood Pressure Reduction in Acute Cerebral Haemorrhage Trial (INTERACT) was carried out primarily in China and demonstrated that blood pressure could be lowered in the acute setting with relative safety in comparison with a control group. A pivotal trial is under way.

Some researchers suggest that the goal for mean arterial blood pressure (MAP) should be gradually lowered to less than 130 mm Hg but that reductions of more than 20% should be avoided, and mean arterial blood pressures should not be reduced to less than 84 mm Hg.[19,20] Current guidelines suggest a target of 160 mm Hg systolic/90 mm Hg diastolic or MAP of 110 unless there is increased ICP (see later discussion, "Intracranial Pressure Considerations").[3] When ICP is elevated, it takes higher MAPs to drive cerebral perfusion pressure. Choice of agent may be important.[21] Intravenous labetalol[22] or nicardipine may provide smooth onset of action and allow physician to control blood pressure in patients without cardiac contraindications to these agents. Labetalol is begun as 10 to 20 mg intravenous (IV) push over 1 to 2 minutes. Doses can be increased to up to 40 to 80 mg every 10 minutes, or a continuous infusion starting at 2 mg/minute can be used if needed. Maximum dose is 300 mg/day. Nicardipine infusions are begun at 5 mg/hour. The dose can be increased by 2.5 mg/hour every 10 minutes if needed. Maximum dose is 15 mg/hour. Nitrates theoretically may worsen cerebral edema owing to their vasodilatory properties and should probably be avoided, given the other available agents.

Mechanical Ventilation

The decision for mechanical ventilation of patients with ICH or IVH relies on a diverse group of indications. One study found that intubation is five times more common in patients with ICH than in those with ischemic stroke.[23] Hypoxia and hypercarbia can damage neurons, contributing to poor outcome. Pulmonary indications include hypoxia related to pneumonia and exacerbated preexisting pulmonary or cardiac conditions. Hypercarbia may be related to central or pulmonary causes. Airway protection in the obtunded patient is also important to avoid aspiration. Intubation is one way of protecting the airway, but an oropharyngeal or nasopharyngeal airway is less invasive. Such an airway may be adequate for the patient who has good oxygenation and ventilation but impairment of consciousness or brainstem dysfunction that prohibits keeping the airway clear.

Endotracheal intubation has some advantages over simply providing an airway. Intubation further protects against aspiration, allows suctioning of upper respiratory structures, and provides for the administration of some drugs. The stimulation provided during intubation may lead to abrupt elevations in ICP. These elevations may be avoided with a rapid induction procedure using a short-acting neuromuscular blocker, barbiturate, and lidocaine. Supplemental oxygen and the placement of nasogastric or orogastric tubes are important to prevent aspiration.[24]

Deep Vein Thrombosis

Prevention of deep vein thrombosis is critical. Admitted patients should be immediately fitted with pneumatic compression stockings. After documentation of cessation of bleeding, subcutaneous heparin can be added 1-4 days from onset.[3] A study comparing unfractionated heparin with enoxaparin for deep vein prophylaxis in patients with acute ischemic stroke found reduced deep vein thrombosis, as measured by ultrasound, with enoxaparin.[25] This study did not use clinically significant deep vein thrombosis as an endpoint, did not report neurologic outcomes, and found a higher rate of systemic hemorrhage (although not intracranial hemorrhage) in subjects receiving enoxaparin. For these reasons, the fact that the study was done in ischemic stroke, and the relative cost of enoxaparin compared with unfractionated heparin, we use subcutaneous unfractionated heparin in patients with ICH.

Steroids

Two randomized trials have examined the role of steroids in ICH.[26,27] Both failed to demonstrate a benefit for steroids in patients with ICH. In fact, in one study,[26] patients who were treated with steroids had more infectious complications than those who were not.

Anticonvulsants

We reserve the use of anticonvulsants to patients who exhibit a first seizure, to avoid unnecessarily treating patients who will never have a seizure. Prophylactic anticonvulsants are not recommended.[3] If a seizure does occur, we administer a loading dose with IV fosphenytoin 10 to 20 mg phenytoin equivalents/kg, followed by maintenance phenytoin 4 to 7 mg/kg daily. Levetiracetam 500 to 1500 mg twice daily can be considered if drug-drug interactions are an issue.

Antiplatelets

Determining whether to use antiplatelet therapy in patients after initial ICH is an important concern, because many patients with ICH are also at risk for ischemic stroke and myocardial infarction. In one study, patients with ICH had a 2.4% yearly risk of recurrence and a 3.0% risk of subsequent ischemic stroke.[28] In a systematic review, the risk of recurrent ICH was 2.3% per year (95% CI, 1.9%-2.7%), whereas the risk of ischemic stroke was 1.1% per year (95% CI, 0.8%-1.7%). Patients with lobar ICH had double the risk of recurrent ICH than those with deep ICH had.[29] We use antiplatelet treatment following ICH only in patients with high cardiac or ischemic stroke risk, such as the presence of atrial fibrillation.

Other Therapies

Critically ill patients should be monitored for infection, and appropriate antibiotics should be instituted if necessary. Frequent change of positioning reduces pressure sores. Gastrointestinal hemorrhage is common in the high stress of an ICU stay. Use of prophylactic histamine (H_2) blockers is suggested. Early rehabilitation is advisable but has not been well studied. Avoidance of sedation except in patients with documented increased ICP allows the patient to more actively participate in rehabilitation and any neurologic changes to be observed and managed.

Prevention of Rebleeding

Evidence now suggests that much of the morbidity and mortality in ICH stems from early rebleeding. The first report of the regrowth of cerebral hematomas came from Fujii et al.[30] They observed that of their 419 patients with ICH who presented within 24 hours of symptom onset, hematoma growth was observed in 14% when imaging was repeated within 24 hours of admission. Patients who presented earliest with larger hemorrhages were likely to have regrowth. Liver disease, an irregularly shaped hematoma on CT, and coagulation abnormalities were also associated with hematoma expansion.

Kazui et al[31] reported that 36% of 74 patients who underwent imaging within 3 hours had hematoma expansion on later imaging studies. Even after 6 hours, 17% had rebleeding, but none showed rebleeding after 24 hours. This group analyzed potential factors associated with risk of rebleeding.[32] They found that hematoma growth was independently associated with a history of ischemic stroke, liver disease, and interaction of either elevated blood glucose (>141 mg/dL) or glycosylated hemoglobin concentration (>5.1%) with systolic blood pressure (>200 mm Hg).

In another study, Brott et al[33] performed head CT in patients with ICH upon emergency department presentation, 1 hour later, and 20 hours later. These researchers found that 26% of the 103 study subjects experienced rebleeding consisting of more than 33% of the initial hematoma volume within 1 hour of hospital arrival. The mean time from hospital arrival to initial CT scan was 89 minutes. This finding implies that a quarter of patients with ICH or IVH rebleed within 2.5 hours of the initial bleeding. Brott et al[33] reported that 12% of the remaining patients experienced rebleeding between the 1-hour and 20-hour CT scans.

It seems that hematoma growth happens early, in the majority of cases within the first minutes to hours of the initial bleed. Rebleeding after 6 hours is rare. Patients who have coagulation disorders or a hepatic predisposition for coagulation deficits are at risk. An initial large size and irregularity of the hematoma should raise concern about rebleeding. The roles of blood pressure and glucose are also potential factors.

Two trials investigated the effect of recombinant factor VIIa (rfVIIa), which is used in bleeding disorders such as hemophilia, on the prevention of rebleeding in acute ICH. The first was a dose-finding, phase 2b, randomized, controlled trial of 399 patients.[34] The group that received rfVIIa had significantly less hematoma growth and reduced severe disability and mortality than the placebo group. There was a trend to increased thromboembolic complications in the rfVIIa-treated groups. The absolute reduction in hemorrhage growth was quite small (4.5 mL). Unfortunately, the pivotal, phase 3 trial showed absolutely no difference in functional outcome or mortality between rfVIIa-treated and placebo-treated patients, and there was a higher rate of arterial thromboembolic events in rfVIIa-treated patients.[35] Therefore, rfVIIa cannot be recommended for routine use in patients with ICH. Some studies have focused on better patient selection to identify patients who would benefit the most from hemostatic therapy. Until data substantiate the efficacy and safety of rfVIIa in a defined clinical scenario, we do not use it in any off-label circumstance. At this time the only indications for use of rfVIIa approved by the U.S. Food and Drug Administration (FDA) are bleeding prophylaxis and bleeding treatment in known factor deficiencies.

One possible way to directly determine whether hemostasis has occurred is through CT with contrast imaging. Becker et al[36] found that extravasation of contrast material in patients with ICH suggested that the hemorrhage was still growing. Extravasation of contrast material can also be demonstrated on MRI, with the same correlation with rebleeding.[37] CT angiography (CTA) is perhaps the easiest acute vascular imaging test to obtain, and continuous bleeding on CTA has been labeled the "spot sign."[38] This finding suggests that patients with imaging evidence of continued bleeding are candidates for local or systemic therapies to promote clotting, and trials to evaluate this possibility are under way.

The coagulation factors related to the occurrence and growth of hemorrhage remain unknown. Finding specific therapies to intervene in the acute period requires an understanding of the natural phenomena in patients with ICH. One study found that normal systemic hemostatic activation does not occur unless the cerebral hematoma extends into the ventricular system or subarachnoid space.[39] Future areas of research to limit clot enlargement might be preventing lysis of the hemostatic plug, enhancing the formation of the hemostatic plug, and more aggressive lowering of blood pressure during the first 24 hours.[40]

Management of Cerebral Edema, Hydrocephalus, and Intraventricular Hemorrhage

Significant causes of mortality in ICH or IVH are cerebral edema and hydrocephalus. There are therapies for these conditions, and their results are mixed, as discussed here.

Cerebral Edema

Cerebral edema is a well-recognized complication of ICH. Whether the edema is due to an acute space-occupying lesion or the toxic effects of blood is unknown. An intriguing finding is that patients with thrombolysis-related ICH have far less cerebral edema than patients with spontaneous ICH.[41] This finding suggests that something in the clotting process may be directly responsible for the cerebral edema seen in patients with spontaneous ICH. Mass effect and midline shift maximize around 48 hours after symptom onset and, perhaps, during a second peak 2 to 3 weeks after hemorrhage.[42] Despite the success of antiedema therapies in controlling ICP in animal models,[43] the therapeutic value of these agents has not been borne out in human studies. Two randomized trials of therapy for cerebral edema in patients with ICH have been performed. The first utilized intravenous glycerol.[44] A total of 216 patients were randomly assigned to receive either glycerol or a placebo. There was no difference in 6-month mortality rates or functional outcomes between the two groups. A similar trial of hemodilution in ICH compared with the best medical therapy failed to demonstrate an advantage for hemodilution treatment.[45] A link between iron deposition, cerebral edema, and neuronal injury in ICH has been elucidated.[46,47] A pilot trial of iron chelation with deferoxamine in acute ICH is currently under way.[48]

Hydrocephalus and Intraventricular Hemorrhage

Hydrocephalus is an independent predictor of poor outcome from ICH or IVH.[49,50] It can occur because of obstruction of cerebrospinal fluid (CSF) flow in patients with ventricular clot or communicating hydrocephalus from a variety of causes. The treatment is placement of a ventriculostomy for external drainage of CSF and blood in the ventricular system. Most devices now allow simultaneous measurement of ICP. When the device is first placed, measurement of opening pressure is important. The drain is usually set at 15 cm above the ear to facilitate drainage. The risk of infection rises with time, so a ventricular fluid specimen is collected every other day for analysis to monitor cell count, differential cell counts, and glucose and protein levels as well as for bacterial culture. The drain should remain in place until the pressure returns to normal (<20 cm H_2O).

Often, when ventricular blood is copious, hydrocephalus becomes chronic, and the patient is drain dependent. Conversion of the ventriculostomy to an internalized shunt must be timed properly. If the externalized shunt is internalized when too much blood still remains, there is the danger of blockage of the shunt by clotting. Waiting too long, however, raises the risk of ventriculitis. In general, when the CSF visually clears of blood and the CSF protein level has decreased toward the normal range, it is time to consider a shunt in a patient who cannot maintain a normal ICP after a trial of 7 to 10 days.

Observational studies suggest that external CSF drainage is associated with a 25% lower risk of death and poor outcome than conservative treatment.[51] Unfortunately, no trials have been conducted to guide our management of hydrocephalus. Certainly, hydrocephalus is a treatable condition that leads to reductions in consciousness and therefore makes patients look more severely impaired. This appearance may lead to early withdrawal of care and the missed opportunity to intervene and help patients with ICH.[52]

An intriguing possibility is lysis of the clot in the ventricular system to improve hydrocephalus. A systematic review suggested a 92% reduction in risk of death and poor outcome in comparison with conservative treatment.[51] In one study, 10 patients with IVH received direct intraventricular injection of recombinant tissue-type plasminogen activator and subsequent CSF drainage.[53] Forty percent of patients made a good recovery, and only 1 died. In another group of 20 patients treated with intraventricular urokinase, the mortality was 20%, compared with a predicted mortality of 68%.[54] This large reduction in mortality for a modest number of patients has prompted a larger trial of ventricular clot lysis that is currently under way, the Clot Lysis: Evaluating Accelerated Resolution of Intraventricular Hemorrhage (CLEAR-IVH) trial.

Intracranial Pressure Considerations

Cerebral edema and hydrocephalus are two causes of increased ICP. ICP must be maintained below 20 cm H_2O. To accomplish this goal, evaluation of the underlying cause of the elevation in ICP should proceed. If it is not possible to remove the underlying cause (e.g., surgical removal of the hematoma), an algorithm for treatment of ICP should be followed (Fig. 55-1). It is important to remember that cerebral blood flow depends on adequate cerebral perfusion pressure. As discussed earlier, *cerebral perfusion pressure* is the difference between mean arterial blood pressure and ICP. Cerebral perfusion pressure should be kept above 70 mm Hg.[55] If ICP is high, lowering the systemic blood pressure could be deleterious.

When ICP is increased, deterioration in consciousness follows quickly. Patients with elevated ICP should be intubated with ICP precautions, as discussed previously. In general, the goal for the P_{CO_2} is 35 to 40 torr. Hyperventilation to a P_{CO_2} of 30 to 35 torr has a very short-lived effect and should be used only in the period immediately before a definitive therapy such as hematoma evacuation.[56,57] The mechanism of action of hyperventilation is decreased

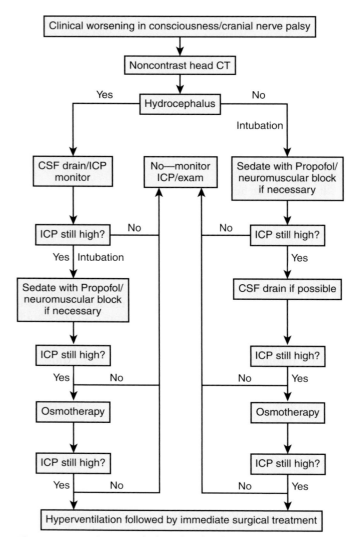

Figure 55-1 Suggested algorithm for the management of intracranial pressure in intracerebral hemorrhage. CSF, cerebrospinal fluid; ICP, intracranial pressure.

cerebral blood flow and edema reduction. The rebound effect from reversal of hyperventilation may dramatically worsen cerebral edema and elevate ICP. Sedation is accomplished with a continuous drip of intravenous propofol, a short-acting agent that can be turned off for intermittent neurologic examinations. Neuromuscular paralysis may be added (vecuronium is a good choice) but should never be given without proper sedation.

When ICP corrections are needed, osmotherapy is often used. Mannitol is the best-known treatment. Therapy is commenced with an infusion of 1 g/kg, followed by 25 to 50 g every 6 hours to titrate the serum osmolality to 310 to 320 mOsm/kg. Mannitol tends to deplete the intravascular space and therefore to lower MAP. An alternative osmotherapy combination is colloid plus furosemide. The choices of colloid are albumin, dextran, and hydroxyethyl starch. The colloid substances allow maintenance of the intravascular space. The risk is pulmonary edema. Careful monitoring of central venous pressures and a critical care specialist consultation are highly recommended. Like that of hyperventilation, the effect of osmotherapy is short-lived, and rebound elevations in cerebral edema and ICP are likely if the therapy is not tapered slowly.

Mechanical devices to measure ICP are controversial.[58,59] Monitoring ICP is necessary when ventricular drainage is proceeding. In patients with a Glasgow Coma Scale (GCS) score less than 9 it is also advisable. Because ICH is an asymmetrical disease, pressures in the skull may vary, unlike in a global condition such as hepatic failure. Patients may undergo various herniation syndromes while the ICP monitor continues to record a "normal" number. The clinical examination should always be the mainstay for detection of progression and institution of emergency imaging and therapy for patients with progressing cerebral edema and mass effect.

Two experimental therapies may hold promise in the future for the management of cerebral edema and increased ICP. Hypothermia dramatically lowers ICP in animal models. Studies show impressive results of hypothermia in the form of improved neurologic outcome in patients who have experienced cardiac arrest.[60,61] Its use in ICH seems a logical next step. One potential side effect of hypothermia is coagulopathy, so studies must be performed before this therapy can be advocated for ICH. The other therapy is hemicraniectomy and duraplasty. This treatment involves removing a large portion of the skull and making a broad incision in the dura to allow the brain to swell without added tissue pressure inside the enclosed skull cavity. A meta-analysis substantiates the benefit of this procedure for malignant hemispheric ischemic stroke.[62] A report of 12 patients with ICH receiving hemicraniectomy shows promise for further investigation.[63]

Special Considerations in Warfarin-Related Intracranial Hemorrhage

Outcome of warfarin-related ICH is tied most to the size of the hemorrhage.[64] Ensuring that the bleeding has stopped is imperative. Emergency hematology consultation should be considered. Vitamin K should be administered urgently, but it takes awhile to work. Fresh-frozen plasma (FFP) has been the "gold standard" of treatment. In a series of 13 patients randomly assigned to receive either FFP or factor IX complex concentrate, coagulopathy reversed significantly faster in the group receiving factor IX than in the group receiving FFP. Neurologic outcomes were the same in the two groups, but the factor IX group had fewer complications.[65] Prothrombin complex concentrates in warfarin-related systemic hemorrhages have received attention.[66] More study is needed to determine the safety and efficacy of these different approaches to warfarin reversal in ICH.[40]

The issue of how to manage anticoagulation in high-risk patients (e.g., those with prosthetic heart valves or atrial fibrillation) who have had an ICH also requires further study. A decision analysis study of patients with nonvalvular atrial fibrillation and ICH suggested that only those with deep ICH who were at especially high risk for ischemic stroke should receive anticoagulation after an ICH.[67] One study found that the risk of ischemic stroke within 30 days after cessation of warfarin was less than 5%, and that in the 35 subjects in whom warfarin was quickly restarted, the risk of recurrent ICH was zero during hospitalization.[68] Another small case series of patients with warfarin-related ICH suggested the pitfalls of withholding warfarin and using it again after the first ICH.[69] If warfarin is to be used again, there is no information on when warfarin may be restarted after an ICH.

Selection of Patients for Surgery

Several small studies and one large study have investigated surgical treatment of ICH. This discussion concentrates on the overall benefits of surgery and on which patients should have surgery. The best reported benefits for hematoma evacuation come from surgical removal of thrombolytic-related ICH. In an observational study, patients treated with surgery had a 65% 30-day survival, compared with a 35% survival for patients treated medically ($P < .001$).[70] For patients with spontaneous hemorrhage, it seems that operating long after symptom onset does not improve outcome. The goals of early surgery are to reduce mortality and to improve functional outcome.[71] One randomized study of 20 patients treated within 24 hours of symptom onset found a nonsignificant trend toward better outcome in those treated medically.[72]

In a randomized trial of 34 patients undergoing either medical treatment or surgery within 12 hours of symptom onset for spontaneous supratentorial ICH, mortality was found to be 24% in the medical group and 19% in the surgical group (the difference was not statistically significant).[73] Functional outcome was unchanged. When these researchers added another surgical arm to the study, involving operation within 4 hours of symptom onset, they found that early postoperative rebleeding was a problem.[74] Figure 55-2 shows examples of a successful clot evacuation and an evacuation complicated by postoperative hematoma reaccumulation. Clearly, residual hematoma volume is directly related to poor outcome,[73] suggesting that if early surgery could be performed with good hemostasis, the procedure might be of benefit. Achieving hemostasis is probably related in part to the compulsiveness of the surgeon in identifying bleeding of microvessels and to careful coagulation.[75,76]

The International Surgical Trial for Intracerebral Hemorrhage (iSTICH) was a herculean effort using a randomized, controlled design to determine whether surgical clot removal was safe and effective.[77] The study found no difference in patients treated surgically and those receiving the best medical treatment. The study had several factors that may have diminished its ability to demonstrate a surgical benefit. Inclusion in the study and randomization to treatment occurred only in patients whom the surgeon wished to enter rather than all eligible subjects. There were many crossovers between treatment arms, and, perhaps most damaging, operations occurred very late (24 hours) post ictus. In a subgroup analysis of iSTICH, patients with hematomas within 1 cm of the brain surface did better with surgery than with medical treatment. A second iSTICH, focusing on these superficial hematomas, is ongoing.

Earlier attempts at synthesizing the evidence to determine the relative value of surgery in spontaneous

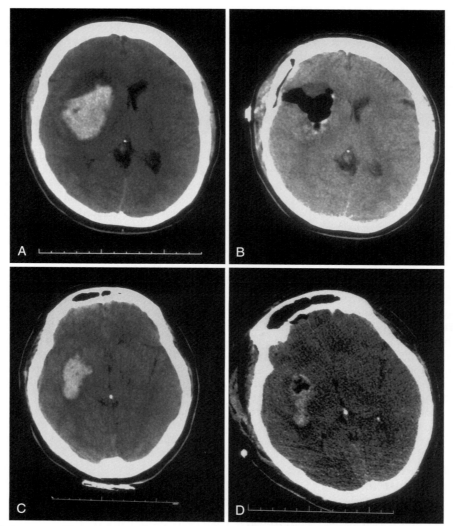

Figure 55-2 Surgical clot removal by craniotomy for intracranial hemorrhage within 4 hours of symptom onset in two patients. Baseline CT scan (A) and 24-hour postoperative CT scan (B) of the head of a patient in whom clot evacuation was successful. Dark areas in the hematoma cavity represent absorbable gelatin sponge (Gelfoam) and air, which subsequently were reabsorbed. Baseline CT scan (C) and 24-hour postoperative CT scan (D) of the head of a patient in whom hematoma regrowth occurred after clot evacuation.

supratentorial ICH usually concluded that the evidence was insufficient to allow any conclusions to be drawn.[78,79]

From the inclusion criteria of these studies, it appears that surgical benefit may be found for patients who (1) receive early treatment, (2) have moderate-size hematomas (20-80 mL in volume), (3) have Glasgow Coma Scale scores greater than 4, (4) are younger, (5) are not very ill with other malignant conditions, (6) do not have large amounts of intraventricular blood, and (7) are treated in centers with "compulsive" surgeons. Surgical technique requires further study to substantiate this claim. Stereotactic and endoscopic approaches allow less disruption of tissue than open craniotomy for deep hemorrhages, but they cannot remove enough hematoma volume in a timely manner. Stereotactic approaches coupled with local thrombolysis may be promising. The Minimally-Invasive Surgery Plus rtPA for Intracerebral Hemorrhage Evacuation (MISTIE) trial uses this combined approach and is ongoing.

For patients with infratentorial hemorrhage, the indications for surgery are different. Patients with cerebellar hemorrhage may experience brainstem compression syndromes quickly at any time within the first 3 weeks after the event. Suboccipital craniotomy with removal of the clot is lifesaving, and patients recover well if the procedure is carried out at the earliest threat of brainstem compression, before frank herniation occurs.[80]

Predictors of Outcome and Withdrawal of Care

Although many researchers have offered complicated formulas, hematoma volume is the most important predictor of outcome for a patient with ICH.[81] Initial Glasgow Coma Scale score is also a potent predictor of outcome.[81,82] In patients with a hematoma volume exceeding 30 mL, both morbidity and mortality rates are high. Some workers have tried to replicate the success of ischemic stroke rating scales, such as the National Institutes of Health Stroke Scale score, with an "ICH Score."[83] This score has been validated.[84] Predicting which patients will experience deterioration after initial presentation is difficult. Studies attempting to identify clinical predictors have been unsuccessful.[82,85]

Becker et al[86] considered the role of withdrawal of care in patients with ICH. They found that the level of medical support was the most important predictor of outcome and that withdrawal of support is likely to bias outcome data and lead to self-fulfilling prophecies. That is, when the predictive models just discussed were constructed, clinicians who saw patients with large-volume ICHs made decisions with the family to withdraw care. The models then linked hematoma volume with ICH mortality. To eliminate this bias from reductions in the level of medical support, it would be necessary to aggressively treat all patients with ICH and determine outcome. This approach has never been studied.

Hemphill et al[87] found that hospitals that use do not resuscitate (DNR) orders more frequently have worse ICH outcomes, even when data are controlled for individual patient factors. Studies from Texas found a high proportion of both do not resuscitate and other withdrawal of care orders and suggested that potentially treatable conditions such as hydrocephalus may, in part, be responsible for early withdrawal of care.[52,88] The American Heart Association/American Stroke Association Guidelines for the Management of Intracerebral Hemorrhage suggest that clinicians not make new "do not resuscitate" orders for patients with ICH within the first 24 hours.[3] This recommendation reflects the true uncertainty we have regarding ICH outcome. Physicians have a difficult time admitting uncertainty. If admitting uncertainty allows us to take more time to make appropriate life-and-death decisions, the guidelines have been successful. New measures of quality of life after ICH are important barometers of recovery and should guide future clinical trial results.[89]

Conclusions

Although ICH is a devastating disease, aggressive medical therapy can make a large difference in outcome. Much of the therapy is "supportive," but it is also intensive and must be started urgently. A nihilistic approach to the care of patients with ICH is quickly dissipating. When care is limited, recovery is all but impossible. Future studies of surgery, neuroprotection, and strategies to prevent rebleeding will likely revolutionize ICH therapy.

In the interim, aggressive but reasonable treatment of the patient with ICH is warranted. Conservative control of blood pressure, treatment of fever, and glucose regulation are important. Patients with ICH or IVH should be cared for in specialized units with well-trained personnel. When elevated ICP is suspected, head CT should be performed, and an ICP treatment algorithm invoked. Early feeding and rehabilitation are also important. Prevention of complications such as pneumonia, ventriculitis, and deep vein thrombosis are necessary. Compulsive attention to these intensive medical therapies are of great value for the patient with ICH, whose life and functional status are clearly related to the level of care provided by the physician in charge of the case.

REFERENCES

1. Marti-Fabregas J, Piles S, Guardia E, et al: Spontaneous primary intraventricular hemorrhage: Clinical data, etiology and outcome, *J Neurol* 246:287–291, 1999.
2. Darby DG, Donnan GA, Saling MA, et al: Primary intraventricular hemorrhage: Clinical and neuropsychological findings in a prospective stroke series, *Neurology* 38:68–75, 1988.
3. Morgenstern LB, Hemphill JC III, Anderson C, et al: American Heart Association Stroke Council and Council on Cardiovascular Nursing: Guidelines for the management of spontaneous intracerebral hemorrhage: A guideline for healthcare professionals from the American Heart Association/American Stroke Association, *Stroke* 41(9):2108–2129, 2010.
4. Langhorne P, Dennis M: *Stroke units: An evidence based approach*, London, 1998, BMJ Publishing Group.
5. Ronning OM, Guldvog B: Stroke units versus general medical wards, I: Twelve- and eighteen-month survival: A randomized, controlled trial, *Stroke* 29:58–62, 1998.
6. Ronning OM, Guldvog B: Stroke unit versus general medical wards, II: Neurological deficits and activities of daily living: A quasi-randomized controlled trial, *Stroke* 29:586–590, 1998.
7. Ronning OM, Guldvog B, Stavem K: The benefit of an acute stroke unit in patients with intracranial haemorrhage: A controlled trial, *J Neurol, Neurosurg Psychiatry* 70:631–634, 2001.
8. Diringer MN, Edwards DF: Admission to a neurologic/neurosurgical intensive care unit is associated with reduced mortality rate after intracerebral hemorrhage, *Crit Care Med* 29:635–640, 2001.
9. Schwarz S, Hafner K, Aschoff A, Schwab S: Incidence and prognostic significance of fever following intracerebral hemorrhage, *Neurology* 54:354–361, 2000.
10. Azzimondi G, Bassein L, Nonino F, et al: Fever in acute stroke worsens prognosis. A prospective study, *Stroke* 26:2040–2043, 1995.
11. Reith J, Jorgensen HS, Pedersen PM, et al: Body temperature in acute stroke: Relation to stroke severity, infarct size, mortality, and outcome, *Lancet* 347:422–425, 1996.
12. Passero S, Ciacci G, Ulivelli M: The influence of diabetes and hyperglycemia on clinical course after intracerebral hemorrhage, *Neurology* 61:1351–1356, 2003.
13. Godoy DA, Pinero GR, Svampa S, et al: Hyperglycemia and short-term outcome in patients with spontaneous intracerebral hemorrhage, *Neurocrit Care* 9:217–229, 2008.
14. Demchuk AM, Morgenstern LB, Krieger DW, et al: Serum glucose level and diabetes predict tissue plasminogen activator-related intracerebral hemorrhage in acute ischemic stroke, *Stroke* 30:34–39, 1999.
15. Qureshi AI, Wilson DA, Hanley DF, et al: Pharmacologic reduction of mean arterial pressure does not adversely affect regional cerebral blood flow and intracranial pressure in experimental intracerebral hemorrhage, *Crit Care Med* 27:965–971, 1999.
16. Hirano T, Read SJ, Abbott DF, et al: No evidence of hypoxic tissue on 18F-fluoromisonidazole PET after intracerebral hemorrhage, *Neurology* 53:2179–2182, 1999.
17. Powers WJ, Zazulia AR, Videen TO, et al: Autoregulation of cerebral blood flow surrounding acute (6 to 22 hours) intracerebral hemorrhage, *Neurology* 57:18–24, 2001.
18. Anderson CS, Huang Y, Wang JG, et al: Intensive blood pressure reduction in acute cerebral haemorrhage trial (INTERACT): A randomised pilot trial, *Lancet Neurol* 7:391–399, 2008.
19. Broderick JP, Adams HP Jr, Barsan W, et al: Guidelines for the management of spontaneous intracerebral hemorrhage: A statement for healthcare professionals from a special writing group of the Stroke Council, American Heart Association, *Stroke* 30:905–915, 1999.
20. Morgenstern LB, Yonas H: Lowering blood pressure in acute intracerebral hemorrhage: Safe, but will it help? *Neurology* 57:5–6, 2001.
21. Kuroda K, Kuwata N, Sato N, et al: Changes in cerebral blood flow accompanied with reduction of blood pressure treatment in patients with hypertensive intracerebral hemorrhages, *Neurol Res* 19:169–173, 1997.
22. Patel RV, Kertland HR, Jahns BE, et al: Labetalol: Response and safety in critically ill hemorrhagic stroke patients, *Ann Pharmacother* 27:180–181, 1993.
23. Gujjar AR, Deibert E, Manno EM, et al: Mechanical ventilation for ischemic stroke and intracerebral hemorrhage: Indications, timing, and outcome, *Neurology* 51:447–451, 1998.

24. Kuzak N, Harrison DW, Zed PJ: Use of lidocaine and fentanyl premedication for neuroprotective rapid sequence intubation in the emergency department, *CJEM* 8:80–84, 2006.

25. Sherman DG, Albers GW, Bladin C, Kuzak N: The efficacy and safety of enoxaparin versus unfractionated heparin for the prevention of venous thromboembolism after acute ischaemic stroke (PREVAIL study): An open-label randomised comparison, *Lancet* 369:1347-1355, 2007.

26. Poungvarin N, Bhoopat W, Viriyavejakul A, et al: Effects of dexamethasone in primary supratentorial intracerebral hemorrhage, *N Engl J Med* 316:1229-1233, 1987.

27. Tellez H, Bauer RB: Dexamethasone as treatment in cerebrovascular disease. 1: A controlled study in intracerebral hemorrhage, *Stroke* 4:541-546, 1973.

28. Hill MD, Silver FL, Austin PC, et al: Rate of stroke recurrence in patients with primary intracerebral hemorrhage, *Stroke* 31:123-127, 2000.

29. Bailey RD, Hart RG, Benavente O, et al: Recurrent brain hemorrhage is more frequent than ischemic stroke after intracranial hemorrhage, *Neurology* 56:773-777, 2001.

30. Fujii Y, Tanaka R, Takeuchi S, et al: Hematoma enlargement in spontaneous intracerebral hemorrhage, *J Neurosurg* 80:51-57, 1994.

31. Kazui S, Naritomi H, Yamamoto H, et al: Enlargement of spontaneous intracerebral hemorrhage. Incidence and time course, *Stroke* 27:1783-1787, 1996.

32. Kazui S, Minematsu K, Yamamoto H, et al: Predisposing factors to enlargement of spontaneous intracerebral hematoma, *Stroke* 28:2370-2375, 1997.

33. Brott T, Broderick J, Kothari R, et al: Early hemorrhage growth in patients with intracerebral hemorrhage, *Stroke* 28:1-5, 1997.

34. Mayer SA, Brun NC, Begtrup K, et al: Recombinant activated factor VII for acute intracerebral hemorrhage, *N Engl J Med* 352:777-785, 2005.

35. Mayer SA, Brun NC, Begtrup K, et al: Efficacy and safety of recombinant activated factor VII for acute intracerebral hemorrhage, *N Engl J Med* 358:2127-2137, 2008.

36. Becker KJ, Baxter AB, Bybee HM, et al: Extravasation of radiographic contrast is an independent predictor of death in primary intracerebral hemorrhage, *Stroke* 30:2025-2032, 1999.

37. Murai Y, Ikeda Y, Teramoto A, et al: Magnetic resonance imaging-documented extravasation as an indicator of acute hypertensive intracerebral hemorrhage, *J Neurosurg* 88:650-655, 1998.

38. Wada R, Aviv RI, Fox AJ, et al: CT angiography "spot sign" predicts hematoma expansion in acute intracerebral hemorrhage, *Stroke* 38:1257-1262, 2007.

39. Fujii Y, Takeuchi S, Harada A, et al: Hemostatic activation in spontaneous intracerebral hemorrhage, *Stroke* 32:883-890, 2001.

40. NINDS ICH: Workshop Participants: Priorities for clinical research in intracerebral hemorrhage: Report from a National Institute of Neurological Disorders and Stroke Workshop, *Stroke* 36:e23-41, 2005.

41. Gebel JM, Brott TG, Sila CA, et al: Decreased perihematomal edema in thrombolysis-related intracerebral hemorrhage compared with spontaneous intracerebral hemorrhage, *Stroke* 31:596-600, 2000.

42. Zazulia AR, Diringer MN, Derdeyn CP, Powers WJ: Progression of mass effect after intracerebral hemorrhage, *Stroke* 30:1167-1173, 1999.

43. Qureshi AI, Wilson DA, Traystman RJ: Treatment of elevated intracranial pressure in experimental intracerebral hemorrhage: Comparison between mannitol and hypertonic saline, *Neurosurgery* 44:1055-1063, 1999.

44. Yu YL, Kumana CR, Lauder IJ, et al: Treatment of acute cerebral hemorrhage with intravenous glycerol. A double-blind, placebo-controlled, randomized trial, *Stroke* 23:967-971, 1992.

45. Italian Acute Stroke Study Group: Haemodilution in acute stroke: Results of the Italian haemodilution trial, *Lancet* 1:318-321, 1988.

46. Huang FP, Xi G, Keep RF, et al: Brain edema after experimental intracerebral hemorrhage: Role of hemoglobin degradation products, *J Neurosurg* 96:287-293, 2002.

47. Nakamura T, Keep RF, Hua Y, et al: Deferoxamine-induced attenuation of brain edema and neurological deficits in a rat model of intracerebral hemorrhage, *Neurosurg Focus* 15:ECP4, 2003.

48. Selim M: Deferoxamine mesylate. A new hope for intracerebral hemorrhage: From bench to clinical trials, *Stroke* 40(Suppl 3):S90-S91, 2009.

49. Diringer MN, Edwards DF, Zazulia AR: Hydrocephalus: A previously unrecognized predictor of poor outcome from supratentorial intracerebral hemorrhage, *Stroke* 29:1352-1357, 1998.

50. Phan TG, Koh M, Vierkant RA, Wijdicks EF: Hydrocephalus is a determinant of early mortality in putaminal hemorrhage, *Stroke* 31:2157-2162, 2000.

51. Nieuwkamp DJ, de Gans K, Rinkel GJ, Algra A: Treatment and outcome of severe intraventricular extension in patients with subarachnoid or intracerebral hemorrhage: A systematic review of the literature, *J Neurol* 247:117-121, 2000.

52. Zahuranec DB, Gonzales NR, Brown DL, et al: Presentation of intracerebral haemorrhage in a community, *J Neurol Neurosurg Psychiatry* 77:340-344, 2006.

53. Goh KY, Poon WS: Recombinant tissue plasminogen activator for the treatment of spontaneous adult intraventricular hemorrhage, *Surg Neurol* 50:526-531, 1998:discussion 531-522.

54. Naff NJ, Carhuapoma JR, Williams MA, et al: Treatment of intraventricular hemorrhage with urokinase: Effects on 30-day survival, *Stroke* 31:841-847, 2000.

55. Diringer MN: Intracerebral hemorrhage: Pathophysiology and management, *Crit Care Medicine* 21:1591-1603, 1993.

56. Fortune JB, Feustel PJ, Graca L, et al: Effect of hyperventilation, mannitol, and ventriculostomy drainage on cerebral blood flow after head injury, *J Trauma Injury Infect Crit Care* 39:1091-1097, 1995:discussion 1097-1099.

57. van Santbrink H, Maas AI, Avezaat CJ: Continuous monitoring of partial pressure of brain tissue oxygen in patients with severe head injury, *Neurosurgery* 38:21-31, 1996.

58. Frank JI: Large hemispheric infarction, deterioration, and intracranial pressure, *Neurology* 45:1286-1290, 1995.

59. Schwab S, Aschoff A, Spranger M, et al: The value of intracranial pressure monitoring in acute hemispheric stroke, *Neurology* 47:393-398, 1996.

60. Mild therapeutic hypothermia to improve the neurologic outcome after cardiac arrest, *N Engl J Med* 346:549-556, 2002.

61. Bernard SA, Gray TW, Buist MD, et al: Treatment of comatose survivors of out-of-hospital cardiac arrest with induced hypothermia, *N Engl J Med* 346:557-563, 2002.

62. Vahedi K, Hofmeijer J, Juettler E, et al: Early decompressive surgery in malignant infarction of the middle cerebral artery: A pooled analysis of three randomised controlled trials, *Lancet Neurol* 6:215-222, 2007.

63. Murthy JM, Chowdary GV, Murthy TV, et al: Decompressive craniectomy with clot evacuation in large hemispheric hypertensive intracerebral hemorrhage, *Neurocrit Care* 2:258-262, 2005.

64. Berwaerts J, Dijkhuizen RS, Robb OJ, Webster J: Prediction of functional outcome and in-hospital mortality after admission with oral anticoagulant-related intracerebral hemorrhage, *Stroke* 31:2558-2562, 2000.

65. Boulis NM, Bobek MP, Schmaier A, Hoff JT: Use of factor IX complex in warfarin-related intracranial hemorrhage, *Neurosurgery* 45:1113-1118, 1999.

66. Kalina M, Tinkoff G, Gbadebo A, et al: A protocol for the rapid normalization of INR in trauma patients with intracranial hemorrhage on prescribed warfarin therapy, *Am Surg* 74:858-861, 2008.

67. Eckman MH, Rosand J, Knudsen KA, et al: Can patients be anticoagulated after intracerebral hemorrhage? A decision analysis, *Stroke* 34:1710-1716, 2003.

68. Phan TG, Koh M, Wijdicks EF: Safety of discontinuation of anticoagulation in patients with intracranial hemorrhage at high thromboembolic risk, *Arch Neurol* 57:1710-1713, 2000.

69. Claassen DO, Kazemi N, Zubkov AY, et al: Restarting anticoagulation therapy after warfarin-associated intracerebral hemorrhage, *Arch Neurol* 65:1313-1318, 2008.

70. Mahaffey KW, Granger CB, Sloan MA, et al: Neurosurgical evacuation of intracranial hemorrhage after thrombolytic therapy for acute myocardial infarction: Experience from the GUSTO-I trial. Global utilization of streptokinase and tissue-plasminogen activator (t-PA) for occluded coronary arteries, *Am Heart J* 138:493-499, 1999.

71. Fujitsu K, Muramoto M, Ikeda Y, et al: Indications for surgical treatment of putaminal hemorrhage. Comparative study based on serial CT and time-course analysis, *J Neurosurgery* 73:518-525, 1990.

72. Zuccarello M, Brott T, Derex L, et al: Early surgical treatment for supratentorial intracerebral hemorrhage: A randomized feasibility study, *Stroke* 30:1833-1839, 1999.

73. Morgenstern LB, Frankowski RF, Shedden P, et al: Surgical treatment for intracerebral hemorrhage (STICH): A single-center, randomized clinical trial, *Neurology* 51:1359-1363, 1998.

74. Morgenstern LB, Demchuk AM, Kim DH, et al: Rebleeding leads to poor outcome in ultra-early craniotomy for intracerebral hemorrhage, *Neurology* 56:1294-1299, 2001.

75. Kaneko M, Koba T, Yokoyama T: Early surgical treatment for hypertensive intracerebral hemorrhage, *J Neurosurg* 46:579-583, 1977.

76. Kaneko M, Tanaka K, Shimada T, et al: Long-term evaluation of ultra-early operation for hypertensive intracerebral hemorrhage in 100 cases, *J Neurosurg* 58:838-842, 1983.

77. Mendelow AD, Gregson BA, Fernandes HM, et al: Early surgery versus initial conservative treatment in patients with spontaneous supratentorial intracerebral haematomas in the International Surgical Trial in Intracerebral Haemorrhage (STICH): A randomised trial, *Lancet* 365:387-397, 2005.

78. Hankey GJ, Hon C: Surgery for primary intracerebral hemorrhage: Is it safe and effective? A systematic review of case series and randomized trials, *Stroke* 28:2126-2132, 1997.

79. Prasad K, Browman G, Srivastava A, Menon G: Surgery in primary supratentorial intracerebral hematoma: A meta-analysis of randomized trials, *Acta Neurol Scand* 95:103-110, 1997.

80. Montes JM, Wong JH, Fayad PB, Awad IA: Stereotactic computed tomographic-guided aspiration and thrombolysis of intracerebral hematoma: Protocol and preliminary experience, *Stroke* 31:834-840, 2000.

81. Broderick JP, Brott TG, Duldner JE, et al: Volume of intracerebral hemorrhage. A powerful and easy-to-use predictor of 30-day mortality, *Stroke* 24:987-993, 1993.

82. Flemming KD, Wijdicks EF, St Louis EK, Li H: Predicting deterioration in patients with lobar haemorrhages, *J Neurol Neurosurg Psychiatry* 66:600-605, 1999.

83. Hemphill JC III, Bonovich DC, Besmertis L, et al: The ICH score: A simple, reliable grading scale for intracerebral hemorrhage, *Stroke* 32:891-897, 2001.

84. Clarke JL, Johnston SC, Farrant M, et al: External validation of the ICH score, *Neurocrit Care* 1:53-60, 2004.

85. Mayer SA, Sacco RL, Shi T, Mohr JP: Neurologic deterioration in noncomatose patients with supratentorial intracerebral hemorrhage, *Neurology* 44:1379-1384, 1994.

86. Becker KJ, Baxter AB, Cohen WA, et al: Withdrawal of support in intracerebral hemorrhage may lead to self-fulfilling prophecies, *Neurology* 56:766-772, 2001.

87. Hemphill JC 3rd, Newman J, Zhao S, Johnston SC: Hospital usage of early do-not-resuscitate orders and outcome after intracerebral hemorrhage, *Stroke* 35:1130-1134, 2004.

88. Zahuranec DB, Brown DL, Lisabeth LD, et al: Early care limitations independently predict mortality after intracerebral hemorrhage, *Neurology* 68:1651-1657, 2007.

89. Hamedani AG, Wells CK, Brass LM, et al: A quality-of-life instrument for young hemorrhagic stroke patients, *Stroke* 32:687-695, 2001.

56

Rehabilitation and Recovery of the Patient with Stroke

BRUCE H. DOBKIN

The rehabilitation of the patient with stroke aims to lessen physical and cognitive impairments, increase functional independence, lessen the burden of care provided by significant others, reintegrate the patient into the family and community, and restore the patient's health-related quality of life. Rehabilitation differs from usual neurologic care in that its long-term goal is to lessen disability and to give patients the opportunity to participate in their typical roles and activities. Despite this soft-sounding edge, neurologic rehabilitation draws heavily from the neuroscientific bases for learning and neural adaptability.

Physicians who consider the management of stroke a "done deal" beyond the first 3 hours or few days after a disabling brain injury are abandoning their obligation to provide best patient care. Along with offering interventions to prevent another stroke, stroke neurologists and other clinicians who treat acute stroke ought to be familiar with the short-term and long-term interventions that may prevent complications of immobility, reduce impairments and disabilities, and improve quality of life for their patients.

Neurologic Rehabilitation

Specialized Assessment and Outcome Measures

To grasp the special concerns of neurorehabilitation services and outcomes, the clinician must be familiar with certain jargon:

Impairments are the physical or psychological abnormalities manifested by an acute neurologic event (e.g., hemiplegia, hemineglect). They are measured by the clinical and neurologic examination or by standard scales such as the National Institutes of Health Stroke Scale (NIHSS) and the Fugl-Meyer Assessment of Sensorimotor Recovery. The Fugl-Meyer Assessment measures both selective and synergistic movements.

Disabilities are the functional restrictions induced by impairments, such as the inability to walk without physical assistance. The Barthel Index (BI) (Table 56-1) and the Functional Independence Measure (FIM) (Table 56-2) are commonly used ordinal scales for the semiquantification of the level of independence in activities of daily living (ADLs). Basic ADLs include bathing, feeding, upper and lower extremity dressing, transfers, toileting, and grooming.

On admission to inpatient rehabilitation, the majority of patients have a moderate level of disability, with a BI of 40 to 60 or a total FIM score of 40 to 80. These impairment and disability scales do not reflect fine motor function, the ease of completion, quality of execution, time for completion of a task, or whether an affected upper extremity is used to carry it out. Patients who score 100 on the BI or more than 60 on the motor subscore of the FIM are continent and can feed, bathe, and dress themselves; get up out of bed and chairs; ambulate household distances with initiation of community distances; and ascend and descend stairs. A maximum score does not imply that such people can cook, keep house, live alone, and meet the public, but they usually get along without attendant care. A BI of less than 60 at hospital discharge predicts a level of dependence that makes discharge to home less likely. Since 2002, scores on the FIM serve as an economic modifying factor in the Medicare payment system for inpatient rehabilitation in the United States.

A general relationship exists between motor impairment and disability scores. The NIHSS score performed 7 days after a stroke forecasts good recovery or severe disability at 3 months.[1] The NIHSS score also describes the severity of impairment observed during inpatient stroke rehabilitation.[2] The Orpington Prognostic Scale is a bit easier to use than the NIHSS and may be modestly better as a predictor of ADLs at 3 to 6 months after a mild to moderate stroke.[3]

Handicaps arise from impairments and disabilities but are driven by barriers in the environment. They include the disadvantages that limit or prevent the fulfillment of a usual role or activity. The scales of handicap describe how well subjects participate in home, work, and community activities, which are called *instrumental ADLs*. Instrumental ADLs are defined as ability to use the telephone, manage money, use transportation, maintain a household or job, and participate in leisure activities. They can be measured, in part, by the Frenchay Activities Index.[4]

Health-related quality of life (QOL), which includes a patient's perception of his or her physical functioning as well as mental, psychosocial, and emotional state, has been measured most often with the Sickness Index Profile and the Medical Outcomes Study Short Form-36 (SF-36).[5] The SF-12 generates the physical and mental component summary scores of the SF-36 in some groups of patients after a stroke.[6] The Stroke-Specific QOL (SS-QOL) scale

TABLE 56-1   THE BARTHEL INDEX

	Needs Help	Independent
1. Feeding (If subject's food must be cut up, score as "needs help").	5	10
2. Moving from wheel-chair to bed and return (includes sitting up in bed).	5-10	15
3. Personal toilet (wash face, comb hair, shave, clean teeth).	0	5
4. Getting on and off toilet (handling clothes, wipe, flush).	5	10
5. Bathing self.	0	5
6. Walking on level surface (or, if unable to walk, propelling wheelchair).	10 / 0*	15 / 5*
7. Ascend and descend stairs.	5	10
8. Dressing (include tying shoes, fastening fasteners).	5	10
9. Controlling bowels.	5	10
10. Controlling bladder.	5	10

*Score only if unable to walk.

TABLE 56-2   FUNCTIONAL INDEPENDENCE MEASURE (FIM) ITEMS

Self-care	Eat
	Groom
	Bathe
	Dress upper body
	Dress lower body
	Toileting
Sphincter	Bladder management
	Bowel management
Mobility	Bed-to-chair and wheelchair-to-chair transfer
	Toilet transfer
	Tub and shower transfer
Locomotion	Walk or use wheelchair
	Climb stairs
Social cognition	Social interaction
	Problem solving
	Memory
	Communication
	Comprehension
	Expression
Score	Burden of care
7	Complete independence (timely, safely)
6	Modified independence (device)
5	Supervision
4	Minimal assistance (subject does at least 75% of task)
3	Moderate assistance (subject does at least 50% of task)
2	Maximal assistance (subject does at least 25% of task)
1	Total assistance (subject does <25% of task)

contains 12 questions about problems walking and using a wheelchair and 9 about functional use of the affected upper extremity.[7] A 54-item QOL scale for young patients who suffer a hemorrhagic stroke (HSQuale) has seven domains, covering work and financial status, social and leisure activities, and relationships.[8] Caregiver strain may be another dimension of QOL for the patient and family.[9,10]

Some scales used in stroke studies, such as the Rankin Scale, mix the domains of impairment, disability, and handicap into five or fewer general outcomes. Such scales are better for large trials than for the assessment of individual patients. The Stroke Impact Scale (SIS) is a self-report measure with 64 item that assess eight domains and covers strength, hand function, ADLs, instrumental ADLs, mobility, communication, memory, emotion, thinking, and participation.[11] Its reliability, validity, and responsiveness between 1 and 6 months after stroke are good, and the tool may not have the floor and ceiling effects of the BI and the SF-36 (see later). A clinically meaningful change in the SIS score is about 10 to 15 points. A 16-item SIS is available.

Another instrument is the American Heart Association's Stroke Outcome Classification (AHA.SOC).[12] This scale rates impairments, basic self-care skills, and instrumental ADLs. The number of impairments and the severity of impairments are graded on a scale of 3 to 0 for motor, sensory, visual, affective, cognitive, and language deficits. Five levels, from independence to complete dependence, are graded for the combination of basic *ADLs* and instrumental ADLs. Many other scales may be of use as assessment and outcome measures for neurorehabilitation interventions.[13]

Mechanisms for Gains

A decrease in impairments and disabilities over the first 3 to 6 months after a stroke is often called *spontaneous recovery*. Resolution of edema, heme, ion fluxes, cell and axon physiologic dysfunction, and diaschisis from trans-synaptic and neurotransmitter dysfunction may lead to *restitutive* intrinsic biologic activity and gains over several weeks. Rehabilitation interventions may aim for *substitutive* extrinsic drives to manipulate biologic activity.[13] Although finger pinch or walking may improve with restitutive mechanisms, the multilevel effects of activity-dependent plasticity associated with practice and learning have become increasingly clear from molecular, electrophysiologic, and morphologic studies in recovering animals as well as from serial functional neuroimaging studies in humans.[14,15] Patients make gains by experience-driven changes within partially spared pathways, within flexible neuronal assemblies that represent movements, sensation, and cognition, and within multiple representational maps in parallel, distributed networks.[13]

Rehabilitation approaches often emphasize *compensatory strategies* for impairments and disabilities. Patients are trained to make a greater effort to employ a defective skill, substitute a latent skill, learn a new way to accomplish a goal or alter the environment to make a task easier, or change their expectations about performing a particular task. Most compensatory approaches require learning, and gains may be reflected in experience-dependent plasticity.

The optimal duration and intensity of training are uncertain for human rehabilitation strategies. More intensive, task-oriented practice seems to enhance learning and performance.[16,17] Most patients, however, receive no more than a few months of formal inpatient and outpatient retraining. *Intensive rehabilitation* often amounts to less than 20 hours of engagement in physical, occupational, or speech therapy. Each therapist works at many tasks for 2 to 4 weeks of inpatient care and 2 to 4 months of outpatient care. This modest amount of practice may be far less than what is needed to, say, regain the ability to walk at a speed that permits community activities or to improve word-finding skills.[18-21]

Organization of Services

The focus of rehabilitation on enhancing gains across a wide range of impairments and disabilities requires a multidisciplinary group of participants, including physicians such as neurologists and physiatrists; nurses with special competence in rehabilitation teaching and care; physical, occupational, recreational, and speech-language therapists; social workers; case managers; neuropsychologists; orthotists; dietitians; and biomedical engineers.

Patients who are at a supervised or minimally assisted level of self-care are usually discharged from the acute hospital setting to the home with either home health or outpatient therapy. By the end of the first 2 weeks after a stroke, from 12% to 20% of patients in the United States are referred for inpatient rehabilitation. These patients need ongoing supervision by physicians and nurses, have enough stamina to participate in rehabilitation therapies for at least 3 hours a day, and have adequate psychosocial supports, so the rehabilitation team can anticipate discharge to the home or to a board-and-care facility. Further criteria for inpatient rehabilitation are adequate motivation and cognition for learning. Patients who do not meet these criteria may receive therapies in a skilled nursing facility.

Although the issue is difficult to study formally, the literature suggests that the earlier the initiation of an inpatient rehabilitation program (within 20 days of onset of stroke, compared with 20 to 60 days in subjects with similar levels of disability), the better the outcomes.[22] Length of stay in inpatient rehabilitation is determined during weekly conferences in which the team reassesses the patient's progress toward reasonable functional goals. The discharge from inpatient or outpatient rehabilitation should be scheduled with adequate notice for the family to make preparations. Patients need appropriate durable medical equipment, such as a lightweight wheelchair, a cane, an ankle-foot orthosis, and a tub bench, along with follow-up medical and disability-oriented community care.

A number of studies have tried to establish the best locus and time for acute and subacute rehabilitation care. At least 20 trials have compared outcomes between patients managed on specialized stroke or rehabilitation units and those receiving standard medical ward care. In general, these subjects were not too low-level or high-level in function for inpatient rehabilitation as practiced in the United States today. The milieu of a dedicated stroke unit that provides rehabilitation or of a dedicated rehabilitation unit appears to improve outcomes. Although some of the benefit relates to acute care interventions,[23] some benefit derives from the focus on prevention of medical complications related to immobility, on retraining in functional activities,[24] on family training, on the intensity of retraining, on early recognition of mood disorders, and on outpatient follow-up.[25] One prospective study showed that patients admitted to a rehabilitation hospital were significantly more likely to return to the community and recover ADLs than patients sent to nursing facilities for therapy.[26] Unfortunately, the role of case management in the multidisciplinary team has yet to be quantified in clinical studies.[27]

Inpatient rehabilitation is expensive and removes patients from their usual psychosocial and physical environment. Studies with good designs for trials of outpatient therapy suggest that the organization and intensity of services may be related to better outcomes. However, several nonrandomized European community studies of all stroke survivors found that patients who receive therapy either in the hospital or through an organized outpatient approach perform, overall, as well as those who receive little or no remedial treatment.[28] This result is likely to vary with the severity of stroke and the availability of medical and home supports. A short-term inpatient stay that enables patients to become independent enough to be treated at home followed by outpatient therapy at home, in a clinic, or in a day program may best meet the functional, cognitive, and psychosocial needs of patients.

One large randomized trial compared patients who had rehabilitation at home after an average 12-day inpatient stay with patients who had an additional week of inpatient care followed by hospital-based outpatient treatment.[29] Subjects who lived alone were independent in transfers when they left the hospital or they were assisted by a caregiver. Similar outcomes at 12 months after stroke were achieved in the two groups, but at lower cost because of less use of hospital beds by the early discharge group. An intention-to-treat randomized trial with 250 subjects showed that rehabilitation on an inpatient unit after a brief stay in an acute stroke unit or general medical ward produced better outcomes in moderate to severely disabled patients (BI < 50) than rehabilitation treatment in the community.[30] No differences in QOL were found, and instrumental ADLs were not measured. Smaller trials confirm similar positive outcomes at 3 to 6 months for home and various forms of outpatient care, with the home groups having fewer in-hospital days[31] and greater gains in instrumental ADLs.

Community mobility, cooking and cleaning skills, leisure activities, social isolation, and support for caregivers often continue to be problematic for 2-year survivors of a stroke.[32] The clinician should either ask about instrumental ADLs or use an assessment that has patients rate the difficulty they perceive in carrying out these tasks,[33] so that an appropriate rehabilitation prescription may be ordered. A pulse of therapy carried out beyond 6 months after stroke, especially if focused on training in specific skills such as walking and using the affected arm, often improves the ADLs that the patient practices.[18,34]

Overview of Practices

At the time of admission to inpatient rehabilitation, the following features are unfavorable prognosticators for functional gains and for a discharge back to the home: advanced age and neurologic impairments such as profound paresis, loss of proprioception, visuospatial hemineglect, gaze palsy, dementia, and bowel and bladder incontinence. Also, the higher the admission BI or FIM score, the higher the discharge score and the greater the likelihood that the patient resumes independence at home.

An epidemiologic report from the Framingham Study is one of the very few studies to compare functional disabilities in survivors of stroke with a control group matched for age and sex.[35] About 80% of the subjects were older than 65 years. Of the 148 patients who had survived for 6 months after stroke, testing with the BI revealed that 20% were dependent in ambulation, one third were dependent in ADLs, and more than two thirds socialized much less than they had before the stroke. These disabilities were significantly greater than any in the stroke-free control subjects. The control subjects, however, had a high level of disability. About 28% did not socialize inside or outside the home, 20% were limited in household tasks, 9% were dependent in self-care activities, and 6% were dependent in mobility. Thus, premorbid functional disabilities may account for limitations in recovery when superimposed upon stroke-induced impairments.

Table 56-3 shows descriptor data and outcomes based on the FIM score for patients admitted for inpatient rehabilitation from more than 500 sites reporting to the Uniform Data Services for Medical Rehabilitation. Most patients had a moderate to maximally assisted level of function and improved to minimally assisted ADLs or better.

Do neurorehabilitation practices lessen residual impairments and disabilities? One may better ask whether global neurorehabilitation services have benefits or whether specific interventions for clearly defined impairments and disabilities really work.[36] After reviewing 124 investigations drawn from a literature search of studies performed from 1960 through 1990, Ottenbacher and Janell[37] carried out a meta-analysis on 36 of them. These trials, which included hemiparetic patients with stroke who were given a rehabilitation service, compared at least two groups or conditions for change in a functional measure that could be quantified.[37] Outcomes included gait, hand function, ADLs, response times, and visuoperception. The average patient who received a program of focused stroke rehabilitation or a particular procedure performed better than about 65% of the patients in the comparison group. Larger treatment effect was associated with an earlier intervention and younger patients. The review could not, however, assess the intensity of the interventions or how well they were carried out, detect systematic biases, or account for missing data.

Rehabilitation-Related Medical Complications

The time from onset of a stroke to transfer to inpatient rehabilitation has decreased by more than half over the past 20 years at centers in the United States. Physicians and nurses are increasingly responsible for managing new medications started during the acute hospitalization, which often means adjusting dosages of anticoagulant, antihypertensive, and diabetes medications, diagnosing a deep vein thrombosis or sleep apnea, and providing therapy to people who have had a myocardial infarction. Medical complications often interfere with a patient's ability to participate in therapy.[38-41] During inpatient rehabilitation, about one third of patients have a urinary tract infection, urinary retention, musculoskeletal pain, or depression. Up to 20% fall, experience a rash, or need continuous management of blood pressure, hydration, nutrition, or glucose levels. About 10% have a transient toxic-metabolic encephalopathy, pneumonia, cardiac arrhythmias, pressure sores, or thrombophlebitis. Up to 5% have a pulmonary embolus, seizures, gastrointestinal bleeding, heart failure, or other medical complications. Prophylactic measures for these potential problems, when feasible, are essential.

Bladder Dysfunction

Urinary incontinence occurs in up to 60% of patients in the first week after a stroke, but the rate tends to decline to less than 25% at hospital discharge without a specific medical treatment.[42] Urinary dribbling and involuntary bladder emptying, however, affect 30% of healthy, noninstitutionalized people older than 65 years. Across studies, about 18% of those who were incontinent at 6 weeks after stroke are still so at 1 year. Urinary tract infections develop in about 40% of patients during acute stroke and rehabilitation care.

In patients with retention of urine volumes greater than 250 mL, intermittent bladder catheterization with a clean technique probably lessens the risk of an infection, although there is no evidence for this claim. Perineal

TABLE 56-3 FIRST ADMISSION FOR STROKE REHABILITATION: TYPICAL FUNCTIONAL INDEPENDENCE MEASURE (FIM) RESULTS, PATIENT CHARACTERISTICS, AND DISCHARGE REPORTS BY UNIFORM DATA SYSTEM FOR MEDICAL REHABILITATION[190]

Average FIM Scores	At Admission	At Discharge
Self-care	3.5	5.2
Sphincter	3.7	5.4
Mobility	3.0	5.0
Locomotion	2.1	4.3
Communication	4.2	5.2
Social cognition	3.5	4.6
Total	62	86
Patient characteristics		
Age (yrs)	70	
Onset (days)	12	
Stay (days)	20	
Discharge destination (%)		
Community	76	76
Long-term care	15	14
Acute care	7	6

Adapted from Iwanenko W, Fielder R, Granger C, et al: The Uniform Data System for Medical Rehabilitation. *Am J Phys Med Rehabil* 80:56-61, 2001.

cleanliness should lessen the risk of infection by fecal contamination. If urinary retention persists, an indwelling catheter is best for the short run. Most patients with incontinence after a hemispheric stroke either have a small bladder and are unable to suppress the micturition reflex or become aware of filling too late to void in a urinal, commode, or toilet. Scheduled voiding is one good approach. Urodynamic testing may point to an abnormality of urine filling and storage, bladder emptying, or a combination of both, making the choice of medication more rational (Table 56-4). Use of an anticholinergic agent such as 5 mg of oxybutynin before sleep may allow greater filling and less urgency or incontinence overnight. Persistent lack of bladder control is often secondary to an unstable detrusor muscle or to detrusor-sphincter dyssynergia.[43] Medications may reduce outlet obstruction in men, but prostatic surgery may be indicated once the patient is a stable outpatient.

Musculoskeletal and Central Pain

Pain is common after a stroke and can limit participation in therapy. Central pain may become a major source of disability, especially after a thalamoparietal stroke, but affects fewer than 5% of all patients with stroke. Some patients only need assurance that the pain or dysesthesia does not represent a serious complication or a warning signal of another stroke. Patients need to assist their physicians in setting goals about moderating the severity, frequency, duration, and time of day of the pain. Musculoskeletal pain is far more common.

Shoulder pain at the hemiparetic arm develops in 5% to 50% of patients.[44] Pain exacerbates hypertonicity and may trigger flexor and extensor spasms and dystonic postures. A painful shoulder may cause the hemiplegic arm to flex at the elbow and wrist. A placebo-controlled, randomized trial of 37 patients with chronic hemiplegic shoulder pain found that three intra-articular injections of triamcinolone over 4 weeks did not produce a statistically significant reduction in pain.[45] The shoulder-hand syndrome with reflex sympathetic dystrophy or complex regional pain[46] has been described in up to 25% of patients in prospective studies.[47] This rate is much higher than expected from clinical experience and may reflect a lack of patient education as well as physician enthusiasm to always manage limb pain immediately with analgesia, anti-inflammatory medication, and range-of-motion exercises.

During rehabilitation and later, many patients suffer with cervical, lumbar, hip, knee, or ankle pain secondary to musculoligamentous injuries, overuse, overstretching, and poor resting postures. Thus, pain may arise from errors of omission and commission by patients, families, and hospital staff. Physical modalities, analgesics, anti-inflammatory agents, and local anesthetics or steroids may reduce most sources of musculoligamentous pain. Examples of prevention of further injury are using an orthotic to hold the wrist and fingers in extension, especially for the patient who has a hemineglect, and controlling hyperextension-induced pain at the knee with an ankle-foot orthosis.

Burning or nonburning spontaneous central pain arises most often from a lesion in the ventroposterolateral nucleus of the thalamus.[48] A variety of drugs may diminish dysesthetic or lancinating pain. In one randomized controlled trial, lamotrigine, 200 mg per day, had a significant, if moderate, effect on reducing symptoms of pain.[49] Tricyclic antidepressants have also shown efficacy in randomized trials.[50] Many anecdotal reports find value in using one or a combination of drugs. The clinician must establish a global pain scale with a patient and initiate trials of medication with a gradual titration of the dosage. If a tricyclic antidepressant such as amitriptyline or desipramine fails to work at doses up to 100 mg, which may not be tolerated, a reasonable series of trials can progress as follows: gabapentin, lamotrigine, carbamazepine, baclofen, clonidine, and mexiletine. Trazodone before sleep or use of a serotonin-specific reuptake inhibitor (SSRI) antidepressant may augment the effectiveness of these drugs.

Depression

Depression is common in late life[51] and after a stroke. The community-based Framingham Study diagnosed depression in 47% of 6-month stroke survivors, with no difference being found in the incidence between subjects with left- and right-sided lesions.[52] Depression was simultaneously diagnosed in 25% of age- and sex-matched controls, however. Other studies suggest a predisposition to depression after left anterior and right posterior infarcts, primarily soon after a stroke.[53] In a population-based cohort of Swedish patients with stroke whose mean age was 73 years, the prevalence of major depression was 25% at hospital discharge, 30% at 3 months after stroke, 16% at 1 year, 19% at 2 years, and 29% at 3 years.[54] A left

TABLE 56-4 PHARMACOLOGIC MANIPULATION OF BLADDER DYSFUNCTION

Medication and Dosage	Indication	Mechanism of Action
Bethanechol, 25 mg bid to 50 mg qid	Facilitate emptying	Increase detrusor contraction
Prazosin, 1 mg bid to 2 mg tid	Decrease outlet obstruction	Alpha blockade of external sphincter to decrease tone
Tamsulosin, 0.4 mg qd	Prostatic hypertrophy	
Oxybutinin, 2.5 mg hs to 5 mg qid	Urge incontinence	Relax detrusor; increase internal sphincter tone
Tolterodine, 2 mg bid	Frequency	
Imipramine, 25-50 mg hs	Urge incontinence Enuresis	Increase internal sphincter tone; decrease detrusor contractions

anterior infarct, dysphasia, and living alone may predict depression. By 3 months after stroke, greater dependence in ADLs and social isolation have been associated with depression. In another large study conducted in Finland, major depression affected 26%, and minor depression 14%, of 486 consecutive patients with stroke from 3 to 4 months after the infarction.[55] Premorbid depression was a strong risk factor for major depression after stroke. Counseling during rehabilitation may lessen the risk for depression, especially when directed toward concerns that patients have about becoming a burden on others.

Clinical trials reveal the efficacy of treatment of depression with tricyclic or SSRI antidepressants. Methylphenidate can also alleviate the mood disorder and improve rehabilitation outcomes.[56-60] The specific medication used depends on the patient's medical risk factors (anticholinergic side effects might cause cardiac arrhythmias, drowsiness, confusion, or urinary retention), the presence of anxiety (some SSRI and tricyclic antidepressants appear to be more useful for this factor), insomnia (a tricyclic antidepressant may aid sleep), and speed of onset (methylphenidate can act within a few days). Small clinical trials reveal the efficacy of citalopram.[56] If depression and apathy limit a patient's participation during inpatient rehabilitation, I most often start with methylphenidate, 10 mg after breakfast, and build up to 20 mg at 8 AM and 2 PM. An SSRI antidepressant such as citalopram, 10 mg, or sertraline, 25 to 50 mg, is started several days later, then increased as needed. Medication may not have to be continued more than 6 months.

Fatigue

The symptom of fatigue after hemiparetic stroke is described by 20% to 40% of community dwellers. Fatigue encompasses feelings of sluggishness, easy tiring, low energy, lack of motivation, impaired endurance, and sleepiness. The source may be a mood disorder or psychological and physical manifestations of disability, medications, cardiovascular fitness, and disease. Patients often cannot distinguish their neurologic impairments and disability from their symptoms of fatigue. Symptoms may also arise from fatigability, meaning diminishing strength that follows repetitive movements, leading to greater weakness superimposed on underlying paresis and deconditioning.[60] For example, central nervous system causes of fatigability may arise from recruitment of higher threshold motor units, reduced numbers of units leading to less drive from cortical pyramidal cells, central conduction block when firing needs to rise above the capacity of residual descending fibers, and metabolically induced afferent inhibition of the spinal and cortical motor network. Interventions for fatigue include antidepressants, stimulants, ruling out a sleep disorder, conditioning and strengthening exercises, and rest periods.

Dysphagia

Swallowing disorders may cause malnutrition, dehydration, and aspiration pneumonia. The stroke and any associated toxic-metabolic encephalopathy may combine to cause lethargy, inattention, poor judgment, and impaired control or sensitivity of the tongue and cheek. These problems often impair the oral stage of swallowing. Patients cannot form a bolus; food is pocketed in the cheek; the swallowing reflex may be delayed; and the bolus slides over the base of the tongue and collects in the valleculae and hypopharynx. In addition, patients may take too much food or liquid in a bolus, which then enters the airway before triggering a swallow reflex. Slow oral intake, a cough or wet voice after swallowing, and a rising blood urea nitrogen level point to the potential for the clinical complications of dysphagia.

A videofluoroscopic modified barium swallow (MBS) study provides the best information about the safety and efficacy of the stages of swallowing. An MBS study performed with less than a teaspoonful of thin barium, the same of thickened barium, and a test of swallowing with a barium-coated piece of cookie help document problems at the oral, pharyngeal, and esophageal stages. The therapist can simultaneously assess the effect of changes in head and neck position on deglutition. During inpatient rehabilitation, an abnormal MBS study result reveals the greater risk for pneumonia in aspirators compared to non-aspirators.[61] Nasogastric feeding tubes and gastrostomies do not appreciably lessen the risk of aspiration, probably because of gastric reflux, aspiration of oral secretions, and errors in tube placement.

Therapy by a speech or occupational therapist is indicated when delayed swallow, cough, residual barium in the vallecula, or aspiration are noted during the MBS study. Therapies include compensatory head repositioning such as flexing or turning to one side, tongue and sucking exercises, double swallowing, and supraglottic and dry coughing. Most patients fed with pureed foods and thickened liquids have adequate nutrition. Nasogastric feedings can supplement oral intake, especially if given after each meal so they do not blunt the patient's appetite. If dysphagia persists near the time of discharge from inpatient rehabilitation, a gastrostomy or gastrojejunostomy tube is a comfortable portal for nutrition. Because a gastrostomy tube must stay in place for at least 6 weeks after insertion, clinicians should be certain that this approach is warranted in the first week after a stroke. Recovery from dysphagia may be associated with a greater motor representation for the pharyngeal muscles in the uninjured hemisphere that evolves over time and with practice in swallowing.[62]

Skin Ulcers

Education in skin management during rehabilitation provides an important opportunity to prevent morbidity and mortality. Ischemia of the skin and underlying tissues occurs particularly in weight-bearing areas adjacent to bony prominences. Sores related to sitting are most commonly associated with the ischial tuberosities, where tissue pressure can exceed 300 mm Hg when the patient sits on an unpadded seat. A 2-inch-thick foam pad may decrease that local pressure to 150 mm Hg. Capillary and venule pressures are 11 to 33 mm Hg.

A four-stage classification for degrees of integument breakdown, prophylactic measures, and wound care is available from the Agency for Health Care Policy and Research.[63]

A stage 1 pressure sore can form within 2 hours. No particular intervention for a pressure sore, other than antibiotics and débridement for stage 3 or 4 ulcers, appears to be better than another.[64]

Sexual Dysfunction

After stroke, sexual desire may persist, but many men and women who had been sexually active experience sexual dysfunction.[65] Premorbid problems from diabetes, medications, vascular disease, and psychogenic causes can be exacerbated by new neural dysfunction, decreased mobility, pain, and polypharmacy. Counseling and education with patient and spouse help. Medication such as sildenafil and prostheses for men assist erectile dysfunction. Such medication may be contraindicated in patients with clinically significant coronary artery disease.

Sleep Disorders

During rehabilitation, insomnia, sleep apnea, and excessive daytime sleepiness can interfere with attention and perhaps with learning.[66] Medications, pain, anxiety, depression, and chronically poor sleep habits contribute to sleep deficits. Reversed sleep-wake cycles are common in patients with cognitive dysfunction in the first days of inpatient rehabilitation. Up to one third of patients receiving inpatient stroke rehabilitation may have a sleep disorder.

Central and obstructive types of sleep apnea have been associated with a higher risk for stroke. Pharyngeal muscle weakness and impairment of neural control of the nasopharyngeal and pharyngolaryngeal muscles due to a stroke contribute to the risk for new onset of obstructive apnea. Polysomnography is indicated when the rehabilitation team observes a hypersomnolent, confused, and snoring or apneic patient. The number of oxygen desaturation events and the oximetry measures during sleep-disordered breathing correlate with poorer functional recovery scores at 1 and 12 months after stroke.[67-69]

Insomnia during the first week or two of rehabilitation can be managed with short-acting hypnotic agents such as temazepam and zolpidem, nighttime nonnarcotic analgesics, and careful positioning in bed. Nocturia more than two times that awakens the patient can be diminished by avoiding liquid intake after dinner and using medications that lessen activation of the bladder detrusor muscle. Melatonin may help correct a reversed day-night sleep cycle. A positive-pressure breathing apparatus prevents the complications of sleep apnea.

Spasticity

A number of still ill-defined mechanisms after stroke alter membrane properties and morphologically and physiologically reorganize spinal circuits, leading to hypertonicity, clonus, spasms, and contractures.[70,71] Spasticity can lead to dystonic postures and, in some instances, limit function. However, the paresis, slowness, and fatigability that accompany an upper motor neuron (UMN) syndrome are usually more serious contributors to impairment and disability than hypertonicity. The difficulty in quantifying spasticity and measuring a functional consequence has made research and drug testing difficult. The Modified Ashworth Scale is most often used, but the score it produces is little more than an extension of the clinical examination of resistance to passive movement. Also, the properties of joints, ligaments, tendons, and muscles change with paresis after a UMN injury and contribute to the alteration in resistance to joint stretch.[72]

The neurophysiologic schools of physical therapy hold that exercise may induce hypertonicity. Small trials of modest exercise therapy have not revealed any increase in tone, however.[73-75] Indeed, clonus and spasms often diminish with weight bearing on the leg or arm. Excessive resistance exercises, however, that only flex the arm, as in performing curls, or that only extend the leg may drive flexor or extensor postures, respectively, and produce a dystonic arm or leg. Nevertheless, experimental studies suggest that hemiparetic subjects can increase force output when pushing against higher loads, such as when pedaling to gain muscular force output, without inducing a decline in motor control.[73,76,77] Use of the large leg muscles by pedaling against resistance at less than 20 cycles per minute or by walking on a treadmill also improves cardiovascular fitness in patients who have at least fair motor control.[78,79]

Pathologically increased muscle tone in patients with hemiplegia can usually be managed by aiming to maintain the normal length of the muscle and soft tissue across a joint and by helping patients avoid abnormal flexor and extensor patterns at rest and during movement. Spasticity should be treated more aggressively when it interferes with nursing care and perineal hygiene or contributes to contractures and pressure sores.

No studies offer convincing evidence of functional benefits on movement from systemic antispasticity medications after a stroke. Dantrolene, baclofen, a benzodiazepine such as clonazepam, and tizanidine[80,81] can reduce hypertonicity-related spasms and flexor postures of the upper limb or extensor postures of the lower extremity (Table 56-5). A clear effect should be evident, and after further physical therapy, attempts should be made to eliminate the drug.

TABLE 56-5 DOSAGES OF MEDICATIONS FOR SYMPTOMATIC SPASTICITY

First Line
Dantrolene, 25 mg bid to 50 mg qid
Baclofen, 5 mg bid to 40 mg qid
Clonidine, 0.05 mg qd to 0.2 mg tid
Tizanidine, 2 mg bid to 8 mg qid
Clonazepam, 0.5 to 2 mg bid to tid
Useful additions
Gabapentin, 300 mg tid to 600 mg qid
Phenytoin, serum concentration 10 to 20 mg/100 mL
Levodopa/carbidopa, 25/100 mg bid to qid
Injectables
Intramuscular botulinum toxin A or B
Intramuscular phenol
Intrathecal baclofen, 50-μg trial dose
Intrathecal clonidine

As a last resort, chemical agents such as phenol have been injected into a nerve, motor point, or muscle to lessen inappropriate muscle co-contraction, spasms, and dystonic postures. Because motor point blocks can partially spare voluntary movement and reduce reciprocal inhibition when given to an antagonist muscle, they may improve some aspects of motor control. Intramuscular injections of botulinum toxin reduce local features of spasticity for about 3 months, especially flexor postures of the arm and hand and equinovarus foot positioning.[82-86] These agents may improve the Modified Ashworth Scale score, but they do not improve motor control or the torque around a joint. Such injections should be followed by physical or occupational therapy to try to maintain range of motion and improve selective motor control. For dystonic postures that do not respond to oral medications, intrathecal baclofen may be of value.[87]

Although surgery is rarely needed after a stroke, a variety of surgical procedures, including tendon lengthening, tenotomy, and tendon transfer, can correct deformities induced by spasticity and sometimes improve function. Tendon lengthening of the hamstrings, Achilles, and toe or finger and wrist flexors is an occasional consideration to improve range of motion. A gait analysis with electromyography (EMG) helps determine which procedure might aid mobility. Physical therapy must be administered after surgery.

Cognitive Rehabilitation

Cognitive impairments may accompany a cortical or subcortical stroke. Disabilities arise from aphasia and hemineglect as well as from faltering attention, visuoperception, memory, and executive functions. Lesions within the frontal-subcortical circuit that include the caudate, basal ganglia, or thalamus may lead to deafferentiation of the dorsolateral prefrontal cortex and impair working memory, judgment, problem-solving skills, and creative thought. Neuropsychological tests help define these problems. A modest number of randomized clinical trials have studied specific interventions for cognitive retraining.[88]

Memory Disorders

Patients are called upon to encode and retrieve new information during rehabilitation. Memory disturbances impede compensatory learning that underlies much of the rehabilitation process. The incidence and risk factors for memory loss and dementia caused by one or more strokes are increasingly being appreciated.[89-93] Up to 30% of all stroke survivors have a disturbance in memory. Community-based studies report dementia in 15% to 30% of patients after stroke within 3 months to 1 year and in 33% within 5 years.[89,94,95]

Cognitive remediation for memory disorders aims to train compensatory strategies such as rehearsal, visual imagery, semantic elaboration, and memory aids, including notebooks, calendars, and electronic devices. In normal subjects who are learning a new skill, constant feedback enhances immediate performance, but an intermittent schedule of reinforcement that allows errors and gradual processing of how to perform may improve long-term retention. The optimal way to enhance learning in a particular person with brain injury may depend on what type of memory, attention, or other cognitive processes have been affected. Amnestic subjects and at least some subjects with impaired episodic memory do worse with trial-and-error training; more frequent feedback and errorless learning may improve retention in these subjects.[96] In general, patients with stroke have good procedural or motor learning abilities.[97,98]

Visuospatial and Attentional Disorders

In one study, visual neglect was found in 38% of 150 consecutive patients with moderate disability after a new stroke, but severe neglect was rare beyond 6 months.[99] Patients with anosognosia, visual neglect, tactile extinction, motor impersistence, or auditory neglect at 10 days after stroke have the lowest BI value at 1 year, even after the data are adjusted for initial ADL scores and for post-stroke rehabilitation.[100] Recovery is most rapid within the first 2 weeks, regardless of the side of the stroke, and visual neglect improves by 3 months in most patients. Many patients have more subtle impairments that are found by testing.

Treatments for left hemi-inattention aim to engage attention to the left, disengage attention to the right, shift spatial coordinates to the left, and increase arousal. Well-described behavioral interventions for visuospatial retraining have been employed to improve attention to the left.[101,102] The techniques include a stimulus such as a red ribbon on the left to anchor attention followed by a gradual withdrawal of left-sided spatial cues, work on sensory awareness to physical stimuli on the left, and tasks to aid spatial organization. Intensive practice involving a variety of pencil-and-paper and physical tasks for left-sided attention may help the subject with moderate to severe neglect.[103,104] Visual scanning training[105] and scanning combined with trunk rotation,[106] self-cuing by movement of the left arm,[99,107] or a warning tone to increase alertness to space have improved scores on tests of left hemispace awareness.[108] These interventions do not necessarily improve left hemiattention during ADLs. Table 56-6 lists

TABLE 56-6 INTERVENTIONS FOR HEMINEGLECT*

Multisensory visual and sensory cues, then fading cues[101]
Verbal elaboration of visual analysis[97]
Visual imagery[191]
Environmental adaptations
Video feedback[192]
Monocular and binocular patches[193-196]
Prisms[195,197]
Left limb movement in left hemispace[99,107]
Head and trunk midline adjustments[106,198,199]
Left cerebral transcranial magnetic stimulation[200]
Vestibular stimulation[201,202]
Optokinetic stimulation[203]
Reduce hemianopic defects[204]
Computer-assisted training[205,206]

*Superscript numbers indicate references.

some of the techniques that have been tried with some success, though usually not in a double-blinded randomized trial.

Pharmacotherapy

Medications that affect neurotransmitters and neuromodulators may have positive or negative effects on domains of cognition. Some may affect general processes like attention and memory. Others, such as stimulants of the noradrenergic projections from the locus ceruleus, may modulate the signal-to-noise ratio for attended stimuli. Other drugs may enable gains in some aspect of cognition when their use is combined with task-oriented practice. Investigators and clinicians have tested many drugs in small trials after stroke and traumatic brain injury. Hemineglect may improve with a dopamine agonist[109] but may make some patients, perhaps those with a striatal lesion, worse.[110] Cholinesterase inhibitors may improve memory in patients with vascular dementia.[111]

Table 56-7 lists some of the adjunct pharmacologic interventions used in patients with stroke and traumatic brain injury that have been found useful in case reports and small series. The number in each column is the order in which I tend to put the drugs into an n-of-1 trial for patients. Therapy specific to targeted goals is provided during these trials. Potential classes of drugs that may contribute to recovery include neurotrophins and molecules associated with the cascades of proteins and genes required for short-term and long-term memory storage and maintenance.[112,113]

Speech and Language Therapies

The Copenhagen Stroke Study was a community-based population study that prospectively monitored about 1200 patients admitted for acute stroke, and nearly all of the 800 survivors. The investigators reported that 38% of 881 patients were aphasic on admission and 20% of the admissions were rated as severe on the Scandinavian Stroke Scale (SSS).[114] Nearly half of the patients with severe aphasia died early after stroke onset, and half of those with mild aphasia recovered by 1 week. Only 18% of community survivors were still aphasic at the time of acute and rehabilitation hospital discharges. Up to 28% received early speech therapy as needed. Patients were retested for 6 months. The investigators found that the best predictor of recovery is a lesser severity of aphasia close to the time of the stroke. Ninety-five percent of subjects with mild aphasia reached their best level of recovery by 2 weeks, those with a moderate aphasia by 6 weeks, and those with severe aphasia by 10 weeks. Only 8% of the severely aphasic patients fully recovered according to the scoring system by 6 months. In this study, mild language deficits and changes undetected by the limited sensitivity of the SSS were not ascertained. Functional communication was not a measured outcome. This natural history data does not imply that aphasic patients cannot improve in aspects of comprehension and expression for months, even years after stroke onset.

Interventions

For the aphasic patient, speech therapists attempt to find ways to circumvent or compensate for impairments in the comprehension and expression of language. Visual and verbal cuing techniques include picture matching and sentence completion tasks. Frequent repetition and positive reinforcement are used as the patient approaches the desired responses. A large variety of approaches for particular language and linguistic impairments have evolved. Melodic intonation therapy for nonfluent aphasics who have good comprehension, for example, may enhance expression.[115]

A meta-analysis performed on 55 interventional trials of speech-language therapy in aphasic patients after stroke offers insights into the effectiveness of language therapies.[116] Significant benefits were found in treated patients in comparison with untreated patients at all stages of recovery. The benefit appeared most evident in patients who started speech therapy soon after stroke. Total treatment amounts of more than 2 hours per week achieved greater gains than lesser amounts. Patients with severe aphasia showed greater improvement when treated by a speech-language pathologist than by family members or assistants. Only one defined intervention, multimodal stimulation, was tested in enough cases to show its greater average effect. Any differential effects of treatment for differing types of aphasia could not be assessed by this analysis because too few studies have been published.[116]

TABLE 56-7 DRUGS THAT MAY ENHANCE ACTIVITY-DEPENDENT GAINS: A CLINICAL ALGORITHM FOR USE

| Drug | Targeted Impairment or Disability | | | | |
	Aphasia	Motor Function	Neglect	Memory	Depression
Amphetamine	3	6	4		
Methylphenidate	4	5	3	2	1
L-Dopa		4	2		
Dopamine agonists	5		1		
Anticholinesterases	2	1		1	
Tricyclics					3
Serotoninergics	6	2	5	3	2
Piracetam	1	3			

1, first choice; 2, second choice; 3, third choice; 4, fourth choice; 5, fifth choice; 6, sixth choice.

The intensity and specificity of practice may be most important in testing a particular therapy. One well-designed study employed a picture card game in which a group of aphasic subjects were prompted to request and provide cards of depicted objects from their hands of cards. The results suggest that behaviorally relevant mass practice for at least 3 hours a day for 10 days that also constrained the use of nonverbal communication and reinforced appropriate responses within a group setting could improve comprehension and naming skills more effectively than less intensive and formalized therapy.[21] The cortical response to an intervention may be monitored during activation studies by means of functional neuroimaging.[117-119]

Computer software offers other forms of practice. An uncontrolled case series of patients with chronic aphasia showed that repetitive practice with a therapist and at home with a microcomputer-based symbolic language device led to improvements on several tests of language function.[120] A visual iconic computer-based interface also improved the ability of subjects with chronic aphasia to relearn the use of past-tense verbs and to comprehend passive-voice sentences, pointing to an approach to lessen agrammatism and syntactic deficits.[121]

Pharmacotherapy

Clinical trials in modest numbers of patients with amphetamine,[122] piracetam,[118,123] and cholinergic[124] and dopaminergic[125,126] agents have suggested efficacy of these agents for particular aphasic syndromes and language impairments. The neurotransmitter systems stimulated by such drugs may affect a variety of pathways for attention, memory, reward, and learning.[127-129] Clinicians can try any of these agents in an n-of-1 series of trials. A few standard tests that can detect changes in perseveration, word finding, simple sentence comprehension, and social communication may serve as measures of efficacy. I tend to start with an anticholinesterase agent in a dose typical for use in patients with Alzheimer's disease and to follow it with levodopa/carbidopa, 25 mg and 100 mg, twice during the day, and then with 10 mg of amphetamine every other day before speech therapy.

Therapeutic strategies are needed that combine analytic approaches from speech pathology, neurolinguistics, neuropsychology, neuroimaging, pharmacology, and computer sciences. Theory-based treatments define the short-term and long-term benefits of a specific

intervention for a particular aspect of language. Single-case studies and clinical trials must also address the optimal intensity, duration, and learning paradigm for a specific intervention.

Mobility Training

Natural History

In the Copenhagen Stroke Study, 51% of patients were initially unable to walk, 12% walked with assistance, and 37% were independent.[130,131] At discharge after acute and rehabilitative care, 22% of survivors could not walk, 14% walked with assistance, and 64% walked independently. About 80% of those who were initially nonwalkers reached their best walking function within 6 weeks, and 95% within 11 weeks. Of patients who initially walked with physical assistance, 80% reached best function within 3 weeks, and 95% within 5 weeks. Independent walking was achieved by 34% of the survivors who had been dependent and by 60% of those who initially required assistance. Recovery of ambulation correlated directly with residual leg strength. Within the first week after onset, patients who improved leg strength by several points on the SSS within the first 2 to 3 weeks after stroke almost always became ambulatory.[132] In general, patients who can flex the hip and extend the hemiparetic knee against gravity after stroke will be able to ambulate without human assistance.

More detailed information about outcomes in relationship to impairment and disability was reported in a prospective study of 95 consecutive inpatients admitted to a rehabilitation center after a hemispheric stroke.[133] Patients were followed up until they reached a plateau of recovery. Life-table analyses of the probability of recovering BI functions were made; patients were divided into three groups according to impairment and examined at 2-week intervals. More than 90% of patients with a pure motor (M) deficit became independent in walking 150 feet by week 14, but only 35% of those with motor and proprioceptive (SM) loss did so by week 24, and 3% of those with motor, sensory, and hemianopic deficits (SMH) did so by week 30. The probability of walking more than 150 feet with assistance increased to 80% by week 8 and to 100% by week 14 in those with M impairment. The probability of walking with physical help exceeded 90% in those with SM and SMH loss by 28 weeks after the stroke. Table 56-8 shows recovery data according to impairment group for another cohort of patients with stroke.

TABLE 56-8   RECOVERY OF WALKING IN PATIENTS GROUPED BY IMPAIRMENTS AT ONSET OF STROKE

Impairment Group	Onset (%)	1 Month (%)	3 Months (%)	6 Months (%)
Motor	18	50	75	85
Sensorimotor	10	48	72	72
Motor, hemianopia	7	28	68	75
Sensorimotor, hemianopia	3	16	33	38

Data from Kaplan-Meier graphs in Patel A, Duncan P, Lai S, et al: The relation between impairments and functional outcomes poststroke. *Arch Phys Med Rehabil* 81:1357-1363, 2000.

Interventions

Sensorimotor impairments and disabilities in mobility and other ADLs are managed by the following four general approaches:

- Exercise and selective muscle group strengthening
- Facilitation and neurophysiologic techniques drawn from various schools of facilitative therapy, including those of Bobath and Brunnstrom
- Compensatory training to adapt to disability
- Task-oriented retraining that emphasizes principles for learning and intensive practice

When the traditional schools of facilitative therapy have been compared with one another, no differences in outcomes have been found among them. Strengthening exercises seem to be mildly more beneficial than facilitation alone.[134] Task-oriented activity with optimal schedules of practice and reinforcement looks promising as part of a physical and occupational therapy strategy.[16,19]

Range of motion in the paretic arm and leg is maintained with positioning, splints, and slow rhythmic rotation and stretch of all joints several times a day, along with weight bearing as soon as possible. Patient and family are taught to assist. Flexion at the hip, knee, and ankle are encouraged by mat exercises that include rolling onto the side and bringing the knee to the chest. Once the patient has adequate endurance and stability to stand in the parallel bars or at a hemibar with the therapist's help to control the paretic leg, gait training begins. The therapist concentrates on the most prominent deviations from normal during the gait cycle, such as circumduction of the hip, pelvic drop, hyperextension or flexor giveway of the knee, inadequate dorsiflexion of the ankle, and toe clawing. The physical therapist also encourages heel strike at initial stance, greater weight bearing on the paretic leg, push-off at the end of stance, at least 5 to 10 degrees of hip extension in late stance, and a longer step length.

The hemiparetic patient who cannot control ankle movement, whose foot tends to turn over during gait, or who lacks enough knee control to prevent the knee from snapping back is fitted with a polypropylene ankle-foot orthosis. As inpatient therapy for gait progresses away from the parallel bars to increasing distances walked with an assistive device such as a quad cane, then to stair climbing and outdoor ambulation on uneven surfaces, therapy continues in the outpatient setting, where mobility in the home and community is stressed.

Task-Oriented Approaches

Treadmill walking is a task-oriented approach for ambulation. Body weight-supported treadmill training (BWSTT), if carried out optimally, allows the spinal cord and supraspinal locomotor regions to experience sensory inputs akin to those of ordinary stepping, unlike the atypical inputs created by compensatory gait deviations and difficulty with loading a paretic limb during conventional locomotor training. The therapist employs different levels of weight support and treadmill speed and, most important, assists the step pattern with physical and verbal cues to optimize the temporal, kinematic, and kinetic parameters of the step cycle. The more normal input may improve the timing and increase the activation of residual descending locomotor outputs on spinal motor pools. Sensory inputs related to the level of loading of the stance leg and to extension of the hip before swing, as well as to treadmill speed, have been shown to modulate the EMG output during BWSTT, even when the legs are fully assisted during the step cycle.[135,136] This finding, which is similar to the results of studies of cats after experimental low thoracic spinal cord transection, points to the powerful modulation by sensory inputs of spinal locomotor neuronal pools and the ability of the spinal cord to learn from rhythmic inputs.[137]

In subjects with a chronic hemiparetic stroke who walk slowly, 12 sessions of BWSTT at 2 mph increases overground walking speed by 30% to 50%.[138] Two randomized trials of ambulatory patients with stroke show that progressive increase in the treadmill speed as physiologically tolerated enables patients to achieve overground walking speeds that are significantly higher than when they are trained at a modest increment of speed or treated with conventional overground training.[138,139] Higher walking speeds are associated with greater likelihood of community ambulation. This approach also leads to a reorganization of activity in the supplementary motor cortex and primary sensorimotor cortex, associated with increases in walking speed and in selective control of ankle dorsiflexion.[140,141] As with any task-oriented approach, the intensity and specificity of practice drive functional gains for the practiced motor skill.

Although small trials suggested that BWSTT is superior to usual care or no intervention in subacutely and chronically slow walkers, well-designed randomized clinical trials show no differences in outcomes with an equal amount of either walking-related therapy or supervised home-based therapy that focuses on balance and strengthening.[137] In addition, treadmill training with weight support that is assisted by a robotic device for stepping appears equal to an equal intensity of more conventional over ground training.[143] No clinically important differences for walking speed, distance, or physical functioning have been found. Another multicenter trial during inpatient stroke rehabilitation found that simply giving patients and their therapists feedback about how fast the person walked 10 m each day, without any other specific intervention, led to improved walking speed at discharge by 24%.[144] Thus, positive feedback about performance may be a critical motivating drive for gains.

EMG, visual, and auditory biofeedback to increase muscle contractions or lessen co-contractions may improve the pattern of arm or leg movements and improve balance,[145] but no technique has come into common usage. Gains during biofeedback sessions may not generalize to movements during walking. Electrical stimulation of leg muscles is sometimes used, mostly to aid ankle dorsiflexion. This peroneal nerve stimulation may improve foot clearance and may modestly improve walking speed. Case reports suggest that some patients may benefit from electrical stimulation of the gluteal and quadriceps muscles for hip stability and knee extension, but this approach is limited to research laboratories.

Selective muscle strengthening,[20] treadmill walking to improve strength and endurance,[146] and rhythmic practice entrained by the temporal elements of music[147] may also improve walking speed and the symmetry of both stance and swing phases of gait.

Upper Extremity and Self-Care Skills

The occupational therapist brings to the rehabilitation team expertise with assistive devices for ADLs and often works with the neuropsychologist in addressing visuospatial inattention, memory loss, apraxia, dysphagia, and difficulties in problem solving. Tables 56-1 and 56-2 provide an overview of the ADL tasks that the therapist addresses, especially during inpatient rehabilitation. Community and leisure activities are addressed during outpatient therapy. Outcomes for prospective studies of patients undergoing rehabilitation, as well as for the overall population of patients admitted for acute care after a first stroke, suggest that 60% to 70% of patients recover the ability to manage basic ADLs, although the majority do not return to their premorbid level of socialization.

Natural History

Using the BI and SSS, the Copenhagen Study graded recovery before and after acute and rehabilitative inpatient stays and at 6 months. Within the same facility, all patients who needed rehabilitation received services for an average stay of 35 days (S.D. 41). By then, 11% had severe impairment, 11% had moderate impairment, and 78% had mild or no deficits. At the same time, 20% had severe, 8% moderate, and 26% mild disability, and 46% had no disability. ADL scores plateaued by 9 weeks in patients with initially mild strokes, within 13 weeks in those with moderate strokes, within 17 weeks in those with severe strokes, and within 20 weeks in those with most severe stroke.[130] The study by Reding and Potes,[133] of patients admitted to one rehabilitation inpatient program, found that 65% of subjects achieved a BI of more than 95 by 15 weeks if they had only M deficits and by 26 weeks with SM loss, but only 10% of those with SMH deficits scored that high by 18 to 30 weeks. However, 100% of patients with M loss achieved a BI higher than 60 by 14 weeks, 75% of those with SM deficits, by 23 weeks, and 60% of those with SMH loss, by 29 weeks.

Functional recovery of the upper extremity was assessed in the Copenhagen Stroke Study with the use of BI subscores for feeding and grooming for the affected arm.[148] Within 9 weeks, 95% of patients achieved their best function. With mild paresis, this was accomplished by 6 weeks after stroke onset. In those with severe paresis, best function was achieved by 11 weeks. The ability to shrug or abduct the affected shoulder within the first few weeks after stroke may predict outcomes better than synergistic hand function.[149] Patients who have no movement of the hand by several weeks after onset of the stroke most often do not recover independent feeding and dressing with that hand. Patients who have some voluntary finger and wrist extension within the first few weeks may show improvement in hand coordination for practiced tasks for 12 months or more.

Interventions

Occupational therapy to improve upper extremity function first puts an emphasis on visually and manually patterning the patient through parts of a task and then through the entire task with frequent positive feedback. Techniques that conserve energy and promote independence in dressing, grooming, bathing, and toileting involve relearning how to carry out the task with compensation when using the unaffected arm and adaptive strategies with the affected arm. The therapist also provides a wheelchair with proper seating, a clear plastic lap board or arm trough to rest the paretic limb where it can be seen by the patient, an arm sling or electrical stimulation if shoulder subluxation or pain arises, a compression glove to reduce hand edema if elevation and massage fail to do so, and static and dynamic splints to maintain wrist and finger position in extension. A visit to the home of a patient who is less than fully independent is the best way to establish the need for assistive devices, such as grab bars, rails, ramps, and environmental controls, as well as architectural changes such as widening a doorway to allow wheelchair access.

Acupuncture appeared to improve motor impairments or functional outcomes in several quasi-experimental and randomized clinical trials.[150] Two well-designed randomized trials that used a sham procedure did not find any improvement in performance of ADLs.[151,152]

Task-Oriented Approaches

Most therapists take a task-oriented approach to retraining ADLs supplemented by Bobath and other techniques. One trial randomly assigned 185 patients within 1 month of stroke to either up to 5 months of home-based therapy with an occupational therapist or no therapy.[17] The number of visits ranged from 1 to 15, with a mean of only 6 visits per patient. None of the subjects had been admitted to a hospital for the stroke, and median BI values were 18 (about 90 on the American version of the test), so they were minimally disabled. Blinded assessment of outcomes revealed significant gains with the therapy. The group that received therapy improved in instrumental ADLs and handicap and made modest gains in ADLs, and caregiver strain decreased in this group.

Failed early attempts to use the affected limb may suppress subsequent use. Forced use of the affected arm and gradual shaping of a variety of functional movements to overcome what is theorized as learned nonuse of the paretic limb may increase the incorporation of the affected arm into daily activities.[153] In one study, 9 patients with chronic stroke who could extend the wrist and fingers at least 10 degrees spent about 7 hours a day for up to 2 weeks practicing a variety of guided upper extremity movements and wore a sling or glove that prevented use of the unaffected upper extremity for the rest of the day. Much of the improvement in daily use of the affected arm was evident within 1 to 2 days of restraint of the unaffected arm plus therapy; this finding suggests that a latent capability had succumbed to learned nonuse.[154,155] Constraint-induced movement therapy (CIMT) is associated with primary motor cortex reorganization in some but not all studies, suggesting that the approach can induce activity-dependent plasticity.[156]

A well-designed randomized trial of 66 subjects with chronic stroke compared CIMT with bimanual hand training based on the neurodevelopmental program developed by Patricia Davies.[157] After 2 weeks of training, the CIMT group scored modestly better in the functional use and amount of daily use of the affected arm. The difference in amount of use did not persist 1 year later. Subjects with sensory loss and hemi-inattention appeared to do better with CIMT, a finding that bears further study. A pilot study of 20 patients with acute stroke compared 2 hours of daily CIMT for 2 weeks with standard occupational therapy that did not emphasize use of the affected arm.[158] Functional outcomes appeared better for the CIMT group. The best designed, randomized trial of CIMT in subjects who, at 3 to 9 months after their stroke, were able to extend several fingers and the wrist at least 10 degrees revealed significantly better outcomes compared to no intervention.[155]

CIMT is a form of intensive, task-oriented practice for patients who have at least modest motor control of the upper extremity. The intervention does not define any particular approach to motor learning. In any controlled trial, CIMT must be compared with an equally active program of upper extremity management. When brief, intensive therapy of various types has been provided to subjects with recent or chronic stroke, aspects of upper extremity function related to the practiced task have usually improved.[16,44,98,159-161] Practice also improves aspects of motor function in the ipsilesional upper extremity,[162] which is often a bit weaker or slow in its movements compared with the upper extremity in normal, healthy subjects.[163]

Robotic and other mechanical assistive training devices have also improved the performance for reaching, usually in the plane of practice or across the joints most used.[164-166] Trials that do not succeed in augmenting the amount of practice time generally produce negative results.[167] In a randomized trial that began about 3 weeks after onset of stroke in 56 subjects undergoing inpatient rehabilitation, robot-trained subjects used a low-inertia, back-drivable device for 25 hourly sessions and 1500 repetitions of assisted movement in the horizontal plane for the shoulder and elbow, whereas the control group used the device for the unaffected arm or for the affected arm without a robotic assist.[168] The robotically trained group, which had significantly less motor and cognitive impairment as indicated by FIM score at the start, had a modest but statistically significant increase in FIM motor score compared with the control group. The FIM tasks were not necessarily carried out by the affected arm, however. A multicenter trial that compared an equal amount of practice using a three-component robotic assistive device to more conventional rehabilitation for the upper extremity found equal, if modest, improvements in highly impaired subjects.[164]

Although available for nearly 20 years, EMG-triggered neuromuscular stimulation procedures that produce modest gains in wrist extensor strength have not come into general use. Two randomized trials provided from 15 to 24 sessions of electrical stimulation of the wrist and finger extensors in response to the feedback of the low-amplitude EMG signal elicited by attempted wrist extension during inpatient rehabilitation for stroke.[169,170] Functional wrist extension improved more in the group undergoing feedback therapy than in those receiving routine therapy, but the positive effects did not persist by 24 weeks after stimulation stopped. A randomized study of 11 subjects with chronic hemiparesis achieved significantly better hand extensor strength and, in a rare demonstration, improved the ability of subjects to pick up small objects.[171] Up to 25% of patients discontinue this form of functional electrical stimulation because the evoked response induces pain.

Five weeks of functional electrical stimulation may also reduce shoulder pain related to subluxation from paresis and may improve shoulder function,[172] perhaps by allowing pain-free practice. Orthotic devices placed across the wrist and designed to electrically stimulate a grasp or pincer movement have not yet been used widely.[173,174] Virtual reality systems that augment feedback about the position of the hand in space represent a potentially powerful form of practice, offering feedback information about knowledge of performance and of results using parameters such as velocity, trajectory, and accuracy of the reaching movement. The optimal style, daily intensity, and overall duration of training and the best outcome measures, in terms of sensitivity to change and relevance to useful movements, are a work in progress for all interventions.

Pharmacotherapy

When combined with physical therapies, several monoaminergic agents have lessened motor impairments and improved ADLs. These attempts to develop a pharmacotherapy for neurorehabilitation are drawn from animal studies of enhanced learning and neuroplasticity,[175-177] although the leap from biologic responses in rats to those in humans after focal brain injury is a precarious one.[178] In small randomized trials, amphetamine,[179,180] methylphenidate,[181] levodopa,[182] and fluoxetine[183,184] have shown modest levels of success for improving strength or motor control, but the trials did not necessarily improve ADLs. No differences in gains were found, however, in an adequately powered trial when upper extremity therapy was provided to chronic, moderately hemiparetic patients randomly assigned to receive ropinirole, a dopamine agonist, or placebo.[185]

Amphetamine has received the most acclaim. Investigators have rejected at least 20 patients for every patient who met the criteria for these trials.[179,180] Best results were achieved when physical therapy relevant to the outcome measure was combined with the drug. Side effects of amphetamine, using 10 mg every other morning, have been minimal, and most studies have probably used exclusion criteria that were too strict. A trial randomly assigned 39 geriatric patients with stroke to 10 therapy sessions combined with 10 mg of amphetamine or placebo during 5 weeks of rehabilitation.[186] No differences between the amphetamine group and the placebo group were found for motor function or ADLs.

A well-designed trial randomly assigned 53 patients admitted for inpatient rehabilitation to 100 mg of levodopa and carbidopa or to placebo.[182] Subjects received their assigned medication every morning before physiotherapy for 3 weeks and then continued therapy for another 3 weeks. Regardless of the initial level of motor dysfunction as indicated by the Rivermead Motor Assessment, subjects receiving levodopa improved a statistically significant 2 points on the 15-point subscale for the arm. Improvement persisted 3 weeks later. The relative improvement, however, does not necessarily correlate with a difference in strength, coordination, or functional use of the arm. Other quasiexperimental studies using, for example, the norepinephrine precursor L-threo-3,4-dihydroxyphenyl-serine,[187,188] reported gains. Drugs that enhance cerebral activation during a task carried out during functional MRI[127,189] may help predict whether an agent is likely to be of benefit in promoting activity-dependent plasticity.

Should clinicians routinely try pharmacologic adjuncts to enhance motor gains? Such an approach may be worthwhile in patients with some sensorimotor function who are undergoing active rehabilitation and in whom motor control lags and limits gains in walking or use of the upper extremity. As shown in Table 56-7, it is best to start with drugs that tend to have the fewest side effects, such as the anticholinesterase inhibitors donepezil or galantamine at typical doses used in Alzheimer's disease, followed by a trial of an SSRI such as sertraline, 50 mg, or the dopaminergic agent levodopa and carbidopa, 25 mg and 100 mg.

Conclusions

The milieu and focus on functional gains provided by an inpatient rehabilitation team lead to better outcomes than those achieved by general medical care and less organized services.

Patients may improve by spontaneous processes at first, but important gains are likely related to intrinsic biologic mechanisms that are driven by external stimuli. Task-oriented practice may be a critical element for successful motor and cognitive retraining. Practice sessions must include learning paradigms and problem-solving techniques with optimal cues and reinforcers. Practice must be relevant to the subject, frequent, and of adequate duration. The goals of therapy include an increase in functional independence and renewed social reintegration into the family and community.

To improve motor performance, practice should engage the patient and aim to improve selective movements, motor control, skill, strength, endurance for an activity, and generalized fitness. This approach to training may lead to synaptic and morphologic changes associated with activity-dependent plasticity at the levels of the spinal cord, brainstem, and cerebral hemispheres.[13] Certain pharmacologic interventions may help drive experience-induced learning and neural adaptations for specific tasks, but clinical trials to date offer only modest support for this theory. The physician with expertise in neurorehabilitation should help therapists develop training paradigms drawn from an integration of basic neuroscience, cognitive neuroscience, clinical neuromedicine, clinical research study designs, and outcomes research.

REFERENCES

1. Adams H, Davis P, Leira E, et al: Baseline NIH Stroke Scale score strongly predicts outcome after stroke, *Neurology* 53:126-131, 1999.
2. Heinemann A, Harvey R, McGuire J, et al: Measurement properties of the NIH Stroke Scale during acute rehabilitation, *Stroke* 28:1174-1180, 1997.
3. Lai S-M, Duncan P, Keighley J: Prediction of functional outcome after stroke: Comparison of the Orpington Prognostic Scale and the NIH Stroke Scale, *Stroke* 29:1838-1842, 1998.
4. Pedersen P, Jorgensen H, Nakayama H, et al: Comprehensive assessment of activities of daily living in stroke: The Copenhagen Stroke Study, *Arch Phys Med Rehabil* 78:161-165, 1997.
5. Golomb B, Vickrey B, Hays R: A review of health-related quality-of-life measures in stroke, *Pharmacoeconomics* 19:155-185, 2001.
6. Pickard A, Johnson J, Penn A, et al: Replicability of SF-36 summary scores by the SF-12 in stroke patients, *Stroke* 30:1213-1217, 1999.
7. Williams L, Weinberger M, Harris L, et al: Development of a stroke-specific quality of life scale, *Stroke* 30:1362-1369, 1999.
8. Hamedani A, Wells C, Brass L, et al: A quality-of-life instrument for young hemorrhagic stroke patients, *Stroke* 32:687-695, 2001.
9. Bugge C, Alexander H, Hagen S: Stroke patients' informal caregivers: Patients, caregiver, and service factors that affect caregiver strain, *Stroke* 30:1517-1523, 1999.
10. Knapp P, Hewison J: Disagreement in patient and carer assessment of functional abilities after stroke, *Stroke* 30:934-938, 1999.
11. Duncan W, Wallace D, Lai M, et al: The Stroke Impact Scale Version 2.0, *Stroke* 30:2131-2140, 1999.
12. Kelly-Hayes M, Robertson J, Broderick J, et al: The American Heart Association Stroke Outcome Classification, *Stroke* 29:1274-1280, 1998.
13. Dobkin B: *The clinical science of neurologic rehabilitation*, New York, 2003, Oxford University Press.
14. Dobkin B: Activity-dependent learning contributes to motor recovery, *Ann Neurol* 44:158-160, 1998.
15. Dobkin B: Functional rewiring of brain and spinal cord after injury: The three R's of neural repair and neurological rehabilitation, *Curr Opin Neurol* 13:655-659, 2000.
16. Kwakkel G, Wagenaar R, Twisk J, et al: Intensity of leg and arm training after primary middle cerebral artery stroke: A randomised trial, *Lancet* 354:191-196, 1999.
17. Walker M, Gladman J, Lincoln N, et al: Occupational therapy for stroke patients not admitted to hospital: A randomised controlled trial, *Lancet* 354:278-280, 1999.
18. Dobkin B: Overview of treadmill locomotor training with partial body weight support: A neurophysiologically sound approach whose time has come for randomized clinical trials, *Neurorehabil Neural Repair* 13:157-165, 1999.
19. Kwakkel G, Wagenaar R, Koelman T, et al: Effects of intensity of rehabilitation after stroke: A research synthesis, *Stroke* 28:1550-1556, 1997.
20. Nugent J, Schurr K, Adams R: A dose-response relationship between amount of weight-bearing exercise and walking outcome following cerebrovascular accident, *Arch Phys Med Rehabil* 75:399-402, 1994.
21. Pulvermuller F, Neininger B, Elbert T, et al: Constraint-induced therapy of chronic aphasia after stroke, *Stroke* 32:1621-1626, 2001.
22. Paolucci S, Antonucci G, Grasso M, et al: Early versus delayed inpatient stroke rehabilitation: A matched comparison conducted in Italy, *Arch Phys Med Rehabil* 81:695-700, 2000.
23. How do stroke units improve patient outcomes? A collaborative systematic review of the randomized trials. Stroke Unit Trialists' Collaboration, *Stroke* 28:2139-2144, 1997.
24. Kalra L, Eade J: Role of stroke rehabilitation units in managing severe disability after stroke, *Stroke* 26:2031-2034, 1995.
25. Indredavik B, Fjaertoft H, Ekeberg G, et al: Benefit of an extended stroke unit service with early supported discharge, *Stroke* 31:2989-2994, 2000.
26. Kramer J, Steiner J, Schlenker R, et al: Outcomes and costs after hip fracture and stroke: A comparison of rehabilitation settings, *JAMA* 277:396-404, 1997.

27. Sulch D, Perez I, Melbourn A, et al: Randomized controlled trial of integrated (managed) care pathway for stroke rehabilitation, *Stroke* 31:1929-1934, 2000.

28. Wade D, Skilbeck C, Bainton D, et al: Controlled trial of a home-care service for acute stroke patients, *Lancet* 1(8424):323-326, 1985.

29. Rudd A, Wolfe C, Tilling K, et al: The effectiveness of a package of community care on one year outcome of stroke patients, *BMJ* 315:1039-1044, 1997.

30. Ronning OM, Guldvog B: Outcome of subacute stroke rehabilitation: A randomized controlled trial, *Stroke* 29:779-784, 1998.

31. Holmqvist L, von Koch L, Kostulas V, et al: A randomized controlled trial of rehabilitation at home after stroke in southwest Stockholm, *Stroke* 29:591-597, 1998.

32. Nilsson A, Aniansson A, Grimby G: Rehabilitation needs and disability in community living stroke survivors two years after stroke, *Top Stroke Rehabil* 6:30-47, 2000.

33. Grimby G, Andren E, Daving Y, et al: Dependence and perceived difficulty in daily activities in community-living stroke survivors 2 years after stroke: A study of instrumental structures, *Stroke* 29:1843-1849, 1998.

34. Taub E, Uswatte G, Pidikiti R: Constraint-induced movement therapy: A new family of techniques with broad application to physical rehabilitation—a clinical review, *Rehabil Res Develop* 36:237-251, 1999.

35. Gresham GE, Phillips TF, Wolf PA: Epidemiologic profile of long-term stroke disability: The Framingham Study, *Arch Phys Med Rehabil* 60:487-491, 1979.

36. Dobkin B: Focused stroke rehabilitation programs do not improve outcome, *Arch Neurol* 46:701-703, 1989.

37. Ottenbacher K, Jannell S: The results of clinical trials in stroke rehabilitation research, *Arch Neurol* 50:37-44, 1993.

38. Dobkin B: Neuromedical complications in stroke patients transferred for rehabilitation before and after DRGs, *J Neurol Rehabil* 1:3-8, 1987.

39. Dromerick A, Reding M: Medical and neurological complications during inpatient stroke rehabilitation, *Stroke* 25:358-361, 1994.

40. Langhorne P, Stott D, Robertson L, et al: Medical complications after stroke: A multicenter study, *Stroke* 31:1223-1229, 2000.

41. Roth E, Lovell L, Harvey R, et al: Incidence of and risk factors for medical complications during stroke rehabilitation, *Stroke* 32:523-529, 2001.

42. Brittain K, Peet S, Castleden C: Stroke and incontinence, *Stroke* 29:524-528, 1998.

43. Gelber D, Jozefczyk P, Good D, et al: Urinary retention following acute stroke, *J Neurol Rehabil* 8:69-74, 1994.

44. Sunderland A, Tinson D, Bradley E, et al: Enhanced physical therapy improves recovery of function after stroke: A randomised controlled trial, *J Neurol Neurosurg Psychiatry* 55:530-535, 1992.

45. Snels I, Beckerman H, Twisk J, et al: Effect of triamcinolone acetonide injections on hemiplegic shoulder pain: A randomized clinical trial, *Stroke* 31:2396-2401, 2000.

46. Rowbotham MC: Complex regional pain syndrome type I (reflex sympathetic dystrophy), *Neurology* 51:4-5, 1998.

47. Werner R, Priebe M, Davidoff G: Reflex sympathetic dystrophy syndrome associated with hemiplegia, *Neuro Rehabil* 2:16-22, 1992.

48. Bowsher D, Leijon G, Thuomos K: Central poststroke pain: Correlation of MRI with clinical pain characteristics and sensory abnormalities, *Neurology* 51:1352-1358, 1998.

49. Vestergaard K, Andersen G, Gottrup H, et al: Lamotrigine for central poststroke pain, *Neurology* 56:184-190, 2001.

50. Leijon G, Boivie J: Central poststroke pain—a controlled trial of amitriptyline and carbamazepine, *Pain* 36:27-36, 1989.

51. Gallo J, Coyne J: The challenge of depression in late life, *JAMA* 284:1570-1572, 2000.

52. Wolf P, Bachman D, Kelly-Hayes M, et al: Stroke and depression in the community: The Framingham Study, *Neurology* 40(Suppl 1): 416, 1990.

53. Robinson R, Kubos K, Starr L, et al: Mood disorders in stroke patients: Importance of location of lesion, *Brain* 187:81-93, 1984.

54. Astrom M, Adolfsson R, Asplund K: Major depression in stroke patients: A 3-year longitudinal study, *Stroke* 24:976-982, 1993.

55. Pohjasvaara T, Leppavuori A, Siira I, et al: Frequency and clinical determinants of poststroke depression, *Stroke* 29:2311-2317, 1998.

56. Andersen G, Vsetergaard K, Lauritzen L: Effective treatment of poststroke depression with the selective serotonin reuptake inhibitor citalopram, *Stroke* 25:1099-1104, 1994.

57. Lazarus L, Moberg P, Langsley P, et al: Methylphenidate and nortriptyline in the treatment of poststroke depression: A retrospective comparison, *Arch Phys Med Rehabil* 75:403-406, 1994.

58. Whooley M, Simon G: Managing depression in medical outpatients, *N Engl J Med* 343:1942-1950, 2000.

59. Wiart L, Petit H, Joseph P, et al: Fluoxetine in early poststroke depression: A double-blind placebo-controlled study, *Stroke* 31:1829-1832, 2000.

60. Dobkin BH: Fatigue versus activity-dependent fatigability in patients with central or peripheral motor impairments, *Neurorehabil Neural Repair* 22:105-110, 2008.

61. DePippo K, Holas M, Reding M, et al: Dysphagia therapy following stroke: A controlled trial, *Neurology* 44:1655-1660, 1994.

62. Hamdy S, Aziz Q, Rothwell J, et al: Recovery of swallowing after dysphagic stroke relates to functional reorganization in the intact motor cortex, *Gastroenterology* 115:1104-1112, 1999.

63. Agency for Health Care Policy and Research: *Pressure ulcers in adults: Prediction and prevention*, Rockville, Md, May 1992, U.S. Department of Health and Human Services, Public Health Service, AHCPR.

64. Epstein F: Cutaneous wound healing, *N Engl J Med* 341:738-746, 1999.

65. Boldrini P, Basaglia N, Calanca M: Sexual changes in hemiparetic patients, *Arch Phys Med Rehabil* 72:202-207, 1991.

66. Maquet P, Laureys S, Peigneux P, et al: Experience-dependent changes in cerebral activation during human REM sleep, *Nature Neurosci* 3:831-836, 2000.

67. Bassetti C, Aldrich M, Quint D: Sleep-disordered breathing in patients with acute supra- and infratentorial strokes: A prospective study of 39 patients, *Stroke* 28:1765-1772, 1997.

68. Good D, Henkle J, Gelber D, et al: Sleep-disordered breathing and poor functional outcome after stroke, *Stroke* 27:252-259, 1996.

69. Mohsenin V, Valor R: Sleep apnea in patients with hemispheric stroke, *Arch Phys Med Rehabil* 76:71-76, 1995.

70. Dietz V: Supraspinal pathways and the development of muscle-tone dysregulation, *Dev Med Child Neurol* 41:708-715, 1999.

71. Hiersemenzel L-P, Curt A, Dietz V: From spinal shock to spasticity, *Neurology* 54:1574-1582, 2000.

72. Hufschmidt A, Mauritz K: Chronic transformation of muscle in spasticity: A peripheral contribution to increased tone, *J Neurol Neurosurg Psychiatry* 48:676-685, 1985.

73. Brown D, Kautz S: Increased workload enhances force output during pedaling exercise in persons with poststroke hemiplegia, *Stroke* 29:598-606, 1998.

74. Sharp S, Brouwer B: Isokinetic strength training of the hemiparetic knee: Effects on function and spasticity, *Arch Phys Med Rehabil* 78:1231-1236, 1997.

75. Smith G, Silver K, Goldberg A, et al: "Task-oriented" exercise improves hamstring strength and spastic reflexes in chronic stroke patients, *Stroke* 30:2112-2118, 1999.

76. Benecke R, Conrad B, Meinck H, et al: Electromyographic analysis of bicycling on an ergometer for evaluation of spasticity of lower limbs in man. In Desmedt J, editor: *Motor control mechanisms in health and disease*, New York, 1983, Raven Press.

77. Brown D, Kautz S, Dairaghi C: Muscle activity adapts to anti-gravity posture during pedalling in persons with post-stroke hemiplegia, *Brain* 120:825-837, 1997.

78. Macko R, Smith G, Dobrovolny C, et al: Treadmill training improves fitness reserve in chronic stroke patients, *Arch Phys Med Rehabil* 82:879-884, 2001.

79. Potempa K, Lopez M, Braun L, et al: Physiological outcomes of aerobic exercise training in hemiparetic stroke, *Stroke* 26:101-105, 1995.

80. Bes A, Eysette M, Pierrot-Deseilligny E: A multi-centre, double-blind trial of tizanidine in spasticity associated with hemiplegia, *Curr Med Res Opin* 10:709-718, 1988.

81. Gelber D, Good D, Dromerick A, et al: Open-label dose-titration safety and efficacy study of tizanidine hydrochloride in the treatment of spasticity associated with chronic stroke, *Stroke* 32:1841-1846, 2001.

82. Bakheit A, Thilmann A, Ward A, et al: A randomized, double-blind, placebo-controlled, dose-ranging study to compare the efficacy and safety of three doses of botulinum toxin type A (Dysport) with placebo in upper limb spasticity after stroke, *Stroke* 31:2402-2406, 2000.

83. Hesse S, Krajnik J, Luecke D, et al: Ankle muscle activity before and after botulinum toxin therapy for lower limb extensor spasticity in chronic hemiparetic patients, *Stroke* 27:455-460, 1996.

84. Reiter F, Danni M, Lagalla G, et al: Low-dose botulinum toxin with ankle taping for the treatment of spastic equinovarus foot after stroke, *Arch Phys Med Rehabil* 79:532-535, 1998.

85. Brashear A, Gordon M, Elovic E, et al: Intramuscular injection of botulinum toxin for the treatment of wrist and finger spasticity after stroke, *N Engl J Med* 347:395-400, 2002.

86. Simpson D, Alexander D, O'Brien C, et al: Botulinum toxin type A in the treatment of upper extremity spasticity: A randomized, double-blind, placebo-controlled trial, *Neurology* 46:1306-1310, 1996.

87. Meythaler J, Guin-Renfroe S, Hadley M: Continuously infused intrathecal baclofen for spastic/dystonic hemiplegia, *Am J Phys Med Rehabil* 78:247-254, 1999.

88. Cicerone K, Dahlberg C, Kalmar K, et al: Evidence-based cognitive rehabilitation: Recommendations for clinical practice, *Arch Phys Med Rehabil* 81:1596-1615, 2000.

89. Desmond D, Moroney J, Paik M, et al: Frequency and clinical determinants of dementia after ischemic stroke, *Neurology* 54:1124-1131, 2000.

90. Gorelick P: Status of risk factors for dementia associated with stroke, *Stroke* 28:459-463, 1997.

91. Moroney J, Bagiella E, Desmond D, et al: Risk factors for incident dementia after stroke, *Stroke* 27:1283-1289, 1996.

92. Rockwood K, Wentzel C, Hachinski V, et al: Prevalence and outcomes of vascular cognitive impairment, *Neurology* 54:447-451, 2000.

93. Tatemichi T, Desmond D, Stern Y, et al: Cognitive impairment after stroke: Frequency, patterns, and relationship to functional abilities, *J Neurol Neurosurg Psychiatry* 57:202-207, 1994.

94. Henon H, Pasquier F, Durieu I, et al: Preexisting dementia in stroke patients, *Stroke* 28:2429-2436, 1997.

95. Pohjasvaara T, Erkinjuntti T, Vataja R, et al: Dementia three months after stroke: Baseline frequency and effect of different definitions of dementia in the Helsinki Stroke Aging Memory Study (SAM) Cohort, *Stroke* 28:785-792, 1997.

96. Wilson B, Baddeley A, Evans J, et al: Errorless learning in the rehabilitation of memory impaired people, *Neuropsychol Rehabil* 4:307-326, 1994.

97. Hanlon R: Motor learning following unilateral stroke, *Arch Phys Med Rehabil* 77:811-815, 1996.

98. Winstein C, Merians A, Sullivan K: Motor learning after unilateral brain damage, *Neuropsychologia* 37:975-987, 1999.

99. Kalra L, Perez I, Gupta S, et al: The influence of visual neglect on stroke rehabilitation, *Stroke* 28:1386-1391, 1997.

100. Marshall R, Sacco R, Lee S, et al: Hemineglect predicts functional outcome after stroke [abstract], *Ann Neurol* 36:298, 1994.

101. Ben-Yishay Y, Diller L: Cognitive remediation in traumatic brain injury: Update and issues, *Arch Phys Med Rehabil* 74:204-213, 1993.

102. Gordon W, Diller L, Lieberman A, et al: Perceptual remediation in patients with right brain damage: A comprehensive program, *Arch Phys Med Rehabil* 66:353-359, 1985.

103. Pizzamiglio L, Antonucci G, Judica A, et al: Chronic rehabilitation of the hemineglect disorder in chronic patients with unilateral right brain damage, *J Clin Exp Neuropsychol* 14:901-923, 1992.

104. Pizzamiglio L, Perani D, Cappa S, et al: Recovery of neglect after right hemisphere damage, *Arch Neurol* 55:561-568, 1998.

105. Young G, Collins D, Hren M: Effect of pairing scanning training with block design training in the remediation of perceptual problems in left hemiplegics, *J Clin Neuropsychol* 5:201-212, 1983.

106. Wiart L, Bon Saint Come A, Debelleix X, et al: Unilateral neglect syndrome rehabilitation by trunk rotation and scanning training, *Arch Phys Med Rehabil* 78:424-429, 1997.

107. Robertson I, North N: Spatio-motor cueing in unilateral neglect: The role of hemispace, hand and motor activation, *Neuropsychologia* 30:553-563, 1992.

108. Robertson I, Mattingley J, Rorden C, et al: Phasic alerting of neglect patients overcomes their spatial deficit in visual awareness, *Nature* 395:169-172, 1998.

109. Fleet W, Valenstein E, Watson R, et al: Dopamine agonist therapy for neglect in humans, *Neurology* 37:1765-1770, 1987.

110. Grujic Z, Mapstone M, Gitelman D, et al: Dopamine agonists reorient visual exploration away from the neglected hemispace, *Neurology* 51:1395-1398, 1998.

111. Erkinjuntti T, Kurz A, Gauthier S, et al: Efficacy of galantamine in probable vascular dementia and Alzheimer's disease combined, *Lancet* 359:1283-1290, 2002.

112. Glazewski S, Giese K, Silva A, et al: The role of alpha-CaMKII autophosphorylation in neocortical experience-dependent plasticity, *Nature Neurosci* 3:911-917, 2000.

113. Kandel E: The molecular biology of memory storage: A dialogue between genes and synapses, *Science* 294:1030-1038, 2001.

114. Pedersen P, Jorgensen H, Nakayama H, et al: Aphasia in acute stroke: Incidence, determinants, and recovery, *Ann Neurol* 38:659-666, 1995.

115. Benson D, Dobkin B, Rothi L, et al: Assessment: Melodic intonation therapy, *Neurology* 44:566-568, 1994.

116. Robey R: A meta-analysis of clinical outcomes in the treatment of aphasia, *J Speech Lang Hear Res* 41:172-187, 1998.

117. Damasio H, Grabowski TJ, Tranel D, et al: Neural correlates of naming actions and of naming spatial relations, *Neuroimage* 13:1053-1064, 2001.

118. Kessler J, Thiel A, Karbe H, et al: Piracetam improves activated blood flow and facilitates rehabilitation of poststroke aphasic patients, *Stroke* 31:2112-2116, 2000.

119. Musso M, Weiller C, Kiebel S: Training-induced brain plasticity in aphasia, *Brain* 122:1781-1790, 1999.

120. Aftonomos L, Steele R, Wertz R: Promoting recovery in chronic aphasia with an interactive technology, *Arch Phys Med Rehabil* 78:841-846, 1997.

121. Weinrich M, Boser K, McCall D, et al: Training agrammatic subjects on passive sentences: Implications for syntactic deficit theories, *Brain Lang* 76:45-61, 2001.

122. Walker-Batson D, Curtis S, Natarajan R, et al: A double-blind placebo-controlled study of the use of amphetamine in the treatment of aphasia, *Stroke* 32:2093-2098, 2001.

123. Huber W, Willmes K, Poeck K, et al: Piracetam as an adjuvant to language therapy for aphasia: A randomized double-blind placebo-controlled pilot study, *Arch Phys Med Rehabil* 78:245-250, 1997.

124. Tanaka Y, Albert M, Yokoyama E, et al: Cholinergic therapy for anomia in fluent aphasia, *Ann Neurol* 50(Suppl 1):S61-S62, 2001.

125. Gold M, VanDam D, Silliman E: An open-label trial of bromocriptine in nonfluent aphasia: A qualitative analysis of word storage and retrieval, *Brain Lang* 74:141-156, 2000.

126. Dobkin B: Greater plasticity through chemicals and practice, *Neurol Network Comment* 2:171-174, 1998.

127. Fried I, Wilson C, Morrow J, et al: Increased dopamine release in the human amygdale during performance of cognitive tasks, *Nature Neurosci* 4:201-206, 2001.

128. Mattay V, Callicott J, Bertolino A, et al: Effects of dextroamphetamine on cognitive performance and cortical activation, *Neuroimage* 12:268-275, 2000.

129. Waelti P, Dickinson A, Schultz W: Dopamine responses comply with basic assumptions of formal learning theory, *Nature* 412:43-48, 2001.

130. Jorgensen H, Nakayama H, Raaschou H, et al: Outcome and time course of recovery in stroke. Part II: Time course. The Copenhagen Stroke Study, *Arch Phys Med Rehabil* 76:406-412, 1995.

131. Jorgensen H, Nakayama H, Raaschou H, et al: Outcome and time course of recovery in stroke. Part I: Outcome. The Copenhagen Stroke Study, *Arch Phys Med Rehabil* 76:399-405, 1995.

132. Wandel A, Jorgensen H, Nakayama H, et al: Prediction of walking function in stroke patients with initial lower extremity paralysis: The Copenhagen Stroke Study, *Arch Phys Med Rehabil* 81:736-738, 2000.

133. Reding M, Potes E: Rehabilitation outcome following initial unilateral hemispheric stroke: Life table analysis approach, *Stroke* 19:1354-1364, 1988.

134. Giuliani C: Strength training for patients with neurological disorders, *Neurol Rep* 19:29–34, 1995.

135. Dobkin B, Harkema S, Requejo P, et al: Modulation of locomotor-like EMG activity in subjects with complete and incomplete chronic spinal cord injury, *J Neurol Rehabil* 9:183–190, 1995.

136. Harkema S, Hurley S, Patel U, et al: Human lumbosacral spinal cord interprets loading during stepping, *J Neurophysiol* 77:797–811, 1997.

137. Duncan P, Sullivan K, Behrman A, Azen S, Dobkin B, et al: Protocol for the Locomotor Experience Applied Post-Stroke (LEAPS) randomized trial, *BMC Neurol* 7:39, 2007.

138. Sullivan K, Knowlton B, Dobkin B: Step training with body weight support: Effect of treadmill speed and practice paradigms on post-stroke locomotor recovery, *Arch Phys Med Rehabil* 83:683–691, 2002.

139. Pohl M, Mehrholz J, Ritschel C, et al: Speed-dependent treadmill training in ambulatory hemiparetic stroke patients, *Stroke* 33:553–558, 2002.

140. Dobkin B, Sullivan K: Sensorimotor cortex plasticity and locomotor and motor control gains induced by body weight-supported treadmill training after stroke, *Neurorehabil Neural Repair* 15:258–259, 2001.

141. Dobkin BH, Functional MRI: A potential physiologic indicator for stroke rehabilitation interventions, *Stroke* 34:23–28, 2003.

142. Hesse S, Bertelt C, Jahnke M, et al: Treadmill training with partial body weight support compared with physiotherapy in nonambulatory hemiparetic patients, *Stroke* 26:976–981, 1995.

143. Hidler J, Nichols D, Pelliccio M, et al: Multicenter randomized clinical trial evaluating the effectiveness of the Lokomat in subacute stroke, *Neurorehabil Neural Repair* 23:5–13, 2009.

144. Dobkin BH, Plummer-D'Amato P, Elashoff R, Lee J: Sirrows Group. International randomized clinical trial: Stroke inpatient rehabilitation with reinforcement of walking speed, improves outcomes, *Neurorehabil Neural Repair* 24:235–242, 2010.

145. Moreland J, Thomson M, Fuoco A: Electromyographic biofeedback to improve lower extremity function after stroke: A meta-analysis, *Arch Phys Med Rehabil* 79:134–140, 1998.

146. Macko R, DeSouza C, Tretter L, et al: Treadmill aerobic exercise training reduces the energy expenditure and cardiovascular demands of hemiparetic gait in chronic stroke patients, *Stroke* 28:326–330, 1997.

147. Thaut M, Kenyon G, Schauer M, et al: The connection between rhythmicity and brain function, *IEEE Eng Med Biol* 18:101–108, 1999.

148. Nakayama H, Jorgensen H, Raaschou H, et al: Recovery of upper extremity function in stroke patients: The Copenhagen Stroke Study, *Arch Phys Med Rehabil* 75:394–398, 1994.

149. Katrak P, Bowring G, Conroy P, et al: Predicting upper limb recovery after stroke: The place of early shoulder and hand movement, *Arch Phys Med Rehabil* 79:758–761, 1998.

150. Johansson K, Lingren I, Widner H, et al: Can sensory stimulation improve the functional outcome in stroke patients? *Neurology* 43:2189–2192, 1993.

151. Gosman-Hedstrom G, Claesson L, Klingenstierna U, et al: Effects of acupuncture treatment on daily life activities and quality of life, *Stroke* 29:2100–2108, 1998.

152. Johannson B, Haker E, von Arbin M, et al: Acupuncture and transcutaneous nerve stimulation in stroke rehabilitation: A randomized, controlled trial, *Stroke* 32:707–713, 2001.

153. Taub E, Wolf S: Constraint induced movement techniques to facilitate upper extremity use in stroke patients, *Top Stroke Rehabil* 3:38–61, 1997.

154. Miltner W, Bauder H, Sommer M, et al: Effects of constraint-induced movement therapy on patients with chronic motor deficits after stroke, *Stroke* 30:586–592, 1999.

155. Wolf SL, Winstein CJ, Miller JP, et al: Effect of constraint-induced movement therapy on upper extremity function 3 to 9 months after stroke: The EXCITE randomized clinical trial, *JAMA* 296:2095–2104, 2006.

156. Liepert J, Bauder H, Miltner W, et al: Treatment-induced cortical reorganization after stroke in humans, *Stroke* 31:1210–1216, 2000.

157. van der Lee J, Wagenaar R, Lankhorst G, et al: Forced use of the upper extremity in chronic stroke patients: Results from a single-blind randomized clinical trial, *Stroke* 30:2369–2375, 1999.

158. Dromerick A, Edwards D, Hahn M: Does the application of constraint-induced movement therapy during acute rehabilitation reduce arm impairment after ischemic stroke? *Stroke* 31:2984–2988, 2000.

159. Butefisch C, Hummelsheim H, Denzler P, et al: Repetitive training of isolated movements improves the outcome of motor rehabilitation of the centrally paretic hand, *J Neurol Sci* 130:59–68, 1995.

160. Dean C, Shepherd R: Task-related training improves performance of seated reaching tasks after stroke, *Stroke* 28:722–728, 1997.

161. Feys H, De Weerdt W, Selz B, et al: Effect of a therapeutic intervention for the hemiplegic upper limb in the acute phase after stroke, *Stroke* 29:785–792, 1998.

162. Pohl P, Winstein C: Practice effects on the less-affected upper extremity after stroke, *Arch Phys Med Rehabil* 80:668–675, 1999.

163. Colebatch J, Gandevia S: The distribution of muscular weakness in upper motor neuron lesions affecting the arm, *Brain* 112:749–763, 1989.

164. Lo AC, Guarino PD, Richards LG, et al: Robot-assisted therapy for long-term upper-limb impairment after stroke, *N Engl J Med* 362:1772–1783, 2010.

165. Volpe B, Krebs H, Hogan N, et al: Robot training enhanced motor outcome in patients with stroke maintained over 3 years, *Neurology* 53:1874–1876, 1999.

166. Whitall J, Waller S, Silver K, et al: Repetitive bilateral arm training with rhythmic auditory cueing improves motor function in chronic hemiparetic stroke, *Stroke* 31:2390–2395, 2000.

167. Lincoln N, Parry R, Vass C: Randomized, controlled trial to evaluate increased intensity of physiotherapy treatment of arm function after stroke, *Stroke* 30:573–579, 1999.

168. Volpe B, Krebs H, Hogan N, et al: A novel approach to stroke rehabilitation: Robot-aided sensorimotor stimulation, *Neurology* 54:1938–1944, 2000.

169. Chae J, Bethoux F, Bohinc T, et al: Neuromuscular stimulation for upper extremity motor and functional recovery in acute hemiplegia, *Stroke* 29:975–979, 1998.

170. Powell J, Pandyan A, Granat M: Electrical stimulation of wrist extensors in poststroke hemiplegia, *Stroke* 30:1384–1389, 1999.

171. Cauraugh J, Light K, Kim S, et al: Chronic motor dysfunction after stroke: Recovering wrist and finger extension by electromyography-triggered neuromuscular stimulation, *Stroke* 31:1360–1364, 2000.

172. Chantraine A, Baribeault A, Uebelhart D, et al: Shoulder pain and dysfunction in hemiplegia: Effects of functional electrical stimulation, *Arch Phys Med Rehabil* 80:328–331, 1999.

173. Jizerman M, Stoffers T, Groen I, et al: The NESS Handmaster orthosis: Restoration of hand function in C5 and stroke patients by means of electrical stimulation, *J Rehabil Sci* 9:86–90, 1996.

174. Popovic D, Stojanovic A, Pjanovic A: Clinical evaluation of the bionic glove, *Arch Phys Med Rehabil* 80:299–304, 1999.

175. Rossignol S, Chau C, Brustein E, et al: Pharmacological activation and modulation of the central pattern generator for locomotion in the cat, *Ann N Y Acad Sci* 860:346–359, 1998.

176. Stroemer R, Kent T, Hulsebosch C: Enhanced neocortical neural sprouting, synaptogenesis and behavioral recovery with *d*-amphetamine therapy after neocortical infarction in rats, *Stroke* 29:2381–2395, 1998.

177. Sutton R, Feeney D: Alpha-noradrenergic agonists and antagonists affect recovery and maintenance of beam walking ability after sensorimotor cortex ablation in the rat, *Restor Neurol Neurosci* 4:1–11, 1992.

178. Dobkin B: Experimental brain injury and repair, *Curr Opin Neurol* 10:493–497, 1997.

179. Crisostomo E, Duncan P, Propst M, et al: Evidence that amphetamine with physical therapy promotes recovery of motor function in stroke patients, *Ann Neurol* 23:94–97, 1988.

180. Walker-Batson D, Smith P, Curtis S, et al: Amphetamine paired with physical therapy accelerates motor recovery after stroke, *Stroke* 26:2254–2259, 1995.

181. Grade C, Redford B, Chrostowski J, et al: Methylphenidate in early poststroke recovery: A double-blind, placebo-controlled study, *Arch Phys Med Rehabil* 79:1047–1050, 1998.

182. Scheidtmann K, Fries W, Muller F, et al: Effect of levodopa in combination with physiotherapy on functional motor recovery after stroke: A prospective, randomised, double-blinded study, *Lancet* 358:787–790, 2001.

183. Dam M, Tonin P, De Boni A, et al: Effects of fluoxetine and maprotiline on functional recovery in poststroke hemiplegic patients undergoing rehabilitation therapy, *Stroke* 27:1211-1214, 1996.

184. Pariente J, Loubinoux I, Carel C, et al: Fluoxetine modulates motor performance and cerebral activation of patients recovering from stroke, *Ann Neurol* 50:718-729, 2001.

185. Reding M, Solomon B, Borucki S: Effect of dextroamphetamine on motor recovery after stroke, *Neurology* 45(Suppl 4):A222, 1995.

186. Sonde L, Nordstrom M, Nilsson C, et al: A double-blind placebo-controlled study of the effects of amphetamine and physiotherapy after stroke, *Cerebrovasc Dis* 12:253-257, 2001.

187. Miyai I, Saito T, Nozaki S, et al: A pilot study of the effect of L-threodops on rehabilitation outcome of stroke patients, *Neurorehabil Neural Repair* 14:141-147, 2000.

188. Nishino K, Sasaki T, Takahashi K, et al: The norepinephrine precursor L-threo-3-4-dihydroxyphenylserine facilitates motor recovery in chronic stroke patients, *J Clin Neurosci* 8:547-550, 2001.

189. Loubinoux I, Carel C, Alary F, et al: Within-session and between-session reproducibility of cerebral sensorimotor activation: A test-retest effect evidenced with functional MRI, *J Cereb Blood Flow Metab* 21:592-607, 2001.

190. Iwanenko W, Fiedler R, Granger C, et al: The Uniform Data System for Medical Rehabilitation, *Am J Phys Med Rehabil* 80:56-61, 2001.

191. Smania N, Bazoli F, Piva D, et al: Visuomotor imagery and rehabilitation of neglect, *Arch Phys Med Rehabil* 78:430-436, 1997.

192. Tham K, Tegner R: Video feedback in the rehabilitation of patients with unilateral neglect, *Arch Phys Med Rehabil* 78:410-413, 1997.

193. Beis J-M, Andre J-M, Baumgarten A, et al: Eye patching in unilateral spatial neglect: Efficacy of two methods, *Arch Phys Med Rehabil* 80:71-76, 1999.

194. Butter C, Kirsch N: Combined and separate effects of eye patching and visual stimulation on unilateral neglect following stroke, *Arch Phys Med Rehabil* 73:1133-1139, 1992.

195. Rossi P, Kheyfets S, Reding M: Fresnel prisms improve visual perception in stroke patients with homonymous hemianopia or unilateral visual neglect, *Neurology* 40:1597-1599, 1990.

196. Serfaty C, Soroker N, Glicksohn J, et al: Does monocular viewing improve target detection in hemispatial neglect? *Restor Neurol Neurosci* 9:7-13, 1995.

197. Rossetti Y, Rode G, Pisella L, et al: Prism adaptation to a rightward optical deviation rehabilitates left hemispatial neglect, *Nature* 395:166-169, 1998.

198. Mennemeier M, Chatterjee A, Heilman K: A comparison of the influences of body and environment centred reference frames on neglect, *Brain* 117:1013-1021, 1994.

199. Simon E, Hegarty A, Mehler M: Hemispatial and directional performance biases in motor neglect, *Neurology* 45:525-531, 1995.

200. Oliveri M, Rossini P, Traversa R, et al: Left frontal transcranial magnetic stimulation reduces contralesional extinction in patients with unilateral right brain damage, *Brain* 122:1731-1739, 1999.

201. Rode G, Charles N, Perenin M-T, et al: Partial remission of hemiplegia and somatoparaphrenia through vestibular stimulation in a case of unilateral neglect, *Cortex* 28:203-208, 1992.

202. Vallar G, Sterzi R, Bottini G, et al: Temporary remission of left hemianesthesia after vestibular stimulation: A sensory neglect phenomenon, *Cortex* 26:123-131, 1990.

203. Pizzamiglio L, Frasca R, Guariglia C, et al: Effects of optokinetic stimulation in patients with visual neglect, *Cortex* 26:535-540, 1990.

204. Kerkhoff G, MunBinger U, Meier E: Neurovisual rehabilitation in cerebral blindness, *Arch Neurol* 51:474-481, 1994.

205. Gray J, Robertson I, Pentland B, et al: Microcomputer-based attentional retraining after brain damage: A randomised group controlled trial, *Neuropsychol Rehabil* 2:97-115, 1992.

206. Robertson I, Gray J, Pentland B, et al: Microcomputer-based rehabilitation for unilateral left visual neglect: A randomized controlled trial, *Arch Phys Med Rehabil* 71:663-668, 1990.

57

Enhancing Stroke Recovery with Cellular Therapies

SEAN I. SAVITZ

Cell-based therapy has taken center stage as a novel investigative approach to enhance recovery from ischemic stroke. The concept of using cells, rather than drugs, as a therapy grew out of an era when transplantation studies were under way in the 1990s for neurodegenerative disorders such as Parkinson's disease. At the time, the rationale for cellular transplantation was restoration of neural connections, particularly in Parkinson's disease, which involves loss of a relatively homogeneous group of neurons, at least in its earlier stages.[1] In an entirely different area of medicine, the relative success of bone marrow transplantation (BMT) for leukemia served as a launching pad to extend BMT to other medical conditions, including neurologic disorders, because BMT is a type of stem cell infusion. In the consideration of BMT for stroke, it was first shown that some types of stem cells from the bone marrow have the capacity to differentiate into neural phenotypes.[2] However, a growing number of studies over the past 5 to 10 years now indicate that newly introduced cells from peripheral sources such as the bone marrow likely exert a number of potentially beneficial effects completely independent of neural replacement.

The introduction of exogenous cells to enhance brain repair has also been supported by our further understanding of the brain's endogenous response to ischemia. Ischemia leads to increased proliferation of neural stem cells (NSCs) along the subventricular zone. As NSCs become activated, they migrate toward the infarct and along their migratory path, differentiating into new neurons with the phenotype of the damaged area.[3,4] However, most of the newly matured neurons die for unclear reasons. Therefore, the brain's intrinsic repair after stroke is limited and insufficient. Cellular therapy might enhance this endogenous response.

Given the wealth of animal data on the potential restorative effects of cellular therapeutics in a range of neurologic disorders, this new approach has grown in momentum to be tested at the bedside. The lack of effective therapies to reduce disability after stroke undoubtedly fuels this momentum.

What Are the Goals of Cell-Based Therapy for Stroke?

The preceding discussion raises the question "What are the real goals of cell-based therapy for stroke?" Initial approaches in the field intended to design a therapy that could replace lost tissue after stroke.[1] Grafting of tissue into the area of an infarct showed promise to reduce deficits and was found to be safe in animal studies.[1] Over the past decade, however, the goals of cellular therapy have entirely changed. Rather than differentiating into new neurons and replacing lost neural connections, most cell-based approaches seek to reduce ongoing injury after stroke, attenuate inflammation, remodel surviving tissue, and enhance endogenous repair such as neurogenesis, angiogenesis, and synaptogenesis. Other mechanisms are possibly decreasing scar formation and reducing inhibitory glycoproteins that prevent axonal regeneration. It is now clear that some type of cellular preparations may even be used as a neuroprotective approach in the acute stroke setting.

The Complexity of Stroke for Cell Therapy

Although we are beginning to learn more about the various mechanisms that cellular therapy may exert in the brain, stroke is far from an ideal clinical condition for which to develop a cell-based therapeutic approach. Ischemic stroke is heterogeneous; infarcts can be small or large, occur in different areas of the brain, and involve different cell types. For example, an occlusion in the posterior cerebral artery can damage at least three different types of neurons in the hippocampus, thalamus, and occipital lobe. Patients with stroke can have a range of deficits with variable rates of recovery, in contrast to patients with an inexorable neurodegenerative disorder. What level of disability and which deficits should be included in clinical studies? Should those with little potential for recovery or those with excellent potential for significant recovery be excluded? When to administer cells after a stroke also remains unclear. In the acute setting, the release of excitotoxic mediators, free radicals, and inflammatory cytokines may threaten the viability of any newly introduced cells. In addition, many stroke patients in the acute setting worsen because of edema, hemorrhagic transformation, and in-hospital medical complications. Waiting weeks to months allows for natural recovery to plateau before consideration of an investigative therapy, but at the same time, gliosis leading to scar formation might inhibit the regenerative capacity of exogenous cells introduced into the infarcted brain. The presence of a persistent vascular occlusive lesion may prevent the passage of cells to the infarcted region if an intraarterial approach is the desired method of delivery.

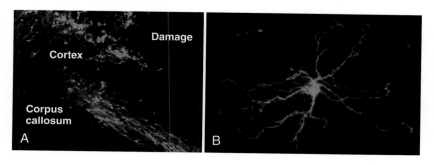

Figure 57-1 Human fetal striatum–derived neural stem cells (NSCs) transplanted in stroke-damaged brain. A, Green fluorescent protein–labeled NSCs migrating across the corpus callosum and populating damaged cortical areas. B, Confocal reconstruction of grafted NSCs exhibiting neuronal morphology. (Courtesy of Zaal Kokaia, PhD, from Lund Stem Cell Center, Sweden.)

The Complexity of Cells

Although stroke is complex, we also face the complexity of an increasing variety of cells that are currently under investigation (Table 57-1), including embryonic stem cells, neural cells, dental cells, and cells from the bone marrow, umbilical cord, placenta, amnion, adipose tissue, and menstrual and peripheral blood.

Embryonic Cells

Theoretically, embryonic stem cells (ESCs) may be ideal to generate all the different types of cells lost in a stroke and to reconstruct lost brain tissue. Studies have even indicated that injection of ESCs to the side of the brain contralateral to a stroke leads to ESC migration to the ischemic lesion. However, it has clearly been shown that the injection of predifferentiated ESCs in the rodent stroke model leads to teratocarcinomas.[5] Therefore, the use of predifferentiated ESCs as a therapy for stroke is not an option at present. Further work must determine how ESCs could be applied as a potential stroke therapy. Other studies have investigated differentiating ESCs to NSCs before administration (see later), but many hurdles remain to establishing the safety of ESC-derived cells administered to the brain.

Neural Cells

Neural cell–based therapies have undergone a more thorough investigation than ESCs and some types have even reached clinical safety testing. Neural cells for stroke can be categorized into three types: neural transplants, NSCs, and immortalized neural stem cell lines.

Neural Transplants

The first neural transplant studies in stroke involved the use of the now largely abandoned NT2N cells. The NT2 cells, derived from a patient with a testicular germ cell teratocarcinoma more than 20 years ago, resemble neural stem cells in that they express cell surface markers and cytoskeletal proteins unique to NSCs.[6] Treatment of NT2 cells with retinoic acid ultimately leads to the production of postmitotic neuron-like cells (called NT2N cells), which express neurotransmitters, functional glutamate receptors, ion channels, synaptic proteins, and secretory proteins.[7-12] Grafted NT2N cells in the recipient rodent brain elaborate processes and release neurotransmitters.[13] In rodent models of ischemic stroke, NT2N cells, injected

TABLE 57-1 DIFFERENT TYPES OF CELLS UNDER INVESTIGATION FOR STROKE

Stem cells
Embryonic
Neural
Bone marrow
Umbilical cord
Placenta, amnion
Menstrual blood
Adipose
Dental
Induced pluripotent stem cells
Heterogeneous
Bone marrow mononuclear
Umbilical cord
CD34+ peripheral blood
Neural stem cell lines
NTera-2 (NT2)
CTX0E03
Fetal brain progenitor cells
Human
Pig (xenografts)

directly to the striatal infarct 1 month after middle cerebral artery occlusion (MCAO), improved neurologic deficits on passive avoidance and elevated body swing test results. Graft survival was dependent on immunosuppression with cyclosporine.[14] These preclinical results led to phase 2 studies testing the safety of NT2N cells in patients with stroke, the results of which are discussed later. Although the animals injected with these cells improved, the mechanism underlying the benefits was not explored. Whether the cells expressed striatal phenotypes, extended processes, and showed evidence for integration in the host brain was not shown.

At the same time as studies were under way on NT2N cells, other investigators turned to neural progenitor cells (NPCs) from the embryonic pig, during an era when fetal xenotransplantation was under active consideration for adult brain disorders. Transplantation of fetal cells from the porcine primordial striatum, called the lateral ganglionic eminence (LGE), was first shown to promote graft integration and to improve deficits in animal models of Huntington's disease and then in stroke.[15,16] LGE cells transplanted 3 to 28 days after MCAO in the rodent led to graft formation within the striatal infarct cavity and the differentiation of donor cells into glial and striatal neurons, some of which elaborated processes and synapses within host brain.[1] These studies also led to one pilot safety study of LGE cells in patients, as discussed later. However, no further work was published on the biologic characterization of the LGE cells in vitro or in vivo, nor were mechanisms ever explored to fully account for the potential benefits seen in the rodent model.

Neural Stem Cells

In contrast to more developed cells or progenitor cells from one area of the brain, NSCs differentiate into all the different brain cell types and therefore have potential to regenerate lost brain tissue. They can be isolated from generative zones of the central nervous system (CNS) in embryonic, fetal, and adult mammals, grown in culture in the presence of growth factors, and engrafted into the brain through various delivery routes. In addition, it is important to point out that NSCs, when expanded as neurospheres, adopt forebrain profiles but can also be differentiated into cell types that are typically lost in ischemic stroke, such as hippocampal neurons, interneurons, and cortical projection neurons. It has even been shown that neurons derived from NSCs generate action potentials.[17] Several studies have shown that transplanted NSCs survive and migrate to the injured brain.[18,19] Kelly et al[18] have been studying fetal human NSCs. When injected at 7 days after cortical stroke, NSCs survive and migrate to the lesion site. Similar cells are currently being tested in patients with neurodegenerative disorders, such as Batten's disease and Pelizaeus-Merzbacher disease.[20,21] Darsalia et al[19] have also been studying NSCs derived from the fetal human cortex or striatum (Fig. 57-1). NSCs from either source directly injected 1 to 2 weeks after stroke into a striatal infarct survive to a similar extent and migrate throughout the injured striatum. Striatal NSCs were found to migrate farther and occupy a greater volume of the infarct than the cortical NSCs.[19] It was also found that striatal and cortical NSCs stopped proliferating and either remained in an undifferentiated state or differentiated exclusively into neurons.[19] Both types of NSCs grafted in damaged brain and generated neurons of different phenotypes.[19] Although these results on the use of NSCs for stroke are intriguing, little information is known on how and to what extent human-derived NSCs integrate with the host brain. Also, few studies to date have been published on whether NSCs reduce neurologic deficits in stroke models. However, it has been shown in a few studies that NSCs can generate neurons that form connections with host cells.[22] ESC-derived NSCs engraft, form all different brain cell types, and elaborate a neuropil when injected into the infarct cavity.[23] ESC-derived neurons have even been shown to exhibit electrophysiologic properties and synaptic connectivity.[24] The derivation and preparation of NSCs are also an important issue. Some studies use specific populations from localized areas of the brain and others use the entire fetal brain. As already discussed, NSCs can be generated from embryonic stem cells. However, a major challenge is the limited in vitro expansion potential of fetal-derived cells. Whether a clinical grade, fetus-derived NSC product can be adequately scaled for clinical application awaits further investigation.

Neural Stem Cell Lines

Partly to address the limitations of the supply of NSCs from fetal and embryonic sources, cell lines exhibiting the properties of NSCs are also being developed. There are several advantages to cell lines. They are homogeneous, being generated from a single source, avoiding the heterogeneity of cell purity and quality in primary human fetal tissue. They are amenable to scalability and stability following good manufacturing production standards. Cells lines can be rapidly generated, are reproducible, and allow for controlled expansion and differentiation. Cell lines also might permit stable expression of genes for therapeutic purposes. Some notable examples are CTX0E03, a cell line derived from fetal brain tissue, infected with c-mycERTAM (Figs. 57-2 and 57-3). CTX0E03, when injected into the brain after stroke, reduces neurologic deficits.[25] These studies have led to approval in the United Kingdom of the first human study assessing the safety of these cells in patients with chronic stroke.

Summary of Neural Cells

Overall, neural stem cells show promise as a potential cell-based approach for stroke. However, if the intended purpose is tissue replacement, before clinical applications, we need a better understanding of how to control stem cell proliferation and differentiation into specific phenotypes, induce their integration into existing neural and synaptic circuits, and optimize functional recovery using animal models of stroke.[1] Otherwise, it appears more likely that NSCs induce recovery through paracrine effects on the host brain, much like other types of stem cells.

Alternative Sources of Adult Stem Cells

Stem cells have been isolated from various tissues throughout the body, including bone marrow, peripheral blood, umbilical cord, and adipose tissue. There are several advantages for these alternative sources. They avoid the political and ethical barriers of fetal tissue, some already have established clinical uses, they permit intravenous administration, some are amenable to autologous transplantation, cells from these sources can be easily obtained, and the intended purpose of using these cells does not involve host integration.

Bone Marrow

Marrow stromal cells. From a historical standpoint, the use of bone marrow cells was one of the first to be investigated as an alternative source of adult stem cells. Adult bone marrow contains not only hematopoietic stem cells but also multipotential mesenchymal stem cells (MSCs).[26,27] A specific group of mesenchymal stem cells reside in the stromal compartment of the bone marrow and have been termed marrow stromal cells. They are fibroblast-like cells that adhere to plastic and are thus easily isolated in culture. They display morphologic and functional heterogeneity, possibly related to variations in tissue source and culture protocols. MSCs display low immunogenicity and powerful immunomodulatory activity, supporting host tolerance toward MSCs as an allogeneic cellular

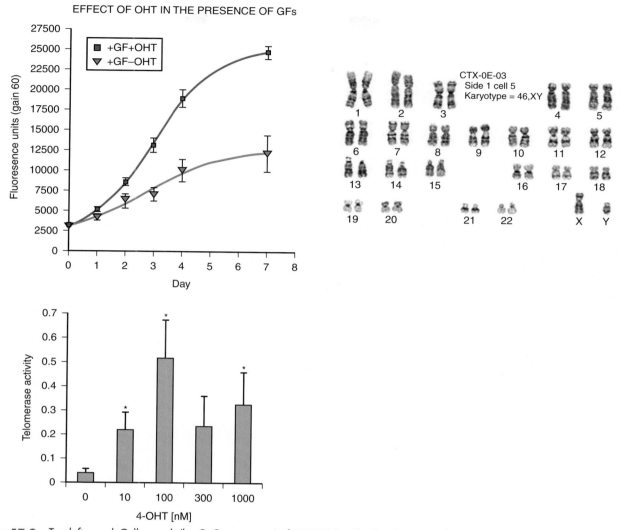

CTX CONDITIONAL PROLIFERATION

Figure 57-2 *Top left panel,* Cell growth (by CyQuant assay) of CTX0E03 cells plated in normal growth media with added growth factors (basic fibroblast growth factor and epidermal growth factor). Note that activation of the c-MycER fusion protein by the addition of 4-hydroxy-tamoxifen (OHT), a minor metabolite of the drug tamoxifen, causes exponential cell growth, permitting scaled-up manufacture of the cell line. *Upper right panel,* The cell line retains a normal (male) karyotype across extended passaging. *Lower left panel,* Activation of the c-MycER fusion protein by addition of 4-hydroxytamoxifen in the CTX0E03 cell line activates hTERT (human telomerase reverse transcriptase) in the cells in a dose-related fashion. (Courtesy of John Sinden, PhD, ReNeuron Group.)

therapy.[28,29] A large body of work has been conducted demonstrating that MSCs, when delivered with intracerebral, intravenous, or intracarotid approaches, enhance recovery from stroke in rat models.[30] MSCs have been shown to reduce neurologic deficits even when administered at 30 days after stroke,[31] although this finding awaits reproducibility. MSCs within the brain exert several different effects that may be termed enhanced repair processes. They stimulate angiogenesis and neurogenesis, promote axonal remodeling and regeneration, and reduce scar formation (Fig. 57-4).

Multipotent adult progenitor cells (MAPCs). The bone marrow also contains stem cells that may be more primitive than MSCs by displaying pluripotent regenerative properties.[32] In 2001, Reyes et al[33] described the isolation from the bone marrow of multipotent adult progenitor cells, which expressed embryonic stem cell markers and demonstrated broad differentiation capability, including epithelial, endothelial, neural, myogenic, hematopoietic, osteogenic, hepatogenic, chondrogenic, and adipogenic lineages (Fig. 57-5). MAPCs share similar features with MSCs with respect to strong immunomodulatory properties[28] but also have distinct phenotypes separate from those of MSCs.[34] In the rat stroke model, stereotactic injection of MAPCs to peri-ischemic regions 1 week after ischemic injury led to significant improvement in limb placement compared with saline and cyclosporine A–treated control animals. The MAPCs had migrated to the site of injury and displayed limited processes and indistinct morphology, with little differentiation.[35]

CTX0E03 CELLS IN BRAIN

Bright field images early after grafting

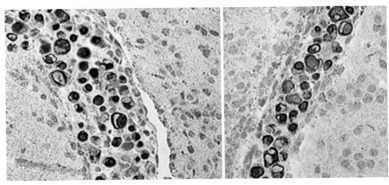

Late time points—showing extensive morphology

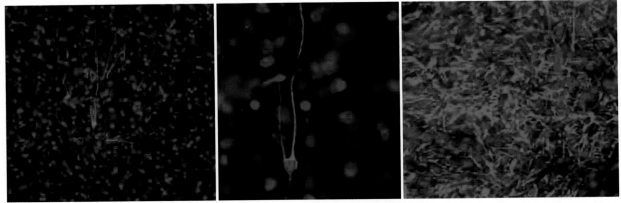

Figure 57-3 CTX0E03 cells implanted in rodent brain can be identified histologically in bright field or fluorescence through the use of antibodies directed against human specific nestin. Note that early after grafting, cells are found close to the injection sites. At later time points, cells are seen to migrate into tissue and adopt a range of morphologies. (Courtesy of John Sinden, PhD, ReNeuron Group.)

Mononuclear cells. Heterogeneous populations of bone marrow have also gained much attention as a potential therapy for stroke. Mononuclear cells (MNCs), as an example, are easily and rapidly separated from bone marrow aspirates by Ficoll density, in contrast to MSCs, which require cell culture and passage. Because MNCs are enriched with hematopoietic and mesenchymal stem cells, many writers have referred to them as stem cells, when in fact they contain a range of different lymphoid and myeloid cells. Nevertheless, a wealth of studies suggests that MNCs enhance left ventricular function after myocardial infarction (MI) in animal models.[36] Furthermore, a meta-analysis of randomized studies shows that MNCs improve cardiac outcomes in patients with MI.[37] Several different laboratories have thus far reported that either intravenous or intraarterial injection of MNCs, both autologous and donor-derived, improve behavioral outcome in animal stroke models.[38-40] Both young and middle-aged animals benefited from autologous MNCs.[41] To a lesser extent, other heterogeneous populations of bone marrow have also undergone testing in animal models. The CD34+/Lin– population of bone marrow, for example, reduces deficits in a mouse model of stroke.[42] Given that they are the two most studied of the cell populations from the bone marrow under investigation for stroke, the potential advantages and disadvantages of MSCs and MNCs are presented in Table 57-2.

Umbilical cord. Cord blood similarly contains an enriched fraction of progenitor cells that are normally found in bone marrow. Several studies have shown that the mononuclear fraction in human umbilical cord blood cells (HUBCs) reduces neurologic deficits in animal models of stroke.[43,44] This is one of the few cellular preparations for which dose response and therapeutic time window have been published. In addition, mesenchymal stem cells have also been isolated from cord blood and are under investigation as a therapeutic for stroke.

Adipose tissue. Studies also suggest that adipose tissue contains pluripotent stromal cells. Primary cultures of adipose tissue are a heterogeneous collection of hematopoietic cells, pericytes, endothelial cells, and smooth muscle cells. Several passages in cultures yield stromal cells that exhibit cell-surface markers consistent with mesenchymal stem cells.[45] Stromal cells can be cultured from human liposuction adipose tissue and is therefore being investigated as a potential autoplastic therapy for stroke. Intracerebroventricular injection of adipose stromal cells 1 day after MCA occlusion in rats was found to lead to migration into the ischemic area, where implanted cells were visualized at the border between intact and injured brain, but cells also traveled far distances, including the contralateral cortex. At 7 days after stroke, transplanted rats had significantly better recovery in motor and somatosensory behavior than animals that received only saline.[46]

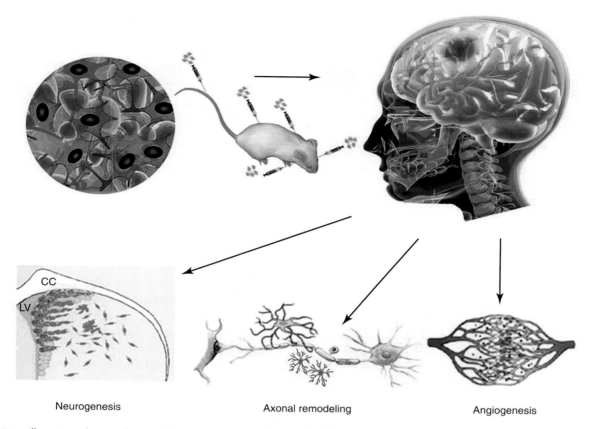

Figure 57-4 Illustration showing how multipotent mesenchymal stromal cells (MSCs) stimulate recovery of neurologic function when used to treat stroke/central nervous system (CNS) disease. MSCs are extracted, separated, and cultured. They are then injected via different local or systemic routes (intracerebrally, intraarterially, intracisternally, intrathecally, or intravenously) into the animal with CNS disease. MSCs selectively migrate and survive in the damaged tissue and the perilesion areas in the animals with stroke. An array of restorative events are stimulated by MSCs. MSCs secrete and induce within the parenchymal cell (including astrocytes, microglia, and oligodendrocytes) secretion of cytokines, growth and trophic factors, and other bioactive factors. These factors increase angiogenesis, neurogenesis, and axonal and dendritic remodeling that improve functional recovery. (Courtesy of Dr. Michael Chopp, PhD, Henry Ford Hospital.)

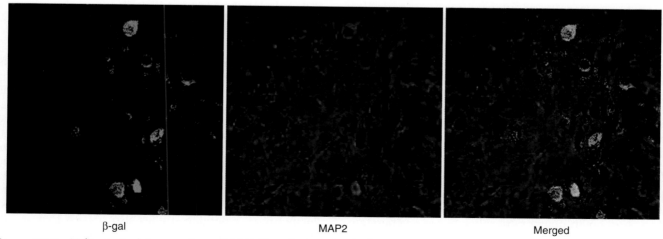

Figure 57-5 Multipotent adult progenitor cell (MAPC) graft survival in the hypoxia-ischemia–injured brain of a neonatal rat that showed behavioral improvement following intravenous delivery of cells. Representative images from the hippocampus following intravenous transplantation of MAPCs is shown. *Left,* Confocal microscopy reveals the presence of intravenously delivered MAPCs tagged with β-galactosidase (β-gal) (AlexaFluor 488/green staining) in the CA3 region of the hippocampus of a neonatal rat after it sustained a hypoxia-induced ischemic injury. *Middle,* Staining for the neuronal marker protein microtubule-associated protein-2 (MAP2) (AlexaFluor 594/red staining) demonstrates the presence of putative neurons in the same field. *Right,* Colocalization (yellow signal) of the β-gal–positive MAPC with MAP2 positive signal is demonstrated. These data indicate that intravenous transplantation of MAPCs results in cell migration into the ischemic hippocampus and subsequent colocalization of the cell tag with a phenotypic neuronal marker, in a rare number of cells. (This work was performed in the laboratory of Dr. Cesar Borlongan as part of an NIH funded Phase I STTR grant to Dr. James Carroll and Athersys Inc. [Grant # NS 055606-01].)

TABLE 57-2 THE TWO MAIN TYPES OF BONE MARROW CELLULAR THERAPIES UNDER INVESTIGATION FOR STROKE

Cell Type	Advantages	Disadvantages
Marrow stromal cells	Most studied; extensive testing in stroke model Permits the possibility of scaling and banking of allogeneic, off-the-shelf product	Culture preparations may influence cell properties Passage influences the extent of cell heterogeneity and cell properties Autologous takes weeks to culture → feasible therapy for acute/subacute stroke or only chronic stroke?
Mononuclear cells	Rapidly prepared in hours from a patient for autologous applications Does not require manipulation or culture Mixed cell types may have combined positive effects Reproducibility of efficacy in multiple animal laboratories	Heterogeneity of different cell populations may vary from patient to patient but whether functionally relevant unknown Bone marrow harvest is invasive Allogeneic not a foreseeable option given major histocompatibility complex incompatibility

Blood. CD34+ selected cells from peripheral blood are currently under clinical investigation in stroke patients in Taiwan. Shyu et al[47] reported that direct intracranial injections stimulate angiogenesis in the brain and enhance recovery in an animal stroke model.

Other sources. Stem cells have been isolated from a range of other tissues, such as amniotic fluid, the placenta, and menstrual blood[48, 49]; emerging studies also suggest that these cells, too, can improve neurologic outcome in rodent stroke models. Like many of the bone marrow–derived stem cells, all of these populations to variable extents may exhibit pluripotent stem cell characteristics, including extensive self-renewal, expression of stem cell markers and in vitro or in vivo differentiation capacity, but all of these possible features are controversial. The different types of cells await further investigation for preclinical development.

Mechanisms

Tissue Replacement

Early work in this field had the intended purpose to restore lost neuronal connections as a true cell transplantation approach.[1] The injection of NT2N cells in animals led to grafts within the host brain, but it was not established whether these grafts integrated into the recipient's CNS. Even the initial work 5 to 10 years ago using marrow stromal cells and other cell types had focused on their potential to differentiate into brain cell types. However, the preponderance of data in the last few years supports a paradigm shift in understanding the way exogenous cells may exert therapeutic effects in the infarcted brain.

Trophicity and Paracrine Effects

The principal mechanisms of action for most types of cells currently being studied occur through trophic influences on the host environment rather than tissue regeneration. Data from various studies indicate that although some types of neural stem cells and MSCs display the capacity for multipotential differentiation in vitro, donor cells in vivo engage in reducing inflammation, inhibiting ongoing apoptosis, protecting peri-infarct tissue, and enhancing repair.[30,41,50,51] All of these mechanisms are likely mediated by the release of trophic and anti-inflammatory factors from the donor cells, but intrinsic factors from the host brain may also be upregulated by donor cells. The

interaction of the microenvironment may heavily influence the behavior of injected cells depending on the timing after the onset of ischemia.[52]

Peripheral Organs as Bioreactors

As we learn more about the migration and fate of intravenously injected cells, we may find that the spleen and other organs such as the lung play pivotal roles in reducing ongoing damage after an acute medical disorder such as stroke.[53] In MI, for example, MSCs promote the secretion of anti-inflammatory mediators within the lung.[54] Nemeth et al[55] have shown that host macrophages are modulated to exert anti-inflammatory effects in a model of shock. And the spleen may be modulated by umbilical cord cells to release interleukin-10 (IL-10).[56] These results raise the intriguing hypothesis that peripheral organs may actively participate to reduce proinflammatory responses after acute injuries. A peripheral rather than central mechanism to explain some of the effects of cell therapy might partially address the disconnect between the benefits seen in animal stroke models and the low percentage of cells entering the brain.

Angiogenesis and Neurogenesis

Various cell types (MSCs, peripheral blood stem cells, HUBCs) have been shown to induce the formation of blood vessels.[47,57,58] One mechanism may be that transplanted cells increase levels of angiogenic factors (e.g., vascular endothelial growth factor, fibroblast growth factor, glial [cell line]–derived neurotrophic factor, brain-derived neurotrophic factor) either by secretion or by stimulating upregulation within the host brain.[57] Such factors may induce the proliferation of vascular endothelial cells (angiogenesis) and cause mobilization and homing of endogenous endothelial progenitors (vasculogenesis). Furthermore, emerging studies also suggest that several different cell types, such as cord blood– and bone marrow–derived cells,[58,59] enhance neurogenesis in the postischemic brain, the significance of which remains unclear.

Upregulating Brain Plasticity

Some cell types, including HUCBCs, increase sprouting of nerve fibers from the contralateral hemisphere to the ischemic hemisphere.[60] The functional significance of these findings remains unclear and awaits further investigation.

Pilot Clinical Trials: Lessons Learned
NT2N Cells

The first clinical trial in the United States was conducted in the late 1990s to assess the safety of intrastriatal transplantation of NT2N cells (produced by Layton Bioscience, Inc., Sunnyvale, CA, and known as LBS neurons for human use) in patients with basal ganglia infarcts and stable motor deficits 6 months to 6 years after stroke. In the first phase 1 study,[61] 12 patients were treated with NT2N cell transplants and immunosuppression using cyclosporine for 9 weeks. On the basis of preclinical safety data, doses of 2 and 6 million cells were considered appropriate. Long-term medical problems since transplantation have been attributed to cardiovascular risk factors and advancing age. Two patients died of unrelated medical illnesses. On autopsy examination of one of these patients, who did not show clinical improvement and died of MI, the graft site showed no signs of inflammation, neoplasia, or infectious disease 27 months after implantation. The detection of grafted neurons, identified at the injection site with fluorescent in situ hybridization, supports the contention that grafts can survive in the human brain 27 months after implantation. Positron emission tomography scanning at 6 months showed greater than 15% relative uptake of fluorodeoxyglucose F18 at the transplant site in six patients. This might have reflected surviving and functioning implanted cells, enhanced host cell activity, or an inflammatory response.

In a phase 2 study,[62] a randomized, open-label trial was undertaken to assess the effects of neuronal cell transplantation in patients with motor deficits 1 to 6 years following basal ganglia infarcts. Fourteen patients were randomly assigned to receive 5 or 10 million implanted cells followed by rehabilitation, compared with four patients who only underwent physiotherapy. Half the patients had an ischemic stroke, whereas the other half had an intracerebral hemorrhage. One patient had a single seizure and another had a subdural hematoma evacuated 1 month after transplantation without new neurologic deficits. There were no cell-associated adverse events. Patients who received transplants showed a trend toward improvement in functional outcomes over baseline measurements obtained before transplantation, but there were no statistically significant trends in comparison with the four control subjects. Several of the transplanted patients with strokes in the nondominant hemisphere showed improvement on tests of memory, recall, and visuospatial/constructional ability 6 months after transplantation. The control subjects did not show such changes.

Porcine Niemann Pick-C1s (NPCs)

In 1998, a pilot safety and feasibility study of intrastriatal transplantation of porcine lateral ganglionic eminence (LGE) NPCs was conducted in five patients with chronic basal ganglia infarcts.[63] Fetal cell suspensions were prepared from dissection of the LGE of porcine embryonic tissue and pretreated in culture with an anti–major histocompatibility complex class I antibody, with the intention to avoid immunosuppression. The patients demonstrated no new neurologic deficits in the acute setting. However, one patient had cortical vein occlusion presumed to be related to the surgery and another had a seizure in the setting of diabetic ketoacidosis. Some of the patients showed sustained improvement in their deficits. There were no long-term adverse events. Together, the clinical trials on NT2 and LGE cells suggest that transplantation is feasible but does pose risks for seizure, subdural hematoma, and venous occlusion. It remains unclear whether implanted cells from these trials led to any sustained long-term benefits.

Recent and Ongoing Studies
Mesenchymal Stem Cells

Given the extensive data on the effects of MSCs in rodent models, more than 5 years ago Korean investigators began a controlled, open-label clinical trial in which they harvested bone marrow from patients who had had MCA ischemic stroke, isolated and purified the MSCs, and re-injected the cells with an intravenous administration.[64] Five patients received 5 million autologous MSCs at 4 to 5 weeks after stroke and another 5 million cells at 7 to 9 weeks after stroke. No adverse effects were seen in the experimental group up to 1 year later. This study illustrated the feasibility of preparing autologous MSCs from five patients with stroke, but it took on average 30 days to grow the cells before injection. There is very limited work on the therapeutic efficacy of MSCs at such late time points, raising the question whether autologous MSCs will be a practical option or whether such cells need to be used at earlier passages in culture. The cell passage and the specific cell culture conditions, including the use of serum, likely will have an impact on the potential efficacy of MSCs in various neurologic disorders. These issues will need to be considered in the planning of future clinical trials in stroke.

Bone Marrow Mononuclear Cells

At the University of Texas in Houston, my colleagues and I are conducting the first U.S. trial on the safety and feasibility of autologous bone marrow mononuclear cells in 10 patients with ischemic stroke.[65] The study design follows from the published data on mononuclear cells in animal models of stroke. Eligible patients must have had an MCA stroke, and cell infusion must occur within 24 to 72 hours of symptom onset. The patients undergo bone marrow aspiration under conscious sedation and receive the MNCs by intravenous infusion within 3 to 6 hours of cell separation in a GMP facility. Patients are being followed for a range of safety and functional outcomes for 2 years. Investigators in Brazil have also been giving MNCs with an intraarterial, catheter-based delivery.[66]

Other Bone Marrow Studies

In the absence of extensive published preclinical data, a range of other bone marrow studies have launched in different countries, including investigation of the

TABLE 57-3 BONE MARROW STUDIES

Location of Study	Study Design	Delivery Route	Sample Number	Cell Type	Inclusion Criteria	Outcomes	Time Window
United States (The University of Texas in Houston)	Single arm	IV	30	Autologous bone marrow mononuclear cells	MCA stroke Age 18-80 yr NIHSS score 6-20	Safety and feasibility	24 to 72 hr
Taiwan (The China Medical University Hospital)	Randomized 2-arm study: cell infusion vs. conventional treatment	IC	30	Autologous peripheral blood CD34+ cells	Age 35-70 yr NIHSS score 9-20	Safety	6 months to 5 yr
Spain (Hospital Universitario Central de Asturias)	Single arm	IA	20	Autologous CD34+ bone marrow cells	MCA stroke Age 18-80 yr NIHSS score ≥8	Safety	5 to 9 days
France (University Hospital of Grenoble)	Randomized, 3 arms: control, 2 dose groups	IV	30	Autologous mesenchymal bone marrow stem cells	Carotid territory stroke Age 18-65 yr NIHSS score >2	Feasibility and tolerability	6 wk
United Kingdom (Imperial College London)	Single arm	IA	10	Autologous CD34+ bone marrow cells	MCA stroke Age 30-80 yr	Safety and tolerability	7 days
Brazil (Federal University of Rio de Janeiro)	2 arms Nonrandomized	IV/IA	15	Autologous bone marrow mononuclear cells	MCA stroke Age 18-75 yr NIHSS score 4-20	Safety	3 hr to 90 days

IA, intraarterial; IC, intracerebral; IV, intravenous; MCA, middle cerebral artery; NIHSS, National Institutes of Health Stroke Scale.

intraarterial delivery of autologous CD34+ cells and the intracerebral injection of CD34+ peripheral blood cells. Table 57-3 shows the various studies registered on the website clinicaltrials.gov. All of these studies are investigator-initiated and involve autologous cells from bone marrow and blood. It is anticipated that industry-sponsored trials will launch in 2011, testing the safety of administering allogeneic cells with intravascular delivery routes in patients with stroke.

Translational Barriers

The wealth of preclinical data on the effects of cell-based therapies for stroke and the emergence of pilot clinical trials have raised a number of pivotal translational questions, as follows.

Delivery Routes

The choice of delivery method depends on the type of cell, location of stroke, patient's comorbidities and prognosis, and intended strategy to promote recovery. The advantage of direct, stereotactic, intracerebral injection is reliable delivery of cells to the damaged area of the brain. The site of injection should correspond to the presumed mechanism by which the cells achieve clinical benefit. Cells that act through a trophic effect might work most effectively in peri-infarct areas, whereas cells designed with replacement and formation of new connections

might work best when injected within the infarct. Certain cell types display significant migratory capacity within the brain and therefore might be appropriate for injection in superficial or relatively silent areas even remote from the stroke. Intracerebroventricular (ICV) injections might spread cells throughout the brain; however, a significant concern is that injected cells could adhere to the ventricular wall and cause obstructive hydrocephalus. It also has not been well established that cells delivered by an ICV route would migrate through the ventricular surface to the damaged brain.

Animal studies also support the selective targeting of cells in the infarcted brain by intracarotid injection of cells. Endovascular drug and device delivery is routinely performed by interventionalists and is less invasive. However, a potential danger of this approach is that cells might obstruct the microvasculature, given that the size of some stem cells are much larger than the diameter of capillaries.[67] Each cell type should be examined for this complication in animal models. In addition, assessing compatibility of cells with catheters is important and may influence maximal cell density for delivery.[68]

Intravenous (IV) administration represents the least invasive method of delivery and in many studies has been shown to target cells to the injured brain. Certain cell types, such as umbilical cord cells, may exert greater benefit when injected intravenously than with direct brain injections.[44] In some cases, cells may enhance recovery through peripheral mechanisms even without direct entry into the brain.[69] To be effective with an IV approach, cells may need a homing signal to travel to injured brain areas. Studies suggest that homing may be mediated by release of chemotactic factors that draw cells to the site of injury.[70] However, the majority of stem cells injected intravenously are trapped by the first-pass filter of the lungs, with only a small percentage traversing to the brain.[67] IV injection also spread cells to perivascular locations of other organs, and it is therefore important to establish that IV delivery does not lead to adverse events of different organ systems.

Allogeneic versus Autologous

Bone marrow permits the possibility of manufacturing autologous cellular preparations, which generally avoid the risks of graft-versus-host disease. Umbilical cord similarly is being studied as an autologous application for neonates with a range of neurologic disorders including hypoxic-ischemic encephalopathy and trauma. However, for disorders of the elderly, concerns have been raised that bone marrow stem cells senesce over time. There may be a decrease in function of some types of bone marrow stem cells with age; however, there is no evidence of differences between human mononuclear cells derived from pediatric patients and those derived from older and elderly patients.[71] Allogeneic cells share a number of other advantages. First, it takes weeks to purify MSCs from patients with stroke,[64] and there remains much less data on the effects of MSCs in animal models of chronic stroke. Second, many adult stem cells from bone marrow and cellular preparations from umbilical cord blood have low immunogenicity. Furthermore, MSCs have been found to modulate and even suppress the immune response. Third, for bone marrow, harvesting a person's own cells requires an invasive procedure. Allogeneic cells are an "off-the-shelf" product; several cellular preparations are being commercialized for this purpose, involving universal allogeneic donors for cell banking and manufacture.

Safety Issues

The safety of cellular therapeutics in stroke can be categorized into acute and chronic effects. In the acute setting, the major concerns are related to acute infusional toxicity, a term describing any potential theoretical effects within peripheral organs known to trap intravenously injected stem cells. Bone marrow transplantation in patients with cancer can cause pneumonitis and even acute respiratory distress syndrome as well as liver injury through veno-occlusive disease. However, these reactions have not been reported in various trials that have been conducted in cancer-free, immunocompetent patients with other medical disorders, particularly with respect to autologous MNCs in cardiac disorders.[37] Another concern is the predisposition of cells to obstruct the microvasculature either because they might clump together or because their cell size is greater than the diameter of the capillary wall.[67] Such a complication has already been shown in an animal stroke model employing an intracarotid injection of MSCs.[72] In the chronic setting, the major concern for

certain types of stem cells is the risk for tumor formation. This concern is underscored by a report that a brain tumor developed in a child with ataxia-telangiectasia who was injected in Russia with fetal neural cells derived from multiple sources.[73] Any intended cellular product needs to be well-characterized and tested in animals with sound rationale before application to patients.

When to Treat

The efficacy of cellular therapy may depend on the pathophysiology and temporal course of the microenvironment within the injured brain after stroke. Reperfusion and neuroprotective strategies are targeted at the acute stage of stroke to minimize the core lesion, whereas the subacute and chronic stages involve infarct expansion, inflammation, apoptosis, and repair processes. Nearly all of the current clinical trials are treating patients days to weeks after stroke, reflecting the belief that cellular therapy may be effective during this time. Although results of several studies suggest that some types of cells are effective in improving recovery when given during the subacute stages of stroke,[40,43] many of the autologous studies (see Table 57-2) have proceeded without extensive published studies characterizing the time window or clear efficacy for late time points in chronic stroke. To the extent possible, guidelines recommend defining the therapeutic time window in animals before proceeding to clinical trial.[74] However, it should also be acknowledged that animal models of chronic stroke with persistent deficits have not been well developed.

Surrogates of Activity and Biologic Potency Assays

The successful development of a cellular therapy for stroke would likely be significantly enhanced with the use of an assay to measure functional effects of the cells. Various biomarkers are under development, including the measurement of cytokines and growth factors in patients' serum, imaging to detect changes to the white matter using diffusion tensor imaging (DTI), and pioneering work on detecting angiogenesis in the brain.[75,76]

Labeling and Tracking of Cells

A critical need in translating cell-based approaches from the laboratory to the clinical area is to track the migration and fate of injected cells. To date, there has been very little clinical work studying labeled cells injected in patients with any medical condition. Iron labeling of cells with iron oxides such as Feridex with the intent to monitor with MRI initially showed much promise, but Feridex is no longer commercially available.[77,78] Radionucleotides such as indium and technetium Tc^{99m} are options actively being explored in stroke,[66] but the effects of these agents on the function of cells still need further study. Various MRI contrast agents linked to labeling reagents are also under development.[77,78] The use of these agents is eagerly anticipated. However, it has already been shown that paracontrast agents might impair the functional effects of the donor cells.[79]

Guidelines: Stem Cell Therapies as an Emerging Paradigm in Stroke

In 1999, investigators in academia, members of the U.S. Food and Drug Administration (FDA) and the National Institutes of Health (NIH), and industry leaders convened the Stroke Therapy Academic Industry Roundtable (STAIR) meeting to draft and publish guidelines on the preclinical development of stroke therapeutics. Following the STAIR format, a similar meeting called Stem Cell Therapies as an Emerging Paradigm in Stroke (STEPS) held in 2007 led to recommendations on developing cell-based therapies for stroke.[74] A second meeting occurred in March 2010 to update these guidelines. These recommendations include testing cell-based therapies in young and old animals, male and female, at least two different species, and multiple animal models. A therapeutic window and dose response need to be defined, and the dosing chosen in initial clinical trials should be guided by animal studies. There is much hope that the STEPS recommendations will guide the preclinical development of specific cellular therapies for stroke.

Conclusion

Cell-based therapy is a rapidly emerging field for the development of novel therapies in stroke. Over the past 10 years, an ever-increasing number of different types of functionally active and potentially therapeutic cells have been identified from various tissues in the body and, at the same time, a paradigm shift has occurred in the rationale and goals of using cells as a potential treatment for stroke. Paracrine and endocrine mechanisms are the main approaches to enhancing recovery with cells, rather than tissue replacement. We have entered a new phase in this field in which the first clinical trials using autologous adult cells are being tested in patients with stroke. And the clinical application of allogeneic cells for stroke is about to begin. As cell-based therapies transition from bench to bedside, it is hoped that clinical studies will follow from sound and robust preclinical data when feasible animal modeling exists.

Disclosures

Dr. Savitz has received a sponsored research grant from Athersys and consulting fees from Johnson and Johnson, Celgene, Aldagen, and Ferrer Grupo.

REFERENCES

1. Savitz SI, Rosenbaum DM, Dinsmore JH, Wechsler LR, Caplan LR: Cell transplantation for stroke, *Ann Neurol* 52:266–275, 2002.
2. Woodbury D, Schwarz EJ, Prockop DJ, Black IB: Adult rat and human bone marrow stromal cells differentiate into neurons, *J Neurosci Res* 61:364–370, 2000.
3. Parent JM, Vexler ZS, Gong C, Derugin N, Ferriero DM: Rat forebrain neurogenesis and striatal neuron replacement after focal stroke, *Ann Neurol* 52:802–813, 2002.
4. Arvidsson A, Collin T, Kirik D, Kokaia Z, Lindvall O: Neuronal replacement from endogenous precursors in the adult brain after stroke, *Nat Med* 8:963–970, 2002.
5. Erdo F, Buhrle C, Blunk J, et al: Host-dependent tumorigenesis of embryonic stem cell transplantation in experimental stroke, *J Cereb Blood Flow Metab* 23:780–785, 2003.
6. Andrews PW, Damjanov I, Simon D, et al: Pluripotent embryonal carcinoma clones derived from the human teratocarcinoma cell line tera-2. Differentiation in vivo and in vitro, *Lab Invest* 50:147–162, 1984.
7. Pleasure SJ, Lee VM: Ntera 2 cells: A human cell line which displays characteristics expected of a human committed neuronal progenitor cell, *J Neurosci Res* 35:585–602, 1993.
8. Pleasure SJ, Page C, Lee VM: Pure, postmitotic, polarized human neurons derived from Ntera 2 cells provide a system for expressing exogenous proteins in terminally differentiated neurons, *J Neurosci* 12:1802–1815, 1992.
9. Guillemain I, Alonso G, Patey G, Privat A, Chaudieu I: Human NT2 neurons express a large variety of neurotransmission phenotypes in vitro, *J Comp Neurol* 422:380–395, 2000.
10. Younkin DP, Tang CM, Hardy M, et al: Inducible expression of neuronal glutamate receptor channels in the NT2 human cell line, *Proc Natl Acad Sci U S A* 90:2174–2178, 1993.
11. Neelands TR, King AP, Macdonald RL: Functional expression of l-, n-, p/q-, and r-type calcium channels in the human NT2-N cell line, *J Neurophysiol* 84:2933–2944, 2000.
12. Hartley RS, Margulis M, Fishman PS, Lee VM, Tang CM: Functional synapses are formed between human Ntera2 (NT2N, HNT) neurons grown on astrocytes, *J Comp Neurol* 407:1–10, 1999.
13. Kleppner SR, Robinson KA, Trojanowski JQ, Lee VM: Transplanted human neurons derived from a teratocarcinoma cell line (Ntera-2) mature, integrate, and survive for over 1 year in the nude mouse brain, *J Comp Neurol* 357:618–632, 1995.
14. Borlongan CV, Saporta S, Sanberg PR: Intrastriatal transplantation of rat adrenal chromaffin cells seeded on microcarrier beads promote long-term functional recovery in hemiparkinsonian rats, *Exp Neurol* 151:203–214, 1998.
15. Isacson O, Deacon TW, Pakzaban P, Galpern WR, Dinsmore J, Burns LH: Transplanted xenogeneic neural cells in neurodegenerative disease models exhibit remarkable axonal target specificity and distinct growth patterns of glial and axonal fibres, *Nat Med* 1:1189–1194, 1995.
16. Deacon TW, Pakzaban P, Burns LH, Dinsmore J, Isacson O: Cytoarchitectonic development, axon-glia relationships, and long distance axon growth of porcine striatal xenografts in rats, *Exp Neurol* 130:151–167, 1994.
17. Englund U, Bjorklund A, Wictorin K, Lindvall O, Kokaia M: Grafted neural stem cells develop into functional pyramidal neurons and integrate into host cortical circuitry, *Proc Natl Acad Sci U S A* 99:17089–17094, 2002.
18. Kelly S, Bliss TM, Shah AK, et al: Transplanted human fetal neural stem cells survive, migrate, and differentiate in ischemic rat cerebral cortex, *Proc Natl Acad Sci U S A* 101:11839–11844, 2004.
19. Darsalia V, Kallur T, Kokaia Z: Survival, migration and neuronal differentiation of human fetal striatal and cortical neural stem cells grafted in stroke-damaged rat striatum, *Eur J Neurosci* 26:605–614, 2007.
20. Selden NR, Guillaume DJ, Steiner RD, Huhn SL: Cellular therapy for childhood neurodegenerative disease. Part II: Clinical trial design and implementation, *Neurosurg Focus* 24, 2008:E23.
21. Taupin P: Hu-CNS-SC (stemcells), *Curr Opin Mol Ther* 8:156–163, 2006.
22. Park KI, Teng YD, Snyder EY: The injured brain interacts reciprocally with neural stem cells supported by scaffolds to reconstitute lost tissue, *Nat Biotechnol* 20:1111–1117, 2002.
23. Wei L, Cui L, Snider BJ, et al: Transplantation of embryonic stem cells overexpressing bcl-2 promotes functional recovery after transient cerebral ischemia, *Neurobiol Dis* 19:183–193, 2005.
24. Buhnemann C, Scholz A, Bernreuther C, et al: Neuronal differentiation of transplanted embryonic stem cell-derived precursors in stroke lesions of adult rats, *Brain* 129:3238–3248, 2006.
25. Pollock K, Stroemer P, Patel S, et al: A conditionally immortal clonal stem cell line from human cortical neuroepithelium for the treatment of ischemic stroke, *Exp Neurol* 199:143–155, 2006.
26. Horwitz EM, Le Blanc K, Dominici M, et al: Clarification of the nomenclature for MSC: The International Society for Cellular Therapy position statement, *Cytotherapy* 7:393–395, 2005.
27. Bianco P, Robey PG, Simmons PJ: Mesenchymal stem cells: Revisiting history, concepts, and assays, *Cell Stem Cell* 2:313–319, 2008.
28. Barry FP, Murphy JM, English K, Mahon BP: Immunogenicity of adult mesenchymal stem cells: Lessons from the fetal allograft, *Stem Cells Dev* 14:252–265, 2005.

29. Le Blanc K, Pittenger M: Mesenchymal stem cells: Progress toward promise, *Cytotherapy* 7:36–45, 2005.

30. Li Y, Chopp M: Marrow stromal cell transplantation in stroke and traumatic brain injury, *Neurosci Lett* 456:120–123, 2009.

31. Shen LH, Li Y, Chen J, et al: Therapeutic benefit of bone marrow stromal cells administered 1 month after stroke, *J Cereb Blood Flow Metab* 27:6–13, 2007.

32. Jiang Y, Jahagirdar BN, Reinhardt RL, et al: Pluripotency of mesenchymal stem cells derived from adult marrow, *Nature* 418:41–49, 2002.

33. Reyes M, Lund T, Lenvik T, et al: Purification and ex vivo expansion of postnatal human marrow mesodermal progenitor cells, *Blood* 98:2615–2625, 2001.

34. Anjos-Afonso F, Bonnet D: Nonhematopoietic/endothelial SSEA-1+ cells define the most primitive progenitors in the adult murine bone marrow mesenchymal compartment, *Blood* 109:1298–1306, 2007.

35. Zhao LR, Duan WM, Reyes M, et al: Human bone marrow stem cells exhibit neural phenotypes and ameliorate neurological deficits after grafting into the ischemic brain of rats, *Exp Neurol* 174:11–20, 2002.

36. Brehm M, Stanske B, Strauer BE: Therapeutic potential of stem cells in elderly patients with cardiovascular disease, *Exp Gerontol* 43:1024–1032, 2008.

37. Lipinski MJ, Biondi-Zoccai GG, Abbate A, et al: Impact of intracoronary cell therapy on left ventricular function in the setting of acute myocardial infarction: A collaborative systematic review and meta-analysis of controlled clinical trials, *J Am Coll Cardiol* 50:1761–1767, 2007.

38. Baker AH, Sica V, Work LM, et al: Brain protection using autologous bone marrow cell, metalloproteinase inhibitors, and metabolic treatment in cerebral ischemia, *Proc Natl Acad Sci U S A* 104:3597–3602, 2007.

39. Giraldi-Guimaraes A, Rezende-Lima M, Bruno FP, Mendez-Otero R: Treatment with bone marrow mononuclear cells induces functional recovery and decreases neurodegeneration after sensorimotor cortical ischemia in rats. *Brain Res* 2009 Feb 9 [epub ahead of print].

40. Iihoshi S, Honmou O, Houkin K, et al: A therapeutic window for intravenous administration of autologous bone marrow after cerebral ischemia in adult rats, *Brain Res* 1007:1–9, 2004.

41. Brenneman M, Sharma S, Harting M, et al: Autologous bone marrow mononuclear cells enhance recovery after acute ischemic stroke in young and middle-aged rats, *J Cereb Blood Flow Metab* 30:140–149, 2010.

42. Schwarting S, Litwak S, Hao W, et al: Hematopoietic stem cells reduce postischemic inflammation and ameliorate ischemic brain injury, *Stroke* 39:2867–2875, 2008.

43. Vendrame M, Cassady J, Newcomb J, et al: Infusion of human umbilical cord blood cells in a rat model of stroke dose-dependently rescues behavioral deficits and reduces infarct volume, *Stroke* 35:2390–2395, 2004.

44. Willing AE, Lixian J, Milliken M, et al: Intravenous versus intrastriatal cord blood administration in a rodent model of stroke, *J Neurosci Res* 73:296–307, 2003.

45. Gronthos S, Franklin DM, Leddy HA, et al: Surface protein characterization of human adipose tissue-derived stromal cells, *J Cell Physiol* 189:54–63, 2001.

46. Kang SK, Lee DH, Bae YC, et al: Improvement of neurological deficits by intracerebral transplantation of human adipose tissue-derived stromal cells after cerebral ischemia in rats, *Exp Neurol* 183:355–366, 2003.

47. Shyu WC, Lin SZ, Chiang MF, et al: Intracerebral peripheral blood stem cell (cd34+) implantation induces neuroplasticity by enhancing beta1 integrin-mediated angiogenesis in chronic stroke rats, *J Neurosci* 26:3444–3453, 2006.

48. Yu SJ, Soncini M, Kaneko Y, et al: Amnion: A potent graft source for cell therapy in stroke, *Cell Transplant* 18:111–118, 2009.

49. Borlongan CV, Kaneko Y, Maki M, et al: Menstrual blood cells display stem cell-like phenotypic markers and exert neuroprotection following transplantation in experimental stroke, *Stem Cells Dev* 19:439–452, 2010.

50. Lee ST, Chu K, Jung KH, et al: Anti-inflammatory mechanism of intravascular neural stem cell transplantation in haemorrhagic stroke, *Brain* 131:616–629, 2008.

51. Janowski M, Walczak P, Date I: Intravenous route of cell delivery for treatment of neurological disorders: A meta-analysis of preclinical results, *Stem Cells Dev* 19:5–16, 2010.

52. Capone C, Frigerio S, Fumagalli S, et al: Neurosphere-derived cells exert a neuroprotective action by changing the ischemic microenvironment, *PLoS One* 2, e373, 2007.

53. Offner H, Subramanian S, Parker SM, et al: Splenic atrophy in experimental stroke is accompanied by increased regulatory T cells and circulating macrophages, *J Immunol* 176:6523–6531, 2006.

54. Lee RH, Pulin AA, Seo MJ, et al: Intravenous HMSCs improve myocardial infarction in mice because cells embolized in lung are activated to secrete the anti-inflammatory protein tsg-6, *Cell Stem Cell* 5:54–63, 2009.

55. Nemeth K, Leelahavanichkul A, Yuen PS, et al: Bone marrow stromal cells attenuate sepsis via prostaglandin E(2)-dependent reprogramming of host macrophages to increase their interleukin-10 production, *Nat Med* 15:42–49, 2009.

56. Vendrame M, Gemma C, Pennypacker KR, et al: Cord blood rescues stroke-induced changes in splenocyte phenotype and function, *Exp Neurol* 199:191–200, 2006.

57. Chen J, Zhang ZG, Li Y, et al: Intravenous administration of human bone marrow stromal cells induces angiogenesis in the ischemic boundary zone after stroke in rats, *Circ Res* 92:692–699, 2003.

58. Taguchi A, Soma T, Tanaka H, et al: Administration of CD34+ cells after stroke enhances neurogenesis via angiogenesis in a mouse model, *J Clin Invest* 114:330–338, 2004.

59. Chen J, Li Y, Katakowski M, et al: Intravenous bone marrow stromal cell therapy reduces apoptosis and promotes endogenous cell proliferation after stroke in female rat, *J Neurosci Res* 73:778–786, 2003.

60. Xiao J, Nan Z, Motooka Y, Low WC: Transplantation of a novel cell line population of umbilical cord blood stem cells ameliorates neurological deficits associated with ischemic brain injury, *Stem Cells Dev* 14:722–733, 2005.

61. Kondziolka D, Wechsler L, Goldstein S, et al: Transplantation of cultured human neuronal cells for patients with stroke, *Neurology* 55:565–569, 2000.

62. Kondziolka D, Steinberg GK, Wechsler L, et al: Neurotransplantation for patients with subcortical motor stroke: A phase 2 randomized trial, *J Neurosurg* 103:38–45, 2005.

63. Savitz SI, Dinsmore J, Wu J, et al: Neurotransplantation of fetal porcine cells in patients with basal ganglia infarcts: A preliminary safety and feasibility study, *Cerebrovasc Dis* 20:101–107, 2005.

64. Bang OY, Lee JS, Lee PH, Lee G: Autologous mesenchymal stem cell transplantation in stroke patients, *Ann Neurol* 57:874–882, 2005.

65. Savitz SI, Misra V: Launching intravenous bone marrow cell trials for acute stroke, *Regen Med* 4:639–641, 2009.

66. Barbosa da Fonseca LM, Gutfilen B, et al: Migration and homing of bone-marrow mononuclear cells in chronic ischemic stroke after intra-arterial injection, *Exp Neurol* 221:122–128, 2010.

67. Fischer UM, Harting MT, Jimenez F, et al: Pulmonary passage is a major obstacle for intravenous stem cell delivery: The pulmonary first-pass effect, *Stem Cells Dev* 18:683–692, 2009.

68. El Khoury R, Misra V, Sharma S, et al: The effect of transcatheter injections on cell viability and cytokine release of mononuclear cells, *AJNR Am J Neuroradiol* 31:1488–1492, 2010.

69. Borlongan CV, Hadman M, Sanberg CD, Sanberg PR: Central nervous system entry of peripherally injected umbilical cord blood cells is not required for neuroprotection in stroke, *Stroke* 35:2385–2389, 2004.

70. Wang Y, Deng Y, Zhou GQ: SDF-1alpha/CXCR4-mediated migration of systemically transplanted bone marrow stromal cells towards ischemic brain lesion in a rat model, *Brain Res* 1195:104–112, 2008.

71. Harting MT, Cox CS, Day MC, et al: Bone marrow-derived mononuclear cell populations in pediatric and adult patients, *Cytotherapy* 11:480–484, 2009.

72. Walczak P, Zhang J, Gilad AA, et al: Dual-modality monitoring of targeted intraarterial delivery of mesenchymal stem cells after transient ischemia, *Stroke* 39:1569–1574, 2008.

73. Amariglio N, Hirshberg A, Scheithauer BW, et al: Donor-derived brain tumor following neural stem cell transplantation in an ataxia telangiectasia patient, *PLoS Med* 6:e1000029 2009.

74. Stem Cell Therapies as an Emerging Paradigm in Stroke (STEPS): Bridging basic and clinical science for cellular and neurogenic factor therapy in treating stroke, *Stroke* 40:510–515, 2009.

75. Seevinck PR, Deddens LH, Dijkhuizen RM: Magnetic resonance imaging of brain angiogenesis after stroke, *Angiogenesis* 13:101–111, 2010.

76. Jiang Q, Zhang ZG, Chopp M: MRI of stroke recovery, *Stroke* 41:410–414, 2010.

77. Liu W, Frank JA: Detection and quantification of magnetically labeled cells by cellular MRI, *Eur J Radiol* 70:258–264, 2009.

78. Arbab AS, Frank JA: Cellular MRI and its role in stem cell therapy, *Regen Med* 3:199–215, 2008.

79. Modo M, Beech JS, Meade TJ, et al: A chronic 1 year assessment of MRI contrast agent-labelled neural stem cell transplants in stroke, *Neuroimage* 47(Suppl 2):T133–T142, 2009.

58 Antiplatelet Therapy for Secondary Prevention of Stroke

MAR CASTELLANOS, BABETTE B. WEKSLER, OSCAR R. BENAVENTE

Stroke is the second-leading cause of death worldwide, after ischemic heart disease, and is the sixth leading cause of adult disability-adjusted life-years worldwide.[1] The predominant mechanisms for ischemic stroke are cardioembolic, thromboembolic, and small vessel disease. The rest are due to unusual mechanisms or are classified as cryptogenic.

Cerebral ischemia tends to recur after a primary episode of either transient ischemic attack (TIA) or stroke. Most commonly, cerebral ischemia is caused by thromboemboli that form on damaged vascular surfaces of extracranial or intracerebral arteries. Local activation of platelets on the walls of diseased arteries initiates thrombus formation under conditions of high flow typical of arteries because activated platelets not only clump together but also directly catalyze thrombin generation. These thrombi are classically considered "white clots"; that is, they are composed mainly of platelets plus some fibrin. These platelet-rich thrombi that form on atherosclerotic plaques may either occlude small arterioles directly or embolize into intracerebral end arteries, producing vascular occlusion that results in neurologic dysfunction.

Because platelet activation is causally linked to episodes of cerebral arterial ischemia, therapies that diminish or block the early steps in hemostasis that are platelet-dependent are used in patients with TIAs or stroke to prevent further episodes of cerebral ischemia.

Stroke prevention can be considered under the rubrics of primary prevention, secondary prevention, and acute stroke. Risk factor management is of the utmost importance in primary prevention of stroke—control of hypertension, for example, is associated with a 30% to 40% reduction in stroke—although antiplatelet use may have a role in primary prevention in certain populations.

However, despite the use of a variety of antithrombotic therapies for secondary prevention of stroke, risk reduction has been disappointing; it has been only about 15% to 20% in most large clinical trials.[2] Increasing the intensity of treatment, either antiplatelet therapy or anticoagulation (or both together), has the important adverse effect of increasing intracerebral and systemic hemorrhage and negates the net therapeutic benefit. The success of antiplatelet drugs in reducing the recurrence of ischemic stroke further incorporates the fact that bleeding is less common during antiplatelet therapy than during anticoagulant therapy.

In contrast to arterial thrombi, venous thrombi form under conditions involving vascular stasis, consist mainly of fibrin and erythrocytes, and are much less dependent on platelet activation. Venous thrombosis, including cerebral venous thrombosis, is thus better prevented by anticoagulation than by antiplatelet therapy.[3] This is also true for cardioembolic strokes associated with atrial fibrillation (AF). However, the distinctions between factors contributing to arterial versus venous thrombi are far from absolute. Both platelet-dependent phases and coagulation factor–dependent phases of hemostasis intermingle to a considerable extent, for example, because of the prominent role played by platelets in catalyzing thrombin generation.

Moreover, combining antiplatelet and anticoagulant agents in the search for more powerful effects during long-term, secondary prevention of cerebral ischemia has been notably unsuccessful because an unacceptably high incidence of intracerebral and extracranial bleeding ensues when the drug combinations are used at doses that effectively block both platelet function and blood coagulation.[4]

Platelet Physiology in the Planning of Antiplatelet Therapy

The evidence is clear that persons at increased risk of stroke have excessively active platelets and that even normal platelet activation in the setting of arterial disease imparts thromboembolic risk. This provides the pathophysiologic basis for antiplatelet therapy in the secondary reduction of stroke risk. To understand the rationale for using particular antiplatelet drugs, it is important first to consider how platelets regulate normal hemostasis. Hemostasis is defined as the appropriate physiologic response to vascular injury that provides prompt control of blood loss. In contrast, thrombosis is excessive or inappropriate blood clotting. Platelet hemostatic function needs then to be contrasted with platelet prothrombotic function, that is, how platelets promote inappropriate formation of blood clots in the setting of arterial vascular disease. Because platelets interact with the blood vessel wall in both hemostasis and thrombosis, the status of the arterial endothelial lining is an important determinant of platelet behavior. Normal vascular endothelium is nonthrombogenic and prevents platelet interactions with it and with other platelets or leukocytes by multiple mechanisms including secretion of prostaglandins and nitric oxide, surface expression of anticoagulant heparan sulfate and adenosine diphosphate (ADP)–metabolizing enzymes, and facilitation of smooth, nonturbulent blood flow.

Normal Functions of Platelets in Hemostasis

Normal platelets circulate for about 7 to 10 days after being released from megakaryocytes in the bone marrow, even though they lack nuclei and are almost incapable of protein synthesis. The youngest platelets are the most hemostatically active. The relatively long life of platelets in the blood has permitted effective, once-daily dosing with several antiplatelet drugs. Circulating platelets do not normally interact with one another, with other blood cells, or with the surface of the normal vascular endothelium. If a blood vessel is injured and endothelial continuity is broken, however, platelets undergo, within seconds, a rapid series of coordinated activation changes that quickly leads to a hemostatic platelet plug. This primary hemostatic plug prevents bleeding at the injury site without blocking blood flow through the vessel (Fig. 58-1).

These activation steps start with adhesion of single platelets to the damaged vessel wall, in which the platelets change in shape from flat, unreactive disks to "spiny spheres" that spread out over the surface. Next is aggregation, in which additional platelets join into masses or clumps on top of the original spread layer of platelets, blocking blood loss. During this process, the now activated platelets release vasoactive substances from storage granules, including adhesive glycoproteins, procoagulants, agonists for platelet activation, enzymes, and inflammatory mediators (Table 58-1). Moreover, once platelets are activated, vasoactive lipids, such as thromboxane A_2 (TXA_2) and leukotrienes, are rapidly synthesized and released. Many of these substances either recruit other platelets or produce vascular contraction, which are functions that help stop bleeding promptly at the injury site. Most importantly, the surface membranes of activated platelets catalyze thrombin generation with great efficiency, such that activated platelets serve to initiate, augment, and localize fibrin formation, further amplifying thrombotic potential as well as participating in clot stabilization.

Participants in the Initial Platelet Response to Vascular Injury

In both hemostasis and thrombosis, the major signal for platelet activation is a local injury to endothelium, which leads to exposure of prothrombotic components to the blood, usually localized in the subendothelial matrix. Whereas normal, intact endothelium displays numerous

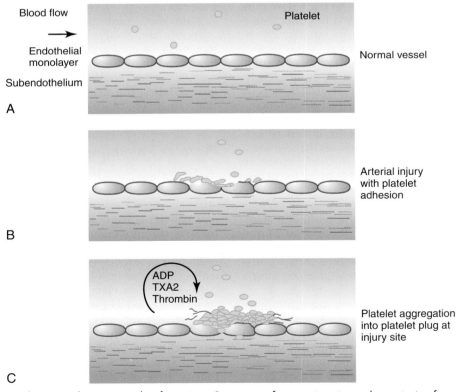

Figure 58-1 Platelets and primary hemostatic plug formation. Sequence of events in primary hemostasis after arterial injury. A, Blood flow over normal arterial endothelium. No interaction of platelets with the vascular wall. B, Immediately after injury that disrupts the arterial endothelium, platelets adhere to the subendothelium exposed at the injury site, forming a platelet monolayer, change shape, spread out, and begin to release vasoactive substances. C, Within a few minutes, activated platelets aggregate on the first layer of spread platelets, clumping together and releasing vasoactive mediators such as adenosine diphosphate (ADP) and thromboxane A_2 (TXA_2), and catalyze generation of thrombin so that fibrin strands (designated by *wavy lines*) form and stabilize the platelet plug.

TABLE 58-1 PLATELET-DERIVED VASOACTIVE MEDIATORS

Dense granule contents	Adenosine diphosphate, adenosine triphosphate, Ca^{2+}, serotonin
Alpha granule contents	Adhesive proteins: fibronectin, fibrinogen, thrombospondin, vitronectin
	Coagulation factors: von Willebrand factor, factor V, factor X
	Growth factors: fibroblast growth factor, platelet-derived growth factor, transforming growth factor-β
	Membrane proteins: P-selectin, amyloid precursor protein
	Others: albumin, immunoglobulin G, antibacterial proteins, platelet inhibitor activator-1
Lysosomes	Acid hydrolases, neutral proteases, elastase, complement-activating enzymes, heparitinase
Peroxisomes	Catalase
Lipid mediators (not preformed)	Prostaglandin endoperoxides, thromboxane A_2, prostaglandin D_2, 12-hydroxy-eicosatetraenoic acid isoprostanes

antithrombotic functions and repels platelets, subendothelium is rich in prothrombotic substances such as collagen and adhesive molecules, including von Willebrand factor (vWF), thrombospondin, and fibronectin. In addition, subtle endothelial dysfunction produced by turbulent blood flow, hyperlipidemia, inflammation, or atherosclerosis—without any physical discontinuity in the endothelial monolayer lining the blood vessels—can also activate platelets. Moreover, once activated, platelets themselves recruit additional platelets by releasing vasoactive mediators and catalyzing thrombin formation; in turn, thrombin is a potent platelet activator. Platelet activation is therefore an exponential and interactive, rather than linear, process.

Platelet Membrane Components Mediating Platelet Activation

Platelet activation involves changes in both the morphologic and biochemical state of the platelet membrane, including conformational changes in adhesion receptors, binding of adhesive proteins, mobilization of intracellular granule contents, interactions with the cytoskeleton, initiation of signaling, and platelet–platelet interaction. Glycoprotein (GP) platelet adhesion receptors mediate attachment of platelets to substrate proteins. Adhesion receptors that are important for normal hemostasis, thus representing potential therapeutic targets for thrombosis prevention, include the following: GPIa, a collagen receptor; GPIb, a receptor for vWF; the GPIIb/IIIa complex, a major receptor for fibrinogen, fibronectin, and vWF; GPIV, a thrombospondin receptor, required for irreversible platelet activation; glycoproteins V and IX; and $\alpha_v\beta_3$, a receptor for vitronectin, fibrinogen, and fibronectin. These receptors are all functional on resting platelets except for GPIIb/IIIa, which requires platelet activation to undergo the conformational change that permits this complex to bind fibrinogen.

Many of the adhesive glycoproteins that are ligands for these receptors share the peptide sequence RGD (R,

arginine; G, glycine; D, aspartic acid), which is directly involved in cell–cell adhesion.

Platelet Adhesion

Adhesion of platelets to other platelets, to the subendothelium exposed by vascular injury, or to activated endothelium is the first major step in the platelet activation sequence. Platelet adhesion is mediated by a complex of GPIb-V-IX, which binds to matrix vWF at high shear rates and is also a binding site for thrombin, thus acting to amplify platelet responses to thrombin.[5,6] GPIb-V-IX is mainly involved in platelet activation resulting from abnormal shear stress, such as is found in arteries narrowed by atherosclerosis. Changes in conformation of the GPIbα component of the complex or of vWF can induce interaction between these two molecules. Binding of vWF to collagen induces small conformational changes in vWF that permit its binding to GPIb. Furthermore, binding of vWF to GPIb causes redistribution of the GPIb-V-IX glycoprotein complex within platelets, linking the complex to the cytoskeleton and activating phosphorylating enzymes that regulate actin polymerization and the activation of the GPIIb/IIIa complex. Therefore, inhibition of platelet adhesion should be antithrombotic. Peptides that block GPIb-V-IX function are under development as novel antiplatelet drugs. Activation of GPIb-V-IX in a thromboxane-independent manner accounts for part of the "resistance" to aspirin that is observed in connection with the presence of atherosclerotic risk factors. Absence or dysfunction of GPIb is characteristic of a rare platelet disorder involving soft tissue bleeding, the Bernard-Soulier syndrome. At low shear, the GPIIb/IIIa complex also participates in platelet adhesion to surfaces through binding of fibrinogen.

Platelet Aggregation

Aggregation is the step in the platelet activation process most relevant to the pathogenesis of occlusive vascular events in an oxygen-sensitive arterial bed. During aggregation, activated platelets clump together atop an initial, adherent layer of platelets deposited at a site of injury or diseased vascular wall. These white thrombi, composed mainly of platelets and fibrin, may be transient or may become stabilized by further fibrin deposition, forming the nidus of bulkier clots in which erythrocytes and leukocytes also become trapped. During normal hemostasis, such platelet plugs halt bleeding from injured microvessels without obstructing blood flow, but in diseased vessels (e.g., in atherosclerosis or vasculitis or after irradiation), excessive platelet plug formation can occlude cerebral vasculature, producing TIA or stroke.

Platelet Membrane Receptors in Aggregation

The most important membrane receptor for aggregation is the integrin GPIIb/IIIa, a bimolecular membrane complex unique to platelets and megakaryocytes. Platelet aggregation by all known pathways depends on conformational changes in GPIIb/IIIa induced by platelet agonists.[7,8] Three main physiologic pathways independently triggered by different ligands can activate the GPIIb/IIIa complex; one pathway is activated by arachidonic acid leading to TXA_2 formation, the second by ADP, and the third by thrombin (Fig. 58-2).[9-11] All of these signaling pathways converge in a final common mechanism to produce a conformational change in GPIIb/IIIa that exposes a high-affinity fibrinogen binding site. The activated GPIIb/IIIa complex thus markedly increases fibrinogen binding, becomes associated with cytoskeletal proteins and signaling kinases (e.g., pp60[c-src]), forms receptor clusters, and becomes phosphorylated. All of these functions favor platelet–platelet interactions. Both outside-inside signaling (e.g., agonist-driven) and inside–outside signaling (i.e., kinase/phosphatase-driven) are involved in this activation process.

Because the final common pathway for platelet activation requires the GPIIb/IIIa complex, therapeutic blockade of the complex inhibits all further platelet activation. In contrast, drugs that inhibit only one of the three pathways, such as aspirin inhibition of the thromboxane pathway or clopidogrel inhibition of the ADP pathway, do not prevent GPIIb/IIIa activation. Drugs that directly block the functions of the GPIIb/IIIa complex thus have profound inhibitory effects on platelet function and are currently used to treat acute cardiac ischemia. Development of the monoclonal antibody abciximab (ReoPro), of peptides such as eptifibatide (Integrilin), and of peptidomimetics

such as tirofiban (Aggrastat), which inhibit GPIIb/IIIa function when administered intravenously, has permitted highly successful antiplatelet therapy in acute cardiac interventions. Used over a short interval in combination with heparin and aspirin, these GPIIb/IIIa inhibitors prevent early thrombosis and deter vascular reocclusion after coronary angioplasty and stent placement. Unfortunately, the use of oral GPIIb/IIIa inhibitors for long-term prevention of cardiac thrombosis has been unsuccessful to date in numerous clinical trials, in which administration of such agents has been accompanied by higher rates of thrombosis or bleeding. A single clinical trial testing the safety of abciximab in treatment of acute stroke has been published (see later). Indeed, the Blockage of the Glycoprotein IIb/IIIa Receptor to Avoid Vascular Occlusion (BRAVO) study of lotrafiban (an oral GPIIb/IIIa inhibitor) and heparin for prevention of cardiovascular and cerebrovascular events, initiated in 2000, had to be discontinued because of excess occurrences of thrombosis.[4]

Multiple Independent Pathways to Aggregation

Each of the three independent biochemical pathways of platelet aggregation provides a separate potential for therapeutic intervention. One major pathway involves metabolism of arachidonic acid, which is released from

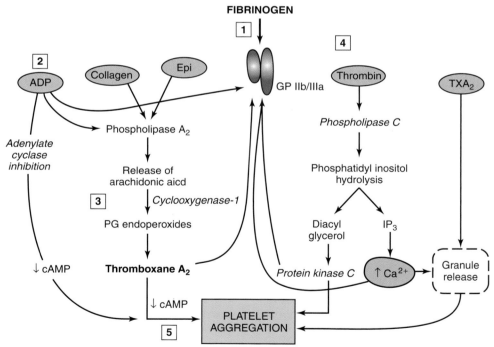

Figure 58-2 Platelet activation pathways and their inhibition. Specific, seven-transmembrane-spanning, G-protein-linked receptors on the platelet surface (depicted as *ellipses*) are activated by binding of their specific ligands and initiate different pathways for platelet activation, which converge on the conformational activation of the glycoprotein (GP) IIb/IIIa receptor complex to increase fibrinogen binding. These pathways lead to activation of the arachidonic acid pathway, hydrolysis of phosphatidyl inositol, increase in intraplatelet calcium ion (Ca^{2+}) concentration, release of vasoactive substances from platelet granules, synthesis of vasoactive lipids, and platelet aggregation. Mechanisms of inhibition of specific activation mechanisms by antiplatelet drugs (numbers in boxes) are (1) blocking of GPIIb/IIIa function and therefore blocking of fibrinogen binding and platelet aggregation; (2) blocking of the adenosine diphosphate (ADP) receptor; (3) inhibition of cyclooxygenase-interrupting arachidonic acid metabolism and prevention of the production of thromboxane A_2 (TXA_2); (4) blocking of thrombin action and thrombin receptor activation; (5) maintenance of high intraplatelet cyclic adenosine monophosphate (cAMP), which prevents platelet aggregation. Not depicted is inhibition of thromboxane A_2 synthase or thromboxane A_2 receptor function because drugs with these activities have not been clinically useful. *Epi,* Epinephrine; *IP₃,* inositol 1,4,5-triphosphate; *PG,* prostaglandin.

membrane phospholipids during platelet activation (see Fig. 58-2, center left). This pathway is sensitive to aspirin and other nonsteroidal anti-inflammatory drugs (NSAIDs). Receptor engagement by various platelet agonists activates phospholipase C to cleave membrane-bound phosphatidyl inositol to inositol 1,4,5-triphosphate (IP_3) and diacylglycerol. IP_3 in turn releases stored calcium ions, permitting activation of platelet phospholipase A_2, which releases esterified arachidonic acid from membrane phospholipids. The enzyme cyclooxygenase-1 in platelets rapidly converts the released arachidonic acid to prostaglandin endoperoxides that are isomerized to thromboxane A_2 (TXA_2), a potent platelet agonist and vasoconstrictor. The TXA_2 diffuses from the platelets and binds to its specific seven-transmembrane receptor on the platelet surface, signaling further activation of phospholipase C. Concomitantly, the liberated diacylglycerol activates protein kinase C, which translocates to the platelet plasma membrane and triggers activation of GPIIb/IIIa, exposing its fibrinogen binding site, thereby permitting platelet aggregation and secretion of platelet granule contents (see Fig. 58-2, right side). Aspirin, which irreversibly binds to cyclooxygenase-1, blocks the formation of TXA_2 for the entire life span of circulating platelets because platelets are incapable of synthesizing new cyclooxygenase protein.

Platelets that cannot produce TXA_2 can still be activated via the ADP-dependent and thrombin-dependent activation pathways. Platelet aggregation can be initiated via two interacting ADP receptors by ADP that is released by platelets or derived from extraplatelet sources such as red blood cells, even in the presence of aspirin.[10,11] Thrombin acts on several specific protease-activated membrane receptors (PARs) that signal the activation of phospholipase C and irreversible platelet aggregation and the release reaction that is independent of arachidonic acid metabolism.[9] Similarly, platelet activation by the phosphorylcholine derivative platelet-activating factor (PAF), which is produced by leukocytes or by disturbed endothelial cells, is also aspirin-insensitive. The existence of these separate pathways for platelet aggregation may be regarded as representing fail-safe or redundant mechanisms to avoid hemorrhages.

Platelet Release Reaction

Release of vasoactive contents of platelet storage granules normally accompanies platelet activation, augments platelet aggregation, and accelerates localized clot formation, vasoconstriction, and the initiation of wound healing. Not only are preformed glycoprotein mediators, ADP, vasoactive amines, growth factors, calcium ions, and serotonin released into the blood or displayed on the surface membrane, but short-lived lipid mediators are also synthesized and released during platelet activation. The extent of the release reaction can be modulated by antiplatelet drugs.

Several types of granules rich in substances that participate in blood coagulation, cell–cell interactions, and wound repair are present in platelets (see Table 58-1). The different granule types—dense granules, alpha granules, lysosomes, and peroxisomes—can be morphologically distinguished and are also functionally characterized by

their contents and the ease of release of their contents. For example, weak platelet stimuli, such as ADP, adenosine triphosphate (ATP), serotonin, and calcium—all of which participate in potentiating irreversible platelet aggregation—release the contents of the dense granules. By contrast, strong stimuli are required for release of alpha granule contents: fibrinogen, fibronectin, vWF, platelet-derived growth factor (PDGF), epidermal growth factor (EGF), transforming growth factor-β (TGF-β), platelet factor-4 (PF-4) and β-thromboglobulin. Alpha granules also contain albumin, immunoglobulins, antibacterial proteins, and a complement inhibitor. The membrane of the alpha granules contains P-selectin and the amyloid precursor protein; on platelet activation, P-selectin is transferred to the surface of the platelets, where it mediates cell–cell interactions with leukocytes and plays an important role in inflammatory reactions. Platelet lysosomes, the last granule type to be released, contain acid hydrolases, neutral proteases, elastase, enzymes that activate complement, and a heparitinase. Peroxisomes contain catalase.

In general, release of components of both dense bodies and alpha granules usually accompanies platelet aggregation but may also occur from platelets that are adherent to damaged endothelium or subendothelium, even without formation of platelet aggregates.

Platelet Synthesis of Vasoactive Lipid Mediators

In contrast to the release of preformed proteins or amines from platelet granules, vasoactive lipid mediators are not stored by platelets but instead are rapidly synthesized and released on platelet activation. Most of these lipids are oxygenated metabolites of arachidonic acid, which is mobilized from membrane phospholipids when agonists interact with platelet membrane receptors. The released arachidonate is the substrate for several different metabolic pathways producing eicosanoids and hydroxylated fatty acids. TXA_2 is the major platelet product of arachidonic acid metabolism by the eicosanoid pathway, and its synthesis occurs very rapidly—within seconds—on platelet activation. G-protein linked, seven membrane-spanning receptors for TXA_2 are present on platelets, leukocytes, and vascular cells.[12] These receptors bind TXA_2 and also its endoperoxide precursors, which have similar vasoconstrictor properties. Signal transduction via TXA_2 receptors initiates platelet activation and causes vasoconstriction.

Platelets also synthesize hydroxylated fatty acids from arachidonate via a separate enzymatic pathway involving lipoxygenase. The major product of this pathway in platelets is 12-hydroxyeicosatetraenoic acid (12-HETE), an inflammatory mediator that is chemotactic for leukocytes, stimulates vascular smooth muscle proliferation, and can be converted to additional inflammatory mediators, di-HETEs, by leukocytes. In contrast to the rapid burst of TXA_2 synthesis by activated platelets, the production of 12-HETE occurs continuously over a long period. Nonenzymatic, vasoactive metabolites of arachidonate, isoprostanes are also formed by oxidation; they can inactivate vascular or platelet nitric oxide (NO).

Interactions among different cell types can produce additional arachidonic acid products via transcellular metabolism, yielding products that are not made by a single cell type alone. Thus, platelet-released arachidonic acid can be converted into other vasoactive products by leukocytes or endothelial cells in close proximity. As mentioned previously, leukocytes can convert 12-HETE into various di-HETEs that have chemotactic and inflammatory properties. Endothelial cells can convert platelet-derived arachidonic acid or endoperoxide into prostacyclin, an antiplatelet substance that is a vasodilator. Similarly, endoperoxides released by endothelial cells can be converted by normal or aspirin-treated platelets into TXA_2.

How Platelet Activation Promotes Blood Coagulation

Platelets responding to strong agonists such as collagen, TXA_2, and thrombin accelerate both primary hemostatic plug formation and catalysis of blood coagulation, efficiently localized on the surface of the activated platelets. By providing specific sites, receptors, procoagulant factors, and lipid cofactors for the assembly of the key complexes of procoagulant enzymes, the activated platelet surface markedly accelerates the rate of localized thrombin generation, increasing by more than 200,000-fold the reaction rate in the fluid phase. Furthermore, activated platelets themselves contribute coagulation factors such as factor V and factor X released from their granules into a local clot as well as antifibrinolytic factors such as plasminogen activator inhibitor-1 (PAI-1). Because thrombin is a strong stimulus for platelet activation, the release reaction, and TXA_2 formation, the initial production of trace amounts of thrombin at the site of vascular injury directly stimulates further platelet activation and promotes coagulation. Microparticles shed from activated platelets also catalyze thrombin generation. Platelets additionally participate in clot stabilization by releasing the fibrin cross-linking protein factor XIII and by supporting clot retraction.

Platelet Participation in Fibrinolysis and Thrombolysis

During fibrinolysis, blood clots are dissolved by the protease plasmin, which cleaves insoluble fibrin. Platelets both promote and inhibit fibrinolysis, and the products of fibrinolysis can affect platelet function.[13,14] Activated platelet surfaces favor fibrinolysis by localizing plasminogen and promoting its activation. Thus, platelets bind plasminogen and plasminogen activators (both urokinase and tissue-type activators) via the GPIIb/IIIa complex. Thrombospondin released from platelet granules and then displayed on the platelet surface also binds plasminogen and enhances the activation of bound plasminogen. Because plasmin is more efficiently formed on a surface than in the fluid phase, activated platelets provide an alternative surface for promoting fibrinolysis. Platelet-bound plasminogen therefore is more readily activated by either tissue plasminogen activator or streptokinase than is free plasminogen, which suggests a mechanism by which platelets can enhance local fibrinolysis. In turn, plasmin at low concentrations enhances and at high concentrations depresses platelet activation.[15]

Platelets also contain and secrete two fibrinolytic antagonists, PAI-1 and α_2-antiplasmin. The net effects of these different platelet activities are that platelet-rich thrombi resist fibrinolysis and thrombolysis and that platelets become activated during therapeutic thrombolysis.[16]

Physiologic Mechanisms That Limit Platelet Activation

For clinical practice, the coexistence of multiple pathways mediating platelet activation means that drugs inhibiting only one pathway—for example, aspirin inhibiting cyclooxygenase, thus blocking TXA_2 formation—only partially block platelet activation. The existence of multiple pathways of platelet activation thus protects against hemorrhage but permits thrombosis. Several natural mechanisms exist in normal blood vessels to limit the extent of platelet activation. These mechanisms are also vasodilatory. They are (1) plasma ADPase enzymes and endothelial ectoADPases that metabolize ADP to adenosine, a vasodilator and inhibitor of platelet activation, (2) prostacyclin, the vasodilator metabolite of arachidonic acid released by endothelial cells, which stimulates platelet adenylate cyclase, raising intraplatelet cyclic adenosine monophosphate (cAMP) levels, blocking calcium release, and inhibiting platelet aggregation and secretion, and (3) NO produced by endothelial cells, platelets, and monocytes via NO synthases.[17-19]

NO stimulates platelet guanylate cyclase and raises levels of cyclic guanosine monophosphate (cGMP), thus inhibiting platelet activation. It also relaxes vascular smooth muscle via stimulation of cGMP in the vessel wall. NO is formed from L-arginine, an amino acid that has been shown to inhibit platelet aggregation. In arterial vascular disease, it is clear that NO-mediated mechanisms are diminished. At present, development of soluble ADPases and stimulators of NO synthase or NO donors as clinical antithrombotic agents is being actively pursued, but such drugs have not yet entered the clinical trial phase of development.

Platelet Activation as a Link between Hemostasis and Inflammation

Activated platelets recruit leukocytes to sites of vascular injury, setting up an inflammatory response that assists in repair of damaged tissue after hemostasis but promotes atherosclerotic progression in vascular disease. Numerous substances released from platelets are directly chemotactic for neutrophils (12-HETE), monocytes (PF-4, PDGF), or both. Platelet proteases release chemotactic complement fragment C5a from plasma C5 and potentiate C3 activation, enhancing leukocyte function. Platelet P-selectin translocated to the surface membrane of activated platelets mediates interactions between platelets and leukocytes, including initial leukocyte rolling on vascular endothelium, and P-selectin also augments leukocyte activation. Activated platelets remain coated with P-selectin, which permits long-lasting inflammatory effects in the vicinity of platelet plugs, whereas display of P-selectin on activated endothelium is a transient phenomenon. Activation of endothelium, however, induces platelet thrombus formation.[20]

Adhesive proteins released by platelets promote inflammation as well as hemostasis; therefore, they contribute to thrombosis. Circulating levels of vWF, fibrinogen, thrombospondin, and PDGF rise during inflammation and are chronically elevated in patients with occlusive vascular disease. The growth factors released by aggregating platelets are chemotactic for leukocytes, smooth muscle cells, and endothelial cells and, during wound healing, stimulate cell division of smooth muscle cells and fibroblasts. Among these factors is TGF-β. Platelets are a major source of circulating TGF-β, which is released on their activation. TGF-β stimulates the synthesis of matrix proteins, a component of atherosclerotic lesions. Because these growth factors can also be released by single platelets adhering to an abnormal vascular wall, they can stimulate excessive proliferative responses in the vessel wall that favor both restenosis after revascularization and progression of atherosclerosis. Platelets are rich in cholesterol, which is also released during platelet activation and can be incorporated into the arterial wall. Therefore, antiplatelet therapy that depresses release of platelet granule contents has potential antiatherosclerotic as well as direct antithrombotic value.

Platelet Function in Patients at Risk of Occlusive Stroke

Factors Contributing to Platelet Hyperactivity

Patients at risk of occlusive stroke often have activated platelets.[21-23] Their platelet hyperreactivity most likely reflects the interactions between platelets and an abnormal vascular surface. Most frequently atherosclerosis but also vasculitis, infection, trauma, or congenital anomaly may lead to vascular endothelial dysfunction. Stroke risk factors such as hypertension, hypercholesterolemia, smoking, diabetes mellitus, and inflammation contribute both to increased platelet reactivity and to abnormal endothelial behavior with consequently higher risk of arterial thrombosis.[24] In addition, turbulent blood flow that accompanies atherosclerotic or hypertensive arterial changes (e.g., endothelial dysfunction, stiff vascular wall, atherosclerotic plaque, or altered pressure gradients) further contributes to increased platelet reactivity in the absence of actual breaches in the endothelium. High levels of platelet activation markers have been associated with carotid artery wall thickening.[25]

Plasma factors may also contribute to increased platelet reactivity in stroke-prone patients. The higher levels of circulating catecholamines associated with advancing age and with stress contribute to platelet reactivity. Catecholamines are weak direct platelet agonists but augment platelet aggregation by other agonists, oppose the effects of natural antiplatelet factors such as prostacyclin and NO, and offset some of the antiplatelet efficacy of aspirin. A circadian rhythm in acute myocardial infarction (MI), stroke, and sudden death has been observed in which the peak incidence is seen in the early morning, soon after patients awaken.[26,27] Platelet aggregability is highest soon after waking and correlates with elevations in plasma catecholamines and free fatty acids.[26] A diminution in the

morning excess of cardiovascular events in patients who take aspirin points to platelet involvement in the process.

In clinical settings marked by stress, in which catecholamine levels are increased, plasma fibrinogen and vWF–factor VIII are also elevated, which contributes to platelet activation.[27] Elevated plasma fibrinogen by itself is an independent risk factor for stroke and is known to increase platelet aggregability.[28] Recent infection may also contribute to the risk of recurrent cerebral ischemia.[29] In the elderly, a seasonal rise in stroke incidence during the winter months may reflect a higher incidence of infection.[30,31]

Role of Platelet Count

High platelet counts may but do not necessarily represent a stroke risk factor. In situations in which platelet turnover is continually enhanced, a compensatory increase in megakaryocyte size may result in release of platelets that are "younger," larger, and more hemostatically active than usual. Young platelets have been found to be larger than average, to produce more prothrombotic factors, and to aggregate in response to lower concentrations of agonists. Large platelets are a risk factor for death and recurrent vascular events after MI.[32] Platelet volume is greater in patients with acute stroke than in age- and sex-matched control subjects, and the high platelet volume may persist for months.[33]

In myeloproliferative diseases, platelets are often very large, and platelet mass is increased even more than platelet count; platelet numbers therefore underestimate total platelet mass. The greater platelet mass probably contributes to the higher thrombotic risk observed in these diseases. High platelet counts in a setting of myeloproliferative disease are associated with increased risk of thrombosis, including cerebral thrombosis, and lowering the platelet count with chemotherapy appears to reduce the risk of both stroke and thrombosis in these diseases.[34] Low-dose aspirin therapy also decreases stroke risk in patients with myeloproliferative diseases, especially if the platelet count has been normalized. In contrast, secondary thrombocytosis that accompanies inflammation or follows splenectomy, for example, is not usually associated with a higher risk of thrombosis or stroke.

Chronic Changes in Platelet Reactivity

The question of whether greater platelet reactivity in patients with stroke merely reflects the body's inflammatory response to tissue damage is, however, clearly answered with a no. Increases in platelet activation not only may follow an acute stroke for many months but also may be chronically present before an episode of cerebral ischemia. In adults, increased platelet aggregability after atherosclerotic stroke has been demonstrated to continue for at least 3 to 9 months after the acute event in 60% of patients; this time extends well beyond that required for resolution of the acute inflammatory changes typical of cerebral tissue damage.[24,35] Similar changes in platelet aggregability are not observed after stroke caused by cardiac emboli, even though brain tissue damage may be extensive. A long-term increase in platelet aggregation after acute cerebral ischemia correlates with a poorer outcome. In some unusual circumstances, oxidative stress has been correlated with chronic platelet activation. In familial stroke, infants seen with stroke can be shown to have a chronic platelet hyperreactivity that is not blocked by NO; such infants lack the plasma enzyme glutathione peroxidase and, therefore, have low blood antioxidant potential that counters the protective effect of NO on platelets.[36] In most cases of adult ischemic stroke, however, no such simple correlation between oxidative stress and platelet hyperreactivity can be made.

The pathologic consequences of greater platelet reactivity in stroke-prone patient clearly show that more is not better. In normal arteries, hemostasis rapidly controls bleeding, and the damaged area is soon precisely repaired, whereas in a diseased arterial bed, even this normal hemostatic response may have the unwanted consequences of arterial thrombosis. This dysequilibrium between hemostasis and thrombosis appears to be particularly true in vessels vulnerable to even temporary occlusion, such as the end arteries of the brain. Furthermore, normal platelet contributions to wound repair can similarly be detrimental in stroke-prone patients, in whom platelet-derived mediators promote excessive vascular cell proliferation that accelerates intimal hyperplasia and vascular narrowing.[24,37]

Antiplatelet Drugs and Prevention of Stroke

The sequential steps in platelet activation are sensitive to different pharmacologic interventions. Antiplatelet drugs that mainly affect platelet aggregation and mediator release tend to block platelet-initiated thrombosis without much depression of hemostasis and, therefore, involve a smaller chance of hemorrhagic complications. On the other hand, antiplatelet drugs that block platelet adhesion, the initial step in platelet activation at a vascular surface, or the GPIIb/IIIa complex and, thus, all aggregation pathways are highly effective in preventing thrombosis; thus far, however, they continue to impose an unacceptable risk of bleeding, particularly in the brain. Only direct inhibitors of thrombin, factor Xa, or both block the capacity of platelets to catalyze thrombin generation. Such agents might pose a major bleeding risk with long-term use in secondary prevention of cerebral ischemia and have not been tested for prevention of noncardioembolic stroke.

Antiplatelet drugs in current use for secondary prevention of stroke include aspirin, clopidogrel, dipyridamole, and various combinations of these agents (Table 58-2). In clinical settings in which platelets are not major factors in the production of vasoocclusive arterial emboli, anticoagulation is an effective form of

TABLE 58-2 ACTIONS OF ANTIPLATELET DRUGS

Activity	Effect on Platelets	Drug
Inhibition of membrane GPIb receptor	Block GPI-V-IX function, prevent adhesion and aggregation	S-nitroso-AR545C*
Inhibition of membrane GPIIb/IIIa receptor	Prevent bending of fibrinogen Prevent platelet–platelet interaction	Abciximab RGD peptide analogues Disintegrins
Inhibition of membrane ADP P2Y$_{12}$ receptor	Prevent binding of ADP Prevent ADP-mediated aggregation Decrease GPIIb/IIIa activation	Ticlopidine, clopidogrel AR-C69931 MX†
Inhibition of membrane ADP P2Y$_1$ receptor	Prevent binding of ADP	Adenosine 3'-phosphate, 5'-phosphosulfate†
Catabolism of ADP	Prevent calcium mobilization Prevent ADP-mediated aggregation Foster disaggregation	Soluble recombinant CD39*
Inhibition of cyclooxygenase-1	Prevent TXA$_2$ generation Inhibit arachidonic acid–mediated platelet aggregation and secretion	Aspirin (irreversible effect) NSAIDs (competitive effect)
Stimulate adenylate cyclase	Raise platelet cAMP, preventing aggregation and secretion	Epoprostenol, Iloprost Fish oils, ω3 fatty acids*
Inhibition of phophodiesterase	Maintain elevated cAMP once raised	Dipyridamole Methylxanthines*
Stimulate guanylate cyclase	Raise platelet CGMP, preventing aggregation and secretion	NO, NO donors (e.g., S-nitrosoglutathione, nitroglycerin)
Inhibit calcium flux	Prevent calcium mobilization Decrease aggregation and secretion	Ca^{2+} channel blockers* Local anesthetics* Beta-blockers*
Inhibit thrombin generation or action	Inhibit aggregation and secretion Inhibit procoagulant activity	Heparins, hirudin Antithrombin peptides†

*Weak or adjunctive effect.
†Under development.
ADP, Adenosine diphosphate; Ca^{2+}, calcium ion; cGMP, cyclic guanosine monophosphate; NO, nitric oxide; NSAID, nonsteroidal anti-inflammatory drug; TXA$_2$, thromboxane A$_2$.

secondary prevention of stroke. The foremost of settings is cardioembolic stroke associated with nonvalvular AF and valvular heart disease. Other important causes of stroke that are relatively independent of platelets are cholesterol emboli released from ulcerated atherosclerotic plaques, patent foramen ovale, fibrin-rich emboli from intracardiac mural thrombus, "bland" cardiac valve vegetations in inflammatory disease, thalassemia, and sickle cell disease[38-42]; these causes together represent about 15% of cerebral ischemic episodes. Even in some of these settings, antiplatelet agents may have a role in stroke prevention if anticoagulation alone does not suffice or if the patient also has atherosclerotic risk factors for stroke.

Aspirin

Mechanism of the Antiplatelet Effect of Aspirin

Aspirin has long been known to prolong bleeding time. That the lengthened bleeding time involves decreased platelet aggregation was first demonstrated in the 1960s. In 1971, aspirin was first shown to affect platelet function by irreversible acetylation and thus inactivation of the platelet enzyme cyclooxygenase-1 (prostaglandin endoperoxide synthase-1), thus preventing the addition of molecular oxygen to arachidonic acid to form prostaglandin endoperoxides G_2 and H_2 and blocking downstream formation of TXA_2 from endoperoxides.[43-45] Because platelets do not synthesize proteins, platelet functions that depend on TXA_2 activity are inhibited for the life span of the platelet. The separate peroxidase function of cyclooxygenase, not involved in eicosanoid synthesis, remains unaffected by aspirin. Very small doses of aspirin rapidly (within minutes) block platelet cyclooxygenase in vivo.[46] Certain peculiarities of platelet kinetics favor the profound and long-lasting effect of aspirin. Platelets circulate for 7 to 10 days, but once exposed to aspirin, they are permanently unable to produce TXA_2. Because only about 10% of circulating platelets are replaced each day by new platelets released from bone marrow megakaryocytes, a single daily dose of aspirin produces virtually complete inhibition of platelet cyclooxygenase. Therefore, high, persistent blood levels of aspirin are not required for the inhibitory effect on platelet function, even in patients with cerebral ischemia.[47]

In contrast to platelets, other cells in vascular endothelium, cells in kidney or lung epithelium, and monocytes are capable of rapid resynthesis of cyclooxygenase. The inhibitory effect of aspirin on eicosanoid synthesis in cells other than platelets is therefore much briefer. Moreover, these other tissues also synthesize cyclooxygenase-2, a related isoform inducible by inflammatory stimuli and cytokines. Platelets neither contain nor synthesize cyclooxygenase-2. Cyclooxygenase-2 is also inhibited by aspirin, but because of its rapid resynthesis in many cell types (i.e., monocytes, vascular endothelium, and smooth muscle), net eicosanoid production by these cells is less durably inhibited by aspirin.[48] In terms of the vascular bed, once-daily dosage with aspirin selectively inhibits platelet function, usually without impairing production of vasoprotective prostaglandins such as prostacyclin and prostaglandin (PG) E_2 by the blood vessel wall.

Pharmacokinetics

After oral administration, aspirin is rapidly absorbed from the stomach and upper small intestine, reaching a peak plasma level 30 minutes after a single dose. It is rapidly deacetylated in the liver to salicylate. Although salicylate has little or no antiplatelet efficacy, it does have independent anti-inflammatory effects through modulation of NFκB-regulated genes. By 3 hours after oral ingestion of aspirin, the plasma acetylsalicylate level is negligible. However, because aspirin exposure inactivates platelet cyclooxygenase within minutes, even a brief exposure of circulating platelets to aspirin produces full inactivation of cyclooxygenase and depresses platelet function. Intravenous aspirin works even faster.[49]

As little as 1 mg aspirin taken orally per hour—a dose completely deacetylated on first pass through the liver—fully inhibits platelet cyclooxygenase within about 12 hours because platelets traveling through the portal circulation encounter sufficient newly absorbed aspirin to inhibit their cyclooxygenase.[46] In clinical studies, an initial dose of 162 mg fully blocks platelet cyclooxygenase in an adult, and 81 mg/day (one pediatric aspirin tablet) maintains full inhibition.[50] As little as 30 mg taken once daily for several days builds to the same net effect within a week because the antiplatelet effects of aspirin are cumulative over time.[51] Effects of enteric-coated aspirin are similar to those of plain aspirin, except for a slightly slower onset of action.[52]

Dose-Response Effects

Antiplatelet effects of aspirin usually maximize at 81 to 325 mg/day, and higher doses do not inhibit platelet function any further.[53] Only in persons with a very rapid rate of platelet turnover are higher or more frequent doses needed for full effect (see later). TXA_2 synthesis must be decreased by 95% for full inhibitory effects of aspirin on platelet function to be achieved.[46] Aspirin was approved by the U.S. Food and Drug Administration (FDA) in 1980 for the prevention of TIAs and stroke and in 1985 for the prevention of unstable angina and secondary prevention of MI; the recommended dosage is 50 to 325 mg/day.

At these doses, the bleeding time lengthens to about double the baseline time in at least 60% of individuals; larger doses of aspirin do not prolong bleeding time further. Indeed, very high doses may slightly shorten the bleeding time because of inhibition of vascular cyclooxygenase. Prolongation of bleeding time by aspirin correlates poorly with either gastric irritation or gastrointestinal bleeding. After aspirin is stopped, bleeding time returns to normal within 1 to 2 days regardless of the dose administered. Concomitant alcohol ingestion can further lengthen aspirin-induced prolongation of bleeding time and slows recovery; this factor may contribute to the incidence of gastrointestinal bleeding in aspirin users.

Once aspirin is stopped, platelet aggregation and TXA_2 formation return to normal levels within 7 to 10 days, and linear kinetics after a 1- to 2-day lag likely reflects the acetylation of megakaryocyte cyclooxygenase, resulting in release of aspirin-impaired platelets during the first 2 days. In patients at major risk of stroke, such as those with high-grade carotid stenosis, doses of aspirin up to 1300 mg/day have been tried, but the data obtained do not show greater clinical efficacy of doses higher than 325 mg (see later).[54-56]

NSAIDs inhibit platelet cyclooxygenase in a reversible, competitive manner, so their antiplatelet effects all depend on maintenance of a high blood level of drug. Therefore, their duration of antiplatelet activity is relatively brief. However, the coadministration of an NSAID, such as ibuprofen or naproxen, with low-dose aspirin can decrease the irreversible effects of aspirin on platelet cyclooxygenase by competition and may impair the antiplatelet efficacy of aspirin.[57]

In contrast, the "coxib" cyclooxygenase-2 inhibitors do not block the ability of aspirin to acetylate platelet cyclooxygenase-1 and so do not diminish the antiplatelet effects of aspirin.[58] No definitive data are currently available on the incidence of cardiovascular events and stroke, in particular, in patients taking both aspirin and cyclooxygenase-2 inhibitors, although patients taking only the latter have been reported in some studies to have a higher incidence of MI; more information is clearly needed.[59]

Range and Limits of Aspirin Effects on Platelet Function

The effects of aspirin on platelet activation all result from cyclooxygenase inhibition. These effects include blocking of TXA_2 production, complete inhibition of arachidonate-induced platelet aggregation, a decreased release reaction that is reflected in diminished and slowed platelet responses to collagen and epinephrine, and reduced platelet aggregation to low-dose ADP. In contrast, aspirin does not affect platelet adhesion, prolong the shortened platelet life span, decrease secretion of vascular growth factors from platelets, or block thrombin-induced platelet activation. Because TXA_2, the major eicosanoid produced by blood platelets, is a strong stimulus for platelet aggregation and release and a powerful vasoconstrictor, all of the aspirin-induced changes in platelet activation previously listed are related to blocking of the TXA_2 pathway of platelet activation.

Because thrombin affects platelets in a cyclooxygenase-independent manner, activation of platelets by thrombin is not inhibited by aspirin. Even so, use of aspirin (325 to 500 mg/day) has been reported to reduce platelet-dependent thrombin generation in vitro and in vivo.[60] The inhibitory effect of aspirin on thrombin generation is weaker in hypercholesterolemic patients, who are known to have a hypercoagulable state and who often show enhanced platelet TXA_2 generation.[61] It is postulated that the antithrombinogenic effect of aspirin may involve acetylation of platelet membrane proteins, but the mechanism is not yet clear. The clinical relevance of aspirin-induced impairment of thrombin generation remains to be assessed.

Aspirin has little or no effect on the lipoxygenase pathway of arachidonic acid metabolism; thus, 12-HETE production by platelets is not altered. Production of epoxyeicosatrienoic acids and isoprostanes, which are formed nonenzymatically, is also unaltered by aspirin.

Aspirin Resistance

In spite of the well-reported efficacy of aspirin in the secondary prevention of cardiovascular disease,[2,62] recurrent vascular events are not uncommon in patients prescribed aspirin. The recurrence of coronary heart disease, stroke, and peripheral vascular disease syndromes under prescription of a regular therapeutic dose of aspirin defines what is known as clinical aspirin resistance or aspirin treatment failure. This may or may not be accompanied by biochemical aspirin resistance, a phenomenon of persistent platelet activation, measured by platelet function tests, despite prescription of a regular therapeutic dose of aspirin.[63] Whereas the incidence of aspirin resistance by the clinical definition has been estimated at 12.9% with a range from 10.9% to 17.3% depending on the dosage,[62] the estimated incidence of biochemical resistance ranges from as little as 5.2% to as much as 60% depending on the studied population and the platelet function assay used.[64] At present, no standardized definition or test can be used to quantify either type of aspirin resistance. A few studies have attempted to quantify both clinical and pharmacologic resistance, but the reported data are hampered by internal and external validity concerns including small sample sizes, lack of agreement between different platelet function tests, different dose regimens and nonadherence, and insufficient information about measurement stability over time. Moreover, none of the available platelet aggregation assays have convincingly been shown to predict clinical events, and the results between different assays have also been discordant. However, it is clear that there is individual biochemical variability in the response to aspirin administration, which may be responsible for treatment failures and secondary vascular clinical events. Research into the mechanisms involved in the aspirin resistance phenomenon is necessary for development of more accurate platelet function tests and correlation of their results with clinical event occurrence.

Measurement of aspirin effects on platelets. Because platelet activation leads to a change in platelet shape and aggregation as well as the release of different platelet constituents, the examination of these changes and/or the analysis in blood and urine of the metabolic products of platelets is the basis for determining the degree of platelet function,[65,66] which can be evaluated by different in vivo and in vitro tests.

In Vivo Tests:

1. Measurement of TXA_2 pathway end products. The analysis of TXA_2 metabolites, which include serum thromboxane B_2[67] and urinary 11-dehydrothromboxane B_2,[68,69] has been used to determine aspirin resistance. However, these tests seem to reflect the contribution of monocyte/macrophages to TXA_2 synthesis as well as the cyclooxygenase-2 linked pathway of arachidonic acid but not specifically platelet activity.[70] The levels of 11-dehydrothromboxane B_2 in urine are highly dependent on the renal function, and ex vivo platelet activation during blood sample collection, storage, and processing may also interfere with the results of these tests.

2. Expression of P-selectin on platelet membranes. P-selectin moves to the plasma membrane when platelets are activated and degranulated; thus increased P-selectin expression on the platelet surface is indicative of platelet activation. However, selectins are also expressed on all blood cell types,[71] which is a fact that results in conflicting data when this marker is used to assess aspirin

efficacy.[72,73] In addition, testing is not easy because it requires expensive equipment and carefully controlled test conditions.[74]

3. Analysis of soluble P-selectin in plasma. Plasma levels of P-selectin increase as a result of platelet activation; thus, this marker may be useful in determining platelet status.[74,75] The test is simple to perform but relatively expensive. Moreover, because of its stability, the sample can be stored for long periods. However, the same concerns regarding the validity of the expression of P-selectin on platelet membranes as a marker of platelet activation also apply for the analysis of P-selectin in plasma.

In Vitro Tests:

1. Optical platelet aggregation tests. These tests measure optical changes in plasma caused by platelet aggregation induced by the addition of various substrates including arachidonic acid, ADP, collagen, epinephrine, and thrombin, in the absence of erythrocytes and blood flow.[76] The induction of platelet aggregation results in a decrease in the turbidity of the solution as the platelets crosslink and clump together. The amount of platelet aggregation is directly related to the amount of light that is allowed to be transmitted through the solution. Aspirin almost completely inhibits platelet aggregation induced by arachidonic acid and collagen, but aggregation in response to ADP and epinephrine is only partially inhibited.[76,77] Moreover, platelet aggregation is sensitive to changes in temperature and pH and so must be carried out within hours of sample collection.[77] In addition, these tests do not correlate well with other indicators of platelet function.[65] Finally, although these tests have been the most widely used to date, the technical difficulties of the tests, which require a specialized laboratory setting, make them unsuitable for routine clinical practice.

2. PFA-100 (Dade-Behring Inc). The PFA-100 is a whole blood, point-of-care, platelet aggregometer that functions by aspirating a blood sample through a capillary tube at a high shear rate and through a small slit aperture that is cut into a membrane coated with either collagen-epinephrine or collagen-ADP platelet agonists.[78,79] Given that measurement is performed in the presence of erythrocytes and at a high shear rate, it can be considered more clinically relevant than platelet aggregometry, which is conducted in the absence of erythrocytes and blood flow. The time for a platelet plug to occlude the slit aperture, reported in seconds as the closure time, is inversely related to platelet activity. A closure time value of 193 seconds is considered normal and a closure time of more than 300 seconds is considered as nonclosure.[78,79] This test is easy to perform, requires only a small volume of blood (800 µL), is quick, and has good sensitivity and reproducibility. However, the PFA-100 test is quite expensive, depends on plasma vWF and hematocrit levels, and testing must be done within 4 hours of blood collection.

3. VerifyNow Aspirin Assay (Accumetrics Inc). Another point-of-care, easy-to-use, and rapid test for measuring platelet-induced aggregation is the VerifyNow Aspirin Assay (formerly called the Ultegra Rapid Platelet Function Analyzer). Unlike the PFA-100, VerifyNow is designed only to detect platelet dysfunction as the result of exposure to antiplatelet agents, including aspirin, clopidogrel, and glycoprotein IIb/IIIa inhibitors. The VerifyNow Aspirin Assay originally used a proprietary platelet agonist consisting of metallic cations and propyl gallate, but this has recently been substituted by an arachidonic acid agonist (Accumetrics Inc, VerifyNow Aspirin Assay package insert, San Diego, Calif; 2004).[80] Platelet aggregation detection is based on the agglutination of platelets on fibrinogen-coated beads detected by an optical turbidimetric method.[80] Platelet inhibition measured by the VerifyNow Aspirin Assay in response to single-dose aspirin has correlated well with measurements by the PFA-100 (r^2 = 0.73–0.86) and with traditional optical platelet aggregation (r^2 = 0.902).[80,81] Platelet responsiveness is expressed in aspirin response units (ARU) with a cutoff for aspirin resistance at 550 ARU. The most important limitation of this test relates to its diagnostic criteria because these were set in comparison with optical aggregation in response to adrenaline after only a single 325-mg dose of aspirin.[70]

Mechanisms of aspirin resistance. Several factors have been mentioned and investigated as related to aspirin resistance, but so far, the exact mechanism responsible for this phenomenon is not known.

A reduction in the bioavailability secondary to lack of adherence to the treatment, low dosage of aspirin, or concurrent intake of NSAIDs such as ibuprofen, naproxen, and indomethacin, which appear to antagonize the antiplatelet effects of aspirin by blocking its union to the cyclooxygenase-1 binding site, may explain the lack of efficacy of the drug in some cases.[63] In fact, it has been reported that about 10% of outpatients who are prescribed aspirin or ticlopidine are noncompliant with their medication and showed a decreased inhibition of platelet aggregation on repeated testing.[82,83]

The activation of platelet function by the stimulation of alternative pathways that are not blocked by aspirin such as red cell–induced platelet activation, stimulation of collagen, ADP, epinephrine, and thrombin receptors on platelets, and the biosynthesis of thromboxane by pathways not inhibited by aspirin has also been mentioned as a possible cause of aspirin nonresponsiveness.[84]

The existence of comorbid conditions increasing vascular risk such as smoking habit, hyperlipidemia, ischemic heart disease, prosthetic heart valves, or arteritis also explain the recurrence of stroke in patients taking aspirin. In one large study, 5.7% of patients consecutively admitted for ischemic stroke were classified as aspirin nonresponders as they had been taking aspirin at the time of stroke. Pertinent characteristics of these patients included significant hyperlipidemia, ischemic heart disease, and lower dose of aspirin, which suggests that individuals with greater risk factors for occlusive vascular disease might benefit less from aspirin.[85]

Moreover, some patients seem to develop aspirin resistance over time. In a study including poststroke patients prescribed aspirin who were repeatedly tested at 6-month intervals to observe the effect of aspirin on platelet aggregation,[86] 75% of 306 patients were found to have a maximum effect and 25% a partial effect of aspirin at the initial testing, but on repeated testing, only 33% continued to show good inhibition. Increasing the aspirin dose restored maximum inhibition in about two thirds of those who had experienced a reduced effect, but this improvement was only temporary. Patients were reminded to take aspirin on the day of testing, but neither compliance with dosing nor lipid status was directly assessed in this study. Overall, about 8% of patients showed aspirin resistance, even at 1300 mg/day. Interestingly, eight patients experienced a stroke during follow-up, all of whom had previously been classified as having aspirin resistance during at least one study visit.

Finally, genetic factors also seem to be involved in aspirin resistance. Several single nucleotide polymorphisms that have been linked to changes in platelet function and thrombosis, including a polymorphism on the cyclo-oxygenase-1 gene, overexpression of cyclooxygenase-2 mRNA on platelets and endothelial cells, the platelet allo-antigen A1/A2 of the gene encoding glycoprotein IIIa, and the homozygous 807T (873A) polymorphism allied with increased density of platelet glycoprotein Ia/IIa collagen-receptor gene, may contribute to aspirin resistance and increased risk of vascular events.[87] However, the effect of these polymorphisms on the antithrombotic effects of aspirin is only based on measurements of platelet function; thus, studies are needed to characterize the prevalence of these polymorphisms fully and, especially, to elucidate whether their presence can influence clinical outcomes.

Aspirin resistance and stroke recurrence. Data regarding the percentage recurrence of ischemic stroke in patients treated with aspirin are scarce. Grotemeyer et al[88] studied the prevalence of aspirin resistance in 174 poststroke patients treated with 1500 mg of aspirin daily, who were followed up for a period of 2 years. Twenty-nine of the 174 patients had major vascular events: 16 patients (9.2%) had MI, and 13 (7.5%) had a second stroke. The authors specified that, of the 29 patients with major events, only 4.4% (5 of 114) belonged to the aspirin responder group as compared with 40% (24 of 60) of the secondary aspirin nonresponder group (P < 0.0001). However, no specific data as to the prevalence of the different major vascular events in the group of responders versus nonresponders were supplied.

As has been mentioned earlier, in Bornstein et al,[85] 129 of 2231 consecutive patients (5.7%) admitted over a 4-year period with ischemic stroke were found to have had a recurrent ischemic stroke while already taking aspirin. The authors found that the average period until stroke was longer for patients taking higher aspirin doses and suggested that doses of 500 mg daily or more should be used in secondary stroke prevention. Moreover, comparison of patients resistant to aspirin with a control group matched for age, sex, date of first ischemic stroke, and aspirin dose demonstrated that these patients more often had statistically significant hyperlipidemia and ischemic heart disease, which confirms the importance of adequate control of vascular risk factors related to stroke, regardless of aspirin intake. Eikelboom et al[69] analyzed the levels of 11-dehydrothromboxane B_2 in urine from 488 patients with MI, stroke, or cardiovascular death during a period of 5 years. Whereas baseline urinary

concentrations of 11-dehydrothromboxane B_2 were significantly higher in patients with MI and in those who died of a cardiovascular cause, the levels were not significantly different between case patients who subsequently had a stroke and their matched control group. The adjusted odds for the composite outcome of MI, stroke, or cardiovascular death increased with each increasing quartile of baseline urinary 11-dehydrothromboxane B_2 concentrations, and patients in the highest quartile had a risk 1.8-fold higher than those in the lowest quartile. A similar association was seen with MI and cardiovascular death but not for stroke. Andersen et al[89] analyzed aspirin resistance using the PFA-100 system in a total of 202 patients with acute MI who were randomly assigned to aspirin 160 mg/day (n = 71), aspirin 75 mg/day together with warfarin (international normalized ratio [INR], 2.0 to 2.5) (n = 58), or warfarin alone (INR, 2.8 to 4.2) (n = 73). Although the authors reported a higher incidence of vascular events, including MI, stroke, and revascularization procedures, over a period of 4 years in the group of patients with aspirin resistance, the results were not statistically significant. Data about the separate prevalence of stroke recurrence in the group with aspirin resistance were not supplied in the article. Using the same system to evaluate platelet function, Grundmann et al[90] reported that 12 of 35 patients (34%) who had a stroke recurrence had evidence of aspirin resistance, whereas none of the patients without further cerebrovascular events had evidence of biochemical aspirin resistance. Gum et al[91] used platelet aggregation to analyze platelet function in a group of 326 prospective stable cardiovascular patients receiving aspirin 325 mg/day for at least 7 days and followed them up for a mean of 679 days. Clinical endpoints included the composite of death, MI, or cerebrovascular accident. Of the patients studied, 17 (5.2%) were classified as having aspirin resistance by optical aggregation and 309 (94.8%) were classified as aspirin sensitive. During follow-up, aspirin resistance was associated with an increased risk of death, MI, or stroke compared with patients who were aspirin sensitive (24% versus 10%; hazard ratio [HR], 3.12; 95% confidence interval [CI], 1.10–8.90; P = 0.03). However, despite there being a consistent trend, the association between aspirin resistance and individual clinical events including stroke did not reach statistical significance (12% aspirin resistant versus 1% aspirin sensitive, P = 0.09).

In spite of these data, the association between aspirin resistance and stroke recurrence as well as other cardiovascular events still remains uncertain. Comparison between studies is difficult because of differences in the platelet function tests used and the studied populations. None of these studies assessed other potential causes of aspirin failure, such as treatment adherence, and most only included a single measurement of aspirin function, which makes it difficult to assess the validity of the data over time. Composite endpoints, which did not allow associations between platelet function and individual clinical events to be established, were typically used. Moreover, the number of events was low in comparison with the prevalence of aspirin resistance, which throws into doubt whether aspirin resistance is the real cause of the recurrence of stroke and other cardiovascular events.

Therapeutic management of aspirin resistance. Because aspirin resistance seems to be a multifactorial phenomenon, different factors need to be addressed when clinical vascular events occur in patients already being treated with this drug. Therapeutic compliance as well as the adequate control of vascular risk factors related to cerebrovascular events may increase the efficacy of aspirin administration.[85,86] However, the decision to increase aspirin dosage has to be considered individually. In fact, it has recently been reported that, in patients with diabetes mellitus, a high dosage of aspirin seems to be neither effective nor safe.[92]

The association between different antiplatelet drugs appears to be the best therapeutic approach in case of aspirin resistance. In fact, patients with aspirin resistance have been shown to have increased platelet sensitivity to ADP[93] as well as increased plasma levels of this agonist.[94] Moreover, those patients with a very low sensitivity to the effect of aspirin on the arachidonic acid pathway appear to be highly sensitive to the $P2Y_{12}$ platelet ADP receptor antagonist clopidogrel,[95] which suggests that the association of both drugs might have a greater effect on platelet action. In an attempt to clarify this question, several clinical trials have tested the efficacy of combining aspirin and clopidogrel in the secondary prevention of stroke.[96,97] However, some recent data seem to demonstrate the existence of clopidogrel resistance[98] and even a dual aspirin–clopidogrel resistance,[99-101] although this deserves further investigation. The combination of different dosages of aspirin and 400 mg extended-release dipyridamole (ERDP) daily has been found to be more effective than aspirin alone in the secondary prevention of stroke.[102,103] However, the combination of 25 mg aspirin and 200 mg ERDP twice a day has been reported to be equally effective as 75 mg clopidogrel daily in secondary stroke prevention.[104] The design and results of these clinical trials are discussed in another section of this chapter.

Finally, the administration of new antiaggregants that modify platelet aggregation by a different mechanism than aspirin can be an alternative for patients who have a recurrent stroke while receiving aspirin. Among these drugs, cilostazol, which is a phosphodiesterase 3 inhibitor, seems to be at least as effective as aspirin in the secondary prevention of stroke. In a pilot study of 720 Chinese patients randomly assigned to receive 100 mg aspirin daily or 100 mg cilostazol twice a day, no differences were found in the rate of stroke recurrence between the two groups. Moreover, the lower rates of ischemic and hemorrhagic stroke in the group of patients treated with cilostazol suggest that this drug might be a more effective and safer alternative to aspirin.[105]

Aspirin Toxicity

Gastrointestinal irritation and bleeding, well-known side effects of aspirin, can cause major or fatal bleeding, partly through a direct irritant action and partly through blocking the production of protective prostaglandins in the gastric mucosa. Risk increases with dose and duration of use.[2,46] Reexamination of the occurrence of hemorrhagic stroke, the major central nervous system toxicity of aspirin as an antithrombotic agent, in a meta-analysis of more than 55,000 subjects enrolled in 16 clinical trials

of secondary prevention of vascular events showed that aspirin use gave an absolute risk reduction per 10,000 persons of 137 MIs and 39 ischemic strokes, which was offset by an absolute risk increase of 12 hemorrhagic strokes.[106] These were all statistically significant effects (in each case, $P < 0.001$). The risk of hemorrhagic stroke did not depend on aspirin dose.[106] Thus, in this later, more focused analysis, as in the analysis by the Antiplatelet Trialists' Collaboration,[2] a real increase in hemorrhagic stroke was clearly observed in patients taking aspirin; this adverse effect was considerably less, however, than the decreases in both MI and ischemic stroke seen when patients with extensive vascular disease took aspirin prophylactically.

Clopidogrel, a Thienopyridine Inhibitor of ADP-Mediated Platelet Activation

Mechanism of Action

Thienopyridine drugs, specifically ticlopidine (Ticlid) and a closely related compound, clopidogrel (Plavix, Iscover), have been clinically tested as antiplatelet agents that are chemically and functionally unrelated to prior classes of antiplatelet drugs.[107,108] These drugs block the binding of ADP to one specific type of purinergic receptor on platelets ($P2Y_{12}$) and therefore inhibit ADP-mediated platelet activation and G_i protein association with platelet membranes.[11] Thienopyridines therefore prevent the activation of GPIIb/IIIa, the fibrinogen receptor, to its high-affinity form but do not inhibit ADP-induced calcium flux or changes in platelet shape. Ticlopidine and clopidogrel have similar antiplatelet effects but differ in potency and pharmacokinetics.[108]

Bleeding time is prolonged much more by thienopyridines than by aspirin, and the prolongation is dose-dependent.[108] When ticlopidine or clopidogrel is given together with aspirin, the effects on bleeding time are additive. The prolongation of bleeding time due to thienopyridines can be reversed by the administration of corticosteroids, although the antiplatelet effects are not reversed. In emergency situations—for example, when urgent surgery is required in a patient taking a thienopyridine—the prolongation of bleeding time can be reversed quickly by desmopressin or by a bolus dose of dexamethasone (20 mg). Clopidogrel is more potent, can be rapidly effective, and is safer than ticlopidine; thus, it is rapidly taking the place of ticlopidine in clinical practice.

In addition to decreasing binding of ADP and fibrinogen to platelet membranes, thienopyridines decrease platelet adhesion to artificial surfaces, reduce platelet deposition on atheromatous plaque,[109] and restore abnormally short platelet survival toward normal. In contrast, they do not affect platelet arachidonic acid metabolism or decrease TXA_2 synthesis. Thienopyridines also reduce plasma fibrinogen levels and blood viscosity and enhance red cell deformability, which suggests possibly beneficial rheologic properties.[108] They can oppose the action of several vasoconstrictors, such as endothelin and TXA_2, presumably by acting on vascular purinergic receptors.[110] In many different experimental thrombosis systems, these drugs have been shown to reduce thrombosis and improve outcomes regardless of whether platelets are important in the pathogenesis of the thrombosis. There is no gender or age difference in response to the drugs.

Pharmacokinetics and Dosing

Clopidogrel is administered orally at 75 mg/day. Clopidogrel blocks ADP-mediated platelet activation processes in vivo; however, it is a prodrug inactive in vitro, which indicates that its antiplatelet activity depends on drug metabolites. The prodrug is activated by hepatic metabolism. Clopidogrel is converted to active metabolites on first pass through the liver and therefore develops antiplatelet efficacy within a few hours when a loading dose (300 mg) is used. The antiplatelet effects last for up to a week after administration is stopped because its effect on circulating platelets is not reversible and active metabolites are slowly cleared.

Clopidogrel Resistance

The concept of clopidogrel resistance has emerged as a possible explanation for the continued occurrence of ischemic events despite the adequate dosage of the antiplatelet agent and proper compliance. *Resistance* is the term used to reflect failure to inhibit platelet function in vitro, and failure of therapy reflects patients who have recurrent events while receiving therapy. The prevalence of clopidogrel nonresponse in different populations has been described as between 4% and 30%. The reason for the response variability among different studies depends on the technique used to evaluate platelet aggregation. In addition, the definition of nonresponders is not standardized or validated.[111,112]

The potential mechanisms of clopidogrel resistance are multiple and can be divided into two main groups: (1) extrinsic mechanisms, that is, drug interactions involving CYP3A4 and (2) intrinsic mechanisms, that is, polymorphisms of $P2Y_{12}$ receptor and CYP3As.

Regarding drug interactions, any medication that interacts with (either inhibiting or increasing) CYP3A4 can potentially block the conversion of clopidogrel into its active metabolite. Among these drugs, statins, except pravastatin, might interfere with clopidogrel metabolism. Also, the antiplatelet activity has been shown to be reduced in persons receiving omeprazole, which is a CYP2C19 inhibitor. However, other studies have not confirmed this observation.

Recently, several reports indicate that certain polymorphisms in the hepatic cytochrome P450 system are associated with an excess of vascular events. Patients who are carriers of a loss-of-function of CYP2C19 allele (including the *2 and *3 alleles), might have a reduced rate in the conversion to an active metabolite, thus resulting in decreased inhibition of platelets. Compared with noncarriers, carriers of loss-of-function alleles showed a significant increase in the risk of major vascular events.[113,114] However, these data were obtained only from clopidogrel-treated patients. Despite the potential limitations of this data, the FDA issued a black box warning about the potential reduced effectiveness of clopidogrel in patients who are carriers of two loss-of-function alleles (poor metabolizers) and has suggested that these patients receive a higher dose of clopidogrel or other antiplatelet agent. A recent analysis of data among 5059 patients with acute coronary syndromes or AF showed that the response to clopidogrel compared with placebo was consistent, irrespective of CYP2C19 loss-of-function carrier status.[115] Therefore, it is possible that loss-of-function variants do not directly alter the efficacy and safety of clopidogrel. Consequently, clopidogrel should be used regardless of the carrier status until further studies can elucidate this paradox.

Currently, the management of clopidogrel resistance is a challenge, and there are no standardized guidelines. Until new data are available, it seems prudent to avoid interactions of drugs with a well-known effect on hepatic cytochrome P450 that might affect the metabolism of clopidogrel.

Antiplatelet Agents in Primary Prevention of Stroke

The role of aspirin versus control for primary prevention of stroke, MI, or vascular death has been studied in six major trials—the British Doctors Study (BDS),[116] US Physicians Study (PHT), Thrombosis Prevention Trial (TPT),[117] Hypertension Optimal Treatment Study (HOT),[118] Primary Prevention Project (PPP),[119] and Women's Health Study (WHS)[120]—and in meta-analyses.[121,122] No other antiplatelet agent has been widely investigated for primary prevention of cerebrovascular disease.

In meta-analyses by the Antithrombotic Trialists' Collaboration (ATTC), the trials, which followed up 95,000 patients and accounted for 660,000 patient-years, showed a 12% reduction in overall events with a small but significant benefit in favor of aspirin. There were 0.51% events per year versus 0.57% in the control group (rate ratio [RR], 0.88; 95% CI, 0.82-0.94). The authors attributed this effect largely to a 23% reduction in nonfatal MI with 0.18% events per year versus 0.23% in the control group (RR, 0.77; 95% CI, 0.67-0.89). There was no significant benefit in reduction of vascular death, with 0.19% events per year in both groups (RR, 0.97; 95% CI, 0.87-1.09). Subgroup analysis revealed no benefit in the aspirin group for primary stroke prevention, with 0.20% events per year versus 0.21% in the control group (RR, 0.95; 95% CI, 0.85-1.06). There was no significant difference when these events were subdivided into fatal and nonfatal stroke or ischemic and hemorrhagic stroke. Major extracranial bleeding was increased in the aspirin group (0.10% versus 0.07% per year; RR, 1.54; 95% CI, 1.30-1.82; $P < 0.0001$).[122]

In Women

Three of the six trials included women: PPP, HOT, and WHS. WHS, with 39,876 subjects, accounted for 74% of female subjects. The results in WHS showed no benefit in the aspirin group for primary prevention of fatal or nonfatal MI with 198 events versus 193 events in the control group (relative risk, 1.02; 95% CI, 0.67-0.97). Aspirin did, however, confer a significant protective benefit against stroke with a 17% reduction in events, that is, a total of 221 events versus 266 in the control group (relative risk, 0.83; 95% CI, 0.69-0.99; $P = 0.04$). Rates of ischemic stroke showed a greater reduction in the aspirin group with 170 events versus 266 in the control group (RR, 0.76; 95% CI, 0.63-0.93; $P = 0.009$), but the benefit was reduced by a nonsignificant increase in hemorrhagic stroke, with 51 versus 41 events (RR, 1.24; 95% CI, 0.82-1.87; $P = 0.31$).[120]

Patients aged 65 or older comprised 10% of the study population but experienced 30% of events. Analysis of this subgroup found a significant reduction in MI, ischemic stroke, and vascular death in the intervention group that was counterbalanced by an increase in gastrointestinal bleeding requiring transfusion.

In Diabetic Patients

Diabetic patients experience MI and cerebral ischemia at a rate of two to five times that of their age-and sex-matched counterparts. The role of aspirin in primary prevention in this susceptible patient group has been investigated in independent prospective trials, in subgroup analyses of other primary prevention trials, and in meta-analysis.

The Prevention of Progression of Arterial Disease and Diabetes (POPADAD) trial, a prospective population-based trial of antiplatelet agents in diabetic patients to prevent stroke and other vascular death, found no benefit for aspirin in the primary prevention of vascular events. A total of 1276 patients with type 1 or type 2 diabetes and asymptomatic peripheral vascular disease as determined by an ankle-brachial index of 0.99 or less were randomly assigned to aspirin or placebo and antioxidant or placebo in a 2 × 2 fashion. Over 6.7 years of follow-up, there was no significant difference in the number of primary vascular events between groups, with 116 in the aspirin group and 117 in the control group (HR, 0.98; 95% CI, 0.76–1.26). There was no significant benefit seen in the stroke subgroup, nor was there a difference seen when patients were subdivided by gender or by age older than or younger than 60.[123]

The Japanese Primary Prevention of Atherosclerosis with Aspirin for Diabetes (JPAD) trial enrolled 2539 diabetic patients without a history of atherosclerotic disease. Patients were randomly assigned to daily aspirin (81 to 100 mg), and the median follow-up was 4.37 years. With respect to the primary endpoints of MI, stroke, and peripheral vascular disease, there was no significant difference between groups (13.6 events/1000 patient-years in the aspirin group versus 17.0 in control group; HR, 0.80; $P = 0.16$). There was no significant difference in the rates of fatal and nonfatal ischemic stroke, nor was there a significant difference in composite rates of major bleeding.[124]

The rates of vascular events for both JPAD and POPADAD were much lower than predicted, which is an effect that the authors of POPADAD suggested may have been due to statin use. The ongoing Aspirin and Simvastatin Combination for Cardiovascular Events Prevention Trial in Diabetes (ACCEPT-D), which aims to enroll more than 5000 patients, may further clarify the role of aspirin versus placebo for primary prevention in diabetic patients taking daily simvastatin.[125]

Prevention of Early Stroke Recurrence

Aspirin given within 48 hours after an ischemic stroke has been documented to decrease stroke recurrence in two very large studies, the Chinese Acute Stroke Trial (CAST, 20,655 patients)[126] and the International Stroke Trial (IST, 19,435 patients).[127] In the CAST, patients were randomly assigned to receive either 160 mg/day aspirin or placebo starting within 48 hours of the stroke (in some, as early as 6 hours) and continuing for 4 weeks. Death or recurrent nonfatal stroke occurred in 5.3% of aspirin-treated patients and in 5.9% of patients receiving placebo, which translates into a significant absolute risk reduction (0.68%; $2P = 0.03$)—in other words, a decrease of seven strokes per 1000 patients treated. The absolute risk reduction for ischemic stroke (0.47%; $2P = 0.01$) was offset by a small excess of hemorrhagic strokes (0.21%; $2P > 0.1$), that is, 2 per 1000 patients treated.[126]

The IST examined the safety and efficacy of 300 mg/day aspirin, subcutaneous unfractionated heparin, or both drugs together in preventing recurrent stroke; treatment was started within 48 hours of the first ischemic event and continued for 14 days. Aspirin therapy in the IST led to an absolute reduction of 1.1% ($2P < 0.001$) for recurrent ischemic strokes without an increase in the risk of hemorrhagic stroke, although the risk of other bleeding rose significantly. Heparin use significantly increased the risk of hemorrhagic stroke or fatal extracranial bleeding, and although it did reduce the risk of recurrent ischemic stroke, this benefit was negated by an equal increase in hemorrhagic stroke. Functional status at 6 months was not altered by early poststroke use of aspirin in either CAST or IST.

A later analysis combined data from both CAST and IST to evaluate the effects of early aspirin use after ischemic stroke on the balance between reduced risk of recurrent ischemic stroke and risk of hemorrhagic stroke.[128] Among all treated subgroups examined, the absolute risk reduction of about seven recurrent ischemic strokes per 1000 was similar (1.6% recurrent strokes with aspirin versus 2.3% without aspirin; $2P < 0.01$), and the benefit from early aspirin treatment did not vary with respect to patient age or sex, level of consciousness, computed tomographic (CT) findings, blood pressure, stroke subtype, prognostic category, or concomitant heparin use. Neither AF nor treatment assignment without a prior CT scan (which occurred in 9000 patients, or 22%) altered the net benefit of aspirin treatment. The risk reduction for those taking aspirin was similar regardless of whether they also received heparin. Overall, there was an absolute decrease of four deaths per 1000 without further stroke, and the increase in hemorrhagic stroke averaged about two per 1000. In aspirin-treated patients, there was a 1.0% rate of hemorrhagic stroke or hemorrhagic transformation, whereas the placebo group had a rate of 0.8% ($2P = 0.07$). Extracranial bleeding that required transfusion was significantly more common in patients receiving aspirin, especially in those also receiving heparin (1.8% of those taking aspirin plus heparin versus 0.9% of those taking aspirin alone; excess bleeding occurred in 9 per 1000 treated; $2P = 0.0001$). Most of the cases of hemorrhage were nonfatal. Indeed, among 800 patients inadvertently randomly assigned to receive aspirin after a hemorrhagic stroke, there was no evidence of net hazard, including further stroke and death. The conclusions of this meta-analysis of the CAST and IST data are that low-dose aspirin started early after an acute ischemic stroke produces a definite reduction of recurrent ischemic stroke that is of net benefit to a wide range of patients. Of particular interest is that the benefit was also observed in patients who started aspirin therapy without a prior CT scan, who might have been expected to have a higher incidence of intracranial bleeding. Patients of both sexes, older patients, patients with AF, and hypertensive patients all benefited. It was also concluded that the reduction of further stroke or death from early aspirin use within 1 month of the first event compared favorably with the monthly benefits previously reported for long-term antiplatelet therapy.

In the Fast Assessment of Stroke and TIA to prevent Early Recurrence (FASTER) trial, patients with minor stroke or TIA were given antiplatelet therapy within 24 hours of symptom onset.[129] All patients enrolled received 81 mg of aspirin daily for the study duration, and patients received a loading dose of 162 mg if they were naive to aspirin before study enrollment. They were then randomly assigned to receive either placebo or a 300-mg clopidogrel loading dose immediately followed by 75 mg clopidogrel daily or to receive placebo or 40 mg simvastatin immediately followed by 40 mg daily in the evening. The primary endpoint of the study was total stroke (ischemic and hemorrhagic) within 90 days. Although the trial was prematurely terminated because of failure to recruit patients at the prespecified minimum enrollment rate, which was caused by a generalized use of statins in cardiovascular prevention, the results of this pilot study showed a reduction in stroke recurrence in patients who had received clopidogrel together with aspirin. In fact, 7.1% of patients treated with clopidogrel had a stroke within 90 days compared with 10.8% of patients in the placebo group (RR, 0.7; 95% CI, 0.3-1.2; absolute risk reduction −3.8%; 95% CI, −9.4 to 1.9; $P = 0.19$). Despite the increased rate of bleeding complications with clopidogrel, the authors concluded that in patients with minor stroke or TIA the addition of this drug to aspirin within 24 hours of onset might reduce the risk of stroke recurrence. The data come from a pilot study and thus cannot be taken as proof of clinical utility, but they do provide strong support for undertaking a large clinical trial.

The ongoing National Institutes of Health-National Institute of Neurological Diseases and Stroke (NIH-NINDS)–sponsored Platelet-Oriented Inhibition in New TIA and Minor Ischemic Stroke (POINT) Trial (NCT00991029) plans to enroll 5000 patients with minor stroke (NIH Stroke Scale < 3) or high-risk TIA (as determined by a simple clinical score of age, blood pressure, clinical features, symptom duration, and diabetes [ABCD2] > 4). This study may further clarify the benefit of short-term combined antiplatelet therapy. Patients receiving 50 mg to 325 mg aspirin daily are being randomly assigned within 12 hours of symptom onset to a 600-mg clopidogrel loading dose, then 75 mg daily, or placebo. The primary outcome is a composite of ischemic stroke, MI, or vascular death at 90 days. The trial started enrollment in early 2010 and is anticipated to be completed by 2016.[130]

Antiplatelet Agents in Secondary Prevention of Noncardioembolic Stroke

Antiplatelets in Comparison with Warfarin

To date, large trials have failed to show the superiority of warfarin over aspirin in secondary prevention of noncardioembolic stroke. Various INR targets have been investigated; the specific indication of intracranial stenosis has been studied, and the indication for high-risk aortic atheroma is currently under investigation.

The Stroke Prevention in Reversible Ischemia Trial (SPIRIT) compared 30 mg daily aspirin against high-target dose-adjusted warfarin (INR target, 3.0 to 4.5) in an open randomized trial. Over 14 months, 1316 patients were enrolled. Because of a high rate of hemorrhagic complications in the warfarin group, the study was terminated early: hemorrhagic events increased by a factor of 1.46 (95% CI, 0.96–2.13) for every increase in INR of 0.5. Major systemic and intracranial hemorrhage rates were 8.1% in the warfarin group and 1.0% in the aspirin group (HR, 9.3; 95% CI, 4.0–22). There was no significant difference between groups (4.1% in both groups; HR, 1.03; 95% CI, 0.6–1.75) in the number of ischemic events, including vascular death, nonfatal ischemic stroke, and nonfatal MI.[131]

More conservative INR targets have also failed to show a benefit for warfarin. The Warfarin–Aspirin Recurrent Stroke Study (WARSS), which compared dose-adjusted warfarin with an INR target of 1.4 to 2.8 with 325 mg daily aspirin in 2206 patients without a cardioembolic source, perioperative stroke, or carotid stenosis requiring operative intervention, found no significant difference between death or recurrent stroke or major hemorrhage in the two groups. The daily INR remained within the target range for 70.7% of patients; 16.3% of INR values were subtherapeutic.[132]

Warfarin with an INR target of 2.0 to 3.0 was compared with 30 to 325 mg daily aspirin in the European and Australasian Stroke Prevention in Reversible Ischemia Trial (ESPRIT). In a separate arm, aspirin was compared with or without 200 mg twice daily dipyridamole. Treatment was randomized but open; outcome event assessment was blinded. A total of 1068 patients with stroke or TIA were enrolled within 6 months of their index event. After combination antiplatelet therapy was found to be more effective than aspirin monotherapy, the warfarin versus aspirin monotherapy arm was terminated early. Patients were within the INR target 70% of the time, and the median INR was 2.57. There was no significant difference found in the rate of primary outcomes of nonfatal stroke, MI, vascular death, or major bleeding in the aspirin group as compared with warfarin, with an 18% event rate in the aspirin group and a 19% event rate in the warfarin group (HR, 1.02; 95% CI, 0.77–1.35). There was a nonsignificant trend toward a lower rate of ischemic stroke in the warfarin group (7.6% versus 10.0%; HR, 0.76; 95% CI, 0.51–1.15), which was counterbalanced by a significantly higher rate of major bleeding in this group (8.4% versus 3.4%; HR, 2.56; 95% CI, 1.48–4.43). In post-hoc analysis, there were no significant differences between the combination antiplatelet group and the warfarin group (HR, 1.31; 95% CI, 0.98–1.75).[133]

The Warfarin-Aspirin Symptomatic Intracranial Disease (WASID) trial compared high-dose daily aspirin (1300 mg) with dose-adjusted warfarin with an INR target of 2.0 to 3.0 for secondary stroke prevention in 569 patients with intracranial stenosis of 50% to 99%. There was no significant difference in the recurrent stroke rate: 22.1% recurrence rate over 1.8 years of follow-up in the aspirin group and 21.8% in the warfarin group

(HR, 1.04; 95% CI, 0.73–1.48). Enrollment was stopped early because of high rates of adverse events in the patients receiving warfarin, including death (4.3% in the aspirin group versus 9.7% in the warfarin group; HR, 0.46; 95% CI, 0.23–0.90; $P = 0.02$), major hemorrhage (3.2% versus 8.3%; HR, 0.39; 95% CI, 0.18–0.84; $P = 0.01$), and MI and sudden death (2.9 versus 7.3%; HR, 0.40; 95% CI, 0.18–0.91; $P = 0.02$). Warfarin patients were within the target range 63% of the time.[134]

Antiplatelets as Monotherapy and in Combination for Secondary Stroke Prevention

Commonly utilized antiplatelet drugs are aspirin, dipyridamole, and clopidogrel. Aspirin is an irreversible inhibitor of cyclooxygenase-1, which in turn inhibits the formation of TXA_2. Dipyridamole increases cAMP by inhibiting platelet phosphodiesterase E5. Clopidogrel is a thienopyridine $P2Y_{12}$-ADP receptor blocker.

Antiplatelet drugs under investigation include cilostazol, an inhibitor of TXA_2 and phosphodiesterase 3; triflusal, a cyclooxygenase-1 inhibitor; sarpogrelate, a 5-hydroxytryptamine receptor agonist; and terutroban, a thromboxane–prostaglandin receptor antagonist.

Several large trials comparing alternative antiplatelet therapies have demonstrated a modest benefit in favor of clopidogrel or combination aspirin and dipyridamole over aspirin for long-term secondary stroke prevention. In direct comparison, combination aspirin and dipyridamole failed to demonstrate noninferiority to clopidogrel, mainly because of problems with tolerability. The minimal benefits of the alternatives over aspirin in addition to their higher cost and tolerability issues allows aspirin to remain the most commonly prescribed first-line antiplatelet for secondary prevention. Combination aspirin and clopidogrel has not proven to be superior to aspirin monotherapy for secondary prevention but is still under investigation for specific indications including subcortical stroke and for short-term secondary prevention immediately after the index event.

Aspirin. In meta-analysis by the ATTC, aspirin was associated with a 23% reduction in the combined events of stroke, MI, and vascular death. Aspirin was associated with a 22% reduction in stroke in secondary prevention trials (2.08% versus 2.54% per year; RR, 0.78; 0.61–0.99, $P = 0.002$). There was a nonsignificant increase in hemorrhagic stroke in the aspirin group.[122]

Aspirin has been shown to be effective in secondary prevention of ischemic events in doses from 30 to 1300 mg daily.[51,62,135,136] Higher doses cause an increased rate of gastrointestinal upset, peptic ulcer disease, and gastrointestinal bleeding.

Aspirin + dipyridamole. The European Stroke Prevention Study (ESPS)-2 randomly assigned patients with ischemic stroke or TIA into one of four groups with twice-daily dosing within 3 months after their index event: placebo, 25 mg aspirin, 200 mg ERDP, or combination aspirin and dipyridamole (aspirin-ERDP, same dose and formulation). A total of 6602 patients were followed up for 2 years. The stroke rate in the placebo group was 15.8%. Both aspirin and dipyridamole were independently associated with a reduced rate of stroke (12.9%: odds ratio [OR], 0.79; 95% CI, 0.65–0.97; 13.2%: OR, 0.81; 95% CI, 0.67–0.99, respectively); the effect was most marked in the combination group (9.9%: OR, 0.59; 95% CI, 0.48–0.73), with a 23% relative risk reduction and 3% absolute risk reduction in stroke between the aspirin monotherapy and the combination group over 2 years of follow-up.[102]

Aspirin monotherapy was compared with aspirin-ERDP in the ESPRIT trial, the results of which echoed that of ESPS-2. A separate arm, already discussed, examined warfarin for secondary prevention. Patients were randomly assigned to 30 to 325 mg aspirin daily with or without 200 mg ERDP twice daily within 6 months of stroke or TIA. A total of 2739 patients were followed up over a mean of 3.5 years. The median aspirin dose was 75 mg, although 44% took 30 mg. There were major ischemic events (vascular death, nonfatal ischemic stroke, and nonfatal MI) in 12.6% of the aspirin group and in 10.3% of the combination group. The absolute risk reduction of major ischemic events was 7% in the combination group (aspirin: HR, 0.81; 95% CI, 0.65–1.01; aspirin-ERDP: HR, 0.88; 95% CI, 0.69–1.02). There was no significant difference in the rates of major bleeding between the two groups (RR, 1.03; 95% CI, 0.84–1.25), although a larger proportion (34%) of the combination group discontinued therapy, mostly because of headaches.[103]

Clopidogrel. The Clopidogrel versus Aspirin in Patients at Risk of Ischaemic Events (CAPRIE) trial investigated the effects of clopidogrel. A total of 19,185 patients with a history of stroke, MI, or peripheral vascular disease were randomly assigned to 75 mg daily clopidogrel or 325 mg aspirin. Over a mean follow-up of 1.91 years, the annual rate of nonfatal stroke, nonfatal MI, and vascular death was 5.83% in the aspirin group and 5.32% in the clopidogrel group (relative risk reduction [RRR], 0.087; 95% CI, 0.003–0.165; $P = 0.043$). In the stroke subgroup, however, this trend was not significant. The annual rate of vascular events was 7.71% in the aspirin group and 7.15% in the clopidogrel group (RRR, 0.073; 95% CI, −0.057–0.187; $P = 0.26$). There was no significant difference in major hemorrhage rates between groups.[137]

Aspirin + dipyridamole versus clopidogrel. Before the Prevention Regimen for Effectively Avoiding Second Strokes (PRoFESS) trial, a study designed to test the noninferiority of aspirin-ERDP against clopidogrel for secondary stroke prevention, the only means of comparing the efficacy of the two regimens was through the indirect comparison of their performance in previous trials against aspirin. In a 2 × 2 factorial double-blinded trial, 20,332 patients were randomly assigned to 75 mg daily clopidogrel or 25 to 200 mg twice-daily aspirin-ERDP in combination with telmisartan or placebo. The mean follow-up was 2.5 years. Recurrent stroke occurred in 9.0% of patients in the aspirin-ERDP group and in 8.8% of the clopidogrel group (HR, 1.01; 95% CI, 0.92–1.11). Stroke, MI, and vascular death occurred at 13.1% (HR, 0.99; 95% CI, 0.92–1.07; RRR, 1%; 95% CI, 7%–8%). Major hemorrhage rates, including intracranial hemorrhage, were higher in the aspirin-ERDP group (HR, 1.15; 95% CI, 1.00–1.32). Rates of discontinuation were higher with aspirin-EDRP than with clopidogrel (29.1% versus 22.6%; 6.5% difference; 95% CI, 5.3%–7.7%), most often because of headache[104] (Table 58-3).

TABLE 58-3 RECENT RANDOMIZED CLINICAL TRIALS TESTING ANTIPLATELET AGENTS FOR SECONDARY STROKE PREVENTION

Study	Year of Completion	Sample Size	Intervention	Results
ESPS-2	1996	6602	ASA 25 mg bid vs. ERDP 200 mg bid vs. ASA–ERDP 25/200 mg bid vs. placebo	ASA-ERDP vs. placebo: 24% RRR ASA-ERDP vs. ASA: 13% RRR Primary outcome: stroke/death
CAPRIE	1996	19,185*	ASA 325 mg vs. clopidogrel 75 mg	Clopidogrel vs. ASA: 9% RRR Primary outcome: stroke/MI/vascular death
MATCH	2004	7599	Clopidogrel 75 mg vs. ASA + clopidogrel	Nonsignificant difference Primary outcome: stroke/MI/vascular death
ESPRIT	2006	2739	ASA 30-325 mg vs. ASA/ ERDP 30-325/200 mg bid	ASA + EDRP vs. ASA: 20% HR Primary outcome: vascular death, stroke, major bleeding
CHARISMA	2006	15,603#	ASA 75-162 mg vs. ASA + clopidogrel 75 mg qd	No significant difference Primary outcome: MI, stroke, vascular death
PRoFESS	2008	20,332	ASA-ERDP 25-200 mg bid vs. clopidogrel 75 mg	No significant difference Primary outcome: stroke

ASA, Acetylsalicylic acid; bid, twice a day; CAPRIE, Clopidogrel versus Aspirin in Patients at Risk of Ischaemic Events [trial]; CHARISMA, Clopidogrel for High Atherothrombotic Risk and Ischemic Stabilization, Management, and Avoidance; ERDP, extended-release dipyridamole; ESPRIT, European and Australasian Stroke Prevention in Reversible Ischemia Trial; ESPS, European Stroke Prevention Study; HR, hazard ratio; MATCH, Management of Atherothrombosis with Clopidogrel in High-Risk Patients with Recent Transient Ischaemic Attack or Ischaemic Stroke; MI, myocardial infarction; PRoFESS, Prevention Regimen for Effectively Avoiding Second Strokes; qd, every day; RRR, relative risk reduction.

Antiplatelet Agents in Secondary Prevention of Cardioembolic Stroke

Oral anticoagulants remain the treatment of choice for secondary prevention of cardioembolic stroke. Antiplatelet therapy, however, provides an alternative when oral anticoagulation is contraindicated or when patient choice or compliance limits choice of therapy.

The superiority of warfarin over combination antiplatelet therapy for stroke prevention in nonvalvular AF has been shown in several trials and in meta-analyses. A meta-analysis of 29 trials incorporating 28,044 patients found a 64% reduction in stroke in the warfarin group as compared with 22% (95% CI, 0.49-0.74) in the antiplatelet groups (95% CI, 0.06-0.35) for a relatively risk reduction of 39% (95% CI, 0.22-0.52).[138] The Atrial Fibrillation Clopidogrel Trial with Irbesartan for Prevention of Vascular Events (ACTIVE)-W trial, which compared warfarin to combination aspirin-clopidogrel in 6706 patients, was terminated early because of a clear benefit in the warfarin group, who had a 3.93% annual event rate versus 5.60% in the control group (RR, 1.44; 95% CI, 1.18-1.76; $P = 0.0003$).[139]

The ACTIVE-A trial enrolled patients with cardioembolic stroke deemed unsuitable for warfarin therapy because of risk of bleeding, physician's judgment, or patient preference. The effects of combination aspirin and clopidogrel versus aspirin and placebo on secondary stroke prevention were compared in 7554 patients over a mean follow-up of 3.6 years. The majority of patients had no history of cerebrovascular disease; 13.2% of patients in the clopidogrel group and 13% of control patients had a history of stroke or TIA. The clopidogrel group experienced major vascular events at a rate of 6.8% per year, as compared with 7.6% per year in the control group (RR, 0.89; 95% CI, 0.81-0.98). The risk reduction was largely due to a significant reduction of ischemic strokes, with rates of 1.9% versus 2.8% per year in the clopidogrel and control groups, respectively (RR, 0.68; 95% CI, 0.57-0.80). This therapeutic benefit, however, was greatly reduced by rates of systemic and intracranial hemorrhages. Annual rates of any major bleeding in the clopidogrel and control groups, respectively, were 2.0% versus 1.3% (RR, 1.57; 95% CI, 1.29-1.92), and rates of intracranial bleeding were 0.4% versus 0.2% (RR, 1.87; 95% CI, 1.19-2.94).[140]

Combinations of Antiplatelet Agents

Aspirin and Thienopyridines

Given that aspirin and the thienopyridines have quite different modes of action, there has been considerable interest in combining these drugs to improve antiplatelet activity. In particular, there has recently been a significant increase in the simultaneous use of aspirin and clopidogrel.[141] However, completed studies in which aspirin and clopidogrel have been combined are few and mainly concern acute cardiac procedures rather than stroke prevention.[142]

Ischemic Strokes

Favorable results of combination aspirin-clopidogrel for prevention of vascular events in patients with percutaneous coronary intervention in the PCI-CURE and TRITON-TIMI 38 trials and acute MI in the CURE and CREDO trials prompted an interest in investigating this combination in other types of vascular disease.

Clopidogrel (75 mg daily) and placebo versus aspirin-clopidogrel (75/75 mg daily) were compared in the

Management of Atherothrombosis with Clopidogrel in High-Risk Patients with Recent Transient Ischaemic Attack or Ischaemic Stroke (MATCH) trial. A total of 7599 patients with previous stroke or TIA and at least one other vascular risk factor were randomly assigned and followed up for 18 months. Nearly a third were randomly assigned more than 1 month after their index event. There was no significant difference in the two groups with regard to all ischemic strokes (11% in both groups; RRR, 0.066; 95% CI, −0.07-0.185; $P = 0.324$), nor was there a difference in the combined endpoints of nonfatal stroke, nonfatal MI, or vascular death (12% in both groups; RRR, 0.059; 95% CI, −0.071-0.173; $P = 0.360$). The rates of major and life-threatening bleeding (1.3% versus 2.6%; AR increase, 1.3%; 95% CI, 0.6-1.9) were significantly increased in the aspirin-clopidogrel group, although there was no increase in rates of mortality.[143]

The Clopidogrel for High Atherothrombotic Risk and Ischemic Stabilization, Management, and Avoidance (CHARISMA) trial randomly assigned 15,603 patients with a history of vascular disease or multiple vascular risk factors to daily aspirin (75 to 162 mg) and placebo or combination aspirin-clopidogrel (75 mg to 162/75 mg). Over the 5 years before enrollment, 27% of patients had a history of stroke and 10% of patients had a history of TIA. Rates of MI, stroke, or vascular death were 7.3% in the control group and 6.8% in the aspirin-clopidogrel group (RR, 0.93; 95% CI, 0.83-1.05; $P = 0.22$). There was a nonsignificant trend toward a reduction in ischemic events in the subgroup with previous stroke (HR, 0.13, 95% CI). There was a nonsignificant reduction in nonfatal ischemic stroke (2.1% control, 1.7% clopidogrel; RR, 0.81; 95% CI, 0.64-1.02; $P = 0.07$) and a significant reduction in all nonfatal stroke in the clopidogrel group (2.4% control, 1.9% clopidogrel; RR, 0.79; 95% CI, 0.64-0.98; $P = 0.03$). Dual antiplatelet therapy was associated with a nonsignificant increase in severe and fatal bleeding and a significant increase in moderate bleeding (1.3% control, 2.1% clopidogrel; RR, 1.62; 95% CI, 1.27-2.08; $P < 0.001$). In the asymptomatic subgroup, there was an unanticipated increase in ischemic events and vascular death in addition to the significant increase in severe bleeding in this group. The phenomenon is yet to be fully explained. Proposed explanations have included a higher proportion of diabetic patients in this group and a theoretical risk of platelet hyperaggregability with medication noncompliance.[97]

Based on the results of the MATCH and CHARISMA trials, the combination of aspirin-clopidogrel should not be routinely indicated for secondary stroke prevention.

The ongoing NIH-NINDS Secondary Prevention of Small Subcortical Strokes (SPS3) (www.sps3.org) trial,[130] is investigating whether daily combination aspirin-clopidogrel (325/75 mg) is superior to aspirin monotherapy for reducing stroke, cognitive decline, and major vascular events in 3000 patients with lacunar stroke. Patients are also being randomly assigned in a 2 × 2 factorial design to two targets of blood pressure control: "usual" (systolic, 130 to 149 mm Hg) or "intensive" (<130 mm Hg). At present the study has enrolled 2700 participants, and the final results are anticipated by mid-2012.

Carotid Endarterectomy and Carotid Artery Stenting

On the basis of the results of the Aspirin and Carotid Endarterectomy (ACE) trial,[56] it is recommended that patients undergoing carotid endarterectomy receive 81 to 325 mg aspirin. Recent data suggest that dual antiplatelet therapy in the preoperative phase of patients undergoing this procedure may be more effective in the reduction of vascular events than aspirin alone. In a study including 100 patients randomly assigned to receive aspirin and concomitant clopidogrel or placebo before carotid endarterectomy, the association of clopidogrel and aspirin reduced the platelet response to ADP by 8.8% while conferring a tenfold decrease in the RR of those patients having more than 20 emboli in the postoperative period. Moreover, this reduction in risk occurred without a significant increase in the risk of bleeding complications.[144] More recently, Markus et al have also reported that combination clopidogrel-aspirin therapy is more effective than aspirin alone in reducing asymptomatic embolization in patients with a recent diagnosis of symptomatic carotid stenosis.[145] Dual antiplatelet therapy was reported to reduce the number of microembolic signals (MES) (RR reduction, 39.8%; 95% CI, 13.8-58.0; $P = 0.0046$) as well as the frequency of MES per hour both at day 2 (RR reduction, 61.6%; 95% CI, 34.9-77.4; $P = 0.0005$) and day 7 (RR reduction, 61.4%; 95% CI, 31.6-78.2; $P = .0013$) of randomization. Moreover, the frequency of stroke and TIA was also lower in the group receiving clopidogrel-aspirin: there were four recurrent strokes and seven TIAs in the monotherapy group compared with no stroke and four TIAs in the dual-therapy group.

With respect to the efficacy of associating thienopyridines and aspirin in patients undergoing carotid artery stenting (CAS), dual antiplatelet therapy also seems to be associated with lower rates of ischemic events. In a study by Bhatt et al, results with clopidogrel-aspirin in 139 consecutive patients undergoing this procedure at a single center were compared with those in 23 similar patients who received ticlopidine-aspirin.[146] The cumulative 30-day rate of death, stroke, TIA, or MI was 5.6% in patients who received an ADP antagonist (clopidogrel or ticlopidine) and aspirin. There were no cases of stent thrombosis in patients who were treated with clopidogrel/ticlopidine and aspirin, but one of five patients who did not receive an ADP antagonist did develop in-stent thrombosis. Dual antiplatelet therapy did not increase the incidence of bleeding events. When the association of ticlopidine or clopidogrel with aspirin was compared, the 30-day rate of death, stroke, TIA, or MI was significantly higher in patients receiving clopidogrel-aspirin than in those receiving ticlopidine-aspirin (4.3% versus 13%; $P = 0.01$). Although these data might suggest that the use of clopidogrel-aspirin in patients with CAS is associated with a low rate of ischemic events and that clopidogrel might be better than ticlopidine in this high-risk group, these are the results of a small, unblinded study, so caution is important. McKevitt et al[147] also carried out a clinical trial comparing aspirin and 24-hour heparin with aspirin-clopidogrel for patients undergoing CAS; they found that the frequency of neurologic complications was much higher in the heparin group than in the clopidogrel group

(25% versus 0%, $P = 0.02$). The 30-day 50% to 100% stenosis rates were also higher in the heparin group, although the differences did not reach statistical significance. Bleeding complications were also similar in both groups. More recently, Dalainas et al[148] reported the results of a study comparing two groups of 50 patients each undergoing CAS who were randomly assigned to receive heparin for 24 hours together with 325 mg of aspirin or 250 mg ticlopidine twice a day together with 325 mg of aspirin. Neurologic complications were significantly more frequent at day 30 in the group with heparin (16% versus 2%, $P < 0.05$); there were no significant differences in the rates of bleeding complications or thrombosis/occlusion between the two groups of treatment.

Similar to the recommendation in patients undergoing percutaneous coronary intervention, the presented data support the administration of dual antiplatelet therapy for patients undergoing CAS. With regard to the duration of dual antiplatelet therapy, it seems that, beyond the periprocedural period, the prolongation of this therapy might also be beneficial in patients undergoing CAS,[149] although additional studies are necessary to determine the optimal duration.

Antiplatelet Agents and Anticoagulants

Anticoagulation has traditionally been used to prevent cardioembolic stroke in patients with AF. Several Stroke Prevention in Atrial Fibrillation (SPAF) trials have compared both the efficacy and safety of aspirin and warfarin. Results of SPAF I suggested that warfarin was more effective, but the overall number of cerebral ischemic events was small, which makes interpretation difficult.[150,151] SPAF II examined age effects of these two regimens (warfarin to maintain INR at 2.0 to 4.5 or 325 mg aspirin per day) in patients younger than and older than 75 years in the prevention of ischemic stroke and systemic embolism.[3] The absolute rate of the primary events varied with age. In treated low-risk patients younger than 75 years, the primary event rate per year was 1.3% for those taking warfarin and 1.9% for those taking aspirin (RR, 0.67; $P = 0.24$). In treated patients older than 75 years, the primary event rate was 3.6% per year with warfarin and 4.8% with aspirin (RR, 0.73; $P = 0.39$). However, for the older group, despite greater effectiveness of anticoagulation in preventing thromboembolic stroke, the rate per year of all strokes (ischemic plus hemorrhagic) with residual deficit was 4.6% with warfarin and 4.3% with aspirin. Thus, although warfarin may be more effective than aspirin for preventing ischemic stroke in older patients with AF or in high-risk younger patients, the overall rate of stroke in warfarin-treated patients remains high, reflecting bleeding complications due to the intervention itself. These results in patients with AF are similar to those observed several decades ago in the Sixty Plus Reinfarction Study, in which elderly patients who received anticoagulation therapy after one MI were observed to have fewer ischemic strokes but more hemorrhagic strokes, so that no net benefit in stroke prevention resulted, whereas the incidence of recurrent MI was clearly decreased.[152]

Many clinical trials have assessed whether the combination of an antiplatelet agent with an anticoagulant improves secondary protection against stroke, but the results have been disappointing. Either no benefit has ensued, or the combination results in increased intracerebral bleeding, negating the benefit. Dose is an important consideration in these studies. For example, the Coumadin Aspirin Reinfarction Study (CARS, 2028 subjects) showed that fixed-dose warfarin (1 or 3 mg) plus aspirin (80 mg/day) after an MI was no better than aspirin alone for the prevention of recurrent MI, stroke, or cardiovascular death.[55] In particular, the incidence of ischemic stroke was lower in patients treated with 160 mg aspirin per day than in those treated with 1 mg warfarin plus 80 mg aspirin per day (0.6% versus 1.1%; $P = 0.0534$). The highest risk group, male patients with Q-wave MI, had greater benefit from aspirin alone. This clinical trial was prematurely discontinued for lack of efficacy.

In SPAF III (1085 subjects), patients with AF who had at least one thromboembolic risk factor had a worse outcome if they took a combination of fixed-dose warfarin plus aspirin than if they took adjusted-dose warfarin alone.[153] This trial was stopped because of the higher rate of strokes and systemic embolism in the combined-therapy group (7.9% per year) compared with the adjusted-dose warfarin group (1.9% per year), although the incidences of bleeding were similar in the two groups.

More recently, the results from the Stroke Prevention Using Oral Thrombin Inhibitor in Atrial Fibrillation (SPORTIF) program, which was designed to investigate the safety and efficacy of ximelagatran for the prevention of stroke in patients with AF, also seem to demonstrate the lack of efficacy of the association of aspirin and warfarin in these patients. Data about concurrent medications were available from 7304 patients. Of these, aspirin was prescribed to 531 patients in the ximelagatran group and 481 patients in the warfarin group, which allowed comparison between four different groups of treatment at baseline: ximelagatran (n = 3120), ximelagatran-aspirin (n = 531), warfarin (n = 3172), and warfarin-aspirin (n = 481). After adjustment for baseline differences, aspirin use during therapy with either ximelagatran or warfarin was not associated with reduced rates of either primary events or stroke as an isolated endpoint. With respect to bleeding, there was significant interaction between aspirin use and therapy with either warfarin or ximelagatran, and the combination of warfarin and aspirin was associated with particularly high risk. The use of aspirin with warfarin was independently associated with an increased risk of major bleeding (HR, 1.58; 95% CI, 1.01–2.49; $P = 0.05$), yet major bleeding was not increased by the combination of aspirin with ximelagatran. When overall (major and minor) bleeding was considered, aspirin was associated with an increased risk when given in combination with either ximelagatran or warfarin.[154]

Risk stratification of patients with nonvalvular AF indicates that patients who can be prospectively identified as having a low risk of stroke, particularly disabling ischemic stroke, benefit from aspirin therapy and so may not require anticoagulation with its higher adverse event rates. Specifically, in patients with AF who have no history of hypertension and none of the following four thromboembolic risk factors, the ischemic stroke risk is no greater than that of the general population of similar age (namely, ≈1%/year): (1) recent congestive heart failure or left ventricular dysfunction, (2) prior thromboembolism, (3) systolic blood pressure higher than 160 mm Hg, and (4) female sex and age greater than 75 years. Although patients with nonvalvular AF are usually considered to be at increased risk of cardioembolic stroke—for which anticoagulation is clearly indicated—they may also be at risk of ischemic stroke. Further modulating factors for stroke risk in patients from the aspirin-only arm of SPAF trials I through III (2012 subjects) were consumption of 14 or more alcoholic drinks per week (decreased stroke risk), prior stroke or TIA (increased stroke risk), and estrogen hormone replacement therapy (increased stroke risk).[155] So far, there is no evidence that combining anticoagulation with an antiplatelet agent reduces the risk of stroke compared with anticoagulant therapy alone in patients with AF.[156]

The combination of anticoagulants with antiplatelet drugs has been beneficial in several clinical settings that do not directly involve the cerebral circulation, heart valve replacements, coronary stent thrombolysis, or angioplasty.[157] Benefit in terms of reduced mortality rates, especially from vascular causes, and decreased embolic rates, without a severe increase in bleeding, was achieved in the patients with prosthetic heart valves.[158] A comparison of the results of four separate trials of patients treated with aspirin (doses between 75 and 1000 mg/day combined with moderate anticoagulation to an INR of 1.5 to 4.5) indicated that the rate of bleeding complications correlated more with a higher aspirin dose than with INR level, which suggested that the aspirin dose should be kept low if the combination is to be used.[159] However, later studies have clearly shown that this combination cannot be used for stroke prevention without incurring unacceptable rates of intracerebral hemorrhage. In the current American Heart Association guidelines for the prevention of stroke, adding aspirin (81 mg daily) is recommended for patients with ischemic stroke or TIA with rheumatic mitral valve disease, regardless of whether AF is present, and a recurrent embolism while receiving warfarin.[156] For patients with mechanical prosthetic heart valves who have an ischemic stroke or systemic embolism despite adequate therapy with oral anticoagulants, 75 to 100 mg/day aspirin in addition to oral anticoagulants and maintenance of the INR at a target of 3.0 (range, 2.5 to 3.5) is a reasonable treatment.[156]

Other Antiplatelet Agents

Current data suggest that triflusal, cilostazol, and sarpogrelate have shown equal efficacy to aspirin, although their performance in phase 3 trials has yet to be seen.

A meta-analysis of five trials comparing 325 mg aspirin daily with triflusal for secondary prevention of stroke and TIA (four trials, 2944 patients; follow-up, 6-47 months) or MI (one trial, 2275 patients; follow-up, 35 days) showed no significant difference in the number of serious vascular events (OR, 1.04; 95% CI, 0.87-1.23). Triflusal had a lower risk of major (OR for aspirin, 2.34; 95% CI, 1.58-3.46) and minor hemorrhage (OR for aspirin, 1.60; 95% CI, 1.31-1.95) but more nonhemorrhagic adverse gastrointestinal events than aspirin (OR for aspirin, 0.84; 95% CI, 0.75-0.95).[160]

Cilostazol has been investigated in two trials for secondary stroke prevention. The first, which randomly assigned 1067 patients with ischemic stroke, compared cilostazol with placebo and found a 41.7% reduction in ischemic stroke (3.37%/year in cilostazol, 5.78% placebo; 95% CI, 10.3%–62.9%; P = 0.0127).[161] The second, which compared 100 mg daily aspirin with 100 mg twice daily cilostazol, had 720 patients enrolled in a pilot study within 1 to 6 months of their index event who were then followed up for 12 to 18 months. There was no significant difference in rates of recurrent stroke (HR, 0.62; 95% CI, 0.30-1.26; P = 0.185) between the treatment groups. There were more intracranial hemorrhages in patients who were taking aspirin (seven aspirin versus one cilostazol; P = 0.034).[105]

The Sarpogrelate-Aspirin Comparative Clinical Study for Efficacy and Safety in Secondary Prevention of Cerebral Infarction (S-ACCESS) trial randomly assigned 1510 patients with stroke within 1 week to 6 months after their event. Patients received 100 mg S three times a day or 81 mg daily aspirin and were followed up for a mean of 1.59 years. There was no significant difference in the number of strokes (6.09%/year S, 4.86%/year aspirin; HR, 1.25; 95% CI, 0.89-1.77; P = 0.19) or vascular events in either group (7.61%/year S, 7.12%/year aspirin; HR, 1.07; 95% CI, 0.80-1.44; P = 0.65). There were fewer hemorrhagic events in the S group (11.9% S, 17.3% aspirin; P < 0.01).[162]

The Prevention of Cerebrovascular and Cardiovascular Events of Ischemic Origin with Terutroban in Patients with a History of Ischemic Stroke or Transient Ischemic Attack (PERFORM) trial investigated the antiplatelet agent terutroban in prevention of stroke, MI, or vascular death. Patients with an index TIA within 8 days or stroke within 3 months were randomly assigned to either 100 mg day aspirin or to 30 mg of the thromboxane–prostanoid receptor agonist.[163,164]

Antiplatelet and Cerebral Microbleeds

Although the benefit of antiplatelet agents for the secondary prevention of stroke has been clearly demonstrated, it is also good evidence for the increased risk of hemorrhagic complications related to the administration of antiaggregants. Cerebral microbleeds (CMB) are deposits of hemosiderin in the brain that are identified in T2*-weighted gradient-echo magnetic resonance imaging (MRI) sequences because they are residues of small hemorrhages.[165,166] They are currently regarded as evidence of small artery disease[167,168] because they are associated with leukoaraiosis and frequently observed in patients with recurrent ischemic and hemorrhagic strokes.[169,170] Moreover, previous use of antithrombotic drugs has been found to be an independent factor for the presence of CMB.[171,172]

Because of the increased risk of hemorrhagic side effects including intracranial hemorrhage (ICH), considerable debate has occurred about the possible increased risk of ICH in patients with CMB who are also receiving antiplatelet therapy. CMB prevalence rates are more than 10 times higher among patients with spontaneous ICH. There is some evidence for a topographic association of lobar and nonlobar ICH with the distribution of

CMB, which suggests that CMB and ICH share an etiologic basis; that is, CMB represents indicators of imminent ICH.[173] Two prospective studies with baseline and follow-up T2*-weighted MRI have reported data about the significance of CMBs for the future development of ICH. In the study of Fan et al,[174] 121 patients with acute ischemic stroke were followed up for a mean of 27 months. Among them, 36% were found to have CMBs, and five patients developed ICH during the follow-up period (all taking antithrombotic medication). Four of the five patients had CMBs at the baseline MRI study, and in two cases the ICH was located at the same sites where the CMBs had been found. Greenberg et al[175] studied 94 consecutive survivors of primary lobar ICH who had been studied with gradient-echo MRI sequences. Seventeen of 34 patients who had a second MRI after a stroke-free interval of 15.6 months were found to have new CMBs, and the authors found that these were associated with an increased risk of subsequent symptomatic ICH (3-year cumulative risk: 19%, 42%, and 67% for subjects with 0, 1 to 3, or ≥4 CMBs; $P = 0.02$). A case-control study by Wong et al[176] investigated whether asymptomatic CMBs were a risk factor for ICH among aspirin users in a Chinese population. Twenty-one patients with ICH and 21 controls with no ICH were compared. CMBs were present in 19 patients (90%) with ICH, whereas only seven patients (33%) in the control group were found to have CMBs ($P < 0.001$). Moreover, the number of CMBs was also significantly higher in the group of patients with ICH (mean number of CMBs, 13 versus 0.2; $P < 0.001$). On the other hand, patients with CMBs also have a higher risk of recurrent ischemic stroke,[177] which might be decreased by the use of antiplatelets; thus, larger studies are needed to confirm these data. So far, recommendations about the use of antithrombotic therapy based on the detection of CMBs are not justified.

Conclusions

Effective primary prevention of stroke depends chiefly on risk factor management. However, based on the current data, aspirin can be considered for primary prevention in women older than 65 years who are at a risk of ischemic events that exceeds their risk of intracranial or extracranial hemorrhage. Aspirin has not been shown to be of significant benefit in primary prevention of stroke in men or in diabetic patients.

Antiplatelet drugs are the current gold standard for secondary prevention of noncardioembolic stroke. There is no current indication for anticoagulants in secondary prevention of atherothrombotic stroke. Aspirin (50 to 325 mg/day) is commonly used given its lower cost, although clopidogrel and aspirin-ERDP are also acceptable options. Clopidogrel is better tolerated than aspirin and offers greater benefit in noncerebrovascular events. Aspirin-ERDP is superior to aspirin alone in preventing stroke recurrence; however, it may be more poorly tolerated than aspirin-clopidogrel. There is no current indication for long-term combination of aspirin-ERDP plus clopidogrel or aspirin-clopidogrel use in atherothrombotic stroke, although the use of combination aspirin-clopidogrel is under investigation

for short-term use and long-term secondary prevention in patients with lacunar stroke. Tests for resistance to aspirin and clopidogrel are not standardized, and their results are not yet validated. Therefore, selection of an antiplatelet agent should not be based on the results of these tests.

Oral anticoagulants are the gold standard for secondary prevention of cardioembolic stroke, although aspirin-clopidogrel confers additional protection over aspirin alone in patients with nonvalvular AF who are not suitable for anticoagulation.

REFERENCES

1. Donnan GA, Fisher M, Macleod M, Davis SM: Stroke. *Lancet* 371(9624):1612-1223, 2008.
2. Antiplatelet Trialists' Collaboration : Collaborative overview of randomised trials of antiplatelet therapy. I: Prevention of death, myocardial infarction and stroke by prolonged antiplatelet therapy in various categories of patients, *BMJ* 308:81-106, 1994.
3. Stroke Prevention in Atrial Fibrillation Investigators: Warfarin versus aspirin for prevention of thromboembolism in atrial fibrillation: Stroke Prevention in Atrial Fibrillation II study, *Lancet* 343:687, 1994.
4. Bousser M-G: Antithrombotic strategy in stroke, *Thromb Haemost* 86:1, 2001.
5. Andrews RK, Shen Y, Gardiner EE, et al: The glycoprotein Ib-IX-V complex in platelet adhesion and signaling, *Thromb Haemost* 82:357, 1999.
6. Fitzgerald DJ: Vascular biology of thrombosis: The role of platelet-vessel wall adhesion, *Neurology* 57:S1, 2001.
7. Shattil SJ, Brass LP: Induction of the fibrinogen receptor on human platelets by intracellular mediators, *J Biol Chem* 262:992, 1987.
8. Plow EF, Cieniewski CS, Xiao Z, et al: $\alpha_{11b}\beta_3$ and its antagonism at the new millennium, *Thromb Haemost* 86:34, 2001.
9. Coughlin SR: Thrombin signalling and protease-activated receptors, *Nature* 407:258, 2000.
10. Gachet C: ADP receptors of platelets and their inhibition, *Thromb Haemost* 86:222, 2001.
11. Hollopeter G, Jntwen HM, Vincent D, et al: Identification of the platelet ADP receptor targeted by antithrombotic drugs, *Nature* 409:202, 2001.
12. Shen RF, Tai HH: Thromboxanes: Synthase and receptors, *J Biomed Sci* 5:153, 1998.
13. Hajjar KA: Cellular receptors in the regulation of plasmin generation, *Thromb Haemost* 74:294, 1995.
14. Miles LA, Ginsberg MH, White JG, Plow EF: Plasminogen interacts with human platelets through two distinct mechanisms, *J Clin Invest* 77:1986, 2001.
15. Schafer AI, Adelman B: Plasmin inhibition of platelet function and of arachidonic acid metabolism, *J Clin Invest* 75:456, 1985.
16. Fitzgerald DJ, Wright F, FitzGerald GA: Increased thromboxane biosynthesis during coronary thrombolysis: Evidence that platelet activation and thromboxane A₂ modulate the response to tissue-type plasminogen activator in vivo, *Circ Res* 65:83, 1989.
17. Marcus AJ, Broekman MJ, Drosopoulos JHF, et al: Thromboregulation by endothelial cells: Significance for occlusive vascular diseases, *Arterioscler Thromb Vasc Biol* 21:178, 2001.
18. Loscalzo J: Nitric oxide insufficiency, platelet activation, and arterial thrombosis, *Circ Res* 88:756, 2001.
19. Yao S-K, Ober JC, Krishnaswami A, et al: Endogenous nitric oxide protects against platelet aggregation and cyclic flow variations in stenosed and endothelium-injured arteries, *Circulation* 86:1302, 1992.
20. Zwaginga JJ, Sixma JJ, DeGroot PG: Activation of endothelial cells induces platelet thrombus formation on their matrix, *Arteriosclerosis* 10:49, 1990.
21. Feinberg WM, Erickson LP, Bruck D, Kittelson J: Hemostatic markers in acute ischemic stroke: Association with stroke type, severity and outcome, *Stroke* 27:1296, 1996.
22. Uchiyama S, Yamazaki M, Hara Y, et al: Alteration of platelet, coagulation and fibrinolysis markers in patients with acute ischemic stroke, *Semin Thromb Hemost* 23:535, 1997.

23. Zeller T, Tschoepe D, Kessler C: Circulating platelets show increased activation in patients with acute cerebral ischemia, *Thromb Haemost* 81:373, 1999.

24. Folsom AR, Rosamond WD, Shahar E, et al: Prospective study of markers of hemostatic function with risk of ischemic stroke. The Atherosclerosis Risk in Communities (ARIC) study investigators, *Circulation* 100:736, 1999.

25. Haddar HB, Cortes J, Salomaa V, et al: Correlation of specific platelet activation markers with carotid arterial wall thickness, *Thromb Haemost* 74:943, 1995.

26. Tofler GH, Brezinski D, Schafer AI, et al: Concurrent morning increase in platelet aggregability and the risk of myocardial infarction and sudden cardiac death, *N Engl J Med* 316:1514, 1987.

27. Marler JR, Price TR, Clark GL, et al: Morning increase in onset of ischemic stroke, *Stroke* 20:473, 1989.

28. Ernst E, Resch KL: Fibrinogen as a cardiovascular risk factor: A meta-analysis and review of the literature, *Ann Intern Med* 118:956, 1993.

29. Becher H, Grau A, Steindorf K, et al: Previous infection and other risk factors for acute cerebrovascular ischemia: Attributable risks and the characterisation of high risk groups, *J Epidemiol Biostat* 5:277, 2000.

30. Woodhouse PR, Khaw K, Plummer M, et al: Seasonal variations of plasma fibrinogen and factor VII activity in the elderly: Winter infections and death from cardiovascular disease, *Lancet* 343:435, 1994.

31. Grau AJ, Buggle F, Becher H, et al: Recent bacterial and viral infection is a risk for cerebrovascular ischemia, *Neurology* 50:196, 1998.

32. Kristensen SD, Roberts KM, Kishk YT, Martin JF: Accelerated atherogenesis occurs following platelet destruction and increases in megakaryocyte size and DNA content, *Eur J Clin Invest* 20:239, 1990.

33. O'Malley T, Langhorne P, Elton RA, Stewart MD: Platelet size in stroke patients, *Stroke* 26:995, 1995.

34. Cortelazzo S, Finazzi G, Ruggeri M, et al: Hydroxyurea for patients with essential thrombocythemia and a high risk of thrombosis, *N Engl J Med* 332:1132, 1995.

35. van Kooten F, Ciabattoni G, Koudstall PJ, et al: Increased platelet activation in the chronic phase after cerebral ischemia and intracerebral hemorrhage, *Stroke* 30:546, 1999.

36. Kenet G, Freedman J, Shenkman B, et al: Plasma glutathione peroxidase deficiency and platelet insensitivity to nitric oxide in children with familial stroke, *Arterioscler Thromb Vasc Biol* 19:2017, 1999.

37. Knapp HR, Reilly IA, Alessandrini P, FitzGerald GA: In vivo indexes of platelet function and vascular function in patients with atherosclerosis, *N Engl J Med* 314:937, 1986.

38. Amarenco P, Cohen A, Tzourio C, et al: Atherosclerotic disease of the aortic arch and the risk of ischemic stroke, *N Engl J Med* 331:1474, 1994.

39. Orgera M, O'Malley P, Taylor AJ: Secondary prevention of cerebral ischemia in patent foramen ovale: Systematic review and meta-analysis, *South Med J* 94:699, 2001.

40. Gunning AJ, Pickering GW, Robb-Smith AH, Russell RR: Mural thrombosis of the internal carotid artery and subsequent embolization, *Q J Med* 33:155, 1964.

41. Eldor A, Rachmilewitz EA: The hypercoagulable state in thalassemia, *Blood* 99:36, 2002.

42. Barnett JHM, Eliasziw M, Meldrum HE: Drugs and surgery in the prevention of ischemic stroke, *N Engl J Med* 332:238, 1995.

43. Smith JB, Willis AL: Aspirin selectively inhibits prostaglandin production in human platelets, *Nature* 231:235, 1971.

44. Vane JR: Inhibition of prostaglandin synthesis as a mechanism of action for aspirin-like drugs, *Nature* 231:232, 1971.

45. Roth GJ, Stanford N, Majerus PW: Acetylation of prostaglandin synthetase by aspirin, *Proc Natl Acad Sci U S A* 72:3073, 1975.

46. Patrono C, Coller B, Dalen JE, et al: Platelet-active drugs: The relationships among dose, effectiveness and side effects, *Chest* 114:S470, 1998.

47. Weksler BB, Kent JL, Rudolph D, et al: Effects of low-dose aspirin on platelet function in patients with recent cerebral ischemia, *Stroke* 16:5, 1985.

48. Weksler BB, Tack-Goldman K, Subramanian VA, et al: Cumulative inhibitory effect of low dose aspirin on vascular prostacyclin and platelet thromboxane production in patients with atherosclerosis, *Circulation* 71:332, 1985.

49. Goertler M, Baemer M, Kross R, et al: Rapid decline of cerebral microemboli of arterial origin after intravenous acetylsalicylic acid, *Stroke* 30:66, 1999.

50. Kyrle PA, Eichler HG, Jager U, Lechner K: Inhibition of prostacyclin and thromboxane A_2 generation by low-dose aspirin at the site of plug formation in man in vivo, *Circulation* 75:1025, 1987.

51. The Dutch TIA Trial Study Group: A comparison of two doses of aspirin (30 mg vs 283 mg a day) in patients after a transient ischemic attack or minor ischemic stroke, *N Engl J Med* 325:1261, 1991.

52. Ali M, McDonald JWD, Thiessen JJ, Coates PE: Plasma acetylsalicylate and salicylate and platelet cyclooxygenase activity following plain and enteric-coated aspirin, *Stroke* 11:9, 1980.

53. Patrono C, Roth GJ: Aspirin in ischemic cerebrovascular disease: How strong is the case for a different dosing regimen? *Stroke* 27:756, 1996.

54. Tohgi H, Konno S, Tamura K, et al: Effect of low-to-high doses of aspirin on platelet aggregability and metabolites of thromboxane A_2 and prostacyclin, *Stroke* 23:1400, 1993.

55. O'Connor CM, Gattis WA, Hellkamp AS, et al: Comparison of two aspirin doses on ischemic stroke in post-myocardial infarction patients in the warfarin (Coumadin) Aspirin Reinfarction Study (CARS), *Am J Cardiol* 88:541, 2001.

56. Taylor DW, Barnett JHM, Haynes RB, et al: Low-dose and high-dose acetylsalicylic acid for patients undergoing carotid endarterectomy: A randomized clinical trial. ASA and Carotid Endarterectomy (ACE) Trial Collaborators, *Lancet* 353:2178, 1999.

57. Catella-Lawson F, Reilly MP, Kapoor S, et al: Cyclooxygenase inhibitors and the antiplatelet effects of aspirin, *N Engl J Med* 345:1809–1817, 2001.

58. Ouellet M, Riendeau D, Percival MD: A high level of cyclooxygenase-2 inhibitor selectivity is associated with a reduced interference of platelet cyclooxygenase-1 inactivation by aspirin, *Proc Natl Acad Sci U S A* 98:14583, 2001.

59. Cardiovascular safety of COX-2 inhibitors, *Med Lett* 43:99, 2001.

60. Szeczklik A, Krzanowski M, Gora P, Radwan J: Antiplatelet drugs and generation of thrombin in clotting blood, *Blood* 80:1992, 2006.

61. Szeczklik A, Musial J, Undas A, et al: Aspirin inhibits thrombogenesis in normocholesterolemic but not in hypercholesterolemic man, *Thomb Haemost* 69:798, 1993.

62. Collaborative meta-analysis of randomised trials of antiplatelet therapy for prevention of death, myocardial infarction, and stroke in high risk patients, *BMJ* 324(7329):71–86, 2002.

63. Sanderson S, Emery J, Baglin T, Kinmonth AL: Narrative review: Aspirin resistance and its clinical implications, *Ann Intern Med* 142(5):370–380, 2005.

64. Mueller MR, Salat A, Stangl P, et al: Variable platelet response to low-dose ASA and the risk of limb deterioration in patients submitted to peripheral arterial angioplasty, *Thromb Haemost* 78(3):1003–1007, 1997.

65. Kamath S, Blann AD, Lip GY: Platelet activation: Assessment and quantification, *Eur Heart J* 22(17):1561–1571, 2001.

66. Kottke-Marchant K, Corcoran G: The laboratory diagnosis of platelet disorders, *Arch Pathol Lab Med* 126(2):133–146, 2002.

67. Hart RG, Leonard AD, Talbert RL, et al: Aspirin dosage and thromboxane synthesis in patients with vascular disease, *Pharmacotherapy* 23(5):579–584, 2003.

68. Bruno A, McConnell JP, Cohen SN, et al: Serial urinary 11-dehydro-thromboxane B_2, aspirin dose, and vascular events in blacks after recent cerebral infarction, *Stroke* 35(3):727–730, 2004.

69. Eikelboom JW, Hirsh J, Weitz JI, et al: Aspirin-resistant thromboxane biosynthesis and the risk of myocardial infarction, stroke, or cardiovascular death in patients at high risk for cardiovascular events, *Circulation* 105(14):1650–1655, 2002.

70. Gasparyan AY, Watson T, Lip GY: The role of aspirin in cardiovascular prevention: Implications of aspirin resistance, *J Am Coll Cardiol* 51(19):1829–1843, 2008.

71. Carlos TM, Harlan JM: Leukocyte-endothelial adhesion molecules, *Blood* 84(7):2068–2101, 1994.

72. Choudhury A, Chung I, Blann AD, Lip GY: Platelet surface CD62P and CD63, mean platelet volume, and soluble/platelet P-selectin as indexes of platelet function in atrial fibrillation: A comparison of "healthy control subjects" and "disease control subjects" in sinus rhythm, *J Am Coll Cardiol* 49(19):1957–1964, 2007.

73. Nadar S, Blann AD, Lip GY: Effects of aspirin on intra-platelet vascular endothelial growth factor, angiopoietin-1, and p-selectin levels in hypertensive patients, *Am J Hypertens* 19(9):970–977, 2006.

74. Serebruany VL, Kereiakes DJ, Dalesandro MR, Gurbel PA: The flow cytometer model markedly affects measurement of ex vivo whole blood platelet-bound P-selectin expression in patients with chest pain: Are we comparing apples with oranges, *Thromb Res* 96(1):51–56, 1999.

75. O'Connor CM, Gurbel PA, Serebruany VL: Usefulness of soluble and surface-bound P-selectin in detecting heightened platelet activity in patients with congestive heart failure, *Am J Cardiol* 83(9):1345–1349, 1999.

76. De Gaetano G, Cerletti C: Aspirin resistance: A revival of platelet aggregation tests? *J Thromb Haemost* 1(9):2048–2050, 2003.

77. Yardumian DA, Mackie IJ, Machin SJ: Laboratory investigation of platelet function: A review of methodology, *J Clin Pathol* 39(7):701–712, 1986.

78. Jilma B: Platelet function analyzer (PFA-100): A tool to quantify congenital or acquired platelet dysfunction, *J Lab Clin Med* 138(3):152–163, 2001.

79. Kundu SK, Heilmann EJ, Sio R, et al: Description of an in vitro platelet function analyzer: PFA-100, *Semin Thromb Hemost* 21(Suppl 2):106–112, 1995.

80. Coleman JWJ, Simon JI: Determination of individual response to aspirin therapy using the Accumetrics Ultegra RPFA-ASA System, *Point Care* 3:77–82, 2004.

81. Malinin A, Spergling M, Muhlestein B, et al: Assessing aspirin responsiveness in subjects with multiple risk factors for vascular disease with a rapid platelet function analyzer, *Blood Coagul Fibrinolysis* 15(4):295–301, 2004.

82. Komiya T, Kudo M, Urabe T, et al: Compliance with antiplatelet therapy in patients with ischemic cerebrovascular disease. Assessment by platelet aggregation testing, *Stroke* 25(12):2337–2342, 1994.

83. Sappok T, Faulstich A, Stuckert E, et al: Compliance with secondary prevention of ischemic stroke: A prospective evaluation, *Stroke* 32(8):1884–1889, 2001.

84. Hankey GJ, Eikelboom JW: Aspirin resistance, *BMJ* 328:477–479, 2004.

85. Bornstein NM, Karepov VG, Aronovich BD, et al: Failure of aspirin treatment after stroke, *Stroke* 25(2):275–277, 1994.

86. Helgason CM, Bolin KM, Hoff JA, et al: Development of aspirin resistance in persons with previous ischemic stroke, *Stroke* 25(12):2331–2336, 1994.

87. Cambria-Kiely JA, Gandhi PJ: Aspirin resistance and genetic polymorphisms, *J Thromb Thrombolysis* 14(1):51–58, 2002.

88. Grotemeyer KH, Scharafinski HW, Husstedt IW: Two-year follow-up of aspirin responder and aspirin non responder. A pilot-study including 180 post-stroke patients, *Thromb Res* 71(5):397–403, 1993.

89. Andersen K, Hurlen M, Arnesen H, et al: Aspirin non-responsiveness as measured by PFA-100 in patients with coronary artery disease, *Thromb Res* 108(1):37–42, 2002.

90. Grundmann K, Jaschonek K, Kleine B, et al: Aspirin non-responder status in patients with recurrent cerebral ischemic attacks, *J Neurol* 250(1):63–66, 2003.

91. Gum PA, Kottke-Marchant K, Welsh PA, et al: A prospective, blinded determination of the natural history of aspirin resistance among stable patients with cardiovascular disease, *J Am Coll Cardiol* 41(6):961–965, 2003.

92. Campbell CL, Smyth S, Montalescot G, et al: Aspirin dose for the prevention of cardiovascular disease: A systematic review, *JAMA* 297(18):2018–2024, 2007.

93. Macchi L, Christiaens L, Brabant S, et al: Resistance to aspirin in vitro is associated with increased platelet sensitivity to adenosine diphosphate, *Thromb Res* 107:45–49, 2002.

94. Borna C, Lazarowski E, van Heusden C, et al: Resistance to aspirin is increased by ST-elevation myocardial infarction and correlates with adenosine diphosphate levels, *Thromb J* 3:10, 2005.

95. Eikelboom JW, Hankey GJ, Thom J, et al: Enhanced antiplatelet effect of clopidogrel in patients whose platelets are least inhibited by aspirin: A randomized crossover trial, *J Thromb Haemost* 3(12):2649–2655, 2005.

96. Diener HC, Bogousslavsky J, Brass LM, et al: Management of atherothrombosis with clopidogrel in high-risk patients with recent transient ischaemic attack or ischaemic stroke (MATCH): A study design and baseline data, *Cerebrovasc Dis* 17(2-3):253–261, 2004.

97. Bhatt DL, Fox KA, Hacke W, et al: Clopidogrel and aspirin versus aspirin alone for the prevention of atherothrombotic events, *N Engl J Med* 354(16):1706–1717, 2006.

98. Snoep JD, Hovens MM, Eikenboom JC, et al: Clopidogrel non-responsiveness in patients undergoing percutaneous coronary intervention with stenting: A systematic review and meta-analysis, *Am Heart J* 154(2):221–231, 2007.

99. Wang TH, Bhatt DL, Topol EJ: Aspirin and clopidogrel resistance: An emerging clinical entity, *Eur Heart J* 27(6):647–654, 2006.

100. Michos ED, Ardehali R, Blumenthal RS, et al: Aspirin and clopidogrel resistance, *Mayo Clin Proc* 81(4):518–526, 2006.

101. Lev EI, Patel RT, Maresh KJ, et al: Aspirin and clopidogrel drug response in patients undergoing percutaneous coronary intervention: The role of dual drug resistance, *J Am Coll Cardiol* 47(1):27–33, 2006.

102. Diener HC, Cunha L, Forbes C, et al: European Stroke Prevention Study. 2. Dipyridamole and acetylsalicylic acid in the secondary prevention of stroke, *J Neurol Sci* 143(1-2):1–13, 1996.

103. Halkes PH, van Gijn J, Kappelle LJ, et al: Aspirin plus dipyridamole versus aspirin alone after cerebral ischaemia of arterial origin (ESPRIT): Randomised controlled trial, *Lancet* 367:1665–1673, 2006.

104. Sacco RL, Diener HC, Yusuf S, et al: Aspirin and extended-release dipyridamole versus clopidogrel for recurrent stroke, *N Engl J Med* 359(12):1238–1251, 2008.

105. Huang Y, Cheng Y, Wu J, et al: Cilostazol as an alternative to aspirin after ischaemic stroke: A randomised, double-blind, pilot study, *Lancet Neurol* 7(6):494–499, 2008.

106. He J, Whelton PK, Vu B, et al: Aspirin and risk of hemorrhagic stroke: A meta-analysis of randomized controlled trials, *JAMA* 280:1930–1935, 1998.

107. Schror K: The basic pharmacology of ticlopidine and clopidogrel, *Platelets* 4:252, 1991.

108. Sharis PJ, Cannon CP, Loscalzo J: The antiplatelet effects of ticlopidine and clopidogrel, *Ann Intern Med* 129:394, 1998.

109. Isaka K, Kiurma K, Etani H, et al: Effect of aspirin and ticlopidine on platelet deposition in carotid atherosclerosis, *Stroke* 17:1215–1220, 1986.

110. Yang IJ, Hoppensteadt D, Fareed J: Modulation of vasoconstriction by clopidogrel and ticlopidine, *Thromb Res* 92:83, 1998.

111. Nguyen TA, Diodati JG, Pharand C: Resistance to clopidogrel: A review of the evidence, *J Am Coll Cardiol* 45(8):1157–1164, 2005.

112. Sugunaraj JP, Palaniswamy C, Selvaraj DR, et al: Clopidogrel resistance, *Am J Ther* 17(2):210–215, 2010.

113. Collet JP, Hulot JS, Pena A, et al: Cytochrome P450 2C19 polymorphism in young patients treated with clopidogrel after myocardial infarction: A cohort study, *Lancet* 373:309–317, 2009.

114. Shuldiner AR, O'Connell JR, Bliden KP, et al: Association of cytochrome P450 2C19 genotype with the antiplatelet effect and clinical efficacy of clopidogrel therapy, *JAMA* 302(8):849–857, 2009.

115. Pare G, Mehta SR, Yusuf S, et al: Effects of CYP2C19 genotype on outcomes of clopidogrel treatment, *N Engl J Med* 363:1704–1714, 2010.

116. Peto R, Gray R, Collins R, et al: Randomised trial of prophylactic daily aspirin in British male doctors, *BMJ (Clin Res Ed)* 296:313–316, 1988.

117. Thrombosis Prevention Trial: Randomised trial of low-intensity oral anticoagulation with warfarin and low-dose aspirin in the primary prevention of ischaemic heart disease in men at increased risk, *Lancet* 351:233–241, 1998.

118. Hansson L, Zanchetti A, Carruthers SG, et al: Effects of intensive blood-pressure lowering and low-dose aspirin in patients with hypertension: Principal results of the Hypertension Optimal Treatment (HOT) randomised trial, *Lancet* 351:1755–1762, 1998.

119. Roncaglioni MC: Low-dose aspirin and vitamin E in people at cardiovascular risk: A randomised trial in general Practice, *Lancet* 357:89–95, 2001.

120. Ridker PM, Cook NR, Lee IM, et al: A randomized trial of low-dose aspirin in the primary prevention of cardiovascular disease in women, *N Engl J Med* 352(13):1293–1304, 2005.

121. Eidelman RS, Hebert PR, Weisman SM, et al: An update on aspirin in the primary prevention of cardiovascular disease, *Arch Intern Med* 163(17):2006–2010, 2003.

122. Antithrombotic Trialists (ATT) Collaboration: Aspirin in the primary and secondary prevention of vascular disease: Collaborative meta-analysis of individual participant data from randomised trials, *Lancet* 373:1849–1860, 2009.

123. Belch J, MacCuish A, Campbell I, et al: The prevention of progression of arterial disease and diabetes (POPADAD) trial: Factorial randomised placebo controlled trial of aspirin and antioxidants in patients with diabetes and asymptomatic peripheral arterial disease, *BMJ* 337:a1840, 2008.

124. Ogawa H, Nakayama M, Morimoto T, et al: Low-dose aspirin for primary prevention of atherosclerotic events in patients with type 2 diabetes: A randomized controlled trial, *JAMA* 300:2134–2141, 2008.

125. De Berardis G, Sacco M, Evangelista V, et al: Aspirin and Simvastatin Combination for Cardiovascular Events Prevention Trial in Diabetes (ACCEPT-D): Design of a randomized study of the efficacy of low-dose aspirin in the prevention of cardiovascular events in subjects with diabetes mellitus treated with statins, *Trials* 8:21, 2007.

126. Chinese Acute Stroke Trial Collaborative Group: CAST: A randomised placebo-controlled trial of early aspirin use in 20,000 patients with acute ischemic stroke, *Lancet* 349:1641, 1997.

127. International Stroke Trial Collaborative Group : The International Stroke Trial (IST): a randomized trial of aspirin, subcutaneous heparin, both or neither among 19,435 patients with acute ischemic stroke, *Lancet* 349:1569, 1997.

128. Chen Z-M, Sanderock P, Pan H-C, et al: Indications for early aspirin use in acute ischemic stroke: A combined analysis of 40,000 randomized patients from the Chinese Acute Stroke Trial and the International Stroke Trial, *Stroke* 31:1240, 2000.

129. Kennedy J, Hill MD, Ryckborst KJ, et al: Fast assessment of stroke and transient ischaemic attack to prevent early recurrence (FASTER): A randomised controlled pilot trial, *Lancet Neurol* 6(11):961–969, 2007.

130. Johnston SC, Easton JD: Platelet-oriented inhibition in new TIA and minor ischemic stroke (POINT) trial, a randomized, double-blind, multicenter clinical trial: http://clinicaltrials.gov. Accessed.

131. Group SS: A randomized trial of anticoagulants versus aspirin after cerebral ischemia of presumed arterial origin, *Ann Neurol* 42:857–865, 1997.

132. Mohr JP, Thompson JLP, Lazar RM, et al: A comparison of warfarin and aspirin for the prevention of recurrent ischemic stroke, *N Engl J Med* 345(20):1444–1451, 2001.

133. Algra A: Medium intensity oral anticoagulants versus aspirin after cerebral ischaemia of arterial origin (ESPRIT): A randomised controlled trial, *Lancet Neurol* 6:115–124, 2007.

134. Chimowitz MI, Lynn MJ, Howlett-Smith H, et al: Comparison of warfarin and aspirin for symptomatic intracranial arterial stenosis, *N Engl J Med* 352(13):1305–1316, 2005.

135. The SALT Collaborative Group: Swedish Aspirin Low-Dose Trial (SALT) of 75 mg aspirin as secondary prophylaxis after cerebrovascular ischaemic events, *Lancet* 338:1345–1349, 1991.

136. Sze PC, Reitman D, Pincus MM, et al: Antiplatelet agents in the secondary prevention of stroke: meta-analysis of the randomized control trials, *Stroke* 19(4):436–442, 1988.

137. A randomised, blinded trial of clopidogrel versus aspirin in patients at risk of ischaemic events (CAPRIE), *Lancet* 348:1329–1339, 1996.

138. Hart RG, Pearce LA, Aguilar MI: Meta-analysis: Antithrombotic therapy to prevent stroke in patients who have nonvalvular atrial fibrillation, *Ann Intern Med* 146:857–867, 2007.

139. ACTIVE Investigators: Clopidogrel plus aspirin versus oral anticoagulation for atrial fibrillation in the Atrial Fibrillation Clopidogrel Trial with Irbesartan for Prevention of Vascular Events (ACTIVE W): A randomised controlled trial, *Lancet* 367:1903–1912, 2006.

140. ACTIVE SPIRIT Study Group Investigators: Effect of clopidogrel added to aspirin in patients with atrial fibrillation, *N Engl J Med* 360:2066–2078, 2009.

141. Brinker AD, Swartz L: Growth in clopidogrel-aspirin combination therapy, *Ann Pharmacother* 40:1212–1213, 2006.

142. Cadroy Y, Bossavy JP, Thalamas C, et al: Early potent antithrombotic effect with combined aspirin and a loading dose of clopidogrel on experimental arterial thrombogenesis in humans, *Circulation* 101:2823, 2001.

143. Diener PH-C, Bogousslavsky PJ, Brass PLM, et al: Aspirin and clopidogrel compared with clopidogrel alone after recent ischaemic stroke or transient ischaemic attack in high-risk patients (MATCH): Randomised, double-blind, placebo-controlled trial, *Lancet* 364:331–333, 2004.

144. Payne DA, Jones CI, Hayes PD, et al: Beneficial effects of clopidogrel combined with aspirin in reducing cerebral emboli in patients undergoing carotid endarterectomy, *Circulation* 109(12):1476–1481, 2004.

145. Markus HS, Droste DW, Kaps M, et al: Dual antiplatelet therapy with clopidogrel and aspirin in symptomatic carotid stenosis evaluated using Doppler embolic signal detection: The Clopidogrel and Aspirin for Reduction of Emboli in Symptomatic Carotid Stenosis (CARESS) trial, *Circulation* 111:2233–2240, 2005.

146. Bhatt DL, Kapadia SR, Bajzer CT, et al: Dual antiplatelet therapy with clopidogrel and aspirin after carotid artery stenting, *J Invasive Cardiol* 13:767, 2001.

147. McKevitt FM, Randall MS, Cleveland TJ, et al: The benefits of combined anti-platelet treatment in carotid artery stenting, *Eur J Vasc Endovasc Surg* 29:522–527, 2005.

148. Dalainas I, Nano G, Bianchi P, et al: Dual antiplatelet regime versus acetyl-acetic acid for carotid artery stenting, *Cardiovasc Intervent Radiol* 29:519–521, 2006.

149. Hirsh J, Bhatt DL: Comparative benefits of clopidogrel and aspirin in high-risk patient populations: Lessons from the CAPRIE and CURE studies, *Arch Intern Med* 164:2106–2110, 2004.

150. Muller TH: Inhibition of thrombus formation by low-dose acetyl-salicylic acid, dipyridamole and their combination in a model of platelet-vessel wall interaction, *Neurology* 57:S8, 2001.

151. Stroke Prevention in Atrial Fibrillation Study Group Investigators: Preliminary report of the Stroke Prevention in Atrial Fibrillation study, *N Engl J Med* 322:863, 1990.

152. A double blind trial to assess long-term oral anticoagulant treatment in elderly patients after myocardial infarction. Report of the Sixty Plus Reinfarction Study Research Group, *Lancet* 2:989, 1980.

153. Adjusted-dose warfarin versus low-intensity fixed-dose warfarin plus aspirin for high-risk patients with atrial fibrillation: Stroke Prevention in Atrial Fibrillation III randomised clinical trial, *Lancet* 348:633, 1996.

154. Flaker GC, Gruber M, Connolly SJ, et al: Risks and benefits of combining aspirin with anticoagulant therapy in patients with atrial fibrillation: an exploratory analysis of stroke prevention using an oral thrombin inhibitor in atrial fibrillation (SPORTIF) trials, *Am Heart J* 152:967–973, 2006.

144. Hart RG, Pearce LA, McBride R, et al: Factors associated with ischemic stroke during aspirin therapy in atrial fibrillation. The Stroke Prevention in Atrial Fibrillation (SPAF) Investigators, *Stroke* 30:1223, 1999.

156. Sacco RL, Adams R, Albers G, et al: Guidelines for prevention of stroke in patients with ischemic stroke or transient ischemic attack: A statement for healthcare professionals from the American Heart Association/American Stroke Association Council on Stroke: Co-sponsored by the Council on Cardiovascular Radiology and Intervention: The American Academy of Neurology affirms the value of this guideline, *Stroke* 37:577–617, 2006.

157. Cappelleri JC, Fiore LD, Brophy MT, et al: Efficacy and safety of combined anticoagulant and antiplatelet therapy versus anticoagulant monotherapy after mechanical heart-valve replacement: A meta-analysis, *Am Heart J* 130:547, 1995.

158. Turpie AG, Gent M, Laupacis A, et al: A comparison of aspirin with placebo in patients treated with warfarin after heart-valve replacement, *N Engl J Med* 329:524, 1993.

159. Fiore LD, Ezekowitz M, Brophy MT, et al: Department of Veterans Affairs Cooperative Studies Program clinical trial comparing combined warfarin and aspirin with aspirin alone in survivors of acute myocardial infarction: Primary results of the CHAMP study, *Circulation* 105:557, 2002.

160. Hankey GJ, Costa J, Ferro JM, et al: Triflusal for preventing serious vascular events in people at high risk, *Stroke* 37:2193–2195, 2006.

161. Gotoh F, Tohgi H, Hirai S, et al: Cilostazol stroke prevention study: A placebo-controlled double-blind trial for secondary prevention of cerebral infarction, *J Stroke Cerebrovasc Dis* 9:147–157, 2000.

162. Shinohara Y, Nishimaru K, Sawada T, et al: Sarpogrelate-Aspirin Comparative Clinical Study for Efficacy and Safety in Secondary Prevention of Cerebral Infarction (S-ACCESS): A randomized, double-blind, aspirin-controlled trial, *Stroke* 39:1827-1833, 2008.

163. Bousser MG, Amarenco P, Chamorro A, et al: The Prevention of Cerebrovascular and Cardiovascular Events of Ischemic Origin with Terutroban in Patients with a History of Ischemic Stroke or Transient Ischemic Attack (PERFORM) study: Baseline characteristics of the population, *Cerebrovasc Dis* 27:608-613, 2009.

164. Hennerici MG: Rationale and design of the Prevention of Cerebrovascular and Cardiovascular Events of Ischemic Origin with Terutroban in Patients with a History of Ischemic Stroke or Transient Ischemic Attack (PERFORM) study, *Cerebrovasc Dis* 27:28-32, 2009.

165. Fazekas F, Kleinert R, Roob G, et al: Histopathologic analysis of foci of signal loss on gradient-echo T2*-weighted MR images in patients with spontaneous intracerebral hemorrhage: Evidence of microangiopathy-related microbleeds, *AJNR Am J Neuroradiol* 20:637-642, 1999.

166. Tanaka A, Ueno Y, Nakayama Y, et al: Small chronic hemorrhages and ischemic lesions in association with spontaneous intracerebral hematomas, *Stroke* 30:1637-1642, 1999.

167. Roob G, Fazekas F: Magnetic resonance imaging of cerebral microbleeds, *Curr Opin Neurol* 13(1):69-73, 2000.

168. Kato H, Izumiyama M, Izumiyama K, et al: Silent cerebral microbleeds on T2*-weighted MRI: Correlation with stroke subtype, stroke recurrence, and leukoaraiosis, *Stroke* 33:1536-1540, 2002.

169. Naka H, Nomura E, Wakabayashi S, et al: Frequency of asymptomatic microbleeds on T2*-weighted MR images of patients with recurrent stroke: Association with combination of stroke subtypes and leukoaraiosis, *AJNR Am J Neuroradiol* 25:714-719, 2004.

170. Imaizumi T, Horita Y, Hashimoto Y, et al: Dotlike hemosiderin spots on T2*-weighted magnetic resonance imaging as a predictor of stroke recurrence: A prospective study, *J Neurosurg* 101: 915-920, 2004.

171. Nighoghossian N, Hermier M, Adeleine P, et al: Old microbleeds are a potential risk factor for cerebral bleeding after ischemic stroke: A gradient-echo T2*-weighted brain MRI study, *Stroke* 33:735-742, 2002.

172. Hanyu H, Tanaka Y, Shimizu S, et al: Cerebral microbleeds in Binswanger's disease: A gradient-echo T2*-weighted magnetic resonance imaging study, *Neurosci Lett* 340:213-216, 2003.

173. Koennecke HC: Cerebral microbleeds on MRI: Prevalence, associations, and potential clinical implications, *Neurology* 66:165-171, 2006.

174. Fan YH, Zhang L, Lam WW, et al: Cerebral microbleeds as a risk factor for subsequent intracerebral hemorrhages among patients with acute ischemic stroke, *Stroke* 34:2459-2462, 2003.

175. Greenberg SM, Eng JA, Ning M, et al: Hemorrhage burden predicts recurrent intracerebral hemorrhage after lobar hemorrhage, *Stroke* 35:1415-1420, 2004.

176. Wong KS, Chan YL, Liu JY, et al: Asymptomatic microbleeds as a risk factor for aspirin-associated intracerebral hemorrhages, *Neurology* 60:511-513, 2003.

177. Imaizumi T, Horita Y, Chiba M, et al: Dot-like hemosiderin spots on gradient echo T2*-weighted magnetic resonance imaging are associated with past history of small vessel disease in patients with intracerebral hemorrhage, *J Neuroimaging* 14:251-257, 2004.

59

Secondary Prevention of Cardioembolic Stroke

MARIA I. AGUILAR, OSCAR R. BENAVENTE

Cardioembolic stroke is an important stroke subtype, accounting for approximately one fifth of all ischemic strokes, and it is expected that the frequency will rise with the aging of the general population.[1] Advances in imaging techniques have led to easier recognition of cardiac disorders potentially responsible for embolic stroke. Because the underlying cardiac condition is often evident before stroke occurs and antithrombotic therapies are notably effective, cardiogenic emboli to the brain are among the most preventable causes of stroke.

With a thorough cardiac evaluation, a potential source of cardiogenic emboli can be identified in at least 30% of all patients with ischemic stroke.[2,3] However, potential cardioembolic sources often coexist with other cardiovascular disease risk factors.[4-6] During the past two decades, new and better noninvasive cardiac imaging became available; therefore new potential cardioembolic sources have been recognized. This situation is reflected in the increased frequency of cardioembolic stroke over time. Aggregate data from stroke registries conducted between 1988 and 1994 show mean frequency of cardioembolic stroke to be 20% (range, 17% to 28%).[4,7-11] Data from later stroke registries (1995 to 2001) showed a higher mean prevalence of cardioembolic stroke, 25% (range 16% to 38%).[12-17]

Cardioembolic stroke is caused by a variety of cardiac disorders, each with a unique natural history and a variable response to antithrombotic therapy (Fig. 59-1).

The embolic material originating from the heart and proximal aorta can be quite diverse. The thrombi may be composed of varying proportions of platelets and fibrin, cholesterol fragments, tumor particles, or bacterial clusters. The natural history and response to antithrombotic therapy of each of these conditions are unique, and consequently, each source of cardioembolic strokes should be considered separately. Thus cardioembolic stroke is not a single disease; it is a syndrome with diverse causes (see Fig. 59-1).

The incidence of ischemic stroke associated with cardioembolic sources varies greatly. Cardioembolic sources of stroke can be divided according to their stroke risk potential as "major-risk sources," for which the risk for stroke is well established, or "minor-risk sources," for which the risk for stroke has been incompletely established (Table 59-1). The major-risk cardioembolic sources carry a substantial annual risk of emboli and a high risk of recurrence, and usually, antithrombotic therapy is warranted for stroke prevention. Conversely, the so-called minor sources of emboli can cause stroke but have a low or uncertain risk of embolism and are more often coincidental than casual; therefore, antithrombotic therapy is usually reserved for selected cases.

Atrial Fibrillation

Atrial fibrillation (AF) is the most common cardiac arrhythmia, affecting 0.7% of the general population of the United States (2.5 million people). Its prevalence increases with age, being present in about 5% of persons at age 65 years and in 10% at age 80 years. AF is equally distributed in men and women, and the mean age of individuals affected is about 75 years (Fig. 59-2).[18]

The following are the forms of AF as proposed by the American College of Cardiology (ACC)/American Heart Association (AHA)/European Society of Cardiology (ESC)[19]:

- *Paroxysmal AF (PAF)*: Self-terminating AF, in which the episodes generally last less than 7 days, usually less than 24 hours. It may be recurrent.
- *Persistent AF:* Fails to self-terminate and lasts longer than 7 days.
- *Permanent AF:* Lasts for more than 1 year.
- *Lone AF:* Paroxysmal, persistent, or permanent AF in the absence of structural heart disease. This term was coined before echocardiography became widely available and most cardiologists consider it now outdated. Whether or not left atrial enlargement and hypertensive heart disease fall under the definition of "structural heart disease" is unclear.
- *Nonvalvular AF:* Cases without rheumatic mitral valve disease, prosthetic heart valve, or valve repair.

Nonvalvular AF is responsible for about 16% (range, 11% to 29%) of all ischemic strokes.[4,5,20-23] AF is present in more than one third of patients older than 70 years with ischemic stroke.[24] Nonvalvular AF is a recognized independent powerful risk factor for ischemic stroke.[25] The risk of ischemic stroke increases fivefold (from 1% to 5% per year) in elderly patients (mean age, 70 years) with nonvalvular AF, and about 18-fold in patients with AF and rheumatic mitral stenosis.[25] AF accounts for about half of presumed cardioembolic strokes. Patients with AF are typically older and have large middle cerebral artery

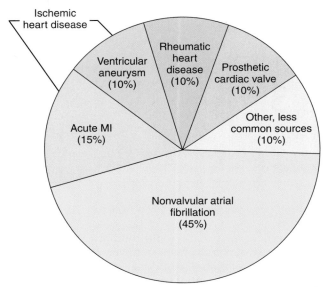

Figure 59-1 Sources of cardioembolic stroke. MI, myocardial infarction.

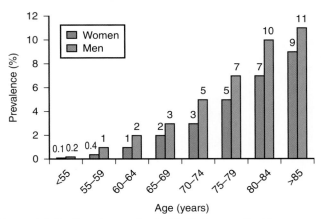

Figure 59-2 Prevalence of atrial fibrillation stratified by age and sex.

TABLE 59-1 CARDIOEMBOLIC SOURCES

Location	Major-Risk Sources	Minor-Risk Sources
Atrial	Atrial fibrillation Left atrial thrombus Left atrial myxoma Sustained atrial flutter	Patent foramen ovale Atrial septal aneurysm
Valvular	Mitral stenosis Prosthetic cardiac valves Infective endocarditis calcification Marantic endocarditis	Mitral valve prolapse Calcific aortic stenosis Mitral annular Fibroelastoma Giant Lambl's excrescences
Ventricular	Left ventricular thrombus (mobile or protruding) Recent anterior wall myocardial infarction Nonischemic dilated cardiomyopathy	Left ventricular regional wall abnormalities Congestive heart failure Akinetic ventricular wall segment

strokes associated with a high mortality rate during the first 30 days (Table 59-2).[26,27]

Most embolic strokes in patients with AF are caused by the embolization of thrombi forming in the appendage of the left atrium. About 70% of ischemic strokes in patients with AF are embolic, but up to 30% are secondary to intrinsic cerebrovascular disease, atheromas of the proximal aorta, or other cardioembolic sources.[28-32] The formation of thrombi in the left atrium appendage in patients with AF is precipitated by the sluggish flow from ineffective atrial contraction. However, AF alone may not be enough to promote thrombi formation. Other factors may also contribute, because associated cardiovascular disease and age appear to influence the stroke risk in AF and, hence, also to influence the formation of atrial appendage thrombi. This variable risk is reflected by the

wide range of stroke risk in patients with AF ("lone AF") unlike in other "high-risk" groups. Temporal variation in factors that influence thrombus formation may explain the intermittency of embolism in different patients with AF and even within each patient. Embolic events are intermittent in AF, sometimes separated by years. A balance between the formation and inhibition of clot is likely present in the atrial appendage of such patients. This balance is influenced by atrial size, appendage flow velocities, and coagulation factors. Therefore, the type and intensity of antithrombotic therapy needed to inhibit appendage thrombi may differ among patients with AF and over time for the same patient.

The overall incidence of ischemic stroke among people with AF is about 5% per year. The rate of stroke varies widely, however, ranging from 0.5% per year in young patients with "lone AF" to 12% per year in those with prior transient ischemia attack (TIA) or stroke. This variation depends on coexisting cardiovascular disorders.[28,32,33] Identification of subgroups of patients with AF with relatively high versus low absolute rates of stroke is important for selecting prophylactic antithrombotic therapy.[34-36] Prospective studies have shown that hypertension, prior TIA or stroke, and left ventricular systolic dysfunction are independently predictive of stroke in patients with AF.[37,38] Echocardiographic studies identified left ventricular systolic dysfunction to be strongly, consistently, and independently associated with subsequent stroke in patients with AF.[34] Stratification schemes are particularly important for the identification of appropriate antithrombotic therapy.[39] The CHADS2 score is widely used as the most reliable scheme of stratification that allows the separation of AF patients according to the risk of stroke.[40] This scheme was validated in an independent cohort. The acronym stands for

- C = congestive heart failure (1 point).
- H = hypertension (1 point)
- A = age older than 75 (1 point)
- D = DM (1 point)
- S2 = history of stroke or transient ischemic attack (TIA) (2 points).

The estimated risk of stroke per year based on the CHADS2 score and the number needed to treat (NNT) with anticoagulation instead of aspirin are shown in Table 59-3.

TABLE 59-2 STROKE RISK IN RELATION TO ATRIAL FIBRILLATION*

Study	Mean Age (yrs)	Stroke Rate %/yr AF	Stroke Rate %/yr Non-AF	Increased Relative Risk
Framingham (USA) (Wolf, 1991)	70	4.1	0.7	× 6
Shibata (Japan) (Nakayama, 1997)	65	5.0	0.9	× 6
Reykjavik (Iceland) (Onundarson, 1987)	52	1.6	0.2	× 7

*Data from epidemiologic studies.

TABLE 59-3 CHADS2 SCORE FOR RISK STRATIFICATION OF STROKE

CHADS2 Score*	Risk	Stroke Rate (%/year)	NNT
0	Low	0.5	417
1	Low	1.5	125
2	Moderate	2.5	81
3	High	5	33
4	High	6	27
5-6	Very high	7	20

*For CHADS2 (congestive heart failure, hypertension, age older than 75 yr, diabetes mellitus) score and validation, see reference 40.
NNT, number needed to treat with anticoagulants instead of aspirin to prevent one stroke per year.

The short-term risk of stroke recurrence after an acute stroke in patients with AF has not been well characterized. However, data from three randomized clinical trials indicate that patients treated with aspirin at different doses administered at different times after stroke have a risk of recurrent stroke of 5% in 2 weeks, a value much lower than previously thought.[41-44]

Stroke Prevention in Atrial Fibrillation

The efficacy of antithrombotic therapies to prevent stroke in nonvalvular AF has been well established by randomized clinical trials. Between 1989 and 2007, 29 randomized trials involving 28,044 patients have been completed, evaluating the efficacy and safety of antithrombotic agents for stroke prevention in AF.[45] An aggregate analysis showed that anticoagulation with warfarin reduces ischemic stroke by 64% in comparison with the rate in untreated patients, and an efficacy analysis indicated an even greater benefit. Warfarin was effective in preventing disabling stroke by 59% and nondisabling stroke by 61%. The absolute risk reduction in all strokes by the use of warfarin was 2.7% per year for primary prevention (NNT for 1 year to prevent one stroke = 37) and 8.4% per year for secondary prevention (NNT = 12).[45] When only ischemic strokes were considered, adjusted-dose warfarin was associated with a 67% relative risk reduction (RRR) (95% confidence interval [CI], 54%–77%). In addition, the increase in rate of major bleeding among elderly patients with AF undergoing anticoagulation in these trials was only 0.3% to 2.0% per year with a target international normalized ratio (INR) of 1.5 to 4.0. Participants in these trials were carefully selected to minimize bleeding risks and were monitored closely by means of clinical trial protocols.[46-49] The risk of major hemorrhage in elderly patients with AF who are taking oral anticoagulants seems to be related to the intensity of anticoagulation, patient age, and fluctuation in INR.[49] The optimal intensity of anticoagulation to prevent ischemic stroke and minimize the risk of bleeding probably varies according to individual stroke risk. Low-intensity anticoagulation (INR target range, 2.0 to 3.0) is effective in primary stroke prevention for patients with AF. However, warfarin proved to be more effective in high-risk patients with prior TIAs or strokes when a higher INR target (2.5 to 4.2) was used.[32,50,51]

The efficacy of aspirin, with doses ranging from 50 to 1300 mg per day, for stroke prevention in patients with AF has been tested in eight trials that included 4876 participants. Comparing aspirin alone with placebo or no treatment, aspirin was associated with a 19% reduction in incidence of stroke (95% CI, 1%–35%). For primary prevention, there was an absolute risk reduction of 0.8% per year (NNT = 125) and for secondary prevention trials a reduction of 2.5% per year (NNT = 40). When only ischemic strokes are considered, aspirin results in a 21% reduction in strokes (95% CI, 1%–38%). When all antiplatelet agents are considered, stroke was reduced by 22% (95% CI, 6%–35%).[45]

Eight trials compared warfarin and other vitamin K antagonists with various dosages of aspirin, other antiplatelet agents in three trials and aspirin combined with low-fixed-dose warfarin in two trials. For the 11 trials that compared adjusted-dose warfarin with antiplatelet therapy alone, warfarin was associated with a 37% reduction in strokes (95% CI, 23%–48%).[45] In the Atrial fibrillation Clopidogrel Trial with Irbesartan for prevention of Vascular Events (ACTIVE-W), anticoagulation therapy was superior to the combination clopidogrel plus aspirin (RRR, 40%; 95% CI, 18%–56%).[52] The risk of intracranial hemorrhage with adjusted-dose warfarin was double that with aspirin. The absolute risk increase, however, was small (0.2% per year).[45]

The higher benefit of warfarin for secondary stroke prevention can be explained by the fact that in patients who have experienced TIA or prior stroke, the underlying mechanism for stroke is more likely an embolus from a thrombus originating in the left atrium.[28,31,32] The effect of antithrombotic therapy varies according to the mechanism of the ischemic stroke in patients with AF. Aspirin reduces the risks of noncardioembolic stroke more than cardioembolic stroke in patients with AF, whereas adjusted-dose warfarin is much more efficacious than aspirin for prevention of cardioembolic stroke.[29-31]

Unquestionably, warfarin is highly efficacious for preventing stroke in patients with AF and relatively safe for selected patients. Aspirin offers less benefit, possibly by decreasing noncardioembolic strokes in these patients.

The choice of antithrombotic prophylaxis is based on the risk stratification (see Table 59-3). Long-term anticoagulation cannot be recommended for all unselected patients with AF, because most of them would not experience strokes even if untreated. Patients with AF with a relatively low risk of subsequent stroke would not substantially benefit from the use of warfarin, because the absolute risk reduction would be small (RRR, 1% per year). In these patients, anticoagulation may not be warranted. On the contrary, patients with AF who have a high risk for ischemic stroke (higher than 7%) because of a history of hypertension, prior TIA or stroke, or ventricular dysfunction would have a significantly lower stroke rate if they received anticoagulation.

High-risk patients who are good candidates for anticoagulation realize remarkable benefit from warfarin. For high-risk patients 75 years or younger, a target INR of 2.5 (range, 2.0 to 3.0) is effective and safe; for those older than 75 years, choosing a slightly lower target (INR, 2.0), with the hope of minimizing bleeding complications, appears appropriate. For secondary prevention, a target closer to an INR of 3.0 may be optimal. Patients younger than 60 years with "lone AF" may not require long-term anticoagulation, and because their intrinsic risk for stroke is small, aspirin may be sufficient. Higher intensities of anticoagulation may be required to prevent ischemic stroke in patients with multiple risk factors.

Paroxysmal atrial fibrillation (PAF), with underlying causes similar to those in sustained or constant AF, constitutes between 25% and 60% of all cases of AF. A clinical concern is whether patients with PAF face the same risk of stroke as those with sustained AF.[53] Epidemiologic data have suggested that the risk of stroke for patients with PAF is intermediate between those of patients with constant AF and patients with sinus rhythm. However, when data are controlled for stroke risk factors, PAF involves a stroke risk similar to that of constant AF.[54,55] Because the awareness of AF among patients with PAF varies greatly, it is difficult to stratify the stroke risk on the basis of the duration of the reported AF episodes; hence every patient with PAF should be assumed to have frequent episodes of AF and should be treated accordingly. The risk-to-benefit ratio for antithrombotic therapy in patients with PAF has not been evaluated in clinical trials. Therefore, the recommendations are based on indirect data from AF trials, so the approach to patients with PAF should be the same as that to patients with sustained AF.[33,53]

It has been theorized that the reversal of AF and maintenance of sinus rhythm might reduce the risk of stroke. The Atrial Fibrillation Follow-up Investigation of Rhythm Management (AFFIRM) study compared the outcomes of patients with AF randomly assigned to treatment with a rhythm-control strategy and with a rate-control strategy.[56] One objective of this study was to describe any differences in stroke occurrence in the two groups. The AFFIRM study was designed to compare mortality rates of patients managed with rate control only and those managed with rhythm control utilizing cardioversion and pharmacologic efforts along with anticoagulation. All patients had AF and at least one additional feature that put them at high risk for stroke. The AFFIRM study enrolled 4060 patients with a mean age of 69 years. Clinical stroke risk factors included hypertension (71%), history of congestive heart failure (CHF) (23%), history of TIA or stroke (13%), and diabetes mellitus (20%). The rate-control and rhythm-control groups did not differ significantly in the primary endpoint, that is, mortality ($P = .078$). Two hundred eleven patients (8%) had at least one stroke event. Ischemic stroke occurred in 6%, primary intraparenchymal hemorrhage in 1.2%, and subdural or subarachnoid hemorrhage in 0.8% of patients.[57] The most common ischemic stroke mechanism was cardioembolic in 37 patients. Eighty-nine patients had an ischemic stroke of unknown mechanism. At 5 years, 94% of patients in both treatment arms remained free of ischemic stroke. Treatment assignment had no significant effect on the occurrence of ischemic stroke. Age, history of TIA or stroke, history of diabetes, AF during follow-up, and absence of warfarin use were positively associated with ischemic stroke. After adjustment of data for other factors, patients with AF at the time of follow-up had a 72% greater chance of having ischemic stroke than those without AF. Taking warfarin reduced the chance of having ischemic stroke by 68%. The AFFIRM study therefore showed that the presence of AF increased ischemic stroke risk and the use of warfarin reduced stroke risk regardless of assigned treatment strategy.

Systemic embolization is the most serious complication of cardioversion of AF. Most of the embolic phenomena occur during the first 72 hours after cardioversion, most likely as a result of emboli arising from the left atrium at the time of cardioversion.[58] Prospective studies have shown an incidence of systemic emboli of 5% in patients with cardioversion who were not receiving anticoagulants versus 0.8% in those who were receiving oral anticoagulants.[59] The current recommendations for patients with AF undergoing cardioversion include anticoagulant therapy (INR, 2.5) for 3 weeks before and at least 4 weeks after the procedure. Alternatively, patients with AF should be started on anticoagulation, undergo transesophageal echocardiogram, and then have cardioversion without delay if no thrombus is seen. Oral anticoagulation should be continued until normal sinus rhythm has been maintained for at least 4 weeks.[33]

Cardiomyopathies

A cardiomyopathy is the second most common cause of cardiogenic stroke after AF, with a threefold increase in relative risk.[60] Cardiac failure affects some 4.5 million Americans, and its prevalence is increasing substantially as the population ages.[61]

The ejection fraction (EF) is a reliable measurement of left ventricular function, with the normal value between 50% and 70%. A decline in EF produces an elevated left ventricular filling pressure and a drop in stroke volume with a consequent reduction of systemic blood flow. The reduced stroke volume creates relative stasis within the left ventricle that promotes thrombus formation and an increased risk of thromboembolic events. Cardiomyopathies can be dilated or hypertrophic. Dilated cardiomyopathy is present if the diastolic dimension of the left ventricle becomes enlarged and hypertrophic when wall thickness is increased.

The relative risk of stroke in patients with heart failure is about 4% at age 60 years and decreases to about 2% by age 80 to 89 years.[60,62] In patients with CHF who are treated with aspirin or warfarin, the aggregate stroke risk per year has been found to be between 1% and 4%.[63-67] The stroke rate was inversely proportional to the EF in two studies.[63,64] In the Survival And Ventricular Enlargement trial (SAVE) trial, patients with EF of 32% had a stroke rate of 1% per year; with an EF of 28% or less, the rate increased up to 2% per year. This translates into an 18% increment in the risk of stroke for every 5% decline in EF.[64] Factors that raise the risk of stroke in patients with ischemic cardiomyopathy are the presence of AF and left ventricular thrombus. Stasis of blood in a poorly functioning left ventricle is thought to predispose to formation of ventricular thrombus; patients with chronic heart failure may also have hemostatic abnormalities.[68]

More than 50 years ago, it was discovered that administration of warfarin reduced the risk of pulmonary embolism, which was a major cause of death in patients with heart failure.[69-71] However, these patients also had a high prevalence of AF and more risks for deep vein thrombosis (DVT) and pulmonary embolism (PE). %. Cerebrovascular reactivity (CVR) also decreases linearly with decreasing left ventricular EF,[72] and reduced regional cerebral blood flow (rCBF) foci seen in patients with heart failure[73] may be a factor predisposing to stroke. Both warfarin and aspirin are effective in reducing stroke risk, but warfarin is associated with more bleeding complications, especially when used with aspirin. Whether antiplatelet or anticoagulant therapy is more beneficial for stroke prevention in patients with heart failure remains uncertain.

Dilated Cardiomyopathy

Ventricular thrombus formation occurs in about 30% to 50% of patients with dilated cardiomyopathy.[74] Systemic embolism occurs in 10% to 20% of patients with dilated cardiomyopathy, representing an annual risk of systemic embolization of 3% to 4%.[75,76] The thrombi present in dilated cardiomyopathy are less well anchored than those in acute myocardial infarction (MI) and often embolize before they can be visualized by echocardiogram. Thrombi in the left ventricle are distributed throughout the diffusely hypokinetic ventricle and are not localized to any particular region, as they are with saccular dyskinetic areas in patients after MI. The underlying mechanism for thrombus formation in patients with dilated cardiomyopathy is probably complex and multifactorial, including mechanical factors such as low velocity in the left ventricle and activation of hemostatic factors.[77,78] The intracavitary flow velocity is chronically reduced in these patients; therefore the risk of thrombus formation is constant.

The Study of Left Ventricular Dysfunction (SOLVD) clarified the relation between embolic stroke risk and worsening ventricular function.[63] Increased stroke risk was seen only in women (2.4 events per 100 patient-years compared with 1.8 events per 100 patient-years in men). In SOLVD, warfarin and aspirin were associated with a lower rate of death or hospitalization for heart failure than aspirin, but only warfarin reduced death from worsening heart failure. Although embolic stroke risk when left ventricular EF declines below 28% is double that for a value of 35%, patients with the lower values also benefit from aspirin alone (56% RRR in SAVE trial[64]) and without the bleeding complications. Owing to the lack of controlled studies of patients with left ventricular dysfunction and anticoagulation,[79] oral anticoagulation (INR intensity, 2.0 to 3.0 range) is recommended in patients with AF, previous episodes of thromboembolism (stroke or systemic or pulmonary embolism), or documented left ventricular thrombus.[80] For patients without these risk factors, there is controversy about whether antiplatelet or anticoagulation therapy should be used.[63,74,81-83]

The Warfarin and Aspirin Therapy in Chronic Heart Failure (WATCH) trial was designed to enroll 4500 patients and compare aspirin 160 mg/day, clopidogrel 75 mg/day, and warfarin (INR 2.5-3.0) in patients with poor LV function.[84] WATCH was terminated 18 months prematurely (June 2003) by the VA Cooperative Study Program because of poor enrollment. The results, presented in 2004,[85] showed that rate of nonfatal stroke was lower with warfarin than with aspirin and clopidogrel ($P = .05$), but the combined endpoint of nonfatal MI or stroke and death did not reach statistical significance ($P = .21$). The Warfarin versus Aspirin in patients with Reduced Cardiac Ejection Fraction (WARCEF) trial is a randomized, double-blind, multicenter trial studying the efficacy of warfarin (INR, 2.5-3.0; target, 2.75) versus aspirin (325 mg per day) in all-cause mortality and stroke (both ischemic and hemorrhagic) in patients with left ventricular EF of 35% or less.[86] The study, which began in 2002, had reached 1693 enrollees out of its goal of 3201 as of April 2008. The results of this study will be useful in determining optimal medical therapy in patients with heart failure and sinus rhythm.

Myocardial Infarction

The stroke rate in survivors of MI is about 1% to 2% per year. Because coronary artery atherosclerosis often coexists with atherosclerotic cerebrovascular disease, not all the strokes in these individuals are cardioembolic.[87,88] The risk of stroke is particularly high during the first 3 months after MI.[89,90]

The use of long-term anticoagulants after MI is associated with a 75% risk reduction in the incidence of stroke; however, this value represents an absolute risk reduction of only 1% per year. At the same time, anticoagulation (INR, 2.5 to 4.5) has an associated tenfold higher risk of intracerebral hemorrhage (ICH), or 0.4% per year. In addition, ICHs have a higher mortality and are more disabling than ischemic strokes.[91] In summary, we would need to treat 1000 unselected MI survivors to prevent approximately 10 strokes per year, and of those 1000 patients treated, 4 would suffer a disabling or fatal ICH; therefore, the net benefit is minimal. The risks and benefits of a lower-intensity anticoagulation (INR, 1.6 to 2.5) have not been tested in this setting.[92] Aspirin reduces the incidence of stroke in patients with prior MI, with an RRR of 30% but a very small absolute risk reduction (less than 0.5%). Because of such small net benefit, oral anticoagulation cannot be routinely recommended to prevent stroke in unselected MI survivors.

There are, however, specific subsets of patients with prior MI who are at higher risk of ischemic stroke and benefit from anticoagulation. Patients suffering anterior wall MI have a higher risk for stroke than patients with MI in other locations.[88,90,93] The presence of left ventricular thrombi after MI is associated with a much higher incidence of embolic stroke (approximately 5% to 10% over the following 6 to 12 months).[1,94] Left ventricular mural thrombus occurs in 20% of all MIs and up to 40% of anterior infarctions involving the apex. Formation of mural thrombi is almost exclusively limited to mural infarctions.[95] More than 90% of mural thrombi involve the left ventricular apex, and in acute MI, the formation of mural thrombi is directly related to the location and size of infarction and to the presence of ventricular failure.[96] Stasis associated with dyskinesias of the ventricle is an essential factor in formation of thrombi. Endothelial injury in the area of the infarction also plays an important role in thrombus formation. Finally, a hypercoagulable state during the acute phase of MI contributes to the development of thrombus.[97,98]

The risk of thromboembolism is greatest in the first week after infarction. Approximately half to two thirds of thrombi are detected within 48 hours of symptom onset, and two thirds of systemic emboli occur in the first 4 weeks after infarction.[94,99] The presence of thrombus mobility, proximity to a hypokinetic segment, and protrusion appear to raise the risk of embolism.[100] Additional risk factors predisposing to thrombus formation are EF less than 35%, apical dyskinesia, and anterior infarction.[94] In about 35% of cases, the thrombus disappears without treatment; however, the use of warfarin for 6 months is associated with thrombus disappearance. Systemic embolization has been documented in 20% of patients with echocardiographically proven thrombi, compared with 2% without visualization of thrombi. In a study from the Mayo Clinic, the presence of thrombus correlated inversely with the duration of anticoagulation. Anticoagulation is associated with a low incidence of embolization because with anticoagulation, the thrombus organizes, becomes endothelialized, and attaches to the ventricular wall.[101-103]

In short, when ventricular thrombus is present, anticoagulants reduce the stroke risk by 60%. Therefore, anticoagulation therapy is indicated for 3 to 6 months after detection of ventricular thrombi. Chronic thrombi (more than 6 months old) have less emboligenic potential, so anticoagulation after this period would be reasonable only for a patient in whom a thrombus is mobile or protruding.[104,105]

The presence of AF in MI survivors markedly raises the risk for embolic stroke.[90,106,107] Therefore, anticoagulation is routinely recommended in this situation. The risk of stroke increases by 1% to 2% per year when CHF is present in MI survivors. Even though the incidence of stroke in patients with CHF is double that in patients without CHF, the risk is still relatively low, and anticoagulation may not be of substantial benefit.[65,82] Patients who experience anterior wall myocardial infarction and are found to have ventricular wall thrombus should receive warfarin therapy, aiming for an INR ranging from 2 to 3, for up to 6 months.[108] Thereafter, aspirin therapy may

be used. Prolonged anticoagulation decreased stroke risk up to 40% over 3 years in the Anticoagulants in the Secondary Prevention of Events in Coronary Thrombosis (ASPECT) trial, although major bleeding complications were increased.[109]

In summary, oral anticoagulation (INR, 2.5 to 4.8) to prevent stroke does not substantially benefit unselected patients with acute MI. The value of lower-intensity anticoagulation (INR, 1.6 to 2.5) and antiplatelet agent therapy for stroke prevention in this setting is still unproven. On the other hand, patients with prior MI and AF or acute left ventricular thrombi are at higher risk of embolic stroke; anticoagulation (INR, 2.0 to 3.0) is routinely recommended for stroke prevention in these patients. On the basis of the available evidence, oral anticoagulation in the patient with left ventricular thrombus should be administered for at least 6 months; the patient should then be reassessed for the presence and characteristics of left ventricular thrombi by means of echocardiography.

Valvular Heart Disease

Before the use of surgical replacement of heart valves, valvular disease, especially rheumatic mitral valve disease, was associated with a very high risk of systemic emboli. Now almost all the patients with congenital or acquired valvular disease undergo surgical implantation of prosthetic heart valves. Hence, for most patients with valvular heart disease, the requirement for antithrombotic therapy depends on the thromboembolic risk associated with valve replacement. Data on antithrombotic therapy in patients with native valvular disease is limited, and all published recommendations are based on clinical experience.

Giant Lambl's excrescence (GLE) consists of valvular abnormalities that have a frondlike appearance and a stalklike attachment that arise mostly from left-sided valvular surfaces (aortic more than mitral) and are of unclear cause (neoplastic, hamartomatous, or reparative).[110] Embolic risk is difficult to quantify for GLE but appears directly proportional to size and mobility. Medical therapy is typically an antiplatelet agent first, and if recurrent cerebral ischemic events occur, anticoagulation or surgical resection is considered for large (more than 1 cm), mobile lesions.[110-112]

Valvular strands[110,113] are common small filiform projections (less than 1 mm in width and 1 cm in length) arising near valve closure lines (mitral more than aortic) that result from traumatic abrasions of the valve surface. Risk factors for valvular strands include age and valvular disease (e.g., rheumatic valve disease). For patients with cerebral ischemic events attributable to valvular strands, antiplatelet therapy is recommended. It is uncertain whether anticoagulation is superior to antiplatelet therapy for stroke prevention in this condition.[113] However, it is reasonable to administer antiplatelet therapy.[79]

Rheumatic Mitral Valve Disease

Of all native valvular diseases, rheumatic mitral valve disease carries the highest risk of systemic emboli. The incidence of systemic emboli ranges from 2% to 5% per year.[114,115] In short, it can be assumed that a patient with rheumatic mitral valve disease has at least one chance in five of having a symptomatic systemic embolus during his or her life.[116] Mitral stenosis carries a higher risk of embolization than mitral regurgitation, and the presence of AF increases the risk of embolism by about sevenfold.[115,117] In addition, the risk of systemic emboli in patients with rheumatic heart disease increases with age and is higher in those with associated low EF.[114,118,119] After a first episode of embolization, recurrent emboli occur in 30% to 65% of patients; more than half of recurrences are seen during the first year, most during the first 6 months.[116,120]

Although long-term anticoagulation was never examined in randomized trials in this population, observational studies have established the effectiveness of this intervention in reducing systemic emboli. Szekely[115] observed a significant reduction in the proportion of emboli in patients receiving anticoagulation in comparison with patients receiving no treatment (3% versus 10% per year, respectively). The annual incidence of systemic emboli in 217 patients who were undergoing anticoagulation and had mitral stenosis was reported to be as low as 0.8% per year.[121,122] In patients with mitral stenosis and ischemic stroke who were monitored for 20 years, there was significant reduction in death associated with cerebral emboli; 13 deaths occurred in the untreated patients, and 4 in the patients receiving anticoagulation.[123]

In view of these data, all patients with rheumatic mitral valve disease and AF should be treated with long-term anticoagulation if possible. Patients with rheumatic heart disease and prior ischemic stroke should also receive anticoagulation in view of the high recurrence rate.[116,120] The recommended intensity of anticoagulation is a target INR of 2.5. If recurrent embolism occurs despite adequate anticoagulation, the target INR should be increased to 3.0 or aspirin, 81 mg per day, should be added. For patients intolerant of aspirin, the addition of clopidogrel could be an option, although there are no data to support this recommendation.[124]

Prosthetic Cardiac Valves

Despite advances in valve design and effective anticoagulant therapy, systemic embolism remains a serious threat in patients who have undergone heart valve replacement. The rate of embolism is high in patients with mechanical prosthetic cardiac valves, being 2% to 4% per year even in those with proper anticoagulation.[125-130] The risk of embolism is higher with tilting disk prosthetic valves in the mitral position than in the aortic position. Embolism occurs at estimated rates of 0.5% per year with prosthetic aortic valves, 1% per year with mitral valves, and 1.5% per year for both.[131] Embolism is more frequent with valves in the mitral position, with multiple valves, and with caged-ball valves. Atrial stasis, a risk factor for thrombogenicity, is influenced by valve type and position, coexistent AF, and ventricular pacemakers. AF and enlargement of the left atrium are more common in patients with mitral valve disease.[123,132]

Permanent anticoagulation is generally recommended to prevent embolic stroke and valve thrombosis with all mechanical prosthetic valves. In addition, anticoagulation

is also recommended for bioprosthetic valves in the mitral position in the patient with AF, enlarged (more than 5.5 cm) left atrium, ventricular pacemakers, or evidence of atrial thrombi or prior thromboembolism.[126]

Long-term anticoagulation may not be required for bioprosthetic valves in the aortic position in patients with sinus rhythm because the stroke rate is relatively low. Warfarin (INR, 2.0 to 3.0) is recommended for a period of 3 months after valve implantation, because the frequency of thromboembolism is increased (about 6%) in patients who do not receive anticoagulation.[124,126]

Thrombogenicity of specific valves varies, as do factors influencing thromboembolic risk; thus, multiple factors should be considered in the selection of prophylactic antithrombotic therapy. In the past, the intensity of anticoagulation for mechanical valves was a target INR between 3.0 and 4.5. Now it is believed that a lower intensity (INR, 2.5 to 3.5) would be as effective; however, this issue remains controversial. Adding an antiplatelet agent such as aspirin or dipyridamole to warfarin further reduces embolism risk; however, this therapeutic strategy may raise the risk of bleeding (mostly minor bleeds when aspirin is added).[127]

The success of antithrombotic therapy in primary stroke prevention in patients with prosthetic valves is influenced by the type of prosthesis, factors associated with left atrial stasis, underlying cardiovascular disease, and tolerability of antithrombotic therapies. The optimal or appropriate intensity of anticoagulation and the decision to use additional antiplatelet agents in individual patients depend on the presence of some of the previously mentioned risk factors and the valve type.

The current recommendations are as follows: Oral anticoagulation with a target INR between 2 and 3 should be used in all patients with mechanical prosthetic valves (St. Jude Medical bileaflet valve or Medtronic ball tilting disk mechanical valve) in the aortic position and with sinus rhythm. For patients with tilting disk valves and bileaflet mechanical valves in the mitral position, the intensity of anticoagulation is a target INR of 2.5 to 3.5. The same intensity of anticoagulation is recommended for patients with AF who are given prosthetic valves in the aortic position. An alternative therapeutic option is to add aspirin, 81 to 100 mg per day, to warfarin (target, INR 2.0 to 3.0) in patients at high risk of embolization (i.e., valves in mitral position, AF, tilting disk valves). For those with caged-ball or caged-disk valves or additional risk factors, a higher target INR (2.5 to 3.5) plus low-dose aspirin is recommended.[124,126]

In patients with full anticoagulation, the incidence of stroke is about 1% per year and most of the emboli are minor, leaving mild residual deficits.[129,130,133] When stroke occurs in patients receiving anticoagulation, transesophageal echocardiography (TEE) should usually be performed to search for infective valve vegetations, thrombi, spontaneous echodensities, and atrial thrombi.[134] Anticoagulation may be increased if embolism from the left atrium is suspected, but adding an antiplatelet agent might be useful if the stroke is attributed to cerebrovascular disease or valve-related thrombi.[127]

In patients at high risk of thromboembolism, the interruption of anticoagulant therapy before invasive procedures often presents a challenge to clinicians. No randomized controlled trial has assessed this situation, but data from small nonrandomized studies favor the use of low-molecular-weight (LMW) heparin for safety and economic reasons.[135-137] It is recommended that warfarin therapy be stopped approximately 4 days before surgery, allowing the INR to return to a normal level. Full-dose LMW heparin is begun as the INR falls (about 2 days before surgery). The LMW heparin can be stopped about 12 hours before surgery and restarted between 8 and 12 hours after the procedure.[138,139]

Nonbacterial Thrombotic Endocarditis

Nonbacterial thrombotic endocarditis (NBTE) or marantic endocarditis is a noninfectious process affecting normal or degenerative cardiac valves that is due to fibrin thrombi deposits in patients with hypercoagulable states associated with adenocarcinomas of the lung, colon, or pancreas that produce mucin.[140] Patients with NBTE may present with arterial and venous thromboembolism and disseminated intravascular coagulation. Heparin but not warfarin has been associated with benefit[140] as well as treatment of the underlying neoplastic disorder.

Libman-Sacks endocarditis is a noninfectious valvular abnormality associated with autoimmune disorders such as systemic lupus erythematosus and the antiphospholipid antibody syndrome. No large-scale, randomized trials exist to provide evidence-based data, but some experts recommend anticoagulation with warfarin as primary treatment to prevent stroke.[141]

Infectious Endocarditis

Infectious seeding of heart valves or endocarditis prior to the advent of antibiotics was associated with a very high cerebral embolic rate (70% to 90%), which decreased (12% to 40%) with the advent of antibiotics.[63,82,140,142-146] Specific antibiotic therapy for endocarditis remains the first-line treatment on the basis of blood culture results, whereas anticoagulation remains controversial or contraindicated,[140,147-152] given the early rates of cerebral hemorrhage and the fact that anticoagulation does not reduce the incidence of embolism in native valve endocarditis. Patients with mechanical prosthetic valves, however, may be at higher risk if anticoagulation is discontinued.[63] Exceptions to this rule include a patient with an infected aortic bioprosthetic valve, a patient who is on antibiotics, or a patient who is in normal sinus rhythm. Controversy remains about the duration and intensity of anticoagulation in patients with prosthetic valve endocarditis, given the risk of embolism versus intracranial hemorrhage.[140,147-152] Prosthetic endocarditis also may embolize to the brain, where an infected microscopic nidus (especially when there is *Staphylococcus aureus*) or microaneurysm that may be prone to cerebral hemorrhage may develop. The patient with prosthetic valve endocarditis may be thought of as an anticoagulation dilemma because the ischemic stroke risk must be balanced against cerebral hemorrhagic risk. We recommend careful consideration of the patient's valve type and location and presence or absence of AF to weigh the ischemic and hemorrhagic

risks. For example, if the patient had a large ischemic stroke from endocarditis, anticoagulation becomes higher risk for brain hemorrhage and may need to be delayed or not administered at all.

Infective endocarditis of a prosthetic heart valve warrants early surgical consultation. Surgical replacement of an infected prosthetic valve carries a high risk for morbidity and mortality especially in the case of mitral position valves. Surgical removal or repair is considered for patients with congestive heart failure, cardiac abscess, or persistently positive blood culture results despite antibiotic treatment. Early surgery is also warranted in the case of fungal endocarditis.

Cardiac Tumors

Primary cardiac tumors are rare (less than 0.2% in unselected autopsy series) and the majority of them benign (50% myxomas and papillary fibroelastoma) but associated with a high frequency of embolic events. Myxomas commonly occur in the left atrium and arise from the interatrial septum. They may embolize to the systemic circulation, particularly to the brain, when tumor pieces break off or there is secondary thrombus formation. TEE is invaluable in defining tumor location, size, and morphology. To prevent embolization, surgical resection of the tumor is recommended in all cases of myxoma.[79,111,112,153]

Papillary fibroelastomas are benign tumors that tend to originate on cardiac valves in single or multiple masses. Embolic events are typically the first clinical manifestation, because they are present on highly mobile valve leaflets. The embolic mechanism is the same as myxomas, being tumor fragmentation or secondary thrombus generation. Surgical resection is also indicated for fibroelastomas.[79,111,112,153]

Metastatic tumors to the heart are 20 to 40 times more frequent than primary cardiac tumors, which are rare (e.g., angiosarcoma, rhabdomyosarcoma).[79,154] Cerebral embolization can occur from these tumors as well. Surgical treatment can be offered but depends on the underlying tumor type and prognosis.

Patent Foramen Ovale

The high frequency of patent foramen ovale (PFO) is in part the result of advances that have been made in cardiac imaging techniques. PFO has been associated with stroke in several case-control studies, particularly in young individuals without an alternative recognized cause of stroke. PFO is a potential conduit for paradoxical embolism.[155-159] However, its relationship to stroke, its prognosis, and the therapeutic implications are not clearly established. Precordial contrast echocardiography detects some interatrial shunting in about 18% of normal controls,[155,160-163] especially during early systole or Valsalva maneuver–provoking activities such as coughing.[164,165] The fossa ovalis and the size of PFO can be directly visualized by TEE, considered the diagnostic "gold standard."[2,3,166] Transcranial Doppler (TCD) ultrasonography can detect injected microbubbles that bypass the pulmonary capillaries and enter the cerebral circulation, an observation that correlates well with the TEE evidence of PFO in the majority of patients.[167-170] The size of the PFO patency varies from 1 to 9 mm at autopsy.[171] The volume of shunting depends on the size of the PFO and the difference in atrial pressures. Contrast-enhanced TCD ultrasonographic assessment of the middle cerebral artery is highly specific compared with contrast TEE in detecting right-to-left shunt.[172]

Several studies have now shown that the prevalence of PFO in young adults with TIA or ischemic stroke is increased (about 40%; range 32% to 48%),[155-159,173] especially among those with cryptogenic ischemic stroke, in whom its prevalence in some series exceeds 50%.[158,163,171] The wide range of PFO prevalence may reflect in part the interobserver variability in the diagnosis of septal abnormalities. Hence, the frequency of PFO is increased twofold to threefold among young adults with cerebral ischemia, and PFO is clearly associated with cryptogenic stroke in young adults, who are less likely to have traditional risk factors for stroke. The difference in risk factors suggests differing stroke mechanisms in patients with and without PFO.[156] In older patients with stroke, the prevalence of PFO is lower, probably because its importance as an independent risk factor is offset by the higher prevalence of other stroke mechanisms.[174-177] In a meta-analysis of case-control studies comparing patients with stroke and control subjects, PFO was significantly associated with ischemic stroke only in patients younger than 55 years. The odds ratio of stroke was 3 (95% CI, 2-4).[178]

Because PFO is also common in normal subjects, it is important to characterize the cases associated with stroke. Therefore, it is possible that patients with PFO plus atrial septal aneurysm (ASA) constitute a subgroup of patients at increased risk of stroke.[156] An ASA is a sustained 15-mm segmental bowing of the interatrial septal membrane in the fossa ovalis of at least 11 to 15 mm beyond the plane of the interatrial septum or may be a phasic excursion to either side of the same distance.[110] Therefore, an ASA may be the substrate for in situ thrombus to form, which later passes through the PFO (right- to left-sided circulation).

The mechanism of PFO-associated stroke is thought to be due to paradoxical embolism in many patients. Paradoxical embolism occurs when embolic material originating in the venous system or right heart chambers migrates into the systemic circulation through vascular shunts that bypass the pulmonary vasculature. However, this mechanism has been well documented in only a few cases, in which the embolus was seen in its passage through a PFO. A venous source of thromboembolism is rarely found in patients with stroke and PFO.[179,180] The failure to document a venous source does not rule out paradoxical emboli, because in many cases, deep venous thrombosis in the pelvis or legs is underrecognized. Another potential mechanism for stroke is direct embolization from thrombi formed locally within the PFO or in an associated ASA.[181] In a prospective study of 503 patients with stroke,[182] PFO or PFO-ASA was detected in 34% and 14% of the patients classified with cryptogenic stroke by Trial of Org 10172 in Acute Stroke Treatment (TOAST) criteria versus 12% and 4%, respectively, with stroke of known type ($P < .001$). The study also compared 131 younger patients (less than 55 years) with 372 older patients (more

than 55 years) and found that the PFO-ASA combination was more strongly associated with cryptogenic stroke in younger ($P < .049$) and older ($P < 0.001$) patients than with known stroke subtype.

It is also postulated that patients with PFO are more prone to development of supraventricular arrhythmias that may predispose to thrombus formation.[163] Emboli can arise from thrombi in the crural pelvic veins or in the right heart chamber; however, the source of embolism is often not found.

Paradoxical embolism then may not be the most common underlying mechanism of stroke in patients with PFO. First, in patients with isolated PFO, the shunting during Valsalva maneuver involves only a small fraction of the cardiac output, and the chances that this level of shunting will result in recurrent emboli is remote.[183] Second, deep venous thrombosis is identified in only about 10% of PFO-associated strokes. Further, PFO is associated with mitral valve prolapse and ASA, both of which are independent potential cardioembolic sources of emboli. ASAs are present in about 25% of young patients with PFO-associated stroke,[156,184] and their presence alone has been associated with a higher risk of embolic stroke. It is possible that in as many as half of patients with PFO-associated stroke, PFO and stroke coexist by chance.

In addition to the unclear mechanism of stroke in patients with PFO, the risk of recurrent stroke remains unsettled owing to the lack of prospective data. Most studies are retrospective and without control subjects.[163,184-186] Two studies reported stroke recurrence between 1% and 2% in patients with PFO.[187,188] A prospective study of 581 patients with cryptogenic stroke treated with aspirin reported that at 4 years, the risk of recurrent stroke was 2% in those with PFO (n = 216), 15% in those with both PFO and ASA (n = 51), and 4% in those with neither. Only 10 patients in the study had ASA alone, and no recurrence was seen in this group. In this study, only the presence of both abnormalities was associated with a significant risk of stroke (relative risk [RR] 4; 95% CI, 1-12). PFO alone, regardless of its size, did not influence the risk of stroke.[189]

Results of the Patent Foramen Ovale in Cryptogenic Stroke Study (PICSS), a substudy of the Warfarin-Aspirin Recurrent Stroke Study (WARSS), were reported in 2002. The 630 patients first underwent TEE, which documented PFO in 34%, and then were randomly assigned to receive either warfarin (INR, 2.0) or aspirin. The stroke rates were similar for the two interventions, and the presence of PFO did not alter the event rate when associated with all or cryptogenic strokes. There was no benefit to using warfarin in patients with large PFO or in those with PFO and ASA (12% of the total).[172]

In short, the role of PFO as a cause of stroke is still unsettled; therefore, the optimal treatment remains undetermined. On the basis of current evidence, every patient with stroke and PFO should receive antiplatelet therapy. In addition, if there is evidence of deep venous thrombosis, pulmonary embolism, or recurrent stroke, the use of long-term anticoagulation seems appropriate.

It is sensible to speculate that closure of PFO by surgical or device-mediated procedures would prevent stroke recurrence in patients with paradoxical emboli. Device closure seems to be effective, safe, and cost effective.[190-195] Its value is still unclear, however, given the uncertainties in pathogenesis, recurrence rate of stroke, and comparative efficacy against antithrombotic agents. Before this procedure is widely used for stroke prevention, it must be compared in randomized clinical trials with medical treatment. No randomized trial has been completed to date despite five ongoing studies recruiting patients for PFO closure in cryptogenic stroke (www.clinicaltrials.gov; identifiers NCT00557479, NCT00196040, NCT00562289, NCT00201461, and NCT00166257). Unfortunately, enrollment has been slow in these studies. Currently, the Randomized Evaluation of recurrent Stroke comparing PFO closure to Established Current standard of care Treatment (RESPECT) trial (AGA Medical Corp) is recruiting patients with prior stroke or TIA and PFO without other known cause. A total of 500 patients will be assigned either to percutaneous closure of PFO using the Amplatzer PFO Occluder device or to best medical treatment (oral anticoagulants or antiplatelet agents), with follow-up for up to 5 years. Until the results of clinical trials are available, patients with PFO should be treated with antithrombotic agents and encouraged to participate in randomized trials testing different interventions.

Because of the lack of randomized trial data comparing PFO closure with standard medical therapy, the American Academy of Neurology issued practice parameters concluding that there was insufficient evidence to recommend routine percutaneous closure of PFOs in patients with cryptogenic stroke.[196]

Aortic Arch Disease

An overlooked but a potentially serious source of embolic stroke is the aortic arch.[197] Aortic embolic events may be misclassified as cryptogenic unless adequate transesophageal echocardiography of the aorta is performed. Patients with ascending aorta or proximal arch plaques of 4 mm thickness are up to seven times more likely to have cerebral infarction than controls (14.4% vs. 2%, P < 0.001).[197,198] For nonmobile aortic plaque, statin therapy may be protective in preventing stroke (level II evidence[199]), whereas uncertainty remains about the optimal antithrombotic therapy, aspirin or warfarin.[199] The Aortic arch Related Cerebral Hazard (ARCH) trial is currently ongoing, comparing the efficacy of anticoagulant therapy (warfarin) with that of antiplatelet therapy (aspirin in combination with clopidogrel) in preventing stroke in high-risk patients with aortic arch atheromas (http://stroke center.org/).

Anticoagulant Agents

Heparin, Low-Molecular-Weight Heparin, and Heparinoids

Heparin is the most commonly used parenteral anticoagulant. Unfractionated heparin is derived from bovine lung or porcine gut tissue. A glycosaminoglycan of varying molecular weight, heparin binds to antithrombin III to inactivate factors IIa and Xa.[2] Its major anticoagulant effect comes from a unique pentasaccharide with high-affinity binding to antithrombin. Unfractionated heparin is quite heterogeneous, containing saccharides ranging in molecular weight from 5000 to 30,000 daltons. Only about one third of the unfractionated heparin molecules have anticoagulant activity. This heterogeneity is one of the reasons for the variability in the anticoagulant effect of heparin administration among individuals.

The most common side effect of heparin administration is bleeding. Other complications are thrombocytopenia, osteoporosis, skin necrosis, alopecia, hypersensitivity reactions, and hypoaldosteronism. Thrombocytopenia is somewhat more common with heparin derived from bovine lung than from porcine gut. The thrombocytopenia is thought to occur because of the binding of immunoglobulin (Ig) G to heparin. Thrombocytopenia occurs in between 0.3% (in prophylactic use) and 2.4% (with higher therapeutic doses) of treated patients.

LMW heparin represents a fragment of a standard heparin with lower molecular weight, higher bioavailability, longer half-life, and more predictable anticoagulant effects. LMW heparin is said to cause fewer bleeding complications and fewer interactions with platelets, but this issue remains somewhat controversial. Heparinoids are analogues of heparin that inhibit factor Xa, have a longer half-life than unfractionated heparin, and cause fewer bleeding complications. LMW heparin is as effective as, if not more effective than, unfractionated heparin, has the advantage of being given in fixed subcutaneous doses, and does not require monitoring or dose adjustment.[200]

Warfarin

Warfarin, an oral anticoagulant, is the most commonly used coumarin. Warfarin acts as a vitamin K antagonist, interfering with the production of vitamin K-dependent proteins, including the coagulation factors II, VII, IX, and X. The dose of warfarin ranges typically between 2 and 10 mg per day and must be individualized and adjusted to achieve the desired INR. Therapy is initiated with an estimated daily maintenance dose, such as 5mg per day. Lower initial doses (3 to 4 mg/day) may be used in elderly and small individuals. The prothrombin time and INR are monitored frequently until values are in the target range and stable. Thereafter, stable patients are typically monitored at least monthly. The target INR for most indications is 2.5 (range, 2.0 to 3.0). The target is increased to 3.0 (range, 2.5 to 3.5) in patients with high-risk mechanical prosthetic cardiac valves and in patients with the antiphospholipid antibody syndrome.[138,139]

Warfarin therapy is contraindicated in patients at risk for major hemorrhage. Commonly acknowledged contraindications include active bleeding, recent surgery, pregnancy, esophageal varices, thrombocytopenia, concurrent use of thrombolytic agents, recent lumbar puncture, and congenital clotting defects. Patients at increased risk for falls or other trauma may not be candidates for long-term anticoagulation therapy. The importance of compliance dictates that unreliable or demented patients should receive warfarin therapy only if their therapy and INR monitoring can be adequately supervised.

Warfarin has the potential to interact with numerous agents (Table 59-4). Some potentiate and others inhibit the anticoagulant effects of warfarin. In addition, foods

TABLE 59-4   NOVEL ANTICOAGULANT AGENTS UNDER EVALUATION FOR PREVENTION OF STROKE IN ATRIAL FIBRILLATION

Drug	Target	Dosing	Onset (h)	Half-Life (h)	Antidote
Apixaban	Factor Xa	Twice a day	3	12	No
Edoxoban	Factor Xa	Once a day	3	9-11	No
Rivaroxaban	Factor Xa	Once a day	3	9	No
Dabigatran	Thrombin	Twice a day	1-2	12-17	No
Tecarfarin	Vitamin K antagonist	Once a day	Unknown	136	Yes; vitamin K
Betrixaban	Factor Xa	Twice a day	Unknown	19	No
Idrabiotaparinux	Factor Xa	Weekly*	1-2	80-130	Yes; intravenous avidin

*Subcutaneous administration. The rest of the agents are administered orally.

high in vitamin K can inhibit the effects of warfarin. Other substances, such as alcohol, may increase bleeding risk. The best course is to monitor the INR after any change in medications in a patient receiving warfarin and adjust the dose as needed. In addition, patient education about the potential effects of over-the counter-preparations and foods is an important element of warfarin management.

The main potential side effect of warfarin is bleeding. The only other serious side effect is skin necrosis. This uncommon complication, seen on the third to eighth day of therapy, is caused by thrombosis of venules and capillaries within the subcutaneous fat. A number of factors influence bleeding risk with warfarin therapy. The intensity of anticoagulation is directly related to bleeding risk, the rate of major bleeds increasing dramatically with INR levels exceeding 4.0. Patients older than 75 years have a higher risk of hemorrhage, particularly ICH. Patients with cerebrovascular disease are at greater risk for ICH than patients without a history of ischemic cerebrovascular disease. Other comorbid conditions that increase bleeding risk are hypertension, heart disease, renal insufficiency, and malignancy. Alcoholism and liver disease are also considered by many to raise the risk of bleeding associated with warfarin therapy.

Oral Anticoagulants Combined with Antiplatelet Agents

The risks and benefits of combination of an oral anticoagulant and an antiplatelet agent compared with an oral anticoagulant alone for secondary prevention of cardioembolic stroke have not been clearly established. Turpie et al[127] studied young patients with prosthetic valves and showed a significant reduction of embolic events in those assigned to combination therapy and no significant increase in the incidence of ICH (7 patients versus 3 patients, respectively).[127] However, in view of the occurrence of only a few events and the patients' ages, these results cannot be generalized to different groups of patients (i.e., elderly with established cerebrovascular disease).

A meta-analysis of six randomized clinical trials that compared warfarin plus aspirin with warfarin alone in different populations found that the addition of aspirin to warfarin significantly increased the risk of ICH (RR, 2.3; 95% CI, 1.1–4.8). The increased risk of ICH was seen even in trials that used lower doses of aspirin.[201] It is possible that the risk-to-benefit ratio of combination therapy

for elderly patients with prior ischemic strokes may be higher than that for young patients with prosthetic valvular disease. For those at high risk of suffering ICH during anticoagulation (i.e., older than 75 years, white matter abnormalities, prior stroke), the addition of aspirin could offset the benefit of reducing ischemic events. Therefore, we recommended that aspirin not be added routinely to oral anticoagulant therapy in elderly patients with established cerebrovascular disease until additional data define the risks and benefits.

New Antithrombotic Agents

Although warfarin is highly efficacious in preventing systemic emboli in AF patients, its use is restricted by the narrow therapeutic window, multiple drug interactions, and the need for permanent INR monitoring.[202] A 2009 survey showed that clearly warfarin is underused in AF patients; fewer than 40% were anticoagulated with only 10% of them with a therapeutic INR. Consequently, owing to the inherent limitations for the use of oral anticoagulants in patients with AF, there is a need to develop and test novel antithrombotic agents with a much safer profile and wider therapeutic window than warfarin.

The results of the RE-LY study showed that dabigatran, a new oral direct thrombin inhibitor, was superior to warfarin in preventing stroke or systemic emboli in patients with AF. Dabigatran was given in fixed doses (110 or 150 mg bid) and warfarin in an adjusted-dose fashion. Patients with AF and a risk of stroke (N = 18,113) were allocated to both interventions. The rate of primary outcome was 1.69% per year in those assigned to warfarin, compared with 1.53% per year in the group that received 110 mg of dabigatran (RR, 0.91; 95% CI, 0.74–1.11; P < .001 for noninferiority) and 1.11% per year in the group that received 150 mg of dabigatran (RR, 0.66; 95% CI, 0.53– 0.82; P < 0.001 for superiority). The rate of intracranial bleeds was significantly lower in patients receiving dabigatran, even in those receiving 150 mg. The rate of systemic major bleeds was higher in patients assigned to dabigatran 150 mg than those treated with warfarin. Patients assigned to dabigatran experienced higher frequency of dyspepsia than those treated with warfarin (11% versus 6%). In short, dabigatran showed different and complementary advantages over warfarin, and it might be a safe and effective alternative to warfarin for patients with AF at risk of stroke. However, the following concerns are still unanswered: (1) the safety and efficacy of dabigatran beyond 2 years (duration of the trial), (2) the lack of antidote to revert anticoagulation, and (3) the cost. One of the potential disadvantages of dabigatran despite the results of the RE-LY study are the presence of dyspepsia and the twice-daily administration, factors that might impact patient adherence to therapy.

A number of novel antithrombotic agents (factor Xa inhibitors) are currently being tested against warfarin in patients with AF (see Table 59-4). The ROCKET-AF study (described as a randomized, double-blind study comparing once-daily oral rivaroxaban with adjusted-dose oral warfarin for the prevention of stroke in subjects with nonvalvular atrial fibrillation) was scheduled to present its results in late 2010.[203] The Apixaban versus Acetylsalicylic Acid to Prevent Strokes (AVERROES) trial compared apixaban with aspirin in patients with AF. The study was terminated prematurely owing to the clinical superiority in stroke or systemic emboli reduction showed by apixaban over aspirin with an excellent safety profile (presented at the European Society of Cardiology Congress 2010). Oral direct thrombin inhibitors and factor Xa inhibitors are an attractive group of agents that do not require the intensive laboratory monitoring and have fewer drug interactions than warfarin.

Intracerebral Hemorrhage Associated with Anticoagulation

ICH is the most serious complication of anticoagulant therapy because of its high associated mortality. Anticoagulation with INR targets between 2.5 and 4.5 increases the risk of ICH 7 to 10 times,[204-206] representing an absolute rate of 1% per year in stroke-prone patients.[49] The mortality related to oral anticoagulants in patients with ICH exceeds 50%. The cerebellum is frequently involved, and simultaneous ICHs at multiple sites can occur, particularly with excessive anticoagulation. One of the unique features of intracerebral hematomas related to anticoagulation is that they can continue to enlarge for 12 to 24 hours; therefore, anticoagulation should be reversed immediately, even in patients with minimal deficits and small hematomas. ICH-related anticoagulation is usually managed by the following approaches:

- Cessation of anticoagulation therapy.
- Administration of vitamin K; the INR is not affected for several hours, and the dose should not exceed 10 mg because higher doses lead to refractoriness to further anticoagulant therapy for days.
- Administration of plasma derivatives containing vitamin K–dependent clotting factors, such as fresh frozen plasma (FFP) and cryoprecipitates.

FFP reverses anticoagulation immediately, but it has the disadvantage of requiring a large infusion to correct the INR, which could be a problem in patients with poor cardiac function. Factor concentrates (factor II, VII, IX, and X) are an alternative for patients who cannot tolerate large volume of fluids but should not be used in patients with liver failure.

The hemostatic agent recombinant activated factor VII (rFVIIa) has been used for the management of hemorrhages in the central nervous system associated with anticoagulation. In the phase 2B randomized controlled trial, Mayer et al[207] and the Novo Nordisk investigators studied the effect of recombinant factor VIIa (rFVIIa) on early hematoma growth. Three hundred and ninety-nine patients with acute ICH were randomly assigned to placebo or to 40 μg/kg, 80 μg/kg, or 160 μg/kg of rFVIIa within 1 hour after a baseline CT scan. The primary outcome of the study was to assess hematoma growth at 24 hours. A dose-dependent effect on reducing hematoma growth was noticed, with a mean increase of 29%, 16%, 14%, and 11% in the placebo, 40 μg/kg, 80 μg/kg, and 160 μg/kg groups, respectively ($P = .01$). The modified Rankin Scale (mRS) performed at 90 days found 69% of placebo-treated patients dead or severely disabled (mRS = 4 to 6), compared with 49% to 55% for the rFVIIa-treated patients ($P = .004$). Mortality at 90 days was 29% for placebo-treated patients, compared with 18% for rFVIIa-treated patients. Thromboembolic events (MI or ischemic stroke) occurred in 7% of rFVIIa-treated patients, compared with 2% of placebo-treated patients ($P = .12$).

To address safety and to find an optimal dose, Novo Nordisk and the NovoSeven Investigators completed the phase 3 Factor Seven for Acute Hemorrhagic Stroke (FAST) study in the United States and Europe, which involved 821 patients randomly assigned to receive placebo or 20 μg/kg or 80 μg/kg of rFVIIa.[208] The investigators reported reduced growth of the hematoma and a safety profile similar to results of the phase 2B study. However, the FAST study failed to confirm that rFVIIa given within 4 hours of onset improves survival or functional outcome in ICH and has not gained a U.S. Food and Drug Administration (FDA) label indication for that purpose. In summary, with the available evidence, the use of rFVIIa for the management of ICH is not indicated outside clinical trials. It remains an off-label indication for this agent.

Well-established risk factors for ICH in patients who have been receiving anticoagulants include advanced age (particularly more than 75 years), hypertension, prior ischemic stroke,[209] and intensity of anticoagulation (perhaps also fluctuations in the level of anticoagulation).[37,206,210] The significance of high INR levels in influencing the development of ICH was demonstrated in an observational study and in the Stroke Prevention in Reversible Ischemia Trial (SPIRIT) study. In this study, the absolute rate of ICH was 3% per year in patients receiving anticoagulation, particularly those with INR values exceeding 4.0.[211,212]

White matter abnormalities, identified by neuroimaging studies in patients with established cerebrovascular disease, were found to be an independent risk factor for ICH associated with anticoagulation.[211,213,214] Small hemosiderin deposits (indicative of asymptomatic "microbleeds") are frequently detected by gradient echo MRI in patients with stroke, particularly those with small vessel disease (i.e., lacunar stroke, primary ICH, and white matter abnormalities).[215,216] It is likely that the presence of microbleeds predisposes to ICH in patients taking anticoagulants; so far, this predisposition has been reported only in patients receiving antiplatelet agents.[217] It is sensible to speculate that white matter abnormalities and microbleeds represent manifestations of a vasculopathy that predisposes to development of ICH in patients receiving anticoagulants.[218] Currently, the presence of white matter abnormalities or microbleeds does not preclude the use of anticoagulants; more data are needed to stratify the risk of ICH on the basis of MRI findings.

Cerebral amyloid angiography (CAA) is characterized by deposition of congophilic amyloid beta protein in cortical and leptomeningeal vessels. ICH associated with CAA is typically seen in an older individual after the age of 55 (predominantly more than 80 years), lobar, often multiple, with a tendency to be located in the posterior half of brain, and prone to recurrence.[219] It is a well-established risk factor for noncoagulopathic ICH, and this information might also apply to WICH.[220]

Anticoagulation in Acute Cardioembolic Stroke

Hemorrhagic transformation is defined as the presence of petechiae or confluent petechial hemorrhage confined to the ischemic zone. It is a relatively common consequence of developing cerebral infarction, being present in about 15% of all ischemic strokes and up to 30% of cardioembolic strokes.[221-223] The proposed mechanism for hemorrhagic transformation is the distal migration or lysis of an embolus resulting in reperfusion of the ischemic tissue, which can become hemorrhagic depending on the extent of the ischemic vascular injury.

Detection of hemorrhagic transformation depends on the neuroimaging technique used. MRI with T2-weighted sequences as well as diffusion- and perfusion-weighted imaging have higher sensitivity than CT for early detection of hemorrhagic transformation.[224,225] A prospective MRI study that imaged patients 3 weeks after cardioembolic stroke reported a 60% incidence of hemorrhagic transformation.[222] Autopsy series showed hemorrhagic transformation in even higher numbers (50% to 70%) of patients undergoing anticoagulation.[226] The great majority of hemorrhagic transformations are asymptomatic in patients not receiving anticoagulants.

The visualization of hemorrhagic transformation in a patient with ischemic stroke is important, in that it may provide guidance as to the possible underlying mechanism of stroke (i.e., cardioembolic) and may influence the selection of antithrombotic therapy. Because of the high incidence of secondary hemorrhagic transformation in patients with cardioembolic stroke, early anticoagulation is potentially risky. At present, it is impossible to formulate firm guidelines for anticoagulation in acute cardioembolic stroke because of a paucity of adequate data. The risk-to-benefit ratio of early anticoagulation is influenced by the specific cardioembolic source of the stroke as well as the size of the infarct.

In the past, the risk of early recurrent stroke or systemic embolism after a recent cardioembolic stroke in untreated patients was estimated to be around 10% during the first week[1] and to be especially high during the first 5 or 6 days after an acute cardioembolic stroke.[227,228] However these data were not supported by later studies, in which the risk of recurrent stroke within the first 14 days of stroke in patients with AF was between 5% and 8% without anticoagulation.[44]

Pooled data from case-series and one small controlled trial suggest that heparin reduces early stroke recurrence by about 70% in patients with cardioembolic stroke.

However, the higher risk of symptomatic ICH in patients in whom anticoagulation is begun early offsets the benefit conveyed by the therapy.[229,230]

The relationship between anticoagulants and clinically significant delayed hemorrhage is controversial. The occurrence and timing of asymptomatic hemorrhagic transformation do not seem to be affected by anticoagulation[231]; however, the magnitude and likelihood of associated clinical deterioration are augmented.[231,232] The incidence of symptomatic hemorrhagic transformation in patients receiving early anticoagulation varies widely (from 1% to 25%).[233,234]

Patients with a large infarct, excessive anticoagulation, and detection of hemorrhagic infarction on initial CT scan are at higher risk for symptomatic hemorrhagic transformation. Small case-series have advocated the use of anticoagulants even in patients with early CT visualization of hemorrhagic infarction.[235,236] It appears that hemorrhagic infarction may not be an absolute contraindication to anticoagulation, especially in individual patients who are at high risk of recurrent embolism. Given the lack of prospective studies and the relatively small number of patients in these case-series, however, early anticoagulation in hemorrhagic infarction cannot be routinely recommended without assessment of the risk of recurrent stroke. Delaying the start of anticoagulation for 1 to 2 weeks after detection of hemorrhagic infarction may be prudent.

For patients at relatively low risk of early stroke recurrence, including those with nonvalvular AF or recent MI without associated ventricular thrombi, deferring anticoagulation for several weeks may reduce the risk of hemorrhagic deterioration, particularly for patients with moderate to large infarcts or uncontrolled hypertension. Initiation of anticoagulation with oral warfarin (without the use of heparin) is an alternative for these patients. Thus, the "typical" patient with ischemic stroke and AF is unlikely to benefit from initiation of anticoagulation within the first day or two, especially if the stroke is large. In the interest of management efficiency, some physicians initiate oral anticoagulation within the first day or two, assuming that therapeutic, and therefore dangerous, levels of anticoagulation will not be achieved for a few days, when the period of increased risk for symptomatic hemorrhage has past. Some patients with AF might benefit from early anticoagulation because their recurrent stroke risk is increased—for example, the patient with documented thrombi in the left atrium. The randomized clinical trials that included patients with AF have not studied this subgroup and other potentially important subgroups to establish with certainty whether atrial thrombi or other predictors might identify a subpopulation at sufficiently increased risk of early stroke recurrence to justify prompt initiation of anticoagulation.[44]

For patients at high risk of recurrent embolization (i.e., mechanical prosthetic valve, intracardiac thrombus, AF with valvular disease or CHF), early anticoagulation is recommended, particularly if there are no associated risk factors for brain hemorrhage. Intravenous boluses of heparin and excessive anticoagulation should be avoided.

The value of antiplatelet agents and low-dose subcutaneous heparin in this setting has not been systematically assessed. Both could be alternatives to intravenous heparin, particularly in patients at low risk of early recurrent stroke (e.g., nonvalvular AF).

Patients with prosthetic valves who are in full anticoagulation at the time of stroke represent a management challenge. Reversing anticoagulation should be considered in patients with large infarcts or with infarcts already visible on early CT scan (less than 6 to 12 hours). Anticoagulation is not indicated for embolic stroke secondary to infective endocarditis of native valves.

Resumption of Anticoagulation in the Presence of Intracerebral Hemorrhage

The risk of ICH in the general population ranges from 0.5% to 2% per year. In patients undergoing anticoagulation, the risk of hemorrhage is about 10 times higher.[49,237] However, the risk of cerebral emboli in patients with major cardioembolic sources (e.g., left ventricular thrombi, prosthetic valve disease) who are without the protection offered by anticoagulation is high. Therefore, it is essential to estimate the risks and benefits of anticoagulation in this particular group of patients. So far, data are insufficient for firm recommendations to be made in these situations. Results of several small series and retrospective studies have suggested that, when absolutely necessary, resumption of oral anticoagulation after 1 or 2 weeks is associated with a low short-term risk of embolism and no major complications, worsening, or recurrence of ICH.[238-244]

The use of intravenous heparin or continuation of oral anticoagulant therapy in a patient who has ICH or a cerebral infarct with hemorrhagic transformation and a high-risk embolic source is less clear and continues to be a challenge for physicians. There are no large, prospective trials addressing the issue of when to restart anticoagulation after warfarin-associated ICH. The literature ranges from recommendations to withhold warfarin anticoagulation for 4 to 6 weeks[238] or 1 to 2 weeks[242,243] and to the use of intravenous heparin immediately after the INR is corrected to normal.[239,241] The risk of thromboembolism (underlying indication to use anticoagulation) and the risk of recurrent ICH (i.e., lobar versus deep location of the initial ICH versus hemorrhagic infarct) are key factors to be considered.

When to initiate anticoagulation and whether to continue anticoagulant therapy in patients with ICH remain controversial, and it is unlikely that these important issues will be settled by a large study.[245] In view of the lack of evidence, we recommend that each case be assessed individually through balancing of the risks and benefits of the intervention.

Summary

Emboli arising from the heart account for at least 20% of ischemic strokes. Cardiac sources of emboli are being detected with increasing ease with modern echocardiography. The common clinical dilemma is whether the detection of one of the "minor" cardiac sources of emboli bears any responsibility for causing a stroke in a given patient. Long-term oral anticoagulation is highly effective in preventing recurrent stroke in patients with "major" cardiac abnormalities, including AF, in patients who have received prosthetic cardiac valves and in patients with intracardiac thrombi due to MI or cardiomyopathy. In the near future, likely novel antithrombotic agents with superior safety and efficacy profile will replace warfarin as alternative agents to prevent cardioembolic stroke.

REFERENCES

1. Cerebral Embolism Task Force: Cardiogenic brain embolism: The second report of Cerebral Embolism Task Force, *Arch Neurol* 46:727–741, 1989.
2. Comess KA, DeRook FA, Beach KW, et al: Transesophageal echocardiography and carotid ultrasound in patients with cerebral ischemia: Prevalence of findings and recurrent stroke risk, *J Am Coll Cardiol* 23:1598–1603, 1994.
3. Albers GW, Comess KA, DeRook FA, et al: Transesophageal echocardiographic findings in stroke subtypes, *Stroke* 25:23–28, 1994.
4. Bogousslavsky J, Cachin C, Regli F, Despland PA, Van Melle G, Kappenberger L: Cardiac sources of embolism and cerebral infarction—clinical consequences and vascular concomitants: the Lausanne Stroke Registry, *Neurology* 41:855–859, 1991.
5. Hornig CR, Brainin M, Mast H: Cardioembolic stroke: Results from three current stroke data banks, *Neuroepidemiology* 13:318–323, 1994.
6. Ramirez-Lassepas M, Cipolle RJ, Bjork RJ: Can embolic stroke be diagnosed on the basis of neurological clinical criteria? *Arch Neurol* 44:87–89, 1987.
7. Foulkes MA, Wolf PA, Price TR, Mohr JP, Hier DB: The Stroke Data Bank: Design, methods, and baseline characteristics, *Stroke* 19:547–554, 1988.
8. Lindgren A, Roijer A, Norrving B, Wallin L, Eskilsson J, Johansson BB: Carotid artery and heart disease in subtypes of cerebral infarction, *Stroke* 25:2356–2362, 1994.
9. Czlonkowska A, Ryglewicz D, Weissbein T, Baranska-Gieruszczak M, Hier DB: A prospective community-based study of stroke in Warsaw, Poland. *Stroke* 25:547–551, 1994.
10. Moulin T, Tatu L, Crepin-Leblond T, Chavot D, Berges S, Rumbach T: The Besancon Stroke Registry: An acute stroke registry of 2,500 consecutive patients, *Eur Neurol* 38:10–20, 1997.
11. Ward G, Jamrozik K, Stewart-Wynne E: Incidence and outcome of cerebrovascular disease in Perth, Western Australia, *Stroke* 19:1501–1506, 1988.
12. Vemmos KN, Takis CE, Georgilis K, et al: The Athens stroke registry: Results of a five-year hospital-based study, *Cerebrovasc Dis* 10:133–141, 2000.
13. Vemmos KN, Bots ML, Tsibouris PK, et al: Stroke incidence and case fatality in southern Greece: The Arcadia stroke registry, *Stroke* 30:363–370, 1999.
14. Lee BI, Nam HS, Heo JH, Kim DI: Yonsei Stroke Registry. Analysis of 1,000 patients with acute cerebral infarctions, *Cerebrovasc Dis* 12:145–151, 2001.
15. Arboix A, Vericat MC, Pujades R, et al: Cardioembolic infarction in the Sagrat Cor-Alianza Hospital of Barcelona Stroke Registry, *Acta Neurol Scand* 96:407–412, 1997.
16. Amarenco P, Cohen A, Hommel M, Bertrand B, Tzouno C: Causes of cerebral infarcts in 250 consecutive elderly patients (abstract), *Stroke* 26:162, 1995.
17. Grau AJ, Weimar C, Buggle F, et al: Risk factors, outcome, and treatment in subtypes of ischemic stroke: The German stroke data bank, *Stroke* 32:2559–2566, 2001.
18. Feinberg WM, Blackshear JL, Laupacis A, Kronmal R, Hart RG: Prevalence, age distribution, and gender of patients with atrial fibrillation. Analysis and implications, *Arch Intern Med* 155:469–473, 1995.
19. Fuster V, Ryden LE, Cannom DS, et al: ACC/AHA/ESC 2006 guidelines for the management of patients with atrial fibrillation—executive summary: A report of the American College of Cardiology/American Heart Association Task Force on Practice Guidelines and the European Society of Cardiology Committee for Practice Guidelines (Writing Committee to Revise the 2001 Guidelines for the Management of Patients With Atrial Fibrillation), *J Am Coll Cardiol* 48:854–906, 2006.

20. Broderick JP, Philips SJ, O'Fallon WM, et al: Relationship of cardiac disease to stroke occurrence, recurrence and mortality, *Stroke* 23:1250-1256, 1992.
21. Mohr JP, Caplan LR, Melski JW: The Harvard Cooperative Stroke Registry: A prospective registry, *Neurology* 28:754-762, 1978.
22. Sandercock P, Bamford J, Dennis M, et al: Atrial fibrillation and stroke: Prevalence in different types of stroke and influence on early and longterm prognosis. Oxfordshire community stroke project, *BMJ* 305:1460-1465, 1992.
23. van Merwijk G, Lodder J, Bamford J, Kester ADM: How often is non-valvular atrial fibrillation the cause of brain infarction, *J Neurol* 237:205-207, 1990.
24. Asplund K, Carlberg B, Sundstrom G: Stroke in the elderly, *Cerebrovasc Dis* 2:152-157, 1992.
25. Wolf PA, Abbot RD, Kammel WB: Atrial fibrillation as an independent risk factor for stroke: The Framingham Study, *Stroke* 22:983-988, 1991.
26. Saxena R, Lewis S, Berge E, et al: Risk of early death and recurrent stroke and effect of heparin in 3169 patients with acute ischemic stroke and atrial fibrillation in the International Stroke Trial, *Stroke* 32:2333-2337, 2001.
27. Lamassa M, Di Carlo AA, Pracucci G, et al: Characteristics, outcome, and care of stroke associated with atrial fibrillation in Europe: Data from a multicenter multinational hospital-based registry (The European Community Stroke Project), *Stroke* 32:392-398, 2001.
28. Hart RG, Halperin JL: Atrial fibrillation and stroke: concepts and controversies, *Stroke* 32:803-808, 2001.
29. Miller VT, Rothrock JF, Pearce LA, et al: Ischemic stroke in patients with atrial fibrillation: Effect of aspirin according to stroke mechanism. Stroke Prevention in Atrial Fibrillation Investigators, *Neurology* 43:32-36, 1993.
30. Miller VT, Pearce LA, Feinberg WM, et al: Differential effect of aspirin versus warfarin on clinical stroke types in patients with atrial fibrillation. Stroke Prevention in Atrial Fibrillation Investigators, *Neurology* 46:238-240, 1996.
31. Hart RG, Pearce LA, Miller VT, et al: Cardioembolic vs. noncardioembolic strokes in atrial fibrillation: Frequency and effect of antithrombotic agents in the stroke prevention in atrial fibrillation studies, *Cerebrovasc Dis* 10:39-43, 2000.
32. Hart RG, Halperin JL: Atrial fibrillation and thromboembolism: a decade of progress in stroke prevention, *Ann Intern Med* 131:688-695, 1999.
33. Albers GW, Dalen JE, Laupacis A, et al: Antithrombotic therapy in atrial fibrillation, *Chest* 119(Suppl):194S-206S, 2001.
34. Flaker GC, Fletcher KA, Rothbart RM, et al: Clinical and echocardiographic features of intermittent atrial fibrillation that predict recurrent atrial fibrillation. Stroke Prevention in Atrial Fibrillation (SPAF) Investigators, *Am J Cardiol* 76:355-358, 1995.
35. The Stroke Prevention in Atrial Fibrillation Investigators: Predictors of thromboembolism in atrial fibrillation: I. Clinical features of patients at risk, *Ann Intern Med* 116:1-5, 1992.
36. The Stroke Prevention in Atrial Fibrillation Investigators: Predictors of thromboembolism in atrial fibrillation: II. Echocardiographic features of patients at risk, *Ann Intern Med* 116:6-12, 1992.
37. Stroke Prevention in Atrial Fibrillation Study: Final results, *Circulation* 84:527-539, 1991.
38. van Latum JC, Koudstaal PJ, Venables GS, et al: Predictors of major vascular events in patients with a transient ischemic attack or minor ischemic stroke and with nonrheumatic atrial fibrillation. European Atrial Fibrillation Trial (EAFT) Study Group, *Stroke* 26:801-806, 1995.
39. Pearce LA, Hart RG, Halperin JL: Assessment of three schemes for stratifying stroke risk in patients with nonvalvular atrial fibrillation, *Am J Med* 109:45-51, 2000.
40. Gage BF, Waterman AD, Shannon W, et al: Validation of clinical classification schemes for predicting stroke: results from the National Registry of Atrial Fibrillation, *JAMA* 285:2864-2870, 2001.
41. Berge E, Abdelnoor M, Nakstad PH, Sandset PM: Low molecular-weight heparin versus aspirin in patients with acute ischaemic stroke and atrial fibrillation: A double-blind randomised study. HAEST Study Group. Heparin in Acute Embolic Stroke Trial, *Lancet* 355:1205-1210, 2000.
42. CAST: randomised placebo-controlled trial of early aspirin use in 20,000 patients with acute ischaemic stroke. CAST (Chinese Acute Stroke Trial) Collaborative Group, *Lancet* 349:1641-1649, 1997.
43. The International Stroke Trial (IST): A randomised trial of aspirin, subcutaneous heparin, both, or neither among 19435 patients with acute ischaemic stroke. International Stroke Trial Collaborative Group, *Lancet* 349:1569-1581, 1997.
44. Hart RG, Palacio S, Pearce LA: Atrial fibrillation, stroke, and acute antithrombotic therapy: Analysis of randomized clinical trials, *Stroke* 33:2722-2727, 2002.
45. Hart RG, Pearce LA, Aguilar MI: Meta-analysis: Antithrombotic therapy to prevent stroke in patients who have nonvalvular atrial fibrillation, *Ann Intern Med* 146:857-867, 2007.
46. Hart RG, Benavente O, McBride R, Pearce LA: Antithrombotic therapy to prevent stroke in patients with atrial fibrillation: a meta-analysis [see comment], *Ann Intern Med* 131:492-501, 1999.
47. Benavente O, Hart R, Koudstaal P, et al: Oral anticoagulants for preventing stroke in patients with non-valvular atrial fibrillation and no previous history of stroke or transient ischemic attacks, *Cochrane Database Syst Rev* (2):CD001927, 2000.
48. Benavente O, Hart R, Koudstaal P, et al: Antiplatelet therapy for preventing stroke in patients with non-valvular atrial fibrillation and no previous history of stroke or transient ischemic attacks, *Cochrane Database Syst Rev* (2):CD001925, 2000.
49. Hart RG, Boop BS, Anderson DC: Oral anticoagulants and intracranial hemorrhage. Facts and hypotheses, *Stroke* 26:1471-1477, 1995.
50. Hart RG: Anticoagulation for nonrheumatic atrial fibrillation, *N Engl J Med* 336:441-442, 1997:discussion 442.
51. Hart RG: Intensity of anticoagulation to prevent stroke in patients with atrial fibrillation, *Ann Intern Med* 128:408, 1998.
52. Connolly S, Pogue J, Hart R, et al: Clopidogrel plus aspirin versus oral anticoagulation for atrial fibrillation in the Atrial fibrillation Clopidogrel Trial with Irbesartan for prevention of Vascular Events (ACTIVE W): A randomised controlled trial, *Lancet* 367:1903-1912, 2006.
53. Lip GY, Hee FL: Paroxysmal atrial fibrillation, *QJM* 94(12):665-678, 2001.
54. Hart RG, Pearce LA, Rothbart RM, et al: Stroke with intermittent atrial fibrillation: Incidence and predictors during aspirin therapy. Stroke Prevention in Atrial Fibrillation Investigators, *J Am Coll Cardiol* 35:183-187, 2000.
55. Risk factors for stroke and efficacy of antithrombotic therapy in atrial fibrillation: Analysis of pooled data from five randomized controlled trials, *Arch Intern Med* 154:1449-1457, 1994.
56. Wyse DG, Waldo AL, DiMarco JP, et al: A comparison of rate control and rhythm control in patients with atrial fibrillation, *N Engl J Med* 347:1825-1833, 2002.
57. Sherman DG, Kim S, Boop BS, et al: The occurrence and characteristics of stroke events in the AFFIRM Study, *Neurology* 60(Suppl 1):A326, 2003.
58. Berger M, Schweitzer P: Timing of thromboembolic events after electrical cardioversion of atrial fibrillation or flutter: A retrospective analysis, *Am J Cardiol* 82:1545-1547, 1998:A8.
59. Bjerkelund CJ, Orning OM: The efficacy of anticoagulant therapy in preventing embolism related to D.C. electrical conversion of atrial fibrillation, *Am J Cardiol* 23:208-216, 1969.
60. Kannel WB, Wolf PA, Verter J: Manifestations of coronary disease predisposing to stroke. The Framingham study, *JAMA* 250:2942-2946, 1983.
61. Pullicino PM, Halperin JL, Thompson JL: Stroke in patients with heart failure and reduced left ventricular ejection fraction, *Neurology* 54:288-294, 2000.
62. Wolf PA, Abbott RD, Kannel WB: Atrial fibrillation: a major contributor to stroke in the elderly. The Framingham Study, *Arch Intern Med* 147:1561-1564, 1987.
63. Dries DL, Rosenberg YD, Waclawiw MA, Domanski MJ: Ejection fraction and risk of thromboembolic events in patients with systolic dysfunction and sinus rhythm: Evidence for gender differences in the studies of left ventricular dysfunction trials, *J Am Coll Cardiol* 29:1074-1080, 1997.
64. Loh E, Sutton MS, Wun CC, et al: Ventricular dysfunction and the risk of stroke after myocardial infarction, *N Engl J Med* 336:251-257, 1997.
65. Katz SD, Marantz PR, Biasucci L, et al: Low incidence of stroke in ambulatory patients with heart failure: A prospective study, *Am Heart J* 126:141-146, 1993.

66. Cioffi G, Pozzoli M, Forni G, et al: Systemic thromboembolism in chronic heart failure. A prospective study in 406 patients, *Eur Heart J* 17:1381-1389, 1996.

67. Effects of enalapril on mortality in severe congestive heart failure: Results of the Cooperative North Scandinavian Enalapril Survival Study (CONSENSUS). The CONSENSUS Trial Study Group, *N Engl J Med* 316:1429-1435, 1987.

68. Sbarouni E, Bradshaw A, Andreotti F, et al: Relationship between hemostatic abnormalities and neuroendocrine activity in heart failure, *Am Heart J* 127:607-612, 1994.

69. Griffith GC, Stragnell R, Levinson DC, et al: A study of the beneficial effects of anticoagulant therapy in congestive heart failure, *Ann Intern Med* 37:867-887, 1952.

70. Harvey WP, Finch CA: Dicumarol prophylaxis of thromboembolic disease in congestive heart failure, *N Engl J Med* 242:208-211, 1950.

71. Anderson GM, Hull E: The effect of dicumarol upon the mortality and incidence of thromboembolic complications in congestive heart failure, *Am Heart J* 39:697-702, 1950.

72. Georgiadis D, Sievert M, Cencetti S, et al: Cerebrovascular reactivity is impaired in patients with cardiac failure [see comment], *Eur Heart J* 21:407-413, 2000.

73. Alves TC, Rays J, Fraguas R Jr, et al: Localized cerebral blood flow reductions in patients with heart failure: A study using 99mTc-HMPAO SPECT, *J Neuroimaging* 15:150-156, 2005.

74. Fuster V, Gersh BJ, Giuliani ER, et al: The natural history of idiopathic dilated cardiomyopathy, *Am J Cardiol* 47:525-531, 1981.

75. Falk RH, Foster E, Coats MH: Ventricular thrombi and thromboembolism in dilated cardiomyopathy: A prospective follow-up study, *Am Heart J* 123:136-142, 1992.

76. Gottdiener JS, Gay JA, VanVoorhees L, et al: Frequency and embolic potential of left ventricular thrombus in dilated cardiomyopathy: Assessment by 2-dimensional echocardiography, *Am J Cardiol* 52:1281-1285, 1983.

77. Randomised trial of late thrombolysis in patients with suspected acute myocardial infarction: EMERAS (Estudio Multicentrico Estreptoquinasa Republicas de America del Sur) Collaborative Group, *Lancet* 342:767-772, 1993.

78. Maze SS, Kotler MN, Parry WR: Flow characteristics in the dilated left ventricle with thrombus: Qualitative and quantitative Doppler analysis, *J Am Coll Cardiol* 13:873-881, 1989.

79. Di Tullio MR, Homma S: Mechanisms of cardioembolic stroke, *Curr Cardiol Rep* 4:141-148, 2002.

80. Koniaris LS, Goldhaber SZ: Anticoagulation in dilated cardiomyopathy.[see comment], *J Am Coll Cardiol* 31:745-748, 1998.

81. Kyrle PA, Korninger C, Gossinger H, et al: Prevention of arterial and pulmonary embolism by oral anticoagulants in patients with dilated cardiomyopathy, *Thromb Haemost* 54:521-523, 1985.

82. Dunkman WB, Johnson GR, Carson PE, et al: Incidence of thromboembolic events in congestive heart failure. The V-HeFT VA Cooperative Studies Group, *Circulation* 87(Suppl):VI94-VI101, 1993.

83. Loh E, Sutton MS: Anticoagulation and left ventricular dysfunction: Friend or foe? *Eur Heart J* 18:1039-1041, 1997.

84. Massie BM, Krol WF, Ammon SE, et al: The Warfarin and Antiplatelet Therapy in Heart Failure trial (WATCH): Rationale, design, and baseline patient characteristics [see comment], *J Cardiac Fail* 10:101-112, 2004.

85. Massie BM: Final results of the Warfarin and Antiplatelet Trial in Chronic Heart Failure (WATCH), New Orleans, La, March 7-10, 2004, Presented to American College of Cardiology Annual Scientific Session.

86. Pullicino P, Thompson JL, Barton B, et al: Warfarin versus aspirin in patients with reduced cardiac ejection fraction (WARCEF): Rationale, objectives, and design, *J Cardiac Fail* 12:39-46, 2006.

87. Stratton JR, Nemanich JW, Johannessen KA, Resnick AD: Fate of left ventricular thrombi in patients with remote myocardial infarction or idiopathic cardiomyopathy, *Circulation* 78:1388-1393, 1988.

88. Martin R, Bogousslavsky J: Mechanism of late stroke after myocardial infarct: The Lausanne Stroke Registry, *J Neurol Neurosurg Psychiatry* 56:760-764, 1993.

89. Dexter DD Jr, Whisnant JP, Connolly DC, O'Fallon WM: The association of stroke and coronary heart disease: A population study, *Mayo Clin Proc* 62:1077-1083, 1987.

90. Tanne D, Goldbourt U, Zion M, et al: Frequency and prognosis of stroke/TIA among 4808 survivors of acute myocardial infarction. The SPRINT Study Group, *Stroke* 24:1490-1495, 1993.

91. Bleeding during antithrombotic therapy in patients with atrial fibrillation: The Stroke Prevention in Atrial Fibrillation Investigators, *Arch Intern Med* 156:409-416, 1996.

92. Long-term anticoagulant therapy after myocardial infarction: United States Veterans Administration, *JAMA* 243:661-669, 1980.

93. Bodenheimer MM, Sauer D, Shareef B, et al: Relation between myocardial infarct location and stroke, *J Am Coll Cardiol* 24:61-66, 1994.

94. Keren A, Goldberg S, Gottlieb S, et al: Natural history of left ventricular thrombi: Their appearance and resolution in the posthospitalization period of acute myocardial infarction, *J Am Coll Cardiol* 15:790-800, 1990.

95. Friedman MJ, Carlson K, Marcus FI, Woolfenden JM: Clinical correlations in patients with acute myocardial infarction and left ventricular thrombus detected by two-dimensional echocardiography, *Am J Med* 72:894-898, 1982.

96. Delemarre BJ, Visser CA, Bot H, Dunning AJ: Prediction of apical thrombus formation in acute myocardial infarction based on left ventricular spatial flow pattern, *J Am Coll Cardiol* 15:355-360, 1990.

97. Merlini PA, Bauer KA, Oltrona L, et al: Persistent activation of coagulation mechanism in unstable angina and myocardial infarction, *Circulation* 90:61-68, 1994.

98. Johnson RC, Crissman RS, DiDio LJ: Endocardial alterations in myocardial infarction, *Lab Invest* 40:183-193, 1979.

99. Stratton JR, Resnick AD: Increased embolic risk in patients with left ventricular thrombi, *Circulation* 75:1004-1011, 1987.

100. Jugdutt BI, Sivaram CA: Prospective two-dimensional echocardiographic evaluation of left ventricular thrombus and embolism after acute myocardial infarction, *J Am Coll Cardiol* 13:554-564, 1989.

101. Reeder GS, Tajik AJ, Seward JB: Left ventricular aneurysm, thrombus, and embolism, *Chest* 79:369, 1981.

102. Reeder GS, Tajik AJ, Seward JB: Left ventricular mural thrombus: two-dimensional echocardiographic diagnosis, *Mayo Clin Proc* 56:82-86, 1981.

103. Reeder GS, Lengyel M, Tajik AJ, et al: Mural thrombus in left ventricular aneurysm: Incidence, role of angiography, and relation between anticoagulation and embolization, *Mayo Clin Proc* 56:77-81, 1981.

104. Ohman EM, Harrington RA, Cannon CP, et al: Intravenous thrombolysis in acute myocardial infarction, *Chest* 119(Suppl):253S-277S, 2001.

105. Cairns JA, Theroux P, Lewis HD Jr, et al: Antithrombotic agents in coronary artery disease, *Chest* 119(Suppl):228S-252S, 2001.

106. Behar S, Tanne D, Zion M, et al: Incidence and prognostic significance of chronic atrial fibrillation among 5,839 consecutive patients with acute myocardial infarction. The SPRINT Study Group. Secondary Prevention Reinfarction Israeli Nifedipine Trial, *Am J Cardiol* 70:816-818, 1992.

107. Komrad MS, Coffey CE, Coffey KS, et al: Myocardial infarction and stroke, *Neurology* 34:1403-1409, 1984.

108. Proceedings of the American College of Chest Physicians 5th Consensus on Antithrombotic Therapy, *Chest* 114(Suppl):439S-769S, 1998.

109. Effect of long-term oral anticoagulant treatment on mortality and cardiovascular morbidity after myocardial infarction: Anticoagulants in the Secondary Prevention of Events in Coronary Thrombosis (ASPECT) Research Group [see comment], *Lancet* 343:499-503, 1994.

110. Kizer JR, Devereux RB: Clinical practice. Patent foramen ovale in young adults with unexplained stroke [see comment; erratum appears in N Engl J Med. 2006;354:2401], *N Engl J Med* 353:2361-2372, 2005.

111. Reynen K: Frequency of primary tumors of the heart, *Am J Cardiol* 77:107, 1996.

112. Castelman B, Roth S: *Tumors of the cardiovascular system*, Washington, DC, 1978, Armed Forces Institute of Pathology.

113. Aziz F, Baciewicz FA Jr: Lambl's excrescences: Review and recommendations, *Texas Heart Inst J* 34:366-368, 2007.

114. Dervall PB, Olley PM, Smith DR: Incidence of stenosis embolism before and after mitral valvotomy, *Thorax* 23:530-540, 1968.

115. Szekely P: Systemic embolism and anticoagulants prophylaxis in rheumatic heart disease, *BMJ* 1:209-212, 1964.

116. Levine HJ: Which atrial fibrillation patients should be on chronic anticoagulation? *J Cardiovasc Med* 6:483-487, 1981.

117. Hinton RC, Kistler JP, Fallon JT, et al: Influence of etiology of atrial fibrillation on incidence of systemic embolism, *Am J Cardiol* 40:509-513, 1977.

118. Daley R, Mattingly TW, Holt C: Systemic arterial embolism in rheumatic heart disease, *Am Heart J* 42:566-581, 1951.

119. Cassella K, Abelmann WH, Ellis LB: Patients with mitral stenosis and systemic emboli, *Arch Intern Med* 114:773, 1964.

120. Carter AB: Prognosis of cerebral embolism, *Lancet* 2:514-519, 1965.

121. Fleming HA, Bailey SM: Mitral valve disease, systemic embolism and anticoagulants, *Postgrad Med J* 47:599-604, 1971.

122. Fleming HA: Anticoagulants in rheumatic heart-disease, *Lancet* 2(7722):486, 1971.

123. Adams GF, Merrett JD, Hutchinson WM, Pollock AM: Cerebral embolism and mitral stenosis: Survival with and without anticoagulants, *J Neurol Neurosurg Psychiatry* 37:378-383, 1974.

124. Salem DN, Daudelin HD, Levine HJ, et al: Antithrombotic therapy in valvular heart disease, *Chest* 119(Suppl):207S-219S, 2001.

125. Saour JN, Sieck JO, Mamo LA, Gallus AS: Trial of different intensities of anticoagulation in patients with prosthetic heart valves, *N Engl J Med* 322:428-432, 1990.

126. Stein PD, Alpert JS, Bussey HI, et al: Antithrombotic therapy in patients with mechanical and biological prosthetic heart valves, *Chest* 119(Suppl):220S-227S, 2001.

127. Turpie AG, Gent M, Laupacis A, et al: A comparison of aspirin with placebo in patients treated with warfarin after heart-valve replacement, *N Engl J Med* 329:524-529, 1993.

128. Butchart EG, Lewis PA, Grunkemeier GL, et al: Low risk of thrombosis and serious embolic events despite low-intensity anticoagulation. Experience with 1,004 Medtronic Hall valves, *Circulation* 78:166-I77, 1988.

129. Kuntze CE, Blackstone EH, Ebels T: Thromboembolism and mechanical heart valves: A randomized study revisited, *Ann Thorac Surg* 66:101-107, 1998.

130. Kuntze CE, Ebels T, Eijgelaar A, Homan van der Heide JN: Rates of thromboembolism with three different mechanical heart valve prostheses: Randomised study, *Lancet* 1(8637):514-517, 1989.

131. Cannegieter SC, Rosendaal FR, Wintzen AR, et al: Optimal oral anticoagulant therapy in patients with mechanical heart valves, *N Engl J Med* 333:11-17, 1995.

132. Coulshed N, Epstein EJ, McKendrick CS, et al: Systemic embolism in mitral valve disease, *Br Heart J* 32:26-34, 1970.

133. Altman R, Rouvier J, Gurfinkel E, et al: Comparison of two levels of anticoagulant therapy in patients with substitute heart valves, *J Thorac Cardiovasc Surg* 101:427-431, 1991.

134. Scott PJ, Essop R, Wharton GA, Williams GJ: Left atrial clot in patients with mitral prostheses: Increased rate of detection after recent systemic embolism, *Int J Cardiol* 33:141-148, 1991.

135. Tinmouth A, Kovacs M, Cruickshank M: Outpatient peri-operative and peri-procedure treatment with dalteparin for chronically anticoagulated patients at high risk for thromboembolic complications, *Thromb Haemost* 82(Suppl):662, 1999.

136. Kearon C, Hirsh J: Management of anticoagulation before and after elective surgery, *N Engl J Med* 336:1506-1511, 1997.

137. Johnson J, Turpie AG: Temporary discontinuation of oral anticoagulants: Role of low molecular weight heparin, *Thromb Haemost* 82(Suppl):62-63, 1999.

138. Ansell J, Hirsh J, Dalen J, et al: Managing oral anticoagulant therapy, *Chest* 119(Suppl):22S, 2001.

139. Hirsh J, Dalen J, Anderson DR, et al: Oral anticoagulants: Mechanism of action, clinical effectiveness, and optimal therapeutic range, *Chest* 119(Suppl):8S-21S, 2001.

140. Salem DN, Levine HJ, Pauker SG, et al: Antithrombotic therapy in valvular heart disease, *Chest* 114(Suppl):590S-601S, 1998.

141. Sila CA: Neurological therapeutics: Principles and practice. In Noseworthy JH, editor: *Cardioembolic stroke*, London, 2003, Martin Dunitz.

142. Caplan L: Posterior circulation ischemia: Then, now, and tomorrow. The Thomas Willis Lecture-2000, *Stroke* 31:2011-2023, 2000.

143. Douglas PS, Khandheria B, Stainback RF, et al: ACCF/ASE/ACEP/ASNC/SCAI/SCCT/SCMR 2007 appropriateness criteria for transthoracic and transesophageal echocardiography: A report of the American College of Cardiology Foundation Quality Strategic Directions Committee Appropriateness Criteria Working Group, American Society of Echocardiography, American College of Emergency Physicians, American Society of Nuclear Cardiology, Society for Cardiovascular Angiography and Interventions, Society of Cardiovascular Computed Tomography, and the Society for Cardiovascular Magnetic Resonance endorsed by the American College of Chest Physicians and the Society of Critical Care Medicine, *J Am Coll Cardiol* 50:187-204, 2007.

144. Drapkin A, Merskey C: Anticoagulant therapy after acute myocardial infarction. Relation of therapeutic benefit to patient's age, sex, and severity of infarction, *JAMA* 222:541-548, 1972.

145. Dressler FA, Craig WR, Castello R, Labovitz AJ: Mobile aortic atheroma and systemic emboli: Efficacy of anticoagulation and influence of plaque morphology on recurrent stroke [see comment], *J Am Coll Cardiol* 31:134-138, 1998.

146. Edvardsson N, Juul-Moller S, Omblus R, Pehrsson K: Effects of low-dose warfarin and aspirin versus no treatment on stroke in a medium-risk patient population with atrial fibrillation, *J Intern Med* 254:95-101, 2003.

147. Dismukes WE: Management of infective endocarditis, *Cardiovasc Clin* 11:189-208, 1981.

148. Fleming HA: General principles of the treatment of infective endocarditis, *J Antimicrob Chemother* 20(Suppl A):143-145, 1987.

149. Hart RG, Foster JW, Luther MF, Kanter MC: Stroke in infective endocarditis, *Stroke* 21:695-700, 1990.

150. Prabhakaran S: Neurologic Complications of Endocarditis, *Continuum Lifelong Learning in Neurology* 14:53-73, 2008.

151. Robbins MJ, Eisenberg ES, Frishman WH: Infective endocarditis: a pathophysiologic approach to therapy, *Cardiol Clin* 5:545-562, 1987.

152. Salgado AV, Furlan AJ, Keys TF, et al: Neurologic complications of endocarditis: A 12-year experience, *Neurology* 39:173-178, 1989.

153. Reynen K: Cardiac myxomas [see comment], *N Engl J Med* 333:1610-1617, 1995.

154. Sastre-Garriga J, Molina C, Montaner J, et al: Mitral papillary fibroelastoma as a cause of cardiogenic embolic stroke: Report of two cases and review of the literature, *Eur J Neurol* 7:449-453, 2000.

155. Di Tullio M, Sacco RL, Gopal A, et al: Patent foramen ovale as a risk factor for cryptogenic stroke, *Ann Intern Med* 117:461-465, 1992.

156. Cabanes L, Mas JL, Cohen A, et al: Atrial septal aneurysm and patent foramen ovale as risk factors for cryptogenic stroke in patients less than 55 years of age. A study using transesophageal echocardiography, *Stroke* 24:1865-1873, 1993.

157. Lechat P, Lascault G, Mas JL, et al: [Prevalence of patent foramen ovale in young patients with ischemic cerebral complications], *Arch Mal Coeur Vaiss* 82:847-852, 1989.

158. Lechat P, Mas JL, Lascault G, et al: Prevalence of patent foramen ovale in patients with stroke, *N Engl J Med* 318:1148-1152, 1988.

159. Webster MW, Chancellor AM, Smith HJ, et al: Patent foramen ovale in young stroke patients, *Lancet* 2:11-12, 1988.

160. Louie EK, Konstadt SN, Rao TL, Scanlon PJ: Transesophageal echocardiographic diagnosis of right to left shunting across the foramen ovale in adults without prior stroke, *J Am Coll Cardiol* 21:1231-1237, 1993.

161. Langholz D, Louie EK, Konstadt SN, et al: Transesophageal echocardiographic demonstration of distinct mechanisms for right to left shunting across a patent foramen ovale in the absence of pulmonary hypertension, *J Am Coll Cardiol* 18:1112-1117, 1991.

162. Konstadt SN, Louie EK, Black S, et al: Intraoperative detection of patent foramen ovale by transesophageal echocardiography, *Anesthesiology* 74:212-216, 1991.

163. Hausmann D, Mugge A, Daniel WG: Identification of patent foramen ovale permitting paradoxic embolism, *J Am Coll Cardiol* 26:1030-1038, 1995.

164. Strunk BL, Cheitlin MD, Stulbarg MS, Schiller NB: Right-to-left interatrial shunting through a patent foramen ovale despite normal intracardiac pressures, *Am J Cardiol* 60:413-415, 1987.

165. Lynch JJ, Schuchard GH, Gross CM, Wann LS: Prevalence of right-to-left atrial shunting in a healthy population: Detection by Valsalva maneuver contrast echocardiography, *Am J Cardiol* 53:1478-1480, 1984.

166. DeRook FA, Comess KA, Albers GW, Popp RL: Transesophageal echocardiography in the evaluation of stroke, *Ann Intern Med* 117:922-932, 1992.

167. Jauss M, Kaps M, Keberle M, et al: A comparison of transesophageal echocardiography and transcranial Doppler sonography with contrast medium for detection of patent foramen ovale, *Stroke* 25:1265-1267, 1994.

168. Jauss M, Schleime C, Hugens-Penzel M, et al: Disclosure of paradoxical brain embolism in two stroke patients with ultrasound test for right-to-left shunt and diffusion-weighted MRI, *Cerebrovasc Dis* 14:267-269, 2002.

169. Karnik R, Stollberger C, Valentin A, et al: Detection of patent foramen ovale by transcranial contrast Doppler ultrasound, *Am J Cardiol* 69:560-562, 1992.

170. Klotzsch C, Janssen G, Berlit P: Transesophageal echocardiography and contrast-TCD in the detection of a patent foramen ovale: Experiences with 111 patients, *Neurology* 44:1603-1606, 1994.

171. Hagen PT, Scholz DG, Edwards WD: Incidence and size of patent foramen ovale during the first 10 decades of life: An autopsy study of 965 normal hearts, *Mayo Clin Proc* 59:17-20, 1984.

172. Homma S, Sacco RL, Di Tullio MR, et al: Effect of medical treatment in stroke patients with patent foramen ovale: Patent foramen ovale in Cryptogenic Stroke Study, *Circulation* 105:2625-2631, 2002.

173. Sacco RL, Homma S, Di Tullio MR: Patent foramen ovale: A new risk factor for ischemic stroke, *Heart Dis Stroke* 2:235-241, 1993.

174. Jones EF, Calafiore P, Donnan GA, Tonkin AM: Evidence that patent foramen ovale is not a risk factor for cerebral ischemia in the elderly, *Am J Cardiol* 74:596-599, 1994.

175. de Belder MA, Tourikis L, Leech G, Camm AJ: Risk of patent foramen ovale for thromboembolic events in all age groups, *Am J Cardiol* 69:1316-1320, 1992.

176. Stollberger C, Finsterer J, Slany J: Why is venous thrombosis only rarely detected in patients with suspected paradoxical embolism? *Thromb Res* 105:189-191, 2002.

177. Stollberger C, Slany J, Schuster I, et al: The prevalence of deep venous thrombosis in patients with suspected paradoxical embolism, *Ann Intern Med* 119:461-465, 1993.

178. Overell JR, Bone I, Lees KR: Interatrial septal abnormalities and stroke: A meta-analysis of case-control studies, *Neurology* 55:1172-1179, 2000.

179. Lamy C, Giannesini C, Zuber M, et al: Clinical and imaging findings in cryptogenic stroke patients with and without patent foramen ovale: The PFO-ASA Study. Atrial Septal Aneurysm, *Stroke* 33:706-711, 2002.

180. Ranoux D, Cohen A, Cabanes L, et al: Patent foramen ovale: Is stroke due to paradoxical embolism? *Stroke* 24:31-34, 1993.

181. Silver MD, Dorsey JS: Aneurysms of the septum primum in adults, *Arch Pathol Lab Med* 102:62-65, 1978.

182. Handke M, Harloff A, Olschewski M, et al: Patent foramen ovale and cryptogenic stroke in older patients, *N Engl J Med* 357:2262-2268, 2007.

183. Falk RH: PFO or UFO? The role of a patent foramen ovale in cryptogenic stroke, *Am Heart J* 121:1264-1266, 1991.

184. Hanna JP, Sun JP, Furlan AJ, et al: Patent foramen ovale and brain infarct. Echocardiographic predictors, recurrence, and prevention, *Stroke* 25:782-786, 1994.

185. Cujec B, Mainra R, Johnson DH: Prevention of recurrent cerebral ischemic events in patients with patent foramen ovale and cryptogenic strokes or transient ischemic attacks, *Can J Cardiol* 15:57-64, 1999.

186. De Castro S, Cartoni D, Fiorelli M, et al: Morphological and functional characteristics of patent foramen ovale and their embolic implications, *Stroke* 31:2407-2413, 2000.

187. Bogousslavsky J, Garazi S, Jeanrenaud X, et al: Stroke recurrence in patients with patent foramen ovale: The Lausanne Study. Lausanne Stroke with Paradoxical Embolism Study Group, *Neurology* 46:1301-1305, 1996.

188. Mas JL, Zuber M: Recurrent cerebrovascular events in patients with patent foramen ovale, atrial septal aneurysm, or both and cryptogenic stroke or transient ischemic attack. French Study Group on Patent Foramen Ovale and Atrial Septal Aneurysm, *Am Heart J* 130:1083-1088, 1995.

189. Mas JL, Arquizan C, Lamy C, et al: Recurrent cerebrovascular events associated with patent foramen ovale, atrial septal aneurysm, or both, *N Engl J Med* 345:1740-1746, 2001.

190. Baker SS, O'Laughlin MP, Jollis JG, et al: Cost implications of closure of atrial septal defect, *Catheter Cardiovasc Interv* 55:83-87, 2002.

191. Bruch L, Parsi A, Grad MO, et al: Transcatheter closure of interatrial communications for secondary prevention of paradoxical embolism: Single-center experience, *Circulation* 105:2845-2848, 2002.

192. Wahl A, Meier B, Haxel B, et al: Prognosis after percutaneous closure of patent foramen ovale for paradoxical embolism, *Neurology* 57:1330-1332, 2001.

193. Wahl A, Windecker S, Eberli FR, et al: Percutaneous closure of patent foramen ovale in symptomatic patients, *J Interv Cardiol* 14:203-209, 2001.

194. Zahn EM, Wilson N, Cutright W, Latson LA: Development and testing of the Helex septal occluder, a new expanded polytetrafluoroethylene atrial septal defect occlusion system, *Circulation* 104:711-716, 2001.

195. Latson LA, Zahn EM, Wilson N: Helex Septal Occluder for Closure of Atrial Septal Defects, *Curr Interv Cardiol Rep* 2:268-273, 2000.

196. Messe SR, Silverman IE, Kizer JR, et al: Practice parameter: recurrent stroke with patent foramen ovale and atrial septal aneurysm: Report of the Quality Standards Subcommittee of the American Academy of Neurology [see comment], *Neurology* 62:1042-1050, 2004.

197. Amarenco P, Cohen A, Tzourio C, et al: Atherosclerotic disease of the aortic arch and the risk of ischemic stroke [see comment], *N Engl J Med* 331:1474-1479, 1994.

198. Fujimoto S, Yasaka M, Otsubo R, et al: Aortic arch atherosclerotic lesions and the recurrence of ischemic stroke, *Stroke* 35:1426-1429, 2004.

199. Tunick PA, Nayar AC, Goodkin GM, et al: Effect of treatment on the incidence of stroke and other emboli in 519 patients with severe thoracic aortic plaque [see comment], *Am J Cardiol* 90:1320-1325, 2002.

200. Hirsh J, Warkentin TE, Shaughnessy SG, et al: Heparin and low-molecular-weight heparin: Mechanisms of action, pharmacokinetics, dosing, monitoring, efficacy, and safety, *Chest* 119(Suppl):64S-94S, 2001.

201. Hart R, Benavente O, Pearce LA: Increased risk of intracranial hemorrhage when aspirin is combined with warfarin: A meta-analysis and hypothesis, *Cerebrovasc Dis* 9:215-217, 1999.

202. Sobieraj-Teague M, O'Donnell M, Eikelboom J: New anticoagulants for atrial fibrillation, *Semin Thromb Hemost* 35:515-524, 2009.

203. ROCKET-AF Study Investigators: Rivaroxaban-once daily, oral, direct factor Xa inhibition compared with vitamin K antagonism for prevention of stroke and Embolism Trial in Atrial Fibrillation: Rationale and design of the ROCKET AF study, *Am Heart J* 159:340-347, 2010.

204. Fogelholm R, Eskola K, Kiminkinen T, Kunnamo I: Anticoagulant treatment as a risk factor for primary intracerebral haemorrhage, *J Neurol Neurosurg Psychiatry* 55:1121-1124, 1992.

205. Franke CL, de Jonge J, van Swieten JC, et al: Intracerebral hematomas during anticoagulant treatment, *Stroke* 21:726-730, 1990.

206. Wintzen AR, de Jonge H, Loeliger EA, Bots GT: The risk of intracerebral hemorrhage during oral anticoagulant treatment: A population study, *Ann Neurol* 16:553-558, 1984.

207. Mayer SA, Brun NC, Begtrup K, et al: Recombinant activated factor VII for acute intracerebral hemorrhage, *N Engl J Med* 352:777-785, 2005.

208. Mayer SA, Brun NC, Begtrup K, et al: Efficacy and safety of recombinant activated factor VII for acute intracerebral hemorrhage [see comment], *N Engl J Med* 358:2127-2137, 2008.

209. Torn M, Algra A, Rosendaal FR: Oral anticoagulation for cerebral ischemia of arterial origin: High initial bleeding risk, *Neurology* 57:1993-1999, 2001.

210. Hylek EM, Singer DE: Risk factors for intracranial hemorrhage in outpatients taking warfarin, *Ann Intern Med* 120:897-902, 1994.

211. A randomized trial of anticoagulants versus aspirin after cerebral ischemia of presumed arterial origin: The Stroke Prevention in Reversible Ischemia Trial (SPIRIT) Study Group, *Ann Neurol* 42:857-865, 1997.

212. Hylek EM, Skates SJ, Sheehan MA, Singer DE: An analysis of the lowest effective intensity of prophylactic anticoagulation for patients with nonrheumatic atrial fibrillation, *N Engl J Med* 335:540-546, 1996.

213. Smith EE, Rosand J, Knudsen KA, et al: Leukoaraiosis is associated with warfarin-related hemorrhage following ischemic stroke, *Neurology* 59:193-197, 2002.

214. Gorter JW: Major bleeding during anticoagulation after cerebral ischemia: Patterns and risk factors. Stroke Prevention In Reversible Ischemia Trial (SPIRIT). European Atrial Fibrillation Trial (EAFT) study groups, *Neurology* 53:1319-1327, 1999.

215. Kato H, Izumiyama M, Izumiyama K, et al: Silent cerebral microbleeds on T2*-weighted MRI: correlation with stroke subtype, stroke recurrence, and leukoaraiosis, *Stroke* 33:1536-1540, 2002.

216. Kim DE, Bae HJ, Lee SH, et al: Gradient echo magnetic resonance imaging in the prediction of hemorrhagic vs ischemic stroke: A need for the consideration of the extent of leukoaraiosis, *Arch Neurol* 59:425-429, 2002.

217. Wong KS, Chan YL, Liu JY, et al: Asymptomatic microbleeds as a risk factor for aspirin-associated intracerebral hemorrhages, *Neurology* 60:511-513, 2003.

218. Hart RG: What causes intracerebral hemorrhage during warfarin therapy? *Neurology* 55:907-908, 2000.

219. Ferro JM: Update on intracerebral haemorrhage, *J Neurol* 253:985-999, 2006.

220. Greenberg SM, Eng JA, Ning M, et al: Hemorrhage burden predicts recurrent intracerebral hemorrhage after lobar hemorrhage, *Stroke* 35:1415-1420, 2004.

221. Hart RG, Easton JD: Hemorrhagic infarcts, *Stroke* 17:586-589, 1986.

222. Hornig CR, Bauer T, Simon C, et al: Hemorrhagic transformation in cardioembolic cerebral infarction, *Stroke* 24:465-468, 1993.

223. Molina CA, Montaner J, Abilleira S, et al: Timing of spontaneous recanalization and risk of hemorrhagic transformation in acute cardioembolic stroke, *Stroke* 32:1079-1084, 2001.

224. Nighoghossian N, Hermier M, Berthezene Y, et al: Early diagnosis of hemorrhagic transformation: diffusion/perfusion-weighted MRI versus CT scan, *Cerebrovasc Dis* 11:151-156, 2001.

225. Hermier M, Nighoghossian N, Derex L, et al: MRI of acute postischemic cerebral hemorrhage in stroke patients: Diagnosis with T2*-weighted gradient-echo sequences, *Neuroradiology* 43:809-815, 2001.

226. Okada Y, Yamaguchi T, Minematsu K, et al: Hemorrhagic transformation in cerebral embolism, *Stroke* 20:598-603, 1989.

227. Immediate anticoagulation of embolic stroke: Brain hemorrhage and management options. Cerebral Embolism Study Group, *Stroke* 15:779-789, 1984.

228. Yasaka M, Yamaguchi T, Oita J, et al: Clinical features of recurrent embolization in acute cardioembolic stroke, *Stroke* 24:1681-1685, 1993.

229. Sandercock P: Full heparin anticoagulation should not be used in acute ischemic stroke, *Stroke* 34:231-232, 2003.

230. Koller RL: Recurrent embolic cerebral infarction and anticoagulation, *Neurology* 32:283-285, 1982.

231. Cardioembolic stroke, early anticoagulation, and brain hemorrhage. Cerebral Embolism Study Group, *Arch Intern Med* 147:636-640, 1987.

232. Calandre L, Ortega JF, Bermejo F: Anticoagulation and hemorrhagic infarction in cerebral embolism secondary to rheumatic heart disease, *Arch Neurol* 41:1152-1154, 1984.

233. Shields RW Jr, Laureno R, Lachman T, Victor M: Anticoagulant-related hemorrhage in acute cerebral embolism, *Stroke* 15:426-437, 1984.

234. Chamorro A, Vila N, Saiz A, Alday M, Tolosa E: Early anticoagulation after large cerebral embolic infarction: a safety study, *Neurology* 45:861-865, 1995.

235. Rothrock JF, Dittrich HC, McAllen S, et al: Acute anticoagulation following cardioembolic stroke, *Stroke* 20:730-734, 1989.

236. Pessin MS, Estol CJ, Lafranchise F, Caplan LR: Safety of anticoagulation after hemorrhagic infarction, *Neurology* 43:1298-1303, 1993.

237. Gebel JM, Broderick JP: Intracerebral hemorrhage, *Neurol Clin* 18:419-438, 2000.

238. Crawley F, Bevan D, Wren D: Management of intracranial bleeding associated with anticoagulation: Balancing the risk of further bleeding against thromboembolism from prosthetic heart valves, *J Neurol Neurosurg Psychiatry* 69:396-398, 2000.

239. Bertram M, Bonsanto M, Hacke W, Schwab S: Managing the therapeutic dilemma: Patients with spontaneous intracerebral hemorrhage and urgent need for anticoagulation, *J Neurol* 247:209-214, 2000.

240. Hacke W: The dilemma of reinstituting anticoagulation for patients with cardioembolic sources and intracranial hemorrhage: How wide is the strait between Skylla and Karybdis? *Arch Neurol* 57:1682-1684, 2000.

241. Leker RR, Abramsky O: Early anticoagulation in patients with prosthetic heart valves and intracerebral hematoma, *Neurology* 50:1489-1491, 1998.

242. Phan TG, Koh M, Wijdicks EF: Safety of discontinuation of anticoagulation in patients with intracranial hemorrhage at high thromboembolic risk, *Arch Neurol* 57:1710-1713, 2000.

243. Wijdicks EF, Schievink WI, Brown RD, Mullany CJ: The dilemma of discontinuation of anticoagulation therapy for patients with intracranial hemorrhage and mechanical heart valves, *Neurosurgery* 42:769-773, 1998.

244. Wijdicks EF, Schievink WI, Brown RD, Mullany CY: Early anticoagulation in patients with prosthetic heart valves and intracerebral hematoma, *Neurology* 52:676-677, 1999.

245. Aguilar MI, Hart RG, Pearce L: Oral anticoagulants versus antiplatelet therapy for preventing stroke in patients with nonvalvular atrial fibrillation and no history of stroke or transient ischemic attacks, *Cochrane Database System Rev* (3):CD006186, 2007.

60

Conduct of Stroke-Related Clinical Trials

BARBARA C. TILLEY, YUKO Y. PALESCH

Drawing from the general literature on the conduct of clinical trials, this chapter addresses the design, data management, analytical, ethical, and regulatory issues relevant to stroke *prevention* and *therapeutic* trials. A *clinical trial* is "an experiment in which a group of individuals is given an intervention and subsequent outcome measures are taken. Results of the intervention are compared to individuals not given the intervention."[1]

Prevention Trials

Primary prevention trials evaluate interventions in participants who have never had a stroke. Pure primary prevention trials are rare, as most "primary" prevention trials include some participants with previous stroke, transient ischemic attack (TIA), or both. A primary prevention trial also may be a trial with a primary outcome such as cardiovascular disease, and stroke as a secondary outcome. *Secondary* prevention trials evaluate interventions in participants who have previously had a TIA or stroke.

Examples of primary prevention trials that include some secondary prevention include the Second Copenhagen Atrial Fibrillation, Aspirin, and Anticoagulation Study (AFASKII),[2] excluding persons who had a stroke or TIA in the previous 6 months but admitting persons who had experienced stroke or TIA before the 6-month period; and the Asymptomatic Carotid Atherosclerosis Study (ACAS), excluding those who had symptoms of stroke or TIA in the randomly chosen artery but otherwise including persons who had previously experienced a stroke or TIA.[3] Seven percent of the participants in the International Cooperative Study of Extracranial-Intracranial Arterial Anastomosis (EC/IC Bypass Study), which compared surgery and medical care, had experienced a stroke or TIA.[4,5]

Examples of true secondary prevention trials include the Warfarin and Aspirin Recurrent Stroke Study (WARSS), comparing warfarin and aspirin in participants with a previous stroke,[6] and the Vitamins To Prevent Stroke (VITA-TOPS) trial of multivitamin therapy[7] in patients with a recent TIA or ischemic stroke. Stroke prevention trials are usually designed with new stroke or stroke-related mortality or overall mortality as the outcome measure, requiring larger numbers of participants and longer follow-up than is usual for therapeutic trials. To increase the potential to observe events in the study cohort and reduce the sample size, the trial may include only those with a risk factor for subsequent events such as atrial fibrillation or some degree of carotid artery stenosis.

Therapeutic Trials

Therapeutic stroke trials are directed at reducing post-stroke–related disability or mortality rather than preventing future second strokes. The International Surgical Trial (IST) in Intracranial Hemorrhage assessed the use of a surgical procedure to reduce mortality from spontaneous intracranial hemorrhage.[8] The National Institute of Neurological Disorders and Stroke (NINDS) studies of recombinant tissue-type plasminogen activator (rt-PA)[9] and the more recent European Cooperative Acute Stroke Study III (ECASS III)[10] were designed to reduce post stroke disability with mortality classification as the more severe disability. Other therapeutic trials may focus on assessing approaches to stroke rehabilitation during and after hospitalization. Sample sizes in most therapeutic trials are usually smaller than those needed for the prevention trials, and follow-up periods tend to be shorter, usually 3 months after stroke. Clinical trials in stroke are infrequently used to determine long-term adverse effects of a treatment. The treatment benefit is assessed to be immediate, and 3 months after stroke is thought to be of sufficient duration to observe intervention and control differences. An exception was the NINDS rt-PA Stroke Study, in which 1-year follow-up on trial participants showed continued treatment benefit.[11]

When Can a Stroke-Related Trial Be Conducted?

Ethical conduct of a randomized clinical trial requires equipoise. A clinical trial can be conducted only at that point in time at which the treatment is acceptable to administer to humans but there is still uncertainty about treatment outcome. If the consensus of potential participants or clinicians is that a treatment or procedure is beneficial (or harmful), randomization becomes impractical and possibly unethical. In the EC/IC Study, some of the original participating centers' investigators decided that they could not ethically randomly assign potential participants away from surgery.[12] Enough centers continued to enroll participants in the trial for it to continue, and at the conclusion, a benefit of surgery over best medical care could not be detected.

Ethical considerations also prohibit conducting a clinical trial using a placebo when a known effective treatment is available. It has been deemed unethical to withhold rt-PA from eligible patients and give placebo in the first 3 hours after stroke onset. Given uncertainty about treatment with rt-PA after 3 hours, ECASS III[11] used a placebo comparison group for their 4 to 6 hours post stroke trial. It is also unethical to evaluate most risk factors in a prevention trial. The magnitude of the stroke-related risk of cigarette smoking cannot be evaluated in the context of a clinical trial with participants randomly assigned to smoking as an intervention. This prohibition does not preclude prevention trials comparing behavioral or therapeutic approaches to modifying stroke-related risk factors.

The Three Phases of Clinical Trials

Although the nomenclature and definition of the phases are, in general, not standardized, the three phases are phase 1 (dose finding and safety), phase 2 (determination of futility, feasibility, and safety), and phase 3 (efficacy or effectiveness). In the development of therapies for stroke, these phases are often not distinct. Phases 1 and 2 or phases 2 and 3 may be combined. After an agent receives approval from the U.S. Food and Drug Administration (FDA) for marketing, phase 4 (post-marketing surveillance) is often conducted, particularly if such a phase is a condition of FDA approval. Phase 4 is a post-marketing surveillance study to assess long-term effects of the new treatment and monitor subsequent adverse reactions, and it can be used for cost-effectiveness assessment and marketing purposes.

Phase 1 Trials

Phase 1 trials establish a safe dose in humans with an acceptable level of toxicity, establish a route of administration, and determine the clinical pharmacology. In studies of cancer chemotherapy, the intent of a phase 1 trial is to discover the maximum tolerated dose (MTD) on the premise that the maximum benefit (efficacy) would be observed with the highest tolerable dose. The occurrence of toxicity that is unacceptable is termed dose-limiting toxicity (DLT). Hence, the MTD is determined by the absence of a DLT, with the MTD being one dose level below a DLT.

In stroke, there is no consensus regarding the need to escalate the dose to the MTD. The level of escalation chosen for a phase 1 trial would be treatment specific. Another ambiguity in phase 1 studies for stroke is the definition of DLT. Oncology clinical trials use standard definitions for the varying levels of toxicity. Stroke has no such guidelines. A phase 1 study funded by NINDS aimed to establish the MTD of human serum albumin as a neuroprotective agent for participants with recent ischemic stroke.[13] A Safety Evaluation Committee, consisting of a team of neurologists and cardiologists, evaluated participants' records at each dose level according to prespecified guidelines to determine whether severe and serious adverse events occurred during the 72 hours after ictus. The existence of DLT was determined by a consensus

after each member of the committee reviewed the charts of all the participants at each dose level.

For the traditional and most often implemented design, the choice of the initial phase 1 dose is based either on animal experiments for a drug that has never been used in humans or on previous studies in humans for an existing drug. The common approach starts from one-tenth of the dose that causes 10% mortality in the rodents (LD_{10}). The dose is increased by a smaller percentage each time, often using a modified Fibonacci scheme. Continual reassessment methods (CRMs) as an alternative design for a phase 1 study can use either the frequentist or bayesian methods. Information gathered in the trial from a previous increase in dose is used to estimate the probability of DLT at the next dose level. Simulation studies show that the MTD may be reached sooner with some CRM methods than with the traditional method putting fewer participants at risk from higher doses.[14]

Phase 2 Trials

Phase 2 studies do not seek to draw definitive conclusions about the treatment effectiveness; instead, they look for evidence to justify proceeding to a phase 3 study. Phase 2 studies primarily rule out clearly ineffective treatments, that is, assess futility, and assess side effects and toxicity, logistics of treatment administration, and project trial costs. Traditional phase 2 trials use data previously collected on historical controls and are considered single-arm studies. Historical placebo data from the NINDS rt-PA Stroke Study trial participants with recent ischemic stroke are available on the Internet from the National Technological Service (http://www.ntis.gov/search/index.aspx; enter PB2006500032 in the search field) and can be obtained by request from numerous other therapeutic stroke trials.

In stroke prevention trials, a surrogate outcome such as reduction in some risk factor would be required in phase 2 because the primary outcome, new stroke or death, generally takes years to ascertain. Therapeutic phase 2 stroke trials generally use outcome measures taken at 3 months and no surrogate is required.

Phase 2 studies have been underutilized in stroke. New therapies often are studied in phase 1 trials and then studied in underpowered phase 3 trials, sometimes called *phase 2B studies*. Traditional phase 2 trials using historical data as a reference have the advantage of requiring smaller sample sizes than a controlled study with the same error and effect size parameters, requiring less time and fewer resources. More new treatments may be explored at this stage of drug development. A single-arm phase 2 design is especially attractive when availability of participants is limited in relation to the rate of development of new treatments. A critical assumption is that the course of the disease has not changed over time and historical controls are an accurate representation of current patients. If there is uncertainty about the validity of historical controls, a comparison group can be included, but the higher alpha level (usually 0.15 to 0.20) and hypothesis being tested will still lead to a reduction in sample size over a phase 2B design.[15,16] A completed phase 2 stroke treatment trial of combined intravenous and intraarterial t-PA was determined to be worthwhile and has moved forward to phase 3.[17] The phase 3 trial is ongoing.

Phase 3 Trials

In a randomized phase 3 clinical trial, whether preventive or therapeutic, each participant is randomly assigned to an intervention or control (placebo, usual care, best medical treatment for the condition, etc.). A well-designed, well-executed, randomized, concurrently controlled phase 3 clinical trial is the ultimate proof (or lack thereof) of the strength of association between the treatment and a clinical effect.

Outcome Measures

All clinical trials must begin with a clear definition of the question to be studied and a definition of the expected outcomes. Most primary and secondary prevention trials use new stroke occurrence and stroke-related mortality or overall mortality because people who experience a stroke frequently die in the first 3 months or even the first year. Thus the outcome measure is unlikely to be mortality alone owing to the length of follow-up required to observe a sufficient number of deaths.

Prevention trials must obtain sufficient information to define new stroke occurrence and, where applicable, stroke-related mortality, at a cost low enough to allow the trial to be conducted. In planning a new trial, investigators can draw on the experience of other large prevention trials. Investigators in the ACAS, for example, devised a symptom-based questionnaire and algorithm for detecting TIAs and other neurologic illness[18] but they recommended that positive results be confirmed by neurologic evaluation. Some trials evaluate participants every 3 months. Reported stroke events are verified and categorized into stroke subtypes (see later section) by a central events committee blinded to treatment assignment who are using a clinical classification scheme. This process of adjudication is costly and time consuming. Classifying deaths as stroke-related adds another level of complexity.

Acute stroke therapeutic trials use some measure of poststroke recovery as the outcome measure rather than mortality or new stroke. Common single measures are the NIH Stroke Scale (NIHSS)[19] and modified Rankin scale,[20] in which participants who have died are given the worst score or some weighted score on an outcome measure. There is no consensus on the best single outcome or on the amount of difference that should be required, and it is clear that no one outcome measures all aspects of recovery after stroke. For example, a participant could obtain a high score on the Barthel Index,[21] which measures performance of activities of daily living, but still have severe aphasia, as indicated by the NIHSS score. In the NINDS rt-PA Stroke Study,[9] to avoid choosing a single outcome measure or an amount of difference to be considered clinically meaningful on a measure, the investigators decided to classify participants as having a favorable or unfavorable outcome through the use of four outcome measures, the modified Rankin Scale (mRS), Barthel Index,[21] NIHSS, and Glasgow Outcome Scale.[22] "Favorable" for each outcome was defined as minimal or no disability at 3 months after stroke. The four outcomes were combined to form a single global outcome. If a trial is planned to use a new outcome measure or to use an existing outcome measure in a new population, the measure should be validated in patients similar to possible trial participants before it is used in the trial. Hanston[23] describes the considerations for and required approaches to validation of new outcome measures for stroke trials.

Sample Size

There are general methods for calculating sample size for most trial outcomes and many software packages, including NQuery Advisor,[24] a user-friendly software package, and free shareware such as that developed by the University of Iowa. Applying these general methods to clinical trials in stroke entails consideration of the distributions of stroke outcomes as well as of the usual parameters required to develop an estimate of sample size.

J-Shaped Distribution

In therapeutic stroke trials, outcome measures are often used as a continuum to increase the power of the test and reduce the required sample size. However if the distribution takes on a J- or U-shaped distribution, the gain from using a continuum is less clear.[25] Figure 60-1 shows a typical example using the Barthel Index. This J- or U-shaped distribution does not lend itself to transformation into a distribution that is less skewed or more normally distributed. An investigator can dichotomize a J- or U-shaped distribution into success or failure by choosing a value or cut point in the distribution, depending on the question of interest. The cut point would be chosen before the start of the study and used in calculating the sample size.

One-Tailed or Two-Tailed Tests

A one-tailed test requires a smaller sample size to achieve the same effect with the same power. Usually investigators design the trial to learn whether the treatment group has an outcome better *or worse* than that of the control group, requiring a two-sided test. In the EC/IC Bypass Study,[4] investigators designed the study using a one-tailed test to compare surgery with best medical care. Because of the cost of surgery, if the trial indicated that surgery was no better than best medical care, surgery would not be recommended in the future.

Power and Alpha Level

In large multicenter phase 3 stroke trials, *power* (1 minus beta, the chance of missing a true difference) is usually set high (90% or greater) to allow interpretation of a negative result or lack of a treatment effect. If the investigators are willing to accept a greater chance of missing a true difference, power can be as low as 80% (i.e., a 20% chance of missing the hypothesized treatment effect). The *alpha level* (chance of calling an ineffective treatment effective) is usually 0.05, but if multiple groups are being compared, the alpha level may be set to a smaller value. See further discussion in the section on data analysis.

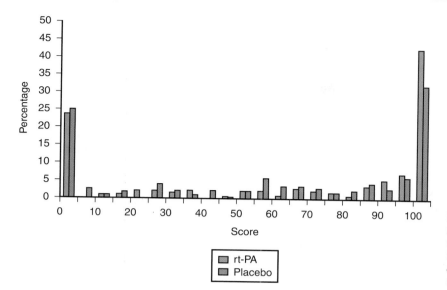

Figure 60-1 Distribution of the Barthel Index. rt-PA, recombinant tissue-type plasminogen activator. (Data from Tissue plasminogen activator for acute ischemic stroke. National Institute of Neurological Disorders and Stroke [NINDS] rt-PA Stroke Study Group. *N Engl J Med* 333:1581-1587, 1995.)

Equivalence or Noninferiority

It may be of interest to show that a treatment is as beneficial as another current treatment, given that the new treatment has fewer side effects or lower cost. Studies to demonstrate the equivalence or noninferiority of one therapy to another require specialized approaches to analysis[26] and high power. If the probability of missing a true difference is high, negative study results are difficult to interpret. The software package NQuery Advisor has the ability to calculate sample size for equivalence studies.[24]

Adjusting for Drop-Outs and Drop-Ins

Drop-outs (patients who are stopping the study therapy) and drop-ins (patients changing over to a study treatment different from their original assignment) must be considered in calculation of sample size. Inflating the sample size by the proportion expected to drop out or drop in may underestimate the size needed. Statisticians often inflate the calculated sample size by using the formula $1/(1-R)$, where R is the drop-out and drop-in rate or a combination of the two. Because the inflation factor greatly enlarges the sample size, efforts should be made to keep these rates as low as possible (see later discussion of adherence).

Adaptive Designs

In an adaptive design, accumulating data are used to make midcourse modifications to the study design while maintaining validity and integrity of study data. For example, designs have been developed to take trials seamlessly from phase 2 to phase 3 using participants from phase 2, to augment the sample size for phase 3, or to take trials from phase 1 to phase 2. The phase 1 to phase 2 design has been applied in ischemic stroke.[27] Adaptive designs have been developed to allow sample size reestimation during the course of the trial and to allow early termination in the face of strong evidence of efficacy or futility. Early termination is described in more detail in the section on interim monitoring. The latter types of design

changes must be prespecified in the protocol for the trial. Other adaptive designs involve concurrent changes during the course of the trial, such as changes in the eligibility criteria, in the length of study follow-up, or in study outcomes—which are changes that can diminish the credibility of the trial.[28]

Inclusion and Exclusion Criteria for Phase 3 Trials

Inclusion and exclusion criteria define the trial population to be studied. Investigators may wish to give a treatment its "best chance to succeed" by excluding participants who do not "do well," such as those who are older or have high NIHSS scores, subtle CT findings, or certain stroke subtypes. If one suspects that patients *with* a risk factor will have a *poorer* outcome with treatment than with placebo and patients *without* a risk factor would have a *better* outcome with treatment than with placebo, a *treatment–risk factor interaction* is implied. It would be difficult to justify randomly assigning treatment for patients with the risk factor. If no interaction with treatment is expected—patients with the risk factor are expected to do worse than those without it, *regardless* of treatment assignment—there is not a strong rationale to exclude these participants.

The more restrictive the criteria for entry into the trial, the less generalizable are the results. Trials that exclude potential participants with specific stroke subtypes or include participants only from large specialty clinics may not provide data applicable to patients seen in the general practice of neurology, and if the treatment appears efficacious, a wider range of patients than used in the trial may receive the treatment. Additionally, because the treatment has not yet been proven to be efficacious (or the trial would not be conducted), there is some uncertainty about the usefulness of the eligibility criteria.

A better approach, unless there are well-documented treatment interactions suggesting harm in one treated subgroup, is to have broad eligibility criteria and include prespecified exploratory post hoc subgroup analyses

TABLE 60-1 PROPORTION OF 3-MONTH FAVORABLE OUTCOMES BY BASELINE NIHSS SCORE, AGE, AND TREATMENT GROUP*

Variable	% Patients with Favorable Outcome	
	t-PA	Placebo
Age ≤60 yr		
Baseline NIHSS score		
0-9 (n = 46)	59	42
10-14 (n = 35)	38	18
5-20 (n = 49)	41	27
>20 (n = 26)	22	12
Age 61-68 yr		
NIHSS score		
0-9 (n = 44)	60	37
10-14 (n = 28)	25	25
15-20 (n = 39)	0	25
>20 (n = 30)	7	0
Age 69-75 yr		
NIHSS score		
0-9 (n = 41)	50	54
10-14 (n = 45)	39	27
15-20 (n = 40)	26	0
>20 (n = 35)	8	0
Age >75 yr		
NIHSS score		
0-9 (n = 46)	67	36
10-14 (n = 28)	27	15
15-20 (n = 43)	23	6
>20 (n = 49)	0	0

*Favorable outcome = NIHSS score of 0 or 1 at 3 months. The categories for age and baseline NIHSS represent quartiles of the range of each variable.
NIHSS, National Institutes of Health Stroke Scale; t-PA, tissue-type plasminogen activator.
Data from The NINDS t-PA Stroke Study Group: Generalized efficacy of t-PA for acute stroke: Subgroup analysis of the NINDS t-PA Stroke Trial. *Stroke* 28:2119-2125, 1997.

(see later discussion of subgroups). Additionally, overly restrictive entry criteria may limit enrollment of older adults and minority populations more likely to have comorbidities and most in need of the new approaches to stroke prevention or therapy. Potential participants at higher risk of unfavorable outcomes are also potential "responders" to treatment.

Table 60-1 shows published data from the NINDS t-PA Stroke Study.[39] The percentage of participants with a favorable outcome decreased with age and with increasing NIHSS score, but the t-PA–treated group had a higher percentage of favorable outcomes in 14 of the 16 age-by-NIHSS subgroups. In the oldest patients with the highest NIHSS scores, there were no favorable outcomes in either treatment group, but 74% of the t-PA–treated patients, versus 86% of the placebo-treated patients, experienced severe disability or death. To minimize problems with missing data (see discussions of adherence and analyses of missing data), investigators may consider excluding potential participants with characteristics that might prevent the participants from completing the study or from complying with the study medication. Stroke trials thus may exclude patients at imminent risk of death such as those with terminal cancer.

Randomization

Randomization is the method of allocating participants to the different treatment arms of a randomized clinical trial. Simple randomization is similar to flipping an unbiased coin and using heads or tails to assign a participant to one of two treatment arms. Using alternating assignment of participants to treatment or control as they come in to a study is not a random assignment: If a participant's treatment assignment in the sequence of alternating assignments is revealed, all other participants' assignments can be ascertained. To ensure randomness, a random number generator, available in most statistical software packages, is generally used to conduct the randomization.

Stratification

Simple randomization may result in imbalances in the risk factors associated with outcome or in the number of participants in each treatment arm. In stroke treatment trials, as in all trials, investigators desire balance in factors associated with treatment outcome such as baseline NIHSS score and age to ensure that one group does not inadvertently have an advantage over another. To obtain balance, one solution is to stratify participants before randomization into specific subgroups and then randomly assign participants to treatment arms within each subgroup. Another goal of stratification is to improve the precision of the statistical analysis.

The EC/IC Bypass Study stratified participants on the basis of clinical center, type of underlying vascular lesion (two categories), presence or absence of a related neurologic deficit; participants with internal carotid occlusion were stratified according to presence or absence of related symptoms after angiographic demonstration of occlusion.[4,5] In therapeutic trials with smaller samples, a smaller number of strata must be used. For the NINDS rt-PA Stroke Study,[9] there was limited knowledge about the predictors of stroke outcome in patients treated soon after stroke (within 180 minutes of stroke onset), so a decision was made to stratify only by clinical site and time from stroke outcome to treatment (0 to 90 minutes or 91 to 180 minutes).

There is a rapid increase in the number of subgroups as the number of variables used for stratification rises. In a trial that is stratified on time from stroke onset (early, late), clinical center (8 locations), NIHSS score (3 levels), and age (3 levels), there would be 144 subgroups. Given a large number of subgroups and a small sample size, participants could be unequally assigned to treatment groups within strata, inducing an overall imbalance in the treatment arms. A complex randomization scheme also makes it more likely that clinics will make errors in the randomization.

Most treatment trials and prevention trials have sufficient sample size to make stratification unnecessary except on the basis of one or two influential variables. There is little gain in statistical precision once the number of participants per group exceeds 50, with the greatest gains from stratification for trials with 20 or fewer participants per treatment arm.[29] Generally, the most important stratifying variable in multiple-site trials is clinical site.

When a study uses stratification, the stratifying variables should be included as covariates in the primary analysis. If the overall sample size is small and there is concern that stratification by site may lead to imbalances in treatment groups, one solution is to use a validated clinical index that takes into account several variables or to use *minimization*, a statistical approach to balancing the treatment arms to the extent possible after each participant's entry criteria are ascertained.[30]

Blocking

Blocking is the process of forcing the proportion in each of the two treatment arms within strata to be fixed through time, usually at 0.5; that is, blocking provides balance on unknown temporal variables. A block size of four in a trial with equal randomization to the two treatment arms would imply that after every four participants are randomly assigned within a block there would be two participants in each treatment arm. Generally, the selected block size is large enough to make it difficult for an investigator to guess the next treatment assignment. Often the block size is randomly chosen from a range of block sizes to make it more difficult to detect the end of a block.

Blinding

Blinding (sometimes referred to as *masking*) is an approach to reduce bias in the assessment of the trial outcome measures. In a single-blind study, either the participant or the investigator is blinded to the treatment assignment before the end of the trial. In the more common double-blind study, neither the participant nor the investigator knows the treatment assignment. When the outcome is death, it is more difficult to introduce bias unless the outcome is classified as stroke-related death. Bias in classifying a participant as having a new stroke (or stroke-related death) could inadvertently be introduced if the rater assessing outcomes knows the treatment assignment or if differing amounts of effort were put into finding information about the event, depending on treatment group. For many of the other outcome measures of poststroke recovery, some inherent subjectivity is built into the scale assessment. Even if the rater does not introduce bias, there can be a perception of bias on the part of those who review the trial report if the study was not blinded.

A traditional approach to blinding is to formulate the intervention in such a way that neither physician nor participant can determine what treatment is being given to the participant. If this approach is not possible (e.g., surgery versus medical care), efforts must be made to collect outcome data in as unbiased a way as possible, such as by using someone not present at the time of treatment, as in the NINDS t-PA stroke trial,[9] or by using an independent adjudicator.

In the WARSS,[6] periodic dose adjustments were needed for many participants receiving warfarin. To maintain the blind, the coordinating center fabricated clinically plausible values for participants in the aspirin-placebo treatment arm. A message to change the placebo dose for some patients was sent from the laboratory to the investigator. The frequency and amount of change for participants receiving placebo was determined through the use of a complex algorithm that mimicked the frequency and direction of changes in the warfarin-treated group.

Recruitment

Proper planning helps ensure recruitment on the timetable projected. This is particularly important for acute stroke therapy trials, in which participant eligibility must be quickly assessed and time from admission to treatment must be minimized. In the NINDS t-PA Stroke Study, methods of total quality improvement were used to flowchart the process in each emergency department and to engage those involved in the process (CT technicians, laboratory technicians, nurses, pharmacists, neurologists, emergency department physicians and staff) in helping determine how to enroll patients more quickly.[31] Another important aspect of recruiting is engagement of the community. For acute stroke trials, cooperation of the community emergency medical services is essential in facilitating prompt arrival of prospective trial participants at participating emergency departments.[32] In acute stroke trials, the yield of participants from community presentations is low, but communication remains important to create a climate of trust. Also, community consent may be needed in order to meet institutional review board (IRB) requirements for randomization in the emergency department (see later section on informed consent). For prevention trials, especially those conducted in groups of participants who are not acutely ill, the special efforts made to engage the community may have a greater effect on recruitment. In particular, some minority groups may be unwilling to participate in prevention trials unless a climate of trust has been developed in the community by the study investigators. There is a growing literature on recruitment of minority participants, but little rigorous research has been conducted to test recruitment methodologies. A 2000 survey of community members in San Francisco[33] identified factors associated with willingness to participate, including altruism and tangible benefits to the participant.

Adherence to Treatment and Trial Follow-Up

Adherence to treatment can be increased by simplifying study procedures and demands on participants, gathering sufficient information to enable close contact with participants after enrollment, and providing the patient, family, or both with sufficient information about the trial and its requirements before randomization. Conducting a "run-in" period that mimics the study before randomization may eliminate "noncompliers" before they are entered into the trial, although using a run-in design could result in enrolling a less generalizable group of participants. A run-in period may be feasible for long-term stroke prevention trials but would not be possible in therapeutic trials for acute stroke, in which treatment must be given as quickly as possible.

In both stroke prevention and therapeutic trials, all participants should be encouraged to return for a final trial visit even if they no longer take study medications or participate in other aspects of the intervention, to avoid the problem of missing outcome data (see later discussion on missing data). For an acute stroke trial with a one-time dose, the possibility of drop-out from therapy is minimal; however, completeness of follow-up remains an important issue.

Measuring Adherence to Treatment

If treatment is an educational intervention to reduce stroke risk factors or an exercise rehabilitation program, a participant's adherence to the regimen can be estimated with process measures (e.g., number of sessions attended) or by changes in knowledge, attitudes, and beliefs. If laboratory tests are applicable, reliable, and affordable, the most accurate assessment of medication compliance may be measurement of blood, saliva, or urine levels of the drug; if, however, a participant is generally noncompliant but takes medication more often close to the next clinic visit, such a measurement does not reflect the true level of adherence. Other standard adherence measures for medication trials include pill counts of returned medication and counting the number of times the pill container was opened by means of a miniaturized electronic device in the lid of the pill bottle. Both methods are only estimates, subject to under- and overcounting or excess opening of the pill container, and can be expensive. Morisky and associates[34] suggest posing a set of questions as a better measure of compliance than a pill count. The usefulness of these questions in stroke trials needs validation, although the approach has been validated in trials of Parkinson's disease treatments.[35] Counts of missed visits, missed forms, and missed items on forms may also be useful in monitoring adherence to treatment.

Data Collection and Quality Assurance

General texts on clinical trials provide detailed plans for study data collection and quality assurance applicable to stroke trials. Key approaches include study documentation, timely applications of range and consistency checks, and prompt communication of data errors to the study coordinators for resolution.

Protocol and Manual of Procedures

A trial has two key documents, the protocol and the manual of procedures. Both are essential to trial management. The *protocol* is the blueprint for the trial. It is the document that is sent to the institutional review board and, when necessary, the FDA. Changes to the protocol and changes in data collected generally require new IRB approval and often notification to the FDA. Protocols should be kept as simple as possible, reflecting the primary aspects of study design with procedures being documented in the *manual of procedures*. Changes to the manual of procedures would not require a protocol change or new approvals. The manual of procedures contains study instruments (i.e., forms for data collection), detailed instructions for completing the study instruments, and other instructions for data collection, follow-up, laboratory procedures, and so on. The manual documents answers to questions raised by investigators conducting the trial in the field so that answers to the same question are consistent over time. The protocol and manual of procedures provide sufficient detail to allow someone who has not been participating in the trial to replicate it in another setting.

Training

An important aspect of quality assurance is training of the people collecting data for the trial. Some trials have developed video training and testing programs for stroke outcomes such as the modified Rankin and NIHSS scales. The training and testing program for the NIHSS scale can be obtained through the National Stroke Association. To maintain consistency of NIHSS measurement over time, investigators are often recertified over the course of the trial.

Data Analyses

Intent to Treat

The guiding principle in clinical trials is the use of intent-to-treat (ITT) analysis. When an ITT analysis is used, all participants undergoing randomization are included in the primary analysis, whether or not they withdraw or deviate from the protocol. In a surgical trial, under an ITT analysis, all participants randomly assigned to surgery would be analyzed in the surgical group, and all participants assigned to medical care would be analyzed in the medical care group. The EC/IC Bypass Study methodology paper describing the design suggested that the intent-to-treat principle would not be followed. However, in the presentation of trial results, the analytic approach was changed, and the intent-to-treat principle was followed.[5]

The terms "completer analysis," "on-treatment analysis," and "analyzable population" are generally used to describe a situation in which participants who stop treatment, did not adhere to protocol, or have incomplete follow-up are excluded. These analyses are often conducted in addition to ITT analyses. If results of these ancillary analyses agree with the analyses of the full trial data set, the interpretation is clear. If results do not agree, emphasis should generally be placed on the ITT analysis.

When some ineligible participants are expected to be enrolled, the effect on the trial sample size should be considered in the trial design. Although some biostatisticians suggest that no withdrawals be allowed and that analyses include all participants who underwent randomization, regardless of the circumstances, there are several other complex situations relevant to stroke trials.[36] For example, if it is necessary to randomly assign participants to treatment before an entry criterion is completely ascertained—for example, before MRI can be performed a large number of participants are enrolled who do not meet the entry criteria. If the eligibility for study is determined on the basis of data collected prior to treatment and eligibility is defined by someone blinded to treatment assignment, the FDA has allowed the ITT analyses to include only eligible participants. Methods for imputing data in order to include participants with missing follow-up and adherence to the ITT principle are described in a later section in the chapter.

General Approaches

Textbooks on clinical trials summarize the analytic approaches used in clinical trials.[1,37] These standard approaches, such as analyses of time to new stroke or death, are generally useful in prevention trials and intervention trials, in which the outcome is usually binary (yes/no; each participant either survived stroke-free or had a new stroke or died). Treatment trials of acute therapy present a special problem. As noted previously, the outcome of therapeutic trials is often recovery from stroke, for which there is no one accepted measure. Thus, trials are usually designed with a set of correlated outcome measures. These measures can be analyzed separately, but interpretation of the set of outcomes with respect to an overall effect of treatment is difficult, particularly if some outcomes show a weak or negative effect. Additionally, having multiple outcome measures generally requires adjustment for multiple comparisons. For this reason some investigators choose a single primary outcome, even though the single outcome does not represent the multiple dimensions of recovery. Others use global tests for multiple outcomes.

Global Tests

A composite outcome can be constructed identifying the results in a subject as a failure if any one of the set of primary outcomes occur.[38] In stroke, the composite outcome is often new stroke or stroke-related death. This approach is most commonly used in cardiovascular disease. Another approach is the use of a global statistical test,[39] such as in the NINDS t-PA Stroke Trial.[9] Investigators chose dichotomization of each of the outcome measures into minimal or no disability (success/failure) to address the question of interest. Dichotomization also solved the statistical issue of the J-shaped distribution of the Barthel Index. When the outcome measures are dichotomous (binary), the global test is reported as an odds ratios. Odds ratios for the individual outcomes were also given to provide an interpretation of the global test outcome.[9]

Multiple Comparisons

An argument has been made[40] that if the comparisons represent separate questions (i.e., assessment of the impact of the intervention on two or three different outcomes), each comparison can be considered a separate experiment with no need for adjustment of the alpha level. When an overall hypothesis and a subgroup hypothesis are being tested (e.g., all patients with stroke and patients with severe NIHSS status at baseline), spending some alpha on this overall comparison (0.04) and less on the subgroups is another approach.[41] When all possible pairwise comparisons are to be made among a series of treatments, a more stringent adjustment of the alpha level for multiple comparisons may be required. Hockberg's correction,[42] a step-down approach, is an example and is less conservative than the traditional Bonferroni approach, which uses alpha divided by the number of comparisons.

Clustering

Special analytic issues arise in the analyses of clustered data when there is some correlation or association among participants, such as a clinical trial in which the unit of randomization is a physician's practice or an emergency department rather than a patient. In the analysis of clustered data, a positive correlation among patients in the provider's practice or clinical site is often assumed, implying that patients in a practice or a clinical site are more like one another than like patients in different practices or sites. In the presence of a positive correlation, the variance unadjusted for clustering underestimates the true variance. Thus, by ignoring the clustering, the investigator may falsely reject a null hypothesis and claim treatment benefit.

Missing Data

Of particular concern in clinical trials is the biased use of only those participants for whom there is complete outcome data. Bias may arise because the participants who provided data may have a better response to treatment than those who did not, even those in the placebo group. Therefore, a subgroup of fully compliant participants ("completers") is not a random sample of the original sample. Patterns of missing data (i.e., rate, time to withdrawal, and reason for withdrawal) may differ among treatment groups, contributing bias to study results. Furthermore, the amount of missing data may differ among treatment groups. If a substantial proportion of data (e.g., >20%) is unobserved, especially in the primary outcome of interest, the integrity and quality of the entire study could be questioned, regardless of the approach taken to adjust for the missing data. When data are missing, a variety of statistical methods may be used to perform an ITT analysis.[37] There are two patterns of missing data in longitudinal clinical trials: intermittent (e.g., due to a single missed clinic visit) and monotone (e.g., due to participant withdrawal or loss to follow-up). Missing data have been classified as follows:

- *Missing completely at random (MCAR):* Data that are missing because of an event, circumstances, or measure completely independent of the outcome of interest or other participant-specific measures collected in the study. For example, the absence of a participant's 3-month NIHSS score is MCAR if (1) the investigational staff simply forgot to evaluate the participant on the NIHSS at 3 months or (2) the participant's car broke down on his/her way to the clinic for the 3-month visit.
- *Missing at random (MAR):* Data that are missing because of an event, circumstances, or measure independent of the outcome of interest but related to another participant-specific measure. If the 3-month NIHSS score is missing because the participant was feeling depressed and did not wish to make the clinic visit, it is MAR (depression is not measured by NIHSS score).

- *Missing not at random (MNAR or nonignorable):* The data are missing because of the unobserved outcome of interest. If the 3-month NIHSS score is missing because the participant's neurologic condition (which is measured by the NIHSS score) had deteriorated to the extent that the participant was unable to travel to the clinic, the missing data are nonignorable.

Statistically, MCAR and MAR data are not problematic because standard statistical methods as well as various imputation methods can be applied with minimal or no bias because the missing data in this case are considered a representative sample of the observed data. If more than a minimal amount of data is missing, this approach leads to reduction in statistical power.

For statistical analysis with MAR data, a multiple imputation method is recommended before analysis, because the method adds some uncertainty to the imputed value, thereby allowing for more appropriate variance estimation. Repeated measures analysis or survival analyses can be conducted with MAR data without imputing, if all other assumptions are met. Nonignorable missing (MNAR) data are more problematic for analysis. Application of standard statistical methods may yield biased results. If there are missing data, various multiple imputation methods are available to substitute values for the missing data items, many of which have good statistical properties.[43] In clinical trials in which an event such as death or recurrent stroke is the primary outcome and are MNAR, using an approach to analysis that censors participants when they are lost to follow-up can introduce bias. Thus, approaches to multiple imputation specifically for survival data have been developed.[44] When the reason for missing data is unknown, the most conservative approach is to assume it is MNAR.

In the WARSS, the primary outcome (recurrent ischemic stroke or death from any cause) for 2173 of the 2206 participants was assessed at the end of the trial. For the remaining 33, an innovative approach to imputation was used. A senior clinician who was blinded to treatment assignments classified the participants with missing outcomes into three categories and the following decisions were made:

1. Endpoint eminent; an endpoint was assumed to have occurred at the time the participant was lost to follow-up (N = 1) (MNAR).
2. Data missing for reason unrelated to study (e.g., participant moved to Puerto Rico with daughter); participant was censored at the date of loss to follow-up (i.e., participant's outcome was considered unknown after the date specified, and participant does not contribute information after that point in time) (N = 20) (MAR or MCAR).
3. Data missing for reason possibly related to study (MNAR). For example, a TIA occurred then a participant was lost to follow-up. For this type of participants, methods of multiple imputation are used to impute a value for time to outcome, taking into account baseline covariates (N = 12). Of the 12 participants for whom multiple imputation was used, a primary outcome was imputed for 2, and an event-free follow-up imputed for 10.[46]

Interim Analysis

Almost all clinical trial participants are enrolled sequentially and followed up over some period. By conducting interim analyses during the course of the trial, investigators are better able to ensure participant safety. Stopping the study early because of overwhelming evidence of the efficacy of a drug means earlier access to an efficacious treatment for patients, less time receiving an ineffective treatment for controls, and earlier profit for the pharmaceutical industry. Stopping a study early because of negative results ensures that participants are not unnecessarily exposed to inferior or ineffective treatment and prevents wasting of resources. Interim analyses also allow the investigators and statisticians to evaluate assumptions made in the design of the trial, such as participant accrual rate and the parameters used for sample size estimation.

Figure 60-2 gives examples of three different guidelines for stopping a trial.[37] Peto et al[46] and O'Brien and Fleming[46] use more conservative guidelines early in their studies, so that the final alpha level for testing is close to the planned overall alpha (0.05). Pocock[48] uses a less conservative guideline, but the final comparison for the trial would be made at an alpha level less than 0.05, potentially less acceptable to investigators.

If all participants are quickly entered into the trial by the time the first or the second interim analysis is to be conducted, further interim analyses may be unnecessary. The Interventional Management of Stroke Study, a phase 2

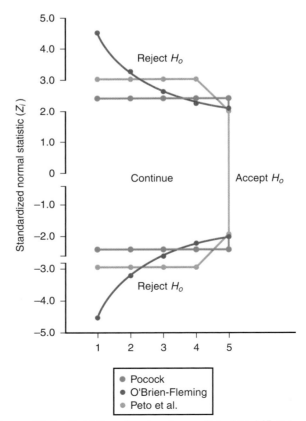

Figure 60-2 Guidelines for stopping a clinical trial.[37] (Adapted from Friedman LM, Furberg CD, DeMets DL: *Fundamentals of clinical trials*, ed 3, New York, 1998, Springer-Verlag.)

trial with a planned sample size of 80, included a planned interim analysis. Trial sites enrolled 10 patients per month and enrollment was completed in 8 months, making the planned interim analyses unnecessary.[17]

Stochastic curtailment originated in the quality control field for manufacturing, in which an entire batch of products would be rejected if a certain number of defective items were found; if and when that number was reached, the rest of the batch was not inspected. In clinical trials, stochastic curtailment is used to determine whether proceeding further with the study would be unlikely to provide a statistically significant result. These analyses are completed separately from analyses of efficacy, and usually implemented using the B statistic.[49] Bayesian rules, derived from subjective prior information, have also been developed for stochastic curtailment and have been used more frequently in trials of cancer therapies than in trials of stroke prevention and therapy. Interim analyses, formal or informal, should be fully described in the study protocol.

Analysis of Covariance

Unless most participants in one treatment arm of a study have the risk factor and most participants in the other arm do not have the risk factor, it is possible to adjust statistically for imbalances between treatment groups by including the risk factor in a model testing for a treatment effect. If the imbalance in the risk factor explains away the treatment benefit, the benefit has been artificially enhanced by the imbalance. If a benefit of treatment remains or is enhanced after adjustment for the risk factor, the imbalance was not artificially inflating the treatment benefit. One danger in such post hoc analyses is that many variables may be tested in an attempt to bring out a positive treatment outcome, making the end result less credible. Investigators can avoid this "data dredging" by prespecifying the variables to be included as covariates.[50]

The odds ratio for a favorable outcome in the second NINDS rt-PA Stroke Study (part II) was 1.7 (95% confidence interval [CI], 1.2–2.6), adjusting for prespecified stratification variables. Post hoc analyses of covariance were also conducted with adjustment for the three variables (age, weight, and aspirin use before stroke) imbalanced ($P < .05$) between the two treatment groups at randomization. These post hoc analyses suggested an even greater benefit of t-PA (odds ratio for a favorable outcome 2.0 (95% CI, 1.3–3.1).[9]

Subgroup Analyses and Interactions

After the completion of a trial, multiple analyses are often performed to determine whether there are subgroups in which the treatment might have been beneficial or harmful. To avoid bias, subgroups should be "proper"—that is, defined by characteristics measured at baseline—before treatment. For example, in the NINDS t-PA Stroke Study, each participant's stroke subtype was determined 7 to 10 days after stroke from CT scans taken 24 hours after thrombolytic treatment and clinical data collected at baseline. The therapy could affect the 24-hour CT findings through both its clot-busting properties and its potential hemorrhagic side effects. The grouping of patients by this postrandomization classification of stroke subtype would not constitute a "proper" subgroup.

The more subgroups examined, the more likely the analyses will lead to an *alpha error,* detection of a difference by chance alone. To protect against bias and alpha errors, the subgroups should be predefined, on the basis of a clearly justified rationale, and specified in the protocol before the start of the trial. These a priori subgroups are less subject to bias than subgroups defined after study results are known (post hoc). Analyses can be adjusted for multiple comparisons, with the potential for greatly reduced power, depending on the number of subgroups. Additionally, to protect against bias and inflated alpha error, particularly in the testing of post hoc hypotheses, testing for a treatment interaction before subgroup analyses are conducted provides a more stringent approach. An interaction between treatment and the subgrouping variable is present if (1) the treatment is harmful in one subgroup but beneficial in another or (2) the magnitude of treatment benefit differs among subgroups.[51] Generally, interactions are tested at the 0.1 rather than 0.05 alpha level in recognition that most studies are not designed with sufficient power to test for interactions effects.

Meade and Brennan[52] conducted subgroup analyses of patients in a thrombosis prevention trial with emphasis on detecting subgroups who might derive the most benefit in terms of stroke prevention. The investigators presented analyses with tests of interactions suggesting that participants who had baseline systolic blood pressures 145 mm Hg and higher and were receiving aspirin therapy were at a higher risk of stroke than those with similar blood pressure levels who were receiving placebo, whereas participants with lower blood pressures experienced a protective effect (P value for the interaction, .006). The time-treatment interaction in the NINDS tPA Stroke Trial[53] (Fig. 60-3) and a study of the effect of apolipoprotein-E on stroke outcomes in participants in the same stroke study[54] provide other examples of treatment by covariate interactions.

Regulations and Guidelines

Federal Regulations

In the United States, the two main federal agencies responsible for regulation of stroke-related clinical trials are the U.S. Department of Health and Human Services (DHHS) and the FDA. Federal regulations apply to all clinical investigations and to studies involving FDA-regulated products. Additional regulations and policies (such as the Good Clinical Practice formulated by the International Conference of Harmonisation of Technical Requirements for Registration of Pharmaceuticals for Human Use, and those of the U.S. Department of Veterans Affairs and the Joint Commission on Accreditation of Health Care Organizations) may also apply, depending on the source of funding or the purpose of the investigation. Federal regulations govern all clinical trials that are funded by federal money or are conducted in institutions that (1) receive federal money, (2) have federal project-wide assurances, or (3) conduct studies of investigational drugs with human participants. Any clinical trial of drugs, biological products, or medical devices involving interstate shipping or marketing requires prior submission to and approval from

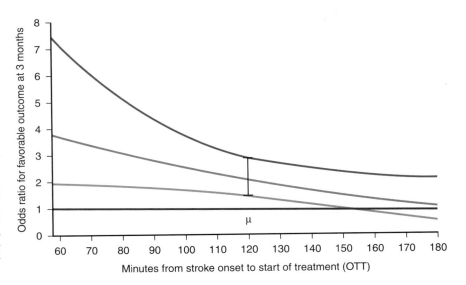

Figure 60-3 Graph of model estimating odds ratio for favorable outcome at 3 months in patients treated with recombinant tissue-type plasminogen activator (rt-PA) and in those given placebo by onset-to-treatment time (OTT) with 95% confidence intervals, after adjustment for the baseline National Institutes of Health (NIH) Stroke Scale score. Odds ratio >1 indicates greater odds that rt-PA–treated patients will have a favorable outcome at 3 months than the placebo-treated patients. Range of OTT was 58 to180 minutes with a mean (μ) of 119.7 minutes. (Aapted from Marler JR, Tilley BC, Lu M, et al: Early stroke treatment associated with better outcome. *Neurology* 55:1649-1655, 2000.)

the FDA. "Interstate shipping" is broadly defined; if the container or label or gel that holds the medication or anything related to the product is shipped across state lines, interstate shipping is considered to be involved.

Ethics and the Protection of Human Subjects

In clinical trials of stroke therapies, the informed consent process may be difficult because stroke may involve an emergency situation in which a participant's life is in peril. In 1996, criteria to waive the informed consent requirement were established for research in emergency settings. These criteria provide exception to the requirement of informed consent from each participant or legally authorized representative before experimental intervention in situations in which the participant cannot provide informed consent because of a life-threatening medical condition and absence of his/her legally authorized representative. The IRB may permit informed consent waiver upon review of the life-threatening situation, existence of clinical equipoise (i.e., the relative benefits and risks of the proposed intervention, as compared with standard therapy, are unknown), and the need for the collection of valid scientific evidence to determine safety and effectiveness of the intervention under study. The IRB must also consider the feasibility, or lack thereof, of obtaining informed consent from the participant or legally authorized representative as well as the prospect of direct benefit to the participant through participation in the trial. Furthermore, for a waiver to be obtained, additional protection of the rights and welfare of participants must be provided, including at least a consultation with the representatives of the communities in which the study is to be conducted and from which the potential participants will be recruited (community consent).

International Guidelines for Conducting Clinical Trials

The International Conference of Harmonisation of Technical Requirements for Registration of Pharmaceuticals for Human Use, established in 1990, is a tripartite harmonization of technical requirements for the registration of pharmaceutical products in the United States, the European Union, and Japan. This Conference is the result of a need to standardize the regulatory requirements among the countries because of globalization of the pharmaceutical industry, arbitrary differences in regulations, and the need for a process to allow more timely access to new drugs for patients. Good Clinical Practice (GCP) is a set of guidelines for design, conduct, analysis, quality control, and reporting of clinical studies to achieve and maintain high-quality clinical research in a responsible and ethical manner. It is a part of the Conference's document (section E6). Compliance with Good Clinical Practice ensures that the rights and safety of trial participants are guaranteed and that the results produced by the clinical trials are credible. All clinical trial personnel (i.e., clinicians, research nurse, study coordinators, statisticians, data managers, project managers, quality assurance personnel) should follow GCP. A copy of the GCP can be obtained online (http://www.fda.gov/oc/gcp/).

REFERENCES

1. Cook TC, DeMets DL, editors: *Introduction to statistical methods for clinical trials*, New York, 2007, Chapman & Hall/CRC.
2. Gullov AL, Koefoed BG, Petersen P, et al: Fixed mini-dose warfarin and aspirin alone and in combination vs adjusted-dose warfarin for stroke prevention in atrial fibrillation, *Arch Intern Med* 158:1513–1521, 1998.
3. Study design for randomized prospective trial of carotid endarterectomy for asymptomatic atherosclerosis. Asymptomatic Carotid Atherosclerosis Study Group, *Stroke* 20:844–849, 1989.
4. The International Cooperative Study of Extracranial/Intracranial Arterial Anastomosis (EC/IC Bypass Study): Methodology and entry characteristics. EC/IC Bypass Study Group, *Stroke* 16:397–406, 1985.
5. EC/IC Bypass Study Group: Failure of extracranial-intracranial arterial bypass to reduce risk of ischemic stroke. Results of an international randomized trial, *N Engl J Med* 313:1191–2000, 1985.
6. Mohr JP, Thompson JLP, Lazar RM, et al: A comparison of warfarin and aspirin for the prevention of recurrent ischemic stroke, *N Engl J Med* 345:1444–1451, 2001.
7. The VITATOPS: (Vitamins to Prevent Stroke) Trial: Rationale and design of an international, large, simple, randomised trial of homocysteine-lowering multivitamin therapy in patients with recent transient ischaemic attack or stroke, *Cerebrovasc Dis* 13:120–126, 2002.

8. Little KM, Alexander MJ: Medical versus surgical therapy for spontaneous intracranial hemorrhage, *Neurosurg Clin North Am* 13:339-347, 2002.

9. Tissue plasminogen activator for acute ischemic stroke: National Institute of Neurological Disorders and Stroke (NINDS) rt-PA Stroke Study Group, *N Engl J Med* 333:1581-1587, 1995.

10. Hacke W, Kaste M, Bluhmki E, et al: *Thrombolysis with alteplase 3 to 4.5 hours after acute ischemic stroke, for the ECASS investigators,* N Engl J Med 359:1317-1328, 2008.

11. Kwiatkowski TG, Libman RB, Frankel M, et al: Effects of tissue plasminogen activator for acute ischemic stroke at one year. National Institute of Neurological Disorders and Stroke Recombinant Tissue Plasminogen Activator Stroke Study Group, *N Engl J Med* 340: 1781-1787, 1999.

12. Goldring S, Zervas N, Langfiti T: The Extracranial-Intracranial Bypass Study: A report of the committee appointed by the American Association of Neurological Surgeons to examine the study, *N Engl J Med* 316:817-820, 1987.

13. Ginsberg MD, Hill MD, Palesch YY, et al: The ALIAS Pilot Trial, A Dose-Escalation and Safety Study of Albumin Therapy for Acute Ischemic Stroke—I: Physiological responses and safety results, *Stroke* 37:2100-2106, 2006.

14. Garrett E-M: The continual reassessment method for dose-finding studies: a tutorial, *Clinical Trials* 3:57-71, 2006.

15. Tilley BC, Galpern W: Screening Potential Therapies: Lessons learned from new paradigms used in Parkinson's disease, *Stroke* 38(Suppl):800-803, 2007.

16. Palesch YY, Tilley BC, Sackett DL, et al: Applying a Phase II Futility Study Design to Therapeutic Stroke Trials, *Stroke* 36:2410-2414, 2005.

17. IMS Study Investigators: Combined intravenous and intra-arterial recanalization for acute ischemic stroke: The Interventional Management of Stroke (IMS), *Stroke* 35:904-911, 2004.

18. Karanjia PN, Nelson JJ, Lefkowitz DS, et al: Validation of the ACAS TIA/stroke algorithm, *Neurology* 48:346-351, 1997.

19. Brott T, Adams HP, Olinger CP: Measurements of acute cerebral infarction: A clinical examination scale, *Stroke* 20:864-870, 1989.

20. Rankin J: Cerebral vascular accidents in patient over the age of 60. II: Prognosis, *Scott Med J* 2:200-215, 1957.

21. Mahoney FI, Barthel DW: Functional evaluation: The Barthel Index, *Md State Med J* 14:61-65, 1965.

22. Jennet B, Bond M: Assessment of outcome after severe brain injury: A practical scale, *Lancet* 1:480-484, 1975.

23. Hanston L: Neurological scales in assessment of stroke. In Grotta J, Miller LP, Buchan AM, editors: *Ischemic stroke: Recent advances in understanding stroke therapy,* Southborough, MA, 1985, International Business Communications, pp 42-54.

24. Elashoff JD: NQuery Advisor® 4.0. Statistical Solutions Ltd, Boston, MA, info@statsolusa.com, 2000.

25. Lesaffre E, Scheys I, Fröhlich J, Bluhmki E: Calculation of power and sample size with bounded outcome scores, *Stat Med* 12:1063-1078, 1993.

26. Ebbutt AF, Frith L: Practical issues in equivalence studies, *Stat Med* 17:1691-1701, 1998.

27. Thall PF, Cook JD: Dose-finding based on efficacy-toxicity trade-offs, *Biometrics* 60:684-693, 2004.

28. Chow SC, Chang M: Adaptive design methods in clinical trials—a review, *Orphanet Journal of Rare Diseases* 3:11, 2008.

29. Grizzle JE: A note on stratifying versus complete random assignment in clinical trials, *Control Clin Trial* 3:365-368, 1982.

30. Scott NW, McPherson GC, Ramsay CR, Campbell MK: The method of minimization for allocation to clinical trials: A review, *Control Clin Trials* 23:662-674, 2002.

31. Tilley BC, Lyden PD, Brott TG, et al: Total quality improvement methodology reduces delays between emergency department admission and treatment of acute ischemic stroke, *Arch Neurol* 54:1466-1474, 1997.

32. National Institute of Neurologic Disorders and Stroke (NINDS) rt-PA Stroke Study Group: A systems approach to immediate evaluation and management of hyperacute stroke: Experience at eight centers and implications for community practice and patient care, *Stroke* 28:1530-1540, 1997.

33. Napoles-Springer AM, Grumbach K, Alexander M, et al: Clinical research with older African Americans and Latinos, *Res Aging* 22:668-691, 2000.

34. Morisky DE, Green LW, Levine DM: Concurrent and predictive validity of a self-reported measure of medication adherence, *Med Care* 24:67-74, 1986.

35. Gillings D, Koch G: The application of the principle of intention-to-treat to the analysis of clinical trials, *Drug Inf J* 25:411-424, 1991.

36. Friedman LM, Furberg CD, DeMets DL: *Fundamentals of clinical Trials,* ed 3, New York, 1998, Springer-Verlag.

37. O'Brien PC, Tilley BC, Dyck PJ: Composite endpoints in clinical trials. In D'Agostino R, Sullivan L, Massaro J, editors: *Wiley encyclopedia of clinical trials,* New York, 2008, John Wiley & Sons.

38. The NINDS t-PA Stroke Study Group: Generalized efficacy of t-PA for acute stroke: Subgroup analysis of the NINDS t-PA stroke trial, *Stroke* 28:2119-2125, 1997.

39. Tilley BC, Huang P, O'Brien PC: Global Assessment Variables. In D'Agostino R, Sullivan L, Massaro J, editors: *Wiley encyclopedia of clinical trials,* Hoboken, NJ, 2008, John Wiley & Sons.

40. O'Brien P: The appropriateness of analysis of variance and multiple comparison procedures, *Biometrics* 39:787-794, 1983.

41. Moye LA: Alpha calculus in clinical trials: Considerations and commentary for the new millennium, *Comment in Stat Med* 19:763-766, 2000.

42. Hochberg Y: A sharper Bonferroni procedure for multiple tests of significance, *Biometrika* 75:800-802, 1988.

43. Schafer JL: Multiple imputation: A primer, *Stat Methods Med Res* 8:3-15, 1999.

44. Taylor JMG, Taylor S, Hsu C- H: Survival estimation and testing via multiple imputation, *Statistics & Probability Letters* 58:221-232, 2002.

45. Thompson JLP, Levin B, Sciacca RR, et al: Statistical Considerations in the WARSS Collaboration. Presented to American Heart Association Stroke Meeting, San Antonio, February 7-9, 2002.

46. Peto R, Pike MC, Armitage P, et al: Design and analysis of randomized clinical trials requiring prolonged observation of each patient. I. Introduction and design, *Brit J Cancer* 34:585-612, 1976.

47. O'Brien PC, Fleming TR: A multiple testing procedure for clinical trials, *Biometrics* 35:549-556, 1979.

48. Pocock SJ: Group sequential methods in the design and analysis of clinical trials, *Biometrika* 64:191-199, 1977.

49. Ellenberg S, Fleming TR, DeMets DL: *Data monitoring committees in clinical trials: A practical perspective,* Hoboken, John Wiley and Sons NJ, 2002, pp 129-133.

50. Koch GG, Davis SM, Anderson RL: Methodological advances and plans for improving regulatory success for confirmatory studies, *Stat Med* 17:1675-1690, 1998.

51. Yusuf S, Wittes J, Probstfield J, Tyroler HA: Analysis and interpretation of treatment effects in subgroups of patients in randomized clinical trials, *JAMA* 266:93-98, 1991.

52. Meade T, Brennan PJ: Determination of who may derive most benefit from aspirin in primary prevention: Subgroup results from a randomised controlled trial, *BMJ* 321:13-17, 2000.

53. Marler JR, Tilley BC, Lu M, et al: Early stroke treatment associated with better outcome, *Neurology* 55:1649-1655, 2000.

54. Broderick J, Lu M, Jackson C, et al: Apolipoprotein E phenotype and the efficacy of intravenous tissue plasminogen activator in acute ischemic stroke, *Ann Neurol* 49:736-744, 2001.

61

Interventional Neuroradiologic Therapy of Atherosclerotic Disease and Vascular Malformations

J MOCCO, STANLEY H. KIM, BERNARD R. BENDOK, ALAN S. BOULOS,
L. NELSON HOPKINS, ELAD I. LEVY

The treatment of vascular disease has undergone a revolution in the past decade. Previously, open surgical techniques were the only treatment modalities available for vascular disease that resulted in ischemic and hemorrhagic neurologic sequelae. Times have changed. Catheter-based treatment modalities have been developed that rival or surpass open surgical techniques for the treatment of these disease entities.

Cerebral revascularization for the treatment of acute ischemic stroke has become a reality within the past decade. Site-specific intraarterial (IA) delivery of thrombolytic agents has enabled recanalization of occlusive lesions in the cerebrovasculature. The application of mechanical techniques to disrupt clot has pushed vessel recanalization rates as high as 90% as a matter of routine. Hemorrhagic complications still diminish the effectiveness of these techniques, yet a reduction in thrombolytic dosing and increased use of mechanical techniques may drive the clinical utility of IA stroke intervention forward. The primary problem is no longer whether a vessel can be recanalized but, rather, *how rapidly* recanalization can be achieved. With improving stroke education of the public ("brain attack"), the future may see relevant reductions in the time to treatment.

Extracranial and intracranial revascularization for atherosclerotic disease has led the vascular revolution for ischemic cerebrovascular disease. Preliminary results suggest that the use of stents for revascularization of the cervical carotid bifurcation will likely supplant carotid endarterectomy (CEA) in the future. Multiple clinical trials are under way to compare the efficacy of stent placement with that of CEA. These trials will provide level 1 evidence within the next few years. Intracranial atherosclerotic disease is being discovered at an alarming rate through the use of noninvasive imaging techniques like MR and CT angiography. The application of angioplasty and stent techniques is gaining acceptance. Balloons and stents initially designed for the coronary circulation are being modified for delivery into the tortuous anatomy of the cerebral circulation. As a result, the location and scope of intracranial lesions that can be treated are increasing.

The findings of initial trials have shown high rates of in-stent restenosis, but the use of drug coatings that inhibit fibrous tissue formation within cerebral vessels after manipulation may pave the way for broad application of these techniques for cerebral ischemia. Additionally, burgeoning technologies, such as flexible intracranial-specific balloon-mounted stents, may improve long-term results.

Results of the initial clinical trial of the Guglielmi detachable coil (GDC, Boston Scientific Target, Fremont, CA) in 1990 led the way for a lasting and irreversible change in methods for the treatment of ruptured and unruptured intracranial aneurysms worldwide. At many centers, coil occlusion has become first-line therapy for all aneurysms. Initially, only one platinum coil was available. Today, several companies offer products used for endovascular treatment of intracranial aneurysms. Additionally, biologic modification of the platinum coil platform has been approved by the U.S. Food and Drug Administration (FDA). Coils with polymer and hydrogel modifications may promote complete aneurysm occlusion by inducing scar formation across the aneurysm neck. Intravascular stents have been used to provide critical assistance to coil techniques, thereby allowing successful treatment of previously untreatable aneurysms. Liquid polymers have been delivered directly into aneurysms to provide atraumatic methods for complete aneurysm filling. Perhaps most excitingly, early data with endoluminal flow diverters also point to an entirely new treatment modality for intracranial aneurysms. All of this explosive development in endovascular techniques comes on the heels of level 1 evidence indicating the superior effectiveness of aneurysm coiling over that of open surgical techniques in the majority of ruptured aneurysms.

The treatment of cerebral arteriovenous malformations (AVMs) has benefited from catheter-based technology. Particles and silk, thread, and muscle fragments have been replaced as embolic agents by liquid polymers and sclerosing agents. Advances in catheter technology have enabled access of distal AVM feeding vessels, thereby enabling safer delivery of these substances. New liquid

TABLE 61-1 OUTCOME OF INTRAVENOUS ALTEPLASE FOR ACUTE ISCHEMIC STROKE

Study*	No. of Patients	% of Symptomatic Intracerebral Hemorrhage	% Mortality or Dependency (modified Rankin Scale Score 2-6)
National Institute of Neurological Disorders and Stroke (NINDS)[1]	312	6.4	61
Second European Cooperative Acute Stroke Study (ECASS II)[3]	409	8.8	60
Standard Treatment with Alteplase to Reverse Stroke (STARS)[2]	389	3.3	57

*Superscript numbers indicate chapter references.

embolic agents show great promise for complete occlusion of AVMs, and multiple studies are now reporting the results of lasting AVM "cure" with the use of solely endovascular techniques, without the need for adjunctive radiosurgery or resection.

This chapter presents advances in the use of catheter-based technology for the treatment of cerebrovascular disease and stroke, highlighting new techniques and recent technologic developments. Although many of the treatment modalities are considered investigational, they represent the current and future treatments for cerebrovascular disease.

Acute Ischemic Stroke

Thrombolysis of Acute Ischemic Stroke

In 1996, the FDA approved the use of intravenous (IV) recombinant tissue plasminogen activator (rt-PA, alteplase) in patients who present within 3 hours of the onset of acute ischemic stroke. This approval was based on the positive results of the National Institute of Neurological Disorders and Stroke (NINDS) study.[1] Currently, IV administration of t-PA within the 3-hour time window is the only treatment for acute ischemic stroke that is supported by level 1 evidence, recommended by the American Heart Association (AHA), and approved by the FDA. However, two major clinical trials and one prospective observational registry have reported outcomes of death or more than 50% functional dependency at the 3-month follow-up evaluation (Table 61-1).[1-3] Moreover, six randomized trials failed to demonstrate a significant benefit for IV thrombolytic therapy initiated within 3 to 6 hours of stroke onset.[3-8] Several randomized trials have evaluated the safety and efficacy of IA thrombolysis administered 3 to 6 hours from symptom onset.[9,10] Additionally, a single-arm, prospective trial funded by the National Institutes of Health (NIH) of IA thrombolysis performed within 6 hours following a bridging dose (2/3 of normal) of IV t-PA within 3 hours demonstrated a benefit in comparison with results in the NINDS–NIH–funded t-PA trial control population and a suggestion of benefit in comparison with results in the NINDS–NIH–funded t-PA trial treatment population.[11,12] In several case series, IA thrombolysis alone or in combination with mechanical thrombolysis has been reported as an alternative modality for treatment of acute ischemic stroke in a select group of patients.[13-19] A randomized study is justified to determine whether IA thrombolysis with or without mechanical thrombectomy is superior to IV thrombolysis for acute ischemic stroke.

The IA approach to thrombolysis has theoretical advantages. First, angiographic evaluation helps determine whether an occlusion exists and local IA therapy is necessary. Second, the IA approach allows delivery of the thrombolytic agent (i.e., t-PA or reteplase [third-generation t-PA]) to the site of occlusion without excessive systemic administration (a lesser amount of the drug can actually be used). Third, the endovascular surgeon can titrate the dose of the agent through angiographic visualization of the clot response to lysis. Fourth, in patients showing a poor response to pharmacologic IA thrombolysis, angiographic evaluation aids in the selection of methods of mechanical thrombolysis or other endovascular intervention. For example, an acute ischemic stroke from occlusion of the M1 segment of the middle cerebral artery (MCA) may occur in the setting of severe pre-existing atherosclerotic stenosis or embolic plaque. A combination of pharmacologic and mechanical forms of IA thrombolysis by use of angioplasty, a stent, or a clot-retrieval device may be required for recanalization (Fig. 61-1). Disadvantages of the IA approach include longer potential time to treatment and significant resource requirements. With better patient education and earlier recognition of stroke symptoms, the time to treatment can be reduced.

Although pharmacologic and mechanical forms of IA thrombolysis are promising novel therapies, patients with acute ischemic stroke still need to be transported expeditiously to an appropriate facility that can provide acute stroke therapy in a timely fashion. Time from onset to treatment is of paramount importance, regardless of the type of thrombolytic therapy used. Furthermore, advancements in imaging techniques, such as diffusion-weighted and perfusion-weighted MRI, xenon-enhanced CT (XeCT), and CT perfusion scanning, may allow improved patient selection for thrombolysis in the future.[20-28]

Intraarterial Thrombolysis Trials

The recanalization efficacy and safety of IA thrombolysis using recombinant pro-urokinase has been evaluated in two randomized, multicenter, placebo-controlled trials.[9,10] In the Prolyse in Acute Cerebral Thromboembolism (PRO-ACT) I and II trials, patients with acute ischemic stroke due to MCA occlusion and onset of symptoms within 6 hours underwent intra-arterial thrombolysis with recombinant pro-urokinase (r-pro-UK).[9,10] The results of these trials are summarized in Table 61-2. Recanalization rates are based on the Thrombolysis in Myocardial

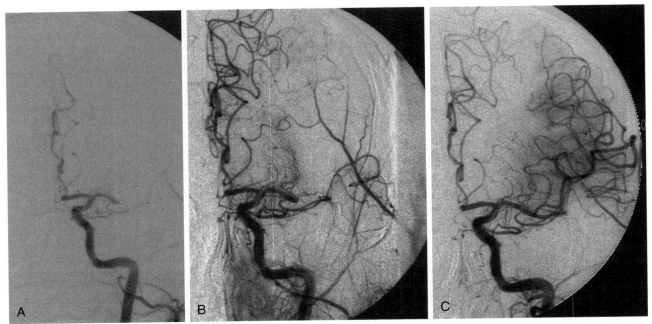

Figure 61-1 A, Cerebral angiogram shows occlusion of the left M1 segment of the left middle cerebral artery (MCA). B, Persistent occlusion of the M1 segment of the left MCA after administration of 4 units of reteplase. C, Recanalization of the left MCA after mechanical thrombolysis was performed via a 4-mm snare (Amplatz Goose-Neck Microsnare, Microvena, White Bear Lake, Minn).

TABLE 61-2   RESULTS OF PROLYSE IN ACUTE CEREBRAL THROMBOEMBOLISM (PROACT) TRIALS I AND II

	PROACT I		**PROACT II**	
No. of patients	40		180	
CT scan exclusion	ICH, mass effect with midline shift, intracranial tumor, early changes of ischemia		Same as PROACT I, hypodensity or effacement of sulci in more than 1/3 of the middle cerebral artery territory	
Median National Institutes of Health Stroke Scale (NIHSS) score	r-Pro-UK, 17; placebo, 19		r-Pro-UK, 17; placebo, 17	
Heparin	All patients received IV heparin; first 16 patients received 100-unit/kg bolus, then 1000-unit/hour infusion during 4 hours; remaining patients received 4000-unit bolus followed by a 500-unit/hour infusion for 4 hours		All patients received 2000-unit heparin bolus IV, then 500-unit/hour infusion for 4 hours	
Agent used	6 mg of r-pro-UK; 9 mg over 2 hours		9 mg of r-pro-UK over 2 hours and heparin	
Placebo group	Saline at 30 mL/hour over 2 hours		IV heparin alone	
Mechanical thrombolysis	Not permitted		Not permitted	
	r-Pro-UK	**Placebo**	**r-Pro-UK**	**Placebo**
% of TIMI grade 2 or 3 recanalization rate	58	14	66	18
% Symptomatic ICH	15	7	10	2
% Outcome at 90 days:				
mRS score 0-1	31	21		
mRS score 0-2			40	25
% Mortality within 90 days	27	43	25	27

ICH, intracerebral hemorrhage; IV, intravenous; mRS, modified Rankin Scale; r-pro-UK, recombinant pro-urokinase; TIMI, Thrombolysis In Myocardial Infarction Study.

Infarction (TIMI) grading system (Table 61-3).[29] Recanalization rates (TIMI 2 or 3) were 58% in the r-pro-UK group and 14% in the placebo group in the PROACT I trial. Because of the low number of patients in PROACT I, clinical efficacy of this treatment modality could not be established. However, because of the safety and recanalization rates observed in PROACT I, PROACT II was performed.

This trial was designed to assess the efficacy of intra-arterial r-pro-UK (9 mg given over 2 hours as opposed to 6 mg in PROACT I) as measured by the modified Rankin scale (mRS) score of 2 or less at 90 days. For the primary outcome measure of efficacy in PROACT II, 40% of patients receiving r-pro-UK and 25% of those receiving placebo achieved an mRS score of 2 or less at 90 days

TABLE 61-3 DEFINITIONS OF PERFUSION IN THE THROMBOLYSIS IN MYOCARDIAL INFARCTION (TIMI) STUDY

Grade	Definition
0 (no perfusion)	There is no antegrade flow beyond the point of occlusion.
1 (penetration without perfusion)	The contrast material passes beyond the area of obstruction but "hangs up" and fails to opacify the entire coronary bed distal to the obstruction for the duration of the cineangiographic filming sequence.
2 (partial perfusion)	The contrast material passes across the obstruction and opacifies the coronary bed distal to the obstruction. However, the rate of entry of contrast material into the vessel distal to the obstruction or its rate of clearance from the distal bed (or both) is perceptibly slower than that of its entry into or clearance from comparable areas not perfused by the previously occluded vessel (e.g., other coronary artery or the coronary bed proximal to the obstruction).
3 (complete perfusion)	Antegrade flow into the bed distal to the obstruction occurs as promptly as antegrade flow into the bed proximal to obstruction and as clearance of contrast material from the involved bed in the same vessel or the opposite artery.

($P = .04$). Recanalization rates (TIMI 2 or 3) were 66% in the r-pro-UK group and 18% in the placebo group in this trial. A 15% absolute increase in favorable outcome was shown with r-pro-UK. For every seven patients treated with r-pro-UK, one would benefit. Despite being associated with an increased frequency of early symptomatic intracranial hemorrhage (ICH), intra-arterial r-pro-UK administered within 6 hours of symptom onset in stroke due to MCA occlusion significantly improved clinical outcome.

PROACT II was a landmark trial in that, for the first time in a randomized study, IA thrombolysis demonstrated clinical efficacy and extended the time window for therapy to 6 hours in a homogeneous group of patients with acute ischemic stroke.[10] This trial was conducted in a standardized fashion in terms of the technique of IA thrombolysis as well as the agent and the dose used. However, the FDA requested additional data to support the clinical efficacy and safety demonstrated in PROACT II before approving IA thrombolysis as a standard therapy for patients with acute ischemic stroke. The success of the PROACT II trial was not sufficient to gain FDA approval for pro-UK, but the trial paved the way for additional studies involving IA thrombolysis (with newer agents) in acute ischemic stroke.

Several studies have evaluated the feasibility, safety, and recanalization rate of a combination of IV and IA pharmacologic thrombolysis in patients with acute ischemic stroke.[11,12,30-34] The results are summarized in Table 61-4. The rationale for the combination approach is based on the fact that clinically severe strokes resulting from occlusion of large intracranial vessels respond poorly to IV thrombolysis. Combining the two therapies

enables patients to receive IV therapy during the time required for initiation of IA thrombolysis, which may be more effective in opening large arteries. Direct comparison of these studies is difficult owing to heterogeneity of the study populations, dosages, and types of thrombolytic agents used as well as of patient selection criteria. Symptomatic ICH rates within 7 days of treatment range from 6% to 16%. Mortality rates range from 15% to 45%. TIMI 3 recanalization rates range from 4% to 55%. The Emergency Management of Stroke (EMS) Bridging Trial was designed to assess safety, feasibility, and recanalization efficacy of this combination approach.[33] However, because of the small sample size (35 patients), the clinical efficacy of this therapy could not be determined. Suarez et al[34] reported that 78% of patients treated by combination therapy had Barthel Index values higher than 95 at 3 months. Ernst et al[30] reported mRS scores of 0 or 1 at or beyond 2-month follow-up for 44% of patients treated with combination therapy. The Interventional Management of Stroke (IMS) study, an NINDS-funded pilot study, was an open-label phase 2 study designed to provide preliminary results on the safety and efficacy of combination IV and IA t-PA therapies in 80 ischemic stroke patients with National Institutes of Health Stroke Scale (NIHSS) scores of 10 or higher.[11] Patients received 0.6 mg/kg of intravenously administered t-PA over 30 minutes (15% as a bolus) followed by intraarterially administered t-PA at a dose of up to 22 mg over 2 hours if thrombus was identified on a cerebral angiogram. The study demonstrated a 16% rate of mortality at 3 months (compared with 24% in the NINDS placebo group) and a 6% rate of symptomatic ICH (compared with 1% in the NINDS placebo group). TIMI 2 and 3 recanalization rates of 40% and 10%, respectively, were observed. Favorable outcome at 3 months, as defined by an mRS score of 0 or 1, was observed in 30% of patients. On the basis of these encouraging results, the IMS II study was undertaken.[12] The protocol was much the same as for IMS, except the use of a catheter with an ultrasonic tip was allowed (EKOS catheter, EKOS Corporation, Bothell, WA). Once again, the results were encouraging, with TIMI 2 or 3 recanalization in 60% of patients and 33% of patients experiencing an mRS score of 0 or 1 at 90 days.

Qureshi et al[19] evaluated the safety and efficacy of reteplase (the only third-generation thrombolytic agent available in addition to alteplase for the IA treatment of acute ischemic stroke) in 16 patients who were considered poor candidates for IV alteplase therapy because (1) the interval from symptom onset to presentation was 3 hours or more or (2) they had severe neurologic deficit on presentation (NIHSS scores ranged from 10 to 26). These investigators used a modified TIMI grading system (Table 61-5) and reported TIMI 3 or 4 (equivalent to the original TIMI grade 3) recanalization rates in 88% of patients. Such a high rate of recanalization was achieved even though 8 of 16 patients presented with occlusion of either the cervical (n = 4) or intracranial (n = 4) internal carotid artery (ICA). Early neurologic improvement (defined as a decrease of 4 or more points in the NIHSS score at 24 hours) was observed in 44% of patients. Qureshi[35] developed a new grading scheme to account for more precise location of occlusion in the cerebral

TABLE 61-4 RESULTS OF COMBINED INTRAVENOUS AND INTRAARTERIAL THROMBOLYSIS

Study*	Study Center	Design	Symptomatic ICH within 7 Days	Outcome Definition	Outcome	Mortality
Emergency Management of Stroke (EMS) Bridging Trial[33]	—	Double-blinded randomized placebo-controlled multicenter study comparing safety and feasibility of two treatment strategies	12% (2/17) IV/IA; 6% (1/18) placebo IA	3-month Glasgow Outcome Scale (GOS) score, Barthel Index, and mRS score	No significant differences in outcome between treatment groups	At 90 days: 45% (5/11) in IV/IA; 10% (1/10) in placebo/IA
Ernst et al[30]	University of Cincinnati	Retrospective study to assess safety and feasibility of IV t-PA/IA t-PA within 3 hours of symptom onset	6% (1/16)	mRS, follow-up range 2-100 months	44% (7/16) had an mRS score of 0 or 1, 19% (3/16) an mRS score of 2, and 25% (4/16) an mRS score of 4 or 5	13% (2/16)
Keris et al[32]	Riga, Latvia	Open-label prospective study to assess safety and efficacy of IV t-PA/IA t-PA within 6 hours of symptom onset	None	mRS scores at 1 month and 12 months: good = mRS 0-3; poor = mRS 4-6	67% (8/12) mRS 0-3 at 1 month, 83% (10/12) mRS 0-3 at 12 months	17% at 12 months
Hill et al[31]	University of Calgary, Alberta	Prospective, open-label study to assess safety and feasibility of IV t-PA/IA t-PA within 3 hours of symptom onset	None	National Institutes of Health Stroke Scale (NIHSS) score <3 at 90 days	67% (4/6) NIHSS score <3 at 90 days	17% (1/6)
Suarez et al[34]	University Hospitals of Cleveland, Case Western Reserve	Pilot study to assess feasibility of IV t-PA/IA UK or t-PA within 3 hours of symptom onset	10% (2/21) in IV t-PA group only	Barthel Index at 90 days: index of 95 or 100 = good outcome	77% good outcome at 3 months, Barthel index >95: 92% (12/13) in IV t-PA/IA UK group, 64% (7/11) in IV t-PA/IV t-PA group, 67% (14/21) in IV t-PA group	16% (7/45)
Interventional Management of Stroke IMS Study[11]	—	Pilot study to assess IA t-PA within 6 hours following bridging dose of IV t-PA within 3 hours	6%	mRS score of 0 or 1 at 3 months	30%	16%
IMS II Trial[12]	—	Single-arm trial to assess IA t-PA within 6 hours following bridging dose of IV t-PA within 3 hours, with or without ultrasound assistance	9.9%	mRS score of 0 or 1 at 3 months	33%	16%

*Superscript numbers indicate chapter references.
IA, intraarterial; IV, intravenous; mRS, modified Rankin Scale; t-PA, recombinant tissue plasminogen activator (alteplase); UK, urokinase.

TABLE 61-5 MODIFIED THROMBOLYSIS IN MYOCARDIAL INFARCTION (TIMI) GRADING SYSTEM

Grade	Definition
0	No flow
1	Some penetration past the site of occlusion but no flow distal to occlusion
2	Distal perfusion but delayed filling in all vessels
3	Distal perfusion with adequate perfusion in less than half of the distal vessels
4	Distal perfusion with adequate perfusion in more than half of the distal vessels

vasculature and the existence of collateral circulation, which are not described in the original and modified TIMI grading schemes. Further studies are needed to evaluate the durability of IA thrombolysis using reteplase in acute ischemic stroke.

Mechanical Thrombolysis

During the last decade, mechanical thrombolysis has evolved into an FDA-approved primary therapy for the treatment of acute ischemic stroke in patients who are ineligible for t-PA therapy and those in whom such therapy has failed to achieve recanalization. The goal of mechanical thrombolysis is to restore cerebral blood flow by means of removing the obstructive thrombus or disintegrating the thrombus to facilitate activation of the thrombolytic agents. This approach may (1) minimize or obviate the use of thrombolytic agents, thereby potentially reducing the risk of ICH associated with pharmacologic thrombolysis, (2) achieve faster recanalization, and (3) extend the window of intervention to 8 hours.

Devices for mechanical thrombolysis have greatly strengthened the armamentarium of the endovascular surgeon in the treatment of acute ischemic stroke. Also, the use of these devices adds another level of skill and resources to the endovascular surgeon's repertoire. Currently, a variety of mechanical devices are either available or being studied. However, as of yet, only two of these devices have been approved by the FDA: the Merci Concentric Retriever System (Concentric Medical, Mountain View, CA) and the Penumbra System (Penumbra, Inc., Alameda, CA). FDA approval for these devices was granted as the result of well-documented recanalization rates of approximately 50% to 70% and demonstration that patients with successful recanalization had better outcomes than those without recanalization.[36-39] However, despite FDA approval and AHA–American Stroke Association recommendations for these tools as a therapeutic option for appropriate patients, there are as yet no randomized data supporting the use of mechanical thrombolysis.[40]

Mechanical thrombolysis was largely developed because approximately 50% of occlusive lesions are resistant to IA pharmacologic thrombolysis.[41,42] This failure of pharmacologic agents in the setting of a tenacious clot may be related to site of occlusion, clot volume, heterogeneous composition of the clot, and underlying atherosclerotic stenosis. Although ranges are wide and variable, lower rates of recanalization are associated with pharmacologic thrombolysis of acute cervical or intracranial ICA occlusions than with distal MCA branch occlusions. In addition, occlusive lesions of the vertebrobasilar artery territory are thought to be more atherothrombotic in nature than MCA occlusions, which may be more embolic.[41,43] As a result, device selection may depend on the occlusion site as well as the vascular pathology.

The Mechanical Embolus Removal in Cerebral Ischemia (MERCI) and Multi-MERCI trials evaluated the safety and recanalization rates of the Merci Concentric Retriever System, without and with or without IV t-PA, respectively.[38,39] These studies established that recanalization rates with the Merci alone range from 46% to 57% but can climb to 69.5% with adjunctive therapy. Overall, a 90-day favorable outcome (mRS score, 0 to 2) was demonstrated in 27.7% and 36% of studied patients, respectively.

With FDA approval of the Merci retrieval device, many efforts have been made to enlarge the armamentarium of mechanical thrombolysis devices. As previously mentioned, the only device to date that has also received approval has been the Penumbra System.[36] It is a mechanical device designed to reduce clot burden in occluded vessels through fragmentation and aspiration of the clot. This publication reports a single-arm 23 patient study wherein 100% of treated vessels (in 20 of 23 patients) were recanalized to TIMI 2 or 3 status. Additionally, 45% of patients had either a 4-point or more improvement in NIHSS score or an mRS score of 2 or less.

Literature is becoming available on the use of stent devices for acute stroke therapy. Several case series have been published that demonstrate high rates of recanalization and promising overall outcomes.[44-47] At present, an FDA-approved pilot trial is under way to evaluate the potential benefit of stent placement for acute stroke.

Physician and Patient Education

Pharmacologic and mechanical approaches for IA thrombolysis are promising interventions in acute ischemic stroke. Patients with "brain attack" must be expeditiously transferred to institutions having the personnel and resources to provide therapies for the treatment of acute ischemic stroke and must be evaluated to determine their eligibility for such therapies. Time is critical for these patients, regardless of the therapy chosen. Newer fibrinolytic agents and mechanical devices may allow faster recanalization, but the safety of these agents and devices requires further evaluation. The precise role and the limits of newer imaging modalities, such as multimodal MR and CT perfusion imaging, need to be defined to aid in selection of candidates for thrombolysis.

Finally, physicians must assume a pivotal role in educating the public about stroke prevention and treatment both locally and nationally. Through the combined efforts of health care professionals, the general public, the AHA, the American Stroke Association, the National Stroke Council, and local and federal governments, management of stroke will improve in the future.

Intracranial Atherosclerotic Disease

Intracranial atherosclerotic disease accounts for 8% of all strokes.[48,49] It is increasingly being discovered with the liberal use of intracranial MR and CT angiography. Both symptomatic and asymptomatic patients are being evaluated more frequently with these noninvasive techniques. Historically, the treatment of these lesions had been principally with either antiplatelet (aspirin) or anticoagulant (sodium warfarin) medications. Randomized trials have demonstrated, however, that aspirin is as effective as warfarin but maintains a safer profile.[50-52] Of equal importance, these investigations have demonstrated a dismal prognosis associated with intracranial atherosclerosis despite medical treatment. Because of the poor outcomes associated with medical therapy, alternative treatment options are being explored. Interventional techniques have revolutionized the treatment of coronary atherosclerotic disease and are similarly leading to significant improvements in the treatment of peripheral atherosclerotic disease. Technologic advancements in angioplasty catheters and stents have driven the application of these devices for revascularization of the intracranial circulation. To date, only patient series have been reported in the literature. An upcoming, NIH-funded, prospective randomized trial—Stent Placement versus Aggressive Medical Management for the Prevention of Recurrent Stroke in Intracranial Stenosis (SAMMPRIS)—will evaluate the benefit of angioplasty and stent placement for intracranial atherosclerotic disease.

Natural History and Medical Management

The management of intracranial atherosclerosis remains perplexing. Unlike for atherosclerosis of the extracranial vasculature, few prospective randomized trials have influenced therapeutic approaches for intracranial disease. The Extracranial-to-Intracranial (EC-IC) Cooperative Bypass Study demonstrated the inefficacy of bypass surgery in preventing recurrence of stroke.[53] This study and other prospective studies have enabled us to define the natural history of intracranial arterial stenosis. In all these studies, patients were enrolled after the occurrence of a defining neurologic event (transient ischemic attack [TIA] or stroke) referable to the vascular distribution of the intracranial stenotic vessel.

In several studies, including the EC-IC bypass study, a subgroup of patients was treated with aspirin alone. In the bypass study, 714 patients with intracranial ICA or MCA stenosis who received aspirin (1300 mg daily) were observed. The annual stroke rate referable to the stenosis was 7%, with an overall stroke rate of 10%. Craig et al[54] followed up 58 patients for 2.5 years and discovered a 43% stroke rate and a 15% mortality rate. Marzewski et al[55] monitored 66 patients with distal ICA stenosis and noted a 3.2% annual stroke rate ipsilateral to the stenosis, with a mortality of 46% over 44 months.[55] Ischemic cerebrovascular disease was responsible for the death of 27% of the patients in these studies.[54,55] A European trial, the Stroke Prevention in Reversible Ischemia Trial (SPIRIT), demonstrated a high hemorrhagic complication rate associated with warfarin therapy in patients who experienced previous cerebral ischemic events.[56] Moreover, in the Warfarin versus Aspirin in the Secondary Prevention of Stroke Study (WARSS), a randomized controlled study of 2206 patients comparing low-dose anticoagulation (international normalized ratio [INR], 1.4 to 2.8) with aspirin (325 mg daily) in patients who had a noncardiogenic source of stroke, warfarin was not proven to be more effective than aspirin in preventing stroke recurrence.[52] Most conclusively though, the Warfarin-Aspirin Symptomatic Intracranial Disease (WASID) study, a prospective randomized, double-blinded, multicenter trial evaluating patients with TIA or stroke secondary to 50% to 99% stenosis of a major intracranial artery, was halted after the enrollment of 569 patients because significantly more adverse events occurred in the warfarin cohort.[51]

For patients who experience neurologic symptoms despite antithrombotic treatment, the risk of recurrent events is very high (47.7% over a mean follow-up period of 14.7 months, with a median time to recurrence of 32 days).[57] There is, therefore, some urgency to change the form of treatment once it has failed. In addition, most patients with intracranial disease are more likely to present with a major event (such as a catastrophic stroke) than with a TIA or a minor stroke.[53] The high risk of a stroke with potentially irreversible neurologic deficits further complicates medical decision-making because the question arises whether medical management should even be attempted initially. It is hoped that the performance and results analysis of the SAMMPRIS study will shed further light on these dilemmas.

An additional confounder to our understanding of the natural history of intracranial stenosis is its apparent dynamic nature, whereby second angiographic imaging can sometimes reveal dramatically different degrees of arterial blockage. Akins et al[58] presented a retrospective series of serial angiographic studies obtained to study the dynamic morphology of asymptomatic intracranial stenosis. In this series of 21 patients with 45 intracranial stenotic lesions, 40% of the lesions progressed and 20% regressed over a 7-year period. The distal ICA did not seem as predisposed to disease progression as the more distal branches (MCA, anterior cerebral artery, posterior cerebral artery). In three patients, regression of the intracranial stenosis was impressive, suggesting that a thrombus was present within the already diseased vessel. In addition, 23% of the patients in this series had strokes during the follow-up period while receiving different regimens of antithrombotic therapy. In a later study, significant angiographic improvement of a stenotic vertebrobasilar artery segment was seen after the administration of high-dose atorvastatin, a potent 3-hydroxy-3 methylglutaryl coenzyme A (HMG-CoA) reductase inhibitor, for a 2-week period.[59] This improvement may have occurred from resolution of thrombus, because statins promote endogenous fibrinolysis and plaque remodeling.

There is considerable debate about the mechanism responsible for large vessel stenosis that leads to stroke. Unlike the extracranial carotid infarctions, in which artery-to-artery embolism is the predominant mechanism, growing evidence in the literature supports a hemodynamic cause for large vessel infarctions. Certainly, a subset of patients has demonstrated a higher rate of stroke recurrence in association with hemodynamic failure.[60-62] More likely, there is an ongoing interaction between the stenosis providing an embolic source and reduced blood flow resulting in diminished ability to clear the emboli. The ischemic events are thus a shift in the balance between embolic load and blood flow.[63]

Endoluminal Revascularization

The methods for achieving endoluminal revascularization are primary angioplasty, primary stenting, direct stenting (stenting without immediate balloon predilation), and provisional stenting. In *primary angioplasty*, the operator places an angioplasty balloon to expand the stenotic segment and has no intention of placing a stent. In *primary stenting*, the operator has the intention of placing a stent and may or may not dilate the lesion with an angioplasty balloon before stent placement. If no previous dilation is required, the procedure is called *direct stenting*. *Provisional stenting* refers to stent placement after unsatisfactory luminal recanalization from angioplasty, or stenting as a "bail-out" procedure.[64,65]

The feasibility and limitations of primary angioplasty were presented in initial patient series.[66-69] The periprocedural risk of stroke or death was 8% to 33%. Later series have documented a lower incidence of complications, demonstrating improving technologies as well as a considerable learning curve for these techniques.[70-73] The periprocedural neurologic event rate in these later angioplasty series, which involved more than 10 patients each, was less than 10%.

The results of these numerous reports are mirrored in the angioplasty series presented by Connors and Wojak.[70] These investigators divided their experience from 1989 to 1998 into three periods. A higher rate of complications was encountered in 17 patients treated during the early and middle periods, from 1989 to 1993; complications included dissection in 82% of patients, neurologic events in 6%, and death in 6%. Subsequent to 1993, the rates among 41 patients were 14% for dissection, 8% for neurologic events (of which 4% were TIAs), and 2% for death. Connors and Wojak[70] attribute the improvements to decreasing the balloon diameter to restore the vessel lumen, very slow inflation of the balloon (over 2 to 5 minutes), and the routine use of glycoprotein IIb/IIIa receptor (GP IIb/IIIa) inhibitors, such as abciximab, during angioplasty. Two hemorrhages (included in the neurologic events rate) occurred during this period. The investigators also avoid crossing a lesion more than once with the angioplasty balloon because that maneuver is likely to raise an intimal flap and cause the vessel to become occluded. One intrinsic advantage of endovascular approaches over surgery is the ability to repeat the angioplasty. A stenotic vessel that has been suboptimally dilated initially can be further dilated on subsequent interventions. Another "pearl" discovered by Connors and Wojak[70] is the use of shorter angioplasty balloons to prevent straightening of the intracranial vessels after balloon inflation, making injury or dissection less likely.

In a single series of clinically symptomatic patients with hemodynamically significant intracranial lesions, Mori et al[72] demonstrated the effectiveness of angioplasty in patients with short (5 mm or less), mildly eccentric or concentric (type A) lesions. In their experience, angioplasty of these lesions resulted in a periprocedural complication rate of 8% (1 stroke in 12). During the 2-year follow-up period, no ipsilateral stroke, neurologic event, or angiographic stenosis occurred; and no bypass surgery or repeat angioplasty was needed. For angiographic lesions that were longer and more eccentric or chronically occluded, the procedure yielded less effective results. For lesions that were either 5 to 10 mm in length or totally occluded and were less than 3 months old (type B), the success rate was 86%. Angiographic restenosis occurred in 33% of lesions within the 2-year follow-up period. Angioplasty attempts were unsuccessful in 2 of 21 patients. Patients with chronically occluded lesions that were 3 months or older or highly angular or long (more than 10 mm) (type C) fared the worst. Angioplasty was associated with an initial success rate of 33% (3 of 9 patients) and a restenosis rate of 100% at 1 year. These results suggest that angiographic characteristics may help determine feasibility and periprocedural risks of angioplasty. One of 9 patients with type C lesions experienced a stroke from abrupt closure of the stenotic vessel, suggesting that vessels harboring these lesions are extremely tenuous.[72] The cumulative risk of ipsilateral stroke was 12% for type B lesions and 56% for type C lesions. Of note, the natural history of these lesions was not delineated according to lesion type in either the WASID study or the EC-IC bypass study. Reports by Mori et al[74,75] suggest that type C and also possibly type B lesions should not be treated by angioplasty alone but rather may benefit from another endovascular technique or surgery.

Marks et al[71] reported a low periprocedural risk of 5% in their intracranial angioplasty series. Like Connors and Wojak,[70] these investigators undersized the balloon and allowed for residual stenosis.[71] They frequently included anticoagulation (warfarin) therapy in their postprocedural regimen (prescribed for 18 of 23 patients), particularly if there was significant (more than 50%) residual stenosis or dissection. Two complications occurred in the immediate postprocedural period among this group of 23 patients. A vessel ruptured, which resulted in death, and an angioplasty site became occluded by a thrombus. The clot was successfully lysed with IA t-PA. Two strokes occurred during the respective follow-up periods of 37 and 32 months. Only one of the strokes involved territory supplied by the treated vessel. This stroke occurred in a vessel with 50% residual stenosis. Including the vessel rupture, the annual rate of stroke in the territory of the previously treated vessel was 3.2%, and the overall rate of stroke during the average 35.4 months of follow-up was 4.8%.

Therefore, it appears that primary angioplasty may provide an effective method of endoluminal revascularization. The intrinsic disadvantages of angioplasty are mirrored in the coronary literature.[76-78] Coronary angioplasty alone resulted in numerous dissections or vessel recoil that would have been resolved with stent placement. Moreover, there was a low incidence of mortality related to vessel rupture during balloon inflation or hemorrhage associated with reperfusion and use of GP IIb/IIIa inhibitors. The vessels at greatest risk for restenosis or further strokes were those with residual stenosis, yet the vessels at greatest risk of rupture or dissection were those inflated with a balloon that was the size of the vessel or larger. In follow-up of angioplasty performed for intracranial atherosclerosis, the results appear durable if minimal residual stenosis is apparent. In almost all series reporting delayed neurologic events, these events occurred in patients in whom residual vessel stenosis was seen immediately after completion of the procedure.

The limitations of primary angioplasty prompted investigators to examine the effectiveness of primary stent placement for the treatment of intracranial atherosclerosis. Stenting for intracranial stenosis was first attempted with the use of balloon-mounted coronary stents, which resulted in superior postprocedure angiographic results—yielding immediate postprocedure stenosis rates typically reported to be less than 10%, versus 40% for angioplasty alone.[79-81] However, the use of coronary stents was associated with higher complication rates than angioplasty alone, and the rigidity of coronary stents provided limited access to the tortuous cerebrovasculature and posed greater technical difficulty.[79]

Self-expanding stents first became available for intracranial applications in 2002.[82] A modified version of the stent, designed for intracranial atherosclerosis treatment, became available in 2005.[83] With increased flexibility, immediate results were encouraging (approximately 30% residual stenosis),[83] and early data were very favorable.[79,83] The flexibility of the self-expanding design greatly improved deliverability and deployment. Typical residual stenosis (approximately 30%) has been demonstrated to be less than that observed after angioplasty alone (approximately 40%), but more than with the balloon-mounted stent (approximately 10%).[84,85] However, midterm results have demonstrated disappointingly high rates of restenosis—up to 45% in patients 55 years or younger.[84,85] The SAMMPRIS multicenter trial, which has begun enrollment, will evaluate the benefit and develop evidence-based recommendations regarding the role of self-expanding stent technology in intracranial stenosis.

Continued development of technology has offered additional interventional options to the armamentarium for intracranial stenosis treatment. Case series have reported results of the use of the Pharos (Micrus Endovascular, San Jose, CA), a highly trackable, balloon-expandable stent mounted on a rapid-exchange percutaneous transluminal angioplasty catheter especially designed for intracranial endovascular applications. Kurre et al[86] reported on 21 patients (7 of whom presented with acute stroke) who were treated with the Pharos at the University of Frankfurt. These researchers found an improvement in stenosis from a preprocedural mean of 85% to a postprocedural mean of 20%. During a mean follow-up period of 7.3 months, no ipsilateral stroke occurred in successfully treated patients (19 of 21). The researchers concluded that treatment of intracranial stenosis with the Pharos is technically feasible. Freitas et al[87] reported a retrospective review of 32 patients treated with the Pharos at six Latin American centers. These investigators observed a 6.2% rate of nonfatal complications and an 8.7% rate of restenosis (more than 50%) over a mean follow-up period of 10.2 months. They concluded that the treatment of intracranial stenosis with the Pharos has a high technical success rate and that their data suggested some efficacy in stroke prevention. Future prospective studies are required to evaluate this and other new technologies.

Ramee et al[88] proposed a combination approach for the treatment of symptomatic intracranial stenosis. They used primary angioplasty for revascularization of lesions classified as Mori type A. If the lesion was complex or long, primary stenting was attempted. If the results of primary angioplasty were suboptimal because of dissection or vessel recoil with residual stenosis, a stent was placed. This approach yielded an excellent short-term outcome with a 93% success rate and a 53% "unexpected benefit" rate in that 8 of 15 patients had reversal of what was initially thought to be a permanent deficit from a previous stroke. Ten of the 15 patients in this series underwent angioplasty alone. Primary stenting was attempted in 4 patients in whom the lesions were complex and long. Stent placement was unsuccessful in 1 of these patients, who then underwent angioplasty alone, which resulted in 30% residual stenosis. Severe elastic recoil encountered during angioplasty of petrous carotid stenosis in 2 patients necessitated stent deployment to achieve a better initial result. As previously mentioned, this method is described in the coronary literature as provisional stenting, and it has become popular for coronary revascularization.

Anatomically, there are several reasons for different responses of intracranial and coronary vessels to endoluminal revascularization. The high incidence of vessel dissection, rupture, and recoil encountered during intracranial revascularization procedures can be explained by these anatomic differences. The histology and physiology of the intracranial vessels change as these vessels course through the skull base. Once within the skull, they become conduit vessels within a space fixed by the skull with a constant total volume occupied by the brain, cerebrospinal fluid, and blood. Thin-walled subarachnoid vessels transport a large volume of circulating blood. Cross-sectional histologic specimens of intracranial vessels demonstrate a paucity of vasa vasorum and absence of external elastic membranes. Near absence of the adventitia is noted. The tunica media is composed of principally smooth muscle cells.[89] Such modified vessels are more likely to rupture or dissect during endoluminal revascularization procedures. Moreover, a more robust smooth muscle cell response to angioplasty or stent placement is likely to occur in these vessels, resulting in intimal hyperplasia.

Ongoing advancements in microcatheters, microwires, angioplasty balloons, and intravascular stents have enhanced our ability to successfully treat intracranial atherosclerotic lesions. A role for endoluminal revascularization of these lesions is apparent, particularly in patients with concentric, short stenoses. Models for intracranial atherosclerosis and endovascular treatments of these stenoses are necessary to gain insight into the vascular responses after endoluminal device placement. Moreover, the potential use of pharmacologically enhanced stent coatings must be tested within the intracranial vasculature, because these materials may significantly impact the long-term effectiveness of stenting for atherosclerotic disease.

Extracranial Carotid Artery Atherosclerotic Disease

Carotid angioplasty and stenting (CAS) is an increasingly popular intervention for carotid artery disease. It is important for clinicians to become familiar with clinical and radiologic factors that determine whether patients should undergo CAS or CEA. More importantly, it is imperative that clinicians understand the risk of stroke associated with treatment in comparison with observation alone. As is the case for most other surgical and interventional procedures, minimizing morbidity is achieved by thoughtful analysis of the patient's neurologic condition and anatomic variables, followed by careful patient selection.

Among the many trials examining stroke risk after treatment of carotid stenosis, the North American Symptomatic Carotid Endarterectomy Trial (NASCET) attempted to quantify stroke risk after CEA in medically treated patients with symptomatic carotid artery disease.[90] At 30 days from the time of surgery, the incidence of death was 1.1%, that of disabling stroke was 1.8%, and that of nondisabling stroke was 3.7%.[91] Among 26 variables evaluated for stroke risk, the following criteria were found to portend increased risk of stroke: contralateral carotid occlusion, hemispheric TIA, left-sided procedure, ipsilateral ischemic lesion on CT scan, and irregular or ulcerated ipsilateral plaque. Other stroke risk factors included diabetes and elevated diastolic blood pressure.[91] Interestingly, previous cardiac intervention for coronary artery disease was found to reduce the risk of stroke. Results from NASCET demonstrated that patients with 70% or more stenosis had a 17% lower incidence in stroke after CEA than with medical treatment alone.[90] Symptomatic stenosis in the range of 50% to 69% was associated with 5-year rates of ipsilateral stroke of 15.7% among patients treated surgically and 22.2% among those treated medically. No benefit of surgery was found for patients with less than 50% stenosis.[91] We caution that these findings, as well as factors that portend increased stroke risk, were found in a post hoc analysis of the NASCET data set.

In an analysis of patients randomly assigned to CEA in the European Carotid Surgery Trial (ECST), the risk of major ischemic stroke or death following surgery was 7% and did not vary substantially with severity of stenosis.[92] Conversely, the risk of major ischemic stroke ipsilateral to the unoperated symptomatic carotid artery did increase with severity of stenosis, most notably with stenosis of 70% to 80%. For patients with more than 80% stenosis, the Kaplan-Meier estimate of the frequency of a major stroke or death at 3 years was 26.5% for the medical treatment group and 14.9% for the surgical group, an absolute benefit from surgery of 11.6%. It is important to note that measurements of 80% stenosis in the ECST corresponded to approximately 60% stenosis in the NASCET.[91]

Treatment of carotid stenosis in asymptomatic patients has been extensively studied. Of the 721 asymptomatic patients with 60% or more carotid stenosis who underwent CEA in the Asymptomatic Carotid Atherosclerosis Study (ACAS), 1 patient died and 10 others had strokes within 30 days (1.5%).[93,94] The estimated 5-year risk of ipsilateral stroke was 11% for the medical group and 5.1% for the surgical group. Risk factors for stroke included diabetes mellitus, contralateral siphon stenosis, radiation-induced stenosis, previous history of stroke, more than 60% contralateral stenosis, and length of external carotid artery plaque.[95] Use of local or regional anesthesia was associated with a higher risk of TIA and myocardial infarction (MI).[95] In another analysis of asymptomatic patients with carotid stenosis, the combined incidence of ipsilateral neurologic events was 8.0% in the surgical group and 20.6% in the medical group ($P < .001$).[96] The incidence of ipsilateral stroke alone was 9.4% in the medical group and 4.7% in the surgical group.

Many factors (mentioned previously) are prognostic for a higher perioperative risk of stroke for patients undergoing CEA. Some of these same risk factors pertain to endoluminal carotid revascularization. Of these, pseudoocclusion, or "slim" sign or "string" sign (angiographic indication of near-complete occlusion of the carotid artery), suggests an increased risk. According to a post hoc analysis of the NASCET data, 106 patients with near-complete occlusion of the carotid artery were subdivided into those with (n = 29) and those without (n = 77) a stringlike lumen. Of patients with near-complete occlusion treated with surgery, 6% had perioperative strokes, as in the group of patients with 70% to 94% stenosis. Only one of the medically treated patients (1.7%) with near-complete occlusion had a stroke within the first month. These data suggest that CEA is not needed on an emergency basis for patients with such lesions and that it does not indicate higher stroke rates for this population than for patients with 70% to 94% stenosis.[97]

Intracranial or extracranial stenoses (such as those found with extracranial tandem lesions) raise the risk of stroke for medically treated patients with carotid stenosis but do not raise the perioperative risk.[98] Although the results from ACAS suggest that contralateral intracranial carotid stenosis increases surgical morbidity, the presence of intracranial stenosis did not increase the surgical risk for a similar subset of patients in the NASCET.

One hundred and fifteen (8.1%) patients enrolled in NASCET had 142 medical complications.[99] The complications were MI and other cardiac disorders (8.1%), respiratory complications (0.8%), transient confusion (0.4%), and other complications (0.7%). Five patients died from these perioperative complications. These results suggest that patients with significant medical comorbidities may be better managed with stent placement than with CAS.

The question arises whether it is possible to identify high-risk patients in need of carotid revascularization who may benefit from CAS and thereby avoid the surgical morbidity of CEA. What is clear are the risk factors that increase the incidence of stroke and the morbidity of CEA, but more evidence is needed to demonstrate whether CAS can significantly decrease the periprocedural morbidity in this subset of patients. Studies are under way to conclusively evaluate the effectiveness of CAS in high-risk patients. In one study of nonrandomized groups with similar patient populations, major ipsilateral stroke and death occurred more frequently in the surgical group (2.9%) than in the stent group (0%), but the difference was not significant.[100] The stent group also had a significantly shorter length of stay in the hospital. In a multicenter registry of 5210 endovascular carotid stent procedures involving 4757 patients, technical success was achieved in 98.4%.[101] TIAs occurred at a rate of 2.82%, with a minor stroke rate of 2.72%. A major stroke rate of 1.49% and a mortality rate of 0.86% were observed. Restenosis rates of carotid stenting were 1.99% and 3.46% at 6 and 12 months, respectively. Roubin et al[102,103] reported their experience of more than 500 carotid stent procedures in a group of asymptomatic and symptomatic patients. They found a 0.6% fatal stroke rate and a 1% death rate from causes other than stroke during the 30-day periprocedural period. The major stroke rate was 1%, and the minor stroke rate was 4.8%. Over the 5-year study period, the periprocedural stroke rate improved from 7.1% to 3.1%.

The CArotid and Vertebral Artery Transluminal Angioplasty Study (CAVATAS), a randomized trial comparing endovascular and surgical treatments for carotid stenosis patients, was published in 2001.[104] This trial included 504 patients enrolled between 1992 and 1997 and was designed to compare balloon angioplasty alone with CEA. Stents, when they became available, were incorporated as well, but accounted for only 26% of the cases. High-risk surgical patients were excluded from enrollment—including those with recent MI, poorly controlled hypertension or diabetes mellitus, renal disease, respiratory failure, inaccessible carotid stenosis, or severe cervical spondylosis. CAVATAS demonstrated no statistically significant difference between endovascular and surgical treatment in the rate of disabling stroke or death within 30 days (6.4% CAS vs. 5.9% CEA) and no significant difference in the 3-year ipsilateral stroke rate. The Wallstent trial,[105,106] a multicenter randomized trial designed to evaluate CEA and CAS equivalence in symptomatic patients, was halted by the Data Safety and Monitoring Committee after an interim analysis demonstrated worse outcomes for the CAS group. It should be noted though that the Wallstent trial did not require the use of distal protection devices. Devices that capture embolic debris released during CAS have significantly improved procedural safety.[107-112]

One of the first trials to use embolic protection was Carotid Revascularization Using Endarterectomy or Stenting Systems (CaRESS), a multicenter, nonrandomized, prospective study comparing CAS with embolic protection (n = 143) and CEA (n = 254) in symptomatic (32%) and asymptomatic (68%) patients with low and high surgical risk.[113,114] The investigators of this study found no statistically significant difference between 30-day and 1-year death or stroke rates in CAS and CEA (2.1% vs. 3.6% and 10.0% vs. 13.6%, respectively), or significant differences for restenosis, residual stenosis, repeat angiography, and need for carotid revascularization. Additionally, overall morbidity and mortality approached NASCET[90,91] and ACAS[94] standards.

Stenting and Angioplasty with Protection in Patients at High Risk for Endarterectomy (SAPPHIRE),[115] a multicenter, randomized trial to determine the noninferiority of CAS to CEA in high-risk patients, demonstrated a 30-day MI, stroke, or death rate of 4.8% for CAS and 9.8% for CEA (P = .09). Much of this difference was due to MIs in the CEA group, and although not reported in SAPPHIRE, the 30-day rates of stroke and death were approximately 4.8% for the CAS group and approximately 5.6%

for the CEA group. At 1 year, 12.2% of patients undergoing CAS had suffered stroke, MI, or death versus 20.1% of patients undergoing CEA (noninferiority analysis: P = .004; superiority analysis: intention-to-treat P = .053; as-treated P = .048). MI and major ipsilateral stroke rates were significantly better following CAS than CEA (2.5% vs. 8.1%, respectively, P = .03; 0% vs. 3.5%, respectively, P = .02). With these encouraging results, the Stent-supported Percutaneous Angioplasty of the Carotid artery versus Endarterectomy (SPACE) trial was established to evaluate noninferiority of CAS compared with CEA in low-risk patients.[116] The 30-day ipsilateral stroke or death rates were 6.84% for CAS and 6.34% for CEA (P value not significant). Embolic protection was not required and was used in only 27% of cases. The SPACE study was halted more than 700 patients shy of its goal enrollment of 1900 patients as the result of an interim analysis demonstrating that 2500 patients would be needed for the trial results to reach significance, given the results up to that point. At its conclusion, "SPACE failed to prove the noninferiority of carotid-artery stenting."[116] However, as evidenced by its early cessation, the study was underpowered to demonstrate noninferiority because of incorrect estimation of the anticipated effect sizes.

An additional multicenter, randomized trial to assess the noninferiority of CAS to CEA, Endarterectomy Versus Angioplasty in Patients with Symptomatic Severe Carotid Stenosis (EVA-3S) trial, was ended after interim analysis demonstrated a 30-day rate of any stroke or death to be significantly higher in the CAS group (9.6%) than the CEA group (3.9%) (P = .01).[117] Once again, the use of embolic protection was not required. Patients treated without embolic protection experienced a 25% 30-day rate of stroke or death (5 of 20 patients), prompting protocol changes by the EVA-3S study safety committee. Additionally, surgeons performing CEA had performed at least 25 endarterectomies in the year before trial entry, yet endovascular physicians were certified after completing as few as 5 to 12 CAS procedures (5 CAS among at least 35 stent procedures of supraaortic vessels or 12 CAS procedures). Endovascular physicians were also allowed to enroll study patients while simultaneously undergoing training and certification. The EVA-3S CAS study results are substantially worse than those of other randomized trials. Therefore, it is likely that such an elevated complication rate is not representative of the practice of CAS in general and that EVA-3S study mainly demonstrates the importance of embolic protection as well as rigorous training and credentialing of CAS physicians. The importance of embolic protection observed in the EVA-3S study is further supported by numerous radiologic studies demonstrating a reduction in the frequency of diffusion-weighted imaging (DWI) lesions with distal embolic protection (49% vs. 67%)[110] and a low frequency of DWI lesions with later embolic protection devices, such as flow-reversal systems.[118]

Both EVA-3S and SPACE have reported equivalent rates of mortality and stroke prevention for CAS and CEA at the 2-year (SPACE[119]) and 4-year (EVA-3S[120]) follow-up periods. With the state of evidence for CAS being subject to conflicting data of variable quality, the results of the Carotid Revascularization Endarterectomy vs. Stenting

Trial (CREST), a prospective, randomized, multicenter, trial funded by the National Institutes of Health (NIH), were anxiously awaited to help determine the potential roles of CAS and CEA in the treatment of patients with extracranial carotid artery atherosclerosis.

The CREST results were published in 2010 and provide the best and most comprehensive data to date regarding CAS and CEA.[121] To avoid the pitfalls of previous studies, CREST utilized a formal lead-in phase to confirm the appropriate quality of the proceduralists.[122] Occurrence of stroke, death, or MI during the periprocedural period and of ipsilateral stroke for up to 4 years was the primary endpoint. The study population included symptomatic patients with more than 50% carotid stenosis and asymptomatic patients with more than 60% stenosis. The inclusion of conventional-risk symptomatic and asymptomatic patients into this randomized prospective design allows for an extremely robust study set, from which a great deal of information will doubtless be gained. Among 2502 patients followed up for a mean of 2.5 years, there was no significant difference in primary endpoint between CAS and CEA (7.2% with CAS vs. 6.8% with CEA; hazard ratio 1.11; 95% confidence interval 0.81–1.51). The rates among symptomatic patients were 8.0% and 6.4% (hazard ratio, 1.37; $P = .14$), respectively; and the rates among asymptomatic patients were 4.5% and 2.7% (hazard ratio, 1.86; $P = .07$), respectively. Periprocedural rates for individual components of the primary endpoint differed between the stenting group and the endarterectomy group for stroke (4.1% vs. 2.3%; $P = .01$) and MI (1.1% vs. 2.3%; $P = .03$) but not for death (0.7% vs. 0.3%; $P = .18$). It should be noted that although the stroke rate was significantly more frequent in patients undergoing CAS and MI was more likely in patients undergoing CEA, the absolute rates were quite low. Perhaps most interesting, there was an effect of age on outcome, wherein CEA would be the favored therapy for patients older than 70 years and CAS would be the favored therapy for those younger than 70 years. Although not necessarily intuitive, these data are consistent with those of the SPACE trial.

Contrasting data to the CREST findings are found in the results of the International Carotid Stenting Study (ICSS), a multicenter randomized trial to evaluate CAS versus CEA in symptomatic patients with more than 50% stenosis, which were published in 2010.[123] In this trial, CAS fared worse than in CREST, with a hazard ratio in favor of surgery of 1.69 (1.16-2.45; $P = .006$) for the risk of stroke death, procedural MI 120 days after randomization. However, there are numerous concerns with this publication. First, the data presented were from an interim analysis and not the final analysis, because the study is still ongoing. Second, the credentialing process required the submission only of a case log demonstrating adequate volume of cases, and in cases in which the volume of cases requirement was not met, a center could still enroll as long as a designated proctor was present. In fact, two centers that were included through this proctoring mechanism were eventually forced to halt enrollment owing to concerns about the quality of CAS performance; however, the data from both of these centers were kept in the cohort for data analysis. Last, the use of distal embolic protection was not required.

Patient selection and timing of carotid stenting may minimize stroke risk. Recent radiographic evidence of a large infarction or a hemorrhage should delay elective carotid stenting for at least 2 weeks. Bovine or tortuous arches with ostial stenoses, inability to tolerate even temporary anticoagulation, severely tortuous carotid arteries, and poor routes of peripheral access (due to severe peripheral vascular disease) are vascular characteristics that may make CEA a more desirable option. Conversely, patients who have restenosis following a previous endarterectomy, contralateral carotid occlusion, a carotid bifurcation at the level of C2 or higher, dissecting lesions, or severe coronary artery disease or who have undergone radiation therapy to the neck may be more likely to derive greater benefit from stenting.

Extracranial Vertebral Artery Stenosis

Atherosclerotic occlusive disease of the extracranial vertebral artery, which is present in approximately 25% to 40% of the population, is an important cause of posterior circulation ischemia.[124,125] The V1 (proximal) segment of the vertebral artery, extending from the origin of the vertebral artery at the subclavian artery to the entrance into the transverse vertebral foramen, is the most common site for atherosclerotic occlusive disease in the vertebral artery.[125] These ostial lesions can serve as not only embolic sources but also flow-limiting stenoses that can produce posterior circulation ischemia. However, the natural history, clinical features, and optimal therapy for atherosclerotic lesions of the extracranial vertebral artery are not clearly defined, particularly because symptoms of posterior circulation ischemia, such as dizziness and ataxia, may be misinterpreted as nonspecific symptoms, leading to misdiagnosis.[126,127] Additionally, no prospective randomized trial has been performed to determine which therapy is optimal for symptomatic stenosis of the extracranial vertebral artery. Surgery of these lesions is technically difficult and associated with significant morbidity and mortality.[128] Medical therapy, consisting of antiplatelet agents, systemic anticoagulation, avoidance of orthostatic hypotension, and elevation of mean arterial blood pressure, remains empiric. In the last decade, angioplasty with or without stenting has been performed as an alternative treatment for extracranial vertebral artery stenosis.[129-131]

We do not recommend routine performance of vertebral artery angioplasty with or without stenting for asymptomatic patients with atherosclerotic stenosis of the extracranial vertebral artery. There are situations, however, for which angioplasty and/or stenting may be indicated for asymptomatic stenosis, such as for stenosis at the vertebral artery origin in a patient with a dominant or single vertebral artery. Further data are needed regarding the natural history of extracranial vertebral artery stenosis as well as the long-term durability of these procedures. Chastain et al[132] reported uncomplicated angioplasty and stenting of extracranial vertebral artery stenosis in 11 asymptomatic patients. These patients were known to have poor intracranial collateral circulation. However, long-term angiographic and clinical follow-up is needed to determine the efficacy of these procedures in this select group of patients.

At this time, we recommend reserving angioplasty with or without stent placement for atherosclerotic extracranial vertebral artery stenosis in the patient whose symptoms fail to respond to medical therapy. Angioplasty with or without stenting may be recommended instead of medical therapy for symptomatic patients who have physiologic evidence of hypoperfusion or inadequate intracranial collateral flow demonstrated by imaging modalities such as MR or CT perfusion imaging and the assessment of the cerebral perfusion reserve. Antiplatelet and anticoagulation therapies may reduce embolic events resulting from vertebral artery stenosis but are unlikely to augment flow distal to these lesions. Wityk et al,[125] reviewing the clinical features and radiographic findings for patients with either occlusion or high-grade stenosis of the V1 segment who were enrolled in the New England Medical Center Posterior Circulation Registry, found that 16% had TIAs resulting from hemodynamic instability. The advantages of a combination angioplasty and stenting procedure over angioplasty alone include prevention of elastic recoil and early restenosis but are, as yet, unproven.

Before vertebral artery stenting was introduced, angioplasty alone for symptomatic stenosis of the extracranial vertebral artery was reported as a safe alternative to medical therapy. Higashida et al[133] reported an 8.8% occurrence of transient neurologic complications among 34 patients in whom proximal vertebral artery stenosis (more than 70% stenosis) was treated with angioplasty alone. However, vertebral angioplasty has several limitations. First, an ostial stenosis can be very difficult to dilate adequately with angioplasty alone. In addition to immediate elastic recoil, an 8.8% rate of restenosis (defined as more than 50% residual luminal stenosis) within 2 to 5 months has been reported.[133] These data have encouraged the use of stents. Mukherjee et al[134] reported symptomatic restenosis in 1 (8%) of 12 patients who underwent vertebral artery origin angioplasty and stenting. Although most studies report a significant benefit of vertebral angioplasty and stenting in alleviating symptoms of posterior circulation ischemia, the series are typically small, retrospective, and nonrandomized. One multicenter, nonrandomized, prospective investigation, the Stenting of Symptomatic Atherosclerotic Lesions in the Vertebral or Intracranial Arteries (SSYLVIA) study, enrolled patients with symptomatic extracranial vertebral artery lesions (n = 18) and demonstrated a high rate of successful deployment, with a 1-year stroke occurrence rate of 11%.[135] However, there was a greater than 50% stenosis rate in 43% of subjects at 6 months. These restenosis, stroke, and technical success rates are comparable to those seen in a number of other series as well.[136] Further study is certainly required to evaluate the efficacy of extracranial vertebral artery stenting.

Subclavian Steal Syndrome

In 1960, Contorni[137] reported the first angiographic demonstration of retrograde flow in the vertebral artery ipsilateral to a proximal subclavian artery stenosis in a neurologically asymptomatic patient. In 1961, Fisher[138] explained that subclavian artery stenosis or occlusion could result in reduction of blood flow to the arm, reversal of flow to the ipsilateral vertebral artery, and claudication or neurologic deficits of the arm when intracranial or extracranial collateral circulation is inadequate; he named this new vascular disease a "subclavian steal syndrome" (SSS). Since the inception of this term, the clinical significance and natural history of subclavian steal have evolved from those of a disease that is morbid with neurologic symptoms, including vertigo, syncope, ataxia, paresthesia, and motor or visual deficits, to those of a condition that is often asymptomatic.[139-145] Moreover, SSS, which until 1980 was treated surgically even in asymptomatic patients, is now considered for treatment only in patients who have symptoms. This syndrome is reported to occur in approximately 6% of patients who have an asymptomatic cervical bruit.[146] Since the late 1980s, noninvasive imaging modalities, such as Doppler ultrasonography, MRI, MR angiography, and XeCT, have complemented angiography as investigative tools.[147,148] A variety of surgical treatments and complications have been reported for SSS over the past four decades.[149-152] Since Bachman and Kim[153] reported the first successful angioplasty for SSS in 1980, subclavian angioplasty with or without stenting has been performed as an alternative to surgery.

Contrary to earlier beliefs that most patients with SSS have symptoms, the subclavian steal alone is rarely a cause of posterior circulation ischemia.[154] The advancement of noninvasive imaging tools has contributed to better understanding of the natural history of a subclavian steal. Bornstein and Norris[155] reported on a 2-year follow-up review of 32 patients with asymptomatic subclavian steal with no cerebrovascular event related to the steal. Using Doppler ultrasonography, Moran et al[156] studied 55 patients with SSS with over a mean follow-up period of 4.1 years, during which only 7.2% of patients experienced symptoms of vertebrobasilar ischemia. No posterior circulation strokes were reported. However, 18% of the patients had symptoms of anterior circulation ischemia or stroke. Hennerici et al[157] reviewed the medical records of 324 patients in whom subclavian steal was detected on the basis of Doppler ultrasonography and reported symptoms of vertebrobasilar ischemia in only 5% of these patients. The majority of patients (64%) were asymptomatic. The remainder had lateralizing hemispheric symptoms. These studies suggested that SSS might become symptomatic when there is hemodynamic insufficiency in the presence of coexisting severe carotid occlusive disease or inadequate intracranial collateralization. For these reasons, revascularization is not advocated for asymptomatic patients.

Subclavian angioplasty with or without stent placement may be indicated for symptomatic SSS in patients who have comorbid medical conditions that raise the risk of perioperative complications. No prospective, randomized study is available to compare the efficacy of surgical versus endoluminal revascularization for SSS. The advantages of an endovascular approach include the avoidance of the complications of general anesthesia and surgery. The disadvantages of angioplasty with or without stenting include potential dissection, thrombosis, and embolization. The durability of patency after subclavian angioplasty is difficult to interpret because, in most series, follow-up angiography was not performed, the investigators having relied on Doppler ultrasonography. However, long-term patency after subclavian angioplasty for stenosis (ranging from 54% to 100% at 2 months to 5 years) appears superior to that for occlusion (less than 50% at 4 to 88 months of follow-up).[158-162]

In an attempt to improve upon the results of angioplasty, subclavian angioplasty-assisted stenting has been popularized for symptomatic subclavian steal and occlusive disease. Case series have reported minimal rates of complications and high rates of technical success.[163-166] However, functional outcome measures have not been consistently reported. Further studies are needed to evaluate the efficacy and long-term patency of angioplasty with stent placement for symptomatic subclavian steal.

The main procedural complications associated with subclavian angioplasty and stenting are hematoma, pseudoaneurysm, and thrombosis at the access site; distal arterial emboli; and arterial dissection. The incidence of these complications ranges from 0% to 11.4%.[158-166] Failure to recanalize an occluded subclavian artery is frequently observed with angioplasty alone; early reocclusion rates as high as 13% have been reported.[167] As a result, subclavian artery stenting for the treatment of occlusions has been evaluated at several institutions. Although many series have reported small numbers of cases, initial success rates as high as 100% and asymptomatic and symptomatic restenosis (>50%) rates of 7% and 3%, respectively, at 1 year have been reported.[158-166]

Rodriguez-Lopez et al[165] reported a 3% incidence of postprocedural TIA in 37 patients after treatment with percutaneous balloon angioplasty and stenting of subclavian artery stenosis. In the occlusion group (15 of 37 patients), no postprocedural cerebrovascular events or deaths occurred. Ringelstein and Zeumer[168] reported that a delay in the reversal of vertebral artery blood flow after percutaneous balloon angioplasty may account for such low rates of neurologic complications. Follow-up ultrasonography in these patients at 9 months showed no restenosis in the occlusion group. Additional studies are needed to determine the long-term morbidity and mortality of subclavian artery stenting for SSS.

Intracranial Aneurysms

Approximately 30,000 Americans are afflicted with aneurysmal subarachnoid hemorrhage (SAH) yearly.[169] The incidence of SAH has been reported to be between 6 and 16 per 100,000 persons in the United States, with higher numbers reported from Japan and Finland.[169-172] Aneurysmal SAH accounts for 25% of cerebrovascular deaths and 8% of all strokes.[173]

Ruptured and unruptured aneurysms carry significantly different natural history risks. The risk of rupture has also been shown to be a function of aneurysm size and tobacco consumption.[174,175] Although the natural history of ruptured aneurysms has been well defined, there is controversy regarding the natural history of unruptured aneurysms, particularly those less than 10 mm in diameter.[169,174] We refer the reader to scholarly reviews of these issues by Weir[169] and by the investigators of the International Study of Unruptured Intracranial Aneurysms (ISUIA).[174]

The most common complication related to cerebral aneurysms is SAH.[176] Other complications are cranial nerve deficits, symptoms related to mass effect,[177] and strokes related to emboli released from thrombus within the aneurysm.[178]

Subarachnoid Hemorrhage

Modern management of patients with SAH in the critical care unit, along with specialized microsurgical and endovascular expertise, contributes significantly to the prevention of recurrent hemorrhage and stroke following aneurysm rupture. Of paramount concern is the prevention of rehemorrhage because it is associated with a case-fatality rate of 70%.[179] Juvela[180] reported a 22.5% incidence of aneurysm rebleeding within 6 months of the primary hemorrhage in 236 untreated patients. Prevention of rebleeding through clip ligation of a ruptured aneurysm or through coil embolization are both accepted techniques for the treatment of ruptured aneurysms; however, with the publication of the results of the International Subarachnoid Aneurysm Trial (ISAT), evidence-based recommendations favor the use of coil embolization, particularly in patients older than 50 years.[181,182]

In addition to the morbidity associated with the initial hemorrhage, SAH can result in vasospasm, which can be neurologically detrimental. Seventy percent of patients with SAH demonstrate angiographic vasospasm; of these patients, approximately 50% have symptoms.[183] Approximately 20% of symptomatic patients will experience stroke or die despite maximal modern therapy.[183] Angiographically evident vasospasm usually peaks during days 5 to 14 after hemorrhage.[179] Hypertension and hypervolemia have emerged as the first line of therapy for symptomatic vasospasm.[184] IA administration of papaverine and balloon angioplasty have been used with some success to treat medically refractory vasospasm.[176] Balloon angioplasty can be used for proximal vessel spasm of the supraclinoid carotid artery, A1 segment of the ICA, M1 segment of the MCA, vertebral artery, or basilar artery.[185] If not performed carefully with avoidance of overdilation, the procedure can be associated with vessel rupture. Improvements in balloon technology may reduce this risk. It has been observed that balloon angioplasty can permanently relieve vasospasm symptoms in 60% to 70% of cases.[185] Papaverine can be used for distal vessel spasm.[186-188] Initial enthusiasm for IA papaverine has waned over the past several years, however, because it has been observed that the effects of papaverine are short lived. An alternative to papaverine, though likely one that is also subject to a short-lived effect, is verapamil.

Mass Effect

In a study by Malisch et al,[177] in which the effect of coiling on symptoms related to the mass effect of aneurysms on cranial nerves was examined, symptoms resolved in 32% of patients and improved in 42% after coiling, with no change in 21% and worsening in 5%. It is believed that removing the pulsatility associated with an aneurysm after coiling may be responsible for symptom improvement.[177]

Ischemic Complications

A paucity of data exists with respect to the embolic risk associated with the presence of an aneurysm. Clot can accumulate in the fundus of an aneurysm as a result of flow stasis, particularly in a large aneurysm. In a study by Qureshi et al,[178] complications associated with embolization from the aneurysm fundus occurred in 3.3% of patients presenting with an unruptured aneurysm. In this study, clipping of the aneurysm was associated with a low risk of symptom recurrence. It should be noted that the presence of clot in an aneurysm might be a risk factor for thromboembolic complications during aneurysm coiling.

Technical Advances in Coil Treatment

Although the results of coil treatment of small aneurysms (diameter less than 12 mm) and aneurysms with small necks (less than 5 mm) appear to be promising, lesser degrees of success have been observed with aneurysms with larger diameter size and wider necks.[189] Technical advances have occurred over the past several years to improve the success rate with coiling of large and wide-necked aneurysms. In the balloon-remodeling technique, which has been championed by Moret et al,[190] more coils can be packed near the aneurysm neck because a balloon is inflated across the neck during coil placement (Fig. 61-2). The balloon is deflated after each coil is deployed to restore flow temporarily. Stent-assisted coiling appears to be another promising technique for certain wide-necked aneurysms (Fig. 61-3).[191,192] The stent serves as scaffolding across the aneurysm neck, holding the coils within the aneurysm sac. Manufacturers have improved coils in an attempt to overcome some of the shortcomings associated with coil technology. Spherical coils (MicruSphere coils, Micrus Endovascular, San Jose, CA) and three-dimensional Guglielmi detachable coils (GDCs) appear to allow certain wide-necked aneurysms to be coiled more effectively. Newer technologies, such as coils made of bioactive materials and endoluminal flow diverters, are demonstrating early promise in continuing to advance endovascular aneurysm treatment.[193-198]

Fusiform Aneurysms

Fusiform aneurysms can lead to mass effect, hemorrhage, or both. The outcomes for patients with fusiform aneurysms remain poor, despite advances in microsurgical and endovascular treatment techniques.[199] The treatment of fusiform aneurysms often requires vessel sacrifice. Over the past several years, stents have emerged as an option to treat certain fusiform aneurysms. Stents offer the advantage of maintaining patency of the parent vessel. Preliminary results suggest that stents may play a significant role in the management of this complex disease.[200] Most excitingly, later case series have reported the use of endoluminal flow diversion, with excellent angiographic and clinical results.[201]

Arteriovenous Malformations

Definition, Pathology, and Epidemiology

An AVM is a congenital lesion that anatomically consists of a collection of abnormal arteries and veins lacking a normal capillary connection. The abnormal arteries form a conglomeration of vessels, which are referred to as the *nidus*. The nidus typically has little to no intervening brain tissue. The lack of a capillary bed causes early venous drainage, venous hypertension, and recruitment of arterial feeders. True arteriovenous shunts are occasionally noted in AVMs. Autopsy data suggest that AVMs occur in 4.3% of the general population.[202] Between 1980 and 1990, the annual incidence of symptomatic AVMs in the Netherlands was 1.1 per 100,000 population.[203]

Aneurysms are commonly associated with AVMs. According to the literature, this association occurs in from 2.7%[204] to 23%[205] of patients. The four types of aneurysms observed in conjunction with AVMs are intranidal aneurysms, pedicular aneurysms, proximal aneurysms, and unassociated. Evidence suggests that the first three types of aneurysms occur as a result of the flow dynamics created by the AVM.

Classification

Although multiple classification systems for AVMs have emerged, the Spetzler-Martin grading system has remained the simplest and most practical to use.[206] The

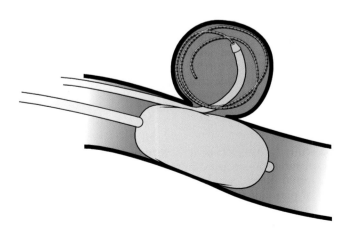

Figure 61-2 Balloon-assisted aneurysm coiling.

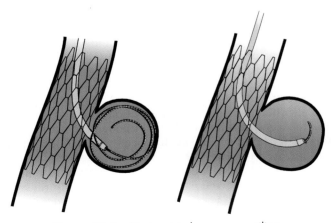

Figure 61-3 Stent-assisted aneurysm coiling.

TABLE 61-6 SPETZLER-MARTIN CLASSIFICATION OF ARTERIOVENOUS MALFORMATIONS OF THE BRAIN*

Feature	Points Awarded
Size	
Small (<3 cm)	1
Medium (3-6 cm)	2
Large (>6 cm)	3
Eloquence of adjacent brain	
Noneloquent	0
Eloquent	1
Pattern of venous drainage	
Superficial only	0
Deep	1

*Grade = [size] + [eloquence] + [venous drainage], that is, [1, 2, or 3] + [0 or 1] + [0 or 1].
Adapted from Spetzler RF, Martin NA: A proposed grading system for arteriovenous malformations. *J Neurosurg* 65:478, 1986.

system assigns AVMs to grades according to size, eloquence of brain surrounding the AVM, and presence or absence of deep venous drainage (Table 61-6). Increased surgical risk is associated with higher AVM grade. The grading system was initially designed to assess the safety and risk of AVM excision but is used by most practitioners regardless of treatment modality. One study suggests that this grading scheme may not have relevance to modern embolization strategies.[207]

Natural History

AVMs have been associated with seizures, hemorrhage, headaches, and ischemia related to steal (see previous discussion of subclavian steal). In children younger than 2 years, congestive heart failure and hydrocephalus are common presentations. For the purpose of this chapter, we focus on the hemorrhagic and ischemic manifestations of AVMs.

Stroke registries indicate that AVMs are responsible for the symptoms in more than 1% of patients who present with stroke.[208] The risk of AVM hemorrhage is approximately 2% to 3% per year.[202,209-212] Mortality from the first hemorrhage varies from 10% to 30%.[199] An estimated 10% to 20% of survivors have long-term disability.[199,212,213] Kondziolka et al[214] proposed the following simplified equation to determine the hemorrhage risk in any given patient:

$$\text{Lifetime risk}(\%) = 105 - \text{patient's age in years}$$

This equation helps put the risk of hemorrhage in perspective when one is considering patients of varying ages. It is important to note, however, that there is a burgeoning belief that such rupture estimates are reflective not of incidental AVMs but rather of those that have previously ruptured only. To evaluate this hypothesis, there is an ongoing NIH-funded trial, A Randomized trial of Unruptured Brain Arteriovenous malformations (ARUBA), that seeks to observe the natural history of unruptured AVMs.[215]

The risk of hemorrhage appears to increase during the first year after a hemorrhage. In two studies, the increase

was 6%,[211,216] and in one study, 17.8%.[210] Certain radiologic findings appear to be associated with an increased hemorrhage risk. Among these findings are central venous drainage, intranidal aneurysm, periventricular or intraventricular location, arterial supply via perforators, multiple aneurysms, vertebrobasilar supply, basal ganglia location, single draining vein, impaired venous drainage, and deep venous drainage alone.[199,217,218]

Treatment

The treatment of AVMs has dramatically evolved within the past 35 years as a result of advances in microsurgery, endovascular techniques (embolization), and radiation therapy. Embolization can play a role as a presurgical tool, as a pre–stereotactic irradiation tool, as sole therapy for a cure, as sole therapy for palliation, and to treat associated aneurysms.

Embolization as a Preoperative Tool

Microsurgery has been shown to be a safe and effective treatment for certain AVMs. The long-term protective effects of AVM surgery against hemorrhage risk have been established. In a study by Heros et al,[219] excellent outcomes were achieved in 98.7% of patients with Spetzler-Martin grade I, II, or III AVMs at a mean follow-up of 3.8 years. Studies and empiric observations have suggested that AVM embolization reduces blood loss and enhances the ease of surgery.[220]

For large AVMs, embolization can achieve the goal of gradually decreasing the volume of the AVM before excision. Although it has never been proven, this strategy is believed to lower the risk of postoperative hemorrhage from normal perfusion pressure breakthrough.[221] According to the normal perfusion pressure breakthrough theory, the increased flow of blood supplying a large AVM deprives the surrounding brain tissue of adequate blood supply. This deprivation creates a chronic ischemic state and loss of autoregulation. When a large AVM is resected, the surrounding tissue, which was previously ischemic, becomes perfused by a larger blood flow. The lack of autoregulation makes the small vessels vulnerable to hemorrhage. Gradual embolization of these large AVMs is thought to allow the surrounding brain tissue to adjust to gradually increasing amounts of perfusion, hence reducing the risk of hemorrhage after eventual resection of the AVM. Endovascular techniques performed before surgery can also be used to treat associated aneurysms, particularly if the aneurysm would be difficult to treat during surgical excision.

Embolization Followed by Stereotactic Irradiation

Radiosurgery has emerged as an attractive option for some AVMs, especially those located in surgically prohibitive deep locations. Stereotactic technology allows the delivery of radiation precisely and directly to the AVM while limiting exposure to surrounding brain tissue. Radiosurgery results in a 78% to 88% obliteration rate of AVMs with volumes equal to or less than 10 mm at 3 years.[222] Lower obliteration rates and higher complication rates are associated with radiosurgery of larger AVMs. Over the past decade, several centers have reported on the strategy of embolization to reduce large AVMs to sizes amenable to radiosurgery.[223,224] This is an attractive strategy for large AVMs for which surgical excision poses a high risk. Long-term outcomes associated with this type of treatment have not yet been determined, and recanalization remains a concern.[224]

Embolization Alone

In the early 1990s only a small percentage of AVMs could be treated by endovascular techniques alone.[225] However, this number has increased dramatically with the advent of the Onyx liquid embolic agent (ev3 Neurovascular, Irvine, CA).[226-229] Such AVMs are typically small (less than 3 cm) and have a limited number (1 or 2) of arterial feeders.

Embolization for Palliation

Palliative embolization can be used in rare situations to decrease symptoms from large AVMs that are deemed untreatable by other means. Embolization can be used to reduce headaches and reversible neurologic deficits attributable to steal or venous hypertension or to occlude associated aneurysms. Embolization for palliation is only temporary, because the AVM can recur over time as a result of recanalization. No evidence exists that partial AVM embolization decreases the long-term risk of AVM hemorrhage.[199]

Conclusion

Endovascular neurosurgery is evolving at a frantic pace. Although endovascular technology is still in its infancy, this field holds the promise to provide minimally invasive therapies for cerebrovascular disease resulting in ischemia and stroke. Clinicians are not yet able to predict the long-term effects of endovascular therapies, such as endoluminal responses to intracranial stent and coil implantations. However, short- and mid-term outcomes of existing technologies show substantial promise. Additionally, future transcatheter technologies may involve processes only hypothesized today, such as the delivery of growth factors able to reconstitute the vessel lumen across an aneurysm or even stem cells with the ability to repair and restore parenchyma destroyed by ischemic stroke. As medicine pushes toward the future, it appears that the most significant limitation of endovascular medicine may be the imagination of its physicians and the industry with which they collaborate.

Disclosures

The authors have the following financial relationships to disclose: Dr. Bendok has received research funding from Cordis; Dr. Mocco serves as a consultant to Actelion, Nfocus, and Lazarus Effect; his employer, The University of Florida, receives research funding from AccessClosure and Codman Neurovascular. Dr. Hopkins receives research study grants from Abbott (ACT 1 Choice), Boston Scientific (CABANA), Cordis (SAPPHIRE WW), and ev3/Covidien Vascular Therapies (CREATE) and a research grant from Toshiba (for the Toshiba Stroke Research Center); has an ownership/financial interest in AccessClosure, Boston Scientific, Cordis, Micrus, and Valor Medical; serves on the Abbott Vascular Speakers' Bureau; receives honoraria from Bard, Boston Scientific, Cordis, and from the following for speaking at conferences—Complete Conference Management, Cleveland Clinic, and SCAI; receives royalties from Cordis (for the AngioGuard device), serves as a consultant to or on the advisory board for Abbott, AccessClosure, Bard, Boston Scientific, Cordis, Gore, Lumen Biomedical, Micrus, and Toshiba; and serves as the conference director for Nurcon Conferences/Strategic Medical Seminars LLC. Dr. Levy receives research grant support (principal investigator: Stent-Assisted Recanalization in acute Ischemic Stroke, SARIS), other research support (devices), and honoraria from Boston Scientific and research support from Micrus Endovascular and ev3/Covidien Vascular Therapies; has ownership interests in Intratech Medical Ltd. and Mynx/AccessClosure; serves as a consultant on the board of Scientific Advisors to Codman & Shurtleff, Inc.; serves as a consultant per project and/or per hour for Micrus Endovascular, ev3/Covidien Vascular Therapies, and TheraSyn Sensors, Inc.; and receives fees for carotid stent training from Abbott Vascular and ev3/Covidien Vascular Therapies. Dr. Levy receives no consulting salary arrangements. All consulting is per project, per hour, or both.

REFERENCES

1. National Institute of Neurological Disorders and Stroke rt-PA Stroke Study Group: Tissue plasminogen activator for acute ischemic stroke, *N Engl J Med* 333:1581–1587, 1995.
2. Albers GW, Bates VE, Clark WM, et al: Intravenous tissue-type plasminogen activator for treatment of acute stroke: The Standard Treatment with Alteplase to Reverse Stroke (STARS) study, *JAMA* 283:1145–1150, 2000.
3. Hacke W, Kaste M, Fieschi C, et al: Randomised double-blind placebo-controlled trial of thrombolytic therapy with intravenous alteplase in acute ischaemic stroke (ECASS II). Second European-Australasian Acute Stroke Study Investigators, *Lancet* 352:1245–1251, 1998.
4. Multicentre Acute Stroke Trial—Italy (MAST-I) Group: Randomised controlled trial of streptokinase, aspirin, and combination of both in treatment of acute ischaemic stroke, *Lancet* 346:1509–1514, 1995.
5. Multicenter Acute Stroke Trial—Europe Study Group: Thrombolytic therapy with streptokinase in acute ischemic stroke, *N Engl J Med* 335:145–150, 1996.
6. Clark WM, Wissman S, Albers GW, et al: Recombinant tissue-type plasminogen activator (alteplase) for ischemic stroke 3 to 5 hours after symptom onset. The ATLANTIS Study: A randomized controlled trial. Alteplase Thrombolysis for Acute Noninterventional Therapy in Ischemic Stroke, *JAMA* 282:2019–2026, 1999.
7. Donnan GA, Davis SM, Chambers BR, et al: Streptokinase for acute ischemic stroke with relationship to time of administration: Australian Streptokinase (ASK) Trial Study Group, *JAMA* 276:961–966, 1996.
8. Hacke W, Kaste M, Fieschi C, et al: Intravenous thrombolysis with recombinant tissue plasminogen activator for acute hemispheric stroke. The European Cooperative Acute Stroke Study (ECASS), *JAMA* 274:1017–1025, 1995.
9. del Zoppo GJ, Higashida RT, Furlan AJ, et al: PROACT: A phase II randomized trial of recombinant pro-urokinase by direct arterial delivery in acute middle cerebral artery stroke. PROACT Investigators. Prolyse in Acute Cerebral Thromboembolism, *Stroke* 29:4–11, 1998.
10. Furlan A, Higashida R, Wechsler L, et al: Intra-arterial prourokinase for acute ischemic stroke. The PROACT II study: A randomized controlled trial. Prolyse in Acute Cerebral Thromboembolism, *JAMA* 282:2003–2011, 1999.

11. IMS Study Investigators: Combined intravenous and intra-arterial recanalization for acute ischemic stroke: The Interventional Management of Stroke Study, *Stroke* 35:904-911, 2004.

12. IMS II Trial Investigators: The Interventional Management of Stroke (IMS) II Study, *Stroke* 38:2127-2135, 2007.

13. Eckert B, Koch C, Thomalla G, et al: Acute basilar artery occlusion treated with combined intravenous abciximab and intra-arterial tissue plasminogen activator: Report of 3 cases, *Stroke* 33:1424-1427, 2002.

14. Endo S, Kuwayama N, Hirashima Y, et al: Results of urgent thrombolysis in patients with major stroke and atherothrombotic occlusion of the cervical internal carotid artery, *AJNR Am J Neuroradiol* 19:1169-1175, 1998.

15. Jahan R, Duckwiler GR, Kidwell CS, et al: Intraarterial thrombolysis for treatment of acute stroke: Experience in 26 patients with long-term follow-up, *AJNR Am J Neuroradiol* 20:1291-1299, 1999.

16. Kim SH, Qureshi AI, Suri MFK, et al: Mechanical thrombolysis using balloon angioplasty and snare with low-dose intraarterial reteplase (third-generation thrombolytic) for ischemic stroke. A prospective study (paper 13), *J Neurosurg* 96:A168, 2002.

17. Nesbit GM, Clark WM, O'Neill OR, Barnwell SL: Intracranial intraarterial thrombolysis facilitated by microcatheter navigation through an occluded cervical internal carotid artery, *J Neurosurg* 84:387-392, 1996.

18. Qureshi AI, Suri MF, Shatla AA, et al: Intraarterial recombinant tissue plasminogen activator for ischemic stroke: An accelerating dosing regimen, *Neurosurgery* 47:473-479, 2000.

19. Qureshi AI, Ali Z, Suri MF, et al: Intra-arterial third-generation recombinant tissue plasminogen activator (reteplase) for acute ischemic stroke, *Neurosurgery* 49:41-50, 2001.

20. Gonzalez RG: Imaging-guided acute ischemic stroke therapy: From "time is brain" to "physiology is brain", *AJNR Am J Neuroradiol* 27:728-735, 2006.

21. Kidwell CS, Saver JL, Mattiello J, et al: Thrombolytic reversal of acute human cerebral ischemic injury shown by diffusion/perfusion magnetic resonance imaging, *Ann Neurol* 47:462-469, 2000.

22. Kidwell CS, Saver JL, Mattiello J, et al: Diffusion-perfusion MRI characterization of post-recanalization hyperperfusion in humans, *Neurology* 57:2015-2021, 2001.

23. Kidwell CS, Saver JL, Villablanca JP, Duckwiler G, Fredieu A, Gough K, Leary MC, Starkman S, Gobin YP, Jahan R, Vespa P, Liebeskind DS, Alger JR, Vinuela F: Magnetic resonance imaging detection of microbleeds before thrombolysis: An emerging application, *Stroke* 33:95-98, 2002.

24. Lansberg MG, Thijs VN, Bammer R, et al: The MRA-DWI mismatch identifies patients with stroke who are likely to benefit from reperfusion, *Stroke* 39:2491-2496, 2008.

25. Lev MH, Segal AZ, Farkas J, et al: Utility of perfusion-weighted CT imaging in acute middle cerebral artery stroke treated with intra-arterial thrombolysis: Prediction of final infarct volume and clinical outcome, *Stroke* 32:2021-2028, 2001.

26. Olivot JM, Mlynash M, Thijs VN, et al: Relationships between infarct growth, clinical outcome, and early recanalization in diffusion and perfusion imaging for understanding stroke evolution (DEFUSE), *Stroke* 39:2257-2263, 2008.

27. Provenzale JM, Shah K, Patel U, McCrory DC: Systematic review of CT and MR perfusion imaging for assessment of acute cerebrovascular disease, *AJNR Am J Neuroradiol* 29:1476-1482, 2008.

28. Rai AT, Carpenter JS, Peykanu JA, et al: The role of CT perfusion imaging in acute stroke diagnosis: A large single-center experience, *J Emerg Med* 35:287-292, 2008.

29. Sheehan FH, Braunwald E, Canner P, et al: The effect of intravenous thrombolytic therapy on left ventricular function: A report on tissue-type plasminogen activator and streptokinase from the Thrombolysis in Myocardial Infarction (TIMI phase I) trial, *Circulation* 75:817-829, 1987.

30. Ernst R, Pancioli A, Tomsick T, et al: Combined intravenous and intra-arterial recombinant tissue plasminogen activator in acute ischemic stroke, *Stroke* 31:2552-2557, 2000.

31. Hill MD, Barber PA, Demchuk AM, et al: Acute intravenous—intra-arterial revascularization therapy for severe ischemic stroke, *Stroke* 33:279-282, 2002.

32. Keris V, Rudnicka S, Vorona V, et al: Combined intraarterial/intravenous thrombolysis for acute ischemic stroke, *AJNR Am J Neuroradiol* 22:352-358, 2001.

33. Lewandowski CA, Frankel M, Tomsick TA, et al: Combined intravenous and intra-arterial r-TPA versus intra-arterial therapy of acute ischemic stroke: Emergency Management of Stroke (EMS) Bridging Trial, *Stroke* 30:2598-2605, 1999.

34. Suarez JI, Zaidat OO, Sunshine JL, et al: Endovascular administration after intravenous infusion of thrombolytic agents for the treatment of patients with acute ischemic strokes, *Neurosurgery* 50:251-260, 2002.

35. Qureshi AI: New grading system for angiographic evaluation of arterial occlusions and recanalization response to intra-arterial thrombolysis in acute ischemic stroke, *Neurosurgery* 50:1405-1415, 2002.

36. Bose A, Henkes H, Alfke K, et al: The Penumbra System: A mechanical device for the treatment of acute stroke due to thromboembolism, *AJNR Am J Neuroradiol* 29:1409-1413, 2008.

37. Flint AC, Duckwiler GR, Budzik RF, et al: Mechanical thrombectomy of intracranial internal carotid occlusion: Pooled results of the MERCI and Multi MERCI Part I trials, *Stroke* 38:1274-1280, 2007.

38. Smith WS, Sung G, Saver J, et al: Mechanical thrombectomy for acute ischemic stroke: Final results of the Multi MERCI trial, *Stroke* 39:1205-1212, 2008.

39. Smith WS, Sung G, Starkman S, et al: Safety and efficacy of mechanical embolectomy in acute ischemic stroke: Results of the MERCI trial, *Stroke* 36:1432-1438, 2005.

40. Adams HP Jr, del Zoppo G, Alberts MJ, et al: Guidelines for the early management of adults with ischemic stroke: A guideline from the American Heart Association/American Stroke Association Stroke Council, Clinical Cardiology Council, Cardiovascular Radiology and Intervention Council, and the Atherosclerotic Peripheral Vascular Disease and Quality of Care Outcomes in Research Interdisciplinary Working Groups: The American Academy of Neurology affirms the value of this guideline as an educational tool for neurologists, *Stroke* 38:1655-1711, 2007.

41. Ringer AJ, Qureshi AI, Fessler RD, et al: Angioplasty of intracranial occlusion resistant to thrombolysis in acute ischemic stroke, *Neurosurgery* 48:1282-1290, 2001.

42. Suarez JI, Sunshine JL, Tarr R, et al: Predictors of clinical improvement, angiographic recanalization, and intracranial hemorrhage after intra-arterial thrombolysis for acute ischemic stroke, *Stroke* 30:2094-2100, 1999.

43. Ueda T, Sakaki S, Nochide I, et al: Angioplasty after intra-arterial thrombolysis for acute occlusion of intracranial arteries, *Stroke* 29:2568-2574, 1998.

44. Levy EI, Ecker RD, Hanel RA, et al: Acute M2 bifurcation stenting for cerebral infarction: Lessons learned from the heart: Technical case report, *Neurosurgery* 58:E588, 2006.

45. Levy EI, Ecker RD, Horowitz MB, et al: Stent-assisted intracranial recanalization for acute stroke: Early results, *Neurosurgery* 58:458-463, 2006.

46. Sauvageau E, Samuelson RM, Levy EI, et al: Middle cerebral artery stenting for acute ischemic stroke after unsuccessful Merci retrieval, *Neurosurgery* 60:701-706, 2007.

47. Zaidat OO, Wolfe T, Hussain SI, et al: Interventional acute ischemic stroke therapy with intracranial self-expanding stent, *Stroke* 39:2392-2395, 2008.

48. Sacco RL, Kargman DE, Gu Q, Zamanillo MC: Race-ethnicity and determinants of intracranial atherosclerotic cerebral infarction. The Northern Manhattan Stroke Study, *Stroke* 26:14-20, 1995.

49. Wityk RJ, Lehman D, Klag M, et al: Race and sex differences in the distribution of cerebral atherosclerosis, *Stroke* 27:1974-1980, 1996.

50. Chimowitz MI, Kokkinos J, Strong J, et al: The Warfarin-Aspirin Symptomatic Intracranial Disease Study, *Neurology* 45:1488-1493, 1995.

51. Chimowitz MI, Lynn MJ, Howlett-Smith H, et al: Comparison of warfarin and aspirin for symptomatic intracranial arterial stenosis, *N Engl J Med* 352:1305-1316, 2005.

52. Redman AR, Allen LC: Warfarin Versus Aspirin in the Secondary Prevention of Stroke: The WARSS Study, *Curr Atheroscler Rep* 4:319-325, 2002.

53. The EC-IC bypass study, *N Engl J Med* 317:1030-1032, 1987.

54. Craig DR, Meguro K, Watridge C, et al: Intracranial internal carotid artery stenosis, *Stroke* 13:825-828, 1982.

55. Marzewski DJ, Furlan AJ, St Louis P, et al: Intracranial internal carotid artery stenosis: Long-term prognosis, *Stroke* 13:821-824, 1982.

56. Gorter JW: Major bleeding during anticoagulation after cerebral ischemia: Patterns and risk factors. Stroke Prevention In Reversible Ischemia Trial (SPIRIT). European Atrial Fibrillation Trial (EAFT) study groups, *Neurology* 53:1319-1327, 1999.

57. Thijs VN, Albers GW: Symptomatic intracranial atherosclerosis: Outcome of patients who fail antithrombotic therapy, *Neurology* 55:490-497, 2000.

58. Akins PT, Pilgram TK, Cross DT III, Moran CJ: Natural history of stenosis from intracranial atherosclerosis by serial angiography, *Stroke* 29:433-438, 1998.

59. Callahan AS III, Berger BL, Beuter MJ, Devlin TG: Possible short-term amelioration of basilar plaque by high-dose atorvastatin: Use of reductase inhibitors for intracranial plaque stabilization, *J Neuroimaging* 11:202-204, 2001.

60. Ozgur HT, Kent Walsh T, Masaryk A, et al: Correlation of cerebrovascular reserve as measured by acetazolamide-challenged SPECT with angiographic flow patterns and intra- or extracranial arterial stenosis, *AJNR Am J Neuroradiol* 22:928-936, 2001.

61. Webster MW, Makaroun MS, Steed DL, et al: Compromised cerebral blood flow reactivity is a predictor of stroke in patients with symptomatic carotid artery occlusive disease, *J Vasc Surg* 21:338-345, 1995.

62. Yonas H, Pindzola RR, Meltzer CC, Sasser H: Qualitative versus quantitative assessment of cerebrovascular reserves, *Neurosurgery* 42:1005-1012, 1998.

63. Caplan LR, Hennerici M: Impaired clearance of emboli (washout) is an important link between hypoperfusion, embolism, and ischemic stroke, *Arch Neurol* 55:1475-1482, 1998.

64. Levy EI, Hanel RA, Bendok BR, et al: Staged stent-assisted angioplasty for symptomatic intracranial vertebrobasilar stenosis, *J Neurosurg* 97:1294-1301, 2002.

65. Levy EI, Hanel RA, Boulos AS, et al: Comparison of periprocedure complications resulting from direct stent placement compared with those due to conventional and staged stent placement in the basilar artery, *J Neurosurg* 99:653-660, 2003.

66. Clark WM, Barnwell SL, Nesbit G, et al: Safety and efficacy of percutaneous transluminal angioplasty for intracranial atherosclerotic stenosis, *Stroke* 26:1200-1204, 1995.

67. Higashida RT, Tsai FY, Halbach VV, et al: Interventional neurovascular techniques in the treatment of stroke—state-of-the-art therapy, *J Intern Med* 237:105-115, 1995.

68. Takis C, Kwan ES, Pessin MS, et al: Intracranial angioplasty: Experience and complications, *AJNR Am J Neuroradiol* 18:1661-1668, 1997.

69. Terada T, Higashida RT, Halbach VV, et al: Transluminal angioplasty for arteriosclerotic disease of the distal vertebral and basilar arteries, *J Neurol Neurosurg Psychiatry* 60:377-381, 1996.

70. Connors JJ III, Wojak JC: Percutaneous transluminal angioplasty for intracranial atherosclerotic lesions: Evolution of technique and short-term results, *J Neurosurg* 91:415-423, 1999.

71. Marks MP, Marcellus M, Norbash AM, et al: Outcome of angioplasty for atherosclerotic intracranial stenosis, *Stroke* 30:1065-1069, 1999.

72. Mori T, Fukuoka M, Kazita K, Mori K: Follow-up study after intracranial percutaneous transluminal cerebral balloon angioplasty, *AJNR Am J Neuroradiol* 19:1525-1533, 1998.

73. Nahser HC, Henkes H, Weber W, et al: Intracranial vertebrobasilar stenosis: Angioplasty and follow-up, *AJNR Am J Neuroradiol* 21:1293-1301, 2000.

74. Mori T, Kazita K, Mori K: Cerebral angioplasty and stenting for intracranial vertebral atherosclerotic stenosis, *AJNR Am J Neuroradiol* 20:787-789, 1999.

75. Mori T, Mori K, Fukuoka M, et al: Percutaneous transluminal cerebral angioplasty: Serial angiographic follow-up after successful dilatation, *Neuroradiology* 39:111-116, 1997.

76. George CJ, Baim DS, Brinker JA, et al: One-year follow-up of the Stent Restenosis (STRESS I) Study, *Am J Cardiol* 81:860-865, 1998.

77. Huang P, Levin T, Kabour A, Feldman T: Acute and late outcome after use of 2.5-mm intracoronary stents in small (< 2.5 mm) coronary arteries, *Catheter Cardiovasc Interv* 49:121-126, 2000.

78. Morice MC, Bradai R, Lefevre T, et al: Stenting small coronary arteries, *J Invasive Cardiol* 11:337-340, 1999.

79. Fiorella D, Woo HH: Emerging endovascular therapies for symptomatic intracranial atherosclerotic disease, *Stroke* 38:2391-2396, 2007.

80. Jiang WJ, Wang YJ, Du B, et al: Stenting of symptomatic M1 stenosis of middle cerebral artery: An initial experience of 40 patients, *Stroke* 35:1375-1380, 2004.

81. Kim JK, Ahn JY, Lee BH, et al: Elective stenting for symptomatic middle cerebral artery stenosis presenting as transient ischaemic deficits or stroke attacks: Short term arteriographical and clinical outcome, *J Neurol Neurosurg Psychiatry* 75:847-851, 2004.

82. Henkes H, Bose A, Felber S, et al: Endovascular coil occlusion of intracranial aneurysms assisted by a novel self-expandable nitinol microstent (Neuroform), *Interv Neuroradiol* 8:107-119, 2002.

83. Henkes H, Miloslavski E, Lowens S, et al: Treatment of intracranial atherosclerotic stenoses with balloon dilatation and self-expanding stent deployment (WingSpan), *Neuroradiology* 47:222-228, 2005.

84. Albuquerque FC, Levy EI, Turk AS, et al: Angiographic patterns of Wingspan in-stent restenosis, *Neurosurgery* 63:23-28, 2008.

85. Turk AS, Levy EI, Albuquerque FC, et al: Influence of patient age and stenosis location on Wingspan in-stent restenosis, *AJNR Am J Neuroradiol* 29:23-27, 2008.

86. Kurre W, Berkefeld J, Sitzer M, et al: Treatment of symptomatic high-grade intracranial stenoses with the balloon-expandable Pharos stent: Initial experience, *Neuroradiology* 50:701-708, 2008.

87. Freitas JM, Zenteno M, Aburto-Murrieta Y, et al: Intracranial arterial stenting for symptomatic stenoses: A Latin American experience, *Surg Neurol* 68:378-386, 2007.

88. Ramee SR, Dawson R, McKinley KL, et al: Provisional stenting for symptomatic intracranial stenosis using a multidisciplinary approach: Acute results, unexpected benefit, and one-year outcome, *Catheter Cardiovasc Interv* 52:457-467, 2001.

89. Lang J: *Clinical anatomy of brainstem vessels*, New Haven, CT, 1981, Miles Pharmaceutical.

90. North American Symptomatic Carotid Endarterectomy Trial Collaborators: Beneficial effect of carotid endarterectomy in symptomatic patients with high-grade carotid stenosis, *N Engl J Med* 325:445-453, 1991.

91. Barnett HJ, Taylor DW, Eliasziw M, et al: Benefit of carotid endarterectomy in patients with symptomatic moderate or severe stenosis. North American Symptomatic Carotid Endarterectomy Trial (NASCET) Collaborators, *N Engl J Med* 339:1415-1425, 1998.

92. Randomised trial of endarterectomy for recently symptomatic carotid stenosis: final results of the MRC European Carotid Surgery Trial (ECST), *Lancet* 351:1379-1387, 1998.

93. Asymptomatic Carotid Atherosclerosis Study Group: Study design for randomized prospective trial of carotid endarterectomy for asymptomatic atherosclerosis, *Stroke* 20:844-849, 1989.

94. Executive Committee for the Asymptomatic Carotid Atherosclerosis Study: Endarterectomy for asymptomatic carotid artery stenosis, *JAMA* 273:1421-1428, 1995.

95. Young B, Moore WS, Robertson JT, et al: An analysis of perioperative surgical mortality and morbidity in the asymptomatic carotid atherosclerosis study. ACAS Investigators. Asymptomatic Carotid Atherosclerosis Study, *Stroke* 27:2216-2224, 1996.

96. Hobson RWI, Weiss DG, Fields WS, et al: Efficacy of carotid endarterectomy for asymptomatic carotid stenosis (Veterans Affairs Cooperative Study Group), *N Engl J Med* 328:221-227, 1993.

97. Morgenstern LB, Fox AJ, Sharpe BL, et al: The risks and benefits of carotid endarterectomy in patients with near occlusion of the carotid artery. North American Symptomatic Carotid Endarterectomy Trial (NASCET) Group, *Neurology* 48:911-915, 1997.

98. Kappelle LJ, Eliasziw M, Fox AJ, et al: Importance of intracranial atherosclerotic disease in patients with symptomatic stenosis of the internal carotid artery. The North American Symptomatic Carotid Endarterectomy Trial, *Stroke* 30:282-286, 1999.

99. Paciaroni M, Eliasziw M, Kappelle LJ, et al: Medical complications associated with carotid endarterectomy. North American Symptomatic Carotid Endarterectomy Trial (NASCET), *Stroke* 30:1759-1763, 1999.

100. Gray WA, White HJ Jr, Barrett DM, et al: Carotid stenting and endarterectomy: A clinical and cost comparison of revascularization strategies, *Stroke* 33:1063-1070, 2002.

101. Wholey MH, Wholey M, Mathias K, et al: Global experience in cervical carotid artery stent placement, *Catheter Cardiovasc Interv* 50:160-167, 2000.

102. Roubin GS, Hobson RW II, White R, et al: CREST and CARESS to evaluate carotid stenting: time to get to work! *J Endovasc Ther* 8:107-110, 2001.

103. Roubin GS, New G, Iyer SS, et al: Immediate and late clinical outcomes of carotid artery stenting in patients with symptomatic and asymptomatic carotid stenosis: A 5-year prospective analysis, *Circulation* 103:532-537, 2001.

104. CAVATAS Investigators: Endovascular versus surgical treatment in patients with carotid stenosis in the Carotid and Vertebral Artery Transluminal Angioplasty Study (CAVATAS): A randomised trial, *Lancet* 357:1729-1737, 2001.

105. Alberts MJ: for the Publications Committee of WALLSTENT: Results of a multicenter prospective randomized trial of carotid artery stenting vs. carotid endarterectomy (abstract 53), *Stroke* 32:325, 2001.

106. Alberts MJ, McCann R, Smith TP, et al: for the Schneider Wallstent Endoprosthesis Clinical Investigators: A randomized trial of carotid stenting vs. endarterectomy in patients with symptomatic carotid stenosis: study design, *J Neurovasc Dis* 2:228-234, 1997.

107. Al-Mubarak N, Roubin GS, Vitek JJ, Iyer SS: Microembolization during carotid stenting with the distal-balloon antiemboli system, *Int Angiol* 21:344-348, 2002.

108. Angelini A, Reimers B, Della Barbera M, Cerebral protection during carotid artery stenting: Collection and histopathologic analysis of embolized debris, *Stroke* 33:456-461, 2002.

109. Kastrup A, Groschel K, Krapf H, et al: Early outcome of carotid angioplasty and stenting with and without cerebral protection devices: A systematic review of the literature, *Stroke* 34:813-819, 2003.

110. Kastrup A, Nagele T, Groschel K, et al: Incidence of new brain lesions after carotid stenting with and without cerebral protection, *Stroke* 37:2312-2316, 2006.

111. Theron JG, Payelle GG, Coskun O, et al: Carotid artery stenosis: treatment with protected balloon angioplasty and stent placement, *Radiology* 201:627-636, 1996.

112. Villalobos HJ, Harrigan MR, Lau T, et al: Advancements in carotid stenting leading to reductions in perioperative morbidity among patients 80 years and older, *Neurosurgery* 58:233-240, 2006.

113. CaRESS Steering Committee: Carotid Revascularization using Endarterectomy or Stenting Systems (CARESS): Phase I clinical trial, *J Endovasc Ther* 10:1021-1030, 2003.

114. CaRESS Steering Committee: Carotid Revascularization Using Endarterectomy or Stenting Systems (CaRESS) phase I clinical trial: 1-year results, *J Vasc Surg* 42:213-219, 2005.

115. Yadav JS, Wholey MH, Kuntz RE, et al: Protected carotid-artery stenting versus endarterectomy in high-risk patients, *N Engl J Med* 351:1493-1501, 2004.

116. Ringleb PA, Allenberg J, Bruckmann H, et al: 30 day results from the SPACE trial of stent-protected angioplasty versus carotid endarterectomy in symptomatic patients: a randomised non-inferiority trial, *Lancet* 368:1239-1247, 2006.

117. Mas JL, Chatellier G, Beyssen B, et al: Endarterectomy versus stenting in patients with symptomatic severe carotid stenosis, *N Engl J Med* 355:1660-1671, 2006.

118. Adami CA, Scuro A, Spinamano L, et al: Use of the Parodi antiembolism system in carotid stenting: Italian trial results, *J Endovasc Ther* 9:147-154, 2002.

119. Eckstein HH, Ringleb P, Allenberg JR, et al: Results of the Stent-Protected Angioplasty versus Carotid Endarterectomy (SPACE) study to treat symptomatic stenoses at 2 years: A multinational, prospective, randomised trial, *Lancet Neurol* 7:893-902, 2008.

120. Mas JL, Trinquart L, Leys D, et al: Endarterectomy Versus Angioplasty in Patients with Symptomatic Severe Carotid Stenosis (EVA-3S) trial: Results up to 4 years from a randomised, multicentre trial, *Lancet Neurol* 7:885-892, 2008.

121. Brott TG, Hobson RW 2nd, Howard G, et al: Stenting versus endarterectomy for treatment of carotid-artery stenosis, *N Engl J Med* 363:11-23, 2010.

122. Hobson RW II: CREST (Carotid Revascularization Endarterectomy versus Stent Trial): Background, design, and current status, *Semin Vasc Surg* 13:139-143, 2000.

123. Ederle J, Dobson J, Featherstone RL, et al: Carotid artery stenting compared with endarterectomy in patients with symptomatic carotid stenosis (International Carotid Stenting Study): An interim analysis of a randomised controlled trial, *Lancet* 375:985-997, 2010.

124. Phatouros CC, Higashida RT, Malek AM, et al: Endovascular treatment of noncarotid extracranial cerebrovascular disease, *Neurosurg Clin North Am* 11:331-350, 2000.

125. Wityk RJ, Chang HM, Rosengart A, et al: Proximal extracranial vertebral artery disease in the New England Medical Center Posterior Circulation Registry, *Arch Neurol* 55:470-478, 1998.

126. Caplan LR, Amarenco P, Rosengart A, et al: Embolism from vertebral artery origin occlusive disease, *Neurology* 42:1505-1512, 1992.

127. Gomez CR, Cruz-Flores S, Malkoff MD, et al: Isolated vertigo as a manifestation of vertebrobasilar ischemia, *Neurology* 47:94-97, 1996.

128. Rocha-Singh K: Vertebral artery stenting: Ready for prime time? *Catheter Cardiovasc Interv* 54:6-7, 2001.

129. Crawley F, Brown MM, Clifton AG: Angioplasty and stenting in the carotid and vertebral arteries, *Postgrad Med J* 74:7-10, 1998.

130. Drescher P, Katzen BT: Percutaneous treatment of symptomatic vertebral artery stenosis with coronary stents, *Catheter Cardiovasc Interv* 52:373-377, 2001.

131. Storey GS, Marks MP, Dake M, et al: Vertebral artery stenting following percutaneous transluminal angioplasty. Technical note, *J Neurosurg* 84:883-887, 1996.

132. Chastain HD II, Campbell MS, Iyer S, et al: Extracranial vertebral artery stent placement: in-hospital and follow-up results, *J Neurosurg* 91:547-552, 1999.

133. Higashida RT, Tsai FY, Halbach VV, et al: Transluminal angioplasty for atherosclerotic disease of the vertebral and basilar arteries, *J Neurosurg* 78:192-198, 1993.

134. Mukherjee D, Roffi M, Kapadia SR, et al: Percutaneous intervention for symptomatic vertebral artery stenosis using coronary stents, *J Invasive Cardiol* 13:363-366, 2001.

135. SSYLVIA Study Investigators: Stenting of Symptomatic Atherosclerotic Lesions in the Vertebral or Intracranial Arteries (SSYLVIA): Study results, *Stroke* 35:1388-1392, 2004.

136. Wehman JC, Hanel RA, Guidot CA, et al: Atherosclerotic occlusive extracranial vertebral artery disease: Indications for intervention, endovascular techniques, short-term and long-term results, *J Interv Cardiol* 17:219-232, 2004.

137. Contorni L: Il circolo collaterale vertebro-vertebrale nella obliterazione dell'arterio subclavia all sua origine, *Minerva Chir* 15: 268-271, 1960.

138. Fisher C: Editorial: A new vascular syndrome: "the subclavian steal.", *N Engl J Med* 265:912-913, 1961.

139. de Bray JM, Zenglein JP, Laroche JP, et al: Effect of subclavian syndrome on the basilar artery, *Acta Neurol Scand* 90:174-178, 1994.

140. Herring M: The subclavian steal syndrome: A review, *Am Surg* 43:220-228, 1977.

141. Piccone VA, Leveen HH: The subclavian steal syndrome, *Ann Thoracic Surg* 9:51-75, 1970.

142. Smith JM, Koury HI, Hafner CD, Welling RE: Subclavian steal syndrome. A review of 59 consecutive cases, *J Cardiovasc Surg (Torino)* 35:11-14, 1994.

143. Thomassen L, Aarli JA: Subclavian steal phenomenon. Clinical and hemodynamic aspects, *Acta Neurol Scand* 90:241-244, 1994.

144. Walker PM, Paley D, Harris KA, et al: What determines the symptoms associated with subclavian artery occlusive disease? *J Vasc Surg* 2:154-157, 1985.

145. Webster MW, Downs L, Yonas H, et al: The effect of arm exercise on regional cerebral blood flow in the subclavian steal syndrome, *Am J Surg* 168:91-93, 1994.

146. Fields WS, Lemak NA: Joint study of extracranial arterial occlusion. VII. Subclavian steal—a review of 168 cases, *JAMA* 222: 1139-1143, 1972.

147. Ackermann H, Diener HC, Seboldt H, Huth C: Ultrasonographic follow-up of subclavian stenosis and occlusion: natural history and surgical treatment, *Stroke* 19:431-435, 1988.

148. Drutman J, Gyorke A, Davis WL, Turski PA: Evaluation of subclavian steal with two-dimensional phase-contrast and two-dimensional time-of-flight MR angiography, *AJNR Am J Neuroradiol* 15:1642-1645, 1994.

149. AbuRahma AF, Robinson PA, Jennings TG: Carotid-subclavian bypass grafting with polytetrafluoroethylene grafts for symptomatic subclavian artery stenosis or occlusion: A 20-year experience, *J Vasc Surg* 32:411-419, 2000.

150. Beebe HG, Stark R, Johnson ML, et al: Choices of operation for subclavian-vertebral arterial disease, *Am J Surg* 139:616-623, 1980.

151. Deriu GP, Milite D, Verlato F, et al: Surgical treatment of atherosclerotic lesions of subclavian artery: Carotid-subclavian bypass versus subclavian-carotid transposition, *J Cardiovasc Surg (Torino)* 39:729-734, 1998.

152. Owens LV, Tinsley EA Jr, Criado E, et al: Extrathoracic reconstruction of arterial occlusive disease involving the supraaortic trunks, *J Vasc Surg* 22:217-222, 1995.

153. Bachman DM, Kim RM: Transluminal dilatation for subclavian steal syndrome, *AJR Am J Roentgenol* 135:995-996, 1980.

154. Taylor CL, Selman WR, Ratcheson RA: Steal affecting the central nervous system, *Neurosurgery* 50:679-689, 2002.

155. Bornstein NM, Norris JW: Subclavian steal: A harmless haemodynamic phenomenon? *Lancet* 2:303-305, 1986.

156. Moran KT, Zide RS, Persson AV, Jewell ER: Natural history of subclavian steal syndrome, *Am Surg* 54:643-644, 1988.

157. Hennerici M, Klemm C, Rautenberg W: The subclavian steal phenomenon: A common vascular disorder with rare neurologic deficits, *Neurology* 38:669-673, 1988.

158. Farina C, Mingoli A, Schultz RD, et al: Percutaneous transluminal angioplasty versus surgery for subclavian artery occlusive disease, *Am J Surg* 158:511-514, 1989.

159. Hebrang A, Maskovic J, Tomac B: Percutaneous transluminal angioplasty of the subclavian arteries: long-term results in 52 patients, *AJR Am J Roentgenol* 156:1091-1094, 1991.

160. Mathias KD, Luth I, Haarmann P: Percutaneous transluminal angioplasty of proximal subclavian artery occlusions, *Cardiovasc Interv Radiol* 16:214-218, 1993.

161. Motarjeme A, Keifer JW, Zuska AJ, Nabawi P: Percutaneous transluminal angioplasty for treatment of subclavian steal, *Radiology* 155:611-613, 1985.

162. Selby JB Jr, Matsumoto AH, Tegtmeyer CJ, et al: Balloon angioplasty above the aortic arch: immediate and long-term results, *AJR Am J Roentgenol* 160:631-635, 1993.

163. Kumar K, Dorros G, Bates MC, et al: Primary stent deployment in occlusive subclavian artery disease, *Cathet Cardiovasc Diagn* 34:281-285, 1995.

164. Queral LA, Criado FJ: The treatment of focal aortic arch branch lesions with Palmaz stents, *J Vasc Surg* 23:368-375, 1996.

165. Rodriguez-Lopez JA, Werner A, Martinez R, et al: Stenting for atherosclerotic occlusive disease of the subclavian artery, *Ann Vasc Surg* 13:254-260, 1999.

166. Sueoka BL: Percutaneous transluminal stent placement to treat subclavian steal syndrome, *J Vasc Interv Radiol* 7:351-356, 1996.

167. Bogey WM, Demasi RJ, Tripp MD, et al: Percutaneous transluminal angioplasty for subclavian artery stenosis, *Am Surg* 60:103-106, 1994.

168. Ringelstein EB, Zeumer H: Delayed reversal of vertebral artery blood flow following percutaneous transluminal angioplasty for subclavian steal syndrome, *Neuroradiology* 26:189-198, 1984.

169. Weir B: Unruptured intracranial aneurysms: A review, *J Neurosurg* 96:3-42, 2002.

170. Broderick JP, Brott T, Tomsick T, et al: Intracerebral hemorrhage more than twice as common as subarachnoid hemorrhage, *J Neurosurg* 78:188-191, 1993.

171. Kiyohara Y, Ueda K, Hasuo Y, et al: Incidence and prognosis of subarachnoid hemorrhage in a Japanese rural community, *Stroke* 20:1150-1155, 1989.

172. Sarti C, Tuomilehto J, Salomaa V, et al: Epidemiology of subarachnoid hemorrhage in Finland from 1983 to 1985, *Stroke* 22:848-853, 1991.

173. Mohr JP, Caplan LR, Melski JW, et al: The Harvard Cooperative Stroke Registry: A prospective registry, *Neurology* 28:754-762, 1978.

174. International Study of Unruptured Intracranial Aneurysms Investigators: Unruptured intracranial aneurysms—risk of rupture and risks of surgical intervention, *N Engl J Med* 339:1725-1733, 1998.

175. Qureshi AI, Suri MF, Yahia AM, et al: Risk factors for subarachnoid hemorrhage, *Neurosurgery* 49:607-613, 2001.

176. Bendok BR, Getch CC, Malisch TW, Batjer HH: Treatment of aneurysmal subarachnoid hemorrhage, *Semin Neurol* 18:521-531, 1998.

177. Malisch TW, Guglielmi G, Vinuela F, et al: Unruptured aneurysms presenting with mass effect symptoms: Response to endosaccular treatment with Guglielmi detachable coils. Part I. Symptoms of cranial nerve dysfunction, *J Neurosurg* 89:956-961, 1998.

178. Qureshi AI, Mohammad Y, Yahia AM, et al: Ischemic events associated with unruptured intracranial aneurysms: Multicenter clinical study and review of the literature, *Neurosurgery* 46:282-290, 2000.

179. Mayberg MR, Batjer HH, Dacey R, et al: Guidelines for the management of aneurysmal subarachnoid hemorrhage. A statement for healthcare professionals from a special writing group of the Stroke Council, American Heart Association, *Circulation* 90:2592-2605, 1994.

180. Juvela S: Rebleeding from ruptured intracranial aneurysms, *Surg Neurol* 32:323-326, 1989.

181. Molyneux A, Kerr R, Stratton I, et al: International Subarachnoid Aneurysm Trial (ISAT) of neurosurgical clipping versus endovascular coiling in 2143 patients with ruptured intracranial aneurysms: A randomised trial, *Lancet* 360:1267-1274, 2002.

182. Molyneux AJ, Kerr RS, Yu LM, et al: International Subarachnoid Aneurysm Trial (ISAT) of neurosurgical clipping versus endovascular coiling in 2143 patients with ruptured intracranial aneurysms: A randomised comparison of effects on survival, dependency, seizures, rebleeding, subgroups, and aneurysm occlusion, *Lancet* 366:809-817, 2005.

183. Biller J, Godersky JC, Adams HP Jr: Management of aneurysmal subarachnoid hemorrhage, *Stroke* 19:1300-1305, 1988.

184. Origitano TC, Reichman OH, Anderson DE: Prophylactic hypervolemia without calcium channel blockers in early aneurysm surgery, *Neurosurgery* 31:804-806, 1992.

185. Newell DW, Eskridge JM, Mayberg MR, et al: Angioplasty for the treatment of symptomatic vasospasm following subarachnoid hemorrhage, *J Neurosurg* 71:654-660, 1989.

186. Coskun E: Papaverine and vasospasm, *J Neurosurg* 96:973-974, 2002.

187. Morgan MK, Jonker B, Finfer S, et al: Aggressive management of aneurysmal subarachnoid haemorrhage based on a papaverine angioplasty protocol, *J Clin Neurosci* 7:305-308, 2000.

188. Ohkuma H, Ogane K, Tanaka M, Suzuki S: Assessment of cerebral microcirculatory changes during cerebral vasospasm by analyzing cerebral circulation time on DSA images, *Acta Neurochir Suppl* 77:127-130, 2001.

189. Turjman F, Massoud TF, Sayre J, Vinuela F: Predictors of aneurysmal occlusion in the period immediately after endovascular treatment with detachable coils: A multivariate analysis, *AJNR Am J Neuroradiol* 19:1645-1651, 1998.

190. Moret J, Cognard C, Weill A, et al: Reconstruction technic in the treatment of wide-neck intracranial aneurysms. Long-term angiographic and clinical results. Apropos of 56 cases, *J Neuroradiol* 24:30-44, 1997.

191. Lanzino G, Wakhloo AK, Fessler RD, et al: Efficacy and current limitations of intravascular stents for intracranial internal carotid, vertebral, and basilar artery aneurysms, *J Neurosurg* 91:538-546, 1999.

192. Mocco J, Snyder KV, Albuquerque FC, et al: Treatment of intracranial aneurysm with the Enterprise stent: A multicenter registry, *J Neurosurg* 110:35-39, 2009.

193. Cekirge HS, Saatci I, Geyik S, et al: Intrasaccular combination of metallic coils and onyx liquid embolic agent for the endovascular treatment of cerebral aneurysms, *J Neurosurg* 105:706-712, 2006.

194. Cekirge HS, Saatci I, Ozturk MH, et al: Late angiographic and clinical follow-up results of 100 consecutive aneurysms treated with Onyx reconstruction: Largest single-center experience, *Neuroradiology* 48:113-126, 2006.

195. Cloft HJ: HydroCoil for Endovascular Aneurysm Occlusion (HEAL) study: periprocedural results, *AJNR Am J Neuroradiol* 27:289-292, 2006.

196. Cloft HJ: HydroCoil for Endovascular Aneurysm Occlusion (HEAL) study: 3-6 month angiographic follow-up results, *AJNR Am J Neuroradiol* 28:152-154, 2007.

197. Fiorella D, Kelly ME, Albuquerque FC, Nelson PK: Curative reconstruction of a giant midbasilar trunk aneurysm with the Pipeline embolization device: Case report, *Neurosurgery* 64:212–217, 2009:discussion 217.

198. Murayama Y, Vinuela F, Ishii A, et al: Initial clinical experience with matrix detachable coils for the treatment of intracranial aneurysms, *J Neurosurg* 105:192–199, 2006.

199. Ogilvy CS, Stieg PE, Awad I, et al: AHA Scientific Statement: Recommendations for the management of intracranial arteriovenous malformations: A statement for healthcare professionals from a special writing group of the Stroke Council, American Stroke Association, *Stroke* 32:1458–1471, 2001.

200. Chiaradio JC, Guzman L, Padilla L, Chiaradio MP: Intravascular graft stent treatment of a ruptured fusiform dissecting aneurysm of the intracranial vertebral artery: Technical case report, *Neurosurgery* 50:213–217, 2002.

201. Fiorella D, Woo HH, Albuquerque FC, Nelson PK: Definitive reconstruction of circumferential, fusiform intracranial aneurysms with the Pipeline embolization device, *Neurosurgery* 62:1115–1121, 2008.

202. Michelson W: Natural history and pathophysiology of arteriovenous malformations, *Clin Neurosurg* 26:307–313, 1978.

203. Jessurun GA, Kamphuis DJ, van der Zande FH, Nossent JC: Cerebral arteriovenous malformations in The Netherlands Antilles. High prevalence of hereditary hemorrhagic telangiectasia-related single and multiple cerebral arteriovenous malformations, *Clin Neurol Neurosurg* 95:193–198, 1993.

204. Patterson J, McKossoch W: A clinical survey of intracranial angiomas with special reference to their mode of progression and surgical treatment: A report of 110 cases, *Brain* 79:233–266, 1956.

205. Lasjaunias P, Piske R, Terbrugge K, Willinsky R: Cerebral arteriovenous malformations (C. AVM) and associated arterial aneurysms (AA). Analysis of 101 C. AVM cases, with 37 AA in 23 patients, *Acta Neurochir* 91:29–36, 1988.

206. Spetzler RF, Martin NA: A proposed grading system for arteriovenous malformations, *J Neurosurg* 65:476–483, 1986.

207. Hartmann A, Pile-Spellman J, Stapf C, et al: Risk of endovascular treatment of brain arteriovenous malformations, *Stroke* 33:1816–1820, 2002.

208. Furlan AJ, Whisnant JP, Elveback LR: The decreasing incidence of primary intracerebral hemorrhage: A population study, *Ann Neurol* 5:367–373, 1979.

209. Brown RD Jr, Wiebers DO, Forbes G, et al: The natural history of unruptured intracranial arteriovenous malformations, *J Neurosurg* 68:352–357, 1988.

210. Fults D, Kelly DL Jr: Natural history of arteriovenous malformations of the brain: A clinical study, *Neurosurgery* 15:658–662, 1984.

211. Graf CJ, Perret GE, Torner JC: Bleeding from cerebral arteriovenous malformations as part of their natural history, *J Neurosurg* 58:331–337, 1983.

212. Ondra SL, Troupp H, George ED, Schwab K: The natural history of symptomatic arteriovenous malformations of the brain: A 24-year follow-up assessment, *J Neurosurg* 73:387–391, 1990.

213. Hartmann A, Mast H, Mohr JP, et al: Morbidity of intracranial hemorrhage in patients with cerebral arteriovenous malformation, *Stroke* 29:931–934, 1998.

214. Kondziolka D, McLaughlin MR, Kestle JR: Simple risk predictions for arteriovenous malformation hemorrhage, *Neurosurgery* 37:851–855, 1995.

215. Hartmann A, Mast H, Choi JH, et al: Treatment of arteriovenous malformations of the brain, *Curr Neurol Neurosci Rep* 7:28–34, 2007.

216. Forster DM, Steiner L, Hakanson S: Arteriovenous malformations of the brain. A long-term clinical study, *J Neurosurg* 37:562–570, 1972.

217. Kader A, Young WL, Pile-Spellman J, et al: The influence of hemodynamic and anatomic factors on hemorrhage from cerebral arteriovenous malformations, *Neurosurgery* 34:801–808, 1994.

218. Miyasaka Y, Yada K, Ohwada T, et al: An analysis of the venous drainage system as a factor in hemorrhage from arteriovenous malformations, *J Neurosurg* 76:239–243, 1992.

219. Heros RC, Korosue K, Diebold PM: Surgical excision of cerebral arteriovenous malformations: late results, *Neurosurgery* 26:570–578, 1990.

220. Jafar JJ, Davis AJ, Berenstein A, et al: The effect of embolization with *N*-butyl cyanoacrylate prior to surgical resection of cerebral arteriovenous malformations, *J Neurosurg* 78:60–69, 1993.

221. Spetzler RF, Wilson CB, Weinstein P, et al: Normal perfusion pressure breakthrough theory, *Clin Neurosurg* 25:651–672, 1978.

222. Pollock BE, Lunsford LD, Flickinger JC, Kondziolka D: The role of embolization in combination with stereotactic radiosurgery in the management of pial and dural arteriovenous malformations. In Connors JJ, Wojak JC, editors: *Interventional Neuroradiology.*, Philadelphia, 1999, WB Saunders, pp 267–275.

223. Fournier D, TerBrugge KG, Willinsky R, et al: Endovascular treatment of intracerebral arteriovenous malformations: experience in 49 cases, *J Neurosurg* 75:228–233, 1991.

224. Gobin YP, Laurent A, Merienne L, et al: Treatment of brain arteriovenous malformations by embolization and radiosurgery, *J Neurosurg* 85:19–28, 1996.

225. Vinuela F, Dion JE, Duckwiler G, et al: Combined endovascular embolization and surgery in the management of cerebral arteriovenous malformations: Experience with 101 cases, *J Neurosurg* 75:856–864, 1991.

226. Jahan R, Murayama Y, Gobin YP, et al: Embolization of arteriovenous malformations with Onyx: clinicopathological experience in 23 patients, *Neurosurgery* 48:984–997, 2001.

227. Song DL, Leng B, Xu B, et al: Clinical experience of 70 cases of cerebral arteriovenous malformations embolization with Onyx, a novel liquid embolic agent, *Zhonghua Wai Ke Za Zhi* 45:223–225, 2007.

228. van Rooij WJ, Sluzewski M, Beute GN: Brain AVM embolization with Onyx, *AJNR Am J Neuroradiol* 28:172–178, 2007.

229. Weber W, Kis B, Siekmann R, Kuehne D: Endovascular treatment of intracranial arteriovenous malformations with Onyx: Technical aspects, *AJNR Am J Neuroradiol* 28:371–377, 2007.

62 Intraarterial Thrombolysis in Acute Ischemic Stroke

ANTHONY J. FURLAN, JITENDRA SHARMA, RANDALL HIGASHIDA

In the 1980s, several reports of intraarterial thrombolysis (IAT) as therapy for acute ischemic stroke were published.[1-3] The thrombolytic agents used in these early series were urokinase (UK) and streptokinase (SK). Two decades later, advances in technique and microcatheter technology now allow superselective catheterization of even distal branches of occluded intracranial vessels. Importantly, rapid technical advances have prompted the Accreditation Council for Graduate Medical Education[4] (ACGME) to standardize the training curricula in endovascular surgical neuroradiology (i.e., interventional neuroradiology) for neuroradiologists, neurosurgeons, and neurologists.

Studies of IAT for acute ischemic stroke were initially limited to uncontrolled protocols.[5,6] There was great variability in technique, and efficacy and complication rates varied among the reported series. As a result, in 1996, an American Heart Association (AHA) Special Writing Group published its recommendations for the use of thrombolytic agents in acute ischemic stroke. On the basis of the strength of the scientific evidence available at that time, the Group concluded that IAT "should be considered investigational and only used in the clinical trial setting," recommending "further testing of" IAT.[7]

Subsequently, the results of the first randomized multicenter controlled trials of IAT, the Prolyse in Acute Cerebral Thromboembolism trials, PROACT I[8] and PROACT II,[9] were reported in 1998 and 1999, respectively. PROACT II remains the only randomized, controlled, multicenter clinical trial to demonstrate the efficacy of IAT in patients with acute ischemic stroke of less than 6 hours' duration due to occlusion of the middle cerebral artery (MCA).

Nonetheless, the U.S. Food and Drug Administration (FDA) has approved two stroke thrombectomy devices, and there is evidence that stroke IAT is being done routinely at most comprehensive stroke centers worldwide.

General Technique of Intraarterial Thrombolysis

In patients with appropriate clinical and CT criteria, a complete four-vessel cerebral angiogram should be performed from a transfemoral approach to evaluate the site of vessel occlusion, the extent of thrombus, the number of territories involved, and the collateral circulation. In this procedure, a diagnostic catheter is guided into the high cervical segment of the vascular territory to be treated, followed by the introduction of a 2.3F coaxial microcatheter with a steerable microguidewire. Under direct fluoroscopic visualization, the microcatheter is gently navigated through the intracranial circulation until the tip is embedded within or through the central portion of the thrombus (Fig. 62-1).

Many variations in catheter design and delivery technique have been described.[10] Two types of microcatheters are being used most often for local cerebral thrombolysis, depending on the extent of clot formation. For the majority of intraarterial procedures, a single–end hole microcatheter is used, whereas for longer segments of clot formation, a microcatheter with multiple side holes is used. Superselective angiography through the microcatheter is performed at regular intervals to assess for extent of clot lysis and to adjust the dosage and volume of the thrombolytic agent.

A superselective angiogram is performed, and if the clot is seen to be partially dissolved, the catheter is advanced into the remaining thrombus, where additional thrombolysis is performed. As the thrombus is dissolved, the catheter is advanced into more distal branches of the intracranial circulation, so that most of the thrombolytic agent enters the occluded vessel and is not washed preferentially into adjacent open blood vessels. The goal is to achieve rapid recanalization with as little thrombolytic agent as possible so as to limit the extent of brain infarction and reduce the risk of hemorrhage. Common experience shows, however, that it can take up to 2 hours to achieve recanalization after the procedure begins, that thrombolytic agents alone (i.e., without mechanical manipulation) rarely achieve recanalization in less than 30 minutes, and that recanalization is often incomplete. Among other factors, clot composition plays a key role in the rapidity and extent of recanalization achieved with IAT.

Thrombolytic Agents

Recombinant pro-urokinase (r-proUK), the thrombolytic agent used in PROACT II (see later), is currently not approved by the FDA and is not yet commercially available. Although some thrombolytic agents have theoretical advantages over others, there is no proof that one thrombolytic agent is superior to another in terms of safety, recanalization rate, or clinical efficacy in acute ischemic

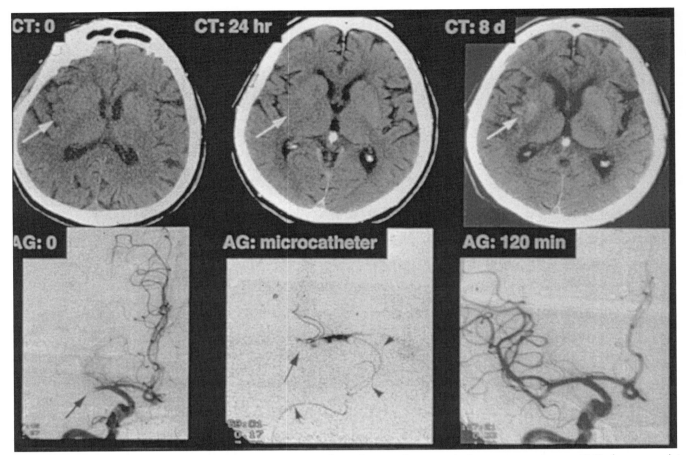

Figure 62-1 Intraarterial thrombolysis, with 9 mg r-proUK, 5.5 hours from stroke onset. A, Diagnostic angiogram (AG) shows complete Thrombolysis in Acute Myocardial Infarction (TIMI) 0 occlusion of the M1 middle cerebral artery; minimal early infarct signs on baseline CT. B, Tip of the microcatheter embedded within proximal thrombus. Partial clot lysis after 1-hour infusion. C, Complete TIMI 3 recanalization at 2 hours. 24-hour CT scan shows minimal infarction. 8-day CT scan shows slight asymptomatic hemorrhagic conversion. (From Furlan A, Higashida R, Wechsler L, et al: Intra-arterial prourokinase for acute ischemic stroke: The PROACT II Study: A randomized controlled trial. *JAMA* 282:2003-2011, 1999.)

stroke. Therefore it is not clear whether the results of PROACT II are applicable when agents other than r-proUK are used for IAT. Commercially available agents include urokinase (UK), tissue-type plasminogen activator (t-PA), reteplase (recombinant t-PA [rt-PA]), and tenecteplase (tNKase). These thrombolytic agents differ in stability, half-life, and fibrin selectivity. UK is not fibrin selective and therefore can cause systemic hypofibrinoginemia. Both t-PA and r-proUK are fibrin selective and are active only at the site of thrombosis. However, r-proUK requires heparin for maximal thrombolytic effect. Newer agents have long half-lives, allowing bolus administration, such as rt-PA, or are more fibrin selective, such as tenecteplase. However, the efficacy of second- and third-generation thrombolytic agents in acute ischemic stroke has not been demonstrated in a randomized controlled trial (RCT).[11]

Adjunctive Therapy

Intravenous (IV) heparin is given by most neurointerventionists during IAT for stroke. Systemic anticoagulation with heparin reduces the risk of catheter-related embolism. Also, the thrombolytic effect of some agents, such as r-proUK, is augmented by heparin. Another rationale for antithrombotic therapy is prevention of early reocclusion, which is probably more common with atherothrombosis than with cerebral embolism. These indications are counterbalanced by the higher risk of brain hemorrhage when heparin is combined with a thrombolytic agent.

The optimal dose of heparin during IAT for stroke has not been established. The PROACT I investigators reported a 27% rate of symptomatic brain hemorrhage when a conventional non–weight-adjusted heparin regimen (100 U/kg bolus followed by 1000 U/h for 4 hours) was used with intraarterial (IA) r-proUK.[8] Subsequently, a low-dose heparin regimen (2000 U bolus followed by 500 U/h for 4 hours) was used with IA r-proUK, which reduced the rate of symptomatic brain hemorrhage to 7% in PROACT I and 10% in PROACT II. Unfortunately, the use of low-dose heparin therapy with IA r-proUK also cut the recanalization rate to half that for the original heparin regimen. Some neurointerventionists now employ the PROACT low-dose heparin regimen during IAT. However, this dose of heparin does not prolong the activated partial thromboplastin time (APTT) or activated clotting time (ACT). Other neurointerventionists employ weight-adjusted heparin dosage, keeping the activated clotting time between 200 and 300 seconds.

The safety and efficacy of platelet glycoprotein (GP) IIb/IIIa inhibitor agents in patients with acute ischemic stroke undergoing IAT are unclear. Coronary doses of IV abciximab appear to be relatively safe in patients with acute ischemic stroke.[12] The risk of brain hemorrhage with the use of combined GP IIb/IIIa inhibitors and reduced-dose thrombolytic agents may be higher in patients older than 75 years.[13] The GP IIb/IIIa inhibitors abciximab and eptifibatide improve the efficacy of acute coronary interventions and have been used in patients undergoing cerebrovascular interventions.[14-16] The GP IIb/IIIa inhibitor dose can be adjusted to keep the platelet inhibition value between 50% and 80% during the intervention through monitoring of the platelet activation units (PAU). However, GP IIb/IIIa inhibitors are not routinely employed during IAT for stroke. Adjunctive use of GP IIb/IIIa inhibition should be considered when the risk of acute reocclusion and endothelial injury is high, as in angioplasty and stenting for basilar artery atherothrombosis. Concomitant use of clopidogrel and aspirin is usually avoided in acute stroke interventions because of the risk of brain hemorrhage.

The Prolyse in Acute Cerebral Thromboembolism Trials

Beginning in February 1994, patients were enrolled in the first placebo-controlled, double-blind multicenter trial of IAT in acute ischemic stroke, PROACT I.[8] The results were published in 1998. The thrombolytic agent used in PROACT I was recombinant prourokinase (r-proUK), which is not yet commercially available. This agent is a recombinant, single-chain zymogen of an endogenous fibrinolytic, either UK or urokinase-type plasminogen activator (u-PA).[17] Infusion of r-proUK does not lead to systemic dysfibrinogenemia with its associated higher risk of hemorrhagic side effects. Another clinically relevant characteristic of r-proUK is the facilitatory effect of coadministered heparin, which when given with r-proUK improves its fibrinolytic efficacy.

In PROACT I, the safety and recanalization efficacy of 6 mg r-proUK given IA were compared with that of IA administration of saline placebo in 40 patients with acute ischemic stroke of less than 6 hours' duration that was due to MCA occlusion. Only patients in whom diagnostic cerebral angiography showed Thrombolysis in Acute Myocardial Infarction (TIMI) grade 0 or grade 1 occlusion of the M1 or M2 segment of the MCA were included. Another major inclusion criterion was a minimum National Institutes of Health Stroke Scale (NIHSS) score of 4 (except for isolated aphasia or hemianopsia) and a maximum score of 30. Major exclusion criteria were uncontrolled hypertension (blood pressure >180 mm Hg systolic/100 mm Hg diastolic), a history of hemorrhage, and recent surgery or trauma. CT evidence of early ischemic changes was not an exclusion criterion. Mechanical disruption of the clot was not permitted because the goal of the trial was to demonstrate the efficacy and safety of r-proUK. Patients also received IV heparin. The first 16 patients received the "high-dose" heparin regimen already mentioned. It consisted of a bolus of 100 IU/kg followed by a 1000 IU/h

infusion for 4 hours; anticoagulation was prohibited for the following 24 hours. On the basis of a recommendation from the external safety committee, the heparin regimen was changed after the first 16 patients to a 2000 IU bolus followed by a 500 IU/h infusion for 4 hours.

The recanalization rate was 57.7% in the r-proUK group and only 14.3% in the placebo group. In the "high-dose heparin" group receiving r-proUK, the recanalization rate was 81.8%, but the rate of symptomatic intracranial hemorrhage (ICH) was 27%. In contrast, the patients receiving r-proUK and "low-dose heparin" had a recanalization rate of 40%, but the ICH rate was only 6%. Overall, symptomatic ICH occurred in 15.4% of patients receiving treatment and in 14.3% of patients receiving placebo. Although PROACT I was not a clinical efficacy trial, there appeared to be a 10% to 12% higher rate of excellent outcomes in the IA r-proUK group than in the control group.

The follow-up clinical efficacy trial, PROACT II, was launched in February 1996, and the results were published in December 1999.[9] PROACT II was a randomized, controlled, multicenter trial but differed from PROACT I in that it employed open-label design with blinded follow-up. Patient selection was essentially the same as in PROACT I, with the major exception that patients with early signs of infarction in more than one third of the MCA territory (the so-called ECASS [European Cooperative Acute Stroke Study] CT criterion)[18] on the initial CT scan were excluded. Additionally, a dose of 9 mg r-proUK was used instead of 6 mg, and "low-dose heparin" was given to both the treatment and control groups. A total of 180 patients were randomly assigned to receive either 9 mg of IA r-proUK plus low-dose IV heparin or low-dose IV heparin alone. Baseline stroke severity in the PROACT II patients was very high, with a median NIHSS score of 17. The median time from onset of symptoms to initiation of IAT was 5.3 hours.

The primary outcome measure was the proportion of patients who achieved a modified Rankin Scale score of 2 or less at 90 days, which signifies slight or no neurologic disability. For the group treated with r-proUK, there was a 15% absolute benefit ($P = .043$). The benefit was most noticeable in patients with a baseline NIHSS score between 11 and 20. On average, seven patients with MCA occlusion would require IAT for one of them to benefit. Recanalization rates were 66% at 2 hours for the treatment group and 18% for the placebo group ($P < .001$). Symptomatic brain hemorrhage occurred in 10% of the r-proUK group and 2% of the control group. Considering the later time to treatment and greater baseline stroke severity in PROACT II, the symptomatic brain hemorrhage rate compared favorably with that in the IV t-PA trials (6% in National Institutes of Neurological Disease and Stroke [NINDS],[19] 9% in ECASS,[18] and 7% in Alteplase Thrombolysis for Acute Noninterventional Therapy in Ischemic Stroke [ATLANTIS]).[20] As in the NINDS trial, patients in PROACT II benefited overall from therapy despite the higher rate of brain hemorrhage, and there was no excess mortality (r-proUK, 24%; control, 27%). Despite these results, r-proUK did not receive FDA approval. However, PROACT II did establish the proof of the principle of IAT and also demonstrated its clinical efficacy up to 6 hours after stroke onset.

Middle Cerebral Artery Embolism Local Fibrinolytic Intervention Trial

The Middle Cerebral Artery Embolism Local Fibrinolytic Intervention Trial (MELT) was a multicenter, randomized trial conducted at 57 centers in Japan (2002 to 2005) to evaluate the safety and efficacy of intraarterial UK to treat patients with MCA occlusion of less than 6 hours' duration.[21] Inclusion criteria were similar to those for PROACT II: age 20 to 75 years, MCA territory stroke within 6 hours from onset, baseline NIHSS score 5 or higher, and CT findings normal or showing only subtle signs of acute stroke in MCA territory. Angiographic inclusion criteria were complete occlusion of the M1 or M2 division of the MCA. Exclusion criteria included NIHSS score higher than 22, baseline modified Rankin Scale (mRS) score higher than 2, patients with high risk of hemorrhagic complication (platelet count < 100,000/mm³, heparin started within 48 hours, International Normalized Ratio [INR] > 1.7), history of head trauma or intracranial hemorrhage, history of stroke in last 3 months, and recent surgery or history of intracranial neoplasm. Clinical outcome was assessed at 7, 30, and 90 days by means of NIHSS, Barthel Index, and mRS. The primary outcome of MELT was favorable outcome at 90 days (mRS ≤ 2). Secondary outcomes were intracranial hemorrhage within 24 hours after start of treatment, death within 90 days, rate of recanalization, NIHSS scores of 0 and 1 at 24 hours, 30 days, and 90 days, Barthel Index more than 95, and mRS score less than 2 at 30 days and 90 days.

MELT was stopped prematurely after approval of intravenous tissue plasminogen activator for stroke in Japan. At the time of discontinuation, 114 patients had been randomly assigned to treatment groups (mean age 66.9 versus 64.90 years, median NIHSS score 14 both arms). A nonsignificant improvement in clinical outcome (mRS score ≤ 2 at 90 days) was seen in the treatment arm over that in the control arm (49.1% and 38.6%, respectively; odds ratio [OR], 1.54; 95% confidence interval [CI], 0.73–3.23; $P = .345$; 73.7% of the patients (42/57) in the treatment arm had partial to complete recanalization. The rate of excellent functional outcome (mRS score ≤ 1 at 90 days) was greater in the treatment arm than in the control arm (41% and 22.8%, respectively; OR, 2.46; 95% CI, 1.09–5.54; $P = .045$). The 90-day mortality rates were 5.3% in the treatment group and 3.5% in the control arm ($P = 1.000$). The rates of intracerebral hemorrhage within 24 hours were 9% in the treatment group and 2% in the control group ($P = .206$).

MELT was not able to show significant results possibly because of early termination of the trial but did suggest better clinical outcome at 90 days (mRS < 1). A meta-analysis that compared PROACT II and MELT showed that the two trials were comparable with slight differences in baseline clinical data (NIHSS scores 14 versus 17; CT signs of early infarct in 47% versus 76%) and time to initiation of therapy (3.8 versus 5.3 hours). MELT prohibited mechanical clot disruption except with the guidewire, but PROACT II allowed only chemical thrombolysis. The earlier start of IAT in MELT was one reason the recanalization rate was better in that trial than in PROACT II (73.7% versus 66%). The rates of intracranial hemorrhages were very similar in the two trials (9% for MELT versus 10% for PROACT II).

Mechanical Thrombectomy in Acute Stroke

Mechanical thrombectomy has become a new treatment option for strokes due to large vessel occlusion. Previous studies have shown that thrombus in large vessels is refractory to intravenous and intraarterial plasminogen activators.[9,19,22,23] Later studies have shown that mechanical thrombectomy can improve recanalization rates, which are associated with better clinical outcomes.[24-26]

The Mechanical Embolus Removal in Cerebral Ischemia and Multi MERCI Trials

The Merci retrieval system (Concentric Medical, Mountain View, Calif) consists of the Merci retriever, the Merci balloon guide catheter, and the Merci microcatheter. In 2004 the Merci retriever was the first device approved by the FDA as a mechanical thrombectomy device to remove clot in patients with acute ischemic stroke. The inclusion criteria specified that the Merci devices were for use in patients who were ineligible for intravenous t-PA or in whom it failed and that the devices could be used up to 8 hours from stroke onset.

The Mechanical Embolus Removal in Cerebral Ischemia (MERCI) trial[25] was a two-part multicenter nonrandomized trial designed to evaluate the safety and efficacy of the Merci retriever device. MERCI part 1[26] enrolled 30 patients in 7 U.S. centers with a baseline NIHSS score of 10 or higher and with stroke presentation more than 3 hours but within 8 hours of symptom onset or within 3 hours but with contraindications to IV thrombolysis. Patients were selected for treatment with the Merci device if brain CT showed early signs of infarction in less than one third of the MCA territory and diagnostic angiography showed an occlusion of the internal carotid artery, M1 segment of the middle cerebral artery, basilar artery, or vertebral artery. Twenty-eight patients were treated, and successful recanalization was achieved in 12 (43%) with mechanical thrombectomy alone and in 18 (64%) when additional intraarterial tissue plasminogen activator was used. At the 30-day evaluation, 50% (9/18) of patients with successful recanalization had made a significant recovery, defined as an mRS score less than 3. There was one procedure-related technical complication with no clinical consequences and 12 (43%) asymptomatic hemorrhages. MERCI part 1 demonstrated that the Merci retrieval system is safe and efficacious for clot removal within 8 hours of stroke symptom onset and suggested that recanalization is associated with improved clinical outcomes.[27]

MERCI part 2[25] was a single-arm prospective multicenter study that evaluated the safety and efficacy of mechanical thrombectomy within 8 hours of acute ischemic stroke onset. It was conducted at 25 centers between May 2001 and December 2003 and enrolled 151 patients. The inclusion criteria were similar to those for MERCI part 1. The primary outcomes for this study were the rates of vascular recanalization and device-related complications. Successful recanalization was defined as TIMI grades 2 and 3 flow assessed immediately after the treatment.

The device was deployed in 141 patients, and recanalization was achieved in 46% (69/151) on intention to treat analysis and in 48% (68/141) in whom the device was actually deployed. Ten patients (7.1%) had clinically significant complications, and symptomatic intracranial hemorrhage occurred in 7.8% (11/141). Although better clinical outcome (mRS score ≤ 2) was seen in patients with successful recanalization, the overall 90-day clinical efficacy for MERCI, reported as 27.7%, was similar to that for placebo in PROACT II, and the mortality rate for MERCI, reported as 43.5%, was higher than that in PROACT II.

The Multi MERCI trial[27] was designed to evaluate the safety and efficacy of a newer-generation thrombectomy device (L5 retriever) and to gain more experience with the first-generation Merci retrievers (X5 and X6). The inclusion criteria for the Multi MERCI trial were the same as those for MERCI, except that patients were also included if IV t-PA within 3 hours of stroke onset failed to open an intracranial large vessel occlusion confirmed by diagnostic angiography. Multi MERCI enrolled 177 patients, and a device was deployed in 164 patients; 131/164 patients were treated with the newer L5 retriever. The mean age was 68 ± 16 years, and the median baseline NIHSS score was 19 (15 to 23). The occlusion sites were internal carotid artery/terminus in 32% of patients, the MCA in 60%, and the posterior circulation in 8%. Forty-eight patients (29.3%) received IV rt-PA before intervention, 11 patients received GP IIB/IIIa antagonists, and 14 received IA thrombolytics before or during mechanical thrombectomy. A 57.3% recanalization rate (75/131) was achieved with the retriever alone; the recanalization rate improved to 69.5% (91/131) with adjunctive IAT. A better recanalization rate was observed with the newer device (57.3%; 75/131) than with the older X5/X6 devices (45.5%; 15/33), but this difference did not reach statistical significance. Favorable outcome (mRS ≤ 2) was seen in 36% of patients, and the mortality rate was 34%. Both outcomes were significantly related to vascular recanalization. Symptomatic intracranial hemorrhage occurred in 16 patients (9.8%), and procedural-related complications occurred in 9 (5.5%) patients.

The Multi MERCI trial showed that the newer device is safe and able to achieve somewhat better recanalization rates. Like MERCI, the Multi MERCI results suggested better outcomes in patients in whom recanalization was achieved. This study also suggested that mechanical thrombectomy after unsuccessful IV rt-PA (so-called rescue IA thrombectomy) is safe.

The Penumbra System

The Penumbra System (Penumbra, Inc., Alameda, CA) is a later-generation device designed to remove clot from large vessels in acute stroke settings.[28] It consists of a reperfusion catheter, a separator, and a thrombus removal ring. The device removes clot by using an aspiration and extraction technique. If any residual thrombus is seen in the vessel after aspiration, a thrombus removal ring is used to remove residual thrombus.

The first study to evaluate the safety and efficacy of the Penumbra System was a prospective multicenter, single-arm study that enrolled 23 patients from seven international centers.[28] The primary endpoint of this study was the ability of the system to recanalize the affected vessel to TIMI grade 2 or higher within 8 hours of stroke onset. A secondary endpoint was clinical outcome 30 days after the procedure using an mRS score or 2 or less or a 4-point improvement in NIHSS score. The inclusion and exclusion criteria were similar to those for the Multi MERCI trial. The Penumbra System was used to treat 21 target vessels in 20 patients. The baseline mean age was 60 years, and the baseline mean NIHSS score was 21. Recanalization was achieved in all treated vessels. At 30-day follow-up, 45% of patients showed improvement in NIHSS score by at least 4 points or an mRS score of 2 or less. The mortality rate was 45%; 70% of deceased patients had a baseline NIHSS score higher than 20 or a basilar artery occlusion. This study demonstrated that the Penumbra System can open large vessel occlusions in acute stroke.

This study was followed by a larger prospective single-arm multicenter trial to further assess the safety and efficacy of the Penumbra System.[29] The baseline mean age was 63.5 years, and the mean NIHSS score was 17.6. The study enrolled 125 patients, and 125 target vessels were treated with the device. The recanalization rate was 81.6%, and the procedural complication rate was 12.8%. Intracranial hemorrhage was seen on 24-hour CT in 28% (35 patients), of which 11.2% (14) were symptomatic. The rate of 90-day mRS of 2 or less was 25%, and the mortality rate was 32.8%. At discharge, 41.6% of patients had good clinical outcome as defined by improvement in NIHSS score by at least 4 points or mRS score of 2 or less at 30-day follow-up. This study further confirmed the safety and efficacy of use of the Penumbra System in acute stroke and led to FDA and Center for Medicaid and Medicare Services (CMS) approval for its clinical use.[29]

Indications for and Drawbacks of Mechanical Thrombectomy

Mechanical thrombectomy can be used in patients with acute stroke who are ineligible for IV or IA chemical thrombolytics, such as patients with recent surgery or other significant risk for hemorrhage. The MERCI trials included patients who were undergoing anticoagulation as long as the INR value was less than 3, the partial thromboplastin time (PTT) was less than 2 times that of controls, and the platelet count was higher than 30,000/mm³. Mechanical thrombectomy can also be used in combination with IV or IA therapy.

The disadvantages of using mechanical thrombectomy include limited access to trained neurointerventionalists, technical difficulty with the navigating wire in delicate intracranial vessels, trauma to vessels, distal embolization, vessel dissection and vasospasm leading to worsening of stroke.

The MERCI, Multi MERCI, and Penumbra studies were able to show that mechanical embolectomy can be effectively and safely used within 8 hours of stroke symptom onset as alternative treatment options for patients who are ineligible for thrombolytics. Because there were no randomized control groups, none of the trials was able to conclusively show that mechanical thrombectomy actually improves stroke clinical outcomes. Despite these limitations, the Merci retriever received approval from both the FDA and the CMS for clot removal up to 8 hours from acute stroke onset.[30]

Ongoing RCTs, including the Interventional Management of Stroke Study III (IMS3) and the Mechanical Retrieval and Recanalization of Stroke Clots Using Embolectomy (MR RESCUE) study, will help answer questions regarding patient selection, comparative efficacy, and clinical outcomes for mechanical thrombectomy and IAT in patients with acute stroke.[31]

Drawbacks of Intraarterial Thrombolysis

Access to facilities and a team of physicians (an interventionist and tertiary stroke team) capable of performing IAT is a limitation to the use of this procedure. Such expertise is not readily available in many developing countries or in communities across the United States, usually being limited to large academic centers. Treatment delays are also inherent to IAT. In PROACT II, the median time from stroke onset to drug infusion was 5.3 hours, and the average time from the patient's arrival at the hospital to the initiation of IA r-proUK was 3 hours. IAT also involves costs and procedural risks not inherent to IV thrombolysis (IVT). However, serious procedural complications were uncommon in PROACT I and II; also, in experienced centers, cerebral angiography is associated with a morbidity of only 1.4% and with rates of permanent complications and death of 0.1% and 0.02%, respectively.[32]

Intraarterial versus Intravenous Thrombolysis

IVT has the important advantages of speed, ease of administration, and widespread availability. Its efficiency is limited, however, by a number of factors. Intravenous thrombolytics achieve arterial recanalization in about 40% of patients. The recanalization rate may decrease with time owing to thrombus formation and growth, as in the proportion of patients with major stroke who have salvageable brain. ECASS I and II excluded patients with extended ischemic edema exceeding one third of the MCA territory.[17,33] In the IVT trials, vascular imaging studies were not performed, so neither the sites of arterial occlusion nor the recanalization rates are known. Patients with ischemic stroke of less than 6 hours' duration have a wide variety of occlusion sites, and 20% have no visible occlusion, despite similar neurologic presentations.[34] Hence, the study populations in the IVT trials were relatively heterogeneous.

Although there have been no randomized studies comparing recanalization rates with outcomes for IVT and IAT, recanalization rates for cerebrovascular occlusions average 70% for IAT and 34% for IVT.[35] These differences in recanalization rates are most apparent with occlusions of large vessels, such as the internal carotid artery (ICA)—which is the vessel most resistant to thrombolysis—the carotid T segment, and the proximal (M1) segment of the MCA.

The greater recanalization efficacy for large vessel occlusions may help explain why the time window for successful IAT may be longer than that for IVT. On the basis of PROACT II, a 6-hour window appears to be a realistic goal for IAT in anterior circulation ischemia. For stroke in the vertebrobasilar circulation, there are some reports of successful therapy up to 48 hours after onset (see later).[3,36] The factors that determine individual susceptibility to ischemia are not completely understood, and there is clearly a great deal of variability in time from onset to irreversible damage among individuals. Even though a longer time window may be offered by IAT, it is critical to understand that urgency is paramount in ischemic stroke intervention and that the earlier recanalization is achieved with either IVT or IAT, the better the neurologic outcome.

IAT may be safer than IVT in patients with an excessive bleeding risk. Katzan et al[37] reported the use of IAT in six patients with acute stroke after open heart surgery. Although this was only a small series, perioperative IAT appeared relatively safe, because only one minor bleeding complication occurred.

There are other special situations in which IAT can be employed. Both Weber et al[38] and Padolecchia et al[39] showed the safety and efficacy of superselective IAT in cases of central retinal artery occlusion. Both studies reported significant improvements in visual acuity with no hemorrhagic complications. In the series reported by Weber et al,[38] 17.6% of patients recovered completely, a rate that is better than that in historical controls.

Combined Intravenous and Intraarterial Thrombolysis

It may be feasible to combine IVT and IAT to take advantage of the early infusion possible with IV administration and the greater recanalization efficacy of IA therapy. Hospital systems are increasingly employing a "drip and ship" strategy, whereby IVT is initiated on site at the local community hospital and the patient is then transported to the regional neurointerventional stroke center for "rescue" IAT. This approach was studied in the pilot Emergency Management of Stroke (EMS) Bridging Trial.[40] Patients with stroke of less than 3 hours' duration were given a loading dose (0.6 mg/kg) of IV t-PA or placebo followed by angiography and IAT if a vascular occlusion remained. In 70% of all patients, angiography showed clot after IV therapy. MCA recanalization improved in patients who then received IA t-PA, but the risk of life-threatening bleeding complications also rose. The results of the follow-up IV plus IA t-PA trial (Interventional Management of Stroke [IMS]) have been reported.[41] Among 62 patients with a baseline NIHSS score of 10 or more entered into the IMS study, 44 (71%) required both IV (0.6 mg/kg) and IA t-PA. The six symptomatic brain hemorrhages in the group receiving IV-IA combination therapy was 6.3%. A good outcome was achieved in 56% of patients younger than 80 years who received combination therapy, compared with 36% of patients with a baseline NIHSS score of 10 or higher who received IV t-PA alone in the NINDS t-PA Stroke Trial, and 40% in the PROACT II patients receiving IA r-proUK alone. Combined IV and IA stroke thrombolysis is still being investigated in the ongoing NIH-supported third Interventional Management of Stroke Study II (IMS3).

Recanalization of Acute Internal Carotid Occlusion

ICA occlusion with distal embolization to the MCA is a common cause of acute stroke. The recanalization rate after IV thrombolytics for large vessel occlusions such as the ICA is generally poor.[36,42-45] Several studies have shown higher mortality and morbidity rates for strokes secondary to large vessel occlusion.[36,42-45]

Jansen et al[42] evaluated the role of early thrombolytics in treating acute carotid occlusion. This study enrolled 32 patients with a mean age of 56 years who were treated with IV alteplase (16), IA alteplase (8), and IA urokinase (8). Recanalization was achieved in only 12.5% of patients, and good clinical outcome was observed in only 16%; 53% had a fatal outcome. None of the therapies—IV or IA alteplase, IA urokinase—was able improve the recanalization rate or clinical prognosis.[42] Zaidat et al[46] reviewed a small series of 18 patients with distal ICA occlusion who were treated with either IA or combined IA-IV thrombolytic therapy. This study showed a higher recanalization rate with combined therapy (82%) than with IV therapy alone (62%) but no difference in the intracranial hemorrhage rate (20% versus 15%, respectively) or improvement in NIHSS score. This study also showed that time to treatment was the most powerful predictor of response to thrombolytic therapy ($P < .001$). Thrombolytics were least effective in patients with carotid T segment occlusion.

Flint et al[47] reviewed the data from the MERCI trial to evaluate the efficacy of mechanical thrombectomy in patients with acute carotid occlusion. Eighty patients with ICA occlusion (mean age 67 years, mean NIHSS score 20, mean time from stroke onset to treatment 4.1 hours) were treated with mechanical thrombectomy. Recanalization with the Merci retriever alone was successful in 53% of patients, and 63% underwent ICA recanalization with Merci retriever plus adjunctive endovascular treatment. Good clinical outcome (mRS ≤ 2 at 90 days) was seen in 39% (19/49 patients) after successful recanalization, but in only 3 of 30 patients without successful recanalization ($P < .001$). Patients with successful recanalization had a lower 90-day mortality rate, 30% (15/50), versus 73% (22/30) in the nonrecanalized group ($P < .001$). This pooled analysis was able to show that mechanical thrombectomy in combination with other endovascular approaches improved the recanalization rate and clinical outcome in patients with internal carotid occlusion.[47]

Jovin et al[48] evaluated the role of emergency stenting in patients with acute stroke secondary to extracranial carotid artery occlusion. This study retrospectively reviewed 25 patients (mean age 62 years, median NIHSS score 14), of whom 15 presented within 6 hours of stroke symptom onset and 10 had fluctuating symptoms secondary to ICA occlusion. Twenty-three patients (92%) underwent recanalization by emergence stenting with only 2 clinically insignificant adverse events (1 asymptomatic ICH and 1 non–flow-limiting dissection). This study suggested that emergence stenting can be a treatment option in patients who present with stroke secondary to ICA occlusion.[48] Acute stenting has also been proposed for MCA occlusion.[49]

"Wake Up" Stroke

Nogueira et al[50] presented preliminary data from the DAWN (DWI/PWI [diffusion/perfusion-weighted imaging] and CTP [CT perfusion] Assessment in the triage of Wake-up and late-presenting strokes undergoing Neurointervention) trial. DAWN is a multicenter RCT that is evaluating the role of acute interventions based on imaging in treating stroke patients who present more than 8 hours after stroke symptom onset. The inclusion criteria for DAWN are a witnessed or nonwitnessed stroke in a patient who was last seen to be normal between 7 and 23 hours earlier, NIHSS score higher than 10, and MRI or angiography findings demonstrating a large vessel occlusion. DAWN requires perfusion imaging with an Albert Stroke Programme Early CT Score (ASPECTS) of 7 or higher on CT perfusion cerebral blood volume maps or a 20% mismatch on MRI. The acute intervention is at the discretion of the neurointerventionalist.

The preliminary study evaluated 193 patients (mean age 64 years, NIHSS score 15, mean time from last seen well 16.3 hours) who were treated for large vessel occlusion: M1 segment of the MCA, 94 patients (49%); M2 segment of the MCA, 19 patients (10%); ICA, 43 patients (22%); and tandem ICA origin/MCA, 25 patients (13%). Multimodality acute interventions were performed to treat these patients with large vessel occlusions: IAT in 92 patients (48%), Merci retriever in 110 patients (57%), and other mechanical modalities in 56 patients (29%). Successful recanalization (TIMI grade 2 or 3) was achieved in 73% of patients (141). Long-term outcomes were available for 151 patients, of whom 45.7% had good outcome and 60.9% had acceptable outcome. The rates of ICH and mortality were 10.3% and 22.2%, respectively. DAWN showed direct significant correlation of favorable outcomes with age (OR, 0.96; 95% CI, 0.93–0.99; $P = .026$), time to treatment (OR, 1.11; 95% CI, 1.01–1.21; $P = .019$), and successful recanalization (OR, 3.21; 95% CI, 1.21–8.51; $P = 0.018$).

Vertebrobasilar Intraarterial Thrombolysis

The natural history of basilar occlusion is extremely poor, with mortality rates ranging from 83% to 91%.[3,47] Because of this poor natural history, IAT has been preferred in patients with acute basilar artery occlusion. Approximately 278 cases have been reported, with an overall basilar recanalization rate of 60%. Basilar artery occlusions have a high incidence of residual stenosis, which often requires adjuvant therapies such as angioplasty and antithrombotic and antiplatelet treatments.

In a compilation of reported cases of vertebrobasilar thrombolysis, the mortality in patients in whom recanalization was not achieved was 90%, compared with 31% in patients in whom at least partial reperfusion was achieved.

Good outcomes are strongly associated with recanalization after thrombolytic therapy. The majority of patients with successful vertebrobasilar recanalization had mild or moderate disability, compared with less than 14% of patients whose vessels remained occluded.[51]

Success of recanalization depends on the location of the vertebrobasilar occlusion. Distal occlusions have higher recanalization rates than proximal occlusions. Emboli, which often lodge in the distal basilar artery, are easier to lyse than atherosclerosis-related thrombi, the usual cause of proximal basilar occlusions.[5,46] Short segment occlusions are easier to lyse than longer segment occlusions.[46] Patients who are younger have higher recanalization rates,[52,53] probably because they have a higher incidence of embolic occlusion.

The time window for thrombolysis may be longer in the posterior circulation. The presence of coma or tetraparesis for several hours portends poor prognosis despite recanalization. However, prolonged vertebrobasilar occlusion symptoms do not preclude survival and recovery. Many series have included patients not treated until 24,[3,54] 48,[46,55] or even 72 hours after symptom onset,[3,52] or patients with prolonged, stuttering courses.[56,57] An association between time to treatment and outcome has been suggested,[58] but other series do not support the finding.[46,59]

This great variability makes it difficult to predict the timing and outcome of thrombolysis in the vertebrobasilar circulation. Patients with vertebrobasilar artery occlusion often have chronic atherothrombotic disease, which allows collateral vessels to develop over time. As hypothesized by Cross et al,[52] there may be two distinct populations of patients with vertebrobasilar occlusion. Paradoxically, patients with a progressive stuttering course may have better collateral circulation and better outcome after IAT despite later treatment than patients with sudden onset of a severe deficit but with poor collateral vessels, who may actually be brought to treatment earlier.

Despite the apparently longer time window, the rate of hemorrhagic transformation after vertebrobasilar thrombolysis appears lower than anterior circulation thrombolysis. The average rate of symptomatic brain hemorrhage after vertebrobasilar IAT is 6.5%, compared with 8.3% for IAT in the anterior circulation. A lower rate of hemorrhagic transformation after vertebrobasilar thrombolysis may be due to higher ischemic tolerance in the posterior circulation, improved collateral circulation, or an increased density of white matter tracts.[60] There is no clear association between hemorrhage risk and time to treatment,[52] although 3 of the 18 symptomatic hemorrhages reported in the literature occurred when thrombolysis was initiated more than 48 hours after symptom onset.[3,59]

Some investigators believe that patients with CT evidence of brainstem infarction are not candidates for thrombolytic therapy,[3,46] but other researchers have found no correlation between this finding and neurologic outcome.[52,59] In two separate series, none of the patients who had CT evidence of ischemia had hemorrhage. However, because of the experience in the anterior circulation, caution should be used when one is considering vertebrobasilar thrombolysis in patients in whom CT reveals signs of early infarction.

Risk Factors for Hemorrhagic Transformation

Several series have found no relationship between recanalization and hemorrhage risk.[61-63] However, these series do not address delayed recanalization or the status of recanalization at the time of brain hemorrhage.[64]

The amount of ischemic damage is a key factor in the development of hemorrhage after thrombolysis. Early extensive CT changes and severity of the initial neurologic deficit, both indicators of the extent of ischemic damage, are the best predictors of risk of hemorrhagic transformation (Fig. 62-2).[63,65] In ECASS I,[18] early CT changes in more than one third of the MCA territory correlated well with the frequency of hemorrhagic infarction. However, the so-called ECASS CT criterion is not present in all cases of hemorrhage, and there is considerable inter-reader variability in the interpretation of early CT changes. Furthermore, extensive early CT changes by themselves may be insufficient to exclude thrombolysis in specific patients.[66,67] An analysis of the PROACT II data indicates that patients with early (i.e., < 6 hours) CT infarct volumes greater than 100 mL do poorly.[68] However, estimated early CT changes (i.e., ECASS CT criterion) appear less predictive of outcome among homogeneous patients with MCA occlusion than in patients with mixed sites of arterial occlusion.[69] Furthermore, time may also be a key factor in interpreting early CT changes. In the NINDS trial, patients with early CT changes still benefited from t-PA administration, perhaps because of the earlier treatment time window.[63] Given the somewhat conflicting data, it would be prudent either (1) to avoid thrombolysis in patients with clear-cut and extensive early signs of infarction on CT and a NIHSS score higher than 20, especially those older than 75 years, or (2) to emphasize to the family of such a patient that the benefit-risk ratio is greatly reduced even if treatment is begun within 3 hours of onset.

The amount of ischemic damage depends on the duration of occlusion and the amount of collateral blood flow. Both of these factors have been associated with increased risk of hemorrhage.[61,63,70] Ueda et al[70] found that the amount of residual blood flow, as determined by single-photon emission CT (SPECT), was associated with hemorrhagic transformation, but they also used results of this assessment to extend the thrombolytic time window beyond 6 hours in three patients. Improved perfusion after 3 hours of IV r-tPA has also been demonstrated with single-photon emission CT.[71]

Other factors that have been associated with hemorrhage after thrombolysis for both stroke and myocardial infarction (MI) are thrombolytic dose,[62,72] blood pressure,[73,74] advanced age, prior head injury,[63,75,76] and blood glucose level.[64] Age was the most important risk factor in one of the largest series of thrombolysis-related ICH. Because of the increased risk in elderly patients, an upper age limit was initially instituted for patients being considered for coronary thrombolysis. Older patients with myocardial infarction were found to benefit from treatment, however, and the generally accepted age limit has been raised. A strong relationship between advanced age and hemorrhage was also demonstrated in the NINDS study and ECASS. Although there is no strict age cutoff, physicians must take into account the greater risk of hemorrhage in patients 75 years and older when choosing to administer thrombolysis for stroke.

ICH after thrombolysis for stroke can occur at sites distant from the ischemic region.[34] Cerebral amyloid angiopathy has been implicated as a causative factor in brain hemorrhages after thrombolysis for myocardial

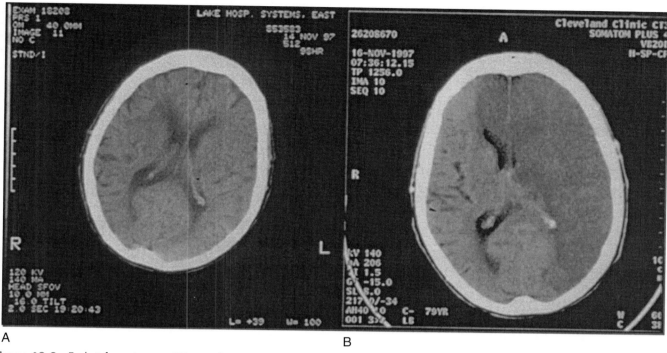

Figure 62-2 Early infarct signs on CT scans from a 67-year-old man with acute right hemiplegia and aphasia, National Institutes of Health Stroke Scale (NIHSS) score 22, and internal carotid artery occlusion. A, Initial CT scan obtained 4 hours after stroke onset shows sulcal effacement, loss of gray-white matter distinction, and loss of insular ribbon in more than one third of the left middle cerebral artery territory (European Cooperative Acute Stroke Study [ECASS] CT criteria). B, Second CT scan obtained at 25 hours shows massive left cerebral and right anterior cerebral artery infarcts.

infarction.[77] Amyloid angiopathy is a well known cause of spontaneous hemorrhage in the elderly and is associated with dementia of the Alzheimer's type. Hence, thrombolytic therapy in elderly demented patients may carry a particularly high risk of brain hemorrhage. Hemorrhage into an arteriovenous malformation and unsuspected ischemic infarction have also been reported as causes of ICH after thrombolysis.[77]

Other Factors Affecting Outcomes with Thrombolysis

Hacke[78] has described the ideal candidate for thrombolysis as follows: a young person with good collateral circulation who has an MCA occlusion distal to the lenticulostriates due to a fresh fibrin-rich thrombus that passed through a patent foramen ovale. The presence of collateral flow is one of the primary determinants of outcome.[79,80] Good leptomeningeal collaterals may limit the extent of ischemic damage and prolong the therapeutic window. Good collateral flow is also associated with higher rates of reperfusion, presumably because it allows a greater amount of thrombolytic agent to reach the clot.

Clot composition is a neglected factor in recanalization success rates.[81] Fresh thrombi, which are rich in fibrin and plasminogen, are easier to lyse than aged atherothrombi, which are more organized and have low fibrin and plasminogen contents and high amounts of platelets and cholesterol. Fresh cardiac emboli may therefore respond better to thrombolysis than atherothrombotic occlusion or calcific embolism.

Angiographic studies indicate that about 20% of patients presenting with a clinical picture consistent with acute ischemic stroke have no visible arterial occlusion.[34] There is controversy regarding the utility of thrombolysis in patients who have no large vessel occlusion.[82] The NINDS trial suggested a benefit of t-PA in patients with small vessel (i.e., lacunar) infarction, and it is possible that thrombolytic therapy may be effective in the recanalization of small vessels that are invisible on angiography. A meta-analysis of thrombolytic trials found no significant differences between results of studies that included patients with lacunar strokes and those of studies that excluded such patients.[83]

New Endovascular Therapies for Acute Stroke

The technique used in IAT, unlike with IV administration, may be critical in achieving success and varies among interventionists. Direct intrathrombus delivery of thrombolytic agent is preferred over regional infusion. However, the infusion process has been variable, ranging from continuous to pulsed infusion both with and without bolus administration. In some series, clot disruption by the microcatheter has been included in the protocol, theoretically to improve exposure of the thrombus to the thrombolytic agent and thereby speed clot lysis. Mechanical clot manipulation was prohibited in PROACT I and PROACT II. In some series, IAT was followed by percutaneous transluminal angioplasty (PTA) of the recanalized vessel.[84,85] To date, however, no prospective comparison of any of these techniques has been conducted, so their relative merits remain unclear.

Several new interventional neuroradiologic techniques designed to improve the speed and completeness of recanalization in acute ischemic stroke have been described. These reports have all been individual case series from single institutions. The techniques include treatment of acute ischemic stroke by direct mechanical balloon angioplasty of the thrombus,[85-88] mechanical snaring of clot from the MCAs,[89] intravascular stenting of underlying occlusive atherosclerosis for restoring vessel patency,[90] use of suction thrombectomy devices for establishing reperfusion, laser-assisted thrombolysis of acute emboli to the brain, and power-assisted Doppler ultrasound thrombolysis.[91] As previously described, intravenous and intraarterial GP IIb/IIIa inhibitors have also been used to enhance the effects of clot lysis during acute stroke.[12,15,16,92] These new technologies are in early feasibility and safety trials in both the United States and Europe and are still investigational. Phase 3 randomized controlled clinical trials must be performed before specific recommendations as to the safety and efficacy of any of these methods can be made.

Current Status of Intraarterial Thrombolysis and Need for More Evidence

The fourth issue of the *Cochrane Database of Systematic Reviews* meta-analysis, which included data from PROACT I and PROACT II, concluded that overall, the risks of thrombolysis are offset by reductions in dependent survival, so that significantly more patients are alive and independent after treatment. Writers of this meta-analysis suggested, "The time window might extend to, or even beyond, six hours in selected patients."[93]

On the basis of this available evidence, the Second American Heart Association International Evidence Evaluation Conference made a "major guideline change"[94]; IAT given within 3 to 6 hours after the onset of stroke symptoms is now a class IIb recommendation (acceptable, clinically useful, alternative or optional treatment supported by good evidence). IAT has also been endorsed by other major medical societies.

Intraarterial stroke thrombolysis using clot retrieval devices is currently being performed routinely at most comprehensive stroke centers worldwide (Fig. 62-3). In the United States, the Merci retriever was used in 2300 ischemic stroke interventions in 2006, and the total number of IA ischemic stroke interventions was estimated to range from 3500 to 7200.[95] Estimates of the potential annual number of IA stroke interventions in the United States alone range from 10,400 to 41,500, and comprehensive stroke centers use a clot retrieval device in approximately 65% of IA interventions. Importantly, although IA stroke intervention typically begins with mechanical clot retrieval, it frequently incorporates thrombolytic agents, antithrombotics, and platelet inhibition. As a result, there are no standard IA protocols or even standard criteria for device selection, and it is routine to make interventional decisions "on the table." This fact reflects the complex technical heterogeneity of acute stroke arterial recanalization and further complicates the design of any potential RCTs.

There is a long history of surgical procedures being done without any RCT data whatsoever.[96] At least for IA stroke thrombolysis, we have one phase 3 RCT demonstrating proof of principle and clinical efficacy.[9] Of course the irony is that PROACT II used an unapproved drug (r-proUK) and specifically prohibited mechanical clot manipulation. The evolution of interventional neuroradiology has now introduced a new "twilight zone" of approved but unproven stroke clot retrieval devices. Both the Merci device and the Penumbra System were approved by the FDA and CMS without an RCT or definitive evidence of clinical efficacy.[97]

The ethics of performing IAT both outside and within a clinical trial have been extensively debated.[98-100] Considering that the criteria for FDA approval were "safety and efficacy" and for CMS reimbursement "reasonable and necessary," the use of stroke clot retrieval devices (in the USA) is not only legal but also ethical outside of a RCT. A compelling case can also be made that universal collective equipoise does *not* exist regarding IAT. U.S. Institutional Review Boards have required the inclusion of the availability of stroke clot retrieval devices in informed consents. This requirement further complicates recruitment into RCTs—the subtleties of clot retrieval versus an improved mRS at 90 days are likely to be lost on patients and families in the throes of dealing with an acute stroke.

In the United States, ethics are conflated by CMS hospital reimbursement policies for IA stroke thrombolysis. CMS policies and off-label use of devices have posed tremendous recruitment barriers for RCTs.[101] Another controversy relates to who should perform acute ischemic stroke interventions. Training and credentialing criteria have been published that have implications for vetting in RCTs.[102] Certainly, clot retrieval devices have different technical training requirements from those of "simple" IAT.

The need for more data is a separate issue from whether usage of clot retrieval devices or IAT should be *restricted* to clinical trials. The painfully slow recruitment in both the Mechanical Retrieval and Recanalization of Stroke Clots Using Embolectomy (MR RESCUE) study and Interventional Management of Stroke Study III (IMS3) indicates how difficult such RCTs are to complete. Recruitment enthusiasm may depend on the clinical trial. For example, IMS3 has no competing trials and avoids the contentious issue of a "placebo." Ten years after PROACT II, what question do we really want to answer? Is it simply "Does IA thrombolysis work?" or has it evolved to "On which patients does it work?" It is not widely known that 10 years ago the FDA approved a protocol for PROACT III with a sample size of 450—why wasn't it done? The issues became cost, the ethics of a "placebo" control, recruitment, and, ultimately, feasibility. Indeed, the task became so daunting that the study's funder, Abbott Laboratories, eventually abandoned the entire arena of stroke thrombolysis. In negotiations with Concentric Medical over the Merci retriever, at least one source reports that the FDA admitted another RCT like PROACT II was not feasible.[103] At a minimum, this suggests that any additional IAT RCT will require international academic-industry collaboration and a novel design.

In addition to recruitment, a major challenge for any new IAT RCT will be to tackle not only the technical

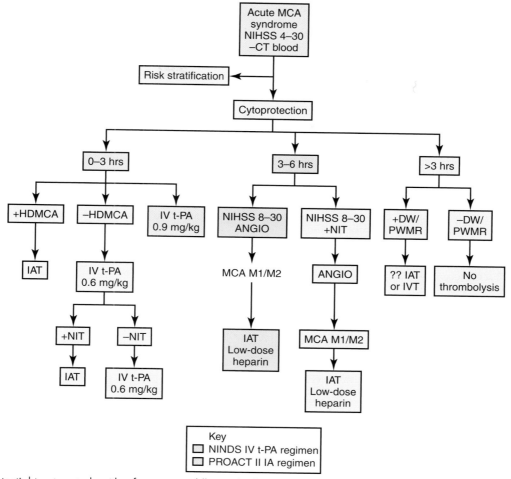

Figure 62-3 Potential treatment algorithm for acute middle cerebral artery syndrome. *Plus sign* indicates positive results, and *minus sign* negative results, of each test. ANGIO, angiography; DW/PWMR, diffusion/perfusion mismatch on MRI of the brain; ECASS, European Cooperative Acute Stroke Study; HDMCA, hyperdense middle cerebral artery; IAT, intraarterial thrombolysis; IV, intravenous; IVT, intravenous thrombolysis; NIHSS, National Institutes of Health Stroke (scale); NIT, noninvasive test; PROACT, Prolyse in Acute Cerebral Thromboembolism study; tPA, tissue-type plasminogen activator.

but also the physiologic heterogeneity of acute ischemic stroke. Recent mismatch imaging–based RCTs—such as the Desmoteplase in Acute Ischemic Stroke phase 2 (DIAS-2) study, the Diffusion and Perfusion Imaging Evaluation for Understanding Stroke Evolution (DEFUSE) study, and the Echoplanar Imaging Thrombolytic Evaluation Trial (EPITHET)—highlight the fact that acute ischemic stroke is even more physiologically heterogeneous than we thought.[104,105] Unfortunately, from the pharmaceutical/medical device industry's perspective, such heterogeneity reduces the potential market and increases the cost of an RCT. Nonetheless, in our view and the placebo issue aside, an IAT RCT that does not adequately account for stroke heterogeneity (both technical and physiologic) either will require a huge (and therefore not feasible) sample size or will be doomed to failure.

Should we therefore put a moratorium on stroke clot retrieval devices and IAT and *restrict* their use to clinical trials? Aside from the fact that in the United States such restricted usage would not be legal, a "yes" answer exposes the conflict between academic altruism and a certain stroke realpolitik. So our answer to this question

is "No, but … we need new data to move beyond old questions." Simply repeating PROACT II but with clot retrieval devices and relying on traditional randomization to account for stroke heterogeneity (both technical and physiologic) has a low probability of successful completion.

REFERENCES

1. Nenci GG, Gresele P, Taramelli M, et al: Thrombolytic therapy for thromboembolism of vertebrobasilar artery, *Angiology* 34:561–571, 1983.
2. del Zoppo GJ, Ferbert A, Otis S, et al: Local intra-arterial fibrinolytic therapy in acute carotid territory stroke: A pilot study, *Stroke* 19:307–313, 1988.
3. Hacke W, Zeumer H, Ferbert A, et al: Intra-arterial thrombolytic therapy improves outcome in patients with acute vertebrobasilar occlusive disease, *Stroke* 19:1216–1222, 1988.
4. Accreditation Council for Graduate Medical Education. Program Requirements for Residence Education in Endovascular Surgical Neuroradiology. Available at www.ACGME.org/RRC_progREQ/.
5. Zeumer H, Freitag HJ, Zanella F, et al: Local intra-arterial fibrinolytic therapy in patients with stroke: Urokinase versus recombinant tissue plasminogen activator (rt-PA), *Neuroradiology* 35:159–162, 1993.

6. Nesbit GM, Clark WM, O'Neil OR, Barnwell SL: Intracranial intra-arterial thrombolysis facilitated by microcatheter navigation through an occluded cervical internal carotid artery, *J Neurosurg* 84:387-392, 1996.

7. Adams HP, Brott TC, Furlan AJ, et al: Guidelines for thrombolytic therapy for acute stroke: A supplement to the guidelines for the management of patients with acute ischemic stroke. A Statement for Healthcare Professionals from a Special Writing Group of the Stroke Council, American Heart Association, *Stroke* 27:1711-1718, 1996.

8. del Zoppo GJ, Higashida RT, Furlan AJ, et al: PROACT: A Phase II randomized trial of recombinant pro-urokinase by direct arterial delivery in acute middle cerebral artery stroke, *Stroke* 29:4-11, 1998.

9. Furlan A, Higashida R, Wechsler L, et al: Intra-arterial prourokinase for acute ischemic stroke—The PROACT II Study: A randomized controlled trial, *JAMA* 282:2003-2011, 1999.

10. Higashida RT, Halbach VV, Tsai FY, et al: Interventional neuro-vascular techniques in acute thrombolytic therapy for stroke. In Yamagushi T, Mori E, Minematsu K, del Zoppo GJ, editors: *Thrombolytic therapy in acute ischemic stroke III. Tokyo*, 1995, Springer-Verlag, pp 294-300.

11. Consensus Conference on Current Strategies for Intracerebral Fibrinolysis for Acute Stroke Therapy, Memphis, TN, January 8-9, 2000, Presented at Centocor.

12. Abciximab in acute ischemic stroke: A randomized, double-blind, placebo-controlled, dose-escalation study. The Abciximab in Ischemic Stroke Investigators, *Stroke* 31:601-609, 2000.

13. Reperfusion therapy for acute myocardial infarction with fibrinolytic therapy or combination reduced fibrinolytic therapy and platelet glycoprotein IIb/IIIa inhibition: The GUSTO V randomised trial. The GUSTO V Investigators, *Lancet* 357:1905-1914, 2001.

14. Wallace RC, Furlan AJ, Moliterno DJ, et al: Basilar artery rethrombosis: Successful treatment with platelet glycoprotein IIb/IIIa receptor inhibitor, *Am J Neuroradiol* 18:1257-1260, 1997.

15. Qureshi AI, Suri MF, Khan J, et al: Abciximab as an adjunct to high-risk carotid or vertebrobasilar angioplasty: Preliminary experience, *Neurosurgery* 46:1316-1324, 2000.

16. McDonald CT, O'Donnell J, Bemporad J, et al: The clinical utility of intravenous Integrilin combined with intra-arterial tissue plasminogen activator in acute ischemic stroke: The MGH experience [abstract], *Stroke* 33:359, 2002.

17. Credo RB, Burke SE, Barker WM, et al: Recombinant glycosylated pro-urokinase: Biochemistry, pharmacology, and early clinical experience. In Sasahara AA, Loscalzo J, editors: *New therapeutic agents in thrombosis and thrombolysis*, New York, 1997, Marcel Dekker, pp 561-589.

18. Hacke W, Kaste M, Fieschi C, et al: Intravenous thrombolysis with recombinant tissue plasminogen activator for acute hemispheric stroke: The European Cooperative Acute Stroke Study (ECASS), *JAMA* 274:1017-1025, 1995.

19. The National Institute of Neurological Disorders and Stroke t-PA Stroke Study Group: Tissue plasminogen activator for acute ischemic stroke, *N Engl J Med* 333:1581-1587, 1995.

20. Clark WM, Wissman S, Albers GW, et al: Recombinant tissue plasminogen activator (alteplase) for ischemic stroke 3 to 5 hours after symptom onset—the ATLANTIS Study: A randomized controlled trial, *JAMA* 282:2012-2026, 1999.

21. Ogawa A, Mori E, Minematsu K, Taki W, et al: for the MELT Japan Study Group: Randomized Trial of Intra-arterial Infusion of Urokinase Within 6 Hours of Middle Cerebral Artery Stroke: The Middle Cerebral Artery Embolism Local Fibrinolytic Intervention Trial (MELT), *Japan Stroke* 38:2633-2639, 2007.

22. Saqqur M, Uchino K, Demchuk AM, et al: Site of arterial occlusion identified by transcranial Doppler predicts the response to intravenous thrombolysis for stroke, *Stroke* 38:948-954, 2007.

23. IMS Study Investigators: Combined intravenous and intra-arterial recanalization for acute ischemic stroke: The Interventional Management of Stroke Study, *Stroke* 35:904-911, 2004.

24. Berlis A, Lutsep H, Barnwell S, et al: Mechanical thrombolysis in acute ischemic stroke with endovascular photoacoustic recanalization, *Stroke* 35:1112-1116, 2004.

25. Smith WS, Sung G, Starkman S, et al: MERCI Trial Investigators. Safety and efficacy of mechanical embolectomy in acute ischemic stroke: Results of the MERCI trial, *Stroke* 36:1439-1440, 2005.

26. Gobin YP, Starkman S, Duckwiler GR, et al: MERCI 1: A phase 1 study of Mechanical Embolus Removal in Cerebral Ischemia, *Stroke* 35:2848-2854, 2004.

27. Smith WS, Sung G, Saver J, et al: Mechanical thrombectomy for acute ischemic stroke: final results of the Multi MERCI trial, *Stroke* 39:1205-1212, 2008.

28. Bose A, Henkes H, Alfke K, et al: Penumbra Phase 1 Stroke Trial Investigators: The Penumbra System: a mechanical device for the treatment of acute stroke due to thromboembolism, *AJNR Am J Neuroradiol* 29:1409-1413, 2008.

29. Penumbra Pivotal Stroke Trial Investigators: The penumbra pivotal stroke trial: safety and effectiveness of a new generation of mechanical devices for clot removal in intracranial large vessel occlusive disease, *Stroke* 40:2761-2768, 2009.

30. Becker K, Brott T: Approval of the MERCI clot retriever: A critical view, *Stroke* 36:400-403, 2005.

31. Tomsick T: Editorial comment—Mechanical embolus removal: A new day dawning, *Stroke* 36:1439-1440, 2005.

32. Waugh JR, Sacharis N: Arteriographic complications in the DSA era, *Radiology* 182:243-246, 1992.

33. Hacke W, Kaste M, Fieschi C, et al: Randomised double-blind placebo-controlled trial of thrombolytic therapy with intravenous alteplase in acute ischaemic stroke (ECASS II), *Lancet* 352:1245-1251, 1998.

34. Wolpert SM, Bruckmann H, Greenlee R, et al: Neuroradiologic evaluation of patients with acute stroke treated with recombinant tissue plasminogen activator, *AJNR Am J Neuroradiol* 14:3-13, 1993.

35. Pessin M, del Zoppo GJ, Furlan AJ: Thrombolytic treatment in acute stroke: Review and update of selective topics. In Moskowitz MA, Caplan LR, editors: *Cerebrovascular diseases: Nineteenth Princeton Stroke Conference*, Boston, 1995, Butterworth-Heinemann, pp 409-418.

36. Hoffman AI, Lambiase RE, Haas RA, et al: Acute vertebrobasilar occlusion: Treatment with high-dose intra-arterial urokinase, *AJR Am J Roentgenol* 172:709-712, 1999.

37. Katzan IL, Masaryk TJ, Furlan AJ, et al: Intra-arterial thrombolysis for perioperative stroke after open heart surgery, *Neurology* 52:1081-1084, 1999.

38. Weber J, Remonda L, Mattle HP, et al: Selective intra-arterial fibrinolysis of acute central retinal artery occlusion, *Stroke* 29:2076-2079, 1998.

39. Padolecchia R, Puglioli M, Ragone MC, et al: Superselective intra-arterial fibrinolysis in central retinal artery occlusion, *AJNR Am J Neuroradiol* 20:565-567, 1999.

40. Lewandowski CA, Frankel M, Tomsick TA, et al: Combined intravenous and intra-arterial r-TPA versus intra-arterial therapy for acute ischemic stroke: Emergency Management of Stroke (EMS) Bridging Trial, *Stroke* 30:2598-2605, 1999.

41. Tomsick T, Broderick JP, Pancioli AP, et al: Combined IV-IA rtPA treatment in major acute ischemic stroke [abstract], *Stroke* 33:359, 2002.

42. Jansen O, von Kummer R, Forsting M, et al: Thrombolytic therapy in acute occlusion of the intracranial internal carotid artery bifurcation, *AJNR Am J Neuroradiol* 16:1977-1986, 1995.

43. Brandt T, von Kummer R, Muller-Kuppers M, et al: Thrombolytic therapy of acute basilar artery occlusion. Variables affecting recanalization and outcome, *Stroke* 27:875-881, 1996.

44. Bruckmann H, Ferbert A, del Zoppo GJ, et al: Acute vertebral-basilar thrombosis. Angiologic-clinical comparison and therapeutic implications, *Acta Radiol Suppl* 369:38-42, 1986.

45. Hacke W, Schwab S, Horn M, et al: "Malignant" middle cerebral artery territory infarction: Clinical course and prognostic signs, *Arch Neurol* 53:309-315, 1995.

46. Zaidat OO, Suarez JI, Santillan C, et al: Response to intra-arterial and combined intravenous and intra-arterial thrombolytic therapy in patients with distal internal carotid artery occlusion, *Stroke* 33:1821-1826, 2002.

47. Flint AC, Duckwiler GR, Budzik RF, et al: Mechanical thrombectomy of intracranial internal carotid occlusion: Pooled results of the MERCI and Multi MERCI Part I trials, *Stroke* 38:1274-1280, 2007.

48. Jovin TG, Gupta R, Uchino K, et al: Emergent stenting of extracranial internal carotid artery occlusion in acute stroke has a high revascularization rate, *Stroke* 36:2426-2430, 2005.

49. Levy E, Siddiqui A, Crumlish A, et al: First Food and Drug Administration-Approved Prospective Trial of Primary Intracranial Stenting for Acute Stroke, SARIS (Stent-Assisted Recanalization in Acute Ischemic Stroke), *Stroke* 40:3552-3556, 2009.

50. Nogueira R, Liebeskind D, Gupta R, et al: Preliminary data for the DAWN trial (DWI/PWI and CTP assessment in the triage of wake-up and late presenting strokes undergoing neurointervention): Imaging based endovascular therapy for proximal anterior circulation occlusions beyond 8 h from last seen well in 193 stroke patients. SNIS Annual Meeting oral abstracts, *J NeuroInterv Surg* 1:85, 2009.

51. Katzan IL, Furlan AJ: Thrombolytic therapy. In Fisher M, Bogousslavsky J, editors: *Current review of cerebrovascular disease*, ed 3, Boston, 1999, Butterworth Heinemann, pp 185-193.

52. Cross DT, Moran CJ, Akins P, et al: Relationship between clot location and outcome after basilar artery thrombolysis, *AJNR Am J Neuroradiol* 18:1221-1228, 1997.

53. Huemer M, Niederwieser V, Ladurner G: Thrombolytic treatment for acute occlusion of the basilar artery, *J Neurol Neurosurg Psychiatry* 58:227-228, 1995.

54. Matsumoto K, Satoh K, et al: Intra-arterial therapy in acute ischemic stroke. In Yamaguchi T, Mori E, Minematsu K, editors: *Thrombolytic therapy in acute ischemic stroke III*, Tokyo, 1995, Springer-Verlag, pp 279-287.

55. Clark W, Barnwell S, Nesbit G, et al: Efficacy of intra-arterial thrombolysis of basilar artery stroke [abstract], *J Stroke Cerebrovasc Dis* 6:457, 1997.

56. Wijdicks EF, Nichols DA, Thielen KR, et al: Intra-arterial thrombolysis in acute basilar artery thromboembolisms: The initial Mayo Clinic experience, *Mayo Clin Proc* 72:1005-1013, 1997.

57. Herderschee D, Limburg M, Hijdra A, et al: Recombinant tissue plasminogen activator in two patients with basilar artery occlusion, *J Neurol Neurosurg Psychiatry* 54:71-73, 1991.

58. Zeumer H, Freitag HJ, Grzyska U, et al: Local intra-arterial fibrinolysis in acute vertebrobasilar occlusion, *Neuroradiology* 31:336-340, 1989.

59. Becker KJ, Monsein LH, Ulatowski J, et al: Intra-arterial thrombolysis in vertebrobasilar occlusion, *AJNR Am J Neuroradiol* 17:255-262, 1996.

60. Becker KJ, Purcell LL, Hacke W, et al: Vertebrobasilar thrombosis: Diagnosis, management, and the use of intra-arterial thrombolytics, *Crit Care Med* 24:1729-1742, 1996.

61. von Kummer R, Hacke W: Safety and efficacy of intravenous tissue plasminogen activator and heparin in acute middle cerebral artery stroke, *Stroke* 23:646-652, 1992.

62. Mori E, Yoneda Y, Tabuchi M, et al: Intravenous recombinant tissue plasminogen activator in acute carotid artery territory stroke, *Neurology* 42:976-982, 1992.

63. Levy DE, Brott TG, Haley EC, et al: Factors related to intracranial hematoma formation in patients receiving tissue-type plasminogen activator for acute ischemic stroke, *Stroke* 25:291-297, 1994.

64. Kase CS, Furlan AJ, Wechsler LR, et al: Hemorrhage after intra-arterial thrombolysis for ischemic stroke: The PROACT II Trial, *Neurology* 57:1603-1610, 2001.

65. Bozzao L, Angeloni U, Bastianello S, et al: Early angiographic and CT findings in patients with hemorrhagic infarction in the distribution of the middle cerebral artery, *AJNR Am J Neuroradiol* 12:1115-1121, 1991.

66. Grotta JC, Choi D, Patel SC, et al: Agreement and variability in the interpretation of early CT changes in stroke patients qualifying for intravenous tPA therapy, *Stroke* 30:1528-1533, 1999.

67. Patel SC, Levine SR, Tilley JC, et al: Lack of clinical significance of early ischemic changes on computed tomography in acute stroke, *JAMA* 286:2830-2838, 2001.

68. Roberts HC, Dillon WP, Furlan AJ, et al: Angiographic collaterals in acute stroke—relationship to clinical presentation and outcome: The PROACT II trial [abstract], *Stroke* 32:336, 2001.

69. Kidwell CS, Saver JL, Duckwiler G, et al: Predictors of hemorrhagic transformation following intra-arterial thrombolysis [abstract], *Stroke* 32:319, 2001.

70. Ueda T, Hatakeyama T, Kumon Y, et al: Evaluation of risk of hemorrhagic transformation in local intra-arterial thrombolysis in acute ischemic stroke by initial SPECT, *Stroke* 25:298-303, 1994.

71. Alexandrov AV, Bratina P, Grotta JC: tPA associated reperfusion after acute stroke demonstrated by HMPAO-SPECT [abstract], *Stroke* 7:101-104, 1998.

72. Gore JM, Sloan M, Price TR, et al: Intracerebral hemorrhage, cerebral infarction, and subdural hematoma after acute myocardial infarction and thrombolytic therapy in the Thrombolysis in Myocardial Infarction Study: Thrombolysis in Myocardial Infarction, Phase II, Pilot and Clinical Trial, *Circulation* 83:448-459, 1991.

73. Selker HP, Beshansky JR, Schmid CH, et al: Presenting pulse pressure predicts thrombolytic therapy-related intracranial hemorrhage. Thrombolytic Predictive Instrument (TPI) Project Results, *Circulation* 90:1657-1661, 1994.

74. Simoons ML, Maggioni AP, Knatterud G, et al: Individual risk assessment for intracranial haemorrhage during thrombolytic therapy, *Lancet* 342:1523-1528, 1993.

75. Gebel JM, Sila CA, Sloan MA, et al: Thrombolysis-related intracranial hemorrhage: A radiographic analysis of 244 cases from the GUSTO-1 trial with clinical correlation, *Stroke* 29:563-569, 1998.

76. Larrue V, von Kummer R, del Zoppo G, et al: Hemorrhagic transformation in acute ischemic stroke, potential contributing factors in the European Cooperative Acute Stroke Study, *Stroke* 28:957-960, 1997.

77. Sloan MA, Price TR, Petito CK, et al: Clinical features and pathogenesis of intracerebral hemorrhage after rt-PA and heparin therapy for acute myocardial infarction: The Thrombolysis in Myocardial Infarction (TIMI) II pilot and randomized clinical trial combined experience, *Neurology* 45:649-658, 1995.

78. Hacke W: Thrombolysis: Stroke subtype and embolus type. In del Zoppo GJ, Mori E, Hacke W, editors: *Thrombolytic therapy in acute ischemic stroke II*, Berlin, 1993, Springer-Verlag, pp 153-159.

79. von Kummer R, Holle R, Rosin L, et al: Does arterial recanalization improve outcome in carotid territory stroke? *Stroke* 26:581-587, 1995.

80. Ringelstein EB, Biniek R, Weiler C, et al: Type and extent of hemispheric brain infarctions and clinical outcome in early and delayed middle cerebral artery recanalization, *Neurology* 42:289-298, 1991.

81. Chimowitz M, Pessin M, Furlan A, et al: The effect of source of cerebral embolus on susceptibility to thrombolysis [abstract], *Neurology* 44(Suppl 2):A356, 1994.

82. Caplan LR, Mohr JP, Kistler JP, Koroshetz W: Thrombolysis—not a panacea for ischemic stroke, *N Engl J Med* 337:1309, 1997.

83. Wardlaw JM, Warlow CP, Counsell C: Systematic review of evidence on thrombolytic therapy for acute ischaemic stroke, *Lancet* 350:607-614, 1997.

84. Gönner F, Remonda L, Mattle H, et al: Local intra-arterial thrombolysis in acute ischemic stroke, *Stroke* 29:1894-1900, 1998.

85. Ueda T, Sakaki S, Nochide I, et al: Angioplasty after intra-arterial thrombolysis for acute occlusion of intracranial arteries, *Stroke* 29:2568-2574, 1998.

86. Mori T, Kazita K, Chokyu K, et al: Short-term arteriographic and clinical outcome after cerebral angioplasty and stenting for intracranial vertebrobasilar and carotid atherosclerotic occlusive disease, *AJNR Am J Neuroradiol* 21:249-254, 2000.

87. Nakayama T, Tanaka K, Kaneko M, et al: Thrombolysis and angioplasty for acute occlusion of intracranial vertebrobasilar arteries: Report of three cases, *J Neurosurg* 88:919-922, 1998.

88. Tsai FY, Berberaj B, Matovich V, et al: Percutaneous transluminal angioplasty adjunct to thrombolysis for acute middle cerebral artery rethrombosis, *AJNR Am J Neuroradiol* 15:1823-1829, 1994.

89. Chopko BW, Kerber C, Wong W, et al: Transcatheter snare removal of acute middle cerebral artery thromboembolism: Technical case report, *Neurosurgery* 40:1529-1531, 2000.

90. Phatouros CC, Higashida RT, Malek AM, et al: Endovascular stenting of an acutely thrombosed basilar artery: Technical case report and review of the literature, *Neurosurgery* 44:667-673, 1999.

91. Alexandrov AV, Demchuk AM, Felberg RA, et al: High rate of complete recanalization and dramatic clinical recovery during tPA infusion when continuously monitored with 2-MHz transcranial Doppler monitoring, *Stroke* 31:610-614, 2000.

92. Lempert TE, Halbach VV, Malek AM, et al: Rescue treatment of acute parent vessel thrombosis with glycoprotein IIb/IIIa inhibitor during GDC coil embolization, *Stroke* 30:693-695, 1999.

93. Cochrane Database Syst Rev (4), 1999.

94. Emergency interventional stroke therapy: A statement from the American Society of Interventional and Therapeutic Neuroradiology and Society of Cardiovascular and Interventional Radiology, *Am J Neuroradiol* 22:54, 2001.

95. Hirsch JA, Yoo AJ, Nogueira RG, et al: Case volumes of intraarterial and intravenous treatment of ischemic stroke in the USA, *J NeuroInterv Surg* 1:27-31, 2009.

96. Spodick DH: Numerators without denominators: There is no FDA for the surgeon, *JAMA* 232:35-36, 1975.

97. Furlan AJ, Fisher M: Devices, drugs, and the Food and Drug Administration: Increasing implications for ischemic stroke, *Stroke* 36:398-399, 2005.

98. Furlan AJ: Ethics and feasibility of placebo-controlled interventional acute stroke trials, *Stroke* 49:e533-e534, 2009.

99. Köhrmann M, Schwab S: Response to letter by Furlan, *Stroke.* Published online before print, July 23, 2009.

100. Grotta J, Barreto: A response to letters by Furlan, and Kohrmann and Schwab, *Stroke.* Published online before print July 23, 2009.

101. Off label practices plague circulatory system device randomized trials. The FDC Reports. The Gray Sheet. Vol 30, May 17, 2004.

102. Meyers PM, Schumacher HC, Alexander MJ, et al: Performance and training standards for endovascular ischemic stroke treatment, *J NeuroInterv Surg* 1:10-12, 2009.

103. Levin S: Concentric Medical: Breaking the stroke device barrier. *In Vivo: The Business and Medicine Report,* Vol 18, No 9, 2004.

104. Liebeskind DS: Reversing stroke in the 2010s. Lessons from Desmoteplase in Acute Ischemic Stroke-2 (DIAS-2), *Stroke* 40: 3156-3158, 2009.

105. Soares BP, Chien JD, Wintermark M: MR and CT monitoring of recanalization, reperfusion, and penumbra salvage: Everything that recanalizes does not necessarily reperfuse! *Stroke* 40: S24-S27, 2009.

63 Endovascular Treatment of Cerebral Aneurysms

AJAY K. WAKHLOO, MATTHEW J. GOUNIS, MICHAEL J. DE LEO III

The field of endovascular surgical neuroradiology has emerged in the past few decades to provide safe and effective options for the treatment of intracranial aneurysms. The primary goal of aneurysm treatment, regardless of the means, is to prevent rupture or rerupture. Before endovascular techniques were developed, craniotomy with clip placement was the only definitive treatment for both ruptured and unruptured aneurysms. But as imaging and device technologies improved, endovascular approaches to intracranial aneurysms became widely available, especially for patients for whom surgery posed high risks.

The first endovascular intracranial aneurysm occlusion was attempted in 1964 by Luessenhop and Velasquez.[1] Though technically unsuccessful, this ground-breaking procedure provided a fundamental shift in the approach to treating intracranial disease. Contemporaries of Lussenhop and Velasquez investigated other technologies for aneurysm occlusion such as metallic[2] and electric current thrombosis.[3,4] However, the work of Fedor Serbinenko in Cold War–era Soviet Russia revolutionized this new field. Inspired by the sight of tethered helium balloons at a 1959 May Day celebration in Moscow's Red Square,[5] Serbinenko pioneered development of the first flow-guided intraluminal balloon catheter.[6] Not long after he performed the first therapeutic vessel occlusion in 1970, Serbinenko used a detachable balloon catheter to embolize an intracranial aneurysm.[7]

Widespread news of Serbinenko's innovations at the Burdenko Neurosurgery Institute reached the West in 1974, when he summarized his experiences in English in the *Journal of Neurosurgery*.[8] Serbinenko's techniques immediately attracted curious minds from around the world. Among the pilgrims was Gerard Debrun, the French neuroradiologist who developed a latex balloon occlusion device.[9] The detachable balloon method of aneurysm embolization underwent a period of growth over the next 15 years in the hands of numerous investigators.[10-12] However, detachable balloon embolization was not without complications. For example, a detached balloon could act as a ball-valve within an aneurysm sac, leading to rapid aneurysm filling and rupture. Furthermore, the balloons would not appropriately appose to the aneurysm boundaries, resulting in dislodgement or suboptimal aneurysm occlusion.

The detachable platinum coil, introduced in the 1990s, was developed to overcome the deficiencies of detachable balloons and represented another fundamental shift in the neurointerventional treatment of intracranial aneurysms. When tightly packed into the aneurysmal sac, the coil mass prevented blood flow into the aneurysm, initiating intraaneurysmal clotting.[13,14] Within days of coil embolization, macrophages and fibroblasts infiltrated into the dome of the aneurysm as endothelial cells began to proliferate across the neck. The long-term histopathologic findings showed that coil embolization promoted a vascularized fibrous connective tissue scar within the aneurysm dome and complete endothelialization of the neck.[15-17] Early experiences with platinum coils revealed that they were difficult to control and that deployment of the coil within the aneurysm sac was unreliable. However, in 1991, Guido Guglielmi published two pivotal articles describing a novel electrolytic coil detachment technique from a stainless steel wire.[18,19] Initial use of Guglielmi detachable coils (GDCs) in 15 patients demonstrated excellent aneurysm occlusion (70% to 100%).[19] Periprocedural complications were limited to a single case of transient aphasia. The first multicenter trial of GDC treatment in 43 posterior circulation aneurysms showed a 7% combined morbidity and mortality, notably better than the 20% combined rate in reports of similarly sized trials that used detachable balloons.[20,21]

Endovascular Treatment of Ruptured Aneurysms: Evidence

Without treatment, patients with aneurysmal subarachnoid hemorrhage (SAH) have a 19% risk of rebleeding within 2 weeks[22] and a greater than 3% annual risk thereafter.[23] Thus, isolating the aneurysm (i.e., the rupture site) from the circulation is the primary goal of treatment. Although endovascular embolization techniques found widespread use in the early 1990s, there was a lack of data comparing surgery with intervention. The International Subarachnoid Aneurysm Trial (ISAT) was the first large-scale prospective randomized trial to compare the safety and efficacy of endovascular coiling with surgical clipping for treatment of ruptured aneurysms.[24] The primary endpoints of this international study were dependency and death at 1 year following treatment. Patient enrollment began in 1994 and was stopped in 2002 after 2143 patients had been randomly assigned to treatments because of significant freedom from death and disability in the endovascular group (22.6% relative risk reduction,

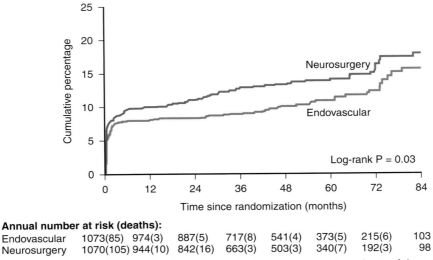

Figure 63-1 Kaplan-Meier graph of cumulative mortality from the surgical and endovascular cohorts of the International Subarachnoid Aneurysm Trial up to 7 years. (From Molyneux AJ, Kerr RS, Yu LM, et al: International subarachnoid aneurysm trial [ISAT] of neurosurgical clipping versus endovascular coiling in 2143 patients with ruptured intracranial aneurysms: A randomised comparison of effects on survival, dependency, seizures, rebleeding, subgroups, and aneurysm occlusion. *Lancet* 366:809-817, 2005.)

6.9% absolute risk reduction). One year after treatment, the absolute risk reduction was 7.4% in the endovascular group in comparison with the clipping group, and the survival advantage continued for 7 years (Fig. 63-1).[25]

The ISAT demonstrated that coil embolization was superior in safety profile to surgical clipping for the treatment of ruptured aneurysms (Fig. 63-2). However, questions remained about the durability of aneurysm occlusion, that is, the efficacy of coils in preventing long-term rebleeding. Previous studies have demonstrated that angiographic follow-up is necessary after aneurysm treatment with detachable coils.[26-28] Although there has been no widely accepted standard for defining recanalization, recanalization rates of aneurysms treated with detachable coils range from 4% to 60% depending on aneurysm size, neck width, and location.[27,28] Recanalization may be associated with an increased risk of rebleeding in patients treated either endovascularly or surgically. The Cerebral Aneurysm Rerupture After Treatment (CARAT) study[29,30] was an ambidirectional cohort study designed to compare rebleeding rates in 1001 patients with aneurysm rupture treated with either coil embolization or surgical clipping with an average of 3.6 years of follow-up. The total risk of rerupture after the initial treatment was 3.4% for coil embolization and 1.3% for surgical clipping.[30] The rebleeding rate as a function of time from both treatments was reported to be 2.2% in the first year, 0.2% in the second year, and 0% thereafter. These findings were similar to those of the ISAT, which found an annual risk of rerupture 1 year after treatment to be 0.21% in the coiling group and 0.03% in the clipping group.[25,31] In both the ISAT and the CARAT study, most rebleeds occurred in the first month after treatment. The latest ISAT analysis reports that with more than 8000 person-years of follow-up, aneurysms treated in the coiling and clipping arms rebled at a rate of 1.3% and 0.3%, respectively, after the first year (treatment received, $P = .023$).[32] Although late rebleeding has been shown to be higher in the endovascular treatment arm

than the surgery arm, the ISAT investigators concluded the risk remains low and similar to the risk for SAH from either an existing or newly formed aneurysm. Long-term rebleeding rates were even lower in an impressive single-center experience of coil embolization of intracranial, berry aneurysms with 1810 patient-years of follow-up.[33] This extensive experience from a Parisian hospital demonstrated that coiled aneurysms have a risk of early rebleeding of 0.94%, and only one case of late aneurysmal rebleed was observed (0.21%).

Subsequent analysis by the CARAT investigators showed that the degree of initial aneurysm occlusion was the strongest predictor of rebleeding. Aneurysms that were completely occluded had a 1.1% risk of rebleeding, whereas the rebleeding risk was 17.6% for aneurysms with only partial initial occlusion.[30] Although total occlusion was achieved in significantly more patients who underwent clipping (92%, compared with 39% with coiling), there were no cases of rerupture following early retreatment if deemed necessary. It should also be noted that retreatment of a previously embolized aneurysm is accompanied by low morbidity (1.1%) and low mortality (0%).[33]

These long-term data on the endovascular treatment of ruptured brain aneurysms confirm that risk of rebleeding from the treated aneurysms is extremely low and that patients have a good clinical outcome in comparison with surgical clipping. However, the recanalization rates have been the impetus for continuous developments in technologies to improve treatment durability. These technologies, which were not available during the ISAT trial, are discussed in subsequent sections.

Endovascular Treatment of Unruptured Aneurysms: Evidence

The management of asymptomatic unruptured aneurysms is controversial.[34-36] Primarily on the basis of the natural history data compiled by the International Study

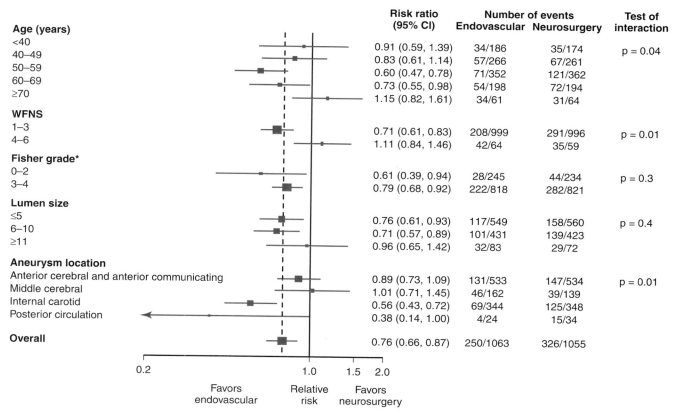

	Risk ratio (95% CI)	Number of events Endovascular	Number of events Neurosurgery	Test of interaction
Age (years)				
<40	0.91 (0.59, 1.39)	34/186	35/174	p = 0.04
40–49	0.83 (0.61, 1.14)	57/266	67/261	
50–59	0.60 (0.47, 0.78)	71/352	121/362	
60–69	0.73 (0.55, 0.98)	54/198	72/194	
≥70	1.15 (0.82, 1.61)	34/61	31/64	
WFNS				
1–3	0.71 (0.61, 0.83)	208/999	291/996	p = 0.01
4–6	1.11 (0.84, 1.46)	42/64	35/59	
Fisher grade*				
0–2	0.61 (0.39, 0.94)	28/245	44/234	p = 0.3
3–4	0.79 (0.68, 0.92)	222/818	282/821	
Lumen size				
≤5	0.76 (0.61, 0.93)	117/549	158/560	p = 0.4
6–10	0.71 (0.57, 0.89)	101/431	139/423	
≥11	0.96 (0.65, 1.42)	32/83	29/72	
Aneurysm location				
Anterior cerebral and anterior communicating	0.89 (0.73, 1.09)	131/533	147/534	p = 0.01
Middle cerebral	1.01 (0.71, 1.45)	46/162	39/139	
Internal carotid	0.56 (0.43, 0.72)	69/344	125/348	
Posterior circulation	0.38 (0.14, 1.00)	4/24	15/34	
Overall	0.76 (0.66, 0.87)	250/1063	326/1055	

0.2   1.0   1.5   2.0

Favors endovascular   Relative risk   Favors neurosurgery

* Fisher grade is a measure of the amount of blood on the CT scan.

Figure 63-2 Subgroup analysis from the International Subarachnoid Aneurysm Trial showing the odds ratios of death or dependency after 1 year for the surgical versus endovascular treatment of ruptured brain aneurysms. (From Molyneux AJ, Kerr RS, Yu LM, et al: International subarachnoid aneurysm trial (ISAT) of neurosurgical clipping versus endovascular coiling in 2143 patients with ruptured intracranial aneurysms: A randomised comparison of effects on survival, dependency, seizures, rebleeding, subgroups, and aneurysm occlusion. *Lancet* 366:809-817, 2005.)

on Unruptured Intracranial Aneurysms (ISUIA) investigators,[37,38] clinical decisions usually take into account patient age, the aneurysm size and location, patient attitudes, and the skills of local neurosurgeons and neuroendovascular interventionalists.[39] The ISUIA was designed with both a retrospective arm (1449 patients) and prospective arm (4060 patients). The primary objective for the retrospective arm was to compare the natural history of unruptured aneurysms in patients with and without a history of SAH in an attempt to determine risk of rupture and treatment options. The prospective arm sought to determine morbidity and mortality rates for patients undergoing treatment for unruptured aneurysms. Mean duration of follow-up was 8.3 years. The investigators concluded that in patients without a history of SAH, aneurysms smaller than 7 mm were extremely unlikely to rupture, with a rupture risk of 0.05% per year (Fig. 63-3). Patients with aneurysms similar in size and location but with a history of SAH were 11 times more likely to experience rupture (0.5% per year). Aneurysm size was an important predictor of rupture in patients without a history of SAH, with large (relative risk, 11.6) and giant (relative risk, 59) aneurysms at higher risk of rupture. Posterior circulation (vertebrobasilar) and basilar apex aneurysms were also at higher risk of rupture, having relative risks of 13.6 and 13.8, respectively. In the endovascular cohort, 2% and 5% of patients suffered hemorrhage

and cerebral infarction, respectively, during the procedure. Complete obliteration of the aneurysm was achieved in 55% of the patients, with a partial occlusion in 24%, and no occlusion in 18%. In 3% of the endovascular cases, the status of aneurysm obliteration was not reported. Rupture of the aneurysm during surgical clipping was observed in 6% of the patients, and intracranial hemorrhage and cerebral infarction were seen in 4% and 11% of the patients, respectively. The morbidity and mortality rates in the surgical arm at 1 year were 12.2% and 2.3%, respectively. In the endovascular cohort, the 1-year total morbidity and mortality rates were 9.5% and 3.1%, respectively.

Not long after the first ISUIA study was published in 1998, the Stroke Council of the American Heart Association adopted Recommendations for the Management of Patients with Unruptured Intracranial Aneurysms.[40] The recommendations were criticized because patients in the ISUIA were not representative of the general population,[41] patient follow-up was limited in comparison with other large-scale studies of unruptured intracranial aneurysms,[42,43] and anterior circulation aneurysms were underrepresented. Because patients with unruptured intracranial aneurysms have never been the subjects of a randomized trial, the Trial on Endovascular Aneurysm Management (TEAM) began enrolling patients with unruptured intracranial aneurysms to compare the

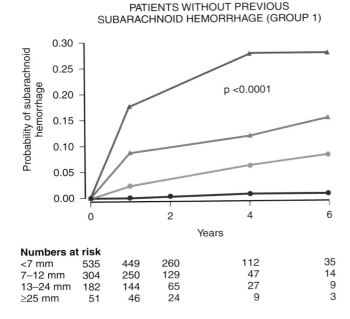

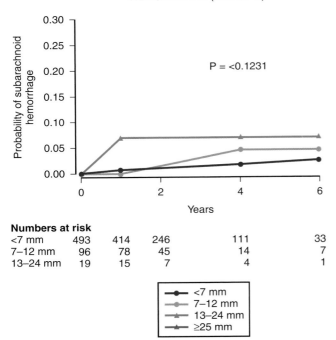

Figure 63-3 Probability of subarachnoid hemorrhage as a function of size separated by previous history of subarachnoid hemorrhage from the International Study of Unruptured Intracranial Aneurysms. The giant aneurysm group is excluded in the analysis of patients with previous subarachnoid hemorrhage because of small sample size. (From Wiebers DO, Whisnant JP, Huston J III, et al: Unruptured intracranial aneurysms: Natural history, clinical outcome, and risks of surgical and endovascular treatment. *Lancet* 362:103-110, 2003.)

combined morbidity and mortality of endovascular treatment with conservative management over a projected 10-year follow-up period.[44] Unfortunately, the low enrollment rate in the TEAM led to its announced cancellation at the 2009 Congress of the World Federation of Interventional Therapeutic Neuroradiology.

Though the controversy over the management of unruptured intracranial aneurysms continues, later studies on the natural history and endovascular treatment outcomes in small unruptured aneurysms prove valuable.[45-47] Six hundred forty-nine patients with a total of 1100 aneurysms were treated endovascularly in 27 Canadian and French neurointerventional centers (Analysis of Treatment by Endovascular approach of Non-ruptured Aneurysms [ATENA]).[45] Aneurysms were treated with coils alone in 54.5% of cases, and in 37.3% and 7.8% of cases, a temporary balloon-assistance or stenting was required, respectively. Endovascular treatment failed in 4.3% of cases. Thromboembolic complications were encountered in 7.1%, intraoperative rupture occurred in 2.6%, and device-related problems were observed in 2.9% of the procedures. Adverse events associated with transient or permanent neurologic deficit or death were encountered in 5.4% of cases. Thirty-day morbidity and mortality rates were 1.7% and 1.4%, respectively. These data demonstrate the safety of the endovascular treatment of unruptured aneurysms, and we await the long-term clinical results from ATENA.

Key developments in the area of unruptured aneurysms involve the identification of the rupture risk of these lesions. Aneurysm wall inflammation has been correlated with ruptured aneurysms,[48] and preliminary research indicates that intraaneurysmal inflammation can be imaged noninvasively.[49] Further development of these techniques may lead to quantitative assays of the risk of rupture in unruptured brain aneurysms that could improve patient selection for endovascular treatment.

Techniques of Endovascular Aneurysm Treatment

The vast majority of endovascular treatments of aneurysms in the previously described clinical trials were performed with the first-generation of embolic coils. These coils, Guglielmi detachable coils (GDCs), are made of a platinum alloy and have a two-dimensional helical shape. Since the early experience, medical devices for the endovascular treatment of aneurysms have dramatically improved. New technologies have facilitated the ability to access the lesion with microcatheters and safely embolize the aneurysm sac with high rates of complete occlusion. Wide-neck aneurysms can now be addressed via the endovascular approach with the use of adjunctive devices such as temporary occlusion balloons or neurovascular stents. Developments in imaging, including flat panel detectors with high spatial and contrast resolution, three-dimensional (3D) reconstruction angiography, and cone-beam CT, offer enhanced visualization of the aneurysm morphology and the medical devices deployed endovascularly. The cumulative effects of these advancements, many of which have occurred in the last 5 years, have not yet been captured in large randomized controlled studies with long-term follow-up. Trials to investigate the impact of various new technologies are ongoing, and to date we rely on single-center studies to demonstrate the positive clinical impact.

Embolic Coil Technology

As noted briefly in the previous section, the major shortcoming of the original two-dimensional GDC bare platinum coils is compaction and aneurysmal recanalization, the rate of which ranges between 21% and 34% of cases and is even higher in subsets of aneurysms, including those that are large or have wide necks[27,28] or large direct blood flow impingement.[50] Nearly 10 years ago, the second generation of bare platinum coils was introduced to the endovascular armamentarium; the 3D shape of the coils were more appropriate to the native aneurysm morphology. These new coils made it possible to achieve a high structural integrity of the coil mass by filling the aneurysm with a high and homogeneous packing density.

Packing density is defined by the ratio of volumes of the coils implanted and the aneurysm. The relation between packing density and compaction in brain aneurysms that were treated with coils has been studied in single-center case series showing that packing densities of more than 20% to 37% resulted in lower rates of coil compaction.[51-54] In one report, packing density higher than 24% was shown to protect against recanalization in aneurysms having volumes smaller than 600 mm³.[52] In another study, 194 coiled aneurysms were followed up angiographically for comparison of recanalization and retreatment rates for aneurysms embolized predominantly with the 3D coil system in comparison with the helical coil system.[54] Approximately 16% of the aneurysms in the 3D coil system cohort were not completely occluded after 6 months, compared with 22% in the helical coil cohort. Retreatment rates were also lower in the 3D coil system group (7.8% versus 13.3% for helical coil). Similarly, our own clinical experience in 77 aneurysms that were treated with only complex 3D coils showed recanalization in 12.9% and retreatment in 6.5% of the aneurysms after an average angiographic follow-up of 10 months.[53]

Very shortly after GDC coil embolization was introduced, basic research to accelerate aneurysm healing by embolic coil surface modifications was undertaken.[55,55a] One of the early surface modifications to reach the clinic involved the impregnation of a hydrogel into the coil (MicroVention, Terumo, Tustin, Calif), which expands after the interaction with blood[56] thereby increasing the packing density in an effort to reduce coil compaction and subsequent recanalization. A prospectively acquired, single-arm registry termed HydroCoil for Endovascular Aneurysm Occlusion (HEAL) failed to demonstrate improvement in recanalization rates, with the recanalization occurring in 28% of the treated aneurysms.[57] However, the HEAL registry also demonstrated a 0% recanalization rate in a small subset of patients in whom more than 75% of the length of coils used had embedded hydrogel. The HydroCoil Endovascular Aneurysm Occlusion and Packing Study (HELPS) is a multicenter randomized controlled trial designed to study the effectiveness of this coil system to reduce recanalization in comparison with bare platinum coils.[58] Recent update on HELPS trial showed no statistical difference in major aneurysm recurrence rate between patients treated with Hydrogel coils versus bare platinum coils.[58a] Although no statistical difference was found, patients treated with Hydrogel coils had a higher rate of hydrocephalus (4.5%) as compared with patients treated with bare platinum coils (0.9%).

Another approach to accelerate aneurysm healing has been to either load into or apply onto the surface of the embolic coil hydrolysable polymers (resorbable sutures) that induce inflammation as they degrade.[59] The working hypothesis was that the induced inflammation would provide a rapid fibrosis of the aneurysm sac, thereby reducing recanalization rates. The first such clinical product was the Matrix coil (Boston Scientific Neurovascular, Fremont, Calif), which had strands of a copolymer (90% polyglycolide, 10% polylactide) covering the external surface of the embolic coil.[60] Single-center case series with Matrix coils did not unequivocally show lower rates of aneurysmal recanalization than seen with bare platinum coils. In particular, Matrix-treated aneurysms recanalized at a rate of 37%, and the retreatment rate was 23%. The recanalization rate for large aneurysms was 75% with a 58% retreatment rate.[61] In another single-center experience, 57% of aneurysms embolized either completely or partially with Matrix coils recanalized over a period of a year (23% retreatment rate), and a high recanalization rate for large aneurysms (82%) was reported.[62] It was hypothesized that the high amount of polymeric coating on the coil produced more friction during deployment and compartmentalization, leading to incomplete aneurysmal packing. Additionally, the loss of occluded volume by the breakdown of the coating, which represented 70% of the cross-section of the coil, actually enhanced coil compaction. In response to these unfavorable clinical data, the manufacturer reduced the fraction of polymer to metallic coil in the second generation of the device.[63]

Alternatively, the polymer can be loaded into the center of the primary coil wind, thereby addressing the aforesaid disadvantages. A polyglycolic acid-loaded coil (Cerecyte, Micrus Endovascular, San Jose, CA) has been developed to deliver aneurysm framing and filling comparable to those in bare platinum coils while delivering the copolymer. Investigators in their early experience with Cerecyte coils described favorable outcome. In 55 prospective aneurysms, the investigators compared the results with a matched (size and location) retrospective group of 55 aneurysms treated with bare platinum coils.[64] Angiographic outcome immediately after embolization and at 6 months showed a recanalization rate of 16% with bare platinum coils and 4% with Cerecyte technology. Retreatment rate at 6 months was 11% and 2% with bare platinum and Cerecyte coils, respectively. In another single-center series that compared retrospectively aneurysms embolized with Cerecyte and with bare platinum coils, the recanalization rates after a minimum of 6 months were 16% and 6% in the bare platinum and Cerecyte groups, respectively.[65] This study showed that packing densities were similar when polymer-loaded and/or bare platinum coils were used (43% in the Cerecyte group versus 40% in the bare platinum groups). In both studies, no rebleeds occurred.

Both polymer-enhanced embolic coils are currently being evaluated in randomized controlled multicenter clinical studies. The Matrix and Platinum Science (MAPS) trial has not completed follow-up at the time this chapter was written. In May 2010 at the Annual Meeting of the American Society of Neuroradiology,[65a] it was announced that the Cerecyte trial demonstrated no difference between bare and coated coils in terms of recanalization or clinical outcomes. It has been generally agreed that these newer coil systems require rigorous clinical study in order to continue to advance coil technology in appropriate directions.

Liquid Embolics

An early technique in the endosaccular embolization of a cerebral aneurysm was performed with the use of cyanoacrylate via needle puncture into the aneurysm dome under direct visualization.[66] It was believed that a liquid that can deform under shear forces can easily conform to the boundaries of the aneurysm and achieve total occlusion. Subsequent polymerization or precipitation of the liquid then led to its solidification. However, even from this early experience the threats of distal emboli generated by fragmentation of the embolic and parent artery occlusion were identified. Because of this limitation, liquid embolics for the treatment of saccular aneurysms of the large arteries were largely abandoned with the exploration of detachable balloons and later detachable coils. It is important to note that excellent results are often obtained when aneurysms associated with arteriovenous malformations and distal traumatic or mycotic aneurysms are treated with liquid embolic agents. One agent, ethylene-vinyl alcohol (Onyx, eV3 Neurovascular, Irvine, CA), was evaluated clinically in the Cerebral Aneurysm Multicenter European Onyx (CAMEO) Trial.[67] This trial was a prospective, nonrandomized, multicenter study to investigate the safety and efficacy of Onyx for the treatment of brain aneurysms. The study reported results in 97 patients with 100 aneurysms. The rate of permanent neurologic morbidity or death related to the procedure or material was 10%. In 9.3% of patients, parent vessel occlusion occurred, which in five cases was asymptomatic. Modifications of Onyx and ancillary devices used to inject the embolic into unruptured wide-neck aneurysms of the internal carotid artery were investigated in a small series of patients at a single center.[68] The rate of parent artery occlusion or stenosis was 13.6% after a mean follow-up of 13 months. Larger single-center series have now shown low rates of recanalization (4.6% to 12.5% after a minimum of 6 months and up to 5 years) and permanent morbidity (7.2% and 8.3%).[69,70] Mortality rates in these reports were 2.9% and 3.2%. In both series, a small percentage of the cases involved ruptured aneurysms (6% and 14%), and thus morbidity and mortality do not appear to compare favorably against endovascular coil embolization in unruptured aneurysms. A randomized controlled multicenter clinical trial comparing the safety and efficacy of Onyx liquid embolic against the standard of care procedure, coil embolization, is needed to determine the long-term viability of this procedure. The key challenge with all liquid occlusive agents is to maintain material stability within the aneurysm sac during injection, which is necessary to prevent embolic complications or obliteration of adjacent perforating arteries secondary to leakage of the embolic material.

Adjunctive Devices

In a landmark paper describing the clinical and technical results from the first series of 403 patients embolized with the GDC coil system by Viñuela et al,[71] it was immediately recognized that aneurysm morphology was critical to complete endovascular occlusion. Aneurysms having a wide neck (>4 mm) or an unfavorable dome-to-neck ratio (<2) were not easily treated with endovascular means because of the lack of mechanical stability of the coil mass within the aneurysm sac. Coil penetration into the parent vessel, or even complete dislodgement of the coil mass, has the potential to produce ischemic stroke complications. An ingenious method to meet this challenge was proposed by several physicians, in which a compliant temporary occlusion balloon was used to bridge the neck of the aneurysm, allowing tight packing of the aneurysm with coils (illustrative case, Fig. 63-4).[72,73] Using this technique in 56 aneurysm embolizations, Moret et al achieved excellent safety results with only a single thromboembolic complication and no deaths.[72] The technical results for this complex aneurysm population were also excellent, with 94% of the aneurysms either completely or partially occluded. Single-center studies with larger patient populations have since reported that the complication rate increases with the use of the balloon remodeling technique.[74,75] Most often, complications involve thromboembolisms, which are likely due to endothelial damage. Consequently, it is necessary to inflate the ultra-compliant balloon cautiously and to maintain satisfactory anticoagulation of the patient during the procedure. There is a small risk of coil mass migration when the balloon is deflated. The latter shortcoming was addressed with the concept of stent-assisted coil embolization, in which the stent deployed into the parent artery serves as a permanent scaffold to retain the coil mass within the aneurysm sac.[76]

Initially, no stents were available for neurovascular stent–assisted coil embolization, and interventionalists were forced to use either coronary balloon–mounted stents or peripheral vascular stents for inoperable wide-neck aneurysms in which parent vessel sacrifice could not be tolerated. Although these procedures were technically difficult because these stents were not designed for the highly tortuous cerebrovasculature, excellent results were obtained.[77,78] A large single-center case series showed that with these suboptimal devices, the stent-assisted coil embolization could be performed successfully in 82% of cases; and complete occlusion persisted at 3- to 6-month angiographic follow-up in 92% of patients with saccular aneurysms and 100% of those with fusiform aneurysms.[77] Long-term data on stent-assisted coil embolization for fusiform aneurysms showed that clinical improvement or stable outcome could be achieved in 89% of patients.[78] Of the 28 patients followed up to 108 months, there were two cases of permanent morbidity, and one patient with a failed treatment died. In this most complex class of aneurysms, 4 (17%) aneurysms recanalized, of which 3 were successfully retreated. The advent of low-profile, microcatheter-delivered, self-expanding stents intentionally designed for the cerebrovasculature have revolutionized stent-assisted coil embolization (Fig. 63-5).[79,80] A single-center experience in 107 wide-neck aneurysms in which stent-assisted coil embolization was performed showed procedure-related morbidity and mortality to be 5.6% and 0.9%, respectively.[81] The researchers reported that favorable clinical outcome (modified Rankin score, 0 to 2) was achieved in 90.7% of the patients after a mean of 47 months. Angiography performed in nearly half of the patients after a mean of 37 months demonstrated a recanalization rate of 13.7%. The largest series

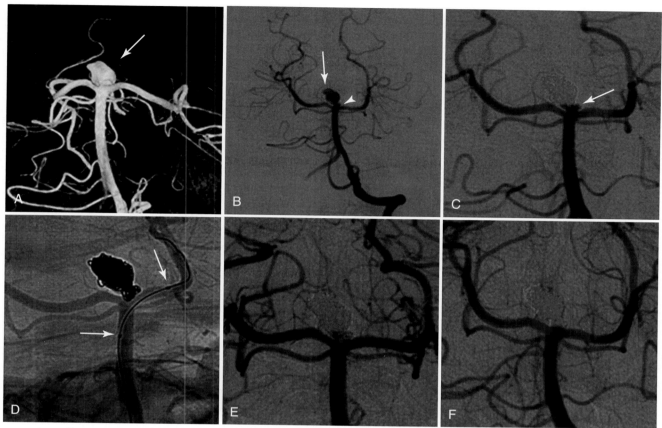

Figure 63-4 Illustrative case of balloon-assisted coil embolization in a 58-year-old man with a ruptured basilar top aneurysm. A, Three-dimensional rotational angiogram in oblique projection demonstrates a 10-mm × 7-mm multilobed basilar tip aneurysm with a 4-mm neck (arrow). B, Angiogram in frontal projection shows the irregularly shaped aneurysm (arrow) and a bleb close to the aneurysm neck (arrowhead). C, Coiling of the aneurysm dome shows the unprotected neck and bleb (arrow). D, A nondetachable, compliant balloon is positioned across the neck of the aneurysm (arrows). With the balloon inflated, additional coils are deployed into the neck and bleb. E, Immediately postoperative angiogram shows contrast penetration between the coils at the neck. F, Follow-up imaging study at 38 months shows angiographic occlusion of the aneurysm.

to date (142 aneurysms) reports 2.8% morbidity and 2% mortality associated with use of latest neurovascular stent technology.[82] We continue to await follow-up data from this multicenter study to see whether the presence of the stent reduces recanalization.

The key disadvantage of stent-assisted coil embolization is the metallic implant that remains within the parent artery, therefore necessitating dual-antiplatelet therapy for a minimum of 3 months to prevent ischemic stroke. This drawback is particularly disconcerting in cases of ruptured aneurysms, in which the risk of rerupture or bleeding from ventriculostomy sites cannot be ignored. Therefore, both adjunctive technologies retain an important place in the endovascular armament to address all brain aneurysms regardless of morphology and presentation.

Periprocedural Management of Patients Undergoing Endovascular Aneurysm Treatment

Preprocedural management of patients undergoing elective endovascular treatment for an unruptured intracranial aneurysm differs from that of a patient with

emergency aneurysmal SAH. Therefore, the two conditions are addressed independently.

Preprocedural Management

Unruptured aneurysms: In patients undergoing elective endovascular embolization of an unruptured intracranial aneurysm, a complete history and physical examination and diagnostic angiogram are required for planning of the intervention. Digital subtraction angiography (DSA) is the traditional gold standard diagnostic test for assessment of intracranial aneurysms.[83,84] However, newer technology, such as 3D rotational angiography (3DRA), allows for more elegant preprocedural planning, especially in anatomically challenging areas such as the middle cerebral artery bifurcation and in small aneurysms (≤3 mm) that may be missed by DSA.[85]

A multidisciplinary approach involving neurosurgery, neurology, and neurointerventional surgeons is recommended for each case (ruptured or unruptured aneurysm). Aneurysm size, location, and morphology are factors to consider in planning of the approach. When endovascular treatment is agreed upon, it is critical to have access to a variety of technology, including various

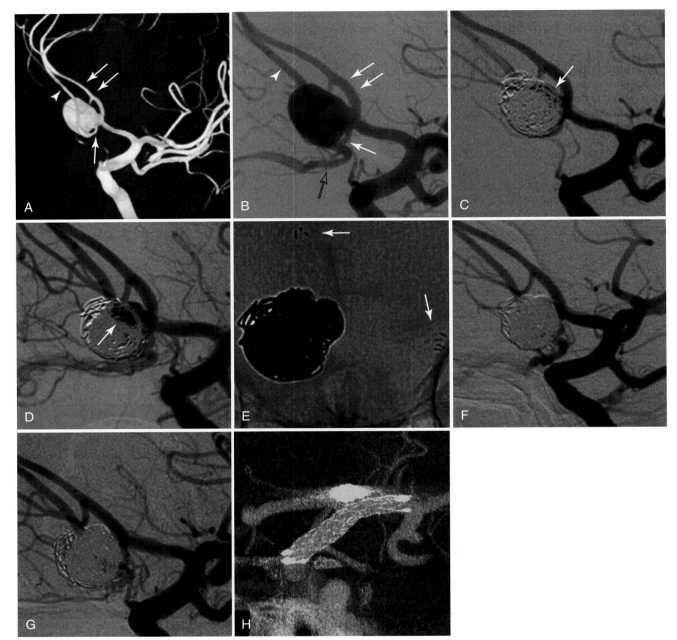

Figure 63-5 A 48-year-old woman presented with chronic headaches. Acute excruciating frontal headaches initiated CT, results of which were negative for subarachnoid hemorrhage. A large anterior communicating artery aneurysm was found. Three-dimensional rotational angiogram (A) and angiogram (B), both left anterior oblique projections, show a 9-mm left A1/A2 anterior cerebral artery (ACA) aneurysm with a 5.2-mm neck; *single arrows* indicate the anterior communicating artery, *arrowheads* indicate the right anterior cerebral artery A2 segment, *open arrow* indicates the right A1 segment with filling of the middle cerebral artery, and *double arrows* indicate the left anterior cerebral artery A2 segment. C, Postembolization angiogram shows a small filling of contrast agent at the superior aspect of the aneurysm dome *(arrow)*. D, One-year follow-up angiogram shows coil compaction and rearrangement with recanalization of the aneurysm *(arrow)*. E and F, Stent-assisted coil embolization, with preservation of both anterior communicating artery and ACAs; *arrows* indicate the stent position in the left ACA. G, Study performed 6 months after retreatment shows complete aneurysm occlusion and no coil compaction. H, A contrast enhanced cone-beam CT of another case of stent-assisted coiling of a left internal carotid artery terminus aneurysm. This imaging modality[80a] delineates simultaneously the stent implant and host vasculature with high spatial resolution.

microcatheters, coil sizes and shapes, and adjunctive devices such as compliant balloons and neurovascular stents. Wide-neck (neck >4 mm, dome-to-neck ratio <2) or fusiform aneurysms often require the use of adjunctive therapies, such as stents. The American Heart Association recommends that dual-antiplatelet therapy commence before and be continued after stenting in patients with coronary artery disease to lower the risk of acute in-stent thrombosis and delayed thrombotic complications and re stenosis.[86] There is, however, no consensus recommendation in cerebrovascular stenting, and the restenosis rate after stenting in intracranial atherosclerosis is reportedly higher.[87,88] One study found that of 55 patients taking clopidogrel after cerebrovascular stent placement, 28 patients (52%) were clopidogrel-resistant.[89] Only 4.2% of patients in the same cohort were aspirin-resistant.[89] In the near future, point-of care tests of platelet function may be feasible so that antiplatelet regimens may be appropriately modified in patients who do not respond to antiplatelet medication.[90] However, stent-assisted coiling of aneurysms, which rarely involves local atherosclerosis, poses a different challenge regarding dual-antiplatelet therapy. Although no specific guidelines for dual-antiplatelet therapy in aneurysm stenting currently exist, most practitioners have adopted the treatment regimen from the coronary stenting literature. All cases, regardless of the use of stent-supported coil embolization, require anticoagulation with heparin to maintain an activated clotting time (ACT) between 250 and 400 seconds. This is accomplished with an intravenous bolus of heparin followed by continuous administration of maintenance doses and ACT monitoring. Furthermore, all endovascular surgeries are performed under general anesthesia for patients' comfort and to prevent complications associated with patient motion. Regardless of the use of adjunctive devices, it has been shown that patients pretreated with oral antiplatelet drugs have a lower incidence of periprocedural thromboembolic events, but consequently a higher rate of intracerebral hemorrhage.[91] There currently is no standard of practice regarding the use of antiplatelet therapy prior to embolization of unruptured aneurysms.

Adverse reactions to contrast agents, although rare, may be life-threatening. To reduce the risk of allergic contrast media reaction and contrast-induced nephrotoxicity, use of low- or iso-osmolar contrast media is supported.[92,93] Furthermore, there is evidence to support pretreatment with corticosteroids[94,95] and antihistamines[96] in patients with suspected or documented history of allergic contrast media reaction. Despite its relatively low incidence (0.03 cases per 1000 patients per year),[97] prophylaxis against contrast-induced nephropathy, especially for patients with elevated serum creatinine levels, is necessary.[93] Preprocedural hydration with isotonic saline (100 mL per hour for up to 24 hours prior) is the pretreatment of choice. Administration of acetylcysteine or sodium bicarbonate 48 hours before coiling may also be beneficial in high-risk patients. In patients taking metformin, the drug should be stopped 24 hours prior to coiling and not resumed until 48 hours after the procedure to minimize the risk of lactic acidosis.[98]

Ruptured aneurysms: Eighty percent of nontraumatic SAHs occur secondary to intracranial aneurysm rupture.[99] Nearly half of all patients with ruptured aneurysm die within the first 30 days,[100] and 46% of survivors suffer long-term disability.[101] Therefore, a rapid neurologic assessment using the World Federation of Neurological Surgeons SAH grade[102] and Hunt and Hess scale[103] is essential. CT of the head without a contrast agent is the first imaging test to confirm the presence and assess the degree of subarachnoid blood.[104] All patients with confirmed SAH should be transferred to a center with dedicated neurologic critical care services.[105,106] The airway should be continuously assessed, and blood pressure maintained within normal limits.[107] Once SAH is confirmed, four-vessel digital subtraction angiography (with 3D rotational angiography if available) is indicated, during which definitive aneurysm treatment may be performed.[108] CT angiography, readily available in most centers, is becoming the choice for first-line diagnostic imaging for aneurysm screening in SAH and for further therapeutic management.[109] Although currently debated, loading doses of aspirin (325 mg) and clopidogrel (300 mg) can be administered through a nasogastric tube,[86] or abciximab can be administered intravenously, if intracranial stent placement in the emergency setting is indicated. Because an increased risk of intracerebral hemorrhage is seen, however, a ventriculostomy should be considered prior to antiplatelet therapy with clopidogrel.[110] Preprocedural decompressive craniotomy in case of a large intracerebral hematoma associated with an aneurysm rupture may be considered before or after the endovascular intervention.

Intraprocedural Management

Endovascular aneurysm treatment requires the careful positioning of microwires and microcatheters into the cerebral blood vessels. Therefore, patients should be kept under general anesthesia with endotracheal intubation to eliminate any movement, thus ensuring accurate imaging and catheter placement.[111] The anesthesiologist can also maintain controlled access over the airway and hemodynamics. Angiography should be performed under apnea conditions to reduce motion artifact.

Thromboembolic complications, including major and minor stroke and transient ischemic attack, occur in between 2.5% and 28% of all patients undergoing aneurysm coiling.[71,112] Thrombi may form on the surfaces of catheters and coils, may be dislodged from the aneurysm sac during coiling, or may occur at sites of catheter-induced vessel injury.[113] In a meta-analysis of 1547 patients from 23 studies treated with GDCs, the majority of thromboembolic complications occurred intraoperatively.[114] Therefore, intraprocedural therapy with a weight-based dosing schedule of heparin[115] is recommended[114] with baseline ACT measured prior to catheter insertion. In the setting of aneurysmal SAH, heparin can be started following placement of the first coil.[116,117] This measure reduces the risk of devastating rebleeding if the coil pierces through the aneurysm rupture site. Intraprocedural ACT should be measured at regular intervals (generally hourly) during the procedure, and heparin dosing titrated to a target ACT of 250 seconds.

Postprocedural Management

Postprocedural use of heparin is controversial and generally not recommended.[114] Aspirin therapy is indicated after coiling for 4 weeks, after which endothelialization of the devices is expected.[118] Thromboembolic complications are very rare after 4 weeks,[114] even if endothelialization is incomplete.[119] For stent-assisted coiling, dual-antiplatelet therapy is recommended for 3 months for the prevention of in-stent stenosis. At some centers, lifelong single-antiplatelet therapy with aspirin is advocated.

Preprocedural and intraprocedural use of heparin and antiplatelets emphasizes the importance of hemostasis at the access site to prevent hematoma formation. A meta-analysis of 4000 patients in 30 trials who underwent percutaneous coronary interventions demonstrated that arterial puncture closure devices (Angio-Seal, St. Jude Medical, St. Paul, MN; Perclose, Abbott Laboratories, Abbott Park, IL) appear to reduce time to hemostasis, but there is no evidence that these devices reduce complication rates or length of hospital stay in comparison with traditional manual compression.[120] To aid effectiveness of manual compression, new glycosaminoglycan-containing matrices have been shown to improve hemostasis in animal models.[121]

Upon hemostasis, controlled extubation should take place in the angiography suite prior to monitored patient transfer to the intensive care unit. If needed, cone-beam CT can be obtained with the newer angiography equipment if acute hydrocephalus necessitating ventriculostomy is suspected. This technology is also useful to evaluate the size and location of hematoma in the case of an intraprocedural aneurysm rupture potentially requiring an emergency decompression. Neurologic examinations are critical in the immediate postprocedural period, because abnormal findings may indicate a need for emergency re-intervention.

Management of Periprocedural Complications during Endovascular Aneurysm Treatment

As with all endovascular approaches, intraoperative complications involve aneurysm or arterial rupture (perforation), nonextravasating damage to the vascular wall (dissection, thrombosis), and cessation of antegrade blood flow (embolus). Unfortunately, the tortuous and fragile cerebrovasculature accentuates the risk of these complications and, at the same time, the brain is the most unforgiving organ when these complications arise. Hence, the need for highly trained and dedicated endovascular interventionalists who specialize in this procedure must be amply emphasized; such specialists must both be capable of preventing complications and know how best to manage them when they occur. Two decades of experience in the endovascular coil embolization of aneurysms have offered valuable techniques and devices to manage these complications in situ, thereby minimizing adverse clinical events.

Thromboembolic Complications

In the absence of class I evidence of a superior anti-platelet regimen for both ruptured and unruptured aneurysms, thromboembolic complications during endovascular aneurysm embolization remain the most common, with a frequency of 2.4% to 5.2%.[26,28] The sources of emboli are platelet aggregation in response to catheters, devices or intimal damage, and intraaneurysmal clot dislodgement. Late thromboembolisms might result from

discontinuation of antiplatelet therapy in patients undergoing stent-assisted embolization or herniation of coils into the parent artery. The safety and efficacy of intraoperative selective administration of abciximab have been demonstrated.[122,123,123a] In addition, stents can be used in the event of coil herniation to trap the extraaneurysmal coil against the vessel wall.[124]

A variety of retrieval systems are now available for use when devices such as embolic coils compromise the parent artery.[125,126] These snares and microforceps are navigated through microcatheters and may be employed to remove foreign bodies. Additionally, devices are now becoming available for mechanical thrombectomy to extract clot that does not respond to lytics.[127,128]

Perforation

Perforation and subsequent hemorrhage due to endovascular devices is more common in patients presenting with SAH (4.1%) than in those with unruptured aneurysms (0.5%).[129] Resulting morbidity and mortality from intraoperative perforation have been reported as 1.8% and 0.2%, respectively. Most aneurysm perforations today do not produce clinical adverse outcomes primarily because of the aggressive and rapid response by experienced interventionalists, which consists of (1) reversal of anticoagulation, (2) using a temporary occlusion balloon to tamponade the bleed site or leaving the perforating instrument in place if surgical repair is needed, and (3) continuation of coil embolization to secure the perforation. Continuous improvements in coil technology have led to reduced incidence of periprocedural aneurysm perforations.

Future of the Endovascular Treatment of Brain Aneurysms

Continuous improvements to imaging, devices, and techniques have made neurointerventional surgery one of the fastest-growing specialties. These improvements are expected to make the procedures even safer and improve the long-term durability of aneurysm obliteration.

Prior to the approval of the GDC coil by the U.S. Food and Drug Administration, researchers were already exploring the concept of flow diversion for the treatment of brain aneurysms.[130,131] Essentially, the concept incorporated two phenomena, the disruption of the fluid momentum transfer into the aneurysm sac and the scaffold that produces a remodeling effect of the vascular wall. The embodiment today of this concept is low-porosity braided stents[132] (Fig. 63-6). The Pipeline braided stent (Chestnut Medical, Menlo Park, CA), and other stentlike devices and stent grafts have potential to represent a paradigm shift in the treatment of intracranial aneurysms away from coil embolization and toward parent vessel reconstruction and flow diversion as well as vessel-preserving strategy for vascular wall lesions. Published preliminary results in human aneurysms are encouraging.[133-135] Perhaps the next decade of development in the endovascular treatment of brain aneurysms will belong to flow diverters and the refinement of these devices to cure a variety of intracranial aneurysms.

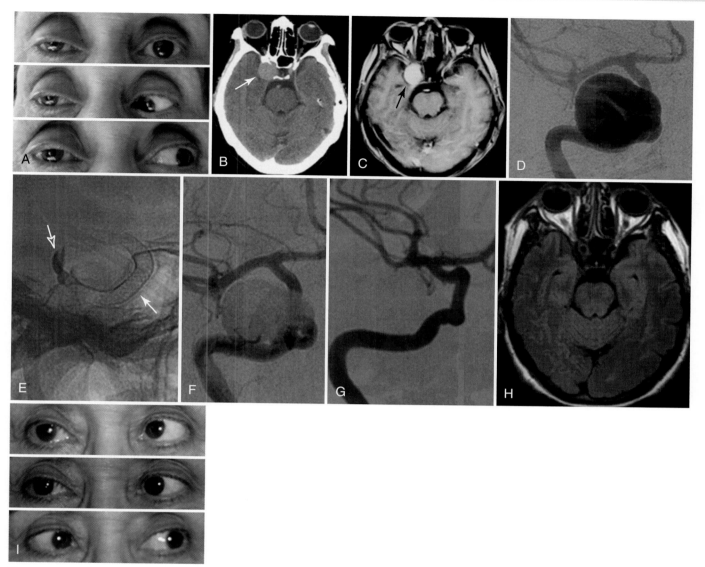

Figure 63-6 A, A 58-year-old woman presents with a right III and VI nerve palsy. CT scan (B) and contrast-enhanced T1-weighted MR image (C) demonstrate a giant (25-mm) right internal carotid artery (ICA) aneurysm of the cavernous segment *(arrows)* with adjacent remodeling of the anterior clinoid (B). D, Right anterior oblique projection from preoperative catheter angiography details a diseased right cavernous ICA with aneurysm formation. E, Two flow-diverting devices are deployed across the neck of the aneurysm *(arrow)*, leading to immediate stagnation of contrast agent in the aneurysm *(open arrow)*. F, Catheter angiography shows disrupted filling of the aneurysm by contrast agent and diversion of the flow from the aneurysm to the distal vasculature. G, Six-month follow-up angiogram, right anterior oblique projection, shows complete obliteration of the aneurysm and remodeling of the treated artery. H, T1-weighted MR image reveals resorption of the obliterated aneurysm with resolution of the mass effect. I, The result was improvement in clinical condition. (Courtesy of Dr. Pedro Lylyk, Buenos Aires.)

REFERENCES

1. Luessenhop AJ, Velasquez AC: Observations on the tolerance of the intracranial arteries to catheterization, *J Neurosurg* 21:85–91, 1964.
2. Alksne JF: Stereotactic thrombosis of intracranial aneurysms using a magnetic probe, *Confin Neurol* 31:95–98, 1969.
3. Mullan S, Beckman F, Vailati G, et al: An experimental approach to the problem of cerebral aneurysm, *J Neurosurg* 21:838–845, 1964.
4. Mullan S, Raimondi AJ, Dobben G, et al: Electrically induced thrombosis in intracranial aneurysms, *J Neurosurg* 22:539–547, 1965.
5. Teitelbaum GP, Larsen DW, Zelman V, et al: A tribute to Dr. Fedor A. Serbinenko, founder of endovascular neurosurgery, *Neurosurgery* 46:462–469, 2000.
6. Serbinenko FA: Catheterization and occlusion of major cerebral vessels and prospects for the development of vascular neurosurgery, *Vopr Neirokhir* 35:17–27, 1971.
7. Serbinenko FA: Balloon occlusion of saccular aneurysms of the cerebral arteries, *Vopr Neirokhir* 8–15, 1974.
8. Serbinenko FA: Balloon catheterization and occlusion of major cerebral vessels, *J Neurosurg* 41:125–145, 1974.
9. Debrun G, Coscas G: Treatment of carotido-cavernous fistulas and intracavernous aneurysms by means of a balloon catheter, which can be inflated and enlarged, *Bull Soc Ophtalmol Fr* 75:857–864, 1975.
10. Higashida RT, Halbach VV, Barnwell SL, et al: Treatment of intracranial aneurysms with preservation of the parent vessel: Results of percutaneous balloon embolization in 84 patients, *AJNR Am J Neuroradiol* 11:633–640, 1990.

11. Debrun G, Lacour P, Caron JP, et al: Detachable balloon and calibrated-leak balloon techniques in the treatment of cerebral vascular lesions, *J Neurosurg* 49:635-649, 1978.

12. Romodanov AP, Shcheglov VI: Endovascular method of excluding from the circulation saccular cerebral arterial aneurysms, leaving intact vessels patent, *Acta Neurochir Suppl (Wien)* 28:312-315, 1979.

13. Bavinzski G, Talazoglu V, Killer M, et al: Gross and microscopic histopathological findings in aneurysms of the human brain treated with Guglielmi detachable coils, *J Neurosurg* 91:284-293, 1999.

14. Stiver SI, Porter PJ, Willinsky RA, et al: Acute human histopathology of an intracranial aneurysm treated using Guglielmi detachable coils: Case report and review of the literature, *Neurosurgery* 43:1203-1207, 1998.

15. Ishihara S, Mawad ME, Ogata K, et al: Histopathologic findings in human cerebral aneurysms embolized with platinum coils: report of two cases and review of the literature, *AJNR Am J Neuroradiol* 23:970-974, 2002.

16. Groden C, Hagel C, Delling G, et al: Histological findings in ruptured aneurysms treated with GDCs: Six examples at varying times after treatment, *AJNR Am J Neuroradiol* 24:579-584, 2003.

17. Castro E, Fortea F, Villoria F, et al: Long-term histopathologic findings in two cerebral aneurysms embolized with Guglielmi detachable coils, *AJNR Am J Neuroradiol* 20:549-552, 1999.

18. Guglielmi G, Viñuela F, Sepetka I, et al: Electrothrombosis of saccular aneurysms via endovascular approach. Part 1: Electrochemical basis, technique, and experimental results, *J Neurosurg* 75:1-7, 1991.

19. Guglielmi G, Viñuela F, Dion J, et al: Electrothrombosis of saccular aneurysms via endovascular approach. Part 2: Preliminary clinical experience, *J Neurosurg* 75:8-14, 1991.

20. Higashida RT, Halbach VV, Dowd C, et al: Endovascular detachable balloon embolization therapy of cavernous carotid artery aneurysms: Results in 87 cases, *J Neurosurg* 72:857-863, 1990.

21. Moret J: Endovascular treatment of berry aneurysms by endosaccular occlusion, *Acta Neurochir Suppl (Wien)* 53:48-49, 1991.

22. Kassell NF, Torner JC: Aneurysmal rebleeding: A preliminary report from the Cooperative Aneurysm Study, *Neurosurgery* 13:479-481, 1983.

23. Jane JA, Winn HR, Richardson AE: The natural history of intracranial aneurysms: Rebleeding rates during the acute and long term period and implication for surgical management, *Clin Neurosurg* 24:176-184, 1977.

24. Molyneux A, Kerr R, Stratton I, et al: International Subarachnoid Aneurysm Trial (ISAT) of neurosurgical clipping versus endovascular coiling in 2143 patients with ruptured intracranial aneurysms: A randomised trial, *Lancet* 360:1267-1274, 2002.

25. Molyneux AJ, Kerr RS, Yu LM, et al: International subarachnoid aneurysm trial (ISAT) of neurosurgical clipping versus endovascular coiling in 2143 patients with ruptured intracranial aneurysms: A randomised comparison of effects on survival, dependency, seizures, rebleeding, subgroups, and aneurysm occlusion, *Lancet* 366:809-817, 2005.

26. Gallas S, Pasco A, Cottier JP, et al: A multicenter study of 705 ruptured intracranial aneurysms treated with Guglielmi detachable coils, *AJNR Am J Neuroradiol* 26:1723-1731, 2005.

27. Raymond J, Guilbert F, Weill A, et al: Long-term angiographic recurrences after selective endovascular treatment of aneurysms with detachable coils, *Stroke* 34:1398-1403, 2003.

28. Murayama Y, Nien YL, Duckwiler G, et al: Guglielmi detachable coil embolization of cerebral aneurysms: 11 years' experience, *J Neurosurg* 98:959-966, 2003.

29. CARAT Investigators: Rates of delayed rebleeding from intracranial aneurysms are low after surgical and endovascular treatment, *Stroke* 37:1437-1442, 2006.

30. Johnston SC, Dowd CF, Higashida RT, et al: Predictors of rehemorrhage after treatment of ruptured intracranial aneurysms: The Cerebral Aneurysm Rerupture After Treatment (CARAT) study, *Stroke* 39:120-125, 2008.

31. Molyneux A, Kerr R, Stratton I, et al: International Subarachnoid Aneurysm Trial (ISAT) of neurosurgical clipping versus endovascular coiling in 2143 patients with ruptured intracranial aneurysms: A randomized trial, *J Stroke Cerebrovasc Dis* 11:304-314, 2002.

32. Molyneux A, Kerr R, Birks J, et al: Risk of recurrent subarachnoid haemorrhage, death, or dependence and standardised mortality ratios after clipping or coiling of an intracranial aneurysm in the International Subarachnoid Aneurysm Trial (ISAT): Long-term follow-up, *Lancet Neurol* 8:427-433, 2009.

33. Holmin S, Krings T, Ozanne A, et al: Intradural saccular aneurysms treated by Guglielmi detachable bare coils at a single institution between 1993 and 2005: Clinical long-term follow-up for a total of 1810 patient-years in relation to morphological treatment results, *Stroke* 39:2288-2297, 2008.

34. Weir B: Unruptured intracranial aneurysms: A review, *J Neurosurg* 96:3-42, 2002.

35. Weir B, Disney L, Karrison T: Sizes of ruptured and unruptured aneurysms in relation to their sites and the ages of patients, *J Neurosurg* 96:64-70, 2002.

36. Komotar RJ, Zacharia BE, Otten ML, et al: Controversies in the endovascular management of cerebral vasospasm after intracranial aneurysm rupture and future directions for therapeutic approaches, *Neurosurgery* 62:897-905, 2008.

37. International Study of Unruptured Intracranial Aneurysms Investigators: Unruptured intracranial aneurysms—risk of rupture and risks of surgical intervention, *N Engl J Med* 339:1725-1733, 1998.

38. Wiebers DO, Whisnant JP, Huston J 3rd, et al: Unruptured intracranial aneurysms: Natural history, clinical outcome, and risks of surgical and endovascular treatment, *Lancet* 362:103-110, 2003.

39. Raymond J, Meder JF, Molyneux AJ, et al: Unruptured intracranial aneurysms: The unreliability of clinical judgment, the necessity for evidence, and reasons to participate in a randomized trial, *J Neuroradiol* 33:211-219, 2006.

40. Bederson JB, Awad IA, Wiebers DO, et al: Recommendations for the management of patients with unruptured intracranial aneurysms: A Statement for healthcare professionals from the Stroke Council of the American Heart Association, *Stroke* 31:2742-2750, 2000.

41. Kobayashi S, Orz Y, George B, et al: Treatment of unruptured cerebral aneurysms, *Surg Neurol* 51:355-362, 1999.

42. Juvela S, Porras M, Heiskanen O: Natural history of unruptured intracranial aneurysms: a long-term follow-up study, *J Neurosurg* 79:174-182, 1993.

43. Juvela S, Porras M, Poussa K: Natural history of unruptured intracranial aneurysms: Probability of and risk factors for aneurysm rupture, *J Neurosurg* 93:379-387, 2000.

44. Raymond J, Molyneux AJ, Fox AJ, et al: The TEAM trial: Safety and efficacy of endovascular treatment of unruptured intracranial aneurysms in the prevention of aneurysmal hemorrhages: A randomized comparison with indefinite deferral of treatment in 2002 patients followed for 10 years, *Trials* 9:43, 2008.

45. Pierot L, Spelle L, Vitry F, et al: Immediate clinical outcome of patients harboring unruptured intracranial aneurysms treated by endovascular approach: Results of the ATENA study, *Stroke* 39:2497-2504, 2008.

46. Ishibashi T, Murayama Y, Urashima M, et al: Unruptured intracranial aneurysms: Incidence of rupture and risk factors, *Stroke* 40:313-316, 2009.

47. Im S, Han M, Kwon O, et al: Endovascular coil embolization of 435 small asymptomatic unruptured intracranial aneurysms: Procedural morbidity and patient outcome, *AJNR Am J Neuroradiol* 30:79-84, 2009.

48. Frösen J, Piippo A, Paetau A, et al: Remodeling of saccular cerebral artery aneurysm wall is associated with rupture; histological analysis of 24 unruptured and 42 ruptured cases, *Stroke* 35:2287-2293, 2004.

49. DeLeo MJ III, Gounis MJ, Hong B, et al: Carotid artery brain aneurysm model: In vivo molecular enzyme-specific MR imaging of active inflammation in a pilot study, *Radiology* 253:9000-9901, 2009.

50. Cha KS, Balaras E, Lieber BB, et al: Modeling the interaction of coils with the local blood flow after coil embolization of intracranial aneurysms, *J Biomech Eng* 129:873-879, 2007.

51. Kawanabe Y, Sadato A, Taki W, et al: Endovascular occlusion of intracranial aneurysms with Guglielmi detachable coils: Correlation between coil packing density and coil compaction, *Acta Neurochir (Wien)* 143:451-455, 2001.

52. Sluzewski M, van Rooij WJ, Slob MJ, et al: Relation between aneurysm volume, packing, and compaction in 145 cerebral aneurysms treated with coils, *Radiology* 231:653-658, 2004.

53. Wakhloo AK, Gounis MJ, Sandhu JS, et al: Complex-shaped platinum coils for brain aneurysms: Higher packing density, improved biomechanical stability, and midterm angiographic outcome, *AJNR Am J Neuroradiol* 28:1395–1400, 2007.

54. Slob MJ, van Rooij WJ, Sluzewski M: Influence of coil thickness on packing, re-opening and retreatment of intracranial aneurysms: A comparative study between two types of coils, *Neurol Res* 27:S116–S119, 2005.

55. Dawson RC III, Krisht AF, Barrow DL, et al: Treatment of experimental aneurysms using collagen-coated microcoils, *Neurosurgery* 36:133–140, 1995.

55a. Szikora I, Wakhloo AK, Guterman LR, et al: Initial experience with collagen-filled Guglielmi detachable coils for endovascular treatment of experimental aneurysms, *AJNR Am J Neuroradiol* 18:667–672, 1997.

56. Deshaies EM, Bagla A, Agner C, et al: Determination of filling volumes in HydroCoil-treated aneurysms by using three-dimensional computerized tomography angiography, *Neurosurg Focus* 18:E5, 2005.

57. Cloft HJ: for the HEAL Investigators: HydroCoil for Endovascular Aneurysm Occlusion (HEAL) Study: 3-6 Month angiographic follow-up Results, *AJNR Am J Neuroradiol* 28:152–154, 2007.

58. White PM, Lewis SC, Nahser H, et al: HydroCoil Endovascular Aneurysm Occlusion and Packing Study (HELPS trial): Procedural safety and operator-assessed efficacy results, *AJNR Am J Neuroradiol* 29:214–223, 2008.

58a. White, P: HELPS Trial. 7th Annual Meeting Society of NeuroInterventional Surgery, Carlsbad, Calif, July 26-30, 2010.

59. Murayama Y, Tateshima S, Gonzalez NR, et al: Matrix and bioabsorbable polymeric coils accelerate healing of intracranial aneurysms; long-term experimental study, *Stroke* 34:2031–2037, 2003.

60. Linfante I, Akkawi NM, Perlow A, et al: Polyglycolide/polylactide-coated platinum coils for patients with ruptured and unruptured cerebral aneurysms, *Stroke* 36:1–6, 2005.

61. Fiorella D, Albuquerque FC, McDougall CG: Durability of aneurysm embolization with matrix detachable coils, *Neurosurgery* 58:51–59, 2006:discussion 51-59.

62. Niimi Y, Song J, Madrid M, et al: Endosaccular treatment of intracranial aneurysms using matrix coils: Early experience and mid-term follow-up, *Stroke* 37:1028–1032, 2006.

63. Ishii A, Muryama Y, Nien YL, et al: Immediate and midterm outcomes of patients with cerebral aneurysms treated with Matrix1 and Matrix2 coils: A comparative analysis based on a single-center experience in 250 consecutive cases, *Neurosurgery* 63:1071–1077, 2008.

64. Bendszus M, Bartsch AJ, Solymosi L: Endovascular occlusion of aneurysms using a new bioactive coil: A matched pair analysis with bare platinum coils, *Stroke* 38:2855–2857, 2007.

65. Linfante I, DeLeo MJ III, Gounis MJ, et al: Cerecyte versus platinum coils in the treatment of intracranial aneurysms: Packing density, clinical and angiographic mid-term results, *AJNR Am J Neuroradiol* 30:1496–1501, 2009.

65a. Moylneux AJ, Coley S, Sneade M, Mehta Z, on behalf of the Cerecyte Coil Trial Investigators. Cerecyte Coil Trial: Clinical outcome of endovascular coiling in patients with ruptured and unruptured intracranial aneurysms treated with Cerecyte coils compared with bare platinum coils. Results of a prospective randomized trial. *Proceedings of the ASNR*, Boston, Mass, May 15-20, 2010, p 228.

66. Sheptak PE, Zanetti PH, Seusen AF: The treatment of intracranial aneurysms by injection with a tissue adhesive, *Neurosurgery* 1:25–29, 1977.

67. Molyneux AJ, Cekirge S, Saatci I, et al: Cerebral Aneurysm Multicenter European Onyx (CAMEO) Trial: Results of a prospective observational study in 20 european centers, *AJNR Am J Neuroradiol* 25:39–51, 2004.

68. Weber W, Siekmann R, Kis B, et al: Treatment and follow-up of 22 unruptured wide-necked intracranial aneurysms of the internal carotid artery with Onyx HD 500, *AJNR Am J Neuroradiol* 26:1909–1915, 2005.

69. Piske RL, Kanashiro LH, Paschoal E, et al: Evaluation of Onyx HD-500 embolic system in the treatment of 84 wide-neck intracranial aneurysms, *Neurosurgery* 64:E865–E875, 2009.

70. Cekirge HS, Saatci I, Ozturk MH, et al: Late angiographic and clinical follow-up results of 100 consecutive aneurysms treated with Onyx reconstruction: Largest single-center experience, *Neuroradiology* 48:113–126, 2006.

71. Viñuela F, Duckwiler G, Mawad ME: Guglielmi detachable coil embolization of acute intracranial aneurysm: Perioperative anatomical and clinical outcome in 403 patients, *J Neurosurg* 86:475–482, 1997.

72. Moret J, Cognard C, Weill A, et al: Reconstruction technic in the treatment of wide-neck intracranial aneurysms. Long-term angiographic and clinical results. Apropos of 56 cases, *J Neuroradiol* 24:30–44, 1997.

73. Mericle RA, Wakhloo AK, Rodriquez R, et al: Temporary balloon protection as an adjunct to endosaccular coiling of wide-necked cerebral aneurysms: Technical note, *Neurosurgery* 41:975–978, 1997.

74. Henkes H, Fischer S, Weber W, et al: Endovascular coil occlusion of 1811 intracranial aneurysms: Early angiographic and clinical results, *Neurosurgery* 24:280–285, 2004.

75. Sluzewski M, van Rooij WJ, Beute GN, et al: Balloon-assisted coil embolization of intracranial aneurysms: Incidence, complications, and angiography results, *J Neurosurg* 105:396–399, 2006.

76. Turjman F, Massoud TF, Ji C, et al: Combined stent implantation and endosaccular coil placement for treatment of experimental wide-necked aneurysms: A feasibility study in swine, *AJNR Am J Neuroradiol* 15:1087–1090, 1994.

77. Lylyk P, Cohen JE, Ceratto R, et al: Endovascular reconstruction of intracranial arteries by stent placement and combined techniques, *J Neurosurg* 97:1306–1313, 2002.

78. Wakhoo AK, Mandell J, Gounis MJ, et al: Stent-assisted reconstructive endovascular repair of cranial fusiform atherosclerotic and dissecting aneurysms: Long-term clinical and angiographic follow-up, *Stroke* 39:3288–3296, 2008.

79. Wanke I, Doerfler A, Schoch B, et al: Treatment of wide-necked intracranial aneurysms with a self-expanding stent system: initial clinical experience, *AJNR Am J Neuroradiol* 24:1192–1199, 2003.

80. Higashida RT, Halbach VV, Dowd CF, et al: Initial clinical experience with a new self-expanding nitinol stent for the treatment of intracranial cerebral aneurysms: The Cordis Enterprise stent, *AJNR Am J Neuroradiol* 26:1751–1756, 2005.

80a. Patel NV, Gounis MJ, Wakhloo AK, et al: Contrast-enhanced angiographic cone-beam CT of cerebrovascular stents: Experimental optimization and clinical application, *AJNR Am J Neuroradiol*, 32:137, 2011.

81. Liang G, Gao X, Li Z, et al: Neuroform stent-assisted coiling of intracranial aneurysms: A 5 year single-center experience and follow-up, *Neurol Res* 32:721–727, 2009.

82. Mocco J, Snyder KV, Albuquerque FC, et al: Treatment of intracranial aneurysms with the Enterprise stent: A multicenter registry, *J Neurosurg* 110:35–39, 2009.

83. Kouskouras C, Charitanti A, Giavroglou C, et al: Intracranial aneurysms: Evaluation using CTA and MRA. Correlation with DSA and intraoperative findings, *Neuroradiology* 46:842–850, 2004.

84. Yoon DY, Lim KJ, Choi CS, et al: Detection and characterization of intracranial aneurysms with 16-channel multidetector row CT angiography: A prospective comparison of volume-rendered images and digital subtraction angiography, *AJNR Am J Neuroradiol* 28:60–67, 2007.

85. van Rooij WJ, Sprengers ME, de Gast AN, et al: 3D rotational angiography: The new gold standard in the detection of additional intracranial aneurysms, *AJNR Am J Neuroradiol* 29:976–979, 2008.

86. Smith SC Jr, Feldman TE, Hirshfeld JW Jr, et al: ACC/AHA/SCAI 2005 guideline update for percutaneous coronary intervention: A report of the American College of Cardiology/American Heart Association Task Force on Practice Guidelines (ACC/AHA/SCAI Writing Committee to Update 2001 Guidelines for Percutaneous Coronary Intervention), *Circulation* 113:e166–e286, 2006.

87. Fiorella D, Levy EI, Turk AS, et al: US multicenter experience with the Wingspan stent system for the treatment of intracranial atheromatous disease: Periprocedural results, *Stroke* 38:881–887, 2007.

88. Henkes H, Miloslavski E, Lowens S, et al: Treatment of intracranial atherosclerotic stenoses with balloon dilatation and self-expanding stent deployment (Wingspan), *Neuroradiology* 47:222–228, 2005.

89. Prabhakaran S, Wells KR, Lee VH, et al: Prevalence and risk factors for aspirin and clopidogrel resistance in cerebrovascular stenting, *AJNR Am J Neuroradiol* 29:281–285, 2008.

90. Lee DH, Arat A, Morsi H, et al: Dual antiplatelet therapy monitoring for neurointerventional procedures using a point-of-care platelet function test: a single-center experience, *AJNR Am J Neuroradiol* 29:1389–1394, 2008.

91. Yamada NK, Cross DT III, Pilgram TK, et al: Effect of antiplatelet therapy on thromboembolic complications of elective coil embolization of cerebral aneurysms, *AJNR Am J Neuroradiol* 28: 1778-1782, 2007.

92. Katayama H, Yamaguchi K, Kozuka T, et al: Adverse reactions to ionic and nonionic contrast media. A report from the Japanese Committee on the Safety of Contrast Media, *Radiology* 175: 621-628, 1990.

93. Thomsen HS, Morcos SK: Contrast media and metformin: Guidelines to diminish the risk of lactic acidosis in non-insulin-dependent diabetics after administration of contrast media. ESUR Contrast Media Safety Committee, *Eur Radiol* 9:738-740, 1999.

94. Lasser EC, Berry CC, Talner LB, et al: Pretreatment with corticosteroids to alleviate reactions to intravenous contrast material, *N Engl J Med* 317:845-849, 1987.

95. Lasser EC, Berry CC, Mishkin MM, et al: Pretreatment with corticosteroids to prevent adverse reactions to nonionic contrast media, *AJR Am J Roentgenol* 162:523-526, 1994.

96. Greenberger PA, Patterson R: The prevention of immediate generalized reactions to radiocontrast media in high-risk patients, *J Allergy Clin Immunol* 87:867-872, 1991.

97. Dachman AH: New contraindication to intravascular iodinated contrast material, *Radiology* 197:545, 1995.

98. Schweiger MJ, Chambers CE, Davidson CJ, et al: Prevention of contrast induced nephropathy: Recommendations for the high risk patient undergoing cardiovascular procedures, *Catheter Cardiovasc Interv* 69:135-140, 2007.

99. van Gijn J, Rinkel GJ: Subarachnoid haemorrhage: Diagnosis, causes and management, *Brain* 124:249-278, 2001.

100. Johnston SC, Selvin S, Gress DR: The burden, trends, and demographics of mortality from subarachnoid hemorrhage, *Neurology* 50:1413-1418, 1998.

101. Mayer S, Kreiter K: Quality of life after subarachnoid hemorrhage, *J Neurosurg* 97:741-742, 2002:author reply 742.

102. Report of World Federation of Neurological Surgeons Committee on a Universal Subarachnoid Hemorrhage Grading Scale, *J Neurosurg* 68:985-986, 1988.

103. Hunt WE, Hess RM: Surgical risk as related to time of intervention in the repair of intracranial aneurysms, *J Neurosurg* 28:14-20, 1968.

104. Claassen J, Bernardini GL, Kreiter K, et al: Effect of cisternal and ventricular blood on risk of delayed cerebral ischemia after subarachnoid hemorrhage: The Fisher scale revisited, *Stroke* 32: 2012-2020, 2001.

105. Bardach NS, Olson SJ, Elkins JS, et al: Regionalization of treatment for subarachnoid hemorrhage: A cost-utility analysis, *Circulation* 109:2207-2212, 2004.

106. Suarez JI, Zaidat OO, Suri MF, et al: Length of stay and mortality in neurocritically ill patients: Impact of a specialized neurocritical care team, *Crit Care Med* 32:2311-2317, 2004.

107. Suarez JI, Tarr RW, Selman WR: Aneurysmal subarachnoid hemorrhage, *N Engl J Med* 354:387-396, 2006.

108. McKinney AM, Palmer CS, Truwit CL, et al: Detection of aneurysms by 64-section multidetector CT angiography in patients acutely suspected of having an intracranial aneurysm and comparison with digital subtraction and 3D rotational angiography, *AJNR Am J Neuroradiol* 29:594-602, 2008.

109. Romijn M, Gratama van Andel HA, van Walderveen MA, et al: Diagnostic accuracy of CT angiography with matched mask bone elimination for detection of intracranial aneurysms: Comparison with digital subtraction angiography and 3D rotational angiography, *AJNR Am J Neuroradiol* 29:134-139, 2008.

110. Tumialán LM, Zhang YJ, Cawley CM, et al: Intracranial hemorrhage associated with stent-assisted coil embolization of cerebral aneurysms: A cautionary report, *J Neurosurg* 108:1122-1129, 2008.

111. Varma MK, Price K, Jayakrishnan V, et al: Anaesthetic considerations for interventional neuroradiology, *Br J Anaesth* 99:75-85, 2007.

112. Pelz DM, Lownie SP, Fox AJ: Thromboembolic events associated with the treatment of cerebral aneurysms with Guglielmi detachable coils, *AJNR Am J Neuroradiol* 19:1541-1547, 1998.

113. Qureshi AI, Luft AR, Sharma M, et al: Prevention and treatment of thromboembolic and ischemic complications associated with endovascular procedures: Part I: Pathophysiological and pharmacological features, *Neurosurgery* 46:1344-1359, 2000.

114. Qureshi AI, Luft AR, Sharma M, et al: Prevention and treatment of thromboembolic and ischemic complications associated with endovascular procedures: Part II: Clinical aspects and recommendations, *Neurosurgery* 46:1360-1375, 2000.

115. Raschke RA, Reilly BM, Guidry JR, et al: The weight-based heparin dosing nomogram compared with a "standard care" nomogram. A randomized controlled trial, *Ann Intern Med* 119:874-881, 1993.

116. Raymond J, Roy D: Safety and efficacy of endovascular treatment of acutely ruptured aneurysms, *Neurosurgery* 41:1235-1245, 1997:discussion 1245-1236.

117. Raymond J, Roy D, Bojanowski M, et al: Endovascular treatment of acutely ruptured and unruptured aneurysms of the basilar bifurcation, *J Neurosurg* 86:211-219, 1997.

118. Van Belle E, Maillard L, Tio FO, et al: Accelerated endothelialization by local delivery of recombinant human vascular endothelial growth factor reduces in-stent intimal formation, *Biochem Biophys Res Commun* 235:311-316, 1997.

119. Ferns GA, Stewart-Lee AL, Anggard EE: Arterial response to mechanical injury: Balloon catheter de-endothelialization, *Atherosclerosis* 92:89-104, 1992.

120. Koreny M, Riedmuller E, Nikfardjam M, et al: Arterial puncture closing devices compared with standard manual compression after cardiac catheterization: Systematic review and meta-analysis, *JAMA* 291:350-357, 2004.

121. Fischer TH, Connolly R, Thatte HS, et al: Comparison of structural and hemostatic properties of the poly-N-acetyl glucosamine Syvek Patch with products containing chitosan, *Microsc Res Tech* 63:168-174, 2004.

122. Ries T, Siemonsen S, Grzyska U, et al: Abciximab is a safe rescue therapy in thromboembolic events complicating cerebral aneurysm coil embolization: Single center experience in 42 cases and review of the literature, *Stroke* 40:1750-1757, 2009.

123. Jones RG, Davagnanam I, Colley S, et al: Abciximab for treatment of thromboembolic complications during endovascular coiling of intracranial aneurysms, *AJNR Am J Neuroradiol* 29:1925-1929, 2008.

123a. Linfante I, Etezadi V, Andreone V, et al: Intra-arterial abciximab for the treatment of thrombus formation during coil embolization of intracranial aneurysms, *J NeuroIntervent Surg* 2:135-138, 2010.

124. Fessler RD, Ringer AJ, Qureshi AI, et al: Intracranial stent placement to trap an extruded coil during endovascular aneurysm treatment: Technical note, *Neurosurgery* 46:248-251, 2000.

125. Henkes H, Lowens S, Preiss H, et al: A new device for endovascular coil retrieval from intracranial vessels: Alligator retrieval device, *AJNR Am J Neuroradiol* 27:327-329, 2006.

126. Wakhloo AK, Gounis MJ: Retrievable closed cell intracranial stent for foreign body and clot removal, *Neurosurgery* 62: ONS390-ONS393, 2007.

127. Smith WS, Sung G, Saver J, et al: Mechanical thrombectomy for acute ischemic stroke: Final results of the Multi MERCI trial, *Stroke* 39:1205-1212, 2008.

128. Grunwald IQ, Walter S, Papanagiotou P, et al: Revascularization in acute ischaemic stroke using the penumbra system: The first single center experience, *Eur J Neurol* 16:1210-1216, 2009.

129. Cloft HJ, Kallmes DF: Cerebral aneurysm perforations complicating therapy with guglielmi detachable coils: A meta-analysis, *AJNR Am J Neuroradiol* 23:1706-1709, 2002.

130. Wakhloo AK, Schellhammer F, Vries JD, et al: Self-expanding and balloon-expandable stents in the treatment of carotid aneurysms: An experimental study in a canine model, *AJNR Am J Neuroradiol* 5:493-502, 1994.

131. Lieber BB, Gounis MJ: The physics of endoluminal stenting in the treatment of cerebrovascular aneurysms, *Neurol Res* 24:S33-S42, 2002.

132. Sadasivan C, Cesar L, Seong J, et al: An original flow diversion device for the treatment of intracranial aneurysms. Evaluation in the rabbit elastase-induced model, *Stroke* 40:952-958, 2009.

133. Lylyk P, Miranda C, Ceratto R, et al: Curative endovascular reconstruction of cerebral aneurysms with the pipeline embolization device: The Buenos Aires experience, *Neurosurgery* 64:632-642, 2009.

134. Szikora I, Berentei Z, Kulcsar Z, et al: Treatment of intracranial aneurysms by functional reconstruction of the parent artery: The Budapest experience with the Pipeline Embolization Device, *AJNR Am J Neuroradiol* 31:1139-1147, 2010.

135. Wakhloo AK, Lylyk P, Hartmann M, et al: A new generation of flow-disruption device for endovascular treatment of intracranial aneurysms—preliminary clinical and angiographic results of a multicenter study [Abstract], *Stroke*, 2011 [in press].

64 Interventional Therapy of Brain and Spinal Arteriovenous Malformations

TIMO KRINGS, SASIKHAN GEIBPRASERT, KAREL TER BRUGGE

One of the basic principles in medicine is that the understanding of a disease should precede its treatment. Unfortunately, in the case of spinal and brain pial arteriovenous malformations (AVMs), too little is known as yet about their etiology, pathophysiology, and natural history for guidelines about their treatment to be given truly and confidently. The numerous different classification schemes that should aid in the understanding of arteriovenous (AV) shunts testify to this lack of knowledge. To additionally complicate matters, advances in diagnostic tools for pretreatment risk assessment as well as continuously improved treatment modalities (catheterization and embolization materials) are likely to further change the way we will manage these vascular malformations. Finally, the skills and experience of the physician performing the endovascular treatment will have a more profound impact on the patient's outcome than any of the aforementioned issues.

We subdivide this chapter into two sections, the first one dealing with the brain, the second one with the spine, and we confine ourselves to the discussion of endovascular treatments of the pial AVMs only, leaving the dural (spinal and cranial) AV shunts for a different chapter. In each subdivision, we describe briefly the classification that we use as an aid in understanding the disease, bearing in mind that this classification may be different from those used by other writers.

Brain Arteriovenous Malformations

Classification of Vascular Malformations in General

A classification of pial brain AVMs that is based on the size, the pattern of venous drainage, and the eloquence of the portions of brain adjacent to the AVM is of limited use when one is considering endovascular treatment, for three reasons. First, such classification cannot predict the natural history of a specific AVM for an individual patient; second, it does not anticipate the risk of treating brain AVMs by endovascular techniques; and third, it does not enhance our understanding of this disease.

Concerning the last, a classification that is based on the etiology of vascular malformations may be a more useful approach to assess vascular malformative diseases in general, of which the AVMs are but a subgroup. This etiologic classification takes into account the target, the timing, and the nature of the triggering event. Because arteries and veins are already differentiated early during vasculogenesis, the target of a triggering event may vary according to its location along the vessel tree: from the arterial side to the arterial-capillary, the venous junction venules, veins, sinuses, and lymphatics.[1] The second determinant is the timing, or when the trigger hits its target: An early hit during vasculogenesis (such as a germinal mutation) affects more cells and leads to a metamerically arranged defect, whereas a late hit (such as a somatic mutation that occurs late during the fetal life or even postnatally) has a more focal impact (such as failed localized remodeling during vascular renewal).[2] Finally, the nature of the triggering event—intrinsic (i.e., genetic vs. extrinsic), environmental, traumatic, or infectious—adds another level of complexity to this schematic approach of classifying brain vascular malformations.[3] Although there is likely to be a continuous spectrum of vascular diseases rather than clear-cut disease entities, the scheme that is based on the previously mentioned assumptions may help to discern vascular malformations from an etiologic standpoint.

Classification of Pial Brain Arteriovenous Malformations in Particular

The main focus of this chapter is on the endovascular treatment of the shunting lesions. Although the previously mentioned classification may be helpful to broadly categorize vascular lesions, the most often encountered shunting lesions, i.e., the pial brain AVMs, deserve further subclassification because the presented classification is too crude to predict the natural history of a specific AVM for an individual patient and is unable to anticipate the endovascular treatment risk.

Natural history. A classification that is able to predict natural history has to distinguish first those AVMs that have bled from those that have not bled, which in most instances is possible through the review of the clinical history. In asymptomatic patients, T2-weighted gradient-echo MRI sequences, which are highly susceptible to depicting signs of old hemorrhage, may assist the identification of those exceedingly rare cases in which a subclinical hemorrhage may have happened (Fig. 64-1). The future risk of bleeding from a brain AVM has been the subject of many studies: In 1983, Graf et al[4] published their results concerning the risk for future hemorrhage, which

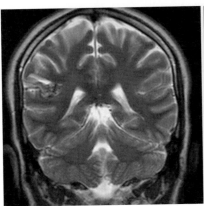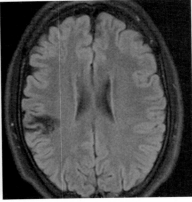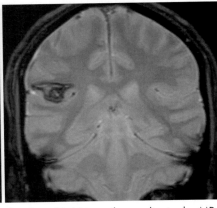

Figure 64-1 Although no bleeding episode was reported by the patient nor was it evident from his history, the gradient-echo MR images demonstrate hemosiderin deposits close to the arteriovenous malformation that testify to a previous bleeding episode.

was calculated to be 37% in 20 years for unruptured AVMs and 47% for ruptured AVMs. Crawford et al[5] found similar 20-year cumulative risks of hemorrhage (33% for unruptured and 51% for ruptured AVMs); however, they added that older age was a major risk factor, with patients older than 60 years harboring a risk for rupture of 90% in 9 years. Both studies demonstrated an annual average risk for hemorrhage of approximately 2%, which was confirmed in the study by Brown et al[6] in 1988, who investigated unruptured AVMs only. These investigators added that the risks for permanent morbidity and mortality following a hemorrhage of a brain AVM were 29% and 23%, respectively. Ondra et al[7] in 1990 calculated a slightly higher risk of 5% per year for unruptured brain AVMs with a mortality risk of 1% per year (i.e., 25% for all hemorrhages) and a morbidity of 2.7% per year (more than 50% for all hemorrhages). In a prospective series published by Mast et al[8] in 1997, the yearly risk of hemorrhage for previously ruptured brain AVMs was calculated as 17% per year, whereas in unruptured AVMs, the risk of hemorrhage was 2% per year. These researchers found male gender, deep vein drainage, and previous hemorrhages to be the major determinants for future hemorrhages.

Pathomechanical classification. Although there is little discussion about the necessity of treating ruptured pial AVMs because of their larger rebleeding risk, unruptured pial AVMs have to be further subdivided to identify those patients in whom therapy is indicated, that is, in whom the risk of treatment is lower than the natural history risk. In our practice, we try to classify these "unruptured" AVMs first according to their **pathomechanism** in relation to the angioarchitecture. Owing to their **high-flow shunt**, fistulous pial AVM (Fig. 64-2), especially when present in childhood, can lead to psychomotor developmental retardation and cardiac insufficiency and, when present later in life, to dementia, and therefore merit treatment.[9] Endovascular treatment should be aimed in these cases to reduce the AV shunt. **Venous congestion** (Fig. 64-3) that can be due to a high input (fistulous lesions) or a reduced outflow (secondary stenosis of the outflow pattern) may go along with a cognitive decline or epilepsy, and we would propose treatment in these cases, with the same aim as stated previously.[10] Even if signs of venous congestion are not present, a long pial course

of the draining vein may indicate that **venous drainage restriction** is present over a large area, increasing the risk of venous congestion and subsequent epilepsy. Conversely, a short vein that drains almost directly into a dural sinus is unlikely to interfere with the normal pial drainage. If a patient were to have epilepsy in this kind of angioarchitecture, MRI should be scrutinized for signs of **perinidal gliosis**. In the former case (epileptic patient harboring an AVM with a long pial draining vein) endovascular treatment is warranted to reduce the interference with the normal pial drainage and is likely to reduce seizure frequency or severity, but in the latter case (epilepsy following perinidal gliosis), endovascular therapies are unlikely to change the seizure frequency or severity, and we would suggest abstention from an endovascular treatment. **Mass effect** is a rare pathomechanism that may result from large venous ectasias or the nidus proper compressing critical structures and may lead to epilepsy, neurologic deficits, and even hydrocephalus (Fig. 64-4).[11] **Arterial steal** has been associated with clinical findings, such as migraine and focal neurologic symptoms, that most often are transitory in nature.[12] With the advent of new imaging modalities such as functional MRI and perfusion MRI, it has now become possible to demonstrate whether the symptoms of a patient can be attributed to a true steal that can be treated by endovascular means, with the aim of reducing the shunt if the symptoms are disabling (Fig. 64-5).

Angioarchitectonic classification. As outlined previously, the first step in nonruptured AVMs is to evaluate whether the specific symptoms of an individual patient can be related to the AVM. Second, one has to evaluate whether the pathomechanism responsible for the symptoms can be treated by endovascular means (as also described previously) (Table 64-1). The third step consists, in our practice, in evaluating the angioarchitecture of the AVM to determine whether endovascular therapies are suitable for a specific brain AVM and whether there are any focal weak points within the AVM of an asymptomatic patient.

The basic principle of the concept of "partially targeted embolization" of brain AVMs is the hypothesis that specific angioarchitectonic features of a pial brain AVM can be regarded as *focal "weak points"* that may

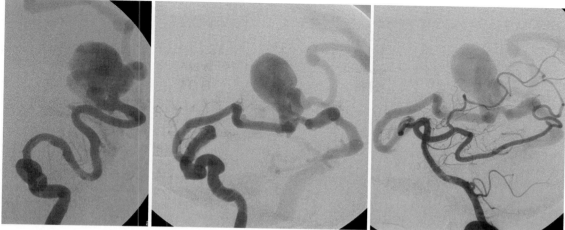

Figure 64-2 Fistulous pial arteriovenous malformation with a high-flow shunt. Such lesions typically manifest in early childhood, can lead to psychomotor developmental retardation or cardiac insufficiency, and should be treated. Multiple shunts of this type are characteristic for hereditary hemorrhagic telangiectasia.

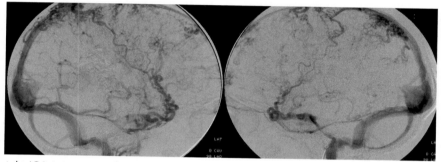

Figure 64-3 Left and right ICA injection in the venous phase of an angiogram demonstrates the classic "pseudophlebitic" aspect of enlarged and tortuous pial veins, which is a sign of long-standing venous congestion that may go along with epilepsy, headaches, cognitive decline, and focal neurologic deficits.

predispose to hemorrhage.[13-15] Although not proven by randomized prospective trials, this principle has been used in our practice over more than 20 years, and we were able to show an improved outcome on follow-up in comparison with the natural history.[16] These angioarchitectonic weak points are (1) intranidal aneurysms and venous ectasias,[17] and (2) venous stenosis.[14] The first to state that specific angioarchitectonic features present in brain AVMs make them more prone to future hemorrhage were Brown et al[6] in 1988, who found that the annual risk of future hemorrhage was 3% in brain AVMs alone, and 7% per year in brain AVMs with associated aneurysms. Meisel et al[16] found that among 662 patients with brain AVMs, 305 patients had associated aneurysms, and there was a significant increase in rebleed episodes in brain AVMs harboring intranidal aneurysms ($P < .002$).[17] In the Toronto series of 759 brain AVMs, associated aneurysms were statistically significantly ($P = .015$) associated with future bleeding.[18] It may be difficult to discern intranidal arterial aneurysms from intranidal venous ectasias, which is why these two angioarchitectonic specificities are grouped as one entity in most series. Venous stenoses, on the other hand, are a separate angiographic weak point and are often seen in ruptured AVMs (Fig. 64-6). The nature of the venous stenosis is not completely understood; most likely high-flow vessel wall changes, failure in

remodeling, or an increased vessel wall response to the shear stress induced by the arterialization may be put forward as potential reasons. A stenotic venous outlet will lead to an imbalance of pressure in various compartments of the AVM, which may induce subsequent rupture of the AVM. The compartment that is drained by the stenotic vessel should be scrutinized for contrast agent stagnation, and if endovascular therapy is contemplated, extreme caution has to be undertaken not to push liquid embolic agent toward the already stenosed vein as doing so may have catastrophic results. In addition to these two angioarchitectonic risk factors, there are also other factors that may lead to an increased risk of hemorrhage. These are: deep venous drainage only, elder age, and male gender.[19]

Angioarchitectonics related to endovascular therapies. Before treatment of an AVM is contemplated, angiography must be scrutinized for the following points: the nature and number of the feeding arteries, the presence or absence of flow-related aneurysms, the number of separate compartments of the malformation, any arterial or venous ectasias near or within the malformation, and the nature of the venous drainage (Table 64-2). On the arterial side, flow-related aneurysms (discussed in greater detail later) are typically present on branching points of the major feeding arteries. They classically resolve following treatment of the AVM and are due to vascular remodeling

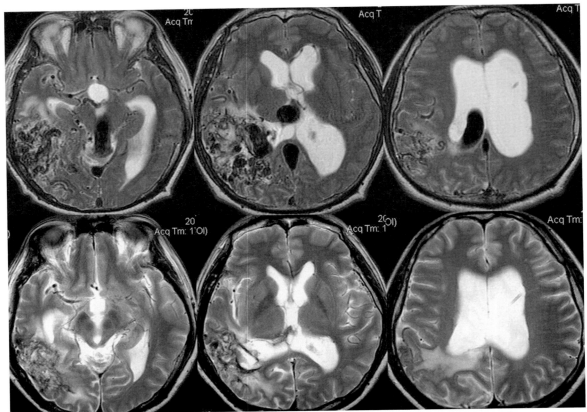

Figure 64-4 In rare cases, mass effect of the nidus proper or, as in this case, of the dilated draining vein on critical structures (aqueduct, third ventricle) may lead to hydrocephalus *(top row)*. Following partial embolization and radiosurgery, the size of the draining vein was reduced, leading to resolution of the mass effect and concomitant resolution of the hydrocephalus *(bottom row)*.

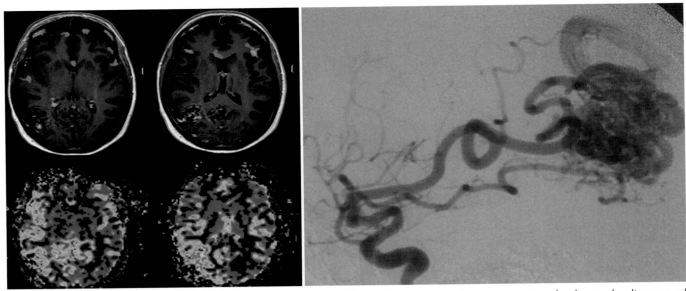

Figure 64-5 The patient complained of repetitive speech arrests without other neurologic signs or symptoms, leading to the discovery of the right parietal arteriovenous malformation (AVM). Functional MRI demonstrates bilateral representation of speech areas. Perfusion MRI was able to show an increased mean transit time in areas remote from the AVM that, however, were active during speech production. Thus the symptoms of the patient could be attributed to the arterial steal effect of the AVM.

after increased shear stress (Fig. 64-7).[20] Although such aneurysms are not a contraindication to endovascular treatment, the neurointerventionalist should take special care, because flow-directed catheters are prone to enter the aneurysm rather than the distal vessels. Concerning the arterial side of the AVM, both the number and the nature of the feeding arteries need to be assessed because they determine whether endovascular approaches will make sense. An AVM with a large number of only slightly dilated feeders will make an endovascular therapy more

TABLE 64-1   PATHOMECHANICAL CLASSIFICATION OF BRAIN ARTERIOVENOUS MALFORMATIONS

Clinical Findings	Angiographic Sign	Additional Imaging Diagnostics	Primary Pathomechanism	Treatment Rationale
Neurologic deficits	Perinidal high flow and associated extranidal (remote) hypoperfusion	Perfusion-weighted MRI, (extranidal hypoperfusion), functional MRI (detection of eloquent tissues)	Steal	Reduce shunting volume
	Venous ectasias/ pouches close to eloquent brain	MRI (compression, focal edema?), functional MRI (detection of eloquent tissues)	Mass effect	Remove mass effect
Headaches	Occipital high-flow arteriovenous malformation	Perfusion-weighted MRI (extranidal occipital hypoperfusion)	Steal	Reduce shunting volume
	Large draining veins	MRI: hydrocephalus with draining veins close to the aqueduct or interventricular foramen	Mass effect	Decrease size of draining vein
	Pseudophlebitic aspect in venous phase, prolonged venous phase	MRI: edema	Venous congestion	Reduce shunt
Epilepsy	Long-standing high-flow shunts, pseudophlebitic aspect in venous phase	CT: calcifications	Venous congestion	Reduce shunt
	Unspecific	MRI: perinidal gliosis	Gliosis	Surgical removal
	Long pial course of draining vein	Unspecific	Venous restriction	Reduce shunt
Cardiac insufficiency	High-flow shunts	MRI/CT: large venous pouches	Right-to-left shunt	Reduce shunt
Psychomotor developmental retardation	High-flow shunts, pseudophlebitic aspect in venous phase, reduced outflow	MRI: melting brain? CT: calcifications	Venous congestion in not fully matured brain	Reduce shunt
Dementia	Pseudophlebitic aspect in venous phase	MRI: edema	Venous congestion	Reduce shunt

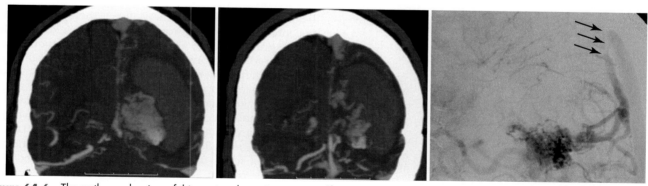

Figure 64-6   The pathomechanism of this ruptured arteriovenous malformation is presumably due to the stenosis of the major venous outlet (*right, arrows*) that led to an increased pressure within the nidus proper. If endovascular therapy is contemplated in cases like these, extreme caution has to be taken that no embolic material penetrates to the venous side.

challenging than an AVM with a single large feeder (Fig. 64-8).[21]

Concerning the nature of the feeding artery, there are two basic types of feeding arteries. *Direct arterial feeders* end in the AVM; *indirect arterial feeders* supply the normal cortex and also supply the AVM "en passage" via small vessels that arise from the normal artery (Fig. 64-9). The nature of arterial feeders may be misdiagnosed because of a high-flow AV fistula that attracts all of the contrast

agent, leaving the en passage arterial branch invisible. Although direct feeders are safe targets for endovascular therapy, the en passage feeder may carry the risk of inadvertent arterial glue migration to distal healthy vessels. In this regard, the "security margin" of the catheter position has to be briefly discussed. Liquid embolic agents may reflux at the end of the injection. Depending on the agent, the microcatheter, the injection technique, and the skills of the operator, this reflux may be as far as 1 cm

TABLE 64-2 FEATURES IMPORTANT FOR A TREATMENT-BASED CLASSIFICATION OF BRAIN ARTERIOVENOUS MALFORMATIONS EMPLOYING ENDOVASCULAR TECHNIQUES

Artery
Flow-related aneurysms
Number of feeders
Type of feeder (direct vs. en passage)

Nidus
Number of compartments
Intranidal aneurysms
Fistulous vs. nidal

Veins
Stenoses
Number of draining veins per compartment

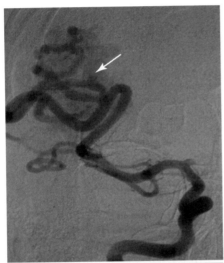
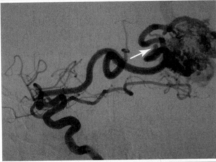
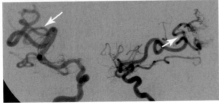

Figure 64-7 In the upper row, pretreatment images demonstrate a prenidal flow-related aneurysm *(arrows)* that following endovascular therapy with flow reduction completely vanished *(lower row)*.

proximal to the tip of the catheter. A safe deposition of liquid embolic agent is therefore possible only if the catheter tip is distal enough to any vessel that supplies normal brain tissue. In case of an en passage feeder, this may not be the case, especially if the catheter is only hooked into

the feeding artery and so will jump backward because of the jet effect of injecting a liquid embolic agent. Intranidal arterial aneurysms and venous varices that indicate weak points must also be recognized as well as the number of compartments and their nature (nidal versus fistulous) (Fig. 64-10). Finally, on the venous side of the AVM, the number of draining veins per compartment (the more the better for endovascular treatment if venous migration should occur), a possible drainage into the deep vein system (higher risk for hemorrhage, more difficult surgical treatment), and stenosis that restricts venous outflow have to be identified to enable full determination of the risk of a specific AVM. At present, this information can be obtained only by conventional digital subtraction angiography that, in our practice, still must precede any treatment decision in AVMs.

Concepts of Treatment

A complete cure of a pial brain AVM by endovascular means is possible in approximately 20% of all AVMs irrespective of their angioarchitecture.[22-24] Those AVMs that are favorable to a complete cure are the small, single-feeder, single-compartment AVMs that have a direct feeding artery (see Fig. 64-8). Because such AVMs are also good candidates for both radiosurgery and open neurosurgery, a tailored team approach for each specific AVM in each individual patient, respecting also the patient's wishes and the peculiarities of the clinical presentation, must be taken. In most instances, endovascular therapies are used to diminish the size of an AVM prior to radiotherapy or surgery, to secure focal weak points in the acute and subacute stages of ruptured AVMs (Fig. 64-11) and in unruptured AVMs for which radiosurgery is contemplated, or to exclude those compartments of an AVM that may be difficult to reach during surgery (see also the discussion of indications and contraindications). It has to be stressed at this point that, once a therapy of an AVM is contemplated, a pathway to its complete exclusion has to be agreed upon by the treatment team, which should include radiosurgeons, vascular neurosurgeons, neurologists, and neurointerventionalists. It does not make sense, in our opinion, to partially treat an AVM without a strategy on how to handle a possible residual of the AVM.

Once endovascular therapy is decided upon, we proceed with a predefined goal, which may mean a partial, targeted embolization. Such rationale is based on the outcomes in a series of more than 600 patients with AVMs that were partially embolized and showed a significant decrease in hemorrhage episodes in comparison with the conservatively treated series reported in the literature.[16] The yearly hemorrhage incidence rate of patients before partial treatment was 0.062 (95% confidence interval [CI], 0.03–0.11). The observed annual rate after the start of this regimen was 0.02 (95% CI, 0.012–0.030).[16] Given the previously mentioned considerations concerning focal weak points, we think that these numbers reflect the benefit of selectively excluding specific weak compartments of an AVM and thereby providing early protection while the patient is scheduled for radiotherapy (the effects of which take more time, but the results of which concerning complete obliteration are better). In these instances the goal is to secure the AVM during its time to complete occlusion

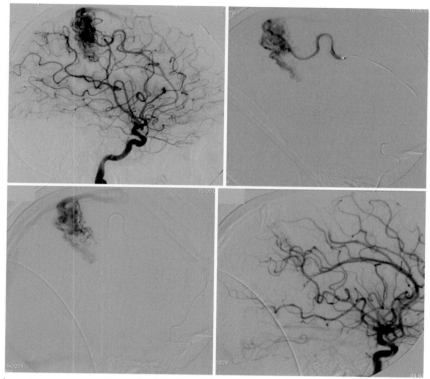

Figure 64-8 Single-feeder arteriovenous malformations (AVMs) are easier to embolize with a higher chance of a complete cure than multiple-feeder AVMs. In this single-compartment AVM, the microcatheter is brought to an intranidal position, where a histoacryl deposition was able to completely occlude the AVM.

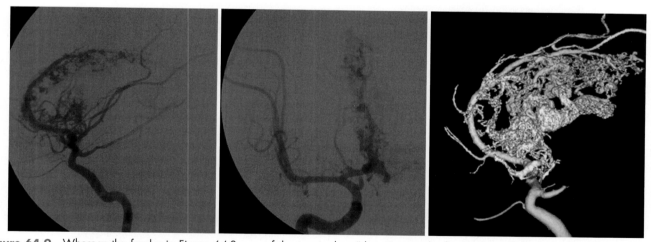

Figure 64-9 Whereas the feeder in Figure 64-8 was of the terminal or "direct" type, the feeder type of this pericallosal arteriovenous malformation is of the "indirect" or "en passage" type. These "en passage" feeders may carry the risk of inadvertent arterial glue migration to distal healthy vessels that in our opinion speaks strongly against an endovascular treatment approach.

(Fig. 64-12). In other instances the goal may be to exclude those compartments that will be difficult to reach prior to surgery or to diminish the size of the AVM prior to radiosurgery. In the latter instance, compartments in the periphery of the AVM have to be targeted, whereas in the former instance, the neurosurgeon has to point out the target of the neurointerventionalist. Because in combined therapies (endovascular + radiotherapy; endovascular + surgery), the relative risks of each procedure are cumulative, embolization makes only sense if a goal is predefined prior to therapy. In most instances, this goal should be reached during a maximum of two or three endovascular sessions.

Liquid embolic materials: For most glomerular pial AVMs, liquid embolic materials are the first choice of treatment. The therapy is done with the patient under general monitored neuroanesthesia. We classically use a 5F guiding catheter that is placed into the distal internal carotid artery (ICA) or vertebral artery (VA). A flow directed microcatheter is then advanced and directed with a microguidewire or gentle contrast agent injections into the feeding artery and into the nidus proper with the use of roadmap or fluoroscopy techniques. Here a wedged position of the catheter tip is sought for, with careful attention to ensure that there are no normal

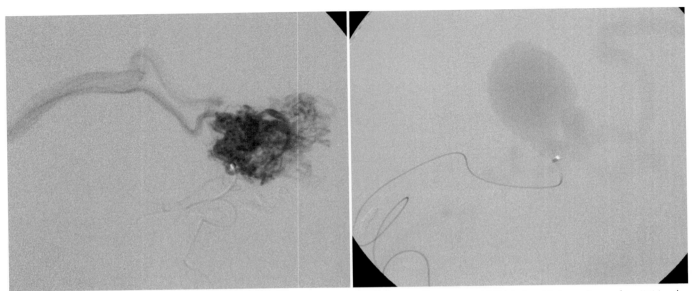

Figure 64-10 Microinjections of nidal versus fistulous types of arteriovenous malformations (AVMs): In nidal or glomerular AVMs, the transit time is slower, unlike the rapid and diluted filling of the fistulous type.

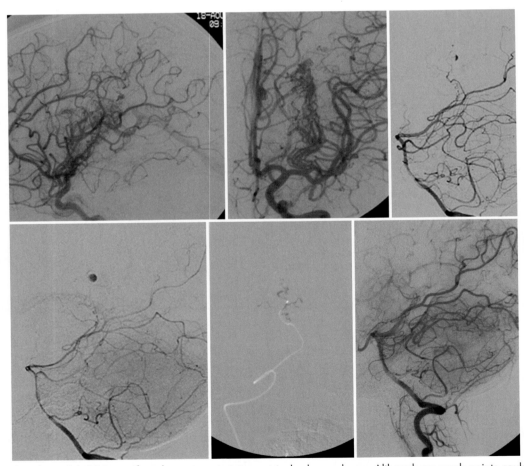

Figure 64-11 This choroidal AVM manifested as an acute intraventricular hemorrhage. Although no weak points could be seen on the ICA injection, injection into the vertebral artery demonstrated a false aneurysm with contrast agent stagnation until late in the venous phase, indicating the point of rupture. These aneurysms have a high propensity to rebleed. In our experience, early treatment is therefore warranted. Superselective catheterization with embolization is in our center the treatment of choice. Control after embolization demonstrates complete occlusion of the false aneurysm.

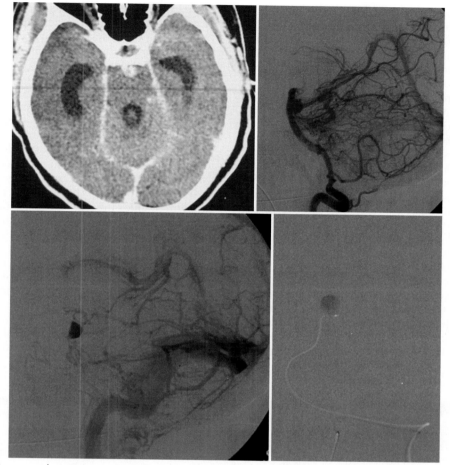

Figure 64-12 As in the example in Figure 64-11, these images demonstrate a false aneurysm as the point of rupture in this small arteriovenous malformation. As previously noted, the target in early embolization has to be the false aneurysm that can be selectively reached by a microcatheter and subsequently treated.

brain-supplying arteries distal or in close proximity to the tip of the catheter. After test injections and preparation of the catheter, the liquid embolic material is injected into the nidus, with careful attention paid to avoid its venous migration. The injection technique will vary with the type of embolic agent and the nature of the nidus (fistulous versus plexiform). To prevent venous migration, temporary lowering of the blood pressure or compression of jugular veins may be done. To date, there is an ongoing debate as to what kind of liquid embolic agent to use. Our personal experience as well as published data demonstrates a higher rate of complete obliteration with the use of Onyx Liquid Embolic System (ev3 Endovascular, Plymouth, MN) (40% to 60%) but with a significantly higher risk for permanent morbidity and mortality (8% to 12%).[25,26] Following an uneventful procedure, the patient is awakened and monitored for 24 hours, after which discharge can be proposed.

Particles/microcoils/coils. A proximal occlusion of feeding arteries without penetration of the embolic material to and just beyond the site of the shunt will lead to reopening of the nidus via leptomeningeal collaterals and may induce a profound neoangiogenesis. Such an occlusion should therefore be avoided, because subsequent endovascular therapies will not be possible. In addition,

the profound neoangiogenesis would make discrimination between the nidus and normal brain-supplying arteries nearly impossible. Coils and microcoils are therefore, in our opinion, not indicated for plexiform AVMs. It is only in certain single-hole macrofistulas that these embolization materials have a place. Likewise, particles, especially if chosen in too large a size, may lead to an occlusion that is too proximal with subsequent neoangiogenesis. In addition, particles do not result in a stable occlusion in pial brain AVMs, and their use at the end of a procedure is more "cosmetically" than predictably occlusive in a stable manner.

Specific Treatment Considerations

Flow-related arterial aneurysms. Redekop et al[27] reported finding that there was no difference in the rate of hemorrhagic occurrence between the overall population of patients with brain AVMs without aneurysms and those with proximal flow–related aneurysms. Likewise, in our experience, proximal flow–related aneurysms are almost never the site of bleeding. Therefore, there is no evidence that treatment of a nonruptured proximal aneurysm associated with an AVM is needed; and we perform treatment of the AVM before a treatment of the proximal aneurysm (only if the latter is still persistent). We have never observed rupture of a proximal aneurysm following embolization of the related contribution to the AVM. As already pointed out, during endovascular treatment of brain AVMs with associated flow-related aneurysms, great caution is needed to avoid entering and rupturing the flow-related aneurysm with the microcatheter.

Fistulous AVMs. Although most AVMs have fistulous and glomerular (plexiform) compartments, a specific subset of purely fistulous pial AV shunts, the pial single-hole macrofistulas, deserve special consideration. They are often present in children and should raise the suspicion of an underlying genetic disease such as hereditary hemorrhagic telangiectasia (HHT).[28] HHT is inherited as an autosomal dominant trait with varying penetrance and expressivity. Cerebral pial AV fistulas in HHT are macrofistulas with a high fistula volume and are of the single-hole type. The feeding arteries drain directly into a massively enlarged venous pouch, and often there is only a single feeding artery. Signs of venous congestion are typically present because of venous overload and are responsible for the patients' symptoms. Associated angiographic abnormalities include venous ectasias, venous stenoses, pial reflux, venous ischemia, calcifications, and associated arterial aneurysms. Patients are typically younger than

16 years but the disease has a propensity for appearing in early infancy; in our series all patients but two were younger than 6 years.[9] Localization of the AVF is either cortical supratentorial or infratentorial, and deep locations are exceptional. Presenting symptoms are intracerebral hemorrhage in the majority of patients; macrocrania, bruit, cognitive deficits, cardiac insufficiency, epilepsy, tonsillar prolapse, and hydrocephalus may also be present.

In our practice, treatment consists of superselective glue embolization to obliterate the fistulous area by pushing the glue via the artery into the venous pouch to establish a mushroom-shaped glue cast that occludes the single-hole fistula. Alternatively, coils may be used to selectively occlude the fistulous site. Because a major problem of glue embolization is the uncontrollable propagation of glue into veins with secondary venous occlusion and hemorrhage, we try to minimize this risk in these macrofistulas by using undiluted glue with tantalum powder at a position close to the venous pouch with the catheter tip pointed against the vessel wall.[9] In selected patients flow reduction with coils may be used prior to glue embolization (Fig. 64-13).

Cerebral proliferative angiopathy (CPA). We have introduced the term cerebral proliferative angiopathy (CPA) to distinguish a specific entity that differs from

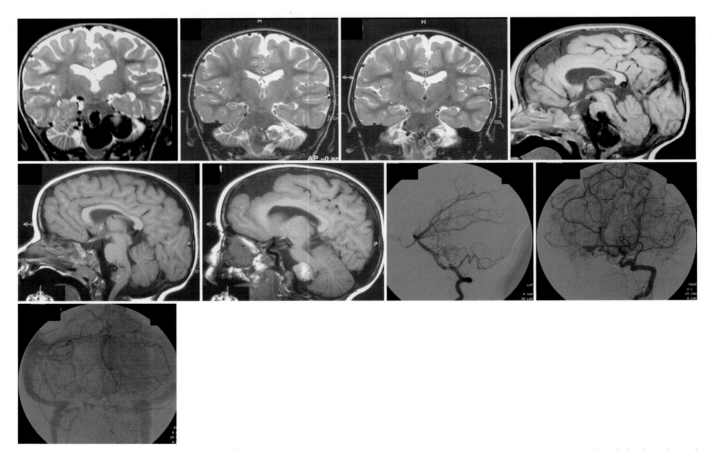

Figure 64-13 Fistulous arteriovenous malformation in a patient with hereditary hemorrhagic telangiectasia treated with both coils and glue. Prior to treatment, the large flow voids seen on MRI testify to the fistulous nature and the concomitant venous pouches. To reduce the flow, coils were deposited via a transarterial route into the venous pouch, followed by glue injection, which led to a nearly complete occlusion as seen on angiography and a progressive thrombosis as seen on MRI.

"classic" pial AVMs in its angiomorphology, histology, presumed pathomechanism, epidemiology, natural history, and clinical presentation.[29]

From an angiomorphologic standpoint, the salient features of CPA, which help discern it from "classic" brain AVMs, are the absence of dominant feeders or flow-related aneurysms, the presence of proximal stenoses of feeding arteries, the extensive transdural supply to both healthy and pathologic tissues, the large size (which might be lobar or even hemispheric), the presence of capillary angioectasia, and the only moderately enlarged veins (compared with the size of the nidus) (Fig. 64-14). Moreover, this special entity of false brain AVM can be suspected when brain tissue is seen on MRI to be intermingled between the vascular spaces (Fig. 64-15). Perfusion MRI indicates an increased blood volume within the nidus with a longer mean transit time (MTT), indicative of capillary and venous ectasias, and an area of hypoperfusion that could be seen throughout the affected hemisphere. This differs from the features of classic brain AVMs, in which the mean transit time is decreased owing to AV shunts and the perinidal areas are not as severely hypoperfused as in CPA. This hypoperfusion trigger might then cause angiogenesis. Whereas transdural supply following iatrogenic ischemia is a normal response to an abnormal demand, the transdural supply in CPA is an abnormal response to an abnormal demand. On histopathology, CPA is characterized by normal brain parenchyma interspersed with the abnormal vascular channels (Fig. 64-16). Brain tissue within the "nidus" of the CPA is therefore functional, similar to brain tissue found in between the abnormal vascular channels present in capillary telangiectasias. Patients (typically, young females) usually do not present with an acute neurologic deficit or hemorrhage, but more commonly with epileptic manifestations, headaches, and progressive neurologic deficits. There is a high rate of strokelike symptoms, transient ischemic attacks (TIAs), and neurologic defects not owing to a hemorrhage that suit the assumption that CPA is a disease related to ischemia rather than hemorrhage. Embolization of these malformations carries an extremely high risk of neurologic deficits, because normal brain tissue is very likely to be embolized owing to the specific histopathology described. We do not recommend endovascular therapy for this condition. Because one of the major pathomechanisms of this disease is ischemia (which in itself is probably multifactorial owing to incompetent angiogenesis, "steal" phenomena, arterial stenosis, and capillary wall involvement), a therapy that enhances cortical blood supply (such as placement of calvarial burr holes) may be adopted.[29]

Cerebrofacial AV metameric syndromes (CAMSs). The association of AVMs of the brain, the orbit (retinal and/or retrobulbar lesions), and the maxillofacial region was originally named after Bonnet-Dechaume-Blanc and Wyburn-Mason. A potential explanation for this striking association is that neural crest and mesodermal cells originating from a given transverse (metameric) level of the embryo finally occupy the same territory in the head and that these embryonic tissues are regionalized in various areas devoted to providing blood vessels to specific regions of the face and brain. Because these fate maps have shown a striking similarity to the distribution of vascular

malformations in the previously mentioned diseases, the term cerebrofacial AV metameric syndrome (CAMS) has been coined, reflecting the putative underlying disorder. Depending on the involved structures, different CAMSs can be differentiated: CAMS 1 is a midline prosencephalic (olfactory) group with involvement of the hypothalamus, corpus callosum, hypophysis, and nose (Fig. 64-17); CAMS 2 is a lateral prosencephalic (optic) group with involvement of the optic nerve, retina, parietotemporooccipital lobes, thalamus, and maxilla; and CAMS 3 is a rhombencephalic (otic) group, with involvement of the cerebellum, pons, petrous bone, and mandible. CAMS 3 is located in a strategic position on the crossroad between the complex cephalic segmental arrangements and the relatively simplified spinal metamers and it may therefore bear transitional characteristics. A more extensive insult will lead to overlapping territories, producing a complete prosencephalic phenotype (CAMS 1+2) or bilateral involvement. The insult producing the underlying lesion would have to develop before the migration occurs and thus before the fourth week of development.[2] The disease spectrum may be incomplete either because some cells are spared or because they have not been triggered to reveal the disease, leading to cases without retinal involvement, cerebral involvement, or facial involvement. Retinal AVM is often the earliest manifestation of a CAMS and it is interesting to note, that in some cases, follow-up showed secondary expression of the full syndrome (Fig. 64-18).

Considered metameric lesions, CAMSs most commonly include intracranial AVMs. Certain angioarchitectural features differentiate cerebral AVMs in CAMS from "classic" AVMs: The AVM nidus in CAMS is a cluster of small vessels with intervening normal brain tissue, some degree of angiogenesis, and a rather small shunting volume. Transdural arterial supply can be present. Progressive enlargement of these cerebral AVMs is one of the special observations in CAMS, suggesting that AVMs in CAMS are not static processes within the segment that carry the embryonic defect. Multifocality is another typical aspect of CAMS AVMs. Despite the common occurrence of cerebral AVMs in CAMS, they are usually clinically silent or asymptomatic at the time of discovery. They rarely manifest as acute neurologic symptoms caused by intracerebral or subarachnoid hemorrhage; rather, they give rise to progressive neurologic deterioration without evidence of intracranial bleeding, most likely owing to a progression in size. About 25% of patients with CAMS-associated AVMs bleed during the course of their disease. Therapeutic management of the cerebral AVMs is particularly challenging. We suggest targeted embolization in an attempt to exclude weak angioarchitectural aspects or to reduce the AV shunt in the least eloquent areas in symptomatic patients who are clinically significantly affected. Brain AVMs associated with CAMS tend to be not easily curable because of their size, location, and evolving natural history.[2]

Indications for and Contraindications to Endovascular Therapies

With the previously described precautions and considerations in mind, in our practice, we see the following indications for endovascular therapies in ruptured brain AVMs:

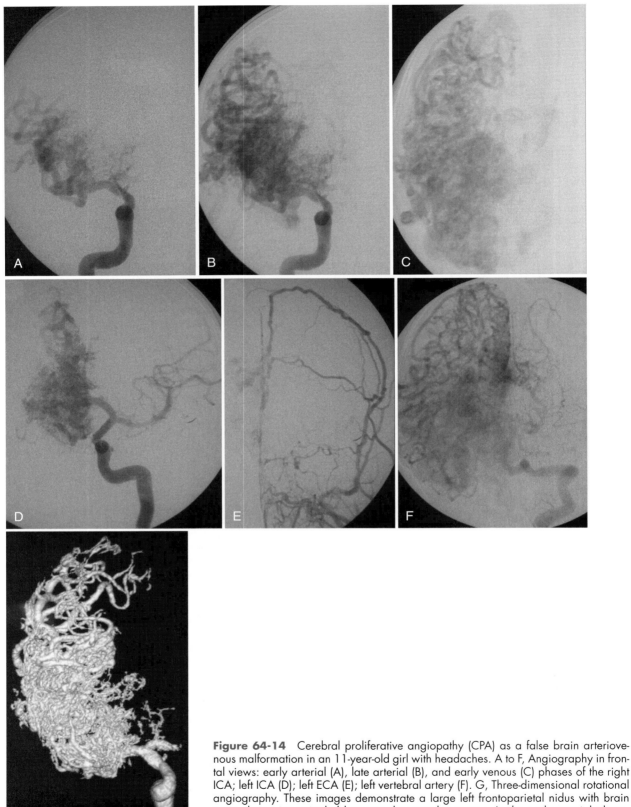

Figure 64-14 Cerebral proliferative angiopathy (CPA) as a false brain arteriovenous malformation in an 11-year-old girl with headaches. A to F, Angiography in frontal views: early arterial (A), late arterial (B), and early venous (C) phases of the right ICA; left ICA (D); left ECA (E); left vertebral artery (F). G, Three-dimensional rotational angiography. These images demonstrate a large left frontoparietal nidus with brain parenchyma intermingled between the vascular spaces. In the early arterial phase, the absence of dominant feeders and the equal contribution of many different arteries can be well perceived. The contrast material dynamics reveal persistence of contrast material in the malformation and hardly any early venous drainage. The transdural supply testifies to the proliferative component of the disease, whereas injection into the vertebral artery demonstrates diffuse neoangiogenesis in other cortical areas.

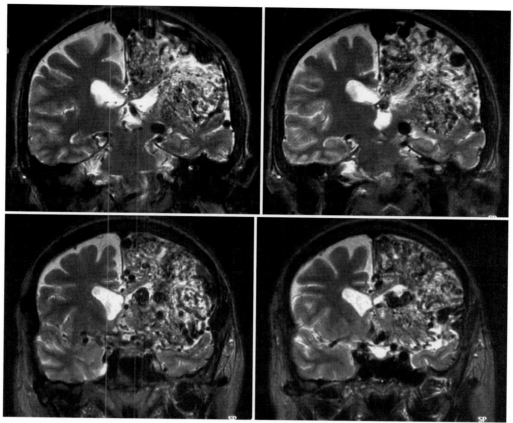

Figure 64-15 Cerebral proliferative angiopathy on T2-weighted coronal MR images, which demonstrate the holohemispheric diffuse nidus type that is characteristic of this kind of vascular malformation.

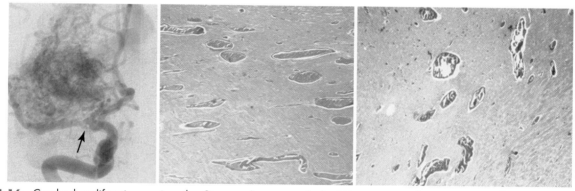

Figure 64-16 Cerebral proliferative angiopathy. Stenoses (as present in the M1 segment in this patient) are often encountered and indicate a failed remodeling of the vessel *(arrow)*. On histologic section (hematoxylin and eosin, and orceine van Gieson stains), proliferation with dilated and irregular arterioles that are histologically otherwise normal can be seen. These dilated vascular channels are located preferentially in regions with low cellular density (white matter tracts and in between the basal ganglia). The venous vessel walls demonstrate collagenous thickening of the veins. Mild perifocal gliosis is seen directly surrounding the vessels; however, normal-appearing neuronal tissue can be seen intermingled between the vascular channels.

(1) ruptured brain AVMs in the hyperacute stage when contrast stagnation in a vessel pouch (pseudoaneurysm) is demonstrated during angiography, because this testifies for a false sac with a large rebleeding rate; (2) ruptured brain AVM in the subacute stage, with intranidal aneurysms being associated with increased risk of rehemorrhage; (3) surgically unfavorable ruptured AVM in the subacute stage when venous stenosis is present; and (4) surgically unfavorable ruptured AVM in elderly men with deep vein drainage.

We see the following indications for endovascular therapies in our practice in unruptured brain AVMs: (1) pial macrofistulas at any age, to reduce venous congestion, especially for the maturing brain; (2) AVMs too large for primary radiosurgery to tailor the size; (3) AVMs with symptoms that are attributable to an endovascularly reachable angioarchitectonic target; and (4) surgically unfavorable AVMs with angioarchitectonic risk factors, especially when other risk factors are present (age, male gender, deep vein drainage).

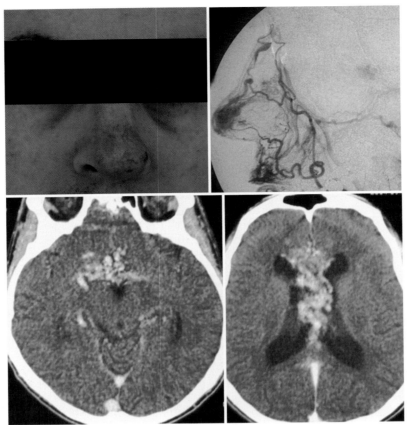

Figure 64-17 Cerebrofacial arteriovenous metameric syndrome type 1 (CAMS 1): Midline or olfactory type with arteriovenous malformation along the nose, hypothalamus, and corpus callosum.

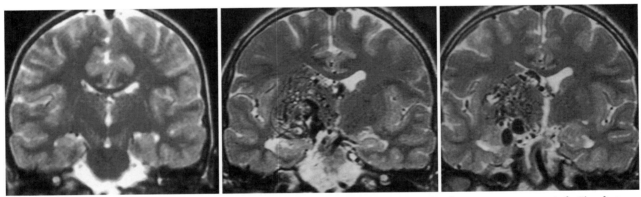

Figure 64-18 Cerebrofacial arteriovenous metameric syndrome type 2 (CAMS 2): development over time. *Left,* The first coronal T2-weighted MR image was performed when the patient, a boy, was at age 10 years, during a work-up for retinal angioma. *Middle* and *right,* Six years later, the patient presented with seizure and progressive weakness. Imaging revealed a newly developed diffuse arteriovenous malformation (AVM) of the thalamic region. The de novo appearance, the aspect of the normal brain tissue intermingled with the pathologic blood channels, and the concurrence with a retinal AVM speak strongly in favor of a lateral prosencephalic cerebrofacial arteriovenous metameric syndrome (CAMS 2).

In our view, there are no true "contraindications" to endovascular therapies; in other words, any AVM can be partially treated by embolization. There are many AVMs, however, in which partial treatment does not make sense. This is particularly true for small unruptured AVMs with no angioarchitectonic risk factors. Finally, the following angioarchitectonic features should make interventional neuroradiologists think twice about endovascular therapy and to strongly consider alternate treatment strategies: en passage feeder, flow-related aneurysms, and diffuse nidus-type AVM.

One should realize that endovascular therapies are rarely complete, but they are fast and efficient and they can and should be targeted to selectively eradicate parts of the AVM. It is inappropriate to simply let the flow or pure chance carry the microcatheter to whatever part of the nidus is desired. Proximal occlusions should certainly be avoided, and more than two embolization sessions should rarely be required when the overall risk management (natural history risk versus treatment-related risk) is kept in mind.

Spinal Arteriovenous Malformations

A classification for spinal AVMs that is based on the same characteristics outlined for brain AVMs is difficult to establish, because of the rarity of the spinal lesions. As in cerebral vascular malformations, there are purely arterial diseases (aneurysms, dissections), AV diseases (i.e., AVMs) and purely venous diseases (cavernomas). In addition, a differentiation between focal (i.e., single spinal AVMs) and metameric diseases can be made, with the latter being similar to the previously mentioned CAM syndromes.[2] Finally, hereditary diseases (such as HHT with its associated spinal neurovascular phenotypes) can be differentiated from nonhereditary lesions.[28] However, for the sake of a treatment-based classification, we use a classification scheme in this chapter that is based on the angioarchitecture in addition to the various pathomechanisms. For an understanding of the rationale for these classifications, it is essential to briefly review the essentials of spinal cord vascularization.

Spinal Cord Vascularization

Segmental arteries supply the spine, including the vertebral bodies, paraspinal muscles, dura, nerve roots, and the spinal cord with blood. Radicular arteries are the first branches of the dorsal division of the segmental arteries. The bony spine is supplied by anterior and posterior central arteries that arise directly from the segmental and radicular arteries. A spinal radicular branch supplying the dura and the nerve root as a radiculomeningeal artery is present at each segment. From these radicular arteries, radiculomedullary and/or radiculopial arteries might branch, following the anterior or posterior nerve roots to reach the anterior or posterior surface of the cord where they form the anterior or posterior spinal arterial systems. In the adult patient, not all lumbar or intercostal arteries have a radiculomedullary feeder and their location for a given patient is not predictable.[30] The anterior and posterior spinal arteries constitute a superficial longitudinal anastomosing system. The anterior spinal artery travels along the anterior sulcus and typically originates from the two vertebral arteries, while the typically paired posterolateral spinal arteries originate from the preatlantal part of the vertebral artery or from the posteroinferior cerebellar artery (PICA). These three arterial systems run from the cervical-medullary junction to the conus medullaris, but are not capable of supplying the entire spinal cord. Instead, they are reinforced by radiculomedullary and radiculopial arteries that derive from various (and unpredictable!) segmental levels. The most known of the anterior radiculomedullary arteries is the artery radiculomedullaris magna (i.e., the Adamkiewicz artery). The anterior radiculomedullary arteries branch in a very typical way to reach the spinal cord. The ascending branch continues along the direction of the radicular artery in the

midline of the anterior surface. The descending branch, being the larger one at thoracolumbar levels, forms a hairpin curve as soon as it reaches the midline at the entrance of the anterior fissure.

The intrinsic network of the spinal cord arteries can be divided into central or sulcal arteries from the anterior spinal artery that supply the gray matter and the central part of the cord on one side or the other.[31] The radiculopial network that is derived from the posterolateral spinal arteries supplies via the rami perforantes of the vasa corona the periphery of the spinal cord (i.e., the white matter). The vasa corona gets a small anterolateral supply from the anterior spinal artery. A multitude of anastomoses is present at the spine and spinal cord: Extradural interconnections between segmental arteries can compensate for a proximal occlusion of a radicular artery, whereas intradurally, both the anterior and posterior spinal arteries represent a system of longitudinal anastomoses that is reinforced from different levels. Moreover, both the posterior and anterior arterial systems are interconnected at the level of the conus via the "basket" anastomosis and via transverse anastomoses of the intrinsic arteries that interconnect by the pial network of the vasa corona. The venous drainage of the cord is via radially symmetrical intrinsic spinal cord veins and small superficial pial veins that open into the superficial longitudinal median anastomosing spinal cord veins, both anterior and posterior to the spinal cord.[32] They may use the nerve roots to reach the epidural plexus and the extraspinal veins and plexus with a reflux-impeding mechanism within the dura mater.[33]

Angiomorphologic Classification

Spinal AV shunting lesions can be differentiated like those of the brain, that is, grossly into those that are supplied by dural (or radiculomeningeal) arteries, that do *not* serve to supply the brain (or spinal cord) under normal circumstances, and those shunting lesions that are supplied by arteries that under normal circumstances also supply the brain or spinal cord (i.e., pial AVMs). Because spinal dural AV fistulas (i.e., those shunting lesions that are supplied by radiculomeningeal arteries) are discussed in a different chapter in this book, we focus here only on those pial AV shunts of the spinal cord that are supplied by cord-supplying—radiculopial or radiculomedullary—arteries.[30]

According to their nidus, these spinal pial AVMs are either glomerular or fistulous in nature, and although the fistulous pial AVMs can be further differentiated into macrofistulas with high fistula volume and microfistulas with small fistula volume, the glomerular (nidus-type of plexiform) AVMs may be further separated into the focal and the diffuse ones. Because the location of the AVM itself (i.e., intramedullary versus perimedullary) depends on the supplying vessel (with AVMs being supplied exclusively by the radiculopial arteries and typically perimedullary in location), we do not use this angiographic feature to further subclassify spinal AVMs.

Fistulous AVMs. Fistulous AVMs (which in some classifications have been called AVMs of the perimedullary fistula type or intradural AV fistulas) are direct AV shunts located superficially on the spinal cord that only rarely possess intramedullary compartments. Feeding vessels are radiculomedullary arteries, radiculopial arteries, or both (differentiating them from the dural AV fistulas). Draining veins are superficial perimedullary veins. The arterialized blood may even ascend via the foramen magnum into the posterior fossa. Fistulous AVMs can be subdivided into two types according to their feeding vessel size, the volume of the shunt, and the drainage pattern (Fig. 64-19). Microfistulas are small AVMs in which both the feeding artery and the draining vein are not markedly dilated and the shunt volume is low. Macrofistulas harbor multiple massively dilated arterial feeders and a large shunt volume. These latter fistulas are typically encountered in HHT. Spinal cord AV fistula in HHT is characterized as an intradural AV malformation with a macrofistula and high fistula volume; the fistula drains directly into

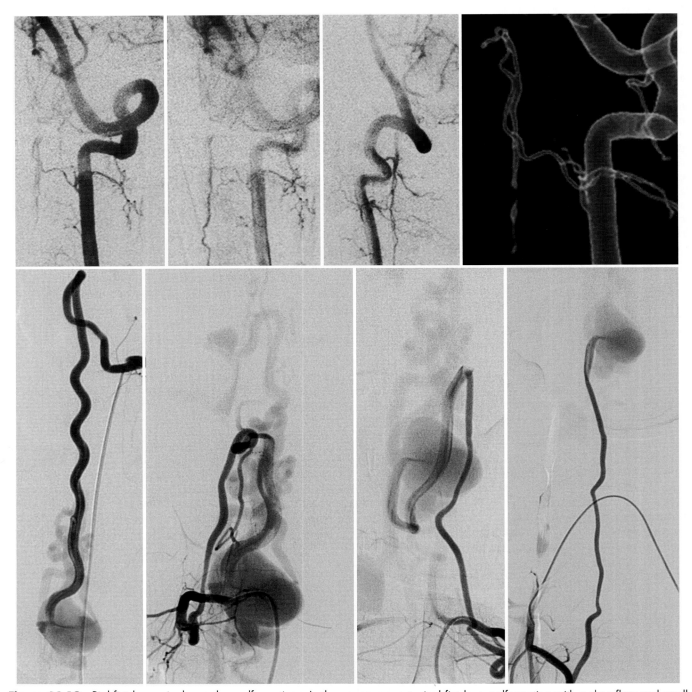

Figure 64-19 Pial fistulous spinal vascular malformations: In the *upper row*, a typical fistulous malformation with a slow flow and small fistula volume is demonstrated. These spinal pial vascular malformations are referred to as microfistulas. In comparison with microfistulas, macrofistulas (as depicted in the *lower row*) are pial vascular malformations that (like microfistulas) have no intervening nidus. Instead, the arteries shunt directly into the veins. Owing to the large shunting volume in macrofistulas, these are typically associated with large venous pouches. The types of fistulas depicted here are extreme variants on the spectrum of pial vascular fistulous malformations.

a massively enlarged venous pouch that can be easily identified on MRI.[28] Feeding vessels might be either the dorsolateral or the anterior spinal arteries or both. Multiple feeders conjoin at the same space into the draining venous pouch. Venous ectasias, stenosis, and pial reflux are present in all patients with these fistulas (Fig. 64-20).

Glomerular AVMs. The *focal type* of glomerular AVM is confined to the spinal cord. It is fed by radiculomedullary and radiculopial (spinal cord feeding) arteries and drained by spinal cord veins. The shunt flow is high but typically not as high as in macrofistulous AVMs. Glomerular AVMs (which are sometimes called plexiform or nidus-type AVMs) are the most often encountered spinal cord AVM, with a nidus resembling closely those of a brain AVM. This type of malformation usually has an intramedullary location, but superficial nidus compartments can also reach the subarachnoid space. Because of the many anastomoses between the anterior and posterior arterial feeding system of the spines, these AVMs typically have multiple artery supply from both the posterior and anterior system. Drainage is into dilated spinal cord veins (Fig. 64-21).

The *diffuse type* of glomerular AVMs is not confined to the spinal cord and, in correlation to its cerebral counterpart has therefore been called spinal AV metameric syndrome (SAMS; previously called Cobb's syndrome or spinal AVM of the juvenile type). SAMS affects the whole myelomere, so affected patients typically present with multiple shunts of the spinal cord, the nerve root, bone, paraspinal, subcutaneous, and skin tissues that share the same myelomere. SAMS can be further subdivided depending on the affected myelomere from 1 to 31 (Fig. 64-22).

Pathophysiologic Classification

As in brain AVMs, a classification of spinal AVMs based on their pathomechanisms and clinical presentations is also possible. The major pathophysiologic mechanisms in spinal cord AVMs are venous congestion and hemorrhage.[34]

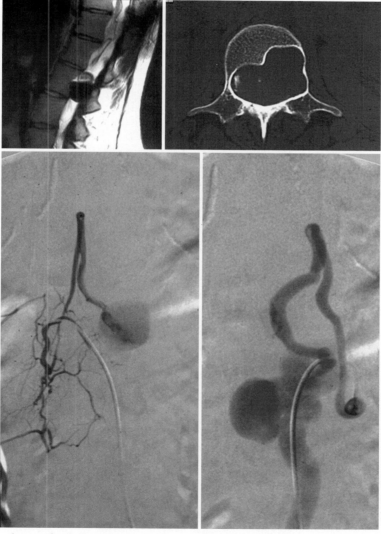

Figure 64-20 Spinal cord pial macrofistulas in a patient with a family history of hereditary hemorrhagic telangiectasia. These spinal malformations are characterized by their high flow and the young age at which they become symptomatic. On T2-weighted MR images, flow voids are present, whereas on CT scans, bony usurpation can be seen in some cases. Feeding vessels might be either dorsolateral or anterior spinal arteries, or both. Multiple feeders conjoin at the same space into an enlarged draining venous pouch.

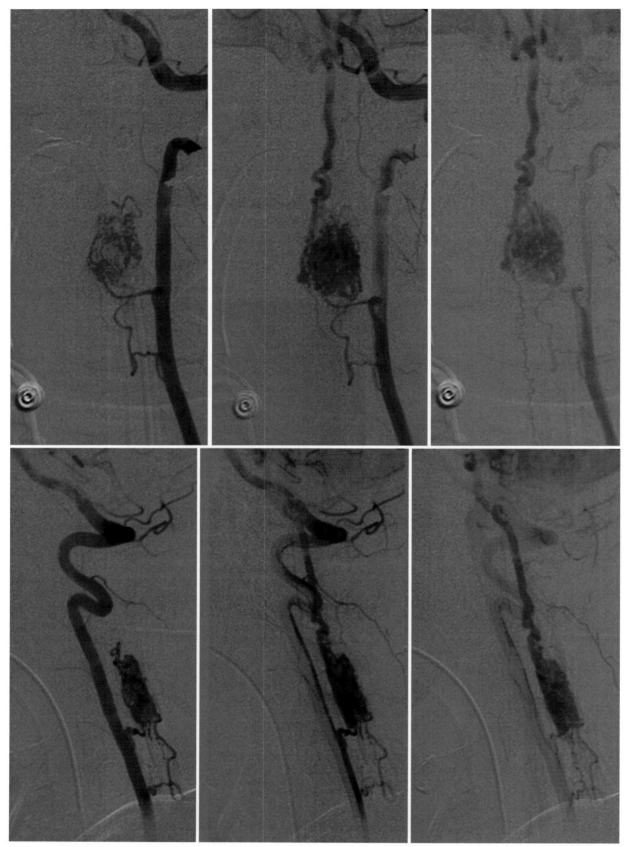

Figure 64-21 Glomerular or nidus-type arteriovenous malformation (AVM). Early arterial to early venous arteriogram phases in antero-posterior views in the *upper row* and the lateral views in the *lower row* demonstrate multiple feeders to an intramedullary AVM that consists of a nidus or glomus of pathologic vessels instead of a single fistula.

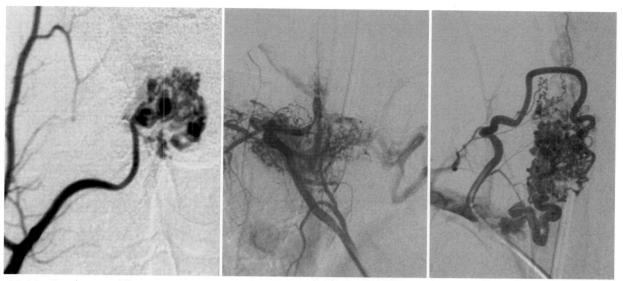

Figure 64-22 Focal versus diffuse type of glomerular arteriovenous malformation (AVM). In the *left* panel, a classic nidus-type or glomerular AVM can be seen, whereas in the *middle* and *right* panels, a diffuse nidus-type AVM that is not confined to the spinal cord but instead extends over the complete metamere is visualized.

Only rarely, space-occupying effects or arterial steal may be present. Acute symptoms may be related to a spontaneous thrombosis of a vein. If the AVM does not manifest initially as acute hemorrhage, symptomatology may be nonspecific. Patients may complain about hypesthesia or paresthesia, weakness, and diffuse back and muscle pain. Progressive sensorimotor symptoms can develop slowly or worsen acutely followed by some improvements over time. Glomerular AVMs tend to become symptomatic in younger children and adolescents, whereas fistulous AVMs become symptomatic in young adults, the latter presenting often with a subarachnoid hemorrhage because of the frequent perimedullary location. Glomerular AVMs can become symptomatic by means of venous congestion alone, intraparenchymal hemorrhage, and/or subarachnoid hemorrhage. Macrofistulas manifest as hematomyelia with acute tetraplegia/paresis in the majority of cases; spinal subarachnoid hemorrhage and venous congestion can also be encountered.[35]

Concepts of Treatment

The therapeutic approach to an asymptomatic AVM is difficult since data concerning the spontaneous prognosis are not available; however, in symptomatic AVMs therapy improves the prognosis of the patient. There are some fundamental differences between brain AVMs and spinal AVMs: First, a hyperacute treatment is rarely indicated because, in our opinion, acute rebleeding of a spinal AVM rarely occurs.[36] Instead, after bleeding of a spinal AVM has occurred, we typically wait for approximately 6 weeks for potential vasospasm to resolve or the hemorrhage to absorb. Second, although brain AVMs have to be completely treated to avoid the risk of rebleeding, this seems not to be the case with spinal AVMs, for which partial treatment appears to be sufficient to dramatically improve the prognosis, especially in those cases in which a complete eradication of the AVM is likely to

produce neurologic deficits. Especially in unruptured spinal AVMs that have become symptomatic with venous congestion rather than hemorrhage,[37] the goal has to be to reduce the shunting volume rather than to make an "angiographically nice" picture that carries a high risk of treatment-related morbidity.[38] Third, because of the low flow in some glomerular AVMs, endovascular therapies with particles seem to have a better and more stable result, if venous stagnation (with subsequent venous thrombosis of the outlet) occurs. Fourth, in our opinion, there is no role for radiosurgery in spinal vascular malformations, and the endovascular route should be the modality of choice in most instances. Surgery remains an option especially when the endovascular route is too long (which may be the case for AV fistulas located at the filum terminale).

Fistulous AVMs. In fistulous AVMs, the aim is to obliterate the point of fistulization. A secure way to reach this goal is to embolize the most proximal venous segment together with the most distal arterial segment. This can be done with either liquid embolic agents or coils. Although the choice of embolization material is of minor importance and merely depends on the interventionalist's preference, the most important (and most difficult) part is to know where the artery stops and where the vein starts. A proximal occlusion of the artery will lead to collateral filling and secondary reopening due to the vast network of anastomoses and may carry the risk of inadvertent occlusion of spinal cord supply. A pure venous occlusion that leaves the fistula open may, on the other hand, result in hemorrhage. The transition between artery and vein may be indicated by a venous aneurysm (which is often the site of rupture) (Figs. 64-23 and 64-24), a large venous pouch (as typically present in the large-volume single-hole fistulas), or a slight change in caliber (Fig. 64-25). A three-dimensional reconstruction of the angiogram is in our opinion particularly helpful to define this fistulous point.[39] Great caution must be taken in identifying the

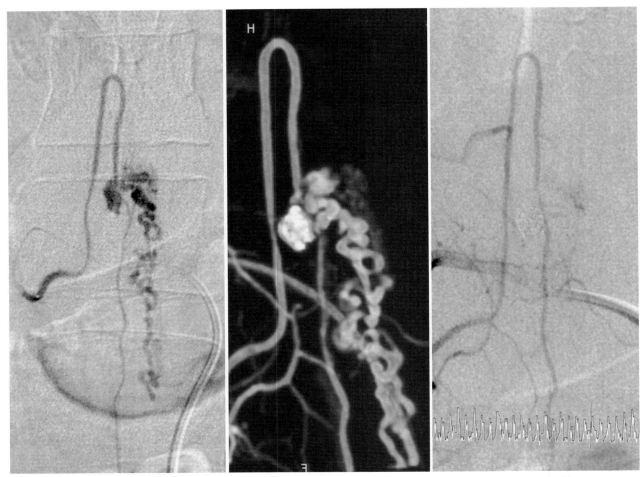

Figure 64-23 Treatment of a microfistula with coils. In this patient the transition between artery and vein was marked by a venous ectasia that was subsequently occluded with coils, leading to complete obliteration of the fistula with preservation of the anterior spinal artery axis.

normal spinal cord arteries (which may be difficult to demonstrate because of the flow being directed primarily into the fistula). Therefore, before therapy is contemplated, complete spinal angiography is done to evaluate potential collaterals to the anterior and posterior spinal arteries. When therapy with a liquid embolic agent is contemplated, the point of security has to be defined because reflux of the embolic agent may occur (especially in small fistulas). Too short a distance between the microcatheter tip and the adjacent anterior spinal arterial system may therefore carry a large risk for the patient. In addition, a too proximal position of the microcatheter tip may prevent the embolic agent from reaching the vein, resulting in a proximal arterial occlusion.[40] In these cases, we rather opt for surgical treatment of the fistula.[41]

In high-flow macrofistulas (which may be indicative of an underlying genetic disease such as HHT), a technique similar to that for single-hole brain AV fistulas has to be adopted: In these types of fistulous AVMs the dilated feeding vessels will allow for superselective catheterization close to the fistula. Closure with highly concentrated glue is therefore possible with the aim to obliterate the fistulous area by pushing the glue via the distal artery into the proximal venous pouch to establish a mushroom-shaped glue cast that occludes the single-hole fistula (Fig. 64-26). This is preferably done via a posterior spinal arterial feeder, with occlusion of the fistula being verified during injection of the other feeders. One important caution has to be kept in mind in this kind of treatment, though. Because the volume of the venous pouch is typically large and may further enlarge following thrombosis (which will happen within the first 24 hours after occlusion), compression of the spinal cord may occur. Such rare evolution may need to be treated with surgical decompression. Given these assumptions, a stepwise approach with reduction of the flow (and subsequently the size of the venous pouch) using coils at the site of the fistula in several sessions may be an alternative treatment strategy.

Glomerular AVMs. In glomerular AVMs, liquid embolic agents (or in rare circumstances particles) can be employed to obliterate the nidus, but even partial embolization seems to improve the natural history of the patient, because in most instances, the pathomechanism can be identified prior to the procedure, leading to an individually tailored therapeutic strategy. In most instances of glomerular AVMs that have become symptomatic with a hemorrhage, a focal weak point can be identified and targeted for embolization (Fig. 64-27).[36]

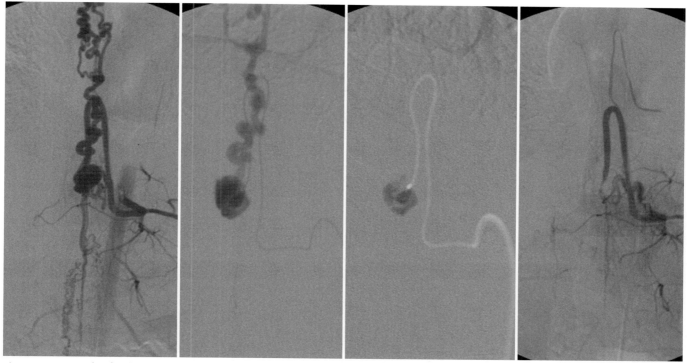

Figure 64-24 This fistulous arteriovenous malformation was characterized by a venous pouch at the transition from the anterior spinal artery to the vein. After selective microcatheterization and glue deposition, the fistula could be completely obliterated with preservation of the anterior spinal artery.

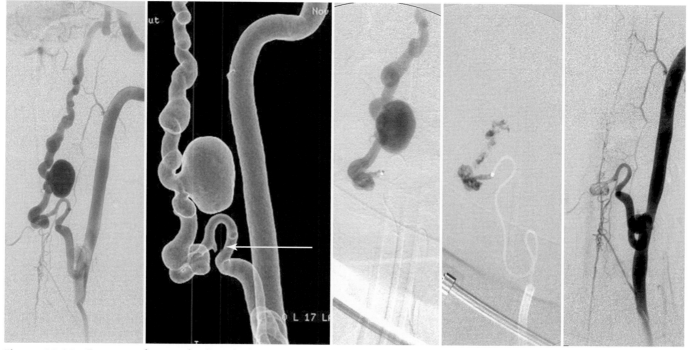

Figure 64-25 Treatment of a microfistula with glue. In this patient, the transition between artery and vein is depicted by the sudden onset of increase in diameter. In addition, the three-dimensional reconstruction demonstrates the further course of the normal anterior spinal artery network *(arrow)*, thereby demonstrating the security margin and the aim of treatment.

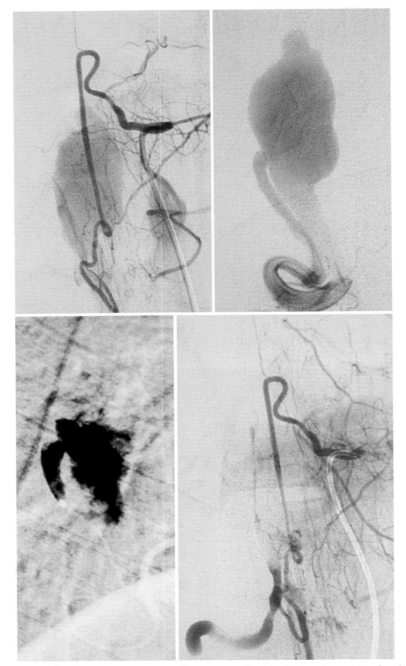

Figure 64-26 Treatment of a macrofistulous arteriovenous malformation with glue. This patient with a family history of hereditary hemorrhagic telangiectasia was found at angiography to have a massively enlarged venous pouch that was predominantly fed by a radiculopial artery, although some supply from the anterior spinal artery converging into the same venous pouch was also noted. Following a mushroom-shaped glue cast via the dorsolateral feeder, complete obliteration of the fistula was obtained with preservation of the anterior spinal artery axis.

On the other hand, in cases in which the symptoms can be attributed to the venous congestion, the aim will be to reduce the shunt as much as possible. As in fistulous AVMs, the first step is to perform complete angiography to determine the collaterals, the main feeders, and the number of different and/or overlapping compartments. Three-dimensional reconstructions will be helpful to demonstrate focal weak points. Conventional series have to include the venous phase because contrast agent stagnation in intranidal outpouchings (pseudoaneurysms) is the classic sign of the point of rupture. With the anatomic characteristics of spinal cord vessels taken into consideration, the safest vessels via which an embolization can be performed are the posterior spinal ones.[42] Because of the vast anastomotic network, compartments belonging to the anterior spinal artery axis can often be reached by the posterior spinal system as well. If treatment with particles is to be performed,

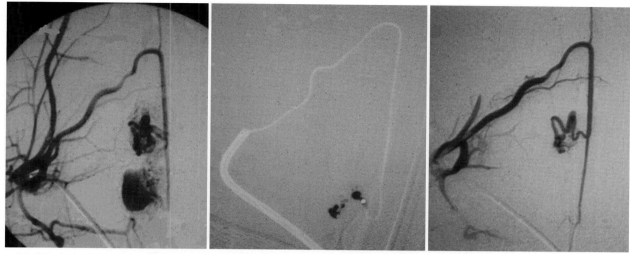

Figure 64-27 In the lower part of this glomerular arteriovenous malformation, a large false aneurysm can be identified with contrast agent stagnation in the venous phase of the arteriogram. After superselective catheterization and glue deposition, the site of bleeding could be secured with preservation of the remainder of the spinal cord vessels.

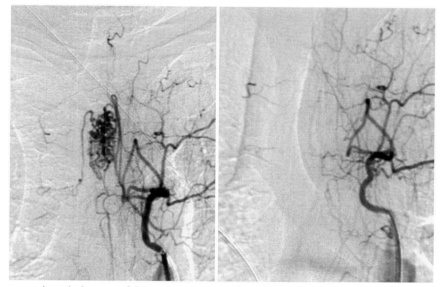

Figure 64-28 Following particle embolization of this arteriovenous malformation (AVM), stable occlusion was obtained. Follow-up images 4 months after embolization demonstrate obliteration of the AVM.

they will have to be very diluted and injected slowly until venous stagnation occurs. In five cases reported by Theron, this approach led to a stable occlusion; likewise, in our practice, several patients had a complete and stable occlusion over time with this approach (Fig. 64-28). Liquid embolic agents have the major advantage of being stable, although their reported complication rates are higher (in the large series, approximately 10%), and only rarely is a complete obliteration possible (Fig. 64-29). In diffuse angiomas (SAMS or juvenile angiomas, Cobb's syndrome), a complete obliteration or resection is almost never possible.[43] In these cases, we again adopt the strategy of a partially targeted embolization to reduce shunting zones and to obliterate potential focal weak points.

Indications for and Contraindications to Endovascular Therapies

As stated in the beginning of this section, a therapy of spinal AVMs improves the prognosis in symptomatic patients, whereas in asymptomatic patients, its use has not been proven. Endovascular therapies are definitely the first line of treatment and should be tailored to the specific individual pathomechanisms and angioarchitectonics. We perceive contraindications to endovascular therapy only in those cases in which a safe catheter position cannot be achieved. The term "safe," however, implies a profound understanding of the angioarchitecture of the spinal cord, which is why, in our opinion, treatment of these rare diseases should be performed exclusively in specialized centers.

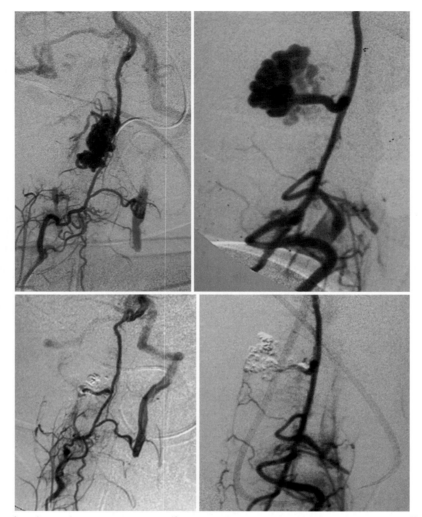

Figure 64-29 Treatment of a glomerular arteriovenous malformation (AVM) employing glue. The patient suffered from a cervical hemorrhage necessitating treatment. Complete occlusion of the spinal nidus-type AVM was possible following superselective catheterization via the ascending cervical artery. No worsening was noted after the embolization, and the patient subsequently recovered from his initial neurologic deficits.

REFERENCES

1. Lasjaunias P: Segmental identiy and vulnerability in cerebral arteries, *Intervent Neuroradiol* 6:113-124, 2000.
2. Krings T, Geibprasert S, Luo CB, et al: Segmental neurovascular syndromes in children, *Neuroimaging Clin North Am* 17:245-258, 2007.
3. Lasjaunias PL, Berenstein A, terBrugge K: Clinical vascular anatomy and variations, *Surgical Neuroangiography*, vol 1, Berlin, 2001, Springer.
4. Graf CJ, Perret GE, Torner JC: Bleeding from cerebral arteriovenous malformations as part of their natural history, *J Neurosurg* 58:331-337, 1983.
5. Crawford PM, West CR, Chadwick DW, et al: Arteriovenous malformations of the brain: Natural history in unoperated patients, *J Neurol Neurosurg Psychiatry* 49:1-10, 1986.
6. Brown RD Jr, Wiebers DO, Forbes G, et al: The natural history of unruptured intracranial arteriovenous malformations, *J Neurosurg* 68:352-357, 1988.
7. Ondra SL, Troupp H, George ED, et al: The natural history of symptomatic arteriovenous malformations of the brain: A 24-year follow-up assessment, *J Neurosurg* 73:387-391, 1990.
8. Mast H, Young WL, Koennecke HC, et al: Risk of spontaneous haemorrhage after diagnosis of cerebral arteriovenous malformation, *Lancet* 350:1065-1068, 1997.
9. Krings T, Chng SM, Ozanne A, et al: Hereditary hemorrhagic telangiectasia in children: Endovascular treatment of neurovascular malformations: Results in 31 patients, *Neuroradiology* 47:946-954, 2005.
10. Alvarez H, Garcia Monaco R, Rodesch G, et al: Vein of Galen aneurysmal malformations, *Neuroimaging Clin N Am* 17:189-206, 2007.
11. Geibprasert S, Pereira V, Krings T, et al: Hydrocephalus in unruptured brain arteriovenous malformations: Pathomechanical considerations, therapeutic implications and clinical course, *J Neurosurg* 110:500-507, 2009.
12. Monteiro JM, Rosas MJ, Correia AP, et al: Migraine and intracranial vascular malformations, *Headache* 33:563-565, 1993.
13. Alexander MJ, Tolbert ME: Targeting cerebral arteriovenous malformations for minimally invasive therapy, *Neurosurgery* 59:S178-S183, 2006:discussion S173-S113.
14. Hademenos GJ, Massoud TF: Risk of intracranial arteriovenous malformation rupture due to venous drainage impairment. A theoretical analysis, *Stroke* 27:1072-1083, 1996.
15. Mansmann U, Meisel J, Brock M, et al: Factors associated with intracranial hemorrhage in cases of cerebral arteriovenous malformation, *Neurosurgery* 46:272-279, 2000:discussion 279-281.
16. Meisel HJ, Mansmann U, Alvarez H, et al: Effect of partial targeted N-butyl-cyano-acrylate embolization in brain AVM, *Acta Neurochir (Wien)* 144:879-887, 2002:discussion 888.

17. Meisel HJ, Mansmann U, Alvarez H, et al: Cerebral arteriovenous malformations and associated aneurysms: Analysis of 305 cases from a series of 662 patients, *Neurosurgery* 46:793-800, 2000.
18. Stefani MA, Porter PJ, terBrugge KG, et al: Angioarchitectural factors present in brain arteriovenous malformations associated with hemorrhagic presentation, *Stroke* 33:920-924, 2002.
19. Hofmeister C, Stapf C, Hartmann A, et al: Demographic, morphological, and clinical characteristics of 1289 patients with brain arteriovenous malformation, *Stroke* 31:1307-1310, 2000.
20. Krings T, Geibprasert S, Pereira V, et al: Aneurysms. In Naidich T, editor: *Neuroradiology of the brain and spine*, New York, 2008, Elsevier.
21. Willinsky R, TerBrugge K, Montanera W, et al: Micro-arteriovenous malformations of the brain: Superselective angiography in diagnosis and treatment, *AJNR Am J Neuroradiol* 13:325-330, 1992.
22. Richling B, Killer M: Endovascular management of patients with cerebral arteriovenous malformations, *Neurosurg Clin North Am* 11:123-145, 2000:ix.
23. Valavanis A, Yasargil MG: The endovascular treatment of brain arteriovenous malformations, *Adv Tech Stand Neurosurg* 24:131-214, 1998.
24. Yu SC, Chan MS, Lam JM, et al: Complete obliteration of intracranial arteriovenous malformation with endovascular cyanoacrylate embolization: Initial success and rate of permanent cure, *AJNR Am J Neuroradiol* 25:1139-1143, 2004.
25. Katsaridis V, Papagiannaki C, Aimar E: Curative embolization of cerebral arteriovenous malformations (AVMs) with Onyx in 101 patients, *Neuroradiology* 50:589-597, 2008.
26. Taylor CL, Dutton K, Rappard G, et al: Complications of preoperative embolization of cerebral arteriovenous malformations, *J Neurosurg* 100:810-812, 2004.
27. Redekop G, TerBrugge K, Montanera W, et al: Arterial aneurysms associated with cerebral arteriovenous malformations: Classification, incidence, and risk of hemorrhage, *J Neurosurg* 89:539-546, 1998.
28. Krings T, Ozanne A, Chng SM, et al: Neurovascular phenotypes in hereditary haemorrhagic telangiectasia patients according to age. Review of 50 consecutive patients aged 1 day-60 years, *Neuroradiology* 47:711-720, 2005.
29. Lasjaunias PL, Landrieu P, Rodesch G, et al: Cerebral proliferative angiopathy: Clinical and angiographic description of an entity different from cerebral AVMs, *Stroke* 39:878-885, 2008.
30. Krings T, Mull M, Gilsbach JM, et al: Spinal vascular malformations, *Eur Radiol* 15:267-278, 2005.
31. Thron A: *Vascular anatomy of the spinal cord: Neuroradiological investigations and clinical syndromes*, Berlin, New York, 1988, Springer.
32. Krings T, Lasjaunias PL, Hans FJ, et al: Imaging in spinal vascular disease, *Neuroimaging Clin North Am* 17:57-72, 2007.
33. Krings T, Mull M, Bostroem A, et al: Spinal epidural arteriovenous fistula with perimedullary drainage. Case report and pathomechanical considerations, *J Neurosurg Spine* 5:353-358, 2006.
34. Rodesch G, Hurth M, Alvarez H, et al: Angio-architecture of spinal cord arteriovenous shunts at presentation. Clinical correlations in adults and children. The Bicetre experience on 155 consecutive patients seen between 1981-1999, *Acta Neurochir (Wien)* 146:217-226, 2004.
35. Ozanne A, Krings T, Facon D, et al: MR diffusion tensor imaging and fiber tracking in spinal cord arteriovenous malformations: A preliminary study, *AJNR Am J Neuroradiol* 28:1271-1279, 2007.
36. Rodesch G, Hurth M, Alvarez H, et al: Spinal cord intradural arteriovenous fistulae: Anatomic, clinical, and therapeutic considerations in a series of 32 consecutive patients seen between 1981 and 2000 with emphasis on endovascular therapy, *Neurosurgery* 57:973-983, 2005.
37. Kataoka H, Miyamoto S, Nagata I, et al: Venous congestion is a major cause of neurological deterioration in spinal arteriovenous malformations, *Neurosurgery* 48:1224-1229, 2001:discussion 1229-1230.
38. Rodesch G, Hurth M, Alvarez H, et al: Embolization of spinal cord arteriovenous shunts: Morphological and clinical follow-up and results—review of 69 consecutive cases, *Neurosurgery* 53:40-49, 2003.
39. Prestigiacomo CJ, Niimi Y, Setton A, et al: Three-dimensional rotational spinal angiography in the evaluation and treatment of vascular malformations, *AJNR Am J Neuroradiol* 24:1429-1435, 2003.
40. Mourier KL, Gobin YP, George B, et al: Intradural perimedullary arteriovenous fistulae: Results of surgical and endovascular treatment in a series of 35 cases, *Neurosurgery* 32:885-891, 1993:discussion 891.
41. Huffmann BC, Spetzger U, Reinges M, et al: Treatment strategies and results in spinal vascular malformations, *Neurol Med Chir (Tokyo)* 38(Suppl):231-237, 1998.
42. Niimi Y, Berenstein A: Endovascular treatment of spinal vascular malformations, *Neurosurg Clin North Am* 10:47-71, 1999.
43. Spetzler RF, Zabramski JM, Flom RA: Management of juvenile spinal AVMs by embolization and operative excision. Case report, *J Neurosurg* 70:628-632, 1989.

65 | Dural Arteriovenous Malformations

J. PAUL ELLIOTT, DANIEL HUDDLE, ISSAM A. AWAD

Arteriovenous malformations (AVMs) affecting the central nervous system include a number of pathologic entities, all characterized by abnormal arteriovenous shunting. The cerebral AVMs (CAVMs) consist of a nidus of arteriovenous shunting within brain parenchyma, supplied by the intracranial anterior and posterior circulation and lacking a normal capillary bed. Pial fistulas are characterized by a direct, high-flow shunt from a pial artery to an enlarged vein or varix. The dural AVMs (DAVMs) are composed of arteriovenous shunts within the dural leaflet, typically supplied predominantly by pachymeningeal arteries and located near a major venous sinus.[1]

Historically, the DAVMs have been a confusing entity, in part because of their multiple names and the difficulty of separating their primary abnormality, dural arteriovenous shunting, from other secondary changes. They are distinct from but are often confused with CAVMs. Some investigators believe that DAVMs should be more appropriately named dural arteriovenous shunts, dural arteriovenous fistulas, or dural arteriovenous fistulous malformations.[2]

DAVMs are distinguished from other intracranial vascular lesions by their nidus, which is composed of arteriovenous shunting localized in the leaflets of the dura mater (Fig. 65-1). They are typically localized adjacent to a major dural sinus, and their arterial supply originates from both intradural arteries and pachymeningeal branches of cerebral arteries. Venous drainage occurs through an adjacent dural sinus, other dural and leptomeningeal venous channels, or both. Although their etiology is controversial, DAVMs appear to be acquired lesions.[3] They may remain asymptomatic or may manifest as a wide range of symptoms, including headache, tinnitus, bruit, cranial neuropathy, seizures, dementia, intracranial hypertension, and focal neurologic deficits from venous congestion.[4-8] DAVMs may also cause life-threatening intracranial hemorrhage.[9] Although it remains difficult to prognosticate for a given lesion, the location (anterior cranial fossa or tentorial incisura) and pattern of venous drainage (retrograde leptomeningeal venous drainage) clearly influence clinical presentation.[10-12] Lesions that manifest as hemorrhages are clearly associated with a significantly higher risk of additional morbidity and mortality. Although many unruptured DAVMs are best treated expectantly, some features identify high-risk lesions, which may be definitively treated with an evolving combination of endovascular, radiosurgical, and surgical techniques.

Clinical Presentation

DAVMs account for 10% to 15% of cranial vascular malformations. There is a 2:1 female preponderance, with typical presentation at 30 to 50 years of age. Typical locations are in proximity to the major sinuses (50% transverse-sigmoid, 15% cavernous, 10% tentorial, 8% superior sagittal). A few DAVMs manifest early in life and are thus thought to be congenital. They are usually associated with complex congenital anomalies, rare phakomatoses, or a vein of Galen malformation—a special form of DAVM.[1] In these cases, there is often gross malformation of dural sinuses with atresia of venous outflow from a region of dura mater involved in the DAVM. The vast majority of DAVMs manifest later in life and are assumed to be acquired.[13,14] Known or suspected etiologic factors include trauma, infection, vascular disease, and tumors. The most important aspect of these etiologic factors may be a shared propensity for sinus thrombosis with a secondary alteration in venous hemodynamics (restricted outflow and venous hypertension) and development of shunting from preexisting physiologic shunts.

Clinical manifestations of DAVMs are highly variable and are related primarily to the location of the fistula and both the arterial supply and venous drainage. The manifestations range from minor symptoms to catastrophic intracranial hemorrhage. The vast majority of symptoms can be attributed to the primary or secondary venous manifestations of the DAVM. More benign symptoms such as pain, tinnitus, and bruit are related to arteriovenous shunting and flow in the DAVM. Manifestation of a DAVM may be sudden or slowly progressive. The severity and type of symptoms are determined by venous topography, the venous flow pattern, and the capacity of surrounding compensatory venous drainage. The most serious neurologic sequelae of DAVMs are associated with retrograde leptomeningeal venous drainage.[15] Focal neurologic deficits likely result from venous hypertension and intracranial hemorrhage from rupture of arterialized leptomeningeal veins.

There are a wide variety of nonhemorrhagic symptoms.[12,16] Pulsatile tinnitus and other subjective auditory symptoms may occur with or without pain. These symptoms are probably related to high flow through dural vascular channels at the base of the skull. Other painful complaints may be related to either orbital congestion or stretching of dural leaflets by engorged vascular channels or to direct compression of the trigeminal nerve

DURAL AVM

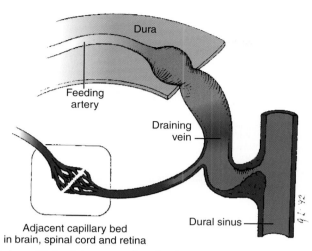

Figure 65-1 Schematic of a dural arteriovenous malformation (AVM). A dural AVM is composed of arteriovenous shunts within the dural leaflet, typically supplied predominantly by pachymeningeal arteries and located near a major venous sinus. Retrograde leptomeningeal venous drainage is associated with a high risk of hemorrhage. (Reprinted with permission of AANS Publications.)

by arterialized venous structures near the petrous apex. Neuroophthalmic manifestations of DAVMs include visual and gaze abnormalities caused by venous hypertension as well as orbital or ocular venous hypertension with resulting orbital crowding, venous stasis retinopathy, and glaucoma. Other cranial DAVMs may manifest as symptoms of increased intracranial pressure (ICP) or a poorly defined headache.[7,17] Although the headaches are nonspecific, they appear to be associated with the dysplastic changes in meningeal vessels, which are often present in DAVMs. There are also a wide spectrum of presenting focal neurologic symptoms, including seizure, hearing loss, cranial nerve palsy, papilledema and other visual symptoms, and focal motor–sensory deficits.[18-20]

DAVMs may also alter the hydrodynamics of cerebrospinal fluid (CSF).[6] Dilated venous structures may act as mass lesions, obstructing the CSF circulation and causing hydrocephalus. In other cases, dural venous hypertension may result in decreased absorption of CSF with secondary intracranial hypertension and papilledema. This latter complication appears to be more common in association with high-flow lesions draining into large dural venous sinuses and in the setting of concomitant dural sinus outflow obstruction.

Particular clinical presentations are associated with DAVMs in specific locations.[2,15,16] DAVMs in the region of the transverse or sigmoid sinus, or near the cavernous sinus, often drain into the associated venous sinuses and may cause a variety of clinical manifestations resulting from flow or local venous engorgement. High flow in the region of the transverse-sigmoid sinus junction, for example, often gives rise to pulsatile tinnitus, headache, and bruit. These lesions do not bleed or cause other deficits unless there is associated retrograde leptomeningeal venous drainage. Lesions at the anterior cranial fossa

or the tentorial incisura rarely drain into a patent dural venous sinus and are more frequently associated with leptomeningeal venous drainage. They are more likely to cause serious clinical sequelae from venous hypertension and hemorrhage. Hemorrhage has not been reported in the absence of this feature; in all published cases with carefully documented diagnostic findings, hemorrhage from DAVMs is associated with rupture of arterialized venous structures. The prognosis of a first hemorrhage from a DAVM is ominous and is associated with a greater than 30% rate of death or serious disability. Hemorrhaging from DAVMs in patients who have undergone anticoagulation has been uniformly fatal.

Pathophysiology and Lesion Evolution

DAVM is usually acquired.[13,14] It is hypothesized to result from altered angiogenesis within the dura after an inciting event such as trauma, surgery, or chronic infection. Altered angiogenesis is often accompanied by sinus thrombosis. In some cases of documented, angiographically proven dural sinus thrombosis, DAVMs subsequently developed in relationship to the obstructed sinus. Initial microshunts are hypothesized to proliferate in association with the venous hypertension, maturing into clinically significant arteriovenous fistulas. The extent of progression or involution determines the significance of the abnormality. The fistulas may result in hemorrhage or have other focal manifestations, including hemodynamic insufficiency. DAVMs cause decreased regional cerebral blood flow in cortical regions where there is retrograde venous drainage.[21]

The development of DAVMs after trauma and surgery is well known.[22,23] These lesions have also been reported in association with chronic infection, vascular disease, and tumors.[24] Other cases of DAVM have no clear association. They may be identified at anatomic sites distinct from the presumed inciting event. The exact mechanism of development remains unclear. It is hypothesized that development of a DAVM in these diverse settings would probably require a common mechanism as well as a possible anatomic or genetic predisposition.[25,26] Experimental work suggests that the diverse clinical associations of DAVM may be explained by the development of venous obstruction and hypertension with aberrant angiogenesis.[27]

An established DAVM may follow one of several natural courses. Some lesions remain asymptomatic or maintain stable clinical symptoms and angiographic features over many years. Others undergo spontaneous regression, involution, and resolution with stabilization or improvement of neurologic symptoms.[11,28-30] Features that may predispose to such spontaneous involution are not known. DAVMs in the region of the cavernous sinus are particularly prone to this phenomenon; as many as 40% of reported cases have undergone spontaneous involution. In contrast, some DAVMs may demonstrate an increase in size from either arterial or venous enlargement.[1,2,15] Pachymeningeal arterial feeders may be progressively recruited and result in enlargement of the nidus. The mechanisms behind this progressive recruitment of arterial feeders from numerous sources have not been elucidated. This phenomenon results in hypertrophy of dural

TABLE 65-1 CLASSIFICATION OF DURAL ARTERIOVENOUS MALFORMATIONS

Type	Djindjian	Cognard	Borden
I	Normal antegrade flow into dural sinus	Normal antegrade flow into dural sinus	Drains directly into venous sinus or meningeal vein
II	Drainage into venous sinus with reflux into adjacent sinus or cortical vein	a. Retrograde flow into sinus b. Retrograde filling of cortical veins only c. Retrograde drainage into sinus and cortical veins	Drains into dural sinus or meningeal veins with retrograde drainage into subarachnoid veins
III	Drainage into cortical veins with retrograde flow	Direct drainage into cortical veins with retrograde flow	Drains into subarachnoid veins without dural sinus or meningeal involvement
IV	Drainage into venous pouch (lake)	Direct drainage into cortical veins with venous ectasia >5 mm and 3× larger than diameter of draining vein	
V		Drainage to spinal perimedullary veins	

arteries and the reappearance of involuted embryonic arteries that may not normally be visible in the adult dura mater.

In some DAVMs, there is also progression of disease on the venous side. Progressive arterialization of the pathologic dural leaflets results in hypertension in adjacent leptomeningeal venous channels; this process may lead to retrograde leptomeningeal venous drainage. Under arterialized pressures, these channels may become tortuous and, eventually, varicose or aneurysmal. Hemorrhage is the unfortunate result. In DAVMs that manifest as intracranial hemorrhage and have retrograde cortical venous drainage, there is a 35% risk of rebleeding within the first 2 weeks.[31]

Diagnosis, Classification, and Indications for Treatment

Diagnosis

Catheter cerebral angiography is the most sensitive and specific diagnostic study for defining DAVMs.[32] In patients with suspected DAVM, the study should include injection of both internal carotid arteries, both vertebral arteries, and both external carotid arteries. In cases of suspected clival or foramen magnum region DAVMs, arch injections may reveal additional ascending muscular or pharyngeal arterial feeders. Imaging should capture the very early arterial phase and continue late into the venous phase. Digital subtraction and magnification techniques and the occasional use of superselective angiography greatly enhance the diagnostic potential of angiography. Cerebral angiography provides the spatial diagnostic detail and dynamic flow information to identify arterial feeders and define the pattern of flow and venous drainage of the DAVM in detail. This information is essential for prognostication and therapeutic decisions.

Other diagnostic modalities such as computed tomography (CT), computed tomography angiography (CTA), magnetic resonance imaging (MRI), and magnetic resonance angiography (MRA) may be useful in the diagnosis and follow-up of DAVM. CT or MRI is often performed as part of the initial investigation of the patient presenting with neurologic symptoms. These studies may reveal thickening of a region of dura mater, tortuosities of leptomeningeal venous drainage, or secondary changes in brain parenchyma reflective of venous hypertension. MRA has

also been used to detect and follow up DAVMs.[33] To maximize the sensitivity of MRI or MRA, the radiologist should have a high index of clinical suspicion for the disorder. At present, these adjuvant diagnostic studies are incapable of totally excluding the presence of a DAVM, and they do not define relevant features of the lesion well enough for prognostic and therapeutic decisions to be based on their findings. However, MRI, MRA, and CTA may be used to screen patients with a low clinical suspicion of a DAVM and to monitor specific features of DAVMs (i.e., development of or enlargement of leptomeningeal venous channels) after baseline correlation with angiography. In the setting of strong clinical suspicion, normal CT or MRI findings should not be used to exclude a DAVM.

Classification

Classification of DAVMs has evolved over time to be useful in guiding therapeutic intervention. Initial attempts were simplistic, emphasizing the anatomic location (e.g., transverse-sigmoid DAVM, cavernous DAVM, and sagittal sinus DAVM). These approaches lacked meaningful information with regard to predicting the nature or outcome of the abnormality or treatment options. Subsequent systems incorporated information from diagnostic angiography (Table 65-1).[34-36]

Perhaps one of the most well-recognized classification schemes specific to DAVMs is that developed by Djindjian et al.[34] This system classifies a lesion as one of four types. Type I DAVMs are characterized by normal antegrade drainage into a venous sinus or meningeal vein; type II lesions drain into a sinus, with reflux into adjacent sinuses or cortical veins; type III DAVMs drain directly into cortical veins with resultant retrograde flow into the cerebral venous compartment; and type IV DAVMs have drainage directly into a venous pouch (venous lake or venous ectasia).

Djindjian et al[34] concluded that type I DAVMs are benign and that types II through IV have gradually more aggressive characteristics. Since the introduction of the Djindjian classification of DAVMs, other studies have been published in which investigators have attempted to correlate certain features of a DAVM with the likelihood of associated hemorrhage or other specific neurologic complications.[9,12,15,37]

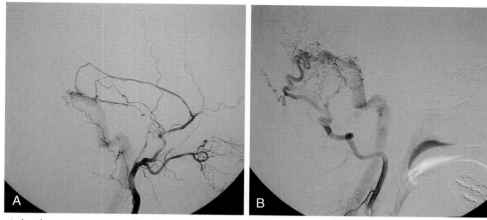

Figure 65-2 Type I dural arteriovenous malformation in a 35-year-old woman with a new-onset bruit behind the right ear. The patient had experienced head trauma requiring hospitalization 13 years before. A, Selective injection of right occipital artery (lateral view). There is arteriovenous shunting via numerous small fistulas from distal arterial branches to the transverse sinus. Venous flow remains antegrade, making this a "benign" lesion. B, Selective right external trunk injection (lateral view) showing additional fistulas from middle meningeal and posterior auricular arteries.

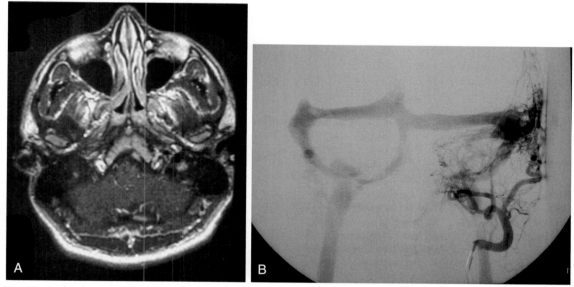

Figure 65-3 Type II dural arteriovenous malformation in a 22-year-old man with a new onset of seizures and no history of head trauma. A, Postcontrast enhancement, T1-weighted axial magnetic resonance image demonstrates increased vascularity along the posteroinferior aspect of the cerebellum. B, Left external carotid injection (frontal view). There is prompt venous opacification during the arterial phase, as well as retrograde filling of the contralateral sinus across the midline. Contribution is primarily from middle meningeal and posterior auricular branches.

With the advent of more effective endovascular therapeutic techniques, a means of predicting lesion risk and management options emerged. Cognard et al[35] developed a classification system derived from a modified version of that published by Djindjian's group, defining five types of DAVMs that are based exclusively on the pattern of venous outflow. Type I DAVMs are characterized by normal antegrade flow into the affected dural sinus (Fig. 65-2). Type II lesions are associated with an abnormal direction of venous drainage within the affected dural sinus (Fig. 65-3). The investigators further categorize type II lesions into three subtypes: type IIa, lesions with retrograde flow exclusively into the sinus or sinuses; type IIb,

lesions with retrograde venous drainage into the cortical veins only; and type IIa+b, lesions with retrograde drainage into both the sinuses and the cortical veins. Type III DAVMs drain directly into a cortical vein or veins without venous ectasia (Fig. 65-4), whereas type IV DAVMs drain into cortical veins with venous ectasia that is greater than 5 mm in diameter and three times larger than the diameter of the draining vein (Fig. 65-5). A type V DAVM drains into spinal perimedullary veins (Fig. 65-6). Correlation with the clinical data of Cognard et al[35] yielded the following conclusions: type I DAVMs are considered benign, and treatment is usually not necessary, except possibly for palliation of symptoms; type IIa lesions are

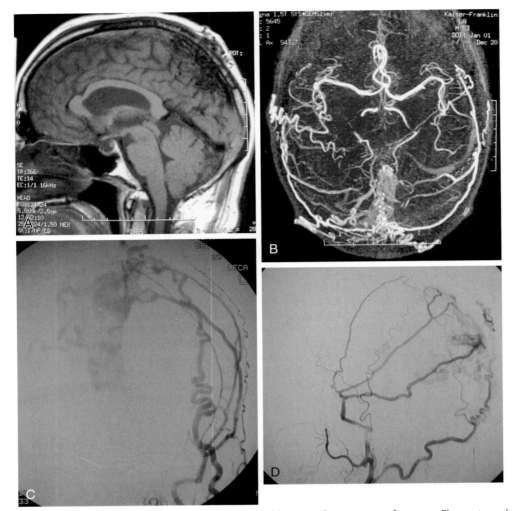

Figure 65-4 Type III dural arteriovenous malformation in a 54-year-old man with new onset of seizure. The patient also noticed a pulsatile mass on his scalp. A, Sagittal T1-weighted, noncontrast magnetic resonance image demonstrates prominent flow voids in the parietal occipital area representing dilated cortical veins. B, Collapsed-view magnetic resonance angiography. Innumerable branches of the external carotid arteries (bilateral) converge near the midline adjacent to the sagittal sinus. Left external frontal (C) and oblique (D) carotid injections. Arteriovenous shunting is noted, with prominent cortical veins to the right of midline and early opacification of the right transverse sinus. Contribution is from superficial temporal, middle meningeal, and occipital arteries.

best treated with arterial embolization; type IIb and type IIa+b lesions usually require both transarterial and transvenous embolization for effective obliteration. For type III through V lesions, transarterial and, occasionally, transvenous embolization aimed at complete occlusion of the fistula is necessary and usually must be combined with surgical techniques to eliminate the dangerous cortical venous drainage.

Borden et al[36] have also proposed a classification system emphasizing venous anatomy. This system is appealing in its simplicity and has only three categories. Type I DAVMs drain directly into dural venous sinuses or pachymeningeal veins. Type II lesions drain into dural sinuses or pachymeningeal veins but also have retrograde drainage into subarachnoid (leptomeningeal) veins. Type III DAVMs drain solely into subarachnoid (leptomeningeal) veins and do not have dural sinus or meningeal venous drainage. The validity of both the Cognard and Borden classification systems was confirmed by examination of 102 intracranial DAVMs in 98 patients.[37]

Indications for Treatment

The Borden classification and others emphasize that the primary determinant of a DAVM's prospective aggressive neurologic course is the presence or absence of leptomeningeal venous drainage. This sole feature also primarily determines whether therapeutic interventions, with their associated risks, are justified for these lesions. Because the clinical presentation and natural history of DAVMs are highly variable, treatment should be individualized on the basis of many factors, including patient age and comorbidities, severity of clinical symptoms, predicted risk of rupture, and risk of potential treatment options. In many cases, an expectant approach may be the best option. In other cases, the goal of treatment is most appropriately palliative, often with a goal of limited or partial treatment. Definitive treatment with its associated risks is usually indicated in lesions that have manifested with intracranial hemorrhage or those considered to be high-risk, that is, DAVMs with leptomeningeal venous drainage

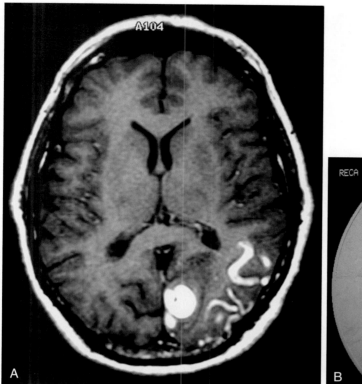

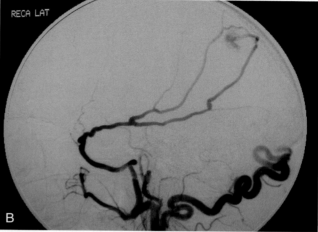

Figure 65-5 Type IV dural arteriovenous malformation in a 57-year-old man whose family noticed personality changes. The patient described intermittent visual changes. A, Axial T1-weighted magnetic resonance image shows prominent cortical veins. High signal represents slow flow status. Note venous varix (pouch) posteriorly, adjacent to the falx. Right external carotid injection, early (B) and late arterial phase. Markedly dilated middle meningeal and occipital arteries. There is early venous opacification with dilated venous varix.

or variceal or aneurysmal changes in the venous circulation. In a study by Van Dijk et al,[38] patients with these high-risk lesions (Borden types II and III) given either no treatment or only partial treatment so that persisting cortical venous involvement persisted had a 10% annual mortality rate and significant additional morbidity.

Treatment Options

Many patients with nonaggressive DAVMs are best treated with only palliation of symptoms, which may consist of reassurance and counseling, biofeedback, and, possibly, jugular massage.[39] The last procedure should be used with caution in the elderly, who might have coexisting carotid disease or may be vulnerable to vasovagal syncope. Patients with dull aching pain or bothersome pulsatile tinnitus may benefit from nonsteroidal anti-inflammatory agents. Carbamazepine may be given for tic-like pain, and short courses of corticosteroids may be particularly effective for retroorbital discomfort. Patients with DAVMs and tic douloureux should not be treated by percutaneous methods involving puncture of the foramen ovale, which might lead to catastrophic hemorrhaging. Once it is decided that a patient with a particular DAVM will benefit from intervention, careful consideration of the available options is required. They include surgery, endovascular treatment, radiosurgery, or a combination of these approaches.

Surgical Technique

The goals of surgical treatment of DAVMs are (1) physical interruption or obliteration of arterialized leptomeningeal venous connections and (2) maximal coagulation or excision of the diseased dura. There is a continuous risk for significant blood loss, particularly early in the procedure, when incomplete surgical exposure may be accompanied by significant bleeding. Beginning with skin infiltration and incision, the operation should proceed a step at a time, and hemostatic control should be achieved before the next step is taken. This approach is indeed more speedy, more efficient, and safer than a faster procedure, which might require the surgeon to spend time controlling brisk bleeding from many sources. As a rule, no incision should be made unless the surgeon is prepared to control catastrophic bleeding from it. A thorough review of preoperative angiography and judicious use of preoperative embolization help limit the risk of bleeding. Continuous communication with the anesthesia team is critical.

Meticulous attention to hemostasis and microsurgical technique throughout the procedure is imperative.[40] After the abnormal dura is identified, its resection is aided by the use of irrigating bipolar cautery forceps. The placement of small permanent vascular clips in tandem alternated with dural transection may be useful. Using aneurysm clips to temporarily occlude variceal veins is

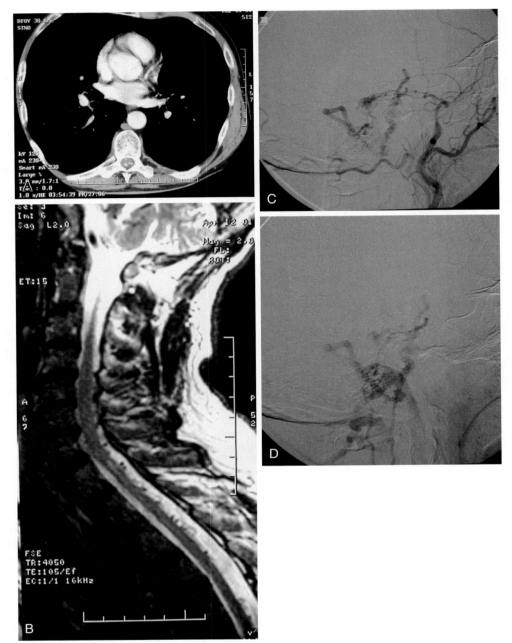

Figure 65-6 Type V dural arteriovenous malformation in a 59-year-old woman with multisystem disease including chronic obstructive pulmonary disease. She had unexplained, progressive difficulty with ambulation. Computed tomography (CT) scanning of the chest was obtained for pulmonary evaluation. A, Postcontrast enhancement CT scan of the chest, axial view. Note the abnormal vascular enhancement within the spinal canal. B, Sagittal T2-weighted magnetic resonance image of the cervical spine. Prominent flow voids are seen dorsal to the spinal cord. These represent prominent venous channels. Left external carotid injection (lateral view), early (C) and delayed (D) images. There is early opacification of venous outflow toward spinal perimedullary veins.

helpful in determining which veins should be coagulated and sectioned because occlusion of some veins may significantly affect adjacent cortical venous circulation. It is sometimes possible to identify discrete arteriovenous connections whose occlusion significantly decreases surrounding subarachnoid venous engorgement.

Direct puncture of large varices with intraoperative placement of obliterating coils has been successful.[41] Both a combination of coils and glue after access has been obtained by craniectomy and direct sinus puncture have also been reported.[42] Resection of the dural sinus can be

accomplished without the risk of venous infarction if the resected segment is arterialized and collateral channels are well developed.[43] In some cases, surgical clipping of the draining vein close to the DAVM, with extensive dural coagulation rather than resection, may be preferred.[44] Presigmoid skull base exposures have also been employed, specifically for access to petrosal and sigmoid lesions.[45] Image-guided frameless navigation is useful for flap design and localization of DAVMs or associated cortical venous drainage. Intraoperative angiography helps ensure complete resection in difficult cases.

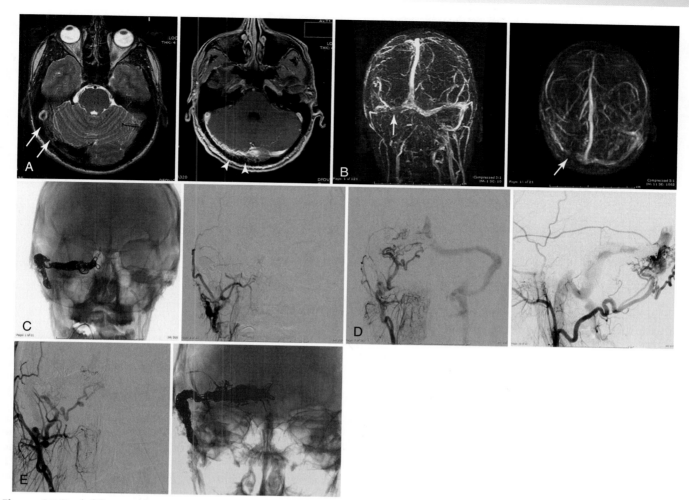

Figure 65-7 A 29-year-old woman presented with progressive headaches and visual difficulty. A, Axial T2 *(left)* shows abnormal flow void in right transverse and sigmoid sinus *(straight arrows)*. Postcontrast T1 *(right)* shows abnormal enhancement along margin of right transverse sinus *(arrowheads)* indicating site of fistulous connections. B, Magnetic resonance venogram (MRV) shows lack of normal flow signal in right transverse sinus, and prominent vascular adjacent to sinus *(arrows)*. C, Transvenous approach for treatment. Conventional coil packing of right transverse/sigmoid sinus with platinum coils *(left)*. External carotid angiogram *(right)* confirms obliteration of shunting. D, Follow-up angiogram at 6 months reveals recurrent fistulas with brisk arterial supply from right occipital artery (selective right external injection). E, Right external carotid angiogram after transarterial embolization of occipital artery with Onyx *(left)*. Spot film *(right)* reveals density of coils in transverse/sigmoid sinus and Onyx within arterial feeders from occipital artery.

Endovascular Treatment

Transarterial embolization has been widely used in the treatment of DAVMs.[1,46,47] The use of flow-guided catheter technology and greater experience with particle and glue embolization as well as detachable coils have greatly improved the safety and efficacy of this method.[48] However, transarterial embolization rarely succeeds in totally eliminating and curing a DAVM, except in rare instances of limited fistulas with a small number of accessible feeding vessels. More commonly, DAVMs involve a multitude of feeders, which often arise as small twigs from major cerebral arteries that are not amenable to embolization. Transarterial embolization may obliterate the filling of the lesion after one injection, but the DAVM often continues to draw feeders from other sources and reappears on subsequent angiography, possibly in a more ominous configuration. DAVMs that are partially treated with transarterial embolization may later recur and progress to catastrophic hemorrhage. More recently, the introduction of ethylene vinyl alcohol copolymer (Onyx-18) has improved the efficacy of DAVM embolization[49,50] (Fig. 65-7). In some cases, an angiographic cure appears possible, although long-term confirmatory follow-up is required.

Transarterial embolization may be effective in palliation of disabling symptoms even when it does not totally "cure" the DAVM. Such a lesion should be monitored as discussed previously. Transarterial embolization also plays an important role in reducing flow through DAVMs before surgical intervention, transvenous obliteration, or radiosurgery.[51-55] This adjunctive, preparatory use of transarterial embolization has greatly enhanced the safety and efficacy of other, more definitive treatment measures.

Symptom palliation may also be accomplished with transarterial embolization of external carotid artery feeders to the DAVM, although such an intervention is not without risk and rarely succeeds in totally eliminating

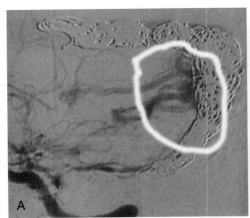 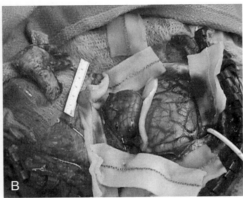

Figure 65-8 Surgical treatment of recurrent dural arteriovenous malformation (DAVM). A, Angiogram of a 17-year-old boy whose symptoms recurred 2 months after endovascular treatment of a DAVM shows reconstitution of arteriovenous channels within the walls of the previously occluded sinus *(white circle)*. B, Surgical excision of the segment of occluded sinus with disconnection of associated arterialized leptomeningeal veins resulted in a cure.

the lesion. Arterial embolization may give a false sense of security that the lesion was "treated," and the DAVM may progress to acquire more aggressive features, including leptomeningeal venous drainage (even in the absence of recurrent symptoms). DAVMs that are observed expectantly or treated palliatively should be monitored closely by means of serial diagnostic studies for the development of leptomeningeal venous drainage, which may occur without a change in clinical symptoms. Noninvasive imaging methods, including CTA, MRI, and MRA, may be used for interval studies, although these modalities may miss the subtle development of leptomeningeal venous drainage, which may be clinically catastrophic. Depending on the clinical situation and the particular lesion, serial MRI may be performed on a yearly basis, and formal angiography may be performed every few years or sooner if symptoms change or if MRI findings suggest new leptomeningeal venous drainage.

Transvenous endovascular obliteration of DAVMs has been used with good results.[54-56] This modality aims at the thrombosis of the venous side of the lesion, often including obliteration of the adjacent dural venous sinus. Occlusion of the venous side of DAVMs is usually well tolerated if the diseased dural sinus is arterialized and does not serve as a site of drainage of cerebrovenous circulation. The diseased dural segment is often associated with harmful retrograde leptomeningeal venous drainage, but these channels are secondarily obliterated with thrombosis of the venous side of DAVMs. This strategy has been used most successfully for the treatment of DAVMs with accessible venous drainage. Transvenous obliteration is particularly effective in the treatment of cavernous sinus DAVMs (access through the inferior petrosal sinus), although these lesions frequently do not require any therapeutic intervention because of their benign clinical symptomatology and tendency for spontaneous regression.

Transvenous obliteration has also been used in cases of transverse-sigmoid sinus DAVMs and may be substantially safer than open surgical approaches to these lesions. However, there may be no accessible transvenous route for many DAVMs, including tentorial incisura DAVMs and anterior cranial fossa DAVMs, which commonly behave

aggressively. Transvenous obliteration may occasionally be performed after open surgical exposure, through puncture of the dural venous sinus or the arterialized venous varix, and the injection of coils or glue.[41] Rarely, transvenous occlusion may result in propagating venous thrombosis or altered hemodynamic patterns with paradoxic clinical deterioration or hemorrhage. Occasionally, a DAVM recurs adjacent to an endovascularly occluded venous sinus; such a development could represent reconstitution of arteriovenous channels within the walls of the occluded sinus or in the organized thrombus within the sinus channel. These cases are amenable to surgical excision of the segment of occluded sinus and disconnection of associated arterialized leptomeningeal veins (Fig. 65-8).

Radiosurgical Treatment

The goal of radiosurgical treatment is sclerosis and obliteration of arteriovenous connections within the diseased dura, which results in secondary thrombosis of the DAVM. Advantages include the noninvasiveness of the treatment, which avoids risks associated with invasive procedures. Disadvantages are a delayed response to treatment and a risk of radiation injury to normal structures in the vicinity of the DAVM.

In a study combining radiosurgery with transarterial embolization, 95% of patients showed symptomatic improvement, and in 87% a cure was demonstrated on angiography performed a median of 12 months after radiosurgery.[57] The complication rate with this treatment strategy was acceptable. Radiosurgery alone was effective when the DAVM was not amenable to embolization, but the time needed for symptom improvement was longer. DAVMs of the transverse-sigmoid sinuses treated with a similar strategy yielded a 96% rate of symptom resolution or significant improvement and a total or near-total obliteration at angiography at a mean of 21 months after radiosurgery.[13] There were no intracerebral hemorrhages or radiation-related complications. Although the ideal treatment parameters and ultimate role of radiosurgery continue to evolve, this method has an established role in the multimodality treatment of DAVMs.

Comprehensive Management Strategy

A DAVM may rarely be discovered on routine imaging studies or on angiograms performed for other indications. Incidental lesions must be carefully assessed for features predisposing to aggressive clinical behavior. Complete angiographic evaluation is indicated in every case of suspected DAVM unless the patient is a poor candidate for therapeutic intervention or refuses invasive diagnostic studies. Lesions should be evaluated specifically for the presence of leptomeningeal venous drainage and for any variceal or aneurysmal changes in the venous circulation. In the absence of these features, the lesion should be observed expectantly. There is little evidence to justify prophylactic treatment of DAVMs that are not associated with leptomeningeal venous drainage. Expectant observation of these lesions should include serial MRI studies for any evidence of development of leptomeningeal venous dilations. Angiographic reexamination of the lesion every few years should be considered, especially for DAVMs at the anterior cranial fossa or the tentorial incisura, which very commonly result in leptomeningeal venous drainage.

Definitive prophylactic treatment should be strongly considered for asymptomatic and incidentally discovered DAVMs that have leptomeningeal venous drainage. The patient should be given the option of open surgical intervention or such alternative radiosurgical or endovascular options as may be appropriate for the lesion's type and location. If treatment does not totally eliminate leptomeningeal venous drainage, either further definitive therapy or very close follow-up of the lesion is indicated. We believe that anticoagulation is contraindicated for DAVMs with leptomeningeal venous drainage.

It appears easiest to justify definitive intervention for DAVMs that have already behaved aggressively. Nevertheless, the morbidity of a first hemorrhage with a DAVM is substantial, and many patients do not survive or do not recover to a condition suitable for therapeutic intervention. Furthermore, little is known about the risk of either subsequent hemorrhage or the progression of neurologic deficits in this clinical setting. However, there are numerous documented cases of progression of focal neurologic symptoms resulting in death or major disability unless the DAVM is obliterated. We recommend that lesions that have hemorrhaged or that cause focal neurologic symptoms due to parenchymal venous hypertension be considered for definitive treatment. Palliative therapy is not sufficient in this setting.

Lesions that manifest as pain or pulsatile tinnitus are evaluated and treated in the same way as incidental lesions. Nonspecific measures aimed at the symptoms are usually sufficient. Palliative treatment of the DAVM may be considered for the control of symptoms. Rarely is definitive treatment indicated solely for pain or pulsatile tinnitus. We do not believe that the risk of definitive treatment is justified in such DAVMs because they do not exhibit leptomeningeal venous drainage.

Lesions associated with ophthalmoplegia are evaluated on a case-by-case basis. Painful ophthalmoplegia often resolves spontaneously, and many such lesions involute after being subjected to angiography for evaluation. In other cases, ophthalmoplegia may be progressive or associated with retinopathy and visual loss; in such cases, treatment of the associated DAVM is justified. Palliative treatment may be sufficient to stabilize visual symptoms. As in other settings, a radical cure of a DAVM should not be pursued at any risk and is generally not warranted unless the symptoms are truly debilitating or the DAVM is associated with leptomeningeal venous drainage.

The management of DAVMs associated with papilledema and increased ICP has been discussed previously. In the absence of leptomeningeal venous drainage, the risk of radical treatment of such lesions may not be justified and may or may not achieve subsequent control of intracranial hypertension. Lumboperitoneal shunting or optic nerve sheath decompression may effectively treat the secondary complications of papilledema, and the DAVM can be observed expectantly or treated palliatively or with radiosurgery.

In summary, clinical symptoms other than hemorrhage and neurologic deficits rarely warrant radical treatment of a DAVM, unless the lesion is particularly accessible or is associated with features predisposing to subsequent aggressive clinical behavior. Patient reassurance, treatment of symptoms, or lesion palliation is often sufficient. For DAVMs with features predisposing to an aggressive clinical course, a more definitive treatment strategy should be adopted. It is obvious that the myriad of clinical manifestations of DAVMs and the wide spectrum of possible angiographic and pathophysiologic scenarios call for highly individualized management strategies. Diagnostic investigation should be thorough so that DAVMs with features predisposing to aggressive clinical behavior are identified. Treatment strategies should include a highly individualized choice of modalities from the available armamentarium of symptom treatment, lesion palliation, transarterial or transvenous endovascular therapy, open surgical invention, and radiosurgery. For the foreseeable future, the treatment of DAVMs should preferably be entrusted to multidisciplinary teams with expertise in the recognition and management of these lesions and with experience in a variety of treatment approaches.

Lesions associated with intracranial hypertension and papilledema require special consideration. Palliation or definitive cure of the DAVM frequently (but not always) results in reversal of papilledema and stabilization of visual symptoms. In other instances, the risks of definitive treatment may not be justified. Intracranial hypertension may be treated by lumboperitoneal shunting. Ventriculoperitoneal shunting may not be possible in the patient with small cerebral ventricles and may be dangerous in the setting of arterialized cortical or subependymal veins. Optic nerve sheath decompression has also been used in cases of progressive papilledema and inoperable DAVMs. CSF diversion or optic nerve sheath decompression may be combined with transarterial embolization, radiosurgery, or both in the management of some lesions. Transvenous occlusion is rarely possible in this setting because it may further compromise intracranial venous outflow.

Summary

Much has been learned about the pathoanatomy, pathophysiology, natural history, and therapeutic options for DAVMs. A better understanding of these lesions has allowed more prompt and precise diagnosis as well as a realistic assessment of features predisposing to an aggressive clinical course. Treatment is guided toward not only the palliation of clinical symptoms but also, just as important, prevention of future sequelae. The therapeutic armamentarium consists of a number of options with varying risk and effectiveness for individual lesions. Transarterial embolization, transvenous embolization, surgical therapy, and radiosurgery can be used alone or in various combinations as required for individual clinical scenarios.

REFERENCES

1. Lasjaunias P, Lopez-Ibor L, Abanou A, et al: Radiological anatomy of the vascularization of cranial dural arteriovenous malformations, *Anat Clin* 6:87-99, 1984.
2. Awad IA, Barrow DL, editors: *Dural arteriovenous malformations*, Park Ridge, IL, 1993, American Association of Neurological Surgeons, pp xi-xii.
3. Lasjaunias P, Berenstein A, editors: *Surgical neuroangiography II: Endovascular treatment of craniofacial lesions*, New York, 1987, Springer-Verlag.
4. Aminoff MJ, Kendall BE: Asymptomatic dural vascular anomalies, *Br J Radiol* 46:662-667, 1973.
5. Fermand M, Reizine D, Melki JP, et al: Long-term follow-up of 43 pure dural arteriovenous fistulas (AVF) of the lateral sinus, *Neuroradiology* 29:348-353, 1987.
6. Gelwan MJ, Choi IS, Berenstein A, et al: Dural arteriovenous malformations and papilledema, *Neurosurgery* 22:1079-1084, 1988.
7. Chimowitz MI, Little JR, Awad IA, et al: Intracranial hypertension associated with unruptured cerebral arteriovenous malformations, *Ann Neurol* 27:474-479, 1990.
8. Hurst RW, Bagley LJ, Galetta S, et al: Dementia resulting from dural arteriovenous fistulas: The pathologic findings of venous hypertensive encephalopathy, *AJNR Am J Neuroradiol* 19:1267-1273, 1998.
9. Malik GM, Pearce JE, Ausman JI, et al: Dural arteriovenous malformations and intracranial hemorrhage, *Neurosurgery* 15:332-339, 1984.
10. Barnwell SL, Malbach VV, Dowd CF, et al: A variant of arteriovenous fistulas within the wall of dural sinuses, *J Neurosurg* 74:199-204, 1991.
11. Bitoh S, Sakaki S: Spontaneous cure of dural arteriovenous malformation in the posterior fossa, *Surg Neurol* 12:111-114, 1979.
12. Lasjaunias P, Chiu M, Bruggs KT, et al: Neurological manifestations of intracranial dural arteriovenous malformations, *J Neurosurg* 64:724-730, 1986.
13. Chardhaury MY, Sachdev VP, Cho SH, et al: Dural arteriovenous malformation of the major venous sinuses: An acquired lesion, *AJNR Am J Neuroradiol* 3:13-19, 1982.
14. Houser OW, Campbell JK, Campbell RJ, et al: Arteriovenous malformation affecting the transverse dural venous sinus: An acquired lesion, *Mayo Clin Proc* 54:651-661, 1979.
15. Awad IA, Little JR, Akrawi WP, et al: Intracranial dural arteriovenous malformations: Factors predisposing to an aggressive neurologic course, *J Neurosurg* 72:839-850, 1990.
16. Vinuela F, Fox A, Pelz D, et al: Unusual clinical manifestations of dural arteriovenous malformations, *J Neurosurg* 64:554-558, 1986.
17. Cognard C, Casasco A, Toevi M, et al: Dural arteriovenous fistulas as a cause of intracranial hypertension due to impairment of cranial venous outflow, *J Neurol Neurosurg Psychiatry* 65:308-316, 1998.
18. Kim MS, Oh CW, Han DH, et al: Intraosseous dural arteriovenous fistula of the skull base associated with hearing loss, *J Neurosurg* 96:952-955, 2002.
19. Rizzo M, Bosch EP, Gross CE: Trigeminal sensory neuropathy due to dural external carotid cavernous sinus fistula, *Neurology* 32:89-91, 1982.
20. Willinsky R, Goyal M, terBrugge K, Montanera W: Tortuous, engorged pial veins in intracranial dural arteriovenous fistulas: Correlations with presentation, location, and MR findings in 122 patients, *AJNR Am J Neuroradiol* 20:103-136, 1999.
21. Iwama T, Hashimoto N, Takagi Y, et al: Hemodynamic and metabolic disturbances in patients with intracranial dural arteriovenous fistulas: Positron emission tomography evaluation before and after treatment, *J Neurosurg* 86:806-811, 1997.
22. Ishikawa T, Houkin K, Tokuda K, et al: Development of anterior cranial fossa dural arteriovenous malformation following head trauma: Case report, *J Neurosurg* 86:291-293, 1997.
23. Nabors MW, Azzam CJ, Albanna FJ, et al: Delayed postoperative dural arteriovenous malformations: Report of two cases, *J Neurosurg* 66:768-772, 1987.
24. Yokota M, Tani E, Maeda Y, Yamaura I: Meningioma in sigmoid sinus groove associated with dural arteriovenous malformation: Case report, *Neurosurgery* 33:316-319, 1993.
25. Singh V, Meyers PM, Halbach VV, et al: Dural arteriovenous fistula associated with prothrombin gene mutation, *J Neuroimaging* 11:319-321, 2001.
26. Yassari R, Jahromi B, Macdonald R: Dural arteriovenous fistula after craniotomy for pilocytic astrocytoma in a patient with protein S deficiency, *Surg Neurol* 58:59-64, 2002.
27. Lawton MT, Jacobowitz R, Spetzler RF: Redefined role of angiogenesis in the pathogenesis of dural arteriovenous malformations, *J Neurosurg* 87:267-274, 1997.
28. Magdison MA, Weinberg PE: Spontaneous closure of a dural arteriovenous malformation, *Surg Neurol* 6:107-110, 1976.
29. Hansen JH, Sogaard I: Spontaneous regression of an extra and intracranial arteriovenous malformation: Case report, *J Neurosurg* 45:338-341, 1976.
30. Olutola PS, Eliam M, Molot M, et al: Spontaneous regression of a dural arteriovenous malformation, *Neurosurgery* 12:687-690, 1983.
31. Duffau H, Lopes M, Janosevic V, et al: Early rebleeding from intracranial dural arteriovenous fistulas: Report of 20 cases and review of the literature, *J Neurosurg* 90:78-84, 1999.
32. Hu WY, terBrugge KG: The role of angiography in the evaluation of vascular and neoplastic disease in the external carotid artery circulation, *Neuroimaging Clin N Am* 6:625-644, 1996.
33. Ikawa F, Uozumi T, Kiya K, et al: Diagnosis of carotid-cavernous fistulas with magnetic resonance angiography demonstrating the draining veins utilizing 3-D time-of-flight and 3-D phase contrast techniques, *Neurosurg Rev* 19:7-12, 1996.
34. Djindjian R, Merland JJ, Theron J, editors: *Superselective arteriography of the external carotid artery*, New York, 1977, Springer-Verlag, pp 606-628.
35. Cognard C, Gobin YP, Pierot L, et al: Cerebral dural arteriovenous fistulas: Clinical and angiographic correlation with a revised classification of venous drainage, *Radiology* 194:671-680, 1995.
36. Borden JA, Wu JK, Shucart WA: A proposed classification for spinal and cranial dural arteriovenous fistulous malformations and implications for treatment, *J Neurosurg* 82:166-179, 1995:erratum appears in *J Neurosurg* 82:705-706, 1995.
37. Davies MA, terBrugge K, Willinsky R, et al: The validity of classification for the clinical presentation of intracranial dural arteriovenous fistulas, *J Neurosurg* 85:830-837, 1996.
38. Van Dijk JM, terBrugge KG, Willinsky RA, Wallace MC: Clinical course of cranial dural arteriovenous fistulas with long-term persistent cortical venous reflux, *Stroke* 33:1233-1236, 2002.
39. Halbach VV, Higashida RT, Hieshima GB, et al: Dural fistulas involving the cavernous sinus: Results of treatment in 30 patients, *Radiology* 163:437-442, 1987.
40. Liu JK, Dogan A, Ellegala DB, et al: The role of surgery for high-grade intracranial dural arteriovenous fistulas: Importance of obliteration of venous outflow, *J Neurosurg* 110:913-920, 2009.
41. Endo S, Kuwayama N, Takaku A, et al: Direct packing of the isolated sinus in patients with dural arteriovenous fistulas of the transverse-sigmoid sinus, *J Neurosurg* 88:449-456, 1998.
42. Houdart E, Saint-Maurice JP, Chapot R, et al: Transcranial approach for venous embolization of dural arteriovenous fistulas, *J Neurosurg* 97:280-286, 2002.
43. Sundt TM Jr, Piepgras DG: The surgical approach to arteriovenous malformations of the lateral and sigmoid dural sinuses, *J Neurosurg* 59:32-39, 1983.
44. Hoh BL, Choudhri TF, Connolly ES Jr, et al: Surgical management of high-grade intracranial dural arteriovenous fistulas: Leptomeningeal venous disruption without nidus excision, *Neurosurgery* 42:796-804, 1998.
45. Kattner DO, Roth TC, Giannotta SL: Cranial base approaches for the surgical treatment of aggressive posterior fossa dural arteriovenous fistulae with leptomeningeal drainage: Report of four technical cases, *Neurosurgery* 50:1156-1161, 2002.

46. Hardy RW Jr, Costin JA, Weinstein M, et al: External carotid cavernous fistula treated by transfemoral embolization, *Surg Neurol* 9:255–256, 1978.

47. Vinuela FV, Debrun GM, Fox AJ, et al: Detachable calibrated-leak balloon for superselective angiography and embolization of dural arteriovenous malformations, *J Neurosurg* 58:817–823, 1983.

48. Nesbit GM, Barnwell SL: The use of electrolytically detachable coils in treating high-flow arteriovenous fistulas, *AJNR Am J Neuroradiol* 19:1565–1569, 1998.

49. Toulgoat F, Mounayer C, Túlio Salles Rezende M, et al: Transarterial embolisation of intracranial dural arteriovenous malformations with ethylene vinyl alcohol copolymer (Onyx18), *J Neuroradiol* 33:105–114, 2006.

50. Cognard C, Januel AC, Silva NA, Tall P: Endovascular treatment of intracranial dural arteriovenous fistulas with cortical venous drainage: New management using onyx, *AJNR Am J Neuroradiol* 29:91–97, 2008.

51. Goto K, Sidipratomo P, Ogata N, et al: Combining endovascular and neurosurgical treatments of high-risk dural arteriovenous fistulas in the lateral sinus and the confluence of the sinuses, *J Neurosurg* 90:289–299, 1999.

52. Collice M, D'Aliberti G, Arena O, et al: Surgical treatment of intracranial dural arteriovenous fistulae: Role of venous drainage, *Neurosurgery* 47:56–66, 2000.

53. Friedman JA, Pollock BE, Nichols D, et al: Results of combined stereotactic radiosurgery and transarterial embolization for dural arteriovenous fistulas of the transverse and sigmoid sinuses, *J Neurosurg* 94:886–891, 2001.

54. Halbach VV, Higashida RT, Hieshima GB, et al: Transvenous embolization of dural fistulas involving the cavernous sinus, *AJNR Am J Neuroradiol* 10:377–383, 1989.

55. Roy D, Raymond J: The role of transvenous embolization in the treatment of intracranial dural arteriovenous fistulas, *Neurosurgery* 40:1133–1141, 1997.

56. Lv X, Jiang C, Li Y, et al: Percutaneous transvenous packing of cavernous sinus with Onyx for cavernous dural arteriovenous fistula, *Eur J Radiol* 71:356–362, 2009.

57. Pollock BE, Nichols DA, Garrity JA, et al: Stereotactic radiosurgery and particulate embolization for cavernous sinus dural arteriovenous fistulae, *Neurosurgery* 45:459–466, 1999.

66 Genetics of Aneurysms and Arteriovenous Malformations

YNTE RUIGROK, CATHARINA J.M. KLIJN

Subarachnoid hemorrhage (SAH) from rupture of an intracranial aneurysm (IA) has a poor prognosis. The case-fatality rate for aneurysmal SAH is around 50%, and another 20% of patients remain dependent in activities of daily living.[1] The incidence of SAH increases with age, but half the patients are younger than 55 years at the time of the SAH.[2] Because of the young age at which SAH occurs and the poor prognosis, the loss of productive life years from SAH in the population is as large as that from ischemic stroke.[3] Risk factors for aneurysmal SAH include smoking, hypertension, and excessive use of alcohol.[4] Besides these acquired risk factors, female sex and familial occurrence are the strongest risk factors for aneurysmal SAH. A higher concordance among relatives has been demonstrated, with first-degree relatives of patients with SAH having a 2.5 to 7 times greater risk for development of SAH than the general population.[5-10] Although it is known that the risk of having an aneurysm is the highest for siblings of patients with SAH,[11] not much is known about the exact relative risk for these siblings (sibs). For the calculation of the sib relative risk (λ_s), which is a commonly used measure to indicate the genetic influence for a disease, this relative risk for these siblings is needed. One screening study identified intracranial aneurysms in 6% of the siblings of patients with SAH.[11] On the basis of this percentage (6%) and a population prevalence of 2%,[12] the estimated sib relative risk (λ_s) for development of intracranial aneurysms is 3. Therefore, for intracranial aneurysms, a genetic influence was suggested, and genetic studies have been undertaken to search for the genetic factors underlying the disease.

The development of intracranial aneurysms and aneurysmal SAH is a complex disease resulting from an interaction between genetic variants and environmental or nongenetic disease risk factors.[13] Because of the multifactorial nature of the disease, each genetic variant generally has only a modest effect, and the interaction of genetic variants with each other (gene-gene interactions) or with environmental factors (gene-environment interactions) may contribute to the observed phenotype.[13] Detailed genetic analyses for genes associated with intracranial aneurysm are described later in this chapter.

Associated Heritable Disorders

Ehlers-Danlos syndrome. Ehlers-Danlos syndrome (EDS) describes a group of heterogeneous disorders with various connective tissue disorders. The most common symptoms are skin abnormalities, joint hypermobility, spontaneous rupture of arteries, and easy bruising.[14] Of the nine recognized types, EDS type IV, also called the vascular type, is one of the more severe types[15] and has been associated with IA formation. The most common neurovascular manifestations are the carotid-cavernous fistulas in EDS type IV,[16] but IAs in patients with Ehlers-Danlos type IV have also been described. The aneurysms are characteristically located at the internal carotid artery and may be saccular or fusiform.[17-19] EDS type IV is caused by an abnormality of type III collagen, and various mutations in this gene have been described thus far.[20] For patients with IAs, molecular analysis of the type III collagen gene has been performed in two studies, and no mutations could be demonstrated.[21,22]

Marfan's syndrome. Marfan's syndrome is an autosomal dominant disorder that affects the cardiac, vascular, ocular, and skeletal systems.[23] It is characterized by diverse clinical symptoms but characteristically patients have a tall stature, joint hypermobility, pectus carinatum or excavatum, scoliosis or spondylolisthesis, and typical facial appearances such as dolichocephaly, retrognathia, enophthalmos, and malar hypoplasia.[23] In classic Marfan's syndrome the disease is caused by mutations in the fibrillin-1 gene, which is located on chromosome 15q21.1.[24] In 2004, *TGFBR2* at chromosome 3p24.1 was newly identified as the cause of the Marfan's syndrome type II.[24] Like the IAs in patients with Ehlers-Danlos type IV, the IAs diagnosed in patients with Marfan's syndrome are often located at the internal carotid artery.[25-27] However, the association of Marfan's syndrome with IA is under debate.[28,29]

Pseudoxanthoma elasticum. Pseudoxanthoma elasticum (PXE), a prototype of heritable multisystem disorders, is characterized by pathologic mineralization of connective tissues, with primary clinical manifestations in the skin, eyes, and cardiovascular system. The causative gene was identified as *ABCC6*, which encodes an

ABC transporter protein (ABCC6).[30] In a longitudinal study of 94 patients with PXE (mean follow-up, 17.1 years; range 1-49 years), none presented with a symptomatic IA, and on the basis of these data, an association between IAs and PXE was considered unlikely.[31]

Autosomal dominant polycystic kidney disease. Autosomal dominant polycystic kidney disease (ADPKD) is characterized by the development of renal cysts, but cysts of the liver, spleen, pancreas, and seminal vesicles may also be found.[32] In 85% of families with ADPKD, the disease is caused by a mutation in the polycystic kidney disease 1 (*PKD1*) gene, located on chromosome 16p13.3.[33] In most of the remaining 15% of families with ADPKD, the cause is a mutation of the *PKD2* gene, situated on chromosome 4q31-23.[33] The prevalence for ADPKD in the general population is 1 per 1000.[34] Many patients with ADPKD and IA have been described,[35,36] and the estimated relative risk of IA in patients with ADPKD is 4.4 (95% confidence interval [CI], 2.7-7.2).[37] IAs arise in about 10% of patients with ADPKD[38] but account for less than 1% of patients with SAH.[38,39] Screening for IA in patients with ADPKD is recommended.[40]

Arteriovenous Malformations of the Brain

Arteriovenous malformations of the brain (BAVMs) are vascular lesions consisting of abnormal direct connections between the arterial and venous systems.[41,42] These direct connections form a vascular mass, called the nidus, and consist of a complex tangle of abnormal, dilated blood vessels that are neither arteries nor veins. The reported point prevalence of BAVMs varies between 15 and 18 per 100,000 adults,[43] with a detection rate of approximately 1 per 100,000 adults per year.[44,45] Asymptomatic BAVMs may have a prevalence of up to 0.1%.[46]

BAVM is a rare cause of stroke in general, accounting for only 1% to 2% of strokes. BAVMs are the cause of only a minority of SAHs and of 4% of primary intracerebral hemorrhages (ICHs). BAVMs are responsible for one third of spontaneous nontraumatic ICHs in young adults. Because BAVMs are most often found in young adults and manifest as ICH in up to 65% of patients, the loss of productive life-years as a result of a BAVM is considerable.[47] Twenty percent of patients with a BAVM present with seizures, and in 15%, the BAVM is an incidental finding. Headache and focal neurologic deficits without ICH are relatively rare.[48] All patients with BAVM have a lifelong risk of ICH with potentially devastating consequences.

The pathogenesis of BAVMs is unknown, but they have long been assumed to be congenital or developmental anomalies.[49] Some investigators have argued that BAVMs are the result of a persistent primitive arteriovenous connection, whereas others have suggested development of such a connection before or after birth.[42,50] Although the increasing application of prenatal ultrasonography and MRI has revealed vein of Galen malformations, there are no reports on the finding of an AVM in utero. If indeed BAVMs develop after birth, it is unclear at what time they are most likely to do so. Most BAVMs are detected in young adults, but they can also be found in children. Growth or spontaneous regression of BAVMs has been described but is very rare.[51,52]

There is a growing body of evidence that genetic factors may play a role in BAVMs and that like IA, BAVM is a complex disease. However, the risk of a BAVM in first-degree relatives of a patient with a BAVM is likely to be much smaller than for IAs. Screening of relatives of patients with BAVM by imaging of the brain has not been reported, but familial clustering of supposedly "sporadic" BAVMs has been described in 53 patients from 25 different families.[53] Further evidence of a genetic contribution to the pathogenesis of BAVMs includes the occurrence of BAVMs in hereditary hemorrhagic telangiectasia (HHT)[54] and hereditary neurocutaneous angiomatous malformations.[55] Twin studies of patients with "sporadic" BAVM have not been reported. Environmental factors influencing the development of BAVMs have not yet been identified.

Associated Heritable Disorders

Hereditary hemorrhagic telangiectasia. HHT is an autosomal dominant disorder characterized by mucocutaneous telangiectasias and AVMs in the lung, the liver, the gastrointestinal tract, and the brain. In 93% of patients a mutation is found in one of two genes. Mutations in the *endoglin* (*ENG*) gene on chromosome 9 lead to HHT1, and mutations in the *activin receptor–like kinase 1* (*ACVRL1* or *ALK1*) gene on chromosome 12 to HHT2.[54] Three more genes have been implicated in HHT[56,57]: an unidentified HHT3 gene linked to chromosome 5q,[57] the *MADH4* families with a combined syndrome of juvenile polyposis and HHT,[56] and another unidentified gene linked to chromosome 7p.[58] Vascular malformations occur in 9% to 21% of patients with HHT1 and rarely in patients with HHT2.[54,59,60] In addition to nidus-type BAVMs, spinal cord arteriovenous fistulas, cerebral arteriovenous fistulas, and micro-AVMs can be found.[61]

Hereditary neurocutaneous angiomatosis. The combination of hemangiomas, AVMs of the skin and brain, and venous malformations in the brain has been described in several families.[55] Autosomal dominant inheritance with variable penetrance has been suggested, but the gene responsible for this disorder has not yet been identified.

Genetic Studies

For the identification of genetic factors responsible for a complex disease such as IAs and AVMs, different approaches can be used. Here we briefly discuss the most widely used approaches.

Linkage Studies

Linkage studies analyze whether cosegregation of a disease phenotype with DNA markers of known location, located throughout the genome, occurs in diseased families. Results of a linkage analysis are expressed in a logarithm of odds (LOD) score. Kruglyak and Lander[62] defined "suggestive evidence for linkage" as a logarithm of odds score greater than 2.2 and "significant evidence for linkage" as a logarithm of odds score greater than 3.6. Linkage of the disease phenotype (and thus the disease-causing gene) with a specific DNA marker means that the marker and the disease-related gene are located in close proximity to each other on the DNA. Linkage studies will identify so-called loci where the disease-related gene is located. Thus, a genome-wide linkage study points only toward the regions in the genome that contain the disease-causing genes and not to these genes themselves.[63] Such chromosomal regions often contain hundreds of genes, many of which may be plausible candidate genes for the disease. Additional studies are needed to identify the disease-causing gene from such a region.[63] One of the most commonly used additional studies is an association study to test genetic variants in candidate genes of the chromosomal region (i.e., positional candidate gene).[13]

Association Studies Using Candidate Genes

Not only are association studies used as a complement to linkage studies, but they can also be performed as independent studies using candidate genes suspected of being involved in the disease on the basis of their function (i.e., functional candidate gene). These studies analyze the association between the disease and genetic variants within the functional candidate gene by comparing patients and controls. The genetic variants most often comprise markers called single nucleotide polymorphisms (SNPs), with an estimated 10 million common SNPs present in the human genome. A disadvantage of this hypothesis-based approach is that genes involved in the pathogenesis of a disease through unknown pathways are overlooked.

Genome-Wide Association Studies

To overcome the drawback just described, genes involved in the development of a disease may be detected through a hypothesis-free approach by whole genome screening with linkage studies (as described previously) or by genome-wide association studies. Genome-wide association studies are made possible by progress such as completion of the International Haplotype Map (HapMap) project and the development of high-throughput, high-density genotyping technology. In this approach, nearly all common variations in the genome (i.e., the 10 million common SNPs) can be screened for association with a disease by investigation of differences in the frequencies of specific alleles between patients and controls.[64]

In addition to variation at the SNP level, genomic copy-number variants (CNVs) are another important source of genetic variation.[65] Copy-number variation is caused by chromosomal rearrangements that result in the loss (deletion) or gain (duplication) of stretches of DNA sequence. CNVs influence gene expression, phenotypic variation, and adaptation by altering gene dosage and can therefore cause a disease.[66] The possible association of CNV markers with the risk of a disease can be analyzed.

Genome-Wide Gene Expression Studies

Another way to identify previously unrecognized associations between genes and a disease is with gene expression studies. Genomic studies can provide important information to understand molecular functions and biologic processes and to characterize unrecognized pathophysiologic pathways. For genomic studies, oligonucleotide microarray technology is frequently utilized to measure genome-wide messenger RNA (mRNA) expression and its changes for diverse biologic samples among diseases.[67] In these studies, the expression of genes in patients' tissue or blood can be studied by analyzing mRNA levels of all genes and comparing their levels with those of normal controls. A disadvantage of the gene expression approach is that besides the primary specific pathophysiologic and genetic factors underlying the disease, secondary molecular factors will also be detected. Discrimination between these factors is not possible.

Genetic Studies of Intracranial Aneurysms

Linkage Studies

Several linkage analyses have been conducted for intracranial aneurysms. A total of nine suggestive linkage regions have been identified to date: chromosomes 1p34.3-p36.13, 5p15.2-p14.3, 5q22-q31, 7q11.2-q22.1, 11q24-q25, 14q23-q31, 17cen, 19q12-q13, and Xp22 (Table 66-1).[68-76] A genome-wide linkage study in the Japanese population analyzing 104 affected sib pairs found three loci with suggestive linkage for intracranial aneurysms on chromosomes 5q22-q31, 14q22, and 7q11. The 7q11.2 is also known as the intracranial berry aneurysm-1 (*ANIB1*) locus in the Online Mendelian Inheritance in Man database.[68] In a study on 13 families with intracranial aneurysms from Utah, linkage to 7q11 was confirmed.[70] In a study in 48 Finish affected relative pairs (i.e., pairs with affected family members other than siblings), linkage was shown to chromosome 19q13.3.[69] In a follow-up study analyzing another 139 affected Finnish sib pairs, along with 83 other affected relative pairs, these results were confirmed.[77] The region at chromosome 19q13.3 that spans 6.6 cM, was designated the *ANIB2* locus. Linkage to this region was also confirmed in two studies from Japan analyzing families with intracranial aneurysms.[71,75] One of these studies analyzing 29 Japanese families revealed linkage not only to 19q13 but also to two additional chromosomal regions on chromosomes 17cen and Xp22.[71]

Four genome-wide linkage studies were performed in single large pedigrees. In a Northern American family with aneurysms segregating as a dominant trait, linkage was found to a locus on chromosome 1p34.3-p36.13, known as the *ANIB3* locus.[72] A Dutch consanguineous family was used to map a susceptibility locus for intracranial aneurysms to chromosome 2p13,[78] but it was subsequently reported that the locus was an artifact because aneurysms developed in some individuals after completion of the study.[76] A follow-up study on this family then showed significant linkage to a locus on chromosome 1p36.11-p36.13 and Xp22.2-p22.32.[76] The locus on chromosome 1 overlaps the 1p34.3-p36.13 locus demonstrated in the Northern American family,[72] whereas evidence for the locus on chromosome X was also found in the 29 Japanese families.[71] In a large Northern American family linkage to chromosome 11q24-25 was shown and analysis of another large Northern American family showed linkage to chromosome 14q23-31.[73] Both loci were also identified in the study analyzing Japanese affected sib pairs, although in this study the threshold levels for "suggestive

TABLE 66-1 IDENTIFIED GENETIC LOCI FOR INTRACRANIAL ANEURYSMS WITH POTENTIAL CANDIDATE GENES FOR WHICH GENETIC ASSOCIATION HAS BEEN DEMONSTRATED*

Genetic Loci	Study Population	Linkage Regions	Potential Candidate Genes within These Loci
1p	Single North American family[72]	1p34.3-p36.13	Perlecan[84]
	Single Dutch family[76]	1p36.11-p36.13	
5p	Single French-Canadian family[74]	5p15.2-14.3	
5q	Japanese sib pairs[68]	5q22-31	Versican[82]
7q	Japanese sib pairs[68]	7q11	Elastin[68,87]
			Collagen type 1 A2[91]
	North American families[70]	7q11	
11q	Single North American family[73]	11q24-25	
14q	Single North American family[73]	14q23-31	Sequence variant rs767603[83]
	Japanese sib pairs[68]	14q23-31	
17 cen	Japanese families[71]	17 cen	TNFRSF13B†[92]
19q	Finnish relative pairs[69]	19q13.3	Kallikrein 8[94]
	Finnish sib pairs and relative pairs[77]	19q13.3	
	Japanese families[71]	19q13	
	Japanese families[75]	19q13.3	
Xp	Single Dutch family[76]	Xp22.2-p22.32	
	Japanese families[71]	Xp22	
	Finnish relative pairs[69]	Xp22	

*Superscript numbers indicate chapter references.
†Transmembrane activator and calcium modulator ligand interactor.

linkage" were not met.[68] Finally, In a large French Canadian family, another susceptibility locus, *ANIB4*, mapping to chromosome 5p15.2-p14.3 was demonstrated.[74]

Association Studies

The results of the association studies of the candidate genes situated in the loci identified by the linkage studies (as previously described) are considered here. The results of association studies in genes that were selected only because of their function and presumed role in the pathogenesis of aneurysms are not reviewed because they have been conflicting or have not been replicated. Most of these studies had small sample sizes, precluding robust results. The results of these studies can be reviewed in three published overviews.[79-81]

A plausible candidate gene in the 1p locus is the perlecan gene, which codes for a heparan sulfate proteoglycan involved in the maintenance of the extracellular matrix of the arterial wall. In a Dutch case-control study analyzing two independent populations, SNPs in the perlecan gene were found associated with intracranial aneurysms ($P = .0005$),[82] further underlining the possible involvement of this gene in the pathogenesis of IAs. In the North American family, other possible candidate genes of the 1p locus, including polycystic kidney disease–like 1, brain-specific angiogenesis inhibitor 2, fibronectin type III domain–containing gene, and collagen type XVI A1, were screened for mutations, but no mutations in these genes segregating on the affected chromosomes could be demonstrated.[81] Also, a study of 29 Japanese patients and 35 controls analyzing SNP markers in the 1p locus showed no association with IAs.[83]

The locus on chromosome 5p15.2-14.3 includes about 25 known genes. Two suggested candidate genes in this locus are catenin delta-2 *(CTNND2)*, which is involved in

neuronal cell adhesion, tissue morphogenesis, and integrity by regulating adhesion molecules and triple functional domain protein.[74] No association studies of these candidate genes have been performed thus far.

The versican gene is an interesting candidate gene located in the vicinity of the locus on 5q22-31, because versican plays an important role in the extracellular matrix. SNPs in strong linkage disequilibrium in the versican gene were found to be associated with aneurysms in the Dutch population ($P = .0006$).[82,84] The linkage region on 5q22-31 also includes several other potential candidate genes, for example, fibroblast growth factor 1, lysyl oxidase, and fibrillin-2. SNPs in these genes were analyzed in 172 Japanese patients with aneurysms and 192 controls, but no associations between these SNPs and aneurysms were observed.[85] Also in two other studies, one with 25 German patients with familial IA and another with two independent populations totaling 692 Dutch patients with aneurysms and 718 controls, no association of SNPs in the lysyl oxidase gene with aneurysms could be demonstrated.[82,86] Finally, in the previously described study of 29 Japanese patients and 35 controls in which also SNP markers in the 5q locus were analyzed, no association with IAs was shown.[83]

In the study that showed linkage to region 7q11, the marker with the best evidence of linkage was in the vicinity of the elastin gene.[68] This gene codes for elastin, which is an important element of the arterial wall, being responsible for its dilatation and recoil. In a further analysis of the elastin gene, a haplotype between the SNPs at intron 20 and intron 23 was strongly associated with aneurysms ($P = 3.81 \times 10^{-6}$).[68] A follow-up study in Japan on the 7q11 locus showed a susceptibility locus covering part of the elastin gene and the entire region of the LIM domain kinase 1 gene, which is positioned close to elastin.[87] An association analysis in 404 patients and 458 controls showed an at-risk haplotype including two functional SNPs, the elastin 3′-UTR (+502) A insertion and the LIM domain kinase 1 promoter C(−187)T SNP.[87] Further analyses demonstrated that both these SNPs are associated with a decrease in transcript levels.[87] In contrast to these findings in Japanese populations, in the Utah population (in which linkage to 7q11 had been confirmed),[70] no mutation in the elastin gene was found segregating in the pedigrees in which linkage was found.[88]

In two German studies comparing 120 patients with IAs and 172 controls,[89] or 205 patients with 235 controls,[90] no allelic association was found with the haplotype associated with IAs in Japanese patients. The differences between the Japanese and European studies may be explained by allelic heterogeneity between Japanese and European populations of patients with aneurysms.

The chromosome region 7q11 also includes the candidate gene collagen type 1 A2. The collagen type 1 fibers together with the collagen type 3 fibers represent up to 90% of the total arterial collagen and are important for the strength of arterial walls. The collagen type 1 A2 gene was analyzed in a Japanese population.[91] Three different SNPs, one of which results in an amino acid substitution, showed significant differences in allelic frequencies between cases and controls, especially the SNP resulting in an amino acid substitution in familial cases ($P = .0009$). This SNP may be a functional variant involved in the development of intracranial aneurysms. However, because the allele frequency of this SNP is low (5.2% in the IA population versus 2.7% in the control population) it may account for only a small proportion of cases. Moreover, this SNP does not seem to play a role in the susceptibility to aneurysms in the Dutch population, because an association of the collagen type 1 A2 gene could not be confirmed in a study from the Netherlands.[82,84] The study of 29 Japanese patients and 35 controls also analyzed SNP markers in the 7q locus, but no association with intracranial aneurysms was shown.[83]

Analysis of SNP markers in the 11q24-25 locus in the study of 29 Japanese patients and 35 controls also showed no association with intracranial aneurysms.[83] In the same study analysis of SNP markers in the 14q23-31 locus showed one variant, rs767603, to be significantly associated with IAs ($P = .00017$). This association was confirmed in the replication cohort of 237 patients and 253 controls ($P = .0046$). Linkage disequilibrium (LD) analysis showed that rs767603 belongs to a large linkage disequilibrium block harboring 13 genes, suggesting that a susceptibility gene might reside within this block. All coding regions of these 13 candidate genes and its flanking regions were sequenced. However, no variants identified through the sequencing were more significantly associated with IAs than rs767603.[83]

Of the 108 genes in the 17cen locus, a selection was screened for mutations in Japanese patients with aneurysms.[92] Mutations were found in *TNFRSF13B*, which codes for the transmembrane activator and calcium modulator ligand interactor, and a haplotype of TNFRSF13B SNPs was found associated with aneurysms ($P = .01$), suggesting that *TNFRSF13B* is a susceptibility gene for aneurysms.[92] No associations were found with the microfibril-associated protein 4 and the inducible nitric oxide synthase genes located in the 17cen locus.[71,82,84,93]

The region on chromosome 19q identified in the Finnish population includes 135 genes, of which 102 have been characterized.[77] One of the genes is apolipoprotein E (*APOE*), but no association of this gene with aneurysms could be demonstrated in two Japanese populations.[71,93] The study of 29 Japanese patients and 35 controls analyzing SNP markers in the 19q locus also showed no association with IAs.[83] The association of SNPs in the kallikrein gene (KLK) cluster with IAs was tested in 266 Finnish patients and 290 Finnish controls.[94] The KLK gene cluster encodes serine proteases known to be involved in a wide range of physiologic processes, including smooth muscle contraction, vascular permeability, cell growth, and tissue remodeling.[95] Two SNPs located in the intronic region of *KLK8* were significantly associated. This association was confirmed in 102 Finnish patients and controls and in 156 Russian patients and 186 controls (combined $P = .0005$), suggesting that the KLK genes are important candidate genes for IAs. The Xp locus contains the angiotensin I-converting enzyme 2 gene, but association with this gene could not be demonstrated in two Japanese studies.[71,93]

Genome-Wide Association Studies

The first genome-wide association study on IAs included Finnish, Dutch, and Japanese cohorts making up over 2100 cases and 8000 controls. Common SNPs on chromosomes 2q, 8q, and 9p showed a significant association with IA, with odds ratios of 1.24 to 1.36.[96] In a follow-up GWAS, additional European case and control cohorts were included and the original Japanese replication cohort was increased, resulting in a cohort of 5891 cases and 14,181 controls.[97] This follow-up study identified three new loci strongly associated with IAs on chromosomes 18q11.2 (odds ratio [OR] = 1.22, $P = 1.1 \times 10^{-12}$, *RBBP8*), 13q13.1 (OR = 1.20, $P = 2.5 \times 10^{-9}$, *KLISTARD13*), and 10q24.32 (OR = 1.29, $P = 1.2 \times 10^{-9}$, *CNNM2*). The prior associations of 8q11.23-q12.1 (OR = 1.28, $P = 1.3 \times 10^{-12}$, *SOX17*) and 9p21.3 (OR = 1.31, $P = 1.5 \times 10^{-22}$, *CDKN2A/CDKN2B*) were replicated.[97] Assuming a fourfold increase in the risk of IA among siblings of cases, the five IA risk loci identified thus far only explain up to 5% of the familial risk of IA.[97]

A second genome-wide association study performed in 497 Japanese patients with ruptured IAs and 497 controls reported not on the SNP analysis but on the CNV analysis instead.[97] In total 597 multiallelic CNV markers for CNV regions in the Japanese population were identified. A case-control association analysis of the identified multiallelic CNV markers with the risk of aneurysmal SAH was performed. One SNP marker (rs1242541) within a CNV region neighboring the Sel-1 suppressor of lin-12-like protein (SEL1L) was significantly associated with a risk of SAH ($P = .0006$).

Genome-Wide Gene Expression Studies

The only whole-genome gene expression study performed thus far included only a small sample of tissue of IAs.[98] The gene expression profiles of tissue samples of six ruptured and four unruptured aneurysms, and four cerebral arteries serving as controls, were analyzed with oligonucleotide microarrays.[98] Analysis of the aneurysmal and control tissues showed 521 differentially expressed genes. Network-based analysis showed evidence for major histocompatibility complex (MHC) class II gene and pathway "antigen presentation" overexpression in aneurysmal tissue. From the results of study, one cannot differentiate whether this overexpression indicates a specific primary pathophysiologic mechanism or a secondary molecular mechanism.

In another gene expression study, gene expression data from tissue of IAs was compared with tissue of non-aneurysmal intracranial arteries.[99] Instead of performing a whole-genome gene expression study, the investigators used a prioritization approach, analyzing the gene expression data of positional candidate genes located in chromosomal loci identified by previous linkage studies. By integrating expression and genetic mapping data, these investigators aimed to identify likely pathways involved in the pathogenesis of IAs. Analysis of the expression profiles showed that the adherens junction, mitogen-activated protein kinase (MAPK), and Notch signaling pathways are likely to play a role in the pathology of IAs.

Genetic Studies of Arteriovenous Malformations of the Brain

Linkage Studies

Genetic studies of BAVM have been hampered by the limited number of families with two or more relatives affected. Review of all reported familial BAVM cases revealed 22 families with two members affected and 3 families with three members with BAVMs.[53] One Japanese group combined linkage and association analyses in a specific community in Japan where clustering of BAVMs has been shown.[100] The genome-wide linkage analysis performed in 12 patients from 6 unrelated families revealed seven candidate regions, but the highest logarithm of odds score at chromosome 6q25 was only 1.88 ($P = .002$). The association studies found four SNPs and two haplotypes associated with BAVM, but none of these were in the regions that were suggested by the linkage study.[100]

Association Studies

Two studies have found an association of an SNP in the *ACVRL1* gene (IVS3-35 A→G polymorphism) with occurrence of sporadic BAVMs, both in a Caucasian population in the United States[101] and in Germany.[102] In the U.S. population, comparison of 177 patients and 129 controls showed that any A (AA or AG) was associated with BAVM with an odds ratio (OR) of 2.47 (95% CI, 1.38-4.44; $P = .002$).[101] In the German study of 101 patients who had a BAVM (94 patients), a dural arteriovenous fistula (DAVF, 3 patients), both (1 patient), or a spinal AVM (3 patients), the IVS3-35A allele was more common than in 202 controls (OR, 1.68; 95% CI, 1.16-2.45; $P = .041$).[102] Results remained essentially unchanged when the patients with dural arteriovenous fistula were excluded. The investigators of the U.S. study commented that the independent replication of the association of the polymorphism in the *ACVRL1* gene in two distinct populations of a disease as rare as BAVM increases the likelihood that the *ACVRL1* gene is truly associated with sporadic BAVM,[103] but confirmation in larger populations is needed. They also suggested that the SNP in the *ACVRL1* gene may have a functional role in BAVM susceptibility, because (1) it is an intronic SNP and intronic SNPs may alter RNA transcription and (2) exons adjacent to the polymorphism code for the extracellular domain of the *ACVRL1* protein and in HHT2 almost half of the mutations are in this part of the gene.[104] Interestingly, patients with HHT2 with a mutation in the *ACVRL1* gene rarely have a BAVM (about 1%), whereas a BAVM is found in approximately 15% of patients with HHT1, who have a mutation in the endoglin (*ENG*) gene.[54] Because of the large variation in phenotype in patients with HHT both within families and between families with mutations in the same gene (*ACVRL1* or *ENG*), it has been suggested that other genes in addition to *ENG* (for HHT1) and *ACVRL1* (for HHT2) may contribute to the phenotype.

Several studies have been performed to assess genetic determinants of behavior of BAVMs, such as the risk of BAVM presentation with ICH[105] and the risk of ICH over time.[106,107] In a study of 180 patients, presentation of BAVM with ICH was associated with a polymorphism in the inflammatory cytokine IL6 gene (*IL6-174GG*), independent of two known predictors of hemorrhagic presentation, small BAVM size and exclusively deep venous drainage.[105] Furthermore, an association was found between specific genotypes of polymorphisms in tumor necrosis factor-α (TNF-alpha-238G→A) and apolipoprotein E (ApoE ε2) and subsequent ICH in a sample of 280 patients with BAVM.[106,108] These genotypes may also play a role in the risk for ICH after initiation of treatment and before complete occlusion is obtained.[107] These results are promising, in that they suggest that in the future, the risk of ICH in an individual patient may be determined from genetic predictors, probably in combination with known angiographic characteristics that predict ICH, but confirmation in larger and different populations is needed.

Genome-Wide Association Studies

To date, genome-wide association studies of BAVM have not been reported.

Genome-Wide Gene Expression Studies

Three studies have assessed gene expression profiles in BAVMs using DNA microarrays.[109-111] In the first study gene expression in four BAVMs and four cerebral cavernous malformations (CCMs) was compared with that in three superficial temporal arteries (STAs), with testing of 12,625 probes. In comparison with CCMs and STAs, 48 genes were upregulated and 59 downregulated in BAVMs.[109] In the second study, gene expression patterns were compared between BAVMs (mainly nidus, 6 patients) and controls (normal brain cortex from 5 patients who underwent surgery because of epilepsy).[110] Of 12,625 probes tested, 1781 showed differential expression in BAVM samples and controls, including genes known to be involved in angiogenesis, the vascular matrix, and apoptosis. Interestingly, the researchers also found increased gene and protein expression of αvβ3 integrin, which has been suggested to play a central role in angiogenesis. In the third study, gene expression levels were compared in the nidus and the draining veins from five patients with BAVMs.[111] Not surprisingly, the number of differentially expressed genes comparing nidus and draining vein was much smaller than in the study comparing BAVM and normal brain. Of 17,086 probes, only 6 genes were upregulated and 13 downregulated. The upregulation of ephrin A1, a gene related to embryogenesis and angiogenesis, was confirmed by real-time reverse transcription polymerase chain reaction analysis. Ephrin A1 was highly expressed in astrocytes and neurons of the perinidal parenchymal tissue, but not in the endothelial or smooth muscle cells of the AVM vessels or in cells of normal brain tissue as assessed by immunohistochemical studies.

These results are promising, but sample sizes have been very small so far. Further insight into the pathobiology of BAVMs may be obtained in genome-wide gene expression studies of larger numbers of patients with careful selection of control tissue.

Conclusion

IAs and BAVMs appear to be complex diseases resulting from an interaction between genetic variants and environmental or nongenetic disease risk factors. Thus far, progress in finding genetic determinants of the development of aneurysms and BAVMs has been modest. Knowledge of the genetic determinants not only may provide insight in the pathophysiology of aneurysms and BAVMs but also may result in diagnostic tools for identification of individuals at increased risk for aneurysm and BAVM formation as well as clues on how to stop aneurysm and BAVM formation. Future studies should also search for genetic determinants of rupture of these vascular lesions. If biomarkers can identify patients who are at high risk for rupture, these patients can be selected for preventive treatment.

REFERENCES

1. Hop JW, Rinkel GJE, Algra A, et al: Case fatality rates and functional outcome after subarachnoid hemorrahge: A systematic review, *Stroke* 28:660-664, 1997.
2. de Rooij NK, Linn FH, van der Plas JA, et al: Incidence of subarachnoid haemorrhage: A systematic review with emphasis on region, age, gender and time trends, *J Neurol Neurosurg Psychiatry* 78:1365-1372, 2007.
3. Johnston SC, Selvin S, Gress DR: The burden, trends, and demographics of mortality from subarachnoid hemorrhage, *Neurology* 50:1413-1418, 1998.
4. Feigin VL, Rinkel GJ, Lawes CM, et al: Risk factors for subarachnoid hemorrhage: An updated systematic review of epidemiological studies, *Stroke* 36:2773-2780, 2005.
5. Norrgard O, Angquist KA, Fodstad H, et al: Intracranial aneurysms and heredity, *Neurosurgery* 20:236-239, 1987.
6. Bromberg JEC, Rinkel GJE, Algra A, et al: Subarachnoid haemorrhage in first and second degree realtives of patients with subarachnoid haemorrhage, *BMJ* 311:288-289, 1995.
7. Schievink WI, Schaid DJ, Michels VV, et al: Familial aneurysmal subarachnoid hemorrhage: A community based study, *J Neurosurg* 83:426-429, 1995.
8. Braekeleer dM, Pérussee L, Cantin L, et al: A study of inbreeding and kinship in intracranial aneurysms in the Saguenay Lac-Saint-Jean region (Quebec, Canada), *Ann Hum Genet* 60:99-104, 1996.
9. Ronkainen A, Hernesniemi J, Puranen M, et al: Familial intracranial aneurysms, *Lancet* 349:380-384, 1997.
10. Teasdale GM, Wardlaw JM, White PM, et al: The familial risk of subarachnoid haemorrhage, *Brain* 28:1677-1685, 2005.
11. Raaymakers TWM: MARS study group: Aneurysms in relatives of patients with subarachnoid hemorrhage. Frequency and risk factors, *Neurology* 53:982-988, 1999.
12. Rinkel GJE, Djibuti M, Algra A, et al: Prevalence and risk of rupture of intracranial aneurysms, *Stroke* 29:251-256, 1998.
13. Newton-Cheh C, Hirschhorn JN: Genetic association studies of complex traits: Design and analysis issues, *Mutat Res* 573:54-69, 2005.
14. Gawthrop F, Mould R, Sperritt A, Neale F: Ehlers-Danlos syndrome, *BMJ* 335:448-450, 2007.
15. Germain DP, Herrera-Guzman Y: Vascular Ehlers-Danlos syndrome, *Ann Genet* 47:1-9, 2004.
16. Desal HA, Toulgoat F, Raoul S, et al: Ehlers-Danlos syndrome type IV and recurrent carotid-cavernous fistula: review of the literature, endovascular approach, technique and difficulties, *Neuroradiology* 47:300-304, 2005.
17. Krog M, Almgren B, Eriksson I, et al: Vascular complications in the Ehlers-Danlos syndrome, *Acta Chir Scand* 149:279-282, 1983.
18. de Paepe A, Van Landegem W, de Keyser F, et al: Association of multiple intracranial aneurysms and collagen type III deficiency, *Clin Neurol Neurosurg* 90:53-56, 1988.
19. Schievink WI, Limburg M, Oorthuys JW, et al: Cerebrovascular disease in Ehlers-Danlos syndrome type IV, *Stroke* 21:626-632, 1990.
20. Malfait F, De Paepe A: Molecular genetics in classic Ehlers-Danlos syndrome, *Am J Med Genet C Semin Med Genet* 139C:17-23, 2005.
21. van den Berg JS, Pals G, Arwert F, et al: Type III collagen deficiency in saccular intracranial aneurysms. Defect in gene regulation?, *Stroke* 30:1628-1631, 1999.
22. Kuivaniemi H, Prockop DJ, Wu Y, et al: Exclusion of mutations in the gene for type III collagen (COL3A1) as a common cause of intracranial aneurysms or cervical artery dissections: Results from sequence analysis of the coding sequences of type III collagen from 55 unrelated patients, *Neurology* 43:2652-2658, 1993.
23. Dean JC: Marfan syndrome: Clinical diagnosis and management, *Eur J Hum Genet* 15:724-733, 2007.
24. Mizuguchi T, Matsumoto N: Recent progress in genetics of Marfan syndrome and Marfan-associated disorders, *J Hum Genet* 52:1-12, 2007.
25. Latter DA, Ricci MA, Forbes RD, et al: Internal carotid artery aneurysm and Marfan's syndrome, *Can J Surg* 32:463-466, 1989.
26. Ohyama T, Ohara S, Momma F: Aneurysm of the cervical internal carotid artery associated with Marfan's syndrome–case report, *Neurol Med Chir (Tokyo)* 32:965-968, 1992.
27. Finney LH, Roberts TS, Anderson RE: Giant intracranial aneurysm associated with Marfan's syndrome. Case report, *J Neurosurg* 45:342-347, 1976.
28. Schievink WI, Parisi JE, Piepgras DG, et al: Intracranial aneurysms in Marfan's syndrome: An autopsy study, *Neurosurgery* 41:866-870, 1997.
29. Conway JE, Hutchins GM, Tamargo RJ: Marfan syndrome is not associated with intracranial aneurysms, *Stroke* 30:1632-1636, 1999.
30. Li Q, Jiang Q, Pfendner E, et al: Pseudoxanthoma elasticum: Clinical phenotypes, molecular genetics and putative pathomechanisms, *Exp Dermatol* 18:1-11, 2009.
31. van den Berg JS, Hennekam RC, Cruysberg JR, et al: Prevalence of symptomatic intracranial aneurysm and ischaemic stroke in pseudoxanthoma elasticum, *Cerebrovasc Dis* 10:315-319, 2000.
32. Grantham JJ: Clinical practice. Autosomal dominant polycystic kidney disease, *N Engl J Med* 359:1477-1485, 2008.
33. Boucher C, Sandford R: Autosomal dominant polycystic kidney disease (ADPKD, MIM 173900, PKD1 and PKD2 genes, protein products known as polycystin-1 and polycystin-2), *Eur J Hum Genet* 1:347-354, 2004.

34. Iglesias CG, Torres VE, Offord KP, et al: Epidemiology of adult polycystic kidney disease, Olmsted County, Minnesota: 1935-1980, *Am J Kidney Dis* 2:630-639, 1983.

35. Schievink WI, Torres VE, Piepgras DG, et al: Saccular intracranial aneurysms in autosomal dominant polycystic kidney disease, *J Am Soc Nephrol* 3:88-95, 1992.

36. Lozano AM, Leblanc R: Cerebral aneurysms and polycystic kidney disease: A critical review, *Can J Neurol Sci* 19:222-227, 1992.

37. Rinkel GJ, Djibuti M, Algra A, et al: Prevalence and risk of rupture of intracranial aneurysms: A systematic review, *Stroke* 29:251-256, 1998.

38. Gieteling EW, Rinkel GJ: Characteristics of intracranial aneurysms and subarachnoid haemorrhage in patients with polycystic kidney disease, *J Neurol* 250:418-423, 2003.

39. Ruigrok YM, Buskens E, Rinkel GJ: Attributable risk of common and rare determinants of subarachnoid hemorrhage, *Stroke* 32:1173-1175, 2001.

40. Rinkel GJ: Intracranial aneurysm screening: Indications and advice for practice, *Lancet Neurol* 4:122-128, 2005.

41. Kaplan HA, Aronson SM, Browder EJ: Vascular malformatons of the brain. An anatomical study, *J Neurosurg* 18:630-635, 1961.

42. Fleetwood IG, Steinberg GK: Arteriovenous malformations, *Lancet* 359:863-873, 2002.

43. Al-Shahi R, Fang JS, Lewis SC, et al: Prevalence of adults with brain arteriovenous malformations: A community based study in Scotland using capture-recapture analysis, *J Neurol Neurosurg Psychiatry* 73:547-551, 2002.

44. Al-Shahi R, Bhattacharya JJ, Currie DG, et al: Prospective, population-based detection of intracranial vascular malformations in adults: The Scottish Intracranial Vascular Malformation Study (SIVMS), *Stroke* 34:1163-1169, 2003.

45. Stapf C, Mast H, Sciacca RR, et al: The New York Islands AVM Study: Design, study progress, and initial results, *Stroke* 34:e29-e33, 2003.

46. Courville CB: *Pathology of the central nervous system: A study based upon a survey of lesions found in a series of fourty thousand autopsies*, ed 3, Mountain View, CA, 1950, Pacific Press Publishing Association, pp 142-152.

47. Brown RD Jr, Wiebers DO, Forbes G, et al: The natural history of unruptured intracranial arteriovenous malformations, *J Neurosurg* 68:352-357, 1988.

48. Al-Shahi R, Warlow C: A systematic review of the frequency and prognosis of arteriovenous malformations of the brain in adults, *Brain* 124:1900-1926, 2001.

49. Young WL, Yang GY: Are there genetic influences on sporadic brain arteriovenous malformations? *Stroke* 35(Suppl 1):2740-2745, 2004.

50. Mullan S, Mojtahedi S, Johnson DL, et al: Embryological basis of some aspects of cerebral vascular fistulas and malformations, *J Neurosurg* 85:1-8, 1996.

51. Du R, Hashimoto T, Tihan T, et al: Growth and regression of arteriovenous malformations in a patient with hereditary hemorrhagic telangiectasia. Case report, *J Neurosurg* 106:470-477, 2007.

52. Buis DR, van den Berg R, Lycklama G, et al: Spontaneous regression of brain arteriovenous malformations—a clinical study and a systematic review of the literature, *J Neurol* 251:1375-1382, 2004.

53. van Beijnum J, van der Worp HB, Schippers HM, et al: Familial occurrence of brain arteriovenous malformations: A systematic review, *J Neurol Neurosurg Psychiatry* 78:1213-1217, 2007.

54. Letteboer TG, Mager JJ, Snijder RJ, et al: Genotype-phenotype relationship in hereditary haemorrhagic telangiectasia, *J Med Genet* 43:371-377, 2006.

55. Leblanc R, Melanson D, Wilkinson RD: Hereditary neurocutaneous angiomatosis. Report of four cases, *J Neurosurg* 85:1135-1142, 1996.

56. Gallione CJ, Richards JA, Letteboer TG, et al: SMAD4 mutations found in unselected HHT patients, *J Med Genet* 43:793-797, 2006.

57. Cole SG, Begbie ME, Wallace GM, et al: A new locus for hereditary haemorrhagic telangiectasia (HHT3) maps to chromosome 5, *J Med Genet* 42:577-582, 2005.

58. Bayrak-Toydemir P, McDonald J, Markewitz B, et al: Genotype-phenotype correlation in hereditary hemorrhagic telangiectasia: Mutations and manifestations, *Am J Med Genet A* 140:463-470, 2006.

59. Sabba C, Pasculli G, Lenato GM, et al: Hereditary hemorrhagic telangiectasia: Clinical features in ENG and ALK1 mutation carriers, *J Thromb Haemost* 5:1149-1157, 2007.

60. Lesca G, Olivieri C, Burnichon N, et al: Genotype-phenotype correlations in hereditary hemorrhagic telangiectasia: Data from the French-Italian HHT network, *Genet Med* 9:14-22, 2007.

61. Krings T, Chng SM, Ozanne A, et al: Hereditary hemorrhagic telangiectasia in children: Endovascular treatment of neurovascular malformations: Results in 31 patients, *Neuroradiology* 47:946-954, 2005.

62. Kruglyak L, Lander ES: Complete multipoint sib-pair analysis of qualitative and quantitative traits, *Am J Hum Genet* 57:439-454, 1995.

63. Dawn TM, Barrett JH: Genetic linkage studies, *Lancet* 366:1036-1044, 2005.

64. Cordell HJ, Clayton DG: Genetic association studies, *Lancet* 366:1121-1131, 2005.

65. Redon R, Ishikawa S, Fitch KR, et al: Global variation in copy number in the human genome, *Nature* 444:444-454, 2006.

66. Lupski JR, Stankiewicz P: Genomic disorders: Molecular mechanisms for rearrangements and conveyed phenotypes, *PLoS Genet* 1:e49, 2005.

67. Stoughton RB, Friend SH: How molecular profiling could revolutionize drug discovery, *Nat Rev Drug Discov* 4:345-350, 2005.

68. Onda H, Kasuya H, Yoneyama T, et al: Genomewide-linkage and haplotype-association studies map intracranial aneurysm to chromosome 7q11, *Am J Hum Genet* 69:804-819, 2001.

69. Olson JM, Vongpunsawad S, Kuivaniemi H, et al: Search for intracranial aneurysm susceptibility gene(s) using Finnish families, *BMC Med Genet* 3:7, 2002.

70. Farnham JM, Camp NJ, Neuhausen SL, et al: Confirmation of chromosome 7q11 locus for predisposition to intracranial aneurysm, *Hum Genet* 114:250-255, 2004.

71. Yamada S, Utsunomiya M, Inoue K, et al: Genome-wide scan for Japanese familial intracranial aneurysms: Linkage to several chromosomal regions, *Circulation* 110:3727-3733, 2004.

72. Nahed BV, Seker A, Guclu B, et al: Mapping a mendelian form of intracranial aneurysm to 1p34.3-p36.13, *Am J Hum Genet* 76:172-179, 2004.

73. Ozturk AK, Nahed BV, Bydon M, Nahed BV: Molecular genetic analysis of two large kindreds with intracranial aneurysms demonstrates linkage to 11q24-25 and 14q23-31, *Stroke* 37:1021-1027, 2006.

74. Verlaan DJ, Dube MP, St-Onge J, et al: A new locus for autosomal dominant intracranial aneurysm, ANIB4, maps to chromosome 5p15.2-14.3, *J Med Genet* 43:e31, 2006.

75. Mineharu Y, Inoue K, Inoue S, et al: Model-based linkage analyses confirm chromosome 19q13.3 as a susceptibility locus for intracranial aneurysm, *Stroke* 38:1174-1178, 2007.

76. Ruigrok YM, Wijmenga C, Rinkel GJ, et al: Genomewide linkage in a large Dutch family with intracranial aneurysms: Replication of 2 loci for intracranial aneurysms to chromosome 1p36.11-p36.13 and Xp22.2-p22.32, *Stroke* 39:1096-1102, 2008.

77. Van der Voet M, Olson JM, Kuivaniemi H, et al: Intracranial aneurysms in Finnish families: Confirmation of linkage and refinement of the interval to chromosome 19q13.3, *Am J Hum Genet* 74:564-571, 2004.

78. Roos YB, Pals G, Struycken PM, et al: Genome-wide linkage in a large Dutch consanguineous family maps a locus for intracranial aneurysms to chromosome 2p13, *Stroke* 35:2276-2281, 2004.

79. Ruigrok YM, Rinkel GJ, Wijmenga C: Genetics of intracranial aneurysms, *Lancet Neurol* 4:179-189, 2005.

80. Krischek B, Inoue I: The genetics of intracranial aneurysms, *J Hum Genet* 51:587-594, 2006.

81. Nahed BV, Bydon M, Ozturk AK, et al: Genetics of intracranial aneurysms, *Neurosurgery* 60:213-225, 2007.

82. Ruigrok YM, Rinkel GJ, Wijmenga C: The versican gene and the risk of intracranial aneurysms, *Stroke* 37:2372-2374, 2006.

83. Mineharu Y, Inoue K, Inoue S, et al: Association analyses confirming a susceptibility locus for intracranial aneurysm at chromosome 14q23, *J Hum Genet* 53:325-332, 2008.

84. Ruigrok YM, Rinkel GJ, van't Slot R, et al: Evidence in favor of the contribution of genes involved in the maintenance of the extracellular matrix of the arterial wall to the development of intracranial aneurysms, *Hum Mol Genet* 15:3361-3368, 2006.

85. Yoneyama T, Kasuya H, Onda H, et al: Association of positional and functional candidate genes FGF1, FBN2, and LOX on 5q31 with intracranial aneurysm, *J Hum Genet* 48:309-314, 2003.

86. Hofer A, Ozkan S, Hermans M, et al: Mutations in the lysyl oxidase gene not associated with intracranial aneurysm in central european families, *Cerebrovasc Dis* 18:189-193, 2004.

87. Akagawa H, Tajima A, Sakamoto Y, et al: A haplotype spanning two genes, ELN and LIMK1, decreases their transcripts and confers susceptibility to intracranial aneurysms, *Hum Mol Genet* 15:1722-1734, 2006.

88. Berthelemy-Okazaki N, Zhao Y, Yang Z, et al: Examination of ELN as a candidate gene in the Utah intracranial aneurysm pedigrees, *Stroke* 36:1283-1284, 2005.

89. Krex D, Konig IR, Ziegler A, et al: Extended single nucleotide polymorphism and haplotype analysis of the elastin gene in caucasians with intracranial aneurysms provides evidence for racially/ethnically based differences, *Cerebrovasc Dis* 18:104-110, 2004.

90. Hofer A, Hermans M, Kubassek N, et al: Elastin polymorphism haplotype and intracranial aneurysms are not associated in central europe, *Stroke* 34:1207-1211, 2003.

91. Yoneyama T, Kasuya H, Onda H, et al: Collagen type I alpha2 (COL1A2) is the susceptible gene for intracranial aneurysms, *Stroke* 35:443-448, 2004.

92. Inoue K, Mineharu Y, Inoue S, et al: Search on chromosome 17 centromere reveals TNFRSF13B as a susceptibility gene for intracranial aneurysm: A preliminary study, *Circulation* 113:2002-2010, 2006.

93. Mineharu Y, Inoue K, Inoue S, et al: Association analysis of common variants of ELN, NOS2A, APOE and ACE2 to intracranial aneurysm, *Stroke* 37:1189-1194, 2006.

94. Weinsheimer S, Goddard KA, Parrado AR, et al: Association of kallikrein gene polymorphisms with intracranial aneurysms, *Stroke* 38:2670-2676, 2007.

95. Clements JA, Willemsen NM, Myers SA, et al: The tissue kallikrein family of serine proteases: Functional roles in human disease and potential as clinical biomarkers, *Crit Rev Clin Lab Sci* 41:265-312, 2004.

96. Bilguvar K, Yasuno K, Niemela M, et al: Identification of susceptibility loci for intracranial aneurysm, *Nat Genet* 40:1472-1477, 2008.

97. Yasuno K, Bilguvar K, Bijlenga P, et al: Genome-wide association study of intracranial aneurysm identifies three new risk loci, *Nat Genet* 42:420-425, 2010.

98. Krischek B, Kasuya H, Tajima A, et al: Network-based gene expression analysis of intracranial aneurysm tissue reveals role of antigen presenting cells, *Neuroscience* 154:1398-1407, 2008.

99. Weinsheimer S, Lenk GM, van der Voet M, et al: Integration of expression profiles and genetic mapping data to identify candidate genes in intracranial aneurysm, *Physiol Genomics* 32:45-57, 2007.

100. Inoue S, Liu W, Inoue K, et al: Combination of linkage and association studies for brain arteriovenous malformation, *Stroke* 38:1368-1370, 2007.

101. Pawlikowska L, Tran MN, Achrol AS, et al: Polymorphisms in transforming growth factor-beta-related genes ALK1 and ENG are associated with sporadic brain arteriovenous malformations, *Stroke* 36:2278-2280, 2005.

102. Simon M, Franke D, Ludwig M, et al: Association of a polymorphism of the ACVRL1 gene with sporadic arteriovenous malformations of the central nervous system, *J Neurosurg* 104:945-949, 2006.

103. Young WL, Kwok PY, Pawlikowska L, et al: Arteriovenous malformation, *J Neurosurg* 106:731-732, 2007.

104. Abdalla SA, Cymerman U, Johnson RM, et al: Disease-associated mutations in conserved residues of ALK-1 kinase domain, *Eur J Hum Genet* 11:279-287, 2003.

105. Pawlikowska L, Tran MN, Achrol AS, et al: Polymorphisms in genes involved in inflammatory and angiogenic pathways and the risk of hemorrhagic presentation of brain arteriovenous malformations, *Stroke* 35:2294-2300, 2004.

106. Achrol AS, Pawlikowska L, McCulloch CE, et al: Tumor necrosis factor-alpha-238G>A promoter polymorphism is associated with increased risk of new hemorrhage in the natural course of patients with brain arteriovenous malformations, *Stroke* 37:231-234, 2006.

107. Achrol AS, Kim H, Pawlikowska L, et al: Association of tumor necrosis factor-alpha-238G>A and apolipoprotein E2 polymorphisms with intracranial hemorrhage after brain arteriovenous malformation treatment, *Neurosurgery* 61:731-739, 2007.

108. Pawlikowska L, Poon KY, Achrol AS, et al: Apolipoprotein E epsilon 2 is associated with new hemorrhage risk in brain arteriovenous malformations, *Neurosurgery* 58:838-843, 2006.

109. Shenkar R, Elliott JP, Diener K, et al: Differential gene expression in human cerebrovascular malformations, *Neurosurgery* 52:465-477, 2003.

110. Hashimoto T, Lawton MT, Wen G, et al: Gene microarray analysis of human brain arteriovenous malformations, *Neurosurgery* 54:410-423, 2004.

111. Sasahara A, Kasuya H, Akagawa H, et al: Increased expression of ephrin A1 in brain arteriovenous malformation: DNA microarray analysis, *Neurosurg Rev* 3:299-305, 2007.

67 Anterior Circulation Aneurysms

BRIAN V. NAHED, CHRISTOPHER S. OGILVY

Anterior circulation aneurysms encompass those that arise from the carotid artery, the anterior and middle cerebral arteries, or their branches. Although these aneurysms have historically been treated surgically, continued advances in endovascular techniques have served to change the treatment paradigms for these lesions. In this chapter, we detail the surgical management of both unruptured and ruptured anterior circulation aneurysms.

Historical Perspective

Intracranial aneurysms were first discovered incidentally during tumor surgery and in postmortem studies. Few dared to treat these lesions until Sir Victor Horsley first ligated the common carotid artery to treat an intracranial aneurysm in 1885.[1] However, the high rate of hemiplegia prompted Harvey Cushing to instead advocate wrapping the aneurysm with muscle. Years later, surgical clips he designed for the occlusion of vessels encountered during tumor surgery would be modified as the first prototype for treating aneurysms.[2] In 1938, Walter Dandy was the first to successfully clip an intracranial aneurysm, pioneering cerebrovascular surgery.[3] Surgical techniques continued to improve, but it was the operating microscope that truly revolutionized aneurysm surgery and led to modern microneurosurgery. Developments in endovascular techniques have now altered the role of surgery in the management of intracranial aneurysms.[4,5]

Intracranial Aneurysms

Asymptomatic unruptured aneurysms are generally managed according to guidelines that carefully consider aneurysm and patient specific risk factors highlighted earlier in this text. The management of unruptured intracranial aneurysms has historically focused on the size of the aneurysm. In 1998, the International Study of Unruptured Intracranial Aneurysms (ISUIA) concluded that aneurysms smaller than 10 mm had a 0.05% per year risk of rupture in patients without previous subarachnoid hemorrhage (group 1).[6] The Stroke Council of the American Heart Association reinforced the ISUIA findings in 2000, recommending that unruptured aneurysms smaller than 10 mm be observed.[7] In 2003, the follow-up report ISUIA study concluded that aneurysms smaller than 7 mm had 0% and 2.5% cumulative rupture risks in the anterior and posterior circulations, respectively, over 5 years.[8] This second study more closely mirrored clinical experience although it was thought to underestimate rupture risk

owing to selection bias and large numbers of patient exclusions. In light of these limitations, many authorities have suggested that aneurysms larger than 5 mm be treated, to expand on the ISUIA study conclusions and account for all patients at highest risk of rupture.[9] We recommend conservatively managing small aneurysms, those smaller than 5 mm. In patients younger than 70 years, we offer treatment for unruptured aneurysms larger than 5 mm and for all aneurysms that produce neurologic symptoms regardless of size.

Anterior circulation aneurysms most often arise from branch points off the anterior communicating or middle cerebral artery (MCA) and can be associated with hypoplastic branches.[10,11] It is unlikely that aneurysms remain static; instead their growth is likely nonlinear, causing fluctuations in rupture risk over time.[12-14] When symptomatic, aneurysms are usually treated because they have a higher annual risk of rupture than asymptomatic lesions (7.3% versus 2.6%, respectively).[15] Anterior circulation aneurysms appear to have a lower annual risk of rupture than posterior circulation aneurysms (1.1 to 1.8% versus 3.2 to 4.4%, respectively).[8,15,16]

The decision whether to clip or coil an aneurysm is complex and involves an evaluation by either a neurosurgeon who performs both open surgical and endovascular treatment or a team comprising subspecialists with both open surgical and endovascular expertise. As endovascular techniques advance, our decision-making process in the management of anterior circulation aneurysms must continuously be updated to reflect the latest data regarding risks and efficacy of open surgical and endovascular treatment of aneurysms. Long-term benefits of higher obliteration rates with open surgery must be weighed carefully against the risks and benefits of the projected durability of endovascular techniques. Depending on the location of the anterior circulation aneurysm, different approaches to therapy may be recommended. Aneurysms of the petrous and intracavernous segments are often managed endovascularly when symptomatic. Paraclinoid aneurysms, which arise as the carotid enters the skull base, require careful analysis to determine the most appropriate therapy. For lesions above the paraclinoid location up to the carotid bifurcation, the choice of surgical and/or endovascular management is based on patient-specific factors, such as age and medical comorbidities, and aneurysm-specific factors, such as calcification, size of aneurysm, thrombus within aneurysm, and relationship of aneurysm neck to parent vessel. MCA aneurysms often require open surgical treatment because

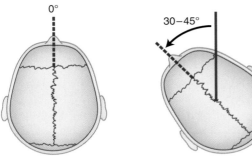

0°

30–45°

Pericallosal aneurysms

Distal anterior cerebral artery aneurysms

Ophthalmic, some anterior communicating and posterior communicating aneurysms, and middle cerebral aneurysms approached through the sylvian fissure

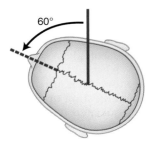
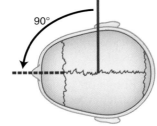

60°

90°

Some anterior communicating and posterior communicating aneurysms, and middle cerebral aneurysms approached through the superior temporal gyrus

Subtemporal approach

Figure 67-1 Head positioning within the Mayfield adapter varies according to aneurysm location to maximize visualization during surgical approach.

of their involvement of the takeoff of MCA branches. In this chapter, we detail the management of anterior circulation aneurysms according to their location.

General Operative Considerations

Operative Setup and Positioning

Patient positioning is integral to a successful surgery because it maximizes surgical exposure while using gravity to minimize retraction of the brain tissue. For anterior circulation aneurysms, the patient is placed supine on the operating table. The patient's head is placed in three-point fixation (Mayfield adapter) and secured to the operating table. Depending on the location of the aneurysm and the surgical approach desired, the head can be rotated to achieve maximal surgical exposure (Fig. 67-1). The head is generally rotated 0, 30, or 60 degrees from midline toward the shoulder of the unaffected side. Anterior communicating artery (ACoA) aneurysms require greatest rotation, while internal carotid artery (ICA) bifurcation and posterior communicating artery aneurysms require the least. Great care should be made to maintain a minimum of two fingerbreadths between the jaw and clavicle to prevent jugular compression, which would increase intracranial pressure (ICP).

The operating room is set up with the operating table in the center of the room and the surgeon and assistant surgeon positioned at the head (Fig. 67-2). The surgical scrub nurse and instruments are located to the right side of the surgeon to facilitate the transfer of instruments. The operating room staff should be experienced in microsurgical technique. The anesthesiologist manages the airway and ventilator from the side of the patient contralateral to the lesion. The operating microscope is powered on, focused, and draped for surgery so that it is ready immediately in the event of an emergency such as intraoperative aneurysm rupture. A special operating chair equipped with foot pedals to maneuver the microscope zoom function allows the surgeon to remain focused on the operative field without interruption.

Surgical Technique

The surgical approach is determined by the location and position of the aneurysm neck and dome (Fig. 67-3). The majority of anterior circulation aneurysms are approached through a pterional craniotomy, which allows access to the circle of Willis and the anterior fossa.[17] The different surgical approaches are discussed in detail in the next section according to aneurysm location.

In general, the surgeon begins by identifying the parent vessel, then carefully dissects along this vessel toward the aneurysm. Subarachnoid adhesions are precisely cut to avoid displacement of tissue, which could tear the aneurysm. Once the aneurysm neck is exposed, its relationship to branching and neighboring vessels can be evaluated. If there is extensive atheromatous disease or the aneurysm has thin and fragile walls, temporary clipping may be used to minimize the chance of intraoperative rupture.

Despite the impaired cerebral autoregulation in patients with subarachnoid hemorrhage (SAH), temporary clipping of the parent artery is a safe alternative to systemic hypotension and can reduce the risk of intraoperative rupture.[18] Many studies have demonstrated that temporary occlusion can be tolerated for between 10 and 20 minutes without infarction.[18-22] A recent study demonstrated neuroprotective agents such as barbiturates can reduce the risk of ischemic injury, particularly when occluded longer than 10 minutes.[19,23-27] Moderate hypothermia ($\approx$34° C), common with general anesthesia, can also lower the risk of infarction. We recommend the following combination of preventive measures during temporary vessel occlusion: (1) elevating blood pressure to 150 to 170 mm Hg systolic if the heart rate is normal, (2) 100 g mannitol, and (3) hypothermia to 33.5° C. Although we encourage minimizing total clamp time, barbiturate protection (5 mg/kg thiopental) is also given by some surgeons if temporary vessel occlusion is expected to be longer than 20 minutes.

The goal of surgical clipping is to obliterate the aneurysm, effectively removing it from the circulation. There are a variety of spring-loaded clip shapes and configurations from which to choose (Fig. 67-4); they consist of (1) straight clips with parallel blades placed directly across the neck of the aneurysm, which come in all lengths, curves, and bayonet shapes, and (2) fenestrated

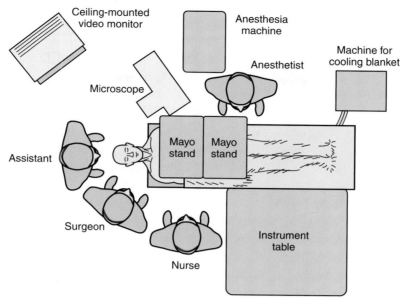

Figure 67-2 Operating room layout for a right-sided pterional craniotomy.

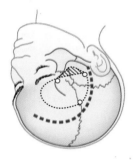

Pterional approach
Aneurysms of internal carotid,
anterior communicating,
middle cerebral arteries,
and some basilar apex

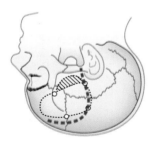

Full frontotemporal approach
Aneurysms of middle
cerebral artery to be done
by the superior temporal
gyrus approach

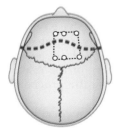

Interhemispheric approach
Aneurysms of distal anterior
cerebral artery

Figure 67-3 Skin incision and bony removal according to aneurysm location.

clips, which combine the parallel, long, thin jaws of the first type with a proximal round aperture through which an artery or nerve may pass.

After the clip is placed, the surgeon assesses the patency of the surrounding vessels using a microvascular Doppler probe to test for flow in the proximal, distal, and branching vessels. The efficacy of surgical clipping is tested by puncturing the aneurysm dome with a 25-gauge spinal needle. If bleeding persists, the clip should be interrogated to determine whether it completely spans the aneurysm neck or the clip is strong enough to occlude the neck. Additionally, intraoperative angiography provides a safe and cost-effective method to detect residual lesions and vascular compromise that may require additional surgical adjustments.[28] Some surgeons have incorporated indocyanine green videoangiography, whereas others use intraoperative angiography (IA).[29-36] Clips that incompletely occlude or inadvertently obstruct adjacent vasculature are identified and adjusted in 8% to 11% of cases in which IA is used.[30,34,35] Given the extremely low complication rate (morbidity less than 1%), low false-negative rate, and near negligible radiation exposure risk to the patient and operator, IA is recommended for complex aneurysms.[30,33,34,36] Indocyanine green videoangiography, although promising, is limited in its evaluation to those vessels within the microscope view and therefore is best used in conjunction with standard intraoperative angiography.

Specific Operative Techniques for Anterior Circulation Aneurysms

Anterior circulation aneurysms arise from the ICA or its two branches, the anterior cerebral and middle cerebral arteries. In this section, we describe the pterional approach and highlight the specific treatment of these aneurysms according to their location. The endovascular treatment of these aneurysms is discussed elsewhere in this text.

Pterional Approach

The pterional (frontotemporal) craniotomy is the standard approach for treatment of anterior circulation aneurysms. The incision begins 1 cm in front of the tragus at the posterior margin of the zygoma, continuing anteriorly and

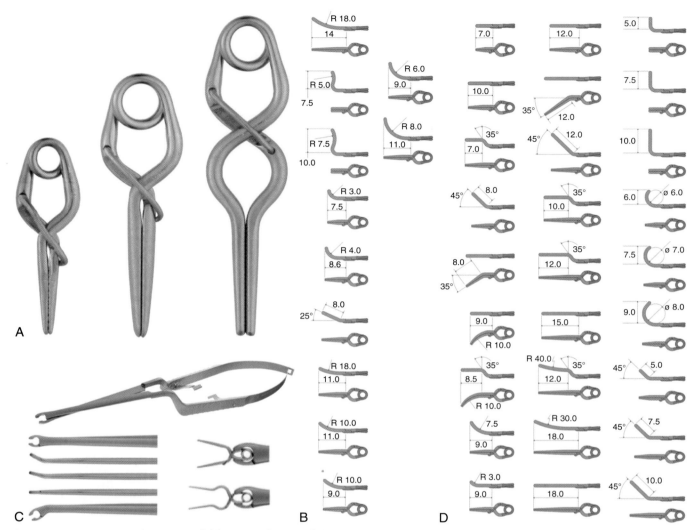

Figure 67-4 Aneurysm clips are available in straight or angled orientations (A to C). Fenestrated clips (D) have an aperture through which an artery or nerve may pass.

superiorly in a curvilinear fashion to just behind the hairline (Figs. 67-5A and 67-6E). The incision is carried down to bone, and the scalp is elevated to reveal the temporalis muscle. This muscular fascia is carefully incised so as to return to its original anatomy upon closing, maximizing cosmesis and mechanical function. The soft tissue and muscle are retracted with use of either fish hooks or simple stitches and elastic bands (Figs. 67-5C and 67-6F). It is imperative to obtain enough of an exposure to adequately access and drill the pterion and the zygomatic process of the frontal bone.

A high-speed drill is used to create three burr holes: The first is placed behind the frontal process of the zygomatic bone; the second is placed at the pterion, a few centimeters behind the first, and the third is placed at the superior temporal line posteriorly (Figs. 67-5C and 67-6G). The burr holes provide a window through which to strip the dura from the skull's inner table and an inlet to insert a craniotome to cut the bone. The cut extends medially 1.5 to 2.0 cm (depending on the specific aneurysm location) and inferiorly to the floor of the anterior cranial fossa. The pterion is then removed with drill or rongeur, and

the lesser wing of the sphenoid bone is flattened to allow for an approach along the base without much retraction. The pterional craniotomy is approximately 6 cm by 6 cm (Fig. 67-6I). Once removed, the outer leaf of the dura is tacked to the periphery of the craniotomy to minimize venous bleeding during the procedure and epidural collection postoperatively.

The dura is incised in a curvilinear flap and retracted inferiorly with sutures over the muscle to minimize obstruction of the surgical view (Fig. 67-6K). The dura is covered with biologic collagen (Bio-Col, Laboratoire Français de Fractionnement et de Biotechnologies, Lille, France) and frequently irrigated to prevent drying. Similarly, the brain parenchyma is covered with cotton fiber/ poly(ethylene terephthalate) (Telfa) strips over which retractors are placed to prevent trauma and drying. The frontal lobe is minimally elevated with a self-retaining retractor (Fig. 67-6N). Maximizing brain relaxation with mannitol, furosemide, and cerebrospinal fluid (CSF) drainage can reduce the amount of brain retraction. Depending on the location, CSF can be drained via the

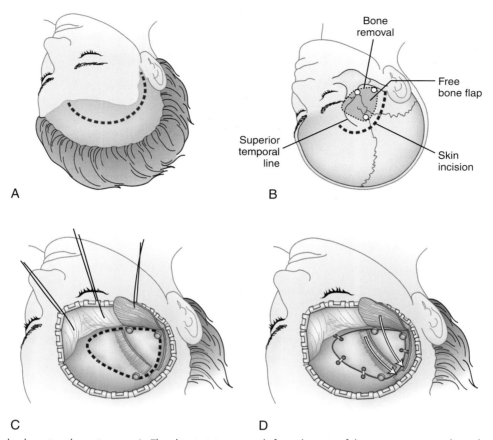

A

B

C

D

Figure 67-5 Standard pterional craniotomy. A, The skin incision extends from the root of the zygoma anteriorly and superiorly to the hairline. B, Relationship of skin incision, bone flap, and craniotomy. C, The scalp and underlying temporalis muscle are elevated and retracted with sutures. Note the outline of the 3 burr holes: the first behind the frontal process of the zygomatic bone, the second at the pterion, a few centimeters behind the first, and the third placed at the superior temporal line posteriorly. D, At the completion of the procedure, the bone flap is replaced and secured with miniplates and screws. The muscular fascia is reapposed (arrows) to allow for cosmetic and functional restoration.

cisterns in the operative field or via ventriculostomy or lumbar drain if needed.

The microscope is brought into the field while the surgical scrub nurse brings the microsurgical instruments, retractors, and suckers to the forefront of the surgical field (Fig. 67-6M). In general, most approaches begin by splitting the sylvian fissure with use of careful arachnoid dissection (Fig. 67-6O). Subarachnoid adhesions are precisely cut with microscissors, giving the surgeon freedom to separate the frontal and temporal lobe with retractors (depending on aneurysm location). Disruption of the venous structures, particularly the transsylvian veins, should be avoided, if possible, especially those that drain into the sphenoparietal sinus. If these veins are sacrificed early in the sylvian fissure dissection, venous congestion may develop, which can cause the frontal and temporal surfaces to become friable and prone to hemorrhage.

Petrous Internal Carotid Artery Aneurysms

Petrous segment aneurysms grow asymptomatically until localized mass effect causes complaints of decreased hearing, ear pain, facial numbness, and/or diplopia. When symptomatic, these aneurysms are initially treated with endovascular occlusion of the ICA or a combination of coiling and stenting to preserve the carotid artery.

Surgical intervention is reserved for aneurysms that fail a test occlusion and for patients who are not candidates for endovascular techniques. Extracranial-to-intracranial (EC-IC) bypass using a superficial temporal artery to MCA anastomosis may be necessary if ICA occlusion is not tolerated. A detailed description of these techniques is discussed elsewhere.

Cavernous Internal Carotid Artery Aneurysms

Cavernous segment ICA aneurysms most often form at the anterior genu of the carotid siphon or the horizontal portion of the carotid artery. Like petrous segment aneurysms, cavernous segment aneurysms grow silently until mass effect affects the adjacent cranial nerves in the cavernous sinus. Patients most often present with a sixth nerve palsy; however, other complaints vary from diplopia and ptosis secondary to third and fourth nerve compression, venous engorgement, and facial pain from compression of the fifth nerve. Ruptured cavernous aneurysms are generally contained within the cavernous sinus and produce a cavernous carotid fistula, leading to pulsatile exophthalmos, scleral injection, and a bruit. Rarely, a ruptured aneurysm can erode through the sinus into the subarachnoid space and may manifest as a surgical hematoma or very rarely as SAH.

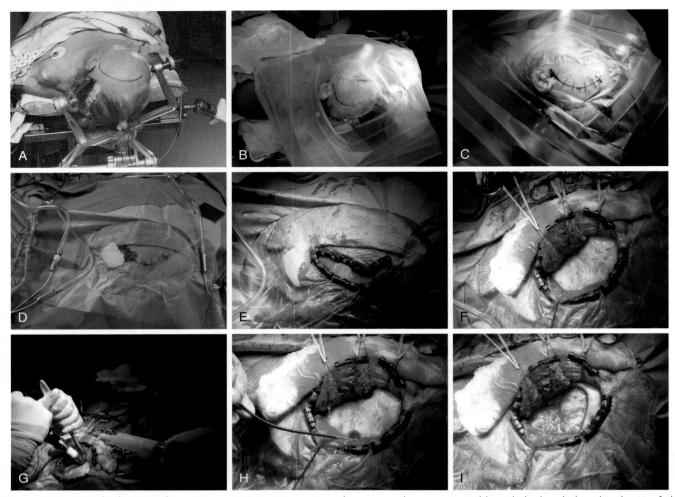

Figure 67-6 Standard pterional craniotomy. A, Patient is positioned supine on the operating table with the head placed in the Mayfield adapter. B and C, The incision is outlined, and self-adhering drapes define the sterile field. D, Surgical field in view covered with sterile drapes with gauze padding covering the ear. E, Incision has been made, exposing underlying fascia. F, The muscle and fascia are elevated and tacked back with sutures and rubber bands to maximize exposure. G and H, A perforator is used to make burr holes to allow for craniotomy. I, The craniotomy bone flap has been completed, exposing the underlying dura. Removal of the lateral wall of the sphenoid wing allows the exposure to be flush along the floor of the frontal fossa.

Unruptured, asymptomatic cavernous aneurysms are managed conservatively and monitored with serial imaging. Treatment is reserved for symptomatic patients and for aneurysms that have enlarged and eroded through the cavernous sinus. Endovascular occlusion of the carotid artery or reconstructive procedures such as stenting and coiling are usually preferred. EC-IC bypass with carotid occlusion is reserved for aneurysms untreatable by endovascular methods.

Paraclinoid ICA Aneurysms

Paraclinoid ICA aneurysms arise from the carotid artery segment as it enters the skull base, following the cavernous sinus and extending up to the region proximal to the posterior communicating artery. They are commonly referred to according to their location from proximal to distal (clinoid, ophthalmic, superior hypophyseal, and posterior wall). They can arise in the carotid cave, at the origin of the ophthalmic artery, at the superior hypophyseal origin, or from the back wall of the carotid artery

without any apparent vessel of origin in association with the lesion (Fig. 67-7). Importantly, the presence of an aneurysm can alter the course of the carotid artery or erode bone at the skull base, either laterally at the base of the anterior clinoid process or medially near the ethmoid sinus. Paraclinoid aneurysms are often found after rupture with SAH. Unruptured aneurysms, however, can cause symptoms including unilateral vision loss from compression of the optic nerve, for which a thorough neuroopthalmologic evaluation is often helpful to characterize visual fields and vision prior to treatment. Many of these lesions are now encountered incidentally during the evaluation of headaches or other neurologic symptoms.

The surgical approach to paraclinoid aneurysms is challenging because of their intradural and extradural location and their proximity to the carotid ring, anterior clinoid process, and optic strut.[44] The anatomy of the aneurysm and the tortuosity of the carotid artery as it enters the skull base must be appreciated by means of CT angiography with three-dimensional reconstructions or three-dimensional

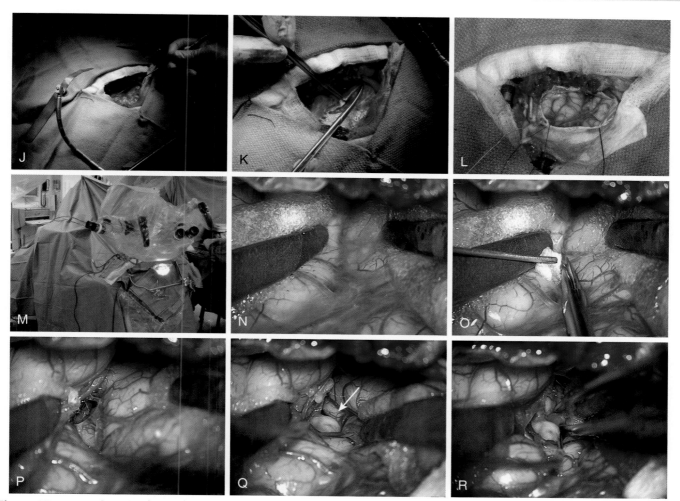

Figure 67-6, cont'd J, Sterile towels are placed, defining the operative field in preparation for the opening of the dura and transition to the microscope. K, The dura is carefully incised so as not to disrupt the underlying pia or inadvertently damage bridging veins or cortical vasculature. L, The dura is opened, revealing the parenchyma with pia and cortical vessels intact. M, Standard operating microscope and setup. N, View through the microscope. Retractors gently separate the frontal and temporal lobes, exposing the pia over the sylvian fissure (corresponds to the schematic drawing in Fig. 67-10). O, Microscissors gently cut the pia, allowing further retraction of the frontal and temporal lobes to expose the sylvian fissure. P and Q, Careful dissection reveals the dome of the aneurysm *(arrow)*. R to T, The aneurysm is carefully dissected free of surrounding vessels, and the middle cerebral artery is exposed proximal and distal to the dome.

Continued

angiography (Fig. 67-8). This operation involves both an intracranial carotid artery approach and a cervical carotid artery exposure for proximal arterial control of the vessel. The patient is placed on a radiolucent operating table with the head turned 30 degrees toward the contralateral shoulder and extended 15 degrees. The patient's head and neck must be optimally oriented for both intracranial and carotid surgical approaches. An external ventricular drain (EVD) is placed for ruptured aneurysms and a lumbar drain is placed for unruptured aneurysms to allow for intraoperative CSF drainage.

Proximal control is established through a neck incision that allows access to the cervical segment of the carotid artery. The common, external, and internal carotid arteries are individually placed in vessel loops to allow for their immediate occlusion in the event of an aneurysmal rupture. Some writers have also described achieving proximal control with endovascular balloon occlusion of the proximal carotid artery, which would also allow for posttreatment angiography.

A pterional craniotomy grants the best surgical exposure to the paraclinoid carotid artery (Fig. 67-9). The dura is incised and dissected from the bone along the medial sphenoid ridge to the tip of the anterior clinoid process and extending medially toward the falciform ligament. Brain relaxation is maximized by draining of CSF after the arachnoid is opened over the optic nerve and carotid artery as well as draining of CSF from the EVD or lumbar drain (Fig. 67-10). The anterior clinoid process and optic strut interfere with exposure and eventual surgical clipping and therefore need to be removed (Fig. 67-11).

For minimal bone removal, intradural drilling of the anterior clinoid process is adequate. However, the majority of these procedures require extradural drilling of the anterior clinoid process and optic strut, and unroofing of the optic canal; this is a modification of the technique initially described by Dolenc.[45] The anterior clinoid process and optic strut are thinned with a high-speed drill, rongeurs, and microdissectors. Bony removal is continued until the aneurysm neck is adequately exposed to allow

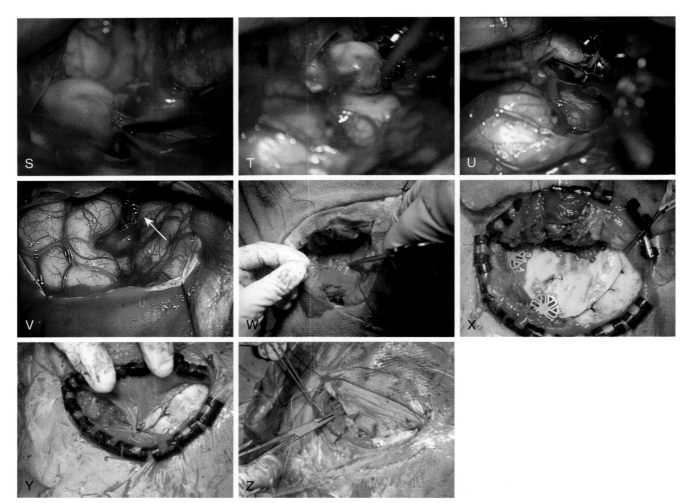

Figure 67-6, cont'd   R to T, The aneurysm is carefully dissected free of surrounding vessels, and the middle cerebral artery is exposed proximal and distal to the dome. U, Aneurysm clip blades are placed across the aneurysmal neck, occluding flow so that the dome collapses. V, After clip application *(arrow)*, the retractors allow the frontal and temporal lobes to relax into original position. W, The dura is reapproximated with sutures. X, The bone flap has been replaced and is secured with titanium plates and screws. Y, The temporalis fascia is reapproximated to ensure functional and cosmetic restoration. Z, The scalp is reapproximated with two layers of sutures.

for clip placement. Ophthalmic and superior hypophyseal aneurysms are predominantly located in the subarachnoid space and therefore require less bony removal than aneurysms located in the carotid cave, which, at times, require both intradural and extradural drilling.

Once the anterior clinoid bony removal is completed, the dura is opened over the bone. The dura propria is then opened over the optic nerve, and the origin of the ophthalmic artery can now be identified. The aneurysm neck is isolated and a direct surgical clip is applied, obliterating the aneurysm. Great care must be taken to ensure that the clip does not displace the optic nerve or occlude the ophthalmic artery. A post-clipping intraoperative angiogram is helpful to ensure complete aneurysm obliteration while also assessing the patency of the ophthalmic artery. During the closure, the sphenoid sinus is occluded with a combination of absorbable gelatin sponge (Gelfoam) and wax to prevent CSF leakage and infection. We also harvest a small fat graft from the neck incision and place it extradurally over the optic nerve region. The patient's visual fields are formally evaluated postoperatively.

Posterior Communicating Artery Internal Carotid Artery Aneurysms

The posterior communicating artery (PCoA) typically originates from the posterior or posterolateral surface of the carotid artery as it bends upward toward the bifurcation (Fig. 67-12). Posterior communicating aneurysms, however, can be divided into the following two subcategories: (1) aneurysms that project laterally and below the tentorial incisura and cause oculomotor nerve compression where the nerve enters the dura at the tentorial edge and (2) aneurysms that project laterally above the tentorium that can manifest as temporal lobe hematoma after they rupture.[46] Patients with ruptured PCoA aneurysms present with SAH and often ipsilateral third nerve paresis that may involve the pupil. As such aneurysms enlarge they may compress against the tentorial edge and reside partially above and below the tentorium. In these cases, great care is utilized in the microdissection of the neck and the dome of the aneurysm. At times, sharp dissection of the tentorium is needed to fully visualize the base of the aneurysm. During this dissection, one must take care

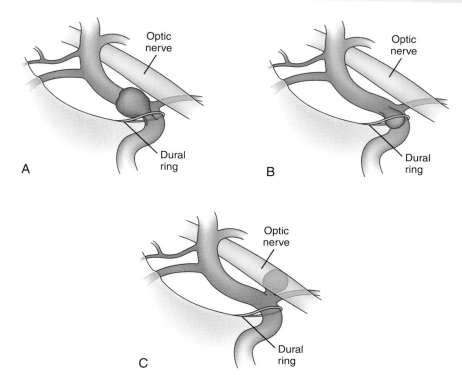

Figure 67-7 A, Paraclinoid aneurysm located in the transition extending superiorly abutting the optic nerve. B, Paraclinoid aneurysm located in the carotid cave projecting inferiorly. C, Ophthalmic artery aneurysm.

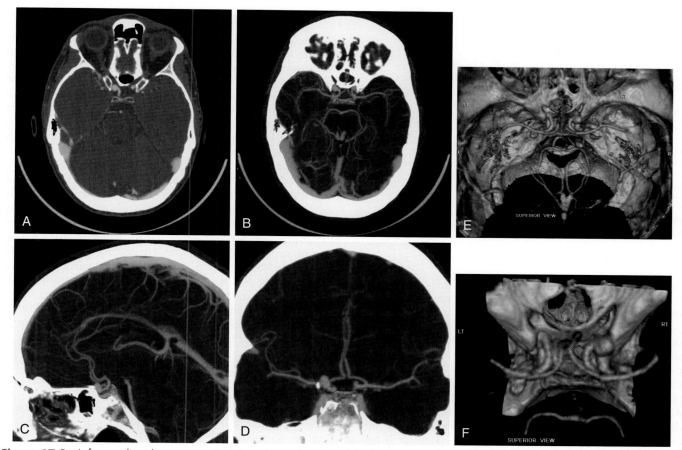

Figure 67-8 Left paraclinoid aneurysm. A, CT angiography scan of the brain in axial section. CT angiography reconstructions demonstrating intracranial vessels in the axial (B), sagittal (C), and coronal (D) sections. E and F, Three-dimensional reconstructions identifying the paraclinoid aneurysm in relation to the surrounding vasculature and bony structures.

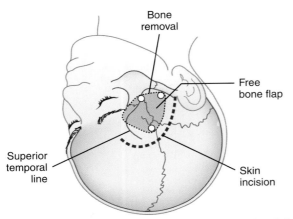

Figure 67-9 Standard pterional craniotomy depicted with location of skin incision, bone flap, and craniotomy. The skin incision is largely behind the hairline but may extend to 1 cm in front of the hairline.

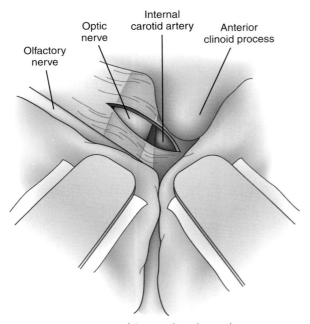

Figure 67-10 Opening of the arachnoid over the optic nerve and the internal carotid artery. With microscissors, a wide opening of the arachnoid is created to allow retraction of the frontal and temporal lobes with undue traction.

to be aware of the fourth nerve, which runs in the fold of the tentorium.

A standard pterional approach is used for surgery. The patient is placed on the operating table with the head slightly turned toward the contralateral shoulder and extended 15 degrees to allow the frontal lobe to fall from the field. The projection of the aneurysm drives the initial dissection. Aneurysms directed laterally or superolaterally are often adherent to the temporal lobe; therefore dissection and retraction are limited to the frontal lobe (Fig. 67-13). Aneurysms projecting posteriorly or inferolaterally are beneath the tentorial edge and unlikely to be adherent to the temporal lobe, so both frontal and temporal retraction can be used.

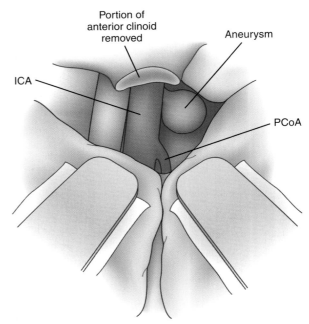

Figure 67-11 Removal of the anterior clinoid process. In an effort to develop adequate exposure, the anterior clinoid process is removed, allowing visualization of the aneurysm dome. The falciform petroclinoid ligament can also interfere with exposure, in which case it can be cut to improve exposure. ICA, internal carotid artery; PCoA, posterior communicating artery.

The arachnoid over the optic nerve, ICA, and medial aspect of the sylvian fissure is first dissected to allow for a wide surgical exposure. Opening the sylvian fissure allows the distal carotid artery at the bifurcation to be visualized. Further dissection along the proximal and distal carotid artery is essential to establish vessel control before further clipping the aneurysm. The plane between the optic nerve and the carotid artery is carefully dissected to establish the inferior and superior aspects of the aneurysm neck. The surgical clip is placed across the neck; a number of clip configurations can be utilized to obliterate the lesion while maintaining the patency of the carotid and posterior communicating artery vessels (Fig. 67-14). After clipping, further dissection is imperative to ensure that the anterior choroidal artery (which may be duplicated), third nerve, thalamoperforators, and PCoA are not occluded or kinked by the blades of the clip. Occlusion of the anterior choroidal artery or perforators is poorly tolerated and leads to infarction. In contrast, occlusion of the PCoA segment may be unavoidable and is tolerated if there is collateral flow to the perforators from the posterior circulation; however, in most cases, the PCoA can be preserved.

Anterior Choroidal Internal Carotid Artery Aneurysms

The anterior choroidal artery stems from the lateral surface of the ICA just distal to the origination of the PCoA, so the hemodynamic factors that lead to aneurysms in the two regions are similar. The choroidal artery proceeds distally along the optic tract, ultimately ending in the choroidal fissure. Anterior choroidal aneurysms often

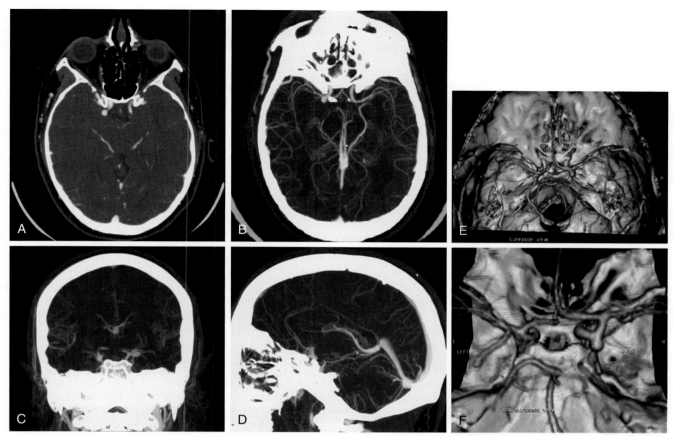

Figure 67-12 Right posterior communicating artery aneurysm. A, CT angiography scan of the brain in axial section. CT angiography reconstructions demonstrating intracranial vessels in the axial (B), sagittal (C), and coronal (D) sections. E and F, Three-dimensional reconstructions identifying the posterior communicating artery aneurysm in relation to the surrounding vasculature and bony structures.

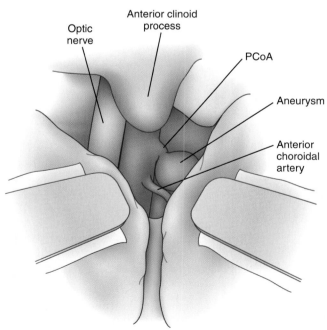

Figure 67-13 Posterior communicating artery (PCoA) aneurysm. The aneurysm dome is depicted projecting laterally into the temporal lobe. As such, frontal lobe retraction is preferred to temporal lobe retraction to avoid damaging the aneurysm dome.

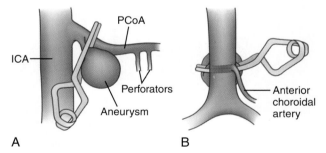

Figure 67-14 Posterior communicating artery aneurysm clipping. Aneurysm clip application for an aneurysm projecting laterally (A) and posteriorly (B). When the aneurysm clip is placed across the aneurysm neck, it is important to separate the neck of the aneurysm from the surrounding vasculature, if possible, so as not to occlude the posterior communicating artery, anterior choroidal artery, or other perforators. ICA, internal carotid artery.

project laterally, superolaterally, and posterolaterally into the temporal lobe and are above the tentorium.

The setup and approach are quite similar to those for PCoA aneurysms; however, the sylvian fissure exposure is extended medially to allow complete visualization of the anterior and middle cerebral arteries at the bifurcation. Anterior choroidal aneurysms often project into the temporal lobe; therefore only frontal lobe retractors are

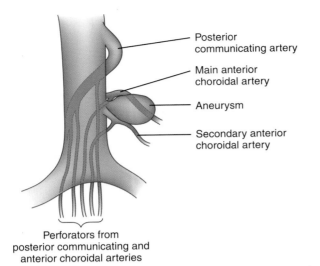

Posterior
communicating artery

Main anterior
choroidal artery

Aneurysm

Secondary anterior
choroidal artery

Perforators from
posterior communicating and
anterior choroidal arteries

Figure 67-15 Anterior choroidal artery aneurysm. When the aneurysm clip is placed across the aneurysm neck, great care must be taken to avoid inadvertently including other vessels, particularly if there is a second anterior choroidal artery, as is drawn in this figure.

used. Upon identification of the anterior choroidal artery, dissection proceeds along the artery medially to its origination from the ICA. The inferior aspect of the aneurysm neck is exposed, allowing for dissection of the superior aspect. Occasionally, there are two or more anterior choroidal arteries. Upon placement of the aneurysm clip, great care must be taken to avoid inadvertently including other vessels, particularly if there is a second anterior choroidal artery (Fig. 67-15). Similarly, caution should be taken in the case of a giant aneurysm because the anterior choroidal artery could be adherent to the aneurysm dome.

Carotid Bifurcation Aneurysms

ICA bifurcation aneurysms project in the direction of terminal carotid flow, either superiorly or posteriorly (Fig. 67-16). When these aneurysms rupture, patients demonstrate SAH and occasionally have a frontal parenchymal clot, which should alert the clinician to aneurysmal rupture. Understanding the projection of the aneurysm dome and its relationship to the anterior and middle cerebral arteries is important in preoperative planning.

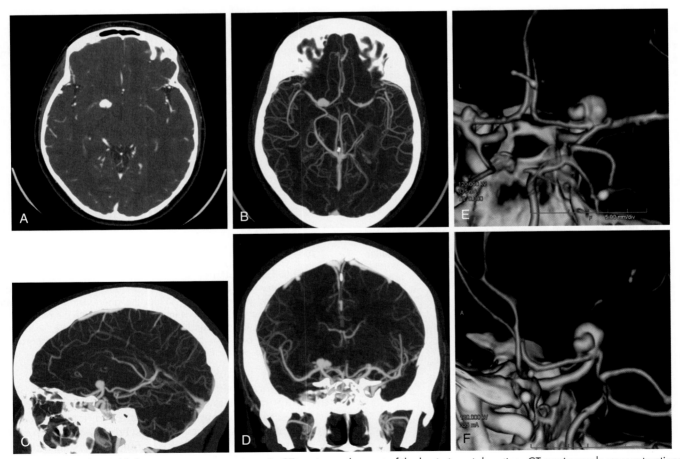

Figure 67-16 Carotid bifurcation artery aneurysm. A, CT angiography scan of the brain in axial section. CT angiography reconstructions demonstrating intracranial vessels in the axial (B), sagittal (C), and coronal (D) sections. E and F, Three-dimensional reconstructions identifying the carotid bifurcation artery aneurysm in relation to the surrounding vasculature and bony structures.

A standard pterional craniotomy is used with the head rotated according to the direction the aneurysm is pointing (Fig. 67-17). Carotid bifurcation aneurysms may point superiorly and medially along the A1 segment. Therefore, the head is rotated 60 degrees as in the approach for an ACoA aneurysm. In contrast, laterally projecting aneurysms course along the MCA into the sylvian fissure and require a 45-degree rotation of the head. Lesions that project distinctly superiorly or posteriorly require a 50-degree rotation of the head to expose the anterior and medial cerebral arteries before the aneurysm neck can be dealt with.

The initial dissection is also determined by the aneurysm projection. Aneurysms that project superiorly into the frontal lobe require a temporal and lateral approach to the internal carotid. Once the ICA is identified, dissection continues along this vessel until the anterior choroidal artery is identified. At this point, the inferior aspect of the anterior and middle cerebral vessels is usually visible. It is essential to expose and define the anterior and middle cerebral arteries prior to dissecting the aneurysm neck to allow for temporary clipping, if needed. The anterior choroidal artery, recurrent artery of Heubner, and branches of the PCoA run posteriorly to the ICA at this level and should not be disturbed. Similarly, venous structures such as the basal vein of Rosenthal and sylvian vein pass posteriorly to the ICA and are equally important. A clip is applied to the aneurysm neck for obliteration with or without the assistance of temporary clips placed on the ICA and/or the anterior and middle cerebral arteries (Fig. 67-18).

Anterior Communicating Artery Aneurysms

ACoA aneurysms arise within the complex of the two anterior cerebral arteries at their anastomosis via the ACoA. They are ensconced by the anterior cerebral arteries and branches leading to a complex and highly variable dissection (Fig. 67-19). ACoA aneurysms can point in any direction, depending on their relationship to the surrounding vasculature that makes up the anterior communicating complex. There is wide variability in the anatomy of the ACoA region. There can be duplications (such as more than one ACoA), deletions (such as only one A2

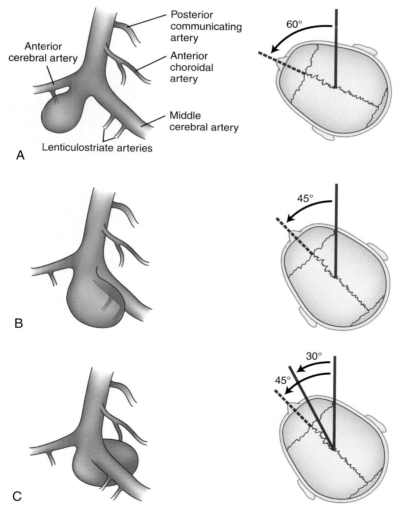

Figure 67-17 Operative positioning depending on internal carotid artery bifurcation aneurysm. A, Medially directed aneurysms require the head to be turned 60 degrees. B, Posteriorly directed aneurysms require 45-degree head turn. C, Inferiorly directed aneurysms require a 30- to 45-degree head turn.

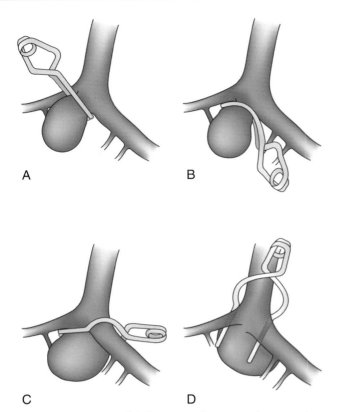

Figure 67-18 Carotid bifurcation clipping techniques. In an effort to occlude the aneurysm neck during reconstruction of the vessel flow, the following surgical clips can be placed: a straight clip (A), a curved clip (B), or a fenestrated clip to avoid occluding the middle cerebral artery (C) or the internal carotid artery (D), depending on the relationship of the aneurysmal dome to the surrounding vasculature.

segment [azygous]), and differences in the number and origins of perforating branches. Despite the marked variability, most ACoA aneurysms are associated with a dominant proximal anterior cerebral artery (A1) segment. Consequently, aneurysms often arise on the dominant side communicating junction and project to the contralateral hemisphere as a continuation of the dominant A1 flow.

In general, the surgeon elects to operate on the side opposite the aneurysm dome; therefore the aneurysm neck is dissected before the aneurysm dome, allowing for proximal control and lower risk of intraoperative rupture (Fig. 67-20). However, if there is a large frontal clot, the surgeon approaches from the side of the clot in order to both evacuate the hemorrhage and clip the aneurysm.

The patient's head is rotated 60 degrees away from the surgical site to allow for a vertical approach. A standard pterional craniotomy is extended to remove additional frontal bone, creating room for a subfrontal approach to both anterior cerebral arteries. The lateral sphenoid ridge is removed to allow a lateral corridor to reach the ipsilateral and contralateral sides of the ACoA complex. Further, the basal cisterns are opened and CSF is drained, promoting brain relaxation. Initial arachnoid dissection starts with the olfactory tract, which is followed to the optic nerve and ultimately the ICA.

Adhesions between the frontal lobe and the temporal lobe sometimes prevent adequate retraction. In this case, the sylvian fissure should be split adequately to detether the frontal lobe. Retractors are carefully applied to separate the frontal lobe from the optic nerve. Great care should be taken during elevation of the frontal lobe in the patient with an inferiorly projecting anterior communicating aneurysm, because the lesion may be inadvertently avulsed. For a superiorly projecting aneurysm, resection of a small portion of the gyrus rectus immediately adjacent to the anterior communicating complex can make visualization and clip placement much easier (Fig. 67-21).

It is imperative to identify the proximal (A1) and distal (A2) branches of both anterior cerebral arteries, the ACoA, the frontopolar branches, and the recurrent arteries of Heubner to both hemispheres prior to final clip placement on the aneurysm neck. Failure to see these vessels and protect them from occlusion can lead to serious neurologic morbidity. Once the ipsilateral A1 segment is identified, the approach differs slightly depending on the projection of the aneurysm dome. Anteriorly projecting aneurysms often block the contralateral A1; therefore the surgeon approaches the vessels in a clockwise fashion as follows: (1) the ipsilateral A1 is followed to the ipsilateral A2, (2) the contralateral A2 is identified, and (3) the contralateral A1 segment is dissected last because this manipulation is associated with the highest risk of aneurysmal rupture. In contrast, posteriorly projecting aneurysms do not obstruct exposure, allowing both A1 segments to be dissected first, and the deeper A2 segments last. Temporary clipping of the parent vessels is encouraged to reduce the risk of intraoperative rupture, particularly in the dissection of the contralateral A1 and A2 segments, which have the greatest risk of rupture during retraction.

Distal Anterior Cerebral Artery Aneurysms

Aneurysms that arise on arteries distal to the ACoA complex are collectively referred to as distal anterior cerebral artery (ACA) aneurysms (Fig. 67-22). Distal ACA aneurysms form at branching points of the artery as it courses over the genu of the corpus callosum, which are (1) the callosomarginal arteries feeding the cingulate sulcus and (2) the pericallosal arteries, which run along the surface of the corpus callosum in the interhemispheric fissure. Ruptured distal ACA aneurysms manifest as SAH and, often, crural monoparesis or contralateral monoparesis from intracerebral hemorrhage.

Distal ACA aneurysms are dissected via an interhemispheric approach. The head is positioned midline in three-point fixation with the head and neck flexed. The bifrontal incision is located behind the hairline and extends laterally as far as needed in each direction to accommodate the bone flap (Fig. 67-23). The craniotomy is typically 2 to 4 cm in size and rectangular, and it remains in front of the coronal suture and extends across the midline. This craniotomy allows for both an anterior and lateral exposure to expose the proximal parent vessels before the aneurysm is encountered. Whenever possible, the nondominant side is preferred.

The dura is opened in a horseshoe fashion and hinged along the edge of the sinus. It is retracted with tacking

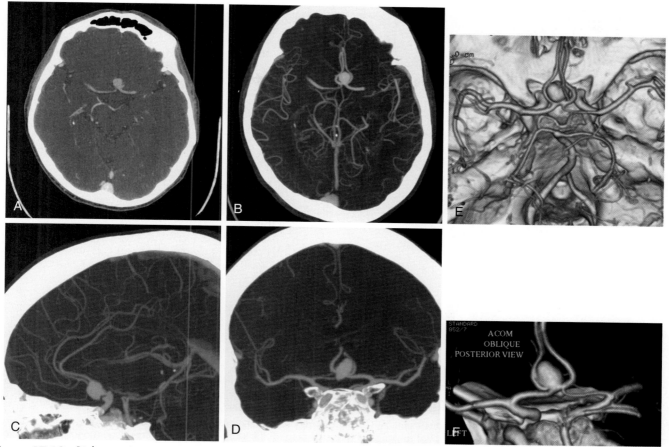

Figure 67-19 Right anterior communicating artery aneurysm. A, CT angiography scan of the brain in axial section. CT angiography reconstructions demonstrating intracranial vessels in the axial (B), sagittal (C), and coronal (D) sections. E and F, Three-dimensional reconstructions identifying the anterior communicating artery aneurysm in relation to the surrounding vasculature and bony structures.

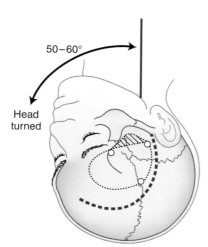

Figure 67-20 Patient positioning for anterior communicating artery aneurysm surgery. In general, the patient's head is rotated 60 degrees to allow the frontal lobe to fall away from the skull base and enable a vertical approach to the aneurysm with the least retraction.

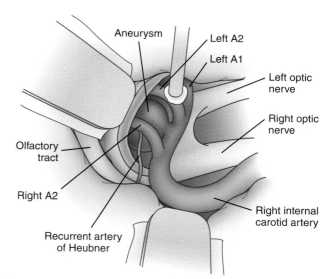

Figure 67-21 Anterior communicating artery complex exposure enhanced after gyrus rectus corticectomy. After a small corticectomy, superior projecting aneurysms and the surrounding anterior communicating artery complex may be better visualized, allowing for easier dissection and clip placement.

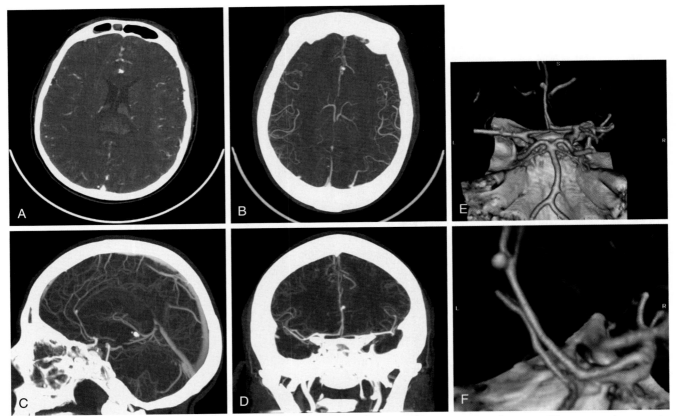

Figure 67-22 Distal anterior cerebral artery aneurysm. A, CT angiography scan of the brain in axial section. CT angiography reconstructions demonstrating intracranial vessels in the axial (B), sagittal (C), and coronal (D) sections. E and F, Three-dimensional reconstructions identifying the distal anterior cerebral artery aneurysm in relation to the surrounding vasculature and bony structures.

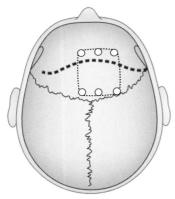

Figure 67-23 Distal anterior cerebral artery aneurysm incision and bone flap. The bifrontal incision is located behind the hairline, extending laterally to allow for exposure of the proximal parent vessels as well as the aneurysm dome.

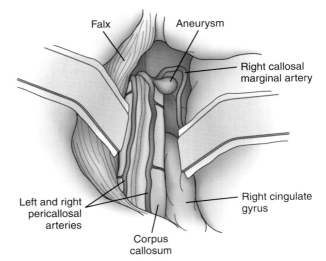

Figure 67-24 Distal anterior cerebral artery aneurysm exposure. Dissection of the interhemispheric fissure and CSF relaxation maximizes the exposure of the anterior circulation arteries. The aneurysm dome can be adherent to parenchyma so proximal vessel control is identified first, before identifying the aneurysm dome.

sutures to maximize midline exposure with minimal frontal lobe retraction. Generally, veins anterior to the coronal suture can be ligated, if needed, without deficit. However, it may be necessary to work between the veins because preservation of these venous structures is preferred. The interhemispheric fissure is carefully dissected while the CSF is drained to maximize relaxation. The operating microscope is used to continue the parasagittal dissection.

The first vessel encountered is often the callosal marginal artery which is followed to the pericallosal artery (Fig. 67-24). Distal ACA aneurysms are often adherent to the parenchyma, and therefore, the dome is avoided until the proximal vessels (which are deep in the dissection) and the aneurysm neck are exposed. Careful dissection along the side of the pericallosal artery eventually allows for visualization and exposure of the parent

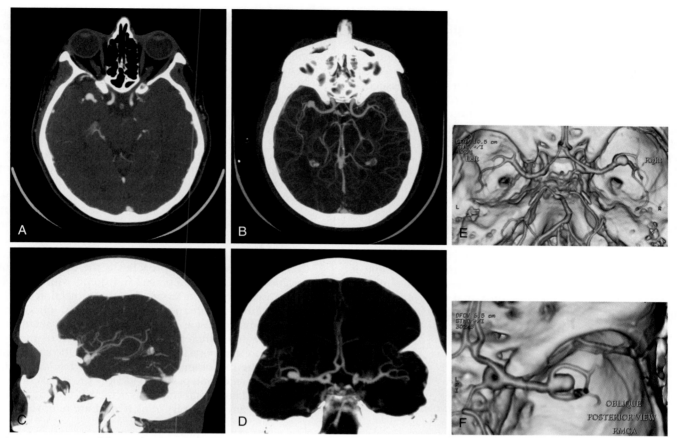

Figure 67-25 Middle cerebral artery aneurysm. A, CT angiography scan of the brain in axial section. CT angiography reconstructions demonstrating intracranial vessels in the axial (B), sagittal (C), and coronal (D) sections. E and F, Three-dimensional reconstructions identifying the middle cerebral artery aneurysm in relation to the surrounding vasculature and bony structures.

vessel proximal to the aneurysm. Upon exposure of both the proximal pericallosal artery and the distal pericallosal branch, the neck is dissected and the surgical clip is placed. Stereotactic navigation to distal ACA aneurysms is preferred by some surgeons.

Middle Cerebral Artery Aneurysms

MCA aneurysms most commonly arise from the bifurcation of the superior and inferior trunks (Fig. 67-25). Additionally, MCA aneurysms can arise from the proximal M1 branch as well as the distal M2/M3 segments (Fig. 67-26). Patients with ruptured MCA aneurysms can have sylvian fissure or anterior temporal lobe hemorrhages, a fact that explains the higher rates of seizure and loss of consciousness with MCA aneurysms than with aneurysms in other locations. Of note, distal aneurysms can be infectious in etiology (mycotic aneurysm), and this diagnosis should be strongly considered if the lesion is more fusiform in appearance.

For surgery of MCA aneurysms, it is important to identify the projection and relationship of the aneurysm dome with the surrounding vasculature. The patient is placed supine with the head rotated 45 degrees to the opposite shoulder. A standard pterional craniotomy is extended posteriorly to provide adequate exposure to the parent and distal branch vessels (Fig. 67-27). There are three commonly used surgical approaches, the

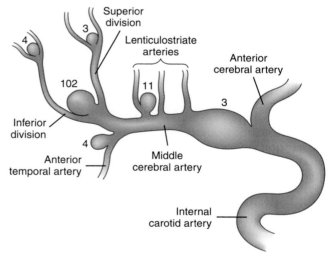

Figure 67-26 Frequency and distribution of middle cerebral artery aneurysms over an 8-year interval.

medial transsylvian, lateral transsylvian, and superior temporal gyrus.

The *medial transsylvian approach* is best tailored for aneurysms located between the proximal M1 trunk and the bifurcation. It is the most commonly used approach, largely because of the high incidence of aneurysms arising from this location. The medial aspect of the sylvian fissure is dissected under the microscope until the origin of the MCA is identified. The proximal MCA is exposed and followed distally until the aneurysm neck is identified. M1 segment aneurysms are quite close to the lenticulostriate arteries, which must not be injured during the dissection or clipping of these aneurysms (Fig. 67-28). Bifurcation aneurysms require additional dissection along the sylvian fissure in order to identify the two or three divisions of the MCA and ultimately the aneurysm neck. Temporary clipping, if needed, can be applied to the distal MCA because it is beyond the lenticulostriate arteries, therefore minimizing the risk of infarction.

The *lateral transsylvian approach* is reserved for distal MCA aneurysms because the sylvian fissure is opened peripherally, avoiding medial dissection and retraction. The initial step involves identifying the distal MCA branch and dissecting along it until the aneurysm is encountered. Unfortunately, in this approach the aneurysm dome is encountered prior to exposure of the proximal parent vessels and establishment of proximal control. As such, upon identifying the aneurysm, the surgeon must dissect

beyond it to establish proximal vessel exposure. Although this approach is less invasive initially, the risk of encountering the aneurysm prior to obtaining proximal control coupled with the additional dissection deep to the aneurysm must be carefully weighed.

The *superior temporal gyrus* approach is ideal for MCA bifurcation aneurysms (Fig. 67-29) that project laterally or when there is a temporal lobe hematoma. The patient is placed supine and the head is rotated approximately 70 degrees to the opposite shoulder. Rather than starting the dissection in the sylvian fissure, the surgeon makes incision in the superior temporal gyrus 1 cm behind the front of the sylvian fissure. The dissection continues until the major division of the MCA branch is identified, at which point the dissection is turned medially along the vessel (Fig. 67-30). As in the lateral transsylvian approach, the aneurysm dome is encountered first and must be carefully passed in order to expose the proximal vasculature for control.

Common to the three approaches is the importance of the relationship of the aneurysm and dome with the surrounding vasculature. Understanding the projection of the aneurysm allows for preoperative planning and intraoperative adjustments to best approach the neck of the aneurysm and avoid the dome, therefore decreasing the risk of intraoperative rupture. Temporary clipping can soften the aneurysm and reduce the risk of aneurysmal rupture while the aneurysm is manipulated and passed to identify proximal control. Once proximal and distal control is achieved, the aneurysm is clipped and any temporary clips, if used, are removed.

Giant Aneurysms

Intracranial aneurysms more than 25 mm in diameter are referred to as giant aneurysms; they arise both in the anterior and posterior circulations. These aneurysms often develop thrombus within the dome as well as atherosclerosis and calcifications within the neck and fundus. The decision to treat asymptomatic giant aneurysms depends on patient and aneurysm specifics, as with nongiant aneurysms. Symptomatic aneurysms should undergo treatment

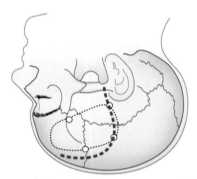

Figure 67-27 Middle cerebral artery aneurysm. The incision and bone flap are extended posteriorly from a standard pterional craniotomy to allow for adequate exposure to the parent and distal branch vessels.

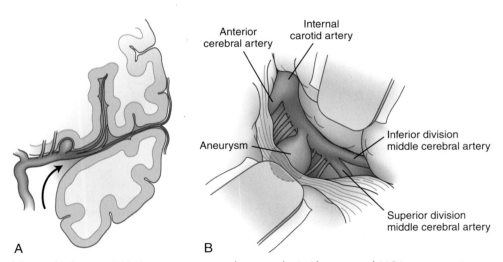

Figure 67-28 Middle cerebral artery (MCA) aneurysm surgical approach. A, The proximal MCA aneurysm is approached by opening the sylvian fissure, following the internal carotid artery (ICA) to the MCA, and then following the MCA distally to the M1 segment. B, Surgical view. The sylvian fissure is opened medially, and retractors are placed in the frontal and temporal lobes to splay the fissure. Upon successful exposure of the proximal and distal vessels, a clip is applied to the aneurysm neck without necessarily exposing the aneurysm dome.

because the mass effect and associated edema can lead to permanent neurologic dysfunction. In addition, rupture risks of giant aneurysm are high.[6] The surgical and endovascular therapies are extremely challenging, and careful consideration must be given to the location of a giant aneurysm and its relationship to the parent vessel and collateral circulation.

Patient positioning for surgery of giant aneurysms is similar to that for surgery of nongiant aneurysms, according to the location of the aneurysm. Owing to the risk of rupture and occasional difficulty in clipping, great care must be taken to establish proximal control. For example, with paraclinoid aneurysms, the neck is prepared and draped in the operative field for immediate access to the carotid artery. The surgical approach depends on the location of the aneurysm, with the goal to establish proximal control as mentioned earlier. If the aneurysm is not amenable to straightforward clipping, the surgeon can use a number of different options such as temporary clipping, aneurysm dome decompression, occlusion of the proximal artery and vessel bypass.

Owing to their size and orientation, giant aneurysms often require special clipping methods to achieve occlusion and reconstruction of the vasculature. Surgical clips can be placed in a variety of orientations, such as side by side or at oblique angles when one clip does not suffice. Furthermore, long surgical clips are used for broad necks or for an aneurysm in a location that restricts the application of a short clip. It is imperative to fully occlude the aneurysm because any residual is at substantial risk for recurrence and rupture. Finally, aneurysms resistant to clipping because of atherosclerosis or calcification of the neck can be occluded with a booster clip. In this method, the initial clip is placed and a second clip is placed over the first to increase the force generated by the first clip so as to close the tips.

The sheer size of giant aneurysms can obstruct the surgical view and prevent visualization of the aneurysm's microenvironment. As with all aneurysm surgery, it is imperative to establish proximal control and identify the relationship of collateral blood vessels. In these circumstances, a 19-gauge needle can be introduced into the

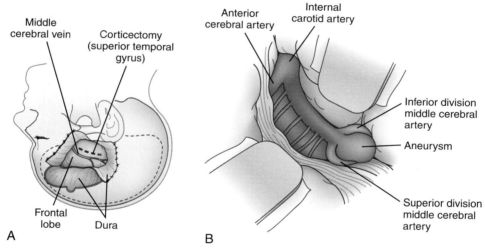

Figure 67-29 Middle cerebral artery (MCA) bifurcation aneurysm. A, The superior temporal gyrus approach is ideal for bifurcation aneurysms of the MCA that point laterally. The incision is made 1 cm behind the sylvian fissure. B, Once the MCA branch is identified, it can be dissected to expose the proximal and distal vessels to the aneurysm dome.

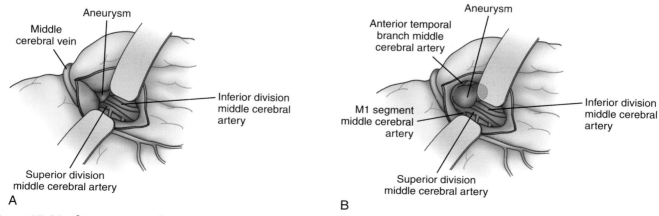

Figure 67-30 Superior temporal gyrus approach. A, Upon entry to the sylvian fissure, the middle cerebral artery branches are identified. B, The branches are then dissected until the aneurysm neck and proximal vessels are exposed.

aneurysm dome to remove obstruction by suction decompression. It is imperative to occlude proximal and especially distal flow with temporary clips to avoid stealing collateral circulation during suctioning. Temporary proximal artery occlusion using temporary clips allows the surgeon to isolate the aneurysm and control blood flow in the event of an aneurysmal rupture. As mentioned earlier the duration of temporary arterial occlusion should be minimized to avoid neurologic deficit.

Giant aneurysms that are not amenable to surgical clipping or endovascular coiling can be treated with permanent occlusion of the proximal vessel and vessel bypass. Prior to any procedure, it is essential to perform a thorough evaluation of the proximal and distal vasculature using CT angiography. Equally as important, one must perform carotid occlusion studies to establish whether the patient would tolerate carotid artery occlusion. In general, when performing an extracranial-to-intracranial (EC-IC) bypass graft, we prefer to use saphenous vein from the cervical carotid artery to the MCA. This graft allows for high-flow hemispheric perfusion.

Postoperative Management

The monitoring and treatment of SAH-induced vasospasm is discussed elsewhere in the text.

Cerebrospinal Fluid Management

Once a ruptured aneurysm is treated, risk of rerupture is thus eliminated and the external EVD can be opened to drain the blood products in the CSF. In general, the EVD is positioned 10 cm above the external acoustic meatus (EAM) and kept there until the CSF output is less than 60 to 80 mL per day, when it can be slowly raised by 5 cm per day during testing for new neurologic deficits. Once the EVD is at 20 cm above the EAM, it is clamped for 24 hours and is opened only if the ICP is greater than 20 cm H_2O or if the patient demonstrates new neurologic deficits. The EVD is removed once the ICP has been 20 cm H_2O or lower for 24 hours and if a CT scan of the head does not demonstrate ventriculomegaly. EVD removal is delayed in patients with active vasospasm in order to allow for continuous ICP monitoring.

Patients who demonstrate either radiographic evidence of or neurologic findings consistent with hydrocephalus often fail the EVD wean and require permanent CSF diversion with a ventriculoperitoneal (VP) shunt. Unfortunately, many patients do not exhibit signs of hydrocephalus until weeks after SAH; therefore the clinician should have a low threshold for obtaining a CT scan of the head or lumbar puncture to assess for it. Radiographic evidence of hydrocephalus (ventriculomegaly, periventricular edema) or a change in neurologic findings (somnolence, neurologic deficits) should prompt evaluation for VP shunt.

Often the ventriculostomy catheter is maintained for weeks; therefore meticulous sterile technique upon placement and tunneling of the catheter a minimum of 4 cm subcutaneously from the incision minimize risk of infection. Prophylactic antibiotics (nafcillin) are initiated prior to incision and continued while the drain is in place. Additionally, the catheter is connected to a drainage system that prevents direct contact during zeroing or for obtaining CSF samples. As monitoring of the shunt, some authorities recommend routine sampling of CSF samples for cell counts and Gram staining and culture, whereas others recommend reserving sampling of CSF only for fever, leukocytosis, or other nonspecific signs of infection.[47-50] Although blood in the subarachnoid space can lead to vasospasm, CSF diversion techniques have been largely unsuccessful in reducing vasospasm. To date, efforts such as cisternal irrigation and combined EVD and lumbar drain placement have produced inconclusive and irreproducible results.

REFERENCES

1. Drake CG: Earlier times in aneurysm surgery, *Clin Neurosurg* 32:41-50, 1985.
2. Cushing H: The control of bleeding in operations for brain tumors. With the description of silver "clips" for the occlusion of vessels inaccessible to the ligature, *Ann Surg* 54:1-19, 1911.
3. Dandy W: Intracranial aneurysm of the internal carotid artery. Cured by operation, *Ann Surg* 107:654-659, 1938.
4. Guglielmi G, Vinuela F, Dion J, Duckwiler G: Electrothrombosis of saccular aneurysms via endovascular approach. Part 2: Preliminary clinical experience, *J Neurosurg* 75:8-14, 1991.
5. Guglielmi G, Vinuela F, Sepetka I, Macellari V: Electrothrombosis of saccular aneurysms via endovascular approach. Part 1: Electrochemical basis, technique, and experimental results, *J Neurosurg* 75:1-7, 1991.
6. Unruptured intracranial aneurysms—risk of rupture and risks of surgical intervention: International Study of Unruptured Intracranial Aneurysms Investigators, *N Engl J Med* 339:1725-1733, 1998.
7. Bederson JB, Awad IA, Wiebers DO, Piepgras D, Haley EC Jr, Brott T, et al: Recommendations for the management of patients with unruptured intracranial aneurysms: a statement for healthcare professionals from the Stroke Council of the American Heart Association, *Stroke* 31:2742-2750, 2000.
8. Wiebers DO, Whisnant JP, Huston J III, et al: Unruptured intracranial aneurysms: Natural history, clinical outcome, and risks of surgical and endovascular treatment, *Lancet* 362:103-110, 2003.
9. Komotar RJ, Mocco J, Solomon RA: Guidelines for the surgical treatment of unruptured intracranial aneurysms: The first annual J. Lawrence Pool Memorial Research Symposium—controversies in the management of cerebral aneurysms, *Neurosurgery* 62:183-193, 2008:discussion 193-184.
10. Bor AS, Velthuis BK, Majoie CB, Rinkel GJ: Configuration of intracranial arteries and development of aneurysms: A follow-up study, *Neurology* 70:700-705, 2008.
11. Kassell NF, Torner JC, Haley EC Jr, et al: The International Cooperative Study on the Timing of Aneurysm Surgery. Part 1: Overall management results, *J Neurosurg* 73:18-36, 1990.
12. Juvela S, Porras M, Heiskanen O: Natural history of unruptured intracranial aneurysms: a long-term follow-up study, *J Neurosurg* 79:174-182, 1993.
13. Juvela S, Porras M, Poussa K: Natural history of unruptured intracranial aneurysms: probability of and risk factors for aneurysm rupture, *J Neurosurg* 93:379-387, 2000.
14. Juvela S, Porras M, Poussa K: Natural history of unruptured intracranial aneurysms: Probability of and risk factors for aneurysm rupture, *J Neurosurg* 108:1052-1060, 2008.
15. Morita A, Fujiwara S, Hashi K, Ohtsu H, Kirino T: Risk of rupture associated with intact cerebral aneurysms in the Japanese population: A systematic review of the literature from Japan, *J Neurosurg* 102:601-606, 2005.
16. Rinkel GJ, Djibuti M, Algra A, van Gijn J: Prevalence and risk of rupture of intracranial aneurysms: A systematic review, *Stroke* 29:251-256, 1998.
17. Yasargil MG, Fox JL: The microsurgical approach to Intracranial aneurysms, *Surg Neurol* 3:7-14, 1975.
18. Batjer H, Samson D: Intraoperative aneurysmal rupture: Incidence, outcome, and suggestions for surgical management, *Neurosurgery* 18:701-707, 1986.

19. McDermott MW, Durity FA, Borozny M, Mountain MA: Temporary vessel occlusion and barbiturate protection in cerebral aneurysm surgery, *Neurosurgery* 25:54-61, 1989:discussion 61-52.

20. Mizoi K, Yoshimoto T: Permissible temporary occlusion time in aneurysm surgery as evaluated by evoked potential monitoring, *Neurosurgery* 33:434-440, 1993:discussion 440.

21. Ogilvy CS, Carter BS, Kaplan S, 50-degree rotation of the head to expose the anterior and medical cerebral arteries: Temporary vessel occlusion for aneurysm surgery: Risk factors for stroke in patients protected by induced hypothermia and hypertension and intravenous mannitol administration, *J Neurosurg* 84:785-791, 1996.

22. Samson D, Batjer HH, Bowman G, et al: A clinical study of the parameters and effects of temporary arterial occlusion in the management of intracranial aneurysms, *Neurosurgery* 34:22-28, 1994:discussion 28-29.

23. Lavine SD, Masri LS, Levy ML, Giannotta SL: Temporary occlusion of the middle cerebral artery in intracranial aneurysm surgery: Time limitation and advantage of brain protection, *J Neurosurg* 87:817-824, 1997.

24. Selman WR, Spetzler RF: Therapeutics for focal cerebral ischemia, *Neurosurgery* 6:446-452, 1980.

25. Selman WR, Spetzler RF, Anton AH, Crumrine RC: Management of prolonged therapeutic barbiturate coma, *Surg Neurol* 15:9-10, 1981.

26. Selman WR, Spetzler RF, Roessmann UR, et al: Barbiturate-induced coma therapy for focal cerebral ischemia. Effect after temporary and permanent MCA occlusion, *J Neurosurg* 55:220-226, 1981.

27. Selman WR, Spetzler RF, Wilson CB, Grollmus JW: Percutaneous lumboperitoneal shunt: Review of 130 cases, *Neurosurgery* 6:255-257, 1980.

28. Stein SC, Burnett MG, Zager EL, et al: Completion angiography for surgically treated cerebral aneurysms: An economic analysis, *Neurosurgery* 61:1162-1167, 2007:discussion 1167-1169.

29. Alexander TD, Macdonald RL, Weir B, Kowalczuk A: Intraoperative angiography in cerebral aneurysm surgery: A prospective study of 100 craniotomies, *Neurosurgery* 39:10-17, 1996:discussion 17-18.

30. Chiang VL, Gailloud P, Murphy KJ, et al: Routine intraoperative angiography during aneurysm surgery, *J Neurosurg* 96:988-992, 2002.

31. de Oliveira JG, Beck J, Seifert V, et al: Assessment of flow in perforating arteries during intracranial aneurysm surgery using intraoperative near-infrared indocyanine green videoangiography, *Neurosurgery* 61:63-72, 2007:discussion 72-63.

32. Derdeyn CP, Moran CJ, Cross DT III, et al: Intracranial aneurysm: anatomic factors that predict the usefulness of intraoperative angiography, *Radiology* 205:335-339, 1997.

33. Klopfenstein JD, Spetzler RF, Kim LJ, et al: Comparison of routine and selective use of intraoperative angiography during aneurysm surgery: A prospective assessment, *J Neurosurg* 100:230-235, 2004.

34. Lopez KA, Waziri AE, et al: Clinical usefulness and safety of routine intraoperative angiography for patients and personnel, *Neurosurgery* 61:724-729, 2007:discussion 729-730.

35. Origitano TC, Schwartz K, Anderson D, et al: Optimal clip application and intraoperative angiography for intracranial aneurysms, *Surg Neurol* 51:117-124, 1999:discussion124-118.

36. Tang G, Cawley CM, Dion JE, Barrow DL: Intraoperative angiography during aneurysm surgery: A prospective evaluation of efficacy, *J Neurosurg* 96:993-999, 2002.

37. Batjer HH, Kopitnik TA, Giller CA, Samson DS: Surgery for paraclinoidal carotid artery aneurysms, *J Neurosurg* 80:650-658, 1994.

38. Cawley CM, Zipfel GJ, Day AL: Surgical treatment of paraclinoid and ophthalmic aneurysms, *Neurosurg Clin North Am* 9:765-783, 1998.

39. Chen F, Oikawa S, Hiraku Y, et al: Metal-mediated oxidative DNA damage induced by nitro-2-aminophenols, *Cancer Lett* 126:67-74, 1998.

40. Day AL: Aneurysms of the ophthalmic segment. A clinical and anatomical analysis, *J Neurosurg* 72:677-691, 1990.

41. Day AL: Clinicoanatomic features of supraclinoid aneurysms, *Clin Neurosurg* 36:256-274, 1990.

42. Gibo H, Lenkey C, Rhoton AL Jr: Microsurgical anatomy of the supraclinoid portion of the internal carotid artery, *J Neurosurg* 55:560-574, 1981.

43. Heros RC, Nelson PB, Ojemann RG, Crowell RM, DeBrun G: Large and giant paraclinoid aneurysms: Surgical techniques, complications, and results, *Neurosurgery* 12:153-163, 1983.

44. Oikawa S, Kyoshima K, Kobayashi S: Surgical anatomy of the juxtadural ring area, *J Neurosurg* 89:250-254, 1998.

45. Dolenc VV: A combined epi- and subdural direct approach to carotid-ophthalmic artery aneurysms, *J Neurosurg* 62:667-672, 1985.

46. Pikus HJ, Heros RC: Surgical treatment of internal carotid and posterior communicating artery aneurysms, *Neurosurg Clin N Am* 9:785-795, 1998.

47. Hader WJ, Steinbok P: The value of routine cultures of the cerebrospinal fluid in patients with external ventricular drains, *Neurosurgery* 46:1149-1153, 2000:discussion 1153-1145.

48. Holloway KL, Barnes T, Choi S, et al: Ventriculostomy infections: the effect of monitoring duration and catheter exchange in 584 patients, *J Neurosurg* 85:419-424, 1996.

49. Lyke KE, Obasanjo OO, Williams MA, et al: Ventriculitis complicating use of intraventricular catheters in adult neurosurgical patients, *Clin Infect Dis* 33:2028-2033, 2001.

50. Rebuck JA, Murry KR, Rhoney DH, Michael DB, Coplin WM: Infection related to intracranial pressure monitors in adults: Analysis of risk factors and antibiotic prophylaxis, *J Neurol Neurosurg Psychiatry* 69:381-384, 2000.

68 Surgical Management of Posterior Circulation Aneurysms

MARK J. DANNENBAUM, ROSE DU, ARTHUR L. DAY

Posterior circulation saccular aneurysms are less common than their anterior circulation counterparts, accounting for approximately 15% of all intracranial aneurysms.[1] They most commonly occur in the upper basilar artery at the basilar apex (7%), followed by those of the basilar-superior cerebellar artery (SCA) (2%) and vertebral-posterior inferior cerebellar artery (PICA) regions (1.8%).[2] As a group, posterior circulation aneurysms appear to have a significantly higher rate of rupture when small (<1 cm) than those arising in the anterior circulation.[3]

In contrast, nonsaccular or fusiform aneurysms occur much more frequently in the vertebrobasilar system than in the anterior circulation. Those that occur at the vertebral artery (VA) independent of the PICA origin are nearly always dissections and carry with them a high risk of intracranial hemorrhage when they form and a high rate of early rebleeding thereafter.[4-7]

As endovascular technologies have evolved, a paradigm shift has occurred in the treatment of most posterior circulation aneurysms. Currently, the primary means of treatment for the majority of posterior circulation aneurysms at most centers is via an endovascular route. Many, however, cannot be treated by current endovascular methodology, and microsurgical management is warranted. Open microsurgical treatment still holds great value in the treatment of many of these lesions, particularly when performed by surgeons experienced in posterior fossa and skull base approaches.[8-13] This chapter discusses the technical considerations in microsurgical clipping for the most common posterior circulation aneurysm sites.

Selection Criteria for Surgical Treatment

Site-specific anatomic and technical details as well as the clinical condition of the patient should form the basis of the decision whether an individual aneurysm should be treated by endovascular or microsurgical means. Patients with poor clinical grade following hemorrhage (as defined by Hunt and Hess Scale score ≥3), those with radiographically or clinically evident vasospasm, or those with high medical morbidity risks are generally considered better candidates for endovascular therapy.[14] Following subarachnoid hemorrhage, the posterior fossa contents and vasculature are often more sensitive to the microsurgical manipulation required for successful aneurysm obliteration. When this sensitivity is combined with the increased technical difficulty often required, the perioperative course and postoperative outcomes are more frequently suboptimal in comparison with those of endovascular treatments. In the nonruptured aneurysm, however, such heightened sensitivity is not as problematic.

Many aneurysms, however, cannot be managed effectively by endovascular means, either because of restricted vascular access or because the shape, size, or other anatomic considerations of the aneurysm are not ideal for such methodology. In such circumstances, open microsurgical obliteration remains a highly effective treatment when performed by a surgeon knowledgeable in and experienced with such approaches and techniques.

Surgical Approaches to the Terminal Basilar Bifurcation (Basilar Apex)

Aneurysms in the basilar apex region, which includes those that arise within the interpeduncular cistern and originate from the terminal basilar bifurcation, the posterior cerebral artery (PCA)/SCA junction, and the proximal P1 segment, represent some of the most difficult technical challenges in neurosurgery (Fig. 68-1). In addition, as endovascular techniques improve, those basilar apex aneurysms referred for surgical treatment are becoming increasingly complex.

The surgeon must be familiar with the microsurgical anatomy of the basilar apex and interpeduncular cistern (IPC) to be successful. The interpeduncular cistern is a midline, unpaired structure that represents the confluence of the supra and infratentorial subarachnoid spaces. It is separated from the chiasmatic cistern by Lilliequist's membrane. This cistern is demarcated by four borders—the clivus and posterior clinoid processes anteriorly, the mesial temporal lobes and tentorial edges laterally, the cerebral peduncles posteriorly, and the mamillary bodies and posterior perforated substances superiorly.

In addition to the basilar apex, the interpeduncular cistern contains the proximal PCA and SCA, the medial posterior choroidal and thalamogeniculate arteries, the basal vein of Rosenthal, and the oculomotor nerve. The basilar bifurcation is most often located at the level of the pontomesencephalic junction. Its location, however, may range from 10 mm below the pontomesencephalic

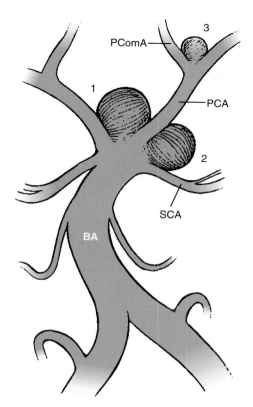

Figure 68-1 Terminal basilar bifurcation aneurysms: type 1 = basilar artery (BA) apex; type 2 = superior cerebellar artery (SCA)–posterior cerebral artery (PCA) junction; type 3 = proximal PCA and/or PCA–posterior communicating artery (PcomA) junction.

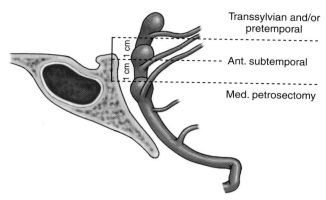

Figure 68-2 The relationship between basilar apex location, posterior clinoid process, and choice of surgical approach.

junction to as rostrally as the mamillary bodies. The basilar apex can be found within 1 cm of the dorsum sella in 87% of patients,[15,16] arising below the dorsum sella in 19% of specimens, at the level of the dorsum sella in 51%, and above it in 30% (Fig. 68-2).

The upper 5 mm of the basilar artery is a source of multiple perforators that generally arise from the posterior and lateral aspects of the parent vessel. Most of these perforators enter the midbrain or pons near the midline; more lateral circumferential branches terminate in the lateral pons, peduncle, and posterior perforated substance.[17] Perforating vessels that arise from the superior and posterior aspects of the P1 segment are termed the posterior thalamoperforators, and they supply the interpeduncular fossa, mamillary bodies, cerebral peduncle, and posterior mesencephalon (Fig. 68-3). Those perforators that arise from the posterior communicating (PcomA) artery are termed the anterior thalamoperforators, and they supply the thalamus, posterior limb of the internal capsule, hypothalamus, subthalamus, substantia nigra, red nucleus, and the oculomotor and trochlear nuclei. The long and short circumflex arteries are brainstem perforators that arise from the distal P1 and proximal P2 segments. The long circumflex arteries supply the quadrigeminal plate, peduncle, geniculate bodies, and tegmentum, whereas the short circumflex vessels pass only a short distance around the perimeter of the brainstem and also supply the peduncle and tegmentum.[17]

The three major surgical approaches to the basilar apex are as follows (1) transsylvian (frontotemporal or pterional), (2) anterior subtemporal, and (3) temporopolar (Fig. 68-4). By nature of their size, anatomy, and location on the terminal bifurcation, some basilar apex aneurysms are more complicated; for safe treatment of these lesions, several modifications have been developed that provide increased exposure. The basic microsurgical approaches to the basilar apex and the factors that determine selection of the optimal approach along with modifications to enhance exposure, so as to allow the surgeon to achieve complete aneurysm obliteration while minimizing risk of brain injury, are discussed here.

Transsylvian (Frontotemporal or Pterional) Approach

The pterional or transsylvian approach to the upper basilar artery (see Fig. 68-5), first advocated by Yasargil et al,[18] was applied to lesions at this site because the basilar bifurcation usually lies only 15 to 17 mm posterior to the intracranial internal carotid artery. A wide incision in the membrane of Lilliequist provides visualization of the basilar apex and the origins of the superior cerebellar and posterior cerebral arteries. Advantages of this approach are its general familiarity to most neurosurgeons, minimal temporal lobe retraction, and less manipulation and injury to the oculomotor nerves. This approach also allows concurrent anterior circulation aneurysms to be clipped during the same procedure.

Several major disadvantages accompany the transsylvian approach. The operative field is deeper and narrower, and visualization may be further impeded by the posterior clinoid process or the internal carotid artery (ICA), its branches, or perforators. The anterosuperior approach to the apex makes visualization and separation of perforators adherent to the posterior aneurysm wall difficult and hazardous. Posterior projecting aneurysms can be quite problematic. Other disadvantages include a limited space and direction for final clip application, and greater difficulty in placing a proximal temporary clip, particularly with low-lying bifurcations.

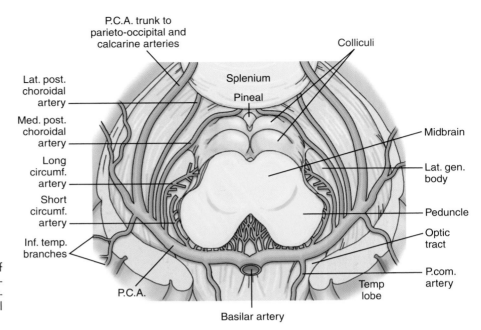

Figure 68-3 Schematic representation of the microsurgical anatomy of the interpeduncular fossa and perforators in the basilar apex region. P.C.A., posterior cerebral artery.

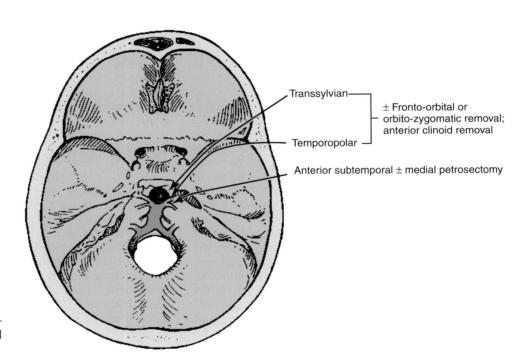

Figure 68-4 Terminal basilar bifurcation aneurysms: surgical approaches (and modifications).

Head Position and Fixation

After induction of general anesthesia, the patient is positioned on a standard operating table. To provide secure fixation without obstruction of the operative field, a radiolucent skull fixation apparatus is applied, during which the blood pressure is carefully monitored and controlled to avoid significant elevations that might precipitate aneurysm rupture. The head is then gently directed vertex down (to facilitate gravitational retraction on the frontal and temporal lobes), elevated slightly higher than the heart (to facilitate venous drainage), and turned 30 to 45 degrees to the left. A roll beneath the ipsilateral shoulder is often useful in allowing gentle neck turning without excessive torque on the airway or cervical vascular structures.

Scalp Incision and Craniotomy

The scalp incision begins at the midline and curves backward and downward just behind the hairline to end at the zygoma 1 cm anterior to the tragus. The temporalis muscle and fascia are reflected posteriorly and inferiorly (interfascial technique), and the desired exposure is maintained with the liberal use of low-profile fishhook retractors.[19] This technique of temporalis mobilization carries a risk of frontalis nerve injury, but the greatly enhanced basal visualization is especially advantageous.

A free bone flap is elevated centered basally around the pterion and sphenoid ridge. The remaining portions of the lateral sphenoid wing and the anterior-inferior temporal squama are removed with the rongeur, with application of bone wax as needed to control osseous bleeding. The medial extension of the sphenoid ridge is removed to leave only a thin rim of superior and lateral posterior orbital wall down to the base of the anterior clinoid process.

Intradural Dissection

The dura is opened in a semicircular fashion over the sylvian fissure, with its base on the drilled-down portion of the sphenoid ridge. A tight brain can be relaxed with hyperventilation, mannitol, or cerebrospinal fluid (CSF) removal through the exposed cisterns, lumbar drain, or ventriculostomy. Brain monitoring with somatosensory evoked potentials is continued throughout the procedure. The sylvian fissure is opened in a lateral-to-medial direction, beginning approximately 2 to 3 cm posterior to the sphenoid ridge on the frontal lobe side of the sylvian veins. This path is continued medially with gentle forceps spreading until the M2 branches of the middle cerebral artery (MCA) are encountered within the insular compartment of the sylvian fissure. The M2 branches are then followed proximally to the genu, and the fissure is opened further in an "inside-to-outside" direction to expose the entire M1 segment and ICA. The basal cisterns surrounding the ICA and optic nerves are opened to further relax and broaden the operative exposure. When the procedure is completed, the frontal and temporal lobes fall away from the sphenoid ridge and orbital roof, and are gently held apart by retractors placed parallel to the brain surface. A broad view of basal structures is provided, without sacrifice of the sphenoparietal veins.

Approaches to the Interpeduncular Cistern

Three routes may be used to access the interpeduncular cistern. The anatomy of the individual patient dictates which approach is most beneficial. The intervals of access are: (1) between the ICA and oculomotor nerve—the carotid-oculomotor interval, (2) between the ICA and optic nerve—the opticocarotid interval, and (3) above the ICA bifurcation (Fig. 68-5). All three routes are at least partially dissected to gain a better conceptualization of the underlying anatomy. In most cases, the best working exposure is achieved through the carotid-oculomotor interval, although in patients with a high basilar bifurcation and a short supraclinoid ICA, the route above the carotid bifurcation may be more advantageous.

The PcomA is identified and followed to and through Lilliequist's membrane to the ipsilateral P1/P2 junction. The oculomotor nerve (cranial nerve [CN] III) and SCA are identified and dissected free of their medial arachnoid attachments, creating enough space to allow the anterior-inferior margin of the P1 segment to be followed proximally. Once the P1 origin is reached, the aneurysm neck becomes visible. The basilar apex is now carefully

exposed, including the origin of the contralateral P1 and a site for a temporary clip below the SCA origins (where there are no perforators). The base of the aneurysm is then dissected, with careful delineation of the relationship of the perforators to the aneurysm. Perforators arising laterally and anteriorly are usually easily separated, but perforators adherent to the posterior wall are often very difficult to visualize and dissect. To separate and preserve these critical vessels, the aneurysm sac must often be displaced laterally and anteriorly, an important maneuver that is hazardous and often best done with use of barbiturate burst suppression and temporary basilar occlusion. Each perforator must be completely free and excluded from the clip.

Modifications to Enhance Pterional Exposure

The "transcavernous-transsellar" modification as described by Dolenc et al[20] was designed to overcome the two major limitations of the standard transsylvian route. In this modification, a standard pterional craniotomy is performed. Alternatively, a frontoorbitozygomatic craniotomy can provide additional exposure, particularly to a high bifurcation. After the lateral sphenoid ridge is removed, a high-speed drill is used to thin the lateral wall of the orbit until the periorbita becomes visible. The posterior lateral orbital wall and roof are removed; both the optic canal and superior orbital fissure are unroofed, and the anterior clinoid process can be removed extradurally. Any cavernous sinus bleeding is easily controlled with gelatin sponge (Gelfoam) or absorbable cellulose fabric (Surgicel).

After the dura is opened in a semicircular fashion based on the exposed periorbita, the sylvian fissure is split in a lateral-to-medial direction, followed by a wide opening of the basal cisterns surrounding the ICA, optic nerve, and oculomotor nerves. The falciform ligament over the optic canal is cut, and the dura over the optic nerve opened in a longitudinal manner along the nerve's lateral margin. The dural ring around the ICA is incised in a circumferential manner, allowing medial mobilization of the ICA and optic nerve. Similarly, the dura that forms the lateral wall of the cavernous sinus is incised, allowing the third nerve to be mobilized and retracted laterally. The space lateral to the carotid artery has now broadened significantly, increasing the exposure for the approach to the basilar apex.

The membrane of Lilliequist is opened, and the dissection of the interpeduncular cisterns proceeds as with the transsylvian approach. If the bifurcation is low and the basilar aneurysm not easily seen or dissected, the posterior clinoid process can be removed for increased exposure. The diaphragma sellae is divided transversely in front of the posterior clinoid process to expose its tip and base, any communications with the cavernous sinus being packed with Surgicel or Gelfoam. The posterior clinoid process is then carefully drilled away with a small diamond burr.

Anterior Subtemporal Approach

The lateral subtemporal approach devised by Drake[21,22] once represented the mainstay of surgical management of basilar apex aneurysms. Although it was initially

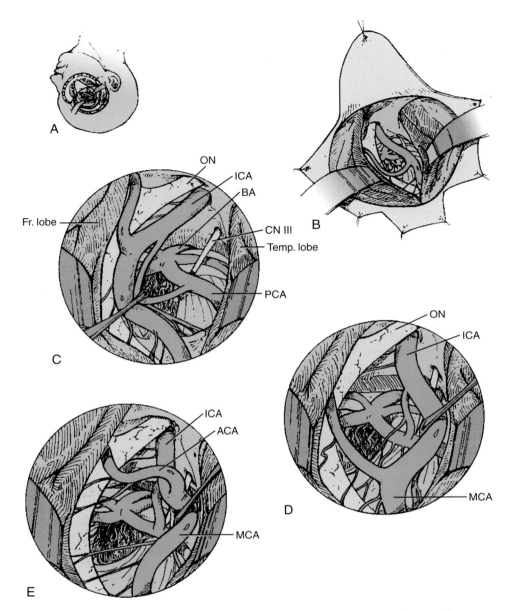

Figure 68-5 Terminal basilar bifurcation aneurysms: transsylvian approach. A, Frontotemporal pterional craniotomy. B, Sylvian fissure broadly split. C, The carotid-oculomotor interval, posterior to the internal carotid artery. D, The opticocarotid interval, medial to the internal carotid artery. E, Above the terminal internal carotid artery bifurcation. ACA, anterior cerebral artery; BA, basilar artery; CN III, cranial nerve III (oculomotor nerve); Fr. Lobe, frontal lobe; ICA, internal carotid artery; MCA, middle cerebral artery; ON, optic nerve; PCA, posterior cerebral artery; Temp Lobe, temporal lobe.

accompanied by a high incidence of temporal lobe contusion or hematoma, subsequent modification to the anterior subtemporal approach now permits the temporal lobe to be gently elevated with a low incidence of damage to the temporal lobe or its venous structures (Fig. 68-6).[23]

The main advantage of this approach is that the basilar apex and aneurysm are viewed from a lateral direction, allowing for easier identification and manipulation of the posterior perforators. This direction of approach also allows the clip to be placed parallel to the plane of aneurysm origin from the parent vessels, a substantial advantage especially for bulbous or broad-based aneurysms. In addition, the working space for dissection and clip application is larger and the working distance more superficial than with the transsylvian route. The main disadvantages are the higher incidence of postoperative third nerve deficits, the inability to clip most concurrent anterior circulation aneurysms, increased difficulty in visualizing the contralateral perforators, and the risk of temporal lobe injury.

Head Position and Fixation

The patient is prepared in a fashion similar to that described for the frontotemporal approach, with use of a lumbar subarachnoid drain and a large shoulder roll beneath the ipsilateral shoulder to bring the head to

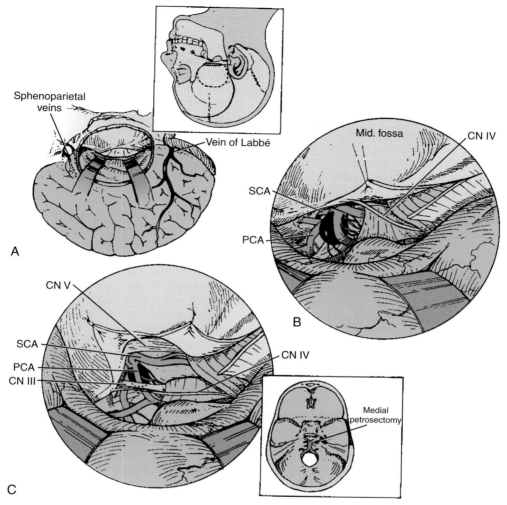

Figure 68-6 Terminal basilar bifurcation aneurysms: anterior subtemporal approach. A, Temporal lobe retraction: The anterior and middle portions of the temporal lobe are slowly elevated in a gentle arch (with use of two narrow retractor blades) between the sphenoparietal veins and vein of Labbé to expose the anterior incisura. Lumbar or ventricular cerebrospinal fluid drainage greatly facilitates temporal lobe relaxation. *Inset,* Note scalp incision, extent of bone removal. B, View of incisura, basilar apex after tentorial section, retraction. The trochlear nerve is identified and followed anteriorly until it enters the tentorium. The tentorium is then sectioned beginning 1 cm posterior to this point and continuing parallel to the superior petrosal sinus for a distance of 2 to 3 cm. Cranial nerve IV (CN IV; trochlear nerve) is then freed of its arachnoid attachments, and the tentorial edge reflected laterally with a dural stitch placed in the middle fossa dura. C, View of incisura, basilar apex after medial petrosectomy. The same temporal bone flap has been removed, followed by extradural removal of the medial petrous apex *(inset)*. The dura can then be coagulated and sectioned across the superior petrosal sinus to greatly enhance exposure to more proximal portions of the basilar artery. CN III, cranial nerve III (oculomotor nerve); CN V, cranial nerve V (trigeminal nerve); PCA, posterior cerebral artery; SCA, superior cerebellar artery.

a horizontal position (90-degree turn), with the vertex gently directed downward.

Scalp Incision and Craniotomy

The scalp incision is similar to that used in the transsylvian approach but extends more posteriorly over the ear and posterior temporal bone. A muscle-splitting temporalis incision mobilizes the bulk of the muscle anteriorly. The free bone flap is centered lower on the temporal bone, and a smaller amount of frontal bone is removed than with the transsylvian route. A temporal craniectomy is performed anteriorly to the temporal pole and inferiorly down to the floor of the middle fossa to expose the anterior and middle portions of the temporal lobe. The

superior half of the zygomatic arch is drilled away to further minimize the amount of brain retraction needed to gain a subtemporal view of the incisura. Although the approach is subtemporal, removal of the lateral aspect of the sphenoid ridge and the posterior-inferior frontal bone is important, because elevation of the temporal lobe can be restricted by these structures.

Intradural Dissection

The dura is opened in an inverted Y fashion, and the dural flap is tightly elevated inferiorly based on the floor of the middle fossa, to secure an unobstructed view to the skull base beneath the temporal lobe. Cerebrospinal fluid is gradually released from the lumbar drain to relax the temporal lobe. Gentle retraction, combined with patience to allow for adequate brain relaxation, is critical to prevent temporal lobe injury. Two parallel self-retaining retractor blades are used to elevate the temporal lobe gently and distribute the retraction force so as to avoid focal angular distortion of the cortical surface. Care is taken to preserve the vein of Labbé. Excessive posterior traction can lead to injury or thrombosis, and this vein must be constantly inspected as the temporal lobe is elevated. Small middle fossa veins draining into the dura may be coagulated if necessary, but the large sphenoparietal veins should be preserved to facilitate anterior temporal lobe venous drainage and minimize postoperative brain swelling.

The surgical route is obliquely oriented across the anterior floor of the middle fossa. When the tentorial edge is reached, the arachnoid is opened inferior to the third nerve, leaving its arachnoidal attachments to the uncus, to release cerebrospinal fluid from the basal cisterns. Further elevation of the temporal lobe and uncus will then gently retract the third nerve superiorly away from the base of the aneurysm. In some cases, particularly with high-riding bifurcations, the third nerve must be separated from the uncus and deflected inferiorly, a maneuver that will invariably produce a postoperative oculomotor deficit. The tentorial edge is incised posterior to the entry point of the fourth cranial nerve, sectioned parallel and posterior to the superior petrosal sinus, and reflected until the superior cerebellar artery is exposed coursing around the peduncle into the ambient cistern. The resultant space allows visualization of a 2.0-cm interval of the anterior superior brainstem and basilar artery centered at the level of the posterior clinoid process.

Approaches to the Interpeduncular Cistern

The anterior-inferior margins of the ipsilateral PCA and SCA are dissected and followed to their origins from the basilar artery. Any cisternal hematoma is evacuated, and the basilar artery below the SCA is prepared for a temporary clip. Anatomic variants, such as a hypoplastic P1 segment with a fetal PCA or duplicate SCAs, are common, and the presence of the third nerve between the SCA and PCA must be absolutely verified. The dissection then proceeds superiorly, with indentification of the basilar bifurcation and the aneurysm neck, and, except in anteriorly projecting aneurysms adherent to the clivus or the dorsum sellae (see later), continues anteriorly across the neck to visualize the contralateral P1 segment. The width of the aneurysm between the two PCA origins is estimated, a critical step when a fenestrated clip encircling the ipsilateral PCA is to be used. Finally, the posterior aspect of the aneurysm is separated from the perforators in the interpeduncular fossa. Coming anterolaterally, both the anterior and posterior walls of the aneurysm are visible with minimal retraction of the sac, allowing easier dissection and precise clip placement to exclude perforators.

The fundus of anteriorly projecting aneurysms is often adherent to the dorsum sellae or clivus, and removal of cerebrospinal fluid through a lumbar drain must be done slowly and carefully, because misdirected shifting of intracranial contents can precipitate premature rupture. The steps of aneurysm dissection proceed in a reverse manner, with the posterior wall exposed first, as the dangers lie on the anterior aneurysm surface. The anterior neck of the aneurysm is exposed just enough to allow clip placement, and the fundus is detached from the dorsum sellae only after the initial clip has been placed. Anteriorly projecting aneurysms are often the easiest basilar apex lesions to clip, because they usually project in a plane free of most perforators.

Modifications to Enhance Subtemporal Exposure (Medial Petrosectomy and Zygomatic Arch Removal)

Low-lying basilar apex or upper basilar trunk aneurysms are difficult to expose with conventional subtemporal approaches, in which visualization is hindered by the bony and dural attachments of the posterior clinoid process, clivus, and petrous apex.[18,21,24,25] An extradural medial petrosectomy followed by a dural incision beneath the trigeminal nerve, as first described by Kawase, can provide access to the midbasilar and upper clival regions.[26-31] The exposure, however, is quite narrow and limited to an interval between the trigeminal and facial nerves, and this corridor is unsuitable for all but the most ideally situated small lesions.

Alternatively, extradural resection of the medial petrous apex can be combined with the anterior subtemporal approach,[27,29,32] creating an exposure that provides access to an additional 1 to 1.5 cm of the basilar artery over that provided by the anterior subtemporal approach alone. This approach is particularly useful for low-lying lesions or for complicated aneurysms in which extra room is needed for a temporary clip of the proximal basilar artery. After a standard subtemporal craniotomy is performed (as outlined previously), the dura is elevated from the floor of the middle fossa to expose the middle meningeal artery at the foramen spinosum. This vessel is divided, and the greater superficial petrosal nerve (GSPN) and the lateral edge of the mandibular division of the trigeminal nerve (V3) are identified medially. A rhomboidal segment of bone is then removed medial to the greater superficial petrosal nerve anterior to the arcuate eminence, all the way to the petrous ridge medially.

Once the bony removal is completed, the dura is opened, the temporal lobe elevated, and the incisura exposed. The tentorial edge is coagulated at a point just behind the entry of the trochlear nerve and then incised laterally and obliquely toward the superior petrosal sinus. A second incision is added perpendicular to the first, oriented anteriorly and laterally to the edge of the trigeminal nerve, traversing the superior petrosal sinus. The trigeminal nerve prolapses into the petrosectomy defect, and the exposure becomes much wider, providing excellent access to the upper half of the basilar artery and clivus and the ventral surface of the mesencephalon and upper pons (Fig. 68-7).

When the basilar bifurcation is particularly high, the temporalis muscle can limit the desired inferior to superior microscope trajectory. In such cases, the zygomatic arch can be removed, and replaced with fixation plates at the end of the procedure.[33] The anterior bony cut must be posterior to the zygomaticofacial foramen, and the posterior cut is made at the root of the zygomatic arch.

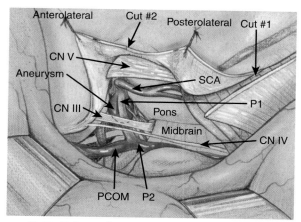

Figure 68-7 Enhanced exposure of the basilar apex region and brainstem after completion of the medial petrosectomy and division of the tentorium. Note the incisions of the tentorium: Cut #1 parallels the petrous apex, and cut #2 is perpendicular to and crosses cranial nerve (CN) V, allowing the anterior limb of the tentorium to be moved forward to expose the clivus and basilar artery well below the oculomotor nerve. PCOM, posterior communicating artery; SCA, superior cerebellar artery.

The temporalis can now be completely reflected inferiorly to facilitate a more superior view into the incisura without further temporal lobe retraction.

Temporopolar Approach

The temporopolar or pretemporal route is in many ways a combination of the pterional transsylvian and anterior subtemporal approaches. First mentioned by Drake[34] as a "half and half" exposure, it was also described by Sano,[35] who coined the term "temporopolar," and Sundt,[36] who called it a modified pterional (anterior temporal) approach. Like the transsylvian approach, the temporopolar approach begins with a pterional craniotomy but includes more inferior and anterior temporal bone removal. As originally described, little dissection of the sylvian fissure is required. Wide splitting of the fissure, however, allows much greater temporal lobe mobility, and is essential when using this approach. After the bridging veins to the sphenoparietal sinus are coagulated and sectioned, the temporal tip is gently retracted posteriorly and laterally to provide a view of the incisura. Adequate exposure to the basilar apex is achieved, but may be limited by the posterior clinoid process and the dorsum sellae when the bifurcation is low.[33,36]

The major advantage of this approach is that posterior retraction of the temporal pole, particularly when accompanied by splitting of the sylvian fissure, produces less temporal lobe swelling than that encountered via the traditional subtemporal approach.[23,26] Like the subtemporal route, a lateral view can be obtained for dissection of the posterior aneurysm wall, but the more anterior view also aids in the visualization of the contralateral P1 segment and the dissection of the opposing aneurysm neck. In addition, concurrent anterior circulation aneurysms can be clipped. The working space is significantly larger than with the pterional transsylvian route. A disadvantage is that the large veins at the temporal pole

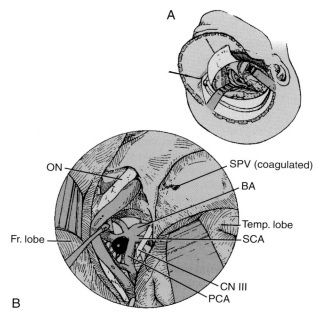

Figure 68-8 Terminal basilar bifurcation aneurysms: temporopolar approach (also referred to as the pretemporal or "half-and-half" approach). A, Frontotemporal pterional craniotomy has been performed, and the sylvian fissure broadly split. B, The sphenoparietal vein (SPV) is coagulated to allow posterior and lateral retraction of the temporal pole. The basilar apex is approached posterior to the internal carotid artery (retracted with suction). BA, basilar artery; CN III, cranial nerve III (oculomotor nerve); Fr. lobe, frontal lobe; ON, optic nerve; PCA, posterior cerebral artery; SCA, superior cerebellar artery; Temp lobe, temporal lobe.

must be sacrificed, and this maneuver is not always well-tolerated. In addition, the posterolateral temporal retraction required places some traction on the ICA, and small branches emanating from the carotid, the anterior choroidal, or the middle cerebral arteries can be avulsed.[36]

Head Position and Fixation

The patient is induced and positioned in the same fashion as for a transsylvian approach with the vertex gently directed downward, but the head is turned more, approximately 60 degrees.

Scalp Incision and Craniotomy

The scalp incision is the same as for a transsylvian approach. Interfascial dissection of the temporalis fascia allows reflection of the temporalis muscle in a postero-inferior direction. A larger pterional craniotomy is made that extends more posteriorly and inferiorly into the temporal bone. A temporal craniectomy is performed anteriorly to the temporal pole and inferiorly to the floor of the middle fossa. The remaining portions of the lateral sphenoid wing are removed, and the superior edge of the zygomatic arch is drilled away similar to the anterior subtemporal approach.

Intradural Dissection

The dura is opened in a semicircular fashion over the sylvian fissure, based on the drilled-down portion of the sphenoid ridge, and is tightly elevated anteriorly and inferiorly to secure an unobstructed view to the skull base along the sphenoid ridge and the anterior margin and floor of the middle fossa. Splitting the sylvian fissure facilitates temporal lobe retraction. The veins from the temporal pole to the sphenoparietal sinus are coagulated and divided, thus allowing a more liberal posterior retraction of the temporal pole. The arachnoidal attachments to the carotid and posterior communicating arteries are cut, and the third nerve dissected from the uncus, thereby exposing the tentorial incisura. The initial view is quite similar to that obtained from the transsylvian approach, but the space is more generous. The head can be turned to a lateral position, using the side tilt on the operating room table, to provide a view similar to that with a subtemporal approach. The tentorium can be incised and reflected if necessary.

Approaches to the Interpeduncular Cistern

The interpeduncular dissection proceeds as described in the sections on the transsylvian and anterior subtemporal routes, depending on the anatomy encountered.

Modifications to Enhance Temporopolar Exposure

When the basilar bifurcation is particularly high, a frontoorbitozygomatic craniotomy or zygomatic arch removal can be used to facilitate a desired inferior to superior microscope trajectory.[24,33] Extradural resection of the sphenoid greater and lesser wings, both above and below the superior orbital fissure down to the base of the anterior clinoid process, can further reduce the extent of temporal lobe retraction and its subsequent venous congestion.[27,37]

Selection of Surgical Approach

Each route to the basilar apex has advantages and disadvantages, with no one approach being applicable for every aneurysm. We prefer the anterior subtemporal route for most lesions, as the lateral view facilitates the most important and hazardous portions of the aneurysm and perforator dissection. With gentle elevation, temporal lobe injury has not been a deterrent.

Any deviation from the standard subtemporal route is determined chiefly by the level of the basilar bifurcation relative to the posterior clinoid process, a relationship that can best be assessed from a lateral angiogram. A lesion lying at the level of the posterior clinoid can be adequately reached by the anterior subtemporal route. For particularly high-riding bifurcation lesions (>1 cm above the posterior clinoid process), the requisite detachment of the oculomotor nerve from the uncus and more extensive temporal lobe retraction make the anterior subtemporal route less attractive. In such situations, a temporopolar route combined with removal of the zygoma, or a transsylvian approach with the "transcavernous-transsellar" modification, is more appropriate. For low-lying bifurcations, we combine the anterior subtemporal approach with a medial petrosectomy.

Aneurysm projection can also affect the choice of routes. Most basilar apex aneurysms project superiorly. When the aneurysm projects posteriorly, a purely transsylvian approach is difficult, because the posterior-inferior aspect of the aneurysm neck and any posteriorly located perforating arteries are obstructed from view by the basilar artery. Similarly, anteriorly projecting aneurysms are often adherent to the dorsum sellae, and a transsylvian route risks premature aneurysm rupture before the dissection is completed. We prefer to approach such lesions through a lateral approach, by either a subtemporal or temporopolar route.

For most solitary basilar apex aneurysms, a right-sided approach is favored. Brain retraction can be confined to the nondominant frontal and/or temporal lobes, thereby limiting the potential for speech deficits. A left-sided approach is preferable in several circumstances: (1) patients presenting with a left CN III palsy or right hemiparesis, (2) coexistent basilar and left-sided anterior circulation aneurysms, and (3) lateral orientation of the basilar aneurysm toward the left side. Any laterality (as seen in a SCA/PCA junction lesion) places the aneurysm neck closer to the ipsilateral incisura, thereby facilitating visualization and clip application from that side. Because the aneurysm is projecting laterally to some degree, the posterior thalamoperforating arteries arising from the contralateral P1 segment are often more easily seen, separated, and preserved.

Surgical Approaches to Distal Posterior Cerebral and Superior Cerebellar Artery Aneurysms

Aneurysms involving the SCA and PCA are much less commonly encountered than aneurysms arising from the basilar bifurcation. The majority of these lesions involve the basilar apex, at the SCA/PCA junction or P1 segment, and approaches to them are considered in the previous discussion. When encountered, more distal SCA or PCA aneurysms can represent fusiform dissections, flow-related aneurysms associated with arteriovenous malformations (SCA), or mycotic lesions associated with subacute bacterial endocarditis. The exact surgical approach taken to these lesions depends on the segment and cisternal location of the aneurysm.

Fusiform and mycotic lesions invariably require sacrifice of the parent vessel, as the entering and exiting vessels arise at opposite ends of the aneurysm. Endovascular sacrifice often requires sacrifice of the parent vessel proximal to the aneurysm, and that segment may harbor important perforators. Clipping, however, offers the advantage of accurate obliteration of the parent vessel right at the aneurysm origin, allowing the perforators to be spared more easily.

Many distal SCA (S2 segment) or PCA (anterior P2 segment) aneurysms in the anterior portions of the ambient cistern are usually approached through an anterior subtemporal route (see previous description), with the tentorium being split over a longer interval to provide the necessary posterior exposure. When a PCA aneurysm lies further back in this cistern toward the quadrigeminal cistern (posterior P2 segment), however, its position lies superior to the undersurface of the temporal lobe, making this approach untenable without resection of the parahippocampal gyrus. Furthermore, elevation of the posterior temporal lobe is difficult without injury of the vein of Labbé, a hazardous maneuver often accompanied by temporal lobe venous infarction or hemorrhage. In such situations, a transtemporal (through the inferior temporal gyrus) transventricular (through the temporal horn) approach, followed by splitting of the choroidal fissure, exposes this vessel segment (Fig. 68-9).

A PCA aneurysm arising after the vessel has encircled the brainstem and is nearing the midline in the quadrigeminal cistern (P3 segment) or a lesion arising along the calcarine fissure can be approached through an occipital posterior interhemispheric route (Fig. 68-10). After induction of general anesthesia, a lumbar subarachnoid drain is placed, and the patient is positioned prone on large rolls on a standard operating table, leaving the abdomen free of compression to minimize venous pressure. The prongs of the clamp are placed anteriorly in the frontal and parietal bone, leaving the occipital region clear for the operative approach. The head is elevated slightly higher than the heart (to facilitate venous drainage) with use of a reverse Trendelenburg position. The head is initially pointed straight down, and the entire body can then be rotated 15 degrees towards or away from the side of the approach to facilitate turning of the scalp and bone flap, and later to allow gravitational retraction of the ipsilateral occipital lobe.

An inferiorly based horseshoe flap is made, beginning just below the inion and 1 cm across the midline. The incision proceeds superiorly to a position approximately 1 to 2 cm above the lambda, then turns laterally for 5 to 6 cm. The occipitalis muscle is cut with the skin incision and reflected in a single layer with the scalp. A rectangular craniotomy is made, and enlarged with a craniectomy to expose the superior sagittal sinus, the transverse sinus, and the torcular Herophili. The dura is opened in a cruciate manner, with the medial inferior leg pointing toward the confluence of the sinuses.

Because the posterior segment of the superior sagittal sinus usually does not contain significant cortical draining veins, the occipital lobe can be separated from the falx and the tentorium and gently retracted superiorly and laterally. The dissection proceeds more deeply anteriorly until the splenium of the corpus callosum is encountered, and just below it, the quadrigeminal cistern. The tentorial incisura is identified, and the tentorium is split lateral and parallel to the straight sinus to widen the deeper exposure. For a PCA aneurysm in the calcarine fissure, the PCA is identified as the vessel enters the fissure (for proximal control), and then followed distally until the aneurysm is

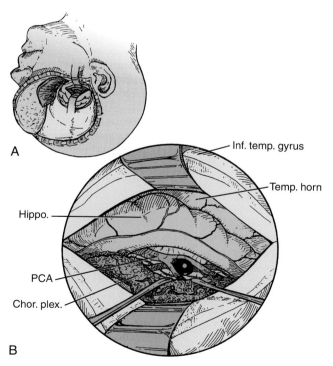

Figure 68-9 Distal posterior cerebral artery aneurysm: transventricular transchoroidal approach. The scalp incision and temporal bone removal are the same as for the anterior subtemporal approach. The temporal horn is entered through the inferior temporal or fusiform gyrus, and the choroidal fissure split to visualize the posterior cerebral artery lateral to the brainstem. Chor. plex., choroidal plexus; Hippo., hippocampal gyrus; Inf. temp gyrus, inferior temporal gyrus; PCA, posterior cerebral artery; Temp. horn, temporal horn of ventricular system.

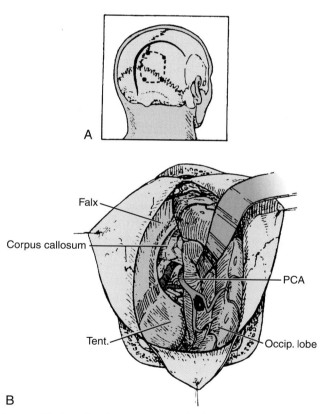

Figure 68-10 Distal posterior cerebral artery aneurysm: posterior interhemispheric approach. The scalp incision and bone removal allow exposure of the occipital lobe (Occip. lobe) along the superior sagittal and transverse sinuses. The occipital pole is retracted laterally and superiorly to expose the tentorium (Tent.), which may be split parallel to the straight sinus to broaden the view. The posterior cerebral artery (PCA) enters the calcarine sulcus just posterior to the splenium of the corpus callosum. This vessel may be followed distally or traced proximally to the posterolateral surface of the mesencephalon, until the aneurysm is encountered.

identified. If the aneurysm is in the quadrigeminal cistern (P3 segment), the dissection proceeds into the ambient cistern, lateral to the dorsal midbrain, until the lesion is identified and proximal control is assured.

Very distal SCA aneurysms posterior to the trigeminal nerve exit from the pons can also be approached through a superior-lateral suboccipital craniectomy, similar to that used for microvascular decompression for trigeminal neuralgia (Fig. 68-11).

Surgical Approaches to Vertebral Artery and Posterior Inferior Cerebellar Artery Aneurysms

The vertebral arteries enter the dura at the foramen magnum laterally and then course superiorly and medially, ventral to the brainstem, to merge at the pontomedullary junction into the basilar artery. The PICA is its principal named branch. The PICA has the most complex and variable course of the cerebellar arteries, and a clear understanding of its anatomy is fundamental to recognizing the clinical features and planning of surgical approaches to treat peripheral aneurysms in this region. The vessel's origin at the VA may vary from below the foramen magnum to the

vertebrobasilar junction. The PICA usually originates from the intracranial portion of the VA (80% to 95% of cases), on average 8.6 mm above the foramen magnum and approximately 1 cm proximal to the vertebrobasilar junction.

The PICA can be divided into five segments and two loops, on the basis of its relationship to the medulla oblongata and the cerebellum (Fig. 68-12). The name of each segment defines the anatomic structures and relationships that contribute to the presentation and management of aneurysms arising along its course. The segments and their distal limits are as follows: (1) anterior medullary, extending from the origin of the PICA at the VA to the inferior olivary prominence, (2) lateral medullary, extending to the origins of the ninth, 10th, and 11th cranial nerves, (3) tonsillomedullary, extending to the level of the tonsillar midportion (includes the caudal loop), (4) telovelotonsillar, extending to the cortical surface of the cerebellum (includes the cranial loop), and (5) cortical, extending to the cerebellar vermis and hemisphere.

This surgical anatomic classification scheme is a critical concept for surgical planning, in deciding whether the PICA can be potentially sacrificed. The proximal segments (anterior and lateral medullary) invariably contribute brainstem perforators; a transitional (tonsillomedullary) segment may or may not contribute perforating vessels to the brainstem; and distal segments (telovelotonsillar and cortical) do not supply blood supply to the brainstem.

Far Lateral Suboccipital Craniotomy

Positioning

Most VA and proximal PICA aneurysms are best approached with a far lateral suboccipital craniotomy combined with removal of the arch of C1. The patient is

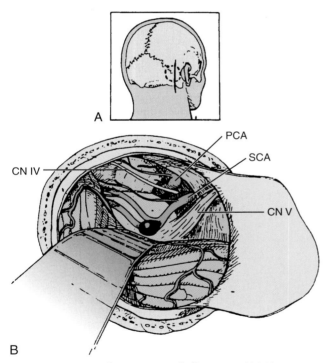

Figure 68-11 Distal superior cerebellar artery (SCA) aneurysm: lateral supracerebellar approach A, The scalp incision and bone removal allow exposure of the superior and lateral cerebellar surfaces along the transverse and sigmoid sinuses. B, The cerebellum is retracted medially and inferiorly, following the tentorial insertion into the petrous apex, until the superior petrosal vein is encountered. The vein is coagulated and sectioned, and the direction of dissection continued until the trigeminal nerve is encountered. The SCA can be identified just superior to this nerve and can be followed until the pathology is identified. More proximal portions of the SCA can be easily visualized via an anterior subtemporal approach. CN IV, cranial nerve IV (trochlear nerve); CN V, cranial nerve V (trigeminal nerve); PCA, posterior cerebral artery.

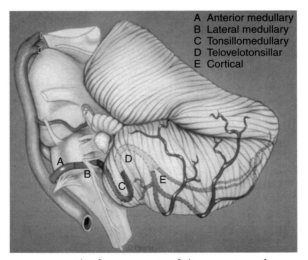

A Anterior medullary
B Lateral medullary
C Tonsillomedullary
D Telovelotonsillar
E Cortical

Figure 68-12 The five segments of the posterior inferior cerebellar artery (PICA) are demonstrated. Aneurysms proximal to the PICA origins are invariably fusiform dissections and require parent vessel sacrifice to be satisfactorily treated. Those that arise at the vertebral artery–PICA junction are almost always saccular. Distal PICA aneurysms may be saccular or fusiform and are not infrequently flow related, arising in association with a more distal arteriovenous malformation.

positioned in the three-quarters-prone lateral decubitus position, with the head rotated 30 degrees toward the floor and slightly flexed at the chin (Fig. 68-13). The ipsilateral shoulder is taped and gently retracted inferiorly to create a more comfortable working space. This head position provides a wide exposure of the cervicomedullary junction and facilitates excellent visualization of the entire intracranial course of the proximal VA without need for brainstem retraction.

Scalp Incision and Craniotomy

The incision generally starts in a vertical paramedian plane centered midway between the midline and the mastoid process. To facilitate a broader view laterally and inferiorly, the incision is curved laterally at its superior end, and medially at its inferior end, in an elongated S configuration.

The craniotomy should expose the transverse and sigmoid sinuses superiorly and laterally and should extend to the midline inferiorly. For optimal access, the ipsilateral bony rim of the foramen magnum and posterior arch of C1 up to the sulcus arteriosus underlying the VA should be removed.[38] The most essential component of the exposure is the aggressive removal of the occipital condyle in order to facilitate better access to the anterolateral margin of the foramen magnum and brainstem.

Intradural Dissection

The dura is opened in a curvilinear fashion starting superolaterally and moving down toward the midline at the craniocervical junction down to the level of C1. The cisterna magna is the opened widely, and the thickened arachnoid boundaries of the cisterna are dissected far laterally to permit unimpeded exposure of the lateral aspect of the brainstem out to the point of VA entry into the subarachnoid space (Fig. 68-14).

After cerebellar relaxation has been achieved, a self-retaining retractor is placed beneath the cerebellar tonsil and elevated in order to expose the lower cranial nerves, the distal PICA, and the VA in the depths of the field. The ascending root of the spinal accessory nerve should be identified, and the arachnoid dissection should be carried more deeply down to the lateral medulla in order

to expose the VA for proximal control if temporary clip application becomes necessary. The ipsilateral cerebellar tonsil is mobilized and its arachnoid attachments are sectioned, following which the lateral inferior surface of the hemisphere is gently elevated superiorly and medially to visualize the lateral cisterns. The arachnoid veil overlying the glossopharyngeal, vagus, and spinal accessory nerves at the jugular foramen, as well as the facial and auditovestibular nerves more superiorly, is opened to facilitate the exposure.

The VA is followed on its lateral and superior surface superiorly until the PICA origin is visualized, often obscured by branches of the hypoglossal nerve.

The final stages of exposure involve dissecting the medial aspect of the VA and completely defining the aneurysm neck. The final completed exposure allows the surgeon to place a clip parallel with the VA axis, sometimes using a fenestrated clip to encircle the origin of PICA. When the aneurysm is large or complex, temporary clips placed on the VA proximally are often helpful to reduce premature rupture risks.

The proximal portions of PICA must be preserved; whenever its origin is potentially compromised by direct clipping, a more proximal VA sacrifice or some type of flow augmentation procedure, such as an occipital artery–PICA or PICA-PICA bypass, should be considered.[39]

For vertebrobasilar junction (VBJ) aneurysms, the positioning, scalp, and bony exposure are the same as those used for the far lateral suboccipital approach. After the VA is dissected distal to the PICA origin, the space between the ninth, tenth, and eleventh cranial nerves and the seventh and eighth nerves is more aggressively expanded to provide visualization of the vertebrobasilar junction.

Suboccipital Craniotomy

For distal PICA aneurysms that arise behind the brainstem, a standard suboccipital craniotomy and C1 arch removal are usually sufficient. For those aneurysms located beneath the tonsil, where mobilization of this structure may be associated with risk of premature

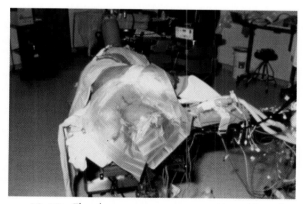

Figure 68-13 The three-quarters-prone position. Note that the ipsilateral shoulder is moved forward toward the floor, so as to not interfere with the surgeon's hands or view.

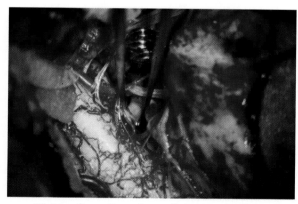

Figure 68-14 Operative view of brainstem, lower cranial nerves, vertebral artery, and posterior inferior cerebellar artery. Note that the lateral rim of the foramen magnum has been extensively removed, allowing an excellent view into the space ventral to the brainstem.

rupture, a subpial tonsillar resection may be preferred to gain exposure. When applicable, direct clip placement across the neck of the aneurysm is performed. Additional techniques to direct clipping with parent vessel preservation include PICA clip reconstruction, resection (end-to-end anastomosis or placement of an interposition graft [superficial temporal artery or occipital artery]), and flow reversal by either proximal ligation or trapping, clip occlusion and vessel reconstruction, distal PICA sacrifice, PICA resection with end-to-end anastomosis, and PICA resection with occipital artery–PICA anastomosis (Fig. 68-15).[39]

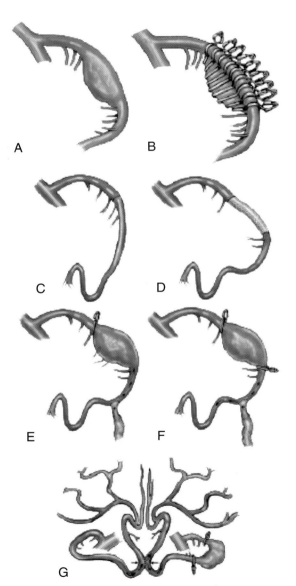

Figure 68-15 Drawings depicting surgical strategies used to treat "unclippable" distal posterior inferior cerebellar artery (PICA) aneurysms. A, Fusiform distal PICA aneurysm. B, Clip reconstruction achieved using stacked fenestrated clips. C, Aneurysm resection and direct reanastomosis. D, Aneurysm resection and interposition graft. E, Proximal ligation (flow reversal) and distal bypass. F, Aneurysm trapping and distal bypass. G, Aneurysm trapping and PICA-PICA anastomosis.

Surgical Approaches to Basilar Trunk Aneurysms

Aneurysms of the basilar trunk are exceedingly rare and are defined anatomically as arising between the vertebrobasilar junction and the superior cerebellar artery. Most commonly they arise at the origin of the anterior inferior cerebellar artery (AICA), in close association with the sixth cranial nerve. Surgical approaches to these lesions may include those described in previous sections, sometimes in association with a lateral suboccipital/retrosigmoid opening. A lateral petrosal presigmoid approach with or without venous sinus sacrifice may be considered in some circumstances, but the operating space and view are usually quite limiting.

REFERENCES

1. Fox JL: *Intracranial aneurysms*, New York, 1983, Springer-Verlag.
2. Redekop G, Ferguson G: Intracranial aneurysms. In Carter LP, Spetzler RF, editors: *Neurovascular surgery*, New York, 1996, McGraw Hill, pp 625–648.
3. Wermer MJ, van der Schaaf IC, Algra A, et al: Risk of rupture of unruptured intracranial aneurysms in relation to patient and aneurysm characteristics: An updated meta-analysis, *Stroke* 38: 1404–1410, 2007.
4. Aoki N, Sakai T: Rebleeding from intracranial dissecting aneurysm in the vertebral artery, *Stroke* 21:1628–1631, 1990.
5. Kawaguchi S, Sakaki T, Tsunoda S, et al: Management of dissecting aneurysms of the posterior circulation, *Acta Neurochir (Wien)* 131:26–31, 1994.
6. Mizutani T, Aruga T, Kirino T, et al: Recurrent subarachnoid hemorrhage from untreated ruptured vertebrobasilar dissecting aneurysms, *Neurosurgery* 36:905–911, 1995:discussion 912-903.
7. Yamaura A, Watanabe Y, Saeki N: Dissecting aneurysms of the intracranial vertebral artery, *J Neurosurg* 72:183–188, 1990.
8. Sanai N, Tarapore P, Lee AC, et al: The current role of microsurgery for posterior circulation aneurysms: A selective approach in the endovascular era, *Neurosurgery* 62:1236–1249, 2008.
9. Krisht AF, Krayenbühl N, Sercl D, et al: Results of microsurgical clipping of 50 high complexity basilar apex aneurysms, *Neurosurgery* 60:242–250, 2007:discussion 250-252.
10. Bendok BR, Getch CC, Parkinson R, et al: Extended lateral transsylvian approach for basilar bifurcation aneurysms, *Neurosurgery* 55:174–178, 2004:discussion 178.
11. Gonzalez LF, Amin-Hanjani S, Bambakidis NC, et al: Skull base approaches to the basilar artery, *Neurosurg Focus* 19:E3, 2005.
12. Lozier AP, Kim GH, Sciacca RR, et al: Microsurgical treatment of basilar apex aneurysms: Perioperative and long-term clinical outcome, *Neurosurgery* 54:286–296, 2004:discussion 296-299.
13. Krisht AF, Kadri PA: Surgical clipping of complex basilar apex aneurysms: A strategy for successful outcome using the pretemporal transzygomatic transcavernous approach, *Neurosurgery* 56(Suppl):261–273, 2005:discussion 261-273.
14. Suzuki S, Jahan R, Duckwiler GR, et al: Contribution of endovascular therapy to the management of poor-grade aneurysmal subarachnoid hemorrhage: Clinical and angiographic outcomes, *J Neurosurg* 105:664–670, 2006.
15. Saeki N, Rhoton AL Jr: Microsurgical anatomy of the upper basilar artery and the posterior circle of Willis, *J Neurosurg* 46:563–578, 1977.
16. Zeal AA, Rhoton AL Jr: Microsurgical anatomy of the posterior cerebral artery, *J Neurosurg* 48:534–559, 1978.
17. Wascher TM, Spetzler RF: Saccular aneurysms of the basilar bifurcation. In Carter LP, Spetzler RF, editors: *Neurovascular surgery*, New York, 1996, McGraw Hill, pp 729–755.
18. Yasargil MG, Antic J, Laciga R, et al: Microsurgical pterional approach to aneurysms of the basilar bifurcation, *Surg Neurol* 6:83–91, 1976.
19. Yasargil MG, Reichman MV, Kubik S: Preservation of the frontotemporal branch of the facial nerve using the interfascial temporalis flap for pterional craniotomy. Technical article, *J Neurosurg* 67:463–466, 1987.

20. Dolenc VV, Skrap M, Sustersic J, et al: A transcavernous-transsellar approach to the basilar tip aneurysms, *Br J Neurosurg* 1:251-259, 1987.

21. Drake CG: Bleeding aneurysms of the basilar artery. Direct surgical management in four cases, *J Neurosurg* 18:230-238, 1961.

22. Drake CG: Gordon Murray lecture: Evolution of intracranial aneurysm surgery, *Can J Surg* 27:549-555, 1984.

23. Heros RC, Lee SH: The combined pterional/anterior temporal approach for aneurysms of the upper basilar complex: Technical report, *Neurosurgery* 33:244-250, 1993:discussion 250-241.

24. Al-Mefty O: Supraorbital-pterional approach to skull base lesions, *Neurosurgery* 21:474-477, 1987.

25. Malis L: The petrosal approach, *Clin Neurosurg* 37:528-540, 1990.

26. Al-Mefty O, Fox JL, Smith RR: Petrosal approach for petroclival meningiomas, *Neurosurgery* 22:510-517, 1988.

27. Day JD, Fukushima T, Giannotta SL: Microanatomical study of the extradural middle fossa approach to the petroclival and posterior cavernous sinus region: Description of the rhomboid construct, *Neurosurgery* 34:1009-1016, 1994:discussion 1016.

28. Hakuba A, Nishimura S, Inoue Y: Transpetrosal-transtentorial approach and its application in the therapy of retrochiasmatic craniopharyngiomas, *Surg Neurol* 24:405-415, 1985.

29. Kawase T, Shiobara R, Toya S: Anterior transpetrosal-transtentorial approach for sphenopetroclival meningiomas: Surgical method and results in 10 patients, *Neurosurgery* 28:869-875, 1991:discussion 875-866.

30. Kawase T, Toya S, Shiobara R, Mine T: Transpetrosal approach for aneurysms of the lower basilar artery, *J Neurosurg* 63:857-861, 1985.

31. Miller CG, van Loveren HR, Keller JT, et al: Transpetrosal approach: Surgical anatomy and technique, *Neurosurgery* 33:461-469, 1993:discussion 469.

32. MacDonald JD, Antonelli P, Day AL: The anterior subtemporal, medial transpetrosal approach to the upper basilar artery and ponto-mesencephalic junction, *Neurosurgery* 43:84-89, 1998.

33. Sano K, Shiokawa Y: The temporo-polar approach to basilar artery aneurysms with or without zygomatic arch translocation, *Acta Neurochir (Wien)* 130:14-19, 1994.

34. Drake CG: Microsurgical evaluation of the pterional approach to aneurysms of the distal basilar circulation [comment], *Neurosurgery* 3:140-141, 1978.

35. Sano K: Temporo-polar approach to aneurysms of the basilar artery at and around the distal bifurcation: Technical note, *Neurol Res* 2:361-367, 1980.

36. Sundt TM: *Surgical techniques for saccular and giant intracranial aneurysms*, Baltimore, 1990, Williams & Wilkins.

37. Day JD, Giannotta SL, Fukushima T: Extradural temporopolar approach to lesions of the upper basilar artery and infrachiasmatic region, *J Neurosurg* 81:230-235, 1994.

38. Heros RC: Lateral suboccipital approach for vertebral and vertebrobasilar artery lesions, *J Neurosurg* 64:559-562, 1986.

39. Samson DS, Batjer HH: *Intracranial aneurysm surgery—Techniques*, Mount Kisco, 1990, Futura.

Surgery for Intracerebral Hemorrhage

ALEXANDER DAVID MENDELOW, BARBARA A. GREGSON

The key to understanding the therapeutic potential in intracerebral hemorrhage (ICH) lies in understanding those aspects of the etiology, pathophysiology, and consequences of ICH that surgery can influence. The etiologic factors to consider are the so-called ictohemorrhagic lesions that may require simultaneous treatment to prevent recurrence of the hemorrhage (Table 69-1). The specific aspects of pathophysiology that require consideration are clot expansion and the existence of a "penumbra" of functionally impaired but potentially viable tissue around the clot. Of the many consequences of ICH, hydrocephalus is the one that requires rapid and repeated attention. The therapeutic initiatives can be medical, surgical, or both, and there is an important interaction between them particularly with regard to periprocedural care. There is no doubt that the incidence of intracerebral hemorrhage continues to rise because of (1) the more common use of antiplatelet therapy for the primary and secondary prevention of atherosclerosis, (2) the increasing use of anticoagulation, particularly in the elderly population, and (3) the more frequent use of thrombolysis for both myocardial[1] infarction and ischemic stroke, particularly since the Third European Cooperative Acute Stroke Study (ECASS 3) has now extended the time window to 4.5 hours.[2] It has been estimated that between 1% and 2% of the population is now undergoing warfarin therapy.[3] Surgical decision-making therefore must often take place against a background of disturbed coagulation, with careful consideration of the etiology, pathophysiology, and consequences in the individual patient.

There are considerable controversies about the prevention of rebleeding as well as the medical management and surgical treatment of this condition. Surgical indications vary in different countries of the world, with high rates of surgical evacuation for spontaneous ICH found in some centers in Lithuania and Sweden, and low rates in some centers in Hungary (Fig. 69-1).[4] The main controversy is about whether or not to evacuate supratentorial ICH; the randomized International Surgical Trial in Intracerebral Haemorrhage (ISTICH) involved 1033 patients from 27 countries worldwide, but at 6 months there was no overall benefit of early surgery over initial conservative treatment.[5] There was, however, a trend toward better outcomes for early surgery in patients with superficial lobar hematomas. A general trend of better outcomes with surgery is reported in the second edition of the *Cochrane Database of Systemic Reviews* article on surgery for ICH.[6] This finding, coupled with further meta-analysis of other trials, has generated the hypothesis that early

craniotomy for such superficial clots will improve outcome, and this hypothesis is being evaluated in the second Surgical Trial in Intracerebral Haemorrhage (STICH II).[7]

Controversies also relate to cerebellar hemorrhage, treatment of the underlying cause (arteriovenous malformation [AVM] or aneurysm), and initial medical treatment. Cerebellar hemorrhage is a special case because of its more frequent progression to hydrocephalus.

Although the International Subarachnoid Aneurysm Trial (ISAT) examined outcomes related to endovascular versus microsurgical treatment of ruptured cerebral aneurysms,[8,9] the trial did not specifically set out to evaluate endovascular coiling in the context of ICH. Nor has it resolved the issue of the durability of endovascular coiling, particularly in young people who would otherwise have a long life expectancy.[10] Similar uncertainty surrounds the efficacy of treatment for unruptured aneurysms in relation to subarachnoid hemorrhage and ICH.[11,12]

All clinicians who deal with such patients must know the natural history of unruptured aneurysms and must keep up to date with ongoing studies, such as the International Study of Unruptured Intracranial Aneurysms (ISUIA), as the sequential reports appear.[11,12] From these studies, it has now become clear that the critical size is 6 mm; for aneurysms larger than this threshold, the risk of hemorrhage rises toward 1% for each year of future life.

Such ictohemorrhagic lesions play an important role in determining treatment of the ICH itself.[13] For example, Heiskanen et al[14] showed that surgical evacuation of ICH due to an aneurysm was much more effective than conservative treatment. For this reason, management of aneurysmal ICH must be considered separately. Investigation of the ICH must therefore include imaging that elucidates the causes and consequences of ICH. A discussion about the nature and timing of such imaging in relation to surgical decision-making follows.

Imaging in the Diagnosis of Intracerebral Hemorrhage

The difficulty of differentiating ischemic stroke from ICH is well known. Although the sudden onset of severe headache, coma, or epilepsy is more likely to be due to ICH, urgent imaging is essential to avoid the danger of using thrombolytic therapy in a patient with an ICH. CT is perfectly adequate for diagnosing ICH, although MRI is similarly diagnostic in the acute phase. MRI has the advantage of defining underlying ictohemorrhagic lesions better without the need for intravenous contrast agents. Because of the dynamic nature of the pathophysiology and consequences of ICH, repeated imaging must be tailored to the clinical status of the patient; hydrocephalus may develop or progress rapidly over just a few hours, so that monitoring of these patients in a critical care area is essential.

Computed Tomography

In the acute phase, spontaneous ICH is easy to recognize on CT as a high-density mass. Subsequently, the area around the ICH develops low-density changes as a result of brain edema. The volume of the hematoma can be calculated with the use of the approximation of an ellipse, from the following equation described by Broderick et al[15]:

$$\frac{4}{3}\pi r^2 = \frac{A \times B \times C}{2}$$

where r is the radius, and A, B, and C are the diameters in three planes.

The volume of the hematoma determines the outcome, larger hematomas having a much poorer prognosis than smaller hematomas.[16] Now that CT is performed more frequently in patients with ischemic stroke, a greater number of patients with ICH will be discovered. This trend should help differentiate these two completely different disorders that have, in the past, often been wrongly lumped together as "stroke."

Sites of Hemorrhage

Lesions at certain sites are more likely to be associated with aneurysmal ICH, such as interhemispheric and sylvian fissures (Figs. 69-2 and 69-3). The classic hypertensive ICH occurs in the basal ganglia, whereas lobar hematomas are more likely with amyloid angiopathy. Imaging may also demonstrate evidence of underlying tumor or trauma. Adjacent or remote calcification may also give an indication that there is an underlying cerebral AVM or tumor. Contrast-enhanced imaging and angiography may display aneurysms or cerebral AVMs. Cerebellar hematomas can produce noncommunicating obstructive hydrocephalus, which may need urgent treatment in its own right.

Magnetic Resonance Imaging

MRI easily differentiates ischemic stroke from ICH. However, the MRI appearances will change as the time from ictus increases (Table 69-2). MRI with diffusion-weighted

TABLE 69-1   CAUSES OF INTRACEREBAL HEMORRHAGE

Idiopathic
Hypertension
Amyloid angiopathy
Cerebral aneurysms
Cerebral arteriovenous malformations
Cerebral arteriovenous fistulas
Cavernous malformations
Brain tumors (primary and secondary)
Anticoagulants/antiplatelet agents/tissue-type plasminogen activator
Recreational drugs
Unrecognized trauma
Postoperatively (remote and cerebellar)
Post-infarction (hemorrhagic conversion)
Hereditary hemorrhagic telangiectasia
Blood dyscrasias (e.g., hemophilia, leukemia)

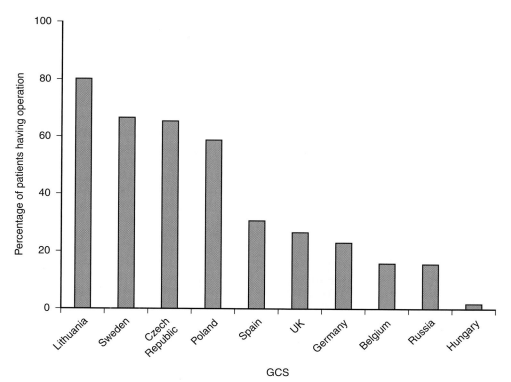

Figure 69-1   Graph showing rates of operation for intracerebral hemorrhage in centers from different countries.

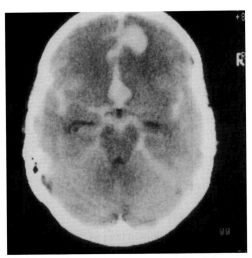

Figure 69-2 CT scan showing interhemispheric hematoma from a ruptured anterior communicating artery aneurysm.

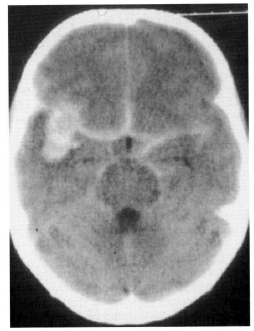

Figure 69-3 CT scan showing intracerebral and subarachnoid hemorrhage from a ruptured middle cerebral artery aneurysm.

imaging (DWI) also displays the development of brain edema. The change in DWI appearance that occurs sequentially following an ICH may provide further insight into the pathophysiology of the penumbra.[1]

Angiography

Some surgeons prefer to obtain an angiogram routinely before undertaking surgery. This step is taken to prevent the unexpected discovery of an otherwise difficult-to-treat AVM. Similarly, for the patient in whom an aneurysm is suspected, most neurosurgeons would recommend angiography to display the aneurysm. CT and MR angiography have now become acceptable alternatives to intra-arterial angiography.

Blood Flow Mapping with Single-Photon Emission CT and Positron Emission Tomography

Single-photon emission CT (SPECT) using technetium hexamethyl-propyleneamineoxime (HM-PAO) has been shown to display a penumbra of functionally impaired but potentially recoverable tissue around an ICH. Through the use of the difference-based region-growing (DBRG) method, the penumbra has been objectively identified in patients with supratentorial ICH.[17] Similarly, positron emission tomography (PET) has been used to identify a penumbra around ICH,[18,19] although this issue remains controversial. Clinical[20,21] and experimental studies[22,23] have indicated that the reduced perfusion in the peri-hematoma region may not be severe enough to induce ischemia and may be secondary to hypometabolism. The importance of demonstrating a penumbra around an ICH is the recognition of the potential for reversal of the oligemic process by either pharmacologic or surgical means. An understanding of this issue is therefore essential to appreciating the possible role for surgery in a particular case; the next section therefore focuses on this important controversy.

Pathophysiology of the Penumbra

Controversy therefore exists as to whether or not there is a penumbra around an ICH.[17,19,23-26] The importance of the issue is that if a penumbra does exist, there is the potential for medical or surgical intervention to minimize the brain damage in the area surrounding the ICH. Histologic studies have unequivocally established that there is

TABLE 69-2   MRI CHARACTERISTICS OF HEMORRHAGE

Time from Ictus	Clinical Phase	Appearance on T1-Weighted Images	Appearance on T2-Weighted Images	Hemoglobin State
Immediate	Hyperacute	Isointense	Bright	Intracellular oxyhemoglobin
6 h	Acute	Isointense	Dark	Intracellular deoxyhemoglobin
6-48 h	Early subacute	Bright	Dark	Extracellular deoxyhemoglobin
2 wk	Late subacute	Bright	Bright	Extracellular methemoglobin
>3 wk	Chronic	Dark	Dark	Hemosiderin

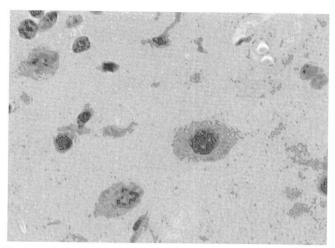

Figure 69-4 Photomicrograph of brain around an intracerebral hemorrhage stained with KU80 antibody to show evidence of apoptosis. (This finding indicates programmed cell death and therefore supports the concept of a penumbra.)

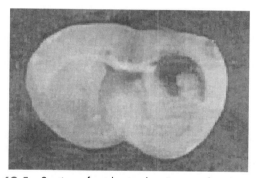

Figure 69-5 Section of rat brain showing caudate intracerebral hemorrhage.

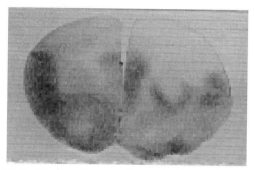

Figure 69-6 Carbon C autoradiograph showing large perfusion defect around caudate intracerebral hemorrhage.

ischemic neuronal damage in the tissue around the ICH. Later studies, using KU80 and fractin antibody stains, have shown that there is apoptosis in the tissue around an ICH (Fig. 69-4). This finding implies that some cells have undergone programmed cell death (apoptosis) and that these cells, having initially survived, may be potential targets for urgent therapeutic intervention.[27]

The first experimental evidence of a large penumbra around an ICH came from experiments in rats in which blood was introduced into the caudate nucleus under arterial pressure (Fig. 69-5).[28,29] Carbon C-14–iodoantipyrene autoradiography demonstrated a large ischemic area (Fig. 69-6). Similarly, in a study using an inflatable and deflatable microballoon (50 μL), deflation of the microballoon 2 hours after inflation produced a much smaller infarct than when the balloon was left inflated for a full 2 hours.[30] These experimental studies provide a background for clinical studies, which have also revealed a penumbra in some patients with ICH. Reduced cerebral blood flow (CBF) has also been demonstrated around ICH in patients by means of dynamic CT perfusion techniques.[19,31] Other clinical studies using MRI and positron emission tomography have similarly demonstrated a penumbra.[17-19]

By contrast, some clinical studies have not shown a penumbra.[32-34] It may well be that a penumbra is present in some patients with ICH but not in others. Therefore, the patient with a penumbra is likely to benefit from surgical decompression; if such patients could be identified, selective surgery could be applied. Kanno et al[35] have shown that the use of hyperbaric oxygen leads to an improvement in the clinical condition of some patients. Microdialysis has also found elevated lactate pyruvate ratios in the penumbra.[16] Heiss[36] has clearly shown that a penumbra does exist in some patients. Also, with time, the penumbra changes and perihematoma edema progresses, adversely affecting outcome.[37,38] As discussed previously, if a penumbra can be identified, surgery is more likely to be beneficial if undertaken rapidly, before permanent secondary processes take place. Such secondary processes include release of cytokines and interleukins as well as the products of the clot itself, including fibrin and metalloproteins. As these inflammatory chemicals are produced, secondary vasogenic brain edema increases, and swelling leads to further brain shift and elevated intracranial pressure (ICP).

Underlying Pathology

In some patients with ICH, the underlying disease (e.g., tumor or cerebral AVM) causes the hemorrhage. Similarly, amyloid angiopathy is associated with amyloid deposits in the area around small cerebral vessels. It is thought that the weakening in the wall associated with this vasculopathic process results in the classic lobar parietooccipital hematomas that occur in the elderly. Of the various tumors, metastatic melanomas are most likely to bleed. For this reason, every ICH should be investigated to exclude underlying disease.

Surgical Treatment

The three objectives of surgical treatment depend on reversal of the pathophysiologic processes, reduction of clot volume, and lowering of ICP. One of the greatest controversies in neurosurgery is whether or not to operate on a patient with a supratentorial ICH. Although it is clear that some patients need surgery and that others do not, there is an area of uncertainty between these extremes. For example, a young patient with ICH in the nondominant hemisphere who is initially conscious and talking but who subsequently

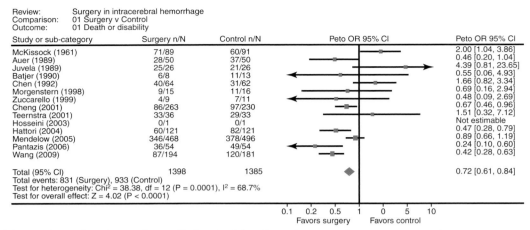

Review:	Surgery in intracerebral hemorrhage				
Comparison:	01 Surgery v Control				
Outcome:	01 Death or disability				
Study or sub-category	Surgery n/N	Control n/N	Peto OR 95% CI		Peto OR 95% CI
McKissock (1961)	71/89	60/91			2.00 [1.04, 3.86]
Auer (1989)	28/50	37/50			0.46 [0.20, 1.04]
Juvela (1989)	25/26	21/26			4.39 [0.81, 23.65]
Batjer (1990)	6/8	11/13			0.55 [0.06, 4.93]
Chen (1992)	40/64	31/62			1.66 [0.82, 3.34]
Morgenstern (1998)	9/15	11/16			0.69 [0.16, 2.94]
Zuccarello (1999)	4/9	7/11			0.48 [0.09, 2.69]
Cheng (2001)	86/263	97/230			0.67 [0.46, 0.96]
Teernstra (2001)	33/36	29/33			1.51 [0.32, 7.12]
Hosseini (2003)	0/1	0/1			Not estimable
Hattori (2004)	60/121	82/121			0.47 [0.28, 0.79]
Mendelow (2005)	346/468	378/496			0.89 [0.66, 1.19]
Pantazis (2006)	36/54	49/54			0.24 [0.10, 0.60]
Wang (2009)	87/194	120/181			0.42 [0.28, 0.63]
Total (95% CI)	1398	1385			0.72 [0.61, 0.84]

Total events: 831 (Surgery), 933 (Control)
Test for heterogeneity: Chi² = 38.38, df = 12 (P = 0.0001), I² = 68.7%
Test for overall effect: Z = 4.02 (P < 0.0001)

0.1 0.2 0.5 1 0 5 10
Favors surgery   Favors control

Figure 69-7 Meta-analysis of randomized controlled trials of the effect of surgery after a supratentorial spontaneous intracerebral hemorrhage, with death and disability combined. (Modified from Fernandes HM, et al: Surgery in intracerebral hemorrhage: The uncertainty continues. *Stroke* 31:2511-2516, 2000.)

deteriorates with a lobar ICH would undoubtedly warrant surgical treatment. By contrast, an elderly dependent patient with a large ICH in the dominant hemisphere and extending into the thalamus who is in coma from the outset has such a poor prognosis that surgery would not be considered. Surgery would also not be considered for the patient with a very small volume ICH who has a minimal focal deficit with no disturbance of consciousness, particularly if the clot is deep-seated. It is, therefore, clear that some patients would not undergo surgery because they are too well and others would not undergo surgery because their prospects are hopeless. These two negative aspects in relation to surgery have resulted in confusion about the indications, particularly because there are some patients, as in the example already given, who would clearly benefit. It is the patients between these extremes for whom uncertainty about performing surgery exists.

Prospective Randomized Controlled Trials and Observational Studies

Class I Evidence

In the original review about surgical treatment for ICH reported by Prasad et al,[60,61] four prospective randomized trials were cited. In a subsequent meta-analysis, Fernandes et al[62] summarized seven prospective randomized controlled trials, results of which have shown that there is no certainty about treatment because most of the trials were too small to produce meaningful conclusions (Fig. 69-7). A further small trial of stereotactic aspiration has also failed to demonstrate improved outcome from thrombolytically assisted aspiration.[63] The second edition of the *Cochrane Database of Systematic Reviews* article on surgery for ICH has now indicated that there is substantial evidence in favor of surgical intervention for ICH.[6] For this reason, the second Surgical Trial in Intracerebral Hemorrhage (STICH II) was begun in 2006, and at the time of writing, recruitment continues. It is likely that the final results of this trial will be known toward the end of 2011. A report of the pooled and blinded results describes the demographic and clinical data so far.[64] The STICH trial

has been misinterpreted by many, and a recent analysis of operation and admission rates for ICH in Newcastle, UK, has shown that there has been a reduction in these rates.[65]

When supratentorial ICH is associated with a ruptured aneurysm, surgical treatment is undoubtedly better, yielding a much lower mortality (27%) than that for conservative treatment (80%).[14] The probability of sudden death from a ruptured intracranial aneurysm has been subject to a systematic review with meta-analysis by Huang and van Gelder.[66]

With cerebellar ICH, no class I evidence exists of the efficacy of any treatment, but it is generally accepted that these patients may do well with surgical intervention. With cerebellar ICH, the treatment of hydrocephalus also must be considered, because hydrocephalus may lead to disturbance of consciousness. Correction of the hydrocephalus with external ventricular drainage may therefore dramatically improve the level of consciousness. Whether or not to remove the cerebellar ICH has been considered, and an algorithm has been offered for its management (Fig. 69-8).[67] In some patients with supratentorial ICH who may have suffered a head injury, it may be difficult to know whether or not the lesion is traumatic or spontaneous. No trials have been conducted to ascertain whether surgical treatment should be undertaken in patients with traumatic ICH. It is clear that patients with traumatic ICH (TICH) differ from patients with spontaneous ICH (SICH), and these differences have been characterized by Siddique and colleagues.[68] By and large, patients with traumatic ICH have better outcomes perhaps because as a group they are younger than patients with spontaneous ICH. A new prospective randomized controlled trial of patients with traumatic ICH (Simplified Treatment Intervention to Control Hypertension [STITCH]) is under way.

Class II and Class III Evidence

Many observational studies (yielding class II and class III evidence) have been performed to examine treatment of ICH. Retrospective studies that either compare results of surgery and nonoperative management or are "pure" surgical series without controls are numerous,

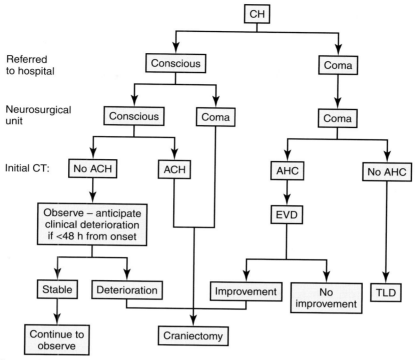

Figure 69-8 Recommendations for neurosurgical management of cerebellar hematomas. ACH, acute hydrocephalus; CH, cerebellar hemorrhage; EVD, external ventricular drainage; TLD, treatment-limiting decision. (Redrawn from Mathew P, et al: Neurosurgical management of cerebellar hematoma and infarct. *J Neurol Neurosurg Psychiatry* 59:287-292, 1995.)

and more than 60 such studies were reported in 2002 by Fernandes.[16] In general, the reports of "new" surgical techniques are encouraging. Such techniques include the well-established and standard craniotomy,[69-72] stereotaxic aspiration,[73-75] and ultrasonic aspirations.[76] Fernandes[16] also summarized the class II evidence, which came from 32 papers comparing medical and surgical treatments prospectively but in a nonrandomized way. The results of these studies were mixed, with some finding better results from surgery,[77] some finding no difference,[78] and others finding surgery worse.[79]

In the largest series to date, Kanaya and Kuroda[80] reported on more than 7000 patients in the Japanese ICH register; these investigators found that patients with deep coma and very large ICHs fared badly with surgical treatment. Craniotomy was better for hematomas larger than 50 mL, whereas aspiration was better for smaller clots. Other studies have similarly concluded that surgical results in patients with large hematomas were poor, particularly because the patients were selected for surgery on the basis of their comatose state and large hematomas. It is possible to draw completely the wrong conclusion from results of these observational studies, however, because they were nonrandomized studies in which the less severely affected patients underwent medical treatment[81] and the most severely affected with a poor prognosis underwent surgery.

Craniotomy

The majority of neurosurgeons around the world still favor craniotomy for the evacuation of a hematoma. Generally, surgeons are more inclined to operate if the ICH is in the nondominant hemisphere, if the patient's condition deteriorates, and if the clot is lobar and near the surface.[82] If the clot is lobar and polar, especially in the nondominant hemisphere, surgery is easier and a larger internal decompression is possible with less risk to neurologic function.

Some surgeons prefer a large craniotomy because it leaves open the option of external decompression for swelling. Although this technique is gaining favor in traumatic ICH and with larger infarcts from ischemic stroke, it has not been formally evaluated in randomized controlled trials. There are no ongoing or planned trials of external decompression for spontaneous supratentorial ICH at present; the technique is therefore unproven in patients with ICH. In a review of the subject of external decompression for ICH, Mitchell et al[84] concluded that there was insufficient evidence to make any recommendation about decompressive craniectomy.

For a craniotomy, the patient is usually positioned supine with the head rotated, but in elderly patients with osteoarthritic necks, the lateral position may be preferred, especially if the clot is occipital as often occurs with amyloid angiopathy in the elderly. A large bolus of intravenous mannitol is given preoperatively; Cruz and Okuchi[50,85] have demonstrated in prospective randomized controlled trials that such a bolus is effective, although these studies have been called into question.[86] A craniotomy is made over the hematoma, with avoidance of eloquent areas of the brain such as the motor strip and speech areas of the cortex. The exact position is facilitated with the use of image guidance.

If the dura is very tight after administration of mannitol, repositioning, and correction of any other problem such as high central venous pressure or hypercapnia, the clot should initially be gently aspirated with a large bore–type cannula so that the dura can be opened without trauma to the cortex, which may otherwise herniate alarmingly through the durotomy. Removal of even a few milliliters of clot by cannula may move the patient's condition down the pressure-volume curve. It is better to correct all of these problems at the earliest opportunity to minimize the oligemia or ischemia which would otherwise persist in any penumbra surrounding the hematoma. In theory, the sooner reperfusion is restored, the smaller the volume of ultimate ischemic damage is likely to be.

Once the dura is open, the clot may be visible or the flattened pale overlying gyri may be obvious. If not, image guidance or ultrasonography may prove helpful. A cortical window that avoids arteries and major venous structures is created, rather than a cortical incision. The window avoids or reduces the need for retraction; and for access through noneloquent cortex, damage is less with a cortical window.

Once located, the clot is entered and easily removed with gentle suction and irrigation, with Hartman's solution rather than saline because it more closely resembles cerebrospinal fluid. Use of the operating microscope, which allows access to all parts of the hematoma through a relatively small cortical window, is highly recommended. Self-retaining retractors facilitate access to all parts of the cavity. Hemostasis is secured with bipolar diathermy. Hemostatic materials can be used, but only after the surgeon has ensured that all arterial and venous bleeding points have been coagulated.

Usually, the brain will have become slack, and the dura can be closed and the bone flap replaced. If the brain is very swollen, however, leaving the dura open with removal of the bone flap is an option. Alternatively, the bone flap can be left riding with the dura open, and the noneloquent cortex covered with a hemostatic material. If the clot has ruptured into the ventricle, it is reasonable practice to leave an external ventricular drain in situ; the drain either can be used to drain cerebrospinal fluid postoperatively or can be connected to a pressure transducer and opened to drainage only if the ICP rises or the CPP drops below an acceptable threshold (e.g., below a CPP of 65 mm Hg in an adult or 55 mm Hg in a child).[87]

Postoperative neurologic monitoring must be continued until the patient shows signs of recovery of consciousness, because the postoperative rebleeding rate is high. In some units, postoperative CT scanning, ICP monitoring, or both are routine, but neither of these critical care measures has yet been formally evaluated in trials.

Endoscopic Removal of Hematoma

In 1989, Auer et al[88] showed, in a single-center prospective randomized controlled trial, that endoscopic removal of hematoma was superior to medical treatment. Other observational reports have also favored endoscopy, and with stereotactic guidance and real-time ultrasonographic imaging, very encouraging results have been obtained with smaller clots (<30 mL). In later studies,

such techniques have been tried with greater success in larger hematomas. This technique is not generally applied at present. Nevertheless, variations on the theme of stereotactic aspiration abound.[89,90] In some reports the laser has been used as a hemostatic tool through the endoscope, again with encouraging results. All these technologic advances have yet to be formally evaluated in prospective randomized controlled trials, although such techniques, including ultrasound dissolution of the clot, are planned in the evaluation that is to become part of the Minimally Invasive Surgery plus t-PA for Intracerebral Hemorrhage Evacuation (MISTIE) trial.[91]

Ultrasonic Aspiration

Hondo et al[76] have reported success with a stereotactic aspiration of supratentorial ICH using an ultrasonic aspirator. Studies of this procedure are observational, and the method has not yet been subjected to prospective randomized controlled trials.

Intracavity Thrombolysis

Blaauw et al undertook a small prospective randomized controlled trial in patients with supratentorial ICH; the investigators introduced urokinase into the cavity of the ICH and, after a specified period, aspirated the contents. This small prospective randomized controlled trial was stopped early; results showed no benefit in terms of mortality,[63,93] although there was a possible benefit in data from a small number of patients analyzed with multivariate analysis.[94] In some patients, in whom ICH has ruptured into the ventricle, external ventricular drainage (EVD) in conjunction with thrombolysis[95] may be useful. These techniques are now being evaluated in prospective randomized controlled trials. The results of the phase 2 trials of intracavity (MISTIE[96]) and intraventricular (Clot Lysis: Evaluating Accelerated Resolution of Intraventricular Hemorrhage [CLEAR IVH][97]) thrombolysis are very encouraging, with low morbidity and mortality reported.[98] Observational studies have highlighted the otherwise poor prognoses in these patients.[99]

Treatment of Intracerebral Hemorrhage Associated with Specific Lesions

Aneurysmal Intracerebral Hemorrhage

Heiskanen et al[14] showed in a prospective randomized controlled trial that the mortality was significantly lower for surgical removal of aneurysmal ICH than for medical treatment. For this reason, it is recommended that for the patient in whom an ICH is associated with aneurysmal rupture, the clot should be removed and the aneurysm should be clipped. Kerr et al[46] reported that endovascular coiling associated with surgical removal of the hematoma is also an option. However, the reporting of good results with endovascular coiling for ICH is anecdotal, and care should be taken in extrapolating these endovascular therapy results to patients with aneurysmal ICH rather than subarachnoid hemorrhage. Also, if the clot is to be removed surgically, clipping the aneurysm at the same time is convenient and efficient, rather than delaying the evacuation to perform the endovascular procedure. Furthermore, removal of the ICH normalizes the ICP, so the need for operative retraction is lessened and access to the aneurysm is facilitated.

Arteriovenous Malformation

Any ICH may be associated with an AVM. If such a lesion is demonstrated, care should be taken in removing the ICH because uncontrollable bleeding from the AVM may be encountered if the anatomy was not clearly defined preoperatively. If the ICH is being treated conservatively and there is an associated AVM, many surgeons prefer to deal with the AVM within 6 to 8 weeks of the ICH, because surgical planes lead easily to the AVM, which is often better visualized within the wall of the ICH. The options for treatment of the underlying AVM are endovascular obliteration, surgical excision, stereotaxic radiosurgery, and a combination of these treatment modalities.

If the ICH is being removed in an urgent procedure, surgical excision of the AVM through the same craniotomy is clearly the preferred method of treatment, provided that it is technically possible and the appropriate inaccessible feeders have been occluded first by endovascular means if time permits. It is not necessary to embolize feeders that are on the surface and that are easily accessible at craniotomy, because they can simply be occluded as the dura is opened. Embolization can usually be achieved if the primary ICH was small and was initially treated conservatively, because the planned surgery at 6 to 8 weeks can be preceded by embolization. The problem occurs when it is deemed necessary to operate on the ICH as an emergency before embolization can be accomplished; in that case, the only option may be to use intraoperative hypotension *after* the ICH has been decompressed, so

as to avoid compromising CPP. After removal of the ICH, the brain should have become slack, with an ICP equal to atmospheric pressure, so that the CPP approximates the blood pressure. Under such circumstances with the dura open, a mean blood pressure of about 60 mm Hg (i.e., a CPP of also about 60 mm Hg mean) would be well tolerated in a previously normotensive individual until the AVM has been excised and hemostasis properly secured.

Cerebellar Hemorrhage

A major difference between supratentorial ICH and cerebellar hemorrhage is the delayed onset of obstructive hydrocephalus that occurs with the latter, often necessitating emergency ventriculostomy. Cerebellar hemorrhage may occur at any site in the cerebellum, but lateral cerebellar hemisphere lesions are more common than midline (vermian) lesions. Clinically, such lesions are more likely to cause ataxia, nystagmus, and varying degrees of brainstem signs with the subsequent onset of deteriorating level of consciousness owing to hydrocephalus.

Serial CT scans may be required to document increasing ventriculomegaly (Fig. 69-9). Cerebellar hemorrhages respond well to surgery, but the effect of hydrocephalus must be considered separately. There are no randomized controlled trials on which to base management decisions. However, Mathew et al[102] have proposed an algorithm for management that is sensible and easy to use (see Fig. 69-8). As with supratentorial ICH, underlying causes of cerebellar hemorrhage should be sought and treated.

With rapid treatment, the outcome of cerebellar hemorrhage with appropriate management of hydrocephalus may be surprisingly good.[102-111] In fact, patients with short-term brainstem compression causing absence of brainstem reflexes may make a gratifying and full neurologic

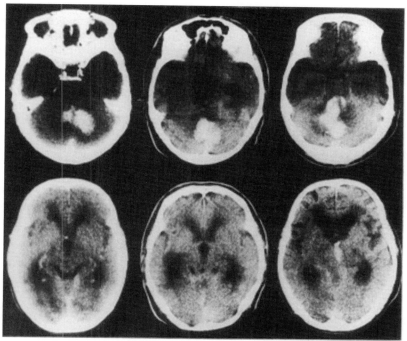

Figure 69-9 CT scans showing cerebellar intracerebral hemorrhage with hydrocephalus.

recovery. Nevertheless, one should not underestimate the morbidity and mortality associated with posterior fossa surgery, which carries a high complication rate compared with ventricular drainage for hydrocephalus, which is relatively straightforward. The counter-argument is that very poor outcomes result from an overly conservative approach.[102,112] Indeed conservative management is condemned by some clinicians, although the series on which arguments are based may have included large hematomas diagnosed in the pre-CT era.[113,114]

Prognosis and Follow-Up

In general, many studies using multivariate analyses of cases of cerebral ICH have shown that patients in deep coma, with advancing age, or with very large hematomas tend to do poorly. Kanaya and Kuroda[115] analyzed more than 7000 patients from Japan and classified them into five groups. They recommended that no surgery should be undertaken in patients in groups IVb and V (patients in coma and patients with herniation).

Our own studies at Newcastle-Upon-Tyne have confirmed that elderly patients in coma with large hematomas fare poorly. We treated 440 patients with spontaneous supratentorial ICHs between May 1993 and August 1999. Of these, only 24% had favorable scores on the Glasgow Outcome Scale (GOS). Multivariate analysis of patients in the prospectively collected database (including patients not in the International Surgical Trial of Intracerebral Hemorrhage) has confirmed these findings (Table 69-3). These adverse prognostic factors have been confirmed in the later, prospectively collected studies and trials.[116-118]

Epilepsy

Patients with ICH may present with epilepsy for the first time, and epilepsy may be the cause of sudden unexplained death.[119] Faught et al[120] reported that in patients with ICH, seizure incidence was more common with cortical lobar hemorrhage than with basal ganglia or subcortical hemorrhage and that no epilepsy was found if the bleed was thalamic.[120] Chronic epilepsy after ICH has been reported in 2.5% to 25% of patients,[121-123] partial seizures being the most common type.[124] The role of

surgery in reducing subsequent seizure frequency after ICH is unknown.

Risk of Rebleeding

Most hematomas enlarge in the first few hours, whatever the cause of the initial bleed,[28] but delayed rebleeding or continued oozing is more likely to occur with a structural vascular cause, such as an aneurysm or AVM, or with an underlying tumor. Emergency angiography is, therefore, necessary if a vascular lesion is suspected. After clot evacuation, delayed angiography should be considered to eliminate an AVM. This step must not be forgotten in a patient who makes a reasonable recovery, because the results of a second hemorrhage are often worse than those of the first.

Assessment of Dependence and Disability

Unfortunately, the quality of life in survivors of ICH is often poor. Most neurosurgeons prefer to use the GOS to quantitate functional outcome.[125] As assessed with this scale, good recovery occurs in only 5% of patients, with 10% moderately disabled (independent) and 40% remaining severely disabled (dependent).[68] Other analyses have employed the Rankin and Barthell scales; very few patients become independent according to ratings on these scales.

The GOS was originally developed by Jennett and Bond[126] for use in head injury studies. "Severe disability" was used for patients who were dependent on daily support because of mental disability, physical disability, or both. Patients with "moderate disability" could travel by public transport and could work in a sheltered environment, could shop independently, and were therefore independent as far as daily life was concerned. Moderately disabled patients could have residual disabilities such as hemiparesis, dysphasia, memory deficits, or personality changes, but this category did not include patients who were able only to care for themselves in their own homes; such patients were described instead as being severely disabled. "Good recovery" implied a resumption of normal life, including the capacity to return to work, to leisure, and family relationships. To compare groups treated in different ways, the scale may be dichotomized into unfavorable

TABLE 69-3 LOGISTIC REGRESSION ANALYSIS OF INDEPENDENT PREDICTORS OF OUTCOME FROM 440 NEWCASTLE PATIENTS WITH INTRACEREBRAL HEMORRHAGE IN THE PROSPECTIVELY COLLECTED DATABASE*

	P	Odds Ratio	95% Confidence Interval Lower Value	Upper Value
Age	<.0001	0.9493	0.9277	0.9715
Verbal Glasgow Coma Scale score	.0013	1.4697	1.1630	1.8574
Location: basal ganglia or lobar	<.0001	7.0618	3.3713	14.7922
Hematoma volume <20 mL compared with >40 mL	<.0001	7.9539	3.3807	18.7132
Hematoma volume 20-40 mL compared with >40 mL	.0035	3.6871	1.5344	8.8598
Basal cisterns (open)	.0251	12.2821	1.3685	110.2258

*December 1993–August 1999.
From Siddique MS: Intracerebral hemorrhage: The global magnitude of the problem and the scientific basis for intervention in the acute phase, Newcastle upon Tyne, UK, 2007, Newcastle University.

OUTCOME BY GCS AT RANDOMIZATION

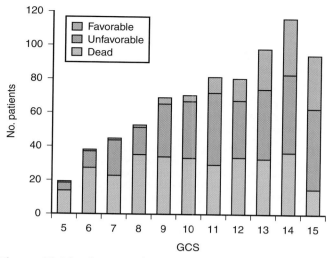

Figure 69-10 Outcome plotted against Glasgow Coma Scale (GCS) score in relation to random assignment to treatment for patients in the Surgical Trial in Intracerebral Hemorrhage (STICH).

outcome (dead, vegetative, or severely disabled) and favorable outcome (moderate disability or good recovery).

With time, the GOS has been used more and more frequently to measure outcome in patients with conditions other than head injury, including stroke, aneurysmal subarachnoid hemorrhage, and spontaneous ICH. The use of this scale in such patient groups must take into account the differences in age, health, and social independence before the event and, hence, the potential for recovery. For many elderly patients, it is clear that independence *within* the home should be regarded as a favorable outcome, but this independence might not include the ability to use public transportation or to shop independently. For patients with ICH, traditional classification to an outcome of severe disability would apply to three quarters of the group, but the category would vary widely from people who were able to look after themselves all day within their own homes to those who were bedridden and needed total care. The GOS should therefore be modified for use in patients with stroke and ICH to take into account these widely differing abilities.

The extended GOS (GOS-E) provides a finer classification of outcome because it subdivides each of the categories into upper and lower levels of disability.[127] It is clear that patients with ICH who are admitted to the hospital in coma very rarely achieve a good recovery or moderate disability whatever treatment they receive, whereas those with ICH and an admission Glasgow Coma Scale score of 14 or 15 may achieve these outcome levels (Fig. 69-10). Thus, a single dichotomous outcome division, uniform for the whole patient group, is less sensitive than measures that take into account the severity of the condition at the outset and the varying potential for improvement in individual patients. A sliding-scale dichotomy has therefore been proposed,[127] with the breakpoints between moderate disability and severe disability for the groups with the best prognoses and between upper and lower severe disability for the groups with the worst prognoses.

REFERENCES

1. Davis S: DWI and perfusion MRI. In Abstracts of the 6th World Stroke Congress and Xth International Symposium on Thrombolysis and Acute Stroke Therapy. September 24-27, 2008 Vienna, Austria and September 21-23, 2008, Budapest, Hungary, *Int Stroke J* 3(Suppl 1):2-474, 2008.
2. Hacke W, Kaste M, Bluhmki E, et al: ECASS Investigators: Thrombolysis with alteplase 3 to 4.5 hours after acute ischemic stroke, *N Engl J Med* 359:1317-1329, 2008.
3. Sudlow M, Thomson R, Thwaites B, et al: Prevalence of atrial fibrillation and eligibility for anticoagulants in the community, *Lancet* 352:1167-1171, 1998.
4. Gregson BA, Mendelow AD: International variations in surgical practice for spontaneous intracerebral hemorrhage, *Stroke* 34:2593-2597, 2003.
5. Mendelow AD, Gregson BA, Fernandes HM, et al: Early surgery versus initial conservative treatment in patients with spontaneous supratentorial intracerebral haematomas in the International Surgical Trial in Intracerebral Haemorrhage (STICH): A randomised trial, *Lancet* 365:387-397, 2005.
6. Prasad K, Mendelow AD, Gregson BA: Surgery for primary supratentorial intracerebral haemorrhage, *Cochrane Database Syst Rev* (4):CD000200, 2008.
7. Mendelow AD. STICH II. In; 2008.
8. Molyneux A, Kerr R, Stratton I, et al: International Subarachnoid Aneurysm Trial (ISAT) of neurosurgical clipping versus endovascular coiling in 2143 patients with ruptured intracranial aneurysms: A randomised trial, *Lancet* 360:1267-1274, 2002.
9. Molyneux A, Kerr R, Sandercock P, et al: International Subarachnoid Aneurysm Trial (ISAT) Collaborative Group: Long term results of ISAT. In Abstracts of the 6th World Stroke Congress and Xth International Symposium on Thrombolysis and Acute Stroke Therapy. September 24-27, 2008 Vienna, Austria and September 21-23, 2008, Budapest, Hungary, *Int Stroke J* 3(Suppl 1):2-474, 2008.
10. Mitchell P, Kerr R, Mendelow AD, et al: Could late rebleeding overturn the superiority of cranial aneurysm coil embolization over clip ligation seen in the International Subarachnoid Aneurysm Trial? *J Neurosurg* 108:437-442, 2008.
11. Brown RDJ: The natural history of unruptured intracranial aneurysms: Prospective data from the International Study of Unruptured Intracranial Aneurysms. In: Abstracts of the 11th European Stroke Conference. Geneva, Switzerland, May 29-June 1, 2002, *Cerebrovasc Dis* (Suppl 3):O146, 2002.
12. Wiebers DO, Piepgras DG, Brown RD Jr, et al: Unruptured aneurysms, *J Neurosurg* 96:50-51, 2002:discussion 58-60.
13. Mitchell P, Mitra D, Gregson BA, Mendelow AD: Prevention of intracerebral hemorrhage, *Current Drug Targets* 8:832-838, 2007.
14. Heiskanen O, Poranen A, Kuurne T, et al: Acute surgery for intracerebral haematomas caused by rupture of an intracranial arterial aneurysm. A prospective randomized study, *Acta Neurochir (Wien)* 90:81-93, 1988.
15. Broderick JP, Brott TG, Duldner JE, et al: Volume of intracerebral hemorrhage: a powerful and easy-to-use predictor of 30-day mortality, *Stroke* 24:987-993, 1993.
16. Fernandes HF: *MD thesis [MD]*, Newcastle upon Tyne, UK, 2002, Newcastle University.
17. Siddique MS, Fernandes HM, Wooldridge TD, et al: Reversible ischemia around intracerebral hemorrhage: A single-photon emission computerized tomography study, *J Neurosurg* 96:736-741, 2002.
18. Heiss W-D, Beil C, Pawlik G, et al: Nontraumatic intracerebral haematoma versus ischaemic stroke. Regional pattern of glucose metabolism, *J Cereb Blood Flow Metab* 5:S5-S6, 1985.
19. Uemura K, Shishido F, Higano S, et al: Positron emission tomography in patients with a primary intracerebral hematoma, *Acta Radiol Suppl* 369:426-428, 1986.
20. Zazulia AR, Diringer MN, Videen TO, et al: Hypoperfusion without ischemia surrounding acute intracerebral hemorrhage, *J Cereb Blood Flow Metab* 21:804-810, 2001.
21. Schellinger PD, Fiebach JB, Hoffmann K, et al: Stroke MRI in intracerebral hemorrhage: Is there a perihemorrhagic penumbra [see comment]? *Stroke* 34:1674-1679, 2003.
22. Orakcioglu B, Fiebach JB, Steiner T, et al: Evolution of early perihemorrhagic changes—ischemia vs. edema: An MRI study in rats, *Exp Neurol* 193:369-376, 2005.

23. Qureshi AI, Wilson DA, Hanley DF, et al: No evidence for an ischemic penumbra in massive experimental intracerebral hemorrhage, *Neurology* 52:266-272, 1999.

24. Zazulia AR, Diringer MN, Videen TO, et al: Hypoperfusion without ischemia surrounding acute intracerebral hemorrhage, *J Cereb Blood Flow Metab* 21:804-810, 2001.

25. Schellinger PD, Fiebach JB, Hacke W: Imaging-based decision making in thrombolytic therapy for ischemic stroke: Present status, *Stroke* 34:575-583, 2003.

26. Orakcioglu B, Fiebach JB, Steiner T, et al: Evolution of early perihemorrhagic changes—ischemia vs. edema: An MRI study in rats, *Exp Neurol* 193:369-376, 2005.

27. Siddique MS: *Intracerebral hemorrhage: The global magnitude of the problem and the scientific basis for intervention in the acute phase [MD thesis]*, Newcastle upon Tyne, UK, 2007, Newcastle University.

28. Mendelow AD, Bullock R, Teasdale GM, et al: Intracranial haemorrhage induced at arterial pressure in the rat: Part 2. Short term changes in local cerebral blood flow measured by autoradiography, *Neurol Res* 6:189-193, 1984.

29. Bullock R, Mendelow AD, Teasdale GM, et al: Intracranial haemorrhage induced at arterial pressure in the rat: Part 1. Description of technique, ICP changes and neurological findings, *Neurol Res* 6:184-188, 1984.

30. Kingman TA, Mendelow AD, Graham DI, et al: Experimental intracerebral mass—time-related effects on local cerebral blood-flow, *J Neurosurg* 67:732-738, 1987.

31. Rosand J, Eskey C, Chang Y, et al: Dynamic single-section CT demonstrates reduced cerebral blood flow in acute intracerebral hemorrhage, *Cerebrovasc Dis* 14:214-220, 2002.

32. Powers WJ, Zazulia AR, Videen TO, et al: Autoregulation of cerebral blood flow surrounding acute (6 to 22 hours) intracerebral hemorrhage, *Neurology* 57:18-24, 2001.

33. Videen TO, Dunford-Shore JE, Diringer MN, et al: Correction for partial volume effects in regional blood flow measurements adjacent to hematomas in humans with intracerebral hemorrhage: Implementation and validation, *J Comput Assist Tomogr* 23:248-256, 1999.

34. Zazulia AR, Diringer MN, Derdeyn CP, et al: Progression of mass effect after intracerebral hemorrhage, *Stroke* 30:1167-1173, 1999.

35. Kanno T, Nonomura K: Hyperbaric oxygen therapy to determine the surgical indication of moderate hypertensive intracerebral hemorrhage, *Minim Invas Neurosurg* 39:56-59, 1996.

36. Heiss WD: Ischemic penumbra: Evidence from functional imaging in man, *J Cereb Blood Flow Metab* 20:1276-1293, 2000.

37. Gebel JM Jr, Jauch EC, Brott TG, et al: Natural history of perihematomal edema in patients with hyperacute spontaneous intracerebral hemorrhage, *Stroke* 33:2631-2635, 2002.

38. Gebel JM Jr, Jauch EC, Brott TG, et al: Relative edema volume is a predictor of outcome in patients with hyperacute spontaneous intracerebral hemorrhage, *Stroke* 33:2636-2641, 2002.

39. Qureshi AI: Antihypertensive treatment of acute cerebral hemorrhage (ATACH), *Neurocrit Care* 6:56-66, 2007.

40. Anderson CS, Huang Y, Wang G, et al: Intensive blood pressure reduction in acute cerebral haemorrhage trial (INTERACT): A pilot randomised trial, *Lancet Neurol* 7:391-399, 2008.

41. Brott T, Broderick J, Kothari R, et al: Early hemorrhage growth in patients with intracerebral hemorrhage, *Stroke* 28:1-5, 1997.

42. Mayer SA, Brun NC, Begtrup K, et al: Recombinant activated factor VII for acute intracerebral hemorrhage, *N Engl J Med* 352:777-785, 2005.

43. Mayer SA, Brun NC, Begtrup K: Efficacy and safety of recombinant activated factor VII for acute intracerebral hemorrhage, *N Engl J Med* 358:2127-2137, 2008.

44. Juttler E, Steiner T: Treatment and prevention of spontaneous intracerebral hemorrhage: Comparison of EUSI and AHA/ASA recommendations, *Expert Rev Neurother* 7:1401-1416, 2007.

45. Pickard JD, Murray GD, Illingworth R, et al: Effect of oral nimodipine on cerebral infarction and outcome after subarachnoid haemorrhage: British aneurysm nimodipine trial, *BMJ* 298:636-642, 1989.

46. Kerr R, et al: Intracerebral hematoma due to aneurysmal rupture: Endovascular treatment followed by clot evacuation. In 12th World Congress of Neurosurgery, 2001, Sydney. Sydney, World Federation of Neurosurgical Societies, 2001.

47. Chandra B: *Small intracerebral bleedings: To treat or not to treat? Paper presented at the XI European Stroke Conference*, Geneva, May 30, 2002, Switzerland.

48. Stevenson J, Jenkins A, Mendelow A: Experimental intracerebral haemorrhage—U74006F (Tirilazad Mesylate) reduces ischaemic neuronal damage, *J Neurosurg* 82:359, 1995.

49. Kane PJ, Cook S, Chambers IR, et al: Cerebral oedema following intracerebral haemorrhage: The effect of the NMDA receptor antagonists MK-901 and D-CCPene, *Acta Neurochir* S60:561-563, 1994.

50. Cruz JMG, Okuchi K: Improving clinical outcomes from acute subdural hematomas with the emergency preoperative administration of high doses of mannitol: A randomized trial, *Neurosurgery* 49:864-871, 2001.

51. Cruz J, Minoja G, Okuchi K: Major clinical and physiological benefits of early high doses of mannitol for intraparenchymal temporal lobe hemorrhages with abnormal pupillary widening: A randomized trial, *Neurosurgery* 51:628-637, 2002:discussion 637-638.

52. Davis M, MA D, Barer D: Age and the risk of stroke progression in the acute stroke monitoring trial, *Cerebrovasc Dis* x:0424, 2002.

53. Fernandes HM, Siddique S, Banister K, et al: Continuous monitoring of ICP and CPP following ICH and its relationship to clinical, radiological and surgical parameters, *Acta Neurochir Suppl* 76:463-466, 2000.

54. Siddique MS: *Intracerebral hemorrhage: The global magnitude of the problem and the scientific basis for intervention in the acute phase [MD thesis]. Newcastle upon Tyne*, 2007, Newcastle University.

55. Meyer JS, Bauer RB: Medical treatment of spontaneous intracerebral haemorrhage by the use of hypotensive drugs, *Neurology* 12:36-47, 1962.

56. Yu YL, Kumana CR, Lauder IJ, et al: Treatment of acute cerebral hemorrhage with intravenous glycerol. A double-blind, placebo controlled, randomized trial, *Stroke* 23:967-971, 1992.

57. Haemodilution in acute stroke: Results of the Italian haemodilution trial. Italian Acute Stroke Study Group, *Lancet* 1(8581):318-321, 1988.

58. Tellez H, Bauer RB: Dexamethasone as treatment in cerebrovascular disease. 1. A controlled study in intracerebral hemorrhage, *Stroke* 4:541-546, 1973.

59. Poungvarin N, Bhoopat W, Viriyavejakul A, et al: Effects of dexamethasone in primary supratentorial intracerebral hemorrhage, *N Engl J Med* 3161:1229-1233, 1987.

60. Prasad K, Browman G, Srivastava A, et al: Surgery in primary supratentorial intracerebral hematoma: A meta-analysis of randomized trials, *Acta Neurol Scand* 95:103-110, 1997.

61. Prasad K, Shrivastava A: Surgery for primary supratentorial intracerebral haemorrhage, *Cochrane Database Syst Rev* (4): CD000200, 1999.

62. Fernandes HM, Gregson B, Siddique MS, et al: Surgery in intracerebral hemorrhage—the uncertainty continues, *Stroke* 31:2511-2516, 2000.

63. Teernstra O, Evers S, Lodder J, et al: Stereotactic treatment of intracerebral hematoma by means of plasminogen activator. A multicentre randomized controlled trial (SICHPA), *Stroke* 34:968-974, 2003.

64. Mendelow AD: STICH II website. In Chilton L, editor: 2007, Newcastle University.

65. Kirkman M, Gregson B, Mahattanakal W, et al: The effect of the STICH trial on management of intracerebral haemorrhage in Newcastle, *Br J Neurosurg* 22:739-746, 2008:discussion 747.

66. Huang J, van Gelder JM: The probability of sudden death from rupture of intracranial aneurysms: A meta-analysis, *Neurosurgery* 51:1101-1107, 2002.

67. Mathew P, Teasdale G, Bannan A, et al: Neurosurgical management of cerebellar haematoma and infarct, *J Neurol Neurosurg Psychiatry* 59:287-292, 1995.

68. Siddique MS, Gregson BA, Fernandes HM, et al: Comparative study of traumatic and spontaneous intracerebral hemorrhage, *J Neurosurg* 96:86-89, 2002.

69. Chen X, Yang H, Cheng Z: The comparative study of the total medical and surgical treatment of hypertensive intracerebral haemorrhage, *Acta Acad Med Shanghai* 19:234-240, 1992.

70. Chen B, Hou D: Surgical treatment of hypertensive intracerebral hemorrhage, *Chin Med J (Engl)* 94:723-728, 1981.

71. McKissock W, Richardson A, Taylor J: Primary intracerebral haemorrhage; a controlled trial of surgical and conservative treatment in 180 unselected cases, *Lancet* 2:221-226, 1961.

72. Pia HW: The surgical treatment of intracerebral and intraventricular haematomas, *Acta Neurochir* 27:149, 1972.

73. Lui ZH, Kang HQ, Chen XH, et al: Evacuation of hypertensive intracerebral hematoma by a stereotactic technique, *Stereotact Funct Neurosurg* 54:451-452, 1990.

74. Niizuma H, Shimizu Y, Yonemitsu T, et al: Results of stereotactic aspiration in 175 cases of putaminal haemorrhage, *Neurosurgery* 24:814-819, 1989.

75. Mohadjer M: Computed tomographic-stereotactic evacuation and fibrinolysis of spontaneous intracerebral haematomas. In Lorenz R, Klinger M, Brock M, editors: *Advances in Neurosurgery*, Berlin, 1993, Springer-Verlag, pp 47-51.

76. Hondo H, Uno M, Sasaki K, et al: Computed tomography controlled aspiration surgery for hypertensive intracerebral hemorrhage. Experience of more than 400 cases, *Stereotact Funct Neurosurg* 54:432-437, 1990.

77. Kanaya H, Yukawa H, Itoh Z, et al: A neurological grading for patients with hypertensive intracerebral hemorrhage and a classification for hematoma location of computer tomography. In 7th conference of surgical treatment of stroke; 1978, Japan; 1978, pp 265-270.

78. Kanno T, Sano H, Shinomiya Y, et al: Role of surgery in hypertensive intracerebral hematoma. A comparative study of 305 nonsurgical and 154 surgical cases, *J Neurosurg* 61:1091-1099, 1984.

79. Coraddu M, Nurchi GC, Floris F, et al: Considerations about the surgical indication of the spontaneous cerebral haematomas, *J Neurosurg Sci* 34:35-39, 1990.

80. Kanaya H, Kuroda K: Intracerebral hematomas. In Kaufman HH, editor: *Development in neurosurgical approaches to hypertensive intracerebral haemorrhage in Japan*, New York, 1992, Raven Press, pp 197-209.

81. Chen X, Yang H, Cheng Z: Comparative study of the internal medical and surgical treatment of hypertensive intracranial haemorrhage, *Acta Acad Med Shanghai* 19:237-240, 1992.

82. Fernandes HM, Mendelow AD: Spontaneous intracerebral haemorrhage: A surgical dilemma, *Br J Neurosurg* 13:389-394, 1999.

83. Taylor ABW, Rosenfeld J, Shann F, et al: A randomized trial of very early decompressive craniectomy in children with traumatic brain injury and sustained intracranial hypertension, *Childs Nerv Syst* 17:154-162, 2001.

84. Mitchell P, Gregson BA, Vindlacheruvu R, et al: Surgical options in ICH including decompressive craniectomy, *J Neurol Sci* 261:89-98, 2007.

85. Cruz JMG, Okuchi K: Major clinical and physiological benefits of early high doses of mannitol for intraparenchymal temporal lobe hemorrhages with abnormal pupillary widening: A randomized trial, *Neurosurgery* 51:628-637, 2002.

86. Roberts I, Smith R, Evans S: Doubts over head injury studies, *BMJ* 334:392-394, 2007.

87. Chambers IR, Treadwell L, Mendelow AD: The determination of threshold levels of cerebral perfusion pressure and intracranial pressure in severe head injury using receiver operator characteristic curves: An observational study on 291 patients, *J Neurosurg* 94:412-416, 2001.

88. Auer LM, Deinsberger W, Niederkorn K, et al: Endoscopic surgery versus medical treatment for spontaneous intracerebral hematoma: A randomized study, *J Neurosurg* 70:530-535, 1989.

89. Marquardt G, Wolff R, Sager A, et al: Manual stereotactic aspiration of spontaneous deep-seated intracerebral hematomas in non-comatose patients, *Br J Neurosurg* 15:126-131, 2001.

90. Marquardt G, Wolff R, Sager A, et al: Subacute stereotactic aspiration of heamatomas within the basal ganglia reduces occurrence of complications in the course of haemorrhagic stroke in non-comatose patients, *Cerebrovasc Dis* 15:252-257, 2003.

91. Zuccarello M. MISTIE Trial. In; 2008.

92. Hanley D. The SLEUTH trial. In; 2008.

93. Teernstra O, Evers S, Lodder J, et al: Stereotactic treatment of intracerebral haematoma by means of a plasminogen activator: A multicentre randomised controlled trial (SICHPA).

94. Teernstra OPM, Blaauw G. SICHPA: Stereotactic Treatment of Intracerebral Hematoma by Means of a Plasminogen Activator: A multicentre randomised controlled trial. In: 12th World Congress of Neurosurgery; 2001; Sydney; 2001.

95. Naff NJ, Hanley DF, Keyl PM, et al: Intraventricular thrombolysis speeds blood clot resolution: Results of a pilot, prospective, randomized, double-blind, controlled trial, *Neurosurgery* 54:577-583, 2004:discussion 583-584.

96. Hanley DF. MISTIE. In; 2007.

97. Hanley DF. CLEAR IVH. In; 2007.

98. Hanley D: Update of Clinical Trials: CLEAR, MISTIE & STICH. In: European Association of Neurosurgery Societies (EANS); 2007 4.9.2007; Glasgow; 2007.

99. Arene NU, Fernandes HM, Wilson S, et al: Intraventricular haemorrhage from spontaneous intracerebral haemorrhage and aneurysmal rupture, *Acta Neurochir Suppl* 79:134-138, 1998.

100. Molyneux AKR, Stratton I, Sandercock P, et al: International Subarachnoid Aneurysm Trial (ISAT) Collaborative Group: International Subarachnoid Aneurysm Trial (ISAT) of neurosurgical clipping versus endovascular coiling in 2143 patients with ruptured intracranial aneurysms: A randomised trial, *Lancet* 360(9342):1267-1274, 2002.

101. Miyamoto S, Hashimoto N, Nagata I, et al: Posttreatment sequelae of palliatively treated cerebral arteriovenous malformations, *Neurosurgery* 46:589-594, 2000:discussion 594-595.

102. Mathew P, Teasdale G, Bannan A, et al: Neurosurgical management of cerebellar haematoma and infarct, *J Neurol Neurosurg Psychiatry* 59:287-292, 1995.

103. Auer LM, Auer T, Sayama I: Indications for surgical treatment of cerebellar haemorrhage and infarction, *Acta Neurochir* 79:74-79, 1986.

104. Donauer E, Loew F, Faubert C, et al: Prognostic factors in the treatment of cerebellar haemorrhage, *Acta Neurochir* 131:59-66, 1994.

105. Dunne JW, Chakera T, Kermode S: Cerebellar haemorrhage: Diagnosis and treatment: A study of 75 consecutive cases, *Q J Med* 64:739-754, 1987.

106. Firsching R, Huber M, Frowein RA: Cerebellar haemorrhage: Management and prognosis, *Neurosurg Rev* 14:191-194, 1991.

107. Gerritsen van der Hoop R, Vermeulen N, van Gijn J: Cerebellar haemorrhage: diagnosis and treatment, *Surg Neurol* 29:6-10, 1988.

108. Heros RC: Cerebellar haemorrhage and infarction, *Stroke* 29:6-10, 1982.

109. Koziarski A, Frankiewicz E: Medical and surgical treatment of intracerebellar haematomas, *Acta Neurochir* 110:24-28, 1991.

110. Lui T, Fairholm DJ, Shu T, et al: Surgical treatment of spontaneous cerebellar hemorrhage, *Surg Neurol* 23:555-558, 1985.

111. Waidhauser E, Hamburger C, Marguth F: Neurosurgical management of cerebellar haemorrhage, *Neurosurg Rev* 13:211-217, 1990.

112. Ott KH, Kase CS, Ojemann RG, et al: Cerebellar hemorrhage: Diagnosis and treatment. A review of 56 cases, *Arch Neurol* 31:160-167, 1974.

113. Brennan RW, Bergland RM: Acute cerebellar haemorrhage. Analysis of clinical findings and outcome in 12 cases, *Neurology* 27:527-532, 1977.

114. Fisher CM, Picard EH, Polak A, et al: Acute hypertensive cerebellar haemorrhage: Diagnosis and surgical treatment, *J Nerv Ment Dis* 140:38-57, 1965.

115. Kanaya H, Kuroda K: Development in neurosurgical approaches to hypertensive intracerebral haemorrhage in Japan. In Kaufman HH, editor: *Intracerebral Hematomas*, New York, 1992, Raven Press, pp 197-209.

116. Mendelow AD, Teasdale GM, Barer D, et al: Outcome assignment in the International Surgical Trial of Intracerebral Haemorrhage, *Acta Neurochir (Wien)* 145:679-681, 2003:discussion 681.

117. Mendelow AD, Gregson BA, Fernandes HM, et al: Early surgery versus initial conservative treatment in patients with spontaneous supratentorial intracerebral haematomas in the International Surgical Trial in Intracerebral Haemorrhage (STICH): A randomised trial, *Lancet* 365:387-397, 2005.

118. Hemphill JC 3rd, Bonovich DC, Besmertis L, et al: The ICH score: A simple, reliable grading scale for intracerebral hemorrhage, *Stroke* 32:891-897, 2001.

119. Black M, Graham D: Sudden unexplained death in adults caused by intracranial pathology, *J Clin Pathol* 55:44-50, 2002.

120. Faught E, Peters D, Bartolucci A, et al: Seizures after primary intracerebral hemorrhage, *Neurology* 39:1089-1093, 1989.

121. Lancman M, Golimstok A, Norscini J, et al: Risk factors for developing seizures after a stroke, *Epilepsia* 34:141-143, 1993.

122. Sung CY, Chu NS: Epileptic seizures in intracerebral haemorrhage, *J Neurol Neurosurg Psychiatry* 52:1273-1276, 1989.

123. Arboix X, García-Eroles L, Massons JB, et al: Predictive factors of early seizures after cerebrovascular disease, *Stroke* 28:1590-1594, 1997.

124. Cervoni L, Delfini R, Santoro A, et al: Multiple intracranial aneurysms: Surgical treatment and outcome, *Acta Neurochir (Wien)* 124:66-70, 1993.

125. Jennett B, Bond M: Assessment of outcome after severe brain damage, *Lancet* 1(7905):480-484, 1974.

126. Jennett B, Bond M: Assessment of outcome after severe brain damage: A practical scale, *Lancet* 1:480-484, 1975.

127. Wilson JT, Pettigrew LE, Teasdale GM: Structured interviews for the Glasgow Outcome Scale and the extended Glasgow Outcome Scale: Guidelines for their use, *J Neurotrauma* 15(8):573-585, 1998.

70 Intraventricular Hemorrhage

J. MAX FINDLAY

Bleeding directly into the ventricles from a source or lesion that is in contact with or is part of a ventricular wall, such as a vascular malformation or neoplasm, is classified as primary intraventricular hemorrhage (IVH). This type of IVH without an associated intracerebral hematoma is rare, accounting for only about 3% of all spontaneous intracerebral hemorrhages (ICHs).[1] Much more commonly, IVH is secondary either to intracerebral bleeding that dissects through brain parenchyma to reach a ventricle or to bleeding into the subarachnoid space that spreads into the ventricles through the fourth ventricular foramina. Primary or secondary IVHs can fill one or more ventricles and, when of sufficient volume and density, can result in formed ventricular blood clots, or hematocephalus. Blood that refluxes into the ventricles from the subarachnoid space often remains unclotted and settles in dependent parts of the ventricular system. Although the presence of IVH per se does not always correlate with neurologic condition or prognosis, IVH is an independent and important clinical problem when clots distend the ventricular system, compress adjacent brain, or obstruct cerebrospinal fluid (CSF) flow to cause hydrocephalus and elevated intracranial pressure (ICP).

There are many causes of spontaneous IVH, but the most common are hypertensive ICH, saccular aneurysms, and arteriovenous malformations (AVMs).[2-8] IVH resulting from germinal matrix hemorrhage in the newborn and traumatic IVH are not discussed in this chapter.

Primary Intraventricular Hemorrhage

Spontaneous IVH with no evidence of associated ICH is most often due either to a vascular malformation that contacts the ependyma of one of the ventricular chambers or to an intraventricular or periventricular neoplasm.[7] There have been rare reports of primary IVH due to ruptured intraventricular aneurysms, which arise from distal lenticulostriate or choroidal arteries that reach the ventricular lining or choroid plexus.[9] Aneurysms have been reported on penetrating arteries enlarged by moyamoya disease.[10-12] In some cases, no cause of primary IVH can be established, although in these instances bleeding may be from rupture of arterioles located in the immediate periventricular region that have been weakened by chronic hypertension. Primary IVH can be due to any type of bleeding disorder, including anticoagulation[8] and fibrinolytic treatment.[13,14]

The most common brain neoplasm that bleeds spontaneously is malignant astrocytoma. Less common tumors to cause primary IVH are ependymoma,[15] subependymoma,[16] choroid plexus papilloma,[17] intraventricular meningioma,[18,19] pituitary tumors that erode through the floor of the third ventricle,[20] neurocytoma,[21] granular cell tumor,[22] metastasis,[23] and craniopharyngioma (Fig. 70-1). It is probable that any cause of spontaneous ICH can be responsible for direct bleeding into the ventricles.

Hypertensive Brain Hemorrhage and Intraventricular Hemorrhage

Spontaneous hypertensive ICHs are associated with secondary IVH in one third to one half of patients.[24] The most significant risk factor for this arteriopathy, which most commonly affects the lenticulostriate and thalamoperforating arterioles, is chronic arterial hypertension; other risk factors are moderate to heavy alcohol intake and anticoagulant treatment.[25] IVH most often complicates thalamic, caudate, or putaminal bleeding that decompresses into the lateral or third ventricles (Fig. 70-2). Not surprisingly, IVH in this setting has been associated with larger parenchymal hematomas, midline shift of brain structures, and worse clinical outcome.[26-28] Patients with spontaneous and deep intracerebral hemorrhages complicated by both IVH and hydrocephalus have a particularly bad prognosis,[29-31] although the associated ICH size probably has the greatest influence on clinical outcome.[32]

Aneurysmal Intraventricular Hemorrhage

Of patients who survive rupture of an intracranial aneurysm, IVH is seen in roughly 15% of the entire group, in 25% of those with severe subarachnoid hemorrhage (SAH), and in 40% of those who subsequently die from the rupture.[33] Aneurysmal IVH is associated with an up to 50% chance of requiring a ventriculoperitoneal shunt.[34-36] Aneurysm rupture can cause IVH through several different mechanisms.[37] Blood can reflux into the ventricular system from an aneurysm in any location, but disproportionate or isolated fourth ventricular hemorrhage in association with SAH is especially suggestive of a posterior circulation aneurysm situated closer to the fourth ventricular foramina. Up to one half of posterior inferior cerebellar artery (PICA) aneurysm ruptures have an accompanying IVH.[38]

Sudden death from aneurysmal SAH is commonly associated with IVH, and in some patients the mechanism may be acute fourth ventricular dilatation causing brainstem compression.[39,40]

Aneurysms also cause IVH when forceful hemorrhage dissects through intervening brain parenchyma to reach the ventricular system. This occurrence is most commonly seen with anterior communicating artery aneurysms.[41] With a 25% incidence of associated IVH, this aneurysm is the most common type to cause IVH. Blood can break directly through the lamina terminalis into the third ventricle or can pass superiorly beneath the rostrum of the corpus callosum to leak through the septum pellucidum into the lateral ventricles. Frontal hemorrhages resulting from anterior communicating or middle cerebral artery aneurysms can spread into the anterior horn of the lateral ventricles.

Internal carotid artery aneurysms, at the origin of either the posterior communicating or the anterior choroidal arteries can rupture into the temporal horn of the lateral ventricles (Fig. 70-3). Basilar apex aneurysms can rupture directly through the hypothalamus to reach the third ventricle, usually with serious clinical consequences.

In large patient series, IVH along with aneurysm rupture is associated with higher intracranial pressures[42] and worse outcome.[43]

Vascular Malformations and Intraventricular Hemorrhage

Cerebral AVMs that are in contact with the ventricular wall and hemorrhage often bleed into the ventricles, and are usually associated with deep cerebral venous drainage (Fig. 70-4). In one prospective AVM database, 16% of first AVM hemorrhages were primarily intraventricular and 31% were combined intracerebral and intraventricular hemorrhages.[44] Periventricular cavernous malformations and dural arteriovenous fistulas with transcerebral venous drainage are less common but can also cause IVH.

Natural Clearance of Intraventricular Hemorrhage

Normally the CSF contains little fibrinolytic activity, although fibrinolysis becomes detectable after bleeding into the CSF. As in plasma, the principal fibrinolytic

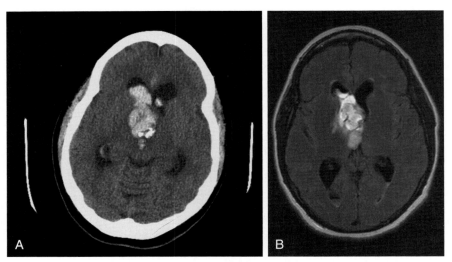

Figure 70-1 A previously healthy 43-year-old woman presented comatose after sudden collapse due to spontaneous intraventricular bleeding from what proved to be a suprasellar craniopharyngioma. A, CT scan; B, MR image. She made a reasonable recovery following ventriculoperitoneal shunting and transcallosal tumor debulking.

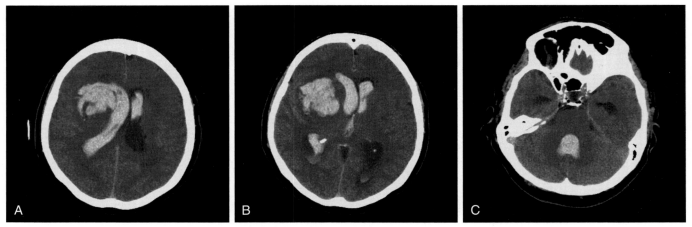

Figure 70-2 A 71-year-old woman presented obtunded and paralyzed on the left side of her body from a right lentiform intracerebral hemorrhage that extended into the ventricular system. See Figure 70-6 for follow-up.

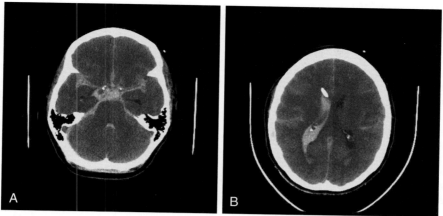

Figure 70-3 A 41-year-old man presented comatose after complaining of a sudden severe headache. CT showed a diffuse subarachnoid hemorrhage from what appeared to be rupture of a right posterior communicating artery aneurysm that bled through the right temporal horn into the lateral ventricular system. The patient deteriorated and died several days later from raised intracranial pressure.

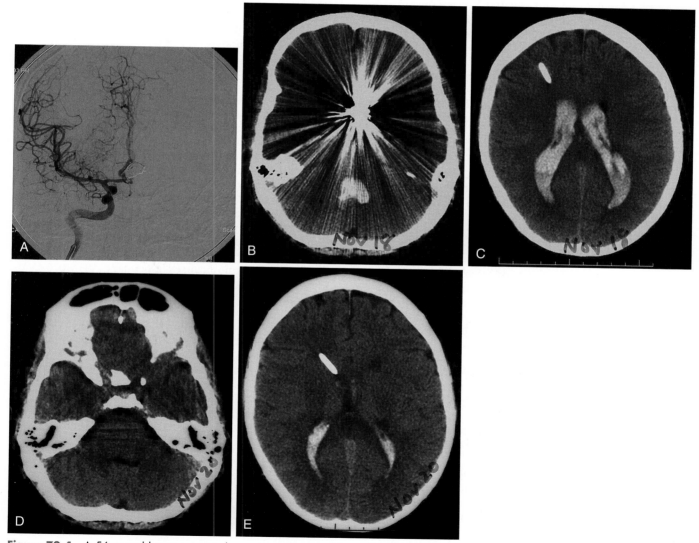

Figure 70-4 A 56-year-old man presented comatose after a sudden collapse. A, A ruptured anterior communicating artery was treated with endovascular coiling. (The patient had a second, small, right middle cerebral artery aneurysm that was not treated.) B and C, CT scanning the next day showed a persistent panventricular hemorrhage that was treated with a single dose of 4 mg of rt-PA via the ventriculostomy catheter. (See text for protocol details.) D and E, CT scans performed 2 days later demonstrate considerable clearance of ventricular clots, and the patient went on to make a good clinical recovery.

enzyme in the CSF is plasmin, carried into the ventricles in its precursor form, plasminogen, as a normal blood constituent. It is converted to its active form by tissue-type plasminogen activator (t-PA). Tissue-type plasminogen activator is released from the endothelium of small vessels in the meninges and ependyma, and leukocytes and platelets within the ventricular thrombi are additional sources of plasminogen activator enzymes. These various activators diffuse into clot, bind to fibrin, and activate plasminogen incorporated into the coagulum. The degree of fibrinolytic activity in "activated" CSF is meager relative to plasma, but is proportional to the volume of blood clot volume. It is also balanced by the presence of inhibitors also released into the CSF by inflamed leptomeninges.[45] Changes in CSF coagulation and fibrinolysis have been studied in the context of SAH and are probably similar to changes following IVH.[46]

The resolution of intraventricular blood clot appears to follow first-order kinetics, such that the daily percentage rate of clot breakdown and clot half-life is constant and the absolute amount of clot broken down per day rises with increasing IVH volume.[47] The clearance of erythrocytes from CSF is accomplished by several mechanisms. The first is hemolysis, which commences within hours and reaches a plateau 2 to 10 days after IVH, depending on the size of the hemorrhage. Another is phagocytosis by macrophages, which occurs both in the leptomeninges irritated by blood and in arachnoid granulations engorged with erythrocytes.

Clinical Features

Spontaneous and primary IVH manifests as sudden headache, vomiting, and sometimes altered mental status.[5,48] A generalized seizure may occur, but without any significant associated ICH, focal signs are generally absent. Symptoms from even a large IVH can sometime be surprisingly minimal, provided that the ventricles have not become distended and ICP remains within normal limits. The total volume of CSF in adults is approximately 150 mL, and the normal ventricular volume is only 20 to 30 mL. Acute fourth ventricular distension after aneurysm or AVM rupture causing brainstem compression is associated with rapid and advanced neurologic deterioration and with sudden death.

With secondary IVH, presenting symptoms are usually due to the associated ICH or SAH, and the nature and magnitude of the symptoms and signs correspond to the location and size of the hemorrhage.

Symptomatic vasospasm of the anterior and middle cerebral arteries after an AVM-related IVH has been described,[49,50] but the complication is exceptional after hemorrhage restricted to the ventricles. Delayed-onset cerebral vasospasm after aneurysm rupture depends on thick blood clots deposited in the basal subarachnoid cisterns and left in prolonged contact with the adventitial surfaces of arteries. The presence of thick subarachnoid hematomas along with blood clots also in both lateral ventricles may predict an especially high risk of delayed cerebral ischemia after aneurysm rupture.[51]

Noncommunicating hydrocephalus can occur acutely after IVH if clots obstruct CSF drainage within the ventricular system, and communicating hydrocephalus may develop more gradually or even in a delayed fashion because of obstruction and then scarring of the arachnoid granulations from blood elements carried to them by CSF flow. The risk of hydrocephalus correlates with the severity of IVH and is greater if there is blood in the third or fourth ventricles or if there is associated SAH. In spontaneous supratentorial ICH, secondary IVH correlates with the presence of acute hydrocephalus and poor outcome.[52] Acute hydrocephalus is seen in roughly 15% of patients with ruptured aneurysms, and its presence is also significantly related to the presence of IVH.[53]

Diagnosis

IVH is diagnosed with CT, and scoring systems have been devised to quantify the extent of IVH seen on CT scan (Table 70-1). Clearly, clinical condition and prognosis are more closely related to ventricular distension, associated parenchymal damage, and the underlying cause of bleeding.

If CT scanning shows IVH secondary to a deep thalamic or ganglionic parenchymal hemorrhage in an adult, and especially an older person, a small vessel cause can usually be assumed, and further investigation is not mandatory. Similarly, if the primary hemorrhage is lobar and is strongly suspected on clinical grounds to be related to a bleeding disorder, amyloid angiopathy, or conversion of a cardioembolic infarction, angiography is again unwarranted. If, after these considerations, the underlying cause of IVH remains uncertain, angiography, MRI, or both are indicated, especially if thrombolytic therapy (discussed in the next section) is being considered. Vascular imaging is recommended for any patient with primary IVH of no apparent cause and for any patient younger than 45 years who has an IVH.[6,48,54] In a 2008 review, nearly 60% of patients with primary IVH had positive angiographic findings of a bleeding source, and the two most common causes of primary IVH were AVMs and aneurysms.[48]

Treatment

Management is directed at any identified underlying cause of IVH (e.g., aneurysm repair, AVM or tumor excision, blood pressure control, correction of bleeding disorder) and external ventricular drainage to relieve any associated hydrocephalus and help manage raised ICP. Surgical evacuation through a frontal corticotomy of lateral ventricles packed with blood clot after aneurysm

TABLE 70-1 GRADING SYSTEM FOR SEVERITY OF INTRAVENTRICULAR HEMORRHAGE*

Score	Criterion
1	Less than half of ventricle filled with blood
2	More than half of ventricle filled with blood
3	Ventricle filled and distended with blood

*Third ventricle, fourth ventricle, and each lateral ventricle are scored separately. All the scores are then summed (maximum total score = 12).

rupture was judged not to be useful,[55] but there has been a report of successful fourth ventricle decompression.[56] Surgery for IVH decompression is not generally recommended.

A regular problem with ventriculostomy for IVH is catheter occlusion with blood clot, necessitating irrigation or replacement of the catheter. With obstruction of the foramen of Monro, bilateral ventricular drainage tubes are sometimes necessary. Infection becomes a risk among patients with IVH in whom prolonged drainage is required.[57] In addition, ventricular drainage alone has a limited ability to relieve cerebral compression due to intraventricular blood clots themselves.

Intraventricular clot breakdown using fibrinolytic enzymes showed promise in animal models of IVH, speeding clearance of ventricular clots, restoring ventricular size, preventing hydrocephalus, and reducing CSF outflow resistance.[58-62] Reports and case series of intraventricular fibrinolysis (IVF) in human patients followed, consisting of either injections or infusions of urokinase or recombinant t-PA (rt-PA) through external ventricular drainage catheters for IVH resulting from aneurysm and AVM rupture, chronic hypertension, ventricular catheter insertion, trauma, and germinal matrix hemorrhage in the newborn.[63-74] Although the type, dose, and duration of fibrinolytic treatment varied, these preliminary studies indicated that IVF accelerated IVH clearance and seemed to have little risk. One case series of mostly aneurysm patients also suggested rt-PA clearance of IVH helped control elevated ICP, especially in younger patients with little intracranial compliance or those in poor neurologic condition due to severe bleeding.[65]

Cohort studies have since compared IVF with external ventricular drainage alone (Table 70-2). All have confirmed that IVF is effective in accelerating intraventricular clot clearance and that it does not appear to induce new or repeated hemorrhages.[73,75-80] Several reviews have reached the same conclusions.[81,82]

Urokinase has been replaced by rt-PA for routine clinical use and is the agent being tested in (Clot Lysis: Evaluating Accelerated Resolution of Intraventricular Hemorrhage (CLEAR IVH) trial, an ongoing (at the time of this writing in April 2008) randomized controlled trial comparing simple external ventricular drainage with IVF (with drainage) in patients with spontaneous, hypertensive ICH complicated by obstructive IVH.[83] This study hopes to determine whether IVF has an impact on clinical outcome, clot reduction, and bleeding events in patients with spontaneous ICH with extension in the ventricles resulting in ventricular obstruction.

On the basis of current evidence, IVF can be considered for patients with large IVHs that expand and occlude the ventricular system but without large parenchymal hematomas or clinical conditions that strongly predict unfavorable outcome regardless of the IVH. Fibrinolytic treatment is not likely to be helpful in patients with extensive deep or dominant brain destruction, those with severely elevated ICP, or those with rapidly failing brainstem activity.

Our protocol is to begin treatment after CT confirmation of results of uncomplicated surgery for aneurysm or AVM repair (if applicable) and satisfactory placement of a ventricular drain catheter. A 2- to 4-mg (1 mg/mL) dose of rt-PA is given slowly through the ventricular catheter with frequent checks of ICP to ensure that it does not reach dangerous levels, which would compromise cerebral perfusion pressure. If the patient tolerates only a portion of the 4-mg dose, the remainder can be given 1 hour later. Care must be taken to ensure that the volume of rt-PA dosage exceeds the CSF-filled tubing "dead" space

TABLE 70-2 COMPARISON STUDIES OF INTRAVENTRICULAR FIBRINOLYSIS WITH EXTERNAL VENTRICULAR DRAINAGE VERSUS EXTERNAL VENTRICULAR DRAINAGE ALONE

Study, Population, Year	No. Patients	Cause of IVH	Fibrinolytic Agent	Main Study Results
Coplin et al,[75] single center, 1998	40 (22 received IVF)	Hypertensive ICH in most	Urokinase	IVF resulted in faster clot clearance, lower mortality rate, trend to better outcomes
Naff et al,[73] multi-center, 2000	20 (16 received IVF, 8 randomized)	Hypertensive ICH in most	Urokinase	IVF was associated with better 30-day survival than predicted
Findlay & Jacka,[76] single-center, 2004	30 (21 received IVF)	Aneurysm rupture	rt-PA	IVF resulted in more rapid ventricular opening, fewer EVD replacements
Naff et al,[77] multi-center, 2004	12 (7 randomized to IVF)	Hypertensive ICH	Urokinase	Randomization to IVF (and female gender) favorably affected clot resolution rate
Varelas et al,[78] single center, 2005	20 (10 received IVF)	Aneurysm rupture	rt-PA	IVF resulted in faster clot clearance, trend to decreased need for shunt placement, better outcome
Torres et al,[79] single center, 2008	28 (14 received IVF)	Hypertensive ICH	Urokinase	IVF resulted in faster clot clearance, fewer catheter obstructions, improved outcome
Huttner et al,[80] single center, 2008	135 (27 received IVF)	Hypertensive ICH	rt-PA	IVF hastened clot clearance, reduced the need for repeated EVD exchanges and permanent shunting, but did not influence long-term outcome

EVD, external ventricular drainage; ICH, intracerebral hemorrhage; IVF, intraventricular fibrinolysis; IVH, intraventricular hemorrhage; rt-PA, recombinant tissue-type plasminogen activator.

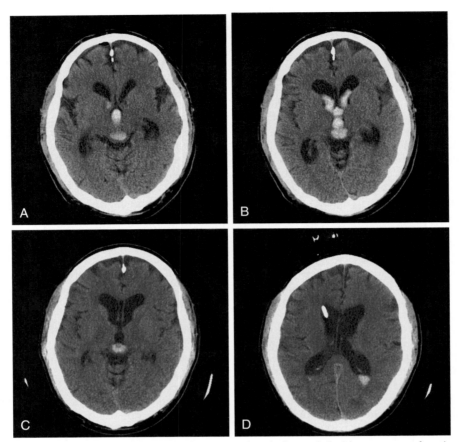

Figure 70-5 A 32-year-old cocaine abuser presenting with a severe headache and double vision was found to have third and lateral ventricular bleeding, along with global cerebral atrophy on CT scan (A and B). Cerebral angiography findings were normal. Following administration of 4 mg of intraventricular recombinant tissue-type plasminogen activator (rt-PA), the ventricles cleared and it became apparent that there was an underlying midbrain hemorrhage in the tectum (C and D). The patient was left with a permanent paralysis of upgaze, skew deviation, and a right trochlear nerve palsy (components of Parinaud's syndrome), resulting in constant diplopia.

between injection port and ventricle to ensure that the rt-PA reaches the ventricles.

Following rt-PA injection the ventricular drain is closed for 1 hour and is then opened to drain against a pressure gradient of 1 to 2 cm (above the level of the external auditory canal) for 1 hour. The drain is then opened and closed during alternating hours for the next 24 hours. CT scanning is performed daily for the first several days, and additional rt-PA can be given if necessary, the goal being to open ventricular pathways, restore normal ventricular size, reduce intracranial hypertension, and maintain catheter patency. Complete clearance of clot settled in dependent parts of the lateral ventricles is not necessary.

We have administered IVF after endovascular coiling of ruptured aneurysms without subsequent bleeding complications (see Fig. 70-4), a therapeutic maneuver reported by others in several patients.[84,85] Interference of aneurysm thrombosis in the coil mass by the administration of rt-PA and the potential risk of aneurysm rebleeding remains a concern. Risks and potential benefits must be taken into account under these circumstances. All of the patients described in the literature who had aneurysm coiling followed by IVF had high-grade aneurysm ruptures with massive IVH, and one of our own patients went on to die from severe subarachnoid hemorrhage;

another made a good recovery. Several examples of rt-PA treatment are shown in Figures 70-5 and 70-6.

Prognosis

The presence of IVH does not necessarily portend a poor prognosis in every patient, as was once thought. Even quite large primary IVHs can be associated with a good clinical condition and good outcome.[86,87] However, secondary IVHs associated with large subarachnoid hemorrhage or ICH or anticoagulant treatment are associated with poorer neurologic condition on presentation and a worse outcome.[88-90] Massive IVH that produces fourth ventricular distension and periventricular cerebral compression is an especially ominous sign associated with early death (Fig. 70-7).[38]

Patients with large IVHs who survive hemorrhage without vital brain destruction are potential candidates for IVF. Intraventricular fibrinolysis helps maintain ventriculostomy blockage with blood clot, promotes rapid IVH clearance, and, we believe, facilitates ICP management, all of which are of great practical help in the intensive care management of patients with severe IVH. It is not currently known whether IVF by itself improves long-term clinical outcome, but this is a subject of ongoing study.

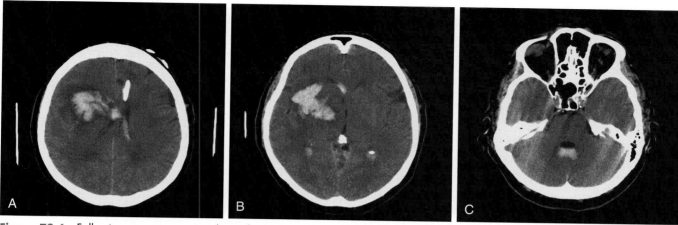

Figure 70-6 Following two consecutive days of intraventricular fibrinolysis (rt-PA, 4 mg per day via the external ventricular drain), a 71-year-old woman with a right-sided lentiform hemorrhage with intraventricular extension (see Fig. 70-2) had considerable clot clearance from the ventricular system. A ventriculoperitoneal shunt was not required. She recovered to her baseline cognition but had a permanent left hemiparesis that prevented her from ambulation.

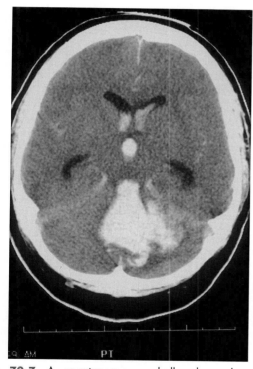

Figure 70-7 A spontaneous cerebellar hemorrhage in a 31-year-old man with intraventricular extension resulted in rapid progression to brain death.

REFERENCES

1. Darby DG, Donnan GA, Saling MA, et al: Primary intraventricular hemorrhage: Clinical and neuropsychological findings in a prospective stroke series, *Neurology* 38:68-75, 1988.
2. Pia HW: The surgical treatment of intracerebral and intraventricular haematomas, *Acta Neurochir* 27:149-164, 1972.
3. Little JR, Blomquist GA Jr, Ethier R: Intraventricular hemorrhage in adults, *Surg Neurol* 8:143-149, 1977.
4. Donauer E, Reif J, Al-Khalaf E, et al: Intraventricular haemorrhage caused by aneurysms and angiomas, *Acta Neurochir* 122:23-31, 1993.
5. Angelopoulos M, Gupta SR, Azat KB: Primary intraventricular hemorrhage in adults: Clinical features, risk factors, and outcome, *Surg Neurol* 44:433-436, 1995.
6. Chang DS, Lin CL, Howng SL: Primary intraventricular hemorrhage in adult—an analysis of 24 cases, *Kao Hsiung I Hsueh Ko Hsueh Tsa Chih* 14:633-638, 1998.
7. Marti-Fabregas J, Piles S, Guardia E, et al: Spontaneous primary intraventricular hemorrhage: Clinical data, etiology and outcome, *J Neurol* 246:287-291, 1999.
8. Taheri SA, Wani MA, Lewko J: Uncommon causes of intraventricular hemorrhage, *Clin Neurol Neurosurg* 92-3:195-202, 1990.
9. Bergsneider M, Grazee JG, DeSalles AA: Thalamostriate artery aneurysm within the third ventricle, *J Neurosurg* 81:463-465, 1994.
10. Hamada J, Hashimoto N, Tskukahara T: Moyamoya disease with repeated intraventricular hemorrhage due to aneurysm rupture, *J Neurosurg* 80:328-331, 1994.
11. Newman P, Al-Menar A: Intraventricular hemorrhage in pregnancy due to moyamoya disease, *J Neurol Neurosurg Psychiatry* 64:686, 1998.
12. Larrazabal R, Pelz D, Findlay JM: Endovascular treatment of a lenticulostriate artery aneurysm with *N*-butyl cyanoacrylate, *Can J Neurol Sci* 28:256-259, 2001.
13. Szabo K, Sommer A, Gass A, et al: Rapid resorption of intraventricular hemorrhage after thrombolytic therapy of ischemic stroke, *Cerebrovasc Dis* 12:144, 2001.
14. Gebel JL, Sila CA, Sloan MA, et al: Thrombolysis-related intracranial hemorrhage: A radiographic analysis of 244 cases from the GUSTO-1 trial with clinical correlation, *Stroke* 29:563-569, 1998.
15. Toffol GJ, Biller J, Adams HP Jr: Nontraumatic intracerebral hemorrhage in young adults, *Arch Neurol* 44:483-485, 1987.
16. Lindboe CF, Stolt-Nielsen A, Dale LG: Hemorrhage in a highly vascularized subependymoma of the septum pellucidum: Case report, *Neurosurg* 31:741-745, 1992.
17. Matsushima M, Yamamoto T, Motomochi M, Ando K: Papilloma and venous angioma of the choroid plexus causing primary intraventricular hemorrhage, *J Neurosurg* 39:666-670, 1973.
18. Lang I, Jackson A, Strang FA: Intraventricular hemorrhage caused by intraventricular meningioma: CT appearance, *AJNR Am J Neuroradiol* 6:1378-1381, 1995.
19. Murai Y, Yoshida D, Ikeda Y, et al: Spontaneous intraventricular hemorrhage caused by lateral ventricular meningioma—case report, *Neurol Med Chir (Tokyo)* 36:586-589, 1996.
20. Challa VR, Richards F II, Davis CH Jr: Intraventricular hemorrhage from pituitary apoplexy, *Surg Neurol* 16:360-361, 1981.
21. Okamura A, Goto S, Sato K, Ushio Y: Central neurocytoma with hemorrhagic onset, *Surg Neurol* 43:252-255, 1995.
22. Graziani N, Dufour H, Figarella-Branger D, et al: Suprasellar granular-cell tumor, presenting with intraventricular haemorrhage, *Br J Neurosurg* 9:97-102, 1995.

23. Mandybur TI: Intracranial hemorrhage caused by metastatic tumors, *Neurology* 27:650-655, 1977.

24. Young WB, Lee KP, Pessin MS: Prognostic significance of ventricular blood in supratentorial hemorrhage: A volumetric study, *Neurology* 40:616-619, 1990.

25. Juvela S, Hillbom M, Palomäki H: Risk factors for spontaneous intracerebral hemorrhage, *Stroke* 26:1558-1564, 1995.

26. Broderick JP, Brott TG, Duldner JE, et al: Volume of intracerebral hemorrhage: A powerful and easy-to-use predictor of 30-day mortality, *Stroke* 24:987-993, 1993.

27. Ruscalleda J, Peiró A: Prognostic factors in intraparenchymatous hematoma with ventricular hemorrhage, *Neuroradiology* 28:34-37, 1986.

28. Hallevi H, Albright KC, Aronowski J, et al: Intraventricular hemorrhage: Anatomic relationships and clinical implications, *Neurology* 70:848-852, 2008.

29. Phan TG, Koh M, Vierkant RA, et al: Hydrocephalus is a determinant of early mortality in putaminal hemorrhage, *Stroke* 31:2157-2162, 2000.

30. Liliang PC, Liang CL, Lu CH, et al: Hypertensive caudate hemorrhage prognostic predictor, outcome, and role of external ventricular drainage, *Stroke* 32:1195-1200, 2001.

31. Bhattathiri PS, Gregson B, Prasad KS, et al: Intraventricular hemorrhage and hydrocephalus after spontaneous intracerebral hemorrhage: Results from the STICH trial, *Acta Neurochir Suppl* 96:65-68, 2006.

32. Huttner HB, Kohrmann M, Berger C, et al: Influence of intraventricular hemorrhage and occlusive hydrocephalus on the long-term outcome of treated patients with basal ganglia hemorrhage: A case-control study, *J Neurosurg* 105:412-417, 2006.

33. Findlay JM: Intraventricular hemorrhage, *Neurosurg Q* 10:182-195, 2000.

34. Vale FL, Bradley EL, Fisher WS III: The relationship of subarachnoid hemorrhage and the need for postoperative shunting, *J Neurosurg* 86:462-466, 1997.

35. Graff-Radford NR, Torner J, Adams HP Jr, Kassell NF: Factors associated with hydrocephalus after subarachnoid hemorrhage, *Arch Neurol* 46:744-752, 1989.

36. de Oliveira JG, Beck J, Setzer M, et al: Risk of shunt-dependent hydrocephalus after occlusion of ruptured intracranial aneurysms by surgical clipping or endovascular coiling: A single-institution series and meta-analysis, *Neurosurgery* 61:924-934, 2007.

37. Inagawa T, Hirano A: Ruptured intracranial aneurysms: An autopsy study of 133 patients, *Surg Neurol* 33:117-123, 1990.

38. Ruelle A, Cavazzani P, Andrioli G: Extracranial posterior inferior cerebellar artery aneurysm causing isolated intraventricular hemorrhage: A case report, *Neurosurgery* 23:774-777, 1988.

39. Schievink WI, Wijdicks EFM, Parisi JE, et al: Sudden death from aneurysmal subarachnoid hemorrhage, *Neurology* 45:871-874, 1995.

40. Shapiro SA, Campbell RL, Scully T: Hemorrhagic dilation of the fourth ventricle: An ominous predictor, *J Neurosurg* 80:805-809, 1994.

41. Mohr G, Ferguson G, Khan M, et al: Intraventricular hemorrhage from ruptured aneurysm: Retrospective analysis of 91 cases, *J Neurosurg* 58:482-487, 1983.

42. Heuer GG, Smith MJ, Elliott JP, et al: Relationship between intracranial pressure and other clinical variables in patients with aneurysmal subarachnoid hemorrhage, *J Neurosurg* 101:408-416, 2004.

43. Rosengart AJ, Schultheiss KE, Tolentino J, et al: Prognostic factors for outcome in patients with aneurysmal subarachnoid hemorrhage, *Stroke* 38:2315-2321, 2007.

44. Hartmann A, Mast H, Mohr JP, et al: Morbidity of intracranial hemorrhage in patients with cerebral arteriovenous malformation, *Stroke* 29:931-934, 1998.

45. Findlay JM, Weir BKA, Kanamaru K, et al: Intrathecal fibrinolytic therapy after subarachnoid hemorrhage: Dosage study in a primate model and review of the literature, *Can J Neurol Sci* 16:28-40, 1989.

46. Ikeda K, Asakura H, Futami K, et al: Coagulative and fibrinolytic activation in cerebrospinal fluid and plasma after subarachnoid hemorrhage, *Neurosurgery* 41:344-350, 1997.

47. Naff NJ, Williams MA, Rigamonti D, et al: Blood clot resolution in human cerebrospinal fluid: Evidence of first-order kinetics, *Neurosurgery* 49:614-621, 2001.

48. Flint AC, Roebken A, Singh V: Primary intraventricular hemorrhage: yield of diagnostic angiography and clinical outcome, *Neurocrit Care* 8:330-336, 2008.

49. Yanaka K, Hyodo A, Tsuchida Y, et al: Symptomatic cerebral vasospasm after intraventricular hemorrhage from ruptured arteriovenous malformation, *Surg Neurol* 38:63-67, 1992.

50. Maeda K, Kurita H, Nakamura T, et al: Occurrence of severe vasospasm following intraventricular hemorrhage from an arteriovenous malformation: Report of two cases, *J Neurosurg* 87:436-439, 1997.

51. Classen J, Bernardini GL, Kreiter K, et al: Effect of cisternal and ventricular blood on risk of delayed cerebral ischemia after subarachnoid hemorrhage: The Fisher Scale revisited, *Stroke* 32:2012-2020, 2001.

52. Diringer MN, Edwards DF, Zazulia AR: Hydrocephalus: A previously unrecognized predictor of poor outcome from supratentorial intracerebral hemorrhage, *Stroke* 29:1352-1357, 1998.

53. Mohr G, Ferguson G, Khan M, et al: Intraventricular hemorrhage from ruptured aneurysm: Retrospective analysis of 91 cases, *J Neurosurg* 58:482-487, 1983.

54. Graeb DA, Robertson WD, Lapointe JS, et al: Computed tomographic diagnosis of intraventricular hemorrhage, *Radiology* 143:91-96, 1982.

55. Shimoda M, Oda S, Shibata M, et al: Results of early surgical evacuation of packed intraventricular hemorrhage from aneurysm rupture in patients with poor-grade subarachnoid hemorrhage, *J Neurosurg* 91:408-414, 1999.

56. Lagares A, Putman CM, Ogilvy CS: Posterior fossa decompression and clot evacuation for fourth ventricle hemorrhage after aneurysmal rupture: Case report, *Neurosurgery* 49:208-211, 2001.

57. Mayhall CG, Archer NH, Lamb VA, et al: Ventriculostomy-related infections: A prospective epidemiologic study, *N Engl J Med* 310:553-559, 1984.

58. Pang D, Sclabassi RJ, Horton JA: Lysis of intraventricular blood clot with urokinase in a canine model: Part 1: Canine intraventricular blood cast model, *Neurosurgery* 19:540-546, 1986.

59. Pang D, Sclabassi RJ, Horton JA: Lysis of intraventricular blood clot with urokinase in a canine model: Part 2: In vivo safety study of intraventricular urokinase, *Neurosurgery* 19:547-552, 1986.

60. Mayfrank L, Kissler J, Raoofi R, et al: Ventricular dilatation in experimental intraventricular hemorrhage in pigs: Characterization of cerebrospinal fluid dynamics and the effects of fibrinolytic treatment, *Stroke* 28:141-148, 1997.

61. Brinker T, Seifert V, Stolke D: Effect of intrathecal fibrinolysis on cerebrospinal fluid absorption after experimental subarachnoid hemorrhage, *J Neurosurg* 74:789-793, 1991.

62. Brinker T, Seifert V, Dietz H: Subacute hydrocephalus after experimental subarachnoid hemorrhage: Its prevention by intrathecal fibrinolysis with recombinant tissue plasminogen activator, *Neurosurgery* 31:306-312, 1992.

63. Shen PH, Matsuoka Y, Kawajiri K, et al: Treatment of intraventricular hemorrhage using urokinase, *Neurol Med Chir (Tokyo)* 30:329-333, 1990.

64. Todo T, Usui M, Takakura K: Treatment of severe intraventricular hemorrhage by intraventricular infusion of urokinase, *J Neurosurg* 74:81-86, 1991.

65. Findlay JM, Grace MGA, Weir BKA: Treatment of intraventricular hemorrhage with tissue plasminogen activator, *Neurosurgery* 32:941-947, 1993.

66. Findlay JM, Weir BKA, Stollery DE: Lysis of intraventricular hematoma with tissue plasminogen activator, *J Neurosurg* 74:803-807, 1991.

67. Mayfrank L, Lippitz B, Groth M, et al: Effect of recombinant tissue plasminogen activator on clot lysis and ventricular dilatation in the treatment of severe intraventricular hemorrhage, *Acta Neurochir* 122:32-38, 1993.

68. Rhode V, Schaller C, Hassler WE: Intraventricular recombinant tissue plasminogen activator for lysis of intraventricular haemorrhage, *J Neurol Neurosurg Psychiatry* 58:447-451, 1995.

69. Akdemir H, Selcuklu A, Pasaoglu A, et al: Treatment of severe intraventricular hemorrhage by intraventricular infusion of urokinase, *Neurosurg Rev* 18:95-100, 1995.

70. Rainov NG, Burkert WL: Urokinase infusion for severe intraventricular haemorrhage, *Acta Neurochir* 134:55-59, 1995.

71. Grabb PA: Traumatic intraventricular hemorrhage treated with intraventricular recombinant-tissue plasminogen activator: Technical case report, *Neurosurgery* 43:966–969, 1998.

72. Goh KY, Poon WS: Recombinant tissue plasminogen activator for the treatment of spontaneous adult intraventricular hemorrhage, *Surg Neurol* 50:526–531, 1998.

73. Naff NJ, Carhuapoma JR, Williams MA, et al: Treatment of intraventricular hemorrhage with urokinase: Effects on 30-day survival, *Stroke* 31:841–847, 2000.

74. Haines SJ, Lapointe M: Fibrinolytic agents in the management of post hemorrhagic hydrocephalus in preterm infants: The evidence, *Childs Nerv Syst* 15:226–234, 1999.

75. Coplin WD, Vinas FC, Agris JM, et al: A cohort study of the safety and feasibility of intraventricular urokinase for nonaneurysmal spontaneous intraventricular hemorrhage, *Stroke* 29(8):1573–1579, 1998.

76. Findlay JM, Jacka MJ: Cohort study of intraventricular thrombolysis with recombinant tissue plasminogen activator for aneurysmal intraventricular hemorrhage, *Neurosurgery* 55(3):532–537, 2004.

77. Naff NJ, Hanley DF, Keyl PM, et al: Intraventricular thrombolysis speeds blood clot resolution: Results of a pilot, prospective, randomized, double-blind, controlled trial, *Neurosurgery* 54(3):577–584, 2004.

78. Varelas PN, Rickert KL, Cusick J, et al: Intraventricular hemorrhage after aneurysmal subarachnoid hemorrhage: Pilot study of treatment with intraventricular tissue plasminogen activator, *Neurosurgery* 56(2):205–213, 2005.

79. Torres A, Plans G, Martino J, et al: Fibrinolytic therapy in spontaneous intraventricular haemorrhage: Efficacy and safety of the treatment, *Br J Neurosurg* 22(2):269–274, 2008.

80. Huttner HB, Tognoni E, Bardutzky J, et al: Influence of intraventricular fibrinolytic therapy with rt-PA on the long-term outcome of treated patients with spontaneous basal ganglia hemorrhage: A case-control study, *Eur J Neurol* 15(4):342–349, 2008.

81. Nieuwkamp DJ, de Gans K, Rinkel GJE, et al: Treatment and outcome of severe intraventricular extension in patients with subarachnoid hemorrhage: A systematic review of the literature, *J Neurol* 247:117–121, 2000.

82. Engelhard HH, Andrews CO, Slavin KV, et al: Current management of intraventricular hemorrhage, *Surg Neurol* 60:15–21, 2003.

83. Johns Hopkins University: CLEAR IVH: Clot Lysis: Evaluating Accelerated Resolution of Intraventricular Hemorrhage (IVH). Available at www.clearivh.com.

84. Azmi-Ghadimi H, Heary RF, Farkas JE, et al: Use of intraventricular tissue plasminogen activator and Guglielmi detachable coiling for the acute treatment of casted ventricles from cerebral aneurysm hemorrhage: Two technical case reports, *Neurosurgery* 50:421–424, 2002.

85. Hall B, Parker D Jr, Carhuapoma JR: Thrombolysis for intraventricular hemorrhage after endovascular aneurysmal coiling, *Neurocrit Care* 3:153–156, 2005.

86. Verma A, Maheshwari MC, Bhargava S: Spontaneous intraventricular haemorrhage, *J Neurol* 234:233–236, 1987.

87. Roos YB, Hasan D, Vermeulen M: Outcome in patients with large intraventricular haemorrhages: A volumetric study, *J Neurol Neurosurg Psychiatry* 58:622–624, 1995.

88. De Weerd AW: The prognosis of intraventricular hemorrhage, *J Neurol* 222:45–51, 1979.

89. Juvela S: Risk factors for impaired outcome after spontaneous intracerebral hemorrhage, *Arch Neurol* 52:1193–2000, 1995.

90. Sjoblom L, Hårdemark HG, Lindgren A, et al: Management of prognostic features of intracerebral hemorrhage during anticoagulant therapy: A Swedish multicenter study, *Stroke* 32:2567–2574, 2001.

71

Surgical Decision Making, Techniques, and Periprocedural Care of Cerebral Arteriovenous Malformations

ROBERT M. STARKE, RICARDO J. KOMOTAR, E. SANDER CONNOLLY

The goal of definitive arteriovenous malformation (AVM) treatment is to eliminate the risk of intracerebral hemorrhage and to preserve or improve functional status. The benefits of intervention must be carefully weighed against the risks of treatment. There are currently four major treatment options. The lesion can be monitored expectantly with the understanding that the patient has a risk of hemorrhage, neurologic deficit, or seizure. Microsurgery, radiosurgery, and embolization have all been used successfully in various combinations, each with associated risks. Intervention can be carried out as long as the goal is complete obliteration, because subtotal treatment does not provide protection from hemorrhage. Treatment planning is based on selecting a modality or a combination of modalities with the greatest success rate according to patient characteristics and AVM morphology.[1-5] Treatment efficacy is a critical outcome parameter (total/permanent angiographic obliteration of the lesion and time required for therapeutic response). Successful microsurgery results in immediate abatement of hemorrhage risk. For patients with small lesions in noneloquent locations, microsurgery has demonstrated excellent results.[4,6-8] However, microsurgery is not indicated for all patients with AVMs. Patient characteristics, AVM morphology, and limitations of available treatment options dictate whether the risk involved with resection is acceptable.[1-5] Complete resection of AVMs in deep or eloquent areas may result in high morbidity and mortality.[9] Interventional planning must determine the modality or combination of modalities with the greatest success rate according to patient characteristics, AVM architecture, and the capabilities of the treatment option to fulfill the goals of treatment.[1-5]

Patient-Related Factors

The analysis of treatment begins with patient-related factors such as symptoms, past medical history, psychological status, and familial and social background. As in any other therapeutic decision making, the choice of intervention with all the risks included must be assessed in light of the patient's needs.

As with any type of surgical planning, the patient's age, comorbidities, and functional status must be taken into account to assess operative risks. The patient with AVM tends to present at a younger age and with fewer medical conditions than patients requiring other vascular surgery but may have serious comorbidities owing to the AVM itself. Particular attention must be paid to the mode of presentation, and the highest priority is often the estimated risk of intracranial hemorrhage or rebleeding. Approximately 50% of patients with AVMs present with hemorrhage, and the others with seizure or headache.[10] The annual risk of hemorrhage is 2% to 4%, with a lifetime risk of rebleeding between 17% and 90%.[7,9,11-17] Each episode of hemorrhage is associated with a 10% risk of mortality and a 30% to 50% morbidity rate.[7] The lifetime risk for intracranial hemorrhage in a person with an AVM is approximated by the following formula[13,15]:

$$\text{Lifetime risk } (\%) = 105 - \text{the patient's age in years}$$

This is an estimated starting point, as many other factors must be assessed in the overall risk of hemorrhage. The risk for recurrent intracranial hemorrhage is elevated after the first hemorrhage and has ranged from 6% to 18% in the first year after bleeding. In one study the risk of hemorrhage after the second bleed was 25% in the first year.

Obliteration of the AVM may also alleviate focal neurologic deficits or reduce the incidence of seizure, the two other most common presentations in patients with AVMs. In one series of 102 patients with AVMs who had presented with seizures, 83% were seizure free over a 2-year minimum follow-up. Of these patients, 48% no longer received anticonvulsant therapy. Although 17% suffered intermittent seizures, 13 of these patients reported improved control than before surgery.[18] Other surgical series report similar results and suggest that seizure control may correlate with age at seizure onset, duration of seizures, and location of lesion and cortical excision.[19] In general, surgical treatment of AVMs can be expected to reduce seizure incidence. Unfortunately, there is a

1358

paucity of data regarding duration or type of anticonvulsant prophylaxis after treatment.

AVM Architecture

Patient characteristics must be used in conjunction with AVM architecture to formulate a treatment plan. Along with a detailed clinical examination, all patients with AVMs must undergo detailed preoperative radiographic clarification of AVM anatomy, architecture, and associated aneurysms with MRI and digital subtraction angiography. After the comprehensive evaluation has been performed, decisions can be made regarding the best management approach through comparison of the natural history of the lesion with the intervention-related morbidity and mortality.

A number of radiologic variables have been associated with an increased risk of hemorrhage, including small AVM size, elevated feeding artery pressure, periventricular or intraventricular location, basal ganglia location, deep venous drainage, impaired venous drainage, single draining vein, intranidal aneurysm, multiple aneurysms, and vertebrobasilar blood supply.[7,20-27]

Data from the New York Islands AVM Hemorrhage Study, an ongoing, prospective, population-based survey determining the incidence of AVM-related hemorrhage and the associated rates of morbidity and mortality in a zip code–defined population of 10 million people, showed that increasing age (hazard ratio [HR], 1.05; 95% confidence interval [CI], 1.03–1.08), initial hemorrhagic AVM presentation (HR, 5.38; 95% CI, 2.64–10.96), deep brain location (HR, 3.25; 95% CI, 1.30–8.16), and exclusive deep vein drainage (HR, 3.25; 95% CI, 1.01–5.67) were independent predictors of subsequent hemorrhage. Annual hemorrhage rates on follow-up ranged from 0.9% for patients without hemorrhagic AVM presentation, deep AVM location, or deep vein drainage to as high as 34.4% for those harboring all three risk factors.[10,16,17] The investigators in this study also evaluated predictors of residual dysplastic vessels on cerebral angiography after AVM surgery. The number of cases showing angiographic evidence for dysplastic vessels was significantly associated with increasing size of the AVM, and symptomatic postoperative intracerebral hemorrhage was associated with dysplastic vessels on the postoperative angiogram.[28]

When information about the natural history of AVMs is combined with knowledge of a patient's characteristics and AVM morphology, a risk profile for future hemorrhage or rebleeding may be developed. A critical question is how the risks associated with the natural history for a patient of a given age with specific AVM architecture compares with the risk of treatment. The answer to this dictates the recommendation whether to treat the AVM, and if so, with which treatment option.

Timing of Surgery

Surgical resection of an AVM should generally be elective in a stable patient. In contrast, patients presenting with intracranial hemorrhage and hydrocephalus due to life-threatening hematoma are treated with emergency surgery. Patients should receive surgical resection with clot removal only in superficial AVMs in which the anatomy can be fully elucidated. Otherwise it is best to allow the patient to recover and obtain angiography to delineate all elements of the lesion.

In patients presenting with acute hydrocephalus as a result of intraventricular hemorrhage and clot formation or compression of the aqueduct of Sylvius by a large draining vein, a ventricular catheter may be necessary to monitor and relieve intracranial pressure. Following microsurgical AVM removal, patients may experience hydrocephalus and should receive the same treatment. Patients with shunt-dependent hydrocephalus may eventually require a ventriculoperitoneal shunt.

Operative Risks

In conjunction with patient characteristics and AVM architecture, the operative risks must be analyzed. In recent years, a number of studies have suggested complex classifications, including not only AVM architecture but also other diagnostic features, such as findings of transcranial Doppler ultrasonography[29] and hemodynamic and clinical elements.[30] Grading scales have incorporated a number of variables, such as size, number of feeding arteries, velocity of flow through the lesion, degree of steal from surrounding brain, location (including surgical accessibility), eloquence of adjacent brain, presence of associated aneurysms, pattern of venous drainage, and patient age. The system developed by Spetzler and Martin[4] remains the most frequently employed classification system. This grading scale is used to predict surgical outcome and stratify AVMs for radiosurgical, endovascular, and combined therapy.[7,31,32]

The Spetzler-Martin (SM) grading system has been widely validated both prospectively and retrospectively as a practical and reliable method for predicting patient outcomes after AVM microsurgery.[5,8,29,33,34] This simplified scoring system was developed to approximate potential risks on the basis of three categories: AVM size, location (eloquence of adjacent brain), and pattern of venous drainage (Table 71-1). It is generally accepted that the majority of patients with SM grade I and II AVMs should be treated with microsurgical resection,[2] although some patients may be medically unfit for or may decline surgery.[35] Grade III lesions are typically treated with microsurgery or radiosurgery, often with adjunctive

TABLE 71-1 SPETZLER-MARTIN CLASSIFICATION OF ARTERIOVENOUS MALFORMATIONS

Characteristic		Point(s) Assigned
Size	Small (<3 cm)	1
	Medium (3-6 cm)	2
	Large (>6 cm)	3
Eloquence*	No	0
	Yes	1
Venous drainage	Superficial only	0
	Any deep	1

*Sensorimotor, language, or visual cortex, hypothalamus or thalamus; internal capsule; brainstem; cerebellar peduncles; or cerebellar nuclei.

embolization. An individualized, multimodal approach is recommended for select grade IV/V lesions in which intervention is deemed beneficial.[2]

Surgical outcomes in patients with grade I AVMs are typically excellent, with a reported range of favorable outcome in the literature of 92% to 100%.[4,5,8] Similarly, grade II lesions have an excellent prognosis with microsurgical resection (94% to 95% chance of excellent or good outcome).[4,5] In grade III lesions, the rate of excellent or good outcome ranges from 68% to 96%.[5,8] For grade IV lesions, the rate of excellent outcome ranges from 71% to 75%.[4,5,29] In patients with grade V AVMs, the reported good/excellent rate is 50% to 70%, with a 14% to 25% rate of poor outcome and a 0 to 5% mortality rate in longer-term follow-up.[5,8,29,36] Despite the heavy selection bias of these surgical series, these studies provide a framework within which to consider operative risks.

The SM grading scale may produce errors in patient selection due to oversimplification.[37] The Modified Spetzler-Martin (mSM) grading system was put forth to address discrepancies between the SM grade and patient outcomes, specifically with regard to grade III lesions.[36,38] The mSM system recognizes that grade III AVMs present unique challenges according to their location/size and introduces two subgroups: grade IIIA (grade III due to size > 6 cm) and grade IIIB (grade III due to venous drainage and/or eloquence). In one study, 4.5% and 30% of grade IIIA and IIB lesions, respectively, had fair or bad outcomes.[38] Recommended treatment plans for grade IIIA lesions should involve embolization to reduce AVM size and facilitate microsurgery, whereas radiosurgery should be seriously considered for grade IIIB lesions, with or without embolization as necessary.[36] Other modifications of SM grade III lesions have been suggested to better define appropriate surgical treatment.[39]

Although the SM grading system is generally considered an accurate method to predict patient outcomes after microsurgery, it may be less predictive of radiosurgical outcomes.[2,32,34,40-42] The system fails to take into account a number of prognostic factors that have been associated with successful radiosurgery, such as radiation dose, AVM volume, specific location, and patient age.[32,40,43] Radiosurgical treatment of AVMs is considered in detail elsewhere in this volume. In addition, the nature, complications, and patient selection criteria for the two treatment modalities markedly differ.[44] In order to address the shortcomings of surgical grading scales, the Radiosurgery-Based AVM Grading System (RBGS) was proposed.[32] The RBGS, composed of patient and AVM variables, is based on factors that are shown to be specifically predictive of AVM radiosurgery: patient age and AVM volume and location. Despite the drawbacks of the SM and mSM, these grading systems are easy to use and have been shown to be relatively predictive of radiosurgical outcome in a number of studies.[45-47] Continued investigation, however, is necessary to validate the efficacy of the SM grading scale and incorporate other prognostic factors.

Current guideline recommendations are that microsurgical resection should be considered the primary mode of therapy for SM grade I and II lesions, unless patient characteristics or wishes do not allow surgical therapy. For patients with small lesions in which surgery confers increased risk based on patient characteristics or AVM morphology, radiosurgery should be considered. In grade III lesions, radiosurgery or a combined-modality approach, in which embolization is followed by either surgery or radiosurgery, is often recommended. Numerous studies have demonstrated an overwhelming increase in morbidity and mortality with SM grade IV and V lesions, and many studies have argued against treatment in these AVMs unless necessary to evacuate hemorrhage or reduce mass effect.[2,4,48] Treatment of patients with such lesions must be undertaken in an individual manner and with multimodality therapy (see later).

Anesthetic Considerations for Microsurgery

Principles of anesthesia for AVM resection follow the recommendations for neuroanesthetic management of intracranial lesions regarding choice of monitoring, vascular access, anesthetic agents, vasoactive drugs, and muscle relaxants.[49] As surgery is often not emergency, medical conditions should be optimized and current neurologic dysfunction should be considered in the management plan. In AVMs, choices of intraoperative monitoring and adequate amounts of transfusion blood must be taken into account, because there is always the risk for massive and rapid hemorrhage.

The risk of AVM rupture during induction is low, but 7% to 41% of patients harbor intracranial aneurysms that may rupture with increases in blood pressure.[50,51] For this reason there should be prudent use of anesthetics and vasoactive agents that cause cerebral vasodilatation—that is, high inspired concentrations of volatile anesthetics and high doses of vasodilators that directly relax vascular smooth muscle. The choice of anesthetic agent must be consistent with safe conduct of intracranial surgery, including brain relaxation, excellent blood pressure control, and rapid emergence from anesthesia. Euvolemia, normotension, isotonicity, normoglycemia, and mild hypocapnia are recommended.[2]

Following resection of the AVM, a brief intraoperative elevation of blood pressure may be beneficial in confirming complete obliteration of the AVM. If the AVM is completely removed, increasing the patient's blood pressure should not result in bleeding in the surgical field. Additionally, blood pressure must be closely controlled when general anesthesia is concluded, during which a spike in the patient's blood pressure and hemorrhage from any residual AVM may occur. Complete AVM obliteration must be confirmed with angiography after surgery.

Microsurgical Resection

In AVM surgery, the operative field must be large enough to expose the AVM as well as a portion of the normal brain. Large craniotomies expose cerebral fissures and cisterns through which the AVM can be approached. The sentiment that surgery of AVMs produces profuse bleeding is inaccurate, and with careful surgical management and bipolar cauterization, a clean operative field can be maintained. Along with minimizing bleeding, as well as opening cisterns and fissures to allow ample access, there should be minimal retraction and limited or no damage to normal brain parenchyma or vessels.

It is important to preserve the arachnoid plane in order to avoid entering the nidus of the AVM before adequate exposure is achieved. Once the lesion is outlined, vessels around the AVM are dissected, and proximal control is attained, the surgeon may begin to obliterate the lesion. Bipolar cauterization is used to coagulate feeding arteries, with special care taken to obliterate only those feeding the AVM and to preserve vessels supplying normal parenchyma. Venous drainage from the AVM, especially the major draining veins, is not ligated until the arterial supply is completely removed.

The greatest challenge lies in coagulation of the deep feeding vessels, which are usually small, fragile, and difficult to obliterate. Application of temporary clips may be beneficial prior to coagulation to help control bleeding from these fragile vessels. Following coagulation of most feeding arterial vessels, the arteriovenous shunt is interrupted, the venous drainage is ligated, and the lesion can be resected.

Posterior Fossa Arteriovenous Malformations

Arteriovenous malformations involving the cerebellum and brainstem are relatively rare lesions that most often manifest as hemorrhage (Fig. 71-1). Bleeds within the smaller confines of the cerebellum or brainstem can have severe consequences, carrying a worse prognosis than supratentorial lesions. Although current management of these lesions often involves preoperative embolization and stereotactic radiosurgery, surgical resection remains the treatment of choice, conferring immediate protection from the risk of future hemorrhage. Most symptomatic AVMs that involve the cerebellum and the pial or ependymal surfaces of the brainstem are candidates for surgical resection.[52,53] It must also be taken into account that rates of obliteration in brainstem AVMs following radiosurgery are significantly lower than supratentorial AVMs because of the inherent risks of radiation necrosis or cyst formation within the brainstem, leading to lower delivered doses. As with all AVMs, the architecture defined by angiography and MRI is critical to determine suitability for resection and choice of operative exposure. In addition to the location of the nidus, arterial supply, and predominant

venous drainage, the surgical approach must also be selected with consideration of the small confines of the posterior fossa and eloquence of the brainstem, cranial nerves, and deep cerebellar nuclei.

Basal Ganglia Region Arteriovenous Malformations

AVMs in the region of the basal ganglia carry a considerable risk of morbidity and mortality with any treatment option. Precise localization of such lesions in conjunction with a thorough understanding of the anatomy allows certain AVMs in proximity to the basal ganglia to receive surgical treatment with acceptable postoperative morbidity. In the majority of these lesions, radiosurgery and adjunctive embolization are the preferred treatments.

Associated Aneurysms

Intracranial aneurysm is found in 7% to 41% of patients with AVMs and may occur within the nidus, in close proximity to the AVM (see Fig. 71-1), in the feeding artery, or at some distance from the AVM in more typical locations of saccular aneurysms.[12,31,50,54] If located in the surgical field, these lesions should be obliterated via direct surgical clipping; if intranidal in location, they should be obliterated during removal of the AVM. If possible, the symptomatic lesion should be treated first, and a careful radiographic review is necessary to best elucidate which lesion may have caused intracranial hemorrhage. Aneurysms in proximity to AVMs may involute after resection of the AVM when normal flow has been resumed.

Multimodality Treatment

Multimodality treatment may occur through planned staged therapy or as the result of treatment failure. In planned multimodality staged therapy, the goal is to combine the advantageous elements of each tool in order to increase procedural safety and efficacy. Combined therapies lead to the accumulation of risk, so each element should be used in the most beneficial manner to decrease the overall complication rate. Despite a number of large studies,[55,56] patients must be evaluated on a case-by-case basis, and general extrapolation of results is difficult. In the event of a failed treatment (radiosurgery or

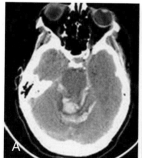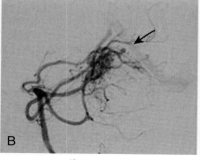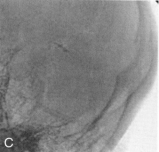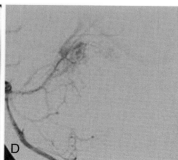

Figure 71-1 Vermian arteriovenous malformation manifesting with intracerebral/intraventricular hemorrhage secondary to a ruptured perinidal aneurysm. A, Non–contrast-enhanced CT scan. B, Lateral vertebral angiogram (aneurysm indicated by *arrow*). C, Post-embolization glue cast. D, Post-embolization lateral vertebral angiogram.

microsurgery), the next modality of treatment is selected according to inherent benefits.[1,55,56] A small portion of an AVM in an eloquent location left after microsurgery may be best obliterated via radiosurgery, but the risk of hemorrhage in the interim must be considered. Conversely, a portion of an AVM left unobliterated after radiosurgery may be best managed with microsurgery and/or embolization. Regardless, multimodality therapy should be considered only when the plan is complete AVM eradication.

Postoperative Care

Angiography—intraoperative, postoperative, or both—should be used in all patients to confirm complete obliteration, and patients with partial obliteration should return to the operating room until complete obliteration is attained. Studies have confirmed that the risk of hemorrhage remains high in those patients receiving only partial AVM obliteration.[17,38,57]

Following microsurgical resection, all patients should be managed in a neurologic intensive care unit for at least 24 hours, to undergo blood pressure control with an arterial catheter and urine output monitoring with an indwelling catheter. Patients are typically kept normotensive and euvolemic. Tight blood pressure control with agents that do not act in the central nervous system may be appropriate for selected individuals. Perioperative antibiotics, steroids, and seizure medications are used variably.

Brain Edema and Hemorrhage

Patients with new neurologic deficits after surgery should be investigated with CT scan to rule out hemorrhage and hydrocephalus and with MRI using diffusion-weighted imaging to evaluate for possible cerebral ischemia. There are two common hypotheses to explain the etiology of brain edema occurring during or after surgery: normal perfusion pressure breakthrough (NPPB) and occlusive hyperemia. According to the theory of normal perfusion pressure breakthrough, chronic hypoperfusion in brain tissue surrounding the AVM results in maximal vasodilation and an inability of the vessels to vasoconstrict in response to the resumption of normal perfusion pressure after AVM resection. This results in hemorrhage and/or edema due to failure of autoregulation. The normal perfusion pressure breakthrough theory supports the use of staged endovascular embolization and surgical ligation of feeders, with operative intervention occurring several days after embolization.[58-62]

A number of studies demonstrate maintained autoregulation in the region surrounding an AVM both before and immediately after its resection, even in cases subsequently complicated by edema and hemorrhage.[63-70] This finding has led to the theory that postoperative edema and hemorrhage are due to "occlusive hyperemia." According to this hypothesis, complications are the result of arterial stagnation and obstruction and/or venous outflow obstruction due to AVM resection.[66,71,72] This theory does not support staged resection and/or hypotensive therapy in the management of postoperative edema, which may be harmful.[71] Because the exact cause of postoperative hemorrhage and edema is currently inconclusive, the impact of these theories on AVM management is only speculative.[2]

Embolization

Embolization is used as an adjunct to microsurgery or radiosurgery to eliminate deep-feeding arteries, occlude feeding vessels not readily accessible during surgery, reduce AVM size, and obliterate associated aneurysms (see Fig. 71-1). Although there have been no prospective randomized trials to assess whether preoperative embolization has a beneficial effect on outcome in patients with AVMs, several studies have demonstrated that use of this adjunctive modality leads to decreases in operative time, blood loss, morbidity, and mortality.[73-75] Further advantages of embolization include the ease of obliteration of strategically targeted vessels by microsurgery and the theoretical benefits of staged flow reduction.[73] Current indications include either preoperative embolization or palliative embolization in large nonsurgical or nonradiosurgical AVMs in patients presenting with progressive neurologic deficit secondary to high flow or venous hypertension. In this group of patients, the goal is flow reduction in an attempt to minimize or halt symptom progression.[2] Embolization as a primary modality leads to a low rate of obliteration and so is not defined as a primary modality of therapy, except as explained previously. In a series of 405 patients, complete cure was achieved in only 9.9% of cases. This was chiefly in small and medium AVMs with fewer than four pedicles.[56] Furthermore, embolization is not without risk. The rate of hemorrhagic complications associated with embolization ranges from 2% to 5%, new neurologic deficits occur in 10% to 14% of patients, permanent deficits occur in 2% to 5% of patients, and death occurs in approximately 1% of patients.[50,56,74,76-79]

Pediatric Lesions

AVMs account for 30% to 50% of hemorrhagic strokes in children, and pediatric patients are more likely to present with hemorrhage than adults.[80-82] Neonates and infants may present with cardiac failure from arteriovenous shunting.[83] As in adults, the remaining pediatric patients present with seizures, headache, or neurologic alterations. Because of the longer life expectancy of pediatric patients and the higher mortality associated with hemorrhage (25%), treatment is warranted when possible.[13,15,84] Pediatric AVMs are more commonly found in eloquent locations; therefore there is increased risk of morbidity and mortality from intervention. In contrast, certain population studies have reported that 10% to 42% of children with AVMs may be managed conservatively, although geographic regions have different referral patterns and treatment biases.[80,85-87] In the largest surgical series of 160 pediatric AVMs, the morbidity and mortality rates were 18% and 11%, respectively. In the largest endovascular series, the morbidity and mortality rates were 28% and 16%, respectively. It is also important to note that AVM recurrence is possible, even after definitive treatment and confirmatory postoperative angiogram.[81,85] This fact suggests a different pathophysiology behind pediatric AVMs, potentially owing to unique vascular growth factors or immature vessels. Although the recurrence of pediatric AVMs after complete surgical excision may be an indication for postoperative radiographic follow-up, there have been no prospective studies to support this step.

Pregnant Patients

The current recommendations for the treatment of AVMs in pregnant patients remain inconclusive. Some studies report that pregnancy does not increase the risk of hemorrhage.[88,89] In a study of 451 patients who had 540 pregnancies, the incidence of hemorrhage was found to be 3.5% during the 52 weeks after the patient's last menstrual period and 5.8% in the year after the last menstrual period in patients with a prior history of hemorrhage.[90] Patients who present with hemorrhage may be at increased risk of rebleeding in comparison with nonpregnant patients. The rebleeding rate of those who present with hemorrhage during pregnancy appears to be substantially elevated (26%).[88,91] The available data suggest that vaginal delivery does not carry a higher risk for hemorrhage than delivery by cesarean section or that increased venous pressure during a Valsalva maneuver is directly transmitted to the draining veins.[2,51,90]

Current recommendations are for pregnant patients with a known AVM to consider treatment prior to pregnancy. Lesions discovered during pregnancy should be managed by comparing the treatment risks for the mother and fetus with the risk of hemorrhage.[2]

Other Vascular Malformations

This chapter specifically addresses the surgical management of intracranial parenchymal AVMs and does not address spinal AVMs, cavernous malformations, dural AVMs, or dural fistulas (including vein of Galen malformations). These other lesions reflect unique considerations of epidemiology, diagnostic evaluation, natural history, risk-benefit analysis, and therapeutic strategies, and are considered elsewhere in this volume.

Conclusion

In summary, management paradigms should determine the modality, or combination of modalities, with the greatest therapeutic success rate according to patient characteristics and AVM architecture. Despite its simplicity, the Spetzler-Martin grading scale provides a framework to begin treatment planning. Current guideline recommendations are that microsurgical resection should be considered the primary mode of therapy for SM grade I and II lesions, unless patient characteristics or wishes do not allow surgical therapy. For patients with small lesions for which surgery offers increased risk on the basis of patient characteristics or AVM morphology, radiosurgery should be considered. In grade III lesions, radiosurgery or a combined-modality approach, with embolization followed by either surgery or radiosurgery, is recommended. Treatment of Spetzler-Martin grade IV and V lesions must be undertaken on a case-by-case basis and involve multimodality therapy.

REFERENCES

1. Richling B, Killer M, Al-Schameri AR, et al: Therapy of brain arteriovenous malformations: Multimodality treatment from a balanced standpoint, *Neurosurgery* 59:S148-S157, 2006:discussion S143-S113.
2. Ogilvy CS, Stieg PE, Awad I, et al: A scientific statement: Recommendations for the management of intracranial arteriovenous malformations: A statement for healthcare professionals from a special writing group of the stroke council, american stroke association, *Stroke* 32:1458-1471, 2001.
3. Batjer HH, Devous MD Sr, Seibert GB, et: Intracranial: Arteriovenous malformation: Relationship between clinical factors and surgical complications, *Neurosurgery* 24:75-79, 1989.
4. Spetzler RF, Martin NA: A proposed grading system for arteriovenous malformations, *J Neurosurg* 65:476-483, 1986.
5. Hartmann A, Stapf C, Hofmeister C, et al: Determinants of neurological outcome after surgery for brain arteriovenous malformation, *Stroke* 31:2361-2364, 2000.
6. Sisti MB, Kader A, Stein BM: Microsurgery for 67 intracranial arteriovenous malformations less than 3 cm in diameter, *J Neurosurg* 79:653-660, 1993.
7. Hartmann A, Mast H, Mohr JP, et al: Morbidity of intracranial hemorrhage in patients with cerebral arteriovenous malformation, *Stroke* 29:931-934, 1998.
8. Heros RC, Korosue K, Diebold PM: Surgical excision of cerebral arteriovenous malformations: Late results, *Neurosurgery* 26:570-578, 1990.
9. Hamilton MG, Spetzler RF: The prospective application of a grading system for arteriovenous malformations, *Neurosurgery* 34:2-6, 1994:discussion 6-7.
10. Stapf C, Mast H, Sciacca RR, et al: Predictors of hemorrhage in patients with untreated brain arteriovenous malformation, *Neurology* 66:1350-1355, 2006.
11. Ondra SL, Troupp H, George ED, et al: The natural history of symptomatic arteriovenous malformations of the brain: A 24-year follow-up assessment, *J Neurosurg* 73:387-391, 1990.
12. Brown RD Jr, Wiebers DO, Forbes G, et al: The natural history of unruptured intracranial arteriovenous malformations, *J Neurosurg* 68:352-357, 1988.
13. Mast H, Young WL, Koennecke HC, et al: Risk of spontaneous haemorrhage after diagnosis of cerebral arteriovenous malformation, *Lancet* 350:1065-1068, 1997.
14. Stapf C, Labovitz DL, Sciacca RR, et al: Incidence of adult brain arteriovenous malformation hemorrhage in a prospective population-based stroke survey, *Cerebrovasc Dis* 13:43-46, 2002.
15. Kondziolka D, McLaughlin MR, Kestle JR: Simple risk predictions for arteriovenous malformation hemorrhage, *Neurosurgery* 37:851-855, 1995.
16. Berman MF, Sciacca RR, Pile-Spellman J, et al: The epidemiology of brain arteriovenous malformations, *Neurosurgery* 47:389-396, 2000:discussion 397.
17. Stapf C, Mohr JP, Pile-Spellman J, et al: Epidemiology and natural history of arteriovenous malformations, *Neurosurg Focus* 11:e1, 2001.
18. Piepgras DG, Sundt TM Jr, Ragoowansi AT, et al: Seizure outcome in patients with surgically treated cerebral arteriovenous malformations, *J Neurosurg* 78:5-11, 1993.
19. Yeh HS, Tew JM Jr, Gartner M: Seizure control after surgery on cerebral arteriovenous malformations, *J Neurosurg* 78:12-18, 1993.
20. Batjer H, Suss RA, Samson D: Intracranial arteriovenous malformations associated with aneurysms, *Neurosurgery* 18:29-35, 1986.
21. Kader A, Young WL, Pile-Spellman J, et al: The influence of hemodynamic and anatomic factors on hemorrhage from cerebral arteriovenous malformations, *Neurosurgery* 34:801-807, 1994:discussion 807-808.
22. Miyasaka Y, Yada K, Ohwada T, et al: An analysis of the venous drainage system as a factor in hemorrhage from arteriovenous malformations, *J Neurosurg* 76:239-243, 1992.
23. Turjman F, Massoud TF, Vinuela F, et al: Correlation of the angioarchitectural features of cerebral arteriovenous malformations with clinical presentation of hemorrhage, *Neurosurgery* 37:856-860, 1995:discussion 860-852.
24. Marks MP, Lane B, Steinberg GK, et al: Hemorrhage in intracerebral arteriovenous malformations: Angiographic determinants, *Radiology* 176:807-813, 1990.

25. Duong DH, Young WL, Vang MC, et al: Feeding artery pressure and venous drainage pattern are primary determinants of hemorrhage from cerebral arteriovenous malformations, *Stroke* 29:1167-1176, 1998.

26. Waltimo O: The change in size of intracranial arteriovenous malformations, *J Neurol Sci* 19:21-27, 1973.

27. Graf CJ, Perret GE, Torner JC: Bleeding from cerebral arteriovenous malformations as part of their natural history, *J Neurosurg* 58:331-337, 1983.

28. Stapf C, Connolly ES, Schumacher HC, et al: Dysplastic vessels after surgery for brain arteriovenous malformations, *Stroke* 33:1053-1056, 2002.

29. Hamilton MG, Spetzler RF: The prospective application of a grading system for arteriovenous malformations, *Neurosurgery* 34:2-7, 1994.

30. Pellettieri L, Carlsson CA, Grevsten S, et al: Surgical versus conservative treatment of intracranial arteriovenous malformations: A study in surgical decision-making, *Acta Neurochir Suppl (Wien)* 29:1-86, 1979.

31. Brown RD Jr, Wiebers DO, Forbes GS: Unruptured intracranial aneurysms and arteriovenous malformations: Frequency of intracranial hemorrhage and relationship of lesions, *J Neurosurg* 73:859-863, 1990.

32. Pollock BE, Flickinger JC: A proposed radiosurgery-based grading system for arteriovenous malformations, *J Neurosurgery* 96:79-85, 2002.

33. Pik JHT, Morgan MK: Microsurgery for small arteriovenous malformations of the brain: Results in 110 consecutive patients, *Neurosurgery* 47:571-577, 2000.

34. Schaller C, Schramm J: Microsurgical results for small arteriovenous malformations accessible for radiosurgical or embolization treatment, *Neurosurgery* 40:664-674, 1997.

35. Pollock BE, Lunsford LD, Kondziolka D, et al: Patient outcomes after stereotactic radiosurgery for "operable" arteriovenous malformations, *Neurosurgery* 35:1-8, 1994.

36. de Oliveira E, Tedeschi H, Raso J: Multidisciplinary approach to arteriovenous malformations, *Neurol Med Chir (Tokyo)* 38(Suppl):177-185, 1998.

37. Du R, Keyoung HM, Dowd CF, et al: The effects of diffuseness and deep perforating artery supply on outcomes after microsurgical resection of brain arteriovenous malformations, *Neurosurgery* 60:638-646, 2007:discussion 646-638.

38. de Oliveira E, Tedeschi H, Raso J: Comprehensive management of arteriovenous malformations, *Neurol Res* 20:673-683, 1998.

39. Lawton MT: Spetzler-Martin grade III arteriovenous malformations: Surgical results and a modification of the grading scale, *Neurosurgery* 52:740-749, 2003.

40. Pollock BE, Kondziolka D, Lunsford LD, et al: Repeat stereotactic radiosurgery of arteriovenous malformations: Factors associated with incomplete obliteration, *Neurosurgery* 38:318-324, 1996.

41. Pollock BE, Flickinger JC, Lunsford LD, et al: Factors associated with successful arteriovenous malformation radiosurgery, *Neurosurgery* 42:1239-1247, 1998.

42. Maruyama K, Kondziolka D, Niranjan A, et al: Stereotactic radiosurgery for brainstem arteriovenous malformations: Factors affecting outcome, *J Neurosurgery* 100:407-413, 2004.

43. Meder J-F, Oppenheim C, Blustajn J, et al: Cerebral arteriovenous malformations:The value of radiologic parameters in predicting response to radiosurgery, *Am J Neuroradiol* 18:1473-1483, 1997.

44. Liscak R, Vladyka V, Simonova G, et al: Arteriovenous malformations after Leksell gamma knife radiosurgery: Rate of obliteration and complications, *Neurosurgery* 60:1005-1014, 2007:discussion 1015-1006.

45. Ellis TL, Friedman WA, Bova FJ, et al: Analysis of treatment failure after radiosurgery for arteriovenous malformations, *J Neurosurgery* 89:104-110, 1998.

46. Friedman WA, Bova FJ, Bollampally S, et al: Analysis of factors predictive of success or complications in arteriovenous malformation radiosurgery, *Neurosurgery* 52:296-308, 2003.

47. Andrade-Souza YM, Zadeh G, Ramani M, et al: Testing the radiosurgery-based arteriovenous malformation score and the modified Spetzler-Martin grading system to predict radiosurgical outcome, *J Neurosurg* 103:642-648, 2005.

48. Heros RC, Korosue K, Diebold PM: Surgical excision of cerebral arteriovenous malformations: Late results, *Neurosurgery* 26:570-577, 1990:discussion 577-578.

49. Szabo MD, Crosby G, Sundaram P, et al: Hypertension does not cause spontaneous hemorrhage of intracranial arteriovenous malformations, *Anesthesiology* 70:761-763, 1989.

50. Hartmann A, Pile-Spellman J, Stapf C, et al: Risk of endovascular treatment of brain arteriovenous malformations, *Stroke* 33:1816-1820, 2002.

51. Young WL, Kader A, Pile-Spellman J, et al: Arteriovenous malformation draining vein physiology and determinants of transnidal pressure gradients. The Columbia University AVM Study Project, *Neurosurgery* 35:389-395, 1994:discussion 395-386.

52. Sinclair J, Kelly ME, Steinberg GK: Surgical management of posterior fossa arteriovenous malformations, *Neurosurgery* 58: ONS-189-ONS-201, 2006:discussion ONS-201.

53. Nozaki K, Hashimoto N, Kikuta K, et al: Surgical applications to arteriovenous malformations involving the brainstem, *Neurosurgery* 58:ONS-270-ONS-278, 2006:discussion ONS-278-ONS-279.

54. Cunha e Sa MJ, Stein BM, Solomon RA, et al: The treatment of associated intracranial aneurysms and arteriovenous malformations, *J Neurosurg* 77:853-859, 1992.

55. Lawton MT, Hamilton MG, Spetzler RF: Multimodality treatment of deep arteriovenous malformations: Thalamus, basal ganglia, and brain stem, *Neurosurgery* 37:29-36, 1995.

56. Vinuela F, Dion JE, Duckwiler G, et al: Combined endovascular embolization and surgery in the management of cerebral arteriovenous malformations: Experience with 101 cases, *J Neurosurg* 75:856-864, 1991.

57. Blount JP, Oakes WJ, Tubbs RS, et al: History of surgery for cerebrovascular disease in children. Part III: Arteriovenous malformations, *Neurosurg Focus* 20:E11, 2006.

58. Drake CG: Cerebral arteriovenous malformations: Considerations for and experience with surgical treatment in 166 cases, *Clin Neurosurg* 26:145-208, 1979.

59. Mullan S, Brown FD, Patronas NJ: Hyperemic and ischemic problems of surgical treatment of arteriovenous malformations, *J Neurosurg* 51:757-764, 1979.

60. Nornes H, Grip A: Hemodynamic aspects of cerebral arteriovenous malformations, *J Neurosurg* 53:456-464, 1980.

61. Sarwar M, McCormick WF: Intracerebral venous angioma. Case report and review, *Arch Neurol* 35:323-325, 1978.

62. Wilson CB, Hoi Sang U, Domingue J: Microsurgical treatment of intracranial vascular malformations, *J Neurosurg* 51:446-454, 1979.

63. Barnett GH, Little JR, Ebrahim ZY, et al: Cerebral circulation during arteriovenous malformation operation, *Neurosurgery* 20:836-842, 1987.

64. Batjer HH, Devous MD Sr: The use of acetazolamide-enhanced regional cerebral blood flow measurement to predict risk to arteriovenous malformation patients, *Neurosurgery* 31:213-217, 1992:discussion 217-218.

65. Batjer HH, Devous MD Sr, Meyer YJ, et al: Cerebrovascular hemodynamics in arteriovenous malformation complicated by normal perfusion pressure breakthrough, *Neurosurgery* 22:503-509, 1988.

66. Hassler W, Steinmetz H: Cerebral hemodynamics in angioma patients: An intraoperative study, *J Neurosurg* 67:822-831, 1987.

67. Young WL, Kader A, Prohovnik I, et al: Pressure autoregulation is intact after arteriovenous malformation resection, *Neurosurgery* 32:491-496, 1993:discussion 496-497.

68. Young WL, Pile-Spellman J, Prohovnik I, et al: Evidence for adaptive autoregulatory displacement in hypotensive cortical territories adjacent to arteriovenous malformations. Columbia University AVM Study Project, *Neurosurgery* 34:601-610, 1994:discussion 610-611.

69. Young WL, Prohovnik I, Ornstein E, et al: The effect of arteriovenous malformation resection on cerebrovascular reactivity to carbon dioxide, *Neurosurgery* 27:257-266, 1990:discussion 266-257.

70. Young WL, Solomon RA, Prohovnik I, et al: Xe^{133} blood flow monitoring during arteriovenous malformation resection: A case of intraoperative hyperperfusion with subsequent brain swelling, *Neurosurgery* 22:765-769, 1988.

71. al-Rodhan NR, Sundt TM Jr, Piepgras DG, et al: Occlusive hyperemia: A theory for the hemodynamic complications following resection of intracerebral arteriovenous malformations, *J Neurosurg* 78:167-175, 1993.

72. Wilson CB, Hieshima G: Occlusive hyperemia: A new way to think about an old problem, *J Neurosurg* 78:165-166, 1993.

73. Jafar JJ, Davis AJ, Berenstein A, et al: The effect of embolization with *N*-butyl cyanoacrylate prior to surgical resection of cerebral arteriovenous malformations, *J Neurosurg* 78:60-69, 1993.

74. Spetzler RF, Martin NA, Carter LP, et al: Surgical management of large AVMs by staged embolization and operative excision, *J Neurosurg* 67:17-28, 1987.

75. DeMeritt JS, Pile-Spellman J, Mast H, et al: Outcome analysis of preoperative embolization with *N*-butyl cyanoacrylate in cerebral arteriovenous malformations, *AJNR Am J Neuroradiol* 16:1801-1807, 1995.

76. Ledezma CJ, Hoh BL, Carter BS, et al: Complications of cerebral arteriovenous malformation embolization: Multivariate analysis of predictive factors, *Neurosurgery* 58:602-611, 2006:discussion 602-611.

77. Hartmann A, Mast H, Mohr JP, et al: Determinants of staged endovascular and surgical treatment outcome of brain arteriovenous malformations, *Stroke* 36:2431-2435, 2005.

78. Purdy PD, Batjer HH, Samson D: Management of hemorrhagic complications from preoperative embolization of arteriovenous malformations, *J Neurosurg* 74:205-211, 1991.

79. Purdy PD, Batjer HH, Samson D, et al: Intraarterial sodium amytal administration to guide preoperative embolization of cerebral arteriovenous malformations, *J Neurosurg Anesthesiol* 3:103-106, 1991.

80. Celli P, Ferrante L, Palma L, et al: Cerebral arteriovenous malformations in children. Clinical features and outcome of treatment in children and in adults, *Surg Neurol* 22:43-49, 1984.

81. Kader A, Goodrich JT, Sonstein WJ, et al: Recurrent cerebral arteriovenous malformations after negative postoperative angiograms, *J Neurosurg* 85:14-18, 1996.

82. Locksley HB: Hemorrhagic strokes. Principal causes, natural history, and treatment, *Med Clin North Am* 52:1193-1212, 1968.

83. Cronqvist S, Granholm L, Lundstrom NR: Hydrocephalus and congestive heart failure caused by intracranial arteriovenous malformations in infants, *J Neurosurg* 36:249-254, 1972.

84. Kondziolka D, Humphreys RP, Hoffman HJ, et al: Arteriovenous malformations of the brain in children: A forty year experience, *Can J Neurol Sci* 19:40-45, 1992.

85. Humphreys RP, Hoffman HJ, Drake JM, et al: Choices in the 1990s for the management of pediatric cerebral arteriovenous malformations, *Pediatr Neurosurg* 25:277-285, 1996.

86. Lasjaunias P, Hui F, Zerah M, et al: Cerebral arteriovenous malformations in children. Management of 179 consecutive cases and review of the literature, *Childs Nerv Syst* 11:66-79, 1995:discussion 79.

87. Malik GM, Sadasivan B, Knighton RS, et al: The management of arteriovenous malformations in children, *Childs Nerv Syst* 7:43-47, 1991.

88. Robinson JL, Hall CJ, Sedzimir CB: Subarachnoid hemorrhage in pregnancy, *J Neurosurg* 36:27-33, 1972.

89. Robinson JL, Hall CS, Sedzimir CB: Arteriovenous malformations, aneurysms, and pregnancy, *J Neurosurg* 41:63-70, 1974.

90. Horton JC, Chambers WA, Lyons SL, et al: Pregnancy and the risk of hemorrhage from cerebral arteriovenous malformations, *Neurosurgery* 27:867-871, 1990:discussion 871-862.

91. Sadasivan B, Malik GM, Lee C, Ausman JI: Vascular malformations and pregnancy, *Surg Neurol* 33:305-313, 1990.

72 Spinal Arteriovenous Malformations

SHERVIN R. DASHTI, LOUIS J. KIM, UDAYA K. KAKARLA, MIN S. PARK, MICHAEL F. STIEFEL, ROBERT F. SPETZLER

Spinal arteriovenous lesions are a collection of disparate and diverse entities. Our understanding of their pathophysiology has evolved significantly over the past century. This chapter discusses significant microsurgical and endovascular advances made in the treatment of spinal arteriovenous malformations (AVMs). Before an effective treatment strategy can be selected, these lesions must first be characterized accurately. To do so, we use the classification system developed by the senior author (RFS) as summarized here.[1,2] This system is based on specific anatomic and pathophysiologic factors. Lesions are divided into arteriovenous fistulas (AVFs) and AVMs (Table 72-1). AVFs are subdivided anatomically into extradural and intradural. Intradural AVFs are further divided into dorsal and ventral types based on their location. Ventral dural AVFs are subdivided into types A, B, and C on the basis of the size and number of feeding branches. AVMs include extradural-intradural and intramedullary lesions.

Treatment Strategies

In contemporary neurosurgical settings, these lesions should be approached in a team-oriented fashion. Optimal patient care depends on direct collaboration between open vascular and endovascular neurosurgeons. The role of each half of this neurovascular team depends on the lesion, and treatment must be individualized to the specifics of each situation. The following surgical strategies and technical consideration serve only as a guide.

At our institution, monitoring somatosensory and motor evoked potentials has become a routine part of spinal AVM surgery. Intraoperative angiography should be used in selected cases when residual AVM may remain. More often, however, we use indocyanine green (ICG) fluorescent angiography, which is usually followed by postoperative catheter-based angiography. Radiosurgery for spinal AVMs is considered elsewhere in this volume.

Extradural Arteriovenous Fistulas

Extradural AVFs (Fig. 72-1) represent an abnormal communication between an extradural arterial branch that usually arises from a branch of a radicular artery and an epidural venous plexus. This entity results in significant engorgement of the venous system, leading to subsequent compression from mass effect on adjacent nerve roots and spinal cord. Venous hypertension and vascular steal also may contribute to myelopathic symptoms. In our experience, the purely extradural fistula is an extremely uncommon lesion. These lesions are primarily treated by endovascular techniques.[3-8] The role of surgery in treating these lesions is limited to cases requiring reduction of local compression after embolization.

Intradural Dorsal Arteriovenous Fistulas

Intradural dorsal AVFs (Fig. 72-2A and B), which correlate with type I dural AVFs, are composed of a radicular feeding artery that communicates abnormally with the venous system of the spinal cord at the dural sleeve of the nerve root. Inherent to their pathophysiology is obstruction of spinal cord venous outflow, which ostensibly contributes to the formation of the fistula. In turn, arterialization of the coronal venous plexus, venous hypertension, and myelopathy ensue.

Dorsal AVFs can be treated endovascularly, but the safety and permanence of treatment heavily favor surgery. The surgery is relatively straightforward and low risk. Successful surgical management, however, requires careful and thorough catheter-based spinal angiography to identify the arterial feeder(s) and artery of Adamkiewicz. Although angiographic visualization is paramount, angiographically occult lesions in patients in whom there is high clinical suspicion for intradural dorsal fistulas have been associated with successful surgical exploration and fistula disruption.[9]

Once the appropriate spinal level has been identified, the surgical strategy involves its posterior exposure. We favor a posterior approach and laminoplasty. High-powered magnification and illumination with the operating microscope are used to perform intradural dissection along the appropriate nerve root. Typically, an arterialized vein is identified along the nerve root and can be sharply dissected to its exit point at the margin of the dural root sleeve. Nonstick bipolar cauterization and microscissors are used to interrupt the fistula. The advantage of surgical disruption is the relative ease of exposure and direct visualization of the vascular anatomy.[9-14] We routinely measure the venous pressure of an AVF before and after its interruption by direct puncture of the venous side with a 27-gauge needle attached to a digital manometer. With complete disruption of the fistula, venous pressure should decrease significantly. However, venous pressure will still be higher than systemic venous pressure because of obstruction of venous outflow (Table 72-2).

Intradural Ventral Arteriovenous Fistulas

Intradural ventral AVFs (Fig. 72-3) are ventral midline lesions located in the subarachnoid space. The fistulous site occurs between the anterior spinal artery (ASA) and an enlarged venous network. The lesions have been subclassified as types A, B, and C.[15] Type A intradural ventral AVFs are small, type B lesion size is intermediate, and type C lesions are giant. Extraordinarily high flow through these lesions leads to the phenomenon of vascular steal from the intrinsic arterial supply to the spinal cord and to the sequelae of ischemic symptoms.

The difficulty in approaching intradural ventral AVFs endovascularly is that catheterization of the ASA feeders is a relatively high-risk procedure. Small intradural ventral

---

TABLE 72-1 CLASSIFICATION OF SPINAL ARTERIOVENOUS LESIONS

Arteriovenous fistula (AVF)
Extradural
Intradural
Dorsal AVF
Ventral AVF
Types A, B, C

Arteriovenous malformations
Extradural-intradural
Intramedullary
Conus medullaris

Modified from Spetzler RF, Detwiler PW, Riina HA, et al: Modified classification of spinal cord vascular lesions. *J Neurosurg* 96: (2 suppl) 145-156, 2002. Used with permission from *Journal of Neurosurgery*.

AVFs (types A and B) are therefore managed surgically.[15-18] These lesions may require an anterior or anterolateral approach for adequate exposure; however, posterolateral approaches are feasible for ventrolateral lesions.[19,20] Therefore, a thorough understanding of complex spinal approaches is essential for both the operative approach and spinal stabilization. Key to surgical success is preservation of the ASA branches during obliteration of the fistula. Giant (type C) lesions, however, are best treated with endovascular embolization techniques because of their complex angioarchitecture and multipedicled feeders.[15,18,21-24] Surgery can then be performed as an adjunct to embolization.

Extradural-Intradural Arteriovenous Malformations

Extradural-intradural AVMs (Fig. 72-4) correspond to juvenile or metameric AVMs. These formidable lesions are invested along a discrete somite level. Typically, they involve bone, muscle, skin, spinal canal, spinal cord, and nerve roots. Complete involvement of an AVM along an entire somite level has been described as Cobb's syndrome.

Extradural-intradural AVMs are technically challenging lesions to treat. They are treated primarily with endovascular embolization; postembolization surgery is reserved for decompression of mass effect along the nerve roots and spinal cord.[7,12,20,22,25,26] Although treatment cures have been reported,[20,26,27] the realistic goal in most cases is reduction of mass effect, venous hypertension, and vascular steal to ameliorate the patient's neurologic deficits.

Intramedullary Arteriovenous Malformations

Intramedullary AVMs, which are analogous to intracranial AVMs, are located entirely in the spinal cord parenchyma. These lesions may have single or multiple feeding arteries from branches of the ASA and posterior spinal artery (PSA). They are further classified as compact or diffuse

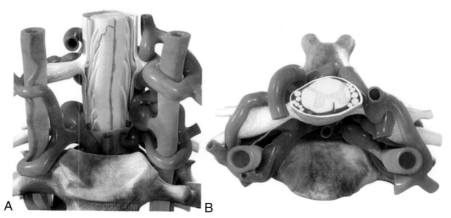

Figure 72-1 A, Posterior illustration shows that engorgement of epidural veins can have a symptomatic mass effect on adjacent nerve roots and spinal cord. B, Axial illustration of an extradural arteriovenous fistula along a perforating branch of the left vertebral artery *(arrow).* (Used with permission from Barrow Neurological Institute.)

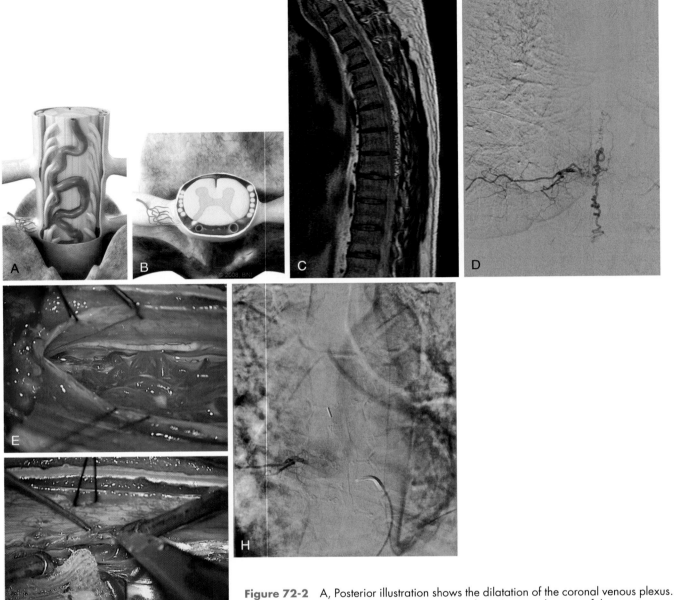

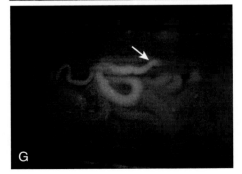

Figure 72-2 A, Posterior illustration shows the dilatation of the coronal venous plexus. In addition to venous outflow obstruction (not shown), arterialization of these veins produces venous hypertension. Focal disruption of the point of the fistula by endovascular or microsurgical methods will obliterate the lesion. B, Axial illustration of an intradural dorsal arteriovenous fistula (AVF) shows an abnormal radicular feeding artery along the nerve root on the right. The glomerular network of tiny branches coalesces at the site of the fistula along the dural root sleeve. C, Illustrative case of a 55-year-old man with progressive myelopathy and bowel and bladder incontinence. Sagittal T2-weighted MR image of the thoracic spine reveals serpiginous vessels dorsal to the spinal cord. D, Selective injection of right T7 segmental vessel shows a dorsal intradural AVF. Angiographic examination of the entire spine showed no other feeder vessels. E, Intradural view at surgery shows multiple dilated vessels over the dorsal aspect of the spinal cord. F, A single feeding arterial pedicle is isolated exiting at the right T7 nerve root sleeve, as expected. G, Indocyanine green angiography confirms the fistula site *(arrow)*. H, Repeat right T7 segmental artery injection after surgical interruption of the fistula site shown in F shows the absence of fistula. (Used with permission from Barrow Neurological Institute.)

TABLE 72-2 INTRAOPERATIVE PRESSURE MEASUREMENTS IN 22 PATIENTS

Measurement Site	Intraoperative Pressure (mm Hg)	
	With Fistula Open	With Fistula Closed
Feeding artery	44 ± 17	82 ± 12
Draining vein	44 ± 1	23 ± 9
Epidural vein	11 ± 4	11 ± 4

(Figs. 72-5 and 72-6), depending on the angioarchitecture of the nidus. The size of the nidus is an important determinant of treatment success. AVMs with a compact nidus are more amenable to both endovascular embolization and surgical resection.

Intramedullary AVMs have been treated successfully with embolization procedures.[28] We have found the embolic agent Onyx (ev3 Inc., Irvine, Calif) to be particularly useful. However, the mainstay of treatment remains surgical extirpation.[1,29] We recommend

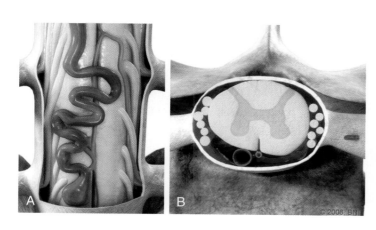

Figure 72-3 A, Anterior illustration shows the arteriovenous fistula (AVF) along the anteroinferior aspect of the spinal cord. Proximal and distal to this type A lesion, the course of the anterior spinal artery is normal. B, Axial illustration of an intradural ventral AVF, a midline lesion derived from a fistulous connection between the anterior spinal artery and coronal venous plexus. (Used with permission from Barrow Neurological Institute.)

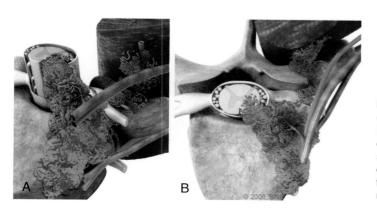

Figure 72-4 (A) Posterior and (B) axial illustrations of an extradural-intradural arteriovenous malformation. Such treacherous lesions can encompass soft tissues, bone, spinal canal, spinal cord, and spinal nerve roots along an entire spinal level. Considerable involvement of multiple structures makes these entities extremely difficult to treat. Although cures have been reported, the primary goal of treatment is usually palliative. (Used with permission from Barrow Neurological Institute.)

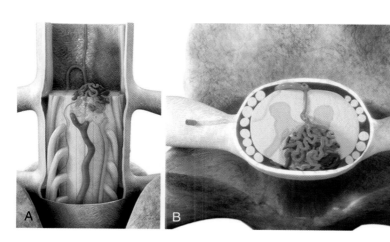

Figure 72-5 A, Posterior illustration shows additional feeding branches from the posterior spinal artery and reemphasizes the compact nature of this type of spinal arteriovenous malformation (AVM). Portions of the AVM are evident along the surface of the spinal cord. Surgical resection is the mainstay of treatment. Preoperative embolization is reserved for select cases only. B, Axial illustration of a compact intramedullary AVM. An arterial feeder from the anterior spinal artery can be identified. Note the discrete, compact mass of the AVM. (Used with permission from Barrow Neurological Institute.)

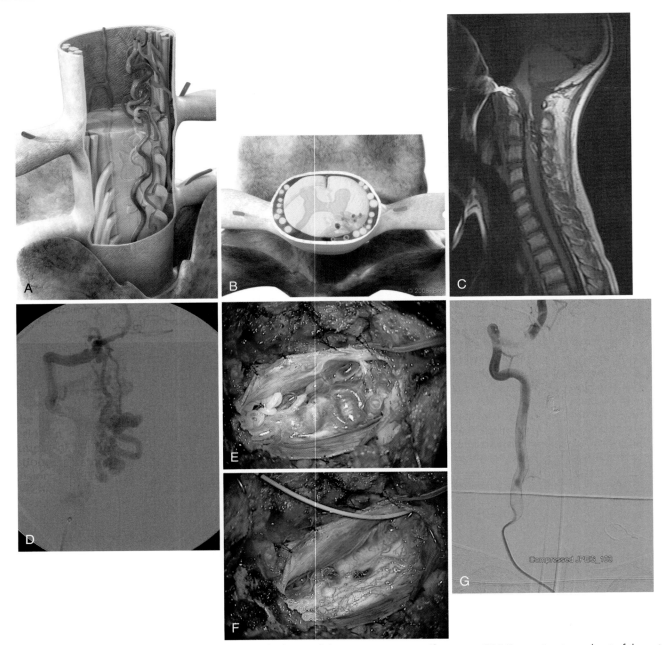

Figure 72-6 A, Oblique posterior illustration shows the loops of the arteriovenous malformation (AVM) coursing in and out of the spinal cord. Normal neural tissue is evident between intraparenchymal portions of the AVM. This view accentuates the diffuse character of such lesions. B, Axial illustration of a diffuse intramedullary AVM shows areas of intervening neural tissue between the intraparenchymal loops of the AVM. Portions of the AVM also course along the pial surface and subarachnoid space. C, Illustrative case of a 12-year-old boy with a history of subarachnoid hemorrhage. Sagittal T1-weighted MR image of the cervical spine reveals abnormal vessels in the spinal cord. D, Right vertebral artery injection shows a diffuse cervical intramedullary AVM with feeders from the anterior spinal artery and muscular branches. E, Intradural view through the operating microscope shows the diffuse cervical intramedullary nidus. Most of the vessels are thrombosed from multiple sessions of endovascular embolization. F, View of the cervical cord after surgical resection of the AVM. G, Repeat angiography with injection of the right vertebral artery shows no residual AVM. (Used with permission from Barrow Neurological Institute.)

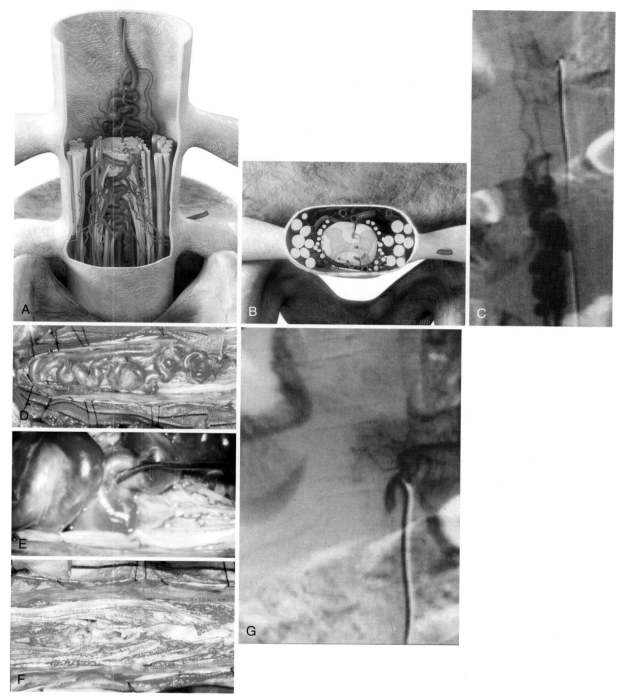

Figure 72-7 A, Posterior illustration recapitulates the complexity of the angioarchitecture of spinal arteriovenous malformations (AVMs). Anterior and posterior spinal arteries, radicular arteries, and anteriorly and posteriorly draining veins are involved simultaneously. Portions of the AVM can consist of direct AV shunts as well as regions of true AVM nidus. During endovascular treatment, surgical treatment, or both, identification of the en passage branches of the anterior and posterior spinal arteries is crucial. B, Axial illustration of a conus medullaris AVM shows the feeding arteries and draining veins from both the anterior and posterior aspects of the spinal cord. Note the proximity of the AVM to branches of the cauda equina. C, Illustrative case of a 15-year-old boy who experienced the acute onset of back pain and subarachnoid hemorrhage. Angiogram shows the AVM with large draining vein at the thoracolumbar junction. D, Intradural view of tortuous arterialized draining vein. E, Intradural view of the nidus at the conus. F, A view of the conus after complete resection of the AVM. G, Postoperative angiography confirms no residual AVM. (A and B used with permission from Barrow Neurological Institute. C through G from Koos W, Spetzler RF, Lang J, et al: *Color atlas of microneurosurgery,* ed 2, vol 3: Intra- and extracranial revascularization and intraspinal pathology, 2000, New York, Thieme. Used with permission from Thieme.)

preoperative embolization in selected cases, particularly for patients with complex, multipedicled, or diffuse lesions. Typically, a posterior or posterolateral approach is suitable, but an anterior approach may be warranted in selected cases.[20,29,30] For diffuse lesions (see Fig. 72-6A and B) situated superficially on the spinal cord, it is prudent to avoid "chasing" vascular loops of AVM that may invaginate into the spinal cord parenchyma. Because the pathophysiology of these lesions defines them as superficial entities, it is best to truncate vessels embedded in the parenchyma at the pial surface. This strategy minimizes trauma to the tissue that could lead to inadvertent neurologic injury yet still permits complete obliteration of the lesion. Postoperative spinal angiography is essential to demonstrate any residual AVM. Repeat or staged operations are common. We have achieved gross total resection of 92% of the intramedullary AVMs that we have treated.[1]

Conus Medullaris Arteriovenous Malformations

Conus medullaris AVMs (Fig. 72-7) occupy a separate category.[1] Conus lesions typically exhibit multiple feeders from the anterior and posterior spinal arteries with direct arteriovenous shunts as well as a diffuse AVM. The pathophysiology underlying neurologic decline includes venous hypertension, ischemia, hemorrhage, and mass effect from hugely dilated venous structures. Because the location and angioarchitecture of these lesions are unique, both upper and lower motor neuron symptoms can occur.

Conus medullaris AVMs are treated with a combined endovascular and microsurgical approach. Careful identification of anterior and posterior spinal artery branches separate from the lesion is crucial. Because the venous structures associated with conus AVMs are so dilated, surgical decompression of adjacent spinal cord and nerve roots can significantly relieve neurologic symptoms. Conus AVMs are usually easily accessible from a posterior approach. Our continuing experience with these entities has demonstrated that aggressive combined treatment can achieve good outcomes.[1] Despite aggressive treatment, however, these lesions can recur. Therefore, patients with conus medullaris AVMs must be followed up closely.

Conclusions

Our ability to identify and treat spinal AVMs and AVFs has advanced tremendously in the last several decades. This chapter describes the contemporary treatment of spinal arteriovenous lesions, which combines endovascular and microsurgical approaches.

REFERENCES

1. Spetzler RF, Detwiler PW, Riina HA, et al: Modified classification of spinal cord vascular lesions, *J Neurosurg* 96(Suppl):145-156, 2002.
2. Kim LJ, Spetzler RF: Classification and surgical management of spinal arteriovenous lesions: Arteriovenous fistulae and arteriovenous malformations, *Neurosurgery* 59(Suppl 3):S195-S201, 2006.
3. Arnaud O, Bille F, Pouget J, et al: Epidural arteriovenous fistula with perimedullary venous drainage: Case report, *Neuroradiology* 36(6):490-491, 1994 August.
4. Graziani N, Bouillot P, Figarella-Branger D, et al: Cavernous angiomas and arteriovenous malformations of the spinal epidural space: Report of 11 cases, *Neurosurgery* 35:856-863, 1994.
5. Heier LA, Lee BC: A dural spinal arteriovenous malformation with epidural venous drainage: A case report, *AJNR Am J Neuroradiol* 8:561-563, 1987.
6. Miyagi Y, Miyazono M, Kamikaseda K: Spinal epidural vascular malformation presenting in association with a spontaneously resolved acute epidural hematoma. Case report, *J Neurosurg* 88:909-911, 1998.
7. Niimi Y, Berenstein A: Endovascular treatment of spinal vascular malformations, *Neurosurg Clin N Am* 10:47-71, 1999.
8. Scully R, Mark E, McNeely W, McNeely B: Case records of the Massachusetts General Hospital, *N Engl J Med* 326:816-824, 1992.
9. Oldfield EH, Di Chiro G, Quindlen EA, et al: Successful treatment of a group of spinal cord arteriovenous malformations by interruption of dural fistula, *J Neurosurg* 59:1019-1030, 1983.
10. Anson J, Spetzler R: Spinal dural arteriovenous malformations. In *Dural arteriovenous malformations*, Park Ridge, IL, 1993, American Association of Neurological Surgeons, pp 175-191.
11. Mourier KL, Gelbert F, Rey A, et al: Spinal dural arteriovenous malformations with perimedullary drainage. Indications and results of surgery in 30 cases, *Acta Neurochir (Wien)* 100:136-141, 1989.
12. Ommaya AK, Di Chiro G, Doppman J: Ligation of arterial supply in the treatment of spinal cord arteriovenous malformations, *J Neurosurg* 30:679-692, 1969.
13. Rosenblum B, Oldfield EH, Doppman JL, et al: Spinal arteriovenous malformations: A comparison of dural arteriovenous fistulas and intradural AVMs in 81 patients, *J Neurosurg* 67:795-802, 1987.
14. Symon L, Kuyama H, Kendall B: Dural arteriovenous malformations of the spine. Clinical features and surgical results in 55 cases, *J Neurosurg* 60:238-247, 1984.
15. Anson J, Spetzler R: Classification of spinal arteriovenous malformations and implications for treatment, *BNI Quarterly* 8:2-8, 1992.
16. Glasser R, Masson R, Mickle JP, et al: Embolization of a dural arteriovenous fistula of the ventral cervical spinal canal in a nine-year-old boy, *Neurosurgery* 33:1089-1093, 1993.
17. Halbach VV, Higashida RT, Dowd CF, et al: Treatment of giant intradural (perimedullary) arteriovenous fistulas, *Neurosurgery* 33:972-979, 1993.
18. Riche MC, Melki JP, Merland JJ: Embolization of spinal cord vascular malformations via the anterior spinal artery, *AJNR Am J Neuroradiol* 4:378-381, 1983.
19. Hida K, Iwasaki Y, Ushikoshi S, et al: Corpectomy: A direct approach to perimedullary arteriovenous fistulas of the anterior cervical spinal cord, *J Neurosurg* 96(Suppl):157-161, 2002.
20. Martin NA, Khanna RK, Batzdorf U: Posterolateral cervical or thoracic approach with spinal cord rotation for vascular malformations or tumors of the ventrolateral spinal cord, *J Neurosurg* 83:254-261, 1995.
21. Gueguen B, Merland JJ, Riche MC, et al: Vascular malformations of the spinal cord: Intrathecal perimedullary arteriovenous fistulas fed by medullary arteries, *Neurology* 37:969-979, 1987.
22. Heros RC, Debrun GM, Ojemann RG, et al: Direct spinal arteriovenous fistula: a new type of spinal AVM. Case report, *J Neurosurg* 64:134-139, 1986.
23. Merland J, Reizine D: Treatment of arteriovenous spinal-cord malformations, *Semin Intervent Radiol* 4:281-290, 1987.
24. Mourier KL, Gobin YP, George B, et al: Intradural perimedullary arteriovenous fistulae: results of surgical and endovascular treatment in a series of 35 cases, *Neurosurgery* 32:885-891, 1993.
25. Malis L: Arteriovenous malformations of the spinal cord. In Youmans J, editor: *Neurological surgery. A comprehensive reference guide to the diagnosis and management of neurological problems*, Philadelphia, 1982, WB Saunders, pp 1850-1874.
26. Spetzler RF, Zabramski JM, Flom RA: Management of juvenile spinal AVMs by embolization and operative excision. Case report, *J Neurosurg* 70:628-632, 1989.
27. Touho H, Karasawa J, Shishido H, et al: Successful excision of a juvenile-type spinal arteriovenous malformation following intraoperative embolization. Case report, *J Neurosurg* 75:647-651, 1991.

28. Ausman JI, Gold LH, Tadavarthy SM, et al: Intraparenchymal embolization for obliteration of an intramedullary AVM of the spinal cord. Technical note, *J Neurosurg* 47:119-125, 1977.

29. Connolly ES Jr, Zubay GP, McCormick PC, et al: The posterior approach to a series of glomus (type II) intramedullary spinal cord arteriovenous malformations, *Neurosurgery* 42:774-785, 1998.

30. Williams FC, Zabramski JM, Spetzler RF, et al: Anterolateral transthoracic transvertebral resection of an intramedullary spinal arteriovenous malformation. Case report, *J Neurosurg* 74:1004-1008, 1991.

73 Radiosurgery for Arteriovenous Malformations

WILLIAM A. FRIEDMAN, FRANK J. BOVA

*S*tereotactic radiosurgery is the term coined by Lars Leksell[1] to describe the application of a single, high dose of radiation to a stereotactically defined target volume. In the 1970s reports began to appear documenting the successful obliteration of arteriovenous malformations (AVMs) with radiosurgery. When an AVM is treated with radiosurgery, a pathologic process appears to be induced that is similar to the response-to-injury model of atherosclerosis. Radiation injury to the vascular endothelium is believed to induce the proliferation of smooth muscle cells and the elaboration of extracellular collagen, which leads to progressive stenosis and obliteration of the AVM nidus,[2-5] thereby eliminating the risk of hemorrhage.

The advantages of radiosurgery—compared with microsurgical and endovascular treatments—are that it is noninvasive, has minimal risk of severe complications, and is performed as an outpatient procedure requiring no recovery time for the patient. The primary disadvantage of radiosurgery is that a cure is not immediate. Thrombosis of the lesion is achieved in the majority of cases, but it commonly does not occur until 2 or 3 years after treatment. During the interval between radiosurgical treatment and AVM thrombosis, the risk of hemorrhage remains. Another potential disadvantage of radiosurgery is possible long-term adverse effects of radiation. Finally, radiosurgery has been shown to be less effective for lesions more than 10 mL in volume. For these reasons, selection of the optimal treatment for an AVM is a complex decision requiring the input of experts in endovascular, open surgical, and radiosurgical treatment.

In the pages below, we will review the world's literature on radiosurgery for AVMs. Topics reviewed will include the following: radiosurgical technique, radiosurgery results (Gamma Knife radiosurgery, particle beam radiosurgery, linear accelerator radiosurgery), hemorrhage after radiosurgery, radiation-induced complications, repeated radiosurgery, and radiosurgery for other types of vascular malformation.

Radiosurgery Technique

The radiosurgical paradigm has been described at length in other publications,[6] but a brief description of radiosurgical techniques—with emphasis on points specifically applicable to AVM treatment—is in order. The fundamental elements of a successful radiosurgical treatment are

the same regardless of the system (i.e., linear accelerator, Gamma Knife, or particle beam) being used to deliver the stereotactically focused radiation. They include

1. Appropriate patient selection
2. Application of a stereotactic head ring
3. Acquisition of quality three-dimensional stereotactic images and transfer of this image database to a dose-planning computer
4. Use of the computer to formulate an optimal plan (dose distribution) for radiation delivery
5. Selection of an appropriate treatment dose
6. Precision radiation delivery that faithfully executes the plan
7. Careful clinical and radiographic follow-up

All these elements are critical, and poor performance of any step will result in suboptimal results.

Patient Selection

Open surgery is generally favored if an AVM is amenable to low-risk resection (e.g., low Spetzler-Martin grade or a young, healthy patient) or is believed to be at high risk of hemorrhage during the latency period between radiosurgical treatment and AVM obliteration (e.g., associated aneurysm or venous outflow obstruction).

Radiosurgery is favored when the AVM nidus is small (<3 cm) and compact, when surgery is judged to carry a high risk or is refused by the patient, or when the risk of hemorrhage is not believed to be extraordinarily high.

Endovascular treatment, although rarely curative alone, may be useful as a preoperative adjunct to either microsurgery or radiosurgery. If radiosurgery can be used alone, embolization should be avoided (see further on): embolic material typically makes radiosurgical targeting much more difficult and almost certainly reduces the success rate.

The pretreatment evaluation of an AVM should ideally be a team effort: surgeons comfortable and experienced with open cerebrovascular surgery, endovascular surgery, and radiosurgery should jointly determine the best method or combination of methods for each patient.

Head Ring Application

Radiosurgical treatment using a linear accelerator (LINAC) or Gamma Knife starts with head ring application; Cyberknife radiosurgery does not require a head ring. The rigidly attached ring enables the acquisition of spatially accurate information from angiography, computed tomography (CT), and magnetic resonance imaging (MRI). The images obtained with the ring in place (and an attached stereotactic localizer) establish fixed relationships between the ring and the target lesion. These spatial relationships provide the substrate for computer-based treatment planning and are later translated from radiographic (virtual) space into real space so that the treatment target can be accurately placed at the precise isocenter of the radiation delivery device. Of equal importance, because the stereotactic head ring is bolted to the treatment delivery device, it also immobilizes the patient during treatment. Most patients find it very difficult to remain motionless in frameless stereotactic systems, which limits their accuracy and utility.

In most centers, patients are premedicated with 10 mg of oral diazepam approximately a half hour before ring application. No skin shaving or scalp preparation is required. The ring and posts are assembled and positioned to fit the patient, and care should be taken to avoid accidental placement of pins into a burr hole, over a shunt path, or onto a bone flap from a prior craniotomy. The pin sites are anesthetized with a local injection of lidocaine plus bupivacaine, and the aluminum-tipped (CT-compatible) pins are hand-tightened with a wrench that is then attached to the ring so that its ready availability for ring removal is ensured. At the conclusion of this procedure, the patient is transferred to a wheelchair and transported to the radiology department for the next step (imaging) in the radiosurgery process.

Stereotactic Image Acquisition

The most problematic aspect of AVM radiosurgery is target identification. In some series (see further on), targeting error is listed as the most frequent cause of radiosurgical failure. The problem lies with imaging. While angiography very effectively defines blood flow (feeding arteries, nidus, and draining veins), it does so in only two dimensions. Using the two-dimensional data from stereotactic angiography to represent the three-dimensional target results in significant errors of both overestimation and underestimation of AVM nidus dimensions (Fig. 73-1).[7-11] Underestimation of the nidus size may result in treatment failure, whereas overestimation results in the inclusion of normal brain tissue within the treatment volume. This can cause radiation damage to normal brain, which—when affecting an eloquent area—may result in a neurologic deficit. A true three-dimensional image database is required so that such targeting errors are avoided. Both contrast-enhanced CT and MRI are now commonly used for this purpose.

Diagnostic (nonstereotactic) angiography is used to characterize the AVM, but because of its inherent inadequacies as a treatment planning database, stereotactic angiography has been largely abandoned at our institution. We use contrast enhanced, stereotactic CT as a targeting image database for the vast majority of AVMs. Our CT technique employs rapid infusion (1 mL/s) of contrast while scanning through the AVM nidus with 1-mm slices. This technique yields a very clear three-dimensional

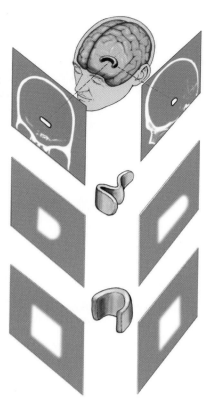

Figure 73-1 The two-dimensional nature of angiography makes it impossible to understand the true three-dimensional shape of an arteriovenous malformation (AVM) nidus as shown in the three examples above.

picture of the nidus. Alternative approaches use MRI/MR angiography as opposed to CT.

The images are transferred via Ethernet to the treatment-planning computer. The fiducial markers on the stereotactic localizer are automatically identified in each image, and the dose planning software uses these reference points to define a three-dimensional Cartesian coordinate system relative to the head ring. Spatial coordinates are assigned to each point (pixel) in each CT slice. Because the ring remains fixed relative to the patient's skull during treatment, any point in the virtual volume defined by the CT scan (including the entire head, and, most importantly, the AVM nidus) can be mapped precisely to a point in real space.

Treatment Planning

Once the necessary stereotactic images have been acquired and transferred to the treatment-planning computer, treatment planning begins; a computer workstation and specialized treatment-planning software "tools" are used. The methodology of treatment-planning varies somewhat depending on the radiosurgery system and software employed, but the objectives and basic principles of radiosurgery dose planning are universal.

The fundamental principle of radiosurgery is the delivery of focal, high-dose radiation to a designated intracranial target—in this case, the nidus of the AVM—while sparing the surrounding normal brain tissue (i.e. conformality).

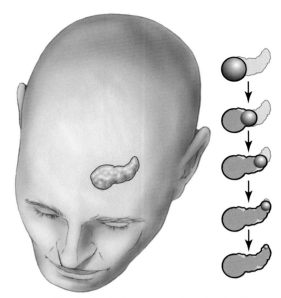

Figure 73-2 The basic dosimetry algorithm for the Gamma Knife and for the University of Florida linear accelerator radiosurgery system is called *sphere packing*. Basically, an irregular target is filled with progressively smaller spheres of tightly focused radiation until a highly conformal radiation shape is developed.

This is accomplished by focusing hundreds of nonparallel radiation beams on a stereotactically defined target. When the effect of these beams is averaged, a very high dose of radiation is delivered to the target volume (where all the beams intersect) while innocuously low doses are delivered to nontarget tissues along the path of any given beam (Figs. 73-2 and 73-3).

The primary goal of AVM radiosurgery treatment planning is to develop a plan with a target volume that conforms closely to the surface of the AVM nidus while maintaining a steep *dose gradient* (the rate of change in dose relative to position) away from the nidal surface so that the radiation dose to surrounding brain tissue is minimized. A number of treatment planning tools can be used to tailor the shape of the target volume to fit even highly irregular nidus shapes. Regardless of its shape, the entire nidus, not including the feeding arteries and draining veins, must lie within the target volume (the "prescription isodose shell"), with as little normal brain tissue included as possible.

Dose planning is ideally a team effort: the treating neurosurgeon, radiation oncologist, and medical physicist should contribute to the development of an optimal plan.

Dose Selection

Once a satisfactory treatment plan has been developed, a dose must be selected. By convention, radiosurgical doses are prescribed to the *isodose shell* (the set of all points in a dose plan that receive the same selected dose) that has been tailored to conform to the surface of the target. Isodose shells are commonly designated as percentages of the maximum dose delivered. For example, a typical AVM dose prescription might read "17.5 Gy to the 70% isodose line." In this case, the 70% isodose shell has been tailored

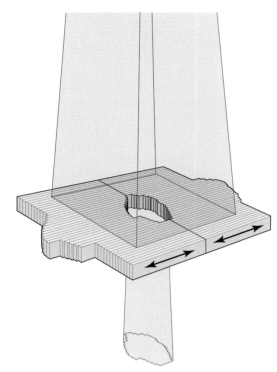

Figure 73-3 An alternative approach to dosimetry, used with some linear accelerator systems, involves a technique called *intensity modulation*. A micromultileaf collimator in the head of the machine is used to generate radiation shapes that are very conformal to the shape of the tumor.

to conform closely to the surface of the AVM nidus, and the minimum target dose of 17.5 Gy is delivered to the periphery of the nidus. Higher doses are delivered within the nidus to a maximum of 25 Gy (17.5 = 70% of 25).

Various analyses of AVM radiosurgery outcomes (described further on) have elucidated an appropriate range of doses for the treatment of AVMs. Minimum nidal doses less than 17.5 Gy have been associated with a significantly lower rate of AVM obliteration, whereas doses more than 20 Gy have been associated with a higher rate of permanent neurologic complications. We prescribe 20 Gy to the margin of the AVM nidus, whenever we believe it can be done safely, to optimize the chances of AVM obliteration. We choose the 80% isodose line for single isocenter plans and the 70% isodose line for multiple isocenter plans because these prescription isodoses are associated with the steepest dose gradients. As our experience has grown, the technology has evolved, and our ability to design very conformal plans has improved, we have used this "optimal" dose on most AVMs less than 3 cm in diameter, provided the nidus is well-defined. Lower doses may be selected for larger AVMs, AVMs in very eloquent locations, or AVMs with more diffuse nidus morphology.

Radiation Delivery

The next step in the process is the execution of the treatment plan. The patient is placed supine on the couch of the treatment device, and the head ring is secured to an immobilizing bracket. The patient's head is positioned so that the focal point of the radiation delivery device coincides with the first isocenter in the treatment plan. An appropriately sized collimator is installed to determine the diameter of the beams; then many beams of radiation are directed at the isocenter from various directions. In the case of a LINAC-based system, this is accomplished by rotating the radiation source in several concentric arcs around the isocenter. The Gamma Knife achieves the same result by exposing the target simultaneously to 201 intersecting radiation beams from independent cobalt sources that are precisely aligned in a hemispheric array around the isocenter.

If the treatment plan includes multiple isocenters, the patient's head is repositioned for each isocenter. Treatment of each isocenter typically takes about 5 minutes. Total treatment time is determined by the number of isocenters needed to achieve conformality (more are needed for irregular shapes). An alternative approach to treatment delivery with some LINAC systems involves the use of a computer-driven "micromultileaf collimator" and a radiation-shaping method called intensity modulation. In general, intensity modulation is faster than multiple isocenter treatment but not quite as conformal. Careful attention to detail and the execution of various safety checks and redundancies (now usually entirely electronic) are necessary to ensure that the prescribed treatment plan is accurately and safely delivered. When radiation delivery has been completed, the head ring is removed, the patient is observed for approximately 30 minutes, and is then discharged to resume her/his normal activities.

Follow-up

Standard follow-up after AVM radiosurgery typically consists of annual clinic visits and MRI/MR angiography to evaluate the effect of the procedure and to monitor for neurologic complications. If the patient's clinical status changes, she/he is followed up more closely at clinically appropriate intervals.

Each patient is scheduled to undergo cerebral angiography 3 years after radiosurgery, and a definitive assessment of the success or failure of treatment is made based on the results of angiography (see further on). If no flow is observed through the AVM nidus, the patient is pronounced cured and is discharged from follow-up. If the AVM nidus is incompletely obliterated, appropriate further therapy (most commonly repeated radiosurgery on the day of angiography) is prescribed, and the treatment/follow-up cycle is repeated.

Reported Efficacy of AVM Radiosurgery

Gamma Knife Radiosurgery

The Gamma Knife is a dedicated radiosurgery machine, invented by Lars Leksell and his colleagues in 1968, in Sweden. Current Gamma Knife equipment contains 192 cobalt sources, held in a hemispheric array (Fig. 73-4). These sources emit high-energy photons (called gamma rays). Each source creates an independent beam path through normal brain tissue to the radiosurgery target. All of the beams coincide at the target, delivering a high dose of radiation, but each individual beam path has very

little dose, which creates a very steep dose gradient with little risk to normal tissue.

Steiner pioneered Gamma Knife radiosurgery for AVMs and has published multiple reports.[12-15] He has reported 1-year occlusion rates ranging from 33.7% to 39.5% and 2-year occlusion rates ranging from 79% to 86.5%. However, these results were "optimized" by retrospectively selecting patients who received a high treatment dose. For example, in one report[16] he stated, "...a large majority of patients received at least 20-25 Gy of radiation.... Of the 248 patients treated before 1984, the treatment specification placed 188 in this group." The reported thrombosis rates in this article only applied to these 188 patients (76% of the total series).

Yamamoto et al reported on 25 Japanese patients treated on the gamma unit in Stockholm but followed up in Japan (Table 73-1).[17] The 2-year thrombosis rate in those AVMs that were completely covered by the radiosurgical field was 64%. Complete thrombosis occurred in an additional patient at 3-year angiography and in another at 5-year angiography, for a total cure rate of 73%. In another article,[18] these authors reported angiographic cures in six of nine children (67%) treated in Stockholm or Buenos Aires and followed up in Japan. Yamamoto et al[19] reviewed the long-term follow-up results of a group of 40 Japanese patients undergoing Gamma Knife radiosurgery for AVMs in three different countries (Argentina, Sweden, and the United States). In this group of patients, the mean lesion volume was only 3.7 mL. Twenty-six patients (65%) were subsequently found to have angiographically confirmed nidus obliteration at 1 to 5 years after radiosurgery.

Kemeny et al reported on 52 patients with AVMs treated with Gamma Knife radiosurgery.[20] They all received 25 Gy to the 50% isodose line. At 1 year, 16 patients (31%) had complete thrombosis and 10 patients (19%) had "almost complete" thrombosis. The authors found that the results were better in younger patients and in patients with AVMs with relatively lateral locations. There was no difference in outcomes among small (<2 mL), medium (2 to 3 mL), and large (>3 mL) AVMs.

Lunsford et al reported on 227 patients with AVMs treated with Gamma Knife radiosurgery.[21] The mean dose delivered to the AVM margin was 21.2 Gy. Multiple isocenters were used in 48% of the patients. Seventeen patients underwent 1-year angiography, which confirmed complete thrombosis in 76.5%. As indicated in the article, "this rate may be spurious since many of these patients were selected for angiography because their MR image had suggested obliteration." Among 75 patients who were followed up for at least 2 years, 2-year angiography was performed in only 46 (61%). Complete obliteration was confirmed in 37 of 46 (80%). This thrombosis rate strongly correlated with AVM size as follows: <1 mL, 100%; 1 to 4 mL, 85%; and 4 to 10 mL, 58%. These authors also reported on a group of 65 "operable" AVMs treated with radiosurgery.[22] Of 32 patients who subsequently underwent follow-up angiography, 84% showed complete thrombosis. In a later publication from this group, Pollock et al[23] reported on 313 patients with AVMs in which an angiographic cure rate of 61% was achieved.

Karlsson et al[24] reported on 945 AVMs treated in Stockholm between 1970 and 1990 with the Gamma Knife. The overall occlusion rate was 56%. Shin et al reported on 400 cases treated with Gamma Knife radiosurgery.[25] They reported a 72% obliteration rate 3 years after treatment. Other groups have reported on Gamma Knife radiosurgery results for specific sites, such as brainstem,[26,27] motor cortex,[28] or basal ganglia,[29] or in specific groups, such as in children.[30]

Particle Beam (Proton or Helium) Radiosurgery

Particle beam radiosurgery facilities use cyclotron-like devices to accelerate subatomic particles to very high speeds before aiming them at patients. They have a unique physical property called *the Bragg–peak effect*, which results in the vast majority of the beam's energy being deposited at a predictable depth in tissue, with little exit dose. This property is theoretically ideal for radiosurgery, but its utility has been limited by the need to spread out the Bragg peak to fit anatomic lesions, restrictions in beam number compared with Gamma Knife or LINAC systems, and the very high cost of the facilities needed for such systems.

Kjellberg et al published multiple reports on the use of Bragg peak proton particle radiosurgery for AVMs.[31-33] Their article in 1983 provided details on long-term follow-up of their first 75 patients[32] and included a well-known diagram of doses versus complications. Only 20% of these patients had complete nidus obliteration on follow-up

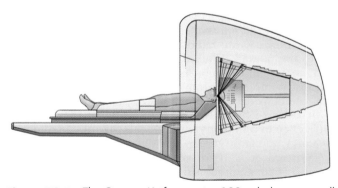

Figure 73-4 The Gamma Knife contains 192 cobalt sources, all of which are focused on the target, generating a highly focused radiosurgical field.

angiography. Seifert et al reported on 63 patients referred to the United States for Bragg peak proton beam therapy and followed up in Europe. Complete nidus obliteration was only seen in 10 patients (15.9%). A number of patients had radiation-induced side effects.

In contrast, Steinberg et al,[34] in an analysis of 86 AVMs treated with a helium particle-beam radiosurgical system, reported 29% 1-year, 70% 2-year, and 92% 3-year thrombosis rates. The best results were obtained with smaller lesions and higher doses. Initially a treatment dose of 34.6 Gy was used, but a higher than expected neurologic complication rate (20% for the entire series) led to lower doses (7.7 to 19.2 Gy). No patients treated with the lower dose range had complications.

Linear Accelerator Radiosurgery

Linear accelerators are devices that use microwave energy to accelerate electrons to very high speeds. The energetic electrons collide with a heavy metal alloy in the head of the machine. Most of the collision energy is lost as heat, but a small percentage results in high-energy photon radiation (called *X rays* because they are electronically produced). These photons are virtually identical to those produced by the spontaneous decay of radioactive cobalt in the Gamma Knife. They are collimated and focused on the radiosurgical target. Linear accelerator systems rotate the beam around the patient, from many different angles, to create the "hundreds of beams" approach used by the Gamma Knife to provide high doses at target but low doses to normal tissues (Fig. 73-5).

Betti et al pioneered LINAC radiosurgery and reported on the results of 66 AVMs treated with a linear accelerator radiosurgical system.[35-37] Doses of "no more than 40 Gy" were used in 80% of patients. The authors found a 66% 2-year thrombosis rate. The percentage of cured patients was highest when the entire malformation was included in the 75% isodose line (96%) or the maximum diameter of the lesion was less than 12 mm (81%).

Colombo et al reported on 97 patients with AVMs treated with a linear accelerator system.[38] Doses from 18.7 Gy to 40 Gy were delivered in one or two sessions. Of 56 patients who were followed up longer than 1 year, 50 underwent 12-month follow-up angiography. In 26 patients (52%), complete thrombosis was demonstrated.

TABLE 73-1   MAJOR AVM RADIOSURGERY SERIES*

First Author	Yamamoto[19]	Pollock[23]	Karlsson[24,60]	Steinberg[34]	Colombo[39]	Friedman[6]
Radiosurgical device	Gamma Knife	Gamma Knife	Gamma Knife	Proton beam	LINAC	LINAC
Number of patients	40	313	945	86	180	388
Angiographic cure rate	65%	61%	56%	92%	80%	67%
Complications						
Permanent radiation induced	3 patients (7.5%)	30 patients (9%)	5%	11%	4 patients (2%)	7 patients (2%)
Hemorrhage	None	8 fatal	55 patients	10 patients	15 patients, 5 fatal	25 patients, 5 fatal

*More than 100 patients. When a group had multiple reports, the most recent results are listed.
LINAC, Linear accelerator.

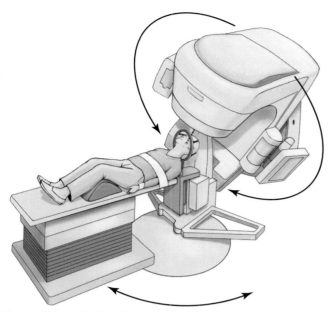

Figure 73-5 Modern linear accelerators rotate small radiation beams around the patient with very high accuracy. This generates multiple noncoplanar arcs of radiation, all intersecting only at the intracranial target point, and allows a highly focused radiation field around the target; only a minimal dose is received by surrounding structures.

Fifteen of 20 patients (75%) undergoing 2-year angiography had complete thrombosis. The authors reported a definite relationship between AVM size and thrombosis rate as follows: lesions less than 15 mm in diameter had a 1-year obliteration rate of 76% and a 2-year rate of 90%. Lesions 15 to 25 mm in diameter had a 1-year thrombosis rate of 37.5% and a 2-year rate of 80%. Lesions greater than 25 mm in diameter had a 1-year thrombosis rate of 11% and a 2-year rate of 40%. In a later article,[39] Colombo et al reported follow-up on 180 radiosurgically treated AVMs. The 1-year thrombosis rate was 46%, and the 2-year rate was 80%.

Souhami et al reported on 33 AVMs treated with a linear accelerator system.[40] The prescribed dose at isocenter varied from 50 to 55 Gy. A complete obliteration rate of 38% was seen on 1-year angiography. For patients whose AVM nidus was covered by a minimum dose of 25 Gy, the total obliteration rate was 61.5%, whereas none of the patients who had received less than 25 Gy at the edge of the nidus obtained total obliteration.

Loeffler et al reported on 16 AVMs treated with a linear accelerator system.[41] The peripheral prescribed dose was 15 to 25 Gy, typically to the 80% to 90% line. The total obliteration rate was 5 of 11 (45%) at 1 year and 8 of 11 (73%) at 2 years after treatment.

Engenhart et al[42] reported on the treatment of 212 patients in Heidelberg. "Above a threshold dose of 18 Gy, the obliteration rate was 72%." Radiation-induced late complications were seen in 4.3%.

Schlienger et al[43] reported on 169 patients treated in Paris. The overall obliteration rate was 64%. Success rates were higher in smaller lesions, in lesions not embolized, in lesions treated with higher doses, and in lesions treated

with one isocenter. Two patients experienced radiation-induced side effects.

Andrade et al[44] reported on 38 rolandic area AVMs treated in Toronto. Complete nidus obliteration was seen in 60.5%. Two patients experienced radiation-induced side effects.

Friedman et al have published multiple reports on the University of Florida experience with radiosurgery for AVMs.[45-49] They have documented occlusion rates of 80% for lesions less than 10 mL in volume, and radiation-induced complications have been in the 2% range. Factors favoring occlusion included smaller AVM size, lower Spetzler-Martin score, higher peripheral radiation dose, and compact nidus morphologic features. Detailed dosimetric analysis suggested that 12-Gy volume and eloquent location correlated with transient radiation-induced complications. Detailed, updated University of Florida results follow.

An angiographic cure required that no nidus or shunting remain on the study, as interpreted by a neuroradiologist and the treating neurosurgeon. Of the 192 follow-up angiograms performed to date, 147 (77%) have demonstrated complete AVM obliteration. With the use of this traditional method of reporting, the following angiographic cure rates were seen in the various size categories: A, 93%; B, 86%; C, 83%; D, 53%. However, angiographic success rates can be misleadingly high because angiography may not be done if MRI shows residual nidus. If angiography or MRI follow-up results at 3 years are accepted, the following results were seen in 367 patients: A, 93%; B, 83%; C, 63%; D, 35%. Finally, if one includes radiosurgical retreatments (which will salvage a number of initial failures, see the next section), the patient success rates were as follows: A, 100%; B, 93%; C, 84%; D, 75%.

Reasons for Radiosurgery Failure

In an effort to clarify the causes of radiosurgical failure, we[46] examined 36 patients who underwent repeated radiosurgery after an initial failure to obliterate their AVMs and compared them to 72 patients who were cured during the same time period. An image fusion methodology was employed to fuse the treatment plan created at the first treatment to the CT scan obtained at the time of retreatment. Two patients were excluded from the targeting error analysis because the nidus was too small to visualize on CT. Of the remaining 34 patients in whom the original treatment failed, 9 (26%) had a partial targeting error at the time of the first treatment.

The retreatment group had statistically significantly higher Spetzler-Martin grade, larger AVM size, and lower treatment dose when compared with the group of patients who were cured. Statistical analysis also demonstrated that patients treated with a peripheral dose less than 15 Gy had a much higher failure rate. In addition, patients with AVM volumes greater than 10 mL had a much higher failure rate.

Other radiosurgery groups have also published analyses aimed at identifying factors that might be predictive of radiosurgical success or failure. Pollock et al[23] found that the following factors predicted success: smaller AVM volume, fewer draining veins, younger age, and more superficial location. Prior embolization of the AVM was a negative predictor. This group also published a review of 45 patients who underwent repeated radiosurgical treatment after an initial treatment failed to obliterate their AVMs.[50] In this study, causes of radiosurgical failure were identified as follows: in five patients (11%), the entire AVM was not visualized secondary to incomplete angiography (two-vessel instead of four-vessel) or inadequate angiographic technique (failure to perform superselective angiography). In three patients (7%), the AVM recanalized after previous embolization. In four patients (9%), the AVM nidus reexpanded after resorption of a prior hematoma that had compressed the vessels within the nidus. In 21 patients (46%), the true three-dimensional shape of the AVM nidus was not appreciated secondary to reliance on biplanar angiography alone. In the remaining patients, a definite cause for failure could not be determined. The authors believed that the AVMs in these patients were exhibiting some form of "radiobiological resistance," that is, resistance to obliteration despite proper planning and adequate dose delivery. In an earlier analysis by the same group,[51] the dose to the periphery (D_{min}) of the target was found to be the most significant predictor of success. In that analysis, neither volume nor maximum dose was found to be predictive. "Problems defining the complete AVM nidus" were cited as significant limitations to successful AVM obliteration.

The Stockholm group published an analysis aimed at defining predictive factors for radiosurgical obliteration of AVMs.[24] Analyzing a 945-patient subset of the 1319 AVM patients treated with the Gamma Knife from 1970 to 1990, they again identified peripheral dose as the most significant predictive factor. The higher the minimum dose, the higher the obliteration rate, up to 25 Gy. The obliteration rate in the 268 cases that received this minimum dose (25 Gy) was 81%. In their analysis, higher average dose and lower AVM volume were also found to predict success. A higher average dose was found to shorten the latency to AVM obliteration. They proposed that the product of the cubed root of the AVM volume and the peripheral dose (the "K index") would serve as a good combined predictor of success and found that a K index of 27 was optimal. Obliteration rates increased with increasing K values up to 27, above which no further improvement was observed.

Yamamoto et al[19] reviewed the long-term follow-up results of a group of 40 patients undergoing Gamma Knife radiosurgery for AVMs. Radiosurgery failed in 13 patients (32.5%) based on follow-up angiography at 3 to 7 years after treatment. In their retrospective analysis, they discovered that the nidus had only partially been covered at the time of the first treatment in six of the 13 patients (46%) whose radiosurgery subsequently failed.

The importance of targeting error as a reason for radiosurgical failure merits brief discussion. In the Pittsburgh series, 67% of all failures were attributed to targeting errors resulting from inadequate imaging or obscuration of the AVM nidus by a hematoma. In Yamamoto's analysis, targeting errors were responsible for 46% of all failures. A similar analysis by Gallina et al[52] attributed 10 of 17 AVM radiosurgery failures (59%) to inadequate targeting. In our experience,[46] targeting errors were also an important

cause of failure, accounting for 26% of failures. This may support the importance of using a three-dimensional database, such as contrast-enhanced CT or MR angiography, for targeting, as opposed to stereotactic angiography alone.

Zipfel et al[53] explored the effect of AVM morphology on radiosurgical success. In 268 patients, they found that "diffuse nidus morphology" and "neovascularity" were a statistically significant predictor of failure. Meder et al, in an earlier study, also documented the importance of angioarchitecture.

Pollock and Flickinger[54,55] have developed an AVM grading system that accurately predicts the chances of an "excellent outcome," meaning occlusion and no radiation-induced side effects after radiosurgery. In a multivariate analysis of 220 patients, five variables were found that related to excellent outcome: AVM volume, patient age, AVM location, previous embolization, and number of draining veins. Further analysis permitted the removal of two variables—embolization and draining veins—yielding the following predictive equation:

$$AVM\ score = 0.1\ (AVM\ volume)$$
$$+ 0.02\ (patient\ age\ in\ years)$$
$$+ 0.3\ (location\ of\ lesion)$$

Location scores are frontal or temporal, 0; parietal, occipital, intraventricular, corpus callosum, cerebellar, 1; basal ganglia, thalamic, brainstem, 2. All patients with an AVM score less than 1 had an excellent outcome compared with only 39% of patients with a score higher than 2. The Spetzler-Martin score and the K index did not correlate with excellent outcome. Subsequently this group showed that the AVM score also predicted the chance of a worsened modified Rankin Scale score after radiosurgical treatment.[56] Andrade-Souza et al[57] have verified the predictive value of the AVM score in 136 patients treated with linear accelerator–based radiosurgery.

Complications

Hemorrhage after Radiosurgery

It should be noted that there are significant pitfalls to be avoided in the analysis of hemorrhage risk after radiosurgery. First, because radiosurgery is usually successful, a large number of patients are eliminated from the at-risk pool during the first and second year after radiosurgery. Failure to adequately account for this fact leads to the false impression that the smaller number of hemorrhages occurring greater than 1 year after treatment are due to some "protective" effect. In fact, the decreasing number of hemorrhages is statistically due simply to the decreasing number of patients at risk.

Second, because there are a significant number of patients seen with hemorrhage in any radiosurgery series and because these patients may have an increased risk of hemorrhage for the first 6 months after hemorrhage, the incidence of bleeding in the first 6 months after treatment may appear, in some series, to be elevated. This is likely not a direct effect of radiosurgery, but rather a reflection of the inclusion of this group of patients with a higher than normal risk of hemorrhage. Series that treat a larger percentage of patients seen with hemorrhages (as opposed to seizures or headaches) might be expected to have an elevated hemorrhage rate during the first 6 months after treatment for this reason.

Third, and most important, the incidence of hemorrhage in patients with AVMs is small. This means that the effect of a slight alteration in the number of hemorrhages over a given period of time may, without the benefit of statistical analysis, significantly skew the conclusions in this type of analysis. Assuming a constant baseline AVM hemorrhage rate of 3 per 100 person-years follow-up (or 3% per year) in untreated patients, 726 person-years of follow-up would be required to have a 95% chance of detecting a reduction in the hemorrhage rate of 1 per 100 person-years of follow-up (or 1% per year) in treated patients at a 0.05 significance level. Given the relatively high cure rate of radiosurgery, a very large number (thousands) of patients treated would be needed to generate a sufficient number of patient follow-up years in years 2, 3, 4, and so on for statistically valid information to be yielded. These factors must be kept in mind when some of the following articles are discussed and interpreted. Any attempt to elucidate the question of AVM bleeding after radiosurgery, without benefit of detailed statistics, must be viewed with some skepticism.

The issue of AVM hemorrhage after radiosurgical treatment was first discussed by investigators using particle beam methodology. Of their first 75 patients, Kjellberg et al initially reported two deaths from hemorrhage in the first year after treatment.[32] In a subsequent report of 389 patients followed up for at least 2 years, eight had died from hemorrhages in the first 2 years after treatment.[31] Only one had died thereafter, which yielded a 0.27% mortality rate in those patients surviving more than 2 years posttreatment. Initially, these investigators suggested that only those patients seen with hemorrhages were at risk for subsequent lethal rebleeding. Later reports, however, document fatal hemorrhages in patients seen with seizures only. It should be emphasized that these authors reported a total hemorrhage rate of 2.4% per year (lethal and nonlethal) for those patients surviving more than 2 years after treatment. Whether this differs from the natural history of the disease is debatable.

Other particle beam proponents have also addressed the hemorrhage question. Steinberg et al reported 10 hemorrhages (two fatal) occurring between 4 and 34 months after radiosurgical treatment in a series of 86 patients (12%).[34] Two of these patients had hemorrhages in the third year after treatment, which suggests no protective effect unless complete obliteration was achieved. Seifert et al analyzed a series of 68 patients treated with proton beam therapy in the United States.[58] Eighteen patients deteriorated neurologically. Five of them had hemorrhages, of which two were fatal.

Gamma knife radiosurgeons have also studied this question. Lunsford et al, in an initial report on AVM treatment with the Pittsburgh Gamma Knife, noted that 10 patients (4%) in a series of 227 patients had experienced hemorrhage.[21] Two of these patients died. Pollock et al, in a study of 65 patients with "operable" AVMs, noted that five patients had hemorrhages (7.7%), all within 8 months of radiosurgery.[22] Two of these patients died. Steiner et al statistically analyzed bleeding in 247 consecutive AVM cases.[59] The Kaplan-Meier approach demonstrated a risk

of nearly 3.7% per year until 5 years after radiosurgery, at which point a plateau was reached. This plateau was believed to be likely owing to the small number of data points for that time period and not indicative of any true protective effect. Karlsson et al reported an analysis of bleeding in 1565 patients treated with the Stockholm Gamma Knife.[60] They believed the risk of hemorrhage was decreased, even with incomplete obliteration. They also reported that increasing age and increasing AVM volume correlated with an increased risk of hemorrhage.

Betti et al, in their pioneering report on LINAC radiosurgery for AVMs, documented hemorrhages in five of 66 (8%) of their patients.[35] These hemorrhages occurred 12, 18, 22, 25, and 29 months after treatment. All had a prior history of hemorrhage. Two of these patients died. Colombo et al also reported a detailed analysis of 180 patients.[39] Fifteen patients had hemorrhages, and five of them died. In cases in which the AVM nidus was totally irradiated, the bleeding risk decreased from 4.8% during the first 6 months to 0% starting at month 12 of follow-up. In partially irradiated cases, the bleeding risk increased from 4% in the first 6 months to 10% in months 6 through 18 and then down to 5.5% from months 18 to 24. No bleeding was observed thereafter.

Our analysis of this issue[61] did not reveal any postradiosurgical alteration in bleeding risk from the 3% to 4% per year expected based on natural history. A similar study by the Pittsburgh group confirmed that "stereotactic radiosurgery was not associated with a significant change in the hemorrhage rate of AVMs during the latency interval before obliteration."[62]

As already discussed, Karlsson et al reported an increased risk of AVM hemorrhage with increasing AVM size. Colombo[38] found a higher incidence in subtotally irradiated AVMs, most of which were presumably larger lesions. He also reported a statistically increased risk in patients treated more inhomogeneously (to a lower isodose line). In a subsequent article,[39] his group attributed this observation to the earlier thrombosis of the portion of the AVM receiving the highest dose of radiation, with shunting of blood into the remaining nidus, increasing the risk of hemorrhage.

In our series,[61] a correlation between AVM volume and the risk of hemorrhage was also found. Ten of the 12 AVMs that bled were greater than 10 mL in volume. In addition, the correlation of hemorrhage with lower dose and lower isodose line treated was likely owing to the deliberate use of lower doses and multiple isocenter treatments (to lower isodose lines) in larger AVMs. Of equal importance are those factors that were found not to statistically correlate with bleeding risk. In this study, neither age nor history of prior hemorrhage correlated with the incidence of hemorrhage.

Pollock et al found a significant correlation between the incidence of postradiosurgical hemorrhage and the presence of an unsecured proximal aneurysm and recommended that such aneurysms be obliterated before radiosurgery. The same group also studied factors associated with bleeding risk of AVMs and found three AVM characteristics to be predictive of greater hemorrhage risk: (1) history of prior bleeding, (2) presence of a single draining vein, and (3) diffuse AVM morphologic features. Nataf et al[63] analyzed bleeding after radiosurgery for 756 patients with AVMs. The actuarial hemorrhage rate was 3.08% per year per patient. It increased from 1.66% the first year to 3.87% in the fifth year after radiosurgery but was never statistically different from the rate before radiosurgery. Intranidal aneurysms, complete coverage, and minimum dose correlated with the risk of hemorrhage.

Maruyama et al[64] performed a retrospective observational study of 500 patients. Compared with the risk in the period between diagnosis and radiosurgery, the risk of hemorrhage decreased by 54% during the latency period and by 88% after obliteration. The risk of hemorrhage was not completely eliminated by angiographic obliteration. Other authors have also reported rare cases of AVM bleeding after documented angiographic obliteration.

In summary, the major drawback of radiosurgical AVM treatment is the risk of bleeding during the latent period (typically 2 years) between treatment and AVM thrombosis. Most studies suggest that the natural history risk of hemorrhage remains unchanged until thrombosis. Some suggest that the bleeding risk decreases somewhat, even before thrombosis. Even after thrombosis occurs, there seems to be a very small risk of continued hemorrhage. At this time only surgery can immediately and completely eliminate the risk of AVM bleeding.

Radiation-Induced Complications

Acute complications are rare after AVM radiosurgery. Several authors have previously reported that radiosurgery can acutely exacerbate seizure activity. Others have reported nausea, vomiting, and headaches occasionally occurring after radiosurgical treatment.[65]

Delayed radiation-induced complications have been reported by all groups performing radiosurgery. In 1984, Steiner reported symptomatic radiation necrosis in approximately 3% of his patients.[13] Statham et al described one patient who developed radiation necrosis 13 months after Gamma Knife radiosurgery for a 5.3-mL AVM with 25 Gy to the margin.[66] In 1991, Lunsford et al reported that 10 patients in the Pittsburgh series (4.4%) developed new neurologic deficits thought to be secondary to radiation injury.[21] Symptoms were location dependent and developed between 4 and 18 months after treatment. All patients were treated with steroids, and all improved. Only two patients were reported to have residual deficits that appeared permanent. In this early analysis, the radiation dose and isodose line treated did not correlate with incidence of complications. As the authors noted, the failure of correlation of dose and complications likely related to the fact that doses had been selected to fall below Flickinger's computed 3% risk line. This is a mathematically derived line that prescribes lower doses for larger lesions and underpins the well-established correlation between increasing radiosurgical target volume and increasing incidence of radiation necrosis.[67-69]

Flickinger et al published an analysis of complications from AVM radiosurgery that emphasized the importance of lesion location and dose.[70] The analysis, which included outcome data from 332 Pittsburgh Gamma Knife AVM radiosurgery cases from 1987 to 1994, found that 30 patients (9%) developed some symptomatic postradiosurgery sequelae (any neurologic problem including headaches). Symptoms resolved in 58% of these patients within 27 months. Statistically, the likelihood of having a transient versus a permanent deficit was dose dependent, and a difference was noted at a peripheral dose of 20 Gy (D_{min}). When D_{min} was less than 20 Gy, 89% of patients who developed deficits experienced complete resolution of their symptoms, whereas only 36% of patients receiving minimum target doses greater than 20 Gy fully recovered. The 7-year actuarial rate for developing a permanent radiation-induced neurologic deficit was 3.8%. The relative risks for various lesion locations were compared, and a postradiosurgery injury expression (PIE) score was assigned to various brain locations. In general, deeper locations had higher PIE scores, which indicates a greater risk of radiation-induced complications. Multivariate statistical analysis identified only PIE location score and 12-Gy volume as significant predictors of radiation-induced symptomatic sequelae. Variables analyzed but found not to be significant predictors of complications included prior neurologic deficit, prior hemorrhage, use of MRI-enhanced treatment planning, prescription isodose line, and number of isocenters. The same group has published numerous other articles documenting the basic value of this approach.[71-73]

The Stockholm group published an analysis of factors associated with complications after AVM radiosurgery.[74] Their report confirms the predictive importance of AVM location and dose. They found that a history of prior hemorrhage was associated with a lower risk of complications in their series, and prior radiation was associated with a higher risk of complications.

Steinberg et al reported a definite correlation between lesion size, lesion dose, and complications.[34] The authors' initial treatment dose of 34.6 Gy led to a relatively high complication rate. Subsequently, patients were treated with a much lower dose and had no radiation-induced complications. In an earlier report on 75 patients with AVMs treated with helium particles at a dose of 45 Gy, seven of 75 patients (11%) experienced radiation-induced complications.[75]

Kjellberg et al,[76,77] using a compilation of animal and clinical data, constructed a series of log–log lines relating prescribed dose and lesion diameter. The group's 1% isorisk line is quite similar to Flickinger's mathematically derived 3% risk line.

In a series published by Colombo et al, nine of 180 patients (5%) experienced symptomatic radiation-induced complications.[39] Four (2.2%) were permanent. Loeffler et al[78] reported that one of 21 patients with AVMs developed a similar problem, which responded well to steroids. Souhami reported "severe side-effects" in two of 33 patients (6%).[40] Marks and Spencer[79] reviewed six radiosurgical series and found a 9% overall incidence of clinically significant radiation reactions. Seven of 23 cases received doses below Kjellberg's 1% risk line.

Chen et al[80] reported a case of aggressive, recurrent cerebral necrosis leading to death, despite surgical intervention. Others have suggested that occlusive hyperemia (due to venous thrombosis), not radiation necrosis, may be responsible for radiation-induced side effects.

At the University of Florida, 12 patients (2.5%) have had permanent radiation-induced side effects. Fifteen (3%)

have had transient side effects. A detailed analysis of dosimetric factors revealed that 12-Gy volume and eloquent brain location correlated with transient complications. No factor was predictive of permanent complications. The University of Florida group has reported one case of symptomatic radiation-induced hemiparesis successfully treated with hyperbaric oxygen.[81]

Very Late Onset Complications

Yamamoto et al have published a series of articles describing radiation-related adverse effects observed on late neuroimaging after AVM radiosurgery.[2,19,82-84] In their study of 53 patients' status after Gamma Knife AVM radiosurgery, MRIs were performed up to 10 years after treatment. In this series, of the five patients (9.4%) who developed delayed neurologic symptoms, three were seen at least 5 years after treatment. One patient with a midbrain AVM had a hemi-Parkinson's syndrome 5.5 years after radiosurgery. Another patient subsequently had gradual visual field narrowing accompanied by signs of increased intracranial pressure 7 years after treatment; MRI revealed a large cyst in the left parietooccipital lobe at the site of the irradiated AVM, and surgery was required. The third patient was seen 7 years after treatment with hemiparesis caused by a diffuse white matter necrotic lesion.

Also concerning were the late development of four additional *asymptomatic* radiologic abnormalities. One middle cerebral artery stenosis of the M1 segment was detected 3 years after irradiation. A dural AV fistula developed 7 years after treatment, and two delayed cysts had formed at 5 and 10 years after treatment.

The lesion volumes and treatment doses used in this series were not unusual (median volume, 1.5 mL; mean peripheral target dose, 21.5 Gy), and careful examination of the cases with complications revealed no obvious deviation from standard radiosurgical practice. Uncommonly meticulous radiologic follow-up may explain some of these unusual findings. Perhaps such abnormalities are not rare but (especially in the cases of asymptomatic patients) simply remain undetected.

Kihlstrom et al also reported a series of late radiologic abnormalities after AVM radiosurgery.[85] MRI scans and follow-up angiography were performed on 18 patients at a mean interval of 14 years (8 to 23 years) after radiosurgical treatment. All patients had previous angiographic documentation of AVM obliteration, and all were clinically asymptomatic. Radiologic findings included cyst formation at the previous AVM site in five patients (28%), contrast enhancement at the former lesion site (without AVM recanalization) in 11 patients (61%), and increased T2 MR signal at the former lesion site in three patients (17%). In this series—unlike the case reported by Yamamoto et al—none of the observed cysts exceeded 2 cm in diameter, all were confined to the volume of the previous AVM nidus, and none caused any mass effect. Because treatment doses used in this study were higher than those currently administered, it is difficult to predict whether similar findings will be reproduced in more recent patient series. The absence of clinical symptoms in these patients may indicate that such late radiographic abnormalities will be of limited clinical importance.

Hara et al has also reported two cases of delayed cyst formation after AVM radiosurgery.[86]

Salvage Retreatment for Failed AVM Radiosurgery

A number of groups have reported on the use of repeated radiosurgery as a salvage technique after failed AVM radiosurgery. The Stockholm radiosurgery group analyzed 101 cases of such salvage retreatment.[87] Obliteration was achieved in 62% of these cases, which is a rate almost identical to that currently reported by this group for primary AVM radiosurgery. The complication rate was 14%, which was significantly higher than that currently reported by this group for primary radiosurgery. The annual risk of hemorrhage during the first 2 years after treatment was 1.8%, which is a value not statistically different from that associated with the natural history of this disease. In a more recent evaluation of 133 patients with an initial nidus volume of 9 mL or more, the estimated obliteration rate was 62% after repeated treatment.[88] Four patients (3%) had radiation-induced side effects, and five others (4%) had cystic changes.

Maesawa et al[89] reported on repeated radiosurgery in 41 patients. The estimated 2-year obliteration rate was 71%. Two patients had radiation-induced side effects.

Mirza-Aghazadeh et al[90] reported on 12 patients undergoing retreatment using a LINAC system. Two thirds were cured, and the radiation-induced complication rate was 13%. Raza et al[91] reported on 14 retreatments. They achieved a complete obliteration rate of 35.7%.

Schlienger et al[92] reported on 41 patients retreated in their Paris unit. The obliteration rate was 59.3%. They had a 9% complication rate. Foote et al[93] reported on 52 patients retreated at the University of Florida. Sixty percent had their AVMs obliterated, as seen on follow-up angiography, with no reported permanent radiation-induced side effects. The current salvage rate at the University of Florida after retreatment is 70%.

In 2000, Pollock et al[94] described an alternative retreatment approach that they called *staged-volume arteriovenous malformation radiosurgery*. The basic idea involves treating only part of the AVM nidus then returning some time later (typically 6 months) and treating the other part. In 2006, Sirin et al[95] reported on 37 patients who had undergone such therapy. The initial AVM volume averaged 24.9 mL. The median marginal dose was 16 Gy at both treatments. Of 14 patients followed up for more than 36 months, 50% had total occlusion and 29% had near total occlusion.

Multimodality AVM Treatment

When an AVM is amenable to safe microsurgical resection, this therapy is preferred because it offers an immediate cure and elimination of hemorrhage risk. When the estimated morbidity of resection is excessive, radiosurgery offers a reasonable chance for a delayed cure. However, some unresectable AVMs, by virtue of their large size, are not candidates for radiosurgery. These problematic lesions may be managed with presurgery or preradiosurgery embolization.

Before radiosurgery, the most important role of embolization is to reduce the size of the lesion. Potential secondary advantages of preradiosurgical embolization are that associated aneurysms may be treated and high-flow arteriovenous fistulas—believed to be less sensitive to radiosurgery—may be identified and occluded.

Dawson et al[96] reported on seven patients with large AVMs who were treated with embolization followed by Gamma Knife radiosurgery. At 2-year follow-up, two AVMs were obliterated, and two others had a 98% reduction in volume. Lemme-Plaghos et al[97] reported their results in 16 patients with high-grade AVMs who were treated with embolization and Gamma Knife radiosurgery. Four cures (25%) were reported. Mathis et al[98] reported on a series of patients with large AVMs (volume >10 mL) who were treated with embolization and radiosurgery. Of the 56 patients treated, 24 were included in their analysis and 12 were cured. Among the analyzed group, two patients (8%) experienced transient neurologic deficits after embolization, and one had mild upper extremity weakness after radiosurgery. Recanalization of previously embolized—but not irradiated—regions of AVM nidus occurred in three patients. Guo et al reported 46 patients treated with embolization and Gamma Knife radiosurgery.[99] In 16 cases, collateral vessels developed that made subsequent delineation of the nidus for radiosurgery difficult. In addition, nine patients had neurologic complications after embolization. Only 19 of 35 large AVMs were reduced in size enough to be subsequently treatable with radiosurgery.

A larger series of patients treated with a combination of embolization and LINAC radiosurgery was reported by Gobin et al.[100] Of the 125 AVMs treated with (usually multiple-session) endovascular treatment, 14 (11%) were completely occluded with embolization alone. Ninety-six AVMs (77%) were reduced in size by embolization enough to be considered for radiosurgery. Of those who underwent postembolization radiosurgery, complete occlusion was achieved in 65%. Embolization resulted in a mortality rate of 1.6% and a morbidity rate of 12.8%. No complications were associated with radiosurgery in this series. The posttreatment AVM hemorrhage rate was 3% per year. Despite the use of cyanoacrylate (the current standard in durable embolic material), a 12% revascularization rate was observed.

Henkes et al[101] reported on 64 patients treated with embolization and radiosurgery. Of 30 patients followed up "beyond the latency interval," 14 (43%) had angiographic cures. Zabel-du Bois et al[102] reported on 50 patients treated with embolization and radiosurgery. The "actuarial obliteration rate" was 67% at 3 years. Smaller AVMs and lower Spetzler-Martin scores were associated with higher obliteration rates.

Embolization is an excellent adjunct to open surgical resection of AVMs, but its role in radiosurgery is less clear. At the University of Florida we try to avoid combining embolization and radiosurgery. Embolization tends to convert a compact nidal target into multiple remaining islands of nidus, which are very difficult to clearly identify and target. Embolic material tends to create artifact on CT and MRI, further reducing radiosurgical targeting ability. Embolic material can wash out, leading to recanalization after radiosurgery. Finally, embolization has a small but real risk of neurologic complications. For these reasons, we prefer to use radiosurgery, with repeated treatment if necessary, for larger AVMs.

Radiosurgery for Other Types of Vascular Malformation
Cavernous Malformations

In general, cavernous malformations have a benign natural history. They frequently are identified incidentally and usually require no treatment. Surgical excision may become the treatment of choice for cavernomas seen with hemorrhages or seizures. Occasionally, cavernous malformations are seen with multiple hemorrhages and are in clearly surgically inaccessible locations (e.g., within the brainstem or the internal capsule). Radiosurgery has been used in such cases in an effort to alter the natural history risk of recurrent bleeding.

In 1995, Kida et al[103] described 20 cases of cavernous malformations treated with radiosurgery. Marginal doses ranged from 15 to 20 Gy. They found "significant control" of both rebleeding and convulsive seizures. Adverse radiation effects occurred in five patients (20%).

In 1998, Karlsson et al[104] reported on the Stockholm experience with 22 cavernous malformations. Nine of the patients experienced postradiosurgery hemorrhages, and six developed radiation-induced complications. They concluded that "the high incidence of radiation-induced complications does not seem to justify the limited protection the treatment may afford."

Chang et al[105] later reported on 57 patients with surgically inaccessible angiographically occult AVMs of the brain treated with helium ion radiosurgery. The mean dose was 18 Gy. Eighteen patients bled symptomatically after radiosurgery, although a significant decrease in the hemorrhage rate was seen in those patients followed up for 3 years or more. Five patients had radiation-induced complications. Eleven patients underwent surgical resection of these lesions. Fibrinoid necrosis was identified, but all lesions still had patent vascular channels—none were completely thrombosed.

Pollock et al[106] reported the Mayo Clinic experience with cavernous malformations. Seventeen patients underwent radiosurgical treatment. The median marginal dose was 18 Gy. In 10 patients (59%), new neurologic deficits developed secondary to radiation-induced side effects. Some reduction in bleeding risk was seen when compared with preoperative bleeding rates.

Hasegawa et al[107] reported the Pittsburgh experience with the treatment of 82 cavernous malformations. Observation before treatment suggested an annual hemorrhage risk (in this highly selected, high-risk group) of 33.9%. After radiosurgery, of 19 hemorrhages identified, 17 were in the first 2 years. The annual hemorrhage risk decreased, therefore, in years 2 to 12, to 0.76% per year. Eleven patients had new neurologic deficits without hemorrhage (13.4%).

The role of radiosurgery in the treatment of cavernous malformations remains uncertain. The use of modern targeting techniques (MRI) and lower marginal doses

(12.5 Gy to 15 Gy) appears to have reduced the previously reported high incidence of neurologic side effects. The Pittsburgh experience suggests that the natural history bleeding risk is reduced after a 2-year latency period.

Venous Malformations

Lindquist et al[108] reported on 13 cases of venous malformations treated with radiosurgery. In two cases, a cavernous malformation was also present. In one case, complete obliteration was achieved. Four patients experienced radiation-induced complications.

Most neurosurgeons currently believe that venous malformations, in isolation, are normal variants of venous drainage anatomy. Treatment, whether surgical or radiosurgical, is likely to result in complications. When they are associated with cavernous malformations, the cavernous malformation may bleed and may, in selected cases, be appropriately treated with surgery (see the section on cavernous malformations).

Telangiectasia

Maarouf et al[109] evaluated the efficacy of radiosurgery for cerebral AVMs in hereditary hemorrhagic telangiectasia (HHT). Two patients with seven HHT AVMs were treated by LINAC radiosurgery. Complete obliteration was achieved 18 to 24 months posttreatment without side effects. They suggested that, because HHT AVMs are small and multiple, radiosurgery might be superior to microsurgery because it is noninvasive and all AVMs can be treated in one session, regardless of their location.

Dural Arteriovenous Malformations

In 1993, Chandler and Friedman[110] first reported the successful treatment of a dural AVM, located near the crista galli, with radiosurgery. Subsequently, Guo et al[111] published their experience treating 18 patients with dural AVMs involving the cavernous sinus. Maximum target doses were 22 to 38 Gy. They achieved an 80% angiographic cure rate. No complications were observed.

Lewis et al[112] described the multimodality treatment of dural AVMs, using endovascular, surgical, and radiosurgical means. Four of nine patients achieved complete AVM obliteration. Link et al[113] described a slightly different approach in 29 patients at the Mayo Clinic. They treated the dural AVM nidus with radiosurgery. Then, within 2 days, 17 patients, who exhibited retrograde pial or cortical venous drainage or who had an audible bruit, underwent embolization. The rationale was to use embolization to control symptoms during the latent period for radiosurgical cure. Angiography 1 to 3 years posttreatment showed total obliteration of 13 fistulas.

Conclusions

1. Surgery is the treatment of choice for AVMs because only surgery can immediately eliminate the risk of hemorrhage. In those lesions that are high risk for surgery, radiosurgery is a very attractive alternative and has high success and low complication rates.

2. When one radiosurgery treatment fails, retreatment frequently produces a cure.
3. The risk of bleeding after radiosurgery appears to fall within the natural history risk range until AVM thrombosis occurs.
4. The risk of permanent radiation-induced side effects after AVM radiosurgery is approximately 2%.
5. The role of radiosurgical treatment in the management of cavernous malformations is less certain. Some series suggest a substantial drop in the hemorrhage rate after a 2-year latent period. Radiation-induced complications are higher than that seen with AVM radiosurgery.

REFERENCES

1. Leksell L: The stereotaxic method and radiosurgery of the brain, *Acta Chir Scand* 102:316, 1951.
2. Yamamoto M, Jimbo M, Ide M, et al: Gamma knife radiosurgery for cerebral arteriovenous malformations: An autopsy report focusing on irradiation-induced changes observed in nidus-unrelated arteries, *Surg Neurol* 44:421, 1995.
3. Szeifert GT, Kemeny AA, Timperley WR, et al: The potential role of myofibroblasts in the obliteration of arteriovenous malformations after radiosurgery, *Neurosurgery* 40:61, 1997.
4. Schneider BF, Eberhard DA, Steiner LE: Histopathology of arteriovenous malformations after gamma knife radiosurgery [see comments], *J Neurosurg* 87:352, 1997.
5. Chang SD, Shuster DL, Steinberg GK, et al: Stereotactic radiosurgery of arteriovenous malformations: Pathologic changes in resected tissue, *Clin Neuropathol* 16:111, 1997.
6. Friedman WA, Buatti JM, Bova FJ, et al: *LINAC radiosurgery—A practical guide*, Berlin, 1998, Springer-Verlag.
7. Spiegelmann R, Friedman WA, Bova FJ: Limitations of angiographic target localization in planning radiosurgical treatment, *Neurosurgery* 30:619, 1992.
8. Kondziolka D, Lunsford LD, Kanal E, et al: Stereotactic magnetic resonance angiography for targeting in arteriovenous malformation radiosurgery, *Neurosurgery* 35:585, 1994.
9. Bova FJ, Friedman WA: Stereotactic angiography: An inadequate database for radiosurgery?, *Int J Radiat Oncol Biol Phys* 20:891, 1991.
10. Blatt DR, Friedman WA, Bova FJ: Modifications based on computed tomographic imaging in planning the radiosurgical treatment of arteriovenous malformations, *Neurosurgery* 33:588, 1993.
11. Aoki S, Sasaki Y, Machida T, et al: 3D-CT angiography of cerebral arteriovenous malformations, *Radiat Med* 16:263, 1998.
12. Steiner L: Radiosurgery in cerebral arteriovenous malformations. In Fein JM, Flamm ES, editors: *Cerebrovascular Surgery* Vol. 4 Wien/New York, 1985, Springer-Verlag, p 1161.
13. Steiner L: Treatment of arteriovenous malformations by radiosurgery. In Wilson CB, Stein BM, editors: *Intracranial Arteriovenous Malformations*, Baltimore/London, 1984, Williams and Wilkins, p 295.
14. Steiner L, Leksell L, Forster DM, et al: Stereotactic radiosurgery in intracranial arteriovenous malformations, *Acta Neurochir (Wien) Suppl* 21:195, 1974.
15. Steiner L, Leksell L, Greitz T, et al: Stereotaxic radiosurgery for cerebral arteriovenous malformations. Report of a case, *Acta Chir Scand* 138:459, 1972.
16. Lindquist C, Steiner L: Stereotactic radiosurgical treatment of malformations of the brain. In Lunsford LD, editor: *Modern stereotactic neurosurgery*, ed 1, Boston, 1988, Martinus Nijhoff, p 491.
17. Yamamoto M, Jimbo M, Kobayashi M, et al: Long-term results of radiosurgery for arteriovenous malformation: Neurodiagnostic imaging and histological studies of angiographically confirmed nidus obliteration, *Surg Neurol* 37:219, 1992.
18. Yamamoto M, Jimbo M, Ide M, et al: Long-term follow-up of radiosurgically treated arteriovenous malformations in children: Report of nine cases, *Surg Neurol* 38:95, 1992.
19. Yamamoto M, Jimbo M, Hara M, et al: Gamma knife radiosurgery for arteriovenous malformations: Long-term follow-up results focusing on complications occurring more than 5 years after irradiation, *Neurosurgery* 38:906, 1996.

20. Kemeny AA, Dias PS, Forster DM: Results of stereotactic radiosurgery of arteriovenous malformations: An analysis of 52 cases, *J Neurol Neurosurg Psychiatry* 52:554, 1989.

21. Lunsford LD, Kondziolka D, Flickinger JC, et al: Stereotactic radiosurgery for arteriovenous malformations of the brain, *J Neurosurg* 75:512, 1991.

22. Pollock BE, Lunsford LD, Kondziolka D, et al: Patient outcomes after stereotactic radiosurgery for "operable" arteriovenous malformations, *Neurosurgery* 35:1, 1994.

23. Pollock BE, Flickinger JC, Lunsford LD, et al: Factors associated with successful arteriovenous malformation radiosurgery, *Neurosurgery* 42:1239, 1998.

24. Karlsson B, Lindquist C, Steiner L: Prediction of obliteration after gamma knife surgery for cerebral arteriovenous malformations, *Neurosurgery* 40:425, 1997.

25. Shin M, Maruyama K, Kurita H, et al: Analysis of nidus obliteration rates after gamma knife surgery for arteriovenous malformations based on long-term follow-up data: The University of Tokyo experience, *J Neurosurg* 101:18, 2004.

26. Maruyama K, Kondziolka D, Niranjan A, et al: Stereotactic radiosurgery for brainstem arteriovenous malformations: Factors affecting outcome, *J Neurosurg* 100:407, 2004.

27. Kurita H, Kawamoto S, Sasaki T, et al: Results of radiosurgery for brain stem arteriovenous malformations, *J Neurol Neurosurg Psychiatry* 68:563, 2000.

28. Hadjipanayis CG, Levy EI, Niranjan A, et al: Stereotactic radiosurgery for motor cortex region arteriovenous malformations. *Neurosurgery* 48:70, 2001.

29. Pollock BE, Gorman DA, Brown PD: Radiosurgery for arteriovenous malformations of the basal ganglia, thalamus, and brainstem, *J Neurosurg* 100:210, 2004.

30. Kiran NA, Kale SS, Vaishya S, et al: Gamma knife surgery for intracranial arteriovenous malformations in children: A retrospective study in 103 patients, *J Neurosurg* 107:479, 2007.

31. Kjellberg RN: Stereotactic Bragg peak proton beam radiosurgery for cerebral arteriovenous malformations, *Ann Clin Res* 18(Suppl 47):17, 1986.

32. Kjellberg RN, Hanamura T, Davis KR, et al: Bragg-peak proton-beam therapy for arteriovenous malformations of the brain, *N Engl J Med* 309:269, 1983.

33. Kjellberg RN, Poletti CE, Roberson GH, et al: Bragg-peak proton beam treatment of arteriovenous malformation of the brain, *Exc Med* 433:181, 1977.

34. Steinberg GK, Fabrikant JI, Marks MP, et al: Stereotactic heavy-charged-particle Bragg-peak radiation for intracranial arteriovenous malformations, *N Engl J Med* 323:96, 1990.

35. Betti OO, Munari C, Rosler R: Stereotactic radiosurgery with the linear accelerator: Treatment of arteriovenous malformations, *Neurosurgery* 24:311, 1989.

36. Betti OO: Treatment of arteriovenous malformations with the linear accelerator, *Appl Neurophysiol* 50:262, 1987.

37. Betti OO, Derechinsky VE: Hyperselective encephalic irradiation with a linear accelerator, *Acta Neurochir Suppl* 33:385, 1984.

38. Colombo F, Benedetti A, Pozza F, et al: Linear accelerator radiosurgery of cerebral arteriovenous malformations, *Neurosurgery* 24:833, 1989.

39. Colombo F, Pozza F, Chierego G, et al: Linear accelerator radiosurgery of cerebral arteriovenous malformations: An update, *Neurosurgery* 34:14, 1994.

40. Souhami L, Olivier A, Podgorsak EB, et al: Radiosurgery of cerebral arteriovenous malformations with the dynamic stereotactic irradiation, *Int J Radiat Oncol Biol Phys* 19:775, 1990.

41. Loeffler JS, Alexander E 3rd, Siddon RL, et al: Stereotactic radiosurgery for intracranial arteriovenous malformations using a standard linear accelerator, *Int J Radiat Oncol Biol Phys* 17:673, 1989.

42. Engenhart R, Wowra B, Debus J, et al: The role of high-dose, single-fraction irradiation in small and large intracranial arteriovenous malformations, *Int J Radiat Oncol Biol Phys* 30:521, 1994.

43. Schlienger M, Atlan D, Lefkopoulos D, et al: LINAC radiosurgery for cerebral arteriovenous malformations: Results in 169 patients, *Int J Radiat Oncol Biol Phys* 46:1135, 2000.

44. Andrade-Souza YM, Ramani M, Scora D, et al: Radiosurgical treatment for rolandic arteriovenous malformations, *J Neurosurg* 105:689, 2006.

45. Friedman WA, Bova FJ, Bollampally S, et al: Analysis of factors predictive of success or complications in arteriovenous malformation radiosurgery, *Neurosurgery* 52:296, 2003.

46. Ellis TL, Friedman WA, Bova FJ, et al: Analysis of treatment failure after radiosurgery for arteriovenous malformations, *J Neurosurg* 89:104, 1998.

47. Friedman WA, Bova FJ, Mendenhall WM: Linear accelerator radiosurgery for arteriovenous malformations: The relationship of size to outcome, *J Neurosurg* 82:180, 1995.

48. Friedman WA, Bova FJ: Radiosurgery for arteriovenous malformations, *Clin Neurosurg* 40:446, 1993.

49. Friedman WA, Bova FJ: Linear accelerator radiosurgery for arteriovenous malformations, *J Neurosurg* 77:832, 1992.

50. Pollock BE, Kondziolka D, Lunsford LD, et al: Repeat stereotactic radiosurgery of arteriovenous malformations: Factors associated with incomplete obliteration, *Neurosurgery* 38:318, 1996.

51. Flickinger JC, Pollock BE, Kondziolka D, et al: A dose-response analysis of arteriovenous malformation obliteration after radiosurgery, *Int J Radiat Oncol Biol Phys* 36:873, 1996.

52. Gallina P, Merienne L, Meder JF, et al: Failure in radiosurgery treatment of cerebral arteriovenous malformations, *Neurosurgery* 42:996, 1998.

53. Zipfel GJ, Bradshaw P, Bova FJ, et al: Do the morphological characteristics of arteriovenous malformations affect the results of radiosurgery?, *J Neurosurg* 101:393, 2004.

54. Pollock BE, Flickinger JC: A proposed radiosurgery-based grading system for arteriovenous malformations, *J Neurosurg* 96:79, 2002.

55. Pollock BE, Gorman DA, Coffey RJ: Patient outcomes after arteriovenous malformation radiosurgical management: Results based on a 5- to 14-year follow-up study, *Neurosurgery* 52:1291, 2003.

56. Pollock BE, Brown RD Jr: Use of the Modified Rankin Scale to assess outcome after arteriovenous malformation radiosurgery, *Neurology* 67:1630, 2006.

57. Andrade-Souza YM, Zadeh G, Ramani M, et al: Testing the radiosurgery-based arteriovenous malformation score and the modified Spetzler-Martin grading system to predict radiosurgical outcome, *J Neurosurg* 103:642, 2005.

58. Seifert V, Stolke D, Mehdorn HM, et al: Clinical and radiological evaluation of long-term results of stereotactic proton beam radiosurgery in patients with cerebral arteriovenous malformations, *J Neurosurg* 81:683, 1994.

59. Steiner L, Lindquist C, Adler JR, et al: Clinical outcome of radiosurgery for cerebral arteriovenous malformations, *J Neurosurg* 77:1, 1992.

60. Karlsson B, Lax I, Soderman M: Risk for hemorrhage during the 2-year latency period following gamma knife radiosurgery for arteriovenous malformations, *Int J Radiat Oncol Biol Phys* 49:1045, 2001.

61. Friedman WA, Blatt DL, Bova FJ, et al: The risk of hemorrhage after radiosurgery for arteriovenous malformations, *J Neurosurg* 84:912, 1996.

62. Pollock BE, Flickinger JC, Lunsford LD, et al: Hemorrhage risk after stereotactic radiosurgery of cerebral arteriovenous malformations, *Neurosurgery* 38:652, 1996.

63. Nataf F, Ghossoub M, Schlienger M, et al: Bleeding after radiosurgery for cerebral arteriovenous malformations, *Neurosurgery* 55:298, 2004.

64. Maruyama K, Kawahara N, Shin M, et al: The risk of hemorrhage after radiosurgery for cerebral arteriovenous malformations, *N Engl J Med* 352:146, 2005.

65. Alexander E III, Siddon RL, Loeffler JS: The acute onset of nausea and vomiting following stereotactic radiosurgery: Correlation with total dose to area postrema, *Surg Neurol* 32:40, 1989.

66. Statham P, Macpherson P, Johnston R, et al: Cerebral radiation necrosis complicating stereotactic radiosurgery for arteriovenous malformation, *J Neurol Neurosurg Psychiatry* 53:476, 1990.

67. Flickinger JC, Lunsford LD, Wu A, et al: Predicted dose-volume isoeffect curves for stereotactic radiosurgery with the ^{60}Co Gamma Unit, *Acta Oncol* 30:363, 1991.

68. Flickinger JC, Schell MC, Larson DA: Estimation of complications for linear accelerator radiosurgery with the integrated logistic formula, *Int J Radiat Oncol Biol Phys* 19:143, 1990.

69. Flickinger JC, Steiner L: Radiosurgery and the double logistic product formula, *Radiother Oncol* 17:229, 1990.

70. Flickinger JC, Kondziolka D, Pollock BE, et al: Complications from arteriovenous malformation radiosurgery: Multivariate analysis and risk modeling, *Int J Radiat Oncol Biol Phys* 38:485, 1997.

71. Flickinger JC, Kondziolka D, Lunsford LD, et al: Development of a model to predict permanent symptomatic postradiosurgery injury for arteriovenous malformation patients. Arteriovenous Malformation Radiosurgery Study Group, *Int J Radiat Oncol Biol Phys* 46:1143, 2000.

72. Flickinger JC, Kondziolka D, Lunsford LD, et al: A multi-institutional analysis of complication outcomes after arteriovenous malformation radiosurgery, *Int J Radiat Oncol Biol Phys* 44:67, 1999.

73. Flickinger JC, Kondziolka D, Maitz AH, et al: An analysis of the dose-response for arteriovenous malformation radiosurgery and other factors affecting obliteration, *Radiother Oncol* 63:347, 2002.

74. Karlsson B, Lax I, Soderman M: Factors influencing the risk for complications following gamma knife radiosurgery of cerebral arteriovenous malformations, *Radiother Oncol* 43:275, 1997.

75. Hosobuchi Y, Fabrikant JI, Lyman JT: Stereotactic heavy-particle irradiation of intracranial arteriovenous malformations, *Appl Neurophysiol* 50:248, 1987.

76. Kjellberg RN, Abbe M: Stereotactic Bragg peak proton beam therapy. In Lunsford LD, editor: *Modern stereotactic neurosurgery*, ed 1, Boston, 1988, Martinus Nijhoff, p 463.

77. Kjellberg RN, Davis KR, Lyons S, et al: Bragg peak proton beam therapy for arteriovenous malformations of the brain, *Clin Neurosurg* 31:248, 1983.

78. Loeffler JS, Rossitch E Jr, Siddon R, et al: Role of stereotactic radiosurgery with a linear accelerator in treatment of intracranial arteriovenous malformations and tumors in children, *Pediatrics* 85:774, 1990.

79. Marks LB, Spencer DP: The influence of volume on the tolerance of the brain to radiosurgery, *J Neurosurg* 75:177–180, 1991.

80. Chen HI, Burnett MG, Huse JT, et al: Recurrent late cerebral necrosis with aggressive characteristics after radiosurgical treatment of an arteriovenous malformation: Case report, *J Neurosurg* 105:455–460, 2006.

81. Lynn M, Friedman WA: Hyperbaric oxygen in the treatment of a radiosurgical complication: Technical case report, *Neurosurgery* 60:E579, 2007.

82. Yamamoto M, Ban S, Ide M, et al: A diffuse white matter ischemic lesion appearing 7 years after stereotactic radiosurgery for cerebral arteriovenous malformations: Case report, *Neurosurgery* 41:1405, 1997.

83. Yamamoto M, Hara M, Ide M, et al: Radiation-related adverse effects observed on neuro-imaging several years after radiosurgery for cerebral arteriovenous malformations, *Surg Neurol* 49:385, 1998.

84. Yamamoto M, Ide M, Jimbo M, et al: Middle cerebral artery stenosis caused by relatively low-dose irradiation with stereotactic radiosurgery for cerebral arteriovenous malformations: Case report, *Neurosurgery* 41:474, 1997.

85. Kihlstrom L, Guo WY, Karlsson B, et al: Magnetic resonance imaging of obliterated arteriovenous malformations up to 23 years after radiosurgery [see comments], *J Neurosurg* 86:589, 1997.

86. Hara M, Nakamura M, Shiokawa Y, et al: Delayed cyst formation after radiosurgery for cerebral arteriovenous malformation: Two case reports, *Minim Invasive Neurosurg* 41:40, 1998.

87. Karlsson B, Kihlstrom L, Lindquist C, et al: Gamma knife surgery for previously irradiated arteriovenous malformations, *Neurosurgery* 42:1, 1998.

88. Karlsson B, Jokura H, Yamamoto M, et al: Is repeated radiosurgery an alternative to staged radiosurgery for very large brain arteriovenous malformations? *J Neurosurg* 107:740, 2007.

89. Maesawa S, Flickinger JC, Kondziolka D, et al: Repeated radiosurgery for incompletely obliterated arteriovenous malformations, *J Neurosurg* 92:961, 2000.

90. Mirza-Aghazadeh J, Andrade-Souza YM, Zadeh G, et al: Radiosurgical retreatment for brain arteriovenous malformation, *Can J Neurol Sci* 33:189, 2006.

91. Raza SM, Jabbour S, Thai QA, et al: Repeat stereotactic radiosurgery for high-grade and large intracranial arteriovenous malformations, *Surg Neurol* 68:24–34, 2007.

92. Schlienger M, Nataf F, Lefkopoulos D, et al: Repeat linear accelerator radiosurgery for cerebral arteriovenous malformations, *Int J Radiat Oncol Biol Phys* 56:529, 2003.

93. Foote KD, Friedman WA, Ellis TL, et al: Salvage retreatment after failure of radiosurgery in patients with arteriovenous malformations, *J Neurosurg* 98:337, 2003.

94. Pollock BE, Kline RW, Stafford SL, et al: The rationale and technique of staged-volume arteriovenous malformation radiosurgery, *Int J Radiat Oncol Biol Phys* 48:817, 2000.

95. Sirin S, Kondziolka D, Niranjan A, et al: Prospective staged volume radiosurgery for large arteriovenous malformations: Indications and outcomes in otherwise untreatable patients, *Neurosurgery* 58:17, 2006.

96. Dawson RC 3rd, Tarr RW, Hecht ST, et al: Treatment of arteriovenous malformations of the brain with combined embolization and stereotactic radiosurgery: Results after 1 and 2 years, *AJNR Am J Neuroradiol* 11:857, 1990.

97. Lemme-Plaghos L, Schonholz C, Willis R: Combination of embolization and radiosurgery in the treatment of arteriovenous malformations. In Steiner L, editor: *Radiosurgery: Baseline and trends*, New York, 1992, Raven Press, p 195.

98. Mathis JA, Barr JD, Horton JA, et al: The efficacy of particulate embolization combined with stereotactic radiosurgery for treatment of large arteriovenous malformations of the brain, *AJNR Am J Neuroradiol* 16:299, 1995.

99. Guo WY, Wikholm G, Karlsson B, et al: Combined embolization and gamma knife radiosurgery for cerebral arteriovenous malformations, *Acta Radiol* 34:600, 1993.

100. Gobin YP, Laurent A, Merienne L, et al: Treatment of brain arteriovenous malformations by embolization and radiosurgery, *J Neurosurg* 85:19, 1996.

101. Henkes H, Nahser HC, Berg-Dammer E, et al: Endovascular therapy of brain AVMs prior to radiosurgery, *Neurol Res* 20:479, 1998.

102. Zabel-du Bois A, Milker-Zabel S, Huber P, et al: Risk of hemorrhage and obliteration rates of LINAC-based radiosurgery for cerebral arteriovenous malformations treated after prior partial embolization, *Int J Radiat Oncol Biol Phys* 68:999, 2007.

103. Kida Y, Kobayashi T, Tanaka T: Treatment of symptomatic AOVMs with radiosurgery, *Acta Neurochir Suppl* 63:68, 1995.

104. Karlsson B, Kihlstrom L, Lindquist C, et al: Radiosurgery for cavernous malformations, *J Neurosurg* 88:293, 1998.

105. Chang SD, Levy RP, Adler JRJ, et al: Stereotactic radiosurgery of angiographically occult vascular malformations: 14-year experience, *Neurosurgery* 43:213, 1998.

106. Pollock BE, Garces YI, Stafford SL, et al: Stereotactic radiosurgery for cavernous malformations, *J Neurosurg* 93:987, 2000.

107. Hasegawa T, McInerney J, Kondziolka D, et al: Long-term results after stereotactic radiosurgery for patients with cavernous malformations, *Neurosurgery* 50:1190, 2002.

108. Lindquist C, Guo WY, Karlsson B, et al: Radiosurgery for venous angiomas, *J Neurosurg* 78:531, 1993.

109. Maarouf M, Runge M, Kocher M, et al: Radiosurgery for cerebral arteriovenous malformations in hereditary hemorrhagic telangiectasia, *Neurology* 63:367, 2004.

110. Chandler HC Jr, Friedman WA: Successful radiosurgical treatment of a dural arteriovenous malformation: Case report, *Neurosurgery* 33:139, 1993.

111. Guo WY, Pan DH, Wu HM, et al: Radiosurgery as a treatment alternative for dural arteriovenous fistulas of the cavernous sinus, *AJNR Am J Neuroradiol* 19:1081, 1998.

112. Lewis AI, Tomsick TA, Tew JM Jr: Management of tentorial dural arteriovenous malformations: Transarterial embolization combined with stereotactic radiation or surgery, *J Neurosurg* 81:851, 1994.

113. Link MJ, Coffey RJ, Nichols DA, et al: The role of radiosurgery and particulate embolization in the treatment of dural arteriovenous fistulas, *J Neurosurg* 84:804–809, 1996.

74 Cerebral Cavernous Malformations and Venous Anomalies: Diagnosis, Natural History, and Clinical Management

CHRISTOPHER S. EDDLEMAN, H. HUNT BATJER, ISSAM A. AWAD

Cerebrovascular malformations are a diverse group of dysmorphic vascular structures associated with distinct pathophysiologic features and clinical behavior. They can manifest in pure or mixed-transitional forms, as solitary or multiple lesions in the same host, and with sporadic or inherited-familial history. In the widely accepted modern classification, as refined by McCormick,[1] the cerebrovascular malformations are of four types: arteriovenous, venous, cavernous, or capillary. Other vascular lesions, such as arterial aneurysms, are typically considered separately, and "varices" are now known to be part of arteriovenous fistulas, another lesion with a distinct pathophysiologic profile. The cerebral arteriovenous malformations (AVMs) traditionally harbor the more dangerous natural history, and capillary malformations (or telangiectasias) are typically viewed as incidental benign lesions. The cavernous and venous malformations can manifest variable and occasionally significant clinical sequelae. It is therefore imperative for the clinician to characterize the lesion with sufficient specificity so as to better predict clinical behavior and more accurately select management strategy. In this chapter, we specifically address approaches to the definition, diagnosis, natural history, and clinical management of the cerebral cavernous malformations (CCMs) and venous anomalies (VAs).

Definition and Pathologic Features

The definition and classification of cerebrovascular malformations have undergone much iteration throughout history.[2-5] Before modern imaging modalities, they were once considered "angiomatous tumors." However, Bailey and Cushing[6] described these lesions as probably arising from cerebral arterial or venous structures, and Wyburn-Mason[7] described several different "phases" of potential development in the same brain suggesting a potential pathologic continuum. However, the development of advanced imaging modalities and, more particularly, MRI (Fig. 74-1), engendered a paradigm shift in our understanding of these lesions and for the first time allowed precise categorization of the distinct lesions during life, the detection of asymptomatic lesions, and the evolution of vascular pathology in association with clinical behavior. The CCMs are mulberry-like clusters of thin-walled vascular sinusoid channels (dilated capillaries or caverns) lined by a layer of endothelium and lacking elements of mature vessel wall (smooth muscle, elastin laminae, etc.).[2,4,8,9] The caverns are filled with blood in a low-flow state or thrombus at varying stages of organization and are separated by a loose collagenous stroma, without intervening neuroglial parenchyma, except in cauliflower-like projections into adjacent brain. Lesions are most often surrounded by hemosiderin deposits and gliosis, representing uniform signatures of previous hemorrhage or ongoing leakage of blood into adjacent brain. There is uniform angiogenic activity within CCMs, the endothelial cells lining the caverns exhibit proliferative activity,[3,10] and the lesions have been shown to exhibit a robust immune response with oligoclonal features.[11] The reddish purple lesions are variable in size, ranging from 1 mm to several centimeters, are multiple or single, and are occasionally calcified or associated with cystic cavities. The CCMs are also known as cavernous hemangiomas, angiomas, or cavernomas.[2-5]

The VAs are venous channels with normal histologic structure but traversing atypical or anomalous transmedullary courses in brain parenchyma rather than the typical superficial and deep venous patterns. They have been described with characteristic "caput medusae" branching and are best viewed as regional venous dysmorphism (Fig. 74-2).[2,5,12] VAs do not manifest any arteriovenous shunting and are typically associated with normal intervening brain tissue, although associated capillary telangiectasias in adjacent brain have been described. They most often lack any evidence of associated hemorrhage, but a small fraction of the lesions is associated with single or multiple hemorrhagic clusters with the typical histology of CCMs. VAs do not exhibit angiogenic or inflammatory activity except within associated CCMs. The VAs are also known as venous developmental anomalies or venous angiomas.[2,5,12]

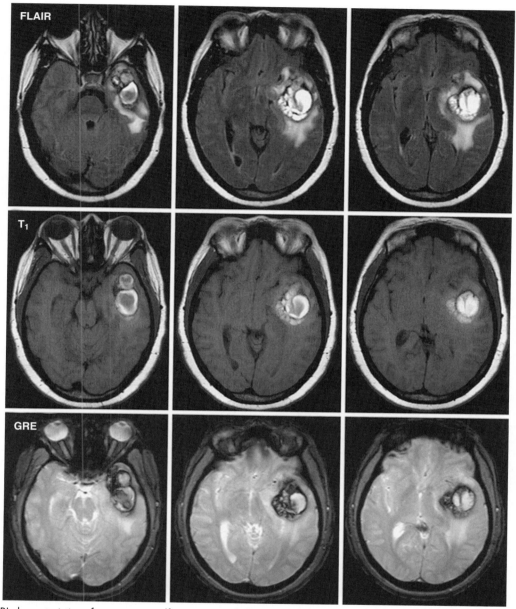

Figure 74-1 MRI characteristics of cavernous malformations with fluid-attenuated inversion recovery (FLAIR), T1-weighted (T1), and gradient echo (GRE) sequence acquisitions. *Top,* The FLAIR sequences demonstrate the possible parenchymal edema that can result from local irritation from the hemosiderin. *Middle and bottom,* The T1-weighted and GRE sequences demonstrate the heterogeneous stages of blood breakdown products within the lesion itself as well as the surrounding hemosiderin layer.

Epidemiology and Genetics

The prevalence estimates for these lesions in the general population have been made on the basis of large autopsy series and large cohorts undergoing MRI.[1,4,13] The VAs are thought to be the most common cerebrovascular malformation, found in up to 2.6% of all autopsied brains.[1,4] CCMs have been reported in 0.3% to 0.5% in autopsy series and of patients undergoing MRI.[1,3,4,13] Female patients with CCM may manifest a more aggressive clinical course, but the prevalence of CCMs and VAs is thought to be approximately equal in males and females.[1,4,13]

Although the cerebrovascular malformations were once thought to be congenital, vascular malformations have been classified according to their now known distinctive pathogenesis. The VAs by their nature likely reflect congenital venous dysmorphism, whereas CCMs have been shown to develop during life.[3,5,8,14-20] The CCMs are known to occur in two forms, namely a non-hereditary (sporadic) form and a hereditary (familial-autosomal dominant) form. The sporadic CCMs are more often associated with a VA (Fig. 74-3), but this association is uncommon in familial CCMs with known gene loci. Sporadic vascular lesions are typically solitary, whereas most familial cases of CCMs have multiple lesions, which are especially evident with more sensitive gradient-echo (GRE) and other magnetic-susceptibility MRI sequences (Fig. 74-4). Multiple CCMs also occur in association with a single VA and in the setting of previous brain irradiation.[2,4,12,17,21-24] Furthermore, some CCMs can exhibit mixed or transitional features of venous, capillary, or arteriovenous histopathology, implying related pathobiologic mechanisms.[2,3,5,12,23]

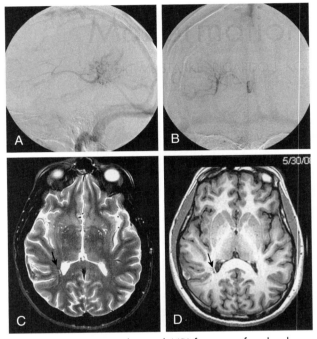

Figure 74-2 Angiographic and MRI features of a developmental venous anomaly (DVA). Lateral (A) and anteroposterior (B) projections of the late venous phase of a right internal carotid artery injection demonstrating the "caput medusae" often seen with DVAs. Axial T2-weighted (C) and T1-weighted (D) MR images demonstrating the subtle appearance of DVAs (arrows) in the brain parenchyma.

To date, three gene loci have been implicated in the pathogenesis of vascular malformations.[3,25-31] By linkage analysis, loci on chromosomal arms 7q (CCM1-KRIT1), 7p (CCM2-Malcavernin), and 3q (CCM3-PDCD10) have been identified and have been shown to have clinical penetrance of 88%, 100%, and 63%, respectively,[32-36] although respective penetrance is likely much higher when magnetic-susceptibility MRI is performed. It has been shown that the KRIT1 protein is expressed by the arterial and microvascular elements but not by the venous elements, with almost 100 distinct mutations identified to date.[32-36] Interestingly, the gene product is also expressed in neuroglial cells, in particular the astrocytes forming the neurovascular unit.[14,25,28,30,37-39] Malcavernin and PDCD10 were also found to have this pattern of expression, with fewer identified mutations.[14,25,27,28,30,31,40] This pattern of gene expression has been invoked to explain lesion predominance in the central nervous system parenchyma. The gene products have been related to common molecular complexes and to related signaling pathways that influence intercellular junctions and vascular permeability.

Natural History and Clinical Manifestations of Cerebral Cavernous Malformations and Vascular Anomalies

The clinical presentation of these cerebrovascular malformations is highly variable, ranging from an asymptomatic incidental discovery through radiographic imaging for nonspecific symptoms or at autopsy to associated headache, hemorrhagic stroke, epilepsy, and focal neurologic deficits.[1,3-5,8,18,21,41] Symptomatic presentation is far more common with CCMs than VAs.[2,4,21] Prospective risks of hemorrhage and new seizures are also more common with CCMs, in the range of 0.5% to 4% per year and 1% to 3% per year respectively, although these complications are rare in VAs except in association with CCMs.[2,12,21,42] Hemorrhage in VAs has been reported in only 0.22% to 0.68% of lesions per year, and most verified cases have included associated CCMs.[2,4,5,21]

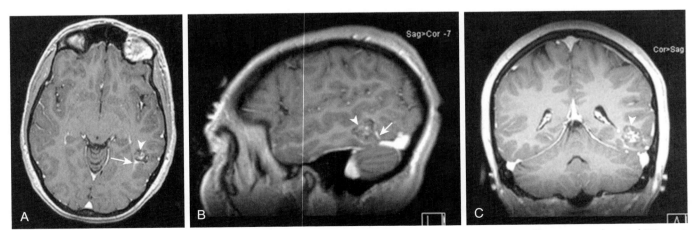

Figure 74-3 MRI appearance of a developmental venous anomaly (DVA) associated with a cavernous malformation in the axial (A), sagittal (B), and coronal (C) planes. The cavernous malformation (arrowheads) lies anterior to the DVA (arrows).

Pediatric presentation of CCMs occurs in a bimodal distribution, normally manifesting in patients either younger than 3 years or in their early teens.[4,22,43] The adult population typically presents with symptoms between the third and fifth decade of life, but the lesions can occur at any point in life.[4,5] Lifetime risk of symptomatic presentation is greater than 30% in CCMs and less than 1% to 2% in pure VAs.[4,5] Deep and infratentorial CCM locations are thought to be associated with greater risk of clinically significant hemorrhage, as are lesions with recent prior hemorrhage—hence the concept of hemorrhage clustering.[4,41,44-48] No known host or extrinsic factor has been demonstrated to impact lesion behavior, although recent trauma and anticoagulation have been linked to symptomatic bleeds.[4,41,44-48] Reports have demonstrated a slightly more benign natural risk in sporadic lesions and in the setting of the CCM1 genotype, as compared with the CCM3 genotype, which apparently demonstrates the most aggressive clinical course.[15,36] The most important risk for clinical manifestations of VAs appears related to the presence of associated CCMs.[2,12,49,50]

Despite the fact that CCMs do not include functional brain tissue, seizures thought to be a result of supratentorial lesions, most commonly frontal or temporal lesions, can be of any type and are believed to be related to multiple factors, including focal irritation and compression from an expanding hematoma, the presence of iron products after red blood cell breakdown secondary to multiple microhemorrhages, the formation of cortical scars, and resultant encephalomalacia.[42,51-57] However, in up to 6% of cases involving CCMs and epilepsy, the lesion itself is found to not be the epileptogenic trigger.[42]

Although virtually all CCMs exhibit some form of microhemorrhaging, clinically significant hemorrhage—either extending beyond the confines of the hemosiderin ring or producing neurologic symptoms—is not common but is thought to be more prevalent in females and

pediatric patients.[4,43,58] A precise definition of clinically significant hemorrhage has been proposed,[59] and findings of the many conflicting clinical series and natural history studies should be interpreted in light of this strict definition.

As with most intracranial lesions, the type of presenting neurologic deficit is related to the location of the lesion. Most vascular malformations that manifest in deep, eloquent brain tissue manifest not with seizure but rather with hemorrhage and focal neurologic deficits, at rates ranging from 15% to 45% of cases, and with more serious neurologic compromise.[4,5,18,20] Presentation of CCMs to the pial surface determines whether safe and effective surgical extirpation is possible.[8,9,41,46-49,60] Otherwise, alternative radiosurgery strategies may help reduce the risk of subsequent hemorrhage in patients with CCMs who have had multiple prior hemorrhages,[3,55,61-64] although this issue is controversial. However, patients may also present with postirradiation neurologic deficits secondary to edema or rehemorrhage.[3,55,61-64]

Cerebral Cavernous Malformations

Diagnostic Imaging

The CCMs have been traditionally considered among angiographically occult or "cryptic" vascular malformations because they are not typically visualized by conventional catheter-based angiography. The nonvisualization is due to their presumed low-flow status and the absence of arteriovenous shunting. CT imaging of CCMs has the ability to demonstrate calcifications, acute or chronic hemorrhage products, and cystic components. However, these findings are nonspecific and can be often observed with numerous other central nervous system lesions, limiting the sensitivity and diagnostic specificity of CT in this pathology. Despite these limitations, CT has been used to follow the size of CCMs after initial hemorrhages as well as to look for new hemorrhage products.

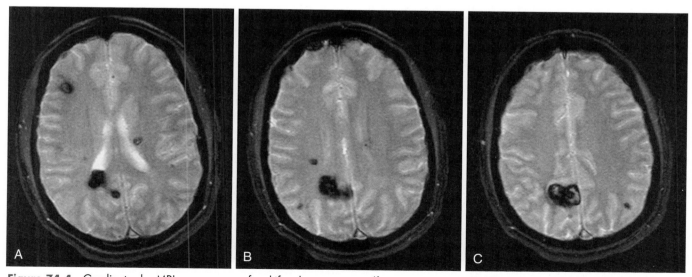

Figure 74-4 Gradient-echo MRI appearance of multifocal cavernous malformations in several different axial planes in the same patient.

MRI has proved to be the superior modality of imaging CCMs owing to the various sequences that can be employed, especially gradient echo and other magnetic-susceptibility sequences, which have been shown to be more sensitive in distinguishing CCMs (see Fig. 74-1).[12,41,49,50,65,66] On the basis of the correlation of MRI characteristics and pathologic specimens, Zabramski et al[67] classified CCMs into four MRI lesion types, although no relation to clinical outcome has been reported. The MRI appearance of CCM is quite specific, but the differential diagnosis may include, but is not limited to, thrombosed AVMs, hematomas, hemorrhagic tumors, and inflammatory lesions mimicking CCM features. The clinical context (including familiality), MRI associations (other lesions, such as VAs and occult CCMs), close imaging follow-up of lesions, which may rarely include catheter angiography (to exclude AVM), or surgical biopsy may be needed to establish a diagnosis.

Clinical Management

The most clinically appropriate treatment for CCMs depends on a multitude of factors regarding the lesion and the patient, including but not limited to natural history, the age and gender of the patient, and the location and clinical manifestations of the lesion. The most common management schemes of CCMs involve expectant follow-up, management of associated seizures, microsurgical excision, and radiosurgery. The generally accepted indications for procedural therapy of CCMs are intractable seizures, worsening neurologic deficits, and symptomatic hemorrhage (acute or recurrent) in both adult and pediatric cases.* Other cases may be treated in consideration of prospective natural risk and lesion accessibility.

Expectant Follow-up and Medical Management

Although fatal events can occur from CCMs, such as intractable seizures and hemorrhages leading to death, their incidence is extremely low.[4,42,53] Therefore, emergency procedural management of CCMs after their detection is not always immediately necessary. Advances in imaging technology have improved the ability not only to detect CCMs but also to follow their natural course in association with clinical symptoms. As such, observation of asymptomatic or mildly symptomatic lesions is feasible and considered first-line management in many cases. However, several situations can dictate more expeditious treatment, including lowering the prospective lifetime hemorrhage risk, decreasing the psychological burden on the patient, and reducing the costs of continued imaging and follow-up. Patient counseling is paramount in these situations and should be extremely detailed regarding the natural history of the lesion, risks of surgery, expectations of surgery, and postprocedural recovery. Patients followed up expectantly typically undergo serial imaging of the lesion, especially in association with new or worsened symptoms.

Expectant management is also indicated in both adults and pediatric patients who have symptomatic lesions that

*See references 4, 13, 20, 41, 43, 44, 46, 48, 51, 55, 56.

are either surgically inaccessible or radiosurgically dangerous. However, the benefits of surgical resection in eloquent areas of the brain may yield significant benefit in younger patients and may thus be justified, as opposed to the small gain in older patients, with lower cumulative prospective risk in their remaining lifetimes.[68]

Patients presenting with seizures are initially treated with anticonvulsants, which have varying degrees of control and side effects, especially when seizures are associated with small or less accessible CCMs, or multiple lesions.[42,68] Later-generation anticonvulsant agents have a better side effect profile but not necessarily greater effectiveness. In patients for whom anticonvulsants are not effective, careful analysis of seizure semiology and electrophysiologic localization might determine whether the CCM is the likely causative factor or merely an incidental association.[42,53-57] This determination may be particularly problematic in patients with multiple CCMs. In cases in which the CCM has been shown to be the epileptogenic factor, the more protracted the seizure history, the less likely the patient will be seizure free after resection.[42,53,56] As such, if the CCM is shown to be the epileptogenic factor, it is recommended that surgical resection be considered earlier rather than later, so as to increase the patient's chances of being seizure free, and possibly off anticonvulsants, and to avoid lesion growth and possible extension or recalcitrant transformation of the epileptogenic region as well as future hemorrhage.[42,53,56] In cases in which other lesions are present with a first seizure in association with overt brain hemorrhage or lesion expansion, excision may be considered (see later).

Microsurgical Excision

As with any intracranial lesion being considered for surgical management, a thorough preoperative assessment must be completed such that the benefits of surgical resection outweigh the potential risks of the procedure. Careful planning should include detailed imaging studies, such as those of the surrounding brain parenchyma and vascular structures in the cases of associated vascular anomalies, as well as functional consideration of eloquence in adjacent brain and in the proposed surgical corridor. Stereotactic guidance should always be considered so that the surgical approach can be most efficiently chosen.[69] In cases of CCMs present in eloquent areas of the brain, functional mapping by MRI activation, electrocorticography, or cortical stimulation, with the patient awake or under general anesthesia, should be carefully considered in order to avoid inadvertent or unnecessary damage to eloquent structures.[64,70]

Timing of surgery should also be carefully considered after hemorrhagic events. Sufficient time should be allowed for the reactive, posthemorrhagic brain to stabilize and for better identification of the CCM lesion. Conversely, the hematoma cavity itself may provide a sufficient surgical conduit for resection (Fig. 74-5). Significant and symptomatic mass effect from resultant hematomas or medically intractable seizures may also dictate an earlier resection.

In most cases of CCM resection, standard surgical approaches are used with the goal of minimizing injury to the surrounding normal parenchyma while maximizing

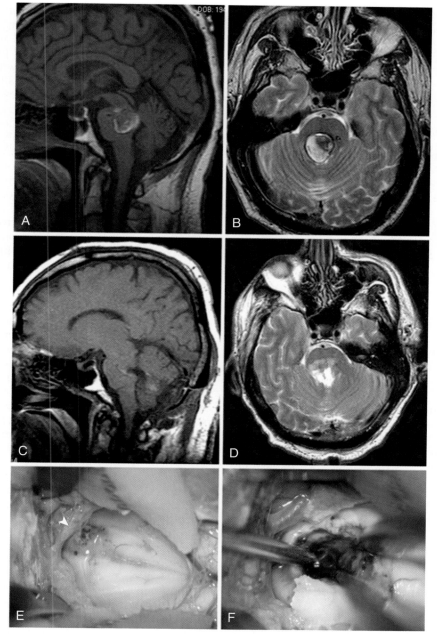

Figure 74-5 Preoperative, postoperative, and intraoperative views of a pontine cavernous malformation. Preoperative sagittal T1-weighted (A) and axial T2-weighted (B) MR images of a large pontine cavernous malformation. Postoperative sagittal T1-weighted (C) and axial T2-weighted (D) MR images from the same patient. Intraoperative image of pial representation of cavernous malformation (E, *arrowhead*) through which the surgical approach was initiated (F).

exposure for an adequate lesion resection. Intraoperative stereotactic guidance has improved over the last decade with the use of frameless tracking systems calibrated to handheld wands and operative microscopes.[69] This adjunct is especially useful for optimizing the planning of the incision and bony exposure, corticectomy, and resection corridor as well as localization of deep lesions. For CCM lesions in noneloquent brain, total resection of the CCM and the accompanying hemosiderin ring is advocated. Any associated VA should not be disturbed because despite being an aberrant vascular structure, it may drain normal brain parenchyma and its destruction could lead to venous infarction and hemorrhage. For CCM lesions in eloquent cortex, deep brain tissue, or brainstem, the gliotic tissue and surrounding hemosiderin ring should often be left undisturbed in order to avoid unnecessary destruction of vital structures and neural pathways. However, it is thought that, in the cases of epileptogenic CCMs, the causative agent may be the hemosiderin material or gliotic scar. Therefore, careful clinical decisions must be made in these cases so as to avoid unnecessary resection. Another adjunct to aid in the monitoring of eloquent areas of the brain is electrophysiologic monitoring and mapping utilizing somatosensory evoked potentials,

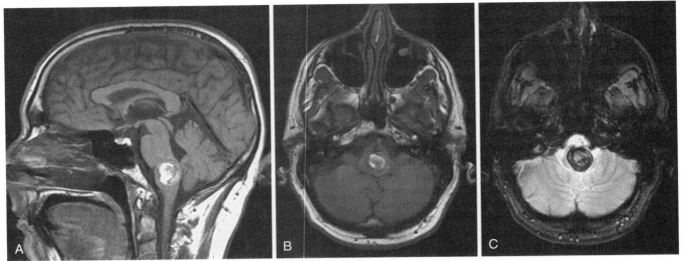

Figure 74-6 Sagittal (A) and axial (B) T1-weighted and gradient-echo (C) MR images of a medullary cavernous malformation without overt pial representation.

brainstem auditory evoked potentials, and lower cranial nerve monitoring.[64,70]

Multiple reports have been published regarding common surgical approaches for CCM resection, which are based on intracranial location and closest area of pial exposure.[4,20,44,46,47,68,71] Resection of superficial lesions of the supratentorial and infratentorial parenchyma often results in 95% to 100% complete removal, with more than 80% of cases having good or excellent outcomes.[4,8,43,46] Deep CCMs present in the brainstem, basal ganglia, and thalamus represent a more formidable challenge and invariably have less favorable outcomes, with 13% to 60% of cases worsening or being associated with serious sequelae (Fig. 74-6).[4,44,46,47,68] However, this fact must be considered in light of similar consequences of hemorrhage in these same locations and the fact that more than 80% of patients ultimately recover to good or better neurologic function despite the initial setback.[4,9,44,47,60] Skull base surgical approaches have been optimized in recent years for various lesion locations presenting to pial or ependymal surfaces, and intraoperative monitoring strategies have been advocated to monitor the function of various associated nuclei and pathways. Studies have also shown that improvements in patient selection and operative approach as well as close postoperative care can result in good long-term results, with about 96% of patients with brainstem, basal ganglia, or thalamic CCMs having excellent or good long-term outcomes.[47,60]

Stereotactic Radiosurgery

The management of CCMs with stereotactic radiosurgery (SRS) remains controversial. Although microsurgical resection of noneloquent, superficial lesions is achievable with acceptable low rates of morbidity, the management of deep-seated lesions, especially in the diencephalon or brainstem, presents a dilemma. The effect of SRS on CCMs is varied. Irradiation itself can cause de novo genesis of CCMs.[17,22] CCMs are not eliminated by SRS, and irradiated CCMs can still grow and hemorrhage.[55,61-63] Furthermore, the continued task of defining the natural history and

relative hemorrhage rates before and after irradiation have further complicated decisions about the potential favorable impact of SRS. SRS management has typically been advocated for progressively symptomatic CCM lesions for which surgical resection was not an option (Fig. 74-7). The aim of treatment is progressive scarring and hyalinization of vascular structures in response to irradiation, ultimately resulting in decreased hemorrhage rates. Kondziolka et al[63] reported that the hemorrhage risk after institution of gamma knife (GK) therapy in patients with at least two prior hemorrhages dropped from 32% to 1.1% per year within 3 years. Huang et al[61] reported a post–linear acceleration (LINAC) treatment hemorrhage rate in 30 CCM patients to be 1.1% per year. No significant difference has been found between gamma knife and linear accelerator radiosurgery in terms of reduction of hemorrhage risk or seizure control,[4,20,61,63] but treatment risks have been closely related to the dose and volume of lesion treated and lesion location, regardless of SRS modality. Post-SRS complications include rehemorrhage, edematous change, temporary neurologic deficit, and posttreatment seizures.[4,20,61,63] It is clear that outcome with microsurgery is better than that with SRS in terms of hemorrhage prevention or seizure control, but SRS remains an unproven option for progressively symptomatic cases in which surgical resection would be unacceptably risky. A more defined role for SRS treatment of CCMs may be determined as more centers report outcomes of various lesions and dosimetries.

Venous Anomalies

Diagnostic Imaging

The VAs can be visualized using multiple imaging modalities. Most lesions are found incidentally in association with frequent complaints of nonspecific symptoms such as headache and dizziness. Although non–contrast-enhanced CT does not visualize a VA unless it is thrombosed or associated with a CCM, contrast-enhanced CT does demonstrate a radial pattern of vessels with a larger

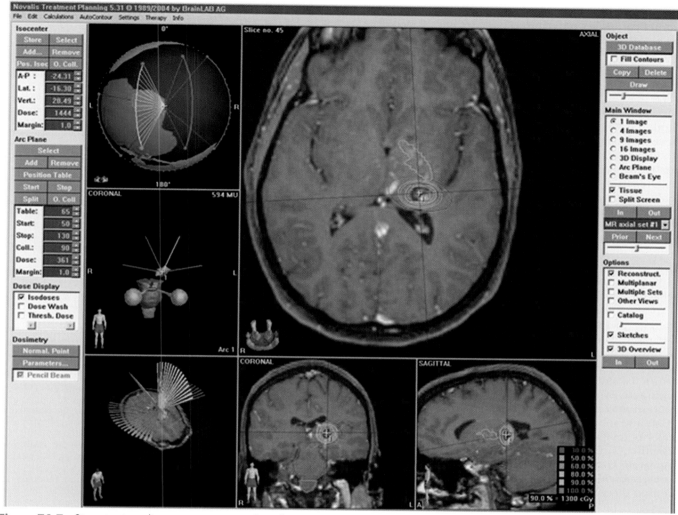

Figure 74-7 Stereotactic radiosurgery treatment plan of a cavernous malformation in the sagittal, axial, and coronal planes showing vital neural structures along with beam trajectories.

central vein, the often reported "caput medusae" pattern.[2,4,24,50] MRI sequences frequently demonstrate the same pattern (see Fig. 74-2) with additional sequences to examine surrounding edema or hemorrhage, potentially suggesting associated capillary telangiectasia (punctate contrast enhancement) or frank CCM (hemosiderin signal on magnetic-susceptibility sequences). Cerebral angiography also demonstrates the lesion and associated venous dysmorphism and excludes arteriovenous shunting but is usually not necessary because noninvasive imaging is sufficient to characterize the lesion.[2,4,24,50] The differential diagnosis of a VA may include prominent venous drainage of an AVM and malignant neoplasm. If either is suspected, repeat imaging or catheter cerebral angiography may be necessary for final diagnostic determination.

Clinical Management

VAs are thought to be associated with an extremely low risk of hemorrhage. As such, their management is most frequently observational and expectant, especially because VAs are thought to arise from dysmorphic venous

drainage of normal brain, interruption of which could lead to venous infarction, hemorrhage, and even death. However, patients with VAs may present with associated hemorrhage, seizures, neurologic deficits, or a combination of these findings.[2,4,24,50] In these cases, an associated CCM or, less likely, an AVM is normally found, whether on radiographic workup or surgical exploration. It is therefore extremely important to preserve the VA at all costs during resection of any associated vascular malformation, most commonly a CCM. In patients who present with seizures and an associated developmental venous anomaly, medical management with anticonvulsants is normally sufficient and does not require surgical management.[2,4,24] Patients with intractable epilepsy may require resection of epileptogenic brain in the region of VA, which can be safe as long as the brain parenchyma drained by the VA is also resected. The use of SRS in VAs is not justified, as the risks of SRS are justified given the benign natural history of VAs. The most important feature of VAs with respect to future hemorrhage risk appears to be the presence of an associated CCM. As such, the use of gradient-echo or magnetic-susceptibility MRI sequences is advocated to identify such lesions, which should be followed expectantly like other CCMs. Other patients with isolated VAs are reassured and cleared to live normal lives without restrictions.

Future Considerations

The natural course of individual CCMs and VAs remains highly variable. Other than lesion excision or irradiation, there is currently no known treatment intervention to modify lesion behavior, and there are no reliable markers predicting aggressive clinical behavior. Scientific knowledge regarding the pathobiology and pathophysiology of cerebrovascular malformations is expected to affect their clinical management. As the genetic signatures of CCMs are becoming more defined, the possibility of large prospective studies of genotype-phenotype associations can be entertained, potentially identifying other genetic modifiers of aggressive clinical course. Host and environmental factors may be identified that may also impact lesion behavior. Furthermore, elucidation of the mechanism(s) of CCM genesis with and without associated VAs should be better defined, including somatic mutations in molecular pathways involving disease genes, the involvement of antigen-driven or inflammatory mechanisms in lesion genesis or progression, and the relationships between neuroglial and vascular mechanisms and enhanced angiogenic activity in CCMs. These studies may also shed some light on why a small fraction of VAs result in associated CCMs and subsequent clinical manifestations but the vast majority remains benign. The convergence of clinical and scientific observations will provide future clinicians the improved knowledge and tools for more specific diagnoses, individual prognostication, and novel and better focused therapeutic interventions.

REFERENCES

1. McCormick W, Hardman J, Boulter T: Vascular malformations ("angiomas") of the brain, with special reference to those occurring in the posterior fossa, *J Neurosurg* 28:241-251, 1968.
2. Abla A, Wait SD, Uschold T, et al: Developmental venous anomaly, cavernous malformation, and capillary telangiectasia: Spectrum of a single disease, *Acta Neurochir (Wien)* 150:487-489, 2008:discussion 489.
3. Awad IA: Unfolding knowledge on cerebral cavernous malformations, *Surg Neurol* 63:317-318, 2005.
4. Brown RD Jr, Flemming KD, Meyer FB, et al: Natural history, evaluation, and management of intracranial vascular malformations, *Mayo Clin Proc.* 80:269-281, 2005.
5. Raychaudhuri R, Batjer HH, Awad IA: Intracranial cavernous angioma: A practical review of clinical and biological aspects. *Surg Neurol* 63:319-328, 2005:discussion 328.
6. Bailey P, Cushing H: Microchemical color reactions as an aid to the identification and classification of brain tumors, *Proc Natl Acad Sci U S A* 11:82-84, 1925.
7. Wyburn-Mason R: Arteriovenous aneurysm of midbrain, retina, facial naevi, and mental changes, *Brain* 66:163-209, 1943.
8. D'Angelo VA, De Bonis C, Amoroso R, et al: Supratentorial cerebral cavernous malformations: Clinical, surgical, and genetic involvement, *Neurosurg Focus* 21:e9, 2006.
9. Jung YJ, Hong SC, Seo DW, et al: Surgical resection of cavernous angiomas located in eloquent areas—clinical research, *Acta Neurochir Suppl.* 99:103-108, 2006.
10. Shenkar R, Shi C, Check IJ, et al: Concepts and hypotheses: Inflammatory hypothesis in the pathogenesis of cerebral cavernous malformations, *Neurosurgery* 61:693-702, 2007:discussion 702-693.
11. Shi C, Shenkar R, Batjer HH, et al: Oligoclonal immune response in cerebral cavernous malformations. Laboratory investigation, *J Neurosurg* 107:1023-1026, 2007.
12. Perrini P, Lanzino G: The association of venous developmental anomalies and cavernous malformations: Pathophysiological, diagnostic, and surgical considerations, *Neurosurg Focus* 21:e5, 2006.
13. Del Curling OJ, Kelly DJ, Elster A, et al: An analysis of the natural history of cavernous angiomas, *J Neurosurg* 75:702-708, 1991.
14. Denier C, Labauge P, Bergametti F, et al: Genotype-phenotype correlations in cerebral cavernous malformations patients, *Ann Neurol* 60:550-556, 2006.
15. Gault J, Sain S, Hu LJ, et al: Spectrum of genotype and clinical manifestations in cerebral cavernous malformations, *Neurosurgery* 59:1278-1284, 2006:discussion 1284-1275.
16. Maiuri F, Cappabianca P, Gangemi M, et al: Clinical progression and familial occurrence of cerebral cavernous angiomas: The role of angiogenic and growth factors, *Neurosurg Focus* 21:e3, 2006.
17. Nimjee SM, Powers CJ, Bulsara KR: Review of the literature on de novo formation of cavernous malformations of the central nervous system after radiation therapy, *Neurosurg Focus* 21:e4, 2006.
18. Revencu N, Vikkula M: Cerebral cavernous malformation: New molecular and clinical insights, *J Med Genet* 43:716-721, 2006.
19. Toldo I, Drigo P, Mammi I, et al: Vertebral and spinal cavernous angiomas associated with familial cerebral cavernous malformation, *Surg Neurol* 71:167-171, 2008.
20. Zhao Y, Du GH, Wang YF, et al: Multiple intracranial cavernous malformations: Clinical features and treatment, *Surg Neurol* 68:493-499, 2007:discussion 499.
21. Beall DP, Bell JP, Webb JR, et al: Developmental venous anomalies and cavernous angiomas: A review of the concurrence, imaging, and treatment of these vascular malformations, *J Okla State Med Assoc* 98:535-538, 2005.
22. Burn S, Gunny R, Phipps K, et al: Incidence of cavernoma development in children after radiotherapy for brain tumors, *J Neurosurg* 106:379-383, 2007.
23. Kovacs T, Osztie E, Bodrogi L, et al: Cerebellar developmental venous anomalies with associated vascular pathology, *Br J Neurosurg* 21:217-223, 2007.
24. Wurm G, Schnizer M, Fellner FA: Cerebral cavernous malformations associated with venous anomalies: Surgical considerations, *Neurosurgery* 57:42-58, 2005.
25. Gianfrancesco F, Cannella M, Martino T, et al: Highly variable penetrance in subjects affected with cavernous cerebral angiomas (CCM) carrying novel CCM1 and CCM2 mutations, *Am J Med Genet B Neuropsychiatr Genet* 144B:691-695, 2007.
26. Gianfrancesco F, Esposito T, Penco S, et al: ZPLD1 gene is disrupted in a patient with balanced translocation that exhibits cerebral cavernous malformations, *Neuroscience* 155:345-349, 2008.
27. Liquori CL, Penco S, Gault J, et al: Different spectra of genomic deletions within the CCM genes between Italian and American CCM patient cohorts, *Neurogenetics* 9:25-31, 2008.
28. Stahl S, Gaetzner S, Voss K, et al: Novel CCM1, CCM2, and CCM3 mutations in patients with cerebral cavernous malformations: In-frame deletion in CCM2 prevents formation of a CCM1/CCM2/CCM3 protein complex, *Hum Mutat* 29:709-717, 2008.
29. Surucu O, Sure U, Gaetzner S, et al: Clinical impact of CCM mutation detection in familial cavernous angioma, *Childs Nerv Syst* 22:1461-1464, 2006.
30. Tanriover G, Boylan AJ, Diluna ML, et al: PDCD10, the gene mutated in cerebral cavernous malformation 3, is expressed in the neurovascular unit, *Neurosurgery* 62:930-938, 2008:discussion 938.
31. Voss K, Stahl S, Schleider E, et al: CCM3 interacts with CCM2 indicating common pathogenesis for cerebral cavernous malformations, *Neurogenetics* 8:249-256, 2007.
32. Brouillard P, Vikkula M: Genetic causes of vascular malformations, *Hum Mol Genet* 16(Spec No. 2):R140-R149, 2007.
33. Dashti SR, Hoffer A, Hu YC, et al: Molecular genetics of familial cerebral cavernous malformations, *Neurosurg Focus* 21:e2, 2006.
34. Guclu B, Ozturk AK, Pricola KL, et al: Cerebral venous malformations have distinct genetic origin from cerebral cavernous malformations, *Stroke* 36:2479-2480, 2005.
35. Hanjani SA: The genetics of cerebrovascular malformations, *J Stroke Cerebrovasc Dis* 11:279-287, 2002.
36. Labauge P, Denier C, Bergametti F, et al: Genetics of cavernous angiomas, *Lancet Neurol* 6:237-244, 2007.

37. Hogan BM, Bussmann J, Wolburg H, et al: CCM1 cell autonomously regulates endothelial cellular morphogenesis and vascular tubulogenesis in zebrafish, *Hum Mol Genet* 17:2424-2432, 2008.

38. Zhao Y, Tan YZ, Zhou LF, et al: Morphological observation and in vitro angiogenesis assay of endothelial cells isolated from human cerebral cavernous malformations, *Stroke* 38:1313-1319, 2007.

39. Shimizu T, Sugawara K, Tosaka M, et al: Nestin expression in vascular malformations: A novel marker for proliferative endothelium, *Neurol Med Chir (Tokyo)* 46:111-117, 2006.

40. Liquori CL, Berg MJ, Squitieri F, et al: Deletions in CCM2 are a common cause of cerebral cavernous malformations, *Am J Hum Genet* 80:69-75, 2007.

41. Cordonnier C, Al-Shahi Salman R, Bhattacharya JJ, et al: Differences between intracranial vascular malformation types in the characteristics of their presenting haemorrhages: Prospective, population-based study, *J Neurol Neurosurg Psychiatry* 79:47-51, 2008.

42. Awad I, Jabbour P: Cerebral cavernous malformations and epilepsy, *Neurosurg Focus* 21:e7, 2006.

43. Lee JW, Kim DS, Shim KW, et al: Management of intracranial cavernous malformation in pediatric patients, *Childs Nerv Syst* 24:321-327, 2008.

44. Batay F, Bademci G, Deda H: Critically located cavernous malformations, *Minim Invasive Neurosurg* 50:71-76, 2007.

45. Chen X, Weigel D, Ganslandt O, et al: Diffusion tensor-based fiber tracking and intraoperative neuronavigation for the resection of a brainstem cavernous angioma, *Surg Neurol* 68:285-291, 2007:discussion 291.

46. de Oliveira JG, Rassi-Neto A, Ferraz FA, et al: Neurosurgical management of cerebellar cavernous malformations, *Neurosurg Focus* 21:e11, 2006.

47. Majchrzak H, Tymowski M, Majchrzak K, et al: Surgical approaches to pathological lesions of the middle cerebellar peduncle and the lateral part of the pons-clinical observation, *Neurol Neurochir Pol* 41:436-444, 2007.

48. Sola RG, Pulido P, Pastor J, et al: Surgical treatment of symptomatic cavernous malformations of the brainstem, *Acta Neurochir (Wien)* 149:463-470, 2007.

49. Jinhu Y, Jianping D, Xin L, et al: Dynamic enhancement features of cavernous sinus cavernous hemangiomas on conventional contrast-enhanced MR imaging, *AJNR Am J Neuroradiol* 29:577-581, 2008.

50. Pozzati E, Marliani AF, Zucchelli M, et al: The neurovascular triad: Mixed cavernous, capillary, and venous malformations of the brainstem, *J Neurosurg* 107:1113-1119, 2007.

51. Baumann CR, Acciarri N, Bertalanffy H, et al: Seizure outcome after resection of supratentorial cavernous malformations: A study of 168 patients, *Epilepsia* 48:559-563, 2007.

52. Baumann CR, Schuknecht B, Lo Russo G, et al: Seizure outcome after resection of cavernous malformations is better when surrounding hemosiderin-stained brain also is removed, *Epilepsia* 47:563-566, 2006.

53. Ferroli P, Casazza M, Marras C, et al: Cerebral cavernomas and seizures: A retrospective study on 163 patients who underwent pure lesionectomy, *Neurol Sci* 26:390-394, 2006.

54. Giulioni M, Zucchelli M, Riguzzi P, et al: Co-existence of cavernoma and cortical dysplasia in temporal lobe epilepsy, *J Clin Neurosci* 14:1122-1124, 2007.

55. Hsu PW, Chang CN, Tseng CK, et al: Treatment of epileptogenic cavernomas: Surgery versus radiosurgery, *Cerebrovasc Dis* 24:116-120, 2007:discussion 121.

56. Noto S, Fujii M, Akimura T, et al: Management of patients with cavernous angiomas presenting epileptic seizures, *Surg Neurol* 64:495-498, 2005:discussion 498-499.

57. Paolini S, Morace R, Di Gennaro G, et al: Drug-resistant temporal lobe epilepsy due to cavernous malformations, *Neurosurg Focus* 21:e8, 2006.

58. Safavi-Abbasi S, Feiz-Erfan I, Spetzler RF, et al: Hemorrhage of cavernous malformations during pregnancy and in the peripartum period: Causal or coincidence? Case report and review of the literature, *Neurosurg Focus* 21:e12, 2006.

59. Al-Shahi R, Bhattacharya JJ, Currie DG, et al: Prospective, population-based detection of intracranial vascular malformations in adults: The Scottish Intracranial Vascular Malformation Study (SIVMS), *Stroke* 34:1163-1169, 2003.

60. Recalde RJ, Figueiredo EG, de Oliveira E: Microsurgical anatomy of the safe entry zones on the anterolateral brainstem related to surgical approaches to cavernous malformations, *Neurosurgery* 62:9-15, 2008:discussion 15-17.

61. Huang YC, Tseng CK, Chang CN, et al: Linac radiosurgery for intracranial cavernous malformation: 10-year experience, *Clin Neurol Neurosurg* 108:750-756, 2006.

62. Iwai Y, Yamanaka K, Yoshimura M: Intracerebral cavernous malformation induced by radiosurgery. Case report, *Neurol Med Chir (Tokyo)* 47:171-173, 2007.

63. Kondziolka D, Flickinger JC, Lunsford LD: Radiosurgery for cavernous malformations, *Prog Neurol Surg* 20:220-230, 2007.

64. Sugano H, Shimizu H, Sunaga S: Efficacy of intraoperative electrocorticography for assessing seizure outcomes in intractable epilepsy patients with temporal-lobe-mass lesions, *Seizure* 16:120-127, 2007.

65. de Souza JM, Domingues RC, Cruz LC Jr, et al: Susceptibility-weighted imaging for the evaluation of patients with familial cerebral cavernous malformations: A comparison with T2-weighted fast spin-echo and gradient-echo sequences, *AJNR Am J Neuroradiol* 29:154-158, 2008.

66. Tong KA, Ashwal S, Obenaus A, et al: Susceptibility-weighted MR imaging: A review of clinical applications in children, *AJNR Am J Neuroradiol* 29:9-17, 2008.

67. Zabramski J, Wascher T, Spetzler RF, et al: The natural history of familial cavernous malformations: Results of an ongoing study, *J Neurosurg* 80:422-432, 1994.

68. Chang H: Surgical decision-making on cerebral cavernous malformations, *J Clin Neurosci* 8:416-420, 2001.

69. Zhao J, Wang Y, Kang S, et al: The benefit of neuronavigation for the treatment of patients with intracerebral cavernous malformations, *Neurosurg Rev* 30:313-318, 2007:discussion 319.

70. Pouratian N, Bookheimer SY, Rex DE, et al: Utility of preoperative functional magnetic resonance imaging for identifying language cortices in patients with vascular malformations, *Neurosurg Focus* 13:e4, 2002.

71. Bizzi A, Blasi V, Falini A, et al: Presurgical functional MR imaging of language and motor functions: Validation with intraoperative electrocortical mapping, *Radiology* 248:579-589, 2008.

Indications for Carotid Endarterectomy in Patients with Symptomatic Stenosis

JONATHAN L. BRISMAN, MARC R. MAYBERG

Symptomatic carotid stenosis or occlusion is, by some estimates, responsible for 25% of all ischemic strokes,[1] with an estimated 6% to 7% estimated annual stroke rate for patients with both symptomatic carotid stenosis and completed occlusion.[2,3] Sufficient evidence is now available from several clinical trials[4-6] showing that carotid endarterectomy (CEA) can reduce the risk of stroke for symptomatic carotid stenosis. This chapter reviews the major clinical trials on CEA as well as some of the post hoc analyses in an effort to best define appropriate candidates for CEA. Guidelines for the use of CEA in patients with symptomatic stenosis published by the American Heart Association/American Stroke Association Council on Stroke as well as the American Academy of Neurology are presented. Data related to the efficacy of carotid artery angioplasty and stenting to prevent stroke in patients with symptomatic carotid stenosis are discussed elsewhere in this volume.

Historical Overview

Clinical trials have achieved a growing role in the contemporary practice of medicine, owing in part to the advent of improved methodology for multicenter studies, increasing public awareness of clinical trials, the role of clinical trials in determining reimbursement policies, and a general consensus in the medical community that any treatment administered should be proven effective according to rigorous scientific criteria.

The evolution of CEA has been predicated on the results of clinical trials, several of which are ongoing.[7] The ECIC Bypass trial[8] introduced the concept of multicenter prospective randomized trials to the cerebrovascular surgical community. The widespread recognition of this trial and its consequences led in part to the development of several studies designed to test the efficacy of CEA. The studies evaluating the use of CEA for symptomatic stenosis are the North American Symptomatic Carotid Endarterectomy Trial (NASCET),[9] the European Carotid Surgery Trial (ECST),[4] and the V.A. Symptomatic Stenosis Trial (VASST).[6] These trials, published in the early 1990s, demonstrated that in patients with symptomatic high-grade (>70%) stenosis, CEA resulted in lower stroke risk

than medical therapy; the benefits of CEA, however, were realized only if the morbidity of surgery could be kept reasonably low (6%). Guidelines for CEA published by the American Heart Association in 1995[10] were updated 10 years later,[11,12] and the number of CEAs performed in this country continue to rise.

Prospective Randomized Trials Using Carotid Endarterectomy for Symptomatic Carotid Stenosis
Early Trials for Carotid Endarterectomy

Results of three randomized trials for carotid endarterectomy were published prior to 1991. The Joint Study of Extracranial Arterial Occlusion[13] involved 24 centers in the United States. From 1962 to 1968, 316 patients with transient ischemic attacks (TIAs) and carotid stenosis were randomized to surgical or nonsurgical therapy. At a mean follow-up of 42 months, stroke occurred in 19 of 167 surgical patients (11%) compared with 18 of 145 nonsurgical patients (12%). In the endarterectomy group, the majority of strokes (13/19) occurred in the perioperative period with a relatively low subsequent stroke rate (approximately 1.5% per year). This study was flawed by a number of methodologic errors, including limited sample size, lack of follow-up for eligible nonrandomized patients, variability in stroke diagnosis, and inconsistency of adjunctive therapies. Shaw et al[14] reported on a limited trial involving 41 symptomatic patients in Great Britain. This trial was terminated because of an excessive perioperative stroke rate (25%) among participating surgeons. In summary, perhaps the only meaningful data from early prospective randomized trials for CEA concerned the relatively low (1% to 2% annual) risk of subsequent stroke in those patients surviving surgery. Because of methodologic flaws, other data involving comparison between surgical and nonsurgical therapies in these studies must be discounted.

The **European Carotid Surgery Trial (ECST)**[4] entered patients with mild (defined as less than 30%), moderate (30% to 69%) or severe (70% to 99%) carotid stenosis, who were then randomly assigned to either surgical or nonsurgical treatment. Interim analysis of 2200 patients (mean follow-up = 2.7 years) led to premature termination of the trial for the mild and severe stenosis groups. Among the 374 patients with mild stenosis, there was no significant difference in ipsilateral stroke between the surgical and nonsurgical groups. There were more treatment failures in the surgical group, which was attributed to the 2.3% risk of death or disabling stroke during the first 30 days after surgery. For severe stenosis, however, surgery was shown to be beneficial in preventing stroke. There was a 7.5% risk of ipsilateral stroke or death within 30 days of surgery. At 3 years of follow-up, there was an additional 2.8% risk of stroke in the surgical group (total = 10.3%) compared with 16.8% in the nonsurgical group ($P < .0001$). More importantly, the risk of death or ipsilateral disabling stroke was 11% in the nonsurgical group compared with 6% in the surgical group.

The **North American Symptomatic Carotid Endarterectomy Trial (NASCET)**[9] prematurely stopped randomly assigning patients with carotid stenosis greater than 70% because of the highly significant stroke risk reduction observed in the surgical group. A total of 659 patients in this category of stenosis were assigned to surgical (N = 331) or nonsurgical (N = 328) therapy. At a mean follow-up of 24 months, ipsilateral stroke was noted in 26% of patients receiving nonsurgical therapy, compared with 9% of patients who had undergone CEA, for an overall risk reduction of 17% (relative risk reduction = 71%). The benefit for surgical patients was highly significant ($P < .001$) for a variety of outcomes, including stroke in any territory, major stroke, and major stroke or death from any cause. A perioperative morbidity/mortality of 5.8% was rapidly surpassed in the nonsurgical group, such that surgical benefit was apparent by 3 months. In addition, the protective effect of surgery was durable over time, with few strokes noted in the endarterectomy group beyond the perioperative period. There was a direct correlation between surgical benefit and the degree of angiographic stenosis.

Enrollment in the **V.A. Symptomatic Stenosis Trial (VASST)**[6] was discontinued in early 1991 on the basis of preliminary data consistent with the NASCET findings. Subsequent analysis demonstrated a statistically significant reduction in ipsilateral stroke or crescendo TIA for patients with carotid stenosis greater than 50% who underwent surgery.[6] A total of 193 men aged 35 to 82 years 9 (mean = 64.2 years) were randomly assigned to surgical (N = 91) or nonsurgical (N = 98) treatment. Two thirds of the patients demonstrated angiographic internal carotid artery stenosis greater than 70%. At a mean follow-up of 11.9 months, there was a significant reduction in stroke or crescendo TIA in patients receiving CEA (7.7%) compared with nonsurgical patients (19.4%), or a risk reduction of 11.7% (relative risk reduction = 60%; $P = .028$). Among subgroups, the benefit of surgery was most prominent in patients with TIA in comparison with those with transient monocular blindness (TMB) or stroke, although these differences were not statistically significant. The benefit for surgery was apparent as early as 2 months after randomization and persisted over the entire period of follow-up. The efficacy of CEA was durable, with only one ipsilateral stroke beyond the 30-day perioperative period. With one preoperative stroke discounted, perioperative morbidity of 2.2% and mortality

of 3.3% (total = 5.5%) were achieved over multiple centers among relatively high-risk patients.

Carotid Endarterectomy Trial Meta-analyses and Other Post Hoc Analyses

Because only three properly powered trials on CEA have been published, considerable attention has focused on the individual results from these trials. However, although the trials had similar outcomes, the inclusion and exclusion criteria and enrollment variables (degree of stenosis measurements, for example) were somewhat different. Nevertheless, because the cohorts in all three trials were relatively homogeneous, it was possible to retrospectively standardize and pool the original data. Additionally, given the volume of pertinent data on demographic and risk indices, it was possible to generate post hoc analyses examining different outcome measures and baseline variables.

In 2003 the investigators of the three CEA trials published a meta-analysis in which raw trial data were pooled and analyzed.[15] Data (6092 patients, 35,000 patient-years of follow-up) included all patients randomly assigned to treatment in one of the three trials in the two decades following trial results publication, which included 95% of patients ever included in CEA trials. Original carotid angiograms were reassessed for degree of stenosis to standardize the data among trials. Outcome events were redefined when necessary for the same purpose. This analysis demonstrated that surgery was associated with a higher 5-year risk of ipsilateral ischemic stroke in patients with less than 30% carotid stenosis, no effect in patients with 30% to 49% risk, and marginal benefit in those with 50% to 69% risk; CEA was highly beneficial in preventing stroke in those with greater than 70% stenosis, provided that there was no near-occlusion. Furthermore, analysis by degree of stenosis showed the benefit proportionately increased within the 70% to 99% range.[15]

Another analysis of pooled data (restricted to the combined ECST and NASCET patient databases) evaluated the risk of ipsilateral stroke with medical therapy, the perioperative risk of stroke and death, and the overall benefit from surgery in relation to seven predefined and seven post hoc–defined subgroups.[16] Predefined variables, that is, those studied in the original trials, were as follows: sex (male, female), age (<65, 65 to 74, >75 years), time since last event (<2, 2 to 4, 4 to 12, >12 weeks), primary symptomatic event (ocular only, cerebral TIA, stroke), presence or absence of diabetes, plaque surface (smooth, irregular, or ulcerated), and contralateral ICA occlusion. Post hoc subgroups were: duration of cerebral TIA (<1 hr, >1 hr), previous TIA or stroke (yes/no), and presence or absence of myocardial infarction, angina, treated hypertension, treated hyperlipidemia, and smoking. Data were analyzed from 5893 patients including 33,000 patient-years of follow-up. In unoperated patients, risk of ipsilateral stroke was found to be higher in close proximity to the last ischemic event and increased with age, male gender, diabetes, in patients with prior hemispheric strokes, and in patients with ulcerated plaques. Perioperative risk was higher in women, diabetics, and patients with hemispheric qualifying events, contralateral carotid occlusion, and ulcerated plaques. In the post hoc subgroups, the perioperative risk was reduced in patients with angina and increased in those with hypertension and previous TIA or stroke.

More specific subgroup correlations identified the highest benefit for surgery in men aged over 75 years operated on within 2 weeks.[16] Benefit fell sharply beyond 2 weeks, such that in order to prevent one ipsilateral stroke in a patient with greater than 50% carotid stenosis at 5 years, one would need to operate on 5 patients if the surgery were done within 2 weeks of random treatment assignment as opposed to 125 patients if surgery were performed beyond 12 weeks.

Several post hoc analyses restricted to the NASCET trial patients have been performed.[17-20] Among 681 patients from the NASCET trial evaluated for the correlation between collateral blood supply (anterior communicating artery, posterior communicating artery, and ophthalmic retrograde flow) and risk of ipsilateral stroke, good collateral formation was found to reduce the risk of stroke in both the medically treated group and patients undergoing CEA.[17] Patients from NASCET who had concomitant intracranial atherosclerotic disease were found to have an increased risk of ipsilateral stroke when treated medically, but not when treated surgically. Furthermore, the stroke risk was reduced for those undergoing CEA.[18] For 193 NASCET patients with leukoaraiosis. Although leukoaraiosis did confer an increased risk of stroke for the medically treated group as well as a higher perioperative risk in the group undergoing surgery, CEA reduced the subsequent stroke risk in this cohort.[20] Analysis of 659 patients with more than 70% stenosis in the NASCET trial revealed an increased risk of stroke in patients found to have an angiographically demonstrated ulcerated plaque who were treated medically. CEA was very successful in this subgroup, reducing the risk of stroke by approximately half at 24 months.[19]

Summary of Trials for CEA and Proposed Indications for Intervention Options

On the basis of the three major trials investigating CEA for symptomatic carotid stenosis, it is clear that CEA provided a profound protection against subsequent ipsilateral stroke or crescendo TIA in patients with high-grade symptomatic stenosis. In addition, CEA moderately reduced stroke risk in comparison with medical therapy in patients with intermediate-grade (>50%) symptomatic carotid stenosis. The stroke risk reduction was realized early after surgery, persisted over extended periods, and was independent of other risk factors. Efficacy for CEA, however, was realized in these trials only when an acceptable level of perioperative morbidity and mortality was achieved (<6%).

As previously mentioned, the American Heart Association published guidelines in 1995 recommending CEA for patients with single or multiple TIAs and ipsilateral carotid stenosis greater than 70% or for symptomatic carotid stenosis in patients found to have an ulcer on angiography and no other source of emboli. Moderate stenosis was considered an indeterminate indication for CEA. Further understanding provided by pooled data and subsequent

post hoc analyses led to newer guidelines for CEA as a treatment for symptomatic carotid stenosis published by the American Heart Association/American Stroke Association Council on Stroke,[11,12] which can be summarized as follows: For patients with recent TIA or ischemic stroke within the last 6 months and ipsilateral severe (70% to 99%) carotid artery stenosis, CEA performed by a surgeon with perioperative morbidity and mortality rates lower than 6% is recommended (class I, level of evidence A; reader is referred to the actual guidelines for definition of level and class of evidence). For patients with recent TIA or ischemic stroke and ipsilateral moderate (50% to 69%) carotid stenosis, CEA is recommended, depending on patient-specific factors such as age, gender, comorbidities, and severity of initial symptoms (class I, level of evidence A). When the degree of stenosis is less than 50%, there is no indication for CEA (class III, level of evidence A). When CEA is indicated for patients with TIA or stroke, surgery within 2 weeks is suggested rather than any delay of the procedure (class IIa, level of evidence B).

The American Academy of Neurology affirmed the preceding recommendations and elaborated on the following points: It is recommended that the patient (undergoing CEA for symptomatic carotid stenosis) have at least a 5-year life expectancy. No recommendation can be provided regarding the value of emergency CEA in patients with a progressing neurologic deficit (level U). Clinicians should consider patient variables in CEA decision making. Women with 50% to 69% symptomatic stenosis did not have clear benefit from CEA in previous trials. In addition, patients with hemispheric TIA/stroke had greater benefit than patients with retinal ischemic events (level C). Clinicians should also consider several radiologic factors in decision making about CEA. For example, contralateral occlusion is associated with increased operative risk but persistent benefit (level C). Symptomatic patients undergoing CEA should be given aspirin (81 or 325 mg/day) prior to surgery and for at least 3 months following surgery (level A). The data are insufficient to recommend the use of other antiplatelet agents in the perioperative setting. At this time the available data are insufficient to declare CEA before or CEA simultaneous with coronary artery bypass grafting (CABG) as superior in patients with concomitant carotid and coronary artery occlusive disease (level U).

Recent Randomized Trials Comparing Carotid Endarterectomy with Carotid Angioplasty and Stenting

Two trials compared the safety and efficacy of CEA relative to carotid angioplasty and stenting (CAS). The International Carotid Stenting Study (ICSS) is an ongoing multicenter, international, randomized trial of CEA versus CAS in carotid stenosis of greater than 50% that has been symptomatic in the last 12 months.[21] Patients for whom CEA posed standard risk were eligible for inclusion in the trial (with only prior CEA as the surgical high-risk exclusionary criterion) and had to be candidates for either CEA or CAS. The 120-day interim analysis of 1713 patients randomly assigned to undergo one of the procedures found no difference in rates of disabling stroke or death between CEA (3.2%) and CAS (4.0%) cohorts, but there was a significantly higher rate of any stroke, myocardial infarction and all-cause death in those patients undergoing CAS (8.5%) than in those undergoing CEA (5.2%; $P = .006$). Thirty day postprocedure rates of any stroke or death were also significantly higher in the CAS cohort. The investigators concluded that CEA for symptomatic carotid stenosis should remain the first-line treatment for patients deemed suitable candidates for surgery.

The Carotid Revascularization Endarterectomy vs. Stenting Trial (CREST) is a North American multicenter, randomized trial comparing CEA with CAS in symptomatic and asymptomatic carotid stenosis.[22] Patients included in CREST were considered symptomatic if they had suffered an event ipsilateral to the carotid artery within 180 days before random treatment assignment and were required to have at least 50% stenosis as shown by angiography or 70% or greater as shown by CT angiography or MR angiography. CREST did not exclude patients deemed to be high-risk surgical candidates. In the initial report of 2502 patients enrolled at 117 sites in the United States and Canada, there was no significant difference between estimated 4-year rates of primary outcome endpoint of stroke, myocardial infarction, or death for CEA (6.8%) and CAS (7.2%). Although there was no significant difference in the composite outcome in the two treatment arms, there was a statistically significant increase in the rates of stroke or death in the CAS cohort (6.4% vs. 4.7% for CE; $P = .03$) and a higher risk of myocardial infarction in the cohort undergoing CEA (2.3% vs 1.1% for CAS; $P = .03$). There was no difference in treatment effect related to presence of symptoms or gender. Although CREST documented acceptable periprocedural stroke rates for both CAS and CEA in experienced hands (4.1% and 2.3%, respectively), it also documented the different relative complication risks of the two procedures (increased risk of stroke for CAS and increased myocardial infarction for CEA) and raises the question of the significance of the relative disability imposed by either type of complication. Further follow-up for both trials as well as additional subgroup analyses will hopefully shed more light on the role of each therapy in carotid revascularization.

Conclusions

Carotid endarterectomy remains an important part of the armamentarium in the treatment of symptomatic carotid stenosis. It is a highly effective modality for treating patients with symptomatic severe carotid stenosis (>70%); there is less compelling but positive evidence supporting its use in patients with moderate (50% to 69%) stenosis. Current guidelines for CEA in symptomatic carotid stenosis reflect a wealth of information derived from analyses subsequent to the publication of the three main CEA trials using pooled data and post hoc analyses. Emerging data have shown that both CEA and carotid angioplasty and stenting are reasonably safe and effective means for treating symptomatic carotid stenosis; each treatment modality has relative risks and benefits in comparison with the other. Future subgroup and meta-analysis will likely identify specific patient cohorts that may preferentially benefit from specific procedural intervention in symptomatic carotid stenosis.

REFERENCES

1. Hanel RA, Levy EI, Guterman LR, et al: Cervical carotid revascularization: The role of angioplasty with stenting, *Neurosurg Clin North Am* 16:263-278, 2005:viii.
2. Grubb RL Jr, Powers WJ: Risks of stroke and current indications for cerebral revascularization in patients with carotid occlusion, *Neurosurg Clin North Am* 12:473-487, 2001:vii.
3. Mayberg MR: Extracranial Occlusive Disease Of The Carotid Artery. In Youmans JR, editor: *Neurological surgery*, ed 4, Philadelphia, 1996, WB Saunders Company, pp 1159-1180.
4. MRC European Carotid Surgery Trial: Interim results for symptomatic patients with severe (70-99%) or with mild (0-29%) carotid stenosis. European Carotid Surgery Trialists' Collaborative Group, *Lancet* 337(8752):1235-1243, 1991.
5. Barnett HJ, Taylor DW, Eliasziw M, et al: Benefit of carotid endarterectomy in patients with symptomatic moderate or severe stenosis. North American Symptomatic Carotid Endarterectomy Trial Collaborators, *N Engl J Med* 339:1415-1425, 1998.
6. Mayberg MR, Wilson SE, Yatsu F, et al: Carotid endarterectomy and prevention of cerebral ischemia in symptomatic carotid stenosis. Veterans Affairs Cooperative Studies Program 309 Trialist Group, *JAMA* 266:3289-3294, 1991.
7. Brisman JL, Mayberg MR: Surgical management of symptomatic carotid disease: Carotid endarterectomy and extracranial-intracranial bypass. In Gillard J, Graves M, Hatsukami T, et al: *Carotid disease: The role of imaging in diagnosis and management*, Cambridge, UK, 2006, Cambridge University Press, pp 72-85.
8. Failure of extracranial-intracranial arterial bypass to reduce the risk of ischemic stroke: Results of an international randomized trial. The EC/IC Bypass Study Group, *N Engl J Med* 313:1191-1200, 1985.
9. Beneficial effect of carotid endarterectomy in symptomatic patients with high-grade carotid stenosis: North American Symptomatic Carotid Endarterectomy Trial Collaborators, *N Engl J Med* 325:445-453, 1991.
10. Moore WS, Barnett HJ, Beebe HG, et al: Guidelines for carotid endarterectomy. A multidisciplinary consensus statement from the Ad Hoc Committee, American Heart Association, *Circulation* 91:566-579, 1995.
11. Adams RJ, Albers G, Alberts MJ, et al: Update to the AHA/ASA recommendations for the prevention of stroke in patients with stroke and transient ischemic attack, *Stroke* 39:1647-1652, 2008.
12. Sacco RL, Adams R, Albers G, et al: Guidelines for prevention of stroke in patients with ischemic stroke or transient ischemic attack: A statement for healthcare professionals from the American Heart Association/American Stroke Association Council on Stroke: co-sponsored by the Council on Cardiovascular Radiology and Intervention: The American Academy of Neurology affirms the value of this guideline, *Stroke* 37:577-617, 2006.
13. Fields WS, Maslenikov V, Meyer JS, et al: Joint Study of Extracranial Arterial Occlusion. V. Progress report of prognosis following surgery or nonsurgical treatment for transient cerebral ischemic attacks and cervical carotid artery lesions, *JAMA* 211:1993-2003, 1970.
14. Shaw DA, Venables GS, Cartlidge NE, et al: Carotid endarterectomy in patients with transient cerebral ischaemia, *J Neurol Sci* 64:45-53, 1984.
15. Rothwell PM, Eliasziw M, Gutnikov SA, et al: Analysis of pooled data from the randomised controlled trials of endarterectomy for symptomatic carotid stenosis, *Lancet* 361(9352):107-116, 2003.
16. Rothwell PM, Eliasziw M, Gutnikov SA, et al: Endarterectomy for symptomatic carotid stenosis in relation to clinical subgroups and timing of surgery, *Lancet* 363(9413):915-924, 2004.
17. Henderson RD, Eliasziw M, Fox AJ, et al: Angiographically defined collateral circulation and risk of stroke in patients with severe carotid artery stenosis. North American Symptomatic Carotid Endarterectomy Trial (NASCET) Group, *Stroke* 31:128-132, 2000.
18. Kappelle LJ, Eliasziw M, Fox AJ, et al: Importance of intracranial atherosclerotic disease in patients with symptomatic stenosis of the internal carotid artery. The North American Symptomatic Carotid Endarterectomy Trial, *Stroke* 30:282-286, 1999.
19. Eliasziw M, Streifler JY, Fox AJ, et al: Significance of plaque ulceration in symptomatic patients with high-grade carotid stenosis. North American Symptomatic Carotid Endarterectomy Trial, *Stroke* 25:304-308, 1994.

20. Streifler JY, Eliasziw M, Benavente OR, et al: Prognostic importance of leukoaraiosis in patients with symptomatic internal carotid artery stenosis, *Stroke* 33:1651–1655, 2002.

21. International Carotid Stenting Study investigators, Ederle J, Dobson J, Featherstone RL, et al: Carotid artery stenting compared with endarterectomy in patients with symptomatic carotid stenosis (International Carotid Stenting Study): An interim analysis of a randomised controlled trial, *Lancet* 375(9719):985–997, 2010.

22. Brott TG, Hobson RW 2nd, Howard G, et al: CREST Investigators: Stenting versus endarterectomy for treatment of carotid-artery stenosis, *N Engl J Med* 363:80–82, 2010.

76

Surgical Management of Asymptomatic Carotid Stenosis

MOHAMED SAMY ELHAMMADY, ROBERTO C. HEROS, JACQUES J. MORCOS

Ischemic stroke remains one of the most common disabling illnesses in developed countries, ranking third as the cause of death.[1] Approximately 795,000 Americans will have a new or recurrent stroke every year, which will result in approximately 143,000 deaths.[1] The permanence of the disability endured by many of the survivors of stroke places a tremendous toll on our socioeconomic system. In 2009, it was estimated that Americans would pay $68.9 billion for stroke-related medical costs and disability.[1] The potential impact of preventive medical or surgical measures is therefore of paramount importance.

The management of asymptomatic carotid artery stenosis (CAS) is based on an understanding of the natural history as well as the risks and long-term benefits of intervention.

Natural History

Patients with asymptomatic carotid stenosis are frequently incidentally identified by noninvasive screening tests such as carotid ultrasonography, by auscultation of a carotid bruit during routine physical examinations, or during evaluation of a contralateral symptomatic carotid stenosis. The prevalence of asymptomatic CAS greater than 50% and greater than 80% has been estimated to be 2% to 8% and 1% to 2%, respectively.[2] The prevalence is higher with advanced age and associated vascular risk factors such as cervical bruits, coronary artery disease, hypercholesterolemia, diabetes, peripheral occlusive disease, and smoking.

Our knowledge of the natural history of asymptomatic CAS has been obtained from screening and follow-up studies, studies comparing carotid endarterectomy (CEA) with medical treatment, and studies in patients undergoing CEA for ipsilateral symptomatic stenosis who have concomitant asymptomatic contralateral disease. Three specific factors have been shown to affect outcome: (1) severity of stenosis (2) progression of stenosis, and (3) presence or absence of plaque ulceration.[3]

Effect of Stenosis Severity

It is clear from the literature that the risk of an ipsilateral neurologic event is directly related to the degree of asymptomatic carotid stenosis. In a review article by Rijbroek et al[2] it was found that the published annual risk of a neurologic deficit for asymptomatic carotid stenosis

of less than 50%, 50% to 80%, and greater than 80% was between 0% to 3.8%, 2% to 5%, and 1.7% to 18%, respectively. It should be noted, however, that the majority of these events were transient ischemic attacks or amaurosis fugax. The annual risk of a stroke was determined to be less than 1%, 0.8% to 2.4%, and 1% to 5% for asymptomatic carotid stenosis of less than 50%, 50% to 80%, and greater than 80%, respectively.

Effect of Stenosis Progression

Although most studies demonstrate an increased rate of ipsilateral neurologic events with stenosis progression, the annual incidence of stroke in the patients who progressed remains low (<5%). This is particularly true for stenosis greater than 80%.[4-6] The risk of progression of an asymptomatic CAS increases with time and is highly unpredictable. Estimated progression rates range anywhere from 4% to 29% per year, depending on the studied population and how stenosis progression is defined.[2]

Effect of Plaque Ulceration

The presence of plaque ulceration as well as the size and extent of the ulcer has been found to be a marker of future cerebrovascular events. Ulcer size can be measured by multiplying the length and the width in millimeters on conventional angiography. On the basis of these measurements, ulcers are classified into small type A (<10 mm^2), large type B (10 to 40 mm^2), and compound type C (>40 mm^2).[7] Independent of associated carotid stenosis, the presence of a type C ulcer has been shown to result in an annual stroke rate of 7.5%.[7] Type A ulcers, on the other hand, have a more benign prognosis: they are associated with an annual stroke rate of 0.4%.[8] The natural history of type B ulcers remains unclear because of conflicting reports regarding the risk of future neurologic events.[3]

Carotid Endarterectomy versus Medical Management

Few conditions have resulted in as much controversy as the management of carotid artery disease. Since the first description of a CEA[9] for the prevention of stroke, there has been doubt as to the effectiveness of the procedure for symptomatic stenosis. The debate has been put to rest after the results of the North American Symptomatic

Carotid Endarterectomy Trial (NASCET)[10,11] and the European Carotid Surgery Trial (ECST),[12,13] which clearly demonstrated the superiority of CEA for symptomatic severe carotid artery disease as compared with best medical therapy (BMT). A similar trend had been observed in a smaller trial involving symptomatic patients in United States Veterans Affairs hospitals before the trial was prematurely terminated because of the conclusions of the North American and European trials.[14] The efficacy of CEA for symptomatic carotid artery disease prompted similar studies to assess the effects of prophylactic CEA for asymptomatic CAS. Five prospective randomized trials were designed to study the efficacy of prophylactic CEA for the treatment of patients with asymptomatic CAS.

The Carotid Artery Stenosis with Asymptomatic Narrowing: Operation Versus Aspirin (CASANOVA) was the first study, published in 1991.[15] This was a multicenter trial consisting of 410 patients with asymptomatic CAS measuring 50% to 90%. Patients were randomly assigned after angiography to surgery versus medical therapy alone. All patients received daily aspirin and dipyridamole. The minimum follow-up period was 3 years. The study demonstrated no significant difference in the number of strokes and death between the surgical and medical groups. Unfortunately, the study had an unusually complicated protocol and excluded patients with greater than 90% stenosis. Furthermore, the combined complication rate of angiography and surgery was exceedingly high (6.9%).

The following year, the Mayo Clinic trial was published.[16] This was a single center study comparing CEA alone with aspirin therapy. The study was terminated early, only after 71 patients had been randomly assigned, because of a significantly higher number of myocardial infarctions and transient cerebral ischemic events in the surgical group. It was presumed that these events were related to the absence of aspirin use in the patients undergoing CEA and therefore reinforced the importance of aspirin administration throughout the perioperative period and beyond. Although there had been more ischemic events in the surgical group than in the medical group, the small number of patients and short follow-up did not allow any conclusions to be drawn.

In 1993 the Veterans Affairs Cooperative Study (VACS) was published and demonstrated a reduction of ipsilateral neurologic events after CEA plus aspirin–antiplatelet therapy as compared with antiplatelet therapy alone (8% versus 20.6%).[17] Unfortunately, the proposed sample size was not large enough to provide statistical power, and the study failed to show a reduction of ipsilateral strokes or death. Nonetheless, after a 4-year follow-up period, the ipsilateral stroke rate in the surgical group was 4.7% in contrast to 9.4% in the medical group. However, when the perioperative mortality (1.9%) was added to the surgical stroke rate, the difference between the two groups did not reach statistical significance. Most deaths were secondary to myocardial infarction. The trial did not include women.

The Asymptomatic Carotid Atherosclerosis Study (ACAS), published in 1995, was a prospective randomized multicenter trial comparing the efficacy of CEA and medical therapy to BMT alone in preventing ipsilateral stroke during a 5-year period.[18] The study consisted of 1662 patients from 39 centers across the United States

and Canada with asymptomatic CAS greater than 60%. The median follow-up was 2.7 years, and 9% of patients completed 5 years of follow-up. The estimated 5-year risk of ipsilateral stroke and any perioperative stroke or death was 5.1% and 11.0% for the surgical and medical groups, respectively. CEA reduced the 5-year stroke risk by 66% in men and by 17% in women. Overall, the risk of ipsilateral stroke was reduced by 53% and remained statistically significant at 3 years' follow-up. CEA, however, did not significantly protect against major strokes or death. The surgical morbidity and mortality rate was surprisingly low: 1.5% and 0.1%, respectively. Approximately half of the total morbidity was related to angiography. A statistical benefit from CEA was seen within less than 1 year after surgery.

The Asymptomatic Carotid Surgery Trial (ACST) was published in 2004 and is the largest multicenter trial to date.[19] The study consisted of 3120 patients with greater than 60% asymptomatic stenosis (diagnosed by duplex ultrasound) randomly assigned to immediate CEA or medical therapy at the discretion of the treating physician. Of the patients randomly assigned to CEA, 50% underwent surgery within 1 month and 88% underwent surgery within 1 year. Exclusion criteria included poor surgical risk, prior ipsilateral CEA, and probable cardiac emboli. Surgeons were required to have a perioperative morbidity and mortality rate of less than 6%. The mean follow-up was 3.4 years. The perioperative morbidity and mortality rate was 3.1%. The net 5-year risk of all strokes and death including perioperative stroke and death was 6.4% and 11.8% in the CEA and medical groups, respectively. Fatal or disabling strokes rates were 3.5% versus 6.1%. Fatal stroke rates alone were 2.1% versus 4.2%. Both men and women benefited from CEA, although there was a greater benefit in men. CEA did not demonstrate a statistically significant benefit for patients older than 75 years. In contrast to the ACAS study, the ACST did not show statistical benefit in the immediate CEA group until nearly 2 years after surgery. This was most likely due to the lower perioperative event rates demonstrated in the ACAS.

Although the ACAS and ACST have shown that CEA is beneficial for asymptomatic CAS greater that 60%, the benefits were not as convincing as the NASCET and ECST results for symptomatic patients. The American Heart Association (AHA) Stroke Council recommended that, for CEA to be efficacious, the combined perioperative death and stroke rate should be less than 3% in asymptomatic patients, 5% for patients with transient ischemic attacks, 7% for patients with a prior stroke, and 10% for patients undergoing surgery for recurrent stenosis.[20]

Carotid Endarterectomy Versus Carotid Artery Stenting

There has been only one randomized trial comparing CEA to carotid artery stenting in asymptomatic "standard risk" patients. In a single institution study, Brooks et al[21] randomly assigned 85 asymptomatic patients with greater than 80% carotid stenosis to CEA or stenting. The follow-up period was 48 months. The postoperative pain, length of hospital stay, return to full activity, and cost were similar in both groups. Furthermore, there was no stroke or death

TABLE 76-1   CRITERIA FOR HIGH RISK IN SAPPHIRE TRIAL*

1. Clinically significant cardiac disease (congestive heart failure, abnormal stress test, or need for open heart surgery)
2. Severe pulmonary disease
3. Contralateral carotid occlusion
4. Contralateral laryngeal nerve palsy
5. Previous radical neck surgery or radiation therapy to the neck
6. Recurrent stenosis after carotid endarterectomy
7. Age >80 years

*At least one factor required.
SAPPHIRE, Stenting and Angioplasty with Protection in Patients at High Risk for Endarterectomy.

in either limb of the trial in the perioperative period or during long-term follow-up. In view of the small number of patients enrolled and the lack of difference in outcomes, the study did not greatly influence current clinical practice.

Very recently, the results of two multicenter RCTs comparing CEA to CAS in "standard risk" patients have become available and are certain to have a marked influence on current practice. The first trial was the interim analysis of the International Carotid Stenting Study (ICSS).[22] This was an international prospective multicenter RCT comparing CEA to CAS in recently (within 12 months) symptomatic patients with greater than 50% by NASCET criteria. Based on the interim analysis, the authors concluded that CEA should remain the treatment of choice for patients suitable for surgery. The second trial was the Carotid Revascularization Endarterectomy versus Stenting Trial (CREST).[22a] This was a prospective multicenter RCT comparing CEA and CAS in both symptomatic (≥50% by angiography, ≥70% by ultrasound, CT, or MR angiography) and asymptomatic patients (≥60% by angiography, ≥70% by ultrasound, ≥80% by CT or MR angiography). The authors concluded that CAS and CEA had similar short- and long-term outcomes.

Based on the available literature, we conclude that there is now level 1 evidence that in "standard risk" patients, the risk of stroke is clearly lower with CEA as compared to CAS. On the other hand, CEA seems to be associated with a higher risk of myocardial infarction. Given the greater impact of stroke on the quality of life of patients as compared to myocardial infarction, CEA should remain the treatment of choice in patients without a significant cardiac history. In the very few months since the publication of the CREST results, we have already witnessed an increase in the proportion of CEA patients.

Decision Making and Patient Selection

The benefit of prophylactic CEA for asymptomatic CAS appears to be low; therefore, it is necessary to identify factors, in addition to the degree of maximal vessel narrowing, that can improve patient selection.

Age and Life Expectancy

Advanced age, itself, is not an absolute contraindication for CEA. Elderly patients should be selected according to the same criteria as their younger counterparts.

Nonetheless, it is important to take into account the patient's life expectancy and associated surgical comorbidities. In the NASCET and ACAS trials, age older than 80 years was considered to be an exclusion criterion.[10,11,18] In the ACST, CEA did not demonstrate a statistically significant benefit for patients older than 75 years.[19] In a multicenter review by Goldstein et al[23] analyzing the impact of potential preoperative risk factors on the frequency of postoperative complications in 463 patients undergoing CEA for asymptomatic CAS, it was found that the postoperative stroke or death rate was 7.8% in patients older that 75 years as compared with 1.8% in patients younger than 75 years.

Gender

Women undergoing CEA for asymptomatic CAS appear to have a higher perioperative risk of stroke than men. In the ACAS, the procedural complication rates were 3.6% for women and 1.7% in males.[18] The overall benefit of CEA was found to be less profound in women: a 5-year stroke risk reduction of 17% was seen in women as compared with 66% in males. Similar findings were reported in the review by Goldstein et al,[23] in which postoperative stroke and death were more frequent in women (5.3% versus 1.6% in men). This raises the question of whether prophylactic CEA should be considered at all for women with asymptomatic carotid artery disease, particularly when the overall benefit of CEA appears to be low.

Carotid Plaque Morphology

There has been interest in carotid plaque morphology as a prognostic marker for future cerebrovascular ischemic events. The degree of plaque echogenicity, based on carotid ultrasonography, has been used as an indicator of plaque stability. Echolucent or hypoechoic plaques suggest greater amounts of lipids and have been associated with symptomatic unstable lesions. On the other hand, echo-rich or hyperechoic plaques have been more commonly seen with asymptomatic lesions.[24,25] Unfortunately ultrasonographic plaque evaluation is highly operator-dependent and therefore should be complemented with or replaced by more objective evaluation methods such as video densitometric analysis, which is commercially available, relatively cheap, and investigator-independent.[26]

The use of spiral CT in assessing plaque morphology has gained interest in recent years. Spiral CT, however, primarily identifies plaque calcification and not the more relevant lipid component; therefore, its significance in preoperative plaque characterization has yet to be determined. In a study comparing the degree of plaque calcification determined by preoperative spiral CT with the histologic extent of plaque macrophage infiltration, it was found that symptomatic plaques were less calcified and more inflamed than asymptomatic plaques and that a strong inverse correlation existed between the extent of carotid plaque calcification and the intensity of plaque fibrous cap inflammation.[27] Although these findings suggest a potential use for spiral CT in preoperative plaque evaluation, larger studies are necessary to investigate the risk of stroke and plaque calcification. Furthermore, spiral CT is time and resource demanding and involves use of both contrast and radiation, which increases the risk of allergic events and, possibly, cancer.[26]

Magnetic resonance imaging (MRI) has emerged as a viable technology for characterizing carotid atherosclerotic lesions with regard to size, composition, and biological activity.[28] The identification of unstable vulnerable plaques on MRI has correlated well with histopathologic sections and has an association with recent ischemic events.[29-31]

Contralateral Carotid Artery Disease

The impact of contralateral carotid artery disease on asymptomatic CAS must be considered with regard to its natural history and the risk of surgical intervention. There are, however, conflicting data in the literature.

In a post hoc analysis of the ACAS that compared 163 patients with baseline contralateral occlusion with 1485 patients with patent contralateral carotid arteries, it was found that the 5-year ipsilateral stroke rate in the surgically treated patients was 5.5% versus 5.0%, which suggests that there is no increased surgical risk in patients with contralateral occlusion.[32] Interestingly, however, medically treated patients *with* contralateral occlusion had a better clinical outcome than those *without* contralateral disease (5-year ipsilateral stroke rate, 3.5% versus 11.7%), which suggests a relatively benign natural history. This was believed to be due to development of collateral circulation secondary to the contralateral occlusion. These findings suggest that prophylactic endarterectomy for asymptomatic CAS in the presence of contralateral occlusion provides no long-term benefit in preventing stroke and death and may actually be harmful.

In contrast, a worse natural history was reported by Irvine et al[33] in a retrospective study consisting of 487 patients with asymptomatic CAS followed up for a mean of 41 months. The presence of bilateral carotid artery disease was found to significantly increase the risk of overall but *not* ipsilateral strokes (relative risk, 2.35). Patients with unilateral asymptomatic carotid artery disease had an overall stroke rate of less than 5% in the first year after presentation as compared with a stroke rate of 9.6% in patients with unilateral asymptomatic CAS and concomitant contralateral stenosis greater than 90%. Similar results were reported by AbuRahma et al[34] in a prospective study consisting of 82 patients with greater than 60% asymptomatic carotid stenosis and contralateral carotid occlusion. Patients were treated with maximal medical therapy for a mean follow-up period of 59.5 months. Late strokes occurred in 33% (23% ipsilateral and 10% contralateral) and transient ischemic attacks occurred in 27% of patients (9% ipsilateral and 18% contralateral), which suggests a higher incidence of ipsilateral stroke than that reported by the ACAS study.

The risk of CEA in the presence of contralateral carotid artery occlusion is debatable. The NASCET reported a combined perioperative stroke and death rate of 14.3% in patients with contralateral carotid occlusion as compared with 4% and 5.1% in patients with patent and mild-moderate stenosis of the contralateral carotid artery, respectively.[35] A similarly higher risk was reported in the

Acetylsalicylic Acid and Carotid Endarterectomy (ACE) trial.[36] This was a multicenter prospective randomized study evaluating the dose and role of acetylsalicylic acid in patients undergoing CEA. The study included 2804 patients, of which 54% (1512) were asymptomatic. Contralateral carotid artery occlusion (n = 236) was found to increase the perioperative risk of stroke and death by 2.3-fold. In a retrospective analysis of 1370 (54% asymptomatic) consecutive CEAs performed at a single institution, Reed et al[37] evaluated the effect of various preoperative risk factors on the incidence of perioperative (30-day) stroke and death. The overall stroke and death rates were 0.8% and 1.2%, respectively. Univariate analysis demonstrated that contralateral carotid occlusion (n = 75) was the only significant predictor of adverse outcome (6.7%) among the variables tested, and the relative risk was 4.3 on multivariate analysis (P = 0.01). Furthermore, the 5-year survival rate in patients with contralateral occlusion was found to be significantly lower than patients with patent contralateral carotid arteries (38% versus 67%). Similar findings were reported by Duncan et al[38] in a single institutional retrospective study consisting of 1609 consecutive CEAs of which 97 had contralateral carotid artery occlusion. The same-admission stroke and mortality rate was 5.2% as compared with 1.3% (P = 0.01) in patients with and without contralateral occlusion, respectively. Despite these findings, several large community observational studies involving both symptomatic and asymptomatic patients demonstrate no early or long-term significant differences between patients with and without contralateral carotid occlusion.[39-43]

In conclusion, although several studies have found no statistically significant difference in the perioperative stroke, death, and survival rates between CEAs in patients with or without contralateral carotid disease, there is a trend toward higher surgical risk in patients with contralateral carotid occlusion. Furthermore, there is a higher incidence of intraoperative electroencephalography (EEG) changes and subsequent shunt requirements in such patients. In two studies the incidence of intraoperative shunting was 46% and 52.9% in patients with contralateral carotid occlusion as compared with 13.5% and 4.8% in patients without contralateral occlusion.[39,40]

Concomitant Operations

At present, there are no clearly defined indications for managing asymptomatic CAS in patients undergoing general and vascular procedures, except in the case of coronary artery bypass grafting (CABG).[44] Three questions must be asked:

1. What is the incidence of perioperative stroke ipsilateral to an asymptomatic carotid stenosis during CABG?
2. Does prophylactic CEA reduce the incidence of perioperative and long-term stroke and mortality rates?
3. What is the appropriate timing of CEA in relation to the surgery in question? Before, simultaneously, or after?

Naylor et al[45] conducted a meta-analysis in an attempt to determine the role of carotid artery disease in the pathogenesis of post-CABG stroke. The perioperative risk of stroke was found to be 1.8% for patients with no significant carotid artery disease (<50% stenosis), 3.2%

in patients with unilateral 50% to 90% stenosis, 5.2% in patients with bilateral 50% to 90% stenosis, and 7% to 12% in patients with unilateral or bilateral carotid occlusion.

Das et al[46] performed a meta-analysis and determined stroke and mortality rates of 1.5% and 5.9%, respectively, in patients undergoing CEA followed by CABG, 3.8% and 4.4% for CABG then CEA, and 3.9% and 4.5% for simultaneous CABG and CEA. The authors concluded that prophylactic CEA before CABG was superior to alternative strategies. Similar findings were reached by Borger et al[47] in their meta-analysis addressing whether surgical staging was of benefit. CEA followed by CABG was found to be associated with stroke and mortality rates of 3.2% and 2.9% as compared with a combined approach that had associated stroke and mortality rates of 6% and 4.7%, respectively. Naylor et al[48] in 2003 conducted a systematic review of 97 published studies comprising 8972 staged or synchronous CEA and CABG operations. Approximately 60% of patients were asymptomatic. The risk rates of stroke for (1) synchronous, (2) staged CEA then CABG, and (3) staged CABG then CEA were 4.6%, 2.7%, and 6.3%, respectively. The operative mortality rates for (1) synchronous, (2) staged CEA then CABG, and (3) staged CABG then CEA were 4.6%, 3.9%, 2.0%, respectively. The authors concluded that overall there were no statistically significant differences in outcomes for staged and synchronous procedures and that there were no comparable data for patients with concomitant cardiac and carotid disease undergoing only CABG. Gaudino et al[49] in 2001 reported the 5-year follow-up of 139 patients with severe (>80%) asymptomatic CAS undergoing CABG at a single institution. Seventy-three patients underwent CABG alone; then there was a change in institutional policy, and 66 patients had synchronous or staged CEA. There was only one perioperative stroke in each group, but by 5 years, 17 (24%) who did not have CEA had a stroke compared with only one patient in the treatment group. In 1998, the AHA guidelines for CEA concluded that, in patients with an operative mortality of less than 3% and a life expectancy of more than 5 years requiring CABG with an asymptomatic CAS of more than 60%, CEA was an acceptable but not a proven indication (Grade C recommendation).[50] Patients with a higher risk of mortality may also have an acceptable indication if bilateral stenoses were present. This was also supported in the 2004 AHA guidelines on CABG, which concluded that CEA is "probably" indicated in asymptomatic stenosis greater than 80% (Grade C recommendation).[51]

In conclusion, low-risk patients with significant asymptomatic CAS should be considered for CEA at some stage. However, there is no strong evidence that indicates that this must be performed before or during CABG.[52] Nowadays, with the availability of stents, we prefer to give such patients stents unless there are anatomic factors preventing endovascular access.

Anesthetic Technique and Neuroprotection

CEAs may be performed under general or local anesthesia. Local anesthesia minimizes the anesthetic risk and potentially reduces the postoperative morbidity and length of hospital stay.[53,54] Furthermore, it allows patient examination during cross-clamping, which has been suggested to be a more reliable method of determining the need for a shunt than other monitoring techniques.[55] General anesthesia, on the other hand, provides a more controlled surgical environment while eliminating the psychological stress that remaining awake imposes on the patient. In a retrospective study comparing EEG changes in 255 consecutive patients undergoing CEA performed by two surgeons, of whom one used local and the other used general anesthesia, it was found that significant EEG changes and a subsequent need for shunting were less frequent with local anesthesia (6.3% versus 15.7%). There were, however, no differences in stroke rates, complications, lengths of hospital stay, or overall outcomes between both groups.[56] In an attempt to determine the impact of local and general anesthetics on clinical outcomes after carotid surgery, Papavasiliou et al[53] retrospectively reviewed their series of 803 consecutive CEAs. Regional and general anesthesia were used in 632 and 171 cases, respectively. The incidence of perioperative stroke and death did not differ significantly between the regional (2.7%) and the general anesthetic groups (2.3%). However, the incidence of nonneurologic, nonfatal complications (i.e., myocardial infarction, postoperative intubation, wound hematomas, cranial nerve injuries, and urinary retention) was significantly less in the regional anesthetic (1.6%) than in the general anesthetic group (14.6%). The results of the General Anesthesia versus Local Anesthesia (GALA) trial for carotid surgery have recently been published.[57] This was a multicenter (95 centers from 24 countries), randomized controlled trial consisting of 3526 patients with symptomatic and asymptomatic CAS. Patients were randomly assigned to CEA under general (n = 1753) or local anesthesia (n = 1773). The primary outcome was stroke (including retinal infarction), myocardial infarction, or death between randomization and 30 days after surgery. No significant difference was found between general and local anesthesia with regard to the primary outcome (4.8% versus 4.5%). Interestingly, a nonsignificant increased rate of myocardial infarction was noted with local anesthesia (0.5% versus 0.2%). Local anesthesia, however, did reduce the need for shunt insertion (14% versus 43%, $P < 0.001$). At our institution, we routinely perform CEA under general anesthesia for the previously mentioned reasons.

Normocapnia and the maintenance of blood pressure at least at preoperative levels are necessary for all patients. The role of preoperative colloid volume expansion in providing neuroprotection has been studied by Gross et al.[58] After the administration of 500 to 1000 mL of 6% hetastarch, the authors found a 40% decrease in incidence of EEG lateralization and a 63% decrease in EEG lateralization refractory to induced hypertension during carotid cross-clamping. The combined perioperative stroke and death rate was 1.3%.

Barbiturates have been used during CEA to increase tolerance to cerebral hypoperfusion. The mechanism of barbiturate neuroprotection is multifactorial and incompletely understood. It is believed to result from reversible, dose-dependent depression of cerebral blood flow and the subsequent reduction in cerebral metabolic rate and intracranial pressure.[59-62] Furthermore, vasoconstriction in normal areas of the brain may result in an inverse steal phenomenon in which cerebral blood flow is redistributed to ischemic tissue.[63] At a cellular level, barbiturates have been demonstrated to reduce ischemic-induced glutamate release,[64] enhance γ-aminobutyric acid (GABA)-ergic transmission,[65,66] and reduce ischemic-induced intracellular calcium levels through inhibition of both voltage-gated calcium channels and N-methyl-D-aspartate (NMDA) receptors.[67] In addition to the previously mentioned neuroprotective properties, barbiturates may also act as a scavenger of membrane-damaging free radicals.[60] Despite the potential benefits, the use of barbiturates is not without hazards. Circulatory and respiratory depression as well as delayed postoperative wakening may be problematic. The use of volume expansion as well as vasopressor agents may prevent or counter any intraoperative hypotension. However, patients with cardiac dysfunction may be better candidates for etomidate, a short-acting agent that results in reversible, dose-dependent reduction of the cerebral metabolic rate and has minimal cardiovascular depressive effects.[68,69] We have not espoused barbiturate or etomidate anesthesia at our institution but rather utilize modest hypothermia and induced hypertension during cross-clamping, unless a decline in somatosensory evoked potentials (SSEPs) or changes on EEG are observed.

Monitoring Techniques

Techniques capable of detecting cerebral ischemia during carotid artery cross-clamping may be classified as follows:
1. Monitoring of cerebral hemodynamics: transcranial Doppler sonography (TCD) and carotid artery stump pressure (SP)
2. Monitoring of cerebral oxygen metabolism: jugular bulb monitoring and near-infrared spectroscopy (NIRS)
3. Monitoring of cerebral functional state: EEG and SSEP

Despite numerous publications, there is little evidence to support the use of one form of monitoring over another in the determination of patients who require a shunt.[70]

TCD is used to continuously insonate the ipsilateral middle cerebral artery (MCA) during CEA. The baseline MCA velocities before carotid cross-clamping as well as the minimum blood flow velocities during clamping are measured, and the percentage of change is calculated. Inadequate temporal bone windows, however, may hinder the utility of TCD in up to 9.1% of patients.[71] In a study comparing the various techniques of cerebral monitoring in 48 patients undergoing CEA under regional anesthesia, Moritz et al[72] were unable to use TCD in 21% of patients because of inadequate bone windows or intraoperative dislocation of the Doppler probe. The proposed minimum MCA velocity cutoff values have widely varied in the literature from 10 cm/s to 25 cm/s.[72-74] Mortiz et al[72] noted that MCA velocities of 25 cm/s provided 100% sensitivity and 69% specificity. The authors also found that the relative change from baseline was more reliable than the absolute value. A 50% reduction in MCA velocities from baseline provided 100% sensitivity and 86% specificity.

SP measurement is a simple and inexpensive monitoring technique. A 22-gauge needle, with the distal third bent at approximately a 60° angle, is inserted into the common carotid artery (CCA) so that the bent portion of the needle parallels the axis of the vessel. The CCA systolic pressure is correlated with the radial artery systolic pressure so that no significant inflow stenosis occurs at the innominate or proximal CCA. The CCA below the needle and the external carotid artery (ECA) are then clamped. The residual pressure measured reflects the back pressure down the internal carotid artery (ICA) and should equal the pressure at the level of the MCA. Despite numerous reports validating SP recording during carotid surgery, there is no consensus on the appropriate cutoff value indicative of cerebral ischemia. Moritz et al[72] found that an SP cutoff of 40 mm Hg provided 100% sensitivity and 75% specificity. In a study correlating SP measurements with neurologic changes in 474 patients undergoing CEA under regional anesthesia, Calligaro et al[75] found that 0.9% of the patients (3 of 335) with SPs more than 50 mm Hg required shunting as compared with 22% (31 of 139) with SPs less than 50 mm Hg. Compared with a threshold of 50 mm Hg, a threshold of greater than 40 mm Hg was associated with a similar need for shunting in patients (1.0% [4 of 402]). However, the need for shunting was almost double (42% [30 of 72]) in patients with SPs less than 40 mm Hg as compared with patients with SPs less than 50 mm Hg. The authors concluded that using a SP threshold of 40 mm Hg resulted in a need for shunting in 15% of cases and a false-negative rate of 1.0% and was equivalent to the results of EEG monitoring during CEA reported in the literature.

Cerebral NIRS is a simple and noninvasive technique that allows continuous monitoring of regional cerebral oxygen saturation (rSo_2). The probe is positioned over the ipsilateral parietotemporal area just above the temporalis muscle. The minimum rSo_2 during carotid cross-clamping and the relative change compared with baseline are determined. Limitations of this technique include its regional nature, the high interpatient variability, and the unclear contribution of noncerebral tissues.[76] Moritz et al[72] found that a minimum rSo_2 of 59 provided 100% sensitivity and 47% specificity, whereas a 20% reduction from baseline was associated with 83% sensitivity and 83% specificity.

SSEPs have been reliably used during CEA to detect cerebral ischemia with 89% to 100% sensitivity and 93% to 100% specificity.[77,78] Recording steel EEG needles are inserted into the scalp above the ipsilateral somatosensory region (C3′ and C4′), and a reference electrode is placed over the forehead. The median nerve at the wrist contralateral to the operated side is then stimulated with an external bipolar electrode. Evoked potentials are recorded over the ipsilateral somatosensory cortex, and the amplitudes are determined as a percent of the baseline.

Intraoperative Carotid Shunting

Indications for carotid artery shunt placement during cross-clamping continue to be debatable. The main debate relates to whether *universal* or *selective* shunting should be used or whether shunting needs to be used at all. Advantages of shunting include a maximal degree of cerebral protection that, in turn, provides extra time for meticulous intimal dissection and arteriotomy closure. Intraoperative shunting, however, is not without risk. There is the potential for embolization of atherosclerotic debris, thrombotic material, or air during shunt placement as well as common carotid or distal ICA intimal damage resulting in postoperative thrombosis and carotid artery dissection. Furthermore, the presence of a shunt increases the technical difficulty during plaque dissection (in particular it increases the difficulty of the dissection of the distal portion of the lesion) and often necessitates a slightly longer arteriotomy than would have been needed otherwise. This is why some surgeons prefer never to use a shunt. At our institution, we selectively shunt when there are major changes in the SSEP or EEG during cross-clamping that cannot be reversed by inducing moderate hypertension. Our incidence of shunting is 5%. We favor using a simple Argyle straight shunt and introduce the proximal (common carotid) end first, bleed out any dislodged plaque material, then introduce the distal (internal carotid) end.

Carotid Patch Grafting

There are three schools of thought regarding the use of carotid patch graft angioplasty: patches should be used in every case, patches should be used in selective cases, and patches should never be used. Advantages of patching include enlargement of the endarterectomized segment, restoration of the normal carotid bulb morphology, and possibly a reduction in the incidence of recurrent stenosis.[79,80] Grafting, however, is not without disadvantages. The need to suture both sides of the graft increases both the operative as well as the cross-clamping time. Furthermore, patching makes the procedure more technically demanding and may be unnecessary in the majority of patients.[81]

Several graft materials have been used including saphenous vein, Dacron, and polytetrafluoroethylene (PTFE). Autologous saphenous vein grafts have the advantage of ease of handling and relative resistance to thrombosis and infection. Potential disadvantages include the increased operative time, limited availability in some patients, and morbidity related to harvesting. Cases of central patch rupture, particularly in women and patients with diabetes, have also been reported.[82] This can be minimized by harvesting the graft more proximally in the thigh rather than the ankle.[83,84] Another complication of vein grafting is postoperative ballooning of the graft, which may predispose to stagnation of blood flow and subsequent mural thrombus formation.[82] Unlike vein grafts, synthetic patches are readily available and avoid the morbidity associated with vein harvesting. Opponents of synthetic grafts, however, fear bleeding through the patch material, intraluminal thrombus formation, and infection.[81] In a single-institution prospective randomized trial consisting of 399 CEAs, AbuRahma et al[85] compared different methods of closure with regard to long-term clinical outcome and recurrent stenosis. In the comparison of primary closure (N = 135), PTFE patch grafting (N = 134), and vein grafting (N = 130), the incidence of ipsilateral stroke was 5%, 1%, and 0%, respectively, and mortality rates were similar at 30 months. The incidence of recurrent stenosis

and occlusion was higher with primary closure (34%) than with PTFE (2%) or vein grafting (9%), especially for women. The authors concluded that PTFE or vein grafting was superior to primary closure with regard to perioperative stroke and late recurrent stenosis, especially in women. Similar findings were noted in a prospective randomized trial of patients undergoing bilateral CEA.[81]

At our institution we generally perform CEA with primary closure of the arteriotomy. We believe that meticulous closure with minimal inclusion of the arterial wall within the 5-0 or 6-0 Prolene suture obviates the need for routine patch grafting. We do, however, reserve patch graft angioplasty for cases of radiation-induced or recurrent postoperative carotid stenosis (although these patients should be treated primarily with stenting today) as well as in patients (especially women) with small ICAs less than 3 mm in caliber.

Surgical Technique

The patient is positioned supine with the head turned slightly to the contralateral side. The degree of head rotation is determined by the relationship of the ECA and ICA on preoperative imaging. Normally the two arteries are nearly superimposed in the anteroposterior plane: the ICA usually lies posterior and slightly lateral to the ECA. Slight head rotation therefore brings the ICA in a more lateral and surgically accessible position. Excessive head rotation, on the other hand, should be avoided as this results in medial rotation of the sternocleidomastoid muscle over the carotid arteries. Occasionally, the ICA lies medial to the ECA, and this must be preoperatively recognized as it increases the technical difficulty. In such cases it may be necessary to extensively dissect the ECA to allow medial mobilization and exposure of the underlying ICA. In addition to head rotation, the neck is slightly extended by placement of an interscapular roll to facilitate deep exposure. A large mouth guard should be avoided so that the available submandibular space is maximized.

A linear skin incision is made along the anterior border of the sternocleidomastoid muscle extending two finger breadths above the clavicle to approximately two finger breadths below the angle of the mandible (Fig. 76-1). It is also acceptable to use a transverse skin crease incision for a slightly improved cosmetic result. If further rostral exposure is necessary, the upper end of the incision may be extended backward in a gentle curve toward the mastoid process so that injury of the mandibular branch of the facial nerve is avoided. Of note, the length of the skin incision should be adjusted appropriately for unusually high or low carotid bifurcations. Meticulous and thorough hemostasis at all stages of the procedure cannot be overstressed because this permits safe anatomic dissection and identification of vital structures and avoids excessive oozing after heparinization.

The platysma is then incised sharply; however, care should be taken to avoid injury to the great auricular nerve, which runs just beneath the muscle at the uppermost aspect of the incision. It is not uncommon to encounter the transverse cervical cutaneous nerve as it crosses the midbelly of the sternocleidomastoid muscle. Transection of this nerve may be necessary for exposure

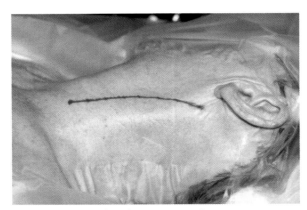

Figure 76-1 Carotid endarterectomy. The patient is positioned supine with the head turned slightly to the contralateral side and the neck slightly extended. The planned skin incision is marked along the anterior border of the sternocleidomastoid muscle, and the upper end should curve slightly toward the mastoid process so that injury of the mandibular branch of the facial nerve is avoided.

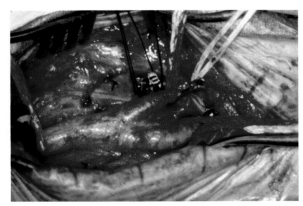

Figure 76-2 Carotid endarterectomy. The common, internal, and external carotid arteries and superior thyroid artery have been isolated, and the appropriate clamps and tapes have been placed.

and results in transient postoperative numbness in the anterior neck that typically disappears within 6 months as the nerve regenerates. The lesser occipital and spinal accessory nerves run along the posterior aspect of the sternocleidomastoid muscle and are rarely encountered or injured during the exposure. Self-retaining retractor blades must always be kept superficial on the medial side so that retraction injury to the laryngeal nerves is prevented; they may, however, be placed more deeply on the lateral side. Excessive retraction should be avoided as this may result in stretch injury of the spinal accessory nerve, which may manifest postoperatively as ipsilateral shoulder and neck pain, in addition to shoulder drooping.

The dissection is then carried along the anterior aspect of the sternocleidomastoid muscle. The carotid sheath is entered, and the internal jugular vein and ansa cervicalis nerve are identified. The ansa cervicalis is formed by the joining of a superior root, which descends from the hypoglossal nerve, and an inferior root, which originates from the ventral rami of C2 and C3, as they cross the internal jugular vein. The dissection is continued between the superior root of the ansa and the internal jugular so as to mobilize the nerve medially and the vein laterally. The medially situated common facial vein is frequently encountered during the dissection and must be ligated and divided so that the internal jugular vein can be mobilized laterally. Rarely, it may be necessary to divide the superior root of the ansa cervicalis so that the hypoglossal nerve can be mobilized medially and access to the carotid artery is improved.

The surgeon should carefully dissect the CCA while avoiding injury to the vagus nerve, which lies along the posterior aspect of the carotid vessels, although a rare anomaly involves an anterior position of the nerve. The dissection is then carried rostrally to free the origin of the ICA, ECA, and superior thyroid artery. The superior laryngeal nerve, which lies along the posterior aspect of the superior thyroid artery, may be injured during the exposure unless one limits the dissection of the superior thyroid artery to its first 1 to 2 mm, enough to place a temporary aneurysm clip or ligature on it. Dissection around

the bifurcation occasionally results in reflex bradycardia and hypotension due to stimulation of the carotid bulb via the nerve of Hering, which may be temporarily blocked with a local injection of 1% lidocaine. As the dissection progresses distally, the hypoglossal nerve should be identified and should be carefully mobilized medially. It is important to have adequate exposure of the ICA distal to the plaque, which can be readily palpated through the artery. Distal exposure can be facilitated greatly by retracting the digastric muscle rostroanteriorly with fish hooks and, occasionally, dividing the digastric muscle. In rare circumstances we have encountered the need to dislocate the temporomandibular joint, divide the sternocleidomastoid muscle, or divide the mandibular ramus. Once the ICA distal to the plaque has been exposed, rubber loops or umbilical tapes are passed around the CCA, ICA, and ECA. We also add Rummel tourniquets to the CCA and ICA loops in preparation for possible shunting. The superior thyroid artery is secured with a temporary aneurysm clip or temporary ligature (Fig. 76-2). At this stage of the procedure the patient is given an intravenous dose of 5000 to 7000 IU heparin, depending on weight, so that intravascular thrombosis does not occur during the period of temporary carotid occlusion. Neuroprotection is achieved with induced moderate hypertension (30% above baseline) and modest hypothermia. Atraumatic vascular clamps are then used in the following sequence: first on the ICA, then on the CCA, and finally on the ECA and superior thyroid artery. This sequence is important to prevent cerebral embolization of plaque or thrombotic material. An arteriotomy is then made with a No. 11 blade in the CCA just below the bifurcation. Some surgeons prefer to make the arteriotomy only down to the plaque and leave the plaque intact during its dissection, whereas others carry the arteriotomy through the plaque into the lumen. The arteriotomy is extended into the internal carotid artery distal to the plaque using Potts scissors. The proximal end of the plaque is circumferentially separated from the wall of the artery with the use of a No. 4 Penfield dissector, which allows complete transection of the plaque proximally (Figs. 76-3 and 76-4). The plaque is then elevated and carefully separated from the wall of the artery at the origin of the ECA through a wall

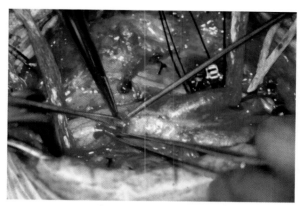

Figure 76-3 Carotid endarterectomy. The arteriotomy incision has been made down to but not through the atheromatous plaque, which is separated from the anterior wall of the artery using a Penfield No. 4 dissector.

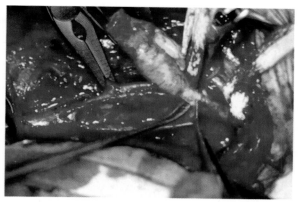

Figure 76-5 Carotid endarterectomy: The plaque has been removed from the external carotid artery and is carefully separated from the internal carotid artery so that it tapers off into the normal intima beyond the plaque.

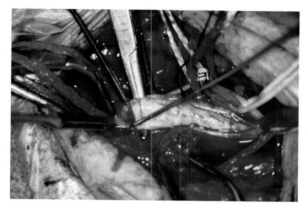

Figure 76-4 Carotid endarterectomy. A right-angled clamp has been placed around the proximal end of the atheromatous plaque, which is then cut sharply with a blade.

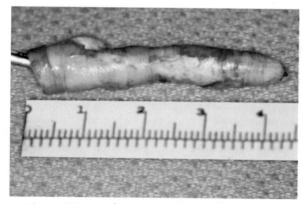

Figure 76-6 Atheromatous plaque after excision.

inversion technique, and the stump is sharply divided. A similar but more delicate technique is used for the distal ICA plaque, where an attempt is made to allow the distal feathery end of the plaque to naturally taper and transition off the normal intima beyond (Figs. 76-5 and 76-6). If the plaque does not separate perfectly, the intima should be trimmed carefully in an effort to prevent any flap formation and, if necessary, tacked down with a horizontal mattress suture, which is rarely needed. The internal surface of the carotid artery is irrigated with heparinized saline and inspected carefully for remaining atheromatous debris.

Once the surgeon is satisfied that the lumen is free of plaque and loose intima, the arteriotomy is closed under the microscope or with loupes with or without a patch from distal to proximal with the use of a running 5-0 or 6-0 Prolene suture, depending on the diameter of the ICA. A second suture is started from proximal to distal, and both sutures are tied together at their meeting point. Before the final tie, the following important sequence of unclamping is necessary. First the ICA is unclamped for 10 seconds to allow backwash of debris, then it is reclamped. Then the ECA and superior thyroid artery are unclamped, followed by the CCA. Ten seconds later,

the ICA is unclamped again, permanently. Cross-tying is performed while some bleeding or air bubbles escape through the arteriotomy.

Slight oozing along the suture line usually stops with pressure and a single layer of a hemostatic agent (Surgicel) over the arteriotomy. A final assessment of vessel patency is made with a handheld Doppler probe or, preferably, with a quantitative flow probe. The wound is copiously irrigated with antibiotic solution and then closed in two layers with absorbable sutures. We do not routinely reverse systemically administered heparin, although this has been advocated by some surgeons.[87]

Indications for shunt placement include a significant change in the EEG after cross-clamping and no improvement with induced hypertension (Fig. 76-7). The shunt is prepared by tying a silk suture around the midportion of the catheter. This serves as a marker so that the tube does not migrate after insertion and assists in shunt removal just before placement of the final arteriotomy sutures. After placement of the arterial clamps, a rapid arteriotomy is made down through the plaque. The length of the arteriotomy is slightly longer than that required for an endarterectomy without a shunt. The shunt tube is first passed proximally into the CCA, followed by tightening of the proximal tourniquet. The shunt is temporarily clamped and then gently passed distally into the ICA; trauma to the intima and formation of a flap by the

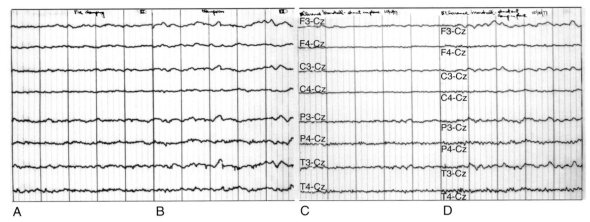

Figure 76-7 Electroencephalographic (EEG) recording during carotid endarterectomy. A, Preclamping EEG, demonstrating a normal tracing. B, Postclamping EEG without shunt, demonstrating slowing and reduced voltage. C, EEG after shunt insertion, demonstrating restoration of normal tracing. D, EEG recording after completion of the endarterectomy and removal of the shunt (with carotid cross-clamping), demonstrating once again slowing and reduced voltage.

catheter tip should be avoided. A tourniquet compresses the arterial wall around the distal end of the shunt, which is then unclamped. Dissection of the plaque commences. The proximal end of the plaque can be cut around the shunt with Potts scissors. Removal of the distal end of the plaque, on the other hand, may require temporary cross-clamping and removal of the distal catheter for meticulous plaque removal and avoidance of the formation of an intimal flap. The arteriotomy is closed with or without the use of a patch graft, as already described. Before placement of the final sutures, the shunt is clamped and removed. Bleeding is initially controlled with a tourniquet, and then clamps are applied to the CCA and ICA. The closure is then completed as usual.

As previously mentioned, removal of the plaque in the presence of a shunt increases the technical difficulty. Therefore an alternative method may be to proceed with plaque removal during cross-clamping, then place a shunt to leisurely remove any residual debris, and then finally close the arteriotomy. This method makes plaque dissection and removal easier and minimizes the risk of embolization or intimal dissection during shunt placement. Plaque removal during cross-clamping usually takes 5 to 10 minutes and is generally unlikely to result in a permanent ischemic deficit.

Complications and Postoperative Care

Basic principles of routine postoperative care should be observed with special attention to the monitoring of neurologic and cardiac status. We are particularly careful to avoid hypotension and order strict blood pressure control parameters aimed at keeping the systolic pressure above 110 mm Hg and below 170 mm Hg. Patients should be monitored in an intensive care or step-down unit overnight. The postoperative neurologic examination includes assessment of speech, motor, and lower cranial nerve function. Patients are usually transferred to a regular care bed and allowed to ambulate the next day. Most patients are discharged 1 to 2 days after surgery.

As previously mentioned, the overall risk of a CEA must be kept at a minimum to maintain its beneficial effect over the natural history. There are, however, definite inherent risks to the procedure.

Thromboembolic Events

Intraoperative ischemic events may occur at several stages during CEA. Extrinsic manual pressure transmitted to the carotid artery during preparation of the surgical field may shower emboli from a fragile plaque. This may also occur as the carotid artery is manipulated during the surgical dissection. Carotid cross-clamping may result in temporary cerebral hypoperfusion, which is frequently unrecognized in the absence of cerebral monitoring. Blood stasis during carotid clamping may also predispose to intravascular thrombosis and subsequent thromboembolic phenomena. Routine heparin administration before cross-clamping helps prevent this complication. Air emboli may occur during carotid artery unclamping if intraluminal air is not completely expelled before the closure of the arteriotomy. Removal of the atherosclerotic plaque exposes the underlying thrombogenic media to subsequent platelet aggregation and activation of the clotting cascade. This results in local platelet aggregation/thrombus formation with a potential for distal emboli and/or carotid occlusion. Preoperative, perioperative, and postoperative administration of aspirin and dipyridamole has been found to significantly reduce the degree of platelet aggregation at the endarterectomy site.[88] We routinely order preoperative daily aspirin for our patients, which is continued indefinitely after surgery.

Postoperative transient or fixed neurologic deficits require rapid assessment of carotid artery patency with duplex ultrasonography or angiography. Intracranial hemorrhage must also be ruled out with a brain CT scan. Any evidence of carotid artery occlusion or partial obstruction during the immediate postoperative period calls, in our opinion, for immediate reexploration.

Wound Hematomas

Postoperative hematomas are relatively common after CEA. In the NASCET study, 5.5% of patients had documented wound hematomas.[10] Fortunately, the majority of postoperative hematomas are small and can be managed conservatively. In 1119 CEAs performed in 1016 patients, reexploration of the wound was only necessary in 1.4% of patients.[89] Large or rapidly expanding hematomas, on the other hand, require surgical evacuation. If there is any evidence of stridor or significant tracheal deviation, the wound must be emergently opened. This can be done at the bedside, but if it can be done very expeditiously, it is best to take the patient to the operating room where the wound can be reopened emergently but under controlled circumstances and with a competent anesthesiologist in attendance. The patient can be quickly intubated if there is no muscle paralysis; however, it is important to never paralyze such patients in respiratory distress because intubation in the presence of major tracheal deviation can be difficult and traumatic, and an emergency tracheostomy, for which the surgeon must be always prepared, may be necessary. This can all be avoided by reopening of the wound under local anesthesia. Disruption of the arteriotomy may be found; however, this would be unusual. We have never encountered this complication. Most frequently, the surgeon finds diffuse oozing and tissue edema and, only occasionally, active arterial bleeding.

Hypertension and Hypotension

Blood pressure is frequently labile in the first 48 hours after a CEA because of the exposure of the carotid bulb to higher blood pressure or from surgically induced carotid baroreceptor dysfunction. It is therefore important to avoid long-acting vasoactive agents. Postoperative hypertension must be managed aggressively because it may predispose to neck hematomas, hyperperfusion syndrome, and intracerebral hemorrhage. In a retrospective review of 100 CEAs, postoperative hypertension (systolic blood pressure [SBP] > 200 mm Hg or diastolic blood pressure [DBP] > 100 mm Hg) was observed in 35% of cases.[90] Towne and Bernhard[91] reported a 19% incidence of postoperative hypertension, defined as a sustained elevation of SBP greater than 200 mm Hg, in 253 carotid procedures. The single most important determining factor for the development of postoperative hypertension was found to be the presence of preoperative hypertension. The incidence of preoperative hypertension in patients who developed postoperative hypertension was 79.6% compared with 57.4% in patients who did not develop this complication. Furthermore, there was a significantly increased incidence of neurologic deficits (10.2% versus 3.4%) and operative mortality in patients who developed postoperative hypertension.

Postoperative hypotension, defined as SBP less than 90 mm Hg, is not an infrequent occurrence and generally responds well to fluids (crystalloids or colloids) and low-dose phenylephrine. In a series of 180 consecutive CEAs reported by Gibbs,[92] postoperative hypotension was seen in 49 patients (27%). All cases had severe (80% to 99%) carotid stenosis preoperatively. Hypotension typically occurred 2 to 4 hours after surgery and resolved within 12 to 24 hours. Patients were rarely symptomatic, and all but one was managed by simple observation; no resulting complications or delay in discharge occurred. The author speculated that the occurrence of postendarterectomy hypotension may actually protect ischemic brain tissue from sudden hyperperfusion and, as such, should not be treated with vasopressor medication unless patients become symptomatic. A similarly benign outcome was reported by Wong et al,[93] who retrospectively reviewed 291 consecutive CEAs and found that the incidence of postoperative hypertension (SBP > 220 mm Hg), hypotension (SBP < 90 mm Hg), and bradycardia (pulse < 60) was 9%, 12%, and 55%, respectively. Only postoperative hypertension was associated with increased stroke, death, and cardiac complications. Although the occurrence of postoperative hypotension is relatively common and generally self-limited, it is still important to rule out myocardial infarction with serial electrocardiography and measurement of cardiac enzyme levels. As already stated, we do not have such a sanguine attitude toward postoperative hypotension and prefer to keep systolic pressure above 110 mm Hg with colloid infusion and vasopressors, if necessary.

Cerebral Hyperperfusion Syndrome

Cerebral hyperperfusion syndrome is a rare but serious complication after CEA. Patients will typically be seen with ipsilateral headaches relieved by upright position, eye pain, and/or seizures. It is believed to occur in patients with chronic cerebral hypoperfusion secondary to high-grade internal CAS. This, in turn, results in maximal vasodilatation in the ischemic brain region in an attempt to maintain cerebral blood flow. Long-standing vasodilatation results in defective cerebrovascular autoregulation and a subsequent inability of these vessels to vasoconstrict after endarterectomy and restoration of normal blood flow. The unprotected cerebral capillary bed is thus exposed to high perfusion pressure resulting in cerebral edema and, possibly, hemorrhage. In a series of 2747 consecutive CEAs performed at the Mayo Clinic, intracerebral hemorrhage occurred in 12 patients (0.4%).[94] All hemorrhages were ipsilateral to the CEA and occurred anywhere from the time of surgery to 8 days later (mean, 3.5 days). All cases had preoperative severe or near-occlusive CAS. Hemorrhages were associated with high mortality and morbidity rates. Seven patients died, and five had a poor outcome (modified Rankin Scale, 3 or more). Cerebral hyperperfusion syndrome, defined as hypertension with typical clinical symptoms or a doubling of intraoperative cerebral blood flow values, was found to be partly responsible in seven of the 12 cases. Other contributing mechanisms included perioperative cerebral ischemia (present in four cases) and anticoagulation therapy (present in six cases).

Seizures

Seizures after CEA are uncommon; the incidence is 0.4%[95] to 1%[96] and may result from postoperative cerebral infarction, intracerebral hemorrhage, or cerebral hyperperfusion syndrome.

Cranial and Sympathetic Nerve Injury

Nerve injuries are an uncommon but potentially serious complication of CEAs and may involve the mandibular branch of the facial nerve, the recurrent laryngeal, the superior laryngeal, spinal accessory, hypoglossal, or sympathetic nerves. Fortunately, the vast majority of cranial nerve palsies resolve over several months, so permanent deficits are rare. Cunningham et al[97] investigated the risk of cranial nerve injuries in patients who underwent CEA in the ECST. The strength of the study was that this was the largest series in which patients underwent neurologic assessments by a neurologist before and after surgery. Cranial nerve injuries were documented, and persisting deficits were identified on follow-up examination at 4 months and 1 year. A total of 88 motor cranial nerve injures (5.1%) occurred among 1739 patients undergoing CEA. In 23 patients, the deficit resolved by hospital discharge, which left 3.7% of patients with a residual deficit. At 4 months' follow-up, only 9 patients (0.5%) had a persisting deficit, from which none recovered.

Myocardial Infarction

Myocardial infarction is one of the most common complications associated with CEA. This is most likely related to the frequent concurrent occurrence of coronary and carotid atherosclerotic disease. The reported general incidence of perioperative myocardial infarction after CEA is approximately 1% to 4%.[98] Operative stress from surgery in addition to perioperative hypertension, increased vascular volume, tachycardia, and the use of intraoperative barbiturates may be predisposing factors. Careful preoperative cardiac evaluation and strict attention to intraoperative and postoperative hemodynamic variables and cardiac monitoring help minimize perioperative cardiac morbidity.

Concluding Remarks and Personal Biases

As discussed at the beginning of this chapter, there is ample scientific support, including Level I evidence, for the performance of CEA in patients with asymptomatic carotid stenosis of more than 60%. Nevertheless, patients with asymptomatic carotid stenosis, while at risk of stroke in the future, do quite well when treated medically; in other words, the natural history of asymptomatic carotid stenosis is relatively benign when compared with, for example, the natural history of symptomatic patients with severe carotid stenosis. Thus, if CEA is to be performed in asymptomatic patients, it must be done with the expectation of minimal morbidity. Additionally, even in the absence of solid scientific evidence, it is logical to assume that the more severe the stenosis in asymptomatic patients, the more likely it is to result in stroke in the future. In other words, we should be particularly cautious in recommending endarterectomy to patients with only a moderate degree of stenosis.

Given the aforementioned considerations, we recommend CEA to asymptomatic patients only when they are relatively young (generally less than 75 or 80 years old) and do not have serious comorbidities that would increase the risk of surgery. In addition, we reserve endarterectomy only for those patients at the upper range of stenosis, generally those with more than 75%. Furthermore, we pay close attention to angiographic and anatomic features that could increase the risk of the operation. In general, we avoid recommending surgery to asymptomatic patients with such conditions as contralateral carotid occlusion, extremely high carotid bifurcation, stenosis due to previous neck irradiation, and delayed recurrent stenosis after endarterectomy. Importantly, we do not limit this risk assessment to the preoperative period, but we continue to assess the risk during the operation until such a point where we commit ourselves by making the arteriotomy. In other words, if additional factors increasing intraoperative risk are encountered during surgery, we abandon the operation.

Finally, the controversial issue of CEA versus carotid angioplasty and stenting is specifically addressed elsewhere in this book. In general, we prefer CEA over angioplasty and stenting in most patients with asymptomatic carotid stenosis. The exception in our practice has been with patients that are relatively young, have very severe asymptomatic carotid stenosis, and yet would be high surgical risks because of serious comorbidities. Of course, a good alternative in these patients is to treat them conservatively given the relatively benign natural history of asymptomatic carotid stenosis. In elderly patients, regardless of the degree of stenosis, we prefer conservative treatment to either endarterectomy or angioplasty and stenting.

REFERENCES

1. American Heart Association: Heart Disease and Stroke Statistics-2009 update: http://www.americanheart.org.
2. Rijbroek A, Wisselink W, Vriens EM, et al: Asymptomatic carotid artery stenosis: Past, present and future. How to improve patient selection? *Eur Neurol* 6:139-154, 2006.
3. Moore WS, Barnett HJ, Beebe HG, et al: Guidelines for carotid endarterectomy. A multidisciplinary consensus statement from the ad hoc committee, American Heart Association, *Stroke* 26:188-201, 1995.
4. Roederer GO, Langlois YE, Lusiani L, et al: Natural history of carotid artery disease on the side contralateral to endarterectomy, *J Vasc Surg* 1:62-72, 1984.
5. Johnson BF, Verlato F, Bergelin RO, et al: Clinical outcome in patients with mild and moderate carotid artery stenosis, *J Vasc Surg* 21:120-126, 1995.
6. Mackey AE, Abrahamowicz M, Langlois Y, et al: Outcome of asymptomatic patients with carotid disease. Asymptomatic Cervical Bruit Study Group, *Neurology* 48:896-903, 1997.
7. Dixon S, Pais SO, Raviola C, et al: Natural history of nonstenotic, asymptomatic ulcerative lesions of the carotid artery. A further analysis, *Arch Surg* 117:1493-1498, 1982.
8. Moore WS, Boren C, Malone JM, et al: Natural history of nonstenotic, asymptomatic ulcerative lesions of the carotid artery, *Arch Surg* 113:1352-1359, 1978.
9. Eastcott HH, Pickering GW, Rob CG: Reconstruction of internal carotid artery in a patient with intermittent attacks of hemiplegia, *Lancet* 267:994-996, 1954.
10. North American Symptomatic Carotid Endarterectomy Trial Collaborators: Beneficial effect of carotid endarterectomy in symptomatic patients with high-grade carotid stenosis, *N Engl J Med* 325:445-453, 1991.
11. Barnett HJ, Taylor DW, Eliasziw M, et al: Benefit of carotid endarterectomy in patients with symptomatic moderate or severe stenosis. North American Symptomatic Carotid Endarterectomy Trial Collaborators, *N Engl J Med* 339:1415-1425, 1998.
12. European Carotid Surgery Trialists' Collaborative Group: MRC European Carotid Surgery Trial: Interim results for symptomatic patients with severe (70-99%) or with mild (0-29%) carotid stenosis, *Lancet* 337:1235-1243, 1991.

13. Randomised trial of endarterectomy for recently symptomatic carotid stenosis: Final results of the MRC European Carotid Surgery Trial (ECST), *Lancet* 351:1379-1387, 1998.

14. Mayberg MR, Wilson SE, Yatsu F, et al: Carotid endarterectomy and prevention of cerebral ischemia in symptomatic carotid stenosis. Veterans Affairs Cooperative Studies Program 309 Trialist Group, *JAMA* 266:3289-3294, 1991.

15. The CASANOVA Study Group: Carotid surgery versus medical therapy in asymptomatic carotid stenosis, *Stroke* 22:1229-1235, 1991.

16. Mayo Asymptomatic Carotid Endarterectomy Study Group: Results of a randomized controlled trial of carotid endarterectomy for asymptomatic carotid stenosis, *Mayo Clin Proc* 67:513-518, 1992.

17. Hobson RW 2nd, Weiss DG, Fields WS, et al: Efficacy of carotid endarterectomy for asymptomatic carotid stenosis. The Veterans Affairs Cooperative Study Group, *N Engl J Med* 328:221-227, 1993.

18. Executive Committee for the Asymptomatic Carotid Atherosclerosis Study: Endarterectomy for asymptomatic carotid artery stenosis, *JAMA* 273:1421-1428, 1995.

19. Halliday A, Mansfield A, Marro J, et al: Prevention of disabling and fatal strokes by successful carotid endarterectomy in patients without recent neurological symptoms: Randomised controlled trial. MRC Asymptomatic Carotid Surgery Trial (ACST) Collaborative Group, *Lancet* 363:1491-1502, 2004.

20. Beebe HG, Clagett GP, DeWeese JA, et al: Assessing risk associated with carotid endarterectomy. A statement for health professionals by an Ad Hoc Committee on Carotid Surgery Standards of the Stroke Council, American Heart Association, *Circulation* 79: 472-473, 1989.

21. Brooks WH, McClure RR, Jones MR, et al: Carotid angioplasty and stenting versus carotid endarterectomy for treatment of asymptomatic carotid stenosis: A randomized trial in a community hospital, *Neurosurgery* 54:318-324, 2004.

22. Ederle J, Dobson J, Featherstone RL, et al: Carotid artery stenting compared with endarterectomy in patients with symptomatic carotid stenosis (International Carotid Stenting Study): an interim analysis of a randomised controlled trial, International Carotid Stenting Study investigators, *Lancet* 375:985-997, 2010.

22a. Mantese VA, Timaran CH, Chiu D, et al: The Carotid Revascularization Endarterectomy versus Stenting Trial (CREST): stenting versus carotid endarterectomy for carotid disease. CREST Investigators, *Stroke* 41:S31-S34, 2010.

23. Goldstein LB, Samsa GP, Matchar DB, et al: Multicenter review of preoperative risk factors for endarterectomy for asymptomatic carotid artery stenosis, *Stroke* 29:750-753, 1998.

24. Grogan JK, Shaalan WE, Cheng H, et al: B-mode ultrasonographic characterization of carotid atherosclerotic plaques in symptomatic and asymptomatic patients, *J Vasc Surg* 42:435-441, 2005.

25. Geroulakos G, Ramaswami G, Nicolaides A, et al: Characterization of symptomatic and asymptomatic carotid plaques using high-resolution real-time ultrasonography, *Br J Surg* 80:1274-1277, 1993.

26. Grønholdt ML: B-mode ultrasound and spiral CT for the assessment of carotid atherosclerosis, *Neuroimaging Clin N Am* 12:421-435, 2002.

27. Shaalan WE, Cheng H, Gewertz B, et al: Degree of carotid plaque calcification in relation to symptomatic outcome and plaque inflammation, *J Vasc Surg* 40:262-269, 2004.

28. Yuan C, Kerwin WS, Yarnykh VL, et al: MRI of atherosclerosis in clinical trials, *NMR Biomed* 19:636-654, 2006.

29. Yuan C, Miller ZE, Cai J, et al: Carotid atherosclerotic wall imaging by MRI, *Neuroimaging Clin N Am* 12:391-401, 2002.

30. Cappeller WA, Schlüter A, Hammer A, et al: Morphologic carotid plaque characteristics in symptomatic and asymptomatic patients on MRI compared to histopathologic and macroscopic criteria, *Chirurg* 74:743-748, 2003.

31. Murphy RE, Moody AR, Morgan PS, et al: Prevalence of complicated carotid atheroma as detected by magnetic resonance direct thrombus imaging in patients with suspected carotid artery stenosis and previous acute cerebral ischemia, *Circulation* 107:3053-3058, 2003.

32. Baker WH, Howard VJ, Howard G, et al: Effect of contralateral occlusion on long-term efficacy of endarterectomy in the asymptomatic carotid atherosclerosis study (ACAS). ACAS Investigators, *Stroke* 31:2330-2334, 2000.

33. Irvine CD, Cole SE, Foley PX, et al: Unilateral asymptomatic carotid disease does not require surgery, *Eur J Vasc Endovasc Surg* 16:245-253, 1998.

34. AbuRahma AF, Metz MJ, Robinson PA: Natural history of > or =60% asymptomatic carotid stenosis in patients with contralateral carotid occlusion, *Ann Surg* 238:551-561, 2003.

35. Gasecki AP, Eliasziw M, Ferguson GG, et al: Long-term prognosis and effect of endarterectomy in patients with symptomatic severe carotid stenosis and contralateral carotid stenosis or occlusion: Results from NASCET. North American Symptomatic Carotid Endarterectomy Trial (NASCET) Group, *J Neurosurg* 83:778-782, 1995.

36. Taylor DW, Barnett HJ, Haynes RB, et al: Low-dose and high-dose acetylsalicylic acid for patients undergoing carotid endarterectomy: A randomised controlled trial. ASA and Carotid Endarterectomy (ACE) Trial Collaborators, *Lancet* 353:2179-2184, 1999.

37. Reed AB, Gaccione P, Belkin M, et al: Preoperative risk factors for carotid endarterectomy: Defining the patient at high risk, *J Vasc Surg* 37:1191-1199, 2003.

38. Duncan JM, Reul GJ, Ott DA, et al: Outcomes and risk factors in 1,609 carotid endarterectomies, *Tex Heart Inst J* 35:104-110, 2008.

39. Mackey WC, O'Donnell TF Jr, Callow AD: Carotid endarterectomy contralateral to an occluded carotid artery: Perioperative risk and late results, *J Vasc Surg* 11:778-783, 1990.

40. Ballotta E, Da Giau G: Baracchini C: Carotid endarterectomy contralateral to carotid artery occlusion: Analysis from a randomized study, *Langenbecks Arch Surg* 387:216-221, 2002.

41. Pulli R, Dorigo W, Barbanti E, et al: Carotid endarterectomy with contralateral carotid artery occlusion: Is this a higher risk subgroup? *Eur J Vasc Endovasc Surg* 24:63-68, 2002.

42. Rockman CB, Su W, Lamparello PJ, et al: Reassessment of carotid endarterectomy in the face of contralateral carotid occlusion: Surgical results in symptomatic and asymptomatic patients, *J Vasc Surg* 36:668-673, 2002.

43. Grego F, Antonello M, Lepidi S, et al: Is contralateral carotid artery occlusion a risk factor for carotid endarterectomy? *Ann Vasc Surg* 19:882-889, 2005.

44. Paciaroni M, Caso V, Acciarresi M, et al: Management of asymptomatic carotid stenosis in patients undergoing general and vascular surgical procedures, *J Neurol Neurosurg Psychiatry* 76:1332-1336, 2005.

45. Naylor AR, Mehta Z, Rothwell PM, et al: Carotid artery disease and stroke during coronary artery bypass: A critical review of the literature, *Eur J Vasc Endovasc Surg* 23:283-294, 2002.

46. Das SK, Brow TD, Pepper J: Continuing controversy in the management of concomitant coronary and carotid disease: An overview, *Int J Cardiol* 74:47-65, 2000.

47. Borger MA, Fremes SE, Weisel RD, et al: Coronary bypass and carotid endarterectomy: Does a combined approach increase risk? A metaanalysis, *Ann Thorac Surg* 68:14-21, 1999.

48. Naylor AR, Cuffe RL, Rothwell PM, et al: A systematic review of outcomes following staged and synchronous carotid endarterectomy and coronary artery bypass, *Eur J Vasc Endovasc Surg* 25:380-389, 2003.

49. Gaudino M, Glieca F, Luciani N, et al: Should severe monolateral asymptomatic carotid artery stenosis be treated at the time of coronary artery bypass operation? *Eur J Cardiothorac Surg* 19:619-626, 2001.

50. Biller J, Feinberg WM, Castaldo JE, et al: Guidelines for carotid endarterectomy: A statement for healthcare professionals from a Special Writing Group of the Stroke Council, American Heart Association, *Circulation* 97:501-509, 1998.

51. Eagle KA, Guyton RA, Davidoff R, et al: ACC/AHA 2004 guideline update for coronary artery bypass graft surgery: A report of the American College of Cardiology/American Heart Association Task Force on Practice Guidelines (Committee to Update the 1999 Guidelines for Coronary Artery Bypass Graft Surgery). American College of Cardiology; American Heart Association, *Circulation* 110:340-437, 2004.

52. Murphy MO, Ghosh J, Omorphos S, et al: In patients undergoing cardiac surgery does asymptomatic significant carotid artery stenosis warrant carotid endarterectomy? *Interact Cardiovasc Thorac Surg* 4:344-349, 2005.

53. Papavasiliou AK, Magnadottir HB, Gonda T, et al: Clinical outcomes after carotid endarterectomy: Comparison of the use of regional and general anesthetics, *J Neurosurg* 92:291-296, 2000.

54. Harbaugh RE, Pikus HJ: Carotid endarterectomy with regional anesthesia, *Neurosurgery* 49:642-645, 2001.

55. Hans SS, Jareunpoon O: Prospective evaluation of electroencephalography, carotid artery stump pressure, and neurologic changes during 314 consecutive carotid endarterectomies performed in awake patients, *J Vasc Surg* 45:511-515, 2007.

56. Wellman BJ, Loftus CM, Kresowik TF, et al: The differences in electroencephalographic changes in patients undergoing carotid endarterectomies while under local versus general anesthesia, *Neurosurgery* 43:769-773, 1998.

57. Lewis SC, Warlow CP, Bodenham AR, et al: General anaesthesia versus local anaesthesia for carotid surgery (GALA): A multicentre, randomised controlled trial. GALA Trial Collaborative Group, *Lancet* 372:2132-2142, 2008.

58. Gross CE, Bednar MM, Lew SM, et al: Preoperative volume expansion improves tolerance to carotid artery cross-clamping during endarterectomy, *Neurosurgery* 43:222-226, 1998.

59. Howe JR, Kindt GW: Cerebral protection during carotid endarterectomy, *Stroke* 5:340-343, 1974.

60. Michenfelder JD, Milde JH, Sundt TM Jr: Cerebral protection by barbiturate anesthesia. Use after middle cerebral artery occlusion in Java monkeys, *Arch Neurol* 33:345-350, 1976.

61. Gross CE, Adams HP Jr, Sokoll MD, et al: Use of anticoagulants, electroencephalographic monitoring, and barbiturate cerebral protection in carotid endarterectomy, *Neurosurgery* 9:1-5, 1981.

62. Imparato AM, Ramirez A, Riles T, et al: Cerebral protection in carotid surgery, *Arch Surg* 117:1073-1078, 1982.

63. Feustel PJ, Ingvar MC, Severinghaus JW: Cerebral oxygen availability and blood flow during middle cerebral artery occlusion: effects of pentobarbital, *Stroke* 12:858-863, 1981.

64. Amakawa K, Adachi N, Liu K, et al: Effects of pre- and postischemic administration of thiopental on transmitter amino acid release and histologic outcome in gerbils, *Anesthesiology* 85:1422-1430, 1996.

65. Buggy DJ, Nicol B, Rowbotham DJ, et al: Effects of intravenous anesthetic agents on glutamate release: A role for GABA(A) receptor-mediated inhibition, *Anesthesiology* 92:1067-1073, 2000.

66. Bieda MC, MacIver MB: Major role for tonic GABA(A) conductances in anesthetic suppression of intrinsic neuronal excitability, *J Neurophysiol* 92:1658-1667, 2004.

67. Zhan RZ, Fujiwara N, Endoh H, et al: Thiopental inhibits increases in [Ca2+]i induced by membrane depolarization, NMDA receptor activation and ischemia in rat hippocampal and cortical slices, *Anesthesiology* 89:456-466, 1998.

68. Milde LN, Milde JH, Michenfelder JD: Cerebral functional, metabolic, and hemodynamic effects of etomidate in dogs, *Anesthesiology* 63:371-377, 1985.

69. Batjer HH, Frankfurt AI, Purdy PD, et al: Use of etomidate, temporary arterial occlusion, and intraoperative angiography in surgical treatment of large and giant cerebral aneurysms, *J Neurosurg* 68:234-240, 1988.

70. Bond R, Rerkasem K, Rothwell PM: Routine or selective carotid artery shunting for carotid endarterectomy (and different methods of monitoring in selective shunting), *Stroke* 34:824-825, 2003.

71. Ghali R, Palazzo EG, Rodriguez DI, et al: Transcranial Doppler intraoperative monitoring during carotid endarterectomy: Experience with regional or general anesthesia, with and without shunting, *Ann Vasc Surg* 11:9-13, 1997.

72. Moritz S, Kasprzak P, Arlt M, et al: Accuracy of cerebral monitoring in detecting cerebral ischemia during carotid endarterectomy: A comparison of transcranial Doppler sonography, near-infrared spectroscopy, stump pressure, and somatosensory evoked potentials, *Anesthesiology* 107:563-569, 2007.

73. Belardi P, Lucertini G, Ermirio D: Stump pressure and transcranial Doppler for predicting shunting in carotid endarterectomy, *Eur J Vasc Endovasc Surg* 25:164-167, 2003.

74. Giannoni MF, Sbarigia E, Panico MA, et al: Intraoperative transcranial Doppler sonography monitoring during carotid surgery under locoregional anaesthesia, *Eur J Vasc Endovasc Surg* 12:407-411, 1996.

75. Calligaro KD, Dougherty MJ: Correlation of carotid artery stump pressure and neurologic changes during 474 carotid endarterectomies performed in awake patients, *J Vasc Surg* 42:684-689, 2005.

76. Davies LK, Janelle GM: Con: All cardiac surgical patients should not have intraoperative cerebral oxygenation monitoring, *J Cardiothorac Vasc Anesth* 20:450-455, 2006.

77. Markand ON, Dilley RS, Moorthy SS, et al: Monitoring of somatosensory evoked responses during carotid endarterectomy, *Arch Neurol* 41:375-378, 1984.

78. Sbarigia E, Schioppa A, Misuraca M, et al: Somatosensory evoked potentials versus locoregional anaesthesia in the monitoring of cerebral function during carotid artery surgery: Preliminary results of a prospective study, *Eur J Vasc Endovasc Surg* 21:413-416, 2001.

79. Archie JP Jr: The geometry and mechanics of saphenous vein patch angioplasty after carotid endarterectomy, *Tex Heart Inst J* 14:395-400, 1987.

80. Wells DR, Archie JP Jr, Kleinstreuer C: Effect of carotid artery geometry on the magnitude and distribution of wall shear stress gradients, *J Vasc Surg* 23:667-678, 1996.

81. AbuRahma AF, Robinson PA, Saiedy S, et al: Prospective randomized trial of bilateral carotid endarterectomies: Primary closure versus patching, *Stroke* 30:1185-1189, 1999.

82. Yamamoto Y, Piepgras DG, Marsh WR, et al: Complications resulting from saphenous vein patch graft after carotid endarterectomy, *Neurosurgery* 39:670-675, 1996.

83. Archie JP Jr, Green JJ Jr: Saphenous vein rupture pressure, rupture stress, and carotid endarterectomy vein patch reconstruction, *Surgery* 107:389-396, 1990.

84. Donovan DL, Schmidt SP, Townshend SP, et al: Material and structural characterization of human saphenous vein, *J Vasc Surg* 12:531-537, 1990.

85. AbuRahma AF, Robinson PA, Saiedy S, et al: Prospective randomized trial of carotid endarterectomy with primary closure and patch angioplasty with saphenous vein, jugular vein, and polytetrafluoroethylene: Long-term follow-up, *J Vasc Surg* 27:222-232, 1998.

86. Spetzler RF, Martin N, Hadley MN, et al: Microsurgical endarterectomy under barbiturate protection: A prospective study, *J Neurosurg* 65:63-73, 1986.

87. Ferguson GG: Extracranial carotid artery surgery, *Clin Neurosurg* 29:543-574, 1982.

88. Findlay JM, Lougheed WM, Gentili F, et al: Effect of perioperative platelet inhibition on postcarotid endarterectomy mural thrombus formation. Results of a prospective randomized controlled trial using aspirin and dipyridamole in humans, *J Neurosurg* 63:693-698, 1985.

89. Ratcheson RA, Grubb RL: Surgical therapy for diseases of the extracranial carotid artery. In Schmidek HH, Sweet WH, editors: *Operative neurosurgical techniques: Indications, methods, and results,* ed 3, Philadelphia, 1995, WB Saunders Co, pp 877-928.

90. Benzel EC, Hoppens KD: Factors associated with postoperative hypertension complicating carotid endarterectomy, *Acta Neurochir (Wien)* 112:8-12, 1991.

91. Towne JB, Bernhard VM: The relationship of postoperative hypertension to complications following carotid endarterectomy, *Surgery* 88:575-580, 1980.

92. Gibbs BF: Temporary hypotension following endarterectomy for severe carotid stenosis: Should we treat it? *Vasc Endovasc Surg* 37:33-38, 2003.

93. Wong JH, Findlay JM, Suarez-Almazor ME: Hemodynamic instability after carotid endarterectomy: Risk factors and associations with operative complications, *Neurosurgery* 1:35-41, 1997.

94. Henderson RD, Phan TG, Piepgras DG, et al: Mechanisms of intracerebral hemorrhage after carotid endarterectomy, *J Neurosurg* 95:964-969, 2001.

95. Reigel MM, Hollier LH, Sundt TM Jr, et al: Cerebral hyperperfusion syndrome: A cause of neurologic dysfunction after carotid endarterectomy, *J Vasc Surg* 5:628-634, 1987.

96. Sundt TM Jr, Sharbrough FW, Piepgras DG, et al: Correlation of cerebral blood flow and electroencephalographic changes during carotid endarterectomy: With results of surgery and hemodynamics of cerebral ischemia, *Mayo Clin Proc* 56:533-543, 1981.

97. Cunningham EJ, Bond R, Mayberg MR, et al: Risk of persistent cranial nerve injury after carotid endarterectomy, *J Neurosurg* 101:445-448, 2004.

98. Guay J: Regional or general anesthesia for carotid endarterectomy? Evidence from published prospective and retrospective studies, *J Cardiothorac Vasc Anesth* 21:127-132, 2007.

77

Extracranial to Intracranial Bypass for Cerebral Ischemia

DAVID W. NEWELL, MARCELO D. VILELA

Providing additional blood supply to the brain in order to treat or prevent stroke has been a goal of neurosurgeons and neurologists for many decades. The concept of an extracranial to intracranial (EC-IC) bypass to increase brain blood flow in patients with symptoms caused by complete carotid artery occlusion was first suggested by Fisher[1] n 1951. The development of the operating microscope and advances in microsurgical techniques led to the field of cerebrovascular microsurgery and the possibility for surgical creation of direct connections between the extracranial and intracranial vasculature. In 1963, Woringer and Kunlin[2] sutured a saphenous vein graft from the cervical portion of the internal carotid artery (ICA) to its intracranial portion (intracranial ICA). The graft remained patent at the time of the patient's death from coronary artery disease a few days later. A subsequent report by Pool and Potts[3] describes an intracranial bypass graft to the anterior cerebral artery for a giant aneurysm. In 1967 the first superficial temporal artery to middle cerebral artery (STA-MCA) bypass was performed in a human by M.G. Yasargil, which led to the development of a series of new procedures for cerebral revascularization. During the decades that followed, this technique and other variations were employed as surgical treatments for occlusive cerebrovascular disease of the extracranial and intracranial cerebral vessels, skull base tumors, aneurysms, cerebral vasospasm, moyamoya disease, and cerebral ischemia from other causes. This chapter reviews the development of EC-IC bypass and the current status of this procedure for the treatment of cerebral ischemia.

Historical Aspects

The introduction of microvascular surgery to neurosurgery was made possible by the combined efforts and ideas of surgeons between 1960 and 1970. Some of the early investigators of the applications of these techniques were surgeons at the University of Vermont in Burlington. Jacobson and Suarez[4] employed the microscope to repair vessels in small animals using the principles and techniques introduced by Alexis Carrel, and were successful in achieving a 100% patency rate after reconstructing carotid arteries in animals using 7.0 atraumatic silk. R.M.P. Donaghy, in the division of Neurosurgery at the University of Vermont, conducted early investigations in the applications of microvascular techniques to the

field of neurosurgery.[5,6] He established a microsurgical laboratory in which he pursued intensive studies on arterial vasospasm and small vessel reconstruction in small animals. Using meticulous techniques, microinstruments and the surgical microscope, he was successful in reconstructing vessels less than 1 mm in diameter.[6]

M.G. Yasargil, working in the department of Neurosurgery in Zurich under Professor Hugo Krayenbuhl, also became interested in neurosurgical applications of microvascular surgery. His enthusiasm to learn techniques of cerebral revascularization increased after the publication of an extracranial to intracranial bypass performed on a patient who had an occluded internal carotid at the neck.[2] In 1965, Yasargil received training in Professor Donaghy's laboratory in Burlington, Vermont, in microvascular techniques utilizing the femoral and carotid arteries of small animals.[7] In 1966, the availability of a bipolar coagulator, together with the use of 9-0 sutures, allowed a major advance in the development of microsurgical revascularization, enabling the dissection of intracranial structures in a clean field and meticulous repair of intracranial vessels.[6] Initially, attempts to create a form of EC-IC bypass in small animals included a technique to interpose a femoral vascular graft from the common carotid artery to the MCA, which frequently led to graft thrombosis after the procedure. An alternative approach of performing a bypass from the STA to the MCA was then utilized. By the end of 1966, more than 30 of such STA-MCA operations in dogs had been performed, and the technique was later published in detail.[8]

Yasargil returned to Zurich and performed the first STA-MCA bypass on October 30, 1967, on a patient with Marfan's syndrome and a complete occlusion of the MCA.[6,9] Another STA-MCA bypass procedure was performed independently one day later by Donaghy. Yasargil later published a manuscript describing a series of nine cases in which STA-MCA bypass had been performed, in seven for occlusion of the internal carotid or middle cerebral artery and in two as an adjuvant to the surgical treatment of complex intracranial aneurysms.[6] The feasibility of creating an EC-IC shunt was thereby demonstrated, and a major step was made into the field of reconstructive intracranial vascular microneurosurgery.

Following these early developments there was great enthusiasm for this new technology, and many neurosurgeons learned to perform the technique. Most EC-IC

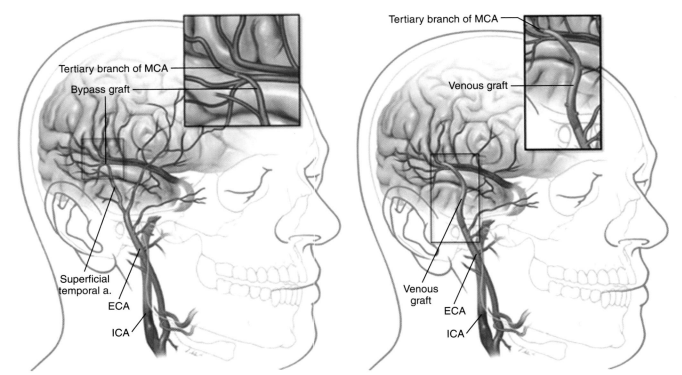

Figure 77-1 *Left,* Illustration of the completed superficial temporal artery (STA) to middle cerebral artery (MCA) (STA-MCA) bypass showing the frontoparietal branch of the STA connected to a distal surface branch of the MCA, immediately after it emerges from the distal portion of the sylvian fissure. *Right,* Illustration of an extracranial to intracranial bypass using a saphenous vein interposition graft from the proximal STA to a distal MCA branch. ECA, external carotid artery; ICA, internal carotid artery.

bypasses in the past were STA-MCA bypasses done for atherosclerotic cerebrovascular disease, but the procedure also became useful as an adjunct in the treatment of certain intracranial aneurysms or tumors that required flow augmentation, for planned vessel sacrifice, in carotid dissections with ischemia (Figs. 77-1 to 77-3), and for moyamoya disease.[10] Subsequently, bypass grafts using other donor arteries and the creation of interposition vein grafts between extracranial and intracranial arteries[11] (Fig. 77-1, *right*) as well as direct intracranial arterial to arterial anastomoses have been developed.[12,13] The use of nonsuture techniques for STA-MCA bypass has also been described.[14]

Initial Experience with Extracranial to Intracranial Bypass in Acute Brain Ischemia

The concept of performing an emergency cerebral revascularization procedure for acute ischemic stroke was reasonable, given the knowledge of ischemic thresholds for infarction and the concept of ischemic penumbra.[15] A method to provide additional blood flow to areas of the brain where the regional cerebral blood flow (rCBF) was low enough to decrease cellular function but not low enough to produce infarction was rational. Some encouraging results were published, but other studies reported that acute cerebral ischemia was a relative contraindication to an emergency bypass owing to poor results and a high rate of complications.[15-17] In reviewing 67 cases in which an emergency STA-MCA bypass

had been performed in the setting of acute cerebral ischemia, Crowell[15] found that 27 patients improved, 26 patients were unchanged, and 11 patients died. This researcher concluded that only those patients with crescendo transient ischemic attacks (TIAs) or mild to moderate deficits of less than 6 hours' duration with no infarct on imaging studies should be considered for an EC-IC bypass.

Subsequently, because of the lack of initial encouraging results using bypass and with the advent of interventional neuroradiology techniques and thrombolytic therapies using tissue plasminogen activator (t-PA) and urokinase,[18,19] the interest in performing emergency EC-IC bypass for acute ischemic stroke decreased.[20]

Experience with Bypass for Ischemia from Cerebral Vasospasm

Cerebral vasospasm is known to cause delayed ischemic neurologic deficit following aneurysmal subarachnoid hemorrhage; STA-MCA bypass has been performed in the past in an attempt to prevent stroke and improve neurologic outcome. Batjer and Samson[21] reported on 11 patients who received an STA-MCA bypass in the setting of symptomatic vasospasm. Six patients improved in the first 24 hours after surgery, and deficits were stabilized in two other patients. Benzel and Kesterson[22] also reported encouraging results and reversal of neurologic deficits in a patient with symptomatic vasospasm refractory to medical therapy who underwent STA-MCA bypass. This indication for the procedure, however, did not gain wide

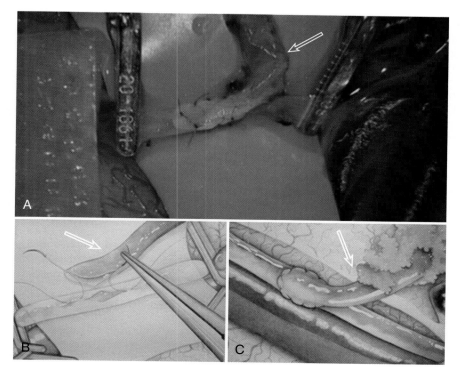

Figure 77-2 Intraoperative photographs (A and C) and drawing (B) of direct superficial temporal (arrows) to middle cerebral artery bypass using a microsuture technique with 10-0 suture to accomplish an end-to-side microvascular anastomosis at a cortical surface branch of the middle cerebral artery.

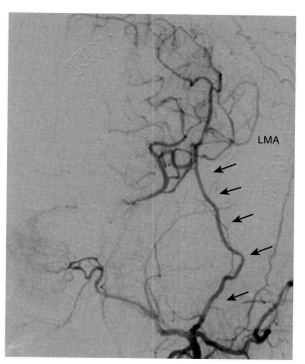

Figure 77-3 Angiogram of a selective injection of the external carotid artery leading to a superficial temporal artery (arrows) to middle cerebral artery bypass showing filling of the middle cerebral artery distribution from the graft. LMA, Left middle cerebral artery.

acceptance. Treatment with calcium channel blockers, triple-H therapy (hypervolemia, hypertension, and hemodilution), and the use of endovascular techniques such as balloon angioplasty are now favored in the management of symptomatic severe vasospasm.[23,24]

Bypass for Occlusive Cerebrovascular Disease Not Amenable to Carotid Endarterectomy

Yasargil's first report of STA-MCA bypass described its use for occlusive cerebrovascular disease of the internal carotid or middle cerebral artery.[6,9] The procedure was still considered experimental at that time, however, because of a lack of proof of efficacy in stroke prevention and uncertain indications.[25] Knowledge of the natural history of occlusive cerebrovascular disease was incomplete, and methods for identification of hemodynamic cerebrovascular insufficiency were still evolving. Moreover, postoperative results had always been compared with the preoperative status of the same patients and not with the natural course of the disease in a randomized, controlled trial.[26]

The North American EC-IC Bypass Study was initiated in 1977, to compare best medical therapy with STA-MCA bypass plus medical therapy for patients with symptomatic occluded or high-grade atherosclerotic stenotic lesions of the MCA or internal carotid artery (ICA) not amenable to endarterectomy.[26] The objective of the study was to determine whether an STA-MCA anastomosis would decrease the incidence of stroke and stroke-related death in those patients. The study randomly assigned 714 patients to best medical treatment and 663 patients to an STA-MCA bypass plus best medical treatment. The 30-day surgical mortality and major stroke morbidity rates were 0.6% and 2.5%, respectively. In the surgical group, fatal and nonfatal strokes occurred earlier and more frequently. The study investigators concluded that the STA-MCA bypass was ineffective in preventing cerebral ischemia in patients with atherosclerotic disease of the MCA and ICA not amenable to endarterectomy.[26] There was no evidence that any subgroup of patients benefited from the procedure. A temporary functional deterioration in several routine daily tasks was also observed during the first months in the surgical group but the difference was not significant at 6-month follow-up.[27] Even though the study was considered well conducted regarding its methodology and follow-up,[28] criticisms of the study included the following issues:

1. Only half of the patients were receiving antiplatelet agents at the time of entry into the study, and the other half was not receiving any medical therapy.[29]
2. Patients were not evaluated preoperatively in terms of their cerebrovascular hemodynamic status. Patients with symptoms due to hemodynamic insufficiency, which would be the group predicted to benefit the most from a bypass augmentation procedure, were not differentiated from patients with symptoms caused by thromboembolic mechanisms.[29,30]
3. Neither the patient nor the therapist was blinded as to the treatment assignment, and therefore the potential for bias was possible.[29]
4. Randomization to treatment bias could have occurred, in which a large number of patients randomly assigned to surgery had major morbidity events that happened before the operation.[29,31]
5. There were no angiographic determinants for entry. The severity of the stenosis was not measured and vertebral angiography was not performed in all patients.[30]
6. A large percentage of patients had no symptoms between the angiographic demonstration of the ICA occlusion and randomization.[29,31]
7. A high number of patients presenting to participating centers underwent surgery outside the study.[30]
8. In a high percentage of patients tandem lesions were demonstrated by angiography, which may be a condition not well suitable for a bypass.[30,31]

Further conclusions from the EC-IC bypass study were subsequently published in a manuscript addressing those criticisms and once more provided evidence to support the results of the trial.[32] Subsequently, a committee appointed by the American Association of Neurological Surgeons was then encouraged to examine the study with emphasis on two aspects: *the randomized trial cohort* and *patients operated on outside the trial*.[33] Within the randomization trial cohort, none of the issues listed was judged to compromise either the design of the trial or any conclusions of the study. Regarding the number of patients operated on outside the trial, a report by Sundt indicated that at least 2500 patients underwent bypass done outside the study in participating centers.[33,34] This fact raised the concern whether the EC-IC bypass trial study conclusions could or could not be generalizable to the entire population at risk for stroke.[34] Owing to lack of sufficient data, this question could not be answered fully.[34] The study investigators also pointed out that randomized trials involve only a small fraction of the population at risk but this fact does not prevent a study from being valid.[35]

Occlusive Cerebrovascular Disease with Hemodynamic Insufficiency

After the EC-IC bypass trial results, a few centers continued to perform EC-IC bypass surgery for the treatment of symptomatic occlusion of the ICA in selected patients, with good outcomes. Indications for the procedure were based on evidence of perfusion abnormalities on imaging studies or presence of symptoms despite maximal medical management.[36-43] This group of patients included those with demonstrated reduced cerebrovascular reserve and either recurrent ischemic symptoms or disabling transient ischemic attacks (TIAs), including limb-shaking TIAs.

The occurrence of ischemic symptoms and stroke in occlusive cerebrovascular disease can usually be attributed to thromboembolic phenomena, a decrease in cerebral perfusion pressure, or a combination of the two mechanisms.[44-46] With advances in neuroimaging, the availability of cerebral blood flow determination, and a better understanding of cerebral metabolism, subsequent investigations were conducted in an effort to determine the natural history of occlusive atherosclerotic carotid disease, the risk of stroke in subpopulations with different states of hemodynamic insufficiency, and whether any of these subpopulations could benefit from a revascularization procedure.[45,47-49]

The overall risk of subsequent stroke in patients with carotid occlusion has been further determined. A prospective study by Powers et al[49] identified stroke risks of 0% at 2 years and 4.4% at 3 years in the group of never-symptomatic patients, in contrast to stroke risks of 7.7% at 1 year, 19% at 2 years, and 21% at 3 years for symptomatic patients with ICA occlusion. Additionally, several studies, using different imaging modalities—xenon CT (Xe-CT), single-photon emission CT (SPECT) or positron emission tomography (PET)—have provided evidence that the presence of hemodynamic impairment of the cerebral blood flow/perfusion is significantly linked to an increased risk of subsequent stroke.[45,50-53]

The St. Louis Carotid Occlusion Study was a prospective blinded study that evaluated the relationship between the state of "misery perfusion," indicated by increased oxygen extraction fraction (OEF) on PET scans, or stage II hemodynamic insufficiency, and stroke risk in patients with symptomatic carotid occlusion.[48,49,54] The 81 patients were divided into two groups: patients with increased OEF (n = 39) and those with normal OEF (n = 42). In all patients with increased OEF, the hemodynamic abnormality was ipsilateral to the occluded carotid artery. At the end of follow-up, in the group with increased OEF, there were 12 total and 11 ipsilateral strokes, in contrast to 3 total and 2 ipsilateral strokes in the group with normal OEF (P = .005 and P = .004, respectively). The risk of ipsilateral stroke in the group with increased OEF was 10.6% at 1 year and 26.5% at 2 years. On the other hand, the group with normal OEF had a risk of stroke of 2.4% and 5.3% at 1 year and 2 years, respectively. The researchers concluded that the state of "misery perfusion" is a significant independent predictor of the subsequent risk of stroke in medically treated patients with carotid occlusion. This study also led to the conclusion that patients with retinal symptoms only were at low risk of subsequent stroke,[49] a result also found in other studies.[55]

Several investigators have described the effects of STA-MCA bypass on improvement of rCBF, regional cerebral metabolic rate for oxygen (rCMRo$_2$), cerebral blood volume (CBV), and OEF, in patients with occlusive cerebrovascular disease. More importantly, there were a demonstrable reversal of the state of "misery perfusion" and marked improvements in regional CBF and CMRO$_2$ in the subpopulation of patients with hemodynamic impairment who underwent a revascularization procedure.[37-40,44,56-62]

The evidence that patients with carotid occlusion and stage II hemodynamic insufficiency have an increased risk of stroke and the substantiation that an EC-IC bypass may reverse this stage of "misery perfusion" have led to a new prospective randomized trial.[48,63]

The Carotid Occlusion Surgery Study (COSS) is a trial that began enrolling patients in 2002, and is currently under analysis at the time of this writing, that will prospectively evaluate the efficacy of the STA-MCA bypass in the prevention of stroke in the subpopulation of patients with symptomatic carotid occlusion and evidence of ipsilateral "misery perfusion" on PET scans.[64,65] COSS is a multicenter randomized trial of EC-IC bypass (primarily STA-MCA bypass), to the cerebral hemisphere that is hemodynamically impaired by an ipsilateral occlusion of the ICA. The trial enrolls only patients with hemispheric ipsilateral symptoms, and all patients receive best medical therapy. The primary outcome event is the occurrence of ipsilateral ischemic hemispheric stroke at any time from the randomization to the end of follow-up at 24 months, or any stroke or death within 40 days of a patient's entry into the trial. Secondary endpoints are any fatal or nonfatal stroke, ipsilateral disabling stroke, death, assessment of quality of life, and function. Other outcome events include TIA, surgical complications other than stroke, perioperative myocardial infarction, and bleeding complications.

Current Trends in the Use of Extracranial to Intracranial Bypass

Basic Surgical Technique

Standard STA-MCA Bypass

The patient is placed in the supine position, with the head turned to the contralateral side and a roll under the shoulder. The hair is shaved in an appropriate distribution along the course of the STA. A selective angiogram with selective external injection of the STA is quite helpful in defining the path of the artery (see Fig. 77-1). Surface mapping with portable continuous-wave Doppler ultrasound is performed to map out the course of the donor branch of the STA. A linear incision is made directly over the artery to its distal portion approximately 4 cm from the midline with use of a needle-point (Colorado tip) cautery unit (Colorado Biomedical, Inc., Evergreen, CO). The STA is then dissected from the surrounding galeal tissue with the needle-point cautery unit. Jeweler's bipolar forceps are also used to coagulate larger branches.

After isolation of the STA, a suitable point for division is identified to ensure that there is an adequate length of the artery for the performance of the bypass. The artery is then divided, temporarily clamped, and then brought down into the lowermost portion of the incision, where it is kept in moist gauze. After the temporalis muscle is divided and mobilized from the bone, a point is selected approximately 6 cm superior to the external auditory meatus for the center of the bone flap, which allows selection of the most appropriate distal branch of the MCA as a recipient artery. The ideal recipient artery is on the surface, has an adequate straight portion without significant branching, and has a diameter of approximately 1.5 mm. The arachnoid is then divided directly over the recipient artery with an arachnoid knife and microscissors. Microjeweler's forceps are used to dissect the arachnoid layer away from the artery, separating it from the surrounding veins. After isolation of the artery, small side branches are cauterized with fine jeweler's forceps under microscopic magnification and then divided with microscissors. A 1.5- to 2-cm segment of the artery is isolated, and a small rubber barrier is placed under the artery, allowing the arteriotomy and the anastomosis to be performed.

Attention is then directed to the distal portion of the STA. The distance between the donor artery and the recipient artery is carefully measured, and approximately 3 cm of redundancy is permitted to facilitate rotating the artery backward and forward to allow sutures to be easily placed on both sides of the arteriotomy. Periadventitial tissue layers are dissected from the divided end of the STA for approximately 2 to 3 cm, to allow an adequate working portion of the donor artery. The soft tissue is then trimmed back, and any small arterial branches are cauterized and divided. A dilute papaverine (Bedford Laboratories, Bedford, OH) solution (15 mg/100 mL of 0.9% saline) is placed on the STA to allow the vessel to dilate and resume its resting caliber. The artery is divided with sharp scissors in an angled fashion and is then spatulated with microscissors (see Fig. 77-2). The length of the spatulation should be approximately two times the diameter of the artery. After preparation of the donor artery, it is then brought onto the rubber barrier, where the recipient artery has been isolated.

After the arteriotomy, the recipient vessel is irrigated with heparinized saline solution, which also prevents sticking from residual blood products. With a tapered needle, a 10-0 microsuture is then used to anchor the spatulated end of the donor artery to the end of the arteriotomy made on the recipient vessel. A second suture is then placed at the distal portion of the vessel, and it is anchored to the contralateral end of the arteriotomy site. Surgeon's knots are tied at both ends to prevent slippage. Interrupted sutures are then placed on each side of the arteriotomy to complete the anastomosis (see Fig. 77-2). Alternatively, a running suture technique can be used to complete the anastomosis. The temporary clips are then removed from the vessels, establishing flow through the anastomosis.

A micro–Doppler ultrasound device (Mizuho America, Inc., Beverly, MA) is used to check the blood flow in the donor artery and in both limbs of the recipient artery. The bone flap is then rongeured around the entry site of the donor artery through the craniotomy to ensure that there is no compression. Occasionally, the inside of the bone flap can be drilled out to create a groove for the artery if this is necessary. A generous space for the artery to pass through the muscle is left. The STA in some patients may be inadequate to serve as donor vessel for an STA-MCA bypass. Several conditions could be responsible for an inadequate STA donor vessel. They include hypoplasia of the artery, previous craniotomy with division of the artery, and damage to the artery during dissection. If no suitable artery exists, using a short vein graft as described by Little et al[11] is a viable option.

Short Saphenous Vein Graft

The incision is made in front of the tragus and is carried down to the base of the ear. The dissection is carried along the tragus down to the tragal point. This step helps locate the facial nerve, which is typically within 1 cm inferior and anterior to the tragal point. The posterosuperior portion of the parotid gland is also typically found in this location. The gland is then mobilized forward so that the trunk of the STA can be identified. Intraoperative Doppler ultrasound is also helpful in locating the artery. The artery is then dissected, and a generous portion is mobilized to allow a 1- to 2-cm working segment.

Preparation of the Saphenous Vein Graft and Anastomosis

A short segment of saphenous vein graft is harvested from the leg for use as an interpositional graft. The distal portion of the saphenous vein is often smaller and more suitable for use than the proximal portion. The standardized technique is to cut down directly over the vein and ligate the branching segments. The vein is then harvested and stored in heparinized saline. The cranial exposure for a recipient vessel is altered slightly so as to facilitate the exposure of the sylvian fissure more proximally than for the standard STA-MCA bypass. The central portion of the craniotomy is moved forward approximately 4 cm so that it is located over the anterior portion of the sylvian fissure. The arachnoid in the sylvian fissure is divided, and the temporal lobe is gently separated from the frontal lobe. The M2 and M3 branches of the MCA are located, and a suitable recipient vessel is found. We prefer performing the distal anastomosis first, a step that allows superior and inferior manipulation of the vessel and an easier placement of the sutures for the end-to-side anastomosis. After completion of the distal anastomosis in a manner similar to the technique described earlier, the vein graft is brought into apposition with the trunk of the STA. The vein is cut to the appropriate length in an angled fashion, and the end is spatulated. The STA trunk is prepared in a similar fashion, with an angled cut and spatulation. A 7-0 running vascular suture is then used to complete the end-to-end anastomosis (see Fig. 77-2B).

Long Saphenous Vein Graft or Radial Artery Graft

EC-IC bypass to the MCA can also be accomplished as described previously, with use of longer grafts, from the external carotid artery, or the stump of the ICA at the bifurcation. These grafts are performed in cases in which there is no suitable STA to serve as a proximal vessel or a larger-capacity graft is required because of the flow demand. The grafts can be created with either the saphenous vein or the radial artery.

Acute Stroke and Emergency Cerebral Revascularization

New imaging modalities were developed for the evaluation of acute stroke during the last decade, and differentiation between regions of acute infarction and potentially salvageable regions with low flow (ischemic penumbra) is now possible with a combination of diffusion-weighted imaging (DWI) MRI, perfusion MRI, perfusion CT/CTA, and PET scans.[66-69] Within the penumbra zone, it may also be possible to differentiate those areas that will infarct without reperfusion from those regions that will most likely survive even without reperfusion.[67,68] Anecdotal case reports on emergency surgical revascularization for acute stroke have demonstrated restoration of normal flow to regions of ischemic penumbra and improvement in perfusion-diffusion mismatch.[70,71] Even though the area of mismatch has been shown to not accurately correspond to the penumbra zone,[68] further developments in imaging modalities and better definitions of ischemic but viable tissue (increased OEF) thresholds will likely help identify selected patients who may be considered for urgent surgical revascularization procedures for acute stroke in whom intraarterial thrombolysis is contraindicated.

Occlusive Cerebrovascular Disease

The current value of EC-IC bypass for stroke prevention in nonacute occlusive cerebrovascular disease remains undefined until data from controlled studies, including the COSS, are available. In addition to the COSS, another randomized study has been conducted in Japan on EC-IC bypass in patients with occlusive disease and demonstrated cerebrovascular insufficiency. The Japanese Extracranial-Intracranial Bypass Trial (JET) included 206 patients who had either carotid occlusion or MCA occlusion or stenosis that was greater than 70% with hemodynamic insufficiency indicated by rCBF of 80% of control or acetazolamide reactivity of less than 10%. They also had to be functionally independent and have small or absent brain infarction. Patients were randomized to best medical treatment (103 patients) or bypass (103 patients) and followed up for 2 years. An early analysis indicated that there was a reduced subsequent stroke risk in the surgically treated patients in comparison with the medically treated patients (6 vs. 15, $P = .0046$).[72]

There are also reports supporting the use of bypass for relief of disabling symptoms in patients with occlusive disease and demonstrated cerebrovascular insufficiency detected with hemodynamic testing.[73] These patients can be evaluated on an individualized basis and offered a good prognosis for relief of their symptoms if their risk for the procedure is judged to be reasonable.

Moyamoya Disease

The first case of moyamoya disease treated with a direct STA-MCA bypass was performed in 1972 by Yasargil on a 4-year-old child, who had remarkable improvement following the procedure.[10] Postoperative angiograms showed patency of the anastomosis and evidence of collaterals from the vertebrobasilar system and other extracranial sources. In 1980 an indirect STA-MCA bypass for bilateral occlusion of the supraclinoid ICA was performed on a patient who had recurrent symptoms of hemiparesis and aphasia.[74] A direct STA-MCA bypass was planned, but at operation no suitable recipient cortical vessel was found and the STA and surrounding tissue were laid over the cerebral hemisphere and sutured to the arachnoid. The patient had a remarkable clinical recovery, and postoperative angiograms showed extensive collateral vessel formation, establishing the effectiveness of an indirect STA-MCA bypass as a form of cerebral revascularization.

In children the benefits of EC-IC bypass for improving symptoms, reversing neurologic deficits, enabling normal intelligence development, preventing further ischemic episodes, decreasing seizure activity, and even disappearance of involuntary movements have been observed.[75-85] Several studies addressing the efficacy of the direct and the indirect bypass techniques have been done in pediatric patients, and better clinical and angiographic results are usually seen when a direct bypass can be performed.[79,84-87]

Various studies have also demonstrated the benefits of STA-MCA bypass in ischemic adult moyamoya disease, preventing further ischemic episodes and improving clinical symptoms and cerebral hemodynamics.[80,88-95] On the other hand, the effectiveness of revascularization in preventing hemorrhage still remains a controversy.[88,90,93,96]

A large retrospective study involving 57 neurosurgical institutions in Japan analyzed 290 patients with the hemorrhagic form of moyamoya disease. Conservative treatment was given to 138 patients, and 152 patients received surgical revascularization. In the nonsurgical group, 28.3% of the patients had a recurrent hemorrhage during follow-up, in contrast to 19.1% in the surgical group. The researchers concluded that prospective studies are needed to clarify the efficacy of the STA-MCA bypass in the prevention of hemorrhage in this disease. A large prospective trial is now under way to evaluate the effectiveness of STA-MCA bypass for the prevention of cerebral hemorrhage in moyamoya disease.[78,97,98]

Aneurysms and Tumors

The use of the STA-MCA bypass as an adjunct for aneurysm treatment is common in most centers that treat complex cerebral aneurysms. This procedure will likely remain a useful option in the future to prevent cerebral ischemia in cases in which there is a high likelihood of vessel sacrifice in order to obliterate certain aneurysms. The procedure has been used successfully as an adjunct to aneurysm or parent vessel occlusion by surgical and endovascular means. The specific threshold of lowered rCBF indicating that the collateral circulation will be inadequate to prevent ischemia after permanent major vessel occlusion remains to be determined.[99] Newer imaging modalities may also allow a more accurate prediction of whether certain aneurysms can be clipped safely or whether wall thickness and the presence of calcification mandate parent vessel occlusion/reconstruction combined with an EC-IC bypass as an adjunct. New STA-MCA bypass techniques[14] may be useful in certain circumstances when a two-limb end-to-end bypass with good blood flow and short anastomotic time are needed.

Conclusions

The EC-IC bypass is a very elegant procedure, and the STA-MCA bypass developed by M.G. Yasargil was first applied on a widespread basis for the treatment of occlusive cerebrovascular disease. The STA-MCA bypass proved to be feasible with a low complication rate, but it has been shown to be ineffective in preventing stroke in nonselected populations harboring occlusive carotid or MCA disease. The demonstration that a subpopulation of patients with symptomatic carotid occlusion and increased oxygen extraction fraction has a higher risk of stroke, together with the evidence that an STA-MCA bypass procedure may reverse the state of misery perfusion, has justified a new trial. The Carotid Occlusion Surgery Study (COSS) will evaluate whether the STA-MCA bypass can decrease the incidence of stroke in patients with evidence of misery perfusion. An international multicenter trial will probably further define the role of the STA-MCA bypass in the setting of hemorrhagic moyamoya disease. This elegant surgical technique will likely remain an important tool in properly selected patients for the management of occlusive atherosclerotic, traumatic cerebrovascular disease, intracranial aneurysms, skull base tumors, moyamoya disease, and possibly, acute stroke.

Acknowledgments and Disclosure Statement

No financial support was provided for the completion of this study. There are no conflicts of interest disclosed by the authors. We would like to thank Raquel L. Abreu for her illustrations in Figure 77-2. Portions of this manuscript appear in the following article by the same authors: Vilela MD, Newell DW: Superficial temporal artery to middle cerebral artery bypass: Past, present, and future. *Neurosurg Focus* 24:E2, 2008.

REFERENCES

1. Fisher CM: Occlusion of the internal carotid artery, *Arch Psychiatry* 65:346, 1951.
2. Woringer E, Kunlin J: Anastomose entre la carotide primitive et la carotide intra-craniene ou la sylvienne par greffon selon la technique de la suture suspendue, *Neuro-Chir* 9:181–188, 1963.
3. Pool JL, Potts DG: *Aneurysms and arteriovenous anomalies of the brain,* New York, 1964, Hoeber, pp 221-222.
4. Jacobson JH, Suarez EL: Microsurgery in anastomosis of small vessels, *Surg Forum* :243–245, 1960.
5. Jacobson JH 2nd, Wallman LJ, Schumacher GA, Flanagan M, Suarez EL, Donaghy RM: Microsurgery as an aid to middle cerebral artery endarterectomy, *J Neurosurg* 19:108–115, 1962.
6. Yasargil M, editor: *Microsurgery applied to neurosurgery,* Stuttgart, 1969, Georg Thieme.
7. Yasargil M: A legacy of microneurosurgery: Memoirs, lessons, and axioms, *Neurosurgery* 45:1025–1092, 1999.
8. Crowell RM, Yasargil MG: End-to-side anastomosis of superficial temporal artery to middle cerebral artery branch in the dog, *Neurochirurgia* 16:73–77, 1973.
9. Yasargil MG, Krayenbuhl HA, Jacobson JH: Microneurosurgical arterial reconstruction, *Surgery* 67:221–233, 1970.
10. Krayenbuhl H: The moyamoya syndrome and the neurosurgeon, *Surg Neurol* 4:353–360, 1975.
11. Little JR, Furlan AJ, Bryerton B: Short vein grafts for cerebral revascularization, *J Neurosurg* 59:384–388, 1983.
12. Newell DW, Skirboll SL: Revascularization and bypass procedures for cerebral aneurysms, *Neurosurg Clin North Am* 9:697–711, 1998.

13. Onesti ST, Solomon RA, Quest DO: Cerebral revascularization: A review, *Neurosurgery* 25:618–629, 1989.

14. Newell DW, Dailey AT, Skirboll SL: Intracranial vascular anastomosis using the microanastomotic system. Technical note, *J Neurosurg* 89:676–681, 1998.

15. Crowell RMJJ: Emergency cerebral revascularization, *Clin Neurosurg* 33:281–305, 1986.

16. Diaz FG, Ausman JI, Mehta B, et al: Acute cerebral revascularization, *J Neurosurg* 63:200–209, 1985.

17. Gratzl O, Schmiedek P, Spetzler RF, et al: Clinical experience with extra-intracranial arterial anastomosis in 65 cases, *J Neurosurg* 44:313–324, 1976.

18. Broderick JP, Hacke W: Treatment of acute ischemic stroke. Part I: Recanalization strategies, *Circulation* 106:1563–1569, 2002.

19. Tissue plasminogen activator for acute ischemic stroke: The National Institute of Neurological Disorders and Stroke rt-PA Stroke Study Group, *N Engl J Med* 333:1581–1587, 1995.

20. Pikus HJ, Heros RC: Stroke: Indications for emergent surgical intervention, *Clin Neurosurg* 45:113–127, 1997.

21. Batjer H, Samson D: Use of extracranial-intracranial bypass in the management of symptomatic vasospasm, *Neurosurgery* 19:235–246, 1986.

22. Benzel EC, Kesterson L: Extracranial-intracranial bypass surgery for the management of vasospasm after subarachnoid hemorrhage, *Surg Neurol* 30:231–234, 1988.

23. Elliot JP, Newell DW, Lam DJ, et al: Comparison of balloon angioplasty and papaverine infusion for the treatment of vasospasm following aneurysmal subarachnoid hemorrhage, *J Neurosurg* 88:277–284, 1998.

24. Eskridge JM, Newell DW, Pendleton GA: Transluminal angioplasty for treatment of vasospasm, *Neurosurg Clin North Am* 1:387–399, 1990.

25. Tew JJ: Reconstructive intracranial vascular surgery for prevention of stroke, *Clin Neurosurg* 22:264–280, 1975.

26. The EC-IC Bypass Study Group: Failure of extracranial-intracranial arterial bypass to reduce the risk of ischemic stroke, *N Engl J Med* 313:1191–1200, 1985.

27. Haynes B, Mukherjee J, Sackett DL, et al: Functional status changes following medical or surgical treatment for cerebral ischemia. Results of the extracranial-intracranial bypass study, *JAMA* 257:2043–2046, 1987.

28. Peerless S: Indications for the extracranial-intracranial arterial bypass in light of the EC-IC bypass study, *Clin Neurosurg* 33:307–326, 1986.

29. Awad IA, Spetzler RF: Extracranial-Intracranial bypass surgery: A critical analysis in light of the International Cooperative study, *Neurosurgery* 19:655–664, 1986.

30. Ausman JI, Diaz FG: Critique of the extracranial-intracranial bypass study, *Surg Neurol* 26:218–221, 1986.

31. Day AL, Rhoton AL, Little JR: The extracranial-intracranial bypass study, *Surg Neurol* 26:222–226, 1986.

32. Barnett HJM, Fox A, Hachinski V, et al: Further conclusions from the extracranial-intracranial bypass trial, *Surg Neurol* 26:227–235, 1986.

33. Goldring S, Zervas N, Langfitt T: The extracranial-intracranial bypass study: A report of the committee appointed by the American Association of Neurological Surgeons to examine the study, *N Engl J Med* 316:817–820, 1987.

34. Sundt TJ: Was the international randomized trial of extracranial-intracranial bypass representative of the population at risk? *N Engl J Med* 316:814–816, 1987.

35. Barnett HJM, Sackett D, Taylor DW, et al: Are the results of the extracranial-intracranial bypass trial generalizable? *N Engl J Med* 316:820–824, 1987.

36. Mendelowitsch A, Taussy P, Rem JA, Gratzl O: Clinical outcome of standard extracranial-intracranial bypass surgery in patients with symptomatic atherosclerotic occlusion of the internal carotid artery, *Acta Neurochir (Wien)* 146:95–101, 2004.

37. Schmiedek P, Piepgras A, Leisinger G, et al: Improvement of cerebrovascular capacity by EC-IC arterial bypass surgery in patients with ICA occlusion and hemodynamic cerebral ischemia, *J Neurosurg* 81:236–244, 1994.

38. Takagi YHN, Iwama T, Hayashida K: Improvement of oxygen metabolic reserve after extracranial-intracranial bypass surgery in patients with severe haemodynamic insufficiency, *Acta Neurochir(Wien)* 139:52–57, 1997.

39. Iwama T, Hashimoto N, Hayashida K: Cerebral hemodynamic parameters for patients with neurological improvements after extracranial-intracranial arterial bypass surgery: Evaluation using positron emission tomography, *Neurosurgery* 48:504–512, 2001.

40. Kobayashi H, Kitai R, Ido K, et al: Hemodynamic and metabolic changes following cerebral revascularization in patients with cerebral occlusive diseases, *Neurol Res* 21:153–160, 1999.

41. Nussbaum ES, Erickson DL: Extracranial-intracranial bypass for ischemic cerebrovascular disease refractory to maximal medical therapy, *Neurosurgery* 46:37–42, 2000.

42. Neff KW, Horn P, Dinter D, et al: Extracranial-intracranial arterial bypass surgery improves total brain blood supply in selected symptomatic patients with unilateral internal carotid artery occlusion and insufficient collateralization, *Neuroradiology* 46:430–437, 2004.

43. Amin-Hanjani SBW, Ogilvy CS, Carter BS, Barker FG 2nd: Extracranial-intracranial bypass in the treatment of occlusive cerebrovascular disease and intracranial aneurysms in the United States between 1992 and 2001: A population-based study, *J Neurosurg* 103:794–804, 2005.

44. Baron JC, Bousser MG, Rey A, et al: Reversal of focal "misery-perfusion syndrome" by extra-intracranial bypass in hemodynamic cerebral ischemia, *Stroke* 12:454–459, 1981.

45. Klijn CJM, Kappelle J, Tulleken CAF, van Gijn J: Symptomatic carotid artery occlusion. A reappraisal of hemodynamic factors, *Stroke* 28:2084–2093, 1997.

46. Powers WJ, Raichle ME: Positron emission tomography and its application to the study of cerebrovascular disease in man, *Stroke* 16:361–376, 1985.

47. Hirano T, Minematsu K, Hasegawa Y, et al: Acetazolamide reactivity on ^{123}I-IMP single photon emission computed tomography in patients with major cerebral artery occlusive disease: Correlation with positron emission tomography parameters, *J Cereb Blood Flow Metab* 14:763–770, 1994.

48. Grubb RL Jr, Derdeyn CP, Fritsch SM, et al: Importance of hemodynamic factors in the prognosis of symptomatic carotid occlusion, *JAMA* 280:1055–1060, 1998.

49. Powers WJ, Derdeyn CP, Fritsch SM, et al: Benign prognosis of never symptomatic carotid occlusion, *Neurology* 54:878–882, 2000.

50. Yonas H, Smith HA, Durham SR, et al: Increased stroke risk predicted by compromised cerebral blood flow reactivity, *J Neurosurg* 79:483–489, 1993.

51. Kuroda S, Houkin K, Kamiyama H, et al: Long-term prognosis of medically treated patients with internal carotid or middle cerebral artery occlusion: Can acetazolamide test predict it? *Stroke* 32:2110–2116, 2001.

52. Ogasawara K, Ogawa A, Yoshimoto T: Cerebrovascular reactivity to acetazolamide and outcome in patients with symptomatic internal carotid or middle cerebral artery occlusion: A xenon-133 single-photon emission computed tomography study, *Stroke* 33:1857–1862, 2002.

53. Yamauchi H, Fukuyama H, Nagahama Y, et al: Evidence of misery perfusion and risk for recurrent stroke in major cerebral arterial occlusive diseases from PET, *J Neurol Neurosurg Psychiatry* 61:18–25, 1996.

54. Derdeyn CP, Yundt KD, Videen TO, et al: Increased oxygen extraction fraction is associated with prior ischemic events in patients with carotid occlusion, *Stroke* 29:754–758, 1998.

55. Klijn CJM, Kappelle J, van Huffelen AC, et al: Recurrent ischemia in symptomatic carotid occlusion: Prognostic value of hemodynamic factors, *Neurology* 55:1806–1812, 2000.

56. Gibbs JM, Wise RJ, Thomas DJ, et al: Cerebral hemodynamic changes after extracranial-intracranial bypass surgery, *J Neurol Neurosurg Psychiatry* 50:140–150, 1987.

57. Grubb RL, Ratcheson RA, Raichle ME, et al: Regional cerebral blood flow and oxygen utilization in superficial temporal-middle cerebral artery anastomosis patients. An exploratory definition of clinical problems, *J Neurosurg* 50:733–741, 1979.

58. Laurent JP, Lawner PM, O'Connor M: Reversal of intracerebral steal by STA-MCA anastomosis, *J Neurosurg* 57:629–632, 1982.

59. Powers WJ, Martin WRW, Herscovitch P, et al: Extracranial-intracranial bypass surgery: Hemodynamic and metabolic effects, *Neurology* 34:1168–1174, 1984.

60. Samson Y, Baron JC, Bousser MG, et al: Effects of extra-intracranial arterial bypass on cerebral blood flow and oxygen metabolism in humans, *Stroke* 16:609-6315, 1985.

61. Tsuda Y, Kimura K, Iwata Y, et al: Improvement of cerebral blood flow and/or CO_2 reactivity after superficial temporal artery-middle cerebral artery bypass in patients with transient ischemic attacks and watershed-zone infarctions, *Surg Neurol* 22:595-604, 1984.

62. Yonas H, Gur D, Good BC, et al: Stable xenon-CT blood flow mapping for evaluation of patients with extracranial-intracranial bypass surgery, *J Neurosurg* 62:324-333, 1985.

63. Grubb RL Jr, Powers WJ: Risks of stroke and current indications for cerebral revascularization in patients with carotid occlusion, *Neurosurg Clin North Am* 12:473-487, 2001.

64. Adams HP, Powers WJ, Grubb RL, et al: Preview of a new trial of extracranial to intracranial arterial anastomosis: The Carotid Occlusion Surgery Study, *Neurosurg Clin North Am* 12:613-624, 2001.

65. Grubb RL Jr, Powers WJ, Derdeyn CP, et al: The Carotid Occlusion Surgery Study, *Neurosurg Focus* 14:e9, 2003.

66. Rohl L, Ostergaard L, Simonsen CZ, et al: Viability thresholds of ischemic penumbra of hyperacute stroke defined by perfusion-weighted MRI and apparent diffusion coefficient, *Stroke* 32:1140-1146, 2001.

67. Schaefer PW, Ozsunar Y, He J, et al: Assessing tissue viability with MR diffusion and perfusion imaging, *AJNR Am J Neuroradiol* 24:436-443, 2003.

68. Sobesky J, Zaro Weber O, Lehnhardt FG, et al: Does the mismatch match the penumbra? Magnetic resonance imaging and positron emission tomography in early ischemic stroke, *Stroke* 36:980-985, 2005.

69. Sobesky J, Zaro Weber O, Lehnhardt FG, et al: Which time-to-peak threshold best identifies penumbral flow? A comparison of perfusion-weighted magnetic resonance imaging and positron emission tomography in acute ischemic stroke, *Stroke* 35:2843-2847, 2004.

70. Ogasawara K, Sasaki M, Tomitsuka N, et al: Early revascularization in a patient with perfusion computed tomography/diffusion-weighted magnetic resonance imaging mismatch secondary to acute vertebral artery occlusion. Case report, *Neurol Med Chir* 45:306-310, 2005.

71. Krishnamurthy S, Tong D, McNamara KP, et al: Early carotid endarterectomy after ischemic stroke improves diffusion/perfusion mismatch on magnetic resonance imaging: Report of two cases, *Neurosurgery* 52:238-241, 2003.

72. Ogawa A: Japanese EC-IC Bypass Trial (JET Study): The interim analysis, *Jap J Stroke* 25:397-400, 2003.

73. Garrett MC, Komotar RJ, Starke RM, et al: The efficacy of direct extracranial-intracranial bypass in the treatment of symptomatic hemodynamic failure secondary to athero-occlusive disease: A systematic review, *Clin Neurol Neurosurg* 111:319-326, 2009.

74. Spetzler RF, Roski RA, Kopaniky DR: Alternative superficial temporal artery to middle cerebral artery revascularization procedure, *Neurosurgery* 7:484-487, 1980.

75. Amine ARC, Moody R, Meeks W: Bilateral temporal-middle cerebral artery anastomosis for moyamoya syndrome, *Surg Neurology* 8:3-6, 1977.

76. Golby AJ, Marks MP, Thompson RC, Steinberg GK: Direct and combined revascularization in pediatric moyamoya disease, *Neurosurgery* 45:50-58, 1999.

77. Holbach KH, Wassman H, Wappenschmidt J: Superficial temporal-middle cerebral artery anastomosis in moyamoya disease, *Acta Neurochir* 52:27-34, 1980.

78. Houkin K, Kuroda S, Nakayama N: Cerebral revascularization for moyamoya disease in children, *Neurosurg Clin N Am* 12:575-584, 2001.

79. Ishikawa T, Houkin K, Kamiyama H, Abe H: Effects of surgical revascularization on outcome of patients with pediatric moyamoya disease, *Stroke* 28:1170-1173, 1997.

80. Karasawa J, Kikuchi H, Furuse S, et al: Treatment of moyamoya disease with STA-MCA anastomosis, *J Neurosurg* 49:679-688, 1978.

81. Karasawa J, Touho H, Ohnishi H, et al: Long-term follow-up study after extracranial-intracranial bypass surgery for anterior circulation ischemia in childhood moyamoya disease, *J Neurosurg* 77:84-89, 1992.

82. Olds MV, Griebel RW, Hoffman HJ, et al: The surgical treatment of childhood moyamoya disease, *J Neurosurg* 66:675-680, 1987.

83. Sakamoto K, Kitano S, Yasui T, et al: Direct extracranial-intracranial bypass for children with moyamoya disease, *Clin Neurol Neurosurg* 99:S128-S133, 1997.

84. Suzuki Y, Negoro M, Shibuya M, et al: Surgical treatment for pediatric moyamoya disease: Use of the superficial temporal artery for both areas supplied by the anterior and middle cerebral arteries. Technique and application, *Neurosurgery* 40:324-330, 1997.

85. Matsushima T, Inoue T, Suzuki SO, et al: Surgical treatment of moyamoya disease in pediatric patients-comparison between the results of indirect and direct revascularization procedures-clinical study, *Neurosurgery* 31:401-405, 1992.

86. Goda M, Isono M, Ishii K, et al: Long-term effects of indirect bypass surgery on collateral vessel formation in pediatric moyamoya disease, *J Neurosurg* 100(Suppl Pediatrics):156-162, 2004.

87. Scott RM, Smith ER: Moyamoya disease and moyamoya syndrome, *N Engl J Med* 360:1226-1237, 2009.

88. Houkin K, Kamiyama H, Abe H, et al: Surgical therapy for adult moyamoya disease. Can surgical revascularization prevent the recurrence of intracerebral hemorrhage? *Stroke* 27:1342-1346, 1996.

89. Houkin K, Kuroda S, Ishikawa T, Abe H: Neovascularization (angiogenesis)after revascularization in moyamoya disease. Which technique is most useful for moyamoya disease? *Acta Neurochir (Wien)* 142:269-276, 2000.

90. Kawagushi S, Okuno S, Sakaki T: Effect of direct arterial bypass on the prevention of future stroke in patients with the hemorrhagic variety of moyamoya disease, *J Neurosurg* 93:397-401, 2000.

91. Kuroda S, Houkin K, Kamiyama H, Abe H: Effects of surgical revascularization on peripheral aneurysms in moyamoya disease: Report of three cases, *Neurosurgery* 49:463-468, 2001.

92. Morimoto M, Iwama T, Hashimoto N, et al: Efficacy of direct revascularization in adult moyamoya disease: Haemodynamic evaluation by positron emission tomography, *Acta Neurochir (Wien)* 141:377-384, 1999.

93. Okada Y, Shima T, Nishida M, et al: Effectiveness of superficial temporal artery-middle cerebral artery anastomosis in adult moyamoya disease. Cerebral hemodynamics and clinical course in ischemic and hemorrhagic varieties, *Stroke* 29:625-630, 1998.

94. Fukui M: Guidelines for the diagnosis and treatment of spontaneous occlusion of the circle of Willis (moyamoya disease). Research Committee on Spontaneous Occlusion of the Circle of Willis (moyamoya disease) of the Ministry of Health and Welfare, Japan, *Clin Neurol Neurosurg* 99:S238-S240, 1997.

95. Han DH, Kwon OK, Byun BJ, et al: A co-operative study: Clinical characteristics of 334 Korean patients with moyamoya disease treated at neurosurgical institutes (1976-1994). *Acta Neurochir (Wien)* 142:1263-1274, 2000.

96. Ikezaki K, Fukui M, Inamura T, et al: The current status of the treatment for hemorrhagic type moyamoya disease based on a 1995 nationwide survey in Japan, *Clin Neurol Neurosurg* 99:S183-S186, 1997.

97. Yoshida Y, Yoshimoto T, Shirane R, Sakurai Y: Clinical course, surgical management and long-term outcome of moyamoya patients with rebleeding after an episode of intracerebral hemorrhage, *Stroke* 30:2272-2276, 1999.

98. Miyamoto S: Japan Adult Moyamoya Trial Group. Study design for a prospective randomized trial of extracranial-intracranial bypass surgery for adults with moyamoya disease and hemorrhagic onset— The Japan Adult Moyamoya Trial Group, *Neurol Med Chir (Tokyo)* 44:218-219, 2004.

99. Latchaw RE, Yonas H, Hunter GJ, et al: Guidelines and recommendations for perfusion imaging in cerebral ischemia, *Stroke* 34:1084-1104, 2003.

78 Cerebral Infarction: Surgical Treatment

ERIC JÜTTLER, WERNER HACKE

Life-threatening space-occupying mass effect is a common finding in various subtypes of cerebral ischemia and intracranial hemorrhages and occurs because of acute intracranial masses such as hematomas, the development of severe brain edema, or both. Independent of the underlying origin, acute intracranial mass represents a potentially life-threatening complication. Irrespective of the underlying cause, transtentorial or transforaminal herniation is the common endpoint and the cause of death in most of these patients and therefore requires prompt and adequate treatment. This chapter deals with the surgical decompression of acute space-occupying middle cerebral artery (MCA) infarction, cerebellar infarction, intracerebral hemorrhage, and cerebral venous thrombosis.

Despite a large body of evidence that decompressive surgery in so-called malignant MCA infarctions effectively lowers mortality, and various studies suggesting improved functional outcome in survivors, the procedure remains an intensely debated issue in neurointensive care medicine. Consequent to this debate, there are large regional differences in its application, especially regarding the treatment of patients with increased age or dominant-hemisphere infarction. For many years the main concern of critics was that by reducing mortality, decompressive surgery may increase severe disability or even result in permanent vegetative states in patients who would otherwise die from herniation. On the basis of data from randomized trials, there is now good evidence that decompressive surgery performed early, within 48 hours, in patients with malignant MCA infarction aged 18 to 60 years decreases mortality and does so without increasing the number of severely disabled survivors. Further open questions concern a generally accepted definition of malignant MCA infarction within the first 12 hours after symptom onset, the optimal timing of surgery, the quality of life in survivors, the impact of aphasia in dominant-hemisphere malignant infarctions, outcome in elder patients and whether there should be an age limit for treatment, and the influence of the premorbid status on decision making.

Pathology

Regardless of the subtype of stroke or the underlying pathology, all types of intracranial masses carry the risk of severe brain tissue shifts and the subsequent compression of formerly healthy brain structures, critical increase in intracranial pressure (ICP), and subsequent complications such as compromise of cerebral blood flow (CBF) and energy supply.

In ischemic stroke, mass effect is due to local brain swelling caused by brain edema. In general, *brain edema* is defined as abnormal accumulation of fluid in the brain parenchyma. Three major subtypes of edema have traditionally been classified: vasogenic, cytotoxic, and interstitial. Cytotoxic edema results from cell swelling after decreased oxygen supply, substrate and energy failure, and the subsequent breakdown of the ion pumps. Vasogenic edema occurs in the context of breakdown of the blood-brain barrier due to increased vascular permeability. Interstitial edema is associated with impaired absorption of cerebrospinal fluid (CSF) and acute hydrocephalus. A combination of these subtypes is found in severe ischemic stroke, with cytotoxic brain edema playing the leading role. However, brain edema formation is a complex molecular and pathophysiologic process that is currently only partly understood.[1-4]

From 1% to 10% of patients with supratentorial ischemic infarcts suffer from subtotal or complete MCA territory infarctions, occasionally with additional infarction of the anterior cerebral artery (ACA) or the posterior cerebral artery (PCA) or both (Fig. 78-1).[5] These infarcts are commonly associated with serious brain swelling, which usually manifests between the second and the fifth days after stroke onset and reaches a maximum at the fourth day in the majority of patients.[6-10] These massive cerebral infarctions are life-threatening events with a uniform natural course and an extremely poor prognosis: Up to 80% of patients with such infarcts die within the first week after symptom onset owing to transtentorial or transforaminal herniation.[5,11,12] For these catastrophic infarcts, the term malignant MCA infarction was coined.[5]

The therapeutic goal is to interrupt the vicious circle of brain swelling, mass effect, increase in ICP, reduced cerebral perfusion and energy supply, and further brain tissue damage that eventually leads to further edema formation. Conservative therapy aims to optimize cerebral perfusion pressure (CPP) and oxygen delivery and to minimize cerebral metabolic demands by general measures such as adequate oxygen supply, maintenance of adequate blood pressure, and optimal body and head positioning, and specific interventions, including deep sedation, barbiturates,

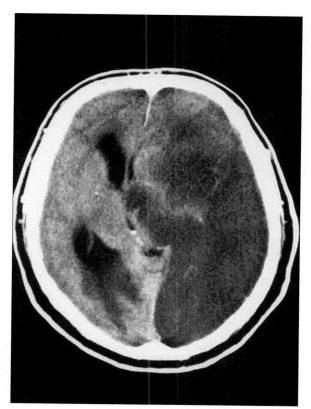

Figure 78-1 Noncontrast CT scan of a patient with malignant left middle cerebral artery (MCA) infarction plus infarction of the left posterior cerebral artery (PCA) 4 days after symptom onset under conservative treatment who died from transtentorial herniation.

TABLE 78-1 PATIENTS WITH ACUTE MIDDLE CEREBRAL ARTERY INFARCTION, WITH A HIGH RISK OF A MALIGNANT COURSE, AND CANDIDATES FOR EARLY (< 48 HOURS) HEMICRANIECTOMY

Age 18 to 60 yr
Severe middle cerebral artery (MCA) syndrome: dense hemiplegia, head and eye deviation, multimodal neglect, global aphasia (in dominant-hemisphere infarction)
National Institutes of Health Stroke Scale (NIHSS) score >15 (in nondominant-hemisphere infarction) or >20 (in dominant-hemisphere infarction)
Level of consciousness: score of ≥1 on item 1a of the NIHSS or <14 on Glasgow Coma Scale (GCS)
Deterioration of consciousness within the first 48 h after symptom onset and/or reduced ventilatory drive
Neuroimaging: definite infarction of ≥2/3 of the MCA territory, at least partially including the basal ganglia; additional infarction of the anterior or posterior cerebral artery optional (CT or MRI using diffusion-weighted imaging [DWI] and perfusion imaging); *and/or* DWI lesion volume >145 mL on DWI *and/or* >82 mL on apparent diffusion coefficient [ADC] maps (MRI)

In contrast to more complex pathophysiologic theories of conservative measures, decompressive surgery is based on pure mechanical thinking: The rationale of removing a part of the neurocranium is simply to create space for the expanding brain. The vector of brain extension is reverted from pressure on midline structures to extension into the newly created compensative spaces, thereby avoiding ventricular compression, reverting brain tissue shifts, and preventing mechanical damage of healthy brain tissue. Decreased ICP and, as a result, restored CBF is more or less a secondary effect, leading to increase in tissue oxygen supply and thereby avoiding secondary damage to the surrounding healthy tissue.[22,23]

Diagnosis

Although the term malignant brain infarction was introduced in 1996, there is currently no generally accepted definition of this condition, especially in the early evaluation of patients with acute MCA infarction.[5] The early prediction of a malignant course of the ischemic lesion would justify early and more aggressive intervention. On the other hand, the majority of patients who have acute MCA infarction do not experience a malignant course and probably do not profit from intensive care treatment or surgery and recover as well under conservative treatment. Currently the diagnosis of malignant brain infarction is based on (1) clinical neurologic findings, (2) a typical clinical course, and (3) neuroimaging findings (Table 78-1), as follows:

1. Clinically, patients with malignant MCA infarctions present with dense hemiplegia, head and eye deviation, multimodal hemineglect, and global aphasia when the dominant hemisphere is involved. It has to be noted that the National Institutes of Health Stroke Scale (NIHSS) underestimates the severity of nondominant infarction, an observation made by Krieger et al,[24] who observed significant differences for NIHSS score as predictor for fatal brain swelling, depending on the

buffers, hypothermia, osmotic therapy, steroids, and controlled hyperventilation.[13,14] However, none of these therapies is supported by adequate evidence from randomized clinical trials of space-occupying cerebral ischemia.[13-15] Several reports suggest that the measures are ineffective or even have harmful effects.[13-20] There are various possible reasons why these therapies often fail or may even be detrimental. It has to be remembered that, for example, osmotic therapy is based on the presence of an intact blood-brain barrier, which, however, is largely disrupted in the infarct territory. From a pathophysiologic point of view, osmotic therapy is therefore of little value. ICP-lowering therapies are often used as escalating treatment options based on ICP measurement and are often not applied until increases of ICP are evident. However, in space-occupying ischemic stroke, early clinical deterioration is usually due not to increases of global ICP but to massive local swelling and brain tissue shifts. Increases of ICP usually occur late, when local mass effect has already led to severe compression and destruction of vital brain structures. Measurement of ICP therefore often does not help prevent these secondary complications, and herniation may occur even without previously increased global ICP. As a result, the value of therapies focusing on lowering ICP is limited and may come too late to be effective. Mild to moderate hypothermia is an exception and represents the most promising alternative treatment option, which, however, is currently not supported by evidence from larger clinical trials.[21]

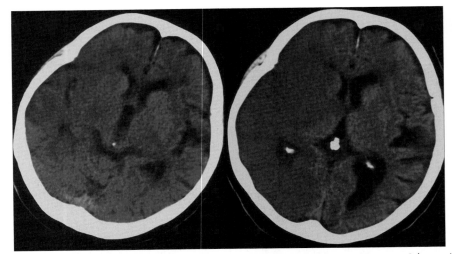

Figure 78-2 Diagnosis of malignant middle cerebral artery (MCA) infarction by noncontrast CT scans, 3 hours *(left)* and 30 hours *(right)* after symptom onset, showing infarction of the complete right MCA territory, including the basal ganglia, plus additional infarctions of the anterior cerebral artery and posterior cerebral artery territories, with incipient space-occupying effect indicated by narrowing of the frontal horn of the lateral ventricle.

side of the lesion. Therefore, NIHSS score typically ranges from higher than 16 to 20 when the dominant hemisphere is involved, and from higher than 15 to 18 when the nondominant hemisphere is involved.[24-27] Furthermore, patients with malignant MCA infarction show an impaired level of consciousness, with score of at least 1 on item 1a of the NIHSS or less than 14 on the Glasgow Coma Scale.[5,24-26]

2. Patients with malignant MCA infarctions show a progressive deterioration of consciousness over the first 24 to 48 hours and frequently a reduced ventilatory drive requiring mechanical ventilation.[5,25]

3. Neuroimaging shows definite infarction of at least two thirds of the MCA territory, including the basal ganglia, with or without additional infarction or perfusion deficit of the ipsilateral ACA or the PCA territory.[25-29] Measurement of early infarct volume in stroke MRI using diffusion-weighted imaging (DWI) or apparent diffusion coefficient (ADC) mapping has shown that early infarct volume has a highly predictive value for the development of a malignant course and may be used for early diagnosis in these patients instead of CT.[27,30,31]

Computed Tomography

In clinical practice CT is widely available and in most cases offers the possibility to detect severe ischemic changes and brain edema formation early enough to predict the probability of a malignant course.[32] In a systematic review by Hofmeijer et al,[29] infarct size was the major determinant of the development of life-threatening edema after MCA infarction. Using noncontrast CT criteria, these researchers reported that infarct size more than 50% of the MCA territory, infarct size more than two thirds of the MCA territory, involvement of the complete MCA territory, involvement of other vascular territories (i.e., ACA and/or PCA), and early mass effect all are highly significant predictors for a malignant course, with infarct

size greater than two thirds of the MCA territory having the highest positive and negative predictive values (86% and 90%, respectively). Additional infarction of the ACA or PCA territory or both also has a high positive predictive value (86%) but a lower negative predictive value (69%) (Fig. 78-2).

Advanced CT technologies using multimodal imaging including CT angiography (CTA) and perfusion CT may also help identify this condition. In studies using perfusion CT, perfusion deficits including more than two thirds of the MCA territory and low perfusion levels in the ACA and/or PCA territory or both were found to predict a malignant course with high positive predictive values of up to 90%, and negative predictive values between 40% and 85%, respectively.[29,33-35] CTA allows fast and reliable evaluation of vessel patency in acute stroke; ICA occlusion is a significant predictor of a malignant course, although it has comparatively low positive predictive values.[29]

Magnetic Resonance Imaging

Using DWI, apparent diffusion coefficient (ADC) mapping, and perfusion imaging, some studies have found early predictors for the development of life-threatening brain edema in acute MCA infarction. In two studies, lesion volume greater than 145 mL on DWI within 14 hours or greater than 82 mL on ADC maps within 6 hours after symptom onset predicted the development of a malignant course with positive predictive values of 91% and 82% and negative predictive values of 100% and 92%, respectively.[30,31] In the Diffusion and Perfusion Imaging Evaluation for Understanding Stroke Evolution (DEFUSE) study, a DWI lesion volume greater than 100 mL also accurately predicted malignant MCA infarction.[36] These positive and negative predictive values may be increased by a combined analysis of DWI and ADC measurements.[30] The value of perfusion imaging for the prediction of a malignant course is still controversial (Fig. 78-3).

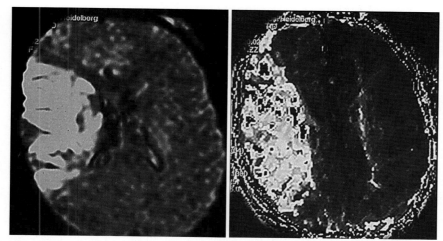

Figure 78-3 Diagnosis of malignant middle cerebral artery (MCA) infarction by MRI. *Left,* Diffusion-weighted imaging (DWI); *right,* perfusion imaging 4 hours after symptom onset. A diffusion lesion of >2/3 of the MCA territory and a perfusion deficit of the complete MCA territory can be seen. This constellation is highly predictive for a malignant course.

Single-Photon Emission Computed Tomography

There are only few studies evaluating single-photon emission CT (SPECT) for the prediction of a malignant course in MCA infarction.[37-39] Berrouschot et al[37] performed CT and technetium Tc 99m–ethylcysteinate dimer (Tc 99m–ECD) SPECT within 6 hours of symptom onset in 108 patients with acute stroke, 11 of whom died owing to MCA infarction. The sensitivity of Tc 99m–ECD SPECT for predicting fatal outcome was 82% in both visual and semiquantitative analyses; specificity was 98% for visual analysis and 99% for semiquantitative analysis. These figures compared favorably with the sensitivity and specificity of baseline CT studies, which were 36% and 100%, respectively.[37] In a study by Lampl et al,[38] who performed Tc 99m diethylenetriaminepentaacetic acid (DTPA) SPECT in 25 patients with MCA infarction at 36 hours after symptom onset, 5 patients died of herniation. Whereas stroke volume on CT was only marginally increased in these 5 patients in comparison with the other 20 patients, the extent of DTPA distribution, including more than one vascular territory, significantly correlated with herniation.[38]

Positron Emission Tomography

Positron emission tomography (PET) still represents the gold standard for defining the ischemic core, penumbra, and oligemia in acute stroke. However, PET is available in very few centers for patients with acute stroke and is therefore currently used mainly for scientific purposes and clinical studies. Only a few studies on malignant MCA infarction involve performance of PET.[40-42]

Dohmen et al[43] investigated 34 patients with acute MCA infarction involving more than 50% of the MCA territory on noncontrast CT performed within 12 hours after symptom onset. PET was performed within 24 hours after symptom onset using flumazenil tagged with radioactive carbon (^{11}C) to assess CBF and irreversible neuronal damage. Results showed significantly larger volumes of the ischemic core and larger volumes of irreversible neuronal

damage in patients with a malignant than in patients with a benign course (144.5 mL versus 62.2 mL and 157.9 mL versus 47.0 mL, respectively). In addition, mean CBF values within the ischemic core were significantly lower and the volume of the ischemic penumbra was significantly smaller in patients with malignant MCA infarction.[40]

Invasive Neuromonitoring

Multimodal invasive monitoring, including the placement of probes allowing measurement of intracranial pressure, (ICP), CPP, microdialysis, and continuous electroencephalography (EEG) monitoring, is an interesting instrument for close observation in patients suffering from severe strokes. Yet, except for ICP and CPP measurement, multimodal invasive monitoring is currently also restricted to a few, mostly academic centers using these tools within clinical studies and is not available for routine use. There are several studies providing data on patients with malignant MCA infarction. Dohmen et al[43] also performed microdialysis in addition to PET. They found close correlations between a number of parameters and the development of a malignant course after MCA infarction. These included increased ICP, decreased CPP and cerebral autoregulation, increased extracellular concentrations of transmitter amino acids and decreased extracellular concentrations of nontransmitter amino acids, increased concentrations of lactate, and decreased partial tissue oxygen pressure. In particular, increased ICP to more than 26.6 mm Hg and decreased CPP to less than 56 mm Hg both showed positive and negative predictive values of 100%.[40,41,43]

Animal Studies

Several animal models of ischemic stroke provide evidence that decompressive surgery improves cerebral perfusion, reduces the volume of infarction, and significantly reduces mortality.[44-49] Using an endovascular occlusion of the MCA technique, Forsting et al[44] demonstrated an

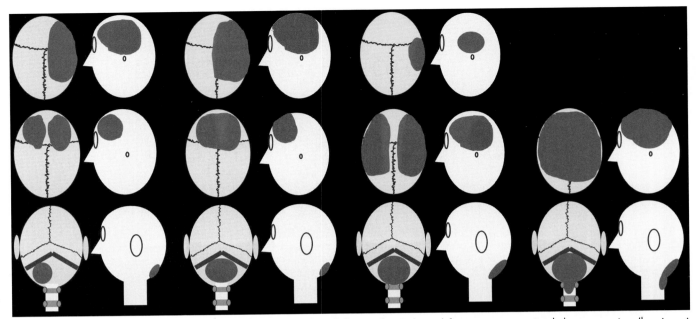

Figure 78-4 Different types of craniectomy: *Upper row, from left to right,* Unilateral frontotemporoparietal decompression (hemicraniectomy) not exceeding the sinus sagittalis superior; frontotemporoparietal decompression exceeding the sinus sagittalis superior; temporal decompression (usually with resection of the temporal lobe). *Middle row, from left to right,* Bifrontal decompression not exceeding the sinus sagittalis superior; bifrontal decompression exceeding the sinus sagittalis superior; bilateral frontotemporoparietal decompression (bilateral hemicraniectomy); total calvarectomy. *Lower row, from left to right,* Unilateral suboccipital decompression; bilateral suboccipital decompression without opening of the foramen magnum; bilateral suboccipital decompression with opening of the foramen magnum; bilateral suboccipital decompression, without opening of the foramen magnum and resection of the atlantic arch.

absolute reduction in mortality of 35% after decompressive craniectomy in a rat model of focal cerebral ischemia. Furthermore, there were marked absolute reductions in average infarct volume compared with controls of 84% in animals subjected to craniectomy 1 hour after MCA occlusion and of 63% in animals subjected to craniectomy at 24 hours.[44]

Engelhorn et al[47] compared reperfusion and craniectomy or both in a rat model of focal ischemia after MCA occlusion. They found significant absolute reductions in infarct volume by craniectomy at 1, 4, and 12 hours after MCA occlusion of 57%, 52%, and 33%, respectively. These results were comparable to those after reperfusion, probably owing to improved cerebral perfusion through collaterals after craniectomy.[49] Interestingly, the combination of reperfusion and craniectomy was not significantly better than one treatment alone.[47,48]

Technical Aspects

There are a variety of techniques for decompressive surgery. External (craniectomy, removal of the cranial vault) is differentiated from internal (removal of nonviable, edematous tissue) decompression. The two can be combined.[50,51] In patients with diffuse brain edema without midline shift, bilateral craniectomy is a reasonable approach, whereas in patients with unilateral swelling of one hemisphere and midline shift, hemicraniectomy is the recommended procedure (Fig. 78-4).

For hemicraniectomy, usually a large question mark–shaped skin incision based at the ear is made, and a

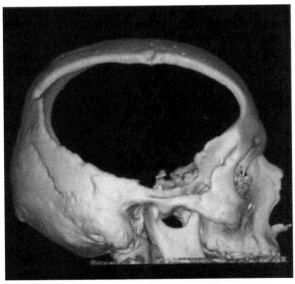

Figure 78-5 Bone defect after hemicraniectomy carried out over the entire lateral temporal lobe down to the floor of the temporal fossa.

bone flap containing parts of the frontal, parietal, temporal, and occipital squama is removed.[52] Alternatively, a T-shaped skin incision can be made in order to protect the occipital artery. Osteoplastic craniectomy should include parts of the frontal, parietal, and temporal squamae and should be performed to the base of the skull (Fig. 78-5). In the past, craniectomies were performed

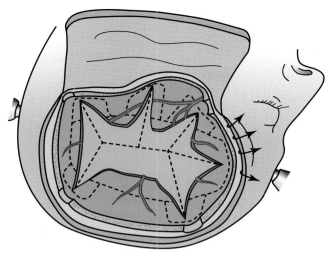

Figure 78-6 The "surgeon's eye view" of the large bone flap removal required in hemicraniectomy and surgical decompression for middle cerebral artery (MCA) territory infarction. Stellate dural incisions permit smooth brain expansion. Areas over the bulged brain are covered with either autologous or artificial dural substitute (duraplasty).

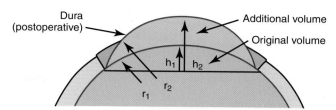

Figure 78-7 Illustration of parameters for estimation of additional volume created outside the skull by craniectomy in middle cerebral artery infarction with space-occupying edema, assuming that the brain takes an approximately spherical shape. h, height; r, radius.

without opening of the dura, but it is now recognized that decompression is achieved mainly by dural opening. Therefore, after dura enlargement, either an autologous or artificial dural patch should be inserted (Fig. 78-6). Some centers prefer to leave the dura open.[53] The need for additional tissue removal (i.e., in the case of malignant MCA infarction, temporal lobectomy) has been discussed over the past years. Although, in theory, resection of the temporal lobe may reduce the risk of uncal herniation, this technique is much more complicated because it is difficult to distinguish between already infarcted and potentially salvageable tissue and a benefit has never been proven by clinical studies. Meanwhile, there is a broad consensus among neurosurgeons that external decompressive surgery by hemicraniectomy is sufficient.[53] The bone flap is stored at −80° C and usually reimplanted after 6 weeks to 3 months. Alternatively, an artificial flap can be inserted.

Serious or life-threatening complications of craniectomy are rare, including postoperative wound and bone infections, epidural or subdural hematomas, hygroma, and hydrocephalus.[50,54-56] The most common, widely underestimated, but potentially detrimental complication of decompressive surgery arises from insufficient craniectomy, which leads to local shear stress and venous problems at the bone margins or, at worst, even to herniation through the craniectomy defect. Wagner et al[57] analyzed postoperative CT scans of 60 patients in order to determine the occurrence of hemicraniectomy-associated infarcts and hemorrhages. Infarcts or hemorrhages of any size occurred in 70% of all patients; most lesions, however, were small (<2 mL). There was a significant association between the frequency of hemorrhage and the size of the bone defect: The smaller the bone defect, the more often lesions were encountered.[57] Therefore, the size of craniectomy is critical, not only to prevent complications but also for craniectomy to be effective, that is, to create enough additional space outside the skull. The volume

of brain tissue to be allowed to shift outside the skull is directly related to the diameter of the removed bone flap and can be estimated using the following formula (Fig. 78-7):

$$\text{Additional volume} = \frac{\pi \times h_2^2}{3} \times (3 \times r_2 - h2) - \frac{\pi \times h_1^2}{3} \times (3 \times r_1 - h_1)$$

It is obvious that in order to compensate additional volumes of 80 to 100 mL, which usually occur in space-occupying malignant infarcts, the diameter of the craniectomy must be at least 12 cm (Fig. 78-8).

Clinical Studies

Hemicraniectomy in space-occupying stroke is by no means new and dates back at least as early as 1935.[58] Up to 2009, more than 100 case reports and case series and three randomized controlled trials involving more than 1800 patients with malignant MCA infarctions had been published (Table 78-2).[25,59]

Clinical Case Series

Most of the clinical case studies and reports are retrospective, with low numbers of patients, using control groups that are often historical and not directly

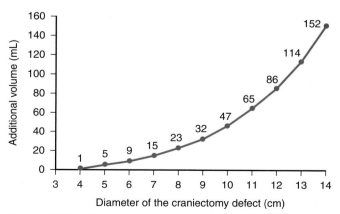

Figure 78-8 Graph demonstrating additional volume outside the skull gained by hemicraniectomy. In malignant middle cerebral artery infarctions, the volume of space-occupying brain edema is usually 80 mL or more. It is obvious that in order to achieve this additional volume, a diameter of at least 12 cm is required to create enough compensating space.

TABLE 78-2 OUTCOME AFTER MALIGNANT MIDDLE CEREBRAL ARTERY (MCA) INFARCTION: COMPARISON OF CONSERVATIVE TREATMENT AND HEMICRANIECTOMY*

	Conservative Treatment	Decompressive Surgery	Absolute Risk Reduction (%)
Nonrandomized studies (all patients)	N = 512	N = 1212	
Independent (%)	1.0	6.1	5.1
Mild to moderate disability (%)	11.2	25.6	14.4
Severe disability (%)	37.8	43.5	5.7
Death (%)	50.0	24.9	−25.1
Nonrandomized studies (individual data)	N = 61	N = 309	
Independent (%)	0.0	5.9	5.9
Mild to moderate disability (%)	0.0	35.6	35.6
Severe disability (%)	17.9	40.7	22.8
Death (%)	82.1	17.8	−64.3
Randomized trials, treatment ≤99 h	N = 65	N = 69	
Independent (%)	0.0	0.0	0.0
Mild to moderate disability (%)	24.6	37.7	13.1
Severe disability (%)	12.3	40.6	28.3
Death (%)	63.1	21.7	−41.4
Randomized trials, treatment ≤48 h	N = 51	N = 58	
Independent (%)	0.0	0.0	0.0
Mild to moderate disability (%)	23.5	39.7	16.2
Severe disability (%)	5.9	39.7	33.8
Death (%)	70.6	20.7	−49.9
Randomized trials, treatment >48-99 h	N = 14	N = 11	
Independent (%)	0.0	0.0	0.0
Mild to moderate disability (%)	28.6	27.3	−1.3
Severe disability (%)	35.7	45.5	9.8
Death (%)	35.7	27.3	−8.4

*Functional outcome classified as (1) independent outcome (modified Rankin Scale [mRS] score 0 to 1; or Glasgow Outcome Scale [GOS] score 5; or Barthel Index [BI] ≥ 90); (2) mild to moderate disability (mRS score 2 to 3; or GOS score 4; or BI 60 to 85); (3) severe disability (mRS score 4 or 5; or GOS score 2 to 3; or BI < 60); and (4) death. In cases in which more than one outcome scale is given, outcome is classified according to the following priority: mRS/GOS/BI.

comparable because of higher age, more frequent lesions of the dominant hemisphere, different comorbidity, largely different conservative treatment concepts, and difference in operation techniques, cooling modes and durations of hypothermia, concomitant therapies, and patient monitoring. Most of all, however, inclusion criteria vary largely among these studies, because there is still no generally accepted definition for malignant MCA infarction.

Clinical Randomized Trials

Five randomized controlled trials were initiated between 2000 and 2004: The American Hemicraniectomy and Durotomy Upon Deterioration from Infarction-Related Swelling Trial (HeADDFIRST), which was completed in 2003, but has not been published yet as a written paper, the German DEcompressive Surgery for the Treatment of malignant INfarction of the middle cerebral arterY (DESTINY) trial, the French DEcompressive Craniectomy In MALignant middle cerebral artery infarcts (DECIMAL) trial, the Dutch Hemicraniectomy After Middle cerebral artery infarction with Life-threatening Edema Trial (HAMLET), and the Philippinian Hemicraniectomy for Malignant Middle Cerebral Artery Infarcts (HeMMI) trial.[25-27,60-62] In 2007 the results of a prospectively planned pooled analysis including all patients from

DESTINY and DECIMAL and 23 patients from HAMLET treated by early hemicraniectomy within 48 hours were published.[63]

Mortality and Functional Outcome

With all the results from nonrandomized studies taken together and reports on hypothermia excluded, hemicraniectomy is shown to reduce early mortality (in hospital) from 66.5% after conservative treatment to about 18.7% (−47.8%). If only patients for whom at least one follow-up is available are considered, this effect decreases, from 50% to 24.9% (−25.1%). If only reports with individual data are considered, 370 patients are available: The effect in reducing mortality after decompressive surgery is more obvious: 81.1% versus 12.6% for early mortality (−68.5%) and 82.1% versus 17.8% after 6 months (−64.3%) (there are no individual patient data after conservative treatment beyond 1 year).[59] These results could be confirmed by the randomized trials: In the pooled analysis (and analyzing all patients from DESTINY, DECIMAL, and HAMLET) including patients treated within 48 hours, mortality at 1 year was significantly decreased from 71.4% (70.6%) in the conservative group to 21.6% (20.7%) in the surgery group (−49.8%; −49.9%).[63] If surgery is delayed more than 48 and up to 99 hours after symptom onset, this effect cannot be observed anymore: Rates are 27.3%

after decompressive surgery and 35.7% after conservative treatment (−8.4%) (see Table 78-2).[25,63]

In nonrandomized studies, 31.7% of all patients undergoing decompressive surgery showed no or mild to moderate disability (modified Rankin Scale [mRS] score 0 to 3; Glasgow Outcome Scale [GOS] score 4 to 5; Barthel Index [BI] 60 or higher) at outcome visits, compared with 12.2% of patients undergoing conservative treatment (+19.5%). Taking into account individual patient data only, 41.5% of patients showed no or mild to moderate disability after decompressive surgery, compared with 0% after conservative treatment (+41.5%).[59] In the pooled analysis of randomized trials on early hemicraniectomy, more patients in the surgery group had an mRS score of 4 or less (74.5% versus 23.8%; +50.7%) and an mRS score of 3 or less (43.1% versus 21.4%; +21.7%). The number needed to treat (NNT) was 2 for survival with a mRS score of 4 or less, 4 for survival with an mRS score of 3 or less, and 2 for survival irrespective of functional outcome.[63] If surgery is delayed more than 48 and up to 99 hours after symptom onset, 67.2% of patients after surgical treatment, compared with 25.5% after conservative treatment, survive with a mRS score of 4 or less (+41.7%), and 39.7% after surgical treatment compared with 23.5% after conservative treatment survive with a mRS score of 3 or less (+16.2%) (see Table 78-2).[25]

However, in the nonrandomized studies, the number of severely disabled patients (mRS score, 4 to 5; GOS score 2 to 3; BI <60) increased after hemicraniectomy from 37.8% to 43.5% (+5.7%) in all patients and from 17.9% to 40.7% (+22.8%) in reports with individual data.[59] In the pooled analysis of the randomized trials, very severe disability (mRS score, 5) was not increased after hemicraniectomy within 48 hours after symptom onset (4% after surgery versus 5% after conservative treatment; −1%), whereas analysis of data from all patients from DESTINY, DECIMAL, and HAMLET shows the number to increase from 3.9 to 12.1% (+8.2%). However, the number of moderately to severely disabled patients (mRS score, 4) increased from 2.4% after conservative treatment to 31.4% after hemicraniectomy (+29.0%) in the pooled analysis, or from 2.0% to 27.6% (+25.6%) in analysis of data from all patients from DESTINY, DECIMAL, and HAMLET. If surgery is delayed more than 48 and up to 99 hours, the number of patients with very severe disability (mRS score, 5) is increased from 3.1% after conservative treatment to 10.1% after hemicraniectomy (+7.0%), and the number of moderately to severely disabled patients (mRS score, 4) is increased from 9.2% after conservative treatment to 30.4% after hemicraniectomy (+21.2%) (see Table 78-2).[25,63]

Assessment of functional outcome remains a fiercely debated issue. Standard outcome measures such as the BI, GOS, and mRS, with their emphasis on motor abilities, may not account for all remaining deficits, particularly cognitive impairments and communication skills in patients with dominant-hemisphere infarctions. Moreover, the dichotomization between favorable and unfavorable outcomes is highly controversial: In this context, it has to be taken into account that according to the results of the randomized trials, after hemicraniectomy, the probability to survive in a condition of being unable to walk and dependent on the assistance of others for most activities of daily living (i.e., mRS score, 4) increases more than 15 times when hemicraniectomy is performed within 48 hours and still increases more than three times when it is delayed up to 99 hours.[25,63] These results have initiated a discussion about which grade of dependency distinguishes between favorable and unfavorable outcomes after malignant MCA infarction.[64,65] There is strong reluctance among many neurologists to regard a score on the mRS of more than 2 as favorable outcome. On the other hand, most neurointensive care physicians agree that in such a life-threatening and primarily severely disabling disease as malignant MCA infarction, an mRS score of 3 may be considered a favorable outcome. There is also agreement that a mRS score of 5 is clearly unfavorable. So the discussion is mainly related to the group of patients surviving with an mRS score of 4. In this group of patients, the terms "favorable" and "unfavorable" do not apply and should rather be replaced by "acceptable" and "unacceptable." It is the patients themselves or eventually their closest relatives or caregivers who should decide what is "acceptable" and what is not. The evaluation of the quality of life and the question of retrospective consent to treatment may help in this issue, with the fact that death is the most probable alternative always being considered.

Quality of Life

There are currently only scarce data on the quality of life of patients after malignant MCA infarction treated by hemicraniectomy, and available studies came to divergent results. Data of these small trials suggest that most survivors of malignant MCA infarction show an average quality of life comparable to patients with other types of stroke.[66-70] One trial revealed a more profound reduction in the quality of life for those surviving MCA infarction.[71] Interpretation of these findings is limited, however, because there are insufficient data on patients treated conservatively.

Treatment of Patients with Dominant-Hemisphere Infarction

The treatment of patients with malignant MCA infarction of the dominant hemisphere is another controversial issue. In many centers decompressive surgery was not warranted in these patients. The inability to communicate and severe hemiplegia, especially of the dominant upper extremity, were considered too disabling, and hemicraniectomy was often restricted to patients with a non-dominant-hemisphere infarction. From the randomized trials and larger prospective case series, there is currently no indication that patients with dominant malignant infarctions do not profit from treatment.[25,63] Neither mortality nor functional outcome depends on the side of the lesion in any of the larger prospective studies.[72] Indeed, the handicap caused by aphasia may be balanced by the neuropsychological deficits, that is, the severe attention deficit, apraxia, and others, in patients with infarction of the nondominant hemisphere.[67,73] In addition, the long-term aphasia in dominant-hemisphere malignant MCA infarction is rarely complete and often shows remarkable improvement.[50,54,67,68,74] So far, there are no indications that surgery should not be considered in patients with dominant-hemisphere infarction.

Timing of Hemicraniectomy

In a review of 138 patients from retrospective and uncontrolled case series, Gupta et al[72] found that neither time to surgery, presence of signs of herniation, nor additional lesions in other vascular territories was an independent predictor for poor outcome.[72] The randomized trials indicate that a benefit of hemicraniectomy can be achieved only when it is performed within 48 hours of symptom onset; however, the numbers of patients randomly assigned to treatment after 48 hours in these trials is too small to allow definite conclusions to be drawn.[25,63] Some studies suggest improved outcome if hemicraniectomy is performed within less than 24 hours after stroke onset in comparison with later surgery, especially when signs of herniation are present.[50,75] On the other hand, in other case series and nonrandomized studies, time to treatment had no influence on outcome.[69,76] Currently, hemicraniectomy should be performed as soon as possible once the decision for surgical intervention has been made.

Treatment of Elder Patients

Although the percentage of young patients with malignant MCA infarction is comparatively high, more than 60% of patients are older than 50 years, and more than 40% are older than 60 years.[77] Several studies indicate unfavorable outcomes and poor quality of life in elder patients, suggesting an age limit of 50, 55, or 60 years.[56,70-72,74,76,78-85] Interpretation of these findings is limited by the fact that in most of these studies, older patients were operated on significantly later and treated less aggressively than younger patients. The subgroup analyses of the randomized trials did not indicate poorer outcome in patients 50 years or older than in younger patients.[25,63] However, the age limit for inclusion in these trials was 60 years, and there are no data from randomized trials of patients older than 60 years. Therefore, from the available data, it is currently impossible to define a certain age limit, where decompressive surgery has no benefit and should not be performed anymore.

Related Disorders

Decompressive Surgery in Space-Occupying Cerebellar Infarction

Space-occupying edema is a common, but frequently overlooked, complication in 8% to 39% of patients with large cerebellar infarction.[86-94] The tight posterior fossa provides only a small space for compensation of mass effect, and life-threatening complications may develop rapidly, including (1) obstructive hydrocephalus due to the blockage of the fourth ventricle, (2) direct compression of the midbrain and pons, (3) upward herniation of the superior vermis cerebelli through the tentorial notch, and (4) downward herniation of the cerebellar tonsils through the foramen magnum.[87,88,94-97] In the case of extensive mass effect, conservative treatment strategies are usually unsuccessful. It is widely accepted among neurosurgeons and neurologists that surgery is the treatment of choice. However, the time point at which to start surgical treatment and which factors should trigger intervention remain unclear. Furthermore, the large number of available procedures—ventriculostomy (either by extraventricular drainage [EVD] or by endoscopic third ventricle ventriculostomy [EVT]), suboccipital decompressive surgery of the posterior fossa with or without resection of necrotic tissue, and a combination of both—have not been tested or compared with another in larger prospective or randomized trials. Most clinicians agree that alert and clinically stable patients should be treated conservatively and monitored closely.[96,98] Others recommend early or preventive intervention, because clinical signs of deterioration are unspecific and neuroradiologic parameters are uncertain or may be detected too late.[99-101] For patients with impaired consciousness or those whose status deteriorates, some authorities recommend ventriculostomy as the first choice, decompressive surgery being considered only when there is further clinical deterioration.[96,102] Others, however, consider this approach to be dangerous because of possible upward herniation and because it does not relieve brainstem compression. In this setting, most surgeons favor suboccipital decompression as first-choice treatment, with or without duraplasty[92,98] and with or without additional resection of infarcted tissue,[96] or a combination of ventriculostomy in addition to decompressive surgery as first choice, especially when occlusive hydrocephalus is present.[88,103,104] As in awake and stable patients, there is evidence showing benefit for surgery on patients who are comatose or show signs of herniation. In one prospective study, 47% of patients who were comatose had a good outcome.[101]

According to the available data, close monitoring and repeated neuroimaging, if possible using MRI to detect brainstem infarction, is the recommended procedure in patients with large cerebellar infarcts. Early surgical intervention is recommended in those patients whose status deteriorates because of mass effect rather than additional brainstem infarction, because brainstem compression, occlusive hydrocephalus, and herniation can most often be reversed or even prevented by suboccipital craniectomy in these patients.

If the decision for suboccipital craniectomy is made, patients should be placed in prone or semiprone (park bench) position. After vertical midline skin incision from the protuberantia occipitalis to the upper cervical spine, separation of skin and subcutaneous tissue from the underlying fascia, which is cut through laterally to the processi spinosi of the upper cervical spine, and disconnection of muscles from the processi spinosi and the occiput, osteoclastic craniotomy should be performed beneath the sinus transversus and enlarged laterally. Great attention must be paid to opening the foramen magnum sufficiently to decompress the cerebellar tonsils. In this context, some neurosurgeons recommend additional laminectomy and resection of the atlantic arch. To maximize the decompressive effect the dura should be opened (Y-shaped) above the cerebellum and the medulla oblongata. After that step, some neurosurgeons recommend resection of necrotic tissue by suction. Finally, duraplasty should be performed with the use of primarily prepared galea strip or artificial dura (see Fig. 78-4). Complications include injury of the vertebral arteries, the induction of major bleeding, as well as epidural and subdural hematoma and hygroma.

Decompressive Surgery in Traumatic Brain Injury

A central pathophysiologic consideration in traumatic brain injury (TBI) is that brain damage does not cease with the impact (primary injury) but continues to proceed over the following days. Apart from mass lesions, particularly focal or diffuse brain edema, subsequent increase in ICP, decrease in blood supply and oxygen delivery, and energy failure resulting in further brain edema are a common cause of death and disability after TBI.[105,106] According to the current guidelines, treatment of intracranial hypertension should be initiated when ICP exceeds the threshold of 20 mm Hg, including osmotic agents, deep sedation, and normothermia. In the case of medically refractory, diffuse cerebral edema and intracranial hypertension, decompressive surgery within 48 hours of injury, consisting of bifrontal craniectomy, may be considered.[107-109] As for malignant ischemic cerebral infarction, there is evidence from animal studies that decompressive surgery in TBI effectively lowers ICP and prevents secondary brain damage, although there are also controversial findings.[110,111] A number of nonrandomized clinical studies demonstrate that decompressive surgery effectively lowers ICP, especially with additional opening of the dura, and suggest favorable outcome in about 50% to 60% of patients.[22,112-122] On the contrary, Munch et al[123] were unable to show that decompressive surgery achieves a significant postoperative reduction of ICP, improvement of cerebral perfusion pressure, or a beneficial effect on patient outcome.[123] It also remains unclear whether the postulated effect on ICP levels is accompanied by better outcome because of the lack of control groups or, at best, the use of historical control groups and/or selection bias in all of these studies, because patients with vast primary lesions, severe hypoxia, severe additional ischemic infarctions, brainstem injuries, or signs of herniation were usually not included into the studies. As with malignant MCA infarction, maximum benefit seems to be obtained by early intervention and before ICP reaches uncontrollably high values.[115] A beneficial effect in routine use, however, has not been consistently demonstrated yet.

Decompressive Surgery in Subarachnoid Hemorrhage

Only a few studies involving very small numbers of patients are available on decompressive surgery in subarachnoid hemorrhage (SAH), demonstrating heterogeneous results.[124-127] Early decompressive surgery seems to be more beneficial,[124] and patients without radiologic signs of ischemia seem to benefit most.[128] The use of prophylactic craniectomy was investigated in one small study of 8 patients with high-grade SAH from MCA aneurysms with associated large sylvian fissure hematomas. In 7 patients, ICP was effectively decreased after decompressive surgery, with favorable outcomes in 5 patients.[125]

Decompressive Surgery for Spontaneous Intracerebral Hemorrhage

There is no convincing evidence for any surgical treatment option in spontaneous ICH. The largest randomized controlled trial so far, International Surgical Trial in Intracerebral Haemorrhage (STICH), included 1033 patients and found no benefit of early hematoma evacuation regarding outcome and mortality.[129] Analogous to malignant MCA infarction and TBI, not only lesion volume but also subsequent edema formation contributes to mass effect and intracranial hypertension in ICH. Perihematomal edema develops immediately after ICH and usually peaks around the third or fourth day but has a very inhomogeneous time course and may increase up to 2 weeks.[130] Whether ICH-associated brain edema is linked to poor outcome, however, remains controversial.[131-134] In concordance with this uncertainty, there is little evidence about decompressive surgery following ICH. Murthy and colleagues report 12 patients with primary supratentorial ICH who underwent hematoma evacuation plus decompressive hemicraniectomy. Of 11 survivors, six had a favorable functional outcome (mRS score ≤3).[135] In another study on clot evacuation in patients with primary supratentorial ICH, 15 patients, in whom progression of brain swelling was anticipated, underwent decompressive craniectomy in addition to clot removal. The combination therapy showed promising results in this subgroup of severely compromised patients.[136]

Decompressive Surgery in Cerebral Venous Thrombosis

In the majority of cases, cerebral venous thrombosis (CVT) naturally takes a benign course, but in a subgroup of patients, large hemorrhagic venous infarctions and brain edema occur, eventually leading to mass effect and intracranial hypertension.[137] These patients may be candidates for more aggressive interventions. In the few reports on craniectomy in the context of CVT, favorable outcomes were reported for most cases: Stefini et al[138] reported experience of performing decompressive craniectomy in 3 patients with dural sinus thrombosis and impending herniation due to large hemorrhagic infarcts. Two patients who underwent operation as soon as signs of herniation developed showed complete functional recovery. One patient who underwent delayed surgery remained severely disabled.[138] In accordance with these results, Coutinho et al[139] reported 3 consecutively treated patients. Two had an excellent outcome. The third patient, who underwent delayed surgery after being comatose for at least 12 hours, died.[139] In a series of 15 patients including 4 with severe CVT, who underwent decompressive craniectomy, all 4 recovered with favorable functional outcomes (GOS score, 4 to 5).[140] However, these case reports are prone to a severe publication bias, and cases with unfavorable outcomes are less likely to be reported. What can be concluded from the available data is that decompressive surgery may be considered in refractory intracranial hypertension in otherwise clinically desperate situations.

REFERENCES

1. Baethmann A, Oettinger W, Rothenfusser W, et al: Brain edema factors: Current state with particular reference to plasma constituents and glutamate, *Adv Neurol* 28:171-195, 1980.
2. Rosenberg GA, Yang Y: Vasogenic edema due to tight junction disruption by matrix metalloproteinases in cerebral ischemia, *Neurosurg Focus* 22:E4, 2007.
3. Liang D, Bhatta S, Gerzanich V, et al: Cytotoxic edema: Mechanisms of pathological cell swelling, *Neurosurg Focus* 22:E2, 2007.
4. Kawamata T, Mori T, Sato S, et al: Tissue hyperosmolality and brain edema in cerebral contusion, *Neurosurg Focus* 22:E5, 2007.
5. Hacke W, Schwab S, Horn M, et al: 'Malignant' middle cerebral artery territory infarction: Clinical course and prognostic signs, *Arch Neurol* 53:309-315, 1996.
6. Silver FL, Norris JW, Lewis AJ, Hachinski VC: Early mortality following stroke: A prospective review, *Stroke* 15:492-496, 1984.
7. Shaw CM, Alvord EC, Berry RG: Swelling of the brain following ischemic infarction with arterial occlusion, *Arch Neurol* 1:161-177, 1959.
8. Frank JI: Large hemispheric infarction, deterioration, and intracranial pressure, *Neurology* 45:1286-1290, 1995.
9. Ropper AH, Shafran B: Brain edema after stroke. Clinical syndrome and intracranial pressure, *Arch Neurol* 41:26-29, 1984.
10. Bounds JV, Wiebers DO, Whisnant JP, et al: Mechanisms and timing of deaths from cerebral infarction, *Stroke* 12:474-477, 1981.
11. Berrouschot J, Sterker M, Bettin S, et al: Mortality of space-occupying ('malignant') middle cerebral artery infarction under conservative intensive care, *Intensive Care Med* 24:620-623, 1998.
12. Kasner SE, Demchuk AM, Berrouschot J, et al: Predictors of fatal brain edema in massive hemispheric ischemic stroke, *Stroke* 32:2117-2123, 2001.
13. Hofmeijer J, van der Worp HB, Kappelle LJ: Treatment of space-occupying cerebral infarction, *Crit Care Med* 31:617-625, 2003.
14. Bardutzky J, Schwab S: Antiedema therapy in ischemic stroke, *Stroke* 38:3084-3094, 2008.
15. Bereczki D, Liu M, Prado GF, et al: Cochrane report: A systematic review of mannitol therapy for acute ischemic stroke and cerebral parenchymal hemorrhage, *Stroke* 31:2719-2722, 2000.
16. Muizelaar JP, Marmarou A, Ward JD, et al: Adverse effects of prolonged hyperventilation in patients with severe head injury: A randomized clinical trial, *J Neurosurg* 75:731-739, 1991.
17. Stringer WA, Hasso AN, Thompson JR, et al: Hyperventilation-induced cerebral ischemia in patients with acute brain lesions: Demonstration by xenon-enhanced CT, *AJNR Am J Neuroradiol* 14:475-484, 1993.
18. Schwab S, Spranger M, Schwarz S, et al: Barbiturate coma in severe hemispheric stroke: Useful or obsolete? *Neurology* 48:1608-1613, 1997.
19. Kaufmann AM, Cardoso ER: Aggravation of vasogenic cerebral edema by multiple-dose mannitol, *J Neurosurg* 77:584-589, 1992.
20. Juttler E, Schellinger PD, Aschoff A, et al: Clinical review: Therapy for refractory intracranial hypertension in ischaemic stroke, *Critical Care* 11:231, 2007.
21. Schwab S, Schwarz S, Spranger M, et al: Moderate hypothermia in the treatment of patients with severe middle cerebral artery infarction, *Stroke* 29:2461-2466, 1998.
22. Yoo DS, Kim DS, Cho KS, et al: Ventricular pressure monitoring during bilateral decompression with dural expansion, *J Neurosurg* 91:953-959, 1999.
23. Jaeger M, Soehle M, Meixensberger J: Improvement of brain tissue oxygen and intracranial pressure during and after surgical decompression for diffuse brain oedema and space occupying infarction, *Acta Neurochir Suppl* 95:117-118, 2005.
24. Krieger DW, Demchuk AM, Kasner SE, et al: Early clinical and radiological predictors of fatal brain swelling in ischemic stroke, *Stroke* 30:287-292, 1999.
25. Hofmeijer J, Kappelle LJ, Algra A, et al: Surgical decompression for space-occupying cerebral infarction (the Hemicraniectomy After Middle Cerebral Artery infarction with Life-threatening Edema Trial [HAMLET]): A multicentre, open, randomised trial, *Lancet Neurol* 8:326-333, 2009.
26. Juttler E, Schwab S, Schmiedek P, et al: Decompressive Surgery for the Treatment of Malignant Infarction of the Middle Cerebral Artery (DESTINY): A randomized, controlled trial, *Stroke* 38:2518-2525, 2007.
27. Vahedi K, Vicaut E, Mateo J, et al: Sequential-design, multicenter, randomized, controlled trial of early decompressive craniectomy in malignant middle cerebral artery infarction (DECIMAL Trial), *Stroke* 38:2506-2517, 2007.
28. Barber PA, Demchuk AM, Zhang J, et al: Computed tomographic parameters predicting fatal outcome in large middle cerebral artery infarction, *Cerebrovasc Dis* 16:230-235, 2003.
29. Hofmeijer J, Algra A, Kapelle LJ, et al: Predictors of life-threatening brain edema in middle cerebral artery infarction, *Cerebrovasc Dis* 25:176-184, 2008.
30. Oppenheim C, Samson Y, Manaï R, et al: Prediction of malignant middle cerebral artery infarction by diffusion-weighted imaging, *Stroke* 31:2175-2181, 2000.
31. Thomalla G, Kucinski T, Schoder V, et al: Prediction of malignant middle cerebral artery infarction by early perfusion- and diffusion-weighted magnetic resonance imaging, *Stroke* 34:1892-1899, 2003.
32. Von Kummer R, Meyding-Lamade U, Forsting M, et al: Sensitivity and prognostic value of early CT in occlusion of the middle cerebral artery trunk, *Am J Neuroradiol* 15:9-15, 1994.
33. Lee SJ, Lee KH, Na DG: Multiphasic helical computed tomography predicts subsequent development of severe brain oedema in acute ischemic stroke, *Arch Neurol* 61:505-509, 2004.
34. Ryoo JW, Na DG, Kim SS, et al: Malignant middle cerebral artery infarction in hyperacute ischemic stroke: Evaluation with multiphasic perfusion computed tomography maps, *J Comput Assist Tomogr* 28:55-62, 2004.
35. Dittrich R, Kloska SP, Fischer T, et al: Accuracy of perfusion-CT in predicting malignant middle cerebral artery brain infarction, *J Neurol* 255:896-902, 2008.
36. Albers GW, Thijs VN, Wechsler L, et al: Magnetic resonance imaging profiles predict clinical response to early reperfusion: The diffusion and perfusion imaging evaluation for understanding stroke evolution (DEFUSE) study, *Ann Neurol* 60:508-517, 2006.
37. Berrouschot J, Barthel H, von Kummer R, et al: 99m technetium-ethyl-cysteinate-dimer single-photon emission CT can predict fatal ischemic brain edema, *Stroke* 29:2556-2562, 1998.
38. Lampl Y, Sadeh M, Lorberboym M: Prospective evaluation of malignant middle cerebral artery infarction with blood-brain barrier imaging using Tc-99m DTPA SPECT, *Brain Res* 1113:194-199, 2006.
39. Limburg M, van Royen EA, Hijdra A, de Bruine JF, Verbeeten BW Jr: Single-photon emission computed tomography and early death in acute ischemic stroke, *Stroke* 21:1150-1155, 1990.
40. Dohmen C, Bosche B, Graf R, et al: Prediction of malignant course in MCA infarction by PET and microdialysis, *Stroke* 34:2152-2158, 2003.
41. Bosche B, Dohmen C, Graf R, et al: Extracellular concentrations of non-transmitter amino acids in peri-infarct tissue of patients predict malignant middle cerebral artery infarction, *Stroke* 34:2908-2913, 2003.
42. Heiss WD, Dohmen C, Sobesky J, et al: Identification of malignant brain edema after hemispheric stroke by PET-imaging and microdialysis, *Acta Neurochir Suppl* 86:237-240, 2003.
43. Dohmen C, Bosche B, Graf R, et al: Identification and clinical impact of impaired cerebrovascular autoregulation in patients with malignant middle cerebral artery infarction, *Stroke* 38:56-61, 2007.

44. Forsting M, Reith W, Schabitz WR, et al: Decompressive craniectomy for cerebral infarction. An experimental study in rats, *Stroke* 26:259-264, 1995.
45. Doerfler A, Engelhorn T, Heiland S, et al: Perfusion- and diffusion-weighted magnetic resonance imaging for monitoring decompressive craniectomy in animals with experimental hemispheric stroke, *J Neurosurg* 96:933-940, 2002.
46. Doerfler A, Forsting M, Reith W, et al: Decompressive craniectomy in a rat model of "malignant" cerebral hemispheric stroke: Experimental support for an aggressive therapeutic approach, *J Neurosurg* 85:853-859, 1996.
47. Engelhorn T, Doerfler A, Kastrup A, et al: Decompressive craniectomy, reperfusion, or a combination for early treatment of acute "malignant" cerebral hemispheric stroke in rats: Potential mechanisms studied by MRI, *Stroke* 30:1456-1463, 1999.
48. Engelhorn T, von Kummer R, Reith W, et al: What is effective in malignant middle cerebral artery infarction: Reperfusion, craniectomy, or both? An experimental study in rats, *Stroke* 33:617-622, 2002.
49. Walberer M, Ritschel N, Nedelmann M, et al: Aggravation of infarct formation by brain swelling in a large territorial stroke: A target for neuroprotection? *J Neurosurg* 109:287-293, 2008.
50. Schwab S, Steiner T, Aschoff A, et al: Early hemicraniectomy in patients with complete middle cerebral artery infarction, *Stroke* 29:1888-1893, 1998.
51. Mori K, Ishimaru S, Maeda M: Unco-parahippocampectomy for direct surgical treatment of downward transtentorial herniation, *Acta Neurochir (Wien)* 140:1239-1244, 1998.
52. Unterberg A, Juettler E: The role of surgery in ischemic stroke: Decompressive surgery, *Curr Opin Crit Care* 13:175-179, 2007.
53. Hutchinson P, Timofeev I, Kirkpatrick P: Surgery for brain edema, *Neurosurg Focus* 22:E14, 2007.
54. Rieke K, Schwab S, Krieger D, et al: Decompressive surgery in space-occupying hemispheric infarction: Results of an open, prospective trial, *Crit Care Med* 23:1576-1587, 1995.
55. Waziri A, Fusco D, Mayer SA, et al: Postoperative hydrocephalus in patients undergoing decompressive hemicraniectomy for ischemic or hemorrhagic stroke, *Neurosurgery* 61:489-493, 2007.
56. Uhl E, Kreth FW, Elias B, et al: Outcome and prognostic factors of hemicraniectomy for space occupying cerebral infarction, *J Neurol Neurosurg Psychiatry* 75:270-274, 2004.
57. Wagner S, Schnippering H, Aschoff A, et al: Suboptimum hemicraniectomy as a cause of additional cerebral lesions in patients with malignant infarction of the middle cerebral artery, *J Neurosurg* 94:693-696, 2001.
58. Greco T: Le thrombosi posttraumatiche della carotide, *Arch Ital Chir* 39:757-784, 1935.
59. Juttler E, Kohrmann M, Aschoff A, et al: Hemicraniectomy for space-occupying supratentorial ischemic stroke, *Future Neurol* 3:251-264, 2008.
60. Frank JI, Krieger D, Chyatte D: Hemicraniectomy and durotomy upon deterioration from massive hemispheric infarction: A proposed multicenter, prospective, randomized study, *Stroke* 30:243, 1999.
61. Frank JI: HeADDFIRST Preliminary results. Presented at the 55th Annual AAN Meeting in Honolulu, Hawaii, April 3, 2003.
62. Stroke Trials Registry. www.strokecenter.org/trials/TrialDetail.aspx?tid=575.
63. Vahedi K, Hofmeijer J, Juettler E, et al: Early decompressive surgery in malignant infarction of the middle cerebral artery: A pooled analysis of three randomised controlled trials, *Lancet Neurol* 6:215-222, 2007.
64. Puetz V, Campos CR, Eliasziw M, et al: Assessing the benefits of hemicraniectomy: What is a favourable outcome?, *Lancet Neurol* 6:580, 2007.
65. Vahedi K, Hofmeijer J, Juettler E, et al: Assessing the benefits of hemicraniectomy: What is a favourable outcome? Authors' reply, *Lancet Neurol* 6:580-581, 2007.
66. Vahedi K, Benoist L, Kurtz A, et al: Quality of life after decompressive craniectomy for malignant middle cerebral artery infarction, *J Neurol Neurosurg Psychiatry* 76:1181-1182, 2005.
67. Walz B, Zimmermann C, Böttger S, et al: Prognosis of patients after hemicraniectomy in malignant middle cerebral artery infarction, *J Neurol* 249:1183-1190, 2002.
68. Woertgen C, Erban P, Rothoerl RD, et al: Quality of life after decompressive craniectomy in patients suffering from supratentorial brain ischemia, *Acta Neurochir (Wien)* 146:691-695, 2004.
69. Curry WT Jr, Sethi MK, Ogilvy CS, et al: Factors associated with outcome after hemicraniectomy for large middle cerebral artery territory infarction, *Neurosurgery* 56:681-692, 2005.
70. Erban P, Woertgen C, Luerding R, et al: Long-term outcome after hemicraniectomy for space occupying right hemispheric MCA infarction, *Clin Neurol Neurosurg* 108:384-387, 2006.
71. Foerch C, Lang JM, Krause J, et al: Functional impairment, disability, and quality of life outcome after decompressive hemicraniectomy in malignant middle cerebral artery infarction, *J Neurosurg* 101:248-254, 2004.
72. Gupta R, Connolly ES, Mayer S, et al: Hemicraniectomy for massive middle cerebral artery territory infarction: A systematic review, *Stroke* 35:539-543, 2004.
73. De Haan RJ, Limburg M, Van der Meulen JH, et al: Quality of life after stroke: Impact of stroke type and lesion location, *Stroke* 26:402-408, 1995.
74. Kastrau F, Wolter M, Huber W, et al: Recovery from aphasia after hemicraniectomy for infarction of the speech-dominant hemisphere, *Stroke* 36:825-829, 2005.
75. Cho DY, Chen TC, Lee HC: Ultra-early decompressive craniectomy for malignant middle cerebral artery infarction, *Surg Neurol* 60:227-232, 2005.
76. Pillai A, Menon SK, Kumar S, et al: Decompressive hemicraniectomy in malignant middle cerebral artery infarction: An analysis of long-term outcome and factors in patient selection, *J Neurosurg* 106:59-65, 2007.
77. Balzer B, Stober T, Huber G, et al: [Space-occupying cerebral infarct], *Nervenarzt* 58:689-691, 1987.
78. Holtkamp M, Buchheim K, Unterberg A, et al: Hemicraniectomy in elderly patients with space occupying media infarction: Improved survival but poor functional outcome, *J Neurol Neurosurg Psychiatry* 70:226-228, 2001.
79. Leonhardt G, Wilhelm H, Doerfler A, et al: Clinical outcome and neuropsychological deficits after right decompressive hemicraniectomy in MCA infarction, *J Neurol* 249:1433-1440, 2002.
80. Maramattom BV, Bahn MM, Wijdicks EMF: Which patient fares worse after early deterioration due to swelling from hemispheric stroke? *Neurology* 63:2142-2145, 2004.
81. Yao Y, Liu W, Yang X, et al: Is decompressive craniectomy for malignant middle cerebral artery territory infarction of any benefit for elderly patients? *Surg Neurol* 64:165-169, 2005.
82. Kilincer C, Asil T, Utku U, et al: Factors affecting the outcome of decompressive craniectomy for large hemispheric infarctions: A prospective cohort study, *Acta Neurochir* 147:587-594, 2005.
83. Harscher S, Reichart R, Terborg C, et al: Outcome after decompressive craniectomy in patients with severe ischemic stroke, *Acta Neurochir (Wien)* 148:31-37, 2006.
84. Rabinstein AA, Mueller-Kronast N, Maramattom BV, et al: Factors predicting prognosis after decompressive hemicraniectomy for hemispheric infarction, *Neurology* 67:891-893, 2006.
85. Chen CC, Cho DY, Tsai SC: Outcome of and prognostic factors for decompressive hemicraniectomy in malignant middle cerebral artery infarction, *J Clin Neurosci* 14:317-321, 2007.
86. Hornig CR, Rust DS, Busse O, et al: Space-occupying cerebellar infarction: Clinical course and prognosis, *Stroke* 25:372-374, 1994.
87. Kase CS, Norrving B, Levine SR, et al: Cerebellar infarction. Clinical and anatomic observation in 66 cases, *Stroke* 24:76-83, 1993.
88. Tohgi H, Takahashi S, Chiba K, et al: Clinical and neuroimaging analysis in 293 patients—Tohoku Cerebellum Infarction Study Group, *Stroke* 24:1697-1701, 1993.
89. Auer LM, Auer TH, Sayama I: Indications for surgical treatment of cerebellar haemorrhage and infarction, *Acta Neurochir* 79:74-79, 1986.
90. Baldauf J, Oertel J, Gaab MR, et al: Endoscopic third ventriculostomy for occlusive hydrocephalus caused by cerebellar infarction, *Neurosurgery* 59:539-544, 2006.
91. Busse O, Laun A: [Therapy of space-occupying cerebellar infarction], *Akt Neurol* 15:6-8, 1988.

92. Chen HJ, Lee TC, Wei CP: Treatment of cerebellar infarction by decompressive suboccipital craniectomy, *Stroke* 23:957-961, 1992.

93. Koh MG, Phan TG, Atkinson JLD, et al: Neuroimaging in deteriorating patients with cerebellar infarcts and mass effect, *Stroke* 31:2062-2067, 2000.

94. Macdonell RAL, Kalnins RM, Donnan GA: Cerebellar infarction: Natural history, prognosis, and pathology, *Stroke* 18:849-855, 1987.

95. Heros RC: Surgical treatment of cerebellar infarction, *Stroke* 23:937-938, 1992.

96. Raco A, Caroli E, Isidori A, et al: Management of acute cerebellar infarction: One institution's experience, *Neurosurgery* 53:1061-1066, 2003.

97. Shenkin HA, Zavala M: Cerebellar strokes: Mortality, surgical indications and results of ventricular drainage, *Lancet* 21:429-432, 1982.

98. Langmayr JJ, Buchberger W, Reindl H: [Cerebellar hemorrhage and cerebellar infarct: Retrospective study of 125 cases], *Wien Med Wochenschrift* 143:131-133, 1993.

99. Busse O, Laun A, Agnoli L: [Obstructive hydrocephalus in cerebellar infarcts], *Neurol Psychiatry* 52:164-171, 1984.

100. Mathew P, Teasdale G, Bannan A, et al: Neurosurgical management of cerebellar haematoma and infarct, *J Neurol Neurosurg Psychiatry* 59:287-292, 1995.

101. Jauss M, Krieger D, Hornig CR, et al: Surgical and medical management of patients with massive cerebellar infarctions: Results of the German-Austrian Cerebellar Infarction Study, *J Neurol* 246:257-264, 1999.

102. Cioffi FA, Bernini FP, Punzo A: Surgical management of acute cerebellar infarction, *Acta Neurochir (Wien)* 74:105-112, 1985.

103. Ho SU, Kim KS, Berenberg RA, et al: Cerebellar infarction: A clinical and CT study, *Surg Neurol* 16:350-352, 1981.

104. Jones HR, Millikan CH, Sandok BA: Temporal profile (clinical course) of acute vertebrobasilar system cerebral infarction, *Stroke* 11:173-177, 1980.

105. Miller JD, Becker DP, Ward JD, et al: Significance of intracranial hypertension in severe head injury, *J Neurosurg* 47:503-516, 1977.

106. Narayan R, Greenberg R, Miller J, et al: Improved confidence of outcome prediction in severe head injury. A comparative analysis of the clinical examination, multimodality evoked potentials, CT scanning, and intracranial pressure, *J Neurosurg* 54:751-762, 1981.

107. Bullock M, Chestnut R, Ghajar J, et al: Guidelines for the Surgical Management of Traumatic Brain Injury. Surgical Management of Traumatic Parenchymal Lesions, *Neurosurgery* 58, 2006.

108. Brain Trauma Foundation; American Association of Neurological Surgeons; Congress of Neurological Surgeons; Joint Section on Neurotrauma and Critical Care, AANS/CNS, Bratton SL, Chestnut RM, Ghajar J, et al: Guidelines for the management of severe traumatic brain injury. VIII. Intracranial pressure thresholds, *J Neurotrauma* 24(Suppl 1):S55-S58, 2007.

109. Brain Trauma Foundation; American Association of Neurological Surgeons; Congress of Neurological Surgeons; Joint Section on Neurotrauma and Critical Care, AANS/CNS, Bratton SL, Chestnut RM, Ghajar J, et al: Guidelines for the management of severe traumatic brain injury. IX. Cerebral perfusion thresholds, *J Neurotrauma* 24(Suppl 1):S45-S54, 2007.

110. Cooper PR, Hagler H, Clark WK, et al: Enhancement of experimental cerebral edema after decompressive craniectomy: Implications for the management of severe head injuries, *Neurosurgery* 4:296-300, 1979.

111. Zweckberger K, Stoffel M, Baethmann A, et al: Effect of decompression craniotomy on increase of contusion volume and functional outcome after controlled cortical impact in mice, *J Neurotrauma* 20:1307-1314, 2003.

112. Polin RS, Shaffrey ME, Bogaev CA, et al: Decompressive bifrontal craniectomy in the treatment of severe refractory posttraumatic cerebral edema, *Neurosurgery* 41:84-92, 1997:discussion 92-84.

113. Stiefel MF, Heuer GG, Smith MJ, et al: Cerebral oxygenation following decompressive hemicraniectomy for the treatment of refractory intracranial hypertension, *J Neurosurg* 101:241-247, 2004.

114. Gower DJ, Lee KS, McWhorter JM: Role of subtemporal decompression in severe closed head injury, *Neurosurgery* 23:417-422, 1988.

115. Kunze E, Meixensberger J, Janka M, et al: Decompressive craniectomy in patients with uncontrollable intracranial hypertension, *Acta Neurochir Suppl* 71:16-18, 1998.

116. Whitfield PC, Patel H, Hutchinson PJ, et al: Bifrontal decompressive craniectomy in the management of posttraumatic intracranial hypertension, *Br J Neurosurg* 15:500-507, 2001.

117. Whitfield PC, Kirkpatrick PJ, Czosnyka M, et al: Management of severe traumatic brain injury by decompressive craniectomy, *Neurosurgery* 49:225-226, 2001.

118. Gaab MR, Rittierodt M, Lorenz M, et al: Traumatic brain swelling and operative decompression: A prospective investigation, *Acta Neurochir Suppl (Wien)* 51:326-328, 1990.

119. Guerra WK, Gaab MR, Dietz H, et al: Surgical decompression for traumatic brain swelling: Indications and results, *J Neurosurg* 90:187-196, 1999.

120. De Luca GP, Volpin L, Fornezza U, et al: The role of decompressive craniectomy in the treatment of uncontrollable post-traumatic intracranial hypertension, *Acta Neurochir Suppl* 76:401-404, 2000.

121. Meier U, Zeilinger FS, Henzka O: The use of decompressive craniectomy for the management of severe head injuries, *Acta Neurochir Suppl* 76:475-478, 2000.

122. Schneider GH, Bardt T, Lanksch WR, et al: Decompressive craniectomy following traumatic brain injury: ICP, CPP and neurological outcome, *Acta Neurochir Suppl* 81:77-79, 2002.

123. Munch E, Horn P, Schurer L, et al: Management of severe traumatic brain injury by decompressive craniectomy, *Neurosurgery* 47:315-322, 2000:discussion 322-313.

124. Schirmer CM, Hoyt DA, Malek AM: Decompressive hemicraniectomy for the treatment of intractable intracranial hypertension after aneurysmal subarachnoid hemorrhage, *Stroke* 38:987-992, 2007.

125. Smith ER, Carter BS, Ogilvy CS: Proposed use of prophylactic decompressive craniectomy in poor-grade aneurysmal subarachnoid hemorrhage patients presenting with associated large sylvian hematomas, *Neurosurgery* 51:117-124, 2002.

126. Mitka M: Hemicraniectomy improves outcomes for patients with ruptured brain aneurysms, *JAMA* 286:2084, 2001.

127. D'Ambrosio AL, Sughrue ME, Yorgason JG, et al: Decompressive hemicraniectomy for poor-grade aneurysmal subarachnoid hemorrhage patients with associated intracerebral hemorrhage: Clinical outcome and quality of life assessment, *Neurosurgery* 56:12-19, 2005.

128. Buschmann U, Yonekawa Y, Fortunati M, et al: Decompressive hemicraniectomy in patients with subarachnoid hemorrhage and intractable intracranial hypertension, *Acta Neurochir (Wien)* 149:59-65, 2007.

129. Mendelow AD, Gregson BA, Fernandes HM, et al: Early surgery versus initial conservative treatment in patients with spontaneous supratentorial intracerebral haematomas in the International Surgical Trial in Intracerebral Haemorrhage (STICH): A randomised trial, *Lancet* 365:387-397, 2005.

130. Hoff JT, Xi G: Brain edema from intracerebral hemorrhage, *Acta Neurochir Suppl* 86:11-15, 2003.

131. Zazulia AR, Diringer MN, Derdeyn CP, et al: Progression of mass effect after intracerebral hemorrhage, *Stroke* 30:1167-1173, 1999.

132. Ropper AH: Lateral displacement of the brain and level of consciousness in patients with an acute hemispheral mass, *N Engl J Med* 314:953-958, 1986.

133. Strbian D, Tatlisumak T, Ramadan UA, et al: Mast cell blocking reduces brain edema and hematoma volume and improves outcome after experimental intracerebral hemorrhage, *J Cereb Blood Flow Metab* 27:795-802, 2007.

134. Gebel JM Jr, Jauch EC, Brott TG, et al: Relative edema volume is a predictor of outcome in patients with hyperacute spontaneous intracerebral hemorrhage, *Stroke* 33:2636-2641, 2002.

135. Murthy JM, Chowdary GV, Murthy TV, et al: Decompressive craniectomy with clot evacuation in large hemispheric hypertensive intracerebral hemorrhage, *Neurocrit Care* 2:258-262, 2005.

136. Maira G, Anile C, Colosimo C, et al: Surgical treatment of primary supratentorial intracerebral hemorrhage in stuporous and comatose patients, *Neurol Res* 24:54-60, 2002.

137. Ferro JM, Canhao P, Stam J, et al: Prognosis of cerebral vein and dural sinus thrombosis: Results of the International Study on Cerebral Vein and Dural Sinus Thrombosis (ISCVT), *Stroke* 35:664-670, 2004.

138. Stefini R, Latronico N, Cornali C, et al: Emergent decompressive craniectomy in patients with fixed dilated pupils due to cerebral venous and dural sinus thrombosis: Report of three cases, *Neurosurgery* 45:626-629, 1999.

139. Coutinho JM, Majoie CB, Coert BA, et al: Decompressive hemicraniectomy in cerebral sinus thrombosis. Consecutive case series and review of the literature, *Stroke* 40:2233-2235, 2009.

140. Keller E, Pangalu A, Fandino J, et al: Decompressive craniectomy in severe cerebral venous and dural sinus thrombosis, *Acta Neurochir Suppl* 94:177-183, 2005.

Cerebellar Infarction and Hemorrhage

TETSUYOSHI HORIUCHI, KAZUHIRO HONGO, SHIGEAKI KOBAYASHI

The management of cerebellar infarction and hemorrhage is a complex matter. The pathophysiology and cause of cerebellar infarction and hemorrhage must be clarified. Acute cerebellar disease is often a life-threatening condition because of the restricted space of the posterior fossa, so appropriate treatment including surgery should be determined on an urgent basis.

Anatomy of the Cerebellum

The cerebellum is located in the posterior cranial fossa, which occupies approximately one eighth of the intracranial space. The posterior fossa extends from the tentorial incisura to the foramen magnum and is formed by the occipital, temporal, parietal, and sphenoid bones. If a mass exists in the cerebellum, upward herniation through the tentorial incisura or downward tonsillar herniation through the foramen magnum may occur.

The cerebellum has afferent connections from the spinal cord, vestibular system, reticular formation, pontine nuclei, inferior olive, raphe nuclei, and locus ceruleus, and efferent connections that terminate in the brainstem and forebrain regions, including the red nuclei and ventrolateral thalami. Many of the efferent fibers are directly or indirectly related to the descending spinal pathway. The loss of muscular coordination is therefore the most common sign in cerebellar disorders. Besides the cerebellum, the posterior fossa contains such important structures as the brainstem, cranial nerves, basilar and vertebral arteries, and outlets of the ventricular system. The brainstem contains pathways regulating consciousness, vital autonomic functions, motor activities, sensory reception, and body coordination. Consequently, in cases of cerebellar hemorrhage or infarction with mass effect, the symptoms are not limited to cerebellar dysfunction. The ventricular system has its outlets only in the posterior fossa: the foramina of Luschka and Magendie from the fourth ventricle. Therefore, when the fourth ventricle is occluded by hematoma or cerebellar edema after the ictus, acute obstructive hydrocephalus occurs.

In the cerebellum, there are three major arteries on each side, the superior cerebellar artery (SCA), anterior inferior cerebellar artery (AICA), and posterior inferior cerebellar artery (PICA). Usually, the cerebellum is supplied predominantly by the SCA, with contributions from the AICA and PICA, but the distribution of flow varies among individuals. There is a rich anastomotic network between the PICA and AICA. The SCA arises near the tip of the basilar artery and passes below the oculomotor and trochlear nerves and above the trigeminal nerve; then it courses along the cerebellomesencephalic fissure, supplying the superior cerebellar peduncle and the tentorial surface of the cerebellum. Spontaneous cerebellar hemorrhage occurs mostly in the area of the dentate nucleus of the cerebellum (see cases 1 and 2, later), which is usually supplied by branches of the SCA. The AICA arises from the lower basilar artery and passes above the abducens nerve. It forms a loop at the facial and vestibulocochlear nerves, supplying the middle cerebellar peduncle and the petrosal surface of the cerebellum. The PICA arises from the vertebral artery and courses in close relation to the glossopharyngeal, vagus, accessory, and hypoglossal nerves. It supplies the inferior cerebellar peduncle and the inferior surface of the cerebellum. The AICA and PICA sometimes have a common trunk. In such cases, acute occlusion of the trunk results in a more extensive infarct of the cerebellum. In addition, unilateral AICA or PICA can occasionally feed bilateral cerebellar hemispheres (see case 4).

Cerebellar Hemorrhage

Clinical Features and Pathophysiology

Spontaneous cerebellar hemorrhage represents approximately 10% of all cases of intracerebral hemorrhage.[1,2] Although the mortality rate is high because of its location, the outcome in survivors with cerebellar hemorrhage is relatively favorable in comparison with outcome in those with supratentorial intracerebral hemorrhage. Although hypertension is the most important causative factor in cerebellar hemorrhage, amyloid angiopathy, arteriovenous malformation, distal PICA aneurysm, and cavernous malformation can cause cerebellar hemorrhage.[3-6]

The symptom onset is often abrupt but may be subacute. Patients present with headache, alterations in level of consciousness, vomiting, and dizziness. Hypertensive cerebellar hemorrhage usually occurs in the dentate nuclei and often extends into the hemispheric white matter and fourth ventricle. Hematoma extension can compress the brainstem and cause obstructive hydrocephalus. Cerebellar hemorrhage rarely involves the vermis only. Although diagnosis of cerebellar hemorrhage is

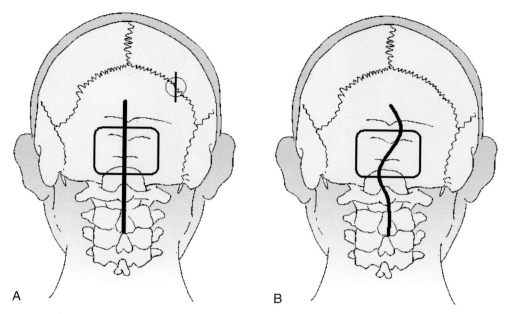

Figure 79-1 Skin incisions for suboccipital craniectomy and ventricular drainage. A, Linear incision. B, Waved skin incision. Note that the waved incision has cosmetic advantages: The postoperative scar is invisible even when the hair is wet.

now made easily with CT and MRI, angiography is still an important modality for investigating the cause of hemorrhage, particularly in a young patient without a history of hypertension. Serial CT scans are also needed to document increasing ventriculomegaly (see case 2).

Damage to the brainstem is the most important factor in predicting the outcome for a patient, and the existence of acute hydrocephalus is also important in the decision to proceed with emergency surgery. Cerebellar hemorrhage can respond well to surgery. Therefore, an overly conservative management results in poor outcome. Surgical options include evacuation of the hematoma and ventricular drainage. Endoscopic hematoma removal through a burr hole has also been introduced.[7]

Indications for Surgery

The key surgical indicators are based on the level of consciousness, the clinical course, and the size of the hematoma. The surgery should be undertaken in patients with large (>3 cm) cerebellar hemorrhage or cerebellar hemorrhage with brainstem compression or hydrocephalus.[1,5,8] Deterioration in the level of consciousness is a strong indication for emergency surgery. For hydrocephalus associated with a lesser degree of "tightness" of the posterior fossa, only ventricular drainage and careful observation are advocated (see case 2).

Surgical Procedure of Hematoma Evacuation

After induction of general anesthesia, the patient is placed in the prone position, and the head is fixed in a head frame with the neck slightly flexed. The head is elevated adequately to avoid development of venous congestion and edema during surgery. *Unilateral* suboccipital craniectomy is usually performed; the extent of the exposure

depends on the location and size of the hematoma. In larger or bilateral hemorrhages, bilateral suboccipital craniectomy with foramen magnum opening is sometimes needed. A linear or curved skin incision is usually placed between 2 cm above the inion and the spinous process of C2 (Fig. 79-1). With a curved skin incision, the postoperative scar is less visible. Other traditional incisions for this approach include hockey-stick and horseshoe incisions. When ventricular drainage is required because of obstructive hydrocephalus, a 3 cm–long linear incision is additionally placed at a point 5 to 6 cm above the orbitomeatal line and 5 cm posterior to the external auditory meatus, to allow insertion of a ventricular catheter (see Fig. 79-1).

Skin flaps are reflected, and the nuchal fascia and muscles are exposed. The trapezius muscle has an attachment to the medial part of the superior nuchal line, and the sternocleidomastoid muscle has an attachment to its lateral part, extending to the mastoid process. An edge of the fascia and muscle is left at the upper incision to facilitate wound closure. The nuchal muscles are split at the midline, and the underlying semispinalis capitis muscle and rectus capitis posterior major and minor muscles are detached from the occipital bone. These muscles are retrogradely dissected from the inferior nuchal line by means of a periosteal elevator with minimum cautery, in the same manner as in a frontotemporal craniotomy.[9] Gentle dissection of these muscles promotes wound healing and prevents postoperative muscle contraction headache.

A craniectomy adequate to the size of the lesion is performed. It is sometimes widened with a drill and a rongeur laterally and superiorly up to the transverse sinus. After craniectomy, we frequently use ultrasonography to determine the location of the hematoma, and color Doppler ultrasonographic imaging with color-flow mapping system is helpful, especially when a vascular anomaly has

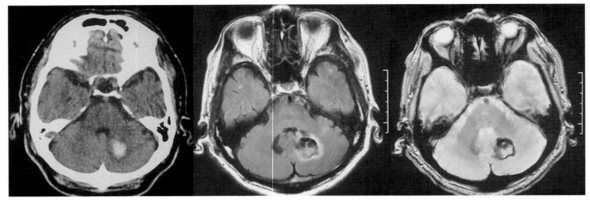

Figure 79-2 CT scan *(left)* and MR images *(center,* fluid-attenuated inversion recovery [FLAIR] image; *right,* T2* image) showing a small cerebellar hematoma in the left dentate nuclei.

caused hematoma.[10] Prior to the dural opening, a small durotomy is made, and a drainage tube is inserted into the hematoma cavity to evacuate the liquid clot. Then, the dura mater is widely opened and the occipital venous sinus is ligated or coagulated and sectioned. After introduction of the operating microscope, the cerebellar surface is inspected for a vascular anomaly. The corticotomy is extended around the drainage tube, and the hematoma is evacuated with suction. The hematoma is removed from the superficial region to the deeper region, and bleeding points are identified and coagulated. The wall of the hematoma cavity is covered with absorbable knitted fabric (Surgicel) to control oozing. After adequate removal of the clot, hemostasis should be completed. To confirm hemostasis, the intratracheal pressure is also raised to 30 cm H_2O for 10 seconds (Valsalva maneuver), and the hematoma cavity is irrigated with saline solution. The dura is closed in a watertight fashion with continuous suture. In cases requiring further decompression, duraplasty is performed with either artificial dura, periosteum, or fascia harvested from the parietal region. To prevent venous sinus bleeding, several suspending dural stitches are placed at the edge of the craniectomy. Then the head frame is loosened and the head is refixed in a neck-extended position to facilitate approximation of the nuchal muscles and fascia easier to the fascia remaining at the superior nuchal line. The muscles are closed in two layers at the midline, and the skin is sutured. Epidural suction drainage is not recommended, so as to avoid accidental forced drainage of cerebrospinal fluid.

Postoperative Management

Many centers perform CT in the operating room immediately after surgery, with general anesthesia maintained, to ensure adequate clot removal. The postoperative patient is managed in the intensive care unit with monitoring of vital signs. Laboratory data and neurologic signs are important. Auditory brainstem response is monitored when brainstem function is severely impaired. A patient who was comatose with or without dyspnea preoperatively is managed postoperatively with mechanical ventilation and short-acting barbiturate therapy. Corticosteroid, mannitol, and a histamine H_2 blocker are administered

intravenously. The systolic blood pressure is maintained at less than 120 mm Hg for 24 hours. A CT scan is taken on day 1 after surgery to rule out rebleeding and cerebellar edema. Barbiturate or propofol is discontinued, and the patient is extubated after neurologic status has stabilized and a follow-up CT scan shows improvement in the "tightness" of the posterior fossa. Rehabilitation should start as soon as possible.

Illustrative Cases

Case 1

A 67-year-old man suddenly complained of vertigo and nausea. CT and MRI showed a cerebellar hematoma (left dentate nucleus) without ventricular perforation (Fig. 79-2). The patient was conservatively treated with full recovery.

Case 2

A 69-year-old man with a history of hypertension and diabetes mellitus had sudden onset of vomiting and ataxia of the right side. The patient was transferred to our hospital, where a CT scan demonstrated cerebellar hematoma extending to the fourth ventricle with mild ventriculomegaly (Fig. 79-3A). The patient became comatose 6 hours later, and a follow-up CT scan disclosed obstructive hydrocephalus (Fig. 79-3B). Emergency placement of a ventricular drain through the right anterior horn of the lateral ventricle was performed (see Fig. 79-3B); hematoma was not evacuated. Postoperative course was uneventful. The patient was sent to a rehabilitation hospital.

Case 3

A 46-year-old man presented to the emergency room with consciousness disturbance following headache and vomiting. A CT scan demonstrated a large high-density area in the right cerebellum (>3 cm) (Fig. 79-4). The patient underwent emergency suboccipital craniectomy with evacuation of the hematoma. At operation, no vascular anomaly was detected. The postoperative CT scan showed complete removal of the hematoma (see Fig. 79-4). The truncal ataxia and right incoordination had resolved within 2 months, and the patient returned to previous daily life.

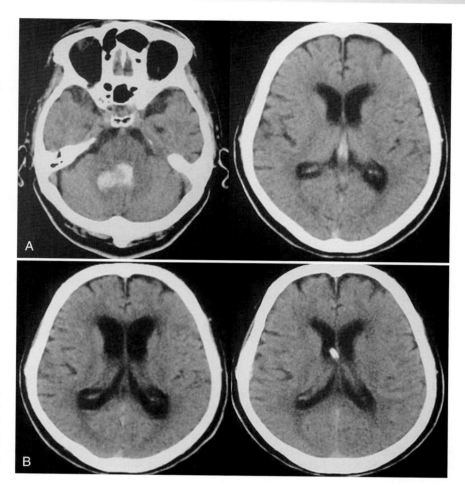

Figure 79-3 A, CT scans on admission demonstrating a cerebellar hematoma extending to the fourth ventricle. B, Follow-up CT scan *(left)*, obtained 6 hours after admission, showing a hydrocephalus. CT scan *(right)* after the placement of ventricular drain tube revealing resolution of the hydrocephalus.

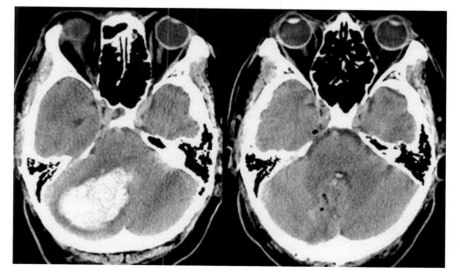

Figure 79-4 CT scan before *(left)* and after *(right)* surgery showing that the right cerebellar hematoma is completely removed.

Cerebellar Infarction

Clinical Features and Pathophysiology

Before the introduction of CT scanning, correct diagnosis of cerebellar infarction was rarely made during life. With the improvement in CT and MRI, however, the diagnosis of cerebellar infarction was greatly facilitated. Amarenco et al[11] studied arterial pathology of 88 cerebellar infarcts in 56 patients. Cardiogenic embolism was the cause in 43% of the patients, and atherosclerotic occlusion in 35%. Emboli tend to lodge in the intracranial vertebral artery, resulting in infarction in the PICA territory; the SCA is rarely affected. The cerebellar infarction sometimes becomes hemorrhagic. Although the infarction is generally unilateral, bilateral cerebellar hemispheres can be affected owing to vascular variation.[12]

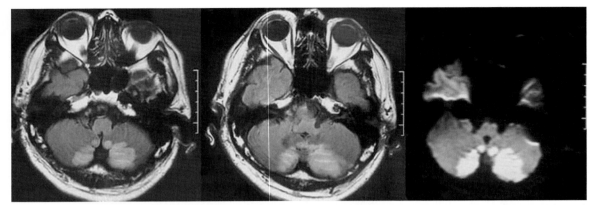

Figure 79-5 Fluid-attenuated inversion recovery (FLAIR) *(left* and *center)* and diffusion *(right)* MR images showing bilateral cerebellar infarction.

The initial symptoms include vertigo or dizziness, headache, nausea and vomiting, ataxia, and dysarthria. Approximately 13% to 39% of all patients with cerebellar infarction demonstrate mass effect in the posterior fossa.[13,14] Large cerebellar infarcts cause edematous changes in the cerebellar hemisphere, resulting in compression of the brainstem typically starting on the third day after the ictus.[15] Initially, sixth nerve palsy is likely to occur ipsilaterally, and facial weakness and Horner's syndrome may be associated. Obstructive hydrocephalus sometimes develops because of compression of the fourth ventricle, leading to disturbance of consciousness that may be rapid. Patients become comatose over several hours once signs of brainstem compression appear and often demonstrate pinpoint pupils and decerebrate posturing from pontine compression. Ataxic respiration and apnea ultimately occur because of medullary compression from tonsillar herniation shortly before death.

Indications for Surgery

Patients with small cerebellar infarcts rarely become candidates for surgical treatment. Surgical treatment is necessary only in the patient with a rapidly progressing disturbance of consciousness caused by brainstem compression and/or fourth ventricle obstruction due to edematous change or hemorrhagic transformation.[14-16] Treatment options are external ventricular drainage, posterior fossa decompressive craniectomy with duraplasty, resection of infarcted cerebellum, and combinations of those treatments.[14-16] Detailed and frequent neurologic monitoring is essential to determine the necessity for surgery.

Surgical Procedure

Surgical decompression with extensive suboccipital craniectomy and duraplasty is the procedure of choice for massive cerebellar infarction. The craniectomy is essentially the same as that described previously for cerebellar hemorrhage. To achieve an effective decompression, the foramen magnum is widely opened, the craniectomy is extended bilaterally, and laminectomy of C1 is performed. When obstructive hydrocephalus is associated,

a ventricular catheter into the occipital horn of the lateral ventricle is placed at this stage. If the dura mater is extremely tense, ventricular drainage is not carried out until the dural opening is large enough to avoid upward herniation. The dura mater is incised first near the foramen magnum to drain the cerebrospinal fluid and then is widely opened. In cases associated with severe edematous change, grossly necrotic tissue of the cerebellum may be resected for internal decompression. Duraplasty is performed with artificial dura or a piece of fascia harvested from the parietal region.

Illustrative Cases

Case 4

A 50-year-old woman was admitted with the complaint of dizziness. MR images revealed bilateral cerebellar infarction (Fig. 79-5). These findings indicated that the right vermian branch might be fed by the left PICA. The symptom disappeared within 2 weeks.

Case 5

A 68-year-old man presented with headache, dizziness, left ataxia, and nausea. MRI showed a high-intensity area in the territory of the left PICA (Fig. 79-6A). The patient was treated conservatively under the diagnosis of left cerebellar infarction. Five days after ictus, the patient progressively deteriorated. A CT scan disclosed a high-density area corresponding to the territory of the PICA (Fig. 79-6B). The fourth ventricle was compressed, and the supratentorial ventricular system dilated. Diagnosis of hemorrhagic infarction was made. The patient underwent emergency surgery (suboccipital decompressive craniectomy with duraplasty, removal of the hemorrhagic portion of the infarcted cerebellum including the tonsil, and ventricular drainage through the right occipital horn). The patient was treated with propofol for 2 days after surgery. The postoperative CT scan showed the posterior fossa to be well decompressed as well as a reduction in ventricular size. The patient's level of consciousness completely recovered, and the patient was discharged with mild ataxia and left dysmetria. Follow-up MRI performed 1 month after surgery showed a normal brainstem with a slack posterior fossa (Fig. 79-6C).

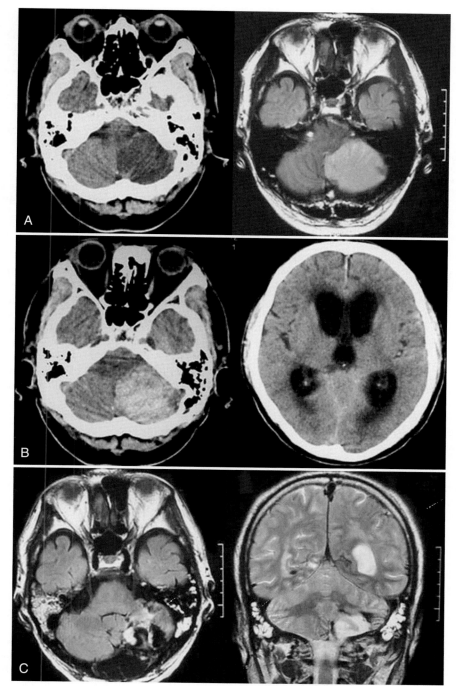

Figure 79-6 A, CT scan *(left)* and fluid-attenuated inversion recovery (FLAIR) MR image *(right)* demonstrating a cerebellar infarction in the left side. B, CT scans obtained at patient deterioration disclosing a hemorrhagic transformation and hydrocephalus. C, Axial FLAIR *(left)* and coronal T2-weighted *(right)* MR images, obtained 1 month after surgery, showing the posterior fossa slack with no evidence of brainstem injury.

Conclusion

Management of cerebellar infarction and hemorrhage is described, with focus on the surgical indications and procedures. To achieve the best surgical outcome, timing of surgery is very important; surgical intervention should be performed without delay when indicated. Perioperative close observation and adequate medical management are important as well.

REFERENCES

1. Kobayashi S, Sato A, Kageyama Y, et al: Treatment of hypertensive cerebellar hemorrhage: Surgical or conservative management? *Neurosurgery* 34:246–251, 1994.
2. Morioka J, Fujii M, Kato S, et al: Surgery for spontaneous intracerebral hemorrhage has greater remedial value than conservative therapy, *Surg Neurol* 65:67–73, 2006.
3. Little JR, Tubman DE, Ethier R: Cerebellar hemorrhage in adults. Diagnosis by computerized tomography, *J Neurosurg* 48:575–579, 1978.

4. Luparello V, Canavero S: Treatment of hypertensive cerebellar hemorrhage: Surgical or conservative management? *Neurosurgery* 37:552-553, 1995.

5. Mayer SA, Rincon F: Treatment of intracerebral haemorrhage, *Lancet Neurol* 4:662-672, 2005.

6. Horiuchi T, Tanaka Y, Hongo K, et al: Characteristics of distal posterior inferior cerebellar artery aneurysm, *Neurosurgery* 53:589-596, 2003.

7. Yamamoto T, Nakao Y, Mori K, et al: Endoscopic hematoma evacuation for hypertensive cerebellar hemorrhage, *Minim Invasive Neurosurg* 49:173-178, 2006.

8. Broderick J, Connolly S, Feldmann E, et al: Guidelines for the management of spontaneous intracerebral hemorrhage in adults: 2007 update: A guideline from the American Heart Association/American Stroke Association Stroke Council, High Blood Pressure Research Council, and the Quality of Care and Outcomes in Research Interdisciplinary Working Group, *Stroke* 38:2001-2023, 2007.

9. Oikawa S, Mizuno M, Muraoka S, Kobayashi S: Retrograde dissection of the temporalis muscle preventing muscle atrophy for pterional craniotomy. Technical note, *J Neurosurg* 84:297-299, 1996.

10. Kitazawa K, Nitta J, Okudera H, Kobayashi S: Color Doppler ultrasound imaging in the emergency management of an intracerebral hematoma caused by cerebral arteriovenous malformations: Technical case report, *Neurosurgery* 42:405-407, 1998.

11. Amarenco P, Hauw JJ, Gautier JC: Arterial pathology in cerebellar infarction, *Stroke* 21:1299-1305, 1990.

12. Han SW, Cho GC, Baik JS, et al: Bilateral cerebellar infarction caused by dominant medial posterior inferior cerebellar artery, *Neurology* 66:1125-1126, 2006.

13. Kase CS, Norrving B, Levine SR, et al: Cerebellar infarction: Clinical and anatomic observation in 66 cases, *Stroke* 24:76-83, 1993.

14. Koh MG, Phan TG, Atkinson JLD, Wijdicks EFM: Neuroimaging in deteriorating patients with cerebellar infarcts and mass effect, *Stroke* 31:2062-2067, 2000.

15. Hornig CR, Rust DS, Busse O, et al: Space-occupying cerebellar infarction: Clinical course and prognosis, *Stroke* 25:372-374, 1994.

16. Adams HP Jr, del Zoppo G, Alberts MJ, et al: Guidelines for the early management of adults with ischemic stroke: A guideline from the American Heart Association/American Stroke Association Stroke Council, Clinical Cardiology Council, Cardiovascular Radiology and Intervention Council, and the Atherosclerotic Peripheral Vascular Disease and Quality of Care Outcomes in Research Interdisciplinary Working Groups: The American Academy of Neurology affirms the value of this guideline as an educational tool for neurologists, *Stroke* 38:1655-1711, 2007.

Page numbers followed by *t* indicate tables; page numbers followed by *f* indicate figures.